Principles and Practice of Surgery for the

Colon, Rectum, and Anus

Principles and Practice of Surgery for the

Colon, Rectum, and Anus

Third Edition

Philip H. Gordon

M.D., F.R.C.S. (C), F.A.C.S., F.A.S.C.R.S., Hon. F.R.S.M., Hon. F.A.C.G.B.I

Professor of Surgery and Oncology, McGill University
Director of Colon and Rectal Surgery
Sir Mortimer B. Davis-Jewish General Hospital and McGill University
Montreal, Quebec, Canada

Santhat Nivatvongs

M.D., F.A.C.S., F.A.S.C.R.S., Hon. F.R.C.S.T. (Thailand), Hon. F.R.A.C.S.

Consultant Surgeon and Professor of Surgery
Mayo Clinic College of Medicine
Rochester, Minnesota, U.S.A.

ILLUSTRATORS

Scott Thorn Barrows, C.M.I., F.A.M.I

Director and Clinical Assistant Professor, Biomedical Visualization
University of Illinois at Chicago Medical Center

with the assistance of

Carla Gunn, Gregory Blew, David Ehlert, Craig Kiefer, and Kim Martens

informa
healthcare

New York London

Informa Healthcare USA, Inc.
270 Madison Avenue
New York, NY 10016

Printed in the United States of America on acid-free paper
10 9 8 7 6 5 4 3 2 1

International Standard Book Number-10: 0-8247-2961-7 (Hardcover)
International Standard Book Number-13: 978-0-8247-2961-5 (Hardcover)

Library of Congress Cataloging-in-Publication Data

Gordon, Philip H.
Principles and practice of surgery for the colon, rectum, and anus / by Philip H. Gordon, Santhat Nivatvongs. -- 3rd ed.
p. ; cm.
Includes bibliographical references and index.
ISBN-13: 978-0-8247-2961-5 (alk. paper)
ISBN-10: 0-8247-2961-7 (alk. paper)
1. Colon (Anatomy)--Surgery. 2. Rectum--Surgery. 3. Anus--Surgery. I. Nivatvongs, Santhat. II. Title.
[DNLM: 1. Colonic Diseases--surgery. 2. Anus Diseases--surgery. 3. Colorectal Neoplasms--surgery. 4. Rectal Diseases--surgery. WI 520 G664p 2006]

RD544.G67 2006
617.5'547--dc22 2006050379

Visit the Informa Web site at
www.informa.com

and the Informa Healthcare Web site at
www.informahealthcare.com

Contributors

Peter A. Cataldo ■ Associate Professor of Surgery, University of Vermont College of Medicine, Fletcher Allen Health Care, Burlington, Vermont, U.S.A.

Jean MacDonald ■ E.T. Nurse Consultant, Sir Mortimer B. Davis–Jewish General Hospital, Montreal, Quebec, Canada

W. Rudolf Schouten ■ Department of Surgery, Division of Colon and Rectal Surgery, University Hospital Dijkzigt, Rotterdam, The Netherlands

Lee E. Smith ■ Clinical Professor of Surgery, George Washington University, Director, Section of Colon and Rectal Surgery, Washington Hospital Center, Washington, D.C.

I am once again deeply indebted to my wife
Rosalie
for her constant patience and understanding through the burden of this third edition.
Her constant life-long support has made all my professional accomplishments possible.

To my wonderful children
Laurel *and* **Elliot**
of whom I am extremely proud.
My love and gratitude to all.
—PHG

To my two angels
Marisa *and* **Nitara**.
Thinking of them makes me smile;
talking to them recharges my energy.
—SN

Preface to the Third Edition

In the first edition of this textbook our goal was to produce a comprehensive book that would encompass the gamit of colon and anorectal diseases. It was not intended to be encyclopedic but to provide information for the busy surgeon who needed to extract information as quickly as possible. With this in mind, the contents were divided into five major sections that we have been told were helpful and so we have maintained the basic format through the second and third editions.

In the eight years that have elapsed since our last edition, the proliferation of information published in the surgical literature makes it necessary to update and elaborate on these developments. Highlights in the revision include a new discussion of fascial attachments of the rectum and relationship to the lateral pelvic wall with specific reference to the application for operations on rectal carcinoma. Newer pharmacologic effects on the internal sphincter and new investigative modalities for anorectal physiology are described. The value and role of virtual colonoscopy is discussed as is the controversy regarding the need for mechanical bowel preparation. There is a detailed description of the newest modality of hemorrhoid therapy, namely the stapler hemorrhoidopexy and its potential role in the armamentarium of hemorrhoid treatment. An extensive section on pharmacologic therapy for fissure-in-ano has been added and the efficacy of various agents for chemical sphincterotomy are described. The value of intra-anal ultrasound and MRI in the diagnosis of complicated recurrent fistula-in-ano have been highlighted as has the efficacy of fibrin glue. A new section on the technique of the repair of rectourethral fistula has been added. Topical agents for condyloma accuminata and drugs and their dosage for various sexually transmitted diseases have been updated. An extensive review on the therapy for fecal incontinence including the artificial sphincter, hyperbaric oxygen, Secca procedure, implantation of silicone biomaterial and detailed description of sacral neuromodulation has been added.

The chapter on the etiology and management of perianal neoplasms and anal carcinoma has been extensively revised reflecting new information, in particular the discussion on anal intraepithelial neoplsia (AIN). This included the new method of diagnosis and management of high grade AIN of the perianal skin or Bowen's disease. In the benign neoplasms chapter, the relatively new interest and better understanding of "serrated" adenoma has been added. The hot topic on the management of malignant polyps of the low rectum has been updated. Information on uncommon benign polyps has been expanded.

New data regarding the incidence, prevalence, and trends in colorectal carcinoma are included. There is an update on the genetics of colorectal carcinoma in general and in particular HNPCC. Extensive discussion of the indications for and interpretation of genetic testing and the invaluable role of genetic counseling are described in detail. There is an update on the propriety of adjuvant therapy with its limitations and complications and possible fine tuning of indications for adjuvant therapy. There is updated information on the treatment of recurrent metastatic carcinoma providing prognostic indicators for recurrence following therapy. A section on intra-luminal stenting for obstruction has been added. There is new information on the staging of rectal carcinoma. There is revised description of sphincter saving operations (pouch, coloplasty, coloanal anastomosis). There is a discussion of total mesorectal excision with results of the use of this technique. There are updated results on the treatment of carcinoma of the rectum with a discussion of the propriety of the use of local excision of rectal carcinoma. There is expansion on the section on palliative management of patients with rectal carcinoma and there is a discussion on the role of preoperative neoadjuvant treatment for rectal carcinoma. A new section on the management of presacral bleeding has been included. Screening, surveillance, and follow-up for large bowel carcinoma continue to evolve rapidly with better understanding. The new algorithm for colorectal carcinoma screening has been revised. The controversy in the surveillance after surgery has been laid out as guidelines from different major societies and institutions.

The controversy on ileal pouch-anal anastomosis (IPAA) as primary treatment of chronic ulcercative colitis has been clarified. A better understanding of the risk of carcinoma in the ileal pouch and the retained anal canal is elucidated. The management of chronic pouchitis now includes immunosuppressive drugs. The long-term outcome of IPAA is now better understood. The Crohn's disease chapter has been extensively revised with an elaborate discussion on the natural history and classification of the disease and an extensive discussion of the medical therapies with their limitations and the consideration of chemoprevention of colorectal carcinoma in inflammatory bowel disease. The changing paradigm regarding the indications for elective operation in diverticular disease has been revisited along with the most recent data on results of the treatment of diverticulitis. The laparoscopy chapter has been totally revised and expanded. The indications for laparoscopic colectomy have been revisited and expanded as newer technology has become available and increased experience has been gained. The new instrumentation of equipment that is available has been outlined including subjects such as handports and robotic surgery. Techniques of laparoscopic colectomy have been added. The results of laparoscopic colectomy, conversion rates, detailed morbidity, and mortality by disease process have been updated. Difficult situations such as obesity, inflammatory masses, and fistulas have been described. Quality of life and cost issues have been included. A major expansion of the complications, including incidence and prevention of complications with laparoscopic colectomy have been described. In the miscellaneous chapter, an entire new section on colon interposition has been added.

The book is replete with color illustrations and photographs adjacent to the text material rather than grouped at the beginning, middle, or end of the book. New illustrations have been added and others redrawn to conform to better understanding and improvement in operative technique. Color has been added to many previous black and white illustrations to enhance the visual image and better display the anatomic details. Each chapter is heavily referenced.

We hope we have accomplished our goal of summarizing the enormous body of knowledge published in the literature and share our personal experience and preferences with our readers. We strove for a book that strikes a balance of being authoritative and detailed without being so inclusive that somewhat irrelevant material and minutia are included. We sincerely hope our efforts will provide the practicing surgeon and surgeon in training, the appropriate information to permit them to provide a rational and up-to-date course of action to the ultimate benefit of each of their patients.

Philip H. Gordon
Santhat Nivatvongs

Preface from the Second Edition

Seven years have elapsed since the first edition of this book was published and we have been amazed at the new developments relevant to diseases affecting the colon, rectum, and anus that have occurred in that relatively short span of time. Some of these developments have been an outgrowth of the increased knowledge of the disease process and the underlying genetic factors that influence it. Others are a reflection of more sophisticated modalities of investigation such as intrarectal ultrasonographic assessment of rectal carcinoma and positron emission tomography (PET) scanning for recurrent carcinoma or improved therapeutic options such as sphincter-saving operations and newer procedures for fecal incontinence. Added to this is the yet undefined and still controversial role of laparoscopic operations to manage a host of colon and rectal disorders. This proliferation of knowledge has prompted a major revision of the last edition of this book. Parts have been entirely rewritten (perianal and anal canal neoplasms, early detection and follow-up of large bowel carcinoma, and ischemic colitis), others have been extensively updated (anal incontinence and adjuvant therapy for colorectal carcinoma), whereas still others have been greatly expanded (fissures and Crohn's disease). An entirely new chapter on laparoscopy has been added in view of the current interest in this technique. The exciting new developments in the genetics of colorectal carcinoma have received the in-depth coverage they deserve.

In our quest to present a balanced view throughout this book, this endeavor has become almost encyclopedic. As a result, this textbook has even grown beyond its original intimidating size. Despite the size, we have tried to make this information readily accessible to our readers while maintaining the author's personal imprint. Therefore, we have preserved our prerogative to state our preferences when applicable and to reflect our individual perspectives. The basic organization of the subject matter has also been maintained to permit ready access to information which we have attempted to present in a systematic format. New illustrations have been added and others have been redrawn to better clarify procedures or disease processes and to further enhance the learning process. A comprehensive bibliography also accompanies each chapter.

We hope we have accomplished our goal of summarizing the staggering body of current knowledge and sharing our own personal experience and preferences with our readers. Our ultimate objective has been to address the needs of practicing surgeons, gastroenterologists, other physicians, residents in training, and medical students so that they can develop a rational course of action for each individual patient.

Philip H. Gordon
Santhat Nivatvongs

Preface from the First Edition

The creation of any medical textbook begins as a labor of love but rapidly takes on a life of its own. This book was no exception. Our goal was to produce a comprehensive textbook that would encompass the gamut of colon and anorectal diseases. Emphasis was placed on the fundamentals of disease, with explanation of etiology and pathogenesis given when applicable, so that the rationale of the proposed treatment would be better understood. In addition to the "what" and "why," the reader will learn "when" and "how" to institute therapy. This book is not simply a revision or extension of our previous book, *Essentials of Anorectal Surgery.* Since the concepts, thoughts, and practices of colon and rectal surgery have changed a great deal during the past decade, current thinking is presented here.

This book was not intended to be encyclopedic. It was written with the busy practicing surgeon in mind—the surgeon who needs to extract information as quickly and easily as possible. Therefore we have divided the contents of the book into five major sections. Since our aim was to be both practical and didactic, we have included theory along with detailed descriptions of operative procedures.

Part I covers anatomy and physiology and discusses the general principles of investigation and preparation of the patient for operation. Part II focuses on anorectal disorders, offering discussions of the various disease entities. It also includes a chapter that highlights outpatient procedures, which play an increasingly important role in the management of patients with anorectal disorders. Part III describes colorectal disorders and their management. Certain subjects that are combined in a miscellaneous chapter in other books have been ascribed chapter status here. We believe that this arrangement offers a great convenience to the reader. Part IV groups a series of subjects related to problem solving. For example, we have chosen to present together the complications of diseases and their management and the complications of colorectal operations rather than to repeat these discussions in several chapters. Part V comprises a group of miscellaneous entities.

A number of this book's special features are worthy of comment. *Principles and Practice of Surgery for the Colon, Rectum, and Anus* is the first textbook on colon and rectal surgery to incorporate the liberal use of color. It contains 956 illustrations—x-rays, photographs, and drawings—300 of which are in color. We strongly believe that the use of color will enhance the reader's understanding of the material. A prime example is the chapter on perianal dermatologic disease, which is greatly strengthened by the addition of color. We realize that the chapters on malignant neoplasms of the colon and the rectum arc lengthy, but the importance of the subject matter mandates the amount of material included. Indeed, certain subsections were intentionally abbreviated but extensively referenced. The chapter on diverticular disease is also long, but because of the controversial nature of the management of this disease, the size was deemed necessary to provide a full account of the problem. One subject that is often not adequately addressed in textbooks is the construction and care of stomas. In contrast, we believe that this topic is important enough to command an entire chapter. Constipation, which is "only" a symptom, may present such a challenge to the treating physician that a separate chapter has been devoted to it. Finally, an innovative chapter on unexpected intraoperative findings was included to help meet those demanding situations that test the skill and ingenuity of the surgeon. In discussions of all controversial issues, an effort was made to present an even-handed and fair presentation of the problem but always to provide the reader with the preference of the author.

We hope that the reader, who might be any surgeon or surgeon-in-training who has an interest in the treatment of colorectal disease, will find both the information in this book and its presentation useful. We trust that the numerous illustrations and the use of color will facilitate understanding and allow us to achieve our goal.

Philip H. Gordon
Santhat Nivatvongs

Acknowledgments

Preparation of a major textbook involves the cooperation and contributions of many people and we would like to acknowledge the assistance of several individuals.

We are most grateful for the continued friendships, contributions, and support of Lee E. Smith, M.D., and W. Rudolph Schouten, M.D., who have provided the time, expertise, and advice through the third edition of this textbook. We are most appreciative of their unwavering help. We are also grateful to Peter A. Cataldo, M.D., and Jean MacDonald, RN CETN for their contributions.

For a book of this magnitude, an enormous amount of skilled secretarial support was required. We would like to thank Lianna Mantley of the Sir Mortimer B. Davis–Jewish General Hospital, Montreal, Canada and Nancy Beckmann of the Mayo Clinic, Rochester, Minnesota, for their care in typing and retyping the manuscript. We wish to thank Silvie D'amico for her secretarial assistance throughout the process and Carmela Masella for handling office duties while the manuscript was being typed. Thanks to Elliot Gordon for gathering the many journal references required for researching the various topics and thanks to Laurel Gordon for her filial words of wisdom. A very special word of thanks to Rosalie Gordon for her unwavering support and advice, and from whom precious hours were stolen to permit the writing of the book. Thanks to Marisa Nivatvongs and Nitara Layton for their good nature and love.

We continue to be blessed and fortunate to have the very talented medical illustrator Scott Barrows provide his expertise to this edition. His enormous skill, cooperation, and ability to convert words into images have greatly enhanced the book. We would also like to thank Joanne Jay of The Egerton Group Ltd. for her efforts in successfully assembling a book of this magnitude and complexity.

Contents

Part II: Anorectal Disorders

I: Essential Considerations

1 Surgical Anatomy

Santhat Nivatvongs and Philip H. Gordon

Although seemingly a single organ, the colon is embryologically divisible into two parts. The transverse colon and portions proximal to it are derived from the midgut and are supplied by the superior mesenteric artery, while the distal half of the colon is derived from the hindgut and receives blood from the inferior mesenteric artery.

The large bowel begins in the right lower quadrant of the abdomen as a blind pouch known as the cecum. The ileum empties into the medial and posterior aspect of the intestine, a point known as the ileocecal junction. The colon proceeds upward and in its course is designated according to location as: ascending colon, hepatic flexure, transverse colon, splenic flexure, descending colon, sigmoid colon, rectum, and anal canal. The colon is approximately 150 cm long, and its diameter gradually diminishes from the cecum to the rectosigmoid junction, where it widens as the rectal ampulla, only to narrow again as the anal canal.

COLON

GENERAL CONFIGURATION

The colon differs from the small bowel in that it is characterized by a saccular or haustral appearance, it contains three taenia bands, and it has appendices epiploicae, a series of fatty appendages located on the antimesenteric surface of the colon. The taenia bands are longitudinal muscle running along the colon from the base of the appendix. They merge in the distal sigmoid colon, where the longitudinal fibers continue through the entire length of the rectum. A study by Fraser et al. (1) has shown that the longitudinal muscle forms a complete coat around the colon but is much thicker at the taeniae. The three taenia bands are named according to their relation to the transverse colon: taenia mesocolica, which is attached to the mesocolon; taenia omentalis, which is attached to the greater omentum; and taenia libera, which has no attachment. These bands are about one sixth shorter than the intestine and are believed to be responsible for the sacculations (2).

The transition from the sigmoid colon to the rectum is a gradual one. It is characterized by the taeniae coli spreading out from three distinct bands to a uniformly distributed layer of longitudinal smooth muscle that is thicker on the front and back than on each side.

COURSE AND RELATIONS

The general topography of the colon varies from person to person, and such differences should be taken into account while reading the following discussion (Fig. 1).

The vermiform appendix projects from the lowermost part of the cecum. From the ileocecal junction the colon ascends on the right in front of the quadratus lumborum and transversus abdominis muscles to a level overlying the lower pole of the right kidney, a distance of about 20 cm. It is invested by peritoneum on its anterior, lateral, and medial surfaces. Superior to the colon is the undersurface of the right lobe of the liver, lateral to the gallbladder, and here the colon angulates acutely medially, downward, and forward, forming the hepatic flexure. Occasionally there is a filmy web of adhesions extending from the right abdominal wall to the anterior taenia of the ascending colon, and this has been referred to as Jackson's membrane.

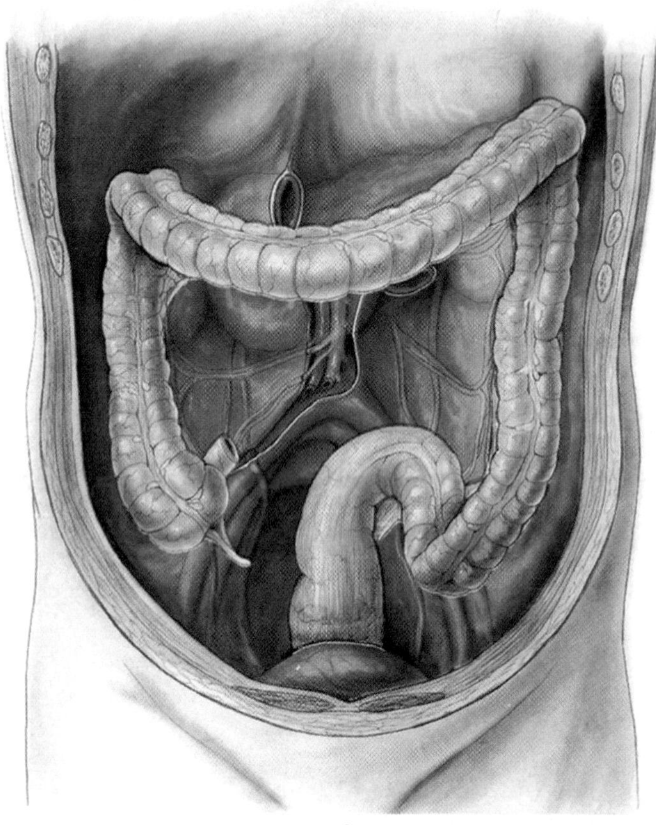

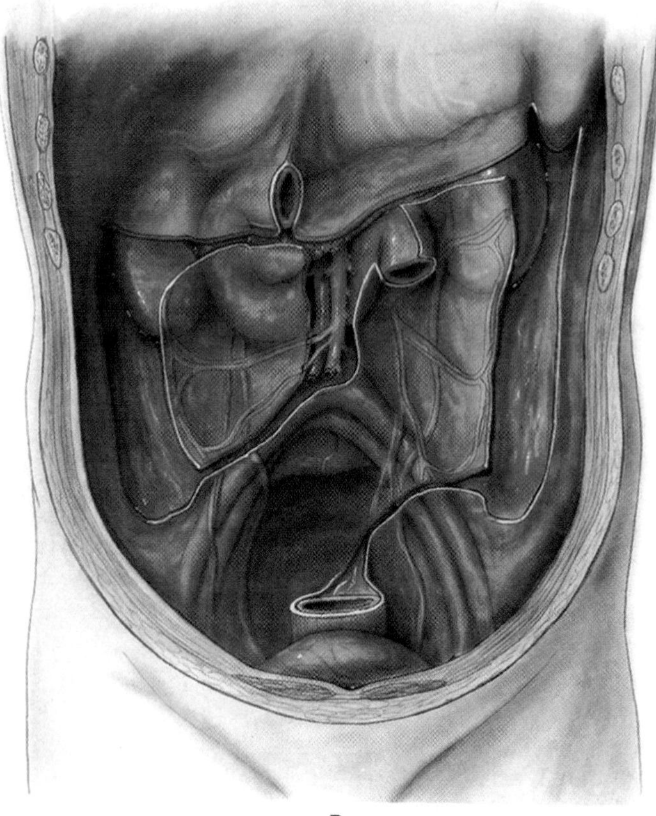

FIGURE 1 ■ General topography of the large bowel. (**A**) Colon. (**B**) Peritoneum and adjacent structures.

The transverse colon is the longest (40–50 cm) segment of colon, extending from the hepatic to the splenic flexure. It is usually mobile and may descend to the level of the iliac crests or even dip into the pelvis. The transverse colon is enveloped between layers of the transverse mesocolon, the root of which overlies the right kidney, the second portion of the duodenum, the pancreas, and the left kidney. It contains the middle colic artery, branches of the right and left colic arteries, and accompanying veins, lymphatic structures, and autonomic nerve plexuses. This posterior relationship is of paramount importance because these structures are subject to injury during a right hemi-colectomy if proper care is not exercised. In the left upper quadrant of the abdomen, the colon is attached to the undersurface of the diaphragm at the level of the 10th and 11th ribs by the phrenocolic ligament. The distal transverse colon lies in front of the proximal descending colon. The stomach is immediately above and the spleen is to the left. The greater omentum descends from the greater curvature of the stomach in front of the transverse colon and ascends to the upper surface of the transverse colon. The splenic flexure describes an acute angle, is high in the left upper quadrant, and therefore is less accessible to operative approach. It lies anterior to the midportion of the left kidney.

The descending colon passes along the posterior abdominal wall over the lateral border of the left kidney, turns somewhat medially, and descends in the groove between the psoas and the quadratus lumborum muscles to its junction with the sigmoid at the level of the pelvic brim and the transversus abdominis muscle (3). Its length averages 30 cm. The anterior, medial, and lateral portions of its circumference are covered by peritoneum. The distal portion of the descending colon is usually attached by adhesions to the posterior abdominal wall, and these adhesions require division during mobilization of this portion of the colon.

The sigmoid colon extends from the pelvic brim to the sacral promontory, where it continues as the rectum. Its length varies dramatically from 15 to 50 cm, and it may follow an extremely tortuous and variable course. It often loops to the left but may follow a straight oblique course, loop to the right, or ascend high into the abdomen. It has a generous mesentery and is extremely mobile. The serosal surface has numerous appendices epiploicae. The base of the mesocolon extends from the iliac fossa, along the pelvic brim, and across the sacroiliac joint to the second or third sacral segment; in so doing, it forms an inverted V. Contained within the mesosigmoid are the sigmoidal and superior rectal arteries and accompanying veins, lymphatics, and autonomic nerve plexuses. At the base of the mesosigmoid is a recess, the intersigmoid fossa, which serves as a valuable guide to the left ureter, lying just deep to it. The upper limb runs medially and upward, crossing the left ureter and iliac vessels; this is an extremely important relationship during resection of this part of the colon. The lower limb extends in front of the sacrum and also may be alongside loops of small bowel, the urinary bladder, and the uterus and its adnexa.

Saunders et al. (4) conducted a novel study in which they investigated possible differences in colonic anatomy and mesenteric attachments between Western (Caucasian) and Oriental patients. Measurements of colonic length and mesenteric attachments were taken according to a set protocol from 115 Western and 114 Oriental patients at laparotomy. Sigmoid adhesions were found more frequently in Western patients (17%) compared to Oriental patients (8%) ($p=0.047$). A descending mesocolon of $\geq$10 cm occurred in 10 (8%) Western patients but only one (0.9%) Oriental patient ($p=0.01$). The splenic flexure was more frequently mobile in Western (20%) compared to Oriental patients (9%) ($p=0.016$). In 29% of Western patients, the midtransverse colon reached the symphysis pubis, or lower when pulled downward, in contrast to that finding in 10% of Oriental patients ($p<0.001$). There was no significant difference in total colonic length when Western patients (median, 114 cm; range, 68–159 cm) were compared with Oriental patients (median, 111 cm; range, 78–161 cm). Western patients have a higher incidence of sigmoid colon adhesions and increased colonic mobility when compared with Orientals. These findings support the observation that colonoscopy is a more difficult procedure to perform on Western patients.

■ PERITONEAL COVERINGS

The antimesenteric border of the distal ileum may be attached to the parietal peritoneum by a membrane (Lane's membrane) (5). The cecum usually is entirely enveloped by peritoneum. The ascending colon is attached to the posterior body wall and is devoid of peritoneum in its posterior surface; thus, it does not have a mesentery. The transverse colon is invested with peritoneum. Its posterosuperior surface, along the taenia band, is attached by the transverse mesocolon to the lower border of the pancreas. The posterior and inferior layers of the greater omentum are fused on the anterosuperior aspect of the transverse colon. To mobilize the greater omentum or to enter the lesser sac, the fusion of the omentum to the transverse colon must be dissected. Because the omental bursa becomes obliterated caudal to the transverse colon and toward the right side, the dissection should be started on the left side of the transverse colon. Topor et al. (6) studied 45 cadavers to elucidate surgical aspects of omental mobilization, lengthening, and transposition into the pelvic cavity. They identified that the most important anatomic variables for omental transposition were three variants of arterial blood supply: (i) In 56% of patients, there is one right, one (or two) middle, and one left omental artery. (ii) In 26% of patients, the middle omental artery is absent. (iii) In the remaining 18% of patients, the gastroepiploic artery is continued as a left omental artery but with various smaller connections to the right or middle omental artery. The first stage of omental lengthening is detachment of the omentum from the transverse colon mesentery. The second stage is the actual lengthening of the omentum. The third stage is placement of the omental flap into the pelvis. The left colonic flexure is attached to the diaphragm by the phrenocolic ligament, which also forms a shelf for supporting the spleen. The descending colon is devoid of peritoneum posteriorly, where it is in contact with the posterior abdominal wall and thus has no mesentery.

The sigmoid colon begins at about the level of the pelvic brim and is completely covered with peritoneum. The posterior surface is attached by a fan-shaped mesentery. The lateral surface of the sigmoid mesentery is fused to the parietal peritoneum of the lateral abdominal wall and is generally known as the "white line of Toldt." Mobilization of the sigmoid colon requires cutting or incising the lateral peritoneal reflection. The sigmoid colon varies greatly in length and configuration.

■ ILEOCECAL VALVE

The superior and inferior ileocecal ligaments are fibrous tissue that helps maintain the angulation between the ileum and the cecum. Kumar and Phillips (7) found these structures to be important in the maintenance of competence against reflux at the ileocecal junction. In an autopsy evaluation, the ascending colon was filled with saline solution by retrograde flow, and in 12 of 14 cases the ileocecal junctions were competent to pressures up to 80 mmHg. Removal of mucosa at the ileocecal junction or a strip of circular muscle did not impair competence to pressures above 40 mmHg, but division of the superior and inferior ileocecal ligaments rendered the junction incompetent. Operative reconstruction of the ileocecal angle restored competence. It therefore appears that the angulation between the ileum and the cecum determines continence.

RECTUM

Although anatomists traditionally assign the origin of the rectum to the level of the third sacral vertebra, surgeons generally consider the rectum to begin at the level of the sacral promontory. It descends along the curvature of the sacrum and coccyx and ends by passing through the levator ani muscles, at which level it abruptly turns downward and backward to become the anal canal. The rectum differs from the colon in that the outer layer is entirely longitudinal muscle, characterized by the merging of the three taenia bands. It measures 12–15 cm in length and lacks a mesentery, sacculations, and appendices epiploicae.

The rectum describes three lateral curves: the upper and lower curves are convex to the right, and the middle is convex to the left. On their inner aspect these infoldings into the lumen are known as the valves of Houston (8,9). About 46% of normal persons have three valves, 33% have two valves, 10% have four valves, 2% have none, and the rest have from five to seven valves (9). The clinical significance of the valves of Houston is that they must be negotiated during successful proctosigmoidoscopic examination and, more importantly, that they are an excellent location for a rectal biopsy, because the inward protrusion makes an easy target. They do not contain all the layers of the bowel wall, and therefore biopsy in this location carries a minimal risk of perforation. The middle fold is the internal landmark corresponding to the anterior peritoneal reflection. Consequently, extra caution must be exercised in removing polyps above this level. Because of its curves, the rectum can gain 5 cm in length when it is straightened (as in performing a low anterior resection); hence, a lesion that initially appears at 7 cm from the anal verge is often found 12 cm from that site after complete mobilization.

In its course the rectum is related posteriorly to the sacrum, coccyx, levator ani muscles, coccygeal muscles, median sacral vessels, and roots of the sacral nerve plexus. Anteriorly in the male, the extraperitoneal rectum is related to the prostate, seminal vesicles, vasa deferentia, ureters, and urinary bladder; the intraperitoneal rectum may come in contact with loops of the small bowel and sigmoid colon. In the female, the extraperitoneal rectum lies behind the posterior vaginal wall; the intraperitoneal rectum may be related to the upper part of the vagina, uterus, fallopian tubes, ovaries, small bowel, and sigmoid colon. Laterally above the peritoneal reflection, there may be loops of small bowel, adnexa, and sigmoid colon. Below the reflection, the rectum is separated from the side wall of the pelvis by the ureter and iliac vessels.

■ PERITONEAL RELATIONS

For descriptive purposes the rectum is divided into upper, middle, and lower thirds. The upper third is covered by peritoneum anteriorly and laterally, the middle third is covered only anteriorly, and the lower third is devoid of peritoneum. The peritoneal reflection shows considerable variation between individuals and between men and women. In men, it is usually 7–9 cm from the anal verge, while in women it is 5–7.5 cm above the anal verge. The middle valve of Houston roughly corresponds to the anterior peritoneal reflection. The posterior peritoneal reflection is usually 12–15 cm from the anal verge (Fig. 2).

The location of the peritoneal reflection has not been extensively studied in living patients. Najarian et al. (10) investigated the location of the peritoneal reflection in 50 patients undergoing laparotomy. The distance from the anal verge to the peritoneal reflection was measured in each patient via simultaneous intraoperative proctoscopy and intra-abdominal visualization of the peritoneal reflection. The mean lengths of the peritoneal reflection were 9 cm anteriorly, 12.2 cm laterally, and 14.8 cm posteriorly for females, and 9.7 cm anteriorly, 12.8 cm laterally, and 15.5 cm posteriorly for males. The lengths of the anterior, lateral, and posterior peritoneal measurements were statistically different from one another, regardless of gender. Their's (10) data indicated that the peritoneal reflection is located higher on the rectum than reported in autopsy studies, and that there is no difference between males and females. Knowledge of the location and position of a rectal carcinoma in relationship to the peritoneal reflection will help the surgeon optimize the use of peranal techniques of resection.

■ FASCIAL ATTACHMENTS

Fascia Propria (Investing Fascia)

The posterior part of the rectum, the distal lateral two thirds, and the anterior one third, are devoid of peritoneum, but they are covered with a thin layer of pelvic fascia, called fascia propria or the investing fascia. At the level of the rectal hiatus, the levator ani is covered by an expansion of the pelvic fascia, which on reaching the rectal wall divides into an ascending component, which fuses with the fascia propria of the rectum, and a descending component, which interposes itself between the muscular coats forming the conjoint longitudinal coat (11). These fibroelastic fibers run downward to reach the dermis of the perianal skin and split the subcutaneous striated sphincter into 8–12 discrete muscle bundles.

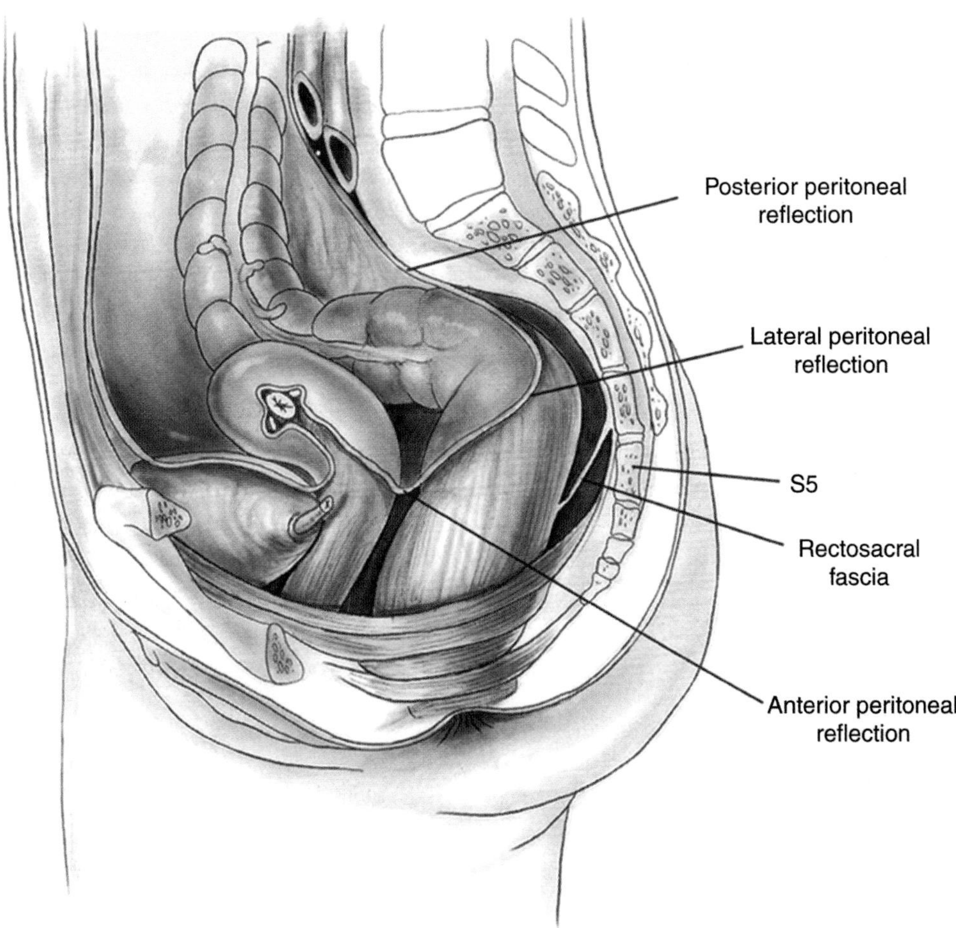

FIGURE 2 ■ Peritoneal relations of the rectum.

Waldeyer's Fascia

The sacrum and coccyx are covered with a strong fascia that is part of the parietal pelvic fascia. Known as Waldeyer's fascia, this presacral fascia covers the median sacral vessels. The rectosacral fascia is the Waldeyer's fascia from the periosteum of the fourth sacral segment to the posterior wall of the rectum (12,13). It is found in 97% of cadaver dissections (13). Waldeyer's fascia contains branches of sacral splanchnic nerves that arise directly from the sacral sympathetic ganglion and may contain branches of the lateral and median sacral vessels. This fascia should be sharply divided with scissors or electrocautery for full mobilization of the rectum (Fig. 3). The posterior space below the rectosacral fascia is the supralevator or retrorectal space (see Fig. 12).

Denonvilliers' Fascia

Anteriorly, the extraperitoneal portion of the rectum is covered with a visceral pelvic fascia, the fascia propria, or investing fascia. Anterior to the fascia propria, or is a filmy delicate layer of connective tissue known as Denonvilliers' fascia (14). It separates the rectum from the seminal vesicles and the prostate or vagina (Fig. 4). Denonvilliers' fascia has no macroscopically discernible layers. Histologically, it is composed of dense collagen, smooth muscle fibers, and coarse elastic fibers (15,16). Its attachments have been surrounded by confusion and debates. Some authors believe it is adherent to the rectum (16–19), others note that it is applied to the seminal vesicles and the prostate (15,20–22).

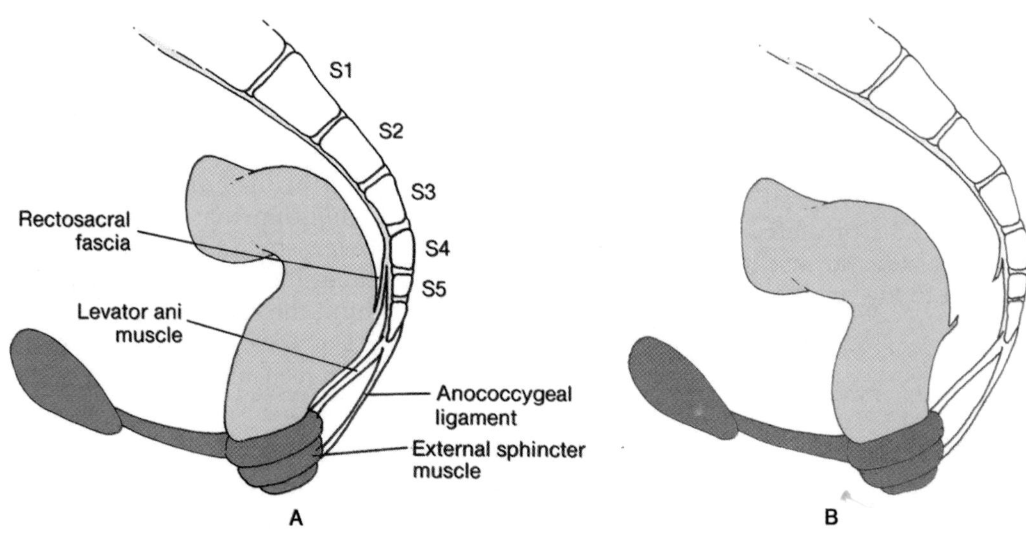

FIGURE 3 ■ (**A**) Rectosacral fascia. (**B**) Sharp division of rectosacral fascia for full mobilization of the rectum.

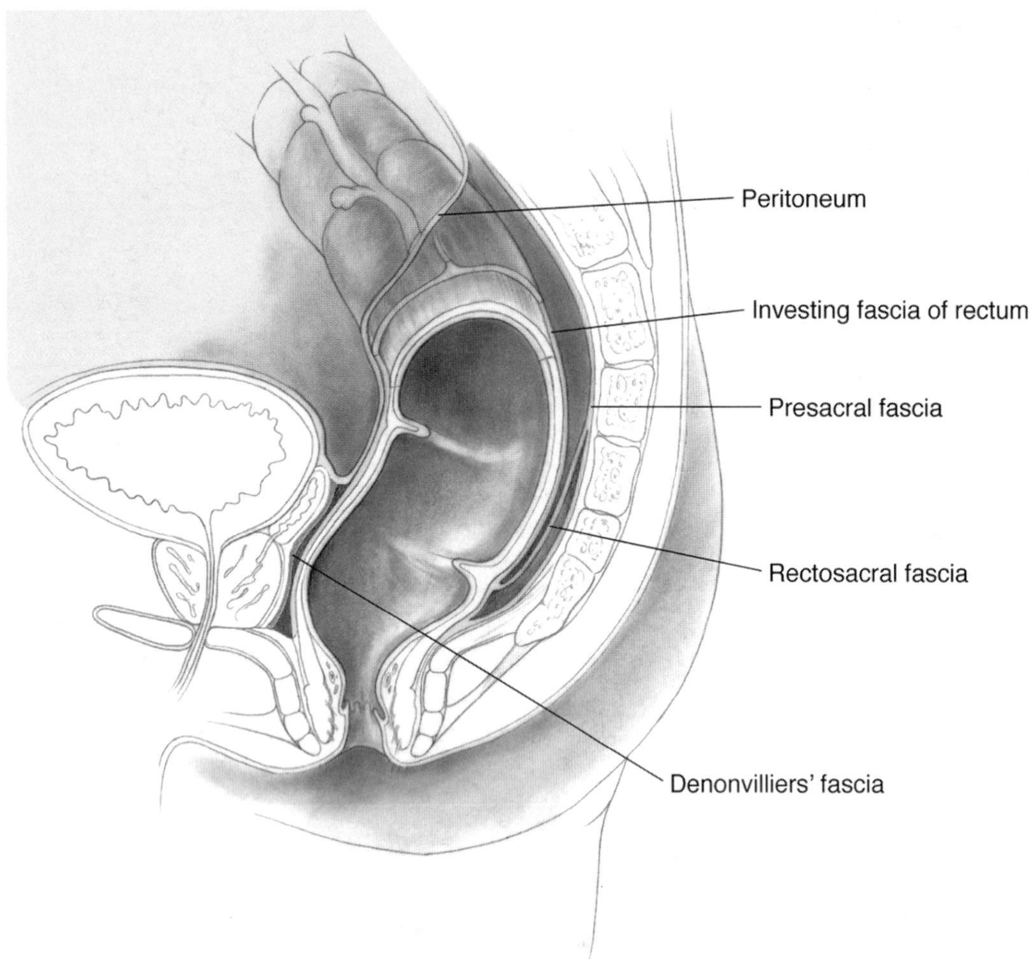

FIGURE 4 ■ Denonvilliers' fascia.

Lindsey et al. (23) designed a study to evaluate the anatomic relation of Denonvilliers' fascia: whether it is attached on the anterior fascia propria of the rectum, or on the seminal vesicles and prostate. They prospectively collected 30 specimens from males undergoing total mesorectal excision for mid and low rectal carcinoma, with a deep dissection of the anterior extraperitoneal rectum to the pelvic floor. The anterior aspects of the extraperitoneal rectal sections were examined microscopically for the presence or absence of Denonvilliers' fascia. In 20/30 patients that the carcinoma involved anteriorly, 55% vs. 45% of the specimens had Denonvilliers' fascia present. On the other hand, when the anterior rectum was not involved with carcinoma (10 patients), 90% of the specimens contained no Denonvilliers' fascia. The authors concluded, "when rectal dissection is conducted on fascia propria in the anatomic plane, Denonvilliers' fascia remains on the posterior aspect of the prostate and seminal vesicles. Denonvilliers' fascia lies anterior to the anatomic fascia propria plane of anterior rectal dissection in total mesorectal excision (TME) and is more closely applied to the prostate than the rectum." This study has put the debates to rest; Denonvilliers' fascia is more closely applied to the seminal vesicles and the prostate than the rectum.

Lateral Ligament

The distal rectum, which is extraperitoneal, is attached to the pelvic side wall on each side by the pelvic plexus, connective tissues, and middle rectal artery (if present) (24). Histologically it consists of nerve structures, fatty tissue, and small blood vessels (25). Recently, the anatomical term of "lateral ligament" has been a subject of debate. In dissection of 27 fresh cadavers and five embalmed pelves, Nano et al. (26) found that lateral ligaments were extension of the mesorectum to the lateral endopelvic fascia. From their experience with anatomic dissection applied to surgery, several conclusion were drawn:

- Lateral ligaments are extensions of the mesorectum and must be cut at their attachment at the endopelvic fascia for TME to take place.
- Lateral ligaments contain fatty tissue in communication with mesorectal fat and possibly some vessels and nerve filaments that are of little importance.
- Insertion of lateral ligaments at the endopelvic fascia is placed under the urogenital bundle.
- The middle rectal artery courses anteriorly and inferiorly in respect to the lateral ligament.
- Lateral ligaments can be cut at their insertion on the endopelvic fascia without injuring the urogenital nervous bundle, which, however, should be kept in view during this procedure, because it crosses the middle rectal artery and fans out behind the seminal vesicles.
- The lateral aspect of the rectum receives the lateral pedicle, which consists of the nervi recti and the middle rectal artery.

A study by Rutegard et al. (25) on 10 patients who underwent total mesorectal excision for rectal carcinoma revealed, "the often thin structures, usually referred to as the lateral ligaments, seem to arise from the pelvic plexuses and bridge over into the mesorectum, ... they can be identified in almost every patient." The authors contend that the lateral ligaments are real anatomical findings. This finding was supported by Sato and Sato (13) in the dissection of 45 cadavers.

On the other hand, Jones et al. (24) meticulously dissected 28 cadaveric pelves; they found insubstantial thin strands of connective tissues traversing the space between the mesorectum and the pelvic side wall. These strands of connective tissues were no different from those one would expect to find in any areolar plane. They were often absent altogether. The pelvic plexuses were distinct from the middle rectal artery (if present) and had no association with the connective tissues. Jones et al. (24) believed that the lateral ligament was nothing more than a surgical artifact that results from injudicious dissection.

When the rectum is pulled medially, the complex of middle rectal artery and vein, the splanchnic nerves, and their accompanying connective tissues form a band-like structure extending from the lateral pelvic wall to the rectum (27). This structure was most likely mistaken as the "lateral ligament" in the past. Whatever one would call the lateral attachment of the low rectum, the tissues need to be divided in full mobilization of the rectum.

MESORECTUM

The posterior rectum is devoid of peritoneum and has no mesorectum. The term mesorectum is a misnomer and does not appear in the Normina Anatomica although it is listed in the Normina Embryologica (28). The word mesorectum was possibly first used by Maunsell in 1892 and later popularized by Heald of the United Kingdom (28). In answering the critique of using this word, Heald answered, "... it was a surgical word used by the foremost of my surgical teachers when I was a young registrar. Mr. Rex Lawrice of Guy's Hospital used to describe the process of dividing the mesorectum as was well described in Rob and Smith's text book of surgery at that time. ... no other word seems readily available to describe it" (29).

Total mesorectal excision implies the complete excision of all fat enclosed within the fascia propria, which Heald calls the "mesorectum." This dissection is performed in a circumferential manner down to the levator muscles (28). Bisset et al. (30) preferred the term "extra fascial excision of the rectum." The term mesorectum has now been used worldwide and appears well entrenched.

Canessa et al. (31) studied the lymph nodes in 20 cadevers using conventional manual dissection. The starting point was at the bifurcation of the superior rectal artery and ending at the anorectal ring. They found an average of 8.4 lymph nodes per rectum; 71% of the lymph nodes were above the peritoneal reflection and 29% were below it. Dissection of seven fresh cadavers on the mesorectum by Toper et al. (32) yielded 174 lymph nodes; over 80% of the lymph nodes were smaller than 3 mm. Fifty-six percent of the nodes were located in the posterior mesentery, and most were located in the upper two thirds of posterior rectal mesentery.

HISTOLOGY

Knowledge of the microscopic anatomy of the large intestine is of paramount importance in understanding the various disease processes. This is especially true in the case of neoplasia, where the depth of penetration will dictate the treatment recommendation. Therefore it is essential to examine histologic features.

The innermost layer is the mucosa, which is composed of three divisions. The first is a layer of columnar epithelial cells with a series of crevices or crypts characterized by straight tubules that lie parallel and close to one another and do not branch (glands of Lieberkühn). The surface epithelium around the openings of the crypts consists of simple columnar cells with occasional goblet cells. The tubules are lined predominantly by goblet cells, except at the base of the crypts where undifferentiated cells as well as enterochromaffin and amine precursor uptake and decarboxylation (APUD) cells are found. The epithelial layer is separated from the underlying connective tissue by an extracellular membrane composed of glycopolysaccharides and seen as the lamina densa of the basement membrane when viewed by electron microscopy (33). Abnormalities classified as defects, multilayering, or other structural abnormalities have been reported in many types of neoplasms, including those of the colon and rectum. These abnormalities are more common in malignant than in benign neoplasms. The second division of the mucosa is the lamina propria, composed of a stroma of connective tissue containing capillaries, inflammatory cells, and lymphoid follicles that are more prominent in young persons. The third division is the muscularis mucosa, a fine sheet of smooth muscle fibers that serves as a critical demarcation in the diagnosis of invasive carcinoma and includes a network of lymphatics (34).

Beneath the muscularis mucosa is the submucosa, a layer of connective tissue and collagen that contains vessels, lymphatics, and Meissner's plexus. It is the strongest layer of the bowel.

The next layer is the circular muscle, which is a continuous sheath around the bowel, including both the colon and the rectum. On the external surface of the circular muscle are clusters of ganglion cells and their ramifications; these make up the myenteric plexus of Auerbach. Unmyelinated postganglionic fibers penetrate the muscle to communicate with the submucosal plexus. The outer or longitudinal muscle fibers of the colon are characteristically collected into three bundles, called the taeniae coli; however, in the rectum these fibers are spread out and form a continuous layer. The muscularis propria is pierced at regular intervals by the main arterial blood supply and venous drainage of the mucosa.

The outermost layer, which is absent in the lower portions of the rectum, is the serosa or visceral peritoneum. This layer contains blood vessels and lymphatics.

ANAL CANAL

The anal canal is the terminal portion of the intestinal tract. It begins at the anorectal junction (the point passing through the levator ani muscles), is about 4 cm long, and terminates at the anal verge (35,36). This definition differs from that of the anatomist, who designates the anal canal as the part of the intestinal tract that extends from the dentate line to the anal verge.

The anal canal is surrounded by strong muscles, and because of tonic contraction of these muscles, it is completely collapsed and represents an anteroposterior slit. The musculature of the anorectal region may be regarded as two tubes, one surrounding the other (Fig. 5) (37). The inner tube, being visceral, is smooth muscle and is innervated by the autonomic nervous system, while the outer funnel-shaped tube is skeletal muscle and has somatic innervation. This short segment of the intestinal tract is of paramount importance because it is essential to the mechanism of fecal continence and also because it is prone to many diseases.

The anatomy of the anal canal and perianal structures has been imaged using endoluminal magnetic resonance imaging (38). Investigators found that the lateral canal was significantly longer than its anterior and posterior part. The anterior external anal sphincter was shorter in women than in men and occupied, respectively, 30% and 38% of the anal canal length. The median length and thickness of the female anterior external anal sphincter were 11 and 13 mm, respectively. These small dimensions explain why a relatively small obstetrical tear may have a devastating effect on fecal continence and why it may be difficult to identify the muscle while performing a sphincter repair after an obstetrical injury. The caudal ends of the external anal sphincter formed a double layer. The perineal body was thicker in women than in men and easier to define. The superficial transverse muscles had a lateral and caudal extension to the ischiopubic bones. The bulbospongiosus was thicker in men than in women. The ischiocavernosus and anococcygeal body had the same dimensions in both sexes.

Posteriorly the anal canal is related to its surrounding muscle and the coccyx. Laterally is the ischioanal fossa with its inferior rectal vessels and nerves. Anteriorly in the male is the urethra, a very important relationship to know during abdominoperineal resection of the rectum. Anteriorly in the female are the perineal body and the lowest part of the posterior vaginal wall.

■ LINING OF CANAL

The lining of the anal canal consists of epithelium of different types at different levels (Fig. 6). At approximately the midpoint of the anal canal there is an undulating demarcation referred to as the dentate line. This line is approximately 2 cm from the anal verge. Because the rectum narrows into the anal canal, the tissue above the dentate line takes on a pleated appearance. These longitudinal folds, of which there are 6 to 14, are known as the columns of Morgagni. There is a small pocket or crypt at the lower end of and between adjacent columns of the folds. These crypts are of surgical significance because foreign material may become lodged in them, obstructing the ducts of the anal glands and possibly resulting in sepsis.

The mucosa of the upper anal canal is lined by columnar epithelium. Below the dentate line the anal canal is lined with a squamous epithelium. The change, however, is not abrupt. For a distance of 6–12 mm above the dentate line there is a gradual transition where columnar, transitional, or squamous epithelium may be found. This area, referred to as the anal transitional or cloacogenic zone, has extremely variable histology.

A color change in the epithelium is also noted. The rectal mucosa is pink, whereas the area just above the

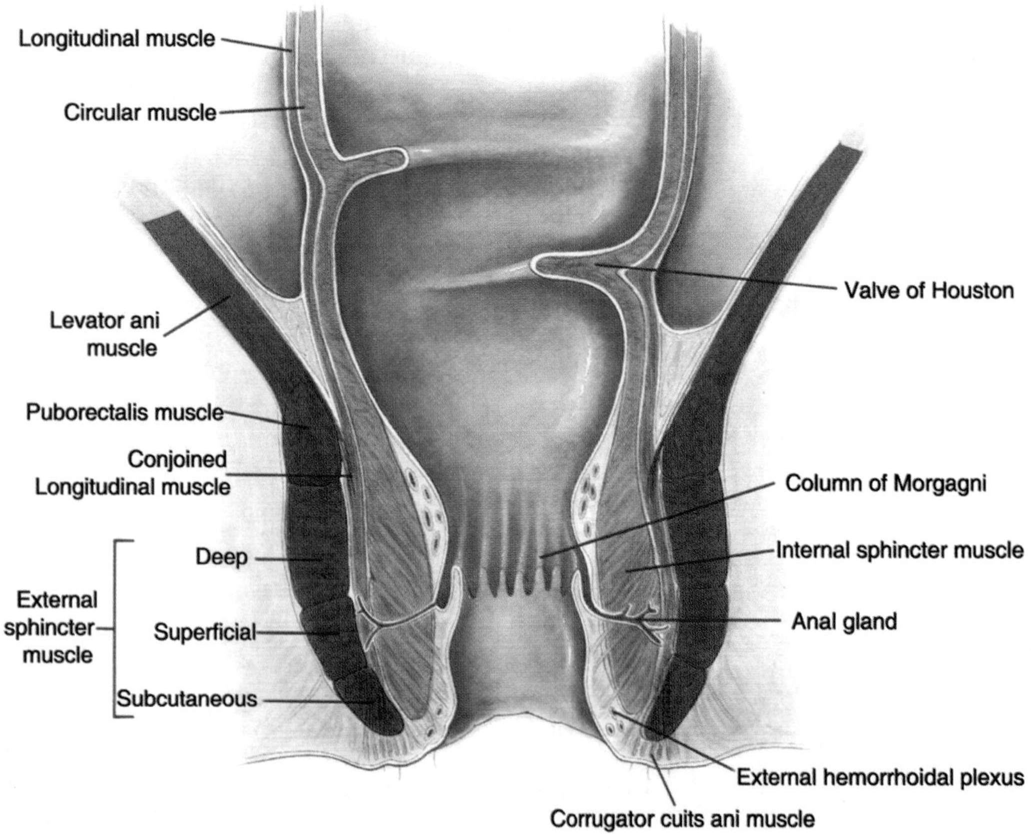

FIGURE 5 ■ Anal canal.

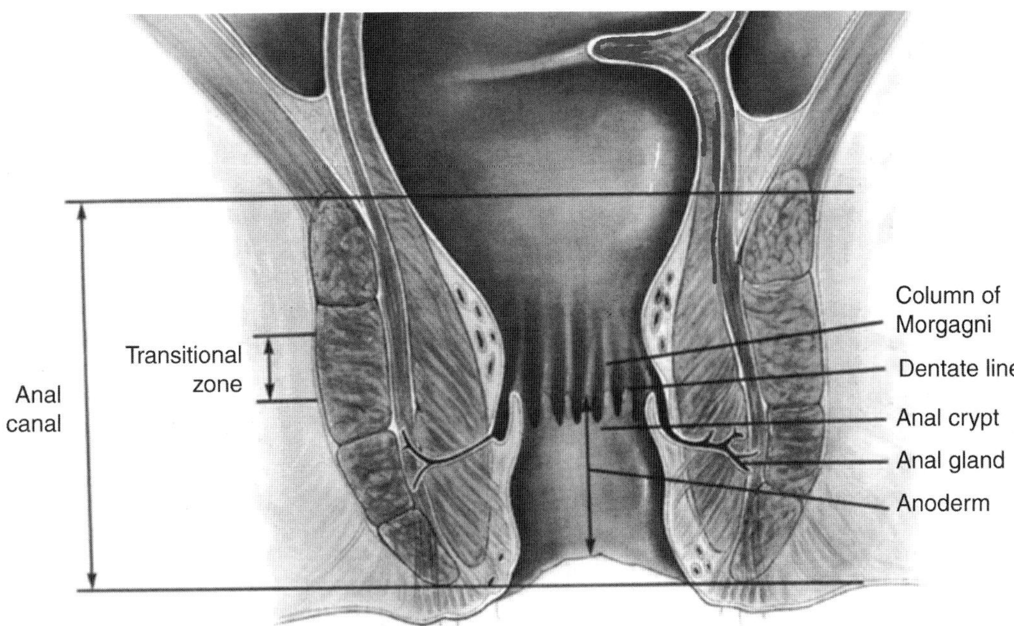

FIGURE 6 ■ Lining of the anal canal.

dentate line is deep purple or plum color due to the underlying internal hemorrhoidal plexus. Subepithelial tissue is loosely attached to and radially distensible from the internal hemorrhoidal plexus. Subepithelial tissue at the anal margin, which contains the external hemorrhoidal plexus, forms a lining that adheres firmly to the underlying tissue. At the level of the dentate line, the lining is anchored by what Parks (39) called the mucosal suspensory ligament. The perianal space is limited above by this ligament and below by the attachment of the longitudinal muscle to the skin of the anal verge. The area below the dentate line is not true skin because it is devoid of accessory skin structures (e.g., hair, sebaceous glands, and sweat glands). This pale, delicate, smooth, thin, and shiny stretched tissue is referred to as anoderm and runs for approximately 1.5 cm below the dentate line. At the anal verge the lining becomes thicker and pigmented and acquires hair follicles, glands, and other histologic features of normal skin (2). In this circumanal area there is also a well-marked ring of apocrine glands, which may be the source of the clinical condition called hidradenitis suppurativa. Proximal to the dentate line the epithelium is supplied by the autonomic nervous system, while distally the lining is richly innervated by the somatic nervous system (40).

■ ANAL TRANSITIONAL ZONE

The anal transitional zone (ATZ) is interposed between uninterrupted colorectal type mucosa (columnar) above and uninterrupted squamous epithelium (anoderm) below, irrespective of the type of epithelium present in the zone itself (41). The ATZ usually commences just above the dentate line. Using computer maps of histology, Thompson-Fawcett et al. (42) found that the dentate line was situated at a median of 1.05 cm above the lower border of the internal sphincter. This is much smaller than the study by Fenger (41), which portrayed the ATZ extending 0.9 cm above the dentate line. Fenger used the traditional Alcian blue stain. This results in overestimation of the length of the ATZ because the pale blue staining is due to staining of superficial nuclei of both squamous anoderm and transitional epithelium rather than staining of mucin-producing cells in the transitional epithelium (42). The ATZ is much smaller than commonly thought.

The histology of the ATZ is extremely variable. Most of the zone is covered by ATZ epithelium, which appears to be composed of four to nine cell layers—the basal cells, columnar, cuboidal, unkeratinized squamous epithelium, and anal glands. The ATZ epithelium contains a mixture of sulphomucin and sialomucin. The mucin pattern in the columnar variant of the ATZ epithelium and in the anal canal is of the same type and differs from that of colorectal-type epithelium. The findings of a similar mucin pattern in mucoepidermoid carcinoma and in some cases of carcinoma arising in anal fistulas as well as in carcinoma suspected of arising in anal glands might indicate a common origin of the neoplasm in the ATZ epithelium.

Histochemical study shows that endocrine cells have been demonstrated in 87% of specimens. Their function is unknown. Melanin is found in the basal layer of the ATZ epithelium in 14% of specimens. Melanin cannot be demonstrated in the anal gland but is a constant finding in the squamous epithelium below the dentate line, increasing in amount as the perianal skin is approached. The melanin-containing cells in the ATZ seem a reasonable point of origin for melanoma, as do the findings of junctional activity and atypical melanocyte hyperplasia in the ATZ.

The ATZ epithelium has a dominating diploid population, although there was a small hyperdiploid peak representing nuclei with a scattered volume considerably higher than that of the main diploid population. This was present regardless of the histologic variant (columnar or cuboid) of the ATZ epithelium. Tetraploid or octoploid populations are not found (41).

■ ANAL GLANDS

The average number of glands in a normal anal canal is six (range, 3–10) (43). Each gland is lined by stratified columnar epithelium with mucus-secreting or goblet cells interspersed within the glandular epithelial lining and has a direct opening into an anal crypt at the dentate line. Occasionally, two glands open into the same crypt, while half the crypts have no communication with the glands.

These glands were first described by Chiari in 1878 (44). The importance of their role in the pathogenesis of fistulous abscess was presented by Parks in 1961 (37).

Seow-Choen and Ho (43) find that 80% of the anal glands are submucosal in extent, 8% extend to the internal sphincter, 8% to the conjoined longitudinal muscle, 2% to intersphincteric space, and 1% penetrate the external sphincter. The anal glands are fairly evenly distributed around the anal canal, although the greatest number are found at the anterior quadrant. Mild to moderate lymphocytic infiltration is noted around the anal glands and ducts; this is sometimes referred to as "anal tonsil."

In an autopsy study of 62 specimens, Klosterhalfen et al. (45) found that nearly 90% of specimens contained anal sinuses. In fetuses and children, more than half the anal sinuses were accompanied by anal intramuscular glands penetrating the internal anal sphincter, whereas in adult specimens, anal intramuscular glands were rare.

MUSCLES OF THE ANORECTAL REGION

■ INTERNAL SPHINCTER MUSCLE

The downward continuation of the circular, smooth muscle of the rectum becomes thickened and rounded at its lower end and is called the internal sphincter. Its lowest portion is just above the lowest part of the external sphincter and is 1–1.5 cm below the dentate line (Fig. 5).

■ CONJOINED LONGITUDINAL MUSCLE

At the level of the anorectal ring, the longitudinal muscle coat of the rectum is joined by fibers of the levator ani and puborectalis muscles. Another contributing source is the pelvic fascia (11). The conjoined longitudinal muscle so formed descends between the internal and external anal sphincters (Fig. 5) (46). Many of these fibers traverse the lower portion of the external sphincter to gain insertion in the perianal skin and are referred to as the corrugator cutis ani (47). Fine and Lawes (48) described a longitudinal layer of muscle lying on the inner aspect of the internal sphincter and named it the muscularis submucosae ani. These fibers may arise from the conjoined longitudinal muscle. Some fibers that traverse the internal sphincter muscle and become inserted just below the anal valves have been referred to as the mucosal suspensory ligament (37). Some fibers may traverse the external sphincter to form a transverse septum of the ischioanal fossa (Fig. 5). In a review of the anatomy and function of the anal longitudinal muscle, Lunnis and Phillips (49) speculated that this muscle plays a role as a skeleton supporting and binding the internal and external sphincter complex together, as an aid during defecation by everting the anus, as a support to the hemorrhoidal cushions, and as a determining factor in the ramification of sepsis.

■ EXTERNAL SPHINCTER MUSCLE

This elliptical cylinder of skeletal muscle that surrounds the anal canal was originally described as consisting of three distinct divisions: the subcutaneous, superficial, and deep portions (36). This account was shown to be invalid by Goligher (50), who demonstrated that a sheet of muscle runs continuously upward with the puborectalis and levator ani muscles. The lowest portion of the external sphincter occupies a position below and slightly lateral to the internal sphincter. A palpable groove at this level has been referred to as the intersphincteric groove. The lowest part (subcutaneous fibers) is traversed by the conjoined longitudinal muscle, with some fibers gaining attachment to the skin. The next portion (superficial) is attached to the coccyx by a posterior extension of muscle fibers that combine with connective tissue, forming the anococcygeal ligament. Above this level, the deep portion of the external sphincter is devoid of posterior attachment and proximally becomes continuous with the puborectalis muscle. Anteriorly, the high fibers of the external sphincter are inserted into the perineal body, where some merge and are continuous with the transverse perineal muscles. The female sphincter has a variable natural defect occurring along its anterior length (51). This makes interpretation of the isolated endoanal ultrasound difficult and explains overreporting of obstetric sphincter defects. The external sphincter is supplied by the inferior rectal nerve and a perineal branch of the fourth sacral nerve. From their embryolic study, Levi et al. (52) demonstrated that the external sphincter is subdivided into two parts, one superficial and one deep without any connection with the puborectalis.

Shafik (46) has suggested that the anal sphincter mechanism consists of three U-shaped loops and that each loop is a separate sphincter and complements the others to help maintain continence (Fig. 7). This concept has not been generally accepted. In fact, more recently Ayoub (56) found that the external sphincter is one muscle mass, not divided into layers or laminae, and that all fibers of the external sphincter muscles retain their skeletal attachment by the anococcygeal ligament to the coccyx. Clinical experience supports Ayoub's concept; we have not been able to identify Shafik's three-part scheme. Indeed, during postanal repairs for anal incontinence, the external sphincter, puborectalis, and levator ani muscles present as one continuous funnel-shaped sheet of skeletal muscle. The currently accepted perception of the arrangement of the external

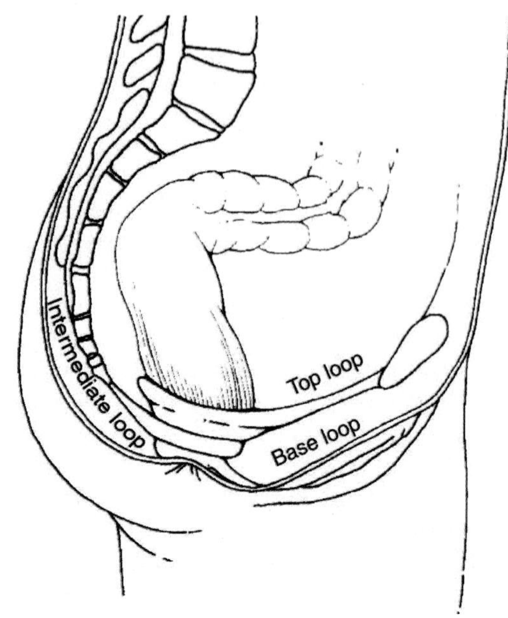

FIGURE 7 ■ Shafik loops. *Source:* From Ref. 46.

sphincter is that it is one continuous circumferential mass, a concept in accordance with a study in which anal endosonography was used (53).

■ PERINEAL BODY

The perineal body is the anatomic location in the central portion of the perineum where the external sphincter, bulbocavernosus, and superficial and deep transverse perineal muscles meet (Fig. 8). This tends to be a tendinous intersection and is believed to give support to the perineum and to separate the anus from the vagina. In patients who have sustained a sphincter injury, an effort should be made to rebuild the perineal body as well as to reconstruct the sphincter.

■ PELVIC FLOOR MUSCLES

The levator ani muscle is a broad, thin muscle that forms the greater part of the floor of the pelvic cavity and is innervated by the fourth sacral nerve (Fig. 9). This muscle traditionally has been considered to consist of three muscles: the iliococcygeus, the pubococcygeus, and the puborectalis (3). Oh and Kark (54) and Shafik (55) suggested that it consists only of the iliococcygeus and pubococcygeus muscles and that the puborectalis is part of the deep portion of the external sphincter muscle, since the two are fused and have the same nerve supply, the pudendal nerve. However, the electrophysiologic study by Percy et al. (57) concluded that in 19 of 20 patients, stimulation of sacral nerves above the pelvic floor resulted in electromyographic activity in the ipsilateral puborectalis but not in the external sphincter. Results of postmortem innervation studies have favored a perineal nerve supply to the puborectalis, but the weight of evidence in favor of a pudendal nerve supply has been challenged by in vivo studies. Levi et al. (52) believe that the puborectalis muscle must be considered part of the levator ani because it is never connected with the external sphincter in different steps of embryonic development.

In a neuroanatomy study Matzel et al. (58) dissected cadavers and traced the sacral nerves from their entrance into the pelvis through the sacral foramina throughout their branching to their final destinations and found that the neural supply of the levator ani was distinct from that of the external anal sphincter. The levator is supplied by branches from the sacral nerves proximal to the sacral plexus and running on the inner surface; the external anal sphincter is supplied by nerve fibers traveling with the pudendal nerve on the levator's undersurface. To document the functional relevance of these anatomic findings, stimulation of the pudendal and sacral nerves was performed. The former increased anal pressure, whereas stimulation of S3 increased anal pressure only slightly but caused an impressive decrease of the rectoanal angle. When S3 was stimulated after bilateral pudendal block, anal pressure did not change, but the decrease in rectoanal angulation persisted. The authors concluded from their anatomic dissection and neurophysiologic study that two different peripheral nerve supplies are responsible for anal continence, that one muscle complex is innervated mainly by the third sacral nerve and another by the pudendal nerve. Further investigation will be required to clarify this point.

Puborectalis Muscle

The puborectalis muscle arises from the back of the symphysis pubis and the superior fascia of the urogenital diaphragm, runs backward alongside the anorectal junction, and joins its fellow muscle of the other side immediately behind the rectum, where they form a U-shaped loop that slings the rectum to the pubes (Fig. 10).

Iliococcygeus Muscle

The iliococcygeus muscle arises from the ischial spine and posterior part of the obturator fascia, passes downward, backward, and medially, and becomes inserted on the last two segments of the sacrum, the coccyx, and the anococcygeal raphe. There are no connections to the anal canal (11).

Pubococcygeus Muscle

The pubococcygeus muscle arises from the anterior half of the obturator fascia and the back of the pubis. Its fibers are directed backward, downward, and medially where they decussate with fibers of the opposite side (11,56). This line of decussation is called the anococcygeal raphe (Fig. 9). Some fibers, which lie more posteriorly, are attached directly to the tip of the coccyx and the last segment of the sacrum. This muscle also sends fibers to share the formation of the conjoined longitudinal muscle (Fig. 5). The muscle fibers of the pubococcygeus, while proceeding backward, downward, and medially, form an elliptical space, called the "levator hiatus" (Fig. 9), through which pass the lower part of the rectum and either the prostatic urethra and dorsal vein of the penis in men or the vagina and urethra in women. The intrahiatal viscera are bound together by part of the pelvic fascia, which is more condensed at the level of the anorectal junction and has been called the "hiatal ligament" (Fig. 10) (56). This ligament is believed to keep the movement of the intrahiatal structures in harmony with the levator ani muscle. The crisscross arrangement of the anococcygeal raphe prevents the constrictor effect on the intrahiatal structures during levator ani contraction and causes a dilator effect (56). The puborectalis and the levator ani muscles have a reciprocal action. As one contracts, the other relaxes. During defecation there is puborectalis relaxation accompanied by levator ani contraction, which widens the hiatus and elevates the lower rectum and anal canal. When a person is in an upright position, the levator ani muscle supports the viscera.

■ ANORECTAL RING

"Anorectal ring" is a term coined by Milligan and Morgan (36) to denote the functionally important ring of muscle that surrounds the junction of the rectum and the anal canal. It is composed of the upper borders of the internal sphincter and the puborectalis muscle. It is of paramount importance during the treatment of abscesses and fistulas because division of this ring will inevitably result in anal incontinence.

■ ANORECTAL SPACES

Certain potential spaces in and about the anorectal region are of surgical significance and will be briefly described (Figs. 11–13).

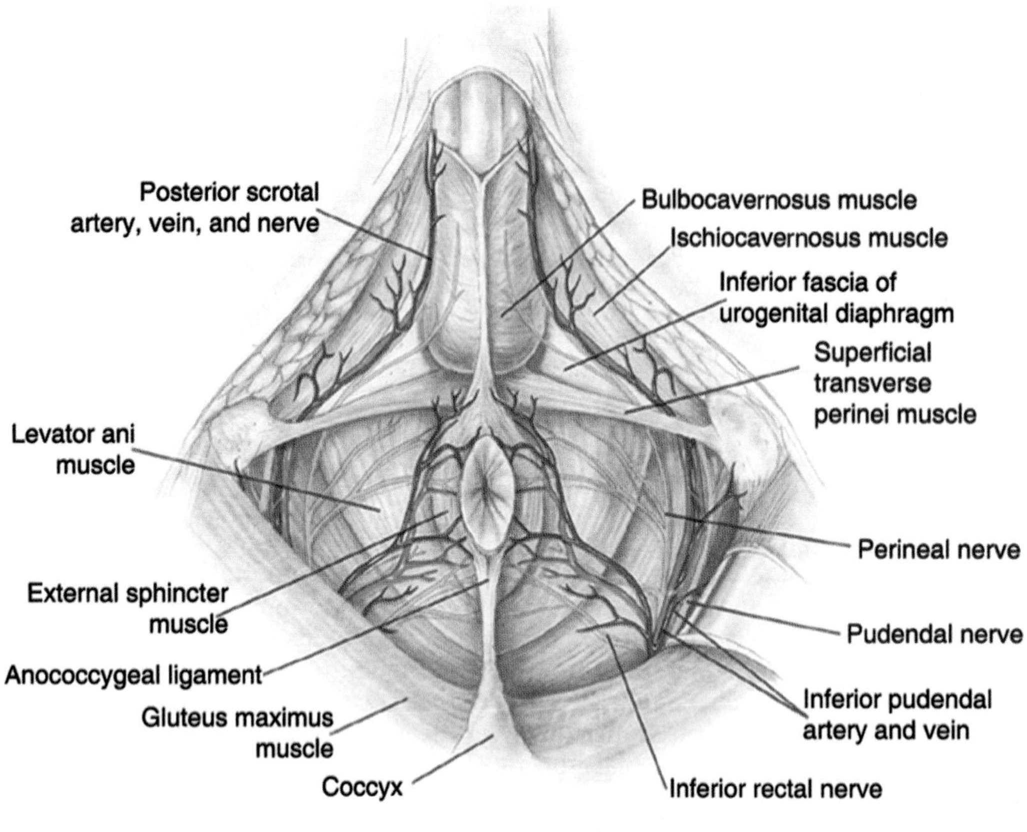

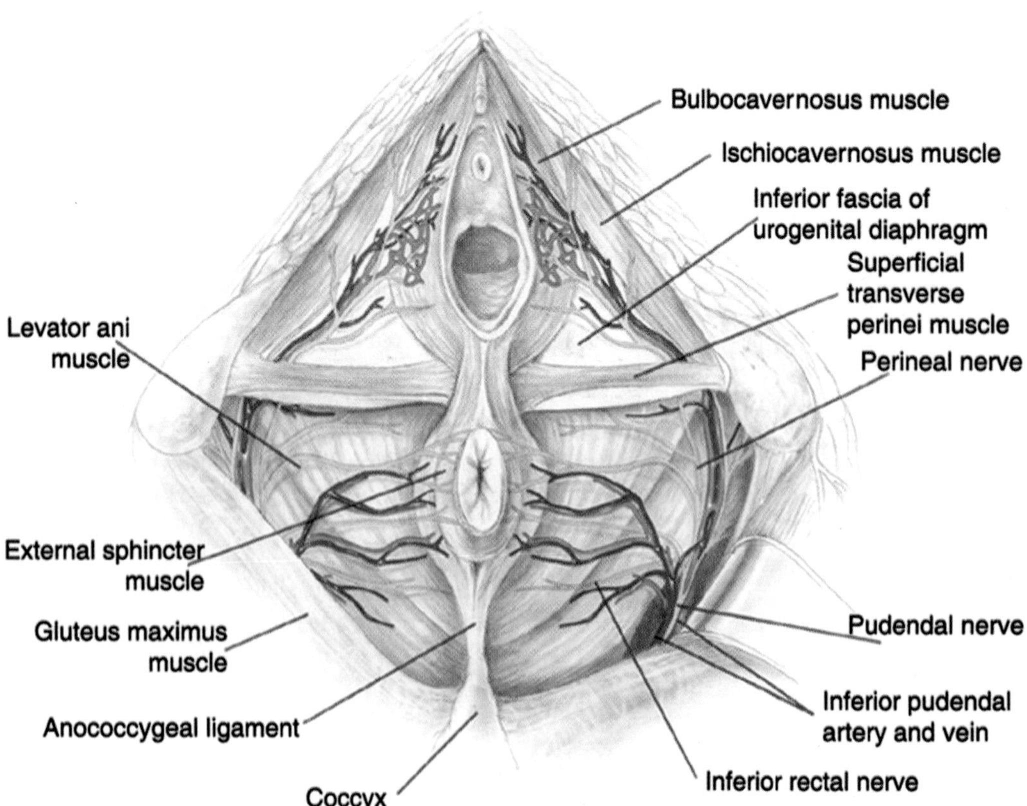

FIGURE 8 ■ Perineal view. (**A**) Male perineum. (**B**) Female perineum.

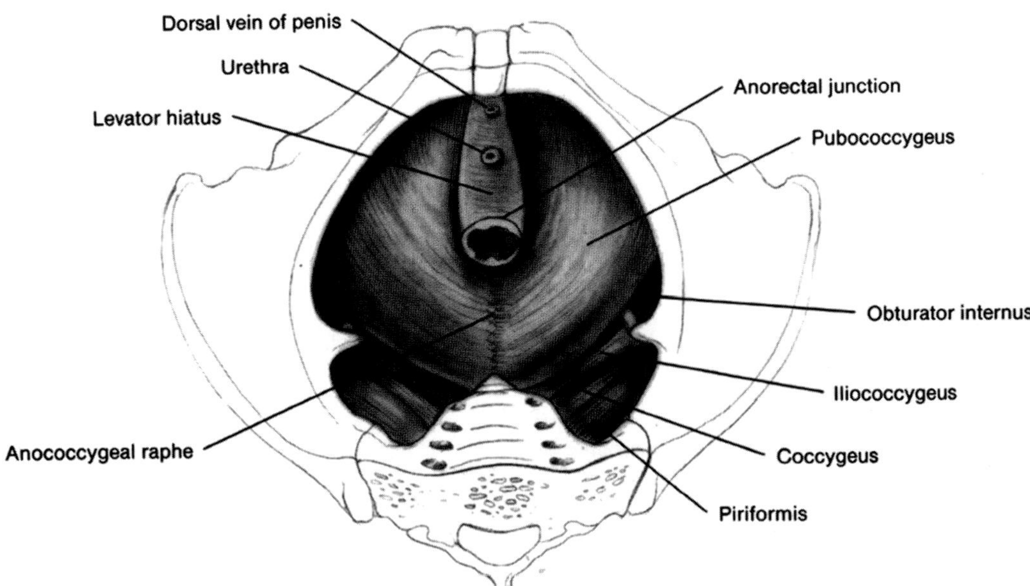

FIGURE 9 ■ Levator muscles.
Source: From Ref. 46.

■ PERIANAL SPACE

The perianal space is in the immediate area of the anal verge surrounding the anal canal. Laterally it becomes continuous with the subcutaneous fat of the buttocks or may be confined by the conjoined longitudinal muscle. Medially it extends into the lower part of the anal canal as far as the dentate line. It is continuous with the intersphincteric space. The perianal space contains the lowest part of the external sphincter, the external hemorrhoidal plexus, branches of the inferior rectal vessels, and lymphatics. The radiating elastic septa divide the space into a compact honeycomb arrangement, which accounts for the severe pain produced by a collection of pus or blood.

■ ISCHIOANAL SPACE

The ischioanal fossa is a pyramid-shaped space. The apex is formed at the origin of the levator ani from the obturator fascia, and the inferior boundary is the skin on the perineum. The anterior boundary is formed by the superficial and deep transverse perineal muscles and the posterior boundary of the perineal membrane. The posterior boundary is the gluteal skin. The medial wall is composed of the levator ani and the external sphincter muscles. The lateral wall is nearly vertical and is formed by the obturator internus muscle and the ischium and by the obturator fascia. The base or inferior boundary is the transverse septum, which divides this space from the perianal space (59). In the obturator fascia, on the lateral wall, is the Alcock's canal, which contains the internal pudendal vessels and the pudendal nerve. When the ischioanal and perianal spaces are regarded as a single tissue space, it is called the ischioanal fossa (60). The contents of the ischioanal fossa consist of a pad of fat, the inferior rectal nerve coursing from the back of the ischioanal fossa forward and medially to the external sphincter, the inferior rectal vessels, portions of the scrotal nerves and vessels in men and the labial nerves and vessels in women, the transverse perineal vessels, and the perineal branch of the fourth sacral nerve running to the external sphincter from the posterior angle of the fossa (61). Anteriorly the ischioanal space has an important extension forward, above the urogenital diaphragm, which may become filled with pus in cases of ischioanal abscesses.

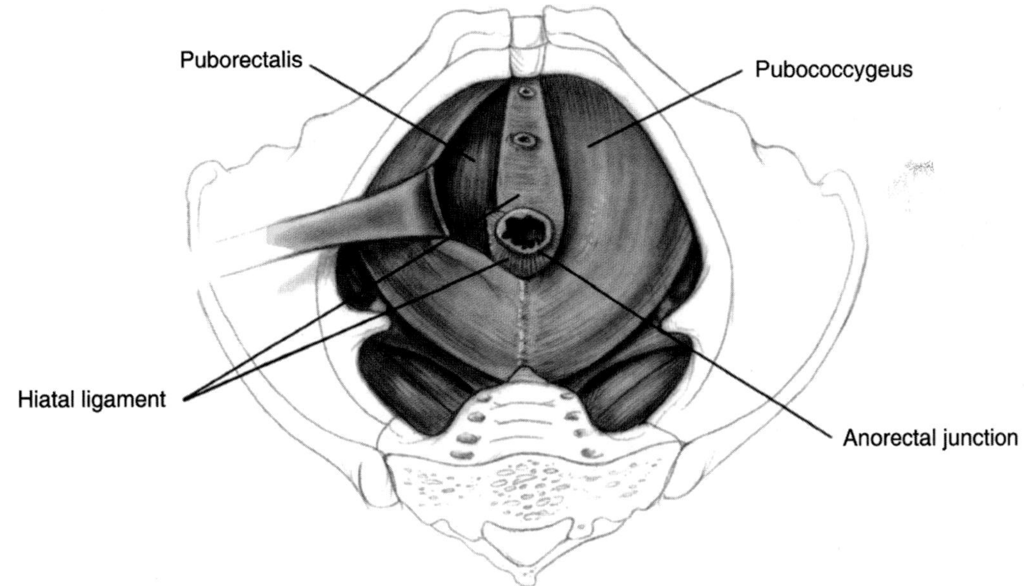

FIGURE 10 ■ Hiatal ligament.
Source: From Ref. 46.

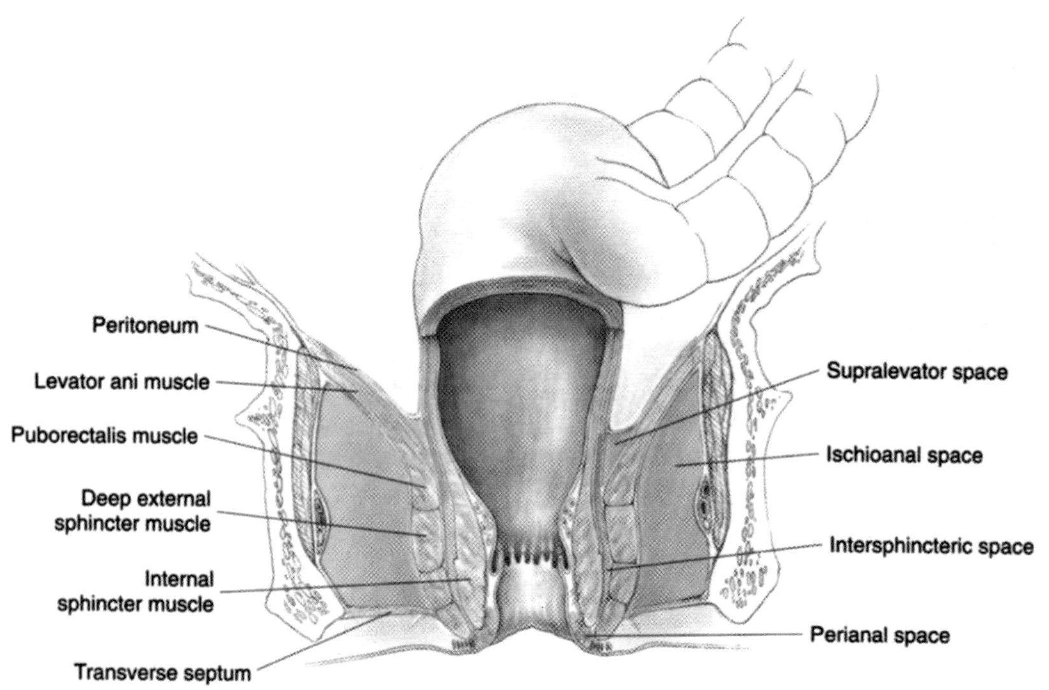

FIGURE 11 ■ Perianal and perirectal spaces (*frontal view*). *Source:* After M. Finch.

■ INTERSPHINCTERIC SPACE

The intersphincteric space lies between the internal and external sphincter muscles, is continuous below with the perianal space, and extends above into the wall of the rectum.

■ SUPRALEVATOR SPACE

Situated on each side of the rectum is the supralevator space, bounded superiorly by the peritoneum, laterally by the pelvic wall, medially by the rectum, and inferiorly by the levator ani muscle. Sepsis in this area may occur because of upward extension of anoglandular origin or from a pelvic origin.

■ SUBMUCOUS SPACE

Between the internal sphincter and the mucosa lies the submucous space. It extends distally to the dentate line and

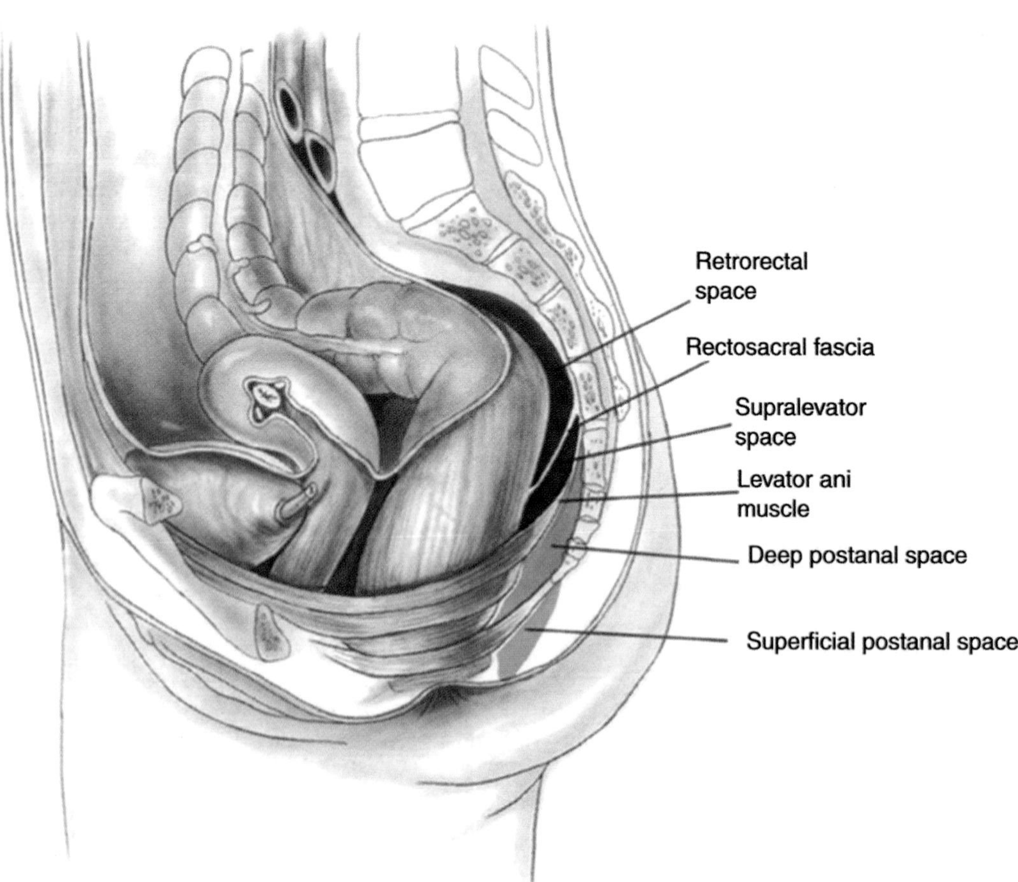

FIGURE 12 ■ Perianal and perirectal spaces (*lateral view*). *Source*: After M. Finch.

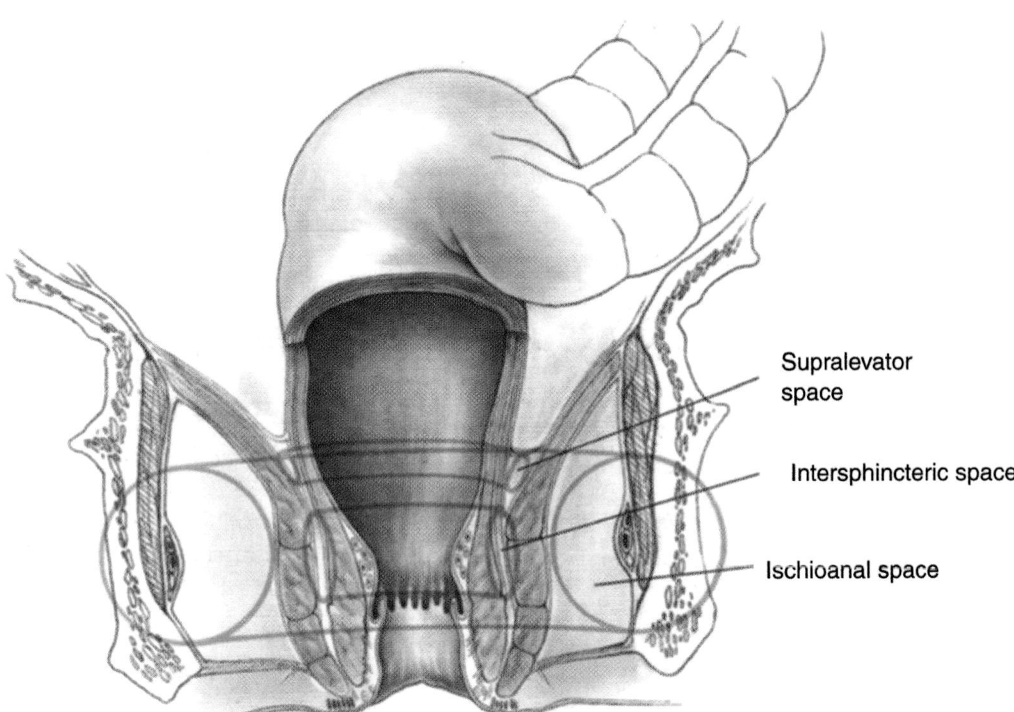

FIGURE 13 ■ Horseshoe-shaped connections of the anorectal spaces.

proximally becomes continuous with the submucosa of the rectum. It contains the internal hemorrhoidal plexus. Although abscesses in this space have been described, they are probably of little clinical significance and have been mistaken for what, in fact, were intersphincteric abscesses.

■ SUPERFICIAL POSTANAL SPACE

The superficial postanal space connects the perianal spaces with each other posteriorly below the anococcygeal ligament.

■ DEEP POSTANAL SPACE

The right and left ischioanal spaces are continuous posteriorly above the anococcygeal ligament but below the levator ani muscle through the deep postanal space (Fig. 12), also known as the retrosphincteric space of Courtney (62). This postanal space is the usual pathway by which purulent infection spreads from one ischioanal space to the other, which results in the so-called horseshoe abscess (Fig. 13).

■ RETRORECTAL SPACE

The retrorectal space lies between the upper two-thirds of the rectum and sacrum above the rectosacral fascia. It is limited anteriorly by the fascia propria covering the rectum, posteriorly by the presacral fascia, and laterally by the lateral ligaments (stalks) of the rectum. Superiorly it communicates with the retroperitoneal space, and inferiorly it is limited by the rectosacral fascia, which passes forward from the S4 vertebra to the rectum, 3–5 cm proximal to the anorectal junction.

Below the rectosacral fascia is the supralevator space, a horseshoe-shaped potential space, limited anteriorly by the fascia propria of the rectum and below by the levator ani muscle (Fig. 12 and Fig. 1 of chap. 17). The retrorectal space contains loose connective tissue. The presacral fascia protects the presacral vessels that lie deep to it. The presacral veins are part of the extensive vertebral plexus and are responsible for the major bleeding problems encountered in this area during operation. In addition to the usual tissues from which neoplasms can arise, this is an area of embryologic fusion and remodeling; thus it is the site for persistence of embryologic remnants from which neoplasms also can arise.

The perianal, ischioanal, and supralevator spaces on each side connect posteriorly with their counterparts on the opposite side, forming a horseshoe-shaped communication (Fig. 13).

ARTERIAL SUPPLY

Because the arterial supply of the large bowel is variable, the following descriptions are presented with the full recognition that they represent only the most frequently encountered patterns. However, they do serve as a basis on which a host of variations will be observed. In general, the right colon is served by branches of the superior mesenteric artery, while the left colon is served by the inferior mesenteric artery.

■ ILEOCOLIC ARTERY

The ileocolic artery is the last branch of the superior mesenteric artery, arising from its right side and running diagonally around the mesentery to the ileocecal junction. It is always present and as a rule has two chief branches. The ascending branch anastomoses with the descending branch of the right colic artery, and the descending branch anastomoses with the ileal artery. Others include anterior and posterior cecal branches and an appendicular branch (Fig. 14A).

■ RIGHT COLIC ARTERY

The origin of the right colic artery varies greatly from person to person. This artery may arise from the superior

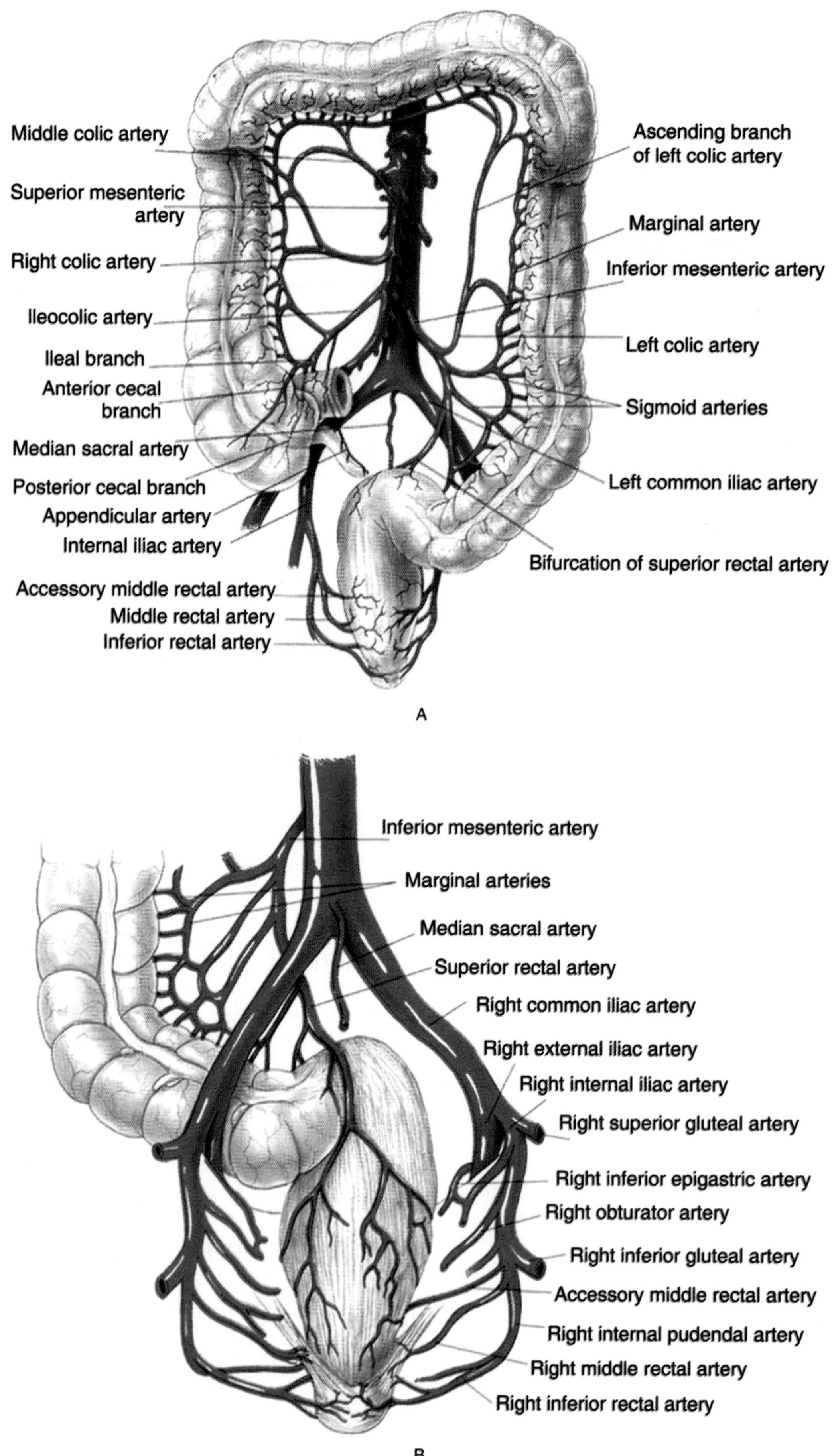

FIGURE 14 ■ Arterial supply. (**A**) Supply to the colon. (**B**) Supply to the rectum (*posterior view*).

mesenteric artery, the middle colic artery, or the ileocolic artery (Fig. 14A). In the series of Steward and Rankin (63), the right colic artery was absent in 18% of cases, whereas in the series of Michels et al. (64) it was absent in only 2% of cases. In a detailed dissection of 56 human cadavers, Garcia-Ruiz et al. (65) found an ileocolic artery in all cases, a middle colic in 55 of 56 cases, and a right colic artery in only six (10.7%) cadavers. Conventionally the right colic artery is described as dividing into a descending branch that anastomoses with colic branches of the ileocolic artery and an ascending branch that anastomoses with the right branch of the middle colic artery.

■ MIDDLE COLIC ARTERY

The middle colic artery normally arises from the superior mesenteric artery either behind the pancreas or at its lower border (Fig. 14A). It frequently shares a common stem with the right colic artery. The artery curves toward the hepatic flexure, and, at a variable distance from the colonic wall, it divides into a right branch that anastomoses with the ascending branch of the right colic artery and a left branch that anastomoses with the ascending branch of the left colic artery. Although Griffiths (66) found the middle colic artery to be absent in 22% using arteriography and dissection, other investigators using cadaver dissection found it to be present in 96–98% (63,67,68).

■ INFERIOR MESENTERIC ARTERY

The inferior mesenteric artery arises from the abdominal aorta approximately 3–4 cm above the aortic bifurcation, about 10 cm above the sacral promontory, or 3– 4 cm below the third part of the duodenum (66). The first branch is the left colic artery, arising 2.5–3 cm from its origin (Fig. 14A). It bifurcates, and its ascending branch courses directly toward the splenic flexure and anastomoses with the left branch of the middle colic artery. The descending branch anastomoses with sigmoid vessels. According to Griffiths (66), the sigmoid arteries exhibit two principal modes of origin. In 36% of cases they arise from the inferior mesenteric artery, and in 30% of cases the first sigmoid artery arises from the left colic artery. The second and third branches of the sigmoid arteries usually come directly from the inferior mesenteric artery. The number of sigmoidal branches may vary up to six.

■ SUPERIOR RECTAL ARTERY

The inferior mesenteric artery proceeds downward, crossing the left common iliac artery and vein to the base of the sigmoid mesocolon to become the superior rectal artery. The superior rectal artery starts at the last branch of the sigmoid artery. It lies posterior to the right of the sigmoid colon, coming in close contact with the posterior aspect of the bowel at the rectosigmoid junction. It forms a rectosigmoid branch, an upper rectal branch, and then divides into left and right terminal branches. The terminal branches extend downward and forward around the lower two-thirds of the rectum to the level of the levator ani muscle. Tortuous small branches ascend subperitoneally to the anterior aspect of the upper third of the rectum and anastomose with the upper rectal branch (Fig. 14B) (67).

The rectosigmoid branch arises at the rectosigmoid junction and divides directly into two diverging branches. One ascends to the sigmoid colon and anastomoses with branches of the last sigmoid artery, and the other descends to the rectum and anastomoses with the upper rectal branch. The upper rectal branch arises from the superior rectal artery before its bifurcation. It makes an extramural anastomosis with the lower branch of the rectosigmoid artery and the terminal branch of the superior rectal artery (Fig. 14B) (67).

■ MIDDLE RECTAL ARTERIES

Most middle rectal arteries arise from the internal pudendal arteries (67%). The rest come from inferior gluteal arteries (17%) and internal iliac arteries (17%) (13). A middle rectal artery of appreciable diameter (1–2 mm) is observed on both sides in only 4.8%, on the right side in 4.8%, and on the left side in 2.4% in the cadaver dissection by Ayoub (68). Sato and Sato (13) find middle rectal arteries in 22% of the specimens. Their terminal branches pierce the wall of the rectum at variable points but usually in the lower third of the rectum. The presence of the middle rectal artery can be anticipated if the diameter of the terminal branches of the superior rectal artery is smaller than usual. Conversely, when the middle rectal arteries are absent, the superior rectal artery has larger size than usual (68).

There is considerable controversy in the literature regarding the presence and origin of this vessel. Other series found the middle rectal artery to be present in 47–100% of cases (69–71). Sato and Sato (13) believe that discrepancies, for the most part, result from incomplete dissection. The origin and course of several arteries, those from inferior vesical arteries, arteries to the ductus deferens, and uterine or vaginal arteries (13), are almost indistinguishable from the middle rectal arteries, which enter the rectum via the lateral stalks. In the presence of occlusive vascular disease, Fisher and Fry (72) believe that collateral circulation develops between superior and middle rectal arteries.

■ INFERIOR RECTAL ARTERIES

The inferior rectal arteries, which are branches of the inferior iliac arteries, arise from the pudendal artery (in Alcock's canal). They traverse the ischioanal fossa and supply the anal canal and the external sphincter muscles. There is no extramural anastomosis between the inferior rectal arteries and other rectal arteries. However, arteriography demonstrates an abundance of anastomoses among the inferior and superior rectal arteries at deeper planes in the walls of the anal canal and rectum (68).

The superior rectal artery is the chief blood supply of the rectum. The middle rectal arteries are inconsistent and cannot be relied on after ligation of the superior rectal artery. Although there is no extramural anastomosis among the superior rectal artery, middle rectal arteries, and inferior rectal arteries on cadaver dissection, arteriography shows abundant intramural anastomosis among them, particularly in the lower rectum (66,67). When a low anterior resection for carcinoma of the rectum is performed in which the superior rectal artery and the middle rectal arteries are ligated, the rectal stump relies on the blood supply from the inferior rectal arteries. It may be safer to perform the anastomosis lower rather than higher, provided there is no tension.

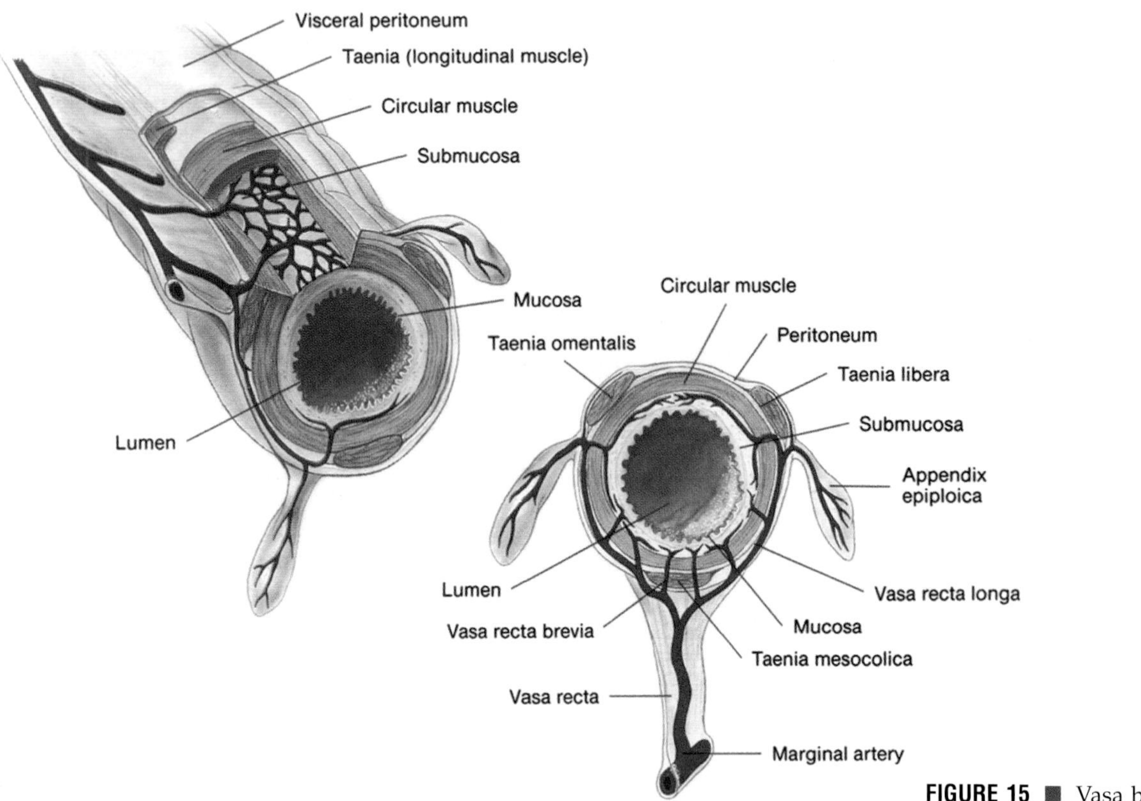

FIGURE 15 ■ Vasa brevia and vasa recta.

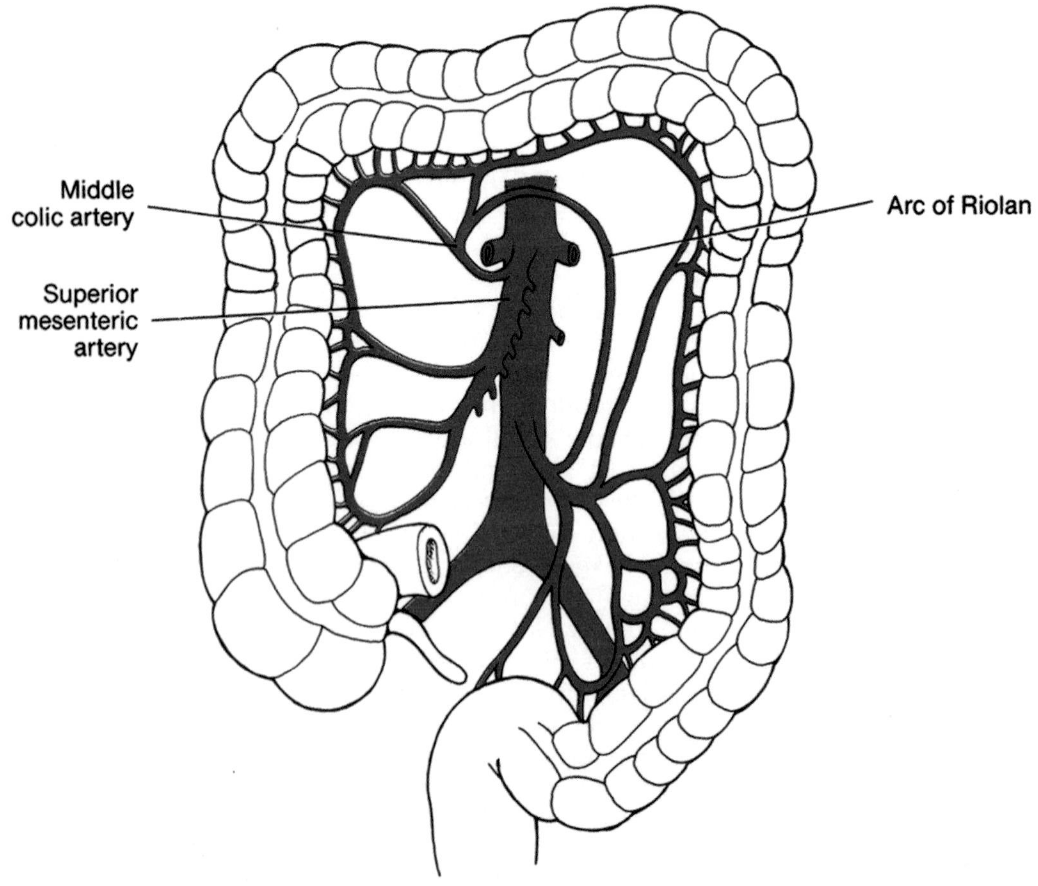

FIGURE 16 ■ Arc of Riolan.

■ MEDIAN SACRAL ARTERY

The median sacral artery arises from the back of the aorta at 1.5 cm above its bifurcation, descends over the last two lumbar vertebrae, the sacrum and the coccyx, and behind the left common iliac vein (Fig. 14A). Twigs of arteries form the median sacral artery. The terminal part of the anterior division of the internal iliac artery, the internal pudendal artery, arteries of the levator ani, and the inferior vesical artery in males and the vaginal artery in females are frequently found. These twigs are distributed mainly to pararectal tissues and sparsely to the wall of the rectum. No obvious anastomosis exists between these twigs and other rectal arteries. They are the major source of oozing during mobilization of the rectum (68). The surgical significance of the median sacral artery is that during rectal excision it is exposed on the front of the sacrum, and when the coccyx is disarticulated, this vessel may demonstrate troublesome bleeding. The presence of this artery is inconsistent (often it is absent), and it probably is insignificant in providing the blood supply to the lower rectum.

■ COLLATERAL CIRCULATION

The marginal artery, generally known as the marginal artery of Drummond, is a series of arcades of arteries along the mesenteric border of the entire colon. It is the branch that connects the superior and the inferior mesenteric arteries. The arcades begin with the ascending colic branch of the ileocolic artery and continue distally to the sigmoid arteries (Fig. 14A). The arcades are constant and rarely incomplete. Ligation of the inferior mesenteric artery in performing a rectosigmoidectomy can keep the left colon viable via the marginal artery.

Slack (73) attributed our current understanding of the distribution of vessels around the colon to the classic paper by Drummond in 1916. That description remains generally accepted today. By using injection studies, Slack determined the exact relationship of the blood vessels supplying the colon to the muscle layers and the position of diverticula. His findings supported those of Drummond. As soon as the vasa recta arise from the marginal artery, they divide into anterior and posterior branches, except in the sigmoid colon, where they may form secondary arcades (Fig. 15) (74). They initially run subserosally in the wall, and just prior to the taeniae they penetrate the circular muscle and continue in the submucosa toward the antimesenteric border (3). The vasa brevia are smaller arteries arising from the vasa recta, and some originate from the marginal artery (75). They supply the mesocolic two-thirds of the circumference.

However, a truly critical point exists at the splenic flexure, where the marginal artery is often small. As noted in 11% of the subjects in a series studied by Sierocinski (75), an area from 1.2 to 2.8 cm in the splenic flexure is devoid of vasa recta. This "weak point" is prone to a compromised blood supply. In the absence of the left colic artery, the marginal artery in this region is larger than usual (50).

The "arc of Riolan" is found in about 7% of individuals. It is a short loop connecting the left branch of the middle colic artery and the trunk of the inferior mesenteric artery (Fig. 16). The term frequently has been misquoted for the marginal anastomosis at the left colic flexure. The arc of Riolan also has been referred to as the "meandering mesenteric artery." It courses in the left colon mesentery roughly parallel to the mesenteric border of the colon. Its size enlarges when a significant arterial occlusion is present. If the arc of Riolan is present in patients undergoing operations to correct aneurysms, consideration should be given to reimplantation of the inferior mesenteric artery. If the superior mesenteric artery is stenotic, the celiac and inferior mesenteric arteries provide the main collateral flow necessary for viability of the small intestine and the right colon (Fig. 17A) (72). If the inferior mesenteric artery is stenotic, the superior mesenteric artery provides the main collateral flow necessary for the viability of the left colon and the rectum (Fig. 17B) (72).

The inferior mesenteric artery also can function as an important collateral vessel to the lower extremities (72). In instances of distal aortic occlusion, the trunk of the inferior mesenteric artery, the internal iliac artery, and the external iliac artery frequently remain patent. In this circumstance blood flowing antegrade through the meandering mesenteric artery flows into the superior rectal artery, which then forms a collateral network with the middle rectal artery, an anterior division branch of the internal iliac artery. Blood can flow from the middle rectal artery into the internal iliac artery and from there into the external iliac artery. Obviously, incorrect ligation of the inferior mesenteric artery or ligation of the meandering mesenteric artery would not only threaten the viability of the rectum but may cause acute ischemia of the lower extremity (Fig. 17C).

The significance of the meandering mesenteric artery is that, during operation on the aorta, if flow is from the superior mesenteric artery to the inferior mesenteric artery, the inferior mesenteric artery may be ligated at its origin; however, if flow direction is the reverse, the inferior mesenteric artery must be reimplanted to avoid necrosis of the left colon (Fig. 17A and B). For operations planned on the left colon, major mesenteric resection must be avoided because, by necessity, the meandering mesenteric artery will be divided. If flow is from the superior mesenteric artery to the inferior mesenteric artery, necrosis of the sigmoid or rectum or even vascular insufficiency of the lower limb may occur. If flow is from the inferior mesenteric artery to the superior mesenteric artery, necrosis of the proximal colon and small bowel may occur.

In 1907 Sudeck (77) described an area in the rectosigmoid colon where the marginal artery between the lowest sigmoid and the superior rectal arteries is absent. Under these circumstances, ligation of the last sigmoid artery was believed to account for the occasional necrosis of part of the sigmoid and rectum during a rectal resection through a perineal or presacral approach. Most recent experiences with transabdominal rectosigmoid resection and dye injection studies have shown that the anastomosis between the superior artery and the last sigmoid artery is always adequate (66,78). Thus Sudeck's critical point does not have the surgical importance that was previously emphasized. With the use of an aortogram, Lindstrom (79) found that there is an important anastomosis between the superior and middle rectal vessels that potentially can prevent gangrene of pelvic organs when the distal aorta is occluded.

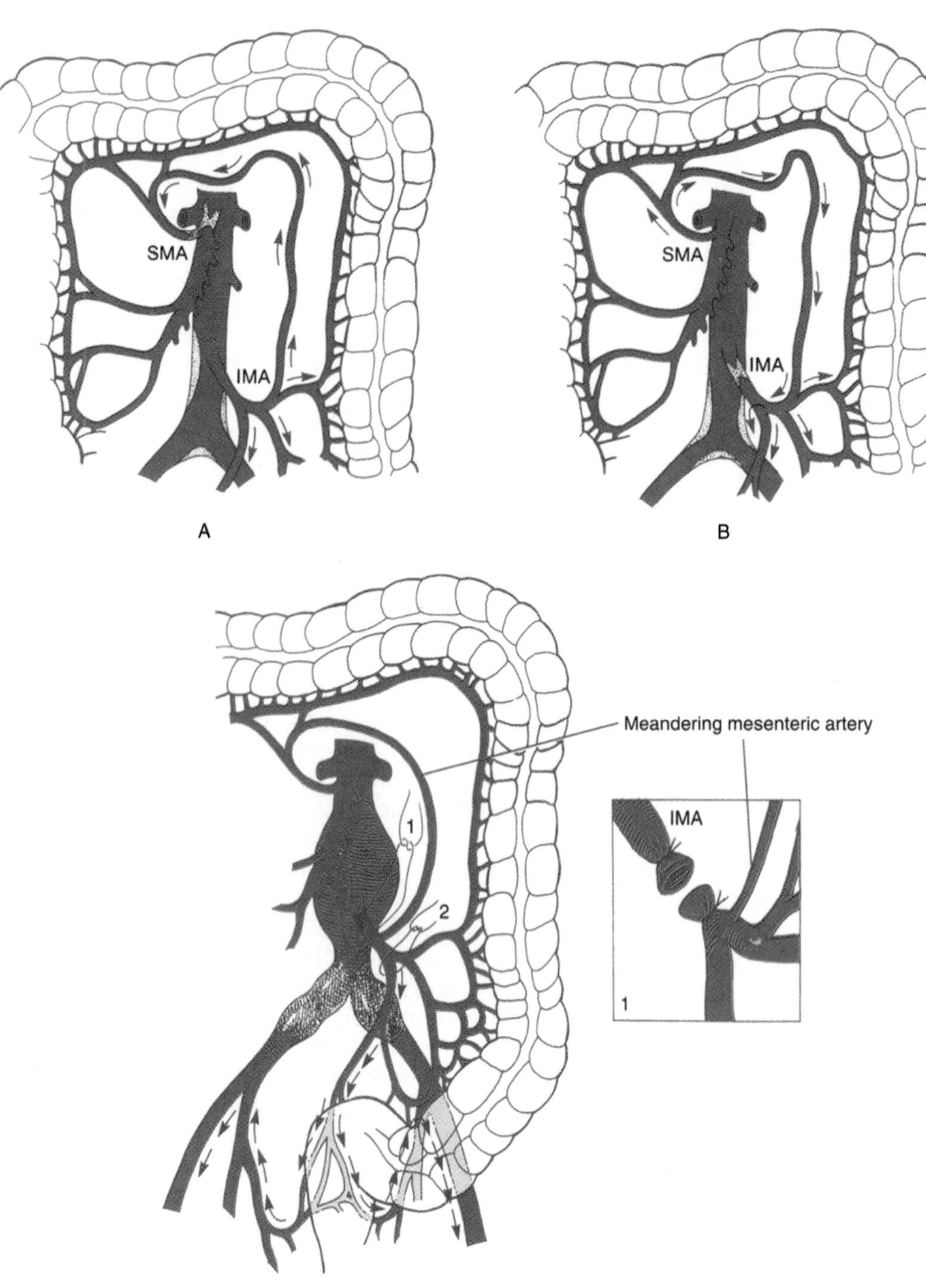

FIGURE 17 ■ Pathologic anatomy and occlusion of the superior mesenteric artery (SMA) and the inferior mesenteric artery (IMA). (**A**) Occlusion of SMA. (**B**) Occlusion of IMA. (**C**) Location for ligating IMA: (1) correct location of ligation (*see inset*); (2) incorrect location of ligation. *Source:* After Fry.

VENOUS DRAINAGE

The veins of the intestine follow their corresponding arteries and bear the same terminology.

■ SUPERIOR MESENTERIC VEIN

The veins from the right colon and transverse colon drain into the superior mesenteric vein. The superior mesenteric vein lies slightly to the right and in front of the superior mesenteric artery. It courses behind the head and neck of the pancreas, where it joins the splenic vein to form the portal vein (Fig. 18).

In the cadaver dissection, Yamaguchi et al. (80) found highly variable venous anatomy of the right colon: all ileocolic veins drained into the superior mesenteric vein. The right colic vein, if present, joined the superior mesenteric vein in 56% and gastrocolic trunk in 44%. The middle colic vein, which was the most variable, and the right colic vein, occasionally formed a common trunk with the right gastroepiploic vein and/or the pancreaticoduodeinal vein. This common trunk was defined as the gastrocolic trunk. The middle colic vein drained into the superior mesenteric vein in 85% and the rest drained into the gastrocolic trunk.

■ INFERIOR MESENTERIC VEIN

The inferior mesenteric vein is a continuation of the superior rectal vein. It receives blood from the left colon, the rectum, and the upper part of the anal canal. All the tributaries of the inferior mesenteric vein closely follow the corresponding arteries but are slightly to the left of them. At the level of the left colic artery, the inferior mesenteric vein follows a course of its own and ascends in the

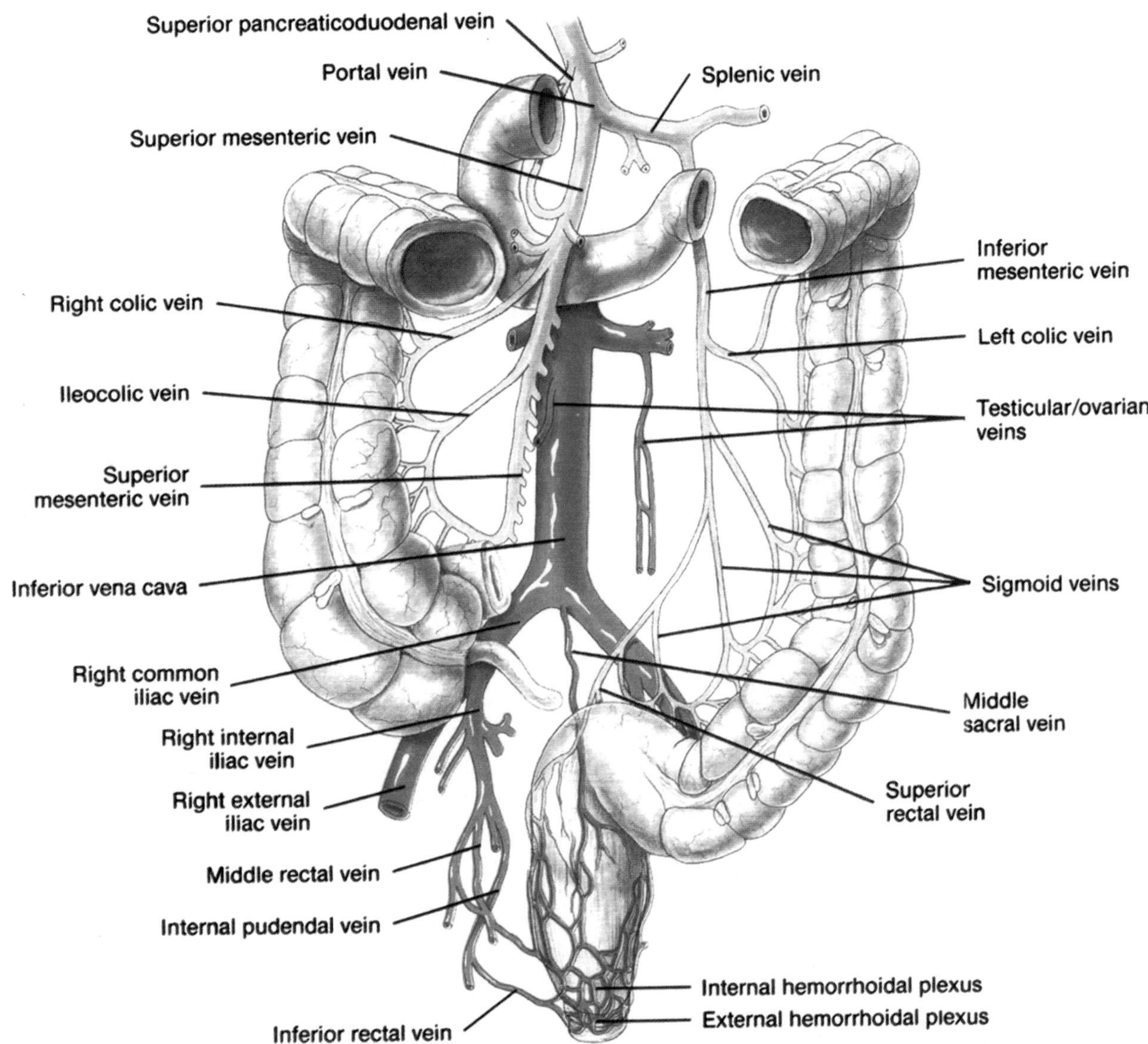

FIGURE 18 ■ Venous drainage of the colon and rectum. (Dark blue represents systemic venous drainage. Light blue shows portal venous drainage.)

extraperitoneal plane over the psoas muscle to the left of the ligament of Treitz. It continues behind the body of the pancreas to enter the splenic vein (Fig. 18).

In the conduct of an extended low anterior resection of the rectum or a coloanal anastomosis, division of the inferior mesenteric vein just inferior to the duodenum prior to its union with the splenic vein may be necessary to ensure adequate mobilization of the colon to permit a tension-free anastomosis. Access to the vessel is facilitated by incising the peritoneum at and just to the left of the ligament of Treitz.

Blood return from the rectum and anal canal is via two systems: portal and systemic. The superior rectal vein drains the rectum and upper part of the anal canal, where the internal hemorrhoidal plexus is situated, into the portal system via the inferior mesenteric vein. The middle rectal veins drain the lower part of the rectum and the upper part of the anal canal into the systemic circulation via the internal iliac veins. The inferior rectal veins drain the lower part of the anal canal, where the external hemorrhoidal plexus is located, via the internal pudendal veins, which empty into the internal iliac veins and hence into the systemic circulation (Fig. 18). Controversy exists regarding the presence or absence of anastomoses formed by these three venous systems. Current thinking supports the concepts of free communication among the main veins draining the anal canal and that of no association between the occurrence of hemorrhoids and portal hypertension (81).

LYMPHATIC DRAINAGE

Lymphatic drainage of the large intestine starts with a network of lymphatic vessels and lymph follicles in the lower part of the lamina propria, along the muscularis mucosa, but becomes more abundant in the submucosa and muscle wall (34). These vessels are connected with and drain into the extramural lymphatics. Although some lymphatic channels exist in the lamina propria above the muscularis mucosa, carcinomas that are confined to the lamina propria have not been known to metastasize (34,82,83). On this basis, the term "invasive carcinoma" is used only when the malignant cells have invaded through the muscularis mucosae (34). Knowledge of the lymphatic drainage is essential in planning operative treatment for malignancies of the large intestine.

■ COLON

The extramural lymphatic vessels and lymph nodes follow the regional arteries. Retrograde flow is retarded by numerous semilunar valves. Jameson and Dobson (84) conveniently classified colonic lymph nodes into four groups: epicolic, paracolic, intermediate, and main (principal) glands (Fig. 19).

Epicolic Glands

The epicolic glands lie on the bowel wall under the peritoneum and in the appendices epiploicae. In the rectum they are situated on the areolar tissue adjacent to the outer longitudinal muscular coat and are known as the "nodules of Gerota." The epicolic glands are very numerous in young subjects, but decrease in number in older patients. Although found on any part of the large intestine, they are especially numerous in the sigmoid colon.

Paracolic Glands

The paracolic glands lie along the inner margin of the bowel from the ileocolic angle to the rectum, mainly between the intestine and the arterial arcades along the marginal artery and on the arcades. The paracolic glands are believed to be the most important colonic lymph glands and to have the most numerous filters.

Intermediate Glands

The intermediate glands lie around the main colic arteries before their point of division.

Main Glands

The main (principal) glands lie along the origins of the superior and inferior mesenteric vessels and their middle and left colic branches. The main glands receive the efferents of the intermediate glands, from efferents of the paracolic glands, and frequently from vessels directly from the bowel.

■ RECTUM AND ANAL CANAL

Lymph from the upper and middle parts of the rectum ascends along the superior rectal artery and subsequently drains to the inferior mesenteric lymph nodes. The lower part of the rectum drains cephalad via the superior rectal lymphatics to the inferior mesenteric nodes and laterally via the middle rectal lymphatics to the internal iliac nodes (Fig. 20).

Studies of the lymphatic drainage of the anorectum in women have shown that when dye is injected 5 cm above the anal verge, spread of the dye occurs to the posterior vaginal wall, uterus, cervix, broad ligament, fallopian tubes, ovaries, and cul-de-sac. When the dye is injected at

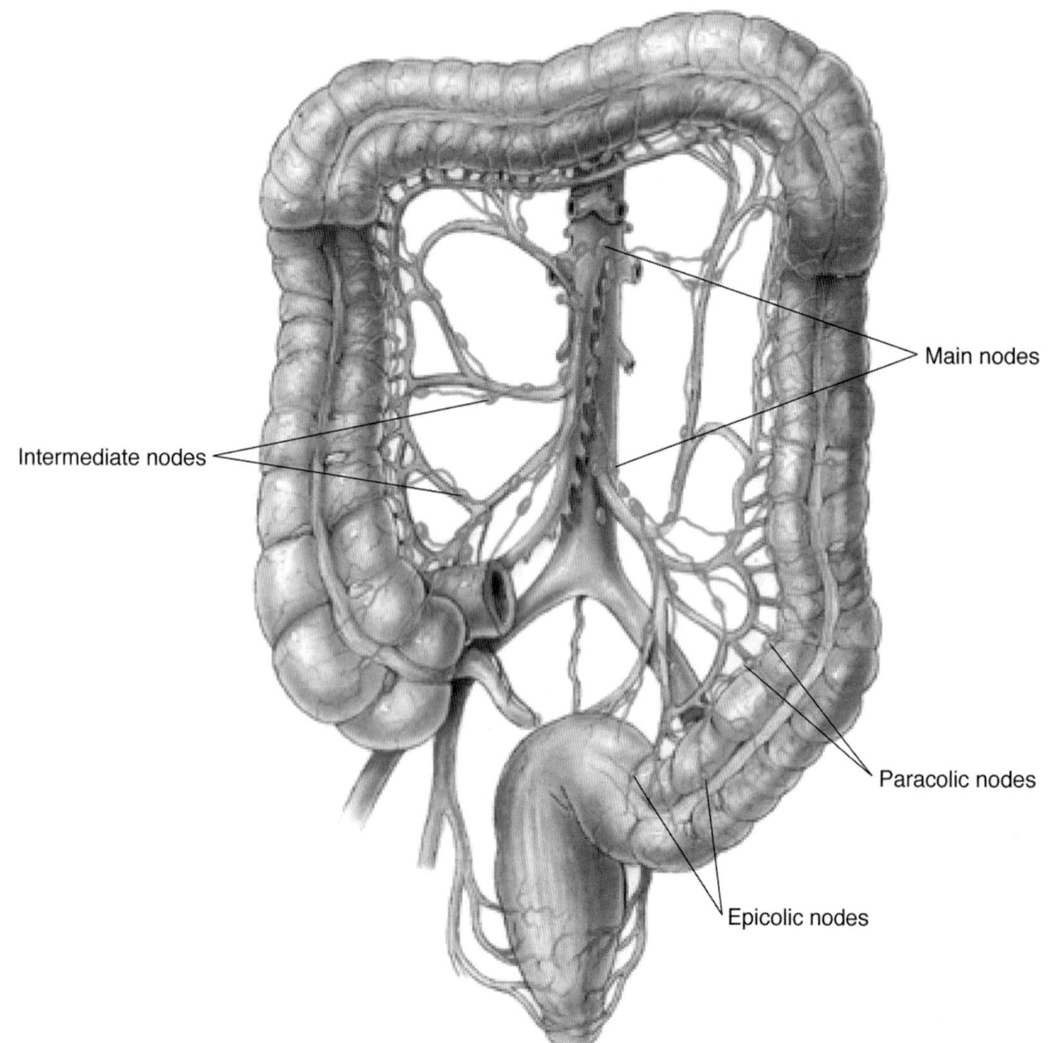

FIGURE 19 ■ Lymphatic drainage of the colon.

10 cm above the anal verge, spread occurs only to the broad ligament and cul-de-sac, whereas injection at the 15 cm level shows no spread to the genital organs (85). It generally has been known that retrograde lymphatic spread in carcinoma of the rectum and anal canal occurs only after there has been extensive involvement of the perirectal structures, serosal surfaces, veins, perineural lymphatics, and proximal lymphatic channels (86). This information obviously is helpful in planning a curative operation for a patient with a rectal or anal canal malignancy.

The most modern study of lymphatic drainage of the rectum and anal canal has used lymphoscintigraphy. Following injection of a radiocolloid (rhenium sulfide labeled with technetium-99m), lymphatic drainage was detected by means of a computerized gamma camera. The lymphatic drainage of both the intraperitoneal and extraperitoneal rectum occurs along the superior rectal and inferior mesenteric vessels to the lumboaortic nodes. There is no communication between these vessels and the vessels along the internal iliac nodes (87).

Canessa et al. (88) performed a systematic examination of the number and distribution of lateral pelvic lymph nodes using 16 cadaveric dissections (19). Dissection fields were divided according to the three surgical groups of pelvic wall lymph nodes: presacral, obturator, and hypogastric. A total of 458 lymph nodes were found, with a mean of 28.6 nodes per pelvis (range, 16–46). Lymph node size ranged from 2 to 13 mm. The highest number of lymph nodes was found in the obturator fossa group (mean, 7; range, 2–18). Hypogastric lymph nodes were found lying predominantly above the inferior hypogastric nerve plexus but reaching the deep pelvic veins. Complete excision of hypogastric lymph nodes demands a deep pelvic dissection of neurovascular structures.

Lymphatics from the anal canal above the dentate line drain cephalad via the superior rectal lymphatics to the inferior mesenteric nodes and laterally along both the middle rectal vessels and the inferior rectal vessels through the ischioanal fossa to the internal iliac nodes. Lymph from the anal canal below the dentate line usually drains to the inguinal nodes. It also can drain to the superior rectal lymph nodes or along the inferior rectal lymphatics through the ischioanal fossa if obstruction occurs in the primary drainage (Fig. 20).

INNERVATION

The large intestine is innervated by the sympathetic and parasympathetic systems, the distribution of which follows the course of the arteries. The peristalsis of the colon and rectum is inhibited by sympathetic nerves and is stimulated by parasympathetic nerves. A third division of the autonomic nervous system is the enteric nervous system, which is described in Chapter 2.

■ COLON

Sympathetic Innervation

The sympathetic fibers are derived from the lower thoracic and upper lumber segments of the spinal cord. They reach the sympathetic chain via corresponding white rami. The thoracic fibers proceed to the celiac plexus by way of the lesser splanchnic nerves. From here they proceed to the superior mesenteric plexus. Nerve fibers from the superior mesenteric ganglia supply the right colon

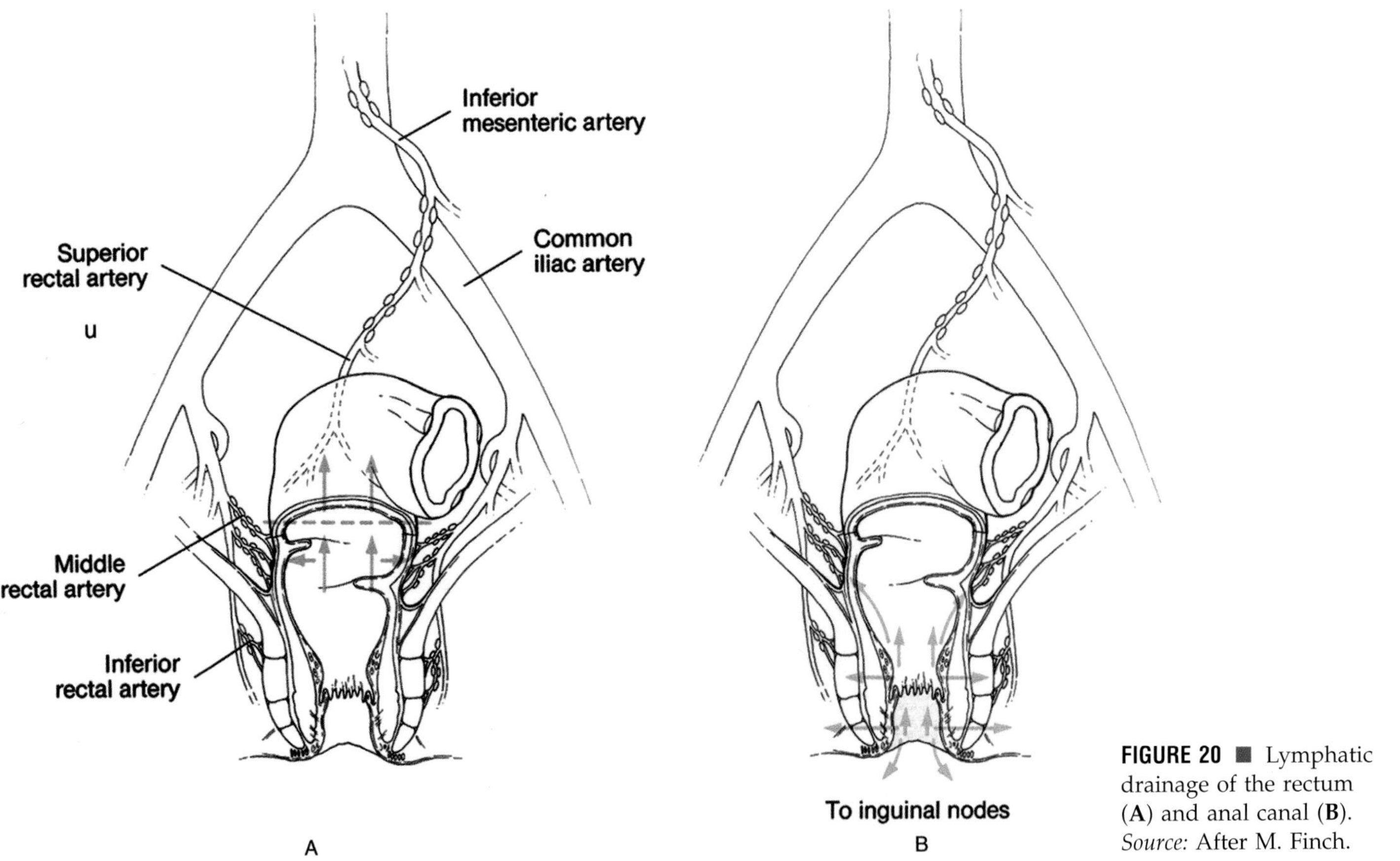

FIGURE 20 ■ Lymphatic drainage of the rectum (**A**) and anal canal (**B**). *Source:* After M. Finch.

including the appendix. The lumbar sympathetic nerves leave the sympathetic chain via the lumbar splanchnic nerves and join the mesenteric nerves. The fibers to the descending colon, the sigmoid colon, and the upper rectum originate in the inferior mesenteric plexus. A lumbar or sacral sympathectomy is often followed by increased tone and contraction of the colon.

Parasympathetic Innervation

Parasympathetic innervation of the colon derives from two levels of the central nervous system: vagus nerve and sacral outflow (5). The vagus nerves descend to the preaortic plexus and then are distributed along the colic branches of the superior mesenteric artery that supply the cecum, the ascending colon, and most of the transverse colon (89). These nerves are secretomotor to the glands, motor to the muscular coat of the gut, but inhibitory to the ileocolic sphincter (89). Administration of parasympathomimetic drugs such as prostigmine usually causes vigorous intestinal contraction and diarrhea. Fibers of the sacral outflow emerge in the anterior roots of the corresponding sacral nerves, then emerge as the nervi erigentes, which in turn join the hypogastric plexuses. The uppermost fibers of the sacral outflow are believed to extend as high as the splenic flexure. The preganglionic parasympathetic fibers entering the colon form synapses in ganglia clustered in the myenteric plexus of Auerbach and Meissner's plexus. There are numerous intricate connections between postganglionic fibers of adjacent myenteric and submucosal ganglia. Postganglionic parasympathetic fibers are cholinergic (Figs. 21 and 22).

■ RECTUM

Sympathetic Innervation

The sympathetic fibers to the rectum are derived from the first three lumbar segments of the spinal cord, which pass

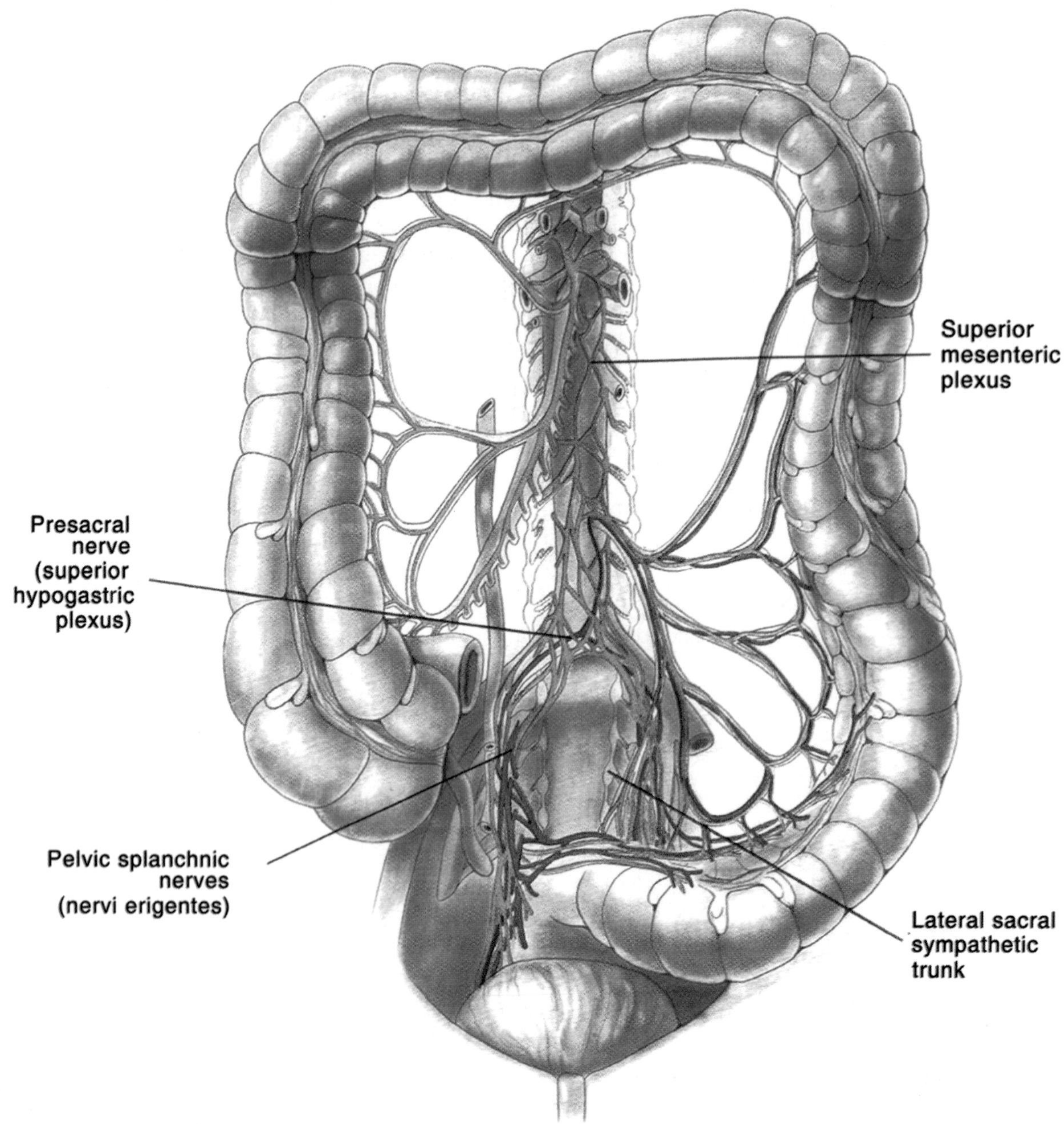

FIGURE 21 ■ Nerve supply to the rectum (*frontal view*).

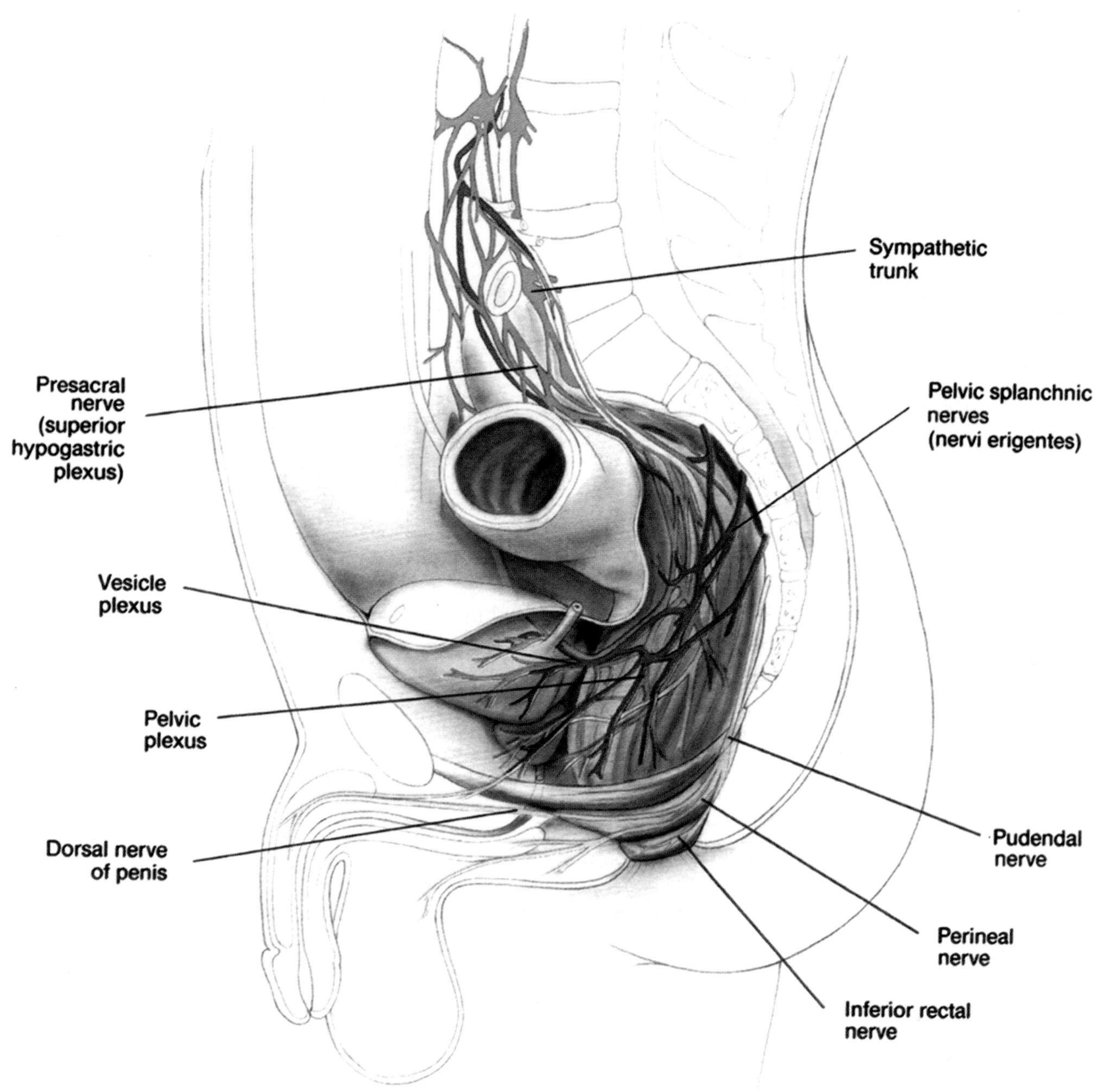

FIGURE 22 ■ Nerve supply to the rectum (*lateral view*).

through the ganglionated sympathetic chains and leave as a lumbar sympathetic nerve that joins the preaortic plexus. From there, a prolongation extends along the inferior mesenteric artery as the mesenteric plexus and reaches the upper part of the rectum. The presacral nerve or superior hypogastric plexus arises from the aortic plexus and the two lateral lumbar splanchnic nerves (Figs. 21 and 22). The plexus thus formed divides into two hypogastric nerves. The hypogastric nerves are identified at the sacral promontory, approximately 1 cm lateral to the midline and 2 cm medial to each ureter on cadaver dissection (71). The hypogastric nerve on each side continues caudally and laterally following the course of the ureter and the internal iliac artery along the pelvic wall. It joins the branches of the sacral parasympathetic nerves, or nervi erigentes, to form the pelvic plexus.

During mobilization of the rectum after the peritoneum on each side of the rectum is incised, the hypogastric nerves along with the ureters should be brushed off laterally to avoid injury. The key zones of sympathetic nerve damage are during ligation of the inferior mesenteric artery and high in the pelvis during initial posterior rectal mobilization adjacent to the hypogastric nerves.

Parasympathetic Innervation

The parasympathetic nerve supply is from the nervi erigentes, which originate from the second, third, and fourth sacral nerves on either side of the anterior sacral foramina. The third sacral nerve is the largest of the three and is the major contributor (71). The fibers pass laterally, forward, and upward to join the sympathetic nerve fibers to form the pelvic plexus on the pelvic side walls (Figs. 21 and 22). From here, the two types of nerve fibers are distributed to the urinary and genital organs and to the rectum. In

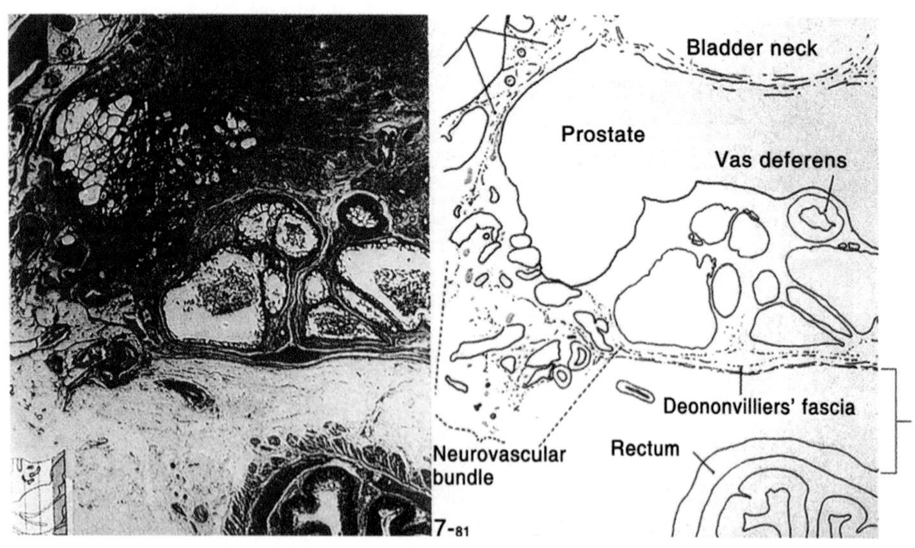

FIGURE 23 ■ Section shows the avascular areolar space between rectum and seminal vesicles and the location of the neurovascular bundle. *Source:* From Ref. 94.

women the sympathetic nerve fibers from the presacral nerve pass toward the uterosacral ligament close to the rectum. In men the nerve fibers from the presacral nerve pass immediately adjacent to the anterolateral wall of the rectum in the retroperitoneal tissue (90,91).

The pelvic plexus supplies the prostate, seminal vesicles, corpora cavernosa, terminal parts of vasa deferentia, prostatic and membranous urethra, ejaculatory ducts, and bulbourethral glands (92).

The pelvic plexus also provides visceral branches that innervate the bladder, ureters, seminal vesicles, prostate, rectum, membranous urethra, and corpora cavernosa. In addition, branches that contain somatic motor axons travel through the pelvic plexus to supply the levator ani, coccygeus, and striated urethral musculature. The pelvic plexus on each side is encased in the mid-portion of the lateral ligament which is located just above the levator ani muscle. To avoid nerve injury in full mobilization of the rectum, the lateral ligament should be cut close to the rectal side wall (91,93).

The branches of the pelvic plexus along with the blood vessels (neurovascular bundle) that supply the male genital organs are located posterolateral to the seminal vesicles (Fig. 23) (94).

The nerves innervating the prostate, the membranous urethra, and the corpora cavernosa travel dorsolaterally in the lateral pelvic fascia between the prostate and rectum. The bulk of the pelvic plexus is located lateral and posterior to the seminal vesicles, which can be used as an intraoperative landmark. Near the apex of the prostate, the nerves course slightly anteriorly to travel on the lateral surface of the membranous urethra. After piercing the urogenital diaphragm, they pass behind the dorsal penile artery and dorsal penile nerve before entering the corpora cavernosa.

Both sympathetic and parasympathetic nervous systems are involved in erection. The nerve impulses from the parasympathetic nerves that lead to erection produce arteriolar vasodilatation and increase blood in the cavernous spaces of the penis. Activity of the sympathetic system inhibits vasoconstriction of the penile vessels, thereby adding to vascular engorgement and sustained erection. Moreover, sympathetic activity causes contraction of the ejaculatory ducts, seminal vesicles, and prostate, with subsequent expulsion of semen into the posterior urethra (95). Depending on which nerves have been damaged, certain deficiencies may occur, including incomplete erection, lack of ejaculation, retrograde ejaculation, or total impotence. Injury to nervi erigentes may occur during division of the lateral ligaments.

Anterior mobilization should start at the avascular plane between the rectum and the seminal vesicles in the midline. The incision is carried laterally to the lateral border of the seminal vesicle. At this point the incision should curve downward (posteriorly) to avoid injury to the neurovascular bundles. Injury to the neurovascular bundle (Fig. 23) probably causes ejaculation problems. Key zones of risk to parasympathetic nerves are during lateral dissection in the pelvis near the pelvic plexus and during the anterolateral dissection deep in the pelvis while mobilizing the rectum from the seminal vesicles and the prostate.

Pudendal Nerve

The pudendal nerve arises from the sacral plexus (S2 to S4). It leaves the pelvis through the greater sciatic foramen, crosses the ischial spine, and continues in the pudendal canal (Alcock's canal) toward the ischial tuberosity in the lateral wall of the ischioanal fossa on each side. Three of its important branches are the inferior rectal, perineal, and dorsal nerves of the penis or clitoris (Fig. 22). The main pudendal nerve is anatomically protected from injury during mobilization of the rectum. Sensory stimuli from the penis and clitoris are mediated by the branch of the pudendal nerve and are preserved after proctectomy.

■ ANAL CANAL

Motor Innervation

The internal anal sphincter is supplied by both sympathetic and parasympathetic nerves that presumably reach the muscle by the same route as that followed to the lower rectum. The parasympathetic nerves are inhibitory to the internal sphincter. The action of sympathetic nerves to the internal sphincter is conflicting. Shepherd and Wright (96) and Lubowski et al. (97) found it to be inhibitory whereas Carlstedt et al. (98) found it to be stimulating.

The external sphincter is supplied by the inferior rectal branch of the internal pudendal nerve and the perineal branch of the fourth sacral nerve. The pudendal nerve passes through the greater sciatic foramen and crosses the sacrospinous ligament accompanied by the internal pudendal artery and vein. The pudendal nerve lies on the lateral wall of the ischioanal fossa, where it gives off the inferior rectal nerve, which crosses the ischioanal fossa with the inferior rectal vessels to reach the external sphincter. Gruber et al. (99) studied the topographic relationship of the pudendal nerve to the accompanying pudendal vessels and the ischial spine. In 58 left and 58 right pelves the course of the pudendal nerve and vessels at the ischial spine were evaluated. Multi-trunked pudendal nerves were found in 40.5% with a left-vs-right ratio of 1:1.5. The diameters of the single-trunked nerves ranged from 1.3 to 6.8 mm. In 75.9% the pudendal nerve was found medial to the accompanying internal pudendal artery. The distance to the artery ranged from 17.2 mm medial to 8 mm lateral. The distance to the tip of the ischial spine ranged from 13.4 mm medial to 7.4 mm lateral. Knowledge of the close spatial relationship between the pudendal nerve and the internal pudental artery is important for any infiltration technique and even surgical release. In 31% of cases, an additional direct branch from the fourth sacral nerve innervates the external sphincter. This is important because it helps to explain why a bilateral pudendal block produces complete paralysis of the external sphincter in only about half the subjects, despite loss of sensation in the area innervated by the pudendal nerves (100). The puborectalis muscle is supplied not by the pudendal nerves, but by a direct branch of the third and fourth sacral nerves, which lie above the pelvic floor (57). The levator ani muscles are supplied on their pelvic surface by twigs from the fourth sacral nerves, and on their perineal aspect by the inferior rectal or perineal branches of the pudendal nerves.

Sensory Innervation

The sensory nerve supply of the anal canal is the inferior rectal nerve, a branch of the pudendal nerve. The epithelium of the anal canal is profusely innervated with sensory nerve endings, especially in the vicinity of the dentate line. Pain sensation in the anal canal can be felt from the anal verge to 1.5 cm proximal to the dentate line (40). The anal canal can sense touch, cold, and pressure.

REFERENCES

1. Fraser ID, Condon RE, Schulte WJ, Decosse JJ, Cowles VE. Longitudinal muscle of muscularis externa in human and non-human primate colon. Arch Surg 1981; 116:61–63.
2. Morson BC, Dawson IMP. Gastrointestinal pathology. Oxford: Blackwell Scientific Publications, 1972:603–606.
3. Goligher JC. Surgery of the anus, rectum, and colon. 4th ed. London: Bailliere Tindall, 1980:14–15.
4. Saunders BP, Masaki T, Sawada T, et al. A preoperative comparison of Western and Oriental colonic anatomy and mesenteric attachments. Int J Colored Dis 1995; 10:216–221.
5. Haubrich WS. Anatomy of the colon. In: Bockus HL, ed. Gastroenterology. 3rd ed. Philadelphia: WB Saunders, 1976:781–802.
6. Topor B, Acland RD, Kolodko VS, Galandiuk S. Omental transposition for low pelvic anastomoses. Am J Surg 2001; 182:460–464.
7. Kumar D, Phillips SF. The contribution of external ligamentous attachments to function of the ileocecal junction. Dis Colon Rectum 1987; 30:410–416.
8. Houston J. Observation on the mucous membrane of the rectum. Dullin Hospital Resp 1830; 5:158–165.
9. Abramson DJ. The valves of Houston in adults. Am J Surg 1978; 136:334–336.
10. Najarian MM, Belzer GE, Cogbill TH, Mathiason MA. Determination of the peritoneal reflection using intraoperative proctoscopy. Dis Colon Rectum 2004; 47:2060–2085.
11. Garavoglia M, Borghi F, Levi AC. Arrangement of the anal striated musculature. Dis Colon Rectum 1993; 36:10–15.
12. Crapp AR, Cuthbertson AM. William Waldeyer and the rectosacral fascia. Surg Gynecol Obstet 1974; 138:252–256.
13. Sato K, Sato T. The vascular and neuronal composition of the lateral ligament of the rectum and the rectosacral fascia. Surg Radiol Anat 1991; 13:17–22.
14. Walsh PC. Anatomic radical retropubic prostatectomy. In: Walsh PC, Gittes RF, Perlmutter AD, Stamey TA, eds. Campbell's urology. Vol. 3. 5th ed. Philadelphia: WB Saunders, 1986:2754–2755.
15. Lindsey I, Guy RJ, Warren BF, Mortensen NJ Mc C. Anatomy of Denonvilliers' fascia and pelvic nerves, impotena, and implications for the colorectal surgeon. Br J Surg 2000; 87:1288–1299.
16. Aigner F, Zbar AP, Ludwikowski B, et al. The rectogenital septum: morphology, function, and clinical relevance. Dis Colon Rectum 2004; 47:131–140.
17. Goligher JC. In: Surgery of the anus, rectum and colon. 4th ed. London: Bailliere Tindal, 1980:6.
18. Moriya Y, Sugihara K, Akasu T, Fujita S. Nerve sparing surgery with lateral node dissection for advanced lower rectal cancer. EW J Cancer 1995; 31A:1229–1232.
19. Heald RJ, Meran BJ. Embryology and anatomy of the rectum. Semin Surg Oncol 1998; 15:66–71.
20. Church JM, Raudkivi PJ, Hill GL. The surgical anatomy of the rectum—a review with particular relevance to the hazards of rectal mobilization. Int J Colorectal Dis 1987; 2:158–166.
21. Nano M, Levi AC, Borghi F, Bellora P, Bogliatto F, Garbossa D. Observations on surgical anatomy for rectal cancer surgery. Hepatogastroenterology 1998; 45:717–726.
22. Arndt VD, Roth S. The anatomy and embryological origins of the fascia of Denonvilliers: a medico-historical debate. J Urol 1997; 157:3–9.
23. Lindsey I, Warren BF, Mortensen NJ. Denonvilliers' fascia lies anterior to the fascia propria and rectal dissection plane in total mesorectal excision. Dis Colon Rectum 2005; 48:37–42.
24. Jones OM, Smeulders N, Wiseman O, Miller R. Lateral ligaments of the rectum: an anatomical study. Br J Surg 1999; 86:487–489.
25. Rutegard J, Sandzen B, Stenling R, Wiig J, Heald RJ. Lateral rectal ligaments contain important nerves. Br J Surg 1997; 84:1544–1545.
26. Nano M, Dalcorso HM, Lanfranco G, Ferromato N, Hernung JP. Contribution to the surgical anatomy of the ligaments of the rectum. Dis Colon Rectum 2000; 43:1592–1598.
27. Havenga K, DeRuiter MC, Enker WE, Welvaart K. Anatomical basis of autonomic nerve-preserving total mesorectal excision for rectal cancer. Br J Surg 1996; 83:384–388.
28. Chapuis P, Bokey L, Fahrer M, Sinclair G, Bogduk N. Mobilization of the rectum. Anatomic concepts and the bookshelf revisited. Dis Colon Rectum 2002; 45:1–9.
29. Margado PJ. Total mesorectal excision: a misnomer for a sound surgical approach [letter to the editor]. Dis Colon Rectum 1998; 41:120–121.
30. Bisset IP, Chau KY, Hill GL. Extrafascial excision of the rectum, surgical anatomy of the fascia propria. Dis Colon Rectum 2000; 43:903–910.
31. Canessa CE, Badia F, Fierro S, Fiol V, Hayek G. Anatomic study of the lymph nodes of the mesorectum. Dis Colon Rectum 2001; 44:1333–1336.
32. Toper B, Acland R, Kolodko V, Galandiuk S. Mesorectal lymph nodes: their location and distribution within the mesorectum. Dis Colon Rectum 2003; 46:779–785.
33. Frei JV. Objective measurement of basement membrane abnormalities in human neoplasms of colorectum and of breast. Histopathology 1978; 2: 107–115.
34. Fenoglio CM, Kay Gl, Lane N. Distribution of human colonic lymphatics in normal, hyperplastic, and adenomatous tissue: its relationship to metastasis from small carcinomas in pedunculated adenomas, with two case reports. Gastroenterology 1973; 64:51–66.
35. Nivatvongs S, Stern HS, Fryd DS. The length of the anal canal. Dis Colon Rectum 1982; 24:600–601.
36. Milligan ETC, Morgan CN. Surgical anatomy of the anal canal: with special reference to anorectal fistulae. Lancet 1934; 2:1150–1156.
37. Parks AG. Pathogenesis and treatment of fistula-in-ano. Br Med J 1961; 1:463–469.
38. Morren Gl, Beets-Tan RGH, van Engelshoven Jma. Anatomy of the anal canal and perianal structures as defined by phased-array magnetic resonance imaging. Br J Surg 2001; 88:1506–1512.
39. Parks AG. The surgical treatment of hemorrhoids. Br J Surg 1956; 43:337–351.
40. Duthie HL, Gairns FW. Sensory nerve endings and sensation in the anal region of man. Br J Surg 1960; 47:585–594.

41. Fenger C. The anal transitional zone. Acta Pathol Microbiol Immunol Scand 1987; 85(suppl 289):1–42.
42. Thompson-Fawcett MW, Warren BF, Mortensen NJMc C. A new look at the anal transitional zone with reference to restorative proctocolectomy and the columnar cuff. Br J Surg 1998; 85:1517–1521.
43. Seow-Choen F, Ho JMS. Histoanatomy of anal glands. Dis Colon Rectum 1994; 37:1215–1218.
44. Chiari H. Über die Nalen Divertikel der Rectumschleimhaut und Ihre Beziehung zu den Anal Fisteln. Wien Med Press 1878;19:1482.
45. Klosterhalfen B, Offher F, Vogel P, Kirkpatrick CJ. Anatomic nature and surgical significance of anal sinus and intramuscular glands. Dis Colon Rectum 1991; 34:156–160.
46. Shafik A. A new concept of the anatomy of the anal sphincter mechanism and the physiology of defecation. The external anal sphincter: a triple-loop system. Invest Urol 1975; 12:412–419.
47. Goligher JC, Leacock AG, Brossy JJ. The surgical anatomy of the anal canal. Br J Surg 1955; 43:51–61.
48. Fine J, Lawes CHW. On the muscle fibres of the anal submucosa with special reference to the pecten band. Br J Surg 1940; 237:723–727.
49. Lunnis PJ, Phillips RKS. Anatomy and function of the anal longitudinal muscle. Br J Surg 1992; 79:882–884.
50. Goligher JC. The blood supply to the sigmoid colon and rectum. Br J Surg 1949; 37:157–162.
51. Bollard RC, Gardiner A, Lindows S, Phillips K, Duthie GS. Normal female anal sphincter. Difficulties in interpretation explained. Dis Colon Rectum 2002; 45:171–175.
52. Levi AC, Borghi F, Garavoglia M. Development of the anal canal muscles. Dis Colon Rectum 1991; 34:262–266.
53. Nielson MB, Pedersen JF, Hauge C, Rasmussen OO, Christiansen J. Normal endosonographic appearance of the anal sphincter: longitudinal and transverse imaging. Am J Radiol 1991; 157:1199–11202.
54. Oh C, Kark AE. Anatomy of the external sphincter. Br J Surg 1972; 59:717–723.
55. Shafik A. A new concept of the anatomy of the anal sphincter mechanism and the physiology of defecation. II. Anatomy of the levator ani muscle with special reference to puborectalis. Invest Urol 1975; 13:175–182.
56. Ayoub SF. Anatomy of the external anal sphincter in man. Acta Anat 1979; 105:25–36.
57. Percy JP, Swash M, Neill ME, Parks AG. Electrophysiological study of motor nerve supply of pelvic floor. Lancet 1981; 1:16–17.
58. Matzel KE, Schmidt RA, Tonaglo EA. Neuroanatomy of the striated muscular anal continence mechanism. Implications for the use of neurostimulation. Dis Colon Rectum 1990; 33:666–673.
59. Netter F. The Ciba collection of medical illustrations. Digestive system. Part II. Lower digestive tract. Vol. 3. New York: Color Press, 1962:32.
60. Lilius HG. Investigation of human fetal anal ducts and intramuscular glands and a clinical study of 150 patients. Acta Chir Scand Suppl 1968; 383:1–88.
61. Brasch JC, ed. Cunningham's manual of practical anatomy. 12th ed. London: Oxford University Press, 1958:383.
62. Courtney H. Posterior subsphincteric space. Its relation to posterior horseshoe fistula. Surg Gynecol Obstet 1949; 89:222–226.
63. Steward JA, Rankin FW. Blood supply of the large intestine. Its surgical considerations. Arch Surg 1933; 26:843–891.
64. Michels NA, Siddharth P, Kornblith PL, Parks WW. The variant blood supply to the small and large intestines: its importance in regional resections. A new anatomic study based on four hundred dissections, with a complete review of the literature. J Int Coll Surg 1963; 39:127–170.
65. Garcia-Ruiz A, Milsom JW, Ludwig KA, Marchesa P. Right colonic arterial anatomy. Implications for laparoscopic surgery. Dis Colon Rectum 1996; 39:906–911.
66. Griffiths JD. Surgical anatomy of the blood supply of the distal colon. Ann R Coll Surg Engl 1956; 19:241–256.
67. Sonneland J, Anson BJ, Beaton LE. Surgical anatomy of the arterial supply to the colon from the superior mesenteric artery based upon a study of 600 specimens. Surg Gynecol Obstet 1958; 106:385–398.
68. Ayoub SF. Arterial supply of the human rectum. Acta Anat 1978; 100:317–327.
69. Boxall TA, Smart PJG, Griffiths JD. The blood supply of the distal segment of the rectum in anterior resection. Br J Surg 1962; 50:399–404.
70. Didio LJA, Diaz-Franco C, Schemainda R, Bezerra AJC. Morphology of the middle rectal arteries: a study of 30 cadaver dissections. Surg Radiol Anat 1986; 8:229–236.
71. Havenga K, De Ruiter MC, Enker WE, Welvaart K. Anatomical basis of autonomic nerve-preserving total mesorectal excision for rectal cancer. Br J Surg 1996; 83:384–388.
72. Fisher DF, Fry WI. Collateral mesenteric circulation. Surg Gynecol Obstet 1987; 164:487–492.
73. Slack WW. The anatomy, pathology and some clinical features of diverticulitis of the colon. Br J Surg 1962; 50:185–190.
74. Griffiths JD. Extramural and intramural blood supply of the colon. Br Med J 1961; 1:323–326.
75. Sierocinski W. Arteries supplying the left colic flexure in man. Folia Morphol (Warsz) 1975; 34:117–124.
76. Moskowitz M, Zimmerman H, Felson H. The meandering mesenteric artery of the colon. AJR 1964; 92:1088–1099.
77. Sudeck P. Füber die Gefassversorgung des Mastdarmes in Hinsicht auf die Operative Gangran. Munch Med Wochenschr 1907; 54:1314.
78. Goligher JC. The adequacy of the marginal blood supply to the left colon after high ligation of the inferior mesenteric artery during excision of the rectum. Br J Surg 1954; 41:351–353.
79. Lindstrom BL. The value of the collateral circulation from the inferior mesenteric artery in obliteration of the lower abdominal aorta. Acta Chir Scand 1950; 1:677–685.
80. Yamaguchi S, Kuroyanagi H, Milson JW, Sim R, Shimada H. Venous anatomy of the right colon. Precise structure of the major veins and gastrocolic trunk in 58 cadavers. Dis Colon Rectum 2002; 45:1337–1340.
81. Bernstein WC. What are hemorrhoids and what is their relationship to the portal venous system? Dis Colon Rectum 1983; 26:829–834.
82. Okike N, Weiland LH, Anderson MJ, Adson MA. Stromal invasion of cancer in pedunculated adenomatous colorectal polyps. Arch Surg 1977; 112:527–530.
83. Whitehead R. Rectal polyps and their relationship to cancer. Clin Gastroenterol 1975; 4:545–561.
84. Jameson JK, Dobson JF. The lymphatics of the colon. Proc R Soc Med (Surg Section) 1909; 2:149–172.
85. Block IR, Enquist IF. Lymphatic studies pertaining to local spread of carcinoma of the rectum in females. Surg Gynecol Obstet 1961; 112:41–46.
86. Quer EA, Dahlin DC, Mayo CW. Retrograde intramural spread of carcinoma of the rectum and rectosigmoid. A microscopic study. Surg Gynecol Obstet 1953; 96:24–29.
87. Miscusi G, Masoni L, Dell'Anna A, Montori A. Normal lymphatic drainage of the rectum and the anal canal revealed by lymphoscintigraphy. Coloproctology 1987; 9:171–174.
88. Canessa CE, Miegge LM, Bado J, Siveri C, Labandera D. Anatomic study of lateral pelvic lymph nodes: implications in the treatment of rectal cancer. Dis Colon Rectum 2004; 47:297–303.
89. Siddharth P, Ravo B. Colorectal neovasculature and anal sphincter. Surg Clin North Am 1988; 68:1195–1200.
90. Bauer JJ, Gelernt IM, Salky B, Kreel I. Sexual dysfunction following proctectomy for benign disease of the colon and rectum. Ann Surg 1983; 197:363–367.
91. Schlegal PN, Walsh PC. Neuroanatomical approach to radical cystoprostatectomy with preservation of sexual function. J Urol 1987; 138:1402–1406.
92. Weinstein M, Roberts M. Sexual potency following surgery for rectal carcinoma. A follow-up of 44 patients. Ann Surg 1977; 185:295–300.
93. Pearl RK, Monsen H, Abcarian H. Surgical anatomy of the pelvic autonomic nerves. A practical approach. Ann Surg 1986; 52:236–237.
94. Lepor H, Gregerman M, Crosby R, Mostofi FK, Walsh PC. Precise localization of the autonomic nerves from the pelvic plexus to the corpora cavernosa: a detailed anatomical study of the adult male pelvis. J Urol 1985; 133:207–212.
95. Babb RR, Kieraldo JH. Sexual dysfunction after abdominoperineal resection. Am J Dig Dis 1977; 22:1127–1129.
96. Shepherd JJ, Wright PG. The response of the internal anal sphincter in man to stimulation of the presacral nerve. Am J Dig Dis 1968; 13:421–427.
97. Lubowski DZ, Nicholls RJ, Swash M, Jordan MJ. Neural control of internal anal sphincter function. Br J Surg 1987; 74:668–670.
98. Carlstedt A, Nordgren S, Fasth S, Appelgren L, Hulten L. Sympathetic nervous influence on the internal anal sphincter and rectum in man. Int J Colorectal Dis 1988; 3:90–95.
99. Gruber H, Kovacs P, Piegger J, Brenner E. New, Simple, ultrasound-guided infiltration of the pudendal nerve: topographic basics. Dis Colon Rectum 2002; 44:1376–1380.
100. Rasmussen O. Anorectal function. Dis Colon Rectum 1994; 37:386–403.

2 Physiology

W. Rudolf Schouten and Philip H. Gordon

COLONIC PHYSIOLOGY

Major functions of the colon include storage and absorption of digestive material. By absorbing most of the water and salt presented to it, the colon responds to body requirements and plays an essential role in protecting the body against dehydration and electrolyte depletion. The absorptive capability enables the colon to reduce the volume of fluid material received from the small bowel and to transform it into a semisolid mass suitable for defecation. The propulsion of feces toward the rectum and the storage of this material between defecations are the result of complex and poorly understood patterns of motility. Other functions of the large bowel include digestion of carbohydrate and protein residues and secretion of mucus.

FUNCTIONS

Absorption and Secretion

Physiologic control of intestinal ion transport involves an integrated system of neural, endocrine, and paracrine components (1). Endogenous mediators, including neurotransmitters and peptides, act on enterocytes through membrane receptors coupled to energy-requiring "pumps" or "channels" through which ions flow passively in response to electrochemical gradients.

In healthy individuals, the colon absorbs water, sodium, and chloride, while secreting potassium and bicarbonate. It receives approximately 1500 mL of fluid material from the ileum over a 24-hour period. From this input the large bowel absorbs approximately 1350 mL of water, 200 mmol of sodium, 150 mmol of chloride, and 60 mmol of bicarbonate (2). It has been estimated that the colon possesses enough reserve capacity to absorb an additional 3.5–4.5 L of ileal effluent, a feature that allows the large bowel to compensate for impaired absorption in the small intestine (3). Several factors that determine colonic absorption include the volume, composition, and rate of flow of luminal fluid. The success of whole gut irrigation capitalizes on this principle. The absorptive capacity is not homogeneous throughout the large intestine due to significant differences in the colonic segments. It has been shown that more salt and water are absorbed from the right colon than from the distal colon (3). Thus a right hemicolectomy is more likely to result in diarrhea than is a left hemicolectomy. Whenever ileocecal flow exceeds the capacity of the colon to absorb fluid and electrolytes, an increase in fecal water excretion (diarrhea) will ensue.

Sodium is absorbed by active cellular transport against concentration and electrical gradients. The average concentration of sodium in the fluid chyme accepted by the colon from the terminal ileum is 130–135 mmol/L and in the stool is approximately 40 mmol/L. When the luminal concentration of sodium is high, more is absorbed; no absorption occurs when the luminal concentration is below 15–25 mmol/L (4). In this way there is a linear relationship between the luminal concentration of sodium and sodium absorption.

Across the colonic mucosa, there is an electrical potential difference of approximately 20–60 mV^2. The basolateral membrane of the mucosal cell is electrically positive, whereas the apical membrane along the luminal border is electrically negative (Fig. 1). It is believed that this negativity is created by the active transport of sodium and by the secretion of anions. Initially sodium moves passively across the apical membrane into the mucosal cell because the intracellular sodium concentration is lower there than in the colonic lumen and because the cell interior is negatively charged with respect to the lumen (5). Sodium is then removed from the cell in exchange for potassium. This mechanism can be considered a sodium pump controlled by Na^+, K^+-ATPase at the basolateral membrane (Fig. 1).

Mineralocorticoids and glucocorticoids stimulate sodium absorption and potassium secretion by increasing Na^+, K^+-ATPase activity. Short-chain fatty acids such as acetate, butyrate, and propionate, which are produced by bacterial fermentation, are the main anions in the colon, and they also promote sodium absorption (6).

Water absorption is intimately related to sodium absorption. The active transport of sodium creates an osmotic gradient across the colonic mucosa, and this initiates the passive cellular transport of water. Like sodium, water also can move backward into the colonic lumen (Fig. 1).

Potassium transport in the human colon is mainly passive, along an electrochemical gradient generated by the active transport of sodium. Potassium moves into the colonic lumen through both cellular and paracellular pathways (Fig. 1). Experimental studies have demonstrated that the secretion of potassium will continue when the luminal concentration is less than 15 mmol/L, but with higher luminal concentrations, the absorption of potassium occurs (5). It has been suggested that potassium also might be secreted actively because potassium equilibrates across the colonic mucosa only when the luminal concentration is between 30 and 50 mmol/L (3). However, the origin and mechanism of this secretion is still unclear. The secretion of potassium into the colonic lumen along electrochemical gradients cannot explain the net fecal loss of potassium.

Because the distal colon is relatively impermeable to potassium, the luminal concentration may increase by the continued absorption of water. It has been suggested that there may be active secretion of potassium in the human rectum (7). The presence of potassium in fecal bacteria and colonic mucus, as well as from desquamated cells, also may contribute to the high concentration (50–90 mmol/L) of potassium in human stool (6,8).

Chloride concentrations are high in ileal effluent but fall markedly during passage through the large intestine. Chloride and bicarbonate are exchanged by an electroneutral mechanism (9). Like sodium, chloride is actively absorbed against concentration gradients, mainly through the cellular pathway. The reciprocal exchange between chloride and bicarbonate takes place at the luminal border of the mucosal cell (Fig. 1). Chloride absorption is increased by a low luminal pH. The presence of chloride in the colonic lumen facilitates the secretion of bicarbonate. This is clinically evident in patients with ureterosigmoidostomy, who may develop hyperchloremia and secrete excessive amounts of bicarbonate (10).

Urea is another constituent of the fluid secreted into the colonic lumen. Of the urea synthesized by the liver, about 6–9 g/day (20%) is metabolized in the digestive tract, mainly in the colon (2). Because the maximum amount of urea entering the colon from the ileum is about 0.4 g/day (11), the bulk of urea hydrolyzed in the large bowel by bacterial ureases must be secreted into the lumen. The metabolism of urea in the colon gives rise to 200–300 mL of ammonia each day. Since only a small amount of ammonia (1–3 mmol) can be found in the feces, most must be absorbed across the colonic mucosa. Although the production of ammonia in the large bowel can be abolished by neomycin, the absorption of ammonia is not affected by this antibiotic.

Ammonia absorption probably occurs by passive coupled nonionic diffusion in which bicarbonate and ammonium ions form ammonia and carbon dioxide (2). The nonionized ammonia can freely diffuse across the colonic mucosa. This process is partially influenced by the pH of the luminal contents; as the luminal pH falls, the absorption of ammonia decreases (2). Although urea is the most important source of ammonia, the ammonia in the colon also may be derived from dietary nitrogen, epithelial cells, and bacterial debris.

Mucus is another product secreted into the colonic lumen. Throughout the entire length of the large bowel, the epithelium contains a large number of mucus-secreting cells, and it has been shown that nerve fibers come close to these goblet cells. Stimulation of the pelvic nerves increases mucus secretion from the colonic mucosa, as has been confirmed histologically. There is evidence for such a nerve-mediated secretion of mucus in the large bowel (12).

The colon is able to absorb amino acids and fatty acids, but only by passive mechanisms. Bile acids also can be reabsorbed.

Digestion

A little recognized function of the colon is the role it plays in digestion. Digestion of food begins in the stomach and is almost accomplished when transit to the end of the small intestine is complete. However, a small amount of protein and carbohydrate is not digested during transit through the small bowel. The colon plays a role in salvaging calories from malabsorbed sugars and dietary fiber (13). In the colon some of the protein residues are fermented by anaerobic bacteria into products such as indole, skatole (β-methylindole), phenol, cresol, and hydrogen sulfide, which create the characteristic odor of feces. The carbohydrate residues are broken down by anaerobic bacteria into short-chain fatty acids (SCFAs) such as acetic 60%, propionic 20%, and butyric acid 15% (14). It has been estimated that 100 mmol of volatile fatty acids are produced for each 20 g of dietary fiber consumed.

Most of these SCFAs, which constitute the major fecal anion in humans (15), are absorbed in a concentration-dependent way. Their absorption is associated with the

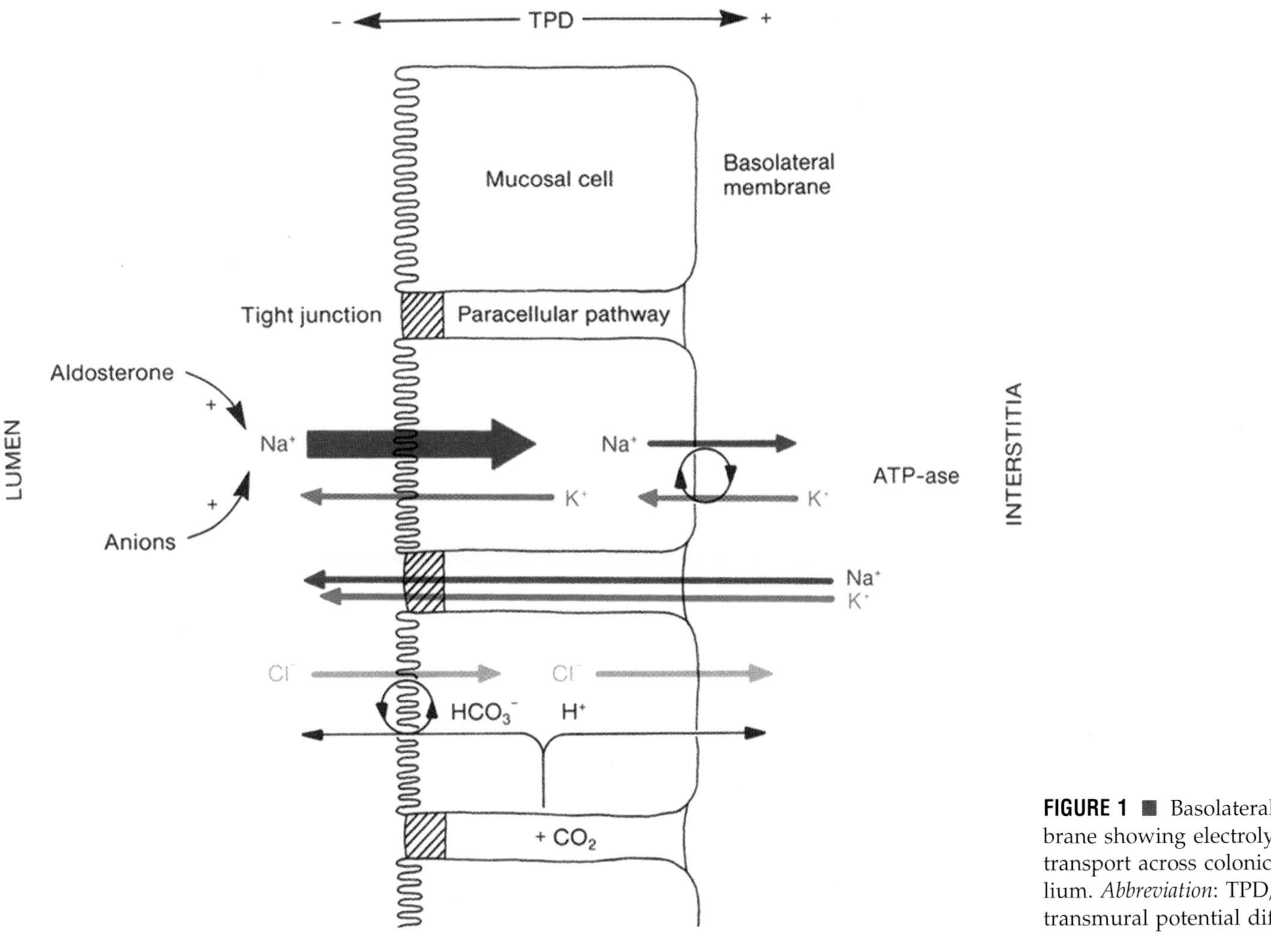

FIGURE 1 ■ Basolateral membrane showing electrolyte transport across colonic epithelium. *Abbreviation*: TPD, transmural potential difference.

appearance of bicarbonate in the lumen, which in turn stimulates the absorption of sodium and water (1). Other end products of fiber fermentation are hydrogen and methane.

About 70% of colonic mucosal energy supply is derived from SCFAs originating in the lumen (14). The functions of the colonocytes, mainly dependent on the absorption and oxidation of SCFAs, include cellular respiration, cell turnover, absorption, and numerous enzyme activities. Furthermore, SCFAs are used by the colonocytes not only as a source of energy but also as substrates for gluconeogenesis, lipogenesis, protein synthesis, and mucin production.

Propulsion and Storage

The main functions of colonic and anorectal motor activity are to absorb water, to store fecal wastes, and to eliminate them in a socially acceptable manner (16). The first is achieved by colonic segmentation and motor activity that propels colonic material forward and backward over relatively short distances. The second is facilitated by colonic and rectal compliance and accommodation, whereas the third is regulated by the coordination of anorectal and pelvic floor mechanisms with behavioral and cognitive responses (16).

Distinct patterns of mechanical activity are required for the normal propulsion and storage of colonic contents. The rate and volume of material moved along a viscus also is related to the pressure differential, the diameter of the tube, and the viscosity of the material. Observation of transit does not necessarily reflect the contractile activity responsible for transit. Although the investigation of colonic motility in vivo has proved to be difficult because of the relative inaccessibility of the colon, new data have been revealed through the use of modern recording techniques. This information provides a better understanding of normal colonic motility in humans.

Assessment and Control of Motility

RADIOLOGIC EVALUATION ■ Early efforts to investigate colonic motility involved radiographic studies in which the colon was filled with barium from either above or below. These studies could demonstrate only organized movements of the colon, represented by changes in contour, and were not helpful in the detailed examination of colonic motility. Moreover, the well-known side effects of radiation have limited the possibilities of radiologic observations, even with such sophisticated techniques as time-lapse cinematography (17).

At the beginning of the 20th century, radiographic studies revealed three types of colonic motility: retrograde movement, segmental nonpropulsive movement, and mass movement. Retrograde movements were identified as contractions originating in the transverse colon and traveling toward the cecum (18,19). Later, studies with cinematography also demonstrated a retrograde transportation of colonic contents (20). These retrograde movements are believed to delay the transit in the right colon, resulting in greater exposure of colonic contents to the mucosa to allow sufficient absorption of salt and water (21).

Segmental nonpropulsive movements are the type more frequently observed during radiologic investigation. These segmental movements are caused by localized, simultaneous contractions of longitudinal and circular muscles, isolating short segments of the colon from one another. Adjacent segments contract alternately, pushing the colonic contents either anterograde or retrograde over a short distance (17). Although segmental movements occur mainly in the right colon, they also have been observed in the descending colon and the sigmoid colon. Like retrograde movements, segmental contractions also might slow colonic transit.

The third type of colonic motility identified from radiographic observations is mass movement (22). It occurs three or four times a day, primarily in the transverse and descending colon, but it also occurs in the sigmoid colon during defecation. Colonic contents are propelled by mass movement over a long distance at a rate of approximately 0.5–1 cm/sec (23,24). Using a microtransducer placed via a sigmoid colostomy, Garcia et al. (25) recorded activity over a 24-hour period. They documented a series of contractions and spiking potentials averaging 5.6 minutes, following which a "big contraction" appeared with mean pressure values of 127 mmHg and mean electric values of 10.6 mV. The duration of this phenomenon averaged 24.93 seconds and corresponded to an observed intense evacuation via the colostomy. They believe this electropressure phenomenon represents the mass movement.

Radiologic assessment can demonstrate only changes in contour. For detailed examination of colonic motility other techniques must be employed, such as isotope scintigraphy, the measurement of intracolonic pressure, the investigation of colonic and rectal wall contractility with barostat balloons, and the examination of myoelectrical activity of colonic smooth muscle.

ISOTOPE SCINTIGRAPHY ■ Although evacuation proctography and isotope proctography with radiolabeled material inserted into the rectum allow the description of rectal emptying, neither technique provides any information about transport of colonic contents during defecation. Colorectal scintigraphy after oral intake of isotopes is a physiological technique and allows accurate assessment of colorectal transport during defecation. Utilizing this technique, Krogh and co-workers observed an almost complete emptying of the rectosigmoid, the descending colon, and part of the transverse colon after normal defecation (26).

MEASUREMENT OF INTRACOLONIC PRESSURE ■ Pressure activity of the large bowel has been intensively studied with many different devices, including water- or air-filled balloons, perfused catheters, radiotelemetry capsules, and microtransducers. The measurement of intracolonic pressure presents special problems. First, the colonic contents may interfere with recording by changing the basal physiologic state of the colon or plugging or displacing the recording device. Second, problems of retrograde introduction of recording devices and difficulty in maintaining them at a constant site may be encountered.

Initially, manometric recordings were limited to the rectum and distal sigmoid colon. Most studies were static and manometry was performed with a retrogradely placed assembly in the prepared left hemicolon. To avoid the potential pertuberation of motor patterns by colonic cleansing and to permit ambulation, several authors have adopted an antegrade approach via nasocolonic intubation of the unprepared colon. To capture all the relevant activity throughout the entire colon with sufficient spatial resolution it is necessary to use an assembly with multiple, closely spaced recording sites (27). Studies utilizing this technique have revealed two major pressure patterns. The most prevalent pattern is non-propagating. This non-propagating activity appears to exhibit the same characteristics as the recurrent bursts of rectal motor activity, termed rectal motor complexes. This type of activity is suppressed during the night and increases after awakening and within 60 minutes after a meal. Non-propagating activity is more predominant in the distal colon (27). Less frequent are the pressure waves constituting propagating sequences. The majority of these propagating sequences consist of isolated monophasic pressure waves with a relatively low amplitude ($\leq$60 mm Hg). These pressure sequences migrate both in antegrade and retrograde directions, with antegrade propagating sequences being more frequent and of greater amplitude. Retrograde propagating waves arise from all colonic regions and demonstrate no regional differences with respect to velocity and extent of propagation. Although antegrade propagating waves also arise in all colonic regions, the majority of them arise in the cecum. In contrast to the retrograde propagating waves, they show regional differences regarding velocity, extent of propagation, and amplitude. The extent of propagation varies between 15 and more than 22.5 cm and is higher the more proximal the site of origin. The amplitude increases as the waves propagate distally, reaching their peak in the descending colon. The velocity also increases as the waves propagate distally. The highest velocity has been found in the rectum ($\geq$4cm/sec).

Less frequent are propagating pressure waves with a high amplitude ($\geq$100 mm Hg). Most of these pressure waves arise in the cecum and ascending colon, especially after awaking and after a meal. According to some workers they migrate caudally over the entire colon with a progressive velocity from proximal to distal (28). Recent work, however, has revealed that high-amplitude pressure waves do not display regional variation in conduction velocity (27). There is evidence that they propagate further and more slowly than the non-high amplitude pressure waves. It has been reported that the high-amplitude pressure waves represent the manometric equivalent of mass movements (29). They may be induced by laxatives, cholinergic agents, stimulation of the pelvic nerves and colonic distension (29,30). Based on previous work it has been suggested that the high-amplitude pressure waves are associated with defecation. Crowell et al. found that 41 percent of these pressure waves occur in the hour before defecation (31). The relationship between high-amplitude pressure waves and defecation has been confirmed by others (29,32,33). Bampton et al. studied the spatial and temporal organization of pressure patterns throughout the unprepared colon during spontaneous defecation (34). They were able to demonstrate a pre-expulsive phase commencing up to 1 hour before stool expulsion. This phase is characterized by a distinctive biphasic spatial and temporal pattern with an early and a late component. The early component is characterized by an array of antegrade propagating sequences. The site of their origin migrates distally with each subsequent sequence. The late component, in the 15 minutes before stool expulsion, is characterized by an array of antegrade propagating sequences. The site of their origin migrates proximally with each subsequent sequence. The amplitude of the pressure waves, occurring in this late phase, increases significantly. Many of them are real high amplitude pressure waves. They are associated with an increasing sensation of urge to defecate. Some of the last propagating sequences, prior to stool expulsion, commence in the ascending colon (Fig. 2). This latter finding illustrates that the entire colon is involved in the process of defecation.

Hirabayashi et al. investigated colorectal motility in adult mongrel dogs before and during spontaneous defecation with the help of force strain-gauge transducers implanted in the proximal, distal, and sigmoid colon, as well as in the rectum and the anal canal. During defecation giant contractions were detected, running from the distal colon into the rectum. It seems likely that these giant contractions are the myoelectric equivalent of the high-amplitude pressure waves (36).

The factors that initiate and modulate the propagating wave sequences are only partially understood. Because these wave patterns disappear during sleep and arousal from sleep is a potent and immediate stimulus, it seems likely that extrinsic neural pathways are involved in their modulation and activation. Chemical stimuli, such as rectal installation of bisacodyl or chenodeoxycholic acid initiate propagating pressure waves in the proximal colon, whereas mechanical stimulation by rectal distension suppresses these pressure waves. It is likely that this rectocolonic inhibitory reflex prevents further passage of stool to a loaded rectum. The responses to chemical and mechanical stimuli are presumed to be mediated by long colocolonic pathways (37). Further recordings have added to our understanding of normal colonic and rectal motility patterns and have provided useful information about different pathologic conditions. It has been shown, for example, that constipated subjects display significantly fewer high-amplitude contractions than healthy volunteers (38–40). Using an ambulatory system Kumar et al. (41) described recurrent bursts of rectal motor activity termed the "rectal motor complexes." They theorized that these runs of rectal contractions represent periodic activity similar to phase III of the small intestinal migrating complex. Other workers have observed similar contractile activity in the human rectum (42,43). However, they were not able to show an association with the migrating motor complex cycle. Orkin et al. (42) suggested that this recurrent phasic activity might act to keep the rectum empty. This view is not supported by others, who found that the phasic rectal motor activity is segmental rather than propelled. Prolonged anorectal pressure recordings have revealed that rectal motor activity is reduced during sleep, whereas a meal provides a stimulus for increased activity in fully ambulant subjects (44). Despite their unknown origin, the rectal motor complexes might be of clinical importance, since it has been shown that women with slow-transit constipation display fewer complexes than control subjects (45).

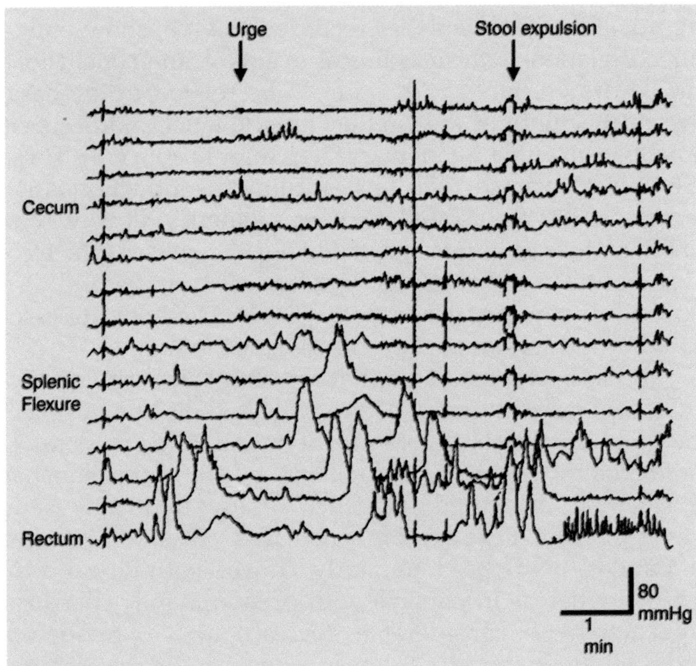

FIGURE 2 ■ Manometric trace of spontaneous defecation. This trace demonstrates an array of propagating sequences with site of origin becoming more proximal with each subsequent sequence. Note that the propagating pressure waves in the the sequences immediately before defecation exhibit a slower velocity and greater amplitude than pressure waves in earlier sequences, and in this example stool expulsion follows immediately after a propagating sequence. *Source*: From Ref. 35.

CONTRACTILE ACTIVITY ■ It has been reported that barostat balloons have the potential to explore variations in the contractile state of the colonic and rectal wall. Barostat balloons are infinitely compliant plastic bags. The barostat assembly moves air in and out to maintain a constant preset pressure in the balloon. Changes in tone are reflected by changes in bag volume. A significant reduction of bag volume has been documented immediately after the ingestion of food, indicating a sustained increase in colonic tone in the postprandial period. During overnight sleep colonic tone decreases (46,47). The increase in colonic tone in response to feeding shows remarkable regional differences. Assessing the contractile activity in the transverse and sigmoid colon using a barostat assembly, Ford et al. (48) found that the mean increase in colonic tone after the ingestion of food was significantly greater in the transverse than in the sigmoid colon. The contractile responses in the human colon are mediated by a $5HT_3$ mechanism (49). It has been reported that hypocapnic hyperventilation produces an increase in colonic tone. This finding suggests that autonomic mechanisms are also involved in the control of the contractile state of the large bowel (50). Grotz et al. (51) reported that changes in rectal wall contractility in response to feeding, to a cholinergic agonist, and to a smooth muscle relaxant are decreased in constipated patients. Gosselink and Schouten used a barostat assembly to investigate the tonic response of the rectum to a meal in healthy volunteers and in 60 women with obstructed defecation. Total colonic transit time was normal in 30 patients and prolonged in the other 30. Following the meal all controls showed a significant increase in rectal tone. A similar response was found in the patients with a normal colonic transit time. In the patients with a prolonged colonic transit the increase in rectal tone was significantly lower (52). It has been stated that intracolonic barostat balloons are more sensitive than manometric probes in the detection of nonoccluding contractions. Using a combined barostat–manometry assembly, von der Ohe et al. (49) found a significant decrease of bag volume consistent with an increment in colonic tone after the ingestion of a 1000 kcal meal. This response was not associated with concomitant changes in intracolonic pressure. In addition, they also reported that the barostat balloon measurements indicated 70% more phasic events than the manometric sideholes located 2 cm proximal to 7 cm distal to the balloon. This finding illustrates that the data obtained from intraluminal pressure recordings should be interpreted with caution and that barostat balloons are far more sensitive in detecting variations in colonic tone.

MYOELECTRICAL ACTIVITY ■ Integration of smooth muscle contractions of the colon is necessary for the orderly progression of intraluminal contents. The basic electrical rhythm in the proximal part of the gastrointestinal tract consists of regular omnipresent slow waves. These slow waves are the manifestation of cyclic depolarization and repolarization of the intestinal smooth muscle cell membrane. The slow waves are generated in a group or in a single smooth muscle cell, which has the characteristics of a coupled oscillator. They act as coupled electrical oscillations leading to control in time and space of the excitability of smooth muscle cells (53). Generally, slow waves are thought to coordinate gastrointestinal motility; therefore slow wave activity is also called electrical control activity.

Many attempts have been made to record in vitro the myoelectrical activity in the human colon. Slow wave activity in human colonic smooth muscle exists in 20–50% of the preparations examined (54,55). Slow wave activity has been recorded from the circular and longitudinal muscle layers in 94% and 100%, respectively, of the muscle strips studied (56). The slow waves of the circular muscle layer, as recorded in vitro, occur at a variable frequency [4–60 cycles per minute (cpm)], while those of the longitudinal muscle layer present a more constant frequency (24–36 cpm). The amplitude is relatively low in both muscle layers (57). The slow wave activity of human colonic smooth muscle in vitro shows an irregular pattern, with bursts of relatively high-amplitude slow waves. The frequency as well as the amplitude of the slow waves are highly sensitive to intrinsic and extrinsic stimuli. A second type of myoelectrical activity is the spike potential activity, which represents summated action potentials; this can result in contraction of smooth muscle cells. Spike potentials occur singly or in bursts and are always superimposed on slow waves. Like slow wave activity, spiking activity also is sensitive to intrinsic and extrinsic stimuli (58).

The technique most often described for the in vivo investigation of large bowel myoelectrical activity uses monopolar or bipolar electrodes mounted on intraluminal tubes. After introduction of the tube into the colon, the electrodes are clipped to the mucosa or attached to the mucosal surface by suction. Alternatively, the electrodes can be implanted under the serosal coat. Some researchers have used silver/silver chloride electrodes placed on the skin of the abdominal wall and overlying the large bowel. With this technique, only the frequency and regularity of the colonic slow waves can be determined (59).

The in vivo investigation of large bowel myoelectrical activity poses many problems. First, it is very difficult with intraluminal recording techniques to obtain a continuous and stable contact between electrode and mucosal surface and to eliminate the effects of colonic contents and/or transit. Second, none of the recording devices is capable of measuring all the activity actually generated. Serosal electrodes record a greater number of spike potentials and a higher proportion of the longitudinal muscle activity than do mucosal electrodes (58). Third, it is not possible to differentiate between the myoelectrical activity generated by the two muscle layers. Finally, the reliability of the recording techniques and the comparability of methods have yet to be evaluated. Differences in recording techniques undoubtedly account for the conflicting results reported in the literature.

There has been much controversy about the exact nature of the myoelectrical activity in the human colon as recorded in vivo. Only in 1982 was it shown that slow waves could be recorded in a continuous manner (60). Two types of slow wave activity have been described: slow waves with a low frequency of 3–4 cpm and slow waves with a higher frequency of 6–12 cpm, the latter being more common (59,61,62). The predominant high-frequency slow waves show a frequency gradient between the proximal and distal part of the colon (59). The physiologic basis for this differentiation between the two slow wave frequencies is disputed (58). Spike potentials in the human colon may occur during any phase of the slow wave cycle (60). Spikes may occur without contractions (60,61,63), and contractions may occur without spikes (59–62). In the human colon, spike potentials can be recorded as short spike bursts (SSBs), lasting only a few seconds, and as long spike bursts (LSBs), which last approximately 30 seconds (64). Although the myoelectrical events, as recorded in vivo, show only a fair correlation with mechanical events, some conclusions can be drawn. First, SSBs seem to be related to the basal electrical activity of the circular muscle layer and occur as slow waves with a frequency of less than 13 cpm (58). These SSBs are associated with low-amplitude contractions (64). Second, LSBs are related to high-frequency slow waves, which appear in bursts and are likely to represent the electrical control activity of the longitudinal muscle and also periodically the circular muscle (58–65). The LSBs are associated with high-amplitude contractions (64).

It has been postulated that abnormal slow wave activity, as well as changing ratios of SSBs to LSBs, might reflect colonic dysfunction. Myoelectrical investigation of rectosigmoid activity in cases of irritable bowel syndrome has revealed an increased incidence of low-frequency slow waves (66,67). Furthermore, increased SSBs were found in patients with predominantly constipation-type bowel activity, whereas in patients with predominantly diarrhea-type activity, a considerable decrease in SSB frequency, and LSB frequency to a lesser extent, could be demonstrated (64). An increased incidence of SSBs also was found in patients with slow-transit constipation, whereas a short colonic transit time (as in patients with diarrhea) seems to be correlated with a preponderance of LSBs (Fig. 3) (68,69). Although these findings strongly suggest that myoelectrical activity of the colon reflects its function, the exact nature of this relationship is still unclear.

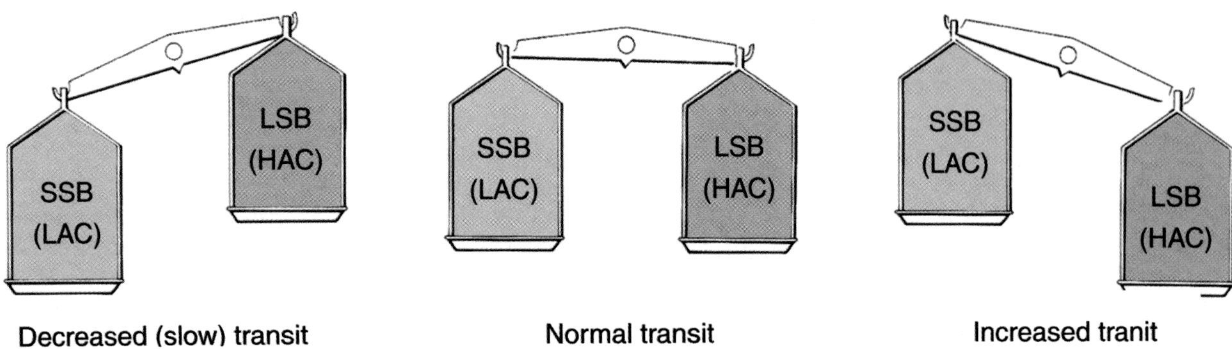

FIGURE 3 ■ Balance between short and long spike bursts in normal and abnormal colonic transit. *Abbreviations*: SSB, short spike burst; LSB, long spike burst; LAC, low-amplitude contraction; HAC, high-amplitude contraction.

NEUROGENIC CONTROL OF MOTILITY ■ Colonic motility is controlled by extrinsic and intrinsic neuronal systems. Considering the influence of these systems, it must be remembered that they are acting on a background of fluctuating intrinsic changes in smooth muscle cell membrane excitability (70). The extrinsic system consists of preganglionic parasympathetic neurons and postganglionic sympathetic neurons. The intrinsic (or enteric) nervous system may be defined as that system of neurons in which the cell body is within the wall of the colon. The extrinsic innervation of the colon is described in chapter 1. The pathways are summarized in Figures 4 and 5.

The enteric nervous system plays a major role in the regulation of secretion, motility, immune function, and inflammation in the small and large bowels (71). The intrinsic nervous system of the colon consists of a number of interconnected plexuses. Within these networks, small groups of nerve cell bodies or enteric ganglia can be seen. The 80–100 million enteric neurons can be classified into functionally distinct subpopulations, including intrinsic primary afferent neurons, interneurons, motor neurons, secretomotor and vasomotor neurons. The enteric nerve cells are organized in two main plexuses, the myenteric plexus of Auerbach and the submucosal plexus of Meissner. In the past it was thought that the deep muscular plexus, described by Cajal, also consisted of neurons. It has been shown, however, that the cells of Cajal are neither neurons nor Schwann cells (72). These cells, located within the inner layers of the circular muscle, are now commonly referred to as interstitial cells of Cajal (ICC). There is growing evidence that ICC are probably pacemakers in the generation of the autorhythmicity of the circular muscle. They also serve as conductors of excitable events and may be mediators of enteric neurotransmission (71).

Studies with the aid of zinc-iodide osmium-impregnated colon have revealed that the structural organization

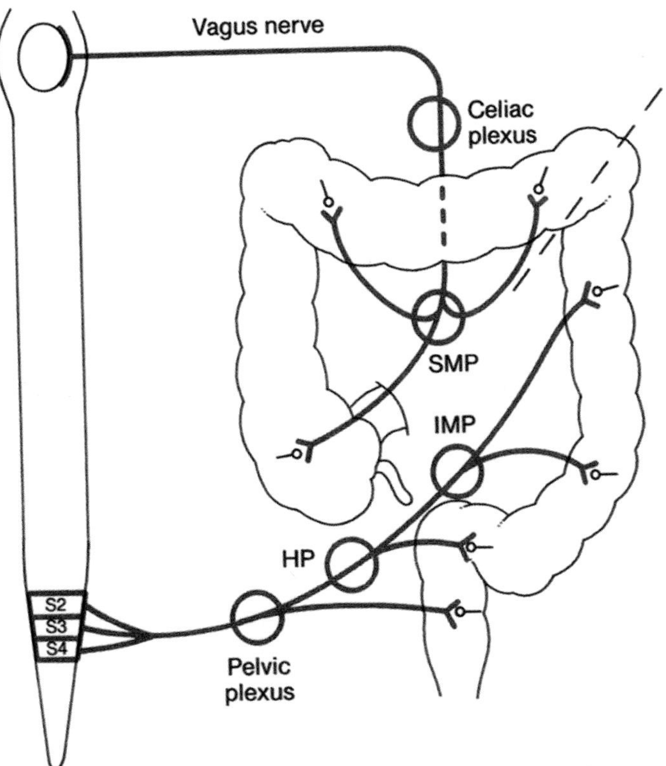

FIGURE 4 ■ Parasympathetic pathways. *Abbreviations*: HP, hypogastric plexus; IMP, inferior mesenteric plexus; SMP, superior mesenteric plexus.

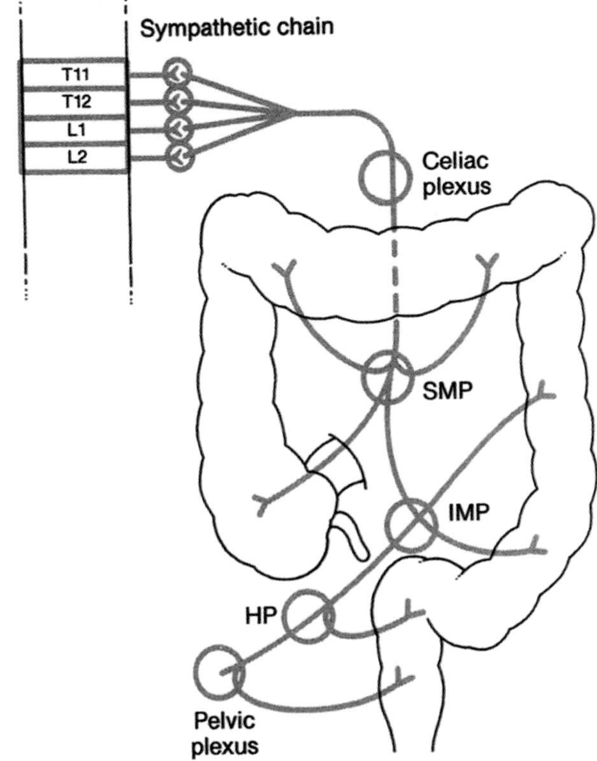

FIGURE 5 ■ Sympathetic pathways. *Abbreviations*: HP, hypogastric plexus; IMP, inferior mesenteric plexus; SMP, superior mesenteric plexus.

of the enteric nervous system is far more complex than previously thought (73). In the mucosal plexus, fine nerve fibers were evident in the connective tissue of the lamina propria among the tubular glands, close to the glandular epithelium and encircling their fundus like a nest to form the interglandular, periglandular, and subglandular networks, respectively. No ganglia were found in the mucosal plexus. The muscularis mucosae plexus appeared as a fine felt made up of a nonganglionated nervous network in which nerve bundles ran mostly parallel to the long axes of the smooth muscle cells. Ganglia of the submucosal plexus appeared arranged along three different planes. The innermost network was composed of small-sized, regularly arranged ganglia in a single row immediately below the muscularis mucosae. Nerve strands from these ganglia ran toward the mucosal plexus and the middle part of the submucosa. A second series of ganglia was deeply located, often at the same level as the large blood vessels, and a third was closely opposed to the circular muscle layer. Nerve strands connected all these ganglia to each other. The intramuscular nerve fiber bundles run parallel to the long axes of the smooth muscle cells and form the nonganglionated circular and longitudinal muscular plexuses, respectively. Large caliber nerve fibers pass through the serosa and penetrate the longitudinal muscle layer. The subserosal plexus at all colonic levels except the sigmoid has no ganglia, and all nerve fibers are amyelinated.

Three groups of neurons can be distinguished in the enteric nervous system: (1) sensory neurons, (2) associative neurons or interneurons, and (3) motor neurons. The sensory neurons play an important role in local reflex pathways, monitoring the chemical nature of the colonic contents as well as the tension in the wall of the large bowel. For example, localized radial distention of the colon evokes an ascending excitatory reflex (i.e., contraction of the circular muscle on the proximal side) and a descending inhibitory reflex (i.e., relaxation of the circular muscle on the distal side) (Fig. 6) (70). These reflexes also can be elicited by mechanical and chemical irritation of the mucosa. Some of the sensory neurons for these reflexes have their endings in the mucosa (Fig. 7). The associative neurons or interneurons form information links between enteric neurons (70). There is some evidence that 5-hydroxytryptamine is the neurotransmitter of these associative neurons (70,74). The most important enteric neurons are the motor neurons, of which different groups can be distinguished: excitatory motor, inhibitory motor, secretomotor, and enteric vasodilator (70). The excitatory and inhibitory motor neurons play an important role in controlling colonic motility.

Excitatory motor neurons of the enteric nervous system are mainly postganglionic parasympathetic neurons. The cell bodies of these cholinergic neurons, which supply the longitudinal and circular muscle cells, are located in the myenteric and submucosal plexuses (Fig. 7). The most important excitatory neurotransmitter is acetylcholine, for which receptors on colonic smooth muscle cells are of the muscarinic subtype. They are blocked by muscarinic antagonists such as atropine and scopolamine, but not by nicotinic antagonists (70). The receptors for acetylcholine also have been found on the membrane of myenteric ganglion cells. Therefore, acetylcholine might have a direct as well as an indirect effect on colonic motility. There is evidence that other noncholinergic agents play an excitatory role in the control of colonic motility. One of these agents is probably substance P, which could be released by cholinergic neurons, because those neurons are known to contain substances other than acetylcholine. It also has been suggested that some of the excitatory motor neurons are noncholinergic (70).

Inhibitory motor neurons of the enteric nervous system are noncholinergic and nonadrenergic. The cell bodies of these inhibitory neurons are located in the myenteric plexus (Fig. 7). They predominantly supply the circular muscle and to a lesser extent the longitudinal muscle. Because adenosine triphosphate or a related purine nucleotide has been proposed as a possible transmitter of these neurons, they have been called purinergic neurons (75). It has been suggested that the transmission of the inhibitory motor neurons also might be peptidergic. There is much evidence that the vasoactive intestinal polypeptide might be the most important inhibitory neuropeptide (70). The inhibitory motor neurons are involved in the mediation of the descending inhibitory phase of the peristaltic reflex (Fig. 7) (70).

More than 40 regulatory peptides have now been isolated from the gastrointestinal tract. Most of these are present in the peptidergic neurons of the enteric nervous system (ENS) (71). Mulvihill and Debas (71) published an excellent review of the role of the ENS and the following draws heavily from their dissertation. Functionally, four categories of peptidergic neurons of the ENS have been identified: (1) motor neurons (2) secretory neurons, (3) interneurons, and (4) sensory neurons, the cell bodies of which lie in the dorsal ganglia.

Histochemically, the neurons of the ENS may be classified by the substances they contain and their use as neurotransmitters. Five types of neurons have been identified: (1) classic cholinergic (acetylcholine), (2) classic adrenergic (norepinephrine), (3) serotoninergic (5-hydroxytryptamine), (4) GABA-ergic (γ-aminobutyric acid), and (5) peptidergic. Of these, the peptidergic neurons are by far the largest group. A wide variety of peptides have been identified as neurotransmitters in the ENS.

Peptides identified in neurons of the enteric nervous system include vasoactive intestinal peptide, peptide histidine isoleucine, substance P, substance K (neurokinin A), cholecystokinin, somatostatin, neurotensin, neuropeptide Y, enkephalins, dynorphin, galanin, calcitonin gene-related peptide, and gastrin-releasing peptide.

The ENS regulates the relaxation and contraction of the sphincters of the gut, including those of the ileocecal valve and anus. Both cholinergic and excitatory adrenergic nerves from the pelvic plexus and pudendal nerves are responsible for contraction of the internal anal sphincter. The mediators for these neurons are acetylcholine and noradrenaline, respectively. The major relaxant of the internal anal sphincter is vasoactive intestinal polypeptide (VIP). Recent evidence suggests that mechanisms involving nitric oxide are also important.

Abnormalities of this regulation are probably the cause of gastrointestinal symptoms in a wide variety of intestinal disorders including gut endocrine neoplasms, Hirschsprung's disease, irritable bowel syndrome, pseudo-obstruction, scleroderma, diverticulosis, chronic constipation, and inflammatory bowel disease.

A

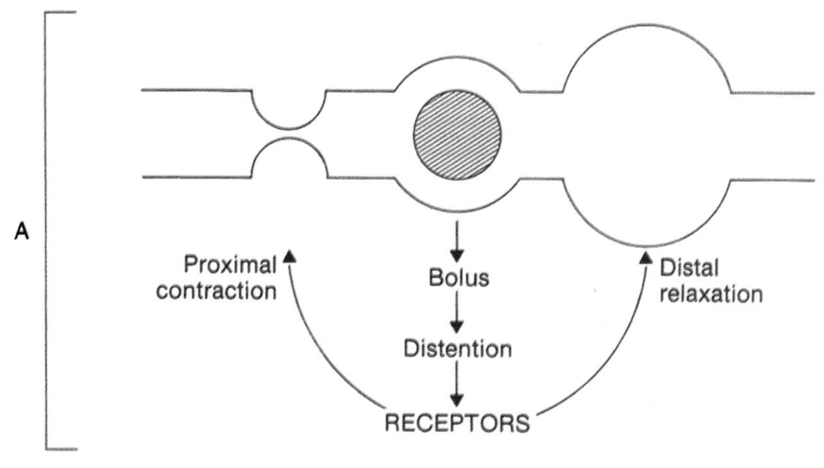

B

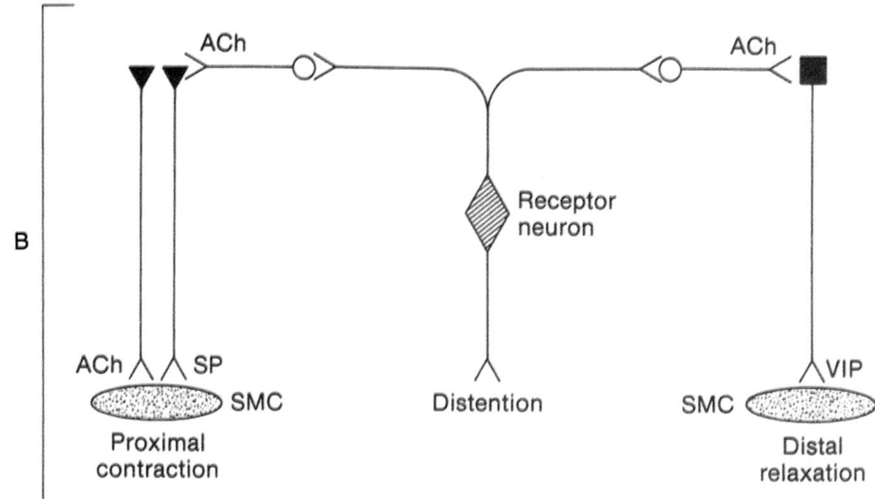

FIGURE 6 ■ Peristaltic reflex arc. (**A**) Proximal contraction is mediated by acetylcholine and substance P. (**B**) Descending inhibitory phase (distal relaxation) is mediated by the vasoinhibitory peptide. *Abbreviations*: ACh, acetylcholine; SMC, smooth muscle cell; SP, substance P; VIP, vasoactive intestinal polypeptide.

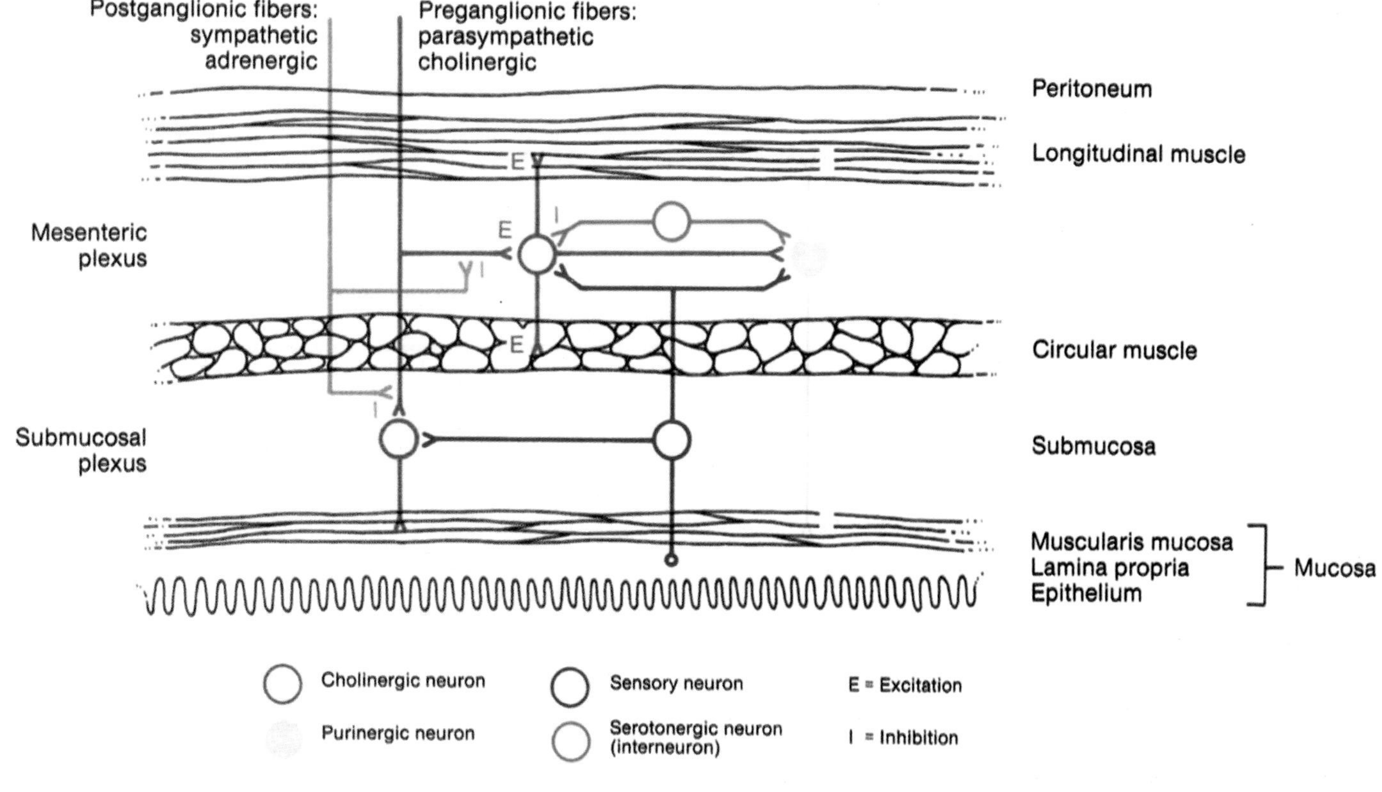

FIGURE 7 ■ Enteric nervous system (ENS).

HORMONAL CONTROL OF MOTILITY ■ Colonic function is affected by an extensive endocrine system. Approximately 15 different gastrointestinal hormones have been identified (76). These gut hormones are synthesized in endocrine and paracrine cells. Many of these substances also are found in enteric neurons; therefore, they are potential neurotransmitters. The pharmacokinetics, catabolism, and release of these hormones are very complex, and their exact role in the regulation of large bowel motor activity is undetermined. The role of only a few hormones, such as gastrin and cholecystokinin, is known. These hormones are synthesized and released in the upper part of the gastrointestinal tract. Because they can reach the colon through the bloodstream, they might be able to control colonic motility.

Investigators have shown that spike potential activity of the colon does increase following the administration of gastrin and pentagastrin (61,77). However, the gastrocolic reflex (i.e., increased colonic motility during and after a meal) is unlikely to be due to gastrin, because this reflex is still present in patients with total gastrectomy and because plasma levels of gastrin peak much later than the postprandial increase in colonic motility (78). More likely, cholecystokinin is the mediator of this postprandial colonic activity. Cholecystokinin is a well-known colonic stimulant, increasing colonic spike activity at physiologic concentrations and in a dose-dependent manner (79).

Other upper gastrointestinal hormones such as glucagon and somatostatin have inhibitory effects (77). It has been reported that secretin also inhibits colonic motility (80), but this effect could not be demonstrated by others (61). Therefore it is not clear whether secretin has an inhibitory effect or no effect at all on colonic motility.

Present knowledge indicates that these hormones play their major role in the control of secretion and absorption.

PHARMACOLOGIC INFLUENCE ■ In a study of the effects of morphine and the opiate antagonist naloxone on human colonic transit, Kaufman et al. (81) found that morphine significantly delayed transit in the cecum and ascending colon and decreased the number of bowel movements per 48 hours. Naloxone accelerated transit in the transverse colon and rectosigmoid colon but had no effect on the number of bowel movements per 48 hours. These results suggest that narcotic analgesics may cause constipation in part by slowing colonic transit in the proximal colon and by inhibiting defecation. Acceleration of transit by naloxone suggests that endogenous opiate peptides may play an inhibitory role in the regulation of human colonic transit. Of immediate practical significance is the fact that it thus may be inadvisable to prescribe morphine as a postoperative analgesic following colonic operations.

■ MICROFLORA

Common Microflora

The bacterial population of the gastrointestinal tract is a complex collection of aerobic and anaerobic micro organisms. Distal to the ileocecal valve, the bacterial concentrations increase sharply, rising to 10^{11}–10^{12} colony forming units (cfu) per milliliter. Nearly one third of the fecal dry weight consists of viable bacteria, with as many as 10^{11}–10^{12} microorganisms present per gram of feces (83). Stephen and Cummings (83) reported that bacteria comprises 55% of the total fecal solids. Anaerobic bacteria outnumber aerobes by a factor of 10^2–10^4. Typically, *Bacteroides* species are present in numbers of 10^{10}–10^{12}/g of feces, and *Escherichia coli* are present in numbers of 10^8–10^{10}/g of feces. The predominant isolates are listed in Table 1. Dunn (85) has summarized the microbial flora that are found in conventional ileostomies and ileal reservoirs (Table 2).

TABLE 1 ■ Colonic Flora

Organism	Concentration (cfu/mL)
Aerobic or facultative organisms	
Microorganisms	10^7–10^{12}
Enterobacteria	10^4–10^{10}
Streptococci	10^5–10^{10}
Staphylococci	10^4–10^7
Lactobacilli	10^6–10^{10}
Fungi	10^2–10^6
Anaerobic bacteria	
Bacteroides spp.	10^{10}–10^{12}
Bifidobacterium spp.	10^8–10^{10}
Streptococci[a]	10^8–10^{11}
Clostridium spp.	10^6–10^{11}
Eubacterium spp.	10^9–10^{12}

[a]Includes *Peptostreptococcus* and *Peptococcus* spp.
Source: From Ref. 84.

It is self-evident that the nature of colonic bacteria is of paramount importance to the surgeon. Knowledge of the type of resident bacteria serves as a useful guide to the rational selection of appropriate antibiotic therapy, both in the prophylactic and therapeutic settings.

Microflora Activity

Guarner and Malagelada conducted an extensive review of gut flora in health and disease in which they summarize the major functions of the gut microflora including metabolic activities that result in salvage of energy and absorbable nutrients, important trophic effects on intestinal epithelia and on immune structure and function, and protection of the colonized host against invasion by alien microbes (86). Much of the following information has been

TABLE 2 ■ Microbial Flora Found in Conventional Ileostomies and Ileal Reservoirs

	Total No. of Organisms	Aerobes	Anaerobes
Normal individual			
Upper small intestine	0–10^5	0–10^5	Few
Lower small intestine	10^4–10^9	10^4–10^9	10^4–10^9
Conventional ileostomy			
Upper small intestine	0–10^5	0–10^5	Few
Lower small intestine	10^7–10^9	10^4–10^{10}	10^4–10^{11}
Continent ileostomy			
Upper small intestine	0–10^5	0–10^5	Few
Lower small intestine	10^7–10^9	10^3–10^{10}	10^6–10^{10}
Ileal ileoanal reservoir			
Upper small intestine	10^3–10^5	10^3–10^5	10^2–10^4
Lower small intestine	10^6–10^{11}	10^6–10^{11}	10^7–10^{11}

Source: From Ref. 85.

derived from their comprehensive review. Gut microflora might also be an essential factor in certain pathologic disorders including multi-system organ failure, colon carcinoma, and inflammatory bowel diseases. Several hundred grams of bacteria living within the colonic lumen affect host homeostasis. Some of these bacteria are potential pathogens and can be a source of infection and sepsis when the integrity of the bowel barrier is physically or functionally breached. Bacteria are also useful in promotion of human health. The constant interaction between the host and its microbial guests can infer important health benefits to the human host. Probiotics and prebiotics are known to have a role in the prevention or treatment of some diseases.

Metabolic Functions

A major metabolic function of the colonic microflora is the fermentation of non-digestible dietary residue which is a major source of energy in the colon. Non-digestible carbohydrates include large polysaccharides (resistant starches, cellulose, hemicellulose, pectins, and gums), some oligosaccharides that escape digestion, and unabsorbed sugars and alcohols. The metabolic endpoint is generation of short-chain fatty acids. Anerobic metabolism of peptides and proteins (putrefaction) by the microflora also produces short-chain fatty acids but, at the same time, it generates a series of potentially toxic substances including ammonia, amines, phenols, thiols, and indoles. Available proteins include elastin and collagen from dietary sources, pancreatic enzymes, sloughed epithelial cells and lysed bacteria. Substrate availability in the human adult colon is about 20 to 60 g carbohydrates and 5 to 10 g protein per day.

Colonic microorganisms also play a part in vitamin synthesis and in absorption of calcium, magnesium, and iron. Absorption of ions in the cecum is improved by carbohydrate fermentation and production of short-chain fatty acids, especially acetate, propionate, and butyrate. All of these fatty acids have important functions in host physiology. Butyrate is almost completely consumed by the colonic epithelium, and it is a major source of energy for colonocytes. Acetate and propionate are found in portal blood and are eventually metabolized by the liver (propionate) or peripheral tissues, particularly muscle (acetate). Acetate and propionate might also have a role as modulators of glucose metabolism: absorption of these short-chain fatty acids would result in lower glycemic responses to oral glucose or standard meal—a response consistent with an ameliorated sensitivity to insulin. Foods with a high proportion of non-digestible carbohydrates have a low glycemic index. Vitamin K is produced by intestinal microorganisms (84).

The enterohepatic circulation of many compounds depends on flora that produce bacterial enzymes, such as B-glucuronidase and sulfatase. Some of the endogenous and exogenous substances that undergo an enterohepatic circulation include bilirubin, bile acids, estrogens, cholesterol, digoxin, rifampin, morphine, colchicine, and diethylstilbestrol (87). The main role of anerobes appears to be the provision of catabolic enzymes for organic compounds that cannot be digested by enzymes of eukaryotic origin. They are needed for the catabolism of cholesterol, bile acids, and steroid hormones; they hydrolyze a number of flavonoid glycosides to anticarcinogens; and they detoxify certain carcinogens (88).

Trophic Functions

All three short-chain fatty acids stimulate epithelial cell proliferation and differentiation in the large and small intestine in vivo in rats. A role for short-chain fatty acids in prevention of some human pathological states such as chronic ulcerative colitis and colonic carcinogenesis has been long suspected although, conclusive evidence is still lacking (86). Short-chain fatty acids butyrate, propionate, and acetate produced during fiber fermentation promote colonic differentiation and can reverse or suppress neoplastic progression. Basson et al. (89) sought to identify candidate genes responsible for short-chain fatty acid activity on colonocytes and to compare the relative activities of independent short-chain fatty acids. A total of 30,000 individual genetic sequences were analyzed for differential expression among the three short-chain fatty acids. More than 1000 gene fragments were identified as being substantially modulated in expression by butyrate. Butyrate tended to have the most pronounced effects and acetate the least.

Host Immunity Functions

The intestinal mucosa is the main interface between the immune system and the external environment (86). Gut-associated lymphoid tissues contain the largest pool of immunocompetent cells in the human body. The dialogue between host and bacteria at the mucosal interface seems to play a part in development of a competent immune system. The immune response to microbes relies on innate and adaptive components, such as immunologlobulin secretion. Most bacteria in human feces are coated with specific IgA units. Innate responses are mediated not only by white blood cells such as neutrophils and macrophages that can phagocytose and kill pathogens, but also by intestinal epithelial cells, which coordinate host responses by synthesizing a wide range of inflammatory mediators and transmitting signals to underlying cells in the mucosa. The innate immune system has to discriminate between potential pathogens from commensal bacteria, with the use of a restricted number of preformed receptors. The system allows immediate recognition of bacteria to rapidly respond to an eventual challenge.

Protective Functions

Anerobes are usually seen as destructive creatures without any redeeming virtues.. Resident bacteria are a crucial line of resistance to colonization by exogenous microbes and, therefore, are highly relevant in prevention of invasion of tissues by pathogens (86). Colonisation resistance also applies to opportunistic bacteria that are present in the gut but have restrictive growth. Use of antibiotics can disrupt the ecological balance and allow overgrowth of species with potential pathogenicity such as toxigenic clostridium difficile, associated with pseudomembranous colitis. Benefits we derive from anerobes include their probable function in restraining growth of *Clostridium Difficile* in human carriers (88).

Bacterial Translocation

The passage of viable bacteria from the gastrointestinal tract through the epithelial mucosa is called bacterial translocation. Translocation of endotoxins from viable or dead bacteria in very small amounts probably constitutes a physiologically important boost to the reticuloendothelial system, especially to the Kupffer cells in the liver. However, dysfunction of the gut mucosal barrier can result in the translocation of many viable microorganisms, usually belonging to gram-negative aerobic genera (*Escherichia, Proteus, Klebsiella*). After crossing the epithelial barrier, bacteria can travel via the lymph to extraintestinal sites, such as the mesenteric lymph nodes, liver, and spleen. Subsequently, enteric bacteria can disseminate throughout the body producing sepsis, shock, multisystem organ failure, or death of the host (86).

The three primary mechanisms in promotion of bacterial translocation in animals are overgrowth of bacteria in the small intestine; increased permeability of the intestinal mucosal barrier, and deficiencies in host immune defences. Bacterial translocation can occur in human beings during various disease processes. Indigenous gastrointestinal bacteria have been cultured directly from the mesenteric lymph nodes of patients undergoing laparotomy. Data suggest that the baseline rate of positive mesenteric lymph node culture could approach 5% in otherwise healthy people. However, in disorders such as multisystem organ failure, acute severe pancreatitis, advanced liver cirrhosis, intestinal obstruction, and inflammatory bowel diseases, rates of positive culture are much higher (16%–50%) (86).

Colon Carcinogenesis

Intestinal bacteria could play a part in the initiation of colon carcinoma through production of carcinogens, cocarcinogens, or procarcinogens. In healthy people, diets rich in fat and meat but poor in vegetables increases the fecal excretion of *N*-nitroso compounds, a group of genotoxic substances that are known initiators and promoters of colon carcinoma. Such diets also increase the genotoxic potential of human fecal water. Another group of carcinogens of dietary origin are the heterocyclic aromatic amines that are formed in meat when it is cooked. Some intestinal microorganisms strongly increase damage to DNA in colon cells induced by heterocyclic amines, whereas other intestinal bacteria can uptake and detoxity such compounds (86). Bacteria of the bacteroides and clostridium genera increases the incidence and growth rate of colonic neoplasms induced in animals, whereas other genera such as lactobacillus and bifidobacteria prevent carcinogenesis. Although the evidence is not conclusive, colonic flora seem to be an environmental factor that modulates risk of colonic carcinoma in human beings (86).

Role in Inflammatory Bowel Diseases

Resident bacterial flora have been suggested to be an essential factor in driving the inflammatory process in human inflammatory bowel diseases. In patients with Crohn's disease, intestinal T lymphocytes are hyperactive against bacterial antigens (86). Patients with Crohn's disease or ulcerative colitis have increased intestinal mucosal secretion of IgG type antibodies against a broad-spectrum of commensal bacteria. Patients with inflammatory bowel diseases have higher amounts of bacteria attached to their epithelial surfaces than do healthy people. Unrestrained activation of the intestinal immune system by elements of the flora could be a key event in the pathophysiology of inflammatory bowel disease. Some patients with Crohn's disease (17–25%) have mutations in the *NOD2/CARD15* gene, which regulates host responses to bacteria (90).

In inflammatory bowel diseases in human beings, direct interaction of commensal microflora with the intestinal mucosa stimulates inflammatory activity in the gut lesions. Fecal stream diversion has been shown to prevent recurrence of Crohn's disease, whereas infusion of intestinal contents to the excluded ileal segments reactivated mucosal lesions (91). In ulcerative colitis, short-term treatment with an enteric-coated preparation of broad-spectrum antibiotics rapidly reduced mucosal release of cytokines and eicosanoids and was more effective in reduction of inflammatory activity than were intravenous steroids (92). However, antibiotics have limited effectiveness in clinical management of inflammatory bowel disease, since induction of antibiotic resistant strains substantially impairs sustained effects.

Probiotics and Prebiotics

Bacteria can be used to improve human health. A bacterium that provides specific health benefits when consumed as a food component or supplement would be called a probiotic. Oral probiotics are living microorganisms that upon ingestion in specific numbers exert health benefits beyond those of inherent basic nutrition (86). According to this definition, probiotics do not necessarily colonise the human intestine. Prebiotics are non-digestible food ingredients that beneficially affect the host by selectively stimulating growth, or activity, or both, of one or a restricted number of bacteria in the colon. For example, coadministration of probiotics to patients on antibiotics significantly reduced antibiotic-associated diarrhea (93,94) and can be used to prevent such antibiotic-associated diarrhea (95). Examples of such bacteria include various strains of lactobacillus GG, bifidibacterium bifidum, and streptococcus thermophilus.

Probiotics and prebiotics have been shown to prevent colon carcinoma in several animals, but their role in reduction of risk of colon carcinoma in human beings is not established (96). However, probiotics have been shown to reduce the fecal activity of enzymes known to produce genotoxic compounds that acts as initiators of carcinoma in human beings (86).

■ INTESTINAL GAS

Intestinal gas may be endogenous or exogenous. Five gases—nitrogen, oxygen, carbon dioxide, hydrogen, and methane—make up 99% of all the gas in the gut. Only nitrogen and oxygen are found in the atmosphere and therefore can be swallowed. Hydrogen, methane, and carbon dioxide are produced by bacterial fermentation of carbohydrates and proteins in the colon. Approximately one third of the human population produces methane. Small amounts of hydrogen sulfide are also produced. Levitt (97), in his extensive studies of this subject, found that patients who complain of excessive flatus almost invariably have high concentrations of hydrogen and carbon dioxide. Hydrogen is cleared by the lungs. Since carbon dioxide is a result of fermentation, therapy consists of diet manipulation with a decrease in the amount of carbohydrate, especially lactose, wheat, and potatoes.

The most dramatic and important point for the surgeon regarding intestinal gas is the fact that explosions may occur during electrocautery in the colon. Because both hydrogen and methane are explosive, intestinal gases should be aspirated before electrocautery is used.

ANORECTAL PHYSIOLOGY

The physiology of the anorectal region is very complex, and it is only recently that detailed investigations have given us a better understanding of its function.

The methods that are used for the systematic and fundamental study of anorectal physiology include anorectal manometry, defecography, continence tests, electromyography of the anal sphincters and the pelvic floor, and nerve stimulation tests. Moreover, combining proctography with simultaneous pressure recordings and electromyographic measurements permits these investigations to present a more dynamic and physiologic account of the state of the anorectal region. Modern imaging techniques furnish a clearer picture of the mechanisms of anal continence and defecation and demonstrate pathophysiologic abnormalities in patients with disorders of continence and defecation.

ANAL CONTINENCE

It is difficult to give a clear definition of anal continence. Complete control or complete lack of control is easy to define; however, while varying degrees of lack of control of flatus and fecal soiling may seem like major disabilities to some patients, other less fastidious individuals may be unconcerned by them. Maintaining anal continence is a complex matter because it is controlled by local reflex mechanisms as well as by conscious will. Normal continence depends on a highly integrated series of complicated events. Stool volume and consistency are important because patients who have weakened mechanisms may be continent for a firm stool but incontinent for liquid feces. Also significant is the rate of delivery of feces into the rectum, which emphasizes the reservoir function of the rectum. Other important factors include the sphincteric component, sensory receptors, mechanical factors, and the corpus cavernosum of the anus (Box 1).

BOX 1 ■ Mechanisms of Anal Continence

- Stool volume and consistency
- Reservoir function
- Sphincteric factors
  - Internal sphincter
  - External sphincter
- Sensory components
  - Rectal sensory perception
  - Anal sensory perception
  - Neuropathways
  - Reflexes
- Mechanical factors
  - Angulation between rectum and anal canal
  - Flutter valve
  - Flap valve
- Corpus cavernosum of anus

Mechanisms of Continence

Stool Volume and Consistency

Stool weight and volume vary from individual to individual, from one time to another in a given individual, and from one geographic region to another. The frequency of passing stool may play some role in continence in that colonic transit time is rapid when the large bowel content is liquid because the left colon does not store fluid well. Stool consistency probably is the most important physical characteristic influencing anal continence (98). The ability to maintain normal control may depend on whether the rectal contents are solid, liquid, or gas. Some patients may be continent for solid stool but not for liquid or gas, or continent for stool but not for gas. This fact is important in the management of patients with anal incontinence because the maneuver of changing stool consistency from liquid into solid may be enough to allow the patient to recapture fecal control.

Reservoir Function of Rectum

The distal part of the large intestine has a reservoir function that is important in the maintenance of anal continence and depends on several factors. First, the lateral angulations of the sigmoid colon and the valves of Houston provide a mechanical barrier and retard progression of stool (99). The weight of the stool tends to accentuate these angles and enhances their barrier effect (Fig. 8) (100).

It has been suggested that a pressure barrier exists at the junction of the rectum and sigmoid colon (a concept referred to as O'Beirne's sphincter); however, evidence for such a pressure barrier is lacking. It also has been proposed

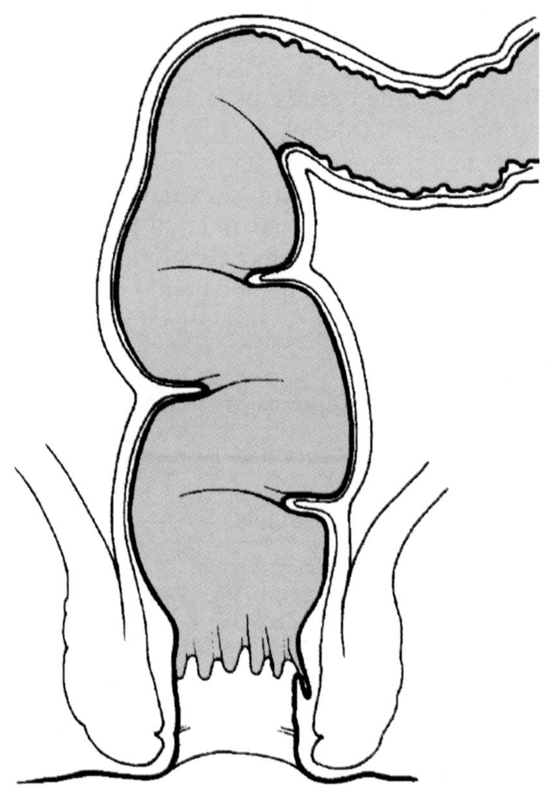

FIGURE 8 ■ Mechanical reservoir function.

that differences in motor activity and myoelectrical activity between the rectum and the sigmoid colon provide a barrier that resists caudad progression of stool (59). Motor activity is more frequent and contractile waves are of higher amplitude in the rectum than in the sigmoid colon. This mechanism may account for the cephalad movement of retention enemas or suppositories (100). A more recent study, however, has disputed the pathophysiologic significance of this phenomenon (58).

The adaptive compliance of the rectum along with rectal capacity and distensibility also are important factors for effective reservoir function. Differences in pressure patterns between the distal and proximal levels of the anal canal result in the development of a force vector in the direction of the rectum. This continuous differential activity may be important in controlling the retention of small amounts of liquid matter and flatus in the rectum. Furthermore, the angulation between the rectum and anal canal, which is due to the continuous tonic activity of the puborectalis muscle, as well as the high-pressure zone in the anal canal contribute to the reservoir function of the rectum.

Sphincteric Factors

Activity of the anal sphincters is generally believed to be the most important factor in maintaining anal continence. Within the anal canal, the sphincters are responsible for the high-pressure zone. The maximum anal resting pressure varies between 40 and 80 mmHg (101) and appears to provide a barrier against intrarectal pressure. The high-pressure zone, as demonstrated by pull-through recordings, has an average length of 3.5 cm (102–104) and results mainly from the continuous tonic activity of both sphincters. Variation in sphincter length at rest has been 3.5, 3.0, and 2.8 cm, and with squeeze 4.2, 3.7, and 3.8 cm for males, parous, and nulliparous females, respectively (105).

INTERNAL SPHINCTER ■ The major contribution to the high-pressure zone comes from the internal anal sphincter, estimated to account for 52–85% of the pressure recorded (Table 3). In a detailed study of factors that contribute to anal basal pressure, Lestar et al. (109) concluded that when a 0.3 cm diameter probe was used, 30% of the maximum anal basal pressure is made up by striated sphincter tonic activity, 45% by nerve-induced internal sphincter activity, 10% by purely myogenic internal sphincter activity, and 15% to the expansion of the hemorrhoidal plexus. The overlapping of the sphincters has generated controversy regarding the relative importance of the internal and external sphincters in maintaining anal continence. However, when the external sphincter is paralyzed, the pressure is not significantly changed, so that the resting pressure would seem to be due largely to the internal sphincter (106). Normally the internal sphincter is in a continual state of tonic contraction, only relaxing in response to rectal distention. The basal tone of the internal sphincter is controlled by both intrinsic and extrinsic neuronal systems and probably is also myogenic in origin. Frenckner and Ihre (110) believed that internal sphincter tone was controlled only by sympathetic (i.e., hypogastric) pathways, but Meunier and Mollard (111) have shown that the sacral parasympathetic pathways also are involved and clinical evidence supports their findings (112).

TABLE 3 ■ **Contribution of Internal Anal Sphincter (IAS) to High-Pressure Zone**

Author(s)	Recording Device	Contribution of IAS (%)
Duthie and Watts (106) (1965)	Balloon catheter	60
	Perfused catheter	68
Frenckner and Euler (107) (1975)	Balloon catheter	85
Schweiger (108) (1982)	Balloon catheter	74
Lestar et al. (109) (1989)	Balloon catheter	55
Cali et al. (105) (1992)	Perfused catheter	
	Males	52
	Females, parous	59
	Females, nulliparous	65

EXTERNAL SPHINCTER ■ Continuous tonic activity at rest and even during sleep has been recorded in the pelvic floor muscles and in the external sphincter (113). The external sphincter is unique in this regard because other striated muscles are electrically silent at rest. Although activity is always present in the external sphincter, its basal tone shows considerable variations, determined by postural changes. For example, external sphincter activity will increase when an individual is in an upright position. The activity also is augmented by perianal stimulation (anal reflex) and by increases in intra-abdominal pressure, such as coughing, sneezing, and the Valsalva maneuver. Rectal distention with initial small volumes also will result in increased activity. The permanent activity of the external sphincter is modulated by the second sacral spinal segment (114). In patients with tabes dorsalis, the external sphincter shows no activity at all because this spinal reflex pathway is disturbed as a result of degeneration of the posterior root. The same phenomenon has been demonstrated in patients with cauda equina lesions. Although the external sphincter will be completely paralyzed following transection of the spinal cord, the tonic activity of the sphincter will return after a period of spinal shock in cases where transection has occurred above the second sacral spinal segment. The external sphincter is unique in that it does not degenerate even when separated from its nerve supply. Although activity always is present in the external sphincter and the pelvic floor muscles, these muscles can be contracted voluntarily for only 40–60 second periods; then both electrical activity and pressure within the anal canal return to basal levels (115).

In contrast to other skeletal muscles, the fiber distribution in the external sphincter is the result of a developmental process (116). The predominance of type II (twitching) fibers explains the state of reflex continence of the young infant. With increasing maturation of tonic type I fibers, an additional voluntary component to continence is made possible with the help of the supporting pelvic musculature. This maturation is determined by the increasing strain on the pelvic floor as the child learns to sit and walk. With increasing age, the number of type II fibers again increases, so that at the age of approximately 75 the reflex component of continence again becomes important.

Rectal Sensory Perception

The conscious sensation of urgency is mediated by extrinsic afferent neurons. These neurons are activated by mechanoreceptors. Although it has been suggested that these receptors are located in the pelvic floor (117), there is growing evidence that the rectal wall itself contains many mechanoreceptors. According to Rühl et al. the sacral dorsal roots contain afferents from low-threshold mechanoreceptors located in the rectal wall. These afferents monitor the filling state and contraction level of the rectum (118). These receptors are very rare or absent more proximally in the colon (119). They do not act simply as tension and stretch receptors. They also detect mechanical deformation, such as flattening of myenteric ganglia. Furthermore, they are able to encode the contractile activity of smooth muscle cells. Activation of the rectal mechanoreceptors induces extrinsic and intrinsic reflexes that play a key role in defecation. Some authors distinguish the superficial mucosal mechanoreceptors from the deeper muscular and serosal receptors. It has been suggested that the superficial mechanoreceptors are connected with sacral afferents, which can be stimulated by slow-ramp rectal distensions and that the deeper mechanoreceptors are connected with splanchnic afferents, which can be stimulated by rapid phasic distensions (120). Several lines of evidence support this hypothesis. Topical application of lidocaine decreases the sensation elicited by slow-ramp distension, but has no effect on the sensation elicited by rapid phasic distension. In patients with irritable bowel syndrome abnormal sensory responses have been demonstrated during rapid phasic distension but not during slow-ramp distension. Patients with a complete lesion of the lower spinal cord do not perceive slow-ramp distensions, although they still perceive phasic stimuli (121). Several workers have tried to modulate rectal sensory perception. The 5-HT_1 receptor agonist sumatriptan causes a relaxation of the descending colon, thereby allowing higher volumes to be accommodated before thresholds for perception and discomfort are reached. In contrast to this effect on the descending colon sumatriptan has no influence on distension evoked rectal perception. This finding may reflect a difference in 5-HT_1 receptor location between descending colon and rectum (122). The 5-HT_4 receptor agonist serotonin seems to be a better candidate for the modulation of rectal sensitivity (123). It has been shown that neurotensin also has an effect on perception by intensifying rectal sensation (124). Chenodeoxycholic acid in physiological concentrations reduces sensory thresholds to rectal distension. It is not clear whether this effect is due to chemoreceptor activation or to chemical-induced alterations in tone or compliance (125). Recently it has been shown that the cortical representation of rectal distension differs between males and females. Kern at al. studied 13 male and 15 female volunteers with functional magnetic resonance imaging during barostat controlled rectal distension. The volume of cortical activity during rectal distension was significantly higher in women. They also observed that intensity and volume of cortical activity were directly related to the strength of the stimulus and that rectal distension below perception level still results in cortical activity (126). Most frequently rectal sensory perception is assessed by distension of an intrarectal balloon, either with air or with water. During this procedure the subject is asked to indicate the onset of awareness of distension, the first urge to defecate and finally the maximum tolerable volume, which is characterized by an irresistible and painful urgency. It has been reported that the volumes registered for each sensation do not differ between men and women, irrespective of their age (127). Sloots et al. investigated rectal sensory perception by pressure controlled distension with a barostat assembly. Although males had larger volumes at the same pressures than females, the sensory perception was found to be equal (128). It should be taken into account that the intensity of perceived sensation depends on the distension rate. The distension stimulus is poorly defined when an air-filled or water-filled latex balloon because with increasing distension, varying degrees of balloon elongation occur, depending on the compliance of the rectal wall. For the assessment of rectal sensory perception the use of an electromechanical barostat assembly is more accurate. It enables the measurement of rectal compliance by recording the change in rectal volume per unit change in pressure. It is also important to perform the isobaric distensions in random order and to use a visual analogue scale in order to record the intensity of the perceived sensation in a more objective manner. Reduced rectal sensory perception, diagnosed on the basis of elevated sensory threshold volumes, is not necessarily the result of impaired afferent nerve function alone. In the case of increased rectal compliance greater distension volumes are required to elicit rectal sensations. Rectal hyposensitivity in patients with normal rectal compliance reflects impairment of afferent nerve function, whereas this finding in patients with an increased compliance might be due to other factors such as abnormal rectal wall properties (129). Reduced rectal sensitivity has been demonstrated in patients with slow transit constipation (130). Rectal afferent fibers travel with the parasympathetic nerves to the dorsal roots of S2, S3 and S4. The parasympathetic pelvic nerves might be injured during pelvic surgery such as rectopexy, when afferent fibres in the lateral ligaments may be divided and hysterectomy, when division of the uterine supporting ligamenst may result in nerve injury (131). Gosselink et al. assessed rectal compliance and rectal sensory perception in female patients with obstructed defecation, utilizing a barostat assembly. Most of their patients had a normal colonic transit time. About half of their patients reported onset of symptoms following pelvic surgery, such as hysterectomy and rectopexy. Rectal compliance was found to be normal, whereas rectal sensory perception was blunted or absent in the majority of their patients. Both findings indicate that impairment of afferent nerve function contributes to obstructed defecation (132,133).

Anal Sensory Perception

A more precise perception of the nature of the rectal content is achieved by sensory receptors within the anal canal. Careful histologic studies have demonstrated an abundance of free and organized nerve endings in the epithelium of the anal canal (134). Several types of sensory receptors have been identified: nerve endings that denote pain (free intraepithelial), touch (Meissner's corpuscles), cold (bulbs of Krause), pressure or tension (Pacini corpuscles and Golgi-Mazzoni corpuscles), and friction (genital corpuscles) (134). These nerve endings are located primarily in the distal half of the anal canal but may extend for

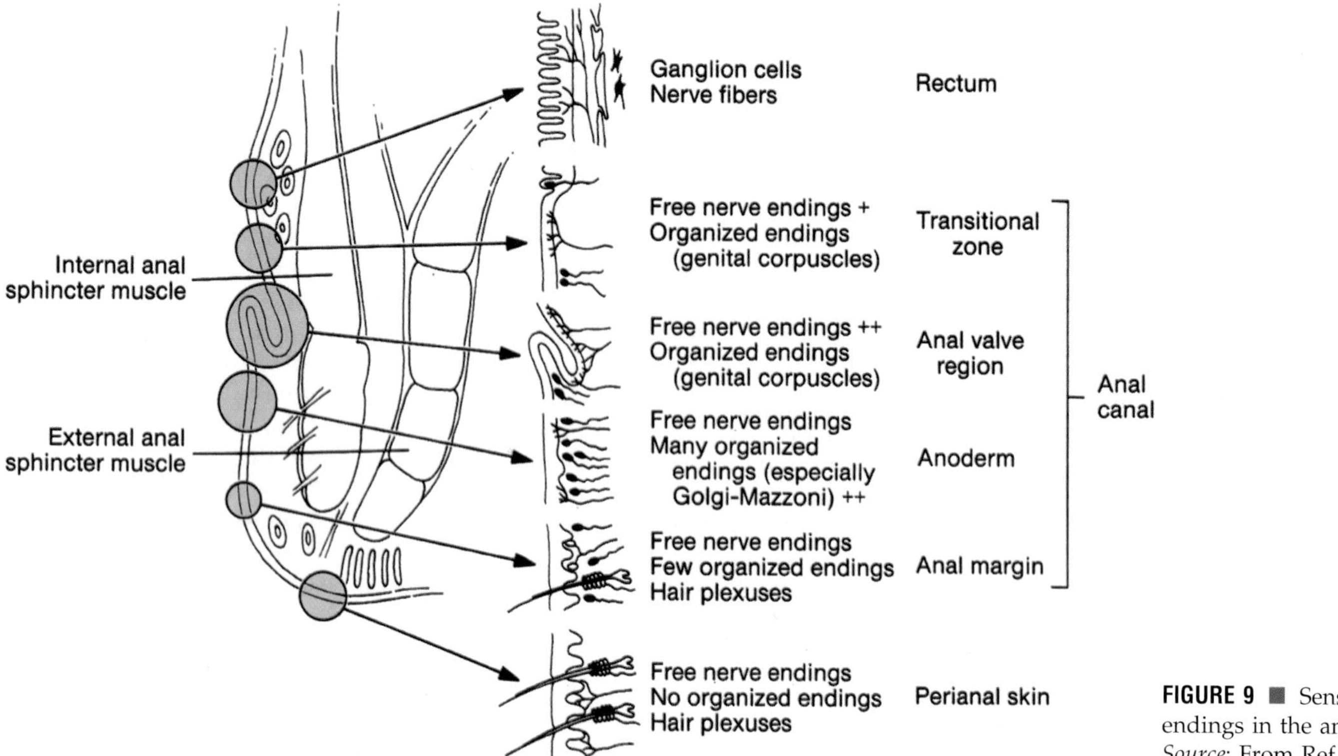

FIGURE 9 ■ Sensory nerve endings in the anal canal. *Source*: From Ref. 134.

5–15 mm above the dentate line (Fig. 9). Pain can be felt as far as 1–1.5 cm above the anal valves; this corresponds with clinical experience, such as the application of rubber band ligation of hemorrhoids. The rectum is insensitive to stimuli other than stretch.

Whether or not this sensory zone is important for anal continence remains controversial. In a study in which a saline continence test was used, no effect could be demonstrated when the anal canal was anesthetized with lidocaine, leading the authors to conclude that anal canal sensation does not play a crucial role in continence (135). However, in a more recent study in which a technique to assess anorectal temperature sensation was used, it has been shown that very small changes in temperature can be detected in the anal canal. The lower and middle parts of the canal were found to be much more sensitive to temperature changes than was the upper part (136). This finding supports the concept of the sampling response and reinforces the role of this sensory zone of the anal canal in maintaining continence.

Neuropathways

The internal sphincter is supplied by a dual extrinsic innervation containing a motor supply from the sympathetic outflow via the hypogastric nerve and an inhibitory supply from the parasympathetic outflow.

The sympathetic pathway to the internal sphincter emerges from the fifth lumbar spinal segment. The preganglionic sympathetic neurons are cholinergic and form synapses on the cell bodies of postganglionic neurons in prevertebral ganglia. The noradrenergic axons of these postganglionic sympathetic neurons run through the hypogastric (presacral) plexus and continue through the pelvic plexuses. The sympathetic nerves have a direct effect on the internal sphincter muscle cells, which possess α- and β-adrenoreceptors (Fig. 10).

The internal sphincter also is supplied by preganglionic parasympathetic fibers that emerge from the second, third, and fourth sacral spinal segments. The cholinergic axons of these preganglionic parasympathetic neurons form synapses on the cell bodies of postganglionic parasympathetic neurons located within the anorectal wall, proximal to the aganglionic sphincteric area. The axons of these neurons run downward to reach the internal sphincter (Fig. 10). In nonsphincteric areas, the sympathetic nerves are inhibitory and the parasympathetic nerves are excitatory to the gastrointestinal smooth muscle cells. It has been proposed that the opposite occurs with the internal sphincter. However, two studies in which electrical stimulation of the hypogastric (presacral) nerves was performed found contradictory results. Lubowski et al. (137) stimulated the presacral plexus in eight patients during abdominal proctopexy or restorative proctocolectomy and found relaxation of the internal sphincter. In contrast, Carlstedt et al. (138) stimulated the presacral hypogastric nerves in patients undergoing operation for rectal carcinoma and elicited a contraction in 13 of 15 patients. In the same study, stimulation of the lumbar nerves elicited clear-cut contraction of the internal anal sphincter, whereas rectal motor response was observed only occasionally. Epidural anesthesia caused a reduction in anal pressure and an increase in rectal tone. Frenckner and Ihre (110) have demonstrated that the internal sphincter retains about 50% of its normal basal tone, even after sympathetic nerve activity is abolished by high spinal anesthesia. The presence of two types of adrenoreceptors on the surface of internal sphincter muscle cells might well explain these conflicting results. Based on data obtained from in vitro studies in experimental animals and one in vivo study in human subjects, it has been suggested that the sympathetic nervous system has a dual influence on internal sphincter activity. These studies show that the

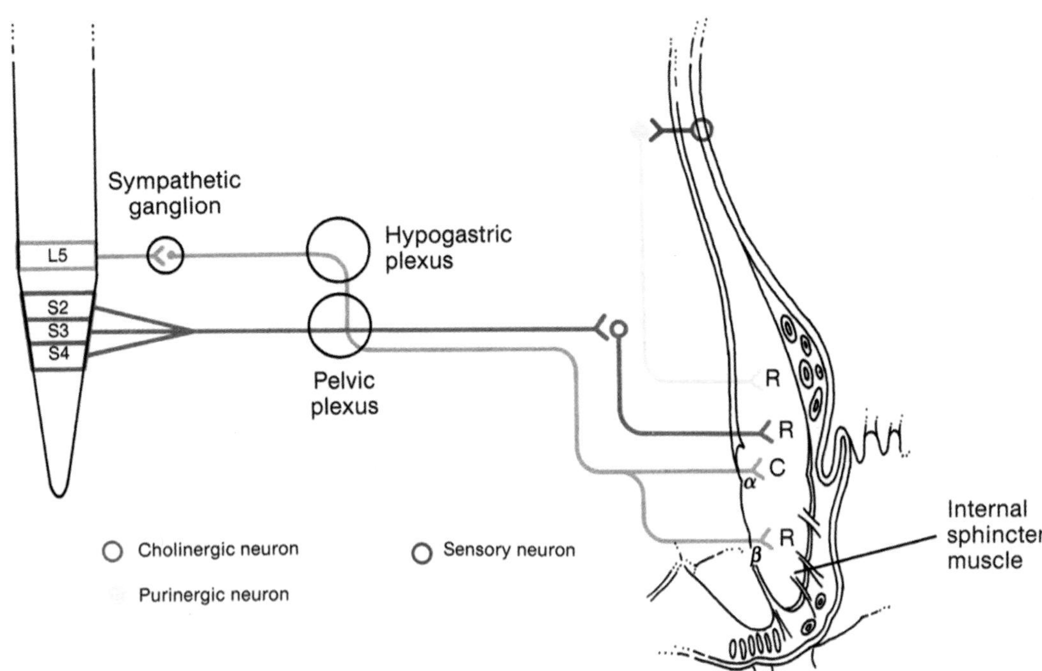

FIGURE 10 ■ Internal sphincter innervation showing muscle in state of relaxation (*R*) or contraction (*C*).

α-adrenoreceptors mediate contractions, whereas the β-adrenoreceptors mediate relaxation (139).

It has been suggested that there is a dominant population of excitatory α-adrenoreceptors on the smooth muscle fibers of the internal sphincter, which might explain the overall excitatory effect of the sympathetic nervous system. Investigation of the effect of acetylcholine has shown that this parasympathetic neurotransmitter has a predominantly inhibitory effect (139–141).

The effects of adrenergic and cholinergic agonists and antagonists on internal sphincter activity, as represented by changes in maximal anal resting pressure, illustrate the complex extrinsic innervation of the internal sphincter (Table 4).

Gunterberg et al. (112) reported that anorectal function was seriously impaired in patients following major sacral resections that resulted in bilateral loss of sacral nerves. Preservation of the first and second sacral nerves bilaterally was not sufficient to permit discrimination of different qualities of rectal content passing the anal canal. The sensation of rectal distention also was impaired. The reflex pattern of the internal sphincter was intact. The external sphincter displayed a weak spontaneous myoelectrical activity in patients who had at least one intact second sacral nerve. However, the normal transient increase of myoelectrical discharge from the external anal sphincter in response to rectal distention could not be elicited. In patients with unilateral loss of the sacral nerves, no significant impairment of anorectal function was noted. Total one-sided denervation implied deficient sensibility of the anal canal unilaterally but no disturbance of sphincter function, as judged from the reflex response of the internal and external sphincters to rectal distention.

TABLE 4 ■ **Effects of Adrenergic and Cholinergic Agonists and Antagonists on Human Internal Sphincter in Vivo**

Pharmacologic Agent	Maximal Anal Resting Pressure
Methoxamine (α_1-receptor agonist)	Increase
Phentolamine (α_1- and α_2-receptor antagonist)	Decrease (50%)
Isoproterenol (β_1- and β_2-receptor agonist)	Decrease
Bethanechol (cholinergic agonist)	Decrease
Atropine (cholinergic antagonist)	Increase

Source: From Ref. 139.

Localio et al. (142) reviewed their experience in the treatment of sacral chordoma and reported that resection of the sacrum, preserving S3 bilaterally, was associated with normal continence. At the S2 level, continence was preserved but voluntary function was less than perfect. There was no fecal soiling, but enemas were necessary every one to two days.

Reflexes

The classic anal reflex is elicited by pricking the perianal skin; the response is contraction of the external sphincter as evidenced by skin dimpling. The reflex has its afferent and efferent pathway in the pudendal nerve and uses sacral segments S1–S4. The reflex responses of both sphincters are essential for the maintenance of anal continence. Rectal distention results in transient relaxation of the internal sphincter and simultaneous contraction of the external sphincter (Fig. 11).

The reflex response of the external sphincter represented by a transient increase in activity can be initiated by a number of stimuli, such as postural changes, perianal scratch, and increased intra-abdominal pressure. The reflex response of the internal sphincter, which consists of transient relaxation, can be stimulated by rectal distention or the Valsalva maneuver. Although this reflex occurs almost immediately after material enters the rectum, peristalsis is not involved because the sphincter relaxes at the moment of rectal distention before the peristaltic wave of contraction reaches the sphincter (143). The transient relaxation

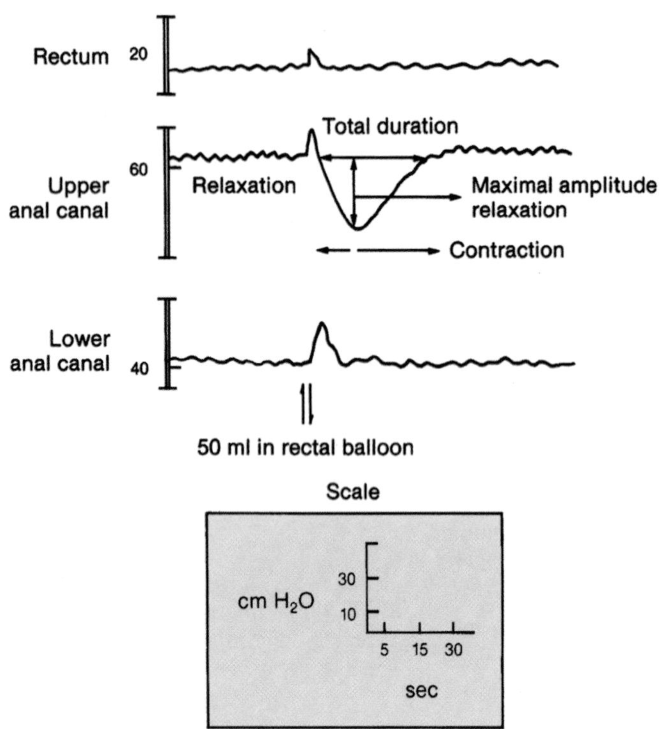

FIGURE 11 ■ Anorectal reflex.

of the internal sphincter allows the rectal contents to come into contact with the sensory epithelium of the anal canal to assess whether the contents are solid, liquid, or gas. During this sampling response, continence will be maintained by synchronous contraction of the external sphincter, which allows time for impulses to reach conscious awareness; thus having determined the nature of the material, the individual can decide what to do about it and then take appropriate action. Voluntary contraction of the external sphincter can extend the period of continence and allow time for compliance mechanisms within the colon to provide for adjustment to increased intrarectal volumes. As the colon accommodates to its new volume, stretch receptors are no longer activated, and afferent stimuli and the sensation of urgency disappear. Further rectal distention leads to inhibition of the external sphincter. Recognizing the nature of the rectal contents is not only a conscious process but also a subconscious one, since flatus can be passed safely during sleep. Conscious sampling is done by slightly increasing intra-abdominal pressure and maintaining, by voluntary control, an increase in the activity of the external anal sphincter. In this way solids can be retained while gas can be passed, thereby relieving the intrarectal pressure.

The inhibition induced by rectal distention was thought to be under parasympathetic control via the sacral nerves. However, evidence now suggests that the reflex is predominantly an intramural one (109), although subject to some sacral control. It is not necessarily abolished by spinal anesthesia, and it disappears in experimental animals after the rectal application of cocaine and after transection of the lower rectum (110). Internal sphincter relaxation is modulated by the spinal cord, since no reflex is found in spinal shock and there is no relationship between the degree of distention and the amplitude of relaxation in patients with meningocele (111). The internal sphincter reflex is a neurogenic response, initiated by sensory neurons located in the rectal wall. The cell bodies of these inhibitory neurons are located in the myenteric plexus, and their axons run downward to the aganglionic part of the internal sphincter where they supply the smooth muscle cells (Fig. 10). These inhibitory nerves are noncholinergic and nonadrenergic. Nitric oxide has been identified as the chemical messenger of the intrinsic, nonadrenergic, and noncholinergic pathway mediating relaxation of the internal anal sphincter (144–147). It has been shown that the axons of nitric oxide-producing nerve cell bodies, located in the distal part of the rectum, descend into the anal canal where they ramify into and throughout the internal anal sphincter (148). Without these inhibitory neurons the reflex response of the internal sphincter on rectal distention is impossible, as shown in patients with congenital and acquired aganglionosis. In patients with an anastomosis between the site of distention and the sphincters, the internal sphincter reflex also is abolished. In one study the internal sphincter reflex could be demonstrated despite such an anastomosis, probably because of regeneration of descending axons of the inhibitory neurons across the anastomosis. It is likely that external sphincter reflexes are initiated by receptors in the levator muscles rather than in the gut. For good functional results, the anatomic relationships must not be distorted by pelvic sepsis.

Ferrara et al. (149) studied the relationship between anal canal tone and rectal motor activity. They noted that rectal motor complexes were invariably accompanied by a rise in mean anal canal pressure and contractile activity such that pressure in the anal canal was always greater than pressure in the rectum. Anal canal relaxation never occurred during a rectal motor complex. The onset of rectal contractions was accompanied by increased resting pressure and contractile activity of the anal canal. They concluded that this temporal relationship represents an important mechanism preserving fecal continence.

Mechanical Factors

ANGULATION BETWEEN RECTUM AND ANAL CANAL ■ Without doubt, the most important component for the conservation of gross fecal continence is the angulation of the anorectal system, which is due to the continuous tonic activity of the puborectalis muscle.

As measured by defecography, the angle between the axis of the anal canal and the rectum in the resting state is about 90°. Radiographic studies have elucidated changes in this angle during defecation (Fig. 12).

FLUTTER VALVE ■ It has been suggested that additional protection of continence might be afforded by intra-abdominal pressure being transmitted laterally to the side of the anal canal just at the level of the anorectal junction. The anal canal is an anteroposterior slit-like aperture, and any increased intra-abdominal pressure tends to compress it in a fashion similar to a flutter valve. This flutter valve mechanism is controversial because the highest pressure is found in the middle part of the anal canal rather than in the upper part, and therefore intra-abdominal forces would need to act at an infralevator level (Fig. 13) (150).

FLAP VALVE THEORY ■ According to the flap valve theory advanced by Parks et al. (151), any increase in

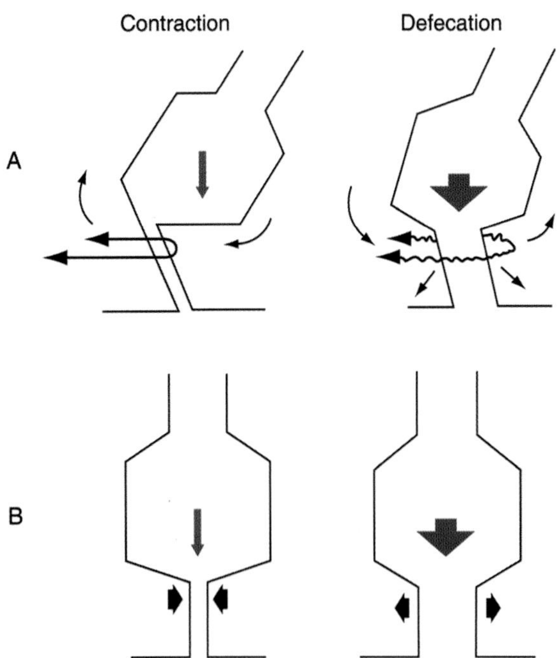

FIGURE 12 ■ Angulation between the rectum and the anal canal. (A) Lateral view. (B) Anteroposterior view.

intra-abdominal pressure (weight lifting, straining, laughing, coughing) tends to accentuate the anorectal angle and force the anterior rectal wall to lie firmly over the upper end of the anal canal, which produces an occlusion or a flap valve effect. For defecation to occur the flap valve must be broken. This breakage takes place by lengthening the puborectalis, lowering the pelvic floor, and obliterating the angle (Fig. 14).

The importance of the flap valve mechanism has been questioned. It was pointed out that a valve operates only if it separates compartments of different pressures. Thus, if a flap valve is responsible for preservation of anal continence during increases in intra-abdominal pressure, the anal pressure should be lower than intra-abdominal pressure. A study that measured anal and rectal pressures during serial increases in intra-abdominal pressure found that anal pressure always remained higher than intrarectal pressure, and this pressure gradient was the reverse of what would be found if a flap valve maintained continence. Based on this finding, it was concluded that anal continence is maintained by reflex contraction of the external sphincter rather than by a flap valve mechanism (152).

In another study anal and rectal pressures were measured simultaneously with external sphincter and

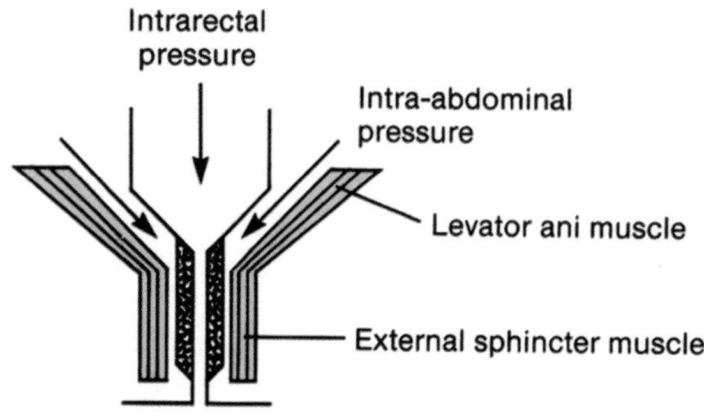

FIGURE 13 ■ Flutter valve mechanism.

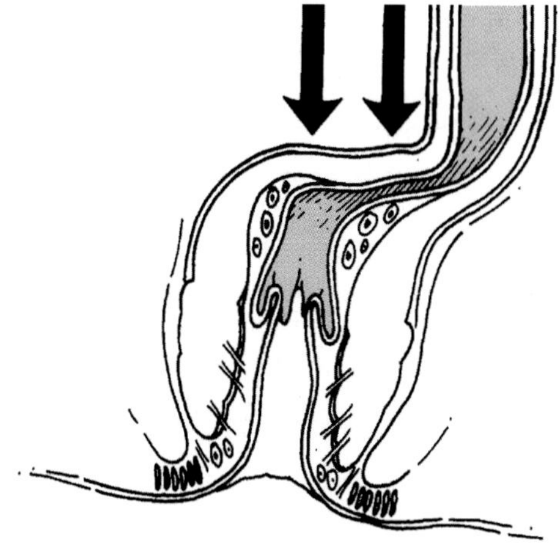

FIGURE 14 ■ Flap valve mechanism.

puborectalis electromyography and synchronously superimposed on an image intensifier displaying the rectum outlined by barium. The anterior rectal wall always was clearly separated from the upper part of the anal canal despite maximal effort to raise intra-abdominal pressure (153). The results of this dynamic study also called into question the flap valve theory because during Valsalva maneuvers (while the rectum was filled with liquid contrast material) continence was maintained by sphincteric activity with no evidence of a valve. The authors of this study commented that normal defecation would require the anterior rectal wall to be lifted away from the upper part of the anal canal. Therefore, they consider a valvular occlusion to be more likely to lead to obstructed defecation (153). Nevertheless, clinical experience with the postanal repair suggests that this mechanism indeed may play some role in continence. However, the modest success this surgical procedure enjoys may be the result of elevated intra-anal pressures.

Corpus Cavernosum of Anus

Stelzner (154) postulated that the vascular architecture in the submucosal and subcutaneous tissues of the anal canal really represents what he called a corpus cavernosum of the rectum. These cushions consist of discrete masses of blood vessels, smooth muscle fibers, and elastic and connective tissue. They have a remarkably constant configuration and are located in the left lateral, right anterolateral, and right posterolateral segments of the anal canal. These vascular cushions have the physiologic ability to expand and contract and to take up "slack," and hence they contribute to the finest degree of anal continence. This theory might be supported by the fact that certain patients who have undergone a formal hemorrhoidectomy have minor alterations in continence, a situation that may be the result of excision of this corpus cavernosum.

■ DEFECATION

Usual Sequence of Events

The stimulus for initiating defecation is distention of the rectum. This in turn may be related to a critical threshold of sigmoid and possibly descending colon distention. As long as fecal matter is retained in the descending and sigmoid colon, the rectum remains empty and the individual feels no urge to defecate. This reservoir type of continence does not depend on sphincter function. Distention of the left colon initiates peristaltic waves, which propel the fecal mass downward into the rectum.

Normally this process occurs once or several times a day. The timing of the act is a balance between environmental factors, since the urge may be suppressed by a complex cortical inhibition of the basic reflexes of the anorectum. Many people establish a pattern whereby the urge is felt either on arising in the morning, in the evening, or after ingestion of food or drink. This balance can be altered by travel, by admission to a hospital, or by changes in diet.

Rectal distention induces relaxation of the internal sphincter, which in turn triggers contraction of the external sphincter. Thus sphincter continence is induced. If the individual decides to accede to the urge, a squatting position is assumed. This causes the angulation between the rectum and the anal canal to straighten. A Valsalva maneuver is the second semivoluntary stage. This overcomes the resistance to the external sphincter by voluntarily increasing the intrathoracic and intra-abdominal pressure. The pelvic floor descends, and the resulting pressure on the fecal mass in the rectum increases intrarectal pressure. Inhibition of the external sphincter permits passage of the fecal bolus. Once evacuation has been completed, the pelvic floor and the anal canal muscles regain their resting activity, and the anal canal is closed.

Responses to Entry of Material into the Rectum

Duthie (155) conducted extensive studies on the dynamics of the rectum and anus and concluded that most dynamic changes in the anorectum are in response to two stresses: (1) the change in intra-abdominal pressure, and (2) entry of material from the colon into the rectum. There is considerable variation in the rate and timing of the entry of feces and flatus into the rectum in different individuals. Colonic transit is accelerated by engaging in physical activity and by eating meals. Local reflexes may be inhibited by cortical inhibition, which is a feature of social training. Afferent nerve impulses, which signal the entry of material into the rectum, proceed at a subconscious level, with the accommodation and sampling responses taking place reflexly. In support of this contention, clinical findings show that patients admitted for routine clinical examination of the rectum often have, unknown to them, a considerable amount of feces in the rectum.

Accommodation Response

The accommodation response is said to consist of receptive relaxation of the rectal ampulla to accommodate the fecal mass. Studies with a rectal balloon show that after inflation of the balloon to approximately 10 mL, the external anal sphincter shows a transient increase in electromyographic activity, while in the internal sphincter a similar short-lived reduction in its pressure activity can be measured within the lumen. With persistent inflation of the balloon, an increase in pressure within the rectal ampulla is maintained for 1–2 minutes and then decreases to preinflation level (Fig. 15). This is the accommodation response. With increasing volume, there is a gradual stepwise increase in rectal pressure, and depending on the age of the patient, an urge to defecate is experienced. This urge abates in a few seconds as the rectum accommodates to the stimulus. When volume increases rapidly over a short period, the accommodation response fails, leading to urgent emptying of the rectum.

The afferent nerve endings for the accommodation reflex are in the rectal ampulla and in the levator ani muscle. The nerve center for the spinal part of the reflex is in the lumbosacral cord with higher center control to permit suppression of the urge to defecate.

Sampling Response

The sampling response consists of transient relaxation of the upper part of the internal sphincter, which permits rectal contents to come into contact with the somatic sensory epithelium of the anal canal for assessment of the nature of the contents. Conscious sampling is done by slightly increasing abdominal tension and maintaining, by voluntary control, an increase in the activity of the external sphincter. Thus, solids can be retained while gas can be passed, thereby relieving the intrarectal pressure. If fluid is present in the rectum, contact with the sensory area in the anal canal excites conscious activity of the external sphincter to maintain control until the rectal accommodation response occurs, and so continence is maintained.

Commencement of Defecation

The method of beginning the act of defecation varies from person to person. If one is exerting anal control during an urge, merely relinquishing this voluntary control will allow the reflex to proceed. However, if the urge abates, voluntary straining with increased intra-abdominal pressure is necessary before defecation can begin. Once begun, the act will follow either of two patterns: (1) expulsion of the rectal contents, accompanied by mass peristalsis of the distal colon, which clears the bowel in one continuous movement, or (2) passage of the stool piecemeal with several bouts of straining. The pattern followed is largely determined by the habit of the individual and the consistency of the feces. Using scintigraphic assessment, after oral intake of isotopes, Lubowski at al. (156) demonstrated that normal defecation is not a process of rectal emptying alone but also includes colonic emptying. This process of colorectal emptying has been quantified by Krogh and co-workers. During normal defecation colorectal emptying varied between 60% emptying of the rectosigmoid to complete emptying of the rectosigmoid, descending colon and transverse colon and 19% emptying of the ascending colon. They observed large inter- and intraindividual variations. They also detected retrograde movements, mainly from transverse and descending colon, during normal defecation. It is not known whether these retrograde movements are caused by contractile activity of the colonic wall or by Valsalva manoeuvres supporting the defecation (26). Kamm et al. reported that defecation, evoked by bisacodyl, is preceded by propagating pressure waves arising in the cecum (157). These pressure waves also occur in dogs prior to defecation evoked by guanethidine, neostigmine, glucose and castor oil (158). Bampton et al. performed prolonged multi-point recordings of colonic pressure after nasocolonic intubation of the unprepared colon. They were able to demonstrate a pre-expulsive phase commencing up to one hour before

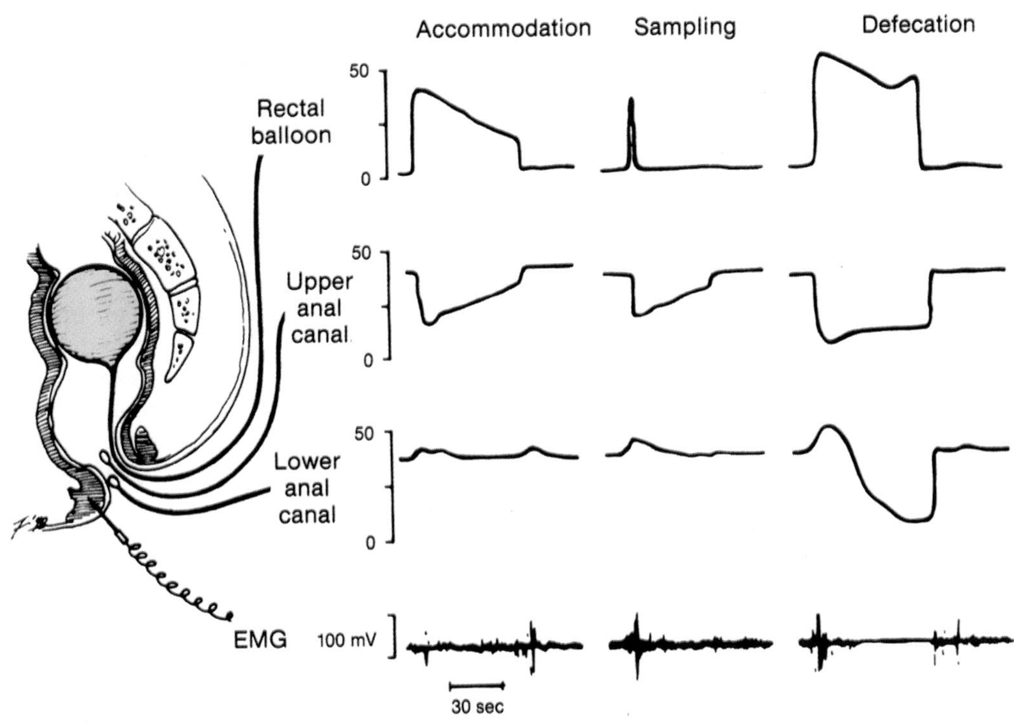

FIGURE 15 ■ Accommodating and sampling response.

stool expulsion. This phase is characterized by a distinctive biphasic spatial and temporal pattern with an early and a late component. The early component is characterized by an array of antegrade propagating sequences. The site of their origin migrates distally with each subsequent sequence. The late component, in the 15 minutes before stool expulsion, is characterized by an array of antegrade propagating sequences. The site of their origin migrates proximally with each subsequent sequence. The amplitude of the pressure waves, occurring in this late phase, increases significantly. Many of them are real high amplitude pressure waves. They are associated with an increasing sensation of urge to defecate. Some of the last propagating sequences, prior to stool expulsion, commence in the ascending colon. This latter finding illustrates that the entire colon is involved in the process of defecation (27). Hagger et al. also detected clusters of high amplitude propagated contractions prior to defecation (159). These contractions were associated with a sensation of an urge to defecate. Similar giant contractions, migrating distally into the rectum, have been observed in mongrel dogs prior to spontaneous defecation (36). These giant contractions could be evoked by electrical stimulation of the sacral nerves. All these findings indicate that high amplitude propagating contractions are necessary for an effective expulsion of stool. Recently it has been shown that patients with obstructed defecation lack the normal predefecatory augmentation in frequency and amplitude of these propagating pressure waves (39).

The high amplitude propagating contractions arise especially after awaking and after a meal. It has been shown that rectal tone increases after a meal (52,160,161). This gastrorectal reflex probably contributes to postprandial defecation. It has been postulated that the increase in rectal tone, as a result of this reflex, results in a greater incremental pressure from the fecal mass on the rectal wall, providing a heightened sensation. This assumption is supported by the observation that distension volumes needed to elicit an urge to defecate are significantly reduced after a meal (162). This suggests that the increased tension in the rectal wall following a meal results in a change in the set point at which the mechanoreceptors are stimulated. Many women with obstructed defecation apply digital pressure upon their perineum in order to facilitate defecation. Recently it has been shown that this manoeuvre results in an increase in rectal tone (163). This observation has been confirmed by others (164). All these findings and data illustrate that the defecatory act is far more complex than previously thought.

The importance of these findings is twofold: (1) proctography is an inadequate method of studying patients with defecation disorders since it examines the rectum in isolation, and (2) disorders of defecation may occur in some patients as a result of a disorder of colonic function rather than a disorder of the rectum or pelvic floor muscles.

Urgent Defecation

If large volumes of fecal material are introduced rapidly into the rectum, the accommodation response may be overcome and cortical inhibition may be unavailing. In this situation the urgency can be controlled for only 40–60 seconds by the voluntary external sphincter complex. This may be enough time to allow for some accommodation; if not, leakage will temporarily relieve the situation.

Pathologic Conditions

During the period of "spinal shock," which supervenes for some weeks immediately after transection of the spinal cord above the origin of the fifth lumbar segment, the rectum and sphincters are completely paralyzed and the patient is incontinent. Frenckner (165) revealed that in these patients there is a cessation of all electrical activity from the striated muscles in response to rectal distention and also a less-pronounced inflation reflex. Thereafter, the tonus of the sphincter returns, and defecation occurs reflexly from the lumbosacral center through pelvic and pudendal nerves.

Because voluntary contraction of the external sphincter is no longer possible and because distention of the rectum is no longer perceived, the patient has no control over the act of defecation. This poses a difficult problem in paraplegic patients, in whom defecation generally must be managed by the regular use of enemas and digital evacuation of the rectum. In some of these patients, the defecation mechanism can be triggered by stimulating the somatic innervation, such as by stroking the thigh or the perianal region.

When the cord lesion involves the cauda equina with destruction of the sacral innervation, the reflexes are abolished, and defecation then becomes automatic (i.e., dependent entirely on intrinsic neural mechanisms). In these circumstances the rectum still responds, although with little force to distention, and the reciprocal relaxation of the already patulous sphincters enables feces to be extruded.

Internal sphincter relaxation can persist with spinal cord transection and occurs if the presacral sympathetic nerves are stimulated. Possibly this mechanism is some form of local muscular reflex (155).

The accumulation of a large fecal mass in a greatly dilated rectum (as occurs especially in the elderly) suggests the abnormal condition known as rectal dyschezia, which results from a loss of tonicity of the rectal musculature. It may be due to a long-standing habit of ignoring or suppressing the urge to defecate or to degeneration of the neural pathways concerned with defecation reflexes. When further complicated by weakness of the abdominal muscles, defecation becomes a chronic problem. In these cases, evacuation may be obtained only by a mechanical washing out of the mass with enemas or by the administration of cathartics that keep the stools semiliquid.

Painful lesions of the anal canal, such as ulcers, fissures, and thrombosed hemorrhoids, impede defecation by exciting a spasm of the sphincters and by causing voluntary suppression to avoid the resulting pain.

A constant urge to defecate in the absence of appreciable content in the rectum may be caused by external compression of the rectum, by intrinsic neoplasms, and particularly by inflammation of the rectal mucosa. This mucosa is normally insensitive to cutting or burning; however, when inflamed it becomes highly sensitive to all stimuli, including those acting on the receptors mediating the stretch reflex.

■ INVESTIGATIVE TECHNIQUES

Techniques have been developed to physiologically assess disorders of function of the anal sphincters, rectum, and pelvic floor. These techniques are used to establish a diagnosis, provide an objective assessment of the function, or identify the anatomic site of a lesion. Sophisticated tests are designed to complement but not to substitute for good clinical examination and sound surgical judgment. Well-established laboratories from around the world have made significant contributions in this area (98,100,155,166). A leader in the field was the late Sir Alan Parks, in whose name a physiology unit was established at St. Mark's Hospital, London.

Manometry

Anorectal manometry is a means of quantifying the function of the internal and external sphincters. A more dynamic and physiologic investigation can be achieved by combining proctography with simultaneous pressure recordings and electromyographic measurements.

There is no standardized method of performing anorectal manometry. Of the many methods available for measuring anorectal pressure, each has its own particular advantages and disadvantages; hence, none has emerged as a gold standard. Until recently, techniques available to perform anorectal manometry have included closed balloon systems and perfused fluid-filled open-tipped catheters. Air-filled balloon systems have a poor frequency response due to the compressibility of air, but one report has suggested that air-filled microballoon manometry gives results similar to those of a water-filled microballoon system (167). Nevertheless, it is more advisable to use a noncompressible medium such as water. However, even water-filled balloon catheters have disadvantages. The relatively large balloons, varying in diameter from 3 to 15 mm, disturb the resting state of the sphincters to some extent; it is a well-known fact that anal pressure rises with an increase in the diameter of the recording device. Another disadvantage of balloon catheters is that reliability depends on the balloon's elasticity; each balloon catheter shows a considerable baseline drift due to a gradual change in its compliance (168).

Perfused open-tipped catheters are smaller than balloon catheters and therefore cause less disturbance of the sphincter muscles. Nevertheless, perfused manometry has been criticized on practical and theoretical grounds because it also has disadvantages. The pressure recorded with a perfused system depends on the compliance of the catheter system and the perfusion rate, as well as on the site and location of the opening (169). In the case of a side opening, the recorded pressure depends on the distance between the opening and the distal end of the tube. Continuous perfusion of water results in leakage from the anal canal with stimulation of the perianal skin, sometimes causing reflex activity of the sphincters. Because the lumen of the anal canal is flattened from side to side rather than circular in cross section, open-tipped tubes are less suitable (170).

Microtransducers are used to overcome the measurement problems and errors associated with perfused open-tipped catheters and closed balloon systems. These modern recording devices, which consist of a miniature pressure sensor located at the tip of the catheter, offer many advantages in anorectal manometry (Fig. 16). The direct connection to a chart recorder obviates the need for fluid-filled tubes, thereby eliminating all the associated artifacts. The small diameter of the catheter minimizes stimulation of the sphincters because it does not distend the anal canal. Most microtransducers have good thermal stability, and therefore the rise in temperature between calibration and actual measurement does not affect the recording. There

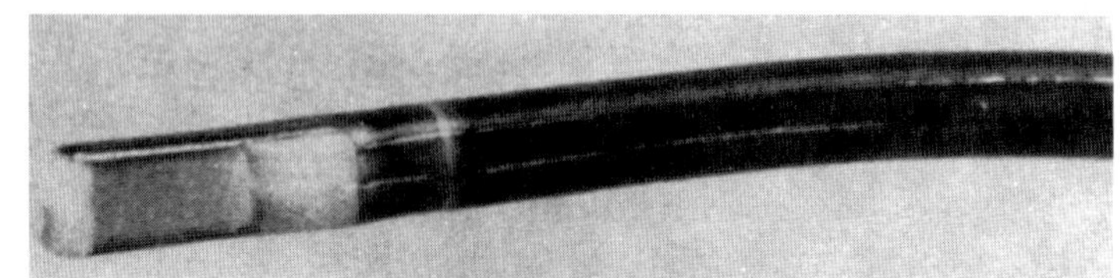

FIGURE 16 ■ Microtransducer catheter. Note the miniature silicone strain gauge located at the tip.

is no problem of perianal skin irritation caused by continuous perfusion and leakage from the anal canal. Furthermore, recordings are not influenced by hydrostatic factors, compliance, or perfusion rate. The high-frequency response of the transducer registers sudden pressure changes. However, the microtransducer-tipped catheters are much more expensive than conventional recording devices.

For the assessment of an anal pressure profile, the recording probe must be withdrawn from the rectum, either stepwise or continuously at a constant rate. Although the step-by-step pull-through technique provides reliable measurements of resting anal canal pressure, the continuous pull-through technique allows a more appropriate assessment of the anal pressure profile and functional sphincter length (104). With the latter technique, the length of the high-pressure zone varies between 2.5 and 5 cm and is shorter in women than in men (103,104,171,172). Most of the difference in functional sphincter length between men and women is attributed to a shorter length of the anterior axis of the anal canal in women (104).

The highest pressure of a pull-through profile is defined as the maximal resting anal pressure (MRAP) (Fig. 17). Normal values of the MRAP are poorly defined because (1) a variety of techniques have been used, (2) "normal" values have been reported only for small control populations, and (3) there is a large range of MRAP in the normal population. McHugh and Diamant (173) have suggested that normal values for MRAP, as determined in 157 healthy subjects, can be constructed only for each sex on a decade basis. Their study revealed that the process of aging in both men and women is associated with a marked decrease in MRAP and that this age-related reduction is more significant in women than in men (172,173).

In another study no change in MRAP could be noted in subjects until the eighth and ninth decade, at which time a sudden decrease occurred (174). However, because a closed balloon system was used, it may have detected only the more marked decrease in MRAP seen in the very aged population. It has been suggested that the age-related reduction in MRAP that occurs in women might be attributed to previous childbearing (175). However, such a relationship has not been demonstrated by other researchers (173). Jameson et al. (172) conducted a study to determine the effects of age, sex, and parity on anorectal function. They found that parity leads only to lower squeeze pressure and does not result in a decrease in anal canal resting pressure.

In yet another study in women, maximum resting anal pressure and maximum squeeze pressure declined with age more rapidly after menopause (176). Closing pressure (i.e., the difference between maximum resting anal pressure and rectal pressure), an important determinant of anal continence, was more markedly reduced with age than was maximum resting anal pressure. Parity and anal pressures were unrelated. Women are more frequently affected by anal incontinence than are men. The more rapid decline of anal pressure after menopause might imply that anal sphincter tissue is a target for estrogen.

Pregnancy itself does not have a significant effect on anal sphincter morphology or function. Sultan et al. (177) conducted manometric and anal endosonographic studies on patients during pregnancy and six weeks after cesarean section and found no differences in pressures or muscle thickness, indicating that any change in sphincter function is caused by mechanical trauma rather than by hormonal factors.

Resting pressure in the anal canal exhibits regular fluctuations that vary from day to night by the presence or absence of fecal material in the rectum and by posture (178). Most of these fluctuations present as slow waves with a frequency between 10 and 20/min and an amplitude varying between 5 and 25 cm H_2O (Fig. 18A). Although these slow waves can be found in all normal subjects, they are not present continuously. Less frequently observed are the ultraslow waves, with an amplitude varying between 30 and 100 cm H_2O and a frequency of <3/min (Fig. 18B). These ultraslow waves seem to be associated with high resting anal pressures (178). Slow and ultraslow waves represent regular fluctuations in internal sphincter activity, as demonstrated by electrical recordings from the internal sphincter (179).

Based on the results of a manometric study with a rigid recording device and a step-by-step pull-through technique, it has been concluded that intra-anal pressure exhibits longitudinal and radial variations (175). In the proximal part of the anal canal, the pressure recorded in the dorsal segment is higher than the pressure in the anterior segment. This finding has been ascribed to the activity of the puborectalis muscle. In the middle anal canal the pressure is equally distributed in all segments, whereas in the lower anal canal the pressure is highest anteriorly (175). However, a more recent study has not been able to demonstrate this radial asymmetry (104). In contrast, significant differences in radial symmetry were found between the two sexes. In

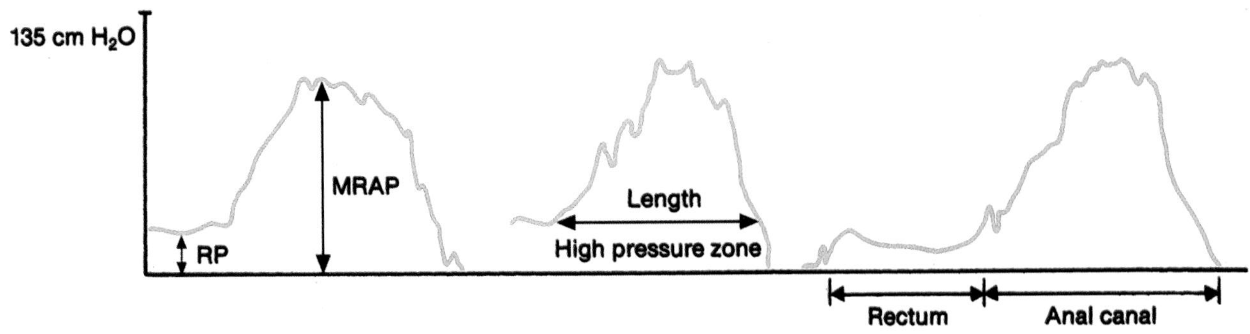

FIGURE 17 ■ Anal pressure profile recorded by the pull-through technique, repeated three times to obtain mean values. Rectal pressure (RP) and maximal resting anal pressure (MRAP) are indicated.

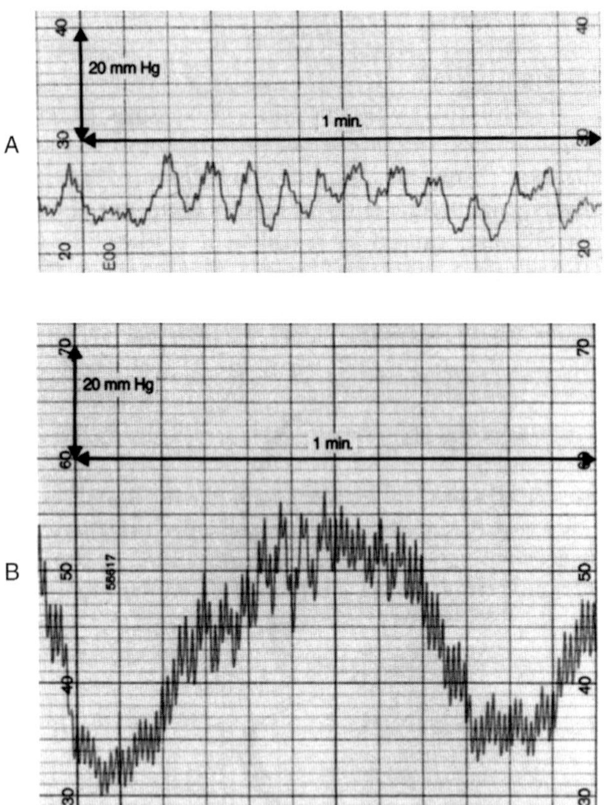

FIGURE 18 ■ Resting pressure variations. (**A**) Slow wave. (**B**) Ultra-slow wave.

women the pressure in the anterior segment of the anal canal was higher distally, while in men the pressure in the anterior and lateral segments was higher proximally (104).

With the aid of a microcomputer and an eight-channel multilumen probe, Coller (171) determined the pressures at each point along the length of the anal canal. The typical resting pressure profile during continuous pullout describes the length and distribution of pressure along the longitudinal axis of the sphincter. The normal MRAP will range from 65 – 85 mmHg above the rectal intraluminal pressure and is located 1–1.5 cm from the distal end of the sphincter. The range of normal sphincter length is 2.5–5 cm. With the same sophisticated equipment, Coller calculated the radial cross-sectional pressure in five segments of the sphincter and found a gradient of pressure that changes from the posterior to lateral to anterior as one proceeds from the proximal end to the distal end.

Williamson et al. (180) reported a comparison of simultaneous longitudinal and radial recordings of anal canal pressures. The catheter they used had the capability of making simultaneous linear longitudinal pressure measurements. An asymmetry of basal, squeeze, and relaxation pressures was found. The highest basal pressures were in the middle of the anal canal, regardless of quadrant orientation. With the radial perfusion catheter, the squeeze pressure profile was consistent with a double-loop external sphincter mechanism. With the linear perfusion catheter, the internal sphincter relaxation pressures showed a greater negative deflection at the proximal portions of the sphincter, which was not achieved at points distally in the same quadrant. This implies that during reflex relaxation pressure is maintained in the distal anal canal; hence patients remain continent during sensory sampling of rectal contents.

Voluntary contraction of the external sphincter gives an increase in anal pressure that is superimposed on the basal tone. This increase in pressure is maximal in the distal part of the anal canal where the bulk of the external sphincter is situated. To determine the functional activity of the different parts of the external sphincter, the recording device has to be withdrawn stepwise. After each step, the patient is asked to squeeze at full strength. In this way, it is possible to measure the maximal squeeze anal pressure (MSAP) at every level of the anal canal (Fig. 19). It has been shown that MSAP is higher in male than in female subjects and is reduced as subjects get older (173,174,181). This age-related reduction of MSAP is most noticeable in women (172,173).

The internal sphincter reflex in response to rectal distention can be elicited by inflation of a rectal balloon. Transient inflation of a balloon with relatively small volumes of air results in an initial rise in pressure, caused by a transient contraction of the external sphincter. Almost immediately after this initial increase in pressure, a transient reduction in anal canal pressure can be observed as a result of relaxation of the internal sphincter (Fig. 20). It has been reported that the transient inflation of a rectal balloon with 30 cc of air results in a pressure reduction of approximately 50% for a mean duration of 19 seconds (182). However, as the balloon is inflated with larger volumes, the amplitude as well as the duration of the relaxation reflex increases. Not only does the relaxation of the internal sphincter result in a pressure reduction, but it also abolishes the pressure fluctuations (slow and ultraslow waves) within the anal canal.

The effect of body position on anal canal pressures was studied by Johnson et al. (183), who used a probe in which were embedded four transducers oriented radially, 90° apart. They concluded that (1) transducer manometry recorded

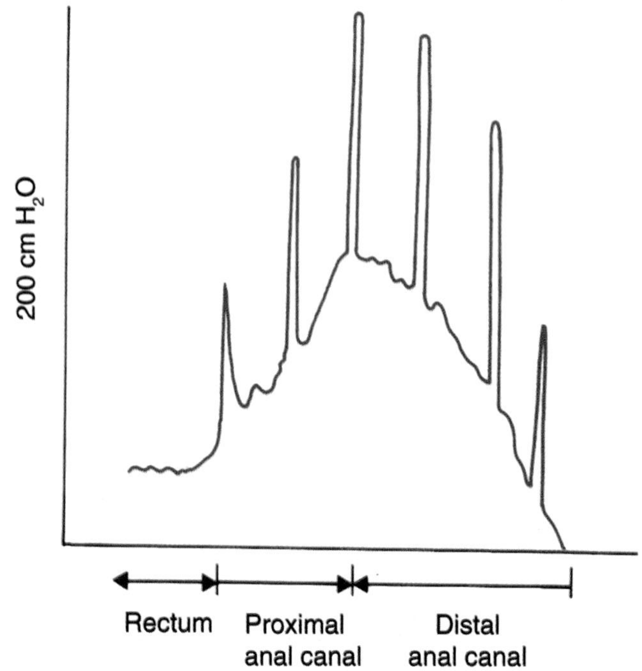

FIGURE 19 ■ Maximal squeeze anal pressure: maximal voluntary contraction of the external sphincter muscle indicated by increase in pressure superimposed on the anal resting pressure.

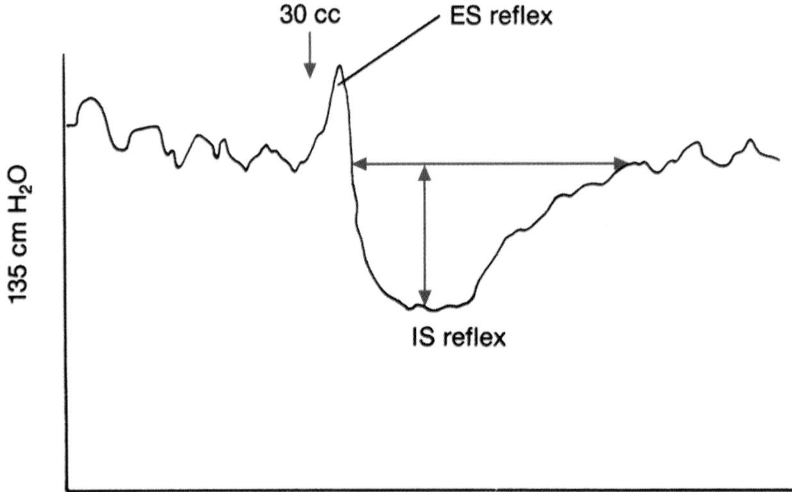

FIGURE 20 ■ ES reflex in response to rectal distension with 30 cc of air followed by IS reflex. *Abbreviations*: ES, external sphincter; IS, internal sphincter.

similar resting pressures but higher squeeze pressures as compared with perfused manometry; (2) transducer manometry recorded the same radial variation in anal canal resting and squeeze pressures as that recorded by the perfused manometer; and (3) standing and sitting caused a fourfold rise in intrarectal pressure, which was associated with a concomitant rise in resting anal canal pressure.

In an effort to correctly interpret manometric results, Cali et al. (105) noted that manometric values for normal patients cover a wide range but categorized definable distinctions among subgroups of patients. They found mean maximal squeeze pressures and length of the anal sphincter at rest and with squeezing are significantly greater in men than women. Parous females have a significant decrease in mean maximal resting pressures compared with nulliparous females. They found no difference in resting pressures of males and nulliparous females. These authors concluded that patients must be compared with their normal subgroups to correctly identify manometric abnormalities. Felt-Bersma et al. (101) also tried to determine normal values in anal manometry. They found that maximal basal pressure was not significantly different in men and women (68 vs. 63 mmHg) but that maximal squeeze pressure (MSP) was significantly different (183 vs. 102 mmHg). Both maximal basal pressure (MBP) and MSP decreased significantly with age. Sphincter length was longer in men than women (4.1 vs. 3.5 cm).

Defecography, Balloon Proctography, and Dynamic MRI

In the 1960s, cineradiography was developed for the dynamic investigation of the defecation mechanism. Some of the techniques used in that period were complex and time consuming and required sophisticated radiologic equipment. Now, however, simplified techniques such as defecography and balloon proctography are available.

Defecography can be performed with different contrast media. A liquid barium suspension might be adequate and convenient for demonstrating specific abnormalities, such as rectal prolapse. A semisolid medium is required for detailed investigation of the physiologic aspects of normal continence and defecation. A contrast medium with a semisolid consistency can be prepared by heating potato starch or rolled oats with barium sulfate and water. After this mixture is introduced into the rectum, the subject is seated on a radiolucent commode to void the contrast medium (184). It has been argued, however, that such a semisolid mixture does not simulate the inspissated feces frequently seen in patients with obstructed defecation, so it is questioned whether the use of a semisolid paste is relevant for the defecographic investigation of patients with evacuation difficulties (185).

Defecography can be used to measure the anorectal angle. This angle depends on the tone of the puborectalis muscle and is normally $92 \pm 1.5^\circ$ at rest and $137 \pm 1.5^\circ$ during straining (186). Another application of defecography is determination of the position of the pelvic floor by calculating the distance between the anorectal junction and the pubococcygeal line. In this way perineal descent at rest and during straining can be measured. The pubococcygeal line is drawn from the tip of the coccyx to the posteroinferior margin of the pubic ramus; normally the pelvic floor lies at a plane approximately 1 cm below that of the pubococcygeal line. Other determinations that can be made include the distance between the anorectal junction and the lower end of the coccyx, the presence of a rectocele, and the ability of the patient to expel rectal contents.

Balloon proctography has been developed to afford a more simplified procedure and make it more acceptable for the patient (187). It provides a visual assessment of the pelvic floor both in the resting state and during defecation. The examination is conducted by inserting into the rectum a special shaped balloon filled with a barium suspension. With the patient seated on a commode, lateral radiographs are taken and the rectum and anal canal can be outlined at rest and during straining. Evacuation of the balloon rather than feces is more esthetically acceptable for both patient and staff. The examination is well tolerated, is quick and clean, and involves a relatively low dose of radiation.

Agachan et al. (188) assessed the incidence and clinical significance of defecographic findings in patients with possible evacuation disorders. Of 744 patients, 60% were diagnosed who complained of constipation, 16.5% of fecal incontinence, 5.6% of rectal prolapse, 11% of rectal pain, and 6.9% of a combination of more than one of these diagnoses. Although 12.5% of these evaluations were considered normal, 8% revealed rectal prolapse, 25.7% rectocele, 11% sigmoidocele, 12.6% intussusception, and 30% a combination of these findings. Patients with paradoxic puborectalis contraction had an extremely high frequency of constipation compared with other symptoms. The authors caution against treating patients strictly on the basis of radiographic findings.

A further refinement in the assessment of rectal evacuation was described by Lestar et al. (189). In what they termed "defecometry," they reported the ability to quantify the maximum rectal pressure increase during straining, the duration of effective evacuation, and the work performed to evacuate a simulated stool. Simultaneous anal pressure records (permitted by the incorporation of a catheter into the balloon device) demonstrate the nature of the sphincter activity during simulated defecation. They believe that defecometry permits more adequate identification and characterization of the outlet-obstruction type of constipated patient than does the single-balloon expulsion test.

The largest series from a single institution was reported by Mellgren et al. (190). They analyzed the results of 2816 patients who underwent defecography for defecation disorders. Their findings included normal, 23%; rectal intussusception, 31%; rectal prolapse, 13%; rectocele, 27%; and enterocele, 19%. A combination of one or more of these diagnoses was present in 21% of patients studied.

For the evaluation of disorders such as anterior rectal wall prolapse, incomplete or complete rectal prolapse, rectocele, and solitary rectal ulcer syndrome, defecography seems to be more sensitive than balloon proctography. With regard to rectoceles, defecographic criteria are used to select which patients should undergo surgical repair. These criteria are rectocele size and retention of barium within the rectocele at the end of attempted evacuation. Although many surgeons use these proctographic selection criteria, it has been shown that they fail to predictwho will and who will not benefit from rectocele repair (191).

A scintigraphic method using a balloon filled with technetium-99m (^{99m}Tc)-labeled suspension has been developed. With this method the anorectal angle can be measured accurately with minimal radiation exposure (192). To reduce radiation exposure, Hutchinson et al. (193) believe this to be the investigation of choice for objective and dynamic assessment of anorectal function.

In summary, defecography is a useful imaging modality for detecting anorectal functional and anatomic abnormalities as possible causes of defecation disturbances and for anatomically guided anorectal surgery (194). The main contribution of defecography is its specific ability to reveal rectal intussusception and enterocele as well as sigmoidocele. Other diagnoses that can be made by defecography include non-relaxing puborectalis syndrome, perineal descent, and rectocele (195).

With the advent of open-configuration magnetic resonance (MR) imaging systems, MR defecography with the patient in the sitting position has become possible. This nonradioactive imaging technique is a promising modality to investigate structural and functional disturbances in patients with defecatory problems (196). MR defecography permits analysis of the anorectal angle, the opening of the anal canal, the function of the puborectalis muscle, and the descent of the pelvic floor during defecation. (197) Good demonstration of the rectal wall permits visualization of intussusceptions and rectoceles. Excellent demonstration of the perirectal soft tissues allows assessment of spastic pelvic floor syndrome and descending perineum syndrome and visualization of enteroceles. MR defecography with an open-configuration magnet allows accurate assessment of anorectal morphology and function in relation to surrounding structures without exposing the patient to harmful ionizing radiation.

The wide range of morphologic variations among healthy individuals and a large interobserver variation in measurements prevent defecography from being an ideal examination of anorectal defecation disturbance. Nevertheless, some patients with clinically occult disorders of anorectal function can be diagnosed with dynamic defecography (198).

Another imaging technique is dynamic transperineal ultrasound. Recent studies suggest that this ultrasound modality is an attractive alternative for defecography with opacification of the small bowel, bladder and vagina (199–201). Beer-Gabel et al. compared dynamic transperineal ultrasound with defecography in 33 women with obstructed defecation. In all these patients the small bowel was opacified following ingestion of Gastrografin®. They found good agreement for the assessment of rectocele, intussusception and rectal prolapse. There was also agreement with regard to the measurement of the anorectal angle at rest, the position of the anorectal junction at rest and the movement of this junction during straining (202).

Simultaneous Dynamic Proctography and Peritoneography

It is believed that simultaneous dynamic proctography and peritoneography identifies both rectal and pelvic floor pathologic conditions and provides a qualitative assessment of severity, allowing for better treatment planning in selected patients with obstructed defecation, pelvic fullness and/or prolapse, and/or chronic intermittent pelvic floor pain (203). As described by Sentovich et al. (203), the method consists of injection of 50 mL of nonionic contrast (Renograffin-60, Squibb Diagnostics, Princeton, New Jersey, U.S.A.) intraperitoneally along the lateral border of the rectus muscle using fluoroscopy. Patients are asked to perform Valsalva's maneuver, and anteroposterior and lateral pelvic radiographs are obtained. Patients are immediately given 100–120 mL of barium and instant mashed potato mixture as an enema and 20–25 mL of liquid barium intravaginally. On a radiolucent commode, lateral radiographs are taken with the patient at rest and during maximal anal squeeze. Patients are asked to evacuate the rectal contrast material, which is observed on videotape using fluoroscopy. A final static radiograph is obtained while the patient strains to evacuate any residual rectal contrast. The initial static radiographs are taken when patients have been given only peritoneal contrast to evaluate for pelvic floor hernias. Radiographs taken on the commode at rest, squeeze, and strain are used to determine the anorectal angle and perineal descent. The evacuation videotape is used to identify rectoceles, enteroceles, and rectal prolapse. An enterocele is present if peritoneal contrast separates the rectum from the vagina, either at rest or during strain.

Sentovich et al. (203) identified clinically suspected and nonsuspected enterocele in 10 of the 13 patients studied. An enterocele or other pelvic floor hernia was ruled out by the technique in three of the women studied. Findings affected operative treatment planning in 85% of patients studied. Women with rectoceles and suspected enteroceles confirmed by dynamic proctography with peritoneography underwent abdominal rectopexy and colopexy rather than per anal repair of their rectocele. In one woman, dynamic proctography with peritoneography ruled out a clinically suspected enterocele, and subsequently she underwent a successful perineal repair of her rectal prolapse. Operation was avoided in women in whom dynamic proctography and peritoneography identified no enterocele or pelvic floor hernia or only a small, nonobstructing enterocele. Complications occurred in two patients (15%)—a vasovagal reaction and postprocedure abdominal pain.

To identify enterocele, some authors have recommended giving patients oral barium 1–3 hours before defecography so that small bowel herniating into an enterocele sac can be easily identified (204). Other authors have given substantial amounts of barium paste intrarectally so that sigmoidoceles can be identified (205). Although both these techniques have been found to be useful, neither directly visualizes the enterocele sacs that may, in fact, be filled with omentum rather than with small bowel or sigmoid colon. In addition, neither technique adequately visualizes potential pelvic floor hernias such as obturator, sciatic, or perineal hernias.

Peritoneography outlines both enterocele and pelvic floor hernia sacs and thus more completely and efficiently evaluates pelvic floor anatomy (203). Other investigators have also found this technique useful (206). A variation of the theme was reported by Altringer et al. (207) who used complete visceral opacification of the small bowel and bladder and vaginal and rectal contrast to improve diagnostic accuracy beyond that provided by physical examination alone. These authors believe that fluoroscopic assessment of the female pelvis is frequently needed to evaluate chronic pain, urinary tract symptoms, vaginal eversions, rectal prolapse, and obstructed defecation. Therefore contrast defecography changed the diagnosis in 75% of the 46 patients studied.

Balloon Expulsion Test

Rectal balloon expulsion may be used as an alternative to defecography, as the inability to expel an intrarectal balloon can point to impaired rectal evacuation. This simple method has been adopted by many units as a test for anismus (208). It is questionable, however, whether the inability to expel a balloon represents paradoxic contraction of the puborectalis muscle during attempted evacuation. Dahl et al. (209) reported that 13 of 14 patients with electromyographic evidence of anismus were able to pass an inflated balloon. They concluded that the balloon expulsion test is not a useful marker of inappropriate contraction of the pelvic floor.

In contrast with this finding, Minguez and co-workers reported that 87% of their patients with manometric and defecographic signs of anismus were not able to expel a balloon. Only 12 of 102 patients (11%), admitted with functional constipation without signs of anismus, showed the same inability to expel an intrarectal balloon. According to these authors the specificity and negative predictive value of the balloon-expulsion test for excluding anismus was 89% and 97% respectively (210).

It has been argued that the failure to expel an inflated balloon might be due to structural abnormalities of the rectum. This seems unlikely, since it has been shown that the ability to pass a balloon is not impaired, neither by the presence and size of a rectocele nor by the presence of a rectal intussusception (185). It might be possible that the inability to expel a balloon represents insufficient colonic and rectal contractility or the failure to adequately increase intrarectal pressure by inappropriate contraction of the diaphragm and abdominal muscles.

Saline Continence Test

The saline continence test provides a more dynamic assessment of the fecal continence mechanism (211). The ability of an individual to retain 1500 mL of saline solution infused into the rectum at a rapid rate (60 mL/min) can provide insights into the strength of the sphincteric barrier against the physical stress of fluid in the rectum. Simultaneous measurements of anorectal pressure and electrical activity of the external sphincter have revealed that rectal infusion of saline induces a regular series of events: rectal contractions, relaxations of the internal sphincter, and contractions of the external sphincter.

The initial phasic contraction of the external sphincter in response to rectal infusion occurs both before the deepest relaxation of the internal sphincter and also before rectal peak pressure, which in normal subjects is lower than anal pressure. Based on these findings, it has been concluded that this brief phasic contraction of the external sphincter contributes little to continence during saline infusion. However, the initial response of the external sphincter is followed by an increased activity that remains continuously above basal values as long as the rectum remains distended. It has been suggested that this compensatory activity of the external sphincter is the major contribution to continence during rectal infusion of saline.

In continent patients, two distinct patterns of anorectal activity have been demonstrated using the saline continence test. In some patients, rectal infusion results in normal rectal contractions and internal sphincter relaxations but little or no compensatory activity of the external sphincter. Although this defective response of the external sphincter may be the result of neuropathic weakness, it also may be caused by diminished anorectal sensation (212). In contrast, other patients with fecal incontinence present a sustained reduction of resting anal pressure soon after saline infusion is begun, whereas the external sphincter of these patients shows irregular contractions, as demonstrated in integrated electromyography (212). These findings suggest that there is a functional weakness of the internal sphincter in this subgroup of patients.

Colonic Transit Studies

Although constipation is not directly related to anorectal function in all cases, colonic transit studies are helpful in understanding the constipated patient. Details are described in Chapter 33.

Anorectal Electrosensitivity

In recent years, there has been a growing interest in the physiologic significance of anorectal sensation. Roe et al. (213) have described a method for the quantitative assessment of anorectal sensation that involves placing a bipolar ring electrode into the rectum or the anal canal and incrementally increasing the current until a threshold of sensation is reported by the patient. They found no significant differences in electrosensitivity thresholds between the two sexes and no relationship between age and anorectal sensory function (213). In contrast, Jameson et al. (172) demonstrated that midanal and rectal electrosensitivity decline with increasing age and that midanal sensitivity is affected by parity. A similar finding has been reported by Broens at al. (214).

Chan et al. found that strong correlation between heat thresholds and balloon distention to maximum tolerable volumes and defecatory desire suggest a common sensory afferent pathway excitation (215). Heat stimulation is a simple technique that has a high degree of repeatability and may be an objective assessment of polymodal nociceptor function in the rectum.

Rectal Compliance

Rectal compliance reflects the distensibility of the rectal wall (i.e., the volumetric response of the rectum to stretch when subjected to an increase of intraluminal pressure). It has been shown that an ultrathin and infinitely compliant polyethylene bag is the most suitable device with which to measure rectal compliance (216). The balloon should be tied at both ends to prevent longitudinal extension during distention. After introduction into the rectum, the balloon is continuously inflated to selected pressure plateaus. The volume changes at the various levels of distending pressures are recorded. Next, a volume–pressure curve is plotted. The slope of this curve (dV/dP) represents compliance. There is growing evidence that the elastance and the compliance of the rectum are closely interwoven with rectal sensation.

Measurements of rectal volumes in response to cumulative pressure steps with an electromechanical barostat system, have revealed a characteristic tri-phasic compliance curve (132). During the first phase, the increase of pressure only gives rise to a small increase of volume, probably reflecting an initial resistance of the rectal wall. The second phase of the compliance curve is characterized by a larger increase of volume, presumably reflecting an adaptive relaxation of the rectal wall. The last phase of the curve is more flattened and probably represents increasing resistance of the rectal wall against further distension. Control subjects experience an initial perception of distension during the first phase of the compliance curve. An urge to defecate is experienced during the second phase. It has been reported that among patients with obstructed defecation the call to stool is encountered much later, at the end of the third phase of the compliance curve (132). This finding does suggest that rectal sensory perception is interwoven with rectal compliance.

There are some conflicting data regarding rectal compliance in patients with obstructed defecation. Varma observed an increased compliance in women with obstructed defecation after hysterectomy (217), whereas Rasmussen et al. noted a decreased compliance. (218). In a more recent study, conducted by Gosselink et al., no difference was found between controls and patients with obstructed defecation regarding their rectal compliance (132). The discrepancy among these three studies is assumed to be the result of variations in recording techniques and differences in defining compliance. This controversy and the reported inter- and intraindividual variations in pressure-volume profiles in normal subjects (219), indicate that compliance measurements should be interpreted with caution. Alstrup et al. (220) reported an endosonographic method that they believe provides a more precise and reproducible estimation of rectal compliance.

Electromyography

Electromyography (EMG) records action potential derived from motor units within contracting muscle. The external sphincter and probably the puborectalis are unique skeletal muscles because they show continuous tonic contractions at rest, with activity present even during sleep. Sphincter activity ceases during defecation.

Conventional Concentric EMG

Various electrophysiologic techniques are available for the investigation of myoelectrical activity generated by the external sphincter and the puborectalis muscle. Some investigators have used silver/silver chloride electrodes applied to the perianal skin. Although these surface electrodes are well tolerated by patients and cause only slight disturbance of the sphincter muscles, they have the disadvantage of recording potentials summated from multiple motor units. Because bipolar concentric needle electrodes have the advantage of recording potentials summated from only a limited number of muscle fibers (±30), they are the type most often used.

Bowel preparation is not necessary before the examination. With the patient lying in the left lateral position, the needle electrode is inserted directly into the external sphincter or the puborectalis muscle without a local anesthetic. The needle is inserted posterior to the anal verge at an angle of 45°. The position of the tip of the needle electrode in the puborectalis can be controlled with a finger hooked into the rectum. Normally with the muscles at rest, a basal low-frequency activity will be recorded that consists of low-amplitude potentials varying between 2 mV and 50 mV (221). This phenomenon usually is not displayed by skeletal muscle, which is characteristically silent at rest. During squeezing and coughing, a burst of electrical activity, which is the consequence of increased frequency of motor unit firing and recruitment of new motor units, is recorded (Fig. 21). Contraction of the external sphincter and puborectalis, reflexly induced by balloon distention, saline infusion of the rectum, or perianal pinprick, also can be recorded electromyographically.

Single-Fiber EMG

Single-fiber EMG is an even more sophisticated technique for identifying the muscle action potential from a single muscle fiber. The technique provides a means of assessing innervation and reinnervation of the muscle under investigation (221). The assessment can be made quantitatively using the fiber density, which represents the mean of a number of muscle fibers supplied by one motor unit within the uptake area of the electrode averaged from 20 different electrode positions (221). Normal fiber density is 1.51 ± 0.16. A raised fiber density can be used as an index of collateral

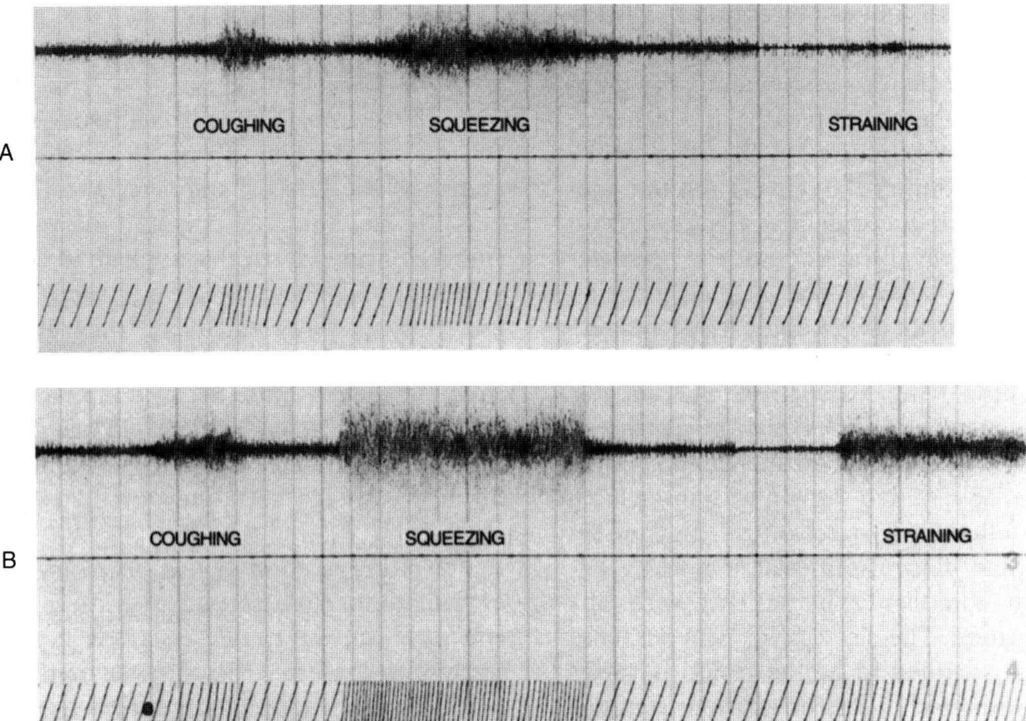

FIGURE 21 ■ Electromyography. (**A**) Normal activity of puborectalis muscle at rest and during coughing, squeezing, and straining. (**B**) Recording of the puborectalis in patient with spastic pelvic floor syndrome. Note the paradoxical increase of activity during straining.

sprouting and reinnervation of denervated muscle fibers. A raised fiber density has been demonstrated in the majority of patients with primary "idiopathic" anal incontinence and in patients with incontinence secondary to neurologic disorders (221).

In the past, the most useful clinical application of EMG was anal mapping for incontinent patients. Now other techniques such as endoanal sonography and endoanal MRI seem to be more accurate in the detection of sphincter defects. Furthermore, the latter techniques obviate the need for the painful insertion of a needle at several locations around the anal canal.

However, Jost et al. (222) reported on the use of surface versus needle electrodes in the determination of motor conduction time to the external anal sphincter. Mean latency in the group with surface electrodes was 19.4 m sec and in the group with needle electrodes, 23.4 m sec. The authors believe that the surface electrodes are preferable.

Nerve Stimulation Techniques

Even more sophisticated techniques have been described to develop a better understanding of perineal functional abnormalities that may be of neurogenic origin. The techniques of nerve stimulation provide objective assessment of neuromuscular function as well as more precise identification of the anatomic site of the nerve or muscle lesion. Also, both the distal and proximal motor innervation of the perianal striated sphincter muscle can be evaluated.

Spinal Nerve Latency

The central component of the motor innervation of the pelvic floor can be studied by transcutaneous spinal stimulation. With the patient in the left lateral position, a stimulus electrode is placed vertically across the lumbar spine (Fig. 22). This special device stimulates the spinal cord, usually at the level of L1 and L4. The induced response of the puborectalis or external sphincter can be detected either by a surface anal plug electrode located at the top of a transrectal finger glove or by an intramuscular needle electrode (221). The normal values of motor latency following transcutaneous spinal cord stimulation are shown in Table 5.

The difference in the latencies from L1 and L4 has been called the spinal latency ratio. This ratio is increased in patients with anal incontinence caused by a proximal lesion in the innervation (223). Such a proximal lesion may be the result of damage to the motor nerve roots of S3 and S4 from disk disease. Stenosis of the spinal canal from osteoarthritis also may disturb proximal motor conduction. Innervation of the puborectalis probably is not derived from the pudendal nerves but rather from direct branches of the motor roots of S3 and S4 (224). Therefore, latency measurements of this muscle can be performed only by spinal cord stimulation.

Pudendal Nerve Terminal Motor Latency

External sphincter motor latencies can be recorded after both spinal cord stimulation and pudendal nerve stimulation.

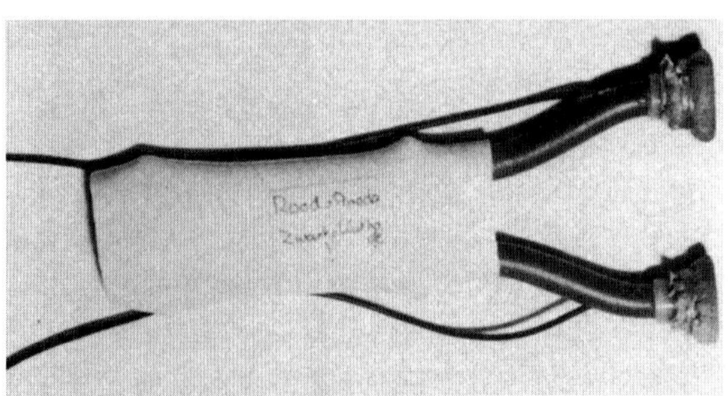

FIGURE 22 ■ Spinal cord stimulator.

TABLE 5 ■ Normal Values of Motor Latency After Spinal Cord and Pudendal Nerve Stimulation

Stimulation	Contraction Response	Latency (millisecond)
L1 nerve	Puborectalis	4.8±0.4
	External sphincter	5.5±0.4
L4 nerve	Puborectalis	3.7±0.5
	External sphincter	4.4±0.4
Pudendal nerve	External sphincter	1.9±0.2

Source: From Ref. 213.

Pudendal and perineal nerve stimulation techniques are used to assess the distal motor innervation of the pelvic floor musculature (i.e., the external anal sphincter and periurethral striated sphincter muscles). The terminal motor latency of the pudendal nerve can be determined by a transrectal stimulation technique, with a special pudendal nerve stimulator. That device consists of two stimulating electrodes located at the tip of the second finger of a rubber glove and two recording electrodes incorporated into its base (Fig. 23). With the patient in the left lateral position, the fingered glove containing the electrodes is introduced into the rectum, and the tip is brought into contact with the ischial spine on each side. After a square wave stimulus is delivered, a tracing is examined for evidence of contraction in the external sphincter as detected by the recording electrodes, thereby indicating accurate localization of the pudendal nerve. A supramaximal stimulus of about 50 Volts is delivered, and the latency between stimulus and external sphincter contraction is measured (Fig. 24). The terminal motor latency of a normal pudendal nerve is of the order of 1.9 ± 0.2 m sec (Table 5). It is increased in patients with pelvic floor disorders, such as anal incontinence with or without rectal prolapse, solitary rectal ulcer syndrome, and traumatic division of the external sphincter. The same phenomenon has been found in patients with intractable constipation. However, this increase in pudendal nerve latency is most impressive in patients with fecal incontinence (221). This technique also can detect occult pudendal nerve damage, which usually is symptomless.

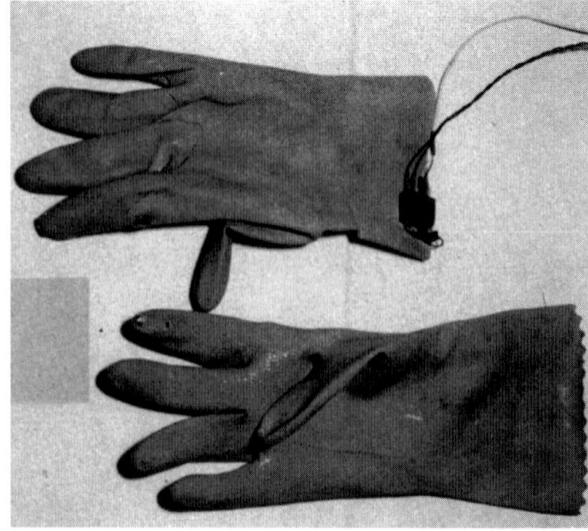

FIGURE 23 ■ Gloves for transrectal stimulation of pudendal nerve. Note stimulating electrodes at tip of index finger and recording electrodes incorporated into the base of the glove.

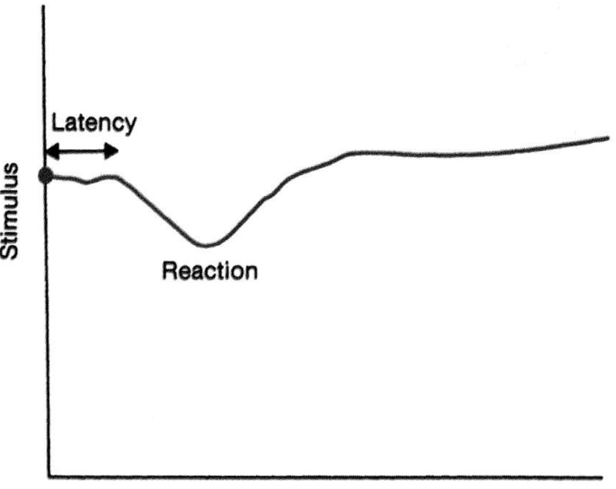

FIGURE 24 ■ Recording of pudendal nerve latency.

Perineal Nerve Terminal Motor Latency

A similar technique can be used to determine the distal motor latency in the perineal branch of the pudendal nerve by measuring the latency from pudendal nerve stimulation to the periurethral striated muscles. The response to the periurethral sphincter muscle is recorded by intraurethral electrodes mounted on a Foley catheter. Nerve stimulation techniques have been used in studies of patients with pelvic floor disorders, especially anal incontinence. They have proved useful in determining the site of conduction delay and in investigating the differential innervation of the puborectalis and the external sphincter.

Ultrasonography

Ultrasonography combined with manometry is another method of assessing anorectal angles and puborectalis function (225). The technique involves ultrasonographic measurement of the anorectal angles at rest and with maximal voluntary contraction of the puborectalis, using a water-filled Lahr balloon in the rectum as contrast, and a vaginal ultrasound probe on the posterior wall of the vagina. The angles are measured with the patient in the 45° supine position on a gynecologic examination table. Significantly different results have been noted in incontinent patients and in control subjects. Advantages of this technique are that it avoids radiation exposure and allows for a longer viewing time. It is less expensive compared with radiographic proctography, and the data are complementary.

Anal endosonography can reveal sphincter defects after anorectal surgery. Felt-Bersma et al. (226) studied 50 patients after hemorrhoidectomy (24), fistulectomy (18), and internal sphincterotomy (eight). In 23 patients (46%), a defect of the anal sphincter was found (13 patients had an internal sphincter defect, one had an external sphincter defect, and nine had a combined sphincter defect). In 70%, the sphincter defect did not produce symptoms. This has clinical implications in the evaluation of patients with fecal incontinence.

■ CLINICAL APPLICATION

Physiologic studies of the anorectal region play an increasingly important role in the diagnosis and management of a number of anorectal disorders. Schuster (100) pointed out that rectosphincteric studies can be used (1) to investigate physiology and pathophysiology, (2) as a sensitive tool to detect functional abnormalities that represent early signs of disease, (3) for the differential diagnosis of clinical disorders, (4) to assess immediate response to some clinical modality, (5) to evaluate long-term progress, and (6) as an integral part of treatment itself (as in operant conditioning). On the other hand, it has been argued that anorectal physiology measurements fail to meet the criteria of a useful clinical test because (1) they are not widely available to clinicians, (2) it is not possible to establish a reproducible normal range, (3) abnormal measurements do not always correlate with disease entities or explain symptoms, (4) the results are often unhelpful in diagnosis and management, and (5) clinical outcome after intervention does not correlate with alteration in the measurements obtained (227). Furthermore, treatment of a disorder may be empiric or rational. Rational treatment relies on the understanding of basic physiology and pathophysiology. With this in mind, specific applications and potential clinical implications are outlined. Details of abnormalities of specific disorders in which physiologic information may assist in management are described in their respective chapters. Wexner and Jorge (228) assessed the value of physiological tests in 308 patients with functional disorders of defecation. Definitive diagnoses were made after history and physical examination alone in 8% with constipation, 11% with incontinence, and 23% with intractable rectal pain. The figures after physiologic tests were 75%, 66%, and 42%, respectively. Treatable conditions were diagnosed by physiologic testing in 67% of patients with constipation and in 55% of patients with incontinence.

Anal Incontinence

This socially crippling disorder has been studied via a number of investigative techniques including manometry, electromyography, and nerve stimulation techniques to better define the exact cause of incontinence. For example, anal manometry may distinguish which of the two sphincters is principally responsible for the incontinence. This is important because if symptoms are due to internal sphincter dysfunction alone, a sphincter repair may not benefit the patient.

The clinical value of manometry in patients with fecal incontinence has been questioned. For example, one study found that 43% of incontinent subjects had "normal" values for both MRAP and MSAP. In contrast, a low MSAP was demonstrated in 9% of normal continent individuals (173). Based on these results, the authors concluded that anal incontinence cannot be assessed by anorectal manometry alone.

Penninckx et al. (229) described the balloon-retaining test, which consists of progressive filling of a compliant intrarectal balloon in a patient in the sitting position. The pressure inside the balloon is monitored, and the patient is asked to retain the balloon as long as possible and to report first, constant, and maximal tolerable sensation levels. The balloon is used to simulate semisolid and solid stool. The authors believe this test to be a more realistic approach to the evaluation of fecal continence than the rectal saline infusion test and anal manometry. The test evaluates the rectal reservoir function, sensation, and sphincter competence simultaneously and also permits objective evaluation of the effect of different treatments in incontinent patients.

In a sophisticated computer model, Perry et al. (230) developed a manometric technique of anal pressure vectography for the detection of anal sphincter injuries. Abnormal symmetry indices exposed even occult anal sphincter injuries. Perry et al. believe that the vector symmetry index may be useful in determining which incontinent patients should have sphincter repair.

Endoanal sonography facilitates the detection of occult sphincter defects. Since the introduction of this investigative technique, opinions about the pathogenesis, investigation, and management of fecal incontinence have changed dramatically. It is well known that 0.5–2% of women delivering vaginally will sustain a third-degree tear. Primary repair of such injury is often inadequate. Sultan et al. (231) reported that half the women with a repaired third-degree tear have symptoms of fecal incontinence or urgency and that sphincter defects can be identified with endoanal sonography in 85% of these women. Sonographic investigations have also revealed that one of three primipara who deliver vaginally develop a permanent defect involving one or both sphincters (232) and that 90% of incontinent women, in whom the only apparent factor is obstetric damage, have a structural abnormality of one or both sphincters (233). It is now agreed that childbirth is the most common cause of fecal incontinence in healthy adult women.

In many patients, biofeedback therapy has been effective in correcting or at least improving anal incontinence.

Constipation

The use of intestinal transit studies and anal manometry has allowed a better definition of the extent of dysfunction of patients having severe chronic constipation, megarectum, megacolon, or Hirschsprung's disease. Biofeedback has been used in the treatment of some patients with constipation.

Rectal Procidentia

A number of manometric and electromyographic abnormalities have been described, but there has not been uniform agreement about their value. The contradictory reports have been discussed by Hiltunen et al. (234).

Rectocele

Cinefluoroscopic studies in women with a rectocele demonstrate a blind pouch that fills like a hernial sac during efforts at defecation.

Solitary Ulcer Syndrome

Electromyographic abnormalities characterized by overactivity in the puborectalis and no reflex relaxation during straining have been demonstrated.

Descending Perineum Syndrome

Several manometric abnormalities have been described. On radiographic examination the perineal floor can be seen to descend and the anorectal angle is more obtuse. Caution should be exercised in interpreting the results. Skomorowska et al. (235) have noted that patients with normal position of the pelvic floor during rest may exhibit considerable descent during straining, whereas those patients who have abnormal position of the perineum during rest may show normal descent during straining. This observation may indicate that the first sign of abnormal function is an increased descent during straining and that only later will it be followed by descent during rest.

Fissure-in-Ano

High anal pressure that is due to increased activity of the internal anal sphincter is found in almost all patients with a chronic anal fissure. Ambulatory anorectal manometry has revealed that the internal anal sphincter hypertonia in fissure patients is sustained during daytime and disappears during sleep (236). Ultraslow wave pressure fluctuations are another manifestation of increased myogenic activity of the internal anal sphincter. These ultraslow waves disappear when high anal pressure is reduced either by manual dilatation (237) or by lateral internal sphincterotomy (238). There is mounting evidence that increased internal sphincter tone reduces microvascular perfusion at the fissure site and that reduction of anal pressure improves anodermal blood flow at the posterior midline and finally results in fissure healing (239). These findings provide evidence for the ischemic nature of anal fissure.

Hemorrhoids

Electrophysiologic and manometric investigations in patients with internal hemorrhoids have suggested that the pathogenesis of this condition may be due to a dysrhythmia within the internal sphincter (240).

Anorectal Malformations

Electromyographic techniques have been used preoperatively to determine the location of the external sphincter in infants with imperforate anus and thus can assist in appropriate placement of the rectum if a pull-through operative procedure is planned. Spina bifida and cauda equina lesions may be accompanied by malfunction of visceral and striated muscle.

Aging

Balloon studies have shown a progressive decrease in rectal sensitivity to distention in the aging population.

Coloanal Anastomosis

Sphincter-saving operations with very low anastomoses have been associated with varying degrees of alteration in continence. This has been attributed to a number of factors including decreased bowel distensibility, varying degrees of ischemia, and decreased anal pressures. The fact that incontinence is temporary in some patients has been attributed to the initial loss of the rectoanal inhibitory reflex that reappears later, possibly associated with improved neorectal compliance with time.

Fistula-in-Ano

Anal manometry has been used in studies of patients undergoing operations for fistula-in-ano repair. A significantly lower pressure was measured in patients in whom the external sphincter had been divided when compared with those in whom the muscle had been preserved. Disturbance of continence was related to abnormally low resting pressures (241,242).

Trauma

In the planning of a sphincter repair, electromyographic studies and sonographic investigations can be used to determine whether there is adequate muscle mass to accomplish a satisfactory repair.

Pelvic Pouches

Preoperative study of the sphincter mechanism might help to determine whether a patient will be continent after a pouch-anal anastomosis. Pouch volumes have been studied and correlated with stool leakage (243). Defecography (evacuation pouchography) has been used to study postoperative function (244). Poorer results were caused by rapid pouch filling and impaired pouch evacuation, which led to increased stool frequency (245). Poor continence after ileoanal anastomosis correlates with an abnormal EMG of the external sphincter (246). From their studies of patients undergoing ileoanal procedures, Beart et al. (247) believe that in the presence of normal sphincter function, which they found to be preserved with this operation, continence is not dependent on the presence of normal mucosa or the anal inhibitory reflex but correlates with reservoir capacity, compliance, and the frequency and strength of intrinsic bowel contractions.

Inflammatory Bowel Diseases

Patients with inflammatory bowel diseases, especially those in the active phase, have a decreased distensibility of the rectum, which could be the result of either decreased muscle compliance or increased sensitivity. Knowledge of this decreased rectal capacity may be of practical value in predicting which patients with Crohn's disease would benefit from an ileorectal anastomosis (98).

Ischemic Fecal Incontinence

Devroede et al. (98) described the disorder of fecal incontinence due to ischemia. They used a combination of patient history, anal manometry, arteriography, barium enema, and biopsy to define this entity.

Spinal Cord Lesions

Bowel dysfunction is common in patients with spinal cord lesions. Tjandra et al (248) studied 12 patients with significant spinal cord lesions who had mixed symptoms of constipation, fecal impaction, and fecal incontinence. None of the patients had a sphincter defect as evaluated by endoanal ultrasonography. Eight of them had traumatic spinal cord injuries while other lesions included spina bifida, syringomyelia, arachnoid cyst, and spinal cord ischemia after abdominal aortic aneurysm repair. In patients with spinal cord lesions, the mean resting anal canal pressure and maximum squeeze anal canal pressure were 46 mmHg and 76 mmHg respectively compared with 62 mmHg and 138 mmHg respectively, in healthy controls. Eleven patients had prolonged pudendal nerve terminal motor latency (9 bilateral and 2 unilateral) whereas rectoanal inhibitory reflex was abolished in all 9 patients tested.

Miscellaneous

Rare conditions such as scleroderma, dermatomyositis, and myotonic dystrophy also may be studied.

REFERENCES

1. Gaginella TS. Absorption and secretion in the colon. Curr Opin Gastroenterol 1995; 11:2–8.
2. Duthie HL, Wormsley KG. Absorption from the human colon. Shields R, ed. Scientific Basis of Gastroenterology. Edinburgh: Churchill Livingstone, 1979.
3. Pemberton JH, Phillips SF. Colonic absorption. Perspect Colon Rectal Surg 1988; 1(1):89–103.
4. Devroede GJ, Phillips SF. Conservation of sodium, chloride and water by the human colon. Gastroenterology 1969; 56:101–109.
5. Cummings JH. Colonic absorption: The importance of short chain fatty acids in man. In: Polak JM, Bloom SR, Wright NA, Butler AG, eds. Basic Science in Gastroenterology. Physiology of the Gut. Ware, Herts, U.K.: Glaxo Group Research Limited, Royal Postgraduate Medical School, 1984.
6. Giller J, Phillips SF. Electrolyte absorption and secretion in the human colon. Am J Dig Dis 1972; 17:1003–1011.
7. Agarval R, Afzalpurkar R, Fordtron JS. Pathophysiology of potassium absorption and secretion by the human intestine. Gastroenterology 1994; 107:548–571.
8. Binder HJ, Sandle GI. Electrolyte absorption and secretion in the mammalian colon. Johnson LR, ed. Physiology of the Gastrointestinal Tract. 2nd ed. New York: Raven Press, 1987:1389–1418.
9. Powell DW. Transport in the large intestine. Giebisch G, Tosteson DC, Ussing HH, eds. Membrane Transport in Biology. New York: Springer-Verlag, 1978:781–809.
10. McConnel JB, Morrison J, Stewart WK. The role of the colon in the pathogenesis of hyperchloremic acidosis in ureterosigmoid anastomosis. Clin Sci 1979; 57:305–312.
11. Gibson JA, Sladen GE, Dawson AM. Studies in the role of the colon in urea metabolism. Gut 1973; 14:816.
12. Phillips TE, Phillips TH, Neutra ME. Regulation of intestinal goblet cell secretion. Electrical field stimulation in vitro. Am J Physiol 1984; 247:G682–G687.
13. Bond IR, Currier B, Buchwald H, Levitt MD. Colonic conservation of malabsorbed carbohydrates. Gastroenterology 1980; 78:444–447.
14. Latella G, Caprilli R. Metabolism of large bowel mucosa in health and disease. Int J Col Dis 1991; 6:127–132.
15. Kerlin P, Phillips SF. Absorption of fluids and electrolytes from the colon: With reference to inflammatory bowel disease. Allan RN, Keighley MRB, Alexander-Williams J, Hawkins C, eds. Inflammatory Bowel Diseases. Edinburgh: Churchill Livingstone, 1983.
16. Wald A. Colonic and anorectal motility testing in clinical practice. Am J Gastroenterol 1994; 89:2109–2115.
17. Ritchie JA. Movements of segmental constrictions in the human colon. Gut 1971; 12:350–355.
18. Cannon WB. The movements of the intestine studied by means of roentgen rays. Am J Physiol 1902; 6:251–277.
19. Elliott TR, Barclay-Smith E. Antiperistalsis and other muscular activities of the colon. J Physiol (Lond) 1904; 31:272–304.
20. Ritchie JA, Truelove SC, Ardran GM, Tuckey MS. Propulsion and retropulsion of normal colonic content. Dig Dis Sci 1971; 8:697–703.
21. Cohen S, Snape WJ. Movement of the small and large intestine. Fordtran J, Sleisinger M, eds. Gastrointestinal Disease. 3rd ed. New York: McGraw-Hill, 1983:859–873.
22. Herz AF. The passage of food along the human alimentary canal. Guy's Hospital Reports 1907; 61:389–427.
23. Ritchie JA. Mass peristalsis in the human colon after contact with oxyphenisatin. Gut 1972; 13:211–219.
24. Torsoli A, Ramorino ML, Ammaturo MV, Capurso L, Paoluzi P, Anzini F. Mass movements and intracolonic pressures. Am J Dig Dis 1971; 16:693–696.
25. Garcia D, Hita G, Mompean B, Hernandez A, Pellican E, Morales G, Parilla P. Colonic motility: electric and manometric description of mass movement. Dis Colon Rectum 1991; 34:577–584.
26. Krogh K, Olsen N, Christensen P, Madsen JL, Laurberg S. Colorectal transport in normal defecation. Colorectal Disease 2003; 5:185–192.
27. Bampton PA, Dinning PG, Kennedy ML, Lubowski DZ, Cook IJ. Prolonged multi-point recording of colonic manometry in the unprepared human colon: providing insight into potentially relevant pressure wave parameters. Am J Gastroenterology 2001; 96:1838–1846.
28. Lemann M, Flourie B, Picon L, Coffin B, Jian R, Ramboud JC. Motor activity recorded in the unprepared colon of healthy humans. Gut 1995; 37:649–653.
29. Narducci R, Bassotti G, Gaburi M, Morelli A. Twenty-four hour manometric recording of colonic motor activity in healthy man. Gut 1987; 28:17–25.
30. Narducci R, Bassotti G, Gaburri M, Solines A, Fiorucci S, Morelli A. Distention stimulated motor acitivity of the human transverse descending and sigmoid colon [abstract]. Gastroenterology 1985; 88:1515.
31. Crowell M, Bassotti G, Cheskin LJ, Shuster MM, Whitehead WE. Method for prolonged ambulatory monitoring of high-amplitude propagated contractions from colon. Am J Physiol 1991; 261:G263–G268.
32. Soffer EE, Scalabrini P, Wingate DL. Prolonged ambulant monitoring of human colonic motility. Am J Physiol 1988; 257:G601–G606.
33. Herbst F, Kamm MA, Morris GP, Britton K, Woloszko J, Nicholls RJ. Gastrointestinal transit and prolonged ambulatory colonic motility in health and fecal incontinence. Gut 1997; 41:381–389.
34. Bampton PA, Dinning PG, Kennedy ML, Lubowski DZ, deCarle D, Cook IJ. The spatial and temporal organization of pressure patterns throughout the unprepared colon during spontaneous defecation. Am J Gastroenterol 2000; 95:1027–1035.
35. Bampton PA, Dinning PG, Kennedy ML, et al. Spatial and temporal organization of pressure patterns throughout the unprepared colon during spontaneous defecation. Am J Gastroenterol 2000; 95:157.
36. Hirabayashi T, Matsufuji H, Yokoyama J, Hagane K, Hoshino K, Morikawa Y, Kitajima M. Colorectal motility induction by sacral nerve electrostimulation in a canine model: implications for colonic pacing. Dis Colon Rectum 2003; 46:809–817.
37. Bampton PA, Dinning PG, Kennedy ML, Lubowski DZ, Cook IJ. The proximal colonic motor respons to rectal mechanical and chemical stimulation. Am J Physiol Gastrointest Liver Physiol 2002; 282:G443–G449.
38. Bassotti G, Gaburri M, Imbimba BP, Rossi L, Farroni F, Pelli MA. Colonic mass movements in idiopathic chronic constipation. Gut 1988; 29:1173–1179.
39. Dinning PG, Bampton PA, Andre J, Kennedy ML, Lubowski DZ, King DW, Cook IJ. Abnormal predefecatory colonic motor patterns define constipation in obstructed defecation. Gastroenterology 2004; 127:49–56.
40. Hervé S, Savoye G, Behbahani A, Leroi AM, Denis P, Ducrottû P. Results of 24-h manometric recording of colonic motor activity with endoluminal installtion of bisacodyl in patients with severe chronic slow transit constipation. Neurogastroenterol Motil 2004; 16:397–402.
41. Kumar D, Williams NS, Waldron D, Wingate DL. Prolonged manometric recording of anorectal activity in ambulant human subjects: Evidence of periodic activity. Gut 1989; 30:1007–1011.
42. Orkin BA, Hanson RB, Kelly KA. The rectal motor complex. J Gastrointest Motility 1989; 1:5–8.
43. Prior A, Fearn UJ, Read NW. Intermittent rectal motor activity: A rectal motor complex? Gut 1991; 32:1360–1363.
44. Auwerda JJ, Bac DJ, Schouten WR. Circadian rhythm of rectal motor complexes. Dis Colon Rectum 2001; 44:1328–1332.
45. Bassotti G, Betti C, Pelli MA, Morelli A. Prolonged manometric recording of rectal contractile activity in patients with slow transit constipation. Digestion 1991; 49:72–77.
46. Bell AM, Pemberton JH, Hanson RB, Zinsmeister AR. Variations in muscle tone of the human rectum: Recordings with an electromechanical barostat. Am J Physiol 1991; 260:17–25.
47. Steadman CJ, Phillips SF, Camilleri M, Haddad AC, Hanson RB. Variation of muscle tone in the human colon. Gastroenterology 1991; 101:373–381.
48. Ford MJ, Camilleri M, Wiste JA, Hanson RB. Differences in colonic tone and phasic response to a meal in the transverse and sigmoid human colon. Gut 1995; 37:264–269.
49. von der Ohe MR, Hanson RB, Camilleri M. Serotonergic mediation of postprandial colonic tonic and phasic responses in humans. Gut 1994; 35:536–541.
50. Ford MJ, Camilleri MJ, Hanson RB, Wiste JA, Joyner MJ. Hyperventilation, central autonomic control and colonic tone in humans. Gut 1995; 37:499–504.
51. Grotz RL, Pemberton JH, Levin KE, Bell AM, Hanson RB. Rectal wall contractility in healthy subjects and in patients with chronic severe constipation. Ann Surg 1993; 218:761–768.
52. Gosselink MJ, Schouten WR. The gastrorectal reflex in women with obstructed defecation. Int J Colorectal Dis 2001; 16:112–118.
53. Daniel EE. Electrophysiology of the colon. Gut 1975; 16:298–329.
54. Van Merwijk AJ, Duthie HL. Characteristics of human colonic smooth muscle in vitro. Christensen J, ed. Gastrointestinal Motility. New York: Raven Press, 1979:473–478.
55. Kubota M, Ito Y, Ikeda K. Membrane properties innervation of smooth muscle cells in Hirschsprung's. Am J Physiol 1983; 244:G406–G415.
56. Huizinga JD, Stern H, Chow E, Diamant NE, El-Sharkawy TY. Electrophysiological control of motility in the human colon. Gastroenterology 1985; 88: 500–511.
57. Chambers MM, Bowes KL, Kingma YL, Bannister C, Cote KR. In vitro electrical activity in human colon. Gastroenterology 1981; 81:502–508.
58. Huizinga JD, Daniel EE. Control of human colonic motor function. Dig Dis Sci 1986; 31:865–877.
59. Taylor I, Duthie HL, Smallwood R, Linkens D. Large bowel myoelectrical activity in man. Gut 1975; 16:808–814.
60. Sarna SK, Latimer P, Campbell D, Waterfall WE. Electrical and contractile activities in the human rectosigmoid. Gut 1982; 23:698–705.
61. Snape WJ, Carlson GM, Cohen S. Human colonic myoelectrical activity in response to Prostigmin and the gastrointestinal hormones. Am J Dig Dis 1977; 22:881–887.
62. Frieri G, Parisi F, Corazziari E, Caprilli R. Colonic electromyography in chronic constipation. Gastroenterology 1983; 84:737–740.

63. Snape WJ Jr, Matarazzo SA, Cohen S. Abnormal gastrocolonic response in patients with ulcerative colitis. Gut 1980; 21:392–396.
64. Bueno L, Fioramonti J, Ruckebusch Y, Frexinos J, Coulom P. Evaluation of colonic myoelectrical activity in health and functional disorders. Gut 1980; 21:480–485.
65. Waterfall WE, Shannon S. Human colonic electrical activity: transverse and human colons [abstr]. Clin Invest Med 1985; 8:A104.
66. Snape WJ, Carlson GM, Cohen S. Colonic myoelectric activity in the irritable bowel syndrome. Gastroenterology 1976; 70:326–330.
67. Taylor I, Darby C, Hammond P. Comparison of rectosigmoid myoelectrical activity in the irritable colon syndrome during relapses and remissions. Gut 1978; 19:923–926.
68. Bueno L, Fioramonti J, Frexinos J, Ruckebusch Y. Colonic myoelectrical activity in diarrhoea and constipation. Hepatogastroenterology 1980; 27: 381–389.
69. Schang JC, Devroede G, Duguay C, Hemond M, Hebert M. Constipation par inertie colique et obstruction terminate: Étude électromyographique. Gastroenterol Clin Biol 1985; 9:480–485.
70. Furness JB, Costa M. The enteric nervous system. Edinburgh: Churchill Livingstone, 1987.
71. Mulvihill SJ, Debas HT. Neuroendocrine regulation of intestinal function. Perspect Colon Rectal Surg 1992; 5:221–234.
72. Sanders KM. A case for interstitial cells of Cajal as pacemakers and mediators of neurotransmission in the gastrointestinal tract. Gastroenterology 1996; 111:492–515.
73. Ibba-Manneschi L, Martihi M, Zecchi-Oriandini S, Faussone-Pellegrini MS. Structural organization of enteric nervous system in human colon. Histology and Histopathology 1995; 10:17–25.
74. Gershon MD. The enteric nervous system. Annu Rev Neurosci 1981; 4: 227–272.
75. Burnstock G. Neural nomenclature. Nature 1971; 229:282–283.
76. Bloom SR, Polak JM. Gut hormones. Edinburgh: Churchill Livingstone, 1981.
77. Taylor I, Duthie HL, Smallwood R, Brown BH, Linkens D. The effect of stimulation on the myoelectrical activity of the rectosigmoid in man. Gut 1974; 15:599–607.
78. Dockray GJ, Taylor IL. Heptadecapeptide gastrin: Measurement in blood by specific radioimmunoassay. Gastroenterology 1976; 71:971–977.
79. Weber J, Ducrotte P. Colonic motility in health and disease. Dig Dis 1987; 5: 1–12.
80. Kinoso VP, Meshkinpour H, Lorber SH, Gutierrez JG, Chey WY. Motor responses of the sigmoid colon and rectum to exogenous cholecystokinin and secretin. Gastroenterology 1973; 65:438–444.
81. Kaufman PN, Krevsky B, Matmud LS, Maurea AH, Somers MB, Siegal JA, Fisher KS. Role of opiate receptors in the regulation of colonic transit. Gastroenterology 1988; 94:1351–1356.
82. Moore WEC, Moore LVH, Cato EP. You and your flora. US Fed Culture Collect Newslett 1988; 18:7–22.
83. Stephen AM, Cummings JH. The microbial contribution to human faecal mass. J Med Microbiol 1980; 13:45–56.
84. Simon GL, Gorbach SL. Intestinal flora and gastrointestinal function. Johnson LRPhysiology of the gastrointestinal tract. 2nd ed New York: Raven Press, 1987:1729–1747.
85. Dunn DL. Autochthonous microflora of the gastrointestinal tract. Perspect Colon Rectal Surg 1989; 2(2):105–119.
86. Guarner F, Malagalade JR, Gut Flora in health and disease. Lancet 2003; 361:512–519.
87. Plaa GL. The enterohepatic circulation. In: Gillete JR, ed. Handbook of Experimental Pharmacology. New York: Springer-Verlag, 1975; 28:130–149.
88. Bokkenheuser V. The friendly anaerobes. Clin Infect Dis 1993; 16(suppl 4): S427–S434.
89. Basson MD, Liu YW, Hanly AM, Emenaker NT, Shenoy SG, Gould Rothberg BE. Indentification and comperative analysis of human colonocyte short-chain fatty acid response genes. J Gastrointest Surg 2000; 4:501–512.
90. Hampe J, Cuthbert A, Croucher PJ, et al. Association between insertion mutation in NOD2 gene and Crohn's disease in German and British populations. Lancet 2001; 357:1925–1928.
91. D'Haens GR, Geboes K, Peeters M, Baert F, Penninckx F, Rutgeerts P. Early lesions of recurrent Crohn's disease caused by infusion of intestinal contents in excluded ileum. Gastroenterology 1998; 114:262–267.
92. Casellas F, Borruel N, Papo M, et al. Anti-inflammatory effects of enterically coated amoxicillin-clavulanic acid in active ulcerative colitis. Inflamm Bowel Dis 1998; 4:1–5.
93. McFarland LV, Surawicz CM, Greenberg RN, et al. Prevention of beta-lactam-associated diarrhea by Saccharomyces boulardii compared with placebo. Am J Gastroenterol 1995; 90:439–448.
94. Armuzzi A, Cremonini F, Bartolozzi F, et al. The effect of oral administration of Lactobacillus GG on antibiotic-associated gastrointestinal side-effects during Helicobacter pylori eradication therapy. Aliment Pharmacol Ther 2001; 15:163–169.
95. D'Souza AL, Rajkumar C, Cooke J, Bulpitt CJ. Probiotics in prevention of antibiotic associated diarrhoea: Meta-analysis. BMJ 2002; 324:1361–1366.
96. Burns AJ, Rowland IR. Anti-carcinogenicity of probiotics and prebiotics. Curr Issues Incest Microbiol 2000; 1:13–24.
97. Levitt MD. Intestinal gas production—Recent advances in flatology. N Engl J Med 1980; 302:1474–1475.
98. Devroede G, Arhan P, Schang JC. Orderly and disorderly fecal continence. Kodner I, Fry RD, Roc JP, eds. Colon, Rectal and Anal surgery. St. Louis: CV Mosby, 1985:40–62.
99. Schuster MM, Mendeloff AJ. Characteristics of rectosigmoid motor function; Their relationship to continence, defecation and disease. Glass CBJ, ed. Progress in gastroenterology. New York: Grune & Stratton 1970:Vol. 2.
100. Schuster MM. The riddle of the sphincters. Gastroenterology 1975; 69:249–262.
101. Felt-Bersma RJF, Gort G, Meuwissen SGM. Normal values in anal manometry and rectal sensation: A problem of range. Hepatogastroenterology 1991; 38:444–449.
102. Varma JS, Smith AN. Anorectal profilometry with the micro-transducer. Br J Surg 1984; 71:867–869.
103. Nivatvongs S, Stern HS, Fryd DS. The length of the anal canal. Dis Colon Rectum 1981; 24:600–601.
104. McHugh SM, Diamant NE. Anal canal pressure profile: A reappraisal as determined by rapid pullthrough technique. Gut 1987; 28:1234–1241.
105. Cali RL, Blatchford GJ, Perry RE, Pitsch RM, Thorson AG, Christiansen MA. Normal variations in anorectal manometry. Dis Colon Rectum 1992; 35: 1161–1164.
106. Duthie HL, Watts JM. Contribution of the external anal sphincter to the pressure zone in the anal canal. Gut 1965; 6:64–68.
107. Frenckner B, Enler CV. Influence of pudendal block on the function of the anal sphincters. Gut 1975; 16:482–489.
108. Schweiger M. Funktionelle Analsphinkteruntersuchungen. Berlin: Springer-Verlag, 1982.
109. Lestar B, Penninckx F, Kerremans R. The composition of anal basal pressure. An in-vivo and in-vitro study in man. Int J Colorectal Dis 1989; 4:118–122.
110. Frenckner B, Ihre T. Influence of autonomic nerves on the internal anal sphincter in man. Gut 1976; 17:306–312.
111. Meunier P, Mollard P. Control of the internal anal sphincter (manometric study with human subjects). Pflügers Arch 1977; 370:233–239.
112. Gunterberg B, Kewenter J, Petersen J, Stener B. Anorectal function after major resections of the sacrum with bilateral or unilateral sacrifice of sacral nerves. Br J Surg 1976; 63:546–554.
113. Kumar D, Waldron D, Williams NS, Browning C, Hutton MR, Wingate DL. Prolonged anorectal manometry and external sphincter electromyography in ambulant human subjects. Dig Dis Sci 1990; 35:641–648.
114. Varma KK, Stephens D. Neuromuscular reflexes of rectal continence. Aust N Z J Surg 1972; 41:263–272.
115. Parks AG, Porter NH, Melzak J. Experimental study of the reflex mechanism controlling the muscles of the pelvic floor. Dis Colon Rectum 1962; 5: 407–414.
116. Lierse W, Holschneider AM, Steinfield J. The relative proportions of Type I and Type II muscle fibers in the external sphincter ani muscle of different ages and stages of development—Observations on the development of continence. Eur J Pediatr Surg 1993; 3:28–32.
117. Stephens FD, Smith ED. Anorectal malformations in children. Chicago: Year Book Medical Publishers, 1971:p. 28.
118. Rühl A, Thewisen M, Ross HG, Cleveland S, Frieling T, Enck P. Discharge patterns of intramural mechanoreceptive afferents during selective distension of the cat's rectum. Neurogastroenterol Motil 1998; 10:219–25.
119. Lynn PA, Olsson C, Zagorodnyuk V, Costa M, Brookes SJ. Rectal intraganglionic laminar endings are transduction sites of extrinsic mechanoreceptors in the guinea pig rectum. Gastroenterology 2003; 125:786–794.
120. Sun WM, Read NW, Prior A, Daly JA, Cheah SK, Grundy D. Sensory and motor responses to rectal distension vary according to rate and pattern of balloon inflation. Gastroenterology 1990; 99:1008–1015.
121. Sabate JM, Coffin B, Jian R, Le Bars D, Bouhassira D. Rectal sensitivity assessed by a reflexologic technique: further evidence for two types of mechanoreceptors. AJP Gastrointest Liver Physiol 2000; 279:G692–G699.
122. Coulie B, Tack J, Demedts I, Vos R, Janssens J. Influence of sumatriptan on rectal tone and on the perception of rectal distension in man. Neurogastroenterol Motil 1998; 10:66.
123. Schkowski A, Thewissen M, Mathis C, Ross HG, Enck P. Serotonin type-4 receptors modulate the sensitivity of intramural mechanoreceptive afferents of the cat's rectum. Neurogastroenterol motil 2002; 14:217–219.
124. van der Veek PPJ, Schots EDCM, Masclee AAM. Effect of neurotensin on colorectal motor and sensory function in humans. Dis Colon Rectum 2004; 47:210–218.
125. Bampton PA, Dinning PG, Kennedy ML, Lubowski DZ, Cook IJ. The proximal colonic motor response to rectal mechanical and chemical stimulation. AJP Gastrointest Liver Physiol 2002; 282:G443-G449.
126. Kern MK, Jaradeh S, Arndorfer RC, Jesmanowicz A, Hyde J, Shaker R. Gender differences in cortical representation of rectal distension in healthy humans. AJP Gastrointest Liver Physiol 2001; 281:G1512-G1523.
127. Sorensen M, Rasmussen O, Tetzscher T, Christiansen J. Physiological Variation in rectal compliance. Br J Surg 1992; 79:1106–1108.

128. Sloots CEJ, Felt-Bersma RJF, Cuesta MA, Meuwissen SGM. Rectal visceral sensitivity in healthy volunteers: influences of gender, age and methods. Neurogastroenterol Motil 2000; 12:361–368.
129. Gladman MA, Dvorkin LS, Lunniss PJ, Williams NS, Scott SM. Rectal hyposensitivity: A disorder of the rectal wall or the afferent pathway? An assessment using the barostat. Am J Gastroenterol 2005; 100:106–114.
130. De Medici A, Badiali D, Corazziari E, Bausano G, Anzini F. Rectal sensitivity in chronic constipation. Dig Dis Sci 1992; 34:747–753.
131. Gladman MA, Scott SM, Williams NS, Lunniss PJ. Clinical and physiologic findings and possible aetiological factors of rectal hyposensitivity. Br J Surg 2003; 90:860–866.
132. Gosselink MJ, Hop WCJ, Schouten WR. Rectal compliance in women with obstructed defecation. Dis Colon Rectum 2001; 44:971–977.
133. Gosselink MJ, Schouten WR. Rectal sensory perception in women with obstructed defecation. Dis Colon Rectum 2001; 44:1337–1344.
134. Duthie HL, Gairns FN. Sensory nerve endings and sensation in the anal region of man. Br J Surg 1960; 47:585–595.
135. Read MG, Read NW. The role of ano-rectal sensation in preserving continence. Gut 1982; 23:345–347.
136. Miller R, Bartolo DCC, Cervero F, Mortensen NJ McC. Anorectal temperature sensation: A comparison of normal and incontinent patients. Br J Surg 1987; 74:511–515.
137. Lubowski DZ, Nicholls RJ, Swash M, Jordan MJ. Neural control of internal anal sphincter function. Br J Surg 1987; 74:668–670.
138. Carlstedt A, Nordgren S, Fasth S, Appelgren L, Hulten L. Sympathetic nervous influence on the internal anal sphincter and rectum in man. Int J Col Dis 1988; 3:90–95.
139. Gutierrez JG, Shak AN. Autonomic control of the internal anal sphincter in man. van Trappen G, ed. Fifth International Symposium on Gastrointestinal Motility. Herentals, Belgium: Typoff Press, 1975:363–373.
140. Burleigh DE, D'Mello A, Parks AG. Responses of isolated human internal anal sphincter to drugs and electrical field stimulation. Gastroenterology 1979; 77:484–490.
141. Paskins JR, Clayden GS, Lawson JON. Some pharmacological responses of isolated internal anal sphincter strips from chronically constipated children. Scand J Gastroenterol 1982; 17:155–156.
142. Localio SA, Eng K, Ranson JHC. Abdominosacral approach for retrorectal tumors. Ann Surg 1980; 191:555–558.
143. Burleigh DE, D'Mello A. Physiology and pharmacology of the internal anal sphincter. Henry MM, Swash M, eds. Coloproctology and the Pelvic Floor. London: Butterworths, 1985.
144. Tottrup A, Glavind EB, Swane D. Involvement of the L-arginine-nitric oxide pathway in internal anal sphincter relaxation. Gastroenterology 1992; 102:409–415.
145. Chakder S, Rattan S. Release of nitric oxide by activation of nonadrenergic, noncholinergic neurons of internal anal sphincter. Am J Physiol 1992; 264:G7–G12.
146. Rattan S, Chakder S. Role of nitric oxide as a mediator of internal anal sphincter relaxation. Am J Physiol 1992; 262:G107–G112.
147. O'Kelly TJ, Brading AF, Mortensen NJ McC. Nerve mediated relaxation of the human internal anal sphincter. Gut 1993; 34:689–693.
148. O'Kelly TJ, Davies JR, Brading AF, Mortensen NJ McC. Distribution of nitric oxide synthase containing neurons in the rectal myenteric plexus and anal canal. Dis Colon Rectum 1994; 37:350–357.
149. Ferrara A, Pemberton JH, Levin KE, Hanson RB. Relationship between anal canal tone and rectal motor activity. Dis Colon Rectum 1993; 36:337–342.
150. Duthie HL. Anal continence. Gut 1978; 12:844–852.
151. Parks AG, Porter NH, Hardcastle J. The syndrome of the descending perineum. Proc R Soc Med 1966; 59:477–482.
152. Bannister JJ, Gibbons C, Read NW. Preservation of fecal continence during rises in intra-abdominal pressure: Is there a role for the flap valve? Gut 1987; 28:1242–1245.
153. Bartolo DCC, Roe AM, Locke-Edmunds JC, Virjee J, Mortensen NJ McC. Flap valve theory of anorectal continence. Br J Surg 1986; 73:1012–1014.
154. Stelzner F. The morphological principles of anorectal continence. Rickham PP, Hecker WCh, Prévot J, eds. Anorectal Malformations and Associated Diseases. Progress in Pediatric Surgery Series. Munich: Urban und Schwarzenberg1976; (9):1–6.
155. Duthie HL. Dynamics of the rectum and anus. Clin Gastroenterol 1975; 4:467–477.
156. Lubowski DZ, Meagher AP, Smart RC, Batleo SP. Scintigraphic assesment of colonic function during defecation. Int J Colo rectal Dis 1995; 10:91–93.
157. Kamm MA, van der Sijp JR, Lennard-Jones JE. Colorectal and anal motility during defecation. Lancet 1992; 339:820.
158. Karaus M, Sarna SK. Giant migrating contractions during defecation in the dog colon. Gastroenterology 1987; 92:925–933.
159. Hagger R, Kumar D, Benson M, Grundy A. Periodic colonic motor activity identified by 24-h pancolonic ambulatory manometry in humans. Neurogastroenterol Motil 2002; 14:271–278.
160. Bell AM, Pemberton JH, Hanson RB, Zinsmeister AR. Variations in muscle tone of the human rectum: recordings with an electromechanical barostat. Am J Physiol 1991; 260:G17-G25.
161. Leroi AM, Saiter C, Roussignol J, Weber J, Denis P. Increased tone of the rectal wall in response to feeding persists in patients with cauda equina syndrome. Neurogastrolenterol Motil 1999; 11:243–245.
162. Musial F, Crowell MD, Kalveram KTh, Enck P. Nutrient ingestion increases rectal sensitivity in humans. Physiol Behav 1994; 55:953–956.
163. Gosselink MJ, Schouten WR. The perineo-rectal reflex. Dis Colon rectum 2002; 45:370–376.
164. Shafik A, Ahmed I, El-Sibai O. Effect of perineal compression on rectal tone: A study of the mechanism of action. Dis Colon rectum 2003; 46:1366–1370.
165. Frenckner B. Function of the anal sphincters in spinal man. Gut 1975; 16:638.
166. Henry MM, Snooks SJ, Barnes PRH, Swash M. Investigation of disorders of the anorectum and colon. Ann R Coll Surg Engl 1985; 67:355–360.
167. Miller R, Bartolo DCC, James D, Mortensen NJ McC. Air-filled microballoon manometry for use in anorectal physiology. Br J Surg 1989; 76:72–75.
168. Jonas U, Klotter HJ. Study of three urethral pressure recording devices: Theoretical considerations. Urol Res 1978; 6:119–125.
169. Hancock BD. Measurement of anal pressure and motility. Gut 1976; 17: 645–651.
170. Schouten WR, van Vroonhoven Th JMV. A simple method of anorectal manometry. Dis Colon Rectum 1983; 26:721–724.
171. Coller JA. Clinical application of anorectal manometry. Gastroenterol Clin North Am 1987; 16:17–33.
172. Jameson JS, Chia YW, Kamm MA, Speajman CTM, Chye YH, Henry MM. Effect of age, sex and parity on anorectal function. Br J Surg 1994; 81: 1689–1692.
173. McHugh SM, Diamant NE. Effect of age, gender and parity on anal canal pressures. Contribution of impaired anal sphincter function to fecal continence. Dig Dis Sci 1987; 32:726–736.
174. Matheson DM, Keighley MRB. Manometric evaluation of rectal prolapse and fecal incontinence. Gut 1981; 22:126–129.
175. Taylor BM, Beart RW, Phillips SF. Longitudinal and radial variations of pressure in the human anal canal. Gastroenterology 1984; 86:693–697.
176. Haadem K, Dahlström JA, Ling L. Anal sphincter competence in healthy women: Clinical implications of age and other factors. Obstet Gynecol 1991; 78:823–827.
177. Sultan AH, Kamm MA, Hudson CN, Bartram CI. Effect of pregnancy on anal sphincter morphology and function. Int J Colorectal Dis 1993; 8:206–209.
178. Schouten WR, Blankensteijn JD. Ultraslow wave pressure variations in the anal canal before and after lateral internal sphincterotomy. Int J Colorectal Dis 1992; 7:115–118.
179. Bouvier M, Gonella J. Nervous control of the internal sphincter in the cat. J Physiol (Lond) 1981; 310:457–469.
180. Williamson JL, Nelson RL, Orsay C, Pearl RK, Abcarian H. A comparison of simultaneous longitudinal and radial recordings of anal canal pressures. Dis Colon Rectum 1990; 33:201–206.
181. Read NW, Harford WV, Schmulen AC, Read MC, Santa Ana C, Fordtran JS. A clinical study of patients with fecal incontinence and diarrhoea. Gastroenterology 1979; 76:747–756.
182. Schouten RW, van Vroonhoven Th JMV. Lateral internal sphincterotomy in the treatment of hemorrhoids. A clinical and manometric study. Dis Colon Rectum 1986; 29:869–872.
183. Johnson GP, Pemberton JH, Ness J, Samson M, Zinsmeister AR. Transducer manometry and the effect of body position on anal canal pressures. Dis Colon Rectum 1990; 33:469–475.
184. Womack NR, Williams NS, Holmfield JHM, Morrison JFB, Simpkins KC. New method for dynamic assessment of anorectal function in constipation. Br J Surg 1985; 72:994–998.
185. Halligan S, Thomas J, Bartram C. Intrarectal pressure and balloon expulsion related to evacuation proctography. Gut 1995; 37:100–104.
186. Mahieu P, Pringot J, Bodart P. Defecography. I. Description of a new procedure and results in normal patients. Gastrointest Radiol 1984; 9:247–251.
187. Preston DM, Lennard-Jones JE, Thomas BM. The balloon proctogram. Br J Surg 1984; 71:29–32.
188. Agachan F, Pfeifer J, Wexner SD. Defecography and proctography. Results of 744 patients. Dis Colon Rectum 1996; 39:899–905.
189. Lestar B, Penninckx FM, Kerremans RP. Defecometry. A new method for determining the parameters of rectal evacuation. Dis Colon Rectum 1989; 32:197–201.
190. Mellgren A, Bremmer S, Johansson C, Dolk A, Uden R, Ahlback SO, Holmstrom B. Defecography. Results of investigations in 2816 patients. Dis Colon Rectum 1994; 37:1133–1141.
191. Stojkovic SG, Balfour L, Burke D, Finan PJ, Sagar PM. Does the need to self-digitate or the presence of a large or nonemptying rectocele on proctography influence the outcome of transanal rectocele repair? Colorectal Disease 2003; 5:169–172.
192. Barkel DC, Pemberton JH, Pezim ME, Phillips SF, Kelly KA, Brown ML. Scintigraphic assessment of the anorectal angle in health and after ileal pouch-anal anastomosis. Ann Surg 1988; 208:42–49.
193. Hutchinson R, Mostafa AB, Grant EA, Smith NB, Deen KI, Harding LK, Kumas D. Scintigraphic defecography: Quantitative and dynamic assessment of anorectal function. Dis Colon Rectum 1993; 36:1132–1138.

194. Yang XM, Partanen K, Farin P, Soimakallio S. Defecography. Acta Radiol 1995; 36:460–468.
195. Jorge JM, Habr-Gama A, Wexner SD. Clinical applications and techniques of cinedefecography. Am J Surg 2001; 181(1):93–101.
196. Fletcher JG, Busse RF, Riederer SJ, Hough D, Gluecker T, Harper CM, Bharucha AE. Magnetic resonance imaging of anatomic and dynamic defects of the pelvic floor in defecatory disorders. Am J Gastroenterology 2003; 98: 399–411.
197. Roos JE, Weishaupt D, Wildermuth S, Willmann JK, Marincek B, Hilfiker PR. Experience of 4 years with open MR defecography: Pictorial review of anorectal anatomy and disease. Radiographics 2002; 22:817–832.
198. Karasick S, Karasick D, Karasick SR. Functional disorders of the anus and rectum: Findings on defecography. AJR 1993; 160:777–782.
199. Rubens DJ, Strang JG, Bogineni-Misra S, Wexler IE. Transperineal sonography of the rectum: Anatomy and pathology revealed by sonography compared with CT and MR imaging. Am J Roentgenol 1998; 170:637–642.
200. Kleinübing H, Jannini JF, Malafaia O, Brenner S, Pinho M. Transperineal ultrasonography: new method to image the anorectal region. Dis Colon Rectum 2000; 43:1572–1574.
201. Piloni V. Dynamic imaging of the pelvic floor with transperineal sonography. Tech Coloproctol 2001; 5:103–105.
202. Beer-Gabel M, Teshler M, Schechtman E, Zbar AP. Dynamic transperineal ultrasound vs. defecography in patients with evacuatory difficulty: A pilot study. Int J Colorectal Dis 2004; 19:60–67.
203. Sentovich SM, Rivela LJ, Thorson AG, Christensen MA, Blatchford GJ. Simultaneous dynamic proctography and peritoneography for pelvic floor disorders. Dis Colon Rectum 1995; 38:912–915.
204. Ekberg O, Nylander G, Fork FT. Defecography. Radiology 1985; 155:45–48.
205. Jorge JM, Yang YK, Wexner SD. Incidence and clinical significance of sigmoidoceles as determined by a new classification system. Dis Colon Rectum 1994; 37:1112–1117.
206. Bremmer S, Ahlback SO, Uden R, Mellgren A. Simultaneous defecography and peritoneography in defecation disorders. Dis Colon Rectum 1995; 38:969–973.
207. Altringer WE, Saclarides TJ, Dominguez JM, Brubaker LT, Smith CS. Four-contrast defecography: Pelvic "floor-oscopy." Dis Colon Rectum 1995; 38: 695–699.
208. Beck DE. Simplified balloon expulsion test. Dis Colon Rectum 1992; 35: 597–598.
209. Dahl J, Lindquist BL, Tysk C, Leissner P, Philipson L, Järnerot G. Behavioral medicine treatment in chronic constipation with paradoxical anal sphincter contraction. Dis Colon Rectum 1990; 34:769–776.
210. Minguez M, Herreros B, Sanchiz V, Hernandez V, Almela P, Anon R, Mora F, Benages A. Predictive value of the balloon expulsion test for excluding the diagnosis of pelvic floor dyssynergia in constipation. Gastroenterology 2004; 126:57–62.
211. Bartolo DCC, Read MG, Read NW. The saline continence test. Dynamic studies in fecal incontinence, hemorrhoids and the descending perineum syndrome. Acta Gastroenterol Belg 1985; 48:39–50.
212. Read NW, Haynes WG, Bartolo DC, Hall J, Read MG, Donnelly TC, Johnson AG. Use of anorectal manometry during rectal in fusion of saline to investigate sphincter function in incontinent patients. Gastroenterology 1983; 85:105–113.
213. Roe AM, Bartolo DCC, Mortensen NJ McC. New method for assessment of anal sensation in various anorectal disorders. Br J Surg 1986; 73:310–312.
214. Broens PMA, Penninckx FM. Relation between anal electrosensitivity and rectal filling sensation and the influence of age. Dis Colom rectum 2005; 48:127–330.
215. Chan CL, Scott SM, Birch MJ, Knowles CH, Williams NS, Lunniss PJ. Rectal heat thresholds: A novel test of the sensory afferent pathway. Dis Colon Rectum 2003; 46:590–595.
216. Toma TP, Zighelboim J, Phillips SF, Talley NJ. Methods for studying intestinal sensitivity and compliance: in vitro studies of balloons and a barostat. Neurogastroenterol Motility 1996; 8:19–28.
217. Varma JS. Autonomic influences on colorectal motility and pelvic surgery. World J Surg 1992; 16:811–819.
218. Rasmussan O, Sorensen M, Tetzschor T, Christiansen J. Dynamic and manometry in the assessment of patients with obstructed defecation. Dis Colon Rectum 1993; 36:901–907.
219. Kendell GPM, Thompson DG, Day SJ, Lennard-Jones JE. Inter- and intra individual variation in pressure volume relations of the rectum in normal subjects and patients with the irritable bowel syndrome. Gut 1990; 31:1062–1068.
220. Alstrup NI, Skjoldbye B, Rasmussen OØ, Christensen NEH, Christiansen J. Rectal compliance determined by rectal endosonography. A new application of endosongraphy. Dis Colon Rectum 1995; 38:32–36.
221. Snooks SJ, Swash M. Electromyography and nerve latency studies. Gooszen HG, ten Cate Hoedemaker HO, Weterman IT, Keighley MRB, eds. Disordered Defecation. Dordrecht, The Netherlands: Nyhoff, 1987.
222. Jost WH, Ecker KW, Schimrigk K. Surface versus needle electrodes in determination of motor conduction time to the external anal sphincter. Int J Colorectal Dis 1994; 9:197–199.
223. Snooks SJ, Swash M. Slowed motor conduction in the lumbosacral nerve roots in cauda equina lesions. J Neurol Neurosurg Psychiatry 1986; 49:808–816.
224. Percy JP, Neill ME, Swash M, Parks AG. Electrophysiological study of motor nerve supply of pelvic floor. Lancet 1981; 1:16–17.
225. Pittman JS, Benson JT, Summers JE. Physiologic evaluation of the anorectum: A new ultrasound technique. Dis Colon Rectum 1990; 33:476–478.
226. Felt-Bersma RJF, van Baren R, Koorevaar M, Strijers RL, Cuesta MA. Unsuspected sphincter defects shown by anal endosonography after anorectal surgery. Dis Colon Rectum 1995; 38:249–253.
227. Carty NJ, Moran B, Johnson CD. Anorectal physiology measurements are of no value in clinical practice. True or false? Ann R Coll Surg Engl 1994; 76:276–80.
228. Wexner SD, Jorge JMN. Colorectal physiological tests: use or abuse of technology? Eur J Surg 1994; 160:167–174.
229. Penninckx FM, Lestar B, Kerremans RP. A new balloon-retaining test for evaluation of anorectal function in incontinent patients. Dis Colon Rectum 1989; 32:202–205.
230. Perry RE, Blatchford GJ, Christensen MA, Thorson AG, Attwood SE. Manometric diagnosis of anal sphincter injuries. Am J Surg 1990; 159:112–117.
231. Sultan AH, Kamm MA, Bartram CI, Hudson CN. Third-degree obstetric anal sphincter tears: risk factors and outcome of primary repair. BMJ 1994; 308: 887–891.
232. Sultan AH, Kamm MA, Hudson CN, Bartram CI. Anal sphicter disruption during vaginal delivery. N Engl J Med 1993; 329:1905–1911.
233. Deen KI, Kumar D, Williams JG, Olliff J, Keighley MRB. The prevalence of anal sphincter defects in fecal incontinence: A prospective endosonic study. Gut 1993; 34:685–688.
234. Hiltunen KM, Matikainen M, Auvinen O, Hietanen P. Clinical and manometric evaluation of anal sphincter function in patients with rectal prolapse. Am J Surg 1986; 151:489–492.
235. Skomorowska E, Hegedus V, Christiansen J. Evaluation of perineal descent by defaecography. Int J Colorectal Dis 1988; 3:191–194.
236. Farouk R, Duthie GS, MacGregor AB, Bartolo DCC. Sustained internal sphincter hypertonia in patients with chronic anal fissure. Dis Colon Rectum 1994; 37:424–429.
237. Hancock BD. Internal sphincter and the nature of haemorrhoids. Gut 1976; 18:651–656.
238. Schouten WR, Blankensteijn JD. Ultra slow wave pressure variations in the anal ianal before and after lateral internal sphincterotomy. Int J Colorectal Dis 1992; 7:115–118.
239. Schouten WR, Briel JW, Auwerda JJA, de Graaf EJR. Ischaemic nature of anal fissure. Br J Surg 1996; 83:63–65.
240. Duthie HL. Defecation and the anal sphincters. Clin Gastroenterol 1982; 11:121–131.
241. Belliveau P, Thomson JP, Parks AG. Fistula-in-ano: A manometric study. Dis Colon Rectum 1983; 26:152–154.
242. Sainio P, Husa A. A prospective manometric study of the effect of anal fistula surgery on anorectal function. Acta Chir Scand 1985; 151:279–288.
243. Heppell J, Kelly KA, Phillips SF, Beart KW, Telander RL, Perrault J. Physiologic aspects of continence after colectomy, mucosat proctectomy, and ileoanal anastomosis. Ann Surg 1982; 195:435–443.
244. Lindquist K, Liljeqvist L, Sellberg B. The topography of ileoanal reservoirs in relation to evacuation patterns and clinical functions. Acta Chir Scand 1984; 150:573–579.
245. Stryker SJ, Kelly KA, Phillips SF, Dozois RR, Beart RW Jr. Anal and neorectal function after ileal pouch-anal anastomosis. Ann Surg 1986; 203:55–61.
246. Stryker SJ, Daube JR, Kelly KA, Telander RI, Phillips SF, Beart RW Jr, Dozois RR. Anal sphincter electromyography after colectomy, mucosal rectectomy, and ileoanal anastomosis. Arch Surg 1985; 120:713–716.
247. Beart RW Jr, Dozois RR, Wolff BG, Pemberton JH. Mechanisms of rectal continence. Lessons from the ileoanal procedure. Am J Surg 1985; 149:31–34.
248. Tjandra JJ. Ooi BS, Han WR. Anorectal physiologic testing for bowel dysfunction in patients with spinal cord lesions. Dis Colon Rectum 2000; 43:927–931.

3 Diagnosis

Santhat Nivatvongs

PATIENT HISTORY

Specific history taking is an important aspect in the diagnosis of colorectal and anal disorders. Because there are myriad signs and symptoms in these diseases, physicians should ask questions in a way that will pinpoint the diagnosis or narrow the differential diagnosis.

■ SYMPTOMS

Bleeding per Anus

In an extensive and thorough review of the literature, Fijten et al. (1) set out to determine the occurrence and clinical significance of overt blood loss per rectum in the general population and in medical practice. The incidence of this symptom in the general population was approximately 20 per 100 people per year, the "consultation" incidence in general practice was approximately six per 1000, and the incidence of referral to a medical specialist about seven per 10,000 per year. The predictive value of anorectal blood loss for colorectal malignancy was estimated to be less than one in 1000 in the general population, approximately two per 100 in general practice, and as many as 36 per 100 in referral patients.

The differential diagnosis of an anorectal condition frequently can be made by the accurate delineation of the type of bleeding experienced by the patient. The types of issues regarding bleeding to be determined are: Is the patient passing clots or is it true melena? Is the blood mixed with or separate from the stool? Does the blood appear on the toilet tissue or does it drip into the toilet bowl?

Blood that drips into the toilet bowl and is bright red, free, and separate from the stool is frequently associated with bleeding internal hemorrhoids. Blood that is on the toilet tissue tends to be associated with anal fissures or an abrasion of the anal canal. Although melena can be caused by any pathologic process higher up in the gastrointestinal (GI) tract, it also can come from the right colon. The association of blood and mucus usually indicates a low-lying carcinoma or, more frequently, an inflammatory condition, such as ulcerative colitis or Crohn's disease. If blood clots are being passed, the source usually is of colonic origin. A rare cause of "bleeding" that frequently is misdiagnosed comes from eating beets. The main coloring matter in beets is from betacyanins, which are violet-red pigments that can mimic blood in the toilet water.

Pain

ANORECTAL PAIN ■ Anorectal pain that occurs during and following a bowel movement and that is described as sharp in nature usually is associated with an anal fissure or an abrasion in the anal canal. Tenesmus, which is a symptom complex of straining and the urge to defecate, frequently is associated with inflammatory or neoplastic conditions of the anorectum. Because the lower anal canal obtains its innervation from the somatic nervous system, any pain-producing lesion in the anal canal is likely to be described as sharp, burning, or stinging. The pain associated with a perianal abscess usually is described as throbbing in nature. Pain that increases in intensity when the patient coughs or sneezes often is associated with an intersphincteric abscess.

Because anorectal pain may be referred to the sacral region, great care must be taken in eliciting the history as it relates to a bowel movement. The classic history of levator ani muscle spasm, better known as proctalgia fugax, frequently is misdiagnosed as hemorrhoidal or fissure pain. Referred pain to the rectum may occur from aneurysmal dilatations in the pelvic vascular tree or from retrorectal tumors. Usually, this condition is described as a feeling of fullness in the area.

Coccygeal pain rarely is anal in origin; most patients who complain of this type of pain have sustained some trauma to the ligaments or periosteum of the coccyx. Occasionally when a presacral cyst is inflamed, the pain may be referred to the coccyx.

ABDOMINAL PAIN ■ Abdominal pain tends to be nonspecific. Pain from the cecum usually is located in the right lower quadrant, while pain from the sigmoid colon is located in the left lower quadrant. Pain experienced in the lower rectum may be referred pain from the sigmoid colon, whereas pain originating in the rectum itself usually is experienced in the perineum and rarely in the hypogastrium. Obstruction of the left colon may manifest as pain in the right lower quadrant because of the distention of the cecum. The character and duration of pain and its relation to meals should be determined.

Abdominal pain that originates from the colon may be crampy in nature when related to an intramural lesion or to excessive colonic contraction or distention, or it may be associated with peritoneal irritation when related to any inflammation in the colon. When the mesentery of the colon is stretched, pain will be experienced, and this can be duplicated in the process of performing a proctosigmoidoscopic or colonoscopic examination. Peritoneal pain may be secondary to colonic disease when there are adhesions between the colon and the parietes. Sites of referred pain to the body surface are determined by the same principles as referred pain elsewhere; pain from the colon is referred to just above the symphysis pubis, and rectal pain can go directly to the sacral area.

Abdominal pain may be a manifestation of anorectal disease when the supralevator space is involved. Because this space has peritoneum as its "roof," a suppurative process may result in signs of peritoneal irritation.

Change in Bowel Habits

CONSTIPATION ■ A normal person should have at least three bowel movements per week (2). To a patient, constipation may mean a variety of conditions, such as stools that are infrequent, hard, small, or difficult to pass. To determine the necessity for further investigation, it is important to know the duration of the constipation, whether the onset is recent or if the condition is a chronic one. Constipation can be the result of a pelvic floor disorder. Appropriate investigation can reveal the location of the problem (3).

DIARRHEA ■ Diarrhea is a symptom of many gastrointestinal diseases. The duration, amount, character, and frequency of the diarrhea should be determined. Clear watery diarrhea may be from a large secretory rectal villous adenoma. A bloody mucous diarrhea may indicate inflammatory bowel disease. Operative procedures such as vagotomy, cholecystectomy, or small bowel resection may alter gastrointestinal motility, absorption, and secretion, and consequently will alter bowel habits. Patients who have had a jejunoileal bypass for morbid obesity are subject to many anorectal problems associated with diarrhea.

Discharge

MUCUS ■ Mucus is secreted by the goblet cells of the colonic and rectal mucosa and may be seen in the stool under many different circumstances. It may be either (1) the result of normal production of mucus, (2) the early sign of a villous adenoma of the rectum, (3) the indication of an early colitic condition, or (4) caused by chemical irritants. The packaged buffered phosphate enemas (e.g., Phospho-soda) can elicit a tremendous response from the bowel, and one is immediately impressed with the amount of mucus seen on endoscopic examination of the bowel after administration of such an enema. If the mucus is associated with bleeding, it may be the sign of a neoplasm or an inflammatory process.

Normally, mucus should not leak through the anus unless the patient is incontinent. Soiling of underwear may be a sign of rectal mucosal prolapse, ectropion from a previous hemorrhoidectomy, or overproduction of mucus, such as occurs with a villous adenoma.

PURULENT DISCHARGE ■ Purulent discharge is indicative of an infectious process. A history of purulent discharge and pain is characteristic for an anorectal abscess, whereas a painless purulent discharge more likely is due to a fistula-in-ano. Passing pus per rectum may indicate a gonococcal proctitis or a spontaneously drained intersphincteric abscess.

FECAL SOILING ■ Fecal soiling of underwear usually is asymptomatic. However, it may be a consequence of early postoperative anorectal procedures, such as hemorrhoidectomy, internal sphincterotomy, and fistulotomy. Fecal soiling is relatively common in the elderly. Fecal soiling must not be mistaken as fecal incontinence.

Perianal Swelling

One must always determine whether or not a perianal swelling is painful and whether it has discharged blood or pus. The swelling also might be intermittent as would be expected with a prolapsing hypertrophied anal papilla. If the swelling is associated with fever and chills, an anorectal abscess should be suspected. The common swelling at the anal verge usually is a thrombosed external hemorrhoid, which develops rather quickly and, if ulcerated, is associated with pain and occasional bleeding.

Pruritus

Pruritus ani, intense itching, is a common symptom associated with anorectal pathology. Most often it occurs in patients who have loose stools and are unable to properly cleanse the anal area. Pruritus also may be associated with the healing phase of an anal condition. Severe pruritus ani usually is associated with a mucoid discharge, which may be blood tinged from the open ulceration of the perianal skin. The patient always should be questioned regarding the use of antibiotics, because these drugs may be the cause of the pruritus ani. In rare cases, pruritus ani in adults may be caused by *Enterobius vermicularis* (pinworms).

Prolapse

In questioning the patient who presents with a protrusion from the anal aperture, it should be determined whether the prolapse occurs only at the time of defecation or whether it occurs independently. Independent prolapsing is more suggestive of a hypertrophied anal papilla or a complete rectal procidentia. Does the prolapse reduce itself spontaneously, or must it be replaced manually? This may suggest the magnitude of the problem. Frequently the patient can give an idea of the relative size of the prolapsing mass; this information often helps in making the diagnosis. The most common prolapsing condition is rectal mucosal prolapse associated with prolapsing hemorrhoids. This must be differentiated from true procidentia of the rectum. Large hypertrophied anal papillae also are known to prolapse from the anal canal. Polyps in the rectum can prolapse; however, this usually is seen in a child with juvenile polyposis or in an elderly patient with a massive villous adenoma.

Incontinence

When a patient presents with a history of incontinence following a previous anorectal surgical procedure, the details of that procedure must be elicited to evaluate the complaints completely. In a parous woman, a good obstetric history should be obtained regarding the nature of an episiotomy and any complications associated with it, as well as the nature and type of delivery. In bedridden elderly patients, fecal impaction may be the cause of overflow incontinence.

Loss of Weight

With the current fad of staying slim, it should be determined that weight loss is not the result of a dieting program. It is important to note the amount of weight loss occurring over a given time period. Rapid loss of weight without obvious reasons may indicate gastrointestinal disease or malignancy.

Flatulence

Because everyone passes gas through the rectum, it should be determined whether this is actually an excessive passage of flatus or merely an unusual sense of awareness of the normal passage. Most patients with increased flatulence are found to have a dietary indiscretion in the form of excessive intake of gas-producing substances, rather than a specific malady of the gastrointestinal tract. Patients are not aware that fermentation is taking place all the time in the bowel. A simple test is to have the patient intake only a clear liquid diet for 24 hours and observe the amounts of flatus following this therapeutic test. Frequently the patient will learn that very little gas is formed when there is not an excessive amount of food in the gastrointestinal tract. Another simple test is to ask the patient if flatus was experienced on the day of a barium enema study. Often the patient will indicate that there was freedom from flatus for the first time when the gastrointestinal tract was cleaned out for the x-ray study.

Elegant studies by Levitt (4) have shown that hydrogen and methane are produced solely by bacteria and are not a product of human cellular metabolism. Levitt also has shown that hydrogen production is negligible in the fasting state; it appears that colonic bacteria are dependent on ingested fermentable substrates (carbohydrates) for hydrogen production. Certain vegetables, particularly legumes, contain a high concentration of indigestible oligosaccharides, which are nonabsorbable even by normal subjects, and these oligosaccharides account for the notorious gaseous properties of legumes. Carbon dioxide can be produced by bacterial fermentation or by the reaction of bicarbonate and acid. Digestion of an average meal could theoretically produce several hundred milliequivalents of acid, thus yielding 4000 cc of carbon dioxide. Although excessive gas is assumed to be a common cause of "functional abdominal complaints," there are little hard data to support this assumption.

Passing gas through the vagina or through the urethra usually is indicative of a fistula to the gastrointestinal tract. Occasionally, gas-forming organisms in the bladder may give rise to pneumaturia without a fistula, but this is rare except in the diabetic patient. A complete gastrointestinal evaluation is mandatory if a history of pneumaturia or flatus per vagina is obtained.

Anorexia

Anorexia is a lack or loss of appetite for food. Frequently this appetite change is psychogenic in origin, as with depression, worry, and boredom; or it may be caused by drugs such as digitalis preparations, sulfasalazine, and antihypertensive agents. Anorexia is a common symptom for patients with an acute viral hepatitis and/or carcinoma. Numerous signals have been implicated in the short-term control of appetite. These include changes in blood glucose, free fatty acid, and amino acid concentrations; altered neuronal activity resulting from distention of the gastrointestinal tract; or alterations in the concentrations of various hormones such as insulin, glucagon, bombesin, and cholecystokinin (5). Other clinical factors that may contribute to the development of anorexia and reduced food intake in patients with carcinoma include intestinal obstruction, radiation therapy, chemotherapy-induced nausea and vomiting, altered taste sensitivity, and oral ulceration.

■ ASSOCIATED ILLNESSES

Inflammatory bowel disease is well known for its associated anorectal problems. A history of this condition should be pursued in any patient with an anorectal complaint. Diabetes mellitus occasionally is associated with nocturnal diarrhea. The patient with peptic ulcer disease may be taking antacids, some of which increase the firmness of the stool and may cause anorectal pain and bleeding, while others may cause loose stools.

■ MEDICATIONS

The use of laxatives is common. Therefore, to evaluate symptoms completely, one must ascertain the medications (both prescribed and over-the-counter) that a patient is ingesting. A detailed laxative history is mandatory for any patient with a bowel complaint. A complete history of drug allergies also should be obtained.

■ FAMILY HISTORY

Often a patient's bowel habits will be very similar to those of the patient's parents. It is amazing how often there will be a familial history of hemorrhoids in patients who are suffering from a rectal mucosal prolapse. A pertinent family history of carcinoma should be sought. In a case-control study in which data from a Utah population database were used, patients with first-degree relatives with colon carcinoma had an increased risk of developing colon carcinoma (6); in men the odds ratio (OR) was 2.51, and in women the OR was 2.90. A second- or third-degree relative with colon carcinoma increased the risk from 25% to 52%. Risk associated with family history was greater in those patients diagnosed before age 50 than in those diagnosed at age 50 or older. Women were at an increased risk of colon carcinoma if they had a first-degree relative with breast (OR = 1.59), uterine (OR = 1.50), ovarian (OR = 1.63), or prostate (OR = 1.49) carcinoma. Men were at increased risk of colon carcinoma if they had a first-degree relative with breast (OR = 1.30), uterine (OR = 1.96), or ovarian (OR = 1.59) carcinoma.

A study from Melbourne, Australia, by St. John et al. (7) also found that first-degree relatives of patients with colorectal carcinoma had an increased risk for colorectal carcinoma. This risk was greater if the diagnosis was made at an early age and was greater when other first-degree relatives were affected. From the National Polyp Study Work Group (8) in the United States, the relative risk of colorectal carcinoma for siblings of patients in whom adenomas were diagnosed before 60 years of age was 2.59, as compared with the risk for siblings of patients who were 60 years or older at the time of diagnosis. The risk increased with decreasing age at the time of the diagnosis of adenoma (p for trend, <0.001). The relative risk for the siblings of patients who had a parent with colorectal carcinoma, as compared with those who had no parent with carcinoma, was 3.25. Thus siblings and parents of patients with colorectal adenomatous polyps are at increased risk for colorectal carcinoma, particularly when the adenoma is diagnosed before the age of 60 or, in the case of siblings, when a parent has had colorectal carcinoma (8). These data support the recommendations that individuals who have an increased risk of colon and rectal carcinoma should have regular screening.

■ BLEEDING TENDENCY

If a surgical procedure is necessary, a history of a bleeding tendency should be ruled out. A simple question may reveal a diagnosis of hemophilia. The patient should also be asked if he or she is taking medications that cause bleeding, such as aspirin, warfarin (Coumadin), and nonsteroidal anti-inflammatory drugs (NSAIDs).

■ EXPOSURE

Travel

In taking a history, one also must be cognizant of the fact that the patient may have returned recently from a tropical country and may have been exposed to certain parasitic diseases.

Sexual Contacts

A history of sexual exposure is important, especially if the patient has had anal intercourse. This may lead to the diagnosis of venereal diseases and/or acquired immunodeficiency syndrome (AIDS).

PHYSICAL EXAMINATION

The precise organization of the consulting room, examining room, and endoscopy suite will vary from one institution to another. It is understood that some office examining rooms are designed primarily for diagnostic evaluation and that others are equipped for the performance of minor operative procedures. Nevertheless, in some room, be it office examining room, clinic examining room, or endoscopy suite, the appropriate stage must be set to accomplish the required objective of a complete colorectal examination.

■ ROOM

The room should be equipped with essential items for the examination: a suction system, a good portable or head light, a toilet, and a washing sink. It is important that instruments be within easy reach of the surgeon, but they should be kept covered and out of view of the patient, who may find them to be a source of unnecessary anxiety.

■ EQUIPMENT

Examining Table

Ideally a proctoscopic table should be used. The table either can be put in the jackknife position or laid flat, with the height of the table adjusted as desired. If this is not available, any flat table (at least 3 ft high) or a litter or stretcher can be used.

Lighting

A good light is important for an efficient anorectal examination. Several types of lamps are commercially available for this purpose. A head lamp is convenient and saves space; a tall lamp on a stand with wheels also is excellent.

Anoscope

A Vernon-David anoscope is an ideal size for anorectal examination (Fig. 1). It is not quite as large as a standard anoscope, which stretches the anal canal and hence results in an underestimation of hemorrhoid size. A medium-size Hinkel-James anoscope is an excellent instrument for rubber band ligation of hemorrhoids, but it is a poor scope for examining the anal canal (Fig. 2) (9).

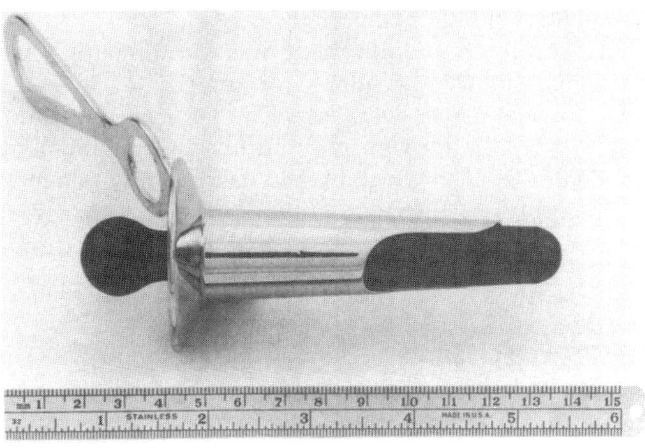

FIGURE 1 ■ Vernon-David anoscope.

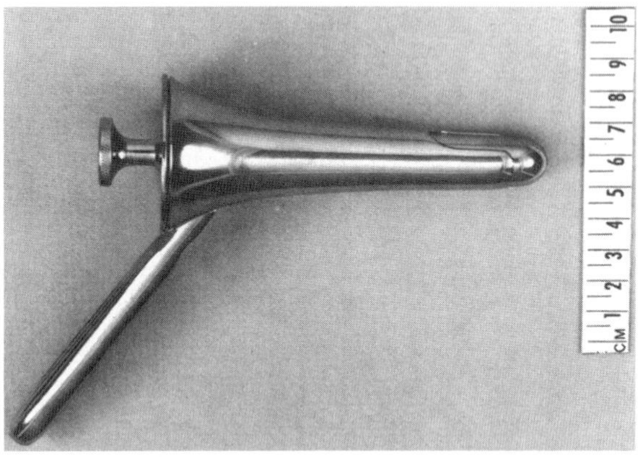

FIGURE 2 ■ Hinkel-James anoscope.

Proctosigmoidoscope

Three sizes of proctosigmoidoscopes are available (Fig. 3). A 19 mm × 25 cm scope is the standard size and should be used for polypectomy or electrocoagulation. A 15 mm × 25 cm scope is an ideal size for general examination. It is much better tolerated by the patient, causing less spasm of the rectum and thus minimal air insufflation, yet enables as adequate an examination as the standard-size scope. An 11 mm × 25 cm scope should be available for examining the patient who has an anorectal stricture, such as in Crohn's disease. More recently, a disposable standard-size proctosigmoidoscope has become popular for routine examination.

Flexible Sigmoidoscope

The standard flexible sigmoidoscope is 60 cm long (Fig. 4). It has all the features of a colonoscope. Due to the shorter length of the flexible sigmoidoscope, its cost, maintenance, and durability are considerably better than those of the colonoscope.

Colonoscope

Colonoscopy was introduced to clinical practice in 1970 and is now an established procedure. The cost of the instrument and its maintenance are expensive, but this cost

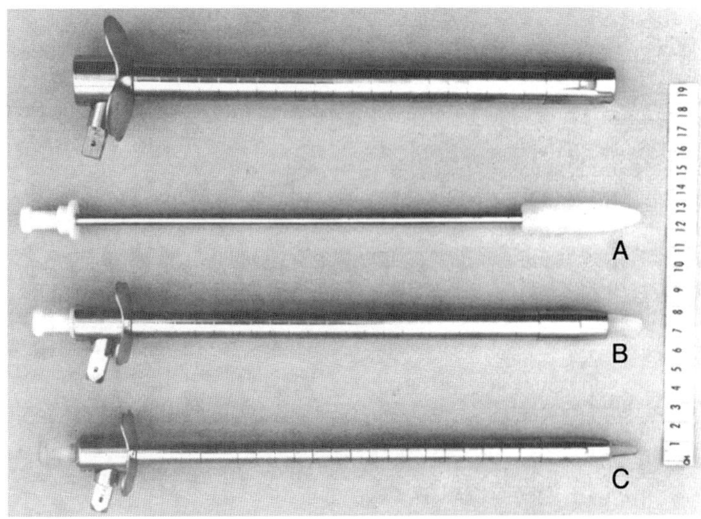

FIGURE 3 ■ Proctosigmoidoscopes. **(A)** 19 mm × 25 cm. **(B)** 15 mm × 25 cm. **(C)** 11 mm × 25 cm.

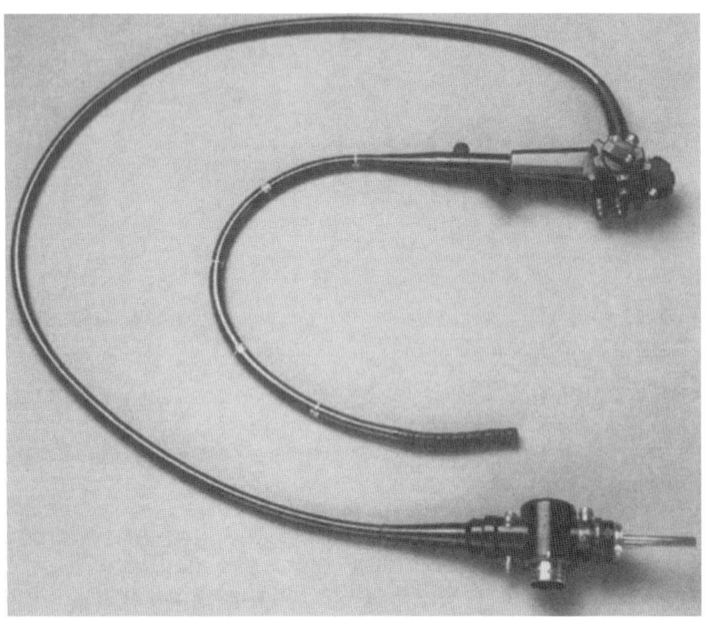

FIGURE 4 ■ Flexible video sigmoidoscope (60 cm).

is offset by its accuracy in diagnosis; its use has avoided numerous unnecessary operations and delays in patient management. The colonoscope is 160 cm (Fig. 5). It should be purchased with the necessary accessories, such as a light source, biopsy forceps, and snare wire. The video colonoscope has become the standard model for general use. In contrast to the fiberoptic scope in which the image is transmitted from the objective lens via optic fibers, the videoscope contains a chip camera at the tip of the scope that transmits the image to the video processing unit and sends it to the monitoring screen. The videoscope is also equipped with a keyboard for entering patients' profiles and data. Still photography and videotape are also available.

Electrocautery Machine

An endoscopy room cannot be complete without an electrocautery unit. Although biopsy performed by colonoscopy or flexible sigmoidoscopy almost never requires electrocautery to stop the bleeding, in many instances a "hot biopsy" technique is used (10). Electrocautery usually is needed for biopsy performed with the proctosigmoidoscope. For polypectomy, an electrocautery unit is an essential piece of equipment. There are many good units on the market, and the choice is a personal one.

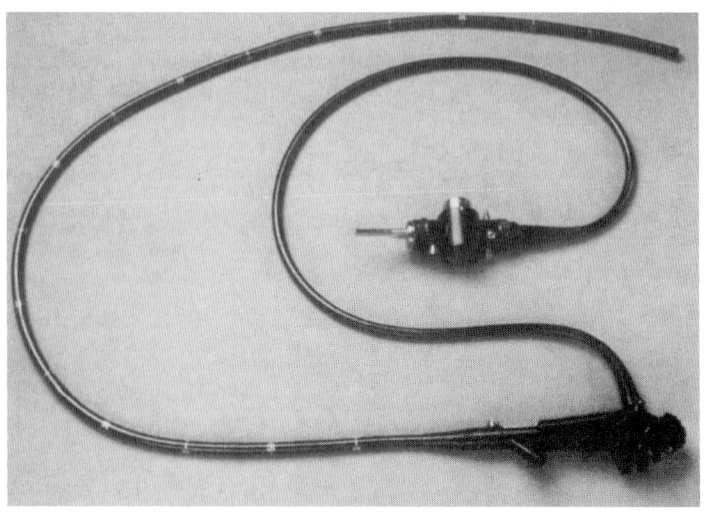

FIGURE 5 ■ Videocolonoscope (160 cm).

Electrocoagulation Electrodes

A ball-tip electrode with an insulated shaft works well for coagulating a small rectal or sigmoid polyp (Fig. 6A). A suction–coagulation electrode is ideal for coagulating a bleeding area, such as after biopsy of rectal mucosa or a lesion (Fig. 6B). It is more versatile because the oozing of blood can be sucked dry during the coagulation, and the gas and smoke that are produced can be readily eliminated. A piece of wire or a needle always should be available to push the plug of tissue or blood out of the insulated shaft.

Electrocautery Snares

There are two types of electrocautery snare wires available commercially (Fig. 7). A rigid-wire snare, known as the Frankfeldt snare, has been in use for a long time and is good for snaring small- or medium-size polyps. A soft-wire snare has a larger loop and is easier to use, especially for larger polyps or for piecemeal snaring; however, the problem with this type of wire is that it is too soft and bends easily. Several snare wires should be available as spare parts.

Biopsy Forceps

There are basically two types of biopsy forceps for use with the proctosigmoidoscope—the cup-shaped forceps and the Turrell biopsy forceps. Both types are excellent for biopsy of lesions or rectal mucosa. The size of the specimen obtained is between 5 and 8 mm. Because of the relatively large size, electrocoagulation usually is required to stop the bleeding. Alligator-type forceps for retrieval of polyps or foreign bodies should be available (Fig. 8).

Probes

Because anorectal probes for fistula-in-ano or sinus tracts cause considerable pain, they should only be used in the operating room when the patient is under anesthesia. The grooved Lockhart-Mummery fistula probes are suitable for diagnosis and fistula surgery (Fig. 9).

Rubber Band Ligation Equipment

Rubber band ligation equipment, including ligator, O ring, and forceps, should be available for immediate use (Fig. 10). Several forceps have been advocated for this technique; however, an Allis forceps may suffice. A suction hemorrhoid ligator is also available. It has the advantage that one can apply the ligation without needing an assistant (Fig. 11). Another advantage is that only the redundant mucosa is sucked into the cup for ligation.

Sclerosing Equipment

Sclerosing procedures require a syringe loaded with a solution of either 5% phenol and vegetable oil or 5% quinine and urea hydrochloride. However, sclerosing of hemorrhoids has been replaced largely by rubber band ligation.

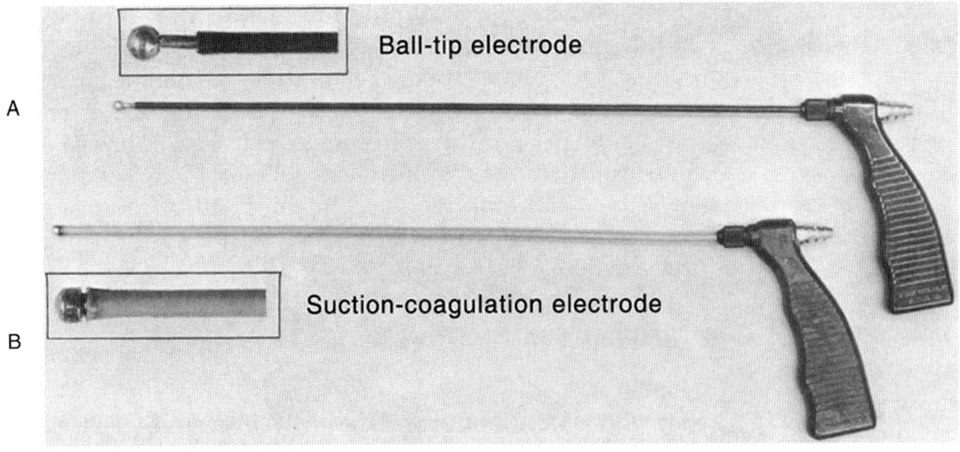

FIGURE 6 ■ Electrocoagulation electrodes. (A) Ball-tip electrode; (B) Suction-coagulation electrode.

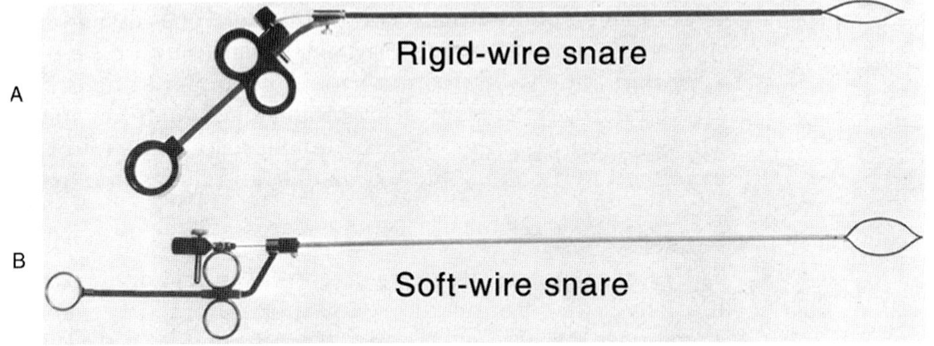

FIGURE 7 ■ Snaring devices for polypectomy via proctosigmoidoscope.

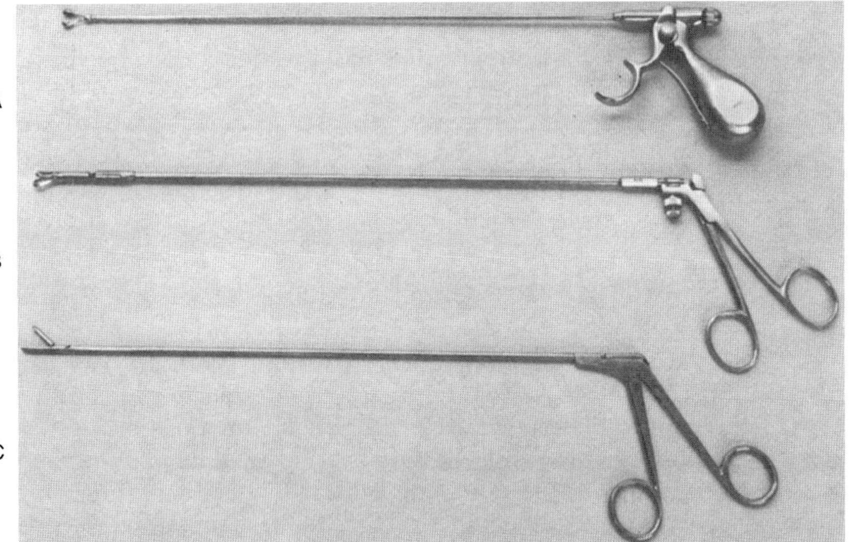

FIGURE 8 ■ Biopsy instruments. (**A**) Cup-shaped biopsy forceps. (**B**) Turrell biopsy forceps. (**C**) Alligator-type biopsy forceps.

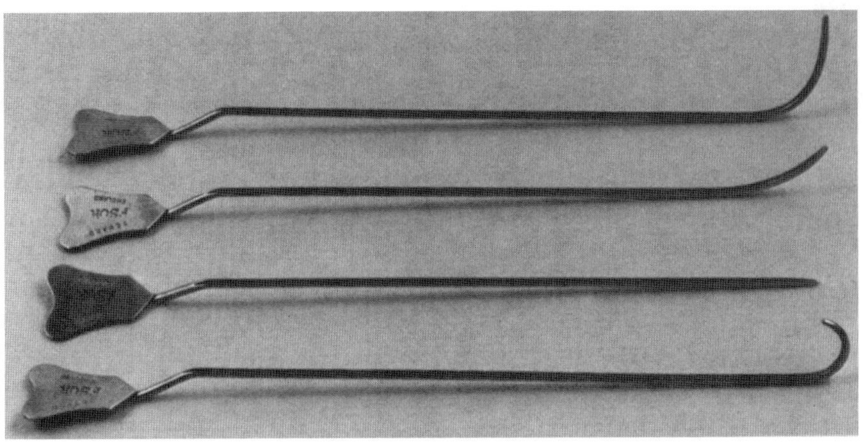

FIGURE 9 ■ Lockhart-Mummery fistula probes.

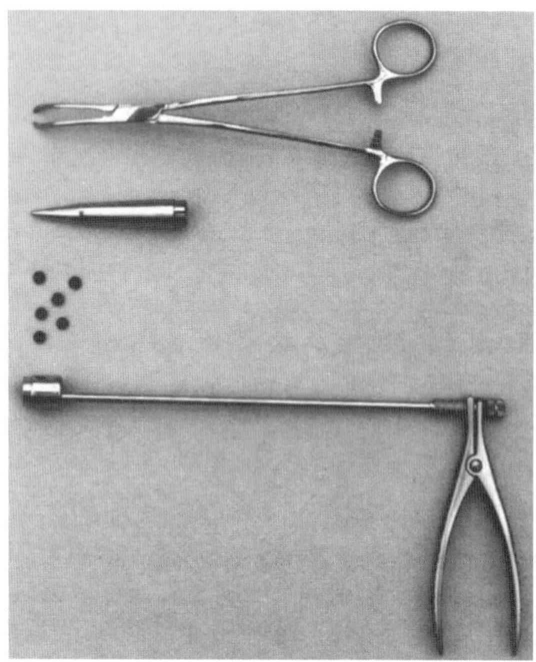

FIGURE 10 ■ Rubber band ligation equipment.

Miscellaneous Items

The room used for colon and anorectal examinations need not be fancy or expensive. However, it needs organization to make it clean and efficient. Along with the necessary equipment already described there are accessories essential for the examination.

A good suction system (either water or motor suction) is indispensable. A long metal or plastic suction rod must be available. Lubricant jelly is required in every case. A 2% lidocaine (Xylocaine) jelly also should be available, especially for patients with anal fissures or abrasions. Rubber or plastic gloves are essential. (Some people are allergic to rubber gloves.) A 1½ to 2-in. 27-gauge needle, a 3 mL syringe, and a local anesthetic should be available. Scalpels, scissors, needle holders, tissue forceps, and suture materials also should be on hand. An irrigating syringe or bottle for irrigating via the proctosigmoidoscope also is needed. A pulsating water injection device (i.e., WaterPik®) can be easily adapted for irrigating via the colonoscope or flexible sigmoidoscope and should be available. An area with proper antiseptic solution must be arranged for cleaning the instruments after they are used. Disposable buffered phosphate enemas should be available for use when the rectum is loaded with stool. Ideally, a toilet should be in or near the examining room. Soft paper tissues are needed to wipe the lubricant jelly from the anal area after the examination. Basic resuscitation equipment should be available, especially when minor surgical procedures are being performed.

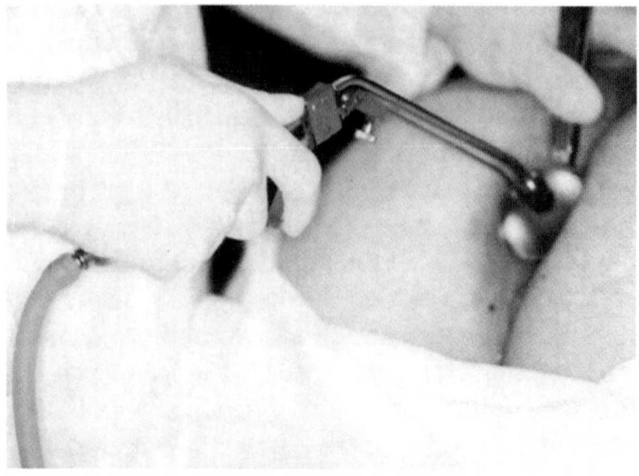

FIGURE 11 ■ A suction hemorrhoid ligator.

■ GENERAL EXAMINATION

Abdomen

Inspection of the abdomen may reveal asymmetrya suggestive of a neoplastic mass or enlargement of the internal organs. Distended abdominal veins suggest portal hypertension or obstruction of the inferior vena cava. Pulsation from an abdominal aortic aneurysm may be seen in very thin patients. Palpation should be aimed at detecting any tenderness, peritoneal irritation, or abdominal mass. The scar from a previous large bowel resection should be examined for healing, sinus or fistula, and metastatic mass.

Perineum

The most common site of recurrence of rectal carcinoma is the pelvis and perineum. Follow-up examination should encompass the perineal wound to determine if it has healed completely or has any evidence of sinus, mass, or tenderness.

Groin

Anorectal carcinoma that has invaded into or below the dentate line may metastasize to the inguinal lymph nodes. Therefore the presence or absence of enlarged inguinal nodes should be recorded. Enlargement of these nodes before or after excision of an anorectal lesion requires further management or a change in management approach.

■ ANORECTAL EXAMINATION

Positioning

Although the inverted prone jackknife position on a proctoscopic table is most popular and is extensively used in the United States (Fig. 12), the left lateral position with the buttocks projecting slightly beyond the edge of the examining table is as good for examination and is much more acceptable to the patient (Fig. 13). It is a myth that the prone jackknife position straightens the rectosigmoid colon and

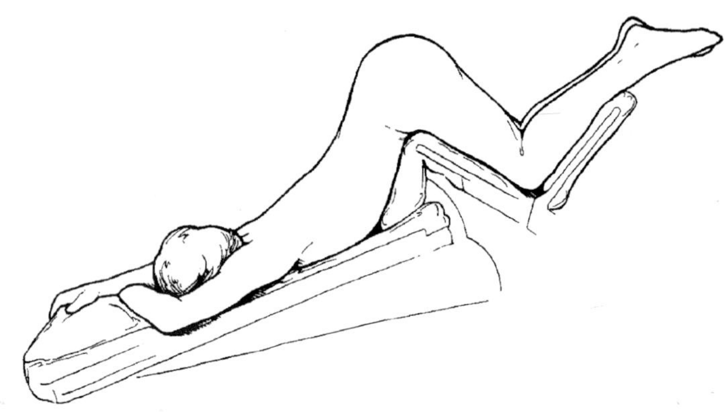

FIGURE 12 ■ Prone jackknife position.

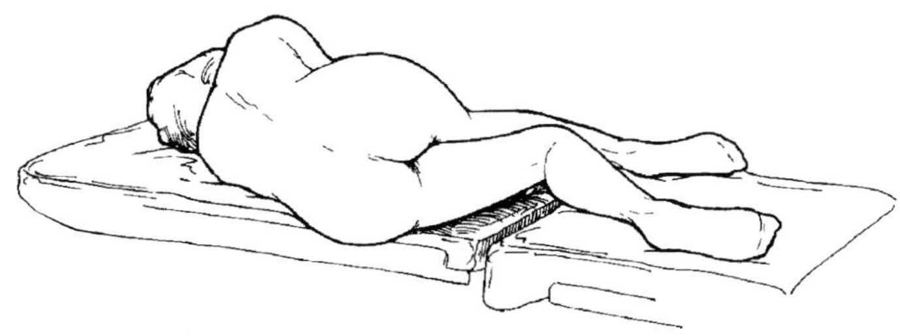

FIGURE 13 ■ Left lateral position (note that the buttocks project slightly beyond the edge of the examining table).

therefore that the proctosigmoidoscope can be passed higher. Altering the patient's position or inducing general anesthesia does not help in negotiating an acute angle that is impassable in the original position. The inverted jackknife position should not be used in various conditions: acute glaucoma, retinal detachment, severe cardiac arrhythmia, severe debilitation, late pregnancy, and recent abdominal surgery.

Inspection

Inspection of the anal area always should precede any other examination, and for this, good lighting is essential. The shape of the buttocks should be noted, because this information can be useful in determining the position in which to place the patient for the operation and the type of anesthetic to use (11). The cheeks of the buttocks are gently spread to gain exposure. Skin tags, excoriation, and change in color or thickness of the anal verge and perianal skin can be detected quickly. A scarred, patulous, or irregularly shaped anus may give clues to the cause of anal incontinence. Particularly in multiparous women, the anal verge may be pushed down too far during straining—a feature of the perineal descent syndrome (12). Prolapse of the rectum (procidentia) is best demonstrated by asking the patient to strain while in a lateral position or sitting on the toilet. When the anal verge is pricked with a needle, the external sphincter visibly contracts because of anal reflex. It is useful for testing the sensibility of the anal canal, which may be absent in areas of a previous scar or defect, or in patients with an underlying neuropathy.

Digital Examination

To begin the digital examination, the index finger should be well lubricated with a lubricant jelly, and the finger pressed on the anal aperture to "warn" the patient. Then the finger should be gradually inserted and swept all around the anal canal to detect any mass or induration. In men the prostate should be felt. In women the posterior vaginal wall should be pushed anteriorly to detect any evidence of a rectocele. Anal tone, whether tight or loose, can be easily estimated. A stricture or narrowing from scarring or a defect in the internal or external sphincters from a previous operation can be felt. A fibrous cord or induration in the anal area and anal canal may indicate a fistulous track.

The external sphincter, puborectalis, and levator ani muscles can also be appreciated by digital examination. When the puborectalis is pulled in the posterior quadrant, the anus will gape but will close immediately when the traction is released (13,14). Persistence of the gaping indicates an abnormal reflex pathway in the thoracolumbar region, commonly seen in paraplegic patients. The finger should press gently on these muscles for signs of tenderness. When a person with good sphincter function is asked to contract the muscles, the examiner not only feels the squeeze of the muscle on the examining finger but also feels the finger pulled forward by the puborectalis muscle.

Anoscopy

Anoscopy, as the name implies, is the examination of the anal canal. The anoderm, dentate line, internal and external hemorrhoids, and lower part of the rectal mucosa can be seen through the anoscope. Anoscopy should not begin until a digital examination has been completed. For most cases, an enema is not required. Insertion of the anoscope always should be done with the obturator in place. The obturator is removed during examination and reinserted to rotate the instrument to another area. If an inverted jackknife position is used, the examination table should not be tipped down more than 10 to 15°. If a left lateral position is used, an assistant needs to pull up the right cheek of the buttocks for exposure. During examination the patient is asked to strain, with the anoscope sliding out to detect any prolapse of the rectal mucosa and the anal cushion. Excoriation, metaplastic changes, and friable mucosa indicate a prolapsed hemorrhoid.

Proctosigmoidoscopy

Although a standard proctosigmoidoscope is 25 cm in length, the average distance that the scope can be passed is 20 cm. In men the scope can be passed to 21 to 25 cm half of the time, and in women it can be passed that distance one third of the time (15). Proctosigmoidoscopy is suitable only to examine the rectum and in some persons, the distal sigmoid colon. The pain experienced from proctosigmoidoscopy is from stretching the mesentery of the rectosigmoid colon when the scope is pushed against the rectal wall and from the air insufflation. When properly performed, proctosigmoidoscopy should produce no pain at all or only mild discomfort. Most patients are fearful of the examination because of past bad experience with the procedure or from what they have heard. A few words of reassurance will be helpful. Since many patients feel undignified in the "bottom up" positioning, a left lateral position can be used instead to alleviate this feeling.

Technique: With the obturator in place and held steady with the right thumb, the proctoscope is gently inserted into the anal canal, aiming toward the umbilicus for a distance of about 4 to 5 cm. Then the scope is angled toward the sacrum and advanced another 4 to 5 cm into the rectum. The obturator is removed, and the bowel lumen is negotiated under direct vision. Air insufflation is limited to the amount necessary to open the lumen. When an angle is encountered, the scope is withdrawn 3 to 4 cm and then readvanced. This may be repeated several times to straighten the angulation. If further advancement is unsuccessful, the procedure is terminated at this point. Careful examination is done as the instrument is withdrawn. It usually is necessary to insufflate a small amount of air for good visualization of the lumen. The instrument should be rotated on withdrawal to ensure examination of the entire circumference. The mucosal folds (valves of Houston) can be flattened with the tip of the scope to see the area behind them.

The length of insertion should be measured from the anal verge without stretching the bowel wall. Some physicians measure it in relation to the dentate line. This is more cumbersome because one also needs to measure the distance to the dentate line and subtract from it the distance to the anal verge. The appearance of the mucosa and depth of insertion should be accurately described. If a lesion is seen, the size, appearance, location, and level must be recorded. If a biopsy is performed, the location, level, number of biopsies, and whether electrocoagulation is necessary should be noted.

Ideally, a phosphate enema should be given within two hours of the examination. If the patient has had a bowel movement that morning, an enema usually is unnecessary. Mucus and watery stool can be easily aspirated. Even if there is some formed stool, the scope can be slipped between the fecal mass and the colonic wall. However, a large amount of solid or soft stool can impede further passage of the scope; in this situation, a phosphate enema should be given in the examining room, or the patient should return at some later date with better preparation.

Flexible Sigmoidoscopy

A flexible sigmoidoscope is no longer fiberoptic but contains a videochip at the tip of scope. This videochip transmits the image through the processing unit of the monitor. The entire sigmoid colon can be reached by the flexible sigmoidoscope in 45% to 85% of cases, and in a few, the splenic flexure also can be visualized (16,17). The discrepancies in success depend on patient selection and the experience of the endoscopist. For selective screening examination, flexible sigmoidoscopy has a three to six times greater yield than does proctosigmoidoscopy in detecting colonic and rectal abnormalities, especially neoplasms (18,19). Because of this higher yield, proponents of flexible sigmoidoscopy have discarded proctosigmoidoscopy (20). With the advance in technology of colonoscopy and because large bowel carcinomas have shifted proximally during the last few decades, the role of proctosigmoidoscopy is now limited to examination of the rectum and is no longer adequate for the screening of large bowel neoplasms.

The role of flexible sigmoidoscopy is difficult to define. Although this type of sigmoidoscopy detects more lesions than proctosigmoidoscopy, flexible sigmoidoscopy cannot be considered adequate when a complete colonic examination is indicated. However, it plays a superior role to proctosigmoidoscopy in case finding. Because barium enema studies miss some lesions in the rectosigmoid and sigmoid colon, a successful flexible sigmoidoscopy that is followed by an air-contrast barium enema gives a more accurate examination than an air-contrast study alone or an air-contrast barium enema combined with rigid proctosigmoidoscopy (21). Although the flexible sigmoidoscope is easier to handle and learn to use than the fiberoptic colonoscope, proper training is nevertheless necessary. The basic principles of technique, the limitations, and the risk of complications must be fully understood.

Technique: Because flexible sigmoidoscopy is designed for examination of the left colon, a formal bowel preparation with laxatives is unnecessary. Normally one or two phosphate enemas before the examination are adequate. The examination is best performed with the patient in a left lateral position, although a prone position is sometimes preferred by some examiners. Sedation is unnecessary. The anal canal is lubricated by digital examination. A well-lubricated flexible sigmoidoscope then is inserted. Advancement of the scope is performed under direct vision. Pushing the scope through a bend in the bowel is a poor technique. Instead, the scope should be withdrawn to straighten the bowel. The key to success is short withdrawal and advancement of the scope or a to-and-fro movement, together with rotating the instrument clockwise and/or counterclockwise as needed. Use of air insufflation should be kept to a minimum. The procedure should be completed within 5 to 10 minutes. If a lesion is detected and proved by biopsy to be a neoplasm, a complete colonic investigation may be indicated ideally by total colonoscopy at some later date. A polyp up to 8 mm in size can be sampled with coagulation (hot) biopsy forceps or biopsy and electrocoagulated. A larger polyp should be reserved for colonoscopy and polypectomy. To prevent possible gas explosion due to hydrogen or methane gas in the lumen, air should be exchanged in the colon and rectum with repeated insufflation and suction.

RADIOLOGIC EXAMINATION

PLAIN FILMS OF ABDOMEN

Radiographic examination of the abdomen is indicated whenever there is clinical evidence of an acute intra-abdominal condition. Although plain x-ray films of the abdomen are generally nonspecific, they often give clues to the underlying problems and lead to further, more specific investigations. Because the intra-abdominal organs change with position, interpretation of the findings must correlate with the position used. The standard techniques are the supine and upright radiographs of the abdomen, with a lateral decubitus included as indicated. Plain abdominal films give useful information regarding the gas pattern in the intestinal tract; masses and fluid also may be appreciated.

Normally there is a variable amount of gas in the large bowel and only a minimal amount in the small bowel. Interpretation of the plain abdominal film is made by the evidence of an abnormal pattern or amount of gas, as in mechanical bowel obstruction or ileus. Displacement of gas is a sign for a mass effect. The presence of gas in organs in which it does not belong indicates a fistula with the bowel, such as air in the biliary tree in a choledochoduodenal fistula or air in an abscess cavity produced by bacteria. Free air in the abdominal cavity is best seen when the patient is upright. Frequently upright chest radiography provides a better picture. Chen et al. (22) found that patients with severe ulcerative colitis have a poor response to medical treatment if three or more loops of small bowel distended with gas are noted on plain abdominal films.

Intraperitoneal fluid usually collects in the pelvis, which is the most dependent area. With negative pressure from the diaphragm, fluid may ascend along the paracolic gutters to the subphrenic areas (23). An early roentgenographic sign of peritoneal effusion is fluid density. A large amount of fluid may displace the right and left colon medially or separate loops of small bowel.

Extraperitoneal fluid in perirenal and pararenal spaces also can be detected in the same manner.

Organ enlargement (particularly the kidneys, spleen, and liver) can be detected easily by a plain abdominal radiograph. Mass densities in cysts or solid tumors can be outlined or detected by displacement of gas-containing structures such as the stomach, small bowel, and large bowel. Plain abdominal radiographs may reveal calcification in various stones, appendicolith, and calcified atheromatous plaques in abdominal aneurysms.

■ BARIUM ENEMA STUDIES

Barium sulfate enema has been the principal method for detecting large bowel neoplasms. When properly performed, the accuracy is high and the detection of large bowel polyps approaches the rate found at colonoscopy (24). Most radiologists now agree that the air-contrast barium enema is superior to the single-column enema (25–27). With good bowel preparation and technique, 4 to 5 mm polyps in the large bowel are detectable. Most missed lesions are the result of poor bowel preparation, faulty technique, and inadequate attention to detail rather than invisibility of the lesion. A good-quality air-contrast barium enema also is accurate and useful in diagnosing inflammatory bowel diseases. It is essential that different views and angles at different anatomic areas be taken to produce a complete colonic examination. The report on the barium enema study should read "positive," "negative," or "must be repeated" (28).

Barium enema study generally is safe if there are no contraindications. Cardiac arrhythmia, believed to be caused by stress, occurs in 40% of patients during the procedure (29), but rarely causes damage. Although the significance of this fact is not known, it suggests that a barium enema should be performed with cautious indications in patients with severe myocardial ischemia. Perforation of the colon and rectum from too much pressure and from the enema tip can be prevented by careful technique. If the patient has had a biopsy specimen taken from a neoplasm, it is not contraindicated to have a barium enema study. However, if a rectal mucosal biopsy is done via a proctosigmoidoscope or a flexible scope, the study should be postponed for at least one week (30). Because the biopsy specimen from colonoscopy or flexible sigmoidoscopy is small and superficial, a barium enema study can be performed safely without delay, provided there is no evidence of inflammatory bowel disease (31). It should not be performed after a recent snare polypectomy or a hot biopsy. In partial colonic obstruction and acute diverticulitis, the use of a barium sulfate enema is contraindicated; instead, an enema study using water-soluble material should be done. In fulminating colitis and in toxic megacolon, a barium enema study is both unnecessary and unwise (29). In children, barium enema has been used successfully to reduce an intussusception.

■ WATER-SOLUBLE CONTRAST MEDIA STUDIES

Many acute or subacute conditions, such as sigmoid and cecal volvulus, pseudo-obstruction of the colon, colonic obstruction, and anastomotic leak, require a "rule in" or "rule out" diagnosis, but do not require a detailed evaluation of the colonic mucosa. Because these conditions may necessitate an operation or colonoscopy, it is best that the colon not be full of barium. In such circumstances, a water-soluble contrast medium should be used. These media also have been shown to be safe in evaluating the postoperative anastomotic leak (32).

The most commonly used water-soluble contrast media are diatrizoate meglumine and diatrizoate sodium (i.e., Gastrografin, Hypaque). These aqueous agents have the following advantages over barium sulfate. They are readily absorbed from the peritoneal cavity in the event of perforation (33), and they are clear liquids and therefore do not interfere with visualization in colonoscopy or fill the bowel lumen if bowel resection is required. They also help to clean and empty the colon. The potential danger associated with the use of water-soluble contrast media is related to their high osmolarity, which may cause serious dehydration in the already dehydrated patient. The aqueous contrast media also have an irritant effect on gastrointestinal mucosa, and this may lead to severe hemorrhage or inflammation (34,35). Water-soluble contrast media should be used with caution, particularly in cases of partial bowel obstruction, which may lead to a prolonged retention of the medium in the viscus. Water-soluble contrast material has been found to be a helpful diagnostic tool in postoperative small-bowel obstruction; however, it does not help to relieve small bowel obstruction (36).

■ BARIUM ENEMA VS. COLONOSCOPY

The choice between colonoscopy and barium enema has been a subject of debate for years. Prospective studies comparing the two methods for detecting colonic neoplasms have been biased because expertise in radiologic and colonoscopic procedures has not been equal. In the diagnosis of colonic neoplasms, most studies have reported a sensitivity of 76% to 98.5% for barium enema and 86% to 95% for colonoscopy (37–39). Most reports conclude that when properly performed, both barium enema and total colonoscopy are highly sensitive in the detection of colorectal neoplasms.

The advantages of colonoscopy are that when polyps or carcinomas are seen, a biopsy can be done or the neoplasms can be removed; also, stool sometimes can be irrigated or aspirated for an adequate examination. The disadvantages of colonoscopy are its higher cost, its time-consuming nature, its inability to allow passage of the scope all the way to the cecum in all cases, and the risk of complications.

The advantages of barium enema are its lower cost, more rapid performance, and greater suitability for mass screening. The disadvantages are that it is difficult to differentiate between stool and neoplasm, there must be an absolutely clean colon, and it requires proctosigmoidoscopy or flexible sigmoidoscopy for rectum and sigmoid colon examination because these areas are not visualized well on barium enema study.

A prospective study by Rex et al. (40) compared examinations of experienced radiologists with those of experienced gastroenterologists. The radiologists were blinded to flexible sigmoidoscopic findings and the colonoscopists were blinded to the barium enema results but not to the flexible sigmoidoscopic findings. The radiologists did not find additional lesions that were not detected during flexible sigmoidoscopy, but nine of 114 patients (8%) had additional polyps found at colonoscopy that were not detected by flexible sigmoidoscopy and barium enema. All nine carcinomas of the distal colon and rectum were found by both barium enema studies and flexible sigmoidoscopy.

With the wide availability of colonoscopy, it has become the first line of diagnostic examination of the colon and rectum. Barium enema is reserved for the situation when a complete colonoscopy could not be accomplished or resources limit the availability of colonoscopy.

■ GENITOURINARY EXAMINATION

Intravenous Urography

There have been controversies about the value of routine intravenous urography (IVU) in preoperative assessment of patients with colon and rectal diseases. Some series have found significant numbers of urologic abnormalities (41); others have found a low yield of abnormal findings. In London, a prospective multicenter study of IVU in the preoperative assessment of patients with adenocarcinoma of the large bowel showed a low incidence of significant associated abnormalities; these results have raised questions about the rationale of a routine use of IVU (42). However, in selected cases IVU is valuable, and in many cases it is essential. One argument for not doing routine IVU is the small but definite risk of a patient having an anaphylactic reaction to the contrast medium; this can be fatal, particularly in the patient with a history of the reaction (43).

Use of IVU is highly advisable in cases with a large colonic or rectal mass, such as a carcinoma or a diverticular abscess, where the lesions might become adherent to the ureter, or in cases in which a large lesion is identified in the splenic or hepatic flexure, that may require a concomitant nephrectomy. IVU may show deviations or obstructions of the ureters and may call for the placement of ureteral catheters to promote a safer operation. It also gives useful information on the function of the opposite kidney in the event one ureter is injured. In a large series from The Cleveland Clinic, the incidence of hydroureter and hydronephrosis in patients with Crohn's disease was 5%; IVU is advised in such patients (44).

Cystography

Urinary symptoms of blood in the urine and of pneumaturia require cystoscopy, followed by a cystogram if indicated. A biopsy should be performed to reveal the nature of the disease and, in particular, to rule out malignancy. The cystogram may reveal the anatomic features of the fistula to the bladder, although, in general, barium enema studies have a higher yield in demonstrating the fistula.

■ FISTULOGRAPHY

Barium enema studies are highly successful in demonstrating coloenteric fistulas (45). However, in colocutaneous fistulas, although the underlying pathology usually is revealed by barium enema, the most useful information is obtained from fistulography, provided care is taken to achieve a leakproof seal around the mouth of the fistula and the investigation is carefully planned. For a gastrointestinal tract fistula, thin barium is superior to water-soluble contrast media. The contrast medium is injected via a soft rubber catheter that can be introduced down the tract or by a Foley catheter in which the balloon can be inflated to occlude the mouth of the orifice. Every orifice that can be found is cannulated, the flow of contrast medium is examined under fluoroscopy, and films are taken in two directions. Fistulography is not worth attempting in patients who have large defects in the abdominal wall and very high outputs; fistulas in such cases usually are better demonstrated by conventional contrast studies (46).

Simple fistula-in-ano does not require a fistulogram. However, in a highly placed and complicated anorectal fistula, fistulography can reveal the depth and branches of the tracts and is valuable in planning the surgical approach.

■ ARTERIOGRAPHY

Since the introduction of percutaneous catheterization angiography by Seldinger in 1953 (47), tremendous improvements in knowledge, technique, and equipment have been made. Arteriography currently is available in more medical centers for the diagnosis and treatment of gastrointestinal bleeding.

Bleeding from the colon can be massive and life threatening. At the present time, selective arteriography is the procedure of choice. Not only is it highly successful in identifying the exact location of bleeding, but it can be used to control bleeding with the infusion of vasopressin or, in some circumstances, with transcatheter emboli to occlude the bleeding vessel (48). A vasopressin (Pitressin) drip via a selective arteriographic catheter is highly successful in controlling lower gastrointestinal bleeding (48,49). It should be tried before a surgical procedure is begun, unless an angiography team is not available or if the procedure is contraindicated. To avoid the loss of valuable time in identifying the source and location of the bleeding, indiscriminate and inappropriate procedures must not be done.

Barium enema studies and colonoscopy should not be used in the patient with acute life-threatening bleeding. Barium may obscure the extravasation of contrast medium and must not be used before arteriography. However, once the bleeding has slowed or stopped, the entire large bowel should be examined by colonoscopy or barium enema or both. The "blind subtotal colectomy," popularly used in the 1970s, will not solve the problem if the bleeding site is not in the resected segment (50). A vigorous attempt should be made to find the precise anatomic site of the bleeding; also one must not overlook bleeding from the anorectum, which can be verified by proctoscopy or anoscopy.

To be successful in identifying the site of the bleeding, selective arteriography of appropriate vessels is required. Bleeding from the small intestine and the ascending and transverse colon is studied by superior mesenteric arteriography. Bleeding from the descending colon, sigmoid, and rectum is evaluated by inferior mesenteric arteriography. A bleeding aortoenteric fistula is the only type of gastrointestinal bleeding for which selective arteriography is not appropriate; rather aortography is needed. Selective arteriography is indicated only if there is continued evidence of bleeding. The rate of bleeding necessary to permit detection by arteriography is at least 0.5 mL/min. Clinically, if a patient requires 500 mL of blood transfusions every eight hours (1 mL/min) to maintain hemodynamic stability, then selective arteriography is indicated (49).

Arteriography is an invasive procedure, but the advantages outweigh the risks. In experienced hands and with proper application, arteriography has a small incidence of complications. Fatal complications have been reported in <0.1% of cases. Major complications such as hematomas, infection, false aneurysms, and arterial thromboses occur in 0.7% to 1.7% of cases and for the most part are localized to the arterial puncture site. Minor complications occur in approximately 5% of cases, and most represent puncture-site hematomas (49).

■ RADIONUCLIDE STUDIES

Radionuclide studies for the detection of gastrointestinal bleeding were first introduced in 1954, but the early studies did not permit localization of the bleeding source (51). With improvement in radionuclide imaging techniques, it became possible to detect and localize active gastrointestinal bleeding (52–54). The technetium-99m (^{99m}Tc) sulfur colloid scan has since been abandoned and has been replaced by the red blood cell–tagged scan.

Bleeding sites in the colon that overlap the liver or spleen may be obscured by the uptake in the reticuloendothelial of the organs.

^{99m}Tc-Labeled Red Blood Cells

In this technique, the circulating ^{99m}Tc-labeled red blood cells are extravasated during bleeding (Fig. 14). Focal accumulation of the radioactivity is interpreted as the site. The advantage of this technique is that the activity remains in the blood pool for a longer time; therefore, intermittent bleeding in a patient may be detected by performing the imaging over several hours. The disadvantage is that, if imaging is not performed precisely when extravasation occurs, the radioactive agent may move with the bowel peristalsis, which may result in erroneous localization of the bleeding site. For patients who are actively bleeding, ^{99m}Tc sulfur colloid scans, which are now largely abandoned by nuclear radiologists, can identify small amounts of bleeding in a rapid fashion (within 5 minutes). The disadvantage of this imaging technique is that the window of opportunity for diagnosis is short (10 to 15 minutes) because the agent is rapidly taken up by the liver.

Radionuclide studies are noninvasive procedures. Some authors use them in a secondary role to arteriography, especially in cases of massive lower gastrointestinal bleeding (49). Some investigators use them as initial diagnostic procedures for localizing bleeding during conservative therapy of patients with mild or intermittent gastrointestinal bleeding. When a radionuclide test reveals no bleeding, no further immediate diagnostic studies are required and subsequent elective studies can be scheduled for further management. When, on the other hand, the radionuclide study shows active bleeding, arteriography should be performed immediately to confirm the bleeding site (48).

■ DIAGNOSTIC IMAGING

Currently, there are several imaging procedures used to detect intra-abdominal diseases: liver scintigraphy, ultrasonography, computed tomography (CT), magnetic resonance imaging (MRI), endorectal ultrasonography, positron emission tomography (PET), and radiolabeled antibody imaging.

Liver Scintigraphy

Scintigraphy is widely accepted as a valuable tool for detecting metastatic malignant disease in the liver. The liver scintiscan is obtained after an intravenous injection of ^{99m}Tc sulfur colloid, and the images are collected on nuclear medicine films. Detection of focal masses by this method depends on the lack of uptake of ^{99m}Tc sulfur colloid by the lesions (Fig. 15), Most reports demonstrate a sensitivity of 80% to 85%, but a significant false-negative and false-positive rate of 15% to 25% has been observed (55). Radionuclide scanning is inexpensive and relatively

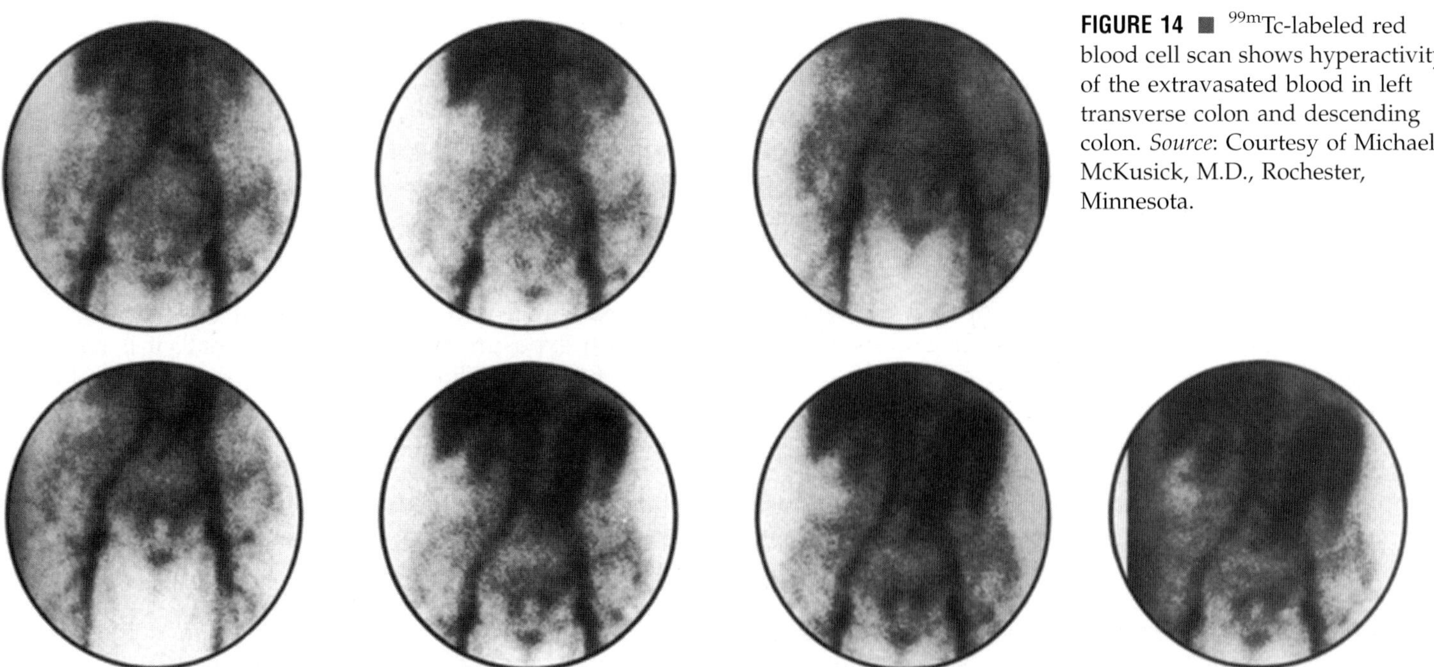

FIGURE 14 ■ ^{99m}Tc-labeled red blood cell scan shows hyperactivity of the extravasated blood in left transverse colon and descending colon. *Source*: Courtesy of Michael McKusick, M.D., Rochester, Minnesota.

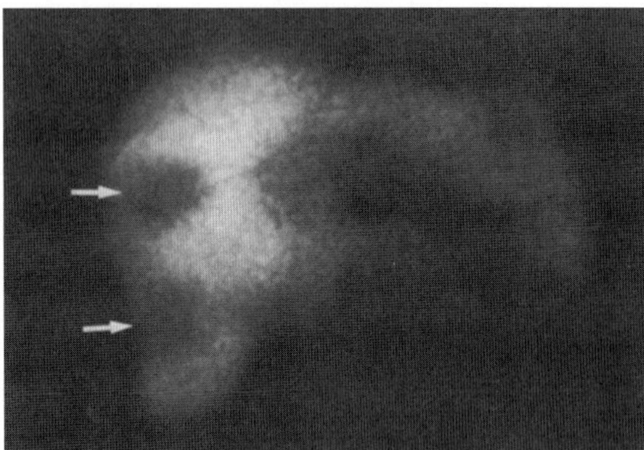

FIGURE 15 ■ Liver scintiscan showing multiple filling defects from metastasis (*arrows*).

easy to perform, but it is nonspecific. The average size of a metastasis detected by radionuclide scintigraphy is 2 cm or larger. Also, most detectable lesions are peripherally located; a large lesion centrally located may not be detected (54). A study by Tempero et al. (56) suggested that metastatic disease in the liver that causes no biochemical abnormalities may be too subtle or small to create focal changes on the liver scan. For practical purposes, a liver scintiscan should be obtained only when the liver function tests are abnormal (56). Liver scintiscan is largely replaced by computed tomography (CT).

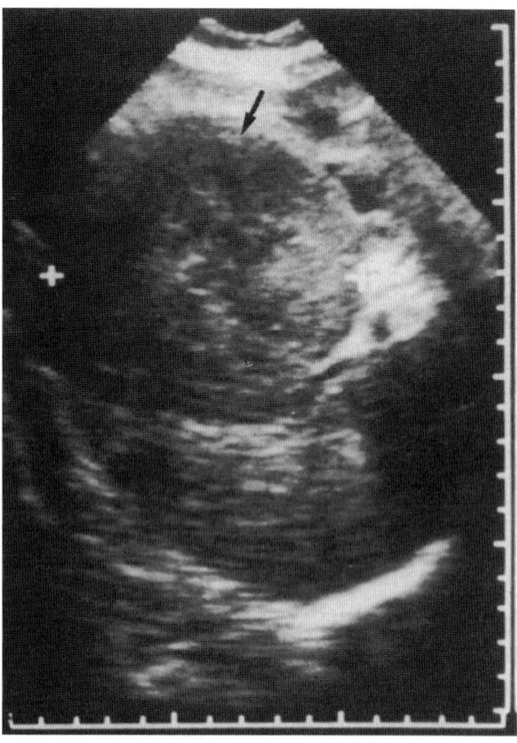

FIGURE 16 ■ Ultrasound image of the liver. A large mass from metastasis is shown (*arrow*).

Ultrasonography

Ultrasonography is a noninvasive imaging technique that uses high-frequency sound waves. A transducer acts as a receiver to record echoes reflected back from the body. The transducer is applied directly to the skin surface, with mineral oil or a water-soluble gel used as a surface couplant. A striking feature of ultrasonographic imaging is that it distinguishes clearly between solid- and fluid-filled structures (Fig. 16). The important feature of ultrasonography is its safety; there is no risk of radiation exposure, which makes it ideal for studies in children and pregnant women. Its limitations are the acoustic barriers such as intestinal gas, bone, excessive fat deposits, and barium. Because the sonic probe must be in direct contact with the skin, it is difficult to apply to postoperative patients who have dressings, retention sutures, drains, and open wounds. As with CT and scintigraphy, the accuracy of ultrasonographic detection of liver metastatic carcinoma is high, but it is not better than palpation on celiotomy (57). Ultrasonography is an extremely sensitive tool for detecting fluid collections in the abdomen and pelvis; however, its limitations make the findings nonspecific, and its accuracy is inferior to that of the CT scan (58). At the present time the limited sensitivity in identifying the large bowel process precludes the use of ultrasonography in screening for abnormalities of the gut. Ultrasonography of the liver is complementary to the CT scan in detecting liver metastasis.

Intraoperative sonography has served to detect the liver metastasis that cannot be appreciated by inspection and palpation. The liver is surveyed by placing the ultrasonographic probes directly over the liver. Multiple investigators consider intraoperative sonography to be the modality of choice for hepatic surgery because lesions have been detected that were not identified by preoperative imaging studies or by the surgeon at the time of operation. With the wide use of laparoscopic evaluation and laparoscopic surgery, laparoscopic sonographic probes have been developed and applied in hepatobiliary and gastrointestinal surgery. It is anticipated that laparoscopic sonography may lead to a less invasive manner of staging colon and rectal carcinoma and to providing pathologic confirmation (59).

Computed Tomography

Computed tomography (CT) is a technique that uses a computer to construct an image from radiographic attenuation data. These data are then converted into either a numeric printout or a cross-sectional image of the anatomic part studied. Depending on the attenuation or absorption values, the image produced varies in density (Fig. 17). More than 2000 density differences can be appreciated by CT, rather than the four (air, bone, fat, and soft tissue) seen by conventional radiography. This accounts for the exquisite density discrimination of CT, which is fundamental to its ability to detect small lesions. The CT scan uses x-rays but the radiation exposure to the patient is small; it is equivalent to one minute of fluoroscopy or one third to one fifth the radiation exposure of standard radiographic studies, such as barium enema or excretory urography (60).

Barium contrast will cause artifacts and distort the image. Large numbers of metal clips in the abdominal cavity cause severe streaking and often lead to a nondiagnostic study. Abdominal fat, because of its low computed tomographic number, helps to outline organs (61). It is helpful, especially in thin patients, to use a diluted oral contrast agent such as 2% diatrizoate meglumine (Gastrografin) to

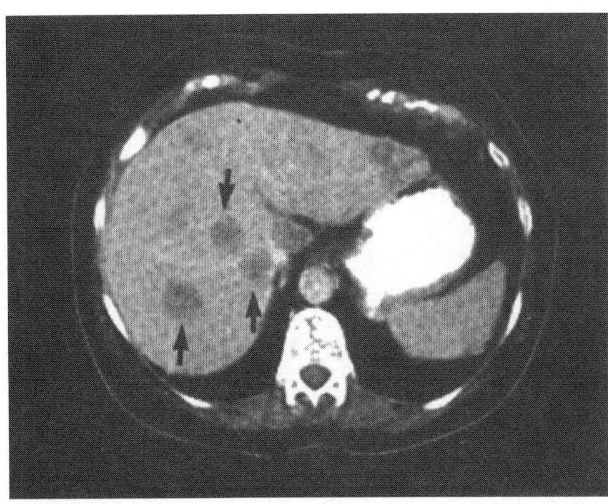

FIGURE 17 ■ Computed tomography scan of the liver. Multiple filling defects from metastases are shown (*arrows*).

provide sufficient enhancement of the density of the luminal contents. This will allow distinction between loops of bowel and solid structures within the abdomen.

The CT scan is commonly used for the diagnosis of diverticulitis, Crohn's disease, and small and large intestinal obstruction (62). It has also played an important role in the early detection of strangulation in small intestinal obstruction (63). CT scan is also useful in diagnosing an intra-abdominal abscess and in investigating carcinoma of the colon and anorectum. With CT as a guide, many intra-abdominal abscesses can be drained percutaneously (64). For large bowel carcinoma, although the diagnosis should be made by barium enema studies or colonoscopy, CT scanning is of great value because it permits direct visualization of the bowel wall, mesentery, and extension of a malignancy into the surrounding organs. In many instances, a CT scan can be used to stage the disease without the need for exploratory celiotomy (60).

The most frequent CT finding in primary colonic carcinoma is focal thickening of the colonic wall. Retroperitoneal adenopathy, liver metastasis, and direct invasion of pelvic muscles, prostate, uterus, bladder, ureter, and spine may be seen. The accuracy of CT scan for staging of colorectal carcinoma is between 77% and 100%. The high accuracy rates result from the more advance cases of the series (65). The newer technique of CT arterial portography has a positive predictive value of 96% for liver metastases (66). CT offers comparable potential in detecting recurrent rectal carcinoma. Ideally, a baseline CT scan should be performed 6 to 9 weeks after surgery, then every 6 to 12 months for 2 to 3 years as indicated. A metastatic lesion to the liver can be detected by CT scan because the lesion has a lower attenuation value than normal hepatic parenchyma. However, in most cases the CT scan is incapable of suggesting a histologic diagnosis. For instance, a primary hepatoma cannot be distinguished from a solitary metastasis (60). Metastatic lesions are less well circumscribed and less uniform in density than cysts.

The prospective study by Smith et al. (67) showed that there is no statistical difference in either the sensitivity or overall accuracy among any of the imaging modalities for detecting metastatic lesions in the liver. Liver scintiscan is the most sensitive test (79%), ultrasonography has the greatest specificity (94%), and CT is the most accurate overall (84%). It is interesting to note that the majority of lesions 2 cm in diameter or smaller are missed by all three modalities, while virtually all lesions 4 cm or larger are detected. In spite of technologic advances in CT scanning, no imaging test available today allows accurate resolution of metastatic lesions that are smaller than 2 cm in diameter.

Magnetic Resonance Imaging

Magnetic resonance imaging (MRI) is a technique for making pictures of internal organs by using the special properties of atoms inside the body and magnetic force. Because no ionizing radiation is used, MRI is potentially safer than studies that use x-rays or injected radionuclides. It is important to note that patients with ferrous metal appliances must be excluded from study.

MRI can detect liver metastases from carcinoma as accurately as contrast-enhanced CT scanning, but it is expensive for routine use. The only advantage of MRI over CT is that it avoids irradiation. The accuracy of MRI for staging of carcinoma of rectum has not reached a clinically useful level (68). MRI is found to be useful and accurate in demonstrating complicated anal fistulas (69).

Endorectal Ultrasonography

In 1956 Wild and Reid (70) used an ultrasonographic probe in the rectal lumen to visualize the rectal wall. The equipment at that time was inadequate, and the method was neglected until 1983 (71) when an improved and more powerful transducer became available. Endorectal ultrasonography can identify different layers of the rectum, and it is included in the armamentarium for preoperative staging of rectal carcinoma. Endorectal ultrasonography is more accurate than CT scanning and MRI in preoperative assessment of carcinoma of the rectum (72). Endorectal ultrasonography, however, cannot evaluate a lesion that causes stenosis or stricture of the rectum. It can determine the depth of malignant infiltration with an accuracy of 85% to 95% (Fig. 18), and in the detection of lymph node metastasis, with an accuracy of 60% to 85% (73–75).

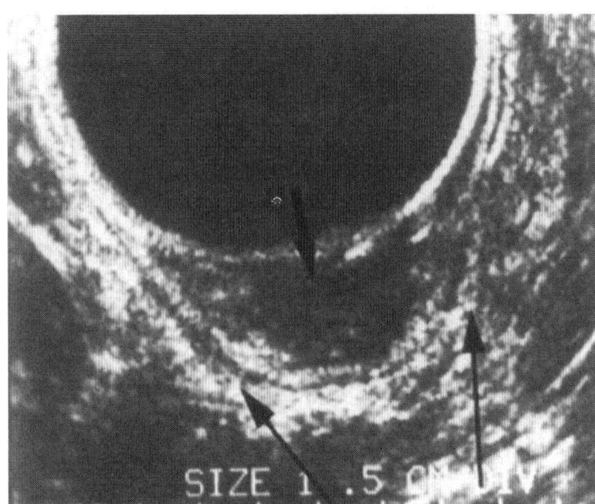

FIGURE 18 ■ Endorectal ultrasound image showing a lesion limited to the rectal wall (*arrows*). Note that the muscularis propria is intact.

Currently, endorectal ultrasound the best tool for preoperative staging of rectal carcinoma. However, endorectal ultrasound identified only one-third asymptomatic local recurrences that were missed by digital, or proctoscopic examination (76). This is probably of the interference of postoperative scars or radiation reactions. Poor results are also observed in detection of recurrences after chemoradiation for squamous cell carcinoma of the anal canal (77). More recently, endorectal ultrasonography has been used to identify the anal sphincter defects in cases of anal incontinence and in the evaluation of a fistula-in-ano (78,79).

Positron Emission Tomography

Positron emission tomography (PET) is a new method of imaging in which a positron-emitting isotope–labeled compound is used. In PET studies, functional images of colorectal neoplasms are obtained by taking advantage of the increase in anaerobic glycolysis that occurs in malignant cells. Fluorine-18 deoxyglucose (FDG), like glucose, is phosphorylated intracellularly. When injected intravenously, this substance is used by all cells with variable uptake, depending on cellular metabolism. Increased uptake of FDG has been noted in cases of colorectal carcinoma (Fig. 19) (80,81).

PET is performed by injecting FDG intravenously. After one hour, emission imaging of the abdomen and pelvis is performed. The PET-FDG images are oriented into sagittal, coronal, and transverse views. Qualitative image analysis for the presence of hypermetabolic regions is performed for each of the views (82). PET scanners are now available in most major metropolitan centers in the United States and PET use is expected to continue to grow despite the expensive equipment (83). In a pilot study performed by Falk et al. (82), metabolic imaging using PET-FDG appeared to be more sensitive and accurate than CT scanning in the preoperative detection of colorectal carcinoma. PET-FDG can detect both locally recurrent and distant metastatic disease. It may detect additional metastatic disease not seen on CT scan (84). It is particularly useful for detecting recurrence at the site of resection because CT scans often show postoperative changes that cannot be differentiated from recurrent carcinoma (85).

A metaanalysis of 11 published studies showed that PET-FDG had an overall sensitivity for recurrent colorectal carcinoma of 97% and specificity of 76% and that PET-FDG findings led to clinical management changes in 29% of cases (86). PET-FDG imaging is less sensitive in the assessment of mucinous carcinoma and neuroendocrine neoplasmas of the gastrointestinal tract. This is possibly related to the low metabolic rate of the malignancies. PET is limited by its poor sensitivity for detecting small lesions (<1 cm) and its inability to discriminate between lesions close to one another as well as between malignant necrotic lesions. False-positive lesions may be caused by inflammatory disease especially granulomatous lesions which can accumulate significant FDG because of activated macrophage (86).

One of the important indications for PET-FDG is the rising carcinoembryonic antigen (CEA) and negative CT scans; PET scan detects recurrent disease in 68% of cases (87). Flanagan et al. (88) showed a positive-predictive value for PET of 85% and a negative-predictive value of 100%.

A

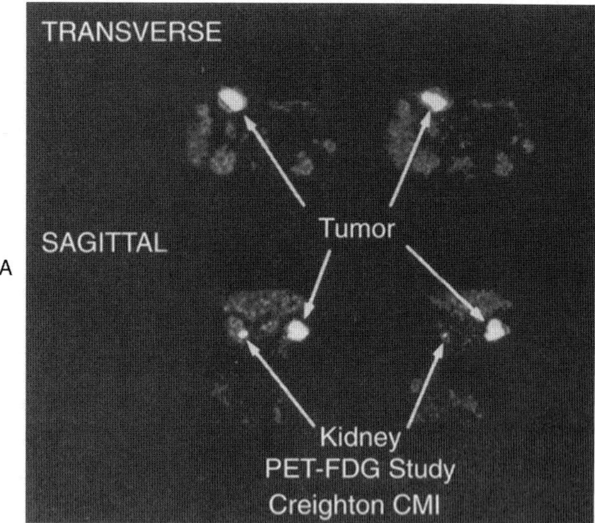

B

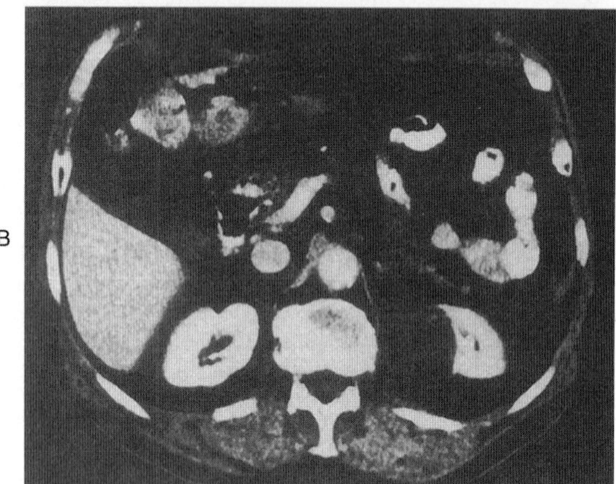

FIGURE 19 ■ (**A**) PET transverse and sagittal views detect a lesion in the hepatic flexure of the colon. Normal renal uptake seen. (**B**) The lesion visualized by PET was not detected on CT scan. *Abbreviations*: PET-FDG, positron emission tomography-fluorine-18 deoxyglucose; CT, computed tomography. *Source*: From Ref. 82.

Another usefulness of PET is to follow patients after radiation therapy and after chemotherapy. However, immediately after radiation therapy, FDG uptake may be associated with inflammatory changes and not necessarily residual carcinoma for approximately six months (85).

Radioimmunoscintigraphy

CT scanning and MRI are limited in their ability to detect the location and extent of metastatic disease, particularly extrahepatic metastases. They are unable to detect metastases in lymph nodes of normal size or <2 cm. Furthermore, they cannot distinguish between postoperative changes from scar tissue or postoperative radiation changes from recurrent carcinoma.

Radioimmunoscintigraphy (RIS) uses monoclonal antibody labeled with radionuclides such as ^{111}Indium or ^{99m}Technitium that produces gamma radiation detectable by a gamma camera. The antibody is targeted against antigen sites found on malignant cells, in this instance CEA. Hepatic metastasis may appear as areas of increased isotope activity or photoperic areas. CT is more accurate in the detection of hepatic metastasis (89).

The major role of RIS is in the detection of metastatic disease. Numerous studies have reported on the usefulness of RIS in identifying pelvic recurrence (90,91). Both RIS and PEI are useful in detecting occult disease and local recurrence. They offer an important adjuvant to conventional imaging.

■ COMPUTED TOMOGRAPHY COLONOGRAPHY

Computed tomography colonography (CTC) (virtual colonoscopy) is a novel technique for colorectal examination. CTC examinations are performed with a helical CT scanner to create high-quality axial and reformatted two-dimensional (2-D) (Fig. 20A) and three-dimensional (3-D) (Fig. 20B) simulated images of the colon and rectum. A bowel preparation similar to that for colonoscopy is required. Because the average colon length is 1400 mm, approximately 560 reformatted images are produced (Fig. 20) (92). It is a relatively new technique, first described by Vinning et al. (93) in 1994. It was first successfully applied in clinical trials by Hara et al. (92) in 1996.

Potential advantages for CTC as a screening study for colorectal carcinoma are:

A

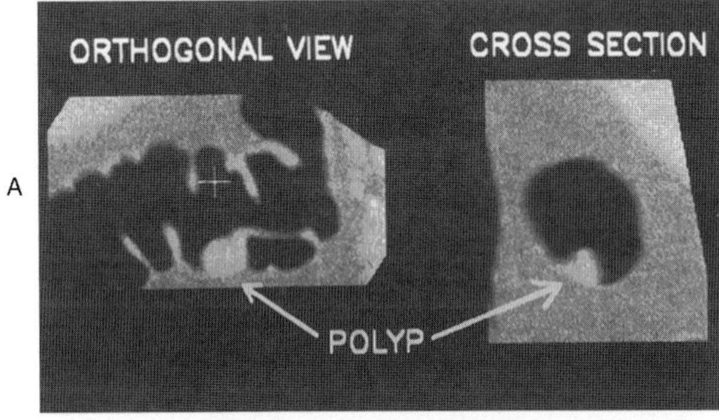

B

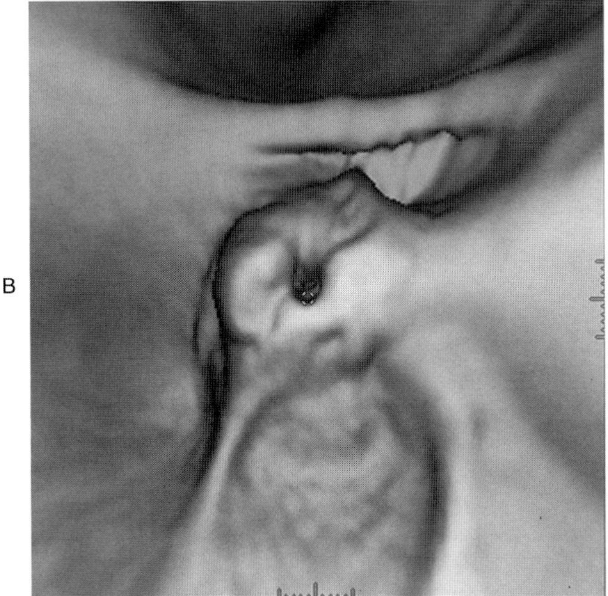

FIGURE 20 ■ (**A**) A pedunculated colonic polyp detected by 2-D CT colonography. *Source*: Courtesy of C. Daniel Johnson, M.D., Mayo Clinic, Rochester, Minnesota. (**B**) A large, ulcerated carcinoma of the cecum detected by 3-D endoluminal CT colonography. *Source*: Courtesy of Robert L. MacCarty, M.D., Mayo Clinic, Rochester, Minnesota.

1. The possibility that this study one day may be performed without prior bowel preparation;
2. The possibility of greater patient acceptability (not yet proven); and
3. The potential for screening of important disease outside the colon (94).

The accuracy of CTC varies widely among reported series depending on how the studies were performed. Pickardt et al. (95) reported a prospective evaluation of CTC as a colorectal carcinoma screening test. The study included 1233 asymptomatic adults who underwent CTC and same-day colonoscopy. More than 97% of subjects were at average risk for colorectal neoplasia. Radiologists used the 3-D endoluminal display for the initial detection of polyps on CTC. They found that the sensitivity of CTC for polyps size ≥1 cm, ≥8 mm, and ≥6 mm was 93.8%, 93.9%, and 88.7% compared to 87.5%, 91.5%, and 92.3%, respectively, for colonoscopy. The authors concluded that CTC with the use of 3-D approach is an accurate screening method for the detection of colorectal neoplasia in asymptomatic average risk adults and compares favorably with colonoscopy.

Pineau et al. (96) conducted a similar prospective study of 205 patients with average risk of colorectal neoplasia using oral contrast with CTC. They showed the sensitivity of 84.4% and specificity of 83.1% for lesions ≥6 mm and 90% and 94.6%, respectively, for lesions ≥10 mm. Of note was the negative predictive value of 95% for a 6 mm cutoff size and 98.9% for a 10 mm cutoff.

In contrast, Cotton et al. (97) found the sensitivity of CTC to be low compared to colonoscopy and the accuracy varied considerably between centers. In this report, a nonrandomized evaluator blinded, noninferiority study design of 615 participants aged 50 years or older who were referred for routine clinically indicated colonoscopy in nine major hospital centers. The CTC was performed by using multislice scanners immediately before standard colonoscopy. The results showed that the sensitivity of CTC for detecting lesions size at least 6 mm was 39% (95% CI, 29.6% to 48.4%), and for lesions at least 10 mm was 55% (95% CI, 39.9% to 70.0%). These results were significantly lower than those for conventional colonoscopy, with sensitivities of 99.0% (95% CI, 97.1% to 99.9%), and 100%, respectively.

Johnson et al. (98) prospectively evaluated the performance of CTC in a large asymptomatic population with low disease prevalence. As such, the study population represents a sample of patients likely to undergo CTC screening. Seven hundred and three asymptomatic persons underwent CTC followed by same-day colonoscopy. Diagnostic review of each study was performed by two of three experienced radiologists in the blind fashion. With colonoscopy serving as gold standard, CTC detected 34%, 32%, 73%, and 63% of the 59 polyps ≥1 cm for readers 1, 2, 3, and double-reading, respectively; and 35%, 29%, 57%, 54% of 94 polyps 5 to 9 mm for readers 1, 2, 3, and double-reading, respectively. The results from this low lesion prevalence study (5% of patients had polyps ≥1 cm) differ from reports of other medical centers including their own previous reports. Technical and perceptual errors accounted for polyps missed by CTC. Causes of error are multifactorial. Technical errors were defined as polyps missed by both observers. This error accounted for 46% of the polyps 5 to 9 mm in diameter and 37% of polyps ≥1 cm. If a lesion was identified by one observer and missed by another, these were classified as perceptive errors. Perceptive errors accounted for 27% of polyps 5 to 9 mm and 34% of polyps greater than 1 cm. Polyp morphology such as sessile polyps, but not location, influenced detection rates.

Limitation in evaluating the current state of CTC technique includes a wide variation in results of clinical trials. There are as yet insufficient data on the use of CTC in routine clinical practice such as screening colorectal carcinoma (99).

At present, CTC seems reasonable in the patients with incomplete colonoscopy or who is a poor candidate for colonoscopy, although double-contrast barium enema is also a good choice and costs less. It also makes sense to do CTC (with IV contrast) in patients with obstructive colon carcinoma (100).

CAPSULE ENDOSCOPY

This is the new diagnostic tool to image the entire small bowel without pain. The imaging system consists of a single-use capsule endoscope. Although the capsule measures only 11 × 26 mm, it packs a color camera, light sources, a radiotransmitter, and batteries. The patient swallows the capsule, and relies on peristalsis to advance it through the digestive tract. The system allows five hours of continuous recording. Patients do not need to be hospitalized for the study (101). The capsule has been recently cleared by the Federal Drug Administration for clinical use in the United States, but the data on its efficiency is still scant. In a report by Appleyard et al. (102) on four patients with recurrent small bowel bleeding capsule endoscopy identified angiodysplasias in the stomach and small bowel. All four patients described the capsule as easy to swallow, painless, and preferable to conventional endoscopy.

Selby (103) evaluated 42 patients (24 men, 18 women) who had gastrointestinal (GI) bleeding of obscure origin, and 50 patients (25 men, 25 women) who had anemia alone. Clinical and other data were collected prospectively. Patients had at least upper endoscopy and colonoscopy which were negative and were referred for capsule endoscopy. The results showed a definite or probable cause of GI blood loss in 60 of 92 patients (65%). The nature of the abnormality was similar between those who presented with overt bleeding and those with anemia. The majority were angiodysplasia (47 of 60), 45 of which were in the small intestine, the most common site was the jejunum (40 patients). Seven patients had small bowel neoplasms, five presented with anemia alone, and two presented with overt bleeding. Three patients had ulcers in the small intestine (two Crohn's, one anastomotic ulcers). One patient had radiation enteritis with active bleeding. Two patients had gastric antral vascular ectasia, a finding not identified at prior endoscopies. Given its diagnostic superiority for examination of the small intestine, capsule endoscopy should be used as the next investigation after a non-diagnostic endoscopy and a colonoscopy in patients with GI bleeding of obscure origin.

Capsule endoscopy has the advantage over push enteroscopy, which is limited to only a few feet beyond the ligament of Treitz. Sonde enteroscopy (Sonde, in French for probe) can endoscopically examine the entire small intestine, but it is time consuming and inefficient for an accurate examinations (104). Most major centers have abandoned this technique. Capsule endoscopy will likely become an essential tool for small bowel examination (105).

COLONOSCOPY

Colonoscopy was introduced for clinical use in 1970. Originally it was used as a diagnostic aid to barium enema studies. Lesions or mucosal abnormalities could be visualized and confirmed by biopsy. At the outset, success in reaching the cecum was only 30% to 50%. The first colonoscopic polypectomy was performed by Hiromi Shinya (106) of New York in 1969. Progress and advancement in technology, both in the technique of passing the scope and in improvement of the instrument, have been rapid. At the present time, colonoscopy is the ultimate procedure for the detection of colonic diseases. When the procedure is properly performed, the complication rates are low (107,108). Almost all pedunculated polyps can be removed via the colonoscope. Most benign large sessile polyps can be removed piecemeal, often in more than one session (109,110). The indications for colonoscopy include almost unlimited colonic problems, and there are only a few contraindications. In fact, the most common excuses for not doing fiberoptic colonoscopy are the cost of the procedure and the unavailability of experienced colonoscopists. Colonoscopy has revolutionized the approach in the management of large bowel diseases.

To become a competent colonoscopist, intensive training in colonoscopy is essential. There are only a few basic principles of colonoscopy, but learning proper technique invariably requires considerable practice. The skill can be acquired only by actual performance. There is no single best method of teaching colonoscopy, but a one-person technique in a one-to-one teaching session is the most effective way. With the improvements in technique and instrumentation, a well-trained colonoscopist can reach the cecum in over 90% of cases (111).

HOW DIFFICULT IS COLONOSCOPY?

Although world-class colonoscopists can reach the cecum as much as 98% of the time (112), a significant number of the procedures are difficult and require good techniques and "tricks" that must be acquired. Williams (113) indicates that 25% of the attempted colonoscopies prove to be quick and easy. Fifty percent are more troublesome but well-tolerated and can be completed in 15 to 20 minutes, but 25% are difficult, painful, or even impossible. Hull and Church (114) find no difficulty in passing the scope to the cecum in 25% of cases, mild difficulty in 33%, moderate difficulty in 28%, and severe difficulty in 14%. A retrospective review of 2194 colonoscopies performed by an expert colonoscopist showed that 31% of examinations in women are technically difficult compared with 16% in men (115). The most common cause of difficulty in colonoscopy is recurrent looping or bowing of the colonoscope in a long or mobile colon. Measurement of colonic length on barium enema films reveals that total colonic length is greater in women (median, 155 cm) compared to men (median, 145 cm) ($p = 0.005$), despite the smaller stature of women ($p < 0.0001$). The particular difference is in the transverse colon, where the colonoscope reaches the true pelvis more often in women (62%) than in men (26%) ($p < 0.001$) (115).

Although we generally regard the descending colon, splenic flexure, hepatic flexure, and ascending colon as fixed structures, measurement and observation of the mobility of different segments of the large intestine conducted by Saunders et al. (116) during a celiotomy have dispelled this belief. They found that 8% of the descending colons and 9% of the ascending colons were mobile because of the mesocolon. Twenty percent of the patients studied had mobile splenic flexure, and in 29% of the cases studied the mid-transverse colon reached the symphysis pubis or lower when pulled downward. In addition, in 20% of cases, the sigmoid colon had adhesions from diverticular disease, previous abdominal operations, or congenital adhesions. Findings such as these add to the difficulty in performing colonoscopy, although they do not necessarily prevent successful colonoscopy to the cecum. Another difficulty in passing the colonoscope successfully is the narrow base of the sigmoid mesentery (Fig. 21). In this situation, it is impossible to straighten the sigmoid colon, and the scope is passed through the left colon as an N configuration (Fig. 22).

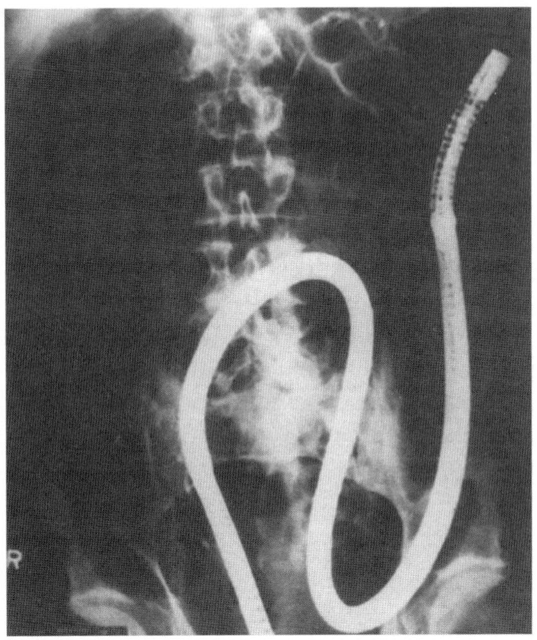

FIGURE 22 ■ N-shaped configuration of colonoscope passed through the left colon.

■ BOWEL PREPARATION

The first rule in colonoscopy is that the patient must have a clean colon. This is essential for ease in passing the scope and for minimizing air insufflation. Polyethylene glycol solution (PEG, Colyte, or GoLytely) was popularized in the 1980s because of its rapid overnight action and because it results in a clean colon in >90% of cases (117,118). However, a significant number of patients (5% to 20%) cannot tolerate the 4 L solution that has to be taken orally within 3 to 4 hours. Adams et al. (119) found that bisacodyl (Dulcolax) reduces the volume of PEG solution required to be taken. A modification of bowel preparation can be done as follows: PEG solution, 250 mL, taken orally every 10 to 15 minutes for 2 L starting at 5 PM the day before colonoscopy, and Dulcolax, 5 mg, three tablets taken orally at 10 PM. The patient may have a low-residue diet at lunch the day before and clear liquids in the evening meal.

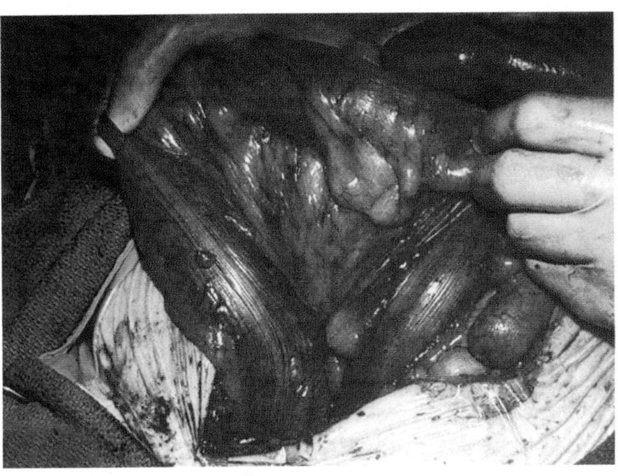

FIGURE 21 ■ Narrow base of the sigmoid mesentery.

In recent years, numerous studies have been conducted comparing the results of oral sodium phosphate (Fleet) to those of PEG. In most studies, the sodium phosphate acts as rapidly as the PEG, provides superior cleaning of the colon and rectum, is better tolerated, is preferred by patients, and is much cheaper than PEG (120–123). To be effective for colonoscopy, 45 mL sodium phosphate should be given in two doses (121). For an early morning or later start of the procedure, preparation at 5 pm followed by a second dose at 10 pm the evening before gives excellent results (124). In a randomized study using carbohydrate-electrolyte rehydration solution (Gatorade®) to mix with sodium phosphate versus water, the Gatorade group had superior visualization ($p < 0.01$), less intravascular contraction ($p < 0.03$), and similar tolerability of preparation ($p = 0.2$) (125).

Patients are allowed a low residue diet for lunch, and liquid diet for dinner. At 2 or 3 PM, they should drink sodium phosphate 45 mL mixed with three glasses of Gatorade or other sports drink. This should be followed by drinking three more glasses of Gatorade. Repeat the preparation at 10 PM.

A new option of bowel preparation is the sodium phosphate tablets (Visicol®, Inkine Pharmacevtical Co., Blue Bell, Pennsylvania, U.S.A.). It has been shown to be better tolerated by patients over sodium phosphate solution and PEG and produces equivalent colon cleansing for colonoscopy (126,127). However, it requires 20 tablets for two doses and the cost is higher. It has not been popularly used.

The Federal Drug Agency has conducted a safety review on oral sodium phosphate using the Agency's databases and medical literature (128). The review shows that serious electrolyte disturbances (hypernatremia, hypokalemia, hyperphosphatemia, and hypocalcemia), dehydration, metabolic acidosis, renal failure, tetany, and death have been attributed to patients receiving more than a 45 mL dose of sodium phosphate (usually minimum of 90 mL during 24-hour period).

In a review of 26 clinical trials with oral sodium phosphate for colonoscopy cleaning in adults conducted by Hookey et al. (129), all the studies use 45 mL sodium phosphate twice per day, dosing at intervals between three and 14 hours. In most series, comorbidities were excluded such as congestive heart failure, chronic renal failure, ascites, myocardial infarction (MI), bowel obstruction, etc. The cumulative series included 2496 patients; in addition, 526 patients received oral sodium phosphate tablets. None of these patients experienced a major adverse event because of sodium phosphate.

Serum potassium levels were reported in 12 studies and hypokalemia was noted in small numbers of patients, with the lowest reported value after oral ingestion of sodium phosphate solution of 2.9 mEq/L. Change in the serum sodium levels were also reported for 13 studies. Six demonstrated a statistically significant increase in values, but the magnitude of these changes was small and did not lead to clinical sequelae. The maximum reported value for serum sodium was 150 mEq/L. Serum calcium has been measured in 654 patients, receiving oral sodium phosphate solution in 12 trials. A decrease in mean serum calcium levels has been observed in most trials. The absolute changes in serum calcium after ingestion of sodium phosphate solution were minor. None of the 3022 patients who participated in clinical trials were reported to have experienced any symptoms attributable to hypokalemia.

Review of the adverse events in 29 adult patients showed that the majority of adverse events in these cases occurred when physicians ordered doses considerably higher than the recommended level (single 90 mL or total 135–360 mL dose).

The safety data reviewed by Hookey et al. (129) showed that sodium phosphate 45 mL dose given 5–12 hours apart in patients without major comorbid conditions would appear to be safe. In addition to encouraging patients to drink fluids liberally, intravenous rehydration should be considered in selected cases where adequate hydration is an issue.

All patients with comorbid conditions who are risking to have an adverse event should be considered contraindication to the use of sodium phosphate as bowel preparation for colonoscopy. These include acute diarrhea with dehydration, renal insufficiency, known electrolyte imbalances, inability to maintain adequate fluid intake, interic fistulas, malabsorption, significant gastrointestinal motility in either upper or lower gastrointestinal tract, congestive heart failure, myocardial infarction or unstable angina, ascites, ileus, peritonitis, megacolon, and bowel obstruction (124,129,130).

Between 1997 and August 2002, the FDA received 139 adverse event reports for sodium phosphate. Of these events, 18 were considered serious, including eight fatalities. For comparison, the FDA received 100 reports for polyethylene glycol solution, of which 30 were considered serious, including six fatalities (129).

None of the 3022 patients who participated in clinical trials were reported to have experienced any symptoms attributable to hypokalemia.

Frizelle et al. (131) reported three patients who developed seizures secondary to hyponatremia following ingestion of sodium phosphate or sodium picosulfate/magnesium citrate combination. Two of the three patients were on long term use of diuretics. They noted that the FDA received five reports of seizures associated with hyponatremia of whom 4 had taken 20 Visicol ™ tablets (1.5 grams sodium phosphate per tablet). In Canada, the Canadian adverse drug reaction monitoring program received 13 reports of suspected serious adverse reaction to oral sodium phosphate between 1994 and 2002 and reports of suspected serious adverse reactions to PEG between 1988 and 2002 (129).

Ayus et al. (132) reported 3 patients who developed severe dysnatremia after receiving 4 litres of an isosmotic PEG solution. Two of the patients suffered nausea, abdominal distention and diarrhea. One patient developed tonic-colonic convulsions leading to status epilepticus. She made a full recovery but the other two patients with end stage renal failure and diabetes mellitus had a fatal outcome. A fourth patient with a fatal outcome was also encountered.

To study the hypothesis that carbohydrate-electrolyte oral rehydration would attenuate the hypovolemic changes associate with administration of sodium phosphate, Barclay et al. (133) randomized patients to ingest either regular clear fluids (81) or carbohydrate-electrolyte rehydration solution (87) during pre-colonoscopy purgation by ingestion of aqueous sodium phosphate. By comparison with clear fluids rehydration resulted in significantly less intravascular volume contraction. Changes in estimated central venous pressure and orthostatic pulse were significantly greater in the clear fluid group versus the rehydration group. Changes in biochemical parameters after purgation also suggested a greater degree of volume contraction in the clear fluid versus rehydration group. Colonoscopic visualization was superior in the rehydration versus clear fluid group; tolerability in the preparations was similar between groups. Tjandra and Tagkalidis (134) conducted a randomized controlled trial to evaluate whether carbohydrate-electrolyte (E-lyte) solution enhanced bowel preparation and improved patient acceptance with oral sodium phosphate. A total of 187 consecutive adults undergoing colonoscopy were randomized to receive two packets of oral sodium phosphate (Fleet phospha-soda) with (90) or without (94) additional supplement of a carbohydrate-electrolyte (E-lyte solution). Patients taking E-lyte supplement had significantly less dizziness (none, 80 vs. 56%) and a trend toward less nausea (none, 70 vs. 56%). All patients in the carbohydrate-electrolyte group completed the bowel preparation as opposed to 3% of patients without the carbohydrate electrolyte being unable to complete the preparation. Hypokalemia was significantly more frequent in patients without E-lyte supplements. More patients without E-lyte supplement needed intravenous rehydration (11 vs. 4%). Differences in serum creatinine and urine-specific gravity suggested possibly a lesser degree of hypovolemia in patients taking E-lyte supplements. The quality of bowel cleansing in patients taking E-lyte supplements was considered better by both the endoscopists and patients. They concluded carbohydrate electrolyte solution protects against hypokalemia, improves patient tolerability, and may enhance use of oral sodium phosphate as a bowel preparation agent.

In a superb editorial on the appropriate use of sodium phosphate oral solutions, Love (135) put the concerns in perpective. Many colonoscopists and surgeons follow the regimen of two 45 ml of oral sodium phosphates solutions 12 hours apart as first described by Vanner et al. (136). Many subsequent trials and millions of doses of clinical experience have confirmed the initial results; it is highly effective, well tolerated, inexpensive and safe when given to appropriately selected and properly instructed patients. The risks and benefits must be kept in perspective, as with all medications. Wholesale abandonment of a useful product is not in our patients' best interest.

The main concern of most physicians is that the recommended maximum total daily dose for any indication in adults is 45 ml of sodium phosphates oral solution in a 24 hour period (137,138). The justification for this warning was statistically significantly electrolyte shifts (hypocalcemia, hyperphosphatemia, hypematremia, hypokalemia and acidosis) that are more likely to occur with more than one 45 ml dose per 24 hours. As noted above, a recent review of the literature by Hookey et al. (129) concluded that most reported adverse events using sodium phosphate oral solutions were due to inappropriate dosing. For normal healthy adults, the benefits far outweigh the risks (less than one in one million doses results in a serious adverse event). The superior cleansing action of sodium phosphate facilitates effective screening colonoscopies. Furthermore, superior patient acceptance of sodium phosphates commonly leads to completion of the appropriate cleansing regimen which is critical to provide a clean field of view for the colonoscopist. The bowel cleansing regimen described by Vanner et al. (136) is safe and effective and offers an alternative to patients. The denominator in the risk benefit ratio should not be forgotten because compliance and adequate cleansing of the bowel for a proper examination may be lifesaving.

A final comment regarding the use of sodium phosphate solution as a colon cleansing agent involves three important issues. The first relates to dosing and we are unaware of any evidence to suggest that spacing of two consecutive doses more than 5–6 hours apart is any more beneficial or less detrimental than shorter intervals. A second issue relates to hydration and it would seem prudent that patients imbibe adequate liquids to follow the oral laxative solution. And finally, patient selection is of paramount importance. As noted above, patients with chronic renal failure and congestive failure would not be candidates for this bowel preparation. Patients with co-morbid diseases who are on ACE inhibitors and diuretics are at increased risk for adverse reactions. The reality is that with current practice in the USA, more than half the physicians ordering bowel preparations use a sodium phosphate solution (two doses of 45 ml. within a 24 hours period) for the cleaning of the colon. Since it is being used anyway, education as to the proper use of the agent would appear to be in order. In so doing the sodium phosphate solution is a safe agent.

It is important that physicians need to be aware of the comorbid conditions that put patients at risk for complications. Physicians should make the decision which patients should not go through any bowel preparation at all. There are currently no substantive reports to suggest the availability of effective agents, or combinations of agents that are without risk.

■ SEDATION

Colonoscopy can be performed without medications in selected patients, but this technique requires a skillful and gentle colonoscopist who also has good techniques (139). Most colonoscopists, however, prefer to give preprocedural medications. Diazepam (Valium) or midazolam (Versed) alone or in combination with meperidine (Demerol) or fentanyl citrate (Sublimaze) are most suitable. The dosage of these drugs varies widely depending on the patient's size and general health. The endoscopist must be familiar with these medications. Naloxone hydrochloride (Narcan), an antidote for meperidine and fentanyl, and flumazenil (Romazicon), an antidote for midazolam and diazepam, should be available. Bradycardia from insufflation and overstretching of the sigmoid mesentery can be easily controlled by aspirating the air and pulling back the scope. Vasovagal reaction from diazepam and midazolam also causes bradycardia and is not uncommon. Atropine, 0.4 to 0.6 mg given intravenously, will quickly correct the problem and should be available. Diazepam may cause phlebitis and must be given slowly, preferably in a larger vein. Substituting midazolam for diazepam essentially eliminates this problem. In difficult cases, medications make the procedure easier for both the patient and the colonoscopist.

It is advisable to simultaneously monitor the patient's blood pressure, heart rate, and oxygen saturation using oximetry. Waye et al. (140) performed colonoscopy in 2097 patients under conscious sedation and removed 2019 polyps. No monitoring equipment or pulse oximetry was used for any patient. Three patients (0.1%) developed hypotension during diagnostic colonoscopy, identified by nurses who noted the patients' pallor and diaphoresis. All patients were resuscitated with naloxone, oxygen, and intravenous fluids. One patient experienced a short period of apnea during which mouth-to-mouth resuscitation was given. All the patients recovered without sequelae. It appears that unless one has an experienced and competent assistant, continuous and simultaneous monitoring of blood pressure, heart rate, and oxygen saturation is prudent.

The newest version of sedation for colonoscopy is propofol (Diprivan). The randomized study by Sipe et al. (141) comparing propofol to midazolam and meperidine showed that sedation was faster in propofol ($p < 0.001$), depth of sedation was greater ($p < 0.0001$), recover and discharge was faster ($p < 0.001$), and patients' satisfaction was greater ($p < 0.05$). There was no significant complication in either group of the series. The propofol was delivered by a designated nurse. Propofol is a respiratory and cardiovascular depressant with no antagonist. In fact it is an anesthetic agent; patients who receive propofol may lapse from the moderate sedation achieved under conscious sedation conditions to deep sedation or even anesthesia; endotracheal intubation may occasionally be necessary (142). Local rules and/or state laws in the United States usually prevent its independent administration by colonoscopists at this time. Cost effectiveness of administration of sedation by an anesthesia specialist for routine cases has not been evaluated. This practice is not recommended at present (143).

■ ANTIBIOTIC PROPHYLAXIS

The role of antibiotic prophylaxis is to reduce the possibility of a significant infectious complication. Randomized, double-blind, placebo-controlled trials, however, will likely never be performed. Despite the large number of endoscopic procedures performed annually, there are few case reports of bacterial endocarditis seen after the procedure. The rate of bacteremia associated with flexible sigmoidoscopy was 0–1%. Rates of bacteremia associated with colonoscopy ranged from 0% to 25%, with a mean frequency of 4.4%. Bacteremia usually was short lived (less than 30 minutes) and was not associated with any infectious complications (144). No studies, to date, that used antibiotic prophylaxis have demonstrated a clinically meaningful reduction in infectious complications during endoscopic procedures. In addition, antibiotic prophylaxis for infectious endocarditis in patients undergoing gastrointestinal endoscopic procedure is not always successful (144).

Antibiotic guidelines established for prophylaxis against infective endocarditis should be reserved for those patients with highest risk for infection. Indiscriminative use of antibiotic associated with gastrointestinal endoscopic procedures is to be discouraged, as it adds unnecessary cost and the potential for adverse reactions (144).

Recommendations for antibiotic prophylaxis for colonoscopy with or without biopsy or polypectomy are given in Table 1.

The Standard Task Force of the American Society of Colon and Rectal Surgeons (ASCRS) recommends prophylaxis for only the high-risk group (145).

The regimen of antibiotic use for the prevention of bacterial endocarditis (in adults) is as follows (144):

TABLE 1 ■ Antibiotic Prophylaxis for Colonoscopy with or without Biopsy

Patient Condition	Antibiotic Prophylaxis
High risk:	Prophylaxis optional
Prosthetic valve	
History of endocarditis	
Systemic pulmonary shunt	
Synthetic vascular graft (<1 yr old)	
Complex cyanotic congenital heart disease	
Moderate risk:	Not recommended
Most other congenital abnormalities	
Rheumatic heart disease	
Hypertrophic cardiomyopathy	
Mitral valve prolapse with regurgitation or thickened leaflets	
Low risk:	Not recommended
Coronary artery bypass graft, septal defect, patent ductus	
Heart murmurs	
Pacemakers, implantable defibrillators	
Ascites	Not recommended
Prosthetic joints	Not recommended
Immunocompromised patients	Not recommended

Source: From Ref. 144.

- Orally one hour before, IM or IV 30 minutes before the procedure
- Amoxicillin, 2 gm by mouth, or ampicillin, 2 gm IV
- Penicillin allergic: Vancomycin, 1 gm IV(7)
  or clindamycin, 600 mg IV
  or cephalexin or cefadroxil, 2 gm IV
  or azithromycin or clarithromycin, 500 mg IV
  or cefazolin, 1 gm IV or IM

■ INDICATIONS

Total colonoscopy is indicated (1) whenever the diagnosis cannot be resolved by air-contrast barium enema combined with flexible sigmoidoscopy or proctoscopy, (2) when a colon and rectal adenoma is detected, (3) for surveillance of chronic ulcerative colitis and Crohn's colitis, (4) for preoperative and postoperative examination in patients with carcinoma of the large bowel, and (5) screening for average and high-risk patients for colorectal carcinoma. Colonoscopy has now become the procedure of choice to decompress acute pseudo-obstruction of the colon (146–149).

■ CONTRAINDICATIONS

For the experienced colonoscopist, the contraindications to colonoscopy have become fewer. A patient with poor bowel preparation should be reprepared and rescheduled. The procedure should not be pursued if there is a fixed angle that cannot be straightened, even though passing of the scope does not cause severe pain. Total colonoscopy should not be performed in patients with acute inflammatory bowel disease and in those with acute diverticulitis; however, with care, the scope can be passed safely to the sigmoid colon for diagnostic purposes in those patients. Colonoscopy should not be performed in patients with large and small bowel obstruction and anal diseases that cause stricture or severe pain. If the patient is too weak, too sick, or too unstable to undergo bowel preparation, such as those who have experienced a recent myocardial infarction, colonoscopy should not be performed.

■ BASIC CONCEPTS IN TECHNIQUE

With the patient in the left lateral position, insertion of the colonoscope is preceded by digital examination to "forewarn" the anal sphincter. The distal 10–15 cm tip of the scope may be lubricated with 2% lidocaine jelly to prevent a burning sensation. Thereafter, a lubricant jelly should be used liberally. Throughout the entire procedure, the scope should be passed under direct vision. The procedure should be performed in a stepwise manner: advance the scope, straighten the scope, exert abdominal compression, change the patient's position. Not all patients require abdominal compression or a change in position. The ultimate goal of the colonoscopist is to pass the colonoscope to the cecum with "quality," without looping or bowing. Properly performed, a question mark configuration is achieved (Fig. 23). In this situation the scope can be advanced, withdrawn, turned left, turned right, and turned all around on command.

The pain caused by colonoscopy is from stretching of the colonic mesentery and/or an excessive amount of air insufflation, and these must be avoided. Pushing the scope forward stretches the mesentery, whereas pulling it back releases it.

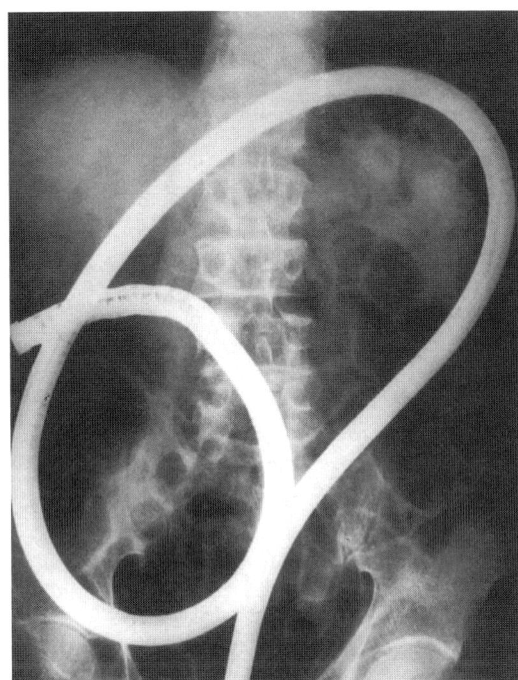

FIGURE 23 ■ Question mark configuration of a properly performed colonoscopy with tip of colonoscope intubated into the terminal ileum.

A spasm of the colon often is due to stretching of the mesentery rather than irritability of the colon. The pain will be alleviated if the scope is pulled back to release the stretching.

Air insufflation should be used only to open the collapsed bowel. Not only is a distended bowel painful, but it makes the angle more acute. Air in the distended bowel should be aspirated from time to time.

Passing the tip of the scope into the sigmoid colon by slightly withdrawing the scope and then gradually torquing or rotating it clockwise will not only straighten the sigmoid colon but will press it against the posterior abdominal wall. The scope can then be advanced without a looping or bowing formation, The sigmoid-descending angle is best passed by a to-and-fro motion, frequently requiring clockwise torquing of the scope (Fig. 24). A "slide by" technique, often needed when older model scopes are used, is occasionally necessary with the much improved current models. The same is true for an α-maneuver, which is quite painful for the patient (150). Turning the patient to a supine position after the scope has passed the sigmoid colon frequently makes passing the scope easier. Sometimes turning the patient or their right side is helpful to advance the scope. If an α-loop is formed in the sigmoid colon, it must be reduced before the scope can be advanced beyond the splenic flexure; this is accomplished by withdrawing and gradually rotating the scope clockwise (Fig. 25). An α-loop formation is suspected if advancing the scope causes more severe pain than it should, or when there is a paradoxical motion at the tip of the scope (i.e., the tip of the scope advances when it is withdrawn and recedes when it is pushed up). Feeling the scope on the anterior abdominal wall indicates that a looping or bowing of the sigmoid colon is being formed.

The same basic principles are applied to passing the scope into the transverse colon and the right colon. Abdominal compression and changes in patient's positioning are helpful. In a study by Waye et al. (151), the application of abdominal pressure or a change of the patient's body position was used 619 times in 165 patients (82% of patients examined). The authors noted an average of 3.75 pressure applications per colonoscopy, most lasting <30 seconds. Pressure is most commonly used when the colonoscope tip is at the splenic flexure followed by when the tip is at the hepatic flexure. Abdominal compression helps splint the colonoscope to prevent a looping or bowing formation. In the right colon, suction of the distended colon often produces an accordion-like bowel, which allows the scope to advance into the cecum. The new variable stiffness colonoscope has yet been shown to make a substantial difference in cecal intubation rates or speed of intubation for routine colonoscopy (152).

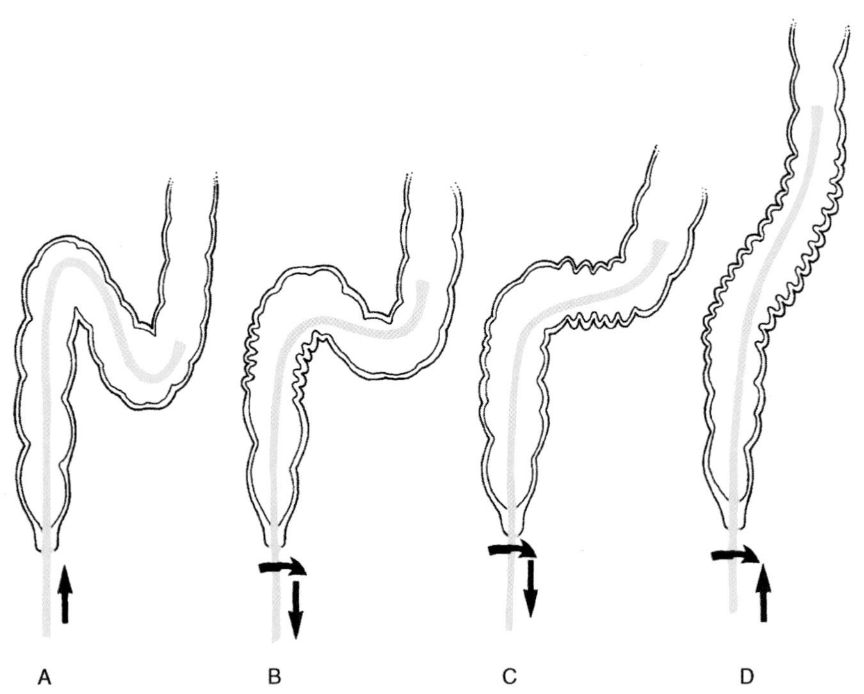

FIGURE 24 ■ Angulations of the sigmoid colon. (**A**) Advancement of the colonoscope causing N-shaped configuration with sharp angles between rectum and sigmoid and sigmoid and descending colon. (**B**) Withdrawal of the scope and clockwise rotation to widen the angles. (**C**) Further withdrawal and clockwise rotation to straighten the sigmoid colon. (**D**) While clockwise rotation is maintained, the scope can be advanced through the straightened sigmoid colon. *Source*: From Ref. 106.

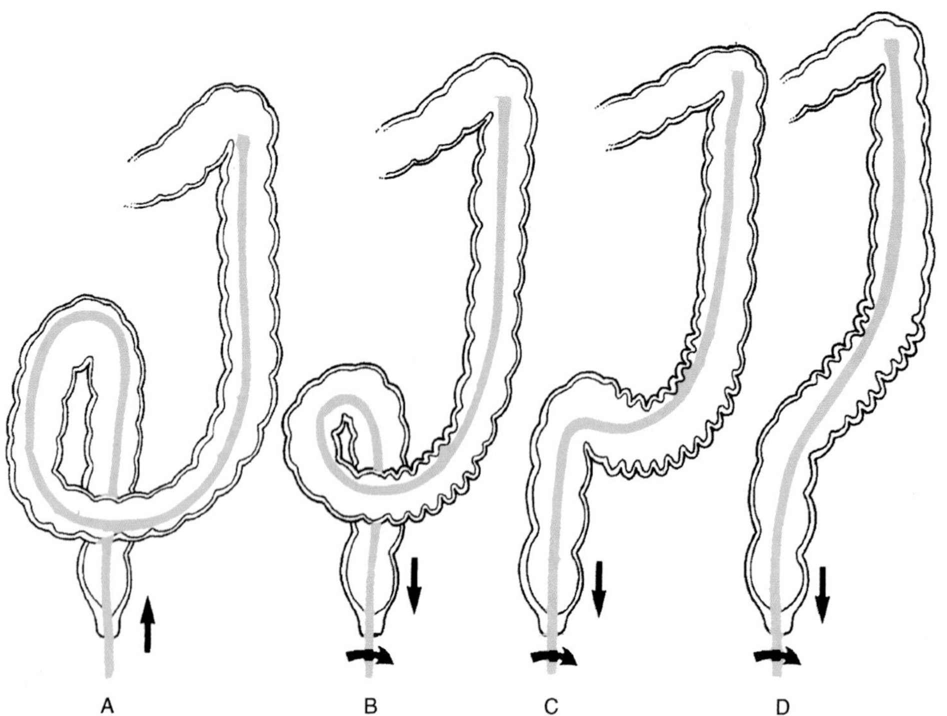

FIGURE 25 ■ α-Loop of the sigmoid colon. (**A**) An α-loop formation of sigmoid colon during colonoscopy. (**B–D**) Withdrawal of the scope with clockwise rotation will eliminate the α-loop and straighten the sigmoid colon. *Source*: From Ref. 106.

■ COMPLICATIONS

Although the complication rate in diagnostic colonoscopy is low, its importance is magnified by the large number of patients undergoing the procedure. Perforations, the most common and the most important complication, are caused by forceful passage of the colonoscope through a loop, bowing of the sigmoid colon, narrowing from diverticular disease, or adhesions from previous pelvic operation. The spectrum of perforations ranges from "silent" pneumoperitoneum to serosal tear, extraperitoneal perforation, and intraperitoneal perforation. Retroperitoneal perforations are usually difficult to assess clinically and may not be detected until the appearance of subcutaneous emphysema. The air may track along the retroperitoneal planes, up to the flank, mediastinum, neck, and around the eyes or down to the scrotum. The most frequent site of perforation is in the intraperitoneal sigmoid colon. Although the incidental finding of "silent" pneumoperitoneum can be observed, operation is indicated in most perforations that occur during diagnostic colonoscopy because those perforations are generally large. If the operation for colonoscopic perforation is performed early, a primary repair can be performed. If generalized peritonitis has already occurred, resection without anastomosis is the safest procedure.

Splenic injury from colonoscopy is uncommon, most likely occurring from pulling down the colonoscope from the transverse colon with the tip of the scope in a locked position. Abdominal pain is the most common symptom, usually within 24 hours. CT scan of abdomen is helpful to confirm the diagnosis. Most patients refuse a splenectomy (153).

The complication rate in diagnostic colonoscopy can be kept to a minimum by use of proper technique, knowledge of when to stop the procedure, and appreciation of the causes and mechanisms.

■ COLONOSCOPIC POLYPECTOMY

Techniques

Colonoscopic polypectomy is potentially dangerous, and patients must be selected carefully. When visualizing the gross appearance of the lesion through the scope, the colonoscopist must decide whether to perform a biopsy, electrocoagulate, excise, or leave the lesion alone. Sessile polyps with a base larger than 2 cm should be removed piecemeal in 1 to 1.5 cm increments each, occasionally in more than one session. Sessile polyps with induration and ulceration are signs of invasive carcinoma. Colonoscopy has no place in removing a frank carcinoma; for those lesions, a biopsy should be done.

Pedunculated Polyps

Almost all pedunculated polyps of any size can be safely snared in one piece because the stalk rarely is larger than 1.5 cm. Usually the snare wire can be manipulated to loop around the polyp, even when it is larger than the size of the wire loop itself. The basic principles of snaring a pedunculated polyp are first to place the snare wire around the head of the polyp and then to manipulate the scope and/or wire toward the stalk. Once the wire is in the desired position just below the head of the polyp, the snare or the scope is advanced so that the base of the wire loop or the plastic sheath is in contact with the stalk. At this point the snare wire is closed snugly, and the electric current is activated (Fig. 26). The level of coagulating current should be set according to the size of the tissue being cut. A large tissue requires a higher setting. For large polyps, it may be wise to cinch the snare around the stalk snugly and wait for a couple of minutes to give the feeding vessels in the stalk a chance to thrombose prior to transection. With optimum setting on the electrocautery machine, the snare wire should cut through the polyp within 4–5 seconds. If this

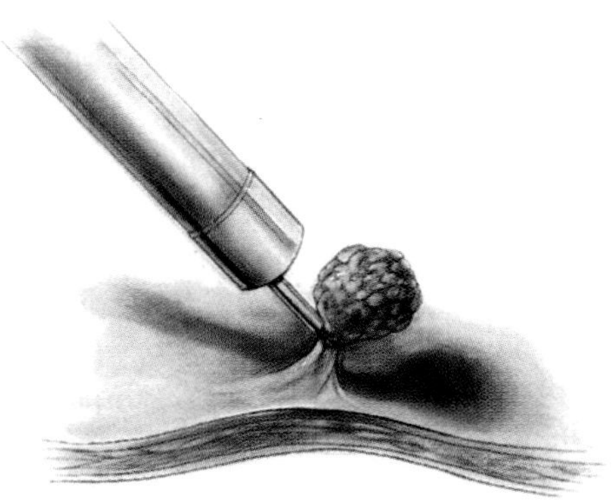

FIGURE 26 ■ Snare wire around the stalk of a polyp.

is not accomplished, the following should be rechecked: possible malfunction of the machine, too low heat, or too much tissue incorporated in the snare wire. Only pure coagulation current is used.

Sessile Polyp

Sessile polyps smaller than 2 cm usually can be snared in one piece. The technique is the same as for a pedunculated polyp, except that the wire is placed flush on the mucosa. When the snare wire is closed, the mucosa and the submucosa are squeezed into the snare wire. Before electrocautery is applied, the polyp should be lifted slightly from the bowel wall to minimize the chance of burning into the colonic wall (Fig. 27). A larger polyp should be snared piecemeal in 1 to 1.5 cm pieces (Fig. 28). It is important that an effort be made to retrieve each piece of the transected polyp for histopathologic examination, because any of these pieces may harbor a focal area of an invasive carcinoma. Depending on the size and difficulty in snaring, some large polyps should be snared in more than one session. Some authors recommend injection of saline with or without epinephrine into the submucosa beneath the polyp (154). The "saline cushion" elevates the polyp from the muscularis propria and renders it safer and more successfully snared. This technique is recommended for large sessile polyps (155,156). Hydroxypropyl methylcellulose or artificial tear (Gonak, Akorn, Inc., Buffalo Grove, Illinois, U.S.A.) is excellent for submucosal injection (157). The bottle of 15 mL should be diluted with 60 mL normal saline solution. Very large polyps (especially those in the right colon) should be reserved for colonic resection.

Diminutive Polyp

Diminutive polyps are defined as polyps that are smaller than 5 mm in diameter. Contrary to past beliefs that most small polyps of the large bowel were of the hyperplastic type and were confined primarily to the rectum, in the era of colonoscopy, diminutive polyps have been found throughout the entire large bowel, and the incidence of neoplastic types is over 50%. In themselves, diminutive polyps have no clinical significance, and most of them probably grow very slowly (158–160). However, it is impossible to predict which ones will grow to sizes that are of clinical significance. A diminutive neoplastic polyp seen in the colon or rectum may be a clue that additional polyps are in the more proximal colon. This calls for a complete colonic examination.

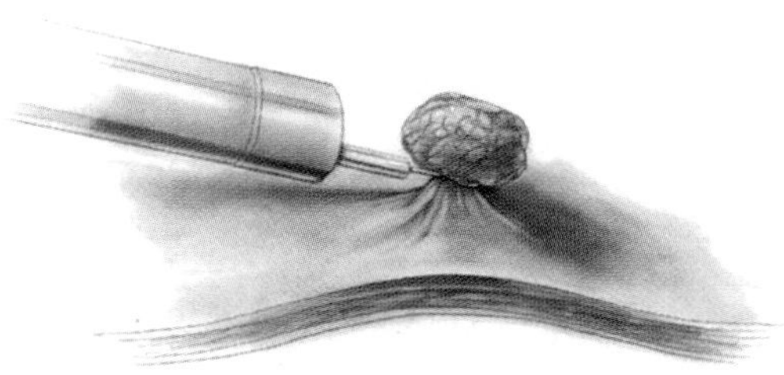

FIGURE 27 ■ Snare wire at the base of a sessile polyp. Note tenting of the mucosa.

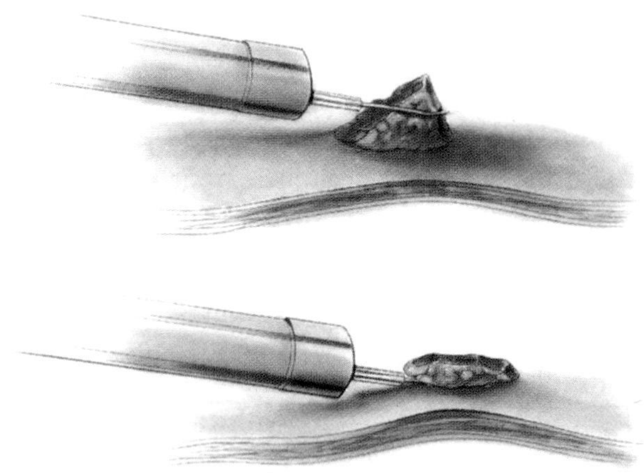

FIGURE 28 ■ Piecemeal snaring of a large sessile polyp.

The importance of destroying diminutive polyps of the large bowel is arguable. There are many advantages in removing these small polyps. The histologic type is known from the biopsy, appropriate endoscopic surveillance can be planned, and the follow-up with a barium enema study every one or two years can be eliminated. Small polyps are best treated by a biopsy followed by electrocoagulation or by using a "hot biopsy" forceps (161). If preferred, the polyp can be excised with a snare wire (162). For practical purposes, many diminutive polyps can be electrocoagulated without biopsy (163).

Risk of Bowel Gas Explosion

Two explosive gases in the colon are hydrogen and methane, both of which are formed by colonic bacteria. To produce hydrogen, colonic bacteria require a constant supply of exogenous substrate, primarily unabsorbed carbohydrate (164). Hence, a good bowel cleansing followed by an overnight fast markedly reduces hydrogen production. In contrast, methane is produced from an exogenous carbon source; thus its production has no clear-cut relation to diet (165). However, the vigorous bowel cleansing required for colonoscopy reduces by tenfold the amount of hydrogen and methane liberated in the colon (166). The risk of bowel gas explosion can be reduced further by exchanging gas and air in the bowel lumen by air insufflation, alternated with several aspirations before the snaring is performed. It is not necessary to use carbon dioxide to prevent gas explosion in the well-prepared colon unless it is done to decrease abdominal distention (167). The tragic case report of a bowel gas explosion was attributed to preparation of the bowel with mannitol, a potent substrate in which bacteria produce hydrogen (168).

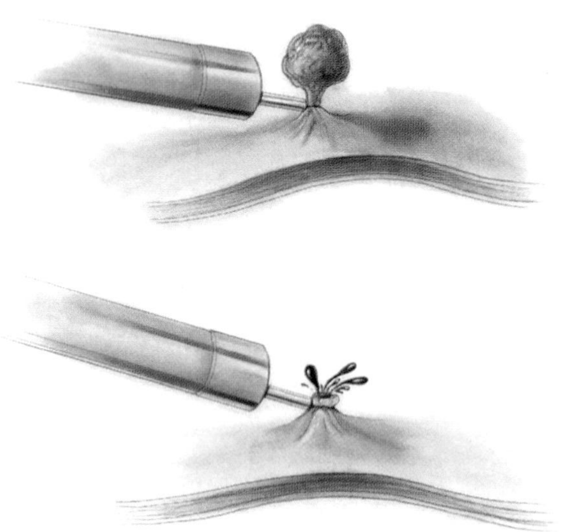

FIGURE 29 ■ Bleeding stump of a polyp is strangulated by the snare.

Mannitol preparation should not be used in patients who require snaring or electrocoagulation of a large bowel polyp.

Complications

The reported complication rates from colonoscopic polypectomy have been low, ranging from 0.7% to 3% (106,107, 169,170). The importance of the rates is magnified by the large number of patients undergoing the procedure. These figures probably do not represent the true incidence of complications because most of the reports come from individuals or institutions with extensive experience. Colonoscopic polypectomy is a potentially dangerous procedure. Bleeding is the most common complication, followed in frequency by transmural burn and free perforation (96,97,140,169,171). Other complications are "silent" perforation, snare entrapment, and ensnarement of the bowel wall. Early recognition of manifestations and understanding of proper treatment are crucial. Management may vary from observation to immediate exploratory celiotomy.

Bleeding

A pedunculated polyp with a thick stalk is the most dangerous with respect to immediate bleeding. It is important to leave enough stalk so that when bleeding occurs, the remnant of the stalk can be resnared and strangulated with the wire without electrocoagulation and can be held for 15–20 minutes (Fig. 29) (106). Immediate bleeding from removal of a sessile polyp can be controlled with injection of diluted epinephrine solution at the site of the bleeding or by the use of hemoclips (172). Delayed bleeding can occur from a few hours to several days after the procedure. Selective arteriography with a vasopressin drip effectively stops the bleeding that occurs (Fig. 30). Selective arteriography with Gelfoam emboli is not recommended because of the danger of ischemia of the colon (Fig. 31); however, it can be used as the last resort. On some occasions, an exploratory celiotomy may be necessary.

Transmural Burn

Transmural burn occurs when excessive heat burns through the bowel wall or when the snare wire is too close to the bowel wall. The classic symptoms are fever, localized abdominal pain, rebound tenderness, and leukocytosis. Once the diagnosis has been made, the patient should be admitted to the hospital, given nothing by mouth, and given intravenous fluids and antibiotics. In patients who do not have fever or leukocytosis, antibiotics are not necessary.

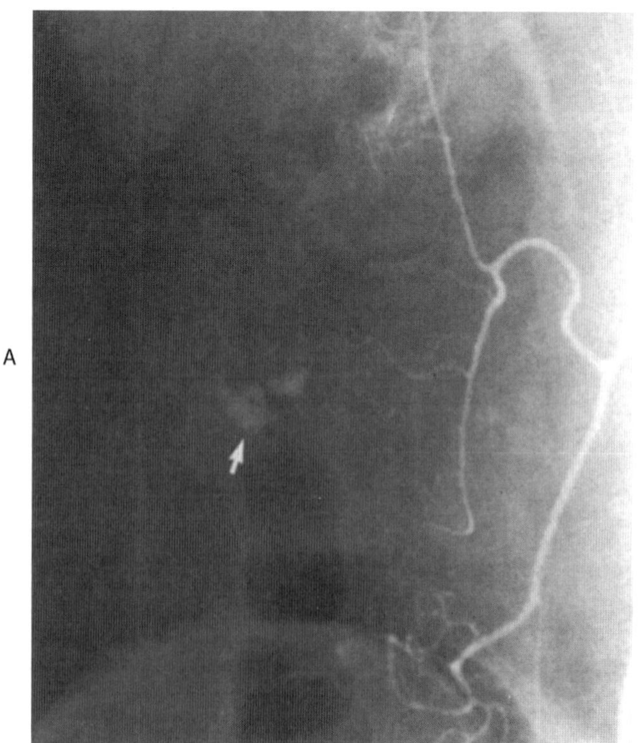

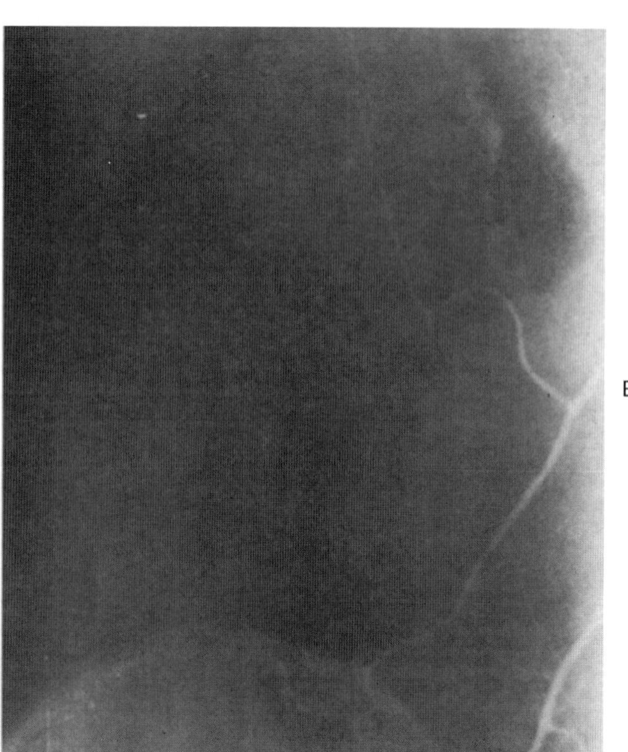

FIGURE 30 ■ Bleeding in the ascending colon after colonoscopic polypectomy. (**A**) Superior mesenteric arteriography showing bleeding (*arrow*). (**B**) Bleeding stopped after vasopressin drip. *Source*: From Ref. 169.

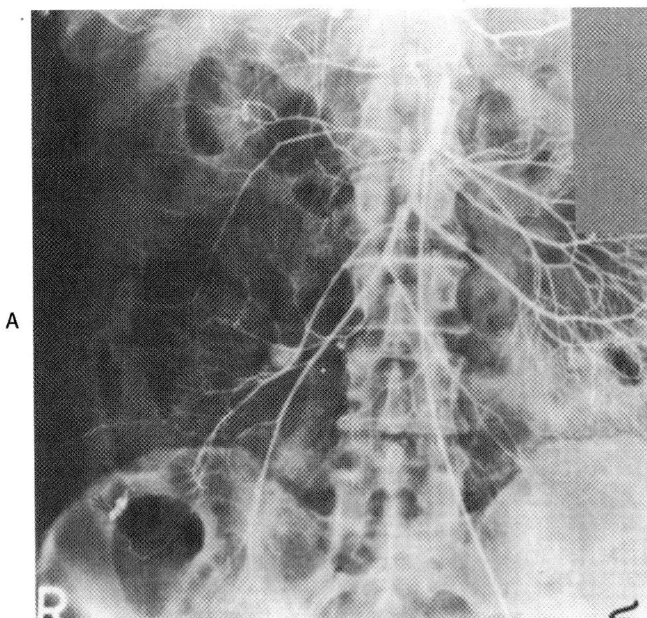

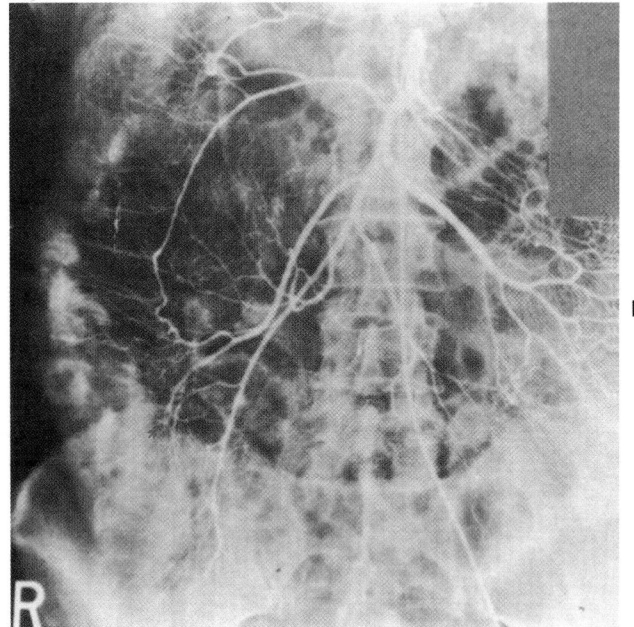

FIGURE 31 ■ Bleeding in the cecum after colonoscopic polypectomy. (**A**) Superior mesenteric arteriography showing bleeding (*arrow*). (**B**) Bleeding stopped after introduction of Gelfoam emboli (*arrow*). *Source*: From Ref. 169.

Intra-abdominal Abscess

This is the progression of transmural burn. The patient should be admitted to the hospital to receive antibiotics followed by a CT-guided percutaneous drainage.

Free Perforation

Unlike the usually large perforation caused by injury from the colonoscope, perforation from polypectomy may vary from "silent" asymptomatic air under the diaphragm (Fig. 32) to a large perforation that causes generalized peritonitis. No treatment is needed to correct asymptomatic air under the diaphragm, but the patient must be observed to detect any development of peritonitis (173). If there is a large symptomatic perforation associated with signs and symptoms of peritonitis, an immediate exploratory celiotomy is required. Perforation in colonoscopic polypectomy is caused by snaring too large a piece, applying too much heat, or snaring tissue that is too deep or too close to the bowel wall.

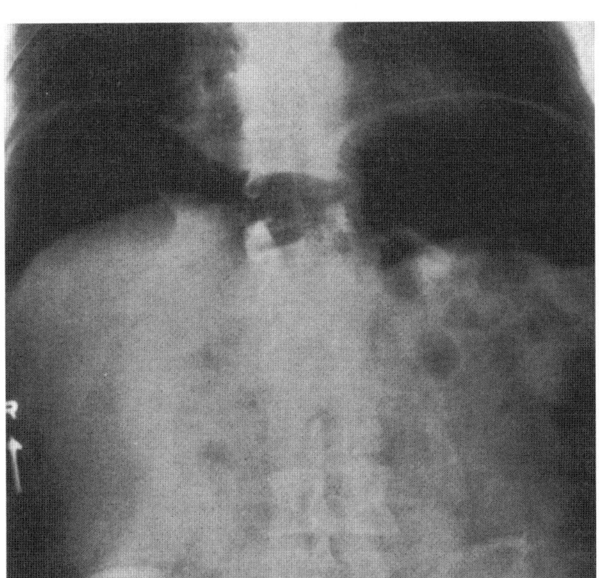

FIGURE 32 ■ Asymptomatic free air under diaphragm after colonoscopic polypectomy. *Source*: From Ref. 169.

Snare Entrapment

If the snare wire gets caught in the substance of a polyp, it may be impossible to cut through the polyp or disengage the wire. This problem is caused by too much tissue in the snare, too low a heat setting (causing "charring" of the tissue), or misjudgment in snaring a frank carcinoma. For a benign lesion, the entrapped wire should be tightened and left in place while the colonoscope is removed from the patient. With the strangulation of the wire, the polyp should fall off in a few days. If the entrapment occurs in a frank carcinoma, a colonic resection is done (169).

Ensnared Bowel

If care is not taken during polypectomy, the adjacent bowel wall inadvertently may be incorporated into the wire loop, causing perforation to occur (Fig. 33). Being aware of this possibility may prevent the complication. Difficulty in transecting the polyp, as evidenced by unusually high current requirements, may indicate that too much tissue is within the wire loop.

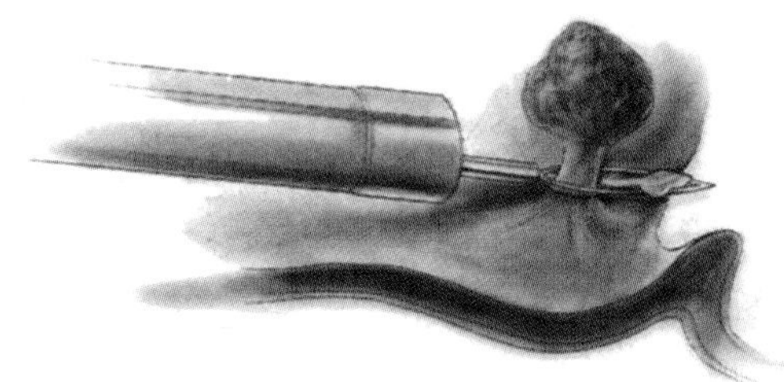

FIGURE 33 ■ Inadvertent ensnarement of adjacent bowel wall.

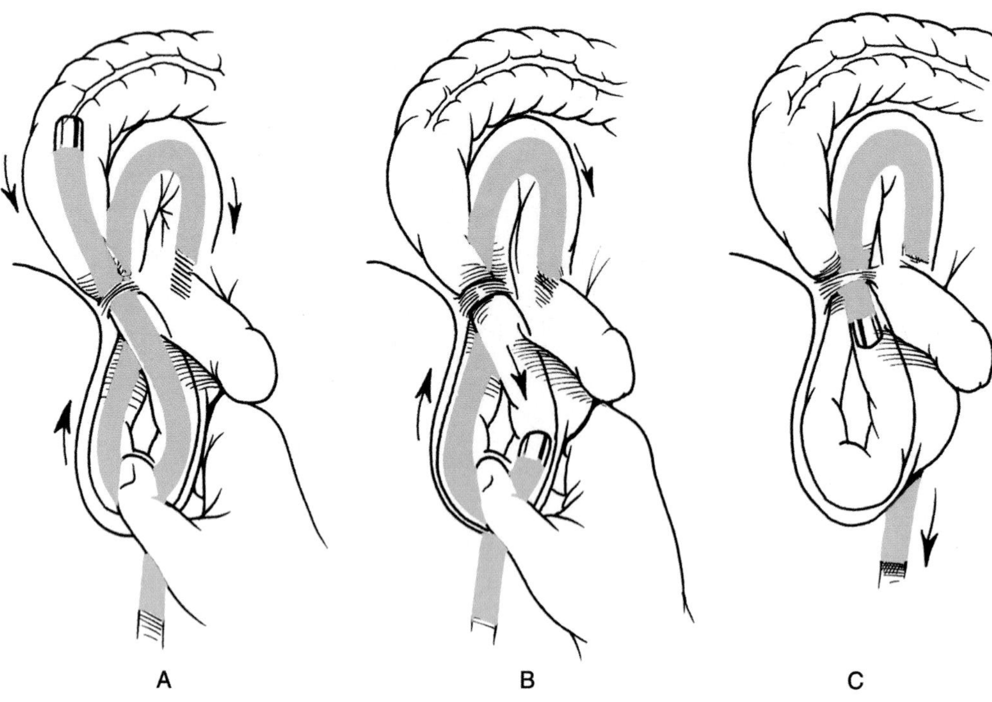

FIGURE 34 ■ "Pulley" technique of removal. (**A**) Scope held along inner edge of loop. (**B** and **C**) Instrument exits one limb at a time; thumb and finger are used as the "pulley." *Source*: From Ref. 174.

Incarceration of the Colonoscope in an Inguinal Hernia

Hernial incarceration of the colonoscope is an unusual complication. Incarceration can be avoided by considering the presence of a large sliding inguinal hernia as an absolute contraindication to colonoscopy. The risk of incarceration can be minimized by reducing the hernia before the procedure and by maintaining reduction while the colonoscope is advanced. If inadvertent incarceration occurs, however, simple traction on the colonoscope should not be used to remove the instrument. Instead, the "pulley" technique, in which the colonoscope is extricated one limb at a time, should be applied (Fig. 34A–C) (174).

Basic Principles for Achieving a Safe Procedure

DO NOT OVERDISTEND THE COLON ■ A colon distended with air causes discomfort to the patient and thins out the bowel wall, making it more susceptible to transmural burn. Aspiration of air to slightly collapse the colonic lumen, while still providing adequate exposure for snaring, will eliminate this problem.

HAVE FULL COMMAND OF THE COLONOSCOPE ■ The snare wire should not be placed around a polyp until the colonoscopist is in complete control of the colonoscope. A looping or a bowing of the scope can be corrected by pulling down the scope and turning it clockwise. Once the scope has been straightened, a 1:1 ratio of movement can be recognized. With the scope under full control, it can be turned to the left and right, advanced, or withdrawn as required.

SNARE THE POLYP AT 5–6–7 O'CLOCK ■ The channel for the snare coming out at the tip of the colonoscope is at the 5 o'clock position. It is safer and easier to snare the polyp in the lower half of the bowel lumen. With complete control of the scope, the polyp in the upper half of the bowel lumen can be rotated to the lower half without much difficulty.

ADJUST THE SETTING OF THE ELECTROCAUTERY UNIT ■ Different cautery units have different intensities. The amount of electrocauterization should vary according to the size of the tissue to be snared. A pure coagulation current should be used. The larger the tissue to be cut, the higher the intensity. In patients with a juvenile polyp, the heat should be turned down to approximately half. The stalk in a juvenile polyp has no muscularis mucosa, and very little coagulation current is needed to cut through it. On the other hand, entrapment of the snare wire into the substance of the polyp can occur when the current density is set too low, causing charring of the tissue. A lipoma contains 90% water and requires a tremendous amount of heat to transect it. Polypectomy for a large sessile lipoma should be avoided.

DO NOT REMOVE A FRANK CARCINOMA AT COLONOSCOPY ■ A frank carcinoma is usually firm or ulcerated. Once the snare wire is closed around the carcinoma, it may not be possible to cut through it or disengage the wire.

DISSIPATE THE HEAT PASSING THROUGH THE POLYP TO THE OPPOSITE BOWEL WALL ■ In the case of a large polyp, the tip of the polyp frequently touches the opposite bowel wall, and heat from the snare at the base of the polyp can be transmitted to this opposite wall (Fig. 35). When such heat

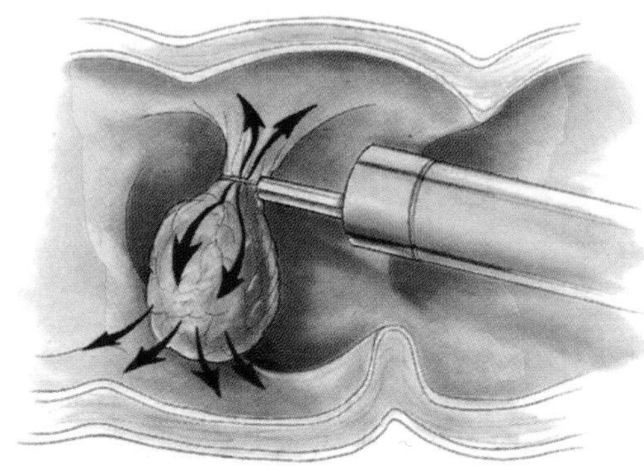

FIGURE 35 ■ Transmission of heat through polyp to opposite bowel wall.

transmission occurs, the burn rarely is severe. Jiggling the polyp head to and fro during snaring will prevent this type of damage by moving a small point of contact to various areas on the wall. An alternate method is to allow the entire head of the polyp to touch the bowel wall, thus distributing the heat to a larger area.

■ INTRAOPERATIVE COLONOSCOPY

Colonoscopy has become a standard procedure for diagnosing colonic diseases and for removing colonic polyps. In skilled hands, total colonoscopy can be achieved more than 90% of the time. However, certain conditions make total colonoscopy impossible, including severe sigmoid diverticular disease, acute and fixed colonic angles from adhesions, an unusually tortuous colon, pelvic inflammation, and irradiation. The only way for colonoscopy to be successful in these situations is by performing an intraoperative colonoscopy (i.e., passing the scope through the rectum with the abdomen open). This procedure has never become popular, and the number of cases in which it has been used is small. The reasons are obvious—the procedure is at best a nuisance, a colonoscopy setup is required in the operating room, the procedure requires two teams of surgeons or a surgeon and an endoscopist, it consumes additional operative time, and there may be considerable colonic distention from air insufflation.

Intraoperative colonoscopy may have a definite place in a small number of cases. One example is to locate the site of the lesion when it cannot be identified by palpation. When properly performed, it is safe (175–177). However, it must be performed with care and by personnel familiar with the technique. Cohen and Forde (178) reported two cases of splenic capsular tear. Another potential danger is serosal tear of the colon or even perforation.

Polypectomy

Intraoperative colonoscopic polypectomy generally is indicated only if the polyp cannot be reached by the conventional method. The techniques of polypectomy are the same as those of the conventional method. Another indication is to locate the site from which the malignant polyp was previously removed and for which colonic resection was required. This can be achieved only if the scar from the polypectomy is not completely healed, usually within two weeks.

Bleeding

Chronic blood loss from the gastrointestinal tract can be very difficult to detect by colonoscopy, barium enema, upper intestinal and small bowel barium studies, and arteriography. Intraoperative enteroscopy in conjunction with intraoperative colonoscopy can help identify the bleeding source (175). The techniques consist of passing the colonoscope orally and advancing it all the way to the ileocecal junction. An alternative is to pass a sterile colonoscope via an upper jejunal enterotomy. The mucosa of the entire small bowel is examined. At the same time, the serosa is examined via the transillumination for vascular abnormalities. The final step is to pass the colonoscope through the anal canal and advance it to the cecum. The entire large bowel is examined in the same manner.

Acute or massive colonic bleeding may be another indication for intraoperative colonoscopy, when all other methods, including preoperative colonoscopy, have failed to localize the source of the bleeding. Intraoperative colonoscopy has the advantages of both intraluminal and extraluminal examination (179). Intraoperative colonic lavage via a catheter inserted into the appendiceal base or a cecostomy has been shown to improve the quality of the examination (180,181).

Carcinoma

Patients with carcinoma of the large bowel require a complete colonic investigation to detect a synchronous carcinoma or adenoma (182). Ideally the examination should be completed before the operation. However, if an examination is not performed, one can proceed with the operation and perform an intraoperative colonoscopy. I prefer to perform colonoscopy before the abdominal incision is made. Intraoperative colonoscopy also is indicated in cases in which the lesion shown on barium enema cannot be palpated at exploration. For patients with obstructive carcinoma in whom preoperative colonoscopy could not be performed, intraoperative colonoscopy immediately following colonic resection may be an option (175). This indication is not advisable because colonoscopy may damage the freshly constructed anastomosis.

EXAMINATION OF STOOL

■ OCCULT BLOOD TESTING

Guaiac Test

Hemoccult is a commercial guaiac-impregnated filter paper used to detect occult blood in the stool. It has good sensitivity, but the specificity is poor. The test can be done by the individual at home by smearing stool on the paper slides provided. Basically, the test detects peroxidase in the hemoglobin; after application of a reagent, the chemically impregnated filter paper will turn blue. The reason the Hemoccult test is not specific is that many foods also contain peroxidase (raw meat, pheasant, salmon, sardines, turnips, radishes, cherry tomatoes, and many fruits and vegetables) (183,184). These foods may cause a false positive result. Vitamin C is known to give a false negative test, whereas iron and aspirin give false positive results (185). During the time of stool collection, these factors must be avoided. A restricted diet is recommended for two to three days before the test and should be continued during the test. At the present time, Hemoccult II and the more sensitive Hemoccult II Sensa are available. The sensitivity of the Hemoccult test varies from series to series. In the series of Allison et al. (186), the sensitivity of Hemoccult II was 37% compared with a sensitivity of 79% for Hemoccult II Sensa.

Heme-Porphyrin Assays

HemoQuant, which differs from Hemoccult, is a newer test for occult fecal blood. It removes the iron from hemoglobin heme and measures the fluorescence of the derived porphyrin (187). Although pseudoperoxidase activity does not affect the assay, a strict diet in which nonhuman heme is excluded is essential (188). The HemoQuant test is quantitative. It measures both degraded and intact hemoglobin, in contrast to a guaiac test. It is more sensitive than the Hemoccult test (189). HemoQuant has not been widely used for fecal occult blood screening because of its complex processing.

Immunologic Test

HemeSelect is an immunologic test based on anti-human hemoglobin. It is specific to human hemoglobin and therefore avoids the problems of dietary interference. The likelihood of false positive results from upper gastrointestinal blood loss is also reduced, because the immunoreactive hemoglobin is rapidly degraded before it reaches the large bowel (188). The sensitivity of HemeSelect is 69% in the series by Allison et al. (186). This test has not been widely used.

■ DIARRHEAL STOOL EXAMINATION

Examination of the feces in diarrhea, especially in the acute phase, often gives clues to the underlying disease.

WET-MOUNT EXAMINATION ■ Wet-mount examination of diarrheal stool stained with Wright's stain or methylene blue is a rapid and reliable procedure for aiding in the early diagnosis of the cause of diarrhea. A large number of white blood cells suggest inflammation. In acute or traveler's diarrhea, pus in the stool suggests invasion of the large bowel mucosa by bacteria, such as invasive *Escherichia coli, Escherichia histolytica, Shigella, Salmonella, Campylobacter,* gonococci, and other invasive organisms (190–192). Diarrhea caused by noninvasive organisms that produce enterotoxin by viruses and by *Giardia lamblia* is not associated with pus in the stool. Simple Gram staining of direct stool smears frequently can provide an accurate and rapid diagnosis of enteritis caused by *Campylobacter* bacteria. Typically, a vibrio-shaped gram-negative organism is seen (193). In some health centers acute diarrhea with wet-mount evidence of fecal leukocytes and darting forms has become pathognomonic of *Campylobacter enteritis* (192).

Examination of a wet-mount or a stained smear of stool usually is adequate for detecting ova, cysts, or trophozoites of parasites. Because most parasites are passed intermittently with variable numbers into the stool, examining three specimens collected at intervals of two to three days will improve the yield substantially. Collected intestinal aspirates or soft-to-watery fecal specimens should immediately be placed in a preservative, such as polyvinyl alcohol, to prevent rapid disintegration of fragile protozoan trophozoites and to allow the preparation of permanently stained smears. Protozoan cysts and helminthic ova in formed stool will survive for one to two days at room temperature and indefinitely if placed in 5% formaldehyde.

The presence of *Candida* organisms in feces of persons with no underlying disease invariably has been considered nonpathogenic. However, *Candida* proliferation in the gastrointestinal tract may be responsible for diarrhea. The common presentation is multiple loose or watery bowel movements without blood or mucus, but sometimes associated with abdominal cramps, and lasting as long as three months. Direct microscopic examination of stool, suspended in saline or iodine solutions, gives precise information. Yeast forms with budding and often mycelial forms are predominant. Once the condition has been diagnosed, antifungal therapy gives a rapid resolution (194).

Stool Cultures

A stool culture should be obtained in patients with acute and severe diarrhea to determine the common infectious diseases. *Campylobacter* bacteria require a selective isolation medium containing antibiotics, and the plates are grown at 43°C under carbon dioxide or reduced oxygen condition. *Yersinia* is an important intestinal pathogen that causes a spectrum of severe illness. It requires a special culture condition for its isolation (195,196). The laboratory must be informed of the suspicion of this organism. Gonococci require Thayer–Martin medium for the culture.

The preferred method of establishing the diagnosis of colitis caused by *Clostridium difficile* is the detection of enzyme immunoarrays for the presence of toxin A and/or B in the stool. The specificity of these tests is very high but false-negative results are not uncommon (197). Although tissue culture assay is accurate and specific, its use may pose a problem to centers where the testing facilities are not available.

■ EXAMINATION FOR STEATORRHEA

Most patients with clinically relevant malabsorption have steatorrhea. Consequently, documentation of steatorrhea is important and is the cornerstone of diagnostic evaluation.

Steatorrhea is defined as excretion in the stool of >7% of ingested fat (198). Steatorrheic stool is bulky and has a grayish cast or silvery sheen. It may have a soft, sticky consistency with a rancid odor; it may be liquid, frothy, and notable for floating oil droplets. However, steatorrheal stool also may be formed and may appear to be normal (199).

Microscopic examination of the stool for excessive fat has been shown to be a rapid, inexpensive, sensitive, and specific screening test for steatorrhea and pancreatic insufficiency. To detect neutral fat, the stool is stained with Sudan III in 80% alcohol and is examined microscopically. The test is termed positive when 10 or more orange-colored globules that are 10 µm in size are present. To detect split fat, 36% acetic acid is added to the stool along with Sudan III, heated until boiling to melt fatty acid crystals, and then examined under the microscope while still warm. The result is positive if 10 or more orange-colored globules that are 20 µm in size or larger are present (199).

The only truly reliable means of documenting steatorrhea is with quantitative chemical analysis of fat in a 72-hour stool collection while the patient is ingesting a high-fat diet (at least 100 g/day). On such a diet normal subjects excrete <7 g of fat/day (coefficient of absorption of >93%). Unfortunately, the quantitative fecal fat determination is cumbersome to perform and difficult to obtain in most hospitals. Furthermore, the documentation of steatorrhea indicates only that the patient has the malabsorption syndrome. It does not indicate pathophysiology or confer a specific diagnosis (191).

The breath test is a more recent approach to the diagnosis of fat malabsorption. This test is based on the measurement of $^{14}CO_2$ in expired air following the ingestion of various ^{14}C-labeled triglycerides (triolein, tripalmitin, and trioctanoin). Steatorrhea from either pancreatic insufficiency or other causes results in a decreased absorption of triglycerides by the digestive system. This in turn results in a decrease in expired CO_2 derived from metabolism of triglyceride fatty acids (200).

REFERENCES

1. Fijten G, Blijham GH, Knottncrus JA. Occurrence and clinical significance of overt blood loss per rectum in the general population and in medical practice. Br J Gen Pract 1994; 44:320–325.
2. Martelli H, Devroede G, Arhan P, Duguay C. Mechanisms of idiopathic constipation: outlet obstruction. Gastroenterology 1978; 75:623–631.
3. Bartolo DCC. Pelvic floor disorders: incontinence, constipation, and obstructed defecation. Perspect Colon Rectal Surg 1988; 1(1):l–24.
4. Levitt MD. Intestinal gas production—recent advances in flatology. N Engl J Med 1980; 302:1474–1475.
5. Fearon KCH, Carter DC. Cancer cachexia. Ann Surg 1988; 208:1–5.
6. Slattery ML, Kerber RA. Family history of cancer and colon cancer risk: the Utah population database. J Natl Cancer Inst 1994; 86:1618–1626.
7. St. John DJB, McDermott FT, Hopper JL, Debney EA, Johnson WRB, Hughes ESR. Cancer risk in relatives of patients with common colorectal cancer. Ann Intern Med 1993; 188:785–790.
8. Winawer SJ, Zauber AG, Gerdes H, et al. Risk of colorectal cancer in the families of patients with adenomatous polyps. N Engl J Med 1996; 334:82–87.
9. Nivatvongs S, Goldberg SM. An improved technique of rubberband ligation of hemorrhoids. Am J Surg 1982; 144:378–380.
10. Waye JD. Techniques of polypectomy: hot biopsy forceps and snare polypectomy. Am J Gastroenterol 1987; 82:615–618.
11. Nivatvongs S, Fang DT, Kennedy HL. The shape of the buttocks. A useful guide for selection of anesthesia and patient position in anorectal surgery. Dis Colon Rectum 1983; 26:85–86.
12. Oettle GJ, Roe AM, Bartolo DCC, Mortensen NJ. What is the best way of measuring perineal descent? A comparison of radiographic and clinical methods. Br J Surg 1985; 72:999–1001.
13. Porter NH. A physiological study of the pelvic floor in rectal prolapse. Ann R Coll Surg Engl 1962; 31:379–404.
14. Sullivan ES, Corman ML, Devroede G, Rudd WH, Schuster MM. Symposium on anal incontinence. Dis Colon Rectum 1982; 25:90–107.
15. Nivatvongs S, Fryd DS. How far does the proctosigmoidoscope reach? A prospective study of 1000 patients. N Engl J Med 1980; 303:380–382.
16. Lehman GA, Buchner DM, Lappas JC. Anatomical extent of fiberoptic sigmoidoscopy. Gastroenterology 1983; 84:803–808.
17. Ott DJ, Wu WC, Gelfand DW. Extent of colonic visualization with the fiberoptic sigmoidoscope. J Clin Gastroenterol 1982; 4:337–341.
18. Marks G, Boggs HW, Castro AF, Gathright JR, Ray JF, Salvati E. Sigmoidoscopic examinations with rigid and flexible fiberoptic sigmoidoscopes in the surgeon's office. A comparative prospective study of effectiveness in 1012 cases. Dis Colon Rectum 1979; 22:162–168.
19. Winnan G, Berci G, Parrish J, Talbot TM, Overholt BF, McCallum RW. Superiority of the flexible to the rigid sigmoidoscope in routine proctosigmoidoscopy. N Engl J Med 1980; 302:1011–1012.
20. Traul DG, Davis CB, Pollock JC, Scudamore HH. Flexible fiberoptic sigmoidoscopy—the Monroe Clinic experience. A prospective study of 5000 examinations. Dis Colon Rectum 1983; 26:161–3.
21. Farrands PA, Vellacott KD, Amar SS, Balfour TW, Hardcastle JD. Flexible fiberoptic sigmoidoscopy and double-contrast barium-enema examination in the identification of adenomas and carcinomas of the colon. Dis Colon Rectum 1983; 26:725–727.
22. Chen CN, Nolan DJ, Jewell DP. Small bowel gas in severe ulcerative colitis. Gut 1991; 32:1535–7.
23. Hau T, Ahrenholz DH, Simmons RL. Secondary bacterial peritonitis: the biologic basis of treatment. Curr Probl Surg 1979; 16:1–65.
24. Warden MJ, Petrelli N, Herrera L, Mittelman A. Endoscopy versus double-contrast enema in the evaluation of patients with symptoms suggestive of colorectal carcinoma. Am J Surg 1988; 155:224–246.
25. Kelvin FM. Radiologic approach to the detection of colorectal neoplasia. Radiol Clin North Am 1982; 20:743–759.
26. de Roos AD, Hermans I, Shaw PC, Kroon H. Colon polyps and carcinomas: prospective comparison of the single and double contrast examination in the same patients. Radiology 1985; 154:11–13.
27. Young J. The double contrast barium enema: Why bother? South Med J 1982; 75:46–55.
28. Miller RE. Detection of colon carcinoma and the barium enema. JAMA 1974; 230:1195–1198.
29. Amberg JR. Complications of colon radiology. Gastrointest Endosc 1980; 26(suppl 2):15S–17S.
30. Merrill CR, Steiner GM. Barium enema after biopsy: current practice and opinion. Clin Radiol 1986; 37:89–92.
31. Maglinite DD, Strong RC, Strate RW, et al. Barium enema after colorectal biopsies: experimental data. AJR 1982; 139:693–697.
32. Shorthouse AJ, Bartram CI, Eyers AA, Thomson JP. The water soluble contrast enema after rectal anastomosis. Br J Surg 1982; 69:714–717.
33. Ott DJ, Gelfand DW. Gastrointestinal contrast agents: indications, uses, and risks. JAMA 1983; 249:2380–2384.
34. Gallitano AL, Kondi ES, Phillips E, et al. Near-fatal hemorrhage following gastrografin studies. Radiology 1976; 118:35–36.
35. Lutzger LG, Factor SM. Effects of some water-soluble contrast media on the colonic mucosa. Radiology 1976; 118:545–548.
36. Feigin E, Seror D, Szold A, et al. Water-soluble contrast material has no therapeutic effect on postoperative small-bowel obstruction: results of a prospective, randomized clinical trial. Am J Surg 1996; 171:227–229.
37. Bolin S, Franzen L, Nilsson E, Sjodahl R. Carcinoma of the colon and rectum. Tumors missed by radiologic examination in 61 patients. Cancer 1988; 61:1999–2008.
38. Reiertsen O, Bakka A, Trønnes S, Gauperaa T. Routine double contrast barium enema and fiberoptic colonoscopy in the diagnosis of colorectal carcinoma. Acta Chir Scand 1988; 154:53–55.
39. Irvine EJ, O'Conner J, Frost RA, et al. Prospective comparison of double contrast barium enema plus flexible sigmoidoscopy v. colonoscopy in rectal bleeding. Gut 1988; 29:1188–1193.
40. Rex DK, Mark D, Clarke B, Lappas JC, Lehman GA. Flexible sigmoidoscopy plus air-contrast barium enema versus colonoscopy for evaluation of symptomatic patients without evidence of bleeding. Gastrointest Endosc 1995; 42: 132–138.
41. Peel AL, Benyon L, Grace RH. The value of routine preoperative urological assessment in patients undergoing elective surgery for diverticular disease or carcinoma of the large bowel. Br J Surg 1980; 67:42–45.
42. Phillips R, Hittinger R, Saunders V, Blesovsky L, Stewart-Brown S, Fielding P. Preoperative urography in large bowel cancer: a useless investigation? Br J Surg 1983; 70:425–427.
43. Madowitz JS, Schweiger MJ. Severe anaphylactoid reaction to radiographic contrast media. Recurrence despite premedication with diphenhydramine and prednisone. JAMA 1979; 241:2813–2815.
44. Siminovitch JM, Fazio VW. Ureteral obstruction secondary to Crohn's disease: a need for ureterolysis? Am J Surg 1980; 139:95–98.
45. Abcarian H, Udezue N. Coloenteric fistulas. Dis Colon Rectum 1978; 21: 281–286.
46. Alexander-Williams J, Irving M. Intestinal fistulas. Bristol, Great Britain: John Wright & Sons, 1982:60–61.
47. Seldinger SI. Catheter replacement of needle in percutaneous arteriography. A new technique. Acta Radiol 1953; 39:368–376.
48. Athanasoulis CA. Angiography in the management of patients with gastrointestinal bleeding. Maclean LD, ed. Advances in Surgery. Chicago: Year Book Medical Publishers1983:16:1–20.
49. Kadir S, Ernst CB. Current concepts in angiographic management of gastrointestinal bleeding. Curr Probl Surg 1983; 10:281–343.
50. Gianfrancisco JA, Abcarian LI. Pitfalls in the treatment of massive lower gastrointestinal bleeding with "blind" subtotal colectomy. Dis Colon Rectum 1982; 25:441–445.
51. Owen CA Jr., Cooper M, Grindlay JH, Bollman J. Quantitative measurement of bleeding from alimentary tract by use of radiochromium-labelled erythrocytes. Surg Forum 1954; 5:663–667.
52. Alavi A. Detection of gastrointestinal bleeding with ^{99m}Tc-sulfur colloid. Semin Nucl Med 1982; 12:126–138.
53. Markisz JA, Front D, Royal HD, Sacks B, Parker JA, Kolodny GM. An evaluation of ^{99m}Tc-labeled red blood cell scintigraphy for detection and localization of gastrointestinal bleeding sites. Gastroenterology 1982; 83:394–398.
54. Winzelberg GG, McKusick KA, Fröelich JW, Callahan RJ, Strauss HW. Detection of gastrointestinal bleeding with ^{99m}Tc-labeled red blood cells. Semin Nucl Med 1982; 12:139–146.
55. Bernardino ME, Thomas JL, Barnes PA, Lewis E. Diagnostic approaches to liver and spleen metastases. Radiol Clin North Am 1982; 20:469–485.
56. Tempero MA, Petersen RJ, Zetterman RK, Lemon HM, Gurney J. Detection of metastatic liver disease. Use of liver scans and biochemical liver tests. JAMA 1982; 248:1329–1332.
57. Grace RH, Hale M, Mackie G, Marks CG, Bloomberg TJ, Walker WJ. Role of ultrasound in the diagnosis of liver metastasis before surgery for large bowel cancer. Br J Surg 1987; 74:480–481.
58. Mueller PR, Simeone JE. Intra-abdominal abscess. Diagnosis by sonography and computed tomography. Radiol Clin North Am 1983; 21:425–443.
59. Tempero M, Brand R, Holderman K, Metamoros A. New imaging techniques in colorectal cancer. Semin Oncol 1995; 22:448–471.
60. Gore RM, Moss AA, Margulis AR. The assessment of abdominal and pelvic neoplasia: the impact of CT. Curr Probl Surg 1982; 19:493–552.
61. Isikoff MB, Guter M. Diagnostic imaging of the upper part of the abdomen. Surg Gynecol Obstet 1979; 149:161–167.
62. Taourel P, Pradel I, Fabre J-M, Cover S, Seneterre E, Bruel J-M. Role of CT in the acute nontraumatic abdomen. Semin Ultrasound CT MR 1995; 16:151–164.
63. Ha HK. CT in the early detection of strangulation in intestinal obstruction. Semin Ultrasound CT MR 1995; 16:141–150.
64. Bernini A, Spencer MP, Wong WD, Rothenberger DA, Madoff RD. Computed tomography-guided percutaneous abscess drainage in intestinal disease. Factors associated with outcome. Dis Colon Rectum 1997; 40:1009–1013.
65. Thoeni RF, Rogalla P. CT for the evaluation of carcinomas in the colon and rectum. Semin Ultrasound CT MRI 1995; 16:112–126.
66. Beasley HS. MR and CT imaging of intraabdominal spread of colorectal cancer. Semin Colon Rectal Surg 2002; 13:105–118.

67. Smith TJ, Kemeny MM, Sugarbaker PH, et al. A prospective study of hepatic imaging in detection of metastatic disease. Ann Surg 1982; 195:486–491.
68. Hadfield MB, Nicholson AA, MacDonald AW, et al. Preoperative staging of rectal carcinoma by magnetic resonance imaging with pelvic phased-array coil. Br J Surg 1997; 84:529–531.
69. Lunniss PJ, Barker PG, Sultan AH, et al. Magnetic resonance imaging of fistula-in-ano. Dis Colon Rectum 1994; 37:708–718.
70. Wild JJ, Reid JM. Diagnostic use of ultrasound. Br J Phys Med 1956; 19: 248–257.
71. Hildebrandt U, Feifel G, Schwarz HP, Scherr O. Endorectal ultrasound: instrumentation and clinical aspects. Int J Colorectal Dis 1986; 1:203–207.
72. Thaler W, Watzka S, Martin F, et al. Preoperative staging of rectal cancer by endoluminal ultrasound vs. magnetic resonance imaging. Dis Colon Rectum 1994; 37:1189–1193.
73. Wong WD, Orrom WJ, Jensen LL. Preoperative staging of rectal cancer with endorectal ultrasonography. Perspect Colon Rectal Surg 1990; 3:315–334.
74. Harewood GC, Wiersema MJ, Nelson H, et al. A prospective, blinded assessment of the impact of preoperative staging on the management of rectal cancer. Gastroenterology 2002; 123:24–32.
75. Yoshida M, Tsukamoto Y, Niwa Y, et al. Endoscopic assessment of invasion of colorectal tumors with a new high-frequency ultrasound probe. Gastrointest Endosc 1994; 41:587–592.
76. Hernandez de Anda E, Lee SH, Finne CO, Rothnberger DA, Madoff RD, Garcia-Aguilar S. Endorectal ultrasound in the follow-up of rectal cancer patients treated by local excision or radical surgery. Dis Colon Rectum 2004; 47:818–824.
77. Lund JA, Sundstrom SH, Haaverstad R, Wibe A, Srinsaas M, Myrvold HE. Endoanal ultrasound is of little value in follow-up of anal carcinomas. Dis Colon Rectum 2004; 47:839–842.
78. Gold DM, Halligan S, Kmiot WA, Bartram CI. Intraobserver and interobserver agreement in anal endosonography. Br J Surg 1999; 86:371–375.
79. Cheong DMO, Nogueras JJ, Wexner SD, Jagelman DG. Anal endosonography for recurrent anal fistulas: image enhancement with hydrogen peroxide. Dis Colon Rectum 1993; 36:1158–1160.
80. Kim EE, Tilbury RS, Haynie TR, Podoloff DA, Lamki LM, Dodd GD. Positron emission tomography in clinical oncology. Cancer Bull 1988; 40:158–164.
81. Tempero M, Brand R, Holderman K, Metamoros A. New imaging techniques in colorectal cancer. Semin Oncol 1995; 22:448–471.
82. Falk PM, Gupta NC, Thorson AG, et al. Positron emission tomography for preoperative staging of colorectal carcinoma. Dis Colon Rectum 1994; 37:153–156.
83. Arulampalam THA, Costa DC, Loizidou M, Visvikis D, Ell PJ, Taylor I. Positron emission tomography and colorectal cancer. Review. Br J Surg 2001; 88:176–189.
84. Strasberg SM, Dehdashti F, Siegel BA, Drebin JA, Linehan D. Survival of patients evaluated by FDG-PET before hepatic resection for metastatic colorectal carcinoma: a prospective database study. Ann Surg 2001; 233:293–299.
85. Pham KH, Ramaswamy MR, Hawkins RA. Advances in positron emission tomography imaging for the GI tract. Gastrointest Endosc 2002; 55(suppl): 553–563.
86. Huebner RH, Park KC, Shepherd JE, Schwimmer J, Czermin J, Phelps ME. A meta-analysis of the literature for whole-body FDG-PET detection of recurrent colorectal cancer. J Nucl Med 2000; 41:1177–1189.
87. Valk PE, Abella-Columma E, Haseman MK, Pounds TR, Tesar RD, Meyers RW. Whole body PET imaging with (18F) fluorodeoxyglucose in the management of recurrent colorectal cancer. Arch Surg 1999; 134:503–511.
88. Flanagan FL, Dehdashti F, Ogunbiyi OA, Kodner IJ. Utility of FDG-PET for investigating unexplained plasma CEA elevation in patients with colorectal cancer. Ann Surg 1998; 227:319–323.
89. Saunders TH, Mendes Ribeiro HK, Gleeson FV. New techniques for imaging colorectal cancer: the use of MRI, PET and radioimmunoscintigraphy for primary staging and follow-up. Br Med J 2002; 64:81–99.
90. Lunnis PJ, Skinner S, Britton KE, Granowska M, Morris G, Northover JMA. Effect of radioimmunoscintigraphy on the management of recurrent colorectal cancer. Br J Surg 1999; 86:244–249.
91. Corman ML, Galandiuk S, Block GE, et al. Immunoscintigraphy with In-111 satumomab pendetide in patients with colorectal adenocarcinoma: performance and impact on clinical management. Dis Colon Rectum 1994; 37:129–37.
92. Hara AK, Johnson CD, Reed JE, et al. Detection of colorectal polyps by computed tomographic colography: feasibility of a novel technique. Gastroenterology 1996; 110:284–290.
93. Vinning DJ, Gelfand DW, Bechtold RE, Scharling ES, Grishaw EK, Shifrin RY. Technical feasibility of colon imaging with helical CT and virtual reality. Ann J Roentgenol 1994; 162:S104.
94. Rex DK. Barium studies/virtual colonoscopy: the gastroenterologist's perspective. Gastrointest Endoscopy 2002; 55(suppl):S33–S36.
95. Pickhardt PJ, Choi JR, Hwang I, et al. Computed tomographic virtual colonoscopy to screen for colorectal neoplasia in asymptomatic adults. NEJM 2003; 349:2191–2200.
96. Pineau BC, Paskett ED, Chen GJ, et al. Virtual colonoscopy using oval contrast compared with colonoscopy for the detection of patients with colorectal polyps. Gastroenterology 2003; 125:304–310.
97. Cotton PB, Durkalski VL, Pineau BC, Palesch YY, et al. Computed tomographic colonography (virtual colonoscopy). A multicenter comparison with standard colonoscopy for detection of colorectal neoplasia. JAMA 2004; 291:1713–1719.
98. Johnson CD, Harmsen WS, Wilson LA, et al. Prospective blinded evaluation of computed tomographic colonography for screen detection of colorectal polyps. Gastroenterology 2003; 125:311–319.
99. Van Dam J, Cotton P, Johnson CD, et al. AGA future trends report: CT colonography. Gastroenterology 2004; 127:970–984.
100. Rex DK. Is virtual colonoscopy ready for widespread application? Editorial. Gastroenterology 2003; 125:608–614.
101. Weinstein LS, Timmcke AE. Future technology: colography and the wireless capsule. Clin Colon Rectal Surg 2001; 14:393–399.
102. Appleyard M, Glukhovsky A, Swain P. Wireless-capsule diagnostic endoscopy for recurrent small-bowel bleeding. N Engl J Med 2001; 344: 232–233.
103. Selby W. Can clinical features predict the likelihood of finding abnormalities when using capsule endoscopy in patients with GI bleeding of obscure origin? Gastrointest Endosc 2004; 59:782–784.
104. Lewis BS. The history of enteroscopy. Gastrointest Endosc Clin North Amer 1999; 9:1–11.
105. Adler DG, Knipschield M, Gostout C. A prospective comparison of capsule endoscopy and push enteroscopy in patients with GI bleeding of obscure origin. Gastrointest Endosc 2004; 59:492–498.
106. Shinya H. Colonoscopy. Diagnosis and Treatment of Colonic Diseases. New York: Igaku-Shoin, 1982.
107. Jentschura D, Raute M, Winter J, Henkel TH, Kraus M, Manegold BC. Complications in endoscopy of the lower gastrointestinal tract. Therapy and prognosis. Surg Endosc 1994; 8:672–676.
108. Nivatvongs S. Colonic perforations during colonoscopy. Perspect Colon Rectal Surg 1988; 1(2):107–112.
109. Nivatvongs S, Snovcr DC, Fang DT. Piecemeal snare-excision of large sessile colon and rectal polyps: is it adequate? Gastrointest Endosc 1984; 30:18–20.
110. Shinya H, Wolff WI. Morphology, anatomic distribution and cancer potential of colonic polyps. An analysis of 7000 polyps endoscopically removed. Ann Surg 1979; 190:679–683.
111. Nivatvongs S. How to teach colonoscopy. Clin Colon Rectal Surg 2001; 14: 387–392.
112. Waye JD, Bashkoff E. Total colonoscopy: is it possible? Gastrointest Endosc 1991; 37:150–154.
113. Williams CB. Colonoscopy. Br Med Bull 1986; 42:265–269.
114. Hull T, Church JM. Colonoscopy—how difficult, how painful? Surg Endosc 1994; 8:784–787.
115. Saunders BP, Fukumoto M, Halligan S, et al. Why is colonoscopy more difficult in women? Gastrointest Endosc 1996; 43:124–126.
116. Saunders BP, Philips RKS, Williams CB. Intraoperative measurement of colonic anatomy and attachments with relevance to colonoscopy. Br J Surg 1995; 82:1491–1493.
117. Ernstoff JJ, Howard DA, Marshall JB, Jumshyd A, McCullough AJ. A randomized blinded clinical trial of a rapid colonic lavage solution (Golytely) compared with standard preparation for colonoscopy and barium enema. Gastroenterology 1983; 84:1512–1516.
118. Beck DE, Fazio VW, Jagelman DG. Comparison of oral lavage methods for preoperative colonic cleansing. Dis Colon Rectum 1986; 29:699–703.
119. Adams WJ, Meagher AP, Lubowski DZ, King DW. Bisacodyl reduces the volume of polyethylene glycol solution required for bowel preparation. Dis Colon Rectum 1994; 37:229–234.
120. Hsu CW, Imperiale TF. Meta-analysis and cost comparison of polyethylene glycol lavage versus sodium phosphate for colonoscopy preparation. Gastrointest Endosc 1998; 48:276–282.
121. Linden TB, Waye JD. Sodium phosphate preparation for colonoscopy: onset and duration of bowel activity. Gastrointest Endosc 1999; 50:811–813.
122. Young CJ, Simpson RR, King DW, Lubowski DZ. Oral sodium phosphate solution is a superior colonoscopy preparation to polyethylene glycol with bisacodyl. Dis Colon Rectum 2000; 43:1568–1571.
123. Zmora O, Wexner SD. Bowel preparation for colonoscopy. Clin Colon Rectal Surg 2001; 14:309–315.
124. Clarkston WK, Tsen TN, Dies DF, Schratz CL, Vaswani SK, Bjerregaard P. Oral sodium phosphate versus sulfate-free polyethylene glycol electrolyte lavage solution in outpatient preparation for colonoscopy: a prospective comparison. Gastrointest Endosc 1996; 43:42–48.
125. Barclay RL, Depew W, Vanner SJ. Carbohydrate-electrolyte rehydration protects against volume contraction during colonic cleansing with orally administered sodium phosphate. Gastrointest Endosc 2002; 56:633–638.
126. Aronchick CA, Lipshutz WH, Wright SH, Dugrayne F, Bergman G. A novel tableted purgative for colonoscopic preparation: efficacy and safety comparisons with colyte and fleet phospho-soda. Gastrointest Endosc 2000; 52:346–352.
127. Kastenberg D, Chasen R, Choudhary C, et al. Efficacy and safety of sodium phosphate tablets compared with PEG solution in colon cleansing: two identically designed randomized, controlled, parallel group, multicenter phase III trials. Gastrointest Endosc 2001; 54:705–713.
128. Schwetz BA. Oral sodium phosphate. JAMA 2001; 286:2660.

129. Hookey LC, Depew WT, Vanner S. The safety profile of oral sodium phosphate for colonic cleansing before colonoscopy in adults. Gastrointest Endosc 2002; 56:895–902.
130. Huynh T, Vanner S, Paterson W. Safety profile of 5-h oral sodium phosphate regimen for colonoscopy cleansing: lack of clinically significant hypocalcemia or hypovolemia. Am J Gastroenterol 1995; 90:104–107.
131. Frizelle FA, Colls BM. Hyponatremia and seizures after bowel preparation: report of three cases. Dis Colon Rectum 2005; 48:393–396.
132. Ayus JC, Levine R, Arieff AI. Fatal dysnatraemia caused by elective colonoscopy. BMJ 2003; 326:382–384.
133. Barclay RL, Depew WT, Vanner SJ. Carbohydrate-electrolyte rehydration protects against intravascular volume contraction during colonic cleansing with orally administered sodium phosphate. Gastrointest Endosc 2002:633–638.
134. Tjandra JJ, Tagkalidis P. Carbohydrate-electrolyte (E-Lyte) solution enhances bowel preparation with oral fleet phospho-soda. Dis Colon Rectum 2004; 47:1181–1186.
135. Love J. The appropriate use of sodium phosphates oral solutions. Am J Gastroenterol 2003; 17:531.
136. Vanner SJ, MacDonald PH, Paterson WG, Prentice RS, DaCosta LR, Beck IT. A randomized prospective trial comparing oral sodium phosphate with standard polyethylene glycol-based lavage solution (Golytely) in the preparation of patients for colonoscopy. Am J Gastroenterol 1990; 85:422–427.
137. Health Canada. Oral sodium phosphates solutions: electrolyte disturbances. < http"//www.hc-sc.gc.ca/hpfb-dgpsa/tpd-dpt/fleet-phospho-soda_e.html and http://www.hc-sc.gc.ca/hpfb-dgpsa/tpd-dpt/sodium_phosphates_e.html > (Version current at August 21, 2003.).
138. US Food and Drug Administration. Food and drug administration science backgrounder: safety of sodium phosphates oral solution. < http://www.fda.gov/cder/drug/safety/sodiumphospate.htm > (Version current at August 21, 2003.).
139. Cataldo P. Colonoscopy without sedation. A viable alternative. Dis Colon Rectum 1996; 39:257–261.
140. Waye JD, Lewis BS, Yessayan S. Colonoscopy: a prospective report of complications. Endoscopy 1992; 15:347–351.
141. Sipe BW, Rex DK, Latinovich D, et al. Propofol versus midazolam/meperidine for outpatient colonoscopy: administration by nurses supervised by endoscopists. Gastrointest Endosc 2002; 55:815–825.
142. Byrne MF, Baillie J. Propofol for conscious sedation? Editorials. Gastroenterology 2002; 123:373–378.
143. Rex DK, Bond JH, Winawer S, et al. Quality in technical performance of colonoscopy and the continuous quality improvement process for colonoscopy: recommendations of the U.S. multi-society task force on colorectal cancer. Ann J Gastroenterol 2002; 97:1296–1308.
144. American Society for gastrointestinal endoscopy. Guidelines for antibiotic prophylaxis for GI endoscopy. Gastrointest Endosc 2003; 58:475–482.
145. American Society of Colon and Rectal Surgeons. Practice parameters for antibiotic prophylaxis—supporting documentation. Dis Colon Rectum 2000; 43:1194–1200.
146. Nivatvongs S, Vermculen PD, Fang DT. Colonoscopic decompression of acute pseudo-obstruction of the colon. Ann Surg 1982; 196:598–600.
147. Dorudi S, Berry AR, Kettlewell MGW. Acute colonic pseudo-obstruction. Br J Surg 1992; 79:99–103.
148. Jetmore AB, Timmcke AE, Gathright JH Jr, Hicks TC, Ray JE, Baker JW. Ogilvie's syndrome: colonoscopic decompression and analysis of predisposing factors. Dis Colon Rectum 1992; 35:1135–1142.
149. Sgambati SA, Armstrong DN, Ballantyne GH. Management of acute colonic pseudo-obstruction. (Ogilvie's syndrome). Perspect Colon Rectal Surg 1994; 7:77–96.
150. Sakai Y. The technique of colonofiberoscopy. Dis Colon Rectum 1972; 15:403–412.
151. Waye JD, Yessayan SA, Lewis BS, Fabry TL. The technique of abdominal pressure in total colonoscopy. Gastrointest Endosc 1991; 37:147–151.
152. Shumaker D, Zaman A, Katon RM. A randomized controlled trial in a training institution comparing a pediatric variable stiffness colonoscope, a pediatric colonoscope, and an adult colonoscope. Gastrointest Endosc 2002; 55:172–179.
153. Ahmed A, Eller PM, Schiffman FJ. Splenic rupture. An unusual complication of colonoscopy. Ann J Gastroenterol 1997; 92:2101–2104.
154. Karita M, Tada M, Okita K, Kodoma T. Endoscopic therapy for early colon cancer: the strip biopsy resection technique. Gastrointest Endosc 1991; 37:128–132.
155. Waye JD. Saline injection colonoscopic polypectomy. Ann J Gastroenterol 1994; 89:305–306.
156. Kanamori T, Itoh M, Yokohama Y, Tsuchida K. Injection-incision-assisted snare resection of large sessile colorectal polyps. Gastrointest Endosc 1996; 43:189–195.
157. Feitoza AB, Gastout CJ, Burgart LJ, Burkert A, Herman LJ, Rajan E. Hydroxypropyl methylcellulose: a better submucosal fluid cushion for endoscopic mucosal resection. Gastrointest Endosc 2003; 57:41–47.
158. Ryan ME, Norflect RG, Kircliner JP, et al. The significance of diminutive colonic polyps found at flexible sigmoidoscopy. Gastrointest Endosc 1989; 35:85–89.
159. Tedesco FJ, Hendrix JC, Pickens CA, Brady PG, Mitls LR. Diminutive polyps: histopathology, spatial distribution, and clinical significance. Gastrointest Endosc 1982; 28:1–5.
160. Feczko PJ, Bernstein MA, Halpert RD, Ackerman LV. Small colonic polyps: a reappraisal of their significance. Radiology 1984; 152:301–303.
161. Waye JD. Techniques of polypectomy—hot biopsy forceps and snare polypectomy. Ann J Gastroenterol 1987; 82:615–618.
162. Tappero G, Gaia E, DeGiule P, Martini S, Gubetta L, Emanuelli G. Cold snare excision of small colorectal polyps. Gastrointest Endosc 1992; 38:310–313.
163. Spencer RJ, Melton LJ III, Ready RL, Ilstrup DM. Treatment of small colorectal polyps: a population-based study of the risk of subsequent carcinoma. Mayo Clin Proc 1984; 59:305–310.
164. Levitt MD. Production and excretion of hydrogen gas in man. N Engl J Med 1969; 281:122–127.
165. Bond JH, Levitt MD. Factors influencing pulmonary methane excretion in man. J Exp Med 1971; 133:572–588.
166. Bond JH, Levitt MD. Factors affecting the concentration of combustible gases in the colon during colonoscopy. Gastroenterology 1975; 68:1445–1448.
167. Phaosawasdi K, Cooley W, Wheeler J, Rice P. Carbon dioxide-insufflated colonoscopy: an ignored superior technique. Gastrointest Endosc 1986; 32: 330–333.
168. Bigard MA, Gaudier P, Lassallc C. Fatal colonic explosion during colonoscopic polypectomy. Gastroenterology 1979; 77:1307–1310.
169. Nivatvongs S. Complications in colonoscopic polypectomy. An experience with 1555 polypectomies. Dis Colon Rectum 1986; 29:825–830.
170. Walsh RM, Ackroyd FW, Shellito PC. Endoscopic resection of large sessile colorectal polyps. Gastrointest Endosc 1992; 38:303–309.
171. Garbay JR, Rotman SC, Fourtanier G, Escat J. Multicentre study of surgical complications of colonoscopy. Br J Surg 1996; 83:42–44.
172. Binmoeller K, Bohnacker S, Seifert H, Thonke F, Valdeyar H, Soeliendra N. Endoscopic snare excision of "giant" colorectal polyps. Gastrointest Endosc 1996; 43:183–188.
173. Lo AY, Beaton HL. Selective management of colonoscopic perforation. Int Am Coll Surg 1994; 179:333–337.
174. Koltun WA, Coller JA. Incarceration of colonoscope in an inguinal hernia. "Pulley" technique of removal. Dis Colon Rectum 1991; 34:191–193.
175. Bowden TA Jr. Intraoperative endoscopy of the gastrointestinal tract: clinical necessity or lack of preoperative preparation? World J Surg 1989; 13:186–189.
176. Saclarides T, Wolff BG, Pemberton JH, Devinc RM, Nivatvongs S, Dozois RR. Clean sweep of the colon. The use of intra-operative colonoscopy. Dis Colon Rectum 1989; 32:864–866.
177. Whelan RL, Buls JG, Goldberg SM, Rothenberger DA. Intra-operative endoscopy. University of Minnesota experience. Am Surg 1989; 55:281–286.
178. Cohen JL, Forde KA. Intraoperative colonoscopy. Ann Surg 1988; 207: 231–233.
179. Rossinni FP, Ferrari A, Spandrc M, et al. Emergency colonoscopy. World J Surg 1989; 13:190–192.
180. Campbell WB, Rhodes M, Kettlewell MG. Colonoscopy following intraoperative lavage in the management of severe colonic bleeding. Ann R Coll Surg Engl 1985; 67:290–292.
181. Scott HJ, Glynn MJ, Theodorou NA, Lloyd-Davies E, Reynolds KW, Parkins RA. Colonic hemorrhage: a technique for rapid intraoperative bowel preparation and colonoscopy. Br J Surg 1986; 73:390–391.
182. Langevin JM, Nivatvongs S. The true incidence of synchronous cancer of the large bowel. A prospective study. Am J Surg 1984; 147:330–333.
183. Bassett ML, Goulston KJ. False positive and negative Hemoccult reactions on a normal diet and effect on diet restriction. Aust N Z J Med 1980; 10:1–4.
184. Caligtore P, Macrae FA, St. John DJB, Rayner LJ, Lcgge JW. Peroxidase levels in food: relevance to colorectal cancer screening. Am J Clin Nutr 1982; 35: 1487–1489.
185. Lifton LJ, Kreiser J. False-positive stool occult blood tests caused by iron preparations. A controlled study and review of literature. Gastroenterology 1982; 83:860–863.
186. Allison JE, Tekawa MA, Ransom LJ, Adrian AL. A comparison of fecal occult-blood tests for colorectal cancer screening. N Engl J Med 1996; 334:155–159.
187. Ahlquist DA, Wieand HS, Moertel CG, et al. Accuracy of fecal occult blood screening for colorectal neoplasia. A prospective study using Hemoccult and Hemoquant tests. JAMA 1993; 269:1262–1267.
188. Bennett DH, Hardcastle JD. Early diagnosis and screening. Williams NS, ed. Colorectal cancer. New York: Churchill Livingstone, 1996:21–37.
189. Ahlquist DA, McGill DB, Fleming JL, et al. Patterns of occult bleeding in asymptomatic colorectal cancer. Cancer 1989; 63:1826–1830.
190. Gertler S, Pressman J, Cartwright C, Dharmsathaphorn K. Management of acute diarrhea. J Clin Gastroenterol 1983; 5:523–534.
191. Harris B, Dupont HL, Hornick RB. Fecal leukocytes in diarrheal illness. Ann Int Med 1972; 76:697–703.
192. Murray BJ. *Campylobacter* enteritis [letter]. Ann Int Med 1983; 98:1029–1030.
193. Sazic ESM, Titus AE. Rapid diagnosis of *Campylobacter* enteritis. Ann Int Med 1982; 96:62–63.
194. Kane JG, Chretien JH, Garagusi VF. Diarrhea caused by *Candida*. Lancet 1976; 1:335–356.

195. Kohl S. *Yersinia enterocolitka*: a significant "new" pathogen. Hosp Pract 1978; 13:81–85.
196. Saebo A. The *Yersinia enterocolitica* infection in acute abdominal surgery. Ann Surg 1983; 198:760–765.
197. Fekety R. Pseudomembranous colitis. In: Goldman L, Bennett JC, eds. Cecil Text Book of Medicine. 21st ed. Philadelphia: Saunders JB, 2000: 1670–1673.
198. Wilson FA, Dietschy JM. Differential diagnostic approach to clinical problems of malabsorption. Gastroenterology 1971; 61:911–931.
199. Drummey GD, Benson JA Jr, Jones CM. Microscopical examination of the stool for steatorrhea. N Engl J Med 1961; 264:85–87.
200. Heisig DG, Threatte GA, Henry JB. Laboratory diagnosis of gastrointestinal and pancreator disorders. Henry JB, ed. Clinical Diagnosis and Management by Laboratory Methods. 12th ed. Philadelphia: Saunders WB, 2001:462–476.

4 Preoperative and Postoperative Management

W. Rudolf Schouten and Philip H. Gordon

GENERAL CONSIDERATIONS

PREOPERATIVE DISCUSSION

Recommendations for elective colorectal surgery can be made properly only when they are based on clinical history, physical examination, and diagnostic evaluation. As with any well-planned operation, the patient undergoing an elective colorectal procedure should be given general information regarding preoperative preparation, in-hospital stay, postoperative period at home, and overall recovery time.

At the outset the surgeon should discuss the goals of the proposed intervention. The type of incision, the extent of the wounds to be created, and the anatomy involved should be outlined in addition to various aspects of normal wound healing. Where appropriate, the possibility of a laparoscopic approach should be included. When anticipated, the possibility of decision making at the time of operation should be mentioned. The surgeon also should be willing to discuss potential complications. The patient should be afforded the opportunity to ask questions regarding potential risks of the operation as well as alternative therapy. A forewarning that substantial postoperative pain will be experienced will prevent the patient from believing that something has gone wrong. At the same time the patient should be reassured that every effort will be made to relieve pain with the liberal use of analgesics and that considerate and empathetic nursing care will be offered. Realistic expectations should be given regarding the functional results after "reconstructive" colorectal operations, such as ileoanal procedures, coloanal anastomoses, and anal sphincter repair.

The patient should be reassured that all measures will be taken to bring about an uneventful postoperative course. At the same time the patient's need to cooperate with postoperative care, especially with regard to pulmonary care and ambulation, must be stressed. Finally, all aspects of daily activities pertinent to recovery should be discussed.

ASSESSMENT OF OPERATIVE RISK

Before any elective colorectal operation, the patient should be assessed and prepared carefully. Special attention should be given to previous exposure to anesthetic agents and medication and to allergies, personal habits (alcohol and drug abuse), and concurrent systemic illness. Since abnormalities in systemic functions may affect the uptake and action as well as the distribution and elimination of anesthetic drugs, the patient should be in the best possible state of fitness consistent with his systemic disease. Therefore the operative risk is assessed in the following areas: cardiovascular status, pulmonary function, renal status, hepatic function, hematologic status, nutritional status, obesity, age, and psychologic status.

Cardiovascular Status

Patients with a history of myocardial infarction are prone to experience another infarction during or following subsequent operations. The incidence of perioperative myocardial infarction was recently reviewed by Roizen and Fleischer (1) who reported the overall re-infarction rate ranged from 1.9% to 15.9% mostly in the 7–9% range with mortality ranging from 1.1% to 5.4%, mostly in the 3–4% range. In the first three months following a myocardial infarction, the numbers are much higher with reported reinfarction rates ranging from 0% to 86% mostly in the 20–40% range with mortality ranging from 0% to 86% mostly in the 23–38% range. With time the numbers improve so that at 4 to 6 months following myocardial infarction, reinfarction rates range from 0% to 26% mostly in the 6–16% and the corresponding mortality rates range from 0% to 5.9%. After six months, reinfarction and mortality rates continue to decrease. Since postoperative myocardial infarction is associated with a high mortality rate, it is wise not to schedule an elective operation within six months of a previous infarction.

Several drugs used in the treatment of cardiovascular disorders may interfere with anesthesia. For example, diuretics used in the treatment of hypertension can cause hypokalemia. As a result, the action of nondepolarizing muscle relaxants is prolonged and the heart is more irritable. Therefore when possible, serum potassium concentrations below 3 mEq/L should be corrected before operation. Interaction between β-adrenergic antagonists and anesthetic drugs can result in bradycardia, hypotension, and congestive heart failure (2). In preparing patients with hypertension, associated organic dysfunctions such as nephropathy and heart failure should be brought under control. If blood pressure is optimal, patient medication can be continued until the time of the operation because circulatory complications due to interaction between antihypertensive drugs and anesthetic agents are now rare.

The patient's cardiovascular status should also be reviewed when a laparoscopic colorectal procedure is considered, since the maintenance of increased intra-abdominal pressure during prolonged periods of time is not without adverse hemodynamic effects. The extent of the cardiovascular changes depends on several factors such as the level of the insufflation pressure and the volume of carbon dioxide absorbed. Usually cardiac index and central venous blood pressure remain relatively unchanged (3). The increased intra-abdominal pressure, however, leads to splanchnic vasoconstriction and a considerable reduction in inferior vena cava, renal, and portal vein blood flow. Due to these changes, the venous return to the heart decreases, which finally results in reduction in stroke volume (4). The heart rate will rise to compensate for this reduction in stroke volume. At higher-than-normal insufflation pressures, the cardiac output will decline because of failure of this compensation mechanism. The rise in abdominal venous pressure results in a significant increase in systemic vascular resistance and mean arterial blood pressure (5).

Pulmonary Function

The pulmonary function of patients with chronic obstructive lung disease may deteriorate further as a result of ventilatory depression and ventilation–perfusion disturbances occurring during anesthesia. Moreover, postoperative hypoventilation due to residual anesthetic effects and the recumbency and diminished breathing resulting from a painful operative wound may result in pulmonary complications such as retention of secretions, atelectasis, and pulmonary infection. Patients with chronic obstructive lung disease might benefit from admission for adequate pulmonary preparation in advance of the operation. Preoperative examination of these patients might include obtaining chest radiographs, arterial blood gas measurements, and pulmonary function tests. Breathing exercises, postural drainage, inhalation therapy with a mucolytic agent or bronchodilator, and administration of corticosteroids may be helpful in improving respiratory function.

Patients with chronic respiratory disease are also at risk during laparoscopic colorectal surgery. The pneumoperitoneum pushes the diaphragm upward and leads to a reduction in pulmonary function. This situation is aggravated when the Trendelenburg position is used. The physiologic dead space will increase and a ventilation–perfusion mismatch will occur (6). During insufflation with carbon dioxide, the arterial partial pressure of carbon dioxide ($Paco_2$) rises with a resultant respiratory acidosis. The decrease in pH can be compensated by increasing the ventilation rate. A rise in $Paco_2$, however, may occur in patients with chronic respiratory disease despite an increase in ventilation, causing a reduction in stroke volume and cardiac arrhythmia (7).

Renal Status

Patients with renal insufficiency are prone to sustain intraoperative and postoperative complications, especially if the renal disorder is associated with hypertension, severe anemia, and electrolyte disturbances. Fortunately, many affected patients tolerate chronic anemia of renal origin relatively well. The introduction and clinical use of erythropoietin has facilitated a more effective treatment of this type of anemia. Therefore, in this group of patients anemia is not a contraindication to anesthesia and operation. In patients with hyperkalemia, the administration of succinylcholine may result in a further increase in serum potassium concentration. Anesthetic drugs, which are entirely dependent on the kidney for elimination, and nephrotoxic agents are contraindicated in patients with chronic renal insufficiency.

Hepatic Function

Although intravenous anesthetics and narcotic analgesics are largely eliminated by the liver, the detoxification and excretion of these agents is still adequate in most patients with liver disease, unless liver damage is severe. Special attention should be given to biochemical abnormalities such as hyperbilirubinemia, hypoalbuminemia, and elevated levels of liver enzymes and ammonia. The hypoalbuminemia and the reversed albumin/globulin ratio in liver disease are associated with altered sensitivity to drugs bound to albumin and to globulin.

Attention should be directed to the correction of electrolyte disturbances such as dilutional hyponatremia in patients with ascites and hypokalemia due to excessive urinary loss resulting from secondary aldosteronism. In many patients chronic liver disease is associated with anemia that is due to hemolysis or blood loss from esophageal varices. Thrombocytopenia caused by hypersplenism secondary to portal hypertension may occur in addition to decreased levels of clotting factors II, V, VII, IX, and X. Both abnormalities result in a coagulopathy, which should be corrected by platelet transfusion and administration of fresh frozen plasma. Finally, it should be noted that potentially hepatotoxic agents such as halothane are best avoided.

Hematologic Status

Patients with a low hemoglobin concentration have a decreased oxygen transport capacity. To maintain adequate oxygen delivery, cardiac output is increased in patients with anemia. However, many anemic patients tolerate an operation quite well, unless they present with a concurrent systemic disorder. Furthermore, in many patients admitted for a colorectal operation, a low hemoglobin concentration may be the manifestation of the underlying disease itself, and the proposed intervention may be curative. Although it is generally advocated to correct anemia before operation in patients with a hemoglobin concentration below 10 g, many patients with lower values will tolerate operation. Although arbitrary, surgically acceptable ranges for hematocrit are 29% to 57% for men, and 27% to 54% for women and for white blood counts 2400–16,000/mm^3 for both men and women (8).

Nutritional Status

Assessment of the patient's nutritional status is an important part of the preoperative evaluation since there is a strong clinical impression that malnourished patients suffer a higher risk of complications such as anastomotic dehiscence and wound infection. Physical examination is the first step in nutritional assessment. A low triceps skinfold thickness and a decreased midarm muscle circumference, for example, indicate fat and muscle wasting, respectively. A body weight loss >10% within six months of presentation may be a sign of moderate or severe malnutrition. Other more objective criteria are based on biochemical parameters such as anemia, low serum albumin level (<35 g/L), low serum transferrin level, and deficiencies of vitamins, minerals, and trace elements. Inadequate nutritional supply will delay and decrease collagen synthesis. As a result, the balance between collagen lysis and collagen synthesis will be disturbed and there will be deteriorating effects on wound healing and anastomotic repair (9).

The suggestion that preoperative improvement of the nutritional status, through the use of total parenteral nutrition or elemental diet, may have a beneficial effect on postoperative morbidity is based largely on data obtained from retrospective uncontrolled studies (10). In a survey of the literature, Reilly and Gerhardt (10) documented only one prospective randomized study showing a favorable effect of preoperative parenteral feeding on wound healing and anastomotic repair. Based on their survey, these authors concluded that preoperative nutritional support has not been definitively proven to have a beneficial impact and should be reserved primarily for severely malnourished patients.

Braga et al. (11) reported that preoperative oral arginine and *n*-fatty acids improves the immunometabolic response and decreases the infection rate from 32% to 12%. Postoperative prolongation with such supplemented formula has no additional benefit.

Obesity

Obesity may be associated with endocrine abnormalities, hypertension, heart failure, a smaller-than-normal functional residual capacity, and other complications. Therefore, for markedly obese patients, arterial blood gas and pulmonary function studies and examination for endocrine dysfunction should be part of the preoperative evaluation. Because the obese patient is at increased risk for postoperative complications such as deep vein thrombosis, pulmonary embolism, and respiratory failure, adequate preoperative and postoperative measures are necessary to minimize these complications. Such measures are effective only in patients who are willing to cooperate, and therefore the potential complications and the necessity to cooperate should be explained to patients prior to operation.

Age

In assessing operative risk, age is another aspect that needs to be taken into account since an increasing number of older patients are requiring major operations. On admission, older patients frequently present with concurrent systemic disorders and inadequate nutrition. As already mentioned, both factors have a negative impact on intraoperative and postoperative morbidity and mortality. Age alone, however, is not a contraindication to operation. Nevertheless, in an older patient with less than optimal fitness, the surgeon may, for example, modify a recommendation for an abdominoperineal resection and opt for a local procedure. With greater age, for example, "reconstructive" procedures such as ileoanal and coloanal anastomoses are relatively contraindicated because both procedures are associated with a functional outcome that is not as good in older patients compared to younger ones.

Psychologic Status

Most patients who have had an operation recommended to them will become anxious. Sometimes the degree of anxiety will be out of all proportion to the magnitude of the proposed operation. For example, a patient may be offered an anal operation when he or she expects a simple pill or cream to solve the problem. On the other hand, the patient may be seeking help for hemorrhoids and, after examination, learn that the problem is a carcinoma of the rectum for which a proctectomy is being recommended. Clearly, a patient in the latter situation requires considerable reassurance about the change in lifestyle that a stoma may create, along with potential complications such as impotence. Explanation of reasonable expectations from the operation, such as duration of hospitalization and estimated time off from work, as well as reassurance that the patient can return to his former type of work, may do much to calm the patient confronted with this totally unexpected diagnosis.

COLON OPERATION

PREOPERATIVE PREPARATION

Colorectal operations are associated with a high potential for septic complications that most commonly manifest as wound infection or as intra-abdominal sepsis. Endogenous bacterial contamination is the most important factor in the development of postoperative wound infection after elective colorectal procedures. However, exogenous contamination and patient-related factors such as age, nutritional status, and other disorders also can contribute to the development of wound infection.

Intra-abdominal sepsis after a colorectal operation is most commonly due to anastomotic dehiscence. Uneventful anastomotic healing depends on many variables, such as the skill of the surgeon and the use of excellent operative techniques. The method by which the anastomosis is made (one vs. two layers), the use or nonuse of drains, the construction of a defunctioning stoma, and the use of peritoneal lavage are other factors that may influence the outcome.

It is generally agreed that antimicrobial preparation is required in order to reduce the incidence of septic complications after elective colorectal surgery. Since most surgeons believe that fecal loading interferes with healing of colonic anastomoses, mechanical bowel preparation has become a traditional ritual. Proponents of mechanical cleansing justify their practice by referring to a paper published by Irvin and Goligher (12) in 1973. Based on their retrospective study, these authors concluded that poor mechanical bowel preparation is associated with a significantly higher incidence of anastomotic dehiscence. They assumed that mechanical cleansing minimizes the risk of fecal impaction at the anastomotic site, thereby reducing undue tension and local ischemia at the suture line. An early randomized clinical trial questioned this view and concluded that vigorous mechanical bowel preparation is not necessary (13). In 1987, Irving and Scrimgeour (14) also questioned the efficacy of mechanical bowel cleansing. They argued that preoperative bowel cleansing is time-consuming, expensive, unpleasant for the patient, and even dangerous on occasion. The editor criticized the work of both authors: "This paper, which challenges accepted surgical practice, is a veritable little bomb of paper, brief, iconoclastic and disrespectful of hallowed tradition in colorectal surgery." During the last decade, more surgeons have challenged the dogma of mechanical bowel preparation. Brownson et al. (15) examined the value of mechanical bowel preparation in a prospective randomized study in 179 patients undergoing elective colorectal surgery. The rate of intra-abdominal infection as well as the rate of anastomotic breakdown was significantly higher in those patients who received mechanical bowel preparation. In an experimental study, Schein et al. (16) found no evidence of anastomotic leakage in dogs with an unprepared or loaded colon. Santos et al. (17) conducted a prospective randomized trial in 149 patients who were admitted for elective colorectal surgery. They observed that the incidence of wound infection was significantly higher in the patients who received preoperative mechanical bowel preparation. Comparing patients who did and did not receive mechanical bowel preparation, they found a similar incidence of anastomotic leakage. All patients received microbial prophylaxis with cephalothin and metronidazole. Based on these data the authors concluded that "mechanical bowel preparation is not necessary and may be harmful in patients undergoing elective colorectal surgery." Burke et al. (18) conducted a randomized study of 186 patients undergoing elective left colonic or rectal resection and found no difference in overall morbidity or anastomotic leak rate between the group of patients who had received bowel preparation and those who had not.

Van Geldere et al. (19) investigated the outcomes of 250 colorectal operations of which 79.6% were elective without mechanical bowel preparation. Colectomies were left sided in 65.6%. Anastomoses were ileocolic in 32%, colocolic in 20.8%, colorectal intraperitoneal in 34.4%, and extraperitoneal in 12.8%. No patient suffered from fecal impaction. Follow-up was complete in 97.2%. Superficial wound infections developed in 3.3% of patients. The overall anastomotic failure rate was 1.2%. The in-hospital mortality rate was 0.8% and was not related to abdominal or septic complications. They concluded that mechanical bowel preparation is not a sine qua non for safe colorectal surgery. Bucher et al. (20) conducted a literature review of prospective randomized clinical trials evaluating mechanical bowel preparation versus no mechanical bowel preparation for elective colorectal surgery. Data were extracted by two independent observers from seven randomized clinical trials. The total number of patients in these trials was 1297 (642 received mechanical bowel preparation and 655 had not). Among all the randomized clinical trials reviewed, anastomotic leak was significantly more frequent in the mechanical bowel preparation group, 5.6%, compared with no mechanical bowel preparation group, 2.8%. Intra-abdominal infection (3.7% for the mechanical bowel preparation group vs. 2% for the no mechanical bowel preparation group), wound infection (7.5% for the mechanical bowel preparation vs. 5.5% for the no mechanical bowel preparation group), and reoperation (5.2% for the mechanical bowel preparation group vs. 2.2% for the no mechanical bowel preparation group) rates were nonstatistically significantly higher in the mechanical bowel preparation group. General morbidity and mortality rates were slightly higher in the mechanical bowel preparation group. They concluded that there was no evidence to support the use of mechanical bowel preparation in patients undergoing elective colorectal surgery.

In 2003, Wille-Jorgensen and coworkers (21) presented a systemic review regarding the clinical value of preoperative mechanical bowel cleansing in elective colorectal surgery. Recently the same authors published their review in the Cochrane Database of Systematic Reviews (22).

They reviewed nine randomized clinical trials including 1592 patients. In group A 789 patients were allocated to mechanical bowel preparation, whereas group B consisted of 803 patients who were allocated to no preparation. The authors stratified their analyses for colon and rectal surgery separately. Comparing group A and B anastomotic leakage after low anterior resection was reported in 9.8% and 7.5% of the patients, respectively. After colonic surgery these percentages were 2.9 and 1.6, respectively. The overall leakage rate was 6.2% in group A and 3.2% in group B. This was a statistically significant difference. The wound infection rate was 7.4% in group A and 5.4% in group B. Based on this review, the authors concluded that there is no convincing evidence that mechanical bowel preparation is associated with reduced rates of anastomotic leakage after elective colorectal surgery. On the contrary, the data obtained from several studies do suggest that this intervention may be associated with an increased rate of anastomotic leakage and wound infections. According to the authors the dogma that mechanical bowel preparation is necessary prior to elective colorectal surgery should be reconsidered.

The most recent publication on the subject was by Bucher et al. (23) who conducted a randomized clinical trial to compare the outcome of patients who underwent elective left-sided colorectal surgery with (78) or without (75) mechanical bowel preparation. The overall rate of abdominal wound infectious complications (anastomotic leak, intra-abdominal abscess, peritonitis, and wound infection) was 22% in patients with a mechanical bowel preparation and 8% in patients without mechanical bowel preparation. Anastomotic leaks occurred in 6% in the group with a mechanical bowel preparation and 1% in patients without a mechanical bowel preparation. Extra-abdominal morbidity rates were 24% and 11%, respectively. Hospital stay was longer for patients who had a mechanical bowel preparation (14.9 vs. 9.9 days). They concluded elective left-sided colorectal surgery without mechanical bowel preparation was safe and was associated with reduced postoperative morbidity. Slim et al. (24) also conducted a meta-analysis of seven clinical trials containing 1454 patients to assess whether a mechanical bowel preparation may safely be omitted before elective colorectal surgery. Significantly more anastomotic leakage was found after mechanical bowel preparation (5.6% vs. 3.2%). All other endpoints (wound infection, other septic complications, and nonseptic complications) also favored the no preparation regimen, but the differences were not statistically significant. Sensitivity analysis showed that these results were similar when trials of poor quality were excluded. Subgroup analysis showed that anastomotic leakage was significantly greater after bowel preparation with polyethylene glycol compared with no preparation but not after other types of preparation. They concluded there is good evidence to suggest a mechanical preparation using polyethylene glycol should be omitted before elective colorectal operations.

Notwithstanding these publications many surgeons still prefer thorough mechanical bowel preparation. It would appear counterintuitive that the presence of stool does not have potential deleterious effects and hence many surgeons are still convinced that a colon loaded with stool may predispose the patient to postoperative impaction or obstruction and that cannot be healthy for a freshly created anastomosis. As van Geldere et al. (19) poignantly pointed out, a mechanical bowel preparation remains mandatory in certain cases. This is especially true when intraoperative colonoscopy is undertaken, when careful palpation of the bowel is indicated, when the loaded bowel can interfere with the use of stapling instruments, when control of the bowel contents will be difficult as in laparascopic surgery, or when resection margins are limited as in low anterior resections or when it is desired to prevent contamination during operations for colonic fistulas. Therefore, the senior author continues to adopt the practice of mechanical bowel preparation. Indeed, a survey by Zmora et al. (25) of the members of the American Society of Colon and Rectal Surgeons practicing in the United States revealed that although 10% of the surgeons question the importance of mechanical bowel preparation more than 99% routinely used it.

Although the total number of colonic micro-organisms is reduced by mechanical cleansing, it must be stressed that mechanical bowel preparation alone does not alter the concentration of residual bacteria (26,27). Therefore no decreased incidence of postoperative wound infections is to be expected from mechanical bowel preparation alone. In a prospective randomized study by Weidema and van den Bogaard (27), the incidence of wound infections following elective colorectal surgery was found to be 50% after whole gut irrigation alone and 10% when whole gut irrigation was combined with the administration of antibiotics.

Adequate mechanical bowel preparation requires total emptying of the colon with no liquid feces remaining in the large bowel. It is more difficult to prevent spillage where there is liquid stool, which has been shown to contain large numbers of bacteria. Furthermore, the ideal method of mechanical preparation should be simple, inexpensive, without distress to the patient, and without side effects such as fluid and electrolyte imbalance. However, such an ideal method does not exist. The various techniques of mechanical bowel preparation currently available will be discussed with respect to patient acceptability, efficiency, influence on fluid and electrolyte balance, and influence on fecal microflora.

When logistically possible, it is best to do skin shaving just before the operation. This will reduce the incidence of wound infection. It also has been suggested that electric clippers are preferable to razor blades because they produce fewer skin injuries, which are believed to be one factor that predisposes the patient to wound infections.

■ MECHANICAL BOWEL PREPARATION

Conventional Method

The traditional technique of mechanical bowel preparation involves a low-residue or clear liquid diet combined with purgation using laxatives and enemas. Such conventional mechanical bowel preparation seems to provide a satisfactory cleansing in about 70% of patients (Table 1). Major

TABLE 1 ■ Efficiency of Mechanical Bowel Preparation

Method	Author(s)	Satisfactory Cleansing (%)
Conventional mechanical bowel preparations	Keighley (28)	66
	DiPalma et al. (29)	69
Elemental diets	Keighley (28)	17
Whole bowel irrigation		
Saline	Keighley (28)	83
	Weidema and van den Bogaard (27)	86
	Beck and Fazio (30)	90
Mannitol	Keighley (28)	82
	Beck and Fazio (30)	75
Polyethylene glycol (PEG)	DiPalma et al. (29)	92
	Beck and Fazio (30)	90
Picolax	Takada et al. (31)	46
Sodium phosphate	Vanner et al. (32)	80
	Lee et al. (33)	84

drawbacks include poor patient compliance, exhaustion for the patient, diminished nutritional status, a high incidence of abdominal pain, and fatigue (28). These disadvantages stimulated the development of more efficient and quicker methods of reliable bowel preparation.

Elemental Diets

Low-residue liquid diets or elemental diets have been used as a means of bowel preparation. Although the use of an elemental diet results in a low fecal bulk, it does not empty the colon. In a consecutive series of patients in whom an elemental diet was used preoperatively, Keighley (28) demonstrated satisfactory cleansing of the colon in only 17% of the patients (Table 1). Although elemental diets are well tolerated, evidence is lacking to advocate these elemental diets as a sole means of bowel preparation.

Whole Gut Irrigation

The technique of whole gut irrigation was introduced as a means of bowel preparation by Hewitt et al. (34) in 1973 and by Crapp et al. (35) in 1975.

Since whole bowel irrigation with saline is associated with water and sodium retention, it might be hazardous for the elderly and for patients with cardiopulmonary and renal disease because of the risk of cardiac failure. Because of the risk of electrolyte disturbance, use of balanced electrolyte solutions has been advocated, for example, solutions containing 125 mmol/L sodium, 35 mmol/L chloride, 20 mmol/L bicarbonate, and 10 mmol/L potassium. Usually the irrigant is warmed to 37°C and introduced via a nasogastric tube at a constant rate of 50–75 mL/min. Most patients begin to pass their first bowel movement 40 to 60 minutes after the start of irrigation, which should be continued until the rectal effluent is completely free of fecal debris. Whole gut irrigation usually takes about four hours, and it requires 10 to 14 L of perfusate.

Irrigation of the bowel with saline provides satisfactory cleansing of the colon in approximately 90% of patients (Table 1) (27,28,30). Many patients complain about abdominal distension, nausea, and vomiting (27). Whole gut irrigation is contraindicated in patients with gastrointestinal obstruction or perforation and in patients with severe toxic colitis. One of its major disadvantages, however, is the necessity for a nasogastric tube. The technique is rarely used.

Mannitol

Mannitol acts as an osmotic agent by pulling fluid into the bowel and produces a purgative effect by irrigating the colon. It can be administered as an isotonic solution (5% = 200 g/4 L) or as a hypertonic solution (10% = 200 g/2 L or 20% = 200 g/1 L). Usually, mannitol is taken on the day before operation over a four-hour period. If an isotonic solution (5%) is used, at least 4 L must be ingested to achieve adequate cleansing of the colon (36). Such a large volume is difficult to drink in a relatively short time and often results in abdominal discomfort and nausea. Oral mannitol bowel preparation provides a satisfactory cleansing of the colon in almost 80% of patients (Table 1) (28,37).

Two major drawbacks associated with oral mannitol bowel preparation should be recognized. First, it predisposes the patient to postoperative infection. In a prospective randomized study, Hares and Alexander-Williams (38) demonstrated a wound infection rate of 41% following mannitol preparation, compared to an infection rate of 16% after whole bowel irrigation with saline, despite perioperative antibiotic prophylaxis in both treatment groups. Beck et al. (37) also found a higher wound sepsis rate after preparation with mannitol.

A second reason for not recommending oral mannitol bowel preparation is the production of potentially explosive gas within the colonic lumen. Keighley et al. (39) and Taylor et al. (40) found a marked increase of explosive mixtures of gases such as methane and hydrogen following bowel preparation with 5% mannitol. Following mannitol preparation, colonic explosions have been reported after colonoscopic polypectomy and after incision of the colon by diathermy (41,42). Because of these serious considerations mannitol is rarely, if ever, used in current clinical practice.

Polyethylene Glycol

Davis et al. (43) introduced an isotonic lavage solution containing polyethylene glycol (PEG) 3350 mmol/L in a balanced electrolyte solution. PEG acts as an osmotic purgative and is marketed under the names GoLytely, Colyte, Klean-prep and NuLytely. GoLytely, for example, contains PEG (3350 mmol/L), sodium (125 mmol/L), sulfate (40 mmol/L), chloride (33 mmol/L), bicarbonate (22 mmol/L), and potassium (10 mmol/L). The osmolarity of this solution is 280 mosm/kg, and the pH varies between 5.5 and 7.5.

To achieve adequate cleansing of the colon, an average of 4 L of PEG solution must be ingested within four hours. The salty taste is not pleasant but the solution is more palatable if chilled or flavored with tea or lemon. Adams et al. (44) reported that the addition of three tablets of bisacodyl (15 mg) taken the morning before 2 L of PEG is more acceptable to patients than a 4 L regimen and is equally effective in cleansing the colon.

PEG solutions have been evaluated in several prospective randomized trials, and it has been shown that they provide satisfactory cleansing in more than 90% of patients (29,37) (Table 1). The use of PEG preparations is not associated with hazardous levels of explosive gas because PEG does not deliver fermentable substrates to colonic bacteria (29).

Picolax

Picolax (sodium picosulfate plus magnesium citrate) was introduced in 1982 by De Lacey et al. (45) as a means of bowel preparation before radiologic examinations. Sodium picosulfate is a stimulant purgative that mainly acts on the left colon after activation by colonic bacteria, whereas magnesium citrate is an osmotic laxative that cleanses the proximal colon as well. Originally two sachets containing 10 mg sodium picosulfate and 13 g magnesium citrate were administered on the day before the examination. Dietary restriction was recommended to improve effectiveness. In most studies Picolax seems to provide adequate bowel preparation for barium enema and colonoscopy with acceptable results (45–48). In a prospective study investigating the metabolic sequelae of Picolax administered either 24 or 48 hours before elective colonic resection, Takada et al. (31) demonstrated acceptable bowel preparation in only 46% of patients (65% in the 24-hour group and 28% in the 48-hour group). Picolax was well accepted and produced few side effects. However, in the 48-hour group, there was significant electrolyte loss with associated serum electrolyte disturbances and acid–base changes. Based on these findings, the authors concluded that Picolax preparation is a poor mechanical bowel cleansing method associated with unacceptable electrolyte disturbance, especially if given two days before operation.

Schmidt et al. (49) conducted a randomized single-blinded prospective trial comparing sodium picosulfate (Picoprep-3) to sodium phosphate (Fleets) with respect to efficacy and patient tolerance for bowel preparation for colonoscopy. With 200 patients assigned to each group sodium picosulfate was found to be better tolerated, and better tasting than sodium phosphate. Patients in the sodium picosulfate group reported significantly less nausea, vomiting, dizziness, abdominal pains, and thirst associated with the preparation. There was no significant difference in visualization of the colon between the two groups. Hamilton et al. (50) conducted a prospective randomized trial of 59 patients comparing a polyethylene glycol bowel lavage solution (Klean Prep) to a sodium picosulfate solution (Picolax) considering their efficacy, patient acceptability, and plasma biochemical changes. The sodium picosulfate solution was more acceptable to patients than the polyethylene glycol, and resulted in significantly less nausea and vomiting. Mean plasma biochemical changes were significantly different for magnesium, chloride, and potassium. Because neither lavage solution displayed a marked advantage for the colonoscopist or radiologist and sodium picosulfate was more acceptable to patients, they concluded sodium picosulfate is the preferred solution for bowel preparation.

Oral Sodium Phosphate

In an ongoing quest to find the "ideal" or at least a better bowel preparation, a growing number of colorectal surgeons/colonoscopists have turned to an oral sodium phosphate preparation, a highly osmotic cathartic. Patients receive 45 mL of sodium phosphate diluted in a half glass of liquid (carbonated or flavored to mask the saltiness) at 2 PM and 8 PM on the day before the procedure or at 7 PM the day before and 6 AM the day of the procedure if it is being performed mid-morning or later. Cited advantages include a greater patient acceptance, superior rapid colonic cleansing, safety, and the fact that it is significantly less expensive than PEG-based solutions. Potential disadvantages include the concern of hypovolemia so patients should be encouraged to drink more liquids. Concern for the use of this agent has been fully discussed in chapter 3.

In a randomized prospective trial comparing oral sodium phosphate with standard PEG-based lavage solution (GoLytely) in the preparation of 102 patients for colonoscopy, Vanner et al. (32) found that patients tolerated the sodium phosphate preparation and that it was easier to complete. Colonoscopists scored the degree of colonic cleansing significantly higher for the sodium phosphate-prepared colon. Serial measurements of blood tests and postural, pulse, and blood pressure changes did not reveal clinically significant changes in intravascular volume. Hyperphosphatemia was noted after sodium phosphate administration but was transient, and no concomitant decrease in calcium was seen. Histologic assessment for possible preparation-induced changes revealed no difference between the two agents. Of the patients who had undergone a previous colonoscopy with a GoLytely preparation, all those who received oral sodium phosphate found it easier to complete.

Ehrenpreis et al. (51) reviewed the possible serum electrolyte abnormalities secondary to Fleet's Phospho-soda colonoscopy preparation and noted cases of hypernatremia, hyperphosphatemia, hypokalemia, hypomagnesemia, and hypocalcemia. They therefore caution its use in patients with renal insufficiency and congestive heart failure.

Frommer (52) undertook a study to compare three bowel preparations—(group A) 3 L of PEG solution taken at 2 PM the day before examination; (group B) 45 mL of sodium phosphate solution taken at 7 AM and 7 PM the day before examination; and (group C) 45 mL of sodium phosphate solution taken at 6 PM the day before and 6 AM on the morning of examination. Cleanliness scores for the three groups were 3.34, 3.22, and 4.11, respectively. Predominance of material in the right side of the colon was found in 13.7%, 29.8%, and 4.2% of groups A, B, and C, respectively. In the three groups, nausea alone occurred in 3.8%, 13.7%, and 16.3% of patients; vomiting occurred in 0.6%, 7.4%, and 5.4% of patients; and dryness/thirst occurred in 1.9%, 17.4%, and 20.4% of patients, respectively. A total of 80.6% and 82.6% of those in groups B and C who had previously used PEG expressed a preference for taking sodium phosphate.

Frommer concluded that the regimen of group C was significantly better than the regimens of groups A or B in bowel cleansing. The regimens of groups A and B did not differ in efficacy of cleansing. It is the timing of taking sodium phosphate in the regimen of group C rather than its composition that is responsible for its superior cleansing ability compared with that of PEG. Overnight deposition of small intestinal material in the right colon is partly responsible for the inferior cleansing ability of regimens that involve taking the solution on the day before colonoscopy. Although sodium phosphate produced a higher incidence of minor side effects than PEG, a significantly higher proportion of patients preferred sodium phosphate.

Outpatient Preparation

Spurred by the pressures of cost containment and the recognition that satisfactory bowel preparation can be obtained for outpatient colonoscopy, efforts have been directed toward outpatient bowel preparation for patients about to undergo colorectal operations. Frazee et al. (53) conducted a prospective randomized trial of inpatient versus outpatient bowel preparation for elective colorectal surgery. In the 100 patients studied, adequacy of bowel preparation as graded by the primary surgeon was good in 84% in the outpatient group. There were no differences in the rate of wound infections, anastomotic leak, or intra-abdominal abscesses in the two groups. They concluded that outpatient bowel preparation is as effective as inpatient bowel preparation and offers the advantage of cost savings and shorter hospitalization. Lee et al. (33) also conducted a nonrandomized trial of inpatient versus outpatient preparation on 188 patients about to undergo elective colorectal operations. In that study, outpatients received an oral sodium phosphate solution while inpatients received 4 L of a PEG solution. The outpatient bowel preparation group had a shorter length of stay in the hospital, whereas the complication rate was similar in the two groups. Outpatient bowel preparation had significantly higher perioperative fluid requirements. It appears that in selected patients, an outpatient bowel preparation may be safe and effective but that in patients with multiple medical problems who may not tolerate extensive fluid shifts, inpatient monitoring would be more appropriate.

Summary

It is difficult to be dogmatic regarding the best mechanical bowel preparation if indeed it is mandatory. Some surgeons have favored the use of the PEG solutions and have considered them the preparation of choice. Despite the fact that a PEG solution generally produces a clear bowel for operation, the patients, who must consume large volumes of the salty solution, are less enthusiastic about that method than the surgeons recommending it. Furthermore, PEG solutions are not appropriate for use in patients with an impending obstruction because of the possibility of producing a complete obstruction. In such a situation, it is probably better to pursue a more conventional method with repeated small doses of a laxative such as magnesium citrate administered over a longer period. In recent years, oral sodium phosphate has received increased attention, and at the present time it is the preparation routinely used by the senior author to prepare patients for colonoscopy and colon surgery. Nivatvongs believes the goal should be to rid the colon of solid stool to prevent impaction or eliminate obstruction and not necessarily rid the colon of every speck of stool.

■ ANTIBIOTIC BOWEL PREPARATION

No reduction of colonic bacterial concentration or decrease in postoperative septic complications is to be expected from mechanical bowel preparation alone. According to the standards of the American National Research Council, elective colorectal operations can be classified as clean-contaminated operative procedures. Because these procedures always result in bacterial contamination of the operative site, the addition of antibiotics is required. Without antimicrobial preparation the overall wound infection rate after elective colorectal operations varies between 30% and 60% (54,55).

The rationale for perioperative administration of antibiotics is either to reduce the colonic bacterial concentration or to obtain sufficient tissue levels of these drugs during and shortly after operation. Reduction of the extent of bacterial colonization of the large bowel can be achieved by oral administration of antimicrobial agents. Because the aerobic species *E. coli* and the anaerobic species *Bacteroides fragilis* are the organisms that are most frequently involved in septic complications following colorectal operations, oral antibiotics active against both types of bacteria must be given.

Matheson et al. (56) reported that oral administration of neomycin and metronidazole during the 48 hours before operation results in a significant reduction of *E. coli* and *Bacteroides* organism concentrations within the colon at the time of operation. Although this oral regimen did not alter the concentration of the other colonic bacteria, the partial decontamination of the large bowel was associated with a significant reduction in the incidence of postoperative sepsis (42% in the placebo group vs. 18% in the oral antibiotics group).

In a prospective randomized trial, Clarke et al. (55) showed that the wound infection rate after elective colorectal procedures was 35% in the placebo group and 9% in those patients receiving oral antibiotics (neomycin plus erythromycin, 1 g each at 1, 2, and 11 PM the day before operation). Similar results have been reported by others. Oral administration of antibiotics initiated postoperatively is not effective at all (57).

The systemic administration of antibiotics is another method of antimicrobial preparation. Since parenteral antibiotics are effective only when adequate tissue levels are present at the time of contamination, systemic administration should be started immediately before the operation.

Whether antibiotic bowel preparation should be oral, systemic, or both is still a controversial issue. Comparing oral with systemic administration of kanamycin and metronidazole, Keighley et al. (58) found a wound infection rate of 36% in the oral group and 6.5% in the parenteral group. Comparable results have been reported by Lau et al. (59). These findings suggest that suppression of intracolonic microorganisms by the oral administration of antibiotics is probably unnecessary. However, several clinical trials revealed no beneficial effects at all with parenteral antibiotics when compared with oral antimicrobial agents (60,61).

Other studies have addressed the issue of whether simultaneous oral and systemic administration might be more efficacious. In one report Playforth et al. (62) described the results of a prospective randomized trial comparing patients receiving only parenteral antibiotics with those having a combined oral and parenteral regimen. The wound infection rate in the parenteral group was significantly higher than that in the combined group (28% vs. 14%). In contrast, Condon et al. (63) could not demonstrate a discernible benefit from adding parenteral to oral antibiotics. These conflicting results do not afford the opportunity for reaching a definite conclusion about the ideal antibiotic bowel preparation for colorectal operations (Table 2).

Many satisfactory combinations of antibiotics have been advocated and successfully used. Most surgeons use both oral and systemic antibiotics. As for specific agents, the oral administration of the combination of erythromycin base and neomycin is the most popular. For systemic usage, agents covering aerobes and anaerobes should be chosen. The senior author has used a combination of oral erythromycin base and neomycin with systemic carbenicillin preoperatively and two doses postoperatively and have been pleased with the results (65), but oral neomycin is no longer available to us and we employ only systemic antibiotics.

Solla and Rothenberger (74) reported on a survey of colon and rectal surgeons in the United States and Canada.

TABLE 2 ■ Comparison of Wound Infection Rate in Elective Colorectal Operations After Different Kinds of Prophylaxis

	Wound Infection Rate (%)		
Author(s)	Combined Oral and Parenteral	Oral	Parenteral
Condon et al. (63) (1983)	6	8	
Coppa et al. (64) (1983)	7	18	
Portnoy et al. (65) (1983)	2–5	27	
Lau et al. (59) (1988)	11	29	
	11		11
Petrelli et al. (66) (1988)	0	3	
Playforth et al. (62) (1989)	14	28	
Hall et al. (67) (1989)			15
Periti et al. (68) (1989)			9–11
Schoetz et al. (69) (1990)	5	15	
Stellato et al. (70) (1990)	6	7	4
Skipper et al. (71) (1992)			14
Matikainen and Hiltunen (72) (1993)			3–12[a]
Morris (73) (1993)			6–17[a]
Santos et al. (17) (1994)			17
Mosimann et al. (76) (1998)			11
Mecchia (75) (2000)			7–11[a]
Rau et al. (77) (2000)	3		4–18[a]
Zanella and Rulli (78) (2000)			7
Lewis (60) (2002)	5		17

[a]Different parenteral antibiotic regimens.

All respondents used a mechanical preparation and some form of antibiotics. The most favored antibiotic regimen was oral antimicrobials combined with systemic antibiotics (88%). Concomitant administration of oral neomycin–erythromycin base and a systemic second-generation cephalosporin active against both anaerobic and aerobic colonic bacteria together with oral PEG electrolyte mechanical cleansing was the most popular method of preoperative bowel preparation (58%). The second most frequently used method of mechanical bowel cleansing consisted of conventional enemas, dietary restrictions, and cathartic preparations (36%). Mannitol solution (5%) and whole gut irrigation per nasogastric tube (1%) were the least popular methods of mechanical bowel cleansing. The authors concluded that the literature supports the methods of preoperative bowel preparation most commonly used by the vast majority of surgeons surveyed.

Using quantitative and qualitative bacterial cultures as well as scanning electron microscopy to study mucosa-associated flora, Smith et al. (79) found that anaerobic and aerobic counts were suppressed the greatest in patients receiving both oral and parenteral antibiotics. Their study documented the effectiveness of oral neomycin–erythromycin in suppressing mucosa-associated flora and suggested that parenteral antibiotics suppress the mucosa-associated bacteria in addition to providing therapeutic serum levels. To learn more about the mucosal microflora at the time of elective operation, Bleday et al. (80) obtained quantitative cultures of the mucosa-associated bacteria in the mechanically prepared colon and rectum. There was a significant increase in aerobes, anaerobes, enterics, gram-positive stains, *B. fragilis*, and *E. coli* mucosal counts with proximal progression. Aerobes showed a steady gradient, while anaerobes demonstrated an increase from the rectum to the transverse colon but no change between the transverse colon and cecum.

Lewis (81) performed a meta-analysis of randomized studies to compare the efficacy of combined oral and systemic antibiotics versus systemic antibiotics alone in preventing surgical site infection in elective surgery of the colon. The summary weighted risk difference in surgical site infections between groups favored combined prophylaxis (relative risk = 0.51). For surgeons adopting parenteral antibiotics, controversy centers around single versus multiple dosing. The review by Chapman and Harford (82) of four studies from 1987 to 1995 found that patients receiving a single preoperative dose had a similar wound infection rate to those patients receiving 2 to 4 doses. Similarly, the review by Platell and Hall (83) documents the considerable support from clinical trials and meta-analysis for the prophylactic use of a single dose of a suitable parenteral antimicrobial agent.

■ POSTOPERATIVE CARE

Laboratory Tests

In the early postoperative period fluid and electrolyte balance must be monitored carefully. The preoperative bowel preparation and the operative procedure itself may be associated with a significant loss of fluid and electrolytes, and these need to be restored. Special attention should be given to hemodynamic parameters such as pulse rate, blood pressure, hemoglobin concentration, and urine output to detect early signs of intra-abdominal hemorrhage or sepsis. The frequency of the laboratory work will depend on the complexity of the operation performed and any preexisting associated medical problems.

Brandstrup et al. (84) investigated the effect of a restricted intravenous fluid regimen on complications after colorectal resection. In a randomized observer-blinded multicenter trial, 172 patients were allocated to either restricted or a standard intra-operative and post-operative intravenous fluid regimen. The restricted regimen aimed at maintaining pre-operative body weight; the standard regimen resembled every day practice. The restricted intravenous fluid regimen significantly reduced postoperative complications both by intention-to-treat (33% vs. 51%) and per-protocol (30% vs. 56%) analyses. The numbers of both cardiopulmonary (7% vs. 24%) and tissue healing complications (16% vs. 31%) were significantly reduced. No patients died in the restricted group compared with four deaths in the standard group (0% vs. 4.7%). No harmful adverse effects were observed.

Nasogastric Intubation

Like most abdominal procedures, colorectal operations are associated with paralytic ileus in the early postoperative period. Intestinal motor dysfunction is a normal physiologic response to operative trauma.

The mean duration of the paralytic state varies between 0 and 24 hours in the small bowel, 24 and 48 hours in the stomach, and between 48 and 72 hours in the colon. The effective duration of postoperative ileus is mainly dependent on the return of colonic motility (85,86).

Although it has been suggested that recovery of intestinal motor function is not influenced by the operative procedure itself, a more recent study has revealed that the longest duration of postoperative ileus is encountered after operation involving the colon (87). There is growing evidence that postoperative ileus is related to the degree of surgical manipulation and the magnitude of the inflammatory response within the muscle layers of the bowel wall. It has been shown that the activation of macrophages within the muscularis during abdominal surgery initiates an inflammatory cascade of events, finally resulting in extravasation of leukocytes into the circular muscle layer. Various potent leukocytic products, such as nitric oxide, prostaglandins and oxygen radicals, contribute to the inhibition of muscularis function (88). For many years, Taché and coworkers (89) have focused their attention on another mechanism. They have found that surgical stress and manipulation of the large bowel initiate the central release of corticotropin-releasing factor (CRF) in the paraventricular nucleus of the hypothalamus. The subsequent stimulation of efferent inhibitory sympathetic pathways, mediated by the CRF release, seems to be a major contributing factor to the motor alterations induced by abdominal surgery. According to others plasma changes in motilin and substance P are related to depressed gastrointestinal motility after the operation (90).

Somatovisceral and viscerovisceral reflexes also contribute to postoperative ileus. Afferent, inhibitory sympathetic reflexes, involving the spinal cord, are of major importance. Especially these reflexes can be modified by epidural blockade. Based on these data it is obvious that the pathogenesis of postoperative ileus is multifactorial. Because depressed gastrointestinal motility after the operation is thought to be a "physiologic" reaction to surgical stress and manipulation of the bowel, this phenomenon is considered an inevitable consequence of open abdominal surgery. Postoperative ileus is associated with significant discomfort. Furthermore, it delays the resumption of a regular diet as well as the mobilization of the patient, thereby resulting in a prolonged hospital stay. It has been suggested that postoperative ileus is related to complications such as anastomotic dehiscence. The morbidity, associated with postoperative ileus, is widely acknowledged and its economic burden has been estimated at $1 billion per year in the United States (91). Since its introduction by Levin (92), the use of a nasogastric tube has been a routine aspect of postoperative care for almost all surgeons. It was thought to relieve postoperative discomfort and to shorten the duration of ileus, thereby decreasing the length of hospital stay. It was also thought to decrease the incidence of complications. However, nasogastric tubes, which are unpleasant at best and usually distressing to the patient, may cause tube-related complications such as vomiting, nasopharyngeal soreness, coughing, wheezing and sinusitis (93).

In the 1980s, surgeons started to question the efficacy of the use of nasogastric tubes. From a prospective study comparing the postoperative course in patients with and without a nasogastric tube, Bauer et al. (94) concluded that routine use of a nasogastric tube was not needed. In their study most patients with a nasogastric tube suffered discomfort, and the incidence of postoperative complications was not increased in the patients without a nasogastric tube. Furthermore, only 6% of the patients in whom nasogastric tubes were not routinely used required nasogastric intubation during the postoperative period.

Clevers and Smout (95) evaluated the restoration of gastrointestinal motility following abdominal operations in 50 patients. Bowel sounds were heard at auscultation on postoperative day 1 or 2. The passage of flatus was first noted in almost all patients on postoperative day 2, and the first defecation occurred on postoperative day 4 or 5. These physical signs, occurring at relatively predictable times, were not influenced by the type of operation, nor were they predicative of postoperative nausea and vomiting. Because the period of intestinal decompression and the volume of gastric aspirate in patients with postoperative nausea did not differ from those of the patients without nausea, the authors concluded that prolonged gastric decompression is not necessary.

In a prospective randomized trial Colvin et al. (96) compared use of a long intestinal tube (Cantor) placed preoperatively, a nasogastric tube placed intraoperatively, and no tube at all. With respect to the length of hospital stay, duration of postoperative ileus, adequacy of intraoperative intestinal decompression, gastric dilatation, and operative complications, there was no significant difference between the patients with tubes and those without tubes. The authors concluded that the routine practice of employing nasointestinal tubes should be abandoned in elective colonic operations. Others have come to the same conclusion (97,98).

In 1995, Cheatham et al. (99) performed a meta-analysis of the results obtained from 26 trials including almost 4000 patients. These trials compared selective versus routine nasogastric decompression. Although patients managed without a nasogastric tube encountered more frequently abdominal distension, nausea, and vomiting, this was not associated with an increased number of complications or a prolonged hospital stay. They also showed that for every patient who needed postoperative gastric decompression, 20 patients did not. Based on these data the authors concluded that routine use of a nasogastric tube was not supported by their meta-analysis. In a randomized controlled trial, comparing early versus regular feeding, Reissman et al. (100) also demonstrated that after elective colorectal surgery patients can be safely managed without nasogastric tubes. In the early feeding group and in the regular feeding group, the tube reinsertion rate was almost equal (11% vs. 10%). In a similar study Feo et al. (101) observed that tube reinsertion was necessary in 20% of their patients because of vomiting. Based on all these data it is apparent that routine use of a nasogastric tube is not needed following elective colorectal surgery.

Foley Catheter

All patients undergoing colorectal operations require a urethral catheter for intraoperative decompression and for postoperative monitoring. Following hemicolectomy and segmental colectomies, the Foley catheter is usually left in place for 2 days. Since micturition difficulties frequently occur after rectal excision, removing the catheter is not advocated until day 4 or 5 after proctectomy. Retention or incontinence after catheter removal requires continuous bladder drainage for another 3 to 5-day period until the patient is fully mobile. Opiates may cause urinary retention by inhibition of detrusor contraction and impaired bladder sensation, resulting in an increased maximum bladder capacity and overdistention (102). The changes are rapidly reversed by therapeutic doses of intravenous naloxone. When retention persists despite subcutaneous injection of carbachol, urologic examination, including cystoscopy and urodynamic investigation, is indicated. Micturition difficulties after colorectal operations most frequently occur in elderly men because of obstruction by prostatic hypertrophy. Bladder dysfunction as a result of pelvic nerve injury during rectal excision is another potential causative factor.

The reported incidence of urinary dysfunction following conventional procedures for rectal carcinoma varies between 30% and 70% (103). In many patients with postoperative urinary dysfunction, sexual function is also affected. In male patients impotence and/or disturbed ejaculation occur in about 30 to 40% (104). In female patients sexual function may be affected, resulting in dyspareunia, loss of lubrication of the vagina, and the inability to achieve orgasm (105). In contrast to voiding disturbances, sexual difficulties rarely disappear. To reduce the incidence of these disabling complications, nerve-sparing operation techniques have been developed that do not compromise adequate clearance of the malignancy (106).

Repeated removal and reinsertion of a transurethral catheter is unpleasant and may be associated with increased risk of urethral trauma and urinary tract infection. Nevertheless some urologists currently prefer repeated straight catheterization rather than prolonged Foley catheterization. Patients can be taught to catheterize themselves. To overcome these problems, in special circumstances, consideration can be given to the use of a catheter inserted into the bladder through the lower abdominal wall. The percutaneous catheter facilitates bladder training since it simply can be locked when left in situ but this option is rarely adopted today.

Analgesia

Adequate pain relief is another important aspect of postoperative care. A pain-free patient will be more cooperative with ambulation and breathing exercises. Although patient comfort is an important goal, acute pain may have harmful physiologic effects because it induces a stress response. Therefore adequate pain control may reduce the incidence of postoperative complications such as impaired pulmonary function (atelectasis and infection), myocardial ischemia and infarction, impaired wound healing, and thromboembolic events (107). Systemic administration of opioids is the method most frequently used to relieve postoperative pain. Intermittent intramuscular injection of morphine is painful and is not always successful because many patients do not receive enough opioid (because of caution about respiratory depression). Epidural infusion of morphine has proved to provide better pain relief when compared with the effect of systemic administration of morphine. When morphine is injected epidurally by continuous infusion, morphine-related side effects, such as pruritus, nausea, urinary retention, and occasionally respiratory depression, are decreased (108).

The benefit of superior pain relief with epidural analgesia must be balanced against the invasive nature of the procedure and its risks, which include respiratory depression, nausea, vomiting, urinary retention, and catheter-related complications. Furthermore, surgeons should be aware of the possible influence of anesthesia and analgesia on postoperative intestinal function, especially the possibility of a prolonged ileus.

Continuous epidural analgesia with a local anesthetic is the most effective technique to shorten the duration of postoperative ileus. This can only be obtained by thoracic application of the local anesthetic, resulting in blockade of afferent and efferent inhibitory reflexes. Lumbar or low-thoracic epidural administration of local anesthetics has no positive effects on postoperative ileus. Holte and Kehlet reviewed 8 randomized controlled studies, comparing epidural thoracic local anesthetics with systemic opioids. Six of these studies revealed that epidural bupivacaine significantly reduced the duration of postoperative ileus (109). Holte and Kehlet also reviewed trials comparing epidural opioid versus epidural bupivacaine alone and epidural bupivacaine combined with a low dose opioid. Based on these studies it is apparent that epidural bupivacaine alone is superior when related to the resolution of postoperative ileus. Continuous epidural analgesia does not increase the risk of anastomotic dehiscence (110). Opioid-sparing analgesia have been developed to avoid the undesirable sequelae of opioid administration in the postoperative period. One technique is pain relief with NSAIDs. It has been reported that the use of these NSAIDs results in a 20–30% sparing of opioids (111). The direct anti-inflammatory effect mediated by the inhibition of prostaglandin synthesis is another advantageous effect of NSAIDs. The disruption of colonic anastomoses has been reported during the use of continuous epidural anesthesia (112). It is difficult to say whether the technique per se may lead to anastomotic breakdown or whether the early clinical presentation may be due to the preserved or increased colonic motility caused by epidural analgesia. Indeed, epidural analgesia may alter the clinical signs of any intra-abdominal complication. A trend suggesting that disruption of colonic anastomoses was more common in patients given morphine during the perioperative period than in those who received pethidine (Demerol) has been reported (113).

Patient-controlled analgesia (PCA) is another method of providing effective pain relief. PCA systems can be set to deliver a bolus of morphine. The maximal dose can be assigned by setting the lockout time. The patient, who is free to use the system as needed, merely presses a button when pain relief is desired. Patients like the security of knowing that they can achieve pain relief quickly and without painful intramuscular injections. According to preliminary results, PCA seems to be an excellent method of obtaining sufficient postoperative pain relief (114). A comparison of the efficacy of analgesia and the extent of sedation showed that PCA allows for analgesia with less sedation and less drug requirement than intramuscular administration (115).

In a prospective randomized study, Cataldo et al. (116) compared the effect of intramuscular ketorolac in combination with PCA (morphine) to that of PCA alone. Narcotic requirements were decreased by 45%. They suggested that this combination may be particularly beneficial in patients especially prone to narcotic-related complications.

A similar finding has been reported by Bradshaw and co-workers (117).

■ PHARMACOLOGIC TREATMENT OF POSTOPERATIVE ILEUS

Postoperative ileus is a significant side effect of abdominal surgery. Without specific treatment, major abdominal surgery causes a predictable gastrointestinal dysfunction which endures for 4 to 5 days and results in an average hospital stay of 7 to 8 days. Ileus occurs because of initially absent and subsequently abnormal motor function of the stomach, small bowel, and colon. This disruption results in delayed transit of gastrointestinal content, intolerance of food, and gas retention. The etiology of ileus is multifactorial, and includes autonomic neural dysfunction, inflammatory mediators, narcotics, gastrointestinal hormone disruptions, and anaesthetics (118). In the past, treatment has consisted of nasogastric suction, intravenous fluids, correction of electrolyte abnormalities, and observation. Currently, the most effect treatment is a multimodal approach. Median stays of 2 to 3 days after removal of all or part of the colon have now been reported.

Opioid Receptor Antagonists

Taguchi at al. studied the effects of an investigational μ-opioid antagonist with limited oral absorption and limited ability to cross the blood-brain barrier, on postoperative gastrointestinal function and length of hospital stay. In a randomized, placebo-controlled study they were able to demonstrate that selective inhibition of gastrointestinal opioid receptors by this antagonist speeds recovery of bowel function and shortens the duration of hospitalisation (119).

Cisapride

Cisapride acts as a serotonin receptor agonist. There is growing evidence that intravenous administration of cisapride reduces the duration of postoperative ileus. However, the reported adverse cardiac effects, will probably limit the widespread use of this agent (109).

Ceruletide

This peptide acts as a cholecystokinin antagonist and may stimulate gastrointestinal activity. In two placebo-controlled studies only a slight affect on postoperative ileus was observed. This finding and the reported side-effects such as nausea and vomiting has limited the use of this agent (120,121).

Erythromycin

This antibiotic acts as a motilin receptor agonist and might be a candidate for the reduction of postoperative ileus. However, such an advantageous effect could not be demonstrated in a randomized controlled trial (122).

Metoclopramide

Metoclopramide acts as a dopamine antagonist and a cholinergic stimulant. Holte and Kehlet have reviewed six controlled trials assessing the effect of metoclopramide. None of these studies has demonstrated a significant effect of this agent on the resolution of postoperative ileus (109).

Early Ambulation

Colorectal surgery is associated with a significant incidence of thromboembolic complications. Immobilization is considered an important causative factor in the pathogenesis of postoperative deep vein thrombosis (DVT). The incidence of pulmonary emboli in patients with DVT varies from 10% to 30%, depending on the location and morphology of the thrombus. One of 10 patients with pulmonary embolism dies within the first hour (123). Therefore ambulation is mandatory as early as possible. Postoperative ambulation can be efficacious only when pain relief is adequate and physiotherapy is added.

The use of compression stockings for both lower extremities during the operation and in the postoperative period until the patient is fully ambulatory will help reduce the incidence of DVT (124). Administration of low-dose heparin is another measure found to be effective in preventing thromboembolic complications.

Using Iodine-125 (^{125}I)-labeled fibrinogen, Törngren and Rieger (125) could detect DVT in 17% of the patients receiving low-dose heparin, whereas the DVT rate was 42% among untreated patients. Although it has been assumed that rectal dissection is associated with an increased risk of DVT, these authors could not demonstrate a significant difference in the frequency of DVT between patients who underwent resections of the colon and those who underwent rectal resections. The incidence of DVT was significantly higher in patients with postoperative infection than among uninfected patients (37% vs. 12%). Based on these findings, Torngren and Rieger concluded that measures aimed at reducing postoperative infection combined with low-dose heparin and adequate ambulation will reduce the incidence of postoperative DVT.

Heparin administration may be associated with an increased incidence of postoperative bleeding. Nevertheless, in high-risk patients, such as those with a previous history of DVT and/or pulmonary embolus, consideration should be given to the subcutaneous administration of low-dose heparin (5000 U every 12 hours). Intermittent pneumatic compression also has been found to be effective in diminishing the incidence of DVT (124).

The reduction in venous return to the heart during laparoscopic procedures suggests that patients undergoing this type of surgery might be at risk for an excess incidence of DVT. However, so far this has not been demonstrated.

Resumption of Diet

Most surgeons have their own idea of when to feed patients after a laparotomy for colorectal disease. Some favor resumption of oral intake at the first sign of a bowel sound. Most, however, would like to witness the return of organized peristalsis, which is recognized by the passage of flatus or a bowel movement. This usually has occurred by the fifth postoperative day. The rationale of such a period of starvation is to prevent nausea and vomiting and to protect the anastomosis, allowing it time to heal. This policy is not really evidence based. Contrary to widespread opinion, there is growing evidence suggesting that early feeding is advantageous. The advent of laparoscopic colorectal surgery has prompted a shift toward early feeding. Several randomized controlled trials comparing laparoscopic and open colonic resections have revealed that minimal invasive surgery is associated with a faster resolution of postoperative ileus, an earlier tolerance of diet, and a faster discharge from the hospital (126). This beneficial effect is probably due to reduction in surgical trauma, resulting in reduced activation of inhibitory reflexes and local inflammation. It has been questioned, however, whether this advantageous effect is a result of the laparoscopic procedure alone or merely reflects a change in postoperative care principles with allowance of earlier transition to a regular diet. Milsom et al. (127) conducted a randomized trial comparing the ileus patterns after laparoscopic and open colorectal surgery. They found a significantly shorter time to first flatus for patients who underwent laparoscopic surgery, but no significant difference in time to first bowel movement. The length of hospital stay was similar in both groups.

Bufo et al. (128) reported on a prospective study of 38 patients undergoing elective open colorectal operations. They found early feeding (ad lib) was tolerated in 86% of patients. They noted that longer operative time and increased blood loss intraoperatively may indicate a more difficult procedure and identify those patients who will not tolerate early feeding. Early feeding also led to shortened length of hospital stay.

Binderow and coworkers randomized 64 patients undergoing open colorectal surgery to either receive a regular diet on the first postoperative day or have their diet held until resumption of bowel movements. There were no differences in the incidence of nasogastric tube reinsertion, vomiting, and the duration of the postoperative ileus (129). In a subsequent group of an additional 161 consecutive patients similar results were demonstrated (130). However, the patients in the early feeding group tolerated a regular diet significantly earlier than the patients in the regular feeding group (2.6 vs. 5 days). It might be noted that the early feeding did not result in any significant shortening of the hospital stay.

Ortiz et al. (131) also conducted a prospective randomized trial and found that 80% of patients tolerated early feeding but 21.5% developed vomiting and required reinsertion of a nasogastric tube. The time until the first bowel movement was similar.

Based on these data, it has been suggested that an early oral feeding regimen consisting of clear liquids on the first postoperative day, followed by a regular diet as tolerated within the next 24 to 48 hours is safe. During the last decade several studies have demonstrated that early oral feeding is indeed permissible after elective open colorectal surgery. Early oral feeding is tolerated by 70% to 80% of the patients (132,133). Lewis et al. (134) performed a systematic review and conducted a meta-analysis of randomized controlled trials comparing any type of enteral feeding started within 24 hours after the operation with nil by mouth management in elective gastrointestinal surgery. Eleven studies, including 837 patients, met their inclusion criteria. Early feeding reduced the risk of any type of infection and the mean hospital stay. Risk reductions were also seen for anastomotic dehiscence, pneumonia, wound infection, intra-abdominal abscess, and mortality. However, these risk reductions failed to reach significance. The risk of vomiting was increased among patients fed early. Even in elderly patients, aged 70 years and older, early postoperative feeding is feasible and beneficial, as shown by DiFronzo et al. (135). Reviewing the literature, it is apparent that 10% to 20% of the patients do not tolerate early feeding. It has been shown that administration of cisapride enhances the tolerance of early postoperative feeding. Camberos et al. (136) used an early feeding protocol in all their patients undergoing open elective colectomy. In group I the patients received early feeding without promotility agents. In group II the patients were treated with metoclopromide, whereas the patients in group III received cisapride. With respect to early feeding the failure rates were 13%, 14%, and 0%, respectively.

Henrik Kehlet (137), from Copenhagen, Denmark, pioneered a more fundamental and multimodal approach to enhance the overall recovery rate after open abdominal surgery. His regimen includes a plan for discharge from the hospital at 48 hours after the operation, optimal pain relief with thoracic epidural anesthesia, limited surgical incision, early postoperative oral intake and early postoperative mobilization. Bradshaw and coworkers (117) from the United States utilized a comparable perioperative regimen, resulting in a faster return of bowel function and a shorter length of hospital stay. With the multimodal approach developed by Kehlet, Basse et al. (138) were able to discharge 32 of 60 patients at 48 hours after open colorectal surgery. In a subsequent report, Basse et al. (139) evaluated the postoperative outcome after colonic resection of 130 consecutive patients receiving conventional care compared with 130 consecutive patients receiving multimodal fast-track rehabilitation. American Society of Anesthesiologist score was significantly higher in the fast-track group. Defecation occurred on day 4.5 in the conventional group and day 2 in the fast-track group. Median hospital stay was eight days in the conventional group and two days in the fast-track group. The use of nasogastric tube was longer in the conventional group. The overall complication rate (26.9%) was lower in the fast-track group, especially cardiopulmonary complications (3.8%). Readmission was necessary in 12% of cases for the conventional group and 20% in the fast-track group. Although other workers were not able to achieve such a short hospital stay, some of them have demonstrated that this approach results in a faster readiness for discharge. In a randomized controlled trial, Delaney et al. (140) demonstrated that patients assigned to a pathway of controlled rehabilitation with early ambulation and early feeding spent less time in the hospital than patients who were assigned to traditional postoperative care (five vs. seven days). Fearon and Luff (141) reported that in their unit hospital stay has been reduced from approximately 10 days with traditional care to seven days with an enhanced recovery program. Smedh et al. (142) were able to discharge their patients after a median postoperative hospital stay of 3.5 days, by using a similar program. Henriksen et al. (143) reported a longer ambulation time and better muscle function after the operation by using this program. The benefits of the multimodal rehabilitation approach cannot be achieved with a unimodal intervention based on early postoperative feeding alone (144,145).

The custom of starting patients on clear fluids and progressing to full fluids and then a "soft" diet seems unnecessary. Once it is deemed permissible to allow oral intake, full fluids may be started and followed shortly thereafter by regular food and a bulk-forming agent such as one of the psyllium seed preparations. This regimen should ensure the passage of a soft stool without straining.

Pulmonary Function

The necessity for aggressive postoperative pulmonary care is unquestioned. Incentive spirometry can help prevent collapse of the bronchoalveolar tree. The development of fever in the first 24 to 48 hours after operation often points to atelectasis as the source, and vigorous chest physiotherapy should be instituted.

ANORECTAL OPERATION

PREOPERATIVE PREPARATION

The preoperative preparation before anorectal operations is straightforward and may be kept to a minimum. In most cases chest radiographs, urinalysis, complete blood count, SMA-12, and electrocardiogram are sufficient to exclude concurrent systemic disorders. In addition, if the patient is taking any medications that prolong bleeding time, coagulation studies should be performed to ensure a near-normal range at the time of operation. Many patients undergoing elective anorectal operations can be admitted on the morning of operation. It is probably prudent to admit elderly patients on the day before operation, which allows a more leisurely evaluation and preparation period.

Almost all anorectal procedures can be performed satisfactorily without routine shaving of the perianal skin. The shaving not only creates minor cuts, which are painful and can become infected, but the itching and irritation following the shaving are most uncomfortable to the patient during healing.

Although routine antimicrobial prophylaxis is not needed for anorectal operations, the administration of antibiotics is advocated in patients with cardiac prosthetic implants as well as in those with impaired immunologic status. The necessity for the use of extensive perianal flaps is another reason for antimicrobial prophylaxis.

Patients undergoing per anal excision of a lesion located high in the rectum, with the possibility of perforation and subsequent intra-abdominal exploration, or those undergoing sphincter repair or rectovaginal fistula repair should have a complete mechanical and antibiotic bowel preparation.

The day before operation the patient is allowed a normal diet. To ensure that the first stool to pass the wound is soft, administration of a bulk-forming agent (psyllium seed preparation) is begun the night before operation. A cleansing enema, such as a sodium phosphate or tap-water enema, is given the morning of operation.

INTRAOPERATIVE FLUID RESTRICTION

Acute urinary retention is a well-recognized complication following anorectal operations. Formerly it occurred so often that it was considered almost a normal part of these operations. The reported incidence of urinary retention ranges from 0% to 52% (146). Repeated catheterization results in urinary tract infection and prolonged hospital stays. The recognition that fluid restriction can dramatically reduce the incidence of urinary retention has made most of these patients more comfortable. In a prospective randomized study, Bailey and Ferguson (147) demonstrated that volume restriction of intravenous fluids during anorectal operations reduced the incidence of bladder catheterization from 26% to 3.5%.

Stimulated by an audit that revealed a 52% incidence of urinary retention after hemorrhoidectomy, Prasad and Abcarian (146) undertook a study of 620 patients who underwent a variety of anorectal operations. By adopting the policy of fluid restriction, these authors realized a remarkable drop in the incidence of urinary retention (1.2%). They found that delaying catheterization until the bladder is obviously distended helps to decrease the incidence of catheterization. Others have encountered a similar experience (148). Obtaining the cooperation of the anesthesiologist in restricting fluids, especially in patients who are undergoing regional anesthesia, is not always an easy task.

WOUND HEALING

Primary Healing

The cosmetic result achieved is important, but the comfort of the healed wound and the curing of the disease are the ultimate criteria on which success in anorectal surgery is judged.

Fortunately, because of the abundant blood supply of the anorectum, primary healing of wounds in this area under normal elective operative conditions is generally not a problem. While the statement made by Hippocrates centuries ago that the "best healing is by the apposition of healthy tissues" still holds true, the medical literature has only a scant amount of research in anorectal wound healing, and most of what is understood about this subject has been derived from clinical experience and observation. Unless unusual circumstances are present, external, perianal, or rectal wounds heal as do any other soft tissue wounds. This healing takes place naturally if mechanical or chemical impediments, such as packs, damaging drugs, improper use of sutures and drains, and improper handling of tissues, are avoided. Occasionally in chronically ill and debilitated patients, mineral or vitamin deficiencies may retard healing.

Critical to the healing of anorectal wounds is the maintenance of a good blood supply and respect for the tissues by gentle manipulation. If these two principles are observed, anorectal wounds created electively can be closed primarily and usually will heal.

Proper healing of anorectal wounds almost never requires the use of antibiotics. This includes topical antibiotic ointments, which have not been shown to decrease healing time. The fallacy of the argument that topical medication reduces inflammation and combats infection is apparent in view of the observed fact that mild or minimal "infection of wounds" is harmless because healthy cells are not only engendered with competent defense mechanisms but also may have their healing ability stimulated by mild infection. The rarity of perianal suppuration following elective anorectal operations raises the question of whether or not this anatomic site has some sort of special environmental immunity. While such factors have not yet been elucidated, future studies may prove revealing.

In summary, the primary healing of anorectal wounds depends on the type of surgical procedure performed, gentleness in handling the tissues during the procedure, and maintenance of an excellent blood supply rather than reliance on any postoperative application of therapeutic agents or the performance of any manipulation such as digital examination or dilatation. Systemic processes such as diabetes mellitus, malignancy, or any form of immunoincompetence may severely retard normal anorectal wound healing and the overall host reaction to healing.

Although it is doubtful that substantial benefit will be reaped by the use of skin grafts in the management of patients with fissures and fistulas, the application of a successful split-thickness skin graft to the perianal region following the excision of a perianal neoplasm or hidradenitis suppurativa undoubtedly will expedite overall healing. Full-thickness skin flaps also can be used to achieve primary healing of anorectal wounds. The Y-V anoplasty, skin advancement flaps, and rotating flaps for S-plasty can be adapted for use in repairing anorectal abnormalities.

As an adjunctive development, Gordon (149) has described the technique of using an elemental diet and codeine to prevent the immediate evacuation of stool through newly closed primary anal wounds. This may add to the effectiveness of primary healing, especially when skin grafts are employed.

BOX 1 ■ Discharge Instructions for Anorectal Operation

1. Medicines or prescriptions to be sent home with the patient: Psyllium seed preparation (two doses daily in one-third glass of liquid of your choice). Non-codeine-containing analgesic (every 3 to 6 hours as needed for pain).
2. Postoperative office visits are essential to ensure proper healing of anal wounds. Please call the office to make your first appointment as instructed.
3. Sitz baths, comfortable and warm, should be taken three times a day, especially after bowel movements. The bath should last no longer than 20 minutes.
4. Some bloody discharge, especially after bowel movements, can be expected after anorectal operations. If there is prolonged or profuse bleeding, call the office at once.
5. Bowel movements after anorectal operations are usually associated with some discomfort. This will diminish as the healing progresses. You should have a bowel movement at least every other day. If two days pass without a bowel movement, take 1 ounce of milk of magnesia. If there are no results, repeat in six hours.
6. Use of dry toilet tissue should be avoided. After a bowel movement, use wet tissue or cotton or medical pads to clean yourself.
7. A general diet including plenty of fruits and vegetables is recommended. Try to drink 6–8 glasses of fluid a day.
8. No strenuous exercise or heavy lifting should be attempted until healing is complete. Climbing stairs, walking, and car driving may be done in moderation.
9. If there are any questions about postoperative care, call the office at any time.

Secondary Healing

One of the major theoretical concerns, which the experience of many surgeons would contradict, is the fallacy that the patient will have sepsis if the wounds are closed primarily. For this reason wounds would be laid open widely at the time of operation and kept open by a suitably applied dressing and dilatations until healing is achieved. Epithelium would eventually cover the surface by growing from the periphery.

From clinical experience it is apparent that reliable healing does take place by secondary intention after treatment of hemorrhoids and fistulas. However, leaving anorectal wounds open to granulate has significant disadvantages. First, complete healing by secondary intention may require a considerable length of time (2 to 3 months). Second, the scarring that results from this type of healing may lead to troublesome stricture and painful scars. Therefore, the surgeon always should strive for primary healing whenever this goal is attainable, as is appropriate in hemorrhoid and fissure operations. Fistula operations do not lend themselves to primary healing. In addition, the drainage of anorectal abscesses should be done by allowing healing by secondary intention.

■ POSTOPERATIVE CARE

The postoperative care of most anorectal patients is routine and uncomplicated. Adequate relief of pain, prevention of constipation, and cleansing of the wound are the most important aspects (Box 1). Sitz baths or tub baths are prescribed as a means of cleansing. These baths are also of great comfort and may allow the patient to void more easily by providing better sphincter relaxation when reflectory spasm prevents spontaneous urination. Micturition difficulties are frequently seen after anorectal procedures, especially in elderly men with prostatic hypertrophy. When simple measures, such as warm sitz or tub baths, or the cautious administration of bethanechol chloride (Urecholine) (if not contraindicated) fail to resolve voiding problems, catheterization is required. If straight catheterization with a persistently high residual volume is required more than two times in a 24-hour period, a Foley catheter is inserted and left in place for at least two days. The urine is cultured at the time of catheter removal, and appropriate antibiotics are administered when necessary.

Although the practice of packing following intra-anal procedures is still performed by some surgeons, its use is not recommended in modern-day surgery. Wounds should be hemostatically dry by the time the operation is completed. Intra-anal packing has no substantial benefit. In fact, it may only mask bleeding, result in significant pain, and increase the incidence of urinary retention. Similarly, rectal tubes are not used. In exceptional cases following anorectal operations, extensive open wounds in the perianal or ischioanal space sometimes require packing to stop oozing. The day after the operation, the dressing is removed.

The archaic practice of postoperative anal dilatation as a means of preventing stricture should be abandoned. Following hemorrhoidectomy, for example, the risk of stricture can be diminished by the use of the closed technique combined with a conservative excision of anoderm.

The patient is encouraged to ambulate within several hours after operation. Liquids are allowed by mouth after the patient has voided. A normal diet combined with stool softeners (in the form of bulk laxatives) is started when it can be tolerated. If the patient does not have a spontaneous bowel movement, a mild oral laxative such as milk of magnesia is recommended; if this preparation is not effective by the third postoperative day, an enema (sodium phosphate or tap water) is administered. The patient is discharged when pain relief no longer requires intramuscular injections and when the patient is comfortable enough to provide self-care at home. Indeed, many anorectal operations are performed on an outpatient basis.

Discharge instructions (Box 1) are given to the patient. The patient is allowed to resume all usual activity two weeks from the day of operation but is told to avoid heavy lifting during this period. Travel may begin when the patient desires. Depending on the procedure performed, the patient visits the office 1 to 4 weeks postoperatively for examination of the anorectal wound. Following a hemorrhoidectomy, a visit one month later is adequate, but a patient undergoing operation for fistula-in-ano should be seen earlier. At the time of initial visit, the wound is inspected and a very gentle anal examination is performed. The patient is reviewed as needed to ensure complete wound healing.

REFERENCES

1. Roizen MF, Fleisher LA. In: Miller RD, ed. Anesthetic implication of concurred diseases in Miller's anesthetic. 6th ed. Chapter 27. Elsevier, 2005:1062–1063.
2. Chang DC, Lam AM, Mezan BJ. Essentials of anethesiology. Philadelphia: WB Saunders, 1983.
3. Liu SY, Leighton T, Davis I, Klein S, Lippmann M, Bongerd F. Prospective analysis of cardiopulmonary responses to laparoscopic cholecystectomy. J Laparoendosc Surg 1991; 1:241–246.
4. Ho HS, Gunther RA, Wolfe BM. Intraperitoneal carbon dioxide insufflation and cardiopulmonary functions. Arch Surg 1992; 127:928–932.
5. Rasmussen I, Berggren U, Arvidsson D, Ljungdahl M, Haglund U. Effects of pneumoperitoneum on splanchnic hemodynamics: An experimental study in pigs. Eur J Surg 1995; 161:819–826.
6. McMahon AJ, Baxter JN, Kenny G, O'Dwyer PJ. Ventilatory and blood gas changes during laparoscopic and open cholecystectomy. Br J Surg 1993; 80: 1252–1254.
7. Baxter JN, O'Dwyer PJ. Pathophysiology of laparoscopy. Br J Surg 1995; 82:1–2.
8. Roizen MF. In: Miller RD, ed. Preoperative evaluate in Millers anesthetic. 6th ed. Chapter 25. Elsevier, 2005:954.
9. Ravo B. Colorectal anastomotic healing and intracolonic bypass procedures. Surg Clin North Am 1988; 68:1267–1294.
10. Reilly JJ, Gerhardt AL. Modern surgical nutrition. Curr Probl Surg 1985; 22: 1–81.
11. Braga M, Gianotti L, Vignali A, Carlo VD. Preoperative oral arginine and n-3 fatty acid supplementation improves the immunometabolic host response and outcome after colorectal resection for cancer. Surgery 2002; 132:805–814.
12. Irvin TT, Goligher JC. Aetiology of disruption of intestinal anastomoses. Br J Surg 1973; 60:461–464.
13. Hughes ESR. Asepsis in large-bowel surgery. Ann R Coll Surg Engl 1972; 51:347–356.
14. Irving AD, Scrimgeour D. Mechanical bowel preparation for colonic resection and anastomosis. Br J Surg 1987; 74:580–581.
15. Brownson P, Jenkins SA, Nott D, Ellenbogen S. Mechanical bowel preparation before colorectal surgery: Results of a prospective randomized trial. Br J Surg 1992; 79:461–462.
16. Schein M, Assalia A, Fldar S, Wittmann DH. Is mechanical bowel preparation necessary before primary colonic anastomosis? An experimental study. Dis Colon Rectum 1995; 38:749–754.
17. Santos JCM, Batista J, Sirimarco MT, Gnimaraes AS, Levy CH. Prospective randomized trial of mechanical bowel preparation in patients undergoing elective colorectal surgery. Br J Surg 1994; 81:1673–1676.
18. Burke P, Mealy K, Gilien P, Joyce W, Traynor O, Hyland J. Requirement for bowel preparation in colorectal surgery. Br J Surg 1994; 81:907–910.
19. van Geldere D, Fa-Si-Oen P, Noach LA, Rietra PJ, Peterse JL, Boom RP. Complications after colorectal surgery without mechanical bowel preparation. J Am Coll Surg 2002; 194:40–47.
20. Bucher P, Mermillod B, Gervax P, Morel P. Mechanical bowel preparation for elective colorectal surgery: a meta-analysis. Arch Surg 2004; 139:1359–1364.
21. Wille-Jorgensen P, Guenaga KF, Castro AA, Matos D. Clinical value of preoperative mechanical bowel cleansing in elective colorectal surgery. Dis Colon Rectum 2003; 46:1013–1020.
22. Guenaga KF, Matos D, Castro AA, Atallah AN, Wille-Jorgensen P. Mechanical bowel preparation for elective colorectal surgery. Cochrane Database Systemic Rev 2005; 1:CDOO1544.pub2.
23. Bucher P, Gervaz P, Soravia C, Mermillod B, Erne M, Morel P. Randomized clinical trial of mechanical bowel preparation versus no preparation before elective left-sided colorectal surgery. Br J Surg 2005; 92:409–414.
24. Slim K, Vicaut E, Panis Y, Chipponi J. Meta-analysis of randomized clinical trials of colorectal surgery with or without mechanical bowel preparation. Br J Surg 2004; 91:1125–1130.
25. Zmora O, Wexner SD, Hajjar L, et al. Trends in preparation for colorectal surgery: Survey of the members of the American Society of Colon and Rectal Surgeons. Ann Surg 2003; 69:150–154.
26. Raahave D, Hansen OH, Carstensen HE, et al. Septic wound complications after whole bowel irrigation before colorectal operations. Acta Chir Scand 1952; 147:215–218.
27. Weidema WF, van den Bogaard AEJM. Whole gut irrigation and antimicrobial prophylaxis in elective colorectal surgery [thesis]. Utrecht, Netherlands: Bohn, Scheltema & Holkema, 1984.
28. Keighley MRB. A clinical and physiological evaluation of bowel preparation for elective colorectal surgery. World J Surg 1982; 6:464–470.
29. DiPalma JA, Brady CK, Stewart DL, et al. Comparison of colon cleaning methods in preparation for colonoscopy. Gastroenterology 1984; 86:856–860.
30. Beck DE, Fazio VW. Current preoperative bowel cleansing methods. Results of a survey. Dis Colon Rectum 1990; 33:12–15.
31. Takada H, Ambrose NS, Galbraith K, et al. Quantitative appraisal of Picolax in the preparation of the large bowel for elective surgery. Dis Colon Rectum 1989; 33:679–683.
32. Vanner SS, MacDonald PH, Paterson WG, Prentice RSA, De-Costa LR, Beck IT. A randomized prospective trial comparing oral sodium phosphate with standard polyethylene glycol-based lavage solution (Golytely) in the preparation of patients for colonoscopy. Am J Gastroenterol 1990; 85:422–427.
33. Lee EC, Roberts PC, Taranto R, Schoetz DJ, Murray JJ, Coller JA. Inpatient vs. outpatient bowel preparation for elective colorectal surgery. Dis Colon Rectum 1996; 39:369–373.
34. Hewitt J, Rigby J, Reeve J, et al. Whole gut irrigation in preparation for large bowel surgery. Lancet 1973; 2:337–340.
35. Crapp AR, Pouis SJA, Tillotsen P, et al. Preparation of the bowel by whole gut irrigation. Lancet 1975; 2:1239–1240.
36. Minervini S, Alexander-Williams J, Donovan I, et al. Comparison of three methods of whole gut irrigation. Am J Surg 1980; 140:400–402.
37. Beck DE, Fazio VW, Jagelman DG. Comparison of oral lavage methods for preoperative colonic cleansing. Dis Colon Rectum 1986; 29:699–703.
38. Hares MM, Alexander-Williams J. The effect of bowel preparation on colonic surgery. World J Surg 1982; 6:175–181.
39. Keighley MRB, Taylor EW, Hares MM, et al. Influence of oral mannitol bowel preparation on colonic microflora and the risk of explosion during endoscopic diathermy. Br J Surg 1981; 68:554–556.
40. Taylor EW, Bentley S, Youngs D, et al. Bowel preparation and the safety of colonoscopic polypectomy. Gastroenterology 1981; 81:1–4.
41. Bigand MA, Gaucher P, Lasalle C. Fatal colonic explosion during colonoscopic polypectomy. Gastroenterology 1979; 77:1307–1310.
42. Zanono CE, Bergamini C, Bertocini M, et al. Whole gut lavage for surgery. A case of intra-operative colonic explosion after the administration of mannitol. Dis Colon Rectum 1982; 25:580–581.
43. Davis GR, Santa Ana CA, Morawski SG, et al. Development of a lavage solution associated with minimal water and electrolyte absorption or secretion. Gastroenterology 1980; 78: 991–995.
44. Adams WJ, Meagher AP, Lubowski DZ, King DW. Bisacodyl reduces the volume of polyethylene glycol solution required for bowel preparation. Dis Colon Rectum 1994; 37:229–234.
45. De Lacey G, Benson M, Wilkins R, et al. Routine colonic lavage is unnecessary for double contrast barium enema in outpatients. Br Med J 1982; 284:1021–1022.
46. Chakraverty S, Hughes T, Keir MJ, Hall JR, Rawlinson J. Preparation of the colon for double-contrast barium enema: comparison of Picolax, Picolax with cleansing enema and Citramag (2 sachets)–a randomized prospective trial. Clin Radiol 1994; 49:566–569.
47. Hawkins S, Bezuiedenhout P, Shorvon P, Hine A. Barium enema preparation: a study of low-residue diet, "Picolax" and 'Kleen-Prep'. Australas Radiol 1996; 40:235–239.
48. Macleod AJ, Duncan KA, Pearson RH, Bleakney RR. A comparison of Fleet Phospho-soda will Picolax in the preparation of the colon for double contrast barium enema. Clin Radiol 1998; 53:612–614.
49. Schmidt LM, Williams P, King D, Perera D. Picoprep-3 is a superior colonoscopy preparation to Fleet: a randomized, controlled trial comparing the two bowel preparations. Dis Colon Rectum 2004; 47:238–242.

50. Hamilton D, Mulcahy D, Walsh D, Farrelly C, Tormey WP, Watson G. Sodium picosulphate compared with polyethylene glycol solution for large bowel lavage: A prospective randomized trial. Br J Clin Pract 1996; 50:73–75.
51. Ehrenpreis ED, Nogueras JJ, Botoman VD. Serum electrolyte abnormalities secondary to Fleet's Phospho-soda colonoscopy preparation. Surg Endosc 1996; 16:1022–1024.
52. Frommer D. Cleansing ability and tolerance of three bowel preparations for colonoscopy. Dis Colon Rectum 1997; 40:100–104.
53. Frazee RC, Roberts J, Symmonds R, Snyder S, Hendricks J, Smith R. Prospective, randomized trial of inpatient vs. outpatient bowel preparation for elective colorectal surgery. Dis Colon Rectum 1992; 35:223–226.
54. Burton RC. Postoperative wound infection in colonic and rectal surgery. Br J Surg 1973; 60:363–365.
55. Clarke JS, Condon RE, Bartlett JG, et al. Preoperative oral antibiotics reduce septic complications of colon operations. Ann Surg 1977; 186:251–259.
56. Matheson DM, Arabi Y, Baxter-Smith D, et al. Randomized multicentre trial of oral bowel preparation and antimicrobials for elective colorectal operations. Br J Surg 1978; 65:597–600.
57. Stone HH, Hooper CA, Kolb LD, et al. Antibiotic prophylaxis in gastric, biliary and colonic surgery. Ann Surg 1976; 184:443–452.
58. Keighley MRB, Arabi Y, Alexander-Williams J, et al. Comparison between systemic and oral antimicrobial prophylaxis in colorectal surgery. Lancet 1979; 1:894–897.
59. Lau WY, Chu KW, Poon GP, et al. Prophylactic antibiotics in elective colorectal surgery. Br J Surg 1988; 75:782–785.
60. Lewis RT, Allan CM, Goodall RG. Are first-generation cephalosporins effective for antibiotic prophylaxis in elective surgery of the colon? Can J Surg 1983; 26:504–547.
61. Figueras-Felip J, Basilio-Bonet E, Lara-Hisman F. Oral is superior to systemic antibiotic prophylaxis in operations upon the colon and rectum. Surg Gynecol Obstet 1984; 158:359–362.
62. Playforth MJ, Smith GMR, Evans M, et al. Antimicrobial bowel preparation. Oral, parenteral or both? Dis Colon Rectum 1988; 31:90–93.
63. Condon RE, Bartlett JG, Greenlee H. Efficacy of oral and systemic antibiotic prophylaxis in colorectal operations. Arch Surg 1983; 118:496–502.
64. Coppa GF, Eng K, Gouge TH, Ranson JH, Localio SA. Parental and oral antibiotics in elective colon and rectal surgery. A prospective randomized trial. Am J Surg 1983; 145:62–65.
65. Portnoy J, Kagan E, Gordon PH, et al. Prophylactic antibiotics in elective colorectal surgery. Dis Colon Rectum 1983; 26:310–313.
66. Petrelli NJ, Conte CC, Herrera L, Stule J, O'Neill P. A prospective randomized trial of perioperative prophylactic cefamandole in elective colorectal surgery for malignancy. Dis Colon Rectum 1988; 31:127–129.
67. Hall C, Curran F, Burdon DW, Keighley MR. A randomized trial to compare amoxycillin/clavulanate with metronidazole plus gentamicin in prophylaxis in elective colorectal surgery. J Antimicrob Chemother 1989; 24(suppl B):1 95–202.
68. Periti P, Mazzei T, Tonelli F. Single-dose cefotetan vs. multiple-dose cefoxitin-antimicrobial prophylaxis in colorectal surgery. Results of a prospective, multicenter, randomized study. Dis Colon Rectum 1989; 32:121–127.
69. Schoetz DJ Jr, Roberts PL, Murray JJ, Coller JA, Veidenheimer MC. Addition of parenteral cefoxitin to regimen of oral antibiotics for elective colorectal operations. A randomized prospective study. Ann Surg 1990; 212:209–212.
70. Stellato TA, Danzinger LH, Gordon N, Han T, Hull CC, Zollinger RM Jr., Shuck JM. Antibiotics in elective colon surgery. A randomized trial of oral, systemic, and oral/systemic antibiotics for prophylaxis. Am Surg 1990; 56: 251–254.
71. Skipper D, Karran SJ. A randomized prospective study of compare cefotetan with cefuroxime plus metronidazole as prophylaxis in elective colorectal surgery. J Hosp Inject 1992; 21:73–77.
72. Matikainen M, Hiltunen K III. Parenteral single dose ceftriaxone with tinidatsole versus aminoglycoside with tinidatsole in colorectal surgery: a prospective single blind randomized multicentre study. Int J Colorect Dis 1993; 8:148–150.
73. Morris WT. Ceftriaxone is more effective than gentamycin/metronidazole prophylaxis in reducing wound and urinary tract infections after bowel operations. Results of a controlled, randomized, blind clinical trial. Dis Colon Rectum 1993; 36:826–833.
74. Solla JA, Rothenberger DA. Preoperative bowel preparation. A survey of colon and rectal surgeons. Dis Colon Rectum 1990; 33:154–159.
75. Mecchia P. Comparative study of ceftriaxone versus cefazolin plus clindamycin as antibiotic prophylaxis in elective colorectal surgery. J Chemother 2000; 12(suppl 3):5–9.
76. Mosimann F, Cornu P, N'Ziya Z. Amoxycillin/clavulanic acid prophylaxis in elective colorectal surgery: a prospective randomized trial. J Hosp Inject 1997; 37:55–64.
77. Rau HG, Mittelkotter U, Zimmermann A, Lachmann A, Kohler L, Kullmann KH. Perioperative infection prophylaxis and risk factor impact in colon surgery. Chemotherapy 2000; 46:353–363.
78. Zanella E, Rulli F. A multicenter randomized trial of prophylaxis with intravenous cefepime + metronidazole or ceftriaxone + metronidazole in colorectal surgery. The 230 Study Group. J Chemother 2000; 12:63–71.
79. Smith MB, Goradia VK, Holmes JW, McClugge SG, Smith JW, Nichols RL. Suppression of the human mucosal-related colonic microflora with prophylactic parenteral and/or oral antibiotics. World J Surg 1990; 14:636–641.
80. Bleday R, Braidt J, Ruoff K, Shellito PC, Ackroyd FW. Quantitative cultures of the mucosal-associated bacteria in the mechanically prepared colon and rectum. Dis Colon Rectum 1993; 36:844–849.
81. Lewis RT. Oral versus systemic antibiotic prophylaxis in elective colon surgery: a randomized study and meta-analysis send a message from the 1990s. Can J Surg 2002; 45:173–180.
82. Chapman S, Harford FJ. Perioperative antibiotics. Clinics in Colon Rectal Surg 2001; 14:7–14.
83. Platell C, Hall JC. The prevention of wound infection in patients undergoing colorectal surgery. J Hosp Infect 2001; 49:233–238.
84. Brandstrup B, Tonnesen H, Beier-Holgersen R, et al. Effects of intravenous fluid restriction on postoperative complications: Comparison of two perioperative fluid regimens: a randomized assessor-blinded multicenter trial. Ann Surg 2003; 238:641–648.
85. Waldhausen JH, Shaffrey ME, Skenderis BS, Jones RS, Schirmer BD. Gastrointestinal myoelectric and clinical patterns of recovery after laparotomy. Ann Surg 1990; 211:777–784.
86. Condon RE, Cowles VE, Ferraz AA, Carilli S, Carlson ME, Ludwig K. Human colonic smooth muscle electrical activity after recovery from postoperative ileus. Am J Physiol 1995; 269:G408–G417.
87. Shibata Y, Toyoda S, Nimura Y, Miyati M. Patterns of intestinal motility recovery during the early stage following abdominal surgery: clinical and manometric study. World J Surg 1997; 21:806–809.
88. Kalff JC, Türler A, Schwarz NT, et al. Intra-abdominal activation of a local inflammatory response within the human muscularis externa during laparotomy. Ann Surg 2003; 237:301–315.
89. Taché Y, Martinez V, Million M, Wang L. Stress and the gastrointestinal tract III: stress-related alterations of gut motor function: role of brain corticotropin-releasing factor receptors. Am J Physiol 2001; 280:G173–G177.
90. Cullen JJ, Eagon JC, Kelly KA. Gastrointestinal peptide hormones during postoperative ileus. Effect of octeotride. Dig Dis Sci 1994; 39:1179–1184.
91. Prassad M, Matthews JB. Deflating postoperative ileus. Gastroenterology 1999; 117:489–492.
92. Levin AL. A new gastroduodenal catheter. JAMA 1921; 76:1007.
93. Burg R, Geigle CF, Faso JM. Omission of routine gastric decompression. Dis Colon Rectum 1978; 21:98–100.
94. Bauer JL, Gelernt IM, Salky BA, et al. Is routine postoperative nasogastric decompression necessary? Ann Surg 1985; 201:233–236.
95. Clevers GJ, Smout JPM. The natural course of postoperative ileus following abdominal surgery. Neth J Surg 1989; 41:97–99.
96. Colvin DB, Lee W, Eisenstat TE, et al. The role of nasointestinal intubation in elective colonic surgery. Dis Colon Rectum 1986; 29:295–299.
97. Wolff BG, Pemberton JM, Van Heerden JA, et al. Elective colon and rectal surgery without nasogastric decompression. A prospective randomized trial. Ann Surg 1989; 209:670–673.
98. Petrelli NJ, Stule JP, Rodriguez-Bigas M, Blumenson L. Nasogastric decompression following elective colorectal surgery. A prospective, randomized study. Am Surg 1993; 59:632–635.
99. Cheatham ML, Chapman WC, Key SP, Sawyers JL. A meta-analysis of selective versus routine nasogastric decompression after elective laparotomy. Ann Surg 1995; 221:469–476.
100. Reissman P, Teoh TA, Cohen SM, et al. Is early oral feeding safe after elective colorectal surgery? A prospective randomized trial. Ann Surg 1995; 222: 73–77.
101. Feo CV, Romanini B, Sortini D, et al. Early oral feeding after colorectal resection: a randomised controlled study. ANZ J Surg 2004; 74:298–301.
102. Wight R, Kennedy H, Abdelal A, Fulton JD. Postoperative urinary retention. Br Med J 1991; 302:1151.
103. Petrelli NJ, Nagel S, Rodriguez-Bigas M. Morbidity and mortality following abdominoperineal resection for adenocarcinoma. Ann Surg 1993; 59:400–404.
104. Havenga K, Welvaart K. Sexual dysfunction in male patients after surgical treatment of rectosigmoid cancer. Neth J Med 1991; 135:710–713.
105. van Driel MF, Weyman-Schultz WCM, van de Wiel HBM. Female sexual function after radical surgical treatment of rectal and bladder cancer. Eur J Surg Oncol 1993; 19:183–187.
106. Schofield JH, Northover JMA. Surgical management of rectal cancer. Br J Surg 1995; 82:745–748.
107. Weitz SR. Management of postoperative pain. Perspect Colon Rectal Surg 1995; 8:66–81.
108. Cullen ML, Staren ED, El-Ganzouri A, et al. Continuous epidural infusion for analgesia after major abdominal operations. A randomized, prospective, double-blind study. Surgery 1985; 98:718–727.
109. Holte K, Kehlet H. Postoperative ileus: a preventable event. Br J Surg 2000; 87:1480–1493.
110. Holte K, Kehlet H. Epidural analgesia and risk of anastomotic leakage. Anesth Pain Med 2001; 226:111.
111. Merry A, Power W. Perioperative NSAIDs: towards greater safety. Pain Rev 1995; 2:268–291.

112. Bigler D, Hjortso NC, Kehlet H. Disruption of colonic anastomosis during continuous epidural analgesia. Anesthesia 1985; 40:278–280.
113. Aitkenhead AR, Wishart HY, Peebles Brown DA. High spinal nerve block for large bowel anastomosis. Br J Anaesth 1978; 50:177–183.
114. McLintock TTC, Kenny GNC, Howie JC, et al. Assessment of the analgesic efficacy of nefopam hydrochloride after upper abdominal surgery: a study using patient controlled analgesia. Br J Surg 1988; 75:779–781.
115. Albert JM, Talbott TM. Patient controlled analgesia vs. conventional intramuscular analgesia following colon surgery. Dis Colon Rectum 31:83–86.
116. Cataldo P, Senagore AJ, Kilbride MJ. Ketorolac and patient controlled analgesia in the treatment of postoperative pain. Surg Gynecol Obstet 1993; 176:435–438.
117. Bradshaw BGG, Liu SS, Thirlby RC. Standardized perioperative care protocols and reduced length of stay after colon surgery. J AM Coll Surg 1998; 186: 501–506.
118. Miedema BW, Johnson JO. Methods for decreasing postoperative gut dysmotility. Lancet Oncol 2003; 4:365–372.
119. Taguchi A, Sharma N, Saleem RM, et al. Selective postoperative inhibition of gastrointestinal opioid receptors. N Engl J Med 2001; 27: 935–40.
120. Sadek SA, Cranford C, Eriksen C, Walker M, Campbell C, Baker PR. Pharmacological manipulation of adynamic ileus: controlled randomised double-blind study of ceruletide on intestinal motor activity after elective abdominal surgery. Aliment Pharmacol Ther 1988; 2:47–54.
121. Madsen PV, Lykkegaard-Nielsen M, Nielsen OV. Ceruletide reduces postoperative intestinal paralysis. A double-blind placebo-controlled trial. Dis Colon Rectum 1983; 26:159–160.
122. Bonacini M, Quiason S, Reynolds M, Gaddis M, Pemberton B, Smith O. Effect of intravenous erythromycin on postoperative ileus. Am J Gastroenterol 1993; 88:208–211.
123. Benotti JR, Dalen ED. The natural history of pulmonary embolism. Chir Chest Med 1984; 5:403–410.
124. Nicolaides AN, Miles C, Hoare M, et al. Intermittent sequential pneumatic compression of the legs and thromboembolism-deterrent stockings in the prevention of postoperative deep venous thrombosis. Surgery 1983; 94:21–25.
125. Törngren S, Rieger A. Prophylaxis of deep venous thrombosis in colorectal surgery. Dis Colon Rectum 1982; 25:563–566.
126. Sands DR, Wexner SD. Nasogastric tubes and dietary advancement after laparoscopic and open colorectal surgery. Nutrition 1999; 15:347–350.
127. Milsom JW, Bohm B, Hammerhofer KA, Fazio V, Steiger E, Elson P. A prospective randomised trial comparing laparoscopic versus conventional techniques in colorectal cancer surgery: a preliminary report. J Am Coll Surg 1998; 187: 46–57.
128. Bufo AJ, Feldman S, Daniels GA, Lieberman RC. Early postoperative feeding. Dis Colon Rectum 1994; 37:1260–1265.
129. Binderow SM, Cohen SM, Wexner SD, Nogueras JJ. Must early postoperative oral intake be limited to laparoscopy? Dis Colon Rectum 1994; 37:584.
130. Reisman P, Teoh TA, Cohen SM, et al. Is early oval feeding safe after elective colorectal surgery? A prospective randomized trial. Ann Surg 1995; 222:23–27.
131. Ortiz H, Armendariz P, Yarnoz C. Is early postoperative feeding feasible in elective colon and rectal surgery? Int J Colorect Dis 1996; 11:119–121.
132. DiFronzo LA, Cymerman J, O'Connell TX. Factors affecting early postoperative feeding following elective open colon resection. Arch Surg 1999; 134: 941–946.
133. Petrelli NJ, Cheng C, Driscoll D, Rodriguez-Bigas MA. Early postoperative oral feeding after colectomy: an analysis of factors that may predict outcome. Ann Surg Oncol 2001; 8:796–800.
134. Lewis SJ, Egger M, Sylvester PA, Topic ST. Early enteral feeding versus "nil by mouth" after gastrointestinal surgery: systematic review and meta-analysis of controlled trials. BMJ 2001; 323:773–776.
135. DiFronzo LA, Yamin N, Patel K, O'Connell TX. Benefits of early feeding and early hospital discharge in elderly patients undergoing open colon resection. J Am Coll Surg 2003; 197:747–752.
136. Camberos A, Cymerman J, DiFronzo LA, O'Connell TX. The effect of cisapride on the success of early feeding after elective open colon resection. Am Surg 2002; 68:1093–1096.
137. Kehlet H. Multimodal approach to control postoperative pathophysiology and rehabilitation. Br J Anaesth 1997; 78:606.
138. Basse L, Hjort Jacobsen D, Billesbolle P, Werner M, Kehlet H. A clinical pathway to accelerate recovery after colonic resection. Ann Surg 2000; 232:51–57.
139. Basse L, Thorbol JE, Lossl K, Kehlet H. Colonic surgery with accelerated rehabilitation or conventional care. Dis Colon Rectum 2004; 47:271–277.
140. Delaney CP, Zutshi M, Senagore AJ, Remzi FH, Hammel J, Fazio V. Prospective, randomised, controlled trial between a pathway controlled rehabilitation with early ambulation and diet and traditional postoperative care after laparotomy and intestinal resection. Dis Colon Rectum 2003; 46:851–859.
141. Fearon KCH, Luff R. The nutritional management of surgical patients: enhanced recovery after surgery. Proc Nutr Soc 2003; 62:807–811.
142. Smedh K, Strand E, Jansson P, et al. Rapid recovery after colonic resection. Multimodal rehabilitation by means of Kehlet's method practiced on Vasteras. Lakartidningen 2001; 98:2568–2574.
143. Henriksen MG, Jensen MB, Hansen HV, Jespersen TW, Hessov I. Enforced mobilization, early oral feeding and balanced analgesia improve convalescence after colorectal surgery. Nutrition 2002; 18:147–152.
144. Bisgaard T, Kehlet H. Early oral feeding after elective abdominal surgery: what are the issues? Nutrition 2002; 18:944–948.
145. Mythen M. Postoperative gastrointestinal tract dysfunction. Anesth Analg 2005; 100:196–204.
146. Prasad ML, Abcarian H. Urinary retention following operations for benign anorectal diseases. Dis Colon Rectum 1978; 21:490–492.
147. Bailey HR, Ferguson JA. Prevention of urinary retention by fluid restriction following anorectal operations. Dis Colon Rectum 1976; 19:250–252.
148. Bowers FJ, Hartmann R, Khanduja KS, et al. Urecholine prophylaxis for urinary retention in anorectal surgery. Dis Colon Rectum 1987; 30:41–42.
149. Gordon PH. The chemically defined diet and anorectal procedures. Can J Surg 1976; 19:511–513.

5 Local Anesthesia in Anorectal Surgery

Santhat Nivatvongs

INTRODUCTION

Local anesthetic agents are unique in that they produce a loss of sensation and muscle paralysis in a circumscribed area of the body by a localized effect on peripheral nerve endings or fibers (1). In spite of being very sensitive areas, the anal canal and the perianal skin can be anesthetized without causing much pain or discomfort, and the success of the anesthetic is predictable. The fully relaxed anal canal then becomes an ideal setting for various surgical procedures.

SELECTION OF PATIENTS

A highly nervous and apprehensive patient or one with a very painful anal canal would not be a good candidate for local anesthesia. For a successful outcome to be achieved, the patient must be completely cooperative. The patient should be given a thorough explanation of the procedure and told what to expect. In addition, the advantages and disadvantages of local anesthesia should be explained.

Since the anesthetic is given by injection into the perianal skin and the anal canal, the local anatomy must be accessible for the procedure; thus patients with deep or high cheeks of the buttocks and obese patients may not be suitable (Fig. 1) (2).

APPLICABLE CONDITIONS

Almost all kinds of simple anorectal conditions are suitable for local anesthesia. These conditions include hemorrhoids (even thrombosed, strangulated, or gangrenous), anal fissure, simple intersphincteric anal fistula, small perianal abscess, pilonidal abscess and sinus, low rectal adenoma, and perianal and anal condyloma acuminatum, as well as in carefully selected cases of sphincter repair and many other anorectal conditions (3).

Most perianal abscesses can be drained with the patient under local anesthesia. However, patients with very large abscesses require an excessive amount of the anesthetic agent because the tissue is acidotic, which causes slower diffusion of the anesthetic solution through the nerve sheath. Patients with scar tissue such as that found in cases of a complicated anal fistula also do not respond well to a local anesthetic. Any anorectal procedure expected to exceed two hours may not be suitable for a local anesthetic because of the discomfort associated with a prone jackknife or lithotomy position. However, a lateral or modified lateral position can be used.

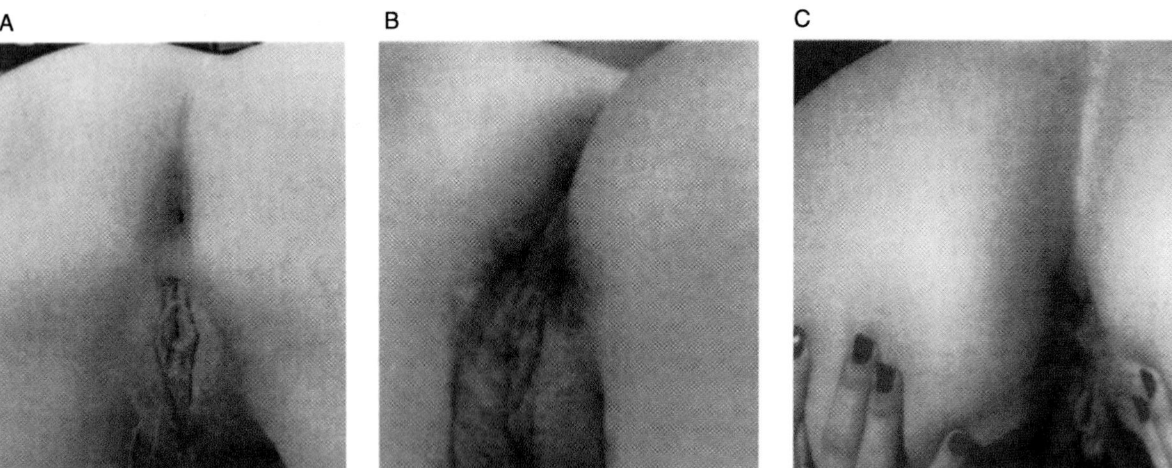

FIGURE 1 ■ Shape of the buttock. (**A**) Flat cheeks, ideal for anesthesia. (**B**) Deep, prominent cheeks, the anal canal is deep, less suitable for local anesthesia. (**C**) Flat cheeks but the anus is more anterior than normal, still suitable for local anesthesia.

ACTIONS OF AGENT

Local anesthetic agents exert their primary pharmacologic action by inhibiting the excitatory process in nerve endings or nerve fibers. They perform in the nerve membrane, which is a highly lipid structure. Thus the intrinsic anesthetic potency of different agents is a function of their lipid solubility. Protein binding is believed to be a primary determinant of anesthetic duration, and the nerve membrane consists of proteins as well as lipids. The greater the binding affinity to nerve proteins, the longer anesthetic activity will persist (1).

Like many drugs, local anesthetics exist in both a charged and an uncharged form, with the equilibrium determined by the pH of the surrounding medium. As the pH of the solution decreases and hydrogen ion concentrations increase, the equilibrium shifts toward the charged cation form, and more cation than free base will be present. Conversely, as the pH increases and hydrogen ion concentrations decrease, the equilibrium shifts toward the free-base form, and more of the local anesthetic agent will exist in that form. The uncharged base form diffuses more readily through the nerve sheath and is reflected clinically in the onset of anesthesia (1). This explains why local anesthesia is not as effective for a large abscess, that is, because the tissue is acidotic.

The susceptibility of nerve fibers to local anesthetics is related to the size of the fiber and its myelin coating. Smaller nerves are blocked first, and lightly myelinated nerves are more susceptible than more heavily coated nerves. In general, the first nerves blocked are the last ones to recover. Sensory nerves are blocked before motor nerves, possibly on the basis of nerve size and myelin thickness. The usual order of sensory loss is pain, temperature, touch, and deep pressure.

DISPOSITION OF AGENT

Knowing the vascular absorption, tissue distribution, metabolism, and excretion of local anesthetic agents is important in understanding their potential toxicity. Absorption varies according to site of injection, dosage, addition of a vasoconstrictor agent, and specific agent used (1).

After their absorption from the injection site, local anesthetic agents distribute themselves throughout total body water. An initial rapid disappearance from blood (alpha phase) occurs because of uptake by tissues with a high vascular perfusion. A secondary slower disappearance rate (beta phase) reflects distribution to slowly perfused tissues and metabolism and excretion of the compound. Although all tissues will take up local anesthetics, the highest concentrations are found in the more highly perfused organs such as the lungs and kidneys. The greater percentage of an injected dose of a local anesthetic agent is distributed to skeletal muscle because of the large mass of tissue in the body (1).

The metabolism of local anesthetic agents varies according to their chemical classification. The ester- or procaine-like agents undergo hydrolysis in plasma by the enzyme pseudocholinesterase. The amide- or lidocaine-like agents undergo enzymatic degradation primarily in the liver. Lidocaine (Xylocaine), mepivacaine (Carbocaine), and etidocaine (Duranest) are intermediate in terms of rate of degradation, whereas bupivacaine (Marcaine) is metabolized most slowly (1).

CHOICE OF AGENT

Although several local anesthetic agents are available for clinical use in anorectal surgery, lidocaine and bupivacaine are most suitable and most widely used (4). Both lidocaine and bupivacaine are amide compounds that undergo enzymatic degradation in the liver. On the other hand, ester compounds such as procaine are metabolized to *para*-amino-benzoic acid. Unlike the ester compounds, the amide groups extremely rarely produce an allergic phenomenon. Lidocaine and bupivacaine are available in various concentrations. The lowest effective concentration should be selected; thus 0.5% lidocaine and 0.25% bupivacaine are the concentrations of choice.

■ EPINEPHRINE

All local anesthetic agents except cocaine cause peripheral vasodilatation by producing a direct relaxant effect on the musculature of the blood vessels. The degree of vasodilator activity appears related to intrinsic anesthetic potency. The more potent and longer acting local anesthetic agents produce a greater degree and longer duration of vasodilatation. Epinephrine incorporated into local anesthetic solutions constricts blood vessels, thereby slowing absorption and minimizing any toxic reaction. Epinephrine accomplishes three purposes: (i) it reduces capillary bleeding; (ii) it prevents rapid absorption of the local anesthetic agent, thus avoiding a high blood level of the anesthetic agent while minimizing any toxic reaction; and (iii) it prolongs analgesia during surgery. Systemic toxic reactions may occur when the epinephrine in the blood reaches a high level. The common signs and symptoms of these reactions are pallor, tachycardia, perspiration, palpitation, apprehension, dyspnea, rapid respiration, and hypertension (5). The side effects are rare when the dilution of 1:200,000 is used.

■ HYALURONIDASE

Hyaluronic acid found in interstitial spaces normally prevents the diffusion of invasive substances. Hyaluronidase (Wydase), a mucolytic enzyme, allows anesthetic solutions to spread in the tissues by inactivating the hyaluronic acid (6). It also tends to reduce swelling and increase the absorption of blood in the subcutaneous tissues. Hyaluronidase is not toxic to tissues and will not cause them to slough. Allergic reactions to hyaluronidase may occur but are insignificant.

Hyaluronidase, 150 IU, can be added to 20 mL of anesthetic solution. Clark and Mellette (7) found that the addition of hyaluronidase reduces tissue edema, enlarges the area of anesthesia, and augments the onset of anesthesia. In a randomized controlled study on the use of peribulbar block during intraocular surgery, the addition of hyaluronidase produced no advantages (8). The disadvantage of using hyaluronidase is that it shortens the duration of analgesia because it enhances absorption, thus defeating the purpose of adding epinephrine to prolong the anesthetic action and to slow down clearance. Therefore there is no reason to add hyaluronidase to the anesthetic solution.

MINIMIZING PAIN IN LOCAL ANESTHESIA

Injection of an anesthetic solution to the perianal skin and anal canal is more painful than "a mosquito bite," a description surgeons use with their patients. There are several useful methods of administration that minimize the pain.

■ METHODS OF INJECTION

The needle should be small and the injecting pressure should be low. For practical purposes and availability, a 1½ inch (3.5 cm) 27-gauge needle with 3 mL disposable syringe works well. The lower the concentration of the anesthetic solution, the less painful it is. Superficial wheal-producing dermal injection is uniformly much more painful than that into the deep dermal-subcutaneous tissue. Rapid injection almost always hurts more than slow infiltration. Warming the solution does not make the injection less painful (9,10).

■ BUFFERING

Most local anesthetic solutions are quite acidic, with a pH ranging from 5.0–7.0. Lidocaine has a pH of 6.8 and bupivacaine is 5.5. Local anesthetic is more soluble and has a shelf life of 3–4 years. Raising the pH to 7.2–7.4 would substantially reduce effective storage shelf life and solubility. Raising the pH above 7.4 increases the risk of precipitation of local anesthetic out of solution. A study by Christoph et al. (11) showed that infiltration of 1% lidocaine is five times more painful than buffered 1% lidocaine, 1% lidocaine with epinephrine is 2.8 times more painful than buffered 1% lidocaine without epinephrine, and 1% mepivacaine (an intermediate action local anesthetic) is 5.7 times more painful than buffered mepivacaine. These results are statistically highly significant.

Buffering can be easily and safely accomplished by the addition of sodium bicarbonate solution so that the resultant ratio of local anesthetic to sodium bicarbonate equals 10:1. In doing so, the efficacy of the local anesthetic is not compromised. Local anesthetic buffering should be performed immediately before its use to eliminate concerns regarding shortened shelf life of the anesthetic caused by the alkalinization (11).

ADVERSE REACTIONS

Toxicity of different anesthetic agents varies, usually in parallel with potency. To some extent the rate of biotransformation will affect toxicity. The rate of absorption also will influence toxicity, and this may be determined by the route of administration. Box 1 lists the signs and symptoms of local anesthetic toxicity.

There are two types of adverse reaction to local anesthetic agents: allergic reaction and toxic reaction.

BOX 1 ■ Signs and Symptoms of Local Anesthetic Toxicity

Central Nervous System Effects	Cardiovascular Effects
Mild	
Lightheadedness	↑ PR interval
Dizziness	↑ QRS duration
Tinnitus	↓ Cardiac output
Drowsiness	↓ Blood pressure
Disorientation	
Severe	
Muscle twitching	↑↑ PR interval
Tremors of face and extremities	↓↓ QRS duration
	Sinus bradycardia
Unconsciousness	Atrioventricular block
Generalized convulsions	↓↓ Cardiac output
Respiratory arrest	↓↓ Hypotension
	Asystole

ALLERGIC REACTIONS

Allergic reaction, a rare occurrence, may be systemic or local. More than 80% of reactions are cell mediated, resulting in contact dermatitis. The remaining reactions are caused by circulating antibodies that give rise to systemic anaphylaxis. Acute anaphylactic reactions are rare, but they are invariably fatal unless promptly treated. Localized systemic anaphylactic reactions manifested by urticaria, laryngeal edema, and extrinsic asthma are less serious and are amenable to treatment. There is no foolproof test for screening susceptible persons. The intradermal test is of no value in determining possible systemic sensitivity. The patch test is useful in the detection of contact allergy (12).

TOXIC REACTIONS

Toxic reactions to local anesthetic agents are far more common than allergic sequelae. The majority of adverse reactions to local anesthetics are due to high plasma levels resulting from the administration of excessive quantities of the drug. The major manifestations of local anesthetic toxicity occur in the central nervous system (CNS) and the cardiovascular system.

Central Nervous System Toxicity

All local anesthetics have the capacity to stimulate the CNS at low toxic doses and suppress the CNS at high toxic doses. Initial signs and symptoms of a high toxic dose are CNS excitation, resulting from the suppression of inhibitory cortical neurons, which permits unopposed functioning of facilitatory pathways. Subsequent signs and symptoms of a high toxic dose include light-headedness, dizziness, nystagmus, sensory disturbances (e.g., visual difficulties, tinnitus, perioral tingling, metallic taste), restlessness, and disorientation or psychosis. Slurred speech and muscle twitching or tremors may immediately precede seizures. If serum levels of the drug continue to increase, generalized depression of the entire CNS occurs, with resultant drowsiness, coma, and respiratory arrest (1,13).

Cardiovascular System Toxicity

The cardiovascular system is relatively resistant to local anesthetic toxicity in comparison with the CNS and does not exhibit toxic reactions until blood levels are much higher. Cardiovascular complications result from negative inotropism, peripheral vasodilatation, and slowing of the myocardial conductive system. The end results of local anesthetic toxicity are hypotension, bradycardia, prolonged electrocardiographic intervals, and cardiac arrest (1,13).

TREATMENT OF ADVERSE REACTIONS

Anaphylactic shock is the least common yet most serious of the allergic reactions. It is characterized by a sudden circulatory and respiratory collapse, loss of consciousness, laryngeal edema, and urticaria. Anaphylaxis must be dealt with promptly. The immediate treatment consists of the subcutaneous injection of 0.5 mL of 1:1000 epinephrine. To increase the rate of absorption, the injection site should be vigorously massaged. Meanwhile, ventilation should be maintained with oxygen under pressure. If the patient does not show rapid improvement, the administration of epinephrine can be repeated in 5–15 minutes. If severe bronchospasm persists, 250–500 mg of aminophylline should be administered intravenously. Once an improvement has been noted, corticosteroids and an antihistamine can be administered intramuscularly to prevent recurrence of symptoms and avoid the use of additional epinephrine (12,14).

Toxic reactions must be recognized and treated as follows without delay:

1. Clear airway (if patient is unconscious).
2. Prevent aspiration.
3. Administer oxygen.
4. Induce intravenous fluid (for administration of intravenous medication).
5. Stop convulsion.
   a. Administration of oxygen alone may stop convulsion.
   b. If oxygen does not stop convulsion, intravenous medications such as thiopental (50–100 mg), midazolam (2–5 mg), and propofol (1 mg/kg) can terminate seizures (15). If seizures fail to respond to such treatment, short-acting neuromuscular blocking agents such as succinylcholine (Anectine) or vecuronium (Norcuron) should be administered until serum levels of local anesthetic agents fall (13).
6. Raise blood pressure by giving a vasopressive drug.
7. Perform cardiac massage if patient's heart has arrested.

PREVENTION OF ADVERSE REACTIONS

Preventing or minimizing the risk of complications is the most important aspect in giving local anesthetic agents. The lowest effective concentration should be used. In anorectal surgery, 0.5% lidocaine and 0.25% bupivacaine are ideal. Unless contraindicated, an addition of 1:200,000 epinephrine should be used to prolong the action and minimize the absorption. The amount injected should not exceed the maximum dose—500 mg lidocaine with 1:200,000 epinephrine (100 mL) and 225 mg bupivacaine with 1:200,000 epinephrine (90 mL). Dosage should be reduced for elderly patients and debilitated patients with cardiac or liver disease. Rapid injection with a large volume of the anesthetic should be avoided; fractional doses should be used when feasible.

Having the patient breathe oxygen during the procedure and avoiding heavy preoperative sedation are helpful. Hypercarbia and acidosis decrease the threshold of local anesthetic agents for convulsive activity. Similarly, hypercarbia, acidosis, and hypoxia tend to increase the cardiodepressant effect of local anesthetic agents (1).

INDUCTION OF ANESTHESIA

The following rules must be observed in inducing local anesthesia[a]:

1. Do not exceed the recommended maximum dosage of the local anesthetic drugs.

[a] Modified from Ref. 5; courtesy of Charles C. Thomas, Publisher.

2. Do not rely on premedication to prevent systemic toxic reactions.
3. Carefully observe the patient after completion of the injection.
4. Objectively evaluate any type of reaction, no matter how mild. Do not treat a reaction without making a definite diagnosis; give only the necessary indicated therapy.
5. Be prepared to treat any type of reaction, for example, convulsion, respiratory collapse, or cardiovascular collapse.
6. Do not overtreat or undertreat the reaction. Some reactions require no treatment; on the other hand, intensive treatment and even closed cardiac massage may be necessary to save the patient's life.

TECHNIQUES OF LOCAL ANESTHESIA

GENERAL CONSIDERATIONS

For good-risk patients, preoperative medication should be given. Both diazepam (Valium) and midazolam (Versed) are excellent agents for blunting consciousness during the procedure. In addition, fentanyl (Sublimaze), a potent but short-acting narcotic drug, may be used as a supplement. For ambulatory short-duration procedures, preoperative sedation is usually not necessary.

A 27-gauge needle with a 3 mL disposable syringe is used for the injection. For most patients the anesthetic solution causes considerable burning pain during the injection. The key is to slowly infiltrate the subdermal plane. Buffering the anesthetic solution with sodium bicarbonate, as described earlier, helps.

CONVENTIONAL TECHNIQUE

The anesthetic solution is infiltrated around the perianal skin and the anal verge (Fig. 2). Next the anal canal is injected subdermally and submucosally in a circumferential manner (Fig. 3). Complete sphincteric relaxation is achieved without having to inject the anesthetic solution directly into the sphincter muscles (16). Some surgeons prefer to inject the muscle and/or the ischioanal fossa directly, but this is not necessary. In most cases, 20–25 mL of the anesthetic solution is used.

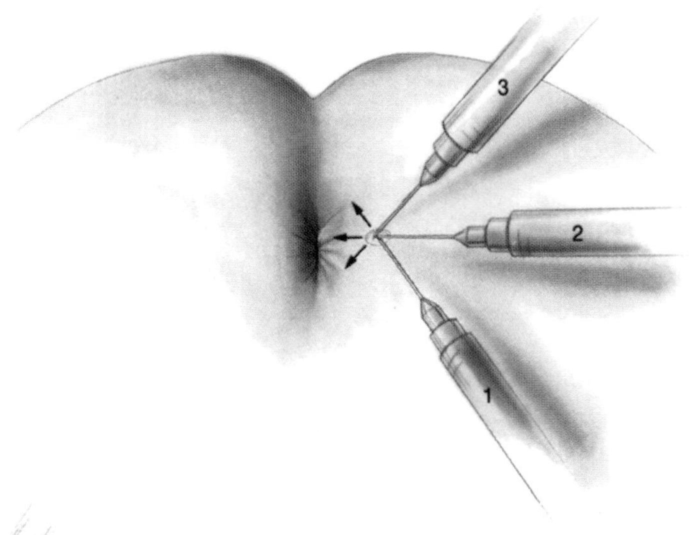

FIGURE 2 ■ Infiltration of the perianal skin and anal verge in a subcutaneous plane.

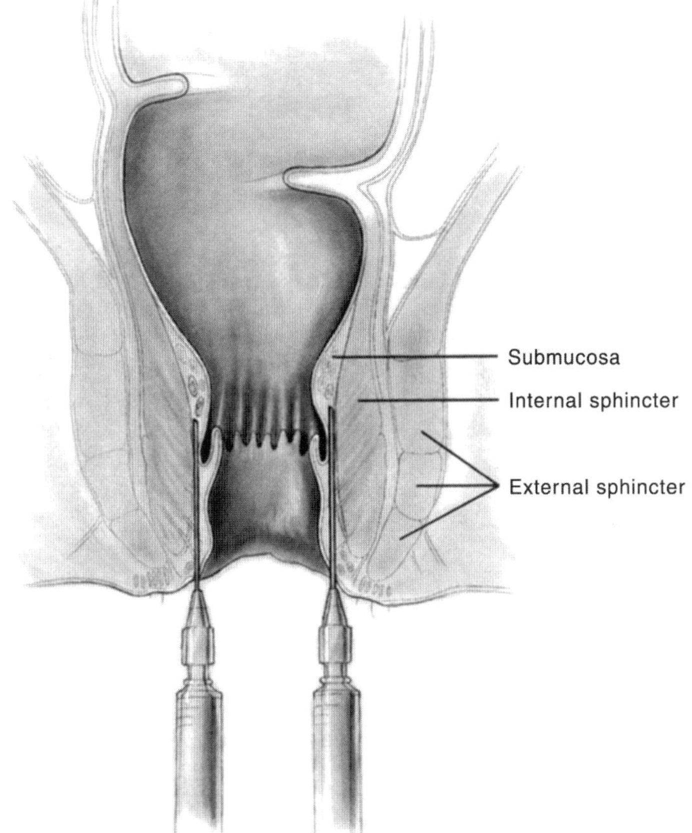

FIGURE 3 ■ Injection of anesthetic into the subdermal and submucosal tissue.

IMPROVED TECHNIQUE

Intraanal Injection

Because the mucosa of the anal canal above the dentate line is less sensitive to pain, injection of anesthetic solution into this area is almost painless. An improved technique has been developed based on this fact (17).

Mild sedation may be used but is not necessary in some patients. Following digital examination of the anal canal with 2% lidocaine jelly, a small anoscope (ideally a Vernon-David anoscope) is inserted into the anal canal. Injection of 2–3 mL of the anesthetic solution makes a submucosal wheal 2 mm above the dentate line (Fig. 4A). If injection at this level still causes pain, the injection site is moved 2 mm higher. The injection is made in four quadrants. The index finger is then inserted into the anal canal, and each wheal of the anesthetic solution is milked into the subdermal plane below the dentate line. This is best accomplished by bending the finger like a hockey stick over the anesthetic wheal and withdrawing it distally (Fig. 4B). The anal canal at this point will be well relaxed to accommodate a large Hill-Ferguson or other suitable anal speculum with ease and without discomfort. Next, with the Hill-Ferguson anal speculum in place for exposure, at 2 mm below the dentate line the anoderm is infiltrated (in the subcutaneous plane) with 2 mL of the anesthetic solution in four quadrants (Fig. 4C). The anal verge and perianal skin are next injected circumferentially.

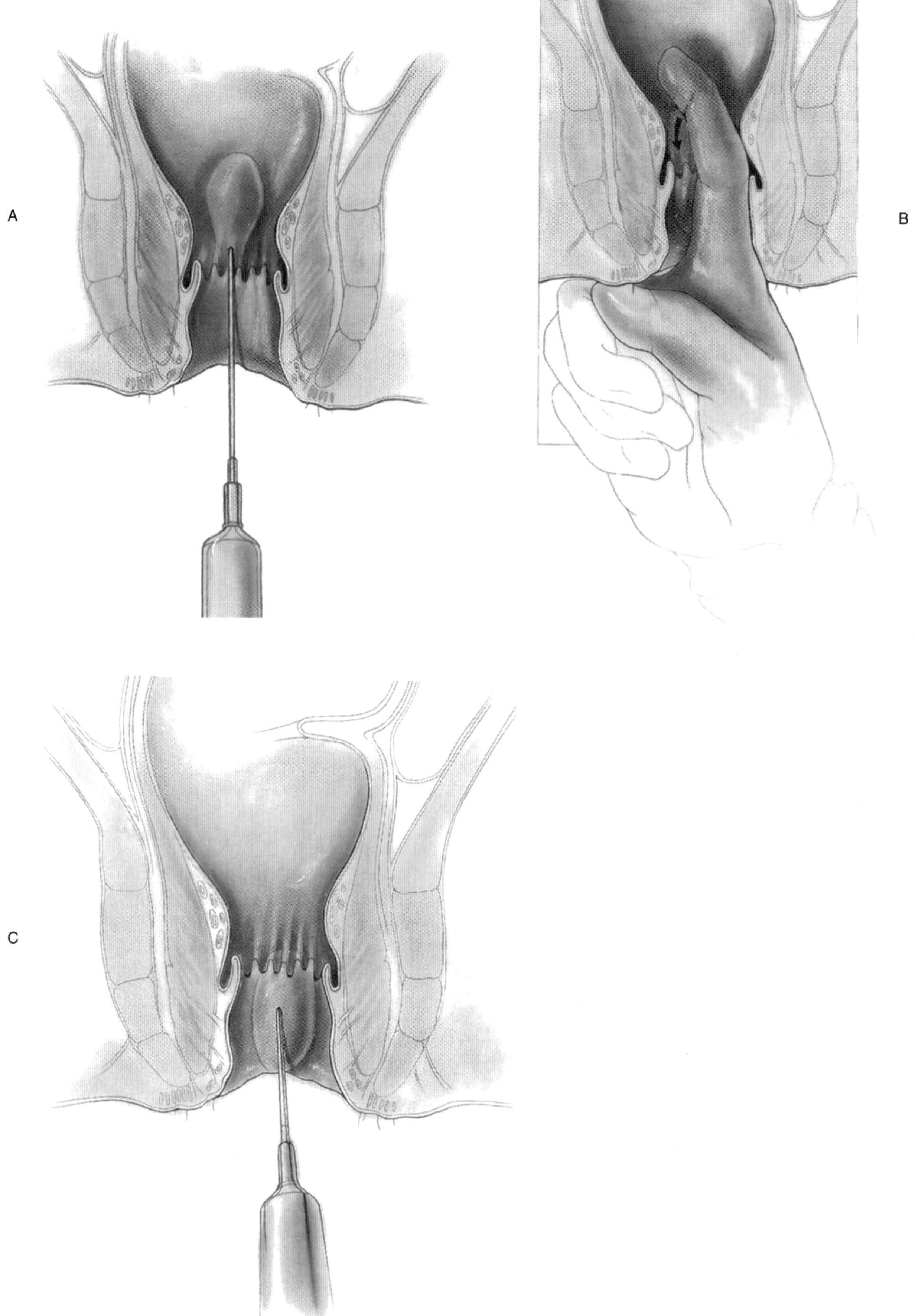

FIGURE 4 ■ Intraanal injection. (**A**) Injection 5 mm above the dentate line in the submucosal plane. (**B**) Milking the anesthetic wheal to below the dentate line. (**C**) Injection 2 mm below the dentate line in the subcutaneous plane.

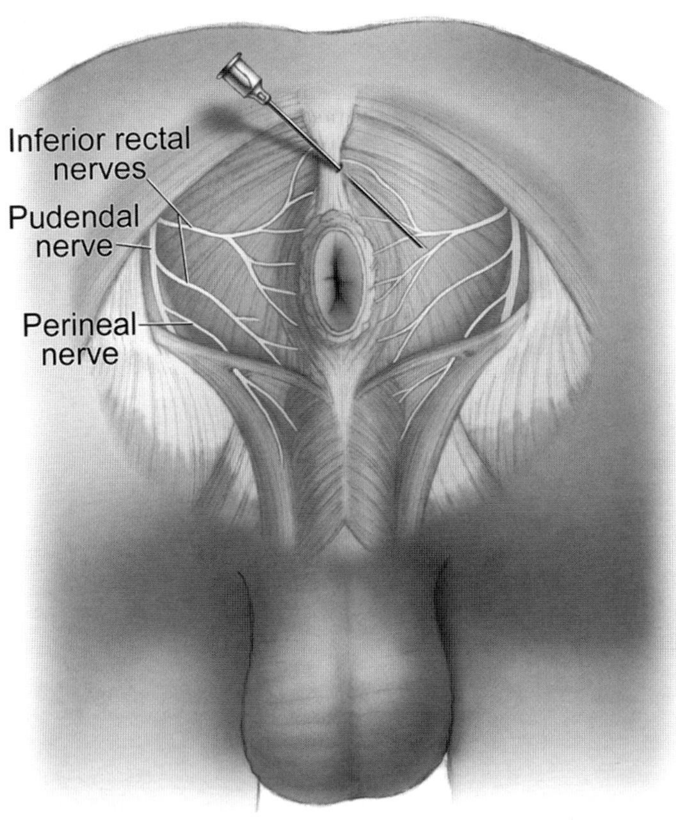

FIGURE 5 ■ Infiltration of the nerves in ischioanal fossa.

The same technique can be applied for a patient with a painful anal fissure, but the injection should start in the quadrant that has the fissure. Such a patient may require heavier sedation.

Posterior Perineal Block

This technique involves infiltration of the anesthetic solution to the inferior rectal nerves, the perineal nerves, and the anococcygeal nerves (18).

First, the surgeon injects 2 mL of the anesthetic solution in the posterior midline of the perianal skin. The needle is then angled 45°, 8–10 cm into each ischioanal fossa to block the inferior rectal and the perineal nerves (Fig. 5). Next, the needle is aimed at the presacral fascia, injecting 5 mL of the anesthetic solution into the presacral space to block the anococcygeal nerves. Finally, about 15 mL of the anesthetic solution are injected into the perianal skin circumferentially to anesthetize the sensitive branches of the superficial perineal nerves. Gabrielli et al. (18) used this technique in 400 hemorrhoidectomies with excellent results.

REFERENCES

1. Philip BK, Covino BG. Local and regional anesthesia. In: Wetchler BV, ed. Anesthesia for Ambulatory Surgery. Philadelphia: JB Lippincott, 1991:309–365.
2. Nivatvongs S, Fang DT, Kennedy HL. The shape of the buttocks—A useful guide for selection of patients for anorectal surgery. Dis Colon Rectum 1983; 26:85–86.
3. Read TE, Henry SE, Hovis RM, et al. Prospective evaluation of anesthetic technique for anorectal surgery. Dis Colon Rectum 2002; 45:1553–1560.
4. Moore DC, Bridenbaugh LD, Thompson GE, Balfour RI, Horton WG. Bupivacaine: A review of 11,080 cases. Anesth Analg 1978; 57:42–53.
5. Moore DC. Regional block. 4th ed. Springfield, I ll.: Charles C Thomas, 1978: 19–43.
6. Clery AD. Local anesthesia containing hyaluronidase and adrenaline for anorectal surgery: experiences with 576 operations. Proc R Soc Med 1973; 66: 680–681.
7. Clark L, Mellette JR Jr. The use of hyaluronidase as an adjunct to surgical procedures. J Dermatol Surg Oncol 1994; 20:842–844.
8. Crawford M, Kerr WJ. The effect of hyaluronidase on peribulbar block. Anaesthesia 1994; 49:907–908.
9. Arndt KA, Burton C, Noe JN. Minimizing the pain of local anesthesia. Plast Reconstr Surg 1983; 72:676–679.
10. Kaplan PA, Lieberman RP, Vonk BM. Does heating lidocaine decrease the pain of injection? AJR 1987; 149:1291.
11. Christoph RA, Buchanan L, Begalla K, Schwartz S. Pain reduction in local anesthetic administration through pH buffering. Ann Emerg Med 1988; 17: 117–120.
12. Andriani J, Zepernick R. Allergic reactions to local anesthetics. South Med J 1981; 74:694–699.
13. Norris RL Jr. Local anesthetics. Emerg Med Clin North Am 1992; 10: 707–716.
14. Laskin DM. Diagnosis and treatment of complications associated with local anesthesia. Int Dent J 1984; 34:232–237.
15. Liu SS, Hodgson PS. Local anesthetics. In: Barash P, Cullen BF, Stoelting RR, eds. Clinical Anesthesia. Philadelphia: JB Lippincott, 2001: 449–469.
16. Ramalho LD, Salvati EP, Rubin RJ. Bupivacaine, a long-acting local anesthetic, in anorectal surgery. Dis Colon Rectum 1976; 19:144–147.
17. Nivatvongs S. An improved technique of local anesthesia for anorectal surgery. Dis Colon Rectum 1982; 25:259–260.
18. Gabrielli F, Cioffi U, Chiarelli M, Guttadauro A, De Simone M. Hemorrhoidectomy with posterior perineal block. Experience with 400 cases. Dis Colon Rectum 2000; 43:809–812.

6 Pharmacology of Anorectal Preparations

Philip H. Gordon

INTRODUCTION

In viewing the spectrum of human illness, there is probably no area in which self-treatment occurs more frequently than in diseases of the anorectal region. Fear and embarrassment associated with this part of the anatomy often result in delay by the affected individual in seeking medical attention. In addition, the ready availability of over-the-counter preparations makes self-treatment easy. The troubled individual often is influenced to a great extent by the unsupported advertising claims that some manufacturers make for the efficacy of their medications. Undue reliance on these preparations, combined with the universal belief that almost all symptoms originate from hemorrhoidal disease, leads to failure to seek medical advice, and this failure may have serious consequences.

Suggested indications for the use of anorectal preparations include the relief of pain and discomfort after anorectal surgery, hemorrhoids (whether or not complicated by thromboses and prolapse), pruritus ani, proctitis, fissures, fistulas, and other congestive, allergic, or inflammatory conditions. These preparations also are suggested for use before rectal examination to anesthetize an area that is too tender or one in which there is too much spasm to admit the examining finger.

The pharmaceutical preparations available are of two types: ointment and suppository. The number of each type exceeds 100 products. In 2003 in Canada, the hemorrhoidal preparations market was worth approximately $24.1 million at the drugstore and hospital acquisition (wholesale) price level (1,2). Other associated products, such as laxatives, topical anesthetics, topical fungicides, anti-infectives and corticoid creams and ointments, amounted to an additional $8.5 million for total wholesale sales of approximately $32.6 million in 2003 for pharmaceutical preparations used for anorectal disease. The corresponding numbers in the United States reached an astounding $142.9 million and $51.7 million, for total sales of $194.6 million. At the retail level, these 2003 figures represent the awesome total of $45.6 million in Canada and $272.4 million in the United States. It should be noted that these numbers might represent an underestimation of the actual amount expended on preparations for anorectal disease because drugstore and hospital audits do not cover all of the over-the-counter market. Of some note also is that data in the United States indicate that the value of sales showed a decrease each year from 1995 to 1999, and has been relatively flat from 2001 to 2003. The retail value in 1995 was $329.8 million in the United States. Possible explanations may be due to lower prices caused by an increase in generic products or a switch to nonprescription status.

The available preparations contain combinations of traditional ingredients, including topical anesthetics and analgesics, antiseptics, mild astringents, anti-inflammatory agents, emollients, and vasoconstrictors in a host of bases and preservatives. Unfortunately, no documented evidence is available about the efficacy of these drugs alone or in combination in relieving the symptoms of anorectal disease.

CLASSIFICATION

TOPICAL ANESTHETICS AND ANALGESICS

Topical anesthetics such as benzocaine (5–20%) or topical analgesics such as diperodon or pramoxine hydrochloride (1%) are included in many ointments and suppositories. Reputedly, pramoxine hydrochloride provides surface analgesia within two to three minutes, lasts up to four hours, and is less toxic and less sensitizing than benzocaine, cocaine, procaine, and dibucaine.

Frequently, dibucaine ointment is recommended as an independent therapeutic agent. Lidocaine hydrochloride ointment has been recommended by its manufacturer for the control of pain, itching, burning, and other unpleasant symptoms caused by inoperable anorectal conditions, hemorrhoids, and fissures. Provided they are active on broken skin and mucous membranes and are present in sufficient concentrations, topical anesthetics can be useful in relieving anal pain and pruritus. Surface or topical anesthetics block the sensory nerve endings in the skin, but to reach these structures the drug must have good powers of penetration. Local anesthetics found in commercial preparations include benzocaine, tetracaine, pramoxine, diperodon, dibucaine, and lidocaine (3). These agents should not be administered intrarectally because mucosal absorption may be quite rapid and can precipitate toxic systemic effects. The risk of contact sensitization and hypersensitivity common to nearly all the drugs must be considered. Of the topical anesthetics used, tetracaine, dibucaine, and benzocaine have caused sensitization most often (3).

The main systemic toxic effect of topical agents is excitation of the central nervous system, manifested by yawning, restlessness, excitement, nausea, and vomiting, and may be followed by depression, muscular twitching, convulsions, respiratory failure, and coma (4). There is simultaneous depression of the cardiovascular system, with pallor, sweating, and hypotension. Arrhythmias may occur. Repeated application to the skin is more likely than systemic administration to give rise to allergic reactions.

In the treatment of fissures, anesthetic ointments, if applied only to the perianal region, are of no help. To have any effect they must be inserted into the anal canal. Since many patients find doing this repugnant and uncomfortable, the success of this treatment is questionable.

ANTISEPTICS

Many preparations also include an antiseptic agent such as phenol, menthol, boric acid, oxyquinoline, or benzethonium chloride. Antiseptics are used to destroy or inhibit the growth of pathogenic micro-organisms. The inclusion of such agents in these preparations in such low concentrations could have only a marginal effect on the constantly renewed bacterial population of the anus and rectum. In all probability these agents are harmless, but the risk of contact sensitization must be taken into consideration.

Boric acid possesses weak bacteriostatic and fungistatic properties. Its use has been superseded by that of more effective and less toxic disinfectants (4). It should be applied only to intact skin, because absorption of boric acid from abraded skin areas and granulating wounds or body cavities can result in systemic toxicity.

ASTRINGENTS

Mild astringents, almost universally incorporated into all anorectal preparations, include substances such as bismuth subgallate, hamamelis water (witch hazel), tannic acid, zinc oxide, calamine, or balsam of Peru. These agents precipitate proteins; when applied to mucous membranes or to damaged skin, they form a protective layer and usually are not absorbed (4). They are designed to contract tissue, harden the skin, and check exudative secretions and minor hemorrhage. In the treatment of a thrombosed hemorrhoid, how they were intended to act is unclear, and in the treatment of fissures, they frequently do not come in contact with the fissure itself.

PROTECTANTS

Protectants act to prevent irritation of the anorectal area and water loss from the skin by forming a physical barrier (5). Protection of the perianal area from irritants such as fecal matter may lead to a reduction in irritation and itching. Absorbents, adsorbents, demulcents, and emollients are included in the protectant classification. Recommended protectants include aluminum hydroxide gel, calamine, cocoa butter, cod liver oil, glycerin, kaolin, lanolin, mineral oil, petrolatum, shark liver oil, starch, wood alcohols, and zinc oxide. Petrolatum is probably the most effective protectant (5).

Emollients are fats or oils used for their local action on the skin and occasionally on the mucous membranes (6). They are used for protection and as agents for softening the skin and rendering it more pliable, but chiefly they act as vehicles for more active drugs. Cocoa butter is a solid that melts at body temperature and hence is widely used as a suppository and an ointment base. Liquid paraffin and other oils also have been included in many products. Because these substances may lubricate the anal canal during defecation, especially in the presence of painful conditions of the anus, they may have some value as soothing agents.

VASOCONSTRICTORS

Agents such as ephedrine and phenylephrine are intended to reduce bleeding from hemorrhoids, but clinical evidence to support this claim is not available. These vasoconstrictors produce capillary and arterial constrictions, but conclusive evidence that they reduce swollen hemorrhoids is lacking (5). In large doses ephedrine can cause side effects such as giddiness, headache, nausea, vomiting, sweating, thirst, tachycardia, hypertension, arrhythmia, precordial pain, palpitations, difficulty in micturition, muscular weakness and tremors, anxiety, restlessness, and insomnia. Some patients exhibit these symptoms with the usual therapeutic dose (4). Manufacturers caution against the use of vasoconstrictors in patients who are sensitive to one of the ingredients and in patients with severe cardiac disease, diabetes mellitus, glaucoma, hypertension, or hyperthyroidism. Vasoconstrictors should not be given to patients being treated with a monoamine oxidase inhibitor.

■ WOUND-HEALING AGENTS

Several ingredients in nonprescription hemorrhoidal products claim to be effective in promoting wound healing or tissue repair in anorectal disease (5,7). In particular, considerable controversy surrounds the substance skin respiratory factor (SRF), a water-soluble extract of brewer's yeast also referred to as live yeast cell derivative. Although some tests have supported the manufacturers' claims, there is no conclusive evidence that products containing SRF promote the healing of diseased anorectal tissue. The Food and Drug Administration advisory review panel on nonprescription hemorrhoidal drug products studied data on live yeast cell derivative as well as cod liver oil, balsam of Peru, shark liver oil, vitamin A, and vitamin D and found them lacking in demonstrated effectiveness as wound healers. One study suggested that SRF could be shown to increase the rate of wound healing in artificially created ulcers in humans, but that study did not address the clinical situation in which the agent is used (8).

■ CORTICOSTEROIDS

Numerous steroid preparations are currently available. These preparations sometimes are used in combination with some of the ingredients already mentioned, whereas on other occasions they are prescribed independently. There is no clinical evidence that corticosteroids relieve hemorrhoids, anal fissures, or posthemorrhoidectomy pain. These agents are available in the following forms for the treatment of anorectal disease: ointments and creams, suppositories, and enemas and foams.

Steroid Ointments and Creams

Steroid ointments and creams frequently are prescribed topically to provide symptomatic relief in the treatment of pruritus ani. However, the side effects of these agents must be recognized, and these are discussed below (9).

Atrophy and Telangiectasia

The long-term use of potent topical corticosteroids in the perianal region may produce an itchy dermatosis. However, when the patient stops applying the drug, the rash and itching recur so that the medication is reinstituted. Atrophy and telangiectasia may take months or years to develop, and their extent and degree vary. In general, the long-term use of fluorinated steroid preparations should be avoided so that this complication will not occur.

Masking or Changing Pre-existing Dermatosis

The anti-inflammatory action of steroids removes or decreases the erythema and other findings in conditions such as scabies and taenia corporis. This effect can make identification of such conditions difficult unless a high index of suspicion is maintained.

Systemic Absorption

After lengthy use of steroids over large areas of the body, systemic absorption may occur, but application of the steroids to the perianal region probably is of limited significance. Since the safety of using topical corticosteroids during pregnancy has not been confirmed, these should not be used in large amounts or for prolonged periods of time by pregnant women.

Jackson (9) classified topical steroids into three groups: weak, medium, and strong. Jackson believes that almost all side effects can be avoided completely by restricting the use of potent topical corticosteroids to small areas for short periods. In many conditions, maintenance therapy with 0.5% hydrocortisone or another weak steroid preparation is adequate. Triamcinolone is more effective than hydrocortisone (4). Jackson points out that potent steroids should not be used to treat undiagnosed conditions. The reader is referred to Jackson's (9) extensive classification for detailed drug names.

Steroid Suppositories

Corticosteroid suppositories may prove of value in treating patients who suffer from distal proctitis. This nonspecific inflammatory condition of the rectum, which involves the distal 8–10 cm of bowel, frequently responds to the administration of hydrocortisone suppositories. Factitial (postirradiation) proctitis may be another indication for the use of such suppositories, although no controlled studies have been done (10).

Steroid Enemas and Foams

Patients who suffer from distal proctitis and do not respond to hydrocortisone suppositories may be helped by steroid enemas. These proprietary enemas are aqueous suspensions of either hydrocortisone or prednisolone. They are administered as retention enemas or foams once or twice daily. They may be effective in treating both distal proctitis and left-sided nonspecific ulcerative colitis. Some systemic absorption occurs with these agents (11). Only a small part of a rectal dose of hydrocortisone acetate foam is absorbed (the mean bioavailability is 2%) (12).

Precautions and Contraindications

General precautions usually mentioned in the pharmaceutical compendia for the use of these agent mixtures include avoidance by patients with a sensitivity to any of the components. Hydrocortisone preparations must not be used in the presence of existing tuberculosis or fungal or viral lesions of the skin.

■ 5-AMINOSALICYLIC ACID PRODUCTS

5-Aminosalicylic acid has been used topically in enema or suppository form for some years for the treatment of distal proctitis or proctosigmoiditis (13). It produces good clinical response; the medication is well tolerated and safe, and few or no side effects are reported. In suppository form spread is limited to the rectum, but in enema form, when administered as recommended clinically, routinely flows retrograde as far as the splenic flexure (13,14).

■ NITROGLYCERIN

Nitric oxide has emerged as one of the most important neurotransmitters mediating internal anal sphincter relaxation. The effect of glyceryl trinitrate, a nitric oxide donor, on anal tone was examined by Loder et al. (15). They found a 27% decrease in sphincter pressure 20 minutes after application of a 0.2% glyceryl trinitrate ointment. Gorfine (16) found that following the topical application of 0.5% nitroglycerin ointment, patients with thrombosed external hemorrhoids and anal fissures reported dramatic relief of anal pain. Side effects were limited to transient headache in seven of 20 patients. Nitroglycerin has also been found to significantly reduce upper anal sphincter pressure in patients with terminal constipation (17).

MISCELLANEOUS

A host of bases and preservatives generally are included in the preparations, and little is known about their effects. Adeps solidus is a range of suppository bases consisting of mixtures of monoglycerides, diglycerides, and triglycerides of saturated fatty acids. Theobroma oil, beeswax, and cetyl alcohol also are used.

DOSAGE FORMS

OINTMENTS

Although from a pharmaceutical point of view there are considerable differences among ointments, creams, pastes, and gels, the therapeutic differences are not significant enough to classify them separately (5). Ointments serve as vehicles for drug use and possess inherent protectant and emollient properties.

SUPPOSITORIES

Suppositories may ease straining at stool by providing a lubricating effect. They are relatively slow acting because they must melt to release the active ingredient.

Occasionally, administration of suppositories results in serious local lesions. Hemet et al. (18) reported a case of ulceration and anorectal stenosis that followed administration of suppositories containing dextropropoxyphene and paracetamol. That complication led to an abdominoperineal resection, and they reported 14 similar cases in the literature.

FOAMS

Hydrocortisone acetate administered as a foam enema is effective in the treatment of distal ulcerative colitis and proctitis. It has been suggested that patients prefer a foam enema to a liquid enema because it causes less interference with social, sexual, and occupational activities. It has been claimed that systemic absorption of foam is extremely low, but Cann and Holdsworth (19) have shown that there is systemic absorption when the hydrocortisone foam is administered intrarectally and the potential for adrenal suppression exists, especially if the foam is used as a long-term treatment.

ENEMAS

Steroid enemas have become an established form of therapy for patients with distal ulcerative colitis and distal proctitis. Different steroid preparations have been advocated, but the important point is that systemic absorption does occur to some degree. There are theoretical advantages in using a poorly absorbed enema to avoid the possibility of systemic steroid effects in patients requiring long-term steroid treatment (20). 5-Aminosalicylic acid is also available in enema form and has been used in the treatment of distal proctosigmoiditis.

PRODUCT SELECTION GUIDELINES

PATIENT CONSIDERATIONS

The patient's general condition and associated diseases may enter the decision-making process. For example, caution should be exercised in prescribing products with vasoconstrictors to patients suffering from cardiovascular disease, diabetes mellitus, hypertension, and hyperthyroidism or patients experiencing difficulty in urination or taking monoamine oxidase inhibitors (5). Patients taking phenothiazines should avoid taking products containing ephedrine. The presence of specific allergies should be determined.

PRODUCT CONSIDERATIONS

Unfortunately, a search of the literature reveals a paucity of definitive information about the efficacy of any of the proprietary medications, either over-the-counter or prescription-only products. An exception to this statement is the use of topical steroids for treating pruritus ani, which does provide symptomatic relief. For physicians uncomfortable in allowing a patient to leave their office without a prescription in hand, prescribing a product with the smallest number of ingredients probably would minimize undesirable effects.

DISCUSSION

Suppositories seldom are helpful in treating the pain of thrombosed hemorrhoids or anal fissure (21). Some commercially available suppositories contain opiates, but the mechanism of their analgesic effect is central and not local. Antibiotic suppositories used to treat inflammatory conditions in the anal canal would appear to be inappropriate because of their ineffectiveness and the potential dangers of inducing local sensitivity.

When suppositories are inserted, they are placed well above the fissure because they must rest above the puborectalis muscle; therefore, they are not in direct contact with the fissure. In addition, many patients complain that insertion is painful. The natural history of a fissure-in-ano is one of healing, and associated treatments such as warm baths to relieve sphincter spasm and stool softeners to avoid straining break the cycle of a hard stool, pain, and reflex spasm.

With the universal prevalence of the anal fissure, it is surprising, if not disconcerting, that prospective trials have not been conducted to evaluate the propriety of using the numerous commercially available prescription and over-the-counter preparations. Supposed reasons for this lack of scientific endeavor are a combination of factors, including the clinician's firm belief in knowing best how to treat the malady and the patient's disappointment if the physician does not prescribe a medication to alleviate the problem. A notable exception was the report by Jensen (22), who conducted a prospective randomized trial to compare the use of lignocaine ointment, hydrocortisone ointment, or warm sitz baths combined with an intake of unprocessed bran. After one or two weeks of treatment, symptomatic relief was significantly better among patients treated with sitz baths and bran than among patients undergoing other types of treatment. After three weeks, there was no difference in symptomatic relief among the three groups, but patients treated with lignocaine had significantly fewer healed fissures (60%) than patients treated with hydrocortisone (82.4%) or warm sitz baths and bran (87%). This study demonstrated that patients treated with medication did not fare as well as those treated with a bulk-forming agent and sitz baths. The latter treatment is inexpensive, produces no side effects, and results in the best and quickest relief of symptoms.

The continued use of the numerous available agents and the credit given to them for their effectiveness are almost certainly functions of the self-limiting nature of the diseases they are treating. The natural history of a thrombosed hemorrhoid is one of resolution, with decreasing pain after two or three days. Patients frequently relate that the suppository or ointment did not work for the first two or three days. By the same token, patients may use a given preparation for two or three days and then switch to a second preparation, which they then praise; again, this healing is almost certainly a function of the natural history of the disease. Had they used the preparations in reverse order, the praise and disdain for the two preparations almost certainly would have been reversed.

REFERENCES

1. IMS Health Canada. Drug store and hospital purchase. Connection Disease and Therapeutic Index, 2003.
2. National Sales perspective. National Disease and Therapeutic Index (NDTI), Diagnosis Value, 2003 (Sales dollars factored by diagnosis).
3. Andrusiak OI. Hemorrhoids. Clarke C, ed. Self medication. A reference for health professionals. Ottawa: Canadian Pharmaceutical Association, 1988:347–354.
4. Reynolds JEF, ed. Martindale: the extra pharmacopoeia. 30th ed. London: Pharmaceutical Press, 1993.
5. Hodes B. Hemorrhoidal products. In: Handbook of non-prescription drugs. 8th ed. Washington, D.C.: American Pharmaceutical Association, 1986: 689–702.
6. Gilman AG, Goodman LS, Rail TW, Murad F, eds. Goodman and Gilman's the pharmacological basis of therapeutics. 7th ed. New York: MacMillan Publishing, 1985.
7. Goodson W, Hohn D, Hunt T, Leung DYK. Augmentation of some aspects of wound healing by a "skin respiratory factor." J Surg Res 1976; 21: 125–129.
8. Subra Manyam K, Patterson M, Gourley WK. Effects of Preparation H on wound healing in the rectum of men. Dig Dis Sci 1984; 29:829–832.
9. Jackson R. Side effects of potent topical corticosteroids. Can Med Assoc J 1978; 118:173–174.
10. Sherman LF, Prem KA, Mensheha M. Factitial proctitis: a re-study at the University of Minnesota. Dis Colon Rectum 1971; 14:281–285.
11. Rodrigues C, Lennard-Jones JE, English J, Parsons DG. Systemic absorption from prednisolone rectal foam in ulcerative colitis [letter]. Lancet 1987; 1:1497.
12. Mollmann H, Barth J, Mollmann C, Tunn S, Kreig M, Derendorf H. Pharmacokinetics and rectal bioavailability of hydrocortisone acetate. J Pharm Sci 1991; 80:835–836.
13. Williams CN, Haber G, Aquino JA. Double-blind, placebo controlled evaluation of 5-ASA suppositories in active distal proctitis and measurement of extent of spread using ^{99m}Tc-labeled 5-ASA suppositories. Dig Dis Sci 1987; 32(suppl):715–755.
14. Chapman NJ, Brown ML, Phillips SF, et al. Distribution of mesalamine enemas in patients with active distal ulcerative colitis. Mayo Clin Proc 1992; 67: 245–248.
15. Loder PB, Kamm MA, Nicholls RJ, Phillips RKS. "Reversible chemical sphincterotomy" by local application of glyceryl trinitrate. Br J Surg 1994; 81:1386–1389.
16. Gorfine SR. Treatment of benign anal disease with topical nitroglycerin. Dis Colon Rectum 1995; 38:453–457.
17. Guillemot F, Leroi H, Lone YC, Rousseau CG, Lamblin MD, Cortot A. Action of in situ nitroglycerin on upper anal canal pressure of patients with terminal constipation. Dis Colon Rectum 1993; 36:372–376.
18. Hemet J, Leroy A, Duprey F, Rocher W, Metayer J, Ducastelle T. Stenose anorectale par suppositoires de dextropropoxythene etparacetamol (Diantalvic). Gastroenterol Clin Biol 1986; 10:517–520.
19. Cann DA, Holdsworth CD. Systemic absorption from hydrocortisone foam enema in ulcerative colitis. Lancet 1987; 1:922–923.
20. McIntyre PB, Macrae FA, Berghouse L, English J, Lennard-Jones JE. Therapeutic benefits from a poorly absorbed prednisolone enema in distal colitis. Gut 1985; 26:822–824.
21. Gordon PH. Anal fissure—diagnosis and treatment. Consultant, Feb 1978, p 73.
22. Jensen SL. Treatment of first episodes of acute anal fissure: prospective randomized study of lignocaine ointment versus hydrocortisone ointment or warm baths plus bran. Br Med J 1986; 292:1167–1169.

7 Electrosurgery and Laser Surgery: Basic Applications

Santhat Nivatvongs and Lee E. Smith

ELECTROSURGERY

The application of diathermy and electrosurgery is based on the fact that with a radiofrequency current >10,000 cycles per second, stimulation of muscle and nerve does not occur (1). When two large (>100 cm^2) electrodes of nearly equal size are used, the current is dispersed evenly within the intervening tissue, and only warm heat is produced (diathermy) (Fig. 1A). On the other hand, when one electrode is large and the other is small, the current is concentrated in the smaller electrode and produces a high concentration of heat, causing destruction of cells (electrosurgery) (Fig. 1B) (1).

DEFINITION

In clinical use electrosurgery consists of electrocutting, electrocoagulation, and fulguration. Electrocutting is the severing of tissue by a blade electrode energized by a high-frequency electrosurgical unit. Electrocoagulation is the heating, desiccation, and destruction of tissue at the point of contact, using a needle-tip, ball-tip, or blade electrode (Fig. 2A) (4). Fulguration is a method of coagulation in which the active electrode is held some distance (e.g., 1–10 mm) away from the tissue and the energy is dissipated in the area by sparking (Fig. 2B). Thus fulguration requires the application of a relatively high voltage to ionize the gas between the electrode and the tissue. Fulguration gives greater depth of penetration and produces more dehydration of the tissue than does electrocoagulation.

The mode of operation [cutting or coagulation or a combined effect (blended)] depends on the waveform of the current. Coagulation current is a high-frequency damped sine wave (Fig. 3). When applied to tissue, the current produces oscillation of the molecules, with heat generation resulting in tissue coagulation and dehydration. This action seals blood vessels (5). Cutting current is a high-frequency sine wave similar to that of coagulation current, but it is undamped. The action of this cutting current on tissue produces a very focused heat build-up, resulting in tissue rupture. There is no coagulating hemostatic action with pure cutting current. A "blend" of cutting and coagulating currents allows execution of the cutting current and obtains the additional benefit of hemostasis (5).

MONOPOLAR AND BIPOLAR ELECTRODES

The terms "monopolar," "bipolar," "monoterminal," and "biterminal" are confusing and are frequently misused in medical literature. These terms are used to describe various forms of high-frequency electrosurgery. However,

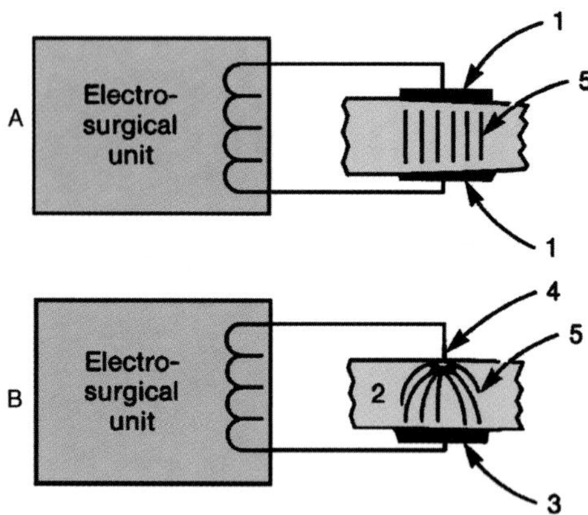

FIGURE 1 ■ Principles of operation of diathermy (**A**) and electrosurgery (**B**). 1, Large electrode; 2, patient; 3, patient plate; 4, active electrode; 5, current flow pattern. *Source*: From Ref. 2.

high-frequency electrosurgery uses alternating current, which does not have positive and negative poles. Only some forms of non–high-frequency electrosurgery, including electrolysis and galvanism, are truly polar. In polar modalities direct current is used, and the negative pole becomes the treatment electrode. The negative electrode releases electrons, which produce hydrogen gas from water, leaving hydroxides for chemical destruction.

The electrical energy of high-frequency electrosurgery alternately enters and exits the tissue through the treatment electrode, which is not polar and should be considered an electrical terminal. Therefore the terms "monoterminal" and "biterminal" are technically more correct than "monopolar" and "bipolar" when reference is being made to high-frequency electrosurgical procedures. However, the "-polar" suffix is much more commonly used in medical terminology than the "-terminal" suffix and is here to stay (6).

Monopolar vs. Bipolar Electrocautery

Electrocautery relies on the principle that high-frequency current can be passed through the body with no effects other than the production of heat. With a monopolar electrocautery probe, one electrode or the ground plate is large (i.e., 100 cm^2) and the other is small (< 1 cm^2). This small or "active" electrode is used to control the current density. It should be pointed out that the term "ground plate" is a misnomer that has been mistermed in the operating room beyond correction. The "ground plate" is actually a dispersive electrode of large surface area that safely returns the generated energy to the electrocautery unit. Because the return plate is large, the current density is low; therefore, no harmful heat is generated and no tissue destruction occurs. The only heat created is at the site of the active electrode that is held by the surgeon (7). In contrast, bipolar electrocautery uses current flow only between two sides of the forceps, with a localization of the tissue effect (Fig. 4).

The main advantages of monopolar over bipolar electrocautery are ease of use and greater effectiveness in cutting tissues and coagulating bleeding points and blood vessels. However, monopolar electrocautery can cause deeper damage. Most of the electrocautery units used in the operating room are monopolar.

The significant advantage of bipolar electrocautery is the reduction in tissue damage. The electrons heat only the tissue interposed within the forceps. This process is self-limiting because, as soon as the cells are charred and completely dehydrated, the current ceases to pass, thus avoiding damage to the surrounding tissues. A monopolar electrode produces an area of coagulation twice that produced by a bipolar electrode, and more than four times that of a carbon dioxide laser (7).

Most of the advantages of bipolar over monopolar electrocautery are the result of the elimination of the ground plate. Bipolar electrocautery operates at lower currents, thereby reducing nerve and muscle stimulation. There is no possibility of sparking. There is also a reduction in the production of smoke, a factor that may be important in accidental intestinal gas explosion.

The main criticism of bipolar electrocautery is that it is more difficult to use. This is the primary reason for using monopolar electrocautery rather than bipolar techniques. Another reason is that the low energy output of a bipolar system may be insufficient to coagulate larger blood vessels. A further drawback to bipolar electrocautery is the adherence of coagulated tissue to the bipolar forceps, which requires repeated cleaning (8).

■ BASIC PRINCIPLES

Tissue, like all other physical substances, offers resistance to the flow of electrical current. As the electrons constituting the current attempt to move through the tissue, they are

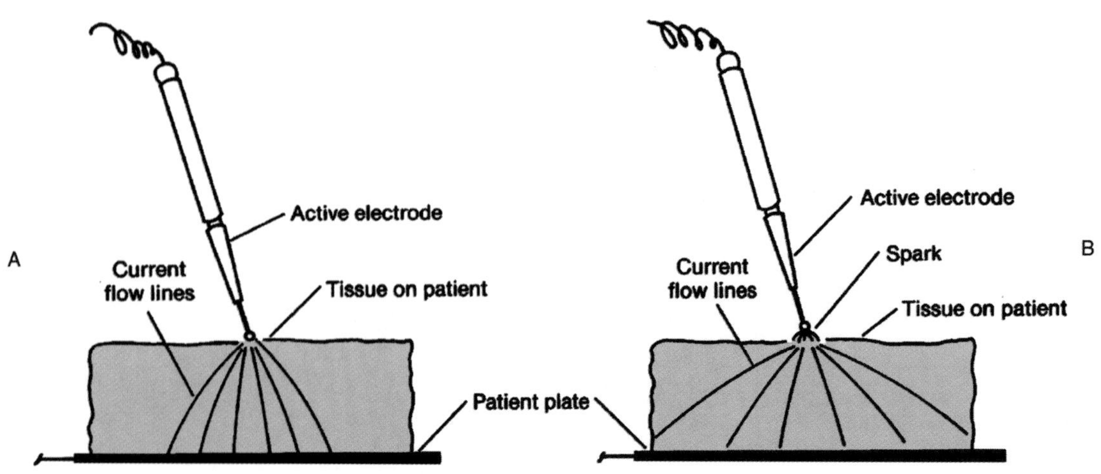

FIGURE 2 ■ (**A**) Electrocoagulation. (**B**) Fulguration. *Source*: From Ref. 3.

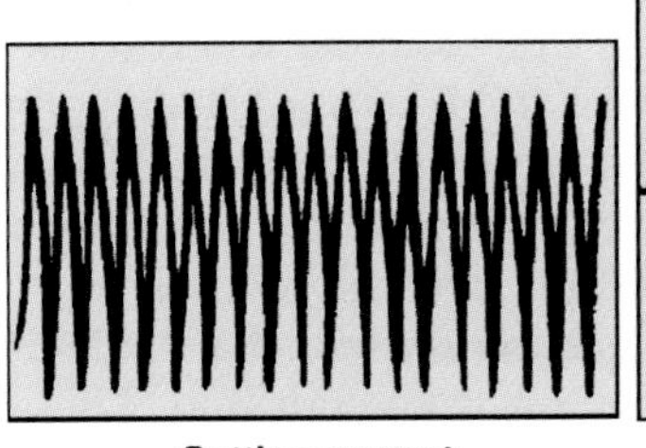
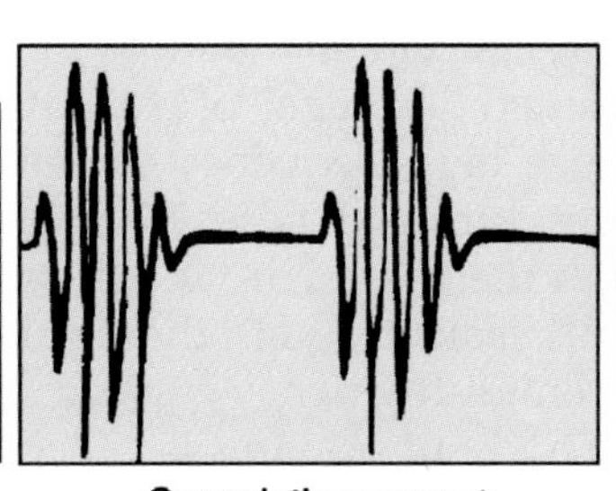
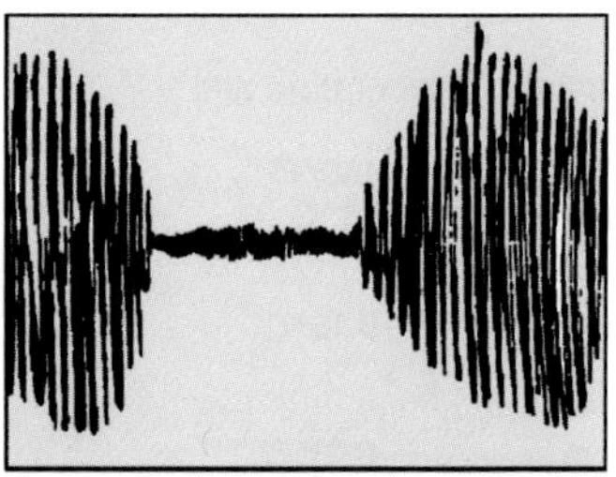

FIGURE 3 ■ Different waveforms of current.

constantly colliding with its molecules. Through these collisions, energy is dissipated in the tissue, causing its temperature to rise. This effect is described by the following equation (9):

$$P = I^2R$$

where

P = the electrical power dissipated in the tissue (watts)
I = the current within the tissue (amperes)
R = the resistance of the tissue to the current (ohms)

Tissue resistance depends, to a large extent, on its vascularity and water content. Bone and fat have higher resistance to the passage of current than skin and muscle. In addition, as tissue dries or is desiccated electrosurgically, its resistance increases greatly, and the current through it falls off. The equation also indicates that the heat produced in tissue is proportional to the square of the current passing through it. Therefore if the current is doubled, the rate of heating increases four times. If it is tripled, heating increases by a factor of nine, and so forth (9). Wet tissue increases the area of contact and reduces the current density or heat production; hence a higher current is required to cut through it. Tissue infiltrated with a local anesthetic agent also requires a higher power setting because the tissue becomes less conductive to electrical current.

Total heat production is also related to the power delivered and the duration of its application. A power of 50 W for one second gives the same total heating as a power of 5 W for 10 seconds, but the distribution of the heat is different. At lower power and longer duration, the temperature is lower near the active electrode, but more heat is generated deeper in the tissue (4). The current density or the total heat generated by electrosurgery is directly related to the surface area of the tissue in contact with the active electrode (4). For example, assuming that a given current passing through a 1 mm^2 cross section results in a temperature rise of 100°C, the same current passing through 2.5 mm^2 gives a rise of 25°C. If the area is increased to 1 cm^2, the temperature rise is only 0.01°C (Fig. 5).

The two electrodes normally used are a large-area patient plate and a small-area active electrode. Use of the patient plate, in good contact with a large area of the skin, ensures a low current density and makes the temperature rise at that electrode negligible.

■ SNARE POLYPECTOMY

Current density or heat production is dependent on the size of the electrode or wire. A very thin snare wire produces more heat and cutting action than thick snare wire does, and it may cut the tissue too quickly if higher current is applied. On the other hand, if a thick snare wire is used, the low current density prolongs the time required to heat the tissue contacting the wire to the point of vaporization, and the tissue will have time to desiccate completely. However, excessive heating of the wall is also possible because there is time to conduct the heat generated in the polyp down the polyp, causing excessive burning of the tissue. Also, the stalk may be desiccated so completely that the tissue does not contain enough water for vaporization (cutting) to take place. As the stalk is dried, its resistance

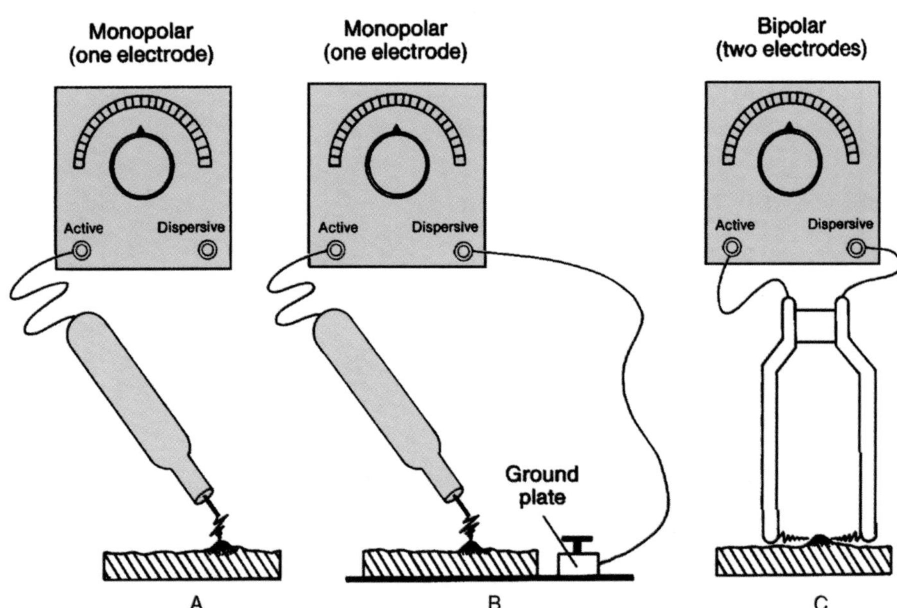

FIGURE 4 ■ Monopolar electrodes can be used without a ground plate (**A**) or with a ground plate (**B**), depending on the type of electrosurgical equipment. Tissue destruction can be deep. Bipolar electrodes require no ground plate. Tissue destruction is confined to the surface (**C**).
Source: From Ref. 4.

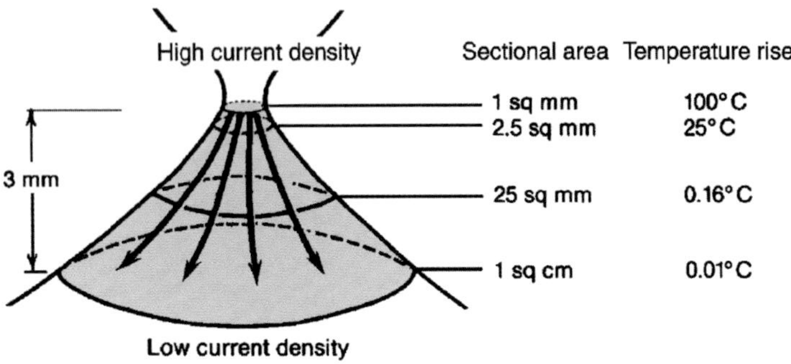

FIGURE 5 ■ Current density and volume of tissue. *Source*: From Ref. 2.

increases, and the amount of current it will conduct drops severely. Because dried tissue is very resistant to current flow, the voltage available is not great enough to drive sufficient current through the polyp to vaporize what little water is left. The desiccated tissue may entrap the snare wire.

The diameters of commercial snare wires are of appropriate size to avoid these two extremes. Therefore, power settings and generator waveforms play important roles in the cutting action of a snare. Generally, only coagulation current is used for snaring polyps. If a typical snare with a very high-powered output is used, it is possible to cut off the polyp with very little hemostatic effect, thus leading to the complication of bleeding. Using the same snare with a very low power setting produces slow heating without causing instantaneous heating to the point of vaporization at the intended incision site and may lead to difficulty in excising the polyp. Snaring larger tissue requires a higher output setting because the tissue's larger cross-sectional area causes a reduction in the current density at the site of the snare wire (9).

■ HAZARDS

Excessive Application of Heat

The dial calibration on each electrosurgery unit is arbitrary and varies widely (Fig. 6). When unfamiliar equipment is used, a lower setting always should be used at the start and should be increased gradually. Short bursts of power are also desirable to minimize the depth of the heat.

Current Leakage and Burn

Unwanted "leakage" of current is unavoidable when working with high-frequency currents. Thus, current leakage is present during all types of electrosurgical procedures. Even though the snare wire is insulated, high-frequency current actually leaks through the insulation. This phenomenon by which high-frequency currents apparently leak across insulators and out of wires is called capacitive coupling. These currents can and have caused burns to both the endoscopist and the patient (9). Burns and shocks to the physician's eyes or hands are possible if the current density at the point of tissue-to-metal contact is great enough. Theoretically, high-frequency currents cannot produce shock; however, a small pinpoint burn often feels like a shock and is described as such. For this reason it is advisable that the metal ocular endoscope be covered with an insulating eyepiece and that surgical gloves be checked for pinpoint holes and small tears. To reduce the risk of shock, the manufacturers provide a safety cord between the endoscope and the patient terminal of the generator. This cord provides a direct low-resistance path for current leakage back to the generator. Therefore all current leakage travels this route rather than the highly resistant routes through the physician and patient (Fig. 7). In any even the patient plate must always be rechecked whenever the patient is repositioned to ensure that it is still in firm contact with the patient and to make certain that cables and connections are intact.

Electrosurgical injuries can occur, particularly during laparoscopic operations, and are potentially serious. The main causes of electrosurgical injuries are inadvertent touching or grasping of tissue during current application, direct coupling (unintended contact) between a portion of intestine and a metal probe that is touching the activated probe, insulation breaks in the electrodes, direct sparking to the intestine from the electrocautery probe, and current passage to the intestine from recently coagulated, electrically isolated tissue. The majority of injuries are caused by monopolar electrocautery (8).

Bowel Gas Explosion

The current widespread use of nonflammable, nonexplosive anesthetic gases allows the safe use of electrosurgery. A more important hazard is explosion caused by bowel gas.

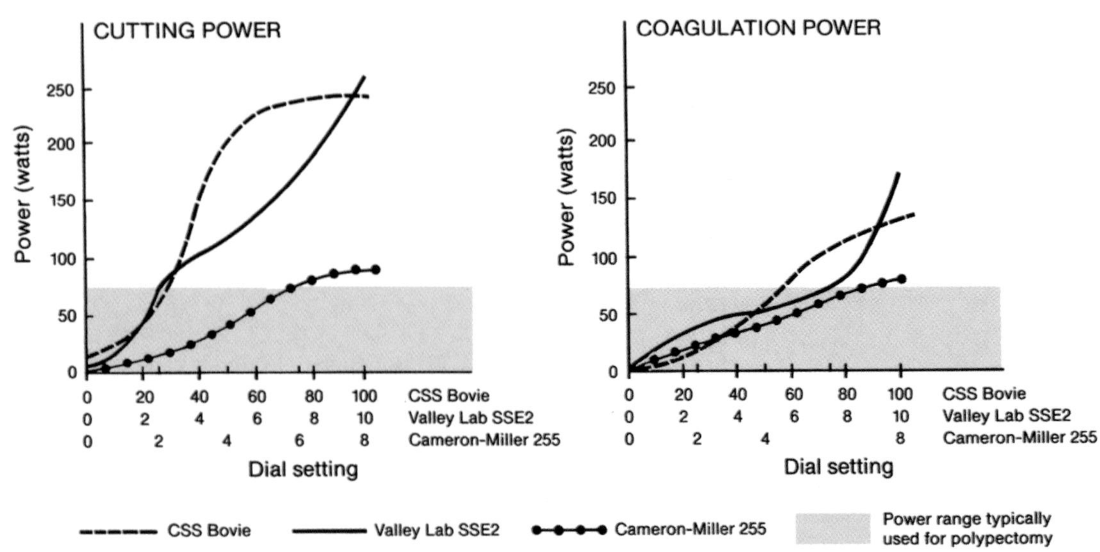

FIGURE 6 ■ Relationship between power and dial setting in different electrosurgical units. *Source*: From Ref. 2.

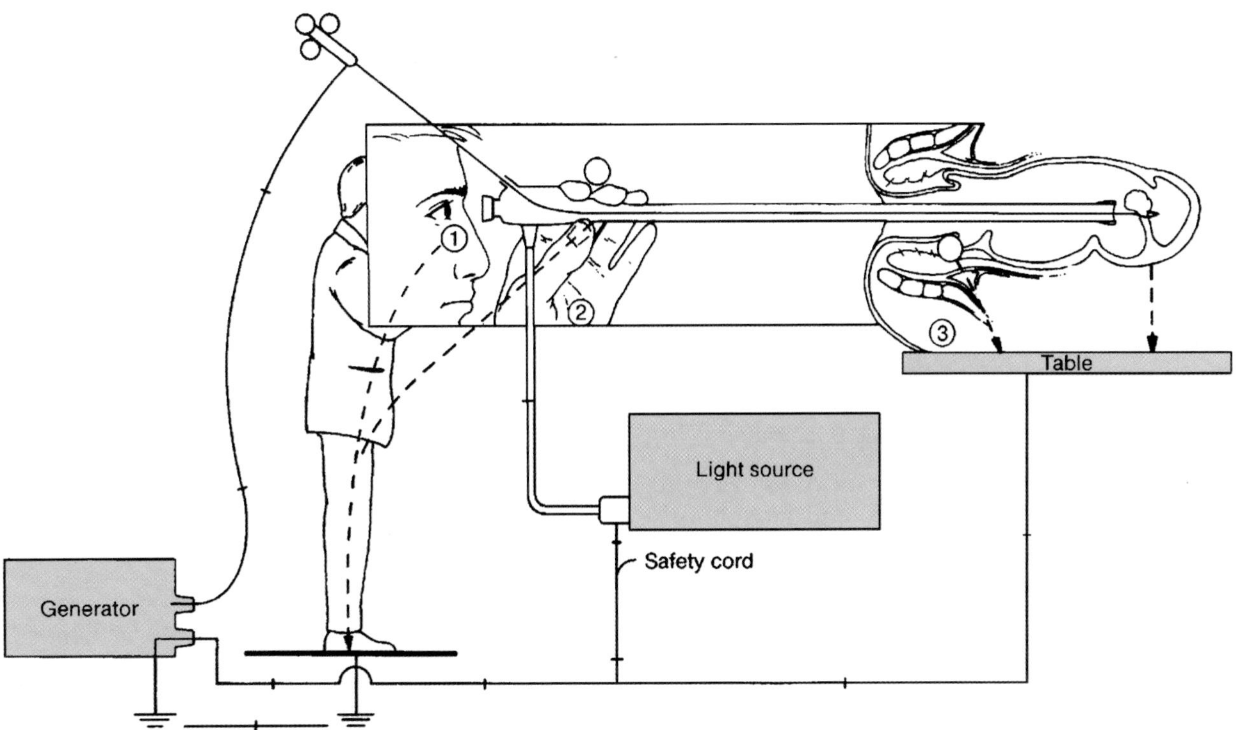

FIGURE 7 ■ Current leaking onto the colonoscope from the snare can flow through the colonoscopist, causing burns to the eye (1) or hand (2). A burn to the patient (3) can result if tissue contacts exposed metal on the scope. Use of a safety cord provides a direct pathway by which current can leak back to the generator, thus avoiding the undesired pathways indicated by the broken lines. *Source*: From Ref. 7.

The bowel's explosive gases are methane and hydrogen, which are liberated by bacteria in the colon (10). When the large bowel is well prepared, such as in preparation for colonoscopy, this hazard is negligible (10,11). However, if it is prepared poorly, serious explosions can occur with other procedures such as electrocoagulation or snaring of rectal polyps through the sigmoidoscope (12). This problem can be eliminated by adequate aspiration of gases from the rectum before each application of the electrical current.

Surgical Smoke

The plume of smoke produced by electrocautery has an unpleasant odor and can induce acute and chronic inflammatory changes in the respiratory tract (13). Airborne particles are not effectively evacuated by operating room filters. Scavenging system and face masks offer protection only from large particles.

In a study by Sagar et al. (14), the chemical composition of electrocautery smoke consisted of five gases (Table 1). Benzene, a known carcinogen, is identified in significant quantities. The recommended amount of exposure to benzene is zero. Other gases are known to cause irritation to the eyes, dermatitis, central nervous system effects, hepatotoxicity, and renal toxicity (14). However, their health risk to operating room personnel is not known at the present time.

Numerous chemicals have been found in the plume generated by laser tissue ablation, including benzene, formaldehyde, acrolein, CO, and hydrogen cyanide. Cellular clumps and erythrocytes have also been found, suggesting the plume's infectious potential. Viable bacteriophage has also been demonstrated to be present in laser plume. Whole intact virions have also been found and their infectivity demonstrated (15).

Ultrasonic (harmonic) scalpel produces a low-temperature vapor, not smoke. One study indicated that the particles created by the ultrasonic scalpel are composed of tissue, blood, and blood by-products but another study noted that very few were morphologically intact and no viable cells were found. This aerosol has not been well studied and no consensus exists regarding its composition (15).

Surgical smoke is a biohazard and cannot be ignored. At a minimum, surgical smoke is a toxin similar to cigarette smoke. Although not a high priority in most surgical cases, surgeons should support efforts to minimize operating room personnel, patients, and their own exposure to surgical smoke (15).

TABLE 1 ■ Chemical Composition of Electrocautery Smoke

	Maximum Level (bg/m^3)
Benzene	71
Ethyl benzene	36
Styrene	21
Carbon disulfide	1.5
Toluene	460

Source: From Ref. 14.

Safety Precautions with Implantable Cardioverter Defibrillator (ICD)

Two potential hazards exist in patients with implantable cardioverter defibrillators (ICDs) or pacemakers when electrocautery is used. One is asystole caused by electrical interference of the sensing circuit in the synchronous type pacemaker. The other hazard is ventricular fibrillation caused by an additional source of electrical energy passing through the body. The first hazard is preventable by converting the pacemaker to a fixed rate since fixed-rate pacemakers are not affected by electrocautery or inactivate the pacemaker. The second hazard is diminished by placing the electrocautery circuit caudad to the level of the pacemaker, such as at the buttock and thigh, and also by using the cautery in very short repetitive bursts (16). Earlier cardiac pacemakers were susceptible to deactivation by external radiofrequency waves, especially electrocautery. Recently, however, implanted pacemakers have been protected by shielding and filtering the layers to reduce the effects of external interference. Nevertheless, electrosurgery can cause significant malfunction of demand pacemaker impulse generation, especially when a cutting current is used (17).

The following are some useful safety guides when electrocautery is used in patients with cardiac pacemakers (18):

1. Inactivate the ICD prior to beginning of the procedure, monitor the patient's cardiac rhythm, and have appropriate resuscitation equipment available.
2. Position the grounding pad on the buttock or thigh, distant from a pacer or ICD generator and their leads.
3. Use electrocautery in short, repetitive bursts rather than longer continuous discharges to minimize periods of pacemaker inhibition.
4. When electrocautery is required in the immediate vicinity of ICD or pacemaker hardware such as a lesion near the splenic flexure of the colon, consider the use of bipolar electrocautery if it is available and applicable.

LASER SURGERY

Lasers are powerful instruments that are standard medical tools. New laser diagnostic and therapeutic modalities will evolve, and the range of uses will expand as military, industrial, and academic scientists explore the properties of various wavelengths. Currently available lasers may not provide the best forms of diagnosis or therapy; in time, new and better lasers will become part of the medical armamentarium.

Lasers have been adapted for medical use, and physicians and surgeons need to learn the principles of laser physics and their current applications; thereafter the laser surgeons must stay abreast of information about the new lasers and the new applications that will influence colon and rectal surgery.

HISTORY

Laser (Light Amplification by the Stimulated Emission of Radiation) was born through the evolution of knowledge about the atom. In the 19th century a young Danish physicist, Niels Bohr, theorized that electrons orbited a positively charged nucleus. When energy is added to a stable atom, the electrons move into an orbital more distant from the nucleus, storing this energy. This energized state is unstable; thus the electrons return to a stable, resting orbital and give up the stored energy, releasing an energy particle (a photon). In 1917 Albert Einstein (19) theorized that activated electron orbitals, exposed to continuing energy input, discharge their stored energy as coherent waves of light and that this cascade of energy release could be harnessed to perform useful work. Forty years later, Gordon et al. (20) carried Einstein's concept of stimulated emission to a working level with their maser (Microwave Amplification by the Stimulated Emission of Radiation). In rapid succession, Maiman (21) in 1960, Johnson (22) in 1961, Bennett et al. (23) in 1962, and Patel et al. (24) in 1964 developed the ruby, neodymium:yttrium-aluminum-garnet (Nd:YAG), argon, and carbon dioxide (CO_2) lasers, respectively. These lasers have been technologically improved and applied within the medical realm.

The electromagnetic spectrum contains all wavelengths of radiant energy. Current medical laser technology includes the visible spectrum of 400 to 700 nm to the infrared spectrum of the CO_2 laser at approximately 10,000 nm. Today medical lasers are designed to produce only one wavelength; technology has not advanced far enough to permit development of an economical multiwavelength machine.

BASIC PROPERTIES OF LASERS

Spontaneous vs. Stimulated Emissions

In contrast to a laser, an ordinary light bulb is an example of a spontaneous emission. Electrical current passes along a filament, raising stable electrons to an energized state. These energized electrons spontaneously emit their photons of energy, producing light and resuming their stable orbitals. Emitted photons collide, causing cancellation or augmentation of the light. The end result is a white light containing all wavelengths of the visible spectrum and whose energy dissipates as the distance from its source increases.

Laser light is generated in a far more complex way. Atoms or molecules of the lasing medium are stored within a containment cylinder, the resonator. At each end of the container are mirrors, one totally reflective and the other partially reflective (i.e., a small hole allows escape of a light beam). Energy, in the form of a flash lamp, electrical charge, or another laser, is pumped into this system. The input energy moves the electrons to a higher orbital, which is called a population inversion when a majority of atoms is energized. Great amounts of energy must be input to achieve a population inversion. The system is extremely inefficient, so much undesired heat is produced as a byproduct. Photons of light characteristic of the lasing medium are emitted. These random emissions collide and further stimulate emissions from adjacent atoms in the energized state. Ultimately, much of this light resonates between the mirrors. This light can be characterized by the following: (1) monochromatism, (4) collimation, and (5) coherence. It is monochromatic in that all the light emitted is of the same wavelength. Collimation refers to the parallel course of all the emissions. Coherence means that all the waves are in phase both temporally and spatially, accounting for the increased power of the system.

The laser light is controlled by a partially reflective mirror that allows a small beam to escape. A series of mirrors on an articulated arm or a conductive fiber delivers light to the target. The articulated mirrors allow air transmission of the laser light. A lens is placed between the target and the mirror so that the collimated beam can be finely focused or defocused to intensify or reduce the effect.

Power Density and Power Energy

The power of the instrument is expressed in watts (W) of energy. The wattage of the laser beam multiplied by the

TABLE 2 ■ Effects of Laser Energy on Tissues

Temperature (°C)	Effect
27–37	Nonthermal biologic effects
37–55	Tissue warming and dehydration
55–60	Tissue welding
60–100	Tissue blanching, denaturing of proteins
100 and above	Boiling and vaporizing of tissue water

number of seconds the beam is activated expresses the unit's power, which is called joules (J). Some lasers provide a digital readout or permanent printout in joules. Power density (PD) is a crucial concept that relates the power of the beam in watts to the area on which the energy is focused:

$$PD = W/cm^2$$

Note that the power density varies directly with the square of the denominator. Therefore if a 1 W beam focused on a 1 cm area has a power density of 1, this same wattage focused to 1 mm size (i.e., 10 times less) produces a power density 100 times greater. Changing power density, either the watts or the area of the spot, changes the physical effect of the energy beam on the target tissue.

Power energy (PE) takes into account the power density and the tissue exposure time in seconds. The longer the laser is directed at a target, the more tissue is damaged.

$$PE = W \times Time/cm^2 = J/cm^2$$

Effects on Biologic Systems

In medicine, laser energy is principally used for its thermal effects. Yet its nonthermal qualities may have a permanent place in medicine. For example, a low laser power may serve as a catalyst for the stimulation of biologic processes, which is called photoactivation. The thermal effects are well described. When laser energy affects a biologic system, the interaction depends on the physical properties of both the wavelength and the target. Various tissues differentially absorb laser light. This interaction is referred to as the coefficient of absorption of the tissue for that specific wavelength of laser. For instance, water or tissue high in water content absorbs the CO_2 laser wavelength, but not the Nd:YAG wavelength, so Nd:YAG is transmitted through water. Chromophores such as hemoglobin or melanin, concentrated in tissues, strongly affect the coefficient of absorption. Additional factors affecting tissue absorption of laser energy include the power energy and the proximity of the large vascular structures, which serve to dissipate the heat by carrying it away from the target area. The stages of tissue heating can be used by knowing the coefficient of absorption of the tissue, the wavelength of the laser, the vascularity of the field, and the power necessary to accomplish the desired result (i.e., cut, coagulate, or weld). Table 2 shows the stages of tissue heating and their biologic effects.

■ COMPARISON OF SURGICAL LASERS

A multitude of commercially available medical lasers include the CO_2, argon, Nd:YAG, copper, krypton, ruby, and alexandrite lasers. The thermal effects are used primarily in surgical applications. For colon and rectal surgery, the CO_2, Nd:YAG, and argon lasers are most often used. This discussion centers on these three lasers. Table 3 compares the three lasers' properties (25,26).

The following discussion centers on the CO_2 and Nd:YAG lasers. Both the CO_2 and Nd:YAG lasers are in the infrared portion of the electromagnetic spectrum. However, their wavelengths are far apart (10,600 nm for the CO_2 laser and 1064 nm for the Nd:YAG laser), and it is the wavelength that determines the specific characteristics. Since they are infrared, neither is visible. Therefore a coaxial aiming beam is part of the delivery system; the helium–neon (HeNe) laser emits a wavelength of 632 nm, which is in the visible spectrum and is seen as red (26). The HeNe beam can be directed through a mirror system or fiber system to coincide closely with a point of high intensity, and the lightspot size provides visual cues about the power density. The CO_2 laser has CO_2 gas as the lasing medium in the resonator cylinder. Nitrogen and helium are added in small quantities to enhance the excitation process (23). The nitrogen is first excited by a powerful electrical discharge, and its energy is transferred to the CO_2 gas, causing a population inversion. After emission, the CO_2 returns to ground state with the aid of collision with the interspersed helium molecules.

TABLE 3 ■ Comparison of CO_2, Nd:YAG, and Argon Lasers

	CO_2	Nd:YAG	Argon
Resonance chamber	CO_2, neon, and nitrogen gases	Solid yttrium–aluminum–garnet crystal doped with 1–3% neodymium gas	Argon gas
Excitation source	Electrical charge	Optical flash lamp	High voltage
Delivery system	Mirror through articulated arm	Fiber	Fiber
Cooling system	Air	Water	Water
Aiming beam	HeNe laser	HeNe laser	Visible
Absorption	Water	Opaque proteins	Hemoglobin, melanin
Penetration (mm)	0.1	4.0–6.0	1.0–2.0
Maximal power (W)	100	100	20
Coagulation	Poor	Good	Fair
Cutting	Good	Poor	Fair
Vessel size	Less than 1 mm	3 mm	1 mm
Spectrum	Infrared	Infrared	Visible
Wavelength (nm)	10,600	1064	488–514

The Nd:YAG laser has a solid crystal of yttrium–aluminum–garnet, which has 1%–3% neodymium ions integrally doped in. This crystal is the lasing material of the resonator. The excitation device is an optical xenon or krypton flash lamp. Because of the inefficiency in delivery of energy, heat is generated as a byproduct; thus a forced water cooling system is an essential part of the laser, without which the laser would quickly lose power. There are some new air-cooled prototypes, but their efficiency is not known. The CO_2 laser is relatively efficient and can be air cooled.

A major difference between the two lasers is the delivery system. A flexible fiber to transmit the CO_2 wavelength has not yet been developed. Recent prototypes are still short and stiff. A mirror system directs the light system through an articulated arm for the CO_2 laser, and this system often gets out of alignment when the laser is jarred. The Nd:YAG laser tolerates jarring and transport much better.

The Nd:YAG beam can be transmitted through a fine quartz fiber, which allows its use through endoscopes. Heat in the fiber is intense, but the fiber is still efficient enough to keep losses at $<20\%$. Use of a catheter as a sheath permits the coaxial flow of air or water to cool the fiber. If the tip is scratched or if it touches debris or tissue, it may burn out, which necessitates cutting off the tip and polishing it again or replacing the fiber. These fibers are expensive and present major technical problems because burns of the tip occur frequently. In addition, a technician must become skilled in cutting and polishing the fiber tips. Sterilization can be achieved only by cold methods, but the fiber may become brittle after repeated cold sterilizations. The hope is for future development of a cheap disposable fiber to circumvent the costly labor needed to repair the fiber tips. The prototypes are promising, but the cost is still high and sterilization is still necessary.

The absorption characteristics determine the degree of tissue penetration. The CO_2 wavelength (10,600 nm) is absorbed by water, and since human cells are 80%–90% water, the light is absorbed superficially. The penetration is <1 mm. The absorption of the CO_2 wavelength by water provides a cutting property. The cells vaporize, and lack of scatter leaves adjacent cells intact. Hence the CO_2 beam may be used as a scalpel, but it is not good for coagulation. The absorption of the Nd:YAG wavelength (1064 nm) is by opaque tissues and minimally by water. As the opaque proteins are hit, there is scatter and wider, deeper thermal destruction. The penetration may be 4–6 mm. The Nd:YAG laser, with lesser absorption, wider scatter, and more necrosis, is a coagulation device.

As is true with water, the CO_2 wavelength is absorbed by glass and plastic, whereas the Nd:YAG wavelength passes through these substances. The safety factors are obvious. The clinician's eyes should be protected by plain glass or plastic when the CO_2 laser is used; even a hit on the eye with a CO_2 laser will cause only a superficial burn because of the absorption by water. However, the Nd:YAG laser can pass through standard operating room windows and will pass through the humors of the eye to the retina. The eyes and skin are the organs at risk when lasers are in use. For use of the Nd:YAG laser, special goggles of high optical density are necessary.

Argon plasma coagulation (APC) is another form of noncontact coagulation. A high-frequency current is transmitted to the tissues by an ionizing gas, argon. Argon is blown from the tip of a catheter where a tungsten electrode conducts a current. The argon jet acts as a current conductor. The electrocoagulation creates a shallow (0.5 to 3.0 mm) necrosis.

Contact tips have appeal for surgeons. The ability to touch tissue with a contact tip has the familiarity of a scalpel for the surgeon, even though it is not drawn through the tissue in the same fashion. Contact tips are made of sapphire or ceramic, which can withstand high temperatures. Temperatures up to 2000°C can be produced at the tip. These tips are designed with different geometrics, and these differences determine whether the tip acts like a scalpel or a coagulator. The long, pointed tip behaves like a scalpel. The blunt, chisel-like tip coagulates more effectively. The contact tip focuses energy to make it more like the CO_2 laser with more precise and superficial cuts.

CLINICAL APPLICATIONS

Endoscopic Laser Therapy

The colonoscope or flexible sigmoidoscope accepts a flexible fiber that will transmit the argon or Nd:YAG laser beams. Other forms of treatment such as the heater probe and bipolar electrocautery are evolving.

The endoscopist uses thermal effects in which temperatures over 100°C will ablate tissue and less than 100°C will coagulate it. The surgical work required dictates which effect is used. In general, the 100 W level is used for ablation and the 50–70 W level for coagulation. Visual cues that denote thermal effect include a white color of the lasered tissue and curling or shrinking of tissue. The colon must be dealt with carefully because perforation may occur. The extraperitoneal rectum can tolerate more energetic treatment.

To be safe, the normal characteristics of the colon, adjacent anatomy, and intraluminal contents must be factored into the choice of power energy and technique. The effects of thermal energy on the colon and other portions of the gastrointestinal tract have been studied (27,28). The colon is thinner than the stomach; thus, less energy density can be exerted. Just as with the use of electrocautery, excellent bowel preparation is needed. Otherwise, direct inspection of the lesion is impaired, and the danger of explosion is enhanced. Normal physiologic mechanisms may interfere with precise application of the laser beam. Peristalsis is expected, and activity increases with endoscopy; intravenous anticholinergics may be used to control motility. The aorta, heart, and larger vessels may pulsate near the colon, moving it at several points and making the task more difficult. Movement caused by respirations must be taken into account, and the patient may need to hold his breath momentarily to allow a short burst of the laser.

Obstruction

The Nd:YAG laser may be used for treating certain obstructive and bleeding lesions or for patients who are at high risk for surgery. Probably the most obvious use for treating obstruction is palliation of obstructive carcinomas that have been determined incurable (29–38). Obstruction in the rectum, where it is easily accessible and where perforation does not result in peritonitis, is ideal for this approach. Usually this procedure is performed on an outpatient basis with the patient under sedation, which makes the procedure cost-effective.

For treatment of rectal carcinoma, the technique usually uses 60–100 W for one second at a distance of 1–2 cm from the neoplasm. In the colon, the time of the pulse is reduced to < 0.5 second. Usually more than one treatment session is required. A more difficult site is the angle of the rectosigmoid colon, where direct vision is impossible. The procedure is performed from the intraluminal surface, preserving a thickness circumferentially to prevent perforation.

Data supporting this approach are sparse in the world literature. Most small series report 100% relief of obstructive symptoms; large series and surveys report more than 85%–90% palliative success for at least three months after the procedure (39). Complications include perforation, hemorrhage, rectovaginal fistula, and stenosis. Presumably edema could worsen an obstruction. Perforation of the extraperitoneal rectum has been reported to result in perirectal abscess. Deaths following complications approach 1%. In time, if the patient survives, reobstruction can be expected.

Obstruction prevents proper bowel preparation, and often two or three surgical stages may follow. To reduce the number of procedures, a new concept has been reported in which the obstructing site is coagulated by laser to open it (40). Thereafter a bowel preparation can be accomplished, allowing a one-stage resection with primary anastomosis. Reports regarding on-the-table bowel preparation indicate that this may be a better alternative for the patient with obstruction. More recently the metal stent applied through a colonoscope provides a better choice.

A less often reported cause of obstruction is benign stricture secondary to an anastomosis in the rectum. A report describes laser incision of two such strictures (41). Fortunately, it is rare for even small anastomoses to become clinically significant.

Hemorrhage

Hemorrhage secondary to incurable colorectal carcinomas responds with an 80%–90% success rate, but the same complications mentioned for obstruction exist (39). Acute massive bleeding is risky to treat because local preparation and visualization are poor.

Vascular ectasias (arteriovenous malformations) are commonly diagnosed as a source of gastrointestinal bleeding. These superficial vascular lesions, measuring 1–2 cm in diameter, may be treated readily by superficial coagulation. Rutgeerts et al. (42) reported on 59 patients with vascular ectasias, noting that 31 of the malformations were in the colon alone. Of the 59 patients, 17 rebled after an 11-month follow-up. In this series the three colonic perforations, two of which required right colectomies, are the focus of great concern. Reduction below 65 W at an application time of less than 0.5 second, plus staying at least 2 cm away from the colon wall, would minimize this complication (42). In smaller studies many perforations have not been reported (43).

The technique for treating tiny lesions is to aim pulses directly on the ectasia. However, lesions > 2 mm should be coagulated around the margins before the middle of the malformation is hit.

Villous Adenomas

The treatment of villous adenomas by laser ablation has been described in several sources (44–46). However, most surgeons argue that this is not good therapy because the disease can be managed effectively and inexpensively with surgical excision; more importantly, with excision a specimen can be inspected for carcinoma by the pathologist.

Intra-abdominal Uses

Surgical Incisions

In the mid-1970s authors touted the advantages of the CO_2 laser for making surgical incisions because of the rapidity with which a laser wound healed when compared with a cold scalpel incision (47–49). The CO_2 laser injury zone can be as little as 50 μm, but even this small injury results in delayed epithelialization and diminished early wound strength for up to 10 to 14 days (50,51). Laser incision has no advantage over scalpel incision except when a coagulopathy or a hypervascular field must be traversed (52). The CO_2 laser may seal vessels 0.5 mm in diameter and may be defocused to coagulate vessels up to 2 mm in size. The ability to achieve superficial cutting that is precise and narrow has made the CO_2 laser the first choice for making an incision. The argon laser, with 1–2 mm penetration of tissue, and a noncontact Nd:YAG laser, which has a 3–4 mm penetration of tissue, leave devitalized margins.

Liver Resection

Wedge resection or lobe resection is sometimes appropriate for solitary liver metastases. Initial enthusiasm for CO_2 and Nd:YAG laser applications in hepatic resection have been replaced by a more practical approach that includes both laser and conventional technologies (53–55). The CO_2 lasers currently in use have an awkward articulating arm that is unwieldy and causes problems in maintaining operating field sterility. However, the contact tip probes are particularly useful for hepatic resection, with operating times and tissue damage decreased by this method. Nevertheless, larger vessels and biliary ducts require clipping or ligature to ensure a dry field. Oozing from resected surfaces can be controlled with either a CO_2 laser or a noncontact Nd:YAG laser. Furthermore, sealing the raw surface reduces protein losses.

Splenic Resection

Iatrogenic splenic injury during mobilization of the splenic flexure of the colon accounts for the majority of splenectomies performed by colon and rectal surgeons. Impaired immune recognition of encapsulated bacteria secondary to splenectomy results in late septic complications; thus efforts should be made to repair or preserve part of this organ (56). Dixon et al. (57) were able to demonstrate the segmental arterial distribution of splenic hilar vessels in freshly removed organs. Using this anatomic data, Dixon constructed three models simulating peripheral organ injury: (1) a rather typical capsular avulsion injury, (4) lacerations to the subsegmental splenic parenchyma, and (5) hilar disruption. Comparison of the Nd:YAG laser with microfibrillar collagen demonstrated that the laser was superior in decreasing volume of blood loss and time to achieve control. In deeper parenchymal and hilar injuries, bleeding in large vessels (2–4 mm) was poorly controlled by both techniques. Surgical clips or ligatures were necessary to secure hemostasis in this type of injury. The ligation of segmental hilar vessels leads to ischemic splenic demarcation in 5–15 minutes. If the line of demarcation is followed, the Nd:YAG laser quickly allows segmental resection. Delayed bleeding from the resected edge has not been a problem. Use of contact Nd:YAG probes for resective techniques promises to improve hemostasis with troublesome vessels in the 2–4 mm range. Clinical data on this subject are not available.

Endometriosis

Sometimes endometriosis causes gastrointestinal blood loss or obstruction that requires operative intervention. Large invading or obstructing lesions require segmental or wedge resection of bowel to correct the problem. However, the small and large bowel may be studded with asymptomatic implants. After the major lesions are corrected, the smaller lesions are vaporized by using the CO_2 laser; satisfactory results can be obtained. Because these lesions are pigmented, an argon laser may be useful, but increased penetrance of this laser on the relatively thin wall merits caution (58).

Perianal and Transanal Uses

Pilonidal Disease

In the treatment of a pilonidal sinus, the CO_2 laser can be used both as a scalpel and as a sterilizer. The surgical procedure consists of cystotomy, excision of the involved tissue, defocused laser application for sterilization of the surface tissues, and primary closure (59,60). The principal advantage of using this laser is a dry, clean wound for primary closure, predicated on a tension-free closure. Even with complete removal of pilonidal tissue, plus a laser-sterilized surface for closure, nonhealing occurs frequently. However, this problem also frequently complicates the closures of pilonidal cystectomies performed by scalpel. Perhaps midline tension, wetness of this area, local contamination, and hirsutism predispose patients to this problem. In addition, epithelialization of laser incisions lags three days behind that of scalpel incisions because of the resorption of the zone of necrosis. Whether this laser application will be an improvement remains to be seen.

Skin Lesions

Hemorrhoidal tags, benign perianal neoplasms and malignant lesions can be vaporized or excised with the laser. For benign lesions the destruction of unwanted tissue is the goal, so obtaining a specimen for pathology is not an issue. The advantages of laser energy are minimization of the associated tissue injury and precise control over the depth of destruction (48). However, vaporization of malignant lesions does not allow pathologic assessment of margins (61). If tumor-free margins are the surgeon's guide to the adequacy of resection, a scalpel or laser excision should be performed. Because standard scalpel wounds heal faster, traditional excision is preferred when excessive blood loss is not a concern. The Nd:YAG contact scalpel has merit in the treatment of vascular lesions because of its coagulation properties (62). For the treatment of contaminated wounds Hinshaw et al. (63) have documented good results with the CO_2 laser.

Condyloma Acuminatum

Spurred by reports of successful treatment using laser to vaporize vaginal, vulvar, and cervical condyloma, many surgeons have applied this modality to the treatment of perianal condyloma acuminatum (64–66). Unfortunately, recurrence rates are high. Billingham and Lewis (67) reported no improvement in recurrence rates when comparing the results of using laser to electrocautery in the same patient. Duus et al. (68) reported no difference between laser and electrocautery in 14 patients when they were analyzed for recurrence, postoperative pain, healing time, and scar formation. It is likely that the discrepancy in reported results is related to the host's immune status and the presence of an associated infection with human immunodeficiency virus (HIV). If the immune mechanism is compromised, recurrence rates will be high, regardless of treatment. The CO_2 laser is preferable when the condylomata are multiple and small because the depth of destruction can be controlled better than with electrocautery. However, large bulky lesions do not lend themselves to laser vaporization.

There have been anecdotal reports of the growth of condylomata on the vocal cords of surgeons who use the CO_2 laser, and viable viral particles have been recovered from the plume generated by the procedure; thus, maintaining good smoke evacuation is essential. Possibly, recurrence rates are lower with electrocautery because of wider lateral zones of necrosis. Condyloma viruses reside in the basal epidermal layer (69). Therefore adequate treatment should ablate the involved tissue to this depth. Additionally, peripheral viruses, which have yet to stimulate growth of the characteristic lesion, must be treated if "recurrence" is to be prevented. Baggish (70) believes that recurrence rates can be decreased by "laser painting" the field of normal-appearing skin with the CO_2 laser to eradicate dormant viruses. Host immune function must be present if there is any hope for cure. The Nd:YAG laser may decrease recurrences by providing a deeper zone of destruction than the CO_2 laser. Since condyloma lesions are infectious and have a malignant potential, patients should be treated aggressively despite a positive HIV titer as long as they have no overt evidence of AIDS (69).

Anal Fistula

In an effort to avoid fistulotomy, Slutzki et al. (71) described a procedure in which the fistulous tract was vaporized over a probe to the internal crypt of origin. This method differs from the standard fistulectomy for muscle conservation in which no effort was made to secure closure of the internal opening. Follow-up was brief, but their apparent success has led the authors to advocate this approach when insertion of a seton would be considered.

Bodzin employed the CO_2 laser for the difficult fistula secondary to Crohn's disease. The laser was used to unroof and sterilize the tracks in seven patients. A seton was used around the external sphincter. The first four healed, but follow-up was too short in the three more recent patients (72).

Hemorrhoids

The CO_2 laser may be used as a scalpel during performance of a hemorrhoidectomy (73). The proximal vascular pedicle of the internal hemorrhoid is suture ligated, and with the handpiece the CO_2 laser is used to incise rectal mucosa, anoderm, and external hemorrhoids. Unfortunately, bleeding is brisk because the CO_2 laser light is absorbed at the surface and will not coagulate the vessels. Reapproximation of tissue edges is performed optionally. Claimed merits of this procedure are rapid healing, less scarring, applicability to outpatient surgery, and the concomitant applicability to ancillary anorectal conditions (i.e., condyloma, skin tags, and fistulas). The same merits can be claimed for a well-performed closed hemorrhoidectomy performed by a skilled surgeon (74). Hemorrhoidectomy with the CO_2 laser has increased operating time and has no perceptible effect on postoperative pain. Healing is good but is comparable to the traditional closed hemorrhoidectomy.

Zahir et al. (75) reported on a series of 50 patients from whom the internal and external hemorrhoids were removed by using contact scalpels with the Nd:YAG laser. With the patient under a local or regional anesthetic, symptomatic first- and second-degree hemorrhoids were treated by applying a coagulating low-power Nd:YAG endoprobe around the periphery of the hemorrhoid, causing coagulation, not vaporization. Then the coagulating probe was applied to the hemorrhoid itself to complete its ablation. Pedicles of third- and fourth-degree hemorrhoids were ligated. With a contact scalpel the mucosa was incised over the internal hemorrhoid and distally to include external hemorrhoidal tissue. Mucosal flaps were elevated with this probe to remove hemorrhoidal tissue. Twenty watts of power was used. Five sutures were used to close the mucosa and skin defects. Blood loss was < 10 mL, operating time was approximately 30 minutes, outpatient surgery was used, and only acetaminophen was required for analgesia. However, only one or two hemorrhoidal columns per patient were treated.

Neoplasms of Anal Canal and Distal Rectum

CO_2 and Nd:YAG lasers can be used to excise pedunculated polyps, sessile polyps, and malignant carcinomas through operating anoscopes. Pfeffermann et al. (76) and Pennino et al. (59) used the CO_2 laser to excise benign adenomas and to vaporize carcinomas. The laser, like standard excision, electrocoagulation, and contact radiation, is used for the treatment of a rectal carcinoma that meets the criteria of being < 3 cm in size, being movable, and not extending over the vagina or peritoneal cavity. Intrarectal ultrasound is an aid in staging the carcinoma to determine whether it is confined to or penetrates the rectal wall. Problems can arise when the CO_2 laser is used intrarectally because vessels with diameters > 0.5 mm bleed briskly and require control by either suture or electrocoagulation. When vaporization is selected as the technique, no specimen is available for pathologic assessment (77). A contact probe used as a scalpel achieves hemostasis of vessels ≤ 3 mm and provides a specimen for pathologic assessment. Noncontact Nd:YAG via a hand-held device may be used for in situ destruction for the cure or palliation of rectal carcinoma, as pointed out by Joffe (77). Gevers et al. reported the use of endoscopic laser therapy for palliation of distal colorectal carcinoma. Two hundred nineteen patients were treated; 198 (92%) had initial successful palliation; however, 160 (75%) had long term palliation (39). Depth of penetration is not as critical in the infraperitoneal rectum as long as the treatment plane does not overlie the vagina. Experience with the electrocautery of neoplasms in the middle and distal thirds of the rectum has demonstrated the safety of such an approach.

Anorectal Stricture

Lasers may be used to open and relieve strictures in the lower rectum, whether it be benign or malignant (78). Vaporization energy levels using the CO_2 or Nd:YAG unit can widen a lumen as long as the natural lumen can be used as a guide. Unfortunately, bleeding can be severe and requires having either a Nd:YAG laser or electrocautery available for hemostasis. The laser's air-transmission characteristics enable the surgeon to work conveniently at a distance from midrectal lesions in which retraction and exposure often prove to be a problem.

Radiation Proctitis

Massive recurrent or chronic bleeding may be an uncontrollable complication of radiation proctitis. Generally seen 2 to 25 years after therapy for gynecologic or prostatic malignancy, bleeding secondary to radiation proctitis necessitates multiple transfusions and eventually proctectomy in many patients. However, performing proctectomy in this group accounts for a mortality rate as high as 47% in some series. Recently, encouraging reports recommend the use of Nd:YAG and argon laser treatments for these vascular lesions (79–81). The most recent technology for control of bleeding secondary to radiation proctitis and has failed topical formalin therapy is the argon plasma coagulator (82,83). Repeated treatments are often necessary. The settings are an argon gas flow of 0.6 L/min with a power setting of 40 W stricture may ensue in some, but the transfusion requirements are significantly reduced. Expected results are 90% improvement and 81% disappearance of bleeding. Also the KTP laser has been used in similar fashion for radiation proctitis (84). Repeated applications at multiple sites via rigid and flexible endoscopes are well tolerated. Long-term efficacy is unknown, but immediate control of bleeding can be achieved.

REFERENCES

1. Glover JL, Bendick PJ, Luik WJ. The use of thermal knives in surgery. Electrosurgery, lasers, plasma scalpel. Curr Probl Surg 1978; 15:1–78.
2. Sittner WR, Fitzgerald JK. High-frequency electosurgery. In: Beric G, ed. Endoscopy. New York: Appleton-Century-Crofts, 1976:215.
3. Sitter WR, Fitzgerald JK. High-frequency electrosurgery. In: Berci G, ed. Endoscopy. New York: Appleton-Century-Crofts, 1976:217.
4. Curtiss LE. High-frequency currents in endoscopy. A review of principles and precautions. Gastrointest Endosc 1973; 20:9–12.
5. Sebben JE. Electrosurgery principles: Cutting current and cutaneous surgery. Part 1. J Dermatol Surg Oncol 1988; 14:29–31.
6. Sebben JE. Electrosurgery: Monopolar and bipolar treatment. J Dermatol Surg Oncol 1989; 15:364–366.
7. Ehrenwerth J. Electrical safety. In: Barash PG, Cullen BF, Stoelting RK, Eds. Clinical Anesthesia. 4th ed. Philadelphia: Lippincot, Williams and Wilkins, 2001:143–163.
8. Nduka C, Super PA, Monson JRT, Darzi A. Cause and prevention of electrosurgical injuries in laparoscopy. J Am Coll Surg 1994; 179:161–179.
9. Barlow DE. Endoscopic application of electrosurgery: A review of basic principles. Gastrointest Endosc 1982; 28:73–76.
10. Bond JH, Levitt MD. Factors affecting the concentration of combustible gases in the colon during colonoscopy. Gastrointest Endosc 1975; 68:1445–1448.
11. Ragins H, Shinya H, Wolff WI. The explosive potential of colonic gas during colonoscopic electrosurgical polypectomy. Surg Gynecol Obstet 1974; 138:554–556.

12. Bond JH, Levy M, Levitt MD. Explosion of hydrogen gas in the colon during proctosigmoidoscopy. Gastrointest Endosc 1976; 23:41–42.
13. Wenig BL, Stenson KM, Wenig BM, Tracey D. Effects of plume produced by the Nd:YAG laser and electrocautery on the respiratory system. Lasers Surg Med 1993; 13:242–245.
14. Sagar PM, Meagher A, Sobezak S, Wolff BG. Chemical composition and potential hazards of electrocautery smoke. Br J Surg 1996; 83:1792.
15. Barrett WL, Garber SM. Surgical smoke—a review of the literature. Is this just a lot of hot air? Surg Endosc 2003; 17:979–987.
16. Erdman S, Levinsky L, Servadio C, Stoupel E, Levy MJ. Safety precautions in the management of patients with pacemakers when electrocautery operations are performed. Surg Gynecol Obstet 1988; 167:311–314.
17. Dresner DL, Lebowitz PW. Atrioventricular sequential pacemaker inhibition by transurethral electrosurgery. Anesthesiology 1988; 68:599–601.
18. American Society of Gastrointestinal Endoscopy Technology Assessment Evaluation: Electrocautery use in patients with implanted cardiac devices. Gastrointes Endosc 1994; 40:794–795.
19. Einstein A. Zur Quantentheorie der Strahlung. Physiol Z 1917; 18:121–128.
20. Gordon JP, Zeigler HJ, Townes CH. The maser: New type of amplifier frequency standard and spectrometer. Physiol Rev 1955; 99:1264–1274.
21. Maiman TH. Stimulated optical radiation in ruby. Nature 1960; 187:493–498.
22. Johnson LF. Optical maser characteristics of rare earth ions in crystals. J Appl Physiol 1961; 34:897–909.
23. Bennett WR, Faust WL, McFarlane RA. Dissociative excitation transfer and optical maser oscillation in NeO_2 and ArO_2 rf discharges. Physiol Rev 1962; 8:470–473.
24. Patel CKN, McFarlane RA, Faust WL. Selective excitation through vibrational energy transfer and optical maser action in $N_2 \cdot CO_2$. Physiol Rev 1964; 13: 617–619.
25. Lipow M. Laser physics made simple. Curr Probl Obstet Gynecol Fertil 1986; 8:445–481.
26. Fuller TA. Fundamentals of lasers in surgery and medicine. Dixon J ed. Surgical Application of Lasers. 2nd ed. Chicago: Year Book, 1987:16–33.
27. Dixon JA, Berenson MM, McCloskey DW. Neodymium:YAG laser treatment of experimental canine gastric bleeding: Acute and chronic studies of photocoagulation, penetration, and perforation. Gastroenterology 1979; 77:647–651.
28. Rutgeerts P, van Trappen G, Geboes K, et al. Safety and efficacy of neodymium:YAG laser photocoagulation: An experimental study in dogs. Gut 1981; 22:38–44.
29. Brown SG, Barr H, Matthewson K, et al. Endoscopic treatment of inoperable colorectal cancers with Nd:YAG laser. Br J Surg 1986; 73:949–952.
30. Brunetaud JM, Maunoury V, Ducrotte P, Cochelard D, Cortot A, Paris JC. Palliative treatment of rectosigmoid carcinoma by laser endoscopic photoablation. Gastroenterology 1987; 92:663–668.
31. Mathus-Vliegen EMH, Tytgat GNJ. Laser ablation and palliation in colorectal malignancy. Results of multicenter inquiry. Gastrointest Endosc 1986; 32: 395–396.
32. Mathus-Vliegen EMH, Tytgat GNJ. Laser photocoagulation in the palliation of colorectal malignancies. Cancer 1986; 57:2212–2216.
33. Morris AL, Krasner N. Laser irradiation of inoperable tumors of the colon and rectum. Br Med J 1985; 80:715–718.
34. Russin DJ, Kaplan SR, Goldberg RI, Barkin JS. Neodymium:YAG laser. A new palliative tool in the treatment of colorectal cancer. Arch Surg 1986; 121: 1399–1403.
35. Hunter JG, Bowers JH, Burt RV, Sullivan JJ, Stevens SL, Dixon JA. Lasers in endoscopic gastrointestinal surgery. Am J Surg 1984; 148:736–741.
36. Wood JW, Innes JW. Tumor ablation by endoscopic Nd:YAG laser. Am J Gastroenterol 1985; 80:715–718.
37. Kiefhaber P, Huber F, Kiefhaber K. Palliative and preoperative endoscopic neodymium:YAG laser treatment of colorectal carcinoma. Endoscopy 1987; 19:43–46.
38. Schwesinger WH, Chumley DL. Laser palliation for gastrointestinal malignancy. Am Surg 1988; 54:100–104.
39. Gevers AM, Macken E, Hiele M, Rutgeerts P. Endoscopic laser therapy for palliation of patients with distal colorectal carcinoma: Analysis of factors influencing long-term outcome. Gastrointest Endosc 2000; 51:580–585.
40. Kiefhaber P, Kiefhaber K, Huber F. Preoperative Nd:YAG laser treatment of obstructive colon cancer. Endoscopy 1986; 18:44–46.
41. Sander R, Poesl H, Spuhler A. Management of non-neoplastic stenoses of the GI tract. Endoscopy 1984; 16:149–151.
42. Rutgeerts P, Van Gompel F, Geboes K, van Trappen G, Broeckaert L, Coreman SG. Long-term results of treatment of vascular malformations of the gastrointestinal tract by neodymium:YAG laser photocoagulation. Gut 1985; 26:586–593.
43. Cello JP, Grendall JH. Endoscopic laser treatment for gastrointestinal vascular ectasias. Ann Intern Med 1986; 104:352–354.
44. Lamber R, Sabben G. Laser therapy in colorectal tumors (villous): Early results. Gastroenterology 1984; 84:1222.
45. Sander R, Poesl H. Treatment of benign gastrointestinal tumors with neodymium:YAG laser. Endoscopy 1986; 18:57–59.
46. Low DE, Kozarek MD, Ball TJ, Ryan JA. Nd:YAG laser photo-ablation of sessile villous and tubular adenomas of the colorectum. Ann Surg 1988; 208:725–732.
47. Kaplan I, Ger R. The carbon dioxide laser in clinical surgery. Isr J Med Sci 1973; 9:79–83.
48. Aronoff BL. CO_2 laser surgery. Kaplan I, ed. Laser Surgery. New York: Academic Press, 1977, pp19–28.
49. Hall RR. The healing of tissues incised by a carbon dioxide laser. Br J Surg 1971; 58:222–225.
50. Ascher PW, Hebner M. Neurosurgical laser techniques. Goldman L, ed. The Biomedical Laser. New York: Springer-Verlag, 1981:224.
51. Sowa D, Masterson BJ, Nealon N, Von Fraunhofer JA. Effects of thermal knives on wound healing. Obstet Gynecol 1985; 66:436–439.
52. Wieman TJ. Lasers and the surgeon. Am J Surg 1986; 151:493–500.
53. Sultan RA, Fallouh H, Lefelvre M. Lasers in surgical tumor vaporization. Proceedings of the Sixth International Congress. Jerusalem: Society for Lasers in Medicine and Surgery, 1985, p9.
54. Meyer HJ, Haverkamp K. Experimental study of partial liver resections with combined CO_2 and Nd:YAG lasers. Lasers Surg Med 1982; 2:149–154.
55. Dixon JA. General Surgical Applications of Lasers. In: Dixon J, ed. Surgical Application of Lasers. 2nd ed. Chicago: Year Book, 1987:119–143.
56. Singer DB. Postsplenectomy sepsis. Perspect Pediatr Pathol 1983; 1:285–311.
57. Dixon JA, Miller F, McCloskey D, Siddorway J. Anatomy and techniques in segmental splenectomy. Surg Gynecol Obstet 1980; 150:516–520.
58. Keye WR, Matson GA, Dixon JA. The use of the argon laser in the treatment of experimental endometriosis. Fertil Steril 1983; 39:26–29.
59. Pennino R, Lanzafame RJ, Herrera HR, Hinshaw JR. Applications of the CO_2 laser in general surgery. Contemp Surg 1986; 28:13–19.
60. Korn A, Glantz GJ. The use of CO_2 laser in general surgery. Proceedings of the Sixth International Congress. Jerusalem: Society for Lasers in Medicine and Surgery, 1985:7.
61. Landthaler M, Haina D, Brunner R, Waidelich W, Braun-Falco O. Laser therapy of bowenoid papulosis and Bowen's disease. J Dermatol Oncol 1986; 12: 1253–1257.
62. Joffe SN, Daikvzono N, Sankar MY, et al. Contact probes for Nd:YAG laser. Optical fibers. Med Biol 1985; 570:42–50.
63. Hinshaw JR, Herrera HR, Lanzafame RJ. The use of carbon dioxide laser permits primary closure of contaminated and purulent lesions and wounds. Proceedings of the Sixth International Congress. Jerusalem: Society for Lasers in Medicine and Surgery, 1985, p49.
64. Ferenczy A. Comparison of 5-fluorouracil and CO_2 laser for treatment of vaginal condylomata. Obstet Gynecol 1984; 64:773–778.
65. Reid R. Superficial laser vulvectomy. Am J Obstet Gynecol 1985; 151:1045–1052.
66. Krebs HB, Wheelock JB. The CO_2 laser for recurrent and therapy-resistant condylomata acuminata. J Reprod Med 1985; 30:489–492.
67. Billingham RP, Lewis FG. Laser versus electrical cautery in the treatment of condylomata acuminata of the anus. Surg Gynecol Obstet 1982; 155:185–187.
68. Duus BR, Philipsen T, Christensen JD, Lundvall F, Sondergaard J. Refractory condylomata acuminata: A controlled clinical trial of carbon dioxide laser versus conventional surgical treatment. Genitourin Med 1985; 61:59–61.
69. Buschke A, Loewenstein LL. Über arcinomihnliche Condylomata Acuminata des Penis. Klin Wochenschr 1925; 4:1726–1729.
70. Baggish MS. Improved laser techniques for the elimination of genital and extragenital warts. Am J Obstet Gynecol 1985; 153:454–460.
71. Slutzki S, Abramsohn R, Bogokowsky H. Carbon dioxide laser in the treatment of high anal fistula. Am J Surg 1981; 141:395–396.
72. Bodzin JH. Laser ablation of complex perianal fistulas preserves continence and is a rectum-sparing alternative in Crohn's disease patients. Am Surg 1998; 64:627–632.
73. Hodgson JB, Morgan J. Ambulatory hemorrhoidectomy with CO_2 lasers. Dis Colon Rectum 1995; 38:1265–1269.
74. Leff EI. Hemorrhoidectomy—laser vs. nonlaser: Outpatient surgical experience. Dis Colon Rectum 1992; 35:743–746.
75. Zahir KS, Edwards RE, Vecchia A, Dudrick SJ, Tripodi G. Use of ND:YAG laser improves quality of life and economic factors in the treatment of hemorrhoids. Connecticut Med 2000; 64(4):199–203.
76. Pfeffermann R, Merhav H, Rothstein J, Simon D. The use of laser in rectal surgery. Lasers Surg Med 1986; 6:467–469.
77. Joffe SN. The neodymium:YAG laser in general surgery. Contemp Surg 1985; 27:17–26.
78. Luck A, Chapuis P, Sinclair G, Hood J. Endoscopic laser stricturotomy and balloon dilatation for benign colorectal strictures. ANZ J Surg 2001; 71(10):594–597.
79. Ventrucci M, Disimone MP, Gulietti P, DeLucca G. Efficacy and safety of Nd:YAG laser for the treatment of bleeding from radiation proctocolitis. Digest Liver Dis 2001; 33(3):230–233.
80. Buchi KN, Dixon JA. Argon laser treatment of hemorrhagic radiation proctitis. Gastrointest Endosc 1987; 33:27–30.
81. Alexander TJ, Dwyer TM. Endoscopic Nd:YAG laser treatment of severe radiation injury of the gastrointestinal tract. Gastrointest Endosc 1985; 31:152.
82. Taieb S, Rolachon A, Cenni JC, et al. Effective use of argon plasma coagulation in the treatment of severe radiation proctitis. Dis Colon Rectum 2001;44(12): 1766–1771.
83. Tjandra JJ, Sengupta S. Argon plasma coagulation is an effective treatment for refractory hemorrhagic radiation proctitis. Dis Colon Rectum 2001; 44(12): 1759–1765.
84. Taylor JG, Disario JA, Bjorkman DJ. KTP laser therapy for bleeding from chronic radiation proctopathy. Gastrointest Endosc 2000; 52(3):353–357.

II: Anorectal Disorders

8 Hemorrhoids

Santhat Nivatvongs

WHAT ARE HEMORRHOIDS?

Hemorrhoids are not varicose veins, and not every one has hemorrhoids. But everybody has anal cushions. The anal cushions are composed of blood vessels, smooth muscle (Treitz's muscle), and elastic connective tissue in the submucosa (Fig. 1). They are located in the upper anal canal, from the dentate line to the anorectal ring (puborectalis muscle).

Three cushions lie in the following constant sites: left lateral, right anterolateral, and right posterolateral. Smaller discrete secondary cushions may be present between the main cushions. The configuration is remarkably constant and apparently bears no relationship to the terminal branching of the superior rectal artery, as previously thought. This vessel and its branches reach the anal canal in a variety of ways. That this arrangement of anal cushions is the normal state of affairs is borne out by the fact that it is present in children and can be demonstrated in the fetus and even in the embryo (1).

Return of blood from the anal canal is via two systems: the portal and the systemic. A connection between the two occurs in the region of the dentate line. The submucosal vessels situated above the dentate line constitute the internal hemorrhoidal plexus from which blood is drained through the superior rectal veins into the inferior mesenteric vein and subsequently into the portal system. Elevations in portal venous pressure may manifest as engorgement and gross dilatation of this internal hemorrhoidal plexus. Vessels situated below the dentate line constitute the external hemorrhoidal plexus from which blood is drained, in part through the middle rectal veins terminating in the internal iliac veins, but mainly through the inferior rectal veins into the pudendal veins, which are tributaries of the internal iliac veins. The veins constituting this external hemorrhoidal plexus are normally small; however, in situations of straining, because communication exists between internal and external hemorrhoidal plexuses, these veins become engorged with blood. If allowed to persist, this condition can lead to the development of combined internal and external hemorrhoids.

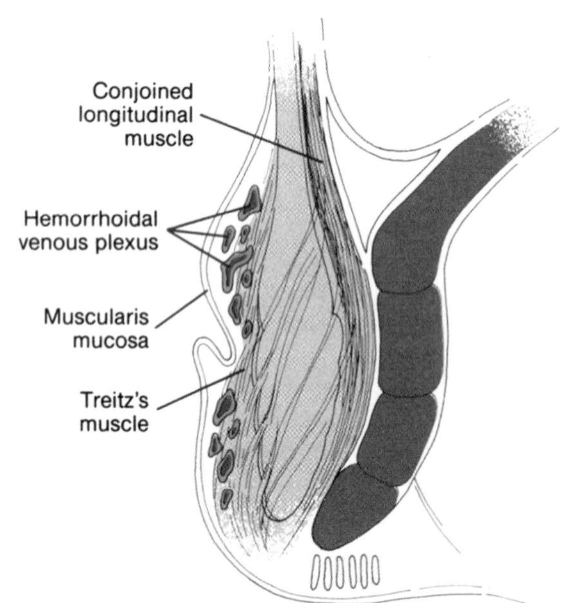

FIGURE 1 ■ Anal cushion showing Treitz's muscle derived from conjoined longitudinal muscle of the anal canal. *Source*: From Ref. 1.

New concepts of the pathophysiology of hemorrhoids have been defined during the past 30 years, yet medical education at the undergraduate and graduate levels has not kept pace with the newer concepts. The traditional concepts of varicose veins are perpetuated in all medical dictionaries and in most textbooks of surgery, medicine, anatomy, and pathology.

PREVALENCE

Using the data from the National Center for Health Statistics, Johanson and Sonnenberg (2) found that 10 million people in the United States complained of hemorrhoids, a prevalence rate of 4.4%. Of them, approximately one-third went to a physician for evaluation, and an average 1.5 million prescriptions were written annually for hemorrhoidal preparations. The rate of hospitalization for patients with hemorrhoids was 12.9 per million people. The age distribution of hemorrhoids demonstrated a hyperbolic pattern, with a peak between age 45 and 65 years and a subsequent decline after age 65 years. The presence of hemorrhoids in patients younger than 20 years old dwas unusual (2). All these figures could have been easily exaggerated, since they are based on complaint. Obviously, not all the complaints are true hemorrhoids. The diagnosis of hemorrhoids is not easy. It requires experienced physicians or surgeons to use a proper anoscope and, if necessary, to ask the patients to strain while sitting on the toilet. Not everyone has "hemorrhoids." A busy colon and rectal surgeon can hear a patient's complaint of "hemorrhoids" or see patients referred by other physicians for "hemorrhoids" only to find that many of these patients have other anal problems, ranging from pruritus ani to anal fissures, fistulas, and skin tags. Some do have true hemorrhoidal symptoms.

The National Hospital Discharge Survey data indicate that an annual average of 49 hemorrhoidectomies per 100,000 people in the United States were performed from 1983 to 1987. Hemorrhoidectomies are performed 1.3 times more commonly in males than in females. Most hemorrhoidectomies are performed in patients 45–64 years old. According to National Hospital Discharge Survey data, a threefold decrease in the number of hemorrhoidectomies is observed, from a peak of 117 per 100,000 in the United States in 1974 to a low of 37 per 100,000 in 1987 (3). This decline does not necessarily reflect a decrease in the occurrence of hemorrhoidal disease. Alternative treatments, particularly increasing bulk in the diet, rubber band ligation (RBL), and electrocautery, have become the standard treatment for grades 1 and 2 hemorrhoids. Hemorrhoidectomies are reserved for grades 3, 4, and some grade 2 hemorrhoids. If the same data were to be updated, the decline would be even more dramatic because most hemorrhoidectomies are now performed as an outpatient procedure.

Assessing the true prevalence of hemorrhoids is virtually impossible. Not surprisingly, the reported prevalence rates have varied widely from 1% to 86%, depending on the method of ascertainment and the definition of "hemorrhoids" (4).

ETIOLOGY AND PATHOGENESIS

Despite the attention it has received for centuries, the cause of hemorrhoids is still unknown. The popular varicose vein theory, stemming from the assumption that dilatations of the veins of the internal rectal venous plexus result from pathologic change, is shown as invalid by confirming that the dilatations are in fact normal (1). The fact that hemorrhoids are no more common in patients with portal hypertension than in the population at large (1,5–7) is additional evidence against the theory, as is the fact that when anal varices occur as the result of portal hypertension (a rare event), the appearance is quite different from that of hemorrhoids. The varicose vein theory also fails to account for the fact that hemorrhoids frequently occur singly and are more common in the right anterior position than elsewhere (1).

The vascular hyperplasia theory is also obsolete. The histologic study of hemorrhoidectomy specimens by Thomson (1) showed no sign of vascular hyperplasia, and they were similar to cadaver specimens in which there was no evidence of hemorrhoids.

From his detailed anatomic study, Thomson (1) concluded that a sliding downward of the anal cushions is the correct etiologic theory. Hemorrhoids result from disruption of the achoring and flattening action of the musculus submucosae ani (Treitz's muscle) and its richly intermingled elastic fibers. Hypertrophy and congestion of the vascular tissue are secondary (1). Hemorrhoids are associated with straining and with an irregular bowel habit, a feature compatible with the sliding anal lining theory (1). Hard, bulky stools as well as tenesmus from diarrhea cause straining, which is more likely to push the cushions out of the anal canal. Furthermore, straining may cause engorgement of the cushions during defecation, making their displacement more likely. Repeated stretching of the submucosal Treitz's muscle causes disruption and results in prolapse (1). Haas et al. (8) and Bernstein (5) found that the anchoring and supporting connective tissue above the anal cushions had disintegrated and fragmented in patients with hemorrhoids.

Technologic advances have made it possible to study abnormalities of the anal canal in patients with hemorrhoids. Many studies consistently show higher anal resting pressures in patients with hemorrhoids (9–12). An increase in resting pressure is reduced to normal after hemorrhoidectomy. Internal sphincter, external sphincter, and pressure within the anal cushions can all account for the increased resting tone. However, it is not possible to distinguish their contributions (13–15). Patients with enlarged hemorrhoids have been found on electromyography to have increased activity (16). Another abnormality found in many of these patients is an ultraslow pressure wave caused by the contraction of the internal sphincter as a whole, but its significance is not known (16). Electrical oscillation frequency of the internal sphincter is not abnormal (17). Anal electrosensitivity and temperature sensation are reduced in patients with hemorrhoids. The greatest change is noted in the proximal anal and mid-anal canals, perhaps because of prolapse of the less-sensitive rectal mucosa. This may also contribute to decreased continence. Rectal sensation to balloon distention is no different from that observed in control subjects (18).

PREDISPOSING AND ASSOCIATED FACTORS

Although chronic constipation has been considered the cause of hemorrhoids, Gibbons et al. (19) cast doubt on this hypothesis. Their studies show that patients with hemorrhoids are not necessarily constipated but tend to have abnormal anal pressure profiles and anal compliance. It is well known, however, that constipation aggravates symptoms of hemorrhoids. A case control study on the risk factors for hemorrhoids by Johanson and Sonnenberg (20) questions the influence of chronic constipation but supports diarrhea as a potential risk factor. The tenesmus from diarrhea does cause straining.

Many other factors have been implicated in the causation of hemorrhoidal disease, notably heredity, erect posture, absence of valves in the hemorrhoidal plexuses and draining veins, and obstruction of venous return from raised intra-abdominal pressure. All these factors may contribute to causing the disease, but these anatomic factors do not account for the differences found in epidemiologic studies. Portal hypertension may lead to venous engorgement of the hemorrhoidal plexus and on rare occasions may result in true varices in this area (e.g., in the lower esophagus and retroperitoneum and around the umbilicus). Pregnancy undoubtedly aggravates pre-existing disease and, by mechanisms not well understood, predisposes to the development of disease in patients who were previously asymptomatic. Furthermore, such patients usually become asymptomatic after delivery, which suggests that hormonal changes, in addition to direct pressure effects, may be involved. Straining in an attempt to overcome this problem in many cases will result in the appearance of hemorrhoidal symptoms. Patients with inflammatory bowel disease may, in fact, present with true hemorrhoidal symptoms or symptoms suggestive of hemorrhoidal disease. This fact always must be considered in the evaluation of all patients with hemorrhoids. Any patient with the combination of diarrhea and hemorrhoids should be viewed with suspicion, and all attempts should be made to exclude inflammatory bowel disease. Operative intervention in such patients may be fraught with greater complications.

FUNCTION OF ANAL CUSHIONS

The function of anal cushions is entirely speculative; however, many reasonable theories have been advanced. Because of their bulk, it is believed that they aid in anal continence. During the act of defecation, when the anal cushions become engorged and tense with blood, they cushion the anal canal lining. Because anal cushions are separate structures rather than a continuous ring of vascular tissue, they allow the anal canal to dilate during defecation without tearing (1).

At low sphincteric pressure, such as at rest, the anal cushions tend to fill with blood and swell, whereas at higher pressures, such as at squeeze, they would be compressed. When the anal sphincter relaxes, this mechanism could maintain closure of the anus by expanding to fill the lumen and could make an important contribution to the resting anal pressure (Fig. 2). These hypotheses may

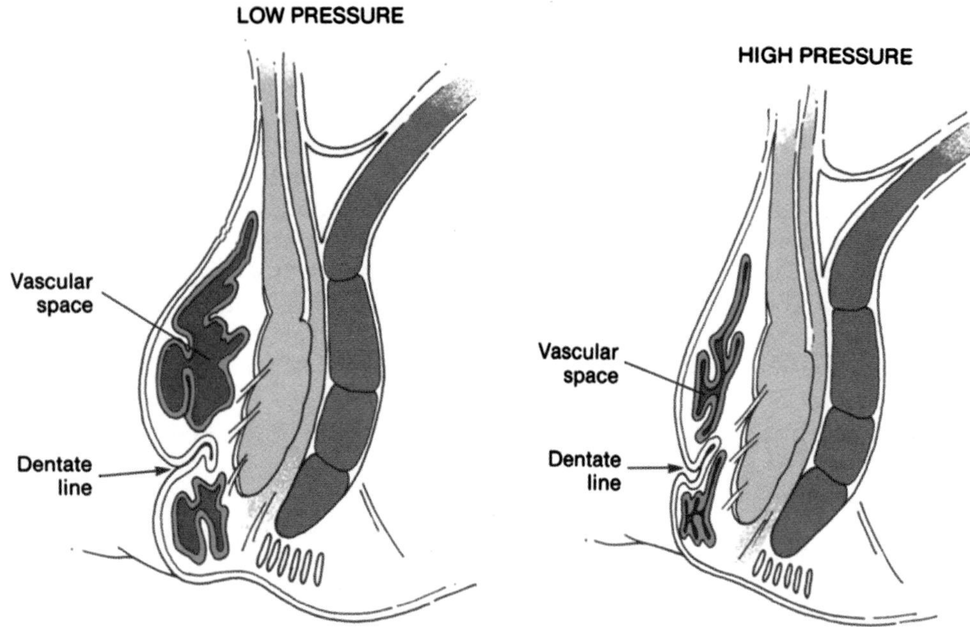

FIGURE 2 ■ Proposed mechanism by which vascular spaces contribute to anal pressure and maintain continence when the sphincters relax and dilate. *Source*: From Ref. 21.

explain why hemorrhoidectomy frequently is associated with minor degrees of incontinence or seepage (21).

On its own the internal sphincter cannot completely close the anal canal. The addition of mucosal fold is still not enough (18). A study of the internal sphincter in vitro and in vivo, including use of MRI, showed a gap of 7–8 mm in diameter that could not be closed by the internal sphincter muscle ring alone (22). This gap must be filled by the anal cushions to maintain fecal continence.

Whatever their contribution to anal resting pressure, the anal cushions also act as a compliant and conformable plug. Hemorrhoidectomy impairs continence to infused saline. An analogy may be drawn between the anal cushions and the washer in a tap; failure of a complete seal results in only minor leakage. However, fluid-filled cushions are not used for such functions. Any conforming tissue (e.g., the thick ileal mucosa of an ileoanal pouch) would do. Nevertheless, the fluid-filled anal cushions may also empty and so may permit easier defecation (18).

The way in which the anal cushions empty and clear the path for defecation is not known. Passive compression by solid stool may contribute, but two active mechanisms may also be involved. First, the formed stool dilating the anus reduces the height of the anal cushions and eases defecation. Second, the subepithelial smooth muscle with its contributions from the conjoined longitudinal layer provides another way of displacing the anal cushions during defecation. The conjoined longitudinal muscle, which consists of both voluntary and involuntary elements, may be particularly important. Just as smooth muscle contraction in the esophagus during swallowing is coordinated with actions beginning in voluntary muscles, so pelvic floor contraction may coordinate the action of rectal and anal smooth muscles during defecation (18).

NOMENCLATURE AND CLASSIFICATION

For clarity of surgical description, the various types and stages of hemorrhoidal disease are defined as follows.

External skin tags are discrete folds of skin arising from the anal verge. Such tags may be the end result of thrombosed external hemorrhoids or may be a complication of inflammatory bowel disease independent of any hemorrhoidal problem.

External hemorrhoids comprise the dilated vascular plexus that is located below the dentate line and covered by squamous epithelium.

Internal hemorrhoids are the symptomatic, exaggerated, submucosal vascular tissue located above the dentate line and covered by transitional and columnar epithelium. Internal hemorrhoids can be divided into categories. Grade 1 internal hemorrhoids are those that bulge into the lumen of the anal canal and may produce painless bleeding. Grade 2 internal hemorrhoids are those that protrude at the time of a bowel movement but reduce spontaneously. Grade 3 internal hemorrhoids are those that protrude spontaneously or at the time of a bowel movement and require manual replacement. Grade 4 internal hemorrhoids are those that are permanently prolapsed and irreducible despite attempts at manual replacement (23).

Mixed hemorrhoids are those in which elements of internal and external hemorrhoids are present. Multiple skin tags are often an accompaniment and most frequently occur with external hemorrhoids but may, on less frequent occasions, be associated with internal hemorrhoids.

In circumstances in which the prolapse cannot be reduced because of swelling and spasm of the sphincter, strangulated hemorrhoids occur. Progression results in gangrenous hemorrhoids.

DIAGNOSIS

DIFFERENTIAL DIAGNOSIS

The examiner should rule out certain disorders before diagnosing hemorrhoids.

Rectal mucosal prolapse is a common condition that frequently is confused with prolapsing hemorrhoids. As the name suggests, patients with this condition present with prolapse of rectal mucosa below the dentate line. Bleeding may occur from trauma to this displaced vascular mucosa. The condition usually results from the same precipitating factors that lead to hemorrhoidal disease, especially chronic straining at stool; however, in many cases the hemorrhoidal cushions are small. Rectal mucosal prolapse also may occur for the same reasons that lead to complete rectal prolapse, and, in fact, may precede the latter condition by some months or even years. Anal sphincter dysfunction, which is either primary or due to trauma (especially surgically induced trauma, such as in a patient with an internal sphincterotomy or maximal anal dilation), also may predispose patients to mucosal prolapse. It is important to recognize this condition as being different from hemorrhoidal disease because the treatment, although similar, must be modified by excision of a more proximal extent of rectal mucosa to achieve satisfactory results without the chance of recurrence.

Hypertrophied anal papillae are present when one or more of the anal papillae situated on the dentate line enlarge. This condition may be secondary to underlying anorectal disease, notably anal fissure, but in most instances no identifiable cause is apparent. The majority of patients with this condition are asymptomatic, and if enlargement is uniform and not gross, it should be considered a variation of normal. Occasionally, a papilla will hypertrophy to large proportions and protrude below the dentate line. In such cases a pedicle is present, and the term "fibrous anal polyp" sometimes is used; however, this condition is in no way similar to true colorectal polyps; hence, it is suggested that this term be abandoned.

Rectal polyps, melanoma, carcinoma, rectal prolapse, fissure, intersphincteric abscess, and perianal endometrioma must be considered in the differential diagnosis of hemorrhoids. These entities are discussed in their respective chapters.

■ EXTERNAL HEMORRHOIDS

External hemorrhoids are covered with anoderm that is distal to the dentate line. The external hemorrhoids may swell, causing some discomfort. Bleeding more frequently is associated with internal hemorrhoids. Treatment is not indicated unless there is an acute thrombosis causing severe pain.

■ INTERNAL HEMORRHOIDS

In the patient with internal hemorrhoids, several symptoms may be present. In the classic case, bleeding is bright red and painless and occurs at the end of defecation. The patient complains of blood dripping or squirting into the toilet bowl. The bleeding also may be occult, resulting in anemia, which is rare, or guaiac-positive stools. In such instances, other causes of bowel bleeding must be excluded before these problems are attributed to hemorrhoids, even if gross hemorrhoidal disease exists.

In a retrospective review of patients seen at the Mayo Clinic and Olmsted Community Hospital in Rochester, Minnesota, the incidence of hemorrhoidal bleeding that causes anemia is 0.5 patient per 100,000 people per year in Olmsted County. The mean age of the patients studied is 50 years (range, 25–72 years). Ninety-three percent of these patients have grade 2 or 3 internal hemorrhoids. The mean hemoglobin concentration before treatment is 9.4 g/dL [±0.97, standard deviation (SD)]. The recovery from anemia after definitive treatment with hemorrhoidectomy is rapid, with a mean hemoglobin concentration of 12.3 g/dL after two months. By six months, the mean hemoglobin concentration is 14.1 g/dL. Of note in the study is the description of hemorrhoidal bleeding that includes blood squirting or clots passing in 84% of patients for whom a description is available (24).

Prolapse of the hemorrhoids below the dentate line usually occurs at the time of straining at defecation. In most instances spontaneous reduction occurs. Occasionally, manual replacement is necessary. In some advanced cases the prolapse is irreducible. Chronic states of prolapse predispose to mucous and fecal leakage, resulting in pruritus and excoriation of the perianal skin with accompanying discomfort.

Pain per se is not a symptom of uncomplicated hemorrhoids. It may indicate associated disease, such as anal fissure, perianal abscess, or, notably, an intersphincteric abscess. If thrombosis occurs, pain becomes a marked feature of the disease. Prolapsed, strangulated hemorrhoids present as an acute problem, with the symptom of pain associated with discharging, edematous, tender, irreducible hemorrhoids. Occasionally, when this state of affairs is left untreated for some time, gangrene and infection with sloughing and secondary bleeding occur. Because of the connection with the portal venous system, infection in this area of venous drainage is possible, and pylephlebitis, although exceedingly rare, is a potential complication.

■ EXAMINATION

Examination of patients with suspected internal hemorrhoids should be aimed at several aspects.

General patient assessment to ascertain the general health status and in particular to exclude associated disease, particularly bleeding disorders and liver disease with portal hypertension, should be the first phase of examination.

Inspection may reveal variable degrees of perianal skin abnormalities, protrusion of internal hemorrhoids, or normal appearance.

Straining while sitting in the toilet is the most useful examination in patients with grades 2, 3, and 4 hemorrhoids. The severity of the prolapse can be easily seen and the degree of descending perineum can be evaluated. It can also differentiate hemorrhoid from rectal prolapse particularly when the true rectal prolapse comes to but not through the anus. Asking the patient to strain while the examiner's index finger is in the anorectum, an enterocele can be detected.

Digital examination will exclude low-lying rectal and anal canal neoplasms and will enable assessment of the tone of the anal sphincter.

Anoscopy is performed to assess the extent of disease. With the anoscope in place, the patient is asked to strain as if having a bowel movement so that the amount of prolapse can be assessed. During anoscopy it is also important to look for and rule out a coexisting anal fissure, especially in patients complaining of pain or those in whom anal sphincter tone is deemed excessive.

Proctoscopy or flexible sigmoidoscopy must be performed in all cases to visualize the rectum and lower colon so that coexisting conditions may be excluded, in particular, carcinoma, adenoma, and inflammatory bowel disease. The latter condition may produce symptoms similar to hemorrhoidal complaints and may potentiate any hemorrhoids present.

Colonoscopy examination should be performed in any patient with unusual symptoms or in whom it is hard to attribute the symptom to the limited degree of confirmed hemorrhoidal disease. This examination must be undertaken before any treatment is commenced since colonic diseases beyond the range of the sigmoidoscope must be excluded first. Patients who fall into the age or family history category of being at risk for colorectal neoplasms also should have a colonoscopy. For practical purposes, this age has been arbitrarily set at 50 years (see Chapter 25).

NONOPERATIVE TREATMENT AND MINOR OPERATIVE PROCEDURES

With the modern concepts of the pathophysiology of hemorrhoids, it is believed that prolapse of anal cushions is initiated by the shearing effect of the passage of a large hard stool or by the precipitous act of defecation, such as that in urgent diarrhea. If the prolapse of the vascular cushions can be prevented or if the congesting effect of a tight anal canal can be abolished, the anal cushions will return to their normal state, and symptoms will be prevented without necessitating the removal of the cushions themselves (25).

DIET AND BULK-FORMING AGENTS

The rationale of adding bulk to the diet is to eliminate straining at defecation. Burkitt and Graham-Stewart (26) observed that stools lacking adequate fiber are small, hard, and difficult to evacuate and thus require prolonged straining. In addition to consumption of plenty of fruits and vegetables, bulk in the diet can be supplemented easily with raw unprocessed wheat or oat bran (1/3 cup per day). An alternative measure is to take psyllium seed (two teaspoons per day). Psyllium seed has been reported in rare cases to cause allergy in some patients (27). An adequate volume of fluids must be consumed each day. A high-fiber diet reduces symptoms of hemorrhoids and is ideal for the treatment of grade 1 and some grade 2 hemorrhoids (28,29). It is important to impress on the patient not to ignore the urge to defecate.

OFFICE, OUTPATIENT, AND MINOR PROCEDURES

Rubber Band Ligation

In 1963, Barron (30) popularized the rubber band ligation of bleeding and prolapsed internal hemorrhoids. Barron reported excellent results in 150 patients; all but seven patients were treated in the outpatient department. Rubber band ligation has proved to be a simple, quick, and effective nonoperative means of treating grades 1 and 2 and selected cases of grades 3 and 4 hemorrhoids (31–34).

The procedure is performed in the office. An enema or a laxative is not necessary. Sedation is also unnecessary. Although others have used rubber band ligation without problems in patients who have been taking aspirin, nonsteroidal anti-inflammatory drugs, or anticoagulants, I ask patients to refrain from these medications at least one week before and two weeks after the procedure. Two rubber bands are used on each drum in case one breaks. The procedure is performed through an anoscope using a rubber band ligator (see Figs. 10 and 11 of Chapter 3). The bands should be placed on the redundant rectal mucosa at the top of the internal hemorrhoids (Fig. 3) (25,35). The external hemorrhoids must be left alone. Traditionally, the ligation is performed at one site at a time. Iyer et al. (36) reported a retrospective series of 805 patients who underwent a single RBL from grades 1 to 4, with a median follow-up of 3.3 years; many return for subsequent RBL (mean 2, range 1–17) with a median time between bandings of 4.7 weeks. The success for improvement of symptoms was 70.5%. The success rates were similar for all grades of hemorrhoids although the patients who required the placement of four or more bands was associated with a trend in higher failure rates and greater need for subsequent hemorrhoidectomy. Complications per treatment series included bleeding (2.8%), thrombosed external hemorrhoids (1.5%), and bacteremia (0.09%). Higher bleeding rates were encountered with the use of aspirin and nonsteroidal anti-inflammatory drugs and warfarin. Ligations of more than one site in a single session have been practiced by many authors with apparently no higher complications than a single site (31,32,37–39). The advantage of multiple applications is that it is more cost effective and one may speculate that the requirement for subsequent bandings may be less.

For grades 3 and 4 hemorrhoids, and for patients with deep cheeks of the buttocks, I prefer to inject the upper anal canal (5 mm above the dentate line) with 1.5 mL each of 0.25% Bupivacaine containing 1:200,000 epinephrine in four quadrants instead of injecting the anesthetic solution into the banded hemorrhoidal tissue as described by Law and Chu (39). This can be performed without pain and the

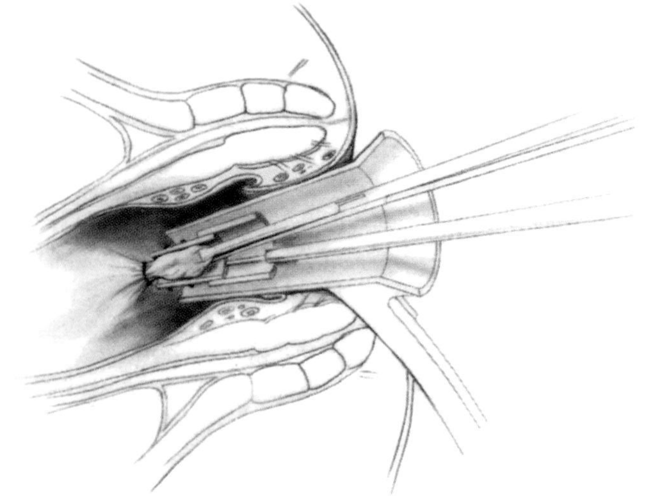

FIGURE 3 ■ Rubber band ligation. Note banding of rectal mucosa just above the apex of the internal hemorrhoid.

entire anal canal is completely relaxed giving patients comfort and making the exposure excellent for the procedure. The key of success in banding severe prolapse is to ligate the redundant rectal mucosa just above the internal hemorrhoids as many sites as required in a single session. I agree with Thomson (40) that rubber band ligation can be performed in most patients with whatever "degree" of their hemorrhoids and that hemorrhoidectomy is seldom required.

Success rates of RBL vary, depending on the grade of hemorrhoids treated, length of follow-up, and the criteria for success. The reported successes range from 80% to 89%. The recurrences at 4–5 years of follow-up is as high as 68% but symptoms usually respond to repeat ligations; only 10% of such patients require excised hemorrhoidectomy (41). The most common complication of RBL is pain, which is reported in 5–60% of treated patients (41,42). Pain following the procedure is usually minor and almost always can be satisfactorily managed with warm sitz baths and over-the-counter analgesics. Immediate severe or progressive pain is an indication of a misplaced rubber band ligation—one that is too close to the dentate line and requires immediate removal. Severe bleeding occasionally requires intervention when the eschar from the band sloughs, usually 1–2 weeks after treatment.

There has been concern about the safety of rubber band ligation because of reports of deaths resulting from acute perianal sepsis (43,44). The clues to severe anal and perianal infection after rubber band ligation are a triad of symptoms: delayed anal pain, urinary retention, and fever (45). Acute awareness of this rare but potentially life-threatening complication is essential, and immediate aggressive treatment is mandatory to prevent death (46,47). Treatment should include administration of antibiotics, drainage of an abscess (if present), and excision of necrotic tissues (if present). Because of possible severe complications, rubber band ligation never should be performed in patients with immunodeficiencies. This procedure could be disastrous in those who have tested positive for the human immunodeficiency virus (HIV) (48).

Infrared Photocoagulation

The infrared photocoagulator produces infrared radiation (Fig. 4). It coagulates tissue protein or evaporates water in the cells, depending on the intensity and duration of application. The unit has an infrared probe that is applied just proximal to the internal hemorrhoids through an anoscope. The recommendation is to use a duration of 1.5 seconds and repeat three times on each hemorrhoid. Infrared photocoagulation does not cause tissue necrosis because of the small amount of heat delivered. It is useful to coagulate the friable blood vessels in first-degree hemorrhoids, but it is not effective in the treatment of second- or third-degree hemorrhoids in which tissue destruction is required. Infrared photocoagulation seldom causes pain or other complications (49). It is not widely used among colon and rectal surgeons.

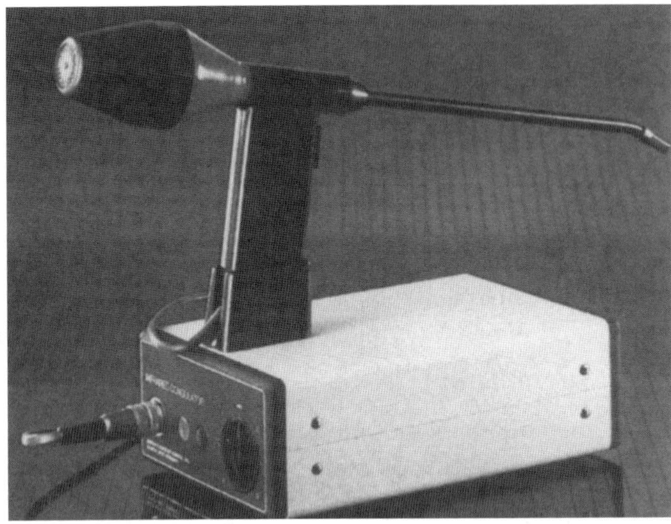

FIGURE 4 ■ Infrared photocoagulation device.

Electrocoagulation

Bipolar (Bicap) coagulation was introduced only recently. This is electrocautery in which heat does not penetrate as deeply as with monopolar electrocoagulation. Its effect is similar to that of infrared photocoagulation, and it is simple to use on an outpatient basis.

Direct current therapy (Ultroit) has been available for several years. The current is applied through a probe placed via an anoscope onto the mucosa at the apex of the hemorrhoid. The current is set to the maximal tolerable level and continued for 10 minutes. Because it is time consuming compared with other simple methods, direct current therapy never has become a popular method. Both methods can be used to treat first- and second-degree hemorrhoids, but some authors have found them effective for treating third-degree hemorrhoids as well (50).

I personally use the ball-tip or spatula-tip monopolar electrocoagulation as an alternative treatment to rubber band ligation in the treatment of second- and early third-degree hemorrhoids. The equipment is readily available in any colon and rectal clinic. The key to success is to coagulate the tops of the internal hemorrhoids until they are charred. The mucosa will be ulcerated as in rubber band ligation and fixed onto the anorectal ring. Because of extensive vascularity, the degree of electrocoagulation must be rather extensive to produce the desired destruction of the submucosa.

Sclerotherapy

The rationale of injecting chemical agents into hemorrhoids is to create fibrosis so that prolapse cannot occur. The solutions used are phenol in oil, quinine urea, and sodium morrhuate. The injection must be made into the submucosa above the internal hemorrhoid at the anorectal ring and not intravascularly. Sclerotherapy formerly was the treatment of choice for grades 1 and 2 hemorrhoids, particularly in the United Kingdom (25,29). It has gradually decreased in popularity in favor of the more effective electrocoagulation and rubber band ligation. Sclerotherapy usually produces dull pain, lasting up to 48 hours. Although it rarely occurs, misplacement of the injection can lead to mucosal ulceration and necrosis. A case of necrotizing fasciitis after injection sclerotherapy for hemorrhoids requiring debridement and defunctioning colostomy has been reported (51).

Anal Stretch

In 1968, Lord reported treating hemorrhoids by manual dilatation of the anus. The procedure is based on the belief that hemorrhoids constitute a reversible condition caused by narrowing of the lower anal canal, leading to abnormal straining that causes venous congestion and eventually hemorrhoids. The narrowing is caused by a fibrous deposit that Lord called the "pecten band." The procedure is performed for grade 3 hemorrhoids. With the patient under intravenous sedation or general anesthesia, the anal canal is stretched maximally until the bands give way. It is usually necessary to stretch the anal canal and the lower rectum until four fingers from each hand are inserted (52). An anal dilator is provided for use at home by patients for the next six months to prevent recurrent anal stenosis. Lord claims that pain and complications are low, and Lord has had no patients with problems of anal incontinence after this treatment. In a trial comparing the results of maximal anal dilatation and hemorrhoidectomy, Lewis et al. (53) found that maximal anal dilatation has good short-term results, but in the long term some patients develop symptoms that require hemorrhoidectomy. Maximal anal dilatation is now rarely performed because of concern about anal incontinence and mucosal prolapse. Another disadvantage of maximal anal dilatation is that the associated external hemorrhoids and skin tags are not treated.

Cryotherapy

Cryotherapy once was advocated by many surgeons who claimed that the procedure produced excellent results, with little pain and few complications. Cryotherapy is based on the concept that freezing at low temperature can destroy the hemorrhoidal tissues. The freezing temperature is achieved by using a special probe through which nitrous oxide at –60°C to –80°C or liquid nitrogen at –196°C is circulated. A study by Smith et al. (54) showed that profuse discharge associated with a foul smell and irritation from the necrosis were the rule. The procedure involves pain, and the healing time is very long. If cryotherapy is not performed properly, destruction of the anal sphincter muscle can cause anal stenosis and incontinence. This technique has fallen into disrepute and should be abandoned.

Lateral Internal Sphincterotomy

Lateral internal sphincterotomy is used widely for the management of patients with anal fissures in whom the underlying problem is thought to be one of "hyperfunction" of the internal anal sphincter. Some authorities claim that similar dysfunction accounts for the occurrence of hemorrhoidal diseases (55,56). Consequently, partial internal sphincterotomy has been advocated to overcome this abnormality. Sun et al. (15) dispute this theory. Combined manometric and ultrasonographic studies of the internal anal sphincter, together with a direct measurement of the anal cushions, revealed that the high anal canal pressure in patients with hemorrhoids is due to high pressure of the anal cushions. The thickness of the internal sphincter is not significantly different from the normal subjects.

Unlike maximal anal dilatation, partial internal sphincterotomy has the advantage of precise division of the sphincter under direct vision. This operation can be performed with the patient under local, regional, or general anesthesia. Incontinence to varying degrees occurs in 25% of patients and is minor in most instances. Prolapse of redundant mucosa is common and usually requires further treatment. Recurrence of symptoms occurs in only 5% of patients (55). This procedure has no effect on external hemorrhoids and skin tags. Postoperative care is simple and is aimed at providing patient comfort and ensuring an early bowel movement.

Although it is a relatively simple technique, partial internal sphincterotomy for the routine treatment of hemorrhoids has not gained general acceptance, but it does have its advocates. In patients with an anal fissure accompanying hemorrhoids or in patients with evidence of a hyperactive sphincter, partial internal sphincterotomy should be part of the therapy undertaken. In a series by Schouten and van Vroonhoven (56), hemorrhoids associated with high anal pressure (>125 cmH_2O) were treated by a lateral internal sphincterotomy under local anesthesia on an outpatient basis. Evaluation of the results six months after the operation showed that 78% of patients with grades 1 and 2 hemorrhoids and 65% of patients with grades 3 and 4 hemorrhoids had excellent or satisfactory results. In spite of the reported excellent results (57), lateral internal sphincterotomy is not considered a standard treatment for hemorrhoids.

HEMORRHOIDECTOMY

Hemorrhoidectomy should be considered when (1) hemorrhoids are severely prolapsed and require manual replacement, (2) patients fail to improve after multiple applications of nonoperative treatments, or (3) hemorrhoids are complicated by associated pathology, such as ulceration, fissure, fistula, large hypertrophied anal papilla, or extensive skin tags. The choice of anesthesia should be individualized. In the majority of cases, hemorrhoidectomy can be performed with the patient under local anesthesia combined with mild sedation. However, in patients with high cheeks of the buttocks, especially in muscular or obese men, using a general or regional block anesthetic is preferable (58). Ultimately, the choice of anesthetic should be made by the patient. Even with general or regional anesthesia, the entire anal canal should be injected with 0.25% bupivacaine (Marcaine) or 0.5% lidocaine (Xylocaine) containing 1:200,000 epinephrine, mainly for hemostatic purposes. I prefer to empty the colon with a laxative such as sodium phosphate 45 mL mixed with three or more glasses of Gatorade or other sport drink the evening before the operation. In this way, the patient does not require a bowel movement for three or four days. Prophylactic antibiotics are not administered. Most hemorrhoidectomies can be performed on an outpatient basis (59).

CLOSED HEMORRHOIDECTOMY

In 1931, Fansler (60) described a technique of hemorrhoidectomy in which the dissection was conducted in an anatomic method (intra-anal anatomic dissection). The

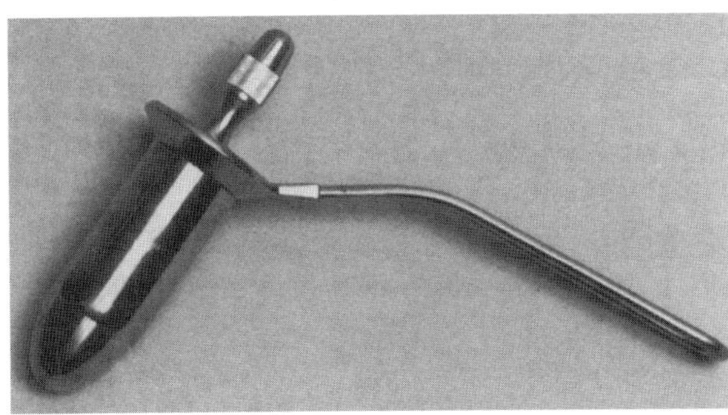

FIGURE 5 ■ Fansler anal speculum measuring 3 cm in diameter, 7 cm in working length.

key to this technique is using the Fansler anal speculum (Fig. 5), which is 3 cm in diameter and 7 cm long. The entire hemorrhoidal tissues, along with the redundant skin, can be dissected easily in their normal anatomic location. There is no need to pull the hemorrhoidal pedicle toward the anus for suturing because the exposure is excellent all the way to the apex of the wound. Thus, prolapse of rectal mucosa or ectropion is almost unknown with this technique. I favor this technique with some modification and have used it with great satisfaction.

Technique

The procedure is performed with the patient in the prone jack-knife position with the cheeks of the buttocks taped apart. Using Lilly Tonsil scissors (V. Mueller Co., McGaw Park, Illinois, U.S.A.), an elliptical excision is begun at the perianal skin to include external and internal hemorrhoids and is ended at the anorectal ring. During the excision, the scissors is pressed firmly on the anal wall. This technique allows excision of a full thickness of mucosa and submucosa without injury to the underlying internal sphincter muscle. The strip of the excision should not be wider than 1.5 cm. Since it is easy to inadvertently cut too high, the top of the internal hemorrhoid should be marked with electrocautery. Unless there is an associated anal stenosis or an anal fissure, internal sphincterotomy is not performed. The entire wound is closed with a running 3–0 chromic catgut suture or a rapid absorbable synthetic suture, 2 mm apart. It is important to use a three-point stitch at the apex of the wound to avoid a mass effect, which can cause a tenesmus (Fig. 6). If too much tissue has been excised, the wound should be marsupialized and left open. The largest and most redundant hemorrhoid should be excised first. With this approach, the original plan to excise three quadrants may be modified so that only a two-quadrant hemorrhoidectomy is necessary. I believe that some anal cushion should be preserved to maintain good anal continence (21), particularly when patients approach the fifth and sixth decades of life. Ideally, the hemorrhoidectomy excision should not be performed in the posterior commissure unless plastic flap procedures are planned, because in this location the wound heals slowly and has a greater tendency to form a fissure.

Ideally, all excised tissues should be labeled properly and submitted separately for microscopic examination. Rarely, unsuspected malignancy or inflammatory bowel

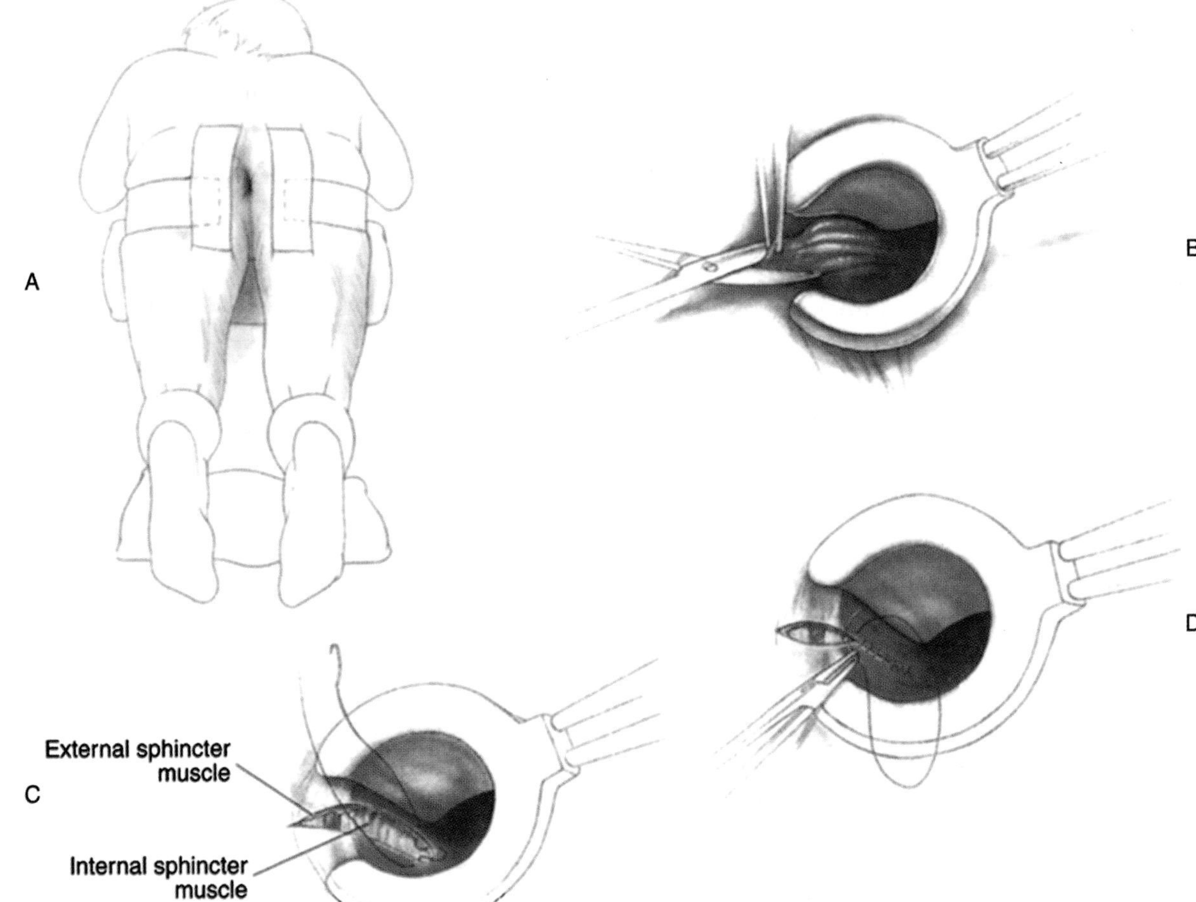

FIGURE 6 ■ Technique of closed hemorrhoidectomy. (**A**) Prone jackknife position. (**B**) Elliptical excision starting at the perianal skin and continuing to the anorectal ring. (**C**) Three-point stitch at the apex of the wound to avoid a mass effect. (**D**) Closure of wound with running 3–0 catgut sutures.

disease may be so diagnosed. Cataldo and MacKeigan (61) reported only one instance of unsuspected anal carcinoma out of 21,257 hemorrhoidectomies. No further treatment is required for the incidental carcinoma found in an excised specimen provided the rest of the anal canal has no high grade and intraepithelial neoplasia (62) (see the section on "Anal Canal Intraepithelial Neoplasia" in Chapter 18).

■ OTHER TYPES OF HEMORRHOIDECTOMY

Excision and Ligation

The procedure known as excision and ligation, also called open hemorrhoidectomy, was originated by Frederick Salmon, the founder of St. Mark's Hospital, London, in the 1830s (63). Milligan et al. popularized and modified the technique, which is widely used in the United Kingdom as well as throughout the world (64–66).

Technique

The procedure is performed with the patient in the lithotomy position. The anal canal is gently dilated with two fingers, and forceps are placed on the perianal skin just outside the mucocutaneous junction at each primary hemorrhoid. As the internal hemorrhoids are pulled down, a second forceps is put onto the main bulk of each hemorrhoidal mass, producing the "triangle of exposure." The hemorrhoid is excised from the underlying sphincter muscle. The dissection is carried out proximally as far as the pedicles, where it is stick-tied with 3–0 chromic catgut. The rest of the wound is left open, and a light dressing is applied to the wound. Other hemorrhoids are treated in a similar manner.

Modified Whitehead Hemorrhoidectomy

In 1882, Whitehead (67) of Manchester, England, described a technique for hemorrhoidectomy. A circular incision was made at the level of the dentate line. The submucosal and subdermal hemorrhoidal tissues then were dissected out. The redundant rectal mucosa was excised and sutured to the anoderm. Although Whitehead called this operation simple, Allingham (63) thought that the operation was rather difficult to perform properly; it was bloody, and the patient was prone to stricture, loss of sensation, and development of ectropion. The technique soon fell out of favor in the United Kingdom, but it has attracted the attention of some surgeons in the United States, where it has been revived with some modifications (68,69).

Technique

The procedure for the modified Whitehead hemorrhoidectomy is performed with the patient in the prone position. Exposure of the anal canal is by the Buie self-retaining anal retractor. An incision is made at the level of the dentate line in one quadrant, and a flap of anoderm is raised. The submucosal and subdermal hemorrhoidal plexuses are excised, and the redundant rectal mucosa is excised transversely. The flap of anoderm is advanced proximally and sutured to the rectal mucosa. Hemorrhoids in other quadrants are removed in a similar manner. The key to the success of this modified technique is suturing the flap of anoderm to the mucosa in the upper anal canal rather than pulling the mucosa down to the anoderm at the dentate line. In a long-term follow-up of 484 patients in the series reported by Wolff and Culp (69), there were no recurrences or ectropions. The cited advantage of this operation is for treatment of extensive circumferential hemorrhoids, but I believe that this procedure should be performed only by surgeons who are thoroughly familiar with the technique.

Laser Hemorrhoidectomy

Laser therapy has been used with success in some patients for the treatment of polyps and rectal carcinomas, although its indications and necessity are quite limited. Laser also has been used for performing hemorrhoidectomy, but reports in the literature are extremely limited. Yu and Eddy (70) reported excellent success with Nd:YAG laser hemorrhoidectomy performed in 134 patients. The procedure was performed on an outpatient basis. Iwagaki et al. (71) reported on 1816 patients who underwent CO_2 laser hemorrhoidectomy with excellent results. These were not controlled studies and are impossible to compare with conventional hemorrhoidectomy.

Senagore et al. (72) conducted a randomized study of the results using the Nd:YAG laser versus a scalpel in the treatment of third- and fourth-degree hemorrhoids, using the closed Ferguson hemorrhoidectomy. The study involved 51 and 35 patients treated with the laser or a scalpel, respectively. The two groups were similar with respect to hospital stay, requirements for parenteral and oral analgesics, as well as time off work. There was a greater degree of wound inflammation and dehiscence at the 10-day postoperative visit for the laser group ($p < 0.05$). The use of the laser was also more expensive. A prospective study by Leff (73) included 170 patients and 56 patients who underwent a closed hemorrhoidectomy using a CO_2 laser or a scalpel, respectively. Outpatient surgery was performed in 72% of the cases studied. There was no difference in postoperative pain, wound healing, and postoperative complications such as urinary retention, bleeding, and fecal impaction in the two groups studied.

At one time, the public demand for laser hemorrhoidectomy was great because of hearsay and rumors that laser hemorrhoidectomy resulted in less pain and produced better results than conventional hemorrhoidectomy. To date, there has been no documentation for such claims.

SPECIAL SITUATIONS

■ THROMBOSED EXTERNAL HEMORRHOIDS

Thrombosed external hemorrhoids are a fairly common complication of hemorrhoidal disease. The condition usually occurs without a known cause. Most patients give no history of straining or physical exertion and do not have a history of hemorrhoidal disease. The typical patient's history is that of a painful mass in the perianal area. The pain usually is described as burning rather than throbbing, and its degree depends on the size of the thrombus. Histopathologic studies reveal an intravascular thrombus of the capillaries that can be stretched to 1 cm in diameter or larger (Fig. 7). The thrombus is confined to the anoderm and does not cross proximally beyond the dentate line.

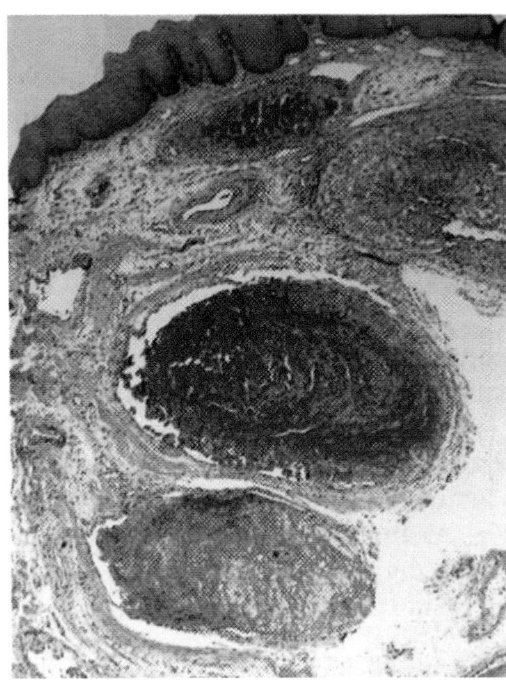

FIGURE 7 ■ Intravascular thrombus in thrombosed external hemorrhoids. Note the greatly dilated capillaries.

The natural history of thrombosed external hemorrhoids is an abrupt onset of an anal mass and pain that peaks within 48 hours. The pain becomes minimal after the fourth day. If left alone, the thrombus will shrink and dissolve in a few weeks. Occasionally, the skin overlying the thrombus becomes necrotic, causing bleeding and discharge or infection, which may cause further necrosis and more pain. A large thrombus can result in a skin tag.

Since thrombosed external hemorrhoids are self-limited, the treatment should be aimed at relief of severe pain, prevention of recurrent thromboses, and residual skin tags. If the patient has intense pain, excision should be offered. On the other hand, if the pain already is subsiding and the thrombosed hemorrhoid has started to shrink, it is wise to manage it nonoperatively (Fig. 8). Management includes prescribing a nonconstipating analgesic drug, warm sitz baths for comfort, proper anal hygiene, and bulk-producing agents such as bran or psyllium seed. Suppositories have not proved helpful in treating this condition.

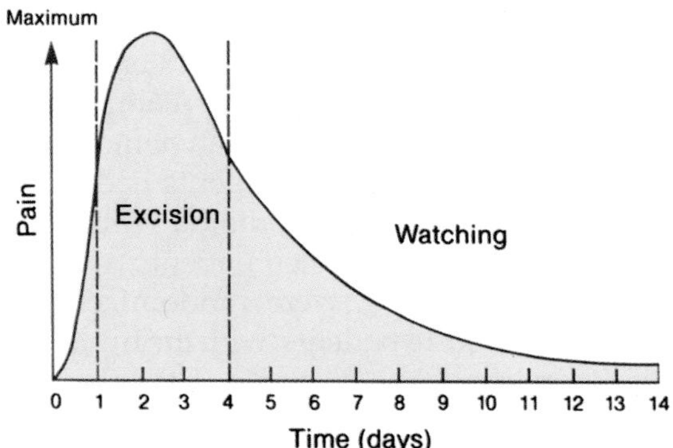

FIGURE 8 ■ The timing of excision of a thrombosed external hemorrhoid.

Proctoscopy or flexible sigmoidoscopy is performed to rule out associated anorectal disease. The procedure can be performed at the time the patient is evaluated initially if the examination can be carried out without undue pain, but usually it is postponed to a later date.

Since the thromboses are intravascular and frequently multiple, the entire thrombus must be excised. The procedure can be performed in the office, clinic, or emergency department with local anesthetic (0.25% bupivacaine containing 1:200,000 epinephrine). It is best to anesthetize the entire anal canal so that a large Hill–Ferguson anal speculum can be used for the exposure. Excising the skin along with the mass is not necessary nor is it desirable. Instead, an incision is made over the mass, and the thrombus can be easily dissected out with a scissors. Excessive skin is trimmed, and the wound is closed with running or interrupted 3–0 chromic catgut or a rapidly absorbable synthetic suture (Fig. 9). The relief of pain usually is immediate provided the wound is closed without tension. Postoperative care, which is simple, is aimed at keeping the wound clean by washing. Warm sitz baths of 10–15 minutes three to four times daily are used only for throbbing pain. An analgesic drug is usually required during the first 24 hours. Excision of thrombosed external hemorrhoids under local anesthesia has been found to have good results (74).

Greenspon et al. (75) retrospectively studied 231 patients with thrombosed external hemorrhoids. Fifty-one percent were managed conservatively; this generally includes sitz bath, dietary changes, stool softeners, and oral and topical analgesics. Forty-nine percent were managed surgically with excision of the thrombosis. The mean follow-up was 7.6 months (up to seven years). The rate of follow-up was 38% for conservative group versus 82% for the surgical group ($p < 0.0001$). Pain was found to be the primary complaint in 99% of the surgical group versus 90% of those managed conservatively ($p < 0.001$).

Time to symptom resolution was 24 days for conservatively managed group versus four days for surgically managed group ($p < 0.001$). The frequency of recurrence was significantly higher for conservative group (25% vs. 6%; $p < 0.001$). Mean time to recurrence was seven months in the conservative group versus 25 months in the surgical group ($p < 0.001$). This study showed that most patients treated conservatively would experience resolution of their symptoms. Excision of thrombosed external hemorrhoids results in more rapid symptom resolution, lower incidence of recurrence, and longer remission intervals.

A conservative treatment of thrombosed external hemorrhoids has been successful using nifedipine gel. Perrotti et al. (76) conducted a prospective, randomized trial of 90 patients. Patients treated with nifedipine ($n = 46$) received topical 0.3% nifedipine and 1.5% lidocaine gel every 12 hours for two weeks. The control group, consisting of 44 patients, received 1.5% lidocaine and 1% hydrocortisone acetate gel during the therapy.

The results showed that relief of pain occurred in 85% in nifedipine group as opposed to 50% of controls after seven days of therapy ($p < 0.01$); oral analgesics were used by 9% of patients in nifedipine group as opposed to 55% of the control group ($p < 0.01$); resolution of thrombosed external hemorrhoids occurred after 14 days of therapy in 91% of nifedipine-treated patients, as opposed to 45% of the controls

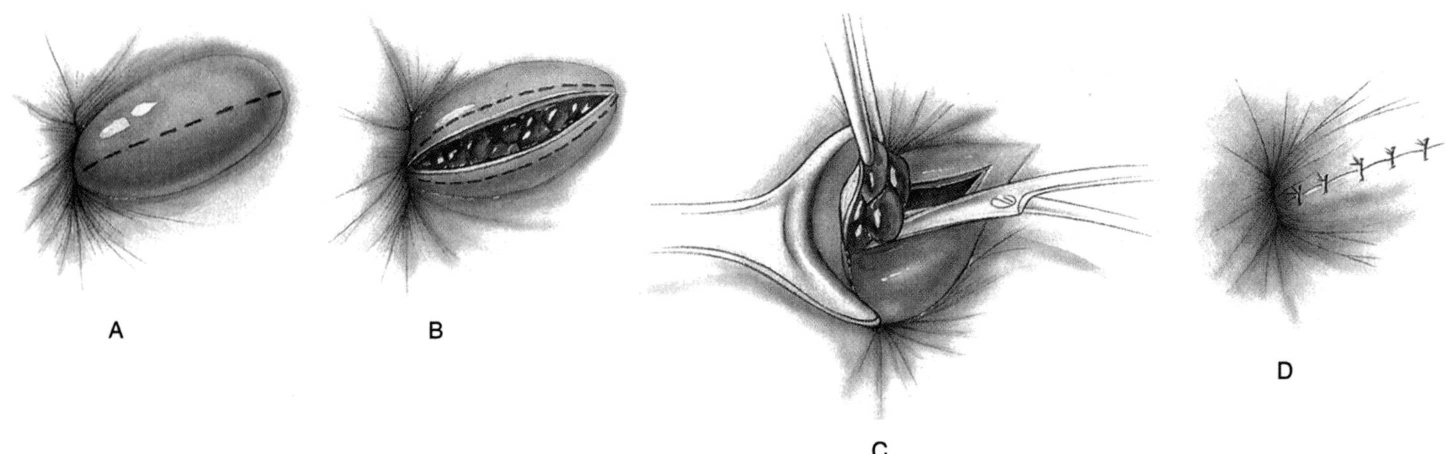

FIGURE 9 ■ Thrombosed external hemorrhoid. (**A**) Line of incision. (**B**) Subcutaneous intravascular blood clots are exposed. (**C**) Lobulated blood clots are dissected with scissors. Note the Hill–Ferguson anal speculum used for exposure. (**D**) Closure of wound with running or interrupted 3–0 chromic catgut or rapidly absorbable synthetic sutures.

($p < 0.01$). No systemic side effects or significant anorectal bleeding were observed in patients treated with nifedipine.

Nifedipine, a hydropiridine, is a calcium antagonist administered only orally for cardiovascular disorders. The effect of topical nifedipine gel is the relaxation of the internal sphincter to relieve pain and improve anodermal blood flow. Other effect may include an anti-inflammatory action (76).

■ STRANGULATED HEMORRHOIDS

Strangulated hemorrhoids arise from prolapsed grades 3 or 4 hemorrhoids that have become irreducible because of swelling (Fig. 10). The patient's history will reveal long-standing hemorrhoidal prolapse on straining. On examination, it is easy to see marked edema of both external and internal hemorrhoids everting through the anus.

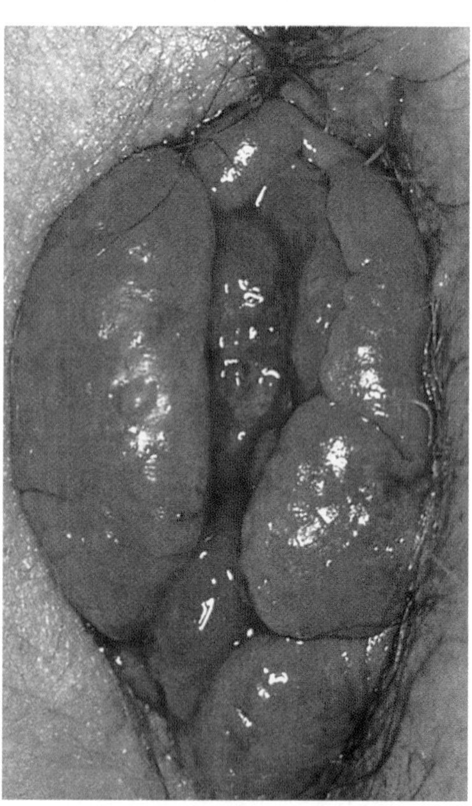

FIGURE 10 ■ Strangulated hemorrhoids.

If untreated, the edema may progress to ulceration and necrosis. Pain is usually severe, and urinary retention is occasionally seen.

Proper treatment requires urgent or emergent hemorrhoidectomy. Because of the severe prolapse, it is usually easy to anesthetize the anal canal with the patient under local anesthesia without causing undue pain. The operation should be performed in the operating room or an ambulatory surgical center. In the presence of a circumferential protrusion, only a standard three-quadrant hemorrhoidectomy is necessary. Unless the tissues are necrotic, mucosa and skin can be closed as in elective hemorrhoidectomy. The patient should be admitted to the hospital after the hemorrhoidectomy and should remain until the pain is minimal or until spontaneous voiding is possible. An antibiotic is not indicated. Hemorrhoidectomy in the presence of strangulation and necrosis is a safe procedure provided that all necrotic tissue is excised (77–79).

Another approach to acute hemorrhoidal disease is to excise only the large blood clots of the external hemorrhoids and incise any large internal clots. All internal hemorrhoids that are prolapsed and reduced are ligated with multiple rubber bandings. The procedure can be performed under local anesthesia. It is important to massage and squeeze the edematous anal tissues until collapse before undertaking any excision or incision if necessary, and banding. When properly performed, the relief is immediate, and later hemorrhoidectomy is seldom necessary (80–82).

Brown et al. (83) conducted a rare study of stapled hemorrhoidopexy on acute strangulated hemorrhoids. This was a prospective randomized study comparing stapled hemorrhoidopexy to a Milligan Morgan hemorrhoidectomy carried out with diathermy. The patients had circumferential, edematous prolapsed hemorrhoids with no evidence of infection or necrosis. Seventeen patients, with mean age of 44 years (range, 32–77), were randomized to stapled hemorrhoidopexy and 18 patients, with mean age of 46 years (range, 16–60), to conventional group. The procedures were performed under general anesthesia within 24 hours of admission. In the stapled group, the thrombosed or the edema was not excised or decompressed. In the conventional group, all of the patients underwent removal of at least three hemorrhoids. No antibiotic was used on either group. The mean postoperative stay was two days in both groups.

The results showed that there was more pain in the immediate postoperative period in the stapled group, with the score of 5 (range, 2–10) compared to 1 (range, 0–10) in the conventional group ($p < 0.02$). However, at two weeks and at six weeks postoperatively, there was no pain in the stapled group compared to the pain score of 5.5 and 5, respectively, in the conventional group ($p < 0.05$). The days off work was 14 days in the stapled group compared to 28 days in the conventional group ($p < 0.05$).

It should be no surprise that the stapled group had more pain in the immediate postoperative period since the authors did not remove the large blood clots or decompress the edematous tissues. These painful masses were probably squeezed by the anal sphincters when they were drawn up as the result of the stapled hemorrhoidopexy. Other than this, the overall results were better in the stapled group.

■ HEMORRHOIDS IN PREGNANCY

Hemorrhoidal symptoms commonly occur and intensify during pregnancy and delivery. In most instances, however, hemorrhoids that intensify during delivery resolve. Hemorrhoidectomy is indicated during pregnancy only if acute prolapse and thrombosis occur. It should be performed with the patient under local anesthesia. In the second and third trimester, a left anterolateral position can be used (84).

Prolapse and thrombosis of hemorrhoids occurring during delivery is an indication for operation in the immediate postpartum period. Similarly, operation is indicated for patients in whom hemorrhoidal disease has been symptomatic before pregnancy, is aggravated during pregnancy, and persists after delivery. In such patients, hemorrhoidectomy is performed best in the immediate postpartum period. Most patients have relief of symptoms the day after the operation (85).

Abramowitz et al. (86) prospectively studied 165 pregnant women during the last three months of pregnancy and after delivery (within two months). Patients underwent perineal and proctoscopic examinations. The results showed that 13 patients (8%) developed external hemorrhoids before delivery. The problems were more frequently observed in females with constipation ($p = 0.023$) than those without constipation.

Thirty-three patients (26%) developed thrombosed external hemorrhoids after delivery; 30 patients (91%) of the external hemorrhoids were observed during the first day after delivery. Constipation and late deliveries were independent risk factors. The most important risk factor was constipation, with an odds ratio of 5.7 (95% CI, 2.7–12). Mild laxatives such as milk of magnesia should be given during the last three months of pregnancy and postpartum period for patients with constipation problems. Late delivery had an odds ratio of 1.4 (95% CI, 1.05–1.9). Patients who delivered after 39.7 weeks of pregnancy were more likely to have thrombosed external hemorrhoids than those who delivered before that time. Traumatic deliveries, such as perineal tear and heavy babies, were associated with thrombosed external hemorrhoids. Cesarean section appears to protect against this problem.

■ HEMORRHOIDS, ANORECTAL VARICES, AND PORTAL HYPERTENSION

The superior rectal vein becomes the inferior mesenteric vein, which drains the upper anal canal, where the internal hemorrhoidal plexus is located, and the rectum into the portal vein. The inferior rectal vein drains the lower part of the anal canal, where the external hemorrhoidal plexus is located, into the internal iliac vein, whereas the middle rectal veins drain the lower part of the rectum and the upper part of the anal canal into the internal iliac veins. Portal hypertension in most patients results in the development of esophagogastric varices that are associated with massive upper gastrointestinal bleeding. Anorectal varices, on the other hand, constitute another collateral pathway in decompressing the portal system into the systemic circulation through the middle and inferior rectal veins (see Fig. 18 of Chapter 1).

Anorectal varices in portal hypertension are quite common. Chawla and Dilawari (87) used a flexible sigmoidoscope to study 72 consecutive patients with portal hypertension, 47 with noncirrhotic portal hypertension (portal vein fibrosis and external hepatic portal vein obstruction), and 25 with cirrhotic portal hypertension (alcoholic, hepatitis B, or cryptogenic). Anorectal varices were observed in 78% of patients studied (89% in noncirrhotic patients and 56% in cirrhotic patients) ($p < 0.01$). Significantly, more patients with noncirrhotic portal hypertension or extrahepatic vein obstruction had large anorectal varices (>5 mm) compared with cirrhotic patients ($p < 0.05$). Esophageal varices were detected in 97% of the patients. Large esophageal varices were significantly more common in patients with noncirrhotic portal hypertension and extrahepatic portal vein obstruction than in cirrhotic patients. None of the patients studied had varices in the sigmoid or descending colon.

In a prospective study by Hosking et al. (6) of 100 consecutive patients with cirrhosis, 44% had anorectal varices, 19% in cirrhotic patients without portal hypertension compared with 59% in those with portal hypertension. This is less than the 78% reported by Chawla and Dilawari (87), probably because of the small numbers of extrahepatic vein obstruction. The presence of anorectal varices probably reflects the later stage in the development of portal hypertension. This is supported by the fact that patients with large esophageal varices have more frequent anorectal varices than patients with small or no esophageal varices. Moreover, the incidence of anorectal varices is significantly higher in patients who have upper gastrointestinal bleeding, which, as a complication, occurs later in the course of portal hypertension (87).

Unlike esophageal varices, anorectal varices rarely bleed. In a large series by Johnson et al. (88), massive bleeding from anorectal varices was reported in five of 1100 patients. Hosking et al. (6) observed bleeding anorectal varices in only two of 100 patients with portal hypertension. In the series of Chawla and Dilawari (87), only one patient with extrahepatic portal vein obstruction bled from anorectal varices.

Despite the communication between systemic and portal systems in the anal canal, the incidence of hemorrhoidal disease in patients with portal hypertension is no greater than in the normal population (5,6). Although massive bleeding from prolapsed hemorrhoids in patients with portal hypertension is uncommon, it can be life threatening. Most commonly it occurs during treatment of encephalopathy, which includes administering nonabsorbable antibiotics along with supplements of potassium. The treatment frequently results in severe diarrhea for the patient. The lining of the anal canal breaks down just below or just above the dentate line, causing a stream of blood. The bleeding can be continuous or intermittent and massive. Anoscopic examination is essential to identify the site of bleeding since proctoscopy or flexible sigmoidoscopy may miss the bleeding point entirely.

Once the bleeding site has been located, the anal canal is anesthetized with 0.25% bupivacaine (Marcaine) containing 1:200,000 epinephrine. A Pratt anal speculum is used to expose the anal canal and a stick-tie figure-of-eight suture of 3–0 synthetic absorbable material is placed (89). The suture must incorporate the mucosa, submucosa, and internal sphincter to arrest the bleeding as well as fix the prolapse. It is important to correct the coagulopathy and control the diarrhea. The anorectal tissues in patients with portal hypertension are engorged and friable. The sutured tissue may slough and necrose several days later, causing secondary bleeding, particularly if coagulopathy persists. In such cases, resuturing is indicated. Hemorrhoidectomy should be reserved for the rare situation in which the stick-tie method fails to control the bleeding. If more than one area is involved, excising the hemorrhoids one quadrant at a time has been recommended (90).

It is possible to rubber band ligated prolapsed hemorrhoids to patients with liver cirrhosis. Konborozos et al. (38) performed multiple bandings in one session to 16 patients with grades 2 and 3 hemorrhoids and with portal hypertension. Six of these patients also had coagulopathy. There was no complications after the bandings.

Bleeding hemorrhoids in patients with portal hypertension must be distinguished from anorectal varices, a true consequence of portal hypertension. Anorectal varices occur in any of three specific zones: the perianal area, anal canal, and rectum (91). The term "anorectal varices" is used because varices have always been present in the anal canal and occasionally extend into the rectum. The site of bleeding is usually at the squamous portion of the anal canal. There are several methods of treatment for bleeding from anorectal varices. Hosking and Johnson (91) successfully used running sutures of synthetic absorbable sutures starting as high as possible in the rectum and continuing to just outside the anus. Usually three to four columns are sutured. This method successfully arrested the bleeding in 13 patients with a median follow-up of seven months (range, 1–36 months). Two early and one late episodes of re-bleeding occurred. Biswas et al. (92) reported a case of portal hypertension with anorectal variceal bleeding requiring multiple units of blood transfusion. A stapled hemorrhoidopexy was performed and successfully stopped the anorectal bleeding problem.

Katz et al. (93) reported the first use of a transjugular intrahepatic portosystemic shunt (TIPS) in a patient with repeated bleeding from anorectal varices. Repeated MRI/MR venography of the abdomen and pelvis 24 hours after placement of the TIPS revealed marked decompression of the anorectal varices. Doppler ultrasonography documented hepatopetal flow through the patent shunt. Repeat flexible sigmoidoscopy seven days after the TIPS placement showed a decrease in the size of the anorectal varices. The patient had no recurrent bleeding over the ensuing six months, when the patient died from a refractory pneumonia. An incidental and useful treatment is reported by Yeh and McGuire (94). They treated a patient with portal hypertension from alcoholic cirrhosis who presented with unrelenting massive bleeding from anorectal varices. The varices were ligated without success as was the rectal packing with gauze. Eventually, the patient was explored to determine the probable success of portosystemic shunt placement. However, because of the extremely dense and vascular retroperitoneal scar, it was impossible to accomplish the planned operation. Instead, the inferior mesenteric vein just beneath the level of the pancreas was ligated. The operation was a success. The anorectal varices promptly disappeared, and there was no recurrence in the following seven months.

■ HEMORRHOIDS IN INFLAMMATORY BOWEL DISEASE

Hemorrhoidal problems are uncommon in patients with inflammatory bowel disease. Most anal problems result from perianal irritation and swelling caused by diarrhea rather than from hemorrhoids themselves. In a study at St. Mark's Hospital from 1935 to 1975, 50,000 patients with hemorrhoids were treated (95). Only 66 patients had inflammatory bowel disease, either ulcerative colitis or Crohn's disease. Hemorrhoids can be treated operatively or nonoperatively in patients with ulcerative colitis. In patients with Crohn's disease, the rate of severe complications was high. Six of 20 patients treated for hemorrhoids required proctectomy for complications apparently relating from their treatment. In contrast, Wolkomir and Luchtefeld (96) reported that 15 of 17 patients had the wounds healed within two months after hemorrhoidectomy for quiescent Crohn's disease of the ileum and large bowel. No patient required a proctectomy as the result of the hemorrhoidectomy. These results suggest that treatment of symptomatic hemorrhoids is usually safe in patients with ulcerative colitis, but is only relatively contraindicated in those with Crohn's disease. If necessary, hemorrhoidectomy can be performed if the Crohn's disease is in a quiescent state.

■ HEMORRHOIDS IN LEUKEMIA

Patients with leukemia or lymphoma or other conditions involving immunosuppression may present with hemorrhoidal disease. In these circumstances, treatment is difficult because the risks from operative intervention are great and poor wound healing and abscesses are common.

Although anorectal problems in patients with leukemia are not uncommon, hemorrhoidal problems are rare. In a series reported from Memorial Sloan-Kettering Cancer Center (97) of 2618 patients hospitalized with leukemia, 151 (6%) had anorectal diseases. Of concern were the 54 patients with leukemia and severe neutropenia; the outcome of their management is depicted in Table 1.

It appears that surgery does not increase the mortality in these very high-risk patients, but nevertheless it should be performed as a last resort to relieve pain and sepsis. *Escherichia coli* and *Pseudomonas aeruginosa* are the most

TABLE 1 ■ **Outcome of Operative vs. Nonoperative Management of 54 Patients with Leukemia and Severe Neutropenia**

Type of Management	Anorectal Infection	Anal Fissure	Anal Fistula	Hemorrhoid
Operative (no.)	11	4	3	2
Death	3	0	0	1
Resolved	5	3	3	1
Recurred	3	1	0	0
Nonoperative (no.)	13	12	2	7
Death	5	0	1	0
Resolved	6	11	0	7
Recurred	2	1	1	0

Source: From Ref. 98.

common bacteria isolated from both blood and anorectal cultures (97). Correction of any coexisting coagulation disorder and administration of appropriate antibiotics are important parts of the management of hemorrhoidal disease in that patient population.

Anal infections in these patients lack classical signs of abscess formation. Fever and local pain along with local tenderness are the most common findings (97). The infected area usually has no pus but rather a cavity of necrotic tissue.

■ HEMORRHOIDS WITH OTHER ANORECTAL DISEASES

If hemorrhoids are associated with other anorectal problems such as anal fissure or fistula-in-ano, hemorrhoidectomy combined with sphincterotomy or fistulotomy can be done without significant added morbidity.

EARLY POSTOPERATIVE PROBLEMS

The problems that are of most concern after hemorrhoidectomy are severe pain, urinary retention, bleeding, and fecal impaction. The most common fear of hemorrhoidectomy patients is the pain. There are many ways that can at least minimize it. With proper management, most patients can be released from the hospital a few hours after the operation.

Ketorolac tromethamine (Toradol) injected into the sphincter muscle at the time of hemorrhoidectomy and taken orally during a five-day postoperative period has been shown by O'Donovan et al. (98) to produce pain control as good as that produced by giving subcutaneous morphine sulfate. An added benefit is the elimination of urinary retention. Injection of the anesthetic agent around the hemorrhoids or into the perianal area prolongs the initial pain relief but does not reduce the overall requirement of pain medication (99,100).

Hoff et al. (101) reduced the urinary retention rate during the postoperative period to 0.5%. Their success is unmatched by other reports of 12–17% (72,73). The methods they used include preoperative instruction to patients to be aware of the pelvic discomfort mimicking voiding and to reduce concern and anxiety about voiding. The patient's intravenous fluid is restricted to about 500 mL, and the postoperative fluid intake is also limited. Adequate analgesics are also prescribed, with the first dose taken before the patient is released from the hospital (3–4 hours postoperatively). Warm sitz baths should be begun the evening of surgery and continued at least three times daily for a few days.

Metronidazole, 500 mg orally three times a day for five days, has been shown to combat inflammation or infection and minimize pain (102). This should be prescribed to patients in cases where the closed wound breaks down causing swelling and pain.

Transdermal fentanyl (Duragesic) has been found to be an effective analgesic alternative for postoperative hemorrhoidectomy (103). However, it is important to note that the pharmaceutical company refutes this report and vigorously labels transdermal fentanyl as contraindicated for postoperative pain control. Hypoventilation and death have been reported from its use (104).

Postoperative bleeding within 24–48 hours after surgery is usually from a technical cause. The anal canal is vascular, and bleeding from the raw surface may not stop spontaneously. The hemorrhoidal wounds should be closed with continuous sutures 1–2 mm apart.

Postoperative fecal impaction can be prevented. Taking a bulk-forming agent or stool softener does not guarantee an adequate bowel movement. The patient should be instructed to take a mild laxative such as milk of magnesia 45–60 mL plus one glass of water if the patient has not had a good bowel movement after the second postoperative day or the third day if the patient had a laxative preoperatively.

■ RECOMMENDATIONS FOR A SMOOTH POSTOPERATIVE COURSE

The technical points for a smooth postoperative hemorrhoidectomy begin in the operating room. A well-performed hemorrhoidectomy with attention to detail or "tricks" can make the difference. Most hemorrhoidectomies can be performed as outpatient procedures, or may require an overnight admission.

- Laxative such as sodium phosphate 45 mL the evening before is useful to delay bowel movement postoperatively to the third day.
- Limit intravenous fluid during the operation to 500 mL.
- When suitable, perform hemorrhoidectomy under local anesthesia. Buffer the anesthetic solution to minimize pain in cases of thrombosed external hemorrhoids (see Chapter 5, p. 119).
- Perform hemorrhoidectomy only to treat severe grades 3 and 4 hemorrhoids, including strangulated hemorrhoids. It is unnecessary to do more than three quadrants. Frequently, only one or two quadrants require surgical treatment.
- Avoid hemorrhoidectomy in the posterior midline. It does not heal well.
- Do not excise a strip >1.5 cm in width. The redundant anoderm and mucosa can be trimmed later. Close the wound 1–2 mm from the edges and 1–2 mm apart. Closure with tension causes pain.
- Do not excise the hemorrhoids above the anorectal ring. Higher excision and suturing frequently cause urinary retention.
- Inject the anesthetic agent into the internal sphincter at completion of the procedure, 3 mL in each quadrant. This will delay the pain for a few hours.
- Provide pre-emptive analgesia with Toradol, 30 mg, intramuscularly just before the patient leaves the operating

room. Reduce the dosage to 15 mg in elderly patients. Toradol is contraindicated in patients with impaired renal and hepatic function.

- Prescribe an analgesic to be taken every six hours for 48 hours. Thereafter it can be taken only as needed.
- Take warm sitz baths to relieve the throbbing pain from the anal spasm; do not exceed 10–15 minutes in the bath for more than three days since water tends to macerate the skin causing separation of the wounds. Wash the anal area by hand with water; do not use a washcloth. This should be done at least twice daily and after each bowel movement.
- Encourage the patient to eat a high-fiber diet and drink plenty of fluid. Supplement the diet with a psyllium seed preparation as indicated. If the patient does not have a good bowel movement two days after surgery, or three days after surgery if the patient had preoperative bowel cleansing, give a mild laxative such as milk of magnesia, 30–45 mL, followed by at least one glass of water. Repeat the next day if there is no result. If the problem continues, the patient should call the surgeon. Fecal impaction is one of the most serious complications after hemorrhoidectomy. It is one of the complications that can be prevented.

STAPLED HEMORRHOIDOPEXY

INTRODUCTION

This is a new and innovative procedure to treat the prolapsed hemorrhoids. Although stapled hemorrhoidectomy is the most popular term, it is literally incorrect since the hemorrhoids are not removed. Other terms that appear in the literature are: stapled anopexy, stapled hemorrhoidopexy, circumferential mucosectomy, rectal prolapsectomy, circular hemorrhoidectomy, circumferential stapled anoplasty, stapled rectal mucosectomy. An international working party experienced in performance of the hemorrhoid operation using circular staple was convened in Missillac, France, in July 2001. The expert panel came up with the term stapled hemorrhoidopexy (105).

The procedure is based on the concept that hemorrhoids occur because of the downward protrusion of the anal cushions resulting from the redundant and loose lower rectal mucosa and that the internal hemorrhoids themselves are histologically normal (1). The goal to this procedure is, in fact, not different from rubber band ligation in which the redundant rectal mucosa at the top of the internal hemorrhoid is ligated. Stapled hemorrhoidopexy resects a much larger redundant rectal mucosa and should be performed only in severe grade 3 or 4 hemorrhoids in which multiple rubber band ligations are not suitable.

In 1990, G. Allegra of the University of Florence, Italy, first used a stapler for hemorrhoidal surgery. The submucosal purse-string was placed at the level of the dentate line and the entire hemorrhoids were excised. This technique was subsequently abandoned, in favor of a higher placed purse-string above the internal hemorrhoids (106).

It was Antonio Longo (107) of the University of Palermo, Italy, who popularized the technique of excising the redundant lower rectal mucosa using a circular stapler for the treatment of patients with prolapsed hemorrhoids. Longo's techniques and results were presented to the World Congress of Endoscopic Surgery in Rome, 1998. Longo's description of the technique using the specially designed circular stapler has become the basis for the present practice.

TECHNIQUE

The preparation of the patient is the same as conventional hemorrhoidectomy. The procedure can be performed under local (108,109) or general or regional anesthesia. The positioning of the patient can be either the prone jack-knife or lithotomy.

The equipment came in as a kit, which consists of a 33 mm stapling gun with a nondetachable anvil, a purse-string speculum, a transparent anal dilator with an operator, and a purse-string suture threader or crochet hook (Fig. 11). The anal dilator is inserted into the anal canal and secured in place with heavy sutures to the perianal skin (Fig. 12A). The purse-string speculum is inserted into the anal dilator. By rotating the speculum, a purse-string of 2–0 Prolene is placed in the rectum 4–5 cm above the dentate line in the rectal ampulla (Fig. 12B). It

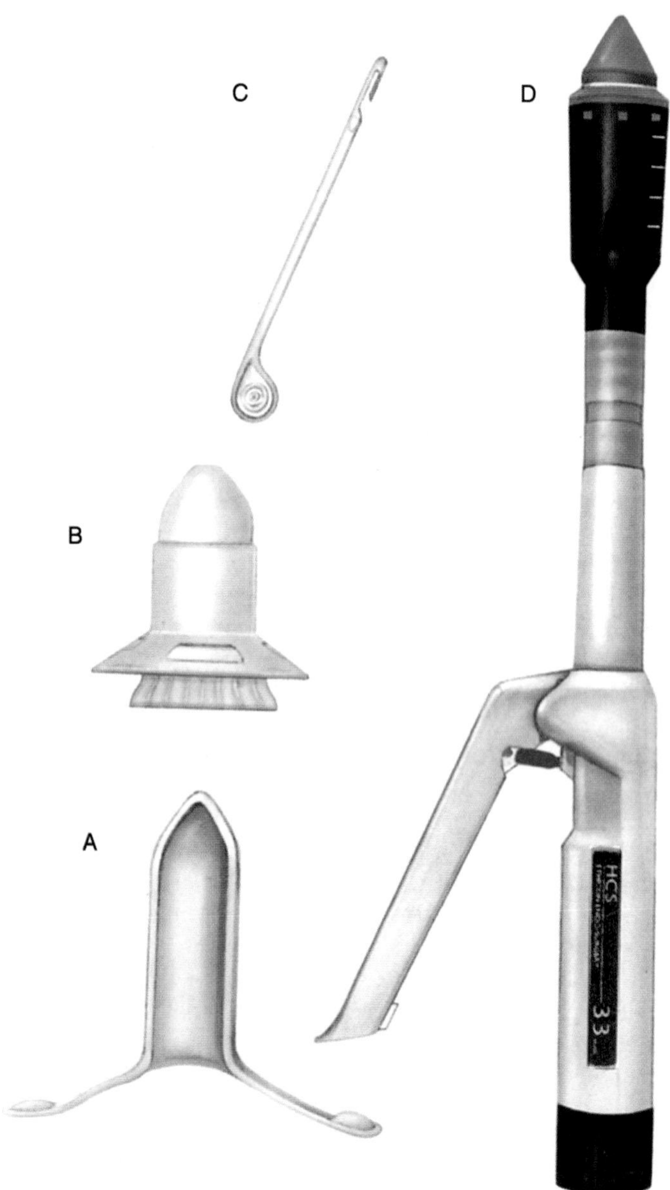

FIGURE 11 ■ Special instruments: (**A**) Purse-string suture anoscope; (**B**) circular anal dilator; (**C**) suture threader (crochet hook); (**D**) 33 mm hemorrhoidal circular stapler.

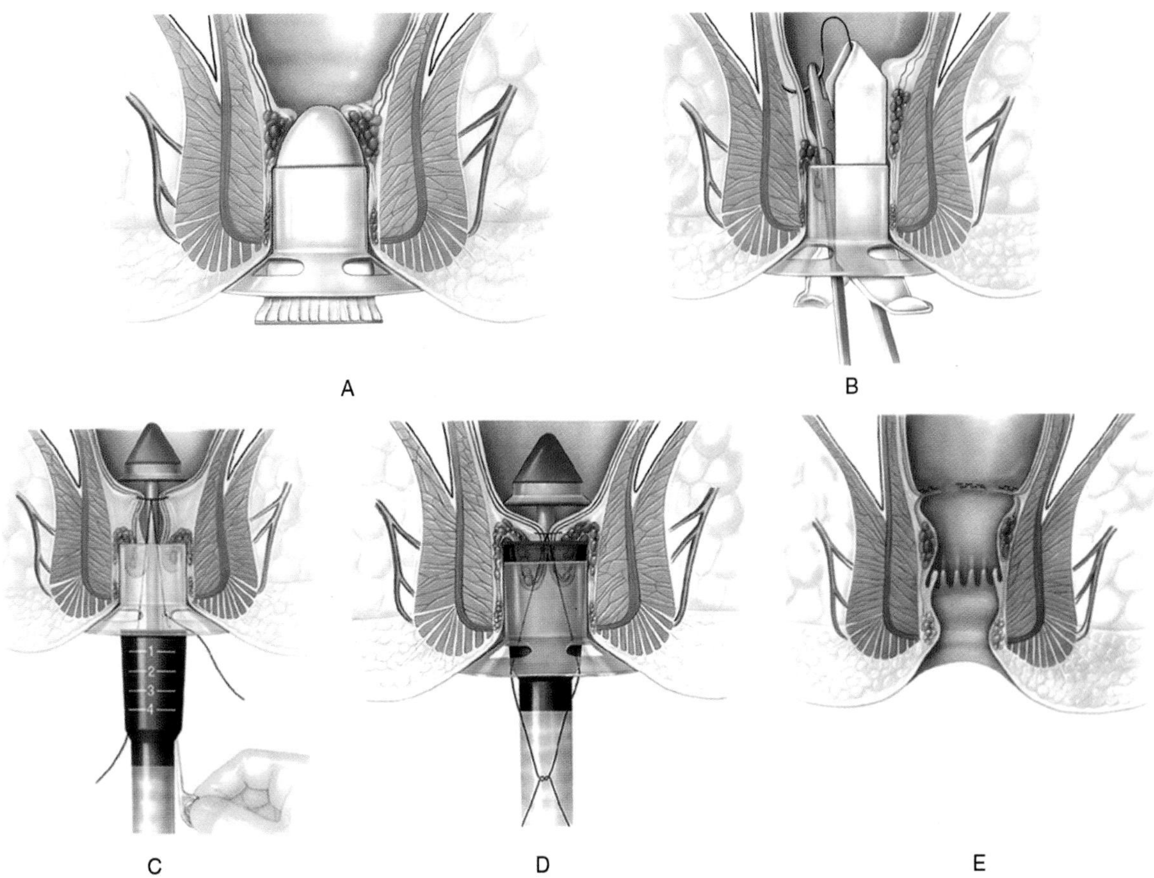

FIGURE 12 ■ (**A**) The anal dilator is inserted into the anal canal and secured to perianal skin with heavy sutures. (**B**) The purse-string suture anoscope is introduced into the anal dilator for placement of a purse-string of 2–0 Prolene in the submucosa, 4–5 cm above the dentate line. (**C**) The hemorrhoidal circular stapler is opened to its maximum position. Its head is introduced and positioned proximal to the purse-string, which is then tied over the shaft of the anvil. With the help of the suture threader (crochet hook), the ends of the suture are pulled through the lateral holes of the stapler. (**D**) The ends of the suture are knotted externally. At this point, the entire casing of the stapler is introduced into the anal canal. The stapler is then closed and fired. (**E**) At completion, the staple line should be about 2 cm above the top of the internal hemorrhoids.

is important to take only the mucosal–submucosal layer. The stapler with the anvil fully extended is inserted and positioned proximal to the purse-string, which is then tied over the shaft of the anvil. The purse-string suture tails are retrieved through the ports in the stapler gun using the crochet hook (Fig. 12C and D). The entire casing of the stapler is introduced into the anal canal. During the introduction, it is advisable to partially tighten the stapler. With moderate traction on the purse-string, a simple maneuver draws the prolapsed mucosa and submucosa into the casing of the stapler. The instrument is then tightened and fired. Compression on the gun is maintained for about 20–30 seconds for hemostasis before the stapler is opened and removed. It is easier to extract the anal dilator and the stapler simultaneously. There is only one donut ring, which should be checked for its completeness. The staple line should lie about 2 cm above the top of the internal hemorrhoids (Fig. 12E). Active bleeding points, which are common, should be stick tied with an absorbable suture.

■ RESULTS

The initial reports from many centers showed that stapled hemorrhoidopexy is safe, effective, rapid, and has minimal pain in most patients (110–114).

In a well-designed prospective, randomized study to evaluate the results of stapled hemorrhoidopexy compared with closed hemorrhoidectomy for grades 3 and 4 hemorrhoids during a 10-month period, Correa-Rovelo et al. (115) showed that stapled hemorrhoidopexy was safe to do. It had less pain and less abling but had higher postoperative bleeding than closed hemorrhoidectomy (Table 2). The majority of patients had a follow-up from seven to 14

TABLE 2 ■ **Stapled Hemorrhoidopexy vs. Closed Hemorrhoidectomy Randomized Controlled Trial**

	Stapled	Closed Hemorrhoidectomy	p
Number of patients	42	42	
Pain first 24 hours (scale 0–10) mean	2.8	5.5	<0.001
Pain at 2 weeks (scale 0–10)	1.1	3.7	<0.001
Days taking Ketorolac (10 mg)	4.9	12.8	<0.001
Disability (days)	6.1	15.2	<0.001
Postop bleeding requiring revision	2.4%	0%	1.0
Wound dehiscence	0	9.5%	0.12
Anal stricture	2.4	2.4	1.0
Dyspareunia	2.4	0	1.0
Fecal incontinence	0	2.4	1.0

Source: From Ref. 115.

TABLE 3 ■ **Stapled Hemorrhoidopexy vs. Open Hemorrhoidectomy Randomized Controlled Trial**

	Stapled	Diathermy Milligan-Morgan	p
Number of patients	62	57	NS
Anesthesia time (minute)	18	11	< 0.001
Pain score at 2 weeks	3	5	< 0.005
Persistent pain at 3 months (%)	1	3	NS
Incontinence at 6 weeks	2	2	NS
Resume work (day)	17	23	< 0.05
Cost ($)	1283	921	NS

Source: From Ref. 117.

months. Another randomized controlled trial conducted by Rowsell et al. (116) comparing stapled hemorrhoidopexy to closed hemorrhoidectomy also showed significant advantages of the stapled technique.

Ho et al. (117) conducted a randomized controlled trial comparing stapled hemorrhoidopexy to diathermy Milligan–Morgan open hemorrhoidectomy. The results showed superiority of stapled hemorrhoidopexy in terms of less painful, less time needed off work, and other parameters (Table 3). Numerous other randomized controlled trials also showed superiority of stapled hemorrhoidopexy to conventional hemorrhoidectomy (Table 4).

■ LONG-TERM FOLLOW-UP

Most series for stapled hemorrhoidopexy have the follow-up from two to six months, with the aim to evaluate its safety, postoperative pain, complications, and duration of disability. The early term of follow-up have shown it to be superior to open or closed hemorrhoidectomy (115,117, 118,121,126,129,130).

A good long-term follow-up (minimum five years) is still not available for stapled hemorrhoidopexy. The true recurrence is the prolapse of anorectal mucosa. In the randomized controlled trial by Ortiz et al. (125) in which the mean follow-up was 15.9 months (range 12.2–24.6 months), the recurrence with prolapse for grade 3 hemorrhoids was two of 17 patients for stapled hemorrhoidopexy and zero of 12 patients for conventional open hemorrhoidectomy ($p = 0.49$). In grade 4 hemorrhoids, the recurrent prolapse was five of 10 patients for stapled hemorrhoidopexy and zero of 16 patients for conventional open hemorrhoidectomy ($p = 0.003$).

■ SELECTION OF PATIENTS

Not all hemorrhoids are suitable for stapled hemorrhoidopexy. Circumferential reducible grades 3 and 4 hemorrhoids are most suitable. Grade 3 or 4 hemorrhoids that protrude in only one or two quadrants should undergo rubber band ligations or a conventional hemorrhoidectomy. Prolapsed hemorrhoids associated with fibrotic skin tags may undergo hemorrhoidopexy with excision of the skin tags at the same or separate operation.

Irreducible grade 4 hemorrhoids is not a candidate for stapled hemorrhoidopexy. Ortiz et al. (131) conducted a randomized trial between stapled hemorrhoidopexy (15 patients) and diathermy Milligan–Morgan hemorrhoidectomy (16 patients) for grade 4 irreducible hemorrhoids. The results showed that from four months after operation, recurrent prolapse was confirmed in eight of 15 patients in the stapled group and none in the conventional hemorrhoidectomy group ($p = 0.002$). Persistent itching occurred in six of 15 patients in the stapled group versus only one in the conventional hemorrhoidectomy group ($p = 0.03$). Six patients in the stapled group and none in the conventional hemorrhoidectomy group experienced tenesmus ($p = 0.007$). From this study, it becomes clear that patients with irreducible hemorrhoids should have an excisional hemorrhoidectomy and not a stapled hemorrhoidopexy.

TABLE 4 ■ **Randomized Controlled Trial Comparing Stapled Hemorrhoidopexy to Conventional Hemorrhoidectomy**

		Number		Pain Score		Disability (days)		Complications	
Author(s)	Year	SH	CH	SH	CH	SH	CH	SH	CH
Bikhehandani et al. (118)	2005	42	42	5.71[a]	7.28	8.12[a]	17.62	NS	NS
Basdanis et al. (119)	2005	50	45	3.0[a]	5.0	6.3[a]	9.8	NS	NS
Senagore et al. (120)	2004	77	79	5[a]	7	—	—	3%[a]	14%
Kairaluoma et al. (121)	2003	30	30	1.8[a]	4.3	NS	NS	NS	NS
Cheetham et al. (122)	2003	15	16	1.3[a]	3.0	NS	NS	NS	NS
Correa-Rovelo et al. (115)	2002	42	42	2.8[a]	5.5	6.1[a]	15.2	NS	NS
Wilson et al. (123)	2002	59	30	—	—	$p < 0.006$[b]	NS	NS	—
Hetzer et al. (124)	2002	20	20	2.7[a]	6.3	6.7[a]	20.7	NS	NS
Ortiz et al. (125)	2002	27	28	11.9[a]	34.6	23.1	26.6	NS	NS
Shalaby and Desoky (126)	2001	100	100	2.5[a]	7.6	8.2[a]	53.9	Lower	Higher
Boccasanta et al. (127)	2001	40	40	3.5[a]	4.5	8[a]	15	NS	NS
Ganio et al. (128)	2001	50	50		$P = 0.03+$	5[a]	13	NS	NS
Ho et al. (117)	2000	57	62	4.5	5.0	17.1[a]	22.9	NS	NS
Mehigan et al. (129)	2000	20	20	2.1[a]	6.5	17[a]	34	NS	NS
Rowsell et al. (116)	2000	11	11	2.5[a]	5.5	8.1[a]	16.9	-	-

[a]Statistically significant.
[b]In favor of stapled hemorrhoidopexy.
Abbreviations: SH, stapled hemorrhoidopexy; CH, conventional hemorrhoidectomy; NS, not statistically significant.

The expert panel (105) were concerned about patients with pre-existing sphincter injury or fecal incontinence because of the insertion of the 33 mm anal dilator during the procedure. This may dilate and impair the sphincter muscle. Anal intercourse is an interesting concern. The staples may not completely bury within the mucosa and submucosa during the first several months and may cause penile injury. Patients may need to be warned.

■ CONTRAINDICATIONS

Contraindications to stapled hemorrhoidopexy are perianal abscess, gangrenous hemorrhoids, anal stenosis, and full-thickness rectal prolapse (105).

■ IS STAPLED HEMORRHOIDOPEXY BETTER THAN RUBBER BAND LIGATION?

W. H. Thomson (40) raised an appropriate question whether stapled hemorrhoidopexy is superior to the simple rubber band ligation in which the action is almost identical. Thomson stated, "in my experience, most of the patients can be rendered symptom-free by it, whatever the "degree" of their hemorrhoids; even fourth degree pile sufferers can readily be relieved of the mucosal contribution to their misery, which may well be enough. Hemorrhoidectomy in my practice is seldom required and then at most as an overnight stay. Stapling may inadvertently incorporate the full rectal wall and even risk vaginal fistulation." Thomson would call for a thorough long-term comparison with banding before the surgeon adopts the stapling treatment. Indeed, major complications have been reported (see section on Complications).

There is a report comparing the two procedures. Peng et al. (132) conducted a randomized controlled trial comparing rubber band ligation to stapled hemorrhoidopexy for symptomatic grade 3 or small grade 4 hemorrhoids. For the rubber band ligation group, three piles were banded, all in one session. There were 25 patients in the rubber band ligation group and 30 patients in the hemorrhoidopexy group. All rubber bands were performed as an outpatient whereas 29 of 30 stapled hemorrhoidopexies stayed in the hospital for 24 hours and one patient stayed longer because of urinary retention. The study demonstrated that both rubber band ligation and stapled hemorrhoidopexy were suitable techniques for the treatment of grade 3 and early grade 4 hemorrhoids. The control of symptoms at the primary end point of six months was similar. Stapled hemorrhoidopexy had more pain both at discharge and at two weeks' follow-up ($p < 0.001$). This difference had reduced to a nonsignificant level by two months follow-up. Postoperative bleeding was significantly more common following rubber band ligation than stapled hemorrhoidopexy ($p = 0.002$), which may be related to the longer time needed for the wound to heal after the tissues slough off. There were six of 30 patients in the stapled group with minor complications (urinary retention—1, bleeding requiring readmission ~2, mild anal stenosis requiring digital dilatation ~3) compared to none in the rubber band ligation group ($p = 0.027$). However, 20% of patients treated with rubber band ligation subsequently required an excisional hemorrhoidectomy for symptom control. There was no difference between the two groups in terms of patient satisfaction or quality of life for the six-month follow-up.

■ COMPLICATIONS

Postoperative Pain

In almost all of the randomized controlled trials, stapled hemorrhoidopexy has significantly less pain than closed or open hemorrhoidectomy in the postoperative period. However, stapled hemorrhoidopexy is not painless, most reported at 0.5–4.5 in a scale of 10 during the first 10 days (115–117,122,127,129). The pain in stapled hemorrhoidopexy is more dull, vague, and deeper in the perineum in the stapled group rather than sharper and more superficial pain in the conventional hemorrhoidectomy group (117). In a survey by Ravo et al. (133) of 20 Italian centers involving 1107 patients, 26% of patients had postoperative pain when there was no muscle incorporated in the donut compared to 66% when the donut contained muscle. Correa-Rovelo et al. (134) had an experience that inclusion of squamous epithelium in the donut is the pain-related factor in the early postoperative period.

Persistent Pain

The effectiveness and successes of stapled hemorrhoidopexy was of concern by the study of Cheetham et al. (135) of St. Mark's Hospital, London. In the randomized controlled trial comparing stapled hemorrhoidopexy to diathermy open hemorrhoidectomy, five of 16 patients in the stapled group (31%, 95% CI, 8.5–54%) developed symptoms of pain and fecal urgency which persisted up to 15 months postoperatively. Because of this, the randomized trial was voluntarily suspended. The mechanism behind this phenomenon was unclear although they speculated that muscle incorporation in the donut might have a role. However, in the series of Correa-Rovelo et al. (134), in spite of 5% of patients had inclusion of transitional and squamous epithelium and 12% had inclusion of external sphincter muscle fibers in the donut, they did not observe cases of persistent or severe anal pain although they identified the inclusion of squamous epithelium as a pain-related factor in the early postoperative period.

Ho et al. (136) reported only one out of 57 patients (1.8%) with persistent pain three months after the operation compared to three out of 62 patients (4.8%) in the conventional open hemorrhoidectomy. Longo (137) quoted his experience of 1404 cases with a follow-up of three months to six years. None of the patients has had persistent postoperative pain, whereas 5% complained of fecal urgency but only for a maximum period of 30 days (mean nine days). Longo believed that persistent pain could be avoided by properly placing the purse-string in the rectal mucosa, not the anal canal.

Thaha et al. (138) reported a unique postdefecation pain syndrome after circular stapled hemorrhoidopexy. Three of the 77 patients who underwent stapled hemorrhoidopexy developed new onset of postdefecation pain. They were all men, with a median age of 38 years (range 37–46). The mean height of the completed staple line from dentate line was 1.5 cm (range 1–2 cm). Postoperative transanal ultrasonography showed that the sphincter complex was intact in all three men. At six weeks follow-up, all three patients reported an incapacitating pain after defecation. Clinical examination ruled out anal fissure or complication at the staple line. Anal manometry showed an abnormally high anal sphincter pressure in all three patients. Nitroglycerin 0.2% ointment was prescribed. Owing to failure of nitroglycerin therapy, oral nifedipine (20 mg twice daily for six weeks) was started as a second-line muscle relaxant. Within one week of commencing nifedipine therapy, all three patients had rapid resolution of symptoms. Repeat anorectal manometry showed no significant reduction in sphincter pressure. A follow-up at a mean of 10.7 months after surgery, the patients remained symptom-free. Because of the clinical response to nifedipine therapy with no concurrent reduction in anal sphincter pressures, together with an absence of structural sphincter damage, the authors suggested that postdefecation pain might be rectal in origin rather than sphincter, as previously thought.

Postoperative Bleeding

Arterial bleedings at the suture line right after the staple excision of the rectal mucosa–submucosa are quite often. In the series of 100 patients, Correa-Rovelo et al. (134) reported that 40% of the patients required 1–3 hemostatic suture points after firing the stapler. Postoperative bleeding that requires operative intervention has been reported at 1–13% (112,115,122,126,139,140). Because of the common bleeding problem, I suture the staple line with running 3–0 absorbable suture.

Urinary Retention

In the randomized controlled trial series, urinary retention after stapled hemorrhoidopexy has been reported between 0% and 6%, which is not statistically significant from open or closed hemorrhoidectomy (115,117,122,128,129).

Anorectal Stenosis

For circular stapling for low anterior resection in which two cut ends of the bowel are stapled together, the incidence of stricture requiring dilatation is fairly common. Most of these problems stem from anastomotic leak, tension, and possible ischemia. For a stapled hemorrhoidopexy, only the mucosa and submucosa layer is cut and stapled. The anorectal wall and the blood supply is not disturbed; ischemia does not occur. However, separation of the staples may cause stenosis from secondary fibrotic healing. In addition, the diameter of the stapler is also larger than the one used for a low anterior resection (33 mm diameter). Symptomatic anal stenosis is uncommon for stapled hemorrhoidopexy. Correa-Rovelo et al. (115) reported only one of 42 patients with mild anal stenosis that did not require dilatation. In a one-year follow-up of 95 patients with stapled hemorrhoidopexy in Shalaby series (126), five patients had anorectal stenosis; three patients responded well to anorectal dilatation, two patients did well after surgical treatment. Ho et al. (117) reported mild stenosis in 12 of 57 patients with stapled hemorrhoidopexy, all occurred in patients who were noncompliant to fiber supplement and were usually detected at six weeks after surgery. They were soft and easily dilated digitally without analgesia.

Anal Sphincter Injuries

With the proper technique of purse-string suture in the mucosal–submucosal layer, at 4–5 cm above the dentate line, mucosectomy should not include a significant amount of muscularis layer of the low rectum. The donut ring should also be above the transitional and squamous epithelium of the anal canal. George et al. (139) microscopically examined the mucosectomy specimens in 26 consecutive patients: 12 of 26 specimens contained columnar, transitional, and stratified squamous epithelium; two of 26 specimens contained columnar and some transitional mucosa; 22 of 26 specimens contained some smooth muscle. Of significance was that two and eight specimens with smooth muscle had overlying transitional and stratified squamous epithelium, respectively. In a prospective study by Correa-Rovelo et al. (134) in 100 patients who underwent stapled hemorrhoidopexy, examination of the donut rings showed that 55% contained smooth muscle from the rectum. In 47%, the transitional epithelium was included and in 5% both transitional and squamous epithelium were included in the specimens. It is obvious from these two studies that the mucosectomy was a little bit too deep and too low in many cases in spite of aiming the purse-string in the submucosa and 4 cm above the dentate line. However, these injuries did not appear to have adverse postoperative outcome.

Ho et al. (136) assessed anal sphincter injuries by means of ultrasound. This was a randomized study comparing 29 patients for stapled hemorrhoidopexy using the standard anal dilator speculum for the procedure compared to 29 patients using Eisenhammer retractor for the purse-string and no retractor or anal speculum to apply the staple gun. Both groups had preoperative ultrasonography. Follow-up ultrasonography was performed at six weeks and 14 weeks after surgery. The results revealed that two of 29 patients using the standard anal dilator speculum had internal sphincter fragmentation compared to none in the no dilator group. There was no damage to the external sphincter in either group. There was no incontinence in either group.

Altomare et al. (141) also studied the anal function after stapled hemorrhoidopexy. Preoperative tests of anal canal sensation showed that seven of 20 patients with grade 3 hemorrhoids had diminished sensitivity of the prolapsed mucosa even without any major impairment of continence. After stapled hemorrhoidopexy, all but one patient had improvement of the sensation. This improvement probably was the result of the prolapsed mucosa pulled up to its normal position in the anal canal after the hemorrhoidopexy. All patients had anal continence after six months of operation. There was no difference in the anal manometry and rectoanal inhibitory reflex between preoperative and postoperative values. Three-dimensional ultrasonography was carried out before and after operation in all 20 patients and showed no fragmentation of internal anal sphincter or other abnormality.

Incontinence

Incontinence for gas or stool is uncommon after stapled hemorrhoidopexy. Most series reported less than 1% (115,117,133).

Pelvic Sepsis

Molloy et al. (142) reported a case that was admitted the evening after discharge after an uneventful stapled hemorrhoidopexy because of passing blood per rectum and mild fever. Computerized tomography of the abdomen showed extensive retroperitoneal gas enveloping the rectum, bladder, kidneys, and pancreas. An exploratory celiotomy showed no intraperitoneal gas or pelvic abscess. The rectum was strikingly edematous and vascular. At a point level with the staple line, a small pocket of pus was seen but the staple line was air tight on testing. The presacral space was drained and an end-colostomy was fashioned. Culture of the pus showed heavy growth of lactose-fermenting coliforms, *Bacteroides fragilis*, and a *Clostridium* (not *C. tatani* or *C. perfringens*). The patient made an uncomplicated recovery.

A similar case was reported by Maw et al. (143) in which the patient was presented with rectal discomfort, lower abdominal pain, fever, and leukocytosis 39 hours after the operation. Abdominal radiograph showed extensive retroperitoneal gas but there was no pneumoperitoneum. Examination showed the staple line to be intact. The patient was successfully treated with antibiotics.

Rectal Perforation

There were two cases reported on this complication (144,145). A full thickness stapled excision of the low rectum was involved in each case. This mistake should be avoided by precisely placing the purse-string suture in the mucosal–submucosal layer. In one of the cases, the donut was only half the circumference, necessitating a second application. This situation may be encountered from time to time but other alternatives can be used: rubber band ligation, open or closed conventional hemorrhoidectomy. In an anonymous survey of 1545 German Departments of Surgery in 1999, Harold and Kirsch (146) quoted 4635 patients with stapler hemorrhoidopexy. There were three rectal perforations requiring two temporary and one permanent stomas, one complete rectal obstruction and one large retrorectal hematoma, one lethal sepsis from Fournier's gangrene.

Acute Rectal Obstruction

Cipriani and Pescatori (147) reported a case of an acute obstruction at the staple line. Of significance was that two purse-string sutures were placed and only one was cut after firing of the gun, leaving one purse-string intact. The authors claimed that the staple line was too high to be examined at the end of the operation. The stricture was released by a per anal cut of the purse-string. Longo (107) used two purse-string techniques when the prolapse of the rectal mucosa is more than 3 cm. Longo describes that the distance between the two purse-string should not be more than 3 cm because excessive quantities of the mucosa cannot be contained in the staple housing. This is a more advanced technique, perhaps one that we all have to learn.

■ CONCLUDING REMARKS

Stapled hemorrhoidopexy is a relatively new procedure. There have been more randomized controlled trials comparing the outcomes of stapled hemorrhoidopexy to conventional hemorrhoidectomy than many other anorectal diseases. All the trials are remarkably consistent in the findings of a safe procedure, less pain and disabled than the conventional hemorrhoidectomy.

The stapled hemorrhoidopexy should not be used to replace rubber band ligation but rather to be used only in patients with severe prolapse that are not suitable for multiple bandings. It is not painless but when properly performed, the pain is minimal and lasts only for a day or two. Serious or even life-threatening complications are rare and can be traced to improper selection of patients or techniques. Because of the rare occurrence of septic complications, perioperative antibiotics are not indicated. It is important to detect signs of sepsis early: abdominal or progressive anorectal pain, fever, unrelenting urinary retention, and leukocytosis.

The critical and the most difficult part of the operation is the placement of purse-string suture. It should be in the submucosal layer, 4–5 cm above the dentate line; it is in the low rectum, not the upper anal canal. A few smooth muscle fibers of the rectal wall included in the donut appear to be unavoidable but it gives no harm to the outcome since this is not internal anal sphincter muscle. Bleeding at the staple line should be sutured with an absorbable suture.

The successes of stapled hemorrhoidopexy rely on excision of the redundant rectal mucosa resulting in pulling up the prolapsed internal and external hemorrhoids to their anatomic location in the anal canal. Prolapsed internal hemorrhoids that are fixed or immobile are not suitable for the stapled procedure. External hemorrhoids may shrink or decrease in size with time; it is wise to wait and see. However, fibrotic anal skin tags should be excised at the same sitting or at a later date if this is indicated.

Stapled hemorrhoidopexy is technically demanding although it is not difficult to learn for a surgeon who is experienced with circular stapling device and anorectal surgery. The expert panel (105) recommends, "the surgeon must attend a formal course. This should include lectures, videos, the application of the instrument in models, and observation of the operation performed by a surgeon recognized by his or her peers leading ultimately to understanding the procedure while being observed by an experienced surgeon."

The last words: A meta-analysis of all randomized controlled trials assessing two or more treatment modalities for symptomatic hemorrhoids, from 1966 to January 2001 was conducted by Macrae et al. (148). The main outcome measures were response to therapy, need for further therapy, complications, and pain. Twenty-three trials were available for analysis. Hemorrhoidectomy was found to be significantly more effective than manual dilatation of the anus ($p = 0.0017$) and associated with less need for further therapy ($p = 0.034$), with no significant difference in complications ($p = 0.60$) but more pain ($p < 0.001$). With short-term follow-up, stapled hemorrhoidopexy was found to be associated with significantly less pain than conventional hemorrhoidectomy, with no significant difference in complication rate or response to treatment. There were no significant differences between open and closed hemorrhoidectomy. Patients who underwent hemorrhoidectomy had a better response to treatment than did patients who were treated with rubber band ligation ($p = 0.001$), although complications were greater ($p = 0.02$), as was pain ($p < 0.00001$). Rubber band ligation was more effective than sclerotherapy and infrared coagulation, without an increase in complications. Rubber band ligation is recommended as the initial mode of therapy for grades 1–3 hemorrhoids. Although hemorrhoidectomy showed a better response, it is associated with more complications and pain than rubber band ligation. Stapled hemorrhoidopexy appears to cause less pain than conventional hemorrhoidectomy. However, further follow-up will be required to assess its effectiveness compared with conventional hemorrhoidectomy and rubber band ligation.

Suggested Plan of Management

Condition	Treatment
Grade 1 hemorrhoids	Exclusion of other causes of bleeding Diet, psyllium seed, or bran Rubber band ligation Electrocoagulation
Grade 2 hemorrhoids	Rubber band ligation Electrocoagulation
Grade 3 hemorrhoids	Rubber band ligation Electrocoagulation Closed hemorrhoidectomy Stapled hemorrhoidopexy
Grade 4 hemorrhoids	Rubber band ligation Closed hemorrhoidectomy Stapled hemorrhoidopexy
Prolapsed strangulated hemorrhoids	Emergency closed hemorrhoidectomy Rubber band ligation Stapled hemorrhoidopexy
Thrombosed external hemorrhoids	If painful, excision of clots with patient under local or general anesthesia
Perianal skin tags	If symptomatic, excision with patient under local or general anesthesia
Hypertrophied anal papillae	Asymptomatic: no treatment Symptomatic: excision

REFERENCES

1. Thomson WHF. The nature of hemorrhoids. Br J Surg 1975; 62:542–552.
2. Johanson JF, Sonnenberg A. Prevalence of hemorrhoids and chronic constipation. An epidemiologic study. Gastroenterology 1990; 98:380–386.
3. Johanson JF, Sonnenberg A. Temporal changes in the occurrence of hemorrhoids in the United States and England. Dis Colon Rectum 1991; 34:585–593.
4. Nelson RL. Editorial comment on time trends of hemorrhoids. Dis Colon Rectum 1991; 34:591–593.
5. Bernstein WC. What are hemorrhoids and what is their relationship to the portal venous system? Dis Colon Rectum 1983; 26:829–834.
6. Hosking SW, Smart HL, Johnson AG, Triger DR. Anorectal varices, hemorrhoids, and portal hypertension. Lancet 1989; 1:349–352.
7. Wang TF, Lee FY, Tsai YT, et al. Relationship of portal pressure, anorectal varices and hemorrhoids in cirrhotic patients. J Hepatol 1992; 15:170–173.
8. Haas PA, Fox TA Jr, Haas GP. The pathogenesis of hemorrhoids. Dis Colon Rectum 1984; 27:442–450.
9. Wexner SD, Baig K. The evaluation and physiologic assessment of hemorrhoidal disease: a review. Tech Coloproctol 2001; 5:165–168.
10. Hiltunen KM, Matikainen M. Anal manometric findings in symptomatic hemorrhoids. Dis Colon Rectum 1985; 28:807–809.
11. Sun WM, Peck RJ, Shorthouse AJ, Read NW. Hemorrhoids are associated not with hypertrophy of the internal anal sphincter, but with hypertension of the anal cushions. Br J Surg 1992; 79:592–594.
12. Lin JK. Anal manometric studies in hemorrhoids and anal fissures. Dis Colon Rectum 1989; 32:839–842.
13. Hancock BD. Internal sphincter and the nature of hemorrhoids. Gut 1977; 18:651–655.
14. Roe AM, Bartolo DCC, Vellacott KD, Locke-Edmunds J, Mortensen NJM. Submucosal versus ligation excision hemorrhoidectomy: a comparison of anal sensation, anal sphincter manometry and postoperative pain and function. Br J Surg 1987; 74:948–951.
15. Sun WM, Read NW, Shorthouse AJ. Hypertensive anal cushions as a cause of the high anal canal pressures in patients with hemorrhoids. Br J Surg 1990; 77:458–462.
16. Waldron DJ, Kumar D, Hallan RI, Williams NA. Prolonged ambulant assessment of anorectal function in patients with prolapsing hemorrhoids. Dis Colon Rectum 1989; 32:968–974.
17. Farouk R, Duthie GS, Pryde A, MacGregor AB, Bartolo DCC. Sustained internal sphincter hypertonia in patients with chronic anal fissure. Dis Colon Rectum 1994; 37:424–429.
18. Loder PB, Kamm MA, Nicholls RJ, Phillips RKS. Hemorrhoids: pathology, pathophysiology and etiology. Br J Surg 1994; 81:946–954.
19. Gibbons CP, Bannister JJ, Read NW. Role of constipation and anal hypertonia in the pathogenesis of hemorrhoids. Br J Surg 1988; 75:656–660.
20. Johanson JF, Sonnenberg A. Constipation is not a risk factor for hemorrhoids: A case-control study of potential etiologic agents. Am J Gastroenterol 1994; 89:1981–1986.
21. Gibbons CP, Trowbridge EA, Bannister JJ, Read NW. Role of anal cushions in maintaining continence. Lancet 1986; 1:886–888.
22. Lestar B, Penninckx F, Rigauts H, Kerremans R. The internal anal sphincter cannot close the anal canal completely. Int J Colorectal Dis 1992; 7:159–161.
23. Cataldo P, Ellis CN, Gregorcyk S, et al. Practice parameters for the management of hemorrhoids [revised]. Dis Colon Rectum 2005; 48:189–194.
24. Kluiber RM, Wolff BG. Evaluation of anemia caused by hemorrhoidal bleeding. Dis Colon Rectum 1994; 37:1006–1007.
25. Alexander-Williams J, Crapp AR. Conservative management of hemorrhoids. Clin Gastroenterol 1975; 4:595–601.
26. Burkitt DP, Graham-Stewart CW. Hemorrhoids—postulated pathogenesis and proposed prevention. Postgrad Med 1975; 51:631–636.
27. Lantner RR, Espiritu BR, Zumerchik P, Tobin MC. Anaphylaxis following ingestions of a psyllium-containing cereal. JAMA 1990; 264:2534–2536.
28. Moesgaard F, Nielsen ML, Hansen JB, Knudsen JT. High fiber diet reduces bleeding and pain in patients with hemorrhoids. Dis Colon Rectum 1982; 25:454–456.
29. Senapati A, Nicholls RJ. Randomized trial to compare the results of injection sclerotherapy with a bulk laxative alone in the treatment of bleeding hemorrhoids. Int J Colorectal Dis 1988; 3:124–126.
30. Barron J. Office ligation treatment of hemorrhoids. Dis Colon Rectum 1963; 6:109–113.
31. Wroblewski DE, Corman ML, Veidenheimer MC, Coller JA. Long-term evaluation of rubber ring ligation in hemorrhoidal disease. Dis Colon Rectum 1980; 23:478–482.
32. Lee HH, Spencer RJ, Beart RW Jr. Multiple hemorrhoidal bandings in a single session. Dis Colon Rectum 1994; 37:37–41.
33. MacRae HM, McLeod RS. Comparison of hemorrhoidal treatment modalities. Dis Colon Rectum 1995; 38:687–694.
34. Jensen SL, Harling H, Arseth P, Tange A. The natural history of symptomatic hemorrhoids. Int J Colorectal Dis 1989; 4:41–44.
35. Nivatvongs S, Goldberg SM. An improved technique of rubber band ligation of hemorrhoids. Am J Surg 1982; 144:379–380.
36. Iyer VS, Shrier I, Gordon PH. Long-term outcome of rubber band ligation for symptomatic primary and recurrent internal hemorrhoids. Dis Colon Rectum 2003; 47:1364–1370.
37. Armstrong DN. Multiple hemorrhoidal ligation. A prospective, randomized trial evaluating a new technique. Dis Colon Rectum 2003; 46:179–186.
38. Konborozos VA, Skrekas GJ, Pissiotis CA. Rubber band ligation of symptomatic internal hemorrhoids: results of 500 cases. Digestion Surg 2000; 17:71–76.
39. Law WL, Chu KW. Triple rubber band ligation for hemorrhoids prospective, randomized trial of use of local anesthetic injection. Dis Colon Rectum 1999; 42:363–366.
40. Thomson WH. Stapled hemorrhoidectomy. Correspondence. Colorectal Dis 2000; 2:310.
41. Madoff RD, Fleshman JW. American Gastrological Association technical review on the diagnosis and treatment of hemorrhoids. Gastroenterology 2004; 126:1463–1473.
42. Hardwick RH, Durdey P. Should rubber band ligation of hemorrhoids be performed at the initial outpatient visit? Ann R Coll Surg Engl 1994; 76:185–187.
43. O'Hara VS. Fatal clostridial infection following hemorrhoidal banding. Dis Colon Rectum 1980; 23:570–571.
44. Russell TR, Donohue JH. Hemorrhoidal banding: a warning. Dis Colon Rectum 1985; 28:291–293.
45. Shemesh EL, Kodner LJ, Fry RD, Neufeld DM. Severe complications of rubber band ligation of internal hemorrhoids. Dis Colon Rectum 1987; 30:199–200.
46. Scarpa FJ, Hillis W, Sabetta JR. Pelvic cellulitis: a life-threatening complication of hemorrhoidal banding. Surgery 1988; 103:383–385.

47. Quevedo-Bonilla G, Farkas AM, Abcarian H, Hambrock TE, Orsay CP. Septic complications of hemorrhoidal banding. Arch Surg 1988; 123:650–651.
48. Buchmann P, Seefeld H. Rubber band ligation for piles can be disastrous in HIV-positive patients. Int J Colorectal Dis 1989; 4:57–58.
49. Johanson JF, Rimm A. Optimal nonsurgical treatment of hemorrhoids: a comparative analysis of infrared coagulation, rubber band ligation and injection sclerotherapy. Am J Gastroenterol 1992; 87:1601–1606.
50. Randall GM, Jensen DM, Machicado GA, Hirabayashi K, Jensen MB, You S, Pelayo E. Prospective randomized comparative study of bipolar versus direct current electrocoagulation for treatment of bleeding internal hemorrhoids. Gastrointest Endosc 1994; 40:403–410.
51. Kaman L, Aggarwal S, Kumar R, Behera A, Katariya RN. Necrotizing fasciitis after injection sclerotherapy for hemorrhoids. Report of a case. Dis Colon Rectum 1999; 42:419–420.
52. Lord PH. A new approach to hemorrhoids. Prog Surg 1972; 10:109–124.
53. Lewis AAM, Rogers HS, Leighton M. Trial of maximal anal dilatation, cryotherapy, and elastic band ligation as alternatives to hemorrhoidectomy in the treatment of large prolapsing hemorrhoids. Br J Surg 1983; 70:54–56.
54. Smith LE, Goodreau JJ, Fouty WJ. Operative hemorrhoidectomy versus cryodestruction. Dis Colon Rectum 1979; 22:10–16.
55. Allgower M. Conservative management of haemorrhoids. Part III: partial internal sphincterotomy. Clin Gastroenterol 1975; 4:608–618.
56. Schouten WR, van Vroonhoven TJ. Lateral internal sphincterotomy in the treatment of hemorrhoids. A clinical and manometric study. Dis Colon Rectum 1986; 29:869–872.
57. De-Roover DM, Hoofwijk AG, van Vroonhoven TJ. Lateral internal sphincterotomy in the treatment of fourth-degree hemorrhoids. Br J Surg 1989; 76: 1181–1183.
58. Nivatvongs S, Fang DT, Kennedy HL. The shape of the buttocks—a useful guide for selection of patients for anorectal surgery. Dis Colon Rectum 1983; 26:85–86.
59. Friend WG, Medwell SJ. Outpatient anorectal surgery. Perspect Colon Rectal Surg 1989; 2:167–173.
60. Fansler WA. Hemorrhoidectomy—an anatomic method. The Journal–Lancet (Minnesota and South Dakota State Medical Association) 1931; 51:529–531.
61. Cataldo PA, MacKeigan JM. The necessity of routine pathologic evaluation of hemorrhoidectomy specimens. Surg Gynecol Obstet 1992; 174:302–304.
62. Foust R, Dean PJ, Stoler HH, Moinuddin SM. Intraepithelial neoplasia of the anal canal on hemorrhoidal tissues: a study of 19 cases. Hum Pathol 1991; 22:528–534.
63. Allingham HW. The diagnosis and treatment of diseases of the rectum. 7th ed. London: Bailliere, Tindall, & Cox, 1901:133–175.
64. Milligan ETC, Morgan CN, Jones LE, Officer R. Surgical anatomy of the anal canal and the operative treatment of hemorrhoids. Lancet 1937; 2:1119–1124.
65. Andrews BT, Layer GT, Jackson BT, Nicholls RJ. Randomized trial comparing diathermy hemorrhoidectomy with scissors dissection. Milligan–Morgan operation. Dis Colon Rectum 1993; 36:580–583.
66. Seow-Choen F, Ho YH, Ang HG, Goh HS. Prospective, randomized trial comparing pain and clinical function after conventional scissors excision/ligation vs. diathermy excision without ligation for symptomatic prolapsed hemorrhoids. Dis Colon Rectum 1992; 35:1165–1169.
67. Whitehead W. The surgical treatment of hemorrhoids. Br Med J 1882; 1: 148–150.
68. Bonello JC. Who's afraid of the dentate line? The Whitehead hemorrhoidectomy. Am J Surg 1988; 156:182–186.
69. Wolff BG, Culp CE. The Whitehead hemorrhoidectomy. An unjustly maligned procedure. Dis Colon Rectum 1988; 31:587–590.
70. Yu JC, Eddy HJ Jr. Laser, a new modality for hemorrhoidectomy. Am J Procto Gastroenterol Colon Rectal Surg 1985; 36:9–13.
71. Iwagaki H, Higuchi Y, Fachimoto S, Orita K. The laser treatment of hemorrhoids: results of a study on 1816 patients. Jpn J Surg 1989; 19:658–661.
72. Senagore A, Mazier WP, Luchtefeld MA, MacKeigan JM, Wengert T. Treatment of advanced hemorrhoidal disease: a prospective, randomized comparison of cold scalpel vs contact Nd:YAG laser. Dis Colon Rectum 1993; 36:1042–1049.
73. Leff EL. Hemorrhoidectomy—laser vs non-laser: outpatient surgical experience. Dis Colon Rectum 1992; 35:743–746.
74. Jongen J, Bach S, Stubinger SH, Bock JU. Excision of thrombosed external hemorrhoid under local anesthesia: a retrospective evaluation of 340 patients. Dis Colon Rectum 2003; 46:1226–1231.
75. Greenspon J, Williams SB, Young HA, Orkin BA. Thrombosed external hemorrhoids: outcome after conservative of surgical management. Dis Colon Rectum 2004; 47:1493–1498.
76. Perrotti P, Antropoli C, Noschese G, et al. Topical nifedipine for conservative treatment of acute hemorrhoidal thrombosed. Colorectal Dis 2000; 2:18–21.
77. Eu KW, Seow-Choen F, Goh HS. Comparison of emergency and elective hemorrhoidectomy. Br J Surg 1994; 81:308–310.
78. Sacco S, Mortilla MG, Tonielli E, Morganti I, Cola B. Emergency hemorrhoidectomy for complicated hemorrhoids. Coloproctology 1987; 9:157–159.
79. Allen PIM, Goldman M. Prolapsed thrombosed piles: a reappraisal. Coloproctology 1987; 9:210–212.
80. Salvati EP. Management of acute hemorrhoidal disease. Perspect Colon Rectal Surg 1990; 3:309–314.
81. Rasmussen OO, Larsen KGL, Naver L, Christiansen J. Emergency hemorrhoidectomy compared with incision and banding for the treatment of acute strangulated hemorrhoids. Eur J Surg 1991; 157:613–614.
82. Eisenstat T, Salvati EP, Rubin RJ. The out patient management of acute hemorrhoidal disease. Dis Colon Rectum 1979; 22:315–317.
83. Brown SR, Ballan K, Ho E, Ho Fams YH, Seow-choen F. Stapled mucosectomy for a cute thrombosed circumferentially prolapsed piles: a prospective randomized comparison with conventional hemorrhoidectomy. Colorectal Dis 2001; 3:175–178.
84. Nivatvongs S. An alternative positioning of patients for hemorrhoidectomy. Dis Colon Rectum 1980; 23:308–309.
85. Salleby RG Jr, Rosen L, Stasik JJ, Riether RD, Sheets J, Khubchandani IT. Hemorrhoidectomy during pregnancy: risk or relief? Dis Colon Rectum 1991; 34:260–261.
86. Abramowitz L, Sobhan I, Benifle JL, et al. Anal fissure and thrombosed external hemorrhoids before and after delivery. Dis Colon Rectum 2002; 45:650–655.
87. Chawla Y, Dilawari JB. Anorectal varices—their frequency in cirrhotic and non-cirrhotic portal hypertension. Gut 1991; 32:309–311.
88. Johnson K, Bardin J, Orloff MJ. Massive bleeding from hemorrhoidal varices in portal hypertension. JAMA 1980; 244:2084–2085.
89. Nivatvongs S. Suture of massive hemorrhoidal bleeding in portal hypertension. Dis Colon Rectum 1985; 28:878–879.
90. Jacobs DM, Bubrick MP, Onstad GR, Hitchcock CR. The relationship of hemorrhoids to portal hypertension. Dis Colon Rectum 1980; 23:567–569.
91. Hosking SW, Johnson AG. Bleeding anorectal varices—a misunderstood condition. Surgery 1988; 104:70–73.
92. Biswas S, George ML, Leather AJM. Stapled anopexy in the treatment of anal varices. Report of a case. Dis Colon Rectum 2003; 46:1284–1285.
93. Katz JA, Rubin RA, Cope C, Holland G, Brass CA. Recurrent bleeding from anorectal varices: successful treatment with a transjugular intrahepatic portosystemic shunt. Gastroenterology 1993; 88:1104–1107.
94. Yeh T Jr, McGuire HH Jr. Intractable bleeding from anorectal varices relieved by inferior mesenteric vein ligation. Gastroenterology 1994; 107:1165–1167.
95. Jeffery PJ, Ritchie JK, Parks AG. Treatment of hemorrhoids in patients with inflammatory bowel disease. Lancet 1977; 1:1084–1085.
96. Wolkomir AF, Luchtefeld MA. Surgery for symptomatic hemorrhoids and anal fissures in Crohn's disease. Dis Colon Rectum 1993; 36:545–547.
97. Grewal H, Guillem JG, Quan SHQ, Enker WE, Cohen AM. Anorectal disease in neutropenic leukemic patients. Dis Colon Rectum 1994; 37:1095–1099.
98. O'Donovan S, Ferrara A, Larach S, Williamson P. Intraoperative use of Toradol facilitates outpatient hemorrhoidectomy. Dis Colon Rectum 1994; 37:793–799.
99. Chester JF, Stanford BJ, Gazet JC. Analgesic benefit of locally injected bupivacaine after hemorrhoidectomy. Dis Colon Rectum 1990; 33:487–489.
100. Pryn SJ, Crosse MM, Murison MSC, McGinn FP. Postoperative analgesia for hemorrhoidectomy. Anaesthesia 1989; 44:964–6.
101. Hoff SD, Bailey HR, Butts DR, et al. Ambulatory surgical hemorrhoidectomy—a solution to postoperative urinary retention? Dis Colon Rectum 1994; 37:1242–1244.
102. Carapeti EA, Kamm MA, McDonald PJ, Phillips RK. Double-blind randomized trial of metronidazole on pain after day-case hemorrhoidectomy. Lancet 1998; 351:169–172.
103. Kilbride M, Morse M, Senagore A. Transdermal fentanyl improves management of postoperative hemorrhoidectomy pain. Dis Colon Rectum 1994; 37: 1070–1072.
104. Bernstein KJ, Klausner MA. Potential dangers related to transdermal fentanyl (Duragesic) when used for postoperative pain. Dis Colon Rectum 1994; 37:1339–1340.
105. Corman ML, Grevie JF, Hager T, et al. Stapled haemorrhoidopexy: a consensus position paper by an international working party—indications, contra-indications and technique. Colorectal Disease 2003; 5:304–310.
106. Pernice LM, Bartalucci B, Bencini L, Borri A, Caterzi S, Kroning K. Early and late (ten years) experience with circular stapler hemorrhoidectomy. Dis Colon Rectum 2001; 44:836–841.
107. Longo A. Treatment of hemorrhoidal disease by reduction of mucosa and hemorrhoidal prolapse with a circular suturing device: a new procedure. Proceeding of the 6th world congress of endoscopic surgery, Rome, 1998:777–784.
108. Esser S, Khubchandani I, Rakhmanine M. Stapled hemorrhoidectomy with local anesthesia can be performed safely and cost-effectively. Dis Colon Rectum 2004; 47:1164–1169.
109. Gahrielli F, Chiarelli M, Cioffi U, et al. Day surgery for mucosa—hemorrhoidal prolapse using a circular stapler and modified regional anesthesia. Dis Colon Rectum 2001; 44:842–844.
110. Senagore A, Abcarian H, Corman M, et al. Safety of stapled hemorrhoidopexy: initial results from a multicenter trial [abstract]. Dis Colon Rectal 2002; 45: A22–A23.
111. Singer MA, Cintron JR, Fleshman JW, et al. Early experience with stapled hemorrhoidectomy in the United States. Dis Colon Rectum 2002; 45:360–369.
112. Arnuad JP, Pessaux P, Huten N, et al. Treatment of hemorrhoids with circular stapler, a new alternative to conventional methods: a prospective study of 140 patients. J Am Coll Surg 2001; 193:161–165.
113. Beattie GC, Lam JPH, Loudon MA. A prospective evaluation of the introduction of circumferential stapled anoplasty in the management of hemorrhoids and mucosal prolapse. Colorectal Dis 2000; 2:137–142.

114. Habr-Gama A, e Sousa JR AHS, Rovelo JMC, et al. Stapled hemorrhoidectomy: initial experience of a Latin American group. J Gastrointest Surg 2003; 7: 809–813.
115. Correa-Rovelo JM, Tellez O, Obregon L, Miranda-Gomez A, Moran S. Stapled rectal mucosectomy vs. closed hemorrhoidectomy. A randomized, clinical trial. Dis Colon Rectum 2002; 45:1367–1375.
116. Rowsell M, Bello M, Hemingway DM. Circumferential mucosectomy (stapled hemorrhoidectomy) versus conventional hemorrhoidectomy: randomized controlled trial. Lancet 2000; 355:779–781.
117. Ho YH, Cheong WK, Tsang C, Ho J, Eu KW, Tang CL. Stapled hemorrhoidectomy—cost effectiveness. Randomized controlled trail including incontinence scoring, anorectal manometry, and endoanal ultrasound assessments at up to three months. Dis Colon Rectum 2000; 43:1666–1675.
118. Bikhehandani J, Agarwal PN, Kant R, Malik VK. Randomized controlled trial to compare the early and mid-term results of stapled vs open hemorrhoidectomy. Am J Surg 2005; 189:56–60.
119. Basdanis G, Papadopoulos N, Michalopoulos A, Apostolodis S, Harlaftis N. Randomized clinical trial of stapled hemorrhoidectomy vs open with ligasure for prolapsed piles. Surg Endosc 2005; 19:235–239.
120. Senagore AJ, Singer H, Abcarian H, Fleshman J, Corman M, Wexner S, Nivatrongs S. A prospective, randomized, controlled multicenter trial comparing stapled hemorrhoidopexy and Ferguson hemorrhoidectomy: Perioperative and I year results. Dis Colon Rectum 2004; 47:1824–1836.
121. Kairaluoma M, Nuorva K, Kellokumpu I. Day-case stapled (circular) vs. diathermy hemorrhoidectomy. A randomized, controlled trial evaluating surgical and functional outcome. Dis Colon Rectum 2003; 46:93–99.
122. Cheetham MJ, Cohen CRG, Kamm MA, Phillips RKS. A randomized, controlled trial of diathermy hemorrhoidectomy vs. stapled hemorrhoidectomy in an intended day-case setting with longer-term follow-up. Dis Colon Rectum 2003; 46:491–497.
123. Wilson MS, Pope V, Doran HE, Fearn SJ, Brough WA. Objective comparison of stapled anopexy and open hemorrhoidectomy. Dis Colon Rectum 2002; 45:1437–1444.
124. Hetzer FH, Demartines N, Handschin A, Clavien PA. Stapled vs excision hemorrhoidectomy. Long-term results of a prospective randomized trial. Arch Surg 2002; 137:337–340.
125. Ortiz H, Marzo J, Armendariz P. Randomized clinical trial of stapled hemorrhoidopexy versus conventional diathermy hemorrhoidectomy. Br J Surg 2002; 89:1376–1381.
126. Shalaby R, Desoky A. Randomized clinical trial of stapled vs. Milligan–Morgan hemorrhoidectomy. Br J Surg 2001; 88:1049–1053.
127. Boccasanta P, Capretti PG, Venturi M, et al. Randomized controlled trial between stapled circumferential mucosectomy and conventional circular hemorrhoidectomy in advanced hemorrhoids with external mucosal prolapse. Am J Surg 2001; 182:64–68.
128. Ganio E, Altomare DF, Gabrielli F, Milito G, Canuti S. Prospective randomized multicenter trial comparing stapled with open hemorrhoidectomy. Br J Surg 2001; 88:669–674.
129. Mehigan BJ, Monson JRT, Hartly JE. Stapling procedure for hemorrhoids versus Milligan–Morgan hemorrhoidectomy: randomized controlled trial. Lancet 2000; 355:782–785.
130. Beattie GC, Loudon MA. Circumferential stapled anoplasty in the management of hemorrhoids and mucosal prolapse. Colorect Dis 2000; 2:170–175.
131. Ortiz H, Marzo J, Armendariz P, De Miguel M. Stapled hemorrhoidopexy vs. diathermy excision for fourth-degree hemorrhoids: a randomized clinical trial and review of the literature. Dis Colon Rectum 2005; 48:809–815.
132. Peng BC, Jayne DG, Ho YH. Randomized trial of rubber band ligation vs. stapled hemorrhoidectomy for prolapsed piles. Dis Colon Rectum 2003; 46: 291–297.
133. Ravo B, Amato A, Bianco V, et al. Complications after stapled hemorrhoidectomy: can they be prevented? Tech Coloproctol 2002; 6:83–88.
134. Correa-Rovelo JM, Tellez O, Obregon L, et al. Prospective study of factors affecting postoperative pain and symptom persistence after stapled rectal mucosectomy for hemorrhoids. A need for preservation of squamous epithelium. Dis Colon Rectum 2003; 46:955–962.
135. Cheetham MJ, Mortensen NJM, Nystrom PO, Kamm MA, Phillips RKS. Persistent pain and focal urgency after stapled hemorrhoidectomy. Lancet 2000; 356:730–733.
136. Ho YH, Scow-Choen F, Tang C, Eu K-W. Randomized trial assessing and sphincter injuries after stapled hemorrhoidectomy. Br J Surg 2001; 88: 1449–1455.
137. Longo A. Pain after stapled hemorrhoidectomy correspondence. Lancet 2000; 356:2189–190.
138. Thaha MA, Irvine LA, Steele RJC, Campbell KL. Post defecation pain syndrome after circular stapled anopexy is abolished by oral nifedipine. Br J Surg 2005; 92:208–210.
139. George BD, Shetty D, Lindsey I, Mortensen NJ, Mc C, Warren BF. Histopathology of stapled hemorrhoidectomy specimens: a cautionary note. Colorectal Dis 2002; 44:473–476.
140. Brusciano L, Ayabaca SM, Pescatori M, et al. Reinterventions after complicated or failed stapled hemorrhoidopexy. Dis Colon Rectum 2004; 47:1846–1851.
141. Altomare DF, Rinaldi M, Sallustio PL, Martino P, De Gazio M, Memeo V. Long-term effects of stapled hemorrhoidectomy on internal anal function and sensitivity. Br J Surg 2001; 88:1487–1491.
142. Molloy RG, Kingsmore D. Life threatening pelvic sepsis after stapled hemorrhoidectomy. Lancet 2000; 355:810.
143. Maw A, Eu KW, Seow-Choen F. Retroperitoneal sepsis complicatory stapled hemorrhoidectomy. Report of a case and review of the literature. Dis Colon Rectum 2002; 45:826–828.
144. Wong LY, Jiang JK, Chang SC, Lin JK. Rectal perforation: a life-threatening complication of stapled hemorrhoidectomy. Report of a case. Dis Colon Rectum 2003; 46:116–117.
145. Ripetti V, Caricato M, Arullani A. Rectal perforation, retropneumoperitoneum, and preumomediastinum after stapling procedure for prolapsed hemorrhoids. Report of a case and subsequent considerations. Dis Colon Rectum 2002; 45:268–270.
146. Harold A, Kirsch JJ. Pain after stapled hemorrhoidectomy. Correspondence. Lancet 2000; 356:2187.
147. Cipriani S, Pescatori M. Acute rectal obstruction after PPH stapled hemorrhoidectomy. Colorectal Dis 2002; 4:367–370.
148. Macrae HM, Teruple LKF, McLeod RS. A meta-analysis of hemorrhoidal treatments. Sem Colon Rectal Surg 2002; 13:77–83.

9 Fissure-in-Ano

Philip H. Gordon

INTRODUCTION

A fissure-in-ano is a painful linear ulcer situated in the anal canal and extending from just below the dentate line to the margin of the anus. It is a very common condition that causes suffering out of proportion to the size of the lesion. In the acute phase, the lesion is often a mere crack in the epithelial surface but may cause much pain and spasm.

CLINICAL FEATURES

The lesion is usually encountered in younger and middle-aged adults but also may occur in infants, children, and the elderly. Fissures are equally common in both sexes. Anterior fissures are more common in women than in men. Occasionally, patients develop anterior and posterior fissures simultaneously. In a review of 876 patients with fissure-in-ano, Hananel and Gordon (1) found the same sex distribution (women, 51.1%; men, 49.9%) with a mean age of 39.9 years (range, 13.5–95 years). The fissure was located in the posterior midline in 73.5%, the anterior midline in 16.4%, and in both in 2.6%. Only tenderness was documented in 7.4% of the patients studied. The fissure was located in the anterior midline in 12.6% of women and 7.7% of men. The authors concluded that anterior fissures are much more common in both men and women than previously reported. Petros et al. (2) also found fissures to be more commonly located in the anterior midline (15% in men and 45% in women). In any event, the length of each fissure is remarkably constant, extending from the dentate line to the anal verge and corresponding roughly to the lower half of the internal sphincter, a point of practical importance when operative therapy is considered.

PATHOLOGY

Acute fissures usually heal promptly with conservative treatment, but they may show considerable reluctance to heal. If the acute fissure does not heal readily, secondary changes develop. One of the most striking features is swelling at the lower end of the fissure, forming the so-called sentinel pile. Often the tag has a very inflamed, tense, and edematous appearance. Later it may undergo fibrosis and persist as a permanent fibrous skin tag, even if the fissure heals. At the proximal end of the fissure at the level of the dentate line, swelling caused by edema and fibrosis occurs; this condition is referred to as a hypertrophied anal papilla. In addition, long-standing cases develop fibrous induration in the lateral edges of the fissure. After several months without healing, the base of the ulcer, which is the internal sphincter, becomes fibrosed, resulting in a rather spastic, fibrotic, tightly contracted internal sphincter. At no time is the fissure in contact with the external sphincter.

At any stage, frank suppuration may occur and extend into the surrounding tissues, forming an intersphincteric abscess or a perianal abscess that may discharge through the anal canal or burst spontaneously externally and produce a low intersphincteric fistula. Usually, the external opening of this fistula is close to the midline and a short distance behind the anus.

ETIOLOGY

All the factors in the causation of anal fissure have not been resolved. Why certain fissures readily heal with no problem and others linger, creating long-standing problems, is not well understood. However, it is generally agreed that the initiating factor in the development of a fissure is trauma to the anal canal, usually in the form of the passage of a fecal bolus that is large and hard.

One of the remarkable features of fissure-in-ano is that it is nearly always located in the midline posteriorly because of the elliptic arrangement of the external sphincter fibers posteriorly. This arrangement offers less support to the anal canal during the passage of a large fecal bolus. Consequently, a tear may develop there more easily than elsewhere in the circumference of the anus.

In a case control study, Jensen (3) found evidence to indicate that anal fissure is likely to result at least partly from an inappropriate diet and that dietary manipulations might reduce the incidence of fissure-in-ano. A significantly decreased risk was associated with frequent consumption of raw fruits, vegetables, and whole-grain bread, and a significantly increased risk was related to frequent consumption of white bread, sauces thickened with roux, and bacon or sausages. Risk ratios for consumption of coffee, tea, and alcohol were not significantly different. No statistical associations were found with particular occupational exposures. However, a history of previous anal surgery was reported significantly more often for cases than for controls.

PREDISPOSING FACTORS

Secondary fissures may occur as a result of either an anatomic anal abnormality or inflammatory bowel disease, particularly Crohn's disease (4). The association of Crohn's disease with anal fissures is well recognized. Previous anal surgery, especially hemorrhoidectomy, may result in anal scarring, skin loss, and stenosis. Fistula-in-ano surgery may result in distortion of the anal canal with scarring and fixation of the anal skin. This decreased elasticity of the anal canal may then predispose to fissure formation. Some of the anterior fissures occurring in women result from childbirth. Perineal trauma leads to scarring and abnormal tethering of the anal submucosa, thus rendering it more susceptible to trauma because of its loss of laxity and mobility. Individuals with a long-standing condition of loose stools, usually resulting from chronic laxative abuse, may develop an anal stenosis with scarring, again predisposing to fissure formation. The presence of hemorrhoids is not likely a predisposing factor; more likely an abnormality of the internal sphincter predisposes the patient to the formation of both hemorrhoids and fissures.

PATHOGENESIS

If the concept that trauma to the anal canal is the initiating factor in the establishment of a fissure-in-ano is accepted, then why certain fissures proceed to and persist in a chronic state must be asked. Perpetuating factors might include infection, for example, but it is unlikely since there is no more florid sepsis in chronic fissures than in the acute ones. Persistently hard bowel movements, in addition to initiating the process, may continuously aggravate the anal canal and result in perpetuation of the fissure. This factor must be taken into account when planning treatment.

Studies have demonstrated that after the initiation of a tear in the anal canal, chronicity is perpetuated by an abnormality in the internal anal sphincter. Most investigators have found that resting pressures within the internal anal sphincter are higher in patients with fissures than in normal controls (5–13). Catheter size does not influence measured maximum resting pressure in fissure patients (14).

Nothmann and Schuster (5) demonstrated that after rectal distention there is a normal reflex relaxation of the internal sphincter. In patients with anal fissures, this relaxation is followed by an abnormal "overshoot" contraction (Fig. 1). This phenomenon could account for the sphincter spasm and explain the pain that results from rectal stimulation during defecation. Furthermore, the authors demonstrated that after successful treatment of the fissure, the abnormal reflex contraction of the internal sphincter

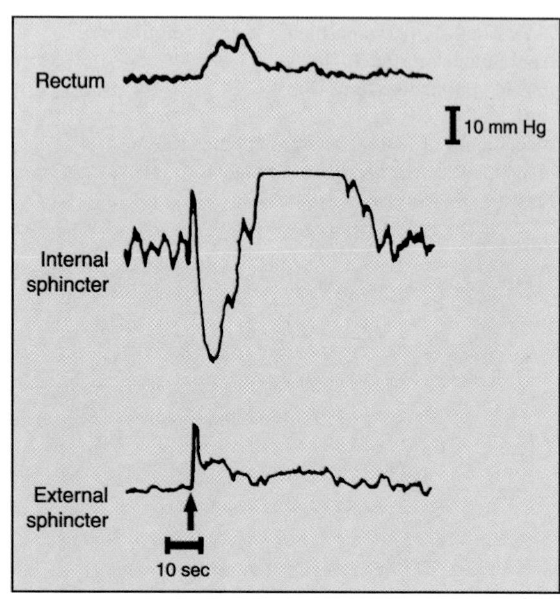

FIGURE 1 ■ "Overshoot" contraction.

vanishes, a finding confirmed by others (15). Keck et al. (11) found the primary abnormality in fissure to be persistent hypertonia affecting the entire internal sphincter, but no overshoot was seen. Chowcat et al. (7) found that after lateral internal sphincterotomy, the pressure dropped by 50% to normal levels and the fissures healed with no change in pressure over a 12-month follow-up. Williams et al. (12) demonstrated a significant reduction in mean resting pressure after lateral sphincterotomy that was maintained five weeks later. Cerdan et al. (15) also have shown that the return to normal pressures persists one year after sphincterotomy. Adequate internal sphincterotomy appears to permanently reduce anal canal pressure, which suggests that abnormal activity in the sphincter contributes to the development of a fissure. Farouk et al. (10) found that following lateral internal sphincterotomy the number of internal sphincter relaxations increased, lending further evidence to the hypothesis that internal sphincter hypertonia may be relevant to the pathogenesis of this disorder. Abcarian et al. (6) have suggested that the beneficial effect of internal sphincterotomy might, at least in part, be due to the anatomic widening of the anal canal, a concept supported by Olsen et al. (16), who failed to find a reduction in resting pressures after lateral sphincterotomy.

Gibbons and Read (17) documented resting pressures that exceeded the normal range within the anal canal, whereas maximal pressures recorded during a voluntary contraction of the sphincter were no higher than in control subjects. They noted that it was unlikely that high resting pressures recorded in patients with chronic anal fissures when probes of varying size were used were caused by spasm but probably represented a true increase in basal sphincter tone. They further proposed that elevated sphincter pressures may cause ischemia of the anal lining, possibly resulting in the pain of anal fissures and their failure to heal. Kuijpers (18), who also found elevated resting anal pressures in patients with fissures, supports the concept of elevated sphincter pressure rather than spasm. Schouten and Blankensteijn (19) studied ultraslow wave pressure variations in the anal canal before and after lateral internal sphincterotomy. Ultraslow waves in the anal canal are discrete pressure fluctuations with a low frequency (1–2/min) and a high amplitude ($\geq$10% above or below baseline resting pressure). These investigators found that these waves are associated with high maximal anal resting pressure and disappear when the high resting pressure is reduced by lateral internal sphincterotomy to a level found in control subjects without ultraslow waves. They concluded that these waves are the manifestation of increased activity of the internal sphincter. Xynos et al. (8) also found the presence of ultraslow waves to be more common in patients with anal fissure. Following internal sphincterotomy, the preoperative elevated resting pressures returned to normal, and the ultraslow waves were significantly reduced postoperatively but did not return to normal. Patients with unhealed fissures showed the same pathologic manometric features as those before operation. Keck et al. (11) found ultraslow waves in 91% of patients and 73% of controls. Ultraslow wave amplitude was 31 mmHg in patients and 15 mmHg in controls.

Using angiographic, histologic, and dissection methods, Klosterhalfen et al. (20) demonstrated that in 85% of specimens the posterior commissure is perfused more poorly than the other portion of the anal canal and postulated that this finding may play a role in the pathogenesis of fissure-in-ano. They suggested that vessels passing through the sphincter muscle are subject to contusion during periods of increased sphincter tone and that the resulting decrease in blood supply might lead to a pathogenetically relevant ischemia at the posterior commissure. In a landmark study, Schouten et al. (21) simultaneously assessed the microvascular perfusion of the anoderm by laser Doppler flowmetry and measured maximal anal resting pressure in 27 patients with anal fissures. Both measurements were repeated 6 weeks after lateral internal sphincterotomy and compared with the measurements of 27 controls. Mean maximum anal resting pressure was significantly higher in those patients with a fissure than in controls, and anodermal blood flow at the fissure site was significantly lower than at the posterior commissure of the controls. In the patients with a fissure, a significant pressure decrease was noted (35%) that was accompanied by a consistent rise in blood flow (65%) at the original fissure site. The increased internal sphincter tone in patients with a fissure reduces anodermal blood flow at the posterior midline. Reduction of anal pressure by sphincterotomy improves anodermal blood flow at the posterior midline, resulting in fissure healing.

A primary internal anal sphincter disturbance may be a contributory etiologic factor. Internal anal sphincter supersensitivity to β_2 (beta-2) agonists has been observed in patients with chronic anal fissure (22). This may be induced by a prolonged absence of the neurotransmitter, by abnormalities at neurotransmitter or metabolic level, or by a modification of cholinergic and adrenergic receptors. Internal anal smooth muscle relaxation can be inhibited by stimulation of nonadrenergic noncholinergic enteric neurones, parasympathetic muscarinic receptors, or sympathetic beta adrenoceptors, and by inhibition of calcium entry into the cell. Sphincter contraction depends on an increase in cytoplasmic calcium and is enhanced by sympathetic adrenergic stimulation (22).

When trying to determine a rational treatment for fissure-in-ano, the surgeon must bear in mind the abnormality in the internal sphincter.

SYMPTOMS

The cardinal symptom of an anal fissure is pain in the anus during and after defecation. The pain usually is described as a sharp, cutting, or tearing sensation during the actual passage of stool. Subsequently, the pain may be less severe and may be described as a burning or gnawing discomfort that may persist from a few minutes to several hours. Because of the anticipated pain, the patient may not defecate when the natural urge occurs. Such procrastination leads to harder stools, with subsequent bowel movements more painful. A relentless cycle may ensue with the individual living from one bowel movement to the next.

Bleeding is very common with fissure-in-ano but is not invariably present. The blood is bright red and usually scant in amount.

Some patients have a large sentinel pile that draws their attention to the anus. In such circumstances, patients usually complain of a painful external hemorrhoid.

Discharge may lead to soiling of the underclothes and to increased moisture on the perianal skin, with resulting pruritus ani, although pruritus may occur independently of any discharge.

Constipation is frequently touted as an accompanying symptom as well as an initiating symptom of anal fissure.

Sometimes patients with a painful fissure develop disturbances of micturition, namely dysuria, retention, or frequency.

Although not usually a presenting complaint, dyspareunia may be caused by an anal fissure.

In a review of 876 patients with fissure-in-ano, Hananel and Gordon (1) found that the dominant presenting symptoms included pain in 90.8% of the patients studied and bleeding in 71.4%. Surprisingly, infrequent hard bowel movements (≥3 days) occurred in only 13.8% of patients. Straining during defecation was reported by 29.3% of patients. They concluded that constipation and hard bowel movements are not universally present in patients with fissure-in-ano. Other presenting symptoms included pruritus (6.2%), swelling (3.3%), prolapse (2.1%), and discharge (1.1%). The duration of symptoms before any treatment was instituted varied widely (<1 month, 22% of patients; 1–6 months, 41.4%; 6–12 months, 7.7%; 1–2 years, 16.6%; >2 years, 12.3%). Associated anorectal problems that needed treatment were diagnosed in 7.3% of patients (mostly hemorrhoids, 6.2%). A history of a previous anal operation was obtained from 5.8% of patients. Previous episodes of the same symptoms were reported by 16.2% of patients; 2.6% reported one episode and 13.6% reported more than one episode.

The clinical entity of painless, nonhealing fissure may be annoying to both patient and surgeon. The patient may experience some bleeding from time to time, but symptoms may not be severe enough to recommend operative treatment. Thirty-two such patients (4.8%) were diagnosed in the study by Hananel and Gordon (1). It should be kept in mind that the lesion may be the progenitor of inflammatory bowel disease.

DIAGNOSIS

The diagnosis of a fissure is usually straightforward and is made from the patient's history alone. A physical examination confirms the suspicion of fissure and rules out other associated disease. The association between fissures and inflammatory bowel disease should always be remembered, and a careful history should be taken and followed, if indicated, by appropriate radiologic, hematologic, and biochemical investigations.

Inspection is by far the most important step in the examination for anal fissure (Fig. 2). If properly sought, most fissures can be seen. Because anal fissures are such extremely painful lesions, special care must be taken to make the examination as gentle as possible. Gentle separation of the buttocks usually reveals the fissure; however, spasm may keep the anal orifice closed, and the finding of spasm of a sphincter is suggestive of a fissure. The coexistence of large hemorrhoids or skin folds may hide the ulcer. Nonvisualization of the lesion does not rule out its presence, and the diagnosis may be made more by history and palpation than by visual appearance. The triad of a chronic fissure includes a sentinel pile, an anal ulcer, and a hypertrophied anal papilla, with the sentinel pile noted first posteriorly.

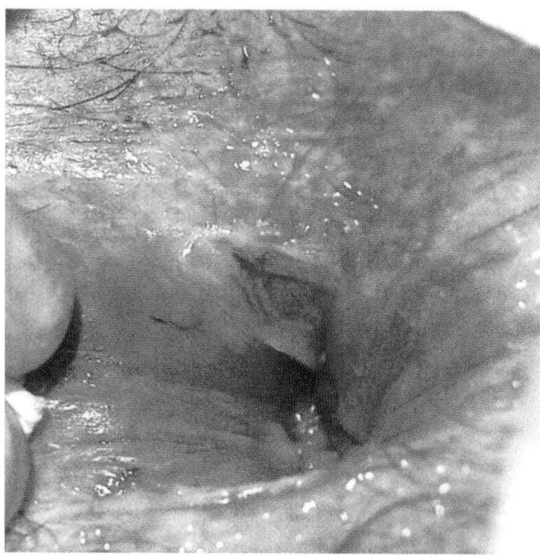

FIGURE 2 ■ A chronic fissure with scarred base, hypertrophied anal papilla, and sentinel pile.

In any patient with a fissure located off the midline, a specific systemic disease should be considered. A full list of the possible diseases is included in the section on differential diagnosis.

Palpation is the next step in the examination and confirms the presence of sphincter spasm. The digital examination is uncomfortable, with maximal tenderness usually elicited in the posterior midline. In fact, the pain may be so intense that a complete digital examination cannot be performed during the initial examination. However, it is essential that the examination be performed later to exclude other lesions of the lower rectum such as carcinoma or a polyp. With a chronic fissure, induration of the base and the lateral edges, as well as a hypertrophied anal papilla, may be palpable.

With an acute fissure, anoscopic examination is usually impossible because of the severe pain. With a chronic fissure, the ulcer itself will be noted as a triangular-shaped slit in the anal canal, with the floor being the internal sphincter. Just proximal to the ulcer, the hypertrophied anal papilla may be identified. A chronic fissure may be associated with anal stenosis of varying severity, especially if the patient has had a previous anal operation such as a hemorrhoidectomy. Evaluation of the chronicity of the process is important. Once the entire internal sphincter is bared with scarring and fibrosis and the history of problems is long-standing, the fissure is unlikely to heal without an operation. Anoscopy may also demonstrate other conditions such as internal hemorrhoids or proctitis.

Sigmoidoscopy likewise may be impossible to perform during the initial examination, but it must be performed at a subsequent visit to rule out an associated carcinoma or inflammatory bowel disease.

A biopsy should be performed on any fissure that fails to heal after treatment. Such biopsy may reveal unsuspected Crohn's disease or an implanted adenocarcinoma.

Squamous carcinoma of the anal canal may be confused with fissure-in-ano.

DIFFERENTIAL DIAGNOSIS

Most conditions in patients presenting with anal pain, swelling, or bleeding are usually easily distinguished. Thrombosed hemorrhoids or perianal abscesses are readily seen. However, certain other conditions may require more careful discrimination (Fig. 3).

■ ANORECTAL SUPPURATION

Of greatest importance is the intersphincteric abscess, which may closely mimic a fissure. An intersphincteric fistulous abscess without an external opening is usually situated posteriorly in the mid-anal canal between the internal and external sphincter. It causes great pain that may last for many hours after defecation. A diagnostic clue to the intersphincteric abscess is that the pain usually does not completely go away. Little if anything is seen externally, but during the examination exquisite tenderness will be elicited over the abscess, which itself may not be palpable. This entity is discussed further in Chapter 10.

■ PRURITUS ANI

Pruritus ani with superficial cracks in the anal skin may sometimes prove a source of difficulty because many patients with anal fissure develop pruritus as a result of the discharge irritating the perianal skin. However, the skin in pruritus ani shows only superficial cracks extending radially from the anus, and these cracks never extend up to the dentate line. Therefore, digital examination of the rectum does not elicit pain, and there is no true anal spasm or tenderness.

■ FISSURES IN INFLAMMATORY BOWEL DISEASE

Anal fissures associated with ulcerative colitis are often situated off the midline and may be multiple. These fissures, as well as being broad, are surrounded with inflamed skin. This inflammation should alert the surgeon to an associated proctocolitis, which can be diagnosed if a view of the rectal mucosa can be obtained through endoscopy.

Anal and perianal ulceration frequently occurs with Crohn's disease. The ulcer is often much more extensive than an idiopathic fissure. If a lesion is suspect, biopsy frequently reveals the histologic features of Crohn's disease. Sigmoidoscopy may, in fact, be normal because the involved intestine may be more proximal. Despite the opinion of some authors, Crohn's fissures are not always painless.

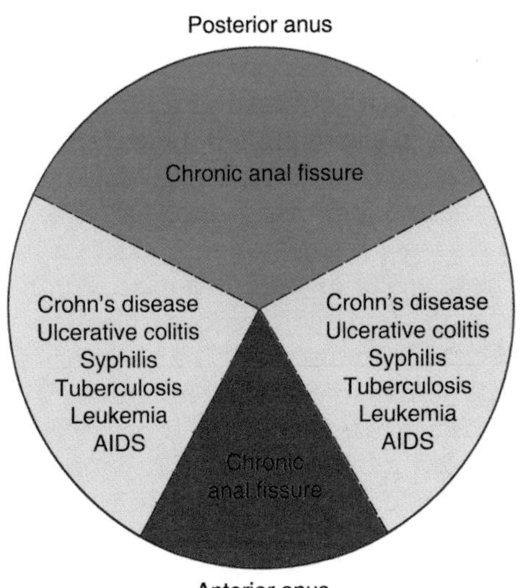

FIGURE 3 ■ Common locations of chronic anal fissures and other anal conditions.

■ CARCINOMA OF ANUS

Squamous cell carcinoma of the anus or adenocarcinoma of the rectum may involve the anal skin, at which time considerable pain with defecation may occur. Palpation, however, may detect a greater degree of induration, and a biopsy should be performed on any suspect lesion (see Chap. 18).

■ SPECIFIC INFECTIOUS PERIANAL CONDITIONS

Syphilitic fissures may be caused by either primary chancres or condylomata lata. In its initial stage, a chancre may closely resemble an ordinary fissure but acquires much induration at its margin, and the inguinal lymph nodes become enlarged. A highly characteristic feature is a symmetric lesion on the opposite wall of the anal canal. Suspect lesions can be diagnosed by a dark-field examination. Anal condylomata lata may occur at the anal orifice, as well as in the perianal region, and may cause multiple anal fissures. Secondary skin lesions and mucous patches, however, are usually present, and the Wasserman reaction is strongly positive. Contrary to popular belief, syphilitic lesions in the anal region are not always painless.

A tuberculous ulcer in the anal region is rare. When it occurs, it tends to enlarge and develop undermined edges. Differentiating this lesion from Crohn's disease may be very difficult; however, the tuberculous ulcer is usually associated with pulmonary tuberculosis. Performing a biopsy and guinea pig inoculations may be necessary. After antituberculous chemotherapy has been administered, these lesions may be treated the same way as an idiopathic fissure.

■ HEMATOLOGIC CONDITIONS

Leukemic infiltration is extremely painful and usually is the sign of the advanced phase of the malignant disease. No treatment is indicated except for drainage of abscesses.

■ MISCELLANEOUS CONDITIONS

An anal abrasion is a rubbing off, or scraping off, of the skin of the anal canal. It is a mild disorder that can be differentiated from a fissure by the features listed in Table 1.

When no local disease is found in the anal region, other diagnoses should be considered, such as proctalgia fugax, coccygodynia, rectal crisis of tabes, or frank psychoneurosis.

Proctalgia fugax may cause severe pain but usually awakens the patient at night, is of short duration, and is not necessarily related to bowel movements (see Chap. 39).

TABLE 1 ■ Fissure-in-Ano vs. Anal Abrasion

Fissure	Abrasion
Deep ulcer	Superficial ulcer
Sentinel pile	No sentinel pile
Anal papilla	No anal papilla
Overhanging edges	Flat edges
Associated scarring	No associated scarring
Rarely lateral	May be lateral
Chronic condition	Transient condition (1–2 days)
Often treated surgically	Not treated surgically

TREATMENT

ACUTE FISSURE

Avoidance of constipation is probably the single most important nonoperative treatment. Patients should be reminded that they must maintain smooth bowel function because bouts of hard stools often result in recurrence of an already healed fissure. The aim of treatment of an acute fissure-in-ano is to break the cycle of a hard stool, pain, and reflex spasm. This result often can be accomplished with simple measures such as warm baths to help relieve the sphincter spasm. Although authors always advise warm baths, the first objective evidence of benefit from this recommendation was described by Dodi et al (23). In a unique study, they manometrically recorded at room temperature (23°C) the resting anal canal pressure of normal controls and patients with anorectal problems such as hemorrhoidal disease, fissures, and proctalgia fugax. Recordings were then made while the anus was immersed in water at varying temperatures (5°C, 23°C, 40°C). Resting pressures were recorded for an additional 30 minutes after immersion at 40°C for 5 minutes. In all subjects, resting anal canal pressures diminished significantly from baseline after immersion at 40°C but remained unchanged in subjects after immersion at 5°C and 23°C. Pinho et al. (24) could find no significant difference between anal pressures in subjects at rest or during voluntary contraction before and after perineal baths at 40°C. However, their study was conducted on normal subjects.

The patient's ingestion of bulk-forming foods (e.g., adequate amounts of unprocessed bran) may be helpful. Alternatively, stool softeners such as psyllium seed preparations can be used to create a soft stool that hopefully will not further tear the anal canal. An additional advantage of a large bulky stool is that it may result in physiologic dilatation of the anal sphincter.

Anesthetic ointments have been used with varying degrees of success. Application only in the perianal region is of no help. The ointment must be inserted into the anal canal to have any effect. Many patients find this procedure rather distasteful and uncomfortable. In addition, a certain number of patients will develop perianal dermatitis.

The use of anal dilators has continued as the mainstay of treatment at St. Mark's Hospital, London. However, the insertion of a cold metal anal dilator through an already extremely painful area is a less than kind form of therapy and is one many patients will probably abandon because of the pain.

Currently, many suppositories are available for the treatment of fissure-in-ano. They contain, in different proportions, sundry combinations of anesthetics, analgesics, astringents, anti-inflammatory agents (usually hydrocortisone), and emollients in a host of bases and preservatives. However, when the suppositories are inserted, they rest well above the area of the fissure because they, by necessity, must rest above the puborectalis muscle and are therefore not in direct contact with the fissure. Many patients complain that the insertion is painful. Credit claimed by the manufacturers for these agents is probably a result of the natural history of the healing of the majority of acute fissures by other measures such as warm baths, stool softeners, and a "tincture of time." Some suppositories may help because of their emollient function.

The many creams and ointments available for treating fissure-in-ano generally contain the same variety of

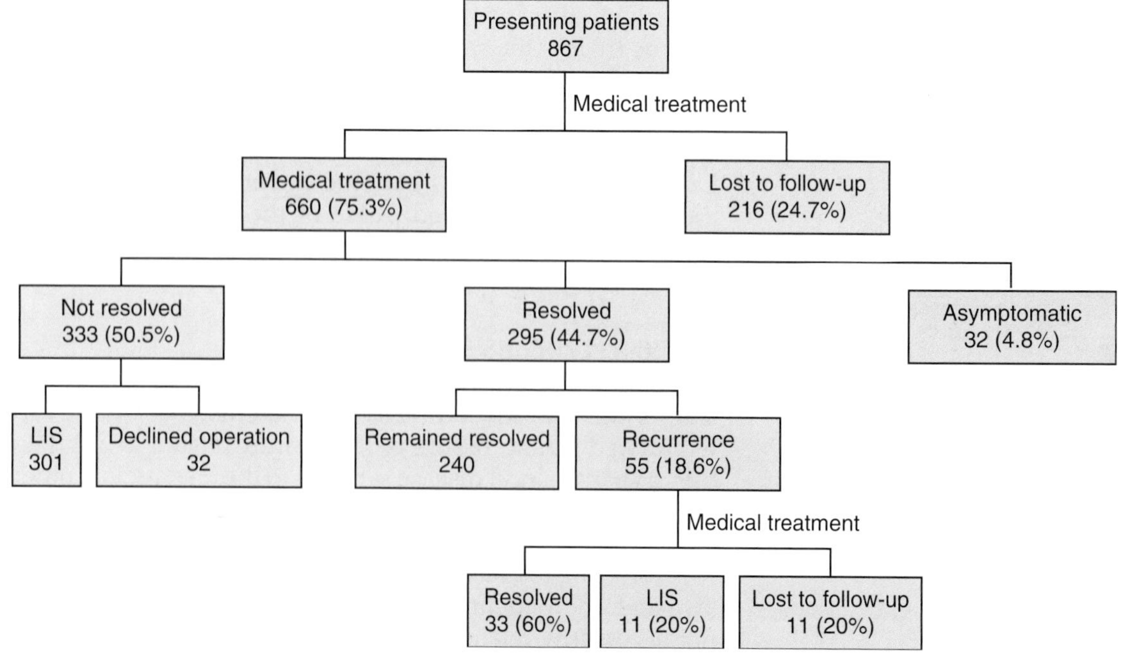

FIGURE 4 ■ Natural history of patients who presented with fissure-in-ano. *Abbreviation*: LIS, lateral internal sphincterotomy.

components as the suppositories. The unproven effectiveness of suppositories applies to those preparations as well.

In a review of 393 patients with fissure-in-ano followed for five years, Shub et al. (25) found that 44% healed within 4–8 weeks with nonoperative treatment consisting of an emollient suppository, a psyllium seed preparation, and sitz baths. The recurrence rate was 27%, and one-third of those lesions healed after further nonoperative treatment. In a review of 137 patients for whom the nonoperative treatment of anal dilators and xylocaine gel was prescribed for an average of 9 weeks, Lock and Thomson (26) reported that one-half were cured, and that the cure was maintained in one-half of these patients at the 4-year follow-up.

In a review by Hananel and Gordon (1) of the response to therapy of 876 patients who presented with fissure-in-ano with a mean follow-up of 26 months (range, 0.5–215 months), 44.7% of patients responded to nonoperative therapy (consisting of bulk-forming agents and sitz baths), 62.4% of them in the first 2 months, and, of those, 18.6% developed recurrent symptoms. Of the latter group, 60% responded to further medical therapy. Of the patients who initially did not respond to medical treatment (50.5%), lateral internal sphincterotomy was recommended (Fig. 4). In an analysis of the time from the initiation of treatment to the resolution of symptoms, it is worthy to note that there was an increase from 62.4% at 2 months to 86.2% at 6 months. Therefore, depending upon the severity of the patient's symptoms, it may be worthwhile to continue medical treatment for up to 6 months if the patient demonstrates steady improvement.

To improve these statistics, Antebi et al. (27) have suggested that for the patient with moderate symptoms who have not responded to other nonoperative methods, the fissure should be injected with 1 mL of a local anesthetic followed immediately by injection of 0.5 mL of the sclerosing agent sodium tetradecyl sulfate (Sotradecol). Pain relief was almost immediate in 96 patients so treated, but four patients developed abscesses, three of which drained spontaneously. When this technique was used, 80% of patients were symptom free at 1-year follow-up.

In a prospective trial, Jensen (28) randomized patients with acute fissure into one of three treatment categories: lignocaine (lidocaine hydrochloride) ointment, hydrocortisone ointment, or warm sitz baths combined with an intake of unprocessed bran. After one and two weeks of treatment, symptomatic relief was significantly better among patients treated with sitz baths and bran than among patients in the other treatment arms. After three weeks there was no significant difference in symptomatic relief among the three groups, but patients treated with lignocaine had significantly fewer healed fissures (60%) than did patients treated with hydrocortisone (82.4%) or warm sitz baths and bran (87%). Jensen's study demonstrated no advantage to the use of proprietary medication; indeed, healing rates were lower in patients receiving such medication.

In another double-blind, placebo-controlled trial, Jensen (29) found that the use of unprocessed bran in doses of 5 g three times daily resulted in a decreased recurrence rate. After a one-year follow-up, the recurrence rate of patients receiving 5 g of bran three times daily was 16%; with patients receiving 2.5 g of bran three times daily, the rate was 60% ($p < 0.01$); and with patients receiving placebo three times daily, the rate was 68% ($p < 0.01$). There was no significant difference in recurrences between patients on 2.5 g of bran and those on placebo. How long should maintenance therapy be continued? In an attempt to answer this question, patients in this study were followed for 6 months after therapy was stopped. Recurrent fissures developed in 25% of patients. This high rate suggests that maintenance therapy should be continued for life.

PHARMACOLOGIC SPHINCTEROTOMY

In recent years, there has been an emerging trend to treat anal fissures by pharmacologic means. Physicians have turned to these methods because of the concern of complications following operation reported by some authors (30–32). Of course, not all authors report high complication rates (see Tables 2 and 3). The new pharmacologic therapies have been used to create a reversible reduction of sphincter pressure until the fissure has healed. Novel agents including glyceryl trinitrate (GTN) and isosorbide dinitrate that results in augmented blood supply to the area, calcium channel blockers such as diltiazem (DTZ) or nifedipine, botulinum toxin that results in chemical denervation of the muscle, muscarinic agonists such as bethanechol, sympathetic neuromodulators such as indoramin, and l-arginine have been studied. A wide variation of results have been reported with the use of these agents and part of the reason for the varied results may be due to the fact that some study patients have included acute fissures, some chronic fissures and often both. The dosage of medication, the frequency of administration of the medication and the length of follow-up also account for the wide variation of results. Indeed, the definition of a chronic fissure has been arbitrary, often considered to be a fissure present for 6–8 weeks (54,55).

Glyceryl Trinitrate

Nitric oxide is the principal neurotransmitter mediating neurogenic relaxation of the internal sphincter. Glyceryl trinitrate (GTN) acts as a nitric oxide donor and when applied as a topical ointment, diffuses across the skin barrier and causes a reduction in internal sphincter pressure as well as improving anodermal blood flow through its vasodilatory effect on the anal vessels. These are the two mechanisms by which it is believed that the glyceryl trinitrate promotes anal fissure healing.

Studies have shown that GTN effectively reduces mean resting anal pressure (54,56,57). In a study of the distribution of nitric oxide synthase containing neurons in the rectal myenteric plexus and anal canal, O'Kelly et al. (58) concluded that their results were consistent with the hypothesis that nitric oxide is the neurotransmitter that mediates the rectoanal inhibitory reflex. In a controlled trial, Loder et al. (57) demonstrated a significant reduction in anal sphincter pressure from the topical application of 0.2% GTN, a finding confirmed by others (59). Lund and Scholefield (54) conducted a prospective randomized double-blind, placebo-controlled study to determine the efficacy of topical GTN 0.2% applied twice a day. After 8 weeks, healing was observed in 68% of patients compared to 8% of controls. Maximum anal resting pressures fell

TABLE 2 ■ Lateral Internal Sphincterotomy

Author(s)	No. of Patients	Impaired Control		Fecal Soiling (%)	Unhealed or Recurrence (%)
		Flatus (%)	Feces (%)		
Abcarian (33)	150	30[d]	0	0	1.3
Lewis et al. (34)	350	17[a]		2.6	6
Hiltunen and Metikainen (35)	65	0	0	0	12.3
Frezza et al. (36)	134	0	0	0	0.6
Xynos et al. (8)	42				4.8
Leong et al. (37)	114	7.9	0	?	2.6
Pernikoff et al. (38)	500	2.8	0.4	4.4	3
Romano et al. (39)	44	9	4.5	4.5	0
Neufeld et al. (40)	112	12.5[d]	0.9	8.9	2.7
Oh, Divino, and Steinhagen (41)	1313	1.5[e]		0	1.3
Usatoff and Polglase (42)	98	7	1	11	3
Garcia-Aquilar et al. (43)	324[b]	30	12	27	14
	225[c]	24	3	16	17
Hananel and Gordon (44)	265	0.4	0.4	0.4	1.1
Farouk et al. (45)	183	?	2.2	?	1.1
Jonas et al. (46)	26	0	0	0	0
Nyam et al. (47)	487	31[d]	23[d]	39[d]	
		6	1	8	8
Argov et al. (48)	2108	1.5[d]		0	1
Richard et al. (49)	38	0	0	0	8
Evans et al. (50)	27	7.4[d]	0	0	3
Mentes et al. (51)	50	16[d]	0	?	6
Arreyo (52)	80	0	4e	?	9
Parelleda (53)	27	15	0	0	0

[a]Impaired control for flatus and feces was combined, but only one-third of these were permanent.
[b]Open sphincterotomy.
[c]Closed sphincterotomy.
[d]Temporary.
[e]Combined flatus and liquid incontinence.

significantly from 115.9 to 75.9 cm H_2O with no change seen after placebo. Watson et al. (60) treated 19 patients with increasing concentrations of GTN (0.2–0.8%) to produce a reduction in maximum resting pressure of > 25%. In an elegant study, Schouten et al. (61) evaluated the influence on the topical application of isosorbide dinitrate on anal pressure, anodermal blood flow, and fissure healing. The 34 patients studied were treated for 6–12 weeks. Before treatment and at three and six weeks, 22 patients underwent conventional anal manometry and laser Doppler flowmetry of the anoderm. Maximum resting anal pressures were significantly reduced; there was a significant increase in anodermal blood flow, and fissure healing occurred in 88% of patients at 12 weeks.

TABLE 3 ■ Immediate or Early Complications of Lateral Internal Sphincterotomy

Author(s)	No. of Patients	Prolapsed Thrombosed Hemorrhoids	Hemorrhage	Perianal Abscess	Fistula-in-Ano
Abcarian (33)	150	0	0	1	1
Lewis et al. (34)	350	0	0	8	4
Hiltunen and Metikainen (35)	65	0	0	0	0
Frezza et al. (36)	134	0	0	0	0
Leong et al. (37)	114	0	5	3	0
Perinikoff et al. (38)	500	0	11	1	3
Romano et al. (39)	44	0	0	1	0
Neufeld et al. (40)	112	0	4	4	1
Oh et al. (41)	1313	0	15	7	3
Hananel and Gordon (44)	265	1	0	0	0
Jonas (46)	26	0	0	0	0
Argov (48)	2108	0	0	21	0
Richard (49)	38	0	0	0	1
Evans (50)	27	0	0	0	0
Mentes (51)	50	0	0	0	0
Arroyo (52)	80	0	1	0	0
Parellada (53)	27	0	0	1	0
Total	5403	1(0.02%)	35(0.7%)	47(0.9%)	13(0.2%)

McLeod and Evans (62) reviewed the literature with respect to the use of nitroglycerin in the management of patients with anal fissure. A total of nine randomized controlled trials have studied the efficacy of GTN in chronic anal fissure. In four out of five trials, GTN was significantly more effective than placebo in healing fissures (54,56,59,63,64). The healing rates in the GTN group varied from 46% to 70% and healing in the placebo group ranged from 8% to 51%. Two trials have reported results of long-term follow-up with symptomatic recurrence rates ranging from 27% to 62% (56,65). Three trials compared 0.2–0.5% GTN to lateral sphincterotomy (49,50,66). Sphincterotomy was superior in two of these trials. Richard et al. (49) conducted a multicenter randomized controlled trial to compare the effectiveness of 0.25% topical GTN with internal sphincterotomy in the treatment of chronic anal fissure. There were 38 patients in the internal sphincterotomy group and 44 patients in the GTN group. At 6 weeks, 34 patients (89.5%) in the internal sphincterotomy group compared with 13 patients (29.5%) in the GTN group had complete healing of the fissure. Five of the 13 patients in the GTN group relapsed whereas none in the internal sphincterotomy group did. At 6 months, fissures in 92.1% of patients in the internal sphincterotomy group compared with 27.2% of patients in the GTN group had healed. In the internal sphincterotomy group, 2.6% patients required further operation for a superficial fistula compared with 45.4% of patients in the GTN group who required an internal sphincterotomy. Of patients in the internal sphincterotomy group, 28.9% developed side effects compared with 84% in the GTN group; 20.5% of patients discontinued the GTN because of headaches or a severe syncopal attack. In each of these trials, healing rates with GTN were much lower than in the other trials with 39–45% eventually having to undergo operation. Follow-up ranged from 4 weeks to 6 months.

Conflicting results with the use of GTN have been reported in the literature with respect to healing rate, recurrence rate, and side effects (Table 4). Differences in reported healing rates may relate to the difficulty in administering a standardized dose to all patients. Most published studies of topical GTN have used 0.2–0.3% preparations. Dosing frequencies varied from two to three times a day and durations vary from 4 to 8 weeks. Healing rates may well be affected by alteration of any of these dosing variables. Zuberi et al. (75) in a randomized trial found the GTN patch to be as effective in treating chronic anal fissures as GTN ointment. The patch offers better compliance and acceptability. Bailey et al. (73) conducted a randomized, double-blind study of intra-anally applied GTN in 17 centers in 304 patients with chronic anal fissures. The patients were randomly assigned to one of eight treatment groups (0.0%, 0.1%, 0.2%, 0.4% GTN ointment applied twice or three times per day) for up to 8 weeks. There were no significant differences in fissure healing among any of the treatment groups. All groups including placebo had a healing rate of approximately 50%. Treatment with 0.4% GTN was associated with a significant decrease in average pain intensity compared with vehicle as assessed with patients with a visual analog scale. At 8 weeks, the magnitude of the difference between 0.4% GTN and control was a 21% reduction in average pain. Treatment was well tolerated with only 3.3% of patients discontinuing treatment because of headaches.

The main concern with GTN is that a significant proportion of patients experience adverse effects. The high incidence of side effects interferes with quality of life and may result in poor patient compliance. Headaches were the primary adverse event and have been reported in 29–72% (56,59). Most were transitory and dose related. Only 3–20% of patients discontinued treatment because of headaches (54,56,66). In the controlled clinical trial of GTN, Altomare et al. (63) failed to demonstrate any superiority of topical 0.2% GTN versus placebo and their high incidences of side effects discouraged the authors from using this treatment as a substitute for operation in chronic anal fissure.

TABLE 4 ■ **Use of Glyceryl Trinitrate in Treatment of Fissure-in-Ano**

Author	Year	*n*	Dose	Frequency	Follow-Up	Healing Rate	Recurrence Rate	Side Effects
Bacher et al. (64)	1997	20	0.2%	t.i.d	1 mo	80%	–	20%
Lund and Scholefield (54)	1997	38	0.2%	b.i.d	2 mo	68%	–	58%
Oettle (66)	1997	12	–	–	22 mo	83%	0	–
Lysy et al. (67)	1998	41	1.25–2.5 mg[a]	t.i.d	11 mo	83%	15%	–
Brisinda (68)	1999	50	0.2%	b.i.d	15 mo	60%	–	10%
Carapeti et al. (59)	1999	70	0.1–0.6	t.i.d	–	67%	33%	72%
Dorfman et al. (69)	1999	31	0.2%	b.i.d	6 mo	56%	27%	78%
Hyman et al. (70)	1999	33	0.3%	t.i.d	–	48%	–	75%
Jonas (46)	1999	49	0.2%	b.i.d	6 wks	43%	2%	4%
Kennedy et al. (56)	1999	43	0.2%	–	29 mo	46%-59%[b]	63%	29%
Altomere et al. (63)	2000	59	0.2%	b.i.d	12 mo	49%	19%	34%
Richard et al. (49)	2000	44	0.25%	t.i.d	6 mo	27%	38%	84%
Evans et al. (50)	2001	33	0.2%	t.i.d	–	61%	45%	–
Gecim (71)	2001	30	0.3%	t.i.d	3–18 mo	80%	25%	7%
Graziano (72)	2001	22	0.25%	b.i.d	0.5–12 mo	77%	53%	–
Pitt et al. (32)	2001	64	0.2%	–	16 mo	41%	46%	–
Bailey et al. (73)	2002	304	01–0.4%	b.i.d–t.i.d	2 mo	50%	–	3%
Kocher et al. (74)	2002	29	0.2%	b.i.d	2 mo	86%	7%	72%
Parellada et al. (53)	2004	27	0.2%	t.i.d	24 mo	89%	11%	30%

[a]Isosorbide dinitrate.
[b]Second treatment with glyceryl trinitrate (GTN).

Pitt et al. (32) conducted a study to identify factors associated with treatment failure of GTN. They cited risk factors of constipation, recent childbirth, colonoscopy and anal receptive intercourse. Fissures were significantly less likely to heal initially, more likely to recur, and more likely to remain unhealed in the long term in the presence of a sentinel pile. Fissures with a history of >6 months were less likely to heal initially. Another reason for the somewhat disappointing results of topical GTN is the frequency of application. Jonas et al. (76) found that GTN 0.2% had a short duration of action (90 minutes) and hence more frequent application of GTN might heal more fissure more rapidly. Duration of treatment has varied from 2 to 12 weeks and this may affect ultimate outcome.

From the reported trials it seems that GTN is effective in healing 1/2 to 2/3 of patients with chronic anal fissure. With long-term follow-up symptoms may recur in 15–63% (Table 4). Despite the initial excitement, the results obtained with GTN have turned out to be rather disappointing with poor patient compliance and high recurrence rates. Randomized trials have also revealed that GTN is inferior to both botulinum toxin (BT) (68) and lateral internal sphincterotomy in providing symptomatic relief and fissure healing (49,50).

Calcium Channel Antagonists

Diltiazem

Diltiazem is a calcium channel blocker, which exerts its effect by lowering the resting anal pressure. Results using this agent are summarized in Table 5. This agent was introduced because of the previously noted side effects of the topical GTN. Jonas et al. (79) conducted a study in patients who failed fissure healing with GTN. Topical use of diltiazem was effective in treating 49% of these patients. Reported side effects included mild perianal itching, headaches, drowsiness, and mood swings. Carapeti et al. (77) compared the use of diltiazem 2% with 0.1% bethanechol tid. Fissures healed in 67% of patients with diltiazem and 60% of those treated with 0.1% bethanechol gel. They found that both diltiazem and bethanechol substantially reduced anal sphincter pressure and achieved fissure healing in a similar degree reported with topical nitrates but without side effects. Jonas et al. (78) evaluated the efficacy of diltiazem for fissures that failed to heal with GTN. Diltiazem 2% was applied twice daily for 8 weeks or until the fissure healed. Fissures healed in 49% of patients within 8 weeks. Side effects occurred in 10% of patients and included perianal itching, but continued with treatment as they were generally well tolerated. Jonas et al. (80) further assessed the effectiveness of oral versus topical diltiazem in the healing of chronic fissures. In a comparison of 60 mg of oral diltiazem with 2% diltiazem gel, healing was noted to be complete in 38% of patients on the oral preparation compared to 65% on those receiving topical treatment. Oral diltiazem caused side effects of headaches, nausea, vomiting, reduced smell and taste, whereas no side effects were seen in those receiving topical therapy. They concluded that topical diltiazem is more effective, achieving healing rates comparable to those reported with topical nitrates with significantly fewer side effects.

Kocher et al. (74) conducted a prospective double-blind randomized trial to compare the incidence of side effects with 0.2% GTN ointment and 2% DTZ cream in the treatment of chronic anal fissure. Treatments were applied perianally, twice daily for 6–8 weeks. There were more side effects with GTN (72%) than with DTZ (42%). In particular, more headaches occurred with GTN (59%) than with DTZ (26%). There were no significant differences in healing and symptomatic improvement rates between patients receiving GTN (86%) and DTZ (77%). DTZ cream caused substantially fewer headaches than GTN ointment and they believe DTZ may be the preferred first-line treatment for chronic anal fissure.

Nifedipine

Nifedipine, a dihydropyridine, is a calcium antagonist that causes smooth muscle relaxation and vasodilatation. Topical application has been shown to lower resting pressure, relieve pain, and heal acute fissures (81). Oral nifedipine and diltiazem have been shown to reduce mean resting pressures between 21% and 36% in healthy volunteers (77,81,82) and in patients with fissures a pressure reduction of 11–36% has been noted (81–83). Results with the use of nifedipine in the treatment of fissure-in-ano both in the cream form as well as the oral form are noted in Table 6.

The principal side effects of oral nifedipine or diltiazem are flushing of the face and limbs, which is usually short lived (82), and mild headaches (77). Proponents of this therapy believe that the few side effects reported with this agent should support its use in the nonoperative treatment of anal fissure. However, Ho and Ho (84) conducted a prospective randomized trial to compare lateral internal anal sphincterotomy with tailored sphincterotomy and oral nifedipine in 132 patients. Lateral internal sphincterotomy was significantly more effective than tailored sphincterotomy in providing pain relief and better patient satisfaction at 4 weeks. Lateral internal sphincterotomy and tailored sphincterotomy were associated with significantly better fissure healing rates and less recurrence than nifedipine. There were substantial problems with compliance in the nifedipine group (41%), related to side effects and slow healing. There were no differences in continence between the three treatment groups. Perrotti et al. (83) performed a prospective randomized double-blind

TABLE 5 ■ Use of Diltiazem in Treatment of Fissure-in-Ano

Author	Year	*n*	Dose	Frequency	Follow-Up	Healing	Recurrence	Side Effects
Carapeti (77)	2000	15	2%	t.i.d		67%		
Knight (55)	2001	71	2%	b.i.d	32 wks	88%	34%	3%
Jonas (78)	2002	39	2%	b.i.d		49%		10%
Kocher et al. (74)	2002	31	2%	b.i.d	3 mo	77%	0	42%

TABLE 6 ■ Use of Nifedipine in Treatment of Fissure-in-Ano

Author	Year	*n*	Dosage	Frequency	Follow-Up	Healing	Recurrence
Antropoli et al. (81)	1999	141	0.2% crm	of12 h	21 days	95%	–
Cook et al. (82)	1999	15	20 mg po	b.i.d	8 wks	60%	–
Perrotti et al. (83)	2002	55	0.3% ungt + 1.5% lidocaine ungt	of12 h	18 mo	95%	6%
Ho et al. (84)	2005	41	20 mg po	b.i.d	16 wks	17%	10%

study in 110 patients to test the efficacy of local application of nifedipine and lidocaine ointment in healing chronic anal fissure. Patients treated with nifedipine ($n = 55$) used topical 0.3% nifedipine and 1.5% lidocaine ointment every 12 hours for 6 weeks. The control group (55) received topical 1.5% lidocaine and 1% hydrocortisone acetate ointment during therapy. Long-term outcomes were determined after a median follow-up of 18 months. Healing of chronic anal fissure was achieved after 6 weeks of therapy in 94.5% of the nifedipine-treated patients as opposed to 16.4% of the controls. Mean anal resting pressure decreased by 11%. They did not observe any systemic side effects in patients treated with nifedipine. After the blinding was removed, recurrence of the fissure was observed in 3 of 52 patients in the nifedipine group within 1 year of treatment and 2 of these patients healed with an additional course of topical nifedipine and lidocaine ointment.

Botulinum Toxin (BT)

Botulinum toxin, a product of clostridium botulinum, produces a potent neuromuscular blockade (51). Several reports have suggested a role for the local muscle relaxant action of this agent in the treatment of anal fissure (68,86,87). The proposed rationale is that it breaks the vicious cycle of inflammation–pain–spasm (87). The toxin inhibits release of acetylcholine into the synaptic gap and causes paresis of the injected muscle that lasts for weeks and allows the fissure to heal. Reinnervation occurs through "sprouting" of the nerve ends.

Many authors have reported on the use of botulinum toxin in the treatment of fissure-in-ano and their results are summarized in Table 7. Temporary incontinence has been reported between 0% and 12%, with complications ranging 0–11% (mostly 0%) and recurrence rates 0–52% (68). Report data are difficult to interpret because of varied dose regimens, different injection sites, and follow-up protocols. In a comparison study of injection of botulinum toxin and topical GTN ointment for the treatment of chronic anal fissure, Brisinda et al. (68) found botulinum toxin more effective (96% vs. 60% healing rate). The optimum dose and method of administration of BT have not been determined. Brisinda et al. (68) conducted a study of 150 patients, half treated with 20 units BT injected into the internal sphincter anteriorly, and if the fissure persisted retreated with 30 units of BT and the other half treated with 30 units BT, and if the fissure persisted retreated with 50 units of BT. After one month, healing in the first group was 73% and in the second group 87%. Five patients in the second group reported incontinence of flatus for 2 weeks. At 2 months, healing in the first group was 89% and in the second group 96%. A relapse of the fissure was observed in 8% in the first group and 2% of patients never healed. A persistent fissure was seen in three patients in the second group. Higher doses appeared more effective in obtaining healing. Lindsey et al. (93) conducted a prospective nonrandomized open-label study of patients with chronic anal fissure failing a course of GTN treated with 20 units of botulinum toxin injected into the internal sphincter. Of 40 patients who underwent BT treatment, 73% were improved symptomatically and avoided operation. Healing occurred in 43% of patients. Of the unhealed fissures, 12% were asymptomatic, 18% were symptomatically improved, and 27% were no better symptomatically and came to operation. Discomfort associated with injection was minimal. Of 34 patients undergoing BT injection, 71% preferred BT, 20% GTN, and 9% were undecided. Transient minor incontinence symptoms were noted in 18%. In their opinion, a policy of first-line GTN, and second-line BT will avoid sphincterotomy in 85–90% of patients. Minguez et al. (92) analyzed the long-term outcome of patients in whom an anal fissure had healed after BT injection and the factors contributing to recurrence. After 42 months of follow-up in the 57 patients

TABLE 7 ■ Use of Botulinum Toxin in Treatment of Fissure-in-Ano

Author	Year	*n*	Dose	Follow-Up	Healing	Recurrence	Temporary Incontinence
Jost (87)	1997	100	2.5–5.0 units	6 mo	79	8%	7%
Fernandez Lopez (88)	1999	76	80 units	–	67%	–	3%
Gonzalez Carro (89)	1999	40	15 units	6	50%	–	–
Maria (90)	1999	50	40 units		60–88%		0
Minguez et al. (91)	1999	23	10 units	1 mo	48%	52%	–
		27	15 units	1 mo	74%	30%	–
		19	21 units	1 mo	100%	37%	–
Gecim (71)	2001	27	5 units	3–18 mo	86%	25%	–
Brisinda (85)	2002	78	20–30 units	2 mo	89%	9.3%	
		75	30–50 units	2 mo	96%	4%	3%
Minguez (92)	2002	57		42 mo		42%	
Montes (51)	2003	61	20–30 units	≥12 mo	75%	11%	

who completely healed six months after injection recurrence developed in 42%. Statistical differences between the permanently healed and the relapsed group were detected when analyzing the anterior location of the fissure (6% vs. 45%), a longer duration of disease (38% vs. 68%), the need for reinjection (26% vs. 59%), a higher total dose injected to achieve definitive healing (13% vs. 45%), and the percentage decrease of maximum squeeze pressure after injection (-28% vs. -13%).

Some reconciliation is necessary between authors recommending injection of toxin into the external sphincter and those advocating injection into the internal sphincter. The mechanism of action must be a diffusion of the toxin into the internal sphincter for those injected into the external sphincter, as the fundamental pathogenesis in chronic fissure formation is an elevated pressure in the internal sphincter. For patients with a posterior fissure, injection of BT results in earlier healing if the injection is made anteriorly (85). This may be due to the scar of the fissure limiting diffusion of the toxin.

Proponents of BT injection state that it is well tolerated, can be performed as an outpatient procedure, and does not cause permanent alteration of continence. However, the safety profile and the ultimate propriety of this form of therapy has not been entirely determined. In an editorial, Brisinda et al. (86) highlighted the popularity of BT treatment and in their review of the literature, cautioned the need for careful review of risks and benefits before extending the approval of BT for widespread use. Following the discovery that BT inhibits neuromuscular transmission, this powerful poison has become a drug with many indications. Controversy exists regarding safety of BT treatment. Effects are seen in autonomic ganglia where it blocks autonomic transmission acutely, producing autonomic symptoms. A study of four patients with botulism found an impairment of heart rate and blood pressure responsivity as well as neuromuscular transmission. The sympathetic tests normalized earlier than the parasympathetic tests on follow-up. Systemic side effects such as skin and allergic reactions, increased residual urine volume, muscular weakness, abnormalities on electromyography of distant muscles, and postural hypotension have been reported and BT diffusion is thought to be responsible for the occurrence of heart block after treatment of esophageal achalasia. Brisinda et al. (86) reported their own experience in an 8-year period, in which up to 1000 patients having pelvic, anorectal, and urologic diseases, such as chronic anal fissure, outlet-type constipation, anterior rectocele, prostatic pain, and benign prostatic hyperplasia have been treated with BT. During this time, none of the patients had systemic complications or severe side effects. Given its effectiveness, they believe that BT seems to be a safe treatment. Nevertheless, more research is needed to optimize the choice of dosage and site of injection.

Muscarinic Agonists

Muscarinic agonists provide nitric oxide synthesis in nonadrenergic, noncholinergic neurons. Bethanechol cream 0.1% decreases sphincter pressure by 24% and has been reported to heal fissures in 60% of patients without side effects (77).

Sympathetic Neuromodulators

Pitt et al. (94) studied the use of alpha-1 adrenoceptor blockade on anal sphincter pressures in patients with fissure. They found that a single oral 20 mg dose of indoramin reduced anal resting pressures by 36%, a reduction that persisted three hours. They proposed that such agents could be suitable for the treatment of fissure-in-ano.

L-Arginine

L-Arginine acts as a substrate for nitric oxide synthase in the production of nitric oxide and has been shown to be effective in the relaxation of the internal anal sphincter. In a placebo-controlled study, Griffin et al. (95) investigated whether topical L-Arginine gel reduces maximal anal resting pressure in volunteers. Anal manometry was performed 2 hours after application of 400 mg of L-Arginine gel in 25 volunteers. Two important findings emerged from this study. First, L-Arginine reduced maximal anal resting pressure by 46%. Second, no side effects occurred. In particular, no episodes of headache were recorded. Since the effects of L-Arginine on sphincter tone is believed to be through the L-Arginine–NO pathway, headaches might be expected. It may be that L-Arginine works through a different mechanism. Its onset of action is rapid and duration is at least two hours. L-Arginine may have therapeutic potential but further evaluation is needed before it can be used as a possible alternative treatment for chronic anal fissure.

Gosselink et al. (96) evaluated the effect of L-arginine on anal resting pressure, anodermal blood flow, and fissure healing in patients with chronic anal fissure in 15 patients, 10 of whom were unsuccessfully treated by local application of isosorbide dinitrate. All patients were treated for at least 12 weeks by local application of a gel containing L-arginine 400 mg/mL five times a day. In patients with a persistent fissure, treatment was continued until 18 weeks. After 12 weeks of treatment, complete fissure healing was observed in 23% of patients and after 18 weeks, the healing rate was 62%. None of the 13 patients experienced typical nitric oxide-induced headache. The pressure recordings showed a significant reduction in maximum anal resting pressure. Recordings of the anal dermal blood flow showed a significant increase in flow.

Gonyautoxin

Garrido et al. (97) studied the efficacy of gonyautoxin infiltration, a paralyzing phytotoxin, in healing anal fissures in 50 patients. Doses of 100 units of gonyautoxin in a volume of 1 mL were infiltrated into both sides of the anal fissure in the internal anal sphincter. Total remission of acute and chronic anal fissures were achieved within 15 and 28 days, respectively. Ninety-eight percent of the patients healed before 28 days with a mean healing time of 17 days. Only one relapsed during 14 months of follow-up. Neither fecal incontinence nor other side effects were observed. The maximum anal resting pressures recorded after two minutes decreased to 56.2% of baseline. Further confirmation of this form of therapy, although promising, must be elucidated as the agent represents a potent toxin and its safety must be established.

Topical Sildenafil

Torrabadella et al. (98) described manometric analysis of the effects of a phosphodiesterase-5 inhibitor, topical sildenafil (Viagra), in 19 consecutive patients with chronic anal fissure with no previous treatment history. Topical administration of 10% sildenafil was accompanied by significant reduction in anal sphincter pressure (18%). Average onset of action was less than 3 minutes, with maximum effect one minute later. No headaches or other side effects were reported.

Summary

With the variety of agents available, it is difficult to make absolute recommendations as to the first-line treatment. Each agent has its proponents. Calcium channel antagonists have growing support because of the response rate and lower recurrence rate with a more favorable side effect profile, but less experience has been gained with these agents. Nitroglycerin is being used with considerable frequency as is botulinum toxin, which is used to treat a whole host of medical conditions. What is clear is when these agents fail, lateral internal sphincterotomy has been proven to be a very effective form of therapy. In an effort to clarify the quagmire of information, Nelson (99) conducted a meta-analysis of randomized, controlled trials to assess the efficacy and morbidity of medical therapies for anal fissure. Medline and Cochrane Controlled Trials Register and the Cochrane Colorectal Cancer Review Groups Controlled Trials Register were searched. Chronic fissure, acute fissure, fissure in children were included in the review; however, atypical fissure associated with inflammatory bowel disease, cancer, or anal infection were excluded. Data were abstracted from published reports and meeting abstracts, assessing method of randomization, blinding, "intention to treat" and dropouts, therapies, supportive measures, dosing and frequency, and crossovers. Outcome measures included nonhealing of the fissure and adverse events. Twenty-one different comparisons of medical therapies to heal anal fissure have been reported in 31 trials, including nine agents—glyceryl trinitrate, isosorbide dinitrate, botulinum toxin, diltiazem, nifedipine, hydrocortisone, lidocaine, bran, placebo—as well as anal dilators and surgical sphincterotomy. Glyceryl trinitrate was favored in the analysis over placebo (odds ratio = 0.55). After excluding two studies from analysis because of placebo response rates >2 standard deviations below the mean for all studies, the advantage of glyceryl trinitrate over placebo was no longer statistically significant (odds ratio = 0.78). Nifedipine and diltiazem did not differ from glyceryl trinitrate in their ability to cure fissure. Botulinum toxin compared with placebo showed no significant efficacy and was also no better than glyceryl trinitrate. Surgery was more effective than medical therapy in curing fissure. It was concluded that medical therapy for chronic anal fissure, acute fissure, and fissure in children might be applied with a chance of cure that was only marginally better than placebo and for chronic fissure far less effective than surgery.

■ CHRONIC FISSURE

There is no precise definition as to what constitutes a chronic anal fissure. From a temporal point of view some have considered a fissure that persists for at least 6–8 weeks. From a pathologic anatomic point of view features of chronicity include exposure of the internal sphincter, induration of the fissure edges, development of a large sentinel pile, and hypertrophied anal papilla. Lock and Thomson (26) reported that once these features were present, it was unlikely that spontaneous healing will occur and early recognition of these associated problems was very important for the institution of the correct treatment.

Simply condensed, the indications for operative repair of a fissure-in-ano are (1) the presence of persistent pain and bleeding, and (2) the lack of response to medical management, which is really a corollary of the first indication.

The clinical entity of a painless, nonhealing fissure may prove annoying to both the patient and the treating physician. The patient may experience some bleeding from time to time, but the symptoms may not be severe enough for the surgeon to recommend operative treatment. A biopsy should be performed on such a lesion, and it should be kept in mind that the lesion might be the prodromal sign of inflammatory bowel disease. Generally, the option of operative treatment would not be entertained, but if symptoms warrant, performing a lateral internal sphincterotomy would be favored.

Once the necessity for operative correction has been determined, the aims of treatment for a chronic fissure must be considered. Based on studies that have demonstrated an elevated "resting" pressure and an exaggerated response to stimulation in individuals with fissures, the first aim should be to modify the function of the internal anal sphincter so that it cannot go into spasm. Second, the diameter of the anal canal should be increased so that there will be less resistance to the passage of stool, thus reducing the degree of anal trauma associated with defecation. There is probably no need to remove either the fissure itself or the sentinel pile. The presence of a large skin tag may warrant its removal for cosmetic or cleansing reasons.

Before advocating any one form of operative treatment, certain factors must be assessed for each modality. Since the chief symptom is pain, how effective a method is in relieving this pain must first be considered. The incidence of failure or recurrence and the incidence of impaired sphincter control are certainly of paramount importance. Also to be considered are the discomfort experienced by the patient during and after the procedure and the healing time of both the fissure and the operative wound. Significant to both the patient and the treating physician is the number of follow-up visits required before healing is complete.

Over the years, various operative procedures have been proposed for the treatment of a chronic or recurrent fissure. They include classic excision of the fissure, with or without sphincterotomy, either partial or complete; V-Y anoplasty with sliding skin graft (advancement flap of anoderm); anal sphincter stretch; and internal sphincterotomy of the posterior and lateral varieties. The Standards Task Force of the American Society of Colon and Rectal Surgeons has addressed the subject in their practice parameters for the management of anal fissure (100).

Classic Excision

The classic excision of a fissure-in-ano is still used by many surgeons and is usually associated with division of varying amounts of sphincter muscle (Fig. 5). The main criticism of this operation is that it leaves the patient with a large, rather uncomfortable external wound that may be difficult to manage on an outpatient basis and requires a long time to heal. Using an excisional technique in 86 patients in the outpatient setting, Badejo (101) reported 100% healing at two weeks, with no complications and no recurrences at 12-month follow-up. Such uniformly excellent results have never been reported by other authors. In his review, Abcarian (33) found that the complication rate ranged from 6% to 50%, some with persistent fecal soilage. Reported recurrences rates were 6–8%.

In an effort to avoid complications reported with other procedures, Engel et al. (102) performed diathermy fissurectomy on 17 patients followed by application of 1% isosorbide cream 4–6 times daily. All wounds were healed within 10 weeks. No fissure recurrences were seen after a mean follow-up of 29 months. They belive the combined therapy may be a sphincter saving technique.

Various complications following excisional surgery for a fissure have been described. These problems, which are common to almost any anorectal procedure, include bleeding, either immediate or delayed, abscess formation, stenosis and strictures, failure to heal, recurrence, and incontinence of varying degrees. Meticulous attention to surgical detail and exacting postoperative care should help keep these complications to a minimum (see Chap. 4).

V-Y Anoplasty (Advancement Flap Technique)

A method using excision of the fissure combined with an advancement flap of anoderm has been referred to as V-Y anoplasty. With this technique, the fissure and the adjacent crypt bearing hemorrhoidal tissue are completely excised. A triangular skin flap based outside the anal canal is elevated in continuity with the excised fissure. A broad base with adequate blood supply to the flap must be ensured. The flap is adequately mobilized to avoid tension on the suture line. Meticulous attention is paid to hemostasis to prevent hematoma formation, which increases tension and the chance of infection. The flap is then advanced, and the defect of the skin and anal canal is closed (Fig. 6).

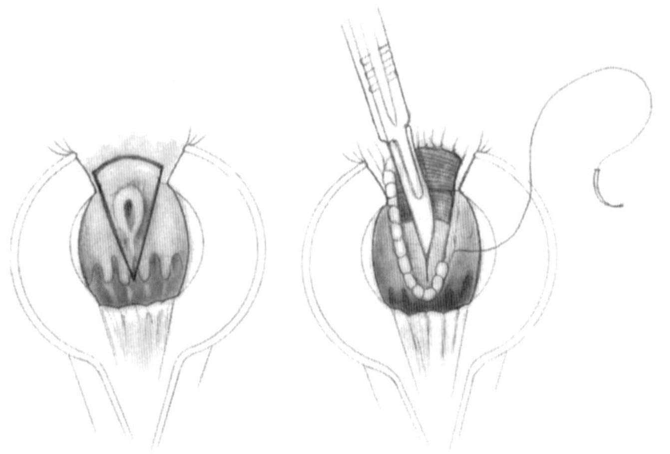

FIGURE 5 ■ Fissurectomy. *Source:* After M. Finch.

Extensive experience with this technique has been reported by Samson and Stewart (104). They state that excision of a chronic fissure-in-ano and coverage of the defect with a sliding, broad-based skin graft offer several advantages over the classic excision. First, postoperative pain is decreased; second, postoperative wound care, both in the hospital and in the office, is decreased; and third, the incidence of postoperative complications is decreased. Of 2072 patients treated in this way, recurrent fissures occurred in 10, and there were only seven cases of mild anal stenosis. Postoperative bleeding occurred in two cases, and their slough rate was 2.4%. The diameter of the anus is actually increased, and this is Samson and Stewart's procedure of choice for treating anal stenosis. A fourth advantage in using this technique is that primary, as opposed to secondary, wound healing occurs, so that healing is more rapid and there is decreased scar tissue and less resultant deformity. The major disadvantages to this method are that it involves considerable dissection and requires increased operative time.

Leong and Seow-Choen (105) conducted a randomized, prospective study to assess the differences between the results of using a rhomboid anal advancement flap and a lateral internal anal sphincterotomy for the treatment of chronic fissure-in-ano. Twenty patients were assigned to each group. The authors found that healing occurred in all patients in the group who underwent sphincterotomy but that there were three failures in the group treated with an advancement flap. Nevertheless, the authors concluded that the flap is an alternative to the sphincterotomy.

Nyam et al. (106) recommended the use of island advancement flaps in the management of anal fissures in patients with weak sphincters. They acknowledge lateral internal sphincterotomy as the treatment of choice for classic high-pressure fissures. Patients fitting into the low-pressure category included those with a failed lateral sphincterotomy, previous obstetric trauma, previous perianal surgery, and other low-pressure fissures-in-ano. Pressure studies in 21 such patients revealed values significantly lower than in controls and those with classic fissure. Endoanal ultrasonography in 15 of those patients showed defects in the anal sphincters. In all, 21 of the patients who underwent flap repair, healing occurred primarily with preservation of sensation, maintenance of continence, and no serious complications. The authors concluded that this procedure provided a useful alternative for the treatment of symptomatic anal fissures in which a sphincter-weakening procedure might jeopardize continence.

Anal Sphincter Stretch

Recamier (107) is credited with first describing anal stretching. The procedure was championed by Lord (108) for various forms of anorectal disease. This method, which is also referred to as manual dilatation of the anus, involves the forceful stretching of the anal sphincter with as many as six or eight fingers. The effect on the internal and external sphincters is to produce a temporary paralysis, usually lasting several days or a week. There may be some incontinence during this time. Because of the nature of the

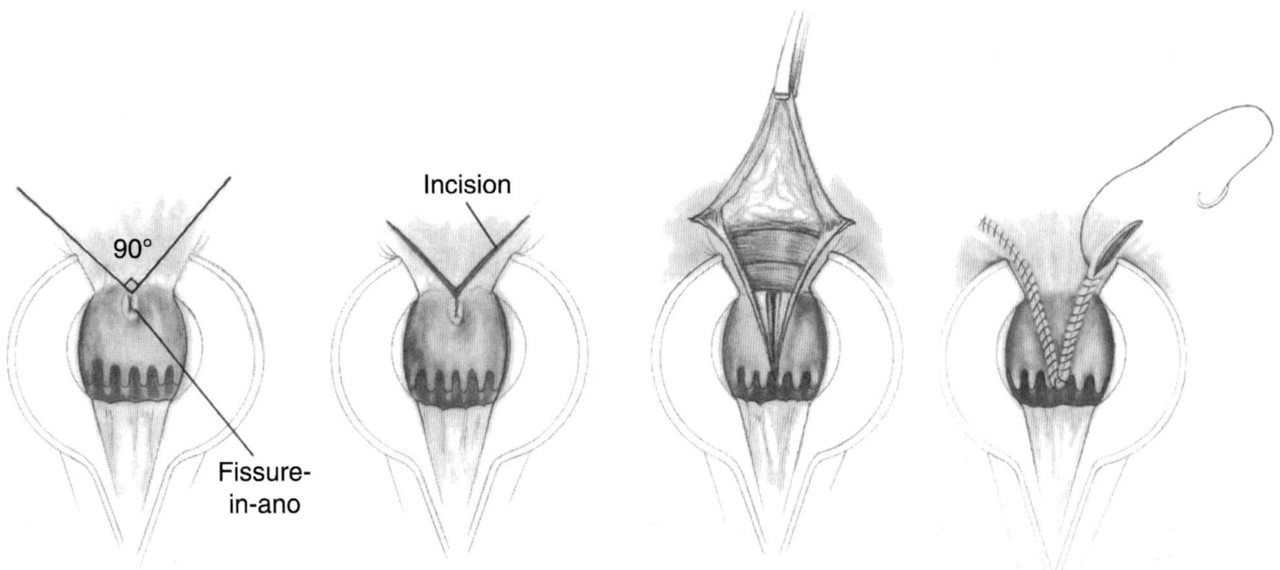

FIGURE 6 ■ V-Y anoplasty. Prone position. *Source:* From Ref. 103.

procedure, sphincter fibers are torn, resulting in extravasation of blood and leading to perianal bruising and discoloration, which may be quite extensive.

Proponents of this method cite as advantages that there is no anal wound and that the patients have an early return to work, both enviable objectives. However, the significant disadvantages of this method must not be overlooked: the incidence of recurrent fissures (10–56%) and the disturbances of anal control (see discussion of results of lateral internal sphincterotomy).

Isbister and Prasad (109) reported on a 15-year experience with a four-finger anal dilatation in 104 patients. There were five failures but no complaints of incontinence. Sohn et al. (110) recommended a precise dilatation performed with a Parks retractor opened to 4.8 cm or with a 40 mm rectosigmoid balloon. In 105 patients so treated, a success rate of 93% was obtained with no incidents of incontinence. Nielson et al. (111) conducted a study to determine the risk of sphincter damage and anal incontinence after anal dilatation for fissure-in-ano. Minor anal incontinence was experienced by 12.5% of 32 patients. Anal endosonographic follow-up demonstrated sphincter defects in 65% of 20 patients studied. Two patients with anal incontinence had internal sphincter defects. Sphincter defects were also found in 11 of the 18 continent patients (nine internal, one external, and one combined). Despite the fact that more than half the patients had sphincter damage, few developed anal incontinence.

Renzi et al. (112) evaluated the clinical, anatomic, and functional pattern in a group of 33 patients with fissure-in-ano treated by pneumatic balloon dilatation. Manometry was accomplished by means of an endoanal 40-mm balloon inflated with a pressure of 1.4 atm that was left in situ for 6 minutes under local anesthesia. The chronic anal fissure healed between the third and fifths weeks in 94% of patients who became asymptomatic 2.5 days after pneumatic balloon dilatation. None of them reported anal pain two years after the treatment ($n = 20$). The first postpneumatic balloon dilatation defecation was painless in 82% of cases. Two multiparous females (6% of the patients) complained of minor transient anal incontinence. Chronic anal fissure recurred in one case (3%) after treatment. At manometry, the preoperative anal resting pressure decreased from 91 to 70.5 and to 78 mmHg, 6 and 12 months after pneumatic balloon dilatation, respectively. Anal ultrasonography did not show any significant sphincter defect.

In a review by Lund and Scholefield (113) of 16 trials examining the use of anal dilatation, reported recurrence rates were 2.2–56.5% and tended to be higher with longer follow-up. Disturbance of continence ranged from 0% to 39.2% for incontinence of flatus or soiling of the underclothes and fecal incontinence was reported in up to 16.2%. Anal dilatation may also be complicated by bleeding, perianal bruising, strangulation of prolapsed hemorrhoids, perianal infection, Fournier's gangrene, bacteremia, and rectal procidentia.

Pressure studies have demonstrated an abnormality in the response of the internal sphincter of patients with fissures, suggesting that a modification in its function is necessary in treating this condition. Nevertheless, a more controlled way of modifying the sphincter function should be used. An eight-finger or even a four-finger dilatation of the anus is hardly a delicate surgical operation. In addition, subsequent prolonged use of an anal dilator is required, and this does not meet with a high degree of patient satisfaction. I personally find no place in the surgical armamentarium for this procedure.

Internal Sphincterotomy

Credit for suggesting the treatment of anal fissure by internal sphincterotomy has been given to Eisenhammer (114) in 1951, but, in fact, this procedure was originally described by Brodie (115) in 1835. The method originally favored by Brodie was division of the lower half of the internal sphincter in the posterior midline through the fissure itself. This procedure resulted in satisfactory results but had two significant disadvantages: the opened wound in the anal canal took a long time to heal, with 4 weeks being the average period and 6–7 weeks being common, and there was a disturbingly high incidence of minor imperfections of anal continence, as shown by occasional lack of control for flatus or feces or an inadvertent slight leakage of fecal matter, leading to soiling of the underwear. Lesser drawbacks included prolonged postoperative pain and prolonged hospitalization. Some of the fecal soiling and minor imperfections in continence are due to the "keyhole" deformity created by a posterior internal sphincterotomy. This abnormality is a groove in the area of the sphincterotomy along, which fecal-stained mucus, and possibly stool as well, escape. Melange et al. (116) studied 76 patients who underwent fissurectomy with posterior midline sphincterotomy for anal fissure. The fissure healed in all cases, but sporadic loss of continence for flatus or for liquid stool occurred in 21 patients (27.6%), and soiling was present in seven other patients (9.2%). Preoperative maximum resting anal pressure was significantly greater in the study group compared to control patients. Postoperative resting anal pressure fell significantly and remained low on long-term assessment. Postoperative maximal squeeze pressure remained unchanged.

The possibility that a lateral sphincterotomy might cause a less prominent groove than a posterior one and be followed by less disturbance of function was suggested by Eisenhammer (117). Parks (118) strongly recommended lateral sphincterotomy. There are variations in the exact details of current forms of performing lateral sphincterotomy. The procedure may be done with the patient under local, regional, or general anesthesia, through a radial or circumferential incision, or using a subcutaneous technique. The muscle may be divided medially to laterally or vice versa.

Technique

Patients may be operated on while under general, regional, or local anesthesia. I prefer the semiprone or jack-knife position. For surgeons less familiar with the anorectal anatomy or those just starting to perform lateral sphincterotomy, the procedure is probably best performed with an open approach.

After the anesthetic is administered, a Pratt bivalve speculum is inserted and the anal pathology is evaluated. The instrument is then rotated to the right or left lateral position, and a linear incision is made from the dentate line to just beyond the anal verge. The internal sphincter and a few fibers of the external sphincter will be exposed. Any bleeding is controlled with electrocautery. The full thickness of the internal sphincter from the level of the dentate line distally is then divided under direct vision. A definite "give" will be noted, and this should correct any element of anal stenosis and cure the fissure. Any adjacent hemorrhoidal tissue can be excised as indicated. Since prolapsing hemorrhoids are a recognized complication after lateral internal sphincterotomy, judicious use of concomitant hemorrhoidectomy should be made in patients with large hemorrhoids to avoid this complication. In such cases, using general or regional anesthesia would be preferable. The wound is then closed with a running absorbable suture such as 3–0 chromic catgut but may be left open if preferred (Fig. 7). The fissure itself need not be treated, but very large sentinel piles or prolapsing, hypertrophied anal papillae might be removed for cosmetic or cleansing purposes. A piece of fluff cotton is then placed between the buttocks to prevent soiling of clothes. Postoperatively, a bulk-forming agent such as a psyllium seed preparation (1 teaspoon twice a day), frequent warm baths, and a non-codeine-containing analgesic are ordered for the patient.

I have adopted the technique described by Sir Alan Parks (Fig. 8) (118). However, I perform this operation as an outpatient procedure in the office, with the patient under local anesthesia, unless there are extenuating circumstances such as an allergy to the local anesthetic.

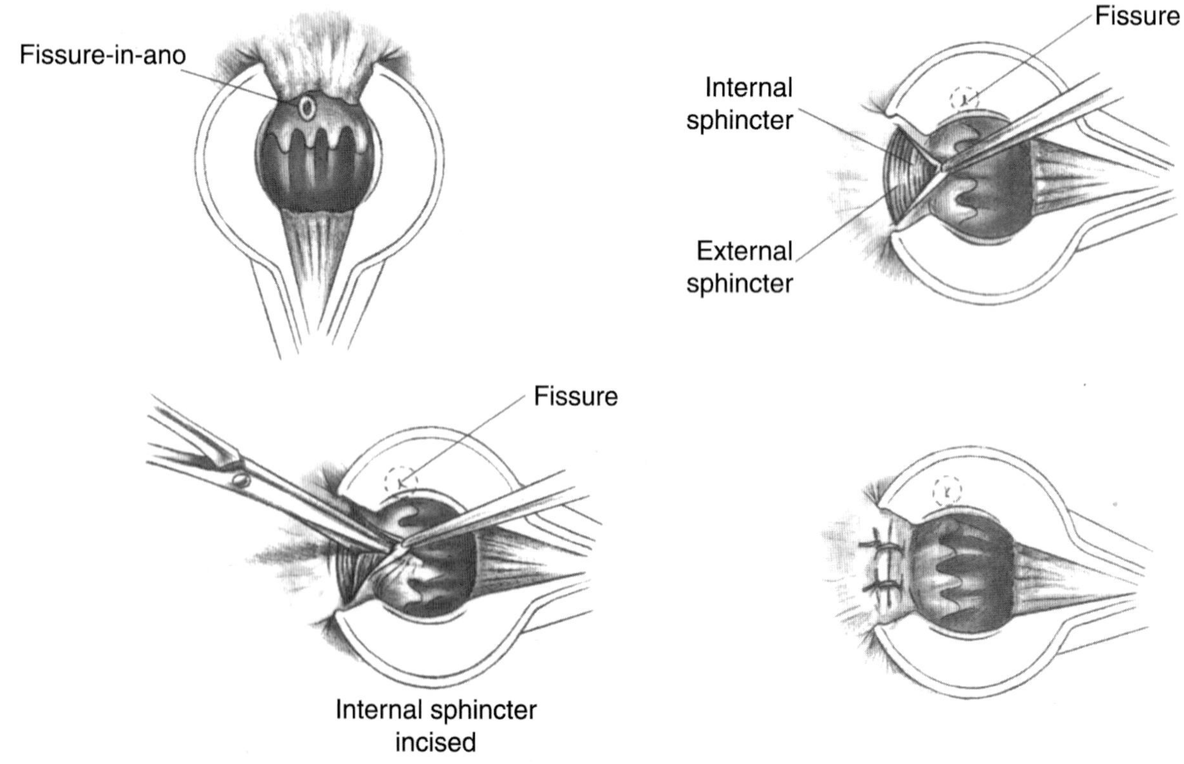

FIGURE 7 ■ Lateral internal sphincterotomy according to Parks.

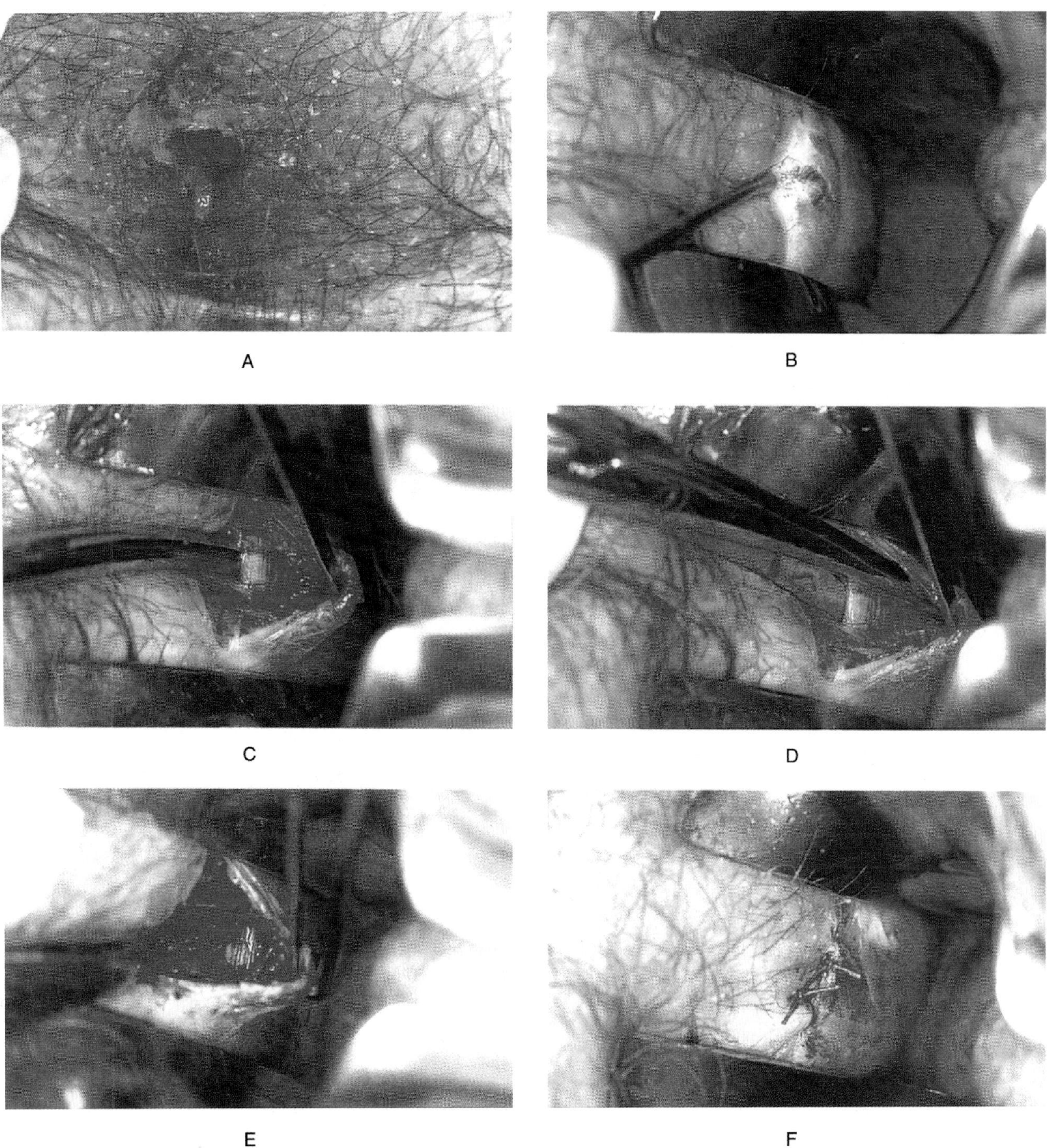

FIGURE 8 ■ (**A**) Posterior midline fissure-in-ano. (**B**) Probe pointing to the intersphincteric groove, indicating the lower end of internal sphincter. (**C**) White fibers of the internal sphincter clearly identified. (**D**) Metzenbaum scissors positioned to divide the lower half of the internal sphincter. (**E**) Lower half of the internal sphincter divided and the new "lower border" of internal sphincter visualized. (**F**) Completed procedure.

With the patient in the prone jack-knife position, the perianal region is prepared with a disinfectant solution and is draped in the usual fashion. A fine needle is used to infiltrate the area of the fissure with an anesthetic solution of 0.5% xylocaine in 1:200,000 epinephrine. The anesthetic solution is next infiltrated into the left lateral aspect near the anal verge, which ensures that the solution is directed to the level of the dentate line. The entire perianal region may be anesthetized. A Pratt bivalve speculum is inserted into the anal orifice. A short incision is made just distal to the intersphincteric groove, which can usually be palpated easily. The anoderm is lifted from the underlying internal sphincter to the level of the dentate line, and the intersphincteric plane is developed. The full thickness of the internal sphincter is divided from its lower edge to the level of the dentate line with either a pair of Metzenbaum scissors or a scalpel. Hemostasis is obtained with cautery, and the wound can be closed with two or three interrupted sutures of 3–0 chromic catgut.

Postoperatively, when patients are discharged home, they are advised to eat a regular diet and to take sitz baths and a psyllium seed preparation as a bulk-forming agent; a non-codeine-containing oral analgesic also is prescribed. Patients are seen 1 month after the procedure.

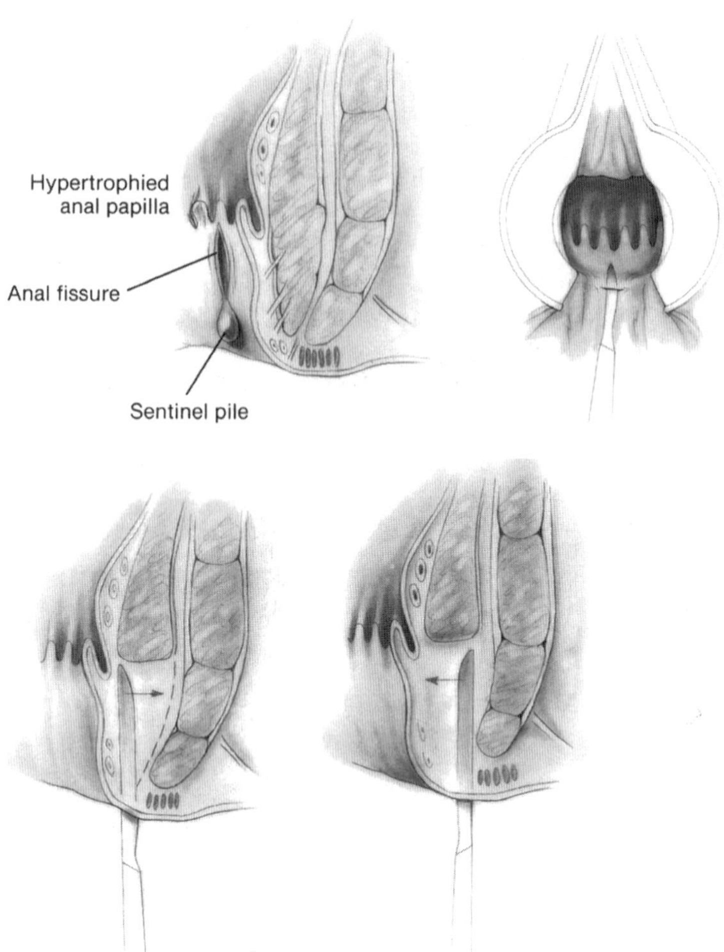

FIGURE 9 ■ Lateral internal sphincterotomy according to Notaras. *Source:* After R.H. Lane.

The great advantage of this method is that it avoids an intra-anal wound. The internal sphincter is divided under direct visual control because the thickness and length of the internal sphincter vary from patient to patient. Bleeding sites can be seen and directly controlled. For these reasons, this technique is my preference.

A minor technical modification is the method of lateral subcutaneous internal sphincterotomy described by Notaras (Fig. 9) (119). This procedure leaves virtually no wound. The operation can be performed in the lithotomy, left lateral, or semi-prone position. Anesthesia is achieved by a bilateral inferior hemorrhoidal nerve block or local anesthetic. An anal speculum such as the Pratt bivalve or Parks retractor is inserted; when the blades are opened, the anus is placed in a slight stretch. The intersphincteric groove and lower edge of the internal sphincter are then palpable. A narrow-bladed scalpel, flat side adjacent to muscle, is introduced through the skin in either lateral position and the tip is advanced submucosally to the dentate line. The sharp edge of the blade is then turned toward the internal sphincter, and the sphincterotomy is performed. When this step is accomplished, a "give" will result in release of the tension of the blades of the anal speculum. Pressure will arrest any bleeding, and the wound is left open to allow any drainage to escape. If preferred, the scalpel blade can be advanced in the intersphincteric plane and turned toward the lumen, thus accomplishing the sphincterotomy. Again, a large sentinel pile and hypertrophied anal papillae can be dealt with appropriately.

■ RESULTS

Among the various operative options available for the treatment of fissure-in-ano, the procedure that has gained the greatest favor is the lateral internal sphincterotomy. Surprisingly, few studies have been conducted comparing the different options, especially comparing lateral internal sphincterotomy with fissurectomy. One surgeon who addressed this issue was Abcarian (33), who conducted a study in which he compared the results of lateral internal sphincterotomy to those of fissurectomy and posterior midline sphincterotomy. Each group contained 150 patients. By almost all the parameters studied, the lateral internal sphincterotomy group fared better. Hospital stay was shorter (1–2 days vs. 3–4 days), pain relief was faster (1–2 weeks vs. 2–3 weeks), and wound healing was quicker (2–3 weeks vs. 6–7 weeks). Although early and temporary loss of continence occurred in 30% of patients with lateral internal sphincterotomy and 40% of patients with fissurectomy and posterior midline sphincterotomy, after 2 weeks persistent loss of control of flatus occurred in 5%, and another 5% experienced fecal soiling after fissurectomy and midline sphincterotomy. On the other hand, none of the patients had these problems with lateral internal sphincterotomy. The recurrence rate, 1.3%, was the same in both groups.

Saad and Omer (120) conducted a prospective randomized study in which anal dilatation, posterior internal sphincterotomy, and lateral internal sphincterotomy were compared. Lateral internal sphincterotomy fared the best with immediate relief of pain, the lowest incidence of complications, and the earliest return to work. Anal dilatation fared the poorest with the main disadvantage being the high rate of postoperative anal incontinence (24.3%).

A wide variation in results has been reported, with recurrence rates ranging from 10% to 56% (mostly in the upper range) after manual dilatation of the anus and from 0% to 15% (the majority in the 1–3% range) after lateral internal sphincterotomy (111,113). Similarly, incontinence is reported in 0–34% of patients after manual dilatation of the anus, as compared with 0–15% (the majority in the 0–3% range) of patients after lateral internal sphincterotomy (Table 2) (111,113). A further caveat was presented by Goldman et al. (121), who found bacteremia in 8% of patients undergoing anal dilatation. They therefore suggested using prophylactic antibiotics in selected patients, that is, patients with cardiac valvular disease, those receiving steroid and immunodepressant treatment, and those known to be immunosuppressed (after splenectomy).

Walker et al. (30) reported on the use of internal sphincterotomy in a variety of circumstances, including the treatment of fissure alone, with or without stenosis, with or without concomitant procedures, and with single or multiple sphincterotomies. There were no fissure recurrences, but an astoundingly high incidence of minor complications (36%) and major complications (3%) and an overall 15% incidence of defects in continence were encountered. The reason for the marked deviation of these data from the experience of most authors (Table 2) is difficult to explain.

In a subsequent report from the same center, 549 patients with chronic fissure-in-ano were assessed to compare the healing rate and long-term effects on continence of open and closed lateral internal sphincterotomy (43). Differences in persistence of symptoms, recurrence of the fissure, and need for reoperation were statistically not significant. However, statistically significant differences were seen in the percentage of patients with permanent postoperative difficulty controlling gas (30.3% vs. 23.6%; $p=0.062$), soiling underclothing (26.7% vs. 16.1%; $p < 0.001$), and accidental bowel movements (11.8% vs. 3.1%; $p < 0.001$) between those who underwent open internal sphincterotomy and those who had closed internal sphincterotomy. They concluded that lateral internal sphincterotomy is highly effective in the treatment of chronic anal fissure but is associated with significant permanent alterations in continence. Closed internal sphincterotomy is preferable to open internal sphincterotomy because it effects a similar rate of cure with less impairment of control.

Khubchandani and Reed (31) also reported on the sequelae of internal sphincterotomy for chronic fissure-in-ano. Their series of 1102 patients from whom surgical data were obtained also noted a complication rate not in keeping with most reports. Alteration in control of flatus occurred in 35.1%, soiling of underclothing in 22%, and accidental bowel movements in 5.3%. Their series contained patients who underwent lateral, posterior, or bilateral sphincterotomy, but the authors state that there were no significant differences between the different groups.

In a prospective study of the extent of internal sphincterotomy, Sultan et al. (122) performed anal endosonography before and two months after operation. In 9 of the 10 female patients, the defect involved the full length of the internal sphincter. This was not true in males. It may be that the high incidence of alterations in continence reported by some of the authors mentioned above may be related to a more extensive division of the muscle than intended. Furthermore, combining the sphincterotomy with other anorectal procedures may explain the increased complication rate.

Factors that may contribute to the wide variation of results include the retrospective analysis used in some studies, the unspecified duration of follow-up, and the lack of a precise definition of incontinence (i.e., for solid stool, liquid stool, or flatus, and whether the problem was temporary or permanent). Some series include patients who have undergone additional anorectal procedures. Thus, the summaries of reports in Tables 2 and 3 are not strictly comparable but present a general overview and acknowledgment of the efficacy of lateral internal sphincterotomy. Many reports on the results of internal sphincterotomy are currently available (Table 2). Early relief of pain is remarkable. Often pain (except for some soreness) disappears by the first bowel movement.

In our review of 265 patients who underwent lateral internal sphincterotomy as a primary and sole procedure, 23 (8.7%) complications occurred in 20 patients (7.5%) (123). Most of the complications were minor and resolved with medical treatment. Delayed wound healing of the sphincterotomy site (>60 days) was recorded in 13 patients (4.9%). One of these patients was re-examined while under general anesthesia, and an unusual finding was demonstrated. The lowermost portion of the internal sphincter had not been divided at the time of the original sphincterotomy; consequently, the wound did not heal (Fig. 10). This problem was easily corrected by completing the incision. Another wound did not heal because the operation was performed on a patient with Crohn's disease. Although the wound did not heal, the patient was asymptomatic. Failure of healing of the fissure or recurrence was noted in 1.1% of the patients. One patient had persistent pain, and the fissure did not heal. Consequently, one month later a lateral internal sphincterotomy was performed on the opposite side, giving prompt relief of symptoms and complete healing of the fissure. Two patients developed a wound infection at the sphincterotomy site that did not necessitate further operation but did cause delayed healing. One patient experienced a temporary loss of control of flatus. Another patient with permanent loss of control of flatus and stool underwent a subsequent postanal repair and regained continence. Permanent fecal soiling was reported by one patient. One patient returned the day after the procedure with a complete ring of prolapsed, thrombosed internal hemorrhoids, and a ring of thrombosed external hemorrhoids. Emergency hemorrhoidectomy was performed, and the postoperative course was smooth. No patient suffered postoperatively from hemorrhage, perianal abscess, or fistula-in-ano. Urinary retention was not encountered. The exact duration of postoperative pain was not documented for each patient, but most had relief within 48 hours and many within 24 hours. The complication rate was substantially higher (20%) in the 21 patients who underwent combined lateral internal sphincterotomy and hemorrhoidectomy and was even higher in the patients who had undergone lateral internal sphincterotomy as a repeated operation. These findings are in direct contrast to those of Leong et al. (37), who found that additional anorectal procedures performed at the same time as internal sphincterotomy do not increase the incidence of postoperative complications.

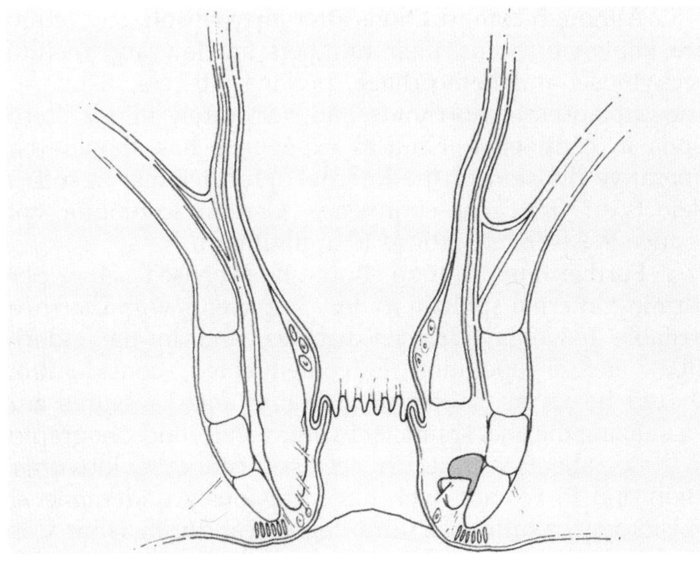

FIGURE 10 ■ Incomplete division of lower portion of the internal sphincter. *Source:* From Ref. 123.

Although complications after internal sphincterotomy are known to occur, their numbers are few and include ecchymosis and hemorrhage, perianal abscess, fistula-in-ano, prolapsed hemorrhoids, and, very rarely, minor alterations in continence. Clinical experience has shown that operative division of the internal sphincter may result in defects of fine anal continence. Careful technique will reduce these complications to a minimum.

Furthermore, caution should be exercised before performing internal sphincterotomy in patients with diarrhea, irritable bowel syndrome, diabetes, and in the elderly (100). Before operation is contemplated, consideration should be given to obtaining resting anal pressures and visualizing the anal sphincter by intra-anal endosonography in those patients with recurrence fissure after previous operation and in women who have previously undergone an episiotomy or suffered a third-degree tear during labor. Cassilas et al. (124) assessed the long-term outcomes and quality of life of patients who have undergone sphincterotomy for chronic anal fissure using the Fecal Incontinence Quality of Life and Fecal Incontinence Severity Index in 298 patients. Recurrence of the fissure occurred in 5.6% of patients of whom 52% were female. Significant factors that resulted in recurrence were initial sphincterotomy performed in the office and local anesthesia. When comparing office records and response to the postal survey, significantly more patients had flatal incontinence than that recorded in their medical records. Twenty-nine percent of females who had a vaginal delivery recorded problems with incontinence to flatus. Temporary incontinence was reported in 31% of patients and persistent incontinence to gas occurred in 30%. Stool incontinence was not a significant finding. The overall quality of life scores were in the normal range, whereas the median Fecal Incontinence Severity Index score was 12. They recommend that females who have two or more previous vaginal deliveries should be warned about possible flatal incontinence. Furthermore, long-term flatal incontinence that is not reported to the caregiver may occur in up to one-third of patients and could be permanent.

The frequency with which complications have been reported is summarized in Tables 2 and 3. As can be seen, the overall immediate or early complication rate is 5%, but if the self-limiting problem of ecchymosis is omitted, the overall complication rate of any consequence is 2.2%.

In the series reported by Abcarian (33), problems relating to the control of flatus and soiling were only temporary. Fecal soiling was reported in some series but varied in degree of concern in different series. Although not a controlled study, Oh et al. (41) pointed out that in their series the incidence of complications and recurrence was higher in patients who had sphincterotomy performed in a subcutaneous blind manner than in those on whom an open technique was used. However, Boulos and Araujo (125) measured anal canal pressures preoperatively and postoperatively and found that lateral internal sphincterotomy performed by the open or subcutaneous method had comparable effects. Kortbeek et al. (126) conducted a prospective randomized study comparing open and subcutaneous lateral internal sphincterotomy. They found no significant difference in acute complications and fissure healing was similar in the two groups. In a retrospective analysis, Lewis et al. (34) found no difference in healing between the open and subcutaneous techniques. Arroyo et al. (52) also reported equivalent results with open and closed lateral anal sphincterotomy performed under local anesthesia. Wiley et al. (127) found that the open versus closed technique did not influence incontinence rates.

The incidence of recurrence may be related to the amount of internal sphincter divided. With this in mind, Littlejohn and Newstead (128) proposed the tailored lateral sphincterotomy, by which they meant that the amount of sphincter division is tailored exactly to the height of the fissure with some recognition of the degree of anal tone, if excessive. In most cases, the vertical height of the sphincter division is between 5 and 10 mm. In a review of 287 patients so treated, recorded complications included imperfect control of flatus, 1.4%; minor staining, 0.35%; and urgency, 0.7%. None experienced incontinence of feces or leakage of stool. Five patients underwent repeat sphincterotomy, four for recurrence, and one for persistent fissure.

Hyman (129) defined the risk of incontinence with sphincterotomy using the Fecal Incontinence Severity Index and assessed the implications of quality of life using the Fecal Incontinence Quality of Life Scale. The Fecal Incontinence Severity Index was measured preoperatively and at six weeks postoperative in 35 patients. Of the evaluable fissures, 94% had healed by 6 weeks, 1 healed by 3 months, and the other required a V-Y anoplasty. There were two minor complications. Three patients had postoperative deterioration in their continence score. Quality of life deteriorated in only 1 patient. Hyman concluded that lateral internal sphincterotomy is a safe and effective treatment for chronic anal fissures that only occasionally impairs continence and rarely diminishes quality of life.

Ellis (130) compared anterior levatorplasty with internal sphincterotomy for the management of anterior anal fissures in females with a rectocele in 54 women. The average length of follow-up was 20 months. Postoperatively, lateral sphincterotomy caused a decrease in the resting pressures and anterior levatorplasty resulted in increased length of the anal canal. Anterior levatorplasty also caused increased postoperative pain scores. There were no differences in fissure healing and patient satisfaction. Ellis suggested that anterior levatorplasty is an option for the management of patients with rectocele, which may avoid the risk of incontinence with lateral internal sphincterotomy.

Nelson (131) conducted a review of the literature of operative procedures for anal fissures. There were 19 publications that fulfilled the criteria of the study encompassing 3083 patients. A total of 11 reports compared anal stretch to internal sphincterotomy; five of these studies were retrospective and six were randomized. Incidence rates for persistence varied widely among reports from 5% to 30% in the anal stretch group and 3% to 29% in the internal sphincterotomy group. The rate of incontinence varied from 0% to 27% in the anal stretch group and from 0% to 20% in the sphincterotomy group. There were seven reports comparing open and closed lateral internal sphincterotomies. Two of these were randomized studies and five were retrospective reviews. The rate of persistence in those reports comparing open and closed sphincterotomies varied from 0% to 9%, although incontinence in these reports varied from 1% to 30%. Six randomized studies compared the efficacy of anal stretch to some form of internal sphincterotomy comprising 385 patients. The overall effect for efficacy became significant favoring sphincterotomy (odds ratio = 3.08). All of these reports looked at minor or flatus incontinence as a complication of each procedure. The Peto odds ratio was 4.22 in favor of sphincterotomy. Two randomized studies compared open partial lateral internal sphincterotomy to closed or subcutaneous partial lateral internal sphincterotomy in a total of 140 subjects. The same two end points were assessed: persistence of fissure and partial or flatus incontinence. The Peto odds ratio for persistence of fissure was 1.63, favoring open sphincterotomy, and for flatus incontinence the odds ratio was 0.77, favoring closed sphincterotomy. The combined overall results of those reports favored sphincterotomy over anal stretch and very little difference in results of open versus closed sphincterotomy. Posterior internal sphincterotomy is more likely to result in persistence (not statistically significant) and incontinence to flatus than lateral sphincterotomy.

Advantages of Lateral Internal Sphincterotomy

Our experience, supported by that of others in the literature, strongly suggests that lateral sphincterotomy is a good operation for patients with a chronic fissure-in-ano. It has several definite advantages. There is no need to hospitalize the patient. The operation can be performed with the patient under local anesthesia. Postoperative discomfort is of short duration, and wounds heal quickly. Fecal soiling is an infrequent problem, and recurrence after this mode of therapy is uncommon. Thus, less time is lost from work, and fewer follow-up visits are required. Careful patient selection, absence of preoperative continence problems, and meticulous attention to operative detail are necessary to achieve excellent results. Because of such excellent results and the fact that the procedure can be performed safely and effectively on an outpatient basis, I believe that lateral internal sphincterotomy is the operative treatment of choice for patients with a chronic anal fissure.

MANAGEMENT OF RECURRENT OR PERSISTENT FISSURE-IN-ANO

In a small percentage of patients in whom the fissure fails to heal or recurrence develops, a number of options are open to the surgeon. In some patients, a recurrent fissure will heal with nonoperative treatment (stool softeners and sitz baths), as described in the section on acute fissure. For the patient with a persistent fissure or a recurrent fissure that does not respond to nonoperative management, a number of options are available. One of the other procedures described earlier in this chapter could be recommended. Since a recurrence of the fissure is generally attributed to an inadequate sphincterotomy, the surgeon could explore the incision and ensure that a complete internal sphincterotomy was accomplished. My own preference is to perform a second lateral internal sphincterotomy on the opposite side, a procedure I have performed with success (123). Xynos et al. (8) also reported that fissures that fail to heal after lateral internal sphincterotomy can be successfully treated by performing an additional internal sphincterotomy on the opposite side.

Failure of lateral internal sphincterotomy may be due to technical failure. Farouk et al. (132) used endoanal ultrasonography and anal manometry to assess 13 patients with persistent anal fissure after sphincterotomy. Endoluminal ultrasonography revealed partial division of the internal sphincter in two patients. The remaining 11 patients had an intact internal anal sphincter but had ultrasonographic evidence of division of the external sphincter at the site of the previous operation. All 13 patients subsequently underwent a second lateral internal sphincterotomy, with resolution of their symptoms. Median preoperative resting pressures of 115 cmH_2O fell to 89 cmH_2O postoperatively. The authors concluded that failure of the original sphincterotomy appears to be related to an inadequate internal sphincterotomy or to inadvertent division of the external anal sphincter. Endoanal ultrasonography allowed accurate assessment to determine why treatment failure occurred.

REFERENCES

1. Hananel N, Gordon PH. Reexamination of the clinical manifestations and responses to therapy of fissure-in-ano. Dis Colon Rectum 1997; 40: 229–233.
2. Petros JG, Rimm EB, Robillard RJ. Clinical presentation of chronic anal fissures. Am Surg 1993; 59:666–668.
3. Jensen SL. Diet and other risk factors for fissure-in-ano. Prospective case control study. Dis Colon Rectum 1988; 31:770–773.
4. Crapp AR, Alexander-Williams J. Fissure-in-ano and anal stenosis conservative management. Clin Gastroenterol 1975; 4:619–628.
5. Nothmann BJ, Schuster MM. Internal anal sphincter derangement with anal fissures. Gastroenterology 1974; 67:216–220.
6. Abcarian H, Lakshmanan S, Read DR, Roccaforte P. The role of internal sphincter in chronic anal fissures. Dis Colon Rectum 1982; 25:525–528.
7. Chowcat NL, Araujo JGC, Boulos PB. Internal sphincterotomy for chronic anal fissure: long-term effects on anal pressure. Br J Surg 1986; 73: 915–916.
8. Xynos E, Tzortzinis A, Chrysos E, Tzovaras G, Vassilakis JS. Anal manometry in patients with fissure-in-ano before and after internal sphincterotomy. Int J Colorectal Dis 1993; 8:125–128.
9. McNamara MJ, Percy JP, Fielding IR. A manometric study of anal fissure treated by subcutaneous lateral internal sphincterotomy. Am Surg 1990; 211:235.
10. Farouk R, Duthie GS, MacGregor AB, Bartolo DCC. Sustained internal sphincter hypertonia in patients with chronic anal fissure. Dis Colon Rectum 1994; 37:424–429.
11. Keck JO, Staniunas RJ, Coller JA, Barrett RC, Oster ME. Computer-generated profiles of the anal canal in patients with anal fissure. Dis Colon Rectum 1995; 38:72–79.
12. Williams N, Scott NA, Irving MH. Effect of lateral sphincterotomy on internal anal sphincter function. A computerized vector manometry study. Dis Colon Rectum 1995; 38:700–704.
13. Prohm P, Bonner C. Is manometry essential for surgery of chronic fissure-in-ano? Dis Colon Rectum 1995; 38:735–738.
14. Horvath KD, Whelan RL, Golub RW, Ahsan H, Cirocco WC. Effect of catheter diameter on resting pressures in anal fissure patients. Dis Colon Rectum 1995; 38:728–731.
15. Cerdan FJ, deLion AR, Azpiroz F, Martin J, Balibrea JL. Anal sphincteric pressure in fissure-in-ano before and after lateral internal sphincterotomy. Dis Colon Rectum 1982; 25:198–201.
16. Olsen J, Mortensen PE, Petersen IK, Christiansen J. Anal sphincter function after treatment of fissure-in-ano by lateral subcutaneous sphincterotomy versus anal dilatation. A randomized study. Int J Colorectal Dis 1987; 2:155–157.
17. Gibbons CP, Read NW. Anal hypertonia in fissures: cause or effect? Br J Surg 1986; 73:443–445.
18. Kuijpers HC. Is there really sphincter spasm in anal fissure? Dis Colon Rectum 1983; 26:493–494.
19. Schouten WR, Blankensteijn JD. Ultraslow wave pressure variations in the anal canal before and after lateral internal sphincterotomy. Int J Colorectal Dis 1992; 7:115–118.
20. Klosterhalfen B, Vogel P, Rixen H, et al. Topography of the inferior rectal artery: a possible cause of chronic, primary anal fissure. Dis Colon Rectum 1989; 32:43–52.
21. Schouten WR, Briel JW, Auwerda JJA, De Graaf E Jr. Ischemic nature of anal fissure. Br J Surg 1996; 83:63–65.

22. Bhardwaj R, Vaizey CJ, Boulos PB, Hoyle CH. Neuromyogenic properties of the internal anal sphincter: therapeutic rationale for anal fissures. Gut 2000; 46:861–868.
23. Dodi G, Bogoni F, Infantino A, Pianon P, Mortellaro LM, Lise M. Hot or cold in anal pain? A study of the changes in internal anal sphincter pressure profiles. Dis Colon Rectum 1986; 29:248–251.
24. Pinho M, Correa JCO, Furtado A, Ramos JR. Do hot baths promote anal sphincter relaxation? Dis Colon Rectum 1993; 36:273–274.
25. Shub H, Salvati E, Rubin R. Conservative treatment of fissure. Dis Colon Rectum 1978; 21:582–583.
26. Lock MR, Thomson JPS. Fissure-in-ano: the initial management and prognosis. Br J Surg 1977; 65:355–358.
27. Antebi E, Schwartz P, Gilon E. Sclerotherapy for the treatment of fissure-in-ano. Surg Gynecol Obstet 1985; 160:204–206.
28. Jensen SL. Treatment of first episodes of acute anal fissure: prospective randomized study of lignocaine ointment versus hydro-cortisone ointment or warm sitz baths plus bran. Br Med J 1986; 292:1167–1169.
29. Jensen SL. Maintenance therapy with unprocessed bran in the prevention of acute anal fissure recurrence. J R Soc Med 1987; 80:296–298.
30. Walker WA, Rothenberger DA, Goldberg SM. Morbidity of internal sphincterotomy for anal fissure and stenosis. Dis Colon Rectum 1985; 28:832–835.
31. Khubchandani IT, Reed JF. Sequelae of internal sphincterotomy for chronic fissure-in-ano. Br J Surg 1989; 76:431–434.
32. Pitt J, Williams S, Dawson PM. Reasons for failure of glyceryl trinitrate treatment of chronic fissure-in-ano. A multivariate analysis. Dis Colon Rectum 2001; 44:864–867.
33. Abcarian H. Surgical correction of chronic anal fissure: results of lateral anal internal sphincterotomy vs. fissurectomy—mid-line sphincterotomy. Dis Colon Rectum 1980; 23:31–36.
34. Lewis TH, Corman ML, Prager ED, Robertson WG. Long-term results of open and closed sphincterotomy for anal fissure. Dis Colon Rectum 1988; 31:368–371.
35. Hiltunen KM, Metikainen M. Closed lateral subcutaneous sphincterotomy under local anesthesia in the treatment of chronic anal fissure. Ann Chir Gynaecol 1991; 80:353–356.
36. Frezza EE, Sander G, Leoni G, Birad M. Conservative and surgical treatment in acute and chronic anal fissure. A study of 308 patients. Int J Colorectal Dis 1992; 7:188–191.
37. Leong AFPK, Husain MJ, Seow-Choen F, Goh HS. Performing internal sphincterotomy with other anorectal procedures. Dis Colon Rectum 1994; 37:1130–1132.
38. Pernikoff MJ, Eisenstat TE, Rubin RJ, Oliver GC, Salvati EP. Reappraisal of partial lateral internal sphincterotomy. Dis Colon Rectum 1994; 37:1291–1295.
39. Romano G, Rotondano G, Santangelo M, Esercizio L. A critical appraisal of pathogenesis and morbidity of surgical treatment of chronic anal fissure. J Am Coll Surg 1994; 178:600–604.
40. Neufeld DM, Paran H, Bendahan J, Freund U. Outpatient surgical treatment of anal fissure. Eur J Surg 1995; 161:435–438.
41. Oh C, Divino CM, Steinhagen RM. Anal fissure 20 years experience. Dis Colon Rectum 1995; 38:378–382.
42. Usatoff V, Polglase AL. The longer term results of internal anal sphincterotomy for anal fissure. Aust N Z J Surg 1995; 65:576–578.
43. Garcia-Aguilar J, Belmonte C, Wong WD, Lowry AC, Madoff RD. Open vs. closed sphincterotomy for chronic anal fissure: Long-term results. Dis Colon Rectum 1996; 39:440–443.
44. Hananel N, Gordon.PH, Lateral internal sphincterotomy for fissure-in-ano revisited. Dis colon Rectum 1997; 40:597–602.
45. Farouk R, Gunn J, Lee PWR, Monson JRT. Failure of lateral internal sphincterotomy for the treatment of chronic anal fissure is due to technical failure. Br J Surg 1996; 83(suppl l):60.
46. Jonas M, Lobo DN, Gudgeon AM. Lateral internal sphincterotomy is not redundant in the era of glyceryl trinitrate therapy for chronic anal fissure. J R Soc Med 1999; 92:186–188.
47. Nyam DCNK, Pemberton JH. Long-term results of lateral internal sphincterotomy for chronic anal fissure with particular reference to incidence of fecal incontinence. Dis Colon Rectum 1999; 42:1306–1310.
48. Argov S, Levandovsky O. Open lateral sphincterotomy is still the best treatment for chronic anal fissure. Am J Surg 2000; 179:201–206.
49. Richard CS, Gregoire R, Plewes EA, et al. Internal sphincterotomy is superior to topical nitroglycerin in the treatment of chronic anal fissure: results of a randomized, controlled trial by the Canadian colorectal Surgical Trials Group. Dis Colon Rectum 2000; 43:1048–1058.
50. Evans J, Luck A, Hewett P. Glyceryl trinitrate vs. lateral sphincterotomy for chronic anal fissure: prospective, randomized trial. Dis Colon Rectum 2001; 44:93–97.
51. Menteş BB, ?körücü O, Akm M, Leventoğlu S, Tatlicioğlu E. Comparison of botulinum toxin injection and lateral internal sphincterotomy for the treatment of chronic anal fissure. Dis Colon Rectum 2003; 46:232–237.
52. Arroyo A, Perez F, Serrano P, Candela F, Calpena R. Open versus closed lateral sphincterotomy performed as an outpatient procedure under local anesthesia for chronic anal fissure: prospective randomized study of clinical and manometric long term results. J Am Coll Surg 2004; 1999:361–367.
53. Parellada C. Randomized, prospective trial comparing 0.2 percent isosorbide dinitrate ointment with sphincterotomy in treatment of chronic anal fissure: a two-year follow-up. Dis Colon Rectum 2004; 47:437–443.
54. Lund JN, Scholefield JH. A randomized, prospective double-blind, placebo-controlled trial of glyceryl trinitrate ointment in treatment of anal fissure. Lancet 1997; 349:11–14.
55. Knight JS, Birks M, Farouk R. Topical diltiazem ointment in the treatment of chronic anal fissure. Br J Surg 2001; 88:553–556.
56. Kennedy ML, Sowter S, Nguyen H, Lubowski DZ. Glyceryl trinitrate ointment for the treatment of chronic anal fissure: results of a placebo-controlled trial and long-term follow-up. Dis Colon Rectum 1999; 42:1000–1006.
57. Loder PB, Kamm MA, Nicholls RJ, Phillips RKS. Reversible chemical sphincterotomy by local application of glyceryl trinitrate. Br J Surg 1994; 81:1386–1389.
58. O'Kelly TJ, Davies JR, Brading AF, Mortensen NJM. Distribution of nitric oxide synthase containing neurons in the rectal myenteric plexus and anal canal. Morphologic evidence that nitric oxide mediates the rectoanal inhibitory reflex. Dis Colon Rectum 1994; 37:350–357.
59. Carapeti EA, Kamm MA, McDonald PJ, Chadwick SJD, Melville D, Phillips RKS. Randomised controlled trial shows that glyceryl trinitrate heals anal fissures, higher doses are not more effective, and there is a high recurrence rate. Gut 1999; 44:727–730.
60. Watson SJ, Kamm MA, Nicholls RJ, Phillips RKS. Topical glyceryl trinitrate in the treatment of chronic anal fissure. Br J Surg 1996; 83:771–775.
61. Schouten WR, Briel JM, Boerma MO, Auwerda JJA, Wilms EB, Graatsma DH. Pathophysiological aspects and clinical outcome of intra-anal application of isosorbide-di-nitrate in patients with chronic anal fissure. Gut 1995; 36:A16–W64.
62. McLeod RS, Evans J. Symptomatic care and nitroglycerin in the management of anal fissure. J Gastrointest Surg 2002; 6:278–280.
63. Altomare DF, Rinaldi M, Milito G, et al. Glyceryl trinitrate for chronic anal fissure-healing or headache? Results of a multicenter, randomized, placebo-controlled, double-blind trial. Dis Colon Rectum 2000; 43:174–181.
64. Bacher H, Mischinger H-J, Werkgartner G, et al. Local nitroglycerin for treatment of anal fissures: an alternative to lateral sphincterotomy? Dis Colon Rectum 1997; 40:840–845.
65. Lund JN, Scholefield JH. Follow-up of patients with chronic anal fissure treated with topical glyceryl trinitrate. Lancet 1998; 352:1681.
66. Oettle GI. Glyceryl trinitrate vs. sphincterotomy for treatment of chronic fissure. Dis Colon Rectum 1997; 40:1318–1320.
67. Lysy J, Israelit-Yatzkan Y, Sestiere-Ittah M, Keret D, Goldin E. Treatment of chronic anal fissure with isosorbide dinitrate: long-term results and dose determination. Dis Colon Rectum 1998; 41:1406–1410.
68. Brisinda G, Maria G, Bentivoglio AR, Cassetto C, Giu D, Albanese A. A comparison of injections of botulinum toxin and topical nitroglycerin ointment for the treatment of chronic anal fissures. N Engl J Med 1999; 341:65–69.
69. Dorfman G, Levitt M, Platell C. Treatment of chronic anal fissure with topical glyceryl trinitrate. Dis Colon Rectum 1999; 42:1007–1010.
70. Hyman NH, Cataldo PA. Nitroglycerin ointment for anal fissures effective treatment or just a headache? Dis Colon Rectum 1999; 42:383–385.
71. Gecim I. Comparison of glyceryl trinitrate and botulinum toxin A in treatment of chronic anal fissure: a prospective, randomized study. Dis Colon Rectum 2001; 44:A5–A26.
72. Graziano A, Svidler Lopez L, Lencina S, Masciangiole G, Gualdrini U, Bisisio O. Long-term results of topical nitroglycerin in the treatment of chronic anal fissures are disappointing. Tech Coloproctol 2001; 5:143–147.
73. Bailey HR, Beck DE, Billingham RP, et al. Fissure study group. A study to determine the nitroglycerin ointment dose and dosing interval that best promote the healing of chronic anal fissures. Dis Colon Rectum 2002; 45(9):1192–1199.
74. Kocher HM, Steward M, Leather AJ, Cullen PT. Randomized clinical trial assessing the side-effects of glyceryl trinitrate and diltiazem hydrochloride in the treatment of chronic anal fissure. Br J Surg. 2002; 89:413–417.
75. Zuberi BF, Rajput MR, Abro H, Shaikh SA. A randomized trial of glyceryl trinitrate ointment and nitroglycerin patch in healing of anal fissure. Int J Colorectal Dis 2000; 15:243–245.
76. Jonas M, Amin S, Wright JW, Neal KR, Scholefield JH. Topical 0.2% glyceryl trinitrate ointment has a short lived effect on resting and pressure. Dis Colon Rectum 2001; 44:1640–1643.
77. Carapeti EA, Kamm Ma, Phillips RKS. Topical diltiazem and bethanechol decrease anal sphincter pressure and heal fissures without side effects. Dis Colon Rectum 2000; 43:1359–1362.
78. Jonas M, Speake W, Scholefield JH. Diltiazem heals glyceryl trinitrate-resistant chronic anal fissures. A prospective study. Dis Colon Rectum 2002; 45(8):1091–1095.
79. Jonas M, Speake W, Simpson J, Varghese T, Scholefield J. Diltiazem heals glyceryl trinitrate (GTN)-resistant chronic anal fissures. Dis Colon Rectum 2001; 44:A5–A26.
80. Jonas M, Neal KR, Abercrombie JF, Scholefield JH. A randomized trial of oral vs. topical diltiazem for chronic anal fissures. Dis Colon Rectum 2001; 44: 1074–1078.

81. Antropoli C, Perrotti P, Rubino M, et al. Nifedipine for local use in conservative treatment of anal fissures: preliminary results of a multicenter study. Dis Colon Rectum 1999; 42:1011–1015.
82. Cook TA, Smilgin Humphreys MM, McC Mortensen NJ. Oral nifedipine reduces resting anal pressure and heals chronic anal fissure. Br J Surg 1999; 86(10):1269–1273.
83. Perrotti P, Bove A, Antropoli C, et al. Topical nifedipine with lidocaine ointment vs. active control for treatment of chronic anal fissure: results of a prospective, randomized, double-blind study. Dis Colon Rectum 2002; 45(11):1468–1475.
84. Ho KS, Ho YH. Randomized clinical trial comparing oral nifedipine with lateral anal sphincterotomy and tailored sphincterotomy in the treatment of chronic anal fissure. Br J Surg 2005; 92:403–408.
85. Brisinda G, Maria G, Sganga G, Bentivioglio AR, Al bonese A, Castagneto M. Effectiveness of higher doses of botulinum toxin to induce healing in patients with chronic anal fissures. Surgery 2002; 131:179–184.
86. Brisinda D, Maria G, Fenici R, Civello IM, Brisinda G. Safety of botulinum neurotoxin treatment in patients with chronic anal fissure. Dis Colon Rectum 2003; 46(3):419–420.
87. Jost WH. One hundred case of anal fissure treated with botulin toxin. Dis Colon Rectum 1997; 40:1029–1032.
88. Fernandez Lopez F, Conde Freire R, Rios Rios A, Garcia Iglesias J, Cainzos Fernandez M, Potel Lesquereux J. Botulinum toxin for the treatment of anal fissure. Dis Surg 1999; 16(6):515–518.
89. Gonzalez Carro P, Perez Rolden F, Legoz Huidobro MZ, Ruiz Corillo F, Pedroza Martin C, Saez Bravo JM. The treatment of anal fissure with botulinum toxin. J Gastroenterol Hepatol 1999; 22:163–166.
90. Maria G, Brisinda G, Bentivoglio AR, Cassetta E, Gui D, Albanese A. Influence of botulinum toxin site of injections on healing rate in patients with chronic anal fissure. Am J Surg 2000; 179(1):46–50.
91. Minguez M, Melo F, Espi A, et al. Therapeutic effects of different doses of botulinum toxin in chronic anal fissure. Dis Colon Rectum 1999; 42:1016–1021.
92. Minguez M, Herreros B, Espi A, et al. Long-term follow-up (42 months) of chronic anal fissure after healing with botulinum toxin. Gastroenterology 2002; 123:112–117.
93. Lindsey I, Jones OM, Cunningham C, George BD, Mortensen NJM. Botulinum toxin as second-line therapy for chronic anal fissure failing 0.2 percent glyceryl trinitrate. Dis Colon Rectum 2003; 46(3):361–366.
94. Pitt S, Craggs MN, Henry MM, Boulos PB. Alpha-1 adrenocepter blockade. Potential new treatment for anal fissure. Dis Colon Rectum 2000; 43:800–803.
95. Griffin N, Zimmerman DDE, Briel JW, et al. Topical l-arginine gel lowers anal resting pressure: possible treatment for anal fissure. Dis Colon Rectum 2002; 45:1332–1336.
96. Gosselink MP, Darby M, Zimmerman DD, Gruss HJ, Schouten WR. Treatment of chronic anal fissure by application of l-arginine gel: a phase II study in 15 patients. Dis Colon Rectum 2005; 48:832–837.
97. Garrido R, Lagos N, Lattes K, et al. Gonyautoxin: new treatment for healing acute and chronic anal fissures. Dis Colon Rectum 2005; 48:335–340.
98. Torrabadella L, Salgado G, Burns RW, Berman IR. Manometric study of topical sildenafil (Viagra) in patients with chronic anal fissure: sildenafil reduces anal resting tone. Dis Colon Rectum 2004; 47:733–738.
99. Nelson R. A systematic review of medical therapy for anal fissure. Dis Colon Rectum 2004; 47:422–431.
100. Standards Task Force, American Society of Colon and Rectal Surgeons, Rosen L, Abel ME, Gordon PH, et al. Practice parameters for the management of anal fissure. Dis Colon Rectum 1992; 35:206–208.
101. Badejo OA. Outpatient treatment of fissure-in-ano. Trop Geogr Med 1984; 36:367–369.
102. Engel AF, Eijsbouts QAJ, Balk AG. Fissurectomy and isosorbide dinitrate for chronic fissure in-ano not responding to conservative treatment. Br J Surg 2002; 89:79–83.
103. Storer EH, Goldberg SM, Nivatvongs S. Colon, rectum, and anus. In: Schwartz ST, ed. Principles of Surgery. New York: McGraw-Hill, 1979:1241.
104. Samson RB, Stewart WRC. Sliding skin grafts in the treatment of anal fissure. Dis Colon Rectum 1970; 13:372–375.
105. Leong AFPK, Seow-Choen F. Lateral sphincterotomy compared with anal advancement flap for chronic anal fissure. Dis Colon Rectum 1995; 38:69–71.
106. Nyam DCNK, Wilson KG, Stewart KJ, Farouk R, Bartolo DCC. Island advancement flaps in the management of anal fissures. Br J Surg 1995; 82:526–528.
107. Recamier JCA. Extension, massage et percussion cadence dansle traitement des contractures musculaires. Revue Medicale 1838; 1:74–89.
108. Lord PH. Diverse methods of managing hemorrhoids: dilatation. Dis Colon Rectum 1973; 16:180–183.
109. Isbister WH, Prasad J. Fissure-in-ano. Aust N Z J Surg 1995; 65:107–108.
110. Sohn N, Eisenberg MM, Weinstein MA, Lugo RN, Ader J. Precise anorectal dilatation—its role in the therapy of anal fissures. Dis Colon Rectum 1992; 35:322–327.
111. Nielson MB, Rasmussen OO, Pedersen JF, Christiansen J. Risk of sphincter damage and anal incontinence after anal dilation for fissure-in-ano. An endosonographic study. Dis Colon Rectum 1993; 36:677–680.
112. Renzi A, Brusciano L, Pescatori M, et al. Pneumatic balloon dilatation for chronic anal fissure: prospective, clinical endosonographic, and manometric study. Dis Colon Rectum 2005; 48:121–126.
113. Lund JN, Scholefield JH. Etiology and treatment of anal fissure. Br J Surg 1996; 83:1335–1344.
114. Eisenhammer S. The surgical correction of chronic anal (sphincteric) contracture. S Afr Med J 1951; 25:486–489.
115. Brodie BC. Lectures on diseases of the rectum. III. Preternatural contraction of the sphincter ani. London Med Gaz 1835; 16:26–31.
116. Melange M, Colin JF, Wymersch TV, Vanheuverzwyn R. Anal fissure: correlation between symptoms and manometry before and after surgery. Int J Colorectal Dis 1992; 7:108–111.
117. Eisenhammer S. The evaluation of internal anal sphincterotomy operation with special reference to anal fissure. Surg Gynecol Obstet 1959; 109: 583–590.
118. Parks AG. The management of fissure-in-ano. Hosp Med 1967; 1:737–738.
119. Notaras MJ. The treatment of anal fissure by lateral subcutaneous internal sphincterotomy—a technique and results. Br J Surg 1971; 58:96–100.
120. Saad AMA, Omer A. Surgical treatment of chronic fissure-in-ano: a prospective randomized study. East Afr Med J 1992; 69:613–615.
121. Goldman G, Zilberman M, Werbin N. Bacteremia in anal dilatation. Dis Colon Rectum 1986; 29:304–305.
122. Sultan AH, Kamm MA, Nicholls RI, Bartram CI. Prospective study of the extent of internal anal sphincter division during lateral sphincterotomy. Dis Colon Rectum 1989; 37:1031–1033.
123. Gordon PH, Vasilevsky CA. Lateral internal sphincterotomy: rationale, technique, and anesthesia. Can J Surg 1985; 28:228–230.
124. Casillas S, Hull TL, Zutshi M, Trzcinski R, Bast JF, Xu M. Incontinence after a lateral internal sphincterotomy: are we underestimating it? Dis Colon Rectum 2005; 48:1193–1199.
125. Boulos PB, Araujo JGC. Adequate internal sphincterotomy for chronic anal fissure: subcutaneous or open technique? Br J Surg 1984; 72:360–362.
126. Kortbeek JB, Langevin JM, Khoo REH, Heine JA. Chronic fissure-in-ano: a randomized study comparing open and subcutaneous lateral internal sphincterotomy. Dis Colon Rectum 1992; 35:835–837.
127. Wiley M, Day P, Rieger N, Stephens J, Moore J. Open vs. closed lateral internal sphincterotomy for idiopathic fissure-in-ano: a prospective, randomized, controlled trial. Dis Colon Rectum 2004; 47:847–852.
128. Littlejohn DRG, Newstead GL. Tailored lateral sphincterotomy for anal fissure. Dis Colon Rectum 1997; 40:1439–1442.
129. Hyman N. Incontinence after lateral internal sphincterotomy: a prospective study and quality of life assessment. Dis Colon Rectum 2004; 47:35–38.
130. Ellis CN. Anterior levatorplasty for the treatment of chronic anal fissures in females with a rectocele: a randomized, controlled trial. Dis Colon Rectum 2004; 47:1170–1173.
131. Nelson R. A review of operative procedures for anal fissure. J. Gastrointest Surg 2000; 6:284–289.
132. Farouk R, Gunn J, Duthie GS. Changing patterns of treatment for chronic and fissure. Ann R Coll Surg Engl 1996; 80:196–197.

10 Anorectal Abscesses and Fistula-in-Ano

Philip H. Gordon

If the theory that both the abscess and the fistula-in-ano have a common cause is accepted, the two conditions can be considered simultaneously. Indeed, the term "fistulous abscess" has been used to describe this problem. The abscess is an acute manifestation, and the fistula is a chronic condition. A fistula is an abnormal communication between any two epithelial-lined surfaces. A fistula-in-ano is an abnormal communication between the anal canal and the perineal skin. Many of these fistulas are easily recognized and readily treated, but others can be very complex and correspondingly difficult to manage.

In a treatise on fistula-in-ano in 1765, Percivall Pott wrote the following:

> Clear and precise definitions of diseases, and the application of such names to them as are expressive of their true and real nature, are of more consequence than they are generally imagined to be: untrue or imperfect ones occasion false ideas; and false ideas are generally followed by erroneous practice.

Thus, the true understanding of a disease is achieved only when its exact cause is identified and the mechanism of the disordered structure or function is established.

ANATOMY

Understanding the anatomy of the pelvic floor is critical to appreciating the origin and ramifications of fistulas. Reduced to its simplest form, the pelvic floor consists of two funnel-shaped structures, one situated within the other. The inner structure is the lower end of the circular muscle of the rectum, which becomes thick and rounded and is referred to as the internal sphincter. Surrounding this sphincter is a funnel of pelvic floor muscle formed by the levator ani, puborectalis, and external sphincter muscles. Between the two structures is the intersphincteric plane. In the middle portion of the anal canal at the level of the dentate line, the ducts of the anal glands empty into the crypts. The greatest concentration of these glands is in the posterior aspect of the anal canal. For further anatomic details, see Chapter 1 and Figure 5 of that chapter.

ETIOLOGY

Numerous conditions, which may be classified as specific or nonspecific, can cause the formation of a fistulous abscess. Nonspecific ones are cryptoglandular in origin. Specific ones include the following: Crohn's disease, chronic ulcerative colitis, tuberculosis (TB), actinomycosis, presence of a foreign body, carcinoma, lymphoma, lymphogranuloma venereum, pelvic inflammation, trauma (impalement, enemas, prostatic surgery, episiotomy, hemorrhoidectomy), radiation, and leukemia.

Other inflammatory conditions associated with fistula-in-ano are mentioned in Chapters 26 and 27. Other causes of these conditions are listed in their respective chapters.

PATHOGENESIS

Evidence suggests that infection of the anal glands is probably the most common cause of fistulous abscess (1–3). In the acute form, such infections are seen as an abscess; in the chronic form the patient presents with a fistula-in-ano. As early as 1878, Chiari first described anal ducts and glands that discharged their contents at the mucocutaneous junction into the anal canal. Chiari's views initially were suspect because of the infrequency with which these structures were found and because of their minute dimensions. In 1956, Eisenhammer (1) ascribed most anorectal abscesses and fistula-in-ano to an anal gland infection in the intersphincteric space; unfortunately, Eisenhammer's papers did not contain pathologic confirmation of his views. However, specimens excised from patients with fistula-in-ano were carefully studied by Parks (3) and Morson and Dawson (4), who after tedious examinations demonstrated infected anal glands in 70% of cases and histologic evidence suggestive of this origin in another 20%, bringing the total attributable to this cause to 90%. Normal anatomy was studied by obtaining material at autopsy and after cases of radical excision for carcinoma of the rectum. The anal glands were found to arise in the middle of the anal canal at the level of the crypts and to pass into, the submucosa, with two-thirds continuing into the internal sphincter and one-half penetrating into the intersphincteric plane (Fig. 1). Obstruction of these ducts, whether secondary to fecal material foreign bodies, or trauma, results in stasis and infection. Morson and Dawson (4) believe that the chronicity of the condition is due to persistence of the anal gland epithelium in the part of the tract joining the internal opening. Such persistent epithelium keeps the opening patent, preventing healing. Lunniss et al. (5) believe that persistence of an anal fistula may be related more to nonspecific epithelialization of the fistula tract from either the internal or external openings than to a chronically infected anal gland. Epithelialization of at least part of a tract was found in 13 of 18 fistulas so studied. Destruction of the anal gland epithelium might explain the occasional spontaneous healing of a fistula.

The concept of a cryptoglandular origin is not universally accepted. In a study of 60 patients with anorectal

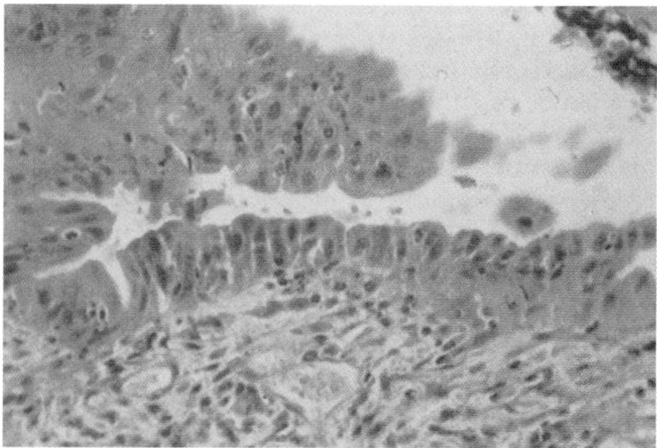

FIGURE 1 ■ Anorectal gland. Section of the anal canal showing duct of anal gland entering at level of the dentate line. Transition from squamous epithelium to transitional epithelium to columnar epithelium can be noted.

abscesses or fistula-in-ano, Goligher, Ellis, and Pissidis (6) found intersphincteric abscesses in only 23%, suggesting that this cause is less often the precursor. Seow-Choen et al. (7) studied the bacteriology of 25 patients who were operated on for anal fistula. Predominant organisms were *Escherichia coli* (22%), *Enterococcus* spp. (16%), and *Bacterioides fragilis* (20%). The majority of growths were obtained only from enrichment. The authors concluded that chronic inflammation in anal fistulas does not seem to be maintained by either excessive numbers of organisms or by organisms of an unusual type. The theory of cryptoglandular origin is, however, supported by the fact that the primary internal orifice is found at the level of the pectinate line.

Sereral predisposing factors may be associated with the initiation of these fistulous abscesses. An acute episode of diarrhea can force liquid feces into the main duct of the intramuscular gland and cause obstructive suppurative adenitis. Trauma, whether in the form of a hard stool or foreign body, also can be a contributing factor. Certain anatomic variations, such as large anal sinuses that collect material and are unable to empty properly because of the pressure on them in the anal canal, may intiate the process. Cystic dilatation also may be a necessary precusor to infection because the disease may not start in a normal gland. Anorectal suppuration may arise in association with a fissure-in-ano, infection of an anal hematoma, Crohn's disease, or tuberculosis and even has been described as caused by *Enterobius vermicularis* or *Trichuris trichiura* (8,9).

AVENUES OF EXTENSION

A fistula most commonly pursues a course from the middle of the anal canal downward in the intersphincteric plane to the anal verge. Infection may overcome the barrier of the external sphincter muscles, thereby penetrating the ischioanal fossa, or it may extend upward in the intersphincteric plane, either remaining in the rectal wall or extending extrarectally (Fig. 2).

In addition to tracking upward and downward, pus may pass circumferentially around the anus. This passage can occur in one of three tissue planes, the most common of which is the ischioanal fossa. This variety commences in the posterior midline of the anal canal, penetrates the sphincteric mass into the deep postanal space, then descends with two limbs, one in each ischioanal fossa. This circumferential spread is referred to as horseshoeing. In addition, circumferential spread may occur in the intersphincteric plane or in the pararectal tissues above the levator muscles (see Fig. 13 of Chap. 1).

DIAGNOSIS

HISTORY

A patient with a fistulous abscess may present with it in either the acute or the chronic phase. The patient with an abscess will present with acute pain and swelling in the anal region. Pain occurs with sitting or movement and is usually aggravated by defecation and even coughing or sneezing. The clinical history may reveal a preceding bout of diarrhea. General symptoms include malaise and pyrexia. In a series of 117 patients with anorectal suppuration reviewed by Vasilevsky and Gordon (10), the most common presenting symptoms included pain (93%), swelling (50%), and bleeding per rectum (16%). Other symptoms included purulent anal discharge, diarrhea, and fever. In the same authors' review of 160 patients with fistula-in-ano, presenting symptoms in decreasing order of frequency were discharge (65%), pain (34%), swelling (24%), bleeding (12%), and diarrhea (5%) (11).

The importance of intersphincteric abscess as a cause of persistent undiagnosed anal pain must be stressed. The pain is generally throbbing in character and remains continuous throughout the day and night. It is aggravated by defecation but may be severe enough to cause fecal impaction. In general, the pain is of longer duration than that in patients with fissures. Minor anal bleeding may occur if the abscess is associated with an opening into the anal canal or a fissure. A discharge, when present, is due to small amounts of pus passing into the anal canal.

In the chronic phase, the patient's history will reveal an abscess that either burst spontaneously or required drainage. The patient will have noticed a small discharging sinus, or the discharge may have caused skin excoriation

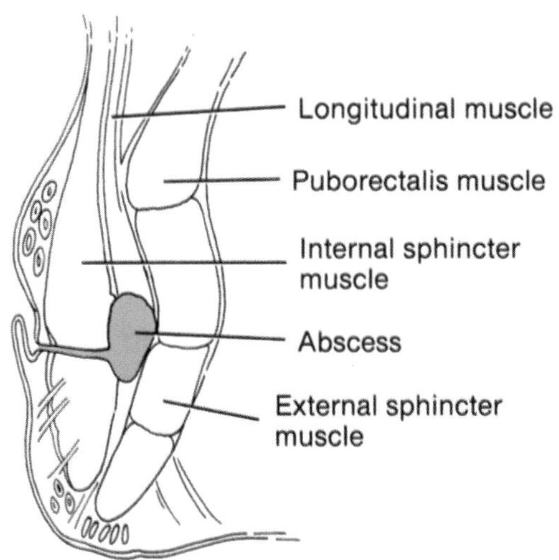

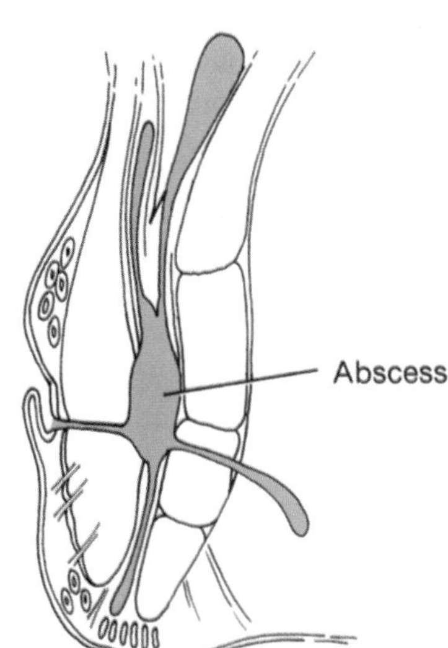

FIGURE 2 ■ Avenues of extension for an anal fistula.

and pruritus. Pain with defecation and bleeding caused by granulation tissue in the region of the internal opening also may be present.

■ PHYSICAL EXAMINATION

In the acute phase of a fistulous abscess, the cardinal signs of inflammation are present with rubor, calor, tumor, dolor, and functio laesa (i.e., redness, heat, swelling, pain, loss of function). Sometimes pus may be seen exuding from a crypt. The swelling may be in either the immediate perianal region or the ischioanal fossa.

Swelling and induration in the perianal region may not occur with an intersphincteric abscess. Rectal examination is exquisitely painful or impossible, but in some cases the suggestion of a mass is present. An opening into the anal canal with or without a fissure may be seen, sometimes with pus exuding (12). The fact that the inguinal lymph nodes may be enlarged and painful with an abscess may help in differentiating between an intersphincteric abscess and an acute fissure-in-ano.

When the patient's pain is severe but its cause is unknown, placing the patient under anesthesia for the examination is not only justified but also indicated. When the abscess is seen, it must be adequately drained. Neglect only allows extension of the abscess and may lead to ischioanal or supralevator abscesses and possibly to horseshoe extensions, with each of these conditions more difficult to manage than the simple intersphincteric abscess. If no abscess is found, another pathologic condition should be found—usually an acute fissure. Treatment of this condition results in dramatic relief of pain (many of such patients probably would not heal completely spontaneously).

An analogy can be drawn with acute appendicitis, in which case whether or not to operate is sometimes a dilemma. Just as it is better to operate on a certain percentage of patients who turn out not to have acute appendicitis rather than expose them to the complications of perforation with abscess and the potential consequences of peritonitis, it is wiser to operate on patients suspected of having an intersphincteric abscess than to allow them to develop more complicated problems. In fact, these patients usually will demonstrate abnormalities amenable to operative treatment.

With the supralevator abscess, a tender mass in the pelvis may be diagnosed by rectal or vaginal examination. Abdominal examination may reveal signs of peritoneal irritation because the pelvic peritoneum forms the roof of the supralevator space.

In the chronic state, an external opening usually can be seen as a red elevation of granulation tissue with purulent serosanguinous discharge on compression. Sometimes, the opening is so small that it can be detected only when palpation around the anus expresses a few beads of pus from an otherwise inconspicuous opening. The internal crypt of origin may not always be patent. The number of external openings and their relationship to the anal canal may reveal much information to the examiner. According to Goodsall's rule, if there is an opening posterior to the coronal plane, the fistula probably originates from the dorsal midline; but if the opening is anterior, it probably runs directly to the nearest crypt. Openings seen on both sides of the anal canal are likely to arise from a midline posterior crypt with a horseshoe type of fistula (Fig. 3).

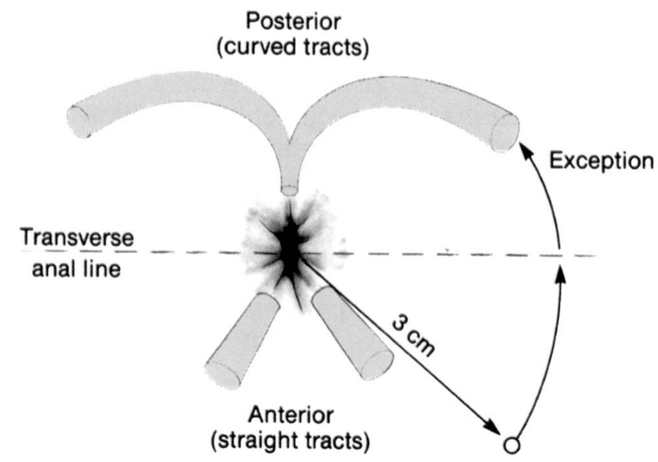

FIGURE 3 ■ Goodsall's rule.

To examine the predictive accuracy of Goodsall's rule, the records of 216 patients who underwent operation for anal fistulas were retrospectively reviewed by Cirocco and Reilly (13). In accordance with Goodsall's rule, 90% of 124 patients with an external opening posterior to the transverse anal line had anal fistulas tracking to the midline. Only 49% of the 92 patients with an external opening anterior to the transverse anal line had anal fistulas that tracked in the radial fashion predicted by Goodsall. Instead, 71% of these patients had anterior fistulas tracking to the midline. Overall, 81% of patients had anal fistulas that coursed to the midline (51% midline posterior and 30% midline anterior). They concluded that Goodsall's rule was accurate only when applied to anal fistulas with posterior external anal openings. The men in this group had anal fistulas that defied Goodsall's rule in an unpredictable manner, whereas 90% of the women had fistulas tracking to a midline anterior origin. In my own series of patients most primary openings (58%) were found in either the posterior or anterior aspects of the anal canal (11).

An external opening adjacent to the anal margin may suggest an intersphincteric tract, whereas a more laterally located opening would suggest a transsphincteric one. The further the distance of the external opening from the anal margin, the greater is the probability of a complicated upward extension. The relationship between increasing complexity and increasing laterality and multiplicity of external openings also has been observed by other authors (14).

The next step is to palpate the skin since with a superficial fistula a cord structure can be felt just beneath the skin leading from the secondary opening to the anal canal. Further palpation may reveal circumferential extension, which would be recognized by a ring of induration hugging the puborectalis sling in a horseshoe fashion. The supralevator spaces then are felt on each side.

In the anal canal, a pit indicative of an internal opening might be palpable. The crypt of origin is often retracted into a funnel by pulling the fibrous tract leading to the internal sphincter; this state is called the funnel, or "herniation sign," of the involved crypt. The latter movement is performed in the operating room. A palpable nodule caused by a chronic intersphincteric abscess occasionally may be felt.

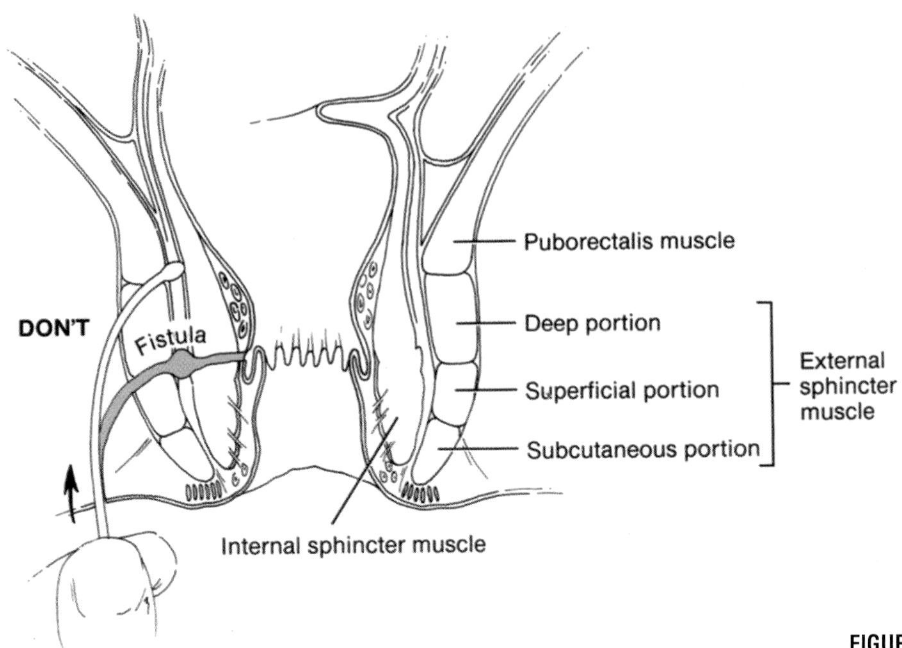

FIGURE 4 ■ Probing of the fistulous tract.

Probing, when done, must be performed with a feather-like touch to prevent false channels; therefore, it is best to avoid such probing outside the operating room. Even in the operating room with the patient under anesthesia, great care must be taken to avoid the creation of false passages into the anal canal or into the rectum (Fig. 4). After a probe has been gently introduced into the tract, it can follow the path of a "low" fistula toward the anus at an angle of approximately 30° to the skin. Passage of the probe at an 80° angle to the skin or almost parallel to the anal canal indicates the presence of a "high" fistula or at least a supralevator or ischioanal extension of a low fistula. Primary openings are successfully located by a probe in two-thirds of patients; in the remainder, a diluted solution of methylene blue dye is used or granulation tissue is pursued.

■ ANOSCOPY AND SIGMOIDOSCOPY

Anoscopy and sigmoidoscopy must be performed for at least three reasons. First, anoscopy can help identify the internal opening in the anal canal. Second, endoscopy can help distinguish between a rectal and an anal canal opening. Third, sigmoidoscopy allows examination of the rectal mucosa to determine the presence of underlying proctocolitis, if it should exist. A rectal biopsy is performed if Crohn's disease is suspected.

■ INVESTIGATION

In the majority of patients who present with a fistula-in-ano, radiologic examination is of limited value. A barium enema study or colonoscopy, however, is indicated in patients with a history of bowel symptoms suggestive of inflammatory bowel disease (IBD). For the same reasons, a small bowel series may be indicated.

Fistulography

Fistulography may help delineate an extrasphincteric fistula of pelvic origin or may help evaluate patients with recurrent fistulas (15). Kuijpers and Schulpen (16) studied 25 patients and compared fistulographic with operative findings; they found fistulography to be inaccurate in 84% of patients. Notwithstanding this discouraging report, a fistulogram on occasion can outline the problem (Fig. 5). Weisman et al. (17) conducted a retrospective review of 27 patients undergoing anal fistulography. Twenty-six fistulograms revealed either direct communication with the anus or rectum, or abscess cavities/tracts, or both. In 13 of the 27 patients (48%), information obtained from the fistulograms revealed either unexpected pathology (seven) or directly altered surgical management (six). They concluded that anal fistulography in properly selected patients might add useful information for definitive management of fistula-in-ano.

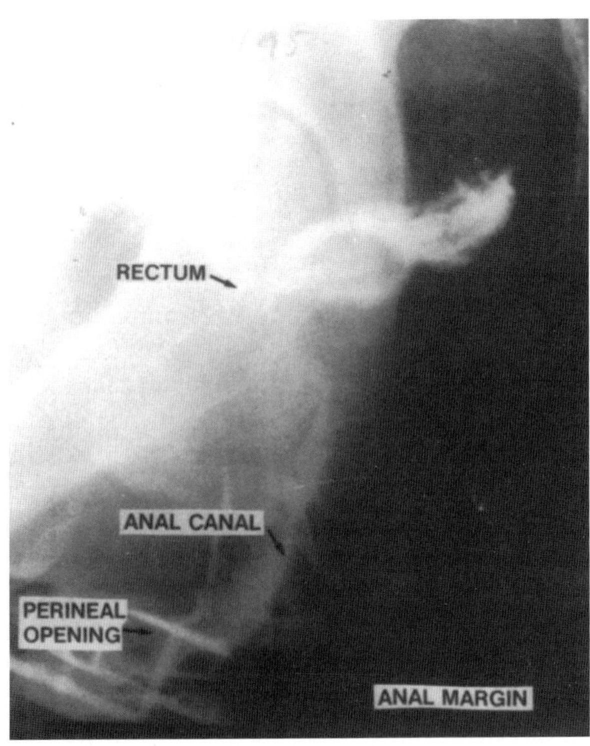

FIGURE 5 ■ Fistulogram demonstrating tract.

Ultrasonography

Anal endosonography has been used to evaluate perianal sepsis and fistula-in-ano. Cataldo et al. (18) evaluated their experience with intrarectal ultrasonography (IRUS) in 24 patients with suspected perianal abscess and fistula. At operation, 19 of 24 patients were found to have perirectal abscesses, with all 19 cases correctly identified preoperatively by IRUS. In 63%, IRUS correctly identified the relationship between the abscesses and sphincters by Parks' classification. At operation, internal openings of fistula tracts were found in 14 of 19 cases but IRUS identified only four of 14 (28%). Certainly, there is no need for IRUS in uncomplicated abscesses, but it may prove to be an adjunct in the evaluation of complex anorectal suppurative disease. Cheong et al. (19) reported that hydrogen peroxide enhancement of the fistula tract is a simple, effective, and safe method of improving the accuracy of endoanal ultrasonographic assessment of recurrent anal fistula. Choen et al. (20) found no statistical difference between consultant assessment and anal ultrasonography in correctly identifying intersphincteric and trans-sphincteric tracts. Ultrasonography was unable to assess primary superficial, suprasphincteric, and extrasphincteric tracts or secondary supralevator and infralevator tracts.

More recently, Chew et al. (21) found Levovist-enhanced ultrasonography better at assessing anal fistula than physical examination and conventional ultrasound. In their pilot study of 15 patients, concordance rate of operation with conventional ultrasound was 69% and with Levovist-enhanced ultrasound was 77%. Detection of the internal opening was 13% on physical examination, 27% on conventional ultrasound, and 60% with Levovist-enhanced ultrasonography. In review of the literature, Zimmerman (22) found that with conventional endoanal sonography correct classification of the fistula ranged from 50% to 94% and correct localization of the internal opening ranged from 5% to 54%. Using hydrogen peroxide-enhanced endoanal sonography, the corresponding rates were 73–95% and 48–96%.

Magnetic Resonance Imaging

Maruyama et al. (23) evaluated the usefulness of magnetic resonance imaging (MRI) for the preoperative diagnosis of deep anorectal abscesses in 21 patients. Sensitivity of ischiorectal abscesses (20 lesions) with digital examination and MRI was 75% and 95%, respectively, and that of pelvirectal abscesses (10 lesions) with digital examination and MRI was 60% and 70%, respectively. Diagnostic accuracy of digital examination and MRI were both 83% in the single abscess group (12 patients), whereas in the double abscess group (nine patients) it was 22% and 78%, respectively. They concluded that MRI was useful for diagnosing and differentiating ischiorectal and pelvirectal abscesses.

In recent years, MRI has been shown to accurately demonstrate pelvic anatomy, in particular, the relationship between anal fistula and the sphincter muscles. Barker et al. (24) conducted a study to prospectively determine the accuracy of MRI in demonstrating the course of fistulas. Concordance rates between MRI and operative findings were 86% for the presence and course of primary tract, 91% for the presence and site of secondary extensions or abscesses, and 97% for the presence of horseshoeing. Although operative findings by an experienced coloproctologist were used as the gold standard, they showed that in 9% of their study group, failure to heal was related to pathology missed at operation that had been documented on preoperative MRI. Chapple et al. (25) conducted a study to determine whether preoperative MRI could predict clinical outcome following operation. In 52 patients available for analysis, dynamic contrast-enhanced MRI had a sensitivity of 81%, a specificity of 73%, and a positive predictive value of 75%. Operation had a sensitivity of 77%, a specificity of 46%, and a positive predictive value of 59%. The authors concluded that MRI better predicted outcome than operative exploration. Buchanan et al. (26) reported that for patients with recurrent fistula-in-ano, further recurrences could be reduced by 75% if the operation is guided by MRI findings. Beets-Tan et al. (27) reported a similar experience in 56 patients with anal fistula who underwent high spatial resolution MRI. Overall benefit was derived in 21% of 56 patients with the greatest benefit in patients with Crohn's disease (40%), then those with recurrent fistulas (24%), and in patients with primary fistulas 8%. Myhr et al. (28) found that saline contrast may improve visualization of fistulas and their relationship to normal anatomic structures. Hussein et al. (29) studied the agreement between endoanal sonography, endoanal MRI, and operative findings in 28 patients undergoing treatment of fistula-in-ano. Sonography classified fistula in 61%, MRI in 89%, and operation in 93% of patients. Concordance between endoanal sonography and MRI occurred in 46% of cases (poor agreement), between sonography and operative findings in 36% (no agreement), and between MRI and operative findings in 64% (moderate agreement). The authors concluded that MRI more accurately allowed depiction and classification of fistula-in-ano than endoanal sonography. Maier et al. (30) also compared anal ultrasonography with MRI in the study of 39 patients when evaluated at the time of operation and ultrasonography showed a sensitivity of 60% compared to 84% for MRI. False positive diagnoses were made in 15% of patients by anal sonography and 26% with MRI yielding a specificity of 68% for MRI and 21% for anal sonography.

West et al. (31) conducted a study to determine agreement between hydrogen peroxide–enhanced three-dimensional endoanal ultrasonography and endoanal magnetic resonance imaging in the preoperative assessment of 21 patients with clinical symptoms of a cryptoglandular perianal fistula and to compare these results with the surgical findings. Each fistula was classified according to the Parks' classification. Agreement for the classification of the primary fistula tract was 81% for hydrogen peroxide–enhanced three-dimensional endoanal ultrasonography and surgery, 90% for endoanal MRI and surgery, and 90% for hydrogen peroxide–enhanced three-dimensional endoanal ultrasonography and endoanal MRI. For secondary tracts, agreement was 67% for hydrogen peroxide–enhanced three-dimensional endoanal ultrasonography and surgery, 57% for endoanal MRI and surgery, and 71% for hydrogen peroxide–enhanced three-dimensional ultrasonography and endoanal MRI in case of circular tracts and 76%, 81%, and 71%, respectively in cases of linear tracts. Agreement for the location of an internal opening was 86% for hydrogen peroxide–enhanced three-dimensional endoanal ultrasonography and surgery, 86% for endoanal MRI and surgery and 90% for hydrogen peroxide–enhanced three-dimensional endoanal ultrasonography and endoanal MRI. They concluded that for evaluation of perianal fistulas hydrogen peroxide–enhanced three-dimensional endoanal ultrasonography and endoanal magnetic resonance imaging had good agreement, especially for classification of the primary fistula tract and the location of an internal opening.

In a study of 42 patients with suspected fistula-in-ano, Beckingham et al. (32) found that dynamic contrast-enhanced MRI had a sensitivity of 97% and a specificity of 100% in the detection of fistula-in-ano. Long-term follow-up revealed that in patients who initially did not have a fistula identified, who had a fistula that failed to heal, or who developed a recurrence and underwent a subsequent operation, the missed fistula was confirmed. This imaging technique was found to be more accurate at identifying secondary tracts and complex fistula than either digital rectal examination alone or operative exploration.

Examples of MRI images are demonstrated in Figures 6–10.

Summary

With the availability of sophisticated imaging, enthusiasm has probably resulted in over-usage of these tools. Certainly, for intersphincteric and low transsphincteric fistula, these imaging devices are not required. They find their place in patients with recurrent and complicated fistulas where both intra-anal sonography and MRI imaging when available may guide the surgeon to previously unsuspected tracts or even hidden abscesses

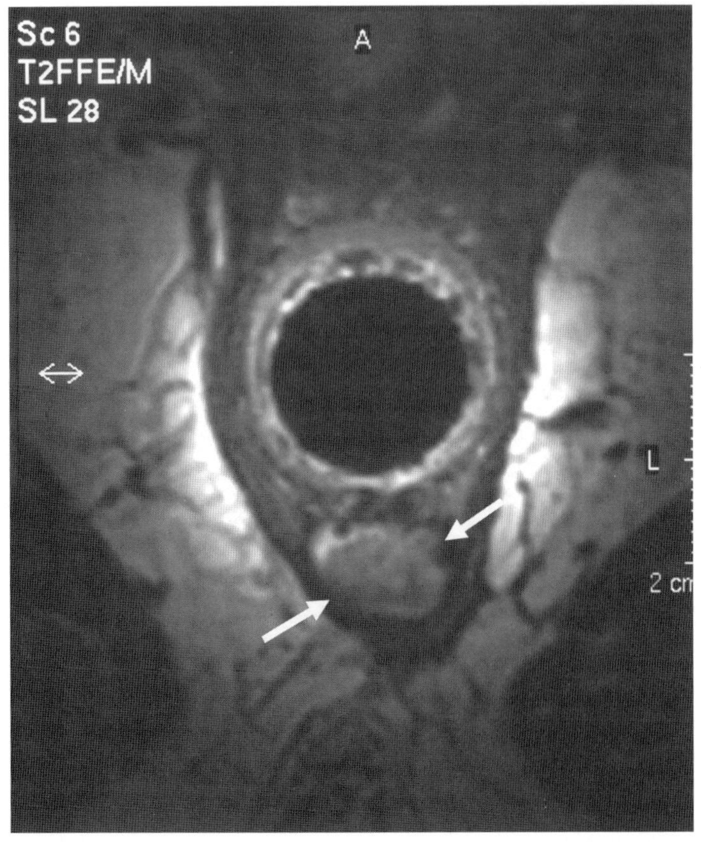

FIGURE 6 ■ MR image of an intersphincteric fistula with supralevator extension. Arrows point to an intersphincteric abscess.
Source: Courtesy of Dr. Ruud Schouten, Rotterdam, The Netherlands.

Differential Diagnosis

A host of conditions might be included in the differential diagnosis of a fistulous abscess, including Bartholin's gland abscess, sebaceous cyst, hidradenitis suppurativa, tuberculosis, actinomycosis, osteomyelitis of the bony pelvis, fissure, urethroperineal fistula, carcinoma or epithelioma, penetrating injuries, pilonidal sinus, retrorectal cyst, folliculitis of the perianal skin, and pruritus ani.

The characteristics of these individual inflammatory processes are dealt with in their respective chapters. In any event, an acute abscess of any cause requires immediate incision and drainage, as described later in this chapter, and the management of the chronic problem depends on the underlying cause. For example, the treatment of a patient with watery purulent material with sulfur granules would consist of antibiotic therapy with ampicillin (33).

ANORECTAL ABSCESS

■ MICROBIOLOGY

Many surgeons believe that identifying the offending organisms in a patient with anorectal sepsis is a waste of time, effort, and money. However, Grace et al. (34) have suggested that it is worthwhile to determine whether the causative bacteria are skin- or bowel-derived organisms, for they believe that the source affects the prognosis with respect to fistula development. In a series of 165 patients, none of the 34 patients from whom the pus grew skin-derived organisms had a fistula-in-ano; in contrast, 54% of the 114 patients from whom the pus grew bowel-derived organisms had a fistula-in-ano. These data are clouded somewhat by the fact that some of the patients had a concomitant fistulotomy at the time of abscess drainage. Fielding and Berry (35) support the contention that the growth of bowel organism can be used to identify patients who will benefit from further examination. In a series of 121 patients undergoing operation for abscess or fistula, they found these organisms in 88% of fistulas, 75% of recurrent abscesses, and 83% of those who subsequently developed fistulas. A subsequent report by Parker and Dale (36) suggested that laying open of a fistula may not be necessary in all patients in which gut-related organisms are identified.

■ INCIDENCE AND CLASSIFICATION

Anorectal abscesses are more common in men than in women, with a ratio of 2:1 (37) to 3:1 (10,38) to 5:1 (39). Since different authors use different classifications, it is difficult to know the exact incidence of each kind, and the need for a uniform system of classification is apparent. As shown in Figure 11, a simple classification that I have used is as follows: perianal, ischioanal, intersphincteric, and supralevator.

In most series, perianal abscesses constitute the predominant type of abscess, but in a review of 117 consecutive patients with anorectal suppuration seen by me, the distribution of abscesses encountered was as follows: perianal, 19%; ischioanal, 61%; intersphincteric, 18%;

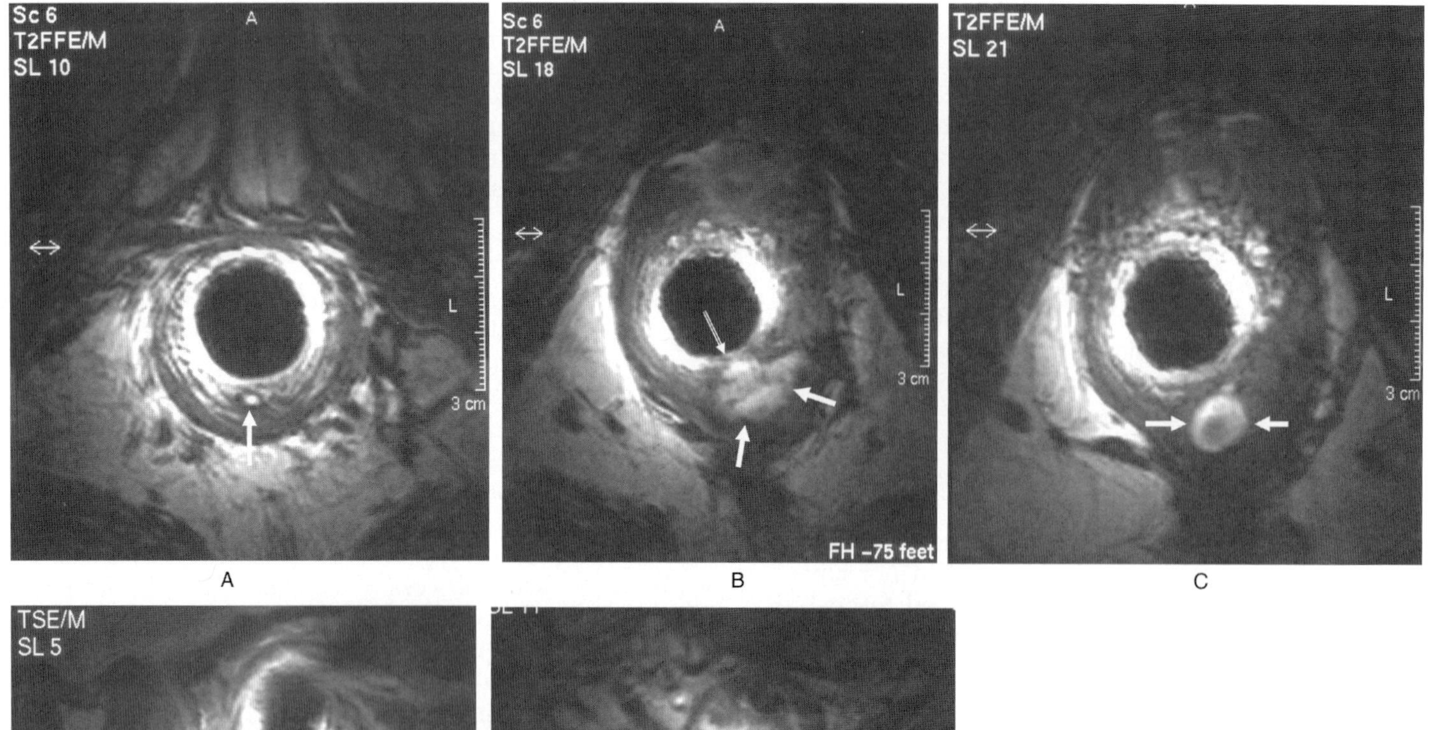

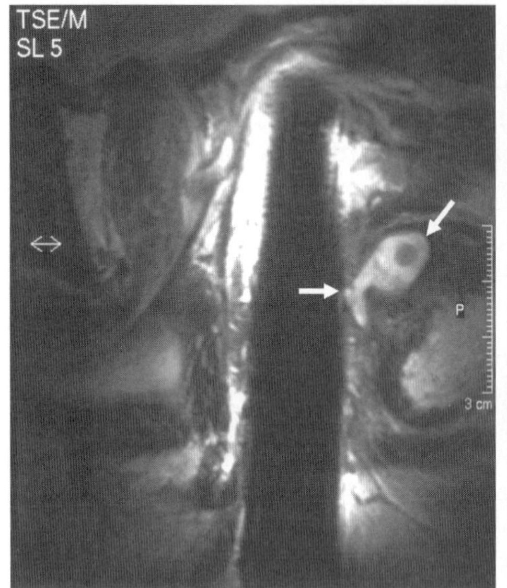

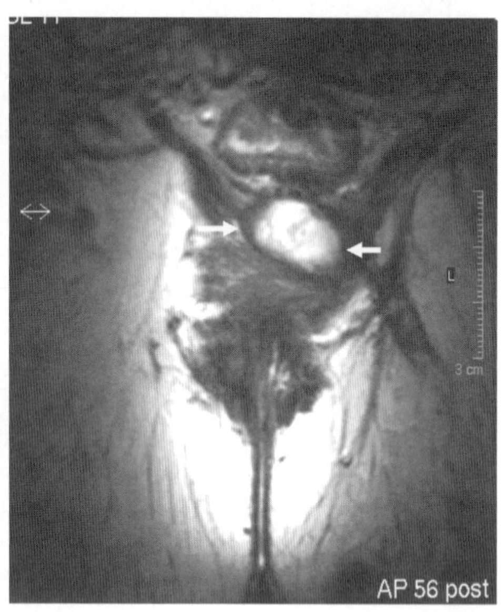

FIGURE 7 ■ MR image of an intersphincteric fistula with a high blind tract ending at the level of the puborectalis muscle. (**A**) Low level-arrow points to intersphincteric tract in posterior midline. (**B**) Higher level-thin arrow points to internal opening, thick arrow points to intersphincteric abscess. (**C**) Higher level-upward extension of the fistulous tract. (**D**) Sagittal plane-arrows point to fistulous tract ending in an abscess cavity in the posterior midline at the level of the puborectalis muscle. (**E**) Coronal plane-upper end of abscess cavity with excellent demonstration of the pelvic floor. *Source*: Courtesy of Dr. Ruud Schouten, Rotterdam, The Netherlands.

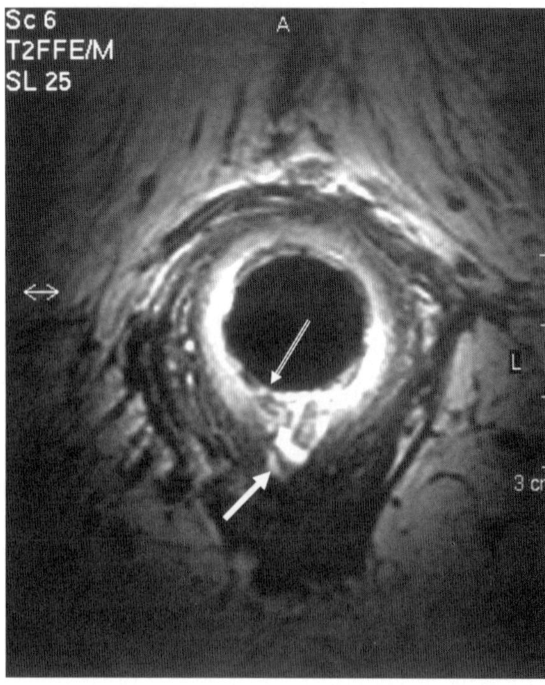

FIGURE 8 ■ MR image of a low transsphincteric fistula passing through the internal sphincter (*pale gray*); thin arrow pointing at internal opening; thick arrow pointing at fistulous tract. *Source*: Courtesy of Dr. Ruud Schouten, Rotterdam, The Netherlands.

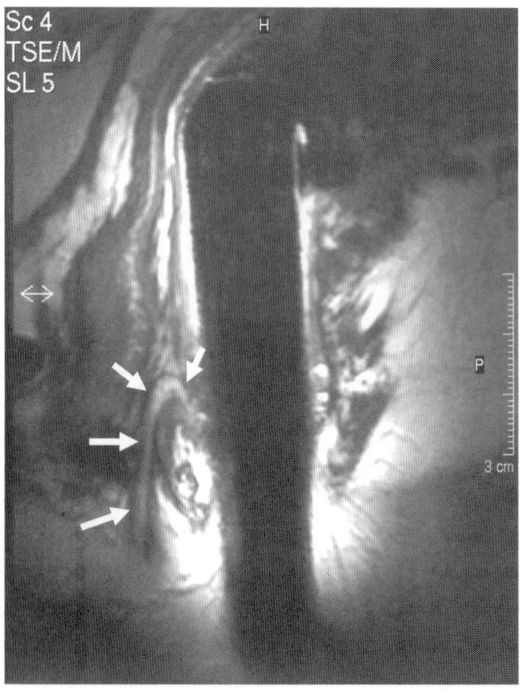

FIGURE 9 ■ MR image in the sagittal plane of an anteriorly located transsphincteric fistula in a female patient. Arrow points to the tract in the rectovaginal septum. *Source*: Courtesy of Dr. Ruud Schouten, Rotterdam, The Netherlands.

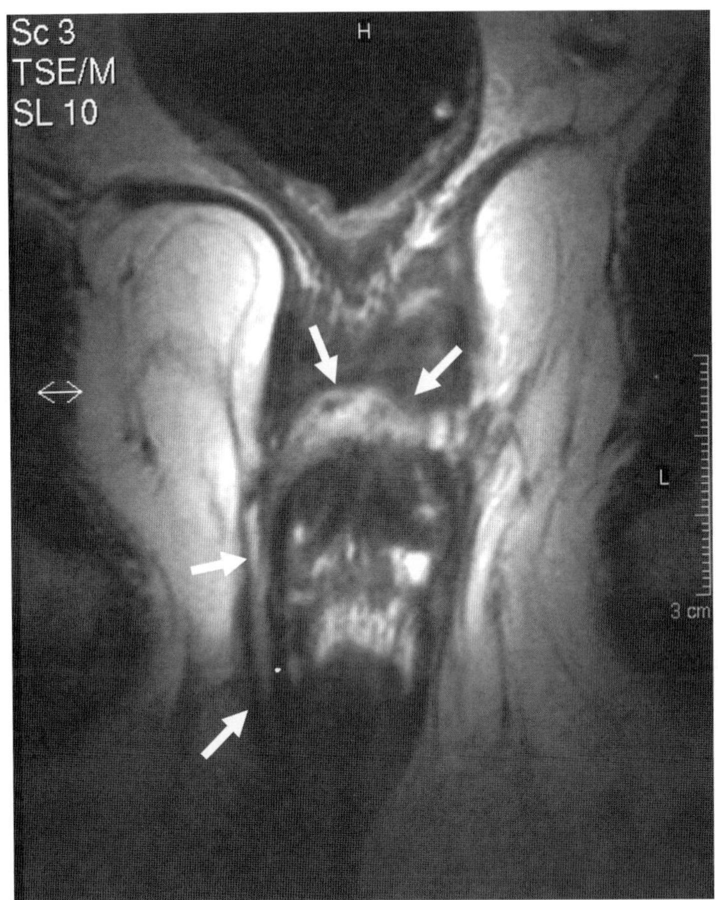

FIGURE 10 ■ MR image in coronal view of a high transsphincteric fistula with horseshoe extension. Arrows point to horseshoe fistulous tracts. *Source*: Courtesy of Dr. Ruud Schouten, Rotterdam, The Netherlands.

and supralevator, 2% (10). Nevertheless, the vast majority was of the perianal or ischioanal variety. (From a descriptive point of view, the term "ischioanal" more accurately describes the location of the septic process.) In this review, an unusually high incidence of intersphincteric abscess was encountered. This higher incidence may be explained by two factors. First, these statistics are from a referral practice; and, second, if the examiner is always conscious of this entity, the diagnosis will be made before the septic process becomes more extensive and points in the perianal region or bursts through the external sphincter and presents as an ischioanal abscess. This diagnosis must be sought.

In a review of 233 abscesses, Winslett et al. (40) found the following frequency: perianal, 136 (58.4%); ischiorectal, 79 (33.9%); and intersphincteric, 4 (1.8%). Fourteen fistulas (6.0%) were included. In a series of 200 patients, Oliver et al. (39) found the following distribution: perianal, 55.5%; ischiorectal, 27.5%; and intersphincteric, 17%. In a study of the anatomic locations of anorectal suppuration in 506 patients, Prasad et al. (41) found the following distribution: perianal, 48%; ischiorectal, 22%; intersphincteric, 12%; supralevator, 9%; intermuscular, 5%; submucosal, 4%. Thus, the distribution of perianal and ischiorectal abscesses reported by the above authors was an almost complete reversal of that seen by Vasilevsky and Gordon (10). No satisfactory explanation can be offered for this observed difference.

■ ROLE OF ANTIBIOTICS

Despite repeated teachings to the contrary, physicians frequently treat patients with anorectal abscesses with antibiotics. Nevertheless, there is little, if any, use for antibiotics in the primary management of para-anal suppuration. Only in the very rare exception will cellulitis in this region be aborted by the use of antibiotics. As a rule, operation will be required, so the sooner it is performed, the better. Adjunctive antibiotic therapy may be indicated in special circumstances. In patients with rheumatic or acquired valvular heart disease and in those who are immunosuppressed, administration of antibiotics would be indicated as an adjunct. When soft tissue infection is unusually extensive, such as with involvement of the perineum, groin, thigh,

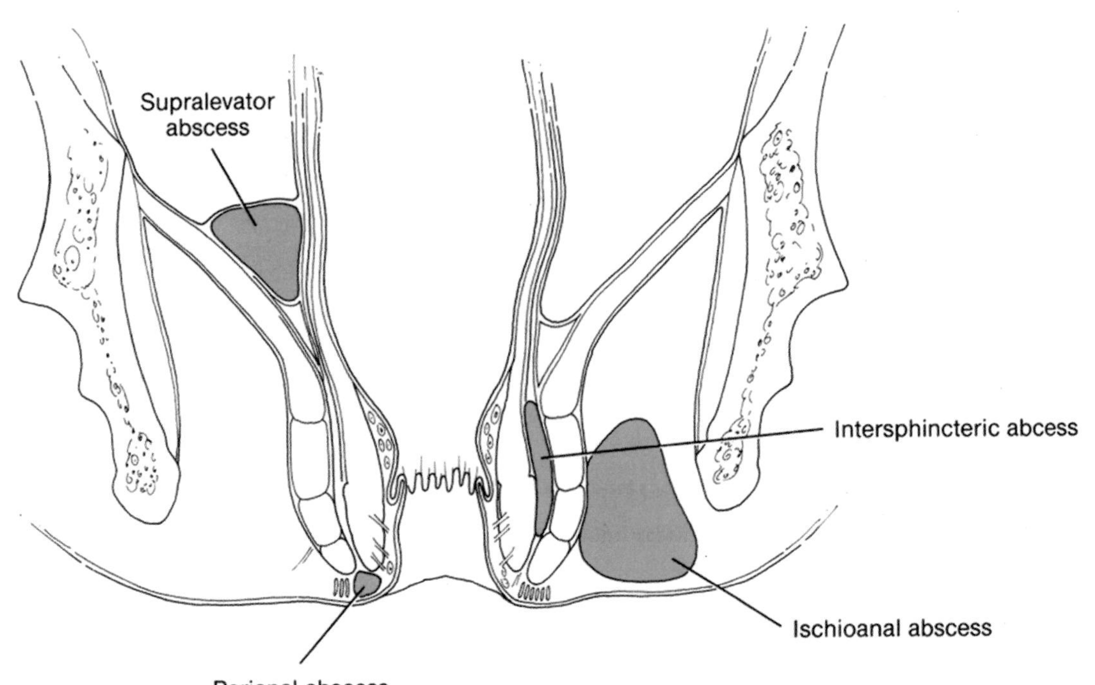

FIGURE 11 ■ Classification of anorectal suppuration.

or abdominal wall, antibiotics should be used. Their use is probably also indicated in patients with diabetes, and extensive adjacent cellulitis. It is neither necessary nor wise to wait until fluctuation can be demonstrated because delay in releasing the pus simply affords the inflammatory process an opportunity to extend and cause damage to the adjacent tissue or, more specifically, the anal sphincter mechanism.

■ TREATMENT

Abscesses in the perineum are treated in the same manner as abscesses in other parts of the body; that is, they must be adequately drained. Drainage usually consists of making a cruciate incision or removing an ellipse of skin over the abscess.

Perianal Abscess

A simple perianal abscess almost always can be drained with the patient under local anesthesia; this procedure can be performed in the office or in the hospital emergency department on an outpatient basis. The skin is usually prepared with an antiseptic solution. The most tender point is determined, and in this region a 2 cm area of skin is anesthetized with 0.5% lidocaine with 1:200,000 adrenaline. A cruciate incision, which will readily allow free drainage of the pus, is made. Skin edges must be excised because if only an incision is made, the edges will fall together readily and seal and the abscess may recur. In general, no packing is inserted since it impedes the drainage of pus and may be painful for the patient. Minor bleeding can be controlled easily by electrocoagulation. If cautery is unavailable, packing for a few hours may be necessary to control bleeding (Fig. 12).

Tonkin et al. (42) designed a study to show that perianal abscess may be safely treated by incision and drainage without packing. Fifty patients were recruited (7 lost to follow-up): 20 in the packing and 23 in the nonpacking arm. Mean healing times, the rate of abscess recurrence, and the postoperative fistula rates were similar. This study confirms in a formal nature what many surgeons have known and practiced for many years.

Ischioanal Abscess

The majority of ischioanal abscesses also can be incised and drained with the patient under local anesthesia and the procedure performed on an outpatient basis. Extensive abscesses might be drained better with the patient under a general or regional anesthetic. Loculations are a rare finding but if present should be sought and broken down to ensure adequate drainage. The same principles of drainage and nonpacking as those for perianal abscess are followed.

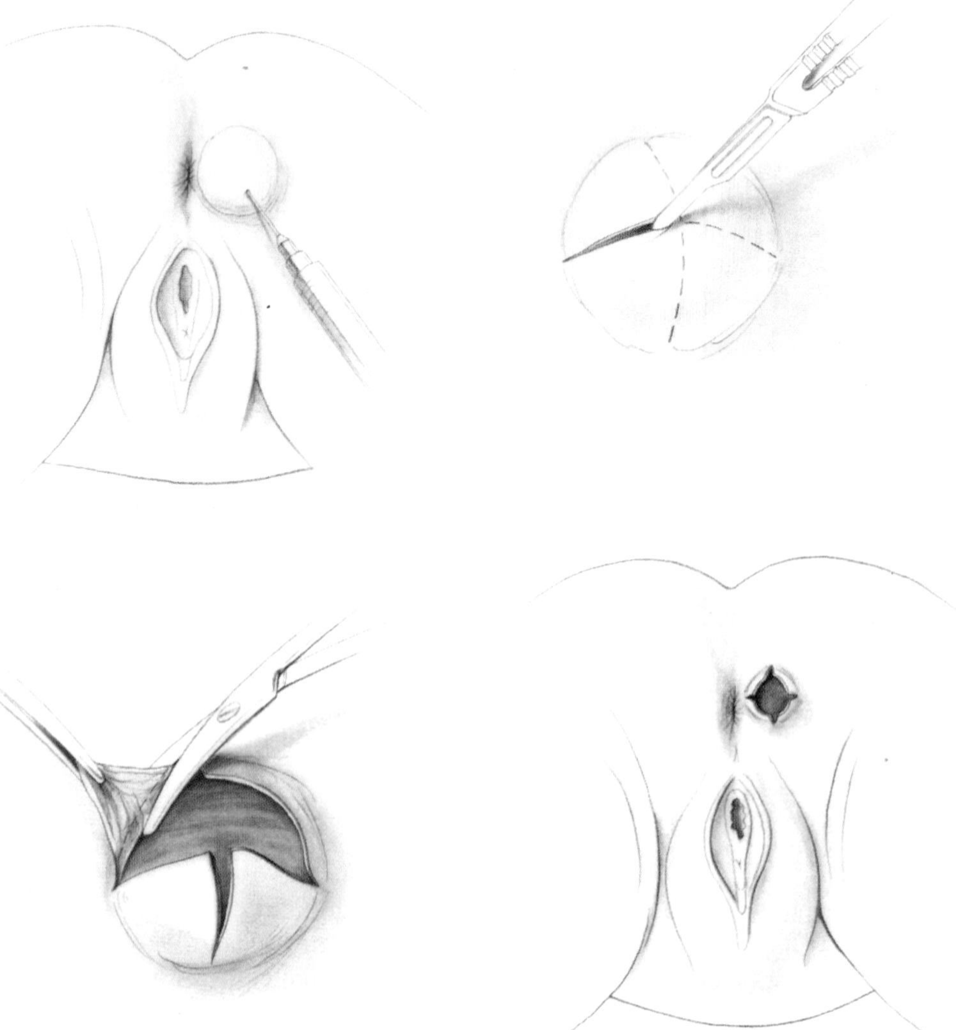

FIGURE 12 ■ Incision and drainage of a perianal or ischioanal abscess.

Some authors have stressed the importance of performing extensive unroofing by excision of enormous amounts of skin over each ischioanal fossa. However, it is necessary to excise only an amount of skin that will allow adequate drainage and prevent the skin edges from falling together too rapidly, thus preventing the reformation of the abscess. If a very large abscess is present, liberal use of one or more counterincisions may be done to drain the cavity satisfactorily.

Intersphincteric Abscess

The diagnosis of an intersphincteric abscess is often missed because the physician may be misled by the absence of external signs of inflammation. It may be necessary to perform an examination with the patient under either a regional or a general anesthetic before the diagnosis is established since adequate exposure cannot be obtained otherwise. Treatment consists of laying open the abscess, with division of the fibers of the internal sphincter from its lower end up to the level of the dentate line, or to a higher level if the cavity extends higher (see Fig. 19). Simply draining the abscess is inadequate therapy, as was clearly demonstrated by Chrabot et al. (43), who, in reviewing recurrent anorectal abscesses, found that all patients with intersphincteric abscesses had a fistula. Thus, it is mandatory that the abscess cavity be unroofed to prevent recurrence.

Supralevator Abscess

Of the various forms of anorectal suppuration, supralevator abscess is the least common and most difficult to recognize, but it probably occurs more commonly than generally recognized. This type of abscess requires proper and aggressive treatment to decrease morbidity and mortality. Because there is no external evidence of disease, its diagnosis may be delayed from a few days to 2–3 weeks. Severe pain in the perianal and gluteal regions is the predominant feature.

If a supralevator abscess is found, its origin, if possible, should be determined before treatment is begun. Such an abscess may arise in one of three ways: (1) from the upward extension of an intersphincteric abscess, (2) from the upward extension of an ischioanal abscess, or (3) from a pelvic disease such as perforated diverticulitis, Crohn's disease, or appendicitis. It may be difficult to distinguish the exact mechanism of origin. One clue is that in the first case there is no tenderness or induration over the ischioanal fossa as may occur in the second scenario. Therapy depends on the presumed origin of the supralevator abscess. If it is secondary to an upward extension of an intersphincteric abscess, it should be drained into the rectum by division of the internal sphincter (see Fig. 20). The cut edges are run with an absorbable suture such as 3–0 chromic catgut to control hemostasis. No packing is used. This abscess should not be drained through the ischioanal fossa because a suprasphincteric fistula may result and become a difficult problem to manage (Fig. 13). If, however, a supralevator abscess arises secondary to the upward extension of an ischioanal abscess, it should be drained through the ischioanal fossa. Attempts at draining this kind of abscess into the rectum will result in an extrasphincteric

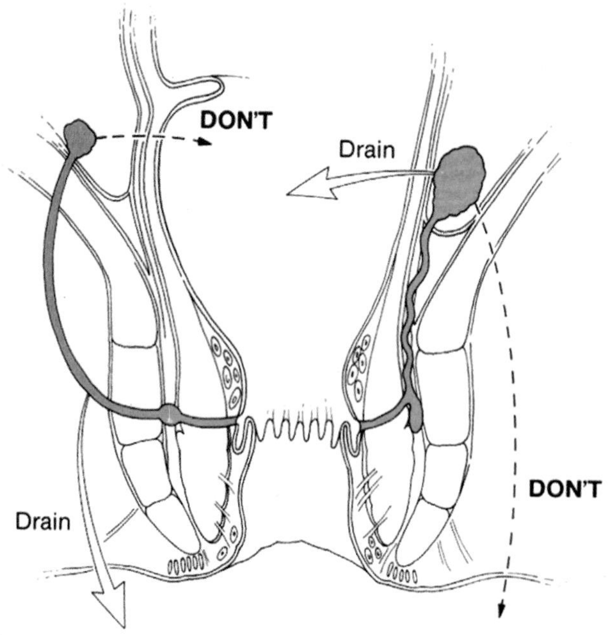

FIGURE 13 ■ Drainage of a supralevator abscess.

fistula and become a much more difficult problem to handle (Fig. 13). In the drainage of supralevator abscesses of pelvic origin, the original disease must be considered. These abscesses can be drained through three routes: (1) into the rectal lumen, (2) through the ischioanal fossa, or (3) through the abdominal wall. The choice of procedure depends on the area to which the abscess points most closely and the general condition of the patient.

Factors to reduce morbidity and prevent mortality in a patient with supralevator abscess include vigorous supportive therapy; treatment of underlying or complicating disorders (e.g., diabetes mellitus); adequate anesthesia; early adequate and dependent drainage; debridement of all necrotic tissue; judicious use of antibiotics; close observation of patients postoperatively, performing drainage again or debridement if necessary; and long-term follow-up to exclude or treat potential fistula (41).

Horseshoe Abscess

Horseshoe-type extensions of anorectal abscesses may occur in the intersphincteric plane, the ischioanal fossa, or the supralevator plane. Use of a general or regional anesthetic is usually necessary to treat sepsis of this nature. The level of circumferential spread will determine the type of therapy. Horseshoe abscesses in the intersphincteric plane usually can be managed by dividing the internal sphincter for the height of the abscess cavity in the portion of the circumference in which the abscess is bulging, thus hopefully exposing the crypt of origin (see Fig. 19).

For "horseshoeing" in the ischioanal fossa, posterior drainage and the liberal use of counterincisions in both ischioanal fossae comprise an ideal treatment. Hanley (44) originally believed that the acute horseshoe abscess should be treated by drainage and primary posterior midline fistulotomy but later modified his thinking, believing that a staged procedure with incision and drainage, preserving all the sphincters of the lower posterior anorectum, should

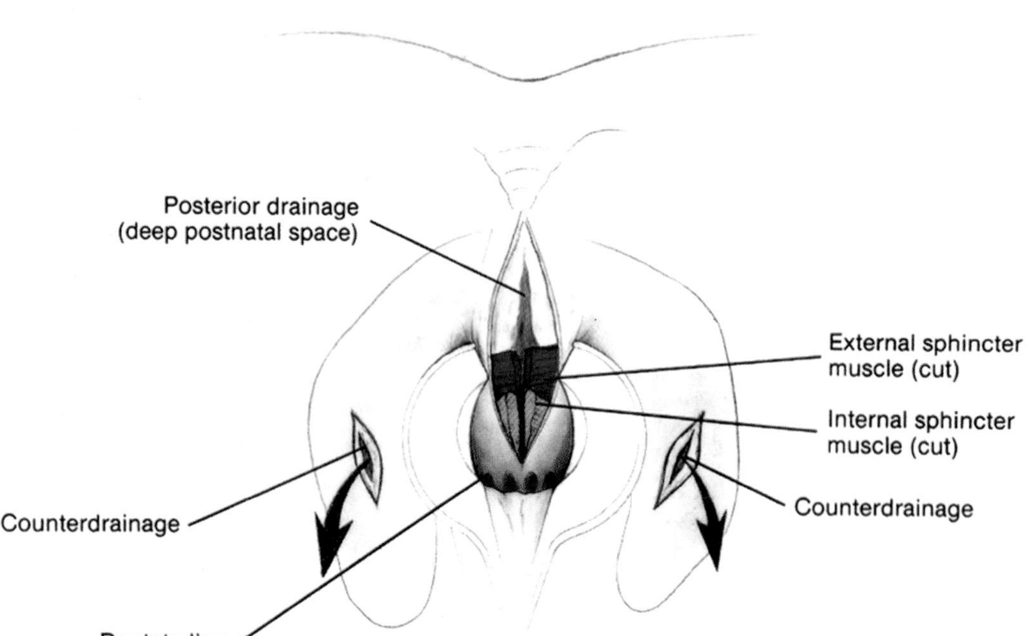

FIGURE 14 ■ Hanley's technique for incision and drainage of a horseshoe abscess.

give better results than the lay-open fistulotomy technique. The deep postanal space abscess would be drained by extending a posterior midline incision from the subcutaneous external sphincter over the abscess to the tip of the coccyx, separating the superficial external sphincter muscle into halves, thus exposing the deep postanal abscess and its communication with the ischioanal spaces (Fig. 14). A probe inserted into the primary opening is directed toward the coccyx, thus passing into the deep postanal space. A rubber seton is drawn through the fistulous tract and is secured around the lower half of the internal sphincter and the lower portion of the external sphincter (45). The separation of the superficial external sphincter near the posterior anorectum is minimal compared with that which occurs with fistulotomy. Para-anal incisions are made to drain the anterior extensions of the abscess in order to drain the abscess completely (Fig. 14). After healing is complete, only a simple fistula around the seton remains. Interval tightening of the seton should result in less separation of the severed sphincter ends and alteration of the anorectum. Hanley et al. (46) believe that this procedure should allow for better results than the operation they previously used. Interestingly enough, all 10 cases treated by Hanley et al. (46) in the original manner healed. Hanley recommends similar management for patients with anterior horseshoe abscesses.

For several reasons, I have not performed immediate fistulotomy. In the acute stage, the tracts do not yet consist of hard fibrous tubes, and definitive fistula surgery would create greater separation of sphincter muscle. A significant number of properly drained abscesses will not result in a fistula. A modification of Hanley's technique might be accomplished by establishing adequate drainage through para-anal incisions and dividing the lower half of the internal sphincter to eradicate the source of the infected gland (Fig. 15). This procedure would preserve the external sphincter and hopefully result in better continence, but it involves the risk of a higher recurrence rate.

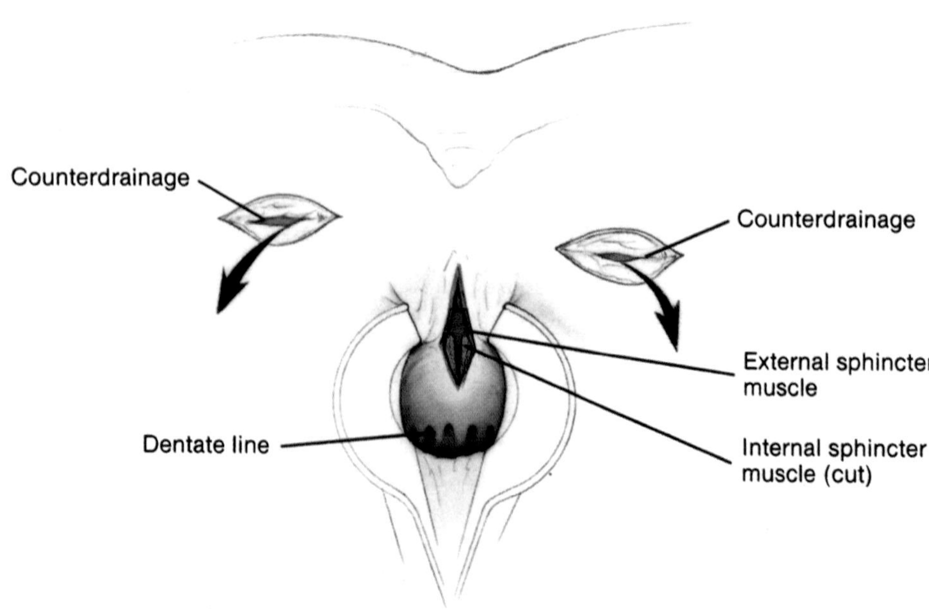

FIGURE 15 ■ Modification of Hanley's technique for incision and drainage of a horseshoe abscess.

Fortunately, horseshoeing in the supralevator plane is exceedingly rare. If the abscess arises because of an upward extension of an ischioanal abscess, bilateral drainage in each ischioanal fossa may be required (see Fig. 23).

Recurrent Abscess

Recurrent anorectal abscesses are often diagnostic and therapeutic dilemmas for the surgeon. Abcarian reported that the major causes of recurrence in anorectal abscesses are failure to provide adequate drainage, presence of undrained pus in adjacent anatomic spaces, and undiagnosed fistulous tracts. Abcarian pointed out that if a patient has a recurrent abscess in the perineum, extra-anal causes must be considered in addition to the usual abscess of cryptoglandular origin. Recurrent abscesses of extra-anal origin most often result from either perianal hidradenitis suppurativa or caudad extension of an infected pilonidal cyst or sinus. For example, in a prospective review of recurrent anorectal abscesses at Cook County Hospital in Chicago, Chrabot et al. (43) noted that one-third of the patients had hidradenitis suppurativa. If the typical appearance of chronic recurrent hidradenitis suppurativa is seen, the entire infected area is excised down to normal fascia. Care must be taken to spare the anoderm and underlying external sphincter. The wound is allowed to granulate. If the tract extends proximally and proves to be associated with pilonidal disease, the appropriate pilonidal operation should be performed.

Onaca et al. (47) analyzed failures in the operative management of 500 consecutive patients who underwent 627 drainage procedures for a perirectal abscess. Reoperation within 10 days of the original procedure was required in 7.6% of patients. The main factors leading to reoperation were incomplete drainage (23 patients), missed loculations within a drained abscess (15 patients), missed abscesses (four patients), and postoperative bleeding (three patients). Incomplete drainage was more common with simple perirectal abscesses, whereas most overlooked collections were located posteriorly. Horseshoe abscesses were associated with a particularly high rate (50%) of operative failures. Neither pre-existing perianal pathology nor systemic immunosuppressive disease contributed to early failures.

Anorectal suppuration of cryptoglandular origin still accounts for the majority of recurrent abscesses. When the abscess or cellulitis appears to be continuous with or leading to the anal canal, the diagnosis of anorectal abscess is more likely, and, like first-time abscesses, it must be unroofed. If this is done with the patient under local anesthesia, a later examination using a general or regional anesthetic should be performed to allow definitive treatment of the underlying problem. The need for additional therapy was clearly demonstrated by Chrabot et al. (43) who found a fistula in 76% of patients with recurrent abscesses. Furthermore, 30% of these patients had had a previous operation; of them, 70% had a previously missed fistula and 30% a previously missed component.

Search for a fistulous tract should be performed gently, and the overlying sphincter mechanism must be assessed to ascertain the safety of performing sphincterotomy. If a fistulous tract traverses only the internal sphincter or the internal sphincter and the distal portion of the external sphincter, sphincterotomy should not result in any functional defect; therefore, fistulotomy is the procedure of choice. If deeper portions of the external sphincter or puborectalis muscle are involved, a two-stage fistulotomy (i.e., dividing only the distal portion of the sphincter mechanism, especially the distal half of the internal sphincter to eradicate the source of the problem, and placement of a seton) is indicated. In dealing with larger horseshoe abscesses, it is preferable to drain the infection through multiple radial incisions rather than through a long circumanal incision. The latter results in retraction of the medial skin margin toward the anus with a "step-off" deformity of the anus. Multiple radial counterincisions tend to heal with virtually no anatomic or functional defect (43).

A diligent search for infection in other anatomic spaces must be carried out during the initial operation. In the study by Chrabot et al. (43), previously missed components accounted for 23% of recurrent infection, and all of the patients were successfully treated by adequate drainage of the missed component.

After an abscess is drained, the patient should be told that this may not be definitive treatment and that the abscess may heal and never trouble him again or may continue to drain, in which case definitive repair of the fistula would be necessary. The patient should also be warned about possible recurrence of the abscess, in which case definitive surgery also would be required.

■ POSTOPERATIVE CARE

Patients whose abscesses were drained should be advised to continue a regular diet, to take sitz baths three or four times daily, and to take a bulk-forming agent such as a psyllium seed preparation. Analgesics should be prescribed as necessary. These patients should be given an appointment for a follow-up examination in one month but should be advised to return promptly if the pain does not diminish.

FISTULA-IN-ANO

■ INCIDENCE

Men predominate in most series with a male-to-female ratio varying from 2:1 to 7:1 (48). Age distribution is spread throughout adult life with a maximal incidence between the third and fifth decades (48).

In a review of 400 fistulas by Parks et al. (49), the following distribution was found: intersphincteric, 45%; transsphincteric, 30%; suprasphincteric, 20%; and extrasphincteric, 5%. However, because of the highly selected patient population in this series, these authors estimated that a more representative incidence of the disease in the general population would be as follows: intersphincteric, 70%; transsphincteric, 23%; suprasphincteric, 5%; and extrasphincteric, 2%.

Marks and Ritchie (14) reviewed a series of 793 consecutive fistulas treated at St. Mark's Hospital, London, including some of the patients reviewed by Parks, Gordon, and Hardcastle, and found the following distribution: superficial, 16%; intersphincteric, 54%; transsphincteric, 21%; suprasphincteric, 3%; extrasphincteric, 3%; and unclassified, 3%. If the superficial and intersphincteric fistulas were combined in this series, the statistics would roughly correspond to Parks, Gordon, and Hardcastle's estimated incidence of the different varieties. A recent report from the same institution reported the following distribution: superficial, 11%; intersphincteric, 31%; transsphincteric, 53%; suprasphincteric, 3%; and extrasphincteric, 2% (50). They classified half these fistulas as complex.

In a series of 375 patients, Garcia-Aguilar et al. (51) found the following distribution: intersphincteric, 48%; transsphincteric, 28.8%; suprasphincteric, 1.6%; extrasphincteric, 1.6%; and unclassified, 20%.

In an analysis of 160 consecutive patients who were classified at the time of operation by the author, the distribution of fistulas was as follows: intersphincteric, 41.9%; transsphincteric, 52.1%; suprasphincteric, 1.9%; and extrasphincteric, 0% (11). A horseshoe extension occurred in 8.8% of the fistulas and 3.8% did not conform exactly to the classification because they were either complex or combinations of more than one type of fistula.

■ INDICATIONS FOR OPERATION

The presence of a symptomatic fistula-in-ano is an indication for operation because spontaneous healing of fistula-in-ano is very rare. Neglected fistulas may result in repeated abscesses and persistent drainage with its concomitant morbidity. Very rarely, malignancy may supervene on a long-standing fistula. Therefore, operation should be recommended unless there are specific medical contraindications to the use of anesthesia. In addition, patients with already compromised anal continence present a relative contraindication since the further division of muscle required in the treatment of the fistula might render the patient totally incontinent. Anal fistulas are sometimes associated with active pulmonary tuberculosis, and the pulmonary disease must be controlled before the tuberculosis fistula is repaired. Since Crohn's disease is associated with anal fistulas, patients with any bowel symptoms suggestive of this condition should have their gastrointestinal tract investigated both endoscopically and radiographically. Control of active Crohn's disease must precede any repair of an anal fistula associated with it (see Chap. 27).

■ PRINCIPLES OF TREATMENT

The objective of fistula surgery is simple: cure the fistula with the lowest possible recurrence rate and with minimal, if any, alteration in continence and do so in the shortest period of time. To approximate this ideal, a number of principles should be observed: (1) the primary opening of a tract must be identified; (2) the relationship of the tract to the puborectalis muscle must be established; (3) division of the least amount of muscle in keeping with cure of the fistula should be practiced; (4) side tracts should be sought; and (5) the presence or absence of underlying disease should be determined. Poor resting tone before operation or diminished voluntary anal contraction indicate a compromised internal or external sphincter function and therefore caution in operation may be necessary to avoid anal incontinence.

■ CLASSIFICATION AND TREATMENT

A number of authors have made significant contributions to the study of fistula anatomy. Eisenhammer (2) stressed the importance of the intersphincteric plane, both in the pathogenesis and spread of a fistula. Steltzner (52) classified fistula-in-ano into three main groups: intermuscular (between the internal and the external sphincter), transsphincteric (spread across the external sphincter into the ischiorectal fossa), and extrasphincteric (a tract passing directly from the perineal skin through the ischiorectal fossa, the levator ani muscles, and pararectal fat into the rectum, outside all the sphincters). Lilius (53) further developed the concept of intermuscular spread, in particular, extension upward into the rectal wall. Finally, Parks et al. (49) described the classification that is presented below.

Over the years, many classifications of fistulas occurring in and surrounding the anorectal region have been described. Some have been very simple but of no help in treatment; others have used terms that have different connotations to different surgeons. The aim of any such classification should be to help the surgeon in the operative cure of the disease. The classification used in this discussion, although very detailed, gives an accurate description of the anatomic course of the fistulous tracts. This knowledge acts as a guide to operative treatment. Although full credit for its description goes to Parks (48), some aspects of this classification of fistula-in-ano (Table 1) were previously described by Steltzner (52).

The following discussion elaborates on this classification and demonstrates the practicality of this detailed classification. Each drawing diagrammatically displays the disease process on the left and the recommended treatment on the right.

Intersphincteric Fistula

The intersphincteric fistula involves only the intersphincteric plane. It is the most common type of fistula-in-ano and is the intermediary form that leads to most other kinds of fistula.

Simple Low Tract

With this type of fistula, after penetrating the internal sphincter at the level of the dentate line, the tract passes from the primary abscess down to the anal verge. Treatment involves eradication of the primary source of

TABLE 1 ■ Parks' Classification of Fistula-in-Ano

Intersphincteric fistulas
Simple low tract
High blind tract
High tract with rectal opening
Rectal opening without a perineal opening
Extrarectal extension
Secondary to pelvic disease
Trans-sphincteric fistulas
Uncomplicated
High blind tract
Suprasphincteric fistulas
Uncomplicated
High blind tract
Extrasphincteric fistulas
Secondary to anal fistula
Secondary to trauma
Secondary to anorectal disease
Caused by pelvic inflammation

Source: From Ref. 49.

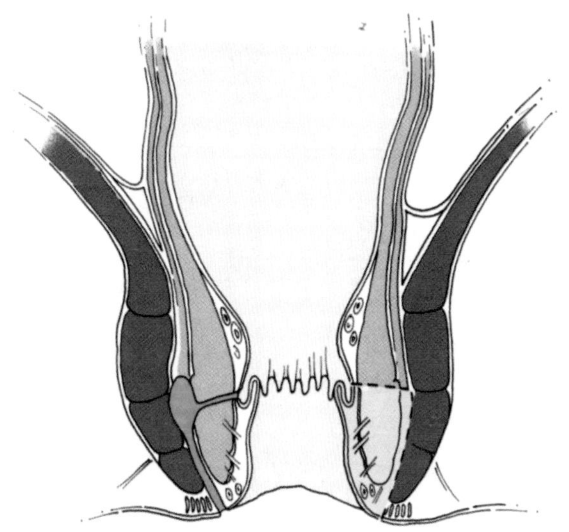

FIGURE 16 ■ Intersphincteric fistula: simple low tract.

disease in the middle of the anal canal by division of the lower half of the internal sphincter. This treatment seldom causes any disturbance of function. In the acute phase, this fistula presents as a perianal abscess (Fig. 16).

High Blind Tract

This kind of fistula, in addition to the downward extension, tracks proximally, resulting in a fistula between the internal sphincter and the longitudinal muscle of the upper anal canal and the rectal wall itself. Treatment consists of dividing the internal sphincter as high as the high blind tract ascends. This procedure will unroof the infected anal gland and the blind extension. Little disturbance of continence will ensue because the edges of the sphincter are held together by fibrosis around the fistulous tract. Failure to recognize this upward extension might result in a recurrence (Fig. 17).

High Tract with Rectal Opening

This type of fistula is an extension of the previous variety, with the fistula breaking back into the lower rectum.

The whole of this tract is intersphincteric, and the tissue medial to it usually can be divided without risk. However, it is easy to believe mistakenly that the tract passes outside the external sphincter. If the probe passes straight upward (i.e., parallel to the anal canal), the direction of this passage often helps in making the diagnosis. With experience, it is not difficult to distinguish between the two because in the case of an intersphincteric tract, the probe passes close to the lumen of the anal canal. If old scarring and previous operations make a distinction difficult, placing an electromyographic needle into the tissue lateral to the tract can be extremely helpful. A potential from the external sphincter will be registered if the fistula is intersphincteric but not if it is extrasphincteric. Alternatively, electrical stimulation can be used to demonstrate contractions in the external sphincter (Fig. 18). EMG for the most part has now been replaced by intra-anal ultrasonography.

High Tract Without Perineal Opening

Infection passes in the intersphincteric plane upward into the rectal wall and terminates as a blind tract or re-enters the gut through a high secondary opening. There is no downward extension to the anal margin and no external evidence of a fistula. In the past, this variety in its acute phase was referred to as a submucous abscess, but since the tract is deep to the internal sphincter, it is, in fact, an intersphincteric abscess. Treatment consists of laying the tract open into the rectum. In addition, the lower portion of the tract must be incised in the middle of the anal canal because it contains the primary source of infection; if this portion is left behind, recurrence will ensue (Fig. 19).

Extrarectal Extension

Infection may spread upward in the intersphincteric plane to reach the true pelvic cavity. At this point, the fistula is above the levator plate. This type is usually encountered with an acute abscess. Correct treatment is drainage into the rectum. Any attempt to drain such an abscess through the ischioanal fossa will result in production of a suprasphincteric fistula, which is a considerably more difficult problem to manage (Fig. 20).

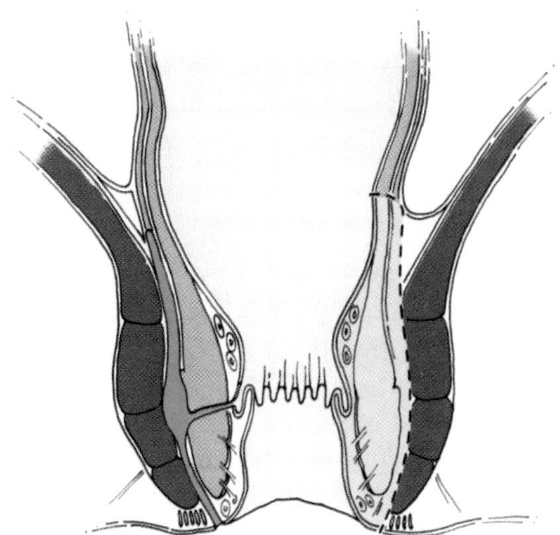

FIGURE 17 ■ Intersphincteric fistula: high blind tract.

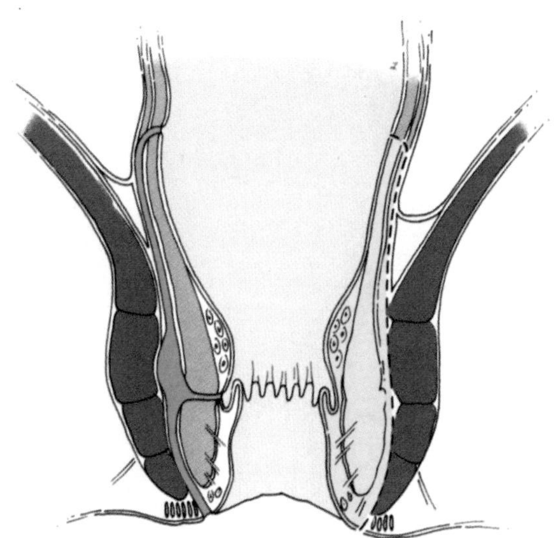

FIGURE 18 ■ Intersphincteric fistula: high tract with a rectal opening.

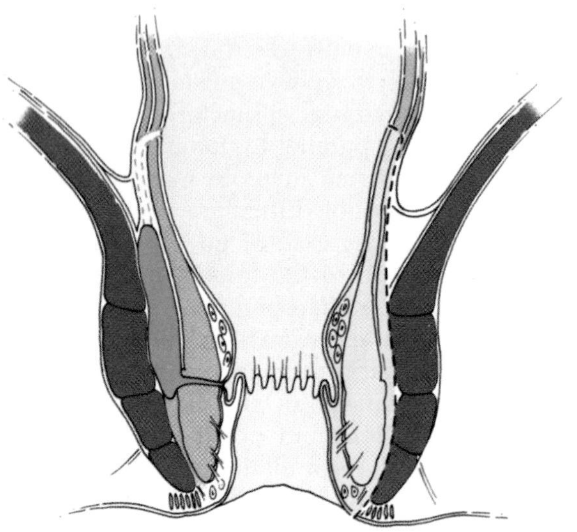

FIGURE 19 ■ Intersphincteric fistula: high tract without a perineal opening.

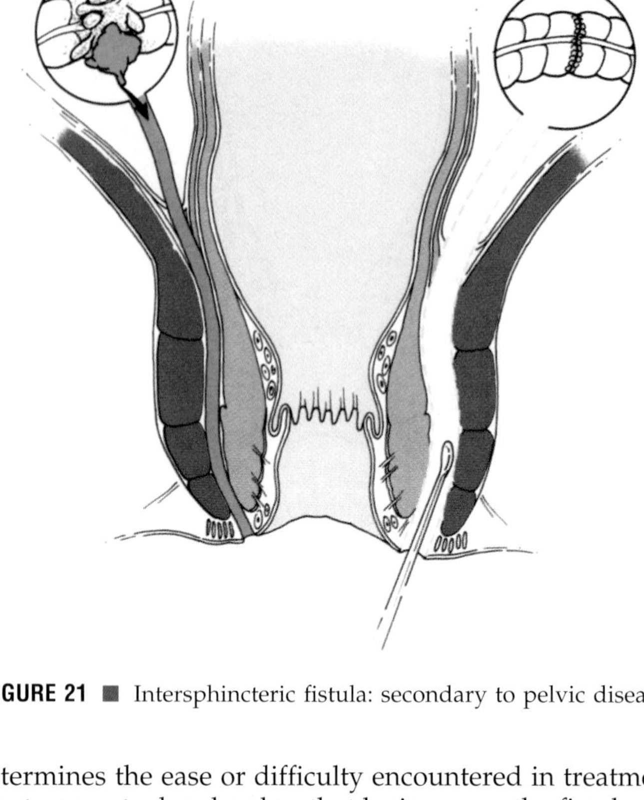

FIGURE 21 ■ Intersphincteric fistula: secondary to pelvic disease.

Secondary to Pelvic Disease

The last category is a fistula that manifests in the perianal region but originates in the pelvis and is caused by processes such as perforated diverticulitis or Crohn's abscess. The prime goal is elimination of the abdominal source, since failure to do so makes cure of the fistula impossible. As a rule, no local treatment other than possible curettage of the tract is necessary because such a fistula usually heals once the pelvic disease has been removed (15). This disorder is not a true anal fistula; therefore, division of the muscle is both unnecessary and potentially dangerous (Fig. 21).

Transsphincteric Fistula

Uncomplicated Type

In the uncomplicated variety of transsphincteric fistula, the tract passes from the intersphincteric plane, through the external sphincter, into the ischioanal fossa, and to the skin. The level at which the tract crosses the external sphincter determines the ease or difficulty encountered in treatment. Most cross at a low level so that laying open the fistula will result in division of only the lower portion of the external sphincter and the lower half of the internal sphincter; consequently, disturbance of function is unlikely. The highest level is just below the puborectalis muscle, at which point all the external sphincter may need to be divided. Even so, enough puborectalis muscle usually remains to maintain near-perfect continence. To preserve sphincter muscle, fistulas with tracts crossing at high levels may be treated by division of the lower half of the internal sphincter, creation of adequate drainage of the fistulous tract, division of only a portion of the external sphincter, and insertion of a seton (Fig. 38). The external portion of the tract may be treated with curettage or "coring out" (Figs. 22,31,32). The latter technique has not met with universal success.

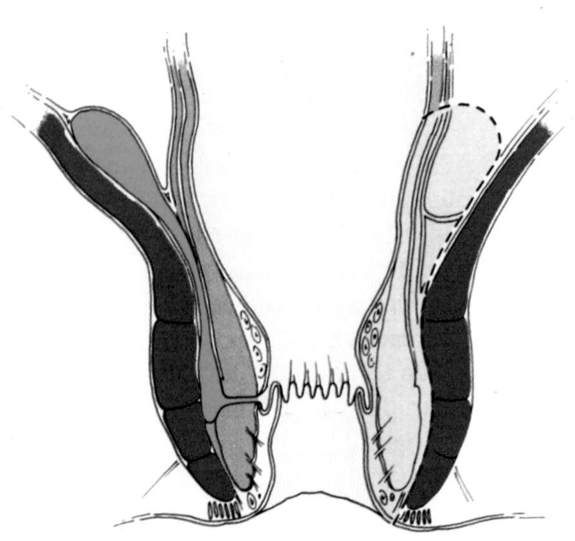

FIGURE 20 ■ Intersphincteric fistula: extrarectal extension.

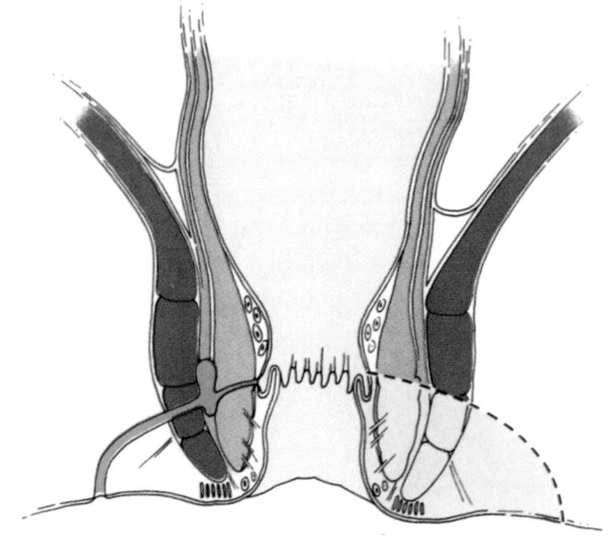

FIGURE 22 ■ Transsphincteric fistula: uncomplicated type.

High Blind Tract

The transsphincteric fistula with a high blind tract is a most important fistula because of the dire consequences that might ensue if it is improperly treated. The tract crosses the external sphincter and then divides into an upper and lower arm. The lower arm extends to the perineal skin; the upper arm may reach the apex of the ischioanal fossa or even pass through the levator ani muscles into the pelvis. A high extension causes induration above the anorectal ring and can be felt digitally through the rectum. If a probe is passed into the external opening, it will go into the upper arm of the tract, and the originating extension from the anal canal will not be demonstrated. The great danger with this procedure is that the tip of the probe may pass through the rectal wall, thus creating an iatrogenic extrasphincteric fistula with its rather grave implications, as discussed later in this chapter. The height and extent of a secondary tract are not of paramount importance, provided that the tract has not ruptured into the rectum. The treatment of this variety consists of finding the primary tract, which passes into the anal canal and laying it open. The high extensions are then provided with adequate drainage. A greater amount of external sphincter possibly will require division, but the amount depends on the level at which the fistulous tract crosses the sphincter. Otherwise, the same considerations pertain as with the uncomplicated variety (Fig. 23).

Suprasphincteric Fistula

Uncomplicated Type

An uncomplicated suprasphincteric fistula starts in the intersphincteric plane in the middle of the anal canal and passes upward to a point above the puborectalis muscle. It tracks laterally over this muscle and downward between the puborectalis and the levator ani muscles into the ischioanal fossa, thus looping over the entire sphincter mass. Treatment of this fistula by a classic lay-open technique would result in division of the external sphincter and the puborectalis muscle, most likely rendering the patient incontinent. Therefore, it is better to use a modification of a lay-open method in which the sphincter mass is divided into successive stages. The fetula itself usually helps provide a solution to the problem. As it passes over the puborectalis muscle, fibrous tissue is created around it. This problem is treated by division of the lower half of the internal sphincter (to eradicate the anal gland of origin), creation of adequate drainage of the secondary limb, and division of variable amounts (approximately half) of the external sphincter. The use of a seton is encouraged, and division of contained muscle, if necessary, is performed in stages. Functional results will be better if muscle can be preserved (Fig. 24). Other treatment options described later in this chapter may replace this techique.

High Blind Tract

This very rare form of fistula, in addition to taking the path of the uncomplicated suprasphincteric fistula, sends an extension into the supralevator compartment. In addition, this variety tends to spread in a horseshoe fashion in the supralevator compartment. The horseshoe extension deposits fibrous tissue above the puborectalis muscle, tissue that can be felt as a rather narrow, sharp ring resembling a crescentic knife edge. Since this fibrous band is above the puborectalis muscle, if the muscle is cut beneath it, the edges of the sphincter will not separate a great deal, and continence will be maintained probably. Treatment is similar to that for the uncomplicated suprasphincteric fistula, but adequate drainage of the abscess in the supralevator compartment also must be established. The supralevator abscess may be bilateral and requires corresponding drainage (Fig. 25).

Extrasphincteric Fistula

An extrasphincteric fistula is most conveniently classified according to pathogenesis. With this type of fistula, a tract passes from the perineal skin through the ischioanal fossa and through the levator ani muscles and finally penetrates the rectal wall. This route lies entirely outside the ring of sphincter muscle. If this tract is laid open, total incontinence will result.

Secondary to Anal Fistula

A trans-sphincteric fistula with a high extension may burst spontaneously into the rectum, although this occurrence is very rare. More commonly, a secondary opening above the puborectalis muscle is iatrogenic because of the surgeon's

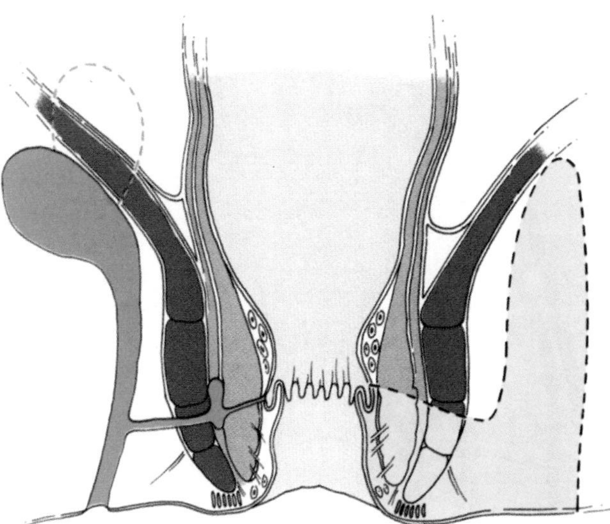

FIGURE 23 ■ Trans-sphincteric fistula: high blind tract.

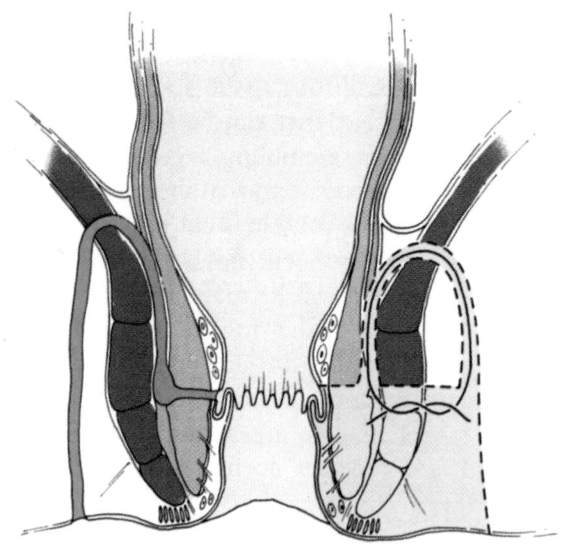

FIGURE 24 ■ Suprasphincteric fistula: uncomplicated type.

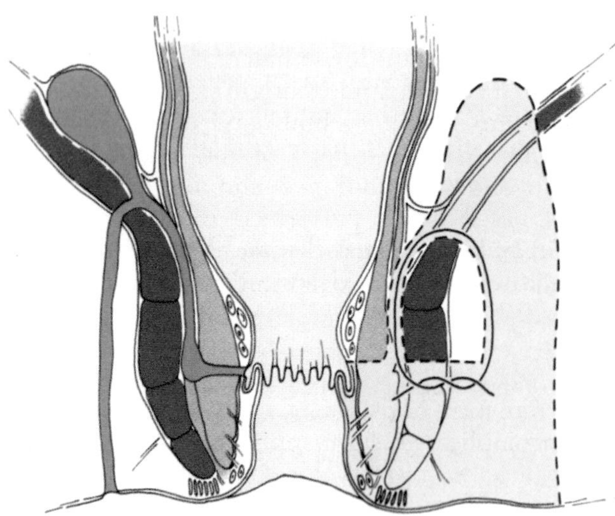

FIGURE 25 ■ Suprasphincteric fistula: high blind tract.

over energetic probing during the repair of a transsphincteric fistula. Once established, this fistula has two factors causing its perpetuation: first, the focus of the disease in the anal canal (i.e., the chronic infection of the anal gland in the intersphincteric plane); and second, the constant contamination of the rectal opening by high intraluminal pressures. These high pressures, which develop in the rectum, force mucus and fecal debris into the internal opening. Both these factors therefore must be eliminated before the fistula can heal. The primary tract in the anal canal must be eradicated by division of the lower half of the internal sphincter. The opening in the rectal wall is closed with two or three interrupted nonabsorbable sutures such as wire ones or with very slowly absorbable sutures such as polyglycolic acid ones. Adequate drainage of the fistulous tract must be achieved with special attention paid to the elimination of pocketing at the apex of the ischioanal fossa or supralevator extension. Preoperatively the patient is given a mechanical bowel preparation and postoperatively is fed an elemental diet, thus effectively creating a "medical colostomy" (54). In this manner, the rectal opening can be sutured without subsequent breakdown, but it may be necessary to create a temporary defunctioning colostomy to reduce rectal pressure before complete healing can occur. The colostomy may be closed three months later (Fig. 26).

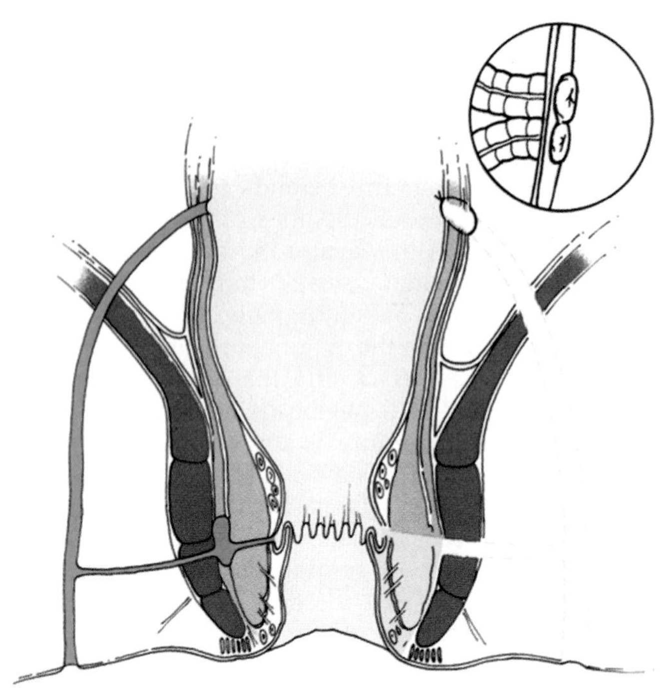

FIGURE 26 ■ Extrasphincteric fistula: secondary to anal fistula.

Secondary to Trauma

A fistula may be caused by trauma in two ways: a foreign body may penetrate the perineum and enter the rectum; or a swallowed foreign body (e.g., fish or chicken bone) may reach the rectum, straddle the sphincters, and be forced through the rectal wall, levator muscles, and ischioanal fossa to the perineum. Treatment consists of removing the foreign body, establishing adequate drainage, and performing a temporary colostomy to reduce the rectal pressure. Cutting any sphincter muscle is not necessary (see Chap. 34) (Fig. 27).

Secondary to Specific Anorectal Disease

Chronic ulcerative colitis, Crohn's disease, and carcinoma may result in gross and bizarre fistulization. These fistulas are not usually amenable to local treatment; thus, the disease itself must be treated, usually with a proctectomy (Fig. 28).

Secondary to Pelvic Inflammation

A pericolic abscess caused by diverticulitis or Crohn's disease may spread through the levator muscles and discharge into the perineum. This type of fistula requires no local treatment and will heal once the pelvic disease has been removed. Once again, no muscle requires division. The same principles pertain as in a patient with intersphincteric fistula secondary to pelvic disease (Fig. 29). For patients with an extrasphincteric fistula associated with severe pelvic sepsis when pelvic dissection would encounter operative danger at the circumferential margins where

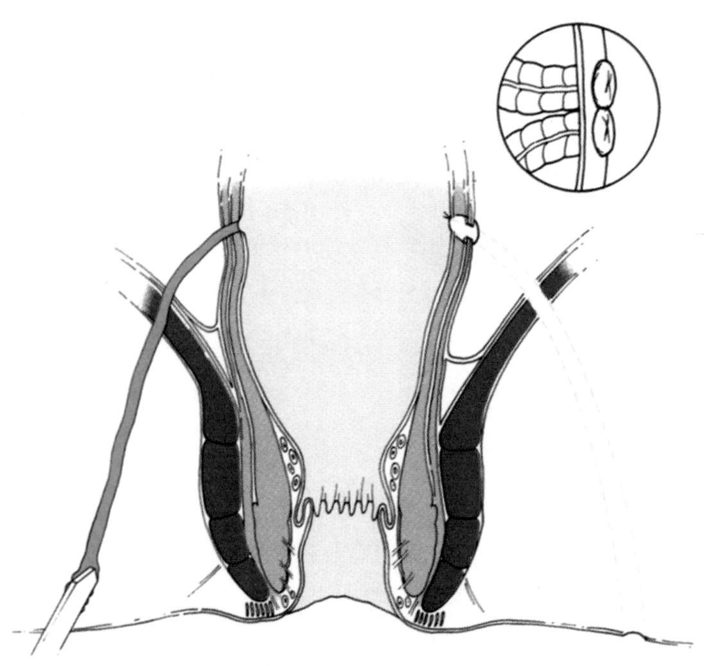

FIGURE 27 ■ Extrasphincteric fistula: secondary to trauma.

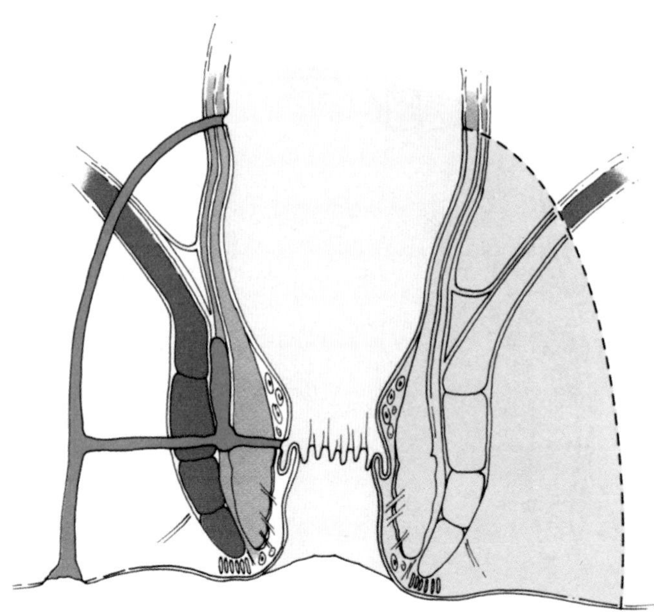

FIGURE 28 ■ Extrasphincteric fistula: secondary to anorectal disease.

ureter, blood vessels, vagina, and prostate can all be damaged, Maxwell-Armstrong and Phillips (55) described the successful use of the Soave procedure. Abdominal dissection proceeds to the point of maximum difficulty, the bowel is transected, a distal mucosectomy is performed from above and/or below and a coloanal anastomosis is performed. If there is a stricture, forced dilatation is performed. If a stricture is found, dilatation is performed with Hegar dilators.

■ TECHNIQUE (OPERATIVE OPTIONS)

Before any operative treatment of fistula-in-ano, it is wise to ascertain whether the patient has normal continence. Fistula surgery has an unenviable reputation because of the risks of recurrence and the possible impairment of anal continence. Therefore, extreme care must be exercised to keep these problems to a minimum, and patients should be told about these possibilities. If the cryptoglandular origin of most fistulas is accepted, using a lay-open technique would be necessary and would require the division of portions of both the internal and external sphincters (Fig. 32). The key landmark is the anorectal ring because dividing this portion of the sphincter mechanism would render the patient incontinent.

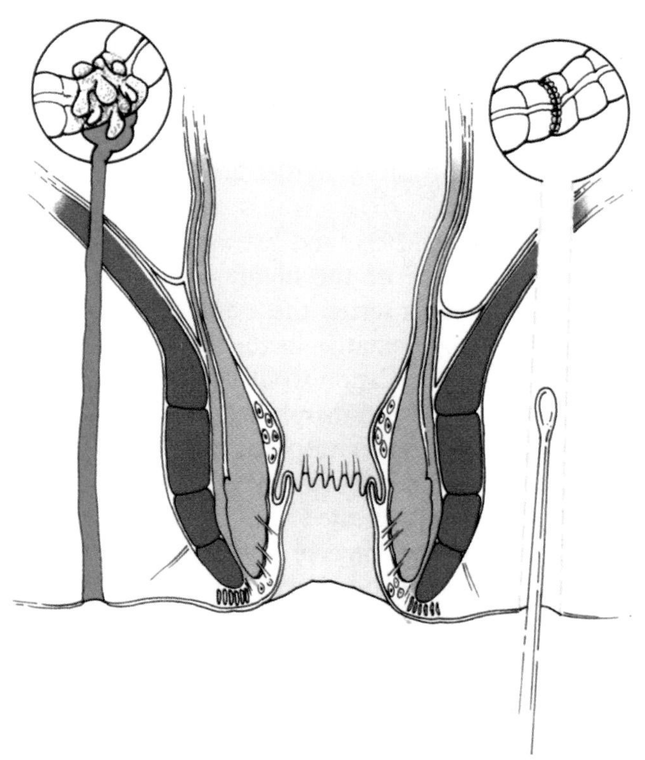

FIGURE 29 ■ Extrasphincteric fistula: secondary to pelvic disease.

Simple Low Fistula

With the patient under a spinal or light general anesthetic and preferably in the prone jack-knife position, the perianal region is prepared and infiltrated with a local anesthetic such as 0.5% lidocaine with 1:200,000 epinephrine. An anal speculum such as the Pratt bivalve is inserted into the anal canal, and any obvious internal opening is identified. A probe (I prefer using a grooved, directional probe) is then inserted into the external orifice and is passed along the distance of the tract (Fig. 30A). In treating a simple intersphincteric and low trans-sphincteric fistula, the tissue over the tract is divided by sliding the scalpel along the grooved probe director (Fig. 30B and C). Granulation tissue is curetted and sent for biopsy (Fig. 30D). Careful examination is made by inspecting and probing the granulating tracts to uncover the side or cephalad branches of the fistulous tracts. Hemostasis is obtained through electrocoagulation. Marsupialization then is accomplished by approximating the skin edges to the edge of the tract with a running absorbable suture such as 3–0 chromic (Fig. 30E and F). This technique is preferred over trimming large amounts of skin and subcutaneous tissue because the wounds appear to heal more quickly. No packing is inserted. Loose cotton dressing is applied to prevent spilling of clothes, and a T-binder or even underpants alone (rather than tape) are used to secure the dressing because tape is uncomfortable to remove, especially from hirsute individuals.

When the probe cannot be advanced along the full distance of the tract, as was the case in 40% of Parks' cases, a weak solution of methylene blue (1:10) is injected. This additional method can reduce to 10% the percentage of cases in which the internal opening cannot be demonstrated. When the primary opening is identified, the technique continues as described above. Although use of methylene blue has been criticized because of staining of tissues, a dilute solution causes no operative inconvenience. Other agents that have been used include hydrogen peroxide, milk, and other dyes. When no such opening can be found, the general direction of the fistulous tracts, as shown by probing from the external opening, will indicate fairly clearly where the connection with the lining of the anal canal is located. The tract can then be laid open and the procedure continued as above.

Ho et al. (57) conducted a randomized controlled trial of 103 consecutive patients with uncomplicated intersphincteric and transsphincteric fistula-in-ano in which half the wounds were laid open and the other half marsupialized. Wounds in the marsupialized group healed faster (6 vs. 10 weeks), incontinence to liquid stool was less (2% vs. 12%) and there was less impairment of maximum anal squeeze pressure.

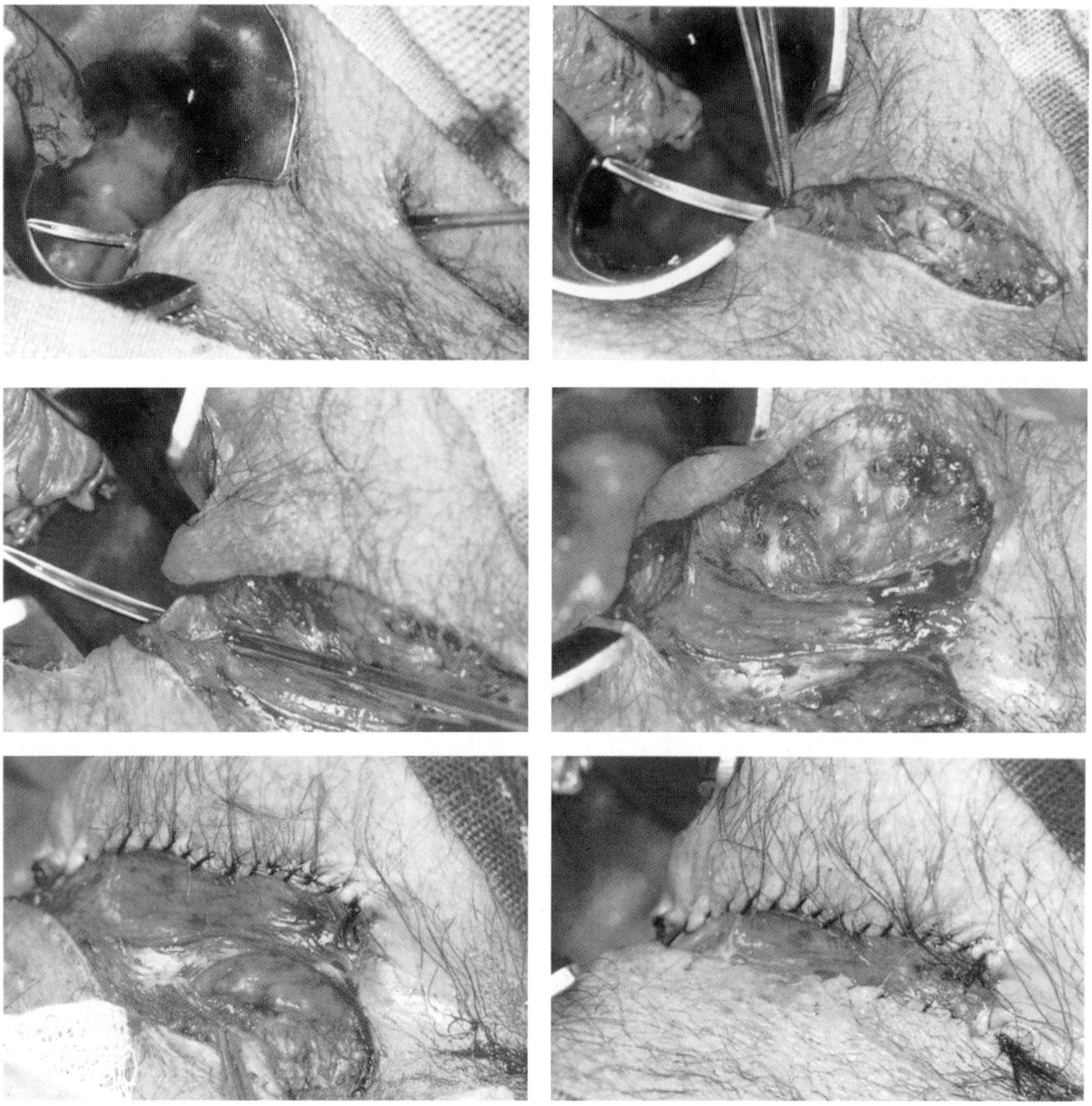

FIGURE 30 ■ Technique for repair of a fistula. (**A**) Lockhart–Mummery probe in fistula. (**B**) Skin and anoderm incised. (**C**) External sphincter incised and internal sphincter exposed. (**D**) Entire tract unroofed and curetted. (**E**) One side of tract marsupialized. (**F**) Marsupialization completed.

Patients with multiple secondary openings generally have tracts that communicate with one another and have a single crypt of origin. Usually, probing demonstrates this condition. It is uncommon for a patient to have entirely separate fistulas.

Parks (3) described a conservative operation in which the lower half of the internal sphincter was divided to eradicate the causative infected anal gland and the peripheral fistula was managed by using coring out, curettage, or incision and curettage. The major advantage of this technique is the preservation of the external sphincter. For fistulas crossing the external sphincter at a high level, the lower portion of this muscle must be divided to allow adequate drainage and healing. Parks believed that it is in these high fistulas that such a conservative approach is advantageous over the classic lay-open technique (Figs. 31 and 32). Few authors have endorsed this method, and even Parks found

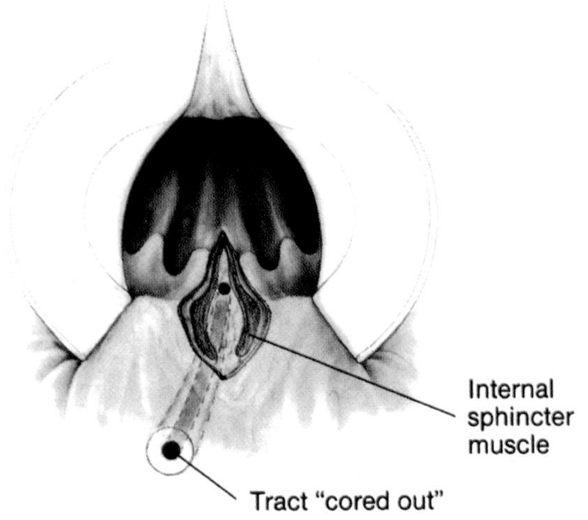

FIGURE 31 ■ Parks fistulectomy. *Source*: From Ref. 3.

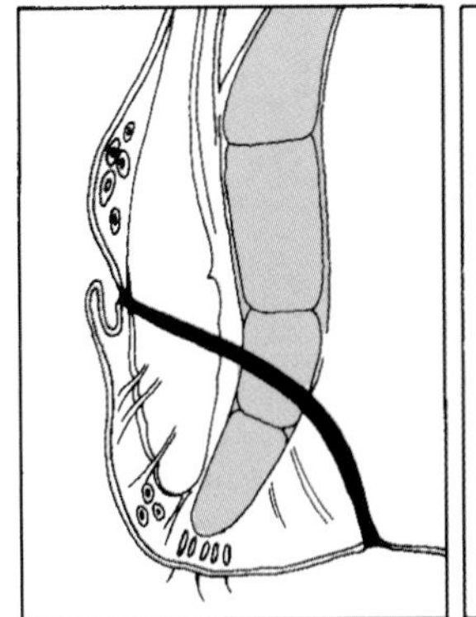
Fistula-in-ano

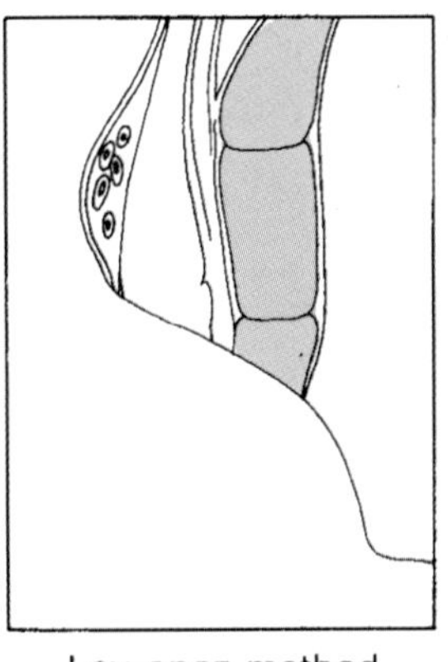
Lay-open method

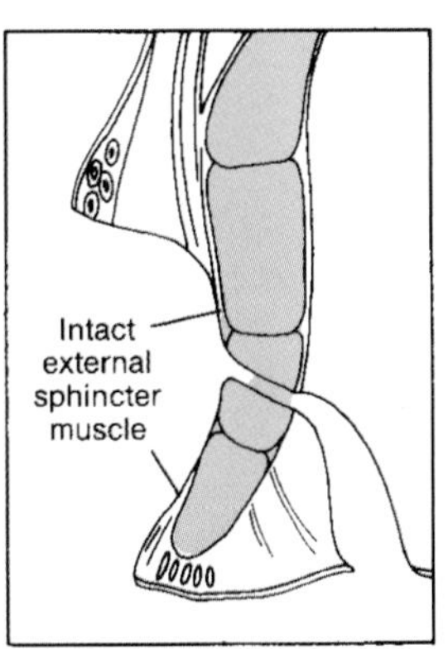

Parks fistulectomy

FIGURE 32 ■ Parks fistulectomy versus. lay-open technique. *Source*: From Ref. 3.

it unsatisfactory for use in many patients. A notable exception is the treatment of patients with Crohn's disease, in whom Sohn et al. (58) reported favorable results.

Buchanan et al. (59) found that the longitudinal direction of a transsphincteric anal fistula tract through the anal sphincter complex may have implications regarding fistulotomy. The angle of the tract of transsphincteric fistula relative to the longitudinal axis of the anal canal was measured before operation by means of MRI in 46 patients. This was compared with the findings at operation. The tract passed cranially as well as laterally at an acute angle (less than 90°) in 23 patients while it passed either transversely or caudally at an obtuse angle (90° or more) in the remaining 23. The internal opening was significantly higher in relation to the dentate line (above in eight patients, at the dentate line in 14 and below in one patient) when the tract was acute than when it was obtuse (above in one, at the dentate line in 17, and below in five patients). Preoperative MRI might alert surgeons to the potential hazard of fistulotomy being more extensive than anticipated from simple palpation at the level of the internal opening.

Horseshoe Fistula

Circumferential spread of the septic process results in the horseshoe fistula, which may have one or several secondary openings. Through probing, it can be seen that these openings are connected with each other. When a complicated fistula is suspected, a preoperative fistulogram may serve as a useful "road map" for the operating surgeon, thus reducing the risk of missing other tracts. Intra-anal ultrasonography has more recently been used to determine the extent of the tracts.

The operation begins with the laying open of a lateral limb of the horseshoe tract. Then the posterior extremity of the tract is exposed, and the other lateral limb is unroofed. The opening into the posterior wall of the anal canal at the level of the dentate line is sought so that the primary source of the fistula is exposed. It is important not to miss such an opening, for to do so inevitably results in recurrence, despite the wide unroofing of the secondary limbs. If no primary internal opening is discovered but the tracts lead to the posterior midline, it is probably wise, based on the assumption that the initiating factor is infection of cryptoglandular origin, to divide the lower half of the internal sphincter posteriorly to expose any such gland. A director can then be passed through the posterior wall of the anal canal from the main wound into the lumen at the level of the dentate line dividing the tissues below it. The granulation tissue is curetted from all tracts, and the patient is carefully examined for further side tracts (Fig. 33).

This large wound can be managed in one of two ways. If feasible, marsupialization is attempted because it will markedly decrease the size of the wound and expedite healing. If this is not possible, the walls of the wound edges are trimmed of both skin and subcutaneous tissue.

A more conservative approach to the management of horseshoe fistulas was described by Hanley. The technique for performing fistulotomy of the portion of the tract from the primary opening to the postanal space is the same as for the acute abscess. The tracts are readily identified by inspection and palpation of the cord-like structures. The single tract, when leaving the deep postanal space, may branch into superficial and deep branches, with numerous ramifications extending to the skin over the ischioanal fossa, perineum, or scrotum and forming many secondary openings. When feasible, Hanley recommends performing partial fistulectomy by excision of 1–1.5 cm of the T-shaped portion of the fistulous tract in the deep postanal space.

The secondary openings are enlarged by incising the opening for 2 cm to permit thorough curettage of the tracts. In well-healed tracts, complete fistulectomies are performed. Hanley cautions against division of the anococcygeal ligament, but Parks et al. (49) believed that this would not affect anal function. Wounds are packed loosely with fine gauze, which is removed in 48 hours. All 31 cases so treated healed with a minimal defect and no problems of incontinence (46).

Once again, I believe that performing fistulectomy is not necessary, but I agree with using a conservative approach, that is, laying open the internal sphincter to eradicate the underlying focus of infection and performing curettage and adequate drainage of tracts without the creation of extensive wounds. This procedure also would preserve the external sphincter and result in better function (Fig. 34).

Anterior horseshoe abscesses or fistulas are quite uncommon, but when they do occur, they are very difficult to manage, especially in women. The process may arise in a crypt in the anterior midline and, after penetrating the internal and external sphincters, may lie deep to the transverse perineal muscles. In planning treatment, it must be recalled that anteriorly there is no puborectalis muscle; therefore, the patient would be rendered incontinent more readily by performing an immediate fistulotomy. In the acute stage, the abscess should only be drained. In the

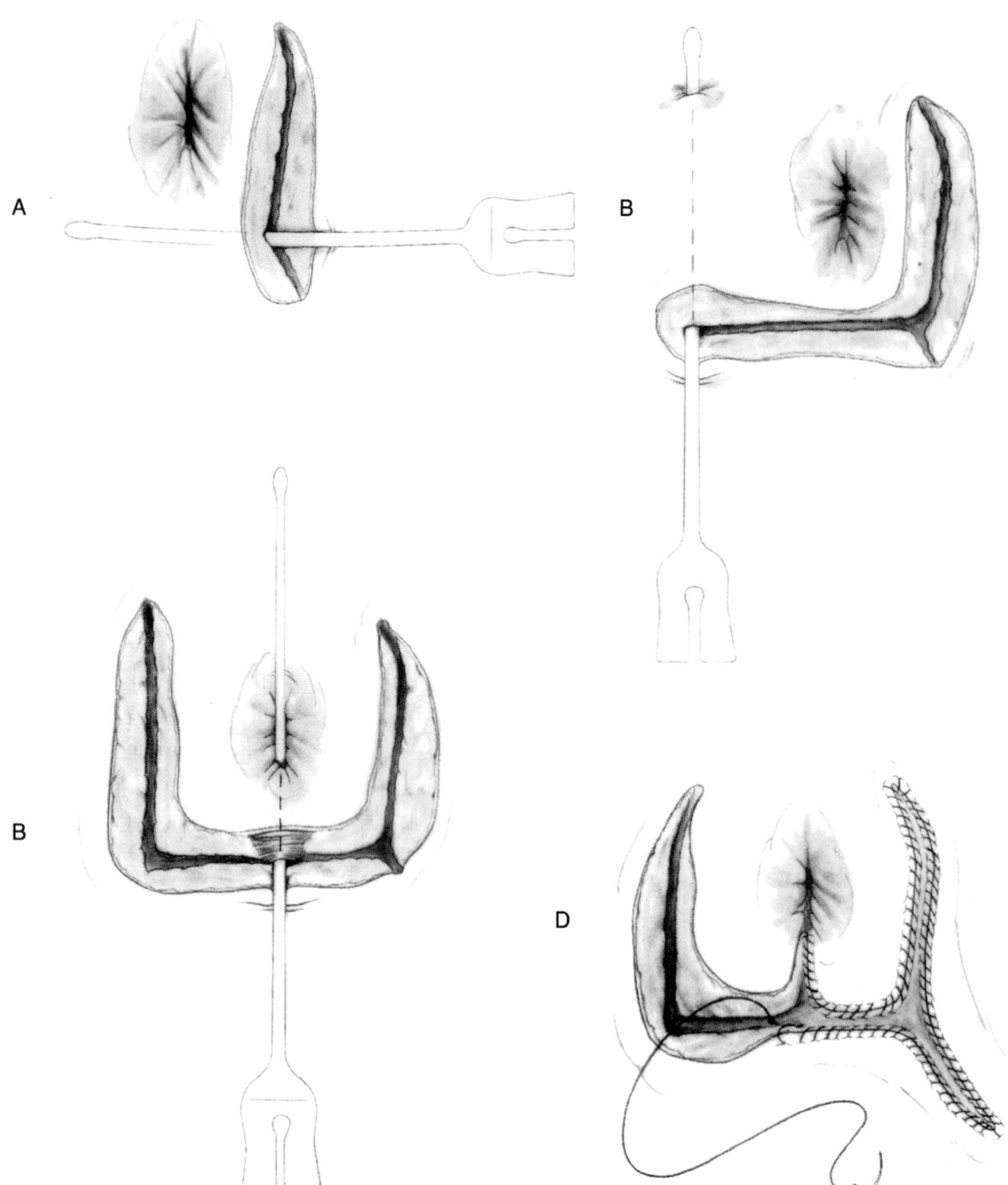

FIGURE 33 ■ Technique for repair of a horseshoe fistula.

fistulous stage, the primary source is handled in the anal canal by division of the lower half of the internal sphincter. Adequate drainage of the secondary tract is then established, and a seton is inserted. If the tract traverses only the lower portion of the external sphincter, repair can be accomplished as described for posterior horseshoe fistulas.

Ustynoski et al. (60) suggested that seton treatment with counter drainage yields a lower rate of recurrence than does primary fistulotomy with counter drainage. A posterior or anterior incision is made to unroof the deep posterior or anterior spaces, respectively, and a seton is passed through to the primary opening in the anal canal. Penrose drains are then passed from the midline incision to the lateral counterincisions. The latter are removed in 24–48 hours. The setons are tightened weekly until the deep space is obliterated. If the latter procedure is not tolerated, a fistulotomy can be performed. Adoption of this management resulted in a recurrence rate of 18.1% in 11 patients.

Pezim (61) believes that successful treatment of a horseshoe fistula requires deroofing the deep postanal space. In 24 patients (three bilateral and 21 unilateral), treatment consisted of deroofing the postanal space with division of overlying external sphincter muscle by section and deroofing lateral wings in 22 patients. With an average follow-up of 23 months, 96% healed and 21% required reoperation. Protective padding was worn by 21% of patients and 64% considered their continence normal.

PMMA Beads

For the management of high and recurrent fistulas, Kupferberg et al. (62) described the technique in which partial excision of the fistula tract is followed by insertion of chains of poly-methyl-meth-acrylate (PMMA) copolymer beads. The wound is closed primarily, and the beads are removed over a period of 7–21 days. In this group's preliminary report, each of the five patients obtained complete healing. The concept is attractive since no muscle requires division, but further experience must be accumulated before it can be generally recommended.

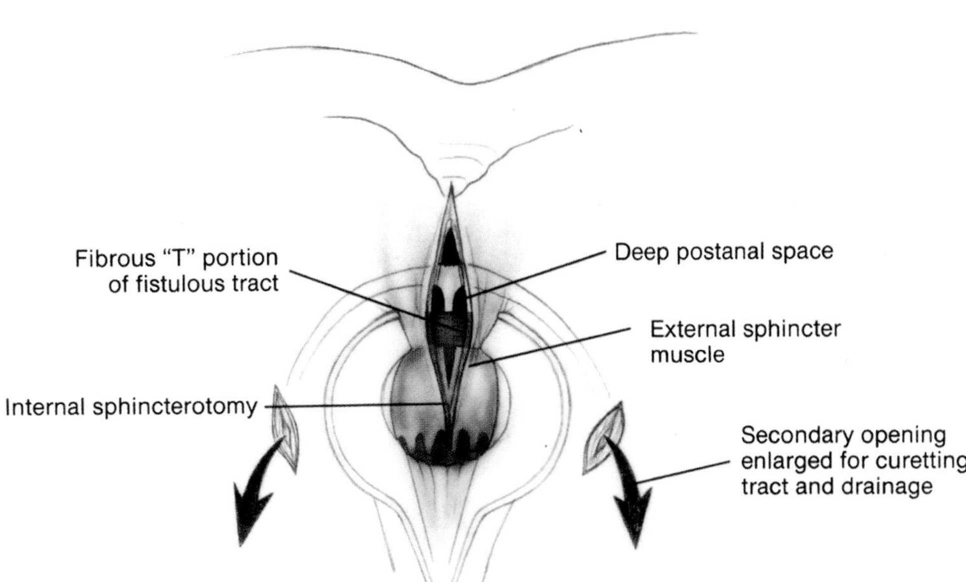

FIGURE 34 ■ Modification of Hanley's treatment of a horseshoe fistula.

Fibrin Glue

Fibrin glue is a novel treatment for anal fistulas. Purported advantages are that it is simple and repeatable; failure does not compromise further treatment options; and sphincter function is preserved (63). MacRae et al. (64) used fibrin glue in the treatment of complex fistula-in-ano. Twelve patients presenting with complex anal fistulas were prospectively treated with curettage and irrigation of the fistulous tract followed by insertion of fibrin glue. The internal opening was managed with an internal sphincterotomy at the fistula site and oversewing of the mucosa in four patients and a mucosal advancement flap in six patients. Two patients had no treatment. Ten patients had fistulas of cryptoglandular origin and two were associated with Crohn's disease. Follow-up was a mean of 7 months. Six of 12 fistulas healed with the first operation. Four were converted to simple fistulas amenable to fistulotomy. Two failed to heal but were successfully treated with repeat instillation of fibrin glue. Complications were minimal. One patient had partial slough of a mucosal flap and one patient had difficulty with urinary retention. There were no complaints of incontinence of either flatus or stool associated with the therapy. How much of the success in this study was due to the internal sphincterotomy performed in half of these patients (to eradicate the source of the problem) and how much of the success was due to the fibrin glue are impossible to know. Even two patients with Crohn's disease healed with this form of treatment. The authors concluded that injection of fibrin glue is a safe, viable form of treatment for complex fistula-in-ano.

Lindsey et al. (63) conducted a randomized control trial of fibrin glue versus conventional treatment for anal fistula. Fibrin glue healed three of six and fistulotomy healed all seven simple fistulas. There was no change in baseline incontinence score, maximum resting pressures, or squeeze pressures between the study arms. Return to work was quicker in the glue arm but pain scores were similar and satisfaction scores higher in the fistulotomy group. Fibrin glue healed 9 of 13 (69%) and conventional treatment healed 2 of 16 (13%) complex fistulas. Satisfaction scores were high in the fibrin glue group. They concluded that no advantage was found for fibrin glue over fistulotomy for simple fistulas but fibrin glue healed more complex fistulas than conventional treatment and with higher patient satisfaction.

The results of various authors are summarized in Table 2. I personally have not been able to achieve healing rates as high as many of those reported in Table 2. These results are not entirely comparable because each series consisted of fistulas of different degrees of complexity, some including patients with Crohn's disease and HIV, all factors that are likely to determine outcome. Patrli et al. (69) found tract length to be important with a recurrence rate of 54% with tracts $<3.5\,cm$ but only 11% for those $>3.5\,cm$. Sentovich (70) used fibrin glue in a two-stage procedure. At the initial operation, Sentovich destroyed the internal gland and placed a seton. About two months later the seton was removed, the internal opening closed, and fibrin glue instilled by way of the external opening to seal the fistula tract. With a median follow-up of 22 months, 60% of the fistulas closed but with retreatment, 69% closed. Failures were treated by fistulotomy or advancement flap. Late recurrence (more than 6 months) developed in 6% of patients. Sentovich found two risk factors for failure—chronic previously treated fistulas and fistulas associated

TABLE 2 ■ **Healing Rates of Fibrin Glue in Treatment of Fistula-in-Ano**

Author		*n*	% Healing
MacRae et al. (64)	1993	12	50
Chiu (65)	1997	25	68
Venkatesh and Ramanujam (66)	1999	21	57
Cintron et al. (67)	2000	79	61
El-Shobaky et al. (68)	2000	30	80
Patrli et al. (69)	2000	69	74
Sentovich (70)	2001	20	85
Chan et al. (71)	2002	10	60
Lindsey et al. (63)	2002	19	63
Buchanan et al. (72)	2003	22	14
Loungnarath et al. (73)	2004	42	31
Singer et al. (74)	2005	24–25–26[a]	21–40–31[a]

[a]Cefoxitin added to sealant-closure internal opening—both.

with an ileal pouch anal anastomosis. Singer et al. (74) examined three modifications of the Tisseel-VH fibrin sealant procedure: the addition of cefoxitin to the sealant, surgical closure of the primary opening, or both. If fistulas failed to heal, patients were offered a single retreatment with sealant. Twenty-four patients were treated in the cefoxitin arm, 25 in the closure arm, and 26 in the combined arm. Median duration of fistulas was 12 months. Patients were followed for a mean of 27 months postoperatively. There was no postoperative incontinence or complications related to the sealant itself. Initial healing rates were 21% in the cefoxitin arm, 40% in the closure arm, and 31% in the combined arm. One of five patients in the cefoxitin arm, one of seven patients in the closure arm, and one of six patients in the combined arm were successfully retreated; final healing rates were 25%, 44%, and 35%, respectively. Treatment of fistula-in-ano

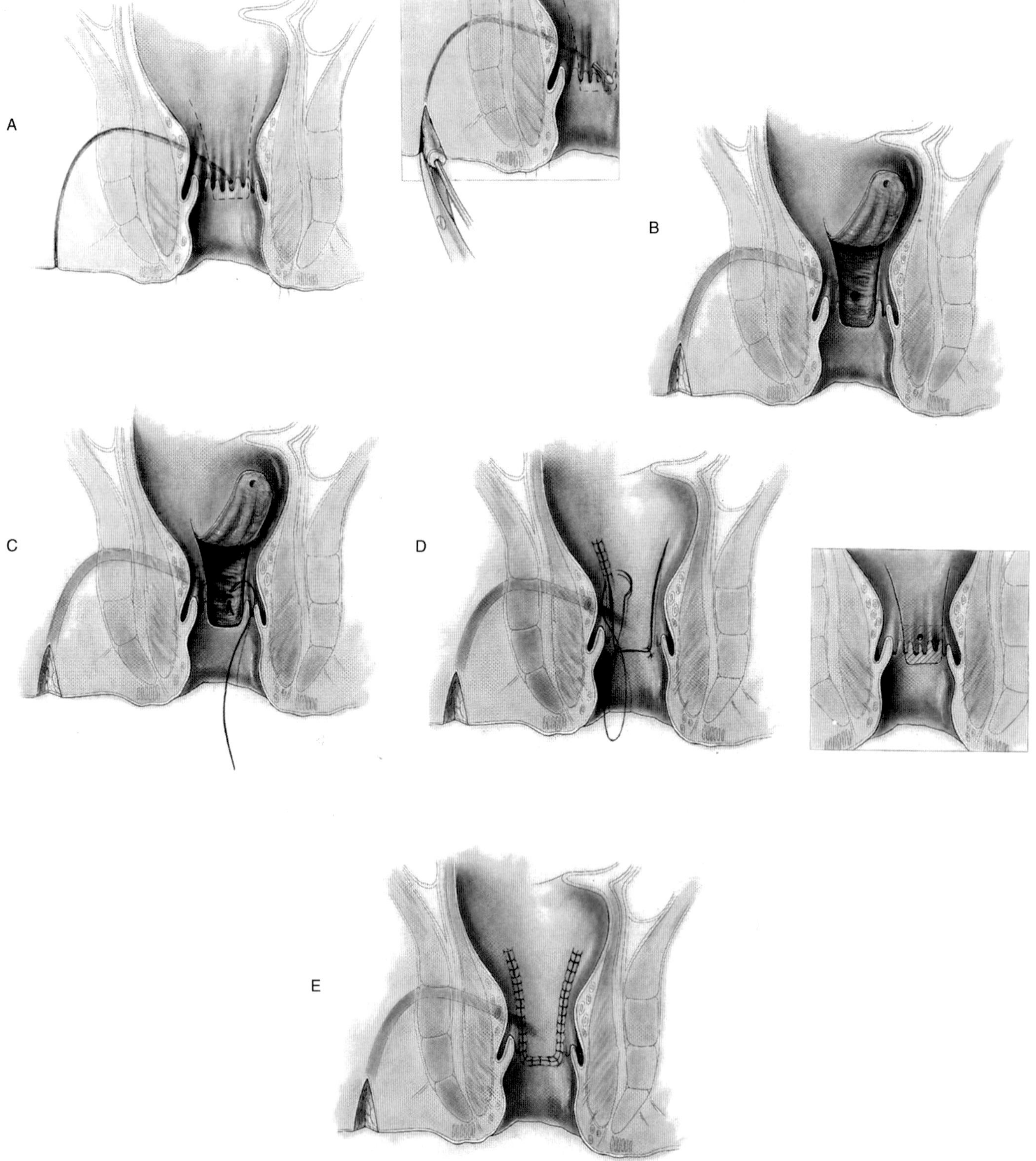

FIGURE 35 ■ Advancement rectal flap X 4. (**A**) Dotted line outlines flap to be raised in repair of high trans-sphincteric fistula-in-ano. Inset indicates beginning of coring-out procedure. (**B**) Fistula is cored out and flap of mucosa, submucosa, and internal sphincter is elevated. (**C**) Opening in anal canal is sutured. (**D**) Flap is drawn down and distal end is excised (*inset*). (**E**) Flap is sutured in place.

with fibrin sealant with closure of the internal opening was somewhat more successful than sealant with cefoxitin or the combination; however, this did not achieve statistical significance. They concluded that the addition of intra-adhesive cefoxitin, closure of the internal opening, or both were not recommended modifications of the fibrin sealant procedure.

It is well recognized that some fistula-in-ano present a major operative challenge to the surgeon. Any method as simple as curettage and injection of a material that results in successful treatment is a most welcome addition to the surgical armamentarium. It may decrease the number of staged procedures. The cost increase is considerable but certainly worthwhile if good success rates can be obtained and the complication rate can be decreased. Even with failure, the patient is left no worse than before. Despite some disappointing results and with recognition that healing success appears to decrease with length of follow-up, fibrin glue installation may be indicated in patients who are already incontinent, those with a major fear of incontinence, those who do not want their seton to remain in place, and patients with an anterior fistula especially in women (72).

Advancement Rectal Flap

For patients whose fistulas cross the sphincter muscle at a high level (e.g., high transsphincteric and suprasphincteric levels), there is always the concern that division of the muscle below the tract will result in significant alterations in continence. Thus, there is renewed interest in the advancement rectal flap technique for treating those patients to preserve fecal continence while eradicating the complex fistula. The procedure has been adopted for repair of the rectovaginal fistula (see Chap. 16). Principles of repair include excision of the internal opening in the anal canal, precise anatomic definition and excision or curettage of the main tracts, advancement of a flap of mucosa and submucosa of rectum beyond the original internal opening, and tension-free suture of the flap to the anal canal distal to the original opening (Fig. 35) (75). Differences exist about the thickness of rectal wall to use, the use of a drain, the level of advancement distally, and the need for temporary fecal diversion. The attractive features of this repair include the fact that no sphincter requires division, contour defects are avoided, the pain is less because there is no perineal wound, and healing is more rapid.

In a series of 109 patients reported by Aguilar et al. (76), the enviable recurrence rate was 1.5%, with no incontinence of solid stool, although incontinence for gas and liquid stool occurred in 7% and 6%, respectively. In 6 patients with suprasphincteric fistulas reported by Ozuner et al. (75), there were no recurrences and no incontinence. In 30 patients treated by Wedell et al. (77), satisfactory results were obtained in 29 patients, with no further alterations in continence and no recurrences during the follow-up period of 18 months to 4 years.

Mizrahi et al. (78) reviewed their results in the management of complex fistula-in-ano with the endorectal advancement flap in 106 procedures performed on 94 patients. At a mean follow-up of 40.3 months, the procedure was successful in 59.6% of patients. Crohn's disease was associated with a significantly higher recurrence rate (57.1%) compared to patients without Crohn's disease (33.3%). In defining predictors of healing, prior attempts at repair, type of fistula, origin, preoperative steroid use, postoperative bowel confinement, use of postoperative antibiotics, or creation of a diverting stoma were not associated with less favorable outcome. The median time to recurrence was eight weeks but recurrences were observed in 15.7% of patients three or more years after repair. In 9% of patients, continence deteriorated after endorectal advancement repair, a more common finding in patients who had undergone previous surgical repairs.

A wide range of results had been reported using this technique and they have been summarized in Table 3. Again, results are not comparable as these series included patients with Crohn's disease, or rectovaginal fistulas, follow-up periods vary, and technique has not been uniform. Reporting of continence is usually related to the tenacity of the investigators seeking this complication. Recurrence rates with 1, 2, 3 previous procedures are 30%, 40%, and 75% (78). In a recent review by Zimmerman (22), healing rates for advancement flap repairs had varied from 68% to 100%. Few authors address the issue of impairment of continence and those who have reported rates from 0% to 10%. Zimmerman et al. (89) also noted that smoking adversely affects healing rates (60% vs. 79% for nonsmokers). In the review by Zimmerman et al. (89) of 105 patients who underwent an advancement flap repair, none of the following variables that were assessed were considered significant: age, sex, number of previous attempts at repair, preoperative seton drainage, fistula type, presence of horseshoe extensions, location of internal opening, postoperative drainage, and body mass index.

For patients in whom conventional techniques are likely to fail, such as those with multiple fistulas, both cryptogenic and rectovaginal involving one-third of the circumference of the anal canal, Berman (90) has recommended the use of

TABLE 3 ■ **Results of Endorectal Advancement Flap for Fistula-in-Ano**

Author		*n*	Success (%)	Incontinence (%)	Mean Follow-Up (mo)
Kodner et al. (79)	1993	107	84	13	8
Athanasiadis et al. (80)	1994	189[a]	89	21	12–96
		35[b]	80	43	
Makowiec et al. (81)	1995	32	66	3	20
Joo et al. (82)	1998	26	71	—	17
Marchesa et al. (83)	1998	13	61	—	15
Kreis et al. (84)	1998	24	63	21	48
Hyman (85)	1999	33	81	0	—
Schouten et al. (86)	1999	44	75	35	12
Ortiz et al. (87)	2000	103	93	8	12
Mizrahi et al. (78)	2002	94	60	9	40
Sonoda et al. (88)	2002	48[c]	77	—	17
		44[d]	50	—	17
Zimmerman (89)	2003	105	69	—	14

[a]Transsphincteric.
[b]Suprasphincteric.
[c]Cryptoglandular origin.
[d]Crohn's disease.

a tubular or sleeve endoanal advancement flap. The operative technique is adapted from the intersphincteric proctectomy. A circumferential incision is made just distal to the internal openings and hence just distal to the dentate line. The uninvolved portion of the circumference need not be mobilized. Fistulous tracts are divided as encountered. Excluded tracts are curetted, disrupting and removing epithelialized or granulation tissue. External openings are enlarged to ensure drainage. The distal diseased tube is amputated and the proximal wall is anastomosed to the initial line of incision. Perioperative antibiotics are advised. Additional applications may include multiple fistulas in patients with Crohn's disease during rectal quiescence and cases of advanced or complicated rectal trauma in which epithelial loss has been significant.

Fistulectomy and Primary Closure

A technique that has not gained a great deal of support is the performance of a fistulectomy and primary closure of the wound. Parkash et al. (91) reported the results of this technique as used in 120 patients; there were only three recurrences and satisfactory functional results in all cases. The addition of a lateral sphincterotomy was done to relieve postoperative pain and to promote good healing. A procedure with coring out of the fistulous tract and closure of internal opening was reported by Takano (92). In 98 patients who underwent this procedure, there were only two recurrences, but alteration in continence was not mentioned. It would seem that the use of primary suture alone is too uncertain to be acceptable as a routine method of treatment. Aguilar et al. (76) reported on 189 patients who underwent anal fistulectomy with mucosal advancement flap. Recurrence developed in 1.6% while 8% of patients reported disturbed continence (minor soiling, incontinence to flatus or incontinence to loose stools). Miller and Finan (93) combined core fistulectomy with a flap advancement for complex fistula. Successful healing occurred in 77% with no disturbance of continence reported with a mean follow-up of 14 months.

Dermal Island Flap Anoplasty

Robertson and Mangione (94) described a technique of cutaneous advancement flap associated with suture closure of the internal opening and external drainage used in 14 patients without inflammatory bowel disease and 6 patients with inflammatory bowel disease. None of the non-IBD patients were diverted but one of the IBD patients was diverted and the other five placed on home TPN in addition to the judicious use of other anti-IBD medication with a follow-up of 18 months. In the non-IBD group, 1 of 14 patients healed with minor incontinence of flatus in one patient. In the IBD group, five fistulas healed, two failed, and one developed a new fistula in a follow-up of 16 months. No conclusion can be gleamed from the IBD patients, as the numbers were small and the treatment heterogeneous.

Nelson et al. (95) reported on their experience with the use of the dermal island flap anoplasty for trans-sphincteric fistulas. Of 73 flaps performed in 65 individuals, recurrence developed 17 times in 13 individuals. Recurrence was more likely to occur in males, patients who have had previous treatments of fistulas, patients with large fistulas requiring combined flaps, and patients who had simultaneous fibrin glue injection. Patients with Crohn's disease and individuals having internal sphincter closure had fewer recurrences. No specific anatomic or demographic characteristic is sufficiently associated with failure to exclude any patient from the operation. Closure of the internal sphincter should be done as part of the procedure and fibrin glue should not be done simultaneously. Perhaps, the most important finding of that study is that the dermal island flap anoplasty can be repeated with a high probability of success if the fistula recurs. The rectal mucosal flap procedure has been technically more difficult to perform than the island flap and may result in a mucosal ectropion because coverage of the internal opening requires a rectal mucosa to be sutured to anoderm beyond the dentate line.

A variety of techniques to accomplish dermal flap anoplasty have been described. One such technique is illustrated in Figure 36.

Amin et al. (96) reported on 18 patients (10 trans-sphincteric, 4 intersphincteric, and 4 suprasphincteric) who underwent core fistulectomy, closure of defect in the internal anal sphincter, and V-Y advancement flap to cover the internal opening leaving the site of the external opening for drainage while preserving the internal and external sphincter. With a median follow-up of 19 months, healing occurred in 85%.

Zimmerman et al. (97) evaluated the healing rate of trans-sphincteric perianal fistulas after anocutaneous advancement flap repair. The crypt bearing tissue around the internal opening as well as the overlying anoderm was excised. An (inverted) U-shaped flap, including perianal skin and fat, was created. The base of the flap was approximately twice the width of its apex. The flap was advanced and sutured to the mucosa and underlying internal anal sphincter proximal to the closed internal opening. The median follow-up time was 25 months. Anocutaneous advancement flap repair was successful in 12 patients (46%). Success was inversely correlated with the number of prior attempts. In patients who had undergone no or only one previous attempted repair ($n=9$), the healing rate was 78%. In patients with two or more previous repairs ($n=17$), the healing rate was only 29%. In seven patients (30%), continence deteriorated after anocutaneous advancement flap repair. Eleven patients (48%) had completely normal continence preoperatively. Two of these patients (18%) encountered soiling and incontinence for gas after the procedure, whereas two subjects (18%) complained of accidental bowel movements. Twelve patients (52%) presented with continence disturbances at the time of admission to hospital. In this group, deterioration was observed in two patients (17%). They concluded, the results of anocutaenous advancement flap in patients with none or only one previous attempt at repair are moderate. For patients who have undergone two or more previous attempts at repair, the outcome is poor. Based on relatively low healing rate and deterioration of continence, this procedure seems less suitable for high trans-sphincteric fistulas than peranal mucosal advancement flap repair.

A recent review by Zimmerman (22) reported healing rates range from 74% to 95%. Few authors address the issue of impairment of continence, but they report rates of 0–7%.

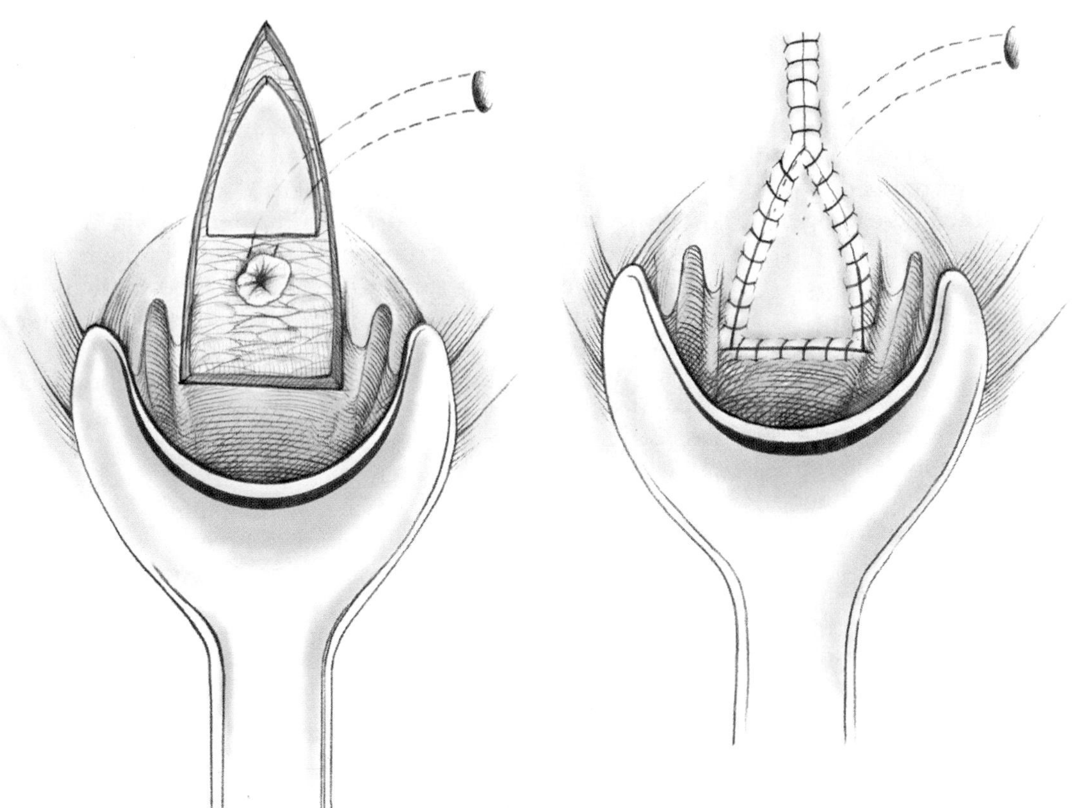

FIGURE 36 ■ V-Y flap anoplasty.

Anal Plug

The newest modality of therapy for the treatment of fistula-in-ano of cryptoglandular origin is the Surgisis AFP (Cook Surgical inc.) anal plug introduced by Armstrong. The plug is cone shaped and made from porcine small intestinal submucosa. When placed in the fistula tract it is proposed to serve as a bioscaffold for native tissue regeneration and hence occlude the fistulous tract. In their most recent study, Champagne et al reported the results of 55 high transphincteric or deeper fistulas in 46 patients (98). Each fistula tract was irrigated with hydrogen peroxide and closed using a rehydrated AFP which was inserted into the primary opening, cut to the length and sutured in place. At a follow up of 1 to 24 months (median 10 months), the complete closure rate was 83%. Failures were due to plug "fall out" (6%), multiple tracts (4%), persistent drainage (4%), and late recurrence (2%) at six months postoperatively. Failures occurred more often in multiple tracts (horseshoe fistulas). They concluded the technique is safe and effective in closing high complex anorectal fistulas. An advantage is that it can be repeated if it fails initially. Armstrong recommends a preoperative bowel preparation but this would not seem to be necessary.

Johnson et al. (99) conducted a prospective cohort study to compare fibrin glue versus the anal plug. Patients with high transphincteric fistulas or deeper were prospectively enrolled. Patients with Crohn's disease or superficial fistulas were excluded. The tract was irrigated with hydrogen peroxide. Ten patients underwent fibrin glue closure, and 15 used a fistula plug. In the fibrin glue group six patients (60%) had persistence of one or more fistulas at three months, compared with two patients (13%) in the plug group. They concluded closure of the primary opening of the fistula tract using a suturable biologic anal fistula plug is an effective method of treating anorectal fistulas. The method seems to be more reliable than fibrin glue closure. Further prospective long-term studies are warranted to determine the efficacy of this latest offering for the treatment of fistula-in-ano.

■ COMPLICATIONS OF OPERATION FOR FISTULOUS ABSCESS

A long list of potential complications may ensue after operation for a fistulous abscess. Excluding urinary retention, which occurred in 25% of his patients, Mazier (56) found that 5.4% of them developed complications, which included hemorrhage, incontinence, acute external thrombosed hemorrhoids, cellulitis, inadequate drainage and pocketing, fecal impaction, recurrent fistulas, rectovaginal fistulas, persistent sinus, bridging, and stricture. However, with caution these complications can be reduced to a minimum. My impression is that avoiding primary fistulotomy surgery helps reduce such untoward events.

■ CAUSES OF RECURRENCE

Anyone treating patients with a fistula-in-ano realizes that in certain instances recurrences will occur despite the most careful operative dissection. The most common cause of recurrence of an anal fistula is failure to identify and treat the primary internal orifice. The result is that the causative infected anal gland in the intersphincteric space is not eradicated. Failure to detect and treat lateral or upward extensions also may be followed by recurrence. Failure to open the fistulous tract for fear of causing incontinence also may result in recurrence. (This statement should not encourage operating with bold recklessness.) Premature closure of fistulotomy wounds may result in early recurrence. Also, when the etiologic factor of the fistula is a specific disease, such as Crohn's disease, recurrences are not infrequent.

In a review of 624 patients who underwent fistula-in-ano operations, Garcia-Aguilar et al. (51) found that factors associated with recurrence included complex type of fistula, horseshoe extension, lack of identification or lateral location of internal opening, previous fistula operation, and the surgeon performing the procedure. Incontinence was associated with female sex, high anal fistula, type of operation, and previous fistula operation.

■ CAUSES OF ANAL INCONTINENCE AFTER OPERATION FOR ANAL FISTULA

Division of Anorectal Muscle

Complete severance of the anorectal ring results in total incontinence. Division of lesser amounts of sphincter muscle may result in varying degrees of partial incontinence, depending on the state of the sphincter muscle at the outset and the location of the myotomy. Lunniss et al. (100) used manometric assessment to study factors affecting continence after operation for anal fistula. They determined that functional deficits are related to low resting pressures, reflecting the change in internal sphincter integrity by its division. In addition, the age of the patient is a factor since the elderly, with a sphincter mechanism already weakened by age, are less likely to tolerate division of even small amounts of muscle.

Severance of Motor Nerve to Sphincter Mechanism

Severing the inferior rectal nerve results in impaired continence, but control may be acceptable with only one nerve functioning. Damage to the nerves bilaterally certainly renders the patient incontinent.

Prolonged Packing After Anorectal Surgery

Packing that is prolonged may be detrimental because it causes fibrosis of the sphincter, which in turn may cause some measure of incontinence as a result of hard scar formation. Mazier (56) found that prolonged packing with iodoform gauze was a factor contributing to incontinence.

van Tets and Kuijpers (101) conducted a study of 312 patients to detect factors that predict the occurrence of continence disorders after anal fistulotomy. The incidence of continence disorders was 27%, whereas incontinence for solid stool did not occur. They found that patients with high openings, posterior openings, or fistula extensions are at high risk to develop continence disorders after anal fistulotomy. Other factors associated with incontinence include female sex, type of operation, and previous fistula operation (51).

■ POSTOPERATIVE CARE

The postoperative care of the wound may be as important as the operative procedure in treating a patient with a fistula-in-ano. The primary goals are sound healing from the depths of the wounds and prevention of the contact and premature healing of opposing skin edges. A regular diet is prescribed, and analgesics are administered as needed. Some physicians prefer to use dressings soaked in solutions of sodium hypochlorite (Milton, Dakin's, or Eusol) to keep the healing edges apart, but this procedure is not often necessary. The patient should take warm baths three times a day for perineal toilet and comfort. A gentle laxative is taken orally until the first bowel movement; a bulk-forming agent is taken until wound healing has been completed. Some authors recommend insertion of an anal dilator, but this is rather harsh treatment. A large stool created by bulk-forming agents effects a physiologic dilatation.

Because of the operative trauma and division of some muscle, patients may experience fecal leaks in the immediate postoperative period, especially if stools are liquid. However, if the anorectal ring has been preserved, after a week or 10 days control approximates normalcy.

The healing time required depends on the complexity of the fistula. A simple fistulotomy may heal in 4 to 5 weeks, whereas a complex one may take several months. Most uncomplicated fistulas heal within 12 weeks of the operation (11). Scrutiny of the healing times discloses a surprisingly long interval needed to accomplish complete healing in many patients, although this finding should probably not be surprising since lengthy healing times have been reported previously by Marks and Ritchie (14) and Parks and Stitz (102).

A number of factors are associated with prolonged healing. Healing time increases with the increasing complexity of the fistula; for example, fistulas characterized by extrarectal extensions or high blind tracts take a long time to heal, as do suprasphincteric or horseshoe fistulas. Delayed healing also occurs in patients with inflammatory bowel disease. This delay may not necessarily be attributable to the presence of inflammatory bowel disease per se since some of these patients have more complex types of fistulas.

■ RESULTS

Results of fistula surgery may vary considerably from surgeon to surgeon. Clearly, results depend on the complexity of the fistula treated.

In general, there is hesitation to report poor results. Often there is a reciprocal relationship between the incidence of recurrence and incontinence, since cure and continence are competing priorities. Reports with low recurrence rates frequently may cite a higher incidence of incontinence, whereas reports with a higher recurrence rate may describe a low rate of incontinence. The results taken from a group of publications are listed in Table 4. However, it is extremely difficult to compare the results of these often different series of patients. Many large series have very inadequate follow-up, with many patients lost to follow-up, whereas others have a very short follow-up period. Since most authors do not define incontinence, the reader often is unaware of whether the problems are temporary or permanent; whether the patient was incontinent for flatus, liquid stool, or solid stool; or whether there was soiling, which unquestionably has a different meaning to different patients and physicians.

The lack of a standard, internationally recognized classification has made it impossible for one surgeon to convey to another the exact nature and extent of the fistulous process. As a consequence, it is impossible to compare the results of one series with those of another. Certain series are reports of only "complex" fistulas (102), whereas other reports may contain a high percentage of simple fistulas. This would explain, at least in part, the enormous range

TABLE 4 ■ Results of Fistula Surgery

Author(s)	No. of Patients	Recurrence Rate (%)	Disturbance of Continence (%)
Hanley et al. (46)	31	0	0
Parks and Stitz (102)	158	9.0 (7.0 unhealed)	17.0,39.0[a]
Marks and Ritchie (14)	793		3.4, 3.9, 25.0, 4.4[b]
Ewerth et al. (103)	143		0.7, 2.8[c]
Adams and Kovalcik (104)	133	3.7	0.8
Kuijpers (105)	51	4.0	9.8
Gingold (106)	74	1.4	
Khubchandani (107)	137	5.0	
Sainio and Husa (108)	199	11.0	34.0
Vasilevsky and Gordon (11)	160	6.3	6.0 (0.7, 2.0, 3.3)[d]
Shouler et al. (109)	115	7.0	1.7, 1.7, 12.0[e]
Dodi et al. (110)	209	3.0	4.3
Girona (111)	437	2.8, 7.6[f]	2.0, 45.5[g]
Parnaud (112)	358	(2.2 unhealed).	0, 20.0[h]
Sangwan et al. (113)	461	6.5	0[i]
Isbister (114)	88	2.3	0
Garcia-Aguilar et al. (51)	375	8.3	45.0[j]
Mylonakis et al. (115)	100	3	0, 6, 3[k]
Malouf et al. (50)	98	4	10
Gupta (116)	210	1.5	0

[a]Seventeen percent without division of seton-contained muscle; 39% with division of seton-contained muscle.
[b]Incontinence (solid stool, liquid stool, flatus, soiling).
[c]Incontinence (flatus, feces).
[d]Incontinence (solid stool, liquid stool, flatus).
[e]Incontinence (feces, flatus, soiling).
[f]At 3 years recurrence rates were 2.8% for transsphincteric fistulas and 7.6% for suprasphincteric fistulas.
[g]Range for first-time operation: 2–6.5%; range for operation for recurrent fistula-in-ano: transsphincteric—solid, 4.3%; liquid, 25.7%; flatus, 21.1%; suprasphincteric—solid, 11.6%; liquid, 34.7%; flatus, 45.5%.
[h]Incontinence (stool, flatus, or soiling).
[i]No incontinence of solid stool.
[j]Soiling, 32%; difficulty holding gas, 31%; accidental bowel movements, 13%.
[k]Incontinence (solid, soiling, gas).

of results reported by different authors. If a standard classification were available, the results of treatment of similar types of fistulas could be compared and, consequently, be more meaningful.

Another problem is the follow-up of patients. Few of the large series have significant follow-up information on their patients [e.g., Mazier (56), 53.4%; Marks and Ritchie (14), 26%]. Vasilevsky and Gordon (11) were fortunate to have a 94% follow-up. The length of follow-up is also important. Often there is no mention of early postoperative problems, so the first area that should be documented is whether trouble with control is temporary or permanent. Also appropriate is recording the degree of difficulty with control, which could be classified as problems with flatus, liquid stool, or solid stool. Possibly, soiling should be a fourth category in this constellation of incontinence problems, but the term "soiling" requires definition. If all series addressed the results of fistula surgery in this manner, valid comparisons of different series could be made.

In an excellent monograph on fistula-in-ano, Lilius (53) reviewed the world literature up to 1964 and discovered an enormous difference in reported results of fistula surgery. Reported recurrence rates varied from 0.7% to 26.5%, and reported disturbances in anal continence varied from 5% to 40%. Lilius's personal study of 150 patients operated on for fistulas revealed a recurrence rate of 5.5%, with disturbances of continence noted in 13.5% of patients.

Marks and Ritchie (14) reviewed 793 patients treated at St. Mark's Hospital, London, and found that follow-up of these patients revealed healing of almost all the fistulas. However, the functional results were less satisfactory, with incontinence of loose stool in 17%, incontinence of flatus in 25%, and soiling in 31%. They point out, however, that there is a definite incidence of these three symptoms in a normal population.

Hanley et al. (46), on the other hand, using techniques described earlier in this chapter, operated on 31 patients with horseshoe fistulas and reported no recurrences and no problems with control. Mazier (56) reported a 3.9% incidence of recurrence in 1000 patients, with 82% of the recurrences developing within 1 year but some recurrences occurring as much as 7 years postoperatively. Reportedly, only one of the 1000 patients had a problem with control. The recurrence rate in the series by Parks and Stitz (102) was 9%, but this was a very selected series of patients and an unusually high percentage of very complex fistulas, hence the unusually high recurrence rate. In a series of 160 patients operated on by me (11), the sole immediate postoperative complication was bleeding, which occurred 1 week postoperatively and ceased spontaneously (0.7%). Alteration in continence occurred in 6% of the patients, with 2.6% experiencing temporary incontinence of flatus, 1.3% of liquid stool, and 0.7% of solid stool. Permanent loss of control for flatus occurred in one patient (0.7%) and for liquid stool in one patient (0.7%). No patients suffered loss of control for solid stool. Recurrence developed in 6.3% of patients, all between 5 and 25 months postoperatively.

Garcia-Aguilar et al. (117) attempted to identify factors that affect patient's lifestyles and may contribute to their satisfaction by a questionnaire mailed to 624 patients treated for cryptoglandular fistula-in-ano. Three hundred and seventy-five patients returned their questionnaire. Patients who were followed up for a minimum of one year were included in this retrospective study. Patient satisfaction was strongly associated with fistula recurrence, difficulty holding gas, soiling of undergarments, and accidental bowel movements. Effects of incontinence on patient quality of life were also significantly associated with patient satisfaction as was the number of lifestyle activities affected by incontinence. Patients with fistula recurrence reported higher dissatisfaction rate (61%) than did patients with anal incontinence (24%), but the attributable fraction of dissatisfaction for incontinence (84%) was greater than that for fistula recurrence (33%). Patient satisfaction was not significantly associated with age, gender, history of previous fistula operation, type of fistula, surgical procedure, time since operation, or operating surgeon. In a study of 110 patients who underwent fistulotomy, Cavanaugh et al. (118) found the Fecal Incontinence Severity Index to be an excellent tool to gauge quality of life after fistulotomy. Fistula Incontinence Severity Index scores greater than 30 predicted detrimental effect on quality of life.

It is difficult to understand why there is such a great variation in the results of fistula surgery. Clearly, one factor is the difference in patient population, with some authors reporting the results of treating mostly simple fistulas and others reporting only the results of treating complex fistulas. The skill of the individual surgeon is also a factor, as is the thoroughness of reporting or at least the intensity of interrogation of the patients during follow-up visits.

SPECIAL CONSIDERATIONS

■ PRIMARY CLOSURE OF ANORECTAL ABSCESS

An unconventional method of handling a perianal and ischioanal abscess is primary suture. A summary of results of this treatment is presented in Table 5. After the purulent material is evacuated with the patient under general anesthesia, the abscess cavity is curetted and sutured primarily while the patient receives systemic antibiotics. The rationale for using curettage is that it allegedly destroys the layer of granulation tissue lining the abscess wall, thereby allowing the antibiotic to penetrate freely. An hour before the operation antibiotics are given by injection. In a controlled trial of the conventional lay-open method compared with incision, curettage, and suture, Leaper et al. (120) administered ampicillin and cloxacillin intramuscularly (500 mg of each) along with the premedication and administered the same amounts orally for 5 days after the treatment. Primary healing occurred in 93% of cases, with a mean healing time of 10 days as compared with 35 days for the open wounds. Their follow-up was short (less than 1 year). Jones and Wilson (119) described a series of patients in whom the antibiotics used were lincomycin along with the premedication and clindamycin for four days postoperatively. Patients were allowed to return home the same day. Follow-up results demonstrated a 14% fistulization rate. In a prospective randomized trial, Kronberg and Olsen (121) compared performing incision and drainage with primary fistulotomy (if found) to performing incision, curettage, and suture with antibiotic cover (clindamycin for 4 days) in 83 patients, all of whom were followed for 3 years. Primary healing occurred in 76% of the 42 patients treated with sutures and did so an average of 3 weeks sooner than in patients who had an incision alone. Recurrences (abscesses or fistulas) tended to occur more frequently with the suture technique (40% vs. 22.5%). Mortensen et al. (123) conducted a randomized study comparing treatment with clindamycin and clindamycin plus Gentacoll (Schering-Plough A/S, DK-3520, Farum, Denmark). The overall incidence of recurrent disease was 19.5%, with no difference in the two groups. Since experience with this technique has been limited, further evaluation is needed to confirm its efficacy.

TABLE 5 ■ Reported Results of Primary Closure of Anorectal Abscesses

Author(s)	No. of Cases	Type of Antibiotic	Recurrence Rate of Abscess or Fistula (%)
Jones and Wilson (119)	23	Lincomycin and clindamycin	14
Leaper et al. (120)	110	Ampicillin and cloxacillin	7
Kronberg and Olsen (121)	42	Clindamycin	49
Lundhus and Gottrup (122)	32	Ampicillin and metronidazole	16
Mortensen et al. (123)	52	Clindamycin	17
	55	Clindamycin and Gentacoll	22

■ SUPERFICIAL FISTULA

A certain number of low fistulas are not associated with anal gland infection. They are the submucous or subcutaneous fistulas that are associated with the bridging of fissure edges in the midline posteriorly or fistulas that occur occasionally in a patient with a hemorrhoidectomy wound. Treatment is accomplished very simply through a lay-open technique or excision and primary closure.

■ PRIMARY VS. SECONDARY FISTULOTOMY

Controversy continues to exist as to whether a primary fistulotomy should be used in the treatment of anorectal abscesses. Some surgeons favor a one-stage procedure in which incision and drainage are combined with fistulotomy (37,44,124,125). They believe that this procedure will eradicate the origin of the infectious process, thereby almost eliminating the development of recurrent abscesses and anal fistulas, which they believe are otherwise inevitable. Proponents of a more conservative approach prefer a two-stage procedure in which incision and drainage are performed initially, followed by fistulotomy at a later date only if necessary. They argue that the need for an operation will not occur for certain; thus, patients would be exposed needlessly to the potential risk of incontinence, a dreaded possible consequence of fistulotomy, especially in the presence of acute inflammation (10,49,126–129).

In a prospective randomized study of 200 consecutive patients with abscesses, Oliver et al. (39) found a 29% recurrence for drainage alone with no incontinence while definitive fistula operation resulted in a 5% rate of recurrence and a 36.7% incidence of incontinence restricted mostly to patients with delayed fistulotomy compared to 2.8% of patients when simple fistulotomy was performed. In this series, patients with high fistulas did not undergo definite fistula operations. They advocate primary fistula operation despite their incontinence rate.

In a review of the subject, Abcarian stated emphatically that one of the reasons for recurrence was an undiagnosed fistula present at the time of abscess drainage. Thus, Abcarian stressed the importance of searching for the fistulous opening at the time of the initial drainage procedure. However, it is not always possible to find an internal opening at that time. In a prospective study of 474 patients with anorectal abscesses, a study in which primary fistulotomy was performed, if the internal opening was discovered at the time of drainage, Read and Abcarian (130) failed to identify such an opening in 66% of their patients. More recently, when 1023 patients with abscesses were studied, a recurrence rate of 3.7% was encountered in the two-thirds of patients undergoing drainage only and 1.8% in the one-third who had a primary fistulotomy along with abscess drainage (37). Despite the fact that primary fistulotomy was advocated, these excellent results could be used to support the use of incision and drainage alone as initial therapy. The recommendation for management may be based on the differences in the patient populations being treated.

Those who favor a more conservative approach believe that performance of a fistulotomy in the presence of acute inflammation is potentially hazardous. Since a fistulous opening may not be seen, overzealous attempts to find one may result in the creation of a false passage, with inadvertent neglect of the true opening, thus leading to persistent suppuration.

The fact that a significant number of patients will not develop fistulas makes primary fistulotomy unnecessary in those cases. If necessary, performing a fistulotomy after the inflammatory action has subsided would be safer. Hanley (44), although a proponent of performing immediate fistulotomy, states that 35–40% of perianal abscesses treated only by incision and drainage will not recur. Scoma et al. (126) demonstrated that 34% would not develop recurrent problems after incision and drainage done with the patient under local anesthesia.

Schouten and van Vroonhoven (131) conducted a prospective randomized trial to determine whether primary fistulotomy should be performed at the time of incision and drainage of anorectal abscesses. They randomly allocated 70 patients to either a group that underwent incision, drainage, and fistulotomy with a partial internal sphincterectomy or a group that underwent incision and drainage alone. After a median follow-up of 42.5 months, the combined recurrence or persistence rate was 2.9% in the former group and 40.6% in the latter. However, scrutiny of anal functional disturbances revealed an incidence of 39.4% in the former and 21.4% in the latter. The authors concluded that the deterioration in functional results overrides the advantage in cure rate and advise using only incision and drainage as the first line of therapy.

In a review of 124 patients who underwent incision and drainage of anorectal suppuration, Winslett et al. (40) found that only 32% of patients required a second procedure, compared with 14% of 109 patients who initially had a definitive operation, with incision and drainage. Seow-Choen et al. (132) reviewed 123 patients with anal abscesses; 74% underwent simple drainage with no anal incontinence and an 11% recurrence rate. Of the 26% who underwent drainage and immediate fistulotomy, 6.5% experienced minor anal incontinence, and 13% developed recurrence. The authors concluded that patients with anal abscesses should be treated with simple drainage. Hamalainen and Sainio (127) followed 146 patients who underwent abscess drainage for an average of 99 months or until a fistula appeared. A fistula developed in 37% and a recurrent abscess developed in 10%. They advocated drainage alone because unnecessary primary fistulotomy could be avoided in more than half of the patients. Vasilevsky and Gordon (10) found that after the drainage of anorectal abscesses, 11% of patients developed recurrent abscesses and 37% of patients were left with an anal fistula, for an overall recurrence or persistence rate of 48%. When looking at the subset of patients in that study who had abscesses drained for the first time, only 5% developed a recurrent abscess, and 31% developed an anal fistula. Thus, only 36% of these patients required a definitive operation. Thus, it would appear that primary fistulotomy is not necessary, especially for patients with an anorectal abscess who are being treated for the first time. In addition, the majority of perianal and ischioanal abscesses can be drained using local anesthesia, obviating the need for general or spinal anesthesia. The use of local anesthetics also removes the temptation to do a fistulotomy. Since one-third to two-thirds of patients will not have a further problem, a primary lay-open technique would be unnecessary in these patients (10,133).

■ HOW MUCH MUSCLE MAY BE DIVIDED?

There is no universal answer to the question of how much muscle can be divided safely. Division of only the lower half of the internal sphincter may result in minor alterations of continence in some individuals, whereas in others division of the internal sphincter and a major portion of their external sphincter may cause no functional deficit. In elderly individuals who already may have a weakened sphincter mechanism, division of only the internal sphincter may result in partial incontinence. Thus, when there is doubt about the competence of the sphincter, it is wise to divide the muscle in successive operations.

In patients with simple intersphincteric or low transsphincteric fistulas, division of the muscle caudad to the tract usually does not significantly jeopardize anal continence. With the more complex fistulas, the dilemma is how to obtain adequate treatment of them without causing incontinence. It must be accepted, however, that to obtain healing in the more complex problems, some loss of muscle function is inevitable; the aim is to minimize this loss.

As a general rule, the whole of the internal sphincter and most of the external sphincter may be cut in the posterior quadrant (with the exception of the puborectalis muscle) without any serious loss of function (49). Unfortunately, this is not true in all cases because sphincter function in all patients is not equal.

In considering the division of the sphincter muscle, it must be remembered that there is no puborectalis muscle anteriorly. Thus, division of muscle in this location is more hazardous than in other portions of the circumference, and appropriate care and attention must be exercised, especially in the female patient.

If the competence of the sphincter is in doubt, it is wise to divide it in stages at successive operations, with a careful assessment made of its state in the conscious patient between each stage.

Using anal manometry, the functional outcome of fistula surgery was quantitated by Belliveau et al. (134). After treatment of intersphincteric fistulas, resting pressure in the distal 2 cm of the anal canal was reduced. In treated trans-sphincteric and suprasphincteric fistulas, anal pressure was reduced in the distal 3 cm. A significantly. lower pressure was measured in patients having the external sphincter divided when compared with those having the muscle preserved. Disturbance of continence was related to abnormally low resting pressures.

In a study of 199 patients at an average of 9 years after fistulotomy, Sainio (135) reported a significant reduction in pressures in 34% of patients with defective anal control. Squeeze pressures were lower in women than in men but were not influenced by age. Resting and squeeze pressures were also much lower after operations for high versus low intermuscular fistulas. Sainio and Husa (136) conducted a prospective study in which 31 patients with fistulas were assessed preoperatively and 7 months postoperatively. Resting pressures in the anal canal as opposed to voluntary contractions were significantly reduced; however, maximal squeeze pressures were greatly reduced in women and after division of the external sphincter muscle. The authors concluded that in selected cases, especially in women, performing preoperative manometry is advisable, and if low pressures are found, division of the external sphincter muscle should be avoided. This recommendation, unfortunately, ignores the pathogenesis of the disease process, for it must be recognized that in most patients with transsphincteric and suprasphincteric fistulas, division of a portion of the external sphincter is necessary for cure. In these situations the use of a seton may prove of value. Also, the most recent offerings for the treatment of fistula-in-ano such as the anal plug may obviate this necessity if they prove to be effective in the long term.

The results of a study by Pescatori et al. (137) suggest that the use of manometry may improve the clinical and functional outcome of patients. They performed anal manometry preoperatively and postoperatively on 96 patients and modified their operative treatment according to the findings. For example, they may have used a seton rather than a lay-open technique. The recurrence rate was 3% in the anal manometry group and 13% in the control group. Postoperative soiling occurred in 14% of patients in the manometry group compared with 31% in the control group. The functional results were also better in the manometry group.

■ FISTULOTOMY VS. FISTULECTOMY

Controversy exists as to whether a fistulotomy or a fistulectomy is the more appropriate operative treatment for a patient with an anal fistula. However, there are a number of reasons supporting a strong recommendation for fistulotomy. First, removal of the complete tract and adjacent scar tissue only results in appreciably larger wounds. Second, fistulectomy results in a larger separation of the ends of the sphincter, leading to a longer healing time and a greater chance of incontinence (Fig. 37) (138). For these reasons, it would appear that no controversy should exist. In a randomized trial to compare lay-open technique with excision of fistula-in-ano, Kronberg (138) determined that healing times were significantly shorter when the fistula was laid open. At 12 months, incontinence of flatus was noted in one of 20 patients in the lay-open group and in three of 17 patients in the excision group. Recurrence rates were similar, and Kronberg concluded that the lay-open operation was superior to using excision and no advantages were apparent from excision.

■ USE OF SETON

When a tract crosses the sphincter at a high level, it may be deemed safer not to divide all the muscle beneath the tract. Only a portion of the muscle is cut, and a seton is inserted. The rationale for this maneuver is threefold. First, it stimulates fibrosis adjacent to the sphincter muscle so that when the second stage, which involves laying open the tract, is completed, the sphincter will not gape. After insertion of a seton, it is anticipated that division of the sphincter will be followed by scar formation proximal to the ligature, thus holding the muscle fibers together, which, may already have been accomplished by fibrosis of the fistulous tract. Another benefit of the seton is that it allows the surgeon to better delineate the amount of muscle beneath the fistulous tract. With the patient anesthetized, the surgeon cannot always be certain of the amount of muscle caudad to the tract. Re-examination in an awake patient may reveal adequate muscle remaining above the level of the fistulous tract. The third advantage of using the seton is that it acts as a drain (Fig. 38).

Actual insertion of the seton through the fistulous tract is usually a simple matter. However, based on the belief that the pathogenesis of most anal fistulas is cryptoglandular disease, the internal sphincter should be divided from the level of the internal opening at the dentate line to its distal end in order to eradicate the source. The overlying skin is divided from this point to the secondary fistulous opening. A nonabsorbable suture is then threaded through the fistulous tract.

Materials for use and their postoperative management have varied widely. Wire has been advocated because it can be twisted gradually until the loop eventually cuts through the muscle; however, it is uncomfortable to sit on wire, so its use is not recommended. I have used a heavy silk seton and have inserted it with a retention needle passed backward through the tract. If used, this needle must not be passed forward because the cutting edge can easily create a false passage. The silk

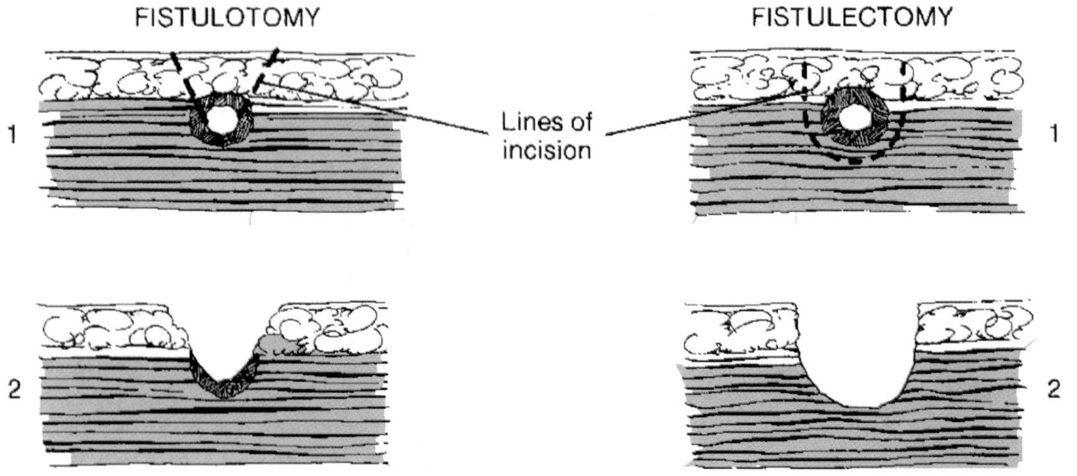

FIGURE 37 ■ Fistulotomy versus fistulectomy. *Source*: After M. Finch.

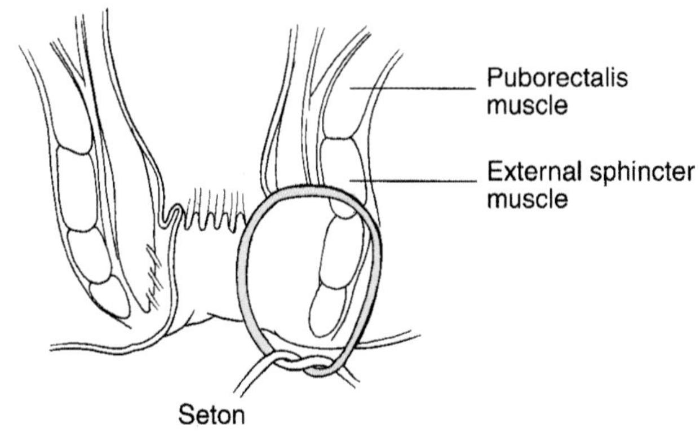

FIGURE 38 ■ Seton insertion.

is then loosely tied with many knots to create a handle for manipulation. For surgeons who believe in a cutting seton, Cirocco and Rusin (139) have described a quick and comfortable approach to seton advancement through the muscle. After initial loose placement, the seton is brought through the drum of a Barron rubber-band ligator (Ford Dixon Co., Dallas, Texas, U.S.) and the instrument is fired, resulting in cinching of the once lax ligature. This enhances advancement of the seton through the external sphincter by pressure necrosis. The procedure may be repeated at 2 to 4-week intervals until the seton has completely cut through the muscle.

Occasionally, because of repeated handling during cleansing, the patient will eventually "saw" through the muscle. Usually, however, the muscle is divided at a second stage 6 to 8 weeks later. Appropriate timing of transection of the sphincter subsequent to seton placement is essential for sufficient fibrosis to ensure sphincter function. When a large portion of muscle is included, it might be wise to divide the remaining muscle in more than one stage. If the wound does heal well, removal of the seton without division of the contained muscle can be considered. Of 34 patients so treated by Thomson and Ross (140), 15 remained healed after seton removal, and 19 required subsequent division of the external sphincter because of persistent or recurrent anal sepsis. In the former group, 83% remained fully continent, whereas in the latter group only 32% remained continent. The authors concluded that cure of transsphincteric fistula with preservation of the external sphincter is possible and may improve continence status but the method prolongs healing time. Buchanan et al. (141) determined the long-term outcome (10 years) after use of the loose-seton technique to eradicate complex fistula-in-ano. Of 20 patients, 18 had a transsphincteric and 2 had a suprasphincteric fistula. There were seven supralevator and 12 ischiorectal secondary extensions. At short-term (6 months) follow-up following seton removal, perianal sepsis had been eradicated in 13 of 20 patients. However, in the long term, 16 patients had persisting or recurrent sepsis, necessitating further operation in 13. In the long term, external sphincter division was necessary to control sepsis in seven of the 20 patients compared with three of 20 patients at short-term follow-up. The rate of relapse in those with Crohn's disease and cryptoglandular fistula-in-ano was similar (5 of 6 vs. 11 of 14). The fistula recurred in 7, 11, and 15 patients at 6, 15, and 60 months, respectively, after seton removal. Counseling before seton removal should emphasize that many patients develop further sepsis that usually require an operation. Hanley (45) advocated the use of a rubber-band seton, with the aim of obtaining a good functional result with minimal deformity of the anus. The elastic seton is tied to a ball-tipped probe and is passed through the tract. The two ends of the seton are tied with a silk suture. At 3 to 4-week intervals, it is tightened by grasping the ends with a forceps, stretching the elastic, and applying another ligature between the first ligature and the muscle. Gradual pressure necrosis will sever the muscle after the seton is tightened three or four times.

Clinical situations in which use of a seton should be considered include high fistulas, anterior fistulas in women, coexistent inflammatory bowel disease (especially Crohn's disease), a markedly, weakened sphincter in elderly individuals, extensive scarring in individuals who have had previous operations, uncertainty about the height of the tract or the amount of muscle previously cut, complex fistulas in AIDS patients, and the presence of simultaneous fistulas. The reported frequency with which setons have been used ranges from 5% to 18% mostly in the 8–10% range (142). van Tets and Kuijpers (143) cautioned against the use of setons for fistulas with high anal or rectal openings. In a review of 34 patients with a two-stage seton procedure (16 extrasphincteric and 18 trans-sphincteric), there were two recurrences but all trans-sphincteric fistulas healed. Of 29 patients with preoperative normal fecal control who were available for follow-up, postoperative continence was normal in 12 patients [category A according to Browning and Parks classification (144)], 5 patients had no control over flatus (category B), 11 were incontinent for liquid stool or flatus (category C), and 1 had continued fecal leakage (category D).

Parks and Stitz (102) assessed function in 68 patients in whom a seton was used. Of those patients who had a seton inserted but removed without further division of muscle, 17% complained of partial loss of control, whereas 39% of patients who later had division of the seton-contained muscle experienced problems with control. Kennedy and Zegarra (145) reported on 32 patients with high trans-sphincteric or suprasphincteric fistulas who underwent incision of skin and subcutaneous tissue overlying the tract along with an internal sphincterotomy and seton placement without external sphincter division. Primary healing after removal of the seton occurred in 78% of patients (66% for posterior fistula and 88% for anterior fistula). Problems controlling flatus occurred in 33%, mucus discharge in 25%, and liquid stool in 4%. The persistence and/or recurrence rate for posterior fistula was 34% and for anterior fistula 12%. These findings support the plan of conserving as much muscle as possible, even though to do so may require repeated procedures to divide the muscle in stages. Nevertheless, this extended healing period seems worthwhile if better continence can be preserved. In view of such data, I believe that it is most reasonable to run the higher risk of recurrence by not dividing the contained muscle in patients in whom the wound is healing satisfactorily.

Ramanujam et al. (146) used setons in 8.5% of their patients. Although the value of using a seton has been questioned, in this report in which all patients had suprasphincteric fistulas, staging the treatment with a seton resulted in only one patient (2.2%) suffering permanent incontinence for flatus and none with fecal incontinence, and the recurrence rate was only 2.2%. It was deemed appropriate to use a seton in 10% of our patients (11). Although 19% of our patients in whom setons were used experienced alterations in continence, this was temporary, and in all cases it was only incontinence of flatus. In addition, setons were used in patients with more complicated fistulas.

A significant difference in seton usage is that Ramanujam et al. (146) prefer to divide the proximal portion of the sphincter mechanism below the tract (deep external sphincter, with or without the puborectalis muscle if involved) and to place the seton around the distal component of the sphincter mechanism, a concept different from that proposed by other seton users (102,138). In a series of 45 patients with suprasphincteric fistulas, use of the latter technique yielded excellent results, with only one patient having incontinence of flatus.

The above discussion highlights the different ways in which setons are used, the different materials employed, and the difference in management after a seton is inserted. Zimmerman (22) reviewed those differences and found that when a cutting seton was used (i.e., loose placement of a seton which is then tightening over several weeks to produce pressure necrosis) the reported incidence of impairment of continence ranged from 0 to 67%, and when a staged seton was employed (i.e., seton placement followed by division of seton-contained muscle 6–8 weeks later) reports of impairment of continence ranged from 3% to 66%. In fact, a direct comparison of the two techniques was reported by Garcia-Aguilar et al. (147) and they found no difference in functional results of recurrence rates.

A summary of results of reported in the literature are recorded in Table 6. The results, of course, are not comparable as some studies report only major fecal incontinence while others report any alteration in fecal continence. Surgeons vary in their indication for seton's usage. The amount of sphincter involved that would otherwise require division will be reflected in the ultimate results. Some authors have combined temporary and permanent incontinence and the results have hot been broken down for incontinence for flatus, liquid, or solid stool; consequently the wide discrepancy in results.

TABLE 6 ■ Results of Use of Seton in Fistula-in-Ano Operations

Author(s)	No. of Patients	Incontinence (%)	Recurrence (%)
Parks and Stitz (102)	68	17–39[a]	
Ramanujam et al. (146)	45	2	2
Vasilevsky and Gordon (11)	16	19[b]	6
Thomson and Ross (140)	34	17–68[c]	
Williams et al. (148)	74	54[d]	18
Pearl et al. (149)	116	5	3
Graf et al. (150)	29	44	8
van Tets and Kuijpers (143)	34	17–38–3[f]	6
Hamalainen and Sainio (151)	35	63	6
Dziki et al. (152)	32	34–38–19–28[i]	0
Garcia-Aguilar (147)	59	53–41–38[h]	8
Balogh (153)	19	0	11
Hasegawa et al. (154)	32	9–32–16[g]	13
Isbister et al. (155)	47	36–9–2[f]	2
Durgun et al. (156)	10	20[e]	—
Theerapal et al. (157)	41	0	2

[a]Seventeen percent incontinent with seton removal; 39% problems with sphincter division.
[b]Temporary incontinence, mostly for flatus.
[c]Seventeen percent incontinent with seton removal; 68% problems with sphincter division.
[d]Patients experienced minor degrees of incontinence.
[e]Incontinence only to flatus (all extrasphincteric fistula).
[f]Incontinence to flatus–liquid stool–solid stool.
[g]Incontinence–major–minor–soiling.
[h]Incontinence to flatus–soiling–solid stool.
[i]Incontinence–flatus-liquid stool-solid stool-soiling.

■ NECROTIZING PERINEAL INFECTION

Key Factors in Morbidity and Mortality

Necrotizing infections of the perineal area are uncommon and may be associated with great morbidity and a high mortality. The incidence of such extensive infection has been estimated as less than 1% of all anorectal sepsis (158). Among English-speaking regions, the highest incidence of the disease occurs in the USA and Canada (159). Many of these infections have been classified into subgroups such as necrotizing fasciitis, clostridial gangrene, synergistic gangrene, and streptococcal gangrene. Heppell and Bénard (160) provided an excellent review of the management of life-threatening perineal sepsis and much of the following information was heavily drawn from that account. They pointed out that a significant number of cases of overwhelming infection have no recognizable cause. Reported causes include genitourinary (24%), anorectal (24%), intra-abdominal (10%), traumatic (2%), and undetermined (38%). The diagnosis is made on clinical grounds. Males outnumber females in a ratio of 10:1 (159). Clinical features may vary from an insidious prodrome consisting of chills, fever, malaise, and local discomfort to an explosive onset with intense pain, followed rapidly by edema, erythema, induration, and finally necrosis and crepitation in a matter of hours. Systemic manifestations of toxicity may include nausea, vomiting, marked tachycardia, high fever, hypotension, and prostration. Important clues to the anorectal origin of the problem may be pain on defecation 2 or 3 days before recognition of swelling, history of previous anorectal operation, infection, or untreated purulent discharge. A delay in diagnosis and treatment of any infection permits wider dissemination of the infection, and morbidity and mortality from infection are usually time and dose related.

Inadequate examination frequently leads to inadequate treatment. The diagnosis of a perianal or ischioanal abscess is straightforward, but in the patient with severe pain who may be harboring an intersphincteric abscess, a general anesthetic may be required for adequate examination. Typically, the perineum and scrotum are painful, edematous, erythematus, warm, and tense. This will progress rapidly to mortification with skin necrosis and induration accompanied by a fetid odor. The typical scrotal black spot described by Fournier is illustrated in Figure 39. Crepitus, the consequence of an infection of gas-producing organisms, may be easily palpated and actual gas and watery pus may be encountered when the surgical incision is made. The area of subcutaneous emphysema will help in delineating the extent of the infectious process and the need for surgical debridement. Polymicrobial cultures of anaerobes and aerobes are the rule. Organisms include clostridia, *Klebsiella*, streptococci, coliforms, staphylococci, bacteroides, and corynebacteria (159).

Predisposing Factors

Every condition that compromises tissue vascularization or alters the immune status has been incriminated as a predisposing factor. Necrotizing perineal infections occur more often in people with poor personal hygiene associated with debilitated states. Poor socioeconomic conditions and alcoholism have also been incriminated (159). Poorly controlled diabetes is the most commonly associated factor. Cortisone therapy, chemotherapy, irradiated tissues, carcinomatosis, malnutrition, sensorineural deficits, polyarteritis nodosa, and hypersensitive vasculitis have also been reported as rare predisposing conditions.

This syndrome has been described in association with various pathologic processes and procedures that are described in Table 7. Local trauma, either thermal, chemical, or mechanical, has been implicated. These fulminating infections may also occur in women during postpartum in episiotomy scars. To this list, Iorianni and Oliver (161) added multiple myeloma, HIV, and a poorly defined immunodeficiency syndrome.

Investigations

Leukocytosis is almost uniformly present, averaging 20,000 leukocytes per μL. Diabetics may present with decompensation and ketoacidosis. Anemia, hyperbilirubinemia, and significant elevations in the blood urea nitrogen to creatinine ratio are sometimes observed. Plain radiography of the pelvis may confirm the presence of subcutaneous gas. The presence of subcutaneous air with normal testicles can also be detected by ultrasonography, which, however, is usually not necessary. CT of the perineum may be useful for detecting perineal abscesses of unusual presentation. Cystourethroscopy, sigmoidoscopy, barium enema, and tissue biopsy to identify or exclude malignancy may be indicated. Examination under anesthesia may be required. Bacteriological examination of pus (preferably syringe aspirate) will determine drug sensitivities.

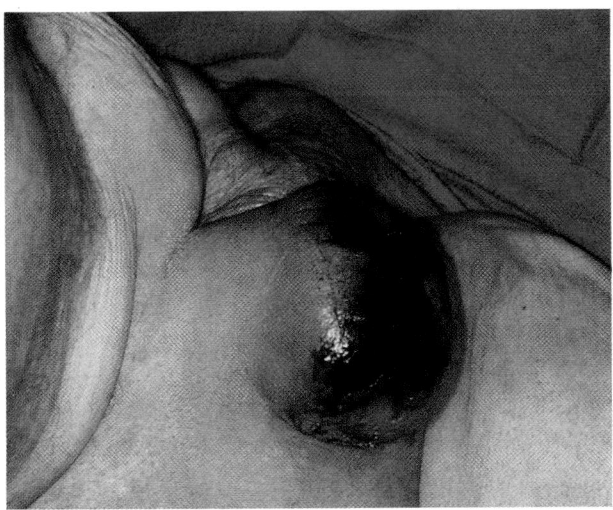

FIGURE 39 ■ Typical scrotal black spot of Fournier's gangrene.

TABLE 7 ■ **Associated Etiologic Factors**

Pathologic Processes	Procedures
Perianal abscess	Leakage after anterior resection
Anal fistula	Indwelling catheter
Retroperitoneal infection	Male sterilization
Complicated diverticulitis	Rubber band ligature
Rectal carcinoma	Thiersch's procedure
Rectal perforation	Rectal mucosal biopsy
Foreign body	Hernia repair
Hemorrhoids	Orchidectomy
Hematologic diseases	Ureterolithotomy
Human bite	Penile prosthetic implant
Heroin injection	Injection of hydrocele
End-stage renal disease	Postpartum

Source: From Ref. 160.

Treatment

After initial fluid and electrolyte corrections and administration of broad-spectrum antibiotics, radical debridement involving extensive excision of all involved skin, fascia, and muscles is performed. Extension may reach the abdominal wall, thighs, chest wall, and axilla (159). Testicular involvement is rare and the only indication for orchiectomy is testicular gangrene. Repeat exploration should be conducted as necessary until the necrotizing process has been interrupted.

In rare instances, anorectal suppuration may assume life-threatening proportions. Abcarian (124) has pointed out that this may be attributed to delay in diagnosis and management; virulence of the organism, especially gas-forming anaerobic bacteria; bacteremia and occurrence of metastatic infections; or underlying disorders (e.g., diabetes mellitus, blood dyscrasias). To this list he later added anorectal trauma (162).

To prevent death, it is recommended to perform immediate incision and drainage and complete debridement, ignoring form and function. Nutritional support may be required. Colostomy also may be indicated. Repeated debridement may be necessary and should be carried out without hesitation. The role of hyperbaric oxygen therapy is of uncertain value (161). Gas gangrene caused by the clostridial group of organisms remains probably the best indication for the use of hyperbaric oxygen (160).

Consten et al. (163) pointed out that in HIV-positive patients with metastatic abscesses, perianal sepsis must always be kept in mind as a possible focus. In their review of 50 HIV-infected patients, seven (14%) had serious septic complications, four with severe necrotizing gangrene and three with abscesses in the mediastinum, liver, and brain. They recommend that although HIV-infected patients have a limited life expectancy, perianal sepsis should be aggressively treated.

Bode et al. (164) addressed three controversial areas in the management of patients with necrotizing perineal infections: fecal diversion, suprapubic cystostomy, and orchiectomy. They consider fecal diversion unnecessary because whole-gut lavage and medical colostomy with total parenteral nutrition or enteral feeding will prevent the morbidity and mortality associated with colostomy and colostomy closure. These measures afford the same advantage as fecal diversion (limitation of perineal soiling) and maintain the patient's nutritional status. They believe that the use of suprapubic catheters is indicated only if urinary tract disease is the source of the sepsis. Because blood supply and venous drainage of the testicles are through the spermatic vessels, testicular necrosis resulting from a fulminant perineal infection is rare. Although scrotal debridement is often necessary, the testicles may be "banked" with their intact blood supply in normal abdominal wall or thigh pockets.

In a report by Abcarian and Eftaiha (162) in which 1020 patients with anorectal infections were treated, 2.3% developed massive tissue necrosis, leaving the anorectum devoid of its anatomic support unilaterally, bilaterally, or circumferentially, thus resulting in "floating" or "free-standing" anus. Despite the extent of the disease, with adoption of aggressive supportive therapy, appropriate use of antibiotics, and early extensive debridement of necrotic tissue, no deaths resulted and a colostomy was not deemed necessary. Even in severely immunocompromised patients, synergistic bacterial gangrene is not inevitably fatal and radical surgery can result in cure (165).

The prognosis of patients with this syndrome remains guarded, with mortality rates reported from 3% to 45% (158,159). These rates can be significantly diminished by early diagnosis and prompt radical operation. Causes of death have included severe sepsis, coagulopathy, acute renal failure, diabetic ketoacidosis, and multiple organ failure (160). In a review by Korkut et al. (166) of 45 patients with Fournier's gangrene, the most prominent associated disease was diabetes. The overall mortality rate was 20% but increased to 36% among diabetics. None of the nondiabetic patients died. Other predictors of outcome were the interval from the onset of symptoms to the initial operative intervention (less than seven days, mortality = 0; more than seven days, mortality = 39.1%) and the need for diversion.

■ REPEAT EXAMINATION WITH PATIENT UNDER ANESTHESIA

In the exceptional patient in whom a fistula is complicated by high upward extensions to the apex of the ischioanal fossa or the supralevator fossa, sound healing occurring from the apex caudad must be ensured. To achieve this goal, the surgeon should not hesitate to re-examine the patient who is under general anesthesia in the operating room one week to 10 days after the initial operation. If at these times healing is progressing satisfactorily, only curettage of excessive granulation tissue that has formed need be done. If pocketing has occurred, it can be corrected, or if further branched tracts are discovered, they can be opened. The upward extension of a tract must heal soundly before the caudad part of the wound is allowed to heal. If at any point the surgeon is dissatisfied with the healing, especially if pus is accumulating, examination in the operating room is indicated, and the wound may need to be enlarged and reshaped. Careful follow-up of extremely complicated fistulas may help prevent recurrence.

■ CARCINOMA ASSOCIATED WITH CHRONIC FISTULA-IN-ANO

Patients with long-standing fistulas or recurrent abscesses around the anus may on exceedingly rare occasions develop carcinoma. The rarity of this entity is underscored by the fact that fewer than 150 cases were reported in the literature up to 1981 (167). Several theories exist about the origin of these neoplasms. It has been suggested that such a carcinoma arises because of the deposition of malignant cells from a carcinoma located more proximally in the gastrointestinal tract and that colloid carcinomas arise in duplications of the lower end of the hindgut (168–172). Carcinoma arising in anal glands is another theory. Such neoplasms may be epidermoid or transitional, with little or no gland formation (173). Others believe that fistulas arise because of mucin production after extension of the carcinoma into perirectal tissues (174). The last theory is that carcinoma may arise in a pre-existing fistula-in-ano (167,175).

Criteria to attribute a carcinoma arising in a fistula-in-ano include that (1) the fistula should predate the carcinoma, (2) there should be no synchronous colorectal carcinoma, and (3) the internal opening of the fistula should be into the anal canal and not the malignancy.

The most common form of carcinoma to arise in a fistula is colloid carcinoma (44%), followed by squamous cell carcinoma (34%), and adenocarcinoma (22%) (176). Patients with this neoplasm usually present with complaints of increasing pain, a perianal mass, or a change in the nature of the fistulous discharge (Fig. 40). The initial diagnosis is often perianal abscess. It is only after a biopsy that the diagnosis is made. A clue to the early recognition of the disease has been described recently: the appearance of mucin globules in fistulotomy or fistulectomy specimens can alert the pathologist to the possibility of perianal mucinous adenocarcinoma, resulting in early diagnosis and treatment (177). Should such

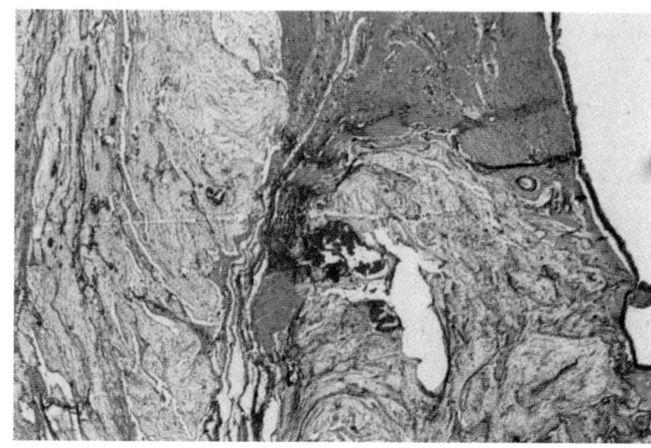

FIGURE 40 ■ Mucinous adenocarcinoma arising in a fistula-in-ano. *Source*: Courtesy of J. Byron Gathright, M.D., New Orleans, Louisiana, U.S.A.

a diagnosis be confirmed, abdominoperineal resection is required (178), but the prognosis is poor. In inoperable cases, radiotherapy may be of some value, especially in patients with squamous epithelioma. A recent report suggests combination chemoradiotherapy in conjunction with an aggressive operative approach may result in long-term survival (179).

■ UNNECESSARY CRYPTOTOMY

In the past, a frequently proposed adjuvant procedure has been the obliteration of the crypts along the dentate line. Cryptotomy or cryptectomy was carried out in the hope of preventing development of inflammation, fissures, or abscesses. However, because of the anatomic features of the anal canal and the pathogenesis of a fistula, as described earlier in this chapter, such manipulation would not prevent disease but might contribute to it. Therefore, since such procedures are in no way helpful and are potentially harmful, they should be abandoned.

■ ASSOCIATED PROCEDURES

A hemorrhoidectomy may be performed in association with the treatment of fistula-in-ano, for example, in a patient who has very large or prolapsing hemorrhoids. However, each case must be individualized. Also, the complication of mucosal prolapse is not an infrequent consequence of extensive muscle division and is easily treated by injection, rubber-band ligation, or operative excision.

■ SEPTIC COMPLICATIONS IN IMMUNOCOMPROMISED PATIENTS

In a patient with leukemia, the occurrence of perianal complications such as ischioanal abscess, fistula-in-ano, fissures, or infected thrombosed ulcerated hemorrhoids poses a very special problem. Performing injudicious incision and drainage procedures in patients with acute leukemia or uncontrolled chronic leukemia can result in necrosis of the perineal area accompanied by uncontrolled septicemia and hemorrhage and may end with sloughing of the whole buttock area and fecal incontinence.

Barnes et al. (180), in a review of the literature, reported that perianal infection in patients with acute leukemia has been associated with mortality rates of 45% to 78%; perirectal infections occurred in 7.9% of their 202 patients with acute leukemia. Lesions were painful, indurated, and associated with urinary retention, peritoneal signs, and extension to genitalia in some cases. Fifteen patients had infections. In 10 the infections were incised, and in 5 they drained spontaneously, and the patients became pain free in <48 hours and afebrile in 2–8 days. Drained lesions all healed. Thirteen of 15 patients left the hospital, whereas 2 died of unrelated causes. The authors believe that their policy of early incision and debridement contributed to their patients' improved survival rate.

Shaked et al. (181) reported on a series of 15 granulocytopenic patients with acute perianal inflammatory disease. Treatment included antibiotic coverage alone or in combination with surgical drainage. This study showed that surgical drainage during agranulocytosis resulted in slow wound healing, prolonged hospitalization, and a higher mortality rate when compared with the group that received antibiotics only (28% vs. 18%). In addition, the authors found that when the incision and drainage were performed after the granulocyte count increased above 1000 cells/mm^3, the postoperative course was uncomplicated, with subsequent good healing. Patients who underwent operations while still granulocytopenic showed no noticeable improvement in their general condition. Carlson et al. (182) also reported that the operative drainage of perianal infection apparently does not increase the survival rate or decrease the morbidity rate in patients with severe granulocytopenia (<500 polymorphonuclear leukocytes/mm^3). Of 20 patients, 9 were treated with operation. The operative mortality was 44.4% vs. 9% in those treated nonoperatively with an overall mortality rate of 25%. It is possible that those patients treated operatively had more extensive infection because progression of local infection occurred in three of them, of whom two required a colostomy.

Chirletti et al. (183) reported their experience in the treatment of patients with septic complications in the presence of a variety of leukemias. The authors stressed the need for prompt operative treatment to prevent the risk of general sepsis, which occurs frequently in immunosuppressed patients, and for early resumption of the antiblastic chemotherapy that is mandatory in these cases. In their review, 38 of 40 patients were cured of their infective complications.

Grewal et al. (184) conducted a retrospective review of 2618 hospitalized patients with leukemia. Concomitant symptomatic anorectal disease was present in 151 (5.8%) patients. Data from 81 patients were available for analysis. Nonoperative treatment was pursued in 52 (64%) patients and 29 (36%) underwent operative therapy. Absolute neutrophil counts of <1000/mm^3 were present in 57 (70.4%) while 54 (66.7%) were severely neutropenic (absolute neutrophil count <500/mm^3). Management and outcomes of 54 severely neutropenic patients were analyzed. In 20 patients who underwent operation, there were 4 deaths (20%) and 4 recurrences (20%), whereas in 34 patients managed nonoperatively, there were 6 deaths (18%) and 4 recurrences (12%). In these patients, anorectal sepsis was a major source of mortality. Their data suggested that anorectal abscesses in neutropenic leukemic patients might be safely drained. Because they did not observe excessive morbidity or mortality (20% vs. 18%) in the operated neutropenic leukemics as compared with the nonoperated patients, they concluded that selected neutropenic leukemic patients should not be denied anorectal operations when otherwise indicated.

Munoz-Villasmil et al. (185) reviewed 83 immunocompromised patients with a diagnosis of perianal sepsis. Associated conditions included HIV+ patients 28%, IBD on steroids 34%, malignancies 20%, and diabetes 18%. Anal fistulas were present in 28%, perianal abscess in 2% and in 40% both were present. The most common procedure performed was a primary fistulotomy. Most wounds (91%) healed within eight weeks. Incontinence (6%) and recurrence (7%) were the most commonly observed complications. They noted that the results were similar to those seen in the general population.

Cohen et al. (186) reviewed their experience of the treatment of perianal infection following bone marrow transplant, a situation often associated with profound neutropenia. Of 963 patients undergoing bone marrow transplants, 24 developed perianal sepsis. Of these 24 patients, 15 did not have purulent collections and were treated with antibiotics and supportive measures alone. The remaining nine patients (38%) required operative intervention at 10–380 days following transplant and a purulent collection was found in seven of these patients. They found that for the most part wound healing was not prolonged.

Nadal et al. (187) compared wound healing after anal fistulotomy in HIV+ and HIV− patients. A fistulotomy for an intersphincteric fistula was performed in 60 patients. For each patient they evaluated the white blood cell count, TCD4 counts, Centre for Disease Control and Prevention classification, and healing duration. There were 31 HIV+ patients. Statistically there was no difference in the healing in HIV+ and HIV− patients. They obtained a significant difference only in those patients classified with clinical AIDS with a WBC <3000 and a CD4 T-cell count <200. They concluded that operation should be done only in emergency cases in the latter situation.

■ INDEPENDENT FISTULAS

It is distinctly uncommon for a patient to have entirely separate fistulas. Should both fistulas be simple and straightforward without involving large portions of the sphincter mechanism, each can be treated as a simple fistula. However, if a larger amount of the sphincter muscle is involved by both fistulas, one may be treated as a straightforward fistula, and the other (the more complex fistula) may be treated with the use of a seton.

■ COMBINATION FISTULAS

Patients may have various combinations of the fistulas described in the classification. Recognition of the various components is mandatory to obtain successful treatment. If one component is not recognized, the patient will be classified as having a recurrent fistula when, in fact, the patient has a persistent untreated fistula.

■ ANOPERINEAL TUBERCULOSIS

Gastrointestinal tuberculosis comprises $<1\%$ of all cases and anoperineal disease (1% of digestive tract incidence) is exceedingly rare (188). Sultan et al. (188) noted in their practice that TB represents 0.31% of anal fistulas and abscesses but in their review noted that in developing countries the incidence is 16%. Much of the following information was extracted from their review. Anoperineal TB is most common in men (77% to 100% of cases) and occurs secondary to a primary site in the lungs. There is no functional sign or preferred site that allows a tuberculosis fistula to be distinguished from a cryptoglandular fistula. A gaping external fistulous orifice with detached margins and highly vascular in nature is suggestive. A higher frequency of complex tuberculous fistula (62% to 100%) sometimes puts the sphincter and continence at risk.

The ulcerated form of anal TB typically presents as a superficial ulceration, not hardened, with a hemorrhagic necrotic base that is granular and covered with thick purulent secretions and mucus. The lesion may be painful or the patient may have few symptoms. Here the diagnosis is based on histology.

The tuberculin skin test remains a valuable guide because it is positive in 75% of cases. A positive diagnosis of anal TB depends on histologic or bacteriologic analysis. The typical histologic lesion is the epitheliod and giant cell tubercle around a zone of caseous necrosis, but the pathognomonic presence of caseation is not constant. The diagnosis can also be made by direct examination (Ziehl Nielsen stain) and culture. More expedient than culture, genomic amplification can detect the presence of the bacterial DNA in 48 hours with high sensitivity and specificity. The diagnosis may also be suspected from clinical symptoms and patients arriving from endemic areas. The differential diagnosis is primarily Crohn's disease (Table 8). Other possible granulomatous diseases of the anus can occur such as amebiasis, reaction to a foreign body, sarcoidosis, syphilis, and venereal lymphogranuloma with chlamydia trachomatis. Anal TB can simulate cancer.

Management consists of specific antituberculous therapy. In some cases, tuberculous fistula-in-ano may heal with antibiotic therapy alone. Should the anal lesion not resolve, conventional management should be instituted as a secondary stage of therapy with drainage of abscesses, and fistula operations as required.

Kraemer et al. (189) reported on 20 patients with anal tuberculous sepsis—abscesses ($n=2$), abscesses and fistulas

TABLE 8 ■ Differential Diagnosis for Crohn's Disease and Anoperineal Tuberculosis

	Crohn's Disease	Anoperineal Tuberculosis
Age (years)	20–30	>50
Gender origin	Same in both genders	Males ++ Immigrant population; bad socioeconomic condition
Clinical aspect	Either typical (deep ulceration) or nonspecific (fissure, abscess, recurring fistula)	Nonspecific in general (recurring fistula, superficial ulceration)
Lung X-ray	Normal in most cases	Tuberculosis (active or sequelae)
Tuberculin skin test	Negative	Positive
Digestive tract affected	Frequent (ileocecal ++)	Rare (ileocecal ++)
Histology	Granuloma without caseation or nonspecific	Granuloma (more numerous, larger, often merging together and rich in multinucleated giant cells; ± caseation; PCR (± ELISA blood)
Culture of Koch's bacillus	Negative	Positive or negative (excised tissue, urine, gastric secretion)
Response to antituberculosis drugs	Rare	Good
Progress after well-managed treatment	Relapse; Crohn's lesions in the digestive tract	Healing; without relapse; no lesions in the digestive tract

Abbreviations: ++, most frequent; PCR, polymerase chain reactor; ELISA, enzyme-linked immunosorbent assay.
Source: From Ref. 188.

($n=6$) or fistulas ($n=12$). All patients had a long history of anal complaints (three months to 20 years), for which 15 patients were operated on previously. Nearly all fistulas (17 out of 18) were complex and secondary tracts or additional complicating features were common, even at first presentation. Eight patients had active concurrent pulmonary tuberculosis, and six showed evidence of previous pulmonary tuberculosis. Recurrence was observed only in cases where tuberculosis was initially not recognized, and antitubercular treatment therefore was not started. They concluded that it should be considered in cases of known pulmonary or extrapulmonary tuberculosis or if anal sepsis is persistent, recurrent, or complex in nature.

■ ANAL FISTULAS ASSOCIATED WITH CROHN'S DISEASE

A major controversy concerns the management of patients with an anal fistula in the presence of Crohn's disease. For a complete discussion, see Chapter 27.

■ RECTOURETHRAL FISTULAS

Rectourethral and prostatic fistulas have been an uncommon but increasingly occurring complication of radical prostatectomy and radiation. In the past, it has been a complication of surgery of benign prostatic obstruction, perineal prostatectomy, and perineal biopsy of the prostate, an etiology that has dramatically shifted during the past two decades due to the unprecedented volume of high dose or salvage brachytherapy, cryotherapy, and radical open and laparoscopic prostatectomy (190). Fistula after radiation therapy is more complex and often has the associated complications of urinary and anal incontinence along with urethral strictures creating a more burdensome reconstructive effort.

Zinman (190) published his extensive experience with this condition. The following information has been extracted from that publication. The descriptions of the operative repairs of complex rectourethral fistulas are those described by him.

The clinical presentation of rectourethral fistula is usually characterized with 90% of the patients initially experiencing rectal passage of urine, 58% noting pneumaturia and fecaluria and a small percentage developing urinary tract infections with multiple organisms or a minor degree of metabolic acidosis with an elevated serum chloride. Fistulas developing after radiation or cyrotherapy for prostatic carcinoma may present initially with severe rectal pain, which is resolved when the radiated walls break open and fistula appears. A small number will present with pelvic or abdominal sepsis requiring urgent drainage and fecal diversion. Retrograde urethrography, voiding cystourethrogram, and urethroscopic cannulation of the fistula with an injection fistulogram may help define some of the more elusive lesions.

Cystourethroscopy with simultaneous digital rectal examination will usually confirm the presence of most fistulas and sigmoidoscopy and colonoscopy will localize the level of the rectal entry, help identify anal sphincter integrity, confirm the absence of other rectal pathology, such as proctitis, or a colonic carcinoma and better define the extent of radiation injury. This information will aid in determining the optimal time for repair and the need and type of fecal diversion required. The lower trans-sphincteric rectourethral fistula secondary to Crohn's disease or any anterior rectal space infection are the most elusive and are best identified by MRI imaging.

The complex rectourethral fistula with an intact anal sphincter can be diverted by a temporary ileostomy, which is readily performed laparoscopically. If there is clearly an irreversible injury to the anal sphincter, then a colostomy would be a better form of permanent diversion. This can be accomplished at the time of the repair unless poorly controlled sepsis, severe rectal pain, or overwhelming urinary and fecal incontinence requires more urgent pre-repair fecal diversion.

The advisability of fecal diversion is not necessarily routine, but should be mandatory in cases of a tenuous repair, prior failed attempts at closure, and complex cases caused by radiation, cryotherapy, or large fistulas that do not lend themselves to primary direct approximation without use of the adjuncts such as a patch graft onlay and an interposition muscle flap. In general, whenever a sound repair has not been achieved, fecal diversion should be an integral part of the reconstruction.

Numerous operative procedures exist for repair of rectourethral fistulas. These include the York-Mason posterior transanosphincteric approach, a transanal advancement flap without rectal wall mobilization, and anterior perineal approaches involving the use of a gracilis muscle buttress. The specific procedure selections are based largely on size, etiology, history of prior failed attempts at closure, and the need to repair concomitant urethral or bladder neck disease.

An anterior transanosphincteric exposure proposed by Gecelter in 1973 has been chosen exclusively for small fistulas of traumatic or surgical origin when a simultaneous urethral reconstruction is planned and there is a normal anal sphincter with no prior anorectal pathology. It also affords wide access, ease of instrument maneuvering, facility to repair the proximal urethra, and ability to transfer buttressing interposition flaps. The technique has been applied to 12 patients whose fistulas occurred following radical retropubic prostatectomy, laparoscopic prostatectomy, pelvic fracture trauma with associated urethral distraction defect and cold knife urethrotomy.

The technique is performed in the dorsal lithotomy using direct O.R. stirrups with anus and rectum exposed. The fistula is catheterized cystoscopically using the ureteral catheter as a guide and an anterior midsagittal incision is made extending from the scrotal base to the anal verge. The dissection is restricted to the midline where the transverse perineal muscles, central tendon and anal sphincter complex are transected inclusive of the internal and external components, including the rectal wall to the fistula site. Strict adherence to a midline approach will prevent anorectal or cavernous nerve injury. The transverse perineal and external sphincter muscle segments are tagged in pairs with silk sutures for subsequent anatomical restoration similar to that manner used in the York-Mason. Any urethral stricture or fistula pathology can be managed at this point by either an anastomotic or substitution procedure or multilayer closure.

A gracilis muscle is harvested from a posterior medial thigh incision and transferred on its proximal dominant pedicle through a capacious (three-finger) tunnel into the anterior perineal space where it is fixed against the urethral closure. The covering epimysium is incised to gain sufficient width so that the muscle will traverse the space and completely separate the rectum from the urethra and prostate. The rectum is closed with a running 3–0 polygalactin suture in two layers. The internal and external anorectal musculatures are approximated using the paired tagging sutures to help prevent the muscle from retracting.

The catheters are removed at three weeks if a voiding cystourethrogram demonstrates a secure closure. The fecal stoma is reversed in 3 months if repeat anal sphincter studies are acceptable and cystourethroscopy confirms an intact rectal and urethral wall. In general, anorectal sphincteric function will permit control of solid stool in 2 to 3 weeks and liquid and gas continence in 3 to 6 weeks after a transsphincteric closure.

An anterior sphincter preserving traditional perineal approach through a classic inverted U-shaped incision has been utilized in the remainder of his patients. Small rectourethral, bladder neck or prostatic fistulas of surgical or traumatic origin less than 1.5–2 cm are repaired through a midline dissection above the external sphincter avoiding lateral and posterior exposure. This type of dissection will prevent injury to the innervation of the rectum, anal sphincter, and penile corpora, thus preventing loss of potency and urinary continence. This technique is particularly applicable to the patient who has a history of failed prior repairs, anorectal pathology (sphincteric), radiation or preoperative studies that reveal any anosphincteric dysfunction and any factors that have potential for permanent anal sphincter injury.

A subset of complex fistulae that were 2 to 6 cm in size and were not amenable to a primary layered closure were also managed through a classic anterior perineal approach with meticulous preservation of the external anal sphincter. This type of fistula occurred following external beam radiation, brachytherapy, cryotherapy, and recurrence following failed prior repairs. These fistulas were complex by virtue of an etiology that created compromised wound healing, size that precluded primary closure by direct approximation, prior failed attempts at closure resulting in fibrous hypovascular space with loss of surgical planes, and the associated comorbidity of urinary and rectal sphincter injury. The reparative procedure is performed in a moderately exaggerated dorsal lithotomy position with an inverted U-shaped incision that may require a vertical midline extension if the urethra requires stricture repair. The rectum, urethra, prostate, and subvesical surfaces are separated with extension of the dissection to the peritoneum and aggressive debridement of the fistula margins. The rectum is widely mobilized and preferentially closed transversely with a two-layer closure to prevent anal stenosis. A tailored buccal graft patch retrieved from the inner cheek is placed on the urethral or prostatic floor defect, as this defect will not usually permit direct approximation of the fistula edges. A radiation bulbomembranous urethral stricture can be repaired at the same time by extending the urethrotomy ventrally and adding a second buccal strip to augment the urethral lumen. These grafts would not survive in this unfavorable radiated and fibrotic, avascular environment without a well vascularized muscle flap. The gracilis muscle, an expendable adductor of the thigh, can be readily transferred through a capacious tunnel into the anterior perineal space where it is securely anchored to the graft in a tension-free state. By incising the surface membrane (epimysium), it can be spread and fixed against the buccal patch graft while simultaneously separating the rectal and urethral suture lines and filling in any existing dead space. The muscle flap becomes, essentially, the recipient bed for the graft and is largely responsible for the consistently successful closure of this complex lesion.

Fecal undiversion has been successfully performed in 24 out of 27 complex rectourethral fistulas at anywhere from 3 months to 2 years when studies to confirm fistula closure were established and rectal continence clearly noted to be intact. Two patients have socially acceptable minor fecal soiling and one had anal stenosis managed by periodic dilations. Four concomitant urethral reconstructions are stable with patent lumens. Two patients with bulbous urethral strictures are being managed conservatively and one has undergone continent stomal urinary diversion. One patient has had a colon conduit with normal rectal function and three have colostomy fecal diversion after repair of the urethral defect with concomitant proctectomy. One patient has had lower rectal excision with urethral repair and a simultaneous in situ coloanal anastomosis. Concurrent urinary incontinence was present in 7 of the 27 patients undergoing repair. Six of these were managed with an artificial urinary sphincter with delayed erosion in the proximal bulbous urethra of one patient who had combined brachytherapy and external beam radiation and a transcorporal placement. One patient had complete wound separation and failure of fistula closure and is waiting for secondary closure.

In conclusion, this heterogeneous group of large complex rectourethral fistulas can be closed successfully with preservation of rectal and urinary function by a wide classic anterior perineal exposure. It requires the use of an aggressive debridement, a buccal mucosal patch graft onlay for the urethral defect, and routine use of interposition gracilis muscle flap to separate suture lines, enhance graft take and bring an unimpaired circulation to this hypovascular space. This reconstructive approach should obviate the need for proctectomy in most complex large rectourethral fistulas of radiation etiology.

REFERENCES

1. Eisenhammer S. The internal anal sphincter and the anorectal abscess. Surg Gynecol Obstet 1956; 103:501–506.
2. Eisenhammer S. A new approach to the anorectal fistulous abscess on the high intramuscular lesion. Surg Gynecol Obstet 1958; 106:595–599.
3. Parks AG. Pathogenesis and treatment of fistula-in-ano. Br Med J 1961; 1: 463–469.
4. Morson BC, Dawson IMP. Gastrointestinal Pathology. London: Blackwell Scientific Publications, 1972.
5. Lunniss PJ, Sheffield JP, Talbot IC, Thomson JPS, Phillips RKS. Persistence of idiopathic anal fistula may be related to epithelialization. Br J Surg 1995; 82:32–33.
6. Goligher JC, Ellis M, Pissidis AG. A critique of anal glandular infection in the etiology and treatment of idiopathic anorectal abscesses and fistulas. Br J Surg 1967; 54:977–983.

7. Seow-Choen F, Hay AJ, Heard S, Phillips RKS. Bacteriology of anal fistulae. Br J Surg 1992; 79:27–28.
8. Mortensen NJ, Thomson JP. Perianal abscess due to *Enterobius vermicularis*. Dis Colon Rectum 1984; 27:677–678.
9. Feigen GM. Suppurative anal cryptitis associated with *Trichuris trichiura*. Dis Colon Rectum 1987; 30:620–622.
10. Vasilevsky CA, Gordon PH. The incidence of recurrent abscess or fistula-in-ano following anorectal suppuration. Dis Colon Rectum 1984; 27:126–130.
11. Vasilevsky CA, Gordon PH. Results of treatment of fistula-in-ano. Dis Colon Rectum 1985; 28:225–231.
12. Parks AG, Thomson JPS. Intersphincteric abscess. Br Med J 1972; 2:537–539.
13. Cirocco WC, Reilly JC. Challenging the predictive accuracy of Goodsall's rule for anal fistulas. Dis Colon Rectum 1992; 35:537–542.
14. Marks CG, Ritchie JK. Anal fistulas at St. Mark's Hospital. Br J Surg 1977; 64:84–91.
15. Parks AG, Gordon PH. Perineal fistula of intra-abdominal or intra pelvic origin simulating fistula-in-ano: report of seven cases. Dis Colon Rectum 1976; 19:500–506.
16. Kuijpers HC, Schulpen T. Fistulography for fistula-in-ano. Is it useful? Dis Colon Rectum 1985; 28:103–104.
17. Weisman RI, Orsay CP, Pearl RK, Abcarian H. The role of fistulography in fistula-in-ano: report of five cases. Dis Colon Rectum 1991; 34:181–184.
18. Cataldo PA, Senagore A, Luchtefeld MA. Intrarectal ultrasound in the evaluation of perirectal abscess. Dis Colon Rectum 1993; 36:554–558.
19. Cheong DMO, Nogueras JJ, Wexner SD, Jagelman DG. Anal endosonography for recurrent anal fistulas: image enhancement with hydrogen peroxide. Dis Colon Rectum 1993; 36:1158–1160.
20. Choen S, Burnett S, Bartram CF, Nicholls RJ. Comparison between anal endosonography and digital examination in the evaluation of anal fistulae. Br J Surg 1991; 78:445–447.
21. Chew SS, Yang JL, Newstead GL, Douglas PR. Anal Fistula: levovist enhanced endoanal ultrasound: a pilot study. Dis colon Rectum 2003; 46:377–384.
22. Zimmerman DDE. Diagnosis and treatment of transsphincteric perianal fistulas. PhD thesis optima, Grafische Communication Rotterdom, 2003.
23. Maruyama R, Noguchi T, Takano M, et al. Usefulness of magnetic resonance imaging for diagnosing deep anorectal abscesses. Dis Colon Rectum 2000; 43(10 suppl):S2–S5.
24. Barker PG, Lunniss PJ, Armstrong P, Reznek RH, Cottam K, Phillips RKS. Magnetic resonance imaging of fistula-in-ano: technique, interpretation, and accuracy. Clin Radiol 1994; 49:7–13.
25. Chapple KS, Spencer JA, Windsor ACJ, Wilson D, Ward J, Ambrose NS. Prognostic value of magnetic resonance imaging in the management of fistula-in-ano. Dis Colon Rectum 2000; 43:511–516.
26. Buchanan G, Halligan S, Williams A, et al. Effect of MRI on Clinical outcome of recurrent fistula-in-ano. Lancet 2002; 360:1661–1662.
27. Beets-Tan RG, Beets GL, van der Hoop AG, et al. Preoperative MR imaging of anal fistulas: does it really help the surgeon? Radiology 2001; 218:75–84.
28. Myhr GE, Myrvold HE, Nilsen G, Thoresen JE, Rinck PA. Perianal fistulas: use of MR imaging for diagnosis. Radiology 1994; 191:545–549.
29. Hussain SM, Stoker J, Schouten WR, et al. Fistula in ano: endoanal; sonography versus endoanal MR imaging in classification. Radiology 1996; 200:475–481.
30. Maier AG, Funovics MA, Kreuzer SH, et al. Evaluation of perianal sepsis: comparison of anal endosonography and magnetic resonance imaging. J Magn Reson Imaging 2001; 14:254–260.
31. West RL, Zimmerman DD, Dwarkasing S, et al. Prospective comparison of hydrogen peroxide-enhanced three-dimensional endoanal ultrasonography and endoanal magnetic resonance imaging of perianal fistulas. Dis Colon Rectum 2003; 46:1407–1415.
32. Beckingham IJ, Spencer JA, Ward JA, et al. Prospective evaluation of dynamic contrast enhanced magnetic resonance imaging in the evaluation of fistula-in-ano. Br J Surg 1996; 83:1396–1398.
33. Coremans G, Margaritis V, Van Poppel HP, et al. Actinomycosis, a rare and unsuspected cause of anol fistulous abscess: report of three cases and review of the literature. Dis Colon Rectum 2005; 48:575–581.
34. Grace RH, Harper IA, Thompson RG. Anorectal sepsis: microbiology in relation to fistula-in-ano. Br J Surg 1982; 69:401–403.
35. Fielding MA, Berry AR. Management of perianal sepsis in a district general hospital. J R Coll Surg Edinb 1992; 37:232–234.
36. Parker SJ, Dale RF. Is perianal sepsis adequately managed? The results of a five-year audit at Royal Naval Hospital, Haslar. J R Nav Med Serv 1994; 80:148–151.
37. Ramanujam PS, Prasad ML, Abcarian H, Tan AB. Perianal abscesses and fistulas. Dis Colon Rectum 1984; 27:593–597.
38. Isbister WH. A simple method for the management of anorectal abscesses. Aust N Z J Surg 1987; 57:771–774.
39. Oliver I, Lacueva J, Perez Vicente F, et al. Randomized clinical trial comparing simple drainage of anorectal abscess with and without fistula track treatment. Int J Colorectal Dis 2003; 18:107–110.
40. Winslett MC, Allan A, Ambrose NS. Anorectal sepsis as a presentation of occult rectal and systemic disease. Dis Colon Rectum 1988; 31:597–600.
41. Prasad ML, Read DR, Abcarian H. Supralevator abscesses: diagnosis and treatment. Dis Colon Rectum 1981; 24:456–461.
42. Tonkin Dm, Murphy E, Brooke-Smith M. et al. Perianal abscess: a pilot study comparing packing with nonpacking of the abscess cavity. Dis colon Rectum 2004; 47:1510–1514.
43. Chrabot CM, Prasad ML, Abcarian H. Recurrent anorectal abscesses. Dis Colon Rectum 1983; 26:105–108.
44. Hanley PH. Reflections on anorectal abscess fistula 1984. Dis Colon Rectum 1985; 28:528–533.
45. Hanley PH. Rubber-band seton in the management of abscess anal fistula. Ann Surg 1978; 187:435–437.
46. Hanley PH, Ray JE, Pennington EE, Grablowsky OM. A ten-year follow up study of horseshoe-abscess fistula-in-ano. Dis Colon Rectum 1976; 19:507–515.
47. Onaca N, Hirshberg A, Adar R. Early reoperation for perirectal abscess: a preventable complication. Dis Colon Rectum 2001; 44:1469–1473.
48. Seow-Choen F, Nicholls RJ. Anal fistula. Br J Surg 1992; 79:197–205.
49. Parks AG, Gordon PH, Hardcastle JE. A classification of fistula-in-ano. Br J Surg 1976; 63:1–12.
50. Malouf AJ, Buchanan GN, Carapeti EA, et al. A prospective audit of fistula-in-ano at St. Mark's hospital. Colorectal Dis 2002; 4:13–19.
51. Garcia-Aguilar J, Belmonte C, Wong WD, Goldberg SM, Ma-doff RD. Anal fistula surgery. Factors associated with recurrence and incontinence. Dis Colon Rectum 1996; 39:723–729.
52. Steltzner F. Die Anorectalen Fisteln. Berlin: Springer-Verlag, 1959.
53. Lilius HG. Fistula-in-ano, an investigation of human fetal anal ducts and intramuscular glands and a clinical study of 150 patients. Acta Chir Scand Suppl 1968; 383:1–88.
54. Gordon PH. The chemically defined diet and anorectal procedures. Can J Surg 1976; 19:511–513.
55. Maxwell-Armstrong CA, Phillips RKS. Extrasphincteric nectal fistula treated successfully by Soave's procedure despite marked local sepsis. Br J Surg 2003; 90:137–138.
56. Mazier WP. The treatment and care of anal fistulas: a study of 1000 patients. Dis Colon Rectum 1971; 14:134–144.
57. Ho YH, Tan M, Leong AF, Seow-Choen F. Marsupialization of fistulotomy wounds improves healing: a randomized controlled trial. Br J Surg 1998; 85:105–107.
58. Sohn N, Korelitz BI, Weinstein MA. Anorectal Crohn's disease: definitive surgery for fistulas and recurrent abscesses. Am J Surg 1981; 139:394–397.
59. Buchanan GN, Williams AB, Bartram CI, Halligan S, Nicholls RJ, Cohen CR. Potential clinical implications of direction of a trans-sphincteric anal fistula track. Br J Surg 2003; 90:1250–1255.
60. Ustynoski K, Rosen L, Stasik J, Riether R, Sheets J, Khubchandani IT. Horseshoe abscess fistula: seton treatment. Dis Colon Rectum 1990; 33:602–605.
61. Pezim ME. Successful treatment of horseshoe fistula requires deroofing of deep post anal space. Am J Surg 1994; 167:513–515.
62. Kupferberg A, Zer M, Rabinson S. The use of PMMA beads in recurrent high anal fistula: a preliminary report. World J Surg 1984; 8:970–974.
63. Lindsey I, Smilgin-Humphrey MM, Cunningham C, Mortensen NJM, George BD. A randomized, controlled trial of fibrin glue vs conventional treatment for anal fistula. Dis Colon Rectum 2002; 45:1608–1615.
64. MacRae H, Weins E, Orrom W. The use of fibrin glue in the treatment of complex fistula-in-ano. Colon Rectal Surg Outlook 1993; 6(10):1.
65. Chiu YSY. Long-term follow up of fibrin glue repair of complex anal fistulas. Perspect Colon Rectal Surg 1997; 10:83–88.
66. Venkatesh KS, Ramanujam P. Fibrin glue application in the treatment of recurrent anorectal fistulas. Dis Colon Rectum 1999; 42:1136–1139.
67. Cintron JR, Park JJ, Orlay CP, et al. Repair of fistulas-in-ano using fibrin adhesive. Long-term follow up. Dis colon Rectum 2000; 43:944–950.
68. El-Shobaky MT, Khafagy W, El-Arody S. Autologous fibrin glue in treatment of fistula-in-ano. Colorectal Dis 2000; 2(suppl):17.
69. Patrli L, Kocman B, Mertinic M, et al. Fibrin glue-antibiotic mixture in the treatment of anal fistulas: experience with 69 cases. Dig Surg 2000; 17:77–80.
70. Sentovich JM. Fibrin glue for anal fistulas. Dis Colon Rectum 2003; 46:498–502.
71. Chan KM, Lau CW, Lai KK, et al. Preliminary results of using a commercial fibrin sealant in the treatment of fistula-in-ano. J R Coll Surg Edinb 2002; 47:407–410.
72. Buchanan GN, Bartram CI, Phillips RK, et al. Efficacy of fibrin sealant in the management of complex anal fistula: a prospective trial. Dis Colon Rectum 2003; 46:1167–1174.
73. Loungnarath R, Dietz DW, Mutch MG, Birnbaum EH, Kodner IJ, Fleshman JW. Fibrin glue treatment of complex anal fistulas has low success rate. Dis Colon Rectum 2004; 47(4):432–436.
74. Singer M, Cintron J, Nelson R, et al. Treatment of fistulas-in-ano with fibrin sealant in combination with intra-adhesive antibiotics and/or surgical closure of the internal fistula opening. Dis Colon Rectum 2005; 48:799–808.
75. Ozuner G, Hull TL, Cartmill J, Fazio VW. Long-term analysis of the use of transrectal advancement flaps for complicated anorectal/vaginal fistulas. Dis Colon Rectum 1996; 39:10–14.
76. Aguilar PS, Plasencia G, Hardy TG, Hartmann RF, Stewart WRC. Mucosal advancement in the treatment of anal fistula. Dis Colon Rectum 1985; 28:496–501.

77. Wedell J, Meier zu Eissen P, Banzhaf G, Kleine L. Sliding flap advancement for the treatment of high level fistulae. Br J Surg 1987; 74: 390–391.
78. Mizrahi N, Wexner SD, Zmora O, et al. Endorectal advancement flap. Are there predictors of failure? Dis Colon Rectum 2002; 45:1616–1621.
79. Kodner IJ, Mazor A, Shemesh EI, Fry RD, Fleshman JW, Birnbaum EH. Endorectal advancement flap repair of rectovaginal and other complicated fistulas. Surgery 1993; 114:682–689.
80. Athanasiadis S, Köhler A, Nafe M. Treatment of high anal fistulae by primary occlusion of the internal ostium, drainage of the intersphincteric space, and mucosal advancement flap. Int J Colorectal Dis 1994; 9:153–157.
81. Makowiec F, Jehle EC, Becker HD, Starlinger M. Clinical course after transanal advancement flap repair of perianal fistula in patients with Crohn's disease. Br J Surg 1995; 82:603–606.
82. Joo JS, Weiss EG, Nogueras JJ, Wexner SD. Endorectal advancement flap in perianal Crohn's disease. Am Surg 1998; 64:147–150.
83. Marchesa P, Hull TL, Fazio VW. Advancement sleeve flaps for treatment of severe perianal Crohn's disease. Br J Surg 1998; 85:1695–1698.
84. Kreis ME, Jehle EC, Ohlemann M, Becker HD, Starlinger MJ. Functional results after transanal rectal advancement flap repair of trans-sphincteric fistula. Br J Surg 1998; 85:240–242.
85. Hyman N. Endoanal advancement flap repair for complex anorectal fistulas. Am J Surg 1999; 178:337–340.
86. Schouten WR, Zimmerman DD, Briel JW. Transanal advancement flap repair of transsphincteric fistulas. Dis Colon Rectum 1999; 42:1419–1423.
87. Ortiz H, Marzo J. Endorectal flap advancement repair and fistulectomy for high transsphincteric and suprasphincteric fistulas. Br J Surg 2000; 87: 1680–1683.
88. Sonoda T, Hull T, Piedmonte MR, Fazio VW. Outcomes of primary repair of anorectal and rectovaginal fistulas using the endorectal advancement flap. Dis Colon Rectum 2002; 45:1622–1628.
89. Zimmerman DD, Delemarre JB, Gosselink MP, Hop WC, Briel JW, Schouten WR. Smoking affects the outcome of transanal mucosal advancement flap repair of trans-sphincteric fistulas. Br J Surg 2003; 90:351–354.
90. Berman IR. Sleeve advancement anorectoplasty for complicated anorectal vaginal fistula. Dis Colon Rectum 1991; 34:1032–1037.
91. Parkash S, Lakshmiratan V, Gajendran V. Fistula-in-ano: treatment by fistulectomy, primary closure and reconstruction. Aust N Z J Surg 1985; 55:23–27.
92. Takano M. Sphincter preserving operation for low intersphincteric fistula: coring out of all the fistulous tract and primary closure of the internal opening. Dig Dis Sci 1986; 31:112S.
93. Miller GV, Finan PJ. Flap advancement and core fistulectomy for complex rectal fistula. Br J Surg 1998; 85:108–110.
94. Robertson WG, Mangione PS. Cutaneous advancement flap closure. Alternative method for treatment of complicated anal fistulas. Dis Colon Rectum 1998; 41:884–887.
95. Nelson RL, Cintron J, Abcarian H. Dermal island-flap anoplasty for transsphincteric fistula-in-ano: assessment of treatment failures. Dis Colon Rectum 2000; 43:681–684.
96. Amin SN, Tierney GM, Lund JN, Armitage NC. V-Y advancement flap for treatment of fistula-in-ano. Dis Colon Rectum 2003; 46:540–543.
97. Zimmerman DD, Briel JW, Gosselink MP, Schouten WR. Anocutaneous advancement flap repair of transsphincteric fistulas. Dis Colon Rectum 2001; 44:1474–1480.
98. Champagne BJ, O'Connor LM, Schertzer ME, Armstrong DN. Efficacy of anal fistula plug in closure of complex cryptoglandular anal fistula. Annual meeting American Society of Colon and Rectal Surgeons, Seattle June 3-7 2006 Abstract book S-30 pg 193.
99. Johnson EK, Gaw JU, Armstrong DN. Efficacy of anal fistula plug vs. fibrin glue in closure of anorectal fistulas. Dis Colon Rectum 2006; 49:371-376.
100. Lunniss PJ, Kamm MA, Phillips RKS. Factors affecting continence after surgery for anal fistula. Br J Surg 1994; 81:1382–1385.
101. van Tets WF, Kuijpers HC. Continence disorders after anal fistulotomy. Dis Colon Rectum 1994; 37:1194–1197.
102. Parks AG, Stitz RW. The treatment of high fistula-in-ano. Dis Colon Rectum 1976; 19:487–499.
103. Ewerth S, Ahlberg J, Collste G, Holmstrom B. Fistula-in-ano. A 6 year follow up study of 143 operated patients. Acta Chir Scand Suppl 1978; 482:53–55.
104. Adams D, Kovalcik PJ. Fistula-in-ano. Surg Gynecol Obstet 1981; 153:731–732.
105. Kuijpers JM. Diagnosis and treatment of fistula-in-ano. Neth J Surg 1982; 34:147–152.
106. Gingold BS. Reducing the recurrence risk of fistula-in-ano. Surg Gynecol Obstet 1983; 156:661–662.
107. Khubchandani M. Comparison of results of fistula-in-ano. J R Soc Med 1984; 77:369–371.
108. Sainio P, Husa H. Fistula-in-ano. Clinical features and long term results of surgery in 199 adults. Acta Chir Scand 1985; 151:169–176.
109. Shouler PJ, Grimley RP, Keighley MR, Alexander-Williams J. Fistula-in-ano is usually simple to manage surgically. Int J Colorectal Dis 1986; 1:113–115.
110. Dodi G, Moretti R, Pianon P, Zaffin M, Lise M. Method for the classification of anal, perianal, and rectal fistulae [abstr]. Gastroenterology 1986; 90:1396.
111. Girona J. Fistula-in-ano. Symposium. Int J Colorectal Dis 1987; 2:51–71.
112. Parnaud E. Fistula-in-ano. Symposium. Int J Colorectal Dis 1987; 2:51–71.
113. Sangwan YP, Rosen L, Riether RD, Staswik JJ, Sheets JA, Khubchandani JT. Is simple fistula-in-ano simple?. Dis Colon Rectum 1994; 37:885–889.
114. Isbister WH. Fistula in ano: a surgical audit. Int J Colorectal Dis 1995; 10: 94–96.
115. Mylonakis E, Katsios C, Godevenos D, Nousias B, Kappas AM. Quality of life of patients after surgical treatment of anal fistula; the role of anal manometry. Colorectal Dis 2001; 3:417–421.
116. Gupta PJ. Radio frequency "sutureless" fistulotomy—a new way of treating fistula in anus. World J Gastroenterol 2003; 9(5):1082–1085.
117. Garcia-Aguilar J, Davey CS, Le CT, Lowry AC, Rothenberger DA. Patient satisfaction after surgical treatment for fistula-in-ano. Dis Colon Rectum 2000; 43:1206–1212.
118. Cavanaugh M, Hyman N, Osler T. Fecal incontinence severity index after fistulotomy: a predictor of quality of life. Dis Colon Rectum 2002; 45: 349–353.
119. Jones NAG, Wilson DH. The treatment of acute abscesses by incision, curettage, and primary suture under antibiotic cover. Br J Surg 1976; 63:499–501.
120. Leaper DJ, Page RE, Rosenberg IL, Wilson DH, Goligher JC. A controlled study comparing the conventional treatment of idiopathic anorectal abscess with that of incision, curettage and primary suture under systemic antibiotic coverage. Dis Colon Rectum 1976; 19:46–50.
121. Kronberg O, Olsen H. Incision and drainage vs. incision, curettage, and suture under antibiotic cover in anorectal abscess, a randomized: study with 3 year follow-up. Acta Chir Scand 1984; 150:689–692.
122. Lundhus E, Gottrup F. Outcome at three to five years of primary closure of perianal and pilonidal abscess. Eur J Surg 1993; 159:555–558.
123. Mortensen J, Kraglund K, Klaerke M, Jaeger G, Suane S, Bone J. Primary suture of anorectal abscess. A randomized study comparing treatment with clindamycin vs. clindamycin and Gentacoll. Dis Colon Rectum 1995; 38: 398–401.
124. Abcarian H. Acute suppurations of the anorectum. Surg Annu 1976; 8: 305–333.
125. Eisenhammer S. A final evaluation and classification of the surgical treatment of the primary anorectal cryptoglandular inter-muscular (intersphincteric) fistulous abscess and fistula. Dis Colon Rectum 1978; 21:237–254.
126. Scoma JA, Salvati EP, Rubin RJ. Incidence of fistulas subsequent to anal abscesses. Dis Colon Rectum 1974; 17:357–359.
127. Hamalainen KP, Sainio AP. Incidence of fistulas after drainage of acute anorectal abscesses. Dis Colon Rectum 1998; 41:1357–1361.
128. Ho YH, Tan M, Chiu CH, Leong A, Eu KW, Seow-Choen F. Randomized controlled trial of primary fistulotomy with drainage alone for perianal abscess. Dis Colon Rectum 1997; 40:1435–1438.
129. Hyman N, Kida M. Adenocarcinoma of the sigmoid colon seeding a chronic anal fistula: report of a case. Dis Colon Rectum 2003; 46:835–836.
130. Read DR, Abcarian H. A prospective survey of 474 patients with anorectal abscesses. Dis Colon Rectum 1979; 22:566–569.
131. Schouten WR, van Vroonhoven TJMV. Treatment of anorectal abscess with or without primary fistulotomy. Results of a prospective randomized trial. Dis Colon Rectum 1991; 34:60–63.
132. Seow-Choen F, Leong AFPK, Goh HS. Results of a policy of selective immediate fistulotomy for primary anal abscess. Aust N Z J Surg 1993; 63: 485–489.
133. Sainio P. Fistula-in-ano in a defined population; incidence and epidemiological aspects. Ann Chir Gynaecol 1984; 73:219–224.
134. Belliveau P, Thomson JP, Parks AG. Fistula-in-ano: a manometric study. Dis Colon Rectum 1983; 26:152–154.
135. Sainio P. A manometric study of the anorectal function after surgery for anal fistula with special reference to incontinence. Acta Chir Scand 1985; 151: 695–700.
136. Sainio P, Husa A. A prospective manometric study of defective anal fistula surgery on anorectal function. Acta Chir Scand 1985; 151:279–288.
137. Pescatori M, Maria G, Anastasio G, Rinallo L. Anal manometry improves the outcome of surgery for fistula-in-ano. Dis Colon Rectum 1989; 32: 588–592.
138. Kronberg O. To lay open or excise a fistula-in-ano: a randomized trial. Br J Surg 1985; 72:970.
139. Cirocco WC, Rusin LC. Simplified seton management for complex anal fistulas: a novel use for the rubber band ligator. Dis Colon Rectum 1991; 34:1135–1137.
140. Thomson JPS, Ross AHM. Can the external sphincter be preserved in the treatment of transsphincteric fistula-in-ano. Int J Colorectal Dis 1989; 4: 247–250.
141. Buchanan GN, Owen HA, Torkington J, Lunniss PJ, Nicholls RJ, Cohen CR. Long-term outcome following loose-seton technique for external sphincter preservation in complex anal fistula. Br J Surg. 2004; 91:476–480.
142. Whitlow CB, Gathright JB. The use of setons in anorectal surgery. Perspect Colon Rectal Surg 1996; 9:100–116.

143. van Tets WF, Kuijpers HC. Seton treatment of perianal fistula with high anal or rectal opening. Br J Surg 1995; 82:895–897.
144. Browning GGP, Parks AG. Postanal repair for neuropathic fecal incontinence: correlation of clinical result and anal canal pressure. Br J Surg 1983; 70:101–104.
145. Kennedy HL, Zegarra JP. Fistulotomy without external sphincter division for high anal fistulae. Br J Surg 1990; 77:898–901.
146. Ramanujam PS, Prasad ML, Abcarian H. The role of seton in fistulotomy of the anus. Surg Gynecol Obstet 1983; 157:419–422.
147. Garcia-Aguilar J, Belmonte C, Wong DW, Goldberg SM, Madoff RD. Cutting seton versus two-stage seton fistulotomy in the surgical management of high anal fistula. Br J Surg 1998; 85:243–245.
148. Williams JG, MacLeod CA, Rothenberger DA, Goldberg SM. Seton treatment of high anal fistulae. Br J Surg 1991; 78:1159–1161.
149. Pearl RK, Andrews JR, Orsay CP, et al. Role of the seton in the management of anorectal fistulas. Dis Colon Rectum 1993; 36:573–9.
150. Graf W, Pahlman L, Ejerblad S. Functional results after seton treatment of high transsphincteric anal fistulas. Eur J Surg 1995; 161:289–291.
151. Hamalainen KPJ, Sainio AP. Cutting seton for anal fistulas. High risk of minor control defects. Dis Colon Rectum 1997; 40:1443–1447.
152. Dziki A, Bartos M. Seton treatment of anal fistula: experience with a new modification. Eur J Surg 1998; 164:543–548.
153. Balogh G. Tube loop (seton) drainage treatment of recurrent extrasphincteric perianal fistulae. Am J Surg 1999; 177:147–149.
154. Hasegawa H, Radley S, Keighley MR. Long-term results of cutting seton fistulotomy. Acta Chir Iugosl 2000; 47:19–21.
155. Isbister WH, Al Sanea N. The cutting seton: an experience at King Faisal Specialist Hospital. Dis Colon Rectum 2001; 44(5):722–727.
156. Durgun V, Perek A, Kapan M, Kapan S, Perek S. Partial fistulotomy and modified cutting seton procedure in the treatment of high extra-sphincteric perianal fistulae. Dig Surg 2002; 10:56–58.
157. Theerapol A, So BY, Ngoi SS. Routine use of setons for the treatment of anal fistulae. Singapore Med J 2002; 43:305–307.
158. Huber P Jr, Kissack AS, Simonton CT. Necrotizing soft tissue infection from rectal abscess. Dis Colon Rectum 1983; 26:507–511.
159. Eke N. Fournier's gangrene: a review of 1726 cases. Br J Surg 2000; 87:718–728.
160. Heppell J, Bénard F. Life-threatening perineal sepsis. Perspect Colon Rectal Surg 1991; 4:1–18.
161. Iorianni P, Oliver GC. Synergistic soft tissue infections of the perineum. Dis Colon Rectum 1992; 35:640–644.
162. Abcarian H, Eftaiha M. Floating free-standing anus: a complication of massive anorectal infection. Dis Colon Rectum 1983; 26:516–521.
163. Consten ECJ, Slors JFM, Danner SA, Sars PRA, Obertop H, van Lanschot JJB. Severe complications of perianal sepsis in patients with human immunodeficiency virus. Br J Surg 1996; 83:778–780.
164. Bode WE, Ramos R, Page CP. Invasive necrotizing infection secondary to anorectal abscess. Dis Colon Rectum 1982; 25:416–419.
165. Williamson M, Thomas A, Webster DJT, Young HL. Management of synergistic bacterial gangrene in severely immunocompromised patients. Report of four cases. Dis Colon Rectum 1993; 36:862–865.
166. Korkut M, Icoz G, Dayangac M, et al. Outcome analysis in patients with Fournier's gangrene: report of 45 cases. Dis Colon Rectum 2003; 46:649–652.
167. Getz SB, Ough YD, Patterson RB, Kovalick PJ. Mucinous adenocarcinoma developing in a chronic anal fistula: report of 2 cases and review of the literature. Dis Colon Rectum 1981; 24:562–566.
168. Jones EA, Morson BC. Mucinous adenocarcinoma in anorectal fistulae. Histopathology 1983; 8:279–292.
169. Thomas DJ, Thompson MR. Implantation metastasis from adenocarcinoma of sigmoid colon into fistula-in-ano. J R Soc Med 1992; 85:361.
170. Gupta R, Kay M, Birch DW. Implantation metastasis from adenocarcinoma of the colon into a fistula-in-ano: a case report. Can J Surg 2005; 48:162–163.
171. Zbar AP, Shenoy RK. Synchronous carcinoma of the sigmoid colon and a perianal fistula. Dis Colon Rectum 2004; 47:544–545.
172. Hyman N, Kida M. Adeno Carcinoma of the sigmoid colon seeding a chronic anal Fistula: report of a case. Dis colon Rectum 2003; 46:835–836.
173. Zaren HA, Delone FX, Lerner HJ. Carcinoma of the anal gland: case report and review of the literature. J Surg Oncol 1983; 28:250–254.
174. Lee SH, Zucker M, Sato T. Primary adenocarcinoma of an anal gland with secondary perianal fistulas. Hum Pathol 1981; 12:1034–1036.
175. Nelson RL, Prasad ML, Abcarian H. Anal carcinoma presenting as a perirectal abscess or fistula. Arch Surg 1985; 120:632–635.
176. Kline RJ, Spencer RJ, Harrison EG Jr. Carcinoma associated with fistula-in-ano. Arch Surg 1964; 89:989–994.
177. Onerheim RM. A case of perianal mucinous adenocarcinoma arising in a fistula-in-ano. A clue to the early pathologic diagnosis. Am J Clin Pathol 1988; 89:809–812.
178. Tan YS, Nambiar R, Sim CS. Adenocarcinoma associated with chronic anal fistula. Ann Acad Med 1989; 18:717–720.
179. Schaffzin DM, Stahl TJ, Smith LE. Perianal mucinous adenocarcinoma: unusual case presentations and review of the literature. Am Surg 2003; 69: 166–169.
180. Barnes SG, Sattler FR, Ballard JO. Perirectal infections in acute leukemia. Improved survival after incision and debridement. Ann Intern Med 1984; 100:515–518.
181. Shaked AA, Shinar E, Freund H. Managing the granulocytopenic patient with acute perianal inflammatory disease. Am J Surg 1986; 152:510–512.
182. Carlson GW, Ferguson CM, Amerson JR. Perianal infections in acute leukemia. Second place winner: Conrad Jobst Award. Am Surg 1988; 54: 693–695.
183. Chirletti P, Bererati M, Apice N, et al. Prophylaxis and treatment of inflammatory anorectal complications in leukemia. Ital J Surg Sci 1988; 18:45–48.
184. Grewal H, Guillem JG, Quan SH, Enker WE, Cohen AM. Anorectal disease in neutropenic leukemic patients. Operative vs. nonoperative management. Dis Colon Rectum 1994; 37:1095–1099.
185. Munoz-Villasmil J. Sands L, Hellinga MI. Management of perianal sepsis in immunosuppressed patients. Am Surg 2001; 67:484–486.
186. Cohen JS, Paz IB, O'Donnell MR, Ellenhorn JOI. Treatment of perianal infection following bone marrow transplantation. Dis Colon Rectum 1996; 39: 381–385.
187. Nadal SR, Manzione CR, Galvao VM, Salim VR, Speranzini MB. Healing after anal fistulotomy: comparative study between HIV+ and HIV− patients. Dis Colon Rectum 1998; 41:177–179.
188. Sultan S, Azria F, Baner P, Abdelnour W, Artienza P. Anoperianal tuberculosis. Diagnostic and management consideration in severe cases. Dis Colon Rectum 2002; 45:407–410.
189. Kraemer M, Gill SS, Seow-Choen F. Tuberculosis and sepsis: report of clinical features in 20 cases. Dis Colon Rectum 2000; 43:1589–1591.
190. Zinman L. The management of the complex recto-urethral fistula. BJU Int 2004; 94:1212–1213.

11 Pilonidal Disease

Santhat Nivatvongs

INTRODUCTION

A.W. Anderson's letter to the editor that appeared in an issue of the *Boston Medical Surgical Journal* of 1847, entitled "Hair Extracted From an Ulcer," is believed to be the first documented case of pilonidal sinus (1). The letter described a young 21-year-old man with pain in his back. Anderson found a "fistula opening" near the coccyx on the left side, which was so small that he could not introduce a probe. Upon opening the cavity, he found a large amount of "very fine, closely matted hairs about 2 in. in length," with very offensive smell. The hairs were removed and the wound healed in three weeks. In 1880, Hodges (2) coined the term "pilonidal sinus" (*pilus,* meaning hair, and *nidus,* meaning nest) to describe the chronic sinus containing hair and found between the buttocks. He believed the condition was congenital in origin, representing an imperfect union of the lateral halves of the body and involving the integument only. Buie (3) called it "jeep disease" because of the frequent reactivation of the quiescent sacrococcygeal sinuses among military personnel who entered training for combat duty, with rugged lifestyle and stresses of driving trucks, tanks, and jeeps. The time loss among patients with pilonidal disease was tremendous, "... a mild ailment, ... it represents one of the most important surgical courses of lost time." Seventy-nine thousand U.S. servicemen were hospitalized, each for an average 55 days, because of pilonidal disease and its treatment during World War II (4).

Pilonidal sinus is a chronic subcutaneous abscess in the natal cleft, which spontaneously drains through the openings. It is not a "cyst," as frequently referred to in many textbooks and articles.

ETIOLOGY AND PATHOGENESIS

The origin of the pilonidal sinus has been a subject of interest for many years. The congenital theory, the remnant of the medullary canal, and the infolding of the surface epithelium, or a faulty coalescence of the cutaneous covering in early embryonic life, were once popular (5). In the modern era, the congenital theory still has its proponents. Lord (6) reasoned that hairs in the pilonidal sinuses are identical in length, diameter, color, and orientation. He said, "It is hard to conceive any other theories that explain how hair can get into the pilonidal sinus from outside, which could possibly explain how 23 hairs should follow each other into a pilonidal sinus and each hair be identical in every respect to the last."

The acquired theory is now widely accepted. Its mechanism, however, is speculative and varied. Bascom (7) believes the affected hair follicles become distended with keratin and subsequently infected, leading to folliculitis and the formation of an abscess that extends down into the subcutaneous fat (Fig. 1). Examination of a section of a pit reveals a distended hair follicle with inflammation (Fig. 2). Once the abscess cavity is formed, hairs can enter through the tiny pit and lodge in the abscess cavity from the suction created by movement of the gluteal area (Fig. 3). Karydakis (8), on the other hand, believes the shaft of loose hair, because of its scales with chisel-like root ends, inserts into the depth of the natal cleft in the midline of sacrococcygeal area (Fig. 4). Once one hair inserts successfully, other hairs can insert more easily. Foreign body tissue reaction and infection follow, and the primary sinus of pilonidal disease forms. Secondary openings often occur because of the self-propelling ability of hair to burrow through the skin, or spontaneous rupture of the abscess. I believe that Karydakis's explanation is the correct one.

Observations, such as isolated reports that pilonidal sinus has occurred in unusual locations, such as the umbilicus, a healed amputation stump, and interdigital clefts, and the recurrence of the disease in an adequately excised area support the acquired theory of this disease particularly Karydakis's concept of hair insertion.

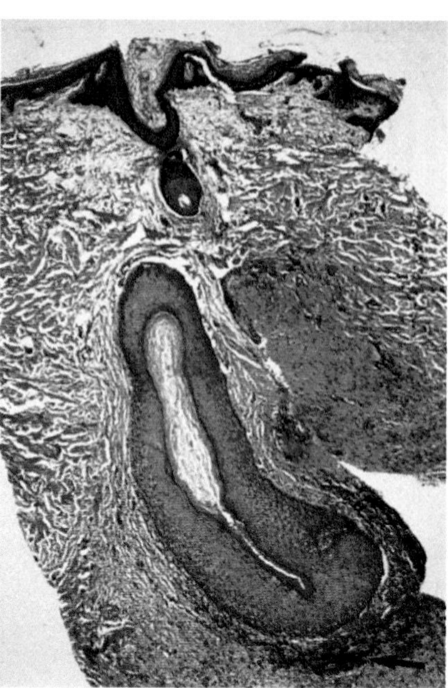

FIGURE 2 ■ Photomicrograph of the pit from midline showing chronic inflammation from infected hair follicle. *Source*: Courtesy of Andrew R. McLeish, M.D., Melbourne, Australia.

SURGICAL PATHOLOGY

The main feature of a pilonidal sinus is the subcutaneous fibrous tract that may be lined with squamous epithelium. This subcutaneous tract extends for a variable distance, usually 2 to 5 cm. A small abscess cavity and branching tracts may come off the primary tract (Fig. 5). Often hairs that are usually disconnected from the surrounding skin are seen entering the midline pit (Fig. 6). As a rule, hair follicles are not identified. The secondary openings have a different appearance from the primary midline ones in that they are marked by elevations of granulation tissue and discharge of seropurulent material. Hairs, if seen, sticking out of the secondary opening are in the abscess cavity that the body tries to spit out (Fig. 6). Most sinus tracts (93%) run cephalad; the rest (7%) run caudad and may be confused with a fistula-in-ano or with hidradenitis suppurativa (9).

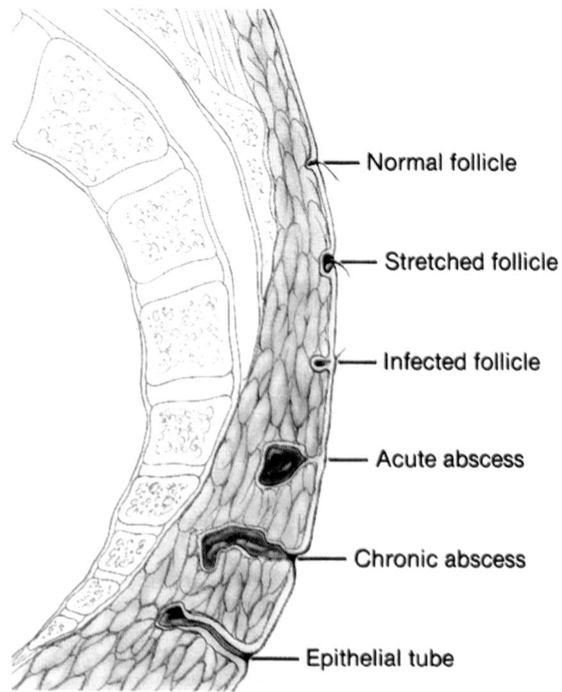

FIGURE 1 ■ Pathogenesis of pilonidal abscess and sinus. *Source*: From Ref. 7.

NATURAL HISTORY

Pilonidal sinus is a chronic disease with a natural regression (10). Usually the disease does not manifest until puberty and seldom occurs after the third decade of life. However, pilonidal sinus may occur at any age. Sagi et al. (11) reported on a seven-year-old patient with a pilonidal sinus that progressed to a squamous cell carcinoma when the patient was 54 years old. Karydakis (8) has seen an increased incidence of pilonidal sinus in the very young, especially girls, as young as 11 years of age. The average age of patients with pilonidal sinus is 32 years in men and 24 years in women (12).

Clothier and Haywood (10) studied 42 military personnel with pilonidal disease. In only 5 of 42 patients (12%), the duration of the disease was less than three weeks, and it presented as an acute abscess. In only two patients (5%), in whom the disease commenced in the third decade, did the disease continue into the fourth decade, suggesting that there tends to be a natural tendency to "burn out" at about 30 years of age. However, there is also a small group of patients who develop the disease for the first time in their fourth decade.

PREDISPOSING FACTORS

Tiny skin dimples in the sacrococcygeal area are common in the normal population (9%), but most never become a

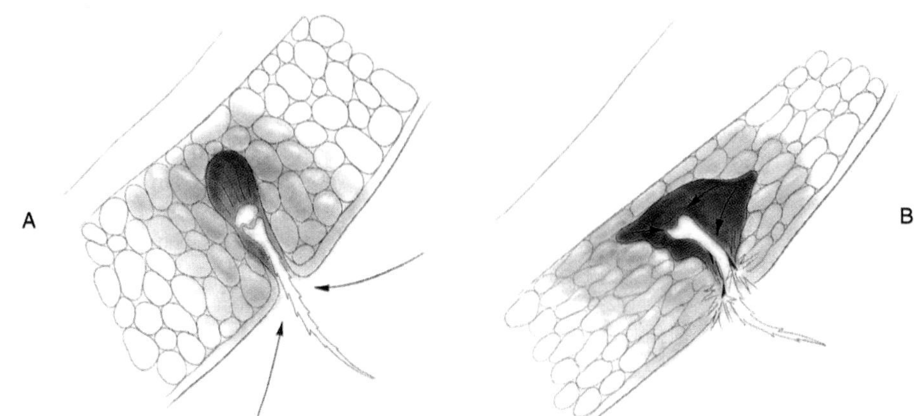

FIGURE 3 ■ Ingestion of hair by a chronic pilonidal abscess cavity. Scales of hair direct the inward movement of hair. Motion causes movement in the cavity. (**A**) Standing, (**B**) sitting. *Source*: From Ref. 7.

problem (13). Because of the common problems of infected pilonidal sinuses among Army and Navy officers, it was speculated that trauma to the sacrococcygeal area was the primary predisposing factor. However, the acquired theory of folliculitis (7) and the spontaneous insertion of hair in the natal cleft (8) refute this theory as the primary cause.

Akinci et al. (14) examined 1000 Turkish soldiers including information on their characters and habits. Eighty-eight (8.8%) of the soldiers had pilonidal sinuses; 48 were symptomatic and 40 were asymptomatic. The factors associated with the presence of a pilonidal sinus were: obesity (weight over 90 kg) ($p < 0.0001$); being the driver of a vehicle ($p < 0.0001$); incidence of folliculitis or furuncle at another site on the body ($p < 0.0001$); and family history of pilonidal sinus ($p < 0.0001$). The history of pilonidal sinus in the family does not mean a congenital tendency but rather, indicating the similar body habitat and hair characteristics.

CLINICAL MANIFESTATIONS

The average patients with pilonidal disease are hirsute and moderately obese in their second decade (15). However, hirsute people or people with dark hairs may have an increased tendency to have pilonidal disease, but the disease is also seen in people who do not (14); people of both sexes and any age can be affected. Pilonidal disease initially may be seen as an acute abscess in the sacrococcygeal area. It frequently ruptures spontaneously, leaving unhealed sinuses with chronic drainage. Once the sinus develops, pain is usually minimal. From 71% to 85% of patients with pilonidal infection are men (5,12).

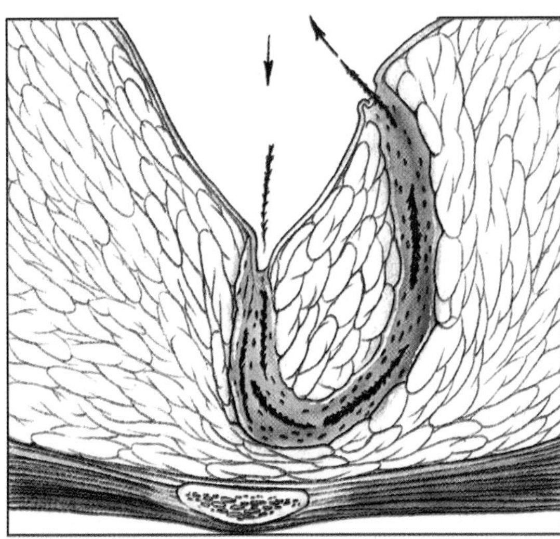

FIGURE 4 ■ Pathogenesis. Insertion of a shaft of loose hair.

DIAGNOSIS

The diagnosis of this condition is usually made quite easily. The patient's history suggests the problem. A painful and indurated swelling is the most common presentation of the acute process. In its earliest stage, only cellulitis may be present. In the chronic state, the diagnosis is confirmed by the sinus' opening in the intergluteal fold approximately 5 cm above the anus. On careful examination, a pit or pits in the midline, which are the main source of the disease, almost always can be found (Fig. 7).

The differential diagnoses that must be considered include any furuncle in the skin, an anal fistula, specific granulomas (e.g., syphilitic or tuberculous), and osteomyelitis with multiple draining sinuses in the skin. Actinomycosis in the sacral region has been described as

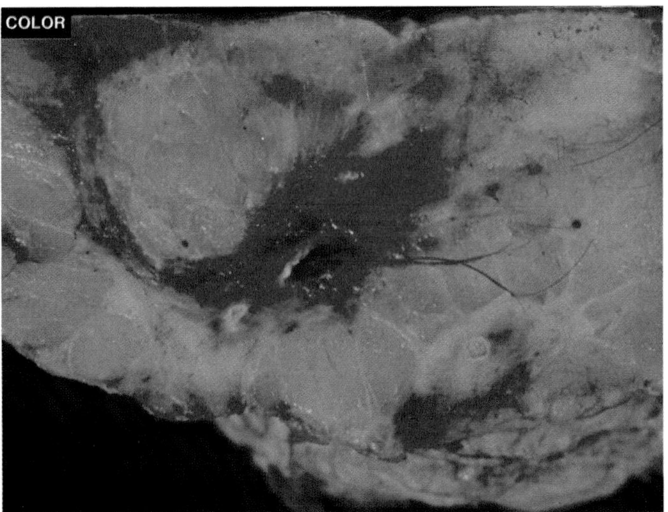

FIGURE 5 ■ Section of an en bloc specimen shows hairs in a chronic abscess cavity and a sinus tract leading to a secondary opening. *Source*: Courtesy of Clyde Culp, M.D., Rochester, Minnesota, U.S.A.

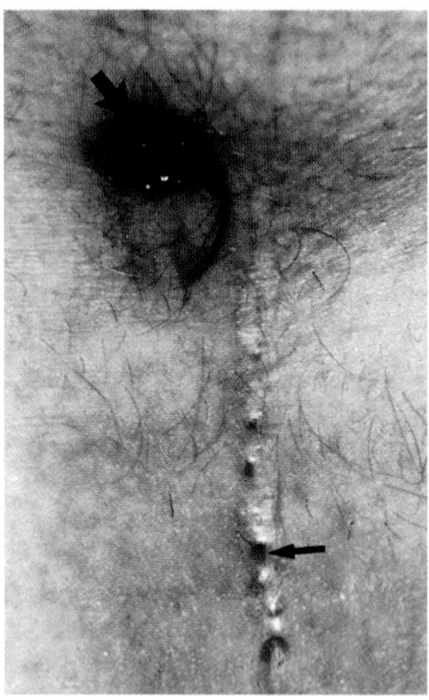

FIGURE 6 ■ Numerous non-inflamed midline pits, the primary source of the disease (*small arrow*). Hairs extrude from the secondary sinus (*large arrow*).

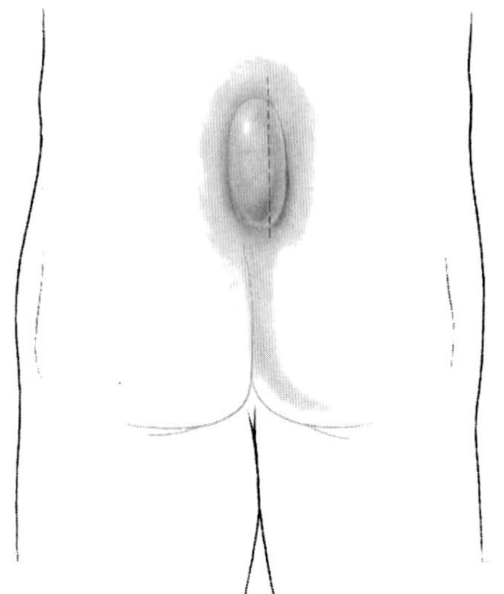

FIGURE 8 ■ A pilonidal abscess. The incision is made off the midline. *Source*: From Ref. 16.

virtually indistinguishable from pilonidal disease. When a fungus is suspected, the diagnosis should be confirmed by the presence of a ray fungus in the smears of the discharge or in a culture.

TREATMENT

PILONIDAL ABSCESS

Although the infected epithelial sinus is in the midline, the abscess is usually lateral on either side and cephalad. It is well known that the midline wound in the intergluteal cleft heals poorly and slowly. Every attempt should be made to avoid the midline wound and, if necessary, to make it small. Drainage of a pilonidal abscess almost always can be performed with the patient under local anesthesia in the clinic, office, or emergency room. A longitudinal incision is made lateral to the midline in the coccygeal area (Fig. 8). The incision is deepened into the subcutaneous tissue, entering the abscess cavity. Hair, if present in the abscess cavity, must be removed. All the infected granulation tissues and necrotic debris are thoroughly curetted. The skin edges are trimmed to make the abscess cavity an open wound. The wound is lightly packed with fine mesh gauge. An antibiotic is not indicated. The patient is instructed to irrigate the wound with diluted hydrogen peroxide (dilution 1:4) twice a day for a few days, if possible. This will effectively remove the residual debris. At the very least, the wound should be washed with soap and water in the shower twice a day. The most important aspect is to prevent hairs from getting into the wound and to remove them from the wound. The hairs around the wound should be shaved or plucked for at least a couple of months. A Cytette brush (Birchwood Laboratories, Inc., Eden Prairie, Minnesota, U.S.A.), which is commonly used for obtaining Papanicolaou (Pap) smears, is an excellent tool for swabbing the hairs and debris from the wound (Fig. 9). With proper care, complete healing is the rule.

PILONIDAL SINUS

Treatment of pilonidal sinus can be done in one of several ways: nonoperative treatment, lateral incision and excision of midline pits, incision and marsupialization, wide local excision with or without primary closure, excision and Z-plasty, or advancing flap operation (Karydakis procedure).

Nonoperative Treatment

Klass (13) believed that the immediate cause of the infection in a pilonidal sinus is a collection of loose hairs and fecal residue in the internatal cleft and that when an abscess has developed, incision and drainage are all that is required.

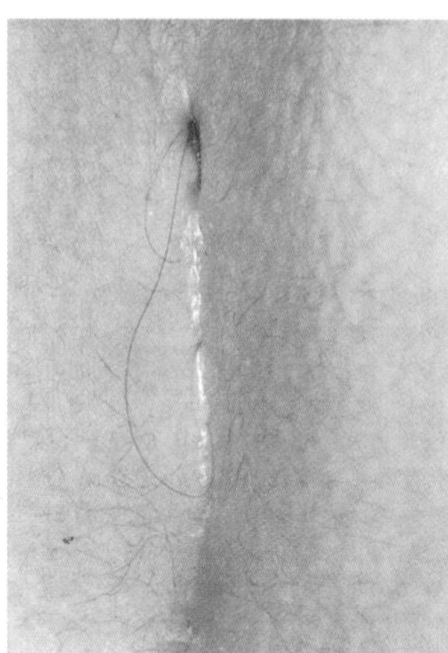

FIGURE 7 ■ A midline pit. Note hairs entering the pit.

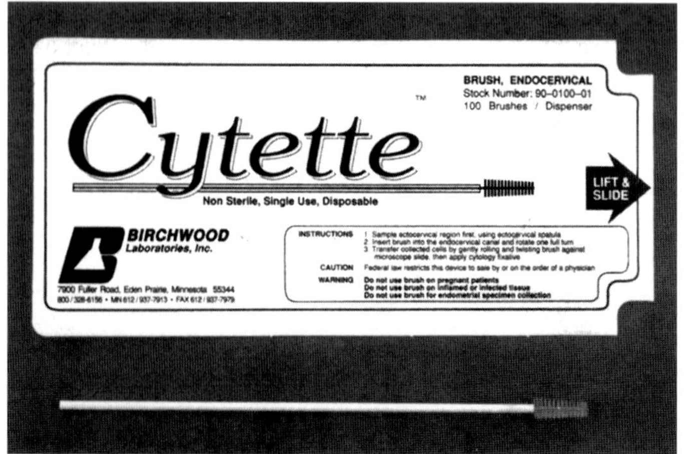

FIGURE 9 ■ Cytette brush, an excellent tool to clean the wound.

He thus treated his patients with strict hygiene by washing with soap and water in the perineal and sacrococcygeal area. An abscess is drained, the sinus is kept open, and the area is cleaned. In a series of 15 patients with chronic discharge from the sinuses, 11 are cured, with follow-up of three years or longer. In another group of 12 patients who required incision and drainage of the abscess, 10 patients healed, and two patients required a second incision and drainage. The follow-up was at least three years.

The most important conservative treatment comes from Tripler Army Medical Center, Hawaii. Armstrong and Barcia (17) treat pilonidal disease mainly by shaving all hairs within the natal cleft, 5 cm from the anus to the presacrum. Visible hairs within the sinus are removed, but no attempt is made to probe for hairs within the sinus. If there is an abscess, a lateral incision for drainage is made. This conservative method was applied to 101 consecutive patients during a one-year period. The wounds healed in all patients. Unfortunately, the length of follow-up and the recurrence rate were not stated in the study.

Injecting phenol into the sinus tract has been advocated by some authors. Schneider et al. (18) studied 45 patients with pilonidal sinuses treated with 1 to 2 mL of 80% phenol injected into the sinus. The injection was performed under local anesthesia. Only 60% of the patients completely healed and it took six weeks on average. Besides, 11% develop abscess requiring excision and drainage, and other patients frequently develop local inflammation caused by the phenol. This method of treatment should not be used.

On the other hand, Dogru et al. (19) used crystallized phenol with success. First, they cleaned out and removed hairs from the abscess cavity and sinus tracts. The surrounding skin was protected before applying the crystals into the wound. The crystallized phenol turned into liquid form quickly at body temperature and filled the sinus. It was left in situ for two minutes and then expressed out. The procedure may be repeated thereafter as indicated. Of 41 patients so treated, two patients had recurrences at five and eight months. The median follow-up was 24 months. The mean recovery time was 43 days. This noninvasive technique may sound good but crystallized phenol is not readily available in most hospitals.

Lateral Incision and Lay Open of Midline Sinus Tracts

Although Lord (6) believes in the congenital theory and Bascom (7) is a strong advocate of acquired etiology, their concept of treatment is remarkably similar. Both advocate excision of the midline pits or sinuses and thorough cleansing of hair and debris from the sinus tract. Bascom (7) emphasizes avoiding midline wounds by using a longitudinal incision off the midline to enter the sinus tract (Fig. 10). In a follow-up of 149 patients, with a mean follow-up 3.5 years (longest, nine years), the cure rate was 84% (20). Senapati et al. (21) reported a success rate of 90%, with a mean follow-up of 12 months (range, 1–60) in 218 patients. Advantages of this technique are minimal surgery and small wounds. It can be done on an outpatient basis. Excision of the midline pits, although small, frequently is slow to heal. A better way is to lay open the midline pits toward the lateral incision. This is an important technique to minimize a recurrence.

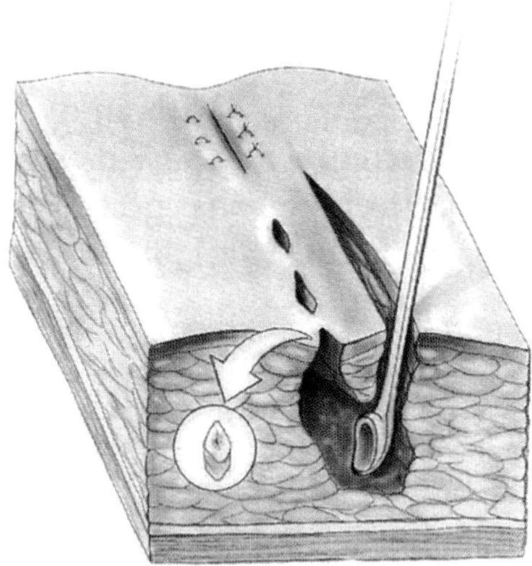

FIGURE 10 ■ Lateral incision to the sinus tract. Granulated tissues are scraped with a curette. *Source*: From Ref. 7.

A case in point is a 20-year-old man who had a pilonidal abscess drained two months ago and was referred for further treatment because of persistent drainage. This patient had an abscess drained in the midline near the anus; there were also several small midline pits cephalad to this unhealed draining site (Fig. 11A). The operation was performed in the clinic under local anesthesia without sedation. An up-and-down incision was made 1 cm lateral to the midline, deepened to the chronic abscess cavity. The incision was extended to the entire length of the abscess cavity, which was lined by gelatinous granulation tissues. All the midline pits were identified with a probe and laid open toward the wound (Fig. 11B). All the granulation tissues and hairs were thoroughly curetted. Note the shaggy edges of the wound that resulted from laying open of the sinus tracts (Fig. 11C). The patient washed the wound at shower and lightly packed it with mesh gauze once or twice daily. A complete healing was achieved in three weeks (Fig. 11D). There was no recurrence at three years follow-up.

Proper packing of the open wound is essential for healing. The patient should be examined one week after surgery. Hypertrophic granulation signifies improper packing and requires cauterization with silver nitrate sticks. The packing should not be tight but the mesh gauze should touch on the entire subcutaneous wound.

Incision and Marsupialization

An open type of operation with marsupialization of the wound was advocated by Buie (3) and later by Culp (22). The technique consists of opening the sinus tract in the midline. The debris and granulation tissues are scraped with a curette. The fibrous tissue in the tract is saved and is sutured to the edges of the wound. This technique not only minimizes the size and depth of the wound but also prevents the wound from premature closure. In addition, it is easy to pack and clean the wound (Fig. 12). In doing so, the size of the wound is reduced 50% to 60% (22). The average healing time is four to six weeks, with prolonged

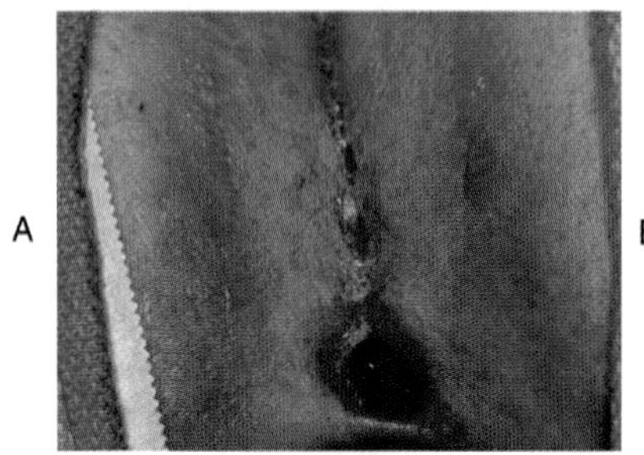

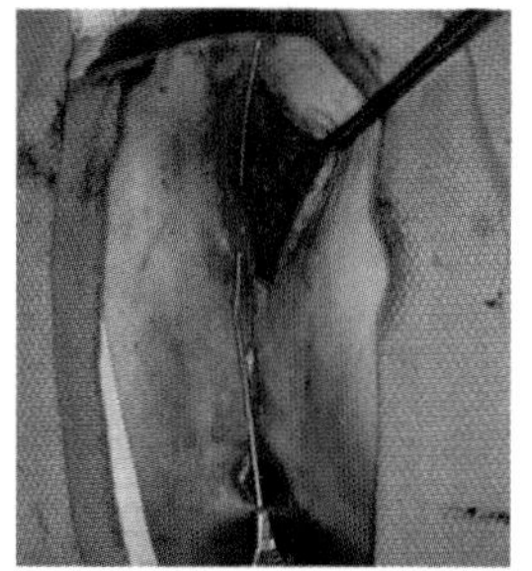

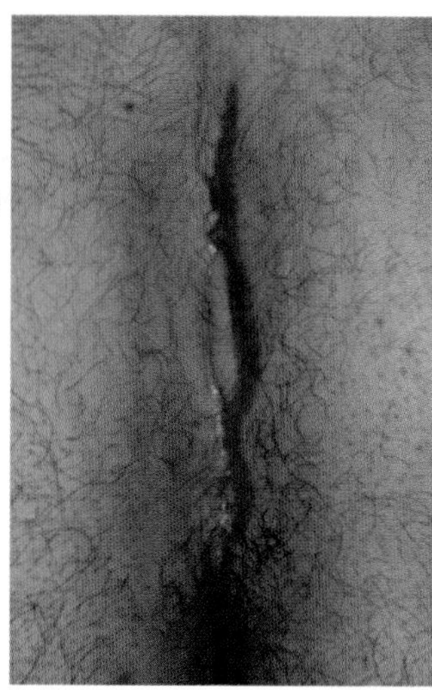

FIGURE 11 ■ (**A**) Several openings in midline sacrococcygeal area. (**B**) An incision is made about 1 cm lateral to the midline, and then dissected to connect with the chronic abscess cavity. A lacrimal probe is used to identify the sinus tracts from the midline pits. (**C**) Note the shaggy edges of the wound resulting from laying open of the sinus tracts. (**D**) Complete wound healing at three weeks.

healing (12–20 weeks) in 2% to 4% and recurrence in 8% (8,23). Although this technique is simple, it is still more extensive than the lateral incision and lay open of the sinus tracts as described above.

Wide Local Excision with or without Primary Closure

An en bloc excision is made around the midline pilonidal, deep down to the sacrococcygeal fascia. The wound is packed with moist saline gauze. In a series of 50 patients, Al-Hassan et al. (24) found that the mean time of healing was 13 weeks (range, 4–78 weeks) and that the recurrence rate was 12% with a mean follow-up of 25 months.

Sondenaa et al. (25) performed a radical excision in 153 patients who had chronic pilonidal sinus. Seventy-eight of those patients received a single dose of 2 g cefoxitin intravenously, and 75 patients received no antibiotic. There was no difference in the rate of wound healing between the two groups. The wounds healed within one month in 69% of patients who received cefoxitin and in 64% of patients who received no antibiotic. The complication rates were 44% and 43%, respectively. Other studies have seen similar problems (26,27). Despite this radical operation, some authors find it to be satisfactory and advocate its use (28–30). In a randomized trial with a three-year follow-up, Kronborg et al. (31) found that excision with primary closure of the wound resulted in a shorter healing time than excision with an open wound, and that the recurrence rate varied from 0% to 38% (32). A randomized trial by Testini et al. (33) also showed a quicker wound healing and a quicker return to normal activity in the primary closure group versus an open technique. This radical technique has no advantages over marsupialization and is seldom necessary.

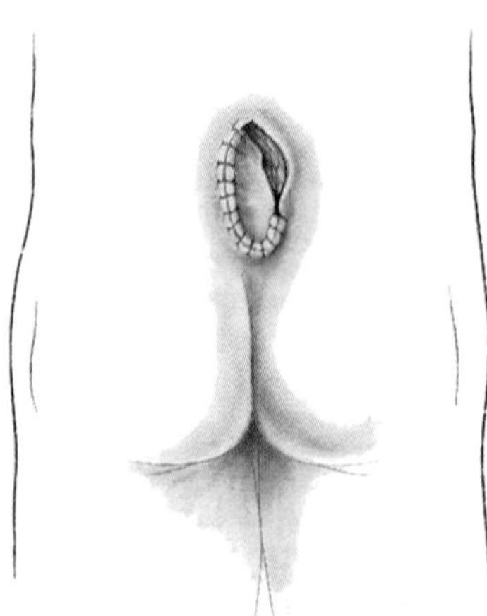

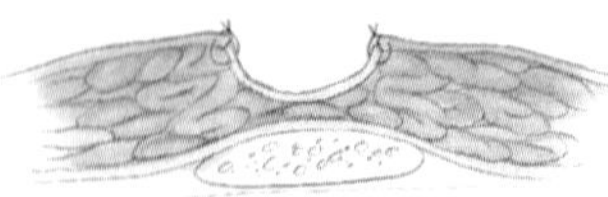

FIGURE 12 ■ Marsupialization. Fibrotic wall at the base of the wound is sutured to the edges of the skin all around with continuous absorbable suture. *Source*: From Ref. 22.

Excision and Z-Plasty

Excision of pilonidal sinuses with primary closure of the wound is simple but has a high recurrence rate. The use of primary closure, however, is appealing because successful wound healing can be accomplished within 7 to 10 days. To avoid recurrence or breakdown of the midline wound, the anatomy of the natal crease must be altered. Z-plasty can be done to achieve this goal. Excision of pilonidal sinuses with primary Z-plasty fills out and flattens the natal crease, directs the hair points away from the midline, largely prevents maceration, reduces suction effects in the soft tissues of the buttocks, and minimizes friction between their adjacent surfaces. The excision is carried down to the subcutaneous tissue. The limbs of the Z are cut to form a 30° angle with the long axis of the wound. Subcutaneous skin flaps are raised, and the flaps are transposed and sutured (Fig. 13). A closed suction drain is placed under the full-thickness flaps. Z-plasty thus avoids the midline wound, which is the main cause of slow healing and recurrences. In a series of 110 patients treated with Z-plasty by Toubanakis (34), there were no recurrences. Mansoory and Dickson (35) reported similar good results. The main disadvantage of this procedure is that it is a rather extensive one for a noncomplicated pilonidal sinus and is not suitable for performance on an outpatient basis. Besides, part of the wound is still in the midline.

Advancing Flap Operation

Karydakis Procedure

Karydakis (8) believes that pilonidal sinuses occur because of the entry of hair into the midline of the intergluteal fold. The hairs are then forced by friction into the depth of the fold. He designed an operative technique to avoid these problems. A "semilateral" excision is made over the sinuses all the way down to the presacral fascia (Fig. 14). Mobilization is carried to the opposite side so that the entire flap can be advanced toward the other side on closure. A closed

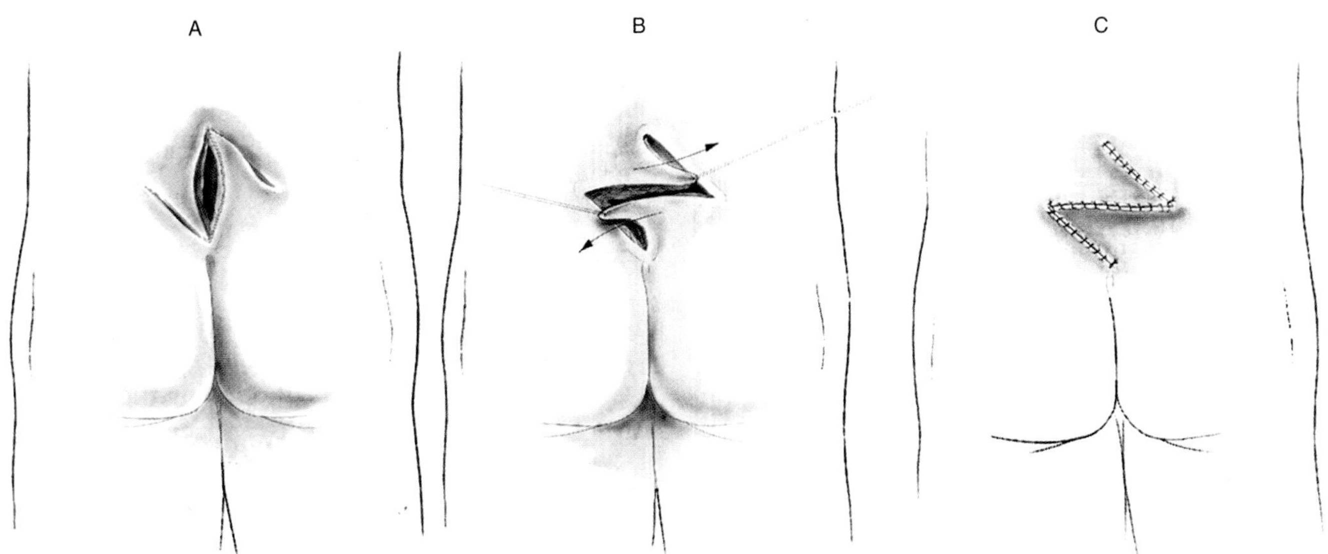

FIGURE 13 ■ Z-Plasty. (**A**) Elliptical excision is made to the pilonidal sinuses. Incisions are made at the limbs of the Z at a 30° angle with the long axis of the wound. (**B**) Subcutaneous skin flaps are raised and transposed. (**C**) Skin is closed.

suction drain is placed. This technique avoids the midline wound. In a series of 7471 patients who received the advancing flap procedure, the complication rate was 8.5%, mainly infection and fluid collection. The mean hospital stay was three days, with many patients requiring one-day hospitalization or the procedure performed on an outpatient basis. The recurrence rate was 1%, with follow-up ranging from 2 to 20 years. In each recurrence, reinsertion of hairs was observed. The Karydakis flap procedure has proved to be effective (8,36,37), but it is a moderately extensive procedure.

Rhomboid Excision with Transposition of Flap

This technique and its results have appeared frequently in the literature recently. It was first reported in French by Dufourmental et al. (38) in 1966 for a sacrococcygeal cyst. Subsequently in 1984, Azab et al. (39) accurately described its construction and used it for the treatment of pilonidal sinuses.

A rhomboid is outlined to encompass the pilonidal sinuses in the midline (Fig. 15A). The lines ab = bc = cd = ad. The line de is drawn to bisect the angle made by bd and cd. The lines de and ef are the same length as ad. The d-e-f angle is the same as the b-a-d angle.

The rhomboid excision is made down to the sacral periosteum in the midline and to the gluteal fascia laterally. The d-e-f flap is made deep to the gluteal fascia to release any tension. The flap is then transposed to cover the rhomboid wound (Fig. 15B). A suction drain is placed under the flap and the wound is closed with sutures (Fig. 15C).

Using rhomboid excision and flap in 67 patients with pilonidal sinuses, Milito et al. (41) reported no recurrence after a mean follow-up of 74 months (range, 8–137 months); primary healing was obtained in all patients except two who developed a seroma and one who had a partial dehiscence of the wound due to a hematoma which necessitated a drainage. The average hospital stay was five days (range, 1–16 days).

Daphan et al. (42) reported a recurrence of 5% in 147 patients, after a mean follow-up of 13 months (range, 1–40 months); 2% of the patients developed a postoperative seroma and 4% had a wound separation.

Urhan et al. (43) and Arumugam et al. (44) reported recurrences of 5% and 7% after a mean follow-up of 36 months and 24 months, respectively.

Topgul et al. (45) reported 200 cases, including 13 cases for recurrences using this technique. Minimal flap necrosis occurred in 3%, seroma in 2%, wound infection in 1.5%, and recurrence in 0.5%; the mean follow-up was five years.

The advantage of rhomboid excision with transposition of flap is appealing because it is easy to perform and the results are as good as any other more complicated flaps.

SUMMARY

Petersen et al. (46) performed a Medline search in February 2001 for a survey of results of different surgical approaches with primary closure techniques. The search identified 74 publications including 1090 patients for primary closure in midline, 35 publications with 2034 patients evaluated, the results of asymmetric or oblique technique (e.g., Karydakis's, Bascom's) were described in 6812 patients of 16 publications whereas for the rhomboid technique, 739 patients in 16 articles were found. For V-Y plasty, 73 patients and 4 publications, and finally for the Z-flap technique, 432 patients in 11 articles were included.

The results showed that overall wound infection occurred in up to 38.5%. The highest pooled infection rate of 12.4% (95% CI, 11.1–13.8) was observed in the midline closure group, and the lowest in the V-Y group. The wound failure appeared in up to 52.4% of all procedures. The lowest pooled failure rates of 3.5% (95% CI, 2.6–4.7) and 3.4% (95% CI, 2.3–4.9) were observed in asymmetric oblique technique group and the rhomboid group, respectively. Recurrence was observed in up to 26.8%, with highest in the midline closure group and lowest in asymmetric oblique group and rhomboid group.

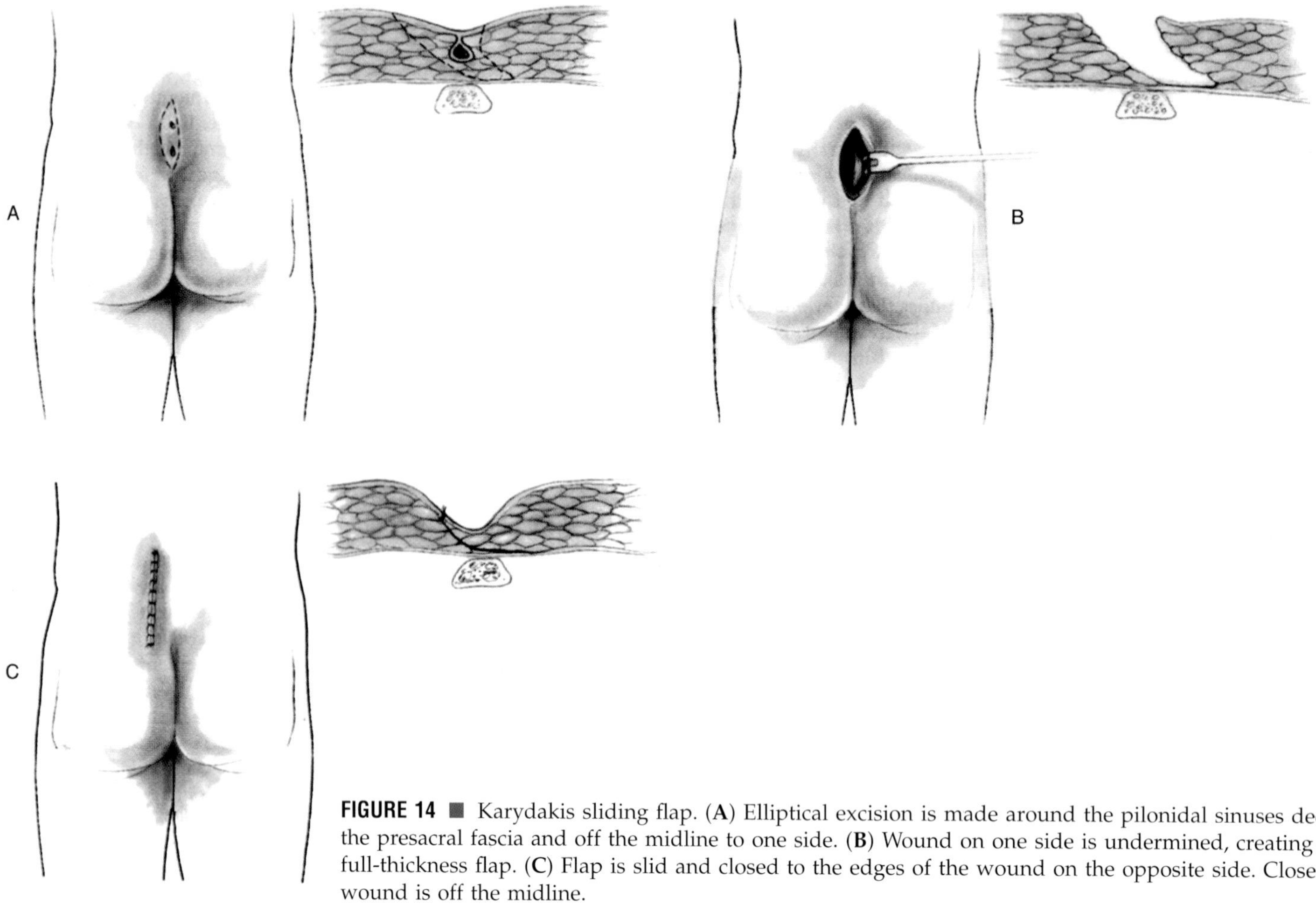

FIGURE 14 ■ Karydakis sliding flap. (**A**) Elliptical excision is made around the pilonidal sinuses deep to the presacral fascia and off the midline to one side. (**B**) Wound on one side is undermined, creating a full-thickness flap. (**C**) Flap is slid and closed to the edges of the wound on the opposite side. Closed wound is off the midline.

Many operations for pilonidal disease end up worse than the disease itself. The treatment of pilonidal disease should be simple and most, if not all, can be performed on an outpatient basis.

A simple incision and drainage off the midline of the abscess, with complete removal of hairs and debris, and shaving hairs around the wound are all that is necessary for an acute pilonidal abscess. The central pit should be searched for and, if identified, should be laid open to the lateral incision. For a chronic pilonidal sinus, the method of choice is a lateral incision into the chronic abscess cavity, with removal of all hairs and granulation tissues. It is to be done along with laying open of the midline pits with their tracts to the lateral wound. If a flap is necessary, the Rhomboid excision with transposition of subcutaneous skin flap is the simplest technique to do.

The surgeon must make it clear to the patients and their families that they are responsible for the second half of the

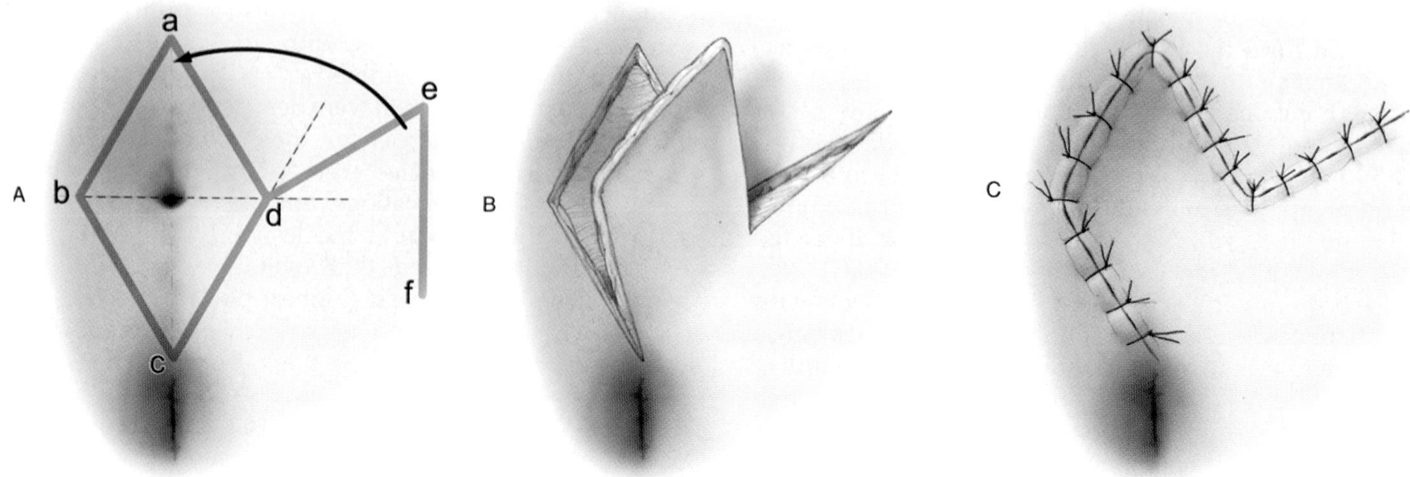

FIGURE 15 ■ (**A**) Outline of rhomboid excision: ab = bc = cd = da; de bisects the angle made by bd and cd. de = ef = ad. (**B**) The flap is made deep into gluteal fascia. The flap is rotated and transposed to cover the rhomboid wound. (**C**) At completion. *Source*: From Ref. 40.

treatment. The open wounds must be irrigated or cleaned in the shower with soap and water. Hairs and debris in the wound must be removed. The wound should be lightly packed to prevent premature closure. The skin around the wound should be shaved or the hairs plucked every 10 to 14 days. The surgeon should check the wound every one to two weeks and cauterize the hypertrophic granulation tissues until proper wound care has been achieved.

ROLE OF HAIR

During the initial operation, all hairs in the pilonidal sinus or the abscess cavity must be removed. The wound will not heal if even one hair is present in or enters the wound. There are three ways in which hair can enter the wound.

INGROWN HAIR

Hairs from the edges of the wound often can be misdirected and grow into the wound. The best way to avoid this problem is to pluck those hairs every 10 to 14 days until the wound is healed completely.

LOCAL HAIR

Hair in the adjacent area, particularly from the perianal area, grows to considerable length, and tips of these hairs can get into the wound causing delayed healing or unhealing of the wound. Shaving or trimming with scissors is required.

LOOSE HAIR

Loose hairs from elsewhere (even dog or cat hairs) are the most common offender. Motion in the intergluteal cleft has been shown to attract loose hair. Packing and cleaning the wound will eliminate this problem. Washing with soap is an easy way to loosen the sticky hairs.

RECURRENT DISEASE

The length of time needed for the pilonidal wound to heal depends on the type of operation and the extent of the disease. The recurrence rate varies widely from series to series (0% to 37%) (8,12,27). Recurrence is caused by reinsertion of the loose hairs into the natal cleft. The mechanism is the same as for primary pilonidal disease, and the treatment is also the same.

UNHEALED WOUND

Not uncommonly, the wound does not heal after operation for a pilonidal sinus. Most often, the base of the wound is filled with gelatinous granulation tissue, which is usually the result of improper postoperative wound care. Hairs may grow into the edges of the wound preventing complete healing. Some wounds are kept clean and yet do not heal. Almost all unhealed wounds are in the midline natal cleft area. The lateral incision technique usually avoids this problem.

CURETTAGE, RE-EXCISION, AND SAUCERIZATION

The hairs around the unhealed wound must be shaved and plucked, after which a complete curettage of the granulation tissue is done. If the shape of the wound appears to fold together causing "pocketing," it should be refashioned and saucerization performed to avoid accumulation of discharge. If the wound is infected with anaerobic bacteria, administering an antibiotic can improve healing. Using a water-pulsating device (e.g., WaterPik®) offers a simple method for irrigation of the wound (47).

REVERSE BANDAGING

Some pilonidal wounds heal well initially but fail to form epithelium. The problem is mainly mechanical when the patients involved are obese and have a narrow intergluteal cleft. The motion of the buttocks traumatizes the wound constantly. Rosenberg (48) has used reverse bandaging with success. A wide piece of adhesive tape is placed on each side of the wound, stretching it outward. The tapes are tied in front of the abdomen (Fig. 16). The net effect is to flatten the wound and remove most of the angle of the intergluteal cleft.

GLUTEUS MAXIMUS MYOCUTANEOUS FLAP

If the wound is extensive and conservative management fails, the wound should be excised. In this situation, use of a gluteus maximus myocutaneous flap offers a secure repair. However, the procedure is rather extensive for a simple disease.

Under general anesthesia, the patient is placed in the prone position. The unhealed wound, along with a scar and the granulation tissue, is excised to reach normal surrounding fat and presacral fascia. A rotational buttock flap is raised, incorporating skin and the underlying superior portion of the gluteus maximus muscle (Fig. 16). After the skin and subcutaneous tissue of the buttock have been traversed, the upper portion of the gluteus maximus is transected to the level of the gluteus medius and piriformis muscles, with care taken to protect the sciatic nerve. The myocutaneous flap is then rotated into place, a closed suction drain is inserted, and the wound is closed in layers (49). The patient is not allowed to lie on the flap for one week. This technique is seldom necessary since I prefer a simpler Bascom's flap as described below.

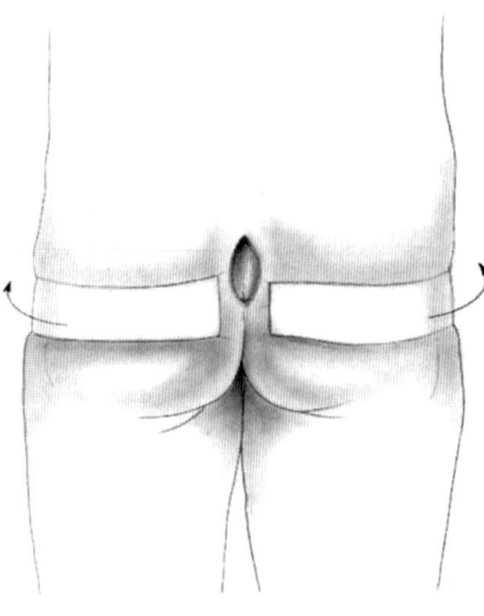

FIGURE 16 ■ Patient's buttocks are strapped with tape in a reverse direction, spreading the wound open.

Z-plasty, V-Y sliding flaps, and rhomboid excision with transposition of flap can also be applied (34,45,50).

■ BASCOM'S FLAP (CLEFT CLOSURE)

This unique method for treating the unhealed wound was devised by Bascom (51). The basic concept is to excise the unhealed skin and the underlying subcutaneous tissue. The natal cleft is eliminated by replacing the defect at the depth of the cleft with a skin flap over the wound. This operation is easier than it appears and is less extensive than the gluteus maximus myocutaneous and other types of flaps. The subcutaneous fat is not mobilized. The flap is a full-thickness skin flap. It is the operation of choice for extensive recurrent pilonidal disease or an unhealed midline wound.

The procedure is performed with the patient under general or spinal anesthesia. A broad-spectrum antibiotic is administered when the patient is called to the operating room and continued until the drain is removed four to five days later. The patient is placed in the prone jackknife position.

With the patient's buttocks pressed together, the lines of contact of the cheeks of the buttocks are marked with a felt-tipped pen (Fig. 17A). The cheeks of the buttocks are then taped apart, and the skin is prepared and draped (Fig. 17B). The skin in this region is infiltrated with 0.25% bupivacaine (Marcaine) containing 1:200,000 epinephrine to decrease bleeding. A triangle-shaped section of skin overlying the unhealed wound is excised, extending above and lateral to the apex of the cleft. The lower end of the incision is curved medially toward the anus to avoid a "dog-ear" upon closure (Fig. 17C). The granulation tissue and hairs are removed. No fat or muscle is mobilized.

After the skin flap (dissected only into the dermis) is raised out to the previously marked line on the left side, the tapes are released. The skin flap is positioned to overlap the edges of the wound on the right side. The excess skin is excised. A closed suction drain is placed in the subcutaneous tissue. The subcutaneous tissue is closed with 3–0 chromic catgut, and the skin is closed with subcuticular 3–0 synthetic monofilament absorbable suture (Fig. 18D and E). The suture line can be reinforced with a running suture, or Steristrips can be applied. The key to this operation is to create the skin flap so that the suture line is off the midline, as seen in Figure 18 E.

It should be noted that Bascom described this technique to treat unhealed wound or recurrent pilonidal sinuses, although it is possible to use it for a complex primary

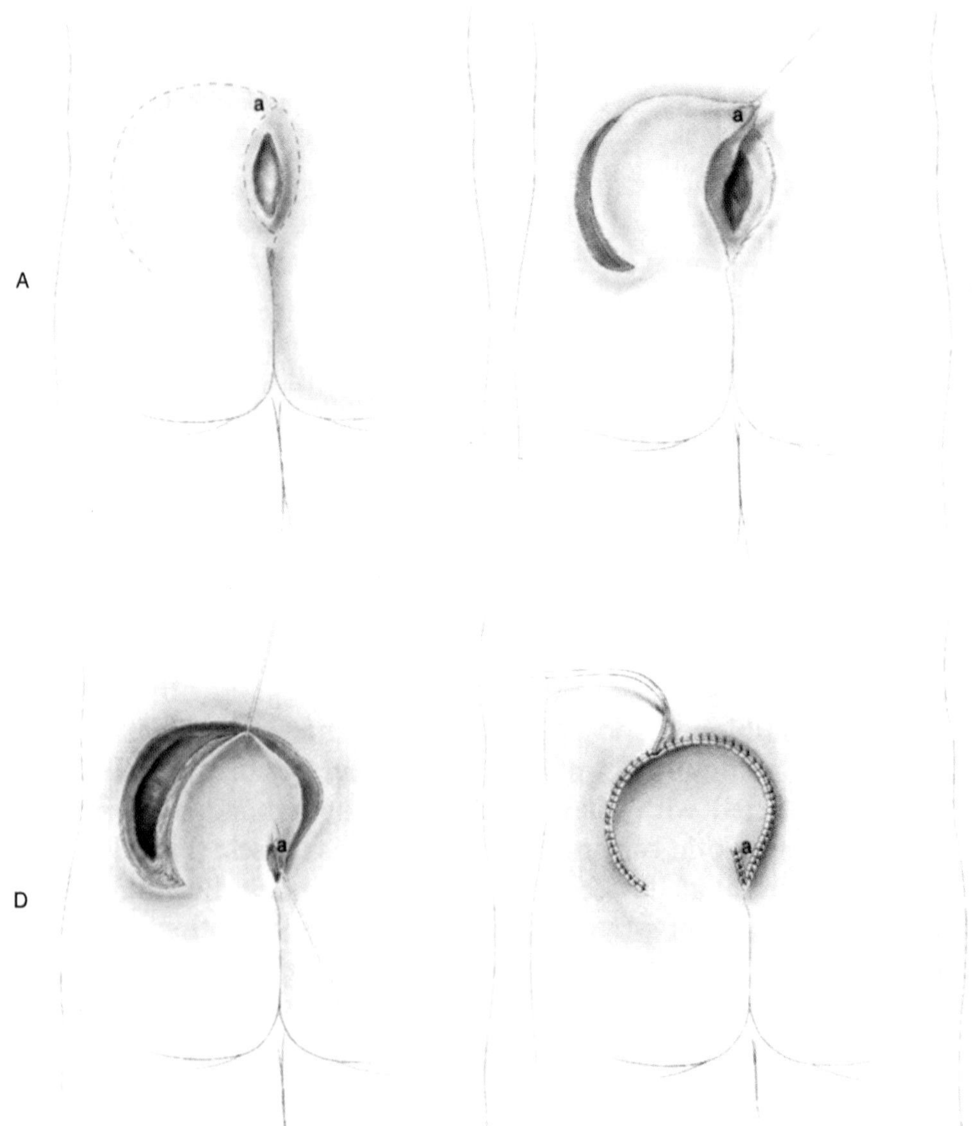

FIGURE 17 ■ Gluteus maximus myocutaneous flap. (**A**) Line of incision for the gluteus myocutaneous flap. (**B**) Chronic wound is excised down to the sacrum, and the flap is created; *a* is apex of the flap. Flap is raised, incorporating superior portion of the gluteus maximus muscle, with great care taken to protect the gluteal vessels and nerve. (**C**) Myocutaneous flap is rotated to cover the presacral defect; *a* is rotated to inferior part of the wound. (**D**) Wound is closed, and a suction drain is placed. *Source*: From Ref. 49.

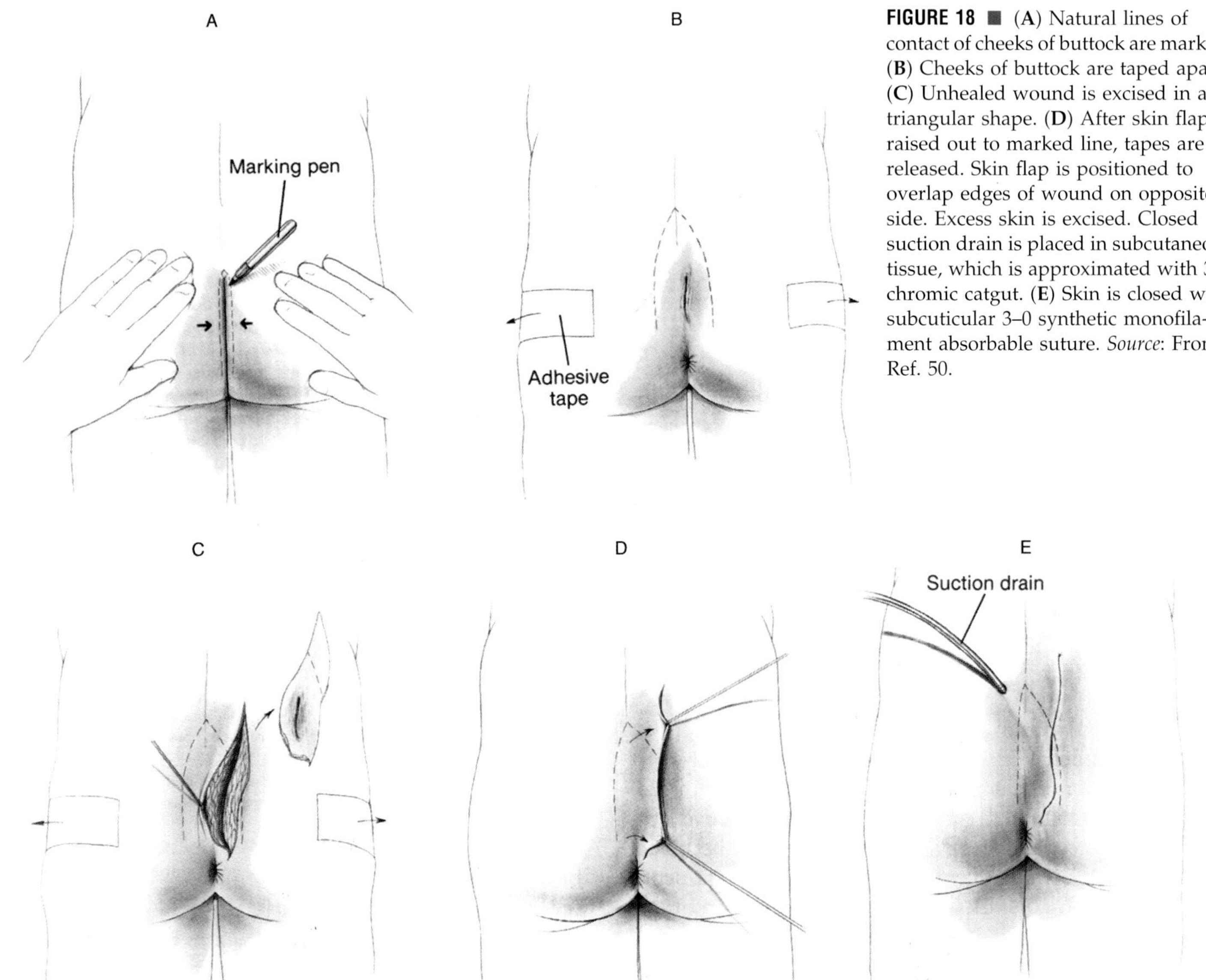

FIGURE 18 ■ (**A**) Natural lines of contact of cheeks of buttock are marked. (**B**) Cheeks of buttock are taped apart. (**C**) Unhealed wound is excised in a triangular shape. (**D**) After skin flap is raised out to marked line, tapes are released. Skin flap is positioned to overlap edges of wound on opposite side. Excess skin is excised. Closed suction drain is placed in subcutaneous tissue, which is approximated with 3–0 chromic catgut. (**E**) Skin is closed with subcuticular 3–0 synthetic monofilament absorbable suture. *Source*: From Ref. 50.

disease. Unlike all other flaps, which are myocutaneous or subcutaneous, Bascom's flap is a full-thickness skin flap. It may look complex, but actually if one follows Bascom's description and drawings, it is quite simple technically.

PILONIDAL SINUS AND CARCINOMA

Carcinoma arising in a chronic pilonidal sinus is rare. In a review of the world literature from 1900 to 1994, only 44 patients were described (Table 1) (52). Thirty-nine cases are squamous cell carcinomas, three are basal cell carcinomas, one is an adenocarcinoma (sweat gland type), and one is an unspecified carcinoma. The cause of pilonidal carcinoma appears to be the same as that by which other chronic inflamed wounds such as scars, skin ulcers, and fistulas undergo malignant degeneration. The average duration of pilonidal disease in the patients is 23 years. Pilonidal carcinoma has a distinctive appearance, and the diagnosis can usually be made on inspection of the patient. A central ulceration is often present, with a friable, indurated, erythematous, and fungating margin. Biopsy confirms the diagnosis. It is usually a well-differentiated squamous cell carcinoma, frequently with focal areas of keratinization and rare mitosis. The carcinoma grows locally before metastasizing to inguinal nodes. Preoperative evaluation of patients with pilonidal carcinoma should include examination of the inguinal areas, perineum, and anorectum. Treatment

TABLE 1 ■ **World Literature on Pilonidal Carcinoma (*n* = 44)**

Male:female ratio	35:9
Age at presentation	50 yr
Mean duration of symptoms	23 yr
Inguinal adenopathy treatment	5 (11%)
Excision	35
Chemotherapy only	1
Radiation only	0
No treatment	2
Excision and radiation	4
Excision and chemotherapy	1
Excision, chemotherapy, and radiation	1
Mean follow-up	29 mo
Recurrence	34%
Time to recurrence	16 mo
Total deceased	12 (27%)
Total deceased with disease	8 (18%)

involves wide local excision to include the presacral fascia. For an extensive wound, a V-Y myocutaneous flap can be performed (53). According to the review of the literature, the recurrence rate is 34%, and death from the disease occurs in 18% of patients on follow-up of 29 months (52).

REFERENCES

1. Anderson AW. Hair extracted from an ulcer. Boston Med Surg J 1847; 36:74.
2. Hodges RM. Pilonidal sinus. Boston Med Surg J 1880; 103:485–486.
3. Buie LA. Jeep disease. South Med J 1944; 37:103–109.
4. Abramson DJ. Outpatient management of pilonidal sinuses: Excision and semi-primary closure technic. Mil Med 1978; 143:753–757.
5. Kooistra HP. Pilonidal sinuses. Review of the literature and report of three hundred fifty cases. Am J Surg 1942; 55:3–17.
6. Lord PH. Etiology of pilonidal sinus. Dis Colon Rectum 1975; 18:661–664.
7. Bascom J. Pilonidal disease: Origin from follicles of hairs and results of follicle removal as treatment. Surgery 1980; 87:567–572.
8. Karydakis GE. Easy and successful treatment of pilonidal sinus after explanation of its causative process. Aust N Z J Surg 1992; 62:385–389.
9. Notaras MJ. A review of three popular methods of postanal (pilonidal) sinus disease. Br J Surg 1970; 57:886–890.
10. Clothier PR, Haywood IR. The natural history of postanal (pilonidal) sinus. Ann R Coll Surg Engl 1984; 66:201–203.
11. Sagi A, Rosenberg L, Greiff M, Mahler D. Squamous cell carcinoma arising in a pilonidal sinus: A case report and review of the literature. J Dermatol Surg Oncol 1984; 10:210–212.
12. Sola JA, Rothenberger DA. Chronic pilonidal disease. An assessment of 150 cases. Dis Colon Rectum 1990; 33:758–761.
13. Klass AA. The so-called pilonidal sinus. Can Med Assoc J 1956; 75:737–742.
14. Akinci OF, Bozer M, Wzankoy A, Duzgun SA, Coskun A. Incidence and etiological factors in pilonidal sinus among Turkish soldiers. Eur J Surg 1999; 165:339–342.
15. Sondenaa K, Andersen E, Nesvik I, Sorlide JA. Patient characteristics and symptoms in chronic pilonidal sinus disease. Int J Colorectal Dis 1995; 10:39–42.
16. Nivatvongs S, Becker ER. The colon, rectum, and anus. In: James EC, Corry KJ, Perry JF Jr., eds. Basic Surgical Practice. Philadelphia: Hanley & Belfus, 1987:339.
17. Armstrong JH, Barcia PJ. Pilonidal sinus disease. The conservative approach. Arch Surg 1994; 129:914–918.
18. Schneider IHF, Thaler K, Kockerling TF. Treatment of pilonidal sinuses by phenol injections. Int J Colorectal Dis 1994; 9:200–202.
19. Dogru O, Camci C, Aygen E, Girgin M, Topuz O. Pilonidal sinus treated with crystallized phenol: An eight-year experience. Dis Colon Rectum 2004; 47: 1934–1938.
20. Bascom J. Pilonidal disease: Long-term results of follicle removal. Dis Colon Rectum 1983; 26:800–807.
21. Senapati A, Cripps NPJ, Thompson MR. Bascom's operation in the day-surgical management of symptomatic pilonidal sinus. Br J Surg 2000; 87: 1067–1070.
22. Culp CE. Pilonidal disease and its treatment. Surg Clin North Am 1967; 47:1007–1014.
23. Bissett IP, Isbister WH. The management of patients with pilonidal disease—a comparative study. Aust N Z J Surg 1987; 57:939–942.
24. Al-Hassan HKL, Francis IM, Neglen P. Primary closure or secondary granulation after excision of pilonidal sinus? Acta Chir Scand 1990; 156:695–699.
25. Sondenaa K, Nesvik I, Gullaksen FP, et al. The role of cefoxitin prophylaxis in chronic pilonidal sinus treated with excision and primary suture. J Am Coll Surg 1995; 180:157–160.
26. Isbiter WH, Prasad J. Pilonidal disease. Aust N Z J Surg 1995; 65:561–563.
27. Allen-Marsh TG. Pilonidal sinus: finding the right track for treatment. Br J Surg 1990; 77:123–132.
28. Spivak H, Brooks VL, Nussbaum M, Friedman I. Treatment of chronic pilonidal disease. Dis Colon Rectum 1996; 39:1136–1139.
29. Fuzun M, Bakir H, Soylu M, Tansug T, Kaymak E, Harmancioglu O. Which technique for treatment of pilonidal sinus—open or closed? Dis Colon Rectum 1994; 37:1148–1150.
30. Dalenback J, Magnusson O, Wedel N, Rimback G. Prospective follow-up after ambulatory plain midline excision of pilonidol sinus and primary suture under local anesthesia—efficient, sufficient, and persistent. Colorectal Dis 2004; 6:488–493.
31. Kronborg O, Christensen K, Zimmermann-Nielsen C. Chronic pilonidal disease: a randomized trial with a complete three-year follow-up. Br J Surg 1985; 72:303–304.
32. Duchateau J, De Mol J, Bostoen H, Allegaert W. Pilonidal sinus. Excision—marsupialization—phenolization? Acta Chir Belg 1985; 85:325–328.
33. Testini M, Piccinni G, Miniello S, et al. Treatment of chronic pilonidal sinus with local anesthesia: A randomized trial of closed compared with open technique. Colorectal Dis 2001; 3:427–430.
34. Toubanakis G. Treatment of pilonidal sinus disease with the Z-plasty procedure (modified). Am Surg 1986; 52:611–612.
35. Mansoory A, Dickson D. Z-plasty for treatment of disease of the pilonidal sinus. Surg Gynecol Obstet 1982; 155:409–411.
36. Kitchen PRB. Pilonidal sinus: Experience with the Karydakis flap. Br J Surg 1996; 83:1452–1455.
37. Akinci OF, Coskun A, Uzunkoy A. Simple and effective surgical treatment of pilonidal sinus. A symmetric excision and primary closure using suction drain and subcuticular skin closure. Dis Colon Rectum 2000; 43:701–707 (commentary by Bascom J in 706–707).
38. Dufourmental C, Mouly R, Beruch J, Banzer P. Sacrococcygeal cysts and fistulas. Pathogenic and therapeutic discussion. Ann Chir Plast 1966; 11:181–186.
39. Azab AS, Kamal MS, Saad RA, Abou al Ata KA, Ali NA. Radical cure of pilonidal sinus by a transposition rhomboid flap. Br J Surg 1984; 71:154–155.
40. Azab ASG, et al. Radical cure of pilonidal sinus by a transposition rhomboid flap. Birt and Surg 1984; 71:154–155, with permission.
41. Milito G, Cortese F, Casciari CW. Rhomboid flap procedure for pilonidal sinus: results from 67 cases. Int J Colorect Dis 1998; 13:113–115.
42. Daphan C, Tekeliogh MH, Sayilgan C. Limberg flap repair for pilonidal sinus disease. Dis Colon Rectum 2004; 47:233–237.
43. Urhan MK, Kucukel F, Topgul K, Ozer I, Sari S. Rhomboid excision and Limberg flap for managing pilonidal sinus. Results of 102 cases. Dis Colon Rectum 2002; 45:656–659.
44. Arumugam PJ, Chandrasekaran TV, Morgan AR, Begnon J, Carr ND. The Rhomboid flap for pilonidal disease. Colorectal Dis 2003; 5:218–221.
45. Topgul K, Ozdemir E, Kilic K, Gokbagir H, Ferahkose Z. Long-term results of Limberg flap procedure for treatment of pilonidal sinus. A report of 200 cases. Dis colon Rectum 2003; 46:1545–1548.
46. Petersen S, Koch R, Stelzuer S, Wendlandt TP, Ludwig K. Primary closure techniques in chronic pilonidal sinus. A survey of the results of different surgical approaches. Dis Colon Rectum 2002; 45:1458–1467.
47. Hoexter B. Use of WaterPik lavage in pilonidal wound care. Dis Colon Rectum 1976; 19:470–471.
48. Rosenberg I. Reverse bandaging for cure of the reluctant pilonidal wound. Dis Colon Rectum 1977; 20:290–291.
49. Perez-Gurri JA, Temple-Walley J, Ketcham AS. Gluteus maximus myocutaneous flap for the treatment of recalcitrant pilonidal disease. Dis Colon Rectum 1984; 27:262–264.
50. Schoeller T, Wechselberger G, Otto A, Papp C. Definitive surgical treatment of complicated recurrent pilonidal disease with a modified fasciocutaneous V-Y advancement flap. Surgery 1997; 121:258–263.
51. Bascom JW. Repeat pilonidal operations. Am J Surg 1987; 154:118–122.
52. Davis KA, Mock CN, Versaci A, Dentrichia P. Malignant degeneration of pilonidal cysts. Am Surg 1994; 60:200–204.
53. Pekmezci S, Hiz M, Saribeyoglu K, et al. Malignant degeneration: an unusual complication of pilonidal sinus disease. Eur J Surg 2001; 167:475–477.

12 Perianal Dermatologic Disease

Lee E. Smith

INTRODUCTION

Patients with primary perianal dermatologic conditions and secondary perianal involvement in systemic diseases are initially seen with a variety of symptoms and macroscopic appearances. Even though patients may have painful, friable, indurated, ulcerated, or raised skin lesions, their most frequent symptom is pruritus (1). For practical purposes the perianal skin conditions may be classified as pruritic and nonpruritic. When no underlying cause for pruritus can be identified, the condition is termed "idiopathic pruritus ani," the most common type. Consequently, it serves as the basis for much of this discussion. In treating this group of conditions, the dermatologist and the surgeon frequently work in concert. The dermatologist, because of his or her visual training, is equipped to diagnose, scrape, culture, and prepare microscopic preparations and perform a biopsy in the office, and the surgeon is able to examine and culture and to perform a biopsy on anorectal pathology through anoscopes and proctoscopes. This chapter reviews the dermatologic conditions with emphasis on diagnosis and treatment from the surgeon's perspective.

PRURITIC CONDITIONS

IDIOPATHIC PRURITUS ANI

Pruritus ani is an unpleasant cutaneous sensation characterized by varying degrees of itching. Men are affected more often than women in a ratio of four to one (1). Idiopathic forms of pruritus ani occur in approximately 50% to 90% of the cases (2,3). The remaining cases of pruritus are symptomatic presentations of either localized or systemic diseases (e.g., hemorrhoids, diabetes), which are considered later in this chapter.

History

Symptoms, which usually start insidiously, are characterized by the occasional awareness of an uncomfortable perianal sensation. The anal skin is richly endowed with sensory nerves, but the perceptions of individual patients vary. Some patients feel an itch, whereas others sense burning. Often the patient is more aware of the problem at night or in hot, humid weather, although this is not always the case. The itching also may be exaggerated by friction from clothing, wool, and perspiration; on the other hand, applying cool compresses counters irritation, and heat avoidance, mental distraction, and lubrication of the skin surface ease the itching. With time, the condition may progress to an unrelenting, intolerably tormenting, burning soreness compounded by the insurmountable urge to scratch, claw, and otherwise irritate the area in a futile effort to obtain relief. The severely afflicted patient is eventually exhausted, and a few have been driven to suicide as a means of obtaining relief.

The patient has usually resorted to self treatment with over-the-counter medications. The patient often overtreats; so a first step for the physician is to stop the acute, contact dermatitis. Poor anal hygiene is often a contributing factor; therefore, questions about the patient's cleansing habits may be important. Specific dietary ingredients and neurogenic, psychogenic, and idiosyncratic reactions with pruritus should be suspected whenever another factor is not readily identified (see specific causes below) (1,4–6). Since the diagnosis is made by exclusion, inquiries about diabetes, psoriasis, family history of atopic eczema, use of local topical medications, seborrhea on other sites on the body, children with similar itching reminiscent of pinworms, antibiotic use, vaginal discharge or infection, acholic stools, dark urine, or anal intercourse may establish the factor or factors responsible for the symptom.

Stress and anxiety may exaggerate pruritus ani. Often personal factors in life are omitted by the patient. When taking a history, the physician may have to encourage the patient to "open up" and to express or consider factors that may be contributing to the discomfort. Common complaints revolve around family, work, and finances (7). Laurent et al. used the Mini-Mult personality test for psychological assessment of patients with idiopathic pruritus ani versus normal controls. They found that the mean hypomania and depression scales were greater and smaller, respectively, in the idiopathic pruritus group. However, the conclusion was that psychological factors are only predisposing factors (8).

Physical Findings

In the early stages of the condition, examination may reveal only minimal erythema and excoriations. As the symptoms progress, the perianal skin becomes thin, friable, tender, blistered, ulcerated, and "weeping" (Fig. 1). In the later stages the skin is raw, red, lichenified, and oozing or pale (Fig. 2), with exaggeration of the radiating folds of anal skin. Often, a secondary bacterial or fungal infection is present. A clinical classification used at Washington Hospital Center, Washington, D.C., is based on the appearance of the skin. Stage 0 skin appears normal. Stage 1 skin is red and inflamed. Stage 2 has white lichenified skin. Stage 3 has lichenified skin as well as coarse ridges of skin and often ulcerations secondary to scratching.

Careful local anorectal examination may distinguish an inciting factor, but a detailed skin examination of the entire body may provide the diagnosis. Adjunctive laboratory and radiologic testing (e.g., determining blood glucose and electrolyte levels or performing a barium enema) may be required to diagnose a primary cause. If a treatment program is begun before the factors that may result in pruritus have been ruled out, a primary cause may be overlooked. Rather than decreasing the misery of the patient, this approach may cause the condition to become worse.

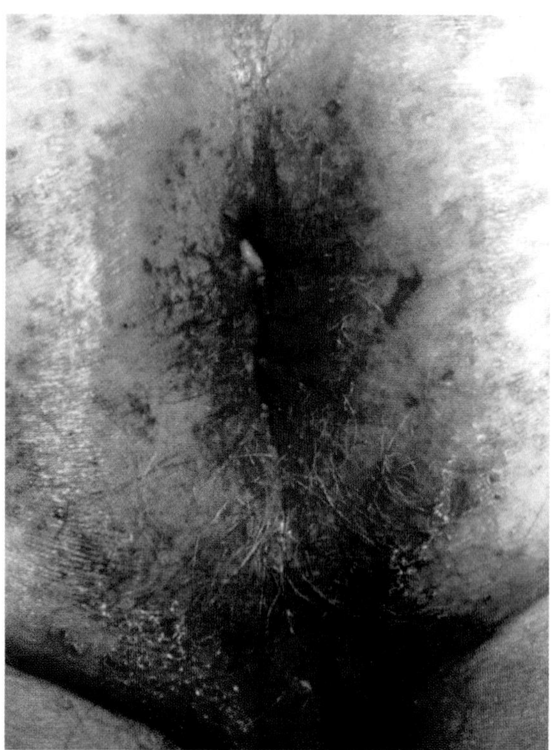

FIGURE 1 ■ Red excoriated skin of stage 1 pruritus ani.

Physiologic Testing

Physiologic studies of patients with pruritus ani have been performed to determine whether disordered function is a causative factor. Manometry, compliance, sensation to rectal balloon, and perineal descent have been measured and were found to be the same as those of controls (9). The exception was a significantly greater fall in anal pressure with rectal balloon distention (2,9). Farouk et al. (10) used computerized ambulatory electromyography and manometry to demonstrate that patients with pruritus ani have an abnormal transient internal sphincter relaxation, one that is greater and prolonged. Thus, occult fecal leakage with

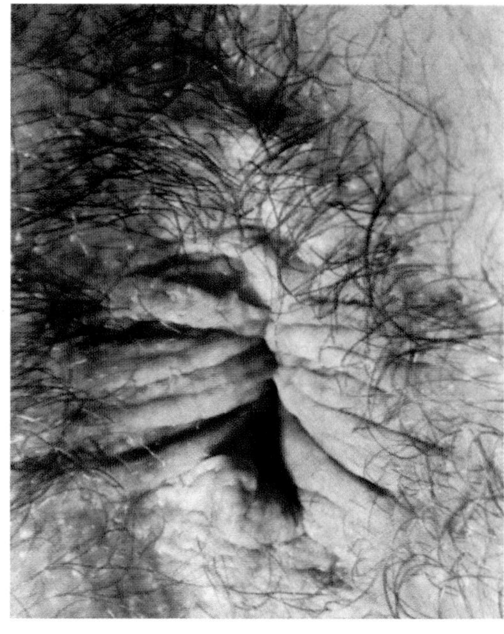

FIGURE 2 ■ Lichenified skin of stage 3 pruritus ani.

subsequent perianal itching results. Others have shown a decreased resting anal pressure by manometric comparison before and after coffee consumption (4). Thus coffee may contribute to a leak.

Saline infusion tests showed early leakage (after 600 mL) as compared to control subjects (after 1300 mL) (9). There is an inverse relationship to the severity of symptoms and the volume of first leakage. Again, leaking and soiling seem to be major factors.

Histopathology

In acute pruritus, epithelial intercellular edema and vesiculation are present. In chronic cases, hyperkeratosis and acanthosis are noted. Atrophy of the outer layers of the epidermis, sebaceous glands, and hair follicles may occur, but in part this may be due to use of potent steroids. Finally, ulceration may supervene.

Treatment

Therapy for idiopathic pruritus ani is nonspecific and often involves changes over the course of time. The treatment is directed at regaining a clean, dry, and intact perianal skin. The following discussion outlines a broad approach to this symptom complex, including reassurance, education, local treatment, and follow-up.

Reassurance

Since, by definition, idiopathic pruritus ani has no identifiable primary cause, treatment is mainly symptomatic and directed toward decreasing moisture in the perianal area. Reassurance to the patient that there is no underlying pathology, particularly carcinoma, is often as effective in producing a "cure" as any of the physical or medicinal modalities used. Often these patients have a long, protracted course of treatment, and a sympathetic, reassuring approach is necessary to achieve ultimate success.

Education and Local Treatment

Providing patient education is very important. Patients are instructed to cleanse several times daily, especially after bowel movements. Although cleanliness is stressed, the use of medicated soaps in the perianal region is discouraged. In the acute, excoriated, weeping, crusting stage, warm wet packs may aid in debridement. The patient can dry him- or herself gently with either a soft towel or, preferably, a hair dryer. A combination of Kerodex 71 and 2.5% hydrocortisone ointment is used as a barrier on the perianal skin and to reduce inflammation. Fluorinated steroid topical preparations should not be used over long periods of time because skin atrophy will ensue and perhaps incite a more unpleasant skin condition. Anesthetic preparations such as Xylocaine ointment may mask the disease or contribute to an allergic dermatitis; thus the use of soothing topical medications is preferred. As the condition improves, or is in milder forms, creams and lotions are replaced with cornstarch powder or talc. A small wisp of absorbent cotton or absorbent paper tissue may be tucked into the anal cleft to help keep the area dry.

Coffee (including decaffeinated blends), tea, colas, chocolate, beer, citrus fruits, alcohol, dairy products, and tomatoes may contribute to idiopathic pruritus (6). Serial elimination of each item for two weeks may help identify the offending substance. If the pruritus disappears, deleted foods are returned to the diet one at a time. If the pruritus recurs, the offending ingredient is withdrawn. Daniel et al. (11) found that coffee directly correlated between the severity of perianal irritation and the amount of coffee consumed daily. If the patient has "after leak," characterized by stinging, burning, or a perianal "crawling" sensation superimposed on the itch after a bowel movement, the patient is instructed to irrigate the rectal ampulla with a small tap-water enema. Following this procedure, the patient needs to cleanse the area with a wet tissue while straining down and opening the anal canal. This process is continued until there is no brown stain left on the tissue. A mucosal prolapse, a rectocele, or a hidden rectal prolapse might be suspected and observed during the physical examination.

Other nonspecific therapy includes shaving hirsute patients. However, as the hair grows back, the short stubble can be a source of irritation and increase the urge to scratch, defeating the original gains. Extreme cases may require sedation and/or antihistamines such as diphenhydramine hydrochloride (Benadryl), 25 mg, four to six times per day. Estrogens may be useful in postmenopausal women. Wearing loose-fitting clothes and undergarments made of cotton may be helpful. Softened fabrics have been shown to reduce frictional effect on skin, especially irritated skin (12). Underwear made of synthetic fibers does not absorb perspiration. If a secondary bacterial or fungal infection is present, topical antibiotics or fungicides may be instituted based on the results from cultures and sensitivity testing. If medical therapy is failing, a biopsy to identify Bowen's or Paget's disease is in order.

In the past various methods such as tattooing with mercury sulfide, sclerotherapy, radiation therapy, and surgical procedures have been used. These methods are generally condemned because permanent cure is seldom reported. However, Eusebio et al. (13) treated 23 patients over a 9½-year period with one intracutaneous injection treatment of the anodermal and perianal skin using intravenous sedation, local anesthesia, and up to 30 mL of 0.5% methylene blue. Of the 23 patients, 10 had complete long-term relief, four had complete relief but were lost to follow-up after 12 weeks, and four had relief for 12 weeks but experienced varying degrees of recurrence. The use of methylene blue was verified by Farouk and Lee (14) in six patients.

Follow-Up

Initially, patients with severe disease may need to be seen as frequently as twice per week. Providing reassurance and visible concern is often the most important part of therapy at this time. As symptoms improve, the time between visits can be gradually lengthened until the patient is seen once every 3 to 4 weeks. It is important not to discontinue seeing a patient using a steroid cream because chronic use can lead to the development of atrophic skin, superinfection, and a secondary pruritus or burning sensation.

Often the symptoms wax and wane, and a cure is based more on a flexible therapy plan coupled with positive psychologic reinforcement than on the actual agent or agents used. Constant reiteration of the desired goals and the methods used to achieve them may be necessary. Finally, the physician should be willing to reassess the patient whenever there is any suggestion that a more specific entity may be responsible for the pruritus.

■ PRIMARY ETIOLOGIES

Poor Hygiene

Poor hygiene is often associated with the diseases discussed in this section. Frequently, this is the only factor identified with cases labeled as "idiopathic." The anatomy of a patient (e.g., a deep intergluteal cleft) may render the perianal region inaccessible to proper cleansing. In other cases, the patient is not fastidious in cleansing, and retained mucus, perspiration, and feces initiate the local irritation process (4). Some disabled patients, such as those with arthritis, strokes, or multiple sclerosis, are physically incapable of performing adequate perianal hygiene. Likewise, the elderly who have even mild incontinence may not cleanse well, such that irritation and pruritus will ensue (15).

Anorectal Lesions

Any lesion in the gastrointestinal tract that can cause excessive moisture in the perianal region may result in pruritus. Hemorrhoids, anal fissures and fistulas, hypertrophied papillae, prolapse, and neoplasms are some of the more frequent anorectal offenders. Rubber band ligation often controls pruritus associated with hemorrhoids (16). Treatment should be directed toward the specific pathology.

Infections

Infections can be caused by parasites, viruses, bacteria, fungi, or yeasts. These pathologies are considered in the following discussion.

Parasites

A common cause of perianal itching in children is infestation with *Enterobius vermicularis*, or pinworms. The child can be the source of infestation in the family. The worms emerge from the anal canal at night and early morning; consequently, pruritus is worst at those times. Scratching tends to scatter the eggs in the bed and wherever the patient disrobes. The diagnosis is made by microscopically identifying the *E. vermicularis* eggs or adult worms (Fig. 3). The specimen is collected by applying clear, adhesive cellulose tape across the anus when symptoms are worst. The tape is then attached to a microscopic slide for examination. The use of lactophenol cotten blue stain enhances the detection of the colorless eggs (17).

If *E. vermicularis* is found, treatment consists of piperazine citrate (Antepar) in doses varied according to the patient's age and weight or, preferably, mebendazole (Vermox), 100 mg for all ages, in a single dose (18). Unfortunately, all family members must be treated because of the frequent cross-spread of eggs to family members. The eggs are everywhere in the household; therefore, after treatment, cleaning all floors, furniture, linens, and beds to eradicate the eggs is important to avoid reinfestation.

Pediculus pubis, a louse, is a parasite visible to the naked eye; under magnification it resembles a crab (Fig. 4).

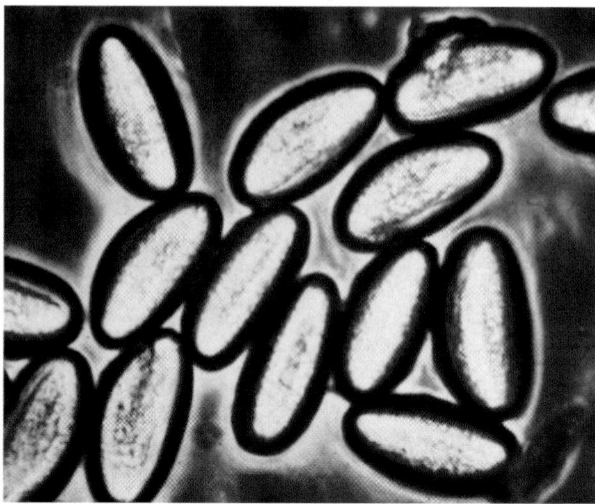

FIGURE 3 ■ Eggs of *Enterobius vermicularis* on clear adhesive tape.

The nits of eggs embedded on the pubic hair can readily be observed. Treatment consists of malathion 0.5% lotion applied to the pubic and perianal hair and then rinsed off after at least two hours. An alternative is permethrin cream 1% applied and washed off after 10 minutes, carbaryl 1% applied and washed out 12 hours later, and phenothrin 0.2% applied and washed out two hours later (19). A second application can be made a week later (20). All sexual partners must be treated. Clothing and bedding can be sterilized by washing in very hot water.

Scabies is estimated to infect over 300,000,000 people worldwide (21). It is a parasitic infestation characterized by itching on the arms, legs, and scrotum before the development of pruritus ani (Fig. 5) (17). As the itch mite, *Sarcoptes scabiei*, burrows, it creates dark punctate lesions, which are readily identified on the trunk and particularly between the fingers and ventral surface of the wrists. The diagnosis depends on demonstration of the parasite in a potassium hydroxide preparation (Fig. 6). Treatment includes topical application of 5% permethrin or 1% lindane (applied as creams or lotions from the neck down, and then washed off in 8 to 12 hours) (20,22). Oral ivermectin (150 to 200 μg/Kg of body weight) given as an initial dose and again in two weeks cures 95%. Good hygiene

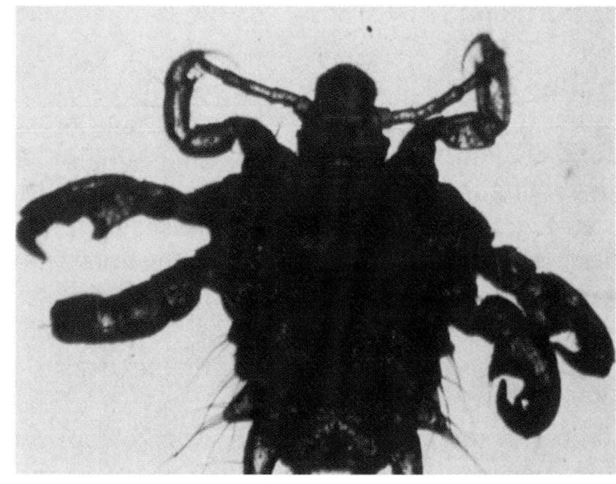

FIGURE 4 ■ *Pediculus pubis* (pubic louse).

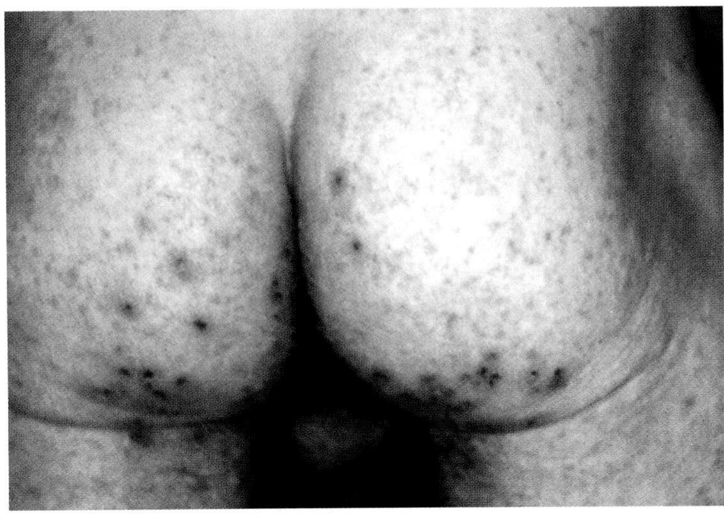

FIGURE 5 ■ Lesions of scabies. *Source*: Courtesy of Milton Orkin, M.D., Minneapolis, Minnesota, U.S.A.

and cleansing of all clothing and bedding by washing in hot water is necessary to avoid reinfestation. Some itching may persist for weeks, due to dead scabies parts, but mild topical steroids and systemic antihistamines control the itching (23). In children, the head also must be treated. Care must be taken to avoid open wounds because absorption may cause convulsions.

Viruses

The most common viral infection in the perianal region is condyloma acuminatum, which is discussed in Chapter 13.

Perianal presentation of herpes simplex virus (HSV-2) is rare; compared to its frequent presentation as genital infection (herpes genitalis), and even less frequently when compared to herpes simplex virus (HSV-1), which presents as the familiar "cold sore" and "fever blister." The mode of infection is usually sexual, but the virus may be spread by direct contact from parent to infant or from the mouth and through the gastrointestinal tract to the perianal site. Unfortunately HSV-1, the nasolabial cold sore type, is becoming a progressively larger proportion of the perineal herpes infections (24).

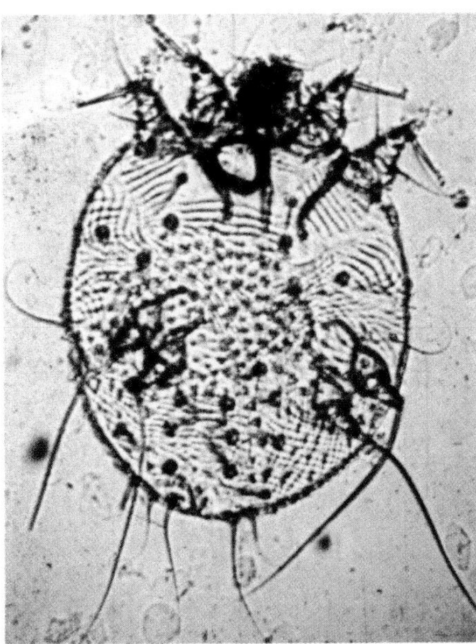

FIGURE 6 ■ *Sarcoptes scabiei* (scabies parasite). *Source*: Courtesy of Milton Orkin, M.D., Minneapolis, Minnesota, U.S.A.

The incubation time is usually 2 to 7 days, but it may last up to three weeks, with prodromal symptoms consisting of minimal burning, irritation, or paresthesias. The infection is characterized by severe pain and pruritus, with a serous or purulent discharge. Tenesmus and secondary spasm are common. The pain may radiate to the groin, thighs, and buttocks.

The initial lesion is a small vesicle with a surrounding erythematous areola (Fig. 7). Within 24 to 48 hours the surface ruptures, and an ulcer results (Fig. 8). In the immunosuppressed patient ulcers may become confluent, appearing as ulcerating cellulitis. The lesions are distributed equally between the perianal skin and the anal canal. If the patient has never had a herpes infection, systemic symptoms (e.g., fever, chills, malaise) are common. Healing leaves scalloped scars. A recurrence may involve only some scattered vesicles.

The diagnosis usually is made by history and physical examination alone. Adjunctive methods include cytology, immunofluorescence, viral culture, and Tzanck test. Currently there are commercial companies vying for a faster, more accurate test, using the new glycoprotein G-based, type-specific HSV serologies (25). If a vesicle or the margin of an ulcer is scraped, the scrapings may be smeared on a slide, heat fixed, stained with methylene blue, and rinsed. Multinucleated giant cells may be seen with this viral disease. Other viral diseases such as herpes zoster or chickenpox also have giant cells.

The disease is usually self-limiting in 1 to 3 weeks if there is no secondary bacterial infection. Symptomatic treatment (see discussion of idiopathic pruritus ani) is the basis for relief. Acyclovir may be used to abort the first attack. Four hundred milligrams five times per day for 10 days, is the usual dose (26). New antiviral agents, famciclovir 250 mg tid for 5 to 10 days, and valacyclovir 1 gm bid for 10 days offer more convenient treatment schedules (26). Recurrence is the rule, and acyclovir, valacyclovir, and famciclovir reduce the duration of viral shedding and time to lesion healing (19). If recurrences are frequent,

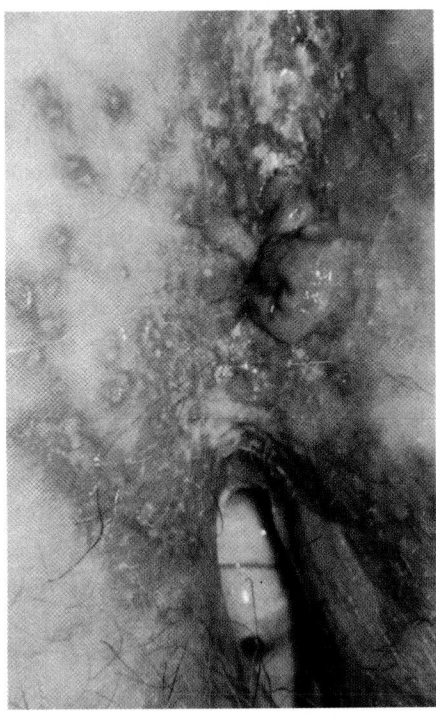

FIGURE 7 ■ Herpes genitalis. Acute vesicles.

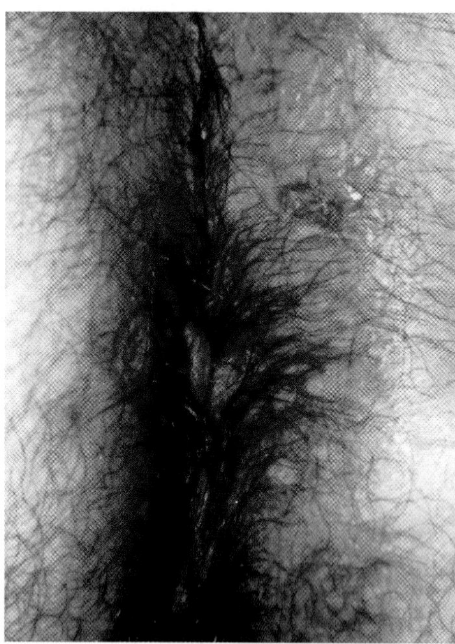

FIGURE 8 ■ Herpes genitalis. Open ulcers.

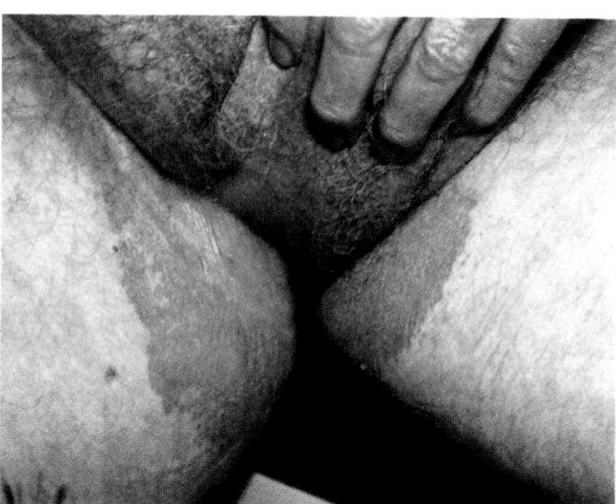

FIGURE 9 ■ Lesions of erythrasma (*Corynebacterium minutissimum*).

prescribing these drugs may be tried as prophylaxis. The prophylactic regimen is acyclovir 400 mg bid, valacyclovir 500 mg po qd, or famciclovir 250 mg po bid for six months. The immunosuppressed patient must be hospitalized for intravenous acyclovir treatment (27). Steroids are never used because they may potentiate the infection. Other specific treatment, such as immunization with vaccines, have been shown to be largely ineffective in the treatment of genital herpes (28).

Lumbosacral dermatomes are involved in 11% of patients infected by herpes zoster (29). The causative virus is *Herpesvirus varicellae*, which has a variable incubation period. The first manifestations are fever, pain, and malaise. After 3 to 4 days, the characteristic closely grouped red papules appear along dermatomes, and they become vesicular and pustular quickly. Lymphadenopathy is common.

Sacral herpes zoster may result in urinary retention and sensory loss in both the bladder and rectum (29). These results can be seen even with unilateral skin involvement, which is somewhat perplexing since hemisection of the cord does not result in detectable sphincter dysfunction.

Treatment is mainly symptomatic. Oral acyclovir and steroids may give early relief and minimize neurologic sequelae (29). Complete spontaneous recovery over 3 to 4 weeks is the usual course. Post-herpetic neuralgia is the most common adverse sequela.

Bacteria

Erythrasma caused by *Corynebacterium minutissimum* may affect the perianal, perineal, and axillary regions but is most common in the toe webs. The characteristic pruritic perianal lesion is a large round patch, initially pink and irregular, but subsequently turning brown and scaly (Fig. 9). The diagnosis is made by examining the lesions under ultraviolet light and observing the characteristic coral-red to salmon-pink fluorescence secondary to porphyrin production by the bacteria (Fig. 10). Occasionally, the visible lesion is non-fluorescent; however, the diagnosis can be made by biopsy of the lesion (30). Treatment consists of 250 mg of erythromycin by mouth, four times per day for a 10 to 14 day period, or chloramphenicol ointment (30).

Patients with syphilis may have pruritus caused by irritation secondary to exudates from the primary chancre or the secondary condyloma latum (Fig. 11). Pruritus is uncommon in the tertiary stage, when there usually is no gross lesion. This disease is more fully discussed in Chapter 14.

Though rare, perianal tuberculosis may be seen initially either as an ulcer with a sharp irregular outline and a grayish granular base or as a purulent ulcerated verrucous lesion. It also may be seen as an extensive perianal inflammation with areas of healing and breakdown, subcutaneous nodules, sinuses, and deformity. Pain is minimal, but local soreness and pruritus are common. Generally the colon is also involved, and the diagnosis is made by having an antecedent history of tuberculosis or a positive chest radiograph or by identifying acid-fast organisms in scrapings from the lesions. With modern day treatments these lesions are relatively rare, but when present they can be readily conquered. The reader is referred to a standard textbook of medicine for details of antituberculosis drug management.

Streptococcus may cause a perianal dermatitis in both children and adults. That dermatitis is a well-defined erythema of the perianal skin that does not respond to the

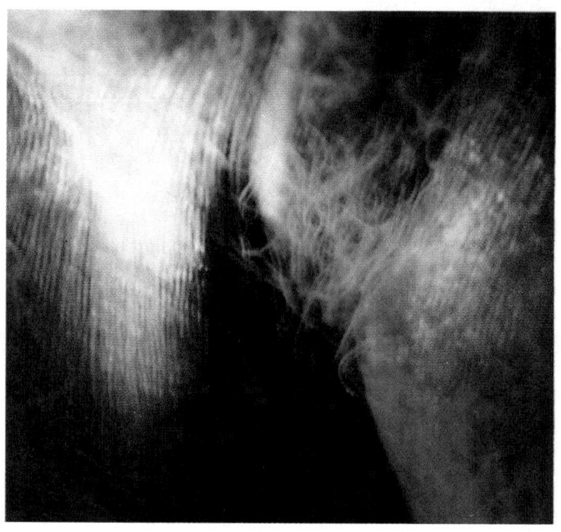

FIGURE 10 ■ Pink fluorescence of erythrasma when viewed under the ultraviolet lamp.

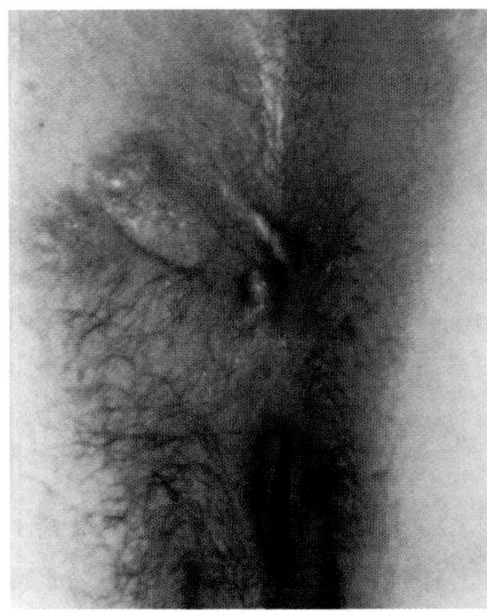

FIGURE 11 ■ Primary chancre of syphilis on white skin. *Source*: Courtesy of Maria Turner, M.D., Washington, D.C.

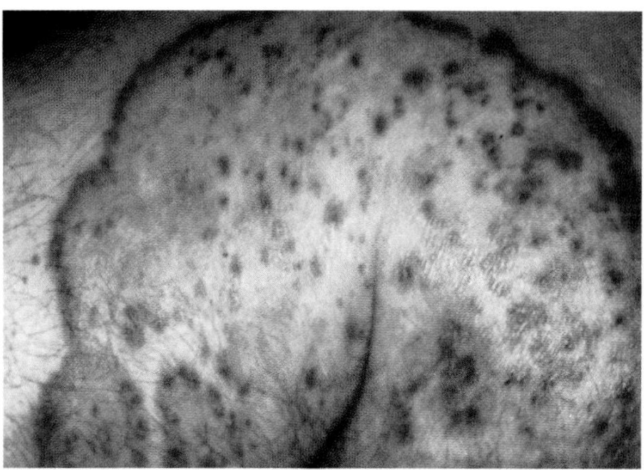

FIGURE 13 ■ *Tinea circinata* (ringworm). *Source*: Courtesy of Maria Turner, M.D., Washington, D.C.

usual topical treatments for anal complaints. Culture of the perianal dermatitis might verify this diagnosis. In therapy-resistant anal redness, streptococcus dermatitis should be considered (31,32). In children, cure is usually obtained by oral penicillin or erythromycin for 10 to 14 days (33). Adults are more difficult to cure, but there has been success with erythromycin, clindamycin, or a dicloxacillin (34).

Fungi and Yeast

Candida albicans, a saprophytic yeast, is normally present in the gut. This yeast can become pathogenic with a change in the patient's resistance or in the normal skin, such as with uncontrolled diabetes mellitus, prolonged antibiotic treatment, or prolonged use of steroids. The infected skin appears moist, red, and macerated (Fig. 12). Pustules form and become confluent, bright red, and scaly, with poorly defined margins and satellite lesions. Under microscopic scrutiny, mycelian forms and spores can be identified from scrapings of the lesion. The microscopic slide is prepared by placing 20% potassium hydroxide on the scrapings and gently warming them; then the slide is examined with 10 and 40 times magnification. Organisms may be grown on Sabouraud's culture medium.

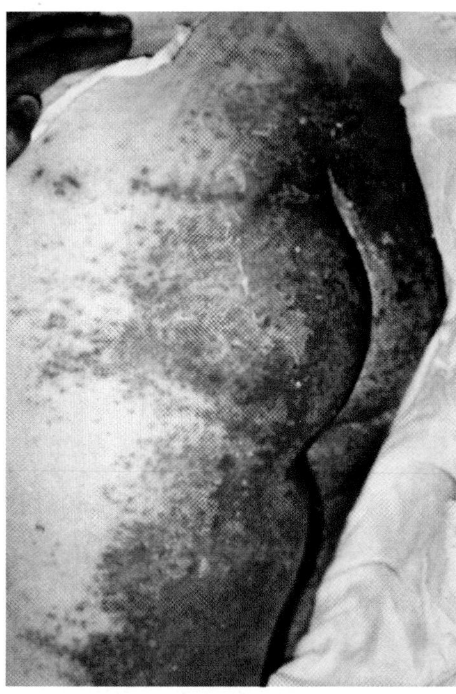

FIGURE 12 ■ Moist, red, macerated lesions of *Candida albicans*. *Source*: Courtesy of Maria Turner, M.D., Washington, D.C.

Treatment consists of applying nystatin (Mycostatin) powder or ointment or imidazole compound several times daily, along with controlling or eliminating the precipitating cause (e.g., control of diabetes, withdrawal of antibiotics and/or steroids). For resistant cases fluconazole (Diflucan) 150 mg po may be tried, and it may be repeated.

Epidermophyton floccosum, *Trichophyton mentagrophytes*, and *Trichophyton rubrum* are fungal infections that are usually seen unilaterally with a scaly, well-defined, circinate margin (Fig. 13). The presence of dermatophytes is always associated with prutitus (35). The dermatophytes begin as a red bump that spreads centrifugally, eventually to give a ring-within-a-ring, or "ringworm," appearance. Often a similar lesion is seen between the toes. Diagnosis is confirmed by culturing scrapings on Sabouraud's medium or by examining them as a potassium hydroxide preparation under the microscope. On low power, strands of fungus may be seen (Fig. 14). Treatment is achieved with various fungicidal preparations such as tolnaftate (Tinactin) or topical imidazole if the lesion is superficial. Deep

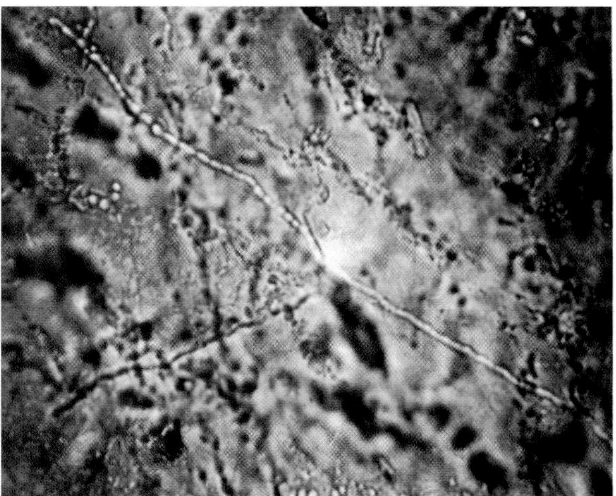

FIGURE 14 ■ Hyphae of a fungus seen in a potassium hydroxide preparation. *Source*: Courtesy of Mervyn Elgart, M.D., Washington, D.C.

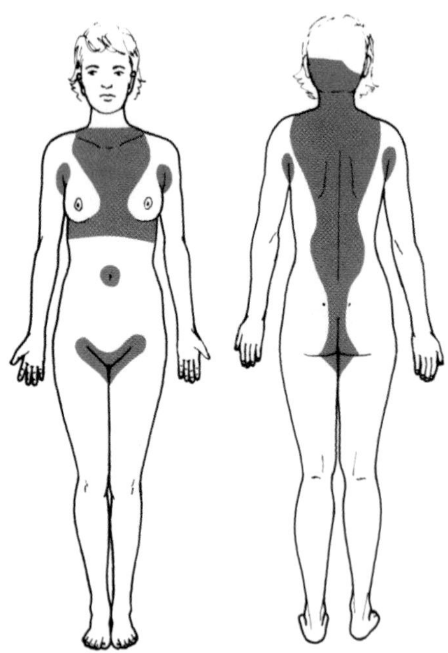

FIGURE 15 ■ Body pattern of seborrhea.

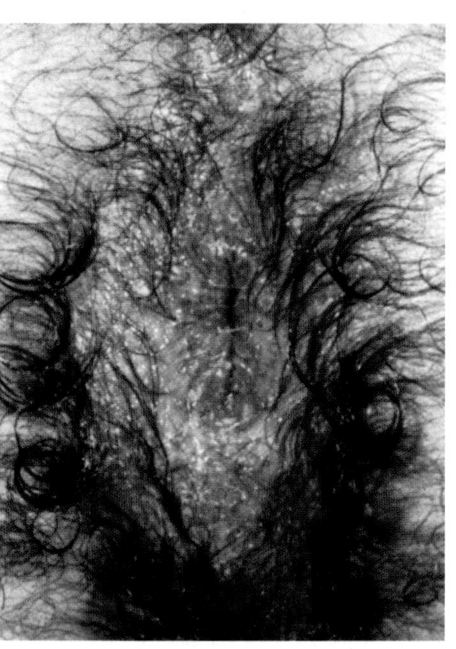

FIGURE 17 ■ Contact dermatitis caused by use of a common over-the-counter hemorrhoidal ointment preparation.

invasion of the follicles may warrant oral therapy with griseofulvin ultrafine, 250 mg twice a day for 3 to 4 weeks; a complete response sometimes requires 6 to 8 weeks of treatment. This drug should be taken with food to minimize gastrointestinal distress and nausea. Ketoconazole (Nizoral) is effective, but occasional deaths resulting from hepatic toxicity have occurred after five months. Any interdigital lesions must also be eradicated to achieve a cure. Terbinafine used orally has been shown to be safe and efficacious (36).

Skin Diseases

Skin lesions may be localized to the perianal region or may be systemic. The patient's entire body must be examined for evidence of further lesions whenever a dermatologic condition is being investigated.

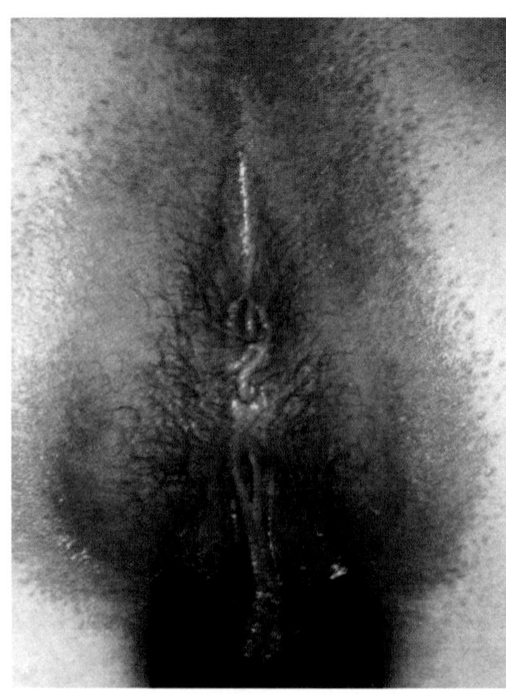

FIGURE 16 ■ Contact dermatitis caused by use of lidocaine.

Seborrhea

Seborrhea, or dandruff, may be found on the perineum. The red color is not bright, but fissuring maybe seen. Pruritus is the chief complaint. Other parts of the body, such as the scalp, chest, ears, suprapubic area, and beard, should be inspected (Fig. 15). Studies of the etiology of seborrheic dermatitis (SD) concentrate on the role of *Pityrasporum ovale* and sebaceous lipids. Patients with SD have lower levels of free fatty acids and higher triglycerides in their skin as compared to patients without SD (37). The treatment is 2% sulfur with hydrocortisone lotion or miconazole lotion, or 2% ketoconazole shampoo (38). Terbinafine solution or 250 mg tablets have been efficacious (39,40). If the patient is immunocompromised, ketoconazole may be used. The response to treatment is usually good.

Contact Dermatitis

The anogenital region is subject to many products that may cause a contact dermatitis, such as douches, dusting powders contraceptives, colored toilet paper, poison ivy, and strong topical medications. The history should include questions about over-the-counter medications and home remedies. The highly irritating, eczematous, ill-defined lesions of contact dermatitis may result from prolonged exposure to topical medications such as lanolin, neomycin, and parabens. Parabens is a preservative that is used in topical preparations; unfortunately, it evokes an allergic reaction in some patients. Topical anesthetics of the "-caine" family may be especially irritating (Fig. 16) (41). Both amide (e.g., lidocaine) and ester (e.g., procaine) topical anesthetics may cause a reaction. A patch test or perhaps intradermal injection tests will show an allergy to lidocaine and a cross-reaction to bupivacaine (42). Quinolones in the anesthetic ointment may results in contact dermatitis. Often the hand with which the patient applies the offending agent is similarly affected. The skin appears intensely erythematous with vesicles and is fragile and macerated.

A common over-the-counter hemorrhoidal preparation that has little efficacy for hemorrhoids causes dermatitis (Fig. 17). Common spices used in cooking may result in anal irritation and inflammation.

Toilet paper can cause an allergy. Euxyl K 400 is a preservative system for cosmetics and toiletries that contains methyldibromoglutaronitrile. This ingredient is a newly recognized allergen contained in moistened toilet paper. Thus anal dermatitis might be tested for with a patch test of 0.3 to 0.5% methyldibromoglutaronitrile in petrolatum.

Cashew nuts, a favorite snack, and oil used to make other foods, unfortunately, belong to the poison oak and poison ivy family. Sensitive people may develop eruptions on the hands, lips, and perianal area when exposed to the cardol oil (43).

The overuse of topical steroids is a problem that results in "steroid skin" (Fig. 18) (44). The perianal skin develops marked striae. Overgrowth with *Candida* organisms is common but can be prevented by limiting the duration of use of and the strength of the steroid ointment. Prolonged use of the fluorinated steroid preparations results in atrophy of the perianal skin, which leads to worse symptoms than those few for which the preparation was initially prescribed (44). Nystatin (Mycolog), a commonly prescribed medication, formerly contained ethylenediamine as a preservative, which frequently caused an allergic reaction. Up to 25% of people exposed to neomycin, which is a constituent of Neosporin, may have an allergic reaction. Poison ivy, sumac, or oak may be the source of acute anogenital eruption if the person has knelt or squatted in the outdoors with an exposed perineum. The vesicles may be debrided.

A patient with severe contact dermatitis may require bed rest for a few days. The skin should be open to air; underwear is not to be worn. A solution of one fourth cup of vinegar in a gallon of tepid water as a sitz bath or applied with a cloth for one hour three times per day will dry, cool, and cleanse the skin. A hair dryer on a cool setting is a good dryer. Applying 1% hydrocortisone or 0.05% flurandrenolide (Cordran) lotion is helpful. Ointments are occlusive and should be avoided. For severe contact dermatitis, oral corticosteroids may be employed. A high dose is rapidly tapered, using 50, 40, 30, 20, and 10 mg for two days each. Antihistamines, such as 4 mg chlopheniramine maleate tablets tid, initially aid in reduction of the inflammation. If the patient follows these instructions, the skin should revert to normal in two weeks.

Unfortunately topical corticosteroids used specifically on anal skin have been shown to be an increasingly recognized cause of contact dermatitis and should be suspected when recalcitrant dermatitis is encountered after application of steroids (45).

Psoriasis

This affliction has no known cause, but genetics may play a role, since 30% of patients have a family history of psoriasis. The lesion is usually a full, red, sharply demarcated, often macerated, scaling plaque. The scales are thick and white and bleeding results if they are removed. Sometimes fissuring is found. The skin may be thickened, and pruritus is common. Because of the moisture in the intergluteal region, the characteristic psoriatic plaque may not be present. Instead, a paler, more poorly defined, nonscaling lesion may result (Fig. 19). A search for diagnostic lesions on other parts of the body should be conducted (Fig. 20). The scalp, penis, elbows, knees, and knuckles should be inspected. The nails may be onycholytic and hyperkeratotic, and pitting and an "oil drop" appearance may be present.

Psoriasis is not curable, but it can be controlled. Applying 1% hydrocortisone and 2% precipitated sulfur lotion in the intergluteal area may be effective. Creams and ointments often cause maceration where the skin is opposed by the gluteal muscles. Anthralin 0.1% salve applied locally twice a day to a site is effective. The lesions also may respond to fluocinolone acetonide 0.025% cream, flurandrenolide, or fluocinolone cream in a coal tar base (46).

Lichen Simplex Chronicus (Neurodermatitis)

Recalcitrant pruritus is a hallmark of lichen simplex, a localized variant of atopic dermatitis. Lichenification is

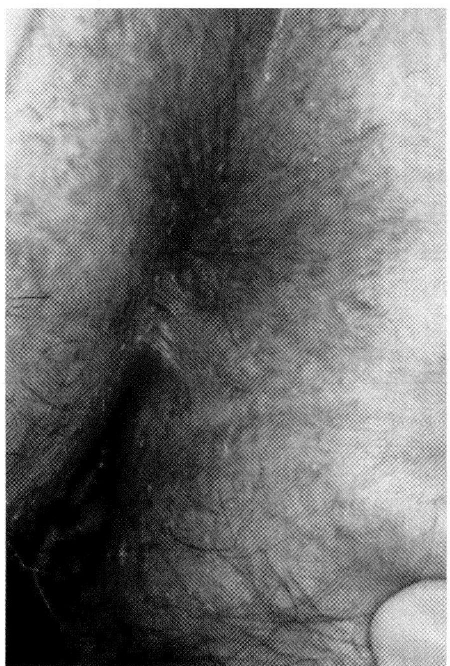

FIGURE 18 ■ Contact dermatitis caused by long-term use of topical steroids.

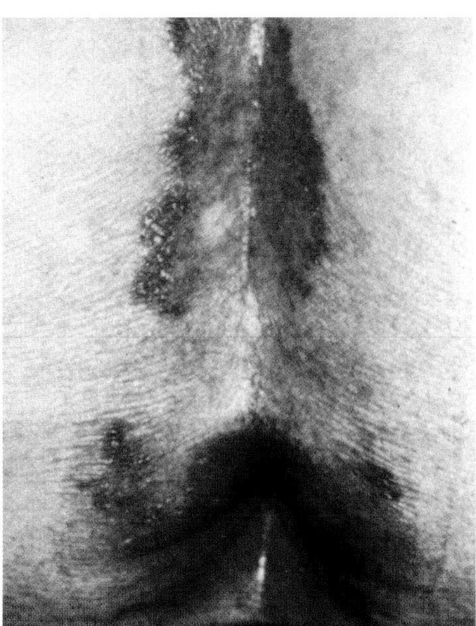

FIGURE 19 ■ Psoriasis. Note intergluteal fold extension.

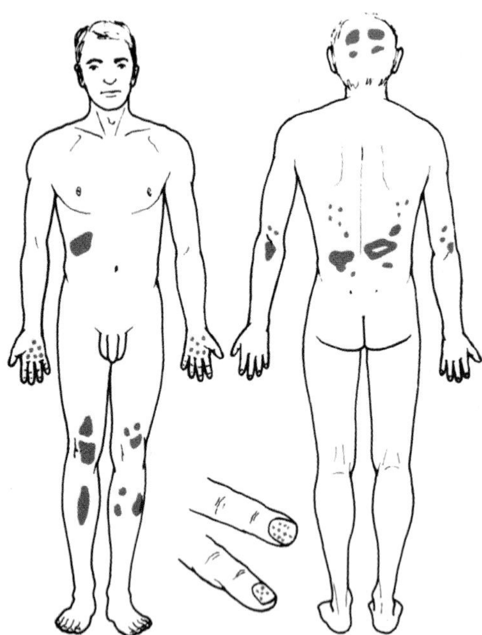

FIGURE 20 ■ Pattern of lesions in psoriasis.

a thickening of all layers of the epidermis. Initially the skin appears red and edematous. In the later stages after cycles of itching and scratching, often at night, the skin lesion evolves into a well-demarcated, erythematous, scaly thickening. The diagnosis is confirmed by performing a biopsy. There is no specific treatment other than the symptomatic methods. Antihistamines reduce itching, and topical steroids reduce inflammation. Unlike atopic dermatitis, there are no familial links.

Atopy

Atopy is an individual's genetic predisposition to develop allergic diseases in response to environmental allergens. Atopic individuals and relatives may have manifestations such as asthma, hay fever, or eczema. Scaling of the face, neck, dorsum of the hands, popliteal fossae, and antecubital fossae may harbor similar eruptions. Soap should be avoided because it is an irritant. Aid is obtained from 5% coal tar solution and 1% hydrocortisone applied topically. Since itching and scratching are worse at night, 50 mg of hydroxyzine aids sleep. This regimen should be tried for two weeks; then a bland ointment such as A and D Ointment or an ointment mixture of cod liver oil, 40% zinc oxide, and talc in a petrolatum-lanolin base (e.g., Desitin) might be used as a barrier. If there is a relapse, the therapy should be reinstituted.

Lichen Planus

This condition has a peak incidence between 30 and 60 years of age. It may have an association with hepatitis; thus, there may be an immunologic basis. This dermatologic condition begins on the genitals and perianal region and subsequently spreads to distant regions in later stages (47). The lesions are shiny, flat-topped papules with a darker pigmentation than is usually seen in the more distant lesions (Figs. 21 and 22). The mouth is checked for white patches, and plaques often are found on the volar aspects of the wrists and forearms. An application of mineral oil to the plaques may demonstrate the intersecting, small gray lines called "Wickham's striae."

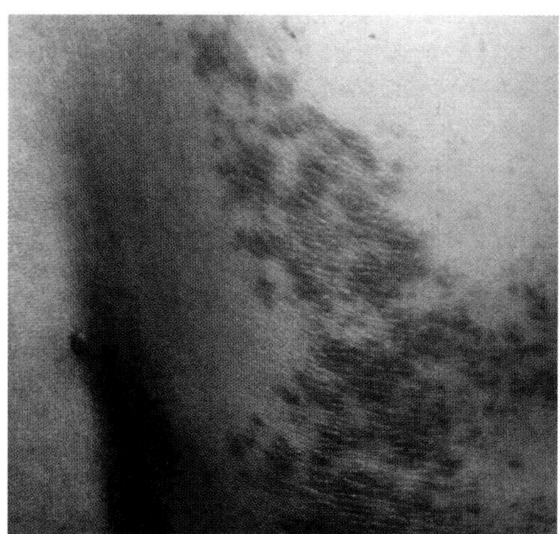

FIGURE 21 ■ Lichen planus on white skin. *Source*: Courtesy of Maria Turner, M.D., Washington, D.C.

The etiology of the lines is not known. Treatment is with bland, wet dressings, sitz baths, and a low-concentration steroid cream. For heavy patches, triamcinolone acetonide (Kenalog), 10 mg/mL mixed one to one with 1% lidocaine hydrochloride (Xylocaine), may be injected into the lesions. Occasionally, very severe eruptions require the use of short courses of systemic corticosteroids. Starting doses of prednisone are 40 to 60 mg/day (48).

Lichen Sclerosus et Atrophicus

This disease predominates in women over men in a ratio of 5:1 (49). Its etiology is unknown; however, a preceding history of vaginitis is often present. Ivory-colored, atrophic papules may break down, exposing a red, edematous, raw surface that causes intense pruritus and soreness (49).

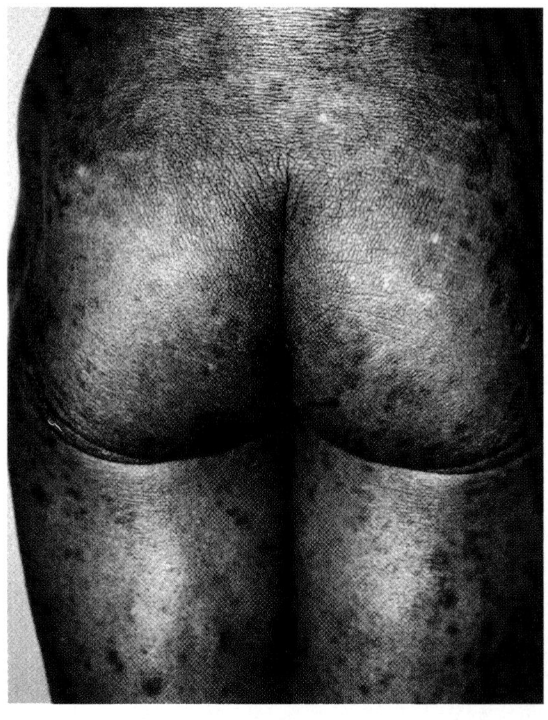

FIGURE 22 ■ Lichen planus on black skin. *Source*: Courtesy of Maria Turner, M.D., Washington, D.C.

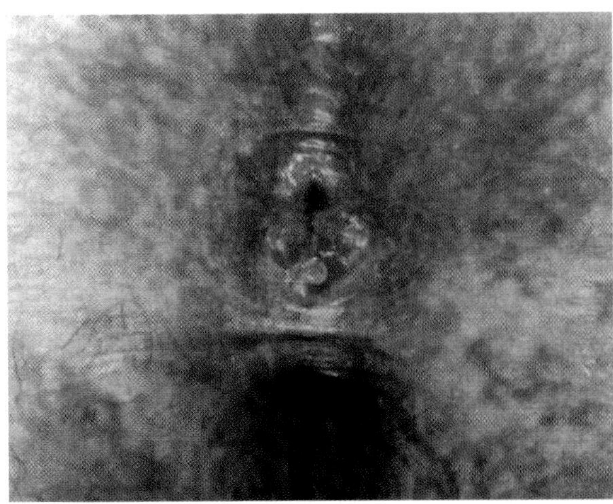

FIGURE 23 ■ Extensive involvement of perianal skin in lichen sclerosus et atrophicus. *Source*: Courtesy of Maria Turner, M.D., Washington, D.C.

As the edema subsides, it is replaced by sclerosis and chronic inflammation (Figs. 23 and 24). Sclerosis around the anus may narrow the stool diameter. The clitoris and labia minora may be absorbed and flattened in the process. White patches in the figure-eight form may be seen over the vulva and anus. The diagnosis is confirmed by performing a skin biopsy. The condition is chronic with exacerbations and remissions, and there is no known effective cure. Potent steroid-containing creams used in short courses along with the usual symptomatic treatments may aid in relieving the pruritus (50). Unfortunately, long-term use of steroids may further thin the skin. Using 2% testosterone cream topically for six weeks allows relief of itching. However, the side effects may be hoarseness, hair growth, acne, and increased libido.

Pemphigus Vegetans

Pemphigus vulgaris is a systemic and usually fatal disease without therapy. It may begin in intertriginous areas as pemphigus vegetans. This variant of pemphigus may be seen initially as either early bullae, later giving way to hypertrophic granulations studded with pustules and blisters, or early pustules, later developing into warty vegetations. The former presentation, which is always accompanied by oral lesions, is known as the Hallopeau type. Both types are treated with oral steroids, with the dosage titrated to the response of the disease and the patient's tolerance.

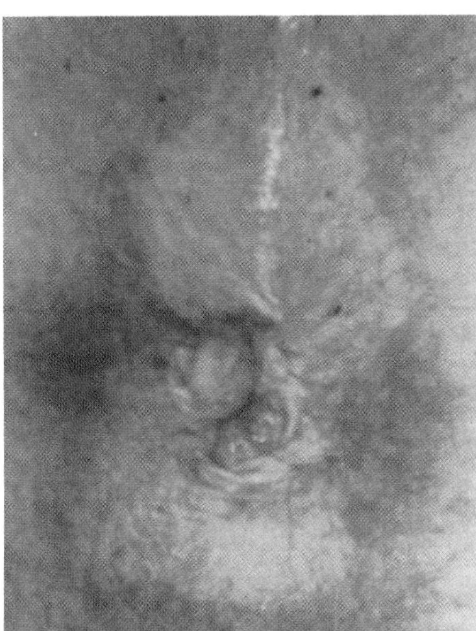

FIGURE 24 ■ Narrowed area of perianal involvement in lichen sclerosus et atrophicus. *Source*: Courtesy of Maria Turner, M.D., Washington, D.C.

Familial Benign Chronic Pemphigus

This is a hereditary dyskeratotic process. The condition is initially seen as erosions and blisters in intertriginous areas and sometimes as perianal irritation. A biopsy showing a pemphigus split in the epidermis and dyskeratotic cells is diagnostic. Local or systemic antibiotics are helpful. Diaminodiphenylsulfone (Dapsone) is frequently effective.

Diarrheal States

Multiple loose stools can produce pruritus by causing a localized skin irritation secondary to the chemistry of the liquid stool itself. Also, trauma from frequent and vigorous cleansing further results in production of excoriating, weeping, itching lesions.

Dietary Factors

Ingredients such as cola, coffee (decaffeinated and caffeinated), chocolate, tomatoes, beer, and tea have been implicated as inciting factors of pruritus (6). Certainly, individual allergies to certain foods can result in itching in various portions of the anatomy (6). Occasionally it is merely the volume of the ingredient ingested that produces loose watery stools and mucous discharge rather than any inherent characteristic of the individual ingredient. This is seen more with liquids than with solids. In a manometric study done by Smith et al. (4), coffee was shown to decrease anal pressure, which might result in soiling.

Gynecologic Conditions

Any inflammatory or ulcerative lesion of the vulva (e.g., Bartholin adenitis, lymphogranuloma venereum, granuloma inguinale, syphilis, lichen sclerosus et atrophicus, or carcinoma) can lead to pruritus. Kraurosis vulvae, a condition in which there is loss of the vulvar fat, is often characterized by itching (50). Irritation secondary to an increased vaginal discharge may lead to pruritus and mandate a workup to identify the underlying cause (e.g., infection, foreign body such as an intrauterine device, or neoplasm).

Antibiotics

The use of antibiotics may lead to pruritus either because of an allergic reaction or by altering the indigenous flora of the bowel or vagina, resulting in an overgrowth of otherwise harmless bacteria or fungi and leading to diarrhea, increased vaginal discharge, or a perianal superinfection, usually candidiasis. Tetracycline is a notable offender (51).

Systemic Diseases

Occasionally pruritus will be the presenting symptom of an otherwise distant or systemic disease. Severe jaundice from any cause is notoriously associated with itching (47). Diabetes, by virtue of its association with candidiasis, frequently has pruritus as its presenting symptom.

Miscellaneous Causes

Any factor that results in irritation to the perianal skin can lead to pruritus. These factors may be quite apparent, such as irradiation, or more nebulous, such as neurogenic, psychogenic, or idiosyncratic reactions (50).

NONPRURITIC LESIONS

Although pruritus ani is the most common presenting symptom of perianal dermatologic conditions, many lesions do not initially present with pruritus, or the pruritus is of minor importance. Some of these diseases are discussed in the following sections.

INFECTIONS

Hidradenitis Suppurativa

An infection of the apocrine glands, hidradenitis suppurativa is fully described in Chapter 39.

Leprosy

Leprosy is endemic in the southern United States and tropical areas the world over. In patients with good resistance to *Mycobacterium leprae*, infection may be confined to local cooler regions of the body. Leprous lesions appear as macules or plaques with healed central areas surrounded by erythematous or copper-colored extensions (51). The lesions usually appear on the face, exterior surfaces of the limbs, the buttocks, and the back and are often preceded by anesthesia secondary to early nerve damage. Recently, molecular mechanisms that are responsible for neuropathy have been discovered. Identification of the endoneural laminin-2 isoform and its receptor alpha-dystroglycan as neural targets of *M. leprae* has opened up scientific inquiry into the pathogenesis of neurological damage (52).

If the individual has poor resistance, the skin lesions can occur anywhere (including the perineum) and appear as small, circular, erythematous or copper-colored, smooth, shiny macules. Nerves are damaged late; consequently, anesthesia follows the development of the skin lesions (51).

The diagnosis is confirmed by skin biopsy. Biologic false-positive tests for syphilis are common. Treatment is with 4-4′ diaminodiphenylsulfone (Dapsone), clofazimine (Lamprene), or rifampin (Rifamate) (53). The genome sequence of *M. leprae* is now understood, which will enable better use of current chemotherapy and lead to new drug targets (53). The reader is referred to textbooks on tropical medicine for further details.

Amebiasis

Amebiasis is caused by the protozoan *Entamoeba histolytica*. Perianal manifestations consist of painful serpiginous ulcers with red, dirty, foul-smelling bases covered by a white pseudomembrane (54). Wet mounting is the simplest and easiest technique to examine the feces for parasites. Lactophenol cotten blue added to the mounting medium stains the trophozoites, cysts, and ova (55). A difficult differential diagnosis is herpes simplex in acquired immunodeficiency syndrome. Therapy is instituted with metronidazole, 750 mg orally three times daily for 10 days. This should be followed by iodoquinol, 650 mg three times daily for 20 days, or paromomycin, 25 mg/kg/day in three doses for seven days, to ensure intestinal cure (18). See Chapter 14 for further details.

Actinomycosis

This rare lesion, actinomycosis, is caused by *Actinomyces israelii*, an anaerobic, non-acid-fast organism. A brawny infiltration of the skin accompanied by proctitis, abscesses, and fistulas is seen. A high degree of suspicion is necessary to recognize an atypical fistula as having an actinomycotic etiology (56,57). The diagnosis is confirmed by identifying characteristic "sulfur" bodies with club-shaped rays in the discharges from the sinus. Treatment consists of penicillin and local symptomatic measures.

Lymphogranuloma Venereum

The disease lymphogranuloma venereum is caused by a sexually transmitted virus. In the advanced stage of the disease, the perianal region is deformed with widespread scarring and vegetating lesions. Periproctitis often results in a stricture 5 to 10 cm from the anal margin, around which fistulas develop (see Chapter 14).

NEOPLASTIC LESIONS

A variety of neoplastic lesions are found in the perianal region. The reader is referred to Chapter 18 for a discussion of specific therapies.

Acanthosis Nigricans

Acanthosis nigricans sometimes may be associated with an underlying bowel carcinoma, obesity, and/or hyperinsulinemia, severe atopic dermatitis, and Down's syndrome (58–60). It appears as a velvety black, acantholytic papillomatous lesion and is found in the axillary region, neck, knuckles, tongue, and perianal region (Fig. 25). It may be benign or malignant. The malignant variety is usually of

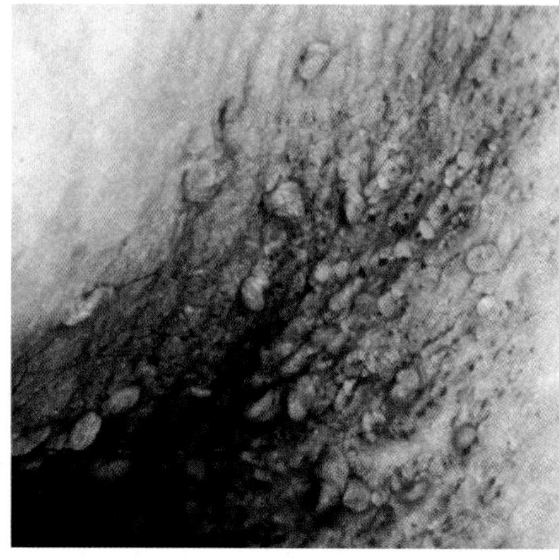

FIGURE 25 ■ Acanthosis nigricans. *Source*: Courtesy of Maria Turner, M.D., Washington, D.C.

sudden onset and is rapidly progressive, but is clinically indistinguishable from the benign form. There is a report of the successful use of a combination of 12% ammonium lactate cream and 0.05% tretinoin cream to treat acanthosis nigricans associated with obesity (61). A complete gastrointestinal workup is warranted to rule out any underlying neoplasm.

Bowen's Disease

Bowen's disease is an intraepidermal carcinoma that appears as a yellowish scale that is easily detached, leaving a reddened granular surface (62). However, there are also reports of hyperpigmented velvety surfaces and well-defined hyperpigmented verrucous patches (Figs. 11 and 26) (see Chapter 18) (44).

Squamous Cell Carcinoma

Squamous cell carcinoma can be misdiagnosed as condyloma acuminatum. It is a warty nodular plaque that may or may not be ulcerated. Maceration and secondary infection are common, often disguising the true nature of the disease. The diagnosis is confirmed by performing a biopsy (see Chapter 18).

Melanoma

Melanoma rarely may occur in the perianal region, the anus, or the rectum. The classic malignant melanoma is a black or purple nodule, but it may be flat or pedunculated. Colors vary from pink to red, tan, brown, or black, or more difficult, have no color, amelanotic. Beware of changes in shape, size, color, erythema, induration, friability, or ulceration. The prognosis, with wide local excision or abdominoperineal resection, is dismal (63–65). More complete discussion of melanoma is found in Chapter 18.

Perianal Paget's Disease

This extramammary presentation of Paget's disease is rare. Helwig and Graham (66) report an 86% association of perianal Paget's disease with subadjacent or bowel carcinomas (67,68). The disease tends to occur later in life, frequently in the seventh decade. The lesion is seen as a progressive, erythematous, eczematoid plaque (Fig. 27). Because of the frequent association of the disease with underlying neoplasms, the prognosis is not good. However, if after wide excision no adjacent or bowel malignancy is found, the prognosis is good, but local recurrence is common (69). Because wide local excision leaves wide defects, special surgical techniques such as V-Y flaps and staged excisions with split thickness grafts are being used (70,71). Close follow-up should continue forever because recurrences have occurred up to eight years after treatment (68).

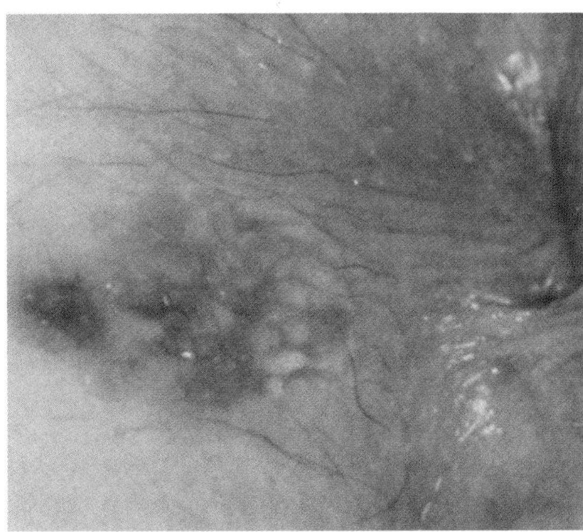

FIGURE 26 ■ Bowen's disease. Squamous cell carcinoma in situ.

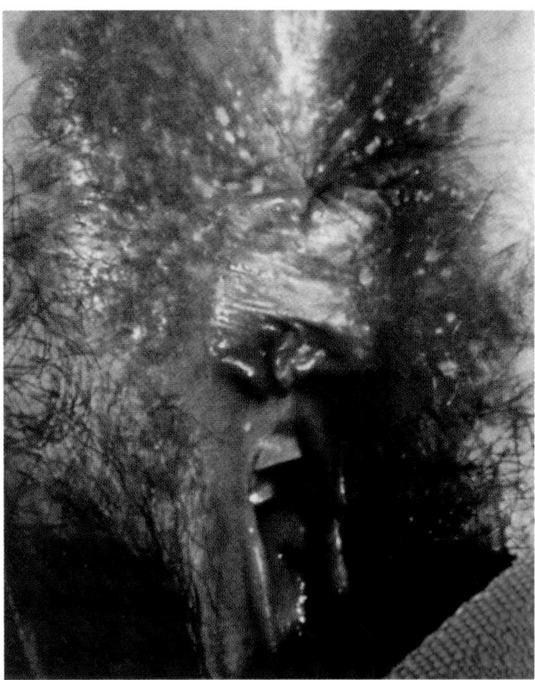

FIGURE 27 ■ Paget's disease.

■ INFLAMMATORY BOWEL DISEASE

Anal lesions are present in approximately 25% of patients with Crohn's ileitis and in 75% of patients with Crohn's colitis; they may precede the intestinal manifestation by several years. Dusky perianal sinuses with undermining ulcers or edema, indolent single or multiple fissures, and fistulas may be some of the early signs. Diagnosis can be made by biopsy, but performing extensive surgical procedures in the presence of active disease is strongly condemned because the healing is notoriously poor (see Chapter 27 on Crohn's disease and Chapter 10 on fistulas for details).

REFERENCES

1. Wexner SD, Dailey TH. Pruritus ani: Diagnosis and management. Curr Concepts Skin Disord 1986; 7:5–9.
2. Eyers AA, Thomson JPS. Pruritus ani: Is anal dysfunction important in aetiology? Br Med J 1979; 2:1549–551.
3. Goldman L, Kitzmiller K. Perianal atrophoderma from topical corticosteroids. Arch Dermatol 1973; 107:611–612.
4. Smith LE, Henrichs D, McCullah RD. Prospective studies on the etiology and treatment of pruritus ani. Dis Colon Rectum 1982; 25:358–363.
5. Alexander-Williams J. Causes and management of anal irritation. Br Med J 1985; 287:1528.
6. Friend WG. The cause and treatment of idiopathic pruritus ani. Dis Colon Rectum 1977; 20:40–42.
7. Mazier WP. Hemorrhoids, fissures, and pruritus ani. Surg Clin North Am 1994; 74:1277–1292.

8. Laurent A, Boucharlat J, Bosson F, Derry A, Imbert R. Psychological assessment of patients with idiopathic pruritus ani. Psychother Psychosom 1997; 66: 163–166.
9. Allan A, Ambrose HS, Silverman S, Keighley MRB. Physiological study of pruritus ani. Br J Surg 1987; 74:576–579.
10. Farouk R, Duthie GS, Pryde A, Bartolo DCC. Abnormal transient internal sphincter relaxation in idiopathic pruritus ani: Physiological evidence from ambulatory monitoring. Br J Surg 1994; 81:603–606.
11. Daniel GL, Longo WE, Vernava AM. Pruritus ani: Causes and concerns. Dis Colon Rectum 1994; 37:670–674.
12. Pierard GE, Arrese JE, Rodriguez C, Daskaleros PA. Effects of softened and unsoftened fabrics on sensitive skin. Contact Dermatitis 1994; 30: 286–291.
13. Eusebio EB, Graham J, Mody N. Treatment of intractable pruritus ani. Dis Colon Rectum 1990; 33:770–772.
14. Farouk R, Lee PW. Intradermal methylene blue injection for treatment of intractable idiopathic pruritus ani. Br J Surg 1997; 84(5):670.
15. Gupta A. Pruritus in the elderly. Practitioner 1999; 243:205–207.
16. Murie JA, Sim JW, MacKenzie I. The importance of pain, pruritus and soiling as symptoms of hemorrhoids and their response to hemorrhoidectomy or rubber band ligation. Br J Surg 1981; 68:247–249.
17. Parija SC, Sheeladevi C, Shivaprakash MR, Biswal N. Evaluation of lactophenol cotten blue stain for detection of eggs of *Enterobius vermicularis* in perianal surface sample. Tropical Doctor 2001; 31(4):214–215.
18. Speck WT. Enterobiasis. Behrman RE, Vaughan VC, eds. Textbook of Pediatrics. 13th ed. Philadelphia: WB Saunders, 1987.
19. Association of Genitourinory Medicine and the Medical Society for the Study of Venereal Disease. Sex Transm Infect 1999; 75(suppl 1):S78–S79.
20. Wendel K, Rompalo. Scabies and pediculosis pubis: An update of treatment regimens and general review. Clin Infect Dis 2002; 35(suppl 2):S146–S151.
21. Hogan DJ, Schachner L, Tagert Sampan C. Diagnosis and treatment of childhood scabies. Pediatr Clin North Am 1991; 38:941–957.
22. Chouela E, Abeldano A, Pellerano E, Hernandez MI. Diagnosis and treatment of scabies. Am J Clin Dermatol 2002; 3(1):9–18.
23. Abramowitz M. Drugs of parasitic infections. Med Lett 1993; 35:111–122.
24. Brugha R, Keersmaekee K, Renton A, Meheus A. Genital herpes infection: A review. Int J Epidemiol 1997; 26:698–709.
25. Ashley RL. Sorting out the new HSV type specific antibody tests. Sex Transm Infect 2001; 77:232–237.
26. Stanberry L, Cunningham A, Martz G, et al. New developments in the epidemiology, natural history and management of genital herpes. Antiviral Res 1999; 42:1–14.
27. Balfour HH, Bean B, Laskin OL. Acyclovir halts progression of herpes zoster in immunocompromised patients. N Engl J Med 1983; 308:1448–1453.
28. Stanberry LR. Control of STD's role of prophylactic vaccines against herpes simplex virus. Sex Transm Infect 1998; 74(6):391–394.
29. Krusinski PA. Herpes zoster. Demis Demis DJ, ed. Clinical Dermatology. Vol. 3. Philadelphia: JB Lippincott, 1989.
30. Mattox TF, Rutgers J, Yoshimari RN, Bhatia NN. Nonfluorescent erythrasma of the vulva. Obstet Gynecol 1993; 81:862–864.
31. Paradisi M, Cianchini G, Angclo C, Conti G, Pudd UP. Perianal streptococcal dermatitis. Minerva Pediatr 1994; 46(6):303.
32. Neri I, Bardazzi F, Marzaduri S, Patrizi A. Perianal streptococcal dermatitis in adults. Br J Dermatol 1996; 135(5):796–798.
33. Kroal AL. Perianal streptococcal dermatitis. Pediatr Dermatol 1981; 27:518.
34. Weismann K, Peterson CS, Roder B. Pruritus ani caused by beta-homolytic streptococci. Acta Derm Venereal 1996; 76:415.
35. Dodi G, Pirone E, Bettin A, et al. The mycotic flora in proctological patients with and without pruritus ani. Br J Surg 1985; 72:907–909.
36. Abdel-Rahman SM, Nahota MC. Oral terbinafine: A new antifungal agent. Ann Pharmacother 1997; 31(4):445–456.
37. Ostlere LS, Taylor CR, Harris DW, Rustin MH, Wright S, Johnson M. Skin surface lipids in HIV-positive patients with and without seborrheic dermatitis. Int J Dermatol 1996; 35(4):276–279.
38. Pierard-Franchimont C, Pierard GE, Arrese JE, DeDancker P. Effect of ketaconazole 1% and 2% shampoo on severe dandruff and seborrheic dermatitis: Clinical, squamometric and mycological assessments. Dermatology 2001; 202(2):171–176.
39. Johnson BA, Nunley JR. Treatment of seborrheic dermatitis. Am Family Phys 2000; 61(9):2703–2710, 2713–4.
40. Scaparro E, Quadri G, Virno G, Orifici C, Milani M. Evaluation of the efficiency and tolerability of oral terbinafine in patients with seborrheic dermatitis. A multicenter, randomized, double-blinded, placebo controlled trial. Br J Dermatol 2001; 144(4):854–857.
41. Fregert S, Tegner E, Thelin I. Contact allergy to lidocaine. Contact Dermatol 1979; 5:185–188.
42. Hardwick N, King CM. Contact allergy to lidocaine with cross-reaction to bupivacaine. Contact Dermatitis 1994; 30:245–246.
43. Rosen T, Fordisc DB. Cashew nut dermatitis. South Med J 1994; 87:543.
44. Adams BB, Sheth PB. Perianal ulcerations from topical steroid use. Cutis 2002; 69(1):67–68.
45. Wilknson SM. Hypersensitivity to topical corticosteroids. Clin Exp Dermatol 1994; 19:1–11.
46. O'Hagen ML. New horizons in the management of psoriasis. Cutis 1998; 61:25.
47. Dilaimy M. Lichen planus subtrophicus. Arch Dermatol 1976; 112: 1251–1257.
48. Oliver GF, Winkelmann RK. Treatment of lichen planus. Drugs 1993; 45:56–65.
49. Rowell NR, Goodfield JMD. The connective tissue diseases. Champion RH, Burton JL, Ebling FJG, eds. Textbook of Dermatology. Oxford: Blackwell Scientific, 1992:2269–2275.
50. Jorizzo JL. The itchy patient. Primary Care 1983; 10:339–353.
51. Goligher JC. Pruritus ani. Surgery of the Anus, Rectum, and Colon. 4th ed. Springfield, Ill.: Charles C Thomas, 1980.
52. Rambukkano A. How does *Mycobacterium leprae* target the peripheral nervous system? Trends Microbiol 2000; 8(1):23–28.
53. Grosset JH, Cole ST. Genomics and the chemotherapy of leprosy. Leprosy Rev 2001; 72(4):429–440.
54. Stanley SL. Amoebiasis. Lancet 2003; 361(9362):1025–1034.
55. Khubnani H, Sivarajan K, Khubnani AH. Application of lactophenol cotten blue for identification and preservation of intestinal parasites in fecal wet mounts. Indian J Pathol Microbiol 1998; 41(2):157–162.
56. Alvarado-Cerna R, Bracho-Riqueline R. Perianal actinomycosis—A complication of a fistula-in-ano. Dis Colon Rectum 1994; 37:378–380.
57. Posnik MR, Potesman I, Abrahamson J. Primary perianal actinomycosis. Eur J Surg 1996; 162(2):153–154.
58. Schwartz RA. Acanthosis nigricans. J Am Acad Dermatol 1994; 31:1–19.
59. Stuart CA, Driscoll MS, Lundquist KF, Gilkison CR, Shaheb S, Smith MM. Acanthosis nigricav. J Basic Clin Physiol Pharm 1998; 9(2–4):407–418.
60. Munoz-Perez MA, Comacho F. Acanthosis nigricans: A new cutaneous sign in severe atopic dermatitis and Down's syndrome. J Eur Acad Dermatol Venereol 2001; 15(4):325–327.
61. Patel P, Starkey R, Maroon M. Topical therapy with tretinoin and ammonium lactate for acanthosis nigricans associated with obesity. Cutis 2003; 71(7):33–34.
62. Kossard S, Rosen R. Cutaneous Bowen's disease. An analysis of 1001 cases according to age, sex and site. J Am Acad Dermatol 1992; 27:406–410.
63. Antoniuk PM, Tjandra JJ, Webb BW, Petras RE, Milsom JW, Fazio VW. Anorectal malignant melanoma has a poor prognosis. Int J Colorectal Dis 1993; 8: 81–86.
64. Cagir B, Whiteford MH, Topham A, Rakinic J, Fry RD. Changing epidemiology of anorectal melanoma. Dis Colon Rectum 1999; 42(9):1203–1205.
65. Bullard KM, Tuttle TM, Rothen Berger DA, et al. Surgical therapy for anorectal melanoma. J Am Coll Surg 2003; 196:206–211.
66. Helwig EB, Graham JH. Anogenital (extramammary) Paget's disease: A clinicopathologic study. Cancer 2001; 16:387–403.
67. Grow JR, Kshirsagar V, Tolentino M, et al. Extramammary perianal Paget's disease: A report of a case. Dis Colon Rectum 1977; 20:436–442.
68. Jensen SL, Sjolin KE, Shoukoun-Amiri MH, Hagen K, Harling H. Paget's disease of the anal margin. Br J Surg 1988; 75:1089–1092.
69. McCarter MD, Quan SHQ, Busam K, Paty PP, Wang D, Guillem JG. Long-term outcome of perianal Paget's disease. Dis Colon Rectum 2003; 46:612–616.
70. Hassan I, Horgan AF, Nivatuongs S. V-Y island flaps for repair of large perianal defects. Am J Surg 2001; 181(4):363–364.
71. Lam DT, Batista O, Weiss EG, Nogueras JJ, Wexner SD. Staged excision and split-thickness skin graft for circumferential perianal Paget's disease. Dis Colon Rectum 2001; 44(6):868–870.

13 Condyloma Acuminatum

Philip H. Gordon

INTRODUCTION

The list of sexually transmitted diseases is lengthy, and among the many conditions condyloma acuminatum stands out and is worthy of separate consideration. Indeed, it has been considered the most common anorectal infection affecting homosexual men (1). Condyloma acuminatum is not usually a serious medical problem, but frequently it causes emotional distress to patient and physician alike because of its marked tendency to recurrence.

CLINICAL FEATURES

ETIOLOGY

The causative agent in condyloma acuminatum is believed to be a papillomavirus that is autoinoculable, filterable, and transmissible (2). At least 66 types of human papillomavirus (HPV) have been identified (3). Certain types of HPV, HPV-6 and HPV-11, are found in benign genital warts (4–6). Syrjanen et al. (7), using a sophisticated in situ hybridization method, detected human papillomavirus agents in 76% of patients with condyloma acuminatum. Furthermore, HPV-16 and HPV-18 behave more aggressively and are more frequently associated with dysplasia and malignant transformation. These observations, revealed in patients with primarily penile warts, may emphasize the necessity of HPV typing to access the malignant potential of HPV lesions. Handley et al. (8) detected HPV deoxyribonucleic acid (DNA) (either 6 or 11, 16 or 18, or 31 or 33 or 35) in 53.3% of anogenital warts.

Using an immunohistochemical stain, Gall et al. (9) found evidence of a papillomavirus in the squamous cell carcinomas of the anal region in five of eight homosexual men (63%) compared with two of six patients of unknown sexual orientation (33%). The significance of the detection of the human papillomavirus antigen in anorectal carcinoma is uncertain; it can be unrelated to the development of malignant neoplasms but represents a biologic marker. The incubation period for this virus is anywhere from one to six months but may be longer (10).

PREVALENCE

The prevalence of condylomata acuminata in the anorectal and urogenital regions points toward a sexual mode of transmission. However, transmission at birth and by close contact with infected individuals has been described (11). These warts occur with greatest frequency in male homosexual patients but also may be seen in heterosexual men, women, and even children (Fig. 1) (11,12). Swerdlow and Salvati (13) reported that 46% of their male patients with condylomata acuminata were homosexual.

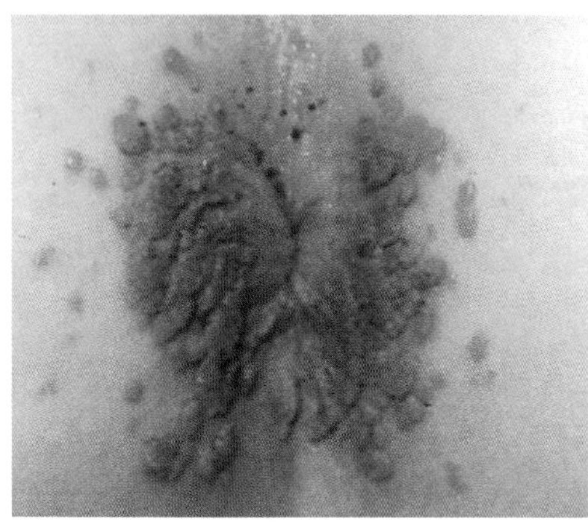

FIGURE 1 ■ Condylomata acuminata in a child.

A study by Carr and William (14) in a population of homosexual men in New York City revealed anal warts to be more frequent among men who practiced anal-receptive intercourse. Of the patients studied, 72% had internal warts during the course of their illness. Anal warts were several times more common than penile warts in homosexual men. A possible explanation for this discrepancy may be that the moist, warm, perirectal area is more conducive to the growth of warts than the drier, cool penile epidermis. Anal intercourse may introduce the virus into the anal region, and concurrent local trauma may impair local defenses. In a study of 58 patients with anogenital warts, Handley et al. (8) found that 37% of men and 25% of women also had warts in the anal canal.

Condylomata acuminata occur more often in immunosuppressed patients than in nonimmunosuppressed patients. Following renal transplantation, the incidence has been reported to be 2.4–4% (15). In this clinical situation, treatment becomes especially difficult. Breese et al. (16) found a strong relationship between the occurrence of anal HPV infections and HIV-associated immunosuppression. Overall, 61% of HIV-positive and 17% of HIV-negative men had anal HPV detected. HPV types 16/18 accounted for more than 50% of infections. Among HIV-positive men, HPV prevalence increased with declining CD4 cell counts: 33% with counts >750, 56% with counts from 200 to 750, and 86% with counts <200. HPV infection was also associated with younger age and increasing numbers of lifetime sexual partners for all men.

Condyloma acuminatum continues to be a significant health problem, with 1 million new cases seen yearly (17). Condyloma acuminatum may be the third most common sexually transmitted disease in the United States after gonorrhea and nongonococcal urethritis. It is the most commonly diagnosed sexually transmitted viral disease in the United States (18).

It has been estimated that 1% of sexually active adults in the United States have visible genital warts (19); however, numerous studies predict an incidence of general HPV infection in women ranging from 15% to 50% as determined by HPV DNA detection (20–22). The highest frequencies of HPV and genital warts have consistently been observed in young adults aged 18–28 years old, particularly young females (19,23–25). In the past few decades the incidence of genital warts appears to have increased, based on studies showing an approximately eight-fold increase in the incidence of genital warts from the 1950s to the 1970s and a similar fold increase again from the 1970s to the 1990s (23,26).

■ LOCATION

Anatomic locations in which condylomata acuminata are found include the perianal region and anal canal, as well as other parts of the perineum, vulva, vagina, and penis.

Treatment of perianal condylomata acuminata without treatment of concomitant anal canal condylomata acuminata is doomed to failure. More than three-fourths of the group of patients studied by Schlappner and Shaffer (27) were found to have internal condylomata acuminata. Sohn and Robilotti (1) found that one-half of homosexual men they studied harbored condylomata. In only 6% were these condylomata confined to the perianal region, while in 84% of the patients, both perianal and intra-anal lesions were present. In 11% of these patients, only intra-anal lesions were found. Thus, failure of the examiner to study the anorectum with an anoscope could have resulted in the failure to diagnose intra-anal lesions in 94% of the patients. Carr and William (14) also found a high percentage of internal warts in men with external warts. In a group of immunocompromised patients, de la Fuente et al. (28) found that condylomata were limited to the anoderm in 27%, located in the anal canal in 20%, and in 53% were in both the anoderm and anal canal.

In men, anal canal condylomata acuminata are frequently associated with penile condylomata; in women, associated condylomata may be found in the vagina, vulva, urethra, and cervix.

PATHOLOGY

■ MACROSCOPIC PATHOLOGY

Condylomata acuminata vary from pinhead-size lesions to projecting cauliflower-like masses. Their surface is papilliform, and they are pink or white in color (Fig. 2A). Individual warts, which may be sessile or pedunculated, have a tendency to grow in radial rows that may become confluent and form almost an entire sheet, around the anal orifice (Fig. 2B). They are almost invariably multiple and may be so numerous as to obscure the anal aperture, which then can be found only with difficulty. In addition, these warts frequently extend into the anal canal and even the rectum. Vulvar warts can grow so luxuriantly as to conceal the introitus. Because of the moisture and warmth in the anal region, the warts may become sodden and white. They may produce an irritating discharge with a disagreeable odor. Anal warts are often soft and friable and therefore may bleed.

■ MICROSCOPIC PATHOLOGY

Microscopically, anal warts show marked acanthosis of the epidermis with hyperplasia of prickle cells, parakeratosis, and an underlying chronic inflammatory cell infiltration. Vacuolation of the cells of the upper prickle layer is present (Fig. 3) (29).

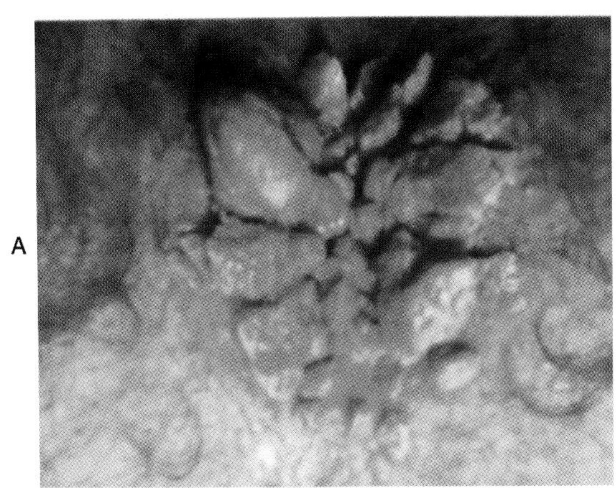

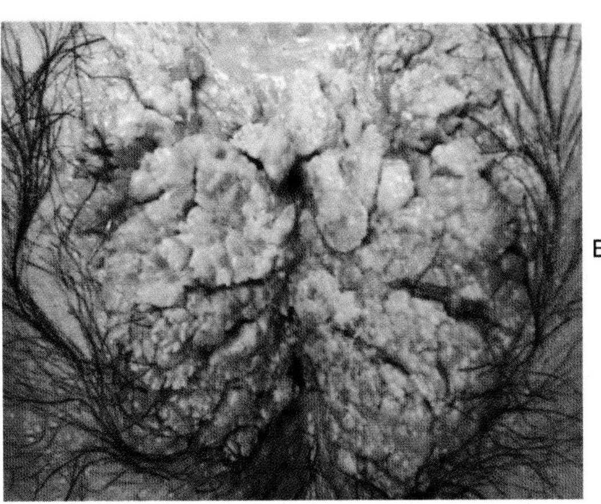

FIGURE 2 ■ Condylomata acuminata in an adult. (**A**) Scattered condylomata. (**B**) A large crop of condylomata encircling the anus.

SYMPTOMS

Patients with condyloma acuminatum present with relatively minor complaints. Almost all note visible perianal warts. Two-thirds of the patients experience pruritus ani, which may be caused by the irritation of the warts themselves or the patient's inability to cleanse the anal area properly after defecation. Approximately one-half of the patients experience some bleeding with defecation because of the friability of some of these warts. Other patients complain of anal wetness. A majority of patients with condyloma acuminatum experience discomfort or pain. Female patients may present with a vaginal discharge.

DIAGNOSIS

In most cases, the clinical appearance of the lesions makes the diagnosis obvious. However, prior treatment with podophyllin may alter the gross morphology of the lesions, and this may adversely affect correct diagnosis. The application of 5% acetic acid may reveal subclinical evidence of HPV infection by the demonstration of acetowhite epithelium (30). It should be stressed that the patient's sexual contacts all should be examined for the presence of warts.

Because of the free association of numerous diseases and the frequent occurrence of condylomata acuminata, other sexually transmitted diseases must be excluded. Sohn and Robilotti (1) have stressed that in addition to the history and physical examination, proctosigmoidoscopy, stool cultures for bacterial pathogens, stool studies for ova and parasites, blood for syphilis serology, and pharyngeal, rectal, and urethral smears for gonococci should be considered. Hillman et al. (31) detected HPV DNA in 96.6% of 116 wart specimens and 22.4% of the men had urethral infection with HPV.

Included in the differential diagnosis are condylomata lata, the lesions of secondary syphilis. However, these are usually fewer in number, smoother, flatter, whiter, and usually more moist than those of condylomata acuminata. It must be remembered that the two lesions may occur concomitantly. A definitive diagnosis is made by the dark-field examination, which will demonstrate the spirochetes.

Another condition that may require differentiation is the squamous cell carcinoma of the anus, but this is more indurated. A biopsy is done to establish this diagnosis.

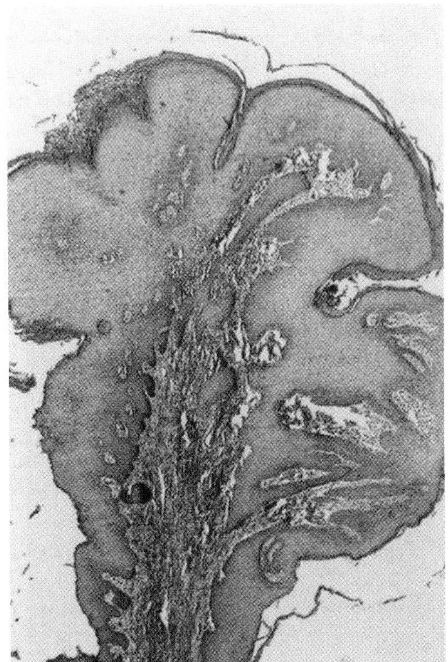

FIGURE 3 ■ Microscopic features of condylomata acuminata. *Source*: Courtesy of H. Srolovitz, M.D., Montreal, Quebec, Canada.

TREATMENT

The presence of condyloma acuminatum mandates treatment. The clinical significance of untreated anogenital HPV includes (1) the transmission of disease to sexual partners, (2) the transmission of viruses to neonates by infected mothers, and (3) the risk of developing invasive squamous cell carcinoma. Many methods of treating condyloma acuminatum have been employed (Tables 1 and 2) (32–46). The topical application of caustic agents such as podophyllin or bichloroacetic acid has been the therapeutic modality of choice for several decades, but such agents have been used with different degrees of enthusiasm. Various methods of local destruction have included surgical excision, electrodessication, cryotherapy, and ultrasonography. The different modes of therapy attempted, in addition to the ones itemized in Table 1, have been listed by Billingham and Lewis (36) and include the use of Fowler's solution, autovaccine, vaccinia, bismuth sodium triglycollamate, ammoniated mercury, chloroquine, sulfonamide cream,

TABLE 1 ■ Treatment of Condyloma Acuminatum

Caustic agents	Cryotherapy
Podophyllin	Liquid air
Bichloroacetic acid	Liquid nitrogen
Trichloroacetic acid	Surgical excision
Nitric acid	Antineoplastic preparations
Imiquimod	5-Fluorouracil
Fulguration	Laser therapy
Cidafovir	Interferon

tetracycline ointment (3%), dinitrochlorobenzene, phenol, colchicine, idoxuridine, dimethyl sulfoxide, and bacille Calmette–Guérin vaccine. Only very rarely will condylomata acuminata regress spontaneously.

■ PODOPHYLLIN

The local application of podophyllin often has been effective treatment. Podophyllin is a cytotoxic agent applied in a vehicle such as liquid paraffin or tincture of benzoin, the latter having the advantage that it adheres better to the warts. Concentrations from 5% to 50% have been used, but a 25% suspension is the one generally employed.

The method of application is to paint the warts accurately, avoiding the adjacent skin because podophyllin is intensely irritating. Dusting powder then is applied to the surrounding skin. Patients are instructed to wash the treated area 6–8 hours after each application to prevent damage to the surrounding skin. This treatment is repeated at weekly intervals as required. Single applications are rarely effective. In some cases, treatment with podophyllin must be abandoned because of the soreness and irritation of the perianal skin.

Podophyllin has several disadvantages (47). It is not a pure compound, and therefore batches may vary in potency. It cannot be applied to perianal or anal warts by patients themselves, so repeated visits to the office may be necessary. Local reactions may be severe and penetration into keratinized warts is poor, so only recently acquired lesions may respond to treatment. In a review, Miller (48) summarized the local side effects reported with the use of podophyllin; these included severe necrosis and scarring of the anogenital area, fistula-in-ano, and dermatitis. The application of large amounts of podophyllin may result in severe systemic toxic effects, which include the hematologic, hepatic, renal, gastrointestinal, respiratory, and central nervous systems (49,50). Karol et al. (51) have recommended the avoidance of treatment with podophyllin during pregnancy because of the possible teratogenic effect and even intrauterine death (49). Finally, prolonged courses of treatment with podophyllin are probably undesirable since it does produce dysplasia. Moreover, treatment with podophyllin may induce temporary cell changes that are difficult to differentiate histologically from carcinoma (Fig. 4). The effects of local application of podophyllin on condylomata are typified by the presence of enlarged, swollen cells with pale, basophyllic cytoplasm, dispersed chromatin material, and large perinuclear and paranuclear vacuolation. Other changes include eosinophilic cells with pyknotic nuclei and various types of nuclear alterations. These histologic abnormalities are temporary and will reverse completely within a few weeks after discontinuation of the drug (10).

Podophyllotoxin, one of the active compounds of podophyllin, has been found to be effective in wart clearance in 45–53% of cases, but wart recurrence has been observed to be as high as 91% (52). The agent is safe and can be self-administered.

■ BICHLOROACETIC ACID

In the absence of a completely satisfactory mode of therapy, Swerdlow and Salvati (13) proposed the use of another caustic agent, bichloroacetic acid. The technique involves cleansing and drying the perianal region with cotton and witch hazel. The caustic agent is spread on with an applicator, with care taken not to apply the chemical to adjacent skin

TABLE 2 ■ Summary of Treatment Modalities for Condylomata Acuminata

Treatment	Advantages	Disadvantages	Results
Podophyllin	Ease of application; no anesthesia; inexpensive	Skin burns; cannot use in anal canal; multiple visits necessary; dysplasia with prolonged use; systemic toxicity	Disappointing; recurrence rate high (30–65%)
Bichloroacetic acid	Ease of application; no anesthesia; inexpensive; can be used in anal canal	Skin burn; multiple visits	25% recurrence
Imiquimod 5% cream	Self-administered; fewer office visits	Local skin reaction, mild to moderate; expensive	13% recurrence
Electrocoagulation	Single-session treatment; effective in anal canal	Anesthesia required; postoperative pain; fumes	May require repeated coagulations; 9% failure rate
Cidofovir topical 1%	Can be used with recurrent condylomata	Mild erosive dermatitis	32% cured; 60% partial regression
Cryotherapy	Single-session treatment; can be used in anal canal	Requires expensive equipment; may require anesthesia	24–37% recurrence rate
Surgical excision	Precise removal; tissue for pathologic study	Anesthesia required; postoperative pain	9–42% recurrence
Laser therapy	Effective for extensive warts; can be used during pregnancy	Requires expensive equipment; requires anesthesia	3–14% recurrence
Interferon	Treatment of recurrent disease	Therapy duration: 2–3 months; systemic side effects; very expensive, discomfort; labor-intensive treatment	36–82% remission

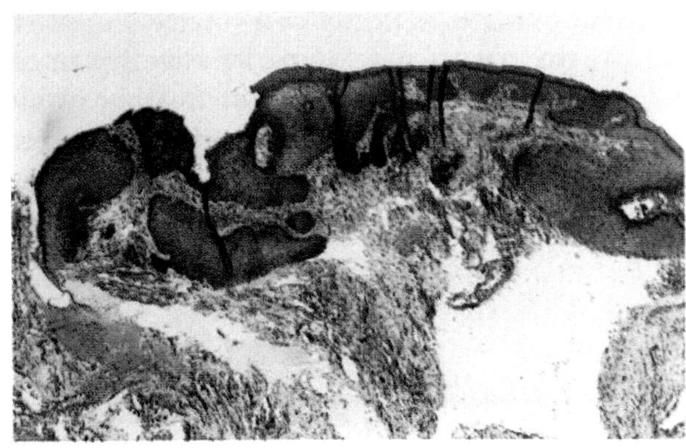

FIGURE 4 ■ Microscopic features of condylomata acuminata with podophyllin changes. *Source*: Courtesy of H. Srolovitz, M.D., Montreal, Quebec, Canada.

because a burn will result. If too much acid is applied, it should be wiped off, the area should be washed with water, and sodium bicarbonate should be applied as a local antidote if necessary. The lesions that are cauterized change from pink to a frosty white color. Lesions within the anal canal are treated similarly but dabbed gently with a cotton ball before the walls of the anal canal are allowed to fall back together.

Analgesic agents are prescribed routinely, but they are necessary only when massive involvement is present. Patients are instructed to keep the perianal area clean and dry. The caustic agent is applied at intervals of 7–10 days to achieve maximum benefit from the treatment. The patient's sexual partners also should be treated.

Approximately 25% of the patients in Swerdlow and Salvati's (13) report had recurrences. These patients were treated with further short courses of therapy. The number of treatments needed varied according to the size and number of warts. It ranged from one to 13 treatments, with most patients receiving four or fewer.

Swerdlow and Salvati (13) noted that when patients treated with bichloroacetic acid as an office procedure were compared to patients treated with other modes of therapy, the former were more comfortable, did not develop post-treatment scars and strictures, and had prompt resolution of warts without losing time from work.

■ IMIQUIMOD (ALDERA®)

Imiquimod (Aldera®) is an imidazoquinoline, a novel synthetic compound which is an immune response stimulator, enhancing both innate and acquired immune pathways (particular T helper cell type 1-mediated immune responses) resulting in antiviral, antineoplastic, and immunoregulatory activities (53). The mechanism of action of imiquimod involves cytokine induction in the skin, which then triggers the host's immune system to recognize the presence of a viral infection or malignancy, ultimately to eradicate the associated lesion. Imiquimod, a patient-applied topical 5% cream, is clinically efficacious and safe in the management of condylomata acuminata and other warty manifestations of human papillomavirus infections. In a randomized, vehicle-controlled, clinical trial conducted in the United States, 50% of patients treated three times per week for up to 16 weeks experienced complete clearance (54). The clinical outcome of imiquimod therapy in this condition is dependent on gender, with a superior efficacy in females compared to males. This is believed to be attributable to the higher degree of keratinization of the skin on the penis compared to the vulva, the most common locations for genital warts in male and female patients, respectively. In this study, 72% of females treated for up to 16 weeks with imiquimod cleared their warts compared to 33% of males, the majority of whom were circumcised. In a recent phase IIIB, international, open-label trial, Garland et al. (55) studied 943 patients from 114 clinic sites in 20 countries with the application of imiquimod 5% cream three times per week for up to 16 weeks. Complete clinical clearance was observed in 47.8% of patients during the initial treatment period, with clearance in an additional 5.5% of patients during the extended treatment period beyond 16 weeks. The overall clearance rate for the combined treatment period was 53.3%. In a treatment failure analysis, the overall clearance rate was 65.5% (female 75.5%, and males 56.9%). Low recurrence rates of 8.8% and 23% were observed at the end of the three- and six-month follow-up periods, respectively. The sustained clearance rates (patients who cleared during treatment and remained clear at the end of the follow-up period) after three and six months was 41.6% and 33.3%, respectively. Local erythema occurred in 67% of patients. The lower degree of keratinization and the semiocclusive effect of the foreskin in uncircumcised males are proposed as possible reasons for the higher clearance rates (62%) observed in a study of uncircumcised males who applied imiquimod three times a week for up to 16 weeks compared to efficacy (33%) in the predominantly circumcised male population in the U.S. trial (56). Another study reported a 50% clearance rate (72% females, 33% males) (57). The low recurrence rate of 13% in the three-month follow-up period after imiquimod treatment is favorable compared to the physician-administered therapies, i.e., cryotherapy, trichloroacetic acid, and podophyllin and the patient-applied therapy podophyllotoxin (54,58).

■ ELECTROCOAGULATION

Electrocoagulation, which necessitates the use of local anesthesia, is an effective means of destroying the small lesions of condyloma acuminatum. The benefits and complications vary according to the skill of the operator, who must control the depth and width of the wound. The aim is to obtain a white coagulum that generally corresponds to a second-degree burn. Such a wound should heal without any significant scarring. However, a black eschar is likely to represent a third-degree burn, which will probably heal with scarring; if such a burn is created circumferentially, a stricture may result. When working on the vital anoderm, the operator must be alert to the potential problems of stenosis and damage to the underlying sphincter. Special care must be taken not to miss any of the warts lying in the anal canal. Extensive warts, both perianal and intra-anal, might require the use of a general anesthetic agent. Postoperative care follows the conventional lines described in Chapter 4.

■ CIDOFOVIR

Coremans et al. (59) studied the efficacy of the topical application of the antiviral agent cidofovir at 1%. Twenty patients treated with coagulation were compared with 27 patients treated with cidofovir. Lesions refractory to cidofovir were cleared up with additional coagulations. Cidofovir alone cured the lesions in 32% of patients and induced partial regression in 60%. However, in smokers, complete resolution of the condylomata occurred only in 16.6% compared with 66% of nonsmokers. The number of coagulation sessions was much lower in the cidofovir-treated group (1% vs. 2.9%). The relapse rate was significantly lower in the cidofovir-treated group (3.7% vs. 55%). All recurrences in the electrocoagulation group occurred within four months of confirmed lesion clearance. Thirty-three percent of the patients reported only mild pain caused by erosive dermatitis. In contrast, coagulations caused painful ulcerations that necessitated the use of analgesics in all patients treated this way.

■ CRYOTHERAPY

Another destructive method used for treatment of condyloma acuminatum is cryotherapy. Various techniques have been advocated, including the use of liquid nitrogen, carbon dioxide snow, and liquefied air. Again, the depth and width of the wound must be carefully controlled. The postoperative course is similar to that of electrocoagulation. A reputed advantage is the lack of need for anesthesia, but this has not been the overall experience. O'Connor (60) reported on 936 patients treated and a total of 2246 cryotherapy sessions. Patients were advised to take sitz baths twice daily. Secondary bacterial infection was not encountered. Recurrences developed in 226 patients, but most patients admitted to re-exposure.

■ SURGICAL EXCISION

When massive involvement is present, surgical excision can be carried out with the use of general or regional anesthesia. A simple enema given the evening before or the morning of treatment is adequate bowel preparation. This method avoids the use of cautery except for controlling bleeding points.

A solution of 1:200,000 adrenaline in saline is injected subcutaneously and submucosally. This separates the warts and allows as much healthy skin and mucosa as possible to be preserved when the individual warts are removed with a pair of fine-toothed forceps and fine-pointed scissors. Good judgment is necessary to gauge the amount of anoderm that may be removed and yet protect the underlying sphincter mechanism. Similarly, the warts are removed from the anal mucosa. The resulting small wounds heal rapidly, but the severity of postoperative pain varies, and prolonged convalescence is common. In the majority of patients, it is possible to remove all the warts in one step, but if there are too many warts, removal may be done in two stages at an interval of approximately one month.

Thomson and Grace (34) reported the results in 75 patients with whom surgical excision was used. Over 75% of these patients had lesions within the anal canal. In 80% the warts were removed in one procedure. Postoperative complications occurred in four patients: bleeding (two), hematoma (one), and previously undetected coagulation defect (one). Relatively little discomfort was experienced, but a 42% recurrence rate was noted. In the majority of patients, recurrent wart formation was detected by the end of the second postoperative month. Gollock et al. (33), in a series of 34 patients treated in the same manner, had a primary success rate of 71.4% and a recurrence rate of 9.3%. Handley et al. (61) reported a 26.3% recurrence rate in 19 children so treated.

Anal stenosis is a well-known complication that may result from removal of anal and perianal warts. However, if adequate normal skin and mucosa are left between the wounds, stenosis should not occur.

A potential advantage of surgical excision over electrocoagulation is that the postoperative wound weeps less, producing a smaller amount of moisture, which is believed to enhance the growth of condylomata.

■ LASER THERAPY

The development of laser technology presents another possible method for decreasing the problem of persistence and recurrence of warts after treatment. Advocates of laser therapy have suggested that there is less postoperative pain and fewer recurrences with this type of therapy. Advantages of laser therapy include the fact that it is rapid and easy to use and that it does not require cleansing of the tip (as does electrical cautery). Significant disadvantages are the fact that the instrument is very expensive, somewhat cumbersome, and requires special instruction in its use (see Chap. 7).

Treating genital condylomata during pregnancy with CO_2 laser, Ferenczy (37) reported only a 5% failure rate and a 14% recurrence rate. In a review of the literature, Schaeffer (38) reported recurrence rates ranging from 3% to 13% after one to three CO_2 laser treatments of urogenital and anal condylomata acuminata, with follow-up periods ranging from 2 to 12 months. Schaeffer concluded that the CO_2 laser is the treatment of choice for condylomata acuminata that are extensive, recurrent, or present during pregnancy. A cure rate of 80% has been reported with the CO_2 laser with up to four laser vaporizations required (62).

Carrozza et al. (63) conducted a questionnaire-based retrospective long-term study on 64 consecutive men. The mean follow-up was 25 months (range 7–75). The overall cure rate after one intervention was 67%. The cure rate in HIV-positive versus HIV-negative patients was 58% versus 71%. Endoanal versus perianal location was associated with a cure rate of 56% versus 84%. After a second treatment session, the cure rate increased to 79% or higher in all subgroups. Painful defecation for an average of 4–5 weeks was the main postoperative complaint.

■ INTERFERON

It has been suggested that interferon may be the most practical way to treat refractory anogenital warts (39). Schonfeld et al. (40) treated 22 patients in a double-blind study of intramuscularly administered natural interferon. Patients with previously untreated condylomata acuminata received 2 million units of interferon beta or placebo for 10 consecutive days. Response to the interferon was measured by decrease in wart size; improvement with complete remission generally was not apparent until 5–8 weeks after treatment. Complete remission occurred in 82% of patients who received interferon but in only 18% of the placebo-treated patients, with follow-up done at 10–12 months. Gall et al. (41) treated refractory condylomata acuminata with intramuscular and intralesional lymphoblastoid interferon. With 5 million units of interferon administered daily for

28 days and then three times a week for 2 weeks, complete responses were obtained in 69% of the patients, partial responses in approximately 25%, and no or minimal response in 6% of patients. Androphy (39) noted that if complete remission is achieved, recurrence rates are very low. The duration of therapy may need to be prolonged 2–3 months. Schonfeld et al. (40) reported slow response for complete remission.

Eron et al. (42) conducted a randomized double-blind trial to compare interferon alpha-2b with placebo in the treatment of condylomata acuminata. The placebo or interferon (1 million IU) was injected directly into one to three warts three times weekly for 3 weeks. Side effects of fever, chills, myalgia, headache, fatigue, and leukopenia rarely disrupted daily routines. Of 257 patients evaluated at 13 weeks, the mean of the wart area decreased 40% below initial size, whereas in the placebo group it increased 46%. All treated warts cleared completely in 36% of interferon recipients and in 17% of placebo recipients, while treated warts progressed in 13% of interferon recipients and in 50% of placebo recipients. Despite the low response rate, the authors concluded that interferon was an effective form of therapy.

Friedman-Kein et al. (64) reviewed 158 patients who received injections of either interferon alpha or placebo into the base of the wart twice weekly for a maximum of 8 weeks or until all treated warts disappeared. Complete elimination of warts was achieved in 62% of patients treated with interferon alpha compared with 21% of placebo-treated patients. Approximately 25% of patients in each group had relapses. A randomized, double-blind, placebo-controlled, international multicenter trial (65) found no difference in efficacy between interferon alpha-2a and-placebo treatment groups.

Fleshner and Freilich (66) conducted a prospective randomized trial with 43 patients comparing surgical excision and fulguration immediately followed by an injection of 500,000 IU (0.1 mL) of interferon alpha-n3 or saline into each quadrant of the anal canal. After a mean follow-up of 3.8 months, 12% of the patients treated with interferon and 39% of the patients treated with saline developed recurrences.

There is growing literature to support the use of interferon in combination with other therapeutic modalities (18). In the treatment of extensive primary or recalcitrant condyloma acuminatum, interferon combined with locally destructive therapy [laser or electrocautery followed by interferon alpha (1–5 million units injected three times a week for 4–8 weeks)] results in a 50–80% response rate. However, The Condylomata International Collaborative Study Group found CO_2 laser ablation combined with systemic recombinant interferon alpha-2a ineffective for anogenital condylomata (67). In a randomized triple-blind placebo-controlled trial involving 250 patients, Armstrong et al. (68) failed to show any therapeutic advantage of adding interferon alpha-2a to placebo and ablative procedures.

Mayeaux et al. (69) compiled information from the literature regarding the efficacy of various forms of therapy. A summary of their findings is presented in Table 3.

■ CLINICAL TRIALS

Each modality of therapy has its advocates, but surprisingly few studies have been conducted comparing different methods of treatment.

TABLE 3 ■ Comparison of Therapies for Condyloma Acuminatum

Method	Success Rate (%)	Recurrence Rate < 6 Months (%)
Cryotherapy	83	28
Podophyllum resin	65	39
Trichloroacetic/bichloroacetic acid	81	36
CO_2 laser	89	8
Electrocautery	93	24
Excision	93	24
5-Fluorouracil	71	13
Interferon alpha	52	25

Source: From Ref. 69.

Simmons (70) randomly allocated 140 patients with anogenital warts to a double-blind study of 10% and 25% podophyllin in tincture of benzoin compound. Of the 109 patients followed up for three months, only 24 (22%) were free of warts, with 12 patients noting clearance after each treatment.

In a trial comparing the use of podophyllin alone, to trichloroacetic acid and podophyllin, Gabriel and Thin (32) found no significant difference between either treatment method at 3 months with a mean clearance rate of 32%.

In a prospective randomized control trial, Jensen (71) compared application of 25% podophyllin (weekly up to 6 weeks) with simple surgical excision in 60 patients with first-episode perianal condyloma acuminatum. Podophyllin completely cleared warts from 77% of patients compared with 93% for surgical excision. Cumulative recurrence rates at 12 months were 29% for surgical excision and 65% for podophyllin ($p < 0.01$). Jensen concluded that surgical excision produces faster clearance and lower recurrence rates of condyloma acuminatum than does application of podophyllin. Similar results were obtained by Khawaja (72), who conducted a prospective study of 37 patients randomly treated by application of 25% podophyllin or by scissor excision. At 6 weeks scissor excision cleared the warts from 89%, compared with 79% treated with podophyllin. The cumulative recurrence rate at 42 weeks was 19% for excision and 60% for podophyllin. Both Jensen (71) and Khawaja (72) believe that scissor excision is preferable to podophyllin application in the treatment of perianal condylomata acuminata.

Simmons et al. (73) randomly assigned 42 patients to receive either cryotherapy or electrocautery for anogenital warts. There was no significant difference in the success rate of these two forms of treatment in patients followed up for 3 months.

Handley et al. (44) found that combination treatment of primary anogenital warts with subcutaneous interferon alpha-2a plus cryotherapy was no more effective than cryotherapy alone. Armstrong et al. (74) found that treatment with interferon alpha-2a in combination with podophyllin was no more effective in the treatment of primary anogenital warts than podophyllin alone and is associated with more adverse events. The Condylomata International Collaborative Study Group (75) found that interferon alpha-2a monotherapy was not as effective as standard therapy of podophyllin 25% application. Vance and Davis (76) compared laser vaporization with laser vaporization followed by a series of, intralesional interferon alpha-2b injections. The former group experienced a 38.2% rate of recurrence or reinfection with a mean follow-up period of 13 weeks. Those treated with lasers and interferon had an 18.5% rate of recurrence or reinfection. Douglas et al. (77) found that the addition of interferon alpha-2b to podophyllin resulted in a wart clearance of 67% compared to 42% with podophyllin alone.

In a novel study to evaluate the claims of advocates of laser therapy, Billingham and Lewis (36) undertook to compare laser therapy with conventional electrical cautery. In 38 patients with extensive warts, all warts on the right half of the anus were treated with conventional electrical cautery, while those on the left side of the anus were cauterized with the CO_2 laser; close follow-up was done. When the patients were questioned postoperatively, it was noted that the laser was associated with either more pain or the same amount of pain in comparison with electrical cautery. Recurrences were first seen more often on the laser side. Billingham and Lewis concluded that laser therapy offered no advantage and, indeed, was less effective in control of the condylomata acuminata.

■ OPERATOR CAUTION

Bergbrandt et al. (78) studied the contamination of personnel and operating theatres with HPV DNA during treatment sessions with the CO_2 laser or electrocoagulation. HPV DNA was found in 32% of specimens collected from nasolabial folds and 16% of nostril cytobrushes. The authors recommend the use of face masks and the evacuation of air in the vicinity of the treatment field.

■ RECOMMENDATIONS FOR THERAPY

From the data available in the literature, it is difficult to make firm recommendations as to the optimal form of therapy.

Alam and Stiller (79) conducted a study to determine which treatment modalities for condyloma acuminata are associated with the lowest direct medical costs in an ambulatory private practice. They constructed a cost effectiveness model. From a literature review, extraction of commonly accepted guidelines regarding duration and frequency, as well as reports of efficacies of typical treatment regimens; from Medicare physician fee schedules, costs of physician visits, and physician-administered treatments; and from published data and average wholesale prices of medication. They found that the mean direct medical costs per complete clearance were lowest for surgical excision ($285). Other low-cost modalities are loop electrosurgical excision procedure ($316), electrodesiccation ($347), carbon dioxide laser ($416), podofilox ($424), and pulsed-dye laser ($479). Higher cost modalities are cryotherapy ($951), trichloroacetic acid ($986), imiquimod ($1255), podophyllum resin ($1632), and interferon alpha-2b ($6665).

It is my practice to manage previously untreated condylomata acuminata with repeated applications of 25% podophyllin in tincture of benzoin. For patients who fail to respond to this therapy or patients referred after failure of other forms of therapy, I use electrocoagulation with repeated electrocoagulation as necessary. Nivatvongs, on the other hand, has abandoned the use of topical agents, and his treatment of choice is surgical excision as recommended by Thomson, followed by electrocoagulation. Nivatvongs believes that the subsequent burning is much less extensive than when electrocoagulation is used alone and that any residual or recurrent disease is less extensive and is more readily re-electrocoagulated. He prefers electrocoagulation for limited disease and imiquinod for extensive disease.

■ MANAGEMENT OF DISEASE IN HIV-POSITIVE PATIENTS

Puy-Montbrun et al. (80) analyzed the anorectal lesions found in 148 HIV-positive patients and found anal condylomata to be the most frequent manifestation, affecting 30% of the patients.

Beck et al. (81) found that anal condylomata are common (18%) in patients who test positive for HIV, and that these patients can be expected to do well with appropriate treatment. With a follow-up of 4–26 months, the recurrence rate for anal condylomata was 26% after local treatment with podophyllin and 4% after fulguration and excision. In patients with symptomatic HIV infection, conservative treatment of condylomata acuminata has been advised because postoperative healing is poor (82).

RECURRENCE

Numerous therapeutic modalities have been used in the treatment of anal condylomata acuminata, with a failure rate ranging from 25% to 70% (13). This recalcitrance to therapy has been associated with several factors, including repeat infection from sexual contact, localization of virus away from lymphatics, and deep or missed lesions (83). Recurrence may also be caused by specific biologic factors, such as a long incubation period for HPV and interactions between HPV and tissue-related local immunity. Indeed, numerous reports have shown that HPV destabilizes local immunity by depleting and altering morphologic aspects of Langerhans cells (84). In HIV-seropositive patients, the infection is further perpetuated by depletion of CD4 cells, CD16 (macrophages/natural killer) cells, and CD1a (Langerhans) cells from the HPV-infected areas, and this local phenomenon correlates well with the systemic immunosuppression characteristic of these patients (85). These patients also may change sexual partners and acquire new infections. Therefore, their partners also should be treated in order to obtain an effective cure. The potentially long incubation period of condylomata acuminata may cause reinfection of sexual partners or delayed recurrence of a new generation of warts. Patients should be forewarned of the marked tendency of the warts to reappear.

de la Fuente et al. (28) investigated risk factors and recurrence rates in immunocompromised patients requiring operation for medically intractable anal condyloma. A retrospective review was performed on 63 consecutive patients who underwent operative intervention for medically intractable anal condyloma. Patient cohorts included immunosuppressed patients (e.g., HIV-seropositive, leukemia, idiopathic lymphopenic syndrome, or transplant patients; $n=45$) and immunocompetent patients ($n=18$). Anal condyloma recurred in 66% of the immunosuppressed patients compared with 27% of the immunocompetent group. Recurrence time was shorter in immunosuppressed patients than in immunocompetent patients (6.8 vs. 15 months). In the subpopulation of HIV-seropositive patients, no association was found between recurrence rates and viral loads; however, CD4 counts were significantly lower in those who had recurrence than those who did not (226 vs. 401 cells/μL).

POSTTREATMENT FOLLOW-UP

Because of the frequency of recurrence, follow-up visits at 4–6-week intervals for at least 3 months while the patient is free of warts are recommended. Small recurrent warts can be treated easily in the office.

RESUMPTION OF SEXUAL INTERCOURSE

Provided that condoms are used prophylactically, sexual activity may be resumed when the patient so desires. Without the use of condoms, sexual intercourse probably may be resumed safely after a 3-month disease-free period has elapsed.

CONDYLOMATA ACUMINATA IN CHILDREN

Condylomata acuminata are known to occur in children, perhaps as a consequence of sexual abuse. They have been reported to be associated with the same HPV types found in adults (86,87). However, Fairley et al. (88) conducted a study of prevalence data to support hand–genital transmission of genital warts. They observed a relatively high proportion of genital warts in children that contain HPV types 1 and 4 (15% in children and 2% in adults): If hand–genital transmission does not occur, the observed difference could only be explained by an eightfold greater probability of transmission to children of types 1–4 than of types 6–11, or by an eight-fold greater duration of infection with types 1 and 4. Handley et al. (89), in a study of 42 prepubertal children, suggested that the majority of children with anogenital warts do not acquire these sexually and that vertical transmission is an important means by which young children acquire anogenital warts. Nevertheless, Gutman et al. (90) believe that considerable evidence suggests that anogenital HPV disease in children that appears after infancy is usually acquired through abusive sexual contact. Derksen (91) also supports that view. Transmission may also be by fomites. HPV typing may help clarify the mode of transmission.

VERRUCOUS CARCINOMA

In 1948, Ackerman (92) published his classic description of a slow-growing, locally aggressive, essentially nonmetastasizing variant of a well-differentiated squamous cell carcinoma and designated it a verrucous carcinoma. Ackerman's original report described the lesion in the oral cavity, but authors subsequently have reported this histologic carcinoma in a wide variety of anatomic locations, including the perianal region and the rectum (93–95).

In 1925, Buschke and Löwenstein (96) described a penile lesion that appeared cytologically benign but behaved in a malignant manner. Due to its histologic similarity to the benign condyloma acuminatum, the lesion was termed a giant condyloma acuminatum or, a Buschke–Löiwenstein tumor. Although no universal agreement has been reached, there is a growing consensus that this entity probably represents a verrucous carcinoma (97–101). What many authors in the past have described as condyloma acuminatum with malignant transformation is now believed to be verrucous carcinoma from the onset.

Creasman et al. (102) summarized the salient features of 20 cases of giant condyloma acuminatum reported in the literature. They found an average age of 43 years, a male-to-female ratio of 2.3:1.0, a recurrence rate of 65%, an overall mortality rate of 30%, an incidence of malignant transformation of 30%, and a mortality rate of 20% in the malignant group.

In a more recent review of the literature, Trombetta and Place (103) identified 51 reported cases of giant condyloma acuminatum. Giant condyloma acuminatum presents with a 2.7:1 male-to-female ratio. For patients younger than 50 years of age, this ratio was increased to 3.5:1. The mean age at presentation is 43.9 years, 42.9 in males and 46.6 in females. The most common presenting symptoms are perianal mass (47%), pain (32%), abscess or fistula (32%), and bleeding (18%). Giant condyloma acuminatum has been linked to human papillomavirus and has distinct histologic features. Foci of invasive carcinoma are noted in 50% of the reports, "carcinoma in situ" in 8%, and no invasion in 42%.

Macroscopically, the lesion presents as an exophytic, warty, gray-white, soft-to-firm mass varying in size from 1 to 10 cm. The cauliflower-like mass may arise in the perianal skin, anal canal, or distal rectum and is frequently indistinguishable from benign lesions. The clinical course of this growth is one of relentless progression and expansion of the neoplasm by extensive erosion and pressure necrosis of surrounding tissues with invasion of the ischioanal fossa, perirectal tissues, and even the pelvic cavity. The invasive nature of the lesion may cause multiple sinuses or fistulous tracts that may invade fascia, muscle, or rectum and may cause inflammation, infection, and hemorrhage. Extent of involvement can be precisely determined by CT examination (Fig. 5A) (104).

Microscopically, the lesion bears a strong resemblance to condyloma acuminatum. It exhibits marked papillary proliferation of well-differentiated, maturing squamous epithelium that projects above the skin or mucosal surface and displays extensive surface keratinization. There is extensive acanthosis, parakeratosis, and vacuolation of the superficial layers (103). Individual cells or groups of cells can have koilocytotic changes as found in condyloma acuminatum. Scattered dyskeratotic and/or slightly atypical squamous cells occur, but a major degree of cytologic atypia or malignancy is not present. There is no evidence of invasion of lymphatics, blood vessels, or other histopathologic criteria of malignancy. The lower borders of proliferating squamous cells are rounded and of the pushing type rather than the kind that infiltrate in narrow cellular cords. Those borders extend below the level of normal adjacent surface epithelium. A heavy inflammatory

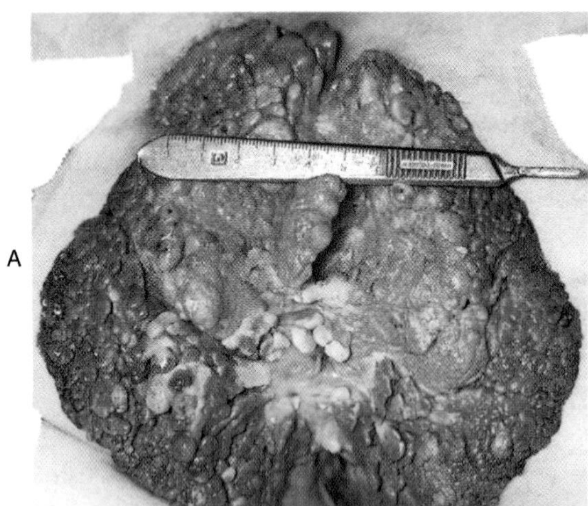
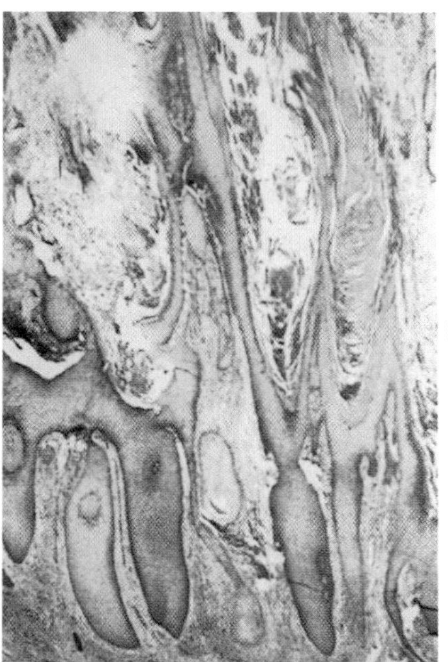

FIGURE 5 ■ Verrucous carcinoma. (**A**) Macroscopic features of a verrucous carcinoma. (**B**) Microscopic features of a verrucous carcinoma demonstrating acanthosis, papillary fronds with rounded bottoms, lack of cytologic atypia, keratin, and lymphoplasma cell infiltrate around bulbous ends of neoplasm. *Source*: (**A**) Courtesy of Charles Orsay, M.D., Chicago, Illinois. U.S.A. and (**B**) H. Srolovitz, M.D., Montreal, Quebec, Canada.

cellular infiltrate made up of lymphocytes and plasma cells lies close to and often permeates the advancing lesion (Fig. 5B).

The extent of operation should be determined for each individual patient. Gingrass et al. (99), who described the lesion as a verrucous carcinoma, recommend wide local excision, with care taken to make certain that the depths of the excision are histologically clear. If the carcinoma involves the anal sphincter, abdominoperineal resection with extended perineal dissection should be performed. Other authors believe that radical surgical excision, which usually means abdominoperineal resection, offers the only hope of eradication of the neoplasm and permanent cure (98). Creasman et al. (102) believe that giant condyloma acuminatum represents an intermediate lesion in a pathologic continuum from condyloma acuminatum to squamous cell carcinoma. They recommend early and radical local excision; in cases of recurrence, invasion, or malignant transformation they recommend abdominoperineal resection. In the review by Trombetta and Place (103), treatment varied greatly from simple excision to complex courses of excisions, fecal diversions, radiation therapy, and chemotherapy. Forty-five of 52 cases underwent primary surgical excision of some kind to include simple excision, wide local excision, wide local excision with fecal diversion, and abdominoperineal resection. Of the seven patients who underwent initial nonsurgical management, two underwent primary radiation therapy, three primary topical therapy with podophyllin, one primary chemotherapy, and one primary interferon therapy. Follow-up period was stated in 41 of 52 cases, and ranged from 3 months to 44 years. Recurrence of GCA was documented in 26 of the 52 cases. Five of the seven patients initially treated with nonsurgical therapy had documented recurrence.

The use of multimodality therapy in the treatment of verrucous carcinoma may obviate the need for radical extirpative surgery. Bjork et al. (105) reported on a case successfully treated with a combination of sphincter-sparing operation, radiotherapy, and adjuvant chemotherapy.

Prasad and Abcarian (10) have termed the clinical situation characterized by ulceration, infiltration, and proliferation into deeper tissues without malignant histologic change as malignant behavior of condylomata. They believed that it was significant that all of their patients with condylomata showing malignant behavior had anal fistulas and that this made the treatment quite difficult. An example of condylomata acuminata growing in a fistulous tract is seen in Figure 6.

CONDYLOMA ACUMINATUM AND SQUAMOUS CELL CARCINOMA

The association between anorectal HPV infection and high-grade anal dysplasia and squamous carcinoma has been well established. Carcinoma is common in males with a history of homosexual intercourse, with estimated incidences as high as 37 per 100,000 (106). The relative risk of anal malignancy among homosexuals with genital warts has been estimated to be 12.6 (107). The risk of anal carcinoma in HIV-seropositive patients is 84-fold higher than in the normal population (108). Prospective cohort studies have shown that among HIV-seropositive patients, the most important risk factors for incidence of anal high-grade squamous intraepithelial lesions are low CD4 cell counts, persistent anal HPV infection, anal infection with multiple HPV types, and higher levels of oncogenic HPV types (109). Malignant transformation, or at least the association of malignancy, with condylomata acuminata has been reported by several authors (10,99,100,110,111). Prasad and Abcarian (10) reported that 1.8% of their 330 patients with anal condylomata acuminata demonstrated malignant potential.

Metcalf and Dean (112) investigated the incidence of dysplasia and risk factors for premalignant and malignant changes in patients with anal condyloma acuminatum. Their study population consisted of 59 heterosexuals and 32 homosexuals or bisexuals. Two heterosexuals (3%) had invasive squamous cell carcinoma, and four (6%) had dysplasia. One homosexual or bisexual (3%) had squamous cell carcinoma in situ, and nine (28%) had dysplasia. The authors concluded that homosexual orientation, disease above the

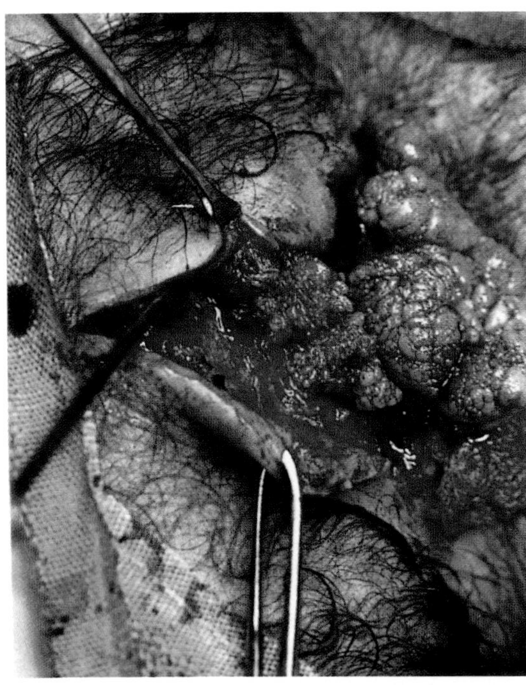

FIGURE 6 ■ Example of condylomata acuminata growing in a fistulous tract.

dentate line, and HIV seropositivity increase the risk of dysplasia in perianal condyloma.

The incidence of anal intraepithelial neoplasia was studied in a group of 210 homosexual and bisexual men (113). The overall incidence was 35%. Anal intraepithelial neoplasia was found in 45% of patients with anal warts and only 7% of patients without anal warts. The relative risk of anal warts on anal intraepithelial neoplasia was 4.70. Although the natural history of anal intraepithelial neoplasia remains unknown, parallels with changes seen in the cervix suggest that, if left untreated, a percentage of patients with high-grade dysplasia will ultimately develop invasive carcinoma. The high relative risk of anal intraepithelial neoplasia in patients with condylomata acuminata is in keeping with the epidemiologic evidence linking condylomata and anal carcinoma (107).

In the most recent report addressing this issue, de la Fuente et al. (28) observed no statistical significance in the incidence of dysplasia or carcinoma between immunocompetent and immunosuppressed patients. Dysplasia was revealed in 23% of the former and 19% of the latter; carcinoma in situ in 5.8% of the former and 11.9% of the latter; and invasive carcinoma in 5.8% of the former and 7.1% of the latter.

Several studies have reported the association of HPV infection with anal carcinoma (114). Beckmann et al. (115) found HPV DNA in 35% of squamous neoplasms of the anus. Palmer et al. (116) found HPV-16 DNA in 56% and HPV-18 DNA in 5% of 45 anal squamous cell carcinomas. No HPV 6 or 11 DNA was detectable. Nonmalignant anal epithelium and malignant rectal mucosa obtained from patients undergoing hemorrhoidectomy and abdominoperineal excision of the rectum did not contain any detectable HPV DNA. In direct contrast, Kirgan et al. (117) found the HPV antigen in 23% of normal colon specimens, 60% of benign neoplasms, and 97% of carcinomas. They believe that HPV also affects the columnar mucosa of the colon, and that an association exists between HPV and colon neoplasia.

In 1986, Longo et al. (118) reported the 14th case of squamous cell carcinoma in situ developing in perianal condylomata acuminata. Salient clinical features of the reported cases included an average age of 39 years and the fact that all patients but one were men, 10 of whom were homosexual. Symptom duration ranged from 3 weeks to 5 years, and five patients had AIDS or developed AIDS shortly after onset of symptoms. Local excision was the recommended treatment.

Operation has been the traditional modality of treatment for carcinoma that arises in condylomata acuminata (10,98,110). Sawyers (119) reported the treatment of four patients with condylomata acuminata who had histologic evidence of squamous cell carcinoma arising in venereal warts. Those patients underwent abdominoperineal resection. Even after aggressive surgical management, local recurrence or distant spread may result in significant morbidity and mortality.

Radiation and chemotherapy also have been used, sometimes in conjunction with operation (97). Butler et al. (120) reported a case of an unresectable squamous cell carcinoma associated with condylomata acuminata rendered operable with chemotherapy (5-fluorouracil and mitomycin C) plus radiation to the primary lesion. An ab dominoperineal resection was performed, and it was noted that the surgical specimen contained no residual carcinoma. This is in keeping with similar findings in patients with squamous cell carcinoma of the anal canal that is not associated with condylomata acuminata treated by combination chemoradiotherapy (121). Therefore, it would appear that combination therapy should be the first line of treatment that is considered for squamous cell carcinoma associated with condyloma acuminatum.

REFERENCES

1. Sohn N, Robilotti JG. The gay bowel syndrome, a review of colonic and rectal conditions in 200 male homosexuals. Am J Gastroenterol 1977; 67:478–484.
2. Oriel JD. Genital warts. Sex Transm Dis 1982; 8:326–329.
3. Sykes NL. Condyloma acuminatum. Int J Dermatol 1995; 34:297–302.
4. Gissmann L, Schwarz E. Persistence and expression of human papillomavirus DNA in genital cancer. Ciba Found Symp 1986; 120:190–207.
5. Parker BJ, Cossart YE, Thompson CH, Rose BR, Henderson BR. The clinical management and laboratory assessment of anal warts. Med J Aust 1987; 147:59–63.
6. Labropoulou V, Balamotis A, Tosca A, Rotola A, Mavromara-Nazos P. Typing of human papillomaviruses in condylomata acuminata from Greece. J Med Virol 1994; 42:254–263.
7. Syrjanen SM, Von Krough G, Syrjanen KJ. Detection of human papillomavirus DNA in anogenital condylomata in men using in-situ DNA hybridisation applied to paraffin sections. Genitourin Med 1987; 63:32–39.
8. Handley JM, Maw RD, Lawther H, Homer T, Bharucha H, Dinsmore WW. Human papillomavirus DNA detection in primary anogenital warts and cervical low-grade intraepithelial neoplasias in adults by in-situ hybridization. Sex Transm Dis 1992; 19:225–229.
9. Gall AA, Meyer PR, Taylor CR. Papillomavirus antigens in anorectal condyloma and carcinoma in homosexual men. JAMA 1987; 257:337–340.
10. Prasad ML, Abcarian H. Malignant potential of perianal condyloma acuminatum. Dis Colon Rectum 1980; 23:191–197.
11. Williams TS, Callen JP, Owen LG. Vulvar disorders in the pre-pubertal female. Pediatr Ann 1986; 8:588–589, 592–601, 604–605.
12. Baruah MC, Sardari L, Selvaraju M, Veliath AJ. Perianal condylomata acuminata in a male child. Br J Venereal Dis 1984; 60:60–61.
13. Swerdlow DB, Salvati EP. Condyloma acuminatum. Dis Colon Rectum 1971; 14:226–229.

14. Carr G, William DC. Anal warts in a population of gay men in New York City. Sex Transm Dis 1977; 4:56–57.
15. Landsberg K, Bear RA. Severe condyloma acuminata in a renal transplant recipient. Am J Nephrol 1986; 6:325–326.
16. Breese P, Judson FN, Penley KA, Douglas JM. Anal human papillomavirus infection among homosexual and bisexual men: prevalence of type-specific infection and association with human immunodeficiency virus. Sex Transm Dis 1995; 22:7–14.
17. Greene I. Therapy for genital warts. Dermatol Clin 1992; 10:253–267.
18. Rockley PF, Tyring SK. Interferons alpha, beta and gamma therapy of anogenital human papillomavirus infections. Pharmacol Ther 1995; 65:265–287.
19. Koutsky L. Epidemiology of genital human papillomavirus infection. Am J Med 1997; 102:3–8.
20. Bauer HM, Hildesheim A, Schiffman MH, et al. Determinants of genital human papillomavirus infection in low-risk women in Portland, Oregon. Sex Transm Dis 1993; 20:274–278.
21. Ho GY, Bierman R, Beardsley L, et al. Natural history of cervicovaginal papillomavirus infection in young women. N Engl J Med 1998; 338: 423–428.
22. Sellors JW, Mahony JB, Kaczorowski J, et al. Prevalence and predictors of human papillomavirus infection in women in Ontario, Canada. Survey of HPV in Ontario Women (SHOW) Group. CAMJ 2000; 163:503–508.
23. Chuang TY, Perry HO, Kurland LT, etal. Condyloma acuminatum in Rochester, Minn, 1950–1978. II. Anaplasias and unfavorable outcomes. Arch Dermatol 1984; 120:476–83.
24. Persson G, Andersson K, Krantz I. Symptomatic genital papillomavirus infection in a community. Incidence and clinical picture. Acta Obstet Gynecol Scand 1996; 75:287–290.
25. Simms I, Fairley CK. Epidemiology of genital warts in England Wales: 1971–94. Genitourin Med 1997; 73:365–367.
26. Lyttle PH. Surveillance report: disease treads at New Zealand sexually transmitted disease clinics 1977-93. Genitourin Med 1994; 70:329–335.
27. Schlappner OLA, Shaffer EA. Anorectal condylomata acuminata, a missed part of the condyloma spectrum. Can Med Assoc J 1978; 118: 172–173.
28. de la Fuente SG, Ludwig KA, Mantyh CR. Preoperative immune status determines anal condyloma recurrence after surgical excision. Dis Colon Rectum 2003; 46:367–373.
29. Morson BD, Dawson IMP. Gastrointestinal pathology. Cambridge, MA: Blackwell Scientific Publications, 1972:623.
30. Petherson CS, Albrectsen J, Larsen J, et al. Subclinical human papilloma virus infection in condylomata acuminata patients attending a VD clinic. Acta Derm Venereol (Stockh) 1991; 71:252–255.
31. Hillman RJ, Botcherby M, Ryait BK, Hanna N, Taylor-Robinson D. Detection of human papillomavirus DNA in the urogenital tracts of men with anogenital warts. Sex Transm Dis 1993; 20:21–27.
32. Gabriel G, Thin RNT. Treatment of anogenital warts. Comparison of trichloroacetic acid and podophyllin versus podophyllin alone. Br J Venereal Dis 1983; 59:124–126.
33. Gollock JM, Slatford K, Hunter JM. Scissor excision of anogenital warts. Br J Venereal Dis 1982; 58:400–401.
34. Thomson JPS, Grace RH. The treatment of perianal and anal condylomata acuminata: a new operative technique. Proc R Soc Med 1978; 71: 180–185.
35. Figuero S, Gennaro AR. Intralesional bleomycin injection in treatment of condyloma acuminatum. Dis Colon Rectum 1980; 23:550–551.
36. Billingham RP, Lewis FC. Laser versus electrical cautery in the treatment of condylomata acuminata of the anus. Surg Gynecol Obstet 1982; 155: 865–867.
37. Ferenczy A. Treating genital condyloma during pregnancy with the carbon dioxide laser. Am J Obstet Gynecol 1984; 148:9–12.
38. Schaeffer AJ. Use of the CO_2 laser in urology. Urol Clin North Am 1986; 13:393–404.
39. Androphy EJ. Papillomaviruses and interferon. Ciba Found Symp 1986; 120:221–234.
40. Schonfeld A, Schattner A, Crespi M, et al. Intramuscular human interferon-B injections in treatment of condyloma acuminata. Lancet 1984; 1: 1038–1041.
41. Gall SA, Hughes CE, Whisnant J, Weck P. Therapy of resistant condyloma acuminata with lymphoblastoid interferon. J Cell Biochem Suppl 1985; 9C:91–92.
42. Eron LJ, Judson F, Tucker S, et al. Interferon therapy for condylomata acuminata. N Engl J Med 1986; 315:1059–1064.
43. Krebs HB. Treatment of genital condylomata with topical 5-fluorouracil. Dermatol Clin 1991; 9:333–341.
44. Handley JM, Maw RD, Horner T, Lawther H, McNeill T, Dinsmore WW. Nonspecific immunity in patients with primary congenital warts treated with interferon alfa plus cryotherapy or cryotherapy alone. Acta Derm Venereol (Stockh) 1992; 72:39–40.
45. Heaton CL, Lichti HF, Weiner M. The revival of nitric acid for the treatment of anogenital warts. Clin Pharmacol Ther 1993; 54:107–111.
46. Damstra RJ, van Vloten WA. Cryotherapy in the treatment of condylomata acuminata: A controlled study of 64 patients. J Dermatol Surg Oncol 1991; 17:273–276.
47. Oriel D. Letter to the editor. Proc Roy Soc Med 1978; 71:234.
48. Miller RA. Podophyllin. Int J Dermatol 1985; 8:491–498.
49. Moher LM, Maurer SA. Podophyllum toxicity: case report and literature review. J Fam Pract 1979; 9:237–240.
50. Montaldi DH, Giambrone JP, Courey NG, Taefi P. Podophyllin poisoning associated with the treatment of condyloma acuminatum: a case report. Am J Obstet Gynecol 1974; 119:1130–1131.
51. Karol MD, Conner CS, Watanabe AS, Murphrey KJ. Podophyllum: suspected teratogenicity from topical application. Clin Toxicol 1980; 16: 283–286.
52. Bonnez W, Elswick RK. Bailey-Farchione A, et al. Efficacy and safety of 0.5% podofilox solution in the treatment and suppression of anogenital warts. Am J Med 1994; 96:420–425.
53. Garland SM. Imiquimod. Curr Opin Infect Dis 2003; 16:85–89.
54. Edwards L, Ferenczy A, Eron L, et al. Self-administered topical 5% imiquimod cream for external anogenital warts. Arch Dermatol 1998; 134:25–30.
55. Garland S, Sellors J, Wikstrom A, et al. Imiquimod 5% cream is a safe and effective self-applied treatment for anogenital warts; results of an open-label, multicentre Phase III trial. International J STD AIDS 2001; 12: 722–729.
56. Gollnick H, Barraso R, Jappe U, etal. Safety and efficacy of imiquimod 5% cream in the treatment of penile genital warts in uncircumcised men when applied three times weekly or once per day. Int J STD AIDS 2001; 12:22–28.
57. Beutner KR, Wiley DJ. Recurrent external genital warts: a literature review. Papillomavirus Report 1997; 8:69–74.
58. Sauder DN, Skinner RB, Fox TL, Owens ML. Topical imiquimod 5% cream as an effective treatment for external genital and perianal warts in different patient populations. Sex Transm Dis 2003; 30:124–128.
59. Coremans G, Margaritis V, Snoeck R, Wyndaele J, De Clercq E, Geboes K. Topical cidofovir (HPMPC) is an effective adjuvant to surgical treatment of anogenital condylomata acuminata. Dis Colon Rectum 2003; 46:1103–1108.
60. O'Connor JJ. Perianal and anal condyloma acuminata. J Dermatol Surg Oncol 1979; 5:276–277.
61. Handley JM, Maw RD, Horner T, Lawther H, Bingham EA, Dinsmore WW. Scissor excision plus electrocautery of anogenital warts in prepubertal children. Pediatr Dermatol 1991; 8:243–245.
62. Peterson CS, Menne T. Anogenital warts in consecutive male heterosexual patients referred to a CO_2-laser clinic in Copenhagen. Acta Derm Venereol (Stockh) 1993; 73:465–466.
63. Carrozza PM, Merlani GM, Burg G, Hafner J. $CO_{(2)}$ laser surgery for extensive, cauliflower-like anogtenital condylomata acuminata: retrospective long-term study on 19 HIV-positive and 45 HIV-negative men. Dermatology 2002; 205:255–259.
64. Friedman-Kein AE, Eron LJ, Conant M, et al. Natural interferon alfa for treatment of condylomata acuminata. JAMA 1988; 259:533–538.
65. The Condylomata International Collaborative Study Group. Recurrent condylomata acuminata treated with recombinant interferon alpha-2a. Acta Derm Venereol (Stockh) 1993; 73:223–226.
66. Fleshner PR, Freilich MI. Adjuvant interferon for anal condyloma. A prospective, randomized trial. Dis Colon Rectum 1994; 37:1255–1259.
67. The Condylomata International Collaborative Study Group. Randomized placebo-controlled double-blind combined therapy with laser surgery and systemic interferon a-2a in the treatment of anogenital condylomata acuminatum. J Infect Dis 1993; 167:824–829.
68. Armstrong DKB, Maw RD, Dinsmore WW, et al. Combined therapy trial with interferon alpha-2a and ablative therapy in the treatment of anogenital warts. Genitourin Med 1996; 72:103–107.
69. Mayeaux EJ, Harper MB, Barksdale W, Pope JB. Noncervical human papillomavirus genital infections. Am Fam Physician 1995; 52:1137–1146.
70. Simmons PD. Podophyllin 10% and 25% in the treatment of anogenital warts. A comparative double blind study. Dr J Venereal Dis 1981; 57: 208–209.
71. Jensen SL. Comparison of podophyllin application with simple surgical excision in clearance and recurrence of perianal condylomata acuminata. Lancet 1985; 2:1146–1148.
72. Khawaja HT. Podophyllin versus scissor excision in the treatment of perianal condylomata acuminata. A prospective study. Br J Surg 1989; 76: 1067–1068.
73. Simmons PB, Langlet F, Thin RNT. Cryotherapy versus electrocautery in the treatment of genital warts. Br J Venereal Dis 1981; 57:273–274.
74. Armstrong DKB, Maw RD, Dinsmore WW, et al. A randomized, double-blind parallel group study to compare subcutaneous interferon alpha-2a plus podophyllin with placebo plus podophyllin in the treatment of primary condylomata acuminata. Genitourin Med 1994; 70:389–393.
75. The Condylomata International Collaborative Study Group. A comparison of interferon alfa-2a and podophyllin in the treatment of primary condylomata acuminata. Genitourin Med 1991; 67:394–399.

76. Vance JC, Davis D. Interferon alpha-2b injections used as an adjuvant therapy to carbon dioxide laser vaporization of recalcitrant anogenital condylomata acuminata. J Invest Dermatol 1990; 95:1465–1485.
77. Douglas JM, Eron LJ, Judson FN, et al. A randomized trial of combination therapy with intralesional interferon α 2b and podophyllin versus podophyllin alone for the therapy of anogenital warts. J Infect Dis 1990; 162:52–59.
78. Bergbrandt IM, Samuelsson L, Olofsson S, Jonassen P, Ricksten A. Polymerase chain reaction for monitoring human papillomavirus contamination of medical personnel during treatment of genital warts with CO_2 laser and electrocoagulation. Acta Derm Venereol (Stockh) 1994; 74:393–395.
79. Alam M, Stiller M. Direct medical costs for surgical and medical treatment of condylomata acuminata. Arch Dematol 2001; 137:337–341.
80. Puy-Montbrun Denis J, Ganansia R, Mathoniere F, Le Marchand N, Arnous-Dubois N. Anorectal lesions in human immunodeficiency virus-infected patients. Int J Colorectal Dis 1992; 7:26–30.
81. Beck DE, Jaso RG, Zajac RA. Surgical management of anal condylomata in the HIV-positive patient. Dis Colon Rectum 1990; 33:180–183.
82. Scholefield JH, Northover JMA, Carr ND. Male homosexuality, HIV infection and colorectal surgery. Br J Surg 1990; 70:493–496.
83. Congilosi SM, Madoff RD. Current therapy for recurrent and extensive anal warts. Dis Colon Rectum 1995; 38:1101–1107.
84. Viac J, Chardonet Y, Euvard S, Chignol MC, Thivolet J. Langerhans cells, inflammation markers and human papillomavirus infection in benign and malignant epithelial tumors from transplant recipients. J Dermatol 1992; 19:67–77.
85. Arany I, Tyring SK. Systemic immunosuppression by HIV infection influences HPV transcription and thus local immune responses in condyloma acuminatum. Int J STD AIDS 1998; 9:268–271.
86. Yun K, Joblin L. Presence of human papillomavirus DNA in condylomata acuminata in children and adolescents. Pathology 1993; 25:1–3.
87. Obalek S, Misiewicz J, Jablonska S, Favre M, Orth G. Childhood condyloma acuminatum: association with genital and cutaneous human papillomaviruses. Pediatr Dermatol 1993; 10:101–106.
88. Fairley CK, Gay WJ, Forbes A, Abramson M, Garland SM. Hand–genital transmission of genital warts? An analysis of prevalence data. Epidemiol Infect 1995; 115:169–176.
89. Handley J, Dinsmore W, Maws R, et al. Anogenital warts in prepubertal children; sexual abuse or not? Int J STD AIDS 1993; 4:271–279.
90. Gutman LT, Herman-Giddens ME, Phelps WC. Transmission of human genital papillomavirus disease. Comparison of data from adults and children. Pediatrics 1993; 91:31–38.
91. Derksen DJ. Children with condylomata acuminata. J Fam Prac 1992; 34: 419–423.
92. Ackerman LV. Verrucous carcinoma of the oral cavity. Surgery 1948; 23: 670–678.
93. Grassegger A, Hopel R, Hussl H, Wicke K, Fritsch P. Buschke–Löwernstein tumor infiltrating pelvic organs. Br J Dermatol 1994; 130: 221–225.
94. Goodman P, Halpert RD. Invasive squamous cell carcinoma of the anus arising in condyloma acuminatum: CT demonstration. Gastrointest Radiol 1991; 16:267–270.
95. Kibrite A, Zeitouni NC, Cloutier R. Aggressive giant condyloma acuminatum associated with oncogenic human papilloma virus: a case report. Can J Surg 1997; 40:143–145.
96. Buschke A, Löwenstein L, Über Carcinomähnliche Condylomata Acuminata des Penis. Klin Wochenschr 1925; 4:1726–1728.
97. Headington JX. Verrucous carcinoma. Cutis 1978; 21:207–211.
98. Elliot MS, Werner JD, Immelman EJ, Harrison AC. Giant condyloma (Buschke–Loewenstein tumor) of the anorectum. Dis Colon Rectum 1979; 22:497–500.
99. Gingrass PJ, Bubrick MP, Hitchcock CR, Strom RL. Anorectal verrucous squamous carcinoma: report of two cases. Dis Colon Rectum 1978; 21: 120–122.
100. Lee SH, McGregor DH, Kuziez MN. Malignant transformation of perianal condyloma acuminatum. A case report with review of the literature. Dis Colon Rectum 1981; 24:462–467.
101. Prioleau PG, Santa Cruz MJ, Meyer JS, Bauer WC. Verrucous carcinoma. A light and electron microscopic, autoradiographic, and immunofluorescence study. Cancer 1980; 45:2849–2857.
102. Creasman C, Haas PA, Fox TA Jr, Balazs M. Malignant transformation of anorectal giant condyloma acuminatum (Buschke–Loewenstein tumor). Dis Colon Rectum 1989; 32:481–487.
103. Trombetta LJ, Place RJ. Giant condyloma acuminatum of the anorectum: trends in epidemiology and management: report of a case and review of the literature. Dis Colon Rectum 2001; 44:1878–1886.
104. Balthazar EJ, Streiter M, Megibow AJ. Anorectal giant condyloma acuminata (Buschke–Loewenstein tumor): CT and radiographic manifestations. Radiology 1984; 150:651–653.
105. Bjork M, Athlin L, Lundskog B. Giant condyloma acuminatum (Buschke–Löwenstein tumor) of the anorectum with malignant transformation. Eur J Surg 1995; 161:691–694.
106. Dailing J, Weiss N, Klopfenestein L, Cochran L, Chow W, Daifuku R. Correlates of homosexual behavior and the incidence of anal cancer. JAMA 1982; 247:1988–1990.
107. Holly E, Whittemore A, Aston D, Nickoloff B, Kristiansen J. Anal cancer incidence: genital warts, anal fissure or fistula, hemorrhoids, and smoking. J Natl Cancer Inst 1989; 81:1726–1731.
108. Melbye M, Cote TR, Kessler L, Gail M, Biggar RJ. High incidence of anal cancer among AIDS patients. The AIDS/Cancer Working Group. Lancet 1994; 343:636–639.
109. Palefsky JM, Holly EA, Ralston ML, Jay N, Michael Berry J, Darragh TM. High incidence of anal high-grade squamous intra-epithelial lesions among HIV-positive and HIV-negative homosexual and bisexual men. AIDS 1998; 12:495–503.
110. Ejeckam GC, Idikio EA, Nayak V, Gardner JP. Malignant transformation in an anal condyloma acuminatum. Can J Surg 1983; 26:170–173.
111. Smedley F, Taube M, Ruston M. Malignant change in perianal condylomata acuminate. J R Coll Surg Edinb 1988; 33:282.
112. Metcalf AM, Dean T. Risk of dysplasia in anal condyloma. Surgery 1995; 118:724–726.
113. Carter PS, de Ruiter A, Whatrup C, et al. Human immunodeficiency virus infection and genital warts as risk factors for anal intraepithelial neoplasia in homosexual men. Br J Surg 1995; 82:473–474.
114. Bradshaw BR, Nuova GJ, DiCostanzo D, Cohen SR. Human papillomavirus type 16 in a homosexual man. Arch Dermatol 1992; 128:949–952.
115. Beckmann AM, Daling JR, Sherman KJ, et al. Human papillomavirus infection and anal cancer. Int J Cancer 1989; 43:1042–1049.
116. Palmer JG, Scholefield JH, Coates PJ, et al. Anal cancer and human papillomaviruses. Dis Colon Rectum 1989; 32:1016–1022.
117. Kirgan D, Manalo P, Hall M, McGregor B. Association of human papilloma virus and colon neoplasms. Arch Surg 1990; 125:862–865.
118. Longo WE, Ballantyne GH, Gerald WL, Modlin M. Squamous cell carcinoma in situ in condyloma acuminatum. Dis Colon Rectum 1986; 29:503–506.
119. Sawyers JL. Squamous cell cancer of the perianus and anus. Surg Clin North Am 1972; 52:935–941.
120. Butler TW, Gefter J, Kleto D, Shuck EH, Ruffner BW. Squamous cell carcinoma of the anus in condyloma acuminatum. Successful treatment with preoperative chemotherapy and radiation. Dis Colon Rectum 1987; 30: 293–295.
121. Nigro ND. An evaluation of combined therapy for squamous cell carcinoma of the anal canal. Dis Colon Rectum 1984; 27:763–766.

14 Sexually Transmitted Diseases

Lee E. Smith

In the classification of infectious disease, sexually transmitted disease (STD), often called venereal disease, is exceeded only by the common cold and influenza. Patients who are infected with STDs often are reluctant to discuss the problem openly and to seek treatment. As sexual freedom has become commonplace and homosexual intercourse has increased, the occurrence of STDs has increased correspondingly. Intestinal disease and anorectal disease among homosexuals and bisexuals have emerged as major public health problems, and physicians and surgeons who deal with gastrointestinal diseases must be prepared to diagnose and treat these diseases (1–4). A list of conditions of the anorectum in homosexuals led to the descriptive term "the gay bowel" (5,6).

Although many of the STDs are treatable, acquired immunodeficiency syndrome (AIDS) has changed both responses and outcomes for many unfortunate patients, a great number of whom are from the homosexual community. In the past 20 years, AIDS has dramatically affected the civilized world with its increasing annual incidence, and there is no cure in sight.

GASTROINTESTINAL SEXUALLY TRANSMITTED DISEASES

EPIDEMIOLOGY

Homosexuality is associated with a higher rate of STD than that of the general population (6–14). The enteric infections are particularly noteworthy, because many STD-infected homosexuals work as food handlers. In San Francisco in 1977, 10% of homosexuals infected with shigellosis, giardiasis, or amebiasis were food handlers (7). Amebiasis and giardiasis have been shown to affect up to 50,000 people in New York City, and most of these were homosexuals (6). The urban setting predisposes to transmission of STD, with the gay community having a much higher rate of STD than urban heterosexuals (10).

As noted by Baker and Peppercorn (3), the penis may serve as a passive conduit for infectious organisms. During intercourse the relatively fragile anorectal mucosa can be abraded, allowing introduction of a pathogen (11). Anilingus (oral–anal contact), practiced by many homosexuals, may be a means of transmitting enteric infections (12).

Promiscuity is another definite risk factor for STD. Monogamous homosexuals have no higher risk than do monogamous heterosexuals. Among promiscuous individuals, however, the number of sexual partners estimated by some studies highlights the vast exposure to STDs. In 1948 Kinsey noted that the average homosexual has 1000 sexual partners during his life (12). In more recent reports moderately active homosexual activity is estimated to involve 100 partners per year (15,16). Since many of these partners are "pickups" or anonymous, their background of sexual activity and risk is unknown to others (17).

The STDs most frequently found in homosexuals are gonorrhea, syphilis, chlamydia, herpes, and condylomata acuminata (genital warts). Presumably, the anoderm and the anal mucosa are quite susceptible to these infections. Heterosexuals are more likely to acquire diseases localized to the genitals (18–20).

■ DIAGNOSIS

Ordinarily, sexual activity is the primary historical incident in STDs. Thus sexual preference and promiscuity provide clues to many STDs and the human immunodeficiency virus (HIV) infections. Questioning the patient about sexual activities is important, because the symptoms and signs may not be specific. Furthermore, a homosexual may not show any characteristics that would suggest his sexual proclivity. Many patients will deny engaging in homosexual activity, and many others are embarrassed to discuss sexual problems. It is important to note that women may engage in anal intercourse; however, the patient must be asked for confirmation or denial.

The history must be taken with discretion and assurance of confidentiality. The type of sexual activity (i.e., oral, anal, vaginal, penile, or manual) will direct the examiner to seek signs at the appropriate sites. Pelvic inflammatory disease, fetal and neonatal infections, vulvovaginitis, urethritis, epididymitis, genital ulcers, arthritis, and conjunctivitis associated with an STD also should increase suspicion of a related gastrointestinal infection. Gastrointestinal manifestations of STDs may be found from the mouth through to the anus. The finding of one STD should prompt a search for others. Ultimately patients with HIV infection can be expected to acquire opportunistic infections.

The colon and rectal surgeon may see the patient for complaints of enteritis, proctitis, or proctocolitis, which are often identified in homosexual men. Amebiasis, giardiasis, and shigellosis are common causes of enteritis. Fecal–oral contact is responsible for this entity as well as hepatitis A. Proctitis is often caused by specific organisms, especially *Neisseria gonorrhoeae, Chlamydia trachomatis, Treponema pallidum*, and herpes virus (herpes simplex). When proctitis, usually associated with anal pain and discharge, is diagnosed, the physician should be prepared to study the patient for other STDs. As part of anoscopy and sigmoidoscopy, smears should be taken for Gram's stain and culture. Serologic tests for syphilis also should be ordered.

Herpetic proctitis, a severely painful condition, is associated with a rectal burning sensation, tenesmus, constipation, fever, and sometimes urinary retention. Anoscopy may reveal internal rectal ulcers that are sometimes confluent. Gonococcal and chlamydial proctitis [not lymphogranuloma venereum (LGV)–type] show friability and erythema of the anal canal with purulent exudate. Strains of *C. trachomatis* may cause LGV and be associated with severe proctocolitis and bloody diarrhea. On examination the mucosa is ulcerated and friable, mimicking acute ulcerative colitis. On biopsy it may be indistinguishable from granulomatous colitis. Therefore a culture for *C. trachomatis* and serologic testing for LGV should be part of the workup. Syphilis may be manifested as a proctitis of variable severity, discrete ulcers, a mass, or friability. Hence the liberal use of the serologic testing for syphilis is warranted in patients presenting with proctitis. Condylomata acuminata sometimes may be noted in these patients during inspection of the anal skin. Bowen's disease and anal cancer may also be present amid the anal warts. Commonly the patient has palpated these warts and may think that they are hemorrhoids. Through anoscopy other warts may be found clustered around the dentate line. A discrete ulcer on the genitals, the perianal skin, or the anorectum should alert the examiner to consider syphilis, chancroid, herpes, and LGV in the differential diagnosis. A mass in the anorectal area should suggest the possibility of abscess, lymphoma, Kaposi's sarcoma (KS), and anal carcinoma.

A laboratory must be available to carry out a panel of studies (Table 1). Basic studies needed include HIV-screening and confirmatory tests for HIV, syphilis serology (both a non-*Treponema* test and a *Treponema* confirmatory test), culture of *N. gonorrhoeae*, antigen test for *C. trachomatis*, Gram's stain capability, dark-field microscopy for *T. pallidum*, and culture for herpes simplex.

Diagnosis must not end with the specific patient presenting with an STD. It is the duty of the physician to report confirmation of an STD to local health officials so that the spread of disease can be controlled. However, strict confidentiality should be maintained. Furthermore, the patients should be counseled about the fact that his or her sexual partners also need to be examined. Preventive measures, especially the use of condoms, should be recommended strongly for all sexual activity.

TABLE 1 ■ **Diagnostic Tests for Enteric STDs**

Pathogen	Test
Spirochete	
Treponema pallidum	Dark-field microscopy, FTA, VDRL serology
Bacteria	
Neisseria gonorrhoeae	Gram's stain, culture
Chlamydia trachomatis	Monoclonal antibody, culture
Shigella spp.	Stool culture
Campylobacter fetus	Stool culture
Salmonella typhimurium	Stool culture, blood culture
Mycobacterium avium	Mucosal biopsy and culture, acid-fast stain of stool
Virus	
Condyloma acuminata	Clinical identification, biopsy
Herpes simplex	Biopsy, culture, monoclonal antibody
Cytomegalovirus	Biopsy, culture
Human immunodeficiency	ELISA, Western blot
Yeast	
Candida	Culture
Cryptosporidiosis	Biopsy, acid-fast stain of stool
Isospora	Biopsy, acid-fast stain of stool
Protozoa	
Entamoeba histolytica	Stool examination
Giardia lamblia	Stool examination

BACTERIAL INFECTION

Neisseria gonorrhoeae

Gonorrhea is the most common reportable infectious disease in the United States. Annually 500,000 people in the United States are infected with gonorrhea, most of whom are in the 15- to 30-year-old age group. Many patients are asymptomatic. In fact, 30% to 50% of males contract the disease from females who have had pelvic inflammatory disease and can be shown to be positive by smear and culture but manifest no symptoms (21). In 75% of infected women gonorrhea is detected by culture only (22).

In males the urethra is the most common site of infection, manifesting after an incubation period of 3 to 5 days. Dysuria is the chief complaint, and a creamy yellow discharge can be expressed from the urethra. Women do not have this type of discharge from the urethra. However, the cervix may be red and have some discharge. This discharge, which should be cultured on a modified Thayer–Martin plate, yields approximately a 70% sensitivity rate. A positive Gram's stain test on a cervical discharge raises suspicion, but the culture is the confirmatory test. Culture of the rectum may be taken by blind anorectal swab insertion with an excellent chance of a correct positive diagnosis (23). However, Gram's stains obtained via anoscopy have been more effective for diagnosis (24). A new assay, Gen-Probe PACE2, is sensitive and specific for detection of rectal and pharyngeal gonorrhea (25). Complications of gonorrhea include Bartholin's gland abscess, epididymitis, pelvic inflammatory disease, pharyngitis, cutaneous abscess, and disseminated infection with chills, fever, joint pain (arthritis), and macular rash.

Gonococcal proctitis results from anogenital sexual exposure. Presenting symptoms include anal itching and irritation, painful defecation, a sensation of rectal fullness, discharge, and constipation. Women who engage in anal sex also may have these symptoms. Janda et al. (26) studied the problems of *Neisseria* infection in homosexual men and found that over a one-year period 33.1% of 315 men developed a gonorrheal infection; of these, 18.5% were urethral, 16.3% rectal, and 5.6% oropharyngeal. All patients with urethritis had symptoms, but 89.1% of oropharyngeal infections and 61.9% of anorectal infections were asymptomatic. On anal examination most patients will have erythema and edema of the crypts from which thick yellow pus may be expressed (27). Sigmoidoscopy may help to exclude ulcerative colitis and Crohn's colitis. Before the advent of antibiotics, local complications were common. Such complications, including anal stricture, fistula, fissure, abscess, and rectovaginal fistula, are rarely found today.

The recommended treatment regimen for proctitis is ceftriaxone, 250 mg administered intramuscularly once, plus doxycycline, 100 mg administered orally twice a day for seven days (28). For those patients who cannot take ceftriaxone, ciprofloxacin, 500 mg orally once, plus doxycycline, 100 mg orally twice a day for seven days, is a good alternative (29). Doxycycline or azithromycin alone is not adequate, but these drugs are added to counteract possible coexisting chlamydial infection. Cultures should be repeated in three months because the failure rate may be as high as 35%. Unfortunately, in recent years, antibiotic-resistant *N. gonorrhoeae* has become endemic in the United States (30,31); hence, a more up-to-date recommendation is treatment with regimens active against the most resistant gonococci. Resistance has been found to penicillin,

TABLE 2 ■ **Areas and Populations for which Fluoroquinolones (FQs) Are *Not* Recommended for the Treatment of Gonorrhea**

Areas
- Asia
- Pacific Islands (including Hawaii)
- India
- Israel
- Australia
- United Kingdom
- United States: California, Washington State, Arizona (Maricopa County), Michigan (Ingham, Clinton, Eaton, Jackson, Livingston, and Shiawassee counties)
- Areas in Canada experiencing rates of FQ resistance greater than 3–5%: check with local public health officials to learn about FQ resistance in your area
- Any area with rates of FQ-resistant *N. gonorrhoeae* greater than 3–5%

Populations
- Men who have sex with men who are epidemiologically linked to the United States (3)
- People with sexual contacts from the areas listed above

TABLE 3 ■ **Recommended Treatment of Urethral, Endocervical, Rectal, or Pharyngeal Gonorrhea in Patients 9 Years of Age and Older (Except Pregnant or Nursing Mothers)**

If there is no suspected resistance to FQs and patient has no cephalosporin allergy or history of immediate or anaphylactic reactions to penicillin:	
Cefixime	400 mg orally in single dose
Ceftriaxone[a]	125 mg intramuscularly in single dose
Ciprofloxacint	500 mg orally in single dose
Ofloxacint	400 mg orally in single dose
If use of FQs is not recommended:	
Cefixime	400 mg orally in single dose
Ceftriaxone[a]	125 mg intramuscularly in single dose
If use of FQs is not recommended and patient has cephalosporin allergy or history of immediate or anaphylactic reactions to penicillin:	
Azithromycin[b]	2 g orally in single dose
Spectinomycin[c]	2 g intramuscularly in single dose (available only through Special Access Programme)
If use of FQs is not recommended but all other treatments are not tolerated or available, FQs may be used. Treatment with FQs must be followed by a test of cure and is acceptable only for patients likely to present for follow-up testing:	
Ciprofloxacin[d]	500 mg orally in single dose
Ofloxacin[d]	400 mg orally in single dose

[a]The preferred diluent for ceftriaxone is 1% lidocaine without epinephrine (0.9 mL/250 mg, 0.45 mL/125 mg) to reduce discomfort.
[b]A 2-g dose of azithromycin is associated with a significant incidence of gastrointestinal adverse effects. Taking the tablet with food may minimize such adverse effects. Antiemetics may be needed.
[c]If spectinomycin is used, a test of cure is recommended. Spectinomycin should not be used to treat pharyngeal infections.
[d]Ciprofloxacin and ofloxacin are contraindicated in pregnant and nursing women. The safety of FQs in children has not been established. Articular damage has been observed in studies of young animals exposed to FQs, although this has not been shown to date in humans. FQs should not be used in prepubertal children. Clinical judgment should be exercised when considering FQ use in postpubertal adolescents under the age of 18.
Abbreviation: FQs, fluoroquinolones.

tetracycline, cefoxitin, and spectinomycin. Other causes of failure include coexistent chlamydial infection, but currently there is no rapid and inexpensive way to test for chlamydial infection. In the most recent publication on the subject of geographic areas of antibiotic-resistant gonorrhea, recommended treatments are summarized in Tables 2 and 3 (32).

Chlamydia trachomatis

Classic lymphogranulomatosis is endemic in tropical countries (33). Yet most *Chlamydia* infections are being diagnosed wherever STDs can be evaluated completely. It is estimated that there are 4 million chlamydial infections each year in the United States and that the incidence is on the increase, making it the most common STD (34). There are 15 immunotypes of *C. trachomatis* (35,36). Trachoma is associated with immunotypes A, B, B-A, and C. Serovars D, E, and F are the most prevalent *C. trachomatis* strains worldwide (37). Types D and K are found most often in patients with genital and anal infections. The more serious venereal lymphogranulomatosis can be linked to serotypes L1, L2, and L3.

The disease is found most often in the urethra, pharynx, and anorectum of male homosexuals. However, 15% of homosexuals are asymptomatic (36). In women chlamydial infections present as cervicitis, urethral syndrome, endometritis, and salpingitis. High-risk groups include teenagers, African-Americans, women taking oral contraceptives, and members of a low socioeconomic class (38).

Once a *Chlamydia* infection has been identified, other STDs should be suspected. Patients with serotypes D and K commonly present with pain, tenesmus, fever, and an erythematous rectal mucosa, but rarely with ulcerations. Inguinal lymph nodes may be large and matted. Venereal lymphogranulomatosis with serotypes L1, L2, and L3 has essentially the same symptoms and signs, but they are dramatically worse. On endoscopic examination the rectal mucosa appears more inflamed and ulcerated with production of purulent and bloody discharge. Biopsy shows crypt abscesses and granulomas (39). As a result of the granulomas, the diagnosis may be confused with that of Crohn's disease. If the disease is untreated, the severity extends by deeper ulcerations, rectovaginal or rectovesical fistulas, abscesses, and rectal stricture (40). Surgery to correct fistulas and strictures is necessary if these problems do not respond to appropriate antibiotic therapy. Bendahan et al. (41) suggested that chlamydia is related to acute hidradenitis; six of seven patients with suppurative hidradenitis had serologic evidence of *C. trachomatis.*

If *C. trachomatis* syndrome is recognized, treatment should be started empirically. The best method for diagnosis is isolating the organism in a cell culture (42). Culture-independent tests have been developed and are quite accurate. Direct immunofluorescent detection of elementary bodies with monoclonal antibodies or detection of chlamydial antigen by enzyme-linked immunosorbent assay (ELISA) are the two tests most often used of the non-culture tests. The ELISA test has more false positive results and a positive result should be checked by another test if there is an adverse social or psychological consequence (43).

For uncomplicated infection, the best treatment is doxycycline, 100 mg twice a day for seven days, or azithromycin, 1 g in a single oral dose (28,34,44). Erythromycin, ofloxacin, and levofloxacin also have been shown to be effective (28).

Campylobacter

Campylobacter species are recognized as a frequent cause of acute diarrhea. *C. jejuni* and *C. coli* cause fever, watery diarrhea, tenesmus, and abdominal pain. *C. fetus* is more likely to cause intravascular, meningeal, or localized infections such as arthritis, cellulitis, and abscess as well as urinary, placental, and pleural infection. *Campylobacter* infections occur predominantly in men, perhaps related to homosexual activity, but whether the source of infection is by sexual transmission is uncertain (45). The *Campylobacter* organism is found in cattle, sheep, swine, fowl, and rodents, but it may be cultured from 4.1% of humans with diarrhea (46). Others sharing the household are exposed and often found to be positive by culture, suggesting a person-to-person transmission. The diagnosis is based on a history of exposure, examination of stool for leukocytes, and stool culture.

Sigmoidoscopy reveals a proctitis. Biopsy shows crypt abscesses and an inflammatory cell infiltration suggestive of ulcerative colitis. With supportive therapy, most cases of diarrhea resolve spontaneously within one week. Severe cases may be treated with erythromycin, 500 mg four times a day for seven days (47). Other antibiotics that eradicate *Campylobacter* infections include tetracycline, chloramphenicol, clindamycin, and aminoglycosides. For severe systemic infections, 2 to 4 weeks of parenteral antibiotic therapy is warranted.

Shigella

In up to 50% of the homosexual population, shigellosis has been recognized as an STD (48–50). The enteric *Shigella* pathogens may be transferred during anilingus or fellatio. The infective dose of this highly communicable organism is less than 10^3, and the incubation time is only 1 to 2 days.

Shigella infections are limited to the gastrointestinal tract, where the mucosa is invaded (51). Crypt abscesses lead to local mucosal necrosis, in turn leading to ulcers, bleeding, and "pseudomembrane" formation, which may be seen by endoscopy. The clinical picture includes abdominal pain, fever, and watery diarrhea. The diarrhea is likely due to an exotoxin. Straining and tenesmus characterize bowel movements. Culturing with a fresh stool specimen is a key to diagnosis. Polymerase chain reaction techniques are being refined and will become tests of choice (52).

The patient should be rehydrated routinely. Opiates should be avoided, because the diarrhea may be a defense mechanism that may decrease exposure of exotoxin to the bowel mucosa (50). Antibiotics are suppressive and often fail to eradicate the organisms. Reports of resistance of *Shigella* to antibiotics have come from many countries. The resistance was to ampicillin, trimethoprim/sulfamethoxazole, chloramphenicol, cephalothin, and amoxacillin/clavulenic acid (53). The current preferred antibiotics are ciprofloxacin, aminoglycosides, and the second- and third-generation cephalosporins. Cultures should be followed until the pathogens are eradicated. Ultimately a vaccine for *Shigella* is expected to be developed (54).

Haemophilus ducreyi

Chancroid was formerly considered to be a disease of underdeveloped countries; however, because of its recent spread, which may be associated with the increasing HIV epidemic, it has become a more important STD (28). The painful ulcers characteristic of chancroid may be found on the genitals or the anorectum. The soft character of the ulcers makes it difficult to differentiate this disease from herpes. Painful lymphadenopathy is present in 50% of patients; some of the lymph nodes may become fluctuant with abscesses (55). Culture of the organism is sometimes possible. There is promise of improved diagnostic accuracy in the future with more recent developments, using polymerase chain reaction testing, and indirect immunofluorescence using monoclonal antibodies.

The recommended treatment is azithromycin, 1 g orally in a single dose, or ceftriaxone, 250 mg administered intramuscularly as a single dose (27). If the organism is sensitive, symptoms improve in three days and the ulcers resolve markedly in seven days. Follow-up is important and failure to improve necessitates a change in antibiotic. Alternative drugs include ciprofloxacin, 500 mg po bid for three days or erythromycin base, 500 mg po tid for seven days (28). Any sexual partner who had contact with the patient within the 10 days preceding the onset of symptoms should also be treated.

Donovania granulomatis

Granuloma inguinale is the chronic granulomatous infection associated with the gram-negative rod, *Donovania granulomatis*. Exuberant masses that are red and shiny appear on the genitals or around the anorectum. Because of slow onset, infection time may have occurred months before appearance of the masses. In time, scarring may lead to marked stenosis of the anorectum. Biopsy is performed to confirm the diagnosis. Confusion in diagnosis is among carcinoma, secondary syphilis, and amebiasis. The Centers for Disease Control and Prevention (CDC) recommends two first-line therapies, trimethoprim-sulfamethoxazole (one double strength tablet bid) or doxycycline (100 mg bid) for three weeks. Alternative drugs include ciprofloxacin 750 mg bid, erythromycin base 500 mg bid, and azithromycin 1 g per week (28). All antibiotics should be continued for three weeks, but continued longer if all ulcers have not completely healed.

■ SPIROCHETE INFECTION

Syphilis

Over 12.2 million cases of syphilis exist worldwide (56). The syphilis rate among African-Americans has doubled since 1986 as compared with that of whites. *T. pallidum*, a spirochete, is the causative agent (57). In 1990 the recorded rate of infection was 20 cases per 100,000 persons, the highest rate reported since 1949 (58).

The infection is transmitted by sexual contact with introduction of the spirochetes through the intact mucous membrane or a break in the skin. The mouth, genitals, and anus are common sites of infections and harbor the primary lesion, the chancre. In 10% to 20% of cases the primary lesion may be hidden within an orifice. After infection the chancre appears within 2 to 10 weeks. The chancre may be either painful or painless. In the differential diagnosis there may be confusion with fissure. However, a lesion situated off the midline, too far out on the anal skin, or too high on the dentate line in addition to irregular configuration is not consistent with the diagnosis of fissure. Compared with HIV-uninfected patients, HIV-infected patients with primary syphilis present more frequently with multiple ulcers (59). Lymphadenopathy is significantly notable. The primary ulcer proceeds to heal spontaneously. However, in 2 to 10 more weeks secondary lesions appear as a red maculopapular rash anywhere on the body. Flat, pale lesions, condylomata lata, may be found around the genitals or the anus. Both primary and secondary lesions are infectious. The exudate of lesions in the early stages (i.e., within one year) may be tested by dark-field examination. The multiple motile spirochetes can be seen through oil emersion technique.

With antibiotic therapy the spirochetes disappear from lesions in only a few hours and thus may interfere with early diagnosis. In one third of patients the condition will proceed to spontaneous cure, and in another one third it will remain latent. Unfortunately the remaining one third of cases will go on to late or tertiary syphilis. Latent or late syphilis, occurring over one year after infection, is detected only by serologic testing because the recognizable primary and secondary lesions are absent. Late disease may lead to cardiovascular, central nervous system, nephritic, and hepatic syphilis. Pregnant women with latent syphilis can pass the disease on to the fetus. Homosexuals develop proctitis and rectal masses, and these lesions are frequently misdiagnosed as lymphomas or neoplasms (60,61). HIV-infected patients more often present with secondary syphilis and persistent chancres. This is true of both homosexuals and heterosexuals who are HIV positive (62).

Presumptive diagnosis of syphilis is made by two serologic tests. The antibody tests remain positive for life, and titers do not correlate with disease activity. Thus they are reported as positive or negative. The most often used specific antibody tests are the fluorescent treponemal antibody absorption test (FTA-ABS) and the microhemagglutination assay for antibody to *T. pallidum* (MHATP). These tests become positive earlier than other blood tests; hence, they should be used in cases suspected to be early. Nontreponemal tests most commonly employed for screening are the Venereal Disease Research Laboratory (VDRL) test and the rapid plasma reagin (RPR). Since both tests vary according to disease activity, titers reflect worsening or response to treatment. Sequential testing to determine disease activity is based on changes of titers of these two tests. Patients who are HIV positive are less likely to experience serologic improvement after recommended therapy than those who are HIV negative (63). More recently a polymerase chain reaction method has been developed which is 95.8% sensitive and 95.7% specific (64).

T. pallidum is still sensitive to penicillin. Benzathine penicillin G, 2.4 million U given intramuscularly, will maintain treponemicidal levels for two weeks. (It is common practice now to give a second injection of 2.4 million units a week later.) For latent syphilis 2.4 million U weekly for two weeks is given (28). The Jarisch-Herxheimer reaction occurs in half the treated patients as the spirochetes are destroyed. The reaction may begin in six hours and be over within 24 hours. The usual manifestations are fever, skin lesions, arthralgia, and adenopathy; these conditions may be treated with analgesics. Patients who are allergic to penicillin may be treated with tetracydine or erythromycin, 500 mg four times a day, or doxycycline 100 mg twice daily for two weeks.

VIRAL INFECTION

Herpes

The herpes simplex virus (HSV) may include several clinical syndromes. HSV type I causes dermatitis, eczema, keratoconjunctivitis, encephalitis, and labialis. HSV type II causes genital and anal infections and neonatal infections. Recently more HSV-1 infections have been identified on genitals, correlating with more orogenital sex (65,66). Manifestations at primary infection include fever, malaise, and lymphadenopathy. Primary infections are usually worse than subsequent recurrent infections.

In homosexuals who present with severe proctitis, 6% to 30% will have a positive culture for HSV (67). In addition, fever is present in 48%, difficulty in urination in 48%, sacral paresthesias in 26%, inguinal adenopathy in 57%, anorectal pain in 100%, tenesmus in 100%, constipation in 78%, and skin ulcerations in 70% (68). A lumbosacral radiculopathy after the acute infection may leave residual deficits such as impotence, bladder dysfunction, and pain in the buttocks and legs.

Recurrences are far different from the primary infection and appear to be due to reactivation of latent HSV. External inspection and sigmoidoscopic examination of the distal 10 cm reveal vesicles and pustules that break and coalesce to become ulcers. The definitive diagnostic laboratory test is viral isolation and tissue culture. A direct fluorescent monoclonal antibody technique will confirm the diagnosis (69,70). In one series serologic testing showed 95% of homosexuals to have been infected with HSV type II (71).

Acyclovir was the first oral antiherpes agent. It is effective, but it is poorly bioavailable. Oral acyclovir, 200 mg five times a day for five days, shortens the duration of virus shedding and thus aids in clearing of the lesions (72,73). Herpes proctitis, likewise, responds to a larger dose of acyclovir, 400 mg, given orally five times a day. Topical acyclovir may be added, but it is less effective than either oral or intravenous administration. Some herpes viruses have become resistant to acyclovir. Recent reports suggest that foscarnet works as an alternative therapy (74). Valacyclovir, using 1 g twice a day for 10 days, was developed to overcome the poor bioavailability of acyclovir (28). Famciclovir is also more bioavailable and may be dosed at 250 mg three times a day for 7 to 10 days (75).

Frequently, recurrent herpes may be suppressed by long-term treatment with acyclovir, 400 mg twice a day (76). Recently, famciclovir 250 mg bid and valacyclovir 500 mg bid have been shown to be effective alternatives (75). However, untreated herpes proctitis is self-limited, resolving completely in approximately three weeks.

Hepatitis

In the United States, 181,000 persons were infected with hepatitis B virus (HBV) in 1998 (28). Hepatitis C (HCV) is the most common blood-borne infection in the United States; 2.7 million persons are infected (28). Hepatitis was not formerly considered to be an STD. Infections by HBV rose from 200,000 in 1978 to 300,000 in 1987 (77). The rise is primarily the result of sexual exposure by chronic carriers. Some decrease can be seen when promiscuous behavior is stopped in the homosexual community. The other large high-risk group is intravenous drug abusers. An excellent vaccination to prevent hepatitis A and B is available. Unfortunately, the vaccination program has reached only health care workers; as a group, homosexuals and drug users have not been treated completely.

The presentation of hepatitis is jaundice associated with nausea, vomiting, anorexia, and fever. Extrahepatic manifestations include a transient serum sickness-like prodrome, polyarteritis nodosa, and glomerulonephritis.

When homosexuals are tested for HBV infection by hepatitis B surface antigen (HB_sAg), a significant number has positive results. Ellis et al. (78) found 5% of 2612 homosexual patients to be HB_sAg positive. Acute hepatitis rarely goes 10 weeks without improvement. Relapses occur in 5% to 20%, as shown by abnormal liver function studies. Up to 10% will become chronic carriers, and 25% of these carriers progress to develop cirrhosis and hepatocellular carcinoma (79).

PARASITIC INFECTION

Entamoeba histolytica

Reports of amebiasis in homosexual patients are numerous (9,17,80–83). Screening stools of homosexual patients has confirmed the presence of amebic cysts in 20% to 30%, thus identifying another STD (80). Fecal-oral transmission by anilingus is the likely cause.

When cysts are swallowed, the trophozoite emerges in the stomach and divides to produce eight smaller trophozoites. These pass to the cecum, where more are produced. The intestinal mucosa is invaded, resulting in clinical disease in 10% of cases. The amebas penetrate through tiny ulcers in the mucosa and dissect laterally above the muscularis mucosa, creating "collar button" ulcers. Eventually there may be healing, or extension deeper into the wall may occur, sometimes leading to perforation. Chronic infection with a resultant inflammatory mass, the ameboma, may form on the intestinal wall. The rectum and the sigmoid often are involved. Mild disease may present with symptoms of diarrhea, urgency, and cramps. The more serious illness has symptoms of severe abdominal pain and dehydrating diarrhea, which may begin as early as the fourth day after exposure. Microemboli of trophozoites may be carried via the portal vein to the liver, where an abscess may begin.

The diagnosis can be made fastest by examination of a fresh stool sample for trophozoites and cysts. Serologic tests are available, but a highly specific antigen is not always present. The indirect hemagglutination test (IHA) is employed when stools are not positive and extraintestinal amebiasis is suspected.

Metronidazole, 750 mg three times a day for 10 days, is the drug of choice followed by a course of diloxanide furoate, 500 mg three times a day for 10 days, or iodoquinol, 650 mg three times a day for 20 days. For severe

TABLE 4 ■ Suggested Treatment for STDs

Organism	Treatment
Neisseria gonorrhoeae	Ceftriaxone, 250 mg, IM once plus doxycycline, 100 mg, PO bid for 7 days
Chlamydia trachomatis	Doxycycline, 100 mg, bid for 21 days, or azithromycin, 1 mg, PO as a single dose
Campylobacter sp.	Erythromycin, 500 mg, qid for 7 days, or ciprofloxadin, 500 mg, q 12 hours for 7 days
Shigella sp.	Trimethoprim-sulfamethoxazole double strength PO bid for 5 days
Haemophilus ducreyi	Azithromycin, 1 g, PO as a single dose, or ceftriaxone, 250 mg, IM one time
Donovania sp.	Trimethoprim-sulfamethoxazole, one double strength tablet bid for 3 weeks
Treponema pallidum	Benzathine penicillin G, 2.4 million U, IM, weekly for 2 weeks, or doxycycline, 100 mg bid for 2 weeks
Herpes virus	Acyclovir, 200 mg, 5 times a day for 7–10 days
Hepatitis virus	Symptomatic
Entamoeba histolytica	Metronidazole, 750 mg, tid for 10 days, plus diloxanide furoate, 500 mg, tid for 10 days
Giardia lamblia	Metronidazole, 250 mg, PO tid for 7 days

disease, emetine, oxytetracycline, and diloxanide furoate followed by chloroquine may be used if the metronidazole fails or is not tolerated.

Giardia lamblia

Giardiasis may be contracted by ingesting fecally contaminated food or water. Homosexuals who practice oral–anal contact often are infected (9,17). Phillips et al. (17) found *Giardia lamblia* or *Entamoeba histolytica* in 21% of homosexuals examined for parasites. Symptoms of malaise, weakness, weight loss, cramps, and flatulence result. The distinctive cysts may be identified in fresh stool samples. The parasites attach to the mucosa of the duodenum and the jejunum. Therefore, sometimes aspiration of the duodenum may be necessary to find the organisms. Metronidazole (250 mg tid for 5 to 7 days) is the best form of treatment (84) but it is not approved by the FDA for use in giardiasis. The approved drug is furazolidone, 100 mg qid for 7 to 10 days Table 4 summarizes the treatments for STDs.

ACQUIRED IMMUNODEFICIENCY SYNDROME

SHORT HISTORY OF AIDS

In 1981, 26 cases of Kaposi's sarcoma (KS) and five cases of *Pneumocystis carinii* pneumonia were reported in young homosexual men in the United States (85). The cause for these diseases was not known or linked to a common etiology. In 1982, the clinical syndrome was characterized, and it was named acquired immunodeficiency syndrome (AIDS). In the same year cases of AIDS were diagnosed in recipients of blood and blood products (86). By 1983, heterosexual transmission had been reported, and the human immunodeficiency virus type 1 (HIV-l) was identified as the cause of AIDS (87).

The antiretroviral activity of zidovudine was recognized by in vitro studies in 1984 (88). This became the basis for azidothymidine (AZT) treatment of AIDS. By 1985 the CDC found a need to broaden the definition of AIDS because a wider range of neoplasms and secondary infections of all types was being linked to this disease. In 1986, the implications of an epidemic out of control prompted the World Health Assembly to recommend a global strategy for AIDS control. HIV encephalopathy and HIV wasting syndrome were added as amendments to the CDC definition of AIDS in 1987. In 1993 the definition was further expanded with the addition of pulmonary tuberculosis, recurrent pneumonia, invasive cervical cancer, and a CD4 count of < 200 (Table 5). This is still the current definition of AIDS. With the new definition using a low CD4 count, survival times have been lengthened. AIDS was the eighth leading cause of death in the United States in 1993 (90). Among men aged 25 to 44 years in 1994, HIV infection was the leading cause of death and for women in this age group the third leading cause of death (91). The concept of prophylaxis for opportunistic pathogens, especially *P. carinii*, delayed onset of terminal infection and has prolonged survival. Monitoring of disease progression was dependent on an indirect marker, the CD4 count. A valuable diagnostic tool, the HIV RNA assay, introduced a means to directly quantitate the viral load (92).

The use of highly active antiretroviral therapy (HAART) became widespread during 1996. Thus, AIDS incidence declined from mid-1990s through 2001. During 1998–2002, the estimated number of deaths declined 14%. However, AIDS prevalence continued to increase, such that an estimated 384,906 persons were known to be living with AIDS. From 1998 through 2002 the number of AIDS diagnoses increased 7% among women and decreased 5% among men; men represent 73% of HIV/AIDS cases (93). Unfortunately, in spite of the large amounts of money, time, and effort towards research in 1999 the World Health Organization lists HIV as the leading infectious cause of

TABLE 5 ■ Diagnosis of AIDS

Cryptosporidiosis
Cytomegalovirus
Isosporiasis
Kaposi's sarcoma
Lymphoma
Lymphoid pneumonia or hyperplasia
Pneumocystis carinii pneumonia
Progressive multifocal leukoencephalopathy
Toxoplasmosis
Candidiasis
Coccidioidomycosis
Cryptococcus
Herpes simplex
Histoplasmosis
Tuberculosis
Other mycobacteriosis
Salmonellosis
HIV encephalopathy
HIV wasting syndrome
Pulmonary tuberculosis
Recurrent pneumonia
Invasive cervical cancer
CD4 T-lymphocyte count < 200

Note: Diagnosis of AIDS is based on HIV infection plus one of the above diseases or conditions.
Source: From Ref. 89.

death in the world of major concern is the emergence of viruses that are resistent to nonnucleoside reverse transcriptase inhibitors (94).

■ PATHOGENESIS

The human immunodeficiency virus is a lentivirus of the human retroviruses (95). The clinical characteristics of the HIV infection that resemble those of a lentivirus are long incubation time, involvement of the central nervous system and hematopoietic system, and association with immune suppression. The HIV infection affects T-helper lymphocytes and macrophages in such a way that there is an absolute reduction in numbers (95,96). Brain cells and bowel epithelium have been shown to contain HIV. In the gut the crypt cells and the enterochromaffin cells are most involved. The enterochromaffin cells influence fluid exchange in the bowel, and the often seen diarrhea may be accounted for by this disturbance (97).

Examination of body fluids has yielded various levels of HIV particles. The virus is easily found in plasma, serum, and cerebrospinal fluid. Low quantities are found in tears, urine, saliva, vaginal secretions, ear secretions, and breast milk. In addition, cells infected with HIV have been identified in saliva, vaginal fluid, semen, and bronchial fluid. Open wounds or venereal ulcers offer an avenue for transmission by exposure to one of these body fluids. The HIV attaches to the cell membrane through a specific antigen complex. After the virus has entered the cell, DNA is produced and integrates the host chromosome, then hiding and remaining latent as a provirius. In the latent state the virus is able to elude the host immune system for years. The host defense against HIV responds by both humoral and cellular immune action. The B-lymphocyte is the primary activator of the humoral response that acts on macrophages and T-helper lymphocytes to create antibodies. T-lymphocytes, macrophages, and killer cells are the primary defenders in the cellular immune response system that perform by suppressing viral replications or by killing infected cells. This cellular response appears to be the most important portion of the host response.

The CD4 counts have been used to indirectly define the state of the immune deficiency. Progressively lower CD4 counts lead to clinicopathologic changes and worsening of the health status. Using CD4 counts, four worsening stages can be delineated:

Stage 1: Primary infection. The virus rapidly proliferates in the blood and lymph nodes. The patient has a seroconversion illness that resolves.

Stage 2: Early immune deficiency (CD4 count > 500/μL). The immune mechanism controls the virus and restricts it to the lymphoid tissue. The patient is asymptomatic.

Stage 3: Intermediate immune deficiency (CD4 count 500 to 200/μL). The immune mechanism is failing. Signs of immunocompromise begin to appear. The risk of opportunistic infection and malignancy is increased.

Stage 4: Advanced immune deficiency (CD4 count < 200/μL). The immune system is overcome by the virus. Major opportunistic infections and malignancies require increasing medical intervention. Death ensues.

Transmission of HIV occurs through sexual contact, exposure to blood or blood products, and mother-to-child perinatal exposure. In the past, 75% of sexual transmissions have been between homosexuals (98). The receptive partner in rectal intercourse is at greatest risk, and practices causing rectal trauma, such as "fisting," increase the risk. During 1994, AIDS cases in 34,974 homosexual men were newly reported to CDC (99). Unsafe sexual behavior and HIV transmissions have increased among homosexual men after a period of decline (100). A substantial proportion of men who have sex with men but do not disclose their sexual orientation, are at high risk for transmitting infections to both male and female sex partners (101). The number of cases of HIV in the heterosexual community is increasing, and this change is presumed to be due to transmission by vaginal intercourse. In fact, in 1994 the incidence of AIDS in women was found to be increasing more rapidly than in men (102). Hemophiliacs and others requiring blood transfusion account for another high-risk group. Drug users, especially those who share needles, account for high rates of infection. Between 1978 and 1993, 14,920 AIDS cases in the United States resulted from transmission from mother to infant (103). Health care workers, on a far lesser scale, may incur accidental needle-stick injuries or wounds during the course of their usual medical activities. Casual contact has no known association with the transmission.

The median time from HIV seroconversion to AIDS was 8.3 years, that from HIV seroconversion to death was 8.9 years, and from AIDS to death was 17 months (104). These data are based on 403 homosexual/bisexual men who seroconverted between 1982 and 1984. In recent years, survival of AIDS-free HIV-1-infected individuals with CD4 cell counts of less than 350 has improved since antiretroviral and HIV prophylactic treatments have become available, but the long-term prognosis remains poor (105).

A large percentage of individuals with HIV infection experienced multiple AIDS-defining opportunistic diseases before death. There is an enhanced transmission of HIV that appears to be caused by other sexually transmitted diseases (106). *P. carinii* pneumonia (45%), mycobacterium avium complex (25%), wasting syndrome (25%), bacterial pneumonia (24%), cytomegalovirus (CMV) (23%), and esophageal and pulmonary candidiasis (22%) account for a substantial proportion of morbidity associated with HIV infection (107).

■ CLINICAL PRESENTATION

The primary illness is characterized by a mono nucleosis-like syndrome associated with seroconversions for HIV antibodies (108). Symptoms include fever, sweats, malaise, myalgia, arthralgia, headache, photophobia, diarrhea, sore throat, lymphadenopathy, and truncal maculopapular rash. The duration of symptoms varies from 3 to 14 days. The central nervous system infection may be manifested by neurologic findings of meningoencephalitis, myelopathy, peripheral neuropathy, and Guillain-Barre syndrome. The incubation period from exposure to onset ranges from five days to three months, with the average between two and four weeks (109). Another terrible fact is that there are a large number of asymptomatic patients who may be found only by detection of an antibody. Unfortunately, general screening is not available or accepted at this time.

The clinical history is a key to developing a case for the diagnosis, especially if the HIV test is not available or is denied. Specifically, questioning must be directed toward aspects that are associated with high risk. Travel to areas in which AIDS is endemic, male-to-male sexual activity, sexual activity when traveling, receipt of blood products, intravenous drug abuse, and a positive venereal disease history raise the index of suspicion.

■ SEROCONVERSIONS

Within two weeks of onset of the acute illness, seroconversion occurs, antibodies against the major proteins of HIV are produced. The antibody then may be detected by an immunofluorescent assay (IFA) for IGM antibody. ELISA detects antibodies in 1 to 2 months. Unfortunately, there are a large number of false positive results. The Western blot test is the most specific test available for practical use.

■ GASTROINTESTINAL MANIFESTATIONS

Symptoms referable to the gastrointestinal tract are frequently encountered, and some can be treated specifically, at least for palliation. Weight loss, anorexia, and diarrhea are nonspecific symptoms, but other symptoms direct attention to a specific segment of the gastrointestinal tract.

The esophagus may be infected initially, and this infection may be manifested by dysphagia, odynophagia, and retrosternal pain (110). Esophagoscopy may reveal discrete ulceration or yellow-white plaques. The symptoms resolve spontaneously within five months as the acute infection resolves. The organism most frequently encountered is *Candida albicans*, which usually can be found in the mouth and esophagus in the form of plaques. *Candida* responds to ketoconazole, 400 mg a day, or fluconazole, 200 mg a day initially followed by 100 mg a day. CMV and herpes are usually responsible for any ulcerations. CMV responds poorly to ganciclovir, but herpes sometimes is limited by acyclovir.

Gastric involvement likewise may be suspected when nausea, vomiting, hematemesis, and early satiety are encountered. However, these symptoms may be related to non-AIDS problems; the workup should be developed to diagnose treatable conditions. Hepatobiliary disease is manifested by abnormal chemical tests, right upper quadrant abdominal pain, and hepatomegaly. Evaluation by ultrasonography and computed tomography should be performed promptly to rule out treatable non-AIDS related disease. The HIV, CMV, *Mycobacterium avium intracellulare* (MAI), or cryptosporidiosis organisms are most often responsible for the liver pathology (111–115). Obstructed ducts may be investigated by endoscopic retrograde cholangiopancreatography (ERCP). Obstructive symptoms due to papillary stenosis may be remedied by sphincterotomy during ERCP.

Small bowel AIDS may be mistaken for a common colonic disease caused by *Salmonella*, *Shigella*, and *Campylobacter* organisms. Symptoms of periumbilical cramping, weight loss, and diarrhea may be associated with AIDS (111). In fact, diarrhea is a significant morbidity in 50% of patients in North America. CMV and MAI have been found in these patients. Parasitic infestations also must be suspected and appropriate stool examination performed.

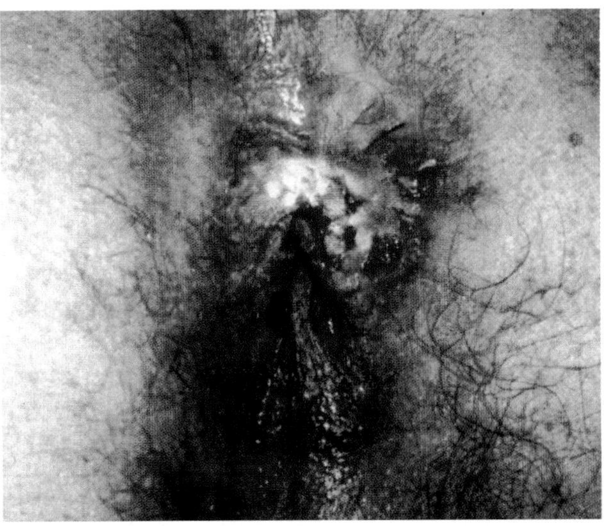

FIGURE 1 ■ Anal disease with AIDS. Note condylomata, scars, and ulcerations. *Source*: Courtesy of Bruce Orkin, M.D., Washington, D.C., U.S.A.

G. lamblia, *E. histolytica*, *Cryptosporidium*, and *Isospora belli* may be isolated (116,117).

Patients with AIDS of the colorectum may present with manifestations of frequent diarrheal stools, lower abdominal cramping, tenesmus, proctalgia, and occasionally blood. Stool for culture and for parasites should be an initial step. CMV and herpes may be responsible for mucosal ulcerations, which can be appreciated by endoscopy of the colorectum (118). *Cryptosporidium* may be diagnosed by obtaining a mucosal biopsy (117).

Individuals who are seropositive for HIV frequently have disorders affecting the anorectum. Orkin and Smith (119) reviewed 40 patients with HIV disease who presented with anorectal pathology. Condylomata were seen in 52% and fistulas or abscesses in 37% (Figs. 1 and 2). Combinations of disease were identified, including symptomatic hemorrhoids, fissures, perianal herpes, and three neoplasms. The same investigators reported on the microbiology of HIV disease found in 47 of 163 seropositive patients. A standard set of cultures was used to study 47 patients

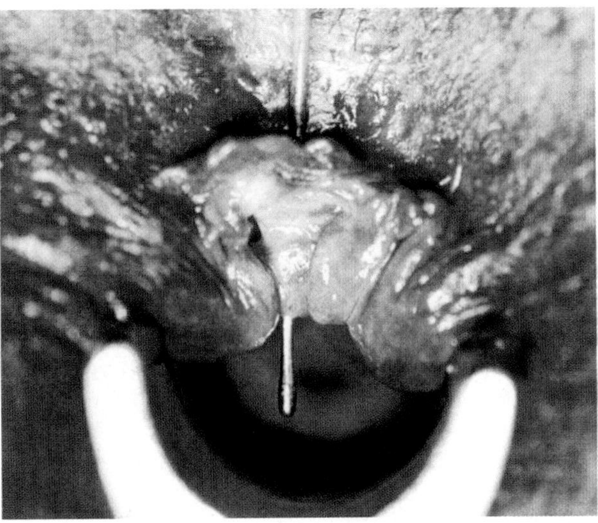

FIGURE 2 ■ Anal disease in AIDS. Note a deep posterior ulcer, herpes, a skin tag, and a fistula. *Source*: Courtesy of Bruce Orkin, M.D., Washington, D.C., U.S.A.

believed to have an infectious process. Thirty-two of the 47 had positive cultures, including herpes, 50%; CMV, 25%; *N. gonorrhoeae*, 16%; *Chlamydia*, 16%; acid-fast bacilli, 2%; and others, 9%. Patients were treated medically only in 50%, surgically only in 25%, and by both medicine and surgery in 25%. Specific pathogens may be identified if they are aggressively sought and thus therapy can be directed (120).

■ OPPORTUNISTIC INFECTION

Protozoans

Pneumocystis carinii. During the first seven years of the AIDS epidemic, *P. carinii* pneumonia accounted for more than 60% of AIDS-defining illnesses and occurred in 80% of persons with AIDS (121–123). Chan et al. (107) report that the most common opportunistic AIDS-defining event before death was *P. carinii* pneumonia in 45% of their patients between 1990 and 1994. The most common presenting symptoms are fever, cough, and shortness of breath. Physical examination is not very helpful. The chest film may be normal, but often interstitial infiltration, consolidation, and pneumatoceles may be seen. Pulmonary function studies and arterial blood gases point out the severity of lung involvement. Gallium lung scans have been very sensitive in defining the site of disease through increased uptake. The cough is usually not productive of sputum, so ultrasonic nebulization may be used to incite sputum for examination or bronchoscopy may be performed to obtain lavage samples. After the specimen has been concentrated, Giemsa or another trophozoite stain will reveal the parasites (124). Biopsy of the lung is seldom indicated. Oral trimethoprim-sulfamethoxazole, dapsone, or aerosolized pentamidine isothionate are effective in 60% to 80% of cases (125,126). The use of these drugs as prophylaxis has markedly reduced the incidence of *P. carinii* pneumonia and has delayed the onset of the first AIDS illness for 6 to 12 months (122).

Toxoplasmosis. *Toxoplasma gondii* is the protozoan responsible for most latent central nervous system infections in AIDS patients (127,128). For those who harbor the latent protozoans, subsequent reactivation often results in encephalitis, which is fatal if not recognized and treated early. Fever, headache, altered mental status, lethargy, focal neurologic defects (often hemiparesis), seizures, and coma are symptoms of this grave disorder (127–129). Laboratory findings are nonspecific. Because of the danger of delay in diagnosis, empiric treatment may be begun on suspicion of the diagnosis. The serologic test to detect IgG toxoplasma antibodies is virtually always positive in these patients (130). However, whether latent or active infection is present, the type cannot be determined by this test. The only definitive diagnosis is achieved by demonstration of the organism in tissue. Treatment with trimethoprim-sulfamethoxazole is the primary therapy for the acute disease (131). Unfortunately, high toxicity rates lead to early discontinuation of therapy in up to 40% of patients (131). If tolerated, these agents in lower doses may be continued as suppressive therapy (132).

Cryptosporidiosis and isosporiasis. AIDS has allowed *Cryptosporidium*, *Isospora belli*, and cyclospora to flourish in the immunocompromised patient and thus become known as a pathogen for man (116,117,133–135). Diarrhea is the symptom that may be profound enough to result in fluid and electrolyte imbalance, finally ending in malnutrition and weight loss. The bacterial and parasitic causes of diarrhea must be suspected and ruled out as well. Cramps, weight loss, anorexia, malaise, vomiting, and myalgia are frequent complaints. Cryptosporidia may be found in the stool specimen when an acid-fast staining technique is applied (136). A new immunofluorescent assay using a monoclonal antibody seems to be more sensitive and specific for detecting the oocytes. More recently, a polymerase chain reaction study may be even more sensitive (137). Unfortunately, there is no specific treatment for cryptosporidiosis. The most common medications used are paromomycin (aminosidine) and azithromycin. On the other hand, isosporiasis responds well to oral trimethoprim-sulfamethoxazole (138).

Fungi

Even common superficial mycotic infections, such as tinea pedis, tinea corpora, and onchomycosis are common in patients with HIV. They respond to the usual antifungal agents (139).

Histoplasmosis and coccidioidomycosis. AIDS patients who are exposed to histoplasmosis or coccidioidomycosis may be infected easily. Probably more likely is the existence of a latent infection from prior exposure, which is unleashed when the immune mechanism fails (CD4 count of $< 200/\mu L$). Thus, the history may reflect recent or remote travel to endemic areas, where these infections may have been acquired (140,141). Patients present with fever, weight loss, and pulmonary symptoms. Disseminated disease may be manifested in any organ system. The diagnosis is made by bone marrow culture and biopsy. Specimens stained with Wright-Giemsa or methenamine silver stain reveal the organism within histiocytes (136). Chest films are nonspecific and resemble those for other pneumonias.

The treatment of these fungi is with amphotericin, 1.0 mg/kg/day until the symptoms abate, usually within 6 to 8 weeks (142,143). Relapses are the rule. Therefore maintenance therapy is instituted for the remainder of the patient's life with itraconazole, 200 mg twice daily (144).

Cryptococcus. Cryptococcus is a frequently encountered opportunistic infection in AIDS patients (145). Dissemination can be expected most often within the central nervous system and second most often in the lungs. However, any organ may be attacked (146). Neurologic and pulmonary symptoms dominate the clinical presentation (147). A latex agglutination (LA) test for cryptococcal antigen is very sensitive, and with the advent of symptoms referable to cryptococcus, the LA test should be done. This test may be applied to any body fluid. Cultures of the body fluids are used to isolate the organism.

Treatment with parenteral amphotericin B, 1.0 mg/kg/day, is mandatory. Maintenance therapy with amphotericin B is warranted to minimize relapse. Unfortunately, overall mortality exceeds 50%, even with treatment (147). An alternative therapeutic agent is fluconazole, 400 mg a day for induction, followed by fluconazole, 200 mg a day, as a maintenance dose.

Bacteria

Although AIDS patients are at higher risk for opportunistic infection by fungi, protozoa, and viruses, bacterial infections also encroach on a compromised immune system. Enteric pathogens, especially *Salmonella*, *Shigella*, and *Campylobacter* species, have been reported in significantly increased numbers (148,149). Schattner et al. (150) proposed that *C. trachomatis* infection might precede HIV infection. They found *C. trachomatis* in three of 10 seroconverters, compared with 5% of matched male homosexuals who remained HIV negative. Bacterial pneumonia may be superimposed on the pulmonary infection caused by other opportunistic organisms, and this condition may not respond to the usual antibiotic therapy. Special mention must be made of *Mycobacterium* infections.

Mycobacteria. The incidence of *Mycobacterium* tuberculosis infections has been increasing in correlation with the increasing AIDS numbers (151). Most cases represent reactivation of latent infection acquired in past years (152). Only up to half of the cases are pulmonary (152,153). Furthermore, the usual apical infiltrates are seen less often than hilar adenopathy or infiltrates of the middle or lower lung fields (154). Any site may be affected, but bone marrow and lymph nodes are noted most frequently. Anal tuberculosis is rare, but must be considered when a perianal ulcer fails to heal (155). Tuberculin skin tests are often negative due to anergy. Culture of appropriate fluids or tissues represents the best possibility of confirming the diagnosis. Therapy for tuberculosis should be begun whenever acid-fast bacteria are identified, and it should be continued until culture results are final (156). The recommended drugs are isoniazid, rifampin, and ethambutol or pyrazinamide. Tuberculous enteritis and peritonitis may result. Surgery is reserved for complications such as obstruction or perforation (157).

Mycobacterium arium intracellulase (MAI) is an unusual infection that occurs rarely outside the AIDS population, and is the most frequent bacterial infection in patients with advanced AIDS (158). In patients with disseminated disease, blood cultures are virtually always positive (148). The clinical syndromes include nonspecific symptoms of fever, malaise, weight loss, or gastrointestinal symptoms of diarrhea, abdominal pain, malabsorption, and extrabiliary jaundice (149). MAI is resistant to antituberculous drugs. For prophylaxis, rifabutin, 300 mg a day, has been well tolerated. For disseminated disease, at least two agents should be used. Every regimen should include either azithromycin or clarithromycin and one of the following agents: clofazimine, rifabutin, rifampin, ciprofloxacin, and amikacin (159). However, curative doses require markedly increased plasma levels that are dangerous (160,161). Surgery is reserved for life-threatening complications such as obstruction, hemorrhage, and perforation (162).

Virus

Condyloma acuminatum is a viral infection frequently noted in homosexuals and HIV-positive patients. (Condyloma acuminatum and resultant anal cancer are discussed in chapters 13 and 18.) This section will specifically review herpes and cytomegalovirus.

Herpes. Ninety-five percent of homosexuals who have AIDS have been infected with an HSV previously (73). Although primary infections are not common, the reactivation of latent infections is common. The severity of the infection is dependent on the degree of immunosuppression.

The incubation period after exposure is 2 to 12 days by herpes virus, type 1 or type 2. A painful vesicular eruption occurs in the affected site, usually the orolabial region, the genitals, the anorectum, or the esophagus (49,68,71,163,164). Encephalitis is rare, but it is the most life-threatening sequela (165). As a cause of proctitis in homosexuals, HSV is second only to gonococcal infections. It is usually due to HSV type 2, which may be diagnosed by HSV culture of the ulcer. HSV-2 reactivation drives the rate of HIV-1 replication higher, suggesting a significant biologic interaction between the two viruses (66).

Acyclovir, famciclovir, and valacyclovir are the preferred drugs for HSV infections in AIDS patients (66). Acyclovir can be given orally, intravenously, or topically. Treatment is continued until all mucocutaneous lesions have crusted over or re epithelialized. Recurrence is frequent and suppressive acyclovir therapy may be necessary (166).

Cytomegalovirus. CMV infects 90% of AIDS patients during their illness (167). However, this rate may reflect the high incidence of CMV identified in homosexuals, a very high-risk group (167). The infection may take the form of chorioretinitis, pneumonia, esophagitis, colitis, encephalitis, adrenalitis, or hepatitis (168). Perianal ulcers may be caused by CMV. CMV colitis is found in up to 10% of AIDS patients (113). Symptoms of diarrhea, hematochezia, fever, and weight loss are predominant (118,169). Diffuse submucosal hemorrhage and mucosal ulcerations as dictated by endoscopy typify the proctocolitis. For the differential diagnosis, consideration must be given to *Clostridium difficile*, ulcerative colitis, and granulomatous colitis, especially if the AIDS diagnosis is uncertain. Biopsy shows CMV inclusions and inflammatory reactions. However, in recent years major progress has been made in developing quantitative detection methods, using polymerase chain reactions (170,171).

The best drugs for use against CMV are ganciclovir or cidofovir. Although similar in formula to acyclovir, ganciclovir is more effective against CMV. Unfortunately resistance has developed to ganciclovir and cross resistance to cidofovir. Thus foscarnet may be used in resistant cases (172). On the horizon is a vaccine against CMV (173).

Pathology due to CMV is the most common indication for emergency laparotomy in AIDS patients. In 1986, Nugent and O'Connell (174) reported on five major abdominal operations in AIDS patients; two of the conditions, a perforation of the colon and a toxic megacolon, were due to CMV. Surgical treatments were colectomy with colostomy and total colectomy. Robinson et al. (175) performed seven emergency operations, and the two celiotomies were for CMV. Colectomy with end colostomy was employed in both cases. Deaths occurred at two weeks and five months in these patients. Eleven AIDS patients underwent 13 emergency celiotomies by Wexner et al. (176); seven of these procedures were due to CMV. Four of the seven had lower gastrointestinal hemorrhage from proctocolitis, and three had perforations. Surgical procedures included three subtotal colectomies, two segmental resections, and two diverting stomas. The mortality rate was 68% in six months. Soderlund et al. (177) reported eight patients with advanced HIV disease and severe CMV enterocolitis. These patients had right ileocolectomies; six had complete or partial palliation for a mean of 14 months, one died of hemorrhage from a Kaposi's sarcoma, and one died three weeks later from unrelated causes.

MALIGNANCIES

One in six patients with AIDS, both in the United States and Europe, develops a malignancy, in particular Kaposi's sarcoma and non-Hodgkin's lymphoma (178). Malignancy is one of the defining characteristics for AIDS. The dominant malignancy is Kaposi's sarcoma, and non-Hodgkin's lymphoma is the second most common. Epidermoid carcinomas are being found in association with condylomata acuminata. The change in rates among never-married men suggests that homosexual men are at special and increasing risk (179). (See chapter 13 on condyloma acuminatum and chapter 18 on anal neoplasms.) In recent studies new malignancies in seropositive patients have increased in statistically significant numbers, including central nervous system lymphoma, nonmelanoma skin carcinomas, seminoma, and Hodgkin's disease (180).

Kaposi's Sarcoma

Kaposi's sarcoma (KS) is the most frequent AIDS-related malignancy; in fact, findings of this disease in a group of young homosexuals led to the original report of AIDS in the United States (181). After an initial rapid increase, the proportion of AIDS patients with KS steadily declined from nearly half of those with diagnosed AIDS in 1981 to 15% in 1986 in the United States, and from 38% in 1983 to 14% in 1991 in Europe (178). Patients coinfected with HIV-1 and human herpes virus 8 (HHV-8) are at accelerated risk for developing KS (182,183). The skin is the most frequent site, and the lesions are multicentric. The nodules are usually 0.5 to 2.0 cm in size and vary in color from purple to black. When the gastrointestinal tract is involved, usually there are few symptoms. However, obstructive symptoms and bleeding have been reported. The gastrointestinal lesions are red, raised, sessile nodules. Since the rectum may be involved, sigmoidoscopy and biopsy should be part of the workup. Pulmonary KS may be debilitating and may lead to death. After the diagnosis has been made, survival past two years is unusual. In fact, these patients usually succumb to opportunistic infections rather than directly to KS. Survival is related to the absolute number of T-helper cells (184). These sarcomas may be staged into four groups as proposed by Mitsuyasu and Groopman (185). Stage I KS has limited (<10) cutaneous lesions; stage II has disseminated (>10) cutaneous lesions; stage III is visceral KS (lymph node and gastrointestinal); and stage IV is cutaneous and visceral KS combined, or pulmonary KS.

The treatment of KS depends on a number of clinical considerations. These include the patient's CD4 count, the total number of lesions, duration of the lesions, the rate of new lesion formation, and the location of individual lesions. Treatment is divided into local management of individual lesions and systemic chemotherapy (186). Local management can be accomplished with five commonly used techniques: observation, intralesional administration of vinblastine, liquid nitrogen, excision, and radiation therapy (187). Minimal KS may be observed expectantly, but with prior opportunistic infections it may be treated with AZT alone or with a chemotherapeutic agent. Rapidly progressing KS may be limited by administration of single or multiple chemotherapeutic drugs. The systemic management of KS is generally achieved using either single-agent vinblastine or a combination of vinblastine and vincristine or a combination of doxorubicin hydrochloride, bleomycin, and vincristine or oral VP-16. The lowest dosages possible should be used, because profound toxicities may result. Interferon alpha has been used with limited success (186). Painful or bulky KS may be palliated by radiotherapy. Surgery is seldom needed. There are only rare reports of indications for surgery for KS because symptoms and mortality are far more likely a result of opportunistic infection.

Lymphoma

Non-Hodgkins lymphoma is often found in immunodeficient patients, including those with AIDS. Most of these lymphomas are of B-cell origin and only a small number are of T-cell origin. A pathologic classification based on the characteristics of lymph cells and nodes is divided into low, intermediate, and high grades (188). Unfortunately, in AIDS patients the disease frequently is found to be present in other organs at the time of presentation. The lymphoma masses sometimes may be found around the anus and the rectum (189–192). Aggressive therapy with cyclophosphamide, doxorubicin, vincristine, and prednisone has been the mainstay of treatment (186). Response rates to chemotherapy by AIDS patients are poorer than those of other groups of immunodeficient patients. Although half of the patients respond to chemotherapy, half of them relapse (186,193). Survival lasts only a few months; the cause of death is usually lymphoma, but almost as often an opportunistic infection supervenes.

COLORECTAL SURGERY IN AIDS PATIENTS

The colon and anorectum are the most common sites requiring surgery in AIDS patients. The aforementioned opportunistic infections and neoplasms lead to hemorrhage, obstruction, and perforation, with either peritonitis or with abscess formation.

Hemorrhage of life-threatening magnitude in AIDS patients is most often due to infectious colitis and enteritis, KS, or lymphoma. The colitis or enteritis is most often due to CMV, which causes well-circumscribed ulcerations that subsequently bleed (194). After resuscitation, the site of bleeding must be localized. Endoscopy has been of little use, because the usual site is the right colon or terminal ileum, and the site may not be visible or even reached by the endoscope. Arteriography will define a rapidly bleeding site. Sharma et al. (195) reported that arteriography was used for nine patients, and the site was localized in seven. Transcatheter intervention was tried; three were embolized, two had vasopressin infusion, and one had both. These six hemorrhages were controlled, but the complications of thrombosis of the femoral artery and a pseudoaneurysm of the femoral artery were encountered.

Patients with HIV disease who develop an acute abdomen from the usual etiologies, as well as those with

TABLE 6 ■ Laparotomy in AIDS Patients

Author(s)	No. of Patients	Operations for Acute Conditions	Complications Associated with Acute Operations	Deaths Associated with Acute Operations
Wolkomir et al. (196)	20	3	0 (0%)	0 (0%)
Deziel et al. (197)	20	10	4 (40%)	2 (20%)
Diettrich et al. (198)	58	12	3 (25%)	3 (25%)
Davidson et al. (202)	28	28	—	3 (11%)
Whitney et al. (199)	57	57	15 (26%)	7 (12%)
Bizer et al. (200)	40	15	20 (50%)	15 (38%)
Samantaray and Walker (201)	24	—	12 (50%)	7 (30%)

etiologies related to opportunistic infections or neoplasms, should be treated appropriately, even though there is greater morbidity and mortality. It can be expected that the mortality will be four times that of otherwise normal patients. A number of series have reported the outcomes of laparotomy for patients with HIV (196–201). Table 6 shows the outcomes. The pathologies include appendicitis, small bowel obstructions, cholecystitis, perforations, gastric lacerations, and mycobacterial or CMV colitis. Bowel obstructions are often associated with KS and lymphomas.

Patients who have an acute abdomen because of an AIDS-related opportunistic disease have a higher incidence of morbidity and mortality. Preoperative factors associated with high mortality include a low CD4 count, decreased total protein, and decreased serum albumin. Wasted patients do less well, and unfortunately, nutritional support has not improved outcomes. Some pathologies more often lead to morbid outcomes. Every attempt should be made to avoid laparotomy for patients with AIDS and lymphoma or MAI. Technically the surgery should be the same as for a non-AIDS patient. However, diverting ostomies might be used more frequently, because leaks are more poorly tolerated in the immunocompromised patient.

CMV is a common, serious, opportunistic infection that is the leading cause of ileocolonic perforation. CMV causes a small vessel vasculitis, which may lead to focal ischemia and necrosis of the bowel wall. The colitis may be either a pancolitis or an inflammation localized to the cecum and terminal ileum. The fever, pain, and hematochezia can progress rapidly to severe hemorrhagic colitis, toxic megacolon, perforation, and death. The CT scan is the best diagnostic tool, showing marked circumferential colonic wall thickening with distortion and ulceration of the mucosal surface and pericolonic inflammation around the cecum, ascending colon, and terminal ileum (203).

Appendicitis is listed high in the differential diagnosis for abdominal pain in a young age group. Whitney et al. (204) in 1992 reviewed the literature and found 30 cases with a 40% perforation rate. Their own series consisted of 28 patients with no deaths and an 18% complication rate. With the exception of diffuse vs. localized abdominal pain, no symptom or sign was useful in differentiating AIDS-related and non-AIDS-related disease.

According to published reports 6% to 34% of HIV-positive patients will develop a significant anorectal problem requiring medical or surgical therapy (205–207). The most frequent surgery performed on HIV patients is to correct a pathologic condition of the anorectum. The usual complaint that brings the patient to the office of the colon and rectal surgeon is pain. Diarrhea, bleeding, and discharge do not prompt a visit with the same urgency. The colorectal disorders may be categorized into three groups: (1) a unique disorder that occurs in only HIV patients, (2) a disorder that is adversely affected by HIV, and (3) a routine anorectal disorder (208). Because of the different categories, general statements cannot be made.

First, the nonsurgical STDs must be diagnosed. In the office, cultures can be taken and biopsies under local anesthesia can be performed. Unfortunately, pain is often so severe that a general anesthesia is necessary to look at and biopsy the anal canal and rectum.

The routine anorectal disorders should be aggressively managed in order to control pain and limit potential extension of sepsis. Anal abscesses tend to be more complex and be chronic, but incision and drainage should be performed when the abscess is recognized. Antibiotics may be an adjuvant therapy, but should not be the only therapy. Healing after incision and drainage is almost normal (205–209).

Anal fistulas tend to be complex in the HIV-positive patient. Furthermore, cutting the sphincter may lead to incontinence when the usual diarrhea must be controlled. Thus being conservative and using setons liberally may be the appropriate choice (120,207,208,210). If fistulotomy is to be performed, it is safer to do it as a second stage after the first-stage seton placement.

Anal fissures are often found in the HIV-positive patient. The problem comes with differentiating them from other ulcerations (Fig. 2). If the sphincter is hypertonic and the fissure resembles a "typical fissure" (i.e., slit-like in the midline and overlying the distal margin of the internal sphincter), it can be treated as any typical fissure. First, a trial of bulk stool softeners, sitz baths, and sphincter relaxing ointment may permit spontaneous healing. Failing conservative medical management, a lateral internal sphincterotomy may be performed. However, if the sphincter is loose, the ulcer is not midline, or it is eroded in appearance, it should not be treated as a typical fissure.

Condylomata are the most common finding in the anal area in these HIV-positive patients. Even though recurrence is common and healing is slow, these lesions should be destroyed by electrocoagulation, laser, etc. Careful follow-up and retreatment have a better chance of success as compared to any less direct management.

Hemorrhoids, if symptomatic, should be treated conservatively, first with bulk stool softeners and sitz baths. Infrared photocoagulation may give some relief. Rubber band ligation has been discouraged because of the fear of Fournier's gangrene. Hemorrhoidectomy may be well tolerated if the patient's immune mechanism is still intact. However, in patients who have a failing immune

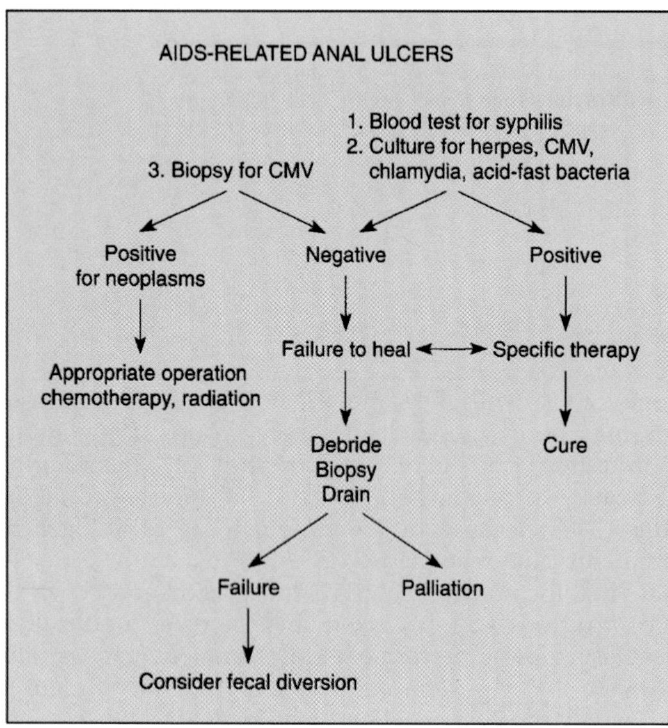

FIGURE 3 ■ AIDS-related anal ulcers.

mechanism, the hemorrhoidectomy incision may be delayed in healing and sepsis may ensue.

Ulcerations in the anal canals of HIV-positive homosexual men are a result of trauma and infection. These ulcers may be large and multiple and may occur anywhere within the anal canal. They are often so painful that general anesthesia is necessary just to examine the patient. Initially cultures, especially for herpes, and a biopsy for CMV and neoplasms are performed (Fig. 3). If a specific organism is identified, specific therapy can be instituted. Reports recently call attention to an ancient disease: tuberculous perianal ulcers (210). If the ulcer persists, total excision has been successful (205). There have been reports of alleviation of pain by administration of Depo-Medrol, but not all investigators are enthusiastic (211). The technique of advancing flaps to cover ulcers has been recommended by Consten et al. (212). However, if poor wound healing is a basic problem, this approach will fare no better. Debridement of overhanging margins to ensure proper drainage is an effective palliative measure.

■ AIDS AND THE HEALTH CARE WORKER

Exposure to blood and blood products places health care workers at risk for being inoculated with HIV. Casual contact does not increase risk. Although saliva, tears, and urine may be weakly infected, no HIV infection of health care workers has been reported from these sources; yet precautions should be taken to minimize exposure. The chance of contracting AIDS by a skin or mucous membrane intrusion is greatest where the exposure is prevalent. The occupational groups that are likely to be at greatest risk can be extrapolated from those at risk for the hepatitis B infection, for example, dentists, surgeons, emergency room personnel, laboratory technicians, obstetric personnel, and bedside nurses.

Numerous reports have been written to assess occupational risks. Kuhls et al. (213) prospectively followed 246 female health care workers of whom 102 had high exposure. After follow-up for 9 to 12 months, no cases of HIV conversion were found. Since 1983 Marcus et al. (214) have conducted a national survey of health care workers. These workers had needlesticks, cuts by sharp objects, and open wound or mucous membrane exposure directly from AIDS patients. Blood samples from those directly exposed to AIDS patients were obtained in 963 of the workers. Of the 963 whose serum was tested, four were positive (0.42%) (214). Two of the four resulted from efforts during resuscitation.

Some precautions have been recommended by the CDC to prevent occupational transmission of HIV infections (215):

1. Hands should be washed before and after each contact.
2. Gloves should be worn when contact with blood or body fluids is likely.
3. Masks and protective eyewear should be worn whenever a splash or spray of blood or body fluid may occur.
4. Masks and eyewear are advisable when working with patients who have pulmonary disease, are coughing, are on mechanical positive pressure, or have copious secretions.
5. Gowns should be worn if clothing is likely to be soiled.
6. Food service should be standard.
7. Private rooms are not absolutely necessary unless there is a personal hygiene problem.
8. Contaminated articles should be bagged with isolation labels for decontamination.
9. Needles and sharp instruments must be handled cautiously. Avoid recapping of needles.
10. Spills of blood or body fluids should be cleaned with a dilute solution of sodium hypochlorite (bleach).
11. Health care workers with open lesions should not participate in invasive procedures.

REFERENCES

1. Weller IVD. The gay bowel. Gut 1985; 26:869–875.
2. Allason-Jones E, Mindel A. Sex and the bowel. Int J Colorectal Dis 1987; 2: 32–37.
3. Baker RW, Peppercorn MA. Gastrointestinal ailments of homosexual men. Medicine 1983; 61:390–405.
4. Quinn TC, Corey L, Chafflee RG, et al. The etiology of anorectal infections in homosexual men. Am J Med 1981; 71:395–406.
5. Kazel HL, Sohn N, Carrasoo JI, et al. The gay bowel syndrome: Clinicopathologic correlation in 260 cases. Ann Clin Lab Sci 1976; 6:184–192.
6. Sohn N, Robilotti JG. Gay bowel syndrome. Am J Gastroenterol 1977; 67: 478–484.
7. Dritz SK, Ainsworth TE, Gayrard WF, et al. Patterns of sexually transmitted enteric disease in a city. Lancet 1977; 2:3–4.
8. Dritz SK. Medical aspects of homosexuality [editorial]. N Engl J Med 1980; 302:463–464.
9. Kean BH, William DC, Luminais SK. Epidemic of amebiasis and giardiasis in a biased population. Br J Venereal Dis 1979; 55:375–378.
10. Willcox RR. Epidemiology of anorectal disease. J Roy Soc Med 1980; 73: 508–509.
11. Owen WF. Sexually transmitted diseases and traumatic problems in homosexual men. Ann Intern Med 1980; 92:805–808.
12. Kinsey AC, Pomeroy WB, Martin CE. Sexual behavior in the human male. Philadelphia: WB Saunders, 1948.
13. Aiigenbraun MH, McCormack WM. Sexually transmitted diseases in HIV-infected persons. Infect Dis Clin North Am 1994; 8:439–448.

14. Modesto VL, Gottesman L. Sexually transmitted diseases and anal manifestations of AIDS. Surg Clin North Am 1994; 74:1433–1463.
15. Gebhard PH. The exposure factor—The VD crisis: Report of International Venereal Disease Symposium. St. Louis, Mo., New York: Pfizer Laboratories, 1976.
16. William DC, Felman YM, Marv JS, et al. Sexually transmitted enteric pathogens in a male homosexual population. NY State J Med 1978; 77:2050–2052.
17. Phillips SC, Mildvan D, William D. Sexual transmission of enteric protozoa and helminths in a venereal disease clinic population. N Engl J Med 1981; 305:603–606.
18. Judson FN, Penley K, Robinson M, et al. Comparative prevalence rates of sexually transmitted diseases in heterosexual and homosexual men. Am J Epidemiol 1980; 112:836–843.
19. British Co-operative Clinical Group. Homosexuality and venereal disease in the United Kingdom. Br J Venereal Dis 1980; 56:6–11.
20. Darrow W, Barre HD, Jay K, et al. The gay report on sexually transmitted diseases. Am J Publ Health 1981; 71:1004–1011.
21. O'Hare PA, Fiumara NJ, McCormack W. PID among women presenting to emergency rooms of hospitals in Massachusetts. Am J Obstet Gynecol 1980; 138:909–912.
22. Fiumara NJ. Gonorrhea and nongonococcal urethritis. Cutis 1981; 27:258–265.
23. Deheragoda P. Diagnosis of rectal gonorrhea by blind anorectal swab compared with direct vision swabs taken via a proctoscope. Br J Venereal Dis 1977; 53:311–313.
24. Daniel DC, Felman YM, Riccardi NB, et al. The utility of anoscopy in the rapid diagnosis of symptomatic anorectal gonorrhea in men. Sex Transm Dis 1981; 8:16–17.
25. Young H, Anderson J, Moyes A, McMillan A. Non-cultured detection of rectal and pharyngeal gonorrhea by the Gen-Probe PACE 2 assay. Genitourinary Med 1997; 73(1):59–62.
26. Janda W, Bohnloff MS, Morella J, et al. Prevalence and site-pathogen studies of *Nisseria meningitis* and *N. gonorrhea* in homosexual men. JAMA 1980; 244:2060–2064.
27. Young H, Moyes A, McKenna JG, et al. Rectal gonorrhea and unsafe sex. Lancet 1991; 337:853.
28. U.S. Department of Health and Human Services. Sexually transmitted diseases treatment guidelines. MMWR 2002; 51(RR-6):1–77.
29. Echols RM, Heyd A, O'Keefe BJ, et al. Single dose ciprofloxacin for the treatment of uncomplicated gonorrhea: A worldwide summary. Sex Transm Dis 1994; 24:345–352.
30. Handsfeld H. Combating syphilis and gonorrhea in the 1990s. JAMA 1990; 264:1451–1452.
31. Schwartz S, Zenilman J, Schnell D, et al. National surveillance of antimicrobial resistance in *Neisseria gonorrhea*. JAMA 1990; 264:1413–1417.
32. Maan J, Kropp R, Wong J, Vanna S, Romonowski B. Gonorrhea treatment guidelines in Canada: 2004 update. CMAJ 2004; 171:0345–0346.
33. Kampmaier R. The establishment of lymphogranuloma inguinale as a sexually transmitted disease. Sex Transm Dis J (Am Venereal Dis Assoc) 1982; 9: 146–148.
34. Centers for Disease Control and Prevention. Recommendations for the prevention and management of *Chlamydia trachomatis* infections. MMWR 1993; 42(RR-12):1.
35. Levine JS, Smith PD, Brugge WR. Chronic proctitis in male homosexuals due to lymphogranuloma venereum. Gastroenterology 1980; 79:563–565.
36. Quinn TC, Goodell SE, Mkrtichian E, et al. *Chlamydia traehomatis* proctitis. N Engl J Med 1981; 305:195–200.
37. Dean D, Millman K. Molecular and mutation trends analyses of amp l alleles for serovar E of *Chlamydia trachomatis*. J Clin Invest 1997; 99(3):475–483.
38. Amaral E. Current approach to STD management in women. Int J Gynecol Obstet 1998; 63(suppl 1):S 183–189.
39. McMillan A, Sommerville RG, McKee PMK. Chlamydial infection in homosexual men. Frequency of isolation of *Chlamydia trachomatis* from urethra and anorectum. Br J Venereal Dis 1981; 57:47–81.
40. Papagrigoriedis S, Rennie JA. *Lymphogranuloma venereum* as a cause of rectal strictures. Postgrad Med J 1998; 74(809):168–169.
41. Bendahan J, Paran H, Kolman S, et al. The possible role of *Chlamydia trachomatis* in perineal suppurative hidradenitis. Eur J Surg 1992; 158: 213–215.
42. Rompalo AM, Price CD, Roberts PF, et al. Potential value of rectal screening cultures for *Chlamydia trachomatis* in homosexual men. J Infect Dis 1986; 153:888–892.
43. Weinstock H, Dean D, Bolan G. *Chlamydia trachomatis* infections. Infect Dis North Am 1994; 8:797–819.
44. Stamm WE, Hicks CB, Martin DH. Azithromycin for empirical treatment of the nongonococcal arthritis syndrome in men: A randomized double-blind study. JAMA 1995; 274:545–549.
45. Blaser MJ. Campylobacter enteritis in the United States. A multicenter study. Ann Int Med 1983; 98:360–366.
46. Walker RI, Caldwell MB, Lee EC, et al. Pathophysiology of campylobacter enteritis. Microbiol Rev 1986; 50:81.
47. Guerrant RL, Bobak DA. Bacterial and protozoal gastroenteritis. N Engl J Med 1991; 325:327.
48. Drusin LM, Genvert G, Topf-Olstein B, et al. Shigellosis, another sexually transmitted disease? Br J Venereal Dis 1976; 52:48–50.
49. Dritz SK, Back AF. Shigella enteritis venereally transmitted. N Engl J Med 1974; 291:1194.
50. Dupont HL, Hornick RB. Adverse effect of lomotil therapy in shigellosis. JAMA 1973; 226:1525–1528.
51. Adam T. Exploitation of host factors for efficient infection by Shigella. Int J Med Microbial 2001; 291(4):287–298.
52. Houng HS, Sethabutr O, Echeverria P. A simple polymerase chain reaction technique to detect and differentiate Shigella and enteroinvasive *E. coli* in human feces. Diagn Microbiol Infect Dis 1997; 28(1):18–25.
53. Jamal WY, Rotimi VO, Chugh TD, Pal T. Prevalence and susceptibility of Shigella species to 11 antibiotics in a Kuwait teaching hospital. J Chemother 1998; 10(4):285–290.
54. Anonymous. Vaccine research and development. New strategies for accelerating Shigella vaccine development. Weekly Epidemiol Record 1997; 72(11):73–79.
55. Catterall RD. Sexually transmitted diseases of anus and rectum. Clin Gastroenterol 1975; 4:659–669.
56. Rompalo AM. Can syphilis be evadicated from the world? Curr OpinInfect Dis 2001; 14:41–44.
57. Clyne B, Jerrard DA. Syphilis testing. J Emerg Med 2000; 18(3):361–367.
58. U.S. Department of Health and Human Services. Primary and secondary syphilis—United States, 2002, MMWR 2003; 52(46):1117–1120.
59. Rompalo AM, Joesoef MR, O'Donnel JA, et al. Clinical manifestations of early syphilis by HIV status and gender: Results of syphilis and HIV study. Sex Transm Dis 2001; 28(3):158–165.
60. Faris MR, Perry JJ, Westermeier TG, et al. Rectal syphilis mimicking histiocytic lymphoma. Am Clin Pathol 1983; 80:719–721.
61. Drusin LM, Singer C, Valenti AJ, et al. Infectious syphilis mimicking neoplastic disease. Arch Intern Med 1977; 132:156–160.
62. Hutchinson CM, Hook EW, Shepherd M, et al. Altered clinical presentation of early syphilis in patients with human immunodeficiency virus infection. Ann Intern Med 1994; 121:94–99.
63. Yinnon AM, Coury-Doninger P, Polito R, Reichman RC. Serologic response to treatment of syphilis in patients with HIV disease. Arch Int Med 1996; 156(3):321–325.
64. Liu H, Rodes B, Chen CY, Steiner B. New tests for syphilis: Rational design of a PCR method for detection of *Treponema pallidum* in clinical specimens. J Clin Microbiol 2001; 39(5):1941–1946.
65. Lowhagen GB, Tunback P, Anderson K, Bergstrom T, Johannissou F. First episodes of genital herpes in a Swedish STD population: A study of epidemiology and transmission by use of HSV typing and specific serology. Sex Transm Infect 2000; 76(3):179–182.
66. Schaoker T. The role of HSV-1 in the transmission and progression of HIV. Herpes 2001; 8:46–49.
67. Peppercorn MA. Enteric infections in homosexual men with and without AIDS. Contemp Gastroenterol 1989; 2:23–32.
68. Goodell SE, Quinn TC, Mkrtichian E, et al. Herpes simplex virus proctitis in homosexual men. N Engl J Med 1983; 308:868–871.
69. Samarasinghe PI, Oates JK, MacLennan IPB. Herpetic proctitis and sacral radiculomyelopathy—a hazard for homosexual men. Br J Med 1979; 2:365–366.
70. Ashley RL. Sorting out new HSV type specific antibody tests. Sex Transm Dis 2001; 77(4):232–237.
71. Nerurkar L, Goedert J, Wallen W, et al. Study of antiviral antibodies in sera of homosexual men. J Fed Proc 1983; 42:6109.
72. deRuiter A, Thin RN. Genital herpes. A guide to pharmacological therapy. Drugs 1994; 47:297–304.
73. Rompalo AM, Mertz GJ, Davis LG, et al. Oral acyclovir for treatment of first episode herpes simplex virus proctitis. JAMA 1988; 259:2879–2881.
74. Chatis PA, Miller CH, Schrager LE, et al. Successful treatment with foscarnet of an acyclovir resistant mucocutaneous infection with herpes simplex virus in a patient with acquired immunodeficiency syndrome. N Engl J Med 1989; 320:297–300.
75. Stanberry L, Cunningham A, Mertz G, et al. New developments in the epidemiology, natural history and management of genital herpes. Antiviral Res 1999; 42:1–14.
76. Mertz GJ, Jones CC, Mills J, et al. Long term acyclovir suppression of frequently recurring genital herpes simplex virus infection. JAMA 1988; 260:201–206.
77. Cates W, Toomey KE. Sexually transmitted diseases. Primary Care 1990; 17:1–27.
78. Ellis WR, Coleman JC, Fluker JL, et al. Liver disease among homosexual males. Lancet 1979; 1:903–904.
79. Beasley KE. Hepatitis B virus as the etiologic agent in hepatocellular carcinoma. Hepatology 1982; 2:21–26.
80. Pomerantz BM, Marr JS, Goldman WD. Amebiasis in New York City 1958–1978—Identification of the male homosexual high risk population. Bull NY Acad Med 1980; 56:232–244.
81. Ainsworth TE, Back A, Baucher LA, et al. Patterns of sexually transmitted enteric diseases in a city. Lancet 1977; July 2.
82. William DC, Shookhoff HB, Felman YM, et al. High rates of enteric protozoal infections in selected homosexual men attending a venereal disease clinic. Sex Transm Dis 1978; 5:155–158.

83. Keystone JS, Keystone DL, Proctor EM. Intestinal parasitic infections in homosexual men—Prevalence, symptoms, and factors in transmission. Can Med Assoc J 1980; 123:512–514.
84. Gardner TB, Hill DR. Treatment of giardiasis. Clin Microbiol Rev 2001; 14(1):114–128.
85. Friedman-Kein A, Laubenstein L, Marmor M, et al. Kaposi's sarcoma and *Pneumocystis* pneumonia among homosexual men—New York City and California. MMWR 1981; 30:305–308.
86. Mosley JW. The Transfusion Safety Study Group. The transfusion safety study [Abstract TH 10.2]. In Abstracts of the Third International Conference on AIDS, Washington, D.C., 1987.
87. Stiegbigel NH, Maude DW, Feiner CJ, et al. Heterosexual transmission of disease by human immunodeficiency virus (HIV) [Abstract W 2,5]. In Abstracts of the Third International Conference on AIDS, Washington, D.C., 1987.
88. Mitsuye H, Weingold KJ, Furman PA, et al. 3′-Azido-3′ de-oxythymidine (BW A509U): An antiviral agent that inhibits the infectivity and cytopathic effect of human T-lymphotropic virus type III/lymphadenopathy associated virus in vitro. Proc Natl Acad Sci USA 1985; 82:7096–7100.
89. Centers for Disease Control and Prevention. 1993 Revised classification system for HIV infection and expanded surveillance case definition for AIDS among adolescents and adults. MMWR 1992;41(17):1–19.
90. Mortality patterns—United States, 1993. MMWR 1996; 45(8):161–164.
91. Update: Mortality attributable to HIV infection among persons aged 25–44 years—United States, 1994. MMWR 1996; 45(6):121–125.
92. O'Brien WA, Hartigan PM, Martin D, et al. Changes in plasma HIV-I RNA and CD4 lymphocyte counts and the risk of progression to AIDS. N Engl J Med 1996; 334:426–431.
93. Nakashima AD, Fleming PL. HIV/AIDS surveillance in the United States, 1998–2001. J Acquir Immune Defic Syndr 2003; 32:68–85.
94. Trachtenberg JD, Sande ME, Emerging resistance to non-nucleoside reverse transcriptase inhibitors. JAMA 2002; 288(2):239–240.
95. Levy JA, Kaminsky LS, Marrow WSW, et al. Infection by the retrovirus associated with the acquired immunodeficiency syndrome. Ann Intern Med 1985; 103:694.
96. Gallo R, Salahuddin S, Popovic M, et al. Frequent detection and isolation of cytopathic retrovirus (HTLV-FII) from patients with AIDS and risk of AIDS. Science 1984; 224:500.
97. Nelson JA, Wiley CA, Reynolds-Kohler C, et al. Detection of the human immunodeficiency virus in bowel epithelium. Lancet 1988; 1:250.
98. Centers for Disease Control. HIV/AIDS surveillance, February 1990.
99. Update: trends in AIDS among men who have sex with men—United States, 1989–1994. MMWR 1995; 44(21):401–404.
100. Evans BG, Catchpole MA, Heptonstall J, et al. Sexually transmitted diseases and HTV-1 infection among homosexual men in England and Wales. BMJ 1993; 306:426–428.
101. Anonymous. HIV/STD risks in young men who have sex with men who do not disclose their sexual orientation—six U.S. cities 1994–2000. MMWR 2003; 52:81–86.
102. Update: AIDS among women in United States, 1994. MMWR 1995; 44(5):81–84.
103. Davis SF, Byers RH, Lindegren ML, et al. Prevalence and incidence of vertically acquired HTV infection in the United States. JAMA 1995; 274:952–956.
104. Veugelers PJ, Page KA, Tindall B, et al. Determinates of HIV disease progression among homosexual men registered in the tricontinental seroconverter study. Am J Epidemiol 1994; 140:747–758.
105. Enger C, Graham N, Peng Y, et al. Survival from early, intermediate, and late stages of HIV infection. JAMA 1996; 275:1329–1334.
106. Wasserheit J. Epidemiological synergy: Interrelationships between human immunodeficiency virus infection and other sexually transmitted diseases. Sex Transm Dis 1992; 19:61–77.
107. Chan ISF, Neaton JD, Saravolatz LD, et al. Frequencies of opportunistic diseases prior to death among HIV-infected persons. AIDS 1995; 9:1145–1151.
108. Centers for Disease Control. Classification system for human T-lymphotropic virus type III/lymphadenopathy—Associated virus infections. MMWR 1986; 35:334–339.
109. Cooper DA, Gold J, MacLean P, et al. Acute AIDS retrovirus infection. Definition of a clinical illness associated with seroconversion. Lancet 1985; 1:537–540.
110. Rabeneck L, Boyko WJ, McLean DM, et al. Unusual esophageal ulcers containing enveloped virus-like particles in homosexual men. Gastroenterology 1986; 90:1882.
111. Wilcox CM, Schwartz DA, Cotsonis G, et al. Chronic unexplained diarrhea in human immunodeficiency virus infection: Determination of the best diagnostic approach. Gastroenterology 1996; 110:30–37.
112. Diettrich DT, Rahmin M. Cytomegalovirus colitis in AIDS. J Acquir Immune Defic Syndr 1991; 4:529–535.
113. Blanshard C, Gazzard BG. Natural history and prognosis of diarrhea of unknown cause in patients with acquired immunodeficiency syndrome. Gut 1995; 36:283–286.
114. Cappell MS. Hepatobiliary manifestations of the acquired immune deficiency syndrome. Am J Gastroenterol 1991; 86:1–15.
115. Schneiderman DJ, Arenson DM, Cello JP, et al. Hepatic disease in patients with acquired immune deficiency syndrome (AIDS). Hepatology 1987; 7:925.
116. Detlovitz JA, Pope JW, Boney M, et al. Clinical manifestations and therapy of *Isospora belli* infection in patients with acquired immunodeficiency syndrome. N Engl J Med 1986; 315:387.
117. Wolfon JS, Richter JM, Waldron MA, et al. Cryptosporidiosis in immunocompetent patients. N Engl J Med 1985; 312:1278.
118. DeRodriguez CV, Fuhrer J, Lake-Bakaar G. Cytomegalovirus colitis in patients with acquired immunodeficiency syndrome. J R Soc Med 1994; 87:203–205.
119. Orkin BA, Smith LE. Perineal manifestations of HIV infection. Dis Colon Rectum 1992; 35:310–314.
120. Goldberg GS, Orkin BA, Smith LE. Microbiology of human immunodeficiency virus anorectal disease. Dis Colon Rectum 1994; 37:439–443.
121. Centers for Disease Control. AIDS weekly surveillance report—United States, October 12, 1987.
122. Hoover DR, Saah AJ, Bacellar H, et al. Clinical manifestations of AIDS in the era of pneumocystis prophylaxis. N Engl J Med 1993; 329:1922–1926.
123. Centers for Disease Control. Recommendations for prophylaxis against *Pneumocystis carinii* pneumonia for adults and adolescents infected with HIV. MMWR 1992; 41(RR4):1–11.
124. Pitchenik AE, Ganjei P, Torres A, et al. Sputum examination for the diagnosis of *Pneumocystis carinii* in the acquired immunodeficiency syndrome. Am Rev Respir Dis 1986; 133:226.
125. Small CB, Harris CA, Friedland GH, et al. The treatment of *Pneumocystis carinii* pneumonia in the acquired immunodeficiency syndrome. Arch Intern Med 1985; 145:837–840.
126. Saah AJ, Hoover DR, Peng Y, et al. Predictors for failure of *Pneumocystis carinii* pneumonia prophylaxis. JAMA 1995; 273:1197–1202.
127. Post MJD, Sheldon JJ, Hensley GT, Tobias JA, et al. Central nervous system disease in AIDS: Prospective correlation using CT, MR imaging and pathologic studies. Radiology 1986; 158:141–144.
128. Frenkel JK, Nelson BM, Arias-Stella J. Immunosuppression and toxoplasmic encephalitis. Hum Pathol 1975; 6:97.
129. Levy RM, Bredesen DE, Rosenblum ML. Neurologic manifestations of the acquired immunodeficiency syndrome (AIDS): Experience at UCSF and review of the literature. J Neurosurg 1985; 62:475–495.
130. Luft BJ, Brooks RG, Conley FK, et al. Toxoplasmic encephalitis in patients with AIDS. JAMA 1984; 252:913.
131. Mariuz P, Bosler EM, Luft BJ. Toxoplasmosis in individuals with AIDS. Infect Dis Clin North Am 1994; 8:365–381.
132. Kovacs JA. Toxoplasmosis in AIDS: Keeping the lid on. Ann Intern Med 1995; 123:230–231.
133. Faust EC, Giraldo LE, Caicedo G, et al. Human isosporosis in the western hemisphere. Am J Trop Med Hyg 1961; 10:343.
134. Sorvillo FJ, Lieb LE, Kerndt PR, et al. Epidemiology of cryptosporidiosis among persons with acquired immunodeficiency syndrome in Los Angeles County. Am J Trop Med Hyg 1994; 51:326–331.
135. Pape JW, Verdier R, Boncy M, et al. *Cydospora* infection in adults infected with HIV. Clinical manifestations, treatment, and prophylaxis. Ann Intern Med 1994; 121:654–657.
136. Ma P, Seave R. Three-step stool examination for cryptosporidiosis in ten homosexual men with protracted watery diarrhea. J Infect Dis 1983; 147:824.
137. Zhu G, Marchewka MJ, Ennis JG. Direct isolation of DNA from patient stools for polymerase chain reaction detection of *Cryptosporidium parrum*. J Infect Dis 1998; 177:1443.
138. Ma P, Kaufmen D, Montana J. *Isospora belli* diarrheal infection in homosexual men. AIDS Res 1984; 1:327.
139. Aly R, Berger R, Common superficial fungal infections in patients with AIDS, Clin Infect Dis 1996; 22(suppl 2):S128–S132.
140. Bonner JR, Alexander WJ, Dismukes WE, et al. Disseminated histoplasmosis in patients with acquired immune deficiency syndrome. Arch Intern Med 1984; 144:2178–218l.
141. Miller RF, Lucas SB, Pinching AJ. Disseminated histoplasmosis in patients with acquired immunodeficiency syndrome. Genitourin Med 1994; 70:132–137.
142. Goodwin RA, Shapiro JL, Thurman GH, et al. Disseminated histoplasmosis: Clinical and pathologic correlations. Medicine 1980; 59:1–33.
143. McNeil MM, Ampel NM. Opportunistic coccidioidomycosis in patients infected with human immunodeficiency virus: Prevention issues and priorities. Clin Infect Dis 1995; 2l(suppl 1):S111–S113.
144. Wheat LJ, Hafner RE, Korzun AH, et al. Itraconazole treatment of disseminated histoplasmosis in patients with the acquired immunodeficiency syndrome. Am J Med 1995; 98:336–342.
145. Zuger A, Louis E, Holzman RS, et al. Cryptococcal disease in patients with acquired immunodeficiency syndrome. Ann Intern Med 1986; 104:234–240.
146. Stevens A. Management of systemic manifestations of fungal disease in patients with AIDS. J Am Acad Dermatol 1994; 31:564–567.
147. Kovaks JA, Kovaks AA, Polis M, et al. Cryptococcus in the acquired immunodeficiency syndrome. Ann Intern Med 1985; 103:533–538.
148. Celum CL, Chaisson RE, Rutherford GW, et al. Incidence of salmonellosis in patients with AIDS. J Infect Dis 1987; 156:998–1002.
149. Moss AR, Osmond D, Bacchetti P, et al. Risk factors for AIDS and HIV seropositivity in homosexual men. Am J Epidemiol 1987; 125:1035–1047.
150. Schattner A, Hanuka N, Sarov B, et al. *Chlamydia trachomatis* and HIV infection. Immunol Lett 1994; 40:27–30.

151. Pitchenik AE, Burr J, Suarez M, et al. Human T-cell lymphotropic virus-III (HTLV-III) seropositivity and related disease among 71 consecutive patients in whom tuberculosis was diagnosed. Ann Rev Respir Dis 1987; 135:875–879.
152. Handwerger S, Mildvan D, Senie R, et al. Tuberculosis and the acquired immunodeficiency syndrome at a New York City hospital. Chest 1987; 91:176–180.
153. Louie E, Rice LB, Holzman RS. Tuberculosis in non-Haitian patients with acquired immunodeficiency syndrome. Chest 1986; 90:542–545.
154. Pitchenik AE, Rubinson HA. The radiographic appearance of tuberculosis in patients with acquired immune deficiency syndrome (AIDS) and pre-AIDS. Am Rev Respir Dis 1985; 131:393–396.
155. Acandela F, Serrano P, Arriero JM, Teruel A, Reyes D, Colpena R. Perianal diseases of tuberculosis origin: Report of a case and review of the literature. Dis Colon Rectum 1999; 42(1):110–112.
156. Sultan S, Azria F, Bauer P, Abdelnour M, Atienza P. Anoperineal tuberculosis: Diagnostic and management considerations in seven cases. Dis Colon Rectum 2002; 45(3):407–410.
157. Sherman S, Rohwedder JJ, Raukrishnan KP, et al. Tuberculosis enteritis and peritonitis. Arch Intern Med 1980, 140:506–508.
158. Shiratsuchi H, Ellner JJ. Expression of IL-18 by *Mycobacterium avium*-infected human manocytes; association with *M. avium* virulence. Clin Exp Immun 2001; 123(2):203–209.
159. Centers for Disease Control. Recommendations on prophylaxis and therapy for disseminated *Mycobacterium avium* complex for adults and adolescents infected with human immunodeficiency virus. MMWR 1993; 42(RR-9):17–20.
160. Heifets LB, Iseman MD, Lindholm-Levy PJ. Ethambutol MICs and MBCs for *Mycobacterium avium* complex and *Mycobacterium* tuberculosis. Antimicrob Agents Chemother 1986; 30:927–932.
161. Yajko DM, Nassos PS, Hadley WK. Therapeutic implications of inhibition versus killing of *Mycobacterium avium* complex by antimicrobial agents. Antimicrob Agents Chemother 1987; 31:117–120.
162. Schneebaum CW, Novick DM, Chabon AB, et al. Terminal ileitis associated with *Mycobacterium avium* intracellular infection in a homosexual man with AIDS. Gastroenterology 1987; 92:1127–1132.
163. Corey L, Spear PG. Infections with herpes viruses. N Engl J Med 1986; 314:649–657.
164. Corey L, Adams HG, Brown ZA, et al. Genital herpes simplex virus infections: Clinical manifestations, course, and complications. Ann Intern Med 1983; 98:958–972.
165. Dix RD, Waitzman DM, Fullansbee S, et al. Herpes simplex virus type II encephalitis in two homosexual men with persistent adenopathy. Ann Neural 1985; 18:203–206.
166. Straus SE, Seidlin M, Takiff H, et al. Oral acyclovir to suppress recurring herpes simplex virus infections in immunodeficient patients. Ann Intern Med 1986; 100:522–524.
167. Lange M, Klein EB, Kornfield H, et al. Cytomegalovirus isolation from healthy homosexual men. JAMA 1984; 252:1908–1910.
168. Armstrong D, Gold JWM, Dryjanski J, et al. Treatment of infections in patients with the acquired immunodeficiency syndrome. Ann Intern Med 1985; 103:738–743.
169. Evans MRW, Booth JC, Wansbrough-Jones MH. Cytomegalovirus viremia in HIV infection: Association with intercurrent infection. J Infect 1995; 31:21–26.
170. Ehrnst A. The clinical relevance of different laboratory tests in CMV diagnosis. Scand J Infect Dis 1996; 100:64–71.
171. Boeckh M, Boivin G. Quantitation of cytomegalovirus: Methodologic aspects and clinical applications. Clin Microbiol Rev 1998; 11(3):533–554.
172. Perez JL. Resistance to antivirals in human CMV: Mechanisms and clinical significance. Microbiologia 1997; 13(3):343–352.
173. Gonezol E, Plotkin S. Development of a cytomegalovirus vaccine: Lessons from recent clinical trials. Expert Opinion on Biological Therapy 2001; 1(3):401–412.
174. Nugent P, O'Connell T. The surgeon's role in treating acquired immunodeficiency syndrome. Arch Surg 1986; 121:1117–1120.
175. Robinson G, Wilson S, Williams RA. Surgery in patients with acquired immunodeficiency syndrome. Arch Surg 1987; 122:170–175.
176. Wexner SD, Smithy WB, Trillo C, et al. Emergency colectomy for cytomegalovirus ileocolitis in patients with the acquired immune deficiency syndrome. Dis Colon Rectum 1988; 31:755–761.
177. Soderlund C, Bratt GA, Engstrom L, et al. Surgical treatment of cytomegalovirus enterocolitis in severe immunodeficiency virus infection: Report of eight cases. Dis Colon Rectum 1994; 37:63–72.
178. Monfardini S, Tirelii V, Vacchert E. Treatment of AIDS-related cancer. Cancer Treat Rev 1994; 20:149–172.
179. Melbye M, Rabkin C, Frisch M, et al. Changing patterns of anal cancer incidence in the United States, 1940–1989. Am J Epidemiol 1994; 139:772–780.
180. Lyter DW, Bryant J, Thackeray R, et al. Incidence of human immunodeficiency virus-related and nonrelated malignancies in a large cohort of homosexual men. J Clin Oncol 1995; 13:2540–2546.
181. Hymes KB, Cheung TL, Green IB, et al. Kaposi's sarcoma in homosexual men—A report of eight cases. Lancet 1981; 2:598–600.
182. Jacobson LP, Jenkins FJ, Springer G, et al. Interaction of HIV type 1 human and human herpes virus type 8 infections on the incidence of Kaposi's sarcoma. J Infect Dis 2000; 181:9.
183. Hengge UR, Ruzicka T, Tyring SK, Stuschke M, Roggendorf M, Schwartz RA, Seeber S. Update on Kaposi's sarcoma and other HHV8 associated diseases. Part 2: Pathogenesis, Castleman's disease, and pleural effusion lymphoma. Lancet Infect Dis 2002; 2(6):344–352.
184. Taylor J, Afrasiabi R, Fahey JL, et al. Prognostically significant classification of immune changes in AIDS with Kaposi's sarcoma. Blood 1986; 67:666–671.
185. Mitsuyasu RT, Groopman JE. Biology and therapy of Kaposi's sarcoma. Semin Oncol 1984; 11:53–59.
186. Conant MA. Management of human immunodeficiency virus-associated malignancies. Recent Results Cancer Res 1995; 139:424–432.
187. Tappero JW, Conant MA, Wolfe SF, et al. Kaposi's sarcoma. J Am Acad Dermatol 1993; 28:371–395.
188. National Cancer Institute. NCI-sponsored study of classification of non-Hodgkin's lymphoma. The Non-Hodgkin's-Lymphoma Pathologic Classification project. Cancer 1982; 49:2112–2135.
189. Burkes RL, Meyer PR, Gill PS, et al. Rectal lymphoma in homosexual men. Arch Intern Med 1986; 146:913–915.
190. Lee MH, Waxman M, Gillooley JF. Primary malignant lymphoma of the anorectum in homosexual men. Dis Colon Rectum 1986; 29:413–416.
191. Ioachim HL, Weinstein MA, Robbtns RD, et al. Primary anorectal lymphoma: A new manifestation of AIDS. Cancer 1987; 60:1449–1453.
192. Gottlieb CA, Meiri E, Marda KM. Rectal non-Hodgkin's lymphoma: A clinicopathologic study and review. Henry Ford Hosp Med J 1990; 38: 255–258.
193. Ziegler JL, Beckstead JA, Vblberding PA, et al. Non-Hodgkin's lymphoma in ninety homosexual men—relation to generalized lymphadenopathy and the acquired immunodeficiency syndrome. N Engl J Med 1984; 311:565–570.
194. Evans JD, Robertson CS, Clague MB, et al. Severe lower gastrointestinal hemorrhage from cytomegalovirus ulceration of the terminal ileum in a patient with AIDS. Eur J Surg 1993; 159:373–375.
195. Sharma VS, Karim V, Bookstein JJ. Gastrointestinal hemorrhage in AIDS: Arteriographic diagnosis and transcatheter treatment. Radiology 1992; 185:447–451.
196. Wolkemir AF, Barone IE, Hardy HW, et al. Abdominal and anorectal surgery and the acquired immunodeficiency syndrome in heterosexual intravenous drug users. Dis Colon Rectum 1990; 33:267–270.
197. Deziel DJ, Hyser MJ, Doolas A, et al. Major abdominal operations in acquired immunodeficiency syndrome. Am Surg 1990; 56:445–450.
198. Diettrich NA, Cacioppo JC, Kaplan G, et al. A growing spectrum of surgical disease in patients with human immunodeficiency virus. Arch Surg 1991; 126:860–865.
199. Whitney TM, Brunei W, Russell TR, et al. Emergent abdominal surgery in AIDS: Experience in San Francisco. Am J Surg 1994; 168:239–243.
200. Bizer LS, Pettorino R, Ashikori A. Emergency abdominal operations in the patient with acquired immunodeficiency syndrome. J Am Coll Surg 1995; 180:205–209.
201. Samantaray DK, Walker ML. Surgery in AIDS patients. Contemp Surg 1996; 49:207–209.
202. Davidson T, Allen-Mersh TG, Miles AJG. Emergency laparotomy in patients with AIDS. Br J Surg 1991; 78:924–926.
203. Wyatt SH, Fishman EK. The acute abdomen in individuals with AIDS. Radiol Clin North Am 1994; 32:1023–1043.
204. Whitney TM, Macho JR, Russell TR, et al. Appendicitis in acquired immunodeficiency syndrome. Am J Surg 1992; 164:467–471.
205. Nadal SR, Manzione CR, Horta SH, Galro V. Management of idiopathic ulcer of anal canal by excision in HIV positive patients. Dis Colon Rectum 1999; 42(12):1598–1601.
206. Safavi A, Gottesman L, Dailey TH. Anorectal surgery in the HIV+ patient: Update. Dis Colon Rectum 1991; 34:299–304.
207. Wexner SD, Smithy WB, Milsom JW, et al. The surgical management of anorectal disease in AIDS and pre-AIDS patients. Dis Colon Rectum 1986; 29: 719–723.
208. Weiss EG, Wexner SD. Surgery for anal lesions in HIV-infected patients. Ann Med 1995; 27:467–475.
209. Burke EC, Orloff SL, Friese CE, et al. Wound healing after anorectal surgery in human immunodeficiency virus infected patients. Arch Surg 1991; 126:1267–1271.
210. Savela AI, Supe AN. Tuberculous perianal ulcers. J R Soc Med 1996; 89(10):584.
211. Viamonte M, Dailey TH, Gottesman L. Ulcerative disease of the anorectum in the HIV+ patient. Dis Colon Rectum 1993; 36:801–805.
212. Consten ECJ, Slors JFM, Danner SA, et al. Local excision and mucosal advancement for anorectal ulceration in patients infected with human immunodeficiency virus. Br J Surg 1995; 82:891–894.
213. Kuhls TL, Viker S, Parris NB, et al. Occupational risk of HIV, HBV and HSV-I1 infection in health care personnel caring for AIDS patients. Am J Publ Health 1987; 77:1306–1309.
214. Marcus R. CDC Cooperative Needlestick Surveillance Group. Surveillance of health care workers exposed to blood from patients infected with the human immunodeficiency virus. N Engl J Med 1988; 319:1118–1123.
215. Centers for Disease Control. Recommendations for prevention of HIV transmission in health care settings. MMWR 1987; 36(2S):1S–18S.

15 Fecal Incontinence

Philip H. Gordon and W. Rudolf Schouten

INTRODUCTION

Anal incontinence is a socially crippling disorder. Soiling, the escape of flatus, or the inadvertent passage of stool are embarrassing situations few people can tolerate. It therefore behooves surgeons who care for these individuals to be familiar with any treatment options that might be available. Anal continence is dependent on a complex series of learned and reflex responses to colonic and rectal stimuli, and the considerable individual variation in bowel habits makes clear distinction of derangement of continence difficult. Normal continence depends on a number of factors: mental function, stool volume and consistency, colonic transit, rectal distensibility, anal sphincter function, anorectal sensation, and anorectal reflexes (1). The patient who has lost complete control of solid feces has complete incontinence. The patient who complains of inadvertent soiling or escape of liquid or flatus has partial incontinence. Less fastidious individuals may not complain of partial incontinence; therefore careful questioning of the patient may be necessary. In an effort to classify the severity of symptoms; Browning and Parks (2) proposed the following criteria: category A, those continent of solid and liquid stool and flatus (i.e., normal continence); B, those continent of solid and usually liquid stool but not flatus; C, acceptable continence of solid stool but no control over liquid stool or flatus; and D, continued fecal leakages. Numerous other grading scales exist. All these severity scores are simple to use. However, they mainly reflect sphincter function. The worse the function, the higher the score. Thus incontinence to solid stool is always considered worse than incontinence for liquid stool. This does not necessarily reflect the subjective experience of the patient. Furthermore, the reliability and validity of these grading scales are questionable. Because of these drawbacks and the lack of precision of the grading scales, they are no longer recommended as the sole method of categorizing patients and monitoring outcome of treatment (3). Some of the deficiencies of grading scales can be addressed by summary scales. These scales produce multilevel summative scores. The values for each type of incontinence are assigned according to the frequency of incontinent episodes. This frequency is one of the factors contributing to the severity of incontinence. Several scales also include items such as urgency, cleaning difficulties, the use of pads and lifestyle alterations. Numerous summary scales have been designed, such as those according to Rockwood, Jorge/Wexner, Pescatori, Vaizey, and many others. The assignment of values to types and frequencies of incontinence varies between scales. The frequently quoted Jorge/Wexner Continence score is outlined in Table 1 (4).

TABLE 1 ■ Jorge/Wexner Continence Grading Scale (0 = Perfect; 20 = Complete Incontinence)

Type of Incontinence	Never	Rarely	Sometimes	Usually	Always
Solid	0	1	2	3	4
Liquid	0	1	2	3	4
Gas	0	1	2	3	4
Wears pad	0	1	2	3	4
Lifestyle alteration	0	1	2	3	4

The continence score is determined by adding points from the table, which takes into account the type of frequency of incontinence and the extent to which it alters the patient's life.
Never = 0 (never); rarely = <1/mo; sometimes = <1/day, ≥1/mo; usually = <1/day, ≥1/wk; always = ≥1/day.

In some summary systems, equal values are assigned to the same frequencies of the different types of incontinence, whereas in other scales variable weights are given. However, the lack of patient perspective in this assignment of values limits the comparability and validity of these summary scales. To address this problem, Rockwood et al. developed the Fecal Incontinence Severity Index (FISI). This index assigns values to various frequencies and types of incontinence on the basis of subjective ratings of severity (5). The matrix includes four types of leakage commonly found in the fecal incontinent population: gas, mucus, and liquid and solid stool, and five frequencies: never, one to three times per month, once per week, twice per week, once per day, and twice per day. Overall patient and surgeon ratings of severity are similar with minor differences associated with the accidental loss of solid stool. Weightings for each of the above categories by patient and surgeon are shown in Table 2.

Given the subjective nature of incontinence, the incorporation of patient values into severity measurement has been a major step forward. Although it is important to know the severity of fecal incontinence, it is also important to measure the impact of incontinence and its treatment on quality of life. To assess quality of life for patients with fecal incontinence, generic quality of life scales such as the SF-36 and condition-specific scales such as the Fecal Incontinence Quality of Life Scale (FIQLS) can be used (6). The FIQLS has been developed by the American Society of Colon and Rectal Surgery. This instrument has been studied well and seems to be very useful.

The FIQLS is composed of a total of 29 items; these items form four scales: Lifestyle (10 items), coping/behavior (9 items), depression/self-perception (7 items), and embarrassment (3 items). Detailed questions are listed in Table 3.

Each of the four scales of the FIQLS is capable of discriminating between patients with fecal incontinence and patients with other gastrointestinal problems. The scales in the FIQLS demonstrated significant correlations with the subscales in the SF-36. The psychometric evaluation of the FIQLS showed that this fecal incontinence–specific quality of life measure produces both reliable and valid measurement. Major incontinence has considerable social consequences and demands an effort at some form of definitive therapy.

The exact incidence of fecal incontinence is unknown. An estimated 2% to 7% of adults are affected with this disorder (7). Groups of individuals at high risk for incontinence include the elderly, the mentally ill, institutionalized patients, those with neurologic disorders, and parous women. The prevalence of fecal incontinence in the community has been estimated as 4.2 per 1000 in men aged 15 to 64 years, 10.9 per 1000 in men aged 65 years or older, 1.7 per 1000 in women aged 15 to 64 years, and 13.3 per 1000 in women aged 65 years or older (8). In a study of community-residing women in The Netherlands, Kok et al. (9) found that 4.2% of women aged 60 to 84 years and 16.9% aged 85 years and older were fecally incontinent. Kemp and Acheson (10) found a prevalence of 9.1% in women older than 75 years of age. Of healthy people aged over 65, who still live in their own home, 7% have fecal incontinence at least once a week or need to wear a pad (11).

In hospitalized geriatric and psychiatric patients, an incidence of 26% and 31%, respectively, has been reported (12). In 30 residential homes for the elderly, fecal incontinence occurred at least once weekly in 10.3% of the residents, of whom 94% had evidence of organic brain damage (13). Thirty-nine percent of Wisconsin nursing home residents have fecal incontinence (14), while a 46% incidence was reported from a Canadian long-term hospital (15). Incontinence of stool is the second most common cause for institutionalizing an elderly person (16,17).

Nelson et al. (14) conducted a community-based study in Wisconsin to determine the prevalence of and characteristics associated with anal incontinence in the general community. The presence of anal incontinence to solid or liquid feces or gas, who suffered from it, the frequency of anal incontinence, and the patient's coping techniques were the main outcome measures.

A total of 2570 households comprising 6959 individuals were surveyed, and 153 individuals (2.2% of the population studied) were reported to have anal incontinence. Thirty

TABLE 2 ■ Surgeon and Patient Ratings of Fecal Incontinence

	Two or More Times per Day		Once a Day		Two or More Times per Week		Once a Week		One to Three Times per Month		Never	
	Patient	Surgeon	Patient	Surgeon	Patient	Surgeon	Patient	Surgeon	Patient	Surgeon	Patient	Surgeon
Gas	12	9	11	8	8	6	6	4	4	2	0	0
Mucus	12	11	10	9	7	7	5	7	3	5	0	0
Liquid	19	18	17	16	13	14	10	13	8	10	0	0
Solid	18	19	16	17	13	16	10	14	8	11	0	0

The various weightings assigned by patients and colorectal surgeons are listed. For the calculation of the FISI score, responses have been coded so that a higher score indicates greater severity, e.g., 1 = least severe condition and 20 = most severe condition. Severity scores ranged from 0 to 61 when using the recommended patient-derived weights and from 0 to 59 when using the surgeon-derived weights.

TABLE 3 ■ Items in the Fecal Incontinence Quality of Life Scale

Scale 1: Lifestyle
- I cannot do many of the things I want to do (agreement, 4 points)
- I am afraid to go out (frequency, 4 points)
- It is important to plan my schedule (daily activities) around my bowel pattern (frequency, 4 points)
- I cut down on how much I eat before I go out (frequency, 4 points)
- It is difficult for me to get out and do things like going to a movie or church (frequency, 4 points)
- I avoid traveling by plane or train (agreement, 4 points)
- I avoid traveling (frequency, 4 points)
- I avoid visiting friends (frequency, 4 points)
- I avoid going out to eat (agreement, 4 points)
- I avoid staying overnight away from home (frequency, 4 points)

Scale 2: Coping behavior
- I have sex less often than I would like to (agreement, 4 points)
- The possibility of bowel accidents is always on my mind (agreement, 4 points)
- I feel I have no control over my bowels (frequency, 4 points)
- Whenever I go somewhere new, I specifically locate where the bathrooms are (agreement, 4 points)
- I worry about not being able to get to the toilet in time (frequency, 4 points)
- I worry about the bowel accidents (agreement, 4 points)
- I try to prevent bowel accidents by staying very near a bathroom (agreement, 4 points)
- I can't hold my bowel movement long enough to get to the bathroom (frequency, 4 points)
- Whenever I am away from home I try to stay near a restroom as much as possible (frequency, 4 points)

Scale 3: Depression
- In general, would you say your health is (excellent–poor 5 points)
- I am afraid to have sex (agreement, 4 points)
- I feel different from other people (agreement, 4 points)
- I enjoy life less (agreement, 4 points)
- I feel like I am not a healthy person (agreement, 4 points)
- I feel depressed (agreement, 4 points)
- During the past month, have you felt so sad, discouraged, hopeless, or had so many problems that you wondered if anything was worthwhile? (extremely so–not at all, 6 points)

Scale 4: Embarrassment
- I leak stool without even knowing it (frequency, 4 points)
- I worry about others smelling stool on me (agreement, 4 points)
- I feel ashamed (agreement, 4 points)

Note: Scoring is calculated by addition of each of the individual items.

percent of the incontinent subjects were older than 65 years of age and 63% were women. Of those with anal incontinence, 36% were incontinent to solid feces, 54% to liquid feces, and 60% to gas. Ten percent had more than one episode of incontinence a week, 33% had restricted their activities due to incontinence, 18% wore protective undergarments, and 36% had consulted a physician about the problem. Independent risk factors for incontinence include female sex, advancing age, poor general health, and physical limitations.

Macmillan et al. (18) conducted a systematic review to investigate fecal incontinence in the community. A total of 16 studies met the inclusion criteria. These could be grouped into the definitions of incontinence that included or excluded incontinence of flatus. The estimated prevalence of anal incontinence (including flatus incontinence) varied from 2% to 24%, and the estimated prevalence of fecal incontinence (excluding flatus incontinence) varied from 0.4% to 18%. The prevalence estimate of fecal incontinence from these studies was 11% to 15%.

Most discussions of etiology of anal incontinence have been based on the assumption that women, particularly women younger than 65 years of age, are more at risk for anal incontinence than men. Obstetric injury to the pudendal nerve or sphincter muscle is described as the primary risk factor, irritable bowel syndrome as second (a disease thought to be more prevalent in women), and other etiologies such as diabetes were listed as a distant third (14). Yet, each population-based survey of anal incontinence prevalence, including that by Nelson et al. (14) has shown a high prevalence in men. Clearly, etiologies other than childbirth must be sought.

Johanson and Lafferty (19) conducted a community-based study to determine the prevalence of what they termed "the silent affliction." Their study comprised two populations: 586 individuals evaluated during a visit to their primary care physician and 295 individuals assessed during a visit to a gastroenterologist. The authors defined incontinence as any involuntary leakage of stool or soiling of undergarments. The overall prevalence of fecal incontinence was 18.4%. When stratified by frequency, 2.7%, 4.5%, and 7.1% of participants admitted to episodes of incontinence daily, weekly, or once a month or less, respectively. The prevalence for individuals younger than 30 years of age was 12.7%, compared with 19.4% in those older than 70 years. Fecal incontinence was 1.3 times more common in men. Only one-third of those with fecal incontinence had ever discussed the problem with a physician. The authors believe that the wide variation in prevalence rates may be due to a variation in the definition of incontinence as well as in a disparity in the methods of data collection.

In an excellent review of the subject, Sangwan and Coller (17) detail the tremendous socioeconomic and psychologic burden of fecal incontinence on society. Their comprehensive but often not discussed list of concerns includes the annual cost to patient, the prevention and management of skin breakdown, the increased incidence of female genital infection, social alienation, a personal sense of inadequacy with depression, pessimism, and low self-esteem, embarrassment about odor, and fear of coital incontinence with decreased libido and sexual dysfunction. The combination of these factors produces a social impact that is impossible to quantitate. In a long-term care hospital, it was estimated that the annual cost of incontinence per patient was $9771 (15). It is reported that over $400,000,000 is spent each year for adult diapers to control incontinence (19). In the United States, the economic impact has been estimated at $16 to $26 billion annually (7).

Therapeutic recommendations for incontinence can be made best when the anatomy and physiology of the anorectal region are understood. (See Chapters 1 and 2 on those subjects for review.)

ETIOLOGY

The exact percentage of incontinence attributable to each of the various causes is unknown. In one series, the most common causes of fecal incontinence were injury sustained to muscles and nerves during operation (48%) and peripheral nerve injuries associated with systemic disease such as diabetes. Spinal cord injuries or defects involving spinal cord injuries accounted for 22% of cases (20). In most series, obstetric and operative injuries account for most cases of incontinence (21,22). The variation often depends on the type of referral practice and the special interests of the authors.

■ PREVIOUS OPERATIVE PROCEDURES

Previous Anal Operations

Lindsey (23) characterized the patterns of anal sphincter injury in 93 patients with fecal incontinence after manual dilatation, internal sphincterotomy, fistulotomy, and hemorrhoidectomy. The internal sphincter was almost universally injured, in a pattern specific to the underlying procedure. One-third of patients had a related surgical external sphincter injury. Two-thirds of women had an unrelated obstetric external sphincter injury. The distal resting pressure was typically reduced with reversal of the normal resting pressure gradient of the anal canal in 89% of patients. Maximum squeeze pressure was normal in 52%. They concluded incontinence after anal operations are characterized by the virtually universal presence of an internal sphincter injury, which is distal to the high-pressure zone, resulting in reversal of the normal resting pressure gradient in the anal canal.

Internal Sphincterotomy

Lateral internal sphincterotomy is highly effective in the treatment of chronic anal fissure. However, this procedure results in a permanent defect in the internal anal sphincter, which may lead to impairment of fecal continence. The exact incidence of this complication is not known. During the first two decades, after the introduction of lateral internal sphincterotomy, several studies have been conducted, aimed at evaluating the sequelae of this procedure. Impaired continence was observed in only a minority of the patients, most of them having temporary incontinence to flatus. In these retrospective studies, the patients were followed by chart review or telephone interview and not by mailed questionnaire. The duration of the follow-up was short. Grading scales and quality of life scales were not used. More recent reviews, emphasizing the importance of long-term follow-up, have shown higher incontinence rates. In the series of Khubchandani and Reed, lack of control of flatus was the most common complaint (35%), followed by soiling of underclothing (22%) and accidental bowel movements (5%) (24). A significantly higher proportion of patients who had accidental bowel movements were aged over 40 years. Similar figures have been reported by Garcia-Aguilar et al. (25). A significant lower incidence of continence disturbances has been reported by others. Pernikoff et al. observed an overall incidence of 8% (26). In their series of 265 patients, Hananel and Gordon encountered impairment of continence in 1.2% of the patients, most of them having only temporarily problems (27). In a prospective study among 35 patients, Hyman assessed continence prior to and six weeks after lateral internal sphincterotomy using the FISI (28). The FIQLS was administered to patients with a FISI score >0. Three patients had worsening of their FISI score after surgery. Only one of them reported an evident deterioration in FIQLS. Based on these data, the author concluded that lateral internal sphincterotomy is a safe procedure. Anecdotal reports illustrate that incontinence for solid stool, although very rare, can occur after lateral internal sphincterotomy. This complication is often attributed to division of an excessive amount of internal anal sphincter or inadvertent injury to the external anal sphincter.

Coexisting occult defects of the external anal sphincter in multiparous women seem to be another risk factor (29). When comparing office records and response to a postal survey, Zutshi et al. found that significantly more patients had incontinence to gas after lateral internal sphincterotomy than that reported in their medical records. This problem was encountered by 29% of the multiparous female patients who underwent this procedure. Incontinece for solid stool was not observed. Among their patients, the overall quality of life scores were in the normal range (30). Sultan et al. performed anal endosonography before and two months after lateral internal sphincterotomy. They found that this procedure in most females tends to be more extensive than intended in contrast to division of the internal anal sphincter in males. According to the authors, this is probably related to the shorter anal canal in females. They also found that lateral internal sphincterotomy may further compromise continence, especially in females with occult sphincter defects (31).

Fistula Surgery

Fistula surgery is the anorectal procedure most commonly followed by postoperative incontinence. Gross incontinence of feces generally may be avoided if the anorectal ring is preserved. However, minor defects in continence may follow if even a small amount of sphincter muscle is severed. This complication can be reduced by avoiding wide separation of the severed ends of the sphincter mechanism. This goal is accomplished either by placing a seton or by "coring out" the fistulous tract, with subsequent sparing of the sphincter mechanism or, in the case of tracts crossing the sphincter mechanism at a high level, by the adoption of the advancement flap technique (see Chapter 10).

Although this transanal advancement flap repair is designed to minimize damage to the anal sphincters, impairment of continence after this procedure has been documented. The reported incidence of this complication varies between 8% and 35% (32–35). It has been suggested that anal stretch caused by the use of a Parks' retractor is a major contributing factor (36). Recently it has been demonstrated that the use of a Parks' retractor has indeed a deteriorating effect on fecal continence.

Because this side effect is not observed after the use of a Scott retractor, this type of retractor has been advised in fistula repairs (37).

Hemorrhoidectomy

In modern surgery for hemorrhoids, incontinence is a rare complication. However, if the sphincter mass is inadvertently injured (e.g., in a blind-clamping technique in which the internal sphincter is grasped by a clamp), incontinence may result. Minor alterations in continence may be due to the removal of the hemorrhoidal tissue, a tissue that has been described as possibly functioning as a corpus cavernosum of the anus (38). When incorrectly performed, the Whitehead operation leads to eversion of the rectal mucosa onto the anoderm. This abnormal anatomy results in incontinence through destruction of the normal sensory mechanism and mucosal leak from the exposed mucosal surface onto the perineum. Rarely, a circumferential scar will form after hemorrhoidectomy. It may lead to improper closure of the anal canal, causing partial incontinence.

Manual Dilatation of Anus

Forceful dilatation of the anal canal for the treatment of any anorectal pathology can result in varying degrees of incontinence. The disadvantages and consequences of this form of treatment are discussed fully in Chapter 9.

Sphincter-Saving Procedures

In the usual anterior resection, normal continence for flatus, liquid, or solid feces is generally maintained. However, when the anastomosis is performed in the distal-third of the rectum, impairment of normal continence is not unusual. Incontinence of liquid or flatus often follows, and the patient may be unaware of a sudden bolus of stool. These problems are frequent in the early postoperative period, but they subside within six months in the great majority of patients. The lower limit at which an anastomosis can be created without interfering with the gross mechanism of incontinence is the uppermost level of the anal canal at the top of the anorectal ring, which in most individuals is approximately 4 cm from the anal verge. Introduction of the circular stapler has made it technically possible to perform extremely low rectal anastomoses. However, if the anorectal ring is disturbed, partial or total incontinence may result. The severity and duration of the dysfunction are not predictable.

Goligher et al. (39) reported that of 62 patients who underwent a low anterior resection, all of the 12 patients with the anastomosis less than 7 cm from the anal verge initially had less than perfect continence. With time, however, 5 developed perfect continence and three nearly perfect continence, but four remained with imperfect continence. In a series of 143 stapled low anterior resections performed by the senior author (40), temporary incontinence was encountered in one patient who had an anastomosis performed 7 cm from the anal verge. It resolved spontaneously within 1 month.

Abdominoanal pull-through resection of the rectum, as popularized by Hughes, results in a high incidence of partial incontinence. In a review of his results with this procedure, he found that only 29% of the patients had normal function postoperatively, 23% had severe incontinence, and the remaining 48% had minor incontinence (41).

Parks and Percy (42) described a coloanal sleeve anastomosis for the treatment of rectal lesions. Of 70 patients who underwent this operation, one was incontinent, whereas 30 others experienced increased frequency of stool. Enker et al. (43) reported that 64% of patients who could be evaluated in their series of 41 patients who underwent coloanal anastomosis had good or excellent function. Vernava et al. (44) reported that 87% of their 16 patients were normally continent.

After ileorectal and ileoanal anastomosis, varying degrees of incontinence may develop. In the former case, the cause is usually the loss of reservoir function, but the situation may be compounded by a weakened sphincter. In the latter case, intraoperative manipulation by necessity may stretch the sphincter mechanism.

■ CHILDBIRTH

Fecal incontinence has a female to male preponderance of 8:1, consistent with childbirth as the principal causative factor.

In 1993 Sultan et al. published their well-known article, entitled "anal sphincter disruption during vaginal delivery." In their paper they described the results of an endosonographic study among 79 primiparous women. Endoanal ultrasound was performed 6 weeks before and 6 months after routine vaginal delivery. After childbirth, sphincter defects were detected in 35% of these females. A similar study was performed in 23 primiparous women, who underwent a cesarean section. None of these women had a sphincter defect after delivery (45). During the last decade, much attention has been focused on this subject. In a study by Eason et al. (46) of 949 pregnant women 3 months after delivery, 3.1% reported incontinence of stool and 25.5% had involuntary escape of flatus. Incontinence of stool was more frequent among women who delivered vaginally and had third- or fourth-degree perineal tears than among those who delivered vaginally and had no anal sphincter tears (7.8% vs. 2.9%). Forceps delivery (relative risk = 1.45) and sphincter tears (relative risk = 2.09) were independent risk factors for incontinence of flatus or stool or both. Anal sphincter injury was strongly and independently associated with first vaginal births (relative risk = 39.2), median episiotomy (relative risk = 9.6), forceps delivery (relative risk = 12.3), and vacuum-assisted delivery (relative risk = 7.4), but not with birth weight (relative risk for birth weight 4000 g or more = 1.4) or length of stage of the second labor (relative risk for second stage 1.5 hours or longer compared with less than 0.5 hours = 1.2).

The reported incidence of occult sphincter defects after normal vaginal delivery varies between 7% and 41% (Table 4).

Oberwalder et al. conducted a meta-analysis in order to determine the incidence of anal sphincter defects after

TABLE 4 ■ Incidence of Occult Sphincter Defects After Normal Vaginal Delivery in Primiparous Women

Author(s)	Year	No. of Subjects	Occult Sphincter Defects (%)
Sultan et al. (45)	1993	79	35
Campbell et al. (47)	1996	88	13
Rieger et al. (48)	1998	53	41
Zetterstrom et al. (49)	1999	38	20
Varma et al. (50)	1999	105	7
Fynes et al. (51)	1999	59	34
Faltin et al. (52)	2000	150	28
Damon et al. (53)	2000	197	34
Abramowitz et al. (54)	2000	202	17
Chaliha et al. (55)	2001	161	38
Belmonte-Montes et al. (56)	2001	98	29
Willis et al. (57)	2002	42	19
Nazir et al. (58)	2002	86	19
Peschers et al. (59)	2004	100	15

vaginal delivery. Their medline search yielded five studies with more than 100 women who underwent endoanal ultrasonography after childbirth. All these women were also questioned about symptoms of fecal incontinence, not including urgency. The incidence of sphincter defects in primiparous women was found to be 27%. In multiparous women, the incidence of new sphincter defects was 8.5%. Overall, 30% of the defects were symptomatic. Only 3% of the women experienced impairment of continence without any sphincter defects. Based on the results of this study, it is clear that sphincter damage during vaginal delivery is quite common in primiparous women. In 70% of these women, the sphincter defects are asymptomatic in the postpartum period (60). The question is whether women with an occult and asymptomatic sphincter defect are at increased risk for fecal incontinence with aging. According to Rieger and Wattchow, it seems likely that many women remain asymptomatic, because the number of occult sphincter defects is far greater than the documented prevalence of fecal incontinence in the community (61). Recently, Oberwalder et al. examined elderly females with late-onset incontinence. All these women had experienced vaginal delivery earlier in life. The authors observed sphincter defects in more than 70% of their patients (62). A similar finding has been reported by others (63). Despite these findings, it is still not possible to determine the exact risk for asymptomatic women with a sphincter defect to develop fecal incontinence later in life. More studies, including control groups of equal parity and age, are mandatory. During the last decade, attention has also been focused on the risk factors for obstetric sphincter defects. Donnelly et al. conducted a prospective study among primiparous women. After cesarian section, even when performed late in labor, none of the women experienced impairment of continence. Neither induction of labor nor its augmentation with oxytocin influenced the risk of sphincter injury or postpartum impairment of continence. Instrumental delivery was associated with a more than eightfold increased risk of anal sphincter damage and a more than sevenfold increased risk of symptoms when compared with unassisted delivery (64). The increased risk of sphincter defects after instrumental vaginal delivery, especially after the use of a forceps, has also been reported by others (Table 5). A recent study, however, does not confirm the previous observations that anal sphincter injury is common after forceps delivery. De Parades et al. observed sphincter defects in only 13% of 93 females after their first forceps delivery. According to the authors, this observation gives support to the conclusion that forceps delivery is still a safe technique (68). However, recruitment bias might be a possible explanation for their contradictory finding, because 60% of their patients did not return for postpartum assessment. Except for this single study, all other reports provide substantial evidence for the detrimental effect of forceps delivery on anal sphincter integrity.

Anal incontinence among primiparous women increases over time and is affected by further childbirth (70). Anal incontinence at nine months postpartum is an important predictor of persistent symptoms. In the study by Pollack et al. (70), among women with sphincter tears, 44% reported anal incontinence at 9 months and 53% at 5 years. Twenty-five percent of women without a sphincter tear reported anal incontinence at 9 months, and 32% had symptoms at 5 years. Risk factors for anal incontinence at five years were age (odds ratio = 1.1), sphincter tear (odds ratio = 2.3), and subsequent childbirth (odds ratio = 2.4). As a predictor of anal incontinence at 5 years after the first delivery, anal incontinence at both 5 months (odds ratio = 3.8) and 9 months (odds ratio = 4.3) was identified. Among women with symptoms, the majority had infrequent incontinence to flatus, whereas fecal incontinence was rare.

TABLE 5 ■ **Incidence of Sphincter Defects After Various Modes of Delivery**

Author(s)	Year	Unassisted (%)	Vacuum (%)	Forceps (%)	Cesarean Section (%)
Sultan et al. (65)	1998	NS	48	81	0
Varma et al. (50)	1999	12	NS	83	NS
Abramowitz et al. (66)	2000	NS	NS	63	0
Damon et al. (53)	2000	29	NS	44	NS
Belmonte-Montes et al. (56)	2001	16	50	76	NS
Bollard et al. (67)	2003	22	NS	44	0
Peschers et al. (59)	2003	10	28	NS	NS
De Parades et al. (68)	2004	NS	NS	13	NS
Pinta et al. (69)	2004	23	45	NS	0

Abbreviation: NS, not stated.

Besides instrumental delivery, other obstetric events are also associated with an increased risk of anal sphincter injury. Prolongation of the second stage of labor due to epidural analgesia, midline episiotomy, and perineal tears are well known independent risk factors. After primary repair of third- or fourth-degree perineal tears, persistent sphincter defects have been reported in up to 85% of the cases (71,72). Nine months after primary repair of perineal tears, Pollack et al. observed impairment of continence in 44% of the women. Five years later 53% of the women suffered from continence disturbances (70). These findings indicate that the damage sustained during third- and fourth-degree tears is much greater than is generally appreciated. Furthermore, it is clear that primary repair does not provide lasting integrity of the anal sphincters. Fernando et al. conducted a systemic review and a national practice survey regarding the management of obstetric anal sphincter injury. They identified 11 studies with long-term follow-up (mean duration: 41 months) after primary repair of third-degree tears. In these studies symptoms of fecal incontinence were reported by 20% to 59% of the women (73).

Sze (74) found the proportion of women who had severe incontinence was significantly higher among women who had undergone at least two additional deliveries after sustaining a fourth-degree sphincter tear as a nullipara. Sze (75) also found the rate of anal incontinence and severe incontinence similar among women who had zero, one, and two or more additional deliveries after sustaining a third-degree perineal laceration and between women who had one sphincter tear and no additional delivery versus those with two tears and more than two subsequent deliveries.

Increasing awareness amongst women and health professionals about the sequelae of obstetric sphincter injury has given rise to a debate regarding the protective role of cesarean delivery.

It has been shown that elective cesarean section at term before the onset of labor protects the anal sphincters and prevents fecal incontinence (76,77). Although cesarean section, performed during labor, also protects the anal sphincters, it does not prevent fecal incontinence. This finding indicates neurologic injury to the sphincters during labor. Fynes et al. (77) followed nulliparous women through two successive vaginal deliveries. A surprising number of women (22%) experienced alteration in fecal continence following their first delivery with eight patients (14%) having persistent symptoms during their second pregnancy. Seven of these eight patients further deteriorated during their second delivery and two of the eight patients who originally recovered became incontinent after their second delivery, whereas another five women developed incontinence for the first time after their second delivery; three of these five women had occult primiparous sphincter injury. Overall, 20 (34%) women, seven of whom had no symptoms, had an anal sphincter injury as a result of their first delivery and two new injuries occurred after the second vaginal delivery. Forty-two percent of women with occult anal sphincter injury during their first delivery developed symptoms of fecal incontinence after a second vaginal delivery.

It is certainly noteworthy that women with transient fecal incontinence or occult sphincter injury after their first delivery are at higher risk of fecal incontinence after a second delivery, but from a practical point of view no change of obstetrical recommendation will be made as women will not be advised to avoid having children based on this information nor would it seem reasonable to recommend a cesarean section on the basis of fear of further alteration in continence. Despite the potential for cumulative sphincter injury or pudendal neuropathy, help is available for those individuals who suffer sphincter damage, and it must be remembered that cesarean section has its own potential immediate complications for mother and baby as well as possible late complications of a laparotomy such as adhesive small-bowel obstruction. Modifying this course of action may be the recognition that injury during the second delivery is primarily neurological with prolonged pudendal nerve terminal motor latency (PNTML). Intra-anal ultrasound has recently been touted as the most accurate method of determining occult injury to the sphincter mechanism, but in the absence of symptoms, a battery of investigative modalities that include intrarectal ultrasound, anorectal manometry, and PNTLML would not likely enthusiastically be endorsed by most postpartum women. Nevertheless, understanding the potential for injury is useful knowledge for the clinician.

Previous Hysterectomy

Patients undergoing abdominal hysterectomy may run an increased risk for developing mild-to-moderate anal incontinence postoperatively, and this risk is increased by simultaneous bilateral salpingo-oophorectomy. In a study by Altman et al. (78), an increased risk of anal incontinence symptoms could not be identified in patients undergoing vaginal hysterectomy.

■ AGING

A very common form of anal incontinence is that associated with old age and general debilitation. Elderly patients with a long-standing history of straining at defecation may cause a stretch injury to the pudendal nerve as well. This often is described as incontinence of neurogenic origin.

■ PROCIDENTIA

In the case of procidentia or complete rectal prolapse, the internal and external sphincter mechanisms may be chronically impaired. Procidentia is associated with incontinence in more than 50% of cases (79). The incontinence has been attributed in part to nerve injury (80). Repair of the procidentia results in improvement of the incontinence in approximately 50% of the patients. Various treatments have been applied in the past, including waiting and hoping that sphincter tone would return, electrical stimulation of the sphincter mechanisms, and various plicating operations.

None of these methods has met with uniform success. Even the well-known Parks postanal repair is not always useful. Biofeedback might be worthwhile in the treatment of persistent incontinence after repair of rectal prolapse. If biofeedback fails, sacral neuromodulation (SNM) is an alternative (81). If incontinence remains a problem, a colostomy is the final option.

■ TRAUMA

In the case of impalement injuries, the sphincter mechanism is often disrupted. Depending on the extent of the injury, primary repair may be achieved without performing a protective colostomy. However, if the tissues are badly destroyed and there has been a delay in recognition, performing a protective colostomy with later definitive repair is preferable. Insertion of foreign bodies or deviant sexual practices may result in sphincter injury.

■ PRIMARY DISEASE

Diarrheal states from any cause at times may overwhelm the normal continence mechanisms and result in temporary transient episodes of anal incontinence. Chronic inflammatory processes of the anorectal region, such as those that occur in patients with ulcerative colitis, amebic colitis, lymphogranuloma venereum, progressive systemic sclerosis, infections, or laxative abuse, can result in local sensory derangement, interference of the sphincter mechanism, and/or mucosal irritability, resulting in a loss of the rectal reservoir function.

A patient with carcinoma of the anal canal may also present with incontinence caused by either infiltration into the sphincter mechanism or failure of the anal canal to close adequately.

■ IRRADIATION

With the treatment of cervical and uterine carcinomas by extracavitary and intracavitary irradiation, varying degrees of destruction of the muscular components of the rectum and anal canal occur, resulting in various degrees of irradiation proctitis. A radiation-induced lumbosacral plexopathy has been reported (82). Although no treatment of irradiation-induced incontinence is uniformly rewarding, two or three daily cleansing enemas are generally recommended along with a high-bulk diet. If the condition becomes intolerable, colostomy is the last recourse. If severe bleeding remains a problem, therapeutic options include the topical application of short-chain fatty acids or 4% formalin. Laser therapy may also prove helpful. In recalcitrant cases, proctectomy may be necessary.

NEUROGENIC CAUSES

In cases of myelomeningocele, the nerve supply, both sensory and motor, is disturbed in a variety of ways, leading to various forms of incontinence. Any form of trauma, neoplasm, vascular accident, infection, or demyelinating disease to the central nervous system or spinal cord can interfere with normal sensation or motor function, leading to incontinence.

Diabetic patients with autonomic neuropathy may have impaired reflex relaxation of the internal sphincter (83). Diabetics with fecal incontinence have a higher threshold of conscious sensation than continent diabetic patients. Late onset of rectal sensation is one cause of anal incontinence in diabetics. Pintor et al. (84) reported that somatic neuropathy plays an important role in fecal incontinence in diabetic patients, combined with sensation threshold impairment as a feature of autonomic involvement.

IDIOPATHIC INCONTINENCE

After the introduction of endoanal ultrasound, it is now possible to identify those incontinent patients who have a sphincter defect. Disruption of the external anal sphincter is the most common surgically correctable cause of fecal incontinence. The prevalence of sphincter defects in patients with fecal incontinence has been assessed with the use of endoanal ultrasound. Deen et al. examined 42 women and 4 men with fecal incontinence. They found sphincter defects in 87% of their patients (85). Karoui et al. observed sphincter defects in 65% of 335 incontinent patients (86). Comparable figures have been reported by others (87,88). Based on these data it is obvious that sphincter defects are present in at least two-thirds of incontinent patients. Less than one-third of the patients do not have any evidence of sphincter defects or other anorectal abnormalities. Their incontinence, formerly termed "idiopathic," is thought to be secondary to pudendal neuropathy, characterized by a slowed conduction in the pudendal nerve. It is most likely that this prolonged latency is due to stretching of the nerve during straining. The question is whether this pudendal neuropathy is the principal cause of "idiopathic" incontinence or not. Ó Súilleabháin and coworkers reported a prolonged latency in only 60% of the incontinent patients without sphincter defects. Furthermore, they were not able to demonstrate a correlation between the PNTML and the maximum squeeze pressure in this group of patients. According to these authors, the etiology of "idiopathic" incontinence is more complex than damage to the pudendal nerve alone. This nerve is probably not the only one to sustain trauma during vaginal delivery. Neuropathic changes in the internal anal sphincter and abnormal sensation in the anal canal as well as in the rectum have been observed in patients with "idiopathic" incontinence. These findings indicate that the neurologic damage associated with vaginal delivery is not limited to the pudendal nerve, but may also involve damage to the autonomic inferior hypogastric nerves (89–91).

CONGENITAL ABNORMALITIES

The various operative procedures designed for treating an imperforate anus are based on the type of deformity. The ultimate goal is to establish a perineal opening with adequate sensory and motor control. Rarely are sensory mechanisms preserved; therefore some defect in continence usually results. Gross incontinence usually can be avoided by careful placement of the colon or rectum through residual sphincter mechanisms (i.e., the puborectalis sling).

MISCELLANEOUS

Overflow secondary to fecal impaction is a frequent cause of incontinence. This problem often is missed because the patient complains of profuse diarrhea. Digital examination usually reveals a rectum full of stool. This problem generally occurs in elderly, in debilitated patients, or in patients and young children recovering from surgical procedures (usually anorectal). Thus physicians must be aware of this potential problem and should routinely institute early preventive measures. In general, hospital patients should be administered a bulk-forming stool softener of a psyllium seed derivative. If impaction occurs, gentle enemas with a combination of tap water, phosphate soda, and hydrogen peroxide may be used. If these measures fail, disimpaction (either with or without administering anesthesia) is the treatment of choice.

In patients with diarrhea, from whatever cause, the normal mechanisms of continence may be overwhelmed, and the patient may experience incontinence.

Soiling rather than complete involuntary loss of rectal contents may occur. For example, large prolapsing third- or fourth-degree hemorrhoids can cause partial incontinence by interfering with the normal closure mechanism of the internal sphincter. This can result in the escape of either flatus or liquid feces or in mucosal irritation. After operations for fistula-in-ano or fissures, soiling may occur as well.

A variety of pelvic floor disorders, including descending perineum syndrome, solitary rectal ulcer syndrome, and a nonrelaxing puborectalis muscle, may be associated with varying degrees of incontinence. Psychiatric problems may predispose the patient to the clinical problem of fecal incontinence.

DIAGNOSIS

HISTORY

As in the investigation of any pathologic condition, obtaining a careful history is necessary. Indeed, treatment recommendations are based on the particular cause of the incontinence together with the assessment of the sphincter status. Particular attention must be paid to the characteristics of the incontinence. Complete incontinence is defined as the uncontrolled passage of solid feces, whereas partial incontinence is defined as the uncontrolled passage of liquid or flatus. True incontinence should be distinguished from perianal leakage, which may be associated with a variety of anorectal disorders. Incontinence also must be distinguished from urgency, in which the patient's diet or individual bowel habits lead to frequent passage of liquid stool accompanied by a great sense of urgency. In such cases, simple dietary change may be all that is necessary. In addition to consistency, knowing the patient's frequency of bowel movements helps determine whether an antidiarrheal agent is required. Urge incontinence has been reported to be a marker of external anal sphincter dysfunction (92). Female patients should be asked about childbirth and type of delivery. It is very important to know whether the delivery was instrumental assisted or not. It is also necessary to obtain a history with regard to episiotomy, perineal tears, and continence in the postpartum period. The patient also should be asked about associated problems or conditions such as urinary incontinence, prolapsing tissue, diabetes mellitus, medications, or radiation treatment.

Patients with congenital abnormalities such as Hirschsprung's disease generally present with some form of constipation and megacolon. An accurate history is necessary to distinguish the condition from acquired megacolon in the adolescent and adult age groups. In a patient with acquired megacolon, soiling of the perineum from the overflow incontinence often is secondary to fecal impaction. With Hirschsprung's disease, incontinence of liquid or flatus is rare because of the constandy closed internal sphincter.

Whether the patient has had a previous anorectal operation or low colon anastomosis must be noted, because these procedures can lead to anal incontinence. Also, beverages such as coffee or beer can lead to frequent loose bowel movements. Any history of remote or recent trauma to the anorectal area may aid in establishing the cause of incontinence. Associated motor or sensory symptoms may point to a neurologic lesion (93). A clue to the severity of the problem is to determine the frequency of the incontinence and the necessity to wear a protective pad.

Grading and scoring the severity of the problem is another important aspect a careful history. It is worthwhile to know the severity of fecal incontinence as well as the impact of this problem and its treatment on the quality of life. Several aspects of grading scales and quality of life scales are discussed in more detail on page 295.

■ PHYSICAL EXAMINATION

It must be noted whether a patient's incontinence is a manifestation of a generalized disease or neurologic disorder or whether it is a local phenomenon. Undergarments should be inspected for staining by stool, mucus, or pus. In addition, the perineum must be inspected. In female patients with a history of vaginal delivery, it is helpful to measure the length of the perineum between anus and vagina. A decreased length of the perineum is frequently associated with a defect of the external anal sphincter. By simple retraction of the gluteal muscles, the large patulous anus that occurs with rectal procidentia can be recognized easily. Also, any large prolapsing hemorrhoids or evidence of pruritus may point to the fact that local anatomic factors may be responsible for the minor soiling by liquid or flatus. Scars from previous operations or episiotomies may also be identified. Sensation to pinprick and the anocutaneous reflex should be checked. The anocutaneous reflex can be checked by stroking the perianal skin and observing the sphincter "wink." On straining, perineal descent or mucosal or full-thickness rectal prolapse may become obvious. Examination while the patient squats may be necessary to demonstrate prolapse.

Digital rectal examination reveals the strength (resting tone and augmentation on squeeze) or discontinuity of the sphincter muscle. Palpation points out any "keyhole" deformity of the anal canal, which might lead to soiling that may be misinterpreted as partial incontinence. The assessment of anal tone is, at best, a very indistinct barometer of sphincter function. The ability to assess the strength of voluntary sphincter contraction is subjective. Contraction of the puborectalis at the tip of the finger versus contraction of the external sphincter over the midportion of the finger may be distinguished. The anorectal angle can be assessed. The patient's complaints should provide a more reliable index of incontinence.

Anoscopic and proctosigmoidoscopic examinations reveal any inflammatory process or neoplasm contributing to the patient's complaint.

Many tests are available for the assessment of fecal incontinence. The need for all those tests has been controversial. In daily practice, most investigations do not influence the choice of treatment. In many centres, for example, the initial steps in the treatment of fecal incontinence consist of medical therapy or biofeedback, irrespective of the underlying cause. However, from a surgical point of view it is essential to know whether the external anal sphincter is damaged or not. Physical examination is unreliable for the detection of sphincter defects. In the past needle electromyography (EMG) has been used to identify defects of the external anal sphincter. The potential discomfort and the inability to identify internal anal sphincter are drawbacks of this type of investigation.

■ SPECIAL INVESTIGATIONS

Anal Endosonography

During the last decade, endoanal ultrasound has supplanted electromyographic mapping. It is easily available and more comfortable for the patient. It has been shown to be superior for the evaluation of sphincter defects with a sensitivity of detecting defects of 100%, compared with 89% for electromyographic mapping, 67% for anorectal manometry, and 56% for physical examination (94). Based on these and other findings, endoanal ultrasound is now considered to be the gold standard as diagnostic tool for the assessment of fecal incontinence (Fig. 1). However, interpretation of ultrasound images of the external anal sphincter is rather subjective, operator dependent, and confounded by normal anatomical variations. Because the external anal sphincter and the perianal fat are both echogenic, it is rather difficult to assess the thickness of the external anal sphincter and to identify atrophy of this muscle. Discrimination of normal variants from sphincter defects is also difficult, especially in the upper part of the anal canal in female patients, due to asymmetry of the external anal sphincter at that level (95). In 75% of asymptomatic nulliparous women, Bollard et al. found a natural gap in the anterior part of the external anal sphincter, just below the

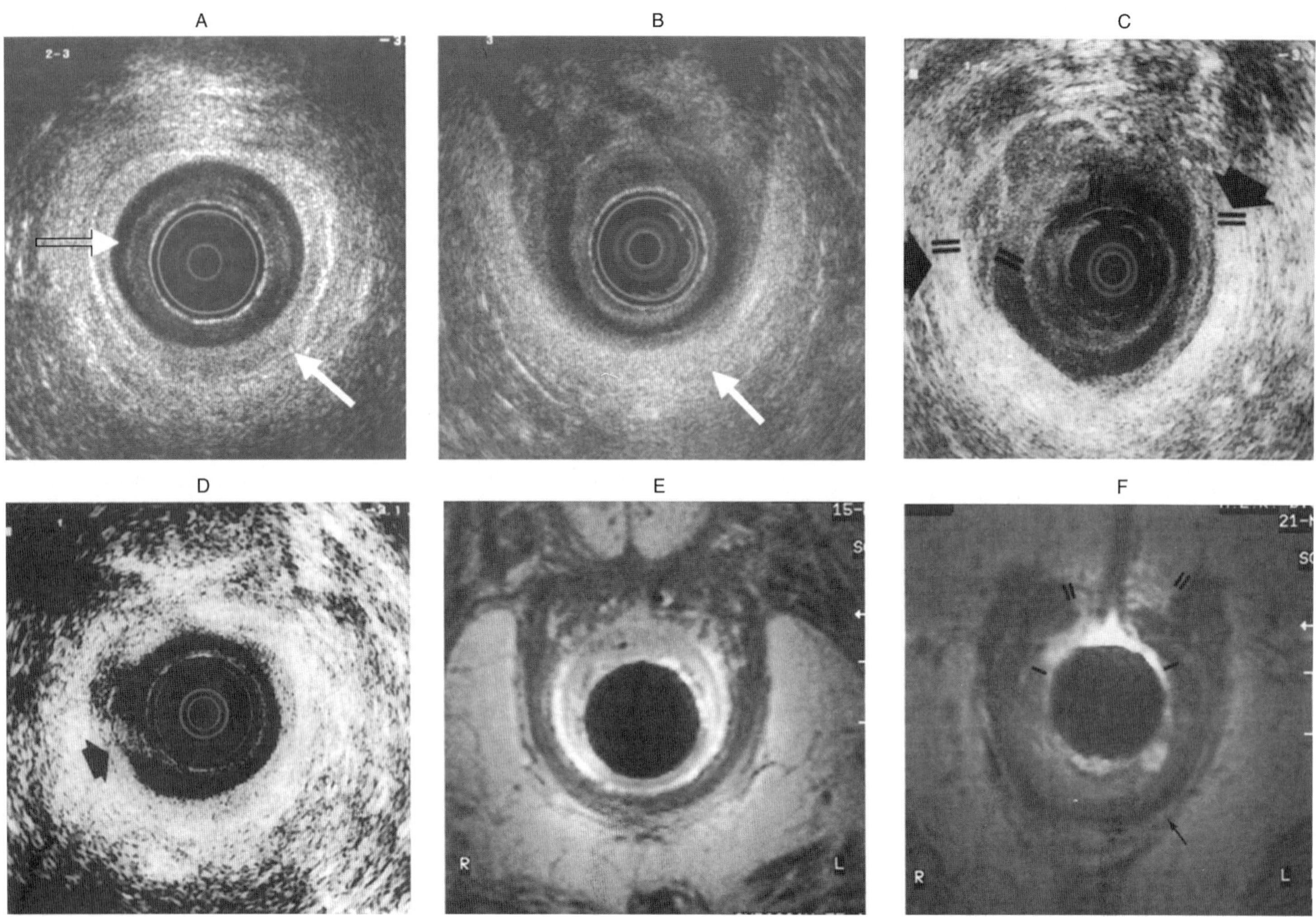

FIGURE 1 ■ Examples of defects demonstrable by endoanal ultrasonography. (**A**) Endoanal ultrasound of the distal part of the anal canal. Internal anal sphincter (*open arrow*) and external anal sphincter (closed arrow). (**B**) Endoanal ultrasound of the proximal part of the anal canal. Puborectal muscle (*closed arrow*). (**C**) Endoanal ultrasonography in patient with fecal incontinence due to obstetric injury. Internal (*black*) and external (*white*) anal sphincter defect. Margins of each defect are outlined (*slashes and arrows*). (**D**) Endoanal ultrasonography in patient presenting with fecal soiling after lateral internal sphincterotomy. Internal (*black*) anal sphincter defect (*arrow*). (**E**) Endoanal magnetic resnonance imaging (MRI) in control subject shows normal internal (*light gray*) and external (*dark gray*) anal sphincter. (**F**) Endoanal MRI in patient with fecal incontinence due to obstetric injury. Internal (*light gray*) anal sphincter defect (*single slashes*) and external (*dark gray*) anal sphincter defect (*double slashes*). Note the rather atrophic external anal sphincter (*arrow*). *Source*: Courtesy of W. Rudolf Schouten, Rotterdam, The Netherlands.

level of the puborectalis sling. According to these authors this gap explains the difficulties in the interpretation of postpartum ultrasounds (96). Sentovich et al. evaluated the accuracy and reliability of endoanal ultrasound for anterior sphincter defects (97). In incontinent, parous women, the sphincter defects, detected by ultrasound, were confirmed at operation in 100% of the cases. A similar accuracy has been reported by others (98). In continent, nulliparous women, the two ultrasonographers identified sphincter defects in 55% and 75%, respectively. This high false-positive rate could be decreased to 40% and 60% by using the video recording of the ultrasounds. The false identification of defects in normal, intact sphincters might be explained by the existence of a natural gap, as described by Bollard et al. It has been suggested that the false-positive rate might be reduced by the measurement of perineal body thickness. Zetterstrom et al. reported that the perineal body thickness was 6 ± 2 mm in patients with an anterior sphincter defect and 12 ± 3 mm in asymptomatic subjects (99). A similar finding has been reported by others (100). Endoanal ultrasound is associated with a substantial interobserver variability with regard to the thickness of the sphincters. It has been shown, however, that the interobserver assessment of sphincter defects is very good (101). Despite several disadvantages, endoanal ultrasound is to date the most optimum diagnostic tool for the assessment of fecal incontinence. The value and clinical relevance of other tests have been questioned. According to some authors most of these investigations lack clinical usefulness because they add little additional information to a complete clinical patient assessment. Furthermore, it is thought to be unlikely that these tests result in a significant alteration in a patient's management plan. Frequently, abnormal values do not correlate with the severity of symptoms. Despite these limitations, several tests are still frequently applied. They have been reported to predict the outcome after medical or surgical treatment, thereby permitting the clinician to provide the patient with sound recommendations and allowing the patient to have realistic expectations (102). In this section the investigations, most frequently used, are highlighted.

The "Enema Challenge"

The simplest and most unsophisticated test for incontinence is administration of an enema. The ability to retain a disposable enema is a very useful clinical guide in the assessment of incontinence. If the patient is able to retain a 100 mL water enema, any surgical correction or prolonged treatment plan is unnecessary. Reassurance that there is not a more serious problem is all that is indicated for such a patient.

Barium Enema

A barium enema will rule out any inflammatory bowel disease or neoplasm, but it is unlikely to contribute to the diagnosis of the source of the incontinence.

Anorectal Manometry

Information derived from manometry includes assessment of the resting and squeeze pressures and the anorectal inhibitory reflex. The presence of the reflex eliminates suspicion of Hirschsprung's disease. Basal pressure is reported to represent mainly the activity of the internal sphincter, and the spontaneous activity of the external sphincter affects maximal basal pressure (103). Squeeze pressure is reported to be the voluntary function of the external sphincter and the pelvic floor muscles (103). If both basal and squeeze pressures are low, patients are prone to be totally incontinent. If only the voluntary function is low, the patients are probably partially incontinent (103). External sphincter function is critical for maintaining continence of solid stool (104).

Penninckx et al. (105) studied the relationship between symptoms and the results of manometric data in incontinent patients. Discriminatory values of greater than 40 mmHg for maximum basal pressure and greater than 92 mmHg for squeeze pressure could identify continent patients with 96% and incontinent patients with 88% accuracy. The uncontrollable evacuation of a balloon, progressively filled with water at 60 mL/min before the maximum tolerable sensation level was reached, was related to the degree of clinical incontinence. Also the maximum retained volume and the interval between the first sensation volume and the maximum retained volume ("perceived rectal capacity") were related to the clinical symptoms. The balloon-retaining test proved to be superior to the rectal saline infusion test for the determination of the severity of incontinence.

Unfortunately, there is a 10% overlap between the manometric values obtained from incontinent and normal persons (104,106). Following childbirth, pudendal nerve damage increases the risk of fecal incontinence in women with anal sphincter rupture, but manometric findings indicate damage to the sphincter apparatus in both continent and incontinent patients (107). However, overlap in anorectal physiologic data between continent and incontinent patients is so great as to make accurate prediction of fecal incontinence impossible. Furthermore, the values do not correlate with the severity of incontinence, nor do they predict postoperative results. No correlation exists between the outcome of the operation and the preoperative anorectal manometric studies (108). Normal manometric findings do not exclude incontinence entirely (103).

In recent years, the relationship between anorectal manometry and endoanal ultrasound has been studied extensively. De Leeuw et al. applied both tests in 34 patients at least 10 years after primary repair of a perineal tear and in 12 asymptomatic women with a history of normal, uncomplicated vaginal delivery. Impaired continence was reported by 22 patients (65%). A persistent sphincter defect was found in 86% of these patients. Because maximum anal squeeze pressure and maximum anal resting pressure showed a considerable overlap between the different groups (with and without impaired continence and with and without a sphincter defect), anorectal manometry provided little additional information (109).

Nazir et al. conducted an observational cohort study among 132 patients after primary repair of a three- or fourth-degree perineal tear. The mean time interval between delivery and evaluation was five months. All women underwent endoanal ultrasound and vector volume manometry. They found no difference in manometric values between females without a defect and those with a less extensive defect. Only in women with a large, extensive defect, the manometric values were significantly lower. Although they observed a correlation between incontinence scores and manometric variables, there was a large overlap between continent and incontinent females regarding manometric values. No cutoff point could be defined to distinguish continent from incontinent females (110). Lieberman et al. designed a study to determine whether anorectal physiology testing alters the management of patients with fecal incontinence. Manometric findings did not change the pretest management plans. No association was found between manometric results and ultrasound findings. Endoanal ultrasound was the only test most likely to change the patient's treatment plan (102). Voyvodic et al. observed a strong correlation between maximum anal squeeze pressure and the presence or absence of an external sphincter defect. The authors classified the defects into partial versus full-length and narrow versus wide-open. This classification appeared to be of little benefit in defining further functional disability because the squeeze pressures in these subgroups were not significantly different. This might imply that the loss of integrity due to disruption of the external sphincter ring is the most important factor in loss of function rather than the degree of separation of the muscle margins (111).

Defecography

The anorectal angle is more obtuse in patients with incontinence (108). Voiding defecography or balloon proctography can demonstrate this increased angle. This examination will probably add little to information regarding the cause of incontinence except perhaps the demonstration of an occult rectal internal procidentia.

Electromyography

In the past, electromyographic mapping of the external anal sphincter with a concentric-needle electrode was widely used in locating defects. During the last decade, endoanal ultrasound has replaced EMG in the assessment of sphincter defects. Now the main purpose of EMG is to identify signs of nerve injury. Single-fiber EMG allows the evaluation of denervation and subsequent reinnervation of individual motor units by the measurement of fiber density.

This fiber density is an index of the number of muscle fibers supplied by one motor unit within the uptake area of the electrode. In patients with fecal incontinence, the fiber density is increased, which is a measure of compensatory reinnervation after previous denervation (112).

Pudendal Nerve Terminal Motor Latency

Although the severity of denervation does not appear to influence the severity of incontinence, it seems to affect the outcome of sphincter repair. Assessment of the PNTML provides a useful tool in defining pathology of the pudendal nerves. Prolongation of PNTML is indicative for pudendal neuropathy and is considered to be a hallmark of "idiopathic" incontinence. Roig et al. (113) found pudendal neuropathy in 70% of their patients with fecal incontinence (59% in patients with a sphincter defect and 94% in patients without a sphincter defect). Based on this finding, it seems likely that pudendal neuropathy is an etiologic or associated factor in fecal incontinence. It is not clear whether a prolonged conduction velocity of the pudendal nerve affects its functional integrity. It has been shown that one out of three patients with bilateral prolonged PNTML have squeeze pressures in the normal range and that almost half of those with a normal PNTML have squeeze pressures below the normal range (114). Although it has been stated that the information obtained by PNTML testing does not contribute to the management of incontinence in individual patients, it might be of prognostic value when surgical treatment is being considered. Laurberg et al. were the first to demonstrate that pudendal neuropathy affects surgical treatment. In their series, the outcome of sphincter repair was successful in 80% of the patients without neuropathy and in only 10% of the patients with neuropathy (115). This finding has been confirmed by others (116). Sangwan et al. reported that the outcome of sphincter repair was good in patients in whom both pudendal nerves were normal, whereas only one out of six patients with a unilateral pudendal neuropathy had such an outcome. According to these authors, both pudendal nerves must be intact to achieve normal continence after sphincter repair (117). The relationship between pudendal nerve integrity and successful outcome after surgical repair is not universally accepted. Rasmussen et al., Chen et al., and Young et al. were unable to identify any relationship between pudendal neuropathy and a poor outcome after sphincteroplasty (118–120).

Osterberg et al. (121) questioned the routine use of PNTML in the assessment of patients with fecal incontinence. They found pudendal neuropathy and increased fiber density are common in patients with fecal incontinence. Fiber density but not PNTML was correlated with clinical and manometric variables. The severity of nerve injury correlated with anal motor and sensory function in patients with neurogenic or idiopathic incontinence.

Rectal Compliance

Rasmussen et al. (122) studied rectal compliance in 31 patients with fecal incontinence. The patients experienced a constant defecation urge at a lower rectal volume and also had a lower maximal tolerable volume and a lower rectal compliance than control subjects (median 126 mL vs. 155 mL, 170 mL vs. 220 mL, and 9 mmHg vs. 15 mmHg, respectively). There was no difference in the parameters between patients with idiopathic fecal continence and patients with incontinence of traumatic origin, indicating that a poorly compliant rectum in patients with fecal incontinence may be secondary to anal incontinence caused by lack of normal reservoir function. The role of compliance is controversial, because some authors have found a decreased rectal compliance and others have not (123,124).

Magnetic Resonance Imaging

Regarding the visualization of anal sphincter defects, magnetic resonance imaging (MRI) is comparable to endoanal ultrasound. However, detailed examination of sphincter morphology is only possible with MRI (Fig. 2A, B). Denervation of the external anal sphincter is associated with fiber type changes and atrophy, characterized by muscle fiber loss with subsequent fat and fibrous tissue replacement. In contrast with ultrasound, MRI allows good distinction

A

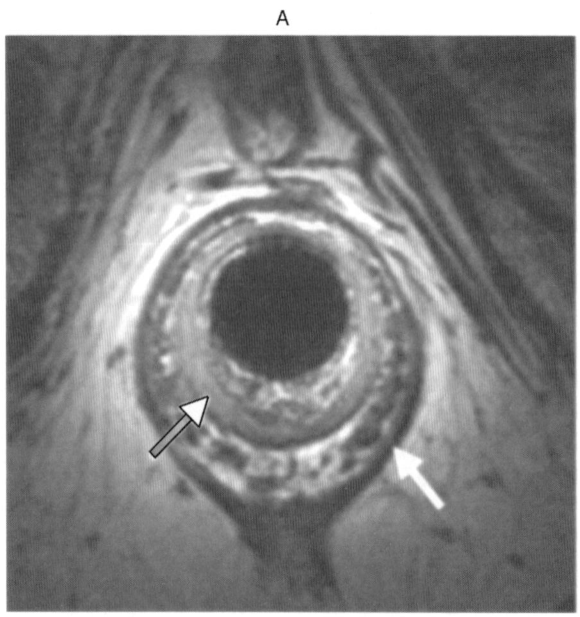

B

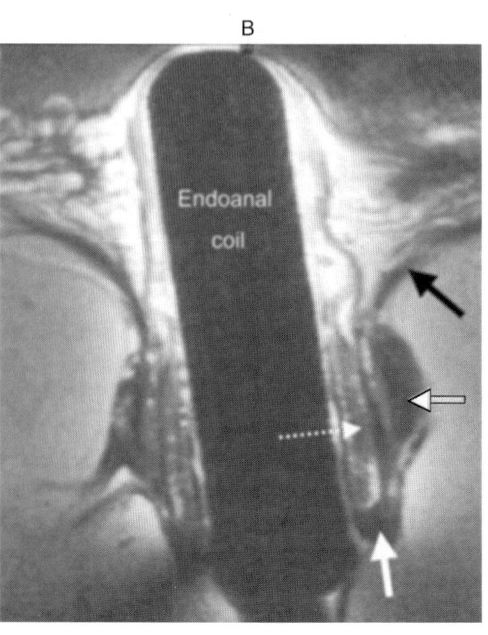

FIGURE 2 ■ (**A**) Endoanal magnetic resonance image, transverse image. Internal anal sphincter (*open arrow*) and external anal sphincter (*closed arrow*). (**B**) Endoanal magnetic resonance image, sagittal image. Levator ani (*black arrow*), puborectal muscle (*open arrow*), distal border of the external anal sphincter, curving around the distal end of the internal anal sphincter (*closed arrow*), and internal anal sphincter (*interrupted arrow*).

between muscle fibers, fibrous tissue, and fat. Williams et al. performed MRI with an endocoil in women with intact sphincters on endoanal ultrasound. Continent women with a normal squeeze pressure had a larger external anal sphincter cross-sectional area with a lower fat content than the incontinent women with a low squeeze pressure. Women with a thin internal anal sphincter and/or a poorly defined external anal sphincter on ultrasound were more likely to have atrophy (125). Briel et al. performed endoanal ultrasound and endoanal MRI in incontinent women with an anterior sphincter defect due to obstetric trauma. Atrophy of the external anal sphincter could only be demonstrated on MRI and was observed in 8 of the 20 patients. The outcome of sphincter repair was significantly better in those without atrophy (126). During sphincter repair, performed in another group of patients, the same authors took biopsy specimens from the left and right lateral parts of the external anal sphincter. Endoanal MRI revealed external anal sphincter atrophy in 36% of the patients. This was confirmed by histopathological examination in all but one. In detection atrophy, endoanal MRI showed 89% sensitivity, 94% specificity, 89% positive predictive value, and 94% negative predictive value (127). Based on these and other findings, it is apparent that MRI provides a powerful tool to detect external anal sphincter atrophy, thereby predicting the outcome of sphincter repair.

TREATMENT

Specific disorders are treated on their own merits (i.e., whatever is appropriate for inflammatory bowel disease, carcinoma, or rectal procidentia). Patients with spinal cord injury can be treated according to the recommendations in Chapter 33.

■ NONOPERATIVE PROCEDURES

Medical Treatment

Dietary changes and perineal exercises are often recommended for patients with anal incontinence, but generally have proved disappointing. Rosen et al. (128) reviewed the various antidiarrheal agents that might be considered in the management of patients with incontinence associated with frequent loose stools. Substances such as kaolin, activated charcoal, pectin, and bulk-forming agents act on the intestinal contents in an effort to solidify them. Agents such as bismuth salts and astringents such as aluminum hydroxide may produce a barrier between intestinal contents and the intestinal wall. Anticholinergic agents such as atropine act as potent inhibitors of intestinal secretion and gut motility. At therapeutic doses, these drugs may produce disconcerting side effects. The opium derivatives such as tincture of opium, paregoric, and codeine act directly on the smooth muscle of the intestinal wall, but the risk of addiction makes them less suitable for long-term use. Diphenoxylate hydrochloride (Lomotil) also has been used. One of the most frequently used drugs is loperamide (Imodium), which inhibits intestinal motility by a direct effect on the circular and longitudinal muscles of the intestinal wall. It solidifies the stool and increases rectal compliance, thereby decreasing urgency. It has also been found to increase resting anal pressures (129) and thus improve anal sphincter function and continence after restorative proctocolectomy (130). For patients with certain neurologic deficiencies, the regular administration of enemas may achieve a certain level of social continence.

Amitriptyline, a tricyclic antidepressant agent with anticholinergic and serotoninergic properties, has been used empirically in the treatment of idiopathic fecal incontinence. Santoro et al. (131) conducted an open study to test the response of amitriptyline 20 mg daily for four weeks by 18 patients with idiopathic fecal incontinence. Amitriptyline improved incontinence scores (median pretreatment score = 16 vs. median posttreatment score = 3) and reduced the number of bowel movements per day. Amitriptyline improved symptoms in 89% of patients with fecal incontinence. The data support that the major change with amitriptyline is a decrease in the amplitude and frequency of rectal motor complexes. The second conclusion is that the drug increases colonic transit time and leads to the formation of a firmer stool that is passed less frequently. These in combination may be the source of the improvement in continence.

Continence Plugs

Mortensen and Humphreys (132) investigated the efficacy of a disposable anal continence plug in patients who were incontinent of both liquid and solid stool. The median wear time for the optimal plug design was 12 hours, and there were no episodes of incontinence in 82% of the periods during which the plug was in place. Patients required a median of 11 plugs per week, and in 82% of cases insertion was as easy as with a suppository. The authors concluded that plugs may have a place in the management of patients with anorectal incontinence.

Christiansen and Roed-Petersen (133) performed a clinical assessment of a polyurethane sponge plug in an ambulatory group of patients incontinent to liquid and solid stool. Nine of 14 patients were continent when they used the plug. In 43% the plug occasionally slipped out, and 71% experienced discomfort to a varying degree. The authors concluded that a majority of patients would use the plug in special circumstances because it eliminates the fear of fecal leakage but that local discomfort would prevent its daily use.

Electrical control of sphincter dysfunction can be provided by direct electrical implants to the muscle tissue or by externally activated "plugs" (134). The electrical implants have the inherent problems of infection and dislodgment, and the continued contraction of those sphincter mechanisms can be sustained for only 40 to 60 seconds. Often this length of time is inadequate to maintain continence. The anal stimulator plug is a more complex apparatus, but it has the advantage of being a noninvasive technique. By gradually decreasing the size of the anal plugs, normal anal tone is gradually returned. Only scattered reports mention the success of this procedure. Most trials are discouraging, perhaps again attributable to the inability of the sphincter mechanism to maintain tonic contraction for any prolonged period.

Biofeedback Training

Engel et al. (135) first described biofeedback training for fecal incontinence, which is achieved by screening patients for incontinence and selecting well-motivated, alert patients for a three-phase instruction of voluntary control mechanisms.

There are at least three components to biofeedback treatment: exercise of the external sphincter muscle, training in the discrimination of rectal sensations, and training synchrony of the internal and external sphincter responses during rectal distention (136). Each of these components may be effective for some patients. The method involves placing a balloon in the rectum and connecting pressure transducers to a graph to give the patient a visual feedback corresponding to his or her sphincter responses to command. Initially, large amounts of air are injected into the rectal balloon; gradually the volume of distention is reduced until the patient can contract the external anal sphincter to small distentions. Subsequently, visual feedback is eliminated, but the patient is checked by a trained observer to see if he or she can respond to rectal sensations alone.

Training occurs at 4- to 8-week intervals and is supplemented by sphincter exercises to increase muscle strength. The goals of this training are to increase the strength of external sphincter contraction and to teach the patient to detect and respond to small volumes of rectal distention.

One major disadvantage is the time involved. Each session takes at least 2 hours and involves a significant amount of sophisticated physiologic monitoring apparatus.

Wald (137) reported that diabetic patients exhibit multiple abnormalities of anorectal sensory and motor functions. Pharmacologic treatment and dietary interventions to modulate diarrhea, as well as biofeedback to improve rectal sensory thresholds and striated muscle responsiveness, may prove successful in the reestablishment of bowel control.

In recent years, several authors have reviewed the literature in an effort to determine the efficacy of biofeedback treatment in the management of fecal incontinence. Norton et al. conducted a Cochrane review of controlled studies of biofeedback and sphincter exercises for fecal incontinence. Only five trials met the inclusion criteria of being a randomized or quasirandomized trial, including a total of 109 participants. The Cochrane review concluded that there is not enough evidence from these trials to judge whether sphincter exercises or biofeedback are effective in reducing fecal incontinence (138). Heymen et al. searched the Medline database for papers published between 1973 and 1999 including the terms "biofeedback and fecal incontinence." Thirty-five studies were reviewed. Only six studies used a parallel treatment design and just three of those randomized subjects to treatment groups. A meta-analysis comparing the treatment outcome of studies using coordination training (i.e., coordinating pelvic floor muscle contraction with the sensation of rectal filling) to studies using strength training (i.e., pelvic floor muscle contraction alone) failed to show any advantage for one treatment strategy over another. The mean success rate was 67% and 70%, respectively. Despite these positive results, the authors state that the conclusions of the reviewed studies are limited by the absence of clearly identified criteria for determining success and by inconsistencies regarding selection criteria, severity of symptoms, duration of treatment, type of biofeedback, and factors predicting outcome (139). Reviewing the literature, Palsson et al. found only a few controlled trials (140). The largest randomized controlled trial has been conducted by Norton et al. They randomly assigned 171 patients with fecal incontinence into four treatment arms: (i) standard care; (ii) standard care plus instruction in sphincter exercises; (iii) same as (ii) plus computer-assisted biofeedback involving coordination techniques; (iv) same as (iii) plus daily use of an EMG home trainer device. About half of the participants in all four groups who completed their treatment protocol showed improvement. This benefit was maintained at 1 year follow-up. These data indicate that improvement can be realized without sphincter exercises and without biofeedback. Patient–therapist interaction and the development of better coping strategies seem to be important factors (141). Another randomized controlled study, conducted by Solomon et al., revealed that instrument-guided biofeedback offers no advantage over simple pelvic floor retraining with digital guidance alone (142). The mechanisms by which biofeedback is effective are still not clear. It has been suggested that biofeedback is beneficial by improving the contraction of the external anal sphincter and the pelvic floor muscles due to strength training. Initial attempts to demonstrate objective manometric changes secondary to biofeedback have proved difficult. Fynes et al. conducted a randomized controlled trial to compare the effects of biofeedback alone with those of biofeedback combined with electrical stimulation. The manometric parameters did not change after the biofeedback alone, whereas anal resting and squeeze pressures increased after combined biofeedback and electrical stimulation (143). Recently Beddy et al. observed a significant improvement in anal resting pressure, duration of the squeeze, and amplitude of the squeeze after EMG-guided biofeedback. There was no improvement in the squeeze pressure (144). Biofeedback might also work by enhancing the ability to perceive and respond to rectal distensions, known as sensory training. Chiarioni et al. reported that sensory retraining is indeed the key to biofeedback treatment of fecal incontinence. Although they observed an increase of maximum squeeze pressure and squeeze duration after biofeedback, the sphincter strength did not separate responders from nonresponders. However, responders had lower thresholds for first sensation at the end of the treatment (145). A better coordination between rectal sensory perception and sphincter activity might also contribute to the effectiveness of biofeedback. Critics of this treatment modality argue that the improvement is a result of the supportive interaction between the physiotherapist and the patient, resulting in decreased anxiety and increased confidence. Despite many unanswered questions, it seems obvious that biofeedback is beneficial for more than half of the patients with fecal incontinence, at least in the short term. The question is whether the outcome of biofeedback can be predicted or not. Data regarding this aspect are scarse. In one study, it has been shown that manometric parameters, except for increased cross-sectional asymmetry, do not predict response to biofeedback therapy (146). Another study revealed that incomplete anal relaxation during straining, especially in patients younger than age 55, adversely affects the outcome of biofeedback (147). The long-term results after biofeedback are also questionable. Most studies offer a follow-up of less than two years. Enck et al. posted a questionnaire to patients who were treated by biofeedback 5 to 6 years earlier. The same questionnaire was also sent to patients who had not entered the treatment program. In both groups 78% of the patients experienced episodes of incontinence. However, the severity of incontinence was significantly less in the treatment group. Five to 6 years after the treatment, the severity of incontinence was similar to that reported immediately after therapy (148). In contrast with this finding, two other studies revealed deterioration over time (149,150). Ryn et al. reported an overall success rate of 60% immediately after the treatment. This dropped to 41% after a median follow-up of 44 months (151). Based on this deterioration over time, it has been suggested that it could be useful to reinitiate biofeedback training. Pager et al. were not able to demonstrate this worsening with time. At a median of 42 months after completion of the training program, 75% of their patients still perceived a symptomatic improvement and 83 reported improved quality of life. They also observed that patients continued to improve during the years following the training, possibly due to the strong emphasis placed on them to continue the exercises on their own (152). Biofeedback treatment is multimodal. More studies are needed to establish selection criteria, to compare different biofeedback techniques and to establish valid end points. Although biofeedback is time consuming and labor intensive, it is noninvasive and safe. Based on the reported outcomes, it should be considered as initial treatment in patients with fecal incontinence. It has been suggested that biofeedback is also beneficial as an adjuvant therapy following anal sphincter repair. Recently Davis et al. evaluated this aspect in a randomized controlled trial. Thirty-eight patients were assigned at random into sphincter repair or sphincter repair plus biofeedback. Shortly after surgery, there was no difference in functional outcome between the two groups. More studies are warranted to elucidate the role of adjuvant biofeedback (153).

■ OPERATIVE PROCEDURES

All operative techniques involve preparing the patient by evacuation of the large bowel with laxatives and enemas or oral lavage solutions. At the time of operation, an indwelling urethral catheter is placed and maintained until decreased pain permits voluntary voiding. Perioperative broad-spectrum antibiotics are administered.

Anterior Anal Sphincter Repair

External anal sphincter defects, most frequently located at the anterior site of the anal canal, are the principal cause of fecal incontinence. These anatomic defects can be treated by an anterior anal sphincter repair, which is the standard surgical procedure. Most surgeons use an overlapping technique to repair the divided external anal sphincter.

The technique of sphincteroplasty, as applied by Fang et al. (154) and Parks and McPartlin (155), provides good-to-excellent results in most patients who have adequate residual muscle mass. The operation is performed with the patient in the prone jackknife position, with the buttocks elevated over a 6-in. roll. Anesthesia may be either regional or general, but the entire operative site is infiltrated with local anesthetic and 1:200,000 epinephrine in order to relax the muscles and improve hemostasis (Fig. 3A).

The first step is the mobilization of the anoderm from the underlying sphincter mechanism and scar. The incision is curvilinear and parallels the outer edge of the external sphincter. The incision should extend for at least 200° to 240° of arc, depending on the amount of scar tissue present (Fig. 3B). Cephalad mobilization should extend approximately to the distal edge of the anorectal ring (Fig. 3C). The entire sphincter mechanism is then dissected widely from its bed (Fig. 3D). Care must be taken to preserve the branches of the pudendal nerves as they enter into the muscle posterolateral. Wide dissection permits approximation without tension. Dissection of two-thirds of the circumference should be adequate in most instances. It is often easiest to begin at the normal muscle and to advance to the scarred area, once a proper plane has been established. The entire sphincter mechanism is sectioned transversely through the middle of the scar tissue, with preservation of this area for suture placement (Fig. 3E). The muscle ends are overlapped to decrease the anal aperture until it fits snugly over the index finger (Fig. 3F).

Six to nine mattress sutures are placed carefully to maintain the desired aperture (Fig. 3G). The material used is generally a 2–0 synthetic absorbable suture. The tendency of the sphincter ends to pull apart must be minimal, because separation of the ends is a sign of inadequate mobilization of the muscle from its bed and will predispose to separation at the suture line. When all sutures have been placed, they are pulled tight, and the orifice is checked again to ensure proper placement of the sutures, which are then tied (Fig. 3H).

Next, an effort is made to reestablish a perineal body. Tissues from each side of the perineum (transverse perinei muscles and/or scar tissue) are approximated in the midline (Fig. 3I). This reconstruction lends support to the anovaginal area and effectively separates the anal orifice from the introitus. The anoderm is sutured carefully over the sphincter with interrupted or running absorbable 3–0 chromic catgut sutures. The horseshoe-shaped defect outside the muscle is partially closed, and the remainder is packed open with fine gauze (Fig. 3J), or a gauze mesh can simply be placed over the wound.

Postoperative management has varied from surgeon to surgeon. The recent trend has been toward early feeding, but we usually still give patients nothing by mouth for three to four days after operation. Although there is concern for the later need for laxatives, we administer opiates to decrease the pain and frequency of bowel movements. Mahony et al. (156) conducted a randomized trial designed to compare a laxative regimen with a constipating regimen in early postoperative management after primary obstetric and anal sphincter repair. A total of 105 females were randomized after primary repair of a third-degree tear to receive lactulose (laxative group, 56) or codeine phosphate (constipated group, 49) for 3 days postoperatively. The first postoperative bowel action occurred at a median of 4 days in the constipated group and 2 days in the laxative group. Patients in the constipated group had a significantly more painful first evacuation compared with the laxative group.

The mean duration of hospital stay was 3.7 days in the constipated group and 3.1 days in the laxative group. Continence scores, anal manometry, and endoanal ultrasound findings were similar in the two groups at 3 months postpartum. Patients in the laxative group had a significantly earlier and less painful bowel motion and earlier postnatal discharge. Sitz baths are given two to three times a day for comfort and to wash away secretions. Some

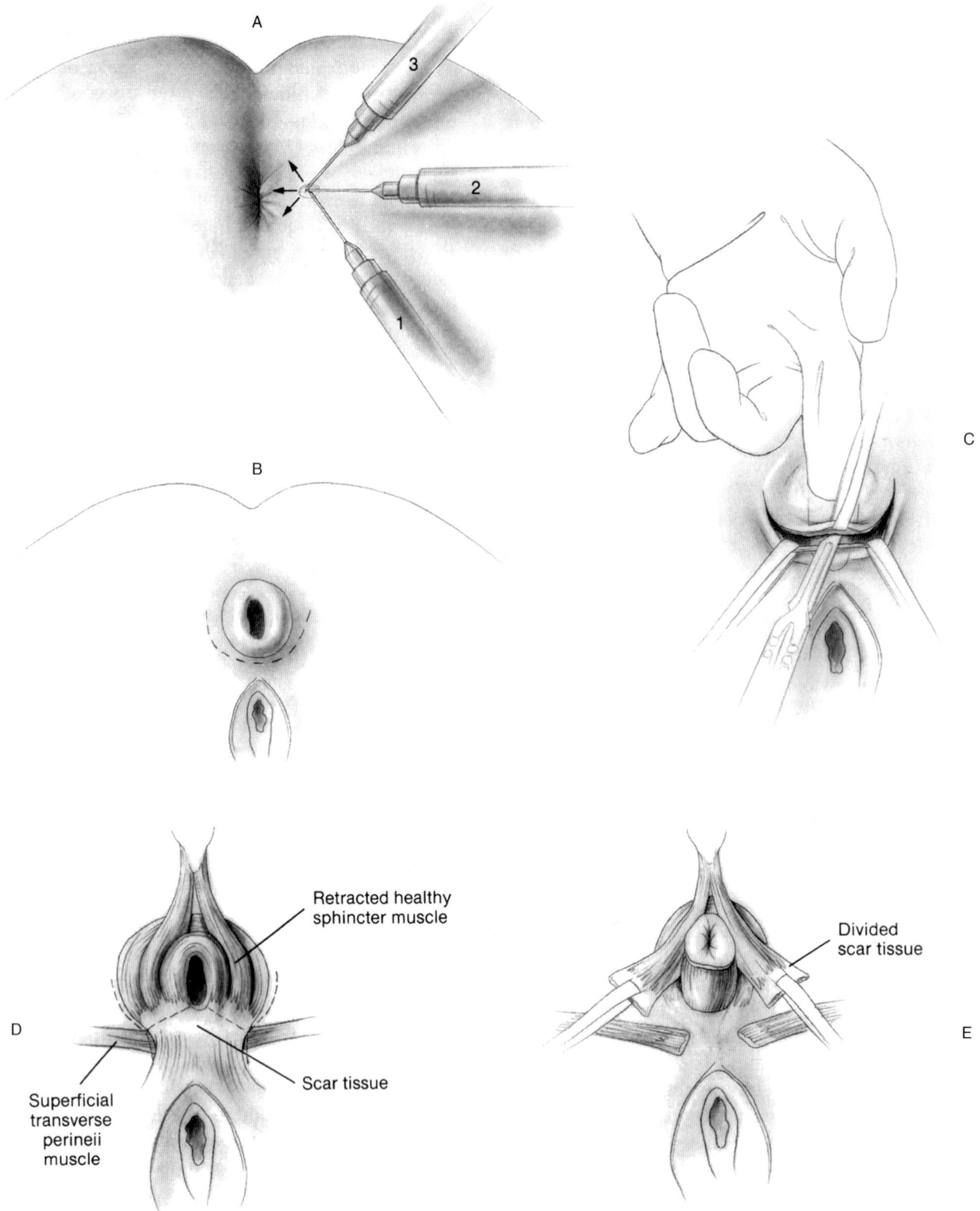

FIGURE 3 ■ Technique of sphincteroplasty. (**A**) Infiltration of local anesthesia. (**B**) Placement of circular incision. (**C**) Mobilization of anoderm. (**D**) Dissection of sphincter muscle. (**E**) Mobilization of severed ends of the sphincter muscle. (**F**) Muscle ends are overlapped. (**G**) Mattress sutures are applied. The scar must be left at each end of the muscle to hold the sutures. (**H**) At completion of suturing, anal canal should admit one finger snugly. (**I**) Perineal body reconstruction is done anterior to the anal canal, and anoderm is sutured to sphincter muscle. Skin edges are partially closed to decrease the size of wound. (**J**) Wound is packed open.

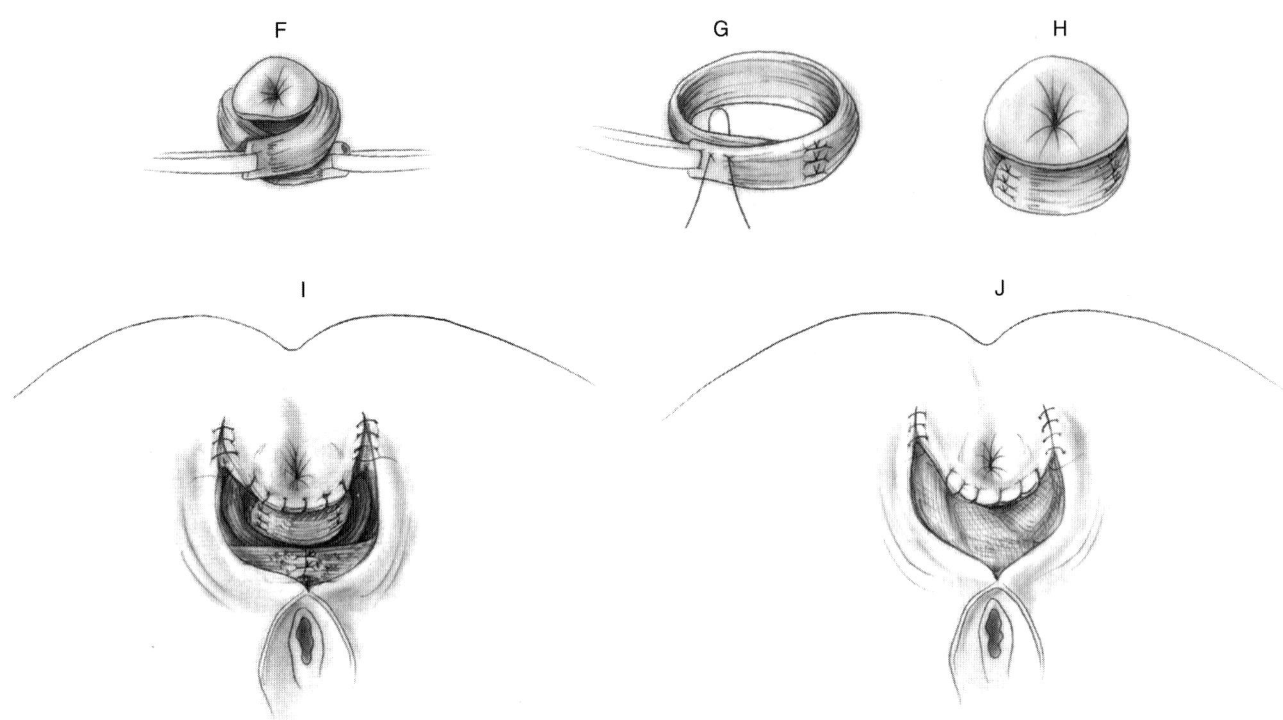

FIGURE 3 ■ (*Continued*)

surgeons are concerned about skin maceration and prefer to irrigate the wound with warm saline solution or even diluted hydrogen peroxide (dilute 1:4) to provide both comfort and cleanliness. With the introduction of food, a psyllium seed preparation is administered twice a day to eliminate any straining at defecation. One preoperative and two postoperative doses of antibiotics are administered. Performing a covering colostomy is not required. Patients usually leave the hospital in 5 to 6 days.

Fang et al. (154) reported on the use of overlapping sphincteroplasty in 79 patients. One postoperative death and 13 complications occurred; the complications included temporary difficulty in voiding (six), excessive bleeding (two), abscess formation (two), fecal impaction (two), and hematoma (one). Results were good-to-excellent in more than 90% of the patients, with an average follow-up of 35 months. The authors concluded that several factors were important for good results: (i) the patient must have an intact neuromuscular bundle with detectable voluntary sphincter contraction; (ii) if a primary repair has failed, a minimum duration of 3 months should elapse before overlapping sphincteroplasty is attempted; (iii) scar tissue from the severed muscles should not be excised; (iv) the internal and external sphincter muscles should not be separated; and (v) a temporary colostomy is not necessary.

Ctercteko et al. (21) studied a number of factors in relation to results of sphincteroplasty. They found that the older the patient, the more likely it was that there would be problems with continence after the operation, the necessity of wearing pads, and dissatisfaction with the result of the operation. The longer the patient had been incontinent before operation, the more likely was a poor result. With respect to etiology, patients with obstetric sphincter injuries were less likely to remain incontinent for solid and liquid stools than patients with operative injury. There was no significant difference between the other etiologic groups. Patients who had had a previous attempt at repairs tended to have worse results.

Hawley (157) reported on a series of 128 patients who underwent repair of sphincter injuries. In that series, 100 repairs were of the overlapping variety and 100 patients had a covering colostomy. Complications occurred in 38 patients; 10 developed fistulas, which usually were treated by laying open the fistula. Partial dehiscence of the wound occurred in 9 patients, infection in 10, and fecal impaction in 2.

For patients with a traumatic cloaca, Abcarian et al. (158) combined the overlapping repair with reconstruction of the perineal body and puborectalis muscle interposition. They used this procedure in 43 patients, with excellent anatomic and physiologic results. Sangalli and Marti (159) reported on 36 patients who underwent sphincter repair following an obstetric injury. Continence was restored in 78% of patients, while six postoperative complications developed—two sphincter breakdowns, two infections, one hematoma, and one skin breakdown.

The recommendation to repair a divided external anal sphincter by an overlapping repair is mainly based on the collective results of the American Proctological Society (now known as the American Society of Colon and Rectal Surgeons). In 1940, this Society reported a failure rate as high as 40% after direct end-to-end sphincter repair. The overlapping technique as described by Parks and McPartlin in 1971 is thought to be better and has been the predominant technique during the last three decades. Arnaud et al. reported on 40 patients who underwent a direct end-to-end repair. Complete continence was obtained in 25 patients (160). Briel et al. investigated the functional outcome after anterior overlapping sphincter repair in a consecutive series of incontinent patients. The functional results were compared with those obtained in a historical group of patients who underwent a direct end-to-end repair. No differences were found (161). In 2003, Tjandra et al. reported the results of a randomized controlled trial, comparing end-to-end repair with overlapping repair. After a median follow-up of 18 months, the outcome after both techniques was similar. This trial, with a rather small sample size, suggests that the overlapping repair has no benefit over the end-to-end repair (162).

Kairaluoma et al. (163) evaluated the medium-term outcome of the overlap sphincteroplasty in the primary repair of obstetric sphincter ruptures in 31 consecutive females who were diagnosed with a complete third-degree or fourth-degree anal sphincter rupture. At a median of 24 months after delivery, 77% were free of symptoms of anal incontinence. Occasional incontinence to flatus and liquid stool occurred in 17% and 7% of patients, respectively.

The failure rate of 40% after end-to-end repair, as reported in 1940, was the main reason to recommend overlapping repair. However, the long-term results of such an overlapping repair are not as good as thought in those early days. In a study from St. Mark's Hospital, the initial success rate of 76% declined to 50% with time (164). This worsening with time has also been reported by others (161,165–169). The data regarding this aspect are summarized in Table 6.

The question is whether a direct failure or a deterioration over time can be predicted. It has been stated that integrity of repair is fundamental for a successful outcome. Several authors have reported that residual external anal sphincter defects are associated with a poor outcome (170,171). Persistent defects also affect the outcome of repeat repairs, as demonstrated by Giordano et al. (172). Another consideration is a history of having undergone a previous repair, (173). However, two recent studies failed to provide evidence for the assumption that previous repairs are a predictor of poor results. Giordano et al. reported a success rate of 62% after repeat sphincteroplasty in patients with one or two previous repairs (172). A similar outcome has been reported by Vaizey et al. (174). It has been suggested that unilateral or bilateral pudendal neuropathy also affects the outcome of sphincter repair (115,175–177). Other workers were not able to demonstrate such a relationship between pudendal neuropathy and outcome of anterior anal sphincter repair (178–181). Recent studies have revealed that advanced age and long-lasting severe incontinence symptoms are significant predictors of a poor outcome (168,169).

Ha et al. (182) determined the parameters that correlate with a successful functional outcome following an overlapping anal sphincteroplasty. In a series of 52 overlapping sphincter reconstructions, 17% had undergone prior sphincter repair. The presence of a rectovaginal fistula, postoperative complications, previous sphincter repair, and increase in PNTML did not affect functional outcome. Patients older than 50 years had a better functional outcome than their younger counterparts, with sphincter repair. Although mean maximal squeeze pressure and mean anal sphincter length increased significantly after sphincter reconstruction, only squeeze pressure difference correlated with functional outcome. Zorcolo et al. (183) recently evaluated the long-term outcome of 93 patients who underwent anterior sphincter repair. Anterior sphincter repair was successful in improving continence in 73% of patients. Long-term results were obtained for 62 patients. Seventy percent had objective clinical improvement based on their questionnaire, but only 55% considered their bowel control had improved and only 45% were satisfied by the operation. Urgency was the most important symptom in determining patient satisfaction; 24 of 46 patients in whom urgency had improved were happy with their outcome. None of the preoperative and operative variables predicted the outcome. They concluded, patients should be warned that complete continence is difficult to achieve and that symptoms tend to deteriorate with time.

Hasegawa et al. (184) conducted a randomized trial to assess whether fecal diversion would improve primary wound healing and functional outcome after sphincter repair. Patients were randomly assigned to a defunctioning stoma ($n=13$) or no stoma ($n=14$). They were assessed by the Cleveland Clinic Continence Score (0–20). Incontinence score improved significantly in both groups (stoma 13.5–7.8; no stoma 14–9.6). No difference was found between the two groups. Maximum resting pressure and maximum squeeze pressure increased significantly only in the no-stoma group. There was no significant difference in the functional outcome or the number of complications of sphincter repair. However, stoma-related complications occurred in 7 of 13 patients having a stoma (parastoma hernia, 2; prolapsed stoma, 1; incisional hernia at the stoma site requiring repair, 5; and wound infection at the closure site, 1). They concluded fecal diversion in sphincter repair is unnecessary, because it gives no benefit in terms of wound healing or functional outcome and it is a source of morbidity.

Lewicky et al. (185) evaluated sexual function following anal sphincteroplasty in 32 women with third- and fourth-degree perineal tear secondary to birth trauma and elected to undergo sphincteroplasty for fecal incontinence. Sexual function is compromised in women with third-and fourth-degree perineal tears. For their patients with this degree of perineal tearing who underwent sphincteroplasty after primary repair, their survey showed consistent improvement in several parameters of sexual function. After sphincteroplasty, physical sensation was higher—much higher in 40%, sexual satisfaction was better—much better in 33.3%, and 28.6% of the patients were more—much more likely to reach orgasm. Libido was improved in 37.5% of the study population, and 20% reported increased partner satisfaction. Before surgery, 23.5% of patients were physically and 31.2% emotionally unable to participate in sexual activity because of fear of incontinence on intimacy; after surgery only 6.3% were

TABLE 6 ■ Short-Term and Long-Term Outcome After Anterior Anal Sphincter Repair

		Successful Outcome by Years of Follow-Up (%)					
Author	Year	0.25	1	2	3	5	10
Briel (161)	1998		70	65		45	
Rothbath (165)	2000	77	62				
Malouf (164)	2000		76			50	
Halverson (167)	2002	80				49	
Karoui (166)	2002	81			51		
Pinta (168)	2002	74		59			
Gutierrez (169)	2004				60		40

Note: Successful outcome = continent for solid and liquid stool with or without incontinence for gas.

physically unable and 0% were emotional unable to engage in sexual activity.

Pinta et al. (186) evaluated the clinical outcome of primary anal sphincter repair caused by obstetric tears and analyzed possible risk factors associated with sphincter rupture during vaginal delivery. A total of 52 females with a third-degree or fourth-degree perineal laceration during vaginal delivery were examined. A control group consisted of 51 primiparous females with no clinically detectable perineal laceration after vaginal delivery. After primary sphincter repair, 31 females (61%) had symptoms of anal incontinence. Fecal incontinence occurred in 10 females (20%). The study group had more severe symptoms of anal incontinence than the control group. In endoanal ultrasound examination, a persistent defect of the external sphincter was found in 75% in the rupture group compared with 20% in the control group. Anal sphincter pressures were significantly lower in the rupture group than in the control group. An abnormal presentation was the only risk factor for anal sphincter rapture during vaginal delivery.

Based on the promising short-term results, anterior anal sphincter repair is still the best first choice of operations in patients with fecal incontinence and a documented external anal sphincter defect. One should realize that it is difficult to compare the different studies. Most studies are retrospective. The definition of incontinence, and the method of data collection may differ from study to study. In almost all studies the outcome is assessed without the use of a standardized incontinence scoring system.

Total incontinence of solid or liquid stool and flatus is easy to categorize, as is full control of solid or liquid stool and flatus. However, many patients fall between these two categories. Some series use type of incontinence as a criterion, whereas others use frequency of incontinence. Furthermore, different series include patients with different causes of incontinence, a factor known to affect outcome. The technique of operation is often not uniform; some series combine more than one technique, and some include patients who have had a covering colostomy. Some authors have reported on a limited number of patients, and some follow-ups have been very brief. Occasionally patients have been included in more than one series when an individual has reported a personal experience and someone else has reported the experience of the institution.

Notwithstanding these considerable difficulties, Table 7 was constructed to provide a general idea of what can be expected from a sphincteroplasty with an overlapping repair.

TABLE 7 ■ **Results of Overlapping Sphincteroplasty**

Author(s)	No. of Patients	Grade of Continence (%)[a] 1	2	3
Browning and Motson (187) (1984)[b]	83	78	13	9
Fang et al. (154) (1984)	76	58	38	4
Hawley (157) (1985)[b]	100	52	30	18
Christiansen and Pedersen (188) (1987)	23	65	30	5
Morgan et al. (189) (1987)[b]	45	82	9	9
Ctercteko et al. (21) (1988)	44	54	32	14
Abcarian et al. (158) (1989)[c]	43	100		
Yoshioka and Keighley (190) (1989)	27	26	48	26
Jacobs et al. (191) (1990)[c]	30	83	17	
Fleshman et al. (192) (1991)	55	51	44	5
Gibbs and Hooks (193) (1993)	33	30	58	12
Engel et al. (194) (1994)	28	57	22	21
Engel et al. (195) (1994)	53	79	17	4
Londono-Schimmer et al. (196) (1994)	94	50	26	24
Sangalli and Marti (159) (1994)	36	78	19	3
Simmang et al. (197) (1994)	14	71	29	—
Oliveira et al. (173) (1996)[d]	55	29	47	29

[a]Grades of continence (see text for explanation of difficulties with table): 1, continent for solid and liquid stool; 2, continent for solid but not always for liquid stool; and 3, little or no continence.
[b]Most patients had a covering colostomy.
[c]Patients had a supplemental anterior puborectalis muscle approximation.
[d]According to study, 55% of patients had previous sphincter repair.

Other Sphincteroplasties

Postanal Repair

Prior to the introduction of endoanal ultrasound, most cases of fecal incontinence were classified as "idiopathic" or neurogenic. For the treatment of patients presenting with this type of incontinence Parks devised the postanal repair. He believed that this procedure works by restoring the anorectal angle and increasing the length of the anal canal. Several studies, however, have revealed that a postanal repair does not result in a significant change of the anorectal angle (198–202). Several studies have revealed an increase in the length of the anal canal after successful postanal repair (2,198,203). Conflicting data have been reported regarding the impact of postanal repair on anal pressure. Some workers have found that resting and squeeze anal pressure increase after successful postanal repair (2,199–201,204). According to others postanal repair does not affect anal pressure (22,198,205). Due to the lack of consistent changes in anatomy and physiology, it is unclear why postanal repair is effective in some patients. Clinical improvement might be the result of lengthening and narrowing of the anal canal. Van Tets and Kuijpers even suggested that this procedure might improve continence by a placebo effect and not by enhanced muscle function (206).

There is much debate about the predictive value of parameters assessed preoperatively. Jameson et al. observed a trend toward a more favorable outcome in patients who presented with a higher squeeze pressure preoperatively (204). Setti Carraro et al. reported that the PNTML was the only preoperative variable that correlated with long-term outcome (203). Other workers, however, were not able to confirm these findings. According to Matsuoka et al. neither prolongation of PNTML nor external sphincter damage or any preoperative manometric parameter correlates with the outcome (207). It has been reported that neurogenic damage to the striated sphincter musculature increases after postanal repair, even in patients with a favorable outcome (205). This phenomenon could not be demonstrated by others (201).

As Parks described the operation, a posterior angular incision is made through the anoderm (Fig. 4A) and proceeds through the intersphincteric plane between the external and internal sphincters (Fig. 4B). This intersphincteric plane is pursued upward until the puborectalis muscle is reached (Fig. 4C). The pelvic cavity is entered by dividing the rectosacral fascia, and the perirectal fat is swept off the levator ani muscles (Fig. 4D). At this point,

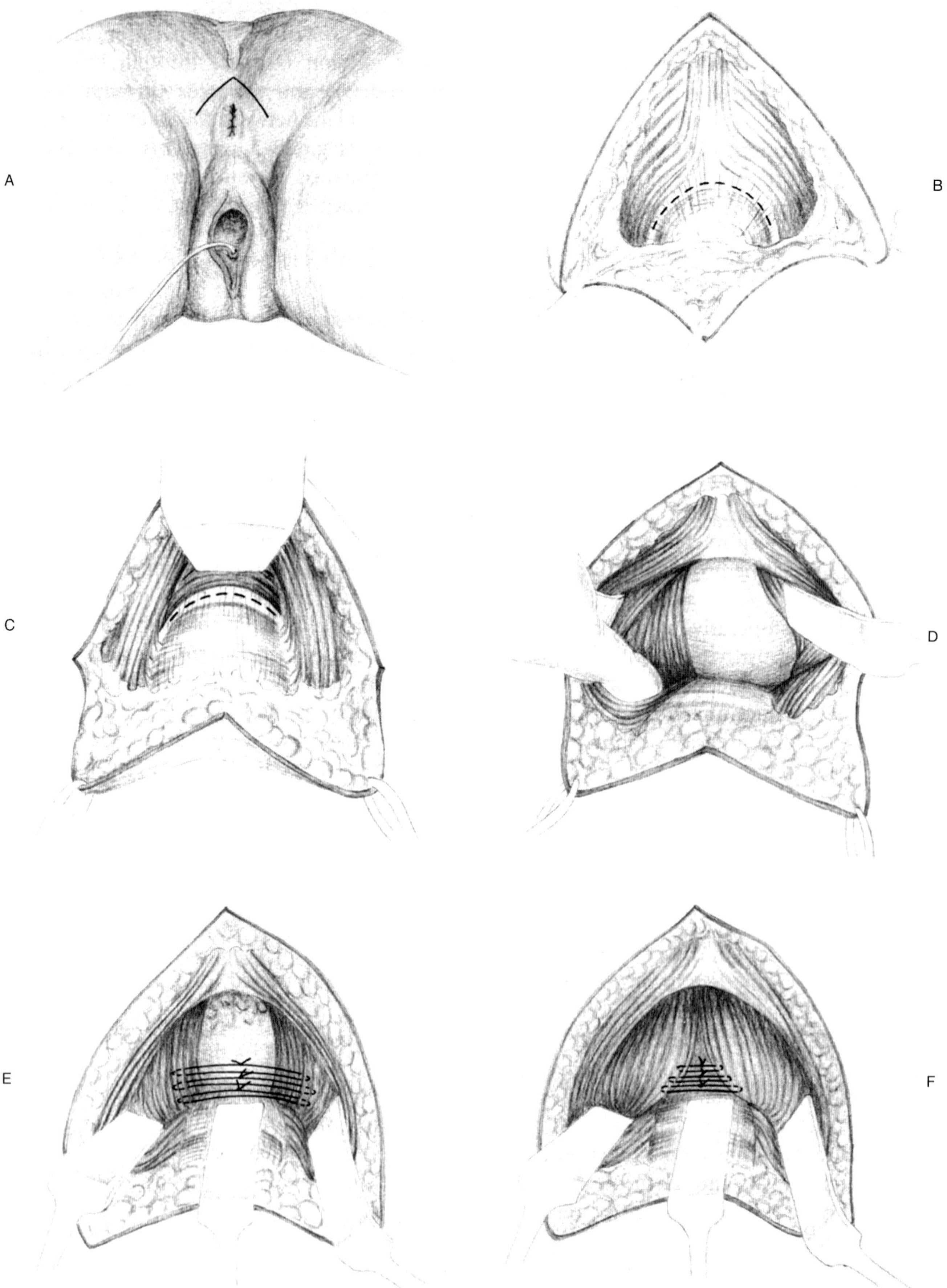

FIGURE 4 ■ Postanal repair. (**A**) Posterior angular incision. (**B**) Identification of intersphincteric plane. (**C**) Dissection to rectosacral fascia (*dotted line*). (**D**) Identification of levator ani muscles. (**E**) Plication of ischiococcygeus muscle. (**F**) Plication of pubococcygeus muscle. (**G**) Plication of puborectalis muscle. (**H**) Plication of external sphincter muscle. (**I**) Skin closure in shape of a Y, with separate stab wound for suction drain.

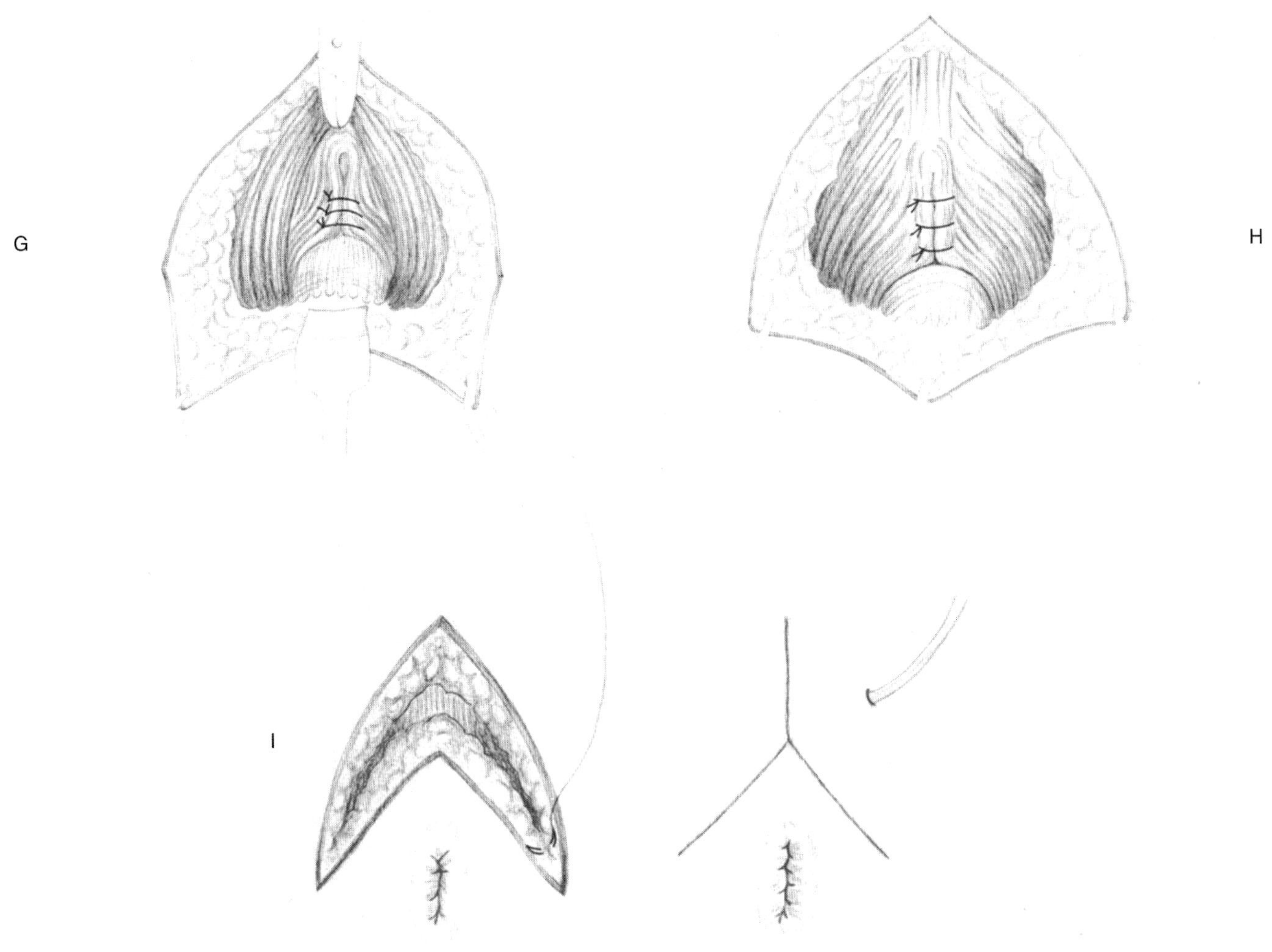

FIGURE 4 ■ *(Continued)*

most of the levator ani muscle can be seen, and sutures can be placed from one side of the pelvis to the other, initially incorporating the ischiococcygeus muscle in the first layer of repair Fig. 4E) and the pubococcygeus muscle in the second layer (Fig. 4F). These muscles will not meet; the sutures only form a lattice. A 0 polyglactin (Vicryl) suture is used.

Next, a row of sutures is placed to oppose the two limbs of the puborectalis muscle, further buttressing the anorectal angle (Fig. 4G). This also makes the pull of the puborectalis muscle more efficient. A suction drain is placed in the presacral space and is brought out through a separate stab wound. Plicating sutures' are placed in the external sphincter muscles to narrow their arc of action (Fig. 4H). By placing a finger in the anal canal, it is possible to determine if the whole area is somewhat stenosed, a state essential for achieving a successful result. The wound is closed with 3–0 chromic catgut sutures for the subcutaneous tissues, and the skin is approximated with 3–0 subcuticular Vicryl sutures (Fig. 4I). Systemic antibiotics are administered, one dose preoperatively and two doses postoperatively. Although Parks recommended purging the patient with magnesium sulfate for a 10-day period to ensure liquid stools, we recommend restriction of the patient's intake orally for five days, during which time the patient is given loperamide and codeine-containing analgesics to quiet the bowel. When diet is reinstituted, the patient is placed on a psyllium seed preparation twice daily.

Browning and the late Sir Alan Parks were the first to describe the functional outcome after postanal repair. According to these authors 86% of their patients became continent for solid stool. In the 1980s and early 1990s, the reported success rates varied between 66% and 94% (Table 8). However, in those days outcome was considered successful not only if patients regained continence for solid and liquid stool, but also if patients experienced improvement despite sporadic episodes of incontinence. Furthermore, most of the studies conducted in that period were retrospective. The definition of incontinence and the method of data collection differed from study to study. In almost all studies, the outcome was assessed without the use of a standardized incontinence scoring system. Furthermore, the duration of follow-up was relatively short or not recorded. During the last decade, several studies have revealed that the long-term results after postanal repair fall short of the short-term results reported in earlier days. This observation is illustrated by the data summarized in Table 9.

These more recent data illustrate that postanal repair is not as good as patients and surgeons would like it to be. The early results are rather disappointing. Moreover, they deteriorate over time. In the past, it was thought that the presence of a neurologic deficit was the principal cause

TABLE 8 ■ Results of Parks Postanal Repair

Author(s)	No. of Patients	Grade of Continence (%)[a]		
		1	2	3
Browning et al. (208) (1984)[b]	140	86	—	14
Van Vroonhoven and Schouten (209) (1984)	16	62	13	25
Henry and Simson (210) (1985)	204	58	12	30
Habr-Gama et al. (211) (1986)	42	52	41	7
Keighley (212) (1987)	114	32	62	6
Miller et al. (199) (1988)	17	59[c]	—	41[c]
Womack et al. (198) (1988)	16	88	—	12
Scheuer et al. (213) (1989)	39	15	54	31
Laurberg et al. (205) (1990)[c]	28	32	43	25
Orrom et al. (200) (1991)	17	76	—	24
Gordon (214) (1993)	23	57	35	8
Carraro et al. (215) (1994)	34	26	56	18
Engel et al. (216) (1994)	38	21	45	34
Jameson et al. (204) (1994)	36	50	33	17

[a]Grades of continence (see text for explanation of difficulties with table; this classification was not used by all authors, but for tabulation purpose, it is a relative approximation): 1, successful—continent for solid stool; 2, significant improvement—sporadic episodes of fecal incontinence; and 3, failure—incontinent for solid stool.
[b]Follow-up of patients operated on by Sir Alan Parks.
[c]It is not clear whether some of these patients should be category 2.

of failure. In a physiologic evaluation of pelvic floor muscles before and after postanal repair, Laurberg et al. found both the fiber density in the external anal sphincter and the PNTML increased after operation (205). They suggested that the progression in neurogenic damage to the pelvic floor muscles may be caused by the operation itself and that it may be responsible for the poor functional outcome noted in many patients. However, this phenomenon could not be demonstrated by others (201). Although progression of neurogenic damage may contribute to the deterioration over time, it provides no explanation for the less favorable early results. Leading the list of reasons for the rather poor outcome is the presence of sphincter defects in at least two-thirds of the patients with fecal incontinence. Most of these defects are located in front of the anal canal and can only be detected by endoanal ultrasound. This imaging technique was not available in the 1980s and early 1990s. In that epoch, many cases of fecal incontinence were classified as "idiopathic." It seems likely that a substantial number of patients, who underwent a postanal repair in that time period, had indeed a hidden sphincter defect. Based on one single study, it has been suggested that a sphincter defect does not influence the outcome of postanal repair (203). This assumption is not supported by other reports. In our opinion, it is unlikely that sphincter defects do not influence the outcome of the procedure.

An anterior anal repair is thereby more appropriate than a postanal repair in patients with an anterior sphincter direct.

Other contributing factors might include failure to obtain an adequate anorectal angle or anal canal length, failure to follow postoperative care, wound sepsis, previous operations, psychiatric illness, irritable bowel syndrome, and purgative abuse.

During the last decade postanal repair is rarely used by most surgeons, not only because of its poor long-term success rate, but also because alternatives are available, such as dynamic graciloplasty and sacral neuromodulation.

In a personal series of 23 patients who underwent a Parks postanal repair between 1976 and 1992, all patients were women and their ages ranged from 32 to 81 years (214). Patients were considered eligible for this operation if they had "idiopathic" fecal incontinence. Furthermore, operations were only offered to patients who were severely distressed by their disability, that is, they were regularly incontinent of solid stool. Individuals who presented with incontinence of flatus or even those who experienced episodes of incontinence with periods of liquid stool were not considered candidates for operation. Patients who suffered fecal incontinence secondary to sphincter disruption because of an obstetric injury, an external trauma, or a fistula-in-ano operation were not included because they had undergone on overlapping sphincter repair. With a follow-up that ranged from 1 month to 173 months (average, 64 months; median, 51 months), 57% of patients were classified as having a successful result (continent of solid stool); 35% as having significant improvement (sporadic episodes of fecal incontinence); and 8% as failures (incontinent of solid stool). A follow-up of this duration provided the opportunity to determine the incidence of late recurrence. Two of the 13 patients with initial good results had late recurrence. The results obtained by patients in the series fall short of the excellent results obtained by the late Sir Alan Parks, but are in the range reported by other authors. If the first two categories are combined, approximately 90% of patients initially have successful results or are significantly improved, and these results may be in part accounted for by the careful selection of patients.

TABLE 9 ■ Relationship Between Length of Follow-Up and Outcome After Postanal Repair

Author(s)	Year	Successful Outcome with Years of Follow-Up (%)							
		0.5	1	2	3	3.5	4	6	8
Setti Carraro et al. (203)	1994	41						26	
Engel et al. (216)	1994					21			
Jameson et al. (204)	1994	50		28					
Athanasiadis et al. (201)	1995						6		
Briel and Schouten (217)	1995		65		46				
Rieger et al. (218)	1997								37
Matsuoka et al. (207)	2000				35				

Note: Successful outcome = continent for solid and liquid stool with or without incontinence for gas.

Muscle Transposition

GRACILIS MUSCLE TRANSPOSITION ■ This procedure is reserved for situations in which massive trauma or infection in the perineum has destroyed the bulk of the patient's sphincter mechanism. A procedure described by Pickrell et al. (219) involves the use of a sling of gracilis muscle still attached to one end of the pubis to encircle the anus; the severed end is reattached to the opposite ischial tuberosity. This might be described as a "living Thiersch procedure" because of the inability of the gracilis muscle or any skeletal muscle other than the external sphincter mechanism to maintain both tonic and phasic contraction necessary for continence. Drawbacks of the procedure include the fact that the transposed muscle does not function as a dynamic sphincter, and patients often must perform awkward movements to achieve imperfect continence (17). Furthermore, the circuitous route adversely affects the efficiency of the neosphincter.

The current champion of this operation is Corman (219), who reported on 22 patients selected on the basis of loss of muscle tissue. Salient features of the operation are to free the tendon as distally as possible, divide it at its point of insertion, and develop a tunnel between the proximal incision and an anterior perianal incision (Fig. 5). The muscle is passed circumferentially around the anus and is sutured to the contralateral ischial tuberosity. If the muscle is taken from the right thigh, it is passed clockwise; if from the left, counterclockwise. The tendon must be anchored while the thighs are adducted, because adduction relaxes the muscle somewhat. Of 14 patients followed for at least five years, Corman reported excellent results in 7, fair in 4, and poor in 3. Christiansen et al. (222) performed 13 procedures. Six achieved satisfactory continence, four were improved, two did not benefit, and one died. From a collected series of publications to 1991, reported postoperative morbidity from the procedure included wound infection in 21%, sling necrosis in 2%, and fecal impaction in 4% (223). With regard to functional outcome, complete continence was reported in 52% of patients, partial continence in 30%, and in 18% the procedure was a failure (223).

Sielezneff et al. (224) reported on eight patients who underwent a gracilis transposition procedure combined with biofeedback training postoperatively. All patients were improved, five achieved normal continence, and three were incontinent to flatus.

Kumar et al. (225) reported on the use of both gracilis muscles to create a neosphincter in 10 patients. The operation was covered by a colostomy. Of the nine patients whose colostomy was closed, all are fully continent at a mean follow-up of 24 months. None of the patients has to wear a pad or is taking constipating agents, and all experience satisfactory evacuation. The authors suggest that this procedure may be an alternative to stimulated dynamic graciloplasty.

DYNAMIC GRACILOPLASTY ■ One of the more exciting developments in the management of patients with intractable fecal incontinence is the concept of the dynamic graciloplasty. One of the drawbacks of the gracilis transposition procedure is the inability of the muscle to simulate sustained contraction, as does the external sphincter. This problem can be solved by stimulating the gracilis muscle electrically with implanted electrodes (226,227). Experimental studies have shown that chronic low-frequency stimulation of skeletal muscle can convert a fast-twitch muscle into a slow-twitch muscle capable of sustained activity. In 1988, Baeten et al. (228) were the first to report the use of the electrically stimulated gracilis muscle. Since then, several investigators have promoted, refined, and modified the procedure (229–233).

Initially Baeten et al. (231) utilized a two-stage technique. During the first operation, the gracilis muscle is mobilized down to its insertion into the tibial tuberosity, and the distal tendon is divided. Proximally, the neurovascular bundle is left intact, and the muscle is transposed around the anal canal and fixed to the ischial spine. During a second procedure, approximately 6 weeks later, intramuscular electrodes (Model SP 5566, Medtronic, Kerkrade, The Netherlands) are implanted at the site of nerve entry and connected through a subcutaneous tunnel to the neurostimulator (Itrel II, Model 7424, Medtronic), which is placed in the abdominal wall (Fig. 6). At present many surgeons implant the stimulator and the intramuscular leads in one stage at the time of the graciloplasty.

With an external magnet, the patient can switch the neurostimulator on (causing the transposed gracilis muscle to contract) and off (causing the muscle to relax). The amplitude, rate, pulse width, polarity, and duty cycle of the stimulation can be programmed telemetrically by the physician. Before continuous stimulation is applied, the transposed gracilis muscle is trained for eight weeks according to a stimulation protocol. All patients receive systemic antibiotic prophylaxis for 24 hours at the time of transposition and implantation. In the last 37 patients to be treated, local antibiotics (gentamicin, Sulmycin Implant, Essex Pharma, Munich, Germany) were administered with the implant.

The technique described by Hallan et al. (229) is very similar. The procedure consists of transposition of the gracilis muscle around the deficient anal sphincter. Then an electrode plate is placed on the main nerve of the muscle, and the electrode is connected to a totally implantable electrical pulse generator, which can be programmed by telemetry and is implanted in the chest wall. The muscle is continually stimulated at a low frequency for a period of 8 to 10 weeks until evidence of transformation from fast-twitch to slow-twitch muscle has been achieved. At this stage, the frequency of stimulation has increased so that the muscle contracts around the anal canal and occludes it continually. When the patient wishes to evacuate, the stimulator can be switched off by passing a powerful magnet over the pulse generator, which contains a magnetic switch. Once evacuation is complete, the stimulator can be turned on again by the magnet.

The stimulator replaces voluntary contraction and exerts a sustained contraction (230,234) that leads to the transformation of type II fatigue-prone muscle fibers into type I fatigue-resistant fibers. Electrical stimulation gives the transposed gracilis muscle the properties required to function as a sphincter (226,227).

In their report, Baeten et al. (231) reported on 52 patients who had undergone dynamic graciloplasty. The clinical results of treatment were evaluated in an interview, by anal manometry and by enema testing. The degree of

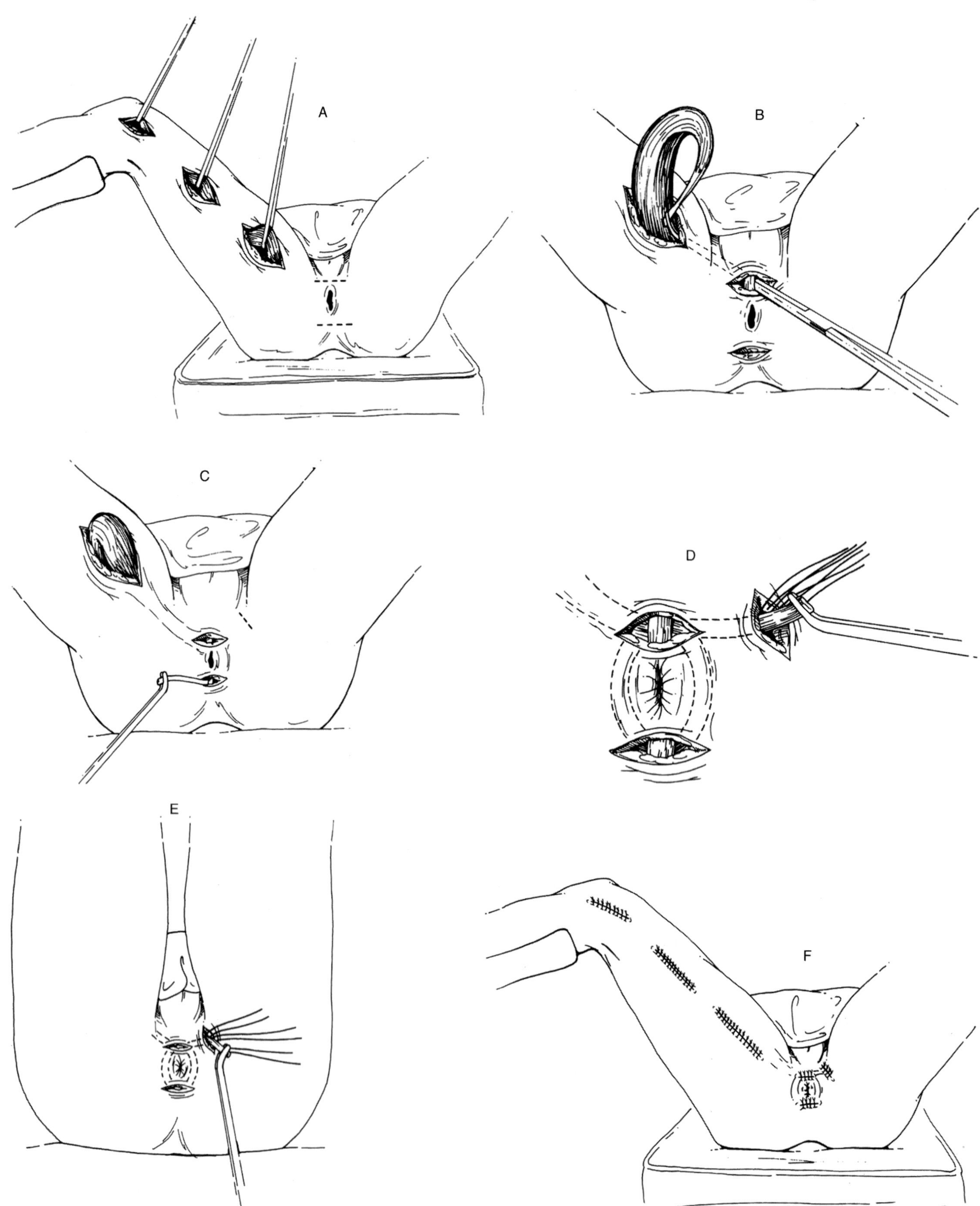

FIGURE 5 ■ Gracilis muscle sling. (**A**) Mobilization of gracilis muscle and division of tendon at its insertion. Locations of anterior and posterior incisions (*dotted lines*). (**B**) Passage of muscle through tunnel to anterior incision. (**C**) Passage of muscle through hemicircumference to posterior incision. Incision over ischial tuberosity (*dotted line*). (**D**) Passage of muscle through opposite hemicircumference of anus and placement of sutures through tendon and fascia of contralateral ischial tuberosity. (**E**) Adduction of thighs prior to tying sutures to ischial tuberosity. (**F**) Completed operation. *Source*: Modified from Ref. 221.

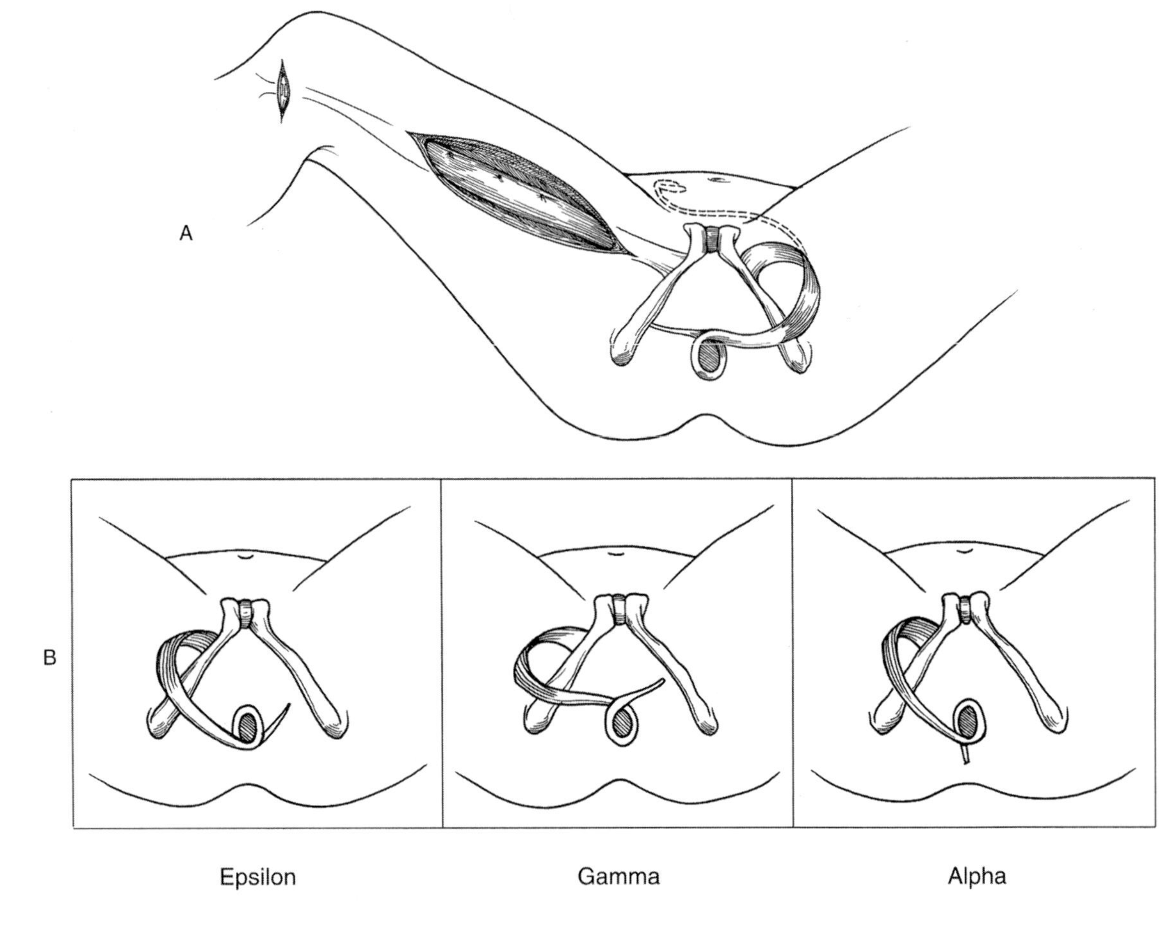

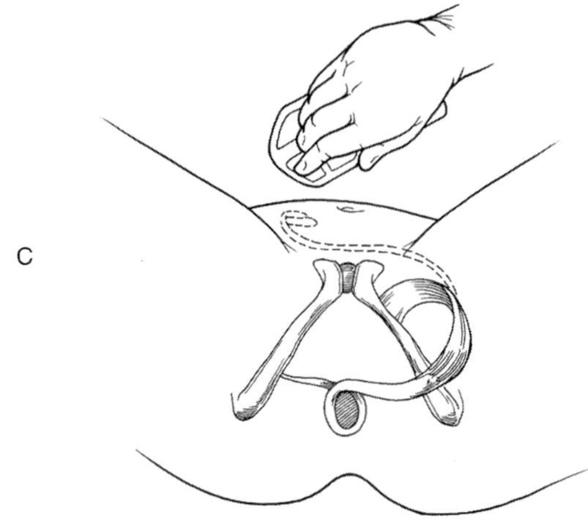

FIGURE 6 ■ Dynamic graciloplasty. (**A**) The incision and dissection of the gracilis muscle (*right leg*). The wrap completed with a Gamma loop (*left leg*). Both leads are depicted (*dotted line*), and the stimulator is located in a pocket in the lower abdomen underneath the rectus fascia. (**B**) Three types of wraps. The Epsilon wrap is used when there is not enough room for the passage of the bulk of the gracilis at the frontal side of the anus. The gamma loop is the configuration most often used. The bulk of the muscle passes first at the frontal side. The alpha loop is used only when the muscle and tendon are not long enough to pass to the contralateral side. The distal tendon is always fixed to the periosteum of the pubic bone, allowing passage of two fingers between the muscle and the anus to prevent too much tension. The construction works by electrically induced contraction of the muscle and not by pretension created during the wrap. (**C**) The stimulator can be put "on" and "off" with the help of a remote control. In older types of stimulators, this was done with a magnet. When the stimulator is deactivated, the muscle relaxes and the patient can defecate. *Soruce*: After Cornelius G. Baeten, M.D., Maastricht, The Netherlands.

continence was scored, and the quality of life was assessed. Of the 52 patients, 73% were continent after a median follow-up of 2.1 years. At 52 weeks, the patients' condition had improved with respect to the median frequency of defecation (from five to two times per 24 hours), the median time defecation could be postponed (from 9 seconds to 19 minutes), and the median time an enema could be retained (from 0 to 180 seconds). Patients in whom the technique was successful became less anxious and less socially isolated than those in whom it failed and improved with regard to effectiveness in their occupations, ability to perform tasks around the home, personal relationships, sexual function, and social life. The authors concluded that dynamic graciloplasty is a safe and reliable technique in patients with severe incontinence and may result in a better quality of life.

Hallan et al. (229) reported on 32 patients who underwent such a procedure—20 for a deficient sphincter mechanism and 12 as part of a total reconstruction following abdominoperineal resection. Of the 20 patients treated with this technique, 12 have a functioning neosphincter, 6 have failed, usually due to sepsis or muscle ischemia, 1 is undergoing muscle transformation, and 1 died of an unrelated cause. The authors state that the initial problem of ischemia has now been eliminated by dividing the distal blood supply to the gracilis several weeks before muscle transposition.

Wexner et al. (235) reported on 17 patients who underwent the procedure. There were two deaths, one from pancreatitis and one from small-bowel carcinoma, 3 and 6 months after the procedure. Three patients required permanent stomas. Other recorded complications in this series included seroma of the thigh incision, excoriation of the skin above the stimulator, fecal impaction, anal fissure, parasternal hernia, rotation of the stimulator, premature battery discharge, fracture of the lead, perineal skin irritation, perineal sepsis, rupture of the tendon, tendon erosion, muscle fatigue during programming sessions, and electrode displacement from the nerve or fibrosis around the nerve. After rectification of these problems, 13 of the 15 eligible patients had stoma reversal. Based on an objective functional questionnaire, 60% of evaluable patients (9 of 15) reported improvement in continence, social interactions, and quality of life. Three of these nine patients require daily enemas.

Geerdes et al. (236) reported on the complications and management of patients who underwent dynamic graciloplasty. Dynamic graciloplasty was performed in 67 patients, with a mean follow-up of 2.7 years. Continence was defined as being continent to solid and liquid stool. The technique was successful in 52 patients (78%), whereas failure occurred in 15 patients (22%). Complications resulted from technical difficulties, infection, and problems attributable to an abnormal physiology of the muscle or an anorectal functional imbalance. In total, 53 complications were identified in 36 patients. Most technical problems concerning the transposition and stimulation of the gracilis muscle could be treated. Failures were attributable to a bad contraction of the distal part of the muscle (four) and perforation of the anal canal during stimulation (one). In eight patients, infection of the stimulator and leads required explanation. Three patients did not regain continence after reimplantation. Apart from moderate constipation, physiologic complications were very hard to treat and resulted in failures in five patients because of overflow incontinence, soiling, a nondistending rectum, strong peristalsis, and strong constipation. In two patients, the technique failed despite a well-contracting graciloplasty; no clear reason for the failure was found. The authors concluded that complications associated with the technique of dynamic graciloplasty such as loss of contraction, infection, bad contraction in the distal part of the muscle, and constipation can often be prevented or treated. Difficulties related to an impaired sensation and/or motility, attributable to a congenital cause or degeneration, are impossible to treat. Thus a good selection of patients is essential to prevent disappointment.

A more recent report from Penninckx, on behalf of the Belgian Section of Colorectal Surgery, indicates that the outcome is less favorable. After a median follow-up of 48 months dynamic graciloplasty had failed in 45% of the patients. The highest rate of failure was observed during the first year after surgery. However, there was also a significant number of failures at a later stage (238). Matzel et al. (239) identified complications associated with dynamic graciloplasty in 121 patients enrolled in a prospective trial of 20 centers. Severe treatment-related complications were defined as those requiring hospitalization or surgical intervention. In 93 patients, 211 complications occurred. Of these, 89 (42%) in 61 patients were classified as severe treatment-related complications and resulted from the following; major infection, 19; minor infection, 10; thromboembolic events, 3; device performance and use, 13; pain, 16; noninfectious gracilis problems, 8; noninfectious wound-healing problems, 3; other surgery-related complications, 3. In addition, severe treatment-related complications resulted from constipation in 10 and stoma creation or closure in 10. The recovery rate (full or partial) was 87% overall and for severe treatment-related complications was 92%. They concluded complications occurred frequently after dynamic graciloplasty, but are usually treatable.

Given the significant morbidity, the high reoperation rate and the necessity for a eight-week training period, it is obvious that patient motivation is essential. Dynamic graciloplasty has also been applied to other situations where patients face a permanent stoma. The concept of total anorectal reconstruction was developed to eliminate the deleterious psychological consequences of abdominoperineal resection of the rectum and permanent colostomy (240). The literature supports the hypothesis that patients suffer less distortion of body image after the creation of a perineal rather than an abdominal stoma (240). The procedure has been applied to patients undergoing abdominoperineal resection for carcinoma of the rectum and in those who had previously undergone an abdominoperineal resection and permanent colostomy (241). In a series of 47 patients reported on by Cavina et al. (233), good function was obtained in 65%, fair in 22.5%, and poor in 12.5%. The seven patients reported by Mercati et al. (242) had an acceptable outcome, but experienced some leakage. Santoro et al. (243) reported good functional results in more than 50% of the 15 cases with complete continence for solid stool. It is important to note that Abercrombie et al. (244) warn that in six patients who underwent objective measurement of anorectal sensory function following abdominoperineal resection and total anorectal reconstruction, none perceived neorectal distention as a desire to defecate or as a feeling of flatus. The loss of rectal sensation suggests that the prime sensor of rectal filling may lie within the rectum itself. Korsgren and Keighley (245) report that only one of their four patients treated with a stimulated gracilis had a functioning neosphincter.

Kennedy et al. (246) reported on the use of the stimulated graciloplasty in 12 patients after abdominoperineal resection for rectal carcinoma. Continence was achieved in seven patients. Complications included deep venous thrombosis, pulmonary embolus, saphenous nerve injury, leg wound hematoma, and late pacemaker infection.

Violi et al. (247) evaluated 23 patients who underwent abdominoperineal resection, coloperineal pull through, double graciloplasty, and loop abdominal stoma. Temporary external source intermittent electrostimulation, biofeedback training, and selective delayed stimulator implantation to improve unsatisfactory results were carried out in the first 13 patients (first series); thereafter second (second series) the stimulator was implanted during graciloplasty. The rate of major and minor postoperative complications was 21.7% and 65%, respectively. Continuous electrostimulation proved effective on resting anal pressure. Early clinical assessment showed satisfactory functional results (considered as having a score equal to 8 or less) in all first-group patients, including five who had stimulator support, and in one half of second-group patients. All functional results improved and became satisfactory from five years on (first series) and from four years on (second series).

Romano et al. (248) reported eight patients who underwent total anorectal reconstruction following abdominoperineal resection, five for a synchronous reconstruction and three cases for a delayed procedure. The follow-up length ranged from 6 to 28 months. Manometry assessed a basal pressure with the ABS cuff inflated between 58 and 62.2 mmHg. All but one patient achieved a good grade of continence with a Wexner score range between 3 and 9. A certain degree of impaired evacuation occurred in three patients but with adequate training this improved and did not affect patient's satisfaction.

Rullier et al. (249) evaluated morbidity and functional results in a homogeneous series of patients undergoing dynamic graciloplasty following APR for rectal carcinoma in 15 patients. All patients had preoperative radiotherapy (45 Gy), 11 with concomitant chemotherapy, 8 with intraoperative radiotherapy (15 Gy), and 10 received adjuvant chemotherapy for six months. The surgical procedure was performed in three stages: APR with coloperineal anastomosis and double graciloplasty (double muscle wrap); implantation of the stimulator 2 months later; and ileostomy closure after a training period. There was no operative death. At a mean of 28 months of follow-up, there was no local recurrence; early and late morbidity occurred in 11 patients, mainly related to the neosphincter (12 of 16 complications). The main complication was stenosis of the neosphincter ($n = 6$), which developed with electrical stimulation. Of 12 patients available for functional outcome, 7 were continent, 2 were incontinent, and 3 had an abdominal colostomy (2 for incontinence and 1 for sepsis). In light of these complications, they suggested that single dynamic graciloplasty should be used for anorectal reconstruction after APR.

GLUTEAL MUSCLE TRANSPOSITION ■ Transposition of the gluteus maximus muscle has been used in situations in which a normally functioning sphincter muscle is absent (250–252). This operation can be used after accidents in which the perineal tissues are avulsed. An excellent review of the subject was conducted by Fleshner and Roberts (223), and the following description is drawn from their dissertation.

The gluteus maximus muscle is ideally suited for transposition to the perianal region. It is a well-vascularized muscle supplied by the inferior gluteal artery (Fig. 7A). It is innervated by the L5 and S1 nerve roots through the inferior gluteal nerve and thus functions despite denervation of the anal sphincter mechanism, which is supplied by the S2 to S4 nerve roots. A potential advantage in using the gluteus maximus muscle rather than the gracilis muscle lies in the fact that it is a large, strong muscle. Its proximity to the anal area eliminates the need for disfiguring thigh incisions. However, because the gluteus maximus muscle is a hip extensor, some theoretical concerns have arisen regarding the impact on hip extension, even though only the inferior portion of the muscle is used.

As with other muscle transposition procedures, transposition of the gluteus maximus muscle is an option of virtually last resort. It is best suited for relatively young, motivated patients with neurogenic fecal incontinence, multiple failed sphincteroplasties, and severe sphincter defects that preclude primary repair. Needless to say, a functioning gluteus maximus muscle is necessary; this may be ascertained by asking the patient to squeeze the muscle. When the integrity of the muscle is in doubt, particularly in a patient who has had a severe traumatic injury or a necrotizing infection requiring debridement, EMG should be performed. Preoperative anal manometry, although not essential, may precisely measure the improvement in anal pressures.

TECHNIQUE ■ After preoperative mechanical and antibiotic bowel preparation, the patient is placed in the prone jackknife position. Bilateral oblique incisions are made lateral to the midline and extending to the ischial tuberosity (Fig. 7B). The inferior border of the gluteus maximus muscle is identified and followed to its sacrococcygeal insertion. The inferior (caudal) portion of the muscle is detached from its sacrococcygeal attachment, ensuring that the dense fascia attaching the muscle to the sacrum is included. The muscle is mobilized laterally, with care to preserve the inferior gluteal artery and nerve (Fig. 7C). A stimulator may be helpful in identifying the nerve (253). The muscle is divided along the direction of its fibers into two equal segments. A similar procedure is carried out on the opposite side.

Two curvilinear incisions are made several centimeters from the anal verge over the left and right ischioanal space. Subcutaneous tunnels are developed anteriorly and posteriorly around the anus. Space is also developed to tunnel the muscle to the perianal area. The ends of the inferior muscle from the right and left side are passed inferiorly toward the perineum, overlapped, and sutured. Similarly, the ends of the superior muscle are passed posteriorly around the rectum, overlapped, and secured, thus creating a valve-like diaphragm around the anus (Fig. 7D). The wounds are closed, and suction drains are left in place.

Postoperative care is routine. Early ambulation is permitted, but sitting is not allowed for several weeks. The patient should avoid climbing stairs for 2 to 3 weeks.

According to a review of the literature by Fleshner and Roberts (223), the most common complication after transposition of the gluteus maximus muscle is infection of the wound (24%). Other complications include skin separation and/or necrosis in 8% and fecal impaction in 8%. Their review of the scant literature on the subject revealed complete continence in 60%, partial continence in 36%, and total failure in 4%.

Pearl et al. (254) reported on seven patients who underwent bilateral gluteus maximus transposition for complete anal incontinence. The indications for operation were sphincter destruction secondary to multiple fistulotomies (four), bilateral pudendal nerve damage (two), and high imperforate anus (one). This procedure was performed without the use of a diverting colostomy. The inferior portion of the origin of each gluteus maximus is detached from the sacrum and coccyx, bifurcated, and tunneled subcutaneously to encircle the anus. The ends are then sutured together to form two opposing slings of voluntary muscle. Postoperatively, six patients regained continence to solid stool, two to liquid stool as well, and only one patient in this group was able to control flatus.

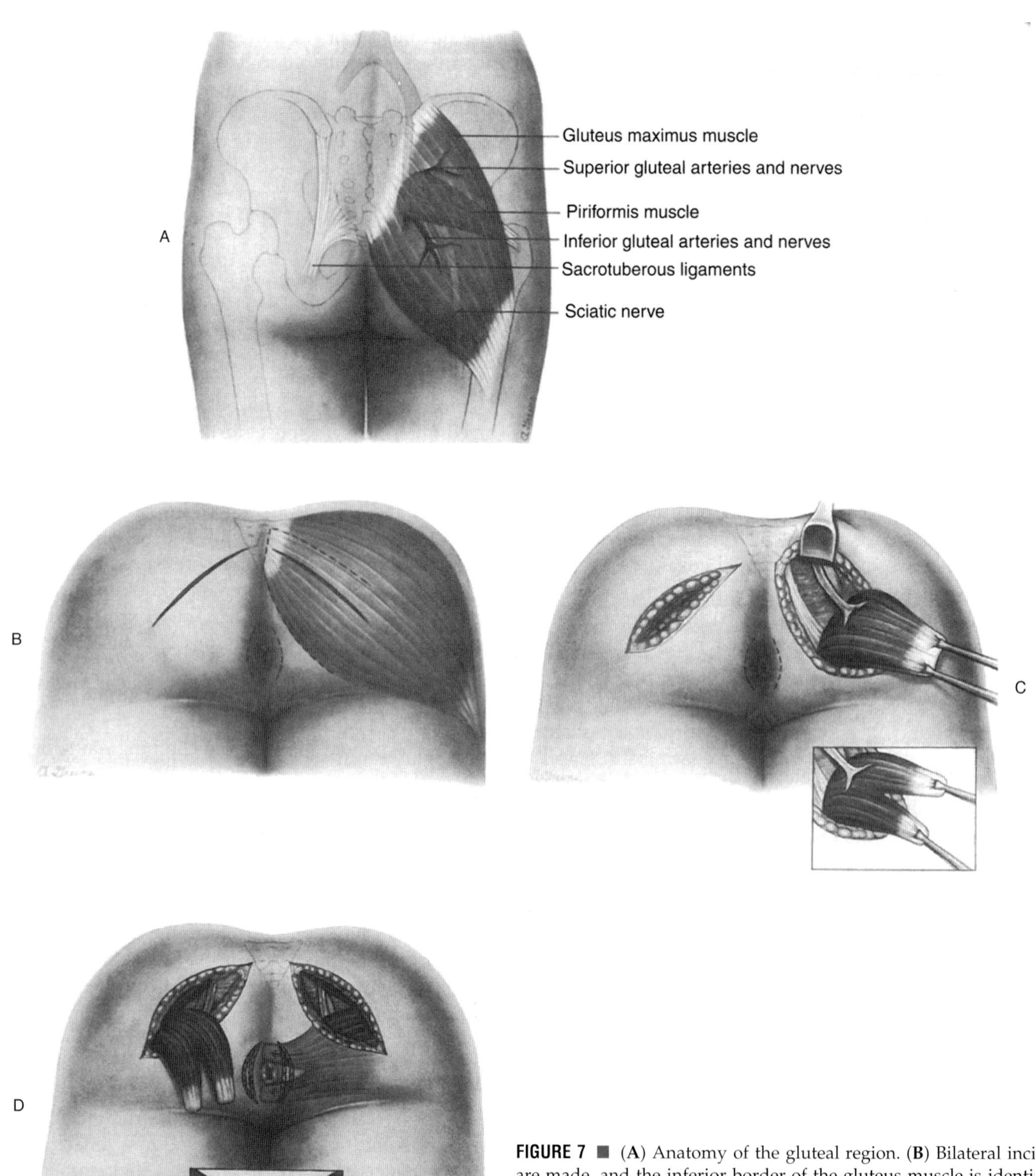

FIGURE 7 ■ (**A**) Anatomy of the gluteal region. (**B**) Bilateral incisions are made, and the inferior border of the gluteus muscle is identified. (**C**) Muscle is detached from the sacrococcygeal attachment, with care to preserve the neurovascular supply. The muscle is split into two sections (*inset*). (**D**) The muscle is tunneled from each side and passed around the anus, overlapped, and sutured. *Source*: From Ref. 223.

Although resting pressures remained unchanged, voluntary squeeze pressures were restored by this operation. In addition, rectal sensation was markedly improved, which helps make this a worthwhile procedure for properly selected patients.

Christiansen et al. (255) used bilateral gluteus maximus transposition to treat seven patients with anal incontinence in whom previous surgery had failed. All patients were incontinent to solid stool. Previous surgery involved postanal repair in four women and secondary overlapping suture for obstetric tear in one. The two men were treated in childhood for anal atresia. No covering stoma was used. Wound infection occurred in three patients, requiring surgical drainage in two. After follow-up of more than one year, three patients experienced improved continence, but in four, continence was unchanged. Anorectal physiologic studies showed moderately increased resting and squeeze pressures in patients in whom continence was improved by the operation, but none could retain more than 200 mL of viscous fluid instilled into the rectum. No change in rectal sensitivity or volume tolerance was found. This preliminary series does not indicate that better results are obtained by gluteus maximus transposition than by unstimulated graciloplasty.

FREE MUSCLE GRAFT ■ Free autogenous muscle transplantation has been used to treat anal incontinence resulting from a traumatized or congenitally absent puborectalis muscle. The palmaris longus or the sartorius muscle transport forms a dynamic ring that becomes innervated from the muscles of the pelvic floor and thus is incorporated automatically in the anal reflex mechanism. This method implies transposition of a striated muscle, two weeks after denervation, to the perirectal area as a U-shaped sling around the rectum corresponding to the location of the so-called puborectalis muscle. Hakelius and Olsen (256) reported on the results in 26 children who underwent this procedure. At follow-up after an average of 11 years and 4 months, 60% of the cases were regarded as good, 16% as fair, 8% as improved, and 16% as failures. In the authors' opinion, free muscle transplant offers a good chance of achieving acceptable continence in a majority of incontinent children.

Artificial Sphincter Implantation

Christiansen and Sparso (257) reported on the implantation of an artificial anal sphincter. Twelve patients with anal incontinence due to neurologic disease or failure of previous incontinence surgery underwent implantation of an artificial anal sphincter. The system used was a modification of the AMS 800 artificial urinary sphincter. In two patients, infection necessitated removal of the system, and in four patients, eight revisional procedures had to be performed because of mechanical failure. Only one case of mechanical failure has occurred. Erosion through the anal canal did not occur. Among 10 patients with the system in function for more than six months, the result was considered excellent in five, with only occasional leakage of flatus, good in three, who occasionally leaked liquid feces and flatus, and acceptable in two, in whom the cuff obstructed defecation. The authors concluded that implantation of an artificial anal sphincter is a valid alternative to permanent colostomy in patients with anal incontinence due to neurologic disorders and in patients in whom other types of incontinence surgery have failed.

Since this report from Christiansen and Sparso, several studies have emerged detailing the preliminary experience of various groups with the artificial sphincter. The modifications of the AMS 800 artificial urinary sphincter culminated in the development of the Action™ neosphincter device, specially designed for fecal incontinence. Wong et al. conducted a multicenter cohort study to investigate the safety and efficacy of this device for fecal incontinence. The Action neosphincter device was implanted in 112 patients (86 females). A total of 384 device-related adverse events were reported in 99 patients. Of these events, 138 required invasive intervention. Infection, necessitating surgical revision, was noted in 25% of the patients. Forty-one patients (37%) have had their device explanted. In patients with a functioning neosphincter, the outcome was successful in 85% of the cases. However, the intention to treat success rate was only 53%. These data illustrate that this procedure, like the dynamic graciloplasty, is associated with a high morbidity and a high reoperation rate (258). Devesa et al. described the functional results and complications among 53 patients who underwent implantation of an Acticon™ neosphincter in one single institution. Normal continence was achieved in 65% of the patients with a functioning device. The device explanation rate was 19%. Sepsis and wound complications were noted in 30% of the patients (259). Lehur et al. assessed quality of life in 12 out of 16 patients with an activated device. They calculated the FIQLS score (according to Rockwood) as well as the Fecal Incontinece Score (also according to Rockwood). Two years after implantation, the mean quality of life scale score was increased from 0.44 to 0.83. The mean fecal incontinence score dropped from 105 to 32. A linear correlation was found between the improvement in quality of life and the better incontinence scores. These results were associated with a significant increase in maximal anal resting pressure (260). Similar figures have been reported by others (261). More recently Mundy et al. performed a systematic review of 14 studies on the safety and effectiveness of artificial bowel sphincters for fecal incontinence. They found that most results were not analyzed on an intention-to-treat basis. Although the patients with a functioning device at the end of the follow-up experienced a better quality of life with improvement of continence, no outcome data were presented for those with a nonfunctioning device or an explanted device. Based on the high rates of adverse events due to infection, device malfunction, ulceration, and pain, it might be possible that patients without a functioning device may have a worsened degree of incontinence or decreased quality of life. The authors concluded that implantation of an artificial sphincter is of uncertain benefit and may possibly harm many patients (262). Based on the outcome of this critical review, the exact role of artificial sphincters in the treatment of fecal incontinence is questionable. Table 10 summarizes the results of the artificial bowel sphincter.

■ NEW DEVELOPMENTS

Hyperbaric Oxygen

Oxygen at pressure has been shown to aid the regeneration of nerves that have been damaged. Other effects that may be useful in the treatment of nerve damage are promotion of angiogenesis and reduction of edema. Because of these effects, Cundall et al. postulated that hyperbaric oxygen might enhance nerve conduction in pudendal neuropathy and thus ameliorate the incontinence (268). They conducted a pilot study in 13 patients with fecal incontinence due to chronic pudendal neuropathy. They received 30 treatments during a period of six weeks. Each treatment was at 2.4 atm breathing pure oxygen for 90 minutes. All patients completed the treatment without major complications. The authors found a consistent improvement of the latencies on both sides. Incontinence scores also improved. These intriguing results justify further trials.

TABLE 10 ■ Results of Artificial Bowel Sphincter

Author(s)	*n*	Complications (%)	Explanted (%)	F/U (mo)	Success: Functioning with Sphincter (%)	Success: Intention to Treat
Christiansen et al. 1999 (263)	17	70	41	84	47	–
O'Brien and Skinner 2000 (264)	13	23	23	–	90	69
Devesa et al. 2002 (259)	53	57	19	27	65	–
Ortiz et al. 2002 (265)	24	42	29	28	27	17
Wong et al. 2002 (258)	112	86	37	12	85	53
Altomare et al. 2004 (266)	28	57	39	50	18	12
Finlay et al. 2004 (267)	12	0	17	59	91	–

Secca® Procedure

Based on the therapeutic effect of temperature-controlled radio frequency (RF) energy delivery to the lower esophageal sphincter for the treatment of gastroesophageal reflux disease, it has been hypothesized that the delivery of RF energy to the anal canal might improve the barrier function of the anal sphincter complex. The Secca procedure can be performed on an ambulatory basis using conscious sedation and local anesthesia. The patient is positioned in the prone-jacknife position. A special RF energy device is used. This instrument comprises an anoscopic barrel with four nickel–titanium curved needle electrodes. Within the tip and at the base of each electrode, thermocouples are present to monitor tissue and mucosal temperature during RF delivery. The instrument is introduced into the anal canal under direct visualization, so that the needle electrodes start to penetrate the tissue 1 cm distal to the dentate line. Additional lesions are created up to 1.5 cm above the dentate line in all four quadrants. Mucosal temperature is cooled by surface irrigation. In this way thermal lesions are created in the muscle below the mucosa, while preserving the mucosal integrity. Takahashi et al. conducted a pilot study in 10 patients with fecal incontinence of varying causes. Twelve months after the procedure, the median Wexner incontinence score was dropped from 13.5 to 5. All parameters in the fecal incontinence–related quality of life were improved. Six months after the procedure, maximum tolerable rectal distension volumes were significantly reduced (269). This therapeutic effect persisted two years after the procedure (270). Similar results have been reported by Efron et al. who conducted a multicenter trial to evaluate the safety and effectiveness of this procedure. Fifty patients were enrolled. Complications included mucosal ulceration in two patients and delayed bleeding in one. Endoanal ultrasound revealed no defects in the underlying sphincters. Pudendal nerve motor latency remained the same and the manometric parameters did not change (271).

Tissue shrinkage with subsequent reduction of compliance, due to heating to approximately 65°C, is one of the possible mechanisms that may explain the therapeutic effect of this procedure. Other possible mechanisms are the observed reduction in tolerable rectal distension volumes and alteration of the sampling reflex.

Implantation of Silicone Biomaterial

Injection of a bulking agent around the internal anal sphincter or into a defect of this sphincter is another new development. In the 1990s, Shafik was the first to inject autologous fat in the perianal region in order to enhance continence (272). This technique was also utilized by Bernardi et al. They observed a short-term improvement that decreased with time and required repeated injections due to migration and absorption on the infected fat (273). Injection of polytetrafluoroethylene and collagen has also been described (274,275). More recently the use of silicone biomaterial has been introduced. For this purpose silicone particles suspended in a bioexcretable carrier hydrogel of polyvinylpyrrolidone are used. Feretis et al. studied six patients who underwent implantation of silicone biomaterial in the submucosa, 1 to 2 cm above the dentate line. The implantation was performed as an outpatient procedure, under intravenous sedation. After a mean follow-up of 8.6 months, the incontinence scores were improved in all the patients. This was not associated with alterations in anal pressure (276). Kenefick et al. reported similar results in patients with incontinence due to an internal anal sphincter dysfunction. They injected the material with a needle, passing through the external anal sphincter into the area of the internal anal sphincter. Three injections were placed circumferentially at or just above the level of the dentate line (277). More recently, Tjandra et al. reported their experience with this technique in 82 patients with disturbed continence caused by a weak or disrupted internal anal sphincter. They also found a marked improvement in fecal continence and quality of life. In addition, their study revealed that injection of the silicone biomaterial is more effective if the particles are implanted with the guidance of endoanal ultrasound (278). The initial results, reported so far, are promising and justify further studies, especially to identify criteria for patient selection.

Sacral Neuromodulation (SNM)

The most exciting new development is SNM. In 1981, Tanagho and Schmidt from the University of California in San Fransisco were the first to implant a pacemaker for SNM in patients with urinary urge incontinence and non-obstructive urinary retention (279). In some patients, a simultaneous improvement in bowel symptoms was observed, prompting the investigation of SNM for the treatment of functional bowel disorders. In 1995, Matzel et al. were the first to report initial results of SNM in three patients with fecal incontinence (280). During the last decade, several studies have revealed that this treatment modality provides a very attractive alternative for the treatment of fecal incontinence. Compared with dynamic graciloplasty and the implantation of an artificial sphincter,

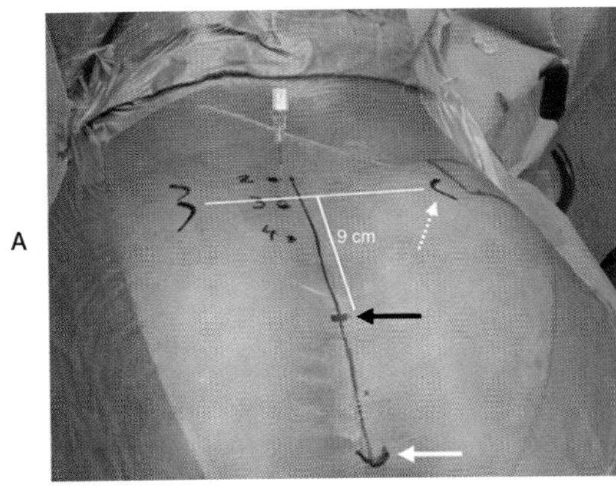

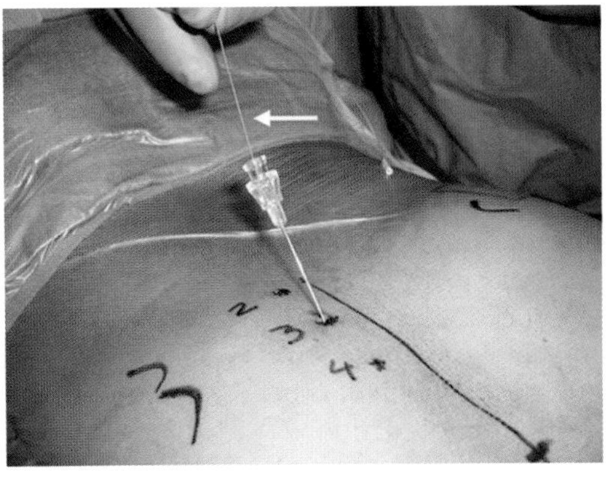

FIGURE 8 ■ (**A** and **B**) Sacrococcygeal junction (*black arrow*), tip of the coccyx (*closed arrow*), and sciatic notch (*interrupted arrow*).

SNM has several advantages. First of all, a test stimulation precedes the definitive implantation of the neurostimulator. The test stimulation, which can be performed under local anesthesia on an outpatient base, enables appropriate selection of patients. With the patient in prone-jacknife position, an insulated needle is inserted perpendicular to the sacrum, with an inclination to the skin of approximately 60° (Fig. 8). Usually the needle is positioned in the third sacral foramen. Stimulation of the third sacral nerve causes a contraction of the pelvic floor and the external anal sphincter and a plantar flexion of the big toe. Once an adequate muscular response is obtained, a temporary stimulator lead is inserted through the needle. Then the needle is removed and the lead is connected to an external stimulator. The patient is subsequently tested for 2 to 3 weeks with low-frequency stimulation, just above the sensory threshold for each patient. If the test stimulation results in a significant reduction in the number of incontinence episodes (at least >50%), a permanent system can be implanted (Fig. 9A–D). An incision over the sacrum allows access to the sacral foramen, and the permanent quadripolar electrode is positioned into the foramen under direct visualization and anchored with sutures to the sacral periosteum. The electrode lead is connected to an extension cable, which is tunnelled subcutaneously to one of the sides of the patient. Finally the extension cable is connected with the neurostimulator, implanted in a subcutaneous pocket in the lower quadrant of the abdomen. Recent technical

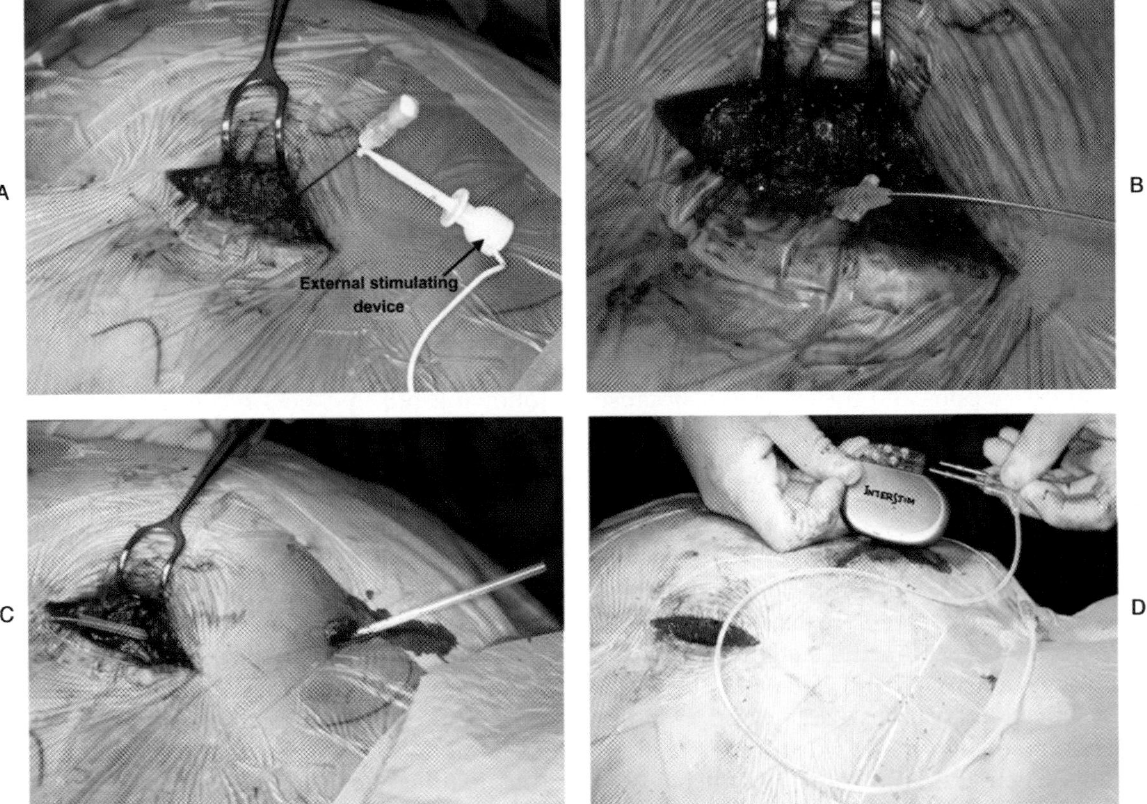

FIGURE 9 ■ Sacral neuromodulation. (**A**) Patient in prone-jackknife position. Placement of needle in sacral foramen through a midline incision. External stimulation to evoke contraction of the external anal sphincter and pelvic floor ("bellow" sign), indicating correct placement. (**B**) Placement of definitive electrode lead into the selected sacral foramen (usually S3). (**C**) Tunneling of the electrode lead in the direction of the subcutaneous pocket at the upper margin of the buttock, created for placement of the permanent stimulator. (**D**) Connection of the electrode lead with the permanent stimulator.

improvements have changed the current technique of implantation. First, there is a new permanent electrode that can be placed percutaneously and is then held in place with barbs, thereby avoiding an operative scar in the natal cleft. Second, it has been shown that the stimulator can be placed in the buttock rather than the abdominal wall. The morbidity, associated with this technique of implantation, is low in comparison with dynamic graciloplasty and implantation of an artificial sphincter. The procedure is easy to learn and not technically demanding. It is not necessary to turn the stimulus off prior to defecation, which can be considered another advantage. The mode of action of SNM is still not elucidated. Vaizey et al. conducted a small double-blind crossover study in two patients. The trial period consisted of two 2-week periods, with the stimulator turned on for 2 weeks and off for 2 weeks. The main investigator and the patients were blinded to the status of the stimulator. There was a dramatic difference between the number and severity of episodes of incontinence when the stimulator was turned on versus turned off. Based on this study, it is unlikely that the beneficial effect of stimulation reflects a placebo effect. Furthermore, this study also demonstrates that the therapeutic effect was unlikely to be caused by a chronic change in the muscles being stimulated, because turning the stimulus off resulted in immediate incontinence (281). Several authors have reported that SNM results in an increase in anal pressure (282,283). Other workers, however, found no significant change, neither in anal resting pressure, nor in anal squeeze pressure (284). These conflicting data are probably due to differences in pacemaker settings. To date, external stimulators are set at an amplitude just below or above the threshold of patient sensation. With this setting, it is unlikely that continence is restored only by a simple direct effect on the efferent motor supply to the sphincters. Increased rectal sensitivity to balloon distension suggests that SNM also affects afferent sensory nerves (285). These nerves have the lowest threshold to stimulation. Malaguti et al. evaluated somatosensory-evoked potentials of the pudendal and posterior tibial nerves in patients with an external stimulator. Their study provides evidence for modulating effects of SNM on the afferent pathways to the central nervous system (286). Probably, this modulation has also a central effect on pons and cortex cerebri, because SNM has been reported to benefit patients with incomplete spinal cord lesions, whereas SNM is not effective in patients with complete spinal cord transection (287,288).

The diminution in urgency, as reported by many patients, suggests that SNM also alters the contractile activity of colon and rectum. Twenty-four-hour ambulatory recordings of rectal and anal pressure have shown that stimulation reduces rectal contractile activity, enhances anal pressure slow-wave activity, and decreases the number of internal sphincter relaxations (289). Laser Doppler flow measurements have shown a rapid increase in rectal mucosal bloodflow when the stimulator is switched on. Because this bloodflow is under the control of autonomic nerve activity, it seems likely that SNM also acts on the extrinsic autonomic nerve system (290). It has been reported that SNM is not successful in patients who became incontinent after low-anterior resection (284). Damage to the nerves innervating the rectum and the pelvic floor seems to be the underlying cause of this failure, indicating that intact reflex arcs are mandatory for a successful outcome of SNM.

Rasmussen et al. (291) studied sacral nerve stimulation in 45 patients with fecal incontinence. If a perineal/perianal muscular response to sacral nerve stimulation could be obtained, electrodes were implanted for a three-week test stimulation period. If sacral nerve stimulation resulted in at least a 50% reduction in incontinence episodes during the test period, a system for permanent sacral nerve stimulation was implanted. Percutaneous electrodes were used in 34 patients, and 23 of these had at least a 50% reduction in incontinence episodes, whereas the electrodes dislocated in seven patients and four had a poor response. Permanent electrodes with percutaneous extension electrodes were used primarily in nine patients and after dislocation of percutaneous electrodes in an additional six patients; 14 of these had good results. A permanent stimulation system was implanted in 37 patients. After a median of 6 months follow-up, 5 patients had the system explanted: three because the clinical response faded out and two because of infection. Incontinence score (Wexner 0–20) for the 37 patients with a permanent system for sacral nerve stimulation was reduced from median 16 before sacral nerve stimulation to median 6 at latest follow-up. There was no difference in effect of sacral nerve stimulation of patients with idiopathic incontinence ($n=19$) compared with spinal etiology ($n=8$) or obstetric cause of incontinence ($n=5$).

More recently, Ratto et al. (292) evaluated fecal incontinence following preoperative chemoradiation and anterior resection for rectal carcinoma in four patients. After device implantation, the mean fecal incontinence scores decreased, and the mean number of incontinence episodes dropped from 12.0 to 2.5 per week. Permanent implant resulted in a significant improvement in fecal continence in three patients, and incontinence was slightly reduced in the fourth. Jarrett et al. (293) also found that sacral nerve stimulation may be effective in the treatment of patients with fecal incontinence following rectosigmoid resection for carcinoma in three patients. One had had a coloanal and two a colorectal anastomosis for rectal carcinoma. Jarrett et al. (294) found sacral nerve stimulation effective in four patients with ongoing fecal incontinence following full thickness rectal prolapse repair.

Initially it was thought that SNM was only effective in patients with fecal incontinence in whom the sphincters were weak but intact. Several anecdotal reports do suggest, however, that SNM is also beneficial for patients with a sphincter defect.

Jarrett et al. (287) conducted a systematic review evaluating sacral nerve stimulation in the treatment of fecal incontinence or constipation. From 106 potentially relevant reports, six patients series and one crossover study of sacral nerve stimulation for fecal incontinence and four patient series and one crossover study for sacral nerve stimulation for constipation were included. After implantation, 41% to 75% of patients achieved complete fecal continence and 75% to 100% experienced improvement in episodes of incontinence. There were 19 adverse events among 149 patients.

The results of SNM, reported so far, are summarized in Table 11. In most papers, the results are quantified by the reduced number of incontinence episodes per week.

TABLE 11 ■ Results of Sacral Neuromodulation

Author(s)	Year	No. of Patients	Follow-Up (Years)	Incontinence Episodes/Wk (Median)	
				Before SNM	At the Last Follow-Up
Rosen et al. (295)	2001	16	1.25	6	2
Ganio et al. (296)	2001	16	1.5	6	0.6
Kenefick et al. (283)	2002	15	2	11	0
Uludağ et al. (284)	2004	50	1	7.5	0.67
Matzel et al. (297)	2004	34	2	16.4	2.0
Jarrett et al. (285)	2004	46	1	7.5	1.0

Abbreviation: SNM, sacral neuromodulation.

■ COLOSTOMY

For patients with anal incontinence so severe that they are disabled by their problem and unable to control their elimination pattern by conventional means, such as medication, diet, and enemas, construction of a colostomy may become necessary. Despite the stoma, the patient's quality of life may be significantly enhanced, and self-imposed ostracization corrected. A colostomy is especially appropriate in patients with irradiation destruction of the rectum. The colostomy must be performed outside the irradiated field to prevent subsequent breakdown or problems with the colostomy. Whether the rectum should be left in situ or removed is a question that can be answered only in a discussion with the patient and by considering the degree of the chance of morbidity that continued rectal discharge might cause. This chance must be balanced with the increased morbidity that accompanies proctectomy.

Norton et al. (298) reviewed the formation of a permanent stoma as a last resort when all other interventions for fecal incontinence have failed. Questionnaires were sent asking about the stoma, previous incontinence, anxiety and depression, and quality of life. A total of 69 replies were received. Respondents were 11 males and 58 females with a median age of 64 years and a median of 59 months since the operation. Rating their ability to live with their stoma now on a scale of 0 to 10, the median response was 8. The majority (83%) felt that the stoma restricted their life "a little" or "not at all," a significant improvement from perceived restriction from former incontinence. Satisfaction with the stoma was a median of 9. Eighty-four percent would "probably" or "definitely" choose to have the stoma again. Quality of life (SF-36) was poor, but neither depression nor anxiety was a prominent feature. They concluded the majority of previous incontinent people were positive about the stoma and the difference it had made to their life. However, a few had not adapted and disliked the stoma intensely.

A novel modification of a colostomy was described by Hughes and Williams (299). A transverse colonic conduit incorporating an intussusception valve and a skin-flapped cutaneous aperture was constructed in nine patients with combined fecal incontinence and disordered evacuation. Intestinal continuity was restored with a colocolonic anastomosis. The median follow-up was 4 months (range, 2–15 months), and daily irrigation with a median 1.2 L (range, 0.3–2.0 L) of water resulted in evacuation in less than 1 hour. At 1 month after operation, there was no leakage of solid or liquid feces from the anus between irrigations. The valve was continent to feces and irrigation fluid, and no stoma appliances were required.

■ SELECTION OF OPERATIVE PROCEDURE

A consensus conference on treatment options of fecal incontinence provided the following conclusions (300): (i) Diarrhea is the most common aggravating factor for fecal incontinence, and antidiarrheal medications such as Loperamide and Diphenoxylate or bile acid binders may help. Fecal impaction, a common cause of fecal incontinence in children and elderly patients, responds to combinations of laxatives, education, and habit training in approximately 60%. These causes of fecal incontinence can usually be identified by history and physical examination alone. (ii) In patients who fail medical management or have evidence of sphincter weakness, anorectal manometry, and endoanal ultrasound are recommended as helpful in differentiating simple morphologic defects from afferent and efferent nerve injuries and from combined structural and neurologic injuries. (iii) Biofeedback is a harmless and inexpensive treatment, which benefits approximately 75% of patients, but cures only about 50%. It may be most appropriate when there is neurologic injury (i.e., partial denervation), but it has been reported to also benefit incontinent patients with minor structural defects. (iv) External anal sphincter plication with or without pelvic floor repair is indicated when there is a known, repairable structural defect without significant neurologic injury. It is effective in approximately 68%. (v) Salvage operations are reserved for patients who cannot benefit from biofeedback or levator-sphincteroplasty. These include electrically stimulated gracilis muscle transpositions and colostomy. (vi) Antegrade enemas delivered through stomas in the cecum or descending colon reduce or eliminate soiling in approximately 78% of children with myelomeningocele; this operation may come to be more widely applied. (vii) Other treatments include implanted nerve stimulators, artificial sphincters, and anal plugs. (viii) Patient characteristics, which influence choice of treatment, include mental status, mobility impairment, and typical bowel habits.

In patients who are incontinent secondary to injury to the external sphincter but in whom innervation to at least one half of the sphincter is intact, we prefer to perform an overlapping sphincteroplasty as described previously. However, if the sphincter is intact and incontinence is secondary to stretching of the puborectalis muscle, with subsequent loss of the normal anorectal angle such as may occur with aging or with rectal procidentia, the Parks post-anal repair is used.

In cases in which the sphincter mechanism is denervated, the use of procedures such as a gracilis muscle transposition, other sphincteroplasties or an artificial sphincter implantation might be considered. The newer developments of silicone implantation and SNM hold promise. In special circumstances, a colostomy may be the only reasonable alternative.

■ "KEYHOLE" DEFORMITY

With the advent of the lateral internal sphincterotomy, the keyhole deformity, fortunately, will become increasingly uncommon. For the patient already afflicted with the problem, instruction in personal hygiene to include careful cleansing, with special attention to cleaning the partially everted anus, should be given. The patient should be counseled to keep the stool formed, because liquid stools are associated with more leakage. A wisp of cotton placed at the anal verge may help prevent skin irritation. An island skin flap has been successfully used to fill the keyhole groove (Fig. 2 in Chap. 36).

■ ANAL SOILING

Anal soiling is often troubling. Felt-Bersma et al. (301) used anorectal function investigations (anal manometry, rectal capacity assessment, and the saline infusion test), to evaluate 45 patients with soiling but not fecal incontinence. The causes of soiling and the effect of treatment on both soiling and anorectal function were studied. The results were compared with a control group of 161 patients without soiling or incontinence. The diagnoses were hemorrhoids in 10 patients, mucosal prolapse in seven, rectal prolapse in six, fistulas in five, proctitis in three, fecal impaction in two, rectocele with intussusception in two, scars after fistulectomy in two, and other causes of soiling in eight patients. Simple inspection and proctoscopy were generally sufficient to establish a diagnosis. For two patients, the diagnosis of rectocele was made after defecography. Anorectal test results did not differ between the two groups, did not contribute to establish a diagnosis, and did not change after treatment. Only patients with a rectal prolapse had abnormal results from anorectal function tests, a low-basal sphincter pressure and a limited continence reserve. Appropriate therapy resulted in complete recovery in 44% of the patients or improvement of symptoms in 29%.

To determine the physiologic alteration resulting in fecal seepage and soiling, Hoffmann et al. (302) evaluated the results of anorectal manometric testing in patients with varying degrees of fecal incontinence. Resting pressures were significantly lower in those with complete incontinence, partial incontinence, and seepage and soiling than in controls. Resting pressures of the "complete incontinence" group were also significantly lower than those of the "partial incontinence" group and "seepage and soiling" group. Squeezing pressures were lower for both the complete incontinence and the partial incontinence groups than in the control group and in the seepage and soiling group, whose results did not differ significantly from controls. The minimum rectal sensory volume was greater in all incontinent groups than in controls. Sensory volume of the seepage and soiling group was significantly greater than that of the complete incontinence and partial incontinence groups. The difference between sensory volume and the volume-producing reflex relaxation was greatest in the seepage and soiling group and differed from that of the partial incontinence and control groups. The authors' findings suggest that the mechanism of incontinence is different in patients who experience seepage and soiling and involves a dyssynergy of rectal sensation and anal relaxation. Patients with the pattern of seepage and soiling may be successfully treated with stool-bulking agents (e.g., psyllium or bran).

Sentovich et al. (303) sought to identify the clinical and manometric characteristics of male fecal incontinence. The clinical charts of 25 men with a chief complaint of fecal incontinence were retrospectively reviewed. Fourteen men (56%) were "leakers," who complained of loss of liquid or solid stool smears that stained their underclothes. Eleven men (44%) had true incontinence, with loss of control of gas, liquid, and/or solid stool. Leakers had lower anal sphincter pressures than normal men but higher pressures than incontinent men. In leakers, the anal sphincter length at rest was longer than in incontinent and normal men. All incontinent men had decreased manometric pressures, abnormal anorectal sensation, or prolonged PNTMLs, whereas only one half of the leakers had physiologic abnormalities. Treatment using dietary manipulation, constipating agents, or cleansing enemas was successful in nearly 90% of incontinent men but in only 55% of the leakers. Whereas true incontinence in men is caused by a short, low-pressure sphincter with altered sensation or innervation, leakage is associated with a long, intermediate-pressure sphincter that frequently has normal sensation and innervation. This long, intermediate-pressure sphincter may predispose these men to leakage.

REFERENCES

1. Madoff RD, Williams JG, Caushaj PE. Fecal incontinence. N Engl J Med 1992; 326:1002–1007.
2. Browning GP, Parks AG. Post anal repair for neuropathic fecal incontinence: correlation of clinical result and anal canal pressures. Br J Surg 1983; 70: 101–104.
3. Baxter NN, Rothenberger DA, Lowry AC. Measuring fecal incontinence. Dis Colon Rectum 2003; 46:1591–1605.
4. Jorge JM, Wexner SD. Etiology and management of fecal incontinence. Dis Colon Rectum 1993; 36:77–97.
5. Rockwood TH,Church JM, Fleshman JW, et al. Dis Colon Rectum 1999; 42:1525–1531.
6. Rockwood TH. Incontinence severity and QOL scales for fecal incontinence. Gastroenterology 2004; 126:S106–S113.
7. Participate 2002; 11:6.
8. Thomas TM, Egan M, Walgrove A, et al. The prevalence of faecal and double incontinence. Community Med 1984; 6:216–220.
9. Kok ALM, Voorhorst FJ, Burger CW, Van Houten P, Kenemans P, Janssens J. Urinary and faecal incontinence in community-residing elderly women. Age Ageing 1992; 21:211–215.
10. Kemp FM, Acheson RM. Care in the community—elderly people living alone at home. Community Med 1989; 11:21–26.
11. Talley NJ, O'Keefe EA, Zinsmeister AR, Melton JL. Prevalence of gastrointestinal symptoms in the elderly. A population based study. Gastroenterology 1992; 102:895–901.
12. Clarke N, Hughes AP, Dodd KJ, et al. The elderly in residential care: Patterns of disability. Health Trends 1979; 11:17.
13. Tobin GW, Brocklehurst JC. Fecal incontinence in residential homes for the elderly: prevalence, etiology, management. Age Ageing 1986; 15:41–46.

14. Nelson R, Norton N, Caudey E, Furner S. Community-based prevalence of anal incontinence. JAMA 1995; 274:559–561.
15. Borrie MJ, Davidson HA. Incontinence in institutions. Costs and contributing factors. Can Med Assoc J 1992; 147:322–328.
16. Whitehead WE, Schuster MM. Behavioral approaches to the treatment of gastrointestinal motility disorders. Med Clin North Am 1981; 65:1397–1411.
17. Sangwan YP, Coller JA. Fecal incontinence. Surg Clin North Am 1994; 74:1377–1398.
18. Macmillan AK, Merrie AE, Marshall RJ, Parry BR. The prevalence of fecal incontinence in community-dwelling adults: a systematic review of the literature. Dis Colon Rectum 2004; 47:1341–1349.
19. Johanson JF, Lafferty J. Epidemiology of fecal incontinence: the silent affliction. Am J Gastroenterol 1996; 91:33–36.
20. Cerulli MA, Nikoomanesh T, Schuster MM. Progress in biofeedback conditioning for fecal incontinence. Gastroenterology 1979; 76:742–746.
21. Ctercteko GC, Fazio VW, Jagelman DG, et al. Anal sphincter repair: a report of 60 cases and review of the literature. Aust N Z J Surg 1988; 58:703–710.
22. Keighley MR, Fielding JW. Management of fecal incontinence and results of surgical treatment. Br J Surg 1983; 70:463–468.
23. Lindsey I, Jones OM, Smilgin Humphreys MM, Cunningham C, Mortensen NJ. Patterns of fecal incontinence after anal surgery. Dis Colon Rectum 2004; 47:1643–1649.
24. Khubchandani IT, Reed JF. Sequelae of internal sphincterotomy for chronic fissure in ano. Br J Surg 1989; 76:431–434.
25. Garcia-Aguilar J, Belmonte C, Wong WD, Lowry AC, Madoff RD. Open vs. closed sphincterotomy for chronic anal fissure: long term results. Dis Colon rectum 1996; 39:440–443.
26. Pernikoff BJ, Eisenstat TE, Rubin RJ, Oliver GC, Salvati EP. Reappraisal of partial lateral internal sphincterotomy. Dis Colon Rectum 1994; 37:1291–1295.
27. Hananel N, Gordon PH. Lateral internal sphincterotomy for fissure-in-ano: revisited. Dis Colon Rectum 1997; 40:597–602.
28. Hyman N. Incontinence after lateral internal sphincterotomy: a prospective study and quality of life assessment. Dis Colon Rectum 2004; 47:35–38.
29. Tjandra JJ, Han WR, Ooi BS, Nagesh A, Thorne M. Fecal incontinence after lateral internal sphincterotomy is often associated with coexisting occult sphincter defects: a study using endoanal ultrasonography. AZN J Surg 2001; 71:598.
30. Zutshi M, Hull L, Casillas-Romero S, Trzoinski R, Bast JF. Incontinence after lateral internal sphincterotomy: are we underestimating it? Dis Colon Rectum 2004; 47:599.
31. Sultan AH, Kamm MA, Nicholls RJ, Bartram CI. Prospective study of the extent of internal anal sphincter division during lateral internal sphincterotomy. Dis Colon Rectum 1994; 37:1031–1033.
32. Aguilar PS, Plasencia G, Hardy TG, Hartman RF, Stewart WR. Mucosal advancement in the treatment of anal fistula. Dis Colon Rectum 1985; 28:496–498.
33. Ortiz H, Marzo J. Endorectal flap advancement repair and fistulectomy for high transsphincteric and suprasphincteric fistulas. Br J Surg 2000; 87:1680–1683.
34. Golub RW, Wise WE, Kerner BA, et al. Endorectal mucosal advancement flap: the preferred method for complex cryptoglandular fistula in ano. J Gastrointest Surg 1997; 1:487–491.
35. Schouten WR, Zimmerman DD, Briel JW. Transanal advancement flap repair of transsphincteric fistulas. Dis Colon Rectum 1999; 42:1419–1423.
36. van Tets WF, Kuijpers JH, Tran K, Mollen R, van Goor H. Influence of Parks' anal retractor on anal sphincter pressures. Dis Colon Rectum 1997; 40: 1042–1045.
37. Zimmerman DDE, Gosselink MP, Hop WCJ, Darby M, Briel JW, Schouten WR. Impact of two different types of anal retractor on fecal continence after fistula repair. Dis Colon Rectum 2003; 46:1674–1679.
38. Stelzner F. The morphological principles of anorectal continence. Prog Pediatr Surg 1976; 9:1–6.
39. Goligher JC, Lee PWR, MacFie J, et al. Experience with the Russian Model 249 suture gun for anastomoses of the rectum. Surg Gynecol Obstet 1979; 148: 516–524.
40. Gordon PH, Dalrymple S. The use of staples for reconstruction after colonic and rectal surgery. Ravitch MM, Steichen FM, eds. Principles and Practice of Surgical Stapling. Chicago: Year Book, 1987:402–431.
41. Kennedy JT, McOmish D, Bennett RC, et al. Abdominoanal pull-through resection of the rectum. Br J Surg 1970; 57:589–596.
42. Parks AG, Percy JP. Resection and sutured coloanal anastomosis for rectal carcinoma. Br J Surg 1982; 69:301–304.
43. Enker WE, Stearns MW, Janov AJ. Peranal coloanal anastomosis following low anterior resection for rectal carcinoma. Dis Colon Rectum 1985; 28: 576–581.
44. Vernava AM, Robbins PL, Brabbee GW. Restorative resection: coloanal anastomosis for benign and malignant disease. Dis Colon Rectum 1989; 32:690–693.
45. Sultan AH, Kamm MA, Hudson CN, Thomas JM, Bartram CI. Anal sphincter disruption during vaginal delivery. N Engl J Med 1993; 329:1905–1911.
46. Eason E, Labrecque M, Marcoux S, Mondor M. Anal incontinence after childbirth. CMAJ 2002; 166:326–330.
47. Campbell DM, Behan M, Donnelly VS, O'Herlihy C, O'Connell PR. Endosonographic assessment of postpartum anal sphincter injury using a 120 degree sector scanner. Clin Radiol 1996; 51:559–561.
48. Rieger N, Schloithe A, Saccone G, Wattchow D. A prospective study of anal sphincter injury due to childbirth. Scand J Gastroenterol 1998; 33:950–955.
49. Zetterstrom J, Mellgren A, Jensen LL, et al. Effect of delivery on anal sphincter morphology and function. Dis Colon Rectum 1999; 42:1253–1260.
50. Varma A, Gunn J, Gardiner A, Lindow SW, Duthie GS. Obstetric anal sphincter injury: prospective evaluation of incidence. Dis Colon Rectum 1999; 42:1537–1543.
51. Fynes M, Donnelly V, Behan M, O'Connell PR, O'Herlihy C. Effect of second vaginal delivery on anorectal physiology and fecal continence. Lancet 1999; 354:983–986.
52. Faltin DL, Boulvain M, Irion O, Bretones S, Stan C, Weil A. Diagnosis of anal sphincter tears by postpartum endosonography to predict fecal incontinence. Obstet Gynecol 2000; 95:643–647.
53. Damon H, Henry L, Bretones S, Mellier G, Minaire Y, Mion F. Postdelivery anal function in primiparous females: ultrasound and manometric study. Dis Colon Rectum 2000; 42:1636–1637.
54. Abramowitz L, Sobhani I, Ganansia R, et al. Are sphincter defects the cause of anal incontinence after vaginal delivery? Dis Colon Rectum 2000; 43: 590–596.
55. Chaliha C, Sultan AH, Bland JM, Monga AK, Stanton SL. Anal function: effect of pregnancy and delivery. Am J Obst Gynecol 2001; 185:427–432.
56. Belmonte-Montes C, Hagerman G, Vega-Yepez PA, Hernandez-de-Anda E, Fonseca-Morales V. Anal sphincter injury after vaginal delivery in primiparous women. Dis Colon Rectum 2001; 44:1244–1248.
57. Willis S, Faridi A, Schelzig S, et al. Childbirth and incontinence: a prospective study on anal sphincter morphology and function before and early after vaginal delivery. Langenbeck's Arch Surg 2002; 387:101–107.
58. Nazir M, Carlsen E, Nesheim BI. Do occult anal sphincter injuries, vector volume manometry and delivery variables have any predictive value for bowel symptoms after first time vaginal delivery without third and fourth degree rupture? Acta Obstet Gynecol Scand 2002; 81:720–726.
59. Peschers UM, Sultan AH, Jundt K, Mayer V, Dimpfl T. Urinary and anal incontinence after vacuum delivery. Eur J Obst Gynecol Reprod Biol 2003; 110:39–42.
60. Oberwalder M, Connor J, Wexner SD. Meta-analysis to determine the incidence of obstetric anal sphincter damage. Br J Surg 2003; 90:1333–1337.
61. Rieger N, Wattchow D. The effect of vaginal delivery on anal function. Aust N Z J Surg 1999; 69:172–177.
62. Oberwalder M, Dinnewitzer A, Baig MK, Thaler K, Cotman K, et al. The association between late-onset fecal incontinence and obstetric anal sphincter defects. Ann Surg 2004; 139:429–432.
63. Damon H, Henry L, Barth X, Mion F. Fecal incontinence in females with a past history of vaginal delivery: significance of anal sphincter defects detected by ultrasound. Dis Colon Rectum 2002; 45:1445–1450.
64. Donnelly V, Fynes M, Campbell D, Johnson H, O'Connell PR, O'Herlihy C. Obstetric events leading to anal sphincter damage. Obstet Gynecol 1998; 92:955–961.
65. Sultan AH, Johanson RB, Carter JE. Occult anal sphincter trauma following randomized forceps or vacuum delivery. Int J Gynaecol Obstet 1998; 61: 113–119.
66. Abramowitz L, Sobhani I, Ganansia R, et al. Are sphincter defects the cause of anal incontinence after vaginal delivery? Dis Colon Rectum 2000; 43:590–596.
67. Bollard RC, Gardiner A, Duthie GS, Lindow SW. Anal sphincter injury, fecal and urinary incontinence: a 34-year follow-up after forceps delivery. Dis Colon Rectum 2003; 46:1083–1088.
68. De Parades V, Etienney I, Thabut D, Beaulieu S, Tawk M, et al. Anal sphincter injury after forceps delivery: myth or reality? Dis Colon Rectum 2004; 47:24–34.
69. Pinta TM, Kylänpää ML, Teramo KAW, Luukkonen PS. Sphincter rupture and anal incontinence after first vaginal delivery. Acta Obstet Gynecol Scand 2004; 83:917–922.
70. Pollack J, Nordenstam J, Brismar S, Lopez A, Altman D, Zetterstrom J. Anal incontinence after vaginal delivery: a five-year prospective cohort study. Obstet Gynecol 2004; 104:1397–1402.
71. Sultan AH, Kamm M, Hudson CN, Bartram CI. Third degree obstetric anal sphincter tears: risk factors and outcome of primary repair. BMJ 1994; 308:887–891.
72. Kumar DK, Stanton SL, Thakar R, Fynes M, Bland J. Symptoms and anal sphincter morphology following primary repair of third-degree tears. Br J Surg 2003; 90:1573–1579.
73. Fernando RJ, Sultan AH, Radley S, Jones PW, Johanson RB. Management of obstetric anal sphincter injury: a systemic review and national practice survey. BMC Health Service Res 2002; 2:9.
74. Sze EH. Prevalence and severity of anal incontinence in women with and without additional vaginal deliveries after a fourth-degree perineal laceration. Dis Colon Rectum 2005; 48:66–69.
75. Sze EH. Anal incontinence among women with one versus two complete third-degree perineal lacerations. Int J Gynaecol Obstet Jun 19 2005 (e-pub ahead of print).

76. Faridi A, Willis S, Schelzig P, Siggelkow W, Schumpelick V, Rath W. Anal sphincter injury during vaginal delivery: an argument for cesarean section on request? J Perinat Med 2002; 30:379–387.
77. Fynes M, Donnelly VS, O'Connell R, O'Herlihy C. Cesarean delivery and anal sphincter injury. Obstet Gynecol 1998; 92:496–500.
78. Altman D, Zetterstrom J, Lopez A, Pollack J, Nordenstam J, Mellgren A. Effect of hysterectomy on bowel function. Dis Colon Rectum 2004; 47:502–508.
79. Parks AG. Anorectal incontinence. Proc R Soc Med 1975; 68:681–690.
80. Snooks SJ, Henry MM, Swash M. Anorectal incontinence and rectal prolapse: differential assessment of the innervation of the puborectalis and external anal sphincter muscles. Gut 1985; 26:470–476.
81. Jarrett MED, Matzel KE, Stösser M, Baeten CGMI, Kamm MA. Sacral nerve stimulation for fecal incontinence following surgery for rectal prolapse repair: a multicenter study. Dis Colon Rectum (published online: 24 March 2005).
82. Igliki F, Coffin B, Ille O, et al. Fecal incontinence after pelvic radiotherapy: evidences for a lumbosacral plexopathy. Dis Colon Rectum 1996; 39:465–467.
83. Schiller LR, Santa Ana CA, Schmulen AC, et al. Pathogenesis of fecal incontinence in diabetes mellitus: evidence for internal anal sphincter dysfunction. N Engl J Med 1982; 307:1666–1671.
84. Pintor MP, Zara GP, Falletto E, et al. Pudendal neuropathy in diabetic patients with fecal incontinence. Int J Colorectal Dis 1994; 9:105–109.
85. Deen KI, Kumar D, Williams JG, Olliff J, Keighley MR. The prevalence of anal sphincter defects in fecal incontinence: a prospective endosonic study. Gut 1993; 34:685–688.
86. Karoui S, Savoye-Collet C, Koning E, Leroi AM, Denis P. Prevalence of anal sphincter defects revealed by sonography in 335 incontinent patients and 115 continent patients. Am J Roentgenol 1999; 173:389–392.
87. Damon H, L, Valette PJ, Mion F. Incidence of sphincter defects in fecal incontinence: a prospective endosonographic study. Ann Chirurgie 2000; 125: 643–647.
88. Nielsen MB, Hauge C, Pedersen JF, Christiansen J. Endosonographic evaluation of patients with anal incontinence and influence on surgical management. Am J Roentgenol 1993; 160:771–775.
89. Swash M, Gray A, Lubowski DZ, Nicholls RJ. Ultrastructural changes in internal sphincter in neurogenic incontinence. Gut 1988; 29:1692–1698.
90. Rogers J, Henry MM, Misiewicz JJ. Combined sensory and motor deficit in primary fecal incontinence. Gut 1988; 29:5–9.
91. Speakman CTM, Hoyle CHV, Kamm MA, Henry MM, Nicholls RJ, Burnstock G. Abnormalities of innervation of internal anal sphincter in fecal incontinence. Dig Dis Sci 1993; 38:1961–1969.
92. Gee ASS, Durdey P. Urge incontinence of faeces is a marker of severe external anal sphincter dysfunction. Br J Surg 1995; 82:1179–1182.
93. Henry MM. Pathogenesis and management of fecal incontinence in the adult. Gastroenterol Clin North Am 1987; 16:35–45.
94. Sultan AH, Nicholls RJ, Kamm MA. Anal endosonography and correlation with in vitro and in vivo anatomy. Br J Surg 1993; 80:508–511.
95. Bharucha AE. Outcome measures for fecal incontinence: anorectal structure and function. Gastroenterology 2004; 126:S90–S98.
96. Bollard RC, Gardiner AB, Lindow S, Phillips K, Duthie GS. Normal female anal sphincter: difficulties in interpretation explained. Dis Colon Rectum 2002; 45:171–175.
97. Sentovich SM, Wong DW, Blatchford GJ. Accuracy and reliability of transanal ultrasound for anterior anal sphincter injury. Dis Colon Rectum 1998; 41:1000–1004.
98. Deen KI, Kumar D, Williams JG, Oliff J, Keighley MR. Anal sphincter defects. Correlation between endoanal ultrasound and surgery. Ann Surg 1993; 218:201–205.
99. Zetterström JP, Mellgren A, Madoff RD, Kim DG, Wong WD. Perineal body measurement improves evaluation of anterior sphincter lesions during endoanal ultrasonography. Dis Colon Rectum 1998; 41:705–713.
100. Oberwalder M, Thaler K, Baig MK, et al. Anal ultrasound and endosonographic measurement of perianal body thickness: a new evaluation for fecal incontinence in females. Surg Endosc 2004; 18:650–654.
101. Gold DM, Halligan S, Kmiot WA, Bartram CI. Intraobserver and interobserver agreement in anal endosonography. Br J Surg 1999; 86:371–375.
102. Lieberman H, Faria J, Ternent CA, Blatchford GJ, Christensen MA, Thorson AG. A prospective evaluation of the value of anorectal physiology in the management of fecal incontinence. Dis Colon Rectum 2001; 44:1567–1574.
103. Hiltunen KM. Anal manometric findings in patients with anal incontinence. Dis Colon Rectum 1985; 28:925–928.
104. Read NW, Bartolo DCC, Read MG. Differences in anal function in patients with incontinence to solids and in patients with incontinence to liquids. Br J Surg 1984; 71:39–42.
105. Penninckx F, Lestar B, Kerremans R. Manometric evaluation of incontinent patients. Acta Gastroenterol Belg 1995; 58:51–59.
106. Kuijpers JHC. Fecal incontinence. Int J Colorectal Dis 1987; 2:177.
107. Tetzschner T, Soronsen M, Rasmussen OO, Lose G, Christiansen J. Pudendal nerve damage increases the risk of fecal incontinence in women with anal sphincter rupture after childbirth. Acta Obstet Gynecol Scand 1995; 74:434–440.
108. Bartolo DC, Jarratt JA, Read MG, et al. The role of partial denervation of the puborectalis in idiopathic fecal incontinence. Br J Surg 1983; 76:664–667.
109. De Leeuw JW, Vierhout ME, Auwerda HJ, Bac DJ, Wallenburg HCS. Anal sphincter damage after vaginal delivery: relationship of anal sonography and manometry to anal complaints. Dis Colon Rectum 2002; 45:1004–1010.
110. Nazir M, Carlsen E, Jacobsen AF, Nesheim BL. Is there a correlation between objective anal testing, rupture grade and bowel symptoms after primary repair of obstetric anal sphincter rupture?: an observational cohort study. Dis Colon Rectum 2002; 45:1325–1331.
111. Voyvodic F, Rieger NA, Skinner S, Schloithe AC, Saccone MR, Wattchow DA. Endosonographic imaging of anal sphincter injury: does the size of the tear correlate with the degree of dysfunction? Dis Colon Rectum 2003; 46:735–741.
112. Dhaenens G, Emblem R, Ganes T. Fibre density in idiopathic anorectal incontinence. Electomyogr Clin Neurophysiol 1995; 35:285–290.
113. Roig JV, Villoslada C, Lledo S, et al. Prevalence of pudendal neuropathy in fecal incontinence. Results of a prospective study. Dis Colon Rectum 1995; 38:952–958.
114. Kouraklis G, Andromanakos N. Evaluating patients with anorectal incontinence. Surg Today 2004; 34:304–312.
115. Laurberg S, Swash M, Henry MM. Delayed external sphincter repair for obstetric tear. Br J Surg 1988; 75:786–788.
116. Baig MK, Wexner SD. Factors predictive of outcome after surgery for fecal incontinence. Br J Surg 2000; 87:1316–1330.
117. Sangwan YP, Coller JA, Barrett RC, Murray JJ, Roberts PL, Schoetz DJ. Unilateral pudendal neuropathy. Significance and implications. Dis Colon Rectum 1996; 39:249–251.
118. Rasmussen OO, Colstrup H, Lose G, Christiansen J. A technique for the dynamic assessment of anal sphincter function. Int J Colorectal Dis 1990; 5:135–141.
119. Chen AS, Luchtefeld MA, Senagore AJ, Mackeigan JM, Hoyt C. Pudendal nerve latency. Does it predict outcome of anal sphincter repair? Dis Colon Rectum 1998; 41:1005–1009.
120. Young CJ, Mathur MN, Eyers AA, Solomon MJ. Successful overlapping anal sphincter repair: relationship to patient age, neuropathy and colostomy formation. Dis Colon Rectum 1998; 41:344–349.
121. Osterberg A, Graf W, Edebol Eeg-Olofsson K, Hynninen P, Pahlman L. Results of neurophysiologic evaluation in fecal incontinence. Dis Colon Rectum 2000; 43:1256–1261.
122. Rasmussen O, Christensen B, Sorenson M, et al. Rectal compliance in the assessment of patients with fecal incontinence. Dis Colon Rectum 1990; 33:650–653.
123. Womack NR, Morrison JF, Williams NS. The role of pelvic floor denervation in the aetiology of idiopathic faecal incontinence. Br J Surg 1986; 73:404–407.
124. Read NW, Haynes WG, Bartolo DC, et al. Use of anorectal manometry during rectal infusion of saline to investigate sphincter function in incontinent patients. Gastroenterology 1983; 85:105–113.
125. Williams AB, Bartram CI, Modhwadia D, et al. Endocoil magnetic resonance imaging quantification of external anal sphincter atrophy. Br J Surg 2001; 88:853–859.
126. Briel JW, Stoker J, Rociu E, Lameris JS, Hop WC, Schouten WR. External anal sphincter atrophy on endoanal MRI adversely affects continence after sphincteroplasty. Br J Surg 1999; 86:1322–1327.
127. Briel JW, Zimmerman DDE, Stoker J, et al. Relationship between sphincter morphology on endoanal MRI and histopathological aspects of the external anal sphincter. Int J Colorectal Dis 2000; 15:87–90.
128. Rosen L, Khubchandani IT, Sheets JA, Spasik JJ, Riether RD. Management of anal incontinence. Am Fam Physician 1986; 33:129–137.
129. Bannister JJ, Read NW, Donnelly C. External and internal anal sphincter responses to rectal distension in normal subjects and in patients with idiopathic fecal incontinence. Br J Surg 1989; 76:617–621.
130. Hallgren T, Fasth S, Delbro DS, Nordgren S, Oresland T, Hulten L. Loperamide improves anal sphincter function and continence after restorative proctocolectomy. Dig Dis Sci 1994; 39:2612–2618.
131. Santoro GA, Eitan BZ, Pryde A, Bartolo DC. Open study of low-dose amitriptyline in the treatment of patients with idiopathic fecal incontinence. Dis Colon Rectum 2000; 43(12):1676–1681.
132. Mortensen N, Humphreys SM. The anal continence plug: a disposable device for patients with anorectal incontinence. Lancet 1991; 338:295–297.
133. Christiansen J, Roed-Petersen K. Clinical assessment of the anal continence plug. Dis Colon Rectum 1993; 36:740–742.
134. Hopkinson BR. Electrical treatment of anal incontinence. Ann R Coll Surg Engl 1972; 50:92–111.
135. Engel BT, Nikoomanesh P, Schuster MM. Operant conditioning of rectosphincteric responses in the treatment of fecal incontinence. N Engl J Med 1974; 290:646–649.
136. Loening-Baucke V. Biofeedback therapy for fecal incontinence. Dig Dis 1990; 7:112–114.
137. Wald A. Incontinence and anorectal dysfunction in patients with diabetes mellitus. Eur J Gastroenterol Hepatol 1995; 7:737–739.
138. Norton C, Hosker G, Brazzelli M. Biofeedback and/or sphincter exercises for the treatment of fecal incontinence in adults. Cochrane Database Syst Rev 2000; 2:CD002111.

139. Heymen S, Jones KR, Ringel Y, Scarlett Y, Whitehead WE. Biofeedback treatment of fecal incontinence: a critical review. Dis Colon Rectum 2001; 44:728–736.
140. Palsson OS, Heymen S, Whitehead WE. Biofeedback treatment for functional anorectal disorders: a comprehensive efficacy review. Appl Psychophysiol Biofeedback 2004; 29:153–174.
141. Norton C, Chelvanayagam S, Wilson-Barnett J, Redfern S, Kamm MA. Randomized controlled trial of biofeedback for fecal incontinence. Gastroenterology 2003; 125:1320–1329.
142. Solomon MJ, Pager CK, Rex J, Roberts R, Manning J. Randomized controlled trial of biofeedback with anal manometry, transanal ultrasound or pelvic floor retraining with digital guidance alone in the treatment of mild to moderate fecal incontinence. Dis Colon Rectum 2003; 46:703–710.
143. Fynes MM, Marshall K, Cassidy M, et al. A prospective randomised study comparing the effect of augmented biofeedback with sensory biofeedback alone on fecal incontinence after obstetric trauma. Dis Colon Rectum 1999; 42:753–758.
144. Beddy P, Neary P, Eguare EI, et al. Electromyographic biofeedback can improve subjective and objective measures of fecal incontinence in the short term. J Gastrointest Surg 2004; 8:64–72.
145. Chiarioni G, Bassotti G, Stegagnini S, Vantini I, Whitehad WE. Sensory retraining is key to biofeedback therapy for formed stool fecal incontinence. Am J Gastroenterol 2002; 97:109–117.
146. Sangwan YP, Coller JA, Barrett RC, Roberts PL, Murray JJ, Schoetz DJ. Can manometric parameters predict response to biofeedback therapy in fecal incontinence? Dis Colon Rectum 1995; 38:1021–1025.
147. Fernández-Fraga X, Azpiroz F, Aparici A, Casaus M, Malagelada JR. Predictors of response to biofeedback treatment in anal incontinence. Dis Colon Rectum 2003; 46:1218–1225.
148. Enck P, Daublin G, Lubke HJ, Strohmeyer G. Long-term efficacy of biofeedback training for fecal incontinence. Dis Colon Rectum 1994; 37:997–1001.
149. Guillemot F, Bauche B, Gower-Rousseau C, et al. Biofeedback for the treatment of fecal incontinence. Dis Colon Rectum 1995; 38:393–397.
150. Glia A, Gylin M, Åkerlund JE, Lindfors U, Lindberg MD. Biofeedback training in patients with fecal incontinence. Dis Colon Rectum 1998; 41:359–364.
151. Ryn AK, Morren GL, Hallböök O, Sjödahl R. Long-term results of electromyographic biofeedback training for fecal incontinence. Dis Colon Rectum 2000; 43:1262–1266.
152. Pager CK, Solomon MJ, Rex J, Roberts RA. Long-term outcomes of pelvic floor exercise and biofeedback treatment for patients with fecal incontinence. Dis Colon Rectum 2002; 45:997–1003.
153. Davis KJ, Kumar D, Poloniecki J. Adjuvant biofeedback following anal sphincter repair: a randomised study. Aliment Pharmacol Ther 2004; 20:539–549.
154. Fang DT, Nivatvongs S, Vermeulen FD, et al. Overlapping sphincteroplasty for acquired anal incontinence. Dis Colon Rectum 1984; 27:720–722.
155. Parks AG, McPartlin JF. Late repair of injuries of the anal sphincter. Proc R Soc Med 1971; 64:1187–1189.
156. Mahony R, Behan M, O'Herlihy C, O'Connell PR. Randomized, clinical trial of bowel confinement vs. laxative use after primary repair of a third-degree obstetric anal sphincter tear. Dis Colon Rectum 2004; 47:12–17.
157. Hawley PR. Anal sphincter reconstruction. Langenbecks Arch Chir 1985; 366:269–272.
158. Abcarian H, Orsay CP, Pearl R, et al. Traumatic cloaca. Dis Colon Rectum 1989; 32:783–787.
159. Sangalli MR, Marti MC. Results of sphincter repair in post obstetric fecal incontinence. J Am Coll Surg 1994; 179:583–586.
160. Arnaud A, Sarles JC, Sielezneff I, Orsori P, Joly A. Sphincter repair without overlapping for fecal incontinence. Dis Colon Rectum 1991; 34:744–747.
161. Briel JW, de Boer LM, Hop WCJ, Schouten WR. Clinical outcome of anterior overlapping external anal sphincter repair with internal sphincter imbrication. Dis Colon Rectum 1998; 41:209–214.
162. Tjandra JJ, Han WR, Goh J, Dwyer P. Direct repair vs. overlapping sphincter repair: a randomized controlled trial. Dis Colon Rectum 2003; 46:937–942.
163. Kairaluoma MV, Raivio P, Aarnio MT, Kellokumpu IH. Immediate repair of obstetric anal sphincter rupture: medium-term outcome of the overlap technique. Dis Colon Rectum 2004; 47:1358–1363.
164. Malouf AJ, Norton CS, Engel AF, Nicholls RJ, Kamm MA. Long-term results of overlapping anterior anal sphincter repair for obstetric trauma. Lancet 2000; 355:260–266.
165. Rothbarth J, Bemelman WA, Meijerink WJHJ, Buyze-Westerweel ME, van Dijk JG, Delemarre JBVM. Long-term results of anterior anal sphincter repair for fecal incontinence due to obstetric injury. Digest Surg 2000; 17:390–394.
166. Karoui S, Leroi AM, Koning E, Menard JF, Michot F, Denis P. Results of sphincteroplasty in 86 patients with anal continence. Dis Colon Rectum 2000:813–820.
167. Halverson AL, Hull TL. Long-term outcome of overlapping anal sphincter repair. Dis Colon Rectum 2002; 45:345–348.
168. Pinta T, Kylänpää-Bäck ML, Salmi T, Järvinen HJ, Luukkonen P. Delayed sphincter repair for obstetric ruptures. Colorectal Dis 2003; 5:73–78.
169. Gutierrez AB, Madoff RD, Lowry AC, Parker SC, Buie WD, Baxter NN. Long-term results of anterior sphincteroplasty. Dis Colon Rectum 2004; 47:727–732.
170. Ternent CA, Shashidharan M, Blatchford GJ, Christensen MA, Thorson AG, Sentovitch SM. Transanal ultrasound and anorectal physiology findings affecting continence after sphincteroplasty. Dis Colon Rectum 1997; 40: 462–467.
171. Savoye-Collet C, Savoye G, Koning E, et al. Anal endosonography after sphincter repair: specific patterns related to clinical outcome. Abdom Imaging 1999; 245:569–573.
172. Giordano P, Renzi A, Efron J, et al. Previous sphincter repair does not affect the outcome of repeat repair. Dis Colon Rectum 2002; 45:635–640.
173. Oliveira L, Pfeifer J, Wexner SD. Physiological and clinical outcome of anterior sphincteroplasty. Br J Surg 1996; 83:502–505.
174. Vaizey CJ, Norton C, Thornton MJ, Nicholls RJ, Kamm MA. Long-term results of repeat anterior anal sphincter repair. Dis Colon Rectum 2004; 47:858–863.
175. Sangwan YP, Coller JA, Barrett RC, et al. Unilateral pudendal neuropathy. Impact on outcome of an anal sphincter repair. Dis Colon Rectum 1996; 39:686–689.
176. Londono-Schimmer EE, Garcia-Duperly R, Nicholls RJ, Ritchie JK, Hawley PR, Thompson JP. Overlapping anal sphincter repair for fecal incontinence due to sphincter trauma: five year follow-up functional results. Int J Colorectal Dis 1994; 9:110–113.
177. Gilliland R, Altomare DF, Moreira H Jr., Oliveira L, Galliland JE, Wexner SD. Pudendal neuropathy is predictive of failure following anterior overlapping sphincteroplasty. Dis Colon Rectum 1998; 41:1516–1522.
178. Simmang C, Birnbaum EH, Kodner IJ, Fry RD, Fleshman JW. Anal sphincter reconstruction in the elderly: does advancing age affect outcome? Dis Colon Rectum 1994; 37:1065–1069.
179. Sitzler PJ, Thompson JP. Overlap repair of damaged anal sphincter: a single surgeons's series. Dis Colon Rectum 1996; 39:1356–1360.
180. Nikiteas N, Korgen S, Kumar D, Keighley MR. Audit of sphincter repair: factors associated with poor outcome. Dis Colon Rectum 1996; 39:1164–1170.
181. Buie WD, Lowry AC, Rothenberger DA, Madoff RD. Clinical rather than laboratory assessment predicts continence after anterior sphincteroplasty. Dis Colon Rectum 2001; 44:1255–1260.
182. Ha HT, Fleshman JW, Smith M, Read TE, Kodner IJ, Birnbaum EH. Manometric squeeze pressure difference parallels functional outcome after overlapping sphincter reconstruction. Dis Colon Rectum 2001; 44:655–660.
183. Zorcolo L, Covotta L, Bartolo DC. Outcome of anterior sphincter repair for obstetric injury: comparison of early and late results. Dis Colon Rectum 2005; 48:524–531.
184. Hasegawa H, Yoshioka K, Keighley MR. Randomized trial of fecal diversion for sphincter repair. Dis Colon Rectum 2000; 43:961–964.
185. Lewicky CE, Valentin C, Saclarides TJ. Sexual function following sphincteroplasty for women with third-and fourth-degree perineal tears. Dis Colon Rectum 2004; 47:1650–1654.
186. Pinta TM, Kylanpaa ML, Salmi TK, Teramo KA, Luukkonen PS. Primary sphincter repair: are the results of the operation good enough? Dis Colon Rectum 2004; 47:18–23.
187. Browning GP, Motson RW. Anal sphincter injury. Management and results of Parks sphincter repair. Ann Surg 1984; 199:351–357.
188. Christiansen J, Pedersen IK. Traumatic anal incontinence results of surgical repair. Dis Colon Rectum 1987; 30:189–191.
189. Morgan S, Bernard D, Tasse D, et al. Results of Parks' sphincteroplasty for post traumatic anal incontinence. Can J Surg 1987; 30:299(R212).
190. Yoshioka K, Keighley MRB. Sphincter repair for fecal incontinence. Dis Colon Rectum 1989; 32:39–42.
191. Jacobs PPM, Scheuer M, Kuijpers JHC, et al. Obstetrical fecal incontinence. Role of pelvic floor denervation and results of delayed sphincter repair. Dis Colon Rectum 1990; 33:494–497.
192. Fleshman JW, Peters WR, Shemesh EI, Fry RD, Kodner IJ. Anal sphincter reconstruction: anterior overlapping muscle repair. Dis Colon Rectum 1991; 34:739–743.
193. Gibbs DH, Hooks VH. Overlapping sphincteroplasty for acquired anal incontinence. South Med J 1993; 86:1376–1380.
194. Engel AF, van Baal SJ, Brummelkamp WH. Late results of anterior sphincter plication for traumatic fecal incontinence. Eur J Surg 1994; 160: 633–636.
195. Engel AF, Kamm MA, Sulton AH, Bartram CI, Nicholls RJ. Anterior anal sphincter repair in patients with obstetric trauma. Br J Surg 1994; 81:1231–1234.
196. Londono-Schimmer EE, Garcia-Duperly R, Nicholls RJ, Ritchie JK, Hawley PR, Thomson JPS. Overlapping anal sphincter repair for fecal incontinence due to sphincter trauma: five-year follow up functional results. Int J Colorectal Dis 1994; 9:110–113.
197. Simmang C, Birnbaum EH, Kodner IJ, Fry RD, Fleshman JW. Anal sphincter reconstruction in the elderly: does advancing age affect outcome? Dis Colon Rectum 1994; 37:1065–1069.
198. Womack NR, Morrison JF, Williams NS. Prospective study of the effects of postanal repair in neurogenic fecal incontinence. Br J Surg 1988; 75:48–52.
199. Miller R, Bartolo DCC, Locke-Edmunds JC, et al. Prospective study of conservative and operative treatment for fecal incontinence. Br J Surg 1988; 75:101–105.

200. Orrom WJ, Miller R, Comes H, Duthie G, Mortensen NJ McC, Bartolo DCC. Comparison of anterior sphincteroplasty and postanal repair in the treatment of idiopathic fecal incontinence. Dis Colon Rectum 1991; 34:305–310.
201. Athanasiadis S, Sanchez, Kuprian A. Long-term follow-up of Parks posterior repair. An elctromyographic, manometric and radiologic study of 31 patients. Langenbecks Arch Chir 1995; 380:22–30.
202. Healy JC, Halligan S, Bartram CI, Kamm MA, Philips RKS, Reznek R. Dynamic magnetic resonance imaging evaluation of the structural and functional results of postanal repair for neuropathic fecal incontinence. Dis Colon Rectum 2002; 45:1629–1634.
203. Setti Carraro P, Kamm MA, Nicholls RJ. Long-term results of postanal repair for neurogenic faecal incontinence. Br J Surg 1994; 81:149–144.
204. Jameson JS, Speakman CT, Darzi A, Chia YW, Henry MM. Audit of postanal repair in the treatment of fecal incontinence. Dis Colon Rectum 1994; 37:369–372.
205. Laurberg S, Swash M, Henry MM. Effect of postanal repair on progress of neurogenic damage to the pelvic floor. Br J Surg 1990; 77:519–522.
206. Van Tets WF, Kuijpers JH. Pelvic floor procedures produce no consistent changes in anatomy and physiology. Dis Colon Rectum 1998; 41:365–369.
207. Matsuoka H, Mavrantonis C, Wexner SD, Oliveira L, Gilliland R, Pikarsky A. Postanal repair for fecal incontinence: is it worthwhile? Dis Colon Rectum 2000; 43:1561–1567.
208. Browning GGP, Rutter KRP, Motson RW, et al. Postanal repair for idiopathic fecal incontinence. Ann R Coll Surg Engl 1984; 66(suppl):30–33.
209. Van Vroonhoven TJMV, Schouten WR. Postanal repair in the treatment of fecal incontinence. Neth J Surg 1984; 36:160–162.
210. Henry MM, Simson JN. Results of postanal repair: a retrospective study. Br J Surg 1985; 72(suppl):S17–S19.
211. Habr-Gama A, Alves PR, da Silva e Sousa AH, et al. Treatment of fecal incontinence by postanal repair. Coloproctology 1986; 8:244–246.
212. Keighley MRB. Postanal repair. How I do it. Int J Colorect Dis 1987; 2:236–239.
213. Scheuer M, Kuijpers HC, Jacobs PP. Postanal repair restores anatomy rather than function. Dis Colon Rectum 1989; 32:960–963.
214. Gordon PH. Parks postanal repair. Perspect Colon Rectal Surg 1993; 6: 241–250.
215. Carraro PS, Kamm MA, Nicholls RJ. Long-term results of postanal repair for neurogenic fecal incontinence. Br J Surg 1994; 81:140–144.
216. Engel AF, van Baal SJ, Brummelkamp WH. Late results of post anal repair for idiopathic faecal incontinence. Eur J Surg 1994; 160:637–640.
217. Briel JW, Schouten WR. Disappointing results of postanal repair in the treatment of fecal incontinence. Ned Tijdschr Geneeskd 1995; 139:23–26.
218. Rieger NA, Sarre RG, Saccone GT, Hunter A, Toouli J. Postanal repair for faecal incontinence: long-term follow-up. Aust N Z J Surg 1997; 67:566–570.
219. Pickrell KL, Broadbent TR, Masters FW, et al. Construction of a rectal sphincter and restoration of anal continence by transplanting the gracills muscle. Ann Surg 1952; 135:853–862.
220. Corman ML. Gracilis muscle transposition for anal incontinence: Late results. Br J Surg 1985; 72(suppl):S21–S22.
221. Corman ML. Colon and Rectal Surgery. 2nd ed. Philadelphia: JB Lippincott, 1989:193–198.
222. Christiansen J, Sorensen M, Rasmussen OO. Gracilis muscle transposition for fecal incontinence. Br J Surg 1990; 77:1039–1040.
223. Fleshner PR, Roberts PL. Encirclement procedures for fecal incontinence. Perspect Colon Rectal Surg 1991; 4:280–287.
224. Sielezneff F, Bauer S, Bulgare JC, Sarles JC. Gracilis muscle transposition in the treatment of fecal incontinence. Int J Colorectal Dis 1996; 11:15–18.
225. Kumar D, Hutchinson R, Grant E. Bilateral gracilis neosphincter construction for treatment of faecal incontinence. Br J Surg 1995; 82:1645–1647.
226. Konsten J, Baeten CG, Spaans F, Havenith MG, Soeters PB. Follow-up of anal dynamic graciloplasty for fecal continence. World J Surg 1993; 17: 404–409.
227. George BD, Williams NS, Patel J, Swash M, Watkins ES. Physiological and histochemical adaptation of the electrically stimulated graciles muscle to neoanal sphincter function. Br J Surg 1993; 80:1342–1346.
228. Baeten C, Spaans F, Fluks A. An implanted neuromuscular stimulator for fecal continence following previously implanted gracilis muscle: report of a case. Dis Colon Rectum 1988; 31:134–137.
229. Hallan RI, George B, Williams NS. Anal sphincter function: fecal incontinence and its treatment. Surg Annu 1993; 25:85–115.
230. Williams NS, Patel J, George BD, Hallon RI, Watkins ES. Development of an electrically stimulated neoanal sphincter. Lancet 1991; 338:1166–1169.
231. Baeten CGMI, Geerdes BP, Adang EMM, et al. Anal dynamic graciloplasty in the treatment of intractable fecal incontinence. N Engl J Med 1995; 332: 1600–1605.
232. Rosen HR, Feil W, Novi G, Zoch G, Dahlberg S, Schlessel R. The electrically stimulated (dynamic) graciloplasty for fecal incontinence—first experiences with a modified muscle sling. Int J Colorectal Dis 1994; 9:184–186.
233. Cavina E, Seccia M, Evangilista G, et al. Perineal colostomy and electrostimulated gracilis "neosphincter" after abdominoperineal resection of the colon and anorectum: a surgical experience and follow-up study in 47 cases. Int J Colorectal Dis 1990; 5:6–11.
234. Baeten CGMI, Konsten J, Spaans F, et al. Dynamic graciloplasty for treatment of faecal incontinence. Lancet 1991; 338:1163–1165.
235. Wexner SD, Gonzalez-Padron A, Ruis J, et al. Stimulated gracilis neosphincter operation. Initial experience, pitfalls, and complications. Dis Colon Rectum 1996; 39:957–964.
236. Geerdes BP, Heineman E, Konsten J, Soeters PB, Baeten CGMI. Dynamic graciloplasty. Complications and management. Dis Colon Rectum 1996; 39:912–917.
237. Rongen MJ, Uludag O, El Naggar K, Gerdes BP, Konsten J, Baeten CG. Long-term follow-up of dynamic graciloplasty for fecal incontinence. Dis Colon Rectum 2003; 46:716–721.
238. Penninckx F on behalf of the Belgian Section of Colorectal Surgery. Belgian experience with dynamic graciloplasty for faecal incontinence. Br J Surg 2004; 91:872–878.
239. Matzel KE, Madoff RD, LaFontaine LJ, et al. Dynamic Graciloplasty Therapy Study Group. Complications of dynamic graciloplasty: incidence, management, and impact on outcome. Dis Colon Rectum 2001; 44:1427–1435.
240. Abercrombie JE, Williams NS. Total anorectal reconstruction. Br J Surg 1995; 82:438–442.
241. Williams NS, Hallan RI, Koeze TH, et al. Restoration of gastrointestinal continuity and continence after abdominoperineal excision of the rectum using an electrically stimulated neoanal sphincter. Dis Colon Rectum 1990; 33:561–565.
242. Mercati U, Trancanelli V, Castagnoli GP, Mariotti A, Ciaccarini R. Use of the gracilis muscles for sphincteric construction after abdominoperineal resection. Technique and preliminary results. Dis Colon Rectum 1991; 34:1085–1089.
243. Santoro E, Santoro R, Santoro E. Perineal reconstruction with continent colostomy after Miles operation. Semin Surg Oncol 1994; 10:208–216.
244. Abercrombie JE, Rogers J, Williams NS. Total anorectal reconstruction results in complete anorectal sensory loss. Br J Surg 1996; 83:57–59.
245. Korsgren S, Keighley MRB. Stimulated gracilis neosphincter— not as good, as previously thought. Report of four cases. Dis Colon Rectum 1995; 38:1331–1333.
246. Kennedy ML, Nguyen H, Lubowski DZ, King DW. Stimulated gracilis neosphincter: a new procedure for anal continence. Aust N Z J Surg 1996; 66:353–357.
247. Violi V, Boselli AS, De Bernardinis M, et al. Surgical results and functional outcome after total anorectal reconstruction by double graciloplasty supported by external-source electrostimulation and/or implantable pulse generators: an 8-year experience. Int J Colorectal Dis 2004; 19:219–227.
248. Romano G, La Torre F, Cutini G, Bianco F, Esposito P, Montori A. Total anorectal reconstruction with the artificial bowel sphincter: report of eight cases. A quality-of-life assessment. Dis Colon Rectum 2003; 46:730–734.
249. Rullier E, Zerbib F, Laurent C, Caudry M, Saric J. Morbidity and functional outcome after double dynamic graciloplasty for anorectal reconstruction. Br J Surg 2000; 87:909–913.
250. Bruining HA, Bos KE, Colthoff EG, et al. Creation of an anal sphincter mechanism by bilateral proximally based gluteal muscle transposition. Plast Reconstr Surg 1981; 67:70–72.
251. Hentz VR. Construction of a rectal sphincter using the origin of the gluteus maximus muscle. Plast Reconstr Surg 1981; 70:82–85.
252. Orgel MG, Kucan JO. A double-split gluteus maximus muscle flap for reconstruction of the rectal sphincter. Plast Reconstr Surg 1985; 75:62–66.
253. Chen Y, Zhang X. Reconstruction of rectal sphincter by transposition of gluteus muscle for fecal incontinence. J Pediatr Surg 1987; 22:62.
254. Pearl RK, Prasad ML, Nelson RL, Orsay CP, Abcarian H. Bilateral gluteus maximus transposition for anal incontinence. Dis Colon Rectum 1991; 34:478–481.
255. Christiansen J, Hanson CR, Rasmussen O. Bilateral gluteus maximus transposition for anal incontinence. Br J Surg 1995; 82:903–905.
256. Hakelius L, Olsen L. Free autogenous muscle transplantation in children. Long-term results. Eur J Pediatr Surg 1991; 1:353–357.
257. Christiansen J, Sparso B. Treatment of anal incontinence by an implantable prosthetic anal sphincter. Ann Surg 1992; 215:383–386.
258. Wong WD, Congliosi SM, Spencer MP, Corman ML, Tan P, et al. The safety and efficacy of the artificial bowel sphincter for fecal incontinence: results from a multicenter cohort study. Dis Colon Rectum 2002; 45:1139–1153.
259. Devesa JM, Rey A, Hervas PL, et al. Artificial anal sphincter: complications and functional results of a large personal series. Dis Colon Rectum 2002; 45:1154–1163.
260. Lehur PA, Zerbib F, Neunlist M, Glemain P, Bruley des Varannes S. Comparison of quality of life and anorectal function after artificial sphincter implantation. Dis Colon Rectum 2002; 45:508–513.
261. Parker SC, Spencer MP, Madoff RD, Jensen LL, Wong WD, Rothenberger DA. Artificial bowel sphincter: long-term experience at a single institution. Dis Colon Rectum 2003; 46:722–729.
262. Mundy L, Merlin YL, Maddern GJ, Hiller JE. Systematic review of safety and effectiveness of an artificial bowel sphincter for fecal incontinence. Br J Surg 2004; 91:665–672.
263. Christiansen J, Rasmussen OO, Lindorff-Larsen K. Long-term results of artificial anal sphincter implantation for severe anal incontinence. Ann Surg 1999; 230:45–48.
264. O'Brien PE, Skinner S. Restoring control: the Acticon Neosphincter artificial bowel sphincter in the treatment of anal incontinence. Dis Colon Rectum 2000; 43:1213–1216.

265. Ortiz H, Armendariz P, DeMiguel M, Ruiz MD, Alos R, Roig JV. Complications and functional outcome following artificial anal sphincter implantation. Br J Surg 2002; 89:877–881.
266. Altomare DF, Binda GA, Dodi G, et al. Disappointing long-term results of the artificial and sphincter for faecal incontinence. Br J Surg 2004; 91:1352–1353.
267. Finlay IG, Richardson W, Hajivassiliou CA. Outcome after implantation of a novel prosthetic anal sphincter in humans. Br J Surg 2004; 91:1485–1492.
268. Cundall JD, Gardiner A, Chin K, Laden G, Grout P, Duthie GS. Hyperbaric oxygen in the treatment of fecal incontinence secondary to pudendal neuropathy. Dis Colon Rectum 2003; 46:1549–1554.
269. Takahashi T, Garcia Osogobio S, Valdovinos MA, et al. Radio-frequency energy delivery to the anal canal for the treatment of fecal incontinence. Dis Colon Rectum 2002; 45:915–922.
270. Takahashi T, Garcia-Osogobio S, Valdovinos MA, Belmone C, Barreto C, Velasco L. Extended two-year results of radio-frequency energy delivery for the treatment of fecal incontinence (Secca® procedure). Dis Colon Rectum 2003; 46:711–715.
271. Efron JE, Corman ML, Fleshman J, et al. Safety and effectiveness of temperature-controlled radio-frequency energy delivery to the anal canal (Secca® procedure) for the treatment of fecal incontinence. Dis Colon Rectum 2003; 46:1606–1616.
272. Shafik A. Perianal injection of autologous fat for treatment of sphincteric incontinence. Dis Colon Rectum 1995; 38:583–587.
273. Bernardi C, Favetta U, Pescatori M. Autologous fat injection for treatment of fecal incontinence: manometric and echographic assessment. Plast Reconstr Surg 1998; 102:1626–1628.
274. Shafik A. Polytetrafluoroethylene injection for the treatment of partial fecal incontinence. Int Surg 1993; 78:159–161.
275. Kumar D, Benson MJ, Bland JE. Glutaraldehyde cross-linked collagen in the treatment of fecal incontinence. Br J Surg 1998; 85:9877–9879.
276. Feretis C, Benakis P, Dailianas A, et al. Implantation of microballoons in the management of fecal incontinence. Dis Colon Rectum 2001; 44:1605–1609.
277. Kenefick NJ, Vaisey CJ, Malouf AJ, Norton CS, Marshall M, Kamm MA. Injectable silicone biomaterial for fecal incontinence due to internal anal sphincter dysfunction. Gut 2002; 55:225–228.
278. Tjandra JJ, Lim JF, Hiscock R, Rajendra P. Injectable silicone biomaterial for fecal incontinence caused by internal anal sphincter dysfunction is effective. Dis Colon Rectum 2004; 47:2138–2146.
279. Tanagho EA, Schmidt RA. Bladder pacemaker: scientific basis and clinical future. J Urol 1982; 20:614–619.
280. Matzel KE, Stadelmaier U, Hohenfellner M, Gall FP. Electrical stimulation for the treatment of fecal incontinence. Lancet 1995; 346:1124–1127.
281. Vaizey CJ, Kamm MA, Roy AJ, Nicholls RJ. Double-blind crossover study of sacral nerve stimulation for fecal incontinence. Dis Colon Rectum 2000; 43:298–301.
282. Ganio E, Luc AR, Clerico G, Trompetto M. Sacral nerve stimulation for treatment of fecal incontinence: a novel approach for intractable fecal incontinence. Dis Colon Rectum 2001; 44:619–631.
283. Kenefick NJ, Vaizey CJ, Cohen RC, Nicholls RJ, Kamm MA. Medium-term results of permanent sacral nerve stimulation for fecal incontinence. Br J Surg 2002; 89:896–901.
284. Uludağ Ö, Koch SMP, van Gemert WG, Dejong CHC, Baeten CGMI. Sacral neuromodulation in patients with fecal incontinence. A single-center study. Dis Colon Rectum 2004; 47:1350–1357.
285. Jarrett ME, Varma JS, Duthie GS, Nicholls RJ, Kamm MA. Sacral nerve stimulation for fecal incontinence in the UK. Br J Surg 2004; 91: 755–761.
286. Malaguti S, Spinelli M, Giardiello G, Lazzeri M, van den Hombergh U. Neurophysiologies evidence may predict the outcome of sacral neuromodulation. J Urol 2003; 170:2323–2326.
287. Jarrett ME, Mowatt G, Glazener CM, et al. Systematic review of sacral nerve stimulation for fecal incontinence and constipation. Br J Surg 2004; 91:1559–1569.
288. Jarrett MED, Matzel KE, Christiansen J, et al. Sacral nerve stimulation for faecal incontinence in patients with previous partial spinal injury including disc prolapse (published online Br J Surg 18 Apr 2005).
289. Vaizey CJ, Kamm MA, Turner IC, Nicholls RJ, Woloszko J. Effects of short term sacral nerve stimulation on anal and rectal function in patients with anal incontinence. Gut 1999; 44:407–412.
290. Kenefick NJ, Emmanuel A, Nicholls RJ, Kamm MA. Effect of sacral nerve stimulation on autonomic nerve function. Br J Surg 2003; 90:1256–1260.
291. Rasmussen OO, Buntzen S, Sorensen M, Laurberg S, Christiansen J. Sacral nerve stimulation in fecal incontinence. Dis Colon Rectum 2004; 47: 1158–1162.
292. Ratto C, Grillo E, Parello A, Petrolino M, Costamagna G, Doglietto GB. Sacral neuromodulation in treatment of fecal incontinence following anterior resection and chemoradiation for rectal cancer. Dis Colon Rectum 2005; 48:1027–1036.
293. Jarrett ME, Matzel KE, Stosser M, Christiansen J, Rosen H, Kamm MA. Sacral nerve stimulation for faecal incontinence following a rectosigmoid resection for colorectal cancer. Int J Colorectal Dis 2005; Apr 21 (e-pub ahead of print).
294. Jarrett ME, Matzel KE, Stosser M, Baeten CG, Kamm MA. Sacral nerve stimulation for fecal incontinence following surgery for rectal prolapse repair: a multicenter study. Dis Colon Rectum 2005; 48:1243–1248.
295. Rosen HR, Urbarz C, Holzer B, Novi G, Schiessel R. Sacral nerve stimulation as a treatment for fecal incontinence. Gastroenterology 2001; 121:536–541.
296. Ganio E, Ratto C, Masin A, Realis Luc A, Doglietto GB, et al. Neuromodulation for fecal incontinence: outcome in 16 patients with definitive implant. Dis Colon Rectum 2001; 44:965–970.
297. Matzel KE, Kamm MA, Stosser M, Baeten CGMI, Christiansen J, et al. Sacral nerve stimulation for faecal incontinence: multicenter study. Lancet 2004; 363:1270–1276.
298. Norton C, Burch J, Kamm MA. Patient's views of a colostomy for fecal incontinence. Dis Colon Rectum 2005; 48:1062–1069.
299. Hughes SF, Williams NS. Continent colonic conduit for the treatment of fecal incontinence associated with disordered evacuation. Br J Surg 1995; 82:1318–1320.
300. Whitehead WE, Wald A, Norton NJ. Treatment options for fecal incontinence. Dis Colon Rectum 2001; 44:131–142.
301. Felt-Bersma RJF, Jansson JJWM, Klinkenberg-Knol EC, Hoitsma HFW, Meuwissen SGM. Soiling: anorectal function and results of treatment. Int J Colorectal Dis 1989; 4:37–40.
302. Hoffmann BA, Timmcke AE, Gathright JB, Hicks TC, Opelka FG, Beck DE. Fecal seepage and soiling: a problem of rectal sensation. Dis Colon Rectum 1995; 38:746–748.
303. Sentovich SM, Rivela LJ, Blatchford GJ, Christensen MA, Thor-son AG. Patterns of male fecal incontinence. Dis Colon Rectum 1995; 38:281–285.

16 Rectovaginal Fistula

Philip H. Gordon

INTRODUCTION

A rectovaginal fistula is a congenital or acquired communication between the two epithelial-lined surfaces of the rectum and the vagina. A fistula between the anal canal distal to the dentate line and the vagina is not a true rectovaginal fistula but an anovaginal fistula.

CLINICAL EVALUATION

Symptoms are dependent on the location, size, and etiology of the rectovaginal fistula and on the woman's perceptiveness and tolerance of the condition. A few patients are asymptomatic, but for most women the symptoms of rectovaginal fistula are distressing and totally unacceptable. Symptoms include the obvious passage of flatus or stool through the vagina. A more subtle presentation is the development of a discharge with fecal odor or recurrent or chronic vaginitis. Stool per vagina may be noted only when the patient has diarrhea. Rectal symptoms of fecal incontinence due to associated sphincter damage or diarrhea or a blood or mucous discharge caused by the underlying disease state may dominate clinical picture. It is important to obtain a history regarding sphincter function as dysfunction will direct the patient to further appropriate investigation and will modify the proposed corrective operation.

Patel, Shrivastav, and Nichols (1) described a unique case of generalized subcutaneous emphysema resulting from a rectovaginal fistula that followed a total abdominal hysterectomy.

Examination is essential to (i) confirm the presence of a rectovaginal fistula, (ii) determine accurately the size and location of the rectovaginal fistula, (iii) assess the state of the anal sphincter, (iv) exclude fistulas involving other organs, and (v) search for signs of an underlying disease state, such as an acute infection, Crohn's disease, irradiation injury, or a neoplastic process. Failure to recognize Crohn's disease as the cause of a rectovaginal fistula may result in inappropriate operative procedures that serve only to make the patient more symptomatic. Most often, the fistula is palpable and/or visualized easily via rectovaginal examination and proctosigmoidoscopy. Stool often is seen in the vagina, which may be the site of active infection. The dark red rectal mucosa contrasts with the lighter vaginal mucosa. If the opening of the fistula is small, it may appear only as a depression or a pit-like defect. Gentle use of a probe may be necessary to reveal the fistula.

Ancillary studies occasionally may be necessary to outline the rectovaginal fistula and to exclude underlying disease states, involvement of other parts of the bowels, or fistulas concomitant with other organs. An elusive rectovaginal fistulous tract can be identified by placing a tampon into the vagina and installing methylene blue into the rectum. The anus is plugged for 15 to 20 minutes; then the vaginal tampon is removed. If the tampon is unstained, the diagnosis of rectovaginal fistula is probably incorrect. A fistula involving other parts of the bowel, such as an ileovaginal fistula, should be excluded. Concomitant vesicovaginal, rectovesical, rectourethral, rectoperineal, and other fistulas should be sought since they may accompany rectovaginal fistulas. Contrast media fistulograms, vaginograms, barium enemas, intravenous pyelograms, and endoscopic procedures may be of value. Endoanal ultrasonography has proven to be a valuable diagnostic modality to establish the status of the sphincter mechanism, an important piece of information required to recommend the appropriate operation (2–4).

CLASSIFICATION

Rectovaginal fistulas may be classified on the basis of location, size, and etiology. Although somewhat arbitrary, such schemata are useful when comparing operative approaches and results of therapy, providing that the definition of terms is standardized.

LOCATION

The anterior rectal wall of the distal two-thirds of the rectum is subjacent to the posterior wall of the vagina. Depending on the underlying etiology, a rectovaginal fistula may occur at any site along this 9 cm rectovaginal septum. For convenience, many surgeons arbitrarily classify a rectovaginal fistula as "low" if it can be corrected surgically from a perineal approach or as "high" if it can be approached only transabdominally.

Basically, a rectovaginal fistula can be classified arbitrarily as "low" when located at or just slightly above the dentate line with the vaginal opening just inside the vaginal fourchette, as "high" when the vaginal opening is behind or near the cervix, and as "middle" when located between the high and low sites (Fig. 1).

SIZE

The size of rectovaginal fistulas varies greatly, although most are < 1 to 2 cm in diameter. They may be classified arbitrarily as "small" if they are < 0.5 cm, "medium" if they are from 0.5 to 2.5 cm, and "large" if they are > 2.5 cm in diameter.

ETIOLOGY

A rectovaginal fistula can result from a congenital malformation or from a variety of acquired disorders (Table 1). The precise incidence of a given etiology is difficult to determine since most series are small and reflect the referral pattern of a particular surgeon or institution. In many series, obstetric injuries account for the majority of rectovaginal fistulas. Examples of incidence by etiology are provided in Table 2.

TRAUMA

Perineal tears during childbirth and obstetric maneuvers such as episiotomies, especially when resulting in episioproctotomy, predispose women to the development of a rectovaginal fistula. Failure to recognize such an injury, inadequate repair, or the development of a secondary infection in a repaired wound virtually ensures the development of a rectovaginal fistula. Prolonged labor with persistent pressure on the rectovaginal septum occasionally causes necrosis with resulting rectovaginal fistula (14). In a review of 28,815 midline episiotomies, Beynon (15) found that the incidence of rectovaginal fistulas was 0.06%. Of the 18 fistulas, 12 healed spontaneously and six required operative repair. Venkatesh et al. (16) studied the incidence of anorectal complications following vaginal delivery in approximately 20,500 women. Episiotomy with third- and fourth-degree tears occurred in 5% of deliveries. Disruption followed in 10% of the repairs, and two-thirds of the failures required operative correction. Complications included anal ulcer, anorectal abscess, sphincter disruption, and rectovaginal fistula. In a review of the literature, Homsi et al. (17) found that rectovaginal fistula was reported to develop in the range of 0.1% of patients who underwent episiotomy during delivery. Further analysis revealed that rectovaginal fistulas develop in 0.05% of patients who undergo a median episiotomy but in 1% of those who suffer third- and fourth-degree lacerations.

Operative trauma is often responsible for development of rectovaginal fistulas. Vaginal or rectal operative procedures can cause them, usually near the dentate line, and pelvic operations can be complicated by the

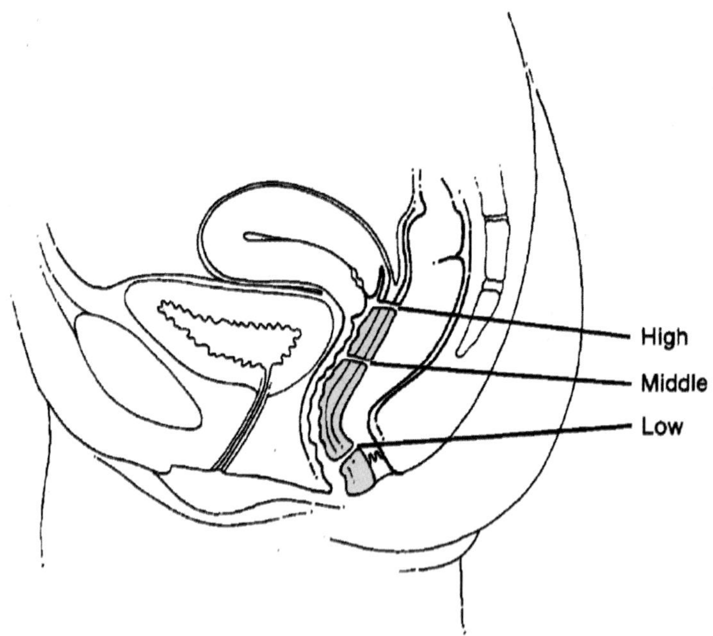

FIGURE 1 ■ Classification of rectovaginal fistula by location.

TABLE 1 ■ **Etiology of Rectovaginal Fistula**

Trauma: Obstetric, gynecologic, colonic, fulguration, violence, foreign body
Inflammatory bowel disease
Pelvic irradiation
Neoplastic (cervix, rectum, vagina) and hematologic (leukemia)
Infection: Anal gland, Bartholin gland abscess
Congenital
Miscellaneous

TABLE 2 ■ Incidence of Rectovaginal Fistula by Etiology

Authors(s)	No. of Patients	Etiology					
		Obstetric Injury (%)	Operative Trauma (%)	Radiation Injury (%)	Inflammatory Bowel Disease (%)[a]	Infection (%)	Miscellaneous (%)
Bandy et al. (5) (1983)	138	20	6	38	11	6	19
Shieh and Gennaro (6) (1984)	22	23		50	23		4
Lowry et al. (7) (1988)	81	74	7			10	
Wise et al. (8) (1991)	40	63	5			20	12
Mazier et al. (9) (1995)	95	81	2	1		16	
Watson and Phillips (10)[b] (1995)	26	50	4			35	11
Yee et al. (4) (1999)	25	76			4	20	
Baig et al. (3) (2000)	19	79				21	
Halverson et al. (11)[c] (2001)	35	43			34	6	17
Soriano et al. (12) (2001)	48	52	6		15	23	4
Zimmerman et al. (13) (2002)	21	43				38	19

[a]Most rectovaginal fistulas in this column reportedly were associated with Crohn's disease.
[b]Most rectovaginal fistulas associated with Crohn's disease or irradiation intentionally omitted.
[c]Recurrent rectovaginal fistula.

development of high rectovaginal fistulas. During creation of an anastomosis with a circular stapling device following a low anterior resection of the rectum, care must be exercised to avoid inclusion of a portion of the posterior vaginal wall, lest a fistula be created between the anastomosis and the vagina (18). With fear of stating the obvious, the perineal operator, must avoid placing the circular stapler in the vagina to avoid anastomosing the colon to the vaginal vault. In a series of 178 low anterior resections for rectal carcinoma (89 of whom were women) performed with the EEA autosuture device, four cases of rectovaginal fistula were reported by Antonsen and Kronberg (19). Rex and Khubchandani (20) surveyed members of the American Society of Colon and Rectal Surgeons and reported 57 patients who developed a rectovaginal fistula, 53 of whom had the anastomosis constructed with a circular stapler.

Violence, either penetrating or blunt, can cause a rectovaginal fistula. Forceful coitus and impalement injuries also have produced fistulas (21). Foreign bodies, such as pessaries or surgical sponges left after a previous procedure, have eroded through the rectovaginal septum, producing a fistula. An unusual case of rectovaginal fistula caused by insertion of a carbonated drink top has been reported (22). Fazio and Tjandra (23) have reported anovaginal fistulas complicating restorative proctocolectomy, sometimes resulting in loss of the pouch.

■ INFLAMMATORY BOWEL DISEASE

Both ulcerative colitis and Crohn's disease can produce a rectovaginal fistula. The reported incidence of rectovaginal fistula associated with inflammatory bowel disease varies considerably, from 6% to 23% (24,25). In a series of 886 women with Crohn's disease, Radcliffe et al. (26) found a 10% incidence of rectovaginal fistulas. Faulconer and Muldoon (27) stated that Crohn's disease, presumably because of its transmural involvement, is much more commonly responsible for rectovaginal fistula than is ulcerative colitis. They reported that 15 of 77 patients (20%) with rectovaginal fistula had associated colitis. One patient had chronic ukerative colitis and 12 patients had Crohn's colitis. Pathology reports for two patients were unavailable. Rectovaginal fistula development has also been described in patients with Behcet's syndrome (28).

Development of a rectovaginal fistula might imply the presence of colitis even in the absence of other signs of the disease. A recurring rectovaginal fistula should suggest inflammatory bowel disease. Buchmann et al. (24) reported an adenocarcinoma arising in a rectovaginal fistula secondary to Crohn's disease. The frequency with which Crohn's disease is associated with rectovaginal fistula is presented in Table 2, but as noted earlier depends on the referral pattern.

■ PELVIC IRRADIATION

Irradiation used in the treatment of pelvic carcinoma, especially carcinoma of the cervix or endometrium, can produce a rectovaginal fistula that generally is located high in the vagina. The incidence of rectovaginal fistula after irradiation for gynecologic malignancy ranges from $<1\%$ to 22%, with the latter figure reported from a highly specialized center (29–33). The incidence depends on the dose of radiation delivered (34). Most irradiation-induced fistulas develop 6 months to 2 years after therapy. The onset of lower bowel symptoms after 2 years is uncommon (34). However, the development of complications secondary to irradiation that may require definitive therapy can occur many years later. Those that develop during therapy are probably due to dissolution of the malignancy that had penetrated the wall of both the vagina and the rectum.

Certain conditions, such as diabetes mellitus, hypertension, and previous abdominal surgery, predispose the bowel to radiation injury (31). The development of irradiation-induced rectovaginal fistula is heralded by increasing looseness of the stool with passage of mucus and blood per rectum. Next, irradiation proctitis, followed by ulceration of the anterior rectal wall 4–5 cm above the dentate line, is noted. One-third to one-half of such ulcers progress to a rectovaginal fistula. When a patient complains of rectal pressure with the constant urge to defecate, fistula formation is imminent. These symptoms abate once the rectovaginal fistula is formed.

It is critical that recurrent carcinoma be distinguished from changes caused by irradiation. A rectal ulcer with a gray, shaggy, friable base and an elevated perimeter is suggestive of carcinoma. Examination with the patient under anesthesia often reveals firm masses or nodules adjacent to normal tissues in a patient with recurrent carcinoma, whereas those in patients with an irradiation-damaged pelvis generally have a uniform tissue texture. If any suspicion of neoplasm exists, appropriate biopsies must be taken and a metastatic investigation instituted.

■ NEOPLASTIC AND HEMATOLOGIC CAUSES

Primary, recurrent, or metastatic neoplasms can cause a rectovaginal fistula. Generally, these processes are extensions of colorectal, cervical, vaginal, or uterine malignancies. Occasionally, leukemias, aplastic anemias, agranulocytosis, and endometriosis have been implicated in the etiology of a rectovaginal fistula (21). Lock et al. (35) reported a case of a giant condyloma of the rectum that produced a rectovaginal fistula.

■ INFECTION

Any infectious process contiguous with the rectovaginal septum can produce a rectovaginal fistula. Diverticular disease, tuberculosis with a perirectal abscess, venereal diseases such as lymphogranuloma venereum, perianal fistulas, and abscesses all have precipitated a rectovaginal fistula. Rectovaginal fistula .on the basis of intestinal amebiosis has been reported (36). A pelvic abscess and Bartholin's abscesses in the pouch of Douglas can present as drainage through the rectovaginal septum. Chemical burns can incite severe inflammatory reaction in local tissues with subsequent development of a rectovaginal fistula.

■ CONGENITAL FISTULA

Since congenital rectovaginal fistula is discussed in various pediatric surgical textbooks, the subject is not discussed here.

■ MISCELLANEOUS

Fecal impaction is associated with many complications, among which rectovaginal fistula has been cited (37). By its pressure and ischemic necrosis of the wall, fecal impaction may cause stercoral ulceration and, when involving the rectum, a rectovaginal fistula may result. Ergotamine suppositories have also been reported to result in rectovaginal fistula (38).

OPERATIVE REPAIR

■ TIMING OF REPAIR

The likelihood of spontaneous or nonoperative healing of a rectovaginal fistula, which is primarily dependent on its etiology and to a lesser extent on its size, will influence the timing of an operative repair. Mattingly stated that one-half of small rectovaginal fistulas secondary to obstetric trauma would heal spontaneously (39). Mattingly therefore recommends waiting at least six months before operative intervention. In their review of the literature, Homsi et al. (17) also found that 52% of fistulas healed spontaneously. Removal of a foreign body is often followed by healing of the rectovaginal fistula. Similarly, proper treatment of an infectious process may allow healing of fistulas without formal operative repair. Once they are formed, irradiation- or neoplasm-induced rectovaginal fistulas rarely heal spontaneously (40).

Operative repair should not be attempted until the patient is in optimal condition, which can be achieved by aggressive treatment of underlying disease states. For some patients, this may involve the use of 5-acetylsalicylic acid preparations, corticosteroids, sulfasalazine (Azulfidine), antibiotics (metronidazole), antidiarrheal agents, immunosuppressive agents, infliximab or hyperalimentation to decrease the risk of operative repair and increase the chances of healing. Fistulas caused by inflammatory bowel disease may fail to heal, even with aggressive medical therapy.

Finally, local tissues should be as close as possible to normal before operative repair. Resolution of pelvic sepsis may require drainage of abscesses, use of antibiotics, warm baths, and other local care. It may be necessary to wait several weeks or months to allow the rectovaginal septum to return to its normal soft, pliable state.

■ PREOPERATIVE CONSIDERATIONS

The bowel preparation, including a mechanical cleansing regimen and the use of perioperative antibiotics, is essential for all transabdominal repairs. A similar preparation is recommended for local operative repairs (39). Vaginal preparation with a mechanical cleansing regimen is advisable. A bladder catheter should be inserted just before the operative procedure. When a difficult pelvic dissection is anticipated, such as in a patient with irradiation enteritis, the use of ureteral catheters may be of value.

Because of the distressing symptoms, some form of operative therapy is indicated in all but extremely poor-risk patients with a rectovaginal fistula. Regardless of the specific repair used, adherence to the operative principles of gentle dissection, full mobilization, excision of the diseased bowel and in most cases the fistulous tract, and accurate apposition of healthy tissues without tension is essential. No attempt will be made here to discuss repairs of congenital rectovaginal fistulas, which are presented well in the pediatric surgical literature.

■ TYPES OF APPROACHES

Rectovaginal fistulas can be corrected through abdominal, rectal, vaginal, perineal, transsphincteric, or transsacral approaches or through a combination of these methods. High rectovaginal fistulas often can be approached only transabdominally. Any of the other approaches may be suitable for low rectovaginal fistulas. However, most gynecologists prefer a vaginal approach.

Hoexter et al. (21) pointed out that a rectovaginal fistula joins the high-pressure system of the rectum (25–85 cmH_2O) with the low-pressure system of the vagina (atmospheric). A rectal approach provides the best exposure of the high-pressure side of the fistula. The literature is replete with various procedures to repair rectovaginal fistulas. All are variations of several basic techniques (Table 3) (41).

Local Repairs

In the past, low rectovaginal fistulas have been treated through simple fistulotomy and drainage, with laying open

TABLE 3 ■ Operative Repair of Rectovaginal Fistula

Local repair
- Conversion to complete perineal laceration with layer closure
- Excision of fistula with layer closure ± muscle interposition
  - Vaginal approach
  - Rectal approach
  - Perineal approach
  - Transsphincteric approach (York-Mason)

Sliding flap advancement
- Mucosa and partial-thickness internal sphincter (Laird)
- Anterior rectal wall (Noble)
- Endorectal type

Sphincter-preserving transabdominal repair
- Mobilization, division, and layer closure without bowel resection ± interposition
- Bowel resection ± interposition
- Pull-through procedures
- Low anterior resection—transsacral, EEA stapler
- Sleeve anastomosis (Parks)
- On-lay patch anastomosis (Bricker)

Miscellaneous
- Sphincter-sacrificing bowel resection
- Colostomy
- Colpocleisis

Source: Modified from Ref. 41 (p. 320).

of the entire tract. This method works well for an anovaginal fistula, but when used to treat a rectovaginal fistula, partial or total incontinence results. Because of such dismal results, simple fistulotomy is not advocated for repair of rectovaginal fistulas.

A commonly used method of local repair is conversion of the fistula to a complete perineal laceration followed by a layer closure (Fig. 2). The entire rectovaginal fistulous tract, including the adjacent sphincters and perineal body, is excised. The vaginal wall is dissected from the remnants of the perineal body, and a two- or three-layer closure is performed. This technique is identical to the classic obstetric repair of a fourth-degree perineal laceration and is described well by many authors (39,42). Soriano et al. (12) perform this as a two-stage procedure (Musset technique) with the initial stage a perineoproctotomy, followed 8 weeks later by a layered closure. Healing rates of 98 to 100% were reported depending upon whether the operation was performed for recurrent disease or as an initial procedure. Functional results were good in 75% of patients and required reoperation.

Tancer et al. (43) reported a 100% success rate in 34 patients who underwent repair by layer closure after conversion of the perineum into a cloaca. Complications were experienced in only three patients: one bleeding, one hematoma, and one small fistula, which was later excised without affecting the rectovaginal repair. Minimum follow-up was three months. In every instance in which the anal sphincter was reunited, a sphincterotomy was performed at the "5 o'clock site." These authors believe that sphincterotomy acts as a safety valve for the anterior repair. It relieves muscle spasm with its attendant discomfort, avoids tension on the suture line when a stool bolus is eliminated; and in the long term prevents anal stenosis. No other authors have made a similar recommendation, and apparently there is no convincing argument for adding a sphincterotomy to the repair. Indeed, it may even prove meddlesome.

A standard method of local repair is excision of the fistula with a layer closure. This can be accomplished through a vaginal, rectal, perineal, or transsphincteric approach, which can be accompanied by the interposition of vascularized pedicles of muscle, if necessary. Using a vaginal approach, Tancer et al. (43) reported 100% success in 10 patients.

Most surgeons do not attempt a local vaginal repair of a high rectovaginal fistula. Lawson (14), however, has used a deep perineal (Schuchardt) incision, which splits the vagina up to the lateral fornix, thus providing access to fistulas located near the cervix. If it is necessary for even greater exposure and mobilization, the pouch of Douglas can be opened behind the cervix and the rectum drawn down for layered repair. Lawson has had good success with this vaginal repair in 42 of 53 cases, opening the pouch of Douglas in 11 cases to facilitate closure of the fistula.

Hoexter et al. (21) reported their updated experience with a method of local repair using a per anal approach (Fig. 3). The repair encompasses total excision of the epithelialized fistula, approximation of the attenuated septal fibers and anal sphincter mechanism, and caudad rectal mucosal advancement that covers and protects the repair from the fecal stream and the high intraluminal pressures of defecation. Thirty-five patients with a rectovaginal fistula involving the middle portions of the rectovaginal septum were treated successfully without a recurrence during a mean follow-up period of four years, with a minimum follow-up of 1 year. Excluded from this report were rectovaginal fistulas arising from neoplasm, irradiation injury, or inflammatory bowel disease and fistulas located more than 6 cm cephalad to the dentate line, although the authors applied the technique in selected cases.

Goligher (42) points out two disadvantages of these methods of local repair: (i) excess tension on the suture line because of inadequate mobilization through the rectal or vaginal approaches, and (ii) direct apposition of the rectal and vaginal suture lines without much intervening tissue, which promotes a high recurrence rate. Goligher therefore proposed another approach involving transperineal dissection of the rectovaginal septum. Through a slightly curved perineal incision, the anal canal and rectum are separated from the vagina. The rectovaginal fistula is divided, and the posterior vaginal and anterior rectal walls are widely mobilized. This approach allows layered closure of both rectal and vaginal fistulous apertures without tension. In addition, by slight rotation of the rectum and the vagina in opposite directions, direct apposition of the suture lines can be avoided.

Wiskind and Thompson (44) also reported good results using a transverse transperineal repair of rectovaginal fistulas. In a series of 21 patients, with a follow-up of 3 months to 8 years, there were no recurrences. The series included seven patients with Crohn's disease and/or previous failed repairs.

The transsphincteric approach provides direct exposure of the anterior rectal wall and rectovaginal fistula, which then can be repaired in layers. York-Mason (45), who developed this approach specifically to deal with a prostatorectal fistula, has used it successfully to repair rectovaginal fistulas in three patients. This approach may obviate the need for transabdominal repairs of middle and high rectovaginal fistulas.

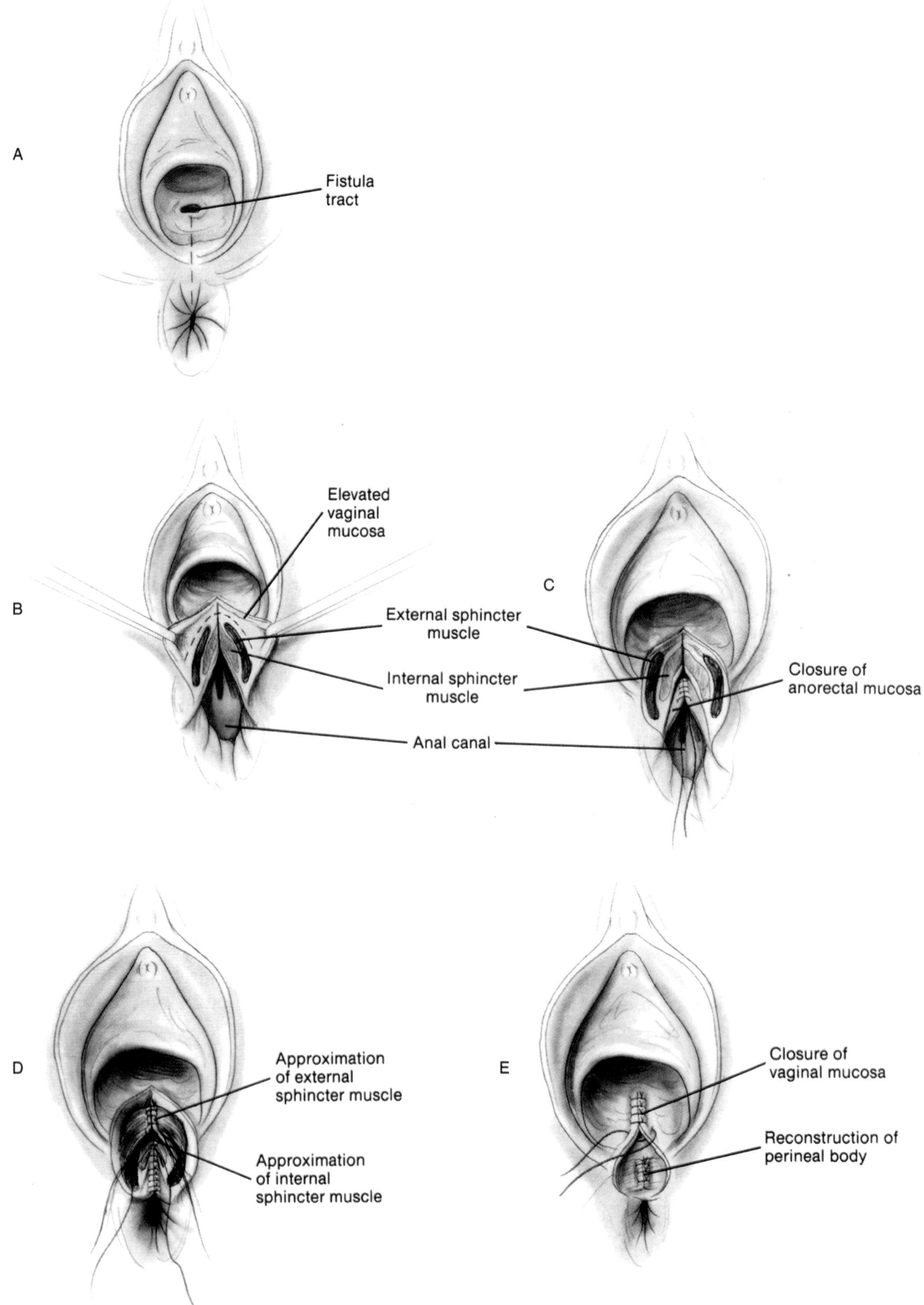

FIGURE 2 ■ Conversion of rectovaginal fistula to complete perianal laceration and layer closure. Transvaginal approach is illustrated. (**A**) Entire rectovaginal fistulous tract, including the sphincters and perineal body, is incised. (**B**) Vaginal wall is dissected from remnants of the perineal body. (**C**) Layered repair of rectal mucosa and external and internal sphincter muscles is begun. (**D** and **E**) Perineal body is reconstructed and vaginal epithelium is approximated.

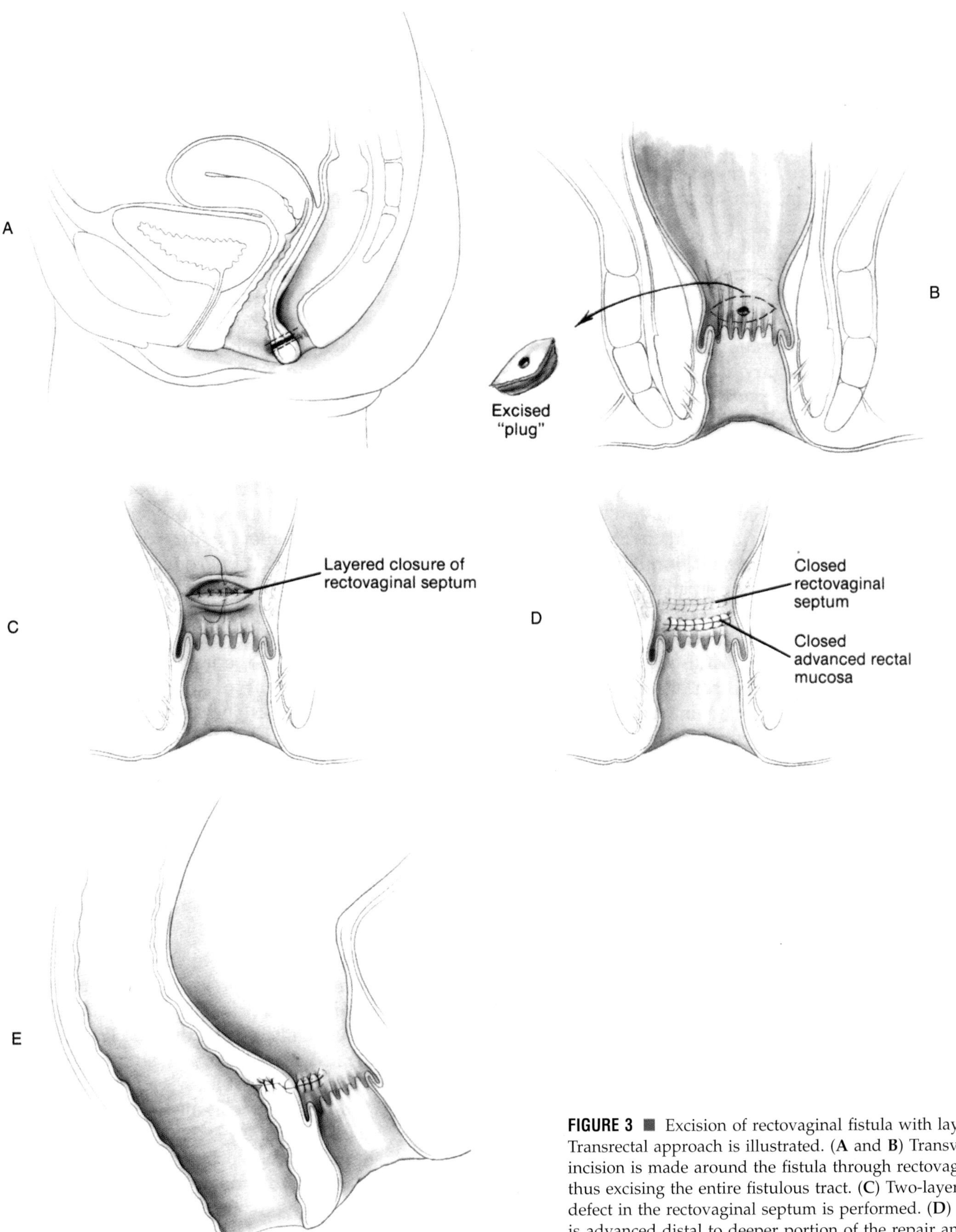

FIGURE 3 ■ Excision of rectovaginal fistula with layer closure. Transrectal approach is illustrated. (**A** and **B**) Transverse elliptical incision is made around the fistula through rectovaginal septum, thus excising the entire fistulous tract. (**C**) Two-layer closure of defect in the rectovaginal septum is performed. (**D**) Rectal mucosa is advanced distal to deeper portion of the repair and is reapproximated. (**E**) Vaginal mucosa is left open for drainage.

Because the difference in recurrence rates among patients with no previous repair and two previous repairs is so striking, Lowry et al. (7) believed that muscle interposition should be considered in patients with a history of multiple previous repairs. Others support this view. Both bulbocavernosus muscle and gracilis muscle interposition have been used successfully (32,46).

Although most local repairs of rectovaginal fistulas secondary to radiation injury are doomed to failure, Boronow (32) has reported exceptionally good results from the repair of the radiation-induced vaginal fistula with the Martius technique. The operation consists of the transposition of a bulbocavernosus-labial fat flap under cover of a colostomy. Successful closure was accomplished in 84% of 16 patients. Colostomy closure was performed within 3–13 months (average, 6 months). No operative mortality and no significant morbidity were reported. Boronow thus recommends the technique as first-line therapy for these extremely difficult management problems.

Sliding Flap Advancement

Various methods of advancing the internal fistulous opening to the anal margin have been described. Many

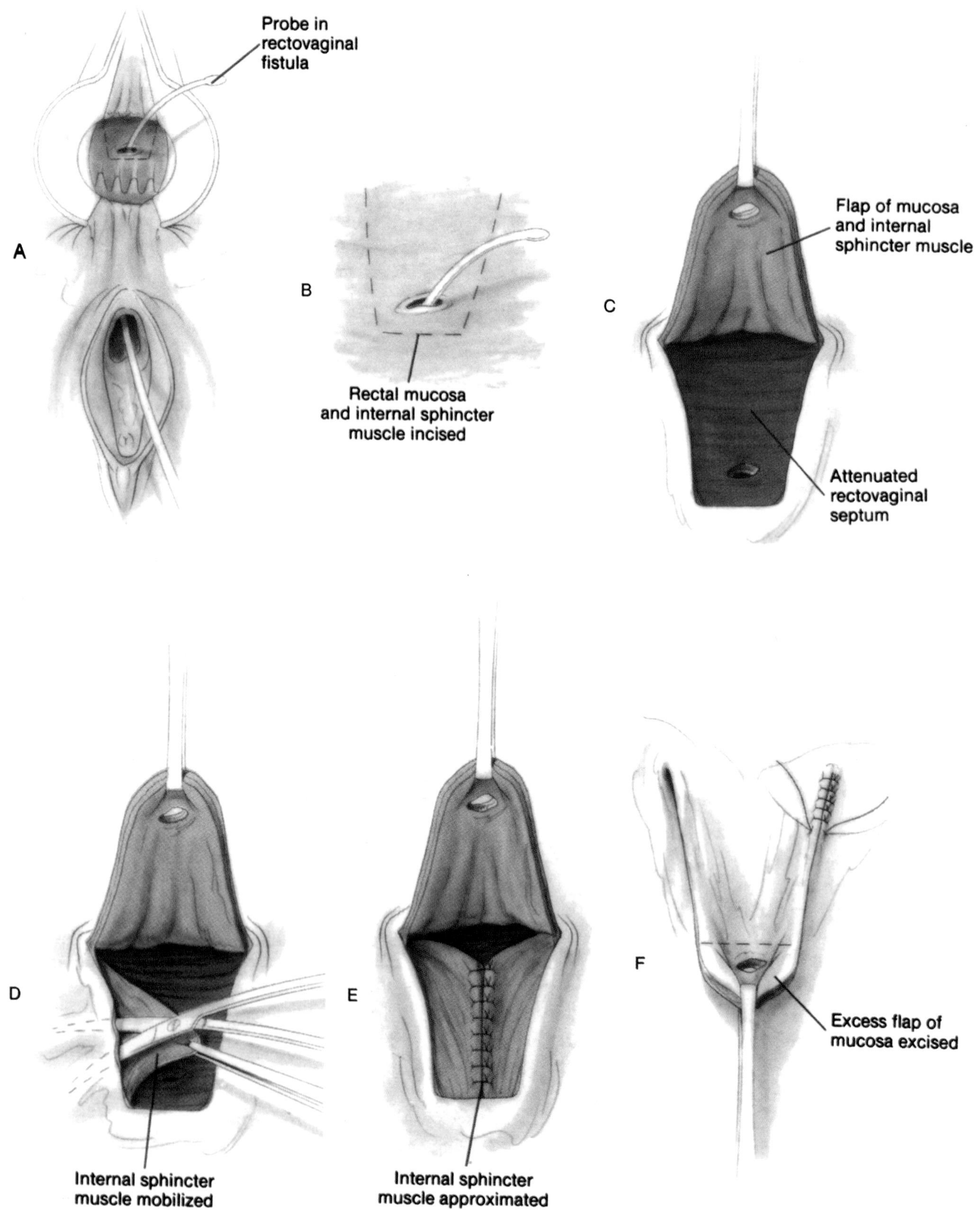

FIGURE 4 ■ Endorectal advancement of rectal flap.

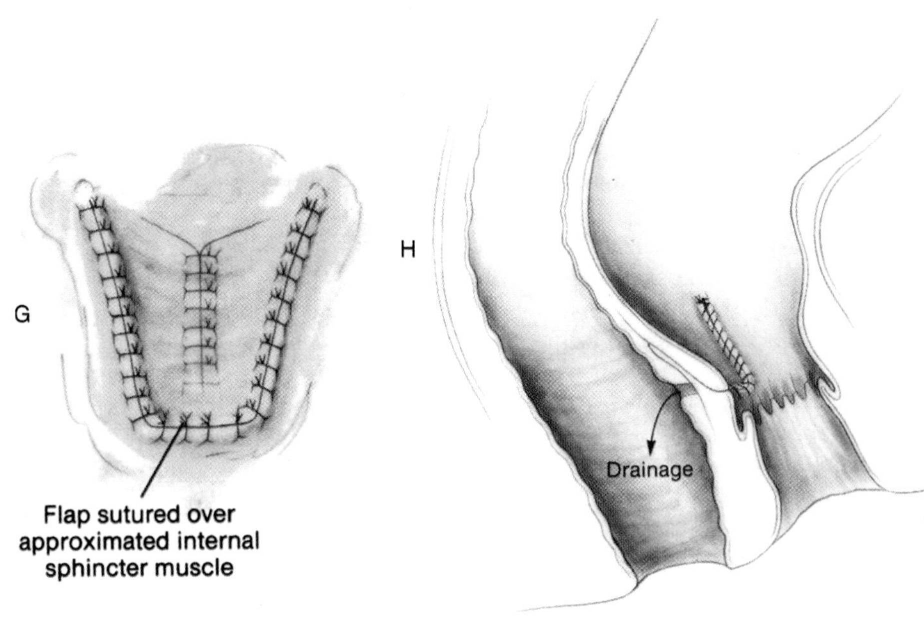

FIGURE 4 ■ (*Continued*)

authors believe that this is the best method of correcting low rectovaginal fistulas. Advancement of the anterior rectal wall is a technique first described by Noble in 1902.

Segmental advancement of the internal sphincter muscle with its attached overlying mucosa and the internal fistulous opening has certain advantages. The approach lessens the need for wide mobilization, has a low incidence of flap retraction, and does not generally interfere with continence since the external sphincter is not disturbed. This approach forms the basis of the technique championed by Lowry et al. (7) and the technique I have adopted for the repair of most patients with rectovaginal fistulas. Preoperatively, a formal bowel preparation is done, and perioperative antibiotics are administered. A colostomy is not used.

The following is a description of the technique previously described (41). Under general or regional anesthesia, the patient is placed in the prone jack-knife position over a hip roll with the buttocks spread by tape. In addition to the perianal field block, injections of 0.5% lidocaine (Xylocaine) or 0.25% bupivacaine with 1:200,000 epinephrine solution are made along the planned routes of dissection. Exposure is gained with the operating anoscope, and the rectovaginal fistula is identified (Fig. 4A). Then the rectal flap is outlined around the fistula, extending approximately 7 cm proximally into the rectum and at least 4 cm cephalad to the fistula. The base of the flap should be approximately two times the width of the apex of the flap to ensure adequate blood supply (Fig. 4B). The flap, consisting of mucosa, submucosa, and circular muscle, is raised from the apex to the base (Fig. 4C). The cut edge of the circular muscle is mobilized laterally so that it can be approximated in the midline without tension. Mobilization is accomplished in both the submucosal and intersphincteric planes (Fig. 4D). Hemostasis is achieved. The mobilized circular muscle then is reconstructed with 2-0 absorbable sutures, which are first placed and then tied serially (Fig. 4E). A final check for hemostasis is made before advancement of the flap. Excess flap, including the rectovaginal fistula, is excised (Fig. 4F). The flap is sutured in place with 3-0 absorbable sutures at the apex and along each side of the flap, thus restoring the normal anatomy (Fig. 4G). Only small bites of the flap should be included in each suture. The vagina is left open for drainge (Fig. 4H).

Postoperatively, oral intake is restricted for approximately 4 days. Not all surgeons believe restriction of oral intake is necessary. The patient is given codeine-containing analgesics and warm baths as needed to control the pain and spasm. Loperamide (Imodium) or diphenoxylate (Lomotil), two tablets four times a day, is added to confine the bowels. When diet is resumed, bulk stool softeners are prescribed to avoid constipation. When the patient is comfortable and after the first bowel movement, the patient is discharged.

Lowry et al. (7) reviewed 81 patients, 25 of whom had a concomitant overlapping sphincteroplasty. The causes were obsteric injury in 74%, perineal infection in 10%, operative injury in 7%, and unknown in 8%. The postoperative complication rate was 10% and included urinary tract infection (four), urinary retention (four), spinal headache (one), and postoperative bleeding that did not require reexploration (two). The overall primary healing rate was 83%. Kodner et al. (47) expanded the application of the sliding flap repair to treat complex anorectal fistulas in addition to rectovaginal fistula. In a series of 107 patients, which lumped the rectovaginal and rectoperineal fistulas from causes including obstetric injury, cryptoglandular abscess, Crohn's disease, and operative trauma, the initial success rate of repair was 84%. With reoperation, the eventual success rate was 94%. Khanduja et al. (48) reported on 25 women managed with an endorectal advancement flap with the addition of sphincteroplasty. Perfect anal continence was restored in 70% of patients. The authors recommend concomitant sphincteroplasty in women with evidence of incontinence. In an effort to improve overall results, Zimmerman et al. (13) added a labial fat flap transposition to the advancement flaps but found that the outcome was not improved (50% vs. 44%). The results reported by other authors are presented in Table 4.

TABLE 4 ■ Results of Advancement Flap Repair for Rectovaginal Fistula

Author(s)	No. of Patients	Success Rate (%)
Hoexter et al. (21)[a] (1985)	35	100
Lowry et al. (7) (1988)	56	78
Venkatesh et al. (16) (1989)	25	92
Kodner et al. (47) (1993)	71	84
Baig et al. (3) (2000)	19	74
Sonoda et al. (49) (2002)	37	43
Zimmerman et al. (13)[b] (2002)	21	48

[a]Layered closure and advancement of only the mucosa.
[b]Labial fat flap transposition added in 12 of the patients.

Repair of Rectovaginal Fistula in Crohn's Disease

Penninckx et al. (50) conducted a Medline review of the literature to compare the healing rate after several types of surgical repair of rectovaginal fistula in Crohn's disease and to identify factors predicting a successful outcome. They further analyzed the results of 32 of their own consecutive patients. All types of repair (rectal, vaginal, anocutaneous advancement flap, or perineoproctotomy with fistula closure) seem to be equally effective. Healing after a first repair is observed in 58% (46–71%). Healing can still be obtained at subsequent attempts in 62% (40–71%) of the patients. The reported overall healing rate is 75% (56–93%) The need for proctectomy after an attempt to repair was 6% (0–27%) in these series. Using a tailored surgical approach, they observed primary healing in 57%, healing after one or more supplementary procedures in 71%, for a total "definitive" closure rate of 75%. Anal continence was never compromised and all temporary stomas could be closed. Univariate analysis identified number of Crohn's sites, presence of extra-intestinal disease and previous Crohn's proctitis to be related with problematic healing after an operative repair. A positive relation was found between extra-intestinal disease and the number of repairs needed to ultimately obtain healing, whereas the relation with previous right hemicolectomy was negative. Multivariate analysis revealed the number of Crohn's sites as the only factor predicting problematic healing. A defunctioning stoma was not related to the healing rate and had its intrinsic morbidity with supplementary hospitalization (9.6 days). After a median follow-up of 40.4 (range, 8–87) months, they observed four late recurrences in 25 patients with healed rectovaginal fistula (16%). They concluded that closure of a rectovaginal fistula in Crohn's disease should not be considered an easy undertaking, especially in patients with several Crohn's sites. In this very heterogeneous group of patients the technique is adapted to the nature and the extent of accompanying anorectal disease. Construction of a temporary stoma is not mandatory and can be limited to complex cases.

Simmang et al. (51) described the use of a rectal sleeve advancement to repair a rectovaginal fistula associated with a stricture in Crohn's disease. Preoperatively, the patient undergoes a standard mechanical and antibiotic bowel preparation. The operation is performed in either the jack-knife or lithotomy position according to the surgeon's preference. Use of a Lone Star retractor (Lone Star Company, Houston, Texas, U.S.A.) facilitates the performance of the stricturectomy. Electrocautery is used to circumferentially incise the mucosa just distal to the palpable stricture. Dissection begins in the submucosal plane and circumferentially extends cephalad and, once above the sphincter complex, may extend outside the longitudinal muscle layer to encompass the full thickness of the rectum. Dissection is continued proximally until enough length has been gained to perform a rectoanal anastomosis without tension. The vaginal fistula is closed posteriorly with interrupted polyglycolic acid sutures; however, the vaginal mucosa is left open for drainage. The rectoanal anastomosis is then performed with interrupted polyglycolic acid sutures. A diverting loop ileostomy is performed. This may be performed in conjunction with a laparotomy and concomitant resection of intra-abdominal Crohn's disease. The loop ileostomy is closed after waiting 3–6 months to ensure that the rectoanal anastomosis has healed without fistula or stricture recurrence. Follow-up in two patients at 12 and 15 months have failed to reveal a recurrence and both patients have good continence of stool although some urgency is present. Both patients have had relief of the perineal pain.

A technique for the rectal sleeve advancement is described in Figure 5.

Sphincter-Preserving Transabdominal Repair

Local repairs and advancements generally cannot be used for high rectovaginal fistulas. In addition, their use may be inappropriate if the fistula is due to irradiation change, neoplasm, or perhaps inflammatory bowel disease, regardless of the location. Concomitant disease states also may warrant a transabdominal approach to a rectovaginal fistula. For such situations, a number of sphincter-preserving repairs have been advocated.

The simplest of these repairs involves mobilization of the rectovaginal septum, division of the fistula, and a layer closure of the rectal and vaginal defects without bowel resection. Interposition of a live pedicle of tissue may be used to supplement this repair (see discussion of ancillary procedures). Goligher (42) has experience with this approach and finds that it works well when normal tissues are available for the layered repair and the fistula can be approached easily from above.

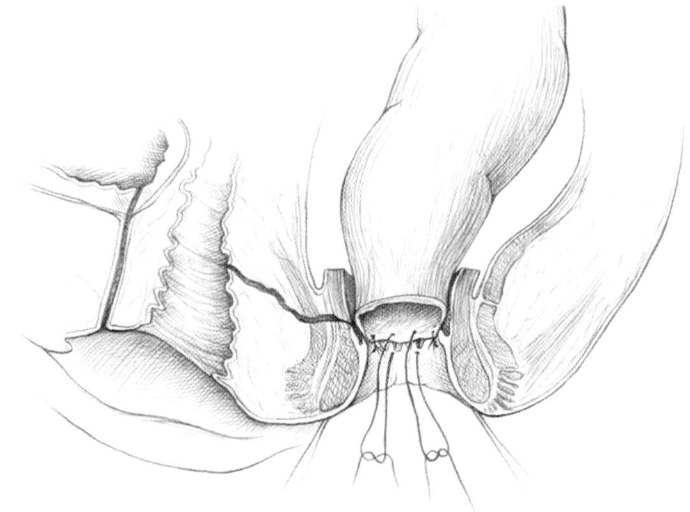

FIGURE 5 ■ Rectal sleeve advancement.

When local tissues are abnormal, whether from irradiation change, inflammatory bowel disease, diverticulitis, or a neoplasm, bowel resection is most often an essential feature of the repair of a rectovaginal fistula. Whenever possible, the anal sphincter should be preserved. Several methods to accomplish this goal are available.

Low anterior resection is another option. In the past, it was often difficult to perform an anastomosis deep in the pelvis at the site where high rectovaginal fistulas occur, although occasionally this was accomplished. Newer techniques make low anterior resection a more attractive choice. Using the circular stapling device to perform a low anterior resection seems preferable. This approach allows resection of the diseased bowel, including that portion involved in the rectovaginal fistula, and preserves continence.

For patients with multiple fistulas, both cryptogenic and rectovaginal involving one-third or more of the circumference, Berman (52) has described a sleeve advancement amputative anorectoplasty. Berman recommends this technique for situations in which conventional operations are likely to predispose to failure, recurrence, diminished continence, or prolonged surgical recovery.

Patients with rectovaginal fistulas secondary to radiation injuries are not amenable to local repair because of vascular damage to the remaining tissues. Therefore, the principle of any repair must provide for the delivery of normally vascularized tissue to the region.

Parks et al. (53) have used a sleeve anastomosis technique to treat postirradiation rectovaginal fistulas in five patients (Fig. 6). This involves complete mobilization of the colon so that nonirradiated bowel can be brought down to the anal canal. The rectum is mobilized down to just beyond the level of the rectovaginal fistula and divided at that point. The irradiated colon is resected. Then, from a perineal approach, the mucosa is stripped off the underlying muscle until the entire remaining rectum is denuded of all mucosa, leaving a rectal muscle tube that may contain the fistula in its most cephalad portion if mobilization of the rectum beyond the fistula was not feasible. Next, the normal colon is threaded through the muscle sleeve, thus covering the fistula. A per anal anastomosis of the colon to the anal canal is performed at the level of the dentate line.

Using the Parks coloanal sleeve anastomosis, Nowacki (54) reported functionally good results in 18 of 23 patients. One postoperative death was observed. Others also have been satisfied with this approach (30).

Cooke and Wellsted (55) reported on Denoon's treatment of radiation-damaged rectum by rectal resection with restoration of continuity by per anal sleeve anastomosis between healthy colon and the rectum stump denuded of its mucosa. The study population consisted of 42 patients with rectovaginal fistulas, 8 with hemorrhage from ulcerative proctitis, 3 with low rectal strictures, 5 with painful rectal ulcers, and 1 with a rectal carcinoma. Technical success was achieved in 93% with no mortality. The functional results were assessed both subjectively and objectively in 46 patients followed up for at least 1 year. Full continence was achieved in 54% initially, improving to 76% at 1 year postoperatively. Of the first 28 patients assessed 1 year after the operation, varying degrees of incontinence for liquid stool persisted in seven of nine patients who had low fistulas with an anastomosis at the dentate line level. When anastomosis was possible at a higher level, all 19 patients were fully continent at one year. Long-term follow-up was possible in 35 of the first 37 consecutive patients, with a mean of 5.1 years (range, 1 to 8 years 9 months). Four patients died of recurrent carcinoma. Twenty-four (77%) of the surviving 31 patients were fully continent, and 3 (9.7%) were reverted to a colostomy because of incontinence or pelvic obstruction. Cuthbertson (56) also has used the pull-through technique in a small number of patients. It is possible that the creation of a colonic J pouch might result in better function than a straight coloanal anastomosis.

Miscellaneous

Sphincter-sacrificing bowel resections such as abdominoperineal resection or even pelvic exenteration may be indicated for patients with neoplasm-induced rectovaginal fistulas. Similarly, patients with active extensive inflammatory bowel disease may require proctectomy and/or colectomy to treat not only the rectovaginal fistula but also the underlying disease. Faulconer and Muldoon (27) reported that 11 of 15 patients with colitis and a rectovaginal fistula were treated by total proctocolectomy and ileostomy and 2 of the 15 by subtotal colectomy with ileostomy and rectal mucous fistula. Patients with irradiation-induced rectovaginal fistulas or rectovaginal fistulas associated with a nonresectable malignancy, especially if they are poor operative risks, may be treated best by a permanent totally diverting colostomy (40). Still another choice for a poor-risk patient is colpocleisis performed with wire or some other permanent suture material to close the vagina at the introitus, thus forming a common chamber consisting of the vagina and the rectum with the anus as the only exit. This approach obviates the need for colostomy in elderly incapacitated patients who would have difficulty dealing with a stoma.

Gorenstein et al. (57) reported the use of a gracilis muscle interposition for the repair of a rectovaginal fistula that occurred after a restorative proctocolectomy with a J-shaped ileal reservoir. Attempts at local repair had failed. Under cover of a diverting ileostomy the fistulas healed and intestinal continuity was restored. These authors believe that this procedure can be useful to salvage a pelvic pouch complicated by a rectovaginal fistula. Harms et al. (58) reported on the management of a rectovaginal fistula associated with chronic ulcerative colitis by performing simultaneous ileal pouch construction and fistula closure.

■ RECURRENT RECTOVAGINAL FISTULA

Recurrent or persistent rectovaginal fistula poses a challenging management problem. The choice of operation should be tailored to the underlying pathology and the type of repair previously done. MacRae et al. (59) reviewed the management of 28 patients with persistent fistula, 14 were secondary to obstetric injury, 5 were caused by Crohn's disease, and 9 had miscellaneous etiologies. Of the 18 patients classified as "simple," 13 healed, 5 after advancement flap, 5 following sphincteroplasty, and 3 after coloanal anastomoses. Of the 10 patients labeled "complex," healing occurred in only 4 patients, 1 following sphincteroplasty, 1 with coloanal anastomosis, and

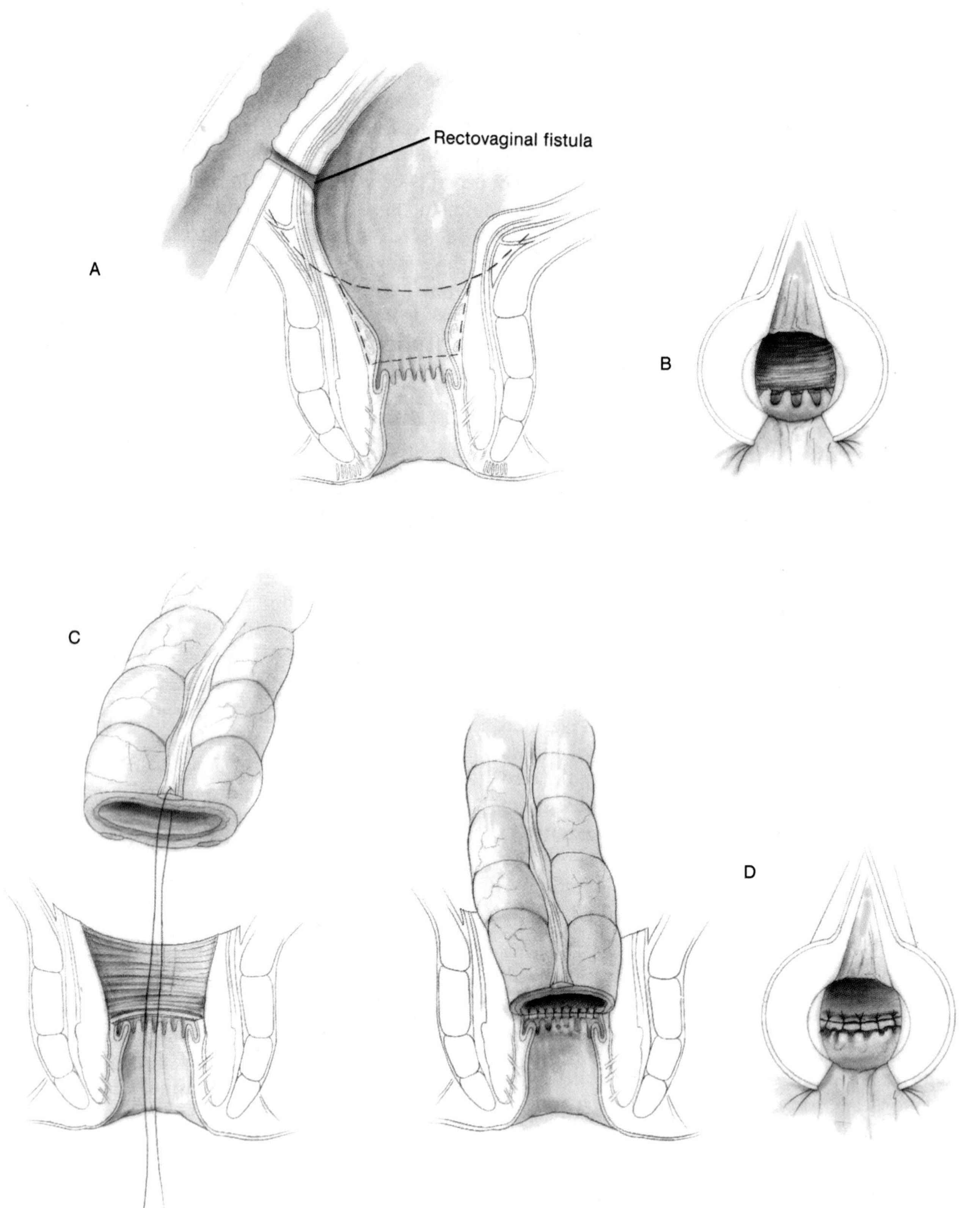

FIGURE 6 ■ Parks' coloanal anastomosis. (**A**) Mobilization of rectum distal to level of the rectovaginal fistula and transection of the rectum distally. (**B**) Removal of mucosa from the anorectal stump. (**C**) Anastomosis between proximal bowel and anal canal at the level of the dentate line. (**D**) Final arrangement of colon within the anal canal.

2 after gracilis muscle transposition. A total of 23 advancement flaps were performed in 17 patients with five patients healing (29%). Sphincteroplasty and fistulectomy were successful in six of seven patients (86%). Coloanal anastomosis resulted in healing in four of six patients (67%) in whom it was attempted. Gracilis muscle transfer was successful in both patients in whom it was tried. Because of the high failure fate, these authors do not generally recommend advancement flap repairs that have previously failed.

The advancement flap, however, has been used successfully for recurrent rectovaginal fistulas. Lowry et al.

(7) reported that after one previous repair an 85% success rate was obtained but this dropped to 55% when used as a third procedure. Repeated failures may be due to sepsis and ischemia and success, therefore, depends on the introduction of new tissue with its blood supply, which can be achieved with sphincteroplasty, labial fat or gracilis muscle interposition, or a coloanal anastomosis.

For the patient with a recurrent rectovaginal fistula, Haray et al. (60) described an operative technique that combines the standard endoanal advancement flap procedure with a diamond-shaped cutaneous flap advancement into the vagina. The wide-based endoanal flap incorporates part of the thickness of the internal sphincter and is sutured to the anal margin. A diamond-shaped incision is made on the skin at the posterolateral margin of the vaginal introitus. This is advanced into the vagina and sutured to the vaginal mucosa above the fistula, thus covering the vaginal opening of the fistulous tract using absorbable interrupted sutures. The skin defect is closed. The procedure is performed under cover of an ileostomy.

Halverson et al. (11) reported on 57 procedures performed in 35 women who presented with recurrent rectovaginal fistula. Median follow-up was 4 months. The causes of recurrent rectovaginal fistula included obstetrical injury ($n=15$), Crohn's disease ($n=12$), fistula occurring after proctocolectomy with ileal pouch-anal anastomosis (for ulcerative colitis, $n=3$; indeterminate colitis, $n=1$; familial polyposis, $n=1$), cryptoglandular disease ($n=2$), and fistula occurring immediately after low anterior resection for rectal cancer ($n=1$). The methods of repair used included mucosal advancement flap ($n=30$), fistulotomy with overlapping sphincter repair ($n=14$), rectal sleeve advancement ($n=3$), fibrin glue ($n=1$), proctectomy with colonic pull-through ($n=2$), and ileal pouch revision ($n=6$). Patients without a diverting stoma underwent bowel preparation with oral lavage before operation. Patients with a diverting stoma received preoperative enemas to eliminate any mucus. All patients received perioperative intravenous antibiotics. Twenty-seven of 34 (79%) patients with adequate follow-up eventually healed after a median of two operations. Crohn's disease, the presence of a diverting stoma, and decreased time interval since prior repair were associated with a poorer outcome.

Pye et al. (61) described a repair for recurrent rectovaginal fistula using a surgical approach that incorporates a Surgisis™ mesh. The operation involves opening the posterior vaginal wall and identifying the fistula tract. The vagina is dissected from the rectum approximately 2 cm above the fistula. The rectal component of the repair is performed with a double layer of PDS 2/0 sutures (Ethicon Endosurgery Inc., Cincinnati, Ohio, U.S.A.) followed by a continuous Lembert suture of number 1 polyglactin (Vicryl™, Ethicon Endosurgery Inc., Cincinnati, Ohio, U.S.), folding the rectal mucosa over the fistula tract. Surgisis mesh is cut to size, approximately 5 cm × 5 cm, placed in the rectovaginal space, and held with five 3–0 PDS sutures at each corner of the mesh and in the middle. Finally, the vaginal mucosa is closed over the mesh using a continuous number 1 polyglactin (Vicryl) suture. Postoperative management involves five days of Lactulosc 10 mg bid and Augmentim 375 mg tid.

■ ANCILLARY PROCEDURES

A wide difference of opinion exists about the need for a temporary colostomy when operative repair of a rectovaginal fistula is contemplated. Goligher (42) routinely established a preliminary temporary colostomy when repairing a rectovaginal fistula, whereas many authors state that a colostomy is unnecessary in most instances. I agree that for most rectovaginal fistulas that are low and/or caused by trauma, infection, or inactive inflammatory bowel disease, a colostomy is unnecessary. However, when dealing with high, complicated rectovaginal fistulas caused by irradiation, neoplasm, active inflammatory bowel disease, and active infectious processes, a colostomy may be a useful adjunct to treatment. In such cases, a staged procedure may be beneficial. After a diverting colostomy has been established, direct repair of the rectovaginal fistula can be deferred as long as 6 to 12 months until local tissues are more normal. Another possible route is the creation of a complementary colostomy at the time of the definitive repair.

Sphincter repair should be performed concomitant with operative correction of the rectovaginal fistula whenever fecal incontinence is associated.

Regardless of the approach used, many authors advocate the interposition of vascularized pedicles of omentum or muscle between the rectum and vagina after division of the fistula, especially when dealing with irradiation-induced rectovaginal fistulas. This avoids direct apposition of the suture lines in the two organs and decreases the chance of recurrence. Goligher (42) has used omental pedicles based on the right gastroepiploic artery.

Several authors had used a Martius graft, originally described as a flap of tissue consisting of the bulbocavernosus muscle and its adjacent labial fat interposed between the rectum and the vagina after a layer closure of the fistulous defects (32,39,62,63). Anatomic studies undertaken of the graft in a cadaver demonstrated that the graft is composed of fibroadipose tissue from the labium majus and not from the bulbocavernosus muscle (62). It receives its blood supply anteriorly from the external pudendal artery and posteriorly from the internal pudendal artery. The technique described by Margolis et al. (63) consists of a vertical incision made over the labia majora and extended ventrally and laterally to include a non-hair-bearing, oval-shaped, patch of skin from the medial thigh. The Martius bulbocavernosus fat pad is then mobilized by grasping the edges of the skin with Allis clamps and sharply dissecting the fat pad from the undersurface of the labia majora. Next, the full-thickness skin patch is elevated and sharply dissected from its bed; however, it is left attached to the bulbocavernosus fat pad. The graft and skin are then passed through the Martius tunnel and attached to the vaginal wall defect with multiple sutures of 3–0 polyglycolic acid. The vulvar and thigh defects are then dosed with interrupted sutures of 2–0 polyglycolic acid after undermining the skin where necessary.

Several advantages have been cited for this technique: (i) skin from the medial thigh is non-hair-bearing, thus avoiding the problems of dyspareunia secondary to hair growth and the higher infection rate associated with wound healing in hair-bearing skin; (ii) much larger patches of skin are available from the medial thigh than can be harvested from the vulva; (iii) blood supply is available from multiple sources; and (iv) swinging the flap adds length to the vascular pedicle, thereby putting less tension on it and the grafted skin.

Aartsen and Sindram (64) reported a relatively poor outcome with the Martius procedure. Of 14 patients who underwent the repair under cover of a colostomy, the initial success rate of 13 out of 14 deteriorated over a 10-year follow-up to only 6 out of 14 who ultimately remained without a colostomy. Unexpected inconveniences and complications following operation included frequent bowel movements, dyspareunia, vaginal stenosis, and sepsis (64). In contrast, White et al. (65) performed 14 Martius procedures on 12 patients with radiation-induced rectovaginal fistulas. There were no postoperative complications, and 11 patients had successful closure. Elkins et al. (62) and Margolis et al. (63) have used the Martius graft to repair a host of vaginal defects, including rectovaginal fistula, and reported an overall success rate of 86.5%.

For repair of chronic radiation wounds of the pelvis, Mathes and Hurwitz (66) described the use of a host of muscle flaps, including the rectus femoris, rectus abdominis, gracilis, and gluteus maximus muscles and musculocutanous flaps and gluteal thigh skin, and fascial flaps. The adductor longus and sartorius muscles have also been used.

Hysterectomy with preservation of the ovaries may facilitate the abdominal repair of a high rectovaginal fistula by improving access to the inferior margin of the fistula. In rare situations when there is dense pelvic fibrosis with obliteration of the pouch of Douglas and fixation of the uterus, cervix, and vaginal vault in solid scar, the only method of exposure may involve a subtotal hysterectomy and midline sagittal split of the cervical stump. This exposes the fistula, which then can be repaired in layers. Five of seven patients were treated successfully in this fashion by Lawson (14). One developed a recurrence, and one died of massive pelvic hemorrhage.

■ SELECTION OF OPERATIVE PROCEDURE

The precise method of operative repair varies with the location, size, and etiology of the rectovaginal fistula; with the number and type of previous repairs; with associated abnormalities such as sphincter damage, rectal or vaginal stricture, or fistulas to other organs; with the patient's operative risk factors; and with the surgeon's training, experience, and interpretation of reported results of similar repairs. Of these many factors, etiology of the rectovaginal fistula is the primary determinant in selection of appropriate repair. Treatment of a rectovaginal fistula produced by a carcinoma, whether primary, metastatic, or recurrent, should not interfere with the appropriate therapy of the underlying neoplasm. In many instances, bowel resection, often with sacrifice of the rectal sphincter, is necessary.

An important consideration in the selection of the appropriate operation is the functional status of the anal sphincter. Tsang et al. (2) conducted a study to determine the effect of a sphincter defect on the outcome of rectovaginal fistula repair. They identified 52 women who underwent 62 repairs of simple obstetrical rectovaginal fistulas. Fourteen patients (27%) had preoperative endoanal ultrasound studies and 25 (48%) had anal manometry studies. Twenty-five patients (48%) complained of varying degrees of fecal incontinence before surgery. There were 27 endorectal advancement flaps and 35 sphincteroplasties (28 with and 8 without levatoroplasty). Success rates were 41% with endorectal advancement flaps and 40% with sphincteroplasties. Endorectal advancement flap was successful in 50% of patients with normal sphincter function but in only 33% of patients with abnormal sphincter function. For sphincteroplasties, success rates were 73% versus 84% for normal and abnormal sphincter function, respectively. Results were better after sphincteroplasties versus endorectal advancement flaps in patients with sphincter defects, identified by endorectal ultrasound (88% vs. 33%) and by manometry (86% vs. 33%). Poor results correlated with prior operations in patients undergoing endoanal advancement flaps (45% vs. 25%) but not sphincteroplasties (80% vs. 75%). They believe that all patients with rectovaginal fistula should undergo preoperative evaluation for occult sphincter defects by endoanal ultrasound or anal manometry or both procedures. Local tissues are inadequate for endorectal advancement flap repairs in patients with sphincter defects and a history of previous repairs. Patients with clinical or anatomic sphincter defects should be treated by sphincteroplasty. Baig et al. (3) found a sphincter defect in 60% of their patients. Yee et al. (4) reported anal incontinence in 40% of their patients.

Irradiation-induced rectovaginal fistulas challenge the judgment and skill of the surgeon because of the generalized nature of the irradiation effect. Diffuse tissue fibrosis makes dissection of the fistula difficult, and diffuse small-vessel endarteritis results in vascular compromise, with subsequent tissue loss from sloughing, and most often precludes the use of local tissues for operative repair. There is often an associated stricture. For these reasons, a frequent method of treatment for irradiation-induced rectovaginal fistulas has been a permanent colostomy. Definitive repair must include the delivery of well-vascularized tissue to the region.

Mazier et al. (9) reviewed their experience with 95 patients operated on for rectovaginal fistulas via septal repair after conversion to a fourth-degree perineal laceration, endoanal flap, or anoperineorrhaphy. Excellent or good results were obtained in 97% of patients. There were no outcome differences between techniques, and similar success occurred in patients with previous failed repairs. The authors believe that the operative technique should be tailored to the anatomic defect and this approach should allow for optimal functional outcome.

In select good-risk patients who apparently are cured of the condition for which they received irradiation but who are plagued by a rectovaginal fistula, various procedures that will preserve normal anorectal function are available. In all such cases, a temporary colostomy is established and maintained for at least 6 months to 1 year to allow necrosis to disappear and the inflammatory reaction to subside. Then, a repair that uses nonirradiated tissue with a normal potential for healing can be undertaken. The fistula, because it is surrounded by abnormal tissue, cannot simply be closed but must be occluded or patched with tissues unaffected by irradiation. Local or transabdominal repairs using vascularized pedicles of omentum or muscle as described above accomplish this goal and are sometimes successful. A unique technique is the on-lay patch anastomosis that was devised by Bricker and Johnston. Still another method of using normal tissue for the repair involves resection of all irradiated bowel with a primary anastomosis of normal bowel. This procedure can be performed as a low anterior resection with the EEA stapler or with the sleeve anastomosis devised by Parks et al. (53).

Rectovaginal fistulas associated with Crohn's disease present a difficult management dilemma. Patients with few symptoms do not require operative care, whereas severely symptomatic patients may require a proctocolectomy. For a small percentage of patients, local repair of the fistula may be warranted. Recurrence during a flare-up of the colitis is not uncommon, however. When a patient has persistently active disease that does not show response to medical therapy or when a patient has associated sphincter destruction and can no longer tolerate the incapacitating symptoms, proctectomy is indicated for treatment of the inflammatory bowel disease and the rectovaginal fistula.

Mixed results have been reported for the local treatment of rectovaginal fistula associated with Crohn's disease. Some authors have reported poor results (27,67). For the patients with quiescent proximal disease and minimal, if any, rectal disease, the recent trend is toward local repair in selected patients (5,26). Bandy et al. (5) performed repair in 10 patients with rectovaginal fistulas associated with Crohn's disease. Their technique was episioproctotomy and layered repair. One patient had diversion of the fecal stream. Healing occurred in nine patients (90%), with a follow-up of 13 to 53 months. Two patients exhibited recurrence of rectovaginal fistulas in association with exacerbation of the Crohn's disease six and 19 months later. Radcliffe et al. (26) used a variety of techniques to repair 12 patients. Primary healing was achieved in eight patients and some patients required multiple attempts at repair. The authors consider the endorectal advancement flap technique the preferred method for local repair.

From a total of 14 patients with rectovaginal fistula associated with Crohn's disease, Cohen et al. (68) reported on the results in seven patients, five of whom underwent staged local repair, with closure of the colostomy in three of them. Two of the three patients have had no evidence of recurrence during follow-up for more than 2 years. The third patient required an ileostomy for intestinal disease and had no recurrence of the fistula. Two patients underwent primary repair of the rectovaginal fistula without fecal diversion; in one of these patients the fistula recurred 10 days after the operation, necessitating a diverting ileostomy. The other patient remained cured 26 months after repair. The technique employed was either a layered closure or the endorectal advancement flap. In this small but carefully studied group of patients, Cohen et al. (68) concluded that in the selected situation of quiescent rectal disease, repair of a rectovaginal fistula can be expected to have a reasonable chance of success, and the presence of a rectovaginal fistula in a patient with Crohn's disease does not mandate removal of the rectum.

Morrison et al. (69) reported their results with the operation for treating rectovaginal fistula in patients with Crohn's disease. Of eight patients who underwent fistula repair, either layered repair or endorectal advancement, complete healing occurred in six. One patient has a persistent fistula that is minimally symptomatic, and the other required proctocolectomy after three unsuccessful repairs. Success of the operations correlated with quiescent intestinal disease and absence of rectal involvement. Morrison et al. believe that in selected patients who have symptomatic fistulas, operative repair is indicated and healing can be anticipated.

For traumatic or infectious rectovaginal fistulas, the surgeon should select a procedure with minimal morbidity and a high likelihood of success. Using a transabdominal approach may be necessary to treat a high rectovaginal fistula near the cervix, although other means of exposure have been described. For low or middle rectovaginal fistulas, local repairs or advancement flaps work well. My preference is the endorectal flap advancement repair for all such fistulas. This procedure has a low morbidity rate because only minimal preoperative preparation is necessary, no colostomy or skin incision is required, operative time is short, postoperative recovery is speedy, and continence is not disturbed. In addition, this procedure allows for concomitant sphincter repair.

RECTOURETHRAL FISTULA

Rectourethral fistulas are a rare but devastating complication of urinary or rectal operations, trauma, or inflammation. Etiologically, these fistulas may arise following prostatectomy, rectal surgery, pelvic radiation, cryotherapy, trauma, perianal abscess, Crohn's disease, or even Kaposi's sarcoma (70,71). The diagnosis of a rectourethral fistula can be suspected from the patient's history. Symptoms of fecaluria, pneumaturia, or leakage of urine from the rectum may be the most common symptoms. A rectourethral fistula causes loss of urine from the rectum only during micturation, while a rectovesical fistula causes a constant escape of urine from the rectum. Rectal examination, urethrocystoscopy, sigmoidoscopy, secretory urography, retrograde urethrography, and voiding cystburethrography may help in the differential diagnosis, as might be rectal contrast (72,73). Historically, repair has posed a challenge because of technical difficulties and the high incidence of recurrent fistulas. The first attempt at repair is the best, and subsequent repair becomes increasingly difficult. An initial trial of fecal and urinary diversion allows spontaneous closure of some fistulas (71).

The variety of options for treatment have been reviewed by Bukowski et al. (71) and the following draws heavily from their account. Garofalo et al. (72) compared the multiple types of repair (perineal, transsphincteric, gracilis muscle transposition rectal advancement flap, abdominoperineal resection, and transanorectal endoscopic microsurgery) and found success rates ranging from 75% to 100%. Most series have few cases.

A transabdominal approach allows the use of omental interposition, as well as an abdominoanal pull-through operation. Most surgeons may be comfortable with this approach, but there may be difficulties due to limited exposure and maneuverability deep in the pelvis, especially in closing the urethra defect. Leaving the prostatic defect open with a fenestrated splinting catheter apposed to the omental flap has been recommended when performing abdominoperineal interposition. This approach has been associated with the complications of any intra-abdominal procedure, as well as increased postoperative recovery time and increased difficulty if adhesions are present due to previous abdominal surgery.

Perineal approaches are used commonly, often with a gracilis or dartos flap to interpose healthy, well-vascularized tissue. However, disadvantages of this approach include the fact that access is through scarred tissue, the approach affords limited exposure, and it may endanger urinary continence. In 1958, Goodwin et al. (74) described several principles important for repair, including excision of the fistula, development of layers on the urinary and rectal sides of the fistula, and closure using nonoverlapping suture lines with interposition of the levator ani muscles when possible.

The anterior transanorectal approach proposed by Gecelter (75) uses a midline perineal incision deepened by incising all structures superficial to the prostatic capsule, including superficial perineal fascia, the central tendon of the perineum, and the external and internal sphincters. This approach affords greater access for repairing complicated membranoprostatic fistulas with reportedly good continence and erectile preservation.

A per anal approach championed by Parks and Motson (76) has the theoretical advantage of minimal scarring and fewer wound infections, although it affords limited exposure and is used infrequently. The authors report five patients with rectoprostatic fistulas repaired per anally using a full-thickness local flap of anterior rectal wall. The repair was protected by a sigmoid loop colostomy. Primary healing occurred in all five patients.

Garofalo et al. (72) reported 23 male patients treated for rectourethral fistula. The cause of the fistula was iatrogenic from prostate or rectal surgery in 10 cases (43%), Crohn's disease in 9 (39%), radiation in 3 (13%), and traumatic (from a motor vehicle accident with severe pelvic trauma in 1 (5%). Fecal diversion alone was performed in seven patients (30%), and urinary diversion alone was performed in one patient (4%). Both fecal and urinary diversions were performed in 12 patients (52%), and no diversion was performed in 3 patients (13%). Four patients were managed conservatively with diversion only. Nineteen patients underwent definitive repair. Rectal advancement flap repair was used in 12 (52%) of the cases.

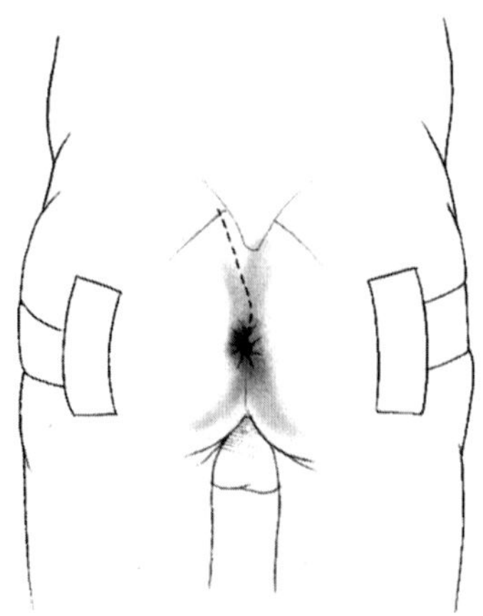

FIGURE 7 ■ Skin incision.

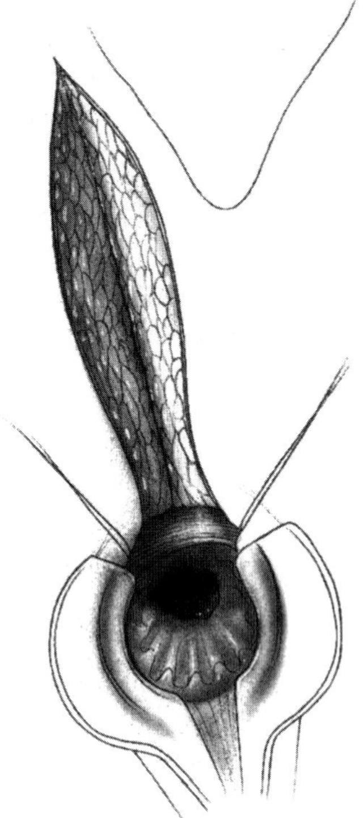

FIGURE 8 ■ Marking mucocutaneous junction with sutures.

Rectal advancement flap repair was typically performed with the patient in the Kraske position. Rectal retractors were placed to expose the fistula opening. A 1:100,000 epinephrine solution was injected submucosally for hemostasis, and a full- or partial-thickness flap was created with a broad proximal base. The fistula tract was excised, and any granulation tissue was removed. The urethral defect was carefully closed with fine absorbable suture. The intervening muscle layer (internal/external sphincter) was reapproximated. The rectal opening of the fistula was excised from the raised flap; the flap was pulled down and sutured in place. Antibiotics were given preoperatively

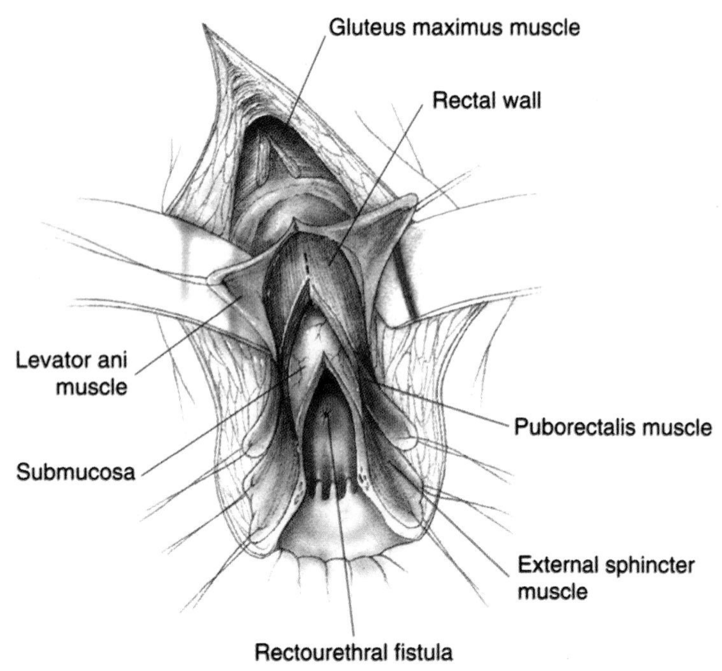

FIGURE 9 ■ Identification of rectourethral fistula.

and postoperatively for a variable amount of time depending on the preference of the attending surgeon. Reversal of any preoperative diversion was performed at a variable amount of time postoperatively (typically 6–12 weeks) after voiding cystogram and rectal contrast studies were performed to rule out persistent or recurrent fistula. Postoperatively length of stay was 4.5 ± 4 days. Patients were followed up for an average of 31 ± 33.4 months. Rectal advancement flap achieved primary closure in 8 (67%) of 12 patients. There were four recurrences. Two patients underwent successful repeat repair, for a final success rate of 83%. Patients with rectovaginal fistula secondary to iatrogenic causes and trauma had a better success rate (7/7) than patients with Crohn's disease 2/5 (40%). Morbidity associated with rectal advancement was 8% (1/12). Dreznik et al. (77) also found success with this technique.

The Kraske laterosacral approach provides excellent exposure and does not divide the anal sphincter mechanism. Its disadvantage is the possible need to excise two to three sacral segments and the muscles, ligaments, and nerves around them.

The posterior midline transsphincteric approach popularized by York-Mason (78) affords rapid, bloodless exposure through unscarred areas and allows complete separation of the urinary and fecal streams. It avoids the neurovascular bundles and the pelvic floor structures that are important for sexual function and urinary continence. The author believes that the initial concern about anal incontinence is unfounded. Using this approach, Prasad et al. (79) successfully repaired three patients with rectoprostatic urethral fistulas. The authors performed their procedure under cover of a colostomy, but mechanical

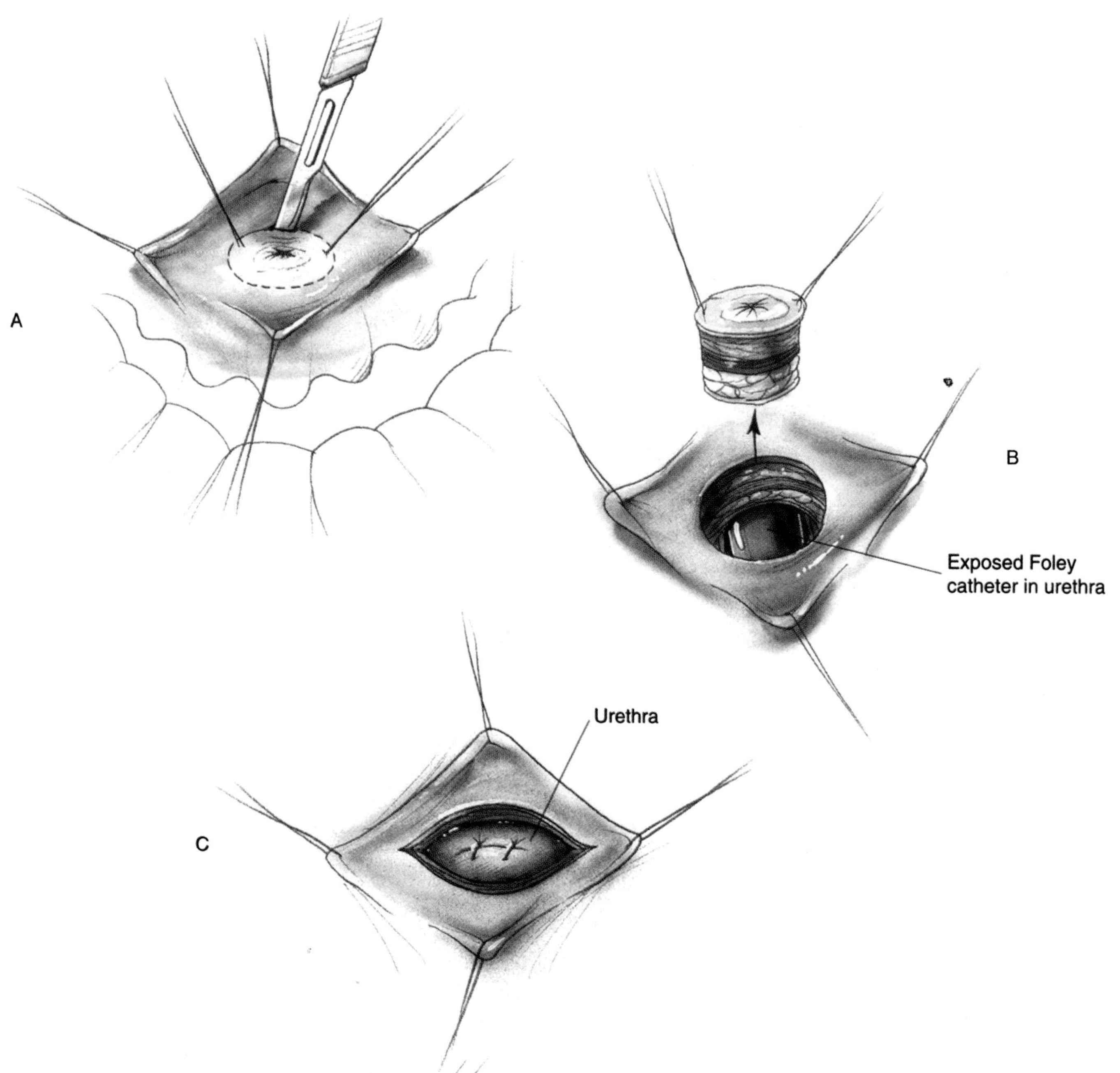

FIGURE 10 ■ (**A**) Coring out fistulous tract. (**B**) Foley catheter exposed in urethra. (**C**) Mobilization of rectal wall and transverse closure of urethral defect.

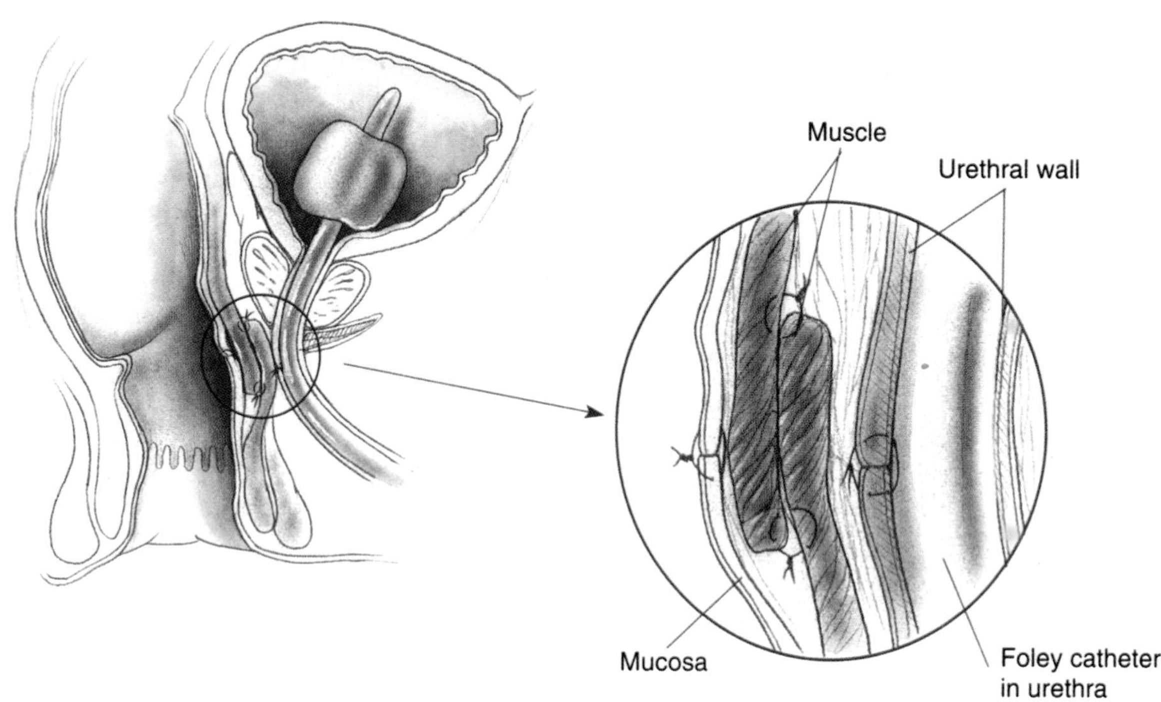

FIGURE 11 ■ Vest-over-pants closure of rectal wall.

bowel preparation and a postoperative elemental diet may obviate the need for a diverting ostomy. Their technique includes placing the patient in a prone jack-knife position with the buttocks strapped apart with adhesive tape. The incision is begun at the level of the anal margin to the left of the midline and extended upward and laterally to the level of the midsacrum (Fig. 7). After the skin incision is made, the rest of the dissection is performed with diathermy to reduce bleeding. Injection of a dilute solution of epinephrine (1:200,000) into the skin and subcutaneous tissue before incision may also help decrease the amount of bleeding. The mucocutaneous junction is marked with stay sutures (Fig. 8). Each layer of sphincter muscle is tagged with suture material of a different color for ease of identification at the time of closure, as the blood stained retracted ends of the sphincter may be difficult to identify at the end of a lengthy operation. The internal sphincter and the superficial or deep portions of the external sphincter, together with the puborectalis muscle, are tagged with sutures and divided. Next, the rectal mucosa is divided to expose the rectoprostatic urethral fistula (Fig. 9). The incision in the rectal wall is extended, if necessary. The fistula is identified in the anterior wall, and the Foley catheter can be seen at the bottom of the fistulous opening. A dilute solution of epinephrine is injected into the tissues around the fistula to decrease the bleeding at the time of dissection. An incision is made around the fistula and its surrounding scar tissue and is deepened with a knife through the posterior wall of the prostatic urethra to excise the fistulous tract (Fig. 10A and B). This incision is then extended transversely in the anterior rectal wall, and full-thickness flaps of the rectal wall are mobilized cephalad and caudad. Whenever possible, the prostatic urethral opening is closed transversely, using absorbable sutures, e.g., Vicryl (Fig. 10C). The rectal flaps are sutured in a "vest-over-pants" technique using polyglactin suture material. Thus, after closure of the fistula, the two suture lines do not overlie each other (Fig. 11). After closing the mucosa with interrupted absorbable sutures, the sphincter muscles, identified by their color-coded suture material, are approximated using polyglactin sutures (Fig. 12). The skin is closed with subcuticular sutures. Drains are not used routinely.

Patients are ambulated the day following the operation. The indwelling urethral catheter is not changed during the first two weeks postoperatively, after which time it is removed. Rectal examination and taking rectal temperature are avoided. Passage of urine through the penile urethra without leakage through the rectum denotes complete healing of the fistula. The colostomy is closed 6 weeks after healing of the fistula.

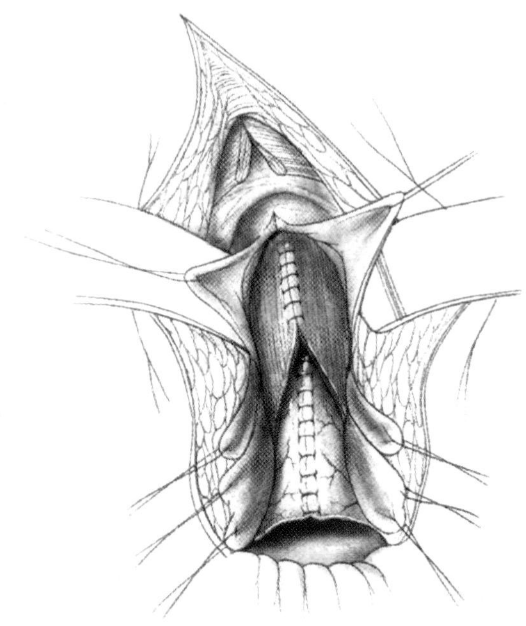

FIGURE 12 ■ Closure of the sphincter mechanism and rectal wall.

Wilbert et al. (80) reported on two patients who successfully underwent transanal endoscopic microscopic microsurgery repair of a rectourethral fistula. The fistula was excised, and a two-layer closure was accomplished.

Some cases may have such a low probability of successful resolution of the fistula, as well as maintenance of urinary continence, that cystostomy and supravesical diversion are appropriate considerations.

REFERENCES

1. Patel DR, Shrivastav R, Nichols J. An unusual complication of rectovaginal fistula: report of a case. Dis Colon Rectum 1971; 17:246–248.
2. Tsang CB, Madoff RD, Wong WD, et al. Anal sphincter integrity and function influences outcome in rectovaginal fistula repair. Dis Colon Rectum 1998; 41:1141–1146.
3. Baig MK, Zhao RH, Yuen CH, et al. Simple rectovaginal fistulas. Int J Colorectal Dis 2000; 1:323–327.
4. Yee LF, Birnbaum EH, Read TE, Kodner IJ, Fleshman JW. Use of endoanal ultrasound in patients with rectovaginal fistulas. Dis Colon Rectum 1999; 42: 1057–1064.
5. Bandy LC, Addison A, Parker RT. Surgical management of recto vaginal fistulas in Crohn's disease. Am J Obstet Gynecol 1983; 147:359–363.
6. Shieh CJ, Gennaro AR. Rectovaginal fistula: a review of 11 years experience. Int Surg 1984; 69:69–72.
7. Lowry AC, Thorson AG, Rothenberger DA, et al. Repair of simple rectovaginal fistula. Influence of previous repairs. Dis Colon Rectum 1988; 31:676–678.
8. Wise WE, Aguilar PG, Padmanabhan A. Surgical treatment of low rectovaginal fistulas. Dis Colon Rectum 1991; 34:271–274.
9. Mazier WP, Senagore AJ, Schiesel EC. Operative repair of anovaginal and rectovaginal fistulas. Dis Colon Rectum 1995; 38:4–6.
10. Watson JJ, Phillips RKS. Non-inflammatory rectovaginal fistula. Br J Surg 1995;82:1641–1643.
11. Halverson AL, Hull TL, Fazio VW, Church J, Hammel J, Floruta C. Repair of recurrent rectovaginal fistulas. Surgery 2001; 130:753–757.
12. Soriano D, Lemoine A, Laplace C, et al. Results of recto-vaginal fistula repair: retrospective analysis of 48 cases. Eur J Obstet Gynecol Reprod Biol 2001; 96: 75–79.
13. Zimmerman DD, Gosselink MP, Briel JW, Schouten WR. The outcome of transanal advancement flap repair of rectovaginal fistulas is not improved by an additional labial fat flap transposition. Tech Coloproctol 2002; 6:37–42.
14. Lawson J. Rectovaginal fistulas following difficult labour. Proc R Soc Med 1972; 63:283–286.
15. Beynon CL. Midline episiotomy as a routine procedure. J Obstet Gynaecol Br Commonw 1974; 81:126–130.
16. Venkatesh KS, Ramanujum PS, Larson DM, et al. Anorectal complications of vaginal delivery. Dis Colon Rectum 1989; 32:1039–1041.
17. Homsi R, Dai Koku NH, Littlejohn J, Wheeless CP. Episiotomy: risks of dehiscence and rectovaginal fistula. Obstet Gynecol Surg 1994; 49:803–808.
18. Sugarbaker PH. Rectovaginal fistula following low circular stapled anastomosis in women with rectal cancer. J Surg Oncol 1996; 61:155–158.
19. Antonsen HK, Kronberg O. Early complications after low anterior resection for rectal cancer using the EEA stapling device. Dis Colon Rectum 1987; 30: 579–583.
20. Rex JC, Khubchandani IT. Rectovaginal fistula: complication of low anterior resection. Dis Colon Rectum 1992; 35:354–356.
21. Hoexter B, Labow SB, Moseson MD. Transanal rectovaginal fistula repair. Dis Colon Rectum 1985; 28:572–575.
22. Anderson PG, Anderson M. An unusual cause of rectovaginal fistula. Aust N Z J Surg 1993; 63:148–149.
23. Fazio VW, Tjandra JJ. Pouch advancement and neoileoanal anastomosis for anastomotic stricture and anovaginal fistula complicating restorative proctocolectomy. Br J Surg 1992; 79:694–696.
24. Buchmann P, Keighley MRB, Allan RN, et al. Natural history of perianal Crohn's disease, ten year follow-up: A plea for conservatism. Am J Surg 1980; 140:642–644.
25. Greenstein AJ, Kark AE, Dreiling DA. Crohn's disease of the colon. I. Fistula in Crohn's disease of the colon, classification, presenting features, and management in 63 patients. Am J Gastroenterol 1974; 62:419–429.
26. Radcliffe AG, Ritchie JK, Hawley PR, et al. Anovaginal and rectovaginal fistulas in Crohn's disease. Dis Colon Rectum 1988; 31:94–99.
27. Faulconer HT, Muldoon JP. Rectovaginal fistula in patient with colitis: review and report of a case. Dis Colon Rectum 1975; 18:413–415.
28. Teh LS, Green KA, O'Sullivan MM, Morris JS, Williams BD. Behcet's syndrome: severe proctitis with rectovaginal fistula formation. Ann Rheum Dis 1989; 48:779–780.
29. Alert J, Jimenez J, Beedarrain L, et al. Complications from irradiation of carcinoma of the uterine cervix. Acta Radiol Oncol 1980; 19:13–15.
30. Allen-Mersh TG, Wilson EJ, Hope-Stone HF, et al. The management of late radiation induced rectal injury after treatment for carcinoma of the uterus. Surg Gynecol Obstet 1987; 164:521–524.
31. Anseline PF, Lavery IC, Fazio VW, et al. Radiation injury of the rectum. Evaluation of surgical treatment. Ann Surg 1981; 194:716–724.
32. Boronow RC. Repair of the radiation-induced vaginal fistula utilizing the Martius technique. World J Surg 1986; 10:237–248.
33. Kimose HH, Fischer L, Spjeldnaes N, et al. Late radiation injury of the colon and rectum. Surgical management, and outcome. Dis Colon Rectum 1989; 32:684–689.
34. Sandeman TF. Radiation injury of the anorectal region. Aust N Z J Surg 1980; 50:169–172.
35. Lock MR, Katz DR, Samoorian S, et al. Giant condyloma of the rectum: report of a case. Dis Colon Rectum 1977; 20:154–157.
36. Fadiran OA, Dare FO, Jeje SA, Nwosu SO, Oyero TO. Amoebic rectovaginal fistula—a case report and review of literature. Cent Afr J Med 1993; 39:172–174.
37. Schwartz J, Rabinowitz H, Rozenfeld V, Leibovitz A, Stelian J, Habot B. Rectovaginal fistula associated with fecal impaction. J Am Geriatr Soc 1992; 40:641.
38. Pfeifer J, Reissman P, Wexner SD. Ergotamine-induced complex rectovaginal fistula. Report of a case. Dis Colon Rectum 1995; 38:1224–1226.
39. Mattingly RF. Anal incontinence and rectovaginal fistulas. In: Mattingly RF, ed. Telinde's Operative Gynecology, 5th ed. Philadelphia: JB Lippincott 1992; 618–626.
40. DeCosse JJ. Radiation injury to the intestine. In: Sabistan D, ed. Davis-Christopher textbook of surgery. Philadelphia: WB Saunders, 1977:1061–1062.
41. Goldberg SM, Gordon PH, Nivatvongs S. Essentials of anorectal surgery. Philadelphia: JE Lippincott, 1980:316–332.
42. Goligher JC. Surgery of the anus, rectum and colon. 5th ed. London: Bailliere Tindall, 1984:208–211.
43. Tancer ML, Lasser D, Rosenblum N. Rectovaginal fistula or perineal and anal sphincter disruption, or both, after vaginal delivery. Surg Gynecol Obstet 1990; 171:43–46.
44. Wiskind AK, Thompson JD. Transverse transperineal repair of rectovaginal fistulas in the lower vagina. Am J Obstet Gynecol 1992; 167:694–699.
45. York-Mason A. Transsphincteric approach to rectal lesions. Surg Ann 1977; 9:171.
46. Zacharain RF. Grafting as a principle in the surgical management of vesicovaginal and rectovaginal fistulae. Aust N Z J Obstet Gynecol 1980; 20:10–17.
47. Kodner IJ, Mazer A, Shemesh EI, Fry RD, Fleshman JW, Birnbaum EH. Endorectal advancement flap repair of rectovaginal and other complicated anorectal fistulas. Surgery 1993; 114:682–690.
48. Khanduja KS, Padmanabhan A, Kerner RA, Wise WE, Aguilar PS. Reconstruction of rectovaginal fistula with sphincter disruption by combining rectal mucosal advancement flap and anal sphincteroplasty. Dis Colon Rectum 1999; 42:1432–1437.
49. Sonoda T, Hull T, Piedmonte MR, Fazio VW. Outcomes of primary repair of anorectal and rectovaginal endorectal advancement flap. Dis Colon Rectum 2002; 4:1622–1628.
50. Penninckx F, Moneghini D, D'Hoore A, Wyndaele J, Coremans G, Rutgeerts P. Success and failure after repair of rectovaginal fistula in Crohn's disease: analysis of prognostic factors. Colorectal Dis 2001; 3:406–411.
51. Simmang CL, Lacey SW, Huber PJ Jr. Rectal sleeve advancement: repair of rectovaginal fistula associated with anorectal stricture in Crohn's disease. Dis Colon Rectum 1998; 41:787–789.
52. Berman I. Sleeve advancement anorectoplasty for complicated anorectal/vaginal fistula. Dis Colon Rectum 1991; 34:1032–1037.
53. Parks AG, Allen CLO, Frank JD, et al. A method of treating postirradiation rectovaginal fistulas. Br J Surg 1978; 65:417–421.
54. Nowacki MR. Ten years of experience with Parks' coloanal sleeve anastomosis for the treatment of post-irradiation rectovaginal fistula. Eur J Surg Oncol 1991; 17:563–566.
55. Cooke SAR, Wellsted MD. The radiation damaged rectum: Resection with coloanal anastomosis using the endoanal technique. World J Surg 1986; 10:220–227.
56. Cuthbertson AM. Resection and pull-through for rectovaginal fistula. World J Surg 1986; 10:228–236.
57. Gorenstein L, Boyd JB, Ross TM. Gracilis muscle repair of rectovaginal fistula after restorative proctocolectomy. Report of two cases. Dis Colon Rectum 1988; 31:730–734.
58. Harms BA, Hamilton JW, Starling JR. Management of chronic ulcerative colitis and rectovaginal fistula by simultaneous ileal pouch construction and fistula closure. Report of a case. Dis Colon Rectum 1987; 30:611–614.
59. MacRae HM, McLeod RS, Cohen Z, Stern H, Reznick R. Treatment of rectovaginal fistulas that has failed previous repair attempts. Dis Colon Rectum 1995; 38:921–925.
60. Haray PN, Stiff G, Foster ME. New option for recurrent rectovaginal fistulas. Dis Colon Rectum 1996; 39:463–464.
61. Pye PK, Dada T, Duthie G, Phillips K. Surgisis trade mark mesh: a novel approach to repair of a recurrent rectovaginal fistula. Dis Colon Rectum 2004; 47:1554–1556.
62. Elkins TE, Delancey JOL, McGuire EJ. The use of modified Martius graft as an adjunctive technique in vesicovaginal and rectovaginal repair. Obstet Gynecol 1990; 75:727–733.

63. Margolis T, Elkins TE, Seffah J, Opuro-Addo HS, Fort D. Full-thickness Martius grafts to preserve vaginal depth as an adjunct in the repair of large obstetric fistulas. Obstet Gynecol 1994; 84:148–152.
64. Aartsen EJ, Sindram IS. Repair of the radiation induced rectovaginal fistulas without or with interposition of the bulbocavernosus muscle (Martius procedure). Eur J Surg Oncol 1988; 14:171–177.
65. White AJ, Buchsbaum HJ, Blythe JG, Lifshitz S. Use of the bulbocavernosus muscle (Martius procedure) for repair of radiation-induced rectovaginal fistulas. Obstet Gynecol 1982; 60:114–118.
66. Mathes SJ, Hurwitz DJ. Repair of chronic radiation wounds of the pelvis World J Surg 1986; 10:269–280.
67. Holland RM, Greiss FC. Perineal Crohn's disease. Obstet Gynecol 1983; 62: 527–529.
68. Cohen JL, Stricker JW, Schoetz DJ, et al. Rectovaginal fistula in Crohn's disease. Dis Colon Rectum 1989; 32:825–828.
69. Morrison JG, Gathright JB, Ray JE, et al. Results of operation for rectovaginal fistula in Crohn's disease. Dis Colon Rectum 1989; 32:497–499.
70. Teichman JMH, Lilly JD, Schmidt JD. Rectourethral fistula caused by Kaposi's sarcoma. J Urol 1991; 145:144–145.
71. Bukowski TP, Chakrabarty A, Powell IJ, Frontera R, Perlmutter AD, Montie JE. Acquired rectourethral fistula: methods of repair. J Urol 1995; 153:730–733.
72. Garofalo TE, Delaney CP, Jones SM, Remzi FH, Fazio VW. Rectal advancement flap repair of rectourethral fistula: a 20-year experience. Dis Colon Rectum 2003; 46:762–769.
73. Trippitelli A, Baobagli S, Lonzi R, Fiorelli C, Masini GC. Surgical treatment of rectourethral fistula. Eur Urol 1985; 11:388–391.
74. Goodwin WE, Turner RD, Winter CC. Rectourinary fistula: principles of management and a technique of surgical closure. J Urol 1958; 80:246–254.
75. Gecelter L. Transanorectal approach to the posterior urethra and bladder neck. J Urol 1973; 109:1011.
76. Parks AG, Motson RW. Perianal repair of rectoprostatic fistula. Br J Surg 1983; 70:725–726.
77. Dreznik Z, Alper D, Vishne TH, Ramadan E. Rectal flap advancements simple and effective approach for the treatment of rectourethral fistula. Colorectal Dis 2003; 5:53–55.
78. York-Mason A. Surgical access to the rectum—a transsphincteric exposure. Proc R Soc Med 1970; 63:91–96.
79. Prasad ML, Nelson R, Hambrick E, Abcarian H. York Mason procedure for repair of postoperative rectoprostatic urethral fistula. Dis Colon Rectum 1983; 26:716–720.
80. Wilbert DM, Buess G, Bichler KH. Combined endoscopic closure of rectourethral fistula. J Urol 1996; 155:256–258.

17 Retrorectal Tumors

Philip H. Gordon

The presacral region is an area of embryologic fusion and remodeling and thus is a common site for embryologic remnants from which neoplasms and cysts may arise. These heterogeneous lesions are categorized as retrorectal tumors. After reviewing the anatomy of the region, this chapter describes these rare but interesting lesions as well as their diagnosis and treatment.

ANATOMY

The retrorectal space lies between the upper two-thirds of the rectum and the sacrum, above the rectosacral fascia. It is limited anteriorly by the fascia propria covering the rectum, posteriorly by the presacral fascia, and laterally by the lateral ligaments (stalks) of the rectum, the ureters, and the iliac vessels. Superiorly, it is bounded by the peritoneal reflection of the rectum and communicates with the retroperitoneal space. Inferiorly, it is limited by the rectosacral fascia, which passes forward from the S4 vertebra to the rectum 3–5 cm proximal to the anorectal junction. Below the rectosacral fascia is the supralevator space, a horseshoe-shaped potential space limited anteriorly by the fascia propria of the rectum and below by the levator ani muscle (Fig. 1).

The retroperitoneal space contains loose connective tissue. The presacral fascia protects the presacral vessels that lie deep to it. These vessels are part of the extensive vertebral plexus and are responsible for the major bleeding problems encountered in this area during surgery.

Teplick et al. evaluated ninety-nine adults with an enlarged retrorectal space on barium enema examination (1). Measurements were based on previously described methods using the lateral view of the barium-filled rectum. In 38.4% of the cases, there was no lesion (normal variations). The rest were classified as inflammatory conditions, tumors, and miscellaneous lesions. It is concluded that an increased width of the presacral space per se does not necessarily connote a lesion. Pathological widening of the space is usually associated with changes of the contour of the rectum, abnormalities of the sacrum, or other alternations of the presacral soft tissues.

CLASSIFICATION

Uhlig and Johnson (2), aided by the composite classification of Freier et al. (3) have proposed the classification outlined in the accompanying Table 1.

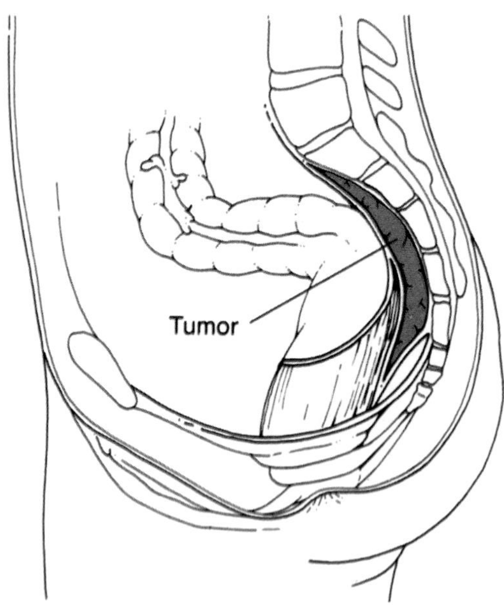

FIGURE 1 ■ Tumor in the retrorectal space.

INCIDENCE

Tumors in the retrorectal region are rare. Uhlig and Johnson (2) reviewed the records of all the patients in local Portland, Oregon hospitals and found a total of 63 cases over a 30-year period. A total of 50 cases of primary sacral and retrorectal tumors were seen at the Cleveland Clinic over a 55-year period (4). Most lesions fell into the categories of teratomas or chordomas, but a host of other miscellaneous lesions were found. The incidence at the Mayo Clinic, as reported by Jao et al. (5), has been found to be approximately one in 40,000 general hospital admissions. These authors reported on 120 patients with retrorectal tumors. Congenital lesions comprised 66% of the total; neurogenic, 12%; osseous, 11%; and miscellaneous, 11%. Metastatic and inflammatory masses were excluded from this report. Cody et al. (6) published a review of 28 years of experience at the Memorial Sloan-Kettering Cancer Center but limited their review to malignant tumors of the retrorectal region. Of the 39 patients, 38% had chordomas; 15% neurogenic tumors; 8% each of chondrosarcomas, hemangiopericytomas, and embryonal adenocarcinomas; and 23% miscellaneous. Stewart et al. (7) summarized reports in the literature and amalgamated reports representing 301 presacral tumors. Congenital lesions comprised 63%; inflammatory, 8%; neurogenic, 10%; osseous, 7%; and miscellaneous, 12%.

Most of these reviews do not include pediatric patients. Sacrococcygeal teratomas, which are the most common retrorectal tumors in the pediatric group, are estimated to occur once in every 40,000 births (8).

TABLE 1 ■ **Differential Diagnosis of Retrorectal Tumors and Cysts**

Congenital	**Osseous**
Developmental cysts (epidermoid, dermoid, and mucus-secreting cysts; teratoma)	Osteoma
Chordoma	Osteogenic sarcoma
Teratocarcinoma	Simple bone cyst, sacrum
Adrenal rest tumor	Ewing's tumor
Anterior sacral meningocele	Chondromyxosarcoma
Duplication of rectum	Aneurysmal bone cyst
	Giant cell tumor
Inflammatory	**Miscellaneous**
Foreign body granuloma	Metastatic carcinoma
Perineal abscess	Liposarcoma
Internal fistula	Hemangioendothelial sarcoma
Retrorectal abscess	Lymphangioma
Chronic infectious granuloma	Extra-abdominal desmoid tumor
Neurogenic	Plasma cell myeloma
Neurofibroma and sarcoma	Malignant neoplasm of unknown type
Neurilemoma	Lipoma
Ependymoma	Fibroma
Ganglioneuroma	Fibrosarcoma
Neurofibrosarcoma	Leiomyoma
	Leiomyosarcoma
	Hemangioma
	Pericytoma
	Endothelioma

Source: From Ref. 2.

PATHOLOGY

An exhaustive review of the pathology of this area is not given here. Many of the tumors have common symptoms and present in a similar manner, and the reader is referred to any standard pathology text. The tumors and cysts discussed here are typical of the retrorectal area. Congenital lesions account for slightly more than half of all presacral tumors, and two-thirds of these are developmental cysts. A postanal dimple is associated with some congenital cysts and may be a clue to the diagnosis.

■ DEVELOPMENTAL CYSTS

As indicated in Table 2, developmental cysts may arise from any of the germ layers (9). A female predominance is associated with congenital cysts (5).

Epidermoid and Dermoid Cysts

These cysts result from closure defects of the ectodermal tube with heterotopic inclusions of skin, sometimes with accessory skin appendages (Table 2). Dermoid and epidermoid cysts found at reoperation for tethered cord following myelomeningocele repair have been attributed to inadequate excision of cutaneous elements and "implantation" in the repair site (10).

The epidermoid cyst is lined with stratified squamous epithelium with keratohyaline granules and intracellular bridges. No skin appendages are found within the epithelium.

In addition to the stratified squamous epithelium seen in epidermoid cysts, dermoid cysts have sweat glands, hair follicles, sebaceous glands, or all three. These appendages characterize dermoid cysts.

Both epidermoid and dermoid cysts tend to be rounded and circumscribed, have a thin connective tissue outer layer, and contain viscid green-yellow material. These cysts can communicate with the skin surface, where they

TABLE 2 ■ Germ Layer Origin of Developmental Cysts

	Epidermoid	Dermoid	Enterogenous	Teratomatous
Tissue of origin	Ectoderm	Ectoderm	Endoderm	All three layers
Histologic characteristics	Stratified squamous	Stratified squamous with skin appendages (sweat glands, sebaceous glands, hair follicles)	Columnar or cuboidal lining; may have secretory function	Varying degrees of differentiation between cysts and cell layers of single cyst
General state	Benign[a]	Benign[a]	Benign	Benign or malignant

[a]Malignant varient is rare.
Source: From Ref. 9.

appear as a postanal dimple. The cysts are more common in women than in men and have a 30% rate of infection (11). In the infected state they may appear as a retrorectal abscess or perirectal suppuration. When the postanal dimple communicates with an infected cyst, a mistaken diagnosis of fistula-in-ano commonly is made.

Enterogenous Cysts

The current belief is that enterogenous cysts result from sequestration of the developing hindgut. On occasion, layers of either squamous or transitional epithelium may be found within the lining of an otherwise mucus-secreting cyst. This is not surprising, since the terminal hindgut, or cloaca, gives rise to rectal and urogenital structures during embryologic development.

Generally, these are thin-walled cysts lined by mucus-secreting columnar epithelium. They tend to be multilocular, usually with one dominant cyst and a series of minor or "daughter" cysts. In the uninfected state, they are filled with a clear to green mucoid material.

Enterogenous cysts are more common in women and, as with epidermoid and dermoid cysts, have a tendency to become infected. In the majority of cases, however, they remain asymptomatic.

The female-to-male ratio of incidence of developmental cysts is 5:1. The majority are asymptomatic and, because tension in the cyst is low, they may be easily missed on rectal examination.

The average age at cyst appearance is in the fourth decade. The duration of symptoms, if they exist, is frequently measured in years.

Rectal Duplication

Intestinal duplications are rare developmental anomalies and only 3–8% of all alimentary tract duplications occur in the rectum (12). They most commonly occur in females and are associated with other congenital defects, especially genitourinary and vertebral anomalies. The diagnosis depends on the fulfillment of three anatomic criteria, namely the cyst must be attached to the alimentary tract, it must be lined by mucous membrane similar to that part of the alimentary tract, and it must possess a smooth muscle coat. Patients may be asymptomatic or present with a perineal mass, constipation, tenesmus, prolapse, lower back pain, urinary symptoms, or recurrent perianal sepsis or fistula formation. Radiologic imaging such as barium enema, computed tomography (CT), magnetic resonance imaging (MRI), or intrarectal ultrasound may help delineate the lesion but the definitive diagnosis is by histologic examination. Malignant change in a rectal duplication in an adult has been reported (13,14). Complete surgical excision is the preferred treatment to prevent recurrence and the risk of malignant degeneration.

Tailgut Cysts

Hjermstad and Helwig (15) collected 53 examples of developmental tailgut cysts in the retrorectal space. The cysts (also called cyst hamartoma) occurred predominantly in women and caused symptoms of mass effect or pain in 51%. Ages ranged from four days to 73 years. The lesions were usually circumscribed, unencapsulated, and multicystic, with an average diameter of 3.9 cm. They were lined by a variety of epithelial types, which included ciliated columnar, mucin-secreting columnar, transitional, and squamous epithelium. The cysts were filled with a colorless to yellow or gray fluid and had no communication with the rectal lumen. Inflammation occurred in 50% of the patients. One patient had a poorly differentiated adenocarcinoma. Glomus bodies were identified in seven patients, a finding reported by other authors (16).

In their review of the literature, Prasad et al. (17) identified 10 cases of malignancy including six adenocarcinomas and four carcinoids and added five further cases, one of which was a neuroendocrine carcinoma. Mourra et al. (18) reported the second case of neuroendocrine carcinoma developing in a tailgut cyst. Complete excision is the recommended treatment. Others have reported adenocarcinomas arising in a tailgut cyst (19,20). A carcinoid arising in a tailgut cyst has also been reported (21).

These cysts are most likely derived from remnants of the embryonic tailgut and differ from teratomas. They have also been described as cystic hamartomas (16,22). Pathologic changes of tailgut cysts are distinctive. The cyst lining is simple and, although a variety of epithelial types almost always lines the cysts, the presence of some glandular or transitional epithelium is required to exclude epidermoid and dermoid cysts. Differential diagnoses from which cysts should be distinguished include teratomas (which always contain elements of three germ cell layers), dermoid cysts (which contain hair and other dermal appendages and are lined with stratified squamous epithelium), enteric cysts, or duplication cysts of the rectum (which are lined with intestinal epithelium with characteristic villi and crypts and contain well-developed layers of smooth muscle, a myoenteric plexus and a serosa), duplications of the anus (which usually appear early in life as chronic draining sinus tracts that open onto the perianal skin), anal gland cysts (which are thought to be acquired lesions located closer to the anal sphincter), and chordomas of the sacrum (which are malignant and arise from the embryonic remains of the notochord, at any age) (23). Complete excision of the multilocular and multicystic process prevents recurrent draining sinuses and eliminates the possibility of malignant change, which is rare.

■ TERATOMA AND TERATOCARCINOMA

These are true neoplasms arising from totipotential cells. Classically, they have representative tissue from each germ cell layer, although the degree of differentiation may vary among the elements. Malignancy, when it occurs, tends to arise from one of the germ cells; however, in the anaplastic variety it may be impossible to distinguish the tissue of origin. The more mature the tissue appears, the more benign the neoplasm tends to be, but all neoplasms should be viewed as potentially malignant. Malignancy is rare beyond the second decade; however, the neonatal malignancy rate is 4% (8).

In a review, Mahour (24) reported that the frequency of malignancy in sacrococcygeal teratomas ranged from 10% to 50%. Of those neoplasms present at birth and not treated immediately, 7% can be expected to be malignant by the fourth month (25). The incidence of malignant degeneration in adult teratomas is approximately 30% (26). Beyond the 20th year, malignancy is less common, as are retrorectal teratomas. Miles and Stewart (27) reported on 11 sacrococcygeal teratomas in adults. All were benign, and all but one occurred in females. The potential for malignant conversion is greatest during the period of growth, in particular during the early years of life. The possibility of malignant conversion significantly decreases, but is still present in adults, hence the need for adequate early surgical removal. Chen (28) reported on a squamous cell carcinoma arising in a sacrococcygeal teratoma. Teratomas are more common in females than males (3:1 to 5:1) and are often associated with anomalies of the vertebrae, urinary tract, or anorectum (4,8,26,27). They tend to be tumors of infancy and childhood (8).

Macroscopic features and the growth pattern of sacrococcygeal teratomas have been described in detail by Pantoja and Rodriguez-Ibanez (8). The lesions are well encapsulated and may be solid or cystic. They may contain all kinds of tissues, the most prominent ones being respiratory, nervous, and gastrointestinal (Fig. 2). Fluid, bones, fingernails, hair, skin derivatives, and sebaceous glands also may be found. A unique case of a rudimentary heart has been reported in a teratoma (29). Teratomas maintain a strong attachment to the coccyx and sometimes the sacrum, but they rarely adhere to pelvic viscera unless previous inflammation has resulted in secondary adhesions. Their blood supply comes mainly from the mid-sacral vessels, but the hypogastric vessels may contribute to the blood supply. A presacral teratoma may remain confined to the pelvis but may extend upward into the retrorectal space or downward, distending the perineum and distorting or displacing the anus and the external genitalia. It may extend into the spinal canal or through the sacrosciatic notch to emerge in the buttocks region.

In neonates, the sacrococcygeal teratoma appears most commonly as an obvious external mass in the perineal area. On the other hand, the only sign of its presence may be skin discoloration or a dimple. Occasionally, the dominant mass is toward the peritoneal cavity. These neoplasms may vary in size from a small retrorectal mass to one that weighs more than the infant and thus is capable of causing pelvic obstruction during labor. Rapid growth after birth may lead to ulceration, infection, bleeding, or urinary retention (8). In children, the female-to-male ratio of teratoma incidence is 2:1.

In adults, teratomas may be associated with infection, and patients may be treated for persistent anorectal fistulas before it is discovered that the underlying disease is a sacrococcygeal teratoma. A teratoma may rupture into the rectum.

The five-year survival rate for children with malignant germ cell tumors is approximately 80% after complete resection (4). Germinomas tend to be radiosensitive, but overall, only approximately 50% of patients can be expected to survive two years (4).

■ CHORDOMA

Chordoma represents the most common malignant neoplasm in the retrorectal region. It arises from the remnants of the fetal notochord (30). The notochord is the primitive flexible vertebral column extending from the basilar portion of the occipital bone to the caudal limit of the embryo. In adults, the only notochordal remnant is found in the nucleus pulposus of the intervertebral disk. The chordoma does not appear to arise from the nucleus pulposus but from the vertebral bodies. Although it can occur anywhere from the hypophysis cerebri to the coccyx, the sacrococcygeal area is the site in approximately 50% of cases (30).

These neoplasms may arise in either sex at any age but are more frequent in men (2:1 to 5:1), and the greatest incidence occurs between 40 and 70 years of age (4,5,31). The preponderance of men is significantly higher in the sacral than in the cranial group. Chordomas represent 3–4% of primary bone neoplasms (32). Patients experience rectal or perineal pain that is often aggravated by sitting and alleviated by standing or walking. Advanced lesions may be associated with constipation, fecal incontinence, urinary incontinence, or impotence (33). The chordoma has been cited as one of the extra-intestinal malignancies associated with colorectal carcinoma (34).

Macroscopically, the chordoma is typically a slow-growing, lobulated, well-defined structure composed of soft gelatinous tissue, often with areas of hemorrhage. It invades, distends, and destroys neighboring bone and extends into adjacent regions. Microscopically, the chordoma is said to resemble the various stages of notochordal development. The cells usually are aggregated in irregular groups separated by stromal tissue. Peripheral cells contain mucous droplets in the cytoplasm. As these cells mature, the droplets coalesce, creating single large vacuoles that comprise the physaliphorous cell typical of chordoma. Toward the center of the neoplasms, cords of cells appear to float in mucus, cell boundaries are indistinct, and the appearance is that of a syncytium.

Physical examination usually reveals a smooth extrarectal mass with intact overlying mucosa. The diagnosis is usually made with plain x-ray film using four criteria: expansion of bone, rarefaction or destruction, trabeculation,

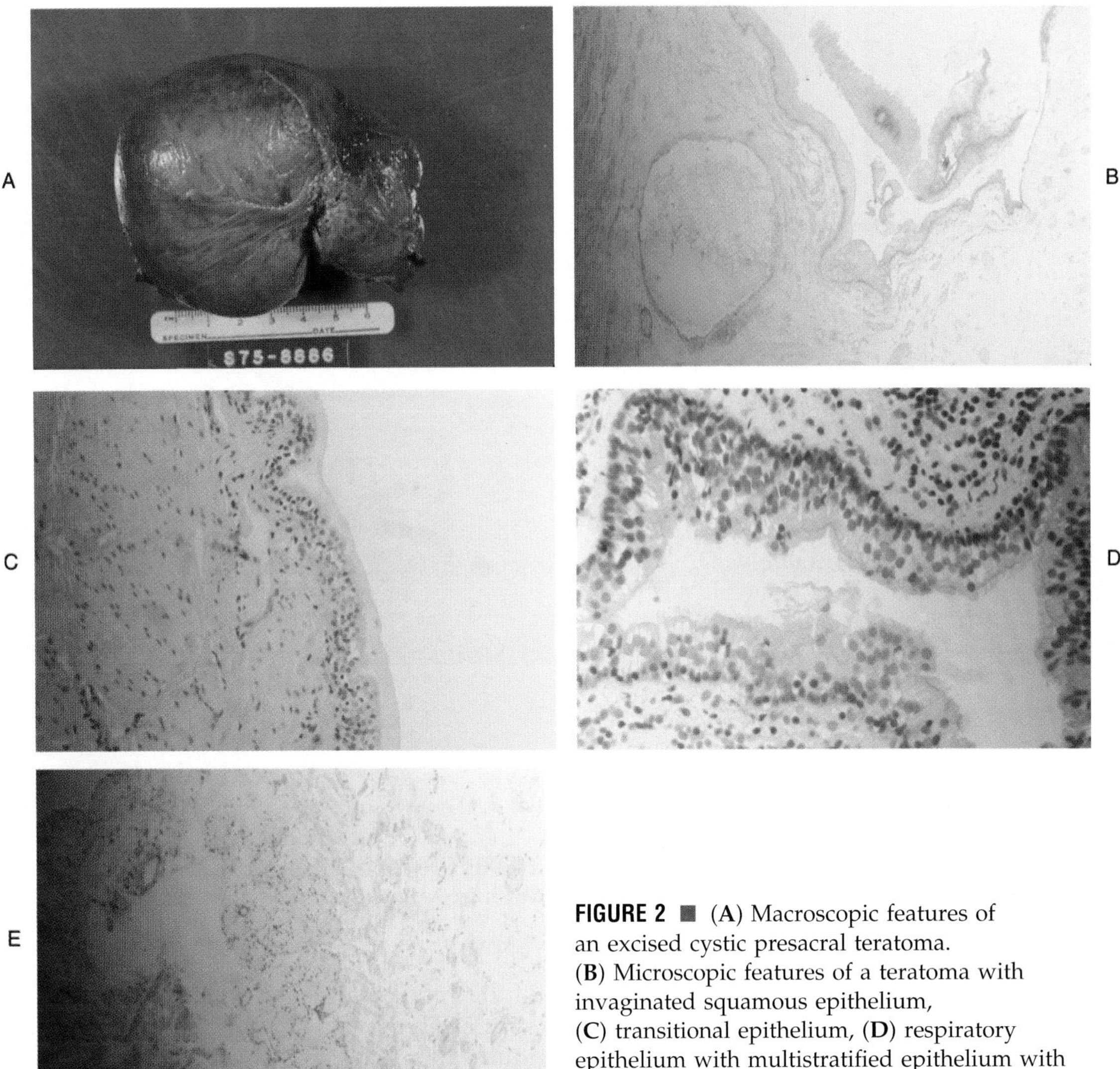

FIGURE 2 ■ (**A**) Macroscopic features of an excised cystic presacral teratoma. (**B**) Microscopic features of a teratoma with invaginated squamous epithelium, (**C**) transitional epithelium, (**D**) respiratory epithelium with multistratified epithelium with cilia, and (**E**) mesodermal components with strands of smooth muscle and submucosa.

and calcification (occasional) (5). A CT scan usually confirms the diagnosis of those neoplasms not seen on plain films (Fig. 3). The recommended treatment requires complete excision to include the preoperative biopsy tracks since implantation along those tracks is known to occur. High-dose radiotherapy may prove palliative for incompletely removed lesions. In a review of the world literature, Finne (26) found only a 4% cure rate out of almost 300 reported patients, with 9% surviving longer than 10 years. A dramatically different result was obtained from the Mayo Clinic, where a 75% five-year survival was reported (5).

In their review, Miyahara et al. (34) found 5- and 10-year survival rates to be 43% to 75% and 22% to 35%, respectively. A possible explanation for the discrepancy in survival rates may be related to the low rates of complete excision, which have been reported to range from 30% to 53% (34).

At the National Cancer Institute of Milan, Baratti et al. (35) reviewed the natural history of 28 patients who underwent resection for sacrococcygeal chordomas. With a median follow-up of 71 months, recurrence developed in 61%. The overall five- and 10-year survival was 88% and 49%, respectively, while disease-free survival was 61% and 24%. Radiotherapy was considered for marginal and intralesional resections.

■ ANTERIOR SACRAL MENINGOCELE

The meningocele is located in the presacral space and contains cerebrospinal fluid. It is more common in women (36). Patients may experience constipation, urinary difficulties, low back or abdominal pain, headaches, meningitis, or dystocia (37). Characteristic physical findings include a pelvic mass and almost unmistakable radiologic changes, but diagnoses tend to be delayed for months or years (38).

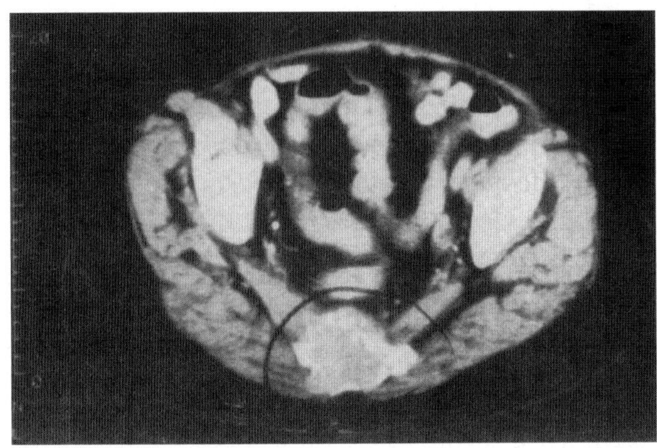

FIGURE 3 ■ CT scan of pelvis showing irregular zone of destruction of sacrum by a chordoma.

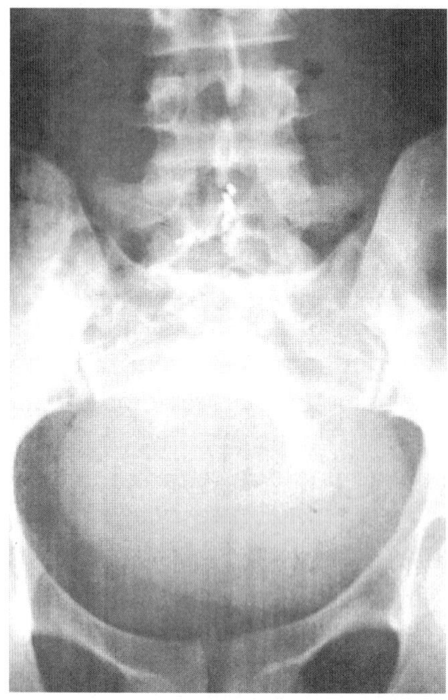

FIGURE 4 ■ "Scimitar" sign of sacrum. *Source*: Courtesy of Charles O. Finne III, M.D., Minneapolis, Minnesota, U.S.A.

The finding of a "scimitar" sacrum, characterized by a rounded, concave border without bone destruction, is pathognomonic (Fig. 4). Myelography with CT scanning is the best way to diagnose the tumor and delineate its exact anatomy to provide optimal operative planning (36). MRI obviates the need for myelography, according to one study (39). Aspiration should be avoided because of the risk of meningitis. Treatment consists of obliterating the neck of the meningocele (4,36). Operative approaches include posterior trans-sacral by laminectomy, perineal, and anterior transabdominal approaches (36,39). The posterior approach allows identification and preservation of the nerve roots, but watertight closure of the pedicle may not be possible. The anterior approach offers easier closure of the neck of the sac, but the nerve roots cannot be protected. Laminectomy yielded a cure without significant complications in 24 out of 28 cases compared with 12 out of 25 for the abdominal approach (40). The mortality after laminectomy was $<4\%$ but increased to 24% after abdominal surgery alone. Two tumors recurred after laminectomy and three after the abdominal operation. Simpson et al. (39) recommend a combined anterior and posterior approach to permit both the protection of the nerve roots and the radical extirpation of the sac.

■ NEUROGENIC NEOPLASMS

Neurogenic lesions are the typical neoplasms of peripheral nerves and arise along the nerve. They constitute 5%–15% of neoplasms in the retrorectal space (4). Benign lesions include neurilemomas and ganglioneuromas, whereas malignant lesions include neuroblastomas, schwannomas, and ganglioneuroblastomas (Fig. 5). Evidence of motor and sensory dysfunction usually is confined to a single peripheral nerve. Because of the cauda equina, a neoplasm arising from a nerve root within the spinal canal may have devastating effects on all the local nerves, even resulting in paraplegia. Neurogenic lesions usually reach a significant size before detection. They are related to the lateral wall of the pelvis, are slow growing, and yield good results with surgical removal. It is rare for a malignant variant to be found here.

A

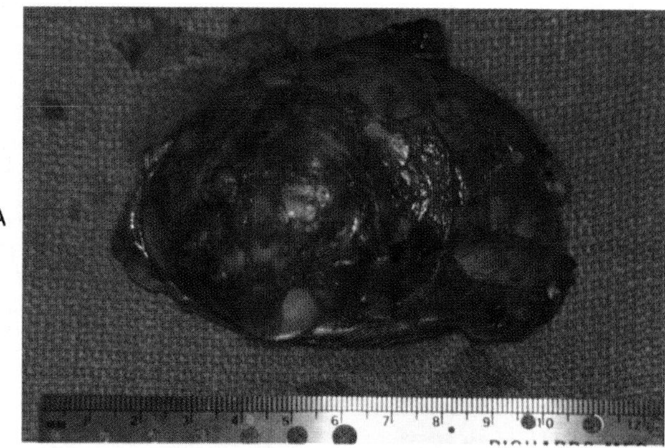

B

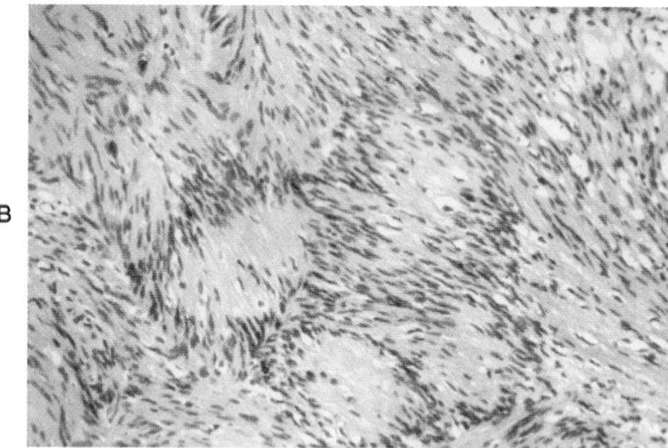

FIGURE 5 ■ (**A**) Macroscopic feature of a presacral schwannoma and (**B**) microscopic feature of a presacral schwannoma.

The most frequent neurogenic neoplasm is the ependymoma (4). Nevertheless, it is rare. A review of the literature by Timmerman and Bubrick (41) revealed only 17 cases of extraspinal postsacral ependymoma and 28 cases of presacral ependymoma. These neoplasms, occurring more often in males, may develop at any age. Metastases may occur. If the lesion is encapsulated and totally excised, long-term survival can be anticipated. Radiotherapy may be palliative. Neoplasms of neural origin should be considered when no obvious cause of perianal discomfort or pain is found in the sacrococcygeal area (42).

In the series reported by Uhlig and Johnson (2), the average age of presentation was 33 years, and, except for one patient with an ependymoma who was paraplegic but stable, the group had good results. The prognosis for life is good with most peripheral nerve neoplasms, but the morbidity can be significant.

■ OSSEOUS LESIONS

Primary bone neoplasms in the retrorectal region, as elsewhere, are far less common than metastatic neoplasms. Despite their rarity, virtually all types of bone lesions, both benign and malignant, have been found in this area. They may arise from bone, cartilage, fibrous tissue, or marrow. Persistent skeletal pain frequently calls attention to these neoplasms, which are usually well advanced when detected. Malignant sarcomas, either of cartilaginous or osseous origin, and other lesions such as Ewing's sarcoma have a disastrous prognosis when they occur. If feasible, wide resection is the recommended treatment, but these malignancies are usually inoperable and widespread. Giant cell neoplasms arise from fibrous tissue and require wide resection.

Benign neoplasms, apart from bone cysts and osteomas, present the problem of recurrence. A block resection is the treatment of choice. Unfortunately, because of the site, the neoplasm is often advanced, requiring an extensive operation that is frequently incomplete. Every attempt must be made to achieve primary resection. Aneurysmal bone cysts may be managed by curettage.

■ MISCELLANEOUS ENTITIES

Connective tissue sarcomas have been reported in the retrorectal space. Examples include liposarcoma, fibrosarcoma, hemangiosarcoma, leiomyosarcoma, and chondromyxosarcoma. Vascular lesions include hemangioendothelioma and hemangiopericytoma. Fortunately, all these sarcomas are rare; the prognosis, as with bone sarcoma, is poor. Lymphoma, myeloma, and metastatic carcinoma can all involve the retrorectal space. Primary adenocarcinoma of the presacral space has been reported (43,44). In Uhlig and Johnson's series (2), nine patients had recurrent or metastatic carcinoma in the presacral area. This should always be kept in mind when the history is being taken. Other miscellaneous entities include myelolipoma, ganglioneuroma, metastatic meningioma to the sacrum, endometrial cyst, sacral perineural cysts, and carcinoids, which may be located in the presacral space or in the coccyx or sacrum in which case coccygectomy or partial sacretomy would be indicated (Fig. 6) (45–53). The unusual development of a hydatid cyst in the presacral space has been reported (54).

Pelvic ectopic kidneys also are included in the differential diagnosis. Inflammatory lesions secondary to Crohn's disease or diverticulitis may present in this area. A posttraumatic, hematoma may appear either acutely as a presacral collection or chronically as a retrorectal mass (55). A presacral mass may even represent extramedullary hematopoiesis (56). Therapy is tailored to the clinical situation and the size of the lesion. The most accurate means of diagnosis is a CT scan.

■ RISK OF MALIGNANCY

Finne (26) noted that presacral lesions diagnosed in the neonatal period carry a malignancy rate of approximately 4%, whereas 95% of those diagnosed in the postnatal and pediatric periods are malignant with a grave prognosis. The incidence of malignancy in the American Academy of Pediatric Surgical Section Survey (57) was only 7% for teratomas present on the first day of life as opposed to 37% for lesions developing at one year of age and 50% for those appearing at two years of age.

In adults, cystic lesions carry a 10% malignancy rate, whereas the malignancy rate for solid lesions approaches 60% (26). The male-to-female incidence of malignancy is equal. This finding is interesting considering the usual female predominance of presacral lesions. The equal incidence among men and women reflects the fact that malignancies always eventually present clinically, whereas benign lesions may remain asymptomatic. Many of the lesions in women are found during the reproductive years, when pelvic examinations are most frequent. Thus, the female predominance may be artificial to some extent. In a review of 120 retrorectal tumors at the Mayo Clinic, 43% of patients had a malignant lesion (5). Stewart et al. (7) reported a 50% incidence of malignancy in 20 cases of presacral tumors in adults. Malignancy was more common in men than in women.

A

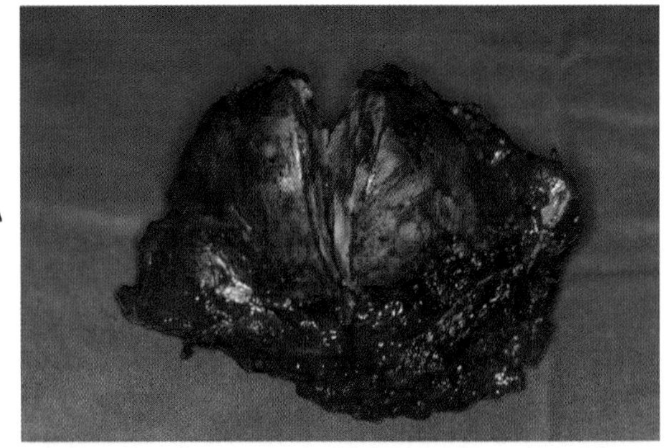

B

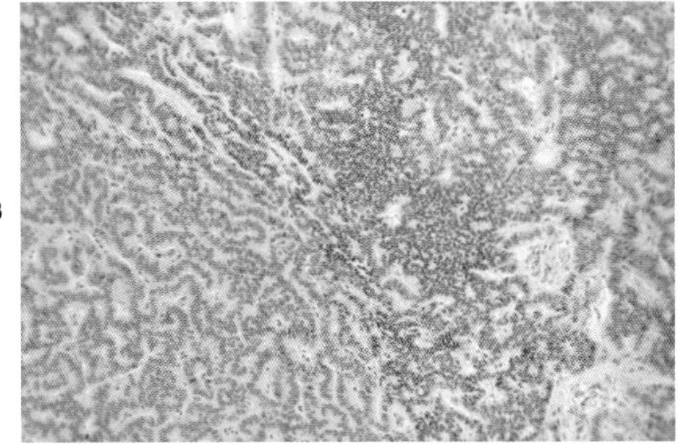

FIGURE 6 ■ (**A**) Excised retrorectal carcinoid that included the sacrum. Lesion and sacrum were excised in continuity. (**B**) Microscopic appearance of presacral carcinoid.

Lack et al. (58) reported a sacrococcygeal adenocarcinoma in a male patient nearly 40 years old following resection of a histologically mature sacrococcygeal teratoma. The adenocarcinoma arose within soft tissue of the presacral area and residual coccyx and extensively invaded the coccygeal stump that had not been removed in toto with the teratoma during initial surgery at two months of age. The patient died nearly two years later with local and regional recurrence and metastases to lymph nodes, liver, lung, bone, and brain. At autopsy, there was no evidence of origin from deep internal organs such as the stomach, pancreas, or other sites. This report supports the concern that microscopic nests of neoplastic cells are commonly found in or immediately adjacent to the coccyx and therefore that coccygectomy in conjunction with tumor resection could theoretically ablate any microscopic residual of totipotential cells.

Yolk sac neoplasms are the most common malignancy arising in sacrococcygeal teratomas, but squamous cell carcinoma also occurs (58). The incidence of malignant change in tailgut cysts is low, with only 1 in 53 cases noted (15).

CLINICAL PRESENTATION

SYMPTOMS

The symptoms caused by retrorectal lesions are related to their site, size, and, in the case of retrorectal cysts, the presence or absence of infection. Benign lesions tend to be asymptomatic and may be detected by complete physical examination or, in the case of women, during childbirth. Malignant lesions are more likely to produce symptoms.

Pain

Pain is common in patients with neoplastic lesions and with infected cysts. It is generally poorly localized as low back or perianal pain, rectal ache, or deep rectal pain. If the sacral plexus is involved, patients may experience referred pain in the legs or buttocks. It is unusual for the pain to be accompanied by paralysis in the early stages.

Characteristically, the pain experienced with retrorectal neoplasms is frequently postural. The patient associates pain with sitting or standing, and often the onset of pain relates to local trauma such as a fall on the sacrum or coccyx.

Infection

Infection may be an isolated event with fever, chills, rigors, and pain, or it may manifest as recurrent episodes of perianal suppuration, frequently with a history of recurrent surgical attempts at treatment. The latter history in a female should always precipitate a careful search to exclude a retrorectal cyst.

Interference with Pelvic Outlet

Constipation

Large masses may interfere with the passage of stool or give the feeling of unsatisfied defecation. Straining may result in the appearance of hemorrhoids, sometimes with rectal bleeding, but as a rule the tumors do not bleed.

Incontinence

Whether from paradoxical diarrhea secondary to obstruction or to interference with sphincter nerve supply, incontinence is an occasional symptom. In the early stages of tumor growth, gross perianal soiling may be the only manifestation of an early loss of fecal control.

Obstructed Labor

Many solid neoplasms first come to light during pregnancy (59). Occasionally, a missed retrorectal tumor appears for the first time as a cause of obstructed labor.

Urinary Symptoms

Disturbances in bladder function are not uncommon and may be caused by interference with the pelvic parasympathetic supply, direct pressure on the bladder or urethra, or obstruction of the pelvic ureters.

Central Nervous System Manifestations

Although rare, anterior sacral meningoceles may present as central nervous system problems. In adults, headache and recurrent episodes of meningitis have been reported to result from recurrent infections of a meningocele (37). The meningomyelocele is a gross disorder of sacral neurogenic and osseous formation, and it occurs with varying degrees of neurogenic disorder in infants.

ASSOCIATED PATHOLOGY

Although not included in this group as retrorectal tumors, two conditions occasionally manifest as retrorectal pathology. The first is a complication of diverticulitis with extension of the suppurative process into the retrorectal space. The second is seen in patients with Crohn's disease, in whom sinus formation and possible fistulization may present as retrorectal induration.

PREVIOUS SURGERY

A history of repeated local operations for perianal suppuration is important in the context of retrorectal cysts. In addition, a history of operations for malignant neoplasms of the genitourinary or gastrointestinal tract—in particular, the bladder, prostate, or rectum—is highly significant in terms of recurrence. The retrorectal space is a common site for metastatic spread.

EXAMINATION

The potential operability of a tumor and the operative approach required can be determined on rectal examination. The examination begins with inspection of the perianal area. A postanal dimple may suggest the presence of a developmental cyst. Soiling and a pouting anus may indicate interference with the nerve supply to the anal sphincters. Laxity of the anal sphincters and saddle anesthesia of the perineum further support involvement of coccygeal nerves.

As the finger passes into the rectum, a solid retrorectal mass should be obvious. In the Mayo Clinic series, 97% of retrorectal tumors were palpable (5). High retrorectal tumors may escape detection unless careful assessment of the sacral curve is made, a sudden anterior angulation being the first indication. Location of the mass should be recorded, as well as whether it is lobulated or solitary, and whether it is possible to define its upper limits. In particular, the mass must be assessed for its relationship to the sacrum and the coccyx. This assessment is important because the location will determine the operative approach (Fig. 7).

Cystic neoplasms may be more difficult to detect since, if flaccid, they tend to feel like mucosal folds. However, if the finger is swept across the posterior mucosal surface, fluid within the cyst will be pushed before the finger into the lateral aspect of the cyst, which becomes tense and distended, thus allowing clear delineation. With tense cysts, it is sometimes difficult to distinguish between a supralevator abscess and a deep posterior space infection. Associated features such as a postanal dimple should be sought in these cases.

An anterior meningocele can be mistaken for a simple cyst. In an infant, pressure over the cysts can cause a rise in fontanelle pressure, which can be palpated. Once the fontanelle has closed, Valsalva's maneuver demonstrates spinal canal cyst continuity.

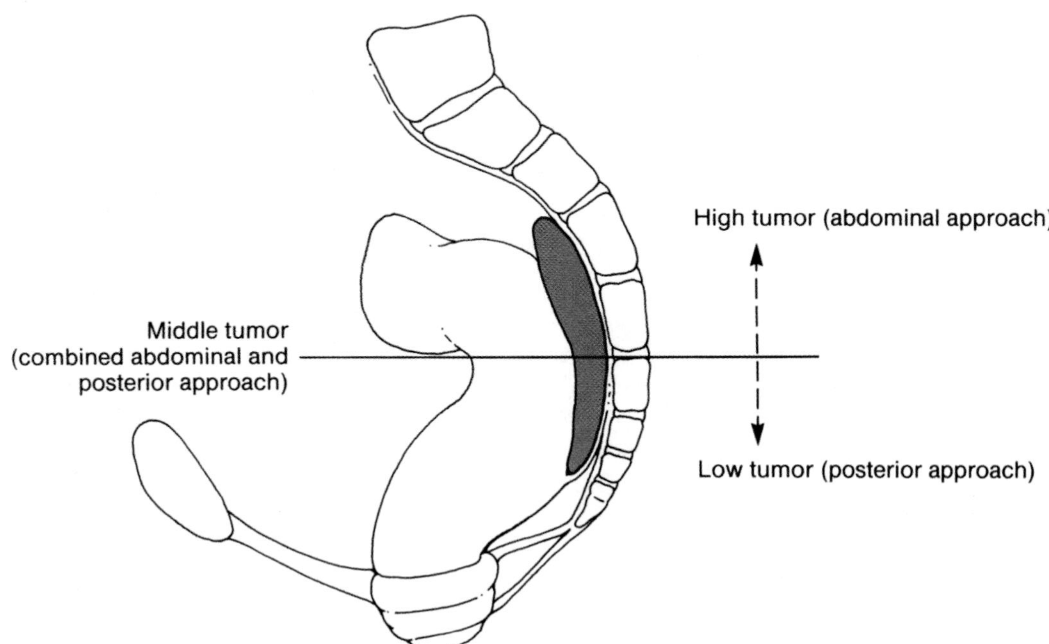

FIGURE 7 ■ Location of retrorectal tumors and operative approach to their treatment. *Source*: After M. Finch.

Sigmoidoscopy should be performed to determine rectal wall involvement. An indentation denoting extrinsic compression may be seen. A note should be made of the state of the overlying rectal mucosa, in particular, the presence of submucosal edema, which may indicate underlying infection. Usually, the mucosa is totally normal.

DIAGNOSTIC MEASURES

■ RADIOLOGY

Plain Films

For solid neoplasms that arise from, compress, invade, or displace the sacrum and coccyx, a plain x-ray film of the pelvis is one of the most useful diagnostic procedures. A soft tissue mass may be identified. However, gas bubbles and fecal matter in the bowel may obscure the bony markings of the sacrum. Anterior sacral meningoceles have a characteristic "scimitar" sacrum caused by the presence of a unilateral sacral defect with increased ossification of the smooth, rounded outer border and no associated bony destruction (37). Bony destruction in the area may indicate a malignancy. Osteoblastic metastases from prostate carcinoma are frequently found in this area and have a characteristic x-ray appearance. Such an appearance must not be confused with Paget's disease of the pelvic bones. With teratomas, the presence of bone or even teeth has been reported as an x-ray finding.

Fistulography

When a chronic fistula is present, particularly after repeated operations, a fistulogram may be extremely useful in defining the presence of a retrorectal cyst and its ramifications, which may not have been recognized previously.

Barium Enema

A barium enema shows an extrarectal mass with anterior displacement of the rectum.

Computed Tomography

CT scans are the most important means of evaluating sacral lesions and planning the operative approach (5,7,22,57). CT scans show whether the lesion is cystic or solid. They define the surface of the tumor in relationship to the sacrum and indicate the degree of invasion or destruction of that structure. CT scanning allows a clearer definition of the extent of the lesion, especially the upper extent, and shows whether structures such as the ureter, bladder, or rectum are involved (Fig. 8).

Burchell (60) reported an example where a CT scan modified the approach to a retrorectal lesion by conclusively demonstrating a communication between the rectum and a retrorectal cyst. A potential rectocutaneous fistula through a previously planned parasacrococcygeal incision was avoided by changing to a peranal approach.

Ultrasonography

The usefulness of abdominal and pelvic ultrasonography in detecting presacral tumors is limited because the presacral tumor lies deep in the pelvis, with overlying bowel and, in women, the genital structures. Bohm et al. (61) have found intrarectal ultrasonography to be a very sensitive method for the assessment of the extent of tumor and infiltration into adjacent pelvic organs. It can also distinguish solid lesions from cysts.

Intravenous Pyelography

For masses located high in the retrorectal space, intravenous pyelography may show ureteral displacement or obstruction, bladder involvement, or ectopic location of a kidney. For small low-lying lesions, intravenous pyelography would not prove helpful.

Angiography

Angiography has provided information on the vascularity of these neoplasms; when such information is required, clearly this modality has a place. Angiography seldom alters

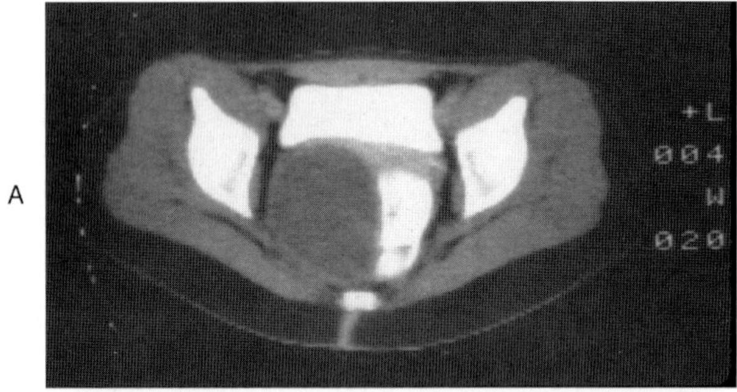

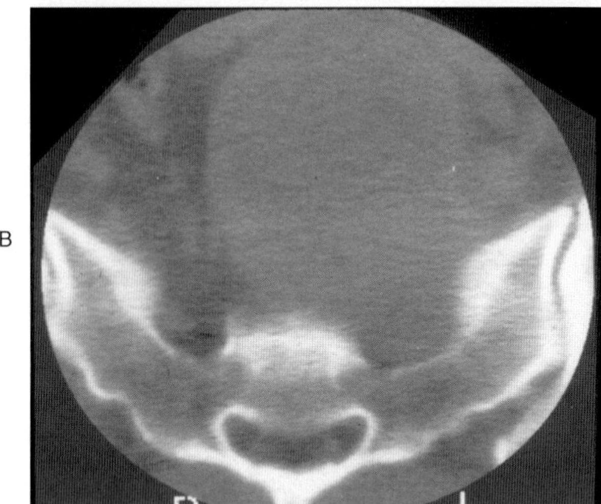

FIGURE 8 ■ (**A**) CT with infusion demonstrating a large homogeneous mass on the right side of the pelvis with density measuring between cystic fluid and solid tissue (presacral teratoma). (**B**) CT demonstrating a large homogenous mass adjacent to left sacral ala from S1 to S4 extending into the anterior sacral foramen. S3 compressing nerve root (presacral schwannoma).

the decision to operate or influences the choice of operative approach. However, the presence of a highly vascularized lesion may lead to the recommendation of preoperative arterial embolization to minimize blood loss (4).

Magnetic Resonance Imaging

MRI provides a detailed image of the anatomic relationship of neoplasms to the bony structures of the pelvis. This modality may be helpful for evaluating central nervous system involvement. For some, MRI has become the preferred imaging modality because of its multiplanar capacity and improved soft tissue resolution defining a plane between the lesion and the presacral fascia (62). MRI defines sacral invasion and the potential for resectability (Fig. 9).

Myelography

When central nervous system involvement is suggested, myelography may prove useful in confirming or excluding the diagnosis.

■ BIOPSY

There is no place for preoperative biopsy of a lesion considered to be operable. If the lesion is solid, a biopsy may cause seeding of malignant cells. If the lesion is a cyst, infection may ensue. If a meningocele is present, meningitis may occur. The best biopsy is total operative excision. When the lesion is considered to be inoperable, then it is necessary to obtain a tissue diagnosis so that adjuvant therapy can be planned. If the diagnosis is in doubt and it is clear that surgical excision cannot be undertaken without significant risk to the patient, a preoperative diagnosis using a biopsy is necessary to prevent inappropriate therapy.

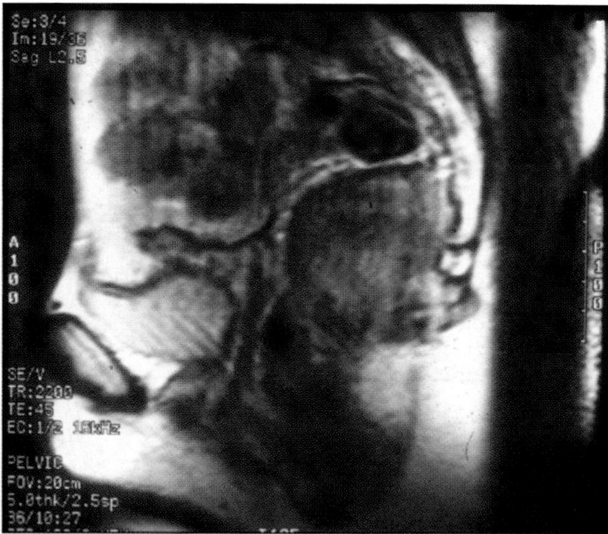

FIGURE 9 ■ MRI of large presacral mass demonstrating invasion and destruction of the distal sacrum.

A biopsy specimen can be obtained by two routes. The first is a direct approach through the posterior wall of the rectum; this is simple and has low morbidity. Prophylactic broad-spectrum antibiotic coverage has been recommended because septicemia has been reported (63). Transrectal biopsy has been condemned because seeding of an un-involved rectum may occur. The second technique is that of an extrarectal presacral approach, with the finger in the rectum directing the needle to the biopsy site. The latter technique is successful in all but a few retrorectal tumors. My preference is for the extrarectal biopsy technique. This can be performed under ultrasonography or CT guidance.

■ THE MISDIAGNOSED ENTITY

The rarity of retrorectal cysts and their nonspecific clinical presentations often lead to misdiagnosis and inappropriate operations. Singer et al. (64) reviewed the medical records of the colorectal surgery divisions at two institutions. Seven patients with retrorectal cysts who had been misdiagnosed before referral were identified. These patients had been treated for fistula-in-ano, pilonidal cyst, perianal abscess; psychogenic, lower back, post-traumatic, or postpartum pain, and proctalgia fugax before the correct diagnosis was made. Patients underwent an average of 4.1 operative procedures. Physical examination in combination with CT scanning made the correct diagnosis in all patients. All patients underwent successful resection through a parasacrococcygeal approach, and six of seven did not require coccygectomy. The resected lesions included four hamartomas, two epidermoid cysts, and one enteric duplication cyst. They concluded that retrorectal cysts are a rare entity that can be difficult to diagnose without a high index of clinical suspicion. A history of multiple unsuccessful procedures should alert the clinician to the diagnosis of retrorectal cyst.

OPERATIVE APPROACHES

Once a retrorectal tumor is diagnosed, resection, even in asymptomatic patients, is recommended for several reasons (5):

1. The lesion may be malignant.
2. With time, a teratoma has a greater chance to become malignant.
3. Cystic lesions may become infected. Once infection occurs, the postoperative recurrence rate is 30%, and repeated operations in the infected area can cause anal incontinence.
4. The mortality associated with untreated anterior sacral meningocele is 30%, chiefly because of infection and meningitis.
5. Young female patients may have dystocia, which increases the risk to mother and fetus.

A multidisciplinary approach to the management of lesions in the area is advisable. Depending on the presumed etiology of the retrorectal tumor, an orthopedic surgeon or a neurosurgeon might be included. Complete mechanical and antibiotic bowel preparation is indicated for operations in the retrorectal space because of the significant risk of rectal injury.

ABDOMINAL APPROACH

Indications for an abdominal approach include the high retrorectal tumors where safe access is not possible from below. This approach is also indicated for extraspinal neurogenic neoplasms. The abdomen is entered through a transverse or midline incision. The sigmoid colon is mobilized, and the rectum is placed on stretch so that the pelvis can be examined and the relationship of the tumor to the rectum determined (Fig. 10). The presacral sympathetic nerves are identified, and the retrorectal space is entered through a plane anterior to these structures. In this way, the rectum is displaced forward and the tumor defined with a minimum of bleeding. The middle sacral vessels are often significantly enlarged in the case of solid retrorectal tumors, and these should be ligated before mobilization is attempted (4). The presacral veins produce the most difficult type of hemorrhage to control because the veins retract when cut and are thus difficult to isolate. Careful dissection with particular attention to hemostasis is essential, and protection of nerve structures should be attempted at all times.

By slow and meticulous dissection, the tumor is mobilized; hemoclips are useful in this procedure. The tumor is then removed. This simplified description should in no way play down the difficulties encountered during dissection. With persistence, provided the tumor is high and the sacrum uninvolved, this procedure can be accomplished.

Malignancies involving the rectal wall require a rectal resection. Depending on the extent of the neoplasm, completion of the operation may require the patient to be repositioned in the prone jack-knife position so that the remainder of the excision can be carried out through a posterior approach. If a biopsy has been performed, the excision should include the skin through which the biopsy was performed. The proximal and lateral extent of the dissection will be determined by the location of the primary lesion. Ideally, a 2 cm margin should be sought. Various bony and nerve structures will be sacrificed, again depending on the location of the lesion. The help of a neurosurgeon or orthopedic surgeon may prove invaluable in these circumstances.

POSTERIOR APPROACH

The posterior approach is useful for low-lying lesions and infected cysts. It is not suited for high lesions or those with high extensions. If the examiner's finger can reach the upper extent of the lesion, the posterior approach should prove successful. If even half of the lesion can be palpated, the lesion can be approached posteriorly.

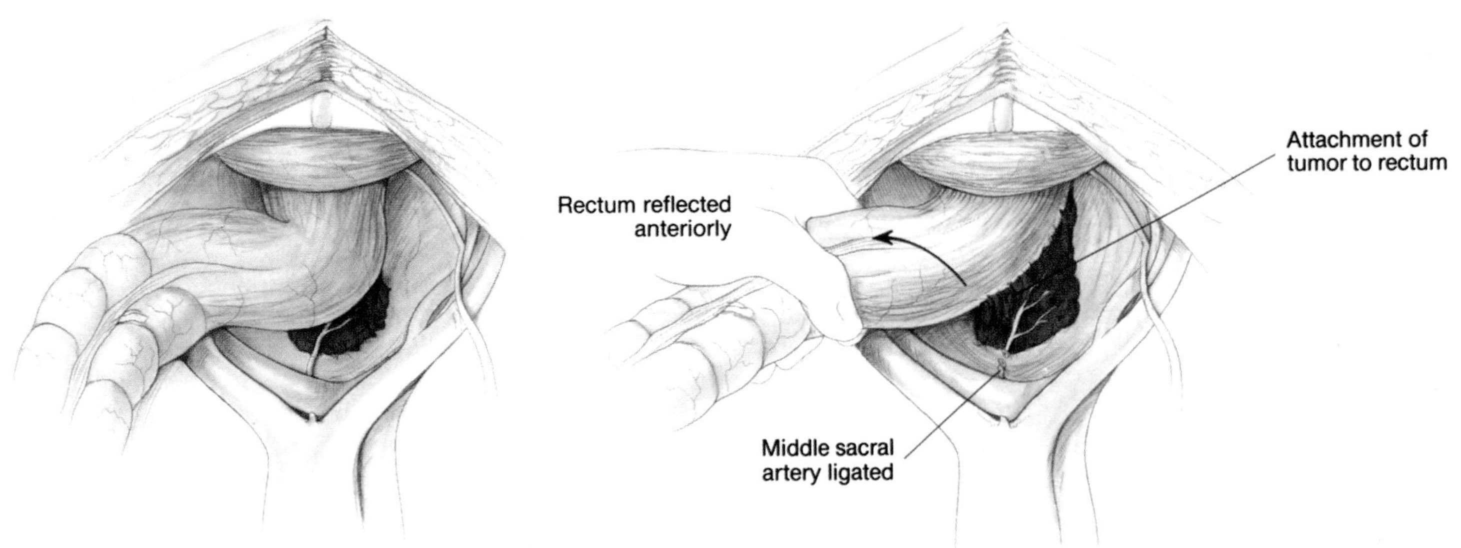

FIGURE 10 ■ Abdominal approach to high retrorectal tumors.

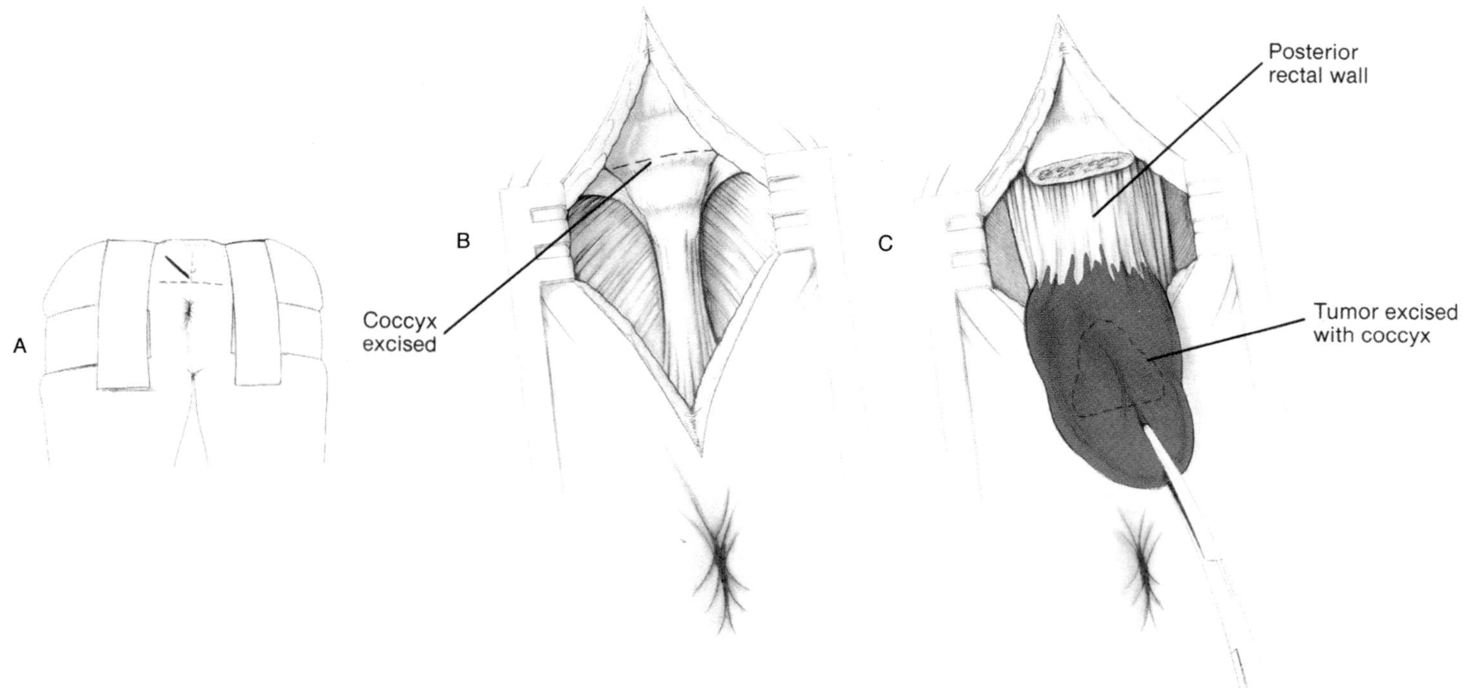

FIGURE 11 ■ Posterior excision of retrorectal tumors. (**A**) Parasacrococcygeal incision. (**B**) Line of disarticulation of coccyx. (**C**) Removed coccyx is attached to mass.

The patient is placed in the prone jack-knife position (Fig. 11). A midline parasacrococcygeal, curvilinear, or horizontal incision is made and deepened to define the sacrum, coccyx, and anococcygeal ligament. The anococcygeal ligament is detached from the coccyx and displaced, revealing the levator ani muscle with the central decussating fibers passing from the rectum to the coccyx. The levator ani muscle is divided, and the supralevator space is entered. The coccyx is disarticulated from the S5 vertebra, allowing entrance into the supralevator space. Varying amounts of levator ani muscle are incised to gain adequate access. The surgeon can double-glove the left hand and insert the index finger in the rectum to push the lesion outward to facilitate excision without injury to the rectal wall. At this point, a decision about whether the distal one or two sacral segments require excision must be made. The decision depends on the size of the lesion, its relationship to the sacrum, and the exposure required. If removing sacral segments is necessary, the gluteus maximus muscle can be detached from each side, and a portion of the sacroiliac ligaments may be incised. The sacral nerves related to the lowest two sacral vertebrae can be divided without fear of significant neurologic deficit. Neither is sacral instability a problem. Bleeding is frequently a problem until the bone has been completely removed. The jack-knife position reduces bleeding to some extent. Removal of a portion of the sacrum is necessary to achieve a block excision of any neoplasm arising from that bone or to achieve greater access to the retrorectal space. Caution, however, must be taken in the presence of a high extension because frequently the vascular supply comes from above, and an uncontrolled vessel in a deep, inaccessible hole proves troublesome. In all cases of retrorectal tumors and cysts, it has been recommended that the coccyx always be sacrificed, not only to achieve better exposure but because the most common factor in recurrence is failure to remove this bone (2). Other authors support this view (5,6). All cystic lesions in this area should be assumed to originate in the coccyx; hence, its removal is believed to be mandatory (Fig. 11C). However, not all authors advocate removal of the coccyx (11). Most of the developmental cysts reported by Bohm et al. (61) were removed without coccygectomy.

The posterior approach is best suited for the removal of cystic lesions, especially precoccygeal cysts. This approach is ideal for all low tumors and for many tumors below the sacral promontory. Preoperative examination is obviously important since a mistake in assessing the upward extent of the lesion can be very difficult to correct in the operating room. Maneuverability through this incision is limited. If significant uncontrolled hemorrhage occurs from deep within the wound, pressure packs should be applied. If hemostasis still cannot be achieved, the patient should be repositioned and the abdominal approach used. After removal of the tumor, wound closure is performed in layers around suction catheters. These catheters ensure elimination of the dead space left when the tumor is removed.

Management of Infected Cysts

Making a differential diagnosis between an infected retrorectal cyst and a retrorectal component of a perianal abscess is difficult (5). Five conditions may indicate a presacral cyst: (1) recurring abscess in the retrorectal space, (2) repeated operations for an "anal fistula," (3) inability to find the primary source of infection at its usual site in a crypt at the dentate margin when an anal, perianal, or rectal sinus is present, (4) the presence of a postanal dimple, and (5) some fixation and fullness in the precoccygeal region.

Unless the cyst has ruptured into the rectum at the time of presentation, the operative approach should be through an extrarectal posterior route. If rupture into the rectum has occurred, however, the posterior approach is clearly contraindicated. In this situation, adequate transrectal drainage should be ensured, curettage of the cavity performed, and expectant treatment adopted with regular follow-up examination.

If the cyst is acutely inflamed, it may be necessary to perform a staged procedure with drainage as the first step. Once inflammation has settled, excision of the cyst will be necessary.

When the chronic sinus tracts are associated with an infected cyst, these tracts should be laid open and the cyst excised. In this situation, the wound should be left open to heal by secondary intention.

■ ABDOMINOSACRAL APPROACH

Localio et al. (65) advocate the following combined approach for the removal of large retrorectal tumors in adults. This approach permits vascular control and provides good exposure for the protection of vital structures and wide resection. Pediatric surgeons have found it a useful approach for large retrorectal teratomas with abdominal extension.

The abdomen is entered through an oblique incision starting between the left iliac crest and costal margin and running parallel to the inguinal ligament. The left colon and rectum are mobilized and displaced anteriorly and to the patient's right. The left ureter is identified. Tapes are placed around the iliac vessels for control. The rectum is dissected from the tumor. The middle sacral vessels and lateral sacral veins, more prominent than usual, are suture ligated. The transverse incision is made over the sacrum posteriorly, and skin flaps are developed. The gluteal muscles are detached from their sacral origins. The anococcygeal ligament is divided, and the presacral space is entered to join the abdominal dissection. The iliac vessels are occluded by traction on the tapes. The sacrotuberous, sacrospinous, and lower sacroiliac ligaments are divided. The piriformis muscles are detached. The sacroiliac articulations are divided at the level determined by the abdominal dissection, and the sacrum is transected. No attempt is made to preserve sacral roots below the level of transection. The specimen is removed, and the wound is closed over suction drainage. This approach does not differ from those performed as isolated operations. The main advantages of the abdominal approach are to perform ligation of the middle sacral vessels, which can be so significant in these tumors, and at the same time to achieve mobilization down to a level that makes lower resection a simpler procedure.

In the case of chordoma, block resection of the tumor and sacral segment is necessary to achieve an adequate resection. Although Localio et al. (65) have recommended a combined abdominosacral approach, chordomas at the Mayo Clinic have been treated using a posterior approach (5).

In the case of chordoma where many surgical disciplines are involved, Dozois (33) advocates the team approach with a combination of specialty surgeons. Dozois further stresses that a defeatist attitude toward the treatment of chordomas is unfounded.

A number of factors have contributed to this negative attitude. First, because chordomas are slow growing and produce vague symptoms, by the time of diagnosis, the size of the mass is intimidating to the surgeon. Second, the misconception that chordomas are entirely benign allowed them to metastasize before definitive treatment was considered. Finally, the size and the location of chordomas resulted in inadequate treatment because of violation of the lesion and fear of neurologic compromise and musculoskeletal instability. For example, Kaiser et al. (66) found that the local recurrence rate increased from 28% to 64% if the chordoma was violated preoperatively.

The clinical features and results of surgical treatment of 13 patients with sacrococcygeal chordoma who were treated as the Chiba Cancer Center and Chiba University were analyzed (67). Intralesional excision was performed in eight patients, marginal excision in two patients, and wide excision in three patients. Local recurrence was observed in six patients, with a high proportion occurring in the gluteal muscles attached to the sacrum. Seven patients died of their disease and six patients were alive with no evidence of disease. The five-year survival rate was 81.8% and the 10-year survival rate was 29.1%.

Curative treatment may necessitate en bloc resection of portions of the sacrum, neural sacrifice, and even loss of the rectum. Gunterberg et al. (68) demonstrated that patients in whom all sacral roots are destroyed unilaterally continue to have normal anorectal function. If the upper three sacral roots on one side and the upper two on the other side are preserved, the patient has near-normal anorectal sphincter function. When both S3 roots are sacrificed, the patient has stool incontinence. Cody et al. (6) believe that if S2 to S4 roots are preserved on one side, bowel and bladder continence may be adequate. Localio et al. (65) have gone as high as transection of the sacrum at the S1–2 interspace with sacrifice of the S2 roots. Patients commonly develop a neurogenic bladder but retain awareness of bladder distention; they initiate voiding by contracting the abdominal muscles. Anal continence was preserved in all patients who were continent preoperatively. Saddle anesthesia occurs with the sacrifice of lower sacral roots, and occasional motor weakness of lower extremities develops. No problems with spinal column stability were reported. Freier et al. (3) agree with this approach and support the results. This is at variance with the writings of other investigators (31). Grundfest-Broniatowski et al. (4) reported that preservation of S1 to S5 nerve roots on one side maintains continence, but with hemisensory loss and some weakness of plantar flexion. If both S3 nerve roots can be preserved, continence and sensation will be near normal. Resection of both S2 nerve roots may require the patient to practice catheterization and bowel training and may cause male patients to suffer impotence. Anson et al. (32) reported that radical excision results in limited postoperative morbidity and excellent preservation of neurologic function, including sphincter control, provided that one S2 nerve root is left intact. Andreoli et al. (69) reported that with unilateral loss of the S2 nerve root, perfect anorectal continence can be expected but that bilateral loss of the S2 nerve root results in incontinence and inability to discriminate rectal contents. Some authors have even resected both S1 nerve roots, but incontinence and some leg weakness have been noted. Preservation of the upper half of the S1 vertebra is generally considered necessary for stability of the spine and pelvis.

When preservation of nervous structures compromises the otherwise successful removal of a tumor, the nerves should be sacrificed and the consequences accepted as a price for cure.

Chordomas not extending above the S3 level can be removed through a posterior approach, whereas large lesions extending above S3 require an anteroposterior approach. The technique was elegantly described by Dozois (33). With the patient in the prone jack-knife position, an incision is made over the sacrum and coccyx. The anococcygeal ligament is transected and the levator ani muscles retracted laterally. The chordoma is separated from the rectum and the gluteus maximus muscles on both sides, the sacrospinous and sacrotuberous ligaments are detached, and the piriformis muscles are serially divided on each side to expose the sciatic nerve. An osteotomy is performed at the S3 level, and the S3 roots are protected. The lesion is removed en bloc, and the wound is closed over suction drainage. It is important at the time of sacral excision to recognize dural injury (61). This may occur in patients with intraspinal extension of the lesion and can lead to a cerebrospinal fluid leak or life-threatening intradural infection. When undertaking sacral resection in the region of S2 to S3 or higher, the dural sac should be searched for and closed with an absorbable suture. For lesions above the S3 level, the presacral space is approached through a laparotomy, and the rectum is mobilized anteriorly. If both S3 roots must be sacrificed, the rectum is transected and an end colostomy is fashioned. Blood loss is reduced by ligation of the middle sacral vessels and the internal iliac vessels on the side of greatest extension of the chordoma. If one S3 root can be preserved, the rectum is left in place. The pelvic floor is reconstructed. The abdomen is closed and the patient repositioned in the prone position. The posterior phase is conducted as previously described.

Postoperative functional outcome and its correlation with nerve root preservation were reported by Baratti et al. (35). No patients with bilateral preservation of S3 experienced urinary or bowel symptoms. The bilateral preservation of S2, although followed in most cases by temporary urinary retention, fecal incontinence, or both, was then characterized by recovery of normal bowel and urinary function in most cases. The preservation of only one S2 root was followed in all cases by urinary and/or bowel symptoms, which were only occasionally recovered. All the patients with preservation of only S1 roots experienced definitive bowel and urinary dysfunction, and nobody recovered.

TRANSRECTAL APPROACH

The transrectal approach has been advocated for the removal of retrorectal cysts in selected patients. We have not used this approach unless the cyst has ruptured at the time of presentation or if the diagnosis was not made preoperatively and the working diagnosis was an intramural lesion that turned out to be a retrorectal lesion.

Pidala et al. (70) reported 14 patients presenting with presacral cystic lesions who were managed over a 20-year period. Forty-three percent presented with pain; half of these patients had infected cysts. Computed tomography identified the cyst in all seven patients in which it was performed. The transrectal approach was used for cyst excision in 10 patients. One patient had transrectal drainage and wall biopsy only. Three patients underwent posterior parasacral excision. Pathologic review demonstrated four dermoid cysts, four epidermoid cysts, four cyst hamartomas, and two benign teratomas. One cyst hamartoma had a focus of invasive adenocarcinoma. Two complications occurred. There were no deaths. Follow-up averaged 39 months, at which time there were no recurrences.

INTERSPHINCTERIC APPROACH

A rarely recognized approach to removal of presacral lesions is via the intersphincteric plane. Access is gained posteriorly between the internal and external sphincter until the retrorectal space is reached. The technique is similar to that described by Parks (71) for postanal repair. Small lesions can be adequately removed in this way.

ADJUVANT THERAPY

RADIOTHERAPY

Radiotherapy is the only modality that can provide adequate palliation for inoperable malignancies. This is particularly true in the case of soft tissue sarcomas since these characteristically appear in an advanced stage.

Chordomas are relatively radioresistant neoplasms, yet high-dose radiotherapy can provide palliation. Amendola et al. (72) used radiation doses ranging from 5000 cGy to 6600 Gy to treat 21 patients with a chordoma. Remission of symptoms was obtained for 1 to 6 years. The authors believe that the combination of high-dose irradiation therapy and complete or subtotal surgical resection offers the best chance for prolonged survival.

Complications related to radiotherapy may be significant. These can manifest as severe skin reactions in the perineal area, severe proctitis, and radiation cystitis. All these conditions are troublesome but can be minimized with modern techniques of radiotherapy.

CHEMOTHERAPY

Few neoplasms in the retrorectal space respond satisfactorily to cytotoxic therapy; this is not, at present, a popular method of therapy. I have been unable to find a satisfactory regimen that can be recommended.

RESULTS

The results of treatment of retrorectal neoplasms and cysts reflect the nature of the tumor and the adequacy of resection. Malignant neoplasms in this area have a poor prognosis; few patients survive five years with either soft tissue sarcomas or teratocarcinomas.

With respect to quality of life, Rintala et al. (73) evaluated 26 adult patients who had undergone resection of a benign sacrococcygeal teratoma in infancy. Good fecal continence was reported by 88% of patients, but only 27% had completely normal bowel habits compared to 77% of a "normal" control population. Deficiencies in anorectal function included soiling, defective rectal sensation, limited ability to hold back defecation, defective discrimination between formed, loose, and gaseous stools, fecal and urinary leakage during sexual intercourse, and the necessity to wear pads.

Gray et al. (31) reviewed 222 patients with sacrococcygeal chordoma from the English-language literature and reported a 10% incidence of metastases and almost universal recurrence of the primary lesion. The five-year survival rates are difficult to interpret because of the slow growth. The 10-year survival rates have varied from a low of 15% to 20% to a high of 76% (4,31).

Localio et al. (65) reported five patients who underwent primary curative resection for chordoma. The treatment of primary sacral sarcoma has not been as successful. At the Mayo Clinic, the five-year survival rate for chordomas was 75%, but for patients with other malignant lesions it was only 17% (5). Postoperative complications in the latter series included neurogenic bladder (15%), wound infection (11%), dysesthesia (7%), stool incontinence (7%), massive bleeding (4%), retrorectal abscess (3%), and fecal fistula (1%). No operative mortalities occurred. For all treated patients with malignant retrorectal tumors at the Memorial Sloan-Kettering Cancer Center, survival rates at 5, 10, 15, and 20 years were 69%, 50%, 37%, and 20%, respectively.

Bohm et al. (61) reviewed their experience with congenital presacral tumors in 24 patients who underwent curative resection. The growths were divided into two broad categories: 20 developmental cysts and four chordomas. Fifteen of 19 developmental cysts were excised by a posterior approach alone, two were excised by an anterior approach alone, and three were treated by a combined approach. Trans-sacral excision was carried out in four patients with developmental cysts. One chordoma was resected posteriorly and the other three through a combined anterior and posterior approach. Three recurrences were diagnosed after excision of developmental cysts eight, 18, and 41 months postoperatively. Recurrence occurred in three of four patients with chordomas after 25, 32, and 55 months. Reexcision was carried out in all patients. None of the patients with a developmental cyst developed a second recurrence, but two of three patients with chordomas have had recurrences, but have undergone local irradiation, which has controlled their disease. The authors believe that in cases of recurrence of both developmental cysts and chordomas, reexcision is a reasonable therapeutic option.

Lev-Chelouche et al. (74) suggested a practical method of classification in 42 patients who underwent operation for presacral tumors. Patients were divided into four groups according to lesion pathology: benign congenital ($n = 12$), malignant congenital ($n = 9$), benign acquired ($n = 9$), and malignant acquired ($n = 12$). Symptoms were nonspecific, and 26% of the cases were completely asymptomatic. Diagnosis was made with rectal examination and confirmed with pelvic computerized tomographic scan. Surgical approach varied among the different groups with the posterior approach used mainly for congenital tumors and the anterior approach for acquired. Complete surgical resection was obtained in all cases of benign tumors and in 76% of malignant tumors. No postoperative mortality was seen and complications occurred in 36%. None of the patients with benign tumors had recurrences. The survival rate of patients with malignant tumors was significantly improved when complete resection was possible.

Benign tumors and congenital cysts can be adequately treated by surgical excision. It is only when the cysts are not recognized, inadequately treated, or, in the case of benign neoplasms, inadequately removed that they recur. The retrorectal region is an area where access is limited; therefore, it is essential that the primary procedure be adequate.

REFERENCES

1. Teplick SK, Slark P, Clark RE, Metz JR, Shapiro JH. The retrorectal space. Clin Radiol 1978; 29:177–184.
2. Uhlig BE, Johnson RL. Presacral tumors and cysts in adults. Dis Colon Rectum 1975; 18:581–596.
3. Freier DT, Stanley JC, Thompson NW. Retrorectal tumors in adults. Surg Gynecol Obstet 1971; 132:681–686.
4. Grundfest-Broniatowski S, Marks K, Fazio VW. Sacral and retro rectal tumors. Fazio VW, ed. Current Therapy in Colon and Rectal Surgery. Toronto: BC Decker, 1990:107–115.
5. Jao SW, Beart RW, Spencer RJ, et al. Retrorectal tumors: Mayo Clinic experience, 1960–1979. Dis Colon Rectum 1985; 28:644–652.
6. Cody HS, Marcove RC, Quan SH. Malignant retrorectal tumors: 28 years' experience at Memorial Sloan-Kettering Cancer Center. Dis Colon Rectum 1981; 24:501–506.
7. Stewart RJ, Humphreys WG, Parks TG. The presentation and management of presacral tumours. Br J Surg 1986; 73:153–155.
8. Pantoja B, Rodriguez-Ibanez I. Sacrococcygeal dermoids and teratomas: Historical review. Am J Surg 1976; 132:377–383.
9. Goldberg SM, Gordon PH, Nivatvongs S. Essentials of Anorectal Surgery. Philadelphia: JB Lippincott, 1980:215–228.
10. Storrs BB. Are dermoid and epidermoid tumors preventable complications of myelomeningocele repair?. Pediatr Neurosurg 1994; 20:160–162.
11. Abel ME, Nelson R, Prasad ML, et al. Parasacrococcygeal approach for the resection of retrorectal developmental cysts. Dis Colon Rectum 1985; 28:855–858.
12. Flint R, Strang J, Bissett I, Clark M, Neill M, Parry B. Rectal duplication cyst presenting as perianal sepsis: Report of two cases and review of the literature. Dis Colon Rectum 2004; 47:2208–2210.
13. Springall RG, Griffiths JD. Malignant change in retrorectal duplication. J R Soc Med 1990; 83:185–186.
14. Michael D, Cohen CR, Northover JM. Adenocarcinoma within a rectal duplication cyst: case report and literature review. Ann R Coll Surg Engl 1999; 81:205–206.
15. Hjermstad BM, Helwig EB. Tailgut cysts: Report of 53 cases. Am J Clin Pathol 1988; 89:139–147.
16. McDermott NC, Newman J. Tailgut cyst (retrorectal cystic hamartoma) with prominent glomus bodies. Histopatology 1991; 18:265–266.
17. Prasad AR, Amin MB, Randolph TL, Lee CS, Ma CK. Retrorectal cystic hamartoma: report of 5 cases with malignancy arising in 2. Arch Pathol Lab Med 2000; 124:725–729.
18. Mourra N, Caplin S, Parc R, Flejou JF. Presacral neuroendocrine carcinoma developed in a tailgut cyst: Report of a case. Dis Colon Rectum 2003; 46: 411–413.
19. Moreira AL, Scholes JV, Boppana S, Melamed J. p53 Mutation in adenocarcinoma arising in retrorectal cyst hamartoma (tailgut cyst): report of 2 cases—an immunohistchemistry/immunoperoxidase study. Arch Pathol Lab Med 2001; 125:1361–1364.
20. Schwarz RE, Lyda M, Lew M, Paz IB. A carcinoembryonic antigen-secreting adenocarcinoma arising within a retrorectal tailgut cyst: Clinicopathological considerations. Am J Gastroenterol 2000; 95:1344–1347.
21. Oyama K, Embi C, Rader AE. Aspiration cytology and core biopsy of a carcinoid tumor arising in a retrorectal cyst: A case report. Diagn Cytopathol 2000; 22:376–378.
22. Gips M, Melki Y, Wolloch Y. Cysts of the tailgut. Two cases. Eur J Surg 1994; 160:1–2.
23. Levert LM, Rooyen WV, Van den Bergon HA. Cysts of the tailgut. Eur J Surg 1996; 162:149–152.
24. Mahour GH. Sacrococcygeal teratomas. Cancer 1988; 38:362–367.
25. Scobie WG. Malignant sacrococcygeal teratoma—a problem in diagnosis. Arch Dis Child 1971; 46:216–218.
26. Finne CO. Presacral tumors and cysts. In: Cameron JL, ed. Current Surgical Therapy. 3rd ed. Toronto: BC Decker, 1989:736–743.

27. Miles RM, Stewart GS. Sacrococcygeal teratomas in adults. Ann Surg 1974; 179:676–683.
28. Chen KJK. Squamous cell carcinoma arising in sacrococcygeal teratoma. Arch Pathol Lab Med 1980; 104:336.
29. Kazez A, Ozercan IH, Erol FS, Faik Ozveren M, Parmaksiz E. Sacrococcygeal heart: a very rare differentiation in teratoma. Eur J Pediatr Surg 2002; 12: 278–280.
30. Rosai J, ed. Ackerman's Surgical Pathology. Vol. 2. St. Louis: CV Mosby, 1989:1507–1509.
31. Gray SW, Singhabhandhu B, Smith RA, et al. Sacrococcygeal chordoma: report of a case and review of the literature. Surgery 1975; 78:573–582.
32. Anson KM, Byrne PO, Robertson ID, et al. Radical excision of sacrococcygeal tumors. Br J Surg 1994; B0:460–461.
33. Dozois RR. Retrorectal tumors: spectrum of disease, diagnosis, and surgical management. Perspect Colon Rectal Surg 1990; 3(2):241–255.
34. Miyahara M, Saito T, Nakashima K, et al. Yokoyama's sacral chordoma developing two years after low anterior resection for rectal cancer. Jpn J Surg 1993; 23:144–148.
35. Baratti D, Gronchi A, Pennacchioli E, Lozza L, Colecchia M, Fiore M. Chordoma: Natural history and results in 28 patients treated at a single institution. Ann Surg Oncol 2003; 10:291–296.
36. Kovalcik PJ, Burke JB. Anterior sacral meningocele and the scimitar sign: report of a case. Dis Colon Rectum 1988; 31:806–807.
37. Oren M, Lorber B, Lee SH, et al. Anterior sacral meningocele: report of five cases and review of the literature. Dis Colon Rectum 1977; 20:492–505.
38. Anderson FM, Burke BL. Anterior sacral meningocele: A presentation of three cases. JAMA 1977; 237:39–42.
39. Simpson BA, Glass RE, Mann CV. Anterior sacral meningocele: Magnetic resonance imaging and surgical management. Br J Surg 1987; 74:1185.
40. Wilkins RH, Odom GL. Anterior and lateral spinal meningocelesIn: Vinkin PJ, Bruyn GW, eds. Handbook of Clinical Neurology. Vol. 32. Amsterdam: Elsevier North-Holland Biomedical Press, 1983; 193–230.
41. Timmerman W, Bubrick MP. Presacral and postsacral extra-spinal ependymoma: report of a case and review of the literature. Dis Colon Rectum 1984; 27:114–119.
42. Ward T, Snooks SJ, Croft RJ. Perianal pain and swelling due to a precoccygeal tumor. J R Soc Med 1987; 80:651–652.
43. Puccio F, Solazzo M, Marciano P, Fadani R, Regtaa P, Benzi F. Primary retrorectal adenocarcinoma: Report of a case. Tech Coloproctol 2003; 7:55–57.
44. Zamir G, Wexner SD, Pizov G, Reissman P. Primary presacral adenocarcinoma. Report of a case. Dis Colon Rectum 1998; 41:1056–1058.
45. Chan YF, Yu SJ, Chan YT, Yik YH. Presacral myelolipoma: case report with computed tomographic and angiographic findings. Aust N Z J Surg 1988; 58:432–434.
46. Horenstein MG, Erlandson KA, Gonzalez-Cueto DM, Rosai J. Presacral carcinoid tumors: report of three cases and review of the literature. Am J Surg Pathol 1998; 22:251–255.
47. Krasin E, Nirkin A, Issakov J, Rabau M, Meller I. Carcinoid tumor of the coccyx; case report and review of the literature. Spine 2001; 26:2165–2167.
48. Marmor E, Fourney DR, Rhines LD, Skibber JM, Fuller GN, Gokaslan ZL. Sacrococcygeal ganglioneuroma. J Spinal Disord Tech 2002; 15:265–268.
49. Rieger N, Munday D. Retrorectal endometrial cyst. Arch Gynecol Obstet 2003; Jul 25.
50. Landers J, Seex K. Sacral perineural cysts: imaging and treatment options. Br J Neurosurg 2002; 16:182–185.
51. Vecchio R, Cacciola RR, Di Martino M, et al. Presacral myelolipoma. A case report. G Chir 2002; 23:93–96.
52. Singla AK, Kechejian G, Lopez MS. Giant presacral myelolipoma. Am Surg 2003; 69:334–338.
53. Lee YY, Wen-Wei Hsu R, Huang TJ, Hsueh S, Wang JY. Metastatic meningioma in the sacrum: A case report. Spine 2002; 27:E100–E103.
54. Baykan A, Yildirim S, Koksal HM, Celayir F, Oner M. Intrapelvic-perianal hydatid disease in an unusual location: Report of a case. Dis Colon Rectum 2004; 47:250–252.
55. Farkas AM, Queveda-Bonilia G, Gingold B, et al. Presacral hematomas: diagnosis and treatment. Dis Colon Rectum 1987; 30:130–132.
56. Sarmiento JM, Wolff BG. A different type of presacral tumor: Extramedullary hematopoiesis: Report of a case. Dis Colon Rectum 2003; 46:683–685.
57. Gross SW. Missed tumors of the sacrum. Bull Clin Neurosci 1983; 48: 106–114.
58. Lack EE, Glaun RS, Hefter LF, et al. Late occurrence of malignancy following resection of a histologically mature sacrococcygeal teratoma: report of a case and literature review. Arch Pathol Lab Med 1993; 117:724–728.
59. Sobrado CW, Mester M, Simonsen OS, et al. Retrorectal tumors complicating pregnancy: report of two cases. Dis Colon Rectum 1996; 39:1176–1179.
60. Burchell MC. Radiologic impact on operative access to a retrorectal cyst. Dis Colon Rectum 1987; 30:396–397.
61. Bohm B, Milson JW, Fazio VW, et al. Our approach to the management of congenital presacral tumors in adults. Int J Colorectal Dis 1993; 8:134–138.
62. Wolpert A, Beer-Gabel M, Lifschitz O, Zbar AP. The management of presacral masses in the adult. Tech Coloproctol 2002; 6:43–49.
63. Verazin G, Rosen L, Khubchandani IT. Retrorectal tumor. Is biopsy risky? South Med J 1986; 79:1437–1439.
64. Singer MA, Cintron JR, Martz JE, Schoetz DJ, Abcarian H. Retrorectal cyst: A rare tumor frequently misdiagnosed. J Am Coll Surg 2003; 196:880–886.
65. Localio SA, Eng K, Ranson JHC. Abdominosacral approach for retrorectal tumors. Ann Surg 1980; 191:555–560.
66. Kaiser TE, Pritchard DJ, Unni KK. Clinicopathologic study of sacrococcygeal teratoma. Cancer 1984; 53:2574–2578.
67. Yonemoto T, Tatezaki S, Takenouchi T, Ishii T, Satoh T, Moriya H. The surgical management of sacrococcygeal chordoma. Cancer 1999; 15:878–883.
68. Gunterberg B, Kewenter J, Peterson I, et al. Anorectal function after major resections of the sacrum with bilateral or unilateral sacrifice of sacral nerves. Br J Surg 1976; 63:546–554.
69. Andreoli F, Balloni F, Bigiotti A, et al. Anorectal continence and bladder function: Effects of major sacral resection. Dis Colon Rectum 1986; 29:647–652.
70. Pidala MJ, Eisenstat TE, Rubin RJ, Salvati EP. Presacral cysts: Transrectal excision in select patients. Am Surg 1999; 65:112–115.
71. Parks AG. Anorectal incontinence. Proc R Soc Med 1975; 68:681–690.
72. Amendola BE, Amendola MA, Oliver E, et al. Chordoma: Role of radiation therapy. Radiology 1986; 158:839–843.
73. Rintala R, Lahdenne P, Lindahl H, et al. Anorectal function in adults operated for a benign sacrococcygeal teratoma. J Pediatr Surg 1993; 28:1165–1167.
74. Lev-Chelouche D, Gutman M, Goldman G, et al. Presacral tumors: A practical classification and treatment of a unique and heterogeneous group of diseases. Surgery 2003; 133:473–478.

18 Perianal and Anal Canal Neoplasms

Santhat Nivatvongs

INTRODUCTION

Perianal and anal canal malignancies are uncommon. Although the literature is replete with reports on this subject, the use of terminology and classification has not been uniform; consequently, interpreting the results of treatment is difficult because the malignant neoplasms at different locations with different behaviors are grouped together.

ANATOMIC LANDMARKS

The anal area, although small, is rather complex due to differences in histologic features, characteristics, and lymphatic spread. Many reports of malignant neoplasms in this region use different terminologies to define the location of the malignancy. To overcome this confusion, the World Health Organization (WHO) and the American Joint Committee on Cancer (AJCC) have developed a universally accepted descriptive terminology for the histologic typing of intestinal neoplasms of the anal region (1,2). According to their terminology, "The anal canal is defined as the terminal part of the large intestine, beginning at the upper surface of the anorectal ring and passing through the pelvic floor at the anus. The lower part extends from the dentate line and downwards to the anal verge" (1). This is essentially the "surgical anal canal." The perianal skin (the anal margin) is defined by the appearance of skin appendages (such as hairs). There exists no generally accepted definition of its outer limit (1). Some authors defined the lateral or distal extent of the perianal skin as 5 to 6 cm from the anal verge (3,4). This definition is in contrast to many series in the literature that use the dentate line as the dividing line describing the anal canal as the area above the dentate line, and the anal margin as the area below the dentate line (5–9). Numerous other reports never define the landmarks.

The area above the dentate line up to the anorectal ring (the first 6–10 mm referred to as the transitional zone) has primarily cephalad lymphatic drainage via the superior rectal lymphatics to the inferior mesenteric nodes. It also has lesser drainage laterally along both the middle rectal vessels and inferior rectal vessels through the ischioanal fossa to the internal iliac nodes. Lymphatic drainage from the anal canal below the dentate line drains to the inguinal nodes. However, secondary drainage can follow the inferior rectal lymphatics to the ischioanal nodes and internal iliac nodes, and along the superior rectal nodes (see Fig. 20B in Chapter 1). Lymphatic drainage of the perianal skin is entirely to the inguinal nodes.

The new edition of the WHO classification, which is similar to the American Joint Committee on Cancer (AJCC), has started to emerge but probably will take years before it is widely used and becomes standardized. Until then, a meaningful comparison of the anal carcinoma presented in different reports in the literature is difficult.

WHO also recommends that the generic term "squamous carcinoma" be used for all subtypes of anal squamous cell (1).

INCIDENCE

In 2001, the new cases of anal carcinomas (anus, anal canal, and anorectum) in the United States was estimated at 3500 cases (2000 female, 1500 male). It accounted for 2.6% of carcinomas of the large bowel (10). In 2005, the new cases of anal carcinomas was estimated at 3990 cases (2240 female, 1750 male). It accounted for 2.7% of carcinomas of the large bowel (11).

If it is accepted that the anal canal extends from the anorectal ring to the anal verge, as defined by WHO, 85% of anal carcinomas arise in the anal canal (12). The mean age of the patient at presentation varies from 58 to 67 years, and the age range is wide: 64 years of age and older, 58%; 45 to 64 years, 37%; and 25 to 44 years, 5%. Anal canal carcinomas show a marked female predominance, with the female-to-male ratio proximately 5:1. However, in areas with a large proportion of male patients at high-risk, the female-to-male ratio may approach 1:1. In contrast, perianal carcinomas are more common in men, with a male-to-female ratio approximately 4:1 (12).

In the United States, the incidence of squamous carcinoma of the anal canal and perianal skin in homosexual men has been estimated to be 11 to 34 times higher than the general male population. Human immunodeficiency virus (HIV)–infected homosexual men appear to be at particular risk. Other factors strongly associated with anal squamous carcinoma include the number of sexual partners, receptive anal intercourse, coexistence of sexually transmitted diseases, history of cervical, vulvar, or vaginal carcinoma, and use of immunosuppression after solid-organ transplantation (1,13).

ETIOLOGY AND PATHOGENESIS

There is strong evidence that human papilloma virus (HPV) infection causes anal carcinoma in a manner that closely parallels the role of HPV infection in the genesis of cervical carcinoma (14,15). Evidence supporting this observation includes the fact that many patients have simultaneous anal and genital viral infections and share common demographic characteristics, including an increased number of sexual partners. Furthermore, both anal and cervical carcinomas are associated with the specific "high-risk" HPV genotypes 16 and 18 (16–18).

Over 60 different HPV genotypes have been identified, approximately 20 of which are known to infect the anogenital region. HPV types 6 and 11 are generally associated with benign lesions such as warts and a low-grade anal intraepithelial neoplasia (AIN) that rarely progress to carcinoma. In contrast, HPV types 16, 18, 31, 33, 34, and 35 are most commonly associated with high-grade dysplastic AIN, carcinoma in situ, and carcinoma of anus and cervix. HPV-6 and -11 are maintained as extrachromosomal episomes, whereas HPV-16 and HPV-18 are integrated into host DNA, thus explaining the different propensity to initiate the development of carcinoma (16,19).

The study by Palmer et al. (17), examining patients with invasive squamous-cell carcinoma of the anus, demonstrated that the majority of lesions in these patients contained HPV 16 and -18 DNA, which is confined to the nuclei of carcinoma cells and is predominantly integrated into the host cell DNA. Their study showed that none of the 56 control samples examined and none of the four nonsquamous cell primary anal malignancies contained any detectable HPV DNA. These observations add considerable weight to the concept of a specific association between HPV-16 and -18 and the development of anal squamous cell carcinoma. The observation that six of seven carcinomas of the upper anal canal contained HPV-16 or -18 DNA while only 8 of 18 carcinomas of the lower anal canal contained HPV-16 or -18 DNA is of interest because the epithelium of the transitional zone of the anal canal has both embryonic and histologic similarities with the transitional zone of the cervix. This study has also demonstrated a significant relationship between the absence of keratin and the presence of HPV DNA. The authors noted that all six carcinomas containing HPV-16 or -18 arising in the anal canal were nonkeratinizing. In contrast, only one of eight heavily keratinized lesions arising in the anal canal below the dentate line contained HPV-16 or -18 DNA. It is possible that these observations indicate a predilection of HPV-16 and -18 for the environment of the less stable epithelium of the upper anal canal rather than the modified skin of the lower anal canal. None of the cases of anal adenocarcinoma contains HPV-16 or -18 DNA (18,20).

Immunocompromised patients such as those with renal transplantation, cardiac allograft recipients, and patients with carcinoma after chemotherapy have increased risk of HPV infection and increased progression to anal squamous cell carcinoma (21,22). They occur at a younger age, are multifocal, persistent, recurrent, and progress rapidly. Approximately 50% of patients positive for HIV have detectable HPV DNA (12). Penn (23) noted 65 anogenital (anal canal, perianal skin, or external genitalia) carcinomas in 2150 renal transplant recipients occurring an average of seven years after transplantation. Two-thirds of the patients were women and one-third men. These patients were much younger than those with similar malignancies in the general population, with the average age of 37 years for women and 45 years for men. Generally, the carcinomas are varieties of squamous cell carcinomas. Thirty two percent of the neoplasms are in situ lesions. Such carcinomas are biologically aggressive despite being histologically low grade. A study by Gervaz et al. (24) on molecular biology of squamous cell carcinoma of the anus between HIV-positive and HIV-negative patients revealed that allelic imbalance on chromosomes 17p, 18q, and 5q differ markedly. The data also demonstrated that DCC and p53 mutations were not required for anal squamous cell carcinoma progression in HIV-positive patients. These data suggest that immunosuppression may promote anal squamous cell carcinoma progression through an alternate pathway and that persistence of HPV infection within the anal canal may play a central role in this process.

In a study on anal squamous cell carcinoma, 47% of patients have a positive history for genital warts. In patients without a history of warts, the carcinoma is associated with a history of gonorrhea, herpes simplex type II virus, and *Chlamydia trachomatis*. Smoking is also a substantial risk factor (25).

Anal intercourse itself does not carry an increased risk of anal squamous carcinomas. Rather, anal sex at young age carries an increased risk. However, most men and women with anal squamous carcinoma do not engage in anal sex. Thus, if HPV is truly a causative agent in anal squamous carcinoma, other modes of transmission to the anal area should be considered (18). Current evidence suggests that the etiology of anal carcinoma is a multifactorial interaction between environmental factors, HPV infection, immune status, and suppressive genes (12).

STAGING

The prognosis for survival in anal carcinoma deteriorates as the primary carcinoma enlarges. It worsens when the carcinoma metastasizes to the regional lymph nodes and to extrapelvic sites (26). Unlike carcinoma of the colon and rectum, the Dukes staging system is irrelevant because part of the lymphatic drainage is in the inguinal region and is outside the extent of the resection. The tumor, node, metastases (TNM) classification system has been proposed. It is important to note that the most recent edition of WHO standards, and the unified AJCC, introduced major changes in the staging of the primary carcinoma. T category is now determined by the largest diameter of the primary carcinoma measured in centimeters. Formerly, it was necessary to estimate clinically the circumferential extent of the anal carcinoma and whether the external sphincter was invaded. The current TNM system is explained in Box 1 (1).

The best means of staging anal carcinoma remains a careful examination and, if necessary, under general anesthesia, supplemented by endorectal ultrasonography, computed tomography (CT), or magnetic resonance imaging (MRI) scanning. These procedures enable good biopsies to be taken and an appropriate decision to be made on the best mode of treatment. If the patient receives radiotherapy (RT) or chemoradiotherapy (CHT), further staging should be carried out eight weeks later to assess the results of treatment (27).

SCREENING FOR ANAL CARCINOMA PRECURSORS

For many years, the approach used to prevent cervical carcinoma has relied on the identification and treatment of cervical intraepithelial neoplasia before its progression to invasive carcinoma. Typically, women are screened at regular intervals using cervical cytology. Women with abnormal results are referred for colposcopy, to permit visualization of the lesion, and biopsy, to precisely ascertain the level of the disease. Based on the biologic similarity between anal and cervical carcinomas and their respective precursors, similar methods might be used to identify the potential anal carcinoma precursors (28).

WHO SHOULD BE SCREENED?

Screening should be considered in the high risk group: (i) a history of homosexual activity in men and/or a history of receptive anal intercourse; (ii) all HIV-positive women, regardless of whether or not they have engaged in anal intercourse; (iii) all women with high-grade cervical or vulvar lesions or carcinoma (29).

In homosexual and bisexual men, Goldie et al. (30) found that screening every two or three years for anal squamous intraepithelial lesions with anal cytology would provide life-expectancy benefits comparable to other accepted preventive health measures, and would be cost effective.

TECHNIQUE OF SCREENING CYTOLOGY TEST

Because it is easy to perform and is relatively inexpensive, cytology remains the screening test of choice. A Cytette brush (Fig. 9 in Chapter 11) is moistened in saline solution or tap water , is rotated on the perianal skin for 10–20 revolutions with firm pressure abrading cells from the area. In the anal canal, very few AIN lesions occur solely in the transitional zone. The cytological preparation should be taken from the anal verge and lower anal canal only, to avoid fecal contamination in the smears. The brush is then smeared across a glass slide and the smear is fixed for standard fixative for Papanicoloau staining. When properly performed, the sensitivity and specificity is over 95% on the presence or absence of abnormal cells (31).

Abnormal anal cytologic results should prompt anoscopic assessment, preferably with magnification and after application of 3% or 5% acetic acid. The identification of one or more well-demarcated lesions that appear white after application of 3% or 5% acetic acid and demonstrate features of vascular punctuation, leukoplakia, papillations, or other topographic irregularities should be biopsied, if (31,32) there is no contraindication, such as a bleeding disorder (29,30).

WHAT TO DO WHEN THE BIOPSIES ARE POSITIVE

Only patients with high-grade AIN should be treated. This approach is based primarily on experience accumulated in natural history studies of cervical intraepithelial neoplasia that suggest that the majority of low-grade lesions regress spontaneously. Currently, it is most often treated with electrocautery or excisional biopsy. Low-grade AIN should be followed by a repeat screening cytology in three to six months (33).

Screening HIV-positive homosexual and bisexual men for anal intraepithelial lesions and squamous cell carcinoma with anal Pap tests offers quality-adjusted life-expectancy benefits at a cost comparable with other accepted clinical preventive interventions (30).

HUMAN PAPILLOMA VIRUS TYPE 16 VACCINE

HPV-16 is most commonly linked with cancer, because it is present in 50% of cervical carcinomas and high-grade cervical intraepithelial neoplasias and in 25% of low-grade cervical intraepithelial neoplasias. A vaccine that prevents

BOX 1 ■ TNM Cancer Staging System

Anal Canal

Primary Carcinoma (T)

Tis	Carcinoma in situ
T0	No evidence of primary carcinoma
T1	Carcinoma 2 cm or less in greatest dimension
T2	Carcinoma more than 2 cm but not more than 5 cm in greatest dimension
T3	Carcinoma more than 5 cm in greatest dimension
T4	Carcinoma of any size invading adjacent organ(s) (e.g., vagina, urethra, bladder); involvement of the sphincter muscle(s) alone is not classified as T4
TX	Primary carcinoma cannot be assessed

Regional Lymph Node(s) (N)

N0	No regional lymph node metastasis
N1	Metastasis in perirectal lymph node(s)
N2	Metastasis in unilateral internal iliac and/or inguinal lymph node(s)
N3	Metastasis in perirectal and inguinal lymph nodes and/or bilateral internal iliac and/or inguinal lymph nodes
NX	Regional lymph nodes cannot be assessed

Distant Metastasis (M)

M0	No distant metastasis
M1	Distant metastasis
MX	Presence of distant metastasis cannot be assessed

Stage Grouping

Stage 0	Tis	N0	M0
Stage I	T1	N0	M0
Stage II	T2	N0	M0
	T3	N0	M0
Stage IIIA	T1-3	N1	M0
	T4	N0	M0
Stage IIIB	T4	N1	M0
	Any T	N2	M0
	Any T	N3	M0
Stage IV	Any T	Any N	M1

Histopathologic Grade (G)

G1	Well differentiated
G2	Moderately differentiated
G3	Poorly differentiated
G4	Undifferentiated
GX	Grade cannot be assessed

Perianal Skin

Primary Carcinoma (T)

T0	No evidence of primary carcinoma
Tis	Carcinoma in situ
T1	Carcinoma 2 cm or less in greatest dimension
T2	Carcinoma more than 2 cm but not more than 5 cm in greatest dimension
T3	Carcinoma more than 5 cm in greatest dimension
T4	Carcinoma invades deep extradermal structure (e.g., cartilage, skeletal muscle, or bone)
TX	Primary carcinoma cannot be assessed

Regional Lymph Node(s) (N)

N0	No lymph node metastasis
N1	Regional lymph node metastasis
NX	Regional lymph nodes cannot be assessed

Distant Metastasis (M)

M0	No distant metastasis
M1	Distant metastasis
MX	Presence of distant metastasis cannot be assessed

Stage Grouping

Stage 0	Tis	N0	M0
Stage I	T1	N0	M0
Stage II	T2–4	N0	M0
Stage III	T4	N0	M0
	Any T	N1	M0
	Any T	Any N	M1

Histopathologic Grade (G)

G1	Well differentiated
G2	Moderately differentiated
G3	Poorly differentiated
G4	Undifferentiated
GX	Grade cannot be assessed

Source: Modified from Ref. 2.

persistent HPV-16 infection could substantially reduce the incidence of cervical carcinoma (34).

In a double-blind study conducted by Koutsky et al. (34), 2392 young women were randomly assigned to receive three doses of placebo or HPV-16 virus-like particle vaccine given at day 0, month 2, and month 6. Genital samples to test for HPV-16 DNA were obtained at enrollment, one month after the third vaccination, and every six months thereafter. Women were referred for colposcopy according to a protocol. Biopsy tissue was evaluated for cervical intraepithelial neoplasia and analyzed for HPV-16 DNA. The primary end point was persistent HPV-16 infection. The primary analysis was limited to women who were negative for HPV-16 DNA and HPV-16 antibodies at enrollment and HPV-16 DNA at month 7.

The women were followed for a median of 17.4 months after completing the vaccination regimen. The incidence of persistent HPV-16 infection was 3.8 per 100 women-years in the placebo group and 0 per 100 ($p < 0.001$) in the vaccine group. All nine cases of HPV-16-related cervical intraepithelial neoplasia occurred among the placebo recipients. The authors concluded that immunizing HPV-16–negative women may reduce their risk of cervical carcinoma but caution that a larger study is required to prove that clinical disease is prevented by vaccination. Its efficacy should also be similar for people with anal HPV-16 and AIN.

If it becomes available, a vaccine to control HPV-16 infection will require universal immunization as opposed to the targeting of "high-risk" persons. Because these are sexually acquired pathogens, immunizing persons before they become sexually experienced will afford the greatest benefit (35).

PERIANAL NEOPLASMS (ANAL MARGIN)

■ ANAL INTRAEPITHELIAL NEOPLASIA (AIN) OF PERIANAL SKIN (BOWEN'S DISEASE)

High-grade AIN of perianal skin is synonymous with the old term perianal Bowen's disease because of their indistinguishable histologic and immunohistochemical features (32). Bowen (36) described an intraepidermal squamous cell carcinoma (carcinoma in situ) in 1912 as a chronic atypical epithelial proliferation.

The term anal canal intraepithelial neoplasia was proposed by Fenger and Nielsen in 1986 (37). Fenger, in 1990 (38) used the term perianal skin intraepithelial neoplasia in lieu of perianal Bowen's disease. Most authors at the present time regard only high-grade AIN as Bowen's disease, which is mostly caused by HPV-16 and -18, in contrast to low-grade AIN which is mostly caused by HPV-6 and -11 (32,39,40). Scholefield et al. (41) found that high-grade AIN had a relatively low potential for malignant transformation in immunocompetent patients.

The natural history of perianal AIN is unknown (42). Most data came from the study of HPV infection. Results from cross-sectional analyses before the era of highly active antiretroviral therapy (HAART) show that nearly all HIV-positive men as well as a substantial proportion of HIV-negative homosexual men harbor the infection (29).

Whether perianal Bowen's disease has higher incidence of malignancy in other organs, particularly internal organs, than the normal population is not clear. Although the studies by Arbesman and Ransohoff (43) and Chute et al. (44) found no increased subsequent risk of internal malignancy, these studies were on Bowen's disease of the skin in general and not perianal Bowen's disease. A survey by Marfing et al. (45) among members of the American Society of Colon and Rectal Surgery in 1987 yielded 106 cases of perianal Bowen's disease. There were two cases of carcinoma of the colon and one case of carcinoma of the anus. Morganthaler et al. (46) reviewed 167 cases (age 34–56 yrs) of perianal Bowen's disease in the literature; there were 31 (19%) associated carcinomas (not limited to internal organs) diagnosed concomitant or after treatment for the perianal Bowen's disease, with a following of one to five years. Morganthaler et al. (46), in the series of 25 patients treated for perianal Bowen's disease, found that five patients (20%) developed malignancy (one sigmoid carcinoma, four carcinoma of the vulva) during the average follow-up of four to seven years. It appears that perianal Bowen's disease has significant associated malignancies, in spite of a relatively young age.

Clinical Features

Grossly, high-grade perianal AIN or Bowen's disease appear as discrete, erythematous, occasionally pigmented,

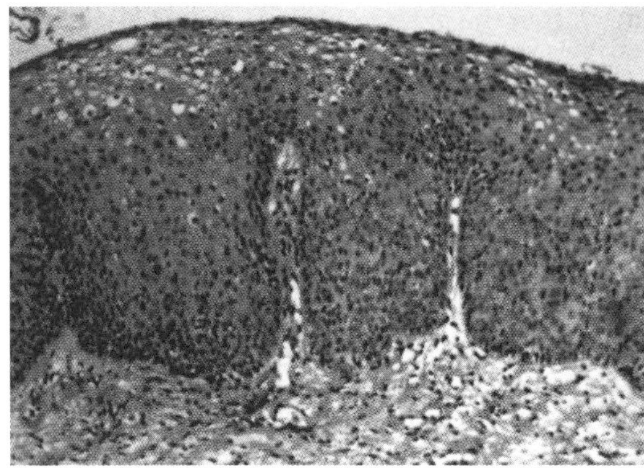

FIGURE 1 ■ Bowen's disease. Note atypical epithelial cells involving full thickness of the epidermis.

noninfiltrating, scaly, or crusted plaques, which sometimes have a moist surface. Foci of ulceration indicate that an invasive carcinoma has developed. Patients may complain of itching, which often is intense, burning, or spotted bleeding, but only a biopsy will confirm the diagnosis. In a series by Marchesa et al. (47), 25.5% of the cases of perianal Bowen's disease were incidental findings, diagnosed after pathologic evaluation of tissue removed from different perianal diseases.

The histologic picture is that of in situ squamous cell carcinoma that may have characteristic bowenoid cells, which are multinucleated giant cells with some vacuolization, giving a "halo" effect (Fig. 1).

Diagnosis

Perianal high-grade AIN can involve perianal skin, anal verge, anoderm, and vulvar. A circumferential involvement of the disease is common (48). Although the gross lesions can be biopsied, their boundary and extent cannot be ascertained. This problem can be overcome by painting the anal canal, perianal region, and in women, including the vulva, with 3% or 5% acetic acid. The abnormal skin and mucosa will be demarcated by whitening of the tissue that should be biopsied. Chang and Welton (32) performed the examination in the operating room under sedation and perianal block. They examined the painted tissue through the operating microscope attached to a real-time video display. Changes in the vascular pattern suggestive of high-grade dysplasia are identified. The same tissue is then painted with Lugol's solution (10% iodine). High-grade AIN does not take up the iodine solution because of the lack of glycogen in the dysplastic cells and they appear yellow or tan, whereas normal tissue or low-grade AIN appears dark brown or black. Lesions suspicious for high-grade AIN are biopsied.

Treatment

Treatment of Bowen's disease or high-grade AIN has changed dramatically. Although the natural history of high-grade AIN is still not known, recent information has played an important role in the current management. High-grade AIN is preinvasive and requires further management. At the time of surgical treatment, 2–28% of patients already have an invasive squamous cell carcinoma (40,47,48). It is well known that the extent of the disease is usually beyond the gross demarcation of the lesion and can only be detected microscopically. Preoperative mappings were used in the past but were plagued with residual disease (39,47,48). Currently, the biopsies are performed with the aid of staining the perianal skin, perineum, and anal canal with 3% or 5% acetic acid (31,32). For low-grade AIN, treatment is not necessary if it is asymptomatic, but the patients should be followed periodically.

There are several options on the treatment of high-grade AIN.

Application of Imiquimod

Imiquimod (Aldara, 3M Pharmaceuticals, St. Paul, Minnesota, U.S.A.) is an immune response modifier with potent antiviral and antitumor activity in animal models. It was approved by the FDA in 1997 for topical treatment of external genital and perianal warts in adults (49). The topical application has also been used for other skin conditions such as basal cell carcinoma, vulva intraepithelial neoplasms, invasive squamous cell carcinoma of skin, herpes simplex virus, and others, with excellent results (44–46). Pehoushek and Smith (50) reported treating an HIV-positive patient with squamous cell carcinoma in situ of perianal skin and the anal canal, with a combination of 5% Imiquimod cream three times a week combined with 5% fluorouracil daily with complete remission of the disease, and had no recurrence after a three-month follow-up. Imiquimod should be used as a preliminary treatment for perianal high-grade AIN (51,52).

Imiquimod is formulated as 5% cream packaged as one box of 12 single-used sachets, each containing 250 mg of cream to cover an area of 20 cm^2. A thin layer should be rubbed in until the cream is no longer visible. The application site should not be occluded. The recommended dosage is three times a week on nonconsecutive days (e.g., Monday, Wednesday, and Friday) at night for up to 16 weeks (49,53).

Most patients tolerate the treatment well. Systemic reactions are rare but may cause fatigue, fever, influenza-like symptoms, headache, diarrhea, nausea, and myalgia. Local reactions are uncommon for applications of three times a week. It may cause itching, burning, and pain at the site of the application (49). In order to minimize local reactions and yet not compromising the therapeutic effects, Chen and Shumack (54) recommended application of Imiquimod three times weekly for three weeks, followed by a rest period of four weeks, to be repeated as necessary. The rest period allows any local skin reactions to subside.

Local application of Imiquimod to a variety of skin diseases is safe and effective but it is new for perianal high-grade AIN. It remains to be seen whether it will become the treatment of choice; the prospect is promising.

Topical 5-Fluorouracil

Topical 5% 5-fluorouracil (5-FU) therapy has been found to be a safe and effective method to treat anal Bowen's disease. Graham et al. (55) conducted a prospective study in 11 patients over a 6-year period. For one-half circumferential disease or greater, patients underwent topical 5% 5-FU therapy for 16 weeks. For smaller involvement, wide surgical excision was performed. All patients underwent anal mapping biopsy one year after the completion of therapy. Of 11 patients, 8 (5 male) received 16 weeks of topical 5% 5-FU therapy. Three patients (3 female) underwent surgical excision for localized disease. All but one patient who was HIV-positive were free of Bowen's disease one year after completion of therapy. One patient underwent total excision of a residual microinvasive squamous carcinoma after circumferential Bowen's disease had resolved. One patient received 8 additional weeks of topical 5-FU therapy for incomplete resolution. All patients were followed yearly, with a mean follow-up of 39 months and the range of 12 to 74 months, and there have been no recurrences. There were no long-term side effects or morbidity from topical 5-FU.

Cautery Ablation

High-grade AIN is still benign and may take a long time to become malignant. Ablation, particularly in extensive disease, is attractive because it is less morbid than an extensive excision. One disadvantage of ablation is the lack of tissue diagnosis and an invasive carcinoma can be overlooked. Cautery ablation is the most convenient because it is available in every operating room compared to cryosurgery or laser vaporization. It should be performed with the aid of acetic acid painting to visualize the extent of the margins. The cauterization should not be too deep to cause a chronic unhealed wound. A circumferential involvement of the disease may require a staging ablation about three months apart to avoid anal stricture. Another drawback of cautery ablation is the findings that high-grade AIN has also the skin appendage involvement: 57% of hair follicles, 16% of sebaceous glands, and 25% of sweat glands (56). These structures can be missed by the cautery ablation.

The most recent advancement in the treatment of high-grade AIN is the use of high-resolution anoscopy (32,57). In this way, change in the vascular pattern suggestive of high-grade dysplasia can be identified. The procedure is performed under 3% acetic acid and Lugol's solution painting to delineate the site of the high-grade lesions. The suspicious lesions are biopsied and ablated with electrocautery.

Using this technique, Chang and Welton (32) have treated over 400 patients. There were no recurrences among HIV-negative patients after 42 months but in the HIV-positive patient group, there was a projected 100% recurrence rate by the end of 60 months. The postoperative pain was significant in half of all patients. There was no sphincter dysfunction or anal stenosis.

High-resolution anoscopy is new to colorectal surgeons and probably will become more popular in its use. Berry et al. (57) recommended, ".... the technique is not particularly difficult to learn, but requires a level of clinical experience. It is important to perform high-resolution anoscopy on a large number of patients with the disease to learn the clinical pathologic correlations that signify high-grade squamous intraepithelial lesions, and potential areas of invasion. We recommend that interested providers first take an introductory colposcopy course. Providers should become familiar with the basics of colposcopy and be able to recognize and distinguish epithelial and vascular changes that are hallmarks of high-grade squamous intraepithelial lesions. To do high-resolution anoscopy well, individuals must be thoroughly trained. It is unlikely that without some training in the basics of colposcopy, one can simply decide to use an operating microscope and recognize the changes that distinguish anal squamous intraepithelial lesions."

As good as it appears, high-resolution anoscopy is not available in most operating rooms and it is not cost effective to buy one to use in a practice that has low volume of this disease.

Excision

A survey of management of perianal Bowen's disease among members of the American Society of Colon and Rectal Surgeons as recent as the year 2000 showed that 87% of the 663 respondents chose a wide local excision as the treatment of choice for a lesion larger than 3 cm (58). This approach has now been challenged because of high residual and recurrence rates, even when mapping biopsies have been used. Marchesa et al. (47) reported a recurrence rate of 34% in 41 patients who underwent local excision, with a median follow-up of 104 months. Samiento et al. (48), in a series of 19 patients, had a recurrence rate of 31% at five-year follow-up. Brown et al. (40) had histologic evidence of incomplete excision at the initial operation in 56% of 34 patients, and the recurrence rate of 40% with a median follow-up of 41 months. Morgenthaler et al. (46), in a series of studies, found that a clear margin was obtained in 23 of the 25 patients (92%), and the recurrence rate was 12% at three years' follow-up; they gave credit for this relatively low residual and recurrence rate to aggressive mapping biopsies and wide margin of excision.

Mapping with the application of 3% or 5% acetic acid followed by Lugol's solution may help to determine the extent of involvement of the disease more accurately. Even with this, if the skin still harbors the HPV, a recurrence can occur later.

For an extensive involvement of the perianal skin, a circumferential excision should include the anoderm up to the dentate line because of its frequent involvement of the disease especially in HIV-positive patients (51). In this situation, V–Y island subcutaneous skin flaps can be performed with good results and avoid the use of a split-thickness skin graft (59).

Evidence now has shown that wide excision of high-grade AIN of perianal area does not preclude a high recurrence rate, even with negative margins. This is partly because it is difficult to accurately determine the margin of the disease, and because the remaining perianal skin may still harbor HPV, especially HPV-16 and -18. Wide excision of perianal skin and anal canal also has high complications, particularly anal stricture, ectropion, and fecal incontinence; some of these patients require a colostomy or a loop ileostomy (39,59).

In a patient who is found to have a high-grade AIN in a routine hemorrhoidectomy specimen or other anorectal procedures, it is necessary to reexamine the area when the wound has had time to heal. Occasionally an invasive lesion is underreported and a persistent ulcerated area two months after the original procedure should lead to rebiopsy of the area. If the area has healed fully, a thorough inspection of the rest of the anogenital region should identify any remaining severely dysplastic lesions, and should be treated accordingly (60).

SUMMARY ■ The management of perianal high-grade AIN or perianal Bowen's disease has changed from the standard, "surgical excision of high-grade AIN remains the treatment of choice" (56) to a more conservative, "close observation with regular biopsy of any suspicious areas to exclude invasive malignancy may be a better treatment option and is the policy currently advocated in this unit" (40). Unless there is an invasive carcinoma, it is reasonable to apply Imiquimod (51) or topical 5-FU (52) as an initial treatment. An alternative option may be cautery ablation. Surgical excision, especially an extensive one, should be reserved for patients with symptomatic disease such as untreatable itching, burning, or crusting of the skin (51). A long-term follow-up is essential because the skin may harbor the virus that perpetuates the disease. Subsequent development of malignancies in other organs should be kept in mind.

■ SQUAMOUS CELL CARCINOMA

General Considerations

Squamous cell carcinomas of the perianal skin resemble those occurring in skin elsewhere in the body. Grossly, they typically have rolled, everted edges with central ulceration (Fig. 2). Any chronic unhealed ulcer should be considered a potential squamous cell carcinoma until proven otherwise by biopsy. Squamous cell carcinomas vary in size from as small as <1 cm to large masses that completely surround and obstruct the anal orifice. The average age of the patient is between 62 and 70 years with a male-to-female ratio approximately equal (61,62).

Clinical Features

Despite their surface location, squamous cell carcinomas are usually diagnosed late; more than 50% of cases are detected more than 24 months after the onset of symptoms (63). The carcinoma is often discovered at a late stage

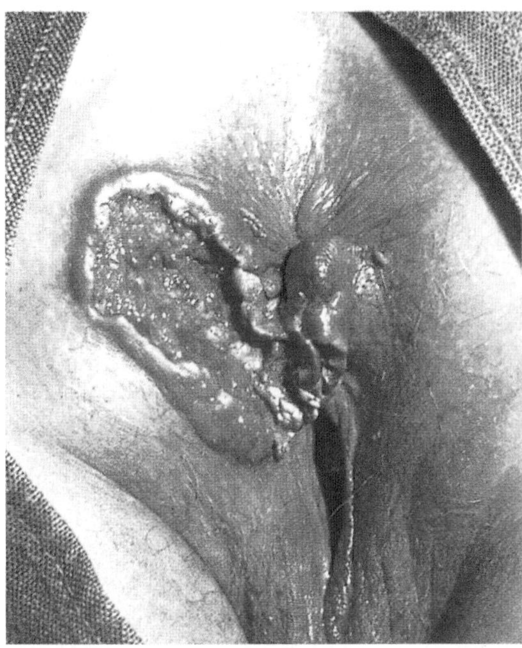

FIGURE 2 ■ Gross appearance of squamous cell carcinoma with rolled everted edges and central ulceration.

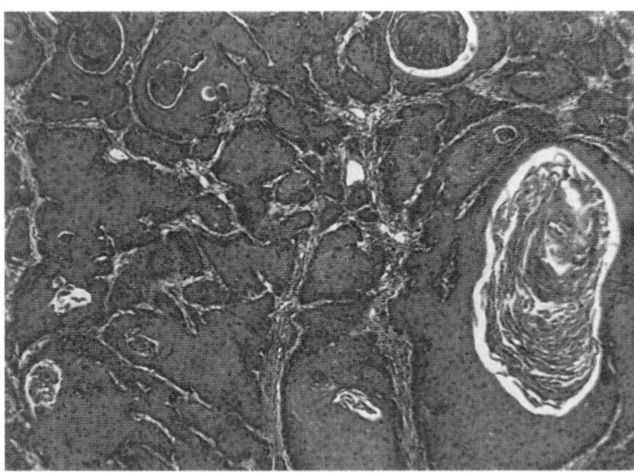

FIGURE 3 ■ Histologic appearance of squamous cell carcinoma. Note the keratinization.

measuring 5 cm or larger in diameter (62). The usual presentations are a lump, bleeding, pain, discharge, and itching (61). On rare occasions, squamous cell carcinoma presents as a perianal abscess (64). Up to 28% of patients with perianal squamous cell carcinoma are misdiagnosed as having hemorrhoids, an anal fissure, an anal fistula, atopic eczema, an anorectal abscess, or a benign neoplasm (4).

Histologically, these carcinomas are usually well differentiated, with well-developed patterns of keratinization (Fig. 3). Local invasion occurs, but the carcinoma is typically slow growing. Lymphatic spread from these carcinomas is directed mainly to the inguinal lymph nodes.

Treatment

There are only a few articles in the literature devoted to perianal squamous cell carcinoma, and it is five times less common than squamous cell carcinoma of the anal canal (62). Only a handful of authors clearly define the perianal region according to the WHO and the AJCC standards.

The treatment of perianal squamous cell carcinoma varies widely among different institutions. One common finding is clear. In advanced cases, local excision and abdominoperineal resection (APR) have high failure rates because of local recurrence, inguinal node metastasis, and distant metastasis (62,65,66).

Wide local excision has remained the cornerstone of the treatment of perianal squamous cell carcinoma, but only in properly selected cases. For in situ or microinvasive carcinoma, local excision has a 100% cure rate (61,67). For superficial well-differentiated or moderately well-differentiated squamous cell carcinoma up to 3 to 4 cm in diameter, Cummings (3) of Princess Margaret Hospital in Toronto has shifted away from radiation therapy toward local excision, supplemented with a skin graft when necessary, provided that the operation is not anticipated to interfere with anal sphincter function. Cummings reasons, "Although severe damage is infrequent following radiation, chronic irritation of the perianal skin and varying degrees of dysfunction of the anal region are common and can be troublesome" (3). For other less favorable lesions, he recommends chemoradiation. Most authors deliver 40 to 70 Gy (62,65,66,68). Chemoradiation has also been shown to be superior to radiation alone in nonrandomized studies (3). Residual or recurrent carcinoma after radiation can be treated with local excision or an APR. Prophylactic radiation to the groin is also recommended, particularly for T2 and T3 lesions (62,66).

In a series of 54 patients who received radiation with or without chemotherapy, Papillon and Chassard (62) achieved a cancer-specific five-year survival rate of 80%. The five- and ten-year cancer-specific survival rates of 86% and 77%, respectively, were reported by Touboul et al. (66) in a series of 17 patients. The size of the carcinoma determined the patient's survival. In that study, 5- and 10-year survival rates for T1 lesions were 100% and 100%, respectively, compared to 60% and 40% for T2 lesions, respectively (4). With proper technique, serious complications from radiation therapy are uncommon. Radionecrosis and fecal incontinence have been claimed to occur only in a few patients (66).

■ PERIANAL PAGET'S DISEASE

General Considerations

Perianal Paget's disease is an intraepithelial neoplasm of the perianal skin. In 1874, Sir James Paget first described this disease in relation to the nipple of the female breast (69). George Thin, in 1881, was the first to describe the cytologic features of Paget's cells, which appeared microscopically as large rounded cells with abundant pale-staining cytoplasm and a large nucleus that is often displaced to the periphery of the cell (70). The first case of perianal Paget's disease was reported by Darier and Couillaud in 1893 (71). Extramammary Paget's disease may be found in the axilla and the anogenital region (labia majora, penis, scrotum, groin, pubic area, perineum, perianal region, thigh, and buttock).

The histogenesis of perianal Paget's disease is not fully understood, but ultrastructural and immunohistochemical studies have helped to clarify the debate. In contrast to Paget's disease of the nipple, which is invariably associated with an underlying invasive or in situ ductal adenocarcinoma, perianal Paget's disease starts out as a benign neoplasm. It may eventually become invasive and give rise to an adenocarcinoma. The immunohistochemical studies show that, in general, Paget's cells stain positive for apocrine cells and in most cases stain negative for colorectal goblet cells (72). Unfortunately, many of the markers expressed by perianal Paget's cells are also expressed by signet ring cell carcinoma of the anorectum (72). However, staining that is negative for all except a marker for anorectal goblet cells almost certainly indicates a spread of Paget's cells from an anorectal mucinous adenocarcinoma. Most authors agree with the concept that Paget's cells are of glandular and probably of apocrine origin (73–75). An alternative hypothesis implicating pluripotential intraepidermal cells cannot be excluded, but the evidence for such a histogenesis is lacking (73).

Clinical Features

Perianal Paget's disease is an uncommon condition that is most commonly found in elderly people with an average age of 66 years. From 1963 to 1995, there have been 194 cases reported in the literature (76). The lesions appear as a slowly enlarging erythematous, eczematous, and often sharply demarcated perianal skin rash that may ooze or scale and is usually accompanied by pruritus. It is normally located outside the anal canal but may extend up to the level of the dentate line. Because of its similarity to other perianal conditions such as idiopathic pruritus ani, hidradenitis suppurativa, condyloma acuminatum, Crohn's disease, Bowen's disease, and epidermoid carcinoma, the diagnosis of perianal Paget's disease is often delayed because of clinical diagnostic error. In almost one-third of the cases in a series by Jensen et al. (77), the lesion involved the entire circumference of the anus.

Diagnosis

The diagnosis must be confirmed by biopsy and by identification of the characteristic Paget's cells through histologic examination (Fig. 4). Paget's cells contain a mucoprotein (sialomucin) which stains with periodic acid-Schiff, and cytokeratin (CK) 7, CK20 immunohistochemical staining (78–80). True Paget's disease of the perianal skin must not be confused with the downward intraepidermal spread of a signet-ring cell carcinoma of the rectum or with Bowen's disease of the perianal skin. Immunohistochemistry for CK7 and CK20 can differentiate between the true perianal Paget's disease and the downward spread of anorectal adenocarcinoma (pagetoid) (76–78). In general, H&E staining is sufficient to diagnose perianal Paget's disease and distinguish it from the grossly similar appearance of perianal Bowen's disease (79).

A complete large bowel investigation with emphasis on thorough examination of the rectum and anal canal should be performed. The coexistence of visceral carcinomas is well known, with an incidence of about 50% (76).

Treatment

In the absence of invasive carcinoma, wide excision is the treatment of choice. A small lesion (< 25% of perianal area or anus) can be excised with the wound left open. Larger defects should be closed with a skin flap. Obtaining an adequate microscopically clear margin is important. Because perianal Paget's disease may extend beyond the gross margin of the lesion, mapping the extent of involvement by obtaining multiple biopsies at least 1 cm from the edge of the lesion in all four quadrants, including the dentate line, the anal verge, and the perineum, is essential (76).

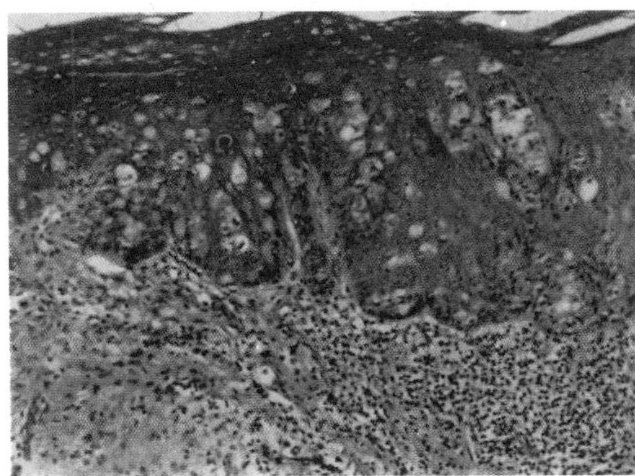

FIGURE 4 ■ Perianal Paget's disease. Paget's cells are found just above the basal layer.

A Case of Circumferential Perianal Paget's Disease

A 65-year-old woman with perianal Paget's disease was prepared for a wide excision (Fig. 5A). The skin about 2 cm from the gross lesion was marked, and multiple small excisional biopsies showed no disease and thus became the lateral extent of the excision. The entire lesion was excised deep to the subcutaneous tissue. The proximal extent of the excision was at the dentate line (Fig. 5B). With the patient in prone position, a V sliding flap was created on each side of the wound. To accommodate the flap into the anal canal, a tongue of skin was excised at the base of each flap (shaded areas in Fig. 5C). The final flaps looked like an arrowhead (Fig. 5D). The flaps were slid into the anal canal and sutured to the mucosa of the anal canal all around, using interrupted 4–0 synthetic monofilament sutures (Fig. 5E). The skin was closed with interrupted subcuticular sutures of the same material in a Y fashion (Fig. 5F). No drain was placed. The same patient is shown 8 years after the operation (Fig. 5G).

The patient should be prepared with the same bowel preparation and antibiotics administered before a colon resection. The results of a circumferential excision of the perianal skin and the anal canal, with bilateral V–Y island flaps are satisfactory. Of the 15 patients undergoing this technique (not all patients had perianal Paget's disease) reported by Hassan et al. (59), none of them had flap loss or infection. Most complications were minor, including superficial wound separation, flap hematoma, and anal stricture. None of the patients had significant fecal incontinences at the time of follow-up, average 45 months. Perineal wound pain was a problem and five of the 15 patients required a diverting ileostomy or colostomy.

Radiation therapy may be an option for perianal Paget's disease. In an extensive review of literature by Brown et al. (81) they had difficulty to confirm or refute the benefit of this mode of treatment. This was because of the rarity of the disease; many were treated for recurrence after a surgical excision, or reserved for the medically unfit patients, lack of standardization, and techniques of radiation therapy. Nevertheless, in a limited cumulative series of nine patients of perianal Paget's disease without invasive carcinoma treated with radiation or chemoradiation, two patients had recurrences at two years and six years. They believed that radiation therapy could be an alternative treatment for noninvasive Paget's disease that has an extensive involvement to require an APR, and for patients who cannot tolerate a general anesthesia. A recurrence after local excision can also be successfully treated with radiation.

Prognosis

In a patient with noninvasive Paget's disease, the lesion can be cured by wide local excision, although recurrence is high. The recurrence can be reexcised. Long-term follow-up is essential to detect local recurrence and development of invasive Paget's disease or intercurrent invasive carcinoma of the rectum and anal canal (82–84). A patient with invasive perianal Paget's disease has a poor prognosis despite APR, and in most cases, distant metastasis has already occurred at the time of diagnosis (56). Adjuvant chemoradiation does not seem to help (81).

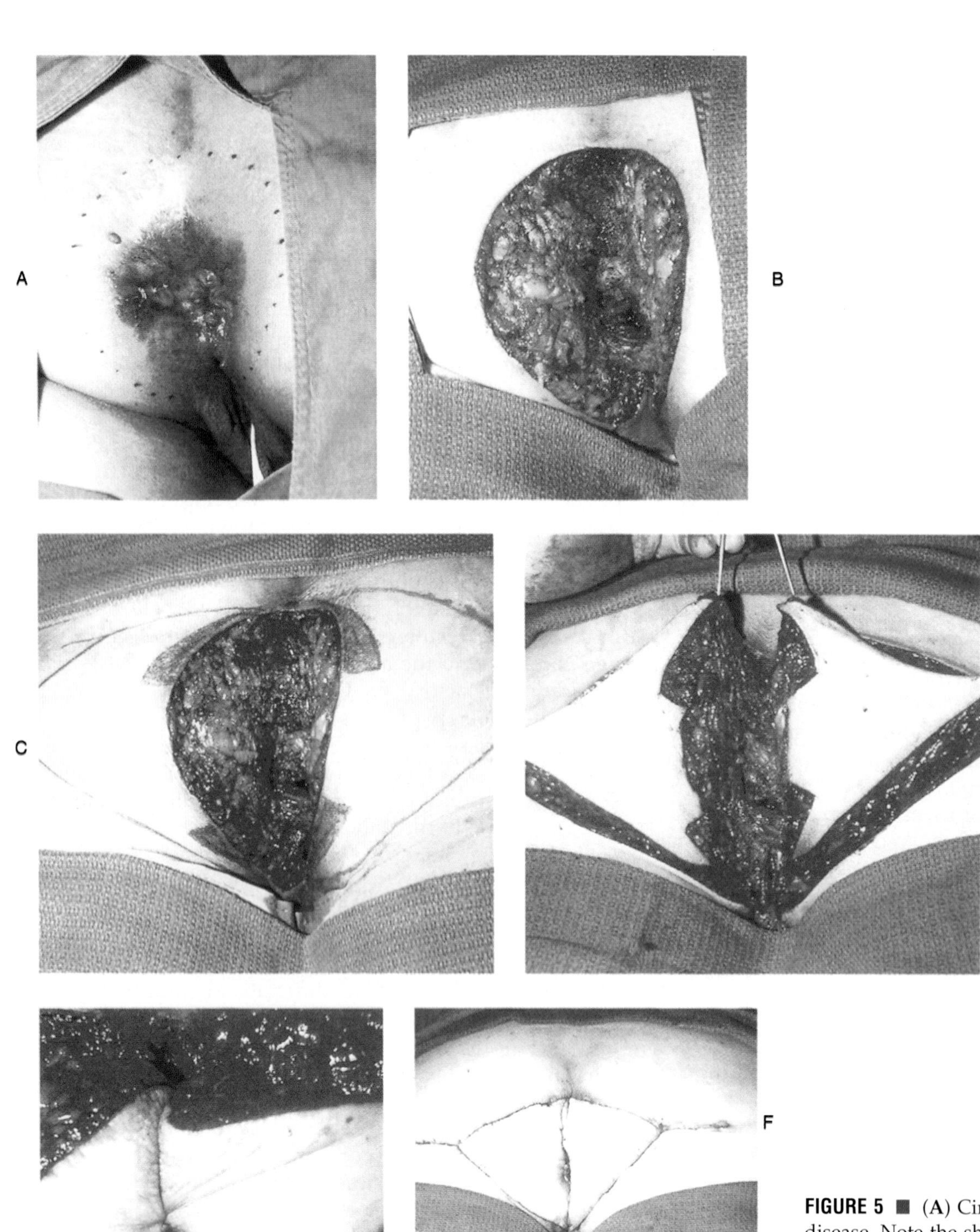

FIGURE 5 ■ (**A**) Circumferential perianal Paget's disease. Note the sharply demarcated erythematous and eczematous skin rash. The dotted line marks the extent of the excision. (**B**) Excision deep to subcutaneous fat was made up to the dentate line. (**C**) V flaps were outlined. Shaded areas were tongues of skin to be excised to accommodate the flaps into the anal canal. (**D**) Sliding flaps were deep down to subcutaneous fat. Note the arrowhead shape of the flaps. (**E**) Note accommodation of the flaps into the anal canal. (**F**) The Y-shaped flaps at completion. (**G**) Ten months after operation. The patient experienced no fecal incontinence and there had been no recurrence after 8 years of follow-up.

■ BASAL CELL CARCINOMA

General Considerations

Basal cell carcinomas of the perianal skin are rare. The Mayo Clinic has listed only 20 patients with this type of neoplasm in the 20 year period ending in 1996 (85). This type of carcinoma occurs more frequently in men than in women, usually appearing in the sixth decade. The etiology is unknown but the most consistent factor was an association with basal cell carcinoma on other cutaneous sites (33% of patients) in the series reported by Paterson et al. (85).

Clinical Features

Basal cell carcinomas are usually 1 to 2 cm in diameter and are localized to the perianal skin, although a large lesion may extend into the anal canal. Grossly, they are similar to cutaneous basal cell carcinomas found elsewhere in the body and are characterized by a central ulceration with irregular and raised edges. These carcinomas remain superficial and mobile and rarely metastasize. Histologically, they are similar to basal cell carcinomas of the skin elsewhere (Fig. 6). They are of long duration, have a low invasive potential, and must be distinguished from squamous cell carcinoma, which have an entirely different origin and behavior.

In the study by Nielsen and Jensen (86), almost one-third of patients with basal cell carcinoma of the anal margin were misdiagnosed as having hemorrhoids, an anal fissure, or perianal eczema. The median delay in treatment caused by an erroneous diagnosis was eight months.

Treatment and Prognosis

Local excision with adequate margins is the treatment of choice for patients with basal cell carcinoma. Local recurrence after local excision is common and accounted for 29% of patients in a series of 27 patients reported on by Nielsen and Jensen (86); they recommend reexcision as treatment. Abdominoperineal resection and radiation therapy are reserved for large lesions. The five-year survival rate in the series by Nielsen and Jensen was 73%, but no patients died as the result of the basal cell carcinoma. In the series reported by Paterson et al. (85), no recurrence or death, occurred from perianal basal cell carcinoma after local excision; however, none of the patients had an invasive carcinoma.

A novel approach is the use of topical Imiquimod 5% cream (Aldara®), an immune response modifier that induces cytokines related to cell-mediated immune response. In the multicenter phase II dose–response open-label trial (87) for small (<2 cm^2) noninvasive basal cell carcinoma of the head, neck, trunk, or limbs, the cream was applied for six weeks, followed by an excision for histologic examination. The complete response was achieved in 100%, 88%, 73%, and 70% for the application of twice daily, daily, three times a week, and daily three times a week, respectively.

All of the patients developed local skin reactions with erythema occurring most often and they were dose-related.

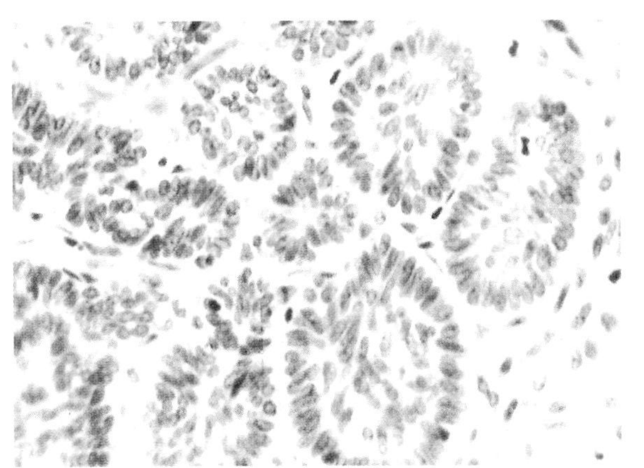

FIGURE 6 ■ Basal cell carcinoma.

In the twice-daily group, all the local skin reactions were assessed as severe in two-thirds of the patients, some of whom had vesicles, ulcerations, and excoriations. However, only one patient of the total of 99 entered the study discontinued because of a medication-related skin reaction at the site of application.

Whether this approach can be used for a large or invasive basal cell carcinoma is not known. It is possible to apply it to the basal cell carcinoma of the perianal skin.

■ VERRUCOUS CARCINOMA

Although there is no universal agreement, there is a growing consensus of opinion that the entity that has been termed a "giant condyloma acuminatum" or a "Buschke–Löwenstein tumor" represents a verrucous carcinoma. Similar to anal warts, verrucous carcinoma is associated with HPV-6 and -11. These lesions typically present as large (8 × 8 cm), slow growing, painful, wart-like growths that are relatively soft and have a cauliflower-like appearance. The lesions may arise in the perianal skin, anal canal, or distal rectum and are frequently indistinguishable from condylomata acuminata. Although they are histologically benign, their behavior is clinically malignant. The clinical course of these lesions is one of relentless progression and expansion of the neoplasm by extensive erosion and pressure necrosis of surrounding tissues with invasion of the ischioanal fossa, perirectal tissues, and even the pelvic cavity. The invasive nature of these lesions may cause multiple sinuses or fistulous tracts, which may invade fascia, muscle, or the rectum and may cause inflammation, infection, and hemorrhage. The extent of involvement can be precisely determined by CT examination. Microscopically, the lesions bear a marked resemblance to condylomata acuminata with papillary proliferation, keratinization, acanthosis, parakeratosis, and vacuolization of superficial layers. Metastasis from these tumors has not been reported to date (88,89).

The basic treatment is wide local excision. If the carcinoma involves the anal sphincters, an APR should be performed. At the present time, there have been no reports regarding the use of multimodality therapy in the treatment of verrucous carcinoma, but such consideration may obviate the need for radical extirpative surgery. Squamous cell carcinoma associated with condyloma acuminatum has been treated effectively with chemoradiation. The difference in the two entities may only be one of nomenclature (88,89).

As an alternative treatment, particularly in unfit patients, Heinzerling et al. (90) reported a successful treatment with Imiquimod followed by CO_2 laser ablation. In this case, 5% Imiquimod was applied to the lesion three times a week and from the second week on once daily. After six weeks of treatment, the persisting residual diseases were removed by CO_2 laser under local anesthesia. To prevent recurrences, treatment with Imiquimod was continued for six weeks after the laser vaporization.

NEOPLASMS OF THE ANAL CANAL

■ ANAL CANAL INTRAEPITHELIAL NEOPLASIA

AIN of the anal canal locates in the anal transitional zone as well as the anoderm below the dentate line. AIN of the anal canal has been found in minor surgical specimens such as hemorrhoidectomy, as well as in females with vulvar and cervical neoplasm. There is considerable evidence that AIN of the anal canal is the precursor of anal canal carcinoma, and possibly has a more aggressive behavior than perianal AIN (38). Similar to perianal AIN, the diagnosis should be confirmed by biopsy, using 3% or 5% acetic acid and Lugol's solution staining as a guide (31,32).

The treatment should be a cautery ablation or local excision. For an extensive involvement of the anoderm, it should be done in stages to avoid anal stricture. AIN of the anal canal found incidentally in hemorrhoidectomy requires no further treatment provided the rest of the anal canal has no high-grade AIN (91); a periodic follow-up with acetic acid staining is indicated.

Using electrocautery ablation directed by high-resolution anoscopy, Chang et al. (92) reported 79% recurrence in HIV-positive patients, with a mean time recurrence of 12 months compared with zero recurrence in HIV-negative patients.

■ SQUAMOUS CELL CARCINOMA

This general category encompasses a number of different microscopic appearances, including large-cell keratinizing, large-cell nonkeratinizing (transitional), and basaloid (Fig. 7). The term "cloacogenic" carcinoma has been used especially for the basaloid and large-cell nonkeratinizing (transitional) forms of squamous carcinoma. Keratinizing squamous cell carcinomas are rare in the anal canal above the dentate line. Mucoepidermoid carcinoma is extremely rare, if it exists at all in this site. Previously reported examples probably represent squamous cell carcinoma with mucinous microcysts (Fig. 8). When carcinomas contain a mixture of cell types, they should be classified according to the appearance that predominates (1). Because of their similar response to treatment, it is reasonable to group them together as squamous cell carcinoma. To comply with the WHO and the AJCC terminology (1,2), we use the term squamous cell carcinoma instead of epidermoid carcinoma.

Clinical Manifestations

The presentation of squamous cell carcinomas generally follows a long history of minor perianal problems, such as bleeding, which occurs in approximately 50% of the

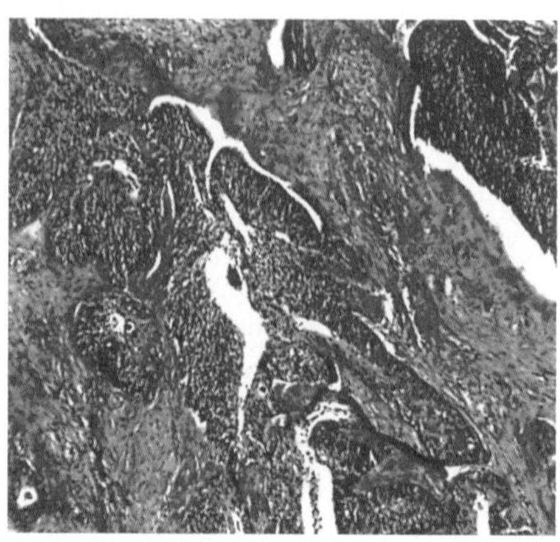

FIGURE 7 ■ Basaloid (cloacogenic) carcinoma. Note the nonkeratinization.

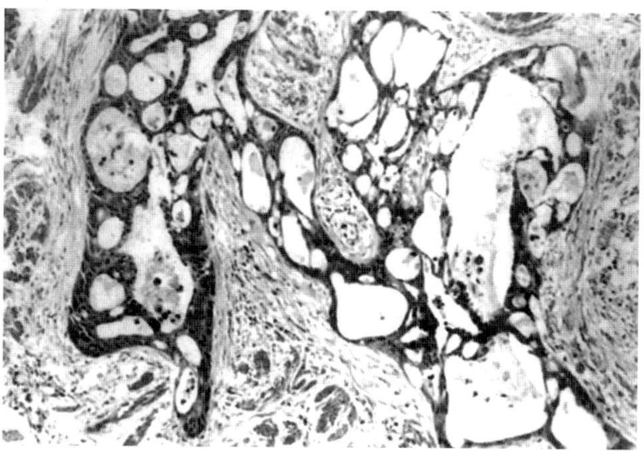

FIGURE 8 ■ Squamous cell carcinoma of anal canal with mucinous microcysts. This is not a mucoepidermoid carcinoma. *Source*: From Ref. 93.

patients (61,94,95). Other signs and symptoms include pruritus, discharge, pain, and an indurated anal mass. Discharge, incontinence, change in bowel habit, pelvic pain, and anovaginal fistula suggest advanced lesions with involvement of the anal sphincter. Almost one-third of the patients in the series study by Stearns and Quan (94) were initially incorrectly diagnosed as having benign or inflammatory disease.

Diagnosis and Workup

The most important part of diagnosis is digital examination of the anal canal. The size, consistency, and fixation of the primary lesion and the presence or absence of pararectal lymph nodes can be determined. Proctoscopy should be done to confirm the digital findings, and the exact location of the neoplasm in relationship to the dentate line should be documented. Biopsy via proctoscope or transanal excision of the neoplasm must be done to determine the histologic type of the carcinoma, thus enabling an appropriate recommendation for treatment. A colonoscopic examination should be done to rule out more proximal associated lesions. Endorectal ultrasonography is useful in evaluating the depth of invasion and detection of lymph node metastasis.

Both groins must be examined carefully to detect any enlargement of lymph nodes. Enlarged or suspicious lymph nodes in the groin area should be assessed by excision or biopsy because inguinal lymphadenopathy caused by reactive hyperplasia is common.

Character of Squamous Cell Carcinoma of Anal Canal

Even though squamous cell carcinoma of the anal canal is within the easy reach of a finger, the carcinoma is seldom diagnosed early. In a series from the Mayo Clinic, 88% of the carcinomas had already invaded beyond the mucosa before diagnosis (96). In approximately 50% of the cases, the carcinoma has penetrated the bowel wall or the perianal skin. Invasion of the vaginal septum is more common than involvement of the prostate or urethra. Extensive carcinoma may invade the muscular or bony walls of the pelvis (97).

The anal canal has extensive lymphatic pathways. If the carcinoma is situated above the dentate line, metastases are found along the superior rectal vessels; if the carcinoma is at the dentate line, the lymphatic drainage is toward the internal pudendal, hypogastric, and obturator nodes; and if the carcinoma is below the dentate line, the lymphatic drainage is via the inguinal nodes. A study of lymph node metastasis of carcinoma of the anal canal has been conducted by Wade et al. (98), who used a clearing technique. Their results showed that 44% of the lymph node metastases were found in lymph nodes measuring < 5 mm in diameter. Analysis of maps of lymph nodes allowed these authors to observe that most lymph nodes were located above the peritoneal reflection and were scant in perianal zones.

Review articles by Cummings (97) revealed that inguinal metastases are found in 15% to 20% of patients at the time of diagnosis and become apparent later in an additional 10% to 25%. The risk of lymphatic metastases is correlated with the depth of the invasion, the size, and the histologic grade. Nodal metastases are present in 30% of the patients when the smooth muscle is infiltrated and in 58% when the infiltration is beyond the external sphincters. Boman et al. (96) found nodal metastases in only 3% of squamous cell carcinomas < 2 cm in diameter but in 25% to 35% of all the larger squamous cell carcinomas. The data from 1973 to 1998 in the Surveillance Epidemiology and End Results (SEER) cancer registry showed the prevalence by stage was localized in 53%, regional in 38%, and distant in 9% (13).

Treatment

Local Excision

This form of therapy should be reserved for early carcinomas or the well-differentiated type that have invaded only the submucosa.

Review of literature reveals that the recurrence rate after local excision is 20% to 78% and the five-year survival rate is 45% to 85% (88,99). However, properly selected, local excision can be highly successful. Of 188 patients with squamous cell carcinoma of the anal canal treated at the Mayo Clinic, 13 patients with a superficially invasive carcinoma and ≤ 2 cm in size were selected for local excision. Although one required an APR for local recurrence, all were cured at a follow-up of five or more years (96). In the series from St. Mark's Hospital, 8 of 145 patients with squamous cell carcinoma of the anal canal were treated by local excision. The cancer-specific five-year survival rate was 100% (8). In general, mobile lesions ≤ 2 cm are suitable for local excision.

Abdominoperineal Resection

In the past, APR with wide excision of perineal tissue formed the basis of treatment (3). Despite this aggressive approach, the results have been disappointing. The local recurrence rate is 27% to 50% and the five-year survival rate ranges from 24% to 62%, with a perioperative mortality rate of 2% to 6% (88). An APR is no longer the primary treatment for invasive squamous cell carcinoma of the anal canal. APR is reserved for those patients who cannot tolerate the chemoradiation and is the primary treatment for failed chemoradiation.

To improve long-term survival and to save some patients from having a colostomy, use of APR as the primary treatment for squamous carcinoma has been challenged by the use of combined modality therapy.

Chemoradiation Regimen

In 1974, Nigro et al. (100) initially attempted giving preoperative 5-FU with mitomycin C (MMC) and radiation in the management of squamous cell carcinoma of the anal canal to enhance the effectiveness of the operation. An APR was performed four to six weeks after the radiation therapy. Subsequently, they found that most of the surgical specimens contained no residual carcinoma. Nigro (9) then dropped the mandatory APR and instead excised the scar for histologic examination. Patients whose carcinoma grossly disappeared after the chemoradiation treatment required no further operation. Nigro's subsequent regime of the chemoradiation is on the accompanying box. It should be noted that currently the dosage used for radiation varies among different practitioners. Review of the literature via MEDLINE search by Sato et al. (102) on the management of carcinoma of the anal canal showed that chemoradiotherapy with 5-FU and MMC was superior in local control, colostomy-free rate, progressive-free survival, and carcinoma-specific survival compared with radiation alone.

Nigro's Chemoradiation Therapy

External Irradiation

- 3000 rads to the primary carcinoma and pelvic and inguinal nodes; start—day 1 (200 rads/day) (101)

Systemic Chemotherapy

- 5-FU 1000 mg/m^2/24 hr as a continuous infusion for four days; start—day 1
- Mitomycin C, 15 mg/m^2 as an intravenous bolus; start—day 1 only
- 5-FU, repeat four-day infusion; start—day 28

There have been questions regarding whether concomitant chemotherapy has the advantage over radiation alone, and whether MMC, which is toxic, is necessary. There were three well-conducted trials to test these questions.

The Radiation Therapy Oncology Group and the Eastern Cooperative Oncology Group trial (103) studied the efficacy of MMC added to 5-FU and radiation. Of 291 assessable patients, 145 received 45 to 50.4 Gy pelvic radiation therapy plus 5-FU; 146 received radiation therapy, 5-FU, and MMC. Patients with residual disease on posttreatment biopsy were treated with a salvage regimen that consisted of additional pelvic radiation therapy (9 Gy), 5-FU, and Cisplatin.

Posttreatment biopsies were positive in 15% of patients in the 5-FU arm versus 7.7% in MMC arm ($p = 0.135$). At four years' follow-up, colostomy rates were lower (9% vs. 22%, $p = 0.002$), colostomy-free survival higher (71% vs. 59%, $p = 0.014$) and disease-free survival higher (75% vs. 51%, $p = 0.0003$) in MMC arm. However, a significant difference in overall survival was not observed at four years.

Toxicity was greater in the MMC arm (23% vs. 7%, Grade 4 and 5 toxicity, $p < 0.001$).

The authors concluded that despite greater toxicity, the use of MMC in a chemoradiation regime for squamous cell carcinoma of the anal canal was justified, particularly in patients with large primary carcinoma. Salvage chemoradiation should be attempted in patients with residual disease following definitive chemoradiation before resorting to radical surgery.

The United Kingdom Coordinating Committee on Cancer Research (UKCCCR) trial (104) was designed to compare combined modality (5-FU + MMC + Radiation) with radiation therapy alone in patients with anal squamous cell carcinoma. In the multicenter trial, 585 patients were randomized to receive 45 Gy RT (290 patients) or radiotherapy (RT) combined with 5-FU + MMC (295 patients). They assessed clinical response six weeks after initial treatment: good responders received a boost RT and the poor responders received a salvage surgery. The main end point was local failure rate (≥6 weeks after initial treatment); secondary end points were overall and cause-specific survival. The results showed that after a median follow-up of 42 months (range 28–62 months) 59% radiation alone group had a local failure compared with 36% of combined modality group. This gave a 46% reduction in the risk of local failure in the patients receiving combined modality (relative risk 0.54, 95% CI 0.2–0.69, $p < 0.0001$). The risk of death from anal canal was also reduced in the combined modality therapy arm (0.71, 0.53–0.95, $p = 0.02$). There was no overall survival advantage (0.86, 0.67–1.11, $p = 0.25$).

Early morbidity was significantly more frequent in the combined modality arm ($p = 0.03$), but late morbidity occurred at similar rates.

They concluded that the standard treatment for most patients with anal squamous cell carcinoma should be a combination of RT and infused 5-FU and MMC, with surgery reserved for those who failed this regimen.

The European Organization for Research and Treatment of Cancer Radiotherapy and Gastrointestinal Cooperative Groups was a prospective randomized trial to validate the use of concomitant RT and chemotherapy in the treatment of squamous cell carcinoma of the anus (105).

The study included 103 patients randomized between RT alone ($n = 51$) and a combination of RT and chemotherapy (5-FU continuous infusion + MMC, $n = 51$). The patients had T3-T4 N0-N3 or T1-T2 N1-N3 squamous cell carcinoma of the anus. The radiation dosage was 45 Gy.

The results showed that at five-year follow-up, the addition of chemotherapy to radiation therapy resulted in a significant increase in the complete remission rate from 54% for RT alone to 80% for chemoradiation therapy, and from 85% to 96%, respectively, if results are considered after surgical resections. Local recurrence improved by 18% while colostomy-free rate increased by 32% in the chemoradiation group. Event-free survival, defined as free of local recurrence, no colostomy, and no severe side effects or death, showed significant improvement in favor of the chemoradiation group ($p = 0.03$). The overall survival rates remained similar in both treatment arms.

Summary of the three randomized trials is in Table 1.

Currently, most investigators recommend combined modality treatment with continuous course radiation (45 Gy in 1.8 Gy fractions) plus two cycles of concurrent continuous infusion 5-FU (weeks 1 and 5) plus MMC (days 1 and 29). This regimen is considered by most to be the standard of care. For patients who have T3 to T4 disease (primary tumors, greater than 5 cm), it is reasonable to provide a radiation boost with an additional 5.4 to 9.0 Gy (106). Doses up to 66 to 70 Gy may be needed to treat patients with radiation alone (107).

The average results of chemoradiation regimen include a complete response rate of 84% (81–87%), a local control rate of 73% (64–86%) and a five-year survival rate of 77% (66–92%). For patients who have T1 to T2 disease, the complete response rates are more than 90%. In patients who have T3 to T4 disease, approximately 50% will require a salvage APR. If they achieve a complete response following completion of combined modality therapy, only 25% will require a salvage APR (106).

An example of chemoradiation treatment of squamous cell carcinoma of the anal canal is illustrated on the study by Myerson et al. (108). During 1975 to 1997, 106 patients with squamous cell carcinoma of the anal canal underwent radiation therapy. The dramatic response to low doses of radiation and concurrent chemotherapy led them to change in policy with most patients receiving chemoradiation, and surgery was reserved for salvage of persistent or recurrent disease. Since 1985, 81 patients have received definitive chemoradiation.

Doses for definitive treatment without chemotherapy were 45 to 50 Gy to the carcinoma and the regional nodes, followed by a boost to a total dose of at least 65 Gy. Substantially lower radiation doses were used with concurrent chemotherapy. A dose of 30 Gy was used for T1/T2, followed by a boost of 10 to 20 Gy (mean 16.19 Gy) and 16 to 30 Gy (mean 23.67 Gy) for T3/T4 lesions. The results of 88 patients that excluded salvage surgery showed: T1-N0 (15 cases, 93 ± 6%); T2-N0 (33 cases, 84 ± 7%); T3-N0 (16 cases, 60 ± 13%); T4-N0 (24 cases, 37 ± 12%)($p = 0.001$) (Fig. 9).

TABLE 1 ■ **Summary of Randomized Controlled Trials on Squamous Cell Carcinoma of the Anal Canal**

Reference (Yr)	Study Group	Statistically Significant	Results
103 (1996)	5-FU + radiation; $n = 145$	Yes: disease-free survival; colostomy-free survival (favoring MMC)	51% vs. 73%, disease-free survival (favoring MMC); follow-up 4 yrs
	5-FU + MMC + radiation; $n = 146$	No: overall survival	
104 (1996)	Radiation alone $n = 285$	Yes: local failure; disease-free survival (favoring chemoradiation)	46% reduction local failure; reduction death from cancer (favoring chemoradiation); follow-up 42 mos
	Radiation + 5-FU + MMC; $n = 292$	No: overall survival	
105 (1997)	Radiation alone $n = 52$	Yes: local failure; cancer-free survival (favoring chemoradiation)	80% vs. 54% complete remission; 18% improve in local recurrence; 32% increase in colostomy-free (favoring chemoradiation); follow-up 5 yrs
	Radiation + 5-FU + MMC; $n = 51$	No: overall survival	

Abbreviations: 5-FU, 5-fluorouracil; MMC, mitomycin C.

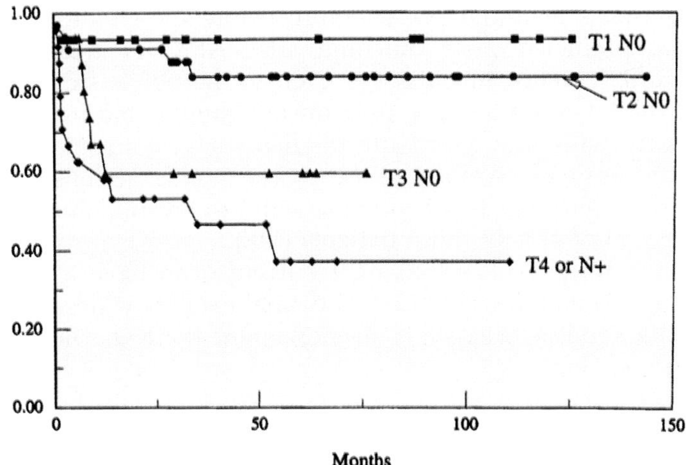

FIGURE 9 ■ Disease-free survival (Kaplan–Meier) vs. clinical stage. The contribution of surgery (planned or salvage) to the ultimate disease status is included in this figure. *Source*: From Ref. 109.

Of importance were the additional malignancies noted by Myerson et al. (108). There were a total of 33 additional malignancies in 26 patients. Nineteen of the lesions antedated the squamous carcinoma of the anal canal, and 14 postdated. Types of the malignancies are on Table 2. With exception of the two sarcomas within the radiation portals occurred 5 and 10 years after radiation without chemotherapy, the additional malignancies were not suggestive of the radiation-induced malignancy.

This information underscores the importance of complete examination in general, in addition to a diligent long-term oncologic screening in patients with squamous cell carcinoma of the anal canal (108).

Brachytherapy

Brachytherapy is an ideal method to deliver conformal radiation for anal carcinoma while sparing the surrounding healthy structures, such as small intestine and bladder. The primary concern is anal necrosis, and anal necrosis rates reportedly vary from 2% to as high as 76% (110). Although there are no randomized data, the phase II Trials suggest that, even in experienced hands, brachytherapy is associated with higher complication rates than in external beam radiation (EBR) therapy (106).

Kapp et al. (111) using brachytherapy to boost during a short split between the EBR ± chemotherapy, gave satisfactory results. The rationale of this combination was to improve tolerance of 50 Gy EBR in the pelvis, perineum, and groin. Intestinal or intraluminal brachytherapy was performed using a single high-intensity (^{192}Ir). Dose calculation for needle implants was 6 Gy. EBR was delivered with one dose 1.8 or 2.0 Gy per day, five days a week. After 30 Gy, an interstitial or intraluminal ^{192}Ir high dose-rate (HDR) boost was performed. Depending on the patient's skin reaction, EBR was resumed within one to two weeks, with an additional 20 Gy. Patients who failed to achieve a complete response received additional brachytherapy.

TABLE 2 ■ **Additional Malignancies in Patients with Squamous Cell Carcinoma of the Anal Canal**

Type	No. of Lesions
Gynecologic	9
Head and neck	6
Lung	5
Colorectal	3
Genitourinary	3
Central nervous system	2
Hematologic	2
Sarcoma	2
Breast	1
TOTAL	33

Follow-up ranged from 3 to 14 months (median 31 months). The median treatment radiation was 56 days. The five-year actuarial rates of locoregional control (LRC) and disease-specific survival (DSS) were 76% and 76%, respectively. The overall anal preservation was 77% and 97% in patients in whom LRC was achieved. Uncompromised anal function was recorded in 93% of these patients.

Although acute toxicity occurred in 89% in radiochemotherapy group and in 64% of RT alone, predominantly the triad of pronounced skin reaction, diarrhea, and nausea, none of these patients required hospitalization. Late complications that required a temporary colostomy occurred in 7.6% of the patients, for pain relief because of ulceration of the lesions.

The authors concluded that the integration of HDR brachytherapy boost in a split-course EBR regimen ± chemotherapy resulted in excellent sphincter function without an increase of severe complications and with rates of locoregional control, disease-specific survival, and cancer-free survival compared favorably with those reported in the literature.

Treatment in HIV-Positive Patients

In general, HIV-positive patients have received lower doses of radiation and chemotherapy because of poorer tolerance to therapy and increased complication rate (106,112,113).

In situ patients with CD-4 counts as low as 105 cells/mL do well with local excision. A low CD-4 count at diagnosis without HAART predicts a poor prognosis because these patients appear to succumb to their HIV status and not the anal disease (112). Even in the era of HAART and with experienced clinicians, treatment of invasive anal squamous-cell carcinoma in HIV-infected patients remains a challenge but the techniques in management will undoubtedly improve in the near future.

Currently, at the University of California, San Francisco (114), HIV-positive patients who had invasive anal squamous cell carcinoma with CD-4 counts greater than 200 cells/mm^3 were treated with CMT in a similar way to patients that were not HIV infected. Patients with CD-4 counts less than 200 cells/mm^3 were treated using more individualized approaches. In general, the dosage was kept tighter, and prophylactic radiation at nodal areas was not used. These patients had a higher rate of colostomies. Cisplatin was used instead of MMC in some cases.

Blazy et al. (115) reported their experience of treating anal canal carcinoma in the era of new antiviral drugs, in patients with HIV-positive. Nine men on highly active antiretroviral therapies with good immune status before chemoradiotherapy received concomitant chemoradiotherapy consisting of 5-FU and Cisplatinum, and high-dose RT (60–70 Gy). Six carcinomas were Stage I, two were Stage II, and one was Stage III. CD-4+ cell counts were less than

200/mL for four patients, between 200/mL and 500/mL for four, and more than 500/mL for one. All patients received the planned dose of radiation (≥60 Gy). The chemotherapy dose was reduced to 25% in six patients. The overall treatment time was 58 days. Grade III hematologic or skin toxicity occurred in four patients. No association was observed between high-grade toxicity and CD-4+ cell count. None of the patients developed opportunistic infections during follow-up. Eight patients were disease-free after a median follow-up of 33 months. Among them, four had no or minor anal function impairment at the last follow-up visit. One patient with T4-N2 disease relapsed locally one year after treatment and underwent salvage abdominoperineal excision. The authors concluded that high-dose chemoradiotherapy for anal canal carcinoma is feasible with low toxicity in HIV-positive patients, treated with highly active antiretroviral therapies.

Toxicity of Chemoradiation

Chemoradiation is not to be taken lightly. Reports of complications vary widely in the literature because they are dose and technique dependent. In general, severe complications are increased when the total dose is >40 Gy. The common complications encountered are dermatitis and mucositis, diarrhea, fecal incontinence, fatigue, bone marrow depression, cystitis, small bowel obstruction, and major arterial stenosis. Death, although very rare, has been reported (116,117).

Anorectal function was preserved in 88% of patients who underwent chemoradiation, as reported in the series of Cummings et al. (116); the dose was 45 to 55 Gy. Those with severe fecal incontinence required a colostomy. Less severe anorectal function, such as fecal urgency and occasional fecal incontinence, can be managed satisfactorily with antidiarrheal medications and the adjustment of diet. Complications of chemoradiation can be minimized by split-course radiation (116). Cisplatin has emerged as a potential replacement for mitomycin in the combination drug regimens. It is a radiation sensitizer and is less myelosuppressive than MMC. However, preliminary results showed the toxicity rate to be similar to MMC regimen (106,107).

Pattern of Failure and Treatment

The predominant sites of failure after chemoradiation are the pelvis, either the anal area or the regional lymph nodes. In a large series of 190 patients reported by Cummings et al. (116), 41% experienced recurrence at one or more sites. Of those recurrences, 62% were confined to the pelvis, 16% were outside the pelvis, and the rest occurred both inside and outside the pelvis.

Those patients with residual or recurrent carcinoma confined to the pelvis or perianal area should undergo a salvage APR with or without a booster dose of radiation. The outcome is significantly related to the extent of the disease at the time of failure. The series from Memorial Sloan-Kettering Cancer Center showed that T stage did not appear to affect survival after APR ($p=0.07$) (118). On the other hand, Nguyen et al. (119) revealed size to be the only significant factor associated with the need for a stoma ($p=0.01$), and that node positivity was the only independent predictor of mortality ($p=0.02$). Inguinal node metastasis at initial presentation, before the chemoradiation, predicted poor outcome after APR for treatment failure. Patients with disease fixed to the pelvic side wall on digital examination at the time of treatment failure fared poorly, with an eight-month median survival and no five-year survival. Among those with mobile lesions, the median survival is 40 months, with an overall five-year survival of 47% of those patients (118).

Salvage APR following recurrence can have a long-term survival rate (120,121). A dismal result was described by the series by Zelnick et al. (122) where there was no five-year survival.

Inguinal Lymph Node

Because of the high morbidity and low yield in the prevention of death from cancer, prophylactic groin dissection is not recommended (94,95).

The simultaneous appearance of inguinal metastasis is an ominous sign. In the series of Gerard et al. (123), of 270 patients with squamous cell carcinoma of the anal canal, synchronous inguinal metastasis occurred in 10%, and metachronous inguinal metastasis in 7.8%. The five-year overall survival in patients without inguinal lymph node involvement was 73% versus 54% in patients with synchronous lymph node metastasis.

For patients with synchronous lymph node metastasis, the authors recommended a unilateral lymph node dissection immediately followed by a cycle of continuous infusion of 5-FU (day 1–4) and bolus of cisplatinum (day 2–5). Radiation to the involved groin was initiated after completion of the chemotherapy. The dose of the radiation was 45 to 50 Gy over five weeks. The results showed local control of the inguinal area in 86%; the five-year overall survival was 54%.

For patients with a metastatic metachronous inguinal lymph node metastasis, the initial treatment was inguinal lymph node dissection. Irradiation started after the wound has healed, delivering 45 to 50 Gy over five weeks. No prophylactic irradiation of the contralateral inguinal area was performed. The local control of the inguinal area was observed in 68% of patients so treated and the five-year overall survival rate was 41% (123).

Whether prophylactic groin radiation should be performed is controversial. Elective radiation of clinically normal inguinal nodes reduces the risk of late node failure and carries little morbidity. Only one of 38 such patients had a late recurrence in the inguinal area after undergoing combination chemotherapy and RT (124). In series in which the inguinal nodes were not treated electively, the late nodal recurrence rate was 15% to 25% (96,125,126).

Ulmer et al. (127) evaluated the feasibility of the sentinel lymph node technique for groin metastasis of anal squamous cell carcinoma. The lesion in the anal canal was injected submucosally or subdermally with 1 mL Tc^{99m} sulfur colloid in four sites, using a 27-gauge needle and an insulin syringe. Scintigraphy was recorded with a gamma camera. Seventeen hours later, patients with detectable radiocolloid enrichment in the groin underwent lymph node biopsy guided by a handheld gamma probe. Sentinel lymph nodes were detected in 13 of 17 patients (76.5%) metastases were found in the sentinel lymph nodes of 5 of 12 biopsied patients (42%); in two patients the metastases were detected by serial sectioning or immunohistochemical staining after H&E results were negative for carcinoma. Compared with staging using ultrasonography and CT, assessment of the sentinel lymph node provides more reliable staging of inguinal lymph nodes because 44% of all lymph nodes metastasis in anal carcinoma are smaller than 5 mm in diameter (127). This technique may prove to be a valuable diagnostic workup for anal squamous cell carcinoma. Further studies are warranted.

Drugs for Metastasis

The most frequent sites of visceral metastasis include the liver, lung, bone, and subcutaneous tissues. The prognosis is poor, with a median survival of approximately nine months. Twenty percent of patients with recurrent carcinoma of the anal canal die from distant metastasis, but most carcinoma-related deaths are secondary to uncontrolled pelvic and perianal disease (128).

Drugs used to treat metastasis include 5-FU, bleomycin, methyl-CCNU, vincristine, doxorubicin, and cisplatin. Combinations of agents such as bleomycin, vincristine, or methotrexate, plus leucovorin, had also been used. All combinations had resulted in only partial responses (129). A phase III randomized study is being completed in the United Kingdom for patients who have locally advanced squamous cell carcinoma of the anal canal using different drugs and radiation, including 5-FU/MMC/radiation; 5-FU/cisplatin/radiation (107).

SUMMARY ■ Surgeons must be familiar with the anatomic landmarks of the anal canal and the perianal skin as defined by the WHO and the AJCC, as well as with TNM staging. Currently, most reports and studies use these systems.

Local excision is still the treatment of choice for carcinoma in situ or microscopic invasive carcinoma that has occurred in the anal canal or the perianal area. Unfortunately, only small numbers of the lesions are suitable for this option because most are too large or too advanced at the time of diagnosis. APR is no longer the primary treatment for invasive carcinoma of the anal canal and most perianal carcinomas. It not only has a high recurrence, but local recurrence after APR has a less favorable prognosis. It responds less favorably to chemoradiation than the primary carcinoma, as 52% of patients have persistent disease after the treatment (130). APR is reserved for local treatment failure of chemoradiation, for anorectal complications of the treatment, especially fecal incontinence, and for those patients who cannot tolerate chemoradiation. Chemoradiation, which was originally used as the primary treatment of anal canal squamous cell carcinoma, is now also applied to its counterpart in the perianal area.

■ ADENOCARCINOMA

Primary adenocarcinomas of the anus are very rare, constituting 3% to 9% of all anal carcinomas (131–133). The WHO classifies these malignancies into the rectal type, the anal glands, and those within an anorectal fistula (1).

Rectal Type

This type is the most common adenocarcinoma found in the anal canal. It arises within the upper zone lined by colorectal-type mucosa. Its histology is that of an adenocarcinoma of the large intestine. It is generally difficult or impossible to separate adenocarcinoma of the anal canal from adenocarcinoma of the lower rectum (1).

Anal Glands

The ducts of the anal glands are lined by squamous epithelium close to their opening in the crypts, by transitional epithelium more deeply, and by mucin-secreting columnar epithelium in the depth of the gland. The histologic picture of these lesions, therefore, may be one of adenocarcinoma or mucoepidermoid carcinoma. It can be differentiated from other types of anal lesions by its haphazardly dispersed, small glands with scant mucin production invading the wall of the anorectal area without an intraluminal component. The glands are positive for CK7 (134).

The most characteristic feature of anal duct carcinoma is its extramucosal adenocarcinoma without the involvement of the surface epithelium, except when the lesion has become advanced (Fig. 10). If there is a break in the surface epithelium, as is often seen clinically, greater perianal involvement or deeper infiltration may provide the only clue to the anal duct origin of these lesions. In a series of 21 patients reported by Jensen et al. (136), nine of the neoplasms were localized in the ischioanal space, seven were in the anal canal, and five were in a fistula-in-ano. Patients usually present with complaints of pain and an extra-anorectal lump, perianal induration, or a perianal abscess. Despite its distal location and its accessibility to digital examination, most anal gland and duct carcinomas are detected late. In the series by Jensen et al. (136), the median duration of symptoms before correct diagnosis was 18 months, the sensation of having a perianal mass, bleeding, pain, soiling, pruritus ani, change in bowel habits, prolapse, and weight loss were common symptoms. Like other malignancies of the anal region, most adenocarcinomas of the anus are diagnosed erroneously by physicians and surgeons, as well as by patients, with a resulting delay in the correct diagnosis. The average size of the carcinoma of the anal canal in the series by Jensen et al. (136) was 5 cm and in the perianal area was 10 cm. Sixty-two percent of the patients already had a regional or distant metastasis. Because of the late stage of the carcinoma 20 of 21 patients died within 18 months after treatment (136).

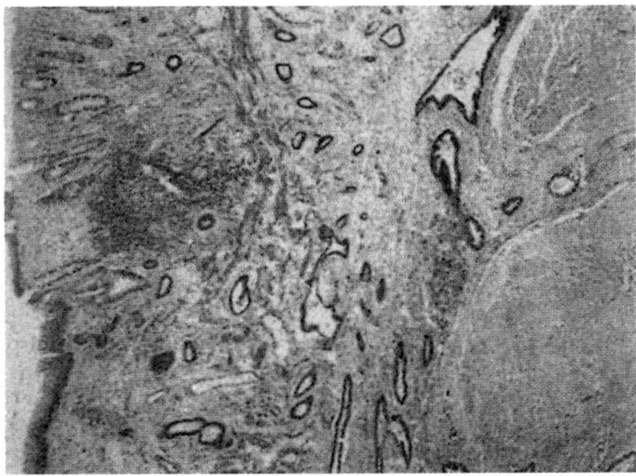

FIGURE 10 ■ Anal duct carcinoma. Note the intact epithelium. *Source*: From Ref. 135.

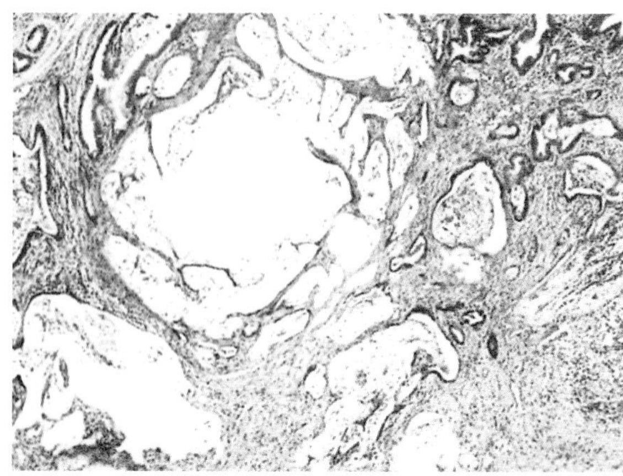

FIGURE 11 ■ Adenocarcinoma in a fistula-in-ano. Note pools of mucin. *Source*: From Ref. 135.

The primary treatment is an APR, with wide excision of the perineal part (137). The role of radiation or chemoradiation is unknown.

Anorectal Fistula

Well-differentiated mucinous adenocarcinomas (Fig. 11) occasionally develop within an anorectal fistula that may be developmental or acquired (1). Most often these carcinomas arise in patients with long-standing perianal disease, especially fistulas (138,139). Some authors believe that they originate in the anal glands and ducts (140,141).

Treatment

For a rectal type or a primary adenocarcinoma of anal canal, a wide local excision can be performed for small and well-differentiated carcinomas that have not invaded the muscular wall of the anorectum. In a multicenter study, data collected for primary adenocarcinoma of the anal canal from patients reported by Belkacemi et al. (142) included: 18 T1 (18%), 34 T2 (42%), 22 T3 (27%), and 11 T4 (13%). There were three treatment categories: radiation and surgery, 45 patients; chemoradiation, 31 patients; and APR, 6 patients.

The patients' characteristics were evenly distributed among the three groups. The results showed that recurrence occurred in 37%, 36%, and 20%, respectively, at four-year follow-up (not statistically significant). Both the overall and the disease-free five-year survival were significantly better in the chemoradiation group (Table 3). Multivariate analysis revealed four independent prognostic factors for survival: T stage, N stage, histologic grade, and treatment modality.

From this study, it is apparent that from Stage T2 onwards, the primary treatment should be chemoradiation and the APR should be reserved for salvage treatment. A small series from Memorial Sloan-Kettering Cancer Center (133) showed that 6 of 13 patients were free of disease after chemoradiation and APR, with a follow-up of 26 months. For adenocarcinomas of the anal gland or an anal fistula, the role of adjuvant therapy is not yet defined due to the uncommon disease. (143). The Nigro chemoradiation regime has been successfully used by Tarazi and Nelson (144). Of nine patients who used this protocol, six patients were free of disease on follow-up of two to four years. Papagikos et al. (145) recommended a preoperative chemoradiation followed by APR.

TABLE 3 ■ **Survival of Three Modes of Treatment of Primary Anal Canal Adenocarcinoma**

Mode of Treatment	Survival	Five Year (%)	Ten Year (%)
RT/APR	Overall	29	23
			$p = 0.02$
RT/CHT	Overall	58	39
APR	Overall	21	21
RT/APR	Disease-free	25	18
			$p = 0.038$
RT/CHT	Disease-free	54	20
APR	Disease-free	22	22

Abbreviations: RT, radiotherapy; CHT, chemotherapy; APR, abdominoperineal resection.

■ SMALL CELL CARCINOMA

This very rare carcinoma may arise in the anorectal region. It is similar in histology, behavior, and histochemistry to small-cell (oat cell) carcinoma of the lung (Fig. 12).

It is a neuroendocrine carcinoma or a Merkel cell carcinoma. The diagnosis can be confirmed by immunohistochemistry and electron microscopy. This type of lesion has been known to have early and extensive dissemination. The case presented by Paterson et al. (146) showed that a 1 cm Merkel cell carcinoma of the anal canal had already metastasized to the liver. Based on Merkel cell carcinoma of other organs, "it is extremely lymphophile; lymph node relapses occur in approximately 80% of the patients with recurrent disease" (147). Merkel cell carcinoma has been known to respond to RT (147). Whether this mode of treatment is useful for Merkel cell carcinoma of the anal canal is not known.

■ UNDIFFERENTIATED CARCINOMA

Also very rare, this type of malignant lesion has no glandular structure or other features to indicate definite differentiation (Fig. 13). Undifferentiated carcinoma may be distinguished from poorly differentiated carcinoma, small-cell carcinoma, lymphoma, or leukemic deposits by the use of mucin stains or immunohistochemical methods (1). The treatment is the same as for adenocarcinomas. The prognosis can be expected to be poor.

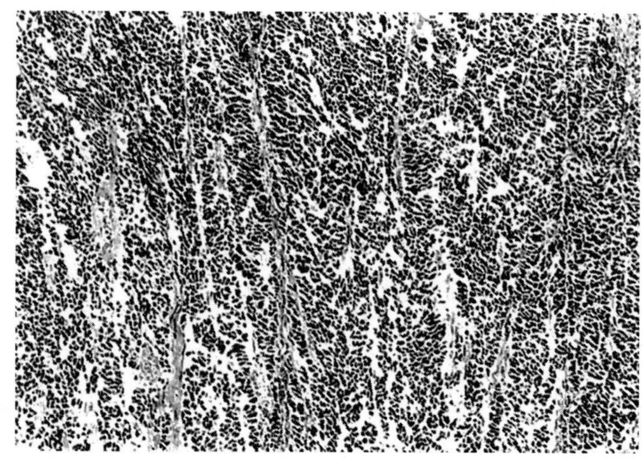

FIGURE 12 ■ Small cell carcinoma of the large intestine. *Source*: From Ref. 93.

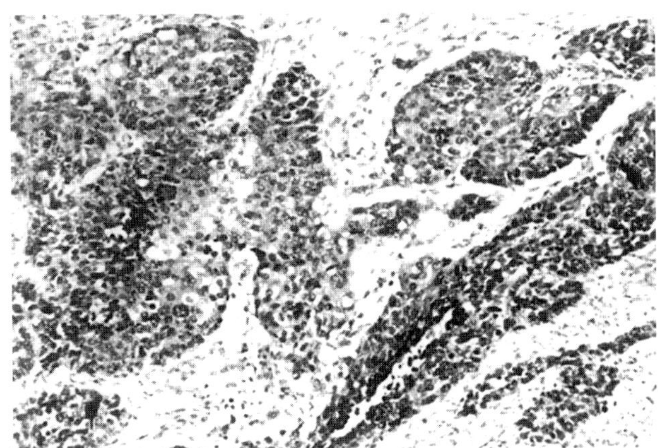

FIGURE 13 ■ Undifferentiated carcinoma of the large intestine. *Source*: From Ref. 93.

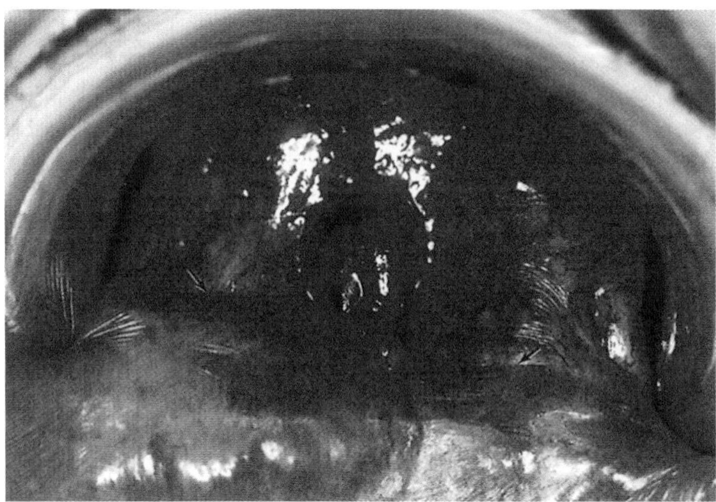

FIGURE 14 ■ Malignant melanoma of the anal canal. The arrows point at the dentate line.

■ MELANOMA

General Considerations

Malignant melanoma is the most depressing of all anorectal malignancies. It is a rare malignant neoplasm of the anorectum that constitutes 1% to 3% of all melanomas. The anal canal is the third most common site, exceeded only by the skin and eyes (148). The female-to-male ratio is approximately 2:1, and the average age at presentation is approximately 63 years (149). Evaluation of the NCI SEER data from 1973 to 1992 showed female-to-male ratio as 1.72:1. The mean age was 66 ± 16 years. Mean age by gender was lower for males (57 years) than for females (71 years; $p < 0.001$). The incidence of anorectal melanoma in young males ages between 25 and 44 years tripled in the San Francisco area when compared with all other locations (14.4 vs. 4.8 per 10 million population; $p = 0.06$). There was indirect evidence that implicated HIV infection as a risk factor (150).

Malignant melanoma arises from epithelium of the anal canal, both above and below the dentate line (151). A few reports describe these lesions as arising from, and being situated in, the rectum (152,153). Electron microscopy shows that normal melanocytes are present in the rectal mucosa (152).

Clinical Features

Rectal bleeding, a mass in the anal canal, and anorectal pain are the three most common, and most consistent signs and symptoms of malignant melanoma (149,154). Only 25% of patients have lesions < 1 cm in diameter. The remainder have melanomas as large as 6 cm in diameter, with an average size of 4 cm (153). Often the mass protrudes through the anus. Weight loss is also a common finding.

Diagnosis

Melanomas are suspected when a pigmented polypoid lesion is noted (Fig. 14). Unless an ulceration with raised edges is present, this disease may be confused with a thrombosed hemorrhoid. The majority of melanomas, however, are only lightly pigmented or nonpigmented and are often misdiagnosed as being polyps or other neoplasms of the anal canal. Between 40% and 70% of melanomas of the anal canal are amelanotic and in only 25% of the pigmented lesions is there abundant melanin (151,155). If melanin is seen on microscopic examination, then the diagnosis is simple. In the amelanotic melanoma, sheets of anaplastic cells may be misinterpreted as undifferentiated squamous cell carcinoma. The most helpful diagnostic feature is the presence of malignant cells in clusters (155). Endorectal ultrasound is useful to determine the depth of invasion and possible adjacent lymph node metastasis (156,157).

Mode of Metastasis

Anal canal melanomas have a marked tendency to spread submucosally along the rectum but rarely invade adjacent organs. Review of the literature by Cooper et al. (158) showed that 46 of 120 patients (38%) had metastasis at the time of diagnosis. Perirectal, perianal, and mesenteric lymph nodes were the most common sites of metastasis, followed by inguinal lymph nodes, liver, and lung. Widespread systemic metastases are early and rapid, most commonly to the liver, lung, and bone.

Wolff (159) raised a question whether, using thickness of the lesion similar to melanoma of the skin can be useful to determine options of treatment and prognosis.

Treatment

There is no survival benefit of adjuvant therapy for melanomas of the anal canal partly because of associated distant metastases in most patients. For the majority of cases, there appears to be no clear-cut choice of surgical treatment between a wide local excision and an APR. Both treatments yield a five-year survival between 0% and 22% (149). In the larger series reported by Brady et al. (160) of 85 cases and Thibault et al. (149) of 50 cases, the five-year survival rates were 17% and 22%, respectively. Both options of treatment have their proponents (Table 4).

Thibault et al. (149) reviewed the series from the Mayo Clinic attempting to find predictive factors of survival, including gender, size of the lesion, presence of melanin, depth of penetration, positive perirectal lymph nodes, wide local excision versus APR, and there was none. This is in contrast to the finding by Brady et al. (160) at Memorial Sloan-Kettering Cancer Center that all long-term survivals

TABLE 4 ■ Selected Series of Anal Melanoma

Author/Reference	No. of Patients	No. Curative WLE and Disease-Free at 5 Yr (%)	No. Curative Abdominoperineal Resection and Disease-Free at 5 Yr (%)	Recommended Treatment
Pessaux et al., 2004 (161)	16	11 (29%)	4 (0%)	WLE
Bullard et al., 2003 (156)	40	21 (16%)	9 (33%)	WLE
Thibault et al., 1997 (149)	50	11 (18%)	26 (19%)	WLE
Ward et al., 1996 (162)	21	3 (0%)	4 (0%)	WLE
Roumen, 1996 (163)	63	16 (13%)	18 (11%)	WLE
Brady et al., 1995 (160)	85	13 (8%)	43 (26%)	APR
Ross et al., 1990 (164)	32	12 (8%)	14 (0%)	WLE
Slingluff et al., 1990 (165)	24	7 (0%)	12 (0%)	Multimodality
Goldman et al., 1990 (166)	49	18 (6%)	15 (7%)	APR

Abbreviation: WLE, wide local excision.

occurred in women. Indeed, in their study, women with operable disease had a five-year survival rate of 29%. Although the authors recommend an APR, only one of nine patients who underwent such an operation had positive mesenteric nodes.

It appears that local control of the disease after the operation is not as much a problem as distant metastasis, which is the major cause of death (156,163). A reasonable approach is to perform local excision of the lesion, only if this can be accomplished with wide margin and full thickness without causing fecal incontinence. Otherwise, an APR should be performed. Pessaux et al. (161) reported 30 patients who underwent APR or wide local excision. Features that showed significantly better results in five-year survival included: negative inguinal node ($p = 0.031$), duration of symptoms less than three months ($p = 0.046$), Stage I versus Stage II ($p = 0.025$), nonmelanomic ($p = 0.033$). Tumor size, depth of invasion (in mm), age, gender, wide local excision versus APR, were not statistically different.

REFERENCES

1. Fenger C, Frisch M, Marti MC, Parc R. Tumors of the anal canal. Hamilton SR, Aaltonen LA, eds. WHO classification of tumors. Pathology and genetics of tumors of the digestive system. Lyon, France: International Agency for Research on Cancer (IARC), 2002:146–155.
2. Green FL, Page DL, Fleming ID, et al. American Joint Committee on Cancer. 6th ed. New York: Springer-Verlag, 2002:139–144, 231–237.
3. Cummings BJ. [Editorial]. Oncology 1996; 10:1853–1854.
4. Jensen SL, Hagen K, Shokouh-Amiri MH, Nielsen OV. Does an erroneous diagnosis of squamous-cell carcinoma of the anal canal and anal margin at first physician visit influence prognosis?. Dis Colon Rectum 1987; 30:345–351.
5. Williams GR, Talbot IC. Anal carcinoma—a histological review. Histopathology 1994; 25:507–516.
6. Brown DK, Ogelsby AB, Scott DH, Dayton MT. Squamous cell carcinoma of the anus. A twenty-five year retrospective. Am Surg 1988; 54:337–342.
7. Greenall MJ, Quan SHQ, Urmacher C, DeCosse JJ. Treatment of epidermoid carcinoma of the anal canal. Surg Gynecol Obstet 1985; 161:509–517.
8. Pintor MP, Northover JMA, Nicholls RJ. Squamous cell carcinoma of the anus at one hospital from 1948 to 1984. Br J Surg 1989; 76:806–810.
9. Nigro ND. Multidisciplinary management of cancer of the anus. World J Surg 1987; 11:446–451.
10. Bal DG. Cancer statistics 2001: quo vadis or whither goest thou? CA Cancer J Clin 2001; 51:11–14.
11. Jemal A, Tiwari RC, Murray T, et al. Cancer statistics 2005. CA Cancer J Clin 2005; 5:10–30.
12. Deans GT, McAlee JJA, Spence RAJ. Malignant anal tumors. Br J Surg 1994; 81:501–508.
13. Maggard M, Beanes SR, Ko CY. Anal canal cancer: a population-based reappraisal. Dis Colon Rectum 2003; 46:1517–1524.
14. Frisch M. On the etiology of anal squamous carcinoma. Dan Med Bull 2002; 49:194–209.
15. Chang GJ, Sheldon A, Welton ML. Epidemiology and natural history of anal HPV infection and ASIL and cancer in the general population. Semin Colon Rect Surg 2004; 15:210–214.
16. Saclarides TJ, Klem D. Genetic alterations and virology of anal cancer. Semin Colon Rectal Surg 1995; 6:131–134.
17. Palmer JG, Scholefield JH, Coates PJ, et al. Anal cancer and human papillomaviruses. Dis Colon Rectum 1989; 32:1016–1022.
18. Shroyer KR, Kim JG, Manos MM, Greer CE, Pearlman NW, Franklin WA. Papillomavirus found in anorectal squamous carcinoma, not in colon adenocarcinoma. Arch Surg 1992; 127:741–744.
19. Bjorget B, Engeland A, Luostarinen T, et al. Human papilloma virus infection as a risk factor for anal and perianal skin cancer in a prospective study. Br J Cancer 2002; 87:61–64.
20. Fisch M, Glimelius B, Van Den Brule AJ, et al. Sexually transmitted infection as a cause of anal cancer. NEJM 1997; 337:1350–1358.
21. Welton ML. Etiology of human papilloma virus infections and the development of anal squamous intraepithelial lesions. Semin Colon Rectal Surg 2004; 15:193–195.
22. Mullerat J, Northover J. Human papilloma virus and anal neoplastic lesions in the immunocompromised (Transplant) patient. Semin Colon Rectal Surg 2004; 15:215–217.
23. Penn I. Cancers of the anogenital region in renal transplant recipients. Analysis of 65 cases. Cancer 1986; 58:611–616.
24. Gervaz P, Hahnloser D, Wolff BG, et al. Molecular biology of squamous cell carcinoma of the anus: a comparison of HIV positive and HIV-negative patients. J Gastrointest Surg 2004; 8:1024–1031.
25. Noffsinger A, Witte D, Fenoglio-Preiser CM. The relationship of human papillomaviruses to anorectal neoplasia. Cancer 1992; 70:1276–1287.
26. Cummings BJ. Anal canal carcinoma. Hermanek P, Gaspodarowicz MK, Henson DE, Hutter RVP, Sobin LH, eds. Prognostic Factors in Cancer. New York: Springer, 1995:80–87.
27. Carter PS. Anal cancer—current perspectives. Dig Dis 1993; 11:239–251.
28. Welton ML, Winkler B, Darragh TM. Anal-rectal cytology and anal cancer screening. Semin Colon Rectal Surg 2004; 15:196–200.
29. Polefsky JM. Anal squamous intraepithelial lesions in human immunodeficiency virus-positive men and women. Semin Oncol 2000; 27:471–479.
30. Goldie SJ, Kuntz KM, Weinstein MC, Freedberg KA, Palefasky JM. Cost-effectiveness of screening for anal squamous intraepithelial lesions and anal cancer in human immunodeficiency virus-negative homosexual and bisexual men. Am J Med 2000; 108:634–641.
31. Sholefield JH, Johnson J, Hitchcock A, et al. Guidelines for anal cytology—to make cytological diagnosis and follow up much more reliable. Cytopathology 1998; 9:15–22.
32. Chang GJ, Welton ML. Anal neoplasia. Seminars Colon Rectal Surg 2003; 14:111–118.
33. Goldstone SE, Winkler B, Wifford LJ, Alt E, Polefsky JM. High prevalence of anal squamous intraepithelial lesions and squamous-cell carcinoma in men who have sex with men as seen in a surgical practice. Dis Colon Rectum 2001; 44:690–698.
34. Koutsky LA, Ault KA, Wheeler CM, et al. A controlled trial of a human papillomavirus type 16 vaccine. NEJM 2002; 347:1645–1651.
35. Stanberry LR. A human papillomavirus type 16 vaccine. Editorial. NEJM 2003; 348:1404.
36. Bowen JT. Precancerous dermatoses: a study of two cases of chronic atypical epithelial proliferation. J Cutan Dis 1912; 30:241–255.
37. Feuger C, Nielsen VT. Intraepithelial neoplasia in the anal canal. The appearance and relation to genital neoplasia. ACTA Pathol Microbiol Immunol Scand 1986; 94:343–349.

38. Feuger C. Intraepithelial neoplasia in the anal canal and perianal area. Curr Topic Pathol 1990; 81:91–102.
39. Halverson AL. Perianal Bowen's disease then and now: evolution of the treatment for anal high-grade intraepithelial neoplasia. Semin Colon Rectal Surg 2003; 14:213–217.
40. Brown SR, Skinner P, Tidy J, Smith JH, Sharp F, Hosie KB. Outcome after surgical resection for high-grade anal intraepithelial neoplasia (Bowen's disease). Br J Surg 1999; 86:1063–1066.
41. Scholefield JH, Castle MT, Watson NFS. Malignant transformation of high-grade anal intraepithelial neoplasia. Br J Surg 2005; 92:1133–1136.
42. Abbasakoor F, Boulos PB. Anal intraepithelial neoplasia. Br J Surg 2005; 92:277–290.
43. Arbesman H, Ransohoff DF. Is Bowen's disease a predictor for the development of internal malignancy? JAMA 1987; 257:516–518.
44. Chute CG, Chuang TY, Bergstralh EJ, Su WPD. The subsequent risk of internal cancer with Bowen's disease. JAMA 1991; 266:816–819.
45. Marfing TF, Abel ME, Gallagher DM. Perianal Bowen's disease and associated malignancies. Results of survey. Dis Colon Rectum 1987; 30:782–785.
46. Morgenthaler JA, Dietz DW, Matthew GM, Birmbaum EH, Kodner IJ, Fleshman JW. Outcomes, risk of other malignancies, and need for formal mapping procedures in patients with perianal Bowen's disease. Dis Colon Rectum 2004; 47:1655–1661.
47. Marchesa P, Fazio VW, Oliart S, Goldblum JR, Lavery IC. Perianal Bowen's disease: a clinico-pathologic study of 47 patients. Dis Colon Rectum 1997; 40:1286–1293.
48. Samiento JM, Wolff BG, Burgart LJ, Frizelle FA, Ilstrup DM. Perianal Bowen's disease. Associated tumors, human pappilloma virus, surgery, and other controversies. Dis Colon Rectum 1997; 40:912–918.
49. Gupta AK, Browne M, Bluhm R. Imiquimod: a review. J Cutan Med Surg 2002; 6:554–560.
50. Pehoushek J, Smith KJ. Imiquimod and 5% fluorouracil therapy for anal and perianal squamous cell carcinoma in situ in an HIV positive man. Arch Dermatol 2001; 137:14–16.
51. Gottesman L. [Editorial]. Dis Colon Rectum 2004; 47:1660–1661.
52. Chang LK, Gottesman L, Breen EL, Bledag R. Anal dysplasia: controversies in management. Semin Colon Rectal Surg 2004; 15:233–238.
53. Nouri K, O'Connell C, Rivas MP. Imiquimod for the treatment of Bowen's disease and invasive squamous cell carcinoma. Case J Drugs Dermatol 2003; 2:669–673.
54. Chen K, Shumack S. Treatment of Bowen's disease using a cycle regimen of imiquimod 5% cream. Clin Exp Dermatol 2003; 28(suppl):10–12.
55. Graham BD, Jetmore AB, Foote JE, Arnold LK. Topical 5-fluorouracil in the management of extensive anal Bowen's disease: a preferred approach. Dis Colon Rectum 2005; 48:444–450.
56. Skinner PP, Ogunbiyio A, Scholefield JH, et al. Skin appendage involvement in anal intraepithelial neoplasia. Br J Surg 1997; 84:675–678.
57. Berry JM, Jay N, Polefsky JM, Welton ML. State-of-the-art of high-resolution anoscopy as a tool to manage patients at risk for anal cancer. Semin Colon Rectal Surg 2004; 15:218–226.
58. Cleary RK, Schaldenbrand JD, Fowler JJ, Schuler JM, Lampman RM. The treatment options for perianal Bowen's disease: survey of American Society of Colon and Rectal Surgeons members. Am Surg 2000; 66:686–688.
59. Hassan I, Horgan AF, Nivatvongs S. V-Y island flags for repair of large perianal defects. Am J Surg 2001; 181:363–365.
60. Scholefield JH. Anal intraepithelial neoplasia. Br J Surg 1999; 86:1364–1364.
61. Beahrs OH, Wilson SM. Carcinoma of the anus. Ann Surg 1976; 184:422–428.
62. Papillon J, Chassard JL. Respective roles of radiotherapy and surgery in the management of epidermoid carcinoma of the anal margin. Dis Colon Rectum 1992; 35:422–429.
63. Moller C, Saksela E. Cancer of the anus and anal canal. Acta Chir Scand 1970; 136:340–348.
64. Nelson RL, Prasad L, Abcarian H. Anal carcinoma presenting as a perianal abscess or fistula. Arch Surg 1985; 120:632–635.
65. Fuchshuber PR, Rodriguez-Bigas M, Weber T, Peorelli NJ. Anal canal and perianal epidermoid cancers. Collective review. J Am Coll Surg 1997; 185:494–505.
66. Touboul E, Schlienger M, Buffat L, et al. Epidermoid carcinoma of the anal margin: 17 cases treated with curative-intent radiation therapy. Radiother Oncol 1995; 34:195–202.
67. Schraut WH, Wang C, Dawson PJ, Block GE. Depth of invasion, location, and size of cancer of the anus dictate operative treatment. Cancer 1983; 51: 1291–1296.
68. Cummings BJ, Keane TJ, Hawkins NV, O'Sullivan B. Treatment of perianal carcinoma by radiation (RT) or radiation plus chemotherapy (RTCT). Int J Radiat Oncol Biol Phys 1986; 12:170–173.
69. Paget J. On disease of the mammary areolar preceding cancer of the mammary gland. St. Bartholomew's Hosp Report 1874; 10:87–89.
70. Tjandra J. Perianal Paget's disease. Report of three cases. Dis Colon Rectum 1988; 31:462–466.
71. Darier J, Couillaud P. Sur un cas de maladie de Paget de la region kerineo-anal et scrotale. Ann de Dermatole et de Syph 1893; 4:25–31.
72. Armitage NC, Jass JR, Richman PI, Thomson JPS, Phillips RKS. Paget's disease of the anus: a clinicopathological study. Br J Surg 1989; 76:60–63.
73. Morson BC, Dawson IMP, Day DW, Jass JR, Price AB, Williams GT. Morson and Dawson's Gastrointestinal Pathology. London: Blackwell Scientific, 1990:673–675.
74. Rosai J. Ackerman's Surgical Pathology. 8th ed. Louis: CV Mosby, 1996: 808–809.
75. Miller LR, McCunniff A, Randall ME. An immunohistochemical study of perianal Paget's disease. Cancer 1992; 69:2166–2171.
76. Beck DE. Paget's disease and Bowen's disease of the anus. Semin Colon Rectal Surg 1995; 6:143–149.
77. Jensen SL, Sjolin KE, Shokouh Amiri MH, Hagen K, Harling H. Paget's disease of the anal margin. Br J Surg 1988; 75:1089–1092.
78. Park JS, Kerner BA. Perianal Paget's disease. Semin Colon Rectal Surg 2003; 14:218–221.
79. Ohnishi T, Watanabe S. The use of cytokeratins 7 and 20 in the diagnosis of primary and secondary extramammary Paget's disease. Br J Dermatol 2000; 142:243–247.
80. Goldblum JR, Hart WR. Perianal Paget's disease. A histologic and immunohistochemical study with and without associated rectal adenocarcinoma. Am J Surg Pathol 1998; 22:170–179.
81. Brown RSD, Lankester KJ, McCormack M, Power DA, Spittle MF. Radiotherapy for perianal Paget's disease. Clin Oncol 2002; 14:272–284.
82. Samiento JM, Wolff BG, Burgart LJ, Frizelle FA, Ilstrup DM. Paget's disease of the perianal region—An aggressive disease? Dis Colon Rectum 1997; 40: 1187–1194.
83. McCarter MD, Quan SHQ, Busam K, Paty PH, Wong D, Guillem JG. Long-term outcome of perianal Paget's disease. Dis Colon Rectum 2003; 46:612–616.
84. Marchesa P, Fazio VM, OliartS, Goldblum JR, Lavery IC, Milsom JW. Long-term outcome of patients with perianal Paget's disease. Am Surg Oncol 1997; 4:475–480.
85. Paterson CA, Young-Fadok TM, Dozois RR. Basal cell carcinoma of the perianal region. 20-year experience. Dis Colon Rectum 1999; 42:1200–1202.
86. Nielsen OV, Jensen SL. Basal cell carcinoma of the anus—a clinical study of 34 cases. BR J Surg 1981; 68:856–857.
87. Marks R, Gebauer K, Shumack S, et al. Imiquimod 5% cream in the treatment of superficial basal cell carcinoma: results of a multicenter 6-week dose-response trial. J Am Acad Dermatol 2001; 44:807–813.
88. Gordon PH. Current status—perianal and anal canal neoplasms. Dis Colon Rectum 1990; 33:799–808.
89. Cintron J. Buschke-Loewenstein tumor of the perianal and anorectal region. Semin Colon Rectal Surg 1995; 6:135–139.
90. Heinzerling LM, Kempf W, Kamarashev J, Hafner J, Nestle FO. Treatment of verrucous carcinoma with Imiquimod and CO_2 laser ablation. Dermatology 2003; 207:119–122.
91. Foust R, Dean PJ, Stoler MH, Monuddin SM. Intraepithelial neoplasia of the anal canal in hemorrhoidal tissue: a study of 19 cases. Hum Pathol 1991; 22:528–534.
92. Chang GJ, Berry JM, Jay N, Polefsky JM, Welton ML. Surgical treatment of high-grade anal squamous intraepithelial lesions. Dis Colon Rectum 2002; 45:453–458.
93. Jass JR, Sobin LH. . Histological Typing of Intestinal Tumors. 2nd Heidelberg: Springer-Verlag, 1989:90.
94. Stearns MW Jr, Quan SHQ. Epidermoid carcinoma of the anorectum. Surg Gynecol Obstet 1970; 131:953–957.
95. Welch JP, Malt RA. Appraisal of the treatment of carcinoma of the anus and anal canal. Surg Gynecol Obstet 1977; 145:837–844.
96. Boman BM, Moertel CG, O'Connell MJ, et al. Carcinoma of the anal canal: a clinical and pathologic study of 188 cases. Cancer 1984; 54:114–125.
97. Cummings BJ. Treatment of primary epidermoid carcinoma of the anal canal. Int J Colorectal Dis 1987; 2:107–112.
98. Wade DS, Herrera I, Castillo NB, Petrelli NJ. Metastases to the lymph nodes in epidermoid carcinoma of the anal canal studied by a clearing technique. Surg Gynecol Obstet 1989; 169:238–242.
99. Jensen SL, Hagen K, Harling H, Shokouh-Amiri MH, Nielsen OV. Long-term prognosis after radical treatment for squamous cell carcinoma of the anal canal and anal margin. Dis Colon Rectum 1988; 31:273–278..
100. Nigro ND, Vaitkevicuis VK, Considine B. Combined therapy for cancer of the anal canal: a preliminary report. Dis Colon Rectum 1974; 17:354–356.
101. Nigro ND. An evaluation of combined therapy for squamous cell cancer of the anal canal. Dis Colon Rectum 1984; 27:763–766
102. Sato H, Koh PK, Bartolo DCC. Management of anal canal cancer. Dis Colon Rectum 2005; 48:1301–1315.
103. Flam M, John M, Pajak TF, et al. Role of mitomycin in combination with fluorouracil and radiotherapy, and of salvage chemoradiation in the definitive nonsurgical treatment of epidermoid carcinoma of the anal canal: results of a phase III randomized intergroup study. J Clin Oncol 1996; 14:2527–2539.
104. UKCCCR Anal Cancer Trial Working Party. Epidermoid anal cancer: results from the UKCCCR randomized trial of radiotherapy alone versus radiotherapy, 5-flourouracil, and mitomycin. UKCCCR anal cancer trial working party. UK Co-ordinating Committee on Cancer Research. Lancet 1996; 348: 1049–1054.
105. Bartelink H, Roelofsen F, Eschwege F, et al. Concomitant radiotherapy and chemotherapy is superior to radiotherapy alone in the treatment of locally

advanced anal cancer: results of a phase III randomized trial of the European organization for research and treatment of cancer radiotherapy and gastrointestinal cooperative groups. J Clin Oncol 1997; 15:2040–2049.
106. Eng C, Abbruzzese J, Minsky BD. Chemotherapy and radiation of anal canal cancer: the first approach. Surg Onc Clin N Am 2004; 13:309–320.
107. Stafford S, Martenson JA. Combined radiation and chemotherapy for carcinoma of the anal canal. Oncology 1998; 12:373–389.
108. Myerson RJ, Kong F, Birnbaum EH, et al. Radiation therapy for epidermoid carcinoma of the anal canal, clinical and treatment factors associated with outcome. Radiother Oncol 2001; 61:15–22.
109. Myerson RJ et al. Carcinoma of the anal canal. Am J Clin Oncol 1995; 18:32–39.
110. Roed H, Engelholm SA, Svendsen LB, et al. Pulsed dose rate (PDR) brachy therapy of anal carcinoma. Radiother Oncol 1996; 41:131–134.
111. Kapp KS, Geyer E, Gebhart FH, et al. Experience with split-course external beam irradiation Ir- chemotherapy and integrated in-192 high dose-rate brachytherapy in the treatment of primary carcinoma of the anal canal. Int J Radiat Oncol Bio Phys 2001; 49:997–1005.
112. Place RJ, Gregory SG, Huber PJ, Simmang CL. Outcome analysis of HIV-positive patients with anal squamous cell carcinoma. Dis Colon Rectum 2001; 44:506–512.
113. Kim JH, Sarani B, Orkin BA, et al. HIV-positive patients with anal carcinoma have poorer treatment tolerance and outcome than HIV-negative patients. Dis Colon Rectum 2001; 44:1496–1502.
114. Berry JM, Polefsky JM, Welton ML. Anal cancer and its precursors in HIV-positive patients: perspectives and management. Surg Onc Clin N Am 2004; 13:355–373.
115. Blazy A, Hennequine, Gornet JM, et al. Anal carcinomas in HIV-positive patients: high-dose chemoradiotherapy is feasible in the era of highly active antiretroviral therapy. Dis Colon Rectum 2005; 48:1176–1181.
116. Cummings BJ, Keane TJ, O'Sullivan B, Wong ES, Cotton CN. Epidermoid anal cancer: treatment by radiation alone or by radiation and 5-fluorouracil with and without mitomycin C. Int J Radiat Oncol Biol Phys 1991; 21:1115–1125.
117. Tanum G, Tveit KM, Karlsen KO. Chemo-radiotherapy of anal carcinoma: tumor response and acute toxicity. Oncology 1993; 50:14–17.
118. Ellenhorn JD, Enker WE, Quan SHQ. Salvage abdominoperineal resection following combined chemotherapy and radiotherapy for epidermoid carcinoma of the anus. Ann Surg Oncol 1994; 1:105–110.
119. Nguyen WD, Mitchell KM, Beck DE. Risk factors associated with requiring a stoma for the management of anal cancer. Dis Colon Rectum 2004; 47:843–846.
120. Longo WE, Vernava AM, Wade TP, Coplin MA, Virgo KS, Johnson FE. Recurrent squamous cell carcinoma of the anal canal. Predictors of initial treatment failure and results of salvage therapy. Ann Surg 1994; 220:40–49.
121. Ghouti L, Houvenaeghel G, Moutardier V, et al. Salvage abdominoperineal resection after failure of conservative treatment in anal epidermoid cancer. Dis Colon Rectum 2005; 48:16–22.
122. Zelnick RS, Hass PA, Ajlouni M, Szilagyi E, Fox TA Jr. Results of abdominoperineal resections for failures after combination chemotherapy and radiation therapy for anal cancers. Dis Colon Rectum 1992; 35:574–578.
123. Gerard JP, Chapet O, Samiei F, et al. Management of inguinal lymph node metastasis in patients with carcinoma of the anal canal. Experience in a series of 270 patients treated in Lyon and review of the literature. Cancer 2001; 92: 77–84.
124. Cummings BJ, Thomas GM, Keane TJ. Primary radiation therapy in the treatment of anal canal carcinoma. Dis Colon Rectum 1982; 25:778–782.
125. Papillon J, Montbarbon JF. Epidermoid carcinoma of the anal canal. A series of 276 cases. Dis Colon Rectum 1987; 30:324–333.
126. Stearns MW, Urmacher C, Sternborg SE, Woodruff J, Attiyeh FF. Cancer of the anal canal. Curr Probl Cancer 1980; 4:1–44.
127. Ulmer C, Bembenek A, Gretschel S, et al. Refined staging by sentinel lymph node biopsy to individualize therapy in anal cancer. Ann Surg Onc 2004; 11(3 suppl):259s–262s.
128. Gupta N, Longo WE, Vernara AM, Wade TP, Johnson FE. Treatment of recurrent epidermoid carcinoma of the anal canal. Semin Colon Rectal Surg 1995; 6:160–165.
129. Gordon PH. Squamous cell carcinoma of the anal canal. Surg Clin North Am 1988; 68:1391–1399.
130. Tanum G, Tveit K, Karlsen KO, Hauer-Jensen M. Chemotherapy and radiation therapy for anal carcinoma. Cancer 1991; 67:2462–2466.
131. Basik M, Rodriguez-Bigas MA, Penetrante R, Pitrelli NJ. Prognosis and recurrence patterns of anal adenocarcinoma. Am J Surg 1995; 169:233–237.
132. Tarazi R, Nelson R. Adenocarcinoma of the anus. Semin Colon Rectal Surg 1995; 6:169–173.
133. Beal KP, Wong D, Guillem JG, et al. Primary adenocarcinoma of the anus treated with combined modality therapy. Dis Colon Rectum 2003; 46: 1320–1324.
134. Hobbs CM, Lowry MA, Owen D, Sobin LH. Anal gland carcinoma. Cancer 2001; 92:2045–2049.
135. Morson BC, Sobin LH. Histologic Typing of Intestinal Tumors. Geneva: World Health Organization, 1976.
136. Jensen SL, Shokouh-Amiri MH, Hagen K, Harling H, Nielsen OV. Adenocarcinoma of the anal ducts: a series of 21 cases. Dis Colon Rectum 1988; 31: 268–272.
137. Perkowski PE, Surrells DL, Evans JT, Nopajaronsri C, Johnson LW. Anal duct carcinoma: case report and review of the literature. Am Surg 2000; 66: 1149–1152.
138. Fenger C. Anal canal tumors and their precursors. Pathol Annu 1988; 23:45–66.
139. Schaffzin DM, Stahl TJ, Smith LE. Perianal mucinous adenocarcinoma: unusual case presentations and review of the literature. Arch Path Lab Med 2001; 125:1074–1077.
140. Jensen SL, Nielsen OV. Anal duct carcinoma [editorial]. Dis Colon Rectum 1989; 32:355–357.
141. Getz SB Jr, Ough YD, Patterson RB, Kovalcik PJ. Mucinous adenocarcinoma developing in chronic anal fistula: report of two cases and review of the literature. Dis Colon Rectum 1981; 24:562–566.
142. Belkacemi Y, Berger C, Poortmans P, et al. Management of primary anal canal adenocarcinoma: a large retrospective study from the rare cancer network. Int J Radiat Oncol Biol Phys 2003; 56:1274–1283.
143. Abel ME, Chiu YSY, Russell TR, Volpe PA. Adenocarcinoma of the anal glands. Results of a survey. Dis Colon Rectum 1993; 36:383–387.
144. Tarazi R, Nelson RL. Anal adenocarcinoma: a comprehensive review. Semin Colon Rectal Surg 1994; 10:235–240.
145. Papagikos M, Crane CH, Skibber J, et al. Chemoradiation for adenocarcinoma of the anus. Int J Radiat Oncol Biol Phys 2003; 55:669–678.
146. Paterson C, Musselman L, Chorneyko K, Reid S, Rawlinson J. Merkel cell (neuroendocrine) carcinoma of the anal canal. Dis Colon Rectum 2003; 46:676–678.
147. Coquard R. Merkel cell carcinoma of the anal canal: importance of radiotherapy [Editorial]. Dis Colon Rectum 2004; 47:256–257.
148. Mason JK, Helwig EB. Anorectal melanoma. Cancer 1966; 19:39–50.
149. Thibault C, Sagar P, Nivatvongs S, Wolff BG. Anorectal melanoma: an incurable disease? Dis Colon Rectum 1997; 40:661--668.
150. Cagir B, Whiteford MH, Topham A, Rakinic J, Fry RD. Changing epidemiology of anorectal melanoma. Dis Colon Rectum 1999; 42:1203–1208.
151. Ward MWN, Romano G, Nicholls RJ. The surgical treatment of anorectal malignant melanoma. Br J Surg 1986; 73:68–69.
152. Werdin C, Limas C, Knodell RG. Primary malignant melanoma of the rectum. Evidence for origination from rectal mucosal melanocytes. Cancer 1988; 61:1364–1370.
153. Quan SHQ. Malignant melanoma of the anorectum. Semin Colon Rectal Surg 1995; 6:166–168.
154. Antoniuk PM, Tjandra JJ, Webb BW, Petras RE, Milsom JW, Pazio VW. Anorectal malignant melanoma has a poor prognosis. Int J Colorectal Dis 1993; 8:81–86.
155. Chiu YS, Unni KK, Beart RW Jr. Malignant melanoma of the anorectum. Dis Colon Rectum 1980; 23:122–124.
156. Bullard KM, Tuttle TM, Rothenberger DA, et al. Surgical therapy for anorectal melanoma. J Am Coll Surg 2003; 196:206–211.
157. Malik A, Hull TL, Milsom J. Long-term survivor of anorectal melanoma. Report of a case. Dis Colon Rectum 2002; 45:1412–1417.
158. Cooper PH, Mills SE, Allen MS Jr. Malignant melanoma of the anus. Report of 12 patients and analysis of 255 additional cases. Dis Colon Rectum 1982; 25:693–703.
159. Wolff BG. Anorectal melanoma [Editorial]. Dis Colon Rectum 2002; 45:1415.
160. Brady MS, Kavolius JP, Quan SHQ. Anorectal melanoma. A 64 year experience at Memorial Sloan-Kettering Cancer Center. Dis Colon Rectum 1995; 38: 146–151.
161. Pessaux P, Pocard M, Elias D, et al. Surgical management of primary anorectal melanoma. Br J Surg 2004; 91:1183–1187.
162. Ward MW, Romano G, Nichollo RJ. The surgical treatment of anorectal malignant melanoma. Br J Surg 1996; 73:68–69.
163. Roumen RMH. Anorectal melanoma in the Netherlands: a report of 63 patients. Eur J Surg Onc 1996; 22:598–601.
164. Ross M, Pezzi C, Pezzi T, Meurer D, Hickey R, Balch C. Patterns of failure in anorectal melanoma. A guide to surgical therapy. Arch Surg 1990; 125: 313–316.
165. Slingluff CL Jr, Vollmer RT, Seigler HF. Anorectal melanoma: clinical characteristics and results of surgical management in twenty-four patients. Surgery 1990; 107:1–9.
166. Goldman S, Glimelius B, Pahlman L. Anorectal malignant melanoma in Sweden. Report of 49 patients. Dis Colon Rectum 1990; 33:874–877.

19 Transanal Techniques

Santhat Nivatvongs

INTRODUCTION

Procedures such as rectal biopsy, electrocoagulation, and snaring of rectal polyps are usually performed in the office or an outpatient clinic. Thus the office or clinic must be well equipped with essential instruments and spare parts, and the clinician should be proficient in the use of these instruments. Providing sedation or anesthesia to the patient is rarely, if ever, necessary. If a barium enema study is indicated, it should be done one day before or three to four weeks after the procedure to avoid the risk of perforation. However, if a biopsy is performed on a carcinoma, a barium enema can be safely performed anytime thereafter because the rectal wall itself is not damaged by the biopsy. Anticoagulants, including aspirin and other nonsteroidal anti-inflammatory drugs (NSAIDs) should be stopped for one week or until the prothrombin time and partial thromboplastin time have reached normal or near-normal values.

In many healthy people the colon contains a variable amount of hydrogen and methane (1). The packaged sodium biphosphate enema (Fleet enema) that is frequently used is not adequate to eliminate these gases, and explosions from electrocoagulation or snaring, although rare, can occur (2,3). Explosions can be prevented by the frequent use of suctioning to evacuate the gases before the electric current is applied.

Patients are usually sent home soon after the procedure. No dietary restrictions are necessary. After removal of larger sessile lesions, a liquid diet may be in order for 24 to 48 hours. The patients are forewarned to report profuse rectal bleeding, persistent abdominal or shoulder pain, or fever. When the patient's status is in doubt, a flat plate, an upright view of the abdomen, and lateral decubitus films should be obtained.

RECTAL BIOPSY

Many local and systemic disorders can be diagnosed by rectal biopsy. Conditions in which rectal biopsy is essential or useful for diagnosis or management include malignant or benign neoplasms of the rectum, chronic ulcerative colitis, Crohn's colitis, ischemic colitis, pseudomembranous colitis, radiation proctitis, collagenous colitis, amebiasis, schistosomiasis, bacillary dysentery, pneumatosis cystoides intestinalis, amyloidosis, solitary ulcer of the rectum, Hirschsprung's disease, and colitis cystica profunda.

Biopsy specimens are inevitably small, rarely >8 mm. However, with an adequate biopsy and proper orientation of the specimen, an accurate interpretation can be achieved.

TECHNIQUE

For a rectal biopsy, the 1.9 × 25 cm proctoscope is used, and the patient is placed in the prone jackknife or a left lateral position. A cup-shaped or an alligator biopsy forceps is suitable (see Fig. 8 in Chapter 3).

BIOPSY OF RECTAL CARCINOMA

The best area for taking a biopsy is the edge of the carcinoma where there is no necrosis. Multiple areas should be sampled. Bleeding is usually minimal but may require electrocoagulation.

BIOPSY OF RECTAL MUCOSA

The lower valve of Houston is frequently thought to be the ideal location for biopsy. Other surgeons believe that the best location for biopsy is the posterior part of the middle valve of Houston. At the middle valve, if bleeding occurs, the proctoscope can be pressed against the sacrum to constrict blood vessels, and electrocoagulation can be applied accurately in a bloodless field (4). Frosted glass, nylon mesh, or filter paper is applied lightly to the submucosal surface of the specimen. The mounted specimen is then dropped into the fixative.

ELECTROCOAGULATION OF RECTAL POLYPS

During a routine proctoscopy it is common to find small rectal polyps, ranging in size from 1 to 5 mm. The majority are hyperplastic polyps or lymphoid hyperplasia and have no malignant potential.

Small adenomatous polyps 1 to 5 mm in size have an extremely low incidence of carcinoma. However, because of the minimal risks of the complications during a properly performed excisional biopsy, all such polyps within the reach of the proctoscope should be obtained for biopsy so that the histologic morphology is known. If several polyps are present, biopsy is performed for one or two and electrocoagulation is performed for the rest.

TECHNIQUE

For electrocoagulation of rectal polyps, the patient is placed in either a prone jackknife position or a Sims' position. A 1.9 × 25 cm proctoscope is suitable for the procedure. A ball-tip or a suction-coagulation electrode, which is connected to the electrocoagulation unit set at an optimal power, is used (see Fig. 6 in Chapter 3). After the biopsy, the electrode is placed directly in contact with the polyp to coagulate it. The duration of each burning should not be more than a few seconds, but this step can be repeated until the entire polyp becomes white. A "pop" noise may be heard, which results from the explosion of the cells due to the pressure of the steam generated within them.

SNARE POLYPECTOMY

The patient is placed in either a prone jackknife or a Sims' position. A 1.9 × 25 cm proctoscope is preferred for snare polypectomy. Different commercial snaring devices are available (see Fig. 7 in Chapter 3). They are connected to the coagulator, which is set at the appropriate power, depending on the size of the polyp. Before transection of a polyp, the stalk or the base must be visualized fully to avoid drawing the bowel wall into the snare. If the polyp is at the limit of the proctoscopic visualization and the base is not adequately visualized, it may be safer to perform a colonoscopic polypectomy.

PEDUNCULATED POLYP

The snare wire is looped around the pedunculated polyp and is positioned onto the stalk a few millimeters from the bowel wall. Once the loop is in a satisfactory position, the snare is pushed cephalad so that the base of the wire loop touches the stalk (Fig. 1A). This fixes the snare wire in the proper position for closing the loop. It always must be ascertained that no mucosal fold has inadvertently been caught in the snare (Fig. 1B). Before coagulation is done, the polyp is manipulated toward the center of the rectal lumen to avert the polyp from resting on the rectal wall. This maneuver avoids the possibility of burning the mucosa of the opposite wall because the current is transmitted through the polyp (Fig. 1C). The coagulator is applied no longer than a few seconds. The snare is gently tightened while the electric current is applied. If the polyp is not cut, approximately 10 to 15 seconds are allowed for the tissue to cool; then coagulation and tightening of the snare are repeated until the stalk of the polyp is completely transected. The polyp can be retrieved easily by using suction or a polyp grasper or a biopsy forceps. The polyp site should be checked for bleeding or perforation.

SESSILE POLYP

A small sessile polyp can be snared in the same way as a pedunculated polyp by including a small part of the underlying mucosa tented as a pseudopedicle. A sessile polyp > 2 cm should be removed piecemeal. The snare wire cuts through the substance of the polyp to divide it into multiple pieces 1 to 1.5 cm in size (Fig. 1D). The residual polyp at the base can be electrocoagulated. It may be necessary to remove a large sessile polyp in more than one session. The patient should return after four to six weeks for examination and removal of any residual polyp.

TRANSANAL EXCISION OF RECTAL ADENOMA

A villous or a tubulovillous adenoma has a characteristic velvety appearance and soft consistency. If the neoplasm is not indurated or ulcerated, the chance that it is benign is 90% (5,6). The entire lesion should be removed in one piece or at least piecemeal in its entirety in the submucosal plane for an adequate histopathologic examination. A preoperative biopsy is unreliable and has high false positive and false negative reports of malignancy (7). It also makes a subsequent transanal excision more difficult. Indurated or ulcerated areas are signs of invasive carcinoma, and it is useful to obtain a biopsy of these areas. An adenoma in the low rectum and in some cases in the midrectum is suitable for transanal excision. The techniques used vary according to the size and site of the lesion (8).

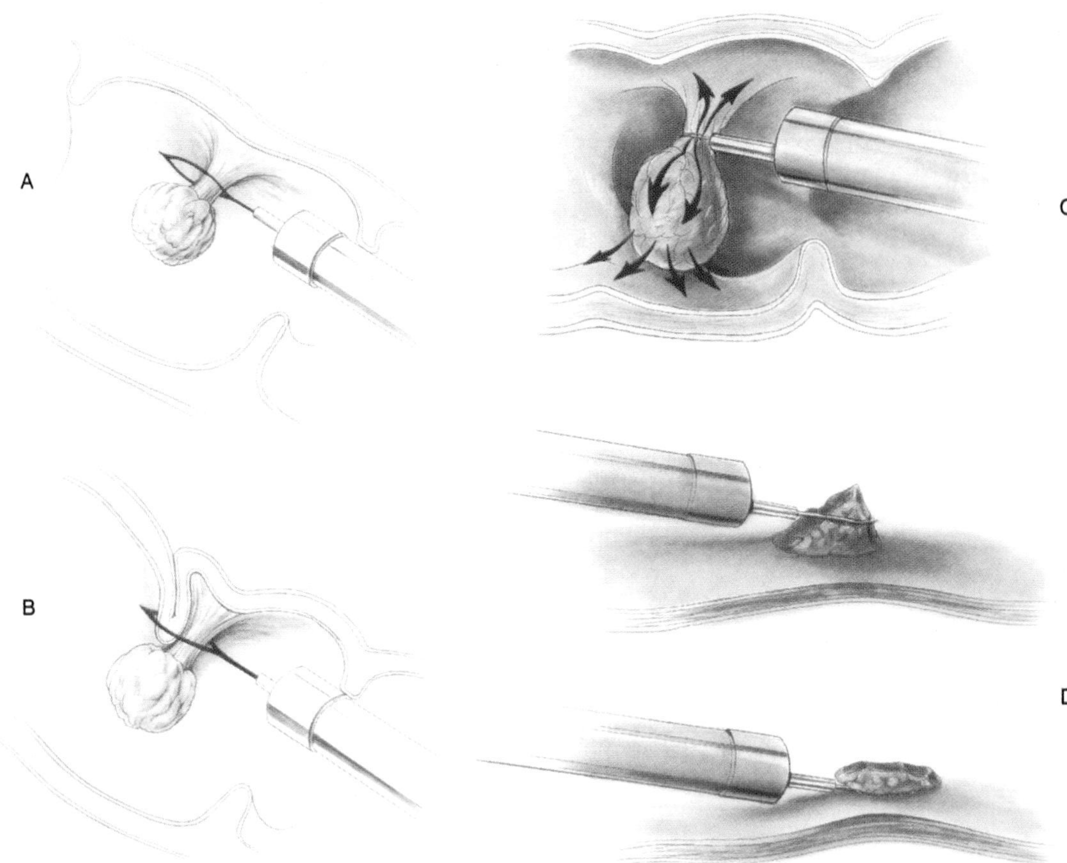

FIGURE 1 ■ Snare polypectomy. (**A**) Base of snare loop is pushed against stalk of the polyp. (**B**) Mucosal fold is entrapped in the snare. (**C**) Electrical current is transmitted through the polyp to opposite bowel wall. (**D**) Piecemeal excision of a large sessile polyp.

■ GENERAL CONSIDERATIONS

All patients who have rectal villous or tubulovillous adenomas should be thoroughly examined by total colonoscopy to rule out other lesions located more proximally. The rectum is prepared with two Phospho-soda enemas. An antibiotic is not indicated. Inducing general or regional anesthesia is preferred, but in selected patients local anesthesia suffices. The patient is placed in the prone jackknife position, but if the adenoma is located on the posterior rectum, a lithotomy position may be preferred. A Pratt anal speculum provides excellent exposure, but other retractors, such as the Fansler anal speculum, the Sawyer anal retractor, the Hill-Ferguson retractor, and the Gelpi retractor should be available and used as appropriate (Figs. 2 and 3).

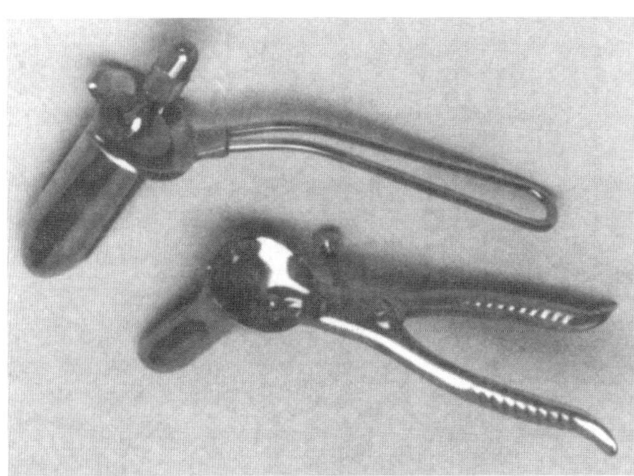

FIGURE 2 ■ Fansler anal speculum (*above*) and Pratt bivalve anal speculum (*below*).

Postoperative care is simple. A clear liquid diet is given for one day to ensure that there are no signs of rectal perforation. The first postoperative check should be in three months. Any residual polyp can be electrocoagulated in the clinic or office. Thereafter, proctosigmoidoscopy or flexible sigmoidoscopy at six months and then annually is desirable.

■ SESSILE ADENOMA OF LOWER RECTUM

A sessile adenoma with the proximal margin up to 7 cm from the anal verge can be excised in one piece. A scissors

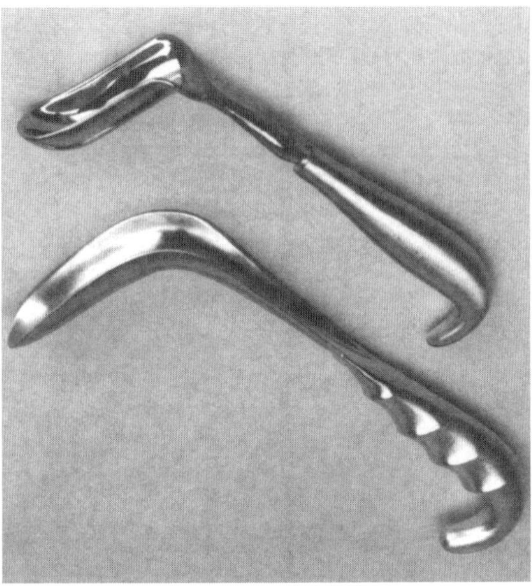

FIGURE 3 ■ Hill-Ferguson anal speculum (*above*) and Sawyer anal speculum (*below*).

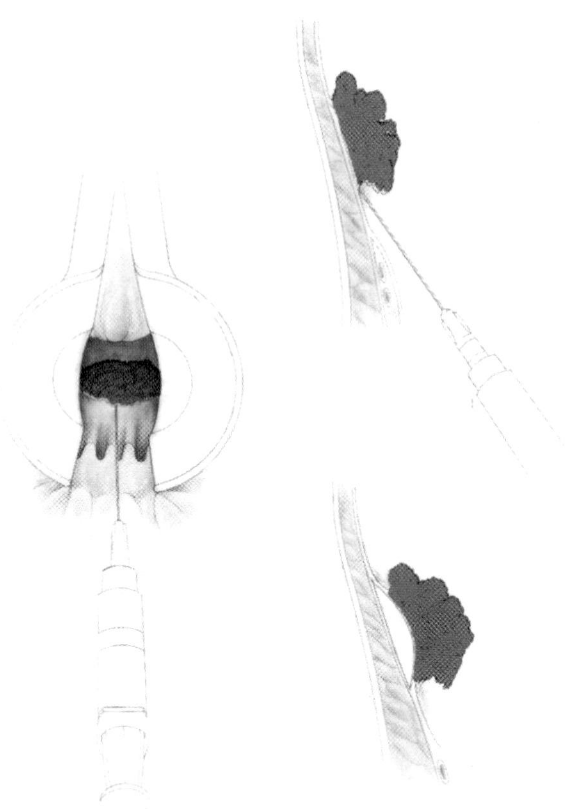

FIGURE 4 ■ Infiltration of a villous adenoma, using 1:200,000 epinephrine solution to raise the submucosa.

or an electrocautery blade is used to raise the mucosa and submucosa from the underlying muscular wall of the rectum. A dilute epinephrine solution (1:200,000) is infiltrated into the submucosa to minimize bleeding (Fig. 4).

A Pratt anal speculum is inserted to expose the anorectum. An incision is made to encompass a margin of about 1 cm of normal mucosa and submucosa. The distal margin of the adenoma is grasped with an Allis forceps for traction. A Sawyer or a Hill-Ferguson retractor may work better at this point to allow prolapse of the rectal wall. The entire lesion is then excised (Fig. 5). Depending on its size and shape, the wound may be completely closed, marsupialized, or left open. Proctosigmoidoscopy is performed at the completion of the procedure to make sure that the lumen is patent. The excised specimen is pinned flat on a piece of cardboard and then placed in a fixative solution (Fig. 6).

■ SESSILE ADENOMA OF MIDDLE RECTUM

Excising a lesion in the middle rectum 7 to 11 cm from the anal verge is difficult, if not impossible, to do per anum. The anal speculum cannot reach the adenoma for adequate exposure. However, if the technique as described by Faivre is used, it is possible to remove such a lesion (9,10).

The anorectal submucosa and the anal canal are infiltrated with 0.25% bupivacaine (Marcaine) or 0.5% lidocaine (Xylocaine) containing 1:200,000 epinephrine to obtain complete relaxation of the anal canal and hemostasis. A Fansler or a Pratt anal speculum is used to expose the anorectum. An elliptical excision is made with a scissors or an electrocautery blade, starting at the dentate line or at the anal verge similar to the technique for hemorrhoidectomy. The mucosa and the submucosa are dissected from their underlying muscle. With this anoderm or submucosal pedicle used as traction, the dissection can be carried up to 8 to 10 cm from the anal verge without much difficulty. When the lower margin of the polyp is reached, the dissection should encompass it with a 1 cm rim of normal mucosa (Fig. 7). If the anorectal wall does not prolapse when the submucosal pedicle is pulled, a Sawyer or Hill-Ferguson retractor should be used instead. The wound is closed with running 3-0 synthetic braided or monofilament sutures. A large wound should be closed transversely. A diverting colostomy is not indicated.

Pigot et al. (10) performed this technique in 207 consecutive patients (100 males), mean age 68 years (range, 24–90 years), for an apparently benign villous rectal adenoma. The mean distance of lower edge of the lesion from the anal margin was 5.6 cm (range, 0–13 cm) and was <10 cm in 82%. Immediate postoperative course was uneventful for 96%. The mean size of the resected lesion was 5.4 cm (range, 1–17 cm).

■ CIRCUMFERENTIAL VILLOUS OR TUBULOVILLOUS ADENOMA OF RECTUM

Good exposure is essential for the removal of a large polyp in the rectum. A Lone Star self-retaining retractor (Fig. 8)

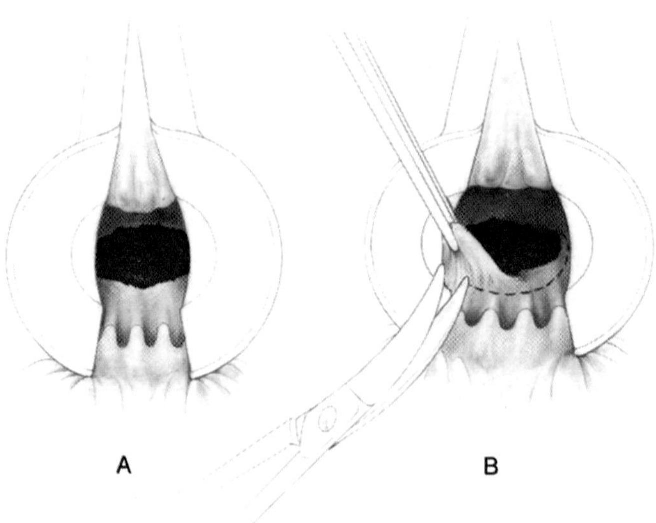

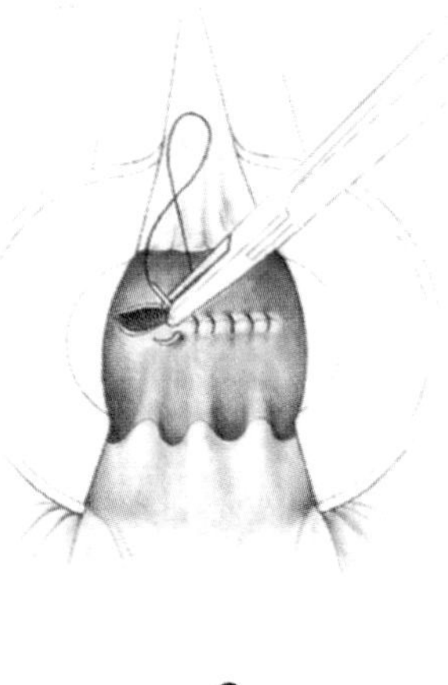

FIGURE 5 ■ (**A**) Flat villous adenoma of the low rectum. (**B**) Dissection of the adenoma in the submucosal plane with 1 cm margin of normal mucosa. (**C**) Transverse approximation of the wound with continuous sutures.

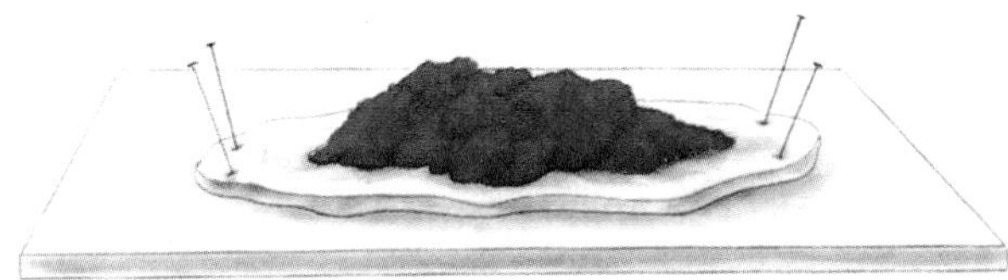

FIGURE 6 ■ Specimen is pinned on cardboard.

helps the exposure tremendously (11). If that instrument is not available, two Gelpi retractors placed at right angles to each other at the anal verge can be used as an alternative. A circumferential villous or tubulovillous adenoma with the lower margin in the lower rectum can be removed even if the proximal margin extends to the midrectum (Fig. 9A). Although Parks and Stuart (12) removed it in three to four longitudinal strips, this type of lesion can be removed in one piece as a submucosal tube.

A circumferential incision is made around the dentate line in the submucosal plane with an electrocautery blade. Diluted epinephrine may be injected to raise the submucosal plane. Using a Pratt anal speculum to stretch the anal canal makes the dissection in the submucosal plane easier, all around up to about 7 cm. The submucosal tube is grasped with an Allis clamp, and a submucosal dissection is carried as far proximally as needed. The circumferential dissection of the submucosa apparently allows the rectum to prolapse during traction. It is relatively easy to dissect the submucosal tube from the dentate line to the anorectal ring. From the anorectal ring to the rectal ampulla (approximately 10 cm from the anal verge), the dissection is difficult, and the submucosal plane may be easily lost. Packing sponges into the submucosal tube facilitates traction on the tube during the dissection. A Pratt speculum, Sawyer or Hill-Ferguson retractor, and a small Deaver retractor should be used freely as appropriate. From the rectal ampulla to upper rectum, dissection is usually easier.

After the entire adenoma has been removed, the proximal cut end of the mucosa and submucosa can be brought down, along with denuded muscle wall, to approximate circumferentially with the lower cut end at the dentate line (Fig. 9B) At the completion of the procedure, the anorectal wall will be imbricated in the longitudinal plane (Fig. 9C). Incontinence of gas and liquid stool may last for a few weeks. Circumferential submucosal dissection of the anorectum can be carried from the dentate line up to 10 cm, and occasionally up to 12 to 15 cm, from the anal verge.

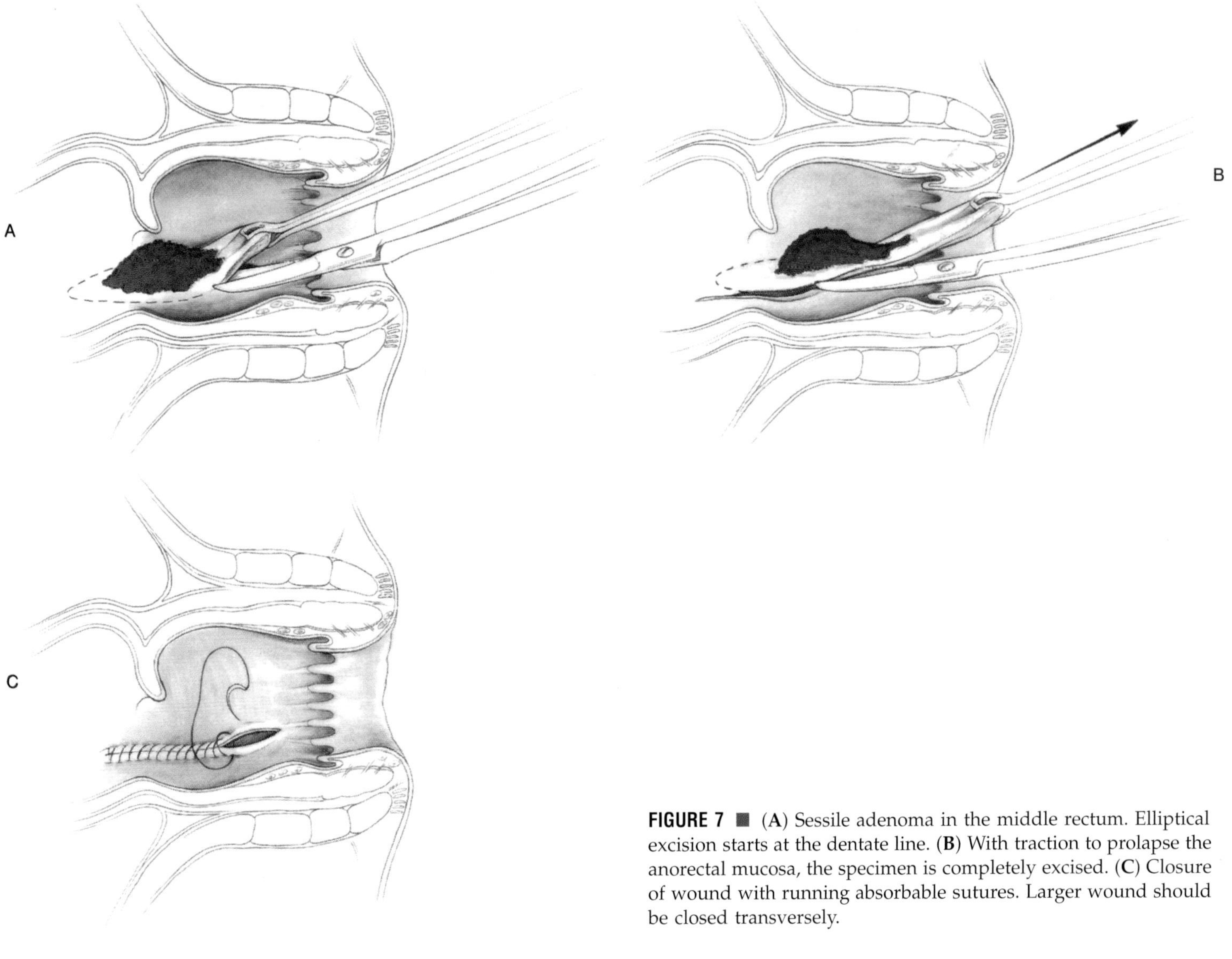

FIGURE 7 ■ (**A**) Sessile adenoma in the middle rectum. Elliptical excision starts at the dentate line. (**B**) With traction to prolapse the anorectal mucosa, the specimen is completely excised. (**C**) Closure of wound with running absorbable sutures. Larger wound should be closed transversely.

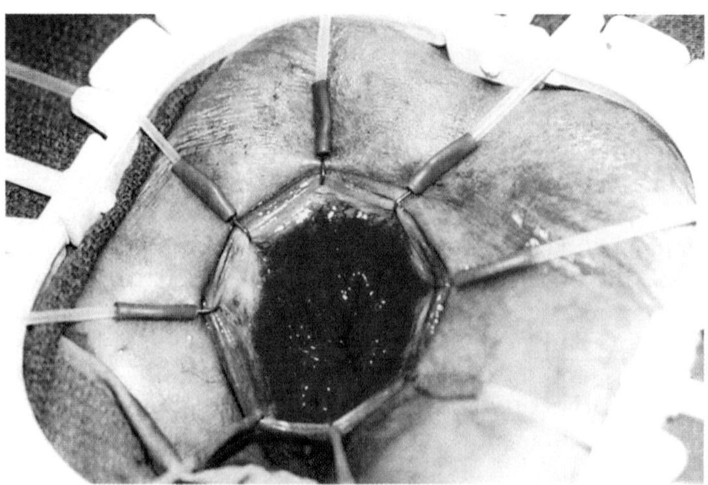

FIGURE 8 ■ An excellent exposure of the anus using a Lone Star self-retaining retractor. Patient is in prone position.

TRANSANAL EXCISION FOR CARCINOMA OF THE LOW RECTUM

Certain carcinomas of the low rectum have not yet spread to the regional lymph nodes at the time of diagnosis. Thus they are amenable to local excision provided the extirpation can be done with adequate margin in all directions. From a technical point of view, suitable lesions are those that are < 3 cm in greatest dimension, invade only the submucosa and have a favorable pathologic grade (grade 1 or 2). Although preoperative intrarectal ultrasonography is useful to determine the depth of the invasion and the lymph node metastasis, the ultimate decision whether additional treatment is indicated relies on the complete histopathologic examination. Approximately 5% of carcinomas of the rectum are suitable for local excision with the intent to cure (13). With proper selection of specific patients in conjunction with meticulous and precise surgical technique, the carcinoma five-year survival rate can be expected to be 74% to 90% (14–17). This approach should be used with caution because it has been recently reported that local recurrence rate is high, between 7% and 29% (14–17) (see Chapters 22 and 24).

■ PREPARATION

The patient should undergo mechanical bowel preparation similar to a colon resection, including prophylactic antibiotics. The prone jackknife position is for lesions in the anterior and lateral locations. For lesions in the posterior rectum, the lithotomy position with candy cane stirrups is preferred.

■ TECHNIQUE

A Foley catheter is placed in the bladder. The anorectum is irrigated with saline solution. Exposure of the anorectum is achieved by a Pratt anal speculum or a Parks retractor. Transanal excision of carcinoma is suitable for an early lesion with an upper margin within 7 cm from the anal verge.

A line of excision is marked around the carcinoma, with at least a 1cm grossly normal margin, using electrocautery (Fig. 10A). The crucial part of the technique is to grasp the internal sphincter muscle at the inferior margin with an Allis clamp (Fig. 10B). An incision is made using an electrocautery blade (coagulation current). The Allis clamp is used for traction and exposure and should be moved around as appropriate. This technique is simpler and more precise than using multiple sutures around the lesion for traction. The tissue is incised all around in the perianorectal plane (deeper then the internal sphincter and rectal wall) until the entire carcinoma is removed. It is important that the excision is full thickness, exposing the fat (Fig. 10C). The wound is closed transversely with running 3-0 or interrupted monofilament or braided synthetic absorbable material (Fig. 10D). No packing or drain is placed.

The electrocautery allows an accurate excision with minimal bleeding. The specimen is carefully placed on a towel and marked for locations, right, left, caudad, and cephalad aspects. The pathologist then checks the margins to determine that they are adequate. If adequate margins cannot be achieved, and if the carcinoma has adverse risk factors a radical resection should be considered in good-risk patients.

Postoperative care is generally simple. The anorectal pain is usually minimal, although mild fever can occur. The Foley catheter is removed on the first postoperative day. Clear liquids are started on the first postoperative day, provided there are no signs of peritoneal irritation, followed by a regular diet the next day and discharge from the hospital. A follow-up proctoscopy or flexible sigmoidoscopy should be performed at three and six months. The patient then begins a routine follow-up schedule appropriate for high-risk patients.

POSTERIOR APPROACH TO THE RECTUM

A large villous or sessile adenoma of the high rectum, with the lower margin more than 10 or 11 cm from the anal verge, is impossible to excise via a transanal approach unless the rectum can be prolapsed through the anus. This higher lesion, however, can be reached by opening the rectum posteriorly. The bowel is prepared as for a colon resection. Because of the potential serious complications, the posterior approach to the rectum should be reserved for cases in which other alternatives are not suitable. In good-risk patients, a low anterior resection can be performed. Other alternatives include piecemeal snaring and electrocoagulation of the adenoma via a proctoscope or a colonoscope and using laser ablation (18). The posterior approach is most useful for local excision of neoplasms in the middle rectum.

■ POSTERIOR PROCTOTOMY APPROACH (KRASKE'S APPROACH)

In 1874 Theader Kocher (19) of Bern recommended excising the coccyx to facilitate access to the rectum when excision of a high rectal neoplasm was contemplated. Kraske, however, found that removal of the coccyx alone is not adequate to expose the upper rectum. In 1885 he reported his posterior approach technique. Kraske found that he could obtain an excellent exposure of the upper rectum by cutting the lower margin of the gluteus maximus muscle and the sacrospinous and sacrotuberous ligaments. The

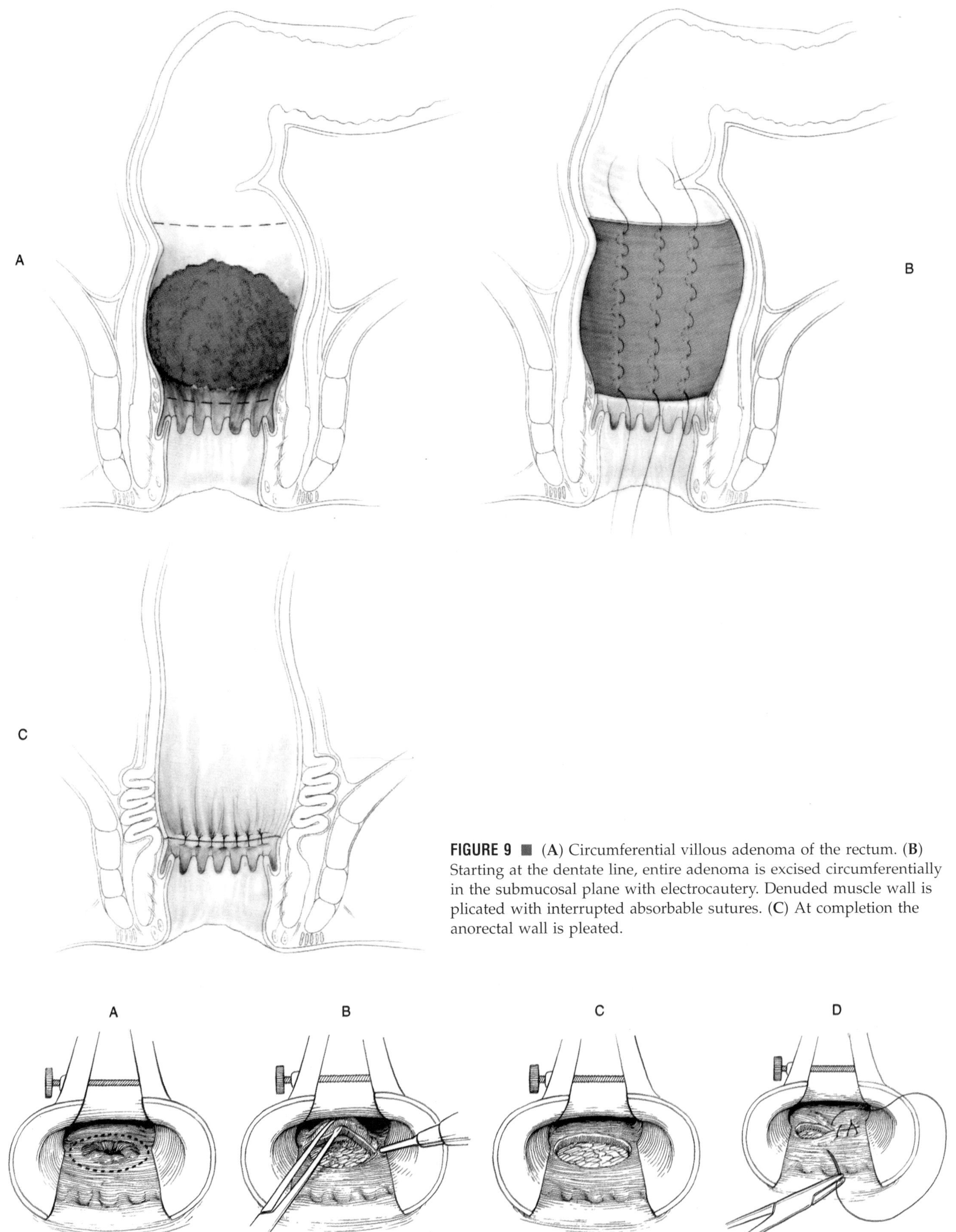

FIGURE 9 ■ (**A**) Circumferential villous adenoma of the rectum. (**B**) Starting at the dentate line, entire adenoma is excised circumferentially in the submucosal plane with electrocautery. Denuded muscle wall is plicated with interrupted absorbable sutures. (**C**) At completion the anorectal wall is pleated.

FIGURE 10 ■ (**A**) The line of excision is outlined with electrocautery. (**B**) Incision is made in full thickness. Allis clamp is used for traction and exposure. (**C**) A full-thickness disk of the lesion is removed, exposing the perirectal fat. (**D**) The defect is closed transversely with running 3-0 monofilament or braided synthetic absorbable material.

exposure was even better when the lowermost part of the left wing of the sacrum was excised (20).

The patient is placed in a prone jackknife position. A transverse or a midline incision is made from the sacrococcygeal joint to a point just proximal to the anus (Fig. 11A). The anococcygeal ligament is separated along the midline (Fig. 11B). If necessary, the coccyx can be excised to gain exposure. The incision is deepened to expose the levator ani muscle, which is incised in the midline to expose the posterior rectal wall (Fig. 11B and C). The rectum is opened through the posterior wall, and the polyp is excised submucosally (Fig. 11D and E). The defect is approximated, if possible, using 3-0 sutures (Fig. 11F). The posterior proctotomy wound is closed vertically or transversely with a

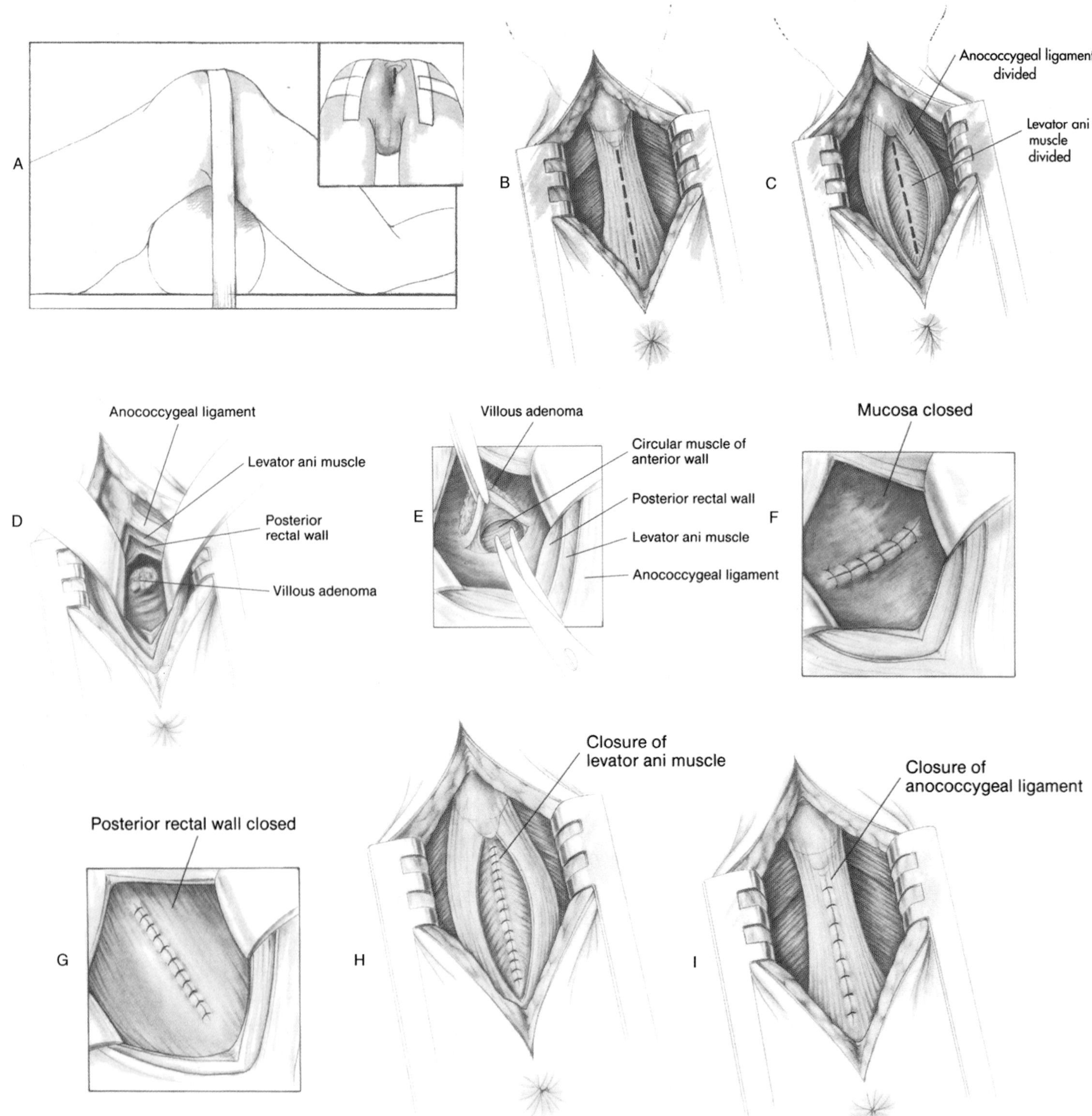

FIGURE 11 ■ Kraske's approach. (**A**) Patient is placed in prone position. A midline or a transverse skin incision is used. (**B**) Incision through skin, with division of anococcygeal ligament. (**C**) Levator ani muscle is divided in the midline plane. Coccyx can be excised as indicated. (**D**) Posterior rectal wall is incised, exposing adenoma in the anterior rectal wall. (**E**) Adenoma is excised in the submucosal plane. (**F**) Closure of anterior rectal mucosa. (**G**) Closure of posterior rectal wall. (**H**) Closure of levator ani muscle. (**I**) Approximation of anococcygeal ligament.

one-layer synthetic absorbable 3-0 suture, depending on which method is easier to accomplish without compromising the lumen (Fig. 11G). A two-layer closure may be performed if desired. Hemostasis is achieved, and the entire wound is irrigated with normal saline solution. A closed suction drain is placed. The muscles are closed in layers using 3-0 sutures (Fig. 11H and I). The skin is closed with a subcuticular 3-0 monofilament synthetic absorbable sutures. A classic Kraske's approach, excising the coccyx and part of the lower sacrum is seldom practiced anymore. However, when needed, one should not hesitate to excise the coccyx.

There have been sporadic reports on Kraske's approach for rectal neoplasm. Arnaud et al. (21) used the modified Kraske's approach in 35 patients with various anorectal diseases, including 24 patients with villous adenomas of the rectum situated between 8 and 15 cm from the anal verge. Significant complications included four patients who developed wound infection, three patients who developed a fistula requiring a sigmoid colostomy, and two patients who developed a perianal hernia that did not require surgical repair. There was no postoperative mortality. Christiansen (22) operated on 17 patients with various neoplasms of the rectum located between 6 and 15 cm from the anal verge. No operative deaths resulted. Two patients developed wound infections, and two had fecal fistulas that spontaneously closed. Bergamaschi and Arnaud (23) successfully resected the midrectum with a circular stapled anastomosis for circumferential adenomas of the midrectum. The coccyx and the fifth and fourth sacrum were osteotomized to fully mobilize the rectum.

■ POSTERIOR TRANSSPHINCTERIC APPROACH (YORK-MASON'S APPROACH)

The posterior transsphincteric approach of the rectum was first introduced by Bevan (24) in 1917 but lacked popular success. In 1970 York-Mason (25) reintroduced this technique and subsequently reported satisfactory results with 89 patients in 1977. He strongly emphasized accurately suturing the divided sphincters, with restoration of the anatomic layers. This enthusiasm was also shared by Allgower et al. (26).

The patient is placed in the prone jackknife position. A left parasacral incision is made from middle sacrum, passing obliquely downward to the anal verge in the midline (Fig. 12A). The exposure can be widened by incising the lower part of the gluteus muscle. The incision is deepened to expose the external sphincteric complex and the puborectalis and levator ani muscles. They are divided along the lines of incision, and the divided edges are tagged step by step (Fig. 12B). It is important to mark each layer and component of the muscles accurately with stay sutures to allow correct identification when reapproximating them. The nerve supply to these muscles lies lateral to the incision and is therefore safe from injury.

Next the internal sphincter is divided, with proximal extension to the thinner muscle wall of the rectum. The submucosa and mucosa are incised to expose the interior of the rectum and the anal canal (Fig. 12C). The lesion is excised (Fig. 12D). The bowel is closed in layers. The mucosa and submucosa are closed with running or interrupted 3-0 synthetic absorbable sutures; the internal sphincter is closed with interrupted or running 3-0 braided or monofilament synthetic sutures (Fig. 12E). The external sphincter and the puborectalis and levator ani muscles are closed with the same kind of sutures. A suction drain is placed in the subcutaneous space, and the skin is closed with subcuticular 4-0 absorbable sutures. York-Mason's approach is used more widely than Kraske's approach because of its superior exposure. Despite cutting the sphincteric muscle during the procedure, anal incontinence has not been a problem.

York-Mason excised or resected carcinomas of the rectum via the transsphincteric approach in 50 patients and removed villous adenomas in another 39 patients. The results were satisfactory, but the outcome of the operation was not given (25). Heij et al. (28) and Bergman and Solhaug (29) used this technique on 6 and 21 patients, respectively. There was no mortality. No patients developed a fecal fistula, sepsis, or anal incontinence. Thompson and Tucker (30) operated on 26 patients; one patient developed temporary anal incontinence. Fecal fistulas occurred in seven patients. Five closed spontaneously and two patients required a temporary colostomy. Allgower et al. (26) reported no deaths in 79 patients, but complications were not mentioned.

The middle and upper rectum can also be mobilized and resected with the York-Mason approach. Either a handsewn or a circular stapled anastomosis can be performed (31).

The posterior approach is seldom required. A low rectal lesion can be excised with a transanal approach. The upper rectal lesion is too high for this approach. The midrectal lesion at the 7 to 10 cm level may be appropriate. I prefer to snare the benign lesion, even a large sessile type, via a colonoscope. For a malignant lesion, a low anterior resection is more appropriate unless there are contraindications.

TRANSANAL ENDOSCOPIC MICROSURGERY

Transanal endoscopic microsurgery (TEM) is a relatively new operative technique to remove sessile lesions of the rectum, developed by Buess et al. (32) of Germany. It has been applied clinically since 1983. The system uses a special rectoscope, 4 cm in diameter and 10 or 20 cm long. The scope is connected to the operative table via a supporting arms system, which can be adjusted to any desired position. The scope has a closed system of sealed caps with individual ports for forceps, suction, scissors, needle holder, and electrocautery. It is connected to a stereoscopic angulated optical system for visualization and can be hooked up to a television screen (Fig. 13). During the procedure, a continuous pressure-controlled insufflation of carbon dioxide keeps the rectum open for exposure. The patient is placed in a prone lateral or lithotomy position, according to the location of the polyp. The procedure is used for lesions in the middle and high rectum and occasionally in the low sigmoid colon up to 20 cm from the anal verge. The excision is done by electrocautery. Lesions located in the extraperitoneal part of the rectum are excised by full thickness. Only adenomas of the anterior wall located higher than 12 cm are excised in the submucosal plane. Invasive carcinomas of this location cannot be adequately treated because a full-thickness excision loses

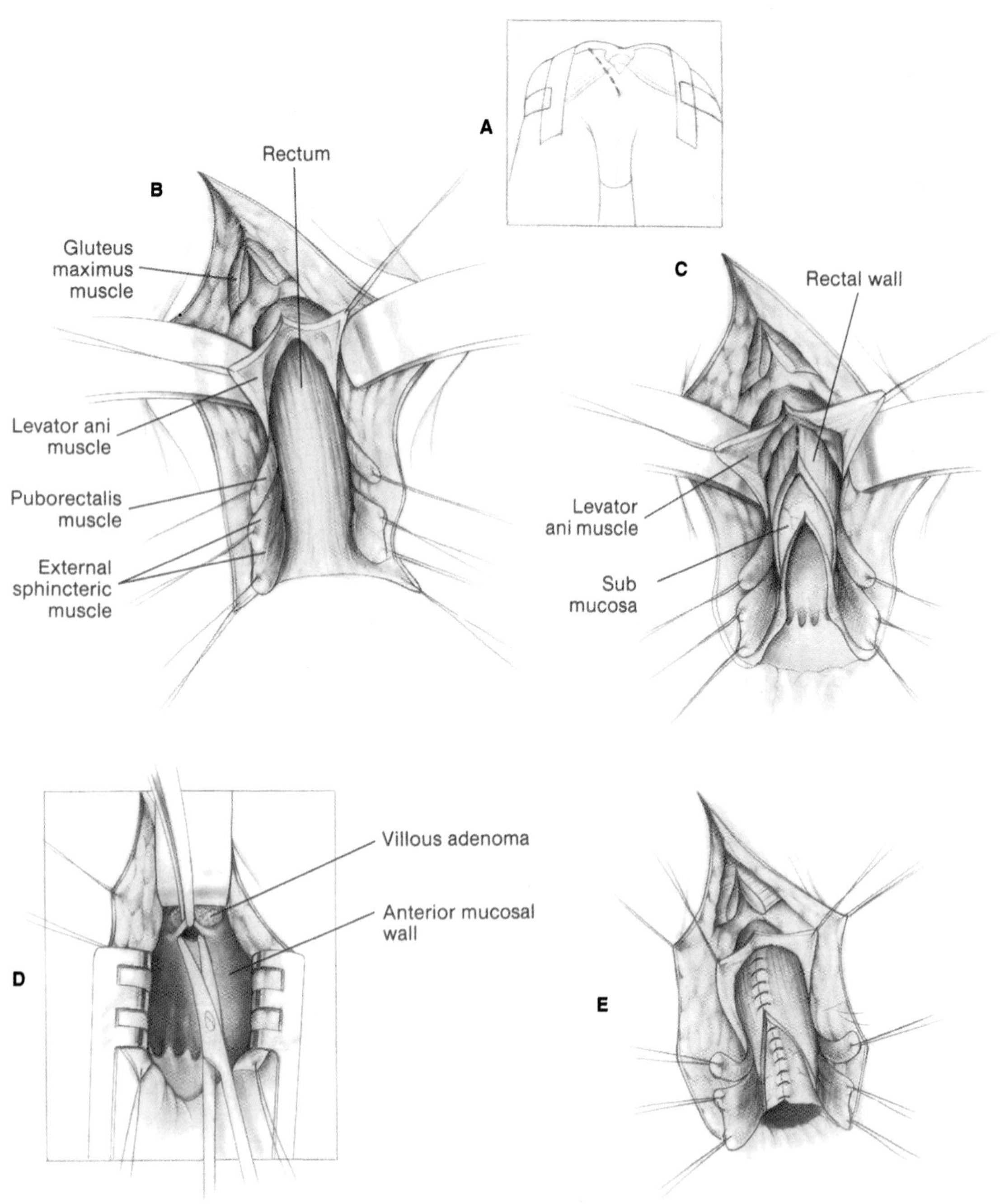

FIGURE 12 ■ York-Mason's transsphincteric approach. (**A**) With patient in prone position, a parasacral skin incision is used. (**B**) Incision is made through subcutaneous tissue, external sphincter muscles, and levator ani muscle. Each pair of muscles is marked on each side with sutures for accurate approximation. Posterior wall of rectum is exposed. Part of the gluteus muscle is incised to gain exposure. (**C**) Posterior wall of rectum is incised to expose the lumen. (**D**) Adenoma is excised in the submucosal plane. (**E**) Posterior wall of rectum is closed with running absorbable sutures, followed by closure of the wound in layers. *Source*: From Ref. 27.

gas into the peritoneal cavity. The defect is closed with 3-0 synthetic monofilament suture, which is cut to 6 cm in length. A silver clip is used instead of tying a knot (Fig. 14). TEM is suitable for a T1 lesion of the rectum.

Buess et al. (33) reported their experience in 326 patients with only one death from a pulmonary embolism. There was no intraoperative complication. Seventy-four patients had an invasive adenocarcinoma. The recurrence rate in the adenoma group was 4%. Twenty-nine of the 74 patients had T1 lesions that did not receive further treatment, and only one patient developed a recurrence. Major complications included breakdown of suture lines and rectovaginal fistulas. Complications occurred in 9% of patients who had invasive carcinoma.

The TEM technique has gained acceptance worldwide, including the United States (34,35). Smith et al. (35) reported the initial registry in the United States from 1990 to 1994. There were 153 patients: 82 with an adenoma, 54 with a carcinoma, and 17 with other entities. Approximately 50% of the lesions were located in the lower half of the rectum (below 8 cm). The sizes of the lesions ranged from 1 to 15 cm. The recurrence rate for adenomas was 11%. According to the TNM staging system, 30 of the malignant lesions were classified as T1, 15 were T2, and 6 were T3 carcinomas. There were three T1 recurrences (10%), six T2 recurrences (40%), and four T3 recurrences (66%). The intraoperative complications were surprisingly low. Eight procedures were converted to celiotomy because of the lack of proximal exposure. There was one perforation and one massive hemorrhage. Early postoperative complications were minor. A review of selected series in the literature by Saclarides (36) on T1 carcinoma of the rectum treated by TEM showed recurrent rates of 0–12.5%, 5-year disease free survival of 96–100%, and 5-year survival of 96-100%.

Middleton et al. (37) conducted a systematic review of comparative studies and the case of TEM from 1980 to 2002.

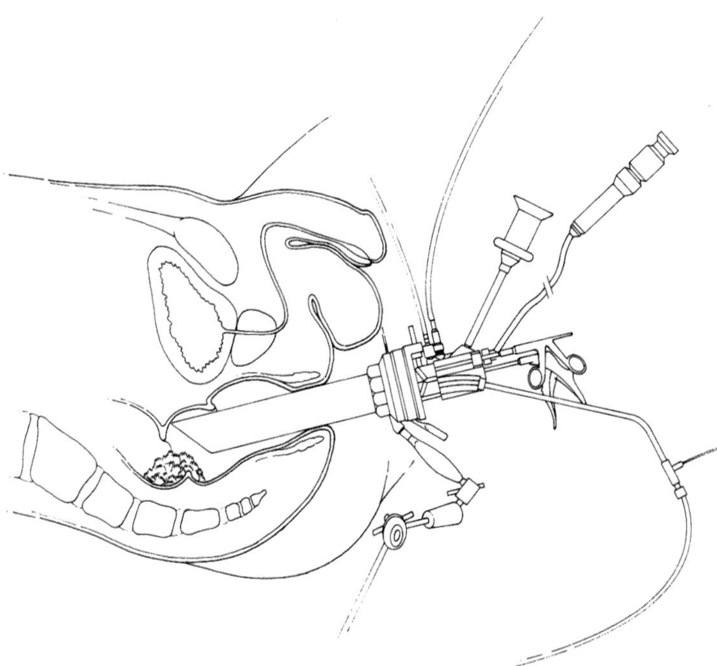

FIGURE 13 ■ Operative system for transanal endoscopic microsurgery.

Three comparative studies (including one randomized, controlled trail) and 55 case series were included. At the first area of study was a safety and efficacy of adenomas. In the randomized, controlled trial, no difference could be detected in the rate of early complications between the TEM (10.3%) and the direct local excision (17%) (relative risk, 0.61; TEM resulted in less local recurrence (6/98; 6%) than direct local excision (20/90; 22%) (relative risk, 0.28). The 6% rate of local recurrence for TEM in this trial is consistent with the rates found in case series of TEM (median, 5%).

The second area of study was a safety and efficacy of carcinomas. In the randomized, controlled trial, no difference could be detected in the rate of complications between TEM and direct local excision (relative risk for overall early complication rates, 0.56).

No difference in survival for local recurrence rate between TEM and anterior resection could be detected in either the randomized, controlled trial (hazard ratio, 1.02 for survival) or nonrandomized, comparative study. There were 2 of 25 (8%) TEM recurrences in the randomized, controlled trial, but no figures were given for recurrence after anterior resection. In the case series, the median local recurrence rate for TEM was 8.4%, ranging from 0% to 50%.

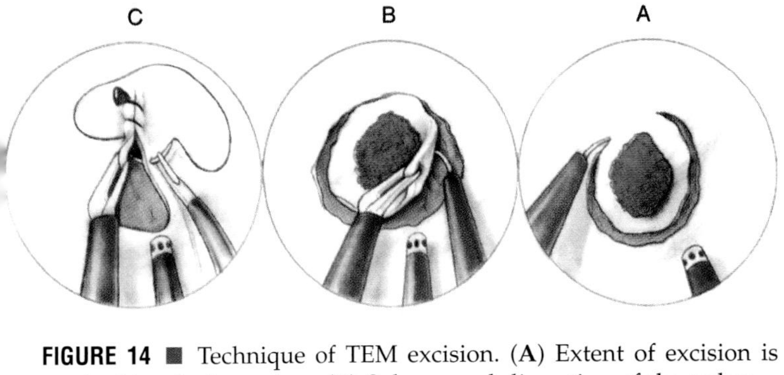

FIGURE 14 ■ Technique of TEM excision. (**A**) Extent of excision is marked by electrocautery. (**B**) Submucosal dissection of the polyp using electrocautery and forceps. A suction tube is placed close at hand. (**C**) Defect is closed with continuous sutures. Note that a silver clip is used as a knot.

The authors concluded that the evidence regarding TEM is very limited, being largely based on a single relatively small randomized, controlled trial.

Despite the large size of the operating scope (4 cm diameter), only three patients had mild incontinence (35). A prospective study to evaluate the anorectal function was conducted by Banerjee et al. (38). The evaluation included the clinical, manometric, and proctographic results of 36 patients presenting for TEM. Anorectal manometry showed no difference in maximal squeeze pressure before and 12 months after operation, but resting pressures were lower after operation (mean, 86.1 vs. 67.2; $p < 0.5$). The rectoanal inhibitory reflex was lost in a significant number of patients (34 of 36 before operation, 27 of 36 after operation, $p < 0.05$). The results of proctography showed no significant difference. Clinically, continence to solid stool or flatus was not affected after the operation. Completeness of emptying was not affected by TEM. This is in agreement with the prospective study by Cataldo et al. (39).

Surgeons who have attempted to learn TEM agree that this is the most difficult technique that they have tried to master (35,40). The problem lies with an inability to use the usual muscles of the arms and shoulders that are used in either open or laparoscopic surgery. In TEM the surgeon's fingers and wrists are the primary movers of the instruments, so a new coordination must be developed (40,41).

Any one wishing to incorporate TEM into their practice must devote significant time and energy to overcome a steep learning curve (40). TEM is a choice in the armamentarium that can obviate the need to perform a more radical operation, such as low anterior resection, and the approaches of Kraske or York-Mason.

According to Saclarides (36), currently, there were about 510 TEM systems in use worldwide. As expected, it was most commonly used in the United Kingdom and Europe where approximately 110 units were present in Germany and 300 were in use in England and remaining areas of the continent. In Japan and Southeast Asia, approximately 58 units were in use. In the United States, 45 systems were functional; however, usage has been slow to catch on for a variety of reasons.

ELECTROCOAGULATION OF CARCINOMA OF THE RECTUM

Since the report by Strauss et al. (42) in 1935 on the excellent results with electrocoagulation of carcinoma of the rectum, there have been sporadic reports of using this approach. In 1957, Madden and Kandalaft (43) reported on a small series of patients with carcinoma of the rectum who were treated by electrocoagulation as the primary and preferred method. Other investigators also reported favorable results in selected cases (44–46). Use of this method of treatment was stimulated by the less than satisfactory long-term survival rate and the high morbidity and mortality rates, especially in the elderly, with abdominoperineal resection. With modern advances in medicine, the morbidity and mortality rates for major operations have dropped dramatically. Indeed, the mortality rate for elective surgery for carcinoma of the rectum is reported as low as <1% (47). Electrocoagulation should be reserved for palliative treatment of rectal carcinoma or for poor surgical risk patients. However, there are proponents who use electrocoagulation as the a primary treatment for care in highly selected patients (46).

SELECTION OF PATIENTS

Chinn and Eisenstat (46) have outlined the criteria for electrocoagulation of distal rectal carcinomas, with the intention for cure:

- Well- or moderately well-differentiated adenocarcinoma
- Located ≤7.5 cm from the anal verge (below peritoneal reflection)
- ≤4 cm in diameter
- Absence of pelvic/pararectal adenopathy
- Stage T1 or T2 on endorectal ultrasonography

The obvious advantages of electrocoagulation for carcinoma of the lower part of the rectum are the 0% mortality rate and the avoidance of a permanent colostomy (48). The disadvantages are that electrocoagulation may fail to eradicate the primary malignancy, and that electrocoagulation fails to cure patients who have lymph node metastasis.

Preparation

Electrocoagulation of rectal carcinoma is not an office procedure. The bowel is prepared in the same manner as for a colonic resection. All patients should be hospitalized after the procedure. Spinal or general anesthesia is required, and the operative time may range from one to two hours.

Technique

The prone jackknife position is used for carcinomas located anteriorly and laterally. The lithotomy position is used for posterior ones. A Pratt speculum is used to visualize low-lying lesions, whereas an operative proctoscope is used for higher ones. Exposure is the key to success. The entire lesion must be seen. In the low-lying region, saline injection into the rectal wall adjacent to the carcinoma is helpful to protect thermal injury. A needlepoint electrode is used in preference to the ball-tip type because of its greater heat production and deeper penetration. A spatula tip, which is available in almost every operating room, is also effective. The coagulator is set at an appropriate power. The cautery tip is embedded in the carcinoma, with the depth dependent on the extent of penetration into the wall. The coagulator is applied repeatedly in an orderly manner until the entire carcinoma becomes flat and soft. Suction is used frequently to evacuate the smoke and the possible explosive gases. A curette or a biopsy forceps can be used to remove the coagulum. Carcinomas located in the posterior or lateral quadrant of the lower and middle portions of the rectum can be coagulated vigorously because they are extraperitoneal, whereas lesions located in the anterior wall of the middle rectum must be treated more cautiously because of their intraperitoneal location. In women, carcinomas of the anterior wall may require coagulation in multiple stages to avoid the development of a rectovaginal fistula.

Postoperative Management

Patients usually have no significant pain following operation. Fever from the reaction to the coagulation may last for several days and should be treated only symptomatically. Only clear liquids are allowed for the first day until it is certain that no perforation has occurred. When the patient has advanced to a regular diet, a bulk-producing agent is prescribed. The patient should be reexamined in the clinic two months after the coagulation. A biopsy should be obtained of any suspicious area. If the area is malignant, repeat coagulation is performed. It may be necessary to repeat the coagulation several times for complete eradication of the malignancy.

Failure of Electrocoagulation

The site of the electrocoagulation must be reexamined by proctoscopy every two to three months during the first year and every three to six months during the second year. If coagulation fails to control the lesion and if digital examination or endorectal ultrasonography strongly suggests lymph node metastasis, an abdominoperineal resection or a low anterior resection is indicated. In the series by Chinn and Eisenstat (46), 31 of 114 patients required conversion to an abdominoperineal resection because of recurrences. The five-year survival rate in that group of patients was 29%, with almost 90% having lesions originally >4 cm, and 21 of 31 patients demonstrating nodal metastasis.

Results

Madden and Kandalaft (48) reported on a series of 204 patients. Electrocoagulation was used as the primary curative method, with a follow-up of 5 to 27 years. The lesions included those in 12 patients with squamous cell carcinoma of the anal canal. The carcinomas were 2 to 10 cm from the anal verge. Fifty-nine percent of the patients required two to four electrocoagulations. No deaths resulted, and the overall complication rate was 24%. Among the frequent complications were bleeding 16%, half of which stopped spontaneously; rectal stricture, 2%; rectovaginal fistula, 2%; and perforation, 1%. The overall five-year survival rate was 64%, with 72% for lesions <3 cm in diameter and 62% for lesions >3 cm.

Of the 81 patients treated with an intention for cure in the study by Chinn and Eisenstat (46), the five-year survival rate was 65%. The complications of electrocoagulation included bleeding, 7%; stricture, 6%; urinary retention, 2.6%; electrical burns, 2.6%; perianal abscess, 0.9%; and perforation; 0.9%. The overall mortality rate was 2.7%.

REFERENCES

1. Levitt MD. Volume and composition of human intestinal gas determined by means of an intestinal washout technic. N Engl J Med 1971; 284:1394–1398.
2. Bond JH, Levy M, Levitt MD. Explosion of hydrogen gas in the colon during proctosigmoidoscopy. Gastrointest Endosc 1976; 23:41.
3. Carter HG. Explosion in the colon during electrodessication of polyps. Am J Surg 1952; 84:514.

4. Nivatvongs S. Technique of rectal biopsy. Dis Colon Rectum 1981; 24:132.
5. Galandiuk S, Fazio VW, Jagelman DG, et al. Villous and tubulovillous adenomas of the colon and rectum. A retrospective review, 1964–1985. Am J Surg 1987; 153:41–47.
6. Nivatvongs S, Nicholson JD, Rothenberger DA, et al. Villous adenomas of the rectum: The accuracy of clinical assessment. Surgery 1980; 87:549–551.
7. Taylor EW, Thompson H, Oates GD, et al. Limitations of biopsy in preoperative assessment of villous papilloma. Dis Colon Rectum 1981; 24:259–262.
8. Sakamoto G, MacKeigan JM, Senagore AJ. Transanal excision of large, rectal villous adenomas. Dis Colon Rectum 1991; 34:880–885.
9. Faivre J. Transanal electro-resection of rectal tumor by means of tractable mucocutaneous anal flap. Coloproctology 1980; 2:77–80.
10. Pigot F, Bouchard D, Mortaji M, et al. Local excision of large villous adenomas. Long-term results. Dis Colon Rectum 2003; 46:1345–1350.
11. Roberts PL. Mucosectomy for treatment of rectal neoplasia. Semin Colon Rectal Surg 1996; 7:210–214.
12. Parks AG, Stuart AE. The management of villous tumors of the large bowel. Br J Surg 1973; 9:688–695.
13. Nivatvongs S, Wolf BG. Technique of per anal excision for carcinoma of the low rectum. World J Surg 1992; 163:447–450.
14. Madbouly KM, Remji FH, Erkek BA, et al. Recurrence after transanal excision of T1 rectal cancer: Should we be concerned: Dis Colon Rectum 2005; 48:711–721.
15. Nascimberi R, Nivatrongs S, Larson DR, Burgart LJ. Long-term survival after local excision for T1 carcinoma of the rectum. Dis Colon Rectum 2004; 47:1773–1779.
16. Paty PS, Nash GM, Barm P, et al. Long-term results of local excision for rectal cancer. Ann Surg 2002; 236:522–530.
17. Mellgren A, Sirivongs P, Rothenberger DA, Modoff RD, Garcia-Aguilar J. Is local excision adequate therapy for early sectal cancer? Dis Colon Rectum 2000; 43:1064–1074.
18. Brunetaud JM, Maunoury V, Cochelard D, Boniface B, Cartot A, Paris JC. Endoscopic laser treatment for rectosigmoid villous adenoma: Factors affecting the results. Gastroenterology 1989; 97:272–277.
19. Kocher TD. Exstirpatic Recti Nach Vorheriger Excision des Steissbeins. Cent Chir 1874; 10:145–147.
20. Perry EG, Hinrichs B. A new translation of Professor Dr. P. Kraske's Zur Exstirpation Hochsitzender Mastdarmkrebse. Aust N Z J Surg 1989; 59:421–424.
21. Arnaud A, Fretes IR, Joly A, Sarles JC. Posterior approach to the rectum for treatment of selected benign lesions. Int J Colorectal Dis 1991; 6:100–102.
22. Christiansen J. Excision of mid-rectal lesion by the Kraske sacral approach. Br J Surg 1980; 67:651–652.
23. Bergamaschi R, Arnaud A. Management of large encircling mid-rectal adenomas in frail patients. Int J Colorectal Dis 1995; 10:53–54.
24. Bevan AD. Carcinoma of the rectum—Treatment by local excision. Surg Clin North Am 1917; 1:1233–1240.
25. Mason AY. Transsphincteric approach to rectal lesion. Surg Annu l977; 9:171–194.
26. Allgower M, Durig M, Hochstetter AV, Huber A. The parasacral sphincter-splitting approach to the rectum. World J Surg 1982; 6:539–548.
27. York-Mason A. In: Malt R, ed. Surgical techniques illustrated. Boston: Little, Brown, 1977, pp 75–77.
28. Heij HA, Tan KG, Houten HV. The transsphincteric approach to rectal villous adenomas. Neth J Surg 1982; 34:4–7.
29. Bergman L, Solhaug JH. Posterior transsphincteric resect small tumors of the lower rectum. Acta Chir Scand 1986; 152:313–316.
30. Thompson BW, Tucker WE. Transsphincteric approach to lesions of the rectum. South Med J 1987; 80:41–43.
31. Kusunoki M, Yanogi H, Shoji Y, Sakanoue Y, Yamamura T, Utsunomiya J. Stapled anastomosis for trans-sphincteric resection of the rectum. Surg Gynecol Obstet 1991; 173:325–326.
32. Buess G, Kipfmuller K, Ibald R, et al. Clinical results of transanal endoscopic microsurgery. Surg Endosc 1988; 2:245–250.
33. Buess G, Mentzes B, Manncke K, Starlinger M, Becker HD. Technique and results of transanal endoscopic microsurgery in early rectal cancer. Am J Surg 1992; 163:63–70.
34. Mayer J, Mortensen NMcC. Transanal endoscopic microsurgery: A forgotten minimally invasive operation. Br J Surg 1995; 821:435–437.
35. Smith LE, Ko ST, Saclarides T, Caushaj P, Orkin BA, Khanduja KS. Transanal endoscopic microsurgery. Initial registry. Dis Colon Rectum 1996; 39:579–584.
36. Saclarides TJ. Transanal endoscopic microsurgery. Semin Colon Rectal Surg 2005; 16:20–25.
37. Middleton PF, Sutherland LM, Madder GJ. Transanal endoscopic microsurgery: A systemic review. Dis Colon Rectum 2005; 48:270–284.
38. Banerjee AK, Jehle BC, Kreis ME, et al. Prospective study of the proctographic and functional consequences of transanal endoscopic microsurgery. Br J Surg 1996; 83:211–213.
39. Cataldo PA, O'Brien S, Oster T. Transanal endoscopic microsurgery: A prospective evaluation of functional results. Dis Colon Rectum 2005; 48:1366–1371.
40. Buess GF, Raestrup H. Transanal endoscopic microsurgery. Surg Oncol Clin N Am 2001; 10:709–731.
41. Smith LE. Transanal endoscopic microsurgery for selected rectal tumors. Semin Colon Rectal Surg 1996; 7:221–226.
42. Strauss AA, Strauss SF, Crawford RA, Strauss HA. Surgical diathermy of carcinoma of the rectum: Its clinical end results. JAMA 1935; 104:1480–1484.
43. Madden JL, Kandalaft S. Electrocoagulation. A primary and preferred method of treatment for cancer of the rectum. Ann Surg 1967; 166:413–419.
44. Crile G Jr., Turnbull RB. The role of electrocoagulation treatment of carcinoma of the rectum. Surg Gynecol Obstet 1972; 135:391–396.
45. Hughes EP Jr., Veidenheimer MC, Corman ML, Collet JA. Electrocoagulation of rectal cancer. Dis Colon Rectum 1982; 25:215–218.
46. Chinn B, Eisenstat TE. Electrocoagulation of selected adenocarcinoma of the distal rectum. Semin Colon Rectal Surg 1996; 7:233–237.
47. Pollard CW, Nivatvongs S, Rojanasakul A, Ilstrup DM. Carcinoma of the rectum: Profiles of intraoperative and early postoperative complications. Dis Colon Rectum 1994; 37:866–874.
48. Madden JL, Kandalaft SI. Electrocoagulation as a primary curative method in the treatment of carcinoma of the rectum. Surg Gynecol Obstet 1983; 157:164–179.

20 Ambulatory Procedures

Peter A. Cataldo and Philip H. Gordon

INTRODUCTION

In 1909, it was reported in the *British Medical Journal* that Dr. James Nicoll had performed more than 1700 operations (1). Although ambulatory surgery may not be a phenomenon of modern surgery, in recent years there has been growing interest in the performance of ambulatory procedures. With health care costs continuing to spiral upward, physicians, hospitals, patients, and third-party carriers are seeking ways to save health care dollars without jeopardizing the patients' safety. The consequence of this search will be the performance of a large number of ambulatory procedures that heretofore have been (and still are, by many) thought to require hospital admission for safe performance. A number of factors have contributed to the acceptance of outpatient procedures. These factors include the development of improved local and general anesthetics, better surgical education encouraging patients to become ambulatory soon after operation, the public's willingness to participate in nursing themselves and their families, the ability to satisfy the unique needs of the patient requiring elective operative care, the public's increased interest in and knowledge of medical matters, and possibly, a healthier public. The changes have been achieved through technological advances, sustained by patient and provider preference, and driven largely by payment system changes (2).

Perhaps the most important are changing surgeon attitudes and changing patient expectations. Surgeons no longer demand their patients be admitted after hemorrhoidectomy, fissure, or fistula surgery. Likewise, patients expect to be released several hours after these operations. In addition, family members now plan (with the encouragement of the government in the form of the Family Leave Act) to be home and available to aid their loved ones through recovery.

Accompanying these changes in expectations, we have developed better outpatient postoperative care systems. This begins with patient and family education. Discharge teams inform family members what to expect with regard to pain, constipation, wound drainage, new medications, and wound care. Home health care and visiting nurses associations have grown exponentially and provide expert care in the patient's homes, and also act as liaisons to the physician should any questions or problems arise.

These factors have lead to a profound increase in ambulatory surgery, particularly in countries where third-party payors provide reimbursement. In the United States, it has been estimated that 90% of anorectal cases can be performed on an outpatient basis (3). Ambulatory surgery continues to increase and the sites where the procedures are performed are also changing.

By definition, ambulatory procedures are those in which the patient returns home on the day of the operation, regardless of whether it was performed with the patient under general or local anesthesia or whether it was performed in a private physician's office, a hospital emergency department, the regular hospital operating room, or a freestanding, independent ambulatory surgery unit. Other terms that have been used to apply to this situation include one-day surgery, same-day surgery, and office-based surgery. In 1999, it was estimated that 65% of surgical procedures in North America were carried out in ambulatory settings (4), but as early as 1986 Smith estimated that 90% of anorectal cases may be suitable for ambulatory surgery (5). In 1994, ambulatory surgery accounted for 50% of all surgery in the United States (2). By contrast, it was estimated that in 1990, same-day surgery constituted only about 10% of all surgical procedures performed in Europe (2). The number of surgical procedures performed annually in hospital outpatient settings between 1980 and 1990 increased from approximately 3.2 million to approximately 11.7 million (1). By contrast, the number of inpatient operations decreased from 16.3 million to 11.4 million over the same period (30%). In 1992, 73% of all ambulatory surgical procedures were conducted in hospital outpatient facilities, 17% in ambulatory surgical centers, and 10% in physician offices. The number of freestanding ambulatory surgical clinics increased 710% from 239 centers in 1983 to 1696 centers in 1992 (1).

Over the prior two decades, there has been a significant shift from inpatient to outpatient surgery. This shift has been stimulated by spiraling health care costs and by the desire of insurance carriers to minimize surgery-related expenses. With this changing paradigm, we have learned that many procedures previously associated with hospital stays can now be accomplished as safely, and sometimes more safely, on an outpatient basis. However, as pressure increases to shorten hospital stays and increase the number of operations done without hospitalization, adverse outcomes may increase along with decreases in patient satisfaction. Not suited for the outpatient environment are those patients who may have postoperative pain unrelieved by oral analgesics, those whose operations are likely to be followed by postoperative bleeding, patients who have severe emotional objections to the idea, or those who live alone (6).

With a better understanding of the anatomy and pathophysiology of anorectal disease, along with acquired technical expertise, a great variety of procedures can be performed safely in the office or outpatient department with the patient under local anesthesia. A well-equipped office, which includes basic resuscitation equipment, permits the surgeon to perform the kind of procedures described below.

In the minds of some surgeons the threat of a malpractice suit for poor results or complications is enough to restrict their office use. However, for selected procedures in an adequately equipped office, this consideration should not be relevant. Recent evidence suggests that ambulatory surgery appears to produce equivalent outcomes (similar or lower mortality and complication rates, if established criteria of selection are followed) and increased levels of patient satisfaction (2).

As we select patients and procedures to be done at outpatient facilities, it is critically important to develop principles on which these decisions can be based. What criteria must be satisfied to perform an operation without overnight hospitalization? And what are the clear contraindications to such procedures?

Certainly patients with significant medical comorbidities requiring postoperative observation, such as cardiac or pulmonary monitoring, must remain inpatients after surgery. Individuals unable to tolerate oral intake, and therefore requiring intravenous hydration must also be hospitalized until they are able to eat and drink well enough to maintain themselves. Patients at significant risk for complications requiring immediate care (such as hemorrhage) must also be hospitalized until this risk has abated. Finally, patients should not be sent home in pain. If intravenous narcotics are necessary to control surgically induced pain, then patients should be treated where intravenous medications are available until oral medications provide adequate pain control.

Who, then, are candidates for outpatient operations? Patients who do not require intensive monitoring, who can tolerate an oral diet, whose pain is well controlled on oral analgesics, and who can care for their surgical wounds. If these criteria are met, outpatient surgery should be uniformly successful. Fortunately the vast majority of patients undergoing anorectal procedures meet these criteria and thus many anorectal operations are performed in an outpatient setting.

Several "gray areas" do, however, exist. How do we treat the patient who travels 3 or 4 hours to the hospital? Or the patient who lives alone and has trouble caring for him- or herself? Or the individual unable to void following operation? All of these are important considerations and must be taken into account when determining the appropriateness of outpatient surgery. In these circumstances, out of hospital support systems such as home health care and/or a visiting nurses association may be of great benefit if they exist in a given community.

Of prime concern in recommending ambulatory surgery is quality assurance. It is important to remember that our primary responsibilities are to our patients and therefore any further shifts to outpatient surgery should be accompanied by scrupulous quality assurance monitoring to ensure that patients are not suffering to satisfy third-party payor demands. In a statement on ambulatory surgery, the American College of Surgeons approved the practice of performing certain operative procedures in ambulatory facilities; however, the College cautioned that such practices require careful patient selection and safe recuperation at home and stated that consideration should be given to the anesthetic risk, age, and general condition of the patient and the time it takes to do the operation. The governing authority of a freestanding ambulatory surgical center should be responsible for maintaining proper standards of surgical care (1). Proper standards include having provisions for utilization review, specified qualifications for personnel using the facility, provisions for medical audits, and access to emergency and ancillary facilities in a nearby hospital. In its 1981 *Accreditation Manual for Hospitals* (7), the Joint Commission on Accreditation of Hospitals stated that when surgical services are provided in an ambulatory care setting, the policies and procedures shall be consistent with those applicable to inpatient surgery, anesthesia, and postoperative recovery. Such recommendations should be self-evident (8). Patient safety should not be compromised for reasons of economy or convenience. Recommendations for ambulatory procedures should be predicated on considerations of the complexity and risks of the procedure, the facility's resources, the availability of quality aftercare, and the physical and emotional state of the patient. Contraindications to outpatient operations include advanced cardiopulmonary disease and other serious medical problems.

PREOPERATIVE ASSESSMENT

PATIENT EVALUATION

The amount of preoperative preparation depends on whether the contemplated procedure will be performed with the patient under local or general anesthesia. For patients having procedures under local anesthesia, a simple history about bleeding diatheses and allergies to local anesthesia or medications such as anticoagulants should be obtained. Particular attention should be focused on comorbid medical conditions and medications (such as cardiac medications and anticoagulants), which may need to be manipulated to maximize patient safety. In addition, disabilities limiting an individual's ability to care for him- or herself (such as blindness, stroke, or dementia) should be evaluated. Bowel preparation comprises only an enema; for some procedures even an enema is not needed.

A preoperative discussion with the patient should describe the procedure and include any of the patient's concerns, such as pain control, complications, and recommended activity at home.

For patients undergoing general anesthesia, a history, physical examination, complete blood count, and urinalysis should be obtained. For patients older than 40 years of age, chest x-ray films and electrocardiograms usually are required. Additional tests such as serum electrolyte values may be indicated in patients taking diuretics. The extensive preoperative testing required in the past has now been deemed unnecessary. There are currently no "routine" preoperative studies. In many centers, anesthesia guidelines recommend cardiograms in males over 50 and females over 55. Some require chest x-rays for all patients over 60. Well-performed studies indicate there is little benefit to unselected, routine preoperative testing (9).

An evaluation of 1200 patients scheduled for outpatient surgery revealed a comprehensive history and physical as the most reliable means for identifying significant abnormalities (10). Despite identification, these abnormalities were not predictive of surgical complications or need for overnight hospitalization.

Macpherson et al. reviewed 1,109 patients undergoing elective surgery and found that 47% of preoperative laboratory tests had been performed in the previous year. Significant changes rarely occurred and were predicted by changes in the patient's history and physical examination (11). In a separate study Turnbull and Buck evaluated 5003 preoperative screening tests and found only 225 abnormal results (12). Of these only 104 had any potential implications and led to changes in evaluation and/or treatment in only 17 cases. The authors concluded that only 4 of the 5003 patients received significant benefit from routine preoperative testing. Many practitioners routinely order coagulation parameters to minimize bleeding risks following surgery. A study looked at a cohort 12,000 individuals subject to invasive procedures. Ninety-two percent were judge by history to be at low risk for bleeding. In this group of patients, clotting studies were of no predictive value (13). Therefore, clotting studies are unjustified preoperatively in individuals without a history of bleeding tendency or of taking anticoagulants.

Based on the above-mentioned studies, a history and physical examination are the most important aspects of the preoperative evaluation. Preoperative testing should be directed by abnormalities identified during this portion of the work-up and not done on a routine basis.

PATIENT PREPARATION

In addition to being diagnosed and evaluated for operation, individuals should be prepared for postoperative discharge at their preoperative visit. Patients and families should be informed as to the nature of the operation including alternative approaches, benefits, and potential complications. The postoperative home course should be detailed including normal pain, wound, and drainage expectations. Alterations in bowel habits (particularly medication-induced constipation) should be predicted and remedies provided. In addition individuals and families should be educated regarding particularly worrisome events, which should prompt calls to their physician, such as high fever, excessive vomiting, inability to void, intractable pain, and significant bleeding. Ideally all of this information should be available in a preprinted postoperative instruction sheet or booklet, and should include a number to call 24-hours a day in case of emergency.

In addition to patient education, office and perioperative medical personnel should be educated regarding their roles in outpatient surgical procedures. Office assistants and nurses will be the first points of contact when patients develop problems or have questions following operation. Therefore, they too should be informed of the normal postoperative course and worrisome complaints that might indicate a significant postoperative complication.

In some institutions, perioperative nursing specialists screen individuals prior to outpatient operation and also provide follow-up phone calls the evening of the operation. This can be reassuring to patients. Educating these nurses to the specific expectations following anorectal procedures can be particularly helpful. Providing serial "in-service" seminars to update office and perioperative personnel will greatly improve the outpatient surgical process and also increase staff satisfaction. Often, inviting team members into the operating room to observe ambulatory anorectal procedures will increase understanding and staff satisfaction as well. The patient must be told to withhold food and drink beginning at midnight before the operation.

OPERATIVE MANAGEMENT

Procedures are most often performed with the patient in the prone jackknife position. Dependable anesthesia that is technically easy to administer and allows rapid recovery with minimal side effects is needed. Anesthetic techniques should have little impact upon the ability to discharge patients following anorectal operations, with a few minor exceptions. For patients undergoing procedures under local anesthesia, some surgeons prefer administering additional sedation, usually a combination of meperidine and diazepam (5). This combination minimizes fluid requirements (vasodilatation, which accompanies spinal anesthesia, is avoided) and can provide extended postoperative analgesia. Local anesthesia technique is described in Chapter 5.

Using regional anesthesia presents a special set of considerations (14). Spinal, epidural, and caudal anesthesia have the following problems in common: time consumed during the block, potential technical difficulties with the block, time consumed waiting for onset, variability in degree of block produced, and problems during the recovery period. Any degree of motor paralysis significantly prolongs time in the recovery room. Although it is possible to send a patient from the recovery room to the surgical ward with a small amount of residual block, the ambulatory patient cannot walk to the car. The problem of postlumbar puncture headache is always a consideration and can significantly complicate the ambulatory surgical patient's course of recovery and early return to work. Therefore, at the Tucson Medical Center perirectal field blocks are used (14).

Long-acting spinal anesthetics, particularly combined with large, intraoperative fluid administration, will increase urinary retention rates and delay discharge (15). Alpha-adrenergic blockers have been administered prophylactically in this setting to decrease the spasm of the autonomically innervated, internal sphincter at the bladder neck in attempts to decrease urinary retention, but have not met with success (16). Limiting postoperative fluids in combination with short-acting spinal anesthetic has, however, decreased urinary retention rates (17).

General anesthesia with heavy emphasis on narcotics may cause postoperative nausea and vomiting leading to prolonged recovery room stay or even overnight hospitalization.

Perianal shaving is not necessary except for patients with pilonidal disease. Some procedures can be performed in the office, whereas others are performed in an operating room setting.

PROCEDURES

The majority of anorectal cases can be performed on an outpatient basis. A large study indicated that 92% of anorectal procedures were performed successfully without hospitalization (5).

Procedures that can be performed on an outpatient basis are discussed in the following sections.

RECTAL BIOPSY

Various forceps and suction biopsy apparatus are available for obtaining specimens from the rectum for histologic evaluation. The forceps technique is probably the best for obtaining localized and proliferative lesions. For the pathologist to provide maximal information to the clinician, a correct anatomic orientation is necessary. Consequently, when the specimen is obtained, it should be submitted with the submucosal surface downward against a flat, ground-glass slide or on paper to which it adheres by its own stickiness. After fixation, the biopsy material is embedded to facilitate detailed assessment of mucosal and submucosal pathology. The advantages of a properly oriented biopsy specimen are apparent and cannot be overemphasized. For biopsies of carcinomas and other localized or proliferative lesions, however, the tissue cannot be fixed and embedded in this way. This method is suitable only for diffuse mucosal conditions, particularly inflammatory diseases.

Morson and Dawson (18) point out that rectal biopsies are becoming more and more useful for a wide range of local and systemic disorders. Performing a biopsy is essential for the diagnosis of neoplasms, particularly malignant ones. Indeed, no major operation should be carried out on the rectum without confirmatory biopsy. Its value is established in the diagnosis of inflammatory conditions, including specific infections such as amebic dysentery. Serial biopsies can be valuable in the diagnosis of ulcerative colitis and Crohn's disease and can be useful in judging the response to treatment. Biopsy may detect changes not apparent to the endoscopist. The correlation between proctosigmoidoscopic observations and the histology of biopsies of the rectal mucosa is not always accurate. For this reason biopsy can, in certain circumstances, add refinement to the clinical opinion. It also confirms the presence of normal rectal mucosa.

Unusual local conditions that can be identified by rectal biopsy include pneumatosis cystoides intestinalis, mucoviscidosis, melanosis coli, oleogranuloma, and parasitic infections such as schistosomiasis (18). Rectal biopsy may be useful in detecting certain systemic conditions such as neurolipidoses, metachromatic leukodystrophy, Hurler's syndrome, amyloidosis, the arteritis of rheumatoid arthritis, periarteritis nodosa, malignant hypertension, cystinosis, and Whipple's disease (18).

HEMORRHOIDS

Excision of Thrombosed External Hemorrhoids

The treatment of a patient with a thrombosed hemorrhoid depends on the severity of pain. If the pain is subsiding, operative treatment is unnecessary. However, if the pain is excruciating or an erosion has developed in the thrombosed hemorrhoid, resulting in persistent bleeding, excision of the involved hemorrhoid is indicated. A complete ring of multiple confluent thrombosed external hemorrhoids is best treated in the operating room by definitive hemorrhoidectomy with the patient under appropriate anesthesia.

Technique for Inducing Local Anesthesia

The skin adjacent to the anus is richly innervated; therefore, injection of a local anesthetic may be a painful procedure. An initial wheal is made with a small needle (25 or 26 gauge), and the anesthetic solution is slowly introduced into the tissue beneath and around the thrombosed hemorrhoid, because injecting the solution rapidly would distend the tissues very quickly and cause increased pain. Lidocaine diffuses rapidly into the tissues, and hyaluronidase may be used to augment this diffusion. The addition of epinephrine aids hemostasis and prolongs the duration of anesthesia.

Technique for Performing Excision

The operative area is prepared with an aqueous antiseptic solution. Alcohol causes a burning sensation and may ignite if cautery is used. An elliptical incision is made to encompass the thrombosed hemorrhoid, and dissection is carried down to the muscle but not into the anal canal. Incisions extended into the anal canal may result in a bleeding point that goes undetected. With the thrombosed hemorrhoid excised, the exposed edge of the external sphincter muscle is noted. Hemostasis is obtained with cautery, and the wound is closed with a continuous absorbable suture such as 3–0 chromic catgut. The wound may be left open for granulation, because the wound margins will fall together anyway. Performing only incision and enucleation of the clot without removal of the hemorrhoid is not advisable, because bleeding and clotting tend to recur within a few hours and the pain may be as intense as before the operation.

Internal Hemorrhoids

The treatment of internal hemorrhoids is done as an office procedure in most situations. Because of the autonomic innervation of the tissues above the level of the dentate line, therapeutic procedures may be performed without anesthesia.

Barron Rubber Band Ligature

The symptoms of bleeding and protrusion usually can be controlled through the Barron rubber band ligation technique. The method is both simple and effective. Details of its application are described in Chapter 8.

Sclerotherapy

Injection of sclerosing agents in the region of the offending hemorrhoidal tissue is effective for treating small internal hemorrhoids. The details of this technique are also included in Chapter 8.

Procedure for Prolapsed Hemorrhoids (PPH)

The most recent operative procedure for internal hemorrhoids via the stapled procedure for prolapsed hemorrhoids (PPH) is also a procedure that can be performed on an ambulatory basis.

Excision of External Hemorrhoidal Skin Tags

External hemorrhoidal tags that annoy patients, mostly because of the inconvenience of cleansing, can be excised simply with no bowel preparation and no admission to the hospital while the patient is under local anesthesia. The tags can be excised in an elliptical manner and the wound edges approximated with an absorbable suture.

Hemorrhoidectomy

Although a one-quadrant hemorrhoidectomy can be performed easily as an outpatient procedure, many believe that in most circumstances a formal three-quadrant hemorrhoidectomy is best performed as an inpatient procedure. Nevertheless, in selected circumstances, hemorrhoidectomies have been performed on an outpatient basis. Definition may be important here because in many institutions, a 23-hour stay is considered ambulatory. With growing experience and confidence, Friend and Medwell (19) have reported an increase in hemorrhoidectomies performed on an outpatient basis from 0% in 1975 to 99% in 1986. Leff (20) reported a more modest 72% of hemorrhoidectomies performed on an outpatient basis.

Certain insurance companies have decreed that when the patients they have insured require hemorrhoidectomy, the operation must be performed on an outpatient basis. Many surgeons fear this policy may compromise the patients' welfare. In response to these pressures, in 1986 an ad hoc committee of the American Society of Colon and Rectal Surgeons formulated the following statement, "Surgical Treatment of Hemorrhoids," which was approved by the Clinical Procedure Review Committee and the Council of the American Society of Colon and Rectal Surgeons:

> Major surgery for external and internal hemorrhoids is appropriately carried out in the hospital because of the necessity of anesthesia and the requirements for postoperative nursing care. Criteria for discharge from hospital care would include institution of urinary and bowel function and absence of complications requiring continuing nursing care.

The statement also notes:

> An over-riding consideration is that the patient and the surgeon must be in agreement on any treatment plan. It is anticipated that governmental agencies and party payers will continue to be in sympathy with this basic requirement.

Nevertheless, there is no doubt that outpatient hemorrhoidectomy can be performed in select situations, contingent on the absence of other overriding medical conditions, whether there is a capable person in the patient's home to take care of him, and how far the patient would have to travel after operation to get home.

■ LATERAL INTERNAL SPHINCTEROTOMY

One of the most painful anorectal conditions is acute fissure. When medical management proves unsatisfactory, a lateral internal sphincterotomy generally produces dramatic and immediate results in relief of pain (21). The operative technique and its numerous advantages are described in detail in Chapter 9.

Associated with a fissure-in-ano may be a large prolapsing, hypertrophied anal papilla. If the papilla is symptomatic, it can be removed easily by infiltrating a small amount of local anesthetic at the base of the pedicle and transecting it flush with the wall of the anal canal. Hemostasis is controlled easily with cautery or suture. Exposure may be obtained either by prolapsing the lesion or visualizing it through a suitable retractor such as a Pratt bivalve.

■ INCISION AND DRAINAGE OF ABSCESSES

Almost all perianal and pilonidal abscesses and most ischioanal abscesses can be drained with the patient under local anesthesia in the outpatient setting. Such treatment immediately relieves the pain. Another advantage of draining abscesses around the anorectal region with the patient under local anesthesia is that the surgeon is not tempted to divide the sphincter muscle initially. Many patients, therefore, will have their sphincter muscle kept intact rather than having portions of it divided during the initial procedure. Details of this technique are described in Chapter 10. A simple incision is inadequate, because the skin edges may coapt within 24 hours and the abscess may recur.

The tiny abscesses and short subcutaneous fistulous tracts associated with hidradenitis suppurativa also may be opened and unroofed with the patient under local anesthesia and treatment handled on an ambulatory basis. However, extensive disease requires more thorough treatment in the operating room.

A patient with an intersphincteric abscess may require admission to the hospital or at least a short hospital stay, because a general or regional anesthetic is required for appropriate drainage.

■ POLYPS AND CARCINOMA

Most pedunculated polyps can be removed on an ambulatory basis. A pedunculated lesion is easily snared, and when the surgeon is familiar with the electrosurgical equipment, bleeding seldom should be a problem. Details of this procedure are outlined in Chapter 19.

A section of an ulcerated or fungating neoplasm can be removed easily for biopsy with a biopsy forceps. Electrocoagulation may be necessary to control bleeding.

Elevations of mucosa less than 5 mm in diameter are frequently seen, and there is a difference in opinion regarding their management. Some surgeons simply destroy such lesions by coagulation, whereas others insist on performance of a biopsy and histologic examination. We strongly favor the latter approach because if the polyp is neoplastic, knowledge of its association with other synchronous and metachronous lesions becomes important and patients require a lifelong follow-up with barium enema and/or preferably colonoscopy. If the lesion proves to be hyperplastic, such close follow-up may not be necessary.

Large sessile lesions are best removed in the operating room by lifting the lesion off the underlying wall in the submucosal plane as described in Chapter 19. If lesions are small, the procedure can be performed on an ambulatory basis.

■ CONDYLOMA ACUMINATUM

Although the application of podophyllin for treating condyloma acuminatum is easily done in the office, its use may be difficult to control and can result in excessive destruction of normal anal canal mucosa.

Electrocoagulation has been an effective means of destroying condyloma acuminatum. This treatment can be performed on an ambulatory basis. Care must be taken to rule out warts within the anal or vaginal canal. Cooperative patients with only a few scattered warts in the anal canal can undergo this procedure under adequately administered local anesthesia. However, patients with extensive warts located within the anal canal and perianal region probably prefer a general or regional anesthetic. Nevertheless, treatment can still be rendered on an outpatient basis.

■ PILONIDAL DISEASE

Incision and drainage of a pilonidal abscess can be accomplished readily as an ambulatory procedure. Indeed, a large percentage of patients can undergo definitive treatment of their pilonidal disease on an outpatient basis while under local anesthesia. If the patient is cooperative and the tracks are not too extensive, they can be unroofed, and their granulation tissue can be curetted and marsupialized or left to heal secondarily. Details of this procedure are described in Chapter 11.

■ ENDOSCOPY

In most circumstances the gamut of diagnostic and therapeutic lower endoscopy can be performed on an ambulatory basis. Rigid sigmoidoscopy has been and will continue to be performed as an outpatient procedure. Similarly, the flexible fiberoptic sigmoidoscope is designed for outpatient use. Colonoscopy, for the most part, can be performed as an ambulatory procedure; only in special circumstances will its use require inpatient care. The details of endoscopy are described in Chapter 3.

■ PERIANAL SKIN LESIONS

Treatment of a host of perianal skin lesions may be handled on an ambulatory basis. A segment of more extensive lesions may be excised for a biopsy, but smaller ones usually can be conveniently excised completely with the patient under local anesthesia.

■ FOREIGN BODY REMOVAL

A host of foreign bodies may be found in the rectum. They often can be removed with the aid of local anesthesia. Occasionally, using a general or regional anesthetic is necessary. Often patients can be discharged after a short period of observation. However, depending on the circumstances, it may be wise to observe these patients for 24 hours to ensure that no bowel perforation has occurred (see Chapter 34).

■ FISTULA SURGERY

Although many patients with simple fistulas can be treated as outpatients, our own preference has been to operate on them as inpatients. Frequently, fistulas that were thought to be simple actually are more complex than originally imagined.

■ EXAMINATION DURING ANESTHESIA

For patients who previously have undergone operations for complicated fistulas with high blind tracts, reexamination with the patient under anesthesia to determine the progress, or lack thereof, of healing may be indicated. When the wounds are not healing well or when pus is reaccumulating, the patient should be reexamined, and this often can be done on an outpatient basis.

Patients who have undergone a proctectomy and experienced poor perineal wound healing may require curettage while under anesthesia, which can be done conveniently as an ambulatory procedure.

POSTOPERATIVE CARE

Patients undergoing procedures under local anesthesia usually can be discharged immediately. Patients having a general anesthetic are monitored in a recovery room, and when vital signs are stable and the level of consciousness returns to normal, they may be discharged. In either case they should be given simple instructions about diet, activity, wound care, and medication. In general, there are no dietary restrictions. Patients are advised to take non-constipating analgesics and bulk stool softeners. Sitz baths are advised for local comfort. Patients are instructed about how to obtain help if any questions or problems arise.

PAIN CONTROL

Essential to discharging a patient in satisfactory condition is adequate pain control. Discharging ambulatory surgery patients who are medically ready but in significant pain may be safe but leads to unnecessary patient discomfort and poor satisfaction ratings. Pain control is best begun immediately prior to initiating surgery.

Preemptive analgesia is pain control originated prior to any surgical tissue injury. Nocioreceptors are receptors that transmit pain signals via the spinothalamic tract to the cerebral cortex. Circulating cytokines, released as the result of tissue injury, either traumatic or surgical, lower the nociceptor threshold thus leading to the perception of pain despite less noxious stimulation. This exaggerated pain response is termed "peripheral sensitization" and may extend for variable periods of time during or following surgery.

Preemptive analgesia involves blocking this response by administering local anesthetic (even if other methods of anesthesia have been employed) prior to initiation of the procedure. Several studies have shown the benefits of this technique in diminishing postoperative pain (22).

Once the patients have entered the recovery room, pain, if present, should be rapidly controlled. Intravenous opioids, including fentanyl, morphine, and Demerol® have a rapid onset of action and are effective in reducing pain. Side effects include respiratory depression (rare postoperatively as pain induces tachypnea), nausea, vomiting, decreased consciousness, and constipation. Nonsteroidal anti-inflammatory drugs (NSAIDS) work by inhibiting cyclooxygenase and subsequently decreasing prostaglandin synthesis, and are known to reduce narcotic requirements. Side effects include gastrointestinal ulcerations, platelet inhibition, and rarely hepatic and renal dysfunction. More recently COX-2 inhibitors (selective inhibition of the cyclooxygenase pathway that mediates pain) have become available and have been associated with minimal platelet dysfunction and gastrointestinal side effects. Preoperative administration may aid in the preemptive analgesia. A combined approach or strategy will maximize pain relief and minimize side effects. One approach is as follows:

1. Administer a COX-2 inhibitor immediately preoperatively with a sip of water.
2. After intravenous sedation (or induction of anesthesia), perform a local field block including blockade of the inferior hemorrhoidal nerve.
3. Administer oral or intravenous opioids at the earliest sign of even minor pain in the recovery room.
4. Discharge when pain has been reasonably controlled on oral analgesics.
5. Prescribe a combination of appropriate opioids and NSAIDS for outpatient pain control with telephone contact for uncontrollable pain.

This strategy should hopefully maximize patient comfort and minimize further hospitalization or visits for poorly controlled pain.

DISCHARGE CRITERIA

In order to ensure a safe and comfortable transition from the post anesthesia care unit (PACU) to home, certain criteria must be met. Many units use an Aldrete Score or Modified Aldrete Score to evaluate a patient's readiness for discharge (Table 1) (23,24). This score is comprised of vital signs, level of consciousness, and activity level with each category being scored from 0 to 2. When a patient's total score is greater than 11 (with no 0 scores in any category), the patient meets the criteria for discharge to an inpatient unit. A second set of "outpatient discharge criteria" must be met prior to discharge home (Table 1). These are comprised of vital signs, level of consciousness, activity level, and logistic arrangements to ensure that the family (and/or professional support services) will be ready to care for postoperative needs once the patient is home.

These criteria act as guidelines and are helpful in minimizing unexpected readmissions or repeat outpatient evaluations.

TABLE 1 ■ **Discharge Criteria**

Inpatient Discharge Criteria	Outpatient Discharge Criteria
1. **Respiratory/Airway** 0-Apnea/Dyspnea or Limited 2-Deep breath/Cough/NL Resp Rate 2. **Circulation** 0-BP +/− 50% preop 1-BP +/− 20–50% preop 2-BP +/− 20% preop 3. **Level of Consciousness** 0-Non-responsive 1-Sleepy but arousable 2-Awake/alert, responds appropriately 4. **Spinal/Activity Level** 0-Unable to lift extremities or head on command/T-9 or above 2-Move 4 extremities/or T-10 spinal level or below 5. **O_2 Saturation Level** 0- < 93% 2- > 93% with O2 6. **Temperature** 0- < 36°C (96.8°-97°F) 1-36°-36.5°C (96.8°-97°F) 2- > 36.5°C (97.7°F) 7. **Pain Assessment** > 4/10 comment Total Score = 12	1. **Vital Signs** -Within 20% of preop status 2. **Activity and Mental Status** -Oriented x3 and a steady gait -Consistent W/developmental age/or preop status 3. **Nausea, and/or Vomiting** -Minimal 4. **Surgical Bleeding** -Minimal-no evidence of progression 5. Tolerating PO fluids 6. Void if spinal anes. or as per surgeon's order (N/A if GU appliance) 7. Responsible adult for transport and to accompany home **Exception**: Local anesthesia/no sedation 8. **Verbal/Written Instructions** -Given/reviewed with patient and family/significant other 9. Arrangements made for post-op prescriptions 10. Arrangements made for follow-up appointment 11. Adequate neurovascular status of operative extremity 12. **Pain Assessment** > 4/10 comment

COMPLICATIONS

Implicit in making a recommendation for an ambulatory procedure is the belief that patient safety and quality of result are as good as with an inpatient service. Several authors have reported on the safety of ambulatory surgery, but these reports have not necessarily been related to anorectal procedures (4,25,26). In the Surgicenter in Tucson Medical Center, more than 47,000 patients have been treated safely without a single death (3). In fact, the types of surgical problems treated have become progressively complex. In another report by Ford (27), in more than 40,000 cases, no deaths or serious medical emergencies have occurred. Mezei and Chung (4) determined the overall and complication-related readmission rates within 30 days after ambulatory surgery at a major ambulatory surgical center. Preoperative, intraoperative, and postoperative data were collected on 17,638 consecutive patients undergoing ambulatory surgery at a major ambulatory surgical center in Toronto, Ontario. With the use of the database of the Ontario Ministry of Health, the authors identified all return hospital visits and hospital readmissions occurring in Ontario within 30 days after ambulatory surgery. There were 193 readmissions within 30 days after ambulatory surgery (readmission rate, 1.1%). Six patients returned to the emergency room, 178 patients were readmitted to the ambulatory surgical unit, and 9 patients were readmitted as inpatients. Twenty-five readmissions were the result of surgical complications, and one resulted from a medical complication (pulmonary embolism). The complication-related readmission rate was 0.15%. Their results support the view that ambulatory surgery is a safe practice.

Encouraging reports about the performance of anorectal surgery on an ambulatory basis have been made (5,19). Friend and Medwell (19), who championed the drive toward ambulatory anorectal surgery, reviewed over 6000 outpatient anorectal operations performed since 1975. They noted that approximately one patient in every 200 is admitted to the hospital from the day-surgery recovery room because of cardiac arrhythmias, anesthetic complications or drug reactions, or postoperative pain or bleeding. Of the first 1433 consecutive patients, only 14 (1%) required catheterization within 24 hours of operation. They found no correlation between catheterization and volume of intravenous fluids, type of anesthesia, age, sex, pathologic condition, or operation. There is no clear explanation for this low rate of urinary retention. In their series of 6000 patients they never had to extract a fecal impaction. Smith (5) reported that less than 1% of the ambulatory population required admission to the hospital after anorectal surgery. The usual reason for admissions is either pain control or urinary retention. Other possible reasons are hemorrhage and infection. In Europe, where ambulatory surgery has not yet been well accepted, Marti and Laverriere (28) reported on 1947 procedures carried out between 1978 and 1990 without any mortality. Complications were observed in 5 of 966 cases—bleeding. No postoperative infection or urinary retention requiring catheterization was seen, and only one case required hospital admission.

Conaghan et al. (29) randomized 100 patients with minor and intermediate surgical emergency conditions to receive standard inpatient care or day surgery. There was a reduction in the number of nights spent in hospital in the day case group (median, 0 vs. 2 nights). The median time from diagnosis to treatment was one day in both groups. There was no significant difference in postoperative outcome or patient and general practitioner satisfaction. The day-case option had no increased impact on primary care services but was associated with a significant saving of about US$ 200 per patient.

BENEFITS

PATIENT

For the patient the advantages of ambulatory operations are numerous. There is no need for a formal hospital admission with its attendant psychologic trauma. Patients may not be as frightened or anxious about an operation if they know they will be home the same day and will not have to spend the night in the hospital. The daily routines and schedules of both patients and their families are less disrupted. Patients have greater accessibility and scheduling convenience, the waiting time for operation is markedly decreased, and there is a considerable cost saving. Patients are not likely to be "bumped" from the operating schedule for "more important" or emergency procedures such as may occur with cases scheduled in the main operating theater.

In general, patients probably convalesce better and are more comfortable in the familiar surroundings of their own homes. In the home environment, patients become mobile, enter the daily routine more rapidly, and return to work sooner. Furthermore, they circumvent exposure to the potential iatrogenic hazards of hospitalization (2).

SURGEON

Ambulatory surgery allows surgeons to use their time better. Fewer hospital visits are required, and less time is needed to complete chart work. In addition, accessibility and scheduling convenience are greater. The turnover time between cases in an outpatient setting is dramatically less than in a hospital setting (27). This factor alone would allow a surgeon to accomplish more in the same time.

HOSPITAL

With ambulatory procedures, hospitals can make better use of their facilities. Because the demand for hospital beds is lessened, use of expensive health care facilities can be handled more efficiently. Pressure on overloaded operating rooms is relieved, thereby freeing more time and space to devote to more complicated procedures. In addition, the need for postoperative nursing care is decreased.

INSURER

Although the list of benefits for third-party carriers is short, the cost for insurance companies has definitely decreased. The daily charge represents the largest single expense saved by same-day operations. This cost saving has led private and public payers to cover ambulatory surgery. In the 1970s only 35% of payers covered such surgery, but by the 1980s fully 96% of payers provided coverage (2). Moreover, third-party payers began to create financial incentives to encourage ambulatory surgery (2). These include reduced reimbursement if the procedure is performed on an inpatient basis and compilation of lists of procedures that will be reimbursed only if they are provided on an ambulatory basis.

COST

Financial incentives have spurred the growth of same-day surgery. At a time when costs for medical care are increasing steadily, great savings can be afforded the patient, third-party carriers, and institutions by performing many anorectal procedures in the office or at least on an ambulatory basis. Although the adoption of ambulatory surgery will decrease the costs per case, it will also lead to greater throughput of patients and thus to total costs (29). This so-called efficiency trap is one greater reason hospital administrators in European countries have been reluctant to adopt ambulatory surgery. This also puts a strain on institutions located in a health care system such as that of Canada, where global budgets are the order of the day. A hospital does not reap any financial reward for improving efficiency. Moving cases to the ambulatory setting and replacing inpatient beds with new and potentially more expensive admissions may provide care for more patients but inevitably creates a budget deficit (30). In certain localities where hospital bed shortages occur, waiting periods are eliminated or reduced by outpatient operations.

Cost analysis is always a difficult subject to evaluate because costs vary considerably from region to region. However, if patients are recovering at home, the cost of hospitalization and ambulatory services is eliminated, and tremendous savings are accrued by both patient and third-party carriers. The exact saving, of course, is difficult to determine. Using the number of inpatient procedures in 1982, obtained from the National Hospital Discharge Survey of the National Center for Health Care Statistics in Hyattsville, Maryland, along with the average cost per day for a hospital bed obtained from the American Hospital Association, Smith (5) estimated that for the procedures hemorrhoidectomy, fistula repair, and fissure operations, a savings of approximately $200 million would have been obtained. A reduction in hospital charges of 25% to 50% has been noted (31).

In a cost analysis, Rhodes (32) calculated that there was a 67% reduction in the cost of a hemorrhoidectomy performed on an ambulatory basis compared with an inpatient procedure. It is, however, clearly stated that a cost comparison between ambulatory surgery and inpatient surgery is confounded by numerous factors that make comparisons difficult to assess.

In a commentary on insights on outpatient surgery, Cannon (33) noted that the dramatic increase in the use of outpatient surgical facilities has been good for society in general and the patient in particular. Outpatient surgery has been the most dramatic cost saving change the medical profession has initiated, and Cannon believes that all areas should be encouraged to introduce this concept to their community. As evidence grows to support the fact that an ever-widening scope of anorectal procedures can be performed safely on an ambulatory basis, this method of management will and in many cases already has become the norm for many patients with anorectal disorders requiring operative intervention. Davis (34) cited four forces that drive this expansion: (i) improved and better operated facilities, (ii) new surgical techniques, (iii) improved anesthetic agents and practices, and (iv) regulations influencing ambulatory surgery. All these forces are strong and appear to be gaining momentum. He believes growth of ambulatory surgery will increase phenomenally in the years ahead.

REFERENCES

1. Stombler RE. What surgeons should know about ambulatory surgery. Bull Am Coll Surg 1993; 78:6–8.
2. Detmer DE, Gelijns AC. Ambulatory surgery. A more cost-effective treatment strategy? Arch Surg 1994; 129:123–127.
3. Detmer DE. Ambulatory surgery. N Engl J Med 1981; 305:1406–1409.
4. Mezei G, Chung F. Return hospital visits and hospital readmissions after ambulatory surgery. Ann Surg 1999; 230:721–727.
5. Smith LE. Ambulatory surgery for anorectal diseases: an update. South Med J 1986; 79:163–166.
6. Reed WA. The concept of the surgicenter. In: Brown BR Jr., ed. Outpatient Anesthesia. Philadelphia: FA Davis, 1978:15–19.
7. Joint Commission on Accreditation of Hospitals. Accreditation manual for hospitals. Chicago, 1981:66.
8. Burns LA, Ferber MS. Ambulatory surgery in the United States Development and prospects. J Ambul Care Manage 1981; 8:1–13.
9. Kaplan EB, Sheiner LB, Brockman AJ, et al. The usefulness of preoperative laboratory screening. JAMA 1985; 253:3576–81.
10. Johnson H, Knee-Ioli S, Butler TA, Munox E, Wise L. Are routine preoperative laboratory screening tests necessary to evaluate ambulatory surgical patients? Surgery 1988; 104:639–645.
11. Macpherson DS, Snow R, Lofgren RP. Preoperative screening: value of previous tests. Ann Intern Med 1990; 113:969–973.
12. Turnball JM, Buck C. The value of preoperative screening in investigators in otherwise healthy individuals. Arch Intern Med 1987; 147:1101–1105.
13. Suchman AL, Mushlin AI. How well does the activated partial thromboplastin time predict postoperative hemorrhage? JAMA 1986; 256:750–753.
14. Putnam LP, Landeen FH. Outpatient anesthesia at the ambulatory surgery center, Tucson Medical Center. In: Brown BR Jr., ed. Outpatient Anesthesia. Philadelphia: FA Davis, 1978:1–14.
15. Petros JG, Bradley TM. Factors influencing postoperative urinary retention in patients undergoing surgery for benign anorectal disease. Am J Surg 1990; 159:375–399.
16. Cataldo PA, Senagore AJ. Does alpha sympathetic blockade prevent urinary retention following anorectal surgery? Dis Colon Rectum 1991; 34:1113–1116.
17. Bailey HR, Ferguson JA. Prevention of urinary retention by fluid restriction following anorectal operations. Dis Colon Rectum 1976; 19:250–252.
18. Morson BC, Dawson IMP. Gastrointestinal Pathology, 4th ed. Eds. Day DW, Jass JR, Price AB, Shepherd NA, Sloan JM, Talbot IC, Warren BF, Williams GT. Blackwell Science, 2003, Malden US, Oxford UK, Carlton, Australia.
19. Friend WG, Medwell SJ. Outpatient anorectal surgery. Perspect Colon Rectal Surg 1989; 2:167–173.
20. Leff EI. Hemorrhoidectomy—laser vs. nonlaser: Outpatient surgical experience. Dis Colon Rectum 1992; 35:743–746.
21. Gordon PH, Vasilevsky CA. Lateral internal sphincterotomy. Rationale, technique, and anesthesia. Can J Surg 1985; 28:228–230.
22. Tong D, Chung F. Postoperative pain control in ambulatory surgery. Surg Clin North Am 1999; 79:401-430.
23. Aldrete JA, Kroulik D. A post-anesthetic recovery score. Anesth Analg 1970; 49:924–934.
24. Aldrete JA. Post-anesthesia recovery score revisited. J Clin Anesth 7 1995 80–91.
25. Freestanding Ambulatory Surgical Association. Statistics reveal top 10 procedures. Same-Day Surg 1981; 5:47–49.
26. Natof HE. Complications associated with ambulatory surgery. JAMA 1980; 244:1116–1118.
27. Ford JL. Outpatient surgery: present status and future projections. South Med J 1978; 71:311–315.
28. Marti JC, Laverriere C. Proctological outpatient surgery. Int J Colorectal Dis 1992; 7:223–226.
29. Conaghan PJ, Figueira E, Griffin MA, Ingham Clark CL. Randomized clinical trial of the effectiveness of emergency day surgery against standard inpatient treatment. Br J Surg 2002; 89:423–427.
30. Maloney S, Helyar C. Measuring opportunities to expand ambulatory surgery in Canada. J Ambul Care Manage 1993; 16:1–7.
31. Place R, Hyman N, Simmang C, Cataldo P, Church J, Cohen J, Denstman F, Kilkenny J, Nogueras J, Orsay C, Otchy D, Rakinic J, Tjandra J; Standards Task Force; American Society of Colon and Rectal Surgeons. Practice parameters for ambulatory anorectal surgery. Dis Colon Rectum 2003; 46:573–576.
32. Rhodes RS. Ambulatory surgery and the societal cost of surgery. Surgery 1994; 116:938–940.
33. Cannon WB. Insights on outpatient surgery. Bull Am Coll Surg 1986; 71(7):9–12.
34. Davis JE. Ambulatory surgery—How far can we go? Med Clin North Am 1993; 77:365–375.

III: Colorectal Disorders

21 Rectal Procidentia

Philip H. Gordon

INTRODUCTION

Rectal procidentia is the protrusion of the entire thickness of the rectal wall through the anal sphincter. It was one of the earliest surgical problems recognized by the medical profession, yet many facets of its etiology and treatment remain controversial.

ETIOLOGY

There are two theories concerning the etiology of rectal procidentia. The first was proposed in 1912 by Moschcowitz (1). His idea was that a rectal procidentia is a sliding hernia through a defect in the pelvic fascia. This theory was based on the observation that an abnormally deep rectovaginal or rectovesical pouch is a striking and constant feature in most patients with complete rectal prolapse (Fig. 1).

The second theory was proposed by Broden and Snellman (2), who demonstrated through cineradiography that the initial step in the genesis of prolapse is circumferential intussusception of the rectum, with its starting point approximately 3 in. from the anal verge (Fig. 2). They believed that they disproved conclusively the theory that herniation of the pouch of Douglas into the rectal lumen is the primary process in the formation of a complete rectal prolapse.

Without trying to cast aspersions on the efforts spent to affirm these two theories, we are constrained to state that it is not difficult to realize that these two processes are really one and the same. The invagination of the anterior rectal wall, classically described as a sliding hernia, might just as well be described as an intussusception that has not yet involved the total circumference of the bowel. On the other hand, during operative correction, when the total circumference is involved, herniation of other viscera has been seen. Thus, instead of arguing about nomenclature, it would be valuable to gain a better understanding of the pelvic musculature. For example, Spencer (3) studied manometric responses in patients with rectal prolapse and noted that the internal sphincteric inhibitory reflex was absent or markedly obtunded. Parks et al. (4) in manometric studies of patients with rectal procidentia, showed decreased anal pressures with normal squeeze sphincteric pressures, indicating internal sphincteric dysfunction but normal external sphincteric function. From the same laboratory, electromyographic and histologic studies of patients with prolapse and incontinence have revealed denervation of the puborectalis and external sphincter muscles, but the pelvic musculature was usually normal in patients with prolapse and no incontinence (5). Sun

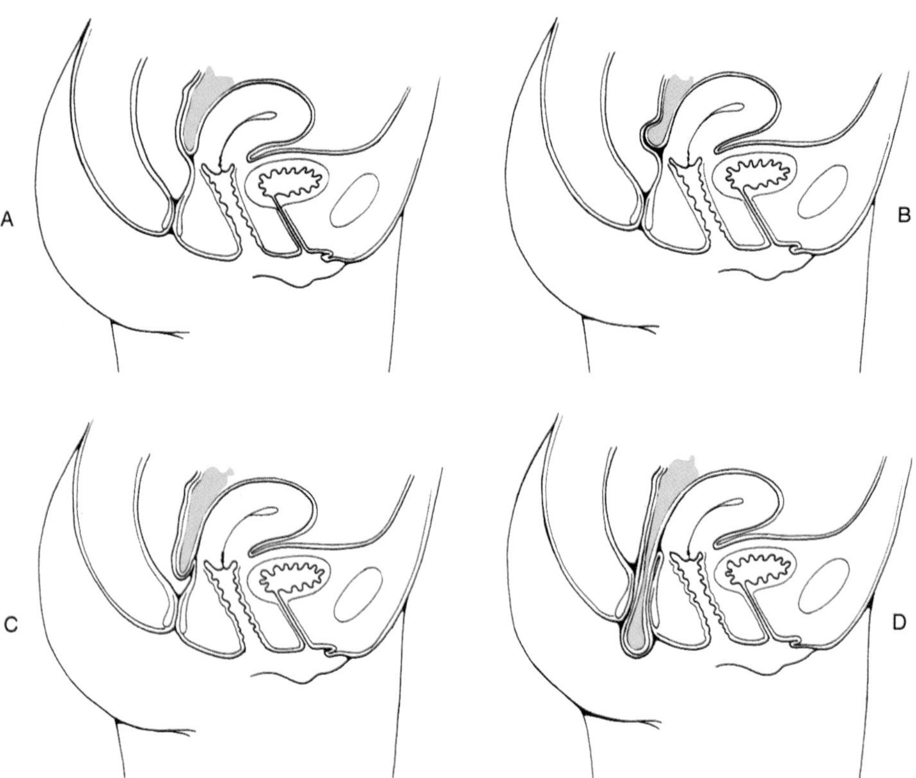

FIGURE 1 ■ Rectal procidentia as conceived by Moschcowitz. (**A**) Incipient procidentia. (**B**) Partial procidentia. (**C**) Incomplete procidentia. (**D**) Complete procidentia.

et al. (6) conducted a detailed study in which they suggested a common pathophysiology for full-thickness rectal prolapse, anterior mucosal prolapse, and solitary rectal ulcer. Anorectal pressures at rest, during conscious contraction of the external sphincter, during serial distention of the rectum, and during straining to inflate a balloon were measured in 56 patients (21 patients with full-thickness rectal prolapse, 24 with anterior mucosal prolapse, and 11 with solitary rectal ulcer) and in 30 normal subjects. Both basal and squeeze pressures were significantly lower in the three groups of patients compared with matched normal controls. During increases in intra-abdominal pressure, anal pressure remained above maximal rectal pressure in normal controls, with the highest anal pressures being recorded in the most caudal anal channels. By contrast, anal pressures tended to be lower than rectal pressures during this maneuver in patients with rectal prolapse, anterior mucosal prolapse, and solitary rectal ulcer, and the highest pressures were recorded in the channels nearest the rectum. During serial distention of the rectum, 64% of patients with solitary rectal ulcer, 75% with anterior mucosal prolapse, and 76% with rectal prolapse, but only 10% of controls, showed repetitive rectal contractions. The highest anal pressure always remained higher than rectal pressure during rectal distention in normal subjects, but not in affected patients. The threshold rectal volume required to cause a desire to defecate and the maximal tolerable volume were significantly lower in each of the patient groups compared with normal subjects. The similarity in the results from patients with rectal prolapse, anterior mucosal prolapse, and solitary rectal ulcer support the hypothesis that they share a common pathophysiology. In each of the groups the rectum is hypersensitive and hyperreactive, and weakness of the anal sphincter creates the conditions in which prolapse of the rectum may occur into or through the anal canal. However, the importance of some subtle disorder of the sphincteric mechanism as the primary causative factor is diminished by the fact that cineradiographically the prolapse starts well above the pelvic floor. Thus laxity of the pelvic musculature cannot be a primary factor in the causation of this condition.

CLASSIFICATION

No efforts made to classify procidentia have yet met with general acceptance. The description by Altemeier et al. (7) was purely anatomic. They believed that either a sliding hernia or an intussusception is present in different patients, a concept that was the apparent basis of their classification of three types of rectal prolapse. Type I is a protrusion of the redundant mucosal layer (labeled as a false prolapse and usually associated with hemorrhoids). Type II is an intussusception with an associated cul-de-sac sliding hernia. Type III is a sliding hernia of the cul-de-sac and is the one that they believed occurs in the vast majority of cases.

Beahrs et al. (8) proposed a clinical classification predicated on the idea that procidentia is an intussusception. They described categories based on gradation of the completeness of the prolapse:

1. Incomplete (mucosal prolapse)
2. Complete (full-thickness wall prolapse): first degree (high or early, "concealed," "invisible"); second degree (externally visible on straining, sulcus evident between rectal wall and anal canal); third degree (externally visible)

Neither of these classifications seriously addresses the ubiquitous problem of incontinence. A more complete and

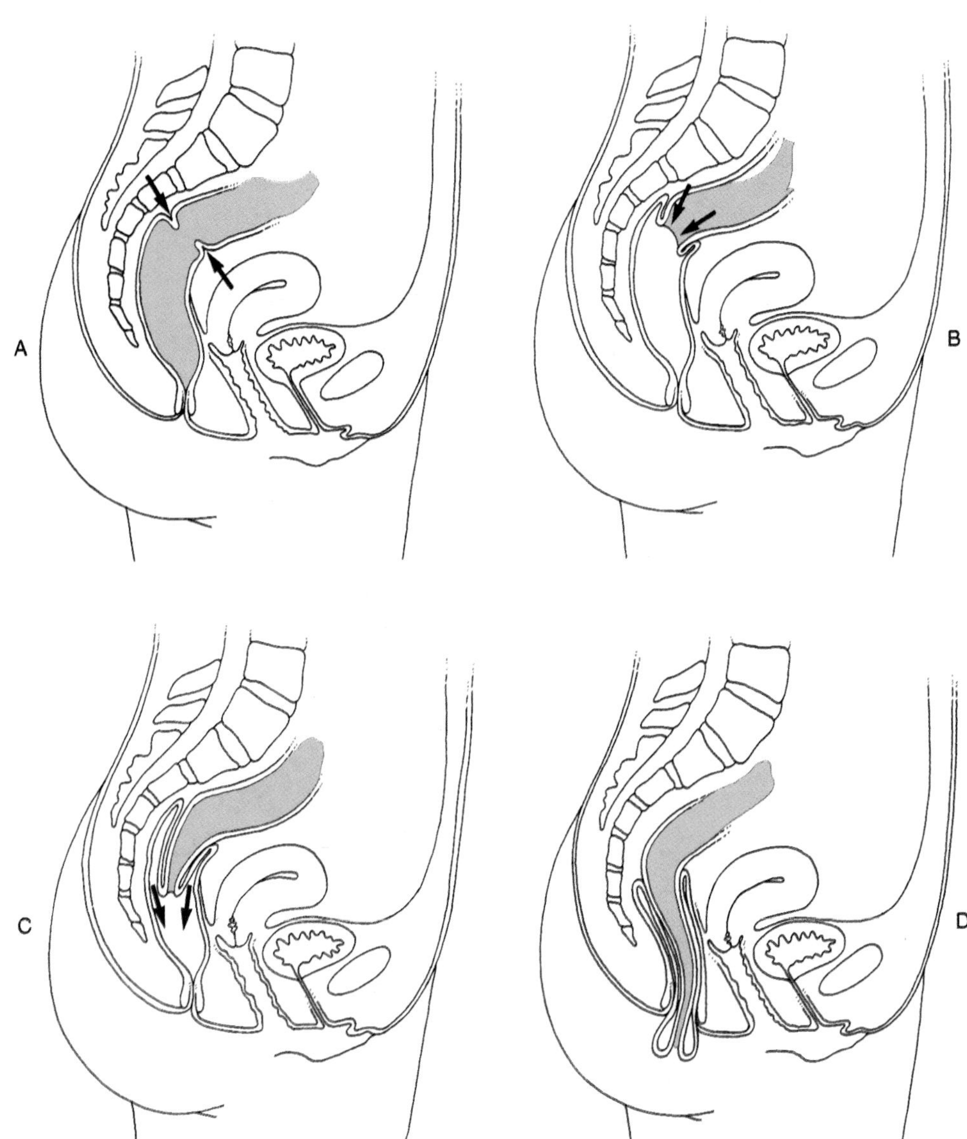

FIGURE 2 ■ Intussusception analogous to Moschcowitz's concept. (**A**) Starting point of intussusception. (**B**) Early point of intussusception. (**C**) Internal procidentia. (**D**) Complete procidentia.

inclusive classification might consider the status of anal control and include information about whether the patient is fully continent or is suffering from varying degrees of lack of control with flatus, liquid stool, or solid stool. A comprehensive classification would prove invaluable when assessing reports of different forms of therapy, a situation in which it becomes important to equate comparable patients.

PREDISPOSING FACTORS

In reviewing 536 cases of rectal prolapse treated at St. Mark's Hospital, London, from 1948 to 1960, Mann (9) reported that 52% of the patients had a history of straining associated with intractable constipation and another 15% experienced diarrhea. Additional contributory causes of anatomic or neuromuscular deficit included pregnancy, previous operations, and neurologic disease. A disproportionately large number of patients with rectal prolapse had a history of psychiatric illness (10). Parks et al. (11) suggested that the pelvic floor weakness is secondary to nerve entrapment or nerve stretching, which leads to a muscular deficiency and complete procidentia. Procidentia has also been associated with progressive systemic sclerosis (12).

PATHOLOGIC ANATOMY

The anatomic defects described as occurring with prolapse of the rectum include the following: (i) a defect in the pelvic floor with diastasis of the levator ani muscles and a weakened endopelvic fascia, (ii) an abnormally deep cul-de-sac of Douglas, (iii) a redundant rectosigmoid colon, (iv) a patulous weak anal sphincter, and (v) loss of the normal horizontal position of the rectum caused by its loose attachment to the sacrum and pelvic walls.

Those who believe that rectal prolapse is primarily an intussusception think that these anatomic changes are secondary to the recurring prolapse (Fig. 3).

PHYSIOLOGIC DYSFUNCTION

Zbar et al. (13) reviewed the physiology and function of rectal prolapse and the following is a summary of their findings. Pre-existing fecal incontinence ranges from 35% to 100% of cases. The etiology of incontinence is multifactorial; in some cases it is secondary to sphincter damage resulting from the prolapse itself while in others it occurs as

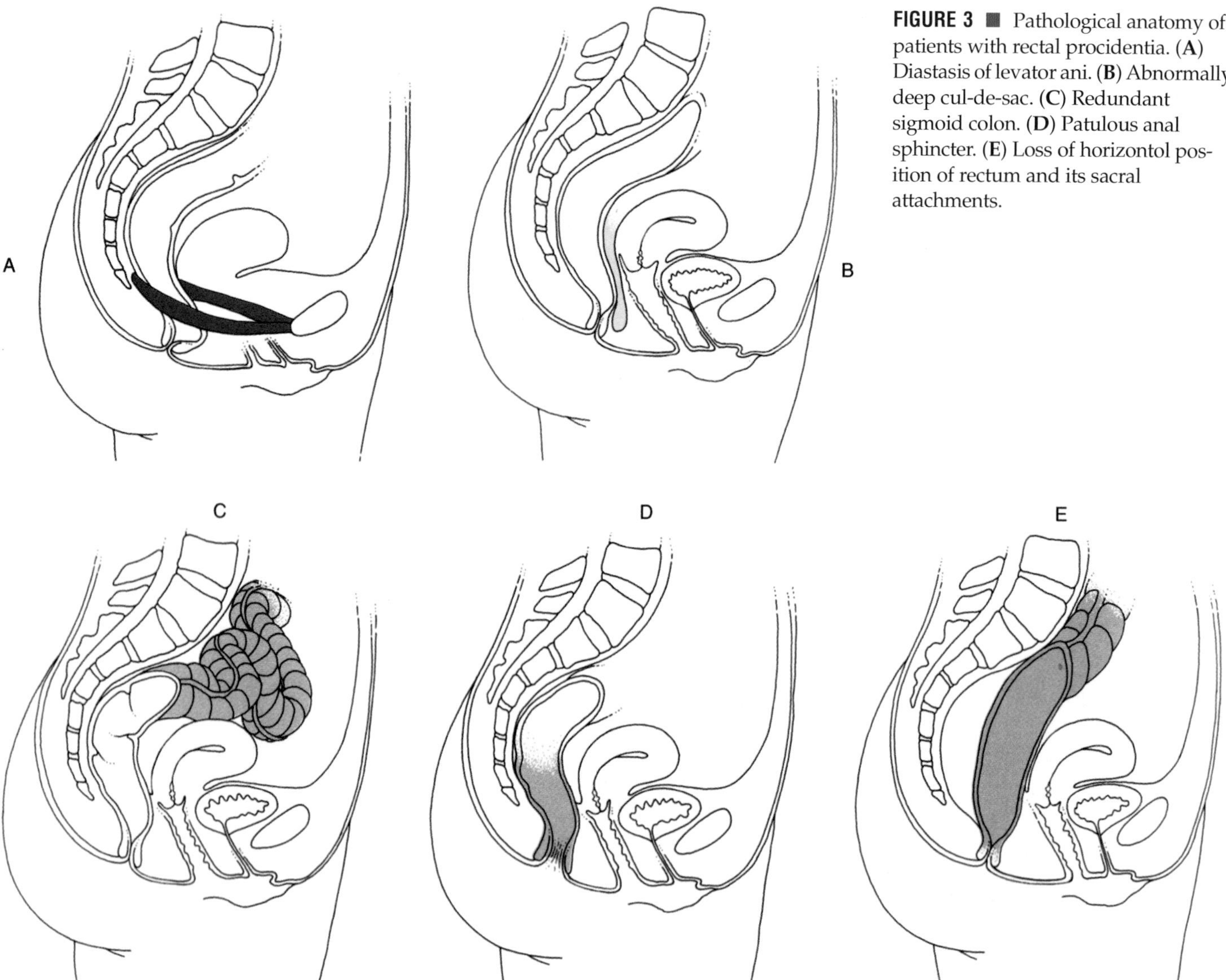

FIGURE 3 ■ Pathological anatomy of patients with rectal procidentia. (**A**) Diastasis of levator ani. (**B**) Abnormally deep cul-de-sac. (**C**) Redundant sigmoid colon. (**D**) Patulous anal sphincter. (**E**) Loss of horizontol position of rectum and its sacral attachments.

a result of internal anal sphincter relaxation induced by the prolapse. The issue is complicated. In many cases, rectal prolapse clearly predates the presence of fecal incontinence and severe incontinence may be clinically present in association with internal ("occult") rectal prolapse unassociated with morphological sphincter damage. The relationship between rectal prolapse and inherent internal anal sphincter function, in particular, is complex. In some patients, there is difficulty in the elicitation of the rectal anal inhibitor reflex (a measure of innate internal sphincter function), accompanied by an absence of internal anal sphincter electromyographic trace. Whereas in patients with idiopathic fecal incontinence, transient internal anal sphincter relaxation correlates with reported episodes of leakage, rectal prolapse patients do not seem to suffer fecal leakage or urgency during anorectal sampling and do not experience major reductions in anorectal pressure of this type. In these patients, it is likely that chronic internal anal sphincter relaxation (secondary to the presence of a prolapse itself) has affected the inherent internal anal sphincter activity, a phenomena which is somewhat disease specific. Most reports have shown a general reduction in rectal tone and compliance (a "rectal adaptation"), following rectal distention in patients with full thickness rectal prolapse.

CLINICAL FEATURES

■ SEX

Women predominate among patients with rectal procidentia with a ratio of 6:1, as shown in the previously mentioned St. Mark's study and by Kupfer and Goligher (14). Parity apparently is not a significant contributory factor (15).

■ AGE

In women, the incidence of this disorder is maximal in the fifth and subsequent decades, but in men, it is evenly distributed throughout the age range (14). Mann (9) reported that in men, the peak incidence declines after the age of 40 years, whereas in women, it climbs steadily to reach its maximal incidence in the seventh decade.

■ SYMPTOMS

Prolapse of the rectum vexes patients with the misery it causes them. The presenting complaints may be related to the prolapse itself or to the disturbance of anal continence that frequently accompanies it. Initially the mass may extrude only with defecation, but in a more advanced form, extrusion occurs with any slight exertion, such as coughing

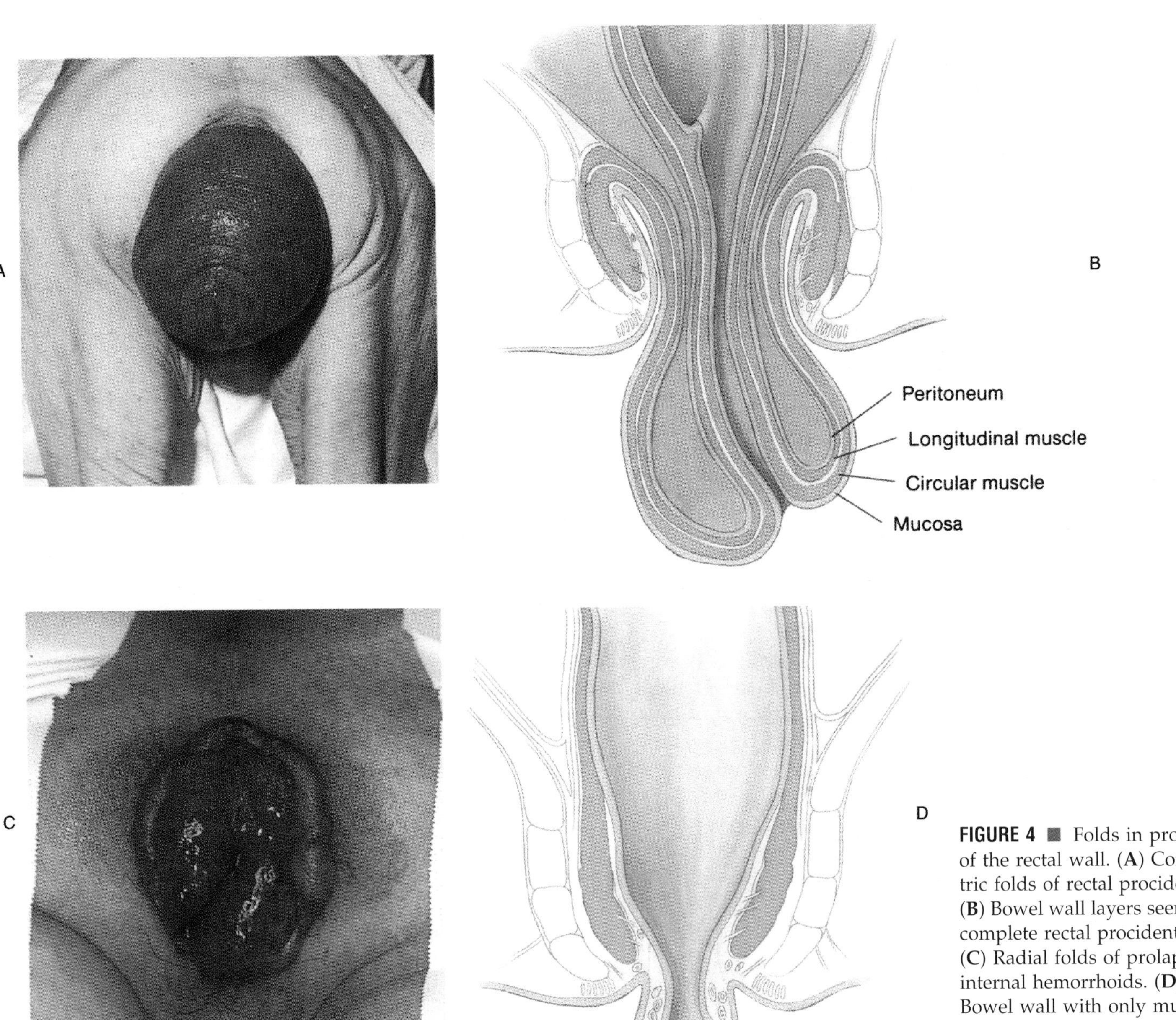

FIGURE 4 ■ Folds in prolapse of the rectal wall. (**A**) Concentric folds of rectal procidentia. (**B**) Bowel wall layers seen with complete rectal procidentia. (**C**) Radial folds of prolapsing internal hemorrhoids. (**D**) Bowel wall with only mucosal prolapse or prolapsing internal hemorrhoids.

or sneezing. In the early stage, symptoms of prolapse may include difficulty in bowel regulation, discomfort, the sensation of incomplete evacuation, and tenesmus. In its florid form this very disabling condition is characterized by a permanently extruded rectum that is excoriated and ulcerated, leading to mucous discharge and bleeding, which cause soiling of the underclothes. Fecal incontinence is very frequently a symptom. Constipation with straining is frequently associated with prolapse. Impairment of anorectal sensation caused by the persistently extruded mass contributes to the incontinence.

In some individuals, associated urinary incontinence may occur, and it may or may not be noted in conjunction with uterine prolapse. The psychologic trauma is formidable, and because of embarrassment, many patients with rectal prolapse avoid all social contact.

■ PHYSICAL EXAMINATION

Inspection

In its florid form, rectal procidentia with its protruding, large red mass is quite unmistakable. During the initial examination, however, the prolapse is frequently reduced. In many cases, the anal orifice is quite patulous. If the patient is asked to bear down, the full thickness of the rectal wall will prolapse, and the concentric folds can be noted readily. This pattern is in marked contrast to the radial folds seen in patients with prolapsing internal hemorrhoids (Fig. 4). Frequently, the mucosa shows superficial ulceration caused by repeated trauma. If the diagnosis is suspected but not readily apparent, the patient may need to sit in the squatting position and bear down to demonstrate the prolapse. An associated uterine prolapse or cystocele may be present (Fig. 5).

Palpation

Digital examination usually demonstrates a diminished tone of the sphincteric muscle. Voluntary contraction of this muscle on the examining finger is either deficient or absent. Another feature is the lack of discomfort experienced by the patient for such an examination. Bidigital palpation of the prolapsing tissue will reveal that the entire bowel wall thickness is involved.

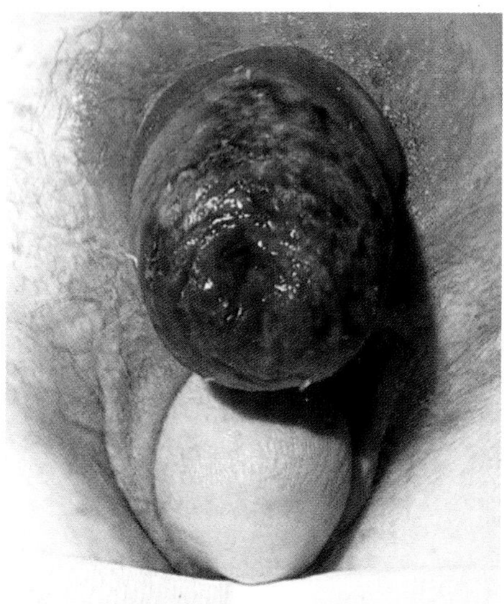

FIGURE 5 ■ Rectal prolapse with superficial ulceration and cystocele.

Sigmoidoscopy

The first 8 to 10 cm on the anterior wall of the rectum may appear red and inflamed, which may be mistaken as a sign of inflammatory bowel disease. On rare occasions granuloma formation may occur and may be the early telltale sign of so-called hidden, or occult, rectal procidentia. Other possible causes of the symptoms, such as a malignancy, should be ruled out. Rashid and Basson (16) reported that the prevalence of rectosigmoid carcinoma with prolapse was 5.7% as opposed to 1.4% in a comparative group. The relative risk for carcinoma was 4.2-fold over the comparative group.

■ DIFFERENTIAL DIAGNOSIS

When the mucosa appears hesitatingly at the anal orifice, distinguishing between a mucosal prolapse or prolapsing internal hemorrhoids from a complete rectal procidentia may be difficult. Helpful points in differentiating the two conditions include the fact that with complete procidentia the furrows are in a concentric ring, whereas with mucosal prolapse they are radial (Fig. 4A and C); with complete procidentia the anus is in a normal anatomic position, whereas with mucosal prolapse it is everted; and with complete prolapse there is a sulcus between the anus and the protruding bowel, whereas no sulcus is present with only a mucosal prolapse (Fig. 4B and D).

Occasionally a large polypoid neoplasm of the rectum or colon may emerge through the anal orifice, giving the impression of a prolapse. However, associated symptoms, digital examination, sigmoidoscopy, colonoscopy, or a barium enema will confirm this diagnosis.

INVESTIGATION

■ RADIOLOGIC EXAMINATION

Barium Enema

A colonic evaluation is indicated to assess for the possible association of another disease process such as a neoplasm, inflammatory bowel disease, or diverticular disease. The presence of another disease process may modify the treatment recommendation. The barium enema has historically been used to gain this information but is often unrewarding as many patients are unable to retain the barium and therefore might better be assessed by colonoscopy.

Spine

Radiographs of the lumbar spine and pelvis may provide a clue to frank neurologic disease (e.g., spina bifida occulta). Such x-ray studies would not be indicated in all cases. If clinically warranted, neurologic consultation might prove to be in order.

Cineradiography

In a patient in whom the diagnosis of procidentia is suspected but cannot be demonstrated, cineradiography may demonstrate the prolapse. Cine-defecography may demonstrate an internal intussusception that starts 6 to 8 cm upward in the rectum. With the use of defecography, Thompson et al. (17) found a 33% incidence of occult rectal prolapse in patients, with clinical rectoceles and defectory dysfunction. Balloon proctography may document some of the anatomic features that are typical of patients who have procidentia, namely loss of the anorectal angle and lax squeeze pressures (see Chapter 2).

Dvorkin et al. (18) characterized clinically and physiologically 896 patients from which three groups were identified: those with isolated rectal intussusception ($n = 125$), those with isolated rectocele: ($n = 100$), and those with both abnormalities ($n = 152$), to test the hypothesis that certain symptoms are predictive of this finding on evacuation proctography. The symptoms of anorectal pain and prolapse were highly predictive of the finding of isolated intussusception over rectocele (odds ratio 3.6 and 4.9) or combined intussusception and rectocele (odds ratio 2.9 and 2.4). The symptom of "toilet revisiting" was associated with the finding of rectoanal intussusception (odds ratio 3.6). Although patients with mechanically obstructing intussusception evacuated slower and less completely than those with nonobstructing intussusception, no symptom was predictive of this finding on evacuation proctography. They concluded subclassifying intussusception morphology seems of little clinical significance, and selection for surgical intervention on the basis of proctographic findings may be illogical.

■ ENDORECTAL ULTRASONOGRAPHY

Dvorkin et al. (19) assessed the morphologic change of the anal canal in 18 patients with rectal prolapse by endo-anal ultrasound scan and compared them with those of 23 asymptomatic controls. The thickness and area of the internal sphincter and submucosa were measured at three levels. Qualitatively, patients with rectal prolapse showed a characteristic elliptical morphology in the anal canal with anterior/posterior submucosal distortion accounting for most of the change. Quantitatively, internal anal sphincter and submucosal thickness and area were greater in all quadrants of the anal canal (especially upper) in patients with rectal prolapse compared with controls. There was statistical evidence of a relationship between increases in all measured variables and the finding of rectal prolapse. The cause of sphincter distortion in rectal prolapse is unknown but may be a response to increased mechanical stress placed on the sphincter from the prolapse or an abnormal response by the sphincter complex to the prolapse. Although a thickened internal anal sphincter has been linked to higher resting pressures, the fact that 53% of their patients suffered from passive fecal incontinence suggested that this thickened internal anal sphincter found in their study was dysfunctional. This is consistent with other studies showing no correlation between internal anal sphincter thickness and function. In addition, the occurrence of sphincter defects in their patients suggest that such defects are not the cause of incontinence in these patients. Patients found to have this feature on endo-anal ultrasound may benefit from defecography to look for rectal wall abnormalities.

■ MAGNETIC RESONANCE IMAGING

A study by Healy et al. (20) found the standard measurements of anorectal configuration made using evacuation proctography and dynamic magnetic resonance imaging (MRI) showed significant correlation. However, in their study, statistical agreement was poor for measurement of anorectal junction descent and anorectal change as seen on imaging obtained with the two techniques. In another study, Healy et al. (21) found MRI clearly shows pelvic visceral prolapse and pelvic floor configuration on straining. Prolapse frequently involves multiple sites in constipated patients that is suggestive of global pelvic floor weakness. In contrast, the weakness is frequently posterior in fecally incontinent patients. Rentsch et al. (22) studied the potential of dynamic MRI defecography to elucidate the underlying anatomic and pathophysiologic background of pelvic floor disorders in 20 proctologic patients with main diagnoses such as rectal prolapse or intussusception, rectocele, descending perineum, fecal incontinence, outlet obstruction, and dyskinetic puborectalis muscle. MRI defecography revealed diagnoses consistent with clinical results in 77.3% and defects in addition to clinical diagnoses in combined pelvic floor disorders in 34%. They believe in complex pelvic floor disorders involving more than a single defect, dynamic MRI represents a convenient diagnostic procedure in females and to a lesser extent in males in terms of dynamic imaging of pelvic floor organs during defecation. Dvorkin et al. (23) investigated whether MR defecography could provide more useful clinical information than evacuation proctography alone in the evaluation of a cohort of 10 patients with full thickness rectal intussusception. There was discordance in the diagnosis of rectal intussusception in three cases. In another two patients MR defecography demonstrated mucosal descent only. MR defecography also showed two patients to have significant bladder descent and two more female patients to have a significant vaginal descent. They concluded evacuation proctography remains the first line investigation for the diagnosis of rectal intussusception but may not distinguish mucosal from full thickness descent. MR defecography further complements evacuation proctography by giving information on movements of the whole pelvic floor, 30% of the patients studied having associated abnormal anterior and/or middle pelvic organ descent. If operation is planned for patients with rectal intussusception, MR defecography provides useful information regarding the presence and degree of anterior pelvic compartment descent that may need to be addressed if a good functional outcome is to be achieved.

■ TRANSIT STUDIES

Watts et al. (24) have suggested that patients with a history of severe constipation should undergo transit studies because an abnormal transit time might influence the choice of operation. If the patient should suffer from total colonic inertia, they would consider performing a proctopexy with total abdominal colectomy and ileorectal anastomosis in a continent patient.

■ COLONOSCOPY

A growing number of colorectal surgeons have adopted colonoscopy to rule out other colonic disease rather than use of barium enema. Certainly for patients ≥ 50 years, screening for colorectal carcinoma would be appropriate in any event.

■ ANORECTAL MANOMETRY

As pointed out in the chapter on physiology (see Chapter 2), patients with rectal procidentia have specific abnormalities detectable through manometry, and such studies may help in the earlier diagnosis of this condition. In one study of patients who have rectal procidentia, physiologic abnormalities included an impaired sphincteric function as manifested by reduced resting and maximal voluntary squeeze pressures and a reduced physiologic rectal capacity as measured by the critical volume and constant relaxation volume (25).

■ ELECTROMYOGRAPHIC STUDIES

Electromyographic studies have demonstrated abnormalities in patients with rectal prolapse. They are also discussed in Chapter 2.

Although it is appropriate to conduct these studies in patients with rectal procidentia in an effort to understand the disease better, the information gathered to date is not sufficient enough to define a treatment strategy based on these physiologic studies alone.

Investigations using cineradiography, transit studies, anorectal manometry, and electromyography are all of interest but, in the usual case of rectal procidentia, do not change the operative plan.

OPERATIVE REPAIR

Rectal prolapse vexes surgeons because of the proliferation of operative techniques that can be used for treatment. A discussion of the operative management naturally centers on the presumed causative factors and the pathologic anatomy. The great number of widely different procedures has been based on the concept of these underlying features. Classification of many of these procedures has been outlined previously (26).

When trying to choose the operative procedure for treating complete prolapse of the rectum, a surgeon must consider the expected mortality and morbidity rates, the

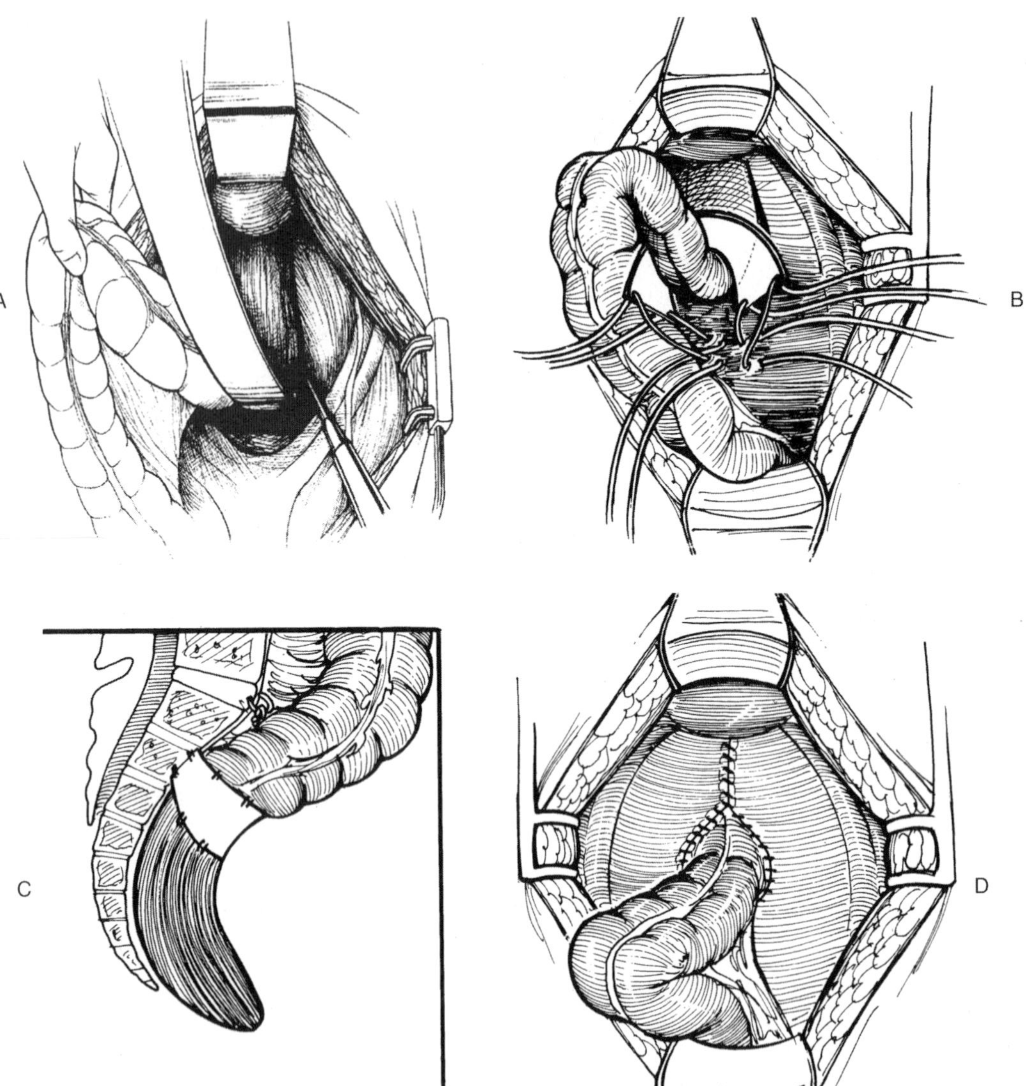

FIGURE 6 ■ Technique of Ripstein repair. *Source*: Modified from Ref. 29.

chance of recurrence, and the probability of restoration of continence or maintenance of continence from each particular operation. In addition, the general health of the patient must be considered.

All patients undergoing operative treatment for rectal procidentia should have mechanical and antibiotic bowel preparation. Postoperative care for abdominal repairs follows the care plan for any patient after laparotomy: intravenous fluids until passage of flatus, then a progressive diet until bowel function returns.

The innumerable proposed procedures have their own advantages and disadvantages. Most procedures have not gained general acceptance and are used almost exclusively by the surgeons who described them; thus the following discussion presents only the more popular techniques in current use. This discussion does not apply to the treatment

TABLE 1 ■ **Results of Ripstein Procedure**

Author(s)	No. of Patients	Recurrence Rate (%)	Mortality Rate (%)	Morbidity Rate (%)	Mean Follow-Up (yr)
Ripstein (31) (1972)	289	0	0.3	–	–
Biehl et al. (32) (1978)	22	10	0	10	–
Gordon and Hoexter (33) (1978)[a]	1111	2.3	–	16.6	–
Eisenstat et al. (34) (1979)	30	0	0	13.3	–
Failes et al. (35) (1979)	53	5.7	0	17	>2
Romero-Torres (36) (1979)	24	0	4.2	–	10
Morgan (37) (1980)	64	1.6	1.6	6	6
Roberts et al. (38) (1988)	135	9.6	0.7	52	3.4
Leenen and Kuijpers (39) (1989)	64	0	0	28	2.5
Tjandra et al. (40) (1993)	134	8	0.6	21	4.2
Winde et al. (41) (1993)	35	0	0	28	4.2
Schultz et al. (42) (2000)	105	2	0	33	7

[a]Collected series.

of mucosal prolapse, because this is a relatively minor problem and its management is dealt with in Chapter 8.

■ ABDOMINAL PROCEDURES

Ripstein Procedure

In the United States, one of the more commonly used techniques for the correction of rectal procidentia is that described by Ripstein and Lanter (27). The authors suggested that massive procidentia is an intussusception that occurs only when the rectum loses its attachment and becomes a straight tube. The pelvic floor defects, they believed, are secondary and not primary in this condition. Therefore, they postulated that if straightening of the rectum can be prevented by keeping it fixed to the sacral hollow, intussusception and hence procidentia would not occur. With the pressures exerted by defecation, the forces acting on the long axis of the tube create an intussusception that begins at the rectosigmoid junction and finally protrudes through the anus. Thus the aim of this operation is to restore the posterior curve of the rectum and maintain it during the act of straining. They believed there was no reason to remove the peritoneal sac or repair the pelvic floor. The only requirement of the operation is to produce a sling that firmly fixes the rectum to the sacrum. The first effective material they used was fascia lata, but to avoid making an extra incision, a Teflon mesh was later substituted. They subsequently used a Marlex mesh; more recently GoreTex has been used (28). Despite the fact that fewer surgeons are performing this procedure, this technique will still be described.

Technique

The Ripstein technique involves mobilization of the rectum down to the tip of the coccyx by opening the lateral peritoneal folds and freeing the bowel from the sacrum (Fig. 6A). It may be necessary to divide the upper portion of the lateral stalks to allow secure placement of the sling. The free ends of a 5-cm band of rectangular mesh (Teflon or Marlex) are placed around the rectum at the level of the peritoneal reflection and are sutured firmly to the presacral fascia approximately 5 cm below the promontory. Nonabsorbable sutures are placed approximately 1 cm from the midline, while presacral blood vessels are carefully avoided. The opposite edge of the synthetic material is then sutured to the presacral fascia 1 cm from the midline on the opposite side (Fig. 6B). The rectum is pulled upward and rendered taut. The upper and lower borders of the sling and an apron-like projection, if desired, are sutured to the rectum with nonabsorbable sutures to prevent the sling from sliding up and down on the bowel (Fig. 6C). Care must be taken not to penetrate the full thickness of the bowel. The sling must be loose enough to allow one or two fingers to pass between the bowel and the sacral fascia, for if it is too snug, it may cause problems ranging from mild constipation to fecal impaction. If angulation of the rectum by the sling is apparent, a "hitch" suture can be placed between the anterior surface of the lumbosacral disk and the mesorectum (Fig. 6C). The sling is then buried beneath the peritoneal floor by suturing the peritoneal defect with a running 3–0 chromic catgut suture (Fig. 6D) (30).

The largest series in which this technique was used was reported by Ripstein (31). He operated on 289 patients; the results included only one death, which was caused by a pulmonary embolus. Only 3% of the patients required resection of the redundant rectosigmoid. Ripstein claimed that his morbidity rate was minimal and that problems such as pulmonary atelectasis, phlebitis, wound infection, and related problems have not been unduly frequent. His results and those of other authors are summarized in Table 1.

Tjandra et al. (40) reported on 142 patients who underwent a Ripstein procedure. Fecal incontinence improved in approximately half the patients. They found that persistence of prior constipation was more common after the Ripstein procedure than after resection rectopexy (57% vs. 17%). Fifteen patients developed constipation for the first time after the Ripstein procedure. The authors suggested that in the presence of constipation, procedures other than the Ripstein might be preferable.

Complications and Prevention

To augment the incomplete information available about the results of using the Ripstein procedure, Gordon and Hoexter (33) polled the members of the American Society of Colon and Rectal Surgeons, obtaining information on a total of 1111 procedures (Table 2). This review revealed a recurrence rate of 2.3%, and complications directly related to placement of the sling occurred in 16.5% of the patients. The overall reoperation rate was 4.1%. Indications for reoperation included fecal impaction, small bowel obstruction, stricture, pelvic abscess, rectal erosion, and hemorrhage. Reoperations for mucosal prolapses and recurrences were not included in this calculation. Possible reasons for recurrence are intraoperative difficulties that result in failure to secure the mesh adequately to the presacral fascia, failure to secure the mesh to the rectum, or inadequate initial mobilization of the rectum, resulting in the presence of prolapsed rectum distal to the point of fixation.

The complication of fecal impaction was not easy to evaluate. Some respondents described severe constipation, which was worse than that in the preoperative phase. Other patients substituted intermittent enemas for prolapse and failed to report their use. However, included in this group were only those patients with fecal impaction who were treated with repeated enemas, disimpaction, or reoperation for release of the fecal impaction. To prevent this complication, considerable care must be exercised to ensure that the sling is not applied too tightly around the rectum.

TABLE 2 ■ Results of 1111 Ripstein Procedures

	No.	%
Recurrences	26	2.3
Complications	183	16.6
Fecal impaction	74	6.7
Presacral hemorrhage	29	2.6
Stricture	20	1.8
Pelvic abscess	17	1.5
Small bowel obstruction	15	1.4
Impotence	9	0.8
Fistula	4	0.4
Miscellaneous	15	1.4

Source: From Ref. 33.

Presacral bleeding ranged from nuisance bleeding to hemorrhages of terrifying proportions. However, only those cases requiring transfusion were included in the review. To minimize this complication, care must be exercised during mobilization of the rectum to ensure that the correct plane is developed. Care must be exerted during the placement of sutures into the presacral fascia. If bleeding occurs in this area, the sutures should be tied immediately; failing this, pressure can be used. If this measure also fails, the use of further sutures may control the bleeding. Thumbtacks, as described by Nivatvongs, may be used to control presacral bleeding refractory to other methods.

Strictures were common, but only those that required further operation, either division or removal of the sling or resection of the segment of bowel, were included (Fig. 7). The patients with narrowing of the rectum documented by a barium enema study who had not undergone operative intervention were excluded from the purview of this review. The treatment for severe symptomatic stricture includes either division or removal of the sling and in some cases may require resection of this segment of bowel (43). When the sling requires division, it should be cut laterally because it is fused anteriorly to the rectal wall and injury may be encountered (44). Prevention consists of avoiding tight application of the sling.

Sepsis referred to the presence of an abscess in the pelvis. Pelvic abscesses were usually relieved by removal of the sling and drainage, but some required diverting colostomies. To prevent this complication, care should be taken to avoid placement of sutures through the full thickness of the rectum. Patients should receive a mechanical bowel preparation, and it is probably wise to administer systemic antibiotics.

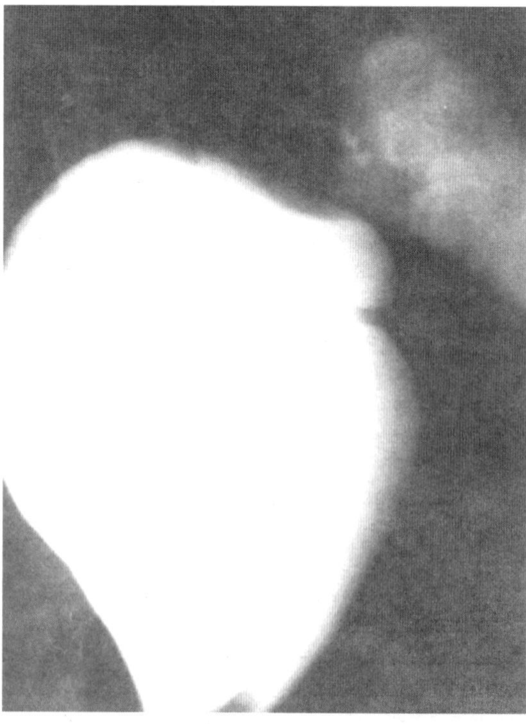

FIGURE 7 ■ Barium enema study showing rectal stricture after a Ripstein repair.

Small bowel obstruction was described as developing from adhesions of the bowel to the site of the placement of the sling. Treatment is by lysis of adhesions. It may be prevented in part by reperitonealizing the pelvic floor and excluding the sling from the remaining peritoneal cavity.

The exact incidence of impotence was impossible to evaluate, especially since the distribution of men and women was not determined and because many of the patients who underwent the procedure were elderly and experienced the problem preoperatively. The chance of causing impotence can be minimized by careful dissection within the pelvis. However, despite meticulous dissection, young male patients were reported to have become impotent.

Fistulas may arise from piercing the bowel with a suture or possibly from erosion of the bowel by the sling, perhaps caused by ischemia of the bowel. The late occurrence of this complication may be due to repeated pressure exerted on the bowel wall by stool as it passes through the sling. Should a fistula arise because of erosion, removal of the sling, closure of the rectum, and a temporary diverting colostomy are required. This complication might be prevented by avoiding excessive tension when placing the sling around the rectum.

One of the most unusual complications was an erosion of the sling into the urinary bladder.

To address the cause of postoperative constipation following rectopexy Selvaggi et al. conducted a randomized study in which 20 patients about to undergo Marlex anterior rectopexy either had division of the lateral ligaments or had them spared. Their data suggested that division of the lateral ligaments is followed by a higher incidence of constipation than when they are preserved. Dolk et al. (45) reported on 18 patients with severe constipation after undergoing a Ripstein procedure. Further investigation revealed that 13 patients had slow-transit constipation. The authors suggest that appropriate preoperative physiologic tests might identify those patients who may benefit from a different operation.

In the most recent review of anterior sling rectopexy, Madiba et al. (46) reported mortality rates ranged between 0% and 2.8%, recurrence rates, between 0% and 13%, there was a trend toward improvement in continence and a mixed response to constipation.

Conclusions

The recurrence rate for this operation, 2.3%, is good. The reported complication rate of 16.5% is related to the specific placement of the sling; if to this are added nonspecific complications such as urinary problems, pulmonary problems, and wound infections, which were reported as approximately 13% at the Lahey Clinic in Boston, the overall complication rate may approximate 30%.

An alternative approach is to place the sling posteriorly. The complication rate might be reduced by half, if the sling were placed posterior to the rectum, leaving the anterior one-fourth to one-third of the circumference of the rectum free to expand, a principle expounded by Wells (47). This speculation is borne out by the reports of Morgan et al. (48) and Penfold and Hawley (49), who used the polyvinyl alcohol (Ivalon) sponge repair when fecal impaction was not a noted postoperative problem. In fact, Ripstein himself has adopted this principle and in his most recent report states that he uses Gore-Tex placed behind the rectum (28).

Ivalon Sponge Wrap Operation

It was Wells who first described the (Ivalon) polyvinyl alcohol sponge wrap operation (47). In the United Kingdom, it has become the treatment of choice in most cases of complete rectal prolapse. In a study using preoperative and postoperative defecography, Kuijpers and de Morree (50) demonstrated that posterior rectopexy corrects rectal dysfunction without creating new functional or anatomic disorders. Postoperative defecography revealed normal evacuation of barium, excellent rectal fixation, maintenance of a straight anterior and posterior rectal wall, absence of an intussuscepted rectum, and no narrowing of rectal lumen at site of fixation.

Technique

There are several variations in the details of the performance of this operation; however, the technique I prefer is as follows (51).

After the bladder has been catheterized, the patient is placed in the supine position, and the skin is prepared with a suitable antiseptic. The abdomen is entered through an infraumbilical transverse incision. With the patient in a Trendelenburg position, the abdominal viscera are packed away in the upper abdomen. Dissection is begun by incising the peritoneum on each side of the rectosigmoid, commencing approximately 5 cm above the pelvic brim (Fig. 8A), with care taken to protect the ureters. The presacral space is entered at the level of the sacral promontory, and the rectum is gently mobilized from the sacral hollow with cautery dissection (Fig. 8B) while the presacral nerves are avoided (Fig. 8C). The rectum is fully mobilized to the level of the coccyx.

Anterior mobilization is begun by continuing the lateral peritoneal incisions distally to join each other in the deepest portion of the cul-de-sac (Fig. 8D). With the rectum grasped in the left hand, this plane can be dissected with cautery dissection. Extensive dissection in this plane is not necessary because in most cases a deep cul-de-sac is a characteristic pathologic anatomic feature of complete rectal procidentia. The seminal vesicles or the vaginal vault can be reached easily. The upper portion of the lateral stalks on each side are divided with cautery. If the rectum is not fully mobilized, leaving redundant rectum below, the point of fixation may lead to recurrence of the prolapse. Throughout the procedure maintaining meticulous hemostasis is essential since hematoma formation may predispose to a purulent collection in the area of the sponge.

A rectangular sheet of previously sterilized Ivalon is then moistened in normal saline solution to make it pliable and easy to handle. Three sutures of a material such as 2–0 Vicryl on a noncutting needle are then passed through the Ivalon sponge and the presacral fascia and back through the Ivalon sponge (Fig. 8E). The distal suture should be placed as low as possible deep in the pelvis. The sponge is then "railroaded" into the pelvis and the sutures are tied (Fig. 8F).

The mobilized rectum is drawn upward and placed on the front of the Ivalon sheet, and the lateral extremities of the sponge are folded around it to encompass approximately three fourths of the circumference of the rectum. A portion of the circumference must be left uncovered to prevent constriction of the lumen. Excess Ivalon is excised. A series of 3–0 Vicryl sutures on each side is used to fasten the lateral limbs of the sponge to the anterior aspect of the rectum (Fig. 8G).

The sponge is extraperitonealized by closing the pelvic peritoneum with continuous 3–0 vicryl (Fig. 8H). No drains are used.

Postoperatively, intravenous fluids are given until the ileus has resolved. Nasogastric suction is ordinarily not necessary. The Foley catheter is removed on the second postoperative day. The patient must not be allowed to strain at defecation. To this end, as soon as the patient has begun oral intake, a bulk-forming agent in the form of a psyllium seed preparation is given and is supplemented by milk of magnesia as necessary.

Complications

Potential complications of the Ivalon sponge wrap operation are identical to those of the Ripstein procedure with the noted exception that fecal impaction and stricture are not observed postoperatively because the entire circumference of the rectum is not enclosed.

A major complication reported with this procedure is the development of pelvic abscesses. This occurrence might be minimized by the use of adequate bowel preparation, by taking care in not transgressing the full thickness of the bowel wall when placing sutures, and by administering prophylactic antibiotics. The treatment of an abscess associated with insertion of the Ivalon sponge requires removal of the sponge and drainage of the abscess. In instances where an abscess does develop, recurrences are unknown, probably because of the development of postinflammatory fibrosis. Pelvic sepsis occurred in 2.6% of the patients in the series reported by Morgan et al. (48). If the bowel is opened or injured during dissection, the Ivalon sponge implant method should be abandoned. If the abscess should point to the vagina or rectum, removal of the sponge through the wall of the viscus may be possible, and complete resolution can be expected. Kupfer and Goligher (14) found a pelvic abscess rate of 16%. Ross and Thomson (52) reported on eight patients who developed sepsis after the Wells' operation. Removal of the infected implant per rectum or per vaginam was successful in four of five attempts and is the recommended initial approach.

The other criterion of effectiveness is the cure rate. Morgan et al. (48) reported cures in 96% of their patients. When recurrent prolapse was noted, it occurred within three years of the operation. Mucosal prolapse occurred in 8.6% of their patients; half of these patients responded to submucosal injections of 5% phenol in almond oil, and the other half required operative excision. Mucosal prolapse causing leakage of fecal-stained mucus results in pruritus and discomfort. Control of the mucosal prolapse will improve the patient's continence.

Mann and Hoffman (53) reported on a modification of the Wells' operation, which they referred to as an extended abdominal rectopexy. The Ivalon prosthesis was attached to the rectum but not to the presacral fascia, and the divided lateral stalks were reattached to the sacral promontory.

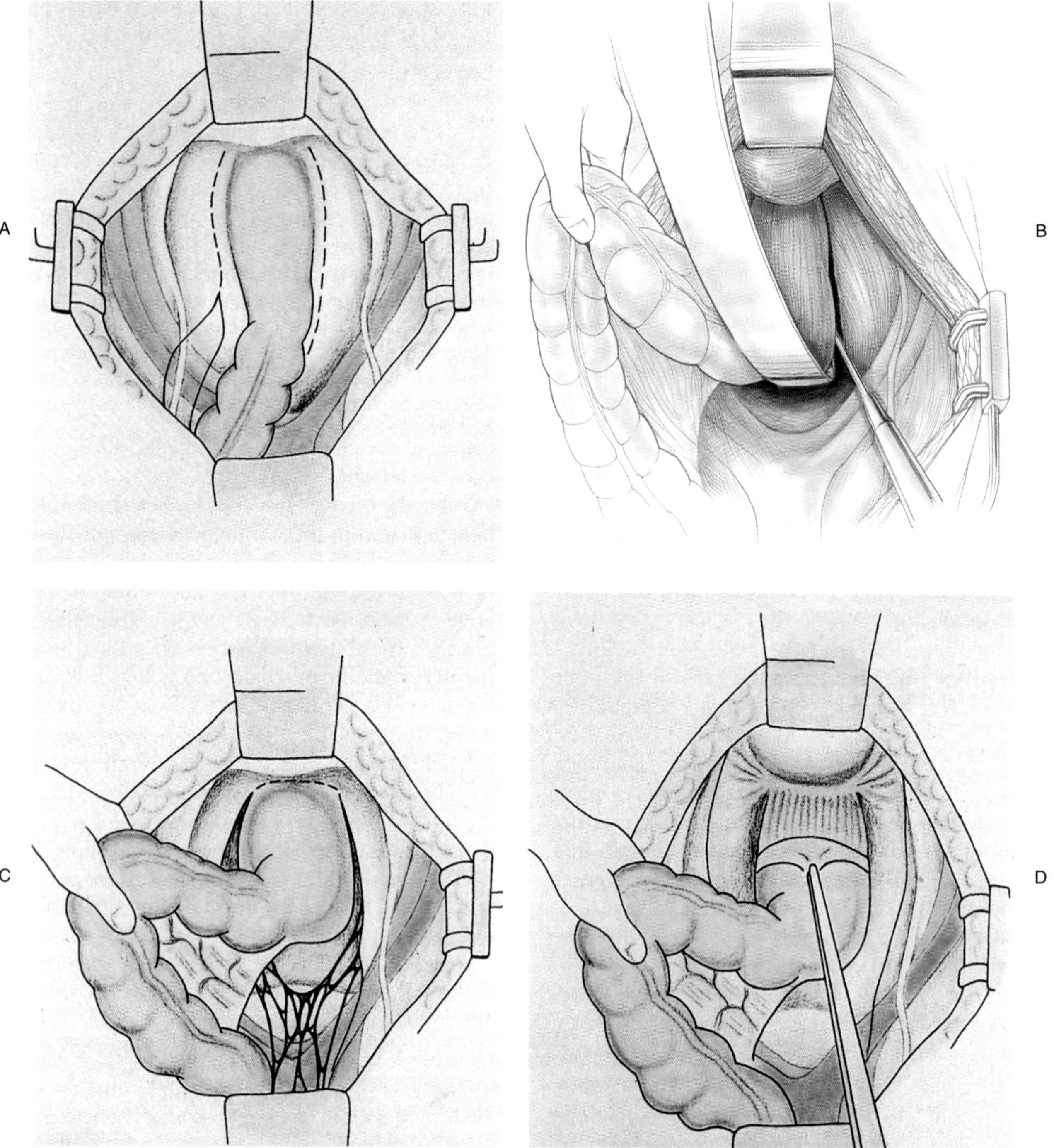

FIGURE 8 ■ Technique of Ivalon sponge repair. *Source*: From Ref. 51.

In 44 patients followed for more than 2 years there were no recurrences and no deaths, and major complications were few; however, constipation (47%) and incontinence (19%) caused serious problems for many patients postoperatively. Allen-Mersh et al. (54) reported that the Ivalon rectopexy increased the prevalence of constipation from 30% before operation to 51% after it. The incidence of incontinence decreased from 49% to 21%.

The published results by various authors are summarized in Table 3.

The polyvinyl alcohol sponge has been shown to produce sarcomas in rats. However, there is no evidence yet that it predisposes humans to malignancy. Ivalon has been found to be present in human tissues for 5 years, producing a foreign body reaction with only moderate fibrosis. Reoperation on patients with previously implanted Ivalon has been surprisingly straightforward. It is believed that the minimal amount of fibrous tissue between the sacrum and the rectum suggests that the success of the operation in controlling prolapse is not due to fixation of the rectum to the sacrum but rather to a stiffening of the rectum itself, thus preventing rectal intussusception (49).

The principle of performing posterior rectopexy has been adopted by other surgeons who have used a variety of materials to accomplish the same goal. Yoshioka et al. (61) reviewed 165 patients who underwent abdominal rectopexy using Marlex mesh. The recurrence rate was 1.5%, with a mucosal prolapse recurrence rate of 7%. Incontinence

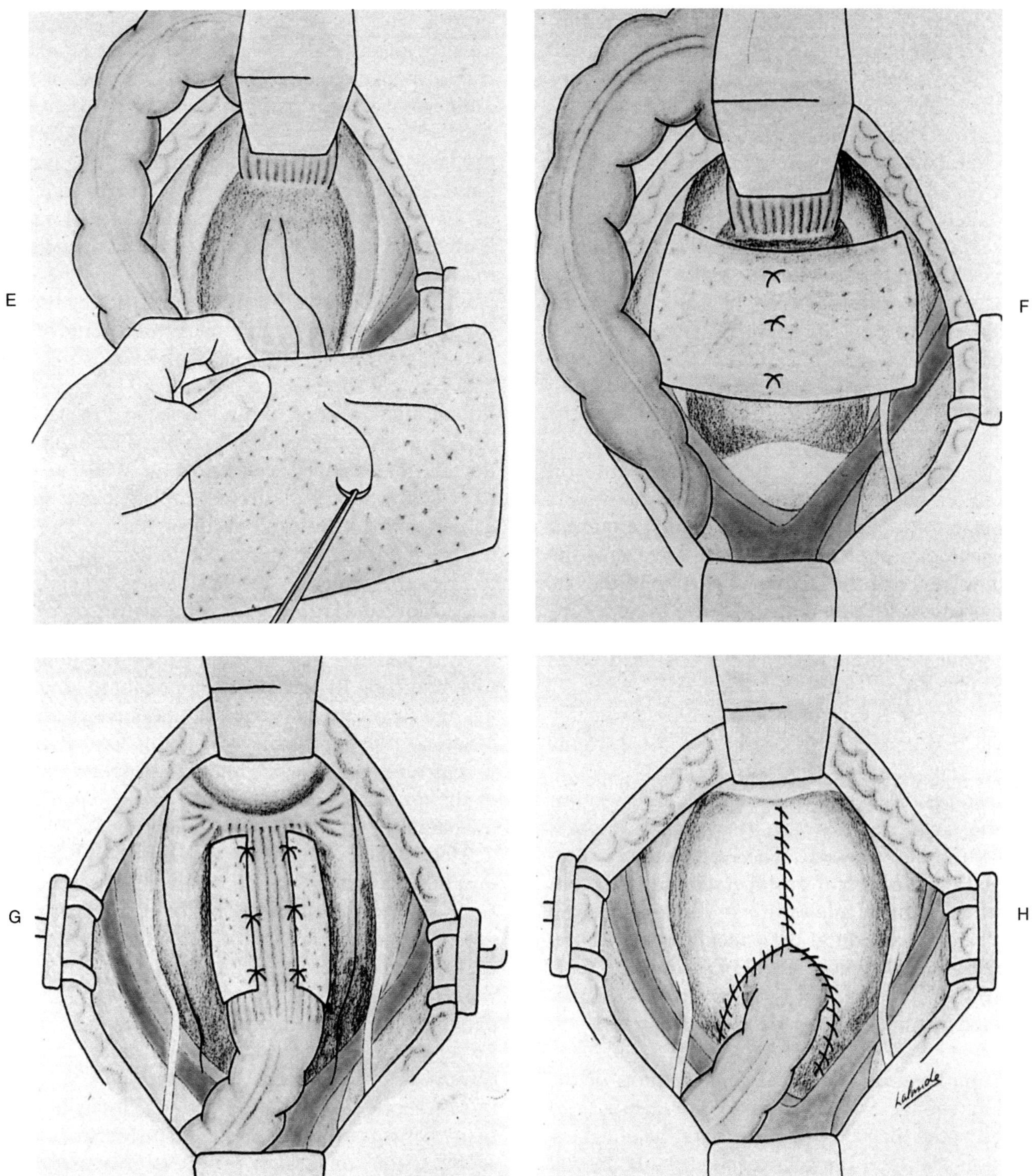

FIGURE 8 ■ *(Continued)*

observed in 58% of patients before operation persisted in only 16% postoperatively while constipation increased from 24% before operation to 44% after rectopexy. Arndt and Pircher (60) reported on the use of an absorbable mesh (Vicryl/Dexon) in 62 patients. There were no deaths, a recurrence rate of 6.4%, and no cases with sepsis. These authors believe that the adoption of an absorbable mesh will decrease the incidence of sepsis.

In a report of 23 patients with rectal procidentia, Delemarre et al. (65) reported that posterior rectopexy offers an 83% chance of regaining full continence or a major improvement and a 17% chance of stabilization of fecal continence.

In the most recent review of the results of posterior mesh rectopexy, Madiba et al. (46) assessed 19 reports and found mortality rates ranged from 0% to 3%, recurrence rates ranged from 3% to 6%, improvement in continence occurred 3% to 40%, but there was conflicting response to constipation with some studies reporting improvement while others noted worsening of symptoms.

Abdominal Proctopexy and Sigmoid Resection

This technique, originally described by Frykman (66) in 1955, is a composite surgical procedure using selected techniques designed to eliminate the abnormal factors that contribute to the formation of rectal procidentia.

TABLE 3 ■ Results of Ivalon Sponge Operation/Posterior Rectopexy

Author(s)	No. of Patients	Recurrence Rate (%)	Mortality Rate (%)	Morbidity Rate (%)	Mean Follow-Up (yr)
Morgan et al. (48) (1972)	150	3.2	2.6	3	–
Penfold and Hawley (49) (1972)	101	3	0	6	6
Stewart (55) (1972)	41	7.3	0	29	5.5
Boutsis and Ellis (15) (1974)	26	11.5	3.8	8	–
Anderson et al. (56) (1981)	37	2.7	2.7	–	7
Anderson et al. (57) (1984	42	2.4	0	–	4
Atkinson and Taylor (58) (1984)	40	10	0	3	2.7
Boulous et al. (59) (1984)	32	15.6	0	3	10
Kuijpers and de Morree (50) (1988)	30	0	–	–[a]	–
Arndt and Pircher (60) (1988)	62	6.4	0	–	3
Yoshioka et al. (61) (1989)	165	1.5	0	19	3
Sayfan et al. (62) (1990)	16	0	0	12.5	–
Luukkonen et al. (63) (1992)	15	0	0	13.3	–
Novell et al. (64) (1994)	31	3.2	0	19	4

[a]Not addressed except to state no infection due to mesh.

Technique

Abdominal proctopexy and sigmoid resection are performed through a transverse or midline abdominal incision and, as described by Frykman (66), consist of the following four essential steps (Fig. 9):

1. *Mobilization of the rectum by the abdominal route.* The dissection of the rectum is carried out exactly as in the abdominal phase of a Miles' abdominoperineal resection except for preserving the blood supply to the rectum and keeping the lateral stalks intact.
2. *Elevation of the rectum as high as possible and fixation of the lateral stalks by suturing them to the periosteum of the sacrum.* The rectum is completely mobilized down to the levator muscles, and the freed rectum is drawn up into the abdomen, which makes the lateral stalks prominent. The stalks are then sutured to the periosteum of the sacrum with silk to hold the organ firmly in this elevated position. Care must be taken not to narrow the bowel by placement of the fixation sutures because this may lead to an obstruction.
3. *Suture of the endopelvic fascia anteriorly to the rectum to obliterate the cul-de-sac.* The excess peritoneum of the cul-de-sac is excised, and the new peritoneal floor is sutured snugly around the elevated intestine with interrupted silk sutures. No attempt is made to approximate the levator muscles anterior to the rectum.
4. *Segmental resection of all the excess sigmoid colon with an end-to-end anastomosis.* The peritoneum lateral to the descending colon is incised up to the splenic flexure, and the entire left colon is mobilized from the retroperitoneal structures. A wedge resection of the colon is then performed, with preservation of the major blood vessels. The redundant colon is resected so that the anastomosis can be accomplished without tension. Alternatively, the fixation sutures can be inserted, the anastomosis accomplished with the intraluminal stapler, and the fixation sutures secured in place. Any convenient site may be selected for the anastomosis. The raw surfaces, except for the left gutter, are reperitonealized.

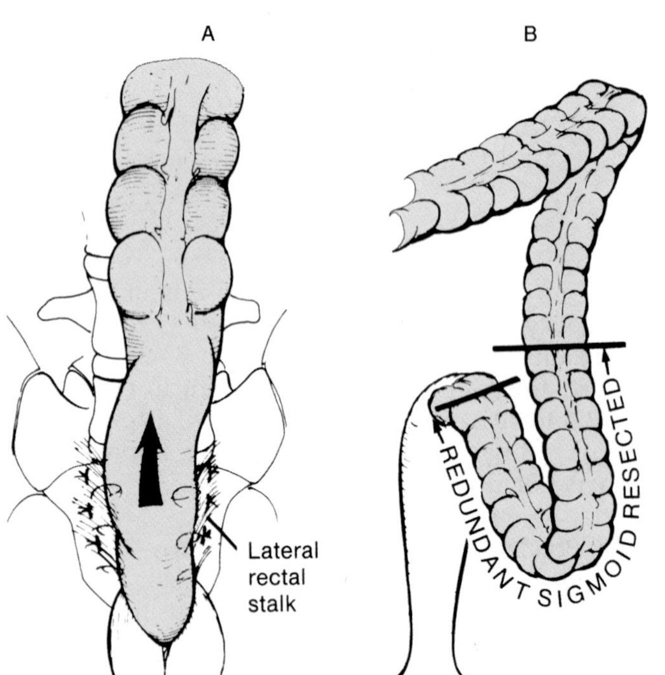

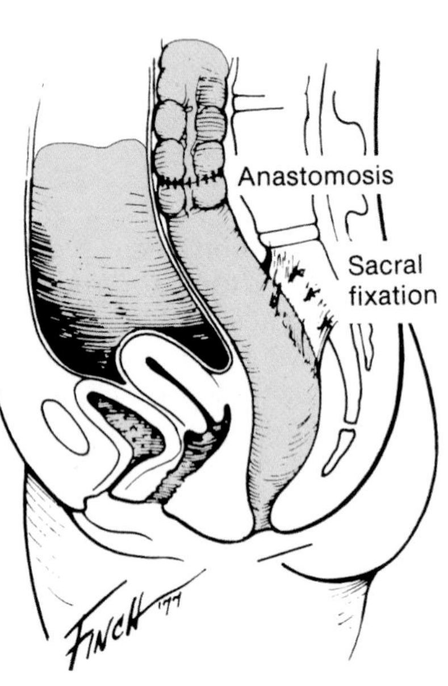

FIGURE 9 ■ Abdominal proctopexy and sigmoid resection. (**A**) After full mobilization by sharp dissection, the tissues lateral to the rectal wall are swept away laterally. (**B**) Resection of the redundant sigmoid colon. (**C**) Anastomosis completed and rectopexy sutures are placed.

Results

Over the 25-year period from 1952 to 1977, 103 patients underwent this operative procedure reported by Goldberg et al. (67). One death occurred. There were no known complete recurrences, although nine patients returned with mucosal prolapses. Initially these prolapses were treated with phenol-in-oil injections, but in recent years rubber band ligatures have been applied with good results. Twelve major complications occurred, for a rate slightly less than 12%. There were three colonic obstructions and one anastomotic leak, each requiring a temporary colostomy. After the closure of one of these colostomies, a fecal fistula developed but closed spontaneously. One patient had severe presacral bleeding, which required six units of blood, and one patient had wound dehiscence. Three patients had a small bowel obstruction, with two requiring operative intervention, and one patient had a cardiac arrest from which she was successfully resuscitated. In addition, there was one patient with acute pancreatitis and one with acute incarceration of a hiatal hernia. An assessment of these patients by Watts et al. (24) included information on 102 of 138 patients who underwent this procedure. Follow-up ranged from 6 months to 30 years, with a recurrence rate of 1.9%. This review focused primarily on postoperative functional results. Before the operation, 40% of the patients experienced varying degrees of incontinence, with 24% reporting major or total incontinence. After the operation, 77% of the patients had perfect continence; 8%, minor incontinence; and only 15%, unacceptable incontinence. A more recent report from this group focused on the long-term functional results in 47 patients followed for more than three years. In this series 33 patients underwent sigmoidectomy, 8 patients subtotal colectomy, and 4 patients sigmoidectomy with subsequent subtotal colectomy. The recurrence rate was 6.3%. Constipation improved in 50%. Incontinence improved in 38% and worsened in 29%. Subsequent stomas were required in 14% of patients (68). These findings might temper some enthusiasm for this procedure.

Husa et al. (69) reported on 48 selected patients who underwent posterior rectopexy and left colon resection, with a 2.1% operative mortality rate and a 9% recurrence rate in 45 patients followed for 1 to 10 years (mean, 4.3 years). No complication was attributable to the bowel resection. All but 2 of the 32 patients with associated incontinence experienced improved anal control after the operation (nine regained normal continence). Bowel habits improved in 56% of the patients. In a series of 39 patients Huber et al. (70) found that constipation complaints improved from 44% to 26%, and incontinence from 67% to 23%. Results of sigmoid resection and rectopexy reported by others are summarized in Table 4. As with other tables, the numbers vary, depending on how the authors of each study viewed morbidity, often ignoring complications not specific to the operation, or including only complications the authors considered to be "major."

In the most recent review by Madiba et al. (46) for patients undergoing suture rectopexy and resection, mortality rates ranged from 0% to 6.7%, recurrence rates, 0% to 5%, with an overall reduction in constipation and improvement in continence in most patients.

Prevention of Complications

The intraoperative complications with abdominal proctopexy and sigmoid resection are similar to those of abdominoperineal resection or low anterior resection and are as follows (44).

BLEEDING ■ Bleeding from the presacral venous plexus can be severe and difficult to control. Cutting the rectosacral fascia with long scissors or cautery instead of tearing it reduces the chance to injure these vessels. The needle used to suture the rectum to the presacral fascia may tear the presacral vessels, causing severe bleeding that usually stops when the sutures are tied.

NEURAL INJURY ■ Injury to the sympathetic and parasympathetic nerves from mobilization of the rectum is difficult to evaluate and is not specifically reported for this procedure in the literature. The incidence should be similar to that for total proctocolectomy in patients with inflammatory bowel disease, which is 0% to 17%.

COMPRESSION ■ Suturing the rectum too close to the wall may cause compression on the anterior wall of the rectum as a result of stretching the visceral peritoneum. Compression must be recognized and corrected by making a vertical incision over the compressed serosa. An alternative method is to place the sutures in the back of the rectum.

Determining Necessity of Colonic Resection

A very pertinent question to ask at this juncture is whether colonic resection is a necessary component in the correction of rectal procidentia. Advocates of this procedure believe that maximal resection of the left colon is an essential step in the treatment of rectal procidentia. It is argued that shortening the left colon should permanently prevent recurrence, irrespective of the type or the multiplicity of causative factors that may be involved, since the straight

TABLE 4 ■ Results of Sigmoid Resection and Proctopexy

Author(s)	No. of Patients	Recurrence Rate (%)	Mortality Rate (%)	Morbidity Rate (%)	Mean Follow-Up (yr)
Watts et al. (24) (1985)	102	1.9	0	4	4
Husa et al. (69) (1988)	48	9	2.1	0	4.3
Sayfan et al. (62) (1990)	13	0	0	23	
McKee et al. (71) (1992)	9	0	0	0	1.8
Luukkonen et al. (63) (1992)	15	0	6.7	20	
Canfrère et al. (72) (1994)	17	0	0	–	2
Huber et al. (70) (1995)	39	0	0	7.1	4.5

left colon firmly supported proximally by the phrenocolic ligament has little mobility and cannot slide. Of all the weaknesses or abnormalities required to produce rectal prolapse, the only factor that can be controlled with any degree of certainty is the length of the colon. Stress and strain may break down the rebuilt rectal support and deepen the cul-de-sac, but the configuration of the straight, short left colon will not change. Without slack and mobility in the left colon, the rectum cannot descend, and rectal prolapse cannot recur.

The low anterior resection as recommended by Muir (73) has the decided advantage of being an operation familiar to all surgeons because of its use in carcinoma of the rectum. However, the low end-to-end anastomosis predisposes to the problems inherent with a low anastomosis, notably a leak and its subsequent complications. Performing resection at any convenient level makes much more sense than performing a low resection. In addition, removal of a large redundant sigmoid will result in smoother bowel function. Less constipation results in less straining, thus decreasing the chance of an anatomic recurrence (74).

A report on 113 patients who under went anterior resection at the Mayo Clinic revealed a 1% mortality rate, a 29% operative complication rate, and a 9% recurrence rate (75). The Mayo Clinic group found that the probability of recurrence was a function of time and that rates at 2, 5, and 10 years were 3%, 6%, and 12%, respectively. They also found that a low anterior resection was associated with a higher morbidity rate than a high anterior resection, with no significant decrease in recurrence rate. They believe that a high anterior resection is preferable to a low anterior resection. Cirocco and Brown (76) reported on 41 patients who underwent anterior resection for rectal prolapse. With an average follow-up of 6 years, the recurrence rate was 7%. Mortality was 0% but morbidity was 15%. McKee et al. (71) concluded that the addition of sigmoidectomy to rectopexy reduces the risk of severe constipation after operation. Baker et al. (77) reported that laparoscopically assisted resection effectively treats rectal prolapse without the morbidity associated with a laparotomy wound and significantly shortens hospitalization.

Although resection of the excess bowel increases the magnitude of the procedure, it provides great potential for permanent cure and hence may be worthwhile. For patients with slow-transit constipation associated with rectal procidentia, Watts et al. (24) recommend performing a subtotal colectomy. Resection, of course, is primarily designed for use in those individuals whose general physical condition justifies an aggressive approach.

Kim et al. (78) reviewed their experience over a 19-year period to assess trends in choice of operation, recurrence rates, and functional results. They identified 372 patients who underwent operation for complete rectal prolapse and had a median follow-up of 64 months with a range of 12 to 231 months. Functional results were obtained from 49% of patients. The median age of patients was 64 years (range, 11–100 years), and female patients outnumbered male patients by nine to one. Perineal rectosigmoidectomy was performed in 49% of patients while 43% of patients underwent abdominal rectopexy with bowel resection. The percentage of patients who underwent perineal rectosigmoidectomy increased from 22% in the first five years of the study to 79% in the most recent five years. Patients who underwent perineal rectosigmoidectomy were more likely to have associated medical problems as compared with patients undergoing abdominal rectopexy (61% vs. 30%). There was no significant difference in morbidity with 14% for perineal rectosigmoidectomy versus 20% for abdominal rectopexy. Abdominal procedures were associated with a longer length of stay as compared with perineal rectosigmoidectomy (8 days vs. 5 days). Perineal procedures, however, had a higher recurrence rate (16% vs. 5%). Functional improvement was not significantly different and most patients were satisfied with treatment and outcome. They concluded that abdominal rectopexy with bowel resection is associated with low recurrence rates. Perineal rectosigmoidectomy provides lower morbidity and shorter length of stay, but recurrence rates are much higher. Despite this, perineal rectosigmoidectomy has appeal as a lesser procedure for elderly patients or those patients in the high surgical risk category. For younger patients, the benefits of perineal rectosigmoidectomy being a lesser procedure must be weighed against a higher recurrence rate.

Rectopexy

Rectopexy alone without resection or insertion of mesh might be adequate therapy for procidentia. Loygue et al. (79) reported on an operation in which, after full mobilization of the rectum, interrupted nonabsorbable sutures or strips of fascia lata were used to secure the rectum to the presacral fascia. In their series of 140 patients, there were two postoperative deaths and, with a follow-up interval of up to 15 years, a remarkably low recurrence rate of 3.6%. Intervertebral disc infection was found in two cases. Of 44 patients in whom incontinence was due solely to loss of tone in the anal sphincter, 41 recovered completely. Blatchford et al. (80) reported on 42 patients who underwent simple posterior suture rectopexy. With a mean follow-up of 28 months, the recurrence rate was 2%. There were no deaths, a morbidity rate of 20%, and an increase in continence from 36% preoperatively to 74% postoperatively.

Douard et al. (81) assessed the functional results after the Orr-Loygue transabdominal rectopexy for complete rectal prolapse in 31 consecutive patients. After a mean follow up of 28 months, no prolapse recurred. Preoperative and postoperative rates of incontinence were 81% and 55%, respectively. Continence improved in 96% of the 25 patients who were incontinent before operation. The mean incontinence score decreased from 11.7 to 3.2 postoperatively. The self reported constipation rate was 61% before operation and 71% after operation. Constipation appeared or worsened in 52% whereas it disappeared or improved in 26%. Evacuation difficulties increased significantly after operation from 23% to 61%. Ninety-seven percent of patients reported good or very good satisfaction.

Madiba et al. (46) recently reviewed the literature on the results of suture rectopexy and found 10 reports in the previous two decades, half of which were performed laparoscopically. There were no deaths, continence was reportedly improved in about two-thirds of cases, constipation was improved in 14% to 83% of cases but made worse in some cases, and recurrence was reported in 3% to 9% of cases.

Novell et al. (63) conducted a prospective randomized trial of the use of the Ivalon sponge versus a sutured rectopexy for full-thickness rectal prolapse and reported that in terms of postoperative complications and function, the two procedures were equivalent, with the exception of a higher rate of wound infection in those undergoing Ivalon rectopexy. The authors suggested that Ivalon rectopexy confers no advantage over the sutured rectopexy.

Abdominal Colorectopexy for Combined Rectal and Vaginal Prolapse

Rectal prolapse and post-hysterectomy vaginal vault prolapse may occur together and constitute a management problem. Collopy and Barham (82) reported on 89 patients presenting with both rectal and gynecologic symptoms to either a colorectal surgeon or a gynecologic surgeon and were found on examination to have overt and/or occult prolapse of the rectum and vaginal vault. Common symptoms were pelvic pain, dragging in type and sometimes associated with dyspareunia; incontinence of urine and/or feces; constipation; or unsatisfied defecation. All patients had undergone hysterectomy and in the majority at least one vaginal repair before their presentation. As described by them, the operation consists of an abdominorectopexy of the Wells type in which a mesh of prosthetic material is attached to the sacral promontory above and extended downward and forward to be attached bilaterally to the mobilized and uplifted rectum. Intravaginal endoscopic transillumination of the vaginal vault is used to define the boundaries of the pelvic cul-de-sac that is then obliterated with a series of abdominally placed concentric pursestring sutures. Finally, the limbs of the same mesh are extended forward and sutured bilaterally to the apex of the obliterated pelvic cul-de-sac, thus performing a colpopexy and further elevating the vaginal vault (Fig. 10). The combined operation was performed on 89 patients. Of these patients, 60 had a concurrent vaginal repair. The mean follow-up time was approximately 5 years. There were no perioperative deaths and the morbidity rate was 9%. No injury occurred to the urinary tract and no wound or pelvic infections were evident. There was no recurrence of either the rectal or vaginal vault prolapse. Improvement occurred in all major symptoms especially in pelvic pain.

Sullivan et al. (83) reported on their total pelvic mesh repair that uses a strip of Marlex mesh secured between the perineal body and the sacrum. Two additional strips attached to the first, are tunneled laterally to the pubis and support the vagina and bladder laterally. Candidates for the procedure have failed previous standard repair or manifest combined organ prolapse on physical and cystodefecography examinations. There were *236* females who had total pelvic mesh repair with an 87% follow-up. Median age was 64 years; median parity 2; and 63% had birth-related complications. Bladder protrusion, vaginal protrusion, or both were the predominant chief complaint (54%) followed by anorectal protrusion (48%). Findings on physical examination showed degrees of prolapse of rectum (74%) and vagina (57%), perineal descent (63%), enterocele (47%), and rectocele (44%). Mean procedure time and length of hospital stay were 3.2 hours and 6 days, respectively. Reoperation rate because of complication of the total pelvic mesh repair procedure was 10%. Marlex erosion into the rectum or vagina occurred in 5% of patients and constituted 46% of the complications requiring reoperation. Additional surgical procedures at various intervals subsequent to a total pelvic mesh repair have been performed in 36% of patients to further improve bladder function and had been performed in 28% of patients to improve anorectal function. There has been no recurrence of rectal or vaginal prolapse to date. Reports of overall satisfaction for correction of primary symptoms for patients grouped into early (0.5–3 years), middle (>3–6 years), and late (>6 years) were 68%, 73%, and 74%, respectively.

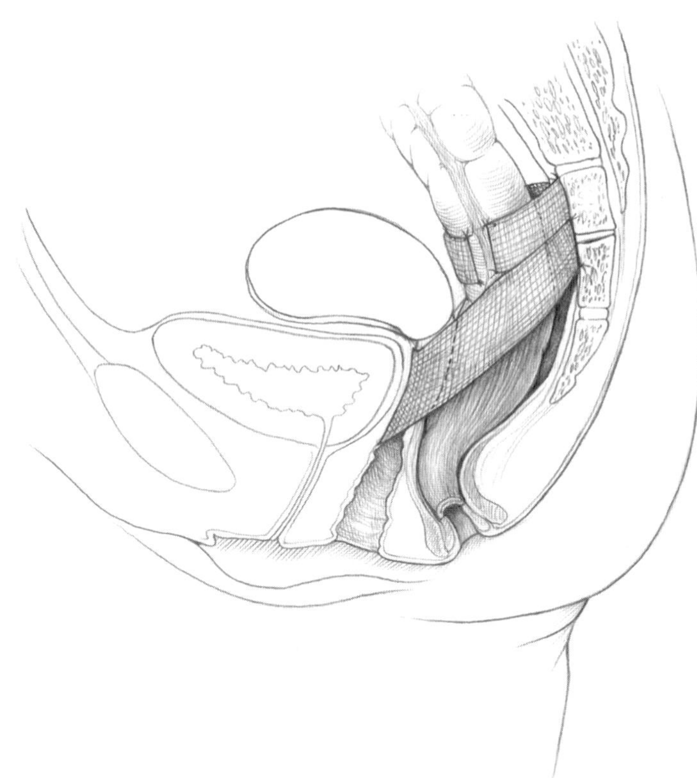

FIGURE 10 ■ Mesh placement for combined rectopexy and colpopexy.

■ PERINEAL PROCEDURES

Perineal Rectosigmoidectomy

Mikulicz first described rectosigmoidectomy in 1889. Miles powerfully advocated the same in 1933, and for many years this remained the favorite method of treatment in Great Britain. This procedure was popularized in the United States of America by Altemeier et al. (7). Recently there has been renewed enthusiasm for this procedure. The operation is recommended for the high-risk population and perhaps also for young men in whom impotence is a concern. It is possible the operation is more accepted now because the recurrence rates in more recently reported series have been dropping.

Technique

Under general or regional anesthesia, the patient is placed in the lithotomy or prone jackknife position and in a slight Trendelenburg position to minimize distention of the hemorhoidal vessels, thus reducing operative bleeding

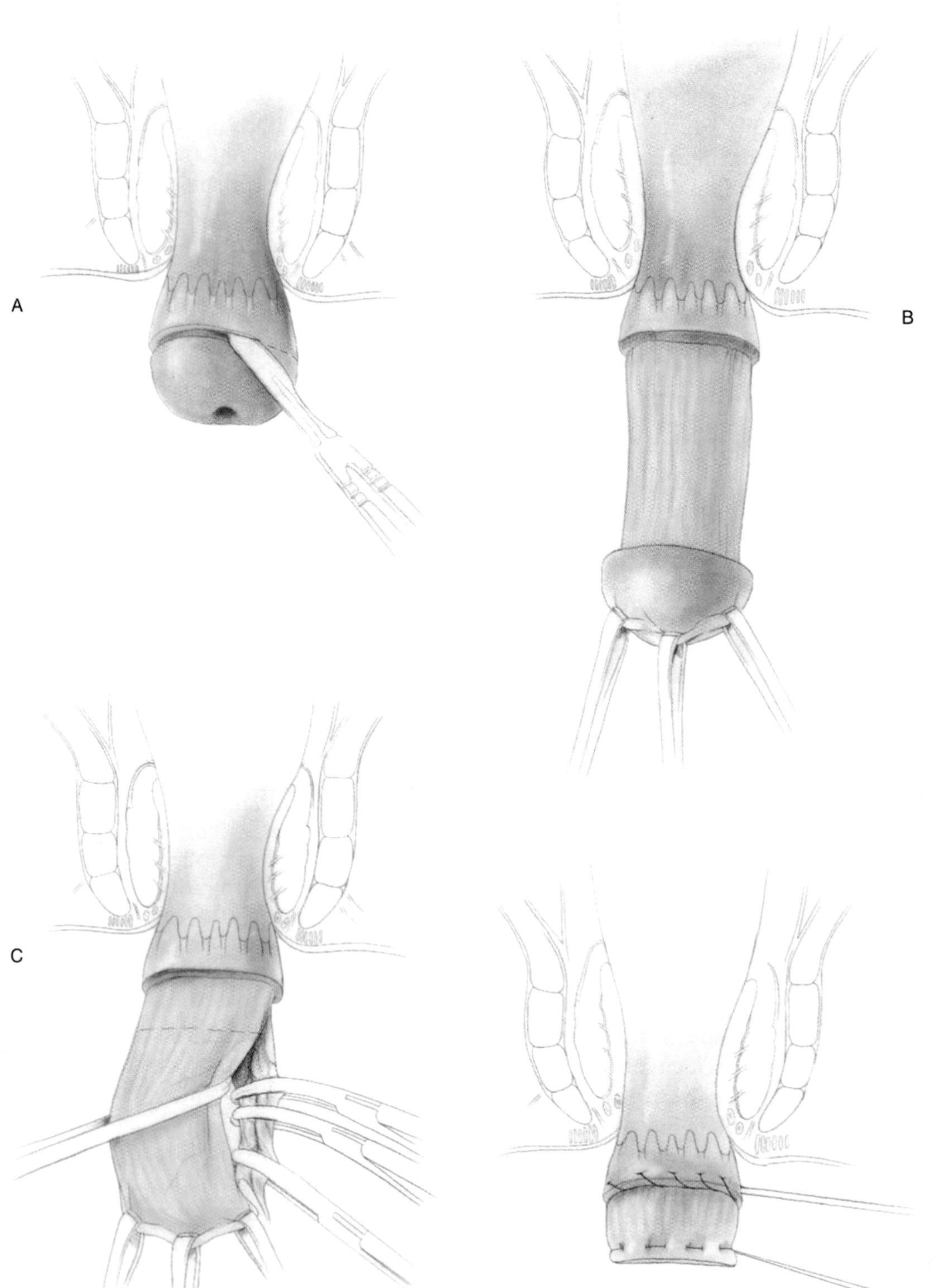

FIGURE 11 ■ Altemeier perineal rectosigmoidectomy. (**A**) Circumferential incision of rectum proximal to dentate line. (**B**) Delivery of redundant rectum and sigmoid colon. (**C**) Ligation of blood supply to rectum. (**D**) Placement of pursestring suture on proximal bowel and excision of redundant colon and rectum. Whipstitch placed on rectal stump.

and allowing the small intestine to retract into the peritoneal cavity (Fig. 11). A circumferential incision through all layers of the rectum is made 1.5 cm proximal to the dentate line when a hand-sutured technique will be used, or approximately 2.5 cm proximal if the stapler will be used. This length is adequate for establishing the anastomosis yet short enough to prevent postoperative protrusion. The anterior wall of the hernial sac is exposed and opened to determine its full extent, and the excess peritoneal reflections are trimmed. The mesentery of the redundant bowel is serially clamped, divided, and ligated until the redundant bowel cannot be pulled down any further. The pouch of Douglas is obliterated by continuous suturing with 2–0 Vicryl. Of unproven efficacy is narrowing of the levator hiatus. At this point in the operation, Altemeier et al. (7) recommended that the medial borders of the retracted levator ani muscles anterior to the rectum be approximated, using the number of sutures required to narrow the defect in the pelvic diaphragm to fit snugly around the surgeon's finger. The value of this plication is controversial. If the patient is incontinent it is reasonable to approximate the puborectalis and even the external sphincter (84). If a hand-sewn anastomosis is to be created, the redundant proximal bowel is transected

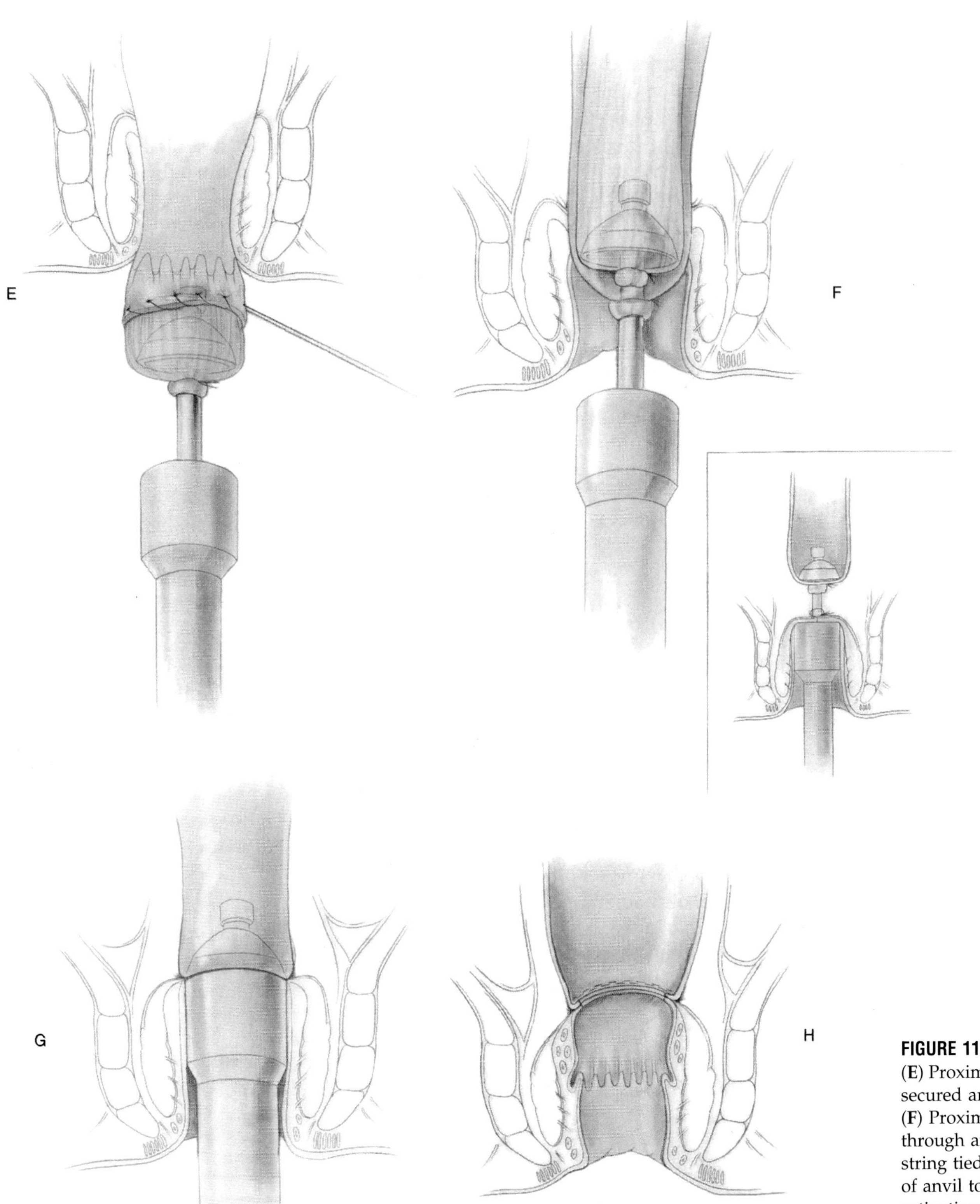

FIGURE 11 ■ *(Continued)* (**E**) Proximal pursestring suture secured around central shaft. (**F**) Proximal bowel advanced through anus and distal pursestring tied. (**G**) Approximation of anvil to cartridge and activation of stapler. (**H**) Completed anastomosis.

serially and grasped with Badcock clamps to prevent retraction. Stay sutures of 2–0 or 3–0 Vicryl are placed full thickness in each quadrant of the proximal and distal ends of the transected bowel. The anstomosis is completed with the same suture material. The everted anastomosis is then reduced.

When the stapler is used, a pursestring clamp is applied to the proximal bowel, a pursestring suture of 2–0 Prolene inserted, and the redundant bowel excised. A whipstitch of 2–0 Prolene is placed on the distal rectal stump. The circular stapler is inserted into the proximal bowel, and the proximal pursestring suture is secured around the central shaft. The instrument is partially advanced through the anus and the distal pursestring suture is tightened. The stapler is closed and activated, thus completing the anastomosis.

Altemeier et al. (7) reported excellent results with perineal rectosigmoidectomy, having only three recurrences after 106 operations. However, these good results generally have not been matched by other surgeons. The technique of perineal rectosigmoidectomy may also induce further damage to the already altered anatomy and physiology.

Kim et al. (85) reported on 183 patients treated with this technique with no associated mortality. Postoperative complications developed in 14% of patients. Anastomotic complications included three leaks, two strictures, and three bleeds. Other complications included pulmonary, cardiac failure, and confusion. Improvement in fecal continence was noted in 20 of 38 patients evaluated.

In a series of 53 patients reported by Agachan et al. (86) significant complications included two leaks, both of which were treated conservatively, one postoperative pelvic hematoma necessitating reoperation and one anastomotic stricture which was treated by dilatation under general anaesthesia. There was one death from a pulmonary embolus. Levatorplasty was associated with marked improvement in postoperative continence from a preoperative incontinence score of 15.7 to a postoperative incontinence score of 4.9.

Kimins et al. (87) reported on 63 patients who underwent a perineal rectosigmoidectomy. Anastomoses were stapled in 83% of cases and 80% of patients were home within 24 hours. Complications occurred in 10% of patients but there were no perioperative deaths. With a median follow-up of 20.8 months, there was a 6.4% recurrence rate. Postoperative bowel function was reported improved in 87% of patients although 32% continued to have problems with constipation and 30% had some degree of incontinence.

Complications and Prevention

ANASTOMOTIC DEHISCENCE ■ Despite the very low anastomosis, leakage is uncommon. If it does occur, it is usually the result of tension and poor blood supply. Therefore extreme care must be taken not to pull the bowel too tightly while transecting it. Good blood supply also should be maintained by not ligating the mesentery too far proximally, especially in a redundant bowel. If an abscess develops, it can usually be drained locally.

POSTOPERATIVE BLEEDING ■ This occurred in 1 of 20 patients undergoing perineal rectosigmoidectomy in which a pelvic hematoma required reoperation (86). Other surgeons have reported lesser degrees of bleeding that stopped spontaneously.

ANASTOMOTIC STRICTURE ■ Most patients have some degree of stricture at the anastomotic site, but it is rare that the strictures require dilatation. Patients should be given a bulk diet as soon as possible.

OTHER POSSIBLE COMPLICATIONS ■ Other complications include injury to the small bowel after the peritoneal sac had been opened and perforation of the posterior vaginal wall during the dissection.

The results of several published series are listed in Table 5.

Perineal Proctectomy, Posterior Rectopexy, and Levator Ani Muscle Repair

Unencumbered by the published reports of poor results with perineal rectosigmoidectomy and the seeming lack of need to approximate the levator ani muscles, Prasad et al. (93) described an innovative operation to address simultaneously the anatomic and functional problems of rectal procidentia: a one-stage perineal proctectomy, posterior rectopexy, and postanal levator ani muscle repair. Cited advantages of the procedure are that it can be performed with the patient under a regional anesthetic, it does not require a laparotomy, and it is well tolerated by poor-risk patients. By combining resection and reconstruction of the anorectal angle, the procedure restores anal continence in addition to correcting the prolapse. After a perineal rectosigmoidectomy is accomplished as described previously, a posterior rectopexy is performed by approximating the seromuscular layers of the bowel to the precoccygeal fascia above the levator ani muscles with 2–0 silk sutures. The levator ani muscles are approximated posteriorly with 4–0 Prolene sutures. This repair pushes the bowel anteriorly to help recreate the anorectal angle. One or two similar sutures are used to approximate the levator ani muscles anterior to the rectum to reinforce the pelvic floor. The redundant bowel is amputated and an anastomosis is constructed (Fig. 12). Of 25 patients so treated, no complications occurred, but there was one death. Remarkably, 88% of the patients became continent within two weeks of the operation, and the remaining ones achieved control within three months. Although follow-up was short, there were no recurrences. Ramanujam and Venkatesh (94) adopted the technique and performed the repair in 72 patients, with acceptable morbidity and no

TABLE 5 ■ Results of Perineal Rectosigmoidectomy

Author(s)	No. of Patients	Recurrence Rate (%)	Mortality Rate (%)	Morbidity Rate (%)	Mean Follow-Up (yr)
Altemeier et al. (7) (1971)	106	3	0	24	–
Friedman et al. (88) (1983)	27	50	0	12	2–17
Gopal et al. (89) (1984)	18	6	6	17	1
Finlay and Aitchison (90) (1991)	17	6	6	18	2
Agachan et al. (86) (1997)	32	13	3	9	26.5 (6–72)
	21[a]	5	0	5	29.6 (6–72)
Kim (85) (1999)	183	16	0	14	47 (12–165) mo
Azimuddin et al. (91) (2001)	36	16	3	6	4.2
Kimmins (87) (2001)	63	16	0	10	21 (6–88) mo
Schutz (92) (2001)	31	0	3	16	7.5 yr
Zbar et al. (13) (2002)	80	4	0	2	22 (6–132) mo

[a]With levatorplasty.

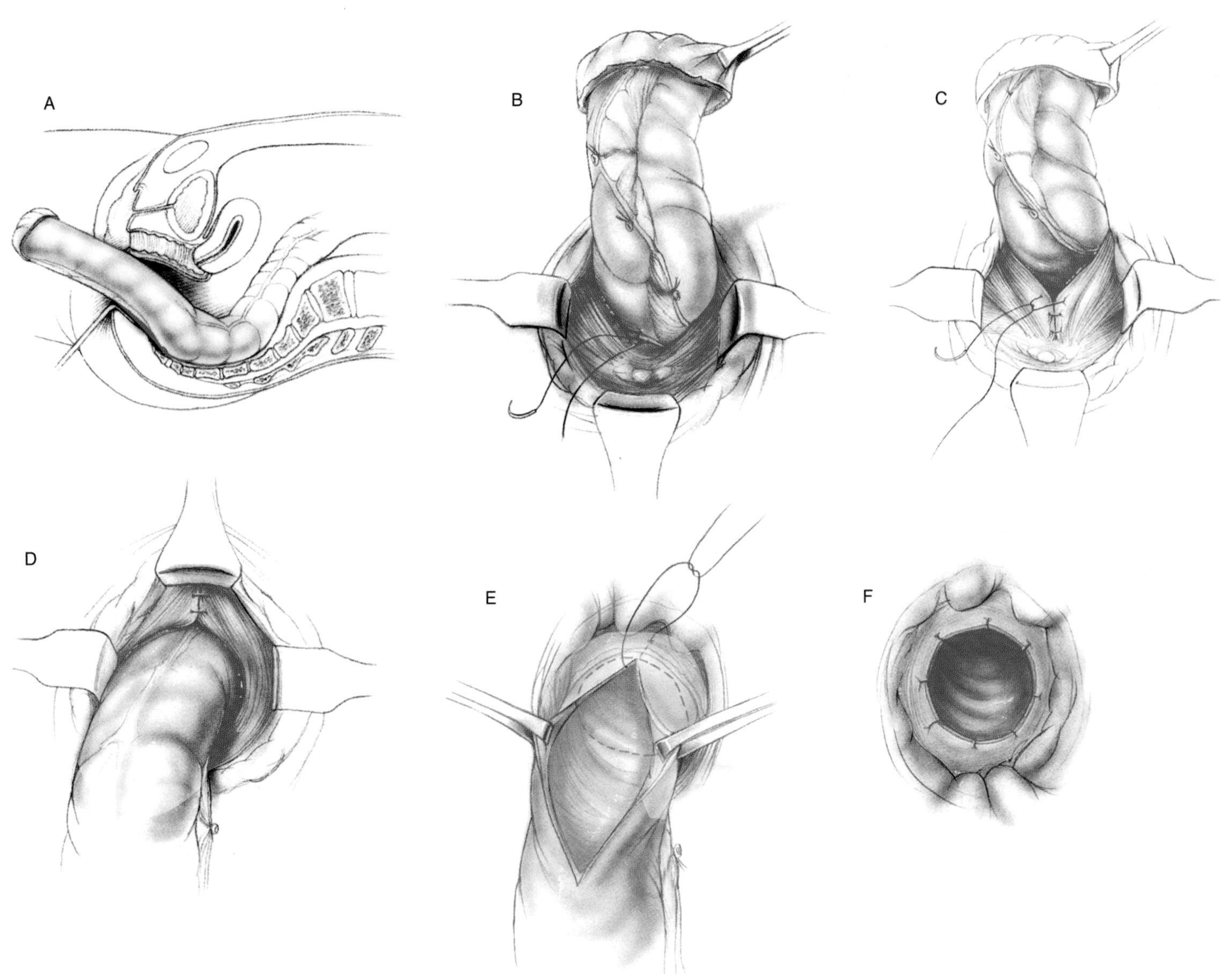

FIGURE 12 ■ A one-stage perineal proctectomy, posterior rectopexy and postanal levator ani muscle repair. (**A**) Mobilized rectosigmoid. (**B**) Suturing seromuscular layer of bowel to precoccygeal fascia above levator ani muscle. (**C**) Approximation of levator ani posteriorly. (**D**) Approximation of levator anteriorly. (**E**) Amputation of redundant bowel. (**F**) Completed anastomosis.

mortality. Significant improvement in continence was seen in 67% of patients, and the recurrence rate was 5.5%.

Kohler and Athanasiadis (95) reported that in 38 patients having posterior levatorplasty, continence improved in 84% of patients. Incontinence scores decreased from 16.4 to 9.4 compared to 15.6 to 11.5 for patients without levatorplasty.

Delorme Procedure

This procedure, originally described by Delorme (96) in 1900, involves stripping the mucosa from the prolapsed bowel, plicating the denuded muscular wall, and re-anastomosing the mucosal rings. Historically, the procedure never gained general acceptance, but a paper by Uhlig and Sullivan (97) rekindled my interest in the operation. In recent years others have supported a renewed popularity.

Technique

The technique, although unfamiliar to many surgeons, is a simple one. After complete bowel preparation, the patient is placed in either the lithotomy or prone jackknife position (the latter being my preference), the perianal region is infiltrated with a local anesthetic such as 0.5% lidocaine (Xylocaine) with 1:200,000 epinephrine (Fig. 12A). A general anesthetic is not necessary, but intravenous sedation is helpful. If not already prolapsed, the rectum can be delivered easily. The submucosa is infiltrated with the same solution to reduce bleeding and facilitate the plane of dissection (Fig. 13B). A circular incision is made through the mucosa approximately 1 cm above the dentate line (Fig. 13C). Initially some bleeding will be encountered, but this is easily controlled by cautery. Through repeated infiltration and scissors or electrocautery dissection, a sleeve of mucosa and submucosa is peeled from the underlying muscle until the point at which there is some tension (Fig. 13D and E). As much as 10 to 25 cm or more of mucosa may be stripped. A rolled gauze inserted into the mucosal-submucosal tube will provide for better traction and identification of plane (97). The denuded muscularis is then pleated in a longitudinal manner by placing sutures of 2–0 polyglycolic acid, polyglactin, or chromic catgut in each quadrant and then placing two more sutures between each quadrant stitch for a total of 12 sutures (Fig. 13F). Each suture is begun just proximal to the incised mucosa, and it is continued proximally to the level at which the mucosa was dissected. The prolapsed bowel is reduced above the anal canal and the sutures tied. Absolute hemostasis must be obtained before tying these sutures. The stripped mucosa is then excised and the proximal mucosa anastomosed to the distal mucosa with a running suture of 3–0 chromic catgut for each half of the circumference of the rectum (Fig. 13G).

For the patient with a minimal prolapse, but nevertheless symptomatic, a modification in the Delorme technique

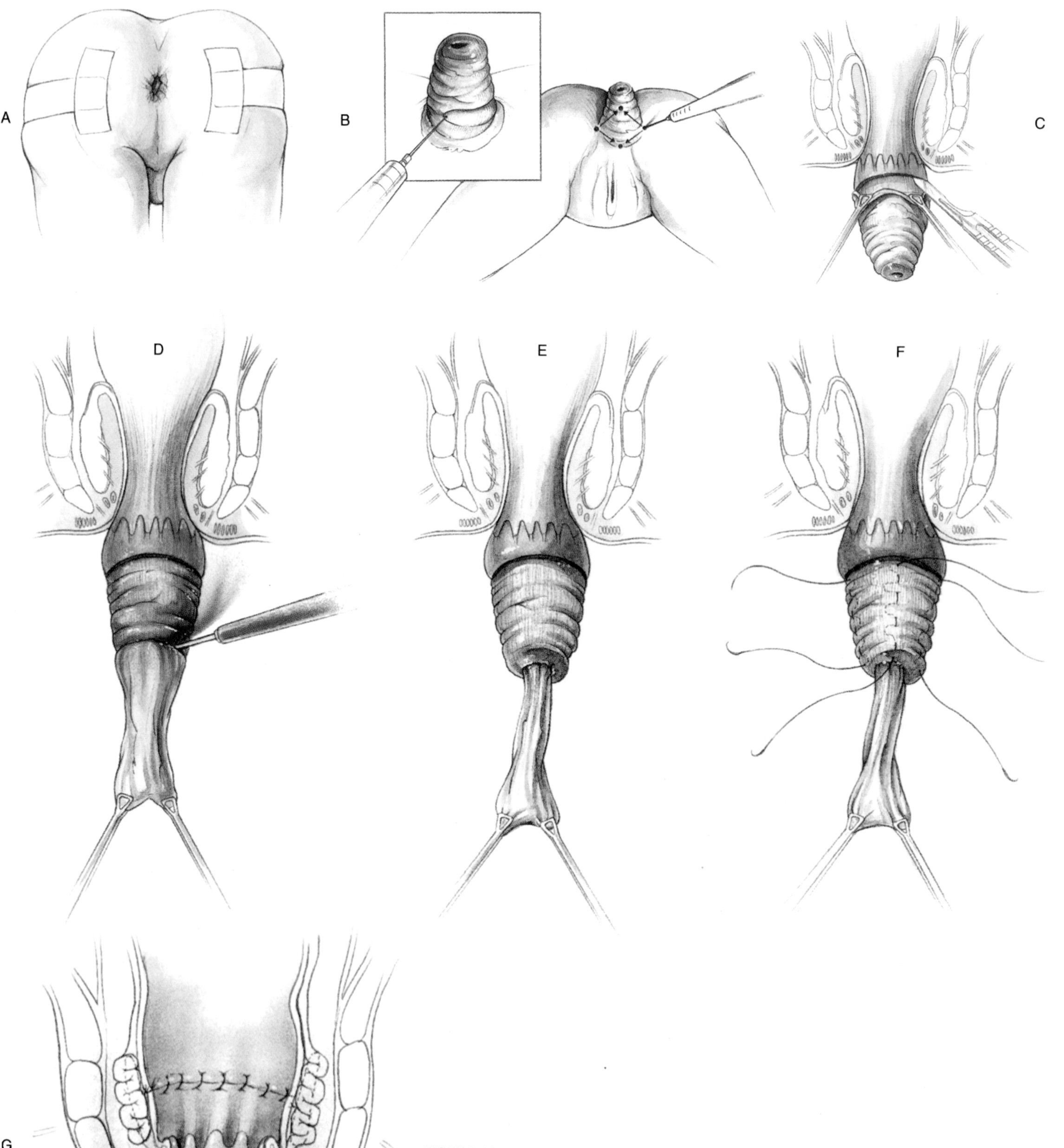

FIGURE 13 ■ The Delorme operation. (**A**) Prone jackknife position. (**B**) Infiltration of submucosa with 0.5% lidocaine with 1:200,000 epinephrine. (**C**) Circular incision 1 cm proximal to the dentate line. (**D**) Dissection of mucosa off the underlying muscle. (**E**) Dissection until tension on mucosal-submucosal tube. (**F**) Plication of muscular tube. (**G**) Reanastomosis of mucosa after redundant sleeve excised.

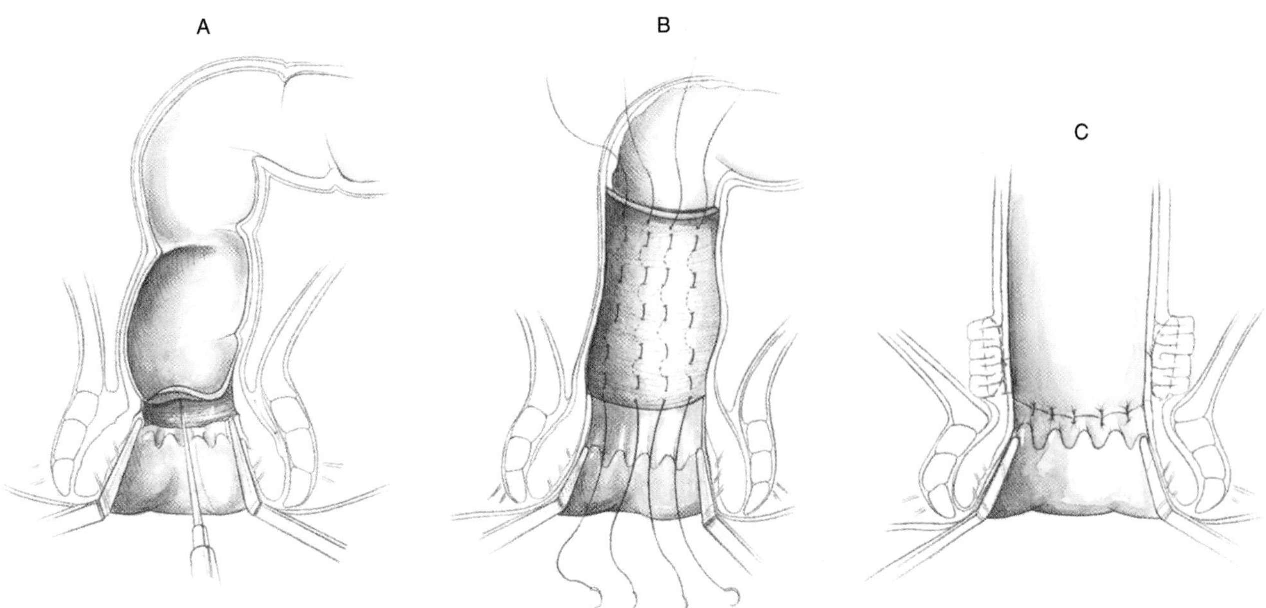

FIGURE 14 ■ Modified Delorme technique. (**A**) Endorectal mobilization of mucosa. (**B**) Plication of muscular wall after redundant mucosa excised. (**C**) Completed muscle plication and reanastomosis of mucosal tube.

has been described in which the mucosal stripping and muscular plication can successfully be carried out using a per anal endoluminal approach. The mucosal stripping is performed per anum (Fig. 14A), followed by muscle plication (Fig. 14B), and finally excision of excess mucosa and reanastomosis of the mucosa (Fig. 14C). Oral intake is allowed on the first postoperative day.

Advantages and Disadvantages

Advantages of the procedure are that it can be performed with the patient under local anesthesia, it is a simple and safe operation to execute, it causes little operative trauma, it can be performed on a patient who is a very poor operative risk but who is distressed with the disabling symptoms of complete rectal procidentia, and it involves neither resection and anastomosis nor an abdominal incision.

The major disadvantages are that it does not correct the underlying anatomic abnormality, and the recurrence rate clearly exceeds that of any intra-abdominal procedure. However, this operation is recommended only for the very poor-risk patient, and the dissection may be tedious, depending on the length of bowel stripped. Watts and Thompson (98) reviewed 126 patients who underwent a Delorme procedure over an 11-year period. Of the 15 patients who underwent a "redo" Delorme procedure, the average follow-up after their first procedure was 24.2 months and the average recurrence-free period 14.9 months. With an average follow-up after the "redo" procedure of 19.5 months, the recurrence rate was 40%, with an average recurrence-free period of 12.7 months. Of three patients who underwent a "re-redo" Delorme procedure, there were no recurrences in 8.3 months. Despite the high recurrence rate the authors concluded that the procedure is beneficial for frail and elderly patients. The results of various authors are summarized in Table 6.

Complications

Complications with the Delorme procedure are uncommon. They include bleeding from wound separation, sepsis, injury to the anal sphincter with resulting incontinence, anal stricture, and pulmonary embolism (44).

Functional results have varied, and reported results are somewhat better than might be expected for a perineal procedure. In a detailed physiologic assessment before and after the Delorme procedure in 19 patients, Plusa et al. (109) attributed improved rectal sensation and lowered rectal compliance to the reduced incidence of defecatory problems after this operation. Sielezneff et al. (111) reported that proximal internal prolapse with rectosacral separation at defecography, preoperative chronic diarrhea, fecal incontinence, and descending perineum (>9 cm on straining) were associated with a poorer outcome.

Not every author has reported continence preoperatively and postoperatively, so the functional results shown in Table 6 most likely are not comparable but do give a rough estimation of success.

Thiersch Operation

Encirclement of the anal orifice with a silver wire, as first described by Thiersch in 1891, is a simple procedure. Occasionally some surgeons have considered using the Thiersch operation in managing patients with complete rectal prolapse, particularly patients considered absolutely unsuitable for any intra-abdominal procedure. In many cases, however, treatment with a Thiersch operation results in as much grief for the patient as the original prolapse. For this reason I have abandoned the procedure in favor of the Delorme operation.

Technique

Although general, caudal, or epidural anesthesia can be used, this procedure is performed only on patients at poor risk, so local anesthesia is the choice. The anesthesia may be supplemented by intravenous sedation such as with diazepam.

Although the procedure may be performed satisfactorily with the patient in the lithotomy position, it is

TABLE 6 ■ Results of Delorme Operation

Author(s)	No. of Patients	Recurrence Rate (%)	Mortality Rate (%)	Morbidity Rate (%)	Functional Results			Mean Follow-Up (Yr)
					E	S	P	
Uhlig and Sullivan (97) (1979)	44	6.8	0	34	55	41	4	2–10
Christiansen and Kirkegaard (99) (1981)	12	16.7	0	0	66	17	17	3
Gunderson et al. (100) (1985)	18	6	0	17	83		6	3.5
Monson et al. (101) (1986)	27	7.4	0	0	83	17	–	–
Houry et al. (102) (1987)	18	16	0	0	72	–	28	1.5
Abulafi et al. (103) (1990)	22	5	0	14 + 14		Improved 75%		3–70 mo (29 mo)
Graf et al. (104) (1992)	14	21	0	–		Improved 55%		1.5
White and Stitz (105) (1992)	17	17.6	0	–	–			2
Oliver et al. (106) (1994)	40	22	2.5	62.5[a]	61	29	10	4
Senapati et al. (107) (1994)	32	12.5	0	6.3	–	–[b]	–	2 (4 mo–4 yr)
Tobin et al. (108) (1994)	43	25.6	0	12.2	53	21	26	3–60 mo (20 mo)
Plusa et al. (109) (1995)	104	25	–	–	–	–[c]	–	2.3
Pescatoria et al. (110)[d] (1998)	33	21	0	45%	79	–	–	39 mo (7–84)
Sielezneff et al. (111) (1999)	20	5	0	37%		No improvement		43 mo (8–73)
Liberman et al. (112) (2000)	34	0	0	35%	76		24	43 mo
Watts et al. (113) (2000)	101	27	4	–	35	40	25	36 (0–139) mo
Watkins et al. (114) (2003)	52	10	0	25%		Improved 83%		61.4 mo

[a]Only one major complication, an anastomotic separation, and hemorrhage.
[b]Incontinence improved in 46%.
[c]Of 13 of 19 patients studied who described themselves as incontinent when presented (before the operation), only four were incontinent to formed stool postoperatively.
[d]Delorme combined with sphincteroplasty.
Abbreviations: E, excellent; S, satisfactory; P, poor.

more comfortable for the operating surgeon, and probably for the patient, to use the semiprone jackknife position (50). The skin around the anus is carefully cleansed and the patient is draped. The perianal region is infiltrated with approximately 20 mL of 0.5% lidocaine with 1:200,000 epinephrine. The initial injection should be made with a fine-gauge needle (25 or less). Short radial incisions 1-cm long are made approximately 2 cm from the anal verge in the left posterolateral and right anterolateral aspects. Incisions are not placed in the midline because the knot resulting when the suture is tied can be buried more adequately in the ischioanal fossa and this will make sitting more comfortable for the patient. Each incision is deepened to 2.5 cm. A curved hemostat or a curved Doyen needle is introduced into the anterior incision and brought out through the posterior incision. In its course it must pass outside the external sphincter (Fig. 15A). In this way the suture will be swept well away from the sphincteric mechanism in the ischioanal fossa. The use of numerous materials has been advocated, but possibly the simplest is a monofilament pliable material such as No. 2 polypropylene. (Included in the host of materials that have been used are silicone rubber suture, Marlex mesh, Silastic-impregnated Dacron, and stainless steel wire.) The suture is drawn through half the circumference of the anus. The hemostat or needle is reintroduced, and the suture is delivered through the other half of the circumference (Fig. 14B). Care must be taken not to break through the posterior vaginal wall or the rectal mucosa. With an index finger in the anal canal, the surgeon ties the suture snugly (Fig. 14C). The knot is buried by approximating the fat in the ischioanal fossa with interrupted 3–0 chromic catgut over the suture. The skin wounds are approximated with 3–0 Vicryl (Fig. 14D).

Postoperative Care

A simple dressing with a Fuller shield is applied since tape is irritating to the skin. Bulk-forming agents should be introduced into the diet because these patients usually have a long-standing history of constipation. In addition, a lubricant such as mineral oil with agar may prove beneficial. Sometimes saline laxatives such as magnesium oxide or a suppository also may be required.

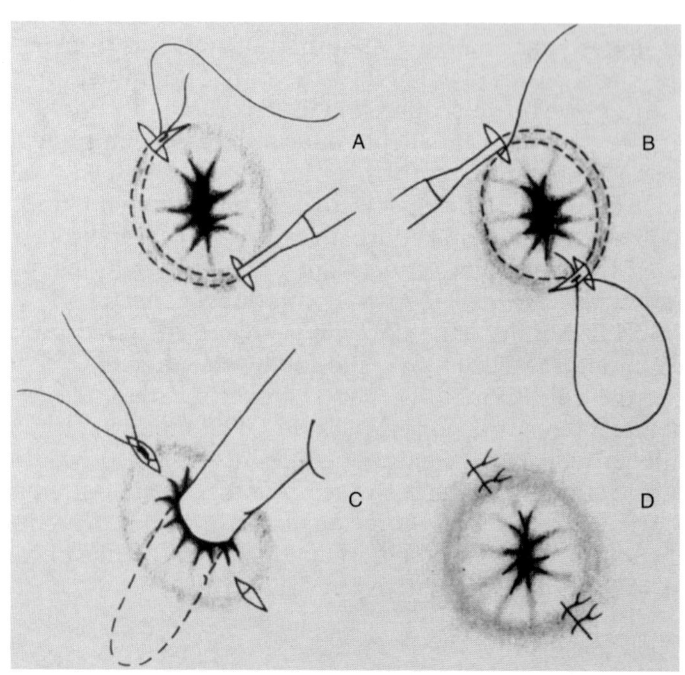

FIGURE 15 ■ Thiersch operation.

Advantages and Disadvantages

Virtues of the Thiersch procedure are that it causes little operative trauma and can be performed easily with the patient under local anesthesia. Also, if the result is not satisfactory, the wire can be withdrawn easily and reintroduced on two or three successive occasions, as is often necessary. The disadvantages of this procedure are that it is palliative and does not cure the prolapse but only prevents the lead point from coming out of the anus, it does not restore continence, and it carries a high degree of recurrence. In a review Fengler and Pearl (115) found procedure-related mortality nonexistent, but recurrence rates range from 0% to 39%, fecal impaction rates from 0% to 22%, infection rates from 6% to 33%, erosion and breakage rates from 7% to 33%, and reoperation rates from 7% to 59%. Mucosal prolapse, rectovaginal fistulas secondary to erosion of the wire and perineal clostridial myonecrosis also have been reported.

Many variations of this technique have been described, with a host of different materials used (i.e., suture material or sheets of mesh, cords or sheets of elastic material), but all have in common the various complications described. Yet sporadic reports still praise the procedure. Earnshaw and Hopkinson (116) reported a 76% success rate using the silicone rubber perianal suture. Labow et al. (117) enthusiastically reported the use of a Dacron-reinforced Silastic sling. Sainio et al. (118) described high anal encirclement with polypropylene mesh in 17 patients. There was a 15% recurrence and 27% improvement in anal incontinence.

SUBSEQUENT MANAGEMENT

POSTOPERATIVE MANAGEMENT

Regardless of which operative procedure is used, the patient must understand that the bowels must move on a regular basis without any straining.

Basse et al. (119) described the results of a multimodal rehabilitation program after abdominal rectopexy. There were 31 consecutive patients with rectal prolapse, median age 69 years, who were scheduled for abdominal rectopexy with the multimodal rehabilitation program including 48 hours of thoracic epidural analgesia or patient-controlled anesthesia, early oral nutrition and mobilization. All patients except one tolerated a normal diet and were mobilized to the same level as before operation on the first postoperative day. Bowel movements were reestablished at a median of day 2 and the median postoperative hospital stay was three days. At two months follow-up, 16% were incontinent versus 74% before operation. Constipation was noted in 43% before operation versus 28% at 2 months follow-up.

RESIDUAL INCONTINENCE AND CONSTIPATION

Perhaps the greatest weakness of the present-day operative treatment for rectal prolapse is its limited capacity to restore normal anorectal function in all patients, despite the excellent anatomic results. The published incidence of residual incontinence varies dramatically from 26% to 81%, but most series report it as 40% to 60% for abdominal repairs and as high as 80% to 90% for perineal repairs (24).

Because of the difficult, if not impossible, task of attempting to classify degrees of incontinence and because individual interpretations are subjective rather than objective, reports of different authors cannot be compared precisely. Morgan et al. (47) defined incontinence as the uncontrolled leak of solid or loose stools and found 80.6% of patients incontinent preoperatively. Almost all of their patients had a variable degree of urgency at defecation, and some restrained the act only with difficulty. In their series 38.8% were incontinent postoperatively; further operative procedures for incontinence were performed in 7.5%.

The exact relationship of prolapse to incontinence is uncertain, for, indeed, some patients with prolapse are not incontinent. Whether the prolonged prolapse of the rectum with mechanical stretching of the sphincter induces the incontinence or whether both are manifestations of the same neuromuscular deficiencies remains open to debate. Parks et al. (4) noted that the pudendal and perineal nerves undergo changes secondary to stretch injuries, with resulting abnormalities of the small nerves supplying the anorectal musculature. Electromyographic studies from the same laboratory showed reduced amplitude of action potentials in the external sphincter and puborectalis muscles in patients with fecal incontinence but not in those with rectal prolapse without incontinence (5).

Yoshioka et al. (120) studied a series of 12 patients who underwent rectopexy, nine of whom were incontinent preoperatively. Preoperative anal pressures were lower and anorectal angles were more obtuse in patients than in controls. These parameters did not change significantly after operation. Parameters that predicted return of continence included delayed leakage during the saline infusion test, a narrow anorectal angle during pelvic floor contraction, minimal pelvic floor descent during contraction, and a long anal canal at rest and during pelvic floor contraction.

Since the return of continence may take as long as 6 to 12 months, demands for further operative treatment for incontinence should be resisted until a year has passed. Improvement in continence may be due to various factors. Patients learn to adjust their aperient regimen better after the operation. The most useful laxative is a bulk-forming agent. An important factor is the absence of continuing dilatation of the anal canal by a large, complete prolapse. To investigate the physiology of improvement in continence following the Ripstein operation, Holmstrom et al. (121) performed preoperative and postoperative anorectal manometry and found the mean maximal anal resting pressure to be increased. This increase probably reflects improved function of the internal anal sphincter, which might contribute to better continence by increasing the closing capacity of the anal canal. In patients with long-standing rectal prolapse and a gaping anal canal, the internal anal sphincter may be so defective that recovery after operation could not be expected. Producing substantial rectal distention may cause constant relaxation of the internal sphincter. Thus a prolapse might inhibit the internal sphincter functionally before it causes mechanical dilatation, and this mechanism could explain how incontinence may develop in patients with internal procidentia. To elucidate the mechanism by which rectopexy restores continence in patients with rectal prolapse, the role of sphincter recovery, rectal morphological changes and improved rectal sensation, Duthie and Bartolo (122) assessed 68 patients undergoing resection rectopexy, anterior and posterior Marlex rectopexy, posterior Ivalon rectopexy, or suture rectopexy. Preoperative and postoperative manometry, radiographic studies, and electrosensitivity measurements were made. Age and duration of follow-up were similar in all groups, and the prolapse was controlled in all patients. Significantly improved continence was seen in all but the Ivalon group. There was no evidence of increasing postoperative constipation. Sphincter length and voluntary contraction were unaltered, but improved resting tone was seen in the resection and suture groups. This was not seen in the prosthetic groups. Improved continence correlated with recovery of resting pressure. Upper anal sensation was improved in all groups. Radiographic changes did not correlate with improved continence. The authors concluded that continence is improved by all rectopexy procedures but seems better without prosthetic material. Sphincter recovery seems to be the most important factor.

Morgan et al. (47) published the results of 150 patients who were operated with the Ivalon sponge method. A number of patients were investigated pre- and postoperatively by means of cineradiography during defecation. Postoperative studies showed good fixation of the rectum in the sacral hollow and improvement in the position of the levator muscular shelf on which the distal portion of the rectum lay. Pre- and postoperative electromyographic studies of the pelvic floor also were performed in some patients. In all these patients there was a gross disturbance of the normal postural pelvic floor reflexes preoperatively, and only two of the patients who were followed postoperatively (both were young) showed any significant recovery in the pelvic muscle function. This indicates that whatever the cause of the prolapse (they believe it is due to a large extent to abnormal habits of defecation), these etiologic factors produce muscle failure in the pelvic floor before prolapse occurs, and this defect is not cured by fixing the rectum in the sacral hollow. These observations are in keeping with those of Parks et al. (11) on the "descending perineum" syndrome. They also contribute toward explaining why correction of the rectal prolapse alone does not entirely solve the functional problems of continence and abnormal bowel habits.

With an increase in the sophistication of the technology available to study anorectal physiology, efforts have been made to determine the reason for improvement in anal continence following a successful anatomic repair of rectal procidentia. In a manometric study of 28 patients undergoing abdominal rectopexy and sigmoid resection, Sainio et al. (123) suggested that recovery of the resting and voluntary contraction functions of the sphincter muscle was the cause of continence improvement after operation. But in a study using manometry, proctometrography, electrosensitivity, and proctography, Duthie and Bartolo (124) concluded that improved continence is not primarily an effect of improved sphincter function or related to constipation. Their study supported the finding of improved sensation as being implicated in the improved continence. Using an ambulatory computerized anal electromyographic and anorectal manometry system, authors from the same center found that median resting anal pressures were 34 cm H_2O in patients with prolapse, 51 cm H_2O in those with neurogenic fecal incontinence, and 94 cm H_2O in controls (125). High pressure rectal waves of median amplitude, 71 cm H_2O lasting 20 to 150 seconds and associated with inhibition of the electromyographic activity of the internal anal sphincter and a fall in anal pressures, were seen in all patients with prolapse but not in controls or those with neurogenic incontinence. These waves were abolished following successful resection and rectopexy. These authors believe recovery of continence occurs by abolition of high-pressure rectal waves, which produce maximal inhibition of sphincter activity before operation. Schultz et al. (126) found that the Ripstein operation often improved anal continence in patients with rectal prolapse and rectal intussusception. This improvement was accomplished by an increased maximal resting pressure in patients with rectal prolapse, indicating recovery of internal anal sphincter function, but no such increase was found in patients with rectal intussusception. This suggests an alternate mechanism of improvement in patients with rectal intussusception. Hiltunen and Matikainen (127) studied 27 patients who underwent a posterior rectopexy. Manometric studies pre- and postoperatively indicated that improved continence was possibly due to improved function in the internal anal sphincter.

Madden et al. (128) also found abdominal rectopexy improves incontinence but worsens constipation. Sayfan et al. (62) compared patients who had a Marlex mesh posterior rectopexy to those who underwent a sigmoidectomy combined with a sutured posterior rectopexy. Restoration of continence occurred in 9 out of 12 incontinent patients after Marlex rectopexy compared with six of nine after sutured rectopexy and sigmoidectomy. Constipation persisted in three patients who were constipated before operation and in 4 of 13 who had previously normal bowel habits but became constipated after Marlex rectopexy. Constipation persisted in one of five previously constipated patients while none of those with previously normal bowel habits became constipated after sutured rectopexy and sigmoidectomy. Significantly fewer patients were constipated after sigmoidectomy than after rectopexy alone.

In the most recent review of the literature, Madiba et al. (46) reported that it would appear that preservation of the lateral ligaments is associated with an improvement in continence and a reduction of constipation. Brown et al. (129) examined the effect of rectal prolapse operation on colonic motility. Patients with rectal prolapse have abnormal colonic motility associated with reduced high-amplitude propagated contraction activity. Rectopexy reduces colonic pressure but fails to restore high-amplitude propagated contractions, reduce constipation or improve colonic transit. These observations help explain the pathophysiology of constipation associated with rectal prolapse.

For patients with residual incontinence after a successful anatomic repair, Parks (130) has described a postanal repair. The technique and results of this operation are described in Chapter 15.

COMPLICATIONS

INCARCERATION, STRANGULATION, AND GANGRENE

Very rarely, a rectal prolapse may become incarcerated (Fig. 16). Reduction can almost always be carried out by

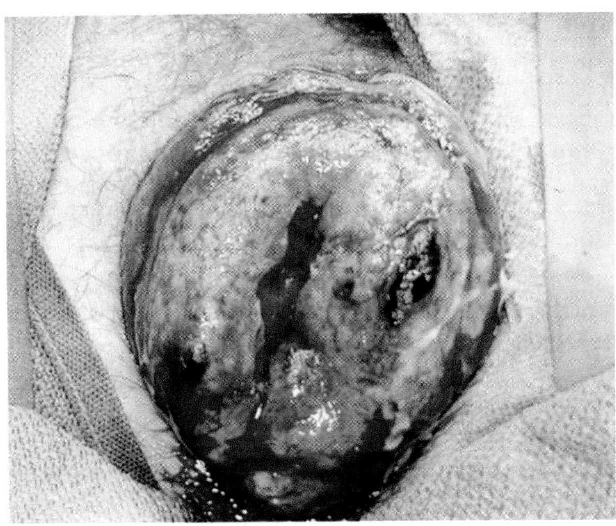

FIGURE 16 ■ A strangulated rectal prolapse.

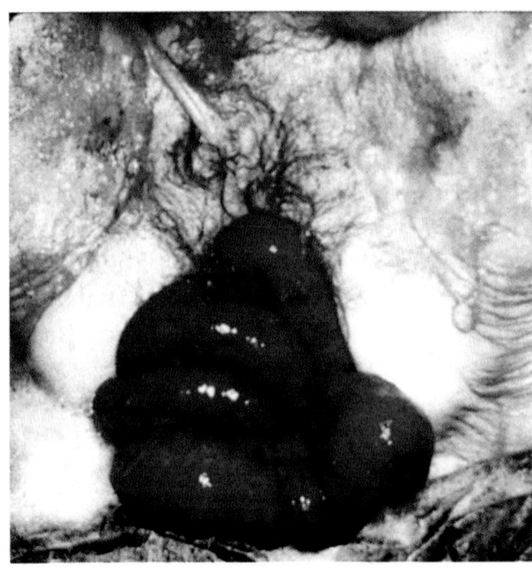

FIGURE 17 ■ A ruptured prolapse.

creating a block with a local anesthetic. In reducing the prolapse, it should be remembered that the last part out should be the first part in. It has also been suggested that sprinkling sugar on the mucosal surface helps reduce edema and thus aids in the reduction (131). Application of ice packs and injection of a mixture of dilute epinephrine and hyaluronidase to reduce edema have also been tried. In circumstances in which the incarceraction is irreducible, and there is doubt about the viability of the bowel, an emergency perineal rectosigmoidectomy should be the treatment of choice. Ramanujam and Venkatesh (132) reported on eight patients with acute incarcerated rectal prolapse, four showing signs of strangulation and areas of gangrene. All underwent emergency perineal rectosigmoidectomy. There were two leaks that required colostomy that was closed at a later date. There were no deaths.

■ ULCERATION AND HEMORRHAGE

Minor ulceration of the exposed mucosa may cause minimal bleeding, but more extensive ulcerations on very rare occasions may cause a severe hemorrhage.

■ RUPTURE OF PROLAPSE

This exceedingly rare complication may occur during straining at defecation with resulting evisceration of small intenstine through the anterior rectal wall (Fig. 17). Until 1994, 57 cases had been reported (133). A case was reported in which a mistaken diagnosis of massive thrombosed hemorrhoid was made and on incision, small intestine appeared (134). So little experience has been obtained with this situation that strong recommendations for treatment are difficult. The patient would clearly require an urgent operation and is probably best handled through an abdominal approach. The tear in the rectal wall is either sutured or partially resected. If the small bowel is viable it can be safely replaced into the periotoneal cavity. Use of a prospthetic material for definitive repair of the prolapse would seem unwise because of the risk of infection. Obliteration of cul-de-sac and simple fixation of the lateral stalks to the presacral fascia may be the simplest procedure in an emergency setting. A colostomy may be advisable if there is doubt about the integrity of the suture line. The mortality rate in 11 cases in the literature was 18% (134).

■ RECURRENT RECTAL PROLAPSE

Hool et al. (135) conducted a study to examine the possible causes of recurrent rectal prolapse, to learn operations performed most frequently, and to examine the outcome following recurrence surgery. The patient population included 24 patients on whom 29 operations were performed. The median duration to recurrence was two years. Recurrent rectal prolapse occurred after 15 abdominal and 9 perineal operations. Treatment included 25 abdominal and 4 perineal operations. Causes for recurrence were identified in 41% of cases and was most often attributable to problems with the mesh following the Ripstein procedure. Preoperative incontinence and constipation were largely unchanged by the operation for recurrent prolapse. They concluded that elimination of prolapse can be obtained but bowel dysfunction still remains in 60% of patients.

Fengler et al. (136) summarized their experience with recurrent rectal prolapse in 14 patients. The average time from initial operation to recurrence was 14 months. Initial operations were perineal proctectomy and levatorplasty (10), anal encirclement (2), Delorme's procedure (1), and anterior resection (1). Operative procedures performed for recurrence were perineal proctectomy and levatorplasty (7), sacral rectopexy [abdominal approach (3)], anterior resection with rectopexy (2), Delorme's procedure (1), and anal encirclement (1). Average length of follow-up was 50 months. No further episodes of complete rectal prolapse were observed during this period. Preoperatively, three patients were noted to be incontinent to the extent that necessitated the use perineal pads. The reoperative procedures failed to restore fecal continence in any of these three individuals. One patient died in the postoperative period after anal encirclement from an unrelated cause. The operative management of recurrent rectal prolapse can be expected to alleviate the prolapse, but not necessarily fecal incontinence.

Pikarsky et al. (137) conducted a study to assess the clinical and functional outcome of operation for recurrent rectal prolapse and compare it with the outcome of patients who underwent primary operation for rectal prolapse. The 27 patients with recurrent prolapse were compared with 27 patients with primary rectal prolapse. In the recurrent rectal prolapse group prior operation included rectopexy in seven patients, Delorme procedure in seven patients, perineal rectosigmoidectomy in seven patients, anal encirclement procedure in four patients and resection rectopexy in two patients. Operations performed for recurrence were perineal rectosigmoidectomy in 14 patients, resection rectopexy in 8 patients, rectopexy in 2 patients, pelvic floor repair in 2 patients and Delorme's procedure in 1 patient. There were no statistically significant differences between the groups in preoperative incontinence score in mortality, in mean hospital stay, in anastomotic complications, in wound infection, and in postoperative incontinence or recurrence rate between the two groups at a mean follow-up of 23.9 and 22 months, respectively. The overall success rate for recurrent rectal prolapse was 85.2%. They concluded the outcome of operation for rectal prolapse is similar in cases of primary or recurrent prolapse and furthermore the same surgical operations are valid in both scenarios.

In the selection of operations for recurrent rectal procidentia, the surgeon must be cautious not to perform an Altemeier procedure following a previous sigmoid resection unless the anastomosis is integrated in the resection and similarly should not perform a sigmoid resection following an Altemeier procedure because of the risk of creating a devascularized segment of bowel. Perineal proctectomies can be safely repeated (136). Non-resectional procedures such as Delorme's procedure should be considered in the management of recurrent rectal prolapse if a resectional procedure was performed initially and failed (136).

PROLAPSE IN CHILDREN

In children, the incidence of prolapse is highest in the first 2 years of life and declines thereafter (10). Boys are affected slightly more frequently than girls. The condition is usually the mucosal type. A predisposing factor generally believed to be important in the development of the prolapse is the absence of the sacral curve, causing the patient's rectum and anal canal in the sitting or standing position to form an almost vertical straight tube. Prolapse may be associated with any illness that leads to excessive straining at stool such as diarrhea, over-purgation, constipation, frequent coughing, or malnutrition. Mucoviscidosis also may be associated with rectal prolapse.

The parent may complain that when the child defecates, the rectum projects from the anus. This projection may be associated with a slight discharge of mucus or blood. Examination may reveal that the ring of prolapsing mucosa projects 2 to 4 cm beyond the anal orifice. Palpation of the prolapsing tissue reveals that only two layers of mucosa are present. Rarely, complete rectal procidentia may occur. Sphincteric tone may be lax.

The differential diagnosis includes a prolapsed rectal polyp or the apex of an intussusception protruding through the anus. In children, prolapsing rectal mucosa is a self-limiting disease. Consequently, treatment should be directed at correcting constipation and instituting proper habits of defecation. Malnutrition, if present, should be addressed. Strapping the buttocks has been advocated, but this probably only buys time until the self-limiting disease resolves. In patients who do not respond to the above forms of therapy, submucosal injection of a sclerosing agent, such as phenol in almond oil, has proved effective (10). For treating a complete rectal prolapse, perirectal injections of sclerosing agents to stimulate periproctitis and to fix the rectum to the sacrum have been advocated. In a review of the literature, Corman (138) found a host of other treatments, including excision of a mucosal prolapse, presacral packing with gauze or Gelfoam, linear cauterization of the anorectum, transsacral rectopexy, transcoccygeal rectopexy, puborectalis plication, perineal proctosigmoidectomy, and transanal rectopexy. Actual surgical resection for prolapse in children is a very rare necessity, but Goligher (10) has had to perform emergency rectosigmoidectomies for large irreducible prolapses in children. For a long-standing prolapse, rectopexy can be performed as it is done in the adult, but rarely is this indicated.

HIDDEN PROLAPSE (INTERNAL PROCIDENTIA)

"Hidden" prolapse refers to the earliest stage of procidentia, when the intussuscepting rectum occupies the rectal ampulla but has not yet continued through the anal canal. The most common complaint is difficulty in emptying the bowel, often described as a sensation of incomplete evacuation or obstruction. The second most common symptom is incontinence (33%). Other symptoms include bloody mucus (51%), perineal pain (16%), and soiling (24%) (139). Digital rectal examination reveals anterior rectal wall prolapse in 84%. Sigmoidoscopic findings include a solitary ulcer (49%) or hyperemia and edema of the mucosa of the anterior rectal wall for a distance of 8 to 10 cm from the anus. Bulging edematous mucosa may be seen. Colitis cystica profunda may be found, and hidden prolapse, a solitary rectal ulcer, and colitis cystica profunda may represent a spectrum of one syndrome (140). Defecography is probably the most useful diagnostic procedure for identifying internal intussusception. Abnormalities may include small residual folds occurring 3 to 7 cm from the anal canal located mainly in the posterior wall, anterior rectal wall prolapse, and circular prolapse creating a funnel-like configuration as seen in complete rectal prolapse (139). van Tets and Kuijpers (139) reported on 37 patients with internal intussusception who underwent rectopexy. The solitary rectal ulcer syndrome was present in 18 and anterior rectal prolapse in 31 patients. All ulcers healed and 26 patients became asymptomatic during a follow-up of from 1 to 9 years.

Fleshman et al. (141) reported on 25 patients with an internal intussusception treated with a Ripstein procedure. Complete resolution of symptoms was achieved in only 20% of patients. Partial improvement of constipation and straining and pain was noted in 32%; but 48% of patients noted no improvement or actual worsening of their symptoms. They therefore recommend conservative management in all but the most severely symptomatic patients.

McCue and Thomson (142) reported on Ivalon rectopexy performed on 12 patients with internal intussusception, of whom 10 had symptoms of obstructive defecation and only three of them were completely continent. Although there were no recurrences over a mean follow-up period of 27 months, functional results were mixed. Only one patient remained incontinent for solid stool, but discomfort and defecatory difficulties persisted. The authors also recommend rectopexy for patients with associated incontinence, significant rectal bleeding, or a solitary rectal ulcer but not for those with obstructed defecation. On the other hand, Berman et al. (143) reported on the performance of the Delorme procedure on 21 patients who also had symptoms of obstructed defecation. They found that 15 had sustained relief from all or most of their preoperative symptoms. No recurrent intussusception developed. Therefore the Delorme procedure may be the indicated operation for patients with an internal intussusception and symptoms of obstructed defecation. Christiansen et al. (144) reported on 24 patients who underwent a Wells rectopexy or Orr's operation. After a follow-up of one to eight years, defecography demonstrated disappearance of the intussusception in 22 patients, but none were completely relieved of their symptoms. The authors therefore counsel a conservative attitude toward operation.

Briel et al. (145) conducted a study to evaluate the clinical outcome of suture rectopexy in a consecutive series of patients with incomplete rectal prolapse associated with fecal incontinence and to compare these results with those obtained from patients with complete rectal prolapse. After a median follow-up of 67 months, continence was restored in 5 of 13 (38%) patients with incomplete rectal prolapse and in 16 of 24 (67%) patients with complete rectal prolapse. In both groups, all male patients became continent. For the majority of incontinent patients with incomplete rectal prolapse, a suture rectopexy is not beneficial. The clinical outcome of this procedure is only good in incontinent patients with complete rectal prolapse. Based on these data it is questionable whether incomplete rectal prolapse plays a causative role in fecal incontinence.

Brown et al. (146) compared the results of operation for "occult" and overt rectal prolapse. Resection rectopexy was the treatment of choice except in patients with fecal incontinence who underwent sutured rectopexy. Those patients who were unfit for an abdominal operation were offered a perineal procedure. Rectal prolapse surgery was undertaken in 69 patients with an overt prolapse and 74 patients with an "occult" prolapse. Patients in the "occult" prolapse group were significantly younger than those with overt prolapse. There were significantly more perineal procedures in the overt prolapse group compared with the "occult" prolapse group (54% vs. 5%). There were no deaths within 28 days of operation. Major surgical complications occurred in 3.5% of patients while 10% of patients experienced recurrent prolapse. Rectal prolapse operation reduced the incidence of St. Mark's grade 4 fecal incontinence from 38% to 19% in the overt prolapse group and from 49% to 29% in the "occult" prolapse group. Following operation, the incidence of constipation increased in the "occult" group from 39% to 50% but decreased in the overt prolapse group from 42% to 35%. They concluded operation for an "occult" rectal prolapse is unlikely to benefit patients whose principle symptom is constipation. Approximately half of those patients whose "occult" rectal prolapse is associated with fecal incontinence will have their bowel habit improved by prolapse operation.

SUMMARY

Bachoo et al. (147) tried to determine the best choice of operation for rectal procidentia. The following specific issues were addressed.

1. Whether surgical intervention is better than no treatment.
2. Whether an abdominal approach to surgery is better than a perineal approach.
3. Whether one method for performing rectopexy is better than another.
4. Whether laparoscopic access is better than open access for operation.
5. Whether resection should be included in the procedure.

All randomized or quasi-randomized trials of operation in the management of rectal prolapse were sought. Two reviewers independently selected studies from the literature. The three primary outcome measures were number of patients with recurrent rectal prolapse, or residual mucosal prolapse or fecal incontinence. Eight trials were included with a total of 264 participants. There were no detectable differences in recurrent prolapses between abdominal and perineal approaches, although there was a suggestion that fecal incontinence was less common after abdominal procedures. There were no detectable differences between the methods used for fixation during rectopexy. Division rather than preservation of the lateral ligaments was associated with less recurrent prolapse but more postoperative constipation although these findings were found in small numbers. There were too few data with which to compare laparoscopic with open operation. Bowel resection during rectopexy was associated with lower rates of constipation but again numbers were small. The small number of relevant trials identified and their small sample sizes together with other methodological weaknesses severely limit the usefulness of this review for guiding practice.

This chapter presents the current information about the more popularly used techniques in the repair of complete rectal procidentia. Each procedure has advantages and disadvantages. The particular method of repair used by a surgeon depends on his previous training and exposure to a certain technique, which is modified by his own personal experience. By and large, the major consideration is the patient's general state of health. At present, for the good-risk patient an abdominal approach is still favored. The recommended procedure would be a pelvic fixation in which the rectum is not completely surrounded anteriorly by a synthetic material. However, a resection might be recommended instead of one of the fixation procedures for an individual who has symptomatic diverticular disease or suffers from severe constipation in association with a very redundant colon. Certainly one would hesitate to insert a foreign body in the pelvis in association with a resection.

For poor-risk patients a perineal approach would be more appropriate, and the Delorme operation or possibly a perineal rectosigmoidectomy is recommended. For intermediate-risk patients a perineal rectosigmoidectomy should be considered. For patients confined to a nursing home, amputation of a massive prolapse definitely would facilitate their care.

Brown et al. (148) described their selective policy based on clinical criteria. Patients were offered operation according the following broad clinical protocol. Those who were unfit for abdominal surgery, were treated with a perineal operation. The remainder had a suture abdominal rectopexy. A sigmoid resection was added for patients in whom incontinence was not a predominant symptom. Operation was performed in 159 patients. Of these, 57 had a perineal operation, 65 had fixation rectopexy, and 37 had resection rectopexy. There were no in-hospital deaths, and major complications occurred in 3.5% of patients. Minimum follow-up was 3 years. Of the 143 patients with long-term follow-up, recurrence occurred in 5%. Constipation increased from 41% to 43% and incontinence decreased from 43% to 19%. They concluded that a selective policy has improved outcome when compared with reports of a single operation.

SOLITARY ULCER SYNDROME OF THE RECTUM

The "solitary ulcer syndrome of the rectum" is a term coined by Madigan (149) in 1964 and elaborated by Madigan and Morson (150) in 1969 to describe unusual rectal ulcerations. The term is not entirely satisfactory since in certain cases there is no ulceration and in other cases there are multiple ulcers. Rutter (151) suggested that the term be discarded and the name "mucosal prolapse syndrome" be adopted, but Martin et al. (152) did not concur, because in most patients with occult rectal prolapse, the rectal mucosa is macroscopically normal. The estimated incidence is 1 to 3.6/100,000/yr (152,153). Curiously, the entity is rarely reported from North American institutions. Its major importance is the fact that it may be confused with carcinoma, leading to an unnecessary radical operation. An extensive review of the subject was made by Rutter (151) and updated by Rutter and Riddell (154). A further review was conducted by Haray et al. (153). The following information was drawn heavily from their comprehensive work.

AGE AND SEX

There is a preponderance of females among patients with solitary ulcer syndrome of the rectum with an estimated preponderance of 3.2:1 (155). The condition has most commonly been reported to occur between 20 and 29 years of age (151,152,156), but a more recent report has cited over 60% of the patients aged over 50 years (153).

SYMPTOMS

The most common symptom is rectal bleeding, which is usually bright red and scant. Rarely, massive hemorrhage requiring transfusion is encountered (150,152). Mucus may be passed with resultant soiling, and a complete rectal prolapse may occur. Pain, if present, is located in the perineum, rectum, anus, the suprapubic, lumbar, or sacral area, or the left iliac fossa. This pain is usually trivial, although it may be continuous or intermittent. Other symptoms include tenesmus and a feeling of anal obstruction, which is manifested by straining and repeated visits to the lavatory. The necessity for straining is almost universal. Martin et al. (152) reported that more than 50% of their patients had partial incontinence to mucus, flatus, and occasionally liquid motions. Prolapse has been reported in a quarter of the cases (153).

Physical Examination

An area of induration can be felt in patients with solitary ulcer syndrome of the rectum, and the ulcers can be visualized on the anterior rectal wall. Solitary rectal ulcers occur most commonly 4 to 12 cm from the anal verge. Characteristically, the ulcer straddles or lies on the side of the rectal fold, and 68% of the lesions occur anteriorly or anterolaterally (81). The diameter of the shallow, well-demarcated ulcers varies in size from 1 to 5 cm, and the base of the ulcers is covered with a grayish-white slough. The ulcers may be round, oval, or linear but are usually irregular with raised, rolled, or polypoid edges. Occasionally, multiple ulcers may be present, or ulceration may be entirely absent (152). The surrounding mucosa is mildly inflamed and may appear nodular as a result of the presence of misplaced mucous membrane in the submucosa at the edge of the ulcer. A complete or incomplete rectal prolapse may be demonstrated during straining. Up to 90% of the patients may have evidence of prolapse if asked to strain (157). An ulcer may be detected on the apex of the complete rectal prolapse. Rectal narrowing may occur, but symptomatic rectal stenosis is rare.

Diagnosis

A delay in diagnosis has ranged from three months to 30 years (155). The diagnosis is usually made through sigmoidoscopy and is confirmed by a rectal biopsy. Blood tests make no contribution. Findings from barium enema studies include rectal stricture, granularity of the mucosa, and thickened rectal folds—all nonspecific (158). The diagnosis rests with the pathologist. The differential diagnosis includes Crohn's disease, ulcerative colitis, villous adenoma, rectal carcinoma, prolapsed hemorrhoids, nonspecific proctitis, ischemic proctitis, and pseudomembranous colitis (151).

Imaging and physiological testing have been utilized but it is doubtful whether they are necessary in majority of the cases as the diagnosis is confirmed by biopsy. Examination of the more proximal colon serves to rule out a coexisting disease state.

Defecography is the investigation of choice and may demonstrate the underlying disorder as either defecation with failure of relaxation of the pelvic floor musculature during straining or an intussusception (159). In a study by Kuijpers et al. (160), 12 of 19 patients with solitary rectal ulcer syndrome had an internal intussusception, and 5 of 19 patients had spastic pelvic floor syndrome. Of 43 patients with biopsy-proven solitary ulcer syndrome of the rectum, Mahieu (161) reported changes in the rectum in all 33 patients who underwent a barium enema study. Thickening of the rectal folds and spasm were the most common changes, followed by ulceration and pseudo-polypoid change. None of these changes is pathognomonic of the solitary ulcer syndrome. During defecography, intussusception of the rectum was observed in 79% of cases—44% with complete rectal procidentia and 35% with internal procidentia.

To determine the proctographic abnormalities and the frequency of rectal prolapse and incomplete or delayed emptying in patients with solitary rectal ulcer syndrome, Halligan et al. (162) reviewed proctographic examinations of 53 patients with histologically proved solitary rectal ulcer syndrome. Comparison was made with a control group of 20 subjects who had no anorectal symptoms. Fourteen patients (26%) had rectal irregularity at rest compared with none in the control group. Rectal prolapse developed on evacuation in 36 patients (68%) with solitary rectal ulcer syndrome: internal prolapse in 24 patients (45%), and external prolapse in 12 (23%). Descent of the pelvic floor on evacuation was greater in the group with solitary rectal ulcer syndrome than in the control group. Thickened rectal folds were seen in 11 of 20 patients (55%) with solitary rectal ulcer syndrome examined with posteroanterior proctography. Evacuation was prolonged and incomplete in patients with solitary rectal ulcer syndrome compared with control subjects. Overall, evacuation proctography disclosed delayed or incomplete emptying and/or rectal prolapse in 40 patients (75%) with solitary rectal ulcer syndrome, compared with two control subjects who showed low-grade internal rectal prolapse only.

Electromyographic abnormalities have been found in patients with solitary ulcer syndrome. The normal response to bearing down is relaxation of the external sphincter and the puborectalis muscle, but Rutter and Riddell (154) found that the puborectalis muscle went into a state of marked activity, with an increase in both the frequency and the amplitude potentials. This response persisted as long as the bearing-down effort was maintained, suggesting that during bearing-down efforts, the puborectalis muscle behaves paradoxically. Instead of undergoing inhibitory lengthening to produce the necessary funnel-shaped anorectum, it goes into a state of tight contraction, tending to maintain the integrity of the flap valve. Thus defecation can occur only after forcible stretching of the puborectalis muscle. The abnormal pelvic floor relaxation has been confirmed by other investigators (152,156,163–165). Jones et al. (164) recorded paradoxic puborectalis muscle contraction in 50% of the patients with the solitary rectal ulcer syndrome. In the series reported by Keighley and Shouler (156), only four of 16 patients exhibited this functional abnormality.

Manometric findings reported by Keighley and Shouler (156) include no differences in resting and squeeze pressures between patients with the solitary ulcer syndrome of the rectum and normal controls. The maximal tolerated volume was decreased in patients with the solitary rectal ulcer syndrome. Some patients exhibited a hyperactive external sphincter. Kang et al. (166) studied the physiologic features of patients with complete rectal prolapse and different degrees of solitary ulcer syndrome. Solitary rectal ulcer patients without prolapse and with internal prolapse had significantly higher anal resting and squeeze pressures than patients with complete rectal prolapse. In contrast, solitary rectal ulcer patients having external prolapse were similar to those with complete rectal prolapse. Solitary rectal ulcer patients without rectal prolapse had significantly decreased anal rectal electrosensitivity when compared to those with healthy controls.

Endoscopic ultrasonography has enabled differentiation of solitary rectal ulcer syndrome from other conditions such as malignancy or Crohn's disease. The five-layer structure of the rectal wall may be completely preserved (167). However, Van Outryve et al. (168) examined 15 patients with endoscopically and biopsy-proved diagnoses of solitary rectal ulcer syndrome. In 13 of the 15 patients, the rectal wall was thicker (mean, 5.7 mm; normal values, 2.8 mm) near the rectal ulcer. In all these cases the muscularis propria layer exceeded the maximum normal diameter of 2 mm. In nine of the 15 patients, the normal rectal wall echostructure with five distinct layers was disturbed and there was fading of the borders between the mucosa and the muscularis propria. Poor relaxation of the puborectalis muscle during straining was seen on ultrasonography in 11 patients, as was intussusception of the rectal wall. The direct visualization of the puborectalis muscle during dynamic transrectal ultrasonography suggests that the fact that it does not relax is an important element in the pathogenesis of solitary rectal ulcer syndrome. In an endosonographic study of 21 patients with solitary rectal ulcer syndrome, Halligan et al. (169) found the submucosa to be inhomogeneous with an increased thickness. The diameter and cross-sectional area of both the internal and external sphincter were increased. The ratio of the external to internal sphincter thickness was reduced.

■ HISTOLOGY

Biopsy reveals a characteristic appearance. There may be some superficial mucosal ulceration; the tubules show structural irregularity, and the epithelium is hyperplastic. The most significant changes are a curious obliteration of the lamina propria by fibrosis and growing by muscle fibers of the muscularis mucosae toward the lumen of the bowel (170) (Fig. 18). Levine et al. (171) have demonstrated a diffuse saffron staining that characteristically fills the full thickness of the lamina propria. This pattern of diffuse excess of mucosal collagen differentiates the solitary rectal ulcer syndrome from other inflammatory bowel diseases. The mucosa may become markedly villous with variable amounts of mucin depletion. Superficial ulceration accompanied by fibrinous and polymorphonuclear leukocytic exudate eventually produces the white floor so characteristic of the true solitary ulcer (151).

The solitary ulcer syndrome tends to give rise to misplaced submucosal glands, which are filled with mucus and lined by normal colonic epithelium. Rutter and Riddell (154) believe that the most common association of this localized form of colitis cystica profunda is with the solitary ulcer syndrome. This situation may lead to the incorrect diagnosis of carcinoma. Invasive carcinoma superimposed

A 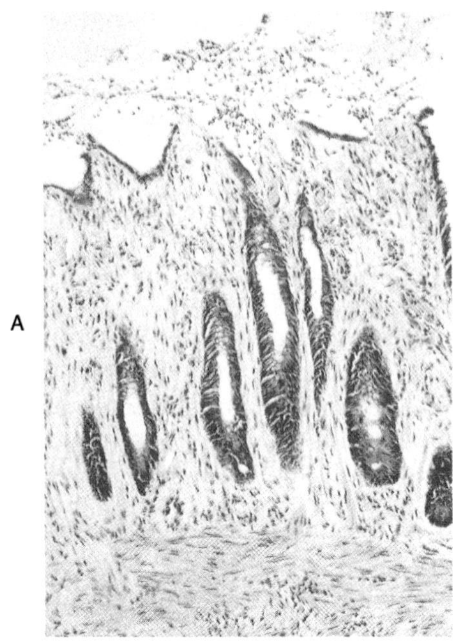

B 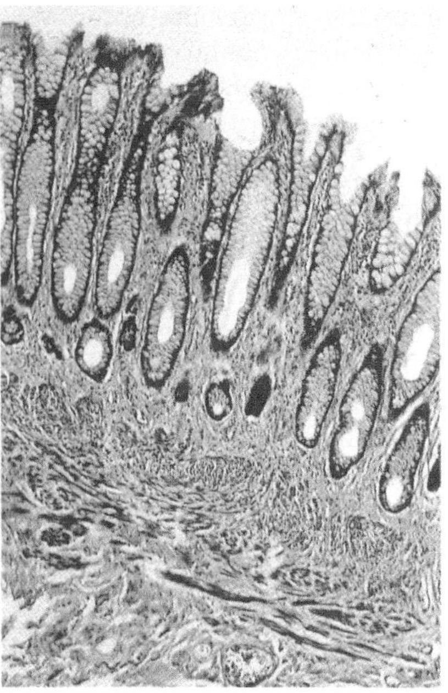

FIGURE 18 ■ (**A**) Sigmoidoscopic rectal biopsy showing microulcers at tip of mucosa, associated acute inflammatory exudate, fibromuscular obliteration of lamina propria, and marked thickening of muscularis mucosa. (**B**) Masson's trichrome stain of rectal mucosal biopsy from solitary rectal ulcer syndrome. Green color represents fibrosis, which is excessive. Fibrosis is seen splaying muscularis mucosa and obliterating lamina propria. *Source*: Courtesy of D.A. Malatjalian, M.D., Halifax, Nova Scotia.

upon a long-standing solitary rectal ulcer has been reported (172,173). Li and Hamilton (174) believe that the histopathology of solitary rectal ulcer syndrome may occasionally represent a nonspecific mucosal reactive change to a deeper seated malignancy.

Kang et al. (175) examined the rectal wall from solitary rectal ulcer syndrome specimens. Unique features included decussation of the two muscular layers, nodular induration of inner circular layer, and grouping of outer longitudinal layer into bundles. These features were not seen in complete rectal prolapse or control specimens and thus suggest a different pathogenesis from these two disorders.

■ ETIOLOGY AND PATHOGENESIS

The etiology of the solitary rectal ulcer syndrome has not been established. This condition is seen in a variety of clinical situations, for example: (i) at the apex of a complete rectal prolapse, (ii) on the anterior mucosal prolapse in patients with the perineal descent syndrome, (iii) at the apex of a prolapsing hemorrhoid, and (iv) occasionally at the tip of a colostomy or ileostomy.

The mechanism of the actual ulceration is postulated as the result of any one or any combination of the following:

1. Ischemia caused by pressure necrosis when the tip of the prolapse becomes impacted in the upper end of the anal canal
2. Trauma if the prolapse is replaced digitally (a proportion of solitary ulcer patients have a habit of passing a finger or instrument into the lower rectum as an aid to defecation, and this may be a contributory factor)
3. Ischemia caused by stretching and possible rupture of the submucosal vessels at the time of maximal prolapse
4. Ischemia caused by obliteration of the mucosal capillaries by the fibrous and muscular tissue filling the lamina propria

Other possible etiologic factors include inflammatory bowel disease, congenital duplication, hamartomatous malformations, and bacterial or viral infections.

The combination of prolonged straining efforts and failure to inhibit the puborectalis muscle results in traumatization of the adjacent anterior rectal mucosa by the posterior bar of the puborectalis muscle. The ulcers appear in the area of mucosa that bears the brunt of that straining effort, the "flap" of the physiologic flap valve. Furthermore, the flap may enter the upper end of the anal canal, where it may be squeezed by an actively contracting sphincter, which may render it relatively ischemic. The long-term result of straining efforts is either a mucosal prolapse of the anterior rectal mucosa or a full-thickness prolapse beginning in the middle rectum. In either case, rectal wall derived from a higher area enters the traumatizing mechanism. Womack et al. (157) found that rectal ulceration occurs when rectal prolapse and high voiding pressures are combined, exposing the prolapsing mucosa to a high transmural pressure gradient, which may lead to rupture of submucosal blood vessels with subsequent sloughing and ulceration of the mucosa. They postulate that the rarity of the solitary rectal ulcer may be explained by the fact that rectal procidentia usually is associated with low voiding pressures. The relative importance of straining, prolapse, trauma, and ischemia in the pathogenesis of the solitary ulcer syndrome of the rectum remains unknown.

■ TREATMENT

The outcome of not treating the solitary rectal ulcer is unpredictable. Spontaneous resolution has been reported in some, whereas other patients may have no change in symptomatology over a period of many years (151). Patients with few symptoms require no specific treatment, for explanation and reassurance may be adequate. If the difficulty is due to faulty bowel training, reeducation and attention to diet, in particular consumption of bran, may be helpful. If the concept of prolapse and eventual pressure necrosis is accepted, healing will not occur until the patient is able to cease straining. If an electromyogram shows the ulcer is caused by a break in the physiologic behavior of the pelvic floor, retraining will be useless. Straining may be reduced by adding bulk-forming agents to the diet and using glycerine suppositories. Molouf et al. (176) reported that the initial improvement in symptoms deteriorates in half the patients by three years. Sulfasalazine and local steroids have been used without obvious or consistent improvement (152,163). The used of 5-ASA enemas has been reported as successful in the treatment of solitary rectal ulcers (177). Complete healing occurs within a few weeks, and recurrent ulcers heal just as readily with renewed therapy. Topical administration of sucralfate, 2 g twice a day for six weeks, has been reported to result in relief of symptoms in four of six patients (178).

Binnie et al. (179) studied 31 patients with solitary rectal ulcer syndrome, 14 treated conservatively or with operation, and had a high recurrence rate. Seventeen patients treated with biofeedback for the associated obstructed defecation (anismus) either before or immediately following operation had a lower recurrence rate but the final symptomatic cure rate was similar in both groups.

For the treatment of distal mucosal prolapse, rubber band ligation has the highest chance of success (151). The technique is similar to that used for the treatment of hemorrhoids, the only difference being that ligation is placed on the areas of maximal prolapse rather than in the classic hemorrhoidal positions. Local excision of the ulcer through the anus usually fails to cure the problem, but some patients may benefit from it (151,152,163).

Argon plasma coagulation has been used to control the bleeding, diminish the pain, and promote healing in a case report (180).

If the ulceration is associated with a complete rectal procidentia, a definitive repair should be performed. Based on the belief in the frequent association of the solitary ulcer with rectal prolapse, the use of a modified Ripstein procedure has met with considerable success (181). Keighley and Shouler (156) stated that rectopexy is a valid method of treatment only if the patient has an established complete procidentia. Excellent results with the use of the Ivalon wrap procedure have also been reported (151,152). van Tets and Kuijpers (182) performed a rectopexy on 18 patients with internal intussusception and solitary rectal ulcer syndrome and, with follow-up of one to nine years, all lesions healed.

Sitzler et al. (183) studied the long-term outcome of operation for solitary rectal ulcer syndrome in 66 patients. Of these, 49 underwent rectopexy, nine Delorme's operation, two anterior resection, and four creation of a stoma as the initial operation. At a median follow-up of 90 months, the rectopexy had failed in 22 of 49 patients; 19 of these patients underwent further operation, including rectal resection with coloanal anastomosis (four with three failures), colostomy (11) and other procedures (4). Ultimately, 14 required a stoma. Constipation was the indication for a stoma in 9 of the 11 patients who had colostomy as the first procedure after failure of rectopexy. Nine patients had Delorme's operation as the first procedure. At median follow-up of 38 months there were 4 failures. Two of these ultimately required a stoma. Of the seven patients who underwent anterior resection as the initial or subsequent procedure, a stoma was finally necessary in four. Anterior resection used as a salvage procedure was not successful. The overall stoma rate was 30% (20 patients). Of 11 symptoms assessed before operation, only incontinence and incomplete evacuation were related to a poor outcome following operation. They concluded anti-prolapse operations result in a satisfactory long-term outcome in about 55% to 60% of the patients having operation for solitary ulcer syndrome. Results of anterior resection are disappointing.

For a patient with massive bleeding secondary to the solitary rectal ulcer, Frizelle et al. (184) performed a high rectosigmoid resection and rectopexy without removal of the ulcer. Although the ulcer did not heal completely, the bleeding was controlled and further treatment was not required.

Despite the controversy in management, it appears that for the symptomatic patient with a solitary rectal ulcer associated with a hidden or overt rectal procidentia, a definitive repair should be offered to the patient with the choices of procedures discussed. In symptomatic patients who have shown recalcitrance to other treatment, it has been recommended that a temporary diverting sigmoid colostomy be constructed, but this treatment would appear rather radical (185).

Marchal et al. (186) reviewed 13 patients operated on for solitary rectal ulcer syndrome. Seven patients had associated internal rectal prolapse (58%), two had associated total rectal prolapse (15%), and two had associated mucosal prolapse (15%). Operations performed included resection of the solitary rectal ulcer in one case (8%), a stoma as primary operation in one (8%), three rectopexies according to Orr-Loygue (23%), and eight Delorme's operation as modified by Bermen (62%). Mean follow-up was in 57 months. Simple resection of the solitary rectal ulcer did not improve symptoms. Colostomy permitted relief of symptoms and healing of the solitary rectal ulcer. Two of the three rectopexies achieved good results and the third patient relapsed at the sixth postoperative month. A secondary modified Delorme's operation permitted relief in symptoms and healing of the solitary rectal ulcer. Five of the eight patients (62.5%) who received modified Delorme's operation had improved at a follow-up of 46 months. They concluded that considering the high postoperative failure rate, operation should be performed only in patients with total rectal prolapse or intractable symptoms not amenable to behavioral therapy. Delorme's operation and abdominal proctopexy helped in about 60% of the cases.

■ CLINICAL REVIEWS

Tjandra et al. (155) conducted a retrospective study of 80 patients with biopsy-proved solitary rectal ulcer. The median follow-up was in 25 months. The female-to-male ratio was 1.4:1.0, and the mean age was 48.7 years (range, 14–76 years). Principal symptoms were bowel disturbances (74%) and rectal bleeding (56%). Twenty-one patients (26%) were asymptomatic and required no treatment. A previous "wrong" diagnosis was made in 25%. Rectal prolapse was identified in 28% (full-thickness, 15%; mucosal, 13%). The macroscopic appearance of the lesion seen in solitary rectal ulcer varied widely and included polypoid lesions in 44% (the predominant finding in the asymptomatic group), ulcerated lesions in 29% (always symptomatic), and edematous, nonulcerated, hyperemic mucosa in 27%. Anorectal manometry provided little helpful information in the patients in whom it was performed. Management by bulk laxatives and bowel retraining led to symptomatic improvement in 19% of cases. In 29% of the cases, symptoms persisted despite endoscopic healing of the lesion. Intractability of symptoms led to operation in only 27 patients (34%). Depending on the presence or absence of rectal prolapse, rectopexy or a conservative local procedure (such as local excision), respectively, appeared to be the optimal operative treatment. The polypoid variety tended to respond to therapy more favorably than nonpolypoid varieties. Thus the macroscopic appearance of the solitary rectal ulcer has a significant bearing on the clinical course, and most cases do not require operation. Halligan et al. (187) investigated the effect of rectopexy on rectal configuration or emptying, or both to identify any preoperative factor associated with a good outcome. Rectal prolapse, demonstrated in 19 of 23 patients before operation (internal in 12, external in seven), was seen in only one patient after operation. The rectal axis became more vertical at rest and on evacuation. Preoperative evacuation time was increased in patients with poor outcome. These features, however, are unrelated to outcome. Prolonged preoperative evacuation time, suggesting a defecatory disorder, may predict poor symptomatic outcome.

REFERENCES

1. Moschcowitz AV. The pathogenesis, anatomy and cure of pro-lapse of the rectum. Surg Gynecol Obstet 1912; 15:7–21.
2. Broden B, Snellman B. Procidentia of the rectum studied with cineradiography: a contribution to the discussion of causative mechanism. Dis Colon Rectum 1968; 11:330–347.
3. Spencer RJ. Manometric studies in rectal prolapse. Dis Colon Rectum 1984; 27:523–525.
4. Parks AG, Swash M, Urich H. Sphincter denervation in anorectal incontinence and rectal prolapse. Gut 1977; 18:656–665.
5. Neill NE, Parks AG, Swash M. Physiological studies of the analsphincter musculature in fecal incontinence and rectal prolapse. Br J Surg 1981; 68:531–536.
6. Sun WM, Read NW, Donnelly TC, Bannister JJ, Shorthouse AJ. A common pathophysiology for full thickness rectal prolapse, anterior mucosal prolapse and solitary rectal ulcer. Br J Surg 1989; 76:290–295.
7. Altemeier WA, Culbertson WR, Schowengerdt CJ, Hunt J. Nineteen years' experience with the one stage perineal repair of rectal prolapse. Ann Surg 1971; 173:993–1006.
8. Beahrs OH, Theuerkauf FJ, Hill JR. Procidentia: surgical treatment. Dis Colon Rectum 1972; 15:337–346.
9. Mann CV. Rectal prolapse. In: Morson BC, Heinemann W, eds. Diseases of the Colon, Rectum and Anus. London: Medical Books, 1969:238–250.
10. Goligher JC. Surgery of the Anus, Rectum and Colon. 4th ed. London: Baillière Tindall, 1980:224–258.
11. Parks AG, Porter NH, Hardcastle JD. The syndrome of the descending perineum. Proc R Soc Med 1966; 59:477–482.
12. Leighton JA, Valdovinos MA, Pemberton JH, Rath DM, Camilleri M. Anorectal dysfunction and rectal prolapse in progressive systemic sclerosis. Dis Colon Rectum 1993; 36:182–185.
13. Zbar AP, Takashima S, Hasegawa T, Kitabayashi K. Perinal rectosigmoidectomy (Altemeier's procedure): a review of physiology, technique and outcome. Tech Coloproctol 2002; 6:109–116.
14. Kupfer CA, Goligher JC. One hundred consecutive cases of complete prolapse of the rectum treated by operation. Br J Surg 1970; 57:481–487.
15. Boutsis C, Ellis H. The Ivalon-sponge-wrap operation for rectal prolapse: an experience with 26 patients. Dis Colon Rectum 1974; 17:21–37.
16. Rashid Z, Basson MD. Association of rectal prolapse with colorectal cancer surgery. 1996; 119:51–55.
17. Thompson JR, Chen AH, Pettit PD, Bridges MD. Incidence of occult rectal prolapse in patients with clinical rectoceles and defecatory dysfunction. Am J Obstet Gynecol 2002; 187:1494–1499.
18. Dvorkin LS, Knowles CH, Scott SM, Williams NS, Lunniss PJ. Rectal intussusception: characterization of symptomatology. Dis Colon Rectum 2005; 48:824–831.
19. Dvorkin LS, Chan CL, Knowles GH, Williams NS, Lunniss PJ, Scott SM. Anal sphincter morphology in patients with full-thickness rectal prolapase. Dis Colon Rectum 2004; 47:198–203.
20. Healy JC, Halligan S, Raznek RH, et al. Dynamic MR imaging compared with evacuation proctography when evaluating anorectal configuration and pelvic floor movement. Am J Roentgenol 1997; 169:775–779.
21. Healy JC, Halligan S, Raznek RH, Waston S, Phillips RK, Armstrong P. Patterns of prolapse in women with symptoms of pelvic floor weakness: assesment with MR imaging. Radiology 1997; 203:77–81.
22. Rentsch M, Paetzel C, Lenhart M, Feuerbach S, Jauch KW, Furst A. Dynamic magnetic resonance imaging defecography: a dianostic alternative in the assesment of pelvic floor disorders in proctology. Dis Colon Rectum 2001; 44:999–1007.
23. Dvorkin LS, Hetzer F, Scott SM, Williams NS, Gedroyc W, Lunniss PJ. Open-magnet MR defactography compared with evacuation proctography in the diagnosis and management of patients with rectal intussusception. Colorectal Dis 2004; 6:45–53.
24. Watts JD, Rothenberger DA, Buls JG, Goldberg SM, Nivatvongs S. The management of procidentia: 30 years experience. Dis Colon Rectum 1985; 28:96–102.
25. Mctcalf AM, Loening-Baucke V. Anorectal function and defecation dynamics in patients with rectal prolapse. Am J Surg 1988; 55:206–210.
26. Goldberg SM, Gordon PH. Operative treatment of complete prolapse of the rectum. Najarian JS, Delaney JP, eds. Surgery of the Gastrointestinal Tract. New York: Intercontinental Medical Book, 1974:423–439.
27. Ripstein CB, Lanter B. Etiology and surgical therapy of massive prolapse of the rectum. Ann Surg 1963; 157:259–264.
28. McMahan JD, Ripstein CB. Rectal prolapse: an update on the sling procedure. Am Surg 1987; 53:37–40.
29. Britten-Jones R. Todd IP, ed. Operative Surgery. London: Butterworth, 1977:226.
30. Britten-Jones R. Complete rectal prolapse: Anterior wrap (Ripstein operation) in operative surgery. In: Rob C, Smith R, eds. Colon, Rectum and Anus. London: Butterworth, 1983:415–420.
31. Ripstein CB. Definitive corrective surgery. Dis Colon Rectum 1972; 15:334–346.
32. Biehl AG, Pay JE, Gathright JB. Repair of rectal prolapse: experience with the Ripstein sling. South Med J 1978; 71:923–925.
33. Gordon PH, Hoexter B. Complications of Ripstein procedure. Dis Colon Rectum 1978; 21:277–280.
34. Eisenstat TE, Rubin RJ, Salvati EP. Surgical treatment of complete rectal prolapse. Dis Colon Rectum 1979; 22:522–523.
35. Failes D, Killingback M, Stuart M, DeLuca C. Rectal prolapse. Aust N Z J Surg 1979; 49:72–75.
36. Romero-Torres R. Sacrofixation with Marlex in massive prolapse of the rectum. Surg Gynecol Obstet 1979; 22:522–523.
37. Morgan B. The Teflon sling operation for repair of complete rectal prolapse. Aust N Z J Surg 1980; 150:121–123.
38. Roberts PL, Schoetz DJ, Coller JA, Veidenheimer MC. Ripstein procedure. Lahey Clinic experience: 1963–1985. Arch Surg 1988; 123:554–557.
39. Leenen LPH, Kuijpers JHC. Treatment of complete rectal prolapse with foreign material. Neth J Surg 1989; 41:129–131.
40. Tjandra JJ, Fazio VW, Church JM, Milson JW, Oakley JR, La-very IC. Ripstein procedure is an effective treatment for rectal prolapse without constipation. Dis Colon Rectum 1993; 36:501–507.
41. Winde G, Reers B, Nottberg H, Berns T, Meyer J, Bunte H. Clinical and functional results of abdominal rectopexy with absorbable mesh graft for treatment of complete rectal prolapse. Eur J Surg 1993; 159:301–305.
42. Schultz I, Mellgren A, Dolk A, Johansson C, Holmstrom B. Long-term results and functional outcome after Ripstein rectopexy. Dis Colon Rectum 2000; 43:35–43.
43. Corman ML. Rectal stricture secondary to Teflon sling repair for rectal prolapse. Dis Colon Rectum 1974; 17:89–90.
44. Goldberg SM, Gordon PH, Nivatvongs S. Complications of surgery after complete rectal procidentia. In: Ferrari BT, Ray JB, Gathright JB, eds. Complications of Colon and Rectal Surgery, Prevention and Management. Philadelphia: WB Saunders, 1985:251–266.
45. Dolk A, Broden G, Holmstrom B, Johansson C, Nilsson BY. Slow transit of the colon associated with severe constipation after the Ripstein operation. A clinical and physiologic study. Dis Colon Rectum 1990; 33:786–790.
46. Madiba TE, Baig MK, Wexner SD. Surgical management of rectal prolapase. Arch Surg 2005; 140:63–73.
47. Wells C. New operation for rectal prolapse. Proc R Soc Med 1959; 52: 602–603.
48. Morgan CN, Porter NH, Klugman DJ. Ivalon (polyvinyl alcohol) sponge in the repair of complete rectal prolapse. Br J Surg 1972; 59:841–846.
49. Penfold JCB, Hawley PR. Experiences of Ivalon-sponge implant for complete rectal prolapse at St. Mark's Hospital, 1960–1970. Br J Surg 1972; 59: 846–848.
50. Kuijpers JHC, de Morree H. Toward a selection of the most appropriate procedures in the treatment of complete rectal prolapse. Dis Colon Rectum 1988; 31:355–357.
51. Gordon PH. Ivalon sponge wrap and Thiersch operations for prolapse. In: Nyhus LM, Baker RJ, eds. Mastery of Surgery. Boston: Little, Brown, 1984:1045–1050.
52. Ross AH, Thomson JPS. Management of infection after prosthetic abdominal rectopexy (Wells' procedure). Br J Surg 1989; 76:610–612.
53. Mann CV, Hoffman C. Complete rectal prolapse: the anatomical and functional results of treatment by an extended abdominal rectopexy. Br J Surg 1988; 75:34–37.

54. Allen-Mersh TG, Turner MJ, Mann CV. Effect of abdominal Ivalon rectopexy on bowel habit and rectal wall. Dis Colon Rectum 1990; 33:550–553.
55. Stewart R. Long-term results of Ivalon wrap operation for complete rectal prolapse. Proc R Soc Med 1972; 65:777–778.
56. Anderson JR, Kinninmonth AWG, Smith AN. Polyvinyl alcohol sponge rectopexy for complete rectal prolapse. J R Coll Surg Edinb 1981; 26:292–294.
57. Anderson JR, Wilson BG, Parks TG. Complete rectal prolapse—the results of Ivalon sponge rectopexy. Post Grad Med J 1984; 60:411–414.
58. Atkinson KG, Taylor DC. Wells procedure for complete rectal prolapse. A 10 year experience. Dis Colon Rectum 1984; 27:96–98.
59. Boulous CD, Stryker ST, Nicholls RJ. The long term results of polyvinyl alcohol (Ivalon) sponge for rectal prolapse in young patients. Br J Surg 1984; 71: 213–214.
60. Arndt M, Pircher W. Absorbable mesh in the treatment of rectal prolapse. Int J Colorectal Dis 1988; 3:141–143.
61. Yoshioka K, Heyen F, Keighley MRB. Functional results after abdominal rectopexy for rectal prolapse. Dis Colon Rectum 1989; 32:835–838.
62. Sayfan J, Pinho M, Alexander-Williams J, Keighley MRB. Sutured posterior abdominal rectopexy with sigmoidectomy compared with Marlex rectopexy for rectal prolapse. Br J Surg 1990; 77:143–145.
63. Luukkonen P, Mikkonen U, Jarvinen H. Abdominal rectopexy with sigmoidectomy vs rectopexy alone for rectal prolapse: a progressive randomized study. Int J Colored Dis 1992; 7:219, 222.
64. Novell JR, Osborne MJ, Winslet MC, Lewis AAM. Prospective randomized trial of Ivalon sponge versus sutured rectopexy for full thickness rectal prolapse. Br J Surg 1994; 81:904–906.
65. Delemarre JBVM, Gooszen HG, Kruyt RH, Soebhag R, Geesteranus AM. The effect of posterior rectopexy on fecal incontinence. A prospective study. Dis Colon Rectum 1991; 34:311–316.
66. Frykman HM. Abdominal proctopexy and primary sigmoid resection for rectal procidentia. Am J Surg 1955; 90:780–789.
67. Goldberg SM, Gordon PH, Nivatvongs S. Essentials of Anorectal Surgery. Philadelphia: JB Lippincott, 1980:248.
68. Madoff RD, Williams JG, Wong WD, Rothenberger DA, Goldberg SM. Long-term functional results of colon resection and rectopexy for overt rectal prolapse. Am J Gastroenterol 1992; 87:101–104.
69. Husa A, Sainio P, Smitten K. Abdominal rectopexy and sigmoid resection (Frykman-Goldberg) operation for rectal prolapse. Acta Chir Scand 1988; 154:221–224.
70. Huber FT, Stein H, Siewert JR. Functional results after treatment of rectal prolapse with rectopexy and sigmoid resection. World J Surg 1995; 19:138–143.
71. McKee RF, Lauder JC, Poon FW, Aichison MA, Finlay IG. A prospective randomized study of abdominal rectopexy with and without sigmoidectomy in rectal prolapse. Surg Gynecol Obstet 1992; 174:145–148.
72. Cannfrère VG, des Varannos SB, Mayon J, Lehar PA. Adding sigmoidectomy to rectopexy to treat rectal prolapse: a valid option? Br J Surg 1994; 581:2–4.
73. Muir EG. Post-anal perineorrhaphy for rectal prolapse. Proc R Soc Med 1955; 48:33–44.
74. Goldberg SM, Gordon PH. Treatment of rectal prolapse. Clin Gastroenterol 1975; 4:489–504.
75. Schlinkert RT, Beart RW, Wolff BG, Pemberton JH. Anterior resection for complete rectal prolapse. Dis Colon Rectum 1985; 28:409–412.
76. Cirocco WC, Brown AC. Anterior resection for the treatment of rectal prolapse: a 20-year experience. Am Surg 1993; 59:265–269.
77. Baker R, Senagore AJ, Luchtefeld MA. Laparoscopic-assisted vs. open resection. Rectopexy offers excellent results. Dis Colon Rectum 1995; 38:199–201.
78. Kim DS, Tsang CB, Wong WD, Lowry AC, Goldberg SM, Madoff RD. Complete rectal prolapase: evolution of management and results. Dis Colon Rectum 1999; 42:460–466.
79. Loygue J, Hugier M, Malafosse M, Biotois H. Complete prolapse of the rectum: a report on 140 cases treated by rectopexy. Br J Surg 1971; 58:847–848.
80. Blatchford GJ, Perry RE, Thorson AG, Christensen MA. Rectorpexy without resection for rectal prolapse. Am J Surg 1989; 158:574–576.
81. Douard R, Frileux P, Brunel M, Attal E, Tiret E, Parc R. Functional results after the Orr-Loygue transabdominal rectopexy for complete rectal prolapse. Dis Colon Rectum 2003; 46:1089–1096.
82. Collopy BT, Barham KA. Abdominal colporectopexy with pelvic cul-de-sac closure. Dis Colon Rectum 2002; 45:522–526.
83. Sullivan ES, Longaker CJ, Lee PY. Total pelvic mesh repair: a ten-year experience. Dis Colon Rectum 2001; 44:857–863.
84. Nivatvongs S. Rectal prolapse: techniques of transperineal repair. Perspect Colon Rectal Surg 1991; 4:101–109.
85. Kim DS, Tsang CB, Wong WD, Lowry AC, Goldberg SM, Madoff RD. Complete rectal prolapase: evoluation of management and results. Dis Colon Rectum. 1999; 42:460–466.
86. Agachan F, Reisman P, Pfeifer J, Weiss EG, Nogueras JJ, Wexner SD. Comparison of three perineal procedures for the treatment of rectal prolapse. South Med J 1997; 90:925–932.
87. Kimmins MH, Evetts BK, Isler J, Billingham R. The Altemeier repair: outpatient treatment of rectal prolapse. Dis Colon Rectum 2001; 44:565–570.
88. Friedman R, Mugga-Sullam M, Freund HR. Experience with the one stage perineal repair of rectal prolapse. Dis Colon Rectum 1983; 26:789–791.
89. Gopal FA, Amshel AL, Shonberg IL, Eftaiha M. Rectal procidentia in elderly and debilitated patients. Experience with the Altemeier procedure. Dis Colon Rectum 1984; 27:376–381.
90. Finlay IG, Aitchison M. Perineal excision of the rectum for prolapse in the elderly. Br J Surg 1991; 78:687–689.
91. Azimuddin K, Khubchandani IT, Rosen L, Stasik JJ, Riether RD, Reed JF III. Rectal prolapse: a search for the "best" operation. Am Surg 2001; 67: 622–627.
92. Schutz G. Extracorporal resection of the rectum in the treatment of complete rectal prolapse using a circular stapling device. Dig Surg 2001; 18:274–277.
93. Prasad ML, Pearl RK, Abcarian H, Orsay CP, Nelson RL. Perineal proctectomy, posterior rectopexy, and postanal levator repair for the treatment of rectal prolapse. Dis Colon Rectum 1986; 29:547–552.
94. Ramanujam PS, Venkatesh KS. Perineal excision of rectal prolapse with posterior levator ani repair in elderly high risk patients. Dis Colon Rectum 1988; 31:704–706.
95. Kohler A, Athanasiadis S. The value of posterior levator repair in the treatment of anorectal incontinence due to rectal prolapase—a clinical and manometric study. Langenbecks Arch Surg 2001; 386:188–192.
96. Delorme E. Sur le traitement des prolapsus du rectum totaux pour l'excision de la muqueuse rectale ou rectocolique. Bull Mem Soc Chir Paris 1900; 26:499–578.
97. Uhlig BE, Sullivan ES. The modified Delorme operation: its place in surgical treatment of massive rectal prolapse. Dis Colon Rectum 1979; 22:513–521.
98. Watts AMI, Thompson MR. High recurrence rates for repeat Delorme's procedure. Int J Colored Dis 1995; 10:241–242.
99. Christiansen J, Kirkegaard P. Delorme's operation for complete rectal prolapse. Br J Surg 1981; 68:537–538.
100. Gunderson AL, Cogbell TH, Landercasper J. Reappraisal of Delorme's procedure for rectal prolapse. Dis Colon Rectum 1985; 28:721–724.
101. Monson JRT, Jones NAG, Vowden P, Brennan TG. Delorme's operation—the first choice in complete rectal prolapse. Ann R Coll Surg Engl 1986; 68: 143–146.
102. Houry S, Lechaux JP, Hugier M, Molkhou JM. Treatment of rectal prolapse by Delorme's operation. Int J Colorectal Dis 1987; 2:1249–1252.
103. Abulafi AM, Sherman IW, Fiddian RV, Rothwell-Jackson RL. Delorme's operation for rectal prolapse. Ann R Coll Surg Engl 1990; 72:382–385.
104. Graf W, Ejerblad S, Krog M, Pahlman L, Gerdin B. Delorme's operation for rectal prolapse in elderly or unfit patients. Eur J Surg 1992; 158:555–557.
105. White S, Stitz R. Rectal prolapse: Delorme or Ripstein repair. Aust N Z J Surg 1992; 62:193–195.
106. Oliver GC, Vachon D, Eisenstat TE, Rubin RJ, Salvati EP. Delorme's procedure for complete rectal prolapse in severely debilitated patients. Dis Colon Rectum 1994; 37:461–467.
107. Senapati A, Nicholls RJ, Thomson JP, Phillips RK. Results of Delorme's procedure for rectal prolapse. Dis Colon Rectum 1994; 37:456–460.
108. Tobin SA, Scott IHK. Delorme operation for rectal prolapse. Br J Surg 1994; 81:1681–1684.
109. Plusa SM, Charig JA, Balaji V, Watts A, Thompson MR. Physiological changes after Delorme's procedure for full-thickness rectal prolapse. Br J Surg 1995; 82:1475–1478.
110. Pescatori M, Interisano A, Stolfi VM, Zoffoli M. Delorme's operation and sphincteroplasty for rectal prolapase and fecal incontinence. Int J Colorectal Dis 1998; 13:223–227.
111. Sielezneff I, Malouf A, Cesari J, Brunet C, Sarles JC, Sastre B. Selection criteria for rectal prolapse repair by Delorme's transrectal excision. Dis Colon Rectum 1999; 42:367–373.
112. Liberman H, Hughes C, Dippolito A. Evaluation and outcome of the Delorme procedure in the treatment of rectal outlet obstruction. Dis Colon Rectum 2000; 43:188–192.
113. Watts AM, Thompson MR. Evaluation of Delorme's procedure as a treatment for full thickness rectal prolapse. Br J Surg 2000; 87:218–222.
114. Watkins BP, Landercasper J, Belzer GE, et al. Long-term follow-up of the modified Delorme procedure for rectal prolapse. Arch Surg 2003; 138: 498–502.
115. Fengler SA, Pearl RK. Perineal approaches in the repair of rectal prolapse. Perspect Colon Rectal Surg 1996; 9:31–42.
116. Earnshaw JJ, Hopkinson BR. Late results of Silicone rubber perianal suture for rectal prolapse. Dis Colon Rectum 1987; 30:86–88.
117. Labow SD, Hoexter B, Moseson MD, Rubin RJ, Salvati EP, Eisenstat TE. Modification of Silastic sling repair for rectal procidentia and anal incontinence. Dis Colon Rectum 1985; 28:684–685.
118. Sainio AP, Halme LE, Husa AL. Anal encirclement with polypropylene mesh for rectal prolapse and incontinence. Dis Colon Rectum 1991; 34:905–908.
119. Basse L, Billesbolle P, Kehlet H. Early recovery after abdominal rectopexy with multimodal rehabilitation. Dis Colon Rectum 2002; 45:195–199.
120. Yoshioka K, Hyland G, Keighley MRB. Anorectal function after abdominal proctopexy. Parameters of predictive value in identifying return of continence. Br J Surg 1989; 76:64–68.
121. Holmstrom B, Broden G, Dolk A, Frenckner B. Increased anal resting pressure following the Ripstein operation. A contribution to continence. Dis Colon Rectum 1986; 29:485–487.

122. Duthie GS, Bartolo DCC. Abdominal rectopexy for lapse: a comparison of techniques. Br J Surg 1992; 79:107–113.
123. Sainio AP, Voutilainon PE, Husa AI. Recovery of anal sphincter function following transabdominal repair of rectal prolapse: cause of improved continence?. Dis Colon Rectum 1991; 34(9):816–821.
124. Duthie GS, Bartolo DCC. A comparison between Marlex and resection rectopexy. Neth J Surg 1989; 41:136–139.
125. Farouk R, Duthie GS, MacGregor AM, Bartolo DCC. Rectoanal inhibition and incontinence in patients with rectal prolapse. Br J Surg 1994; 81:743–746.
126. Schultz I, Mellgren A, Dolk A, Johansson C, Holmstoom B. Continence is improved after the Ripstein rectopexy. Different mechanisms in rectal prolapse and rectal intussusception?. Dis Colon Rectum 1996; 39:300–306.
127. Hiltunen KM, Matikainen M. Improvement of continence after abdominal rectopexy for rectal prolapse. Int J Colorect Dis 1992; 7:8–10.
128. Madden MV, Kamm MA, Nicholls RJ, Santhanam AW, Cabot R, Speakman CTM. Abdominal rectopexy for complete prolapse: prospective study evaluating changes in symptoms and anorectal function. Dis Colon Rectum 1992; 35:48–55.
129. Brown AJ, Nicol L, Anderson JH, McKee RF, Finlay IG. Prospective study of the effect of rectopexy on colonic motility in patients with rectal prolapse. Br J Surg 2005 Sep 26 [Epub ahead of print].
130. Parks AG. Post-anal perineorrhaphy for rectal prolapse. Proc R Soc Med 1967; 60:920–921.
131. Myers JD, Rothenberger DA. Sugar in the reduction of incarcerated prolapsed bowel: report of two cases. Dis Colon Rectum 1991; 34:416–418.
132. Ramanujam PS, Venkatesh KS. Management of acute incarcerated rectal prolapse. Dis Colon Rectum 1992; 35:1194–1196.
133. De Vogel PL, Kamstra PEJ. Rupture of the rectum with evisceration of small intestine through the anus: a complication of advanced rectal prolapse. Case report. Eur J Surg 1994; 160:187–188.
134. Schepens MA, Vandernekan MA, Gerard YE. Herniation of the small intestine through an incised rectal prolapse. Case report. Acta Chir Scand 1989; 155:495–496.
135. Hool GR, Hull TL, Fazio VW. Surgical treatment of recurrent complete rectal prolopase: a thirty-Year experience. Dis Colon Rectum 1997; 40:270–272.
136. Fengler SA, Pearl RK, Prasad ML, et al. Management of recurrent rectal prolapase. Dis Colon Rectum 1997; 40:832–834.
137. Pikarsky AJ, Joo JS, Wexner SD, et al. Recurrent rectal prolapse: what is the next good option? Dis Colon Rectum 2000; 43:1273–1276.
138. Corman ML. Rectal prolapse in children. Dis Colon Rectum 1985; 28: 535–539.
139. van Tets WF, Kuijpers JHC. Internal intussusception—fact or fancy? Dis Colon Rectum 1995; 38:1080–1083.
140. Rutter KRP. Solitary ulcer syndrome of the rectum: its relation to mucosal prolapse. In: Henry MM, Swash M, eds. Coloproctology and the Pelvic Floor. London: Butterworth, 1985:282–298.
141. Fleshman JW, Kodner IJ, Fry RD. Internal intussusception of the rectum: a changing perspective. Neth J Surg 1989; 41:145–148.
142. McCue JL, Thomson JPS. Rectopexy for internal rectal intussusception. Br J Surg 1990; 77:632–634.
143. Berman IR, Harris MS, Rabeler MR. Delorme's transrectal excision for internal rectal prolapse. Patient selection, technique, and three year follow-up. Dis Colon Rectum 1990; 33:573–580.
144. Christiansen J, Zhu BW, Rasmussen OO, Sorensen M. Internal rectal intussusception: results of surgical repair. Dis Colon Rectum 1992; 35: 1026–1029.
145. Briel JW, Schouten WR, Boerma MO. Long-term results of suture rectopexy in patients with fecal incontinence associated with incomplete rectal prolopse. Dis Colon Rectum 1997; 40:1228–1232.
146. Brown AJ, Anderson JH, McKee RF, Finlay IG. Surgery for occult rectal prolapse. Colorectal Dis 2004; 6:176–179.
147. Bachoo P, Brazzelli M, Grant A. Surgery for complete rectal prolapse in adults. Cochrance Database Syst Rev 2000; 2:CD001758.
148. Brown AJ, Anderson JH, Mckee RF, Finlay JG. Strategy for selection of type of operation for rectal prolapse based on clinical criteria. Dis Colon Rectum 2004; 47:103–107. Epub 2004 Jan 2.
149. Madigan MR. Solitary ulcer of the rectum. Proc R Soc Med 1964; 57:403.
150. Madigan MR, Morson BC. Solitary ulcer of the rectum. Gut 1969; 10: 871–881.
151. Rutter KRP. Solitary ulcer syndrome of the rectum; its relation to mucosal prolapse. In: Henry MM, Swash M, eds. Coloproctology and the Pelvic Floor. Pathophysiology and Management. London: Butterworth, 1985:282–298.
152. Martin CJ, Parks TG, Biggart JD. Solitary rectal ulcer syndrome in Northern Ireland. Br J Surg 1981; 68:744–747.
153. Haray PN, Morris-Stiff GJ, Foster ME. Solitary rectal ulcer syndrome—an underdiagnosed condition. Int J Colorectal Dis 1997; 12:313–315.
154. Rutter KR, Riddell RH. The solitary ulcer syndrome of the rectum. Clin Gastroenterol 1975; 4:505–530.
155. Tjandra JJ, Fazio VW, Church JM, et al. Clinical conundrum of solitary rectal ulcer. Dis Colon Rectum 1992; 35:227–234.
156. Keighley MR, Shouler P. Clinical and manometric features of the solitary ulcer syndrome. Dis Colon Rectum 1984; 27:507–512.
157. Womack NR, Williams NS, Holmfield JH, Morrison JF. Anorectal function in the solitary rectal ulcer syndrome. Dis Colon Rectum 1987; 30:319–323.
158. Goei R, Baeten C, Arends JW. Solitary rectal ulcer syndrome: findings at barium enema study and defecography. Radiology 1988; 168:303–306.
159. Goei R, Baeten C, Janevski B, et al. The solitary rectal ulcer syndrome: diagnosis with defecography. AJR 1987; 149:933–936.
160. Kuijpers HC, Schreve RH, ten Cate Hoedemakers H. Diagnosis of functional disorders of defecation causing the solitary rectal ulcer syndrome. Dis Colon Rectum 1986; 29:126–129.
161. Mahieu PHG. Barium enema and defecography in the diagnosis and evaluation of the solitary rectal ulcer syndrome. Int J Colorectal Dis 1986; 1:85–90.
162. Halligan S, Nicholls RJ, Bartram CI. Evacuation proctography in patients with solitary rectal ulcer syndrome: anatomic abnormalities and frequency of impaired emptying and prolapse. Am J Roentgenol 1995; 164:91–95.
163. Ford MJ, Anderson MH, Gilmour HM, et al. Clinical spectrum of "solitary ulcer" of the rectum. Gastroenterology 1983; 84:1533–1540.
164. Jones PH, Lubowski DZ, Swash M, et al. Is paradoxical contraction of puborectalis muscle of functional importance? Dis Colon Rectum 1987; 36:667–670.
165. Levine DS. "Solitary" rectal ulcer syndrome. Are "solitary" rectal ulcer syndrome and "localized" colitis cystica profunda analogous syndromes caused by rectal prolapse. Gastroenterology 1987; 92:243–253.
166. Kang YS, Kamm MA, Nicholls RJ. Solitary rectal ulcer and complete rectal prolapse: one condition or two? Int J Colorectal Dis 1995; 10:87–90.
167. Hizawa K, Iide M, Suekane H, et al. Mucosal prolapse syndrome: diagnosis with endoscopic US. Radiology 1994; 191:527–530.
168. Van Outryve MJ, Pelckmans PA, Fierons H, et al. Transrectal ultrasound study of the pathogenesis of solitary rectal ulcer syndrome. Gut 1993; 34:1422–1426.
169. Halligan S, Sultan A, Rottenberg G, et al. Endosonography of the anal sphincter in solitary rectal ulcer syndrome. Int J Colorectal Dis 1995; 10:79–82.
170. Morson BC, Dawson MP. Gastrointestinal pathology. Oxford: Blackwell Scientific Publications, 1972:587.
171. Levine DS, Surawicz CM, Ajer TN, et al. Diffuse excess mucosal collagen in rectal biopsies facilitates differential diagnosis of solitary rectal ulcer syndrome from other inflammatory bowel diseases. Dig Dis Sci 1988; 33:1345–1352.
172. Tsuchida K, Okayama N, Miyata M, et al. Solitary rectal ulcer syndrome accompanied by submucosal invasive carcinoma. Am J Gastroentrol 1998; 93:2235–2238.
173. Monkemuller KE, Lewis JB Jr, Ruiz F, et al. Association of solitary rectal ulcer syndrome and mucinous adenocarcenoma adenocarcenom of the rectam. Am J Gastroenterol 1996; 91:2031.
174. Li SC, Hamilton SR. Malignant tumors in the rectum simulating solitary rectal ulcer syndrome in endoscopic biopsy speciments. Am J Surg Pathol 1998; 22:106–112.
175. Kang YS, Kamm MA, Engel AF, et al. Pathology of the rectal wall in solitary rectal ulcer syndrome and complete rectal prolapse. Gut 1996; 38:587–590.
176. Malouf AJ, Vaizey CJ, Kamm MA. Results of behavioral treatment (biofeedback) for solitary rectal ulcer syndrome. Dis Colon Rectum 2001; 44:72–76.
177. Malatjalian DA, Williams CN. 5-ASA therapy in solitary rectal ulcer syndrome. Report of three patients. Can J Gastroenterol 1988; 2:18–21.
178. Zargar SA, Khuroo MS, Mahajan R. Sucralfate retention enemas in solitary rectal ulcer. Dis Colon Rectum 1991; 34:455–457.
179. Binnie NR, Papachrysostoman M, Clare N, et al. Solitary rectal ulcer: the place of biofeedback and surgery in the treatment of the syndrome. World J Surg 1992; 16:836–840.
180. Stoppino V, Cuomo R, Tonti P, et al. Argon plasma coagulation of hemorrhagic solitary rectal ulcer syndrome. J Clin Gastroenterol 2003; 37:392–394.
181. Schweizer M, Alexander-Williams J. Solitary-ulcer syndrome of the rectum, its association with occult rectal prolapse. Lancet 1977; 1:170–171.
182. van Tets WF, Kuijpers HC. Internal rectal intussusception—fact or fancy? Dis Colon Rectum 1995; 38:1080–1083.
183. Sitzler PJ, Kamm MA, Nicholls RJ, McKee RF. Long-term clinical outcome of surgery for solitary rectal ulcer syndrome. Br J Surg 1998; 85:1246–1250.
184. Frizelle FA, Santoro GA, Nivatvong S. Solitary rectal ulcer syndrome: stopping the prolapse heals the ulceration. G Chir. 1996; 17:320–322.
185. Stavorovsky M, Weintroub S, Ratan J, Rozen P. Successful treatment of a benign solitary rectal ulcer by temporary diverting sigmoidostomy: report of a case. Dis Colon Rectum 1977; 20:347–350.
186. Marchal F, Bresler L, Brunaud L, et al. Solitary rectal ulcer syndrome: a series of 13 patients operated with a mean follow-up of 4.5 years. Int J Colorectal Dis 2001; 16:228–233.
187. Halligan S, Nicholls RJ, Bartram CI. Proctographic changes after rectopexy for solitary rectal ulcer syndrome and preoperative predictive factors for a successful outcome. Br J Surg 1995; 82:314–317.

22 Benign Neoplasms of the Colon and Rectum

Santhat Nivatvongs

POLYPS OF COLON AND RECTUM

The word "polyp" is a nonspecific clinical term that describes any projection from the surface of the intestinal mucosa regardless of its histologic nature. Polyps can be conveniently classified according to their histologic appearance:

1. Neoplastic tubular adenoma, villous adenoma, and tubulovillous, adenoma and serrated adenoma
2. Hamartomatous—juvenile polyps, Peutz-Jeghers syndrome (PJS), Cronkhite-Canada syndrome, Cowden's disease
3. Inflammatory—inflammatory polyp or pseudopolyp, benign lymphoid polyp
4. Hyperplastic

NEOPLASTIC POLYPS

Adenomas

A neoplastic polyp is an epithelial growth composed of abnormal glands of the large bowel. A neoplastic polyp has been termed an adenoma and is classified according to the amount of villous component. Those with 0% to 25% villous tissue are classified as tubular adenomais, 25% to 75% as tubulovillous adenomas, and 75% to 100% as villous adenomas (1). Tubular adenomas (Fig. 1) account for 75% of all neoplastic polyps; villous adenomas (Fig. 2), 10%; and tubulovillous adenomas (Fig. 3), 15%. The villous growth pattern is most prominent in sessile large adenomas, particularly those located distally in the rectum. There remains considerable uncertainty as to the nature of villous growth, whether it is merely a manifestation of continued growth of tubular adenomas, or whether it is a distinct phenotype that may reflect an acquired genetic change. In favor of the former is the rarity of small villous adenomas and large purely tubular adenomas (1).

Dysplasia describes the histologic abnormality of an adenoma according to the degree of atypical cells, categorized as low-grade (mild), moderate, and high (severe). Thus high-grade dysplasia designates a condition one step away from an invasive carcinoma. The frequency of high-grade dysplasia correlates with the size of the adenoma (Fig. 4). The term carcinoma-in-situ, or "intramucosal carcinoma" should be avoided, since it implies a biological potential for distant spread, which is unwarranted and could result in overtreatment (1).

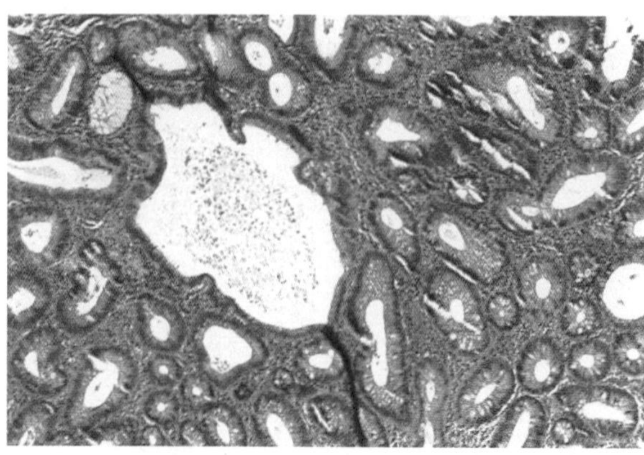

FIGURE 1 ■ Tubular adenoma.

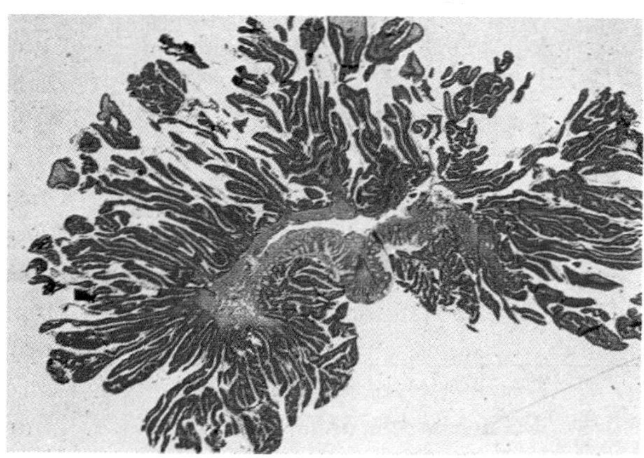

FIGURE 2 ■ Villous adenoma.

Neoplastic polyps are common. Since data on the clinical recording of adenomas may be biased due to selection of patients and diagnostic methods, most accurate epidemiologic data on adenomas are obtained from autopsy studies. In autopsy series adenomas are present in 34% to 52% of males and 29% to 45% of females over 50 years of age. Most adenomas (87–89%) are less than 1 cm in size (2,3). The number, but not the size, of adenomas, increases with age (2). Carcinomas are found in 0% to 4% (2–5). The National Polyp Study, a multicenter randomized clinical trial in the United States, included 3371 adenomas in 1867 patients detected by colonoscopy (6). This study gives valuable information regarding the natural history and characteristics of polyps: 66.5% of polyps were adenomas, 11.2% were hyperplastic, and 22.3% were classified as "other" (normal mucosa, inflammatory and juvenile polyps, lymphoid hamartomas, submucosal lipomas, carcinoids, and leiomyomas). The majority of the adenomas (69%) were in the left colon (Table 1). The sizes of the adenomas were $\leq$0.5 cm, 38% 0.6 to 1 cm, 37% and 1 cm, 25%.

It is important to note that the size, the extent of villous component, and the increasing age are independent risk factors for high-grade dysplasia. The increased frequency of high-grade dysplasia in adenomas located distal to the splenic flexure is attributable mainly to increased size and villous component rather than to location per se. Multiplicity of adenomas affects the risk of high-grade dysplasia but is dependent on size and villous component and thus is not

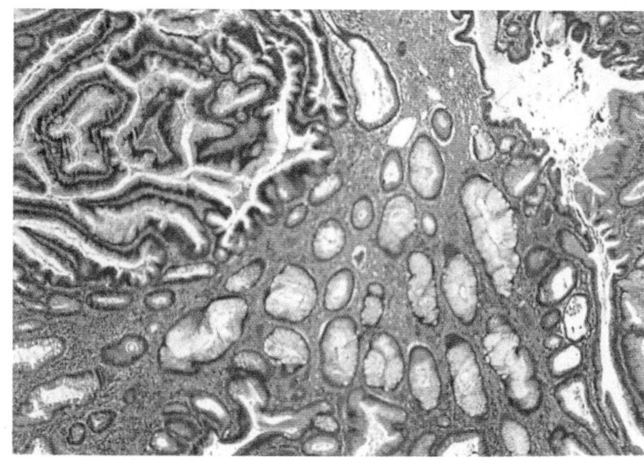

FIGURE 3 ■ Tubulovillous adenoma; mixture of tubular and villous glands.

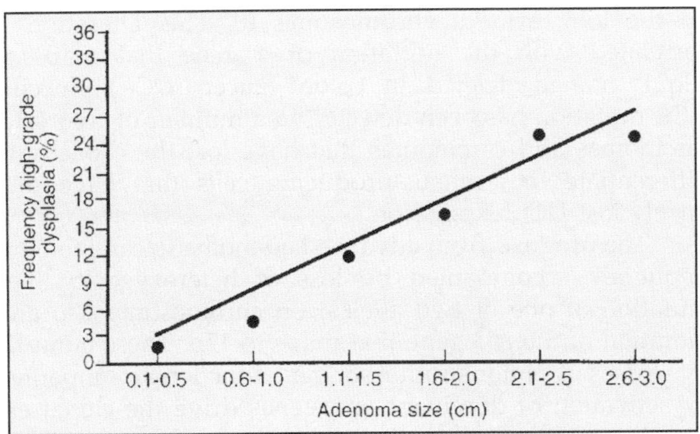

FIGURE 4 ■ Relationship between adenoma size and frequency of dysplasia. *Source*: From Ref. 6.

an independent factor (6). Invasive carcinomas are uncommon in adenomas <1 cm, and the incidence increases with and increased size of the adenomas (Table 2) (7,8).

Adenoma-Carcinoma Sequence

The Observation

The concept that carcinomas of the colon and rectum derived from benign adenoma was observed by Dukes (9) of St. Mark's Hospital, London, in 1926. Jackman and Mayo (10) coined the term adenoma-carcinoma sequence in 1951. After decades of debates and challenges by those who believed that carcinoma of the colon and rectum derived de novo (11,12), the adenoma-carcinoma sequence has finally become widely accepted and currently is the rationale of the approach to the secondary prevention of colorectal carcinoma by colonoscopic polypectomy (1,13–16). Circumstantial evidence supporting the adenoma-carcinoma sequence abounds and explains the high concurrence rate of carcinoma and adenoma and the frequent findings of contiguous benign adenoma in the resected carcinoma (17). Numerous studies (most of which are retrospective), based on tumor registry reports, hospital records, pathology reports, surgical specimens, and colonoscopy show a coexistence of adenomas and adenocarcinomas of the colon and rectum ranging from 13% to 62% (18). The cumulative incidence curve of adenomas based on data from the Norwegian Cancer Registry precedes the corresponding incidence curve of carcinomas by about five years (Fig. 5). It should be kept in mind that adenomas are first diagnosed and reported to the cancer registry simultaneously with the diagnosis of colorectal carcinoma, indicating a longer time span between the two types of lesions than the curve indicates. It is manifested also in the natural history of both familial adenomatous polyposis (FAP) and hereditary nonpolyposis colon cancer (HNPCC) syndrome. The latter was originally thought to offer support to the de novo school of thought but several studies have since demonstrated coexisting and contiguous adenomas associated with HNPCC carcinoma with a frequency similar to that observed with sporadic carcinomas (1). Due to the high prevalence of adenomas and the relatively far less frequent incidence of carcinomas, only a small proportion of adenomas give rise to carcinomas (20).

Although the adenoma-carcinoma sequence concept has been favored by most authors as the main pathogenesis of colorectal carcinoma, the "de novo" origin of carcinoma developing from normal mucosa has received some attention in recent years as an alternative pathway (19). In support of this de novo theory, authors (21–23) reported early colorectal carcinomas without evidence of adjacent adenomatous cells. In the series reported by Stolte and Beckte (22) of 155 such lesions, 59% of the lessions were Polyponl and 34% were flat. However, proponents for the adenoma-carcinoma sequence may argue that these types of lessions are so aggressive that the infiltration destroys the adenomatous remuants. Muto et al. (24)

TABLE 1 ■ **Distribution of Colorectal Adenomas Diagnosed by Colonoscopy**

Site	(%)
Cecum	8
Ascending colon	9
Hepatic flexure	4
Transverse colon	10
Splenic flexure descending colon	4
Descending colon	14
Sigmoid colon	43
Rectum	8
Total	100

Source: From Ref. 6.

TABLE 2 ■ **Relationship Between Size of Adenoma and Carcinoma**

Size (cm)	Adenoma (No.)	Invasive Carcinoma (%)
<0.5	5027	0
0.6–1.5	3519	2
1.6–2.5	1052	19
2.6–3.5	510	43
>3.5	1080	76

Source: From Ref. 7.

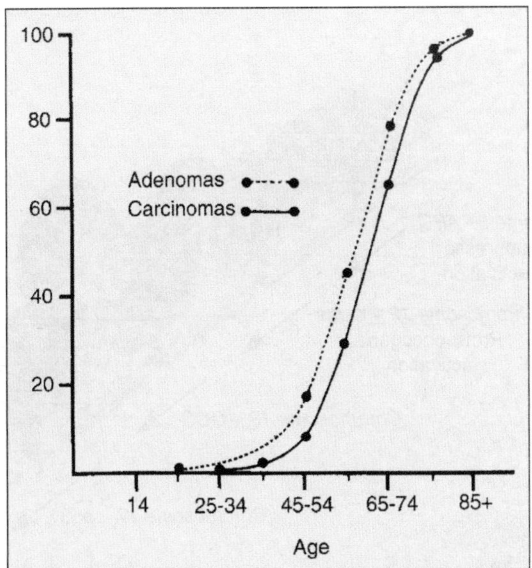

FIGURE 5 ■ Cumulative incidence of colorectal adenomas and carcinomas recorded in the Norwegian Cancer Registry 1983 to 1985. *Source*: From Ref. 19.

thought that all genetic alterations may take place rapidly, one after another, without a chance for morphologic changes to be expressed as seen in the adenoma-carcinoma sequence. They said, "until a specific responsible gene for de novo carcinoma is detected, de novo carcinoma arising directly from normal mucosa is only an imaginary entity. Until then, the term 'de novo' carcinoma is better avoided and instead de novo-type carcinoma should be used."

Molecular Genetics

Molecular genetic discoveries provide substantial support for the adenoma-carcinoma sequence concept (25). An adenoma represents an epithelial proliferation derived from a single cell (crypt). Its de-velopment occurs as a series of genetic mutations. The progression of colorectal epithelium from normal to adenoma to carcinoma can be simplified as in Figure 6.

The initial step in colorectal carcinogenesis is the mutation in the adenomatous polyposis coli (*APC*) gene on chromosome 5q. The *APC* gene is inactivated, causing the affected cells to proliferate. These cells are thus primed for subsequent growth-enhancing mutation, which is more likely because of the increased rate of cell division.

Hypomethylation of DNA has been identified as the next factor involved in colorectal carcinogenesis. Loss of methylation of CpG dinucleotides occurs in cells that are already hyperproliferative because of the inactivation of the *APC* gene. These changes produce a growth of the affected cells resulting in adenoma formation. Hypomethylation of DNA may be directly linked to the K-*ras* (Kirsten rate sarcoma virus) activation that enhances the dysplasia so that the neoplasia can progress.

Because K-*ras* is an oncogene, thus mutation of one allele is enough to produce an effect. K-*ras* mutations can occur in the absence of *APC* gene mutations but, in this case, are usually limited to aberrant crypt foci (ACF) that do not progress to malignancy. In cells that have already suffered *APC* mutation (both alleles need two "hits"), K-*ras* mutation will drive progression. Small adenomas tend to advance to intermediate adenomas.

The transition from intermediate to advanced (or late) adenoma is associated with a distinct genetic alteration on the long arm of chromosome 18. This alteration is correlated with the mutation of a gene that maps to 18q21, named deleted in colon cancer (*DCC*). Specific *DCC* mutation has been detected in a number of colorectal carcinomas and carcinomas that have lost the capacity to differentiate into mucus-producing cells that have uniformly lost *DCC* expression.

The progress from advanced adenoma to carcinoma is frequently accompanied by loss of heterozygosity (i.e., mutation of one of two alleles) on chromosome 17p and mutation of the *p53* gene that maps to 17p. These cumulative losses in tumor suppressor gene function accompanied by activation of dominant oncogenes drive the clonal expression of cells from the benign to the malignant site (25).

A fuller account of molecular genetics of colon and rectal adenocarcinoma is provided in Chapter 23.

Diagnosis of Large Bowel Adenomas

Clinically, there are two morphologic types of polyps, pedunculated and sessile. The pedunculated polyp has a stem lined with normal mucosa, called a stalk or a pedicle, and has the appearance of a mushroom (Fig. 7). A sessile polyp grows flat on the mucosa (Fig. 8). A pedunculated polyp rarely is >4 cm in diameter, whereas a sessile polyp can encompass the entire circumference of the large bowel.

Adenomas of the large bowel are usually asymptomatic and are frequently discovered during routine radiologic studies or endoscopic examinations. Bleeding per rectum is the most common finding if the polyp is situated in the rectum or sigmoid colon. A large pedunculated polyp in the lower part of the rectum may prolapse through the anus. A large villous adenoma may manifest as watery diarrhea; in rare instances it causes fluid and electrolyte imbalance. Intermittent abdominal pain from recurrent intussusception or spasm may occur with a large colonic polyp but is unusual. Mild anemia may follow chronic bleeding from an ulcerative polyp. With a small polyp, up to 8 mm, biopsy and electrocoagulation can be performed, preferably using a "hot" biopsy forceps for histopathologic examination. A large polyp should be completely snared or excised and sent for histopathologic

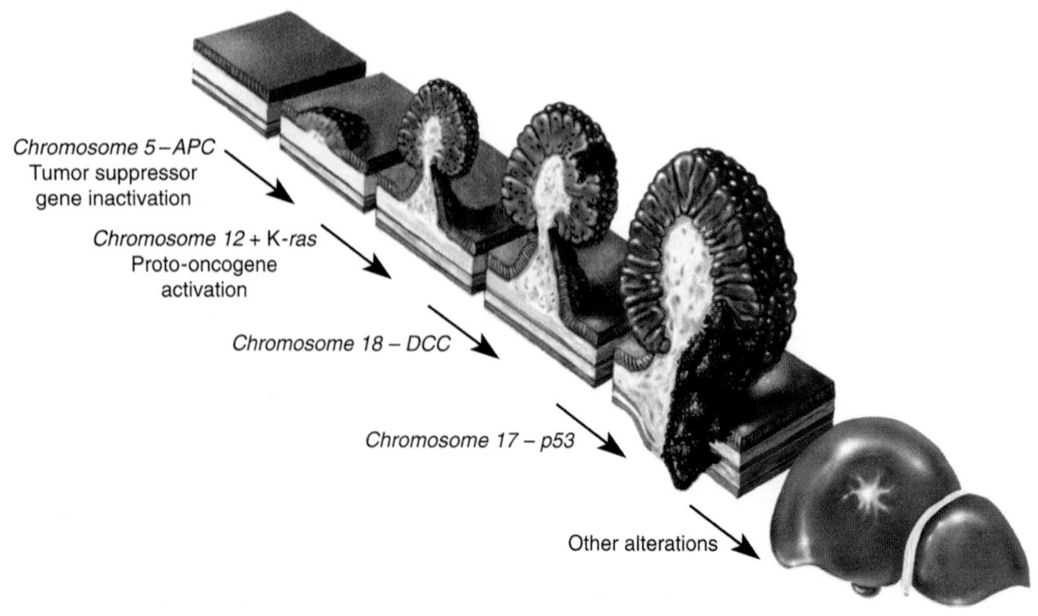

FIGURE 6 ■ A genetic model for the adenoma-carcinoma sequence. Tumorigenesis proceeds through a series of genetic alterations that accumulate. The histopathologic stages of colorectal tumor development are shown with increasing size and dysplasia until an invasive carcinoma is formed. *Abbreviations*: DCC, deleted in colon cancer; APC, adenomatous polyposis coli. *Source*: Modified from Ref. 26.

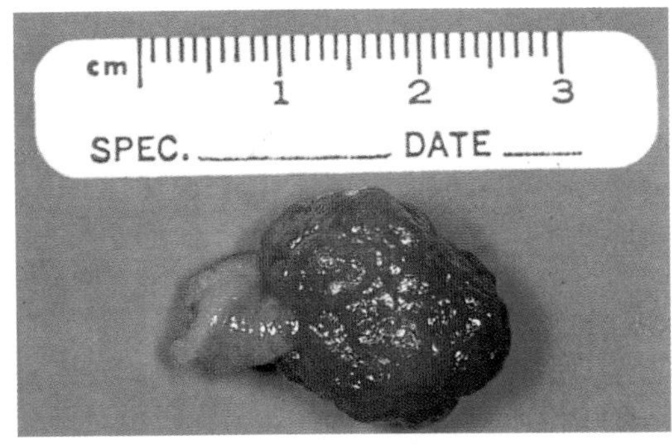

FIGURE 7 ■ Pedunculated polyp.

examination. A biopsy of a large polyp does not represent the entire lesion and presents difficulty in the interpretation of an invasive carcinoma. Occasionally, biopsy may cause displacement of the gland into the submucosa and can be misinterpreted as an invasive carcinoma (27). This pseudoadenomatous invasion can also be caused by trauma from hard feces, repeated twisting of the stalk with subsequent ulceration of the surface (28).

Management of Benign Adenomas

Colonoscopy has revolutionized the management of large bowel polyps. Most polyps throughout the entire colon and rectum can be excised through the colonoscope with minimal morbidity. At the present time, colonic resection or colotomy and polypectomy are reserved for cases in which colonoscopic polypectomy cannot be performed, such as lesions that are too large or too flat, or when the colonoscope cannot be passed to the site of the polyp.

Most pedunculated polyps can be snared in one piece since the pedicles are rarely >2 cm in diameter. Sessile polyps <2 cm usually can be snared in one piece. Large sessile polyps should be snared piecemeal and in more than one session as appropriate. Excised polyps must be prepared properly and sectioned so that all the layers can be examined microscopically and the evidence of invasive carcinoma detected.

Adenomas in the rectum present a unique situation. These lesions can be palpated with finger, suction, or endoscope. If there is no induration, the chance that a lesion is benign is 90% (29,30). There are a number of ways to remove a large adenoma in the rectum, including proctoscope or a colonoscope, per anal excision, trans anal endoscopic microsurgery and posterior proctotomy (see Chapter 19).

Patients with a neoplastic polyp have a higher risk of developing another polyp; so follow-up colonoscopy is advised. After the colon and rectum are cleared of polyps, follow-up colonoscopy every three to five years is adequate. A large sessile polyp, particularly villous type, is prone to recur, and a follow-up check of the polypectomy site should be done every 3 to 6 months the first year, every 6 to 12 months the second year, and every year thereafter to the fifth year. Then colonoscopic examination every three to five years is appropriate.

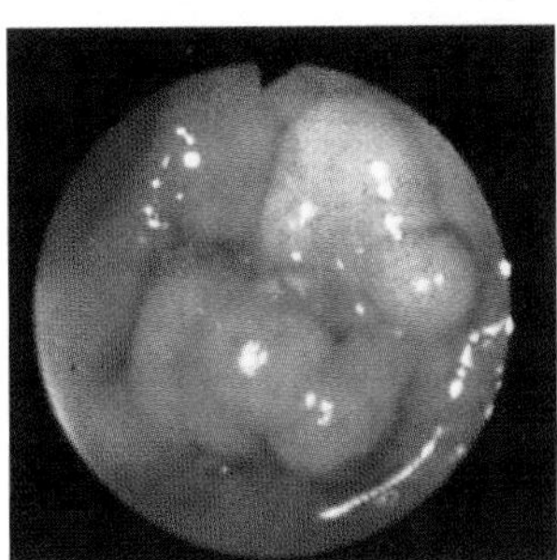

FIGURE 8 ■ Sessile polyp.

The Flat Polyp

In 1985, Muto et al. (31) called attention to a separate type of polyp called a "flat" adenoma. This type of polyp is unique in that it is usually small and flat, often with a central depression, and is difficult to detect with colonoscopy or even with the resected colon and rectal specimens. Ninety percent of flat adenomas are <1 cm and more than half are less than 5 mm (32). The significance of flat adenomas is the high incidence of carcinomas, which occur in 6% of patients, even when the lesions are as small as 2 to 4 mm, and rapidly rise to 36% when the lesions are 9 to 10 mm. Approximately 10% of the adenomas in the Muto series were flat adenomas. They were most frequently located in the left colon and the rectum. Lynch et al. (33) found similar flat adenomas in patients who were members of the same kindred under study for HNPCC. Most of the lesions were in the right colon. The flat adenomas, originally thought to occur mostly among Japanese, have also been found in studies from Australia, Canada, and the United Kingdom (32).

In a prospective study of 1000 executive patients attending for colonoscopy, flat or depressed lesions were examined by Rembacken et al. (34). Patients were not preselected and the indications were similar to other units in the United Kingdom. A flat adenoma was defined as mucosal elevations with a flat or slightly rounded surface and a height of less than half the diameter of the lesion. In practice, most flat adenomas were less than 2 mm in height and only very broad lesions were 5 mm high. During the examination, they used 0.2% indigo carmine dye, 3 to 6 mL, sprayed directly onto suspicious areas. Magnifying colonoscopy was also used.

The authors identified 321 adenomas, 119 (37%) were flat and 4 (1%) appeared depressed. Fifty-four percent of the flat or depressed lesions were situated between splenic flexure and rectum.

Seventy of the flat lesions (59%) were <10 mm in size (mean, 5 mm) and 4% had early carcinoma (invasive into submucosa); 49 flat lesions (41%) were >10 mm (mean, 21 mm), and 29% had early carcinoma. The mean size of the depressed lesions was 9 mm and three of four (75%) had early carcinoma, indicating their aggressiveness compared to other types of lesions.

Rembacken et al. (34) suggested, "Western colonoscopists refuse training in the recognition of flat, elevated and depressed lesion in order to detect colorectal neoplasms in their early stages." The readers should note that in this study, all of the patients had indications for colonoscopic examinations and not as a screening examination for low risk asymptomatic patients. In response to an editorial comment (35), Rembacken et al. wrote (34), "The use of indigo carmine dye is paramount to the detection of flat and depressed lesions and only takes a few seconds. Without the dye, it is difficult to evaluate non-polypoid lesions because they generally appear to be erythematous patches, easily mistaken for scope trauma. The magnifying colonoscope does not help in the initial recognition of lesions but allows the endoscopists to assess the crypt pattern and predict the histology."

Recent molecular analysis of such flat adenomas suggests that they are etiologically distinct from other polypoid adenomas (36). The mutation rate and the K-*ras* gene are both significantly reduced (16% in flat adenomas compared to 50% in ordinary colorectal adenomas) and do not occur in the same codons. The management of flat adenomas is the same as for sessile adenomas.

Why Remove a Polyp?

It has generally been accepted that most colorectal carcinomas are derived from benign adenomas through the adenoma-carcinoma sequence. It takes about five years from a clean colon to the development of an adenoma and about 10 years from a clean colon to the development of invasive carcinoma (13). Thus, removal of an adenoma is prophylactic against the development of colorectal carcinoma. Gilbertsen (37), in a retrospective study, showed that removal of rectal polyps in patients under surveillance with yearly rigid proctosigmoidoscopy results in a lower than expected incidence of rectal carcinoma. This result was confirmed by Selby et al. (38) in a case-control study using rigid proctosigmoidoscopy; screening examination produced a 70% reduction in the risk of death from rectal and distal sigmoid carcinoma. The National Polyp Study also showed that colonoscopic polypectomy results in a lower than expected incidence of colorectal carcinoma (39).

Most adenomatous polyps found on routine examination with rigid proctosigmoidoscopy, or through flexible sigmoidoscopy are small and have a minimal risk of harboring a carcinoma. Because we do not know, whether these small adenomas will continue to grow with eventual degeneration into an invasive carcinoma, their removal is logical provided it can be performed with minimal or no risk of complications. This approach also gives the opportunity to clear the colon and rectum and thus extends the follow-up time to several years. Another point of concern is whether the patient has a synchronous polyp or polyps more proximally and, if so, whether it is important to have it (or them) removed. The incidence of synchronous polyps beyond the reach of the rigid proctoscope or flexible sigmoidoscope is approximately 50% (6). However, most of these polyps are small and have little clinical significance.

It is debatable whether a total colonoscopy should be performed in every person in whom a small polyp is found in the rectum or sigmoid colon. A small hyperplastic polyp frequently found in the rectum or sigmoid has no malignant potential, nor has it been shown to predict an adenoma in the proximal colon (40–42); therefore no further evaluation or follow-up is indicated. Church (43) studied diminutive (1–5 mm) and small (6–10 mm) adenomas of the colon and rectim and found that although the risk of invasive carcinoma was low (0.1 % and 0.2%, respectively) the risk of severe dysplasia was significant (4.4% and 15.6%, respectively). He advised a cold excision or a hot snare as appropriate (Table 3).

A retrospective study using death from carcinoma as the end point, Atkin et al. (44) showed that the risk of development of carcinoma in the proximal colon is significant if the adenoma found in the rectum or sigmoid colon is >1 cm, if the polyp has a villous component, and if there are multiple adenomas. The authors also found that if a tabular adenoma found in the rectum or sigmoid colon is ≤ 1 cm. This risk of carcinoma remote to these sites is insignificant.

TABLE 3 ■ **Risk of Diminutive and Small Adenomas**

Size (mm)	No.	Severe Dysplasia (%)	Invasive Carcinoma (%)
1–5 (diminutive)	2066	4.4	0.1
6–10 (small)	418	15.6	0.2

No effect of age, site, or family history.
Source: From Ref. 43.

Natural History of Untreated Large Bowel Adenomas

A retrospective review of patients from the pre-colonoscopic era by Stryker et al. (45) analyzed 226 patients who had colonic polyps $\geq$10 mm in diameter and in whom periodic radiographic examination of the colon was elected over excision. Twenty-one invasive carcinomas were identified at the site of the index polyp at a mean follow-up of 108 months (range, 24–225 months). The risk of having a polyp $\geq$1 cm in size develop into an invasive carcinoma at 5, 10, and 20 years was 2.5%, 8%, and 24%, respectively.

Further study of this same group of patients by Otchy et al. (46) revealed that the cumulative probability of developing an invasive metachronous carcinoma at a site different from the index polyp was 2% at five years, 7% at 10 years, and 12% at 20 years. Over a median duration of polyp surveillance of 4.8 years (range, 1–27 years), 11 (5%) of the index polyps disappeared, 129 (57%) had no growth noted, and 86 demonstrated growth. Forty-two of the 86 polyps (49%) had at least a twofold increase in size. Seventy-one of the 86 polyps were removed, and 24 (34%) were carcinomatous. Fifteen of the 86 polyps that increased in size were not removed, and none of these patients developed a carcinoma. Forty-three of the 129 polyps that did not grow were eventually removed. Five of those polyps had carcinoma and one of these patients also developed a metachronous carcinoma at a later date. In addition, two of the 43 patients developed a colon carcinoma in areas distant from the site of the index polyp.

These data further support the recommendation for excision of all colonic polyps $\geq$10 mm in diameter and a periodic examination of the entire colon. Although this study has limitations inherent to any retrospective analysis, comparable prospective data are unlikely to be available in the future because of the widespread availability of colonoscopy and the compelling evidence to recommend the removal of neoplastic polyps.

What Happens to Smaller Adenomas?

Hofstad et al. (47) prospectively studied the growth of colorectal polyps. Colonoscopy was performed in 58 subjects. Polyps $\geq$10 mm were removed; polyps <5 mm, and 5 to 9 mm were left behind for a follow-up study. Colonoscopy was followed-up by one investigator once a year. On the third year, polyps were removed by snare or hot biopsy. The measurement of the polyps was performed by a measuring probe plus photography. On the third year, 7 of 58 patients had only hyperplastic polyps. Twenty-nine individuals had one adenoma, 17 individuals had two to three adenomas, 5 individuals had four to five adenomas. Twenty-five percent of all the adenomas were unchanged in size whereas 40% displayed growth and 35% showed regression or shrinking in size. Adenomatous polyps < 5 mm showed a tendency to growth, while the adenomas 5 to 9 mm showed a tendency to reduction in size. The hyperplastic polyps showed a similar pattern. There was a tendency to increase growth in the adenomatous polyps in the younger age groups reaching significance from initial examination to the third year and from the first to the second year of re-examination. Moreover, in the patients with four to five adenomas at the initial examination, the polyps showed larger growth than the polyps in patients with only one or two to three adenomas. There were no differences in polyp growth between the sexes. A similar prospective study by Bersentes et al. (48) on adenomas of the upper rectum or sigmoid colon, size 3 to 9 mm, showed no regression or consistent linear growth rates with a 2 year follow-up.

In the study by Hofstad et al. (47), 86% of the individuals had at least one new polyp during the 3 years and 75% had at least one new adenoma. The newly discovered polyps were significantly smaller than the average size at initial examination. They were also more frequent in the proximal part of the colon (71%) than the polyps discovered at initial examination (38%). There were more new adenomas among those with more than four to five adenomas at initial examination, than those with one adenoma, reaching significance from initial examination to the first year of examination and from initial examination to third year. There were more new adenomas among patients ≥ 60 years of age than those < 60 years. No differences were found between the sexes.

Management of Adenomas with Invasive Carcinoma

The term "invasive carcinoma" is applied only when the malignant cells have invaded the polyp, either sessile or pedunculated, partially or totally, through the muscularis mucosa into the submucosa. Carcinoma superficial to the muscularis mucosa does not metastasize and should be classified as atypia (rather than carcinoma in situ or superficial carcinoma) (13). For this type of lesion, complete excision is all that is necessary. Follow-up of these polyps is the same as for benign polyps.

A polyp with invasive carcinoma or a malignant polyp is an early carcinoma. For the TNM classification, it is a $T_1N_xM_x$. Local excision for a malignant polyp can be curative if the lession can be adequately excised and if the lession has not spread to the regional lymph nodes or if there are no distant metastaces.

In 1985, Haggitt et al. (44) proposed a classification for polyps with adenocarcinoma according to the depth of invasion as follows (Fig. 9):

Level 0—Carcinoma in situ or intramucosal carcinoma. These are not invasive.

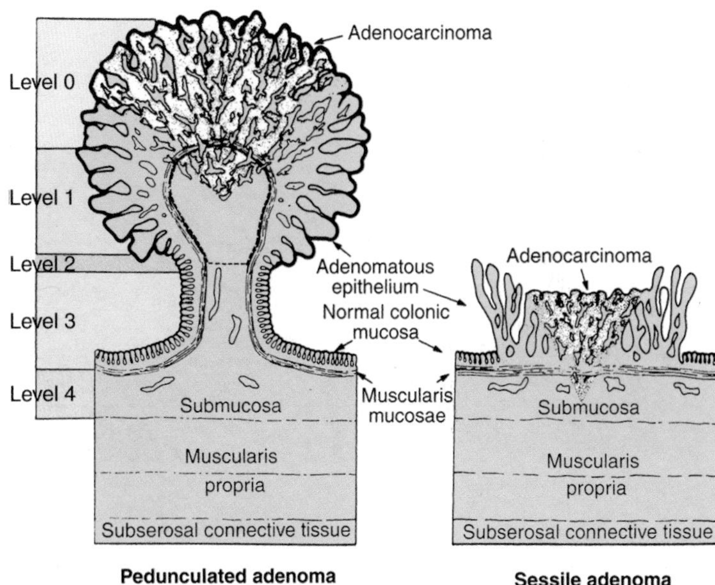

FIGURE 9 ■ Anatomic landmarks of pedunculated and sessile adenomas. *Source*: From Ref. 49.

Level 1—Carcinoma invading through the muscularis mucosae into the submucosa but limited to the head of the polyp (i.e., above the junction between the adenoma and its stalk).

Level 2—Carcinoma invading the level of the neck of the adenoma (junction between adenoma and its stalk).

Level 3—Carcinoma invading any part of the stalk.

Level 4—Carcinoma invading into the submucosa of the bowel wall below the stalk of the polyp but above the muscularis propria. By definition, therefore, all sessile polyps with invasive carcinoma are in level 4.

Pedunculated Polyp with Invasive Carcinoma

Using Haggitt classification, the risk of lymph node metastasis for pedunculated polyp Haggitt level 1, 2, and 3 is low (49–52). For these lesions, a complete snaring or a transanal excision is adequate. A close follow-up examination with endoscopy to detect a local recurrence should be performed every 3 to 6 months for the first year. This period can be extended to every 6 to 12 months in the second year and to every year for the next 2 years. Thereafter, endoscopy every 3 years is adequate. There have been reports in the literature that undifferentiated carcinoma and invasion of the malignancy into the lymphatic or vascular channels have a high risk of lymph node metastasis. In such situations, bowel resection should be performed even though the invasion is limited to the head of the polyp (53–57). A pedunculated polyp with level 4 invasion is treated the same way as a sessile lesion.

Sessile Polyp with Invasive Carcinoma

The Haggitt classification has been widely used for pedunculated polyps with invasive carcinoma in the United States but it is not adequate for sessile lesions. In 1993, Kudo (58) classified the submucosal invasion of the sessile lesions into three levels (Fig. 10):

Sm1—invasion into the upper third of the submucosa.
Sm2—invasion into the middle third of the submucosa.
Sm3—invasion into the lower third of the submucosa.

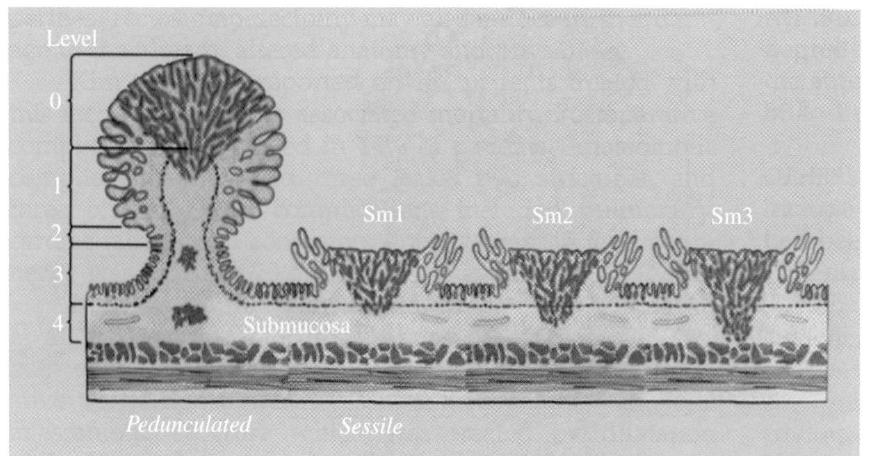

FIGURE 10 ■ Incorporation of Haggitt classification to Sm system. *Abbreviations*: Sm1 = Invasion into upper ⅓ of submucosa. Sm2 = Invasion into middle ⅓ of submucosa. Sm3 = Invasion into distal ⅓ of submucosa. Haggitt's pedunculated levels 1, 2, 3, are all in Sm1; pedunculated level 4 can be Sm1, Sm2, or Sm3. *Source*: With permission from the Mayo Foundation.

The consensus workshop in Paris on November 30 to December 1, 2002, recommended Sm system for early carcinoma of the large bowel (59). The Sm system appears to be effective and practical. In the series by Nascimbeni et al. (60), the pathologist could evaluate the depth of invasion into Sm1, Sm2, and Sm3 in 97% of the cases. In fact, the Haggitt level for the pedunculated lesion can be incorporated into the Sm system (Fig. 10). The endoscopists must properly prepare the specimens and the pathologists must properly section them in order to examine the entire layers.

Among the increased risk factors for early colorectal carcinoma reported in the literature are: lymphovascular invasion, poor differentiation, gender, extensive budding, micro-acinar structure, flat or depressed lesions, and depth of invasion in submucosa (61). Recent studies with multivariate analysis showed the independent risk of lymph node metastasis in early carcinoma of rectum to be: lymphovascular invasion and invasion into the depth of the submucosa (Sm3) (60,62). When the rectum was divided into three levels, Nascimbeni et al. (60) showed that the lower third of rectum had a high risk of lymph node metastasis.

Some sessile lesions with invasive carcinoma < 2 cm in diameter in the colon, upper third and middle third of rectum can be adequately snared in one piece via colonoscopy. A microscopic free margin of at least 2 mm is considered adequate (53). A malignant lesion that is removed piecemeal requires further excision or resection. A sessile lesion that has high risk factors such as lymphovascular invasion and deep invasion into Sm3 level should have an oncologic resection. In case of a lower third rectal lesion, a full thickness transanal excision is required. Some authors advise postoperative radiation or chemoradiation (63–65); some series showed no advantage, or showed high recurrence rate (66,67). Benson et al. (67) reported a series of 21 patients with T1 adenocarcinoma of the lower third of the rectum (median 4 cm from anal verge) underwent radiation therapy without chemotherapy after a local transanal excision, the recurrence at five years was 39% and the disease-free survival at 5 years was 59%.

A sessile polyp with invasive carcinoma or an early carcinoma of the low rectum is unique in that in spite of favorable histopathologic parameters, a full thickness transanal excision has a high recurrence rate from 7% to 29% and a cancer-specific 5-year survival of 74% to 95% (Table 4) (66,68–70). In a retrospective study by Nascimbeni et al. (70) on the outcome comparing transanal local excision to oncologic resection for T1 carcinoma of low rectum revealed that for carcinoma of middle-third rectum or lower-third rectum, the 5-year and 10-year outcomes were significantly better for overall survival and cancer-free survival in the oncologic resection group. Local recurrence and distant metastasis were not significantly different. When it came to T1 carcinoma of the lower-third rectum, the authors showed the oncologic resection group had a trend of improved survival but was not statistically significant, possibly because of low statistical power from the small sample size.

Suitable cases of T1 carcinoma of rectum for a transanal excision are uncommon. Some authors recommended to do it even fewer (69). Transanal excision for a sessile polyp with invasive carcinoma, or a T1 carcinoma of the low rectum has a three to fivefold higher risk of carcinoma recurrence compared with patients treated by radical resection (71). Waiting to perform a radical resection after a local recurrence is a poor choice. In most series, the cancer-free survival for salvage resection in these patients is 50% to 56% (68,69). On the other hand, an immediate radical resection after local excision (within 1 month), gives a better prognosis, 94% cancer-free survival at 10 years and is comparable to primary resection in a case-controlled comparison (72).

In short, local excision for a sessile polyp with invasive carcinoma (T1) of the lower third of rectum has high local recurrence. It appears that the early lesion at this site is a locally disseminated disease. To improve the outcome, the recurrence rate has to be improved: options include doing more radical resection in young and good health patients;

TABLE 4 ■ **Selected Series of Local Recurrence and Survival After Transanal Excision for T1 Carcinoma of the Rectum**

Institution	No.	LR (%)	5-Yr Survival (%, CSS)	F-U (mo)
University of Minnesota (68)	69	18	95	52
Memorial Sloan-Kettering (66)	67	14	74	60
Cleveland Clinic (69)	52	29	75	55
Mayo Clinic (70)	70	7	89	60

Abbreviations: LR, local recurrence; CSS, cancer-specific survival; F-U, follow-up.

finding a better adjuvant therapy; or finding better ways in selection of patients, such as molecular markers in the future.

Serrated Adenoma

This is the term coined by Longacre and Fenoglio-Preiser in 1990 (73) to describe a new entity of mixed hyperplastic polyp/adenomatous polyp. In their study of 110 serrated adenomas, compared to 60 traditional adenomas and 40 hyperplastic polyps, they found that these lesions distributed throughout the colon and rectum, with a slight preponderance of large lesions (> 1 cm) occurred in the cecum and appendix.

There are two types of mixed epithelial polyps: one in which adenomatous and hyperplastic glands are mixed (Fig. 11A), and one in which the adenoma has a serrated appearance on microscopic examination (Fig. 11B). Microscopic examination of the lesions shows goblet cell immaturity, prominent architectural distortion, cytologically atypical nuclei, rare upper zone mitoses, and absence of a thickened collagen table (73,74).

Grossly the lesion is flat and smooth; it may look like a plaque or thickened mucosa on colonoscopic examination (Fig. 12). This type of lesion can be easily missed on colonoscopy if the colon is overdistended stretching it flat or underdistended causing wrinkle on mucosa to mask it. Unlike the classic hyperplastic polyps that are small and restricted to the rectum and rectosigmoid colon, serrated adenomas are larger and occur in both proximal and distal colon and rectum (75). Some of the individuals previously reported as having multiple hyperplastic polyps could instead have had multiple serrated adenomatous polyps (73).

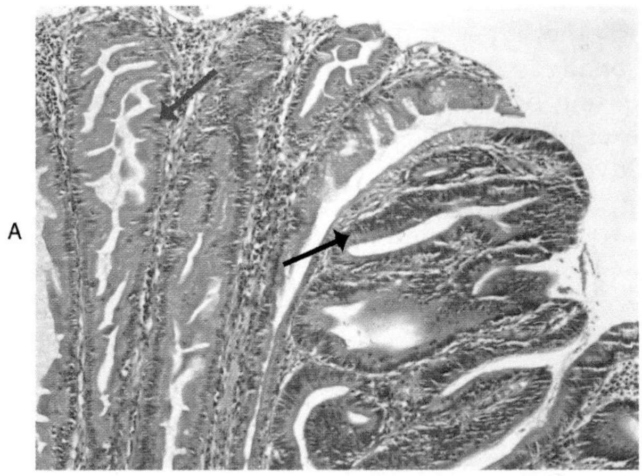

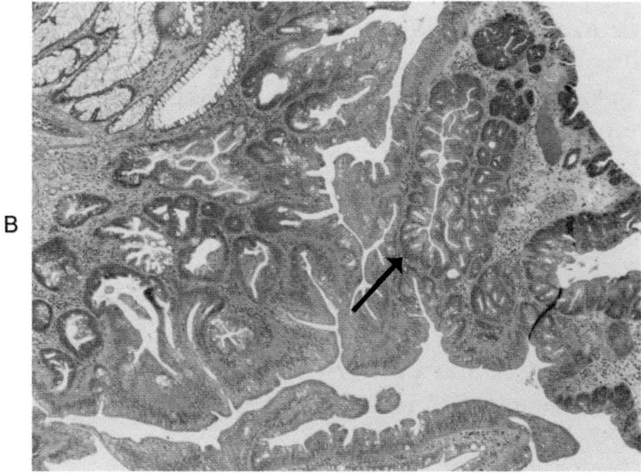

FIGURE 11 ■ (**A**) Mixed hyperplastic gland (*red arrow*) and adenomatous gland (*black arrow*). (**B**) Adenomatous gland with serrated appearance (*arrow*). *Source*: Courtesy of Thomas C. Smyrk, M.D., Mayo Clinic, Rochester, MN, U.S.A.

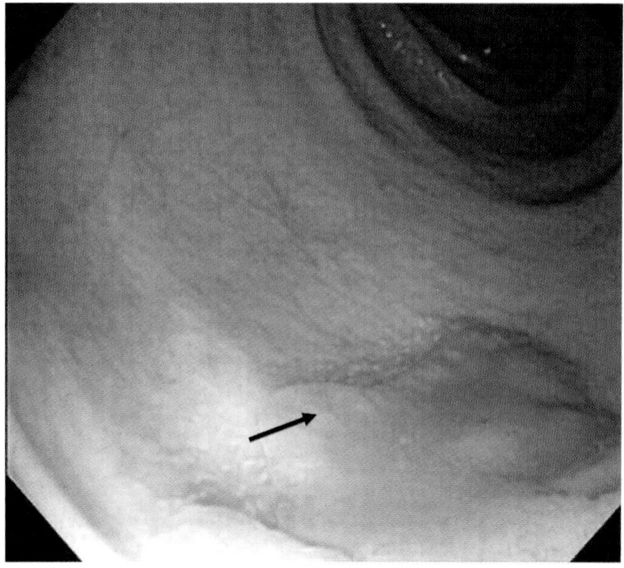

FIGURE 12 ■ Plaque-like serrated adenoma in transverse colon.

Clinical Importance of Serrated Adenoma

Based on the observation that 11% of serrated adenomas in the series of Longacre and Fenoglio-Preiser (73) contained foci of intramucosal carcinoma, it was surmised that an individual lesion would carry a significant malignant potential. Nevertheless, the rarity of serrated adenoma (0.6% of colorectal polyps) would minimize their contribution to the overall burden of colorectal malignancy (76). Torlakovic and Snover (74) reported six patients with serrated adenomatous polyposis. Each patient had at least 50 polyps, ranging from 0.3 to 4.5 cm in size, mostly sessile. Three patients had diffuse polyps, two patients had the polyps in the left colon, and one patient had them in the right colon. Four patients had carcinoma.

Why are serrated adenomas infrequently observed in endoscopic practice? The answer may lie partly in under diagnosis and partly in their rapid evolution to carcinoma. The latter suggestion is supported by the demonstration of DNA microsatellite instability in mixed polyps and serrated adenomas and by analogy with the aggressive adenomas in hereditary nonpolyposis colorectal cancer (HNPCC) (76).

Genetics

The known alterations include K-*ras* mutation, low and occasional high level microsatellite instability, 1pLOH, and methylation of HPP1/TPEF (a putative anti-adhesion molecule). Additional genetic alterations may be observed in neoplastic subclones occurring within or adjacent to hyperplastic polyps. These include loss of expression of MGMT or hMLH1 (77).

Sporadic MSI-L and MSI-H carcinomas may evolve through the serrated adenoma pathway (76). The serrated adenoma pathway is likely to show marked molecular heterogeneity, but patterns are beginning to emerge. The view

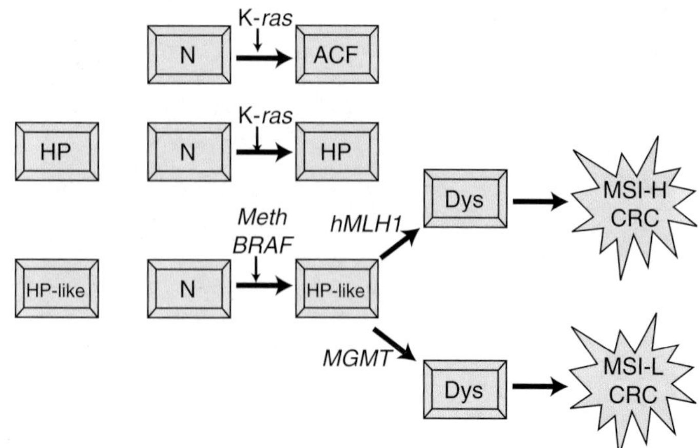

FIGURE 13 ■ Possible key steps in three pathways to aberrant crypt foci (ACF), hyperplastic polyp, and hyperplastic-like polyp or small serrated adenoma. (See details in text.) *Abbreviations*: N, Normal mucosa; HP, hyperplastic polyp; Meth, methylation; BRAF, a gene encoding a kinase that is regulated by K-ras; DYS, dysplasia; MSI-H, microsatellite instability-high; MSI-L, microsatellite instability-low; CRC, colorectal carcinoma. *Source*: From Ref. 77.

that all, or even most, colorectal carcinomas are initiated by mutation of APC gene and evolve through the classical adenoma-carcinoma sequence may no longer be tenable. This understanding will surely transform our approach to the early detection and prevention of colorectal carcinoma (76).

Figure 13 illustrated the possible key steps in three pathways to ACF, hyperplastic polyp, and hyperplastic-like polyp or small, serrated adenoma. The molecular steps that determine growth of ACF into hyperplastic polyp are not known. Colorectal carcinoma is envisioned to arise from hyperplastic-like polyps (or sessile serrated polyps) in which the earliest events might be BRAF mutation synergizing with a methylated and silenced pro-apoptotic gene. Subsequent methylation of hMLH1 or MGMT then predisposes to mutation, dysplastic change, and finally to malignancy that is frequently characterized by MSI-H or MSI-L status. K-*ras* mutation may substitute for BRAF in methylator pathways culminating in MSI-L and some MSS colorectal carcinomas (78).

Management

Serrated adenomas are neoplastic polyps. The treatment is the same as in adenomatous polyps.

■ HAMARTOMATOUS POLYPS

A hamartoma is a malformation or inborn error of tissue development characterized by an abnormal mixture of tissues endogenous to the part, with excess of one or more of these tissues. It may show itself at birth or by extensive growth in the postnatal period.

Juvenile Polyps and Juvenile Polyposis

Juvenile polyps characteristically occur in children, although they may present in adults at any age. This type of polyp is a hamartoma and is not pre-malignant. Macroscopically they are pink, smooth, round, and usually pedunculated. The cut section shows a cheeselike appearance from dilated cystic spaces. Microscopic pictures show dilated glands filled with mucus and an abnormality of the lamina propria, which has a mesenchymal appearance (Fig. 14). The muscularis mucosa does not participate in the structure of the polyp. Bleeding from the rectum is a common finding. A moderate amount of bleeding can occur if the polyp is auto-amputated, a phenomenon not seen in other types of polyps. Intussusception of the colon occasionally occurs if the polyp is large. Treatment is by excision or snaring through a colonoscope or a transanal excision.

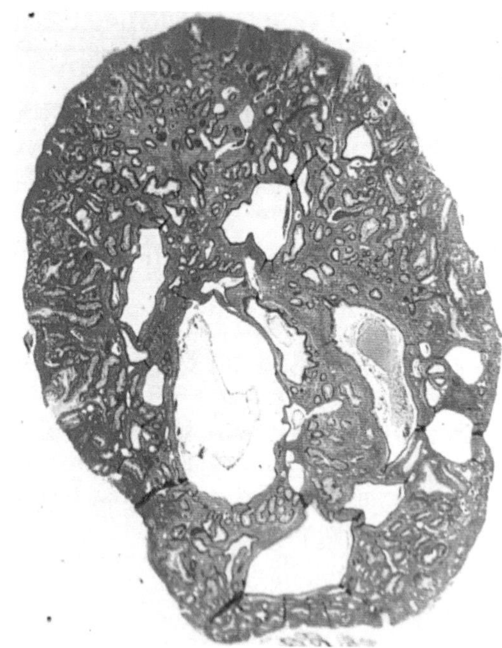

FIGURE 14 ■ Juvenile or retention polyp. Note the Swiss-cheese appearance from dilated glands.

Juvenile polyposis is an entity characteristically and biologically distinct from solitary juvenile polyp or other polyposis. The condition was first observed by McCall et al. in 1964 (79). The term juvenile polyposis rather than juvenile polyposis coli is to be preferred as polyps are also found in the stomach and the small intestine (80). There are two types of juvenile polyposis: in infancy and in other variable age of onset (81).

Juvenile Polyposis of Infancy

Juvenile polyposis of infancy is a rare form. No family history is found. The infant presents with diarrhea, either bloody or mucinous, anemia, protein-losing enteropathy, intussusception; rectal prolapse develops between 8 and 10 months of age and leads to significant morbidity (81,82). The entire gastrointestinal (GI) tract is usually affected; the prognosis depends on the severity and extent of GI involvement. Death occurs before the age of 2 years in severe cases (80).

Surgery is indicated in cases of intussusception, or polypectomies in cases of rectal prolapse to reduce the leading point of the prolapse. Supportive care to replace fluid and electrolytes or total parenteral nutrition as indicated (82).

Juvenile Polyposis in Childhood and Adult

The majority of patients with juvenile polyposis manifest in their first or second decade but in 15% of patients, the diagnosis is delayed until they are adults. They usually present with rectal bleeding and anemia. Family history of juvenile polyposis is found in 20% to 50% of patients. Various extra-colonic abnormalities, described in 11% to 20% of cases, have included digital clubbing, pulmonary arteriovenous fistula, macrocephaly, alopecia, bony swellings, cleft lip, cleft palate, supernumerary teeth, porphyria, arteriovenous malformation affecting the skin, psoriasis, congenital heart disease, malrotation of the gut, abnormalities involving the vitello-intestinal duct, double renal pelvis and ureter, acute glomerulonephritis, undescended testes, and bifid uterus and vagina (80).

Patients with juvenile polyposis usually have 50 to 200 colorectal polyps and a proportion have polyps in the stomach and small intestine. Some patients seem to have relatively few polyps, but these tend to be the parent of the prospectus. It is conceivable that the juvenile polyps are produced only within the first few decades and are subsequently lost through autoamputation. Thus, juvenile polyposis may be diagnosed when a relatively old and asymptomatic parent is screened colonoscopically and the smallest number of polyps found on this basis is 5 (81).

Jass et al. (81) proposed a working definition of juvenile polyposis:

1. More than five juvenile polyps of the colorectum.
2. Juvenile polyps throughout the GI tract.
3. Any number of juvenile polyps with a family history of juvenile polyposis.

On the other hand, Giardiello et al. (83) suggested that the patients with as few as three juvenile polyps should undergo screening for colorectal neoplasm.

A Precancerous Condition

Although there is no evidence that isolated juvenile polyp could be malignant, it is now well established that juvenile polyposis is a precancerous condition (81,84–87). The risk of GI malignancy in affected members of juvenile polyposis kindred exceeds 50% in a series of kindred reported by Howe et al. (84).

In a classic paper on juvenile polyposis, Jass et al. (81) studied 87 patients with juvenile polyposis recorded in the St. Mark's Polyposis Registry, including 1032 polyps and 18 patients with colorectal carcinoma. They found that about 20% of juvenile polyps did not conform to the classical description. Grossly, they formed lobular mass (instead of spherical). These atypical juvenile polyps also revealed relatively less lamina propria and more epithelium than that found in the more typical variety and often adopted a villous or papillary configuration. Epithelial dysplasia occurred in both typical and atypical juvenile polyps but was very much more frequent in the latter. Nearly 50% of the atypical juvenile polyps showed some degree of dysplasia; these resembled adenomatous dysplasia. Eighteen patients in this series had colorectal adenocarcinoma with a mean age of 34 years (range 15–59 years). A high proportion of carcinomas were mucinous and/or poorly differentiated and this is in accord with case reports from other authors.

There is little direct information on the histogenesis of carcinoma in juvenile polyposis. Dysplasia has been shown to occur in two forms: (*i*) a focus of adenomatous change within a polyp, (*ii*) an adenoma showing no residual juvenile features (81).

On the mechanism of polyp-cancer sequence in juvenile polyposis, Kinzler and Vogelstein (85) postulated, "an abnormal stroma can affect the development of adjacent epithelial cells is not a new concept. Ulcerative colitis is an autoimmune disease that leads to inflammation and cystic epithelium in the mucosa of the colon. Initially, the imbedded epithelium shows no neoplastic changes, but foci of epithelial neoplasia and progression to cancer eventually develops in many cases. The regeneration that occurs to replace damaged epithelium may increase the probability of somatic mutations in this abnormal microenvironment. The increased risk of cancer in juvenile polyposis syndrome and ulcerative colitis patients, therefore, seems primarily the result of an altered terrain for epithelial cell growth and can be thought of as a *landscaper defect*."

Genetics

Juvenile polyposis is an autosomal dominant condition (84). The germ-line mutation is in the gene SMAD-4 (also known as DPC-4), located on chromosome 18q21.1 (88,89).

Management and Surveillance

There is no good information about prophylactic colectomy or proctocolectomy to prevent occurrence of carcinoma. The decision on performing the operation should be dictated by the number and the site of the polyps. Polyps of the colon and rectum that are too numerous for colonoscopy and polypectomies should have an abdominal colectomy with ileorectal anastomosis (IRA) or proctocolectomy with ileal pouch-anal anastomosis (IPAA) or an ileostomy (80,86,90,91).

In a series reported by Onsel et al. (90), 5 of 10 patients who underwent colectomy with IRA for juvenile polyposis required a subsequent proctectomy with a mean follow-up of 9 years (range 6–34 years). This and other studies suggest that proctocolectomy with ileoanal pouch procedure may be a better option as an initial operation (90,91).

The proband and relatives of the first degree should be screened, probably starting in the later teen years, by upper and lower GI endoscopy. If this initial screen is negative, a follow-up endoscopy should be performed every 3 years (92). For patients who have had a colectomy or an ileoanal pouch, surveillance should be performed periodically (90,91).

Howe et al. (93) recommended genetic testing as part of the workup. However, given the presumed genetic heterogeneity of this syndrome, failure to show a mutation in SMAD-4 does not support lengthening the surveillance interval to 10 years as they suggested (90).

Peutz-Jeghers Syndrome

PJS is a rare autosomal dominant disease characterized by GI hamartomatous polyposis and mucocutaneous pigmentation. It was originally described by Peutz in 1921 but was not clearly identified until attention was brought to it by Jeghers, McKusick, and Katz (94) in 1949. The syndrome comprises of melanin spots of buccal mucosa arid lips; the face and digits may be involved to a variable extent, but mouth pigmentation is the sine qua non of this portion

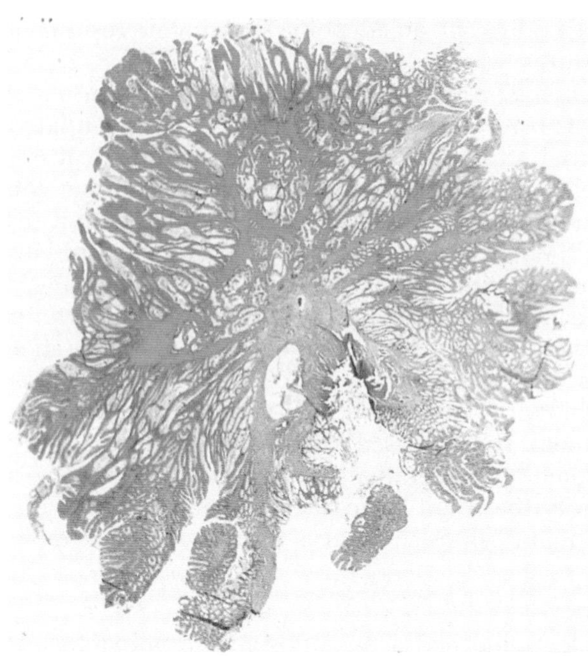

FIGURE 15 ■ Peutz-Jeghers polyp. Note Christmas-tree appearance from branching of muscularis mucosa.

of the syndrome. The presence of polyps in the small bowel is a constant finding of this syndrome, but the stomach, colon, and rectum also may be involved. The characteristic Peutz-Jeghers polyp has an abnormal muscularis mucosa branching into the lamina propria, giving the appearance of a Christmas tree (Fig. 15).

Diagnosis

Giardiello et al. (95) defined a definitive diagnosis of PJS by the presence of histologically confirmed hamartomatous polyps, plus at least two of the following:

1. Family history of the syndrome.
2. Labial melanin deposits.
3. Small bowel polyposis.

The diagnosis is "probable" if two of the three clinical criteria described above are present but without histopathological verification of hamartomatous polyps (95). Genetic testing may then be used to confirm the diagnosis (96).

For patients without a family history of PJS, definitive diagnosis depends upon the presence of two or more histologically verified Peutz-Jeghers type hamartomatous polyps (97). For patients with a first-degree relative with PJS, the presence of mucocutaneous hyperpigmentation is sufficient for presumptive diagnosis (96).

Genetics

To date, the only identifiable mutations causing PJS affect the serine/threonine-protein kinase 11 (STK11, also known as LKB1) gene, located on chromosome 19p13.3. Although PJS is inherited in an autosomal dominant manner, up to 25% of documented cases are not familial. These sporadic cases are felt to be due to de novo mutations in STK11 or low penetrance variance (96).

Genetic testing for STK11 mutations is available but they have variable sensitivity. In familial cases with a known genetic linkage to STK11, testing carries a sensitivity of 70%. In sporadic cases, genetic testing has sensitivity ranging from 30% to 67%. A significant proportion of familial and sporadic Peutz-Jeghers cases may result from mutations in genes other than STK11 (96).

High Risk of Cancers

It is a well-known fact that patients with PJS have high risk of developing cancer in many parts of the body. However, the risk varies depending on how the studies are undertaken. Giardiello et al. (98) conducted an individual patient metaanalysis to determine the relative risk (RR) of malignancy in patients with PJS compared with general population. The authors used strict criteria for the analysis. Searches of MEDLINE EMBASE, and referenced articles yielded 94 articles. Only six publications which consisted of 210 individuals qualified for the study. The results showed that the RR for all carcinomas was 15.2. A statistically significant increase of RR was noted for: esophagus (57.0), stomach (213.0), small intestine (520.0), colon (84.0), pancreas (132.0), lung (17.0), breast (15.2), uterus (16.0), ovary (27.0). There was no risk for testicular or cervical malignancy. The cumulative risk for all malignancy was 93% from age 15 to 64 years old.

Carcinoma in Peutz-Jeghers Polyps

Ordinarily, hamartomatous polyps should not degenerate into malignancy. However, there have been reports of invasive adenocarcinoma in Peutz-Jeghers polyps of the small and large intestine, although the risk is not high. Giardiello et al. (95) did not detect invasive carcinoma within hamartomatous polyps in any of their patients. The polyps containing hamartomatous, adenomatous, and malignant components have been observed in Peutz-Jeghers polyps of the small and large intestine (99–103). Spigelman et al. (102) surveyed 72 patients registered with PJS at St. Mark's Polyposis Registry. Four patients had nine carcinomas in hamartomatous polyps in stomach, duodenum, jejunum, and colon. This observation suggests that a hamartomatous, adenomatous, and carcinomatous progression may be important in the development of malignancy in Peutz-Jeghers polyps.

Genetic analysis showed that STK11/LKB1 acts as a tumor suppressor gene and may be involved in the early stages of PJS carcinogenesis (104,105). The results suggest that Peutz-Jeghers related carcinoma have different molecular genetic alteration compared with those found in sporadic GI carcinomas (103).

Peutz-Jeghers–Like Mucocutaneous Pigmentation

Characteristic mucocutaneous pigmentation is often the clinical clue that heralds the diagnosis of PJS. The melanotic or lentiginous pigmented macules are dark brown, blue, or blue-brown and located on the vermillion border of the lips (>90%), buckle mucosa, digits, and occasionally on the periorbital, auricular, perianal, and vulva skin (106). The relevance of PJS-like hyperpigmentation in the absence of other features of PJS is not known. Boardman et al. (106) coined the terms isolated melanotic mucocutaneous pigmentation (IMMP).

To ascertain the risk of malignancy for patients with IMMP, they identified a group of individuals with mucocutaneous melanotic macules indistinguishable clinically from PJS hyperpigmentation but who did not manifest the other phenotypic characteristics of PJS. To distinguish those patients with possible or definite PJS from those with pigmentation only, the authors applied the diagnostic criteria of Giardiello et al. (95) to define definite PJS. Patients who had PJS-like oral hyperpigmentation only and none of the other criteria of PJS were classified as IMMP. Of 60 patients who had the diagnosis of PJS or PJS-like pigmentation were identified through the patient registry of the Mayo Clinic from 1945 to 1996. Twenty-six unrelated patients were identified with IMMP. There were 16 men and 10 women.

The results showed that 10 individuals developed 12 noncutaneous malignancies including breast ($n = 1$), cervical ($n = 3$), endometrial ($n = 3$), renal ($n = 1$), lung ($n = 2$), colon ($n = 1$), and lymphoma ($n = 1$). The median age of diagnosis of noncutaneous malignancy was 47 years (range 33–84 years); this compared to a median age of carcinoma in the general population of 68 years. In their previous review of carcinoma risk in PJS patients, the median age at diagnosis of carcinoma was 38 years (range 16–59 years) (105). The mean interval from the identification of the pigmentation to the development of carcinoma in IMMP patients was 24.2 years, compared to a mean latency period of 19.9 years in PJS patients (103,106). Although the magnitude and gender associations of carcinomas in patients with IMMP and PJS are remarkably similar, the authors detected no alterations in the LKB1 among IMMP patients. Is IMMP an entity distinct from PJS? The overlap in the two conditions of phenotypic pigmentary features and the increased risk of malignancy, specifically of the breast and gynecologic tract in women, support the notion that they might share a common genetic origin. Though none of nine individuals with IMMP had mutations in LKB1, 14% to 42% of patients with definite PJS lack LKB1 mutations, suggesting that another yet to be identified gene or genes may be responsible for cases of both PJS and IMMP not caused by LKB1 mutations (106). Based on the increased RR for gynecologic and breast carcinomas that they detected in their patient population of IMMP, the authors recommend following current screening guidelines for gynecologic and breast carcinoma with thorough evaluation of PJS-like pigmentation. They recommended examination of the GI tract at age 20 years in asymptomatic individuals with PJS-like hyperpigmentation.

Screening

Given the multitude of carcinomas that these patients are susceptible, aggressive screening protocols are recommended. Upper and lower GI endoscopies are indicated for any adolescent or adult suspected of having PJS. Radiographic studies should also be used to screen for distal small intestinal polyps. Pelvic ultrasound of females and gonadal examination in young men is also recommended.

An at-risk, but unaffected relative is a first-degree relative of an individual with PJS who does not meet clinical criteria for PJS. Guidelines for surveillance of affected patients also apply to these at-risk family members. The current guideline for carcinoma screening is summarized in Table 5.

Management of Peutz-Jeghers Polyps

The clinical course of PJS is characterized by asymptomatic periods interspersed with complications such as abdominal pain, intussusception often leading to frank intestinal obstruction, and hemorrhage that is often occult. Small bowel obstruction is the presenting complaint in half of the cases, and exploratory celiotomy due to polyp-induced complications occurs commonly and may do so at quite short intervals (107). Because this problem is coupled with the significant risk of malignancy in the polyps, the surgical approach is now more aggressive. The current approach is to operate on the patient if the small intestinal polyps are larger than 1.5 cm (107,108).

Endoscopic resection of Peutz-Jeghers polyps throughout the small intestine at double-balloon enteroscopy without exploratory celiotomy has been reported to be successful (109). However, in general, an enteroscopy is performed at the time of exploratory celiotomy with polypectomy or resection of the small bowel (110,111). The indications for surgery included obstructing or intussuscepting polyps, polyps larger than 1.5 cm identified radiologically, or smaller polyps associated with iron deficiency anemia (111).

In order to achieve more complete polyp clearance, Edwards et al. (111) analyzed their experience of using intraoperative enteroscopy in conjunction with explore celiotomy. The enteroscope was introduced through an enterotomy at the site of polypectomy for the largest polyps. Depending on the size of the polyps, snare polypectomy, electrocoagulation, or biopsies were performed. In their experience of 25 patients, enteroscopy identified 350 polyps not detected by palpation or transillumination of the bowel by an operating light. All the polyps were removed. There was one early complication of a delayed small bowel perforation at the site of a snare polypectomy that resulted in an urgent reoperation but no long-term sequelae. No patient in this group had required operative polypectomy within four years of polyp clearance by intraoperative enteroscopy, compared with registry data of 4 of 23 patients who had more than one exploratory celiotomy within a year. It appears that intraoperative enteroscopy for PJS improves polyp clearance without the need for additional enterotomies and may help to reduce the frequency of exploratory celiotomy (112).

TABLE 5 ■ **Screening Recommendations for Peutz-Jeghers Syndrome**

Organs	Age to Begin	Interval (yr)	Procedure
Colon	25	2	Colonoscopy
Gastrointestinal tract	10	2	Upper endoscopy
Pancreas	30	1–2	Endoscopic ultrasound Transabdominant ultrasound
Breast	20	2 1	Mammography Self-breast exam
Uterus	20	1	Transvaginal ultrasound Endometrial biopsy
Cervix	20	1	Pap smear
Testicular	10	1	Physical exam, ultrasound if clinically indicated

Source: From Ref. 96.

Cronkhite-Canada Syndrome

Cronkhite-Canada syndrome is characterized by generalized GI polyposis associated with alopecia, cutaneous pigmentation, and atrophy of fingernails and toenails (Onychotrophia). It was first deducted in two patients and described by Cronkhite and Canada in 1955 (113).

Etiology

The etiology is unknown. There is no familial inheritance pattern and no associated gene or mutation has been identified (114).

Clinical Presentations

Diarrhea is a prominent feature of this syndrome, accounting for 46 of 55 patients in the series of Daniel et al. (115). The cause of diarrhea is unknown. Nardone et al. (116) reported a case of Cronkhite-Canada syndrome associated with achlorhydria and hypergastrinemia causing direct gastric wall invasion by gram-negative *Campylobacter pylori*. This may explain the diarrhea in those patients.

Hair loss was noted in 49 of 55 patients. In most patients, hair loss took place simultaneously from the scalp, eyebrows, face, axillae, pubic areas and extremities, but in some only loss of scalp hair was described (115).

Nail changes were reported in 51 of 55 patients. In most of them, the nails showed varying degrees of dystrophy, such as thinning and splitting, and partial separation from the nail bed (onycholysis). Complete loss of all finger and toenails (onychomadesis), over a period of several weeks, was also noted in some patients (115).

Hyperpigmentation was present in 45 of 55 patients, ranging from a few millimeters to 10 cm in diameter. The distribution of pigmentary skin changes could be anywhere, including extremities, face, palms, soles, neck, back, chest, scalp, and lips (115).

Other manifestations include nausea, vomiting, weakness, weight loss, abdominal pain, numbness and tingling of extremities (115).

Electrolyte disturbances are a prominent feature and appear to reflect malabsorption and losses from the GI tract. Total serum protein is also found to be low in most patients due to excessive enteric protein loss (115).

The Polyps

From radiologic, endoscopic, and autopsy data, the stomach and large intestine were involved in 53 of 55 cases. The actual frequency of small bowel involvement would be inaccurate because the small bowel X-rays and biopsies were not performed in every case, in the series of Daniel et al. (115). From the autopsy data, the number of polyps were greatest in the duodenum, less in the jejunum and proximal ileum, and again increased in the terminal ileum (115).

The polyps consist of cystic dilatation of the epithelial tubules similar to that of juvenile polyps, but the lesions are usually smaller and do not show marked excess of lamina propria (115,117).

Risk of Malignancy in Polyps

The true incidence of GI carcinoma in Cronkhite-Canada syndrome is unknown. In the review of literature by Daniel et al. (115) in 55 cases, they found six cases of carcinoma of the colon and/or rectum, including one case of carcinoma of the stomach. Some of these carcinomas were multiple. Watanabe et al. (118) reported a case of Cronkhite-Canada syndrome associated with triple gastric carcinoma. Histopathologic examination revealed that the polyp underwent malignant transformation without an adenoma component.

Management

There has been no specific treatment. The management is symptomatic and the correction of any deficiencies. A complete spontaneous remission has been reported (119).

Bowel resection is reserved for cases in which complications such as carcinoma, bleeding, intussusception, and rectal prolapse develop (115). Surgery is not usually performed for improvement of protein-losing gastroenteropathy because the protein losing is usually not localized (120). Hanzawa et al. (120) reported a patient with Cronkhite-Canada syndrome with numerous polyps in the stomach, duodenum, and from cecum to transverse colon. The patient had severe hypoproteinemia and peripheral edema, unresponsive to conservative treatment including elemental diet and hyperalimentation. Scintigraphy with technetium TC99m-labeled human albumin (121,122) demonstrated a protein-losing region in the ascending colon. An ileo-right colectomy was performed. After the operation, the protein-losing enteropathy stopped; the ectodermal changes improved, and other polyps that was a secondary cause to malnutrition regressed.

Cowden's Disease

Cowden's disease is an uncommon familial syndrome of combined ectodermal, endodermal, and mesodermal hamartomas. The disease was named after the family name of the propositus by Lloyd and Dennis in 1963 (123).

Eighty percent of patients present with dermatologic manifestations, such as keratosis of extremities, the most common being a benign neoplasm of the hair shaft: a trichilemmoma. If a patient is diagnosed with more than one trichilemmoma, consideration should be given to the diagnosis of Cowden's disease. The second most common area of involvement is the central nervous system. Cowden's disease in concert with cerebella gangliocytomatosis is referred to as the Lhermitte-Duclos syndrome. Approximately 40% of affected individuals have macrocephaly as a component of the syndrome. Only 35% of patients who meet the diagnostic criteria for Cowden's disease have GI polyposis (124).

Polyps in patients with Cowden's disease are small, typically < 5 mm in diameter. Microscopic features are consistent with hamartomas, characterized by disorganization and proliferation of the muscularis mucosa with minimally abnormal overlying mucosa (125).

Genetics

Most patients with Cowden's disease have been shown to subsume germ-line mutations in the PTEN gene located at 10q22 (126). PTEN is a tumor suppressor gene which has been shown to be involved with other forms of carcinoma such as familial thyroid carcinoma, inherited breast carcinoma, prostatic carcinoma, and malignant melanoma (124).

Neoplastic Risk

The majority of patients with Cowden's disease will have some form of benign thyroid or breast disease. In addition, the projected lifetime risk of thyroid malignancy is 10% and of breast malignancy is approximately 30% to 50% (127–129). There has been no reported increased risk of invasive GI malignancy to date (124).

Management and Surveillance

Screening and surveillance for breast malignancies should include a schedule of monthly breast self-examinations. Clinical examination should be undertaken annually, beginning in the late teen years or as clinically warranted by symptoms. Mammography should be implemented at the age of 25. Although no specific recommendations for thyroid surveillance have been published, annual screening by clinical examination should begin in the late teen years or as symptoms warrant. A thyroid ultrasound may be used in parallel every 1 to 2 years (124).

GI polyposis should be addressed by endoscopic surveillance. Although no definitive increased risk of colorectal carcinoma has been documented, the syndrome is rare; thus, the true risk may be unrecognized (124).

Bannayan-Ruvalcaba-Riley Syndrome

This disease encompasses three previously described disorders: Bannayan-Zonana syndrome, Riley-Smith syndrome, and Ruvalcaba-Myhre-Smith syndrome. In 1960, Riley and Smith noted an autosomal dominant condition in which macrocephaly with a slowed cycle motor development, pseudopapilledema, and multiple hemangiomas were observed (130). In 1971, Bannayan noted the congenital combination of macrocephaly with multiple subcutaneous and visceral lipoma as well as hemangiomas (131). In 1980, Ruvalcaba described two males with macrocephaly, hamartomatous intestinal polyposis, and pigmentary spotting of the penis (132). Given the clinical similarities between the conditions and the autosomal dominant pattern of inheritance, geneticists began to accept the notion of combining the disorders into a single entity as Bannayan-Ruvalcaba-Riley syndrome (96). The syndrome gene is located at chromosome 10q23 (133). Intestinal polyposis affects up to 45% of these patients. Usually multiple hamartomatous polyps are identified with the majority limited to the distal ileum and colon, though they may be seen throughout the GI tract. Histologically, they appear similar to the juvenile polyposis-type polyp (96).

Genetics

Bannayan-Ruvalcaba-Riley syndrome is an autosomal dominant condition and, like Cowden's disease, appears to be associated with genetic alterations in the PTEN gene (133).

Neoplastic Risk

There has been no increased risk of colorectal carcinoma, other GI malignancies, or extraintestinal malignancy documented in these patients (124).

■ INFLAMMATORY AND LYMPHOID POLYPS

Inflammatory polyps, or pseudopolyps, may look grossly like adenomatous polyps. However, microscopic examination shows islands of normal mucosa or mucosa with slight inflammation. They are caused by previous attacks of any form of severe colitis (ulcerative, Crohn's, amebic, ischemic, or schistosomal), resulting in partial loss of mucosa, leaving remnants or islands of relatively normal mucosa.

Radiologically, both the acute and chronic forms appear similar. Distinction can be made with the proctosigmoidoscope, but in the chronic stage a biopsy may be necessary to distinguish the condition from familial polyposis. Inflammatory polyps are not premalignant, and their presence in no way influences the potential malignant status of the patient with ulcerative colitis, a development that remains related to the extent, age of onset, and duration of disease. That these polyps are not premalignant in ulcerative colitis is relative; the potential carcinomatous status of the pseudopolyp in this condition is no more or less than that of the adjacent mucosa (134).

Benign lymphoid polyps are enlargements of lymphoid follicles commonly seen in the rectum. They may be solitary or diffuse. Their cause is unknown. Lymphoid polyps must not be confused with familial adenomatous polyposis (FAP).

The histologic criteria set out by Dawson et al. (135) for the diagnosis of benign lymphoid polyps are as follows: the lymphoid tissue must be entirely within the mucosa and submucosa; there must be no invasion of the underlying muscle coat; at least two germinal centers must be present; and if the rectal biopsy fails to include the muscle coat and no germinal centers are seen, the diagnosis is inconclusive.

■ HYPERPLASTIC POLYPS

Hyperplastic polyps, also known as metaplastic polyps, are nonneoplastic polyps commonly found in the rectum as small, pale, and glassy mucosal nodules. Most are 3 to 5 mm located predominately in the left colon (136), although larger ones can be seen in the more proximal part of the colon. Histologic differentiation from neoplastic polyps presents no problem. The characteristic picture is a sawtooth appearance of the lining of epithelial cells, producing a papillary outline (Fig. 16). There is no nuclear dysplasia and thus no potential for malignancy.

Despite the colonoscopic findings of more adenomas than hyperplastic polyps, autopsies from Hawaii, Finland,

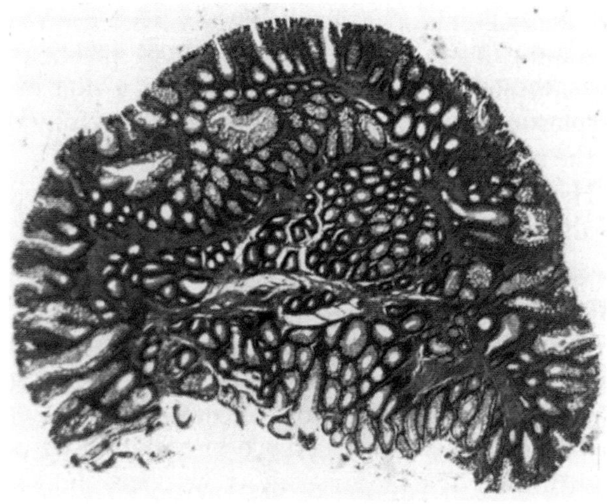

FIGURE 16 ■ Hyperplastic polyp. Note typical sawtooth appearance of the surface epithelium with a papillary appearance.

and England demonstrate hyperplastic polyps in excess upto threefold over adenomas, with the great majority of them occurring in the sigmoid colon and rectum. In contrast adenomas are distributed fairly evenly along the length of the large bowel (137). The possibility of hyperplastic polyps serving as markers for adenomas has been raised in some colonoscopic data. It is clear, though, that the predictive value of the hyperplastic polyp is low, and the clinical usefulness of the marker must be critically questioned (137).

Hyperplastic polyposis is a relatively new entity. The following criteria for hyperplastic polyposis have been proposed: (i) at least histopathologically diagnosed hyperplastic proximal to the sigmoid colon, of which two are greater than 10 mm in diameter; (ii) any number of hyperplastic polyps occurring in proximal to the sigmoid is an individual who has a first-degree relative with hyperplastic polyposis; (iii) more than 30 hyperplastic polyps of any size, but distributed throughout the colon (137). Although Williams et al. (138) found no association between hyperplastic polyposis and colorecal carcinoma, some of the polyps contained mixture of hyperplastic and adenomatous elements which nowadays would have been classified as serrated adenomas. Subsequent case reports and small series recorded the presentation of colorectal carcinoma in patients with hyperplastic polyposis (139,140). Colorectal carcinoma complicating hyperplastic polyposis is characterized by early age at onset multiplicity, frequent location in proximal colon, and greater likelihood of showing the molecular phenotype known as DNA microsatellite instability–high (MSI–H).

The association between colorectal carcinoma and hyperplastic polyposis does not prove that carcinomas orginate within hyperplastic polyposis. Adenomas might coexist with hyperplastic polyposis and might be the precursors of colorectal carcinomas, or these polyposis are infact serrated adenomas.

Little has been reported on the risk of metachronous adenomas in patients with hyperplastic polyps. Benson et al. (141) examined data from two large randomized colorectal chemoprevention trials for possible associations of hyperplastic polyps and adenomatous polyps with subsequent development of these lesions. Of the 1794 patients randomized in two trials, 1583 completed two follow-up colonoscopies, and are considered in their analysis. They computed rates of incidence on hyperplastic polyps and adenomas over the three-year follow-up after the first surveillance examination with polyp status (type and number) at that examination as predictors. During the three-year follow-up, 320 (20%) had one or more hyperplastic polyps detected, and 564 (36%) had one or more adenomas. Patients with hyperplastic polyps at the first surveillance examination had a higher risk of any hyperplastic polyp recurrence on follow-up than those without hyperplastic polyps (odds ratio 3.67). Similarly, patients with adenomas at the first surveillance examination had a higher risk of adenoma recurrence than those without adenomas (odds ratio 2.08). However, the presence of hyperplastic polyps at the first surveillance examination was not significantly associated with adenoma occurrence during follow-up, nor was the presence of adenoma significantly associated with subsequent hyperplastic polyp occurrence.

FAMILIAL ADENOMATOUS POLYPOSIS

DEFINITION AND NATURAL HISTORY

Familial adenomatous polyposis (FAP) is an inherited, non-sex-linked and Mendelian–dominant disease characterized by the progressive development of hundreds or thousands of adenomatous polyps throughout the entire large bowel. The clinical diagnosis is based on the histologic confirmation of at least 100 adenomas (Fig. 17). However, with the widespread practice of family counseling and the genetic testing, this number of adenomas is no longer rigidly applied. In the absence of a family history of FAP, the number 100 or more is still good to entertain the diagnosis. The important feature of the disease is the fact that one or more of these polyps will eventually develop into an invasive adenocarcinoma unless a prophylactic proctocolectomy is undertaken. The disease has high penetrance, with a 50% chance of development of the disease in the affected family. Approximately 20% of patients with FAP have no family history and their condition represents spontaneous mutation (142). The term "FAP" is now used to replace the term "familial polyposis coli" because the disease also affects other organs. The older terms Gardner's syndrome, familial polyposis of the gastrointestinal (GI) tract, familial multiple polyposis, and many other names should be avoided.

The incidence of FAP is one in 7000 live births (143). Although the disease is congenital, there is no evidence that adenomas have ever been present at birth. In his extensive experience with the St. Mark's Hospital, London, Polyposis Registry, Bussey (144) summarized the natural course of FAP in the average untreated patient as follows:

Age of appearance of adenomas:	25 years
Age of onset of symptoms:	33 years
Age of diagnosis of adenomas:	36 years
Age of diagnosis of carcinoma:	39 years
Age at death from carcinoma:	42 years

CLINICAL MANIFESTATIONS AND DIAGNOSIS

Symptoms usually do not develop until there is a full-blown development of polyposis. Bleeding from the rectum and diarrhea are the most common symptoms. The diagnosis is made by endoscopic examination of the colon and rectum or by barium enema studies. It must be confirmed by histologic findings of adenomatous polyps.

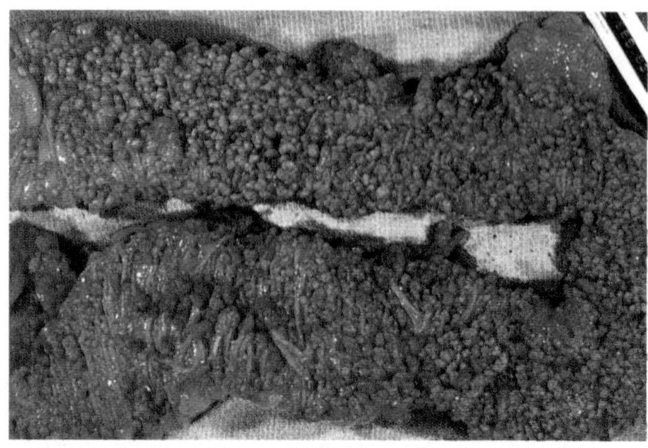

FIGURE 17 ■ Numerous small adenomatous polyps of the colon and rectum in a patient with familial adenomatous polyposis.

Only occasionally are tubulovillous adenomas found and villous adenomas are rare. The smallest possible microadenoma consists of only a single crypt, obviously not visible by examination with the naked eye (145).

The average age at which the disease is diagnosed is 36 years. The adenomas actually appear much earlier, as is seen by comparison with the age of diagnosis in family members called for examination. In this group of patients, the average age is 24 years.

Nearly two of three patients (65%) who were present because of symptoms already have carcinoma. The average age of colorectal carcinoma in these patients is 39 years, compared with 65 years in the normal population.

Since most of the polyps in FAP are small, the best methods of diagnosis are colonoscopy and biopsy. A complete colonic examination has become important since rectal sparing has been reported, even when adenocarcinoma is present in the proximal colon (146).

■ DISTRIBUTION OF POLYPS AND CARCINOMAS

Although the rectum is almost invariably involved with polyps, the number of polyps in each segment of the colon and rectum varies from person to person. In general, the left colon has a higher density of polyps than the right colon (144). In any one patient, the polyps vary in size from barely visible mucosal nodules 1 or 2 mm in diameter, to up to 1 cm or larger. In some patients and families, the adenomas are mostly small, while in others they are large. Most patients with FAP have myriads of polyps, frequently up to 5000 (147). In a series from Denmark, the risk of developing carcinoma was highest in the rectum, followed by the sigmoid colon (Table 6) (147).

TABLE 6 ■ Distribution of Colorectal Carcinoma in 109 Propositions

	No. of Carcinomas	(%)
Right colon	8	6
Transverse colon	6	5
Descending colon	8	6
Sigmoid colon	31	24
Rectum	77	59
Total	130	100

Source: From Ref. 147.

■ ATTENUATED FAMILIAL ADENOMATOUS POLYPOSIS

This is a variant of FAP that has only relatively recently been recognized (148,149). The majority of patients who were present with between 1 and 50 adenomas, primarily located proximal to the splenic flexure and often morphologically flat. The polyps are diagnosed at the mean age of 44 years, and carcinomas at the mean age of 56 years. Thus, diagnosis of polyps and carcinomas in attenuated familial adenomatous polyposis (AFAP) is generally 10 to 15 years later than in FAP. However, because these data are based on when these lesions are detected and not necessarily on when they arise, the true age of development of polyps and carcinomas in AFAP is unclear. Certainly, lack of recognition of AFAP by patients and by physicians results in fewer patients presenting for voluntary surveillance, perhaps contributing to a delay in diagnosis in these patients (150).

Clinical Features

A striking feature of AFAP is the variability in number of polyposis within members of the same kindred. Some affected members have few polyps, while others have several hundred. This variability presents difficulties in classifying members of the same kindred as AFAP or FAP. Similar to FAP, colorectal carcinomas in patients with AFAP are generally accompanied by synchronous adenomas (150). The extracolonic manifestations in AFAP are similar to FAP. Church (151) argues that AFAP is not a distinct clinical entity. It is not distinct generally because a large number of different APC mutations can be expressed as AFAP. It is not distinct clinically because patients with fewer than 100 adenomas may have FAP, HNPCC, or multiple sporadic adenomas. It is not even distinct in a familial sense, because members of AFAP family may vary widely in the severity of their polyposis. The definition of AFAP, multiple but fewer than 100 synchronous colorectal adenomas, is arbitrarily one that suffers from its imposition of a finite number on a disease with a spectrum of subtle variations. He would rather regard AFAP as some patients with FAP with a mild expression of the colonic polyposis. This mild form of the colonic disease is most common with mutations at either end of the gene, and in many cases, the polyps are predominantly right sided. However, the underlying disease remains FAP.

Diagnosis and Genetic Test

The clinical diagnosis of AFAP is more difficult than that of classic FAP because of the wide variability of phenotypic expression, and overall lack of awareness of this syndrome. In addition, screening with flexible sigmoidoscopy, the recommended modality for classic FAP, is inadequate because the majority of colonic lesions in patients with AFAP are right-sided.

For asymptomatic at-risk individuals belonging to known FAP or AFAP kindreds, genetic testing should be ideally performed between the ages of 10 and 15 years to determine the presence or absence of an APC mutation. A baseline colonoscopy and esophagoduodenoscopy at the time of genetic testing or by the age of 15 years should be performed (151). In patients with true-negative APC test results (a mutation has been demonstrated in an affected member but not in an at-risk member), a colonoscopy should be performed at the time of genetic testing or by the age of 15. Although the protein truncation test (PTT) is nearly 100% accurate in this setting, endoscopic evaluation serves as confirmation of a negative test. Because polyps occur later in AFAP individuals than in classic FAP, a second colonoscopy at age 20 should be considered to detect late, appearing polyps. If both examinations are negative, no further surveillance is necessary, and the patient may undergo future colorectal carcinoma screening as an average-risk individual (150). Church (151), however, has the opinion that people who test negative when their affected relatives test positive should be recognized that they do not have FAP and can be excluded from surveillance.

Surgical Management

Patients with AFAP are at increased risk for the development of colorectal carcinoma, although the exact risk remains unknown at this time. They do not have the near certainty of developing colorectal carcinoma that classic patients with FAP have. Thus, the indications for prophylactic colectomy differ between these two entities. In patients with few adenomas, colonoscopic polypectomy is sufficient to clear the affected bowel segments. When multiple polyps are clustered within a single segment of the colon, especially the cecum, resection may be the safest option. When resection is required, a total abdominal colectomy can be performed with an IRA. Because the rectal segment is generally uninvolved in these patients, total proctocolectomy with IPAA does not seem to be required. The rectal segment does need continued surveillance because this mucosa is still at risk. Total abdominal colectomy with IRA may also be required in patients who are difficult to examine fully by colonoscopy and, thus, unable to undergo proper surveillance (151).

AFAP has two forms: patients with mutations at the five prime of APC are at minimal risk for desmoid disease, whereas patients with mutation in exon 15 are at high risk. This risk of desmoids, often manifest in other relatives who have had an operation, may encourage deferment of surgery. The alternative to colectomy, endoscopic polypectomy with or without chemoprevention, is risky especially when the patient has been shown to carry a germline APC mutation. Colonoscopic surveillance does not prevent carcinoma in all patients with HNPCC, the same can be applied to AFAP; this must be reserved for truly compliant patients who realize the risks (151).

■ MOLECULAR GENETICS

Using genetic-linkage analysis, it has been determined that FAP is caused by a mutation in the tumor suppressor gene *APC* located on the long arm of chromosome 5q21–22. The term FAP is not used to describe this gene because familial amyloidotic polyneuropathy takes historical precedence in the genetic literature (152). The genetic alterations found in the FAP patient's colon and rectal carcinoma are similar to those noted in sporadic carcinoma, except that an *APC* mutation is already present constitutionally at birth (a germline mutation).

There are correlations between the location of the APC mutation and the clinical phenotype. Figure 18 (153) shows the correlation between the APC genotype and the clinical phenotype. The 15 exons of the APC gene are shown. The locations of germ-line mutations associated with specific clinical phenotypes indicated by the dark horizontal lines. Thirty-four mutations causing AFAP have been reported to date; these are clustered either at the five prime ends (before codon 436) or at the three prime end (after codon 1596) of the APC gene. In contrast, mutations causing classic FAP are located in the central region, and mutations between codons 1250 and 1464 are associated with particularly severe polyposis. Abdominal desmoid tumors are more likely in persons with mutations between codons 1445 and 1578.

The molecular mechanisms that explain why certain APC mutations result in a classic phenotype and others in an attenuated phenotype are currently being elucidated. Most models are predicated on the "two-hit hypothesis"—which states that both alleles of APC must be inactivated in order to initiate tumorigenesis. In Figure 19 (153), both copies of chromosome 5 are shown. In classic FAP (panel A), the biallelic inactivation of APC is typically achieved by the combination of an inherited germ-line mutation in one allele (black X) and a chromosomal deletion of the remaining wild-type allele; this is called loss of heterozygosity. In some cases, the germ-line APC mutation (red X) can result in the production of a protein that can inhibit the activity of the wild-type protein (white X). This dominant negative effect functionally results in biallelic inactivation.

In AFAP (panel B), the mechanism of APC inactivation is different. Germ-line mutations involved in AFAP may lead to the formation of alternative APC proteins that are initiated from an internal translation site that is located distal to the truncating mutation. This alternative APC protein does have functional activity. Because of this residual gene activity, an additional "hit" is necessary to fully inactivate APC (panel C). This third "hit" is indicated by the blue X. The second hit is often an intragenic mutation (green X) that inactivates the wild-type APC allele, rather than a large

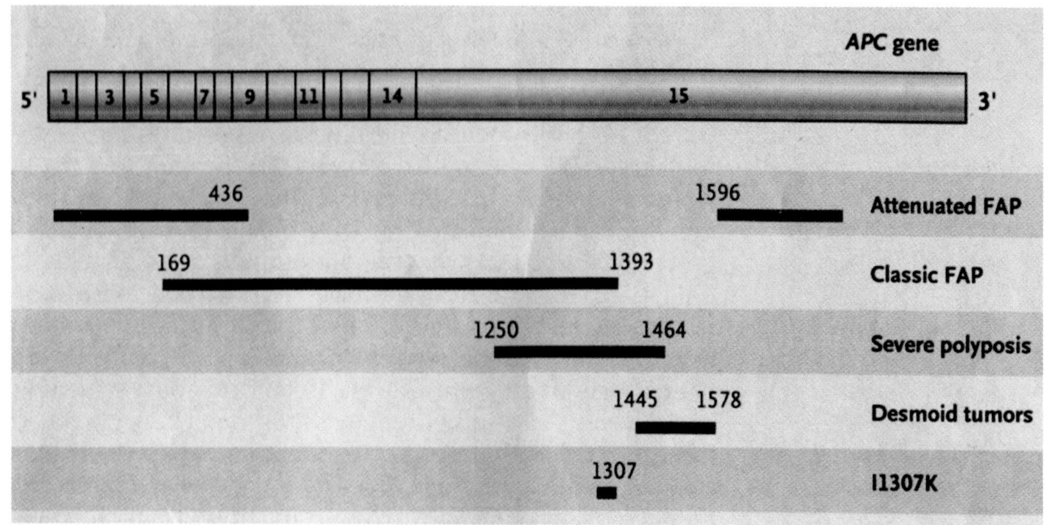

FIGURE 18 ■ Correlation between the APC genotype and the clinical phenotype. (See details in text.) *Source*: From Ref. 153.

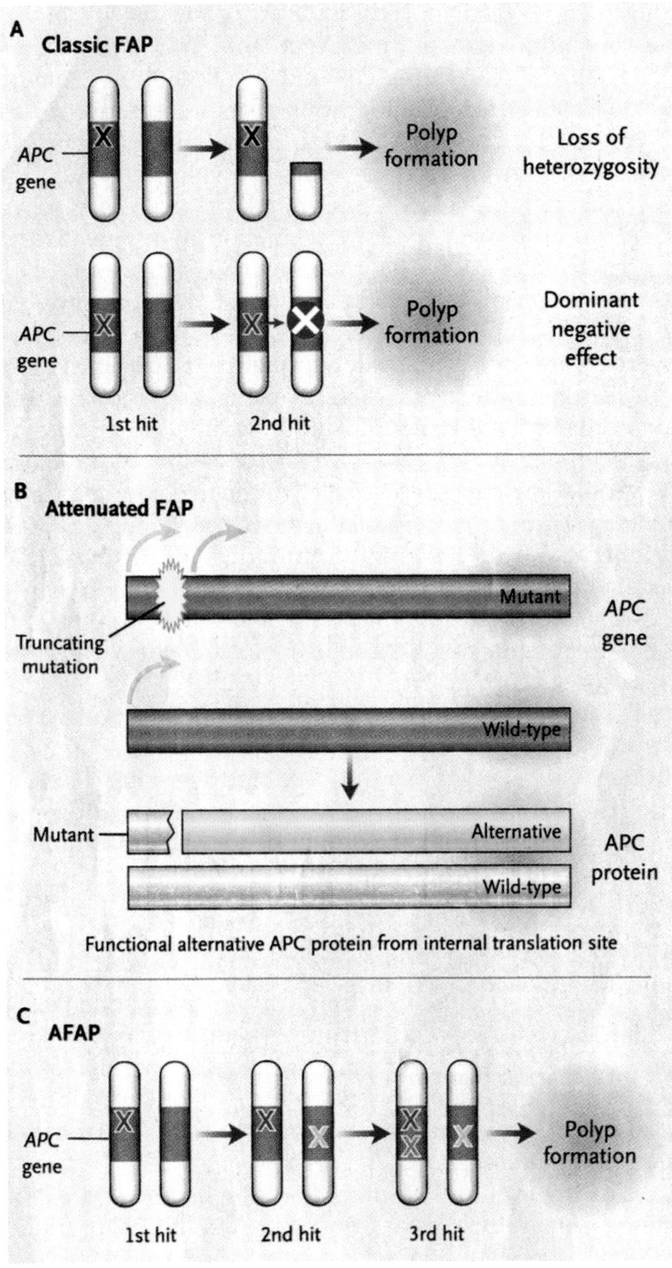

FIGURE 19 ■ Mechanisms of inactivation of the APC gene in classic and attenuated familial adenomatous polyposis (FAP). (See details in text.) *Source*: From Ref. 153.

chromosomal deletion as in classic FAP. The red X represents the inherited APC mutation (153).

■ EXTRACOLONIC EXPRESSIONS

In 1951, Gardner (154) reported finding osteomatosis, epidermoid cysts, and fibromas of the skin, a triad in FAP known as Gardner's syndrome. The detection of identical mutations in individuals with FAP and Gardner's syndrome helps confirm that at the genetic level they are variants of a common entity (155). The disease affects the whole body, involving tissues derived from all three germ layers (145). Factors that contribute to the extracolonic manifestations are unresolved. Modifying genetic factors (e.g., other genes or different genetic backgrounds) or environmental variables probably play a role in the final phenotype. Likewise, the role that APC plays in the development of various extracolonic neoplasms and manifestations remains to be defined. There have been some indications that the location of the APC mutation itself may have an effect on the phenotype, although conclusive evidence for this proposal is lacking (155).

Endodermal Abnormalities

Gastric Polyps

With improved survival rates following colorectal resection, gastric polyps or upper GI lesions have become increasingly important because of the risk of malignant change in duodenal polyps. The introduction of flexible endoscopy has provided more ready access to the upper GI tract, although at present the course of the disease is not precisely known (156).

The prevalence of gastric polyps ranges from 34% to 100%; most of them are hyperplastic type in the fundus of the stomach, and a few adenomatous types have been reported in the anturm (157,158).

Of the 102 patients screened prospectively, in the series of Spigelman et al. (159), 56 had gastric polyps. Gastric fundus polyps were small (mean 4.7 mm) and multiple, whereas antral polyps, when present, were larger (mean 6.4 mm) and less numerous. Only 6 of 73 patients who had gastric biopsy revealed adenoma. When gastric adenomas are present they seem to be in patients who have duodenogastric reflux, in an area, exposed to bile (160).

Duodenal Polyp and Carcinoma

In most series, duodenal adenomas occur in more than 90% of FAP patients, particularly in the periampullary region (161–163). The macroscopic appearance of duodenal polyps is very different to that of colonic polyps. The number of the former varies from invisible to over 100. They may present as multiple discrete adenomas (1–10 mm in diameter) or as flat confluent plagues. Sometimes no lesion can be seen and the only clinical abnormality is a prominent ampulla, or the mucosa may appear pale and seem to have a white covering which cannot be removed by rubbing. Biopsy of apparently normal mucosa frequently showed microadenomas (160). The lifetime risk of adenoma in FAP patients is high. Mutations downstream from coden 1051 seem to be associated with severe periampullary adenomas (164). Spigelman et al. (159) staged the duodenal polyposis according to polyp number, polyp size, and histologic type. The criteria provided a four-stage scoring system (Table 7). The classification allows estimation of the severity of duodenal polyposis.

In a prospective study conducted by Domizio et al. (165), over 102 asymptomatic FAP patients were screened

TABLE 7 ■ **Staging of Duodenal Polyposis**

	Grade Points		
Criteria	1	2	3
Polyp number	1–4	5–20	>20
Polyp size (mm)	1–4	5–10	>10
Histology	Tubular	Tubulovillous	Villous
Dysplasia	Mild	Moderate	Severe

Note: Stage 0, 0 point; stage I, 1–4 points; stage II, 5–6 points; stage III, 7–8 points; stage IV, 9–12 points.
Source: From Ref. 159.

with side-viewing video endoscope, duodenal polyps were found to be multiple in two-thirds of patients, with one-third of patients having more than 20. The average size of a duodenal polyp was 9 mm, but they can be much bigger (2 cm). Duodenal polyps were almost always adenomas. Duodenal adenomas were tabular in architecture in about 70% of patients, tubulovillous in 20% and villous in 10%. Duodenal polyps were not seen in approximately 10% of patients. In just over one-half of these patients, micro adenomas were subsequently found. Presumably, if more random biopsies had been taken, more patients with microadenomas would have been found.

Only 10% of patients had stage IV duodenal polyposis, while just under 20% had stage I disease and the remaining, 35% each, had stage II or stage III duodenal polyposis. Those with stage IV disease were older than the rest, implying that duodenal polyposis is a progressive disorder. Advanced duodenal disease might be a marker for the presence of gastric adenomas, as nearly all those with gastric adenomas had stage III or stage IV duodenal polyposis in their series (165). The risk of duodenal carcinoma in FAP has increased more than 100 times that of the normal population. Of 222 FAP patients who had a colectomy and IRA at St. Mark's Hospital between 1948 and 1990 (inclusive), duodenal carcinoma accounted for 11 deaths, more than twice the number of deaths attributed to carcinoma of the rectal stump (166). A retrospective survey based on 10 polyposis registries in the Leeds Castle Polyposis Group showed duodenal and periampullary carcinoma in 30% of 1225 patients (167). The major causes of death in a series of 36 FAP patients treated with prophylactic proctocolectomy or colectomy with an IRA at the Cleveland Clinic were desmoid tumor (31%), periampullary carcinoma (22%), and rectal carcinoma (8%) (168). The cause of death from extracolonic diseases is also higher than carcinoma of colon and rectum in recent decades in the series of Belchetz et al. (169).

One of the most difficult problems is the treatment of duodenal adenomas. Bile has been implicated in the pathogenesis of duodenal polyps in patients with FAP. FAP bile has been shown to contain an excess of carcinogens able to form DNA adducts. DNA adducts are chemical modification of DNA, formed by covalent binding of electrophilic carcinogens to DNA, which are implicated in the initiation of carcinogenesis because when they are left unrepaired they can lead to mutations. Modification of the action of these carcinogens may reduce the adduct load to the duodenum and so decrease actual duodenal polyp number. However, in the double-blind randomized placebo-controlled trial conducted by Wallace et al. (170), 26 patients with FAP were randomly assigned to ranitidine, 300 mg daily, or placebo for six months after baseline endoscopy. The result showed that acid suppression therapy does not seem to improve duodenal polyposis.

Celecoxib (Celebrex®) has been shown to reduce the number of duodenal polyps. Phillips et al. (171) conducted a randomized, double-blind, placebo controlled study of celecoxib, 100 mg twice daily ($n = 34$), or 400 mg twice daily ($n = 32$), versus placebo ($n = 17$), given orally twice daily for six months to patients with FAP associated with duodenal polyposis. Efficacy was assessed qualitatively by blinded review of shuffled endoscopy videotapes comparing the extent of duodenal polyposis at entry and at six months and quantitatively by measurement of the percentage change in duodenal area covered by discrete and plaque-like adenomas from photographs of high- and low-density polyposis. The results showed a statistically significant effect of 400 mg twice daily celecoxib compared with placebo treatment. Overall, patients taking celecoxib, 400 mg twice daily, showed a 15.5% reduction in involved areas compared with a 1.4% for placebo. The authors suggested that celecoxib might have been indicated in patients with established duodenal disease, particularly when it is severe. However, it is harder to justify its use in patients with lesser duodenal disease, as progression to duodenal carcinoma in these patients with an earlier onset of the disease is unusual.

Some authors successfully eradicated few adenomas of duodenum in FAP patients but the number of these patients had been too small to judge its efficacy (172,173). In general, endoscopic snaring or thermal contact can be performed only in patients with few small lesions as an initial treatment, or in patients who are not a candidate for major surgery.

The natural history of untreated duodenal and ampullary adenomas in patients with FAP has been studied by Burke et al. (174). One hundred fourteen FAP patients who had two or more surveillance examinations were followed for a mean of 51 months (range 10–151 months). Duodenal polyps progressed in size in 26% (25 of 95), number in 32% (34 of 106), and histology in 11% (5 of 45) of patients. Morphology and histology of the main duodenal papilla progressed in 14% (15 of 110) and 11% (12 of 105) of patients, respectively. A minority of FAP patients had progression of endoscopic features and histology of duodenal polyps or the main duodenal papilla when followed over 4 years. An endoscopic surveillance interval of at least 3 years may be appropriate for the majority of untreated patients with FAP.

An operation is indicated if polyps showed villous change, severe dysplasia, rapid growth, and induration at endoscopic probing (162). Duodenectomy or local excision is not preferred because of very high recurrences and complications (161,175–178). A pancreatoduodenectomy, particularly duodenectomy with preservation of pancreas, for patients with severe duodenal polyposis or patients who already had carcinoma appears to be the best option (176,179–181).

The lifetime risk of duodenal adenomas approaches 100% (182). Recommendations concerning the age of initiation of upper tract surveillance are not uniform. Some propose that screening for upper GI disease should start at the time of FAP diagnosis. The National Comprehensive Cancer Network, after review of all case reports of duodenal carcinoma in FAP patients, recommended a baseline upper GI endoscopic examination at 25 to 30 years of age. In general, recommendations include stage 0 every 4 years; stage I every 2 to 3 years; stage II every 2 to 3 years; stage III every 6 to 12 months with consideration for surgery; and stage IV strongly consider surgery (182).

Polyps in the Small Bowel

Adenomas have been detected in the ileum following colectomy and IRA and also in Kock's pouch following proctocolectomy. A small number of cases of malignant neoplasms in the small bowel in association with FAP have been recorded; the risk of developing such a lesion appears minimal. Lymphoid polyps have also been noted in FAP, both in the small bowel and colon. Histological confirmation should be undertaken because presentation may mimic FAP (156).

Mesodermal Abnormalities

Desmoid Tumors

Patients with mutation between codons 1445 and 1578 frequently developed desmoid tumors (183). Desmoid tumors are benign tumors arising from fibroaponeurotic tissue. It is not known whether they are true neoplasms or the result of a generalized fibroblast abnormality; there is increasing evidence to support the former theory (184). Although a benign disease, desmoid tumors are focally invasive. They do not metastasize but can be lethal because of aggressive growth with pressure and erosion causing obstruction of the small bowel (Fig. 20). A report from the Finnish Polyposis Registry included 202 FAP patients, of whom 169 underwent colectomy. Desmoids were observed in 29 patients (14%): 15 (7%) in the mesentery, 10 (5%) on the abdominal wall, and four (2%) in other sites. The cumulative lifetime risk is 21.0%, 1.5%, 3.0%, 8.9%, 16.0%, and 18.0% at ages of 10, 20, 30, 40 and 50 years, respectively (185). Clark et al. (186) studied desmoid tumors from St. Mark's Polyposis Registry Database. Eighty-eight patients had 166 desmoids (median age 32). Eighty-three patients (50%) had the tumor intra-abdominally, with 88% in the small bowel mesentery; 80 patients (48%) had the tumor on the abdominal wall, with 39% in surgical scars; three patients (2%) had the tumor extra-abdominally (chest wall, intra-thoracic). All (82%) but 16 patients had already undergone abdominal surgery.

The behavior of desmoids in FAP ranges from rapid growth with symptoms resulting from visceral compression to a more indolent course, or even spontaneous regression. Plaque-like thickening of the small bowel mesentery and the peritoneum that does not amount to a discrete mass has been described as a relatively common finding at celiotomy in patients with FAP undergoing surgery (187,188).

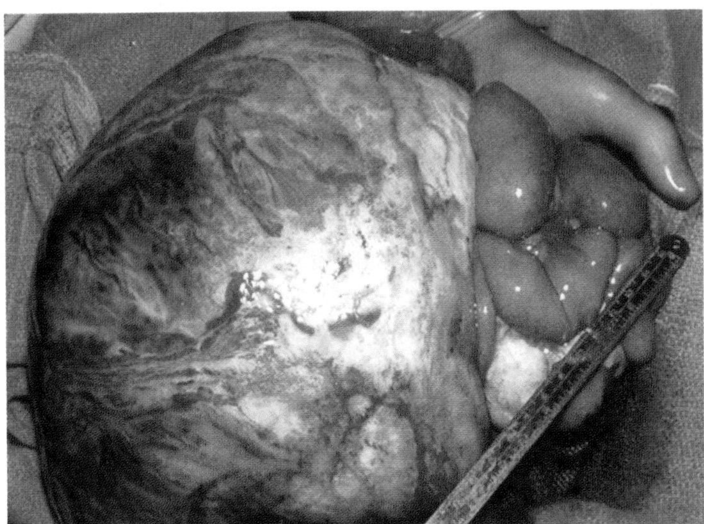

FIGURE 20 ■ Large desmoid tumor of mesentery causing partial small bowel obstruction. *Source*: Courtesy of Roger R. Dozois, M.D., Mayo Clinic, Rochester, MN, U.S.A.

Hartley et al. (187) studied the natural history of these lesions that were incidentally found on celiotomy. A total of 266 patients underwent abdominal surgery for FAP. Incidental intra-abdominal desmoid tumors were identified in 34 patients, eight at the index surgery and 26 at re-celiotomy (median 130 months from the index procedure, range, 23–364 months). Intra-abdominal desmoids identified at the time of index surgery influenced the intended procedure in one of eight cases (6 cm mass in mesentery precluded IPAA). Intra-abdominal desmoids identified at second celiotomy influenced the intended surgery procedure in 10 of 26 cases (38%), including one for Kock pouch, two for IPAA, two difficult pouch reach, two prevented covering stoma, one iliac vein surgery, and two bypass only. Desmoid reaction was found in one of the index and 11 of the re-explore celiotomy group. This type of lesion was not an obstacle to the planned surgery. Desmoid reaction or mesenteric fibromatosis is precursor lesion for subsequent desmoid formation. However, the risk for progression in any individual case is likely to be small (188). Phillips (189) recommended computed tomography (CT) scan of any FAP patients before planned second major surgery, whether for pouch conversion or management of duodenal polyposis.

The most common symptom in patients with intra-abdominal desmoids is a painful abdominal mass (50%). The rest have a painless mass or no palpable mass. The pain is usually caused by bowel obstruction. Other causes of the pain are ureteric obstruction, direct pressure effects of the tumor, or hemorrhage into the tumor (190). The preferred investigation is the CT scan, which permits serial observation of the tumor (156,191). Magnetic resonance imaging (MRI) has been shown to provide adequate images of intra-abdominal soft tissue tumors while sparing the patient's exposure to ionizing radiation (156,192).

Intra-abdominal desmoids are a difficult clinical challenge. Their tendency to recur (65–85%) after removal has encouraged a conservative approach to management (190). Operation should be preferred for patients in whom life-threatening complications have occurred as a result of local invasion (156). In many patients, operation is unavoidable. Middleton and Phillips of St. Mark's hospital (193) were forced to remove a large intra-abdominal desmoid tumor from four patients (three patients had FAP). Three had complete excision their desmoids and all remained well with no recurrence at a median follow-up of 12 (range 7–14) months. Eight of 22 patients who underwent resection of their intra-abdominal desmoids at St. Mark's died in the postoperation period (186). Church (190) cautioned that survey for a large intra-abdominal desmoid is technically extremely difficult, demanding high levels of skill and support. It should only be done in setting of a major medical center. On the other hand, abdominal wall and other superficial desmoids can be often cured by wide excision, especially when the tumor is small.

The tumors are extremely resistant to radio therapy and cytotoxic chemotherapy (156). Encouraging reports have appeared following treatment with sulindac, with or without tamoxifen. Church and Others (190,194) suggested treatment of intra-abdominal desmoid tumors in FAP with sulindac, 150 mg twice daily. If the tumor continues to grow as shown by clinical observation and CT scan, add tamoxifen, 80 mg/day. If the tumor stabilizes, continue the medications but reduce the tamoxifen dose after 6 months and then gradually discontinue therapy. If the desmoid keeps growing or is still symptomatic, consider chemotherapy. If an intra-abdominal desmoid is discovered during operation and can be resected with a minimum of small bowel and low risk of complications, proceed. If complete excision is impossible, obtain tissue for histologic and estrogen-receptor assays.

Using an antisarcoma regimen consisting of doxorubicin and dacarbazine, Möslein and Dozois (195) used this regimen in nine patients with FAP-related desmoid tumor and it led to complete regression in four patients and partial regression in five patients. Poritz et al. (196) treated eight patients with desmoid tumors and FAP who had inoperable GI obstruction and/or uncontrolled pain. The regimen consisted of doxorubicin and dacarbazine followed by carboplatin and dacarbazine. Follow-up at a mean of 42 months in seven patients revealed two patients achieved complete remission after the therapy. Four patients achieved a partial remission after completing or some of the chemotherapy regimen; of these, three remained at stable remission, whereas the other was lost to follow-up. There were two recurrences that required further therapy; one of these patients was treated with further chemotherapy, which induced a second remission, and the other was treated with pelvic exenteration and has subsequently died. This cytotoxic regimen should be considered only for patients with fast-growing, life-threatening mesenteric desmoid tumors.

Church et al. (197) developed a staging system that can be applied to the management of FAP-related desmoid tumor:

Stage I: Asymptomatic, not growing. Asymptomatic desmoids are usually small and are found incidentally either during exploratory celiotomy or on CT scan performed for unrelated reasons. Such tumors can be observed, or, at the most, a relatively nontoxic medication such as nonsteroidal anti-inflammatory drugs (NSAIDs) may be prescribed. If a stage I desmoid is found incidentally at surgery and it is easily resectable without the removal of a significant amount of bowel, resection is appropriate.

Stage II: Symptomatic and 10 cm or less in maximum diameter, not growing. Small desmoids that are causing symptoms (including bowel or ureteral obstruction) need therapy even if they are not obviously growing. If they are resectable with minimal sequelae, then resection is best. If the tumor is unresectable, the addition of tamoxifen or raloxifene to a NSAID offers the possibility of a quicker and more consistent response with low risk of side effects.

Stage III: Symptomatic and 11 to 20 cm, or asymptomatic and slowly growing desmoids. Larger, symptomatic (including bowel or ureteric obstruction) desmoids, or desmoids that are slowly increasing in size (<50% increase in diameter in 6 months), need active treatment. Here the choices include NSAID, tamoxifen, raloxifene, and vinblastine/methotrexate. Antisarcoma chemotherapy can be given if the tumor continues to grow despite less toxic agents.

Stage IV: Symptomatic, >20 cm, or rapid growth, or complicated desmoids. These are the worse desmoids: Large, or growing rapidly (>50% increase in diameter within 6 months), these cause life-threatening complications such as sepsis, perforation or hemorrhage. Here treatment is an urgent necessity and the possibilities are major exenterative surgery likely to result in significant loss of bowel, antisarcoma therapy, and radiation.

The authors noted that one of the most important uses of the staging system is to allow prospective trials of the various treatment options, some of which are inappropriate for certain stages of tumor (197).

Death from desmoid tumors is caused by either direct effects, such as erosion into a blood vessel or sepsis from an enteric fistula, or to secondary effects as the result of desmoid surgery (190).

Osteomas

Osteomas may occur in any bone but they are most commonly located on the facial skeleton, particularly the mandible. These tumors are benign but may cause symptoms following local growth. They are sometimes identified before the diagnosis of FAP is made (156).

Teeth

Teeth are derived from both mesoderm and ectoderm. Dental abnormalities, distinct from osteomas of the jaw, have been described in from 11% to 80% of individuals with FAP. Although slightly less frequent than osteomas of the jaw, their frequency and the fact that they may appear at an early age are sufficient reasons to make them diagnostically useful. The lesions in question are impactions, supernumerary or absent teeth, fused root of first and second molars, and unusually long and tapered roots of posterior teeth (145).

Ectodermal Abnormalities

Eye Lesions

Although the presence of pigmented lesions of the fundus was noted in a patient with the signs of Gardner's syndrome by Cabot (198) in 1935, it was not until 1980, when Blair and Trempe (199) recorded pigmented lesions in three affected members of a kindred with Gardner's syndrome, that the possibility of using this lesion as a marker for FAP was suggested. The abnormality is considered to be congenital hypertrophy of retinal pigment epithelium (CHRPE). The occurrence of CHRPE is restricted to APC mutation in codons 463 to 1444 (183).

The examination is made by indirect ophthalmoscopy, following instillation of 1% tropicamide for pupil dilatation. It normally appears as a round or oval pigmented lesion with a surrounding pale halo (Fig. 21).

Microscopic examination shows that CHRPE is a hamartoma. The acronym, while not strictly correct, has become accepted and has continued in use (156). The incidence of CHRPE in patients with FAP varies widely

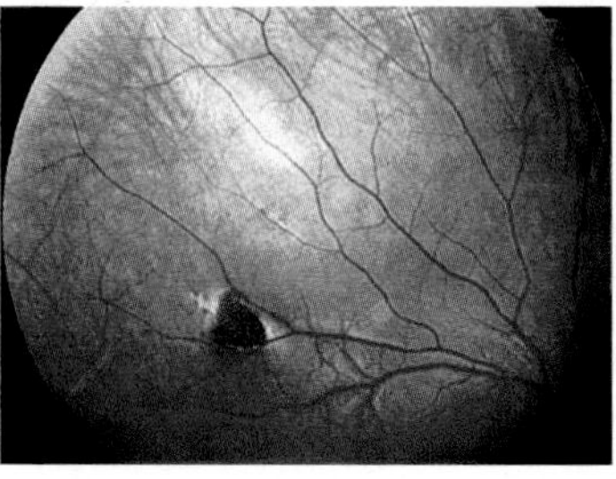

FIGURE 21 ■ Fundus photograph of the pigmented lesion of the retina (CHRPE). *Source*: Courtesy of Helmut Buettmer, M.D., Mayo Clinic, Rochester, MN, U.S.A.

from 50% to 79% (145,156) compared with 7% and 5% in at-risk groups and in age- and sex-matched individuals, respectively. The sensitivity of CHRPE in FAP is 79% and specificity is 95% (156).

The presence of CHRPE in a person who is a member of a kindred of a patient manifesting FAP suggests that he or she has inherited the gene. The absence of the lesion does not, however, indicate that the person has not inherited the gene (156).

Epidermoid Cyst

In patients with FAP, cysts may be found on the limbs, face, and scalp. In the general population they occur predominantly on the back. Leppard and Bussey (200) found epidermoid cysts in 53% of a series of 74 patients affected by FAP. Perhaps the most significant finding related to epidermoid cysts is their rarity in childhood in any condition other than FAP; skin cysts may be evident before the development of colorectal polyps (201). Leppard and Bussey (200) recommend that a child with an epidermoid cyst undergo sigmoidoscopy after the age of 14 years but before attaining 30 years of age.

Brain Neoplasms

In 1949 Crail (202) reported a case of synchronous cerebellar medulloblastoma, colonic polyposis (approximately 100 polyps), and papillary carcinoma of the thyroid. This report did not receive widespread recognition at that time (203). In 1959 Turcot et al. (204) described two siblings who presented with colonic polyposis at the ages of 13 and 15 years, respectively. Both patients went on to develop a glioblastoma of the frontal lobe and a medullary medulloblastoma, respectively. The first sibling also had a chromophobe adenoma of the pituitary gland. The authors suggested that these neoplasms might be another extracolonic manifestation of FAP. These associations bear the name Turcot's syndrome.

Hamilton et al. (205) studied Turcot's syndrome at the molecular level. Fourteen families with Turcot's syndrome were identified. Germ-line mutations in the APC gene characteristic of FAP were evaluated, as well as DNA replication errors and germ-line mutations in nucleotide mismatch-repair genes characteristic of HNPCC.

Genetic abnormalities were identified in 13 of 14 registry families. Germ-line APC mutations were detected in 10. The predominant brain tumor in these 10 families was medulloblastoma (11 of 14 patients, or 79%), and the RR of cerebellar medulloblastoma in patients with FAP was 92 times that in the general population. In contrast, the type of brain tumor in the other four families was glioblastoma multiforme. Germ-line mutations in the mismatch-repair gene hMLH1 or hMMS2 were found in two families.

In the study of the APC gene in 14 families that included at least one affected member, 12 families classified as having polyposis, mutations were found in 10 (83%). All the mutated genes encoded truncated variance of the APC protein, as is true of the vast majority of patients with FAP. The mutations were heterogeneous in type and location, and there was no association between specific mutations and the development of brain tumors. Two families with polyposis and both families without polyposis had no identifiable germ-line APC mutations.

Analysis of the hMSH2, hMLH1, hPMS1, and hPMS2 mismatch-repair genes, which are mutated in HNPCC, was carried out in the three patients with neoplasms that contained replication errors. Two had germ-line alterations: the hPMS2 gene was mutated in one patient and hMLH1 was mutated in another patient. No germ-line APC mutations were detected in these three patients.

The authors concluded that the association between brain neoplasms and multiple colorectal adenomas might result from two distinct types of germ-line defects: mutation of the APC gene or mutation of the mismatch-repair gene. Molecular diagnosis may contribute to the appropriate care of affected patients.

Review of literature by Matsui et al. (206) and Itoh et al. (207) revealed that there were 131 documented cases in the medical literature. Of the 35 cases that they considered having true Turcot's syndrome, the average age of death was 20.3 years. Most (76%) died from brain malignancy, 16% died from colorectal carcinoma, and the rest from other causes. Death at young age has made it difficult to determine whether the mode of inheritance is autosomal recessive or autosomal dominant.

A more complete list of the extracolonic manifestations of FAP is summarized in the Box 1 (203).

■ MANAGEMENT

Histologic verification of adenomas is essential so that confusion with familial juvenile polyposis, hyperplastic polyposis, pseudopolyposis, and lymphoid polyposis is avoided. Performing total colonoscopy arid biopsy is the best choice.

Virtually all patients with FAP will develop carcinoma of the colon and rectum by age 40. For this reason, patients with FAP should have prophylactic colectomy. At present, there are several surgical options, and each has advantages and disadvantages.

Proctocolectomy with Ileostomy

This procedure removes all the disease, but an obvious side effect is the creation of a permanent ileostomy, which is not well accepted by most patients, particularly the young ones. With other alternatives, especially colectomy with IRA and proctocolectomy with an ileoanal pouch procedure, and proctocolectomy with ileostomy are seldom chosen by patients. However, if there is a carcinoma in the rectum or in patients with a desmoid tumor of the small bowel mesentary, a proctocolectomy should be performed.

Proctocolectomy with Continent Ileostomy

This procedure was a popular option in the 1970s. An ileal reservoir with a nipple valve is created from the terminal ileum and is brought out as an ileostomy. Its advantage over the conventional ileostomy is that an ileostomy bag is not required. The pouch must be evacuated four to six times a day with a catheter. Because of the frequent extrusion of the nipple valve, which results in incontinence, use of the procedure has been limited to a small number of patients. The IPAA now has largely replaced this procedure.

Colectomy with Ileorectal Anastomosis

This procedure minimizes the risk of development of carcinoma upto only the last 12 to 15 cm of the rectum. Patients require lifelong close follow-up, at least once or twice a year, with electrocoagulation of the polyps as indicated. It

BOX 1 ■ Extracolonic Manifestations of Familial Adenomatous Polyposis

Ectodermal Origin	Mesodermal Origin	Endodermal Origin
Epidermoid cyst	Connective tissue	Adenomas
Pilomatrixoma	Fibroma	Stomach
Tumors of central nervous system	Fibrosarcoma	Duodenum
Congenital hypertrophy of the retinal pigment epithelium	Desmoid tumors	Hepatopancreatobiliary system
	Diffuse fibrosis mesenteric retroperitoneum	Small intestine
	Excessive intra-abdominal adhesion	Endocrine tissue
	?Lipoma	Adrenal cortex (adenomas)
	Bone	Thyroid gland
	Osteoma	?Parathyroid
	Exostosis	?Pituitary
	Sclerosis	?Pancreatic islets
	Dental	Carcinomas
	Dentigerous cyst	Stomach
	Odontoma	Duodenum
	Supernumerary teeth	Hepatobiliary system
	Unerupted teeth	Small intestine
	Lymphoid	Thyroid gland
	Hyperplasia of ileum	Adrenal gland
		Fundic gland polyp
		Hepatoblastoma

Source: From Ref. 203.

should be selected for patients in whom the rectum is not carpeted with polyps and who are willing to return for follow-up. The main advantages of this choice are that it is a relatively simple procedure familiar to most surgeons and it has excellent functional results.

Controversy exists about the risk of developing carcinoma in the remaining rectum after colectomy and IRA. The risk varies from series to series, from 0% at the Cleveland Clinic (208) to an overall 32% at the Mayo Clinic (209). The discrepancy is not clear, but it appears that the risk of developing carcinoma increases with time (210). The unusually high incidence of carcinoma in the retained rectum in the Mayo Clinic series prompted Bess et al. (209) to reanalyze the series 10 years later, with the aim of identifying factors that may contribute to the risks. The following variables do not cause an increase in the risks: male versus female, number of colonic polyps (≥100 vs. ≤100), family history of polyposis, age at the time of surgery (≥40 years vs. ≤40 years), and level of ileorectal or ileosigmoid anastomosis (≥15 cm vs. ≤15 cm). Factors that contribute to an increase in carcinoma risk include the number of preoperative rectal polyps (the risk is increased if there are more than 20 polyps in the remaining rectum) and colonic carcinoma resected at or before colectomy. Of significance is the cumulative risk of carcinoma in the St. Mark's series, increasing from 10% at 20 years follow-up to more than 30% at 35 years (210).

Risk of Carcinoma in the Retained Rectum

The series from St. Mark's (210) showed that until the age of 50 years, the cumulative risk of carcinoma in the IRA is reasonably low at 10%, increasing sharply to 29% by the age of 60 years. This means that surveillance of the retained rectum in older patients must either be improved or the patients should undergo restorative proctocolectomy in earlier middle age. Nugent and Phillips (211) recommend a flexible videoendoscopy at fixed intervals of four months for all patients at risk over the age of 45 years who wish to retain the rectum. A similar age-dependent rectal carcinoma risk is also reported by Heiskanen and Jarvinen (212) 3.9%, 12.8%, and 25.7% at 40, 50, and 60 years, respectively, and rectal excision rates of 9.5%, 26.3%, and 44.0%, respectively. The authors also reported a cumulative rectal carcinoma risk of 4.0%, 5.6%, 7.9% and 25.0% at 5, 10, 15, and 20 years, respectively, after the ileorectal anastomosis (IRA).

These findings have raised the question of the justification of ileorectal anastomosis (IRA) as the primary treatment of FAP. The planned strategy of two prophylactic operations, first a colectomy with IRA at an earlier age (perhaps 20 years of age), and then a restorative proctectomy at the age of 45 years, doubles the risks of the operations and may also increase the risk of desmoid tumors. Furthermore, a second-stage restorative proctectomy may not result in perfect functional outcome, or is impossible in cases of pelvic fibromatous adhesions or desmoids (212). The previous recommendation by Bess et al. (209) in 1980 is still a good one, that the colon and rectum should be removed but the rectum may be retained if there are fewer than 20 polyps in the rectum.

Heiskanen and Jarvinen (212) now favor proctocolectomy and ileoanal pouch procedure as the primary operation for FAP. A more detailed view of the cumulative rectal carcinoma incidence is shown on Table 8.

A close follow-up of patients with IRA is essential. The retained rectum should be examined, preferably with a flexible sigmoidoscope, once a year or sooner, depending on the number of polyps that should be electrocoagulated. Any time the number of the polyps become too numerous or too large to be safely removed, a proctectomy should be considered. In a series reported by Penna et al. (220) of 148 patients with an IRA, 29 required a secondary proctectomy: 16 because the rectal polyps were too numerous, 8 because the patients wished to discontinue regular surveillance, and 3 because of the discovery of rectal carcinoma (one was Dukes' A 3 years after the IRA, one Dukes' B 14 years after, and one Dukes' C 17 years later). An IPAA was

TABLE 8 ■ Selected Series on Risk of Rectal Carcinoma After Colectomy and Ileorectal Anastomosis

Authors	No. of Patents	Years After IRA	Rectal Carcinoma Rate (%)
Bess et al. (209)	143	19	32
Bulow (147)	58	10	13
Sarre et al. (213)	133	20	12
DeCosse et al. (214)	294	25	13
Nugent and Phillips (211)	224	25	15
Iwama and Mishima (215)	342	15	24
Heiskanen and Jarvinen (212)	100	20	25
Jenner and Levitt (216)	55	10	13
Bjork et al. (217)	195	25	24
Bertario et al. (218)	371	20	23
Church et al. (219)	62	15	13

Abbreviation: IRA, ileorectal anastomosis.

successfully performed in all but three patients who had pelvic desmoid tumors. In a series reported by Nugent and Phillips (211) of 224 patients with IRA, 22 patients developed carcinoma of the rectum. Nine were Dukes' A, four were Dukes' B, and nine were Dukes' C. These carcinomas developed despite a close follow-up; 14 of 22 patients were last examined less than 6 months before. It is essential to realize that despite the close follow-up, surveillance cannot always prevent rectal carcinoma (221).

A Place for Ileorectal Anastomosis

Colectomy with IRA has its strong support. Phillips and Spigelman (222) reason that the ileoanal pouch procedure has high morbidity and does not give perfect functional results and that patients can still succumb to other related diseases of FAP.

Bulow et al. (223) studied 659 patients undergoing IRA. The data was obtained from the National Polyposis Registries in Denmark, Finland, the Netherlands, and Sweden. They found that chronologic age was the only independent risk factor of developing rectal carcinoma. The risk of secondary proctectomy was higher in patients with mutation in codon 1250 to 1500 than outside this region. None of the 18 patients with AFAP (mutation in codon 0–200 or greater than 1500) had a secondary proctectomy.

Church et al. (224) found that the risk of rectal carcinoma after IRA was strongly related to the severity of colorectal polyposis at presentation.

Bertario et al. (218) found independent predictors of rectal carcinoma after IRA in the FAP with mutation between codon 1250 and 1464 (RR = 4.4).

It is, therefore, reasonable to perform colon resection with IRA in young patients with few adenomas (less than 20 rectal adenomas, less than 1000 colonic adenomas) and in FAP with mutation in codon 0 to 200 or greater than 1500 (223,224). These patients must understand their responsibility to have a periodic surveillance with an endoscopy, and that they may require a proctectomy in the future.

Regression of Polyps

A temporary spontaneous regression or disappearance of polyps in the rectum after IRA is a common observation. This gives some comfort to clinicians, a hope that perhaps the risk of developing carcinomas can be minimized as well. A study of the effect of colectomy and IRA on rectal mucosal proliferation in FAP showed a significant reduction in rectal mucosal cell proliferation. However, the mechanism is unknown (225). Sulindac has also been found to markedly reduce epithelial cell proliferation and significant polyp regression, including dysplastic reversion (226,227). This observation must be guarded, since Spagnesi et al. (228) observed the persistence of abnormal rectal mucosal proliferation after sulindac therapy, despite the reduction of number of polyps.

Winde et al. (229) conducted a prospective, controlled, nonrandomized Phase II dose-finding study from sulindac given rectally, and looked at the molecular mechanism by which sulindac worked. The study group ($n = 28$) and the control group ($n = 10$) underwent colectomy and IRA, with repeated proctoscopy with endoluminal ultrasound and biopsies every three months. The treatment group was given sulindac suppositories, 150 mg twice daily, for three months. Visible improvement was followed by a dose reduction to 50 mg daily. Worsening of the polyps required changing to the initial dose level. The results showed that all patients responded to sulindac after 24 weeks (at the latest). Complete reversion was reached with 50 mg/day in 78% of patients. Twenty-two percent had partial reversions of adenomas at latest re-examination and there was no influence on upper GI tract adenomas. There was a permanent antiproliferative effect (Ki-67) of low-dose sulindac, significant blocking of *ras* mutation activation, and a significant difference of untreated and treated mucosa in mutant p53 content. The follow-up was 4 years. The authors concluded that low dose antiproliferative sulindac therapy is highly effective in adenoma reversion in FAP patients. Sulindac shows influence on tumor-suppressor genes and on apoptosis markers. All cases with relapse represented by newly developed flat mucosal elevations respond to dose increases.

Giadiello et al. (230) conducted a randomized, double-blind, placebo-controlled study looking whether sulindac can prevent adenoma rather than causing regression of the polyps. The study consisted of 41 young subjects (age range, 8 to 25 years) who were genotypically affected with familial FAP but phenotypically unaffected. Subjects received either 75 or 150 mg of sulindac orally twice a day or identical-appearing placebo tablets for 48 months. The number and size of new adenomas and the side effects of therapy were evaluated every four months for four years, and the levels of five major prostaglandins were serially measured in biopsy specimens of normal-appearing colorectal mucosa.

The results after 4 years of treatment showed the average rate of compliance exceeded 76% in the sulindac group, and mucosal prostaglandin levels were lower in this group than in the placebo group. During the course of the study, adenomas developed in 9 of 21 subjects (43%) in the sulindac group and 11 of 20 patients in the placebo group (55%). There were no significant differences in the mean number or size of polyps between the groups. The authors concluded that standard doses of sulindac did not prevent the development of adenomas in subjects with FAP.

Evidence that sulindac has a short-lived effect on established polyps in patients with FAP has been reported.

The rate of regression of adenomas was greater after 6 months of sulindac treatment than after nine months has been reported in some patients who had undergone IRA. Long-term use of sulindac resulted in the development of resistance to this medication (230). Moreover, colorectal carcinoma has developed in rectal segment in patients with FAP during maintenance therapy with sulindac (231–233).

The lack of efficacy of primary chemoprevention could have been due to resistance to sulindac. Most results do not provide support for the use of NSAIDs such as sulindac for the primary treatment of FAP. Prophylactic colectomy remains the treatment of choice to prevent colorectal carcinoma in patients with this disorder (230).

Proctocolectomy with Ileal Pouch Procedure

The advantage of the ileal pouch procedure for FAP is its total eradication of the colonic disease. The inconvenience and a small risk of perforation of a long-term or lifetime follow-up of the rectum with proctoscopy or flexible sigmoidoscopy and electrocoagulation in patients who undergo colectomy with IRA thus is eliminated. The argument against its use as the procedure of choice is the fact that it is a more extensive procedure, with high potential for complications, especially sepsis and fecal incontinence more and more authors and medical centers favor the IPAA as the primary treatment for patients with FAP (234,235). Although IPAA is a longer, more bloody, and more complex operation with a longer hospital stay than IRA, no significant difference is found between the two groups in terms of complication rate and quality of life in a series of teenagers. IPAA also has few effects on life activities that are especially important at this age (235,236). The same is true in adult series (234,237,238). In the series of Soravia et al. (239), although IRA had a significantly better functional outcome with regard to nighttime continence and perianal skin irritation, functional results otherwise, and the quality of life were similar, they favor IPAA over IRA because of lower long-term failure rate.

With concern about the increasing risk of carcinoma in the retained rectum, which is 25% at 20 years after the IRA, Heiskanen and Jarvinen (212) the IPAA for their patients with FAP as the primary treatment. This approach eliminates the need for a proctectomy, after an IRA.

Proctocolectomy with IPAA for FAP cannot be considered the end of the patient's management. In these patients, adenomas and carcinomas can develop in the ileal pouch, at the anastomosis, or in the anal transitional zone. Church (240) reviewed these problems, searching the MEDLINE database for studies reporting ileoanal pouch adenomas, ileal pouch-anal anastomotic carcinomas, and ileal pouch carcinomas in patients with FAP. Reports of adenomas in Kock pouches and in Brooke ileostomies in the setting of FAP were also included. The primary end points of the study were the time between pouch (or ileostomy) construction and the diagnosis of neoplasia, the age of the patients at the diagnosis of neoplasia, and the severity of the neoplasia.

The results showed that 18 studies reporting pouch neoplasia, 15 with adenomas (98 patients) and three with carcinomas (three patients). Three prospective studies showed that the incidence of the pouch adenomas increases with time of follow-up and that the severity of the polyposis varies. The median time from pouch construction to diagnosis of pouch adenomas was 4.7 years and the range was 0.5 to 12 years.

A prospective review at the Cleveland Clinic showed a rate of 28% for adenomas 3.5 years after stapled IPAA and 14% at four years after hand-sewn IPAA (241). Similar data had been reported from 97 FAP patients who had an IPAA in a multicenter study by van Duijvendijk et al. (242). At a median follow-up of 78 months (range, 25–137 months), 13 of these patients had adenomas at the anastomosis. The risk for anastomotic adenomas after double-stapled IPAA was 31%, three times that after mucosectomy and hand-sewn IPAA (10%).

There were six studies, reporting eight patients with carcinoma at the IPAA, diagnosed a median of eight years after pouch construction (range, 3 to 20 years). One-half of the carcinomas were locally advanced (T4) and one-half were not (T1 or T2). One-half followed stapled anastomosis and one-half were after mucosectomy. There were eight case reports of carcinoma described in an ileostomy in patients with FAP. The median time for ileostomy construction to the ileostomy carcinomas was 25 years (range, 9–40).

Pouch adenomas are difficult to manage endoscopically because of the thin ileal mucosa and the way it is tethered to the submucosa and underlying muscle. Their propensity to occur on suture lines also makes endoscopic treatment difficult. There are no large studies of endoscopic treatment of pouch adenomas so risks and complication rates are not established. The prospect of coagulating or snaring tens or hundreds of polyps is a concern, however. Pouch excision for uncontrollable polyposis has previously been reported (242) but would be a difficult operation in many patients, usually resulting in an ileostomy and risking complications such as impotence, retrograde ejaculation, ureteric injury, and worsening female fecundity. Chemoprevention of pouch polyposis is, therefore, an attractive alternative.

The role of nonsteroidal anti-inflammatory drugs (NSAIDs) in suppressing colorectal adenomas in FAP is established, and there are anecdotal reports of their use in pouch polyposis. While chemoprevention of colorectal adenomas in FAP using sulindac works only partially and for a limited time, its effectiveness in the ileal pouch has not been systematically studied (240).

Those caring for patients with FAP need to make sure that endoscopic surveillance is continued after IPAA. The endoscopy has to be accurate and the endoscopists must be aware of the increasing risk of pouch and anastomotic neoplasia. Church (240) recommended pouchoscopy to be done yearly for life, initially to look for anastomotic adenomas and then later to check for pouch adenomas. Once neoplasia is seen, appropriate treatment needs to be determined. This includes transanal excision of residual, adenoma-bearing anal transitional zone, transanal polypectomy for isolated large (1 cm) pouch adenomas, or sulindac (150 mg twice daily) for multiple (>10) pouch adenomas.

■ GENETIC COUNSELING AND TESTING

The gene responsible for FAP, known as *APC*, is located on chromosome 5q21. Mutations of the *APC* gene have been found in patients with FAP. These are often insertions, deletions, and nonsense mutations that lead to frameshifts and/or premature stop codons in the resulting transcript of the gene. It is not yet clear how the subsequent truncated protein product causes adenomas to form. Capitalizing on the nature of these mutations has led to the development of molecular genetic tests for FAP (243). It is not carcinoma but the predisposition to carcinoma that is inherited (244). Genetic testing can capture the opportunity for surgeons to prevent the development of the carcinoma.

Genetic Counseling

Genetic counseling is a dynamic communication process between the patient and the counselor who provides education and support within a multidisciplinary team (245). Patients and their families must understand the natural history of the disease, the involvement of other blood relatives, and that carcinomas of the large bowel as well as other organs are, in most cases, preventable.

The decision to undergo genetic testing is a personal one based on informed consent. The elements of informed consent include information on the gene being tested and the implications, limitations, and impact of results for the person being tested and two other family members. It should be emphasized that genetic testing is voluntary and the patients need to be aware of alternatives (245).

The first phase in determining whether genetic testing is appropriate is genetic counseling. This stage educates the patient about the role of inherited causes for developing carcinoma, determines their risk for a malignancy, and provides screening recommendations. The objective is effectively accomplished by understanding the patient's perspective. Education and discussing the benefits and risks of genetic testing through each patient's viewpoint promotes autonomy and lays the foundation for informed consent. An overall general summary of the genetic counseling and testing process is described in Figure 22 (245).

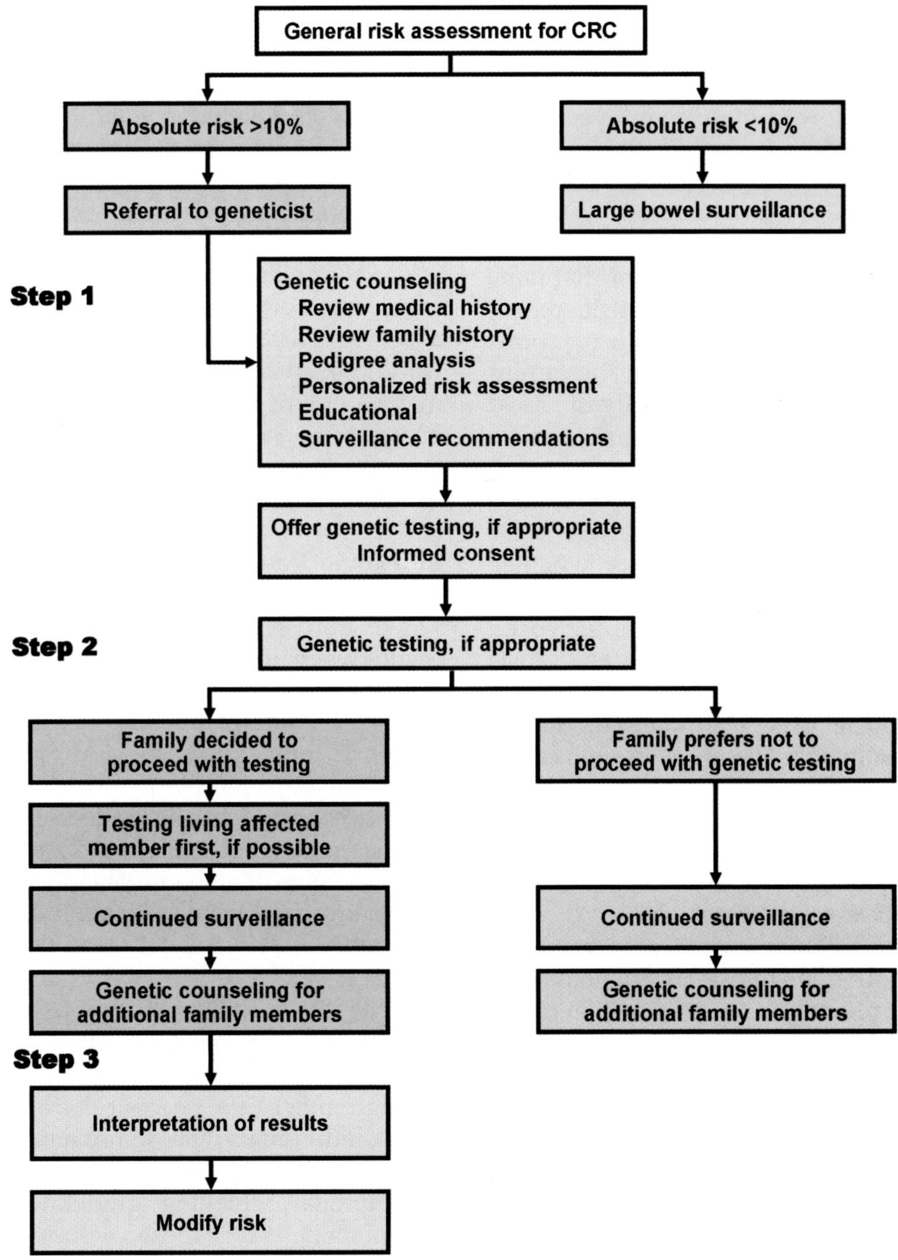

FIGURE 22 ■ General summary of the genetic counseling and testing process. *Abbreviation*: CRC, colorectol carcinoma. *Source*: From Ref. 245.

Genetic Testing

The most important recent development in the management of families of patients with FAP is the use of predictive gene testing. In this context, both children and adults at 50% risk could benefit from genetic testing because of the resultant reduction of uncertainty regardless of test outcome, modifications in screening guidelines for those who do not have the mutant gene, and increased compliance with screening regimens in those who do have the mutant gene (243).

Because approximately 96% of the mutations in FAP lead to a truncated protein, it has become routine to use the in vitro synthesized-protein assay (IVSP). Sometimes this is called a PTT, for mutation detection. When a truncated protein is identified in the assay, it is possible to localize the mutation to a specific segment of the gene and then use DNA sequencing to determine the mutated nucleotides. However, the use of IVSP as the sole genetic test in FAP misses approximately 20% of APC mutations. Another screening technique is based on analysis of electrophoretic migration of small segments of the wild type and mutant gene (SSCA). The sequential use of two molecular diagnostic tests has become a common practice; a simple and less expensive screening technique (of high sensitivity and moderate specificity) followed by a definitive test of high sensitivity, usually DNA sequencing (246).

When the mutation in the family is known from one or more affected members previously studied, only one test, usually IVSP, need be performed, as the expression pattern of the mutation is already established for that family. A positive result in such a test is considered a "mutation-positive" result, and the patient can be counseled as recommended. When the mutation in the family is not known, IVSP is performed. In the majority of cases, mutation will be found in the APC gene that can be further characterized by DNA sequencing. Again, a "mutation-positive" result is obtained leading to the appropriate genetic counseling to the patient. Other options include DNA sequencing and linkage analysis (which tests whether FAP is associated with particular markers in or near APC but requires large families). Even by combining two or more techniques, it is not possible to achieve 100% sensitivity, because the mutations may not be in the coding region of the gene or because a few FAP kindreds do not exhibit linkage to chromosome 5q. Therefore, in such cases, a "no mutation detected" result must not be interpreted as a "negative test" result, with very important considerations for counseling the patient (246).

Implications of a "Mutation-Positive Test" Result (245)

Approximately 75% of individuals who carry an APC germline truncating mutation manifest an adenomatous polyp by age 20. These premalignant lesions inevitably evolve to malignancy, and if untreated, the risk for developing colorectal carcinoma is virtually 100% by age 40. Because polyposis often starts before puberty, flexible sigmoidoscopy beginning at puberty is recommended as a screening procedure by most authors.

Mutation carriers require surveillance by gastroduodenoscopy for extracolonic neoplasms in the upper GI tract. Other variant manifestations in FAP include osteomas, cutaneous cysts, and CHRPE. A phenotype-genotype correlation exists. For example, CHRPE is often present if the mutation is located in exon 9–15e of the APC gene. For families who carry mutation in this region, the presence of CHRPE is a diagnostic indication of FAP.

When a mutation has been identified in the family, direct gene testing of relatives who have not yet been clinically assessed will distinguish between those who carry the mutation and those who do not. However, about 30% of FAP cases are caused by new mutations in the APC gene. In these cases, the parents will not carry this mutation and are not at risk of FAP; only descendants of the proband are at 50% risk.

Implications of a "Negative Test" Result versus "No Mutation Detected" Result (246)

A negative test result is given if the patient does not carry the mutation that is known to exist in their family. In this instance, family members are not at increased risk for developing colorectal carcinoma compared with the general population and should follow guidelines for carcinoma surveillance for that group.

If the patient is affected with FAP and complete coding sequence analysis of the APC gene fails to identify a mutation, this could mean that the APC gene is not responsible for the patient's diagnosis. This is possible because locus heterogeneity has been reported in FAP; not all FAP kindreds are linked to chromosome 5q. In this case, a "no mutation detected" result, APC gene testing has no predictive value for asymptomatic at-risk relatives. In these families, first-degree relatives should continue colorectal surveillance annually between the ages of 12 and 25 years, every other year between the ages of 25 and 35 years, and every third year between the ages of 35 and 50 years. Family members who have not developed multiple adenomatous polyps on colonoscopic examination by the age of 50 years are assumed to be unaffected by FAP.

Caution should be used in interpreting genetic test results when a mutation is not detected, because these results can be misinterpreted as a negative result. This in turn could lead to controversy in the guidelines in the follow-up care for those with a "no mutation detected" result.

A third scenario with a "no mutation detected" result occurs when an unaffected family member of an APC kindred is tested without testing an affected family member. In such a case, the result does not mean that the unaffected person is not at risk for FAP, because it has not been determined that a mutation in APC is present in the family. It is important that the patient not be falsely reassured, because other mechanisms may inactivate the APC gene, or other genes may be involved.

Summary on interpretation of APC genetic testing is in Figure 23 (245).

■ WHEN TO SCREEN AND WHEN TO OPERATE?

Gene test results can change the risk for FAP from a priori 50% to essentially 0% or 100%. Presymptomatic genetic testing removes the necessity of annual screening of those at-risk individuals who do not have the gene, and probably improves compliance in those who do. No change in conventional screening guidelines for colon polyps is recommended for those whose presymptomatic DNA diagnosis indicates that they have the FAP-causing gene. These individuals should have annual colon and rectal

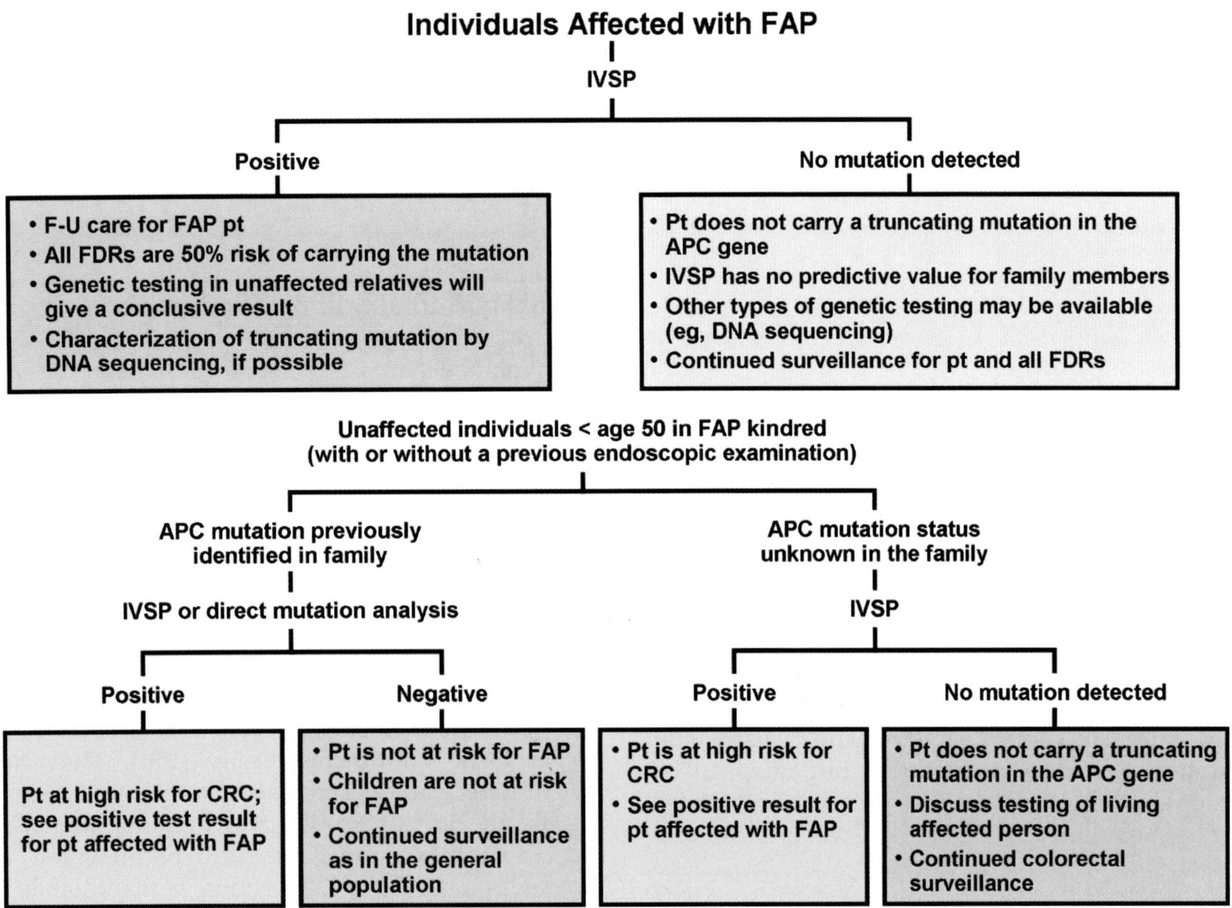

FIGURE 23 ■ Summary interpretation of APC genetic testing. *Abbreviations*: CRC, colorectal carcinoma; FAP, familial adenomatous polyposis; FDR, first degree relative; F-U, follow-up; IVSP, in vitro synthesized protein assay (protein truncation test); pt, patient. *Source*: From Ref. 245.

examinations with at least a flexible sigmoidoscopy beginning at approximately 10 or 11 years' of age (243). The age for the start of screening varies from series to series. The St. Mark's series began at 14 years of age or older (226). Follow-up surveillance for extracolonic neoplasms is also indicated. At this time, the patients should also be counseled to prepare for an eventual prophylactic colectomy and should be given genetic counseling about the risk of FAP for future offspring.

Timing of operation depends on the number of polyps found in the colon and rectum. The natural history of the disease, even though it is highly variable between individual cases, suggests that operation should be performed by 25 years of age, although most of the St. Mark's patients had a colectomy by the age of 20 years. The youngest FAP patient with a carcinoma in the St. Mark's registry is a 17-year-old girl (226).

For those who have not inherited the *APC* mutation, colon screening can be significantly reduced to three or fewer time points: at ages 18, 25, and 35 years. These time points are selected to provide the clinician with a management margin that accommodates false negative results from laboratory error and infrequent phenomena, such as tissue mosaicism or de novo mutations. The individual's lifetime risk of colorectal carcinoma becomes the general population's risk of approximately 3%, and colon carcinoma screening should resume again around age 50, according to conventional guidelines. These individuals can also be assured that their offspring will not be at risk for FAP (243).

■ THE POLYPOSIS REGISTRY

The aims of a polyposis registry are to ensure efficient care of patients and their families and to promote and carry out the research that will advance the knowledge of FAP for physicians and surgeons. Data held in a standardized format on computers assist the day-to-day of those in the registry as well as allow for speedy analysis (244).

A registry deals not only with the patient but also with the patient's family members. Family pedigrees are collected and regularly updated. A counseling team plays an important part of the registry. Early diagnosis, using modern and reliable techniques, timely operation to prevent the onset of carcinoma, and continued surveillance after operation for early detection and treatment of associated carcinomas are key features of a successful registry. The impact of screening on carcinoma incidence in patients with FAP at St. Mark's Registry is shown in Figure 24. It has a remarkable success in preventing the development of colorectal carcinomas (244).

The Leed's Castle Polyposis Group in Kent, United Kingdom, was established in June 1985. The aims of this gathering were to discuss the problems facing those who cared for polyposis patients and to establish an international cooperative organization. In 1992, there were 51 such centers worldwide. The group seeks furtherknowledge of the etiology, clinical features, prevention, and treatment of FAP in all of its manifestations (244).

As outlined by Church and McGannon (247), there are three types of FAP registries.

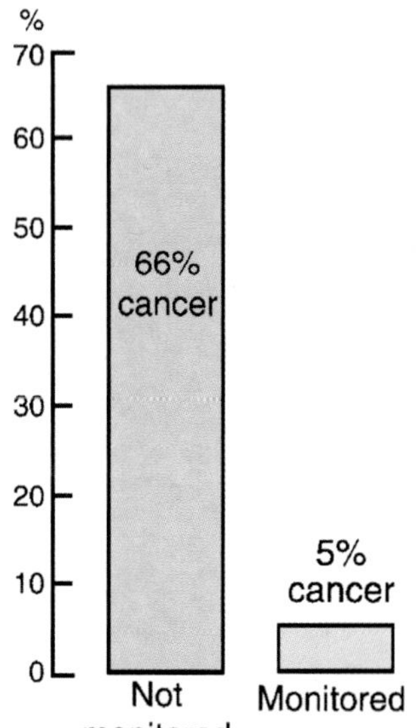

FIGURE 24 ■ The results of screening by the St. Mark's Polyposis Registry. *Source*: From Ref. 244, p. 9.

The Countrywide Registry

In this type of registry, cases of FAP from the entire country are collected into one central registry. The registry staff need not undertake direct patient care but must collect and collate data from everywhere. Examples of countrywide registries are those in Denmark, Sweden, Holland, and Singapore.

The Regional Registry

This type fits well with very large or widespread populations or those without a uniform health care system. Regional registries are miniatures of countrywide registries in which families are collected from a defined region, for example, an area health board or a county. Parish, city, and county records contain extensive information with which to flush out family data, and the registry develops lines of communication with hospitals and physicians in its area. Registry staff need not commit to patient care but can offer specialized counseling and testing services. Regional registries are common in the United Kingdom.

The Tertiary Referral Center

This type develops around one or two physicians of repute who work in a tertiary referral medical center and who have a special interest in FAP. Families are accumulated and a patient base is built. Patients may come from all over a country for treatment and return to the registry for surveillance. An example of such a registry is the Cleveland Clinic Foundation. Minnesota Colorectal Cancer Initiative (248) is a community-based Colorectal Cancer Registry run by two physician groups and the University Cancer Center. It is a not-for-profit organization financially supported by healthcare organizations, pharmaceutical companies, a consulting firm, and other practice groups. It is a model of effective collaboration between an academic tertiary referral center and community healthcare providers. Enrollment is not limited to individuals with an established diagnosis of a hereditary colorectal cancer syndrome, but is most likely to benefit people who may be at increased risk of developing colorectal or other carcinoma because they have a personal or family history of colorectal carcinoma.

Setting up a successful polyposis registry is a large project requiring large sums of funds, space equipment, and personnel. Table 9 shows the organization of a successful registry (247).

HEMANGIOMAS OF LARGE BOWEL

Hemangiomas are rare vascular lesions of the large bowel. More than 200 cases have been documented in the literature from 1931 to 1974, with more than 50% involving the rectum (249). Hemangiomas of the large bowel are congenital, developing from embryonic sequestration of mesodermal tissue. However, whether they represent a simple vascular malformation (hamartoma) or a neoplasm is unsettled.

■ CLASSIFICATION

Capillary hemangiomas consist of a network of fine, newly formed, closely packed capillaries, with a distinct hyperplastic endothelial lining (250). They are usually encountered at operation and are found mainly in the small intestine, appendix, and perianal skin. This type of hemangioma accounts for 10% of all colon and rectal hemangiomas (249). Cavernous hemangiomas are large, thin-walled vessels. The stroma has little connective tissue and muscle.

■ CLINICAL MANIFESTATIONS

The great majority of patients present early in life with recurrent, painless, and sometimes massive hemorrhage. Nine of 15 cases in the report of Londono-Schimmer et al. (251) were first seen at a hospital before the age of 5 years. The age of onset, type, frequency, and severity of bleeding are related to the size, number, and type of vascular malformations.

Capillary hemangiomas are characterized by slow, persistent bleeding, producing dark stools and anemia. Cavernous hemangiomas characteristically present early with moderate to severe, painless hemorrhage. The bleeding recurs and increases in severity with each subsequent episode. In severe cases of profuse and unremitting bleeding, an urgent or emergency bowel resection is necessary. This propensity to bleed has been attributed to the lack of muscular and supporting connective tissue in the wall and around the vessels. Anemia is common and accounts for 43% of patients in the series presented by Allred and Spencer (250). Bowel obstruction accounts for 17% of the

TABLE 9 ■ **Staff for a Successful Registry**

Physicians	Administrative	Research
Gastroenterologist	Secretary	Molecular geneticist
Colorectal surgeon	Statistician	Lab technician
Medical geneticist	Computer technician	Research fellows
Pathologist	Financial counselor	Study assistant/ research nurse
	Marketing	

Source: From Ref. 247.

cases. Diarrhea, tenesmus, rectal prolapse, and sometimes constipation can occur.

■ DIAGNOSIS

Hemangiomas of the large bowel are often misdiagnosed because of the lack of awareness of the clinical features. They are frequently mistaken for hemorrhoids, inflammatory bowel diseases, polyps, carcinomas, and other entities (249). At St. Mark's Hospital, 8 of 10 patients had at least one hemorrhoidectomy before the age of 20 years (252).

Flexible sigmoidoscopy is the most important and most useful part of the workup. The mucosa has a deep blue or dull red color and appears wine or plum colored. The mucosa is usually nodular, with or without dilated viens (Fig. 25). Chronic inflammatory changes may mimic proctitis. Usually there is no mucosal ulceration. Hemorrhoids and ulcerative proctocolitis are the most common misdiagnoses.

Plain abdominal films are useful. Calcification within the venous plexus of the bowel wall repre sents a sequela of thrombosis within the neoplasm caused by perivascular inflammation and sluggish blood flow. Phleboliths also accompany heman giomas at other locations along the GI tract and in venous plexuses of the uterine broad ligament, the urinary bladder, the prostate, and the spleen. Approximately 50% of adults with intestinal hemangiomas are noted to have phlebolith clusters on plain films (249).

In a patient with an extensive hemangioma, barium enema studies reveal a characteristic scalloped contour of submucosal masses, causing narrowing of the colonic and rectal lumen. It can be differentiated from other neoplastic masses by its compressibility and a longer segment of involvement than polyps or carcinomas.

A CT scan of the pelvis may show a large and markedly thickened rectal wall and phleboliths (if present) (Fig. 26).

Selective inferior mesenteric arteriography is valuable to assist in determining the extent of the disease, particularly the less extensive hemangiomas in which localization at operation may be difficult. The delayed phase of arteriography may show large venous pooling within the cavernous hemangiomas (253). Arteriography is also helpful in detecting any abnormal blood vessels in the pelvis.

Hypofibrinogenemia or afibrinogenemia that is caused by a consumptive coagulopathy is occasionally seen in these patients. Isotope studies with ^{51}Cr-labeled platelets suggest sequestration within the hemangiomas. Resection of the hemangiomas has resulted in complete reversal of the coagulopathy (249).

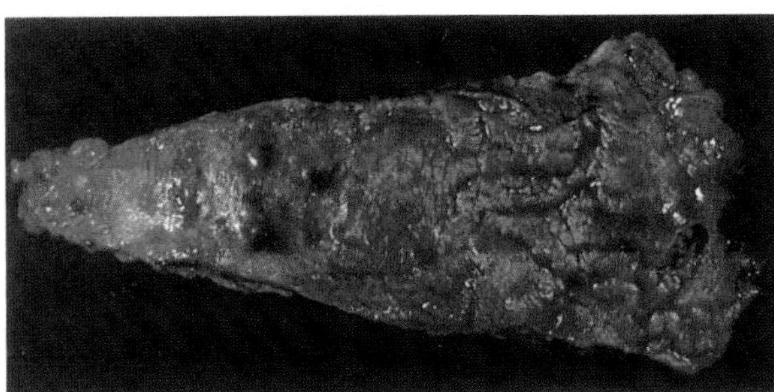

FIGURE 25 ■ Diffuse hemangioma of rectum. Note thickening and irregular mucosa. *Source*: Courtesy of Roger R Dozois, M.D., Mayo Clinic, Rochester, MN, U.S.A.

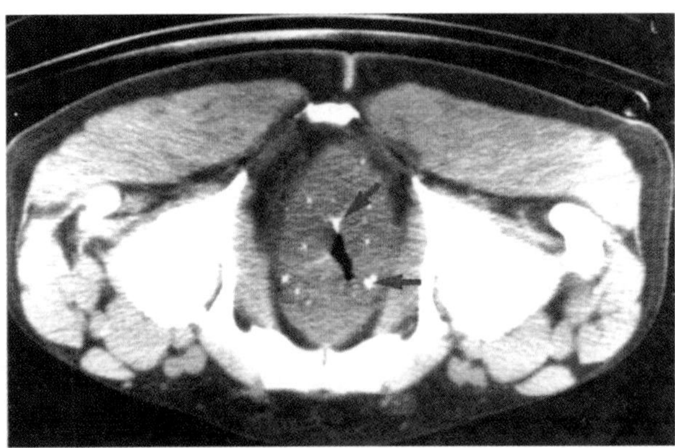

FIGURE 26 ■ Computed tomography scan of pelvis shows calcification of submucosal vascular plexus in diffuse hemangioma of rectum (*arrows*).

■ TREATMENT

Until 1971 abdominoperineal resection was the only definitive treatment for diffuse hemangiomas of the anorectum. Since then, the St. Mark's group has performed a rectosigmoid resection with preservation of the pelvic floor and sphincter muscles. The entire rectum is mobilized and transected at the level just above the levator ani muscle. The anorectal mucosa and submucosa from the dentate line are stripped from underlying muscle up to the level of the transection. The sigmoid colon or the descending colon is then brought through the denuded anorectum and anastomosed to the dentate line. Londono-Schimmer et al. (251) reported success in all 15 patients using this technique and concluded that it is the treatment of choice. Telander et al. (254) successfully performed this operation in four children with rectal hemangiomas associated with Kleppel-Trenaunay syndrome, a congenital venous anomaly manifested by extensive hemangiomatous malformation within the pelvis and extremity, hypertrophy of the extremity, and atypical varicosities. Coppa et al. (253), on the other hand, reported that three of eight patients who underwent coloanal sleeve anastomosis had recurrent episodes of rectal bleeding similar to preoperative symptoms, most likely caused by involvement of the anal canal by diffuse cavernous hemangiomas. Ten of those patients who underwent abdominoperineal resection had no recurrent bleeding.

Many other treatments have been reported in literature, all of which are temporary measures. They include colostomy, injection of sclerosing agents, radium implantation, irradiation, ligation of superior rectal arteries, embolization of inferior mesenteric artery, rectal packing, and cryosurgery. The place for the use of the laser in treating diffuse colon and rectal hemangiomas has not been established, but it is doubtful that it would give a permanent cure.

LEIOMYOMAS OF LARGE BOWEL

Leiomyomas of the large bowel are rare neoplasms of the smooth muscle of the bowel. In a review of 160 cases of smooth muscle neoplasms of the GI tract by He et al. (255) only four cases involved the rectum, and none was in the colon or the anal canal. One hundred thirty-one patients with benign gastrointestinal (GI) smooth muscle neoplasms were treated at the Massachusetts General Hospital between 1963 and 1987: 8% in the esophagus, 61% in the stomach, 19% in the small intestine, 5% in the colon, and 6% in the rectum (256). Kusminsky and Bailey (257) reviewed the world literature from 1959 to 1979 and found 79 cases of leiomyoma of the rectum. Leiomyomas are most commonly found in patients 50 to 59 years old and are rare or absent in children.

Miettinen et al (258) studied all the mesenchymal neoplasms involving the rectum and anus coded as leiomyoma, leiomyosarcoma, smooth muscle neoplasm, schwannomas, neurofibromas, nerve sheath, stromal neoplasm. They used immunonohistochemistry. Antibodies to the antigens were: KIT (CD1147), CD34 α-smooth muscle, desmin D33, keratin 18 and 19, neurofilaments, sglial fibrillary acidic protein, and S-100 protein.

The results showed a total of 133 anorectal GI stromal tumors (GIST). Of these, 50 tumors had been originally diagnosed as lymphosarcomas, 29 as smooth muscle tumors of uncertain malignant potential, 21 as leiomyomas, and 3 as GIST.

Only three patents were diagnosed as leiomyoma. All three patients were women, age 25, 29, and 38 years. Tumor size was 1.5, 2, and 4 cm in diameter. All tumors were positive for desmin, α-smooth muscle acting, or both. They were negative for CD117 and CD34. One should be cautious to interprete the diagnosis of leiomyomas in the older literature where the study for GIST were not performed.

■ CLINICAL MANIFESTATIONS

Leiomyomas of the large bowel usually occur in the rectum and less commonly in the anal canal. The most common finding is the presence of a mass, usually detected as an incidental finding during rectal or proctosigmoidoscopic examination. Most patients with leiomyomas are asymptomatic, but some may present with constipation, bleeding, anorectal pain, and a pressure sensation in the rectum.

■ PATHOLOGY

Leiomyomas may be pedunculated or sessile, submucosal, extrarectal, or dumbbell shaped to involve both intramural and extramural positions (Fig. 27). They may be in the abdomen or may protrude into the retrorectal space. In the anal canal, they may be found submucosally but are most commonly found in the intersphincteric position with a variable relationship to the sphincter muscles (257). Leiomyomas are firm, rounded, sharply circumscribed neoplasms, but they have no definite capsule microscopically. There are few reliable criteria for separating benign from malignant growths. Most malignant neoplasms are judged by metastases and may not be recognized until months or years later. Some pathologists accept more than two mitoses revealed under high power as evidence of malignancy. Morgan et al. (256) concluded that symptomatic gastric and small intestinal leiomyomas with more than two mitoses per 50 high-power field should be suspicious for a malignant potential. Whether this statement can be applied to leiomyomas of the large intestine is unknown. Others do not accept these criteria and do

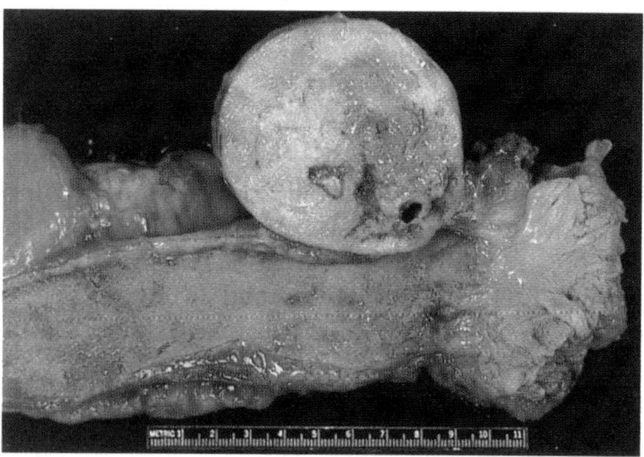

FIGURE 27 ■ Leiomyoma of the rectum of a patient with ulcerative colitis.

not attempt to differentiate between benign and malignant growths at the time of examination (259).

■ ORIGIN

Smooth muscle neoplasms of the large bowel may arise from the muscularis mucosa or the muscularis propria. The division into neoplasms arising from the muscularis mucosa of the rectum, muscularis propria, or internal sphincter is based primarilon microscopic appearance to indicate the layer from which the neoplasm appears to arise. Histologically, all neoplasms arising from the muscularis mucosae of the rectum appear totally benign and arid, while the others vary in degree of differentiation. Of the 48 cases at St. Mark's Hospital, 26 arose from muscularis mucosa, 18 from the muscularis propria, and four from the internal sphincter muscle (259).

■ TREATMENT

Since it may not be known which neoplasm is malignant, the key to successful management is complete removal of the lesion. Walsh and Mann (259) reported local excision of 26 neoplasms arising from the muscularis mucosa and four neoplasms arising from the internal sphincter with no recurrence. However, local excision of 18 lesions arising from the muscularis propria resulted in a 60% recurrence rate. Of significance is that the incidence of recurrence after local excision bears no relationship to the degree of histologic differentiation. It appears that for neoplasms arising from the muscularis propria and those >5 cm in diameter, a radical approach is indicated, that is, bowel resection or even abdominoperineal resection (257). Vorobyov et al. (260) presented their experience of 36 patients with rectal leiomyomas at the Moscow Proctology Institute. The authors recommend electro-excision through the endoscope for a neoplasm <1 cm in diameter. A transanal excision can be performed for a lesion <3 cm in diameter. When the lesion is >5 cm, a resection is advised.

■ LIPOMAS OF LARGE BOWEL

Lipomas of the large bowel are uncommon fatty neoplasms. The Mayo Clinic experience reveals 91 cases of large bowel lipomas during the period from 1976 to 1985 (261).

Approximately 90% of the large bowel lipomas are in the submucosa and 10% in the subserosa (262). In order of frequency, the most common sites are the cecum, ascending colon, and sigmoid colon, with one-third to one-half located in the right colon (261,263) Rare cases of submucosal lipomatous polypors of the colon have been reported (264,265). In one of the reports (265) the number of polyps was between 700 and 1000 (size 1–9 mm) through out the entire colon. A subtotal colectomy was performed in this case because of the frequent bowel movement and inability to rule out neoplastic polyps. The specimen did showed a combination of tabular adenomas, estimated fewer than 60 in number.

■ CLINICAL MANIFESTATIONS

A lipoma < 2 cm rarely causes symptoms. A large lipoma can cause abdominal pain from partial bowel obstruction. Colicky pain may be caused by intermittent intussusception. Lipomas are the most common benign neoplasms that cause intussusception in adults. Bleeding can occur if the mucosa overlying the lipoma is ulcerated, which is usually caused by chronic intussusception.

■ DIAGNOSIS

In the Mayo Clinic series 46% of the large bowel lipomas were discovered incidentally in the specimens removed for other diseases. Eleven percent of them were resected because of a neoplasm suspected as being a carcinoma (263).

Barium enema reveals a filling defect in the colon or rectum. A lipoma appears smooth and radiolucent and changes in shape on compression during examination. Despite these characteristics, the correct radiologic diagnosis is not always made. A CT scan is helpful in confirming the presence of fatty tissue in the mass (266,267). Colonoscopy can confirm the diagnosis in most cases. The lipoma has a characteristic yellowish submucosal soft mass. When pressed with the tip of a biopsy forceps, the lipoma is depressed; this is known as the "cushion sign." A biopsy must include the submucosal layer but seldom is necessary for diagnosis. An ulcerated lipoma can be confused with an adenoma or an adenocarcinoma. Lipomas of the large bowel should not be forgotten in the differential diagnosis of all large bowel neoplasms.

■ TREATMENT

Small and asymptomatic lipomas of the large bowel do not require removal. Colonoscopic polypectomy of a large lipoma should be avoided since a tremendous amount of heat is required to cut through the lipoma because of its high water content. The risk of transmural burn, perforation, or bleeding outweighed the benefits in seven lipomas removed by colonoscopic polypectomy by Pfeil et al. (268); three had perforations (size, 4.2 ± 0.7 cm). The authors warned that a lipoma >2 cm is at the greatest risk for perforation. Symptomatic lipomas should be excised by colotomy or a limited colon resection (269).

REFERENCES

1. O'Brien MJ. Colorectal adenomas: concepts and controversies. Semin Colon Rectal Surg 1992; 3:195–206.
2. Rickert RR, Averbach O, Garfinkel L, Hammond EC, Frasca JM. Adenomatous lesions of the large bowel: an autopsy survey. Cancer 1979; 43:1847–1857.
3. Williams AR, Balasooriya BA, Day DW. Polyps and cancer of the large bowel: a necropsy study in Liverpool. Gut 1982; 23:835–842.
4. Vatn MH, Stalsberg H. The prevalence of polyps of the large intestine in Oslo: an autopsy study. Cancer 1982; 49:819–825.
5. Eide TJ, Stalsberg H. Polyps of the large intestine in northern Norway. Cancer 1978; 42:2839–2848.
6. O'Brien MJ, Winawer SJ, Zauber AG, et al. The National Polyp Study. Patient and polyp characteristics associated with high-grade dysplasia in colorectal adenomas. Gastroenterology 1990; 98:371–379.
7. Nusko G, Mansmann U, Partzsch U, et al. Invasive carcinoma in colorectal adenomas: multivariate analysis and adenoma characteristics. Endoscopy 1997; 29:626–631.
8. Muto T, Bussey HJ, Morson BC. The evolution of cancer of the colon and rectum. Cancer 1975; 36:2251–2270.
9. Dukes C. Simple tumors of the large intestine and their relationship to cancer. Br J Surg 1926; 13:720–733.
10. Jackman RJ, Mayo CW. The adenoma-carcinoma sequence in cancer of the colon. Surg Gynecol Obstet 1951; 93:327–330.
11. Castleman B, Krickstein HI. Do adenomatous polyps of the colon become malignant? N Engl J Med 1962; 267:469–475.
12. Ackerman LV, Spratt JS, Fischel E. Do adenomatous polyps become cancer? Gastroenterology 1963; 44:905–907.
13. Morson BC. The polyp-cancer sequence in the large bowel. Proc R Soc Med 1974; 67:451–457.
14. Jass JR. Do all colorectal carcinomas arise in pre-existing adenomas?. World J Surg 1989; 13:45–51.
15. Nelson RL. Diet and adenomatous polyp risk. Semin Colon Rectal Surg 1991; 2:262–268.
16. Armitage NC. Intervention studies in adenoma patients. World J Surg 1991; 15:29–34.
17. Kronborg O, Fenger C. Clinical evidence of the adenoma–carcinoma sequence. Eur J Cancer Prevention 1999; 8:573–586.
18. Tierney RP, Ballantyne GH, Modlin IM. The adenoma to carcinoma sequence. Surg Gynecol Obstet 1990; 171:81–94.
19. Eide TJ. Natural history of adenomas. World J Surg 1991; 15:3–6.
20. Eide TJ. Risk of colorectal cancer in adenoma-bearing individuals within a defined population. Int J Cancer 1986; 38:173–176.
21. Shimoda T, Ikegami M, Fujisaki J, Matsui T, Aizawa S, Ishikawa E. Early colorectal carcinoma with special reference to its development de novo. Cancer 1989; 64:1138–1146.
22. Stolte M, Beckte B. Colorectal mini–de novo carcinoma: a realty in Germany too. Endoscopy 1995; 27:286–290.
23. Bedenne L, Faivre J, Boutron MC, Piard F, Cauvin JM, Hillon P. Adenoma–carcinoma sequence or "de novo" carcinogenesis? A study of adenomatous remnants in a population-based series of large bowel cancers. Cancer 1992; 69:883–888.
24. Muto T, Nagawa H, Watanabe T, Masaki T, Sawada T. Colorectal carcinogenesis. Historical review. Dis Colon Rectum 1997; 40(suppl):580–585.
25. Church JM, Williams BR, Casey G. Molecular Genetics and Colorectal Neoplasia. A Primer for the Clinician. New York: Igaku-Shoin Medical Publishers, 1996.
26. Nivatvongs S, Dorudi S. Colorectal polyps and their management. In: Williams NS, ed. Colorectal Cancer. London: Churchill Livingstone, 1996:39–54.
27. Dirschmid K, Kiesler J, Mathis G, Beller S, Stoss F, Schobel B. Epithelial misplacement after biopsy of colorectal adenomas. Am J Surg Pathol 1993; 17:1262–1265.
28. Fenoglio-Preiser CM. Colonic polyp histology. Semin Colon Rectal Surg 1991; 2:234–245.
29. Nivatvongs S, Nicholson JD, Rothenberger DA, et al. Villous adenoma of the rectum: the accuracy of clinical assessment. Surgery 1980; 87:549–551.
30. Galandiuk S, Fazio VW, Jagelman DG, et al. Villous and tubulovillous adenomas of the colon and rectum. A retrospective review, 1964–1985. Am J Surg 1987; 153:41–46.
31. Muto T, Kamiya J, Sawada T, et al. Small "flat adenoma" of the large bowel with special reference to its clinicopathologic features. Dis Colon Rectum 1985; 28:847–851.
32. Muto T, Watanabe T. Flat adenomas and minute carcinomas of the colon and rectum. Perspect Colon Rectal Surg 1993; 6:117–132.
33. Lynch HT, Smyrk T, Lanspa SJ, et al. Flat adenomas in a colon cancer-prone kindred. J Natl Cancer Inst 1988; 80:278–282.
34. Rembacken BJ, Fujii T, Cairms A, et al. Flat and depressed colonic neoplasms: a prospective study of 1000 colonoscopies in UK. Lancet 2000; 355:1211–1214.
35. Radaelli F, Minoli G. Editorial comments. Gastrointest Endosc 2001; 53: 689–691.
36. Minamoto T, Sawaguchi K, Mai M, Yamashita N, Sugimura T, Esumi H. Infrequent K-ras activation in superficial-type (flat) colorectal adenomas and adenocarcinomas. Cancer Res 1994; 54:2841–2844.
37. Gilbertsen VA. Proctosigmoidoscopy and polypectomy in reducing the incidence of rectal cancer. Cancer 1974; 34(suppl):936–939.
38. Selby JV, Friedman GD, Quesenberry CP Jr, Weiss NS. A case-control study of screening sigmoidoscopy and mortality from colorectal cancer. N Engl J Med 1992; 326:653–657.
39. Winawer SJ, Zauber AG, Ho MN. Prevention of colorectal cancer by colonoscopic polypectomy. N Engl J Med 1993; 329:1977–1981.

40. Sciallero S, Constantini M, Bertinelli E, et al. Distal hyperplastic polyps do not predict proximal adenomas. Results from a multicentric study of colorectal adenomas. Gastrointest Endosc 1997; 46:124–130.
41. Rex DK, Smith JJ, Ulbright TM, Lehman GA. Distal colonic hyperplastic polyps do not predict proximal adenomas in asymptomatic average-risk subjects. Gastroenterology 1992; 102:317–319.
42. Provenzale D, Garret JW, Condon SE, Sandler RS. Risk for colon adenomas in patients with rectosigmoid hypoplastic polyps. Ann Intern Med 1990; 113: 760–763.
43. Church JM. Clinical significance of small colorectal polyps. Dis Colon Rectum 2004; 47:481–485.
44. Atkin WS, Morson BC, Cuzick J. Long-term risk of colorectal cancer after excision of rectosigmoid adenomas. N Engl J Med 1992; 326:658–662.
45. Stryker SJ, Wolff BG, Culp CE, Libbe SD, Ilstrup DM, Mac-Carty RL. Natural history of untreated colonic polyps. Gastroenterology 1987; 93:1009–1013.
46. Otchy DP, Ransohoff DF, Wolft BG, et al. Metachronous colon cancer in persons who have had a large adenomatous polyp. Am J Gastroenterol 1996; 91:448–454.
47. Hofstad B, Vatri MH, Anderson SN, et al. Growth of colorectal polyps: redetection and evaluation of unresected polyps for a period of three years. Gut 1996; 39:449–456.
48. Bersentes K, Fennerty MB, Sampliner RE, Harinder SG. Lack of spontaneous regression of tubular adenomos in two years of follow-up. Am J Gastroenterol 1997; 92:1117–1120.
49. Haggitt RC, Glotzbach RE, Soffer EE, Wruble LD. Prognostic factors in colorectal carcinomas arising in adenomas: implications for lesions removed by endoscopic polypectomy. Gastroenterology 1985; 89:328–336.
50. Nivatvongs S, Rojanasakul A, Reiman HM, et al. The risk of lymph node-metastasis in colorectal polyps with invasive adenocarcinoma. Dis Colon Rectum 1991; 34:323–328.
51. Pollard CW, Nivatvongs S, Rojanasakul A, Reiman HM, Dozois RR. The fate of patients following polypectomy alone for polyps containing invasive carcinoma. Dis Colon Rectum 1992; 35:933–937.
52. Kyzer S, Begin LR, Gordon PH, Mitmaker B. The care of patients with colorectal polyps that contain invasive adenocarcinoma.Endoscopic polypectomy or colectomy.. Cancer 1992; 70:2044–2050.
53. Muto T, Sawada T, Sukihara K. Treatment of carcinoma in adenomas. World J Surg 1991; 15:35–40.
54. Morson BC, Whiteway JE, Jones EA, Macrae FA, Williams CB. Histopathology and prognosis of malignant colorectal polyps treated by endoscopic polypectomy. Gut 1984; 25:437–444.
55. Richards WO, Webb WA, Morris SJ, et al. Patient management after endoscopic removal of the cancerous colon adenoma. Ann Surg 1987; 205:665–672.
56. Coverlizza S, Risio M, Ferrari A, Fenoglio-Preiser CM, Rossini FP. Colorectal adenomas containing invasive carcinoma. Pathologic assessment of lymph node metastatic potential. Cancer 1989; 64:1937–1947.
57. Cooper HS, Deppisch LM, Gourley WK, et al. Endoscopically removed malignant colorectal polyps: clinicopathologic correlations. Gastroenterology 1995; 108:1657–1665.
58. Kudo S. Endoscopic mucosal resection of flat and depressed types of early colorectal cancer. Endoscopy 1993; 25:455–461.
59. Participants in the Paris Workshop. The Paris endoscopic classification of superficial neoplastic lesions: esophagus, stomach and colon. Gastrointest Endosc 2003; 58:S3–S43.
60. Nascimbeni R, Burgart LJ, Nivatvongs S, Larson DR. Risk of lymph node metastasis in T_1 carcinoma of the colon and rectum. Dis Colon Rectum 2002; 45:200–206.
61. Nivatvongs S. Surgical management of malignant colorectal polyps. Surg Clin North Am 2002; 82:959–966.
62. Kikuchi R, Takano M, Takagi K, et al. Management of early invasive colorectal cancer. Risk of recurrence and clinical guidelines. Dis Colon Rectum 1995; 38:1286–1295.
63. Lamont JP, McCartz TM, Digan RD, Tulanon P, Lichliter WE. Should locally excised T_1 rectal cancer receive adjuvant chemoradiation? Am J Surg 2000; 180:402–406.
64. Bouvet M, Milas M, Giacco GG, Cleary KR, Janjan NA, Skibber JM. Predictors of recurrence after local excision and postoperative chemoradiation therapy of adenocarcinoma of the rectum. Ann Surg Oncol 1999; 6:26–32.
65. Bailey HR, Huval WV, Max F, Smith KW, Butts DR, Zamora LF. Local excision of carcinoma of the rectum for cure. Surgery 1992; 111:555–561.
66. Paty PB, Nash GM, Baron P, et al. Long-term results of local excision for rectal cancer. Ann Surg 2002; 236:522–530.
67. Benson R, Wong CS, Cummings BJ, et al. Local excision and postoperative radiotherapy for distal rectal cancer. Int J Radiat Oncol Biol Phys 2001; 50:1309–1316.
68. Mellgren A, Sirivongs P, Rothenberger DA, Madoff RD, Garcia-Aguilar J. Is local excision adequate therapy for early rectal cancer? Dis Colon Rectum 2000; 43:1064–1074.
69. Madbouly KM, Remzi FM, Erkek BA, et al. Recurrence after transanal excision of T_1 rectal cancer: should we be concerned? Dis Colon Rectum 2005; 48: 711–721.
70. Nascimbeni R, Nivatvongs S, Larson DR, Burgart LJ. Long-term survival after local excision for T_1 carcinoma of the rectum. Dis Colon Rectum 2004; 47: 1773–1779.
71. Bentrem DJ, Okabe S, Wong WD, et al. T_1 adenocarcinoma of the rectum. Transanal excision or radical surgery? Ann Surg 2005; 242:472–479.
72. Hahnloser D, Wolff BG, Larson DW, Ping J, Nivatvongs S. Immediate radical resection after local excision of rectal cancer: an oncologic compromise? Dis Colon Rectum 2005; 48:429–437.
73. Longacre TA, Fenoglio-Preiser CM. Mixed hyperplastic adenomatous polyps serrated adenomas. A distinct form of colorectal neoplasia. Am J Surg Pathol 1990; 14:524–537.
74. Torlakovic E, Snover DC. Serrated adenomatous polyposis in humans. Gastroenterology 1996; 110:748–755.
75. Torlakovic E, Skovlund E, Snover DC, Torlakovic G, Nesland JM. Morphologic reappraisal of serrated colorectal polyps. Am J Surg Pathol 2003; 27:65–81.
76. Jass JR. Serrated route to colorectal cancer: back street or super highway? J Pathol 2001; 193:283–285.
77. Jass JR. Pathogenesis of colorectal cancer. Surg Clin N Am 2002; 82:891–904.
78. Jass JR. Hyperplastic polyps and colorectal cancer: is there a link? Clin Gastroenterol Hepatol 2004; 2:1–8.
79. McCall I, Bussey HJ, Veale AM, Morson BC. Juvenile polyposis coli. Proc R Soc Med 1964; 57:896–897.
80. Desai DC, Neali KF, Talbot IC, Hodgson SV, Phillips RK. Juvenile polyposis. Br J Surg 1995; 82:14–17.
81. Jass JR, Williams CB, Bussey HJ, Morson BC. Juvenile polyposis—a precancerous condition. Histopathology 1988; 13:619–630.
82. Sachatello CR, Hahn IS, Carrington CB. Juvenile gastrointestinal polyposis in a female infant: report of a case and review of the literature of a recently recognized syndrome. Surgery 1974; 75:107–114.
83. Giardiello FM, Hamilton SR, Kern SE, et al. Colorectal neoplasia in juvenile polyposis or juvenile polyps. Arch Dis Child 1991; 66:971–975.
84. Howe JR, Mitros FA, Summers RW. The risk of gastrointestinal carcinoma in familial juvenile polyposis. Ann Surg Oncol 1998; 5:751–756.
85. Kinzler KW, Vogelstein B. Landscaping the cancer terrain. Science 1998; 280:1036–1037.
86. Giardiello FM, Hamilton SR, Kern SE. Colorectal neoplasia in juvenile polyposis or juvenile polyposis. Arch Dis Child 1991; 66:971–975.
87. Jarvinen H, Franssila KO. Familial juvenile polyposis coli; increased risk of colorectal cancer. Gut 1984; 25:792–800.
88. Howe JR, Ringold JC, Summers RW, Mitros FA, Nishimura DY, Stone EM. A gene for familial juvenile polyposis maps to chromosome 18q21.1. Am J Hum Genet 1998; 62:1129–1136.
89. Howe JR, Roth S, Ringold JC, et al. Mutations in the SMAD4/DPC 4 gene in juvenile polyposis. Science 1998; 280:1086–1088.
90. Onsel M, Church JM, Remzi FH, Fazio VW. Colonic surgery in patients with juvenile polyposis syndrome: a case series. Dis Colon Rectum 2005; 48: 49–56.
91. Scott-Conner C, Hausmann M, Hall TJ, Skelton DS, Anglin BL, Subramony C. Familial juvenile polyposis: patterns of recurrence and implications for surgical management. J Am Coll Surg 1995; 181:407–413.
92. Wirtzfeld DA, Petrelli NJ, Rodriguez-Bigas MA. Hamartomatous polyposis syndrome: molecular genetics, neoplastic risk, and surveillance recommendations. Ann Surg Oncol 2001; 8:319–327.
93. Howe JR, Ringold JC, Hughes JH, Summers RW. Direct genetic testing for SMAD4 mutations in patients at risk for juvenile polyposis. Surgery 1999; 126:162–170.
94. Jeghers H, McKusick VA, Katz KH. Generalized intestinal polyposis and melanin spots of the oral mucosa, lips and digits. A syndrome of diagnostic significance. N Engl J Med 1949; 241:993–1005.
95. Giardillo FM, Walsh SB, Hamilton SR, et al. Increased risk of cancer in Peutz-Jeghers syndrome. N Engl J Med 1987; 316:1511–1514.
96. Schreibman IR, Baker M, Amos C, McGarrity TJ. The hamartomatous polyposis syndromes: a clinical and molecular review. Am J Gastroenterol 2005; 100:476–490.
97. Tomlinson IP, Houlston RS. Peutz-Jeghers syndrome. J Med Genet 1997; 34:1007–1011.
98. Giardiello FM, Brensinger JD, Tersmette AC, et al. Very high risk of cancer is familial Peutz-Jeghers syndrome. Gastroenterology 2000; 119:1447–1453.
99. Foley TR, Mcgarrity TJ, Abt AB. Peutz-Jeghers syndrome: a clinicopathologic survey of the "Harrisburg Family" with a 49-year follow-up. Gastroenterology 1988; 95:1535–1540.
100. Narita T, Eto T, Ito T. Peutz-Jeghers syndrome with adenomas and adenocarcinomas in colonic polyps. Am J Surg Pathol 1987; 11:76–81.
101. Perzin KH, Bridge MF. Adenomatous and carcinomatous changes in hamartomatous polyps of the small intestine (Peutz-Jeghers syndrome): report of a case and review of the literature. Cancer 1982; 49:971–983.
102. Spigelman AD, Murday V, Phillips RK. Cancer and Peutz-Jeghers syndrome. Gut 1989; 30:1588–1590.
103. Boardman LA, Thibideau SN, Schaid DJ, et al. Increased risk for cancer in patients with Peutz-Jeghers syndrome. Ann Intern Med 1998; 128: 896–899.

104. Entius MM, Keller JJ, Westerman AM, et al. Molecular genetic alterations in hamartomatous polyps and carcinomas of patients with Peutz-Jeghers syndrome. J Clin Pathol 2001; 54:126–131.
105. Gruber SB, Entius MM, Petersen GM, et al. Pathogenesis of adenocarcinoma in Peutz-Jeghers syndrome. Cancer 1998; 58:5267–5270.
106. Boardman LA, Pittelkow MR, Couch FJ, et al. Association of Peutz-Jeghers like mucocutaneous pigmentation with breast and gynecologic carcinomas in women. Medicine 2000; 79:293–298.
107. Pedersen IR, Hartvigsen A, Hansen BF, Toftgaard C, Konstantin-Hansen K, Bullow S. Management of Peutz-Jeghers syndrome. Experience with patients from the Danish polyposis register. Int J Colorect Dis 1994; 9:177–179.
108. Spigelman AD, Phillips RK. Peutz-Jeghers syndrome. In: Phillips RK, Spigelman AD, Thomson JP, eds. Familial Adenomatous Polyposis and Other Polyposis Syndromes. London: Edward Arnold, 1994:188–202.
109. Ohmiya N, Taguchi A, Shirai K, Mabuchi N, et al. Endoscopic resection of Peutz-Jeghers polyps throughout the small intestine at double-balloon enteroscopy without laparotomy. Gastrointest Endosc 2005; 61:140–147.
110. Oncel M, Remzi FH, Church JM, Connor JT, Fazio VW. Benefits of "clean sweep" in Peutz-Jeghers patients. Colorectal Dis 2004; 6:332–335.
111. Edwards DP, Khosraviani K, Stafferton R, Phillips RK. Long-term results of polyp clearance by intraoperative enteroscopy in the Peutz-Jeghers Syndrome. Dis Colon Rectum 2003; 46:48–50.
112. Oncel M, Remzi FH, Church JM, Connor JT, Fazio VW. Benefits of "clean sweep" in the Pertz-Jeghers patients. Colorectal Dis 2004; 6:332–335.
113. Cronkhite LN Jr, Canada NJ. Generalized gastrointestinal polyposis. An unusual syndrome of polyposis, pigmentation, alopecis and onjehotrophia. N Engl J Med 1955; 252:1011–1015.
114. Hurt S, Mutch MG. The genetic of other polyposis syndromes. Semin Colon Rect Surg 2004; 15:158–162.
115. Daniel ES, Ludwig SL, Lewin KJ, Ruprecht RM, Rajacich GM, Schwale AD. The Croukhite-Canada syndrome. An analysis of clinical and pathologic features and therapy in 55 patients. Medicine 1982; 61:293–309.
116. Nardone G, D'Armiento F, Carlomagno P, Budillon G. Cronkhite Canada syndrome: case report with some features not previously described. Gastrointest Endosc 1990; 36:150–151.
117. Rappaport LB, Sperling HV, Stavirides A. Colon cancer in Cronkhite-Canada syndrome. J Clin Gastroenterol 1986; 8:199–202.
118. Watanabe T, Kudo M, Shirane H, et al. Cronkhite-Canada syndrome associated with triple gastric cancers: a case report. Gastrointest Endosc 1999; 50:688–691.
119. Russell DM, Bhathal PS, St John DJ. Complete remission in Cronkhite-Canada syndrome. Gastroenterology 1983; 85:180–185.
120. Hanzawa M, Yoshikawa N, Tezuka T, et al. Surgical treatment of Cronkhite-Canada syndrome associated with protein-losing enteropathy. Report of a case. Dis Colon Rectum 1998; 41:932–934.
121. Divgi CR, Lisann NM, Yeh SD, Benua RS. Technitium-99 m albumin scintigraphy in the diagnosis of protein-losing enteropathy. J Nucl Med 1986; 27: 1710–1712.
122. Tseng KC, Sheu BS, Lee JC, Tsai HM, Chiu NT, Dai YC. Application of Technetium-99 m-labeled human serum albumin scan to assist surgical treatment of protein-losing enteropathy in Cronkhite-Canada syndrome: report of a case. Dis Colon Rectum 2005; 48:870–873.
123. Lloyd KM II, Dennis M. Cowden's disease: a possible new symptom complex with multiple system involvement. Ann Intern Med 1963; 58:136–142.
124. Wirtzfeld DA, Petrelli NJ, Rodriguez-Bigus MA. Hamartomatous polyposis syndrome: moleculer genetics, neoplastic risk, and surveillance recommendations. Ann Surg Oncol 2001; 8:319–327.
125. Carlson GJ, Nivatvongs S, Snover DC. Colorectal polyps in Cowden's disease (multiple hamartoma syndrome). Am J Surg Pathol 1984; 8:763–770.
126. Nelen MR, Padberg GW, Peeters EA, et al. Localization of the gene for Cowden disease to chromosome 10q22–23. Nat Genet 1996; 13:114–116.
127. Hanssen AM, Fryns JA. Cowden syndrome. J Med Genet 1995; 32:117–119.
128. Starink TM, van der Veen JP, Arwet F, et al. The Cowden syndrome: a clinical and genetic study in 21 patients. Clin Genet 1986; 29:222–233.
129. Longy M, Lacombe D. Cowden disease. Report of a family and review. Ann Genet 1996; 39:35–42.
130. Riley HD, Smith WR. Macrocephaly, pseudopapilledema and multiple hemangioma. Pediatrics 1960; 26:293–300.
131. Bannayan GA. Lipomatosis, angiomatosis, and macrocephaly. A previously undescribed congenital syndrome. Arch Pathol 1971; 92:1–5.
132. Ravalcaba RHA, Myhre S, Smith DW. Sotos syndrome with intestinal polyposis and pigmentary changes of the genitalia. Clin Genet 1980; 18:413–416.
133. Zigman AF, Lavine JE, Jones MC, et al. Localization of the Bannayan-Riley-Ruvalcaba syndrome gene to chromosome 10q23. Gastroenterology 1997; 113:1433–1437.
134. Morson BC, Bussey HJ. Predisposing causes of intestinal cancer. Curr Probl Surg 1970:1–46.
135. Dawson IM, Cornes JS, Morson BC. Primary malignant lymphoid tumors of the intestinal tract: report of 37 cases with a study of factors influencing prognosis. Br J Surg 1961; 49:80–89.
136. Khan A, Shrier I, Gordon PH. The changed histologic paradigm of colorectal polyps. Surg Endosc 2002; 16:436–440.
137. Jass JR. Nature and clinical significance of colorectal hyperplastic polyp. Semin Colon Rectal Surg 1991; 2:246–252.
138. Williams GT, Arthur JF, Bussey HJ, Morson BC. Metaplastic polyps and polyposis of the colorectum. Histopathology 1980; 4:155–170.
139. Hyman NH, Anderson P, Blasyk H. Hyperplastic polyposis and the risk of colorectal cancer. Dis Colon Rectum 2004; 47:2101–2104.
140. Jeevaratnam P, Cottier DS, Browett PJ, Van De Water NS, Pokos V, Jass JR. Familial giant hyperplastic polyposis predisposing to colorectal cancer: a new hereditary bowel cancer syndrome. J Pathol 1996; 179:20–25.
141. Bensen SP, Cole BF, Mott LA, Baron JA, Sandler RS, Halle R. Colorectal hyperplastic polyps and risk of recurrence of adenomas and hyperplastic polyps. Lancet 1999; 354:1873–1874.
142. Rustin RB, Jagelman DG, McGannon E, Fazio VW, Lavery IC, Weakley FL. Spontaneous mutation in familial adenomatous polyposis. Dis Colon Rectum 1990; 33:52–55.
143. Bulow S. The Danish polyposis registry. Dis Colon Rectum 1984; 27:351–355.
144. Bussey HJ. Familial Polyposis Coli. Family Studies, Histopathology, Differential Diagnosis and Results of Treatment. Baltimore: Johns Hopkins University Press, 1975.
145. Talbot IC. Pathology. In: Phillips RK, Spigelman AD, Thomson JP, eds. Familial Adenomatous Polyposis and Other Polyposis Syndromes. London: Edward Arnold, 1994:15–25.
146. Perry RE, Christensen MA, Thorson AG, Williams T. Familial polyposis: colon cancer in the absence of rectal polyps. Br J Surg 1989; 76:744.
147. Bulow S. The risk of developing rectal cancer after colectomy and ileorectal anastomosis in Danish patients with polyposis coli. Dis Colon Rectum 1984; 27:726–729.
148. Spiro L, Olschwang S, Groden J, et al. Alleles of the APC gene: an attenuated form of familial polyposis. Cell 1993; 75:951–957.
149. Lynch HT, Smyrk T, McGinn T, et al. Attenuated familial adenomatous polyposis (AFAP). A phenotypically and genotypically distinctive variant of FAP. Cancer 1995; 76:2427–2433.
150. Hernegger GS, Moore HG, Guillem JG. Attenuated familial adenomatous polyposis. An evolving and poorly understood entity. Dis Colon Rectum 2002; 45:127–136.
151. Church JM. Editorial. Dis Colon Rectum 2002; 45:134–135.
152. Hodgson SV, Spigelman AD. Genetics. In: Phillips RK, Spigelman AD, Thomson JP, eds. Familial Adenomatous Polyposis and Other Polyposis Syndromes. London: Edward Arnold, 1994:26–35.
153. Chung DC, Mino H, Shannon RM. Case 34–2003: a 45-year-old woman with a family history of colonic polyps and cancer. N Engl J Med 2003; 349:1750–1760.
154. Gardner EJ. A genetic and clinical study of intestinal polyposis, a predisposing factor for carcinoma of the colon and rectum. Am J Hum Genet 1951; 3:167–176.
155. Powell SM. Clinical applications of molecular genetics in colorectal cancer. Semin Colon Rectal Surg 1995; 6:2–18.
156. Campbell WJ, Spence RA, Parks TG. Familial adenomatous polyposis [review]. Br J Surg 1994; 81:1722–1733.
157. Utsunomiya J, Maki T, Iwama T, et al. Gastric lesions familial polyposis coli. Cancer 1974; 34:745–754.
158. Arcello PW, Asbun AJ, Veidenheimer MC, et al. Gastroduodenal polyps in familial adenomatous polyposis. Surg Endosc 1996; 40:418–421.
159. Spigelman AD, Williams CB, Talbot IC, Domizio P, Phillips RK. Upper gastrointestinal cancer in patients with familial adenomatous polyposis. Lancet 1989; 2:783–785.
160. Wallace MH, Phillips RK. Upper gastrointestinal disease in patients with familial adenomatous polyposis. Br J Surg 1998; 85:742–750.
161. Bulow S, Alm T, Fausa O, Hulterantz R, Jarvinen H, Vasen H. DAF Project Group. Duodenal adenomatosis in familial adenomatous polyposis. Int J Colorect Dis 1995; 10:43–46.
162. Spigelman AD. Familial adenomatous polyposis and the upper gastrointestinal tract. Semin Colon Rectal Surg 1995; 6:26–28.
163. Church JM, McGannon E, Hull-Boiner S, et al. Gastroduodenal polyps in patients with familial adenomatous polyposis. Dis Colon Rectum 1992; 35:1170–1173.
164. Bjork J, Akerbrant H, Iselius L, et al. Periampullary adenomas and adenocarcinomas in familial adenomatous polyposis: cumulative risks and APC gene mutations. Gastroenterology 2001; 121:1127–1135.
165. Domizio P, Talbot IC, Spigelman AD, Phillips RK, Williams CB. Upper gastrointestinal tract pathology in familial adenomatous polyposis: results from a prospective study of 102 patients. J Clin Pathol 1990; 43:738–743.
166. Kashiwagi H, Spigelman AD, Debuiski HS, Talbot IC, Phillips RK. Surveillance of ampullary adenomas in familial adenomatous polyposis [letter]. Lancet 1994; 344:1582.
167. Jagelman DG, DeCosse JJ, Bussey HJ. the Leeds Castle Polyposis Group Upper gastrointestinal cancer in familial adenomatous polyposis. Lancet 1988; 1:1149–1151.
168. Arvanitis ML, Jagelman DG, Fazio VW, Lavery IC, McGannon E. Mortality in patients with familial adenomatous polyposis. Dis Colon Rectum 1990; 33:639–642.
169. Belchetz LA, Berk T, Bapat BV, Cohen Z, Gallinger S. Changing causes of mortality in patients with familial adenomatous polyposis. Dis Colon Rectum 1996; 39:384–387.

170. Wallace MH, Forbes A, Beveridge IG, et al. Randomized, place co-controlled trial of gastric acid-lowering therapy on duodenal polyposis and relative adduct labeling in familial adenomatous polyposis. Dis Colon Rectum 2001; 44:1585–1589.
171. Phillips RK, Wallace MH, Lynch PH, et al. The FAP study group. A randomized, double blind, placebo controlled study of celecoxib, a selective cyclooxygenase inhibitor on duodenal polyposis in familial adenomatous polyposis. Gut 2002; 50:857–860.
172. Perez A, Saltzman JR, Carr-Locke DL, et al. Benign nonampullary duodenal neoplasms. J Gastrointest Surg 2003; 7:536–541.
173. Alarcon FJ, Burke CA, Church JM, van Stolk RW. Familial adenomatous polyposis. Efficacy of endoscopic and surgical treatment for advanced duodenal adenomas. Dis Colon Rectum 1999; 42:1533–1536.
174. Burke CA, Beck GJ, Church JM, van Stolk RW. The natural history of untreated duodenal and ampullary adenomas in patients with familial adenomatous polyposis followed in an endoscopic surveillance program. Gastrointest Endosc 1999; 49:358–364.
175. Soravia C, Bork T, Haber G, Cohen Z, Gallinger S. Management of advanced duodenal polyposis in familial adenomatous polyposis. J Gastrointest Surg 1997; 1:474–478.
176. Penna C, Bataille N, Balladur P, Tiret E, Parc R. Surgical treatment of severe duodenal polyposis in familial adenomatous polyposis. Br J Surg 1998; 85:665–668.
177. de Vostot Nederveen Cappel WH, Jarvinen HJ, Bjork J, Berk T, Griffioen G, Vasen HF. Worldwide survey among polyposis registries of surgical management of severe duodenal adenomatosis in familial adenomatous polyposis. Br J Surg 2003; 90:705–710.
178. Morpurgo E, Vitale GC, Galandick S, Kimberling J, Ziegher C, Polk HC Jr. Clinical characteristics of familial adenomatous polyposis and management of duodenal adenomas. J Gastrointest Surg 2004; 8:559–564.
179. Mackey R, Walsh RM, Chung R, et al. Pancreas-sparing duodenectomy is effective management for familial adenomatous polyposis. J Gastrointest Surg 2005; 9:1088–1093.
180. Farnell MB, Sakorafas GH, Sarr MG, et al. Villous tumors of the duodenum: reappraisal of local vs extended resection. J Gastrointest Surg 2000; 4:13–23.
181. Ruo L, Coit DG, Brennam MF, Guillem JG. Long-Term follow-up of patients with familial adenomatous polyposis undergoing pancreaticoduodenal surgery. J Gastrointest Surg 2002; 6:671–675.
182. Brosens LA, Keller JJ, Offerhaus GJ, Goggins M, Giardiello FM. Prevention and management of duodenal polyps in familial adenomatous polyposis. Gut 2005; 54:1034–1043.
183. Giardiello FM, Petersen GM, Piantadosi S, et al. APC gene mutations and extra-intestinal phenotype of familial adenomatous polyposis. Gut 1997; 40: 521–525.
184. Clark SK, Phillips RK. Desmoids in familial adenomatous polyposis [review]. Br J Surg 1996; 83:1494–1504.
185. Heiskanen I, Jarvinen HJ. Occurrence of desmoid tumors in familial adenomatous polyposis and results of treatment. Int J Colorect Dis 1996; 11:157–162.
186. Clark SK, Neale KF, Landgrebe JC, Phillips RK. Desmoid tumors complicating familial adenomatous polyposis. Br J Surg 1999; 86:1185–1189.
187. Hartley JE, Church JM, Gupta S, Mcgannon E, Fazio VW. Significance of incidental desmoids identified during surgery for familial adenomatous polyposis. Dis Colon Rectum 2004; 47:334–340.
188. Lofti AM, Dozois RR, Gordon H, et al. Mesenteric fibromatosis complicating familial adenomatous polyposis: predisposing factors and results of treatment. Int J Colorect Dis 1989; 4:30–36.
189. Phillips RK. Editorial. Dis Colon Rectum 2004; 47:339–340.
190. Church JM. Desmoid tumors in patients with familial adenomatous polyposis. Semin Colon Rectal Surg 1995; 6:29–32.
191. Middleton SB, Clark SK, Matravers P, Katz D, Reznek R, Phillips RK. Stepwise progression of familial adenomatous polyposis-associated desmoid precursor lesions demonstrated by a novel CT scoring system. Dis Colon Rectum 2003; 46:481–485.
192. Healy C, Reznek RH, Clark SK, Phillips RK, Armstrong P. MR appearances of desmoid tumors in familial adenomatous polyposis. Am J Roentgenol 1997; 169:465–472.
193. Middleton SB, Phillips RK. Surgery for large intra-abdominal desmoid tumors (Editorial, Church JM). Dis Colon Rectum 2000; 43:1759–1763.
194. Bulow S. Sulindac and tamoxifen in the treatment of desmoid tumors in patients with familial adenomatous polyposis. Colorect Dis 2001; 3:266–267.
195. Möslein G, Dozois RR. Desmoid tumors associated with familial adenomatous polyposis. Perspect Colon Rectal Surg 1998; 10:109–126.
196. Poritz LS, Blackstein M, Berk T, Gallinger S, Melevd RS, Cohen Z. Extended follow-up of patients treated with cytotoxic chemiotherapy for intra-abdominal desmoid tumors. Dis Colon Rectum 2001; 44:1268–1273.
197. Church J, Berk T, Buman BM, et al. Staging intra-abdominal desmoid tumors in familial adenomatous polyposis: a search for a uniform approach to a troubling disease. Dis Colon Rectum 2005; 48:1528–1534.
198. Cabot RC. Case 21061. N Engl J Med 1935; 212:263–267.
199. Blair N, Trempe CL. Hypertrophy of the retinal pigment epithelium associated with Gardner's syndrome. Am J Ophthalmol 1980; 90:661–667.
200. Leppard B, Bussey HJ. Epidermoid cysts, polyposis coli and Gardner's syndrome. Br J Surg 1975; 62:387–393.
201. Campbell WJ, Spence RA, Parks TG. The role of congenital hypertrophy of the retinal pigment epithelium in screening for familial adenomatous polyposis. Int J Colorect Dis 1994; 9:191–196.
202. Crail HW. Multiple primary malignancies arising in the rectum, brain and thyroid. Report of a case. US Navy Med Bull 1949; 49:123–128.
203. Bret MC, Hershman MJ, Glazer G. Other manifestations of familial adenomatous polyposis. In: Phillips RK, Spigelman AD, Thomson JP, eds. Familial Adenomatous Polyposis and Other Polyposis Syndromes. London: Edward Arnold, 1994:143–158.
204. Turcot J, Després JP, St. Pierre F. Malignant tumors of the central nervous system associated with familial polyposis of the colon. Dis Colon Rectum 1959; 2:465–468.
205. Hamilton SR, Liu B, Parsons RE, et al. The molecular basis of Turcots syndrome. N Engl J Med 1995; 332:839–847.
206. Matsui T, Hayashi N, Yao K, et al. A father and son with Turcot's syndrome: evidence for autosomal dominant inheritance. Report of two cases. Dis Colon Rectum 1998; 41:797–801.
207. Itoh H, Hirata K, Ohsato K. Turcot's syndrome and familial adenomatous polyposis associated with brain tumor: review of related literature. Int J Colorect Dis 1993; 8:87–94.
208. Gingold BS, Jagelman DG, Turnbull RD. Surgical management of familial polyposis and Gardner's syndrome. Am J Surg 1979; 137:54–56.
209. Bess MA, Adson MA, Elveback LR, Moertel CG. Rectal cancer following colectomy for polyposis. Arch Surg 1980; 115:460–467.
210. Bussey HJ, Eyers AA, Ritchie SM, Thomson JP. The rectum in adenomatous polyposis. The St. Mark's policy. Br J Surg 1985; 72(suppl):S29–S31.
211. Nugent KP, Phillips RK. Rectal cancer risk in older patients with familial adenomatous polyposis and an ileorectal anastomosis: a cause for concern. Br J Surg 1992; 79:1204–1206.
212. Heiskanen I, Jarvinen HJ. Fate of the rectal stump after colectomy and ileorectal anastomosis for familial adenomatous polyposis. Int J Colorect Dis 1997; 12:9–13.
213. Sarre RG, Jagelman DG, Beck GJ, et al. Colectomy with ileorectal anastomosis for familial adenomatous polyposis: the risk of rectal cancer. Surgery 1987; 101:20–26.
214. DeCosse JJ, Bulow S, Neale K, the Leeds Castle Polyposis Group. Rectal cancer risk in patients treated for familial adenomatous polyposis. Br J Surg 1992; 79:1372–1375.
215. Iwama T, Mishima Y. Factors affecting the risk of rectal cancer following rectum-preserving surgery in patients with familial adenomatous polyposis. Dis Colon Rectum 1994; 37:1024–1026.
216. Jenner DC, Levitt S. Rectal Cancer following colectomy and ileorectal anastomosis for familial adenomatous polyposis. Aust N Z J Surg 1998; 68:136–138.
217. Bjork JA, Akerbrant HI, Iselius L, Hultcrantz RW. Risk factors for rectal cancer morbidity and mortality in patients with familial adenomatous polyposis after colectomy and ileorectal anastomosis. Dis Colon Rectum 2000; 43: 1719–1725.
218. Bertario L, Russo A, Radice P, et al. Genotype and phenotype factors as determinants for rectal stump cancer in patients with familial adenomatous polyposis. Ann Surg 2000; 231:538–543.
219. Church J, Burke C, McGannon E, Pastean O, Clark B. Risk of rectal cancer in patients after colectomy and ileorectal anastomosis for familial adenomatous polyposis. A function of available surgical options. Dis Colon Rectum 2003; 46:1175–1181.
220. Penna C, Kartheuser A, Parc R, et al. Secondary proctectomy and ileal pouch-anal anastomosis for familial adenomatous polyposis. Br J Surg 1993; 80: 1621–1625.
221. Heiskanen I, Matikainen M, Hiltunen KM, Rintala R, Jarvinen HJ. Colectomy and ileorectal anastomosis or restorative for proctocolectomy for familial adenomatous polyposis. Colorect Dis 1999; 1:9–14.
222. Phillips RK, Spigelman AD. Can we safely delay or avoid prophylactic colectomy in familial adenomatous polyposis? Br J Surg 1996; 83:769–770.
223. Bulow C, Vasen H, Jarvinen H, Bjork J, Bisgaard ML, Bulow S. Ileorectal anastomosis is appropriate for a subset of patients with familial adenomatous polyposis. Gastroenterology 2000; 119:1454–1460.
224. Church J, Burke C, McGannon E, Pasteam O, Clark B. Predicting polyposis severity by proctoscopy: how reliable is it? Dis Colon Rectum 2001; 44: 1249–1254.
225. Farmer KC, Phillips RK. Colectomy with ileorectal anastomosis lowers rectal mucosal cell proliferation in familial adenomatous polyposis. Dis Colon Rectum 1993; 36:167–171.
226. Karen P, Nugent MA, Northover J. Total colectomy and ileorectal anastomosis. In: Phillips RK, Spigelman AD, Thomson JP, eds. Familial Adenomatous Polyposis and Other Polyposis Syndromes. London: Edward Arnold, 1994:80–91.
227. Winde G, Schmid KW, Schfegel W, Fischer R, Osswald H, Bunte H. Complete reversion and prevention of rectal adenomas in colectomized patients with familial adenomatous polyposis by rectal low-dose sulindac maintenance treatment. Dis Colon Rectum 1995; 38:813–830.

228. Spagnesi MT, Tonelli F, Dolara P, et al. Rectal proliferation and polyp occurrence in patients with familial adenomatous polyposis after sulindac treatment. Gastroenterology 1994; 106:362–366.
229. Winde G, Schmid KW, Brandt B, Müller O, Osswald H. Clinical and genomic influence of sulindac on rectal mucosa in familial adenomatous polyposis. Dis Colon Rectum 1997; 40:1156–1169.
230. Giadiello FM, Yang VW, Hylind LM, et al. Primary chemoprevention of familial adenomatous polyposis with sulindac. N Engl J Med 2002; 346:1054–1059.
231. Thorson AG, Lynch HT, Smyth TC. Rectal cancer in FAP patients after sulindac. Lancet 1994; 343:180.
232. Yang VW, Geiman DE, Hubbard WC, et al. Tissue prostanoids as biomarkers for chemoprevention of colorectal neoplasia: correlation between prostanoid synthesis and clinical response in familial adenomatous polyposis. Prostaglandins Lipid Mediat 2000; 60:83–90.
233. Niv Y, Fraser M. Adenocarcinoma in the rectal segment in familial polyposis coli is not prevented by sulindac therapy. Gastroenterology 1994; 107:854–857.
234. Kartheuser AH, Parc R, Penna CP, et al. Ileal pouch-anal anastomosis as the first choice operation in patients with familial adenomatous polyposis: a 10-year experience. Surgery 1996; 119:615–623.
235. Ziv Y, Church JM, Oakley JR, McGannon E, Fazio VW. Surgery for the teenager with familial adenomatous polyposis: ileo-rectal anastomosis or restorative proctocolectomy?. Int J Colorect Dis 1995; 10:6–9.
236. Pare YR, Moslein G, Dozois Pamberton JH, Woeff BG, King JE. Familial adenomatous polyposis. Results after ileal pouch-anal anastomosis in teenagers. Dis Colon Rectum 2000; 43:893–902.
237. Ambrose WL, Dozois RR, Pemberton JH, Beart RW, Ilstrup DM. Familial adenomatous polyposis: results following ileal pouch-anal anastomosis and ileorectostomy. Dis Colon Rectum 1992; 35:12–15.
238. Setti-Carraro P, Nicholls RJ. Choice of prophylactic surgery for the large bowel component of familial adenomatous polyposis [review]. Br J Surg 1996; 83:885–892.
239. Soravia C, Klein L, Berk T, Oconnoroz BI, Cohen Z, McLeod RS. Comparison of ileal pouch-and anastomosis and ileorectal amastomosis in patients with familial adenomatous polyposis. Dis Colon Rectum 1999; 42:1028–1034.
240. Church J. Ileoanal pouch neoplasia in familial adenomatous polyposis: an underestimated threat. Dis Colon Rectum 2005; 48:1708–1713.
241. Remzi FH, Church JM, Bast J, et al. Mucosectomy vs stapled ileal pouch-and adenomatous polyposis. Functional outcome and neoplasia control. Dis Colon Rectum 2001; 44:1590–1596.
242. van Duijvendijk P, Varen HF, Bertario L, et al. Cumulative risk of developing polyps or malignancy at the ileal pouch-anal anastomosis in patients with familial adenomatous polyposis. J Gastrointest Surg 1999; 3:325–330.
243. Petersen GM. Genetic counseling and predictive genetic testing in familial adenomatous polyposis. Semin Colon Rectal Surg 1995; 6:55–60.
244. Spigelman AD, Thomson JP. Introduction, history and registries. In: Phillips RK, Spigelman AD, Thomson JP, eds. Familial Adenomatous Polyposis and Other Polyposis Syndromes. London: Edward Arnold, 1994:3–14.
245. Wong N, Lesko D, Rahelo R, Pinsky L, Gordon PH, Foulkes W. Genetic counseling and interpretation of genetic tests in familial adenomatous polyposis and hereditary nonpolyposis colorectal cancer. Dis Colon Rectum 2001; 44:271–279.
246. Rabelo R, Foulkes W, Gordon PH, et al. Role of molecular diagnostic testing in familial adenomatous polyposis and hereditary nonpolyposis colorectal cancer familiar. Dis Colon Rectum 2001; 44:437–446.
247. Church JM, McGannon E. A polyposis registry: how to set one up and make it work. Semin Colon Rectal Surg 1995; 6:48–54.
248. Rotherberger DA, Dalberg DI, Leininger A. Minnesota colorectal cancer initiative: successful development and implementation of a community-based colorectal cancer registry. Dis colon Rectum 2004; 47: 1571–1577.
249. Lyon DT, Mantia AG. Large bowel hemangiomas. Dis Colon Rectum 1984; 27:404–414.
250. Allred HW, Spencer RJ. Hemangiomas of the colon, rectum, and anus. Mayo Clin Proc 1974; 49:739–741.
251. Londono-Schimmer EE, Ritchie JK, Hawley PR. Coloanal sleeve anastomosis in the treatment of diffuse cavernous hemangioma of the rectum: long-term results. Br J Surg 1994; 81:1235–1237.
252. Jefferey PI, Hawley PR, Parks AG. Colo-anal sleeve anastomosis in the treatment of diffuse cavernous hemangioma involving the rectum. Br J Surg 1976; 63:678–682.
253. Coppa GF, Eng K, Localio SA. Surgical management of diffuse cavernous hemangioma of the colon, rectum, and anus. Surg Gynecol Obstet 1984; 159:17–22.
254. Telander RL, Ahlquist D, Blanfuss MC. Rectal mucosectomy: a definitive approach to extensive hemangiomas of the rectum. J Pediatr Surg 1993; 28:379–381.
255. He LJ, Wang BS, Chen CC. Smooth muscle tumors of the digestive tract: report of 160 cases. Br J Surg 1988; 75:184–186.
256. Morgan BK, Compton C, Talbert M, Gallagher WJ, Wood WC. Benign smooth muscle tumors of the gastrointestinal tract. Ann Surg 1990; 211:63–66.
257. Kusminsky RE, Bailey W. Leiomyomas of the rectum and anal canal: report of 6 cases and review of the literature. Dis Colon Rectum 1977; 20:580–599.
258. Miettinen M, Furlong M, Sarlomo-Rikala M, Burke A, Sobin LH, Lasota J. Gastrointestinal stromal tumors, intramural leiomyomas and leiomyosarcomas in the rectum and anus. A clinicopathologic, immunohistochemical, and molecular genetic study of 144 cases. Am J Surg Path 2001; 25:1121–1133.
259. Walsh TH, Mann CV. Smooth muscle neoplasms of the rectum and anal canal. Br J Surg 1984; 71:597–599.
260. Vorobyov GI, Odaryule TS, Kapulter LL, Shelygin YA, Kornyak BS. Surgical treatment of benign, myomatous rectal tumors. Dis Colon Rectum 1992; 35:328–331.
261. Taylor B, Wolff BG. Colonic lipomas. Report of two unusual cases and review of the Mayo Clinic experience, 1976–1985. Dis Colon Rectum 1987; 30:888–893.
262. Gordon RT, Beal JM. Lipoma of the colon. Arch Surg 1978; 113:897–899.
263. Castro EL, Stearns MW. Lipoma of the large intestine: a review of 45 cases. Dis Colon Rectum 1972; 15:441–444.
264. Brouland JP, Poupard B, Nemeth J, Valleur P. Lipomatous polyposis of the colon with multiple lipomas of peritoneal folds and giant diverticulosis. Dis Colon Rectum 2000; 43:1767–1769.
265. Santos-Briz, Garcia JP, Gonzalez C, Colina F. Lipomatous polyposis of the colon. Histopathology 2001; 38:81–83.
266. Zhang H, Cong JC, Chen CS, Qiao L, Liu ES. Submucous colon lipoma: a case report review of the literature. World J Gastroenterol 2005; 11:3167–3169.
267. Liessi G, Pavanello M, Cesari S, Dell'Antonio C, Avventi P. Large lipomas of the colon: CT and MR findings in three symptomatic cases. Abdom Imaging 1996; 21:150–152.
268. Pfeil SA, Weaver MG, Abdul-Karim FW, Yang P. Colonic lipomas: outcome of endoscopic removal. Gastrointest Endosc 1990; 36:435–438.
269. Chung YF, Ho YH, Nyam DC, Leong AF, Seow-Choen F. Management of colonic lipomas. Aust N Z J Surg 1998; 68:133–135.

23 Malignant Neoplasms of the Colon

Philip H. Gordon

CLASSIFICATION

Malignancies of the large intestine assume a major importance because of their frequency in the general population. The types of malignancies that may occur can be classified as follows:

1. Adenocarcinoma
2. Carcinoid
3. Lymphoma
4. Sarcoma
5. Squamous cell carcinoma
6. Plasmacytoma

DiSario et al. (1) reported the review of a population-based registry with complete ascertainment. There were 7422 colorectal carcinomas—4900 (66%) colonic and 2522 (34%) rectal. The breakdown of the 222 (3%) nonadenocarcinoma malignancies was squamous, 75 (34%); malignant carcinoids, 74 (33%); transitional cell-like, 37 (17%); lymphomas, 25 (11%); sarcomas, nine (4%); and melanomas, two (0.9%). Although not stated, the transitional cell-like (including cloacogenic and basaloid carcinomas) and the squamous cell carcinomas (including epidermoid carcinomas) were almost certainly of anal canal origins.

ADENOCARCINOMA

INCIDENCE, PREVALENCE, AND TRENDS

Colorectal carcinoma is the fourth most common internal malignancy; it is second only to carcinoma of the lung as a cause of carcinoma death (2). It was estimated that in 2004, there would be 146,940 new cases of colorectal carcinoma in the United States (estimated to be 11% of all malignancies) and that 56,600 deaths would result from this disease (2). Colorectal carcinoma incidence rates have stabilized since the mid-1990s in males and females. For the same year, it was estimated that there would be 19,100 new cases of colorectal carcinoma in Canada and that 8300 individuals would die of the disease (3). There has been a slight increase in incidence in both men and women annually since 1997 (3). The mortality has continued to decline in both sexes but more so among women. Consensus is emerging internationally about the benefits of population-based screening for colorectal carcinoma. This is under consideration in Canada at both provincial and national levels. However, casual screening is already prevalent in Canada and may have contributed to the most recent increased incidence and decreased mortality rates. At birth, the probability of eventually developing a colorectal carcinoma in women is 5.5% in the United States and 6.5% in Canada and in men, 5.9% and 6.5%, respectively. The probability of dying of the disease in the United States is 2.3% and in Canada is 3.2% in women and in men 2.4% in the United States and 3.6% in Canada.

In the United States, enormous data have been collected in the ongoing SEER program and the following information has been obtained from that database (4). In the last 30 years, the incidence of carcinoma of the colon and rectum has been relatively stable with a 0.8% annual increase from 1975 to 1985, a 1.8% annual decrease from 1985 to 1995, a 1.2% annual increase from 1995 to 1998, and a 2.9% annual decrease from 1998 to 2001. In absolute terms, the age-adjusted incidence has dropped from 59.5 per 100,000 in 1975 to 51.8 per 100,000 in 2001, the greatest decline in the last few years of reporting. Mortality rates have shown a decline over this period with a 0.5% annual decrease from 1975 to 1984 and a 1.9% annual decrease from 1984 to 2001. The largest decrease has been noted with rectal carcinoma 1998 to 2001 when a 3.9% annual decline was reported. Age-adjusted mortality rates for colon and rectal carcinoma have dropped from 28.1 per 100,000 in 1975 to 20.0 per 100,000 in 2001.

The 5-year relative survival rates have improved from 49.8% in 1974–1976 to 63.4% in 1995–2000. The stage distribution of cases during the 1995 to 2000–reporting period was localized (39%), regional (38%), distal (19%), and unstaged (5%) with the corresponding 5-year relative survival rates at 89.9%, 67.3%, 9.6%, and 35.2%, respectively, with an overall survival of 63.4%.

Hayne et al. (5) examined the trends in colorectal carcinoma in England and Wales over the last 30 years. Age-standardized incidence, mortality, and survival rates for colorectal carcinoma based on data from the National Cancer Intelligence Centre at the Office for National Statistics were calculated and trends assessed. Between 1971 and 1997, the total number of cases of colorectal carcinoma increased by 42%. The site distribution of the colorectal carcinomas between 1971 and 1974 was rectum (38%), sigmoid (29%), cecum (15%), transverse colon and flexures (10%), ascending colon (5%), and descending colon (3%). Between 1971 and 1997, the direct age-standardized incidence increased by 20% in males and by 5% in females. The direct age-standardized mortality fell by 24% in males and by 37% in females. Age-standardized relative 5-year survival in adults improved from 22% to 27% for patients diagnosed during 1971 to 1975 to over 40% for those diagnosed during the period of 1991 to 1993. The 5-year survival has improved substantially but rates are still below those in comparable countries, elsewhere in Europe, and in the United States.

EPIDEMIOLOGY

An extensive and comprehensive review of the worldwide information on colon carcinoma was collated by Correa and Haenszel (6). Much of the following information was extracted from their excellent review.

AGE

Carcinoma of the large intestine is predominantly a disease of older patients, with the peak incidence being in the seventh decade. However, it must be borne in mind that the disease can occur at virtually any age and may be seen in patients in their twenties and thirties (7). It has been estimated that only 5% of colorectal carcinomas occur in patients who are younger than 40 years of age (8).

SEX

It was estimated that during 2005 in the United States 71,820 men and 73,470 women would develop carcinoma of the colon and rectum. In Canada, corresponding numbers were 10,600 and 9,000. In the United States it was estimated that 28,540 men and 27,750 women would die from the disease in 2005 (2). In Canada corresponding numbers were 4,500 and 3,900 (3). Carcinoma of the colon and rectum ranks third as a cause of death from carcinoma, surpassed by lung and equalled by prostate carcinoma in men and lung and breast carcinoma in women (2).

FAMILY HISTORY

There have been many reports that indicate an increased incidence of colorectal carcinoma in first-order relatives of patients who have suffered from the disease.

In a prospective study of 32,085 men and 87,031 women, Fuchs et al. (9) found that the age-adjusted relative risk of colorectal carcinoma for men and women with affected first-degree relatives, when compared with those without a family history of the disease, was 1.72. The relative risk among study participants with two or more first-degree relatives was 2.75. For participants younger than 45 years, who had one or more affected first-degree relatives, the relative risk was 5.37.

Slattery et al. (10) assessed the risk of developing multiple primaries after a diagnosis of colon carcinoma and determined the impact that having a family history of carcinoma has on carcinoma risk. Data from the Utah Cancer Registry and the Utah Population Database were used. A cohort of 2236 patients with first primary colon carcinomas was observed for the subsequent development of additional carcinomas. The authors observed a greater than expected incidence of colon, rectal, and pancreatic carcinomas among the cohort. The standardized incidence ratios were 2.77, 2.26, and 2.38, respectively. Having a family history of colon or rectal carcinoma did not greatly influence risk of having a multiple primary carcinoma. However, there was a trend toward increased risk of pancreatic carcinoma (hazard ratio, 1.99), and bladder carcinoma (hazard ratio, 2.35) among patients with a family history of rectal carcinoma. The authors also observed that the risk of uterine carcinoma in a cohort was positively associated with a family history of uterine carcinoma, risk of breast carcinoma was positively associated with a family history of breast carcinoma, and risk of prostate carcinoma was positively associated with a family history of prostate carcinoma.

To compare the risk in relatives of patients with colorectal carcinoma diagnosed at different ages, Hall et al. (11) studied two cohorts of patients, 65 diagnosed when they were younger than 45 years of age and 212 patients of all ages. The overall relative risk of colorectal carcinoma in first-degree relatives was 5.2 in the first group and 2.3 in the second group. The cumulative incidence of colorectal carcinoma for relatives of the young cohort rose steeply from 40 years, reaching 5% at 50 years and 10% at 70 years, compared with the older group, reaching 5% at 70 years and 10% at 80 years.

St. John et al. (12) conducted a case-control family study of 7493 first-degree relatives and 1015 spouses of 523 case-control pairs to determine the relative risk of developing carcinoma. The authors found an odds ratio of 1.8 for one and 5.7 for two affected relatives. The risk

TABLE 1 ■ Estimated Relative and Absolute Risk of Developing Colorectal Carcinoma

Family History	Relative Risk	Absolute Risk by Age 79
No family history	1	4%[a]
One first-degree relative with colorectal carcinoma	2.3	9%[b]
More than one first-degree relative with colorectal carcinoma	4.3	16%[b]
One affected first-degree relative diagnosed with colorectal carcinoma before age 45	3.9	15%[b]
One first-degree relative with colorectal adenoma	2.0	8%[b]

[a]Data from SEER database. *Source*: From Ref. 13.
[b]The absolute risks of colorectal carcinoma (CRC) for individuals with affected relatives was calculated using the relative risks for CRC and the absolute risk of CRC by age 79.

to parents and siblings was 2.1 times greater; 3.7 for patients diagnosed before 45 years and 1.8 times greater for patients diagnosed at the age of 45 years or older. The cumulative incidence was 11.1%, 7.3%, and 4.4% among relatives 55 years and older, between 45 and 54 years, and younger than 45 years, respectively. The most recent summary has shown the risk to be increased 2- to 4-fold (Table 1) (13). Furthermore people who have a first-degree relative with colorectal carcinoma are estimated to have an average onset of colorectal carcinoma about 10 years earlier than people with sporadic colorectal carcinoma (9).

■ SITE

The distribution of carcinoma in the various segments of the large bowel has been the subject of several detailed clinical studies. Each of these studies has shown that over the past 50 years there has been a gradual shift in the location of carcinomas from the rectum and left colon toward the right colon. Our initial account reported a dramatic shift from the rectum to the right colon (14). Our subsequent study has determined that the left-to-right progression has continued (15). Reasons for this shift to the right are not entirely clear. A review of patterns in different countries has revealed an increase in the incidence of colon carcinoma with a corresponding decrease in rectal carcinoma (6). Such findings imply that methods for the early detection and screening of large bowel carcinoma should be directed at the entire colon rather than being limited to the distal 25 cm of the large intestine. Qing et al. (16) in a comparison between American and Chinese patients found lesions in 36.3% of white patients versus 26.0% of Asian patients, while carcinomas of the rectum were found in 63.7% of white patients and 74% of Asian patients. The rightward shift has continued in recent decades in the United States (17) and Japan (18).

■ GEOGRAPHIC DISTRIBUTION

There is a wide variation of the incidence of colorectal carcinoma in different countries. In general, countries of the Western world have the highest incidence of colorectal carcinoma, and these include Scotland, Luxembourg, Czechoslovakia, New Zealand, Denmark, and Hungary. Countries with the lowest incidence include India, El Salvador, Kuwait, Martinique, Poland, and Mexico. The United States and Canada hold an intermediate position (2,6). In large countries extending over a wide range of latitudes, there may be considerable regional differences that mimic international variations (6).

It has been suggested that low-risk populations have a relatively increased incidence of right-sided carcinomas while relatively high-risk communities have an increased risk of left-sided malignancies (6). There is an increased risk of large bowel carcinoma in urban populations when compared to rural populations. The incidence of colorectal carcinoma in Japanese Americans is higher than in Japanese individuals living in Japan. The children of these immigrants have an incidence approximating that of the general U.S. population. The effects of environmental exposure and food habits can be exemplified by a notable occurrence in Israel. Israelis who were born in Europe or North America run roughly 2.5 times, the risk of bowel carcinoma than those born in North Africa or Asia. After their arrival in Israel, the incidence becomes similar (6).

■ RACE AND RELIGION

Black Americans who once enjoyed a lower incidence of colorectal carcinoma than their white counterparts now suffer a similar incidence of the disease (6), but the 5-year survival rate for African-Americans is significantly lower than for whites (19). The risk of large bowel malignancy in American Indians is less than half that for whites in the United States. Individuals of Mexican extraction born in the United States also experience a lower risk for large bowel carcinoma. With respect religion, Jews in the United States have a higher incidence of colorectal carcinoma, while Mormons and Seventh Day Adventists have a lower rate than the general U.S. population (6). Ashkenazi Jews have a lifetime colorectal carcinoma risk of 9% to 15%, which differs strikingly from the 5% to 6% colorectal carcinoma risk for non-Ashkenazi members of the general western populations (20). The lower incidence in Mormons has been attributed to their prohibition of the use of tobacco and alcohol. Self-reported or perceived religiousness has been determined to be a protective factor in the development of colorectal carcinoma (a relative risk of 0.7) (21).

■ OCCUPATION

Vobecky, Devroede, and Caro (22) observed an increased relative risk of three (i.e., a threefold increase) in the incidence of colorectal carcinoma in individuals working in factories that produce synthetic fibers. In the authors' review of the literature, they found that other workers who were at greater risk of developing large bowel carcinoma included metallurgy workers handling chlorinated oil, manufacturers of transport equipment, weavers, firemen, those working with asbestos or coke by-products, and those working in copper smelters. de Verdier et al. (23) found elevated relative risks of colon carcinoma among male petrol station and/or automobile repair workers (2.3) and men exposed to asbestos (1.8), while elevated relative risks of rectal carcinoma were found among men exposed to soot (2.2), asbestos (2.2), cutting fluids and/or oils (2.1), and combustion gases from coke, coal, and/or wood (1.9).

A meta-analysis by Homa et al. (24) suggested that exposure to amphibole asbestos may be associated with colorectal carcinoma but exposure to serpentine asbestos is not. Another study failed to find an association between asbestos exposure and carcinoma of the colon and rectum (25). Cumulative exposure to organic solvents, dyes, or abrasives also may contribute to an increased risk of colorectal carcinoma (26,27). Workers involved in the manufacture of polypropylene also exhibit an increased incidence of colorectal carnicoma (28), but this risk was more recently reported not to exist (29). Workers with intense exposure to ethyl acrylate and methyl methacrylate for 3 years have an increased risk of colon carcinoma two decades later (30).

ETIOLOGY AND PATHOGENESIS

As with other malignancies, neither the etiology nor the pathogenesis of carcinoma of the colon is known. A number of factors have been considered important in its causation, and certain clinical conditions are considered precursors of carcinoma and will be detailed here.

■ POLYP-CANCER SEQUENCE

Considerable evidence has accumulated to suggest that most, if not all, carcinomas develop from a precursor polyp, a situation known as the polyp-cancer sequence. This sequence is described in detail in Chapter 22.

■ INFLAMMATORY BOWEL DISEASE

Although colorectal carcinoma, complicating ulcerative colitis and Crohn's disease, only accounts for 1% to 2% of all cases of colorectal carcinoma in the general population, it is considered a serious complication of the disease and accounts for approximately 15% of all deaths in inflammatory bowel disease patients.

Patients with universal ulcerative colitis, having a more severe inflammation burden and risk of the dysplasia-carcinoma cascade especially those who have had the condition for more than 10 years and those patients who experienced onset in childhood, without doubt are at increased risk of developing carcinoma of the colon or rectum. Lennard-Jones et al. (31) reported that the incidence of colorectal carcinoma (in 22 patients among 401 patients with extensive ulcerative colitis followed over 22 years) was 3%, 5%, and 13% at 15 years, 20 years, and 25 years, respectively. For the 17 patients developing colorectal carcinoma during supervised surveillance (344 patients) Dukes' staging was A or B in 12 patients. In half the carcinoma patients under surveillance, dysplasia signaled the associated carcinoma found only after colectomy in the operative specimens. Others have confirmed the increased risk (32). Of 3117 patients with ulcerative colitis followed for up to 60 years through the Swedish Cancer Registry, the relative risk of colorectal carcinoma was 5.7 (nonsignificant for proctitis), 2.8 for left-sided disease, and 14.8 for pancolitis (33). Recent figures suggest that the risk of colon carcinoma for people with inflammatory bowel disease increases by 0.5% to 1.0% yearly, 8 to 10 years after diagnosis (34). Considering the chronic nature of the disease, it is remarkable that there is such a low incidence of colorectal carcinoma in some of the population-based studies, and possible explanations have to be investigated. One possible carcinoma protective factor could be treatment with 5-aminosalicylic acid preparations (5-ASAs) (34).

Adenocarcinoma of the small bowel is extremely rare, compared with adenocarcinoma of the large bowel. Although only few small bowel carcinomas have been reported at sites of involvement with Crohn's disease, the number was significantly increased in relation to the expected number (34).

The incidence of colorectal carcinoma in patients with Crohn's disease has been reported as being four to 20 times greater than the general population (32). In a study of 1656 patients with Crohn's disease, Ekbom et al. (35) indicated relative risks for colon carcinoma of 3.2 (in Crohn's ileocolitis) to 5.6 (in Crohn's colitis only). With the onset of any Crohn's colitis before the patient was 30 years of age, the relative risk was 20.9, but only 2.2 when diagnosed after age 30.

■ GENETICS

In the last decade and a half, there has been an explosive increase in knowledge about the molecular biology of carcinoma. Publications are legion but often difficult to understand. This not withstanding, the past decade has been witness to unprecedented progress in the comprehension of the basic mechanisms involved in the genesis of colorectal carcinoma. In his outstanding review of the molecular biology of colorectal carcinoma, Allen (36) attempted to make the subject understandable to the clinician, and the following dissertation draws heavily from that review.

Molecular Biology

The codes that control production of protein enzymes and form the basic information needed for life itself are found within the cell nucleus as long strands of deoxyribonucleic acid (DNA) molecules that are, in turn, composed of four nucleotides: adenine (A), guanine (G), thymine (T), and cytosine (C). Under normal circumstances, adenine only pairs with thymine (A:T), and guanine pairs with cytosine (G:C). As a result of base pairing, cellular DNA forms the familiar stepladder configuration that is twisted into a double helix and supercoiled into microscopically visible structures called chromosomes.

Long DNA sequences are subdivided into smaller segments called genes, each of which contains the information needed for a single protein. Genes are composed of hundreds or thousands of nucleotides. In humans, the entire genetic code, termed the genome, is composed of approximately 3 billion nucleotides organized into approximately 100,000 genes contained within 23 pairs of chromosomes (total, 46). One chromosome in each pair is inherited from the mother and one from the father. Thus each gene has another similar (but not identical) gene called an allele on the complementary chromosome. Genes can act in a dominant or recessive fashion. For dominant genes, one allele assumes the responsibility for producing the protein and the other allele remains dormant.

The sequence of nucleotides within cellular chromosomes is reproduced faithfully and is passed down from generation to generation during cell division. A "normal" rate of mutation is estimated to be one mistake in every

10 billion base pairs copied. To correct replication errors, a repair mechanism is dependent on genes called mismatch repair genes. Malignant transformation appears to result from the accumulation of mutations within genes that are critical to cell growth and differentiation caused either by an increase in the mutational rate or because the DNA repair process is compromised. A carcinoma is the end result of four to 12 genetic changes that convey a growth advantage to the mutated cells. During the initiation phase, there is an increase in the mutational rate of DNA. Mutations in some genes become incorporated into an individual's genome and are passed from generation to generation. These "germline mutations" may occur in genes related to carcinoma and, as a result, cause hereditary carcinoma. Other mutations, termed "somatic," cause a sporadic carcinoma. Knudson (37) proposed that inherited carcinomas arise in individuals with germline mutations of one allele of a recessively acting carcinoma gene, after which only one additional somatic alteration is needed to inactivate the gene and initiate carcinogenesis. Sporadic carcinomas require two somatic mutations (or allelic loss).

Mechanisms of Gene Action

Three major categories of genes have been implicated in carcinoma development: (1) oncogenes, (2) tumor suppressor genes, and (3) mismatch repair genes (Table 2). When a proto-oncogene (a normal human growth-related gene) becomes abnormally activated, it drives the cell through the cell cycle facilitating clonal proliferation and is known as an oncogene. Oncogenes act in a dominant fashion because alteration of only one allele is necessary to produce a cellular effect. Oncogenes, however, do not tell the entire story, because only 20% of human carcinomas carry oncogene alterations.

Other genes called tumor suppressor genes can halt the cell cycle even when oncogenes are altered. Tumor suppressor genes act in a recessive manner and promote carcinoma only when they are inactivated by allelic loss or mutations in both alleles. If cells cannot repair DNA damage, tumor suppressor genes such as *p53* drive the cell into a suicide mode called apoptosis. A tumor suppressor gene critical to colorectal carcinoma was described on chromosome 5—the adenomatous polyposis coli (*APC*) gene. It was found to contain an inherited mutation causing truncation of the protein product. Somatic mutations of *APC* are found early during the neoplastic process in most polyps and carcinomas.

TABLE 2 ■ Genes Known to Be Involved in Development of Colorectal Carcinoma

Type	Name	Chromosome
Oncogen	K-*ras*	12
Tumor suppressor gene	*APC*	5
	DCC	18
	p53	17
	MCC	5
	TGF-β-RII	3
Mismatch repair gene	*hMLH1* ✓	3
	hMSH2	2
	hPMS1 ✓	2
	hPMS2	7
	hMSH6 ✓	2
	hMSH3	5
Others (currently of theoretical importance only)	Fat acetylation *p450* genes, etc.	Many

Source: From Refs. 13,36.

The latest genes found to be related to carcinogenesis are called mismatch repair genes, which are needed for cells to repair DNA replication errors and spontaneous base pair loss. The six DNA mismatch repair genes found in humans to date are hMSH2 (chromosome 2p16), hMLH1 (chromosome 3p21), hPMS1 (chromosome 2q31–33), hPMS2 (chromosome 7q11), hMSH6 (chromosome 2p16), and hMSH3 (chromosome 5q11.2-q13.2). When both copies of these genes are inactivated, DNA mismatch repair is defective, and the cell exhibits an increased frequency of mistakes in DNA replication, thereby accelerating the progression to oncogenesis. The first four genes are regarded to contribute to hereditary nonpolyposis colorectal carcinoma (HNPCC) in 31%, 33%, 2%, and 4%, respectively (38).

The founder mutation MSH2*1906G > C is also considered an important cause of HNPCC in the Ashkenazi Jewish population (39). This pathogenic mutation accounting for 2% to 3% of colorectal carcinoma in those whose age at diagnosis is less than 60 years is highly penetrant and accounts for approximately one-third of HNPCC in Ashkenazi Jewish families that fulfill the Amsterdam criteria. This founder mutation MSH2*1906 was found in 8% of 1342 individuals (0.6%) of those of Ashkenazi descent with colorectal carcinoma. A subsequent study (40) sought to characterize the proportion of individuals of Ashkenazi heritage with very early-onset colon carcinoma (diagnosed at age 40 or younger) that could be attributed to MSH2*1906G > C detected the mutation in 3 of the 41 samples (7.14%) of patients who had colorectal carcinoma diagnosed at age 40 years or younger. The incidence is significantly greater than the 8 in 1345 (0.6%) observed for cases of colorectal carcinoma in Ashkenazi Jews not selected for age. These results suggest that consideration for testing for the MSH2*1906G > C mutation should be included in the evaluation of Ashkenazi Jewish individuals diagnosed with early onset of colon carcinoma.

hMSH2 and hMLH1 accounted for 63% of kindreds meeting international diagnostic criteria (41). A recent review by Peltonaki (42) cited germline mutations in one of four major HNPCC-associated mismatch repair genes (MLH1, MSH2, MSH6, and PMS2) detected in up to 70% to 80% of such families. More than 400 different predisposing mismatch repair gene mutations are known with approximately 50% effecting MLH1, about 40% MSH2, and about 10% MSH6 (42). The share of PMS2 is less than 5%. The newly identified human mismatch repair gene MLH3 may account for a small percentage of HNPCC. A germline mutation in PMS1 was originally reported in an HNPCC-like family but there is presently no evidence of PMS1 as an HNPCC predisposition gene. The available data on two additional components of mismatch repair, exonuclease 1 (EXO1) and DNA polymerase, are too limited to allow any reliable assessment of their role in HNPCC predisposition (42).

Genetic Pathways to Colorectal Carcinoma

Traditionally, carcinoma is seen as a three-step process of initiation, promotion, and progression. Colorectal carcinoma

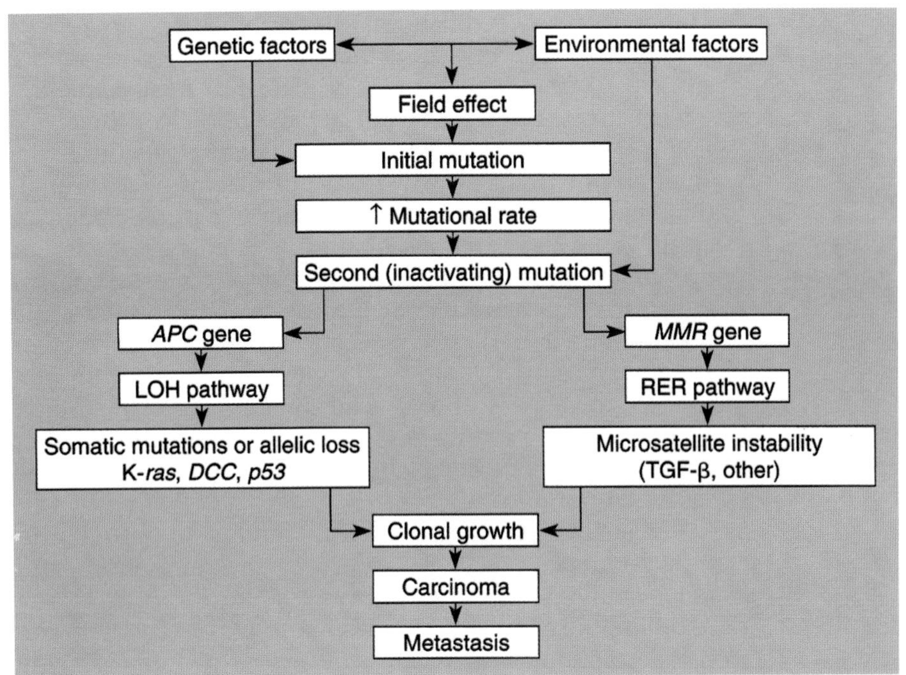

FIGURE 1 ■ Molecular pathway to colorectal carcinoma. The two arrows associated with the box labeled "genetic factors" illustrate the difference between initiation of a sporadic vs. hereditary colon carcinoma. The arrow leading from the box labeled "genetic factors" to "initial mutation" illustrates inheritance of a germline mutation capable of initiating neoplasia. APC = Adenomatous polyposis coli; LOH = loss of heterozygosity; DCC = deleted in colon carcinoma; MMR = mismatch repair; RER = replication error; TGF-β = transforming growth factor-*β*. *Source*: From Ref. 36.

is a genetically heterogeneous disease, and a series of genetic events has been described in the evolution of colorectal carcinoma. The initiation stage (from the beginning to the first mutation) involves a complex (and poorly understood) interplay between environmental factors and host susceptibility (Fig. 1). Specific environmental factors are known to modify colorectal carcinoma (Fig. 2). For patients with hereditary colorectal carcinoma, the influence of environmental factors is small compared with the power of the underlying genetic mutations. Thus the risk of initiating colorectal carcinoma is substantially higher in hereditary conditions (100% in patients with polyposis syndromes and approximately 85% in HNPCC).

A number of early reports tried to relate genetic importance to the etiology of colorectal carcinoma. Burt et al. (43) examined the inheritance of susceptibility to colonic polyps and carcinomas in a large pedigree with multiple cases of colorectal carcinoma. The authors' analysis suggested that the observed excess of discrete adenomatous polyps and colorectal carcinoma was the result of an inherited autosomal-dominant gene for susceptibility rather than an inherited recessive gene for susceptibility. Solomon, Voss, and Hall (44) examined colorectal carcinomas for loss of alleles on chromosome 5. Using a special probe that maps to chromosome 5q, the authors demonstrated that at least 20% of carcinomas lose one of the alleles present in matched normal tissue. They suggested that becoming recessive for this gene may be a critical step in the progression of a relatively high proportion of colorectal carcinomas. No deletions were found in any other chromosome, which indicates that the loss from chromosome 5 is nonrandom. Law et al. (45) reported allelic losses in chromosomes 17 and 18 to be more frequent in colorectal carcinoma than losses on chromosome 5.

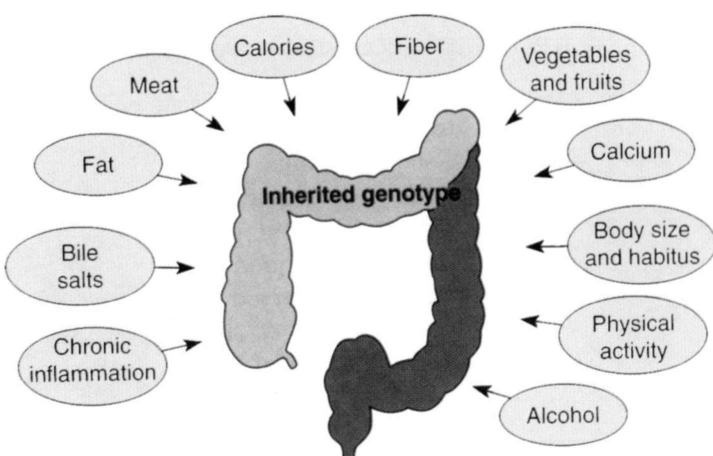

FIGURE 2 ■ Environmental factors that may contribute to altering colonic mucosa to produce a field effect that precedes initiation of neoplasia. Colonic cells respond to each environmental factor based on the genotype of DNA loci associated with metabolic pathways that relate to the various dietary constituents. Genetic polymorphisms are thought to play a role in determining how individuals respond at a cellular level to various environmental factors. *Source*: From Ref. 36.

It is now believed that the mutation that initiates colonic neoplasia is found in one of two gene loci. The 5q21 loci contains the *APC* gene, which is altered in more than 70% of all neoplastic lesions. Other polyps and carcinomas demonstrate micro-satellite instability, a hallmark of mismatch repair gene mutations. Depending upon which type of gene has been inactivated, one of two pathways to colorectal carcinoma is followed (see Fig. 1). In the first pathway, *APC* gene inactivation leads to a pathway termed loss of heterozygosity (LOH). Approximately 70% to 80% of colorectal carcinoma develops through the LOH pathway following inactivation of the *APC* gene. The genes involved in the LOH pathway include K-*ras*, *DCC*, and *p53* in addition to *APC* (Fig. 3). Germline *APC* mutations initiate the neoplastic process in patients with familial adenomatous polyposis (FAP) and endow all colonic crypt stem cells with a high risk for clonal proliferation.

A large body of evidence supports the concept of a multistep process that typically develops over decades and appears to require at least seven genetic events for

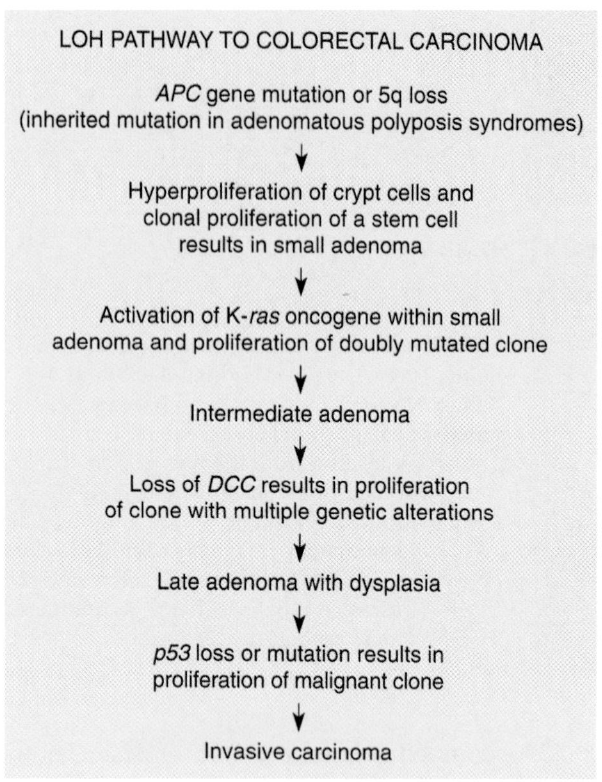

FIGURE 3 ■ LOH pathway to colorectal carcinoma. *Source*: From Ref. 36.

completion. But even single altered genes can result in disease (e.g., FAP, HNPCC). In 1990 Fearon and Vogelstein (46) published the now-classic genetic model for colorectal carcinogenesis. The authors proposed a genetic series of events that corresponded to the apparent ordered sequence from a benign to a malignant lesion in histopathologic recognizable stages. They postulated that colorectal carcinoma arises as a result of mutational activation of oncogenes coupled with the mutational inactivation of tumor suppressor genes. Their original suggestion was that there must be mutations in at least four or five genes, but it is now believed to be at least seven for the formation of a carcinoma. Although the genetic alterations often occur according to a preferred sequence, the orderly sequence (see Fig. 2 and Fig. 3) rarely occurs in any individual carcinoma. It is the total accumulation of genetic alterations rather than their order that is responsible for determining the biologic properties of the carcinoma. The cascade of events described by Fearon and Vogelstein (46) begins with a loss or mutation the FAP gene on chromosome 5q, resulting in a change from normal epithelium to hyperproliferative epithelium. One of these hyperproliferating cells gives rise to a small adenoma in which the genome is hypomethylated. The next event involves activation of the K-*ras* oncogene on the chromosome 12p mutation to form the intermediate adenoma. Unlike oncogenes, tumor suppressor genes are expressed in a recessive manner. Therefore, both allelic copies must be lost or inactivated by point mutations for phenotypic expression to occur. Usually the *DCC* gene on chromosome 18q is next to be deactivated or lost, and results in the development of a late adenoma. The final genetic alteration found consistently in colorectal carcinoma is loss and/or mutation of the *p53* tumor suppressor gene on chromosome 17p. The *p53* gene is altered in 50% of all human carcinomas and in 70% of colorectal carcinomas. Further genetic alterations are required for the development of metastases, subsequently believed to involve the loss of heterozygosity of the *Nm23* gene (47). While there is no obligatory sequence of mutations in the pathway from normal mucosa through adenoma to carcinoma, there is clearly an association of certain types of mutations in specific oncogenes or tumor suppressor genes with early and late states of transformation. This multistep pathway can be observed in sporadic and inherited colorectal carcinoma. Many other genes, such as *MCC, TGF-β, Rb,* and *Myc,* have been implicated in the genesis of colorectal carcinoma. Further study of the molecular events will undoubtedly lead to a better understanding of the multistep carcinogenesis and the relative importance of each.

Mismatch repair gene defects initiate an entirely different sequence of events known as the replication error (RER) pathway. These pathways lead to carcinomas that are biologically quite different. This second pathway to colorectal carcinoma is found in approximately 20% of carcinomas. The RER pathway is similar in both patients with HNPCC and those who develop a spontaneous RER carcinoma. Patients with HNPCC inherit a single defective allele of a mismatch repair gene and require an additional somatic mutation to inactivate the second allele. Spontaneous carcinomas develop after two somatic events inactivate the relevant gene. In either case, inactivation leads to a marked increase in replication errors. As errors accumulate in microsatellites, malfunction of genes that contain or are near affected microsatellites may occur (Fig. 4). Aaltonen et al. (48) found the RER positive phenotype in 77% of colorectal carcinomas from HNPCC patients compared with only 13% of patients with sporadic carcinoma.

How do DNA mismatch repair defects cause carcinoma? The mismatch repair gene defect increases the risk of malignant transformation of the cells, which may ultimately result from the disruption of one or several

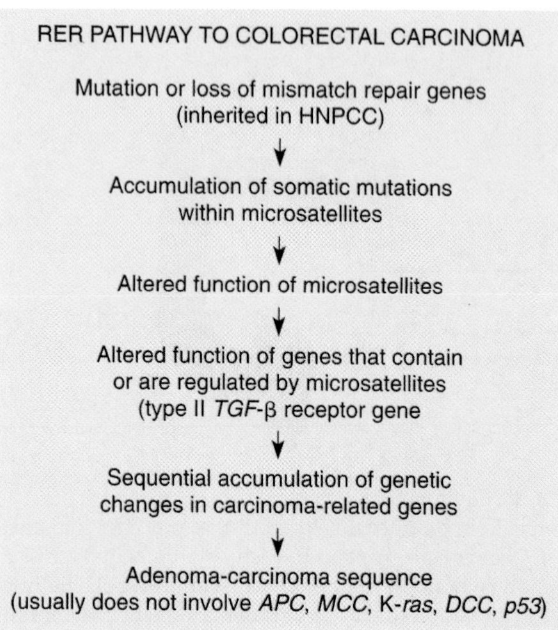

FIGURE 4 ■ Genetic alterations often occur according to a preferred sequence. *Source*: From Ref. 36.

anticarcinogenic functions of the mismatch repair genes. Peltomaki recently summarized these (42). First, malfunction of the mismatch repair system is associated with decreased genomic stability, which may manifest itself as highly elevated rates of subtle mutations (MSI) throughout the genome. Second, although mismatch repair–deficient cells typically have a diploid or near-diploid DNA content, loss of heterology-dependent suppression of recombination in these cells may promote gene conversion and expose tumor suppressor genes in analogy to loss of heterozygosity, or allow chromosomal translocations to occur. Furthermore, increased mutational inactivation of genes involved in DNA double-strand break repair may contribute to an elevated degree of chromosomal aberrations in mismatch repair–deficient cells. Third, besides anonymous microsatellite sequences, critical genes may be affected with mutations, conferring a growth advantage on the cells. Typical "target" genes include those involved in growth suppression, apoptosis, or signal transduction. Fourth, there is evidence that failed protection against endogenous or exogenous DNA damage and the ensuing persistence of mutagenic or premutagenic lesions may contribute to genomic instability/MSI in intestinal cells.

There are examples of non-FAP, non-HNPCC hereditary colorectal carcinomas; a family not meeting the Amsterdam criteria with no deficiency of DNA mismatch repair in the malignancy of the proband was found to have a germline mutation of the TGFBR2 gene that encodes the type II TGF-β receptor; loss of the remaining normal allele was observed in the carcinoma (49). Thus, other biologic mechanisms may underlie non-FAP, non-HNPCC hereditary colorectal carcinoma.

The transition from normal epithelium to adenoma to carcinoma is associated with acquired molecular events. A recent update on the genetic pathway to carcinoma has become available (13). At least five to seven major molecular alterations may occur when a normal epithelial cell progresses in a colonal fashion to carcinoma. There are at least two major pathways by which these molecular events can lead to colorectal carcinoma. About 85% of colorectal carcinomas are due to events that result in chromosomal instability and the remaining 15% are due to events that result in microsatellite instability. Key changes in chromosomal instability carcinomas include widespread alterations in chromosome number (aneuploidy) and detectable losses at the molecular level of portions of chromosome 5q, chromosome 18q, and chromosome 17p; and mutation of the KRAS oncogene. The important genes involved in these chromosome losses are APC (5q), DCC/MADH2/MADH4 (18q), and TP53 (17p), respectively, and chromosome losses are associated with instability at the molecular and chromosomal level. Among the earliest events in the colorectal carcinoma progression pathway is loss of the APC gene, which appears to be consistent with its important role in predisposing persons with germline mutations to colorectal neoplasms. Acquired or inherited mutations of DNA damage repair genes also play a role in predisposing colorectal epithelial cells to mutations. Not every carcinoma acquires every mutation, nor do mutations always occur in a specific order. The key characteristics of microsatellite instability carcinomas are largely intact chromosome complement, but acquisition of defects in DNA repair, such that mutations that may occur in important carcinoma-associated genes are allowed to persist. These types of carcinomas are detectable at the molecular level by alterations in repeating units of DNA that occur normally throughout the genome, known as a DNA microsatellite. Mitotic instability of microsatellites is the hallmark of microsatellite instability carcinomas.

Microsatellite instability, the hallmark of HNPCC, occurs in approximately 15% to 25% of sporadic colorectal carcinomas. According to international criteria, a high degree of microsatellite instability (MSI-H) is defined as instability at two or more of five loci or $\geq$30% to 40% of all microsatellite loci studied, whereas instability at fewer loci is referred to as MSI-low (MSI-L). Colorectal carcinomas with MSI-H encompass a group of malignancies with a predilection for the proximal colon, that have diploid DNA content, that are high grade, that are associated with female sex; and have better survival. These features distinguish MSI-H carcinomas from those without widespread MSI; that is, MSI-L or microsatellite-stable (MSS) carcinomas. A majority of MSI-H colon carcinomas are caused by inactivation of MLH1. Whereas the MSI-L subset of colon carcinomas is as equally prevalent as the MSI-H group, immunohistochemical and mutation studies have found no involvement in MLH1, MSH2, MSH6, or MSH3 in the former carcinomas. The clinicopathological features do not seem to distinguish this group from MSS colon carcinomas either.

Clinical Relevance of Basic Genetic Knowledge

An effort by Allen (36) to reclassify the subtypes of colorectal carcinoma based on their molecular pathogenesis and inheritance pattern is depicted in Table 3. Prior to the definition of molecular pathways to colorectal carcinoma, proximal carcinomas were known to have normal cytogenetics, diploid DNA content, slower growth, less frequent metastasis, and a better prognosis compared to distal carcinomas. In addition, the frequency of extracolonic carcinomas had been found to be higher in both patients with colorectal carcinoma and their first-degree relatives when the index colon carcinoma was proximal.

Most carcinomas that arise in the distal colon develop along the LOH pathway, while most proximal carcinomas are RER (Fig. 5). Clinical characteristics of LOH carcinomas indude a propensity for left-sided location (80%), aneuploidy, a polyp-to-carcinoma ratio of 20:1, and a total developmental period of 7 to 10 years. The exception to this observation is the rare adenomatous polyposis syndrome variant called hereditary flat adenoma syndrome (HFAS) or attenuated adenomatous polyposis coli (AAPC) syndrome associated with *APC* mutations. In this syndrome the inherited point mutation is found upstream from FAP mutations within exons 1 to 4. This subtle difference between FAP and AAPC mutations (sometimes within 10 base pairs of each other) results in dramatically different phenotypes. Patients with AAPC have few polyps (usually fewer than 10); the polyps are diminutive, flat, and located in the proximal colon; and a high proportion of polyps progress to carcinomas and they develop late compared with other hereditary neoplasias related to *APC* mutations. RER carcinomas tend to develop proximal to the splenic flexure (>70%), have a normal (diploid) DNA content, and carry a better prognosis compared to LOH carcinomas. Molecular analysis of resected carcinomas has led to recognition that LOH carcinomas carry a worse prognosis,

TABLE 3 ■ Classification of Colorectal Carcinoma Based on Molecular Pathogenesis, Genetic Pattern, and Clinical Features

Genetic Pattern	Total Colorectal Carcinoma (%)	Clinical Features
LOH		
Sporadic	35	Distal carcinomas (70%), aneuploid DNA, no family history of polyps or colorectal carcinoma, age of colorectal carcinoma older than 60 yr
Familial	25	Distal carcinoma, aneuploid, family history of polyps or colorectal carcinoma in several relatives, age of colorectal carcinomas 50 to 60 yr
Inherited (polyposis syndromes)	1 to 3	More than 100 polyps, early onset of disease (polyps, 10 to 25 yr; colorectal carcinoma, 30 to 40 yr)(except HFAS/AAPC)
FAP		Upper gastrointestinal polyps and carcinoma, retinal findings
Gardner's syndrome		Desmoid neoplasms, bone abnormalities
Turcot's syndrome		Medulloblastoma
HFAS/AAPC		Small flat adenomas of proximal colon, usually fewer than 10, late age of onset (50 yr or older), gastric fundic polyps
RER		
Sporadic	20	Proximal carcinomas (70%), diploid DNA, better prognosis than LOH carcinomas, age of colorectal carcinoma older than 60 yr
Familial	6	Proximal carcinomas, diploid DNA, family history of colorectal carcinoma or polyps, age of colorectal carcinoma 50 to 60 yr
Inherited (HNPCC)	10	
Lynch syndrome I		Colorectal carcinoma only, proximal carcinomas (70%), diploid, 40% have synchronous or metachronous colorectal carcinoma, age of colorectal carcinoma 40 to 45 yr
Lynch syndrome II		Lynch I plus carcinoma of endometrium, ovaries, pancreas, stomach, larynx, urinary system, small bowel, bile ducts (vary with families)
Muir-Torre		Lynch syndromes plus skin lesions
Turcot's syndrome		Glioblastomas

DNA = Deoxyribonucleic acid; FAP = familial adenomatous polyposis; HFAS/AAPC = hereditary flat adenoma syndrome/attenuated adenomatous polyposis coli; HNPCC = hereditary nonpolyposis colorectal carcinoma; LOH = loss of heterozygosity; RER = replication error pathway.
Source: From Ref. 36.

stage-for-stage, than RER carcinomas. To date, the most important molecular marker for prognosis appears to be the *DCC* gene locus on chromosome 18.

Classification based on genetic patterns and specific syndromes reveals three major forms: sporadic, familial, or inherited. The difference appears to be the method by which the initiating mutation occurs. For sporadic carcinomas, there is a period during which environmental factors influence colon mucosa and eventually alter it so that clonal growth can occur. Familial colorectal carcinoma is defined by patients who have several family members with colon or rectal carcinoma but who do not fit a recognized inherited pattern. Familial colorectal carcinoma may include as many as 30% of patients with colorectal carcinoma when both carcinoma and polyps are included in the pedigree. Explanations for familial clustering could be either shared environment, shared genetics, or both.

Liu et al. (50) divided carcinomas with microsatellite instability into three classes. The first subset of colorectal carcinomas occurs in patients without a strong family history of colorectal carcinoma (sporadic cases). These account for 12% to 15% of the total colorectal carcinomas in the United States. The second class comprises colon, endometrial, and ovarian carcinomas that develop in patients with a family history of these forms of carcinoma (HNPCC). Virtually all carcinomas that develop in these patients exhibit microsatellite instability. The third class of RER carcinomas includes a variable fraction of several types of neoplasms, including those of the lung, breast, and pancreas. The magnitude and prevalence of the microsatellite alterations in this class are generally less pronounced than in RER colorectal carcinomas. The results of Liu et al. led to three major conclusions. First, carcinogenesis associated with *MMR* gene defects usually results from the inactivation of

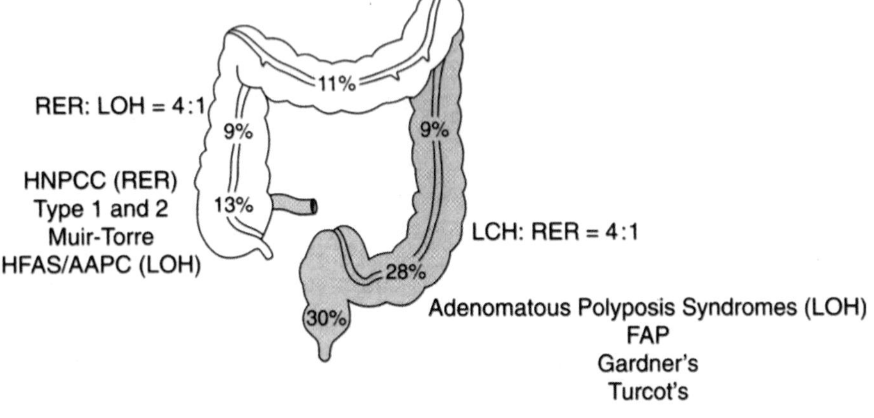

FIGURE 5 ■ The distribution of neoplastic lesions within the colon is depicted by percentages within the colonic diagram. The ratio of LOH to RER carcinomas is given for the proximal and distal colon in addition to the locations of most lesions found in various hereditary syndromes. *Source*: From Ref. 36.

both alleles of the relevant gene. Second, a significant fraction of sporadic RER carcinomas (four of seven in study) arises from mutations in genes other than the four that account for most HNPCC cases. Finally, most sporadic RER carcinomas are not associated with germline mutations of the known match repair genes.

In their review, DeFrancisco and Grady (51) cited the causative genes of HNPCC in decreasing frequency of occurrence to include MLH1, MSH2, MSH6, MLH3, PMS1, PMS2, TGFBR2, and EXO1. Peltomaki summarized the phenotypic features associated with germline mutations manifesting a predisposition to HNPCC (42). MLH1 is mostly associated with typical HNPCC. Approximately 30% of mutations are of the missense type whose phenotypic manifestations may vary. MSH2 is also mostly associated with typical HNPCC. Extracolonic carcinomas may be more common than in MLH1 mutation carriers. It is a major gene underlying the Muir-Torre syndrome. MSH6 is associated with typical or atypical HNPCC. It is often characterized by late onset, frequent occurrence of endometrial carcinoma, distal location of colorectal carcinomas, and low degree of MSI in carcinomas. PMS2 is also associated with typical or atypical HNPCC. The penetrance of mutations may vary. It is a major gene underlying Turcot's syndrome. MLH3 is seen mostly in atypical HNPCC. It may be characterized by distal location of colorectal carcinomas and variable degrees of MSI in carcinomas. EXO1 is mostly seen in atypical HNPCC. It may be associated with MSI in carcinomas.

Lawes et al. (52) reviewed the world literature to determine the clinical importance and prognostic implications of microsatellite instability and sporadic carcinoma. In clinical studies, colorectal carcinomas demonstrating MSI respond better to chemotherapy while in-vitro studies using MSI positive cell lines show resistance to radiotherapy and chemotherapy. They concluded MSI may be a useful genetic marker in prognosis and could be an influential factor in deciding treatment options.

Clinical Syndromes

For many years, FAP was considered the only hereditary variety of colon carcinoma. Now, three types of hereditary colorectal carcinomas are recognized: adenomatous polyposis syndromes (Chapter 22), HNPCC, and familial colorectal carcinoma, a group in which families exhibit aggregation of colorectal carcinoma, and/or adenomas, but with no identifiable hereditary syndrome. Approximately 1% to 3% of all colorectal carcinomas are due to hereditary adenomatous polyposis syndromes that include FAP, Gardner's syndrome, Turcot's syndrome, and HFAS/AAPC, all of which begin with germline mutations in the *APC* gene.

HNPCC

HNPCC is inherited as an autosomal dominant pattern with almost complete penetrance. It is estimated that from 0.5% to 6.0% of all colorectal carcinomas can be attributed to HNPCC (38,53–55).

Based on clinical criteria only, Peltomaki (42) noted the estimated incidence of HNPCC varies between 0.5% and 13% of the total colorectal carcinoma burden. Strictly molecular approaches based on the identification of germline mutation carriers among newly diagnosed colorectal patients whose carcinomas showed MSI have arrived at lower estimates—0.3% to 3% of the total colorectal carcinoma burden.

HNPCC has four major subtypes: (i) Lynch type I (site-specific nonpolyposis colorectal carcinoma); (ii) Lynch type II (formerly called the carcinoma family syndrome), in which carcinomas occur in the colon and related organs (endometrium, ovaries, stomach, pancreas, and proximal urinary tract, among others); (iii) Muir-Torre syndrome, associated with multiple benign and malignant skin neoplasms, sebaceous gland adenomas, carcinomas, and keratoacanthomas (56), and (iv) a variant of Turcot's syndrome (brain neoplasms). HNPCC-related colon carcinomas begin with mutations in the mismatch repair genes and are RER positive.

Clinical criteria were established to confirm the diagnosis of HNPCC at a meeting of the International Collaborative Group on HNPCC in Amsterdam in 1990 (54). The group agreed that minimum criteria should include (i) at least three relatives with histologically verified colorectal carcinoma, one of whom should be a first-degree relative of the other two (those with FAP should be excluded); (ii) at least two successive generations should be affected; and (iii) in one of the relatives, colorectal carcinoma should have been diagnosed when the patient was younger than 50 years of age.

These criteria have not proved to be comprehensive, therefore, in 1999, the International Collaborative Group developed revised criteria and these are known as Amsterdam-II criteria. They are essentially the same except that there should be at least three relatives with HNPCC-associated carcinoma (colorectal, endometrial, small bowel, ureter, or renal pelvis). Even this extension of clinical features fails to identify some families with germline mismatch repair gene mutations so the Bethesda guidelines for testing of colorectal carcinomas for microsatellite instability have been developed. They include:

1. Individuals with carcinoma in families that meet the Amsterdam criteria.
2. Individuals with two HNPCC-related carcinomas, including synchronous and metachronous colorectal carcinomas or associated extracolonic malignancies (endometrial, ovarian, gastric, hepatobiliary or small bowel carcinoma, or transitional cell carcinoma of the renal pelvis or ureter).
3. Individuals with colorectal carcinoma and a first-degree relative with colorectal carcinoma and/or HNPCC-related extracolonic malignancy and/or a colorectal adenoma; one of the malignancies diagnosed at age less than 45 years, and the adenoma diagnosed at less than 40 years.
4. Individuals with colorectal or endometrial carcinoma diagnosed at age less than 45 years.
5. Individuals with right-sided colorectal carcinoma with an undifferentiated pattern (solid/cribriform) on histopathology diagnosed at less than 45 years. (*Note*: solid/cribriform defined as poorly differentiated or undifferentiated carcinoma composed of irregular, solid sheets of large eosinophilic cells and containing small gland-like spaces.)
6. Individuals with signet-ring-cell-type colorectal carcinoma diagnosed at age less than 45 years. (*Note*: composed of 50% signet-ring cells.)
7. Individuals with adenomas diagnosed at age less than 40 years.

TABLE 4 ■ The Revised Bethesda Guidelines for Testing Colorectal Carcinomas for Microsatellite Instability (MSI)

Carcinomas from individuals should be tested for MSI in the following situations:

1. Colorectal carcinoma diagnosed in a patient who is less than 50 yr of age
2. Presence of synchronous, metachronous colorectal, or other HNPCC-associated malignancies[a] regardless of age
3. Colorectal carcinoma with the MSI-H[b] histology[c] diagnosed in a patient who is less than 60 yr of age[d]
4. Colorectal carcinoma diagnosed in one or more first-degree relatives with an HNPCC-related neoplasm, with one of the neoplasms being diagnosed under age 50 yr
5. Colorectal carcinoma diagnosed in two or more first- or second-degree relatives with HNPCC-related malignancies regardless of age

[a]HNPCC-related malignancies include colorectal, endometrial, stomach, ovarian, pancreas, ureter and renal pelvis, biliary tract, and brain (usually glioblastoma as seen in Turcot syndrome) neoplasms, sebaceous gland adenomas, and keratoacanthomas in Muir-Torre syndrome, and carcinoma of the small bowel.
[b]MSI-H = microsatellite instability-high in carcinomas refers to changes in two or more of the five National Cancer Institute–recommended panels of microsatellite markers.
[c]Presence of carcinoma infiltrating lymphocytes, Crohn's-like lymphocytic reaction, mucinous/signet-ring differentiation, or medullary growth pattern.
[d]There was no consensus among the Workshop participants on whether to include the age criteria in guideline 3 above; participants voted to keep less than 60 yr of age in the guidelines.

In 2002 another workshop was held at the NCI in Bethesda and the following revised guidelines were created (Table 4) (57).

It is estimated that 20% to 25% of population-based cases of colorectal carcinoma meet the Bethesda criteria. It is suggested that for all patients who meet these criteria, a search for MSI is indicated. To establish the most effective and efficient strategy for the detection of MSH2/MLH1 gene carriers in HNPCC, Pinol et al. (58) conducted a prospective multicenter nationwide study (the EPICOLON study) in 20 hospitals in the general community in Spain of 1222 patients with newly diagnosed colorectal carcinoma. Microsatellite instability testing and MSH2/MLH1 immunostaining were performed in all patients regardless of age, personal, or family history, and carcinoma characteristics. Patients whose carcinoma exhibited microsatellite instability and/or lack of protein expression underwent MSH2/MLH1 germline testing. The revised Bethesda guidelines were fulfilled by 23.5% of patients and 7.4% had a mismatch repair deficiency, with the carcinoma exhibiting either microsatellite instability or loss of protein expression. Germline testing identified mutations in 0.9% in either MSH2 or MLH1 genes. Strategies based on either microsatellite instability testing or immunostaining previous selection of patients according to the revised Bethesda guidelines were the most effective (sensitivity, 81.8% and 81.8%; specificity, 98.0% and 98.2%; and positive predictive value, 27.3% and 29.0%, respectively) to identify MSH2/MLH1 gene carriers. They concluded the revised Bethesda guidelines are the most discriminating set of clinical parameters (OR 33.3).

In conclusion, MSI and IHC analysis using antibodies against MLH1, MSH2, PMS2, and MSH6 appeared to be equally effective for the identification of mutation carriers.

Despite its name, polyps are a feature of HNPCC, and a review of the literature revealed a polyp incidence in 8% to 17% of first-degree relatives during colonoscopic screening (38).

Carriers of a MMR defect develop adenomas more frequently than controls. The adenomas identified in carriers are larger, and a significantly higher proportion showed histologic features that are associated with a high risk of malignant degeneration, such as a high degree of dysplasia and the presence of more extensive villous architecture (59). A relatively high proportion of patients develop colorectal carcinoma within 3 years after a clean colonoscopy and this suggests that the adenoma-carcinoma sequence is accelerated and that the progression from adenoma to carcinoma may take fewer than 3 years.

Genetically speaking, HNPCC syndromes are dominantly inherited with nearly 100% penetrance reported by one group of investigators (53) but only 70% to 80% (i.e., 20% to 30% of individuals with a predisposing mutation may never develop carcinoma) by others (60) Asymptomatic gene carriers can pass the causative mutation to their children (60). The disease is heterogeneous. All first-degree relatives of a patient with HNPCC have a 50% risk of carrying one of the deleterious genes. Adenomas in patients carrying HNPCC gene mutations display microsatellite instability, suggesting that mismatch repair defects are important early events in colorectal carcinogenesis. Carcinoma formation requires inactivation of both copies of a given mismatch repair gene, one copy by germline mutation and the other by somatic (acquired) mutation (60).

Individuals with the Lynch syndrome differ from patients with sporadic colorectal carcinoma in several ways (38). They show (1) an autosomal dominant mode of inheritance, (2) a predominance of proximal colonic carcinoma (72% of first colon carcinomas were located in the right colon, and only 25% were found in the sigmoid colon and rectum), (3) an excess of multiple primary colonic carcinomas (18%), (4) an early age of onset (mean, 44 years), (5) a significantly improved survival rate compared with family members with distal colonic and rectal carcinomas when compared with right-sided lesions in an American College of Surgeons series (53% vs. 35% 5-year survivals), and (6) 24% developed metachronous colon carcinoma with a risk for the development of metachronous lesions in 10 years of 40% based on life-table methods. In addition to the above features, Lynch type II syndrome is characterized by a high frequency of other adenocarcinomas and the occasional occurrence of cutaneous manifestations in the form of sebaceous adenomas and carcinomas, epitheliomas, or keratoacanthomas. In a study by Mecklin and Jarvinen (61), of 40 HNPCC families with 315 affected members, a total of 472 malignancies was identified. They included colorectal (63%), endometrial (8%), gastric (6%), biliopancreatic (4%), and uroepithelial (2%) carcinomas.

The relative risk of these carcinomas ranges from 3 to 25 times that of the general population (13). The risk of colorectal carcinoma increases 1.6% per year from age 25 to 75 years in patients with these mutations (56). In a detailed pedigree analysis of 40 families with HNPCC Aarnio et al. (62) identified 414 patients affected with carcinoma. The risk of any metachronous carcinoma reached 90% after treatment of colorectal carcinoma and 70% after endometrial carcinoma; the second malignancy was most often a new colorectal carcinoma or endometrial carcinoma (62). Other sites of carcinoma include breast, pancreas, and possible lymphoma and leukemia. The review by De Francisco and Grady (51) found the four most common extracolonic carcinomas include (in descending order) endometrial, ovarian, gastric, and transitional cell carcinoma of the uro-epithelial tract (bladder, kidney, ureter). Women with HNPCC are at a 10-fold increased risk of endometrial carcinoma, which is usually diagnosed between the ages of 40 and 60 years, that is, 15 years earlier than the general population. The estimated cumulative risk at age 70 years is 40% to 50%. With MSH2 and MLH1 mutations the risk of colorectal carcinoma or endometrial carcinoma before age 50 years is 20% to 25% compared with 0.2% for the general population (56). Ovarian carcinoma is less common (incidence approximately 9%). Gastric carcinoma occurs in 5% to 20% of HNPCC families. The relative risk of gastric carcinoma was 19.3 in MSH2 mutation carriers compared with the general population. Transitional cell carcinoma of the uro-epithelial tract occurs in 1% of HNPCC patients. Only the carriers of MSH2 mutations appear to have a significantly increased risk of carcinoma in the urinary tract (relative risk 75.3). Overall, the relative risk of gastric carcinoma, ovarian carcinoma and carcinoma of the urinary tract has been shown to be higher in patients with mutations in the MSH2 as compared with MLH1. Women with MSH6 mutations appear to be more likely to develop endometrial carcinoma. Other HNPCC-associated extracolonic neoplasms include carcinomas of the small bowel, pancreas, hepatobiliary tree, brain, and skin. Muir-Torre's syndrome, first described in 1967 refers to patients with HNPCC who also develop benign or malignant sebaceous skin neoplasms (sebaceous adenomas, carcinomas, squamous or basal cell), and multiple kerato-acanthomas. Muir-Torre's syndrome usually arises from mutations in MSH2. The development of glioblastoma multiforme, in association with HNPCC, is called Turcot's syndrome. Muir-Torre's syndrome is also used to describe central nervous system neoplasms occurring in FAP, although these are usually medulloblastomas instead of glioblastomas. Approximately a third of patients with Turcot's syndrome have mutations in one of the mismatch repair genes. HNPCC is associated with a 50% risk of a second carcinoma within 15 years of the initial carcinoma diagnosis (56) compared with 5% in the general population. Information regarding the cumulative risk of developing various HNPCC-associated malignancies has been summarized from several reports and tabulated in Table 5 (13,51,56,62,63).

Plaschke et al. (64) analyzed the involvement and phenotypic manifestations of MSH6 germline mutations in families suspected of HNPCC. Patients were preselected among 706 families by microsatellite instability, immunohistochemistry, and/or exclusion of MLH1 or MSH2 mutations and were subjected to MSH6 mutation analysis. Clinical and molecular data of MSH6 mutation families were compared with data from families with MLH1 and MSH2 mutations. They identified 27 families with 24 different pathogenic MSH6 germline mutations, representing 3.8% of the total of the families, and 14.7% of all families with DNA mismatch repair gene mutations. The median age of onset of colorectal carcinoma in putative mutation carriers was 10 years higher for MSH6 (54 years) compared with MLH1 and MSH2 (44 years). Relative to other malignancies, colorectal carcinoma was less frequent in MSH6 families compared with MLH1 and MSH2 families. In contrast, the frequency of non–HNPCC-associated neoplasms was increased. Later age of disease onset and lower incidence of colorectal carcinoma may contribute to a lower proportion of identified MSH6 mutations in families suspected of HNPCC. However, in approximately half of these families, at least one patient developed colorectal or endometrial carcinoma in the fourth decade of life. Therefore, a surveillance program as stringent as that for families with MLH1 or MSH2 mutations is recommended.

TABLE 5 ■ Malignancies Associated with Hereditary Nonpolyposis Colorectal Carcinoma

Malignancy	Median Age of Onset (Yr)	Lifetime Risk (%)	General Population (%)[a]
Colorectal	40–45	78–82	5
Endometrial	45	39–61	1.5
Ovarian	47	9–12	1
Gastric	54	13–19	<1
Urothelial (bladder, kidney, and ureter)	60	4–10	<1
Pancreaticobiliary	54	2–18	<1
Brain	43	1–4	<1
Small bowel	49	1–4	<1

[a]From Ref. 56.

Approximately 60% of families that meet the Amsterdam-I criteria (HNPCC) have a hereditary abnormality in a DNA mismatch repair gene. Carcinoma incidence in Amsterdam criteria-I families with mismatch repair gene mutations is reported to be very high, but carcinoma incidence for individuals in Amsterdam criteria-I families with no evidence of a mismatch repair defect is unknown. Lindor et al. (65) conducted a study to determine if carcinoma risks in Amsterdam criteria-I families with no apparent deficiency in DNA mismatch repair are different from carcinoma risks in Amsterdam criteria-I families with DNA mismatch repair abnormalities. Identification of 161 Amsterdam criteria-I pedigrees from multiple population- and clinic-based sources in North America and Germany, were grouped into families with (group A) or without (group B) mismatch repair deficiency by testing. A total of 3422 relatives were included in the analysis. Group A families from both population- and clinic-based series showed increased incidence of HNPCC-related carcinomas. Group B families showed increased incidence only for colorectal carcinoma (SIR, 2.3) and to a lesser extent than group A (SIR, 6.1). Families who have fulfilled Amsterdam criteria-I but who have no evidence of DNA mismatch repair defect do not share the same carcinoma incidence as families with HNPCC with mismatch-repair deficiency. Relatives in such families have a lower incidence of colorectal carcinoma than those in families with HNPCC-Lynch syndrome and incidence may not be increased for other carcinomas. These families should not be described or counseled as having HNPCC. To facilitate distinguishing these entities, the designation of "familial colorectal cancer type X" is suggested to describe this type of familial aggregation of colorectal carcinoma.

Jass (66) dispelled any thoughts that the morphogenetic pathway involved flat adenoma or de novo carcinoma in these cases. In a review of 131 carcinomas, none was small and superficial. Residual adenoma (contiguous with carcinoma) was present in three of three (100%) in situ carcinomas, eight of nine (89%) carcinomas involving only submucosa, four of 14 (29%) carcinomas limited to the muscle coat, and 13 of 105 (12%), carcinomas extending beyond the muscle coat. Lynch type II syndrome colon carcinomas show a significant increase in the proportion of mucinous, poorly differentiated carcinomas, and Crohn's-like lymphoid reaction around the lesion as well as a higher rate of synchronous and metachronous carcinomas (38,67).

Other investigators have also studied HNPCC. Sankila et al. (68) compared the survival rates of 175 patients with *hMLH1*-associated HNPCC with those of 14,000 patients with sporadic colorectal carcinoma diagnosed at <65 years. The overall 5-year cumulative relative survival rate was 65% for patients with HNPCC and 44% for patients with sporadic colorectal carcinoma.

In a series of 1042 Japanese patients who underwent resection for colorectal carcinoma, 3.7% were found to have HNPCC (69). The characteristic early stage of onset, right-sided predominance, and favorable survival were confirmed. Metachronous colorectal carcinoma developed significantly more often in cases with HNPCC (12.8% vs. 1.8%), and metachronous extracolonic malignancies also developed more often (10.2% vs. 3.5%). In cases with HNPCC, the mean interval between initial operation and the diagnosis of the second malignancy was 61 months (range, 12 to 153 months). These findings stress the importance of long-term follow-up.

Rodriguez-Bigas et al. (70) reported the experience from the HNPCC Registry at Roswell Park in Buffalo, New York, which included 301 people in 40 families. In 284 of 301 people, 363 carcinomas were identified. Colorectal carcinomas alone were identified in 64% and in conjunction with extracolonic malignancies in another 11%. Extracolonic malignancies alone were identified in 25%. The median age at diagnosis of colorectal carcinoma was 48 years. Right-sided malignancies predominated (55%), synchronous and metachronous lesions were noted in 33%, and synchronous or metachronous adenomas were documented in 51% of those studied. Generational anticipation was also noted.

Hampel et al. (71) assessed the frequency of the mismatch repair genes MLH1, MSH2, MSH6, and PMS2, in patients with a new diagnosis of colorectal carcinoma to identify patients with the Lynch syndrome. Genotyping of the carcinoma for microsatellite instability was the primary screening method. Among patients whose screening results were positive for microsatellite instability, they searched for germline mutations in the MLH1, MSH2, MSH6, and PMS2 genes with the use of immunohistochemical staining for mismatch repair proteins, genomic sequencing, and deletion studies. Family members of carriers of the mutations were counseled and those found to be at risk were offered mutation testing. Of 1066 patients enrolled in this study, 19.5% had microsatellite instability, and 2.2% of these patients had a mutation causing the Lynch syndrome. Among the 23 probands with the Lynch syndrome, 10 were more than 50 years of age and 5 did not meet the Amsterdam criteria or the Bethesda guidelines for the diagnosis of HNPCC. In the families of 21 of the probands, 117 persons at risk were tested, and of these 52 had Lynch syndrome mutations. They concluded, routine molecular screening of patients with colorectal adenocarcinoma for the Lynch syndrome identified mutations in patients and their family members that otherwise would not have been detected. In most centers it would not seem feasible to test all patients with colorectal carcinoma.

The characteristics of HNPCC mandate the development of surveillance programs. Screening recommendations have varied, but the recommendation by Lynch, Smyrk, and Lynch (72) for gene carriers has been colonoscopy, beginning at age 20 to 25 years or at least 5 years earlier than the earliest age at which colon carcinoma was diagnosed in a particular kindred with the procedure repeated every other year until the patient is 30 years of age and then annually thereafter. The frequency of colonoscopic examination is justified by the finding that HNPCC adenomas have repair deficient cells with rapidly and relentlessly accumulating mutations that support the clinical concept of "aggressive adenomas" and accelerate the adenoma-carcinoma sequence. The authors strongly believe that germline carriers should be offered prophylactic subtotal colectomy.

The importance of screening colonoscopy was underscored by the report of Sankila et al. (68) who compared the colorectal carcinoma death rates of two groups of HNPCC patients—those screened every 3 years and controls who refused screening. The authors' data indicated that one carcinoma was prevented for every 2.8 polypectomies performed. This is in stark contrast to the National Polyp Study data for the general population, which gave a range of 41 to 119 polypectomies per carcinoma prevented.

The importance of screening is further emphasized by the study that compared screened with unscreened (by choice)"controls" evaluated over a 15-year period with 252 relatives at risk for HNPCC, 119 of whom declined screening. In the screened group, 8 of 133 (6%) developed colorectal carcinoma compared to 19 (16%) in the unscreened group (73). de Vos tot Nederveen Cappel and coworkers (74) examined the stage of the screening detected carcinomas in relation to the surveillance interval and to assess the risk of developing colorectal carcinoma while on the program in 114 families in the Dutch Family Registry. A total of 35 carcinomas were detected while on the program. With intervals between colorectal carcinoma and the preceding surveillance examination of two years or less, carcinomas were at Dukes' stage A ($n=4$), B ($n=11$), and C ($n=1$). With intervals of more than two years, carcinomas were Dukes' stage A ($n=3$), B ($n=10$), and C ($n=6$). The 10-year cumulative risk of developing colorectal carcinoma was 10.5% in proven mutation carriers, 15.7% after partial colectomy, and 3.4% after subtotal colectomy. There is a substantial risk of developing colorectal carcinoma while on the program. However, all carcinomas but one of subjects who underwent a surveillance examination two years or less before detection was at a local stage. They therefore recommend surveillance for HNPCC with an interval of two years or less.

For women who are gene carriers, an annual endometrial aspiration curettage should begin at age 30 years. Those patients should be advised of the option of ovarian carcinoma screening with trans-vaginal ovarian ultrasonography, Doppler color blood flow imagery, and CA-125 evaluation. They should be encouraged to have their children early so they can consider the option of undergoing prophylactic total abdominal hysterectomy and bilateral salpingo-oophorectomy between the ages of 35 and 40 years.

Screening for breast and gastric carcinoma should be initiated earlier in life than might otherwise be considered. If at least one family member is affected, gastroscopy beginning at age 30 to 35 years and every one to two years is advised (56). Also, only if at least one family member is affected, ultrasonography of the urinary tract and urine cytology beginning at age 30 to 35 years and every one to two years is advised (56).

Mecklin and Jarvinen (75) analyzed 22 Finnish HNPCC families followed up for 7 years. Metachronous neoplasms were diagnosed in 41% of patients treated by segmental resection and 24% of those treated by subtotal colectomy. Extracolonic carcinoma was diagnosed in 30%. The most common malignancy was biliopancreatic carcinoma, which accounted for all five deaths related to carcinoma. The authors concluded that subtotal colectomy is superior to hemicolectomy or segmental resection in patients with HNPCC and that regular follow-up is necessary for surveillance of remaining bowel and extracolonic malignancies.

Itoh et al. (76) conducted a study of 130 HNPCC kindreds to determine the risk of death from malignancy in first-degree relatives. The authors found a sevenfold increase in the risk of colon carcinoma in both sexes. In women relatives, the risk of breast carcinoma was increased fivefold, and a lifetime risk of breast carcinoma was 1 in 3.7. From these results, the authors recommended a screening program.

Because clinical premonitory signs such as multiple colonic polyps seen in cases of familial polyposis coli are lacking, the clinician must rely on the clinical findings and a family history typical of HNPCC. Disorders that have been considered in the differential diagnosis of HNPCC have included FAP, attenuated FAP, juvenile polyposis coli, and Peutz-Jeghers syndrome (38). Once the diagnosis has been made, the physician is faced with the responsibility of informing the patient that other family members are at risk because the genetic implications for carcinoma expression are profound. Identification of individuals at risk may be aided by inspection of the patient's skin, which may provide clues to the existence of a carcinoma associated with genodermatosis. Criteria providing clues to the diagnosis of Lynch type II syndrome include (1) any patient presenting with an early onset of carcinoma of the colon (particularly of the proximal colon in the absence of multiple polyps), endometrium, or ovaries (particularly when the patient is younger than age 40 years); (2) any patient with multiple primary carcinomas in which the lesions are integral to Lynch type II syndrome (carcinoma of the colon, endometrium, or ovary and other adenocarcinomas); and (3) any patient who states that one or more first-degree relatives manifested early onset of the carcinomas integral to Lynch type II syndrome.

It is important to determine whether an HNPCC syndrome is present because the operative procedure of choice for the index carcinoma is subtotal colectomy as opposed to a more limited resection (38,72). In the case of a woman who has completed her family, the resection may be extended to a prophylactic hysterectomy and bilateral salpingo-oophorectomy because of the patient's inordinately high risk of developement of carcinoma of the endometrium and ovaries.

The lifetime risk of endometrial and ovarian carcinomas in HNPCC is up to 60% and 12%, respectively (77). Watson et al. (78) collected data on 80 ovarian carcinoma patients who are members of HNPCC families, including 31 known mutation carriers, 35 presentive carriers (by colorectal/endometrial carcinomas status), and 14 at-risk family members. Among frankly epithelial cases, most carcinomas were well or moderately differentiated. Ovarian carcinoma in HNPCC differs from ovarian in the general population in several clinically important respects. It occurs at a markedly earlier age (42.7 years). It is more likely to be epithelial (95.6%). If it is a frankly invasive epithelial carcinoma it is more likely to be well or moderately differentiated (85% were FIGO stage I or II at diagnosis). HNPCC patients with ovarian carcinoma are more likely to have a synchronous endometrial carcinoma (21.5%).

Familial Colorectal Carcinoma

Ten to fifteen percent of patients with colorectal carcinoma and/or colorectal adenomas have other affected family members but their family histories do not fit the criteria for either FAP or HNPCC and may not appear to follow a recognizable pattern of inheritance, such as autosomal dominant inheritance. Such families are categorized as having familial colorectal carcinoma. The presence of colorectal carcinoma in more than one family member may be due to genetic factors, shared environmental risk factors or even to chance (13). With a family history the risk of colorectal carcinoma is increased earlier in life than later such that at age 45 years the annual incidence is more than three times higher than average-risk people; whereas at age 70, risk is not significantly different. The incidence in a 35 to 40 year old is about the same as that of an average-risk person at age 50 years. A personal history of adenomatous polyps confers a 15% to 20% risk of subsequently developing polyps. A history of adenomatous polyps in a sibling or parent is also associated with increased risk of colorectal carcinoma. Expert recommendations on screening for such persons are similar to those with a positive family history of colorectal carcinoma. Most experts suggest that screening should begin at age 35 to 40 years when the magnitude of risk is comparable to that of a 50 year old. Because the risk increases with extent of family history there is room for clinical judgment in favor of even earlier screening, depending on the details of the family history. A common but unproven clinical practice is to initiate colorectal carcinoma screening 10 years before the age of the youngest colorectal carcinoma case in the family.

Evidence demonstrates that patients in families with breast and colon carcinoma (hereditary breast and colon carcinoma) may have a carcinoma family syndrome caused by CHEK2 1100delC mutations that are present in a subset of the families (79). The CHECK2 mutation is incompletely penetrant.

Genetic Testing

Genetic testing provides the ability to determine who is and who is not at risk for disease before the onset of symptoms. Such information is becoming essential for proper management of patients and their families. In individuals who inherit mutant genes, simple preventive measures often can reduce morbidity and mortality and allow more thoughtful planning for the future. The benefits of genetic testing are equally important for those families who are found not to carry the relevant mutation; these individuals are spared unnecessary medical procedures and tremendous anxiety. However, genetic testing is not without its problems.

These problems can be broadly divided into psychological or technical in nature. From the societal view, issues related to insurance, employment, discrimination, and privacy have garnered much concern and attention. The technical challenges associated with genetic testing can be just as formidable and are often overlooked. Even when the mutated gene is known, routine genetic testing may fail to identify mutations. As a result of these uncertainties, genetic testing that fails to find the mutation is often inconclusive. Studies have shown that these inconclusive results may be misinterpreted by the patient and physicians and are a source of great anxiety. Because of the complex psychosocial and technical issues, it is clear that genetic testing should never be offered to patients without appropriate genetic counseling.

Prior to embarking upon any genetic testing it is critically important that the individual at risk of developing carcinoma and the referring physician as well have an understanding of what the testing is designed to do. To this end, genetic counseling is of paramount importance for patients to fully understand the limitations of genetic testing and will aid in the management of patients who are susceptible to colorectal carcinoma. The management of individuals who may be at increased risk for an inherited colorectal carcinoma susceptibility is complex. Knowledge about genetic information can contribute to clinical management at several stages during patient care. Obtaining and interpreting genetic information can be a lengthy process but are essential to avoid harm and to heighten the benefits of genetic testing.

Genetic counseling and interpreting genetic test results can be complex but without knowing the limitations of the methods used and the lifetime probability of developing carcinoma in individuals who carry a gene that predisposes to carcinoma, misinterpretation may lead to false assurance. Wong et al. (80) conducted a review of the literature and combined with their clinical and research experience suggested a guide to enable various health care providers to better counsel patients in their quest for advice on prevention, early detection, and surveillance for colorectal carcinoma. Much of the following information was extracted from their review.

Interpretation of genetic tests for colorectal carcinoma is not a straightforward as interpreting a blood sugar test to ascertain whether it is elevated, normal or lowered. Genetic counseling is a dynamic communication process between the patient and the counselor who provides education and support within a multidisciplinary team. Counseling is targeted toward individuals who are interested in having a personal risk estimate. Those at greatest risk for developing malignancy may benefit by assessing current screening tests, whereas those at lower risk will be reassured that their risk for colorectal carcinoma is not as high as they thought. Furthermore, survivors of malignancies may want to know their risk of recurrence or of a second primary neoplasm and the risk for their relatives, especially their children.

Carcinoma is a genetic disease but is not necessarily inherited. Virtually all neoplasms and certainly all malignant ones result in part from genes that mutate somatically (during one's lifetime). In contrast, a minority of neoplasms arises from an inherited gene that confers susceptibility in development. Genetic counseling is appropriate when the family history is suggestive of a heritable predisposition for malignancy. In general, the counseling process is composed of discrete elements: risk assessment, informative counseling, supportive counseling, and follow-up. Before initiating the process it is important for the counselor to gain insight into the action of these components from the perspective of the patient. This is initially obtained by contracting. Contracting allows patients to know what to expect from genetic counseling and ensures their needs will be elicited and addressed by the counselor.

The presence or absence of a family history of benign and malignant neoplasms helps to determine whether a person has an increased probability of having an inherited susceptibility for malignancy. Other familial traits can be characteristic signs of a genetic syndrome and suggestive that an increased risk for carcinoma may be present in a family. Pedigree analysis is multigenerational and includes details from both sides of the proband's family. Current age or age at death is ascertained for everyone, because early death may explain the absence of a positive family history. Genetic counseling is recommended for individuals with an absolute risk greater than 10% (Table 6) for developing carcinoma of the colon and rectum.

Providing risk assessment is only one part of the overall education process in genetic counseling. Explaining what genes are, how they are passed to subsequent generations, and the natural history of the neoplastic disease

TABLE 6 ■ Personal and Family Features that Confer a Higher than Average Risk for Developing Colorectal Carcinoma

	Absolute Risk to Age 70 (%)
Population risk	3–6
Polyps	
Family history	4–7
Personal history	
<1 cm in diameter	3–6
>1 cm in diameter	9–18
Family history of colorectal carcinoma	
1 FDR	
$<$ Age 45	15–30
Age 45–55	6–25
$>$ Age 70	3–6
1 FDR + 1 SDR	10
2 FDR	15–30
ICG-HNPCC (mutation status unknown)	35–45
Mutation carrier in a gene associated with HNPCC	70–90
FAP (not clinically screened and mutation status unknown)	40–45
APC mutation carrier for FAP	80–90

Abbreviations: FDR, first-degree relative; SDR, second-degree relative; FAP, familial adenomatous polyposis; ICG-HNPCC, International Collaborative Group on Hereditary Non-Polyposis Colorectal Cancer.
Source: From Ref. 80.

is an integral part of genetic counseling. Other educational aims include the recommendation or provision of screening modalities for early detection and preventive options. Medical intervention such as prophylactic surgery or chemoprevention, and the possible limitations of these treatments are issues for members of hereditary carcinoma families. Obtaining knowledge may empower the individual and family by dispelling the myths about malignancy and by providing guidelines that help in decision making. It also establishes the foundation of informed consent for genetic testing.

Indications

Genetic testing is discussed when the patient's family history of carcinoma falls in the autosomal dominant mode of inheritance. Appropriate situations include families who carry a mutation in APC, hMLH1, hMSH2, hPMS1, hPMS2, or hMSH6 or in families fulfilling the clinical FAP or ICG-HNPCC criteria. The decision to undergo genetic testing is a personal one based on informed consent. The first phase in determining whether genetic testing is appropriate is genetic counseling.

Among FAP families, who are candidates for genetic testing? The diagnosis of FAP is made because of the presence of polyps on examination of the presenting patient (proband or index case). In autosomal dominant inheritance, on average, 50% of the patient's first-degree relatives (parents, siblings, and offspring) will be at risk. As soon as the FAP diagnosis emerges, either before or after operation, the surgeon should recommend that all first-degree relatives be examined. If a mutation in APC is identified in the patient's germline DNA, the immediate family and other branches of the family can be encouraged to come forward for genetic counseling and to know their risk status if so desired. If a mutation is not detected, further genetic testing for APC mutations in the family is contraindicated and the clinical decision is to monitor first-degree relatives by colonoscopy at recommended intervals. Depending on the expression of colorectal carcinoma in the proband and the pattern of colorectal carcinoma and other malignancies in the family, genetic testing for HNPCC may be advisable. In every case of FAP, a genetic test to pinpoint the heritable, germline APC mutation is justified, with the informed consent of the patient. As far as testing the patient's family is concerned, a common exception (occurring in 30% of probands) is a patient with FAP whose parents are negative on endoscopic examination and who therefore has a "new mutation" in the APC gene. In this instance, the risk for colorectal carcinoma for siblings falls to that of the general population. Nonetheless, children of the patient will require testing (if a mutation was identified in the proband) if so desired, because they are at 50% risk for FAP. The only obvious example in which genetic testing is not recommended would be in an isolated patient with FAP with no living first-degree relatives.

What patients with suspected HNPCC should be referred for genetic counseling and testing? Because HNPCC is not always obvious based on clinical findings, either preoperatively or during resection, the clinical management of a possible HNPCC patient is complex. A detailed family history, with sites of malignancy verified, is critical to determine whether the patient fits the Amsterdam criteria and other associated features of HNPCC. Analysis of neoplastic material would provide assistance in determining whether to test the proband's germline DNA (i.e., a blood sample) for HNPCC mutations (after genetic counseling) and refer the first-degree relatives should a mutation be detected. In the instance of a positive family history it is ideal for testing to be conducted despite microsatellite instablility (MSI) phenotype. The clinical algorithm would be much the same as for FAP, with the exception that the multiple genes might need to be analyzed unless tests on pathogenic samples narrow the search. It is important to point out that at present, detection of a confirmed pathogenic mutation occurs in less than 50% of HNPCC families. In the absence of an identified deleterious mutation, genetic testing is inconclusive, which must be explained to the patient by an individual skilled in genetic counseling. Family members can be given general advice for colorectal carcinoma screening of first-degree relatives of patients with this malignancy.

Techniques

The molecular techniques used in testing for germline mutations in hereditary colorectal carcinoma have been described in detail by Rabelo et al. (81) and the following is a synopsis of that work.

Germline DNA can be tested in three ways:

1. With in vitro–synthesized protein assay (also called protein truncation test or in vitro truncation test), specific gene segments are amplified by polymerase chain reaction (PCR) or reversed transcription (RT) -PCR, transcribed and translated in vitro, and the protein product is analyzed by gel electrophoresis. If the amplified segment has a mutation that causes the production of a truncated protein, its smaller size will allow in it to be more mobile in the gel.
2. Single-stranded conformation analysis (SSCA) is also a mutation detection technique in which specific gene segments are amplified by PCR or RT-PCR, denatured to separate the stands of the DNA product and analyzed by gel electrophoresis. The mutant DNA often migrates differently under certain conditions, allowing the putative localization of mutation within the segment.
3. DNA sequencing is the criterion standard technique for mutation detection, with up to 99% accuracy. It allows the precise identification of the mutation in the DNA sequence by pinpointing any change in the number or identity of bases.

Pathologic specimens are examined in two ways:

1. A clue to identify colorectal carcinoma caused by HNPCC is by an associated alteration in the length stability of repetitive tract DNA in the carcinoma of an affected individual. This is known as microsatellite instability also called replication error positive phenotype. The presence of MSI+ thereby increases the likelihood that direct testing for defects in HNPCC genes will be informative. There are three outcomes of MSI analysis (56).
   a. If at least two markers tested show instability, the result indicates an increased likelihood that the colorectal carcinoma arose due to an HNPCC-associated mutation (MSI-H high).
   b. If no marker shows instability in the absence of a compelling family history the result is usually interpreted as ruling out HNPCC (MSS stable).

c. If instability is seen in only one of the markers the result does not indicate HNPCC. The clinical behavior of MSI-low carcinomas is identical to those with MSS, and does not have the mutational fingerprints of the clinical behavior of MSI-H carcinomas. MSI-L results occur as commonly as do MSI-H results.

2. Immunohistochemistry is a technique for diagnosing a carcinoma that lacks expression of a particular HNPCC gene. It examines either hMLH1 or hMSH2 protein expression in carcinomas by immunostaining using monoclonal antibodies. Formalin fixed, paraffin embedded adenocarcinoma tissue is the sample required for testing with a region of normal mucosa adjacent to the carcinoma for comparison. The absence of hMLH1 or hMSH2 immunostaining shows which gene is defective and should be analyzed for the presence of a germline mutation. Studies have shown that the lack of hMLH1 or hMLH2 immunostaining was associated with the presence of MSI+.

Genetic Testing for FAP

Presymptomatic genetic diagnosis of FAP in at-risk individuals has been feasible with linkage and direct detection of APC mutations (13). If one were to use linkage analysis to identify gene carriers, ancillary family members, including more than one affected individual, would need to be studied. With direct detection, fewer family members' blood samples are required than for linkage analysis, but the specific mutation must be identified in a least one affected person by DNA mutation analysis or sequencing. Because approximately 96% of the mutations in FAP lead to a truncated protein, it has become routine to use in vitro–synthesized protein (IVSP) assay (sometimes called protein truncation test) for mutation detection. When a truncated protein is identified, it is possible to localize the mutation to a specific segment of the gene and then use DNA sequencing to determine the mutated nucleotide(s). The use of IVSP as the sole genetic test in FAP misses approximately 20% of APC mutations. Another screening technique is based on analysis of electrophoretic migration of small segments of the wild-type mutant gene (SSCA). The sequential use of two molecular diagnostic tests has become a common practice: a simple and less expensive screening technique (of high sensitivity and moderate specificity) followed by a definitive test of high sensitivity, usually DNA sequencing.

These mutation search methods, APC protein truncation testing (from lymphocyte RNA) considerably enhance the feasibility of testing at-risk individuals without requiring DNA from multiple affected family members (as linkage requires). In particular, it is useful for testing in small families or in patients with spontaneous or "de novo" mutations (the first occurrence of FAP in a kindred), which may account for as much as one third of incident cases (13). Only about 80% of APC mutations can be detected by this method. Therefore, the clinician cannot rule out FAP on the basis of this molecular test alone if other criteria support the FAP diagnosis. When the mutation in a family is known from one or more affected members, one test, usually IVSP, need be performed, as the expression pattern of the mutation is already established for that family. A positive result in such a test is considered a "mutation-positive" result, and the patient can be counseled as recommended. When the mutation in the family is not known, IVSP is performed. In the majority of cases, a mutation will be found in the APC gene that can be further characterized by DNA sequencing. Again, a "mutation-positive" result is obtained leading to the appropriate genetic counseling for the patient. Other options include DNA sequencing and linkage analysis. Even by combining two or more techniques, it is not possible to achieve 100% sensitivity, because the mutations may not be in the coding region of the gene or because a few FAP kindreds do not exhibit linkage to chromosome 5q. In such case, a "no mutation detected" result must not be interpreted as a "negative test" with the very important considerations for counseling the patient.

For at-risk individuals who have been found to be definitively mutation-negative by genetic testing, there is no clear consensus on the need or frequency of colon screening, though it would seem prudent that at least one flexible sigmoidoscopy or colonoscopy examination should be performed in early adulthood (age 18–25 years) (13).

Molecular Genetic Diagnosis of HNPCC

The HNPCC syndrome is more complex in terms of genetic testing because at least six genes involved in DNA mismatch repair predispose to this syndrome. The two most commonly involved genes are hMSH2 (involved in approximately 45% of cases) and hMLH1 (involved in approximately 49% cases). Protein truncation is observed in >80% of HNPCC cases caused by mutations in hMSH2 and to a lesser degree in hMHL1. Currently, IVSP or SSCA or both are used, followed by DNA sequencing for precise characterization. In the case of a mutation already known in an affected member of the kindred, the same technique used to detect that mutation can be used, and a "mutation-positive" result leads to genetic counseling. If no mutation has been previously described in the kindred, analysis of hMLH1 and hMSH2 in an affected individual by IVSP or SSCA followed by DNA sequencing for confirmation is indicated. If a truncating mutation is found, a causative role can be inferred for the mutation. This "mutation-positive" result allows counseling of the affected individual and further testing of the kindred. If a nontruncating mutation is found, tests such as linkage analysis and functional assays may be required to discriminate between an "inconclusive" and a "mutation-positive" result. It is estimated that approximately 30% of mutations will be missed if IVSP is used as the sole genetic test and that a similar or higher percentage of false negatives may also be expected if SSCA is used instead. Again, even by combining two or more techniques, it is not possible to achieve 100% sensitivity. Other genes may be responsible (locus heterogeneity). A "no mutation detected" result must not be interpreted as a "negative test" result.

Summary

A proposed algorithm for genetic testing of individuals in FAP and HNPCC kindreds is as follows. First, use IVSP to locate the mutation, then use DNA sequencing to characterize it precisely in the first affected family member. If the IVSP test is negative, DNA sequencing of the APC gene is warranted. When the mutation is defined for that kindred, the testing of other family members at risk may be accomplished by using IVSP alone. If the mutation in the first affected individual was identified by DNA sequencing, it is logical to continue to use this method for genetic testing of at-risk individuals. Considering the weighty psychological, ethical, and legal implications of the results of genetic tests, the use of two different techniques, one to detect the mutation and the second to identify and confirm it, is recommended in all cases. DNA sequencing, the most sensitive method for mutation detection, should be one of the techniques used. For HNPCC, two techniques are appropriate for initial testing of mutations in these genes, IVSP and SSCA. Screening with IVSP is recommended but this preference may vary among laboratories. If a mutation is detected by any of these methods, DNA sequencing should be used to identify it precisely in the first affected member of a kindred. If these screening techniques are negative, the sequencing of both hMSH2 and hMLH1 may be warranted. If still negative, in view of the locus heterogeneity seen in HNPCC, the same screening protocol may have to be used for hPMS2, hPMS1, and hMSH6. Again, the use of two different tests in all cases is recommended and DNA sequencing is used and when the pathogenic mutation is defined for that kindred, the testing of other family members at risk may be accomplished with either IVSP or SSCA alone.

When a mutation (a variant gene) is identified by any of the methods, it must be validated as a pathogenic mutation (true-positive result) instead of a polymorphism, a common variant in the protein that does not contribute to the disease phenotype (false positive). When a mutation is not identified ("no mutation detected") the negative result may be a "true negative" (no predisposing mutations in any relevant genes), or a "false negative" (undetected mutation may exist in known or unknown genes). If the person is affected with colorectal carcinoma, this is either a false negative in a familial colorectal carcinoma syndrome or a sporadic case. This "no mutation detected" result is the one most likely to be misinterpreted, leading to inappropriate genetic counseling. The use of two genetic tests decreases the rate of false-negative results. DNA sequencing is the most sensitive technique for this purpose and its use is advocated whenever a negative result is obtained by IVSP or SSCP for affected members with a strong family history. Even if the APC gene or all five DNA mismatch repair genes are fully sequenced, there will still be a residue of false-negative results caused by mutations in the noncoding regions of those genes, locus heterogeneity, or in still-unidentified genes.

A "negative test" in patients at risk for FAP or HNPCC will rule out these disorders only if a mutation has been identified in an affected family member. If tests to identify a mutation in an affected family member are negative, a "no mutation detected" result should be considered as noninformative or inconclusive (as if no test had been performed). The correct interpretation of a negative result in mutation analysis of hereditary colorectal carcinoma syndromes is mandatory to avoid adverse outcomes, because a false-negative result may lead to lack of appropriate endoscopic surveillance. Molecular genetic testing must be coupled with appropriate genetic counseling.

Interpretation of Genetic Test Results

FAP ■ A summary for interpreting APC genetic test results is as follows. The implication of a mutation-positive test result is that APC mutation carriers need to be informed that prophylactic colectomy is necessary when adenomatous polyps become evident. Mutation carriers require surveillance by gastroscopy for extracolonic neoplasms in the upper gastrointestinal tract. Other variant manifestations in FAP include osteomas, cutaneous cysts, and congenital hypertrophy of retinal pigment epithelium (CHRPE). When a mutation has been identified in the family, direct gene testing of relatives who have not yet been clinically assessed will distinguish between those who carry the mutation and those who do not. About 30% of FAP cases are caused by new mutations in the APC gene. In these cases the parents will not carry this mutation and are not at risk of FAP; only descendants of the proband are at 50% risk. *What are the implications of a "negative test" result versus "no mutation detected" result?* A negative test result is given if the patient does not carry the mutation that is known to exist in their family. In this instance family members are not at increased risk for developing colorectal carcinoma compared with the general population and should follow guidelines for carcinoma surveillance for that group. If the patient is affected with FAP and complete coding sequence analysis of the APC gene fails to identify a mutation, this could mean that the APC gene is not responsible for the patient's diagnosis. In this case, a "no mutation detected" result, APC gene testing has no predictive value for asymptomatic at-risk relatives. In these families first-degree relatives should continue colorectal carcinoma surveillance annually between the ages of 12 and 25 years, every other year between the ages of 25 and 35 years, and every third year between 35 and 50 years. Family members who have not developed multiple adenomatous polyps on complete bowel examination by the age of 50 years are assumed to be unaffected by FAP. If a "no mutations detected" result occurs when an unaffected family member from a APC kindred is tested without testing an affected family member, it is important that the patient not be falsely reassured because other mechanisms may inactivate the APC gene or other genes may be involved.

APC I1307K ■ A mutation in the APC gene termed I1307K was found in about 6% of people of Ashkenazi Jewish descent and about 28% of Ashkenazim with a family history of colorectal carcinoma. It appears to be associated with an approximately twofold increase in colorectal carcinoma risk (13). This alteration is a transversion of a single base from thymidine to adenine in codon 1307 of the APC gene. Analysis for this mutation is done by allele specific oligonucleotide analysis (extremely sensitive and specific) and consequently delivers a conclusive positive or negative test result. Genetic testing for this alteration is possible but the clinical utility of such testing is uncertain. The mean age at which colorectal carcinoma occurs in people carrying the I1307K alteration is not known nor has the natural history of colorectal carcinoma in carriers of I1307K been assessed or compared to sporadic colorectal carcinomas. No screening outcomes have been assessed in carriers of I1307K. Therefore, it is not yet known whether the I1307K carrier state should guide decisions about the age at which screening is initiated, the optimal screening strategy or the optimal screening interval (13).

HNPCC. A summary of interpreting HNPCC genetic testing results is as follows. *The implication of a positive mutation result* is that individuals carrying a mutation in a gene that predisposes to HNPCC should be educated on the risk of colorectal carcinoma as well as carcinoma in other sites: endometrium, stomach, small bowel, biliary tract, ovary, pancreas, renal pelvis, and ureter. The risk to age 70 years for developing any neoplasm may be as high as 90% for males and 70% for females (82).

For mutation carriers who develop colorectal carcinoma, total abdominal colectomy with ileo-rectal anastomosis is recommended because the entire colonic mucosa is at risk for malignancy. Proctocolectomy may also be a consideration, because the distal rectum is also a possible site of carcinoma. Prophylactic resection may be an option for mutation carriers unwilling to undergo surveillance or when endoscopic polypectomy is difficult. It should be emphasized that there are no data on whether resection is effective in reducing overall mortality. All first-degree relatives of patients who carry a mutation in one of the mismatch repair genes should be counseled that they have a 50% chance of carrying the same mutation.

What are the implications of a negative test result versus no mutation detected? A patient who tests negative for a known family mutation is not at risk for HNPCC, because it is a conclusive negative test result. Subsequent carcinoma surveillance should be as for the general population. If a mutation in a family with strong circumstantial evidence for HNPCC has not been identified, the interpretation of a "no mutation detected" test result in the HNPCC-associated gene or genes tested is complex. It may be necessary to perform more than one screening test to strengthen the suspicion that a mutation in a mismatch repair gene exists in the family. The difference between a negative test result and a "no mutation detected" result with its subsequent implications is dependent on whether a mutation has been previously identified in the family in HNPCC families. If the person is affected with HNPCC, and no mutation was detected in hMLH1 and hMSH2 with in vitro–synthesized protein assay and single-strand conformation polymorphism, other investigations may be offered to determine whether the patient carries a mutation in a mismatch repair gene. For example, testing for microsatellite instability (MSI) in neoplastic tissue may be a worthy investment before sequencing hMLH1 and hMSH2. If no abnormality in hMLH1 and hMSH2 is found by sequencing, analysis of the rarer HNPCC-causing genes is indicated.

Caution should be exercised in providing genetic risk assessment on the basis of currently used germline mutation detection strategies. While screening for hMSH2 gene mutations in HNPCC kindreds, Xia et al. (83) observed that using RT-PCR and the protein truncation test, the hMSH2 exon 13 deletion variant was found in >90% of individuals. This may lead to a misdiagnosis of HNPCC and has profound implications for counseling and genetic risk assessments of other family members.

Impact of Genetic Testing

Individuals need to know the implications and possible impact of genetic test results before testing. An ambiguous test result may be more distressing than a positive test result. Moreover, genetic testing often yields results that are probabilistic. The psychological burden of knowing that one is at high risk for developing a neoplasm may outweigh the possible benefits from intervention. Results of a study by Keller et al. (84) suggest that expressed intention and attitude toward genetic testing do not reliably predict actual uptake of counseling or testing. Data on the actual uptake of genetic testing for HNPCC in a clinical sample of 140 patients fulfilling clinical criteria of HNPCC, was 26%. Some 60% of participants experienced pronounced distress related to their potential inheritance of the disorder compared to 35% among nonparticipants. Distress reached a clinically significant level in 28% of participants. Restricted communication within the family was observed frequently. Irrespective of groups, a positive attitude toward obtaining a gene test result predominated. Therefore, the benefits and risks of participating in genetic tests must be described before testing is begun. Undergoing early detection of colorectal carcinoma or prophylactic operation or both can save lives. Surveillance or operation can be targeted to specific sites that are more prone to neoplasia, depending on the identity of the gene. For instance, female members of HNPCC families have a 10-fold increased risk for developing endometrial carcinoma, with an age of onset 10 to 15 years earlier than the same disease in the general population. Options for intervention and early detection and provision of knowledge to other family members are common reasons why individuals seek testing for genes predisposing to carcinoma of the colon and rectum.

Gritz et al. (85) examined the impact of HNPCC genetic test results on psychological outcomes among carcinoma-affected and -unaffected participants up to 1 year after results disclosure. A total of 155 persons completed study measures before HNPCC genetic testing, and 2 weeks and 6 and 12 months after disclosure of test results. Mean scores on all outcome measures remained stable and within normal limits for carcinoma-affected participants, regardless of mutation status. Among unaffected carriers of HNPCC-predisposing mutations, mean depression, state anxiety, and carcinoma worries scores increased from baseline to 2 weeks postdisclosure and decreased from 2 weeks to 6 months postdisclosure. Among unaffected noncarriers, mean depression and anxiety scores did not differ, but carcinoma worries scores decreased during the same time period. Affected and unaffected carriers had higher mean test-specific distress scores at two weeks postdisclosure compared with noncarriers in their respective groups; scores decreased for affected carriers and all unaffected participants from 2 weeks to 12 months postdisclosure. Classification of participants into high-versus low-distress clusters using mean scores on baseline psychological measures predicted significantly higher or lower follow-up scores, respectively, on depression, state anxiety, quality of life, and test-specific distress measures, regardless of mutation status. Although HNPCC genetic testing does not result in long-term adverse psychological outcomes, unaffected mutation carriers may experience increased distress during the immediate post-disclosure time period. Furthermore, those with higher levels of baseline mood disturbance, lower quality of life, and lower social support may be at risk for both short- and long-term increased distress.

Examining a person's DNA has the potential for far-reaching consequences beyond the person being tested. Genetic testing can reveal information about relatives with whom we share a common genetic legacy. Despite the possible benefits of testing for susceptibility for malignancy, the uncertainty and limitations of current efforts to lower mortality or morbidity contribute to the psychosocial and ethical complexities. Genetic information must remain confidential. However, breach of confidentiality has been considered permissible if all of the following conditions are met: reasonable effort to encourage disclosure has failed; harm is likely to occur if the information is withheld; the harm is serious and avoidable; and the disease is treatable or preventable (86). Conflict between issues of privacy and duty to forewarn family members arises because genetic information is, at once, individual and familial. Several key issues may be raised in genetic testing. First, at times genetic test results need to be interpreted in the context of the results of other family members. Second, family members should be independently and autonomously counseled. Third, the decision of each member regarding testing should be followed without coercion by other family members. Fourth, genetic test results have familial implications whether results are disclosed to other family members or not.

To provide information useful in the education and counseling in individuals considering genetic testing, Lerman et al. (87) conducted structured interviews with 45 first-degree relatives of colorectal carcinoma patients. Fifty-one percent of respondents indicated that they definitely would want to obtain a genetic test for colon carcinoma susceptibility when it is available. Motivation for genetic testing included the following: to know if more screening tests are needed, to learn if one's children are at risk, and to be reassured. Barriers to testing included concerns about insurance, test accuracy, and how one's family would react emotionally. Most participants anticipated that they would become depressed and anxious if they tested positive for a mutation; many would feel guilty and still worry if they tested negative. These preliminary results underscore the importance of the potential risks, benefits, and limitations of genetic testing with particular emphasis on the possibility of adverse psychological effects and implications for health insurance. Ethical issues of revealing or concealing genetic information will be debated long into the future because the potentially enormous consequences must be carefully considered. Hadley et al. (88) assessed the impact of genetic counseling and testing on the use of endoscopic screening procedures and adherence to recommended endoscopic screening guidelines in 56 symptomatic at-risk individuals in families known to carry an HNPCC mutation. They analyzed data on colonoscopy and flexible sigmoidoscopy screenings collected before genetic counseling and testing and 6 and 12 months postgenetic counseling and testing on 17 mutation-positive and 39 true-negative mutation individuals. Among mutation-negative individuals, use of colonoscopy and flexible sigmoidoscopy decreased significantly between pre- and postgenetic counseling and testing. Among mutation-positive individuals a non-significant increase in use was noted. Age was also associated with use of endoscopic screening after genetic counseling and testing. More mutation-negative individuals strictly adhered to guidelines than did mutation-positive individuals (87% vs. 65%). They concluded genetic counseling and testing for HNPCC significantly influences the use of colonic endoscopy and adherence to recommendations for colon carcinoma screening.

THREAT OF GENETIC DISCRIMINATION ■ Patients considering genetic testing need to be informed about the potential for genetic discrimination. This is of great concern for asymptomatic family members, because disclosure of a positive mutation result to third parties could be used to limit, raise rates for, or deny access to individual health insurance. However, nondisclosure could nullify a patient's insurance contract.

A survey of medical directors of United States life insurance companies indicated that familial colon or breast carcinoma constituted sufficient grounds to deny insurance (1 of the 27) or charge higher premiums (6 of the 27), despite not having actuarial data to support underwriting (calculating premiums) guidelines pertaining to these carcinomas.

In the United States several states have safeguards against the potential misuse of genetic information. The potential for misuse of genetic information has led to federal initiatives in the United States to regulate the use of genetic information. In the context of insurance and employment it is unclear whether the Americans with Disabilities Act of 1990 (ADA) will provide adequate protection to carriers of carcinoma-susceptibility genes, because the Equal Employment Opportunity Commission does not view a person with genetic predisposition for a disease or a carrier of a gene for a late-onset disorder as having a disability. This implies that these persons are not protected under the ADA. Legislation has been introduced to extend the definition of disability to "genetic or medically identified potential of or predisposition toward a physical or mental impairment that substantially limits a major life activity." For now, the ADA has been interpreted to offer protection only to those who develop symptoms.

Health Insurance Portability and Accountability Act (Kennedy-Kassebaum bill) came into effect in the summer of 1997. It defined genetic information as part as an individual's health status. This act was implemented to prohibit employers and insurers from excluding individuals in a group from coverage or charging higher premiums on the basis of health status. Also in 1997 the Genetic Information Nondiscrimination in Health Insurance Act (Slaughter-Snowe bill) called for a ban of the use of "genetic information" in denying or setting rates for group health insurance. In this act genetic information was defined broadly to include genetic tests as well as information about inherited features. This bill called for a limit on the collection or disclosure of genetic information without the written consent of the individual.

Fourteen states have enacted legislation to provide safeguards and to protect misuse of genetic information by insurers and employers. Other states have followed suit, and amendments are being made to those existing laws in some states, as reviewed by Offit (89).

In summary, individuals undergoing genetic testing should understand the advantages and disadvantages of receiving and sharing genetic results. Attempting to protect the individual from genetic discrimination by disseminating results to only a few selected medical staff could impede care. So far, there has been no substantial use of genetic information by health insurers, and laws restricting its use have thus far maintained social fairness in the area of health insurance. When integrated with existing testing protocols for colorectal carcinoma and when applied with appropriate caveats particularly regarding interpretation of negative results, genetic testing can result in improved management of patients and families.

Alternate Pathway of Carcinogenesis

An understanding of the mechanisms that explain the initiation and early evolution of colorectal carcinoma should facilitate the development of new approaches to effective prevention and intervention. Jass et al. (90) have proposed a model for colorectal neoplasia in which APC mutation is not placed at the point of initiation. Other genes implicated in the regulation of apoptosis and DNA repair may underlie the early development of colorectal carcinoma. Inactivation of these genes may occur not by mutation or loss but through silencing mediated by methylation of the gene's promoter region. hMLH1 and MGMT are examples of DNA repair genes that are silenced by methylation. Loss of expression of hMLH1 and MGMT protein has been demonstrated immunohistochemically in serrated polyps. Multiple lines of evidence point to a "serrated" pathway of neoplasia that is driven by inhibition of apoptosis and the subsequent inactivation of DNA repair genes by promoter methylation. The earliest lesions in this pathway are aberrant crypt foci (ACF). These may develop into hyperplastic polyps or transform while still of microscopic size into admixed polyps, serrated adenomas, or traditional adenomas. Carcinomas developing from these lesions may show high- or low-level microsatellite instability (MSI-H and MSI-L, respectively) or may be microsatellite stable (MSS). The suggested clinical model for this alternative pathway is the condition hyperplastic polyposis. Hyperplastic polyposis presents a plausible model for the following reasons:

1. Polyps in this condition may show MSI and silencing of relevant DNA repair genes including hMLH1.
2. Methylation is demonstrated in DNA extracted from hyperplastic polyps in a subset of subjects with hyperplastic polyposis. The finding of methylation is concordant within multiple polyps in such cases, whereas discordant findings occur in subjects with multiple adenomas.
3. The requisite plasticity in methylator pathways is evident in hyperplastic polyposis in which all types of epithelial polyp may occur (hyperplastic, admixed, serrated adenoma, and traditional adenoma), and carcinomas may be MSI-H, MSI-L, or MSS (even within the same subject).
4. The condition hyperplastic polyposis may be familial. Jass et al. (90) believe that molecular and morphologic observations have stripped the hyperplastic polyp of its long-presumed innocence. However, the fact that the vast majority of hyperplastic polyps will never progress to carcinoma has not altered. It is impractical to advocate the removal of every minute hyperplastic lesion. On the other hand, more attention might be given to subjects with "high-risk" hyperplastic polyps. High-risk features would include multiplicity (more than 20), size (greater than 10 mm), proximal location, associated polyps with dysplasia, and a family history of colorectal carcinoma. New diagnostic criteria and markers are required to distinguish innocent hyperplastic polyps from their serrated counterparts with a malignant potential that belies their deceptively bland morphology.

DIETARY FACTORS

Dietary factors have been implicated in the etiology of colorectal carcinoma. Prime candidates are dietary fats and fiber-deficient diets. Studies thus far have been inconclusive with respect to which component is most important. Experimental, epidemiological, and clinical evidence show that diets consumed by Western populations have an important role in the modulation of this disease (91). The diet contains various mutagens and carcinogens that can be classified into three groups: (1) naturally occurring chemicals that include mycotoxins and plant alkaloids, (2) synthetic compounds exemplified by food additives and pesticides, and (3) compounds produced by cooking, which include polycyclic aromatic hydrocarbons and heterocyclic amines (92). Since heterocyclic amines are genotoxic compounds, a causal role in some stage of human colon carcinogenesis is plausible.

Fat

Populations with diets high in unsaturated fat and protein, especially if associated with low-fiber ingestion, are associated with a high incidence of colorectal carcinoma. In a Canadian study, patients with colon carcinoma reported a higher intake of total fat, saturated fat, and dietary cholesterol than controls, with the highest relative risk in saturated fat (93). In a prospective cohort study of diet and colon carcinoma, Willett et al. (94) gathered information on 98,464 nurses. Among the 150 nurses who developed colon carcinoma, the trend for risk with total fat intake ($p < 0.05$) and animal fat ($p < 0.01$) was significant. Animal fat from dairy sources (e.g., butter or ice cream) was not associated with risk. A study by Nigro et al. (95) found that animals fed 35% beef fat develop more colon carcinoma than those fed 5% beef fat. Reddy and Maruyana (96) found that a diet containg 20% of either corn or safflower oil increased the incidence of colon carcinoma in animals much more than in those fed 5% of the same fat. Not only is the amount of fat important, but the type may be equally important. Diets containing high levels of olive oil, coconut oil, or fish oil did not increase the incidence of colon carcinoma more than in animals fed 5% of the same fats. The mechanism of action is believed to be indirect, with the resulting high concentration of fecal bile acids and cholesterol stimulating cell proliferation and acting as promoters of carcinogenesis. However, this seemingly neat hypothesis is not universally accepted. It must be noted that the role of dietary fat is inextricably linked to excretion of bile acids and the ratio of anaerobic to aerobic bacteria.

Meat and Fish

Consumption of red and processed meat has been associated with colorectal carcinoma in many but not all epidemiological studies. Chao et al. (97) examined the relationship between recent and long-term meat consumption and the risk of incident colon and rectal carcinoma. A cohort of 148,610 adults aged 50 to 74 years (median, 63 years), residing in 21 states with population-based registries, who provided information on meat consumption in 1982 and again in 1992/1993 were enrolled in the Cancer Prevention Study II Nutrition Cohort. Follow-up identified 1667 incident colorectal carcinomas. Participants contributed person-years at risk until death or a diagnosis of colon or rectal carcinoma. High intake of red and processed meat reported in 1992/1993 was associated with higher risk of distal colon carcinoma after adjusting for age and energy intake but not after further adjustment for body mass index, cigarette smoking, and other covariates. When long-term consumption was considered, persons in the highest tertile of consumption in both 1982 and 1992/1993 had higher risk of distal colon carcinoma associated with processed meat (RR, 1.50) and ratio of red meat to poultry and fish (RR, 1.53) relative to those persons in the lowest tertile at both time points. Long-term consumption of poultry and fish was inversely associated with risk of both proximal and distal colon carcinoma. High consumption of red meat reported in 1992/1993 was associated with a higher risk of rectal carcinoma (RR, 1.71) as was high consumption reported in both 1982 and 1992/1993 (RR, 1.43). Their results strengthen the evidence that prolonged high consumption of red and processed meat may increase the risk of carcinoma in the distal portion of the large intestine.

Larsson et al. (98) prospectively examined whether the association of red meat consumption with carcinoma risk varies by subsite within the large bowel. They analyzed data from 61,433 women aged 40 to 75 years and free from diagnosed carcinoma at baseline. Diet was assessed at baseline using a self-administered food-frequency questionnaire. Over a mean follow-up of 13.9 years, they identified 234 proximal colon carcinomas, 155 distal colon carcinomas, and 230 rectal carcinomas. They observed a significant positive association between red meat consumption and risk of distal colon carcinoma but not of the proximal colon or rectum. The multivariate rate ratio for women who consumed 94 g/day or more of red meat compared to those who consumed less than 50 g/day was 2.22 for the distal colon, 1.03 for proximal colon, and 1.28 for rectum. Although there was no association between consumption of fish and risk of carcinoma at any subsite, poultry consumption was weakly inversely related to risk of total colorectal carcinoma.

Norat et al. (99) prospectively followed 478,040 men and women from 10 European countries who were free of carcinoma at enrollment. After a mean follow-up of 4.8 years, 1329 incident colorectal carcinomas were documented. Colorectal carcinoma risk was positively associated with intake of red and processed meat [highest (>160 g/day) and lowest (<20 g/day)] intake, HR = 1.35 and inversely associated with intake of fish (>80 g/day vs. <10 g/day, HR = 0.69), but was not related to poultry intake. In this study population, the absolute risk of development of colorectal carcinoma within 10 years for a study subject aged 50 years was 1.71% for the highest category of red and processed meat intake and 1.28% for the lowest category of intake and was 1.86% for subjects in the lowest category of fish intake and 1.28% for subjects in the highest category of fish intake. Their data confirmed that colorectal carcinoma risk is positively associated with high consumption of red and processed meat and support an inverse association with fish intake.

Fiber

Following his observation of the low incidence of colorectal carcinoma in African natives, Burkitt (100) promoted the idea that their high-fiber intake was responsible for this finding. He further deduced that the Western low-fiber diet along with high carbohydrate and animal fat intake was responsible for the higher incidence of maligiiancy of the large bowel. Burkitt also noted that when Africans abandon their customary diet, the incidence of carcinoma of the colorectum progressively increases. Diets with a high roughage content result in the production of soft frequent stools. A potential carcinogen in a patient with infrequent stools remains in contact with the colonic and rectal mucosa longer.

Experimental work by Fleiszer et al. (101) has supported this thesis in that a high-fiber diet resulted in a diminished incidence of dimethylhydrazine (DMH) -induced carcinoma of the colon in rats. Yet the potential protective effect of fiber is controversial. A study by Nigro et al. (102) in which a group of rats was given a 30% beef fat and 10% fiber diet, demonstrated no protective effect from wheat bran or cellulose. Animals fed 5% fat and 20% or 30% fiber developed fewer carcinomas than fiber-free controls. This finding suggests that a large quantity of fat can overcome the protective effect of fiber.

From an epidemiologic point of view, Greenwald, Lanza, and Eddy (103) analyzed 55 original reports and found evidence of an inverse association between a high fiber diet and the risk of colon carcinoma. The same group conducted a meta-analysis of 12 methodologically sound and descriptively complete case-control studies and showed protection with an odds ratio of 0.57 (95% CI, 0.50 to 0.64) (104). Those studies delineating vegetable fiber from total fiber suggested a stronger protective effect from vegetable fiber. Freudenheim et al. (105) conducted a case-control study of 850 pairs in which the fiber source was subdivided from grain, fruit, and vegetables and in which the results of consuming soluble vs. insoluble fiber were also compared. Fruit and vegetable fiber protected against rectal carcinoma in men and women and against colon carcinoma in men. Grain fiber protected against colon carcinoma only. Insoluble fractions of grain fiber were more protective in the colon, with both soluble and insoluble fractions from fruit and vegetables protective in the rectum. In a follow-up of 11 years of a German cohort of 1904 patients, the mortality rate for patients with colon carcinoma was reduced for individuals following a vegetarian lifestyle for over 20 years (106).

A study with contrary findings was reported. Asano and McLeod (107) conducted a systematic review and meta-analysis to assess the effect of dietary fiber on the incidence or recurrence of colorectal adenomas, the incidence of colorectal carcinoma, and the development of adverse events. Five studies with 4349 subjects met the inclusion criteria. The interventions were wheat bran fiber, ispaghula husk, or a comprehensive dietary intervention with high fiber whole food sources alone or in combination. When the data were combined there was no difference between the intervention and control groups. The reviewers concluded there is currently no evidence from randomized clinical trials to suggest that increased dietary fiber intake will reduce the incidence or recurrence of adenomatous polyps within a two- to four-year period. Fuchs et al.

(108) conducted a prospective study of 88,757 women who were 34 to 59 years old and had no history of carcinoma, inflammatory bowel disease, or familial polyposis. During a 16-year follow-up period, 787 cases of colorectal carcinoma were documented. In addition, 1012 patients with adenomas of the distal colon and rectum were found among 27,530 participants who underwent endoscopy during the follow-up period. After adjustment for age, established risk factors, and total energy intake, they found no association between the intake of dietary fiber and the risk of colorectal carcinoma or colorectal adenoma. The same investigators found no protective effect of fruit vegetable consumption (109). On the other hand, Terry et al. (110) found that total fruit and vegetable consumption was inversely associated with the risk of the development of colorectal carcinoma whereas they observed no association between colorectal carcinoma risk and consumption of cereal fiber. Michels et al. (109) prospectively investigated the association between fruit and vegetable consumption and the incidence of colon and rectal carcinoma in two large cohorts; the Nurses' Health Study (88,764 women) and the Health Professionals' Follow-up Study (47,325 men). With a follow-up including 1,743,645 person-years and 937 cases of colon carcinoma, they found little association of colon carcinoma incidence with fruit and vegetable consumption. Although fruit and vegetables may confer protection against some chronic diseases, their frequent consumption did not appear to confer protection from colon and rectal carcinoma in this study. Peters et al. (111) used a 137-item food-frequency questionnaire to assess the relation of fiber intake and frequency of colorectal adenoma. The study was done within the prostate, lung, colorectal, ovarian (PLCO) Cancer Screening Trial, a randomized controlled trial designed to investigate methods for early detection of carcinoma. In their analysis they compared fiber intake of 33,971 participants who were sigmoidoscopy-negative for polyps, with 3591 cases with at least one histologically verified adenoma in the distal large bowel (i.e., descending colon, sigmoid colon, or rectum). High intakes of dietary fiber were associated with a low risk of colorectal adenoma, after adjustment for potential dietary and nondietary risk factors. Participants in the highest quintile of dietary fiber intake had a 27% lower risk of adenoma than those in the lowest quintile. The inverse association was strongest for fiber from grains and cereals than from fruits. Risks were similar for advanced and nonadvanced adenoma. Risk of rectal adenoma was not significantly associated with fiber intake. Why these two studies reached different results is impossible to answer. The use of different types or sources and amounts of fiber may be one explanation.

In a population-based case-control study, Meyer and White (112) found for both sexes that a higher dietary fiber intake was associated with lower relative risks for colon carcinoma. Howe et al. (113) examined the effects of fiber, vitamin C, and beta-carotene intakes on colorectal carcinoma risk in a combined analysis of data from 13 cases-controlled studies previously conducted in populations with differing colorectal carcinoma rates and dietary practices. Original data records for 5287 case subjects with colorectal carcinoma and 10,470 control subjects without disease were combined. Risk decreased as fiber intake increased; relative risks were 0.79, 0.69, 0.63, and 0.53 for the four highest quintiles of intake compared with the lowest quintile. The inverse association with fiber is seen in 12 of the 13 studies and is similar in magnitude for left- and right-sided colon and rectal carcinomas, for men and for women, and for different age groups. In contrast, after adjustment for fiber intake, only weak inverse associations are seen for the intakes of vitamin C and beta-carotene. This analysis provided substantive evidence that intake of fiber-rich foods is inversely related to risk of carcinomas of both the colon and rectum. If causality is assumed, they estimated that risk of colorectal carcinoma in the United States population could be reduced by 31% (55,000 cases annually) by an average increase in fiber intake from food sources of about 13 g/day, corresponding to an average increase of about 70%. Bingham et al. reached the same conclusion. In the biggest study ever published Bingham et al. (114) prospectively examined the association between dietary fiber and incidence of colorectal carcinoma in 519,978 individuals aged 25 to 70 years taking part in a study recruited from 10 European countries. Participants completed a dietary questionnaire in 1992–1998 and were followed up for the incidence of carcinoma. Follow-up consisted of 1,939,011 person-years, and data for 1065 reported cases of colorectal carcinoma were included in the analysis. Dietary fiber in foods was inversely related to the incidence of large bowel carcinoma (adjusted relative risk 0.75 for the highest vs. lowest quintile of intake), the protective effect being greatest for the left side of the colon, and least for the rectum. After calibration with more detailed dietary data, the adjusted risk for the highest versus lowest quintile of fiber from food intake was 0.58. No food source of fiber was significantly more protective than others, and nonfood supplement sources of fiber were not investigated. They concluded, in populations with low average intake of dietary fiber, an approximate doubling of total fiber intake from foods could reduce the risk of colorectal carcinoma by 40%.

Calcium Deficiency

Slattery, Sorenson, and Ford (115) observed that the dietary intake of calcium decreased the risk of development of colon carcinoma. Calcium can bind intraluminally with bile acids and fatty acids, thus reducing their mitogenic effect (116). Calcium salts may have antiproliferative effects in the colon of patients who are predisposed to developing large bowel carcinoma (117). Dietary supplementation with calcium reduces colonic crypt cell production in both normal and hyperplastic mucosa. One of the main pathways used by extracellular calcium to exert its chemopreventive actions is through activation of a calcium-sensing receptor. This results in increased levels of intracellular calcium, inducing a wide range of biological effects, some of which restrain the growth and promote the differentiation of transformed colon cells (91). Calcium likely reduces lipid damage in the colon by complexing with fat to form mineral-fat complexes or soaps (118). It has been shown in an increasing number of animal experiments that calcium has the ability to inhibit colon carcinoma. In limited studies in man, the colonic hyperproliferation associated with increased risk of colon carcinoma has been reversed for short periods by the administration of supplemental dietary calcium. In a population-based case-control study, Meyer and White (112) showed that calcium was associated with a decreased risk of colon carcinoma in women only. Baron et al. (119) conducted a randomized double-blind trial of the effect of supplementation with calcium carbonate on recurrence of colorectal adenomas. They randomly assigned 930 subjects (mean age, 61 years; 72% men) with a recent history of colorectal adenomas to receive either calcium carbonate [3 g (1200 mg of elemental calcium) daily] or placebo, with follow-up colonoscopies one and four years after the qualifying examination. Among the 913 subjects who underwent at least one study colonoscopy, the adjusted risk ratio for any recurrence of adenoma with calcium as compared with placebo was 0.85. At least one adenoma was diagnosed between the first and second follow-up endoscopies in 127 subjects in the calcium group (31%) and 159 subjects in the placebo group (38%). The effect of calcium was independent of initial dietary fat and calcium intake. They concluded calcium supplementation is associated with a significant—though moderate—reduction in the risk of recurrent adenomas. Wu et al. (120) examined the association between calcium intake and colon carcinoma risk in two prospective cohorts, the Nurses' Health Study and the Health Professionals Follow-up Study. Their study population included 87,998 women in the former and 47,344 men in the latter. During the follow-up period, 15 years for the Nurses' Health Study cohort, and 10 years for the Health Professionals Follow-up Study, 626 and 399 colon carcinomas were identified in women and men, respectively. In women and men considered together they found an inverse association between high total calcium intake (>1250 mg/day vs. ≤ 500 mg/day) and distal colon carcinoma (women relative risk ratio 0.73, men relative risk ratio 0.58, and pooled relative ratio 0.65). No such association was found for proximal colon carcinoma (women relative risk ratio = 1.28, men relative risk ratio = 0.92, and pooled relative risk ratio 1.14). The incremental benefit of additional calcium intake beyond approximately 700 mg/day appeared to be minimal.

Wallace et al. (121) examined the effect of calcium on the risk of different types of colorectal lesions. They used patients from the Calcium Polyp Prevention Study, a randomized double-blind, placebo-controlled chemoprevention trial among patients with a recent colorectal adenoma in which 930 patients were randomly assigned to calcium carbonate (1200 mg/day) or placebo. Follow-up colonoscopies were conducted approximately one and four years after the qualifying examination. The calcium risk ratio for hyperplastic polyps was 0.82, that for tubular adenomas was 0.89, and that for histologically advanced neoplasms was 0.65 compared with patients assigned to placebo. There were no statistically significantly differences between the risk ratio for tubular adenomas and that for other types of polyps. The effect of calcium supplementation on adenoma risk was most pronounced among individuals with high dietary intakes of calcium and fiber and with low intake of fat, but the interactions were not statistically significant. Their results suggest that calcium supplementation may have a more pronounced antineoplastic effect on advanced colorectal lesions than on other types of polyps. Taken together the available evidence suggests that increases in the daily intake of calcium in the diet may provide a means of colorectal carcinoma control. Although a positive effect has not been proven, it might be prudent for the public to consume diets that contain adequate amounts of calcium.

Magnesium

Larsson et al. (122) suggested that a high magnesium intake may reduce the occurrence of colorectal carcinoma in women. In a population-based prospective cohort of 61,433 women aged 40 to 75 years without previous diagnosis of carcinoma at baseline and a mean of 14.8 years (911,042 person-years) of follow-up, 805 incident colorectal carcinoma cases were diagnosed. Compared with women in the lowest quintile of magnesium intake, the multivariate rate ratio was 0.59 for those in the highest quintile. The inverse association was observed for both colon (RR, 0.66) and rectal carcinoma (RR, 0.45).

Micronutrients and Chemical Inhibitors

In geographic regions where the trace element selenium is found to be lacking, there is a higher incidence of colorectal carcinoma, while high selenium areas have low colorectal carcinoma rates (123). Significantly decreased selenium concentrations in blood samples from patients with colorectal carcinomas and various adenomas have been found when compared to normal controls (124).

High selenium broccoli decreased the incidence of aberrant crypts in rats with chemically induced colon carcinomas by more than 50% compared with controls (125). In a case-controlled study, Nelson et al. (126) found that higher levels of selenium produced a protective effect against colon polyps or carcinomas. Jacobs et al. (127) conducted a combined analysis of data from three randomized trials—the Wheat Bran Fiber Trial, the Polyp Prevention Trial, and the Polyp Prevention Study—which tested the effects of various nutritional interventions for colorectal adenoma prevention among participants who recently had an adenoma removed during colonoscopy. Selenium concentrations were measured from blood specimens from a total of 1763 trial participants, and quartiles of baseline selenium were established from pooled data. Analyses of the pooled data showed that individuals whose blood selenium values were in the highest quartile (median = 150 ng/mL) had statistically significantly lower odds of developing a new adenoma compared with those in the lowest quartile (OR = 0.66). They concluded the inverse association between higher blood selenium concentration and adenoma risk supports previous findings indicating that higher selenium status may be related to decreased risk of colorectal carcinoma.

A number of micronutrients and chemicals have been shown to have an inhibitory effect on the development of colorectal carcinoma: phenols, indoles, plant serols, selenium, calcium, vitamins A, C, and E, and carotenoids (128). They are present in small amounts in water and in whole grain cereals, fruits, and vegetables. The chemicals in foods that inhibit carcinoma development in laboratory animals have been summarized by Wargovich (129). They include plant phenols (in grapes, strawberries, and apples), dithiothiones and flavones (in cabbage, broccoli, brussels sprouts, and cauliflower), thioethers (in garlic, onions, and leeks), terpenes (in citrus fruits), and carotenoids (in carrots, yams, and watermelon). Some chemicals not present in the average diet affect the carcinogenic process in animals. Prostaglandin inhibitors and chemicals that influence cell proliferation and differentiation are examples (130). Some of these agents may be toxic, so the feasibility of administering a combination of agents was studied experimentally by Nigro et al. (131) By the addition of small nontoxic amounts of selenium, 13-cis-retinoic acid, and β-sitosterol, an additive inhibitory effect resulted in a significant diminution of intestinal carcinoma. Other combinations also have been found effective (128). Ascorbic acid, dialyl sulfide, and thioether found in garlic and onions also may aid in prevention (129,132).

Most of the pleiotropic actions of vitamin D are mediated by binding to a nuclear receptor that interacts with specific consensus sites in promoters of specific genes, resulting in downregulation or upregulation of their expression. The actions of vitamin D involve cross-talk with growth factors/cytokines, inhibitory effects on the cell cycle and stimulation of apoptosis (91).

Folate lies at the intersection of metabolic pathways involved in DNA methylation and biosynthesis. Three main mechanisms by which decreased levels of folate (and of other dietary one-carbon donors) might increase the risk of carcinoma are alteration of the normal DNA-methylation process; imbalance of the steady-state level of DNA precursors, leading to aberrant DNA synthesis and repair; and chromosome and chromatin change (91).

Alcohal Ingestion

A relationship between alcohol ingestion and development of colorectal carcinoma has been reported (OR, 2.6) (112) specifically the development of rectal carcinoma in association with beer consumption (6). Daily alcohol drinkers experience a twofold increase in risk of colorectal carcinomas (133). The positive association had been accounted for primarily by an increased risk of carcinoma in men whose monthly consumption of beer was 15 L or more (134,135). Beer drinking increases the risk 1.3 to 2.4 times (135–138). In a study of 6230 Swedish brewery workers, the relative risk for rectal carcinoma was 1.7 while the risk of colon carcinoma was not significantly increased, supporting the hypothesis that high beer consumption is associated with an increased risk of rectal carcinoma (139). Newcomb, Storer, and Marcus (135) found that high levels of alcohol consumption in women (11 or more drinks per week) were associated with an increased risk of large intestinal carcinoma (RR = 1.47).

Maekawa (140) reported that the heavy cumulative intake of alcohol was associated with significantly higher risk of colorectal carcinoma than in nondrinkers (OR = 6.8). The association of alcohol intake with the risk of colorectal carcinoma was not effected by the type of alcoholic beverage. Sharpe et al. (141) found the daily consumption of alcohol of any type was associated with increased risks of carcinoma of the distal colon (OR = 2.3), and the rectum (OR = 1.6) but not with an increased risk of a carcinoma of the proximal colon (OR = 1.0).

Smoking

The association of smoking (odds ratio for >40 pack years, 3.31) with adenomas (and by implication carcinoma) has been reported (142). Smoking for 20 years has a strong relation to adenomas, but an induction period of at least 35 years is necessary for colorectal carcinoma (143,144).

Chao (145) examined cigarette smoking in relation to colorectal carcinoma mortality, evaluating smoking duration and recency, and controlling for potential confounders in the Cancer Prevention Study II. This prospective nationwide mortality study of 1,184,657 adults (age ≥ 30 years) was begun by the American Cancer Society in 1982. After exclusions, their analytic cohort included 312,332 men and 469,019 women, among whom 4432 colon or rectal carcinoma deaths occurred between 1982 and 1996 among individuals who were carcinoma free in 1982. Multivariate-adjusted colorectal carcinoma mortality rates were highest among current smokers, were intermediate among former smokers, and were lowest in lifelong nonsmokers. The multivariate-adjusted relative rate for current compared with never smokers was 1.32 among men and 1.41 among women. Increased risk was evident after 20 or more years of smoking for men and women combined as compared with never smokers. Risk among current and former smokers increased with duration of smoking and average number of cigarettes smoked per day; risk in former smokers decreased significantly in years since quitting. If the multivariate-adjusted relative rate estimates in this study do, in fact, reflect causality, then approximately 12% of colorectal carcinoma deaths among both men and women in the general U.S. population in 1997 were attributable to smoking.

Clinical Dietary Studies

A number of case control studies have been reported. Jain et al. (146) examined patients with large bowel malignancy and compared them with population and hospital controls. An increased risk was found in persons with an increased intake of saturated fat as well as calories, total protein, total fat, oleic acid, and cholesterol. The strongest effect was that of saturated fat. Potter and McMichael (147) found that dietary protein was the strongest predictor of colon carcinoma with a two- to threefold relative risk. In a review, Kritchevsky (148) reported that studies for specific vegetables have been carried out with carrots, broccoli, cabbage, lettuce, potatoes, and legumes. Of a total of 105 studies, 67% have shown no association.

Prospective studies have examined the relationship between diet and subsequent development of colorectal carcinoma. Phillips and Snowdon (149) found a positive association for the risk of colon carcinoma with egg consumption, coffee intake, and weight greater than 125% of ideal weight. No association was noted for use of meat, cheese, milk, or green salad. Garland et al. (116) failed to note any association between dietary fat, animal or vegetable protein, ethanol, or energy intake and subsequent colorectal carcinoma. The authors did note a negative association between vitamin D and calcium intake and subsequent colorectal carcinoma. Stemmerman Nomura, and Heilbrun (150) studied the relationship between the intake of dietary fat and subsequent colorectal carcinoma during a 15-year follow-up in 7074 Japanese men and found a negative association between dietary total fat and saturated fat intake and colon carcinoma. The strongest effect was found in the right colon, whereas in contrast a weakly positive relationship was found in the rectum. Berry, Zimmerman, and Ligumsky (151), in a study of patients undergoing colonoscopy, analyzed fatty acid and plasma lipid analogs and found that the quality of dietary fat did not influence the development of carcinoma or neoplastic polyps in their population.

The fact that in most high-risk countries there is a positive association between fat or meat intake and risk of large bowel malignancy, but results are inconsistent in low-risk countries, implies that there is perhaps a threshold effect by which a minimal level of fat or meat is necessary to effect the development of colorectal carcinoma. There may be a confounding factor whereby dietary fat or protein increases the risk in persons eating low-fiber diets. In a case-control study of pathologically confirmed, single primary carcinomas of the rectum, the risk of rectal carcinoma increased with an increasing intake of kilocalories, fat, carbohydrate, and iron (152). The risk decreased with an increasing intake of carotenoids, vitamin C, and dietary fiber from vegetables. Fiber from grains, calcium, retinal, and vitamin E were not associated with risk. Associations of intake with risk were generally stronger for men than for women, except with vitamin C. The associations for carotenoids, vitamin C, and vegetable fiber persisted after stratification on intake of either kilocalories or fat.

Giovannucci et al. (153) evaluated the relation between folate intake and incidence of colon carcinoma in a prospect of cohort study of 88,756 women from the Nurses' Health Study. There were 442 with new cases of colon carcinoma. Higher folate intake was related to a lower risk of colon carcinoma (relative ratio 0.69) for intake $>400\,\mu g/day$ compared with intake $\leq 200\,\mu g/day$ after controlling for age; family history of colon carcinoma; aspirin use; smoking; body mass; physical activity; and intake of red meat, alcohol, methionine, and fiber. When intake of vitamins C, D, and E and intake of calcium were also controlled for, results were similar. Women who used multivitamins containing folic acid had no benefit with respect to colon carcinoma after four years of use. After 15 years of use, risk was markedly lower (relative ratio 0.25) representing 15 instead of 68 new cases of colon carcinoma per 10,000 women 55 to 69 years of age. Folate from dietary sources alone was related to a modest reduction in risk for colon carcinoma and the benefit of long-term multivitamin use was present across all levels of dietary intakes. In a large study designed to determine the relationship between fish consumption and risk of the development of carcinoma Fernandez et al. (154) noted a consistent pattern of protection against the risk of selected malignancies; colon OR 0.6 and rectum OR 0.5.

■ IRRADIATION

There have been sporadic reports of carcinoma of the colon and rectum that develops after radiation therapy for a variety of pelvic malignancies (155–160). The average interval between irradiation and the diagnosis of rectal carcinoma is 15.2 years with a range from 14 months to 33 years (158). There is controversy as to whether the relationship is one of cause and effect or purely coincidental. The characteristics are different from ordinary large bowel carcinoma in that there is a high incidence of mucin-producing carcinoma (53%) (159). Radiation injury was observed in 64% of cases (159).

Radiation therapy for prostate carcinoma has been associated with an increased rate of pelvic malignancies, particularly bladder carcinoma. Baxter et al. (161) conducted a retrospective cohort study using Surveillance, Epidemiology, and End Results (SEER) registry data. They focused on men with prostate carcinoma, but with no previous history of colorectal carcinoma, treated with either surgery or radiation who survived at least five years. They evaluated the effect of radiation on development of carcinoma for three sites: definitely irradiated sites (rectum), potentially irradiated sites (rectosigmoid, sigmoid, and cecum), and nonirradiated sites (the rest of the colon). A total of 30,552 men received radiation, and 55,263 underwent surgery only. Colorectal carcinomas developed in 1437 patients: 267 in irradiated sites, 686 in potentially irradiated sites, and 484 in nonirradiated sites. Radiation was independently associated with development of carcinoma over time in irradiated sites but not in the remainder of the colon. The adjusted hazards ratio for development of rectal carcinoma was 1.7 for the radiation group, compared with the surgery only group. Radiation had no effect on development of carcinoma in the remainder of the colon indicating that the effect is specific to directly irradiated tissue.

Tami et al. (157) described some characteristics of radiation-associated rectal carcinoma. All four of their patients presented with chronic radiation colitis. Radiation-associated rectal carcinoma has a tendency to be diagnosed in the advanced stage and to have a poor prognosis. Since there are no reliable clinical or laboratory indicators of the presence of a curable colorectal carcinoma in the setting of chronic radiation proctocolitis, they recommend surveillance with a colonoscope should be done 10 years after irradiation in patients with previous pelvic radiotherapy.

■ URETERIC IMPLANTATION

Several reports have documented the development of neoplasia at or near the site of a ureterosigmoidostomy (162–167). The risk of sigmoid carcinoma has been estimated to be anywhere from 8.5 to 10.5 and 80 to 550 times greater in patients with ureterosigmoidostomy than in the normal population (166,167). Adenomatous polyps at the level of the ureterosigmoidostomy may be precursors of a subsequent carcinoma. The interval between the implanation of ureters and the occurrence of colonic carcinoma varies from 5 to 41 years. Husmann and Spence (168) reviewed the literature to 1990 and found 94 patients who had colonic neoplasia after ureterosigmoidostomy for vesical exstrophy. The average patient age at diagnosis of neoplasia was 33 years with an average latency of 26 years. Blood in the stool and symptoms and signs of ureteral obstruction were cardinal warning signs. Treatment consisted of local extirpation of the lesion with reimplantation of one or both ureters back into the sigmoid in one third of patients. The preferred treatment is either endoscopic destruction of polyps after biopsy or resection of the involved segment with cutaneous loop diversions. If the polyp is located at the mouth of or immediately adjacent to the ureterocolic anastomosis, caution must be exercised to avoid obstruction of the orifice as a result of vigorous electrocautery. Death from carcinoma occurred in 30 of 49 patients. The current trend is away from this type of urinary diversion, but for those individuals who have already had this operation, periodic endoscopic surveillance appears to be in order.

■ CHOLECYSTECTOMY

There is considerable epidemiologic evidence to suggest that bile acids play an important role in the development of colorectal malignancy, but their precise action in the initiation or promotion of the neoplastic process remains to be determined (169). A suggested explanation is that, although before cholecystectomy the bile acid pool circulates two or three times per meal, after cholecystectomy the pool circulates even during fasting. This enhanced circulation results in increased exposure of bile acids to the degrading action of intestinal bacteria, a step in the formation of known carcinogens. Hill (170) has noted a concentration of bile acids in populations of the United States and England that is seven times higher than that in Uganda and India. Populations with a high incidence of colorectal carcinoma have high fecal bile acid concentrations in comparison with those with a low incidence. A high proportion of anaerobic bacteria in these populations caused degradation of bile acids to form known carcinogens. Both deoxycholic and lithocholic acids have been shown to be promoters of colon carcinoma in animal models. These secondary bile acids are the products of bacterial dehydroxylation of the primary bile acids cholic and chenodeoxycholic acid, respectively. The primary bile acids are not promoters of carcinogenesis. Jorgensen and Rafaelsen (171) compared the prevalence of gallstone disease in 145 consecutive patients with colorectal carcinoma with gallstone prevalence in 4159 subjects randomly selected from a population. The group of patients had a significantly higher prevalence of gallstone disease than the population (odds ratio, 1.59), whereas cholecystectomies occurred with equal frequency in the two groups. There was a nonsignificantly trend toward more right-sided carcinomas in patients with gallstones than in patients without gallstones.

Schernhammer et al. (172) conducted a prospective study of 85,184 women, 877 of whom developed colorectal carcinoma. They found a significant positive association between cholecystectomy and the risk of colorectal carcinoma (RR = 1.21). The risk was highest for carcinomas of the proximal colon (RR = 1.34) and the rectum (RR = 1.58). Lagergren et al. (173) evaluated cholecystectomy and risk of bowel carcinoma with a slightly different result. Cholecystectomized patients identified through he Swedish Inpatient Register were followed up for subsequent carcinoma. In a total of 278,460 cholecystectomized patients, contributing 3,519,682 person-years, followed up for a maximum of 33 years. Cholecystectomized patients had an increased risk of proximal intestinal adenocarcinoma which gradually declined with increasing distance from the common bile duct. The risk was significantly increased for carcinoma (SIR 1.77) and carcinoids of the small bowel (SIR 1.71) and right-sided colon carcinoma (SIR 1.16). No association was found with more distal bowel carcinoma.

These results, together with available literature, give substantial evidence for an association between gallstones and colorectal carcinoma, an association that is not due to cholecystectomy being a predisposing factor to colorectal carcinoma. Sporadic findings of an association between cholecystectomy and colorectal carcinoma can be explained by the above relationship. Wynder and Reddy (174) were impressed by the correlation between dietary fat intake and colon carcinoma. These authors reasoned that the dietary fat content raised both the concentration of anaerobic bacteria and the amount of bile acid and cholesterol substrates in the gut, thus enhancing the production of bile acid and cholesterol metabolites, which may be the proximate carcinogens.

Considerable attention has been directed to absence of the gallbladder and its possible relationship to the development of colorectal carcinoma. Many studies have been published offering arguments for and against such an association. In their comprehensive review of the controversy, Moore-head and McKelvey (175) found series that suggested an increased relative risk of developing colorectal carcinoma in the range of 1.59 to 2.27. Higher relative risks have been reported up to 3.5 for right-sided carcinoma in women, with the highest report being 4.5 for sigmoid lesions (176–178). In a total Icelandic population prospective study of 3425 individuals who underwent cholecystectomy and were followed 8 to 33 years, Nielsen et al. (179) found a relative risk of carcinoma in men of 2.73. McFarlane and Welch (180) found an overall odds ratio of 2.78, but it was 6.79 for right-sided lesions. However, this concept is not universally supported. Abrams, Anton, and Dreyfuss (181) found no relationship between cholecystectomy and the subsequent occurrence of proximal colonic carcinoma. Kune, Kune, and Watson (182) and Kaibara et al. (183) found no statistical association between previous cholecystectomy and the risk of colorectal carcinoma, either in general or in any subsite, age, or sex. Ekbom et al. (184), in a population-based study of 62,615 patients who underwent cholecystectomy, found no overall excess risk of colorectal carcinoma but observed an increased risk among women for right-sided colon carcinoma 15 years or more after operation. In a case-control study conducted by Neugent et al. (185), no significant association was found between cholecystectomy and adenomatous polyps or carcinoma. Even if an association between large bowel neoplasia and biliary tract disease were confirmed, it is possible that there is no direct cause-and-effect relationship. It may be that the diet predisposing to one disease increases the risk of developing the other disease. Resolution of this controversy would be of considerable clinical significance by clearly exposing a readily identifiable at-risk group and offering more intensive screening opportunities to them.

■ DIVERTICULAR DISEASE

Most surgeons believe that because of the frequency with which both colon carcinoma and diverticular disease exist, it is not uncommon to see both conditions concomitantly without necessarily invoking a cause-and-effect relationship. A study by Boulos et al. (186) hinted that patients with diverticular disease might constitute a group at higher risk of developing neoplasia. Morini et al. (187) ascertained that adenomas and carcinomas were detected more often in patients with diverticular disease, with an overall odds ratio of 3.0. When examined separately, adenomas maintained their significantly higher frequency but no difference was observed for carcinomas.

■ ACTIVITY AND EXERCISE

Persky and Andrianopoulos (188) reviewed studies examining the relation between exercise levels and risk of carcinoma. The authors found a relative risk increase of 1.3 to 2.0 for individuals with sedentary jobs. This association held true only for colon carcinoma, not for rectal carcinoma. Thune and Lund (189) also found a reduced risk for colon carcinoma for men and women who engaged in physical activity at least 4 hours per week. The reduced risk was more marked in the proximal colon. No association between physical activity and rectal carcinoma was observed in men or women. In a case-control study of men with colorectal carcinoma in Japan, physical inactivity based on occupational category increased the risk from the lowest to the highest levels 1.32 to 1.92 times (rectum and proximal colon, respectively) (136).

In a more recent report contrary results were found by Slattery et al. (190). They conducted a population-based study of 952 incident cases of carcinoma in the rectum and rectosigmoid junction with 1205 age- and sex-matched controls in Utah and Northern California at the Kaiser Permanente Medical Care Program (190). Vigorous physical activity was associated with reduced risk of rectal carcinoma in both men and women (OR = 0.60, for men and 0.59 for women). Among men, moderate levels of physical activity were also associated with reduced risk of rectal carcinoma (OR = 0.70). Participation in vigorous activity over the past 20 years conferred the greatest protection for both men and women (OR = 0.55 for men and 0.44 for women). In another case-controlled study among men, increased physical activity ($\geq$2 hr/wk) was associated with reduced risk for advanced adenomas (OR = 0.4) and for nonadvanced adenomas (OR = 0.8) (191).

Colbert et al. (192) examined the association between occupational and leisure physical activity and colorectal carcinoma in a cohort of male smokers. Among the 29,133 men aged 50 to 69 years in the Alpha-Tocopherol, Beta-Carotene Cancer Prevention study, 152 colon and 104 rectal carcinomas were documented during up to 12 years of follow-up. For colon carcinoma, compared with sedentary workers, men in light occupational activity had a relative risk of 0.60, whereas those in moderate/heavy activity had a relative risk of 0.45. For rectal carcinoma, there were risk reductions for those in light (relative risk 0.71) and moderate/heavy occupational activity (relative risk 0.50). These data provide evidence for a protective role of physical activity in colon and rectal carcinoma. Others support the concept of physical activity as being protective against the development of colon carcinoma (193,194).

Various mechanisms for this protective effect have been extensively cited. Quadrilaters and Hoffman-Goetz (195) reviewed the published evidence of physical activity and the hypothesized mechanisms. These mechanisms included changes in gastrointestinal transit time, altered immune function and prostaglandin levels, as well as changes in insulin levels, insulin-like growth factors, bile acid secretion, serum cholesterol and gastrointestinal and pancreatic hormone profiles. There is currently little data to support any of the hypothesized biological mechanisms for the protective effect of exercise on colon carcinoma. It is likely that no one mechanism is responsible for the risk reduction observed in epidemiological and animal studies and therefore, the observed benefits of physical activity in colon carcinoma may be a combination of these and other factors.

■ OTHER FACTORS

A host of seemingly totally unrelated factors have been suggested to play a role in colorectal carcinoma genesis. Many of these are cited below. The risk of colorectal carcinoma is increased following adenocarcinoma of the small bowel (196).

A factor that has been studied but for which no definitive association has been documented is obesity. With regard to bowel function, a meta-analysis of 14 case-control studies revealed statistically significant risks for colorectal carcinoma associated with both constipation and the use of cathartics (pooled odds ratios, 1.48 and 1.46, respectively) (197).

A meta-analysis of published data revealed that women with a history of breast, endometrial, and ovarian carcinomas have an increased relative risk of developing colorectal carcinoma of 1.1, 1.4, and 1.6, respectively (198). Large bowel malignancy correlates with the distribution of endocrine-dependent neoplasms (e.g., breast, endometrium, ovary, or prostate) and arteriosclerotic heart disease. It would be important to know whether there is a protective effect of hormone replacement therapy against colorectal carcinoma. Increased parity was reported to be associated with a decline in the risk of colon carcinoma (odds ratio, 0.44 for women with five children or more relative to nulliparous women), but not for rectal carcinoma (199). The association with colon carcinoma is restricted to women 50 years of age or older. A population based case-control study of postmenopausal women revealed that when compared with women who never used hormone replacement therapy, recent users had a relative risk of 0.54 for colon carcinoma and a relative risk of 0.91 for rectal carcinoma (200). Estrogen replacement therapy is associated with a substantial decreased risk in colon carcinoma (RR = 0.71) (201). Users of 1 year or less have a relative risk of 0.81, while users of 11 years or more have a relative risk of 0.54. Other investigators found little overall association between colon carcinoma and oral contraceptive use, parity, age at first birth, hysterectomy, oophorectomy status, or age at menopause (202,203).

In a meta-analysis of 18 epidemiologic studies of postmenopausal hormone therapy and colorectal carcinoma Grodstein et al. (204) found a 20% reduction in risk of colon carcinoma and a 19% decrease in the risk of rectal carcinoma for postmenopausal women who had ever taken hormone therapy compared with women who never used hormones. Much of the apparent reduction in colorectal carcinoma was limited to current hormone users (relative risk = 0.66). From a case-control study among women, ever use of hormone replacement therapy was more strongly associated with reduced risk of advanced adenomas relative to polyp-free controls (OR = 0.4) than with reduced risk of nonadvanced adenomas (OR = 0.7) (191). Baris et al. (205) studied the patterns of carcinoma risk in Sweden and Denmark in 177 patients with acromegaly. Increased risks were found for colon (standardized incidence ratio = 2.6) and rectum (standardized incidence ratio = 2.5). Among other risks, the increased risk for several carcinoma sites among acromegaly patients may be due to the elevated proliferative and antiapoptotic activity associated with increased circulating levels of insulin-like growth factor-1.

Bile acids are suspected from both clinical and experimental studies to have a role in colon carcinogenesis. The twofold increased mortality from colorectal carcinoma is apparent only 15 to 20 years after gastric surgery. It is suggested that the increased mortality from colorectal carcinoma after gastric surgery may be due to altered bile acid metabolism. To determine the relationship between bile acids and increased risk of colorectal neoplasms after truncal vagotomy, Mullen et al. (206) conducted a prospective screening study of 100 asymptomatic patients who had undergone truncal vagotomy at least 10 years previously. The patients were investigated by barium enema, colonoscopy, and gallbladder ultrasonography. Control data were obtained from forensic autopsy subjects. The incidence of neoplasms >1 cm in the vagotomized group was 14% (11 adenomas and three carcinomas) and 3% in controls. The authors found increased proportions of chenodeoxycholic acid and lithocholic acid and decreased proportions of cholic acid in the duodenal bile of vagotomized patients and believe that these abnormalities in bile acid metabolism may help to explain the increased risk of colorectal neoplasia 10 years after truncal vagotomy. On the other hand, Fisher et al. (207), in their cohort study of 15,983 males, found no elevation of risk of large bowel carcinoma following gastric surgery for benign disease.

Little et al. (208) tested the hypothesis relating bile acids, calcium, and pH to colorectal carcinoma in a large sample of asymptomatic subjects who had participated in fecal occult blood screening. Fecal samples were obtained from 45 cases of carcinoma, 129 subjects with adenoma, 167 fecal occult blood negative controls, and 155 fecal occult blood positive subjects in whom no-carcinoma or adenoma was found. No association between colorectal carcinoma and fecal bile acids or pH was observed. Although there was no overall association between colorectal adenomas and fecal bile acids or pH, villous adenomas were associated with increasing concentrations of major bile acids and decreasing concentration of minor bile acids, and there was a suggestion of an inverse association with an acid pH. High levels of fecal calcium were associated with a reduced risk of both colorectal carcinoma and adenoma, but this was not statistically significant. Their study does not support an association between colorectal carcinoma and fecal bile acids. However, there is evidence that increases in major bile acids are associated with villous adenomas.

There is diverse evidence suggesting that intracolonic production of oxygen radicals may play a role in carcinogenesis (209). The relatively high concentrations of iron in feces, together with the ability of bile pigments to act as iron chelators that support Fenton chemistry, may very well permit efficient hydroxyl radicals generation from superoxide and hydrogen peroxide produced by bacterial metabolism. Such free radicals generation in feces could provide a missing link in our understanding of the etiology of colon carcinoma: the oxidation of procarcinogens either by fecal hydroxyl radicals or by secondary peroxyl radicals to form active carcinogens or mitogenic neoplastic promoters. Intracolonic free radical formation may explain the high incidence of carcinoma in the colon and rectum compared with other regions of the gastrointestinal tract, as well as the observed correlation of a higher incidence of colon carcinoma with red meat in the diet, which increases stool iron, and with excessive fat in the diet, which may increase the fecal content of procarcinogens and bile pigments.

Epidemiologic studies and laboratory research have indicated an association between the metabolic activity of the intestinal microflora and carcinoma of the large bowel (210). It has been suggested that activation of procarcinogens could be mediated enzymatically by intestinal bacteria. The levels of incriminated colonic bacterial enzymes are increased by dietary fat and inhibited by certain dietary fibers. Organic extracts of feces contain a mutagenic substance, presumably derived from bacterial metabolism in the large bowel. Whether this substance or some other organic chemical is the putative proximate carcinogen remains speculative, but the evidence continues to point to intestinal bacteria as the metabolic intermediary in colon carcinoma.

High iron stores may increase the risk of colorectal carcinoma through their contribution to the production of free oxygen radicals. Knekt et al. (211) studied serum iron, total iron binding capacity, and transferrin saturation levels in a cohort of 41,276 subjects ranging in age from 20 to 74 years. The authors found a relative risk of 3.04 for colorectal carcinoma in subjects with transferrin levels exceeding 60%. Asthmatic patients have a reported elevated relative risk of colon (1.17) and rectum (1.28) carcinoma (212). The prevalence of colon carcinoma in patients with Barrett's esophagus is 7.6% compared with 1.6% in a control population (213). Men with esophageal adenocarcinoma may be more likely to be diagnosed with colorectal carcinoma in their lifetime than expected. The opposite association may exist for women (214). A relative risk of 3.04 has been calculated for colorectal carcinoma as a result of anthranoid laxative abuse (215). Younes, Katikaneni, and Lechago (216) reported that 25% of patients who underwent appendectomy and were found to have mucosal hyperplasia were associated with adenocarcinoma of the colon.

Plasma C-reactive protein concentrations are elevated among persons who subsequently develop colon carcinoma. These data support the hypothesis that inflammation is a risk factor for the development of colon carcinoma in average-risk individuals (217).

Woolcott et al. (218) found colon carcinoma risk was inversely associated with coffee. Relative to those drinking fewer than one cup of coffee per day, the ORs for those drinking two cups was 0.9, for those drinking three to four cups 0.8, and for those drinking five or more cups 0.7. The reduced risk estimates were more pronounced with carcinoma of the proximal colon than the distal colon. Rectal carcinoma risk was not associated with either coffee or tea.

In a study of premorbid and personality factors, aggressive hostility was the only variable found to be significant between colon carcinoma patients and controls (219).

■ JUVENILE VS. ADULT CARCINOMA

To add further confounding information to the matter, two different types of carcinoma may exist. Concerning the wide age range that colorectal carcinoma encompasses, Avni and Feuchtwanger (27) wrote a thought-provoking editorial in which they made a sharp differentiation between "juvenile" and "adult" carcinoma and suggested that a search be made for different etiologies. To support the concept that two different types of colon carcinoma may exist, the authors cited the following observations:

1. In the nonwhite population, the juvenile form occurs up to 16 times more frequently than in the white population, whereas the adult form occurs 10 times more frequently in the white population.

2. Mucinous carcinomas comprise only 5% of all colonic carcinomas, although in the young age group they comprise 76%.
3. In adult patients with colon carcinoma, coexisting polyps can be found in 40% to 50% of patients, whereas in the juvenile group polyps are exceedingly rare.
4. Alleged nutritional factors in the genesis of colon carcinoma must be present for many years, which cannot be the case in the juvenile group. Moreover, diet in the nonwhite population in whom the juvenile type is more frequent differs from that of the white population.
5. In the adult population with colon carcinoma, a family history of disease is found in 20% to 30%, although this factor is almost nonexistent in the juvenile type.

Only further investigation will resolve this issue.

■ PROSPECTS FOR PREVENTION

Epidemiologic evidence suggests that diet is the principal factor in the cause of colorectal carcinoma. Ingestion of excessive amounts of fat appears to be the major factor. Also noteworthy is the interrelationship between the varying relative amounts of fat and fiber in the diet. For example, in an experimental study on colorectal carcinogenesis by Galloway et al. (220), manipulation of diet resulted in significant differences in alteration of the surface architecture of the colonic mucosa. The high-fat, low-fiber diet was associated with the greatest risk for macroscopic malignant production, and the low-fat, high-fiber diet, with the lowest risk. Furthermore, the sources of fat vary in the degree of their promotional effect (128). Fiber is considered to inhibit carcinoma, but only the type of fiber found in whole grain cereals, fruits, and vegetables, which contain large amounts of uronic acid, is effective. The exact nature of fat and fiber sources is yet to be delineated.

An effective prevention strategy should be based on an understanding of the pathogenesis of carcinoma, but no such definitive understanding exists. From the available evidence it appears that a high intake of animal fat and protein promotes the formation of colon carcinoma and that certain cruciferous vegetables exert a protective influence. The two-step concept of carcinogenesis includes (i) initiation, about which little is known in human carcinoma, and (ii) promotion, which presumably takes a long time to complete. We may well be able to capitalize on the latter fact by the administration of inhibitors during the promotional phase, a concept realized experimentally by Nigro and Bull (128). Their studies suggested that an appropriate strategy for prevention of carcinoma of the large bowel would be a program aimed at a 10% reduction of fat consumption (i.e., from 40% to 30% of calories) and adoption of a more varied type of fat. The daily addition of 25 to 30 g of dietary fiber, especially grains and vegetables that contain cellulose and uronic acid, may prove effective. A third recommendation is to include in the diet chemical inhibitors such as selenium, retinoids, and plant steroids. Other studies have suggested that other factors, such as calcium and sulfur compounds present in garlic and onions, may be of value in the inhibition of colon carcinoma (129). Antioxidants such as β-carotene, vitamin C, vitamin E, and folic acid have been assessed (221). Individuals with a significant inheritance factor for colon carcinoma may require a supplement to enhance inhibition.

Cassidy, Bingham, and Cummings (222) reported a strong inverse association and suggested a potentially important role for starch in the protection against colorectal carcinoma. This corresponds with the hypothesis that fermentation in the colon is the mechanism for preventing colorectal carcinoma.

Experiments in animals and two epidemiologic studies in humans suggest that aspirin and other nonsteroidal anti-inflammatory drugs (NSAIDs) may be protective against colon carcinoma. Thun, Namboodiri, and Heath (223) tested this hypothesis in a prospective mortality study of 662,424 adults who provided information in 1982 on the frequency and duration of their aspirin use. Death rates from colon carcinoma were measured through 1988. The possible influence of other risk factors for colon carcinoma was examined in multivariate analyses for 598 case patients and 3058 matched control subjects drawn from the cohort. Death rates from colon carcinoma decreased with more frequent aspirin use in both men and women. The relative risk among persons who used aspirin 16 or more times per month for at least 1 year was 0.60 in men and 0.58 in women. The risk estimates were unaffected when they excluded persons who reported at entry into the study that they had a malignancy, heart disease, stroke, or another condition that might influence both their aspirin use and their mortality. Adjustment for dietary factors, obesity, physical activity, and family history did not alter the findings significantly. No association was found between the use of acetaminophen and the risk of colon carcinoma. The authors concluded that regular aspirin use at low doses may reduce the risk of fatal colon carcinoma.

Rosenberg et al. (224) assessed NSAID use in relation to risk of human large bowel carcinoma in a hospital-based case-control study of 1326 patients with colorectal carcinoma and 4891 control patients. For regular NSAID use that continued into the year before the interview, the multivariate relative risk estimate was 0.5. The inverse association was apparent for both colon and rectal carcinoma in men and women and in subjects younger and older than 60 years. Regular NSAID use that had been discontinued at least 1 year previously and nonregular use were not associated with risk. Almost all regular NSAID use was of aspirin-containing drugs. The present data suggest that the sustained use of NSAIDs reduces the incidence of human large bowel carcinoma.

Smalley et al. (225) studied how patterns of use (duration, dose, and specific drug) of NSAIDs affected the incidence of colorectal carcinoma. The population-based retrospective cohort study of 104,217 persons aged 65 years or older had at least 5 years of enrollment. Incident histologically confirmed colorectal carcinoma was documented. Users of nonaspirin NSAIDs for at least 48 months of the previous 5 years had a relative risk of 0.49 for colon carcinoma when compared with those of no use of NSAIDs. Among those with more than 12 months of cumulative use, those using NSAIDs in the past year (recent users) had a relative ratio of 0.61 whereas those with no recent use had a relative ratio of 0.76. No specific NSAID offered a unique protective effect and low doses of NSAIDs appeared to be at least as effective as higher doses. Protection was most pronounced for right-sided lesions. The relative risk among recent users with more than 12 months of cumulative use was 0.81 for rectal carcinoma and 0.77 for left-sided carcinoma and 0.48 for right-sided colon carcinoma. In this elderly population, long-term use of nonaspirin NSAIDs nearly halved the risk of colon carcinoma. This study was consistent with previous studies that suggest that duration of use but not daily dose of NSAIDs is an important factor for chemoprevention. Their data also suggest that the protective effect is shared by most NSAIDs, and not confined to a small number of these drugs.

Baron et al. (226) performed a randomized double-blind trial of aspirin as a chemopreventive agent against colorectal adenomas. They randomly assigned 1121 patients with a recent history of histologically documented adenomas to receive placebo (372 patients), 81 mg of aspirin (377 patients), or 325 mg of aspirin (372 patients) daily. Follow-up colonoscopy was performed at least one year after randomization in 97% of patients. The incidence of one or more adenomas was 47% in the placebo group, 38% in the group given 81 mg of aspirin per day and 45% in the group given 325 mg of aspirin per day. Unadjusted relative risks of any adenomas (as compared with the placebo group) were 0.81 in the 81-mg group and 0.96 in the 325-mg group. For advanced neoplasms (adenomas measuring at least 1 cm in diameter or with tubulovillous or villous features, severe dysplasia, or invasive carcinoma), the respective relative risks were 0.59 and 0.83. They concluded low dose aspirin has a moderate chemopreventive effect on adenomas in the large bowel. Since adenoma development can be used as a surrogate marker for the development of carcinoma, the reduction in adenoma development by extrapolation would result in a decrease in the incidence of carcinoma.

In contrast to most observational studies, the randomized Physician's Health Study found no association between aspirin use and colorectal carcinoma after 5 years (227). In a randomized prospective cohort study 22,071 healthy male physicians who were 40 to 84 years of age in 1982 were given 325 mg of aspirin every other day. In 1988 the aspirin arm of the randomized trial was stopped early. Participants then chose to receive either aspirin or placebo for the rest of the study. Colorectal carcinoma was diagnosed in 341 patients during the study period. Over 12 years of follow-up, random assignment to aspirin was associated with a relative risk of colorectal carcinoma of 1.03. The relative risk for colorectal carcinoma in persons who used aspirin frequently after 1988 was 1.07. In the Physicians Health Study, both randomized and observational analyses indicate that there is no association between the use of aspirin and the incidence of colorectal carcinoma. In their review, Burke et al. (228) reported that in population-based observational studies, people had lower rates of colorectal carcinoma if they were taking various agents, including nonsteroidal anti-inflammatory drugs, calcium, and folate. In placebo-controlled trials in patients with familial adenomatous polyposis and in patients with sporadic colon adenomas, nonsteroidal anti-inflammatory drugs reduced the rates of adenomas, and there is a biologic rationale that they would be effective in reducing colorectal carcinoma as well.

Large-scale chemoprevention trials sponsored by the National Cancer Institute are under way (229). Agents being evaluated include piroxicam, sulindac, aspirin, acarbose (α-glucosidase) inhibitors, and calcium carbonate. Targeted populations include patients with previous adenoma, FAP, history of multiple polyposis, and subjects at risk for colon carcinoma.

PATHOLOGY

MACROSCOPIC APPEARANCE

On gross examination, adenocarcinoma of the colon appears as one of four fairly distinctive types— ulcerative, polypoid, annular, or diffusely infiltrating. The ulcerative carcinoma, the most common type, presents as a roughly circular mass with a raised, irregular, everted edge and a sloughing base. It is confined to one aspect of the bowel wall but may occupy a larger portion of the bowel circumference (Fig. 6).

The polypoid, or cauliflower-type, carcinoma presents as a large fungating mass that projects into the lumen and is often of a low-grade malignancy. The ascending colon is a site of predilection (230) (Fig. 7). In approximately 10% of cases, the cut surface of the growth may have a gelatinous appearance, due to abundant mucin secretion, and this type has been referred to as a colloid carcinoma (230).

The annular, or stenosing, carcinoma occupies the entire circumference of the bowel wall. The extent in the long axis is variable. The bowel lumen is usually considerably compromised (Fig. 8), and the proximal bowel may demonstrate varying degrees of dilation. Such carcinomas occur with greatest frequency in the transverse and descending colon (230).

The diffusely infiltrating carcinoma produces a diffuse thickening of the intestinal wall and for the most part is covered with intact mucosa. It is extensively infiltrating, although it preserves the layers of the gastrointestinal wall. It occurs more often in the rectosigmoid, but any portion of the colon may be involved. This variety is similar to linitis plastica of the stomach. It is the type of carcinoma commonly associated with ulcerative colitis (Fig. 9). A review of the literature by Papp, Levine, and Thomas (231) revealed only 85 documented cases of primary linitis

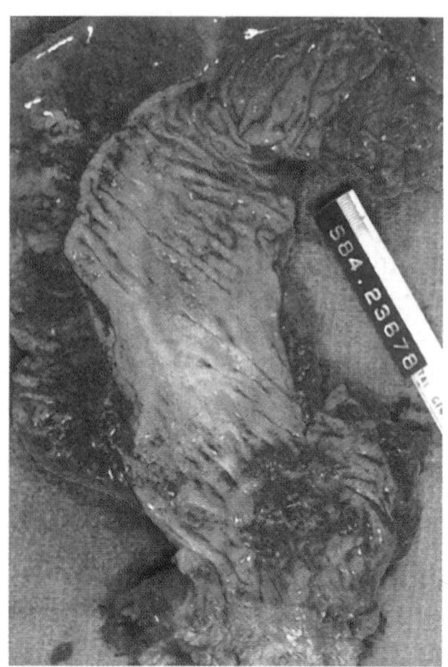

FIGURE 6 ■ Macroscopic features of an ulcerated adenocarcinoma.

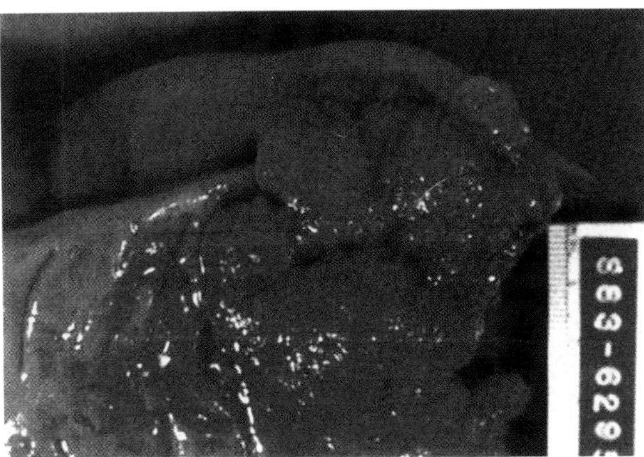

FIGURE 7 ■ Macroscopic appearance of a polypoid adenocarcinoma.

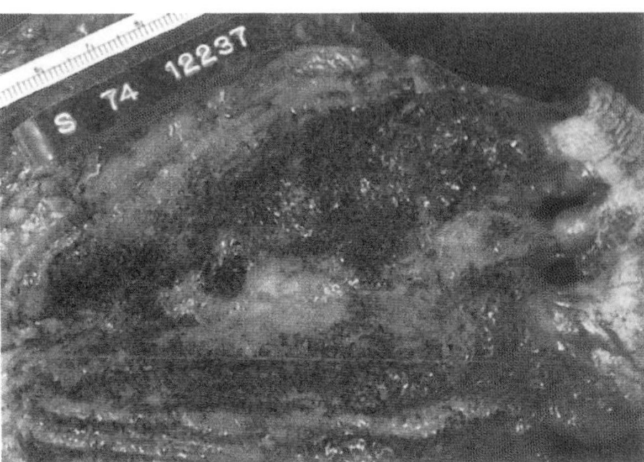

FIGURE 9 ■ Macroscopic appearance of an infiltrating adenocarcinoma.

plastica of the colon and rectum, characterized by presentation in younger patients and associated with metastatic disease, a higher mortality, and insidious growth, often making detection difficult.

■ MICROSCOPIC APPEARANCE

The histological appearance of carcinoma may vary considerably, with the major importance being related to prognosis. The lesion may be well differentiated (20%) (Fig. 10), moderately differentiated (60%) (Fig. 11), or poorly differentiated (20%) (Fig. 12) (231). The incidence of lymph node metastases is about 25%, 50%, and 80% in low-, average-, or high-grade malignancy, respectively. Furthermore, the histologic grade influences survival, with corrected 5-year survival rates of 77%, 61%, and 29%, for low-, average-, and high-grade rectal malignancies, respectively (230). Broders (232) popularized a method that divides adenocarcinoma into four grades. In grade 1, 75% to 100% of the cells are differentiated; in grade 2, 50% to 75%; in grade 3, 25% to 50%; and in grade 4, 0% to 25%. The principle of grading by differentiation is based on the biologic law that the higher the degree of differentiation, the less the power of reproduction; therefore it might be anticipated that well-differentiated carcinomas would proliferate at a slower pace than those that are comparatively undifferentiated. One difficulty in the application of histologic grading is the lack of uniformity in the degree of differentiation throughout the neoplasm. In general, malignant cells are less differentiated at the invading margins than on the surface. Dukes (233) carefully differentiated his classification from that of Broders (232) by noting that the two methods answer different questions. Histologic grade is essentially an estimate of the pace of growth, whereas classification into Dukes' A, B, and C cases is a measurement of the boundaries reached. Both methods permit grouping into cases with favorable and unfavorable outcome. Jass et al. (234) proposed a grading system that includes the parameters of tubule configuration, advancing margin, and lymphocytic infiltration.

Contrary to what might be expected and what is generally believed, Gibbs (235) reported that rare undifferentiated carcinomas of the large intestine tend to spread circumferentially and do not readily give rise to lymphatic or hematogenous metastases. Affected patients may have a good prognosis.

Colloid, or mucus-producing, lesions may present with varying degrees of differentiation and are said by some to have a poor prognosis (Fig. 13). Colloid adenocarcinoma can be classified as extracellular or intracellular, according to the predominant location of the mucin. Most colloid carcinomas are extracellular, with only approximately 2% of all carcinomas of the colon and rectum being the pure signet-ring cell variety. With the latter variety, the patient is unlikely to survive more than 2 years from the time of diagnosis (230). The largest number of mucinous

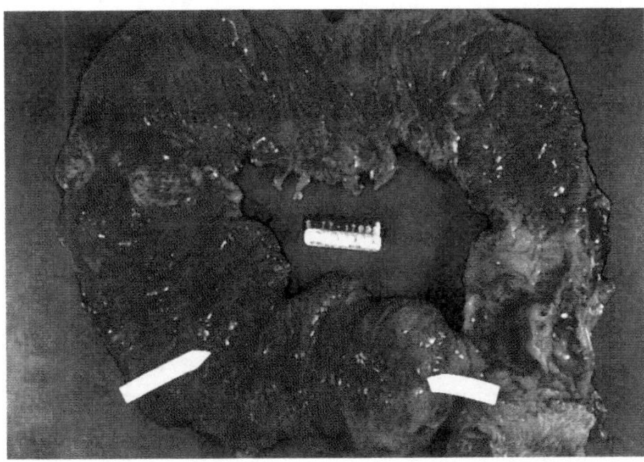

FIGURE 8 ■ Macroscopic features of an annular carcinoma. Arrows indicate associated adenomas.

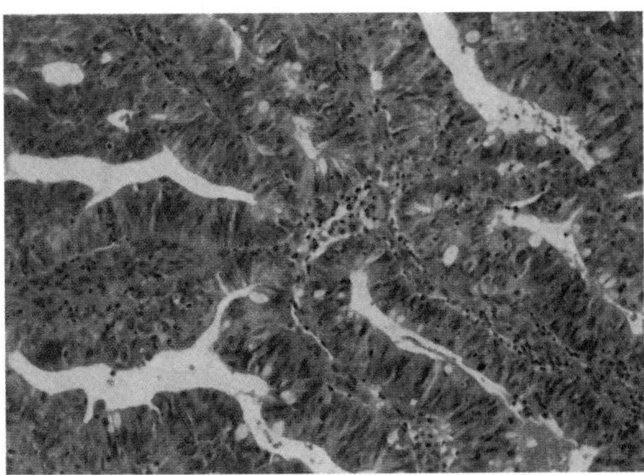

FIGURE 10 ■ Microscopic appearance of a well-differentiated adenocarcinoma with well-developed glands. *Source*: Courtesy of L.R. Bègin, M.D., Montreal, Quebec.

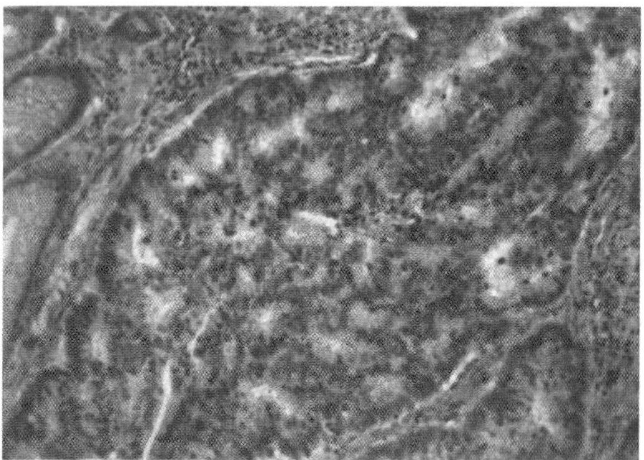

FIGURE 11 ■ Microscopic appearance of a moderately differentiated adenocarcinoma with gland formation that is less well defined. *Source*: Courtesy of L.R. Bègin, M.D., Montreal, Quebec.

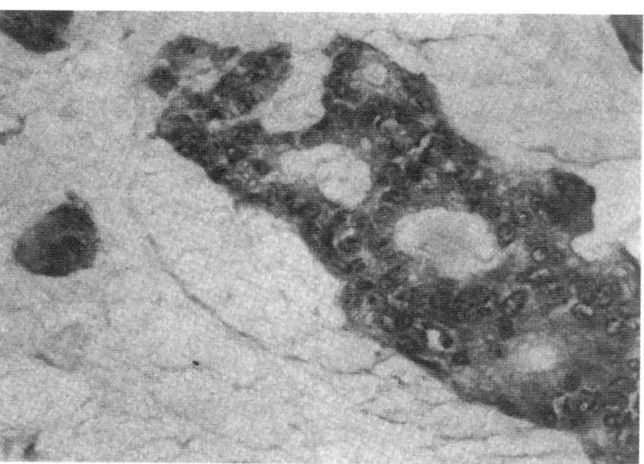

FIGURE 13 ■ Microscopic features of a mucin-producing adenocarcinoma with abundant extracellular mucin. *Source*: Courtesy of L.R. Bègin, M.D., Montreal, Quebec.

carcinomas are found in the rectum, but the relative incidence of mucinous carcinoma is higher in the right colon (236). The primarily intracellular variety of mucinous carcinoma is classified as a signet-ring cell because the mucus pushes the nucleus to the periphery and thereby gives the cells their characteristic appearance. In a review of 426 patients with carcinoma of the rectum and rectosigmoid seen at Memorial Sloan-Kettering Cancer Center, Bonello, Sternberg, and Quan (237) found 4% of the carcinomas to be of the signet-ring cell type, and this accounted for 0.4% of all rectal carcinomas. Umpleby, Ranson, and Williamson (238) compared the clinical and pathologic features of 54 mucinous carcinomas of the large intestine with 576 nonmucinous carcinomas. Lesions were categorized as mucinous if they contained at least 60% mucin by volume. Those with moderate mucin content (60% to 80%) were indistinguishable in behavior from nonmucinous lesions. By contrast, those with a high mucin content (>80%) showed several differences from nonmucinous carcinomas. They had a more proximal distribution through the large intestine, they comprised a greater fraction of carcinomas in the under-50 age group (24% vs. 7%), they were more likely to be Dukes' stage D (58% vs. 31%), and local fixity was more common (70% vs. 37%). Consequently, the overall resection rate was reduced from 90% to 73%, the curative resection rate from 69% to 42%, and the 5-year survival rate from 37% to 18%. Umpleby, Ranson, and Williamson (238) concluded that colorectal carcinomas of high mucin content require wide excision, tend to recur locally, and carry a poor prognosis. The dramatic difference in this report from others in the literature may be due to this study's strict definition of a mucinous carcinoma as one with >80% mucin content.

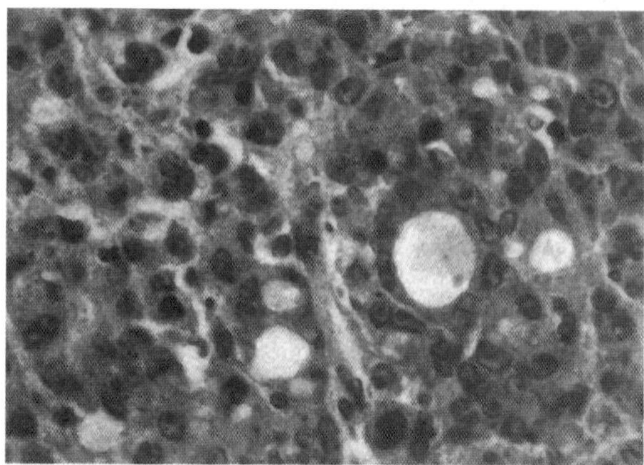

FIGURE 12 ■ Microscopic features of a poorly differentiated adenocarcinoma with pleomorphic cells and little recognizable gland formation. *Source*: Courtesy of L.R. Bègin, M.D., Montreal, Quebec.

In a review of 540 cases of colorectal carcinoma, Okuno et al. (239) found that mucinous carcinomas accounted for 6.4% of cases. Such carcinomas were more common in patients 39 years of age or younger and in women patients. They were most commonly located in the rectum, followed by occurrence in the right colon; however, the relative incidence was higher in the right colon (40.5% vs. 12.5%). These carcinomas were characterized by infiltration of the surrounding tissues (24.3% vs. 7.8%), positive lymph node involvement (75.7% vs. 48.6%), and peritoneal implant (21.6% vs. 4.1%). The cumulative 5- and 10-year survival rates after resection of mucinous carcinoma were 45.5% and 39.8%, respectively; those after curative resection were 77.4% and 63.5%. The authors suggested the need for aggressive lymph node dissection and wide excision of the surrounding tissues for mucinous carcinoma, with special attention paid to local recurrence.

This microscopic variety of carcinoma is associated with a higher incidence of metastases and a higher incidence of associated synchronous polyps and carcinoma than nonmucinous carcinomas. The clinical relevance of this association is that it is necessary to perform colonoscopy on patients with mucinous carcinoma (236).

Anthony et al. (240) reported the largest series of signet cell carcinoma of the colon and rectum. There was equal distribution between the right and left colon. Synchronous carcinomas were present in 14%. Nodal or metastatic disease was present in 72% of patients at the time of diagnosis. The 5-year actuarial survival rate was 22%. Patient mortality was due to carcinomatosis in all 22 patients who died. Parenchymal liver involvement occurred in only two patients (9%). Ovarian metastases have been reported in 25% to 60% of patients at time of diagnosis and hence bilateral salpingo-oophorectomy should probably accompany the original resection.

Primary linitis plastica of the colon and rectum is an uncommon entity with a poor prognosis. Papp, Levine, and Thomas (231) found 85 cases reported in the literature. Shirouza et al. (241) classified linitis plastica into two types according to histologic growth pattern—the more common scirrhous type and the lymphangiosis type. The scirrhous type is composed mainly of poorly differentiated or signet-ring cells and is accompanied by a severe desmoplastic reaction. The lymphangiosis type is composed mainly of moderately differentiated cells, frequently with glandular formation. The characteristic diffuse tubular thickening and rigidity are the result of fibrotic reaction around infiltrating malignant cells, such as in desmoplasia (see Fig. 9). The microscopic appearance is that of poorly differentiated pleomorphic cells (see Fig. 12).

The pathologist can be instrumental in guiding the surgeon to the appropriate clinical management. Surgeons are often reluctant to recommend major operative procedures for patients with "minimally invasive" carcinoma. Hase et al. (242) conducted a study to determine the long-term outcome after curative resection of colorectal carcinomas that extend only into the submucosa. Seventy-nine patients who underwent curative resection were followed for at least 5 years. Formal operation followed attempted endoscopic removal in 25 patients. Lymph node metastases, found in 11 of 79 patients (13.9%), were associated with a worse outcome; 36.4% of node-positive patients developed recurrence vs. only 5.9% of node-negative patients. The cumulative survival rate was also worse in node-positive vs. node-negative patients; 72.7% vs. 91.1% at 5 years and 45.5% vs. 65.3% at 10 years. Five histopathologic characteristics were identified as risk factors for lymph node metastases: (i) small clusters of undifferentiated carcinoma cells ahead of the invasive front of the lesion ("tumor budding"), (ii) a poorly demarcated invasive front, (iii) moderately or poorly differentiated malignant cells in the invasive front, (iv) extension of the carcinoma to the middle or deep submucosal layer, and (v) malignant cells in lymphatics. Whereas patients with three or fewer risk factors had no nodal spread, the rate of lymph node involvement with four or more risk factors was 33.3% and 66.7%, respectively. Appropriate bowel resection with lymph node dissection is indicated if a lesion exhibits more than three histologic risk factors for metastasis.

The coexistence of two or more cell types in colonic malignancy has been reported. Novello et al. (243) reported cases containing areas with clear adenocarcinomatous and squamous differentiation and morphologic as well as histochemical evidence of neuroendocrine differentiation.

■ DEPRESSED CARCINOMA

A unique macroscopic type of carcinoma rarely recorded in the Western world is the superficial depressed type, which represents de novo growth and is clearly different from that usually seen in the polyp-carcinoma sequence. This type of carcinoma, frequently described in the Japanese population, has a strong tendency to develop into invasive and advanced carcinoma. At our institution, Begin, Gordon, and Alpert (244) described a case of endophytic malignant transformation in a flat adenoma of the colon. The deep component was a well-differentiated adenocardnoma extending into the serosa and probably was an example of the depressed carcinomas described in the Japanese literature.

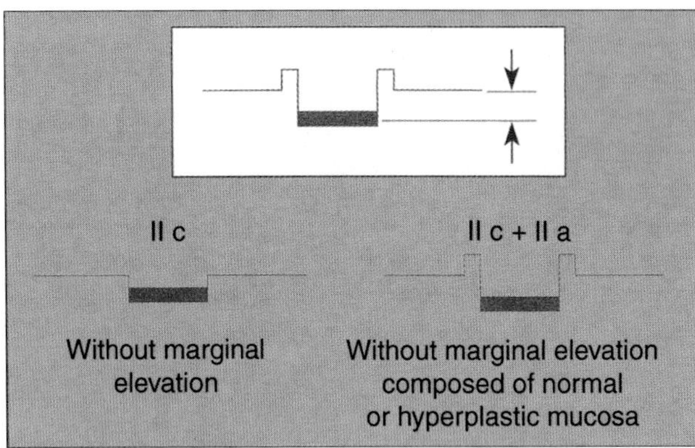

FIGURE 14 ■ Depressed type of colorectal carcinoma. Definition: Carcinoma whose surface is lower than that of neighboring normal mucosa. II c and II c + II a types of carcinoma meet this definition. *Source*: From Ref. 245.

Kudo et al. (245) published an excellent description of the gross and microscopic features with the subtle nuances of making the diagnosis. The authors reported that the depressed type of invasive carcinoma represented 15.5% of all invasive carcinomas diagnosed on 30,311 endoscopic examinations. The definition of a depressed carcinoma is shown in Fig. 14. To detect the depressed type of carcinoma, it is important to pay special attention to slight changes in the mucosal color during endoscopy—slight redness or in some cases, pallor (Fig. 15). The detection rate was about 1 in 1000 endoscopic examinations. Indigo carmine spraying of suspicious areas reveal the underlying pathology of the depressed type of carcinoma (Fig. 16). Histologic confirmation of such a lesion is seen in Fig. 17. The degree of submucosal extension is depicted in Fig. 18. The management of patients with depressed carcinomas is outlined as an algorithm in Fig. 19. In sm 1 a and sm 1 b, extension without vessel invasion, strip biopsy is suitable. For sm 1 b with vessel invasion, resection is recommended because of the risk of lymph node metastases. For sm 2 and sm 3 (see Fig. 18), resection is the preferred treatment.

Kubota et al. (246) examined 300 surgically resected specimens with a dissecting microscope and found 297 adenomas (240 polypoid, 32 flat, and 25 depressed) along with three nonpolypoid carcinomas. Nonpolypoid adenomas were mostly found in the transverse and descending colon. Almost all depressed adenomas were <3 mm in

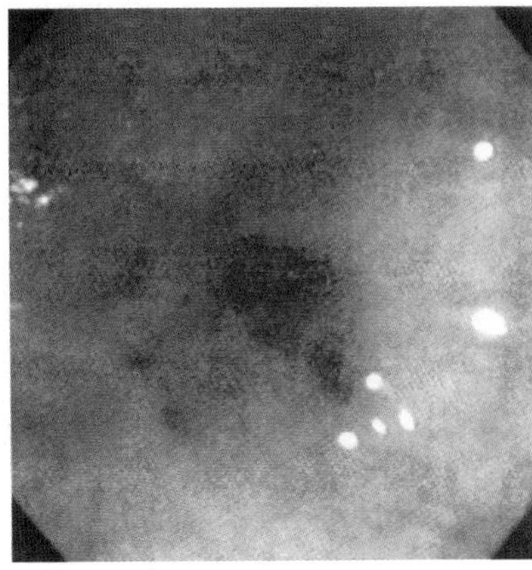

FIGURE 15 ■ Normal endoscopic image after indigo carmine spraying. *Source*: From Ref. 245.

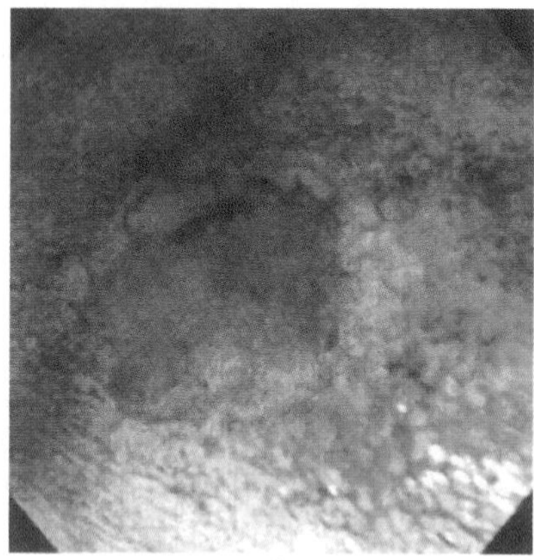

FIGURE 16 ■ Normal endoscopic image. *Source*: From Ref. 245.

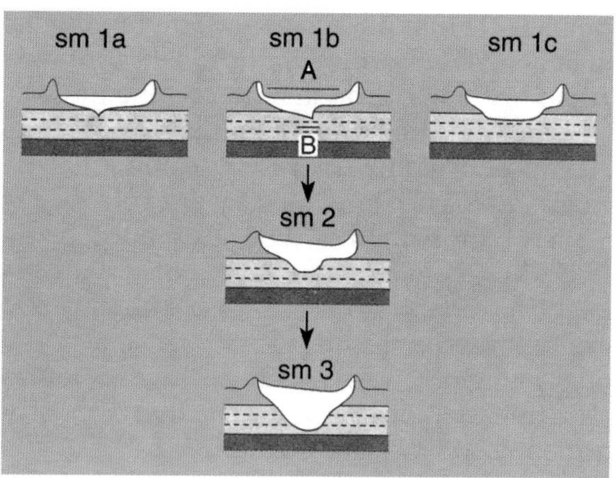

FIGURE 18 ■ Classification of submucosal invasion of early colorectal carcinoma: sm 1 = invasion limited to the upper third of the submucosa; sm 1 a = horizontal invasion limited to less than one quarter of the width of the carcinoma component in the mucosa; sm 1 b = invasion limited to one quarter to half of the width of the carcinoma component in the mucosa; sm 1 c = invasion extending to more than half of the width of the carcinoma component in the mucosa; sm 2 = invasion limited to the middle third of the submucosa; sm 3 = invasion of the lower third of the submucosa. *Source*: From Ref. 245.

dimension (96%), and almost all flat adenomas were < 3.5 mm in dimension (96.9%). The 3 minute carcinomas ranged in size from 2.4 to 2.9 mm. Minamoto et al. (247) suggested that superficial-type adenocarcinomas show rapid growth, aggressive behavior, and may not progress by the adenoma-carcinoma pathway but may rise from a very small superficial-type adenoma.

Tada et al. (248) conducted a clinicopathologic study of 62 flat colorectal carcinomas and 80 polypoid colorectal carcinomas. The authors found the former to be smaller, more often in the proximal colon, and away from the rectosigmoid area, less frequently well differentiated, with fewer adenomatous remnants, and with more frequent deep invasion and lymphovascular permeation.

Iishi et al. (249) reported on a series of 256 early colorectal carcinomas (Dukes' A and B) of which 8% were superficial early carcinomas defined as < 3 mm in height. These lesions were found scattered throughout the large intestine and were often observed as reddish spots that were easily overlooked without careful observation. Histologically, 90% of these were well differentiated, 24% reached the submucosal layer, and 86% were not associated with adenoma.

Flat lesions are being increasingly recognized with new colonoscopic techniques. Togashi et al. (250) reported 10,939 consecutive high-resolution video colonoscopies and indigocarmine spraying to detect flat lesions. All lesions suggesting neoplastic changes were removed by polypectomy or operation. Carcinomas invading beyond the submucosal layer were excluded from this analysis. The gross appearance of flat-type lesions was classified as flat elevated type or flat depressed type based on the presence or absence of central depression. A total of 5408 neoplastic lesions were index lesions, including 5035 adenomas and 373 carcinomas (124 with submucosal invasion). The prevalence of flat depressed and flat elevated lesions were 2.8% and 18.1%, respectively. Submucosal invasion rates were 17.1% in the flat depressed, 0.8% in the flat elevated, 1.6% in the sessile, 4.0% in the pedunculated lesions, and 9% in the creeping lesions. The submucosal invasion rate in the flat depressed lesions was significantly higher than in any others, except for creeping lesions. The percentage of flat elevated and flat depressed carcinomas among all carcinomas invading the submucosa was 6.5% and 21.0%, respectively. They concluded that one-quarter of all colorectal carcinomas may be derived from flat lesions. Training in dye spray technique may result in a higher detection rate of flat colonic lesions.

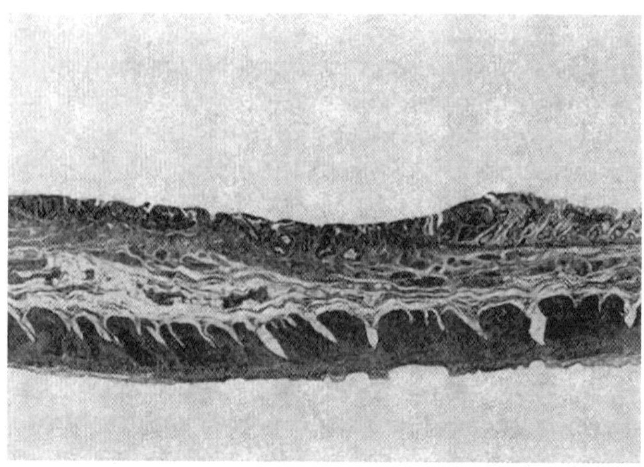

FIGURE 17 ■ Carcinoma invading the submucosal layer (hematoxylin-eosin stain, original magnification X10). *Source*: From Ref. 245.

Nivatvongs (251) reviewed the subject of early colorectal carcinoma. Most such carcinomas can be treated by adequate local excision, such as colonoscopic polypectomy and peranal excision. If there are adverse risk factors, especially poorly differentiated carcinoma, lymphovascular invasion, or incomplete excision, a radical resection is indicated if there is no contraindication. In the case of a low rectal carcinoma, adjuvant chemoradiation should be considered. Recently, a new classification has been developed: sm 1 is invasion to the upper one-third of the submucosa, sm 2 is invasion to the middle one-third, and sm 3 is invasion to the lower one-third. Lesions of sm 1 and sm 2 have a low risk of local recurrence and lymph node metastasis; local excision is adequate. The sm 3 lesions and sm 2 flat and depressed types have a high risk of local recurrence and lymph node metastasis; further treatment is indicated.

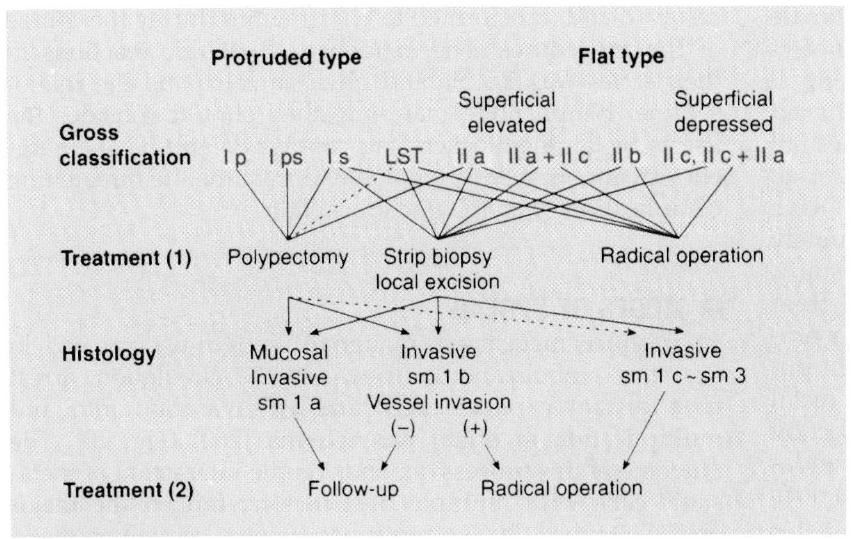

FIGURE 19 ■ Treatment algorithm for colorectal lesions, p = pedunculated; ps = subpedunculated; s = sessile; LST = laterally spreading type. *Source*: From Ref. 245.

■ SENTINEL LYMPH NODE MAPPING

Lymph node involvement with metastatic disease has long been recognized as a prognostic discriminant that decreases survival. Ultrastaging by serial sectioning combined with immunohistochemical techniques, improves detection of lymph node micrometastases. The introduction of sentinel lymph node mapping has provided the potential to facilitate ultrastaging. The impact of staging in the oncologic management of patients may have therapeutic implications. The challenge is to determine the biologic relevance and the prognostic implications. Mulsow et al. (252) reviewed the electronic literature (1996–1993) on sentinel node mapping in carcinoma of the colon and rectum. Lymphatic mapping appears to be readily applicable to colorectal carcinomas and identifies those nodes most likely to harbor metastases. Sentinel node mapping carries a false-negative rate of approximately 10% but will also potentially upstage a proportion of patients from node-negative to node-positive following the detection of micrometastases. The prognostic significance of micrometastases in colorectal carcinoma is required before the staging benefits of sentinel lymph node mapping can be routinely adopted. Bilchik et al. (253) proposed a TNM classification for micrometastases and isolated malignant cells. They studied 120 patients who underwent lymph node mapping before resection of primary colorectal carcinoma. Sentinel nodes were identified using blue dye and/or radiotracer and were examined by hematoxylin-eosin staining, cytokeratin immunohistochemistry, and multilevel sectioning. The comparison group comprised 370 patients whose primary colorectal carcinomas were resected without lymph node mapping during the same period. Lymph node mapping was successfully performed in 96% of patients and correctly predicted the status of the nodal basin in 96% of patients. Nodal involvement was identified for 14.3%, 30%, 74.6%, and 83.3% of T1, T2, T3, and T4 carcinomas, respectively in the study group, and for 6.8%, 8.5%, 49.3%, and 41.8% of T1, T2, T3, and T4 carcinomas, respectively, in the comparison group. The study group had a higher percentage of nodal metastases (53% vs. 36%). They believe lymph node mapping and focused sentinel node analysis should be considered to better stage colorectal carcinoma.

Saha et al. (254) used the combination of isosulfan blue (Lymphazurin) 1% and 99mTc sulfur colloid, to test the feasibility and accuracy of lymphatic mapping for colorectal carcinoma. In 57 consecutive patients, mapping was successful in 100% of patients with isosulfan blue and in 89% with sulfur colloid. Lymphatic mapping was accurate in 93% of patients with isosulfan blue vs. 92% with sulfur colloid. The combined accuracy was 95%. A total of 709 lymph nodes were found (12.4 per patient): 553 nonsentinal lymph nodes (5.6% nodal positivity) versus 156 sentinel lymph nodes (16.7% nodal positivity). Isosulfan blue detected 152 sentinel lymph nodes, sulfur colloid detected 100, and both modalities detected 96. Of the sentinel lymph nodes detected by isosulfan blue only, 10.7% had nodal metastases, whereas 19.8% of sentinel lymph nodes detected with both modalities had nodal metastases. Nodal disease was detected in 41% of patients with invasive carcinoma. Metastases were detected only in the sentinel lymph nodes in 26% and only by micrometastases in 11% of these patients. The metastatic yield is significantly higher in sentinel lymph nodes identified by both modalities compared with isosulfan blue only. A less encouraging report was published by Bembenek et al. (255). They evaluated the feasibility and utility of lymphatic mapping in 48 patients with rectal carcinoma, 37 of whom had already undergone preoperative radiochemotherapy for locally advanced lesions. An endoscopic injection of sulfur colloid into the submucosa adjacent to the carcinoma was performed 15 to 17 hours before the operation. Ex vivo identification of the nuclide-enriched "sentinel lymph nodes" was performed using a hand-held gamma-probe. The selected sentinel lymph nodes were examined using serial sections and immunohistochemistry. One or more sentinel lymph nodes were found in 46 of the 48 patients. The sentinel lymph node detection rate was 96%. Lymph node metastases were present in 35%. A sensitivity of only 44%, and a false-negative rate of 56% were found. Further analysis showed that the method correctly predicted the nodal status only in the small subgroup of patients with early carcinoma without preoperative radiation. They concluded that although lymph node identification shows a relatively high detection rate, the sensitivity in patients with locally advanced irradiated rectal carcinoma is low.

Further studies will be required to determine the ultimate utility of this modality but even this may not be necessary. The results of the Cancer and Leukemia Group B (CALGB) Protocol 80001, a prospective study conducted in 12 institutions, concluded that sentinel lymph nodes fail to predict nodal status in 52% of cases (256). Read et al. (257) reported that sentinel node mapping would have potentially benefited only 3% and failed to accurately identify nodal metastases in 24% of patients in their study. They concluded the fraction of patients benefiting from sentinel lymph node mapping and lymph node ultra processing techniques would be 2%. These studies might put the question of sentinel lymph node mapping for colorectal carcinoma to rest. The most recent review of the subject by Stojadinovic et al. (258), concluded that there are fundamental questions that remain unanswered, namely, (i) does sentinel lymph node mapping significantly upstage or increase staging accuracy? (ii) do patients with H and E negative nodes but nodal metastases have a significantly worse oncologic outcome than those without micrometastases?, and (iii) does treatment of nodal micrometastases with adjuvant chemotherapy translate into meaningful survival benefit? They believe that until these questions are answered, sentinel lymph node mapping for colorectal carcinoma will likely remain investigational.

Cimmino et al. (259), reported that in 267 patients who underwent intraoperative lymphatic mapping with the use of both isosulfan 1% blue dye and radiocolloid injection, five adverse reactions to isosulfan blue were encountered—two cases of anaphylaxis and three cases of "blue hives." The two patients with anaphylaxis experienced cardiovascular collapse, erythema, perioral edema, urticaria, and uvular edema. The blue hives in three patients resolved and transformed to blue patches during the course of the procedures. The incidence of allergic reactions in their series was 2%. Should physicians expand the role of sentinel lymph node mapping, they should consider the use of histamine blockers as prophylaxis and have emergency treatment readily available to treat the life threatening complication of anaphylactic reaction.

■ MODES OF SPREAD

To produce metastases, malignant cells must succeed in invasion, embolization, survival in the circulation, arrest in a distant capillary bed, and extravasation into and multiplication in organ parenchyma (260) (Fig. 20). The outcome of this process depends on the interaction of metastatic cells with multiple host factors. Indeed the major obstacle to the effective treatment of colon carcinoma metastasis is the biologic heterogeneity of neoplasms. Another challenge to therapy is the finding that different organ environments can modify a metastatic malignant cell's response to systemic therapy. Carcinoma of the colon may spread in one of the following ways: direct continuity, transperitoneal spread, lymphatic spread, hematogenous spread, and implantation.

Direct Continuity

Intramural spread of the carcinoma occurs more rapidly in the transverse than the longitudinal axis of the colon and has been estimated to proceed roughly at the rate of one quarter of the bowel circumference every 6 months. It is unusual for microscopic spread to occur more than 1 cm beyond the grossly visible disease. Radial extension

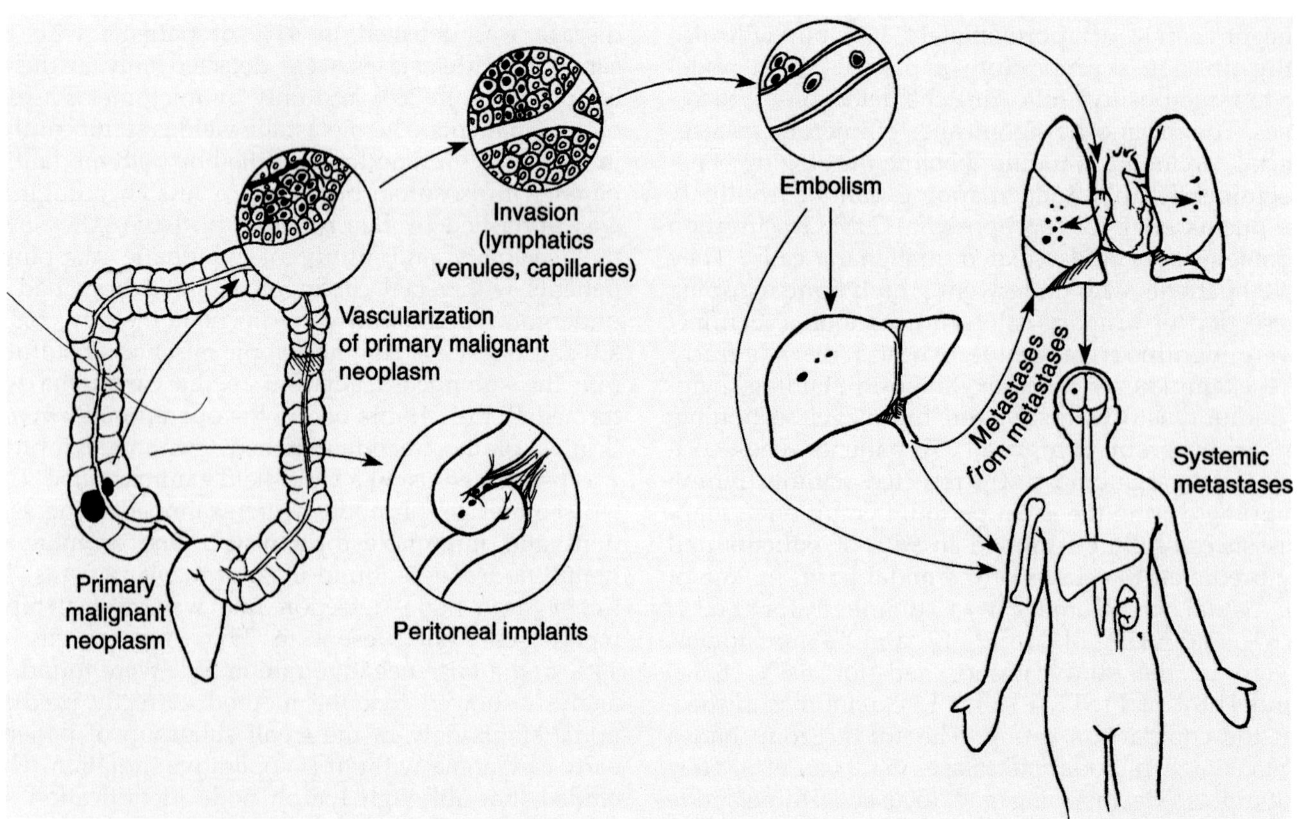

FIGURE 20 ■ Pathogenesis of metastases from colorectal carcinoma, including metastases from metastases.

through the bowel wall may result in adherence to abdominal viscera such as the small or large gut, stomach, pelvic organs, or abdominal parietes. If the lesion is situated on the retroperitoneal aspect, infiltration of the posterior abdominal wall, duodenum, ureter, perirenal fascia, or iliacus or psoas muscles may occur. Knowledge of the degree of extension is necessary to effect a curative resection. As the carcinoma penetrates the bowel wall, neighboring structures are involved in 10% of patients (260). Probably one third to two thirds of such attached viscera are involved with the neoplastic process. An additional pattern of local spread is perineural invasion, which may reach as far as 10 cm from the primary lesion. Mechanisms involved in invasion of host tissues include (i) mechanical pressure produced by a rapidly proliferating neoplasm may force cords of malignant cells along tissue planes of least resistance, (ii) increased cell motility can contribute to malignant cell invasion, and (iii) malignant cells may secrete enzymes capable of degrading basement membranes, breaking down barriers between epithelial cells and the stoma (260).

Transperitoneal Spread

Transmural extension of carcinoma ultimately penetrates the peritoneal surface, following which dissemination may occur in a transcelomic manner, with implants occurring anywhere on the peritoneal surface or omentum. Approximately 10% of patients with colon carcinoma develop peritoneal deposits (230).

Lymphatic Spread

The nature of extramural lymphatic spread is of paramount importance in planning the scope of an operation for carcinoma. Indeed, the extent of involvement of the lymphatic system is related to the prognosis of the patient. First metastases usually take place in the paracolic glands nearest the carcinoma and proceed in a stepwise way from gland to gland; however, exceptions to such an orderly progression do occur, and these glands may be missed with the first deposits detected in a more proximal location. Retrograde lymphatic metastases may occur when anterograde blockage is present.

Hematogenous Spread

Blood-borne metastases result in systemic spread of disease, with the liver being the organ most commonly involved. Circulating malignant cells have been found to occur in 28% of patients during induction of anesthesia and in 50% during laparotomy (261). Surprisingly, follow-up studies of patients with circulating malignant cells during operation have not shown an adverse effect on the ultimate prognosis. Using an experimental melanoma model it was found that $< 1.0\%$ of cells are viable 24 hours after entry into the circulation and $< 0.1\%$ of these cells eventually produce metastases (260). Other sites of hematogenous spread include the lung and, less commonly, bone.

Weiss et al. (262) analyzed the sequence of events in hematogenous metastasis from colonic carcinoma using 1541 necropsy reports from 16 centers. The authors' findings were consistent with the cascade hypothesis that metastases develop in discrete steps, first in the liver, next in the lungs, and finally, in other sites. In only 216 of 1194 cases was there suggestive evidence that metastatic patterns (excluding lymph nodes) were causally related to lymph or nonhematogenous pathways. The concept that extrahepatic metastases arise from liver metastases is also supported by Taylor (263).

Implantation

Several reports have been made concerning instances in which exfoliated malignant cells have implanted on raw surfaces, such as with hemorrhoidectomy wounds, fissures-in-ano, fistulas-in-ano, or along the suture line (264–269). Other forms of implantation may relate to an abdominal scar or at the mucocutaneous margin of a colostomy (260) (Fig. 21).

■ SITE OF SPREAD

For every 100 patients with intestinal carcinoma, approximately one half will be cured by operation and five will die from lymphatic spread, 10 from local recurrence, and 35 from blood-borne metastases. The organs most frequently involved are the liver (77%), lungs (15%), bones (5%), and brain (5%). The spleen, kidneys, pancreas, adrenals (270), breast, thyroid, and skin are rarely involved (230). Even the trachea, tonsils, skeletal muscle, urethra, oral cavity, penis, and nail bed have become involved (230,271–275).

■ STAGING

It is helpful for the treating physician to be aware of the extent of spread of the disease. By definition, the lesion must penetrate through the muscularis mucosa for it to be considered an invasive carcinoma. Cytologic malignant cells superficial to this layer are considered carcinoma-in-situ. Dukes (233) originally proposed a classification based on the extent of direct extension along with the presence or absence of regional lymphatic metastases. Dukes' A lesions are those in which growth is confined to the bowel wall, Dukes' B lesions include those in which direct spread has progressed through the full thickness of the wall involving the serosa or fat, and Dukes' C lesions are those in which

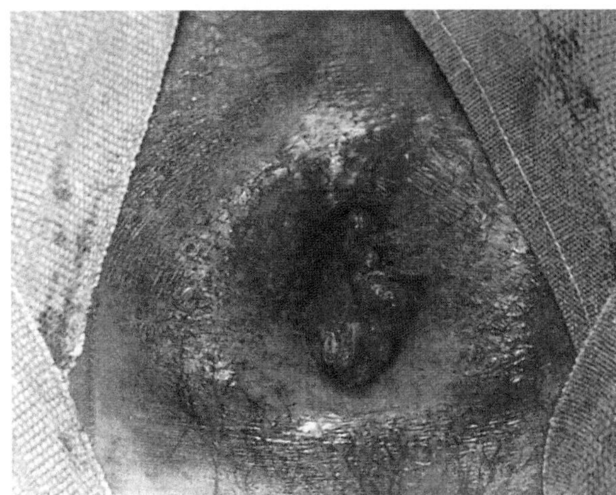

FIGURE 21 ■ Macroscopic appearance of anal implantation from a proximally located adenocarcinoma of the descending colon.

regional lymph node metastases are present. Dukes' C lesions are further divided into C_1, in which lymph nodes are involved near the bowel wall, and C_2, in which there is continuous involvement of nodes up to the point of ligature (276). Not unexpectedly, there is a correlation between histologic grade and the Dukes classification. By common usage, a fourth category, labeled D, has been added. In this group metastatic disease has advanced beyond the confines of surgical resection, as in the case of a patient with distant metastases or an unresectable local lesion (277).

Wong et al. (278) conducted a study to determine the number of nodes that need to be examined to accurately reflect the histology of the regional lymphatics in colorectal carcinoma. Patients undergoing curative resection for T2 and T3 colorectal carcinomas were reviewed. The number of nodes examined ranged from 0 to 78 (mean, 17 nodes). Node-negative patients had fewer nodes examined (mean, 14 nodes) than node-positive patients (mean, 20 nodes). The entire sample had a node-positive rate of 38.8%. When at least 14 nodes were examined, the percent of patients with at least one positive node was 33.3%. They concluded the examination of at least 14 nodes after resection of T2 or T3 carcinomas of the colon and rectum will accurately stage the lymphatic basin.

The staging of large bowel carcinoma remains a confused topic for most and has been discussed at length (279). In an effort to better define or categorize patients in order to achieve better prognostication, numerous eponymous modifications have been introduced, but to my mind these have served only to cloud the issue. Despite the intentions of well meaning physicians, all in the name of progress, few significant advances have been made. Some of the staging systems proposed are remarkably similar to the Dukes staging system, while others are so detailed that they are cumbersome and unmanageable, difficult to recall and apply, and, simply stated, not practical (277,279–289). Further confusion has resulted from the fact that the Dukes staging system is frequently misquoted (287,289).

An ideal staging system would be one that is simple and easy to remember and apply. It should include important prognostic discriminants without becoming too complex. The Australian Clinicopathological Staging (ACPS) system was proposed to incorporate clinical nformation in an effort to better define prognosis (283,285) (see Box 1). The tumor/node/metastasis (TNM) classification was proposed to incorporate findings at laparotomy and provide greater precision in the identification of prognostic subgroups, but its complexity has hindered general acceptance (281). The most current definitions of the TNM classification are depicted in Box 2. The completeness of resection designation is seen in Box 3 (280). The most commonly used classifications are depicted in Fig. 22.

The value of any staging system is its potential application in the treatment of the patient. Since there is not yet an ideal method of definitively staging the patient's disease preoperatively, a study of the resected specimen continues to have merit. Traditional pathologic variables considered important include histologic grading; depth of penetration; cell type; lymph node involvement; lymphatic, venous, or perineural invasion; distal margin of resection; and surrounding inflammatory response. In addition, it has been suggested that certain subsets of patients may benefit from adjuvant therapy. Being able to select appropriate therapy would be advantageous so that the remaining patients would not be subjected to potentially harmful treatments.

Obtaining international agreement on a staging system will prove to be a Herculean task. Proponents of "new" classifications believe their system to be the best and their followers will continue to adhere to those systems. Only if and when a new system is proved to be beneficial from a prognostic or therapeutic viewpoint will

BOX 1 ■ Australian Clinicopathological Staging System

When all known carcinoma has been removed by a "Curative resection," the following categories are used for staging:

ACPS O
The carcinoma is confined to the mucosa in a patient who has undergone a bowel resection.

ACPS A
The carcinoma has spread into the bowel wall but not beyond the muscularis propria. There are no lymph node metastases, nor distant metastases.

ACPS B
The carcinoma has spread beyond the muscularis propria into the adjacent tissues in continuity or into adjacent organs. There are no lymph node metastases, nor distant metastases.

ACPS C
The carcinoma may have spread varyingly into or through the bowel wall, but one or more lymph nodes contain cancer. There are no distant metastases.

ACPS D
This category is used when there is clinical or microscopic evidence of any carcinoma remaining locally or at a distance, whether there has been a "palliative resection," a "palliative operation," a local excision or no operation because of the extent of the carcinoma.
In the event of synchronous carcinomas being present in the resected specimen of bowel, the ACP stage allocated should be that of the most advanced carcinoma.

ACPS X
Category "X" is used where a local excision or other local procedure is done without lymphadenectomy. This may be subdivided into:
XO—The carcinoma is confined to the mucosa.
XA—The carcinoma does not spread beyond the muscularis propria.
XB—The carcinoma spreads beyond the muscularis propria.
Operations may be done with curative or palliative intent in this group.

ACPS Y
This category is used when the pathologic details are, for some reason, not known or are incomplete.

Source: From Davis NC, Newland RC. Terminology and classification of colorectal adenocarcinoma. The Australian Clinicopathological Staging System. Aust N Z J Surg 1983; 53:211–221.

BOX 2 ■ TNM Definitions

Primary tumor (T)

TX	Primary tumor cannot be assessed
T0	No evidence of primary tumor
Tis	Carcinoma in situ: intraepithelial or invasion of the lamina propria*
T1	Tumor invades submucosa
T2	Tumor invades muscularis propria
T3	Tumor invades through the muscularis propria into the subserosa, or into nonperitonealized pericolic or perirectal tissues
T4	Tumor directly invades other organs or structures, and/or perforates the visceral peritoneum**,***

*Tis includes cancer cells confined within the glandular basement membrane (intraepithelial) or lamina propria (intramucosal) with no extension through the muscularis mucosae into the submucosa.

**Direct invasion in T4 includes invasion of other segments of the colorectum by way of the serosa; for example, invasion of the sigmoid colon by a carcinoma of the cecum.

***Tumor that is adherent to other organs or structures, macroscopically, is classified T4. However, if no tumor is present in the adhesion microscopically, the classification should be pT3. The V and L substaging should be used to identify the presence or absence of vascular or lymphatic invasion.

Regional lymph nodes (N)

NX	Regional lymph nodes cannot be assessed
N0	No regional lymph node metastasis
N1	Metastasis in 1 to 3 regional lymph nodes
N2	Metastasis in 4 or more regional lymph nodes

A tumor nodule in the pericolorectal adipose tissue of a primary carcinoma without histologic evidence of residual lymph node in the nodule is classified in the pN category as a regional lymph node metastasis if the nodule has the form and smooth contour of a lymph node. If the nodule has an irregular contour, it should be classified in the T category and also coded as V1 (microscopic venous invasion) or as V2 (if it was grossly evident), because there is a strong likelihood that is represents venous invasion.

Distant metastasis (M)

MX	Distant metastasis cannot be assessed
M0	No distant metastasis
M1	Distant metastasis

STAGE GROUPING

Stage	**T**	**N**	**M**	**Dukes***	**MAC***
0	Tis	N0	M0	–	–
I	T1	N0	M0	A	A
	T2	N0	M0	A	B1
IIA	T3	N0	M0	B	B2
IIB	T4	N0	M0	B	B3
IIIA	T1-T2	N1	M0	C	C1
IIIB	T3-T4	N1	M0	C	C2/C3
IIIC	Any T	N2	M0	C	C1/C2/C3
IV	Any T	Any N	M1	–	D

*Dukes B is a composite of better (T3 N0 M0) and worse (T4 N0 M0) prognostic groups, as is Dukes C (Any TN1 M0 and Any T N2 M0). MAC is the modified Astler-Coller classification.

Note: The y prefix is to be used for those cancers that are classified after pretreatment, whereas the r prefix is to be used for those cancers that have recurred.

BOX 3 ■ Residual Tumor (R)

R0	Complete resection, margins histologically negative, no residual tumor left after resection
R1	Incomplete resection, margins histologically involved, microscopic tumor remains after resection of gross disease
R2	Incomplete resection, margins involved or gross disease remains after resection

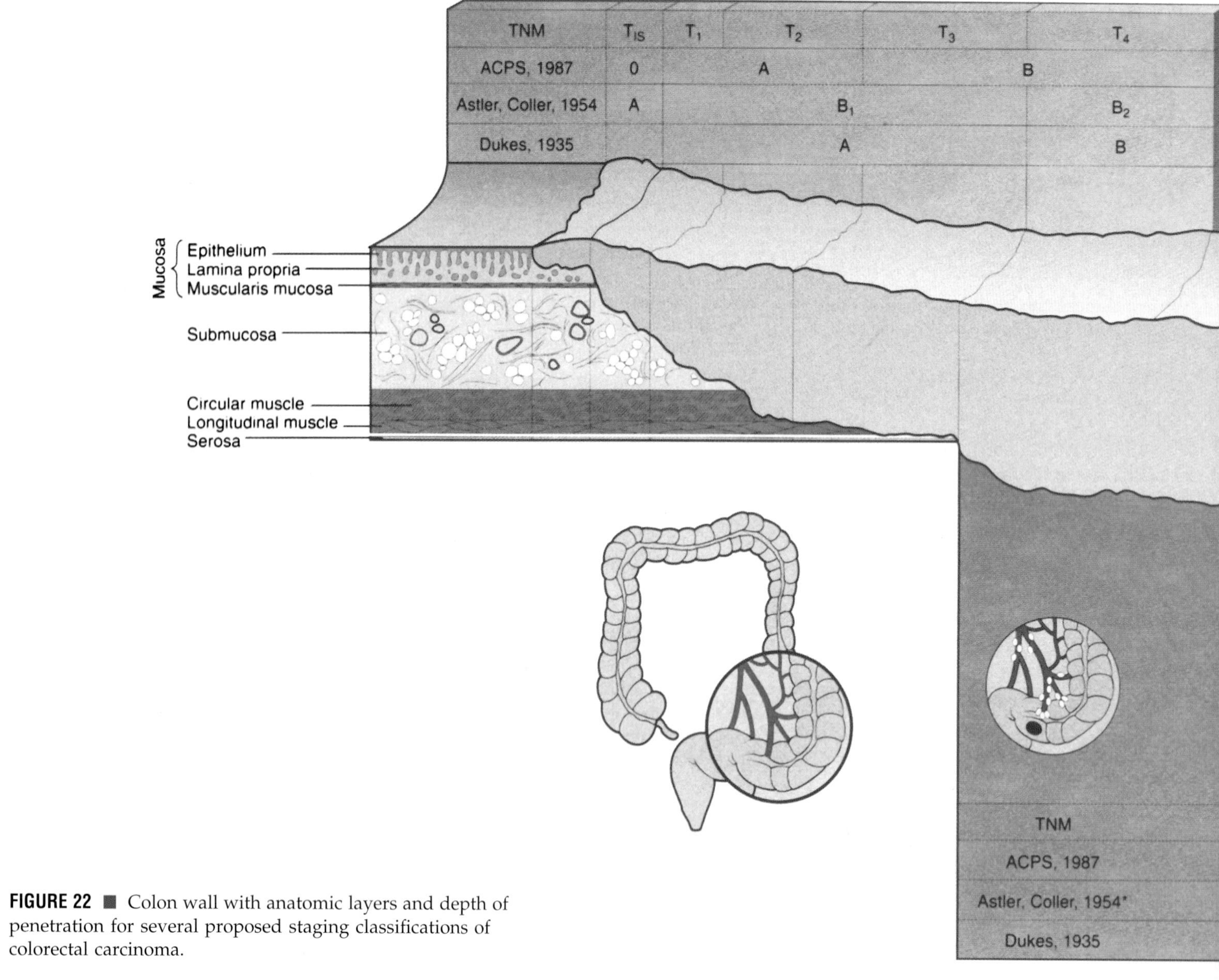

FIGURE 22 ■ Colon wall with anatomic layers and depth of penetration for several proposed staging classifications of colorectal carcinoma.

it stand a chance of acceptance. The objectives of the staging system for carcinoma, succinctly enumerated by Davis and Newland (284), include:

- to aid the physician in planning treatment
- to give some indication of prognosis
- to assist in the evaluation of treatment results
- to facilitate the exchange of information between treatment centers
- and to contribute to the continuing investigation of human cancer.

It provides a method of conveying one group's experience to others without ambiguity.

To achieve these goals, a pilot project confirming their virtues would be necessary to convince the international community of the efficacy of the new system. As one example, from a practical point of view, demonstration of histopathologic penetration may be difficult, but Newland, Chapuis, and Smyth (290) have shown the distinction to be clinically relevant. In a prospective study of 1117 cases, they reported a 77% 5-year survival rate in node-negative patients with carcinoma limited to the bowel wall and a 54% 5-year survival rate when there was serosal penetration. One important advantage of a universal staging system would be to allow new or different modes of therapy or adjuvant therapy from different centers to be compared and a rational interpretation to be made. Indeed, such a system would facilitate or influence the choice of treatment. For example, it could extend the use of sphincter-saving operations, identify patients suitable for local treatment, and define those with considerable risk of local recurrence when combined operation and adjuvant treatment might be considered. Knowing the precise extent of the disease would be helpful for interpreting the influence of treatment on parameters such as disease-free survival so that we can identify small and useful improvements in prognosis. It is likely that much time will elapse before any such system will be accepted universally.

■ BIOLOGY OF GROWTH

The rate of growth of an individual carcinoma is almost certainly the most important prognostic discriminant. Colorectal carcinomas are relatively slow-growing neo-

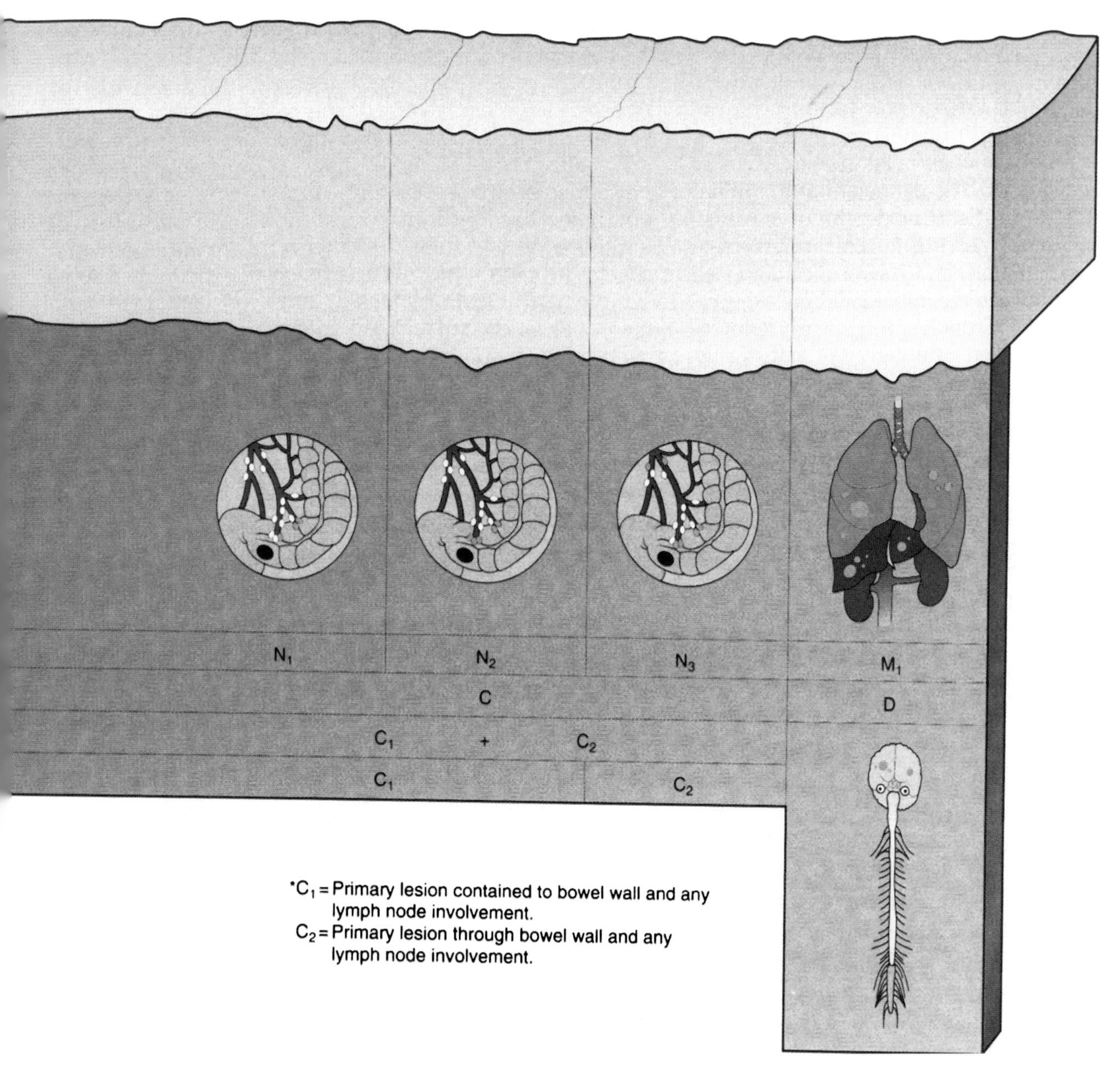

plasms, and metastases occur relatively late. In his summary of the results of several series of studies, Spratt (291), using radiographic measurements, initially calculated a doubling time of 636.5 days in a follow-up of 7.5 years for an unusual case in which a patient was not treated by resection. Similar analysis of 19 other patients revealed a mean doubling time of 620 days, with a 95% range extending from 111 days to 3430 days. Spratt reported the doubling time of pulmonary metastases from colon and rectal carcinoma calculated radiographically to be 109 days, with a 95% range extending from 9 days to 1300 days. He believed that metastatic carcinomas increase their cellular complement six times faster than do primary carcinomas. The doubling time of untreated hepatic metastases has varied between 50 and 95 days (292,293). It has been theorized that the absence of desquamation in the metastatic site accounts for this observed difference. Bolin, Nilsson, and Sjodahl (294) had the opportunity to measure radiographically lesions in 27 patients on two separate occasions, with a median interval of 11 months (4 to 91 months), and found median doubling time to be 130 days (53 to 1570 days). The authors suggested that the high growth rate observed in their investigation was due to the large size of the neoplasm at the time of initial examination. Burnett and Greenbaum (295) believe that although there is little doubt that many colonic carcinomas are slow growing, there is probably a subset of rapidly growing lesions. In a small group of patients, the authors observed doubling times as short as 53 to 150 days. The implication of their report is that a carcinoma seen on a barium enema study at a given time was not necessarily missed by a negative barium enema study reported, for example, 2 years earlier.

Matsui et al. (296) estimated a statistical curve for growth from 31 patients with colorectal carcinoma in which initial lesions were diagnosed as mucosal carcinoma. These lesions were overlooked in the first or second investigations, but were detected later. Initial radiographic features were as follows; 4 pedunculated lesions, 1 semipedunculated lesion, 6 sessile lesions, 9 superficially elevated lesions, and 11 superficially depressed lesions. The diameters of the initial lesions were 12.1 ± 6.1 mm. The final depths of invasion were 6 mucosal carcinomas, 12 submucosal carcinomas, 6 muscularis propria carcinomas, and 7 serosal carcinomas. The observation period between the initial and final examination was 41.5 ± 25.8 months. Growth speed of early colorectal carcinoma was estimated through a statistically significant growth curve. Estimated doubling time of the volume of early colorectal carcinoma was 26 months.

CLINICAL FEATURES

SYMPTOMS

Patients with carcinoma of the large intestine may present in one of three characteristic ways: insidious onset of chronic symptoms, acute intestinal obstruction, or perforation with peritonitis. Aldridge et al. (297) reported that those conditions will occur in 77%, 16%, and 7% of patients, respectively. Mandava et al. (298) reported perforated carcinomas in 51 of 1551 patients (3.3%) with colorectal carcinoma. Localized perforation with abscess formation occurred in 31 patients (61%), and free perforation with generalized peritonitis occurred in 20 patients (39%). Runkel et al. (299), in a review of 923 patients, found the presentation with insidious onset, obstruction, and perforation to occur in 92.0%, 6.0%, and 2.0% of patients, respectively, with a combination of obstruction and perforation occurring in 0.5% of patients. In a report from Scotland of 750 consecutive patients, an unusually high number (33%) presented as an emergency (300).

Depending on the location in the bowel, one or another of the following symptoms may predominate. Bleeding is probably the most common symptom of large bowel malignancy (301). All too often the bleeding is attributed by the patient, and regrettably by the physician as well, to hemorrhoids. Despite the fact that the most common cause of rectal bleeding is hemorrhoids, bleeding cannot be dismissed lightly, especially in a middle-aged or older individual. It has been estimated that visible blood per rectum occurs in 10% of the adult population over the age of 30 years (302). However, Beart et al. (301) found that in patients 40 years of age or older with a history of rectal bleeding and known hemorrhoids, 6% had rectal or colon carcinoma and 14% had colon polyps. This underscores the necessity of taking the symptom of bleeding seriously. Bleeding may be occult, as is often the case in right-sided lesions, or overt, being either bright red, dark purple, or even black, depending on the location in the bowel.

The second most common presenting symptom is probably a change in bowel habits, either constipation or diarrhea (301). The absolute frequency of defecation is not important, but a deviation from what is normal for a given individual may signal the presence of an intestinal neoplasm. Lesions in the proximal colon may not result in a change in bowel symptoms until they are very far advanced. Lesions in the distal colon are more likely to be manifest in symptoms since the stool is more formed in consistency and the bowel lumen is narrower. A progressive narrowing of the caliber of the stool may be reported in the case of a compromised lumen.

Pain may occur with almost equal frequency as the preceding symptom. Abdominal pain may be vague and poorly localized, or it may result from a partially obstructing lesion of the colon. The latter type of pain is generally colicky in nature and may be associated with obstructive symptoms of bloating, nausea, and even vomiting. Rectal pain does not occur with carcinoma unless there is sacral nerve root or sciatic nerve involvement. However, tenesmus may occur with rectal carcinoma. Back pain is a late sign of penetration of retroperitoneal structures.

Other symptoms include mucus discharge, which may coat the stool or be mixed with it. Investigation of weight loss as a solitary complaint only uncommonly yields a large bowel malignancy. However, when associated with a carcinoma, weight loss is usually a sign of advanced disease and bodes a poor prognosis. Nonspecific symptoms of general impairment of health, loss of strength, anemia, and sporadic fever also may be present. Rarely a carcinoma of the cecum obstructs the appendiceal orifice, and the patient presents with the signs and symptoms of acute appendicitis (303). Bladder involvement may result in urinary frequency, suprapubic pressure, and even pneumaturia if a sigmoidovesical fistula has developed. In the report of the Commission on Cancer (304), in which 16,527 patients were diagnosed with carcinoma of the colon, the presenting symptoms in order of frequency were abdominal pain (40.5%), change in bowel habits (33.2%), rectal bleeding (28.5%), occult bleeding (34.3%), malaise (16%), bowel obstruction (14.9%), pelvic pain (3.4%), emergency presentation (6.6%), and jaundice (1%).

Iron deficiency anemia is a recognized complication of colorectal carcinoma especially with right-sided lesions and failure to investigate the anemia in older patients may lead to a delay in diagnosis. Acher et al. (305) conducted a study of all patients presenting with confirmed colorectal carcinoma in a catchment population of 280,000. The criteria for iron deficiency anemia was hemoglobin < 10.1 g. Of 440 patients with colorectal carcinoma, 38% had iron deficiency anemia at diagnosis and of the latter, 12% were known to have iron deficiency anemia for more than 6 months before diagnosis and 6% had iron deficiency anemia more than one year before diagnosis. Iron deficiency anemia was more common in right-sided carcinomas (65%) than those arising in the left side of the colon and rectum (26%). They concluded the investigation of iron deficiency anemia in older patients is important but in order to detect 26 patients with colorectal carcinoma a year earlier, the investigation of approximately 5000 patients would be required—a detection rate of less than 1%.

Church and McGannon (306) performed a study to find out how often and how accurately a family history of colorectal carcinoma was recorded in the charts of 100 in patients on a colorectal surgical floor. The chart review was repeated 4 years later. In the initial review, they found that a family history was recorded in 45 of 100 charts. It was accurate for colorectal carcinoma in 36 charts. Four years later the rate of family history recording increased to 61 of 96, whereas the accuracy rate did not change. Despite improvement during a 4-year period, there is still room for further improvement.

■ GENERAL AND ABDOMINAL EXAMINATIONS

The general examination may be a guide to the patient's state of nutrition. Any obvious excess weight loss may indicate advanced disease. Pallor may be a sign of anemia. The assessment may help in evaluating the patient's fitness for operation.

Usually the general abdominal examination fails to reveal significant abnormalities. Occasionally a mass may be present and may indicate the primary malignancy or possible metastatic disease. The liver may be enlarged, and if it is also umbilicated, this sign would be characteristic of metastatic disease. Ascites may be appreciated. Borborygmi may be present. Abdominal distention may suggest partial obstruction from a constricting lesion. Inguinal and left supraclavicular lymphadenopathy can occur rarely. Peritonitis from a perforated carcinoma may be difficult to differentiate from perforated diverticulitis.

■ DIGITAL RECTAL EXAMINATION

Although a digital rectal examination will not identify the presence of a colon carcinoma, it should reveal the presence of a rectal lesion. The exam is described in detail in Chapter 24. Sometimes a sigmoid carcinoma that hangs down into the cul-de-sac may be palpable.

■ EXTRAINTESTINAL MANIFESTATIONS

Rosato et al. (307) noted a number of cutaneous presentations associated with gastrointestinal malignancy. These included acanthosis nigricans, dermatomyositis, and pemphigoid (see Chapter 12). Halak et al. (308) reported on the incidence of synchronous colorectal and renal carcinomas and reviewed the literature on that issue. Among 103 patients who underwent colorectal surgery in their series, 5 cases of synchronous colorectal and renal carcinomas were detected (4.9%). A review of the literature suggests the incidence of simultaneous colorectal and renal carcinoma to be 0.04% to 0.5%.

■ SYNCHRONOUS CARCINOMAS

Synchronous carcinomas are not uncommon, and in recent reviews the incidence was found to range from 2% to 8% in colon carcinoma patients (309–312). In view of this, it behooves the treating surgeon to evaluate the entire colon, if possible, to determine the presence of other neoplastic lesions. Colonoscopy performed preoperatively in patients undergoing elective resection is the optimal method for assessing the unresected colon for synchronous lesions. In a prospective study of 166 patients, Langevin and Nivatvongs (313) found synchronous carcinomas in eight patients, seven of whom required resection of more colon than was necessary to treat the index carcinoma. In a study of 320 colorectal patients, Evers, Mullins, and Mathews (311) found synchronous carcinomas in different surgical segments in six of 21 patients (38%). Pinol et al. (312) conducted a study designed to identify individual and familial characteristics associated with the development of synchronous colorectal neoplasms in patients with colorectal carcinoma. During a 1-year period, 1522 patients with colorectal carcinoma attended in 25 Spanish hospitals were included. Synchronous colorectal neoplasms were documented in 505 patients (33.2%): adenoma (in 411 patients) (27%), carcinoma (in 27 patients) (1.8%), or both ($n=67$) (44%). Development of these lesions was associated with male gender (OR 1.94), personal history of colorectal adenoma (OR 3.39), proximal location of primary carcinoma (OR 1.4), TNM Stage II (OR 1.31), mucinous carcinoma (OR 1.89), and family history of gastric carcinoma (OR 2.03). Based on individual and familial characteristics associated with synchronous colorectal neoplasms, it has been possible to identify a subgroup of patients with colorectal carcinoma prone to multicentricity of neoplasm with potential implications on the delineation of preventive strategies.

If technically and logistically possible, it would be ideal for all patients about to undergo elective resection carcinoma to have a preoperative colonoscopic examination. If not possible, it is suggested that patients should have postoperative colonoscopy.

■ ASSOCIATED POLYPS

Neoplastic polyps are frequently associated with carcinoma of the colon, and, indeed, on sigmoidoscopic examination, when a patient is found to have a neoplastic polyp, the entire colon should be assessed to rule out the presence of another associated polyp or an associated malignancy. Approximately 7% of patients with polyps will harbor an associated carcinoma of the colon or rectum (314). Slater, Fleshner, and Aufses (315) studied the relationship between the location of a colorectal carcinoma and the existence of adenomas in 591 patients. The overall incidence of adenomas was 29.7%, with resected specimens of right-sided carcinomas containing adenomas in 47% of cases and left-sided specimens having them in 22%. Thus the authors suggested that efforts be made to identify polyps preoperatively in patients with colorectal carcinoma. Also, since patients with carcinoma and associated adenomas are at increased risk of developing metachronous carcinoma, the group with right-sided carcinoma should be part of a particularly active surveillance program.

Chu et al. (316) retrospectively studied the relationship of colorectal carcinoma with polyps in 1202 patients. Synchronous polyps were found in 36% of patients. Synchronous carcinoma was found in 4.4% of patients and metachronous carcinoma developed in 3.5% of patients. The incidence of synchronous carcinoma and a metachronous carcinoma increased with synchronous polyps, and varied according to number, size, and histologic features of the polyps. The adjusted 5-year survival rate was improved in patients with synchronous polyps compared with those without synchronous polyps. The pattern of relapse was the same for the synchronous polyp and nonsynchronous polyp groups. The authors even went so far as to recommend subtotal colectomy for colorectal carcinoma and synchronous polyps in good-risk patients.

There is a general trend for the incidence of multiple carcinomas to rise as the number of adenomas increases whereas in patients in whom there is evidence of only one adenoma being present, the incidence of multiple carcinomas is less than 2%, the figure for those with more than five adenomas rises to 30% (231).

■ OTHER ASSOCIATED MALIGNANCIES

In a review of 9329 cases of colorectal carcinoma from the literature, Lee et al. (317) found that the incidence of primary malignant neoplasms at sites other than the colon ranged from 3.8% to 7.8%. In a series of 14,235 patients with colon and rectal carcinomas followed for an average of 3.6 years, Tanaka et al. (318) observed an elevated risk of second primary malignancies as follows: rectum (observed/expected [O/E] 2.0, men; O/E 4.3, women), corpus uteri (O/E, 8.2), ovary (O/E, 4.3), and thyroid gland (O/E 4.7, women). These observations were more notable in right-sided colon carcinoma patients than left-sided colon carcinoma and in those younger than 50 years. Schoen, Weissfeld, and Kuller (319) also found that women with a history of breast, endometrial, or ovarian carcinoma were at a statistically significant increased risk for subsequent colorectal carcinoma (1.1, 1.4, and 1.6, respectively).

COMPLICATIONS

A number of well-recognized complications of carcinoma of the large bowel may alter its clinical presentation.

■ OBSTRUCTION

Depending on the macroscopic features and location of the malignancy, interference with the passage of intestinal contents may occur. Carcinoma is the most common cause of large bowel obstruction, contributing to 60% of cases in the elderly (320). Ohman (321) summarized the results of 26 series on colorectal carcinoma reported in the literature. The combined total comprised 23,434 patients of whom 15% presented with obstruction. Incidences ranged from 7% to 29%. In the right colon, carcinomas are usually polypoid, and because of the liquid nature of the intestinal contents, obstruction is unlikely unless it involves the critical ileocecal valve, in which case obstruction may supervene. In the left colon, where the intestinal contents are solid and the nature of the malignancy is more inclined to be annular, occlusion is more likely. Complete obstruction of the colon from carcinoma is often entirely insidious in its onset. The patient often has had progressive difficulty in moving his or her bowels and has taken increasing doses of laxatives until the abdomen has become more distended with pain and eventual obstipation. Nausea and vomiting may supervene. Alternatively, the patient may present with sudden, severe, colicky abdominal pain that persists, and investigation may reveal a complete obstruction. The offending lesion may be surprisingly small as seen in Fig. 23. On examination, the patient's general condition usually is found to be good, because dehydration and electrolyte depletion are often late phenomena. Examination of the abdomen reveals that it is distended and tympanitic but not tender. Hyperactive peristalsis may be present. It is unlikely that an abdominal mass will be felt in the presence of a distended abdomen. Digital examination may reveal a balloon-type rectum and, in the exceptional case, a palpable carcinoma may be present. A mass in the cul-de-sac may be appreciated, representing either a sigmoid loop that is hanging down or a cul-de-sac implant. Sigmoidoscopy may reveal the lower edge of a constricting lesion. The diagnosis is usually suggested from a history of intestinal symptoms and physical findings. Plain x-ray films of the abdomen will reveal the presence of obstruction and indicate its level. The amount of small bowel distention will depend on the competence of the ileocecal valve. The presence of an obstructing carcinoma can be confirmed with an emergency barium enema study.

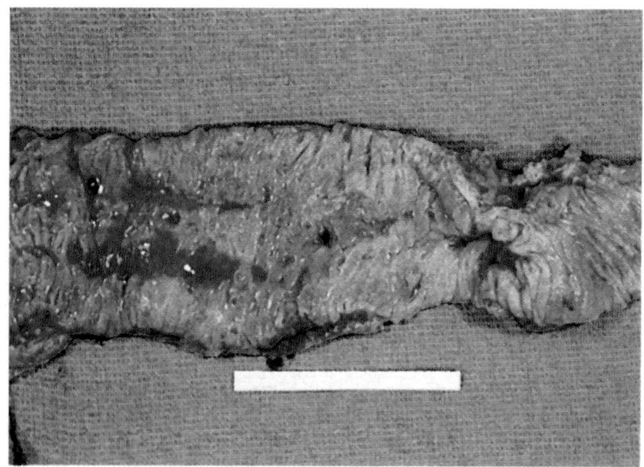

FIGURE 23 ■ Small adenocarcinoma of splenic flexure in patient who presented with acute colonic obstruction.

A nonspecific type of colitis may develop proximal to an obstructing carcinoma of the colon (322,323). It is reported to occur in 2.0% to 7.5% of cases (324,325). In most cases, there is a short segment of normal mucosa immediately proximal to the carcinoma, above which the colitic process appears. The etiology of these changes in the colonic mucosa proximal to the obstructed lesion is obscure, although the gross pathology and microscopic features are consistent with those of ischemic colitis in the subacute or chronic phase (324). The extent of the colitic process varies. It may be unsuspected and discovered only at the time of operation. The extent of resection may be dictated by the length of inflamed bowel. Seow-Choen, Chua, and Goh (325) reported that four of 204 new cases of colorectal carcinoma seen in a 24-month period were proven to have concomitant proximal ischemic colitis. Ischemic colitis associated with obstructing carcinoma of the colorectum may present dramatically with gangrene or colonic perforation if the acute vascular insufficiency is severe. Less severe degrees of ischemic insult must be recognized intraoperatively because the incorporation of ischemic colon in a colonic anastomosis may result in an anastomotic leak.

The National Surgical Adjuvant Breast and Bowel Project (NSABP) trials have suggested that obstructing carcinomas in the right colon carry a more significant risk of recurrence and carcinoma-related mortality than obstructing carcinomas in the left colon (326). The diminished survival rate in patients presenting with obstructing malignancies does not appear to correlate significantly with annularity of the lesion or the presence of lymph node metastases.

PERFORATION

The incidence of perforation associated with carcinoma of the colon is in the 6% to 12% range of all hospital admissions for colon carcinoma (323). A perforation may result in peritonitis, abscess formation, adherence to a neighboring structure, or fistulous communication into a viscus. Perforation is found in conjunction with obstruction in approximately 1% of patients with colorectal carcinoma. In patients with obstruction, concurrent perforation is found in 12% to 19% of patients (323,327). If acute obstruction supervenes in the middle or distal colon, the cecum may perforate. However, the most common form of perforation is associated with the carcinoma itself. Such perforation may develop suddenly with diffuse peritonitis or more gradually with a localized peritonitis; when it occurs in the cecum, it may resemble appendicitis. Patients with obstruction and a proximal perforation present as desperately ill individuals with generalized peritonitis, dehydration, and electrolyte depletion. Immediate exploratory laparotomy is demanded. Patients without obstruction but with perforation of the carcinoma are also gravely ill and require immediate laparotomy after some correction of dehydration and electrolyte depletion. Patients without obstruction but with perforation of a carcinoma may present with a localized peritonitis. Under these circumstances it may be confused with diverticulitis if the sigmoid colon is involved, or with appendicitis or Crohn's disease if the right colon is involved.

BLEEDING

Bleeding is a common symptom of colorectal carcinoma, but massive bleeding is an uncommon presentation.

UNUSUAL INFECTIONS ASSOCIATED WITH COLORECTAL CARCINOMA

Unusual infections associated with colorectal carcinoma may, in some instances, be the sole clue to the presence of a malignancy. The infections are either related to invasion of tissues or organs in close proximity to the neoplasm or secondary to distant seeding by transient bacteremia arising from necrotic carcinomas. Panwalker (328) identified a series of patients whose clinical presentations included endocarditis (*Streptococcus bovis* bacteremia), meningitis (*S. bovis* bacteremia), nontraumatic gas gangrene (*Escherichia coli*), empyema (*E. coli, Bacteroides fragilis*), hepatic abscesses (*Clostridium septicum*), retroperitoneal abscesses (*E. coli, B. fragilis*), clostridial sepsis, and colovesical fistulas with urosepsis (*E. coli*). Panwalker also reviewed the English language literature and identified other infections associated with colon carcinoma, including nontraumatic crepitant cellulitis, suppurative thyroiditis, pericarditis, appendicitis, pulmonary microabscesses, septic arthritis, and fever of unknown origin. Lam, Greenberg, and Bank (329) reported an unusual presentation of colon carcinoma with a purulent pericarditis and cardiac tamponade caused by *B. fragilis*.

With or without endocarditis, septicemia caused by *S. bovis* may be associated with an occult colonic malignancy (330,331). The septicemia also has been described with a variety of gastrointestinal pathologic conditions, such as colonic adenomas, inflammatory bowel disease, and carcinoma of the esophagus. Patients may be entirely asymptomatic, but all patients with endocarditis caused by *S. bovis* should be evaluated for concomitant colon carcinoma.

In a literature review, Panwalker (328) found *S. bovis* bacteremia reported in 467 adults with endocarditis present in 62%, absent in 13%, and of unclear status in the remaining patients. Other organisms associated with endocarditis are *S. salivarius* and enterococcus.

An asymptomatic colonic malignancy has been reported in a patient with meningitis caused by S. *salivarius* (332). *S. bovis* meningitis was reported in 10 adults (328).

Silent colon carcinoma has been reported to present as hepatic abscesses (333,334), and therefore anaerobic hepatic abscesses might alert the physician to the possibility of a malignancy of the large intestine.

Panwalker (328) found 55 patients with the dramatic clinical presentation of gas gangrene associated with colorectal carcinoma (16 of which were cecal). The gas gangrene was metastatic in 10 patients. Sites included the neck, chest wall, upper extremities, shoulders, and axilla. Kudsk (335) subsequently reported five cases of painful, rapidly spreading gas-producing infection of the lower extremity (three cases), upper extremity (one), and pelvis (one), which represented metastatic *C. septicum* infections in diabetic patients. All had occult carcinomas of the right colon. More recently, Lorimer and Eldus (336) reported three cases of invasive *C. septicum* infection associated with colorectal carcinoma. The authors cited a previous review of 162 cases of nontraumatic C. *septicum* infection identified-malignant disease in 81%, approximately half of which were colorectal. The carcinoma is typically right sided and always ulcerated, which can occur in three circumstances: occult carcinoma (80%), anastomotic recurrence, or carcinoma that is unresectable or has been bypassed. In summary, gas gangrene associated with colorectal carcinoma is a catastrophic illness that appears to be clostridial, affects diabetic patients disproportionately, and, in almost 50% of cases, is the result of an otherwise silent cecal carcinoma.

DIAGNOSIS

In a case of carcinoma of the colon the patient's history may not be helpful. Consequently, early diagnosis may depend on screening, which may be directed at the identification of high-risk groups, the use of screening tests, and the investigation of patients with positive screening test results. Early detection is described in Chapter 25. Suffice it to say that a combination of occult blood testing and flexible fiberoptic sigmoidoscopy is the minimum current recommendation (337). Colonoscopy is ideal and preferable. Atypical dyspepsia and vague abdominal symptoms should be investigated since malignancy may be the cause of otherwise un-explained ill health and anemia. Of course, the symptoms suggestive of the disease, as previously described, should be pursued with the appropriate modalities as described in the discussion of investigations.

For *differential diagnosis,* a host of conditions may be considered, depending on the predominant symptom complex with which the patient presents. These include inflammatory bowel disease, either of the nonspecific type, such as ulcerative colitis or Crohn's disease, or of the specific type, such as amebiasis, actinomycosis, or tuberculosis. For patients presenting with narrowed bowel, ischemic strictures may be included in the differential diagnosis. Acute abdomen may be confused with conditions such as diverticulitis or appendicitis with abscess, Crohn's disease, foreign body perforation, or even an infarcted appendix epiploica. If marked bleeding is the prominent feature, vascular ectasis, diverticulosis, or acute ischemia are possibilities. With acute obstruction, volvulus, diverticulitis, and Crohn's disease might be considered. Extrinsic pressure from a metastatic carcinoma, endometriosis, or even pancreatitis are possibilities in appropriate circumstances. Uncommon conditions (e.g., colitis cystica profunda) also can be considered.

INVESTIGATIONS

OCCULT BLOOD TESTING

Occult blood determinations are of value in the screening setting; however, for patients who have symptoms that are suggestive of large bowel disease, occult blood testing is inadequate (337). Certainly patients who relate a history of rectal bleeding do not need occult blood testing to confirm its presence.

ENDOSCOPY

Anoscopy and Sigmoidoscopy

Use of an anoscope to determine the presence of any significant internal hemorrhoids is of value, especially for patients who present with bright-red rectal bleeding.

Sigmoidoscopic examination is an indispensable diagnostic tool in the assessment of rectal carcinoma (338). The appearance of rectal carcinoma is usually quite distinctive. A protruding mass into the lumen may be seen, but more characteristically a raised everted edge with a central, sometimes necrotic, sloughing base will be noted. The distance from the lower edge of the lesion to the anal verge should be carefully determined because it may be crucial in deciding whether intestinal continuity can be restored. Two points also should be noted: which wall the lesion is located on and whether the lesion is annular. In addition, information can be obtained regarding the mobility, of the lesion by placing the end of the sigmoidoscope against the lower margin of the lesion and exerting gentle pressure along the long axis. Mobile carcinomas can be moved and present a quite different sensation from the rigid feel of a fixed carcinoma. The size of the lesion should be recorded, and finally a biopsy should be performed to confirm the diagnosis.

Flexible Fiberoptic Sigmoidoscopy

Flexible fiberoptic sigmoidoscopy has assumed an increasing role in the diagnosis of colon disease (339,340). Because of its greater length and flexibility than the rigid sigmoidoscope, the flexible sigmoidoscope allows for the detection of a larger number of neoplastic lesions. In addition, equivocal lesions seen on a contrast enema can be elucidated if they are within the reach of the scope. Some surgeons have replaced rigid sigmoidoscopy with flexible sigmoidoscopy, but others, including myself, believe that the rigid instrument is still superior for the crucial assessment of the distance of a carcinoma from the anal verge and this judgement cannot be made satisfactorily or accurately with a flexible instrument.

Colonoscopy

The role of colonoscopy also has assumed greater importance in the evaluation of colon disease (Chapter 3). In particular, colonoscopy plays a major role in screening for colorectal carcinoma, especially in high-risk patients, as described in Chapter 25. With specific reference to its value in the assessment of patients with large bowel malignancy, colonoscopy has been recommended as a preoperative examination to detect the presence of synchronous neoplastic polyps or carcinomas. Its necessity in the preoperative or at least perioperative setting has been debated, but growing evidence suggests that it plays an important role (310,341,342). The rationale is that synchronous carcinomas exist in 2% to 7% of cases (313,343,344). It has been suggested that preoperative colonoscopy alters the operative procedure in one third of patients (342). Another group of surgeons, concerned with the potential for implantation of malignant cells, exfoliated by preoperative colonoscopy, has opted for intraoperative palpation to detect synchronous carcinomas and postoperative colonoscopy to clear the colon of polyps (345).

RADIOLOGY

Barium Enema

The method by which the largest number of carcinomas of the colon are diagnosed is the barium enema examination, although in some hands colonoscopy is the preferred investigative modality. Various radiologic features may be demonstrated, such as an annular, or "napkin ring," appearance, as often seen in the left colon (Fig. 24). Features distinguishing it from spasm are the irregular, jagged outline and destruction of the mucosa with a typical "apple

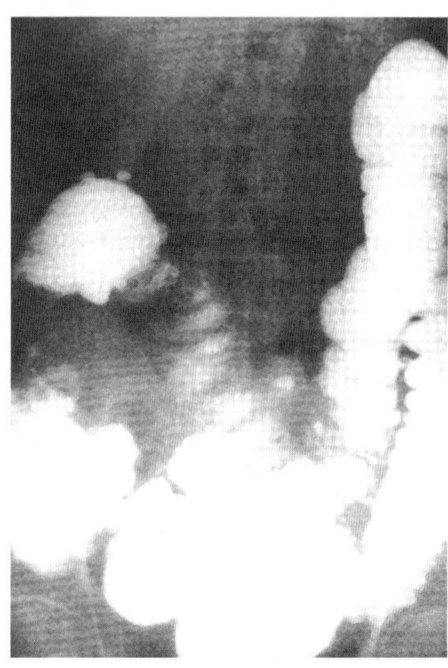

FIGURE 24 ■ Barium enema study appearance of an annular adenocarcinoma of the colon. *Source:* Courtesy of M. Rosenbloom, M.D., Montreal, Quebec.

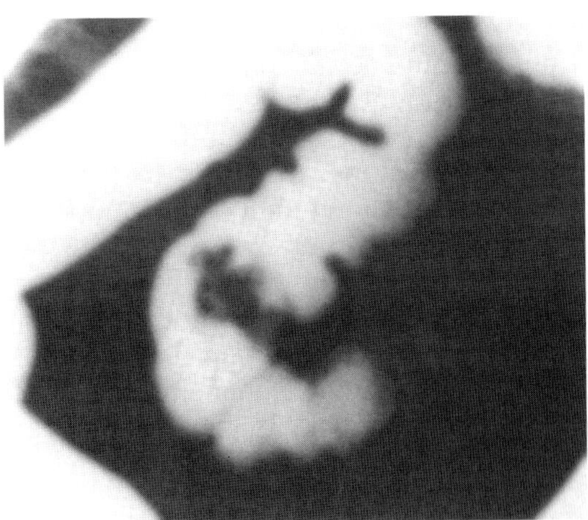

FIGURE 25 ■ Barium enema study appearance of a polypoid adenocarcinoma of the colon. *Source:* Courtesy of M. Rosenbloom, M.D., Montreal, Quebec.

core" appearance and overhanging edges. A large filling defect representing a bulky neoplasm projecting into the lumen is seen more often in the right colon (Fig. 25). A polypoid sessile lesion occupying only one wall of the bowel is demonstrated in Fig. 26. Sometimes a polypoid lesion on a pedicle may be entirely malignant. Occasionally a complete retrograde obstruction may be present (Fig. 27), but this radiologic appearance is not necessarily indicative of a clinically anterograde obstruction.

In an audit of 557 barium enema studies in patients with known carcinomas, a malignant lesion was recorded in 85% (346). Reviewing cases in which there was failure to perceive a demonstrated lesion or failure to analyze a perceived lesion indicated that 94% of carcinomas should have been reported.

The air-contrast barium enema has been considered superior to the full-column barium enema for detection of small polyps. For detection of large constricting lesions, the single-contrast enema is superior to the double-contrast enema.

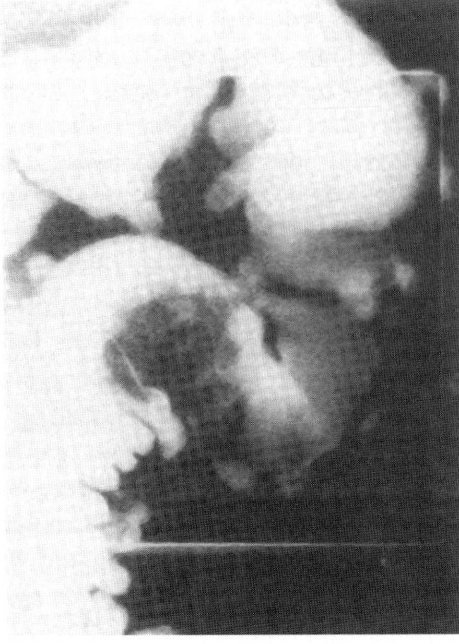

FIGURE 26 ■ Barium enema study appearance of a sessile adenocarcinoma of the colon. *Source:* Courtesy of M. Rosenbloom, M.D., Montreal, Quebec.

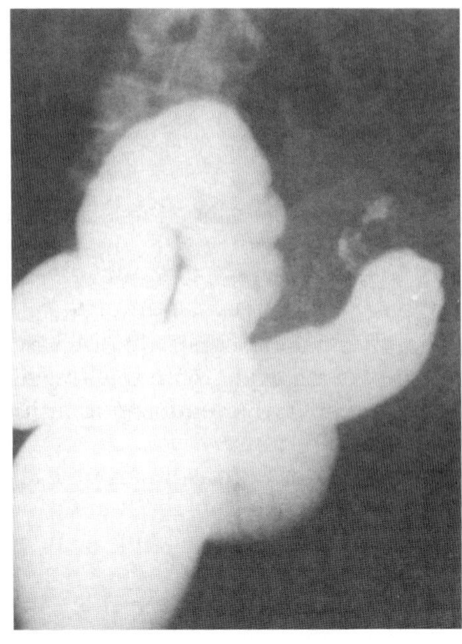

FIGURE 27 ■ Barium enema study appearance of a complete retrograde obstruction due to adenocarcinoma of the colon. *Source:* Courtesy of M. Rosenbloom, M.D., Montreal, Quebec.

In the event of a negative barium enema report, subsequent management will depend on clinical assessment. Should there be a strong degree of clinical suspicion of a carcinoma, colonoscopic evaluation would be in order. If no strong suspicion exists and the barium enema was ordered because of minimal symptoms of constipation, no further investigation may be deemed necessary. If rectal bleeding was the prominent feature and the patient exhibited prominent internal hemorrhoids, hemorrhoid treatment should be performed to eliminate confusion with bleeding of colonic origin. Should bleeding persist after such treatment, colonoscopic examination would be indicated.

Intravenous Pyelography

There is controversy as to whether an intravenous pyelogram is necessary preoperatively. Supporters suggest that it is helpful in advance to know whether the ureters or bladder are involved with the neoplastic process, whether two kidneys are present, or whether additional ureters may be present. Furthermore, in the follow-up of patients who develop urinary tract problems postoperatively, it provides a baseline for differentiating whether these problems are due to a surgical complication or are secondary to preexisting urologic disease (347,348). In one study, abnormalities were found in as many as 26% of patients (348). Adversaries suggest that intravenous pyelography is not cost-effective and is not necessarily reliable in demonstrating the absence of disease involvement (349,350). For the most part, a CT scan will provide the information previously sought by the IVP.

Ultrasonography

Sonographic evaluation of colorectal carcinoma can be performed via trans-cutaneous or intracorporeal approaches. The transcutaneous approach evaluates the liver for metastases and identifies ascites, adenopathy, and an omental cake. Intracorporeal imaging can be performed endoluminally, intraoperatively, or laparoscopically.

Preoperative assessment of the liver by ultrasonography may provide valuable information to consider when recommending the appropriate management of patients with colorectal carcinoma. In a preoperative ultrasonographic study of 195 patients, Grace et al. (351) found a false negative rate of 7.2%.

Both rigid and flexible echoendoscopes are available. Because of the lack of input on the management of the patient with a carcinoma above the peritoneal reflection, endosonography currently finds its role in staging rectal carcinoma. The echo-colonoscope, although available, has not been evaluated extensively. With the advent of laparoscopic colectomy, preoperative endosonography may have an increased role in the future.

Intraoperative liver ultrasonography is currently being touted as the most accurate method for detecting colorectal metastases. It has served to supplement inspection and palpation at the time of laparotomy. The liver can be surveyed by a radiologist experienced in intraoperative sonography in 5 to 10 minutes. Although peripheral lesions are easily palpable by the surgeon, deeper lesions may be missed by manual examination. Additional findings may very well alter the course of management, either extending or eliminating the planned procedure. Rafaelsen et al. (352) compared diagnostic accuracies of measuring liver enzymes, preoperative ultrasonography, manual palpation, and intraoperative ultrasonography in the detection of liver metastases in 295 consecutive patients with colorectal carcinoma. The presence of metastases was further assessed by ultrasonography 3 months postoperatively. The sensitivity of intraoperative ultrasonography (62 of 64) was significantly superior to that of manual palpation (54 of 64) and preoperative ultrasonography (45 of 64). The lowest sensitivity was presented by the measurement of liver enzymes. The authors concluded that intraoperative ultrasonography reduced the number of patients with liver metastases from being subjected to superfluous or even harmful liver surgery and may increase the number in whom liver surgery will prolong life. They cite six other studies that suggest a higher sensitivity of intraoperative ultrasonography than preoperative ultrasonography in the detection of liver metastases. Meijer et al. (353) studied a series of 122 patients who underwent elective resection—34 with suspected liver lesions seen on preoperative computed tomography (CT) and ultrasonography and 88 without suspected lesions. Of the 34 patients with suspected lesions, the diagnosis was confirmed with intraoperative ultrasonography in 21 and, in the remaining 13 patients, the suspected lesion was shown to be benign. Of the 88 patients with normal preoperative imaging, lesions were detected in five patients. During an 18-month follow-up, 6.5% of patients developed liver metastases not recognized during operation. Machi et al. (354) evaluated 189 patients with colorectal carcinoma at the time of operation and revealed that the sensitivity of intraoperative ultrasonography (93.3%) was significantly higher than that of preoperative ultrasonography (41.3%), conventional CT (47.1%), and manual palpation (66.3%). Metastatic liver lesions were detected solely by intraoperative ultrasonography in 9.5% of patients. During the postoperative follow-up period of 18 months or more, liver metastases that were unrecognized during operation appeared in 6.9% of patients. Reevaluation based on these follow-up results indicated that the sensitivity of intraoperative ultrasonography decreased to 82.3%, which was still significantly better than that of other methods. Takeuchi et al. (355) reported on a consecutive series of 119 colorectal carcinoma patients who were studied by preoperative extracorporeal ultrasonography, inspection and palpation of the liver at laparotomy, and intraoperative liver ultrasonography. Hepatic metastases were diagnosed in 19 patients—eight by extracorporeal ultrasonography, seven by palpation, and the last four only after intraoperative ultrasonography. Follow-up for a median of 38 months revealed another eight patients with liver metastases detected at a mean time from operation of 14.7 months. The authors concluded that although intraoperative sonography is a sensitive and useful method in detecting liver metastases, some occult hepatic metastases will remain undetected.

Laparoscopic ultrasonography has been used to image the liver and may lead to a less invasive manner of staging the patient and providing pathologic confirmation.

Computed Tomography

When there is suspicion on ultrasonography of the presence of a hepatic metastatic lesion or if there is clinical suspicion that the primary malignancy has invaded adjacent viscera or anterior or posterior abdominal walls, CT scanning of the abdomen may help delineate the extent of the disease. This may help in the preoperative planning of the extent of the operation. CT scanning of the abdomen is useful in the preoperative investigation of patients to detect occult metastases. Kerner et al. (356) used CT of the abdomen and pelvis to augment the preoperative evaluation of 158 consecutive patients with primary, colorectal carcinoma. In 88 patients findings present on CT were otherwise unknown. Of those, 35% were clinically significant in that they allowed the surgeon to alter the propsed operative procedure or added additional technical information for consideration preoperatively. Findings included liver metastases (26), atrophic kidney (three), and abdominal wall or contigous organ invasion (11). In addition, two other solid organ carcinomas were detected. The authors concluded that CT eliminates the need for a preoperative intravenous pyelogram, improves the preoperative staging of metastatic disease, and provides a baseline for comparison during the postoperative follow-up if recurrence is suspected or adjuvant therapy is planned.

CT has a low accuracy for identifying early stages of primary colorectal carcinoma, but is useful in examining patients suspected of having extensive disease or recurrent disease with an extrinsic component at an anastomosis (357).

Mauchley et al. (358) assessed the clinical utility of the practice of routine preoperative CT scanning and determined its cost-effectiveness in 130 colon carcinoma patients. CT scans provided information that was used in treatment planning in 33% of patients and definitively altered the mode of treatment in 16% of patients. The practice saved the institution US$24,018 over 6 years. They concluded routine preoperative CT scanning-definitively alters treatment in a small number of cases and is cost-effective.

Magnetic Resonance Imaging

Magnetic resonance imaging (MRI) is a technique that creates images by evaluating nuclei for the absorption or emission of electromagnetic energy in the presence of a stable magnetic field (359). It has a greater tissue contrast resolution than CT, is multiplanar, and involves no ionizing radiation. The imaging times are longer, the spatial resolution is less than CT, calcifications and bone detail are not as obvious, and the study is more expensive. Certain patients cannot be safely imaged and these include those with cardiac pacemakers, implanted drug infusion pumps, ferromagnetic vascular aneurysm clips, and ocular foreign bodies.

MRI has limitations in assessing depth of penetration of the bowel wall but this limitation can be partly overcome by the use of an endorectal coil with up to 90% accuracy. The sensitivity for detecting lymph node metastases ranges from 13% to 40%. Initially MRI was believed to be better than CT in distinguishing between fibrotic changes and recurrences, but this is probably not so. MRI can be used to assess hepatic metastases. Metastatic lesions to the lungs are better defined by CT. For metastatic lesions involving osseous structures, especially the spine and central nervous system, MRI should be the imaging modality of choice. Zerhouni et al. (360) evaluated the accuracy of CT and MRI in staging 478 patients with colorectal carcinoma. CT was more accurate than MRI in the definition of penetration of the muscularis propria by rectal carcinoma (74% vs. 58%). Accuracies were equivalent in depiction of transmural extent of colonic carcinoma. CT and MRI exhibited accuracies of 62% and 64%, respectively, in assessment of lymph node involvement with sensitivities of 48% and 22%, respectively. The accuracy of MRI and CT in the evaluation of liver metastases was equivalent (85%).

Positron Emission Tomography

Positron emission tomography (PET) is a method of imaging using a positron-emitting isotope-labeled compound that is incorporated into the biochemical process occurring in organs and tissues of the body. The anatomic and morphologic characteristics are not as well delineated as with other imaging modalities such as CT and MRI, but PET images provide useful information about the nature and physiology of the cellular function of the tissue and have been used to evaluate neoplasms, including colorectal carcinoma. The most widely used isotope is 2-deoxy-2(18F) fluoro-D-glucose, or fluorodeoxyglucose (FDG). Imaging relies on the premise that there is an enhanced rate of glucose in malignant tissue. PET scanning is more accurate than CT scanning in identifying malignancy. This is especially true in the postoperative follow-up in differentiating recurrent carcinoma from fibrosis. Tempero et al. (359) reviewed three studies that compared the results of PET to CT, MRI, and radioimmunoguided scintigraphy (RIGS). In each case PET sensitivity and specificity were very high and better than the other modalities. The major problems are to clarify the role of PET in clinical management and determine who will benefit from this additional expensive, time consuming study. PET scans may have a role in both the diagnosis of and response to therapy of hepatic metastases.

Several studies have been performed comparing computed tomography scan with positron emission tomography scan in clinical decision making. Unfortunately, therapeutic decisions are being made based on positron emission tomography scan data without a clear understanding of how well the diagnostic findings correlate with the clinical findings. Johnson et al. (361) conducted a retrospective review of 41 patients with metastatic colorectal carcinoma. All patients had both a computed tomography scan and a positron emission tomography scan before surgical exploration. PET scan was found to be more sensitive than CT scan when compared with actual operative findings in the liver (100% vs. 69%), extrahepatic region (90% vs. 52%), and abdomen as a whole (87% vs. 61%). Sensitivities to PET scan and CT scan were not significantly different in the pelvic region (87% vs. 61%). They concluded PET scanning is more sensitive than CT scanning and more likely to give the correct result when actual metastatic disease is present.

■ RADIOIMMUNODETECTION

Radioimmunodetection of carcinoma is usually accomplished by obtaining whole-body gamma scans of patients who have been injected intravenously with an antibody labeled or conjugated with a gamma-emitting radionuclide (359). In colorectal carcinoma, a variety of antigens have been targeted (e.g., TAG-72 and carcinoembryonic antigen [CEA]). A variety of radionuclides used include iodine-131 (^{131}I), technetium-11 (^{11}Tc), indium-111 (^{111}In), and iodine-125 (^{125}I). Combined results using a variety of antibodies and radionuclides suggests that the sensitivity and detection are high in selected patients; the reports range from a sensitivity of 60% to more than 90% (359). A number of benefits are attributed to radioimmunodetection. Although it can localize metastases, it is not yet clear whether any changes in management translate into long-term patient benefits. Another goal in monitoring recurrent colorectal carcinoma is to distinguish colorectal carcinoma from benign conditions (e.g., postoperative or radiation changes in the pelvis). False positive rates of antibody imaging may be as high as 13%, and it is thus advisable to pursue positive scans with biopsy confirmation (359). Liver metastases may be diagnosed but the identification of extrahepatic sites might spare the patient an unnecessary liver resection.

Bertsch et al. (362) reported on 32 patients with primary colorectal carcinoma who underwent RIGS after being injected with anti-TAG-72 murine monoclonal antibody CC49 labeled with iodine-125. Sixteen patients had gross disease and RIGS-positive tissue removed (five with en bloc resection and 11 with extraregional tissues resected, two liver resections, and 25 lymphadenectomies— 10 in the gastrohepatic ligament, 5 celiac axis, 6 retroperitoneal, and 4 iliac) and 16 had only traditional extirpation of disease because RIGS-positive tissue was too diffuse. With a median follow-up of 37 months, survival in the former group was 100%, and 14 of 16 patients had no evidence of disease. In the latter group, 14 of 16 patients died and two were alive with disease. The same authors reported that for patients with recurrent disease, the addition of RIGS increased the detection rate at operation from 116 sites without RICS to 184 with RIGS (a 57% increase) (363).

Using murine antibody B72.3 labeled with indium-111 (^{111}In-CYT-103, Cytogen), Dominguez et al. (364) studied 15 patients with recurrent colorectal carcinoma. It was more accurate than a CT scan but when the value of the scan was examined with respect to the potential contribution to patient management, it was beneficial in only 13% of patients.

Moffat et al. (365) assessed the clinical impact of an anti-CEA Fab′ antibody fragment labeled with technetium-99m pertechnetate in 210 patients with advanced or metastatic colorectal carcinoma. When compared with conventional diagnostic modalities, the CEA scan was superior in the extra-hepatic abdomen (55% vs. 32%) and pelvis (69% vs. 48%). Potential clinical benefit was demonstrated in 89 of 210 patients. Corman et al. (366) evaluated the role of immunoscintigraphy with ^{111}Insatumomab pendetide in 103 patients with colorectal carcinoma. In the 84 patients for whom histopathologic information was available, the sensitivity was 73% and the specificity was 100%, with an overall accuracy of 85% for determining the presence and extent of malignant disease. Investigators judged that the antibody imaging mode was a beneficial contribution in 44% and a negative effect in 2% of case studies. Treatment plans were altered in 17 patients.

The exact role of immunoscintigraphy has not yet been defined. Galandiuk (367) suggested three potentially major roles of immunoscintigraphy in the management of patients who have undergone curative resection: (1) the detection of recurrent disease in patients with an elevated CEA level and either a negative investigation or equivocal findings on CT scan, (2) the exclusion of extra-abdominal disease, prior to planned resection of a presumably isolated recurrence, and (3) earlier detection of recurrence in the follow-up of high-risk patients.

Immunoscintigraphy may allow recurrent disease to be detected at a time when curative resection may still be feasible and result in improved survival and/or effective palliation.

Miscellaneous Investigations

The results of hydrocolonic sonography, a technique of trans-abdominal sonography following retrograde installation of water into the colon were compared with conventional transabdominal sonography by Limberg (368). In a study of 29 patients with carcinoma, the diagnosis was correctly made in 97%, compared with only 31% by conventional sonography. Further studies will be required to determine the utility of this technique. Deranged liver blood flow patterns have been detected in patients with hepatic metastases (369). The sugar moiety detected from rectal mucus by the galactose oxidase-Schiff (Sham's test) has been studied in screening for colorectal carcinoma. Dian-Yuan et al. (370) found a sensitivity of 85.7% for colorectal carcinoma and 47.1% for adenomas in a study of 6480 subjects older than 40 years of age. This compared favorably to 90.5% and 41.2% for fecal occult blood testing in the same group of individuals. In a study of 330 asymptomatic individuals, Sakamoto et al. (371) found an overall specificity of Sham's test of 92.2%.

■ CYTOLOGY

The value of cytology in establishing the diagnosis of carcinoma for the most part has been appreciated only in investigational studies. To date, clinical application has been limited. Brush cytology via the colonoscope has been reported to be 86% accurate in establishing the diagnosis preoperatively, a% identical to that of biopsy (372). A special circumstance in which cell brushings may be of value is when a stricture prevents the colonoscope from reaching the lesion, a situation in which a biopsy cannot be performed.

In a study of 33 patients, 15 of whom had proven carcinoma, colonic cytology was positive in 93% of cases, whereas the cytology of control patients was negative (373).

■ BLOOD MARKERS

Liver Function Tests

To determine the presence or absence of anemia, a complete blood count is indicated. Liver function tests often will point to metastatic disease, but a normal liver profile does not rule out hepatic metastases.

Carcinoembryonic Antigen

The initial report of a tumor-specific antigen in human colonic carcinomas by Gold and Freedman (374) heralded a new era in the assessment of the status of patients with colorectal carcinoma. However, CEA evaluation has not fulfilled its promise as a simple blood test that would afford an early diagnosis of carcinoma of the colon.

In a most comprehensive treatise on the subject, Gold (375) described his life's work on CEA. The following information is drawn from that most comprehensive publication.

The CEA molecule is considered an oncodevelopmental human marker of neoplasia initially found in adenocarcinomas of the human digestive system. The molecule has a nominal molecular mass of 180 kDa. The CEA gene family comprises 29 gene-like sequences in two defined clusters on chromosome 19.

It is of interest that human colonic carcinoma develops in mucosal tissue that has already undergone multiple steps of genetic change. It has been postulated that these multiple steps create a field effect that is characterized by morphologically normal, but biologically altered, epithelial cells. CEA has been used as a phenotypic marker of this field effect by examining the immunohistochemical expression of CEA on morphologically normal mucosa adjacent to colonic adenocarcinomas. It has been shown very clearly that CEA expression occurs in 'normal' mucosa adjacent to a carcinoma and that there is a gradient of CEA expression, falling off at increasing distances from the carcinoma. These data are relevant to both the biology of human colorectal carcinoma and, more practically, to the optimal location of surgical resection. Kyzer et al. (376), using statin as a marker, similarly demonstrated that the proliferative rate of mucosa adjacent to a colonic carcinoma is elevated and returns to normal at 5 cm from the carcinoma, even though it is morphologically indistinguishable from its normal counterparts.

The role of CEA in clinical medicine first became a consideration with the development of a radioimmunoassay for circulating CEA. The first series of data, derived from patients with established colonic carcinoma, were most exciting, but more extensive studies revealed the clearly expected false negative assays, particularly in early-stage bowel carcinoma, and false positive results in patients with nonenteric carcinoma as well as in others with nonmalignant conditions. Over the years, suggestions for the use of the CEA assay have included detection, diagnosis, monitoring, staging and classification (prognosis), pathology, localization, and therapy.

Normal concentrations of CEA are 2.5 to 5.0 ng/ml, depending on the assay used. CEA concentrations are in general more often elevated in smokers than in nonsmokers, more frequently elevated in men than in women, and more frequently elevated in older subjects than in younger individuals. Racial differences in the frequency of serum elevations of CEA have been suggested but not established. Elevated CEA levels have been described in advanced breast carcinoma, pancreatic carcinoma, lung carcinoma, and other noncolonic adenocarcinomas, but they do not detect early stages of these diseases. Although 80% or more of patients with advanced colonic adenocarcinoma have circulating CEA, the CEA assay should not be used as the sole diagnostic test for suspected carcinoma. CEA levels are not presently useful for distinguishing locally invasive polyps from benign lesions.

Preoperative serum CEA levels in diagnosed colorectal carcinoma are elevated in 40% to 70% of patients. Preoperative serum CEA concentrations correlate inversely with the grade of the carcinoma and directly with the pathologic stage. The CEA is elevated in 95% of patients with well-differentiated lesions, while it is elevated in as few as 30% of those with poorly differentiated adenocarcinomas. The higher the preoperative CEA level, the greater the likelihood of a postoperative recurrence. A significant negative correlation between preoperative elevated plasma CEA levels and patient survival has been observed. Despite disagreement between various groups that have explored the relationship between preoperative CEA levels and prognoses, most studies report that a high preoperative CEA level is indicative of a poor prognosis. This association is often as discriminating as pathologic staging and grading. It is still uncertain which absolute preoperative CEA value reliably discriminates high-risk from low-risk cases for postoperative recurrence (see discussion of Prognostic Discriminants on p. 590).

An increase in the blood CEA concentration in a patient after apparently successful surgical treatment for carcinoma has repeatedly been shown to signal a recurrence of the carcinoma. After apparently complete surgical resection of colorectal carcinoma, the blood CEA concentration, if elevated before operation, decreases to the normal range in nearly all patients. The decrease usually occurs within 1 month but sometimes takes up to 4 months. If levels fail to decrease to the normal range, it is likely that the resection has been incomplete or that the carcinoma has already metastasized. A sustained and progressive rise is strong evidence for recurrence at the primary area or at distant sites. Serial CEA monitoring is currently considered by some authors as the best noninvasive technique for detecting recurrent colorectal carcinoma.

The debate concerning the merit of postoperative determinations of CEA values in monitoring patients with resected colon carcinoma continues to rage. At one extreme are those who feel that the carcinoma cures attributable to CEA monitoring are too infrequent to justify the substantial costs and physical and emotional stress that this intervention may cause for patients. Others believe that intensive follow-up using CEA assays can identify treatable recurrences at a relatively early stage. It has been suggested that when CEA increases more rapidly than an average of 12.6% per month, recurrence should be strongly suspected. Because the overall prognosis for patients with recurrent disease after surgical resection is dismal, serum CEA determination may offer the only chance of a cure for a select group of individuals.

Immunohistochemically, CEA has been identified in carcinomas of the colorectum, breast, lung, uterine cervix, gallbladder, stomach, pancreas, liver, prostate, urinary bladder, and uterus and in neuroendocrine neoplasms associated with the larynx, lung, and thyroid (377,378). There are good reasons to regard ulcerative colitis and certain colonic adenomas as premalignant lesions. Immunoperoxidase staining for CEA supports the concept of a polyp-adenoma-carcinoma sequence. Both chronic inflammatory bowel disease and colorectal adenomas show higher tissue CEA concentrations than normal colonic mucosa, suggesting that these situations can be regarded biochemically as premalignant conditions. Results concerning the correlation between positive CEA test results in the carcinoma immunohistochemistry and histologic grade, lymph node involvement, locoregional recurrence, disease-free interval, and patient survival remain controversial.

Initial difficulties have been overcome and several, virtually instant, and easy-to-use radiolabeling kits for anti-CEA antibodies are available. The reported sensitivities for the detection of liver metastases have ranged from 0% to 94% in different studies, indicating differences largely due to technical ability and knowledge in avoiding pitfalls. The most complete clinical report so far was conducted in Italy. $F(ab)_2$ fragments of the monoclonal antibodies anti-CEA FO23C5, determined to be more suitable than intact immunoglobulin (IgG) or Fab fragments for immunoscintigraphy, were labeled with either iodine-131 or indium-111. The variation in results reported by various groups reflects the gamut of potential variables, including the radiolabel used, the route of administration of the conjugate, the size and location of the lesion, the vascularity of the lesion, the patient population studied, the imaging technology used, the unavoidable parameter of subjective interpretation of scans, even in blinded situations, and the type of antibody preparation used. On the basis of the foregoing information, it may, therefore, be concluded that primary lesions with a high CEA content have the best anti-CEA antibody uptake and are most easily imaged and that large fungating carcinomas accumulate a high proportion of the injected labeled antibody in contrast to ulcerating carcinomas with poor vascularity. Hepatic metastases have a high CEA content and a high antibody uptake but may not image well because of the relatively high background uptake of the conjugate by the normal liver.

To date, adjuvant chemotherapy has not been very successful in those patients whose carcinomas have seen resected but who are at high risk for recurrence (i.e., Dukes' B and C lesions). The ability to detect carcinomas by radioimmunolocalization raises the possibility of treating such lesions by targeting with the same technology. An even more intriguing approach to the treatment of CEA-producing carcinomas has been developed by incorporating the recombinant CEA gene, in whole or in part, into an appropriate vector, such as the vaccinia virus. This construct, with or without other gene products to enhance immunity, has been shown to enhance cell-mediated anti-CEA immunity in both animal and human studies. Based on the results to date, a clinical trial of this form of therapy has been initiated.

Other Markers

A host of less well-described markers have been reported to have potential screening value. For example, ornithine decarboxylase activity has been found to be significantly lower patients with adenomas than in controls, and even lower in patients with carcinoma (379). Opposite findings were reported by Narisawa et al. (380), who found increased levels in patients with carcinoma. Compared with its activity in control mucosa, urokinase activity has been found to be significantly elevated in adenomas and carcinomas, with levels significantly higher in carcinomas (381). Tissue plasminogen activator activity is reduced in adenomas and carcinomas, with levels significantly lower in carcinomas.

TREATMENT

The evolution of operative treatment for carcinoma of the colon has involved several stages because of the original enormous risk of sepsis. These stages have included initially nothing more than a diverting colostomy, subsequent recommendations for exteriorization and double-barrel colostomy, efforts at reestablishing intestinal continuity with various internal stents, resection and anastomosis with proximal diversion, and ultimately resection and primary anastomosis. The acceptance of a one-stage procedure was achieved through a better understanding of the mechanical and antimicrobial bowel preparation.

■ CURATIVE RESECTION

Preoperative Evaluation

The general assessment of the patient is discussed in Chapter 4. Fazio et al. (382) described a dedicated prognostic index for quantifying operative risk in colorectal carcinoma surgery from data collected from 5034 consecutive patients undergoing major surgery. Primary end point was 30-day operative mortality. The patients' median age was 66 years. Operative mortality was 2.3% with no significant variability between surgeons or through time. Multivariate analysis identified the following independent risk factors: age (OR = 1.5 per 10-year increase), American Society of Anesthesiologists grade (OR for ASA II, III, IV-V vs. I = 2.6, 4.3, 6.8), TNM staging (OR for Stage IV vs. I–III = 2.6), mode of surgery (OR for urgent vs. nonurgent = 2.1), no-carcinoma resection versus carcinoma resection (OR = 4.5), and hematocrit level. The model has implications in every day practice, because it may be used as an adjunct in the process of informed consent and for monitoring surgical performance through time.

Bowel Preparation

Preoperative bowel preparation has been the subject of considerable controversy. It has long been believed that adequate mechanical preparation and antibiotic preparation are necessary. This has recently been brought into question (see Chapter 4). How each of these is accomplished has also been debated. Mechanical cleansing may be accomplished by the use of vigorous laxatives along with repeated enemas until clearing. For a number of years, an oral lavage with a polyethylene glycol hypertonic electrolyte solution, such as GoLytely, was used extensively and still is by some colorectal surgeons. Oral Phospho-soda preparations have become increasingly popular but certain precautions regarding their use are discussed in Chapter 4.

In the area of antibiotics, controversy exists as to whether the patient should receive oral or systemic antibiotics or possibly both. Further, there is the question of which antibiotic is the most appropriate. Clearly, whichever antibiotics are chosen, they should be selected on the basis of gram-positive and gram-negative aerobic and anaerobic coverage. There is no question that there are a number of acceptable combinations. Further argument centers around the timing of antibiotic administration, but it is certain that antibiotics should be started preoperatively. The duration of antibiotic administration is also controversial, but the antibiotic is probably not necessary after the day of operation. Our current antibiotic regimen consists of one preoperative dose and two postoperative doses of systemic ticarcillin (Timentin 3.1 gm) (383).

Exploration of Abdomen

Before operation a Foley catheter is routinely inserted into the bladder. A nasogastric tube is not necessary in the vast majority of cases, but for those cases in which it becomes necessary, the tube can be inserted during the postoperative period.

For access to the abdominal cavity, incisions should be made in a manner that provides maximum exposure for the planned resection. All operations can be performed through a midline incision and this is the access preferred by most surgeons. For a patient about to undergo a right hemicolectomy, an oblique right-sided abdominal incision is usually most adequate; if necessary, the incision can be extended. For transverse colon lesions, a supraumbilical transverse incision places access immediately in the area of the planned operation, and the incision can be extended in either direction if there is any difficulty encountered in taking down the flexures. For splenic flexure lesions, Rubin et al. (384) advocate the use of a left subcostal transverse incision combined with the right lateral position. For left-sided colonic lesions, a subumbilical transverse incision can be used. This permits adequate exposure for even a low anterior resection. For descending colon lesions, an oblique incision may prove very convenient. The use of paramedian incisions appears quite antiquated. For emergency operations, a midline incision seems the access of choice.

When the abdomen has been opened, attention should be directed to ruling out the presence of metastatic disease, with special attention given to the liver and the pelvis. A relatively new technique advocated for the detection of occult hepatic metastases is intraoperative contact ultrasonography (385). Lesions > 1 cm in diameter can be detected in 95% of cases, and those between 0.5 cm and 1.0 cm, in 66% of cases. After assessment of the abdomen, attention is focused on the primary lesion to determine its resectability.

Principles of Resection

Dogma abounds with respect to the technical aspects of operation for colorectal carcinoma. The general principles

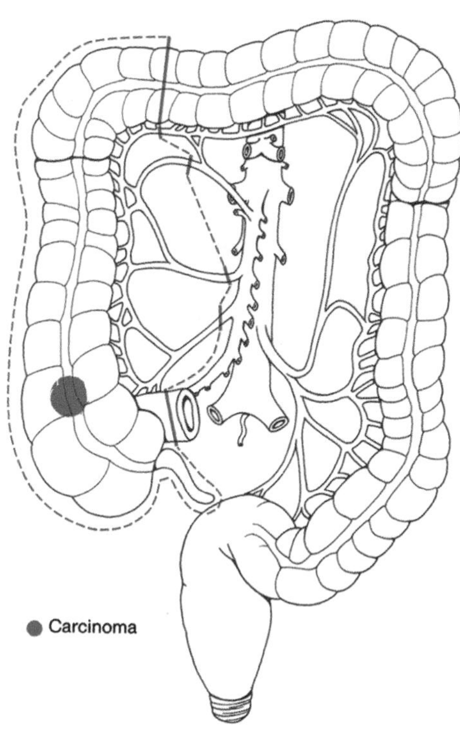

FIGURE 28 ■ Extent of resection for carcinoma in the cecum or ascending colon.

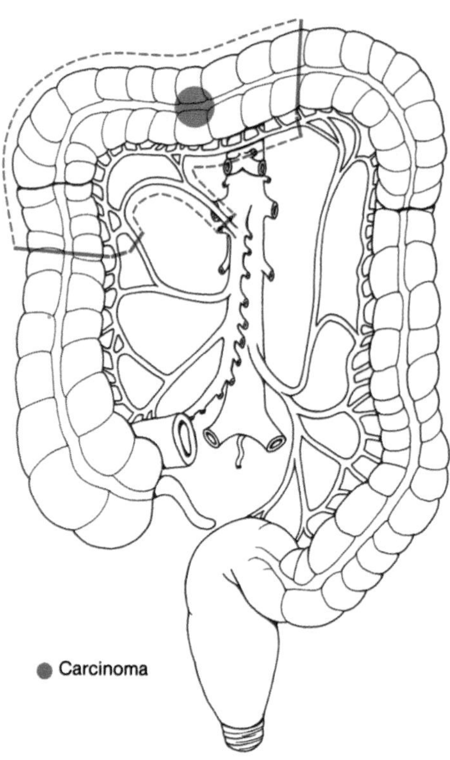

FIGURE 30 ■ Extent of resection for carcinoma in the transverse colon.

advocated for all operations for carcinoma include removal of the primary lesion with adequate margin, including the areas of lymphatic drainage. The definition of an adequate margin especially for rectal carcinoma remains controversial. Approximately one half of the patients seeking operative treatment already have metastatic disease spread to the regional lymph nodes. Controversy exists as to the

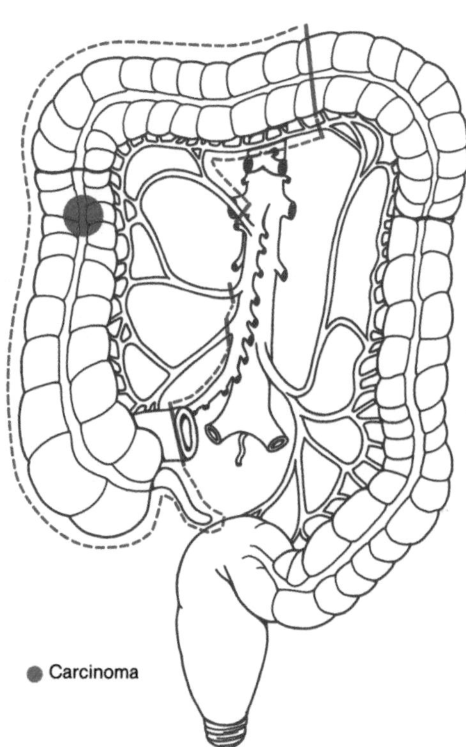

FIGURE 29 ■ Extent of resection for carcinoma in the hepatic flexure.

appropriate extent of lymphatic dissection. Is a segmental resection adequate therapy? Or with a sigmoid carcinoma, for example, should a formal left hemicolectomy be performed? For the most part the literature suggests that no survival advantage can be attributed to extended lymph node dissections for left colon and rectal carcinoma (386–389). An exception is the isolated report by Enker, Laffer, and Black (390). Without doubt this operation does result in increased morbidity, with patients often suffering from impotence, bladder difficulties, and potential vascular problems. Any marginal improvement is outweighed by the considerable morbidity. The principle of en bloc resection of involved structures is firmly established. Continued controversy surrounds radical lymph node dissection, luminal ligation, oophorectomy, and the "no-touch technique." What is becoming increasingly evident is that differences in outcome among different surgeons suggest that technique is important. Whether a properly performed lymphadenectomy may produce a therapeutic benefit or whether it is simply a more accurate staging procedure is unknown.

For lesions located in the cecum or the ascending colon, a right hemicolectomy to encompass the bowel served by the ileocolic, right colic, and right branch of the midcolic vessels is recommended (Fig. 28). For lesions involving the hepatic flexure, a more extended resection of the transverse colon is indicated (Fig. 29). For lesions in the transverse colon, depending on the portion involved, a segment of bowel is removed as shown in (Fig. 30). Splenic flexure lesions require removal of the distal half of the transverse colon and the descending colon (Fig. 31). Sigmoid lesions are appropriately treated by excision of the sigmoid colon (Fig. 32). Some surgeons prefer more radical excisions, but there is no convincing evidence to suggest that prolonged survival or decreased local

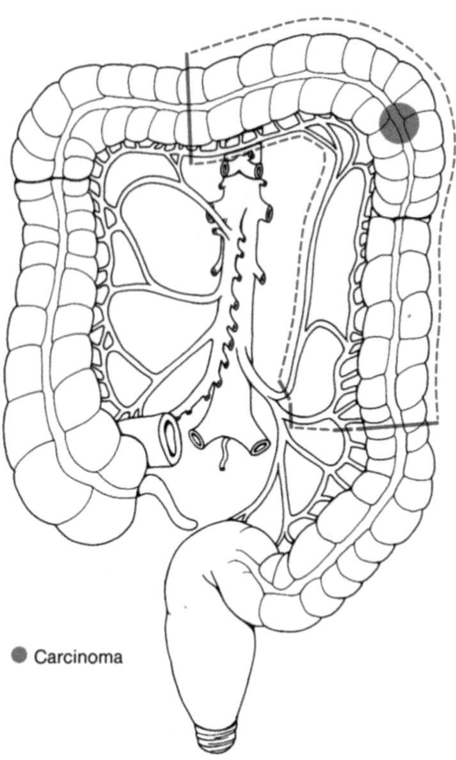

FIGURE 31 ■ Extent of resection for carcinoma in the splenic flexure.

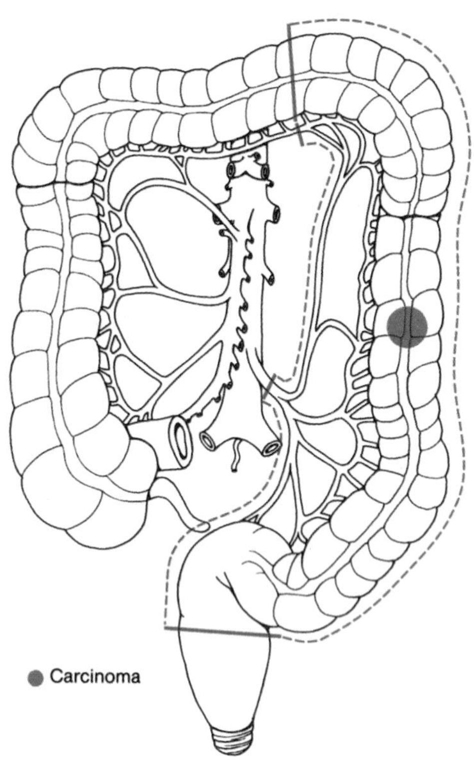

FIGURE 33 ■ Extended resection preferred by some surgeons for carcinoma in the sigmoid colon.

recurrence will result (Fig. 33). Indeed, operative mortality and postoperative complications are reportedly higher (386). For patients who have synchronous carcinomas in different portions of the colon, a subtotal colectomy seems appropriate (Fig. 34). Other suggested indications for subtotal colectomy include associated polyps (not removed by colonoscopy), acute or subacute obstruction, associated sigmoid diverticulosis (symptomatic), prior transverse colostomy for obstruction, young patient age (<50 years) with a positive family history, and adherence of the sigmoid colon to a cecal carcinoma (391).

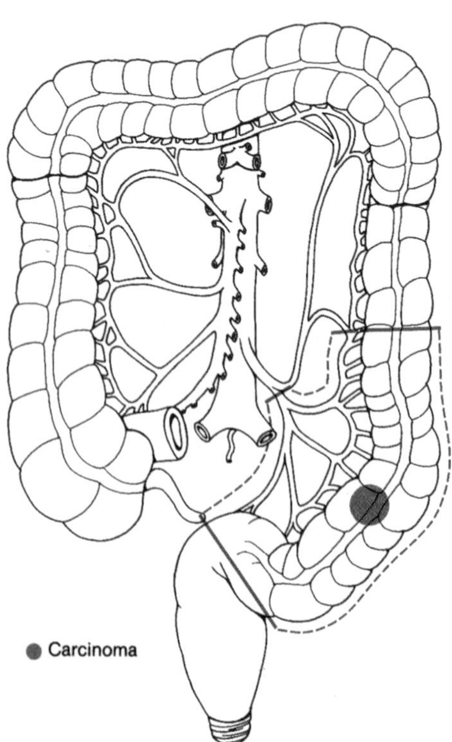

FIGURE 32 ■ Extent of resection for carcinoma in the sigmoid colon.

The techniques described in the following section pertain to good-risk patients. For poor-risk patients or patients undergoing palliative resection, segmental resections are more appropriate.

Certain intraoperative precautions have been proposed to eliminate or at least minimize the dissemination of malignant cells. Concern has been expressed that manipulation of the carcinoma results in blood-borne metastases. There is also the risk of exfoliated malignant cells adjacent to the primary lesion becoming implanted at the suture line, in the peritoneal cavity, or in the wound. It has been postulated that handling of the primary lesion early in the operation promotes such dissemination. This thesis was supported by the demonstration of malignant cell in the circulation (392,393), a finding that led Turnbull et al. (394) to popularize the no-touch technique in which lymphovascular channels were ligated prior to any manipulation of the primary lesion. After using this maneuver, they reported improved survival rates for Dukes' C lesions. However, this was not a controlled trial, and Turnbull's results have not been duplicated. Therefore the technique has not been adopted by most surgeons as standard therapy.

In an effort to avoid implantation of malignant cells shed from the primary carcinoma, Cole, Packard, and Souffiwic (393) recommended encirclement of the bowel lumen proximal and distal to the primary lesion. This is a simple addition to the operation and can usually be performed easily. Wound edges can be covered to prevent malignant cell implantation in the wound. In an effort to diminish the risk of implantation of malignant cells distal to the lesion, a host of cytotoxic agents (e.g., Dakin's

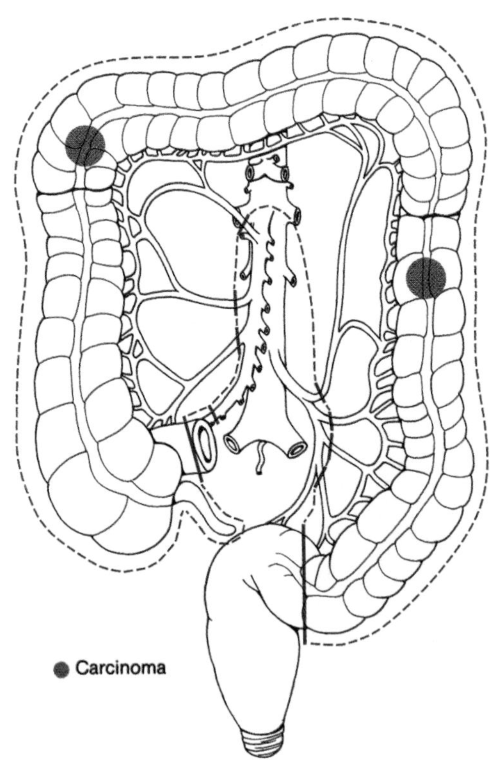

FIGURE 34 ■ Extent of resection for synchronous carcinomas in different portions of the colon.

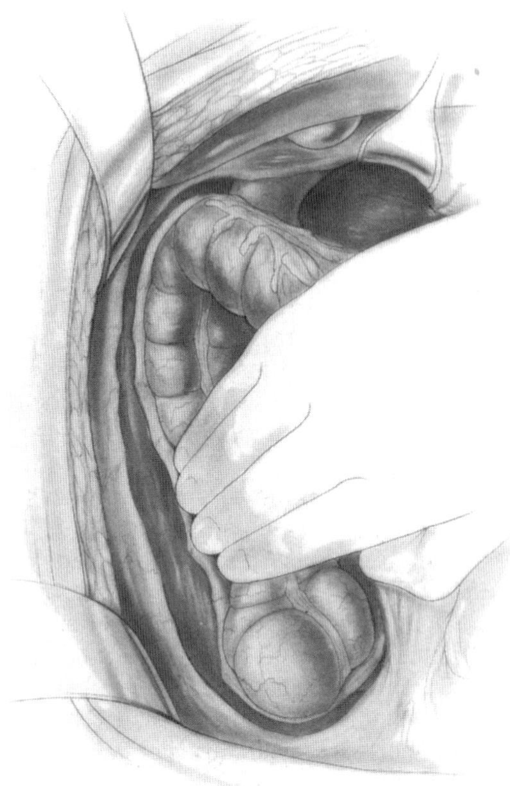

FIGURE 35 ■ Incision of parietal peritoneum.

solution or bichloride of mercury) have been used to irrigate the distal bowel; distilled water has also been used for this purpose. Since none of these cytotoxic agents has been used in a clinical trial setting, their value is in question. As a means of diminishing suture line implantation, iodized catgut was popular for a brief time (395). Another effort is the intraluminal installation of diluted formalin, in which case local recurrence was reportedly reduced to 2.6% from 14.3% for untreated patients (396).

None of the techniques tried thus far, including irrigation of the peritoneal cavity or the use of iodized catgut, has been proven of value. However, proximal and distal ligation of the bowel would appear to be a harmless practice. Adjuvant chemotherapy administered directly into the bowel lumen at the time of operation has been used but not in a trial setting. These empirical maneuvers were the forerunners of the clinical trials currently in progress.

Technique

RIGHT HEMICOLECTOMY ■ With the appropriate retractor in place and the small bowel packed toward the left side of the abdomen, the procedure is begun by incising the parietal peritoneum from just below the terminal ileum toward the hepatic flexure (Fig. 35). This can be done with Metzenbaum scissors or preferably by use of diathermy. If feasible, the colon is encircled above and below the carcinoma with umbilical tapes. This procedure is performed as soon as the lesion is appropriately mobile. The right colon is elevated from the retroperitoneum, with care taken not to injure the ureter, gonadal vessels, or inferior vena cava (Fig. 36). As dissection is carried toward the hepatic flexure, attention is given to avoiding any injury to the duodenum. Peritoneal division is continued around the hepatic flexure and horizontally along the upper border of the transverse colon, with division of any adhesions to the gallbladder. As dissection continues, the lesser sac is opened by dividing the gastrocolic ligament. Mobilization is continued for as far as the resection is planned. During this stage of the operation, the second and third portions of the duodenum are

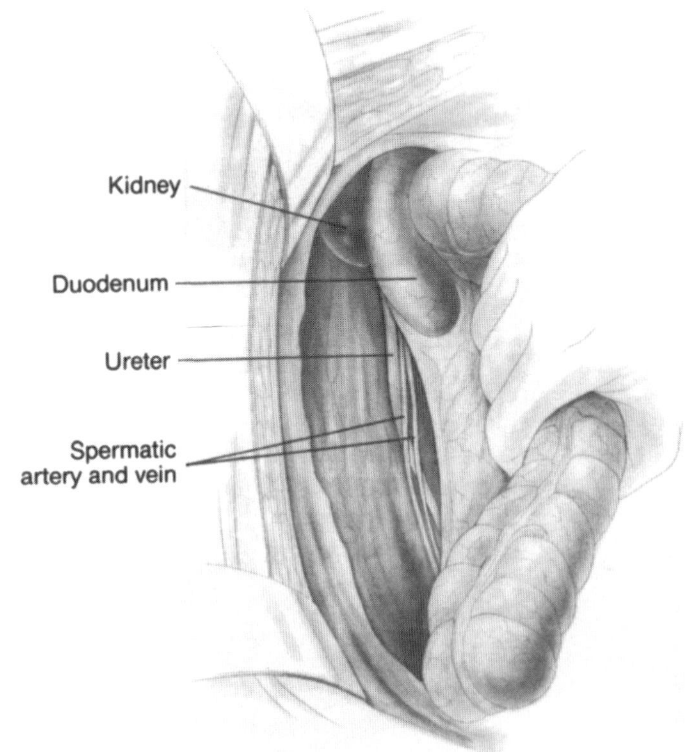

FIGURE 36 ■ Mobilization of the right colon. Exposure of the duodenum with care taken to avoid injury to retroperitoneal structures.

exposed, and caution should be exercised to prevent injury to this structure. Next, the greater omentum is transected vertically (Fig. 37). The medial aspect of the peritoneum then is incised along the planned area of resection. Mesenteric attachments are divided until the vascular anatomy is clear. The vessels are now displayed, and their trunks are triply clamped and divided, and the remaining end is doubly ligated (Fig. 38). The ileocolic, right colic, and right branches of the middle colic artery are divided in turn. The small vessels adjacent to the small bowel and transverse colon at the level of the proposed transection are divided between clamps, and hemostasis is secured. The two ends of bowel are now ready for division (Fig. 39). The technique the surgeon adopts—stapling or suturing—will-direct how the bowel is handled.

Surgeons, who advocate the no-touch isolation technique ligate the lymphovascular structures as the initial maneuver of the operation. An incision is made in the root of the mesentery, and the trunks of the vessels are identified, divided, and ligated prior to any mobilization. The major concern with this method is the potential need to deal with the ureter, gonadal vessels, and duodenum without the benefit of adequate exposure, which may keep these structures out of harm's way. In terms of long-term survival advantage, the efficacy of this method has not been supported in surgical trials against standard operative procedures. In a multicenter prospective randomized controlled trial, Wiggers, Jeekel, arid Arends (397) compared the no-touch isolation technique to a conventional technique. Both overall and corrected survival data did not differ between the two groups, although there was a tendency toward reduction in the number of occurrences and the length of time to the development of liver metastases with the no-touch technique.

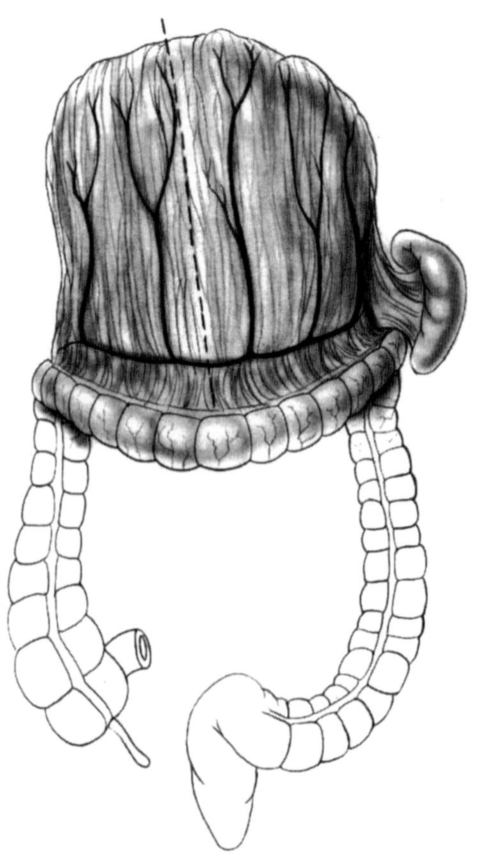

FIGURE 37 ■ Transection of the greater omentum.

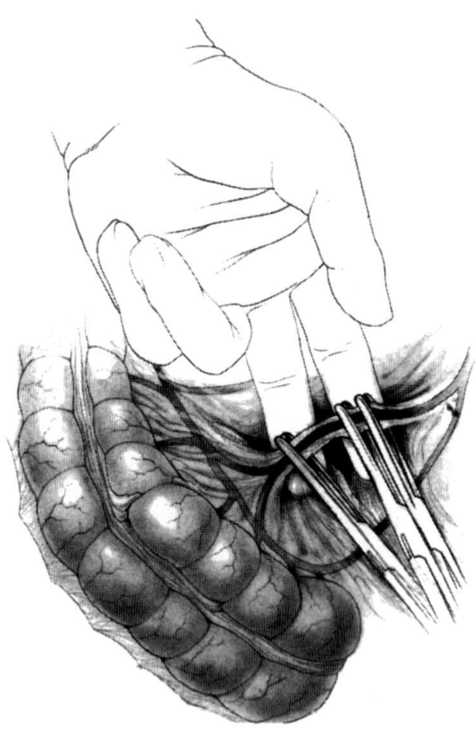

FIGURE 38 ■ Ligation and division of vessels.

For the reestablishment of intestinal continuity, my preference is to use staplers. A functional end-to-end anastomosis is created in the following way (398). Once the site of transection has been selected, a small area (less than that necessary for hand-sutured anastomoses) is cleared. Enough fat is cleared from the edge so that when the bowel opening is closed, there is room for the linear stapler to be applied without inclusion of mesenteric fat or appendices epiploicae. Obesity per se is not a contraindication to the use of staplers. In fact, since less clearing is necessary, staplers may have an advantage in such circumstances. The linear anastomosing instrument is applied in the mesenteric-antimesenteric plane (Fig. 40A). If the bowel diameter is too large to fit within the jaws of the instrument, such as with the transverse colon, the instrument is placed so that

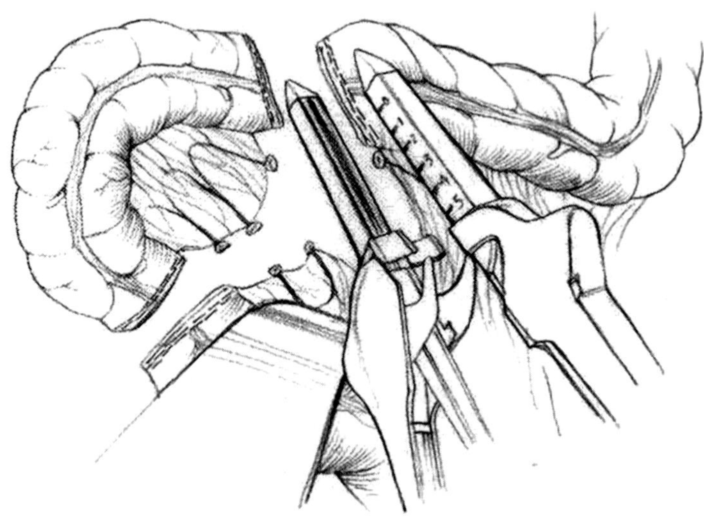

FIGURE 39 ■ Application of stapler to divide the bowel.

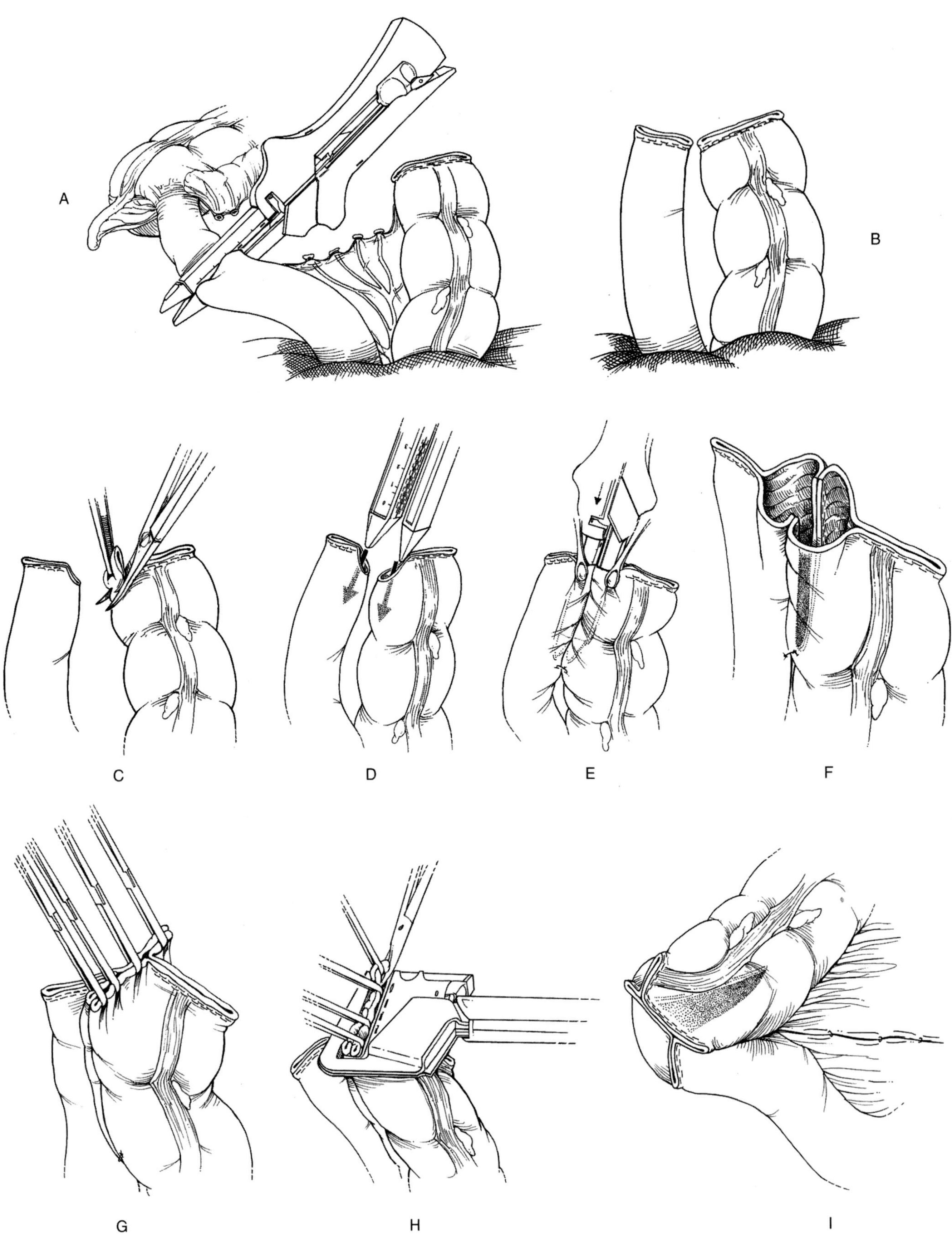

FIGURE 40 ■ (**A**) After complete bowel mobilization, the segment of bowel to be resected is transected with the anastomosing stapling instrument. Meseriteric edges are approximated. (**B**) Alignment of proximal and distal resected ends with closure of the mesentery completed. (**C**) Excision of the antimesenteric corner to accommodate the anastomosing stapler. (**D**) Insertion of each limb of the instrument into the bowel ends to be anastomosed. (**E**) With the bowel ends snugly fitted to the neck of the stapler to-provide maximum length of anastomosis, the instrument is activated and the anastomosis is accomplished. Suture is placed through antimesenteric border of bowel just beyond the bowel anastomosis. (**F**) Staple line is carefully inspected for proper completion and possible bleeding from the line. (**G**) Approximation of the bowel edges performed so that the previous staple lines are staggered and the side-to-side anastomosis created is in the open shape of a V. Application of Allis clamps to include the full thickness of the bowel wall and. the complete circumference of the bowel. (**H**) Application of the linear stapler with excision of excess tissue. Alternatively, bowel opening can be closed with the anastomosing instrument. (**I**) Completed anastomosis with the staple lines clearly demonstrated.

the tips of the instrument are on the antimesenteric border. Then if the bowel is not completely transected and stapled closed, the open area will occur where an opening would have been made to create the functional end-to-end anastomosis. The advantage of a stapled transection is that little or no devascularization of the bowel is necessary. With manual anastomoses too little clearing may make anastomotic suturing insecure, and too much may jeopardize the viability of the bowel ends. Caution, however, must be exercised in patients with diverticular disease.

It is often easier to close the mesentery before the anastomosis is constructed, especially with a right hemicolectomy and with patients who are overweight. Completing this step prior to constructing the anastomosis also will diminish the possibility of the error of rotation of the ileum (Fig. 40B).

The antimesenteric borders are aligned, and at each corner an amount of tissue just adequate to insert the fork of the anastomosing instrument is excised (Fig. 40C). The instrument is inserted to its full length to create a large anastomosis (Fig. 40D). The halves of the instrument are joined and the bowel is drawn up, which ensures an anastomosis that is the full length that the instrument is capable of creating (Fig. 40E). The anastomosis should be checked to see that it is being created through the antimesenteric border and that no fat, omentum, mesentery, sponge, or viscus is trapped. It might be best to insert the "sleeping suture of Steichen" before the instrument is removed. The suture is placed at the end of the anastomosis on the antimesenteric border of the bowel to diminish any possible tension on the anastomosis. It should be noted that the use of this suture is omitted in patients with Crohn's disease for fear of possible development of a fistula. Alternatively, the suture may be placed prior to insertion of the stapler. The halves of the instrument should be gently separated because excessive force may result in disruption of the anastomosis. Some bleeding at the suture line is not uncommon and may be controlled by sponge compression, light cautery, or suture ligature. Excessive cautery may result in a weakened anastomosis and may predispose to leakage. Heavy bleeding should be controlled with fine sutures.

The anastomotic suture lines are held apart in preparation for the application of the linear stapler (Fig. 40F). Welter, Charlier, and Psalmon (399) showed that with the functional end-to-end anastomosis the area of the anastomosis can be increased by up to one third of the original bowel lumen if the linear stapler closing staple line is applied so as to hold the anastomosing staple lines in an open V position. There is also the very remote possibility that if the suture lines remain in apposition, unwanted healing may occur from one to the other.

The staple lines should be staggered when the linear stapler is applied (Fig. 40G). This modification was suggested by Chassin, Rifkind, and Turner (400) to avoid too many intersecting staple lines, which may create an ischemic point with potential for a leak. Allis clamps are applied to the tissues being approximated to prevent a portion of the bowel circumference from slipping back as the jaws of the instrument compress the tissue (Fig. 40H). The instrument is fired, and the excess tissue is cut away prior to release of the instrument to avoid injury to the anastomosis. A fine ooze of blood is reassuring of a good blood supply to the anastomosis, but more brisk bleeding should be controlled with gentle cautery or a fine suture. Alternatively, the bowel opening can be closed with the application of the anastomosing instrument. This technical variation has been suggested to reduce the cost of the anastomosis. If adopted, care should be taken to ensure that the instrument application does not compromise the size of the anastomosis. The anastomosis is checked to ensure that it is complete and no leak is present (Fig. 40I).

To determine the results of our experience with the use of staples for construction of anastomoses following colonic resection, we reviewed a series of 223 anastomoses performed in 205 patients (401). Indications for operation included malignancy, benign neoplasms, inflammatory bowel disease, and several miscellaneous entities. A functional end-to-end anastomoses using the standard GIA cartridge and the TA 55 instruments was performed. The operative mortality rate was 1.5%, with none of the deaths related to the anastomosis. Intraoperative complications encountered included bleeding (21), leak (one), tissue fracture (one), instrument failure (four), and technical error (three). Early postoperative complications related to or potentially related to the anastomosis included bleeding (five), pelvic abscess (one), fistula (one), peritonitis (two), and ischemia of the anastomosis (one).

Late complications included five patients with small bowel obstruction, two of whom required operation. Anastomotic recurrences developed in 5.9% of patients. Our experience with stapling instruments has shown them to be a reliable method for performing anastomoses in the colon in a safe and expeditious manner. Complications after functional end-to-end anastomoses reported by other authors are depicted in Table 7.

A variety of commercial instruments are available for the construction of stapled anastomoses (Fig. 41).

TABLE 7 ■ Complications After Functional End-to-End Anastomosis

Author(s)	No. of Cases	Bleeding (%)	Fistula or Leak (%)	Intraperitoneal Abscess (%)	Obstruction or Stenosis (%)	Operative Mortality (%)
Chassin et al. (402) (1978)	181	0	1.1	1.7	1.1	0.7
Fortin, Poulin, and Leclerc (403) (1979)	118	0	5.0	0	0.8	2.5
Brodman and Brodman (404) (1981)	88	0	0	2.3	*	0
Reuter (405) (1982)	69	0	9.0	*	*	2.9
Scher et al. (406) (1982)	35	*	2.9	*	*	8.6
Steichen and Ravitch (407) (1984)	264	0.4	3.4	*	0.8	*
Tuchmann et al. (408) (1985)	51	2.0	6.0	*	*	0.4
Kyzer and Gordon (401) (1992)	223	2.2	0.9	0.4	0	1.5
Kracht et al. (409) (1993)	106	*	2.8	1.9	*	1.9

*Not addressed.

A
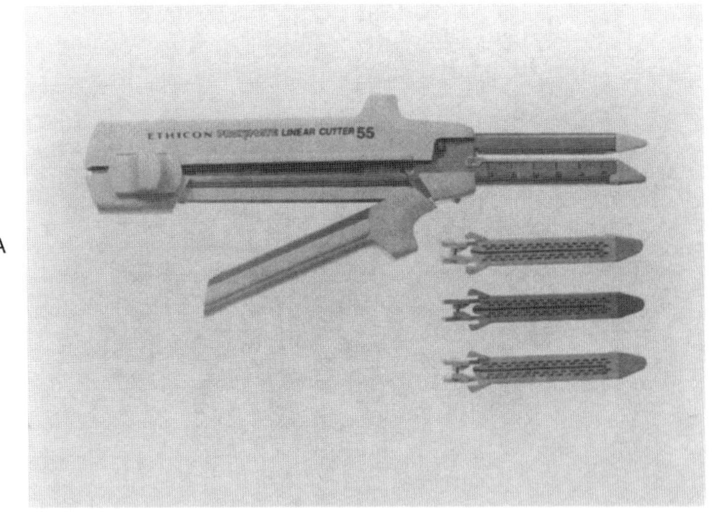

B
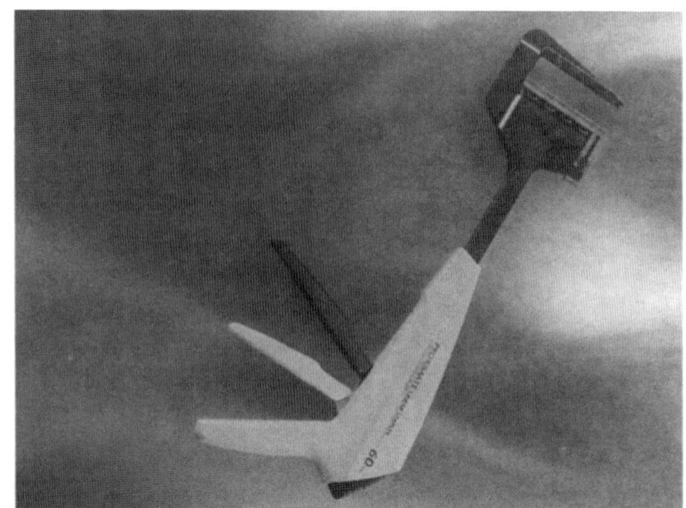

C
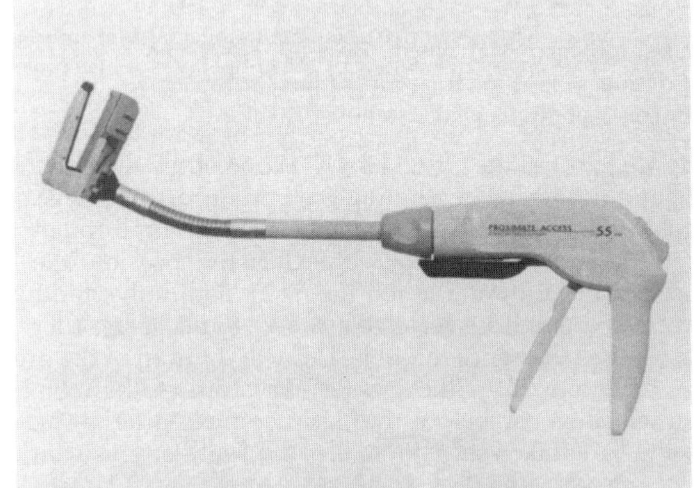

D
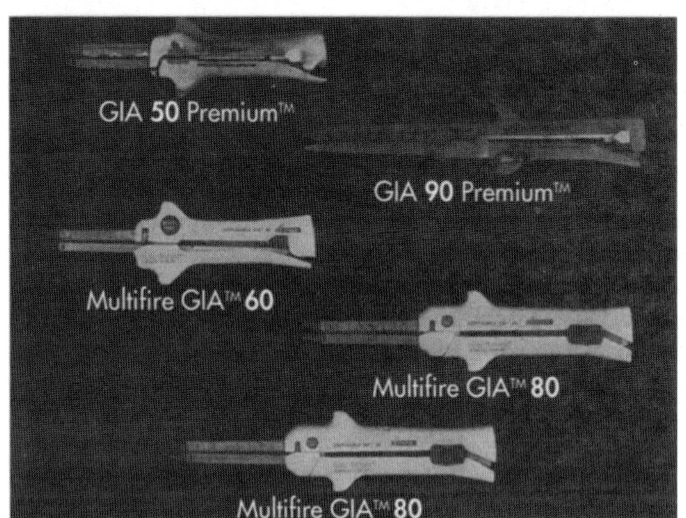

E
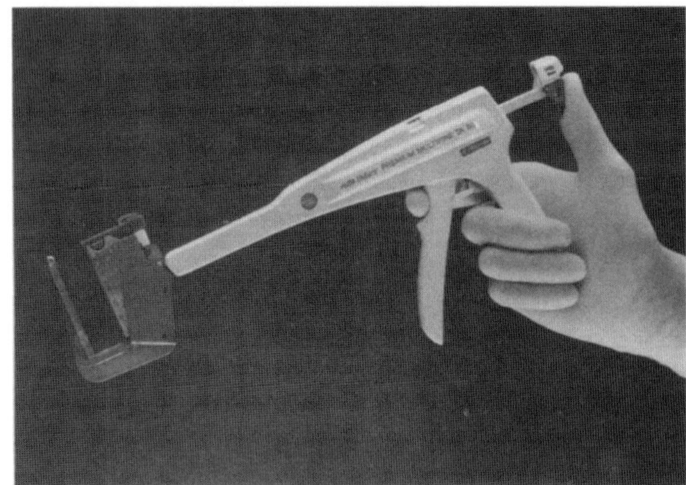

F
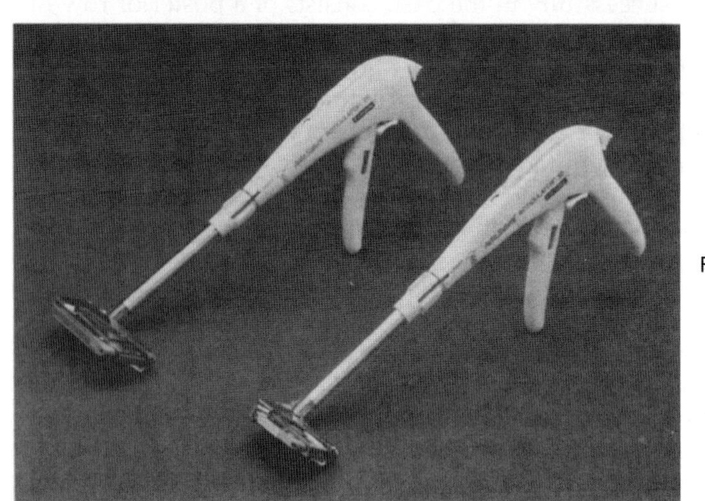

G
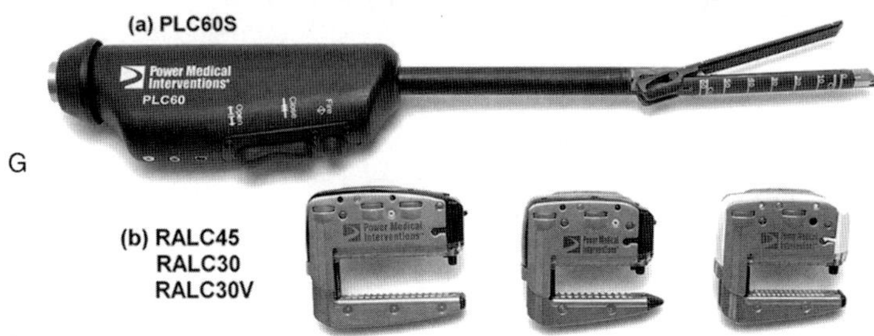

FIGURE 41 ■ Instruments for constructing stapled anastomoses. (**A**) Proximate linear cutter. (**B**) Proximate linear stapler. (**C**) Flexible proximate access stapler. (**D**) GIA staplers. (**E**) TA stapler. (**F**) Roticulator. (**G**) Computer-powered linear surgical stapling products: (*a*) Reusable 60 mm linear cutter, (*b*) right-angle linear cutters: 45 mm, 30 mm, and 30 mm vascular. *Source*: (**A, B, C**): courtesy of Ethicon Inc., Sommerville, NJ; (**D, E, F**): courtesy of U.S. Surgical Corp., Norwalk, CT; (**G**): courtesy of Power Medical Interventions, Langhorne, PA.

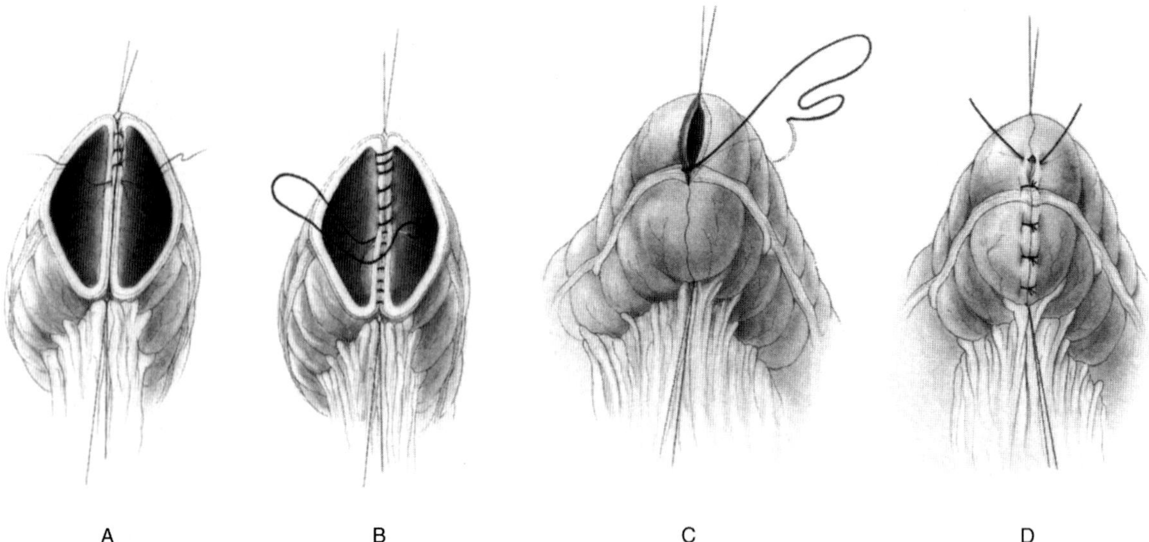

FIGURE 42 ■ (**A**) Posterior placement of outer layer of seromuscular interrupted sutures. (**B**) Placement of continuous inner layer of absorbable sutures. (**C**) Continuation of inner layer of sutures anteriorly. (**D**) Completion of anastomosis by anterior placement of layer of interrupted seromuscular sutures.

When a hand-sutured anastomosis is elected, the bowel edges are transected obliquely to ensure adequate blood supply at the bowel edges to be anastomosed. Today most surgeons prefer end-to-end anastomoses. Even where there is a disparity in size of the bowel lumina, as occurs in anastomoses of the ileum to the transverse colon, the discrepancy can be readily overcome by division of the antimesenteric border of the ileum. Considerable controversy has been engendered about whether to use a one-layer or two-layer anastomosis and the type of suture material to be used. The two-layer technique, which I have used successfully in the past, consists of a posterior row of 4–0 silk or vicryl placed on a fine atraumatic needle into the seromuscular layer. An inner layer of 4–0 chromic catgut or vicryl is placed through the full thickness of the bowel wall, begun on one edge, and continued on the posterior wall in a simple running over-and-over suture but with a change to the Connell suture on the anterior half. The anterior seromuscular layer is then completed with 4–0 silk or vicryl sutures (Fig. 42).

A growing number of surgeons have favored a single-layer inverting interrupted technique. A posterior interrupted single layer of an absorbable suture such as 3–0 or 4–0 Vicryl or Dexon has been used. The suture is then continued on the anterior wall (Fig. 43). Care must be taken not to invert excessive amounts of tissue, thereby causing narrowing of the lumen, but this is true for any type of hand-sutured anastomosis. Some surgeons prefer to use a Gambee suture for the single-layer anastomosis (Fig. 44). Other suture materials such as Prolene and wire have been used.

Copious saline irrigation of the abdominal cavity is performed to remove blood, bacteria, and debris. Drains are not necessary. Wounds are closed with continuous absorbable sutures for the peritoneum and fascia, with staples or subcuticular continuous absorbable material used for the skin.

Resection of Transverse Colon

The appropriate operation for a carcinoma of the transverse colon has been a controversial matter. The reason is the desire to fulfill the criteria for resection of the regional lymphatic drainage. Depending on portion of the transverse colon that is involved, drainage may occur through the middle and/or right colic branches and possibly the left colic branches. For a lesion that is located in the midtransverse colon, a transverse colectomy would be in order.

The procedure might begin with division of the greater omentum from the greater curvature of the stomach, either above or below the gastroepiploic arterial arcade, with care taken not to injure the wall of the stomach

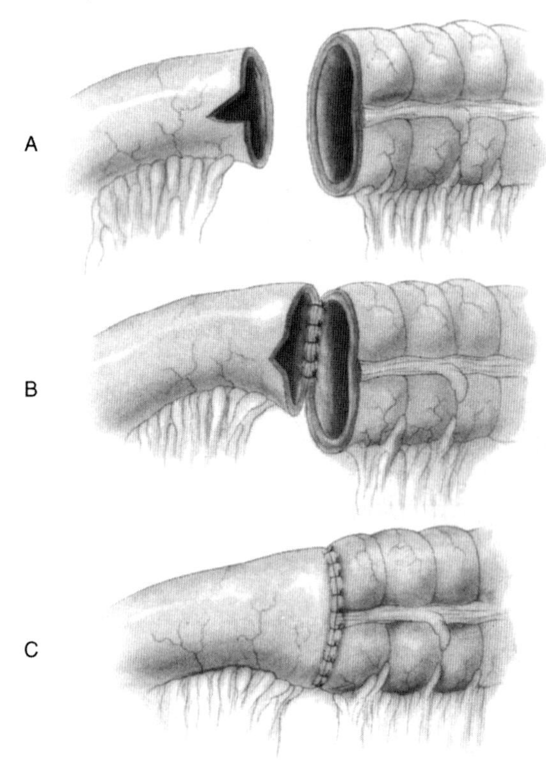

FIGURE 43 ■ (**A**) When disparity in bowel ends exists, smaller end may be fishmouthed. Alignment of bowel ends for anastomosis. (**B**) Placement of single layer of interrupted sutures in a posterior row. (**C**) Completed anastomosis by placement of anterior row of interrupted sutures. *Source:* From Ref. 410.

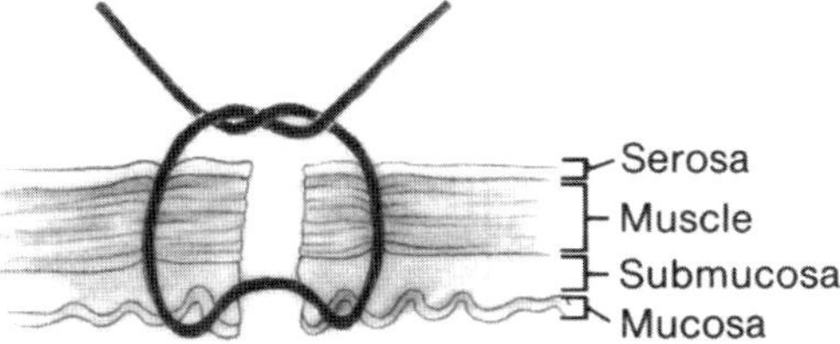

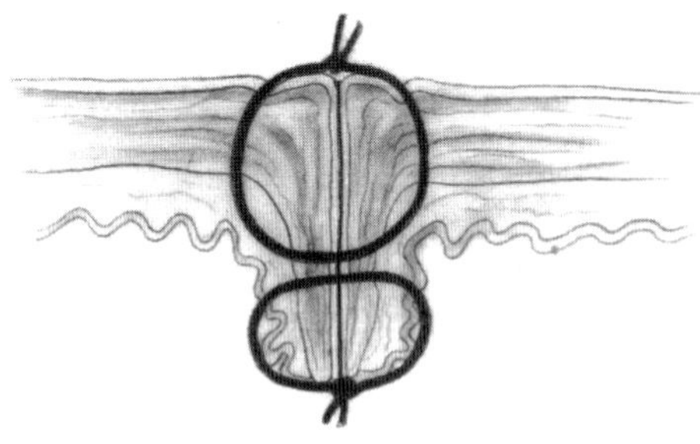

FIGURE 44 ■ Placement of the Gambee suture is begun with the full-thickness bowel and continued with the mucosa and submucosa on the same side. Suturing is continued on the opposite side with the submucosa and mucosa and then the full-thickness wall. Inverted anastomosis is thus created.

(Fig. 45). In the event of a very redundant transverse colon, the omentum may be divided vertically on either side at the proposed proximal and distal lines of resection of the colon. For a short transverse colon, the entire omentum may be included in the resected specimen. To avoid tension on the anastomosis, either one or both of the hepatic and splenic flexures will require mobilization. It is often technically easier to resect the right and transverse colon rather than attempt to mobilize both flexures. The technique of mobilization of the hepatic flexure has been described in the discussion of right hemicolectomy.

Mobilization of the splenic flexure is facilitated by incising the lateral peritoneal attachment along the descending colon (Fig. 46). As the splenic flexure is approached, great care must be exercised to avoid injury to the spleen. The lienocolic ligament can be accentuated by passage of a finger along the colonic wall from the descending colon side toward the splenic flexure. The ligament then can be clamped and divided, or, alternatively, it can be divided with the use of cautery. Great caution should be exercised in this maneuver since there are frequently numerous adhesions to the splenic capsule. The peritoneum is incised on the mesocolon, and in the process the splenic flexure is mobilized downward and to the right, exposing the retroperitoneum. If the greater omentum becomes a limiting factor, division of the omentum is begun. Varying other posterior attachments may require division, with care taken not to incite bleeding in this location. The trunk of the middle colic vessel and smaller vessels are secured (Fig. 47). It should be noted that the origin of the middle colic vessels is quite proximal on the superior mesenteric vessels and must be pursued with extreme caution to prevent injury to these structures. The bowel is divided and an anastomosis is created as previously described. In reconstituting the mesenteric defect between the ileum and the descending colon, care

FIGURE 45 ■ Division of the greater omentum from the greater curvature of the stomach.

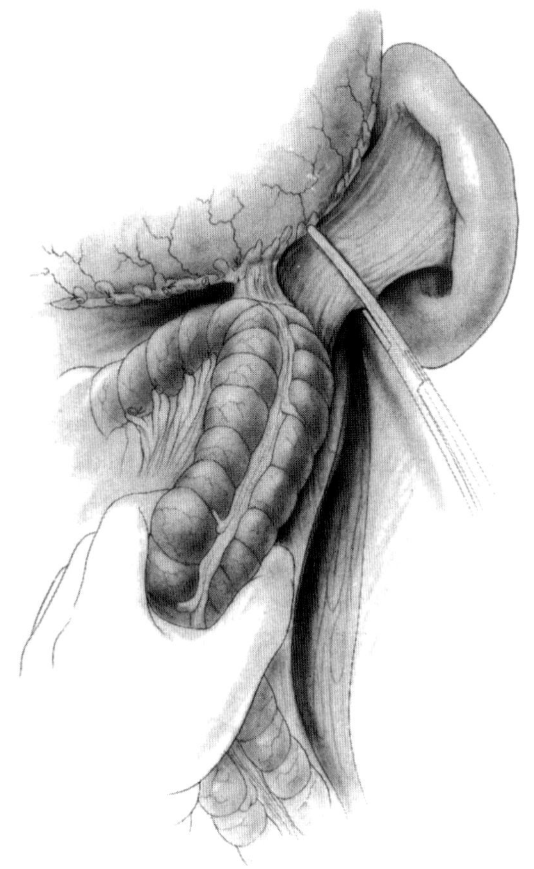

FIGURE 46 ■ Mobilization of the splenic flexure by division of the lienocolic ligament.

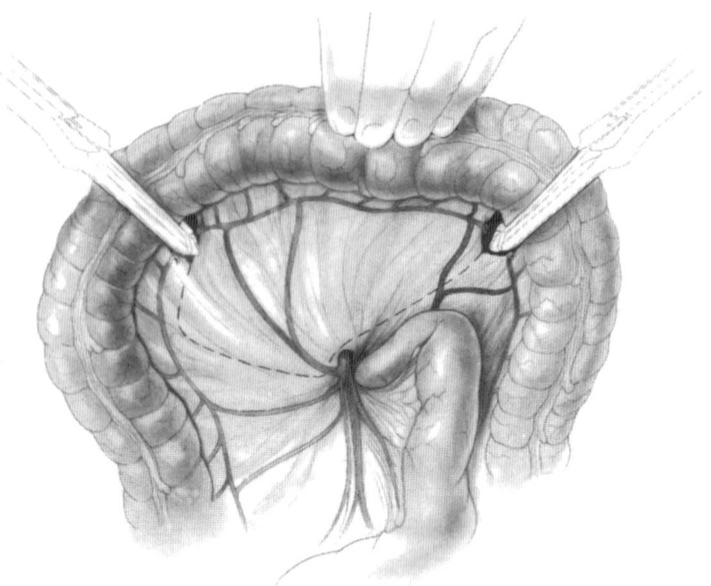

FIGURE 47 ■ Ligation and division of the middle colic and adjacent smaller vessels.

must be exercised to avoid narrowing of the duodenojejunal junction.

For lesions at or near the hepatic flexure or the ascending colon, a right hemicolectomy is performed. For lesions near the splenic flexure, a partial left colectomy with anastomosis of the transverse colon to the proximal sigmoid is performed (Fig. 48). Resection of this type may necessitate division of the left branch of the middle colic and left colic vessels.

Resection of Descending Colon

For lesions of the descending colon, the left branch of the middle colic artery remains intact, but the left colic artery and, depending on the level of the lesion, the first sigmoidal vessels are ligated. The anastomosis is performed between the distal transverse and proximal sigmoid colon. Some surgeons advocate a more formal left hemicolectomy.

Sigmoid Resection

Some controversy exists as to the most appropriate procedure for removal of a sigmoid carcinoma. One school of thought supports the necessity for a radical left hemicolectomy with anastomosis of the transverse colon to the rectum. However, there is a growing number of surgeons who realize that the extended resection has not resulted in increased survival rates. When patients who have lymphatics involved to the root of the inferior mesenteric artery have these resected, no increased survival rate is noted in comparison with patients who have a less radical procedure (388). It would, therefore, seem that the extra mobilization, with its potential risks and prolonged operating time, is not justified. The extent of the resection depends on the portion of the sigmoid colon involved. Lesions of the proximal sigmoid would require an anastomosis performed between the descending colon and the distal sigmoid, those of the distal sigmoid would involve an anastomosis between the proximal sigmoid and the upper rectum, and those of the mid-portion of the sigmoid, depending on the redundancy of the colon, would require an anastomosis between the sigmoid-descending junction and the rectosigmoid. The splenic flexure is not routinely mobilized, but, depending on the location of the lesion and the redundancy of the colon, it may require mobilization to avoid tension on the anastomosis.

The patient may be placed in the supine position, but for more distal lesions it is preferable to have the patient in the modified lithotomy position so that simultaneous access can be obtained through the abdomen and the rectum. This access is necessary to allow use of the circular stapling device or inspection of the anastomosis by proctosigmoidoscopy.

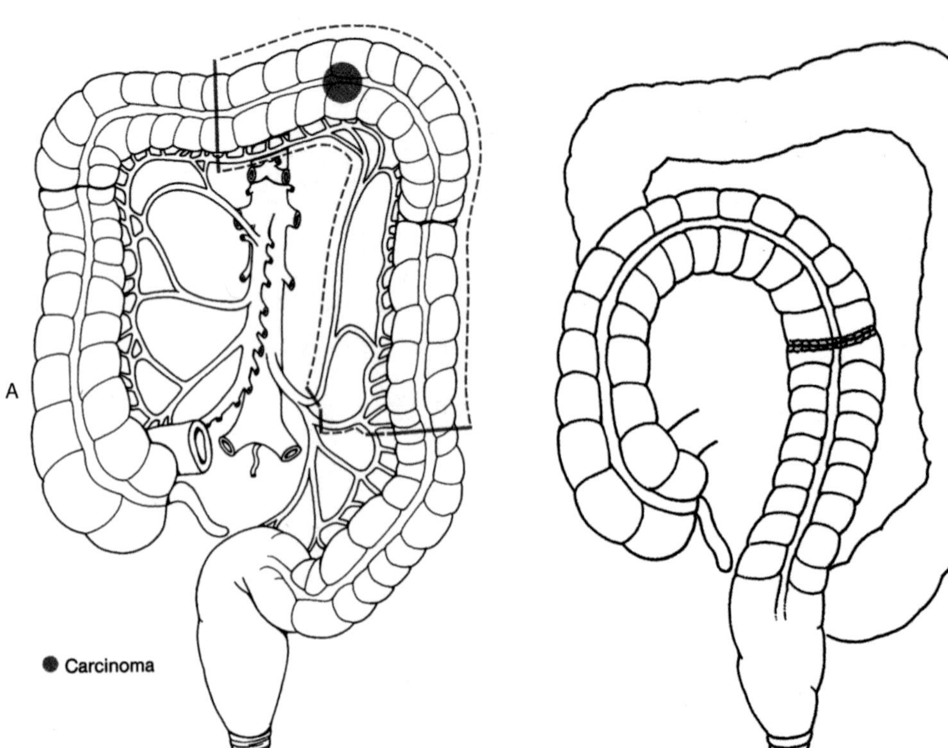

FIGURE 48 ■ (**A**) Extent of resection for carcinoma near the splenic flexure. (**B**) Result after resection.

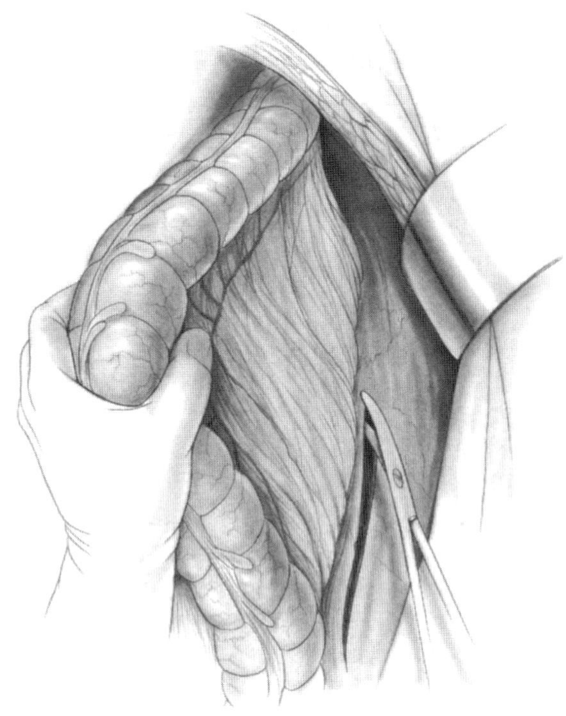

FIGURE 49 ■ Incision of peritoneum along the white line of Toldt.

The procedure is initiated by incising the peritoneum along the white line of Toldt in the left paracolic gutter, freeing the distal descending colon and the sigmoid from their developmental attachments from the splenic flexure to the pelvic brim (Fig. 49). In the midportion of the sigmoid meso-colon is the intersigmoid fossa, a small depression in the peritoneum that acts as a guide to the underlying ureter (Fig. 50). As the sigmoid mesentery is further mobilized, care is taken to displace the mesosigmoid from the left ureter, which is seen coursing over the iliac vessels (Fig. 51). The gonadal vessels should be protected in a similar way because injury will result in troublesome bleeding. After lateral mobilization and determination of the proximal line of resection, the peritoneum over the medial aspect of the mesosigmoid is incised toward the root of the inferior mesenteric artery to the level of the proposed ligation and then downward toward the pelvis. The inferior mesenteric artery, with its left colic and sigmoidal branches, will be identified (Fig. 52). The inferior mesenteric artery distal to

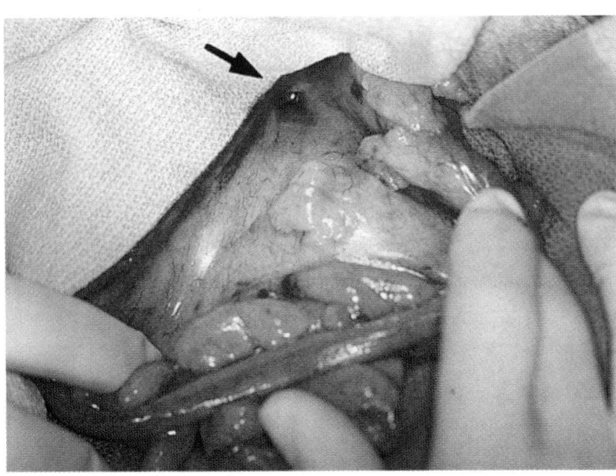

FIGURE 50 ■ Intersigmoid fossa.

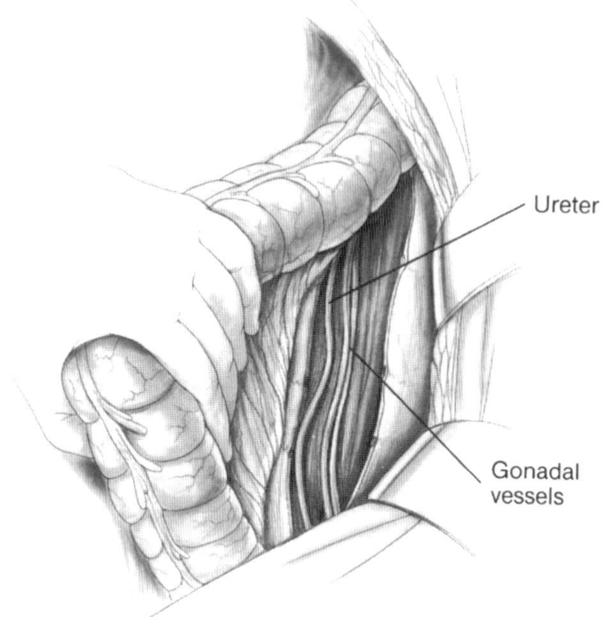

FIGURE 51 ■ Mobilization of the sigmoid colon with care taken not to injure retroperitoneal structures.

the left colic branch is then divided and ligated. Smaller vessels leading toward the planned lines of resection are secured, and the bowel is transected proximally and distally. As with the technique for right hemicolectomy, some surgeons advocate ligation and division of the blood supply prior to any other manipulation, but the same general principles pertain. In such a situation, depending on the extent of resection, the inferior mesenteric artery at its origin from the aorta (or distal to the left colic branch) and the inferior mesenteric vein at the level of the duodenum (or more distally for a lesser resection) require ligation and division. Abcarian and Pearl (411) have described a simple

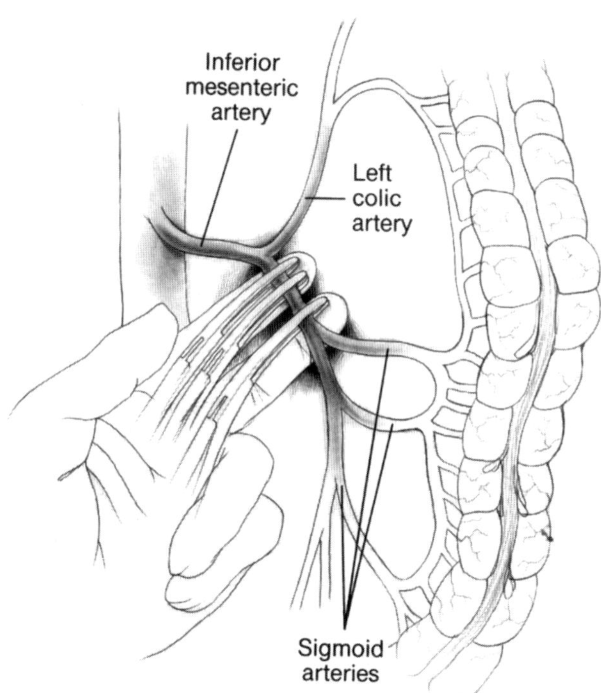

FIGURE 52 ■ Identification of the inferior mesenteric artery and its left colic and sigmoidal branches.

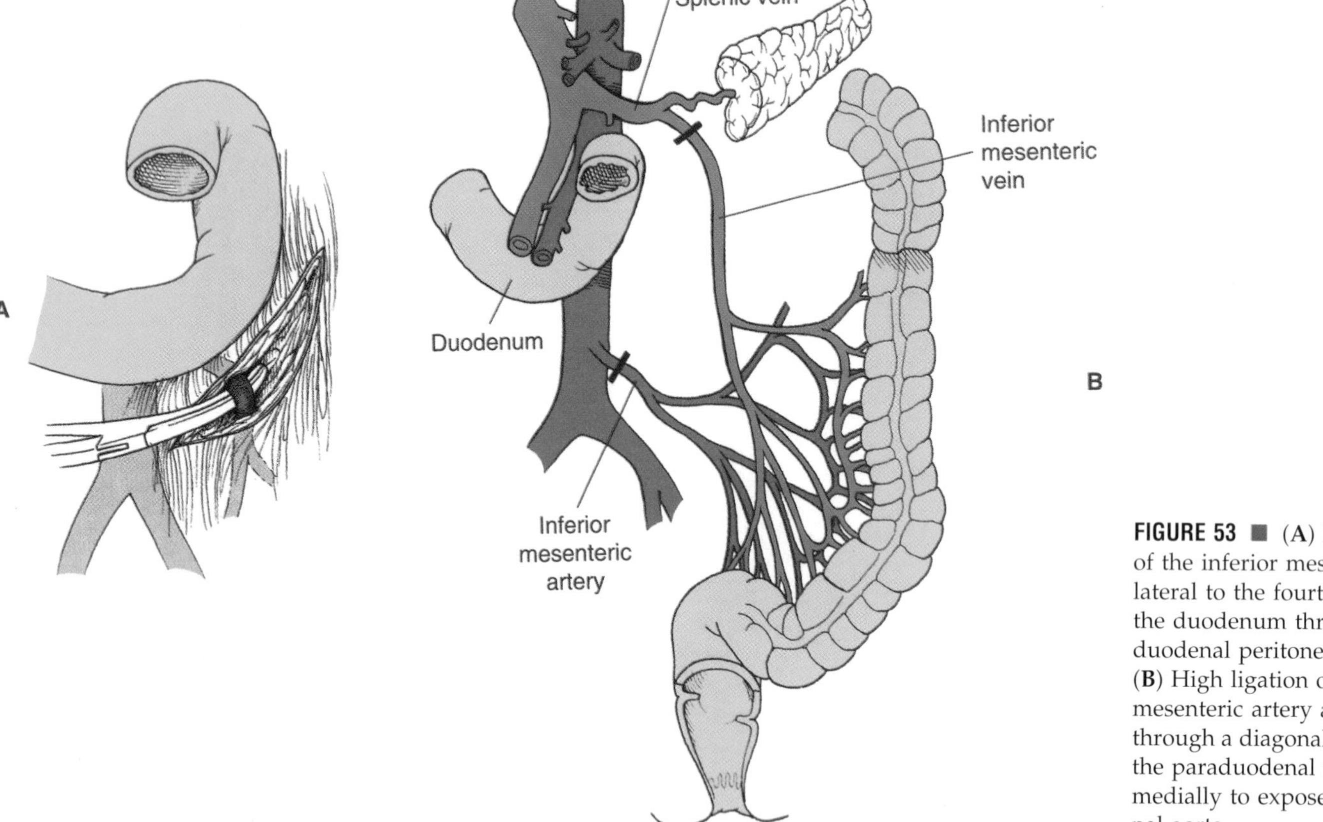

FIGURE 53 ■ (**A**) High ligation of the inferior mesenteric vein lateral to the fourth portion of the duodenum through a paraduodenal peritoneal incision. (**B**) High ligation of the inferior mesenteric artery at its origin through a diagonal extension of the paraduodenal incision medially to expose the infrarenal aorta.

technique for high ligation of the inferior mesenteric artery and vein. After completion of abdominal exploration, the small bowel is packed away toward the right side of the abdominal cavity to expose the duodenojejunal flexure. The peritoneum overlying the lateral border of the fourth portion of the duodenum is incised, exposing the inferior mesenteric vein. The vein is mobilized for 2 to 3 cm, ligated in continuity with non-absorbable suture, and divided. This incision is extended diagonally 5 to 6 cm medially to expose the infrarenal aorta proximal to its bifurcation. The inferior mesenteric artery is easily identified, doubly ligated in continuity, and divided at its origin. The lymph nodes surrounding the takeoff of the inferior mesenteric artery are dissected sharply in a proximal-to-distal manner to allow for their complete excision (Fig. 53). Heald (412) recommends division of the inferior mesenteric artery approximately 2 cm from the aorta to preserve the autonomic nerves, which split around its origin.

The anastomosis is then created according to the surgeon's method of choice. However, if the anastomosis is low, my preference is to use the circular stapler as described in detail in Chapter 24. For surgeons who deem it necessary to perform a radical left hemicolectomy, the operation is conducted in a similar way by combining the mobilization of the sigmoid, the splenic flexure, and the distal transverse colon. The notable difference is the level at which the vessels are secured. To accomplish the radical left hemicolectomy, the posterior parietal peritoneum is incised to expose the inferior mesenteric vessels. The artery is tied flush with the aorta, and the vein is ligated separately at the level of the duodenum (Fig. 54).

Bilateral Salpingo-Oophorectomy

In a review of their experience and the surgical literature, Birnkrant, Sampson, and Sugarbaker (413) found the incidence of ovarian metastases from colorectal carcinoma to be approximately 6% with a range of 1.5% to 13.6%. In a prospective controlled study, Graffner, Aim, and Oscarson (414) detected ovarian metastases in 10.3% of patients undergoing operations on all segments of the large bowel. Since bilateral involvement occurs between 50% and 70% of the time, a bilateral oophorectomy is recommended, especially for postmenopausal women. However,

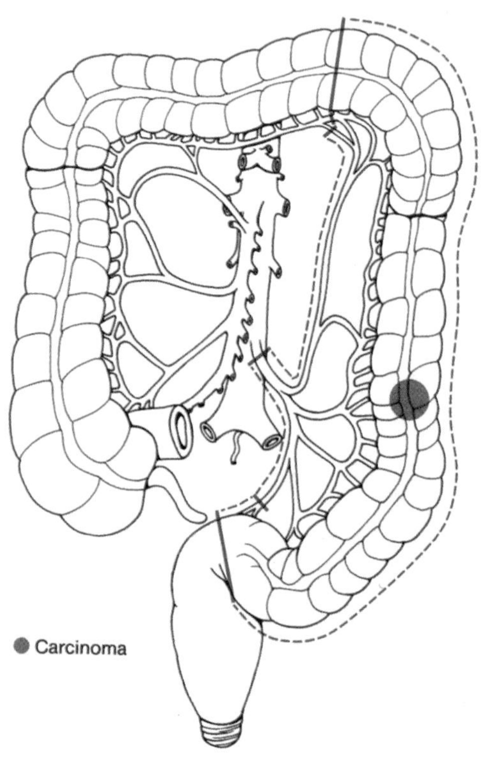

FIGURE 54 ■ High ligation of the inferior mesenteric artery and vein.

controversy exists about the role of prophylactic oophorectomy dunrig resecticin of primary colorectal carcinoma. Sielezneff et al. (415) attempted to prospectively assess the prognostic impact of simultaneous bilateral oophorectomy in postmenopausal women undergoing curative resection for colorectal carcinoma. Ovarian metastases were detected in 2.4% of the operative specimens. Local recurrence or liver metastases rates were not affected by oophorectomy. Five-year actuarial survival rates were not significantly different whether patients had oophorectomy (81.6%) or not (87.9%). Their results suggested that microscopic synchronous ovarian metastases is rare at the time of curative resection of a colorectal carcinoma in postmenopausal women and does not modify prognosis. Young-Fadok et al. (416) conducted a prospective randomized trial of 152 patients to evaluate the influence of oophorectomy on recurrence and survival in patients with Dukes' B and C stage colorectal carcinoma. In 76 patients randomized to oophorectomy, no incidence of gross or microscopic metastatic disease to the ovary was found. Preliminary survival curves suggest a survival benefit for oophorectomy of 2 to 3 years after operation, but this benefit does not appear to persist at 5 years (Fig. 55). There has been no incidence of colorectal carcinoma metastatic to the ovaries in this series of Dukes' B and C stage carcinoma, unlike other nonrandomized studies of all stages, which have reported a 4% to 10% incidence. These authors concluded that the possibility of a survival advantage emphasizes the need to continue this preliminary work.

Concomitant oophorectomy is controversial, and its efficacy in prolonging survival has been questioned since few patients survive 5 years after operation. However, it generally adds little to the operation and will prevent the subsequent development of ovarian carcinoma (417). Removal of the ovaries at the time of bowel resection will eliminate the need for repeat laparotomy to resect an ovarian mass in approximately 2% of women with large bowel carcinoma (413). Oophorectomy is often recommended more strongly for patients who have carcinoma of the rectum, but no site in the colon results in a greater proportion of ovarian metastases. The apparent greater proportion from the left colon is probably due to the fact that this portion of the large bowel harbors the largest number of malignancies.

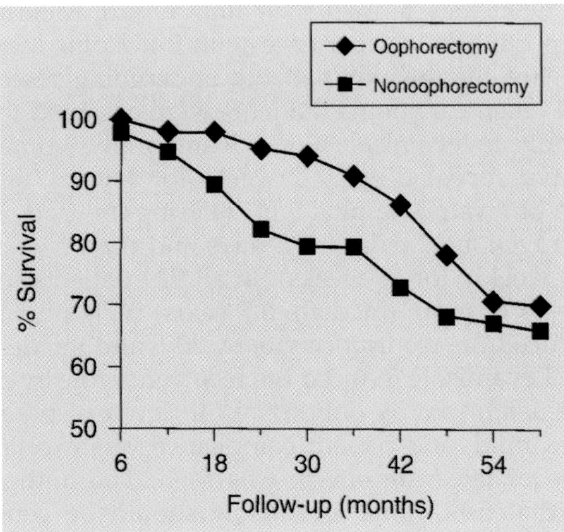

FIGURE 55 ■ Survival curves for prophylactic oophorectomy during resection for primary colorectal carcinoma. *Source*: From Ref. 416.

Oophorectomy should be performed in premenopausal women if any gross abnormality of the ovary is detected (413). Indeed, ovarian metastases of colorectal origin have been reported to occur more commonly in premenopausal women, with rates ranging from 3.8% to 28% (413,418). This finding might support the recommendation for prophylactic oophorectomy regardless of patient age (419). Certainly, contiguous involvement necessitates en bloc resection. Ovarian involvement carries with it a poor prognosis (420).

Postoperative Care

The postoperative care of the patient is discussed in Chapter 4. It should be noted that it is not necessary to use nasogastric suctioning on a routine basis.

■ ADJUVANT THERAPY

In the last half century, there has been very little improvement in the ultimate 5-year survival rate of patients operated on for colorectal carcinoma, and physicians are constantly trying methods that will improve the current results. Five general principles underlie adjuvant therapy (421):

1. There may be occult, viable malignant cells in circulation (intravascular, intralymphatic, or intraperitoneal) and/or established, microscopic foci of malignant cells locally, at distant sites, or both.
2. Therapy is most effective when the burden of malignancy is minimal and cell kinetics are optimal.
3. Agents with reported effectiveness against the carcinoma are available.
4. Cytotoxic therapy shows a dose-response relationship and therefore must be administered in maximally tolerated doses, and the duration of therapy must be sufficient to eradicate all malignant cells.
5. The risk-to-benefit ratio for therapy must be favorable to individuals who may remain asymptomatic for their natural life expectancy after resection of their malignancy.

Radiotherapy

Although radiotherapy has been used extensively in various settings for the treatment of rectal carcinoma, little use has been made of it in the treatment of colon carcinoma. Exceptions relate to the presence of a carcinoma in a portion of the colorectum fixed to the retroperitoneum (cecum, ascending colon, and descending colon) or pelvis (rectosigmoid or rectum). Indications that have been considered appropriate for postoperative radiotherapy include (i) involvement of lymph nodes, (ii) known inadequate margins of resection, (iii) adherence to the retroperitoneum, sacrum, or pelvic side walls, (iv) transmural penetration to a macroscopic degree, and (v) extensive microscopic penetration with the presence of positive lymph nodes (422). Radiotherapy has been used in both the adjuvant setting and in situations of incomplete removal (423–425). In a non-randomized prospective trial, Dutterhaver et al. (423) documented an improved 5-year survival rate in patients with B_3, C_2, and C_3 colon carcinomas (Gunderson and Sosin staging modification) treated with postoperative radiation compared with historical controls. Similarly,

Kopelson (426,427) found postoperative adjuvant pelvic irradiation to be beneficial with respect to disease control in patients with transmural carcinoma of the cecum, ascending colon, descending colon, or sigmoid colon as well as improved survival for these cases. Minsky (428) reviewed the literature on the use of whole abdominal radiation therapy for resectable colon carcinoma. In general, patients received 20 to 30 Gy to the whole abdomen with or without a local boost. Additional 5-fluorouracil (5-FU) was delivered in a variety of doses and schedules. Combined results revealed an in-field failure rate of 12% to 50%. Significant toxicity varied from 5% to 38%. With a median follow-up of 5 years, the 5-year disease-free and overall survival rates were 58% and 67%, respectively.

Chemotherapy

The use of adjuvant chemotherapy is attractive because it may offer the possibility of identifying patients who are likely to have occult, residual, or disseminated disease at the time of operation. Chemotherapy is most effective when the burden of carcinoma is smallest and the fraction of malignant cells in growth phase is the highest (429). Many chemotherapeutic agents have been used singly or in combination in an effort to improve survival rates. A large number of studies have directed enormous energy to the subject of intravenous or oral administration of chemotherapeutic agents beginning 4 to 6 weeks after operation. For the most part, none of the early studies directly indicated that adjuvant chemotherapy was of overall benefit to the survival of patients with colon carcinoma (430–436).

Results were often equivocal. In 1988 a meta-analysis of randomized adjuvant studies using systemic 5-FU for up to 1 year demonstrated a marginal overall reduction in the odds ratio of death of approximately 17% and an absolute 5-year survival benefit of 3.4% (436). Promise was offered by the combination of leucoyorin and 5-FU or levamisole and 5-FU (437). An encouraging publication by Laurie et al. (438) reported that the use of a combination of 5-FU and levamisole administered to patients undergoing curative resection for Dukes' C carcinoma of the colon resulted in a 5-year survival rate of 49% compared with 37% in patients receiving no postoperative treatment.

The North Central Cancer Treatment Group (NCCTG) —Mayo Clinic Trial (Intergroup Study) randomized 1296 patients with Dukes' B and C carcinoma to treatment for 1 year with levamisole and 5-FU or to operation alone (439). Patients with Dukes' C could be assigned to levamisole alone. With a median follow-up of 3 years, Dukes' C patients treated with levamisole and 5-FU had a reduced risk of carcinoma recurrence of 41% (chiefly within the liver) and overall death rate reduced by 33%. This initial improvement corresponded with an absolute survival benefit of approximately 5%, which was maintained at 5 years. Treatment with levamisole alone had no detectable effect. The survival benefit for patients with Dukes' B carcinoma did not reach conventional levels of significance, and there was no reduction in the incidence of liver metastases (440).

In April 1990 the National Institutes of Health (NIH) sponsored a consensus development conference on adjuvant chemotherapy for colorectal carcinoma (421). It was concluded that based on the results of the NCCTG (434) and a subsequent trial by the Intergroup consortium (439), there was compelling evidence to recommend the combination of 5-FU and levamisole as "standard" adjuvant treatment for patients with stage III colon carcinoma (regional lymph node involvement) if they are unable to enter a clinical trial.

However, an update of the Intergroup Trial INT-0089 in which there were four arms [leucovorin and 5-FU vs. leucovorin and 5-FU (different dose and schedule) vs. levamisole plus 5-FU vs. levamisole and leucovorin plus 5-FU] were compared revealed a similar survival (441). Intergroup Trial 0153 (Southwest Oncology Group trial 9415) was developed to compare the efficacy of continuous-infusion FU plus levamisole to FU/LV plus leucovorin plus levamisole in the adjuvant treatment of high-risk Dukes' B2 and C1 or C2 colon carcinomas (442). A total of 1135 patients were registered. At least one grade 4 toxicity occurred in 39% of patients receiving FU/LV and 5% of patients receiving continuous-infusion 5-FU. However, almost twice as many patients receiving continuous-infusion 5-FU discontinued therapy early compared with those receiving FU/leucovorin. The 5-year overall survival is 70% for FU leucovorin and 69% for continuous-infusion FU. The corresponding five-year disease-free survival is 61% and 63%, respectively. For all patients, 5-year overall survival is 83%, 74%, and 55%; five-year disease-free survival is 78%, 67%, and 47% for N0, N1, and N2-3, respectively. They concluded, continuous infusion of 5-FU has less severe toxicity but did not improve disease-free survival or overall survival in comparison with bolus FU/LV.

Thirion et al. (443) presented an update of the meta-analysis with a longer follow-up and the inclusion of 3300 patients randomized in 19 trials on an intent-to-treat basis. Their overall analysis showed a twofold increase in response rates (21% for FU leucovorin vs. 11% for FU alone; OR = 0.53) and a small but statistically significant overall survival benefit for FU leucovorin over FU alone (median survival 11.7 vs. 10.5 months, respectively; hazards ratio 0.9) which were primarily seen in the first year. They observed a significant interaction between treatment benefit and dose of FU with response and overall survival advantage of FU leucovorin over FU alone being restricted to trials in which similar dose of FU was prescribed in both arms.

In what they termed their final report, Moertel et al. (444) reported their experience with 5-FU plus levamisole as adjuvant therapy for patients undergoing resection of stage III colon carcinoma. Patients were assigned to observation only, to levamisole alone (50 mg orally, 3 times a day for 3 days, repeated every 2 weeks for 1 year), or to this regimen of levamisole plus 5-FU (450 mg/m^2 body surface area intravenously daily for 5 days and then beginning at 28 days weekly for 48 weeks). In all 929 patients followed for 5 years or more (median, 6.5 years) 5-FU plus levamisole reduced the recurrence rate by 40% and the death rate by 33%. Levamisole reduced the recurrence rate by only 2% and the death rate by only 6%. With few exceptions, toxicity was mild, and patient compliance was excellent. No evidence of late side effects was seen. The authors concluded that 5-FU plus levamisole should be considered the standard treatment for all patients with stage III colon carcinoma not entered into clinical trials.

In the NSABP Protocol C-01 (445), 1166 patients with Dukes' B and C carcinoma of the colon were randomized to one of three therapeutic categories: (i) no further treatment following curative resection, (ii) postoperative chemotherapy consisting of 5-FU, semustine, and vincristine, or (iii) postoperative bacille Calmette-Guèrin (BCG). With an average study time of 77.3 months, patients in the chemotherapy arm had an overall improvement in disease-free survival ($p = 0.02$) and survival ($p = 0.50$) and 1.31 times the likelihood of dying compared with patients treated by operation alone. Comparison of the BCG-treated group with opertion alone revealed no statistical significance in disease-free survival ($p = 0.90$), but there was a survival advantage in favor of the BCG-treated group ($p = 0.03$). At 5 years the risk of dying in the operation-only group was 1.28 times the risk of the BCG-treated patients. Further analysis disclosed that the survival advantage was the result of a diminution in deaths not related to carcinoma; when these deaths were eliminated, the survival difference was not statistically significant. Findings from the C-01 trial demonstrated a significant disease-free survival and survival benefit that lasted 5 years after colon resection, but at 8 years, the disease-free survival and survival differences were no longer significant. In a subsequent NSABP protocol C-03, Wolmark et al. (446) reported data from 1081 patients with Dukes' B and C carcinoma of the colon. Patients were randomly assigned to receive either lomustine (MeCCNU), vincristine, and 5-FU (MOF), or leucovorin-modulated 5-FU (leucovorin plus 5-FU). The mean time, of the study was 47.6 months. Comparison: between the two groups indicates a disease-free survival advantage for patients treated with leucovorin and 5-FU. The 3-year disease-free survival rate for patients in this group was 73% compared with 64% for patients receiving MOF. The coresponding percentage of patients surviving was 84% for those randomized to receive leucovorin plus 5-FU and 77% for the MOF-treated cohort. At 3 years of follow-up, patients treated with postoperative leucovorin plus 5-FU had a 30% reduction in the risk of developing a treatment failure and a 32% reduction in the mortality risk compared with similar patients treated with MOF. The disease-free survival and survival rates with 5-FU and leucovorin in the NSABP protocol C-03 appear comparable to those with 5-FU and levamisole.

A meta-analysis was performed on nine randomized clinical trials that compared 5-FU with 5-FU plus intravenous leucovorin for the treatment of advanced colorectal carcinoma (447). Therapy with 5-FU plus leucovorin administered either as a weekly or monthly regimen showed a highly significant benefit over single-agent 5-FU in terms of the response rate of the carcinoma (23% vs. 11%). This increase in response did not, however, result in a discernible improvement of overall survival.

In 1989 the NSABP initiated a clinical trial C-04 in which 2151 patients with Dukes' B and C colon carcinoma were randomized to receive 5-FU plus leucovorin, 5-FU plus levamisole, or 5-FU plus leucovorin and levamisole. With an average time on study of 63.4 months, there was no significant difference in disease-free survival or survival rates in the three arms. The authors concluded that when compared with 5-FU plus levamisole, 5-FU plus leucovorin is at least as effective and possibly produces a disease-free survival and survival advantage in patients with Dukes' B and C colon carcinoma (440).

Wolmark et al. (448) reported data presented for 2176 patients with Dukes' stage B or C carcinoma entered into NSABP protocol C-05. Patients were randomly assigned to receive either 5-FU + Leucovorin or 5-FU + Leucovorin and Interferon. The mean time on the study was 54 months. There was no statistically significant difference in either disease-free survival (69% vs. 70%) or overall survival (80% vs. 81%) at four years of follow-up. Toxic effects of grade 3 or higher were observed in 61.8% of subjects in the group treated with 5-FU + LV and in 72.1% of subjects in the group treated with 5-FU + LV + IFN. The addition of Interferon to 5-FU + LV adjuvant therapy conferred no statistically significant benefit but did increase toxicity in this study.

Although the benefit from adjuvant chemotherapy has been established for Dukes' C colon carcinoma patients, many still question the worth of such therapy in patients with Dukes' B disease. Mamounas et al. (449) examined the relative efficacy of treatment observed in four NSABP studies and reported that in patients with Dukes' B disease, the relative reduction of recurrence and mortality was comparable to that in patients with Dukes' C disease. A report from a pooled analyses of 1016 patients from five separate other trials found no significant difference in event-free survival or overall survival. They felt their data did not support the use of chemotherapy in Dukes' B colon carcinoma (450).

Three cooperative groups evaluated 5-FU and leucovorin individually, but because their protocols were so similar, their data were pooled to allow a combined analysis (451). Patients with Dukes' B and C were randomized to operation alone or to operation followed by 5-FU and leucovorin administered for 5 days every 28 days for 6 months. The crude rate of recurrence in the liver was twice as high in the control group compared with the treatment group. The 3-year overall survival rate for patients with Dukes' B disease was not significantly different between the control and chemotherapy groups. There was a statistically significant improvement in overall survival only in patients with Dukes' C lesions (hazard ratio for overall survival, 0.7). Accordingly there is now considerable evidence of a survival benefit produced by systemic chemotherapy in patients with Dukes' C disease, but some uncertainty of benefit in those with Dukes B lesions.

In another review of the efficacy of adjuvant chemotherapy, Dubé, Heyen, and Jenicek (452) conducted a qualitative and quantitative meta-analysis of 39 randomized clinical trials. Patients with colon carcinoma who received chemotherapy could expect an increase of 5% in the survival rate and those with rectal carcinoma a 9% increase. Given the high incidence of colorectal carcinoma, even a small benefit is far from negligible.

In a recent report Sakamoto et al. (453) performed a meta-analysis on individual data from three randomized trials conducted by the Japanese Foundation for Multidisciplinary Treatment for Carcinoma involving a total of 5233 patients with stages I to III colorectal carcinoma to assess the survival and disease-free survival benefits of treating patients after resection of a primary carcinoma with oral fluoropyrimidines for 1 year. Compared to a control group of untreated patients oral therapy reduced the risk of death by 11% and the risk of recurrence or death by 15%. There was no significant difference in benefit of oral therapy with respect to stage (I, II, or III), site (rectum or colon), patient age, or patient sex.

In a recent study, Andre et al. (454) randomly assigned 2246 patients who had undergone curative resection for stage II or III colon carcinoma to receive 5-FU and leucovorin alone or with oxaliplatin for 6 months. After a mean follow-up of 37.9 months, 21% in the group given 5-FU and leucovorin + oxaliplatin had had a carcinoma-related event, as compared with 26.1% in the 5-FU leucovorin group. The rate of disease-free survival at 3 years was 78.2% in the group with 5-FU leucovorin + oxaliplatin and 72.9% in the 5-FU leucovorin group. In the group with 5-FU leucovorin + oxaliplatin, the incidence of febrile neutropenia was 1.8%, the incidence of gastrointestinal adverse effects was low, and the incidence of grade 3 sensory neuropathy was 12.4% during treatment, decreasing to 1.1% at 1 year of follow-up. Six patients in each group died during treatment (death 0.5%). They concluded, adding oxaliplatin to a regimen of 5-FU and leucovorin improved the adjuvant treatment of colon carcinoma.

Martenson et al. (455) conducted a trial to determine whether radiation therapy added to an adjuvant chemotherapy regimen improves outcome in high-risk patients. Patients with resected colon carcinoma with adherence or invasion of surrounding structures or with T3 N1 or T3 N2 carcinomas of the ascending and descending colon were randomly assigned to receive fluorouracil and levamisole therapy with or without radiation therapy (45–50.4 Gy in 25–28 fractions beginning 28 days after starting chemotherapy). Overall five-year survival was 62% for chemotherapy patients and 58% for chemoradiotherapy patients; five-year disease-free survival was 51% for both groups. Toxicity ($\geq$ grade 3) occurred in 42% of chemotherapy patients and 54% of chemoradiotherapy patients. They concluded the overall survival and disease-free survival were similar but toxicity was higher among chemoradiotherapy patients.

Based on the recognition that the liver is usually involved when large bowel malignancy disseminates, present in 25% to 30% of patients on initial diagnosis, and also that the liver is the most frequent site of subsequent metastatic disease (40% to 50% of patients) (456), Taylor et al. (457) proposed the strategy of immediate postoperative portal vein perfusion of chemotherapy. In the update of their randomized trial, in which 127 control patients were compared with 117 patients who received intraportal 5-FU and heparin via an umbilical vein catheter for 7 days after operation, benefit was demonstrated in treated patients, with 5-year survival rates of 70% vs. 45%. When individual groups were analyzed, only patients with Dukes' B carcinoma had a significant improvement in overall survival.

Taylor reported that there have been 10 published series of adjuvant cytotoxic portal vein infusion in patients with primary colorectal carcinoma (263). Portal vein cytotoxin infusion is usually begun at operation or in the immediate postoperative period and given continuously for the first 7 days after operation. This short perioperative therapy is in marked contrast to long-term chemotherapy in which 5-FU is given systemieally for 6 months. Toxicity is reduced as, indeed, is cost. A Swiss group (458) reported a 25% incidence of relapse confined to liver in the control arm compared with an incidence of 12% in the portal vein infusion group in node-positive patients. Overall, portal vein infusion reduced the recurrence by 21% (hazard ratio, 0.90) and the risk of death by 26% (0.74). The major risk reduction was in patients with Dukes' C disease as, indeed, was the overall absolute survival improvement. This differed from the original report of Taylor et al. (457), in which only patients with Dukes' B carcinoma obtained a survival benefit.

In the NSABP protocol C-02, 1158 patients with Dukes' A, B, and C carcinoma of the colon were randomized to either no further treatment following curative resection or to postoperative 5-FU and heparin administered via the portal vein (459). Therapy began on day of operation and consisted of constant infusion for 7 successive days. The average time on study was 41.8 months. A comparison of the two groups of patients indicated both an improvement in disease-free survival (74% vs. 64%) at 4 years, and a survival advantage (81% vs. 73%) at 4 years in favor of the chemotherapy-treated group. When compared with the treated group, patients who received no further treatment had 1.26 times the risk of developing a treatment failure and 1.25 times the likelihood of dying after 4 years. Particularly significant was the failure to demonstrate an advantage produced by 5-FU in decreasing the incidence of hepatic metastases. The liver was the first site of treatment failure in 32.9% of 82 patients with documented recurrences in the control group and in 46.3% of 67 patients who received additional treatment. Therapy is administered via a regional route to affect the incidence of recurrence within the perfused anatomic boundary. Since, in this study, adjuvant portal-vein 5-FU infusion failed to reduce the incidence of hepatic metastases, it may be concluded that the disease-free survival and survival advantages are a result of the systemic effects of 5-FU. This report differs from those of Taylor et al. (457) and Wereldsma et al. (460), who reported a decreased incidence of liver metastases.

A meta-analysis of all 10 published trials of portal vein cytotoxic infusion, including a total of 3499 patients, has provided confirmatory evidence (461). Overall, portal vein infusion was associated with a mean 18% reduction in the annual risk of death from any cause, with a 20% reduction in death from colorectal carcinoma. In this meta-analysis, overall survival at 5 years was 64% in the portal vein infusion group vs. 59% in the operation-only group. The benefit was significantly greater for patients with Dukes' C disease (54.2% vs. 46.6%) than for those with Dukes' B lesions (76.3% vs. 72.1%).

The published results of both adjuvant systemic chemotherapy for 6 to 12 months or portal vein infusion for 1 week are roughly comparable, with an approximate 5% improvement in absolute survival at 3 years (263). The major benefits from both treatments occur in patients with lymph node-positive disease. This is entirely consistent with the hypothesis that chemotherapy inhibits occult hepatic micrometastases rather than producing systemic effects, outside the liver. Subsequent relapse in extra-hepatic organs is also inhibited, since extrahepatic metastases spread from liver metastases.

The adjuvant x-ray and 5-FU infusion study (AXIS) is the largest trial yet reported to determine the efficacy of postoperative portal vein infusion of 5-FU. Consenting patients with colorectal carcinoma were randomized to operation with or without seven days of portal vein infusion (1 g 5-FU plus 5000 units heparin in 1 L per 5% dextrose infused over each 24-hour period). In addition, patients with rectal carcinoma could be randomized to radiotherapy or no radiotherapy to be given either before or after operation. A total of 3583 patients were randomized with respect to portal vein infusion. No survival benefit was seen in the 761 patients randomized with respect to radiotherapy and although not statistically significant, the impact on local recurrence rates was similar to that reported in the literature. No overall benefit of portal vein infusion was established in the AXIS study when colonic and rectal carcinomas were considered together but the evidence suggesting a differential treatment effect according to site of carcinoma in AXIS was strongly supported by a meta-analysis incorporating the previous trials. Combining the data gave hazard ratios of 0.82 and 1.00 for colonic and rectal carcinoma respectively, equating to an absolute survival benefit for patients with colonic carcinoma of 5.8%, a level close to that seen for prolonged systemic therapy.

There is now sufficient evidence to recommend that patients with Dukes' C (stage III) disease who are otherwise sufficiently fit should receive adjuvant chemotherapy (usually a combination o 5-FU plus leucovorin or 5-FU plus levamisole). A recent review noted bolus scheduling of 5-FU + leucovorin is favored in North America while infusion of 5-FU leucovorin is favored in Europe (462). They noted infused 5-FU leucovorin may be safer with new drugs such as oxaliplatin and irinotecan.

A review by Haydon (463) reported that in stage III disease chemotherapy appears to be equally effective whether it is given daily for 5 days per month or on a weekly scheduled. The overall effect is a relative reduction in recurrence of 25% or an absolute improvement in survival of 10%. However, doubt remains as to the role of adjuvant chemotherapy in stage II colon carcinoma. Most of the randomized trials have demonstrated a relative reduction in recurrence but have not shown any significant impact on survival. Even for patients with lymph node involvement the indications may not be uniformly obvious. Chapuis et al. (464) conducted a study to identify patient and carcinoma characteristics that might assist in patient selection for chemotherapy after resection of clinicopathological stage III colonic carcinoma. From an initial 2980 patients, after exclusions, 378 remained who had a potentially curative operation for colonic carcinoma with nodal metastases and did not receive adjuvant chemotherapy. Both overall and colonic carcinoma-specific survival rates were negatively associated with serosal surface involvement, apical node metastasis, high histological grade, and venous invasion. The survival of patients with stage III disease who had none of these adverse features was not significantly different from that of patients with stage II lesions. However, survival diminished significantly when one or more of the adverse features were present. Patients with stage III disease but none of the identified adverse features experience relatively good survival and are unlikely to benefit from adjuvant chemotherapy. In this series such patients accounted for 40.5% of patients with stage III disease.

There is still some uncertainty, however, with regard to the benefits for patients with Dukes' B lesions. Figueredo et al. (465) conducted a systematic review to address whether patients with stage II colon carcinoma should receive adjuvant therapy. Thirty-seven trials and 11 meta-analysis were included. The evidence for stage II colon carcinoma comes primarily from a trial of fluorouracil plus levamisole and a meta-analysis of 1016 patients comparing fluorouracil with folinic acid versus observation. Neither detected an improvement in disease-free or overall survival for adjuvant therapy. A recent pooled analysis of data from seven trials observed a benefit for adjuvant therapy in a multivariate analysis for both disease-free and overall survival. The disease-free survival benefits appeared to extend to stage II patients. A meta-analysis of chemotherapy by portal vein infusion has also shown a benefit in disease-free and overall survival for stage II patients. A meta-analysis was conducted using data on stage II patients where data were available ($n = 4187$). The mortality risk ratio was 0.87. They concluded there is preliminary evidence indicating that adjuvant therapy is associated with a disease-free survival benefit for patients with stage II colon carcinoma but these benefits were small and not necessarily associated with improved overall survival.

An American Society of Clinical Oncology panel in collaboration with the Cancer Care Ontario Practice Guideline Initiative, conducted a literature based meta-analysis to determine whether medically fit patients with curatively resected stage II colon carcinoma should be offered adjuvant chemotherapy as part of routine clinical practice (466). They found no evidence of a statistically significant survival benefit of adjuvant chemotherapy. However, there are populations of patients with stage II disease that could be considered for adjuvant therapy, including patients with inadequately sampled lymph nodes, T4 lesions, perforation, or poorly differentiated histology. The ultimate clinical decision should be based on discussions with the patient about the nature of the evidence supporting treatment, the anticipated morbidity of treatment, the presence of high-risk prognostic features on individual prognosis, and patient preferences.

A refinement of the selection of patients for adjuvant chemotherapy might be devised from the study by Ribic et al. (467) who investigated the usefulness of microsatellite instability status as a predictor of the benefit of adjuvant chemotherapy with fluorouracil in stage II and III colon carcinoma. Specimens were collected from patients with colon carcinoma who were enrolled in randomized trials. Among 287 patients who did not receive adjuvant therapy, those with carcinomas displaying high-frequency microsatellite instability had a better 5-year rate of overall survival than patients with carcinomas exhibiting microsatellite stability or low-frequency instability (hazard ratio for death, 0.31). Among patients who received adjuvant chemotherapy, high-frequency microsatellite instability was not correlated with increased overall survival (hazard ratio for death, 1.07). Adjuvant chemotherapy improved overall survival among patients with microsatellite-stable and low-frequency microsatellite instability carcinomas.

Consideration must be given to the definite toxicities. Treatment is often suspended or modified because of gastrointestinal or marrow complications. These observations emphasize the need to evaluate the potential benefits of chemotherapy in a trial setting. In addition, consideration should be given to absolute survival as well as to the quality of life during and following treatment.

The complication side of chemotherapy was poignantly highlighted in the report by Culakova et al. (468) who reviewed the hospitalization of colorectal carcinoma patients with febrile neutropenia at 115 academic medical centers. Over a 6-year period, 957 patients with colorectal carcinoma experienced 1046 hospitalizations with febrile neutropenia. The mean (median) length of stay was 9.0 days while the average (median) cost per hospitalization was $12,484 ($7153). The 30% of patients hospitalized ≥10 days accounted for 62% of all hospital days and 66% of all costs. Clinical infection was reported in 57% of patients, with microbiological documented infection reported in 31% including gram-negative sepsis in 8.5%, gram-positive in 2.7%, and other bacterial infections in 17.5%. Pneumonia was reported in 5% while 5% presented with hypotension and 34% with evidence of hypovolemia. Death occurred in 8.5% of hospitalizations. Mortality rates were greatest in those with gram-negative sepsis (35%), gram-positive sepsis (23%), hypotension (23%), and pneumonia (32%). One or more major comorbidities were reported in 57% of patients. Mortality rates increased with the number of comorbidities. Significant independent risk factors for mortality in multivariate analysis were gram-negative sepsis (OR = 6.1), gram-positive sepsis (OR = 3.8), hypovolemia (OR = 2.5), pneumonia (OR = 4.9), lung disease (OR = 4.6), liver disease (OR = 4.4), heart disease (OR = 3.9), and other vascular disease (OR = 13.3). One-third of hospitalized patients with febrile neutropenia experienced complicated hospitalizations with significant morbidity and mortality.

Arora and Potter (469) reviewed the literature to determine whether adjuvant chemotherapy was safe and effective in patients > 70 years. Of 3347 patients from 7 randomized trials, 43% had stage II and 57% had stage III disease. The probability of death without recurrence of carcinoma was strongly associated with age. The oldest patients had a higher probability of dying without evidence of recurrence (13%) than the youngest patients (2%). In addition, 32% of deaths of the oldest patients but only 5% of deaths of the youngest patients were due to causes other than the carcinoma. Approximately 30% of the patients in each group died with recurrence of carcinoma over the 8-year follow-up period. The 5-year overall survival was 71% for those who received adjuvant therapy, compared with 64% of those untreated. The 5-year recurrence-free rate was 69% in the treated patients compared with 58% in untreated patients. After five years, patients aged 70 years and older had decreased overall survival because of death from other causes. Patients treated with fluorouracil plus levamisole had significantly more leukopenia and nausea or vomiting, whereas those treated with fluorouracil plus leucovorin had significantly more stomatitis and diarrhea. Leukopenia was significant in patients with levamisole and fluorouracil treatment (31% of subjects ≥70 years vs. 17% of subjects < 70 years) and borderline significantly higher in patients with fluorouracil and leucovorin treatment (8% of subjects ≥70 years vs. 4% of subjects < 70 years). This analysis supports the benefit of adjuvant chemotherapy in patients with resected stage II and III colon carcinoma. The patients enrolled in these trials may not be representative of all older patients with colon carcinoma. Only 0.7% of patients in the trial were aged 80 years or older so caution is advised in extrapolating these findings to the oldest patients. The decision to treat older people who have functional limitations and comorbid conditions should be individualized.

Rothenberg et al. (470) conducted a review to assign attribution for the causes of early deaths on two National Cancer Institute-sponsored cooperative group studies involving irinotecan and bolus fluorouracil and leucovorin. The inpatient, outpatient, and research records of patients treated on Cancer and Leukemia Group B protocol C89803 and on North Central Cancer Treatment Group protocol N9741 were reviewed by a panel of five medical oncologists not directly involved with either study. Each death was categorized as treatment-induced, treatment-exacerbated, or treatment-unrelated. Patients treated with irinotecan plus bolus 5-FU/leucovorin had a threefold higher rate of treatment-induced or treatment-exacerbated death than patients treated on the other arm(s) of the respective studies. For C89803, these rates were 2.5% for irinotecan/fluorouracil leucovorin group versus 0.8% for bolus weekly 5-FU and leucovorin. For N9741, these rates were 3.5% for irinotecan/fluorouracil leucovorin, 1.1% for oxaliplatin plus bolus and infusional 5-FU and leucovorin, and 1.1% for oxaliplatin plus irinotecan. The majority of deaths in both studies were attributed to thromboembolic events or gastrointestinal toxicities.

The colorectal carcinoma chemotherapy study group of Japan (471) reported on the efficacy of postoperative treatment with mitomycin C and oral 5-FU for colorectal carcinoma. They designed a second trial to evaluate the effectiveness of additional preoperative chemotherapy to postoperative treatment with mitomycin C and oral 5-fluorouracil for curatively resected colorectal carcinoma patients. There were 1355 patients (colon 755 and rectum 600) enrolled in this study. The pre- and postoperative chemotherapy group were treated preoperatively with 5-FU (320 mg/m^2/day) by continuous intravenous infusion for 5 days beginning on day 6 before operation and postoperatively with mitomycin C (6 mg/m^2 on days 7 and 14 and in months 2, 4, and 6 by bolus injection), and oral 5-FU (200 mg/day) for 6 months. The postoperative chemotherapy group received postoperative chemotherapy only. In an intent-to-treat analysis, the 5-year survival rate in the pre- and postoperative chemotherapy group and the postoperative chemotherapy group was 77.3% and 75.7% for colon carcinoma and 67.2% and 69% for rectal carcinoma, respectively. In a per-protocol analysis, the five-year disease-free survival rate in the pre- and postoperative group and the postoperative group was 76% and 80.7% for colon carcinoma and 60.5% and 63% for rectal carcinoma, respectively, indicating no significant difference between the two groups.

Douillard et al. (472) compared oral uracil/tegafur and oral leucovorin to conventional intravenous fluorouracil and leucovorin in previously untreated metastatic colorectal carcinoma. Eight hundred sixteen patients were randomized to receive either uracil/tegafur (300 mg/m^2/day) and leucovorin (75 or 90 mg/day for 28 days every

35 days) or IV bolus 5-FU (425 mg/m^2/day) and leucovorin (20 mg/m^2/day) for 5 days every 28 days. Comparable survival was noted in both groups with a median of 12.4 months for the oral group and 13.4 months in the other group. The overall response rate did not differ between treatment arms. Oral uracil provided a safer, more convenient alternative to a standard bolus of intravenous 5-FU leucovorin. Diarrhea, nausea and vomiting and stomatitis and mucositis were significantly less frequent with the oral regimen as was myelosuppression. Patients treated with the oral medication had fewer episodes of febrile neutropenia and documented infections.

Bevacizumab

Bevacizumab (Avastin; Genentech Inc., South San Francisco, California, U.S.A.) is a recombinant humanized antivascular endothelial growth factor monoclonal antibody that inhibits neoplastic angiogenesis, and has demonstrated survival benefit in patients with previously untreated metastatic colorectal carcinoma when combined with irinotecan/fluorouracil/leucovorin (IFL). Kabbinavar et al. (473) combined analysis of data from three randomized clinical studies evaluating bevacizumab in combination with FU/LV alone. The median duration of survival was 17.9 months in 5-FU/LV bevacizumab group compared with 14.6 months in the combined control group, corresponding to a hazard ratio for death of 0.74. The median duration of progression-free survival was 8.8 months in the FU/LV bevacizumab group, compared with 5.6 months in the combined control group, corresponding to a hazard ratio for disease progression of 0.63. The addition of bevacizumab also improved the response rate (34.1% vs. 24.5%).

In a phase III trial, combining bevacizumab with irinotecan, bolus fluorouracil, and leucovorin (IFL) increased survival compared with IFL alone in first-line treatment of patients with metastatic colorectal carcinoma. Hurwitz et al. (474) described the efficacy and safety results of the patient cohort who received bevacizumab combined with fluorouracil leucovorin and compared them with results of concurrently enrolled patients who received IFL. Median overall survivals were 18.3 and 15.1 months with fluorouracil leucovorin bevacizumab ($n = 110$) and IFL/placebo ($n = 100$), respectively. Median progression-free survivals were 8.8 and 6.8 months, respectively. Overall response rates were 40% and 37% and median response durations were 8.5 and 7.2 months, respectively. Adverse events consistent for those expected from the fluorouracil leucovorin or IFL-based regimens were seen, as were modest increases in hypertension and bleeding in the bevacizumab arm, which were generally easily managed. They concluded the fluorouracil leucovorin bevacizumab regimen seems as effective as IFL and has an acceptable safety profile. They further concluded that fluorouracil leucovorin bevacizumab is an active alternative treatment regimen for patients with previously untreated metastatic colorectal carcinoma.

Immunotherapy

Immunotherapy was believed to have some effect on colon carcinoma, but there is no conclusive evidence to indicate significant improvement in survival (445). A review of prospective randomized trials by Lise et al. (475), which included an immunotherapy arm, failed to demonstrate any benefit. A report of a controlled randomized trial consisting of a 2-year program of vaccination with BCG and neuraminidase-treated autologous carcinoma cells at 5-year follow-up failed to alter either the disease-free interval or the survival of patients (476). A controlled clinical trial of interferon-α as postoperative surgical adjuvant therapy for patients with colon carcinoma demonstrated significant enhancement of nonspecific immune function but no significant difference in patient survival (477). A study in which 189 patients with Dukes' C colorectal carcinoma underwent resection for cure were randomized to observation or postoperative treatment with 17-1A antibody. After a median follow-up of 5 years, antibody treatment was reported to have reduced the overall death rate by 30% (478). In the future, genetic engineering techniques may allow generation of substances during the immune response, and these may have therapeutic value by modifying the biologic response to malignancy (479).

■ COMPLICATED CARCINOMAS

Previous studies have reported that emergency presentation of colorectal carcinoma is associated with poor outcome. McArdle and Hole (480) conducted a study aimed to establish, after adjusting for case mix, the magnitude of the differences in postoperative mortality and survival between patients undergoing elective surgery and those presenting as an emergency. Of 3200 patients who underwent surgery for colorectal carcinoma, 72.4% of 2214 elective patients had a potentially curative resection compared with 64.1% of 986 patients who presented as an emergency. Following curative resection, the postoperative mortality rate was 2.8% after elective and 8.2% after emergency operation. Overall survival at five years was 57.5% after elective and 39.1% after emergency curative operation; carcinoma-specific survival at 5 years was 70.9% and 52.9%, respectively. The adjusted hazard ratio for overall survival after emergency relative to elective surgery was 1.68 and that for carcinoma-specific survival was 1.90.

Jestin et al. (481) identified risk factors in emergency surgery for colonic carcinoma in a large population of 3259 patients; 806 had an emergency and 2453 an elective procedure. Patients who had emergency surgery had more advanced carcinomas and a lower survival rate than those who had an elective procedure (5-year survival rate 29.8% vs. 52.4%). There was a stage-specific difference in survival with poorer survival both for patients with stage I and II carcinomas and for those with stage III carcinomas after emergency compared with elective surgery. Emergency surgery was associated with a longer hospital stay (mean 18 days vs. 10 days) and higher costs (relative cost 1.5) compared with elective surgery. The duration of hospital stay was the strongest determinant of cost.

Obstruction

When complete obstruction of the colon arises as a result of a carcinoma, the recommended treatment depends on the level of the colon that is obstructed as well as the beliefs and experience of the treating surgeon (482,483). In their review of 115 obstructing carcinomas, Sjodahl, Franzen, and Nystrom (484) found that 37% were right sided (proximal to splenic flexure) and 63% were left sided. Only 4% were Dukes' A while 15% already had distant metastases.

Interestingly, a study by Nozoe et al. (485) found the mean size of the obstructing carcinoma was 3.7 cm which was significantly smaller than that of nonobstructing carcinomas (5.4 cm). The proportion of lymph node metastases in obstructing carcinomas was 66.9% which was significantly higher than that in nonobstructing carcinomas (42.4%). The proportion of carcinomas classified into Dukes' C or D in obstructing carcinomas was 84.6% and was significantly higher than that in nonobstructing carcinomas (52.5%).

If the patient's condition can be stabilized and there is evidence of resolution of the occlusion, bowel preparation and elective resection is the ideal solution. This clinical course is unusual, and therefore decisions on how to proceed must be made. For right-sided colonic obstructions, it is generally accepted that the treatment of choice is a resection and primary anastomosis with removal of the right and proximal transverse colon (486). Even though the bowel is not prepared, the resection usually can be readily accomplished.

When the obstruction is located in the distal transverse colon, the matter of how to proceed is controversial. Some surgeons believe that the patient should have a proximal diversion followed by a definitive resection. However, under these circumstances a growing number of surgeons have adopted the procedure of an extended right hemicolectomy followed by a primary ileodescending colon anastomosis.

Lee et al. (487) compared the operative results of 243 patients who had emergency operations for right-sided and left-sided obstructions from primary colorectal carcinomas. One hundred seven patients had obstruction at/or proximal to the splenic flexure (right-sided lesions), and 136 had lesions distal to the splenic flexure (left-sided lesions). The primary resection rate was 91.8%. Of the 223 patients with primary resection, primary anastomosis was possible in 88% of patients. Among the 101 primary anastomosis in patients with left-sided obstruction, segmental resection with on-table lavage was performed in 75 patients and subtotal colectomy was performed in 26 patients. The overall operative mortality rate was 9.4%, although that of the patients with primary resection and anastomosis was 8.1%. The anastomotic leakage rate for those with primary resection and anastomosis was 6.1%. There were no differences in the mortality or leakage rates between patients with right-sided and left-sided lesions (mortality 7.3% vs. 8.9% and leakage 5.3% vs. 6.9%). Colocolonic anastomosis did not show a significant difference in leakage rate when compared with ileo-colonic anastomosis (6.1% vs. 6%).

Three-Stage Procedure

For patients with an obstruction of the left colon, greater controversy exists and a larger number of options are available. Traditionally, these patients have undergone a three-stage operation, with the first-stage being a transverse colostomy or possibly a cecostomy, followed by resection and anastomosis, and finally by closure of the colostomy.

In a review of the subject, Deans, Krukowski, and Irwin (488) reported that between 70% and 80% of patients having a transverse colostomy undergo resection of their carcinoma during the first hospitalization, with a hospital stay of 30 to 55 days. Overall, 25% of patients do not undergo closure of their colostomy because they are unfit or unwilling to undergo an additional operation. Overall mortality rates range from 2% to 15%, mostly in the 10% range, with morbidity rates ranging from 20% to 37%, often related to stoma complications, ranging from 6% to 14%. Although many reports show that the combined mortality rate of the three-stage procedure is similar to that of primary resection with delayed anastomosis, there is the suggestion that long-term survival is decreased in the three-stage operation (488). Sjodahl, Franzen, and Nystrom (484) found a modest increase in 5-year survival rate of 38% for immediate resection compared with a rate of 29% for a staged resection. Although proximal decompression is still promoted as a simple, safe initial option, the cumulative morbidity and mortality rates, survival disadvantage, prolonged hospital stay, and necessity of repeated operations make the three-stage procedure most unfavored.

Hartmann's Procedure

Some surgeons have advocated an immediate resection without anastomosis (i.e., a proximal colostomy and mucous fistula or closed rectal stump, Hartmann's procedure). The perceived advantages include immediate removal of the carcinoma, avoidance of an anastomosis in less than ideal circumstances, and more rapid convalescence and shorter hospital stay. In the event it proves to be permanent, a left-sided colostomy is much less of a burden than a transverse colostomy. The overall operative mortality rate has ranged from 6% to 12%, mostly in the 10% range (488), with hospital stay ranging from 17 to 30 days. Rates of colostomy closure of 60% or more are common. It must be remembered that significant morbidity can be associated with colostomy closure. In their report on 130 stomas and their subsequent closure, Porter et al. (489) experienced a complication rate of 44%. Nevertheless, Hartmann's procedure combines primary resection and relief of the obstruction with acceptable morbidity and mortality rates. It is particularly appropriate for a patient with perforation of the left colon and for the elderly unfit patient.

Subtotal Colectomy

More recently, some surgeons have recommended a subtotal colectomy with primary ileosigmoid anastomosis or even ileorectal anastomosis. Advantages offered by this operation include (i) no stoma problems, (ii) a one-stage, procedure with a single hospitalization, (iii) a shorter hospital stay with financial savings, and (iv) removal of synchronous proximal neoplasms and reduced risk of metachronous lesions. Wong et al. (490) reported on 35 patients who presented with left-sided obstructing carcinoma. Unsuspected synchronous proximal lesions occurred in 12 patients (32%)—three carcinomas, eight adenomas, and one with another synchronous carcinoma and polyp. Initial reports stressed the technical demands of this operation but, with care, good results can be obtained. Operative mortality rates of 3% to 11% have been reported and morbidity rates are low, with a leakage rate of 4% and a hospital stay of 15 to 20 days (488). Subtotal colectomy carries a risk of diarrhea and/or fecal incontinence, particularly in elderly patients. However, most reported experience has not rated this a significant problem. The overall morbidity rate (6% vs. 44%) and length of hospital stay (17 vs. 34 days) are significantly less than after combined procedures (491). Perez et al. (492) evaluated the results of emergency subtotal colectomy in 35 patients with obstructing carcinoma of the left colon. The postoperative mortality rate was 6%, and complications were significant:

wound infection, 28%; ileus, 17%; evisceration, 8%; intestinal obstruction, 8%; and anastomotic leak, 11%. In a series of 35 patients, Lau, Lo, and Law (493) reported a complication rate of 31%, which included an anastomotic leak rate of 3%. Their review of the literature revealed leak rates that ranged from 0% to 4.5% for subtotal colectomy and 0% to 14% for colonic lavage methods.

Chrysos et al. (494) reported four patients with obstructing carcinoma of the rectosigmoid junction and upper rectum who underwent a total colectomy followed by construction of a 10 cm ileal-J pouch that was subsequently anastomosed to the distal rectal stump. One year postoperatively, all patients experienced one to three normal bowel motions daily and no episodes of incontinence. They believe total colectomy with ileal-J-pouch-rectal anastomosis is a reasonable operative alternative in cases with obstructing carcinomas of the rectosigmoid junction which necessitate removal of the upper rectum.

On-Table Lavage

Still others have recommended resection of the primary disease combined with on-table lavage and primary anastomosis. A major perceived disadvantage of on-table lavage is that it is time-consuming. The operative technique consists of the mobilization of the appropriate segment of colon according to oncologic principles. In most circumstances, both the hepatic and splenic flexures require mobilization. The bowel at an appropriate distance distal to the carcinoma is divided, as is the proximal bowel 5 to 10 cm distal to the proximal site of the anastomosis, thus removing the carcinoma-bearing portion of colon. A No. 22 or No. 24 Foley catheter is inserted into the cecum through the freshly amputated appendicular stump or through the terminal ileum if the patient has had an appendectomy (Fig. 56). The catheter balloon is inflated and held

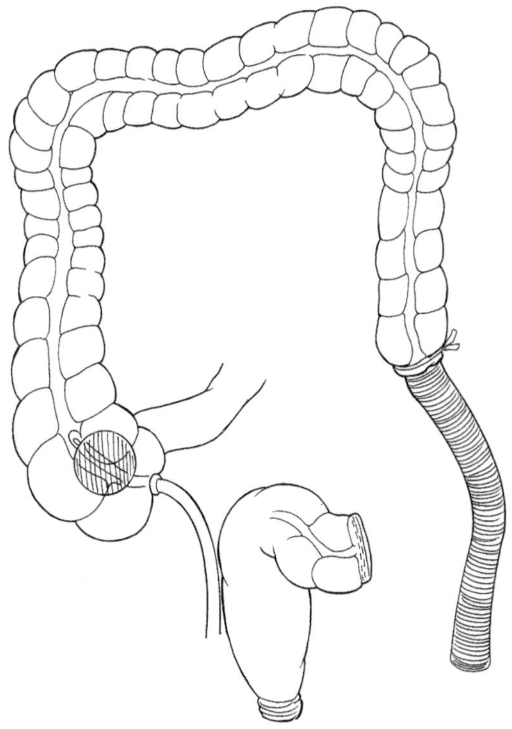

FIGURE 56 ■ On-table colonic lavage.

in place by a pursestring suture. A noncrushing clamp is placed across the terminal ileum to prevent reflux of the irrigation fluid. A standard intravenous infusion set is connected to the Foley catheter. The bowel, having been adequately mobilized, permits the distal portion to be placed in a kidney basin and hard fecal scybala can be "milked" into the kidney basin. A sterile corrugated anesthetic scavenger tube, 22 mm in diameter, is then inserted into the distal bowel and secured in place with strong tapes. The free end of this tube is draped over the side of the patient and secured in an appropriate collecting system. The colon is then lavaged with warm isotonic saline solution until the effluent in the corrugated tube is clear. The volume of lavage solution required is determined by the extent of fecal loading but can usually be accomplished with 3 to 6 L. Lavage time may vary from 20 to 45 minutes. Once the effluent is clear, the Foley catheter is removed, and the appendiceal opening or ileum is closed. A short segment of bowel containing the irrigated tube is resected and an anastomosis created according to the surgeon's preference.

Most series quote an operative mortality rate of approximately 10% (488). Anastomotic leakage rates following primary anastomosis are low. Tan and Nambiar (495) performed 36 primary resections and anastomoses following intraoperative antegrade colonic lavage for left-sided obstructing carcinoma. There were two deaths (one from anastomotic leak). Other complications included chest infection in 11% and wound infection in 19.4%. Others support this form of management (492,496,497). Leakage rates are approximately 4% (488). Wound infection rates remain a problem, with rates of 25% to 60%, and hospital stays around 20 days (488).

The Scotia study group (498) conducted the first multicenter prospective randomized trial comparing subtotal colectomy with segmental resection and primary anastomosis following intraoperative irrigation for the management of malignant left-sided colonic obstruction. Of the 91 eligible patients recruited by 12 centers, 47 were randomized to subtotal colectomy and 44 to on-table irrigation and segmental colectomy. Hospital mortality and complication rates did not differ significantly, but 4 months after operation, increased bowel frequency (three or more bowel movements per day) was significantly more common in the subtotal colectomy group (14 of 35 vs. 4 of 35). More patients in the subtotal colectomy group reported that they had consulted their general practitioner with bowel problems than those in the segmental resection group (15 of 37 vs. 3 of 35). The authors believe that segmental resection following intraoperative irrigation is the preferred option except when there is cecal perforation or if synchronous neoplasms are present in the colon, when subtotal colectomy is more appropriate.

Chiappa et al. (499) reported 39 patients who were treated with intraoperative decompression, on-table lavage, resection, and primary anastomosis. The primary anastomosis was intraperitoneal in 74% and below the peritoneal reflection of the rectum in 26% of patients. Operative mortality was 3% and anastomotic leakage was observed in 6% of patients. Complications included intra-abdominal abscess (3%), and wound infections (8%).

Ohman (321) also found a higher operative mortality rate for primary resection (14%) compared with staged resection (5%) and, although there was an early apparent superior survival rate with the staged procedures, it did not persist into the fourth and fifth years: Umpleby and Williamson (327) reported a better 5-year survival rate following resection and anastomosis (48%) than after staged procedures (18%).

Primary Resection

Rather boldly, some surgeons have performed a resection with primary anastomosis in the absence of bowel preparation (500). An intracolonic bypass has been suggested as treatment (501). Still others have suggested a primary resection with anastomosis and proximal diversion. In an effort to shed light on the issue, Kronborg (502) conducted a randomized trial in which he compared the results of traditional staged procedures with an initial transverse colostomy, followed by curative resection, and subsequent colostomy closure with immediate resection and end colostomy and mucous fistula with subsequent reanastomosis. He found no difference in mortality or carcinoma-specific survival rates between the two treatments.

From this constellation of choices, it becomes difficult to select the best one. Ultimately, the selection depends on the surgeon's experience and preference. An informed decision rests on the recognition of the comparable morbidity and mortality rates for the single procedure compared with the combined morbidity and mortality rates of the multiple operations of the staged procedures. Fielding, Stewart-Brown, and Blesovsky (503) recorded an operative mortality rate of 25% for primary resection and 34% for staged resection. This prospective study compared the outcome of primary staged resection in colonic obstruction and failed to show any difference in mortality rates between these options.

My own preference is to extend the primary resection for, lesions as far as the sigmoid colon. It appears worthwhile to cleanse the bowel distal to the obstruction, and a primary anastomosis then can be effected between the terminal ileum and the sigmoid colon. The morbidity and mortality rates are lower than those found with the staged approach, and the length of hospitalization is shorter. By eliminating a second or third hospitalization and a temporary colostomy, palliation is better for those patients who ultimately die from recurrent disease. Furthermore, those patients who undergo resection for cure may have increased rates of long-term survival. If the lesion is so distal that there would be little remaining reservoir by resecting all the obstructed colon proximal to the carcinoma, a reasonable alternative would be to cleanse the bowel distal to the carcinoma, perform a primary resection, and use on-table lavage, with a primary anastomosis. In the very debilitated patient, consideration should be given to a right transverse colostomy.

In the exceptional case in which the obstructing lesion is deemed unresectable, a bypass should be performed when possible. For right-sided lesions, an ileotransversostomy can be performed. In other circumstances a colocolostomy might be deemed appropriate; in any event, this choice would be preferable to a permanent stoma, which would be the last option.

There have been reports on the role of preresectional laser recanalization for obstructive carcinomas of the colon and rectum. Eckhauser and Mansour (504) reported on use of the neodymium: yttrium-aluminum-garnet (Nd:YAG) laser to successfully accomplish decompression and allow for a formal bowel preparation and a definitive one-stage operation. The authors' experience with 29 patients did not involve compromise of patient safety. In several other series, the success rate for recanalization was 80%, with a 2% to 50% procedure-related morbidity and mortality (488).

Stenting

Intestinal stenting is a procedure that is rapidly coming into more widespread use. It was first introduced by Doharto in 1991 (505) as definitive palliative treatment for patients with obstructive disease where resection for cure was not appropriate due to very advanced local disease, metastatic disease, or because of an unacceptably high operative risk. In 1994 Tejero et al. (506) proposed stent placement as a "bridge-to-surgery" for emergency relief of colonic obstruction with an aim to subsequent elective resection. The technique can be applied in patients who refused operative treatment. Colostomy can be avoided with an improved quality of life especially in the palliative setting.

Suitable lesions for endoluminal colorectal stenting include both obstructing primary left-sided colorectal carcinomas as well as extracolonic malignancies such as prostate, bladder, ovarian, or pancreatic. It is not required for right-sided obstructing carcinomas and it is also not appropriate for lesions less than 5 cm from the anal verge. The actual length of the lesion is not a theoretical limitation. It is contraindicated in the presence of colonic perforation with peritonitis and would not prove effective with multiple sites of obstruction.

Although it is not mandatory, it is probably best that stents be placed under endoscopic guidance with the aid of fluoroscopy. The administration of prophylactic antibiotics is probably wise. The procedure is conducted under conscious sedation. A catheter over a guide wire is advanced through the lesion. Contrast is injected into the proximal lumen. Once deployed, the stents expand and become incorporated into the surrounding tissue by pressure necrosis thus anchoring the stent. Post procedure plain abdominal x-rays are obtained for 3 or 4 days.

Dauphine et al. (507) reviewed their experience with 26 self-expanding metal stents as the initial interventional approach in the management of acute malignant large bowel obstruction. In 14 patients, the stents were placed for palliation, whereas in 12, they were placed as a bridge-to-surgery. In 85%, stent placement was successful on the first occasion. In the remaining four individuals, one was successfully stented at the second occasion, and three required emergency operation. Nine of the 12 patients (75%) in the bridge to surgery group underwent elective colon resection. In the palliative group, 29% had reobstruction of the stents and in 9% the stent migrated. In the remaining 64%, the stent was patent until the patient died or until the time of last follow-up. Colonic stents achieved immediate nonoperative decompression and proved to be both safe and effective.

Since first described, there have been numerous publications on the subject. Khot et al. (508) conducted a systematic review of the published data on stenting for the treatment of colorectal obstruction. A total of 58 publications was found of which 29 case series were included in the analysis. Technical and clinical success, complications, and reobstruction, both in palliation and as a "bridge to surgery" were assessed. Pooled results showed that stent insertion was attempted in 598 instances. Technical success was achieved in 92% and clinical success in 88%. Palliation was achieved in 90% of 336 cases while 85% of 262 insertions succeeded as a "bridge-to-surgery" (95% had a one-stage operative procedure with a mean time to the operating room 8.9 days). Technical reasons for failure included inability to place the guide wire, malposition or perforation. Clinical failures included perforation, persistent obstructive symptoms, or adhesion of colonic wall to the stent. There were three deaths (1%). Perforation occurred 22 times (4%); 1% in balloon dilatation versus 2% in nonballoon dilatation. Stent migration was reported in 10% of 551 technically successful cases. Management included stent removal, stent reinsertion, operation, and no immediate intervention but proceed to planned operation. The rate of stent reobstruction was 10% of the 525, mainly in the palliative group. Reason for obstruction included ingrowth of malignancy, stent migration, and fecal impaction. Bleeding occurred in 5% of patients, the majority requiring no treatment but three patients received transfusions. Another 5% of patients experienced pain, either abdominal or rectal, and this was controlled with oral analgesics. They concluded, that the evidence suggests that colorectal stents offer good palliation, and are safe and effective as a "bridge-to-surgery." Stent usage can avoid the need for a stoma and is associated with low rates of mortality and morbidity. Dilatation of malignant strictures at the time of stent placement appears to be dangerous and should be avoided.

Law et al. (509) evaluated the outcomes of self-expanding metallic stents as a palliative treatment for malignant obstruction of the colon and rectum. The insertion of self-expanding metallic stents was attempted for palliation in 52 patients. Successful insertion of the stent was achieved in 50 patients. The median survival of patients was 88 (range, 3–450) days. Complications occurred in 13 patients (25%). These included perforation of the colon ($n=1$), migration or dislodgement of the stents ($n=8$), severe tenesmus ($n=1$), colovesical fistula ($n=1$), and ingrowth of malignancy ($n=2$). Insertion of a second stent was required in eight patients. Subsequent operations were performed in nine patients, and stoma creation was required in seven patients.

Saida et al. (510) evaluated the long-term prognosis of expandable metallic stent insertion compared with emergency operation without expandable metallic stent. Forty emergency operations and 44 expandable metallic stent insertions were retrospectively compared. Postoperative complications were significantly less frequent in the expandable metallic stent group: wound infection was 14% vs. 2%; leakage following anastomosis was 11% versus 3%, 3-year overall survival rate was 50% vs. 48%; 5-year survival rate was 44% vs. 40% in the emergency operation and expandable metallic stent groups, respectively. They concluded that because preoperative expandable metallic stent insertion for obstructive colorectal carcinoma had good postoperative results and no disadvantages in long-term prognosis, this procedure should be used in preoperative treatments of obstructive colorectal carcinoma.

Martinez-Santos et al. (511) evaluated primary anastomosis and morbidity rates obtained with self-expandable stents in comparison with the results of emergency surgical treatment. Patients with left-sided malignant colorectal obstruction were enrolled. Forty-three patients were assigned to preoperative stent and elective operation or palliative stent (emergency surgical treatment). In the stent group, the obstruction was relieved in 95% after the stent placement. Of 26 patients who underwent operative treatment, a primary anastomosis was possible in 84.6% vs. 41.4% in the immediate operative group, with lower need for a colostomy (15.4% vs. 58.6%) in the immediate operative group. The anastomotic failure rate was similar and the reintervention rate was lower (0% vs. 17%). The total stay (14.2 days vs. 18.5 days), the intensive care unit stay (0.3 days vs. 2.9 days), and the number of patients with severe complications (11.6% vs. 41.2%) were significantly lower in the stent group.

Johnson et al. (512) studied 36 patients of whom 18 had obstructing left-sided colon carcinomas relieved by placement of endolumnal stents. These were compared with 18 historical controls with similar clinicopathological features that were treated more conventionally with palliative stoma formation. Both groups of patients gained relief of obstructive symptoms. There were no differences in survival or in-hospital mortality. The median length of palliation was 92 days for stenting and 121 days for palliative stoma formation. Formation of a stoma required a significantly longer stay in the intensive care unit but hospital stay was similar. They concluded as an alternative to palliative operation, selected patients benefit from colonic endoluminal stenting with relief of obstructive symptoms and no adverse effect on survival. Patients may be spared the potential problems associated with palliative stoma formation and the morbidity of operation. Stenting can be offered to the very frail patient who would otherwise be managed conservatively.

Meisner et al. (513) reported on 104 procedures with self-expanding metal stents performed in 96 patients. The goals of the procedure were either postponement of emergency operation or definitive palliative treatment. Technical success was achieved in 92% and clinical success in 82%. Procedure-related complications included perforation in three patients during stenting and in one instance 6 to 7 hours after. Other technical problems could mainly be overcome by introducing an additional stent. They believe complications seen in the group treated with self-expanding metal stents and subsequent resection (mortality 18% and anastomotic leakage 18%), do not differ from the number of complications usually seen in patients who undergo colorectal resection.

Suzuki et al. (514) reviewed 36 patients with malignant obstruction, and 6 patients with benign obstructive disease who underwent placement of self-expandable stents using a combined endoscopic and fluoroscopic technique. Stent placement was successful in 86%. Complication occurred in 44%, migration ($n=7$), reobstruction ($n=5$), perforation ($n=2$), fistula formation ($n=1$), and stent fracture ($n=1$). Stent placement was successful in 100% of patients with benign strictures but poststent migration was frequent (2/6).

Tomiki et al. (515) compared the clinical outcome of 18 patients who had stent placement and 17 patients who underwent only colostomy. The postoperative hospital stay was 22.3 days for stent placement compared with 47.4 days for colostomy. The duration to readmission was 129.2 days for stent placement and 188.4 days for colostomy. The estimated duration of primary stent patency was 106 days. Mean survival period was 134 days in patients with stent placement and 191 days in patients with colostomy. They concluded, stent placement increases the option of palliative treatment and is an effective treatment contributing to improving quality of life.

Sebastian et al. (516) systematically reviewed the efficacy and safety of self-expanding metal stents in the setting of malignant colorectal obstruction. Fifty-four studies reported the use of stents in a total of 1198 patients. The median technical and clinical success rates were 94% and 91%, respectively. The clinical success when used as a bridge to surgery was 71.7%. Major complications related to stent placement included perforation (3.8%), stent migration (11.8%), and reobstruction (7.3%). Stent-related mortality was 0.58%.

Carne et al. (517) compared the use of expandable metallic stents as a palliative measure to traditional open surgical management. Patients with left-sided (splenic flexure and distal), colorectal carcinoma and nonresectable metastatic disease (stage IV) were treated with expandable metal stents or open resection or stoma. Twenty-two of 25 patients had colonic stents successfully inserted and 19 patients underwent open operation. The malignancies were primary in 22 stent procedures and 18 open operations. The open operations were laparotomy only ($n=2$), bypass ($n=1$), stoma ($n=7$), resection with anastomosis ($n=4$), resection without anastomosis ($n=5$). The complications after open operation were urinary ($n=2$), stroke ($n=1$), cardiac ($n=2$), respiratory ($n=2$), deep venous thrombosis ($n=1$), anastomotic leak ($n=1$). There were no stent-related complications. The mean length of stay was significantly shorter in the stent group (4 vs. 10.4 days). There was no difference in survival between the two groups (median survival: stent group 7.5 months; open operation, 3.9 months). They concluded, patients treated with stents are discharged earlier than after open operation. Stents do not affect survival.

Although stents are expensive, the procedure appears to be cost-effective since emergency operation can be avoided with acute bowel obstruction, and in those with advanced disease no resection of the colon is necessary.

Perforation

Perforation has been reported to occur in 3% to 9% of patients with colorectal carcinomas (299). Patients who develop a free perforation of the colon associated with a carcinoma present with signs and symptoms of generalized peritonitis. The carcinoma itself may be perforated, or there may be a left-sided carcinoma associated with a right-sided perforation. Each situation is handled differently: In the clinical setting, for treatment of a perforated carcinoma, older reports recommended that the perforation be managed by diversion, with a proximal colostomy or cecostomy performed in association with repair of the perforation. However, this treatment does not relieve the septic process, and the aim of therapy should be to remove the diseased segment. Otherwise, contamination will continue from the level of the stoma to the level of the perforation. On completion of the resection, the question arises as to how to handle the bowel ends. If the patient already has generalized peritonitis, it seems inappropriate to perform a primary anastomosis. In this event, the proximal bowel is brought out as a stoma, and the distal bowel is drawn out as a mucous fistula or closed as a Hartmann pouch. For a right-sided perforation, a similar procedure can be performed. Another option is to resect the perforated diseased bowel and perform a primary anastomosis with a proximal diversionary stoma, either a proximal colostomy or a loop ileostomy. If technically feasible, the two ends of bowel should be brought out adjacent to each other as described for the end loop stoma. The advantage of this technique is that bowel continuity can be established at a later date without the need for a formal laparotomy.

When there is an obstructing lesion of the left colon and a perforation of the right colon, a viable option is a subtotal colectomy encompassing removal of the perforated colon and the malignancy in one operation. Saegesser and Sandblom (323) stressed the fact that simple suture repair of an ischemic colon will not hold and that a temporary colostomy placed in an ischemic or inflamed bowel will pull through. The authors believe that the practice of closure of the perforation and relief of obstruction by colostomy or by exteriorization of the perforated cecum is illogical and inadequate. The surgeon should proceed with resection of the carcinoma and the entire distended part of the ischemic and perforated colon. A subtotal colectomy might even be considered if only a left-sided perforation is present, since this operation would fulfill the criteria of removing the diseased and unprepared bowel. Another option for management of the patient with a perforation remote from the diseased segment is to bring out the perforated segment as a stoma, either by colostomy or cecostomy.

For the patient who presents with localized peritonitis on the right side, the diagnosis may be confused with that of appendicitis. If the diagnosis is definite at the time of laparotomy, it is reasonable to proceed with a right hemicolectomy and primary anastomosis. If the localized peritonitis occurs on the left side, the differential diagnosis will include diverticulitis. Resection of the diseased segment is indicated, and management of the ends involves the same considerations as with the obstructed unprepared bowel.

Bleeding

Massive bleeding from a carcinoma is an unusual complication, but when it arises, it offers the built-in advantage of being a colonic cathartic. Therefore, if bleeding is so profuse that urgent operation is required, a mechanical cleansing is automatically present, and the affected portion of bowel can be resected with a primary anastomosis.

Obstructive Colitis

Obstructive colitis is an ulceroinflammatory condition that occurs in a dilated segment of the colon proximal to an obstructing or partially obstructing lesion. The entity is rarely reported in the literature and the following information was drawn from the review by Tsai et al. (518). Obstructive colitis is only encountered in 0.3% to 3.1% of all colorectal carcinomas and affects both men and women over 50 years of age. Minor degrees of obstructive colitis may be overlooked and its prevalence may be as high as

7% when specifically sought. The left side of the colon, especially the sigmoid colon, is usually involved in obstructive colitis. Patients with obstructive colitis usually complain of bleeding per rectum and abdominal pain as well as nausea and vomiting, all of which are indistinguishable from the symptoms of colorectal carcinoma. Regardless of severity and distribution pattern, a diagnostic feature of obstructive colitis is the presence of an intact mucosal segment of about 2- to 6-cm long between the carcinoma and the colitis. The area of colitis is usually a single confluent area, often with regular geographic margins, which is well demarcated from the surrounding normal mucosa.

Microscopically, focal areas of colitis associated with obstructive colitis show replacement of mucosa by active granulation tissue. Acute and chronic inflammatory cells are moderate in amount and seldom extend beyond sites of granulation. Pseudopolyps of granular tissue or edematous mucosa may occur, and crypt abscesses may involve the mucosa at the ulcer margin. The mucosa in the intervening segment and distal to the obstructing lesion is usually normal. It is differentiated from ulcerative colitis which is characterized histologically by an intense inflammation of the mucosa and submucosa in addition to the presence of multiple crypt abscesses. The rectum is always involved and the disease extends proximally for varying distances but always with continuity of involvement to the proximal extent of the disease process.

One suggested pathogenic mechanism of obstructive colitis is that of secondary ischemia caused by hypoperfusion. Additional factors, such as preexisting atheroma, anemia, or a past history of pelvic irradiation may play a role in precipitating the colitis.

Obstructive colitis can cause both diagnostic and therapeutic problems. The signs and symptoms arising from obstructive colitis may be attributed to the primary obstructive lesion, which is usually most obvious on radiological and endoscopic studies. Areas of colitis may be a source of septicemia or may perforate and lead to peritonitis. Anastomoses in the unrecognized area of colitis may break down. Up to 25% of cases of obstructive colitis have been associated with anastomotic complications. Their frequently normal appearance at operation may lead to involved segments of colon being used for anastomoses with consequent complications. Because perforation through a colonic carcinoma is a grim prognostic event with negligible 5-year survival, it is important to distinguish this from perforation through the obstructive colitis, which may have a different prognosis. Awareness of the features and incidence of obstructive colitis should help surgeons avoid these diagnostic and therapeutic problems.

Invasion of Adjacent Viscera

Occasionally a carcinoma becomes attached to the abdominal wall or the adjacent viscera, such as the small bowel, urinary bladder, uterus, stomach, spleen, ureter, or duodenum. It is estimated that such attachment occurs in approximately 10% of all patients with colon carcinomas with a reported range of 3.1% to 16.7% (519). The philosophy of treatment to be followed in these circumstances might best be expressed by the quote attributed to Hippocrates: "To extreme diseases, extreme remedies." In order to perform

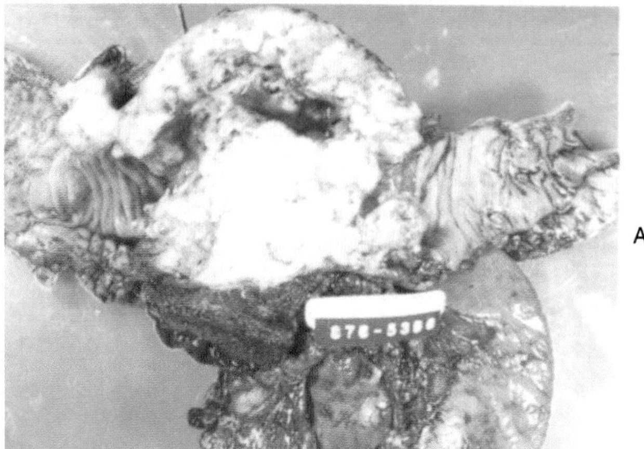

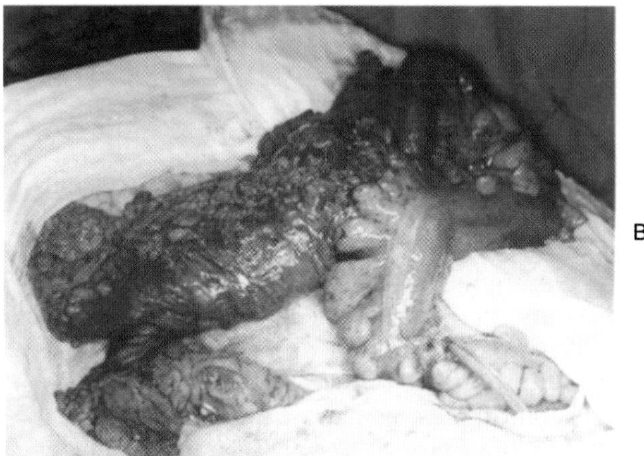

FIGURE 57 ■ (**A**) Carcinoma of the transverse colon attached to the spleen and greater curvature of the stomach resected enbloc. (**B**) Carcinoma of the transverse colon invading the sigmoid colon.

an adequate curative operation, it sometimes becomes necessary to excise en bloc all or part of the attached viscus (Fig. 57). Often these adhesions are inflammatory in nature and not caused by malignant infiltration, so the prognosis frequently is better than might have been anticipated originally (Table 8). With this knowledge, the surgeon should not hesitate to resect attached structures.

An exception to these recommendations might be when the duodenum or bladder base is extensively involved, in which case the primary lesion is removed and the structures at risk are marked with metal clips. Under these circumstances, the morbidity and mortality rates of the radical operation involving an anterior exenteration or Whipple's procedure would probably exceed any possible benefit derived from a very radical operation. However, Curley, Evans, and Ames (530) reported on 12 patients in whom the carcinoma involved the duodenum or pancreatic head and who underwent an en bloc extended right hemicolectomy and pancreaticoduodenectomy. There were no operative deaths, and malignant invasion was confirmed in all patients. At time of report, eight of the 12 patients were alive at a median 42 months.

Similarly Koea et al. (531) reported their experience with 8 patients with bulky primary carcinomas of the right colon infiltrating the duodenum ($n=4$) or pancreatic head ($n=4$) surgically managed at Memorial Sloan-Kettering Cancer Center. Six patients presented with anemia, and one

TABLE 8 ■ Nature of Adhesions Between Colon and Adjacent Viscus

Author(s)	No. of Patients	Adhesions (%) Carcinomatous	Adhesions (%) Inflammatory	5-Year Survival (%)	Operative Mortality (%)
Glass et al. (520) (1986)	69	49	51	70	–
Gall, Tonak, and Altendorf (521) (1987)	121	55	45	52	12
Hunter, Ryan, and Schultz (522) (1987)	28	39	61	61	0
Orkin et al. (523) (1989)	65	57	43	52	0
Eisenberg, Kraybill, and Lopez (524) (1990)	58	84	16	0–76[a]	2
Montesani et al. (525) (1991)	35	71	29	30	0
Curley et al. (526) (1992)	101	70	30	54	4
Izbicki et al. (527) (1995)	83	54	46	44 mo (mean)	1
Rowe et al. (519) (1997)	118	69	31	34–78[b]	4
Carne et al. (528) (2004)	53	38	62	51	–
Nakafusa et al. (529) (2004)	53	53	47	77	0

[a]0% survival for those with lymph node metastases; 76% for those without lymph node metastases.
[b]5 year survival: 78% for inflammatory adhesions plus negative lymph nodes; 58% for inflammatory adhesions plus positive lymph nodes; 34% for invasive adhesions plus positive lymph nodes; 64% for invasive adhesions plus negative lymph nodes; 71% for negative lymph nodes; 47% for positive lymph nodes.

patient each with epigastric pain and an abdominal mass. All patients had T4 lesions, whereas five had lymph node metastases at presentation. All patients were resected with clear pathologic margins either by right colectomy and en bloc duodenectomy ($n=4$) or en bloc pancreaticoduodenectomy ($n=4$). The 30-day mortality rate was 0. Six patients remained alive and free of disease at a median follow-up of 26 months, and there was one long-term survivor who was alive and free of disease at 84 months after resection.

Talamonti et al. (532) reviewed 70 patients who underwent resection of a carcinoma of the colon and rectum with en bloc total cystectomy (36 patients) or partial cystectomy (34 patients). There were three postoperative deaths in the total cystectomy group but none, after partial cystectomy. The 5-year actuarial survival rate for the 64 patients with negative resection margins was 52%. In exceptionally good-risk patients, consideration may be given to a total pelvic exenteration.

In a review of 1918 patients who underwent curative resection for colorectal carcinoma, Gall, Tonak, and Altendorf (521) noted that 121 patients had multivisceral organ involvement. Extended multivisceral radical resections resulted in a postoperative mortality rate of 12% (compared to 6% without such resection), with a 5-year survival rate of 54% for patients with inflammatory adherence and 49% for patients with malignant infiltration. In this series the most frequently used extension of resection was total hysterectomy (39%), small bowel (21%), urinary bladder (16%), and abdominal wall (4%). It is worthy of note that when carcinoma was inadvertently torn or transected during resection, the 5-year survival rate dramatically dropped to 17%. Despite the increased operative mortality with extended resection, the authors of this review believe that the benefit outweighs the disadvantages. Hunter, Ryan, and Schultz (522) reviewed their results of colorectal carcinoma in three treatment groups: standard colectomy, en bloc resection, and colectomy with separation of adherent organs. The 5-year survival rates were 55%, 61%, and 23%, respectively. No operative mortality occurred with en bloc resection. The 5-year survival rate, recurrence rate, and local recurrence rate for standard colectomy were 55%, 33%, and 11%, respectively; for en bloc resection, 61%, 36%, and 18%; and for separation of organs, 23%, 77%, and 69%. The authors concluded that colorectal carcinoma adherent to adjacent organs must be treated by en bloc resection because separation of organs results in unacceptably high local recurrence and poor 5-year survival rates. On the other hand, the results of en bloc resection were comparable to those of standard colectomy for nonadherent carcinomas.

Natafusa et al. (529) evaluated the short-term or long-term outcome of multivisceral resection relative to that of the standard operation. Of 323 patients, 16.4% received multivisceral resection because of adhesion to other organs. Overall, morbidity rates were 49.1% for multivisceral resection versus 17.8% for the standard operation and postoperative mortality was 0% in both groups. Only multivisceral resection (odds ratio, 2.7) was an independent factor for overall postoperative complications. The survival of patients with multivisceral resection was similar to that after the standard operation (5-year rate 76.6% vs. 79.5%). Lymph node metastases (hazard ratio 2.5) and blood transfusion (hazard ratio 2.4) were independently associated with patient survival.

Kroneman, Castelein, and Jeekel (533) evaluated the results of 33 patients who underwent curative en bloc resection. Adherent organs excised included small bowel, urinary bladder, abdominal wall, uterus, duodenum, pancreas, stomach, and kidney. The postoperative morbidity rate was 6%, the mortality was 3%, and the 4-year survival rate was 33%. Poeze et al. (534) reported on 1346 patients with colorectal carcinoma, 144 (11%) of whom underwent multivisceral resections for invasion of adjacent organs. In patients who had disease-free margins, there was no compromise of long-term survival (i.e., local invasion to adjacent organs with or without lymph node involvement was not related to survival). The overall operative mortality rate was 5%. Izbicki et al. (527) reported on 83 patients who underwent en bloc resection. Mean survival was 44 months after extended resection. The postoperative mortality, morbidity, and survival rates were comparable to those in patients who underwent nonextended resections.

Landercasper et al. (535) reported on 54 of 1284 patients (4%) who underwent potentially curative resections of right colon lesions found to be adherent to adjacent organs, abdominal wall, or retroperitoneum. Postoperative complications developed in 24% of patients. The mortality rate was 1.9% and the 5-year survival rate was 31%. Only one of nine patients with pancreatic or duodenal adherence treated with limited resection remained disease free. The authors recommend radical en bloc resection if no distant metastases are present. Adjuvant radiation therapy or chemotherapy did not improve survival.

To determine the perioperative mortality and morbidity and the long-term prognosis of patients undergoing extended pelvic resections for localized advanced primary adenocarcinoma of the rectum, Orkin et al. (523) reviewed their experience with 65 patients. Local invasion without distant metastases was present in all patients at operation and en bloc resection of all involved organs was performed with intent of cure. Average age at operation was 61 years; 23% were men and 77% were women. Operations included abdominoperineal resection in 57%, low anterior resection in 31% and Hartmann procedure in 12%. Additionally, women (81%) with intact uteri underwent en bloc hysterectomy, 77% women with intact ovaries had oophorectomy, and 50% of women had partial vaginal resection. Twenty-six percent of the 65 patients had a cystectomy, and two patients had a portion of small intestine resected in continuity with their carcinoma. Pathologic examination revealed lymph node involvement in 45% and histologic confirmation of adjacent organ extension in 57%. There were no perioperative deaths. Overall, 5-year survival was 52% with 65% of deaths attributable to either recurrent carcinoma or a new primary lesion. The cumulative probability of recurrence at five years was 39%.

Carne et al. (528) reported on multicenter experiences of en bloc bladder resection for colorectal carcinoma adhering to the urinary bladder. Fifty-three patients were identified of which 45 had en bloc partial cystectomy performed, 4 en bloc total cystectomy and four had the adhesions disrupted and no bladder resection. All patients who did not have a bloc resection developed local recurrence and died from their disease. Mean follow-up was 62 months. The extent of bladder resection did not seem important in determining local recurrence. The decision to perform total rather than partial cystectomy should be based on the anatomic location of the carcinoma.

Rowe et al. (519) determined the therapeutic benefit of multivisceral resection in patients with locally advanced colorectal carcinomas. The study population was composed of 118 patients whose resection of the primary lesion included one or more adhesed adjacent secondary organs or structures. Their survival is reported in Table 8 but clinical relevance is that there was no statistically significant difference in the 5-year survival rates when multiple adjacent secondary organs or structures were resected and therefore they believe an aggressive operative approach is warranted.

Yamada et al. (536) reported 64 patients with locally advanced primary or recurrent rectal carcinoma who underwent abdominoperineal resection with sacral resection in 9 patients, anterior pelvic exenteration in 8 patients, total pelvic exenteration in 27 patients, and total pelvic exenteration with sacral resection in 20 patients. Rates of morbidity, reoperation, and mortality were 50%, 4.5%, and 0% in 22 patients with primary carcinoma, and 60%, 2.4%, and 2.4% in 42 patients with recurrent disease, respectively. Major complications, such as sepsis, intra-abdominal abscess, and enteric fistula caused one hospital death and reoperation in two patients. In 21 patients who underwent curative resection for primary carcinoma, the overall 5-year survival rates were 74.1% for Dukes' B and 47.4% for Dukes' C although the difference was not statistically significant. Thirty patients with recurrent carcinoma who underwent curative resection, had significantly improved survival with a 5-year survival rate of 22.9% compared with 12 patients who underwent palliative resection resulting in a survival rate of 0%.

In an excellent clinical review of the role of extended resection in the initial treatment of locally advanced colorectal carcinoma, Lopez and Monafo (537) collated information on the results of multivisceral resection for colorectal carcinoma. In 11 publications in which 609 patients underwent extended resection for colorectal carcinoma, the operative morbidity rate was 27%, the operative mortality rate was 6%, and lymph node metastases occurred in 39%. The 5-year survival rate was 68% for node-negative status and 23% for node-positive status. If adherence to adjacent viscera was benign, the 5-year survival rate was 68% but declined to 40% if the attachment was malignant. Survival in locally advanced colorectal carcinoma is more dependent on lymph node status than on the extent of local invasion (524). In 23 publications in which 248 patients underwent total pelvic exenteration for rectosigmoid carcinoma, the operative morbidity rate was 60% and the operative mortality rate was 12%. The 5-year survival rate was 64% for node-negative status and 32% for node-positive status.

In the unique situation in which there is isolated invasion of the prostate by a rectal carcinoma, Campbell et al. (538) described the use of radical retropubic prostatectomy in conjunction with restorative proctosigmoidectomy for en bloc excision. This novel technique offers an alternative to total pelvic exenteration, thereby obviating the need for urinary and fecal diversion. The expected 5-year survival of patients subjected to en bloc resection ranged from 30% to 79% (see Table 8) and thus justifies an aggressive approach.

Urinary Tract Involvement by Colorectal Carcinoma

McNamara et al. (539) recently reviewed the literature on urinary tract involvement by colorectal carcinoma with the aim of highlighting technical and oncologic issues that should be considered when dealing with this complex problem. From the relevant literature, they identified three distinct clinical scenarios in which the urinary tract may be affected by colorectal carcinoma: involvement by primary colorectal carcinoma, involvement of recurrent carcinoma, and unexpected intraoperative findings of urinary tract involvement. The following information and guidelines draw heavily from their dissertation.

Primary Involvement of the Urinary Tract

Involvement of the urinary tract system occurs in 5% of patients with primary colorectal carcinoma. Any level of the urinary tract can be affected by direct invasion or be involved with an associated inflammatory mass. Three sites are most commonly affected: the dome of the bladder, the lower ureter, and the base of the bladder. Adherence to or invasion of the dome of the bladder is the most common presentation and most frequently occurs in rectosigmoid malignancies. Locally advanced disease with direct invasion of adjacent organs may result in fistula formation, but half of such patients have no symptoms at presentation. Involvement of the trigone may compromise the intramural ureter. Lower third lesions of the rectum may involve the prostate gland and prostatic urethra. A CT is usually performed as part of the standard investigation of patients with sigmoid or rectal carcinoma but is mandatory in patients with urinary symptoms. In addition to staging, CT allows localization of the ureters and confirms bilateral renal function, although it tends to overestimate the need for urinary organ resection. CT is more likely to produce a false-positive diagnosis of pelvic floor or piriform muscle invasion than magnetic resonance imaging and is less likely to identify sacral bone invasion when it is present. Modern high-resolution MRI (sensitivity 97% and specificity 98%) is superior to CT (sensitivity 70% and specificity 85%) in staging locally advanced primary or recurrent rectal carcinomas, with better detection of penetration of the fascia propria and involvement of the potential circumferential resection margin. Cystoscopy diagnoses the cause of genitourinary symptoms in 79% to 87% of patients with rectal carcinoma. Only 57% of patients with a mucosal abnormality at cystoscopy have bladder invasion at final pathology, yet locating the vesical opening of a malignant rectovesical fistula improves identification of patients who require pelvic exenteration for adequate resection.

Bladder Involvement

If involvement of the dome of the bladder is suspected, en bloc resection of the carcinoma and all adherent bladder should be performed, because of the well documented difficulty in distinguishing between adherence and invasion macroscopically and the greatly diminished survival experienced by patients in whom the carcinoma is breached during resection. This policy carries the risk that the adjacent organ in the resected specimen may show no evidence of malignant invasion but is justified because no increase in morbidity is reported following multivisceral resection, especially partial cystectomy. No adverse effect on local recurrence or survival has been demonstrated when partial cystectomy is performed instead of total cystectomy for localized malignant involvement, provided the resection is R0.

Involvement of the trigone is less straightforward, and curative resection requires total pelvic exenteration. Total pelvic exenteration is appropriate for direct invasion of the trigone, vesicoureteric junction, or intramural ureter in the absence of distant metastases and has been used in both primary and locally recurrent disease. Total pelvic exenteration may be combined with sacral resection, especially in patients with local recurrence extending into the presacral space. Bladder reconstruction requires construction of a urinary conduit, of which an ileal conduit is the most common, although cecal or colonic conduits are sometimes used. Supralevator exenteration with double-pouch reconstruction using a colonic J-pouch and a Mainz pouch with sphincter-preserving urethral anastomosis has been described, but long-term results are not available and recurrence in this setting may result in catastrophic complications. Early urologic complications of urinary diversion include ileoureteral anastomotic dehiscence and early hydronephrosis. Late urologic complications include ureteral stenosis and late hydronephrosis. Unsuccessful endoscopic and radiologic management of these complications may lead to the necessity for nephrectomy. Operative mortality rates following total pelvic exenteration ranging between 5% and 33% have been quoted. There is a trend toward increased morbidity in patients who receive preoperative radiotherapy. Review of the literature reveals 3-year survival figures ranging from 30% to 64.5% and 5-year survival figures ranging from 9% to 61%. Some surgeons routinely include intrapelvic dissection of the internal iliac and obturator nodes in their approach to total pelvic exenteration but no convincing survival advantage has been demonstrated. Total pelvic exenteration has been reported to have a sixfold greater mortality than, lesser, exenterative procedures.

Ureteric Involvement

Bilateral involvement of the ureters may occur because of compression from extensive nodal disease at the pelvic brim or by invasion of the trigone by the primary carcinoma but both scenarios usually require total pelvic exenteration if curative resection is desired. In contrast, unilateral ureteric invasion may be approached by en bloc resection of the affected segment followed by appropriate reconstruction. Ipsilateral ureteroureterostomy over a double-J stent is the simplest form of anastomosis but even when combined with use of a vesicopsoas hitch is suitable only for short resections of the distal ureter. Reconstruction following resection of a longer segment may require use of a Boari flap in which a well-vascularized flap of bladder is constructed into a tube to which the proximal ureter may be anastomosed. Cystoureterectomy and ureteric crossover is recommended for unilateral involvement of the ureterovesical junction and may be performed without significantly increasing postoperative morbidity and mortality. Ileal interposition has satisfactory oncologic results and allows resection of a long ureteric segment but may result in renal damage because of transmission of high intravesical pressures and should only be performed in carefully selected patients. Rarely, nephrectomy may be an acceptable option.

Fistula

Rectourinary fistulation is an uncommon event that rarely occurs in females because of the protective effect afforded by the interposition of the female genital tract. The classic triad of pneumaturia, fecaluria, and recurrent urinary tract infection is unusual, and patients more commonly present with fever, a pelvic mass, or cystitis. Most patients have a urinary tract infection, but pneumaturia is reported by only 10% of patients. Only 21% of fistulas associated with a rectal carcinoma contain malignant cells. The remaining 79% result from interventions (including operation, radiotherapy and chemotherapy) for rectal carcinoma. The success rate for initial and reoperative surgery was 21% and 88%, respectively, when malignant cells were identified in the fistula tract as compared with success rates of 44% and 100% for treatment-related fistulas. The decision to administer neoadjuvant chemoradiotherapy must balance the possibility of improved survival and less radical operation against the reported increase in preoperative fistulization and perioperative morbidity and mortality.

Hydronephrosis

In a patient with primary colorectal carcinoma, the most common cause of hydronephrosis is regional nodal disease from a sigmoid or rectal carcinoma at the pelvic brim but direct extension of a primary carcinoma, local inflammation, and isolated ureteric metastases are all possible. Malignant hydronephrosis detected at the time of first diagnosis of colorectal carcinoma is a worrying finding because less than half of such patients have resectable disease.

Radiotherapy

The role of preoperative radiotherapy in rectal carcinoma involving the urinary tract is not yet clear. Downstaging may improve resectability by reducing the extent of operation necessary to obtain negative margins and rendering some inoperable carcinomas resectable.

Unexpected Intraoperative Involvement

A particular difficulty arises when unexpected local extensive disease is identified at operation. Discovery of a rectosigmoid carcinoma adherent to the bladder for which one can envisage a relatively straightforward en bloc resection with primary closure of the bladder clearly differs from a carcinoma likely to require complex reconstruction. Important are issues relating to the quality of the preoperative informed consent, particularly if the proposed resection requires a procedure with the potential for considerably greater morbidity and mortality than anticipated or an unexpected impact on postoperative quality of life such as necessity to create a stoma. In some circumstances, the correct decision is to defer resectional operation in favor of radiotherapy or a subsequent more aggressive one-stage procedure.

Recurrent Colorectal Carcinoma

The finding of hydronephrosis after a previous colorectal resection usually indicates pelvic sidewall disease that precludes resection. It is associated with concomitant metastatic disease in 50% of patients and predicts poor survival, even after salvage operation. Investigation of a patient with suspected recurrence involving the urinary tract should be vigorous to avoid the morbidity and mortality of salvage operation in patients unlikely to benefit. Inoperable metastatic disease should be excluded with spiral CT and MRI or PET. Rarely, urinary and/or fecal diversion may be justified in the presence of metastatic disease in patients who are symptomatic but cannot be successfully palliated with less invasive radiologic or endourologic techniques.

Abnormal Renal Function

Patients with abnormal preoperative renal function require optimization of their condition before operation. An elevated preoperative urea level is independently predictive of increased 30-day mortality, while patients who develop acute renal failure postoperatively have a 30-day mortality in excess of 50%. Patients may require preoperative urinary decompression. Early urinary decompression is a priority to prevent or minimize irreversible renal damage. This may take the form of initial retrograde double-J stenting or percutaneous nephrostomy with subsequent endourologic stent insertion.

Palliation

Treatment of unresectable carcinoma involving the urinary tract or potentially resectable local disease in the presence of unresectable metastases should maximize survival without adverse effects on quality of life. Most malignant strictures of the ureter can be treated by an endourologic approach with minimal morbidity, allowing normal micturition without external drainage and with durable results. Pelvic arterial infusion of 5-FU and mitomycin C may reduce pain and improve hydronephrosis while systemic steroid therapy has also been suggested for the temporary improvement of hydronephrosis in the palliative setting.

Unresectable Carcinoma

In the unusual circumstance in which a lesion is totally unresectable, it usually can be bypassed satisfactorily.

Palliative Resection

One of the most unsatisfying situations facing any surgeon who operates on patients with colon and rectal carcinoma is that of recommending a major abdominal procedure, with its potential complications, to a patient who has definite evidence of incurable disease. The decision regarding operative intervention is usually reached with some trepidation, since many of these patients are in poor physical condition and have a limited life expectancy. However, even for patients with metastatic carcinoma of the large bowel, resection performed to eliminate the symptoms of local disease has been advocated as a worthwhile procedure for avoiding the potential complications of obstruction and massive bleeding and the effects of local invasion of the primary lesion. In general, resections relieve patients of their symptoms and sometimes may even prolong life expectancy (540). The most common symptoms are pain and bleeding (541,542).

It has been estimated that 10% to 20% of patients who are seen with primary operable colorectal carcinoma already have associated liver metastases (540). Unfortunately, not all patients will benefit from resection, and, in fact, some patients will be caused additional morbidity. This morbidity, together with the mortality of the operative procedure, may exceed the benefit of any temporary symptomatic relief. Thus the role of palliative resection for malignant neoplasms has been questioned from time to time. This is especially true for the decision to perform a palliative abdominoperineal resection, an operation that entails not only an operative procedure of considerable magnitude but also the establishment of a permanent colostomy in a patient with only a chance of limited survival.

In the presence of metastatic disease, survival will depend on the nature and extent of the metastases. Indeed, some metastatic lesions should be resected in addition to the primary lesion. Survival depends on the pattern of metastatic disease. For example, Joffe and Gordon (541) noted survival with unilobar liver metastases to be 16.9 months, while with bilobar metastases, survival was only 8.5 months. Cady, Monson, and Swinton (540) noted a survival of 13 months; Takaki, Ujiki, and Shields (543), 12 months; and Goslin et al. (544) a similar length of survival. Under such circumstances, the recommendation for resection should be tempered by a consideration of factors such as extensive hepatic replacement or jaundice, marked ascites, or massive peritoneal seeding, in which case life expectancy is very short and no benefit could be accrued from a resection. The prognosis is poor for patients with extensive liver metastases, patients older than 75, and patients with a previous history of cardiovascular disease (541).

Makela et al. (545) reviewed 96 patients who underwent palliative operations with an 8% postoperative mortality rate (5% for resections and 17% nonresection procedures) and a 24% postoperative morbidity rate. Median survival was 10 months (15 months for resections and 7 months for nonresection procedures) and 5% of patients survived longer than 5 years. The median relief of symptoms related to the malignancy was 4 months (4 months after resection and 1 month after nonresection procedures). Twenty-five patients underwent a second palliative operation.

Liu et al. (542) studied 68 patients with incurable colon carcinoma to try to identify objective criteria that might help surgeons decide which patients will benefit from palliative operations. The postoperative mortality rate was 10% and the complication rate was 10%. The mean survival after palliative resection was 10.6 months, after bypass was 3.4 months, and after diagnosis in patients not operated on was 2.0 months. Of the variables studied, the only factors affecting survival were poorly differentiated lesions and >50% replacement of liver. The authors concluded that although resection carries with it a relatively high postoperative mortality rate, it is worthwhile as long as hepatic metastases occupy <50% of liver volume.

The macroscopic features of the primary disease must be taken into consideration because of the ever-present concern of obstruction. However, the advent of endoscopic, laser therapy appears entirely suited to maintaining an adequate caliber of lumen to prevent obstruction. Endoluminal stenting is another way of dealing with obstructive symptoms.

Synchronous Carcinomas

Recommendations for the appropriate treatment of synchronous carcinomas of the colon are at least in part based on the magnitude of the risk of development of metachronous adenomas and carcinomas after conventional resections. The incidence of synchronous carcinomas has been reported to be 1.5% to 7.6% (546). In a series of 2586 patients, an incidence of 1.8% was reported (546). Bussey, Wallace, and Morson (547) reported on 3381 patients who survived conventional resections for carcinoma of the colon and rectum at St. Mark's Hospital in London and found an overall incidence of metachronous carcinoma of 1.5%. The incidence rose to 3% in those cases followed up for at least 20 years. For those patients in whom an associated adenomatous polyp was found in the original operative specimen, the level rose to 5%. In a more recent study, synchronous carcinomas were found in 4.4% of patients (548). Passman, Pommier, and Vetto (549) reported on an 18-year multi-institutional data base of 4878 patients with colon carcinoma. There were 160 patients (3.3%) with 339 synchronous carcinomas. Eight percent of these patients had more than two lesions at the time of diagnosis. Based on highest stage lesion, 1% of patients were at stage 0, 28% at stage I, 33% at stage II, 25% at stage III, and 11% at stage IV. The disease-specific 5-year survival rate by highest stage was 87% for stage 0 or I, 69% for stage II, 50% for stage III, and 14% for stage IV. These "highest stage" survival rates for patients with synchronous carcinomas were not significantly different from survival of patients with same-stage solitary carcinomas in their data base. In light of this, it seems reasonable that if synchronous carcinomas are located in the same anatomic region, a conventional resection should be performed. When the carcinomas are widely separated, a subtotal colectomy is the operation of choice.

Synchronous Polyps and Carcinoma

Recommendation for the treatment of patients with colon carcinoma and associated polyps involves the same considerations as for synchronous carcinomas. However, it also depends on the number, location, and size of these polyps. For example, if the polyps were confined to the region of the index carcinoma, the conventional operation for that portion of the bowel would be indicated. With the availability of colonoscopy, assessment and possible therapy of associated polyps can be accomplished. If the remaining bowel contains only occasional polyps that can be easily excised with the colonoscope, it would appear reasonable to have these polyps excised and to proceed with a conventional resection of the carcinoma. If one of the excised polyps should contain a carcinoma or if the polyps were of a size deemed in excess of colonoscopic polypectomy, a subtotal colectomy would be appropriate (550). Subtotal colectomy even has been recommended for colon carcinoma and synchronous polyp in good-risk patients (548). An individual who has exhibited the propensity for growth of many polyps in the colon, although not in adequate numbers to be considered familial adenomatous polyposis, would still qualify for a subtotal colectomy and ileorectal, or at least ileosigmoid, anastomosis.

Metachronous Carcinoma

Gervaz et al. (551) assessed the incidence of metachronous colorectal carcinomas in a population-based study of 500,000 residents. Of this total, 5006 patients had sporadic carcinoma of the colon or rectum with 34% being located proximal to the splenic flexure. Occurrence of a second primary colorectal carcinoma was observed in 2.4% of this population. The risk for developing a second incidence of primary colorectal carcinoma was higher in patients whose initial carcinoma was located in the proximal colon (3.4% vs. 1.8%, odds ratio 1.9). The risk for each segment of large bowel was as follows: cecum, 3.4%; right colon, 3%; transverse colon, 3.8%; left colon, 2.8%; sigmoid colon, 1.7%; and rectum 1.8%. By contrast, the risk for developing a second extracolonic carcinoma did not differ between patients with proximal and distal carcinomas (13.7% vs. 13.4%).

Shitoh et al. (552) reported that microsatellite instability can be regarded as an independent marker for predicting the development of metachronous colorectal carcinoma after operation. In a study of 328 colorectal carcinoma patients surveyed by periodic colonoscopy for at least three years after operation, 17 metachronous colorectal carcinomas were detected during the follow-up period. The% of microsatellite instability-positive cases was 26.4%. Incidences of metachronous colorectal carcinomas in microsatellite instability-positive and microsatellite instability-negative cases were 15.3% and 3%, respectively. The cumulative 5-year incidence of metachronous colorectal carcinomas was significantly higher in microsatellite instability positive cases than in microsatellite instability-negative cases (12.5% vs. 2.5%).

Treatment of Metastatic Disease

Liver

Metastases to the liver from carcinoma of the colon or rectum are frequent occurances. Indeed, the liver is the dominant site of treatment failure and the major cause of death in patients with colorectal carcinoma. Studies have demonstrated that up to 30% of patients undergoing apparently curative operation already have hepatic metastases that are not evident to the surgeon at the time of laparotomy (369,553,554). Furthermore, another 50% have recurrent disease develop within the liver (555). Some 90% of patients who die from colorectal carcinoma have liver metastases (264). In a study of doubling times, Finlay et al. (556) determined that the mean doubling time for overt metastases was 155 ± 34 days ($\pm$ SEM) compared with 86 ± 12 days for occult metastases. The mean age of the metastases at the time of operation was estimated by extrapolation of the observed growth curve, assuming Gompertzian kinetics, to be 3.7 ± 0.9 years ($\pm$ SEM) for overt metastases and 2.3 ± 0.4 years for occult metastases.

There is a perception that streamline flow of blood in the portal vein may influence the anatomic distribution of liver metastases, depending on the site of the primary lesion. It has previously been reported that carcinomas arising in the right colon are distributed to the right lobe of the liver 10 times more commonly than to the left lobe, whereas liver metastases from carcinomas arising from the left colon and rectum are believed to be distributed homogenously. Wigmore et al. (557) collected data prospectively on the anatomic site of hepatic metastases in 207 patients with colorectal metastases. This study could not find any evidence to support a differential pattern of metastasis within the liver dependent on the location of the primary colorectal carcinoma.

In an effort to accurately detect liver metastases, Van Ooijen et al. (558) prospectively compared continuous CT angiography to preoperative ultrasonography and conventional CT in 60 patients with primary or secondary colorectal carcinoma. The standard references were palpation of the liver and intraoperative ultrasonography. Continuous CT angiography had a high sensitivity of 94% in contrast to ultrasonography (48%) and conventional CT (52%). However, there was a higher false positive rate because of variations in the perfusion of normal liver parenchyma. Overall, continuous CT angiography had the highest accuracy (74%) compared with ultrasonography (57%) and CT (57%). The low specificity will hamper its routine application.

Strasberg et al. (559) reviewed 43 patients with metastatic colorectal carcinoma referred for hepatic resection after conventional staging with CT. PET scanning was performed on all patients. PET identified additional carcinoma not seen on CT in 10 patients. Operation was contraindicated in six of these patients because of the findings on PET. Laparotomy was performed in 37 patients. In all but two, liver resection was performed. The Kaplan-Meier estimate of overall survival at three years was 77%. This figure is higher than 3-year estimate of survival found in previously published series. They concluded preoperative PET scan lessens the recurrence rate in patients undergoing hepatic resection for colorectal metastases to the liver by detection of disease not found on conventional imaging. Some patients who will not benefit from operation can thus be spared a laparotomy and major resection.

Liver surgeons usually recommend against biopsy of colorectal liver metastases because of the risk of local dissemination. Rodgers et al. (560) conducted a multicenter retrospective review of cases of colorectal liver metastases presenting for operation that had undergone a preoperative biopsy. Of 231 cases of colorectal metastases, 18.6% had undergone a preoperative biopsy. Evidence of dissemination related to the biopsy was 16%. Within the operative period (median 21 months), three of the seven cases with evidence of dissemination and 11 of the 35 without dissemination were alive without disease. They concluded there is a significant risk of local dissemination with biopsy of colorectal liver metastases.

The value of intraoperative hepatic ultrasonography has been discussed in detail on p. 619. Fuhrman et al. (561) reported on the use of intraoperative ultrasonography in the assessment of porta hepatis lymph nodes and the evaluation of resection margins to determine whether this modality would improve the selection of patients likely to benefit from operation. Of 151 patients undergoing exploration, 30 patients were considered unresectable, 14 (9.2%) demonstrated by intraoperative ultrasonography. The authors concluded that intraoperative ultrasonography did, indeed, improve the selection process.

The question of what to do for patients with these metastases has been a matter of controversy. At one point any suggestion of an operative approach to metastatic disease was deemed foolish by some. The natural history of untreated hepatic metastases confirms a median survival of 6 to 12 months and of 4.5 months if metastases are synchronous (562–564). If not resected, 3-year survival rates ranged from 3% to 7% and only 1% to 2% of patients will survive for 5 years (555). Six studies of the natural history of such metastases in a total of 1151 patients described a 5-year survival rate of $\leq$3%. In a study of 484 untreated patients, six independent determinants of survival were identified in the following order: (1)% liver volume replaced by carcinoma, (2) grade of malignancy of the primary lesion, (3) presence of extrahepatic disease, (4) mesenteric lymph node involvement, (5) serum CEA, and (6) patient age (565). The prognosis is closely related to the extent of liver replacement.

A variety of chemotherapeutic regimens, including systemic chemotherapy and direct intraportal and intra-arterial modes of administration, have been attempted, all with limited and short (if any) benefit, but with the cost

TABLE 9 ■ Survival Following Resection of Hepatic Metastases

Author(s)	No. of Patients	Survival (%) 3-Year	Survival (%) 5-Year	Operative Mortality (%)	Complication Rate (%)
Hughes, Scheele, and Sugarbaker (567) (1989)[a]	800		32		
Schlag, Hohenberger, and Herforth (568) (1990)	122	40	30	4	34
Petrelli et al. (569) (1991)	62		26	8	30
Doci et al. (570) (1991)	100		30	5	41
Rosen et al. (571) (1992)	280	47	25	4	
Nakamura et al. (572) (1992)	31	45	45	3	16
Van Ooijen et al. (573) (1992)	118		21	8	35
Grayowski et al. (574) (1994)	204	43	32	1	
Scheele et al. (575) (1995)	434	45	33	4	22
Fuhrman et al. (561) (1995)[b]	107		44	3	
Hananel, Garzon, and Gordon (576) (1995)	26		31	0	66
Rougier et al. (577) (1995)	123	35	21		
Wade et al. (578) (1996)	133		26	4	
Wanebo et al. (579) (1996)	74		24	7	35
Ohlsson et al. (580) (1998)	111		25	4	
Fong et al. (581) (1999)	1001	57	37	3	31
Buell et al. (582) (2000)	110	54	40	2	21
Elias et al. (583) (2003)	111	38	20	4	28
Kato et al. (584) (2003)[c]	585		33		
Teh and Ooi (585) (2003)	96	71		0	7
Weber et al. (586) (2003)	62	45	22	0	36

[a]Tumor registry of 24 institutions (24%, 5-year disease-free survival).
[b]Ultimate patient selection with intraoperative ultrasonography.
[c]Post operative hepatic artery chemotherapy in 33% but no difference in survival noted in those with or without chemotherapy.

of considerable toxicity and anxiety. Systemic chemotherapy has resulted in response rates ranges 18% to 28% (566), and the median survival rate ranges of 8 to 14 months (555). Other efforts have been directed at hepatic artery embolization, hepatic artery ligation, and even irradiation, all without significant worthwhile benefit.

The lack of effective therapeutic alternatives has made hepatic resection the primary treatment consideration. Indeed, worthwhile survival rates in selected patients have been reported (Table 9). The timing and extent of operation varies. In the patient who presents with a synchronous lesion, which is amenable to operation, it appears appropriate to excise the lesion at the time of operation. If the lesion requires a major hepatic resection, the combination of partial hepatectomy and colectomy appears to be too great a task for one operation. After the colonic resection, if there is no other evidence of metastases and if a thorough evaluation, including a CT scan, has demonstrated removable disease, proceeding with resection is the treatment of choice. If the patient presents with metastatic disease at a later date, evaluation is necessary to ensure that the metastatic disease is confined; at the same time evaluation should be performed to rule out the presence of recurrent disease at the area of the index carcinoma. The resection of hepatic metastases in patients with intra-abdominal extrahepatic disease is of no proven benefit (587). Even with preoperative staging, as many as 26% of patients will have intra-abdominal extrahepatic metastases, most commonly in portal and celiac lymph nodes (587). It is necessary to rule out evidence of other metastatic disease. Unfortunately, investigation of patients rarely unveils a solitary lesion. Only approximately 10% of patients develop metastases suitable for operation. In their study of the natural history of hepatic metastases from colorectal carcinoma, Wagner et al. (588) found that the median survival rate for unresected solitary and multiple unilobar metastases was 21 and 15 months, respectively. Earlier series reported untreated patients to have a median survival of 6 to 12 months. It is understandable why hepatic resection became an attractive option.

Surgical resection of primary colorectal carcinoma in patients with stage IV disease at initial presentation remains controversial. Although bowel resection to manage symptoms such as bleeding, perforation, or obstruction has been advocated, management of asymptomatic patients has not been well defined. Patient-dependent factors (performance status, comorbid disease) and extent of distant metastases are among the considerations that have an impact on the decision to proceed with operative management in asymptomatic stage IV colorectal carcinoma. To ascertain the natural history of a group of untreated patients and to evaluate simultaneously in another group whether or not the administration of systemic chemotherapy modifies this natural history, Luna-Perez et al. (589) followed 77 patients with liver metastases from colorectal carcinoma. Untreated patients consisted of 45 patients; 41 developed extrahepatic metastatic disease and their median survival rate was 13 months. The group who received chemotherapy included 32 patients; 29 developed extrahepatic metastatic disease and their median survival was 15 months. There were no differences in overall survival in both groups. The administration of systemic chemotherapy did not modify the natural course of the disease. Dismal results of this nature mandate a better form of therapy, namely, operative. Ruo et al. (590) reviewed 127 patients who underwent elective resection of their asymptomatic primary colorectal carcinoma. Over the same time period, 103 stage IV patients who did not undergo resection were identified. The resected group could be easily distinguished from the nonresected group by a higher frequency of right colon carcinomas and metastatic disease restricted to the liver or one other site apart from the primary carcinoma. Resected patients had prolonged median (16 months vs. 9 months) and two years (25% vs. 6%) survival compared with patients never resected. Univariate analysis identified three significant prognostic variables (number of distant sites involved, metastases to liver only, and volume of hepatic replacement by malignancy) in the resected group. Volume of hepatic replacement was also a significant predictor of survival. Subsequent to resection of asymptomatic primary colorectal carcinoma, 20% developed postoperative complications. Median hospital stay was six days. Two patients (1.6%) died within 30 days of operation. They concluded stage IV patients selected for elective palliative resection of asymptomatic primary colorectal carcinomas had substantial postoperative survival that was significantly better than those never having resection.

A review by Blumgart and Fong (555) revealed an operative mortality of <5% in most series, but complications arose in excess of 20% in most series. Myocardial complications were seen in 1%, pleural effusion requiring thoracostomy in 5% to 10%, pneumonia in 5% to 22%, and pulmonary embolism in 1%. Complications specifically related to liver resection included liver failure (3% to 8%), bile leak and biliary fistula (4%), perihepatic abscess (2% to 10%), and significant hemorrhage (1% to 3%). The most common sites for failure were the liver and lung with the liver involved as a site of recurrence in 45% to 75% of patients having liver resection. In light of this, adjuvant systemic chemotherapy seems to be an attractive option, but to date its role is unproven. Because the liver is the most common site of recurrence and may be the sole site in up to 40% of patients, regional hepatic chemotherapy is theoretically attractive, but studies in this arena have also failed to prove the benefit of that therapy. However, some studies are encouraging.

The prognosis of metastatic carcinoma is grave. Kuo et al. (591) collected data from 74 patients with stage IV colorectal carcinoma to identify prognostic factors for predicting selection criteria for operative treatment in patients with metastatic disease. Overall survival time was 16.1 months. Survival in the curative resection group was significantly longer than in the noncurative groups (31.9 months vs. 12.7 months). The operative mortality and morbidity rates were 5.6% and 21%, respectively. The two most common complications were leakage at the site of anastomosis and urinary tract infection. Based on these results, they concluded that patients older than 65 years with metastases at multiple sites, intestinal obstruction, preoperative carcinoembryonic antigen level ≥500 ng/mL, lactate dehydrogenase ≥350 units/L, hemoglobin <10 mg/dL, or hepatic parenchymal replacement by metastatic disease >25% have poor prognosis for operative intervention. They noted the more aggressively they performed radical resection and metastasectomy in selected patients the more survival benefits the patients obtained.

SIMULTANEOUS COLORECTAL AND HEPATIC RESECTION ■ Weber et al. (586) reported that in selected patients, simultaneous resection of the colorectal primary carcinoma and liver metastases does not increase mortality or morbidity rates compared with delayed resection, even if a left colectomy and/or a major hepatic resection are required. De Santibanes et al. (592) reviewed the results of liver resection performed simultaneously with colorectal resection in 71 cases. The median hospital stay was eight days. Morbidity was 21% and included nine pleural effusions, seven wound abscesses, four instances of hepatic failure, three systemic infections, three intraabdominal abscesses, and one colonic anastomotic leakage. Operative mortality was 0%. Recurrence rate was 57.7% and progression of disease was detected in 33.8%. Overall and disease-free survivals at one, three, and five years were 88%, 45%, and 38% and 67%, 17%, and 9%, respectively. Prognostic factors with notable influence on patient outcomes were nodal stage as per TNM classification, number of liver metastases, diameter (smaller or larger than 5 cm), liver resection specimen weight (lighter or heavier than 90 g) and liver resection margin (smaller or larger than 1 cm).

Chua et al. (593) retrospectively analyzed 96 consecutive patients with synchronously recognized primary carcinoma and hepatic metastases who underwent concurrent (64 patients) or staged (32 patients) colonic and hepatic resections. No significant differences were observed between concurrent and staged in type of colon resection, or hepatic resection, overall operative duration, blood loss, volume of blood products transfused, perioperative morbidity (53% vs. 41%), disease-free survival from date of hepatectomy (median 13 months vs. 13 months) or overall survival from date of hepatectomy (median 27 months vs. 34 months). There was no operative mortality. Overall duration of hospitalization was significantly shorter for concurrent than for staged resection (mean 11 days vs. 22 days). They concluded, concurrent colectomy and hepatectomy is safe and more efficient than staged resection and should be the procedure of choice for selected patients in medical centers with appropriate capacity and experience.

Tocchi et al. (594) reviewed the results of 78 patients who underwent resection of primary colorectal carcinoma and hepatic metastases with curative intent. Adverse predictors of the long-term outcome included the number of metastases (>3), preoperative CEA value >100 ng/mL, resection margin <10 mm, and portal nodal status.

Tanaka et al. (595) reported on 39 consecutive patients with synchronous colorectal carcinoma metastases to the liver who underwent curative simultaneous "one-stage" hepatectomy and resection of the colorectal primary. Only the volume of the resected liver was selected as a risk factor for postoperative complications (350 g mean resected liver volume in patients with postoperative complications vs. 150 g in those without complications). Patient age of 70 years or older and poorly differentiated mucinous adenocarcinoma as the primary lesion predicted decreased overall survival. They concluded, a one-stage procedure appears desirable for synchronous colorectal hepatic metastases except for patients requiring resection of more than one hepatic section, patients aged 70 years or older, and those with poorly differentiated or mucinous adenocarcinomas as primary lesions.

Currently there is no consensus as to which factors are important in selecting patients for operation and which factors are important in determining the patient's prognosis.

For example, Attiyeh and Wichern (596) found no significant difference in the survival rates of patients with a solitary metastasis and in those with multiple lesions, nor was survival influenced by the size of the metastasis. The survival rate was better in patients whose primary colorectal lesion was Dukes' B compared with those whose lesion was Dukes' C. Adson (597) listed several determinants for a favorable prognosis, including (1) primary colorectal carcinoma of limited locoregional extent (Dukes' A or B), (2) presence of fewer than four liver lesions, (3) metastases that appear a long time after the primary lesion was removed, (4) lesions that can be removed with wide margins, and (5) lack of extra-hepatic metastases. Combining their own experience with reports in the literature, Bozzetti et al. (598) found that sites of failure after liver resection were hepatic in 16%, extrahepatic in 15%, and both in 14%. Patterns of recurrence in our patients were hepatic in 31%, hepatic and an extrahepatic site in 15%, and lung in 15% (576). Nagorney (563) reported that the only characteristic associated with prolonged survival was the stage of the primary lesion, with Dukes' B patient survival being greater than Dukes' C. In Nagorney's review, site of origin and degree of differentiation of the primary carcinoma did not correlate with survival rate. Characteristics of metastatic disease that influenced survival included the number of hepatic metastases (one to three are better than four or more), the interval between diagnosis of the primary lesion and hepatic metastases, the resection margin (a margin >1 cm is better), and the presence of extrahepatic disease. The size and distribution of lesions within the liver had no associated with survival. We were also interested in variables related to survival and reviewed 26 selected patients with liver colorectal metastases who underwent hepatic resection (576). The patient's age, sex, site of primary lesion, histologic grade, lymph node involvement, location, size, and number of hepatic metastases, type of hepatic resection, and preoperative CEA blood levels were documented. Complete removal with histologically negative resection margins were accomplished in 24 patients. The extent of resection performed was hepatic lobectomy in 12 patients, segmentectomy in eight patients, and wedge resection in four patients. The 5-year survival rate was 30.5%. Patients with metachronous metastases had a better survival rate than those with synchronous lesions (46.6% vs. 13.6%, respectively). None of the other factors studied showed a significant effect on survival. During a median follow-up of 30.9 months, 20 patients developed recurrence of their disease (60% in the liver). There was no perioperative mortality. Morbidity arose in 66% of patients, with a majority of the complications minor. Wanebo et al. (579) reported a significant relationship with survival and the number of metastases (three or fewer vs. four or more), the presence of bilobar vs. unilobar metastases, and the extent of liver resection (wedge and segmental vs. lobectomy and trisegmentsctomy). They believe that resection of bilobar disease or extended resection should generally be avoided, especially in medically compromised patients. Nakamura et al. (572) adopted a very aggressive approach for patients suffering from liver metastases. Of 31 patients, 22 underwent lymph node dissection of the hepatic hilus, in the minds of most surgeons, a current contraindication to hepatic resection. Six of the 22 patients who underwent lymph node dissection had nodes positive for carcinoma. Ten patients underwent removal of recurrent lesions in the liver, lung, adrenal glands, and brain after initial hepatic resection. Based on an overall 5-year survival rate of 45%, the authors concluded that repeat hepatectomy and dissection of hilar lymph nodes improves prognosis in selected patients with hepatic metastases of colorectal carcinoma.

In an analysis of risk factors, Grayowski et al. (574) found that gender, Dukes' classification, site of primary colorectal carcinoma, histologic differentiation, size of metastatic lesion, and intraoperative transfusion requirement were not statistically significant prognostic factors. In patients 60 years of age or older, an interval of 24 months or less between colorectal and hepatic resection, four or more metastatic lesions, bilobar involvement, positive resection margins, lymph node involvement, and the direct invasion of adjacent organs were significant poor prognostic factors.

Hughes, Scheele, and Sugarbaker (567) collated information from a registry of 24 participating institutions. Factors that they found to affect prognosis detrimentally were (1) more than four metastaltic lesions, (2) a short disease-free interval from initial resection to appearance of metastases (<1 year), (3) a pathologic margin of <1 cm on the liver specimen, and (4) the presence of lymph node metastases at the time of initial resection.

Using a multivariate regression analysis, Scheele et al. (575) found that survival was dependent on the presence of satellite metastases, grade of the primary carcinoma, time of the diagnosis of metastases (synchronous vs. metachronous), diameter of the largest metastases (>5 cm), anatomic vs. nonanatomic approach, year of resection, and mesenteric lymph node involvement. Rougier et al. (577) studied 544 patients with resected hepatic metastases from colorectal carcinoma to determine prognostic factors. Among the 20 variables assessed, eight items were singled out. In decreasing order of relative risk, they included performance status (2 to 4 vs. 0 to 1), alkaline phosphatase level (greater than normal vs. normal), number of involved segments (≥4 vs. ≤3), chemotherapy (no vs. yes), extrahepatic metastases (yes vs. no), primary location (right vs. other), prothrombin time (<75% vs. >75%), and resection of the primary carcinoma (no vs. yes).

Specific criteria for the selection process are constantly evolving. Adson (597) has offered a thoughtful set of guidelines. Patients whose primary colorectal lesions are well confined, who have one to three evident unilobar hepatic metastases that likely can be removed with wide margins, and who have no evidence of extrahepatic metastases should undergo resection. Patients with extrahepatic metastases, numerous hepatic metastases involving more than one half of the liver, large lesions that encroach on major hepatic veins, or contralateral hilar ducts or veins or lesions sited so as to preclude resection with free margins have an unfavorable prognosis and should not undergo resection. Unfortunately, many patients do not fall neatly into one of these categories, and the surgeon must exercise considerable judgment in making a definitive recommendation.

The role of neoadjuvant chemotherapy for patients with multiple (five or more) bilobar hepatic metastases irrespective of initial resectability is still under scrutiny. Tanaka et al. (599) compared the outcome of hepatectomy alone with that of hepatectomy after neoadjuvant chemotherapy for multiple bilobar hepatic metastases from colorectal carcinoma. The outcome of 48 patients treated with neoadjuvant chemotherapy followed by hepatectomy was compared with that of 23 patients treated by hepatectomy alone. Patients who received neoadjuvant chemotherapy had better three and five year survival rates from the time of diagnosis than those who did not (67.0% and 38.9% vs. 51.8% and 20.7%, respectively) and required few extended hepatectomies (four segments or more) (39 of 48 vs. 23 of 23). In patients with bilateral multiple colorectal liver metastases, neoadjuvant chemotherapy before hepatectomy was associated with improved survival and enabled complete resection with fewer extended hepatectomies.

Allen et al. (600) compared the treatment and outcome in patients referred for staged resection of synchronous colorectal liver metastases between patients who did not receive neoadjuvant chemotherapy and had exploratory operations after recovery from colon resection and patients who did receive chemotherapy before liver resection. Neoadjuvant chemotherapy was given to 52 patients; in 29 of them the disease did not progress but in 17 the disease progressed while they were receiving treatment. Median follow-up was 30 months. Five-year survival was statistically similar between patients who did and those who did not receive neoadjuvant therapy (43% vs. 35%). Patients within the neoadjuvant group whose disease did not progress while they were receiving chemotherapy experienced significantly improved survival as compared to patients who did not receive chemotherapy (85% vs. 35%). In the setting of synchronous colorectal metastases the response to neoadjuvant chemotherapy may be a prognostic indicator of survival and may assist in the selection of patients for conventional or experimental adjuvant therapies.

Fong et al. (581) reported on 1001 consecutive patients undergoing liver resection for metastatic colorectal carcinoma. These resections included 237 trisegmentectomies, 394 lobectomies, and 370 resections encompassing less than a lobe. The operative mortality rate was 2.8%. The 5-year survival rate was 37% and the 10-year survival rate was 22%. Seven factors were found to be significant and independent predictors of poor long-term outcome: positive margin, extrahepatic disease, node-positive primary, disease-free interval from primary to metastases <12 months, number of hepatic lesions >1 cm, largest hepatic lesion >5cm, and carcinoembryonic antigen level >200 ng/mL. When the last five of these criteria were used in a preoperative scoring system, assigning one point for each criterion, the total score was highly predictive of outcome. The five-year actuarial survival for patients with 0 points was 60%, 1 point was 44%, 2 points was 40%, 3 points was 20%, 4 points was 25%, and 5 points was 14%. In fact, no patient with 5 points survived five years. Patients with up to two criteria can have a favorable outcome. Patients with three, four, or five criteria should be considered for experimental adjuvant trials.

Iwatsuki et al. (601) examined various clinical and pathologic risk factors in 305 consecutive patients who underwent primary hepatic resection for metastatic colorectal carcinoma. Preliminary multivariate analysis revealed that independently significant negative prognosticators were: (1) positive surgical margins, (2) extrahepatic carcinoma involvement including the lymph nodes, (3) three or more metastatic lesions, (4) bilobar metastases, and (5) time from treatment of the carcinoma to hepatic recurrence of 30 months or less. Because the survival rates of the 62 patients with positive margins or extrahepatic metastases were uniformly very poor, multivariate analysis was repeated in the remaining 243 patients who did not have these lethal risk factors. The reanalysis revealed that independently significantly poor prognosticators were: (1) three or more metastases, (2) metastases size greater than 8 cm, (3) time to hepatic recurrence of 30 months or less, and (4) bilobar metastases. Risk scores (R) for recurrence were divided into five groups: grade 1, no risk factors; grade 2, one risk factor; grade 3, two risk factors; grade 4, three risk factors; and grade 5, four risk factors. Grade 6 consisted of the 62 culled patients with positive margins or extrahepatic metastases. Estimated five-year survival rates of grade 1 to 6 patients were 48.3%, 36.6%, 19.9%, 11.9%, 0%, and 0%, respectively. The proposed risk-score grading predicted the survival differences.

Smith et al. (602) found that in patients who are undergoing curative resection of hepatic colorectal metastases, an elevated expression of the biomarkers hTERT and Ki-67 are better predictors of poor long-term survival than is a score based on clinical features.

Kato et al. (584) reported on 585 patients who underwent hepatectomy at 18 institutions. The 5-year survival rate for those treated by hepatectomy was significantly higher (32.9%) than for those not undergoing hepatectomy (3.4%). After hepatectomy for hepatic metastases, the most prevalent form of recurrence was in the remnant liver (41.4%), followed by recurrence of pulmonary metastases (19.2%), and other (7.2%). Factors of the primary carcinoma adversely affect prognosis included poorly differentiated adenocarcinoma or mucinous carcinoma, depth of invasion, lymph node metastases of Stage n3 and n4 by the Japanese classification of colorectal carcinoma, number of metastatic lymph nodes of more than four, and Dukes' stage D. Factors at the time of hepatectomy adversely affecting prognosis after operation for hepatic metastases included residual carcinoma, extrahepatic metastases, hepatic metastases of degree H3 stipulated by the Japanese classification of colorectal carcinoma, number of metastases of four or more, pathology of hepatic metastases of poorly differentiated carcinoma, resection margin of <10 mm, and carcinoembryonic antigen value higher than normal preoperative and one month postoperative.

Indications for hepatectomy in patients with four or more hepatic colorectal metastases remain controversial. Imamura et al. (603) reviewed data from 131 patients who underwent a total of 198 hepatectomies. Patients were grouped according to the number of metastases. The 5-year survival rate of patients with 1 to 3, 4 to 9, and 10 or more metastases were 51%, 46%, and 25%, respectively. They concluded hepatic resection for patients with four to nine metastases clearly is warranted. On the other hand, for patients with 10 or more nodules operation cannot be insured absolutely to be contraindicated in high volume centers at which the operative mortality rate is nearly zero.

In the review by Jaeck (604) the 5-year survival rate for resection of colorectal liver metastases ranged from 20% to 54%. However, the resectability rate of colorectal liver metastases is reported to be less than 20%. This limitation is mainly due to insufficient remnant liver and to extrahepatic disease. Among extrahepatic locations, lymph node metastases are often considered indications of a very poor prognosis and a contraindication to resection. He found that the presence of hepatic pedicle lymph node metastases ranged from 10% to 20%. When located near the hilum and along the hepatic pedicle, they should not be considered an absolute contraindication to resection and extended lymphadenectomy should be performed. However, when they reach the celiac trunk, there is no survival benefit after resection of colorectal liver metastases.

Elias et al. (605) reported the long-term outcome and prognostic factors of 75 patients who underwent a complete R0 resection of extrahepatic disease simultaneously with hepatectomy for colorectal liver metastases. Extrahepatic disease localization included peritoneal carcinomatosis (limited), hilar lymph nodes, local recurrences, retroperitoneal nodes, lung, ovary, and abdominal wall. The mortality rate was 2.7% and morbidity was 25%. After a median follow-up of 4.9 years, the overall 3- and 5-year survival rates were 45% and 28%, respectively. They concluded extrahepatic disease in colorectal carcinoma patients with liver metastases should no longer be considered as a contraindication to hepatectomy. However, there must be an intended R0 resection and it is inappropriate for patients with multiple extrahepatic disease sites or more than five liver metastases.

The optimal operative strategy for the treatment of synchronous resectable colorectal liver metastases has not been defined. Martin et al. (606) reviewed their experience with 240 patients who were treated surgically for primary adenocarcinoma of the large bowel and synchronous hepatic metastasis. One hundred thirty-four patients underwent simultaneous resection of a colorectal primary and hepatic metastases in a single operation (group 1), and 106 patients underwent staged operations (group 2). Simultaneous resections tend to be performed for right colon primaries, smaller, and fewer liver metastases, and less extensive liver resection. Complications were less common in the simultaneous resection group, with 49% sustaining 142 complications compared with 67% sustaining 197 complications for both hospitalizations in the staged resection group. Patients having simultaneous resection required fewer days in hospital (median 10 days vs. 18 days). Perioperative mortality was similar (simultaneous $n=3$ staged, $n=3$). They believe simultaneous resection should be considered a safe option in selected patients with resectable synchronous colorectal metastases.

Nelson and Freels (607) assessed the effect of post-hepatic resection, hepatic artery chemotherapy on overall survival. Trials were sought in Medline, the Cochrane Controlled Trial Register, the Cochrane Hepatobiliary Group Trials Register, and through contact of trial authors and reference lists using key words. Overall survival at five years in the hepatic artery group was 45% and 40% in the control group. No significant advantage was found in the meta-analysis for hepatic artery and chemotherapy measuring overall survival. Adverse events related to hepatic artery therapy were common including five therapy-related deaths. They concluded that this added intervention for the treatment of metastatic colorectal carcinoma cannot be recommended at this time.

More recently, Clancy et al. (608) conducted a meta-analysis of prospective clinical trials to determine if adjuvant hepatic arterial infusion confers a survival benefit to treat residual microscopic disease after curative hepatic resection for colorectal carcinoma metastases. Prospective clinical trials comparing hepatic arterial chemotherapy after curative hepatic resection for colorectal carcinoma metastases against a control arm were included. The outcome measure was survival difference at one and two years after operation. Seven studies met the inclusion criteria, and all except one were randomized trials. The survival difference in months was not statistically significant at two years. Based on these findings, they concluded routine adjuvant hepatic artery infusion after curative resection for colorectal carcinoma of the liver cannot be recommended.

Bines et al. (609) reported on a review of 131 patients who underwent hepatic resection for metastatic colorectal carcinoma. There were 31 recurrences and, of those, 13 underwent re-resection with a morbidity rate of 23%, a mortality rate of 8%, and a 5-year survival rate of 23%. The authors concluded that in properly selected patients, repeat resection yields results similar to those after initial resection. Wanebo et al. (579) reported that 12% of their patients had repeated resection of metastases, with an overall 5-year survival rate of 43% after the first resection and 22% after the second resection. In their review of 10 reports, Blumgart and Fong (555) noted that between 15% and 40% of patients who undergo resection for hepatic metastases have the liver as the sole site of recurrence, and approximately one third will be candidates for further resection. In the 146 patients collated, the operative mortality rate was 3%, and the complications encountered were similar to those that developed after initial resection. These results were in highly selected patients. The median survival was >30 months when calculated from the time of second liver resection and >47 months when calculated from the time of the first resection. However, there were only four 5-year survivors. Although resection is feasible, only approximately 5% of all patients undergoing further resection will come to a second resection (555). Wanebo et al. (610) reported recurrence rates in from 65% to 85% of patients after initial hepatectomy for metastases for colorectal carcinoma. Approximately one half of these have liver metastases and in 20% to 30%, only the liver is involved. The opportunity for resection is frequently limited because of diffuse liver disease or extrahepatic extension, and only approximately 10% to 25% of these patients have conditions amenable to resection. The authors' comprehensive review of the 28 series showed that the mean interval between the first and second liver resections varied from 9 to 33 months and was approximately 17.5 months in the two largest series. The median survival in the series reporting 10 or more patients was 19 months (mean, 24 months), which is comparable to data in the single resection series. In the large French Association series containing 1626 patients with single resections and 144 patients with two resections, the 5-year survival rates were 25% and 16%, respectively. The recurrence rate after repeat resection was high (>60%), and half of the recurrences were in the liver. The prognostic factors favoring repeat resection are variable,

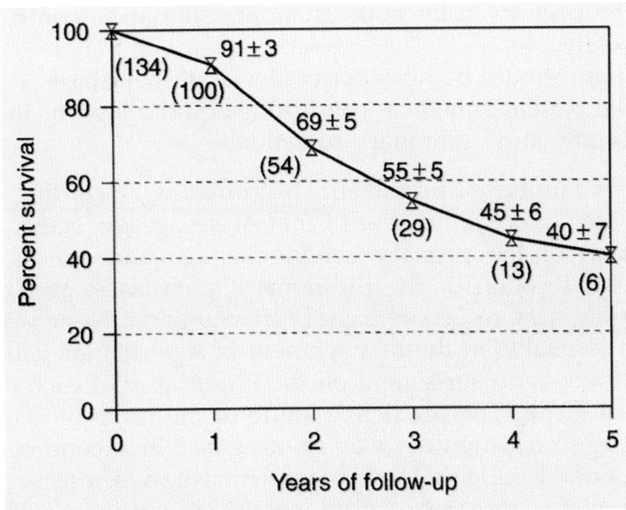

FIGURE 58 ■ Survival curve for 134 patients undergoing second hepatic operations for colorectal metastasis (collected from 15 reports in the literature). *Source*: From Ref. 611.

but they include absence of an extrahepatic extension of carcinoma and a complete resection of liver metastases. The authors concluded that repeat hepatic liver resection for metastatic colorectal carcinoma in carefully selected patients appears warranted. From their own experience and review of the literature, Pinson et al. (611) came to the same conclusion. For patients collected from the literature, the authors constructed a survival curve (Fig. 58). Fernandez-Trigo, Shamsa, and Sugarbaker (612) were also encouraged to perform repeat hepatic resections for colorectal metastases because it remains the only curative treatment. Others concur with this course of management (613).

Takahashi et al. (614) reviewed clinical data of patients undergoing repeat hepatectomy for metastatic colorectal carcinoma compared with those of initial hepatectomy to determine criteria for repeat hepatectomy. For 22 patients who underwent repeat hepatectomy, no mortality and an 18% morbidity rate were observed. The 3-year survival rate after hepatectomy was 49%. The only poor prognostic factor after repeat hepatectomy was a serum carcinoembryonic antigen level greater than 50 ng/mL before initial hepatectomy. Suzuki et al. (615) assessed the risks and clinical benefits of repeat hepatectomy for those patients who underwent hepatectomy for colorectal metastases. There was no operative mortality after repeat hepatectomy in 26 patients. Operative bleeding was significantly increased in the second hepatectomy but operating time, duration of hospital stay, and performance status after the second hepatectomy were comparable with those of the initial hepatectomy. The median survival time from the second hepatectomy was 31 months and the three 3- and 5-year survival rates were 62% and 32%, respectively. A short disease-free interval (six months or less) between the initial hepatectomy and diagnose of hepatic recurrence in the remnant liver was significantly associated with poor survival after the second hepatectomy.

Oshawo et al. (616) conducted a study aimed to compare outcome in patients with solitary colorectal liver metastases treated by operation ($n = 20$) or by radiofrequency ablation. Most patients in both groups also received systemic chemotherapy. Median survival after liver resection was 41 months with a 3-year survival of 55.4%. There was one postoperative death and morbidity was minimal. Median survival after radiofrequency ablation was 37 months with a 3-year survival of 52.6%. In this study, survival after resection radiofrequency ablation of solitary colorectal liver metastases was comparable. The latter is less invasive and requires either an overnight stay or day-case facilities only.

Berber et al. (617) determined the predictors of survival at the time of laparoscopic radiofrequency thermal ablation in 135 patients with colorectal liver metastases who were not candidates for resection. The median survival for all patients was 28.9 months. Patients with a CEA less than 200 ng/mL had improved survival compared with those of a CEA more than 200 ng/mL (34 months vs. 16 months). Patients with the dominant lesion less than 3 cm in diameter had a median survival of 38 months versus 34 months for lesions 3 to 5 cm, and 21 months for lesions greater than 5 cm. Survival approached significance for patients with one to three metastases versus more than three metastases (29 months vs. 22 months). The presence of extrahepatic disease did not affect survival. Only the largest liver metastases more than 5 cm was found to be a significant predictor of mortality with a 2.5-fold increased risk of death versus the largest liver metastases less than 3 cm in size.

Ueno et al. (618) collected data from 68 patients who underwent resection of colorectal liver metastases who might benefit from prophylactic regional chemotherapy. The extrahepatic recurrence rate at three years after hepatectomy was 57.8%. Three variables were independently associated with extrahepatic recurrence including raised serum level of carcinoembryonic antigen after hepatectomy (relative risk 5.4), venous invasion of the primary carcinoma (relative risk 4.0) and high-grade budding of the primary carcinoma (relative risk 3.1). Patients with none of these risk factors had a 3-year extrahepatic recurrence rate of 7.1% compared with 61.6% for those with one risk factor and 100% for those with two or three risk factors. This system might be used on an individual basis to select patients with colorectal liver metastases for regional chemotherapy or systemic chemotherapy after operative intervention. The value of postoperative chemotherapy following resection of hepatic metastases was reviewed by Cohen and Kemeny (619). Two studies compared hepatic artery infusion with no treatment and no overall survival benefit was reported. In one study there was a modest two-year survival improvement from 72% to 86%. Drugs used included FUDR, 5-FU/leucovorin and in light of newer drugs used for systemic chemotherapy, this improvement may not be relevant.

For patients with unresectable liver metastases, Gray et al. (620) reported on the use of embolization of yttrium-90-containing microspheres into the liver via a catheter inserted into the hepatic artery at laparotomy. In 29 patients, the CEA levels fell in the 26 patients in whom this therapy was tested, and there was CT evidence of reduction in 48% of the 22 patients re-examined. Some patients also received continuous chemotherapy infusion to potentiate the radiation effect. Although this is an important first step, there is no evidence that reduction of disease is translated to either improved survival or quality of life. Stubbs et al. (621) treated 50 patients with advanced nonresectable colorectal liver metastases with selective internal radiation therapy. Estimated liver involvement was less than 25% in 30 patients, 25% to 50% in 13 patients, and greater than 50% in 7 patients. A single dose of between 2.0 and 3.0 GBq of 90 yttrium microspheres was injected into the hepatic artery via a subcutaneous port and followed at 4-week intervals by regional chemotheraphy with 5-FU. Treatment-related morbidity did occur including a 12% incidence of duodenal ulceration. Median survival for patients with extrahepatic disease was 6.9 months. For patients with no extrahepatic disease median survival was 17.5 months. Substantial destruction of liver metastases can be achieved in more than 90% of patients with a single treatment. Lang and Brown (622) recommended the selective embolization of doxorubicin and ethiodized oil for unresectable hepatic metastases. In his review, Stuart (623) found that chemoembolization for patients with metastatic colorectal carcinoma appears to be a reasonable alternative for many who are not operative candidates. Response rates of approximately 50% have been reported, with survival longer than would be expected in studies of systemic therapy among patients who had failed standard chemotherapy. Survival may be especially enhanced in treated patients who have no extrahepatic metastases.

Cryoablation has also been used in this clinical setting but has not yet been proven to improve outcome (555). For patients with unresectable hepatic metastases, Weaver, Atkinson, and Zemel (624) reported the use of hepatic cryosurgery with or without resection in 140 patients, 119 of whom had carcinomas that were colorectal in origin. The median number of lesions treated was three. The operative mortality rate was 4%, and complications included coagulopathy, hypothermia, myoglobinuria, pleural effusion, acute tubular necrosis and infection. The median survival rate was 27 months. Ruers et al. (625) reported on the long-term efficacy of cryosurgery as an adjunct to hepatic resection in patients with colorectal liver metastases not amenable to resection alone. Thirty patients met the following inclusion criteria: metastases confined to the liver and judged irresectable, 10 or fewer metastases, cryosurgery alone or in combination with hepatic resection allowed disease clearance. Median follow-up was 26 months. Overall, 1- and 2-year survival rates were 76% and 71%, respectively. Median survival was 32 months. Disease-free survival at one year was 35%, two years 7%. Six patients developed recurrence at the site of cryosurgery; given that the total number of cryosurgery-treated lesions was 69 the local recurrence rate was 9%.

Lung

Pulmonary metastases occur in approximately 10% of all patients with adenocarcinoma of the colon and rectum, and the majority of these are only of one facet of a generalized spread of disease. About 10% of these patients, that is, 1% of the total, will develop solitary pulmonary metastases. The criteria for determining resectability of pulmonary metastases are similar to those applied to resection of hepatic metastases:

1. Ideally the pulmonary metastasis should be solitary. If more than one is involved, the lesions should be confined to one lung; if bilateral, the lesion in each lung must be solitary.
2. The primary colorectal carcinoma should be controlled locally.
3. There should be no other evidence of metastases.
4. The patient's medical condition should allow for thoracotomy and pulmonary resection.

A number of prognostic discriminants, including disease-free interval, number of metastases, grade, stage, and location of the primary carcinoma, age and sex of the patient, location of the pulmonary metastases, and type of pulmonary resection, have been examined. None is uniformly reliable in the management of a particular patient, and there is no agreement on the importance of each individual factor. The predictive value of the route of venous drainage on prognosis was investigated in a consecutive series of 44 patients who underwent curative resection of pulmonary metastases from colorectal carcinoma (626). The primary lesion was located in the colon in 14 patients and in the upper third of the rectum in 11 patients, thus indicating blood drainage directed toward the portal vein (group I). In 10 and nine cases, respectively, the initial growth was in the middle and lower third of the rectum with the venous outflow at least partially directed into the vena cava (group II). There was no obvious difference in the two groups regarding the initial site of carcinoma recurrence. The liver was involved in four of 15 patients failing in group I as opposed to four of 13 patients with hematogenous relapse in group II. Median survival and disease-free survival times were significantly longer in patients in group I (58.4 and 50.2 months, respectively) than in patients in group II (30.9 and 16.8 months, respectively), and, even more pronounced, in colon carcinoma patients (75.4 and 60.2 months, respectively) when compared with rectal carcinoma patients (31.0 and 17.9 months, respectively). In contrast, survival curves did not differ significantly when the two groups with different routes of drainage (5-year survival rate, 53% vs. 38%; 5-year disease-free survival rate, 43% vs. 37%), or carcinomas of the colon and rectum (5-year survival rate, 67% vs. 38%; 5-year disease-free survival rate, 60% vs. 32%) were compared using the log-rank test. The primary carcinoma site does therefore not become a major criterion in selecting patients for surgical resection.

Saclarides et al. (627) reported on 23 patients who underwent 35 thoracotomies for metastatic colorectal carcinoma. The pulmonary disease was diagnosed within an interval of 0 to 105 months (average, 33.4 months) after colon resection. Fifteen patients underwent a single thoracotomy (12 patients had solitary lesions and three patients had multiple nodules). Eight patients underwent multiple thoracotomies. The median survival following thoracotomy was 28 months, the 3-year survival rate was 45%, and the 5-year survival rate was 16%. Factors that had no significant bearing on survival included the origin and stage of the primary carcinoma and the patient's age and sex. An interval before thoracotomy of 3 years had an impact on survival. Patients who underwent multiple thoracotomies had a significantly prolonged survival. Patients who underwent a single thoracotomy for a solitary lesion had a significantly prolonged survival compared with patients who underwent a single thoracotomy for multiple metastases. After thoracotomy, 14 patients eventually developed recurrent disease, which was confined to the lung in only four patients. Of these 14 patients, 11 subsequently died of carcinoma. The authors concluded that thoracotomy for metastatic disease should be considered when the primary carcinoma is controlled, the lungs are the only site of metastatic disease, and there is adequate lung reserve to withstand surgery.

In a review of 12 series of patients, including their own, Brister et al. (628) summarized the results of 335 patients who underwent pulmonary resection. The authors found overall 2-year and 5-year survival rates of 70% and 30%, respectively. In their series the only factor significant in determining survival was a long disease-free interval. It seems logical that a longer disease-free interval reflects a slower growing malignancy and would in turn be associated with a longer postthoracotomy survival. In a series of 76 pulmonary resections, Wade et al. (578) found a projected 5-year survival rate of 36%, a mean survival rate of 38 months, and a 3% operative mortality rate.

Kanemitsu et al. (629) studied factors that might be helpful in predicting survival in 313 patients (the largest number) with pulmonary metastases from colorectal carcinoma who were candidates for thoracotomy. Pulmonary resections included lobectomy 137, partial resection 132, segmentectomy 38, and pneumonectomy 6. Overall survival rates were 90.4% in one year, 53% at three years, and 38.3% at five years. The 1-, 3- and 5-year survival rates of patients with pulmonary metastases from colorectal carcinoma who did not undergo thoracotomy were 58.6%, 8.5%, and 1.9%, respectively. They identified five variables as independent predictors of 3-year survival: prethoracotomy carcinoembryonic antigen level, number of pulmonary lesions, presence of hilar or mediastinal infiltrated lymph nodes, histology of the primary carcinoma and presence of extrathoracic disease. Their model has moderate predictive ability to discriminate between patients who are likely to survive after thoracotomy for pulmonary metastases from colorectal carcinoma.

Watanabe et al. (630) also reviewed 49 patients to identify prognostic factors for overall survival and risk factors for further intrapulmonary recurrence after resection of pulmonary metastases from colorectal carcinoma. Survival after resection of pulmonary metastases was 78% at three years and 56% at five years. Solitary pulmonary metastases were significantly correlated with survival. The pathological features of the primary colorectal carcinoma had no impact on survival. Histologically incomplete resection of pulmonary metastasis significantly correlated with pulmonary re-recurrence.

Negri et al. (631) reported on the development of a preoperative chemotherapy strategy for patients selected to undergo pulmonary metastasectomy from colorectal carcinoma in 31 patients. The median age at operation was 61 years. Twenty (65%) proceeded directly to operation and five of these patients received postoperative chemotherapy. Eleven (35%) received preoperative chemotherapy which consisted of fluoropyrimidine in combination with either Oxaliplatin, or Mitomycin C, except for one patient who received single agent CPT-11; 82% had a partial response and 18% had stable disease. In total, 39 thoracic operations (six bilateral and one incomplete) were undertaken. There were no postoperative deaths. Twenty percent who had initial operation had postoperative complications compared to 18% of the preoperative chemotherapy group. Overall 3- and 5-year survival rates after the first thoracic operation were 65.2% and 26.1%, respectively. Disease-free interval, number of pulmonary metastases, previous resection of hepatic metastases, prethoracotomy carcinoembryonic antigen (CEA), and preoperative chemotherapy were not found to be significant prognostic factors for survival. They concluded resection of lung metastases has a low morbidity and mortality and results in long-term survival for 20% to 30% of patients. Furthermore, in this clinical setting preoperative chemotherapy produced a high response rate with no patients experiencing disease progression prior to operation.

King et al. (632) assessed the safety and efficacy of imaging-guided percutaneous radiofrequency ablation for local control of lung metastases from colorectal carcinoma. Forty-four metastatic lesions in 19 patients were treated successfully at 25 treatment sessions. Five of 19 patients were retreated for new lesions. There were 13 pneumothoraces following the 25 treatments, and six patients required drainage. Six months after treatment CT demonstrated that three lesions had progressed, 25 metastases were stable or smaller, and 11 were no longer visible. At 12 months five metastases had progressed, 11 were smaller or stable and 9 were not visible.

Retreatment for recurrence or new metastases is feasible and occurred in five patients in this series. Some patients also received concomitant chemotherapy. Improving long-term survival is not the only goal of treatment. Relief of symptoms such as cough, hemoptysis, and pain is also beneficial. Furthermore, survival benefit has been shown for repeat pulmonary metastasectomy.

Ike et al. (633) evaluated results of their strategy for intensive follow-up after resection of colorectal carcinoma and aggressive resection of lung metastases. The follow-up program for lung metastases includes a serum CEA assay every two months and chest x-ray every six months. Operative resection of lung metastases was performed if the primary and any nonpulmonary metastases had been controlled, lung metastases numbered four or fewer, and pulmonary functional reserve was adequate. Standard operation for lung metastases was lobectomy and lymph node dissection was added in cases where the metastases were over 3 cm in size. Forty-two patients underwent 50 lung resections for metastatic colorectal carcinoma. Overall five-year survival rate after resection of lung metastases from colorectal carcinoma was 63.7%. Patients with well differentiated primary carcinoma, a solitary metastatic nodule, and disease-free interval of at least two years after initial operation are likely to be long-term survivors.

Ishikawa et al. (634) reviewed retrospectively the clinical course of 37 patients who underwent operative resection of primary colorectal carcinoma and metastatic lung disease. Multivariate analysis indicated that the existence of an extranodal malignant deposit in the primary lesion (hazard ratio = 4.55) and three or more lung metastases (hazard ratio = 2.9) were significant indicators for poor prognosis. They divided the patients into two groups; Goup A ($n = 12$) had neither of these two parameters, and Group B ($n = 25$) comprised all other patients. Survival rate at three and five years were 90.9% and 90.9% in Group A and 16.1% and 8.1% in Group B, respectively; and disease-free survival after thoracotomy (3-year and 5-year disease-free survival rate, 52.9% and 39.7% in Group A and 5.3% and 5.3% in Group B, respectively). They identified an extra nodal malignant deposit at the primary carcinoma site as a new significant prognostic factor after resection of pulmonary metastases from colorectal carcinoma. Resection of pulmonary metastases is expected to be very useful for patients without extra nodal deposits and fewer than three pulmonary metastases.

Zink et al. (635) reviewed medical records of 110 patients operated on pulmonary metastases of colorectal origin. The median time interval between diagnosis of the primary carcinoma and thoracotomy was 35 months. After resection of the pulmonary metastases, the 3- and 5-year post-thoracotomy survival measured 57% and 32.6%, respectively. The overall survival was significantly correlated with the disease-free interval and the number of intrapulmonary metastases. Treatment, stage, and grade of the primary carcinoma, occurrence of liver metastases and local recurrences, mode of treatment of metastases, and postoperative residual stage had no significant correlation with either total or post-thoracotomy survival.

Irshad et al. (636) reviewed 49 patients treated operatively for pulmonary metastases from colorectal carcinoma. The perioperative death rate was 4%. Overall 5- and 10-year survival rates were 55% and 40%, respectively. The mean interval between the initial colonic resection and resection of pulmonary metastases was 36 months. Variables that carried a poor prognosis included more than one pulmonary lesion, a disease-free interval less than two years, and moderately or poorly differentiated colorectal carcinoma. The 16 patients who received chemotherapy after their thoracotomy had a 5-year survival rate of 51% compared with 54% for the 33 patients who did not receive chemotherapy, demonstrating postoperative chemotherapy has no survival benefit.

Vogelsang et al. (637) evaluated clinically relevant prognostic factors to define a subgroup of patients who would most benefit from resection of lung metastases from colorectal carcinoma. There were 75 patients with pulmonary metastases from colorectal carcinoma who underwent 104 R0 lung resections. Patients who had no evidence of recurrent extrathoracic disease, no more than three metastases on either side, lobectomy as the maximum operative procedure, and adequate cardiorespiratory function were eligible for operation. Overall median survival was 33 months with 3- and 5-year survival rates of 47% and 27%, respectively. Prognostic groups included patients with a maximum metastasis size of 3.75 cm or less with a disease-free interval of more than 10 months and patients with larger metastases and a shorter disease-free interval. Median survival and 5-year survival were 45 months and 39% in the former group and 24 months and $< 11\%$ in the latter.

When a solitary pulmonary shadow occurs synchronously with a large bowel carcinoma, the dual problems of the nature of the pulmonary lesion and the priority of management arise. Based on the principles of management of metastatic lesions, this clinical situation should not be a dilemma. The large bowel malignancy should be handled without regard for the pulmonary lesion. If the surgeon achieves a curative resection, thus fulfilling the criterion of control of local disease, and there is no other evidence of metastatic disease, attention then can be directed toward the pulmonary lesion, usually 2 or 3 months later. The pulmonary lesion may, in fact, prove to be a primary lung carcinoma.

Assessment of the contribution of surgery to the treatment of pulmonary metastases from carcinoma of the colorectum demonstrated that it is a valid treatment option with survival benefit. An aggressive operative policy directed toward metastatic carcinoma confined to the lung has resulted in a rewarding rate of disease-free survivals and appreciable palliative benefit for appropriately selected patients. Even multiple metastases may be successfully managed as long as the cardinal principles of patient selection are observed. Pulmonary resection is attended with little risk (operative mortality rates ranging from 0% to 4% and major complication rates from 0% to 12%), the survival results justify an aggressive operative approach (627). Accordingly, patient follow-up should include regular chest x-ray examinations to detect subsequent metastases amenable to operative therapy.

Liver and Lung

Although simple lung or liver metastasectomy from colorectal carcinoma has proved effective in selected patients, the subject of simultaneous bi-organ metastasectomies is seldom addressed. Mineo et al. (638) reported on 29 patients who presented simultaneous ($n=12$) or sequential liver before lung ($n=10$) and lung before liver ($n=7$) metastases. All metastases were successfully resected in a total of 56 separate procedures. In 35 thoracic procedures, 45 metastases were removed by wedge resection ($n=36$) or lobectomy ($n=9$). In addition, 47 liver metastases were resected with wedge ($n=24$), segmentectomy ($n=13$), or lobectomy ($n=10$). There were no perioperative deaths and the morbidity rate was 10.7%. All patients were followed for a minimum of three years. Median survival from the second metastasectomy was 41 months, with a 5-year survival rate of 51.3%. Risk-factor distribution among the three metastatic pattern groups was insignificant. Premetastasectomy elevated levels of both CEA and CA19–9, and mediastinal or celiac lymph node status were significantly associated with survival, although number of metastasectomies, disease-free interval, and simultaneous versus sequential diagnosis were not. In the multivariate analysis, only elevated CEA plus CA19–9 was significantly associated with survival. They concluded that either simultaneous or sequential lung and liver metastasectomy can be successfully treated by operation.

Ike et al. (639) retrospectively analyzed 48 patients who underwent pulmonary resection for metastatic colorectal carcinoma, 27 of whom had lung metastases alone and 15 had previous partial hepatectomy, and 6 had previous resection of local or lymph node recurrence. Five-year survival rates after resection of lung metastases were 73% in patients without preceding recurrence, 50% following previous partial hepatectomy, and 0% after resection of previous local recurrence. There was no significant difference in survival after lung resection between patients who had sequential liver and lung resection versus those who had lung resection alone.

Nagakura et al. (640) analyzed retrospectively a total of 136 patients who underwent resection of hepatic or pulmonary metastases of colorectal origin. Eighty-four patients underwent hepatectomy alone, 25 underwent pulmonary resection alone, and 27 underwent both hepatic and pulmonary resection. The 27 patients undergoing hepatic and pulmonary resection were divided into two groups; 17 patients with sequentially detected hepatic and pulmonary metastases and 10 patients with simultaneous detected metastases. Patient survival after hepatic and pulmonary resection was comparable with that after hepatic alone and that after pulmonary resection alone. Among the 27 patients undergoing hepatic and pulmonary resection, the outcomes after resection were significantly better in patients with sequentially detected metastases (cumulative 5-year survival of 44%) than in those with simultaneously detected ones (cumulative 5-year survival of 0%). They concluded patients with sequentially detected hepatic and pulmonary metastases from a colorectal primary are good candidates for aggressive metastasectomy but simultaneous detection of these metastases does not warrant resection.

Ovary

The mechanism of spread of large bowel carcinoma to ovary is not clear. Postulated methods include implantation from intraperitoneal spread, hematogenous spread, and lymphatic dissemination. Immunostaining for cytokeratin 7 (CK7) (positive in ovarian carcinoma) and cytokeratin 20 (positive in colorectal carcinoma) is a useful technique for making the distinction between the organs of origin (231). The development of ovarian metastases was discussed in the section on treatment. Colon carcinoma may present as metastatic disease to the ovaries in a Krukenberg-like pattern (641). Treatment consists of bilateral salpingo-oophorectomy (Fig. 59). In a study of a series of patients who presented with what appeared to be primary ovarian neoplasms but actually were ovarian metastases from a colonic origin, Herrera-Ornelas et al. (642) found that survival was similar to that of patients who were primarily diagnosed as having large bowel carcinoma and subsequently developed ovarian metastases. Average life expectancy after diagnosis was 16.5 months. In their review of 63 patients with metachronous ovarian metastases, Morrow and Enker (643) found that such disease was part of diffuse intra-abdominal disease in 55% of patients. The mean survival rate following operation was 16.6 months. Ability to remove all gross disease at the time of oophorectomy was the major determinant of survival. Patients rendered disease free had a mean survival of 48 months compared with 9.6 months in patients with unresectable disease. Morrow and Enker believe that bilateral oophorectomy is warranted as part of the palliative treatment of women with metastatic disease to prevent the development of large symptomatic metastases that require further therapy.

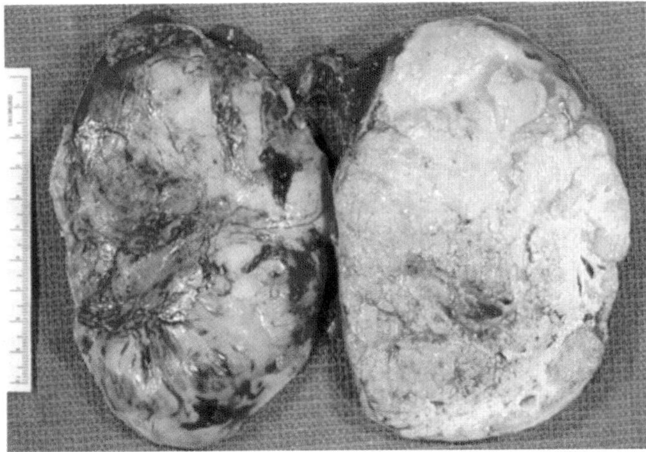

FIGURE 59 ■ Example of bilateral ovarian metastases in a patient presenting with acute colonic obstruction.

Huang et al. (644) reviewed the impact of elective and therapeutic oophorectomy on the natural history of colorectal carcinoma. A total of 155 patients were studied. Synchronous ovarian metastases occurred in 90 patients (58.1%); metachronous ovarian metastases occurred in 41.9%. Estimated 5-year survival for patients with synchronous ovarian metastases was 9% versus 20% for metachronous ovarian metastases. Resection of metastatic disease was associated with an improved 5-year survival for synchronous ovarian metastases (15% vs. 0%) and metachronous ovarian metastases (24% vs. 0%) if patients were disease-free postoperatively. Other clinical characteristics including age, menopausal status, stage, location of primary carcinoma, had no significant impact on survival. Thus, ovarian metastases from colorectal carcinoma are associated with a poor outcome. Although there is no survival advantage associated with resection of occult microscopic disease, long-term survival is possible if patients are rendered surgically disease free.

Bone

Metastases to the bone are usually associated with widely disseminated disease. Besbeas and Stearns (645). reported osseous involvement in 6.9% of patients, 5.1% as part of widespread metastases and 1.8% with skeletal metastases only. Sites of metastatic disease included the skull, scapula, clavicle, ribs, vertebrae, pelvic bones, humerus, and femur. The interval from initial diagnosis to manifestation of osseous metastases ranged from 10 months to 6 years and 11 months in that report. Bonnheim et al. (646) reported a 4% incidence of osseous metastases. Scuderi et al. (647) reported a case of sternal metastases as the initial presentation of an unknown rectal carcinoma. They stated osseous metastases occur in 3.8% to 10.5% of cases of rectal carcinoma. Isolated bony metastases are very rare and usually represent a late manifestation, being part of diffuse metastatic disease. Operation is an option in cases of solitary sternal localization but must be reserved for patients in good general condition. Treatment is directed toward pain control, and this is often achieved through radiotherapy. The mean period from onset of osseous metastases to death was 10 to 13.2 months (645,646).

Brain

Wong and Berkenblit (648) recently reviewed therapeutic options and expected outcomes for patients with brain metastases. They reported that the median survival with no treatment was 1 to 2 months; with steroids 2 to 3 months; with whole-brain radiotherapy 3 to 6 months; with operation and whole-brain radiotherapy 10 to 16 months; with radiosurgery and whole-brain radiotherapy 6 to 15 months; and with chemotherapy 8 to 12 months. Because the majority of cytotoxic agents seem to be unable to penetrate the blood–brain barrier, the role of chemotherapy in the treatment of brain metastases remains controversial. A few of the newly developed cytotoxic agents can cross the blood-brain barrier and may have a role in the treatment of patients with brain metastases. They noted that recent studies have demonstrated the antineoplastic activity of topotecan against brain metastases, with objective response rates ranging from 33% to 63% in patients with various solid malignancies mostly of lung origin. This result may be explained by the lack of exposure of brain metastases to previous cytotoxic agents, suggesting a role for topotecan in patients with brain metastases. Early studies have also suggested that topotecan, an apparent radiosensitizer, may be particularly effective in combination with radiotherapy, the current standard of care for patients with brain metastases. Alden, Gianino, and Saclarides (649) reviewed their experience with brain metastases from colorectal carcinoma. The authors identified 19 of their own patients and collected information from other reports. Fifty-eight percent of the patients had disseminated disease at initial diagnosis. The mean interval between treatment of the primary lesion and the diagnosis of brain metastases was 32.1 months. The brain was the sole site of metastatic disease in 21% of patients. Lesions were solitary in 63%, exclusively cerebral in 53%, cerebellar in 32%, or both in 15%. Presenting complaints ranged from ataxia (63%), headaches (21%), dizziness (26%), and weakness (32%) to seizures (16%), dysphasia (21%), and mental status changes (21%).

Diagnosis is established by CT scanning (Fig. 60) or MRI. Treatment consists of steroids to decrease intracranial swelling and radiation or craniotomy in special circumstances. Survival is dismal with no 1-year survivors in the series of 19 patients reviewed by Alden, Gianino, and Saclarides (649). The median survival rate following craniotomy was 4.9 months and following radiation was 2.6 months. Survival was not affected by the number or location of metastatic lesions or whether the brain was the sole site of metastatic disease. Because of the dismal survival rate, the authors believe that craniotomy is rarely indicated, except in the rare patient who has minimal neurologic impairment, a long disease-free interval, a solitary metastasis, and no extracranial disease. The authors believe that for most patients, radiation is the treatment of choice.

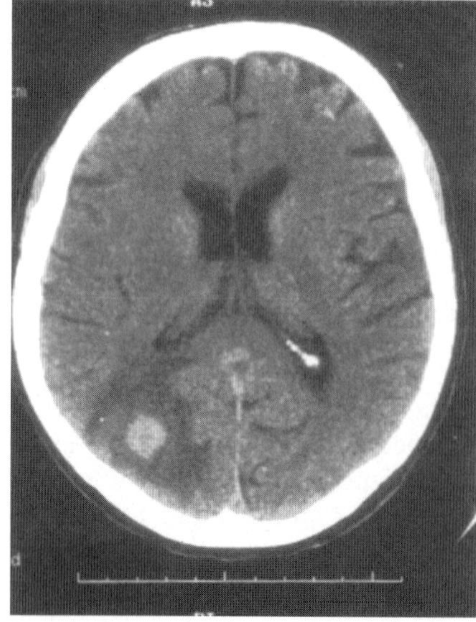

FIGURE 60 ■ CT scan demonstrating metastasis to brain. The hyperdense thick-walled lesion is surrounded by a "halo"—vasogenic (white matter) edema.

Hammond et al. (650) reported on 100 patients with brain metastases secondary to colorectal carcinoma. Of these patients, 36 underwent operation, 57 underwent radiotherapy alone, and the remaining seven received steroids. The median interval between the diagnosis of the primary carcinoma and the diagnosis of brain metastasis was 26 months. The median survival time was 1 month for patients who received only steroids, 3 months for those who received radiotherapy, and 9 months for those who underwent operation. The early onset of brain metastases was associated with a poor prognosis.

Farnell et al. (651) reported that brain metastases occur in 25% to 35% of all patients with malignancies, with colorectal carcinoma accounting for approximately 8% of these. Of 150 patients with brain metastases, 82% had concomitant extracerebral metastases, especially in the lungs. Only 16% of patients survived >1 year. The median survival rates for all patients receiving operation and radiotherapy (39), operation alone (11), radiotherapy alone (79), and supportive care (17) were 42, 45, 16, and 8 weeks, respectively. Of the patients treated with radiotherapy, 30% showed regression and three had complete regression. Given the similar results in patients treated with operation plus radiotherapy and those treated with operation alone, the authors believe that consideration should be given to withholding radiotherapy to obviate its side effects.

Peritoneal Carcinomatosis

Intraperitoneal carcinomatosis accounts for 25% to 35% of recurrences of colorectal carcinoma (652). Studies demonstrate that peritoneal carcinomatosis is not necessarily a terminal condition with no options for treatment for cure. The combination of aggressive, cytoreductive surgery and intra-abdominal hyperthermia chemotherapy improves long-term overall survival in selected patients but is a time-consuming procedure (approximately 12 hours) and entails high mortality (5%) and morbidity (35%) (652). Most commonly used drugs are Mitomycin C and platinum compounds, which have synergistic toxic effects on malignant cells when hyperthermia is applied. The three principal studies dedicated to the natural history of peritoneal carcinomatosis from colorectal carcinoma consistently showed median survival ranging between six and eight months. Glehen et al. (653) conducted a retrospective multicenter study to evaluate the international experience with cytoreductive surgery and perioperative intraperitoneal chemotherapy and to identify the principal prognostic indicators. The study included 506 patients from 28 institutions. The median age was 51 years. The median follow-up was 53 months. The morbidity and mortality rates were 22.9% and 4%, respectively. The overall median survival was 19.2 months. Patients in whom cytoreductive surgery was complete had a median survival of 32.4 months, compared with 8.4 months for patients in whom complete cytoreductive surgery was not possible. Positive independent prognostic indicators by multivariate analysis were complete cytoreduction, treatment by a second procedure, limited extent of peritoneal carcinomatosis, age less than 65 years, and use of adjuvant chemotherapy. The use of neoadjuvant chemotherapy, lymph node involvement, presence of liver metastases, and poor histologic differentiation were negative independent prognostic indicators.

Culliford et al. (654) reported aggressive treatment of peritoneal metastases from colon carcinoma by surgical cytoreduction and infusional intraperitoneal chemotherapy may benefit selected patients. There were 64 patients having surgical debulking and intraperitoneal (FUDR) plus leucovorin for peritoneal metastases. Primary carcinoma sites were 47 in the colon and 17 in the appendix. Peritoneal metastases were synchronous in 48 patients and metachronous in 16 patients. Patients received intraperitoneal FUDR (1000 mg/m^2 daily for three days) and intraperitoneal leucovorin (240 mg/m^2) with a median cycle number of 4. The median number of complications was 1 with no treatment related mortality. Only 9% required termination of intraperitoneal chemotherapy because of complications. The median follow-up was 17 months. The median survival was 34 months; 5-year survival was 28%. The 5-year survival was 54% for complete and 16% for incomplete resection.

Occasionally a few discrete nodules on the peritoneum are present at the time of colonic resection and it would seem appropriate to excise these. Verwaal et al. (655) conducted a randomized trial of cytoreduction and hyperthermia intraperitoneal chemotherapy versus systemic chemotherapy and palliative surgery in patients with peritoneal carcinomatosis of colorectal carcinoma. Of the 105 patients randomly assigned with a median follow-up of 21.6 months, the median 5-year survival was 12.6 months in the standard therapy arm and 22.3 months in the experimental therapy arm. The treatment-related mortality in the aggressive therapy group was 8%. In their review of the literature of 11 other reports on similar therapy, median reported survival ranged from 6 to 39 months mostly in the 15 month rage but the best series reported a 30% 5-year survival. Verwaal et al. (656) reported updated data on 117 patients treated by cytoreduction and hyperthermic intraperitoneal chemotherapy. The median survival was 21.8 months. The 1-, 3-, and 5-year survival rates were 75%, 28%, and 19%, respectively. In 59 patients a complete cytoreduction was achieved, and in 41 patients there was minimal residual disease. The median survival of these patient groups was 42.9 and 17.4 months, respectively. When gross macroscopic disease was left behind, as was the case in 17 patients, the median survival was five months. Involvement of the small bowel before cytoreduction was associated with poor outcome.

In patients with widespread peritoneal deposits, such an approach seems excessively aggressive. Improved outcomes for selected patients with peritoneal spread has been reported. Shen et al. (657) reviewed their experience of cytoreductive surgery and intraperitoneal hyperthermic chemotherapy with mitomycin C in 77 patients. Peritoneal carcinomatosis was synchronous and metachronous in 27% and 73% patients, respectively. Seventy-five percent of patients had received chemotherapy prior to intraperitoneal hyperthermic chemotherapy. Complete resection of all gross disease was accomplished in 48% of patients. Overall survival at one, three, and five years was 56%, 25%, and 17%, respectively. With a median follow-up of 15 months, the median overall survival was 16 months. Perioperative morbidity and mortality were 30% and 12%, respectively. Hematologic toxicity occurred in 19%. Poor performance status, bowel obstruction, malignant ascites, and incomplete resection of gross disease, were independent predictors of decreased survival. Patients with complete resection of all gross disease had a 5-year overall survival of 34% with a median overall survival of 28 months.

Elias et al. (658) conducted a two-center prospective randomized trial comparing postoperative peritoneal chemotherapy plus systemic chemotherapy alone, both after complete cytoreduction surgery of colorectal peritoneal carcinomatosis. Analysis of 35 patients showed that complete resection of peritoneal carcinomatosis resulted in a two-year survival of 60%, far above the classic 10% survival rate among patients with colorectal peritoneal carcinomatosis treated with systemic chemotherapy and symptomatic surgery. In this small series, postoperative intraperitoneal chemotherapy did not demonstrate any advantage for survival.

Other Metastatic Disease

Metastatic carcinoma that involves the spleen is usually a manifestation of widely disseminated disease, but solitary splenic metastases have been reported (659).

Cutaneous metastasis of rectal adenocarcinoma is a rare event occurring in fewer than 4% of all patients with rectal carcinoma (660,661). When present, it typically signifies disseminated disease with a poor prognosis (662). Metastatic colonic carcinoma may present in an old operative scar. Metastases to the glans penis (663), pancreas (664), and vagina (not contiguous disease) (665) have been reported. Metastatic colon carcinoma has even presented as a testicular hydrocele (666) or to the testis (667).

Carcinoma in Young Patients

It has been reported that carcinoma of the colon occurring under the age of 40 carries with it a poor prognosis. It has been suggested that this is due to the fact that patients present at a later stage in their development because the diagnosis had not been suspected. (See page 518.)

In a depressing report by Radhakrishan and Bruce (668), eight children with primary carcinoma of the colon presented with the common symptom being right iliac fossa pain. All children had poorly differentiated, highly aggressive lesions. In spite of operation and adjuvant therapy, all the children died within one year of presentation.

POSTOPERATIVE COMPLICATIONS

The complications that may be encountered following colonic surgery are discussed in detail in chapter 36.

Nevertheless, one very detailed and extraordinarily carefully studied series of cases should be cited. Killingback et al. (669) reviewed 1418 elective resections with anastomoses by a single colorectal surgeon. Postoperative mortality was 1.6%. Significant adverse events which were potentially avoidable occurred in 45.5% of the patients who died. The morbidity rate was (41.6%). Clinical anastomotic leaks occurred more frequently in extraperitoneal anastomoses (4.7%) than in intraperitoneal anastomoses (0.2%). Anastomotic leak caused the death of two

TABLE 10 ■ Results of Curative Operation for Colon Carcinoma

Author(s)	No. of Patients	Resectability Rates (%)	Operative Mortality (%)	5-Year Survival (%) Crude	5-Year Survival (%) Corrected
Corman, Veidenheimer, and Coller (7) (1979)	1,008	95	4		
Pihl et al. (671) (1980)	434		7		76
Stefanini, Castrini, and Pappalardo (672) (1981)	436	81	3		
Zhou, Yu, and Shen (673) (1983)	302	71	2	73	
Umpleby et al. (674) (1984)	439		13	27	59
Isbister and Fraser (675) (1985)	1,505			43	
Wied et al. (676) (1985)	442			47	
Glass et al. (520) (1986)	413		3		82
Davis, Evans, and Cohen (677) (1987)	405		3	38	52
Moreaux and Catala (678) (1987)	646		1	78	
Brown, Walsh, and Sykes (679) (1988)	550	85	7		
Enblad et al. (680) (1988)	38,166		3		46
Jatzko, Lisborg, and Wette (681) (1992)	223	98	2	81	
Clemmensen and Sprechler (682) (1994)	212			47	
Singh et al. (199) (1995)	304	99	3		59 (10 yr)
Carraro et al. (683) (2001)	256	—	4	60	
Read et al. (684) (2002)	316		2	84	
Morin et al. (685) (2006)	310		1	72	

patients (0.14%). Routine prophylactic anticoagulation did not decrease the incidence of pulmonary embolism. Significant thrombophlebitis at the intravenous cannula site occurred in 3.8%, wound infection in 2.1%, and postural peripheral nerve injury in the upper limbs occurred in 0.8%. Unscheduled operations were required in 2.7% of patients. A classification of anastomotic leak is suggested to assist in comparisons of this complication which remains a significant concern following extraperitoneal anastomoses.

RESULTS

In an effort to determine the survival rate following operations for colon carcinoma, review of the plethora of reports makes the reader quickly realize that the literature consists of a maze of information. In attempting to compare the results from various institutions, it rapidly becomes apparent that a host of reporting methods have been used. For example, some authors present overall survival rates of all patients who present with colon carcinoma. Others present data only for those who underwent an operation, while still others present data only for those who presumably had a curative operation. Some authors present survival data for subsets of patients according to the Dukes classification, while others state that they are using the Dukes classification but, in fact, are using some variation of it, and therefore survival data are not comparable. Some reports use actuarial methods correcting the data for the age of the patients, thereby attempting to give a more accurate survival statistic. Some authors have used corrected 5-year survival rates by means of life tables to exclude deaths not due to carcinoma but caused by intercurrent disease. Presumably, this method is being used to increase the precision of reporting rather than making the survival statistics look better because, by definition, the corrected survival rate is always higher than the crude survival rate.

Estimates of survival are commonly used in the literature to describe outcomes in patients treated for carcinoma. Terms such as carcinoma-specific and carcinoma-free survival are frequently quoted although often without clear definitions. Platell and Semmens (670) compared survival estimates on the same population of patients but using different definitions of what constitutes an event. This was to highlight some of the variation that can occur when different techniques are used to perform these calculations. The

TABLE 11 ■ 5-Year Survival According to Dukes' Staging Following Curative Resection

Author(s)	Dukes' A No. of Patients	Dukes' A Survival (%) Crude	Dukes' A Survival (%) Corrected	Dukes' B No. of Patients	Dukes' B Survival (%) Crude	Dukes' B Survival (%) Corrected	Dukes' C No. of Patients	Dukes' C Survival (%) Crude	Dukes' C Survival (%) Corrected
Corman, Veidenheimer, and Coller (7) (1979)	225	81	95	332	62	90	204	35	55
Pihl et al. (671) (1980)	109		88	208		78	90		60
Eisenberg et al. (686) (1982)	101		75–87[a]	274		64–85[a]	501		39–43[a]
Isbister and Fraser (675) (1985)	172	64		427	58		354	32	
Davis, Evans, and Cohen (677) (1987)	24	71	96	125	65	87	85	36	52
Read et al. (684) (2002)	73	99		151	87		92	72	
Staib et al. (687) (2002)	184	82		388	74		246	49	
Morin et al. (685) (2006)	80	84		147	76		79	58	

[a]Range depending on portion of colon affected.

study included 497 patients with a mean age of 68 years, and a male to female ratio of 1.3 to 1. They were followed for a mean of 2.2 years. The various survivals at 5 years were: (1) overall survival, 55.6%; (2) carcinoma-specific survival, 67%; (3) carcinoma-free survival, 49.9%; (4) recurrence-free survival, 43.5%; and (5) relative survival, 73.4%. The 5-year survival calculations for this group of patients with colorectal carcinoma varied by as much as 30% depending on how the data were censored. This highlights that there needs to be a clear and accountable definition on how survival curves are calculated and presented in the literature to allow for meaningful interpretation and comparisons.

It is not unreasonable to assume that figures quoted from major surgical centers would offer better survival rates because a higher standard of care is assumed. However, these figures may not be representative of the majority of regional hospitals. Statistics from tumor registries may be more representative. The crude 5-year survival rates reported from cancer registries have been less impressive, partly because a proportion of these patients almost certainly had only palliative excisions and partly because statistics for those patients who are alive 5 years after operation are expressed as a percentage of those submitted to surgical treatment and not of those surviving that treatment. Thus operative deaths would be included among the nonsurvivors, making the number of 5-year survivors correspondingly less.

A more useful measure of surgical treatment is the overall or absolute survival rate, which expresses the number of patients alive and well after 5 years as a percentage of the total number of patients presenting to hospital with carcinoma of the colon in the first instance, not as a percentage of the immediate survivors of operation. The absolute survival rate automatically takes into account the resectability and operative mortality rates as well as the success of the operation in eradicating the carcinoma.

Despite this confusing information and with full recognition of the limitations of the exercise, an effort has been made to extract a number of representative series of reasonable size, and these are presented in Tables 10 and 11. In a review of 22 series, Devesa, Morales, and Enriquez (688) determined that the corrected 5-year survival rates for patients with large bowel carcinoma operated on for cure varies from 44% to 68%.

The Commission on Cancer Data from the National Cancer Data Base reports time trends in stage of disease, treatment patterns, and survival for patients with selected carcinomas. The 1993 data for patients with colon carcinoma are described (689). Five calls for data yielded 3,700,000 cases of carcinoma for the years 1985 through 1993 from hospital cancer registries across the United States, including 36,937 cases of colon carcinoma from 1988 and 44,812 from 1993. Interesting trends are as follows: (1) the elderly (> 80 years) present with earlier stage disease than do younger patients, (2) the National Cancer Institute recognized that cancer centers have more patients with advanced disease than do other types of hospitals, (3) all ethnic groups have generally similar stages of disease at presentation except for African-Americans, who have a slightly higher incidence of stage IV disease, (4) the proximal migration of the primary carcinoma continues; 54.7% of primary colon carcinoma arose in the right colon in 1993 compared with 50.9% in 1988, (5) an interaction between grade and stage of carcinoma seems present, and (6) patients with stage III colon carcinoma who received adjuvant chemotherapy had a 5% improvement in 5-year relative survival (Fig. 61). The data suggest an important biologic role for grade of carcinoma. They also suggest that African-Americans and other ethnic groups have the same outcome as non-Hispanic whites but that access to medical care may still be less. Finally, the use of adjuvant therapy for stage III colon carcinoma may just beginning to be appreciated. The relative 5-year survival rates for patients with colon carcinoma are depicted in Fig. 62. Comparable data for those with rectal carcinoma are shown in Fig. 63.

Survival rates for patients presenting with obstructing and perforating carcinomas are considerably more dismal. Representative reports are shown in Tables 12,13 and 14. The factors primarily contributing to this distressingly poor outlook are the low curability and survival rates for patients with large bowel obstruction secondary to colorectal carcinoma because of advanced disease at the time of diagnosis and treatment (321). Serpell, McDermott, and Katrivessis (695) reported a reduction in curative resection rate from 71% in patients without obstruction to 50% in those with obstruction. A review of the literature by Smithers et al. (486) revealed an operative mortality of 9% to 35% for emergency right hemicolectomy. Indeed, emergency operations of all kinds carry a higher operative mortality rate than do elective operations. Goodall and Park (500) reported on 40 patients with an obstructed left colon who underwent primary resection and anastomosis with a 5% mortality rate and a 40% complication rate.

Mandava et al. (299) reported that in their series of 51 patients with perforated colorectal carcinoma, if the patients with metastatic disease and operative mortalities were excluded, there was a 58% 5-year survival rate in the remaining 32 patients. Scott, Jeacock, and Kingston (713) reported on risk factors in patients presenting in an emergency with colorectal carcinoma. Of 905 patients with colorectal carcinoma admitted to a single hospital, 272 (30%) were admitted as emergencies. Emergency patients had more advanced lesions (Dukes' B and C, 96% vs. 88% of those admitted electively), a shorter history (median, 3 vs. 11 weeks), were less likely to be fully ambulatory (44% vs. 80%), and more likely to have abdominal pain (74% vs. 51%) and vomiting (40% vs. 10%). More emergency patients were given stomas (56% vs. 35%) and died in hospital (19% vs. 8%). Of those who survived to be discharged, patients admitted as an emergency spent longer in hospital (median stay, 16 vs. 13 days) and had a poor overall 5-year survival rate (29% vs. 39%). Emergency patients were significantly older (median, 74 vs. 72 years) and were much more likely to be widowed (41% vs. 27%) than those admitted for elective surgery. The authors concluded that if the personal and resource disaster of emergency colorectal carcinoma admission is to be reduced, screening strategies targeted by demographic characteristics require investigation.

Anderson, Hole, and McArdle (713) conducted a prospective study of 570 patients presenting with colorectal carcinoma over a 6-year period. Of these, 363 were admitted electively and 207 presented as emergencies. In the elective group, the proportion of resected lesions was greater (77% vs. 64%), the operative mortality rate was

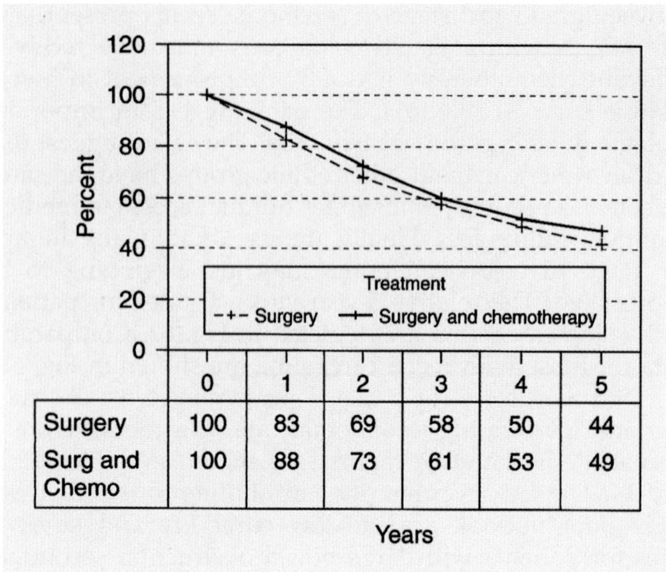

	0	1	2	3	4	5
Surgery	100	83	69	58	50	44
Surg and Chemo	100	88	73	61	53	49

FIGURE 61 ■ Relative survival for 1985 to 1988 colon carcinoma cases (combined AJCC stage group III) by treatment modality. *Source*: From Ref. 689.

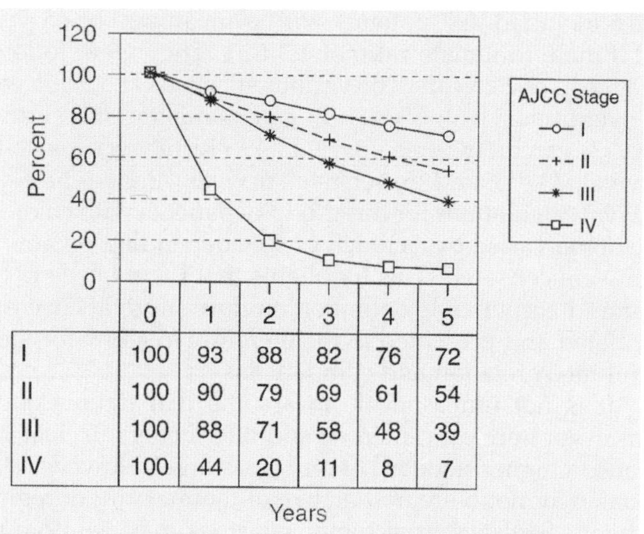

	0	1	2	3	4	5
I	100	93	88	82	76	72
II	100	90	79	69	61	54
III	100	88	71	58	48	39
IV	100	44	20	11	8	7

FIGURE 63 ■ Relative five-year survival rate for carcinoma of rectum by combined pathologic and clinical AJCC staging. Percent survival by stage is shown in boxes below graph. *Source:* From Ref. 304.

lower (9% vs. 19%), and the 5-year disease-related survival rate was higher (37% vs. 19%). These differences may relate to the greater resection rates in the elective situation. Clemmensen and Sprechler (682) reported on the results of 803 patients with colorectal carcinoma, 273 of whom required emergency admission. Immediate operation was performed on 76 of these patients, 37 for obstruction, 15 for perforation, and 24 for other indications. The operative mortality rate for this group was 25%.

Other factors to consider are advanced disease and high-risk elderly patients. Fitzgerald et al. (715) reviewed the perioperative mortality and long-term survival in elderly and high-risk patients with colorectal neoplasia. Elderly high-risk patients with localized disease were compared with those with advanced disease. Over a 5-year period, 82 high-risk (at least one major organ system disease) or elderly (age $\geq$70 years) patients underwent an operation for colorectal neoplasia. Overall 43 of 82 patients (52%) had advanced disease (obstruction, perforation, hemorrhage, or metastatic disease), while 39 of 82 patients (48%) had localized disease. Pre-operative comorbid diseases included coronary atherosclerosis, 59 (72%); previous myocardial infarction, 17 (21%); previous arrhythmia, 10 (12%); emphysema, 32 (39%); renal failure, six (7%); and cirrhosis, three (4%). At the time of operation, 26 patients (32%) had metastatic disease. Six patients (7%) died in the perioperative period. There was no difference in major morbidity between patients operated on for localized and for advanced disease. The mean actuarial 18-month survival rate was less for patients with advanced disease. Sixty-eight patients (83%) were alive at a follow-up of 17.7 $\pm$ 29 months postoperatively. The morbidity and mortality rates associated with resection of colorectal neoplasia in high-risk elderly patients are acceptable even in the presence of advanced disease. In select patients, resection offers the best palliation and may improve the quality of remaining life.

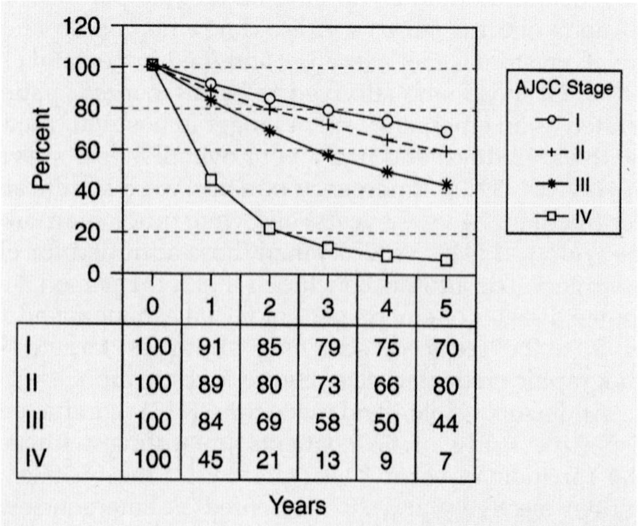

	0	1	2	3	4	5
I	100	91	85	79	75	70
II	100	89	80	73	66	80
III	100	84	69	58	50	44
IV	100	45	21	13	9	7

FIGURE 62 ■ Relative survival for 1985–1988 colon carcinoma cases by combined AJCC stage group. *Source*: From Ref. 689.

Colorectal carcinoma in cirrhotic patients is different from that in patients without the liver disease. Gervaz et al. (716) retrospectively analyzed 72 patients operated on for colorectal adenocarcinoma with confirmed liver cirrhosis at the time of abdominal exploration. There were 43% Child A, 42% Child B, and 15% Child C. The median age was 70 years, and the mean duration of follow-up was 46 months. Postoperative death was 13%. The risk factors were an elevated bilirubin and prolonged prothrombin time. Liver metastases developed in 10%. For the whole group 1-, 3-, and 5-year survival rates were 69%, 49%, and 35%, respectively. Child A patients had a significantly better survival rate than the combined group of Child B and C patients. The risks for long-term survival were decreased albumin and prolonged prothrombin time. The Child's classification, and not the TNM stage of the carcinoma, predicts the risk of postoperative death and long-term survival.

Kotake et al. (717) examined trends of colorectal carcinoma in relation to age, gender, site, and survival during a 20-year period. The multi-institutional registry of the Japanese Society for Cancer of the Colon and Rectum offered 87,695 surgical cases with invasive adenocarcinoma. The number of cases showed a 2.5-fold increase with

TABLE 12 ■ Overall 5-Year Survival for Patients with Obstructing Carcinoma

Author(s)	No. of Patients	Operative Mortality (%)	Survival (%)	
			Crude	Corrected
Kelley et al. (690) (1981)	156	18	18	
Ohman (321) (1982)	148	9	16	
Brief et al. (691) (1983)	41	2	78	
Crooms and Kovalcik (692) (1984)	37	3	33	
Umpleby and Williamson (327) (1984)	124	20	18	
Phillips et al. (693) (1985)	713	23		25
Willett et al. (694) (1985)	77		31	
Serpell et al. (695) (1989)	148	9		
Ueyama et al. (324) (1991)	40	0	52	
Sjodahl, Franzen, and Nystrom (484) (1992)	115	17		
Mulcahy et al. (696) (1996)	92	12	36	
Chen et al. (697) (2000)	120	5	33	
Carraro et al. (683) (2001)	177	10	46	

consistent male predominance confined to the distal colon and rectum. Colon carcinoma in the last 5-year period was more likely right-sided for females (odds ratio, 1.26) and males (odds ratio, 1.16) compared with the first period. Carcinoma in younger patients were more likely at stage III to IV in the late 1990s if the carcinoma were in the distal colon, the rectum (for both genders), or the proximal colon (for females). Survival was improved except for cases with proximal colon carcinoma of stage IV. In the multivariate analysis, hazard ratios for death in the postoperative five years were 0.77, 0.59, and 0.66 for proximal colon, distal colon, and rectal carcinomas respectively in the last period as compared with those in the first period. Reduced hazard ratio for females was the largest for proximal colon carcinoma with stage I and II. Although surgical outcome was largely improved, delayed presentation or diagnosis in younger patients remained a problem.

Wang et al. (718) investigated the clinical features, diagnosis, treatment, and prognosis of 37 patients with multiple primary carcinomas. The incidence of multiple primary colorectal carcinomas was 2.7% in patients with primary colorectal carcinomas, 15 cases were patients with synchronous carcinomas and 22 cases were diagnosed as metachronous carcinomas. Most carcinomas were located in the right colon and rectum. Fifty-five percent of metachronous carcinomas were diagnosed within three years after resection of the initial lesion and 41% of metachronous carcinomas occurred after eight years. Radical resections were performed in all patients except for one case. The five-year survival rate of synchronous carcinomas was 72.7% and that of metachronous carcinomas after the first carcinoma and second carcinoma was 71.4% and 38.9%, respectively. Their results indicate the importance of complete preoperative examination and careful intraoperative exploration and periodic postoperative surveillance.

Immunosuppression used in transplantation is associated with an increased incidence of various carcinomas. Papaconstantinou et al. (719) defined the characteristics and survival patterns of transplant patients developing

TABLE 13 ■ Results of Immediate Resection and Primary Anastomosis for Obstructing Carcinoma of the Left Colon

Author(s)	Procedure	No. of Patients	Operative Mortality (%)	Complication Rate (%)
Amsterdam and Krispin (482) (1985)	Segmental resection	25	12	60
Hughes et al. (698) (1985)	TAC or STC	52	12	
Morgan et al. (699) (1985)	TAC or STC	16	13	
White and Macfie (483) (1985)	LHC or sigmoid resection	35	9	29
Feng, Hsu, and Chen (700) (1987)	STC or segmental resection	15	7	27
Halevy, Levi, and Orda (701) (1989)	STC	22	5	36
Slors et al. (702) (1989)	TAC and IRA	10	10	30
Stephenson et al. (703) (1990)	STC	31	3	6
Runkel et al. (300) (1991)	STC, LHC	21	14	46
Antal et al. (704) (1991)	STC	40	0	25
Brief et al. (391) (1991)	STC	23	4	29
Tan et al. (705) (1991)	Segmental resection	23	9	43
Murray et al. (706) (1991)	Segmental resection	21	0	60
Sjodahl, Franzen, and Nystrom (484) (1992)	Not stated	18	6	17
Stewart, Diament, and Brennan (707) (1993)	Segmental resection	60	7	
Arnaud and Bergamaschi (708) (1994)	STC	44	7	7
Lau, Lo, and Law (493) (1995)	STC or segmental resection	35	6	31
Carraro et al. (682) (2001)	Segmental or STC	107	10	–

Abbreviations: STC, Subtotal colectomy; TAC, total abdominal colectomy; LHC, left hemicolectomy; IRA, ileorectal anastomosis.

TABLE 14 ■ Overall 5-Year Survival for Patients with Perforated Carcinoma

Author(s)	No. of Patients	Operative Mortality (%)	5-Year Crude Survival (%)
Kelley et al. (690) (1981)	27	33	7
Michowitz et al. (709) (1982)	42	38	23
Willett et al. (694) (1985)	34		44
Badia, Sitges-Serra, and Pia (710) (1987)	36	14	40
Runkel et al. (299) (1991)	20	30	
Mandava et al. (298) (1996)	51	12	32
Mulcahy et al. (696) (1996)	13	12	12
Carraro et al. (711) (1998)	54[a]	17	–
Chen et al. (697) (2000)	35[a]	9	–
	13[b]	31	33
	29[b]	48	1
Khan et al. (712) (2001)	48	14	14

[a]Perforation at site of carcinoma.
[b]Perforation proximal to carcinoma.

de novo colorectal carcinomas. A total of 150 transplant patients with de novo colorectal carcinoma were identified: 93 kidney, 29 heart, 27 liver, and 1 lung. Mean age of transplantation was 53 years. Age of transplantation of colorectal carcinoma diagnosis was not significant for gender, race, or stage of disease. Compared to National Cancer Institute Surveillance Epidemiology and End Results database, transplantation patients had a younger mean age of colorectal carcinoma diagnosis (58 years vs. 70 years) and a worse 5-year survival (overall 44% vs. 62%, Dukes' A and B 74% vs. 90%, Dukes' C 20% vs. 66%, and Dukes' D 0% vs. 9%). Their data suggest that chronic immunosuppression results in a more aggressive biology. Frequent posttransplantation colorectal screening program may be warranted.

PROGNOSTIC DISCRIMINANTS

Over, the years, many factors that might influence survival rates have been studied, and different authors have placed varying degrees of confidence in certain ones. For example, in a large prospective analysis of 2524 patients who had undergone curable resection, the prognostic factors in order of importance were (1) lymph node status, (2) mobility of the carcinoma, (3) number of positive lymph nodes, (4) presence of bowel obstruction, and (5) depth of penetration of the primary lesions (720).

In a review of the literature and combined with his experience, Jass (721) summarized the important variables as follows. The pathologist should provide the staging, completeness of excision (resection lines), extent of spread through the bowel wall, lymph node or satellite nodule involvement, especially involvement of nodes at the apex of the vascular pedicle, and the number of nodes. Other variables should be considered. For completeness of documentation, carcinoma of the large bowel should be typed as adenocarcinoma, mucinous adenocarcinoma, signet-ring cell carcinoma, undifferentiated carcinoma, or other. In addition, the grade of differentiation, well, moderate, or poor, should be stated. However, type and grade of carcinoma have little or no independent prognostic value. Classification of carcinoma as expanding or diffusely infiltrating has been shown to be of prognostic importance in a number of multivariate studies. Most large bowel carcinomas are relatively well circumscribed. Approximately 25% show an irregular margin of growth with tongues of neoplastic cells dissecting between the normal structures of the bowel wall, making it difficult to define a clear border of the carcinoma. The term "diffuse infiltration" does not imply massive intramural spread, a type of spread very rarely seen in the large bowel.

The presence of venous invasion by carcinoma should be recorded because this may have a bearing on the documentation of extent of spread. The presence of venous invasion is strongly correlated with distant spread. When cases with distant spread are excluded, the prognostic value of venous spread is greatly diminished and is absent in some multivariate studies. The presence of perineural and lymphatic spread influences prognosis adversely, but these factors were not found to be independent when Jass (721) examined 500 specimens from the prospectively collected Australian series. A conspicuous lymphocytic infiltrate, either within an inflammatory mantle at the growing edge of the carcinoma or arranged within nodular collections around small serosal vessels, confers a favorable prognosis that has been shown to be independent.

The following discussion, although not totally comprehensive, elaborates on the factors that most often have been considered relevant. A survey of prognostic discriminants for colon carcinoma is presented in Table 15.

CLINICAL FEATURES

Age

Survival rates of patients younger than 40 years of age are frequently believed to be lower than overall survival rates. The 5-year survival rates in this group of patients range from 16% to 43% (724–729,856). The poor prognosis in young patients has been attributed to the larger portion of poorly differentiated lesions, a larger number of mucinous lesions, and a lower potential for curative resection (724,725).

Not all authors believe that young patients have a less favorable prognosis (856,857). Svendson et al. (919) reported that patients who are between 40 and 60 years of age at the time of diagnosis have a worse prognosis than both younger and older patients.

TABLE 15 ■ Prognostic Discriminants

Discriminants	Effect on Prognosis[a] Diminished	None	Improved
Clinical Features			
Age			
Young (< 40 years)	421, 722–729	7, 731, 856–863	
Elderly (> 70 years)	674, 731, 732	696, 864–867	738, 894
Sex			
Female	733	7, 696, 731, 738, 747, 775, 793	
Male	734	671, 696, 775	
History			
Asymptomatic			737, 895, 896
Bleeding as presenting symptom			731, 736, 739, 747
> 2 presenting symptoms	735		
Delay in diagnosis (medical)	421		
Long duration of symptoms	736	774, 796, 868, 869	731
Short duration of symptoms	138		
Obstruction	7, 327, 422, 583, 683, 697, 727, 731, 738–743, 922	324	
Perforation	298, 327, 421, 521, 696, 697, 711, 712, 727, 734, 738, 739, 745		
Adjacent organ involvement	422, 731, 747–750		
Presence of metastatic disease	All authors		
Systemic manifestations	422		
Technique of resection			
Left hemicolectomy vs. segmental		752, 870	
No-touch technique		397, 752	
Occlusion of bowel ends		752	
Intraoperative perforation of bowel	745, 747, 752–754		
High volume		872	300, 753, 754, 897–903
Colorectal trained surgeon			754, 871, 904–909
Anastomotic leakage	755–757		
Perioperative blood transfusion	758–763	872–874	
Postoperative fever	764	875	910
Previous appendectomy	765		
Obesity	766		
Pathologic Features			
Location			
Rectum	732, 740, 764, 767	696, 720, 775	735
Right colon	674, 731, 768	739, 775, 876	422, 740, 767
Size	769–772	696, 731, 773, 793, 877	
Configuration			
Ulcerated	769, 773		
Polypoid			769, 773, 911, 912
Annular	740, 774		
Microscopy			
Well differentiated			421, 671, 696, 720, 731, 747, 769
Moderately differentiated			
Poorly differentiated	422, 674, 714, 720, 731, 732, 747, 769, 771, 772, 775		
Mucin producing	237, 238, 696, 725, 776–781	742, 771, 773, 791, 878, 879	
Inflammatory infiltrate			671, 769, 773, 913
Desmoplastic reaction	782		
Linitis plastica	783		
Depth of penetration	720, 727, 732, 772, 782, 784		
Circumferential margin involvement	737		
Micro acinar	785		
"Budding"	786–788		
Signet ring cell	789–791		
Residual disease	792		

(Continued)

TABLE 15 ■ Prognostic Discriminants (*Continued*)

	Effect on Prognosis[a]		
Discriminants	**Diminished**	**None**	**Improved**
Staging			
Dukes A			All authors[b]
Dukes B			
Dukes C	All authors[b]		
Lymph node status			
Positive	All authors[b]		
≥4 nodes	7, 230, 441, 720, 740, 741, 771, 773, 784, 793, 794, 795, 797	732	
Necrosis in metastatic lymph nodes			914
Venous invasion	7, 230, 676, 693, 720, 731, 732, 740, 747, 752, 754, 772, 799–805	771	
Perineural invasion	693, 754, 799, 800, 802, 804, 806, 807		
Perioperative disseminated malignant cells	808	880	
Biochemical and Special Investigations			
Diabetes mellitus	809		
High preoperative CEA levels	747, 810–817	687, 881	
Abnormal liver function tests	818	747	
DNA non-diploid	744, 819–824	772, 775, 882–885	
Low serum protein levels	747		
Hemoglobin levels		747, 775	
White blood cell count		747	
Erythrocyte sedimentation rate		747	
Genetic alteration			
17p deletion	825		
DCC expression		886	
Loss of hMLHI expression			915
Allelic loss chromosome 18q	825–830		
Allelic loss chromosome 5q	826		
p53 overexpression	831–838	886–889	
CD-44 v6 expression	839	772, 890–892	
ras p21 overexpression	840		
high Ki67 expression		888	836
Microsatellite instability			830, 916–918
DNA microarray–based gene expression	841		918
Thymidylate synthetase overexpression	836, 842, 843	893	
Increased EGF expression	844		
Apoptotic index		847	
Sialyl Lewis^x antigen	845–847		
PCNA expression	848, 849		
Sialomucin staining	850–852		
Nuclear morphometry (>0.84)[c]	853		
High u-PA/t-PA (>0.22)	854		
Socioeconomic deprivation	855		

Abbreviations: CEA, carcinoembryonic antigen; DNA, deoxyribonucleic acid; PCNA, proliferating cell nuclear antigen.
[a]All numbers in "Effect" columns correspond to reference numbers for this chapter.
[b]"All authors" refers to unanimous agreement by all authors who address the subject.
[c]See text for explanation.

Cusack et al. (729) conducted a retrospective review of 186 patients younger than 40 years of age. Regional lymph node metastases, distant metastases, or both were seen on first examination in 66% of young patients. The authors identified three biologic indicators of aggressive and potentially metastatic biology: signet-ring cell carcinoma (11.1%), infiltrating edge of the carcinoma (69%), and aggressive (poorly differentiated) grade (41%). Vascular invasion in stage II disease was also a significant negative prognostic variable. These histologic measures of more aggressive disease in part account for the higher rate of advanced disease at presentation in patients younger than 40 years of age.

Liang et al. (859) compared 138 consecutive patients with colorectal carcinoma aged less than 40 years with 339 patients aged 60 years or more. The younger patients with colorectal carcinoma had more mucin-producing (14.5% vs. 4.7%) and poorly differentiated (7.2% vs. 3.3%)

carcinomas, a higher incidence of synchronous (5.8% vs. 1.2%) and metachronous (4.0% vs. 0.6%) colorectal carcinomas, and more advanced stage than older patients. The operative mortality rate was lower (0.7% vs. 5.0%), and carcinoma-specific survival was similar (in stage I, II, and III disease) or better (in stage IV disease). There was a higher% of normal p53 expression (61.1% vs. 46.8%) and high-frequency of microsatellite instability (29.4% vs. 6.3%) and a similar family history of carcinoma (17.5% vs. 14.2%), compared with older patients.

O'Connell et al. (730) performed the most comprehensive systematic review focusing on colorectal carcinoma in the young aiming to (1) characterize the disease in the young population and (2) determine how colorectal carcinoma in this population should be further addressed regarding detection and treatment. A Medline literature search chose 55 studies that examined 6425 patients less than 40 years old. Approximately 7% of all colorectal carcinomas consisted of patients less than 40 years old. They found that colorectal carcinoma in the young population appears to be more aggressive, to present with later stage (66% of patients <40 years old presented with Dukes' C and D lesions compared with 32% to 49% reported for patients >40 years old), and to have poorer pathologic findings (higher prevalence of mucinous or poorly differentiated lesions including signet-ring carcinoma—one of the main distinctions between the disease in older vs. younger patients. Mucinous lesions constituted an average of 21% of carcinoma in younger patients compared with an average of 10% to 15% of patients of all ages with colorectal carcinoma. The average% of lesions found to be poorly differentiated was 27% for the young group compared with 2% to 29% of patients over the age of 40). The average overall 5-year survival for young patients was 33% compared with 61% overall 5-year survival reflecting presentation with later stage disease thus appearing to have a poorer prognosis. However, if detected early, young patients with Dukes' stage A or B lesions have better overall 5-year survival rates. Average-adjusted 5-year survival for Dukes' A 94%; B 77%, and C 39%. A crucial issue is that close attention must be paid to young patients who present with common symptoms of colorectal carcinoma. O'Connell et al. (862) used a national-level, population-based cancer registry to compare rectal carcinoma outcomes between young versus older populations. All patients with rectal carcinoma in the Surveillance Epidemiology and End Results Cancer database from 1991 to 1999 were evaluated. Young (range 20–40 years; $n=466$) and older groups (range 60–80 years; $n=11{,}312$) were compared for patient and carcinoma characteristics, treatment patterns, and 5-year overall and stage-specific survival. Mean ages for the groups were 34.1 and 70 years. The young group was comprised of more black and Hispanic patients compared with the older group. Young patients were more likely to present with late stage disease (young vs. older: stage III, 27% vs. 20% and stage IV, 17.4% vs. 13.6%, respectively). The younger group also had worse grade (poorly differentiated 24.3% vs. 14%, respectively). Although the majority of both groups received surgery (85% for each), significantly more young patients received radiation. Importantly, overall and stage-specific, 5-year survival rates were similar for both groups.

From a group of 2495 patients with malignancies of the colon and rectum, Turkiewicz et al. (860) identified 61 patients with colorectal carcinoma who were aged less than 40 years at presentation. Their clinical data were then compared with the larger group of older patients. A positive family history was the most consistent risk factor, present in 34% of patients. Despite this, only one patient out of 61 had been diagnosed as a result of a screening program. The overall 5-year survival among younger patients was 53%. The 5-year survival rates in younger patients were better than for older patients for the Australian Clinicopathological Staging A and B reaching statistical significance for both of these stages. Their results indicate that young patients with colorectal carcinoma have the potential to do just as well as older ones.

For the prognosis of elderly patients, conflicting reports are found. A common notion is that aged patients have less biologically aggressive neoplasms. Newland et al. (732) found that in patients ≥ 75 years of age, the hazard ratio for survival was 1.98. Coburn, Pricolo, and Soderberg (920) compared 177 cases of colorectal carcinoma in patients >80 years to 623 in patients <80 years. There was no difference in operative mortality between the two groups. Octogenarians and nonagenarians more often displayed obstruction or perforation, elevated preoperative CEA levels, right-sided lesions, and solitary hepatic metastases. The actuarial 5-year survival rate was 32% in the older patients and 48% in the younger group. Others report that the prognosis for the elderly is not different from that of younger patients (864–866).

Sex

Some authors have reported a slightly higher incidence of carcinoma of the colon in women than in men, but the 5-year survival rates are slightly higher in women (3). However, others have reported poorer survival rates in women (735). The hazard ratio for the male gender has been estimated at 1.27 (732).

History

As might be expected, patients who are asymptomatic have better survival rates than symptomatic patients do (736,895,896).

Patients who have rectal bleeding as a presenting symptom have a better prognosis than do those presenting with other symptoms of colonic carcinoma (895). The number of symptoms is also a prognostic discriminant since patients with more than two symptoms have a poorer prognosis (735).

There appears to be no correlation between the duration of symptoms and survival. In a study of 152 patients, Goodman and Irvin (869) found no difference in the survival rate for patients in whom the diagnosis was delayed >12 weeks from the onset of symptoms compared with those who presented early. They did find that patients with anemia and no abdominal symptoms had a significantly higher survival rate than those presenting with abdominal symptoms. Patients who ignore their symptoms tend to have biologically more favorable lesions. Ironically, in patients with a longer history of symptoms, there appears to be either no effect on survival or a better survival rate

(774,796,921). Wiggers, Arends, and Volovics (747) found that patients who had symptoms for a very short time (<1 week) or a very long time (>6 months) had a poorer survival rate than those in the intermediate range, but this was not statistically significant. This apparent paradox may be explained by the fact that patients with aggressive lesions (i.e., annular, constricting, or poorly differentiated) are compelled to seek help early. Patients with less acute symptoms often exhibit lesions of average grade and may ultimately prove to have a better prognosis.

Obstruction

The incidence of intestinal obstruction has been reported to be between 7% and 29% of all patients with colon and rectal cancer (922). The occurrence of acute obstruction diminishes the ultimate survival rate and increases the immediate hazard to the patient (739,740,742,895,922). In a review of 12 reports, Sugarbaker, Gunderson, and Wittes (422) found a median overall survival rate of 20% and a 5-year survival rate of 40% with curative surgery. The authors attributed this dismal prognosis to the fact that only about one half of the patients had potentially curative operations and that the operations were accompanied by high morbidity and mortality rates, with a median hospital mortality rate of 18% and complications occurring in one third to one half of the patients.

Wang et al. (922) conducted a study to assess the long-term prognosis of patients with obstructing carcinoma of the right colon. The 256 patients who were status post-curative resection of right colon adenocarcinoma were classified as obstruction group ($n = 35$) or nonobstruction group ($n = 221$). The overall (49% vs. 22%), distant (40% vs. 18%), and local (14% vs. 5%) recurrence rates were significantly higher in obstructive patients than in nonobstructive patients. Long-term crude (36% vs. 77%) and carcinoma-specific survival rates (46% vs. 83%) were significantly lower in obstructed patients. Multivariate analysis demonstrated that obstruction and stage were both independent prognostic factors.

Carraro et al. (683) reported on a series of 528 patients with colonic carcinoma, 34% of whom presented with obstruction. One-stage primary resection and anastomosis as curative treatment were performed in 107 obstructed and 256 nonobstructed patients. Three hundred thirty-six potentially cured survivors (94 in the former group and 242 in the latter) were followed for a median of 55 months. During follow-up, local recurrence occurred in 37 patients [12 obstructed (12.8%) and 25 nonobstructed (10.4%)], and metastatic disease in obstructed (27.6%) and nonobstructed (17.8%). Multivariate analysis of survival showed that age over 70 years, Dukes' stage, histologic grade, and recurrence were the only prognostic factors. After one-stage emergency curative treatment, patients presenting with obstructing carcinomas of the colon have a smaller survival probability than that of patients with nonobstructing lesions.

Chen et al. (697) reviewed the medical records of 1950 patients with colorectal carcinoma. Patients were grouped as follows: group 1, complete colonic obstruction without perforation ($n = 120$); group 2, complete obstruction with perforation at the site of the carcinoma ($n = 35$); group 3, complete obstruction with perforation proximal to the carcinoma ($n = 13$); and group 4, nonobstructing, nonperforated carcinomas ($n = 1682$). When compared with group 4, group 1 had a more advanced Dukes' stage, older age, greater incidence of colonic versus rectal carcinomas and a poorer carcinoma-free survival. Groups 2 and 3 had a greater incidence of colonic versus rectal carcinomas, and group 3 had a greater operative mortality. No significant differences were found between groups 1, 2, and 3. Independent factors favorable to carcinoma-free survival were female gender, well-differentiated pathology, uncomplicated cases, colon versus rectal location, and early stage. The perioperative mortality rate for perforated colorectal carcinoma at the site of the carcinoma was 9%; for obstructive colorectal carcinoma 5%. Perioperative mortality was much greater for perforations of the colon and rectum occurring proximal to the carcinoma (31%). Survival was worse for patients with obstruction (33%), or perforation proximal to the carcinoma (33%).

Perforation

In comparison with obstruction, perforation has an even greater detrimental effect on the ultimate outcome for the patient. In a review of four reports, Sugarbaker, Gunderson, and Wittes (422) found a median overall 5-year survival rate of only 9% and a 5-year survival rate of 33% with curative surgery. The median curative operative rate was 55%, with a hospital mortality rate of 30%. For patients with a free perforation into the peritoneal cavity, the 5-year survival rate was a dismal 7.3%, whereas for a localized perforation, the 5-year survival rate was 41.4%. Another report shows an even higher postoperative mortality of 52% (327).

Khan et al. (712) reviewed 48 patients presenting with acute colonic perforation associated with colorectal carcinoma. Thirty-six had perforation of the carcinoma, 11 proximal to the carcinoma, and one distal to the primary carcinoma. Patients who perforated proximal to the carcinoma were older (74.5 years vs. 64.7 years) and had a longer length of stay (46.8 days vs. 11.6 days). Fourteen patients had stage II disease, 19 stage III, and 15 stage IV. Thirty-day mortality was 14%. Of the 30-day survivors, 60% had curative resection (21 with local perforation and 9 with proximal perforation). Thirty-three percent had either unresectable or metastatic disease on exploration. One-year survival was 55%. Five-year disease-free survival was 14%. There were no long-term survivors after perforation proximal to the carcinoma although disease stage was comparable in both groups.

Adjacent Organ Involvement

Direct invasion of adjacent viscera does not preclude the possibility of a curative resection, and every effort must be made to perform a resection if technically possible. A review of 25 reports in the literature by Sugar baker, Gunderson, and Wittes (422) noted a median adjacent organ involvement in 9%, an operative mortality rate of 8%, and a salvage rate of 30% to 50%. This includes fistulization into an adjacent viscus such as the urinary bladder. Although adjacent organ involvement represents more advanced disease, curative resection may still be possible. However, extensive operation is associated with a higher morbidity and mortality.

Presence of Metastatic Disease

It is axiomatic that patients with metastatic disease bear a poorer prognosis than those who are free of disseminated disease. The rare exception is the situation in which the metastatic disease can be resected for cure.

Systemic Manifestations

Patients who develop symptoms of weight loss, anorexia, weakness, or anemia frequently do so in the presence of advanced disease, which does not bode well for the patient.

Obesity

To determine the relationship between body mass index and rates of sphincter preserving operations, overall survival, recurrence, and treatment-related toxicities, Meyerhardt et al. (766) evaluated a nested cohort of 1688 patients with stage II and III rectal carcinoma participating in a randomized trial of postoperative fluorouracil-based chemotherapy and radiation therapy. Obese patients were more likely to undergo an abdominoperineal resection than normal-weight patients (odds ratio, 1.77). Increasing adiposity in men was a strong predictor of having an abdominoperineal resection. Obese men with rectal carcinoma were also more likely than normal-weight men to have a local recurrence (hazard ratio 1.61). In contrast, obesity was not predictive of carcinoma recurrence in women nor was body mass index predictive of overall mortality in either men or women. Underweight patients had an increased risk of death (hazard ratio 1.43) compared with normal-weight patients but no increase in carcinoma recurrences. Among all study participants, obese patients had a significantly lower rate of grade 3 to 4 leukopenia, neutopenia, and stomatitis and a lower rate of any grade 3 or worse toxicity when compared with normal-weight individuals.

Technique of Resection

Various efforts have been made to diminish the risk of dissemination of malignant cells during the operation, but for the most part the results have not been conclusive. In their large multicenter trial, Phillips et al. (727) reported considerable surgeon-related variation with respect to local recurrence. The patients of surgeons with considerable experience had fewer recurrences of disease. Possible causes cited for local recurrence include inadequate resection, suture implantation of malignant cells, and development of a second primary carcinoma at the anastomosis site. The authors state that surgeons should be aware that a small group of our colleagues are obtaining results substantially better than those of the majority, and they conclude that these good results have been achieved by meticulous attention to detail.

In a comprehensive review of the literature, Sugarbaker and Corlew (752) analyzed available data and concluded that there was no survival benefit with the use of radical left hemicolectomy instead of segmental resection, the use of the no-touch technique instead of conventional techniques, or the adoption of control of intraluminal spread of malignant cells. En bloc resection of an attached structure did seem important. The inadvertent intraoperative perforation of the bowel during a curative resection has a decidedly detrimental effect, both in terms of survival and local recurrence (745). The 5-year survival rate with bowel disruption was 23%, and the rate fell as low as 14% when the carcinoma itself was disrupted. Local recurrence rose to 67% in Dukes' B cases with spillage and as high as 87% when Dukes' C carcinomas were perforated at the time of operation (745). Other authors have reported that spillage of malignant cells at the time of operation reduces 5-year survival after resection for cure from 70% to 44% (753).

Akyol et al. (754) examined anastomotic leaks as a risk factor for recurrence. At a mean follow-up of 25 months. 46.9% of patients with leaks developed a recurrence compared with 18.5% for those with out a leak. Cancer-specific mortality rates at 24 months were higher for patients with leaks (36.9% vs. 12.6%). Fujita et al. (756) also found that for patients with anastomotic leakage, the incidence of local recurrence was higher (21.2% vs. 2.4%) and the disease-free survival rate was lower in Dukes' A and B patients (55% vs. 80% at 5 years), but not in Dukes' C patients than in patients with no leakage.

In a study of 403 patients, Bell et al. (757) found after adjustment for lymph node metastases, the distal resection margin of resection, nontotal anatomical dissection of the rectum, and the level of the anastomosis, identified a significant association between anastomotic leakage and local recurrence (hazard ratio 3.8). They concluded that leakage following a colorectal anastomosis after potentially curative resection for carcinoma of the rectum is an independent predictor of local recurrence.

Rouffet et al. (870) reviewed 270 consecutive patients randomly allotted to undergo either left hemicolectomy or left segmental colectomy. Left hemicolectomy removed the entire left colon along with the origin of the inferior mesenteric artery and the dependent lymphatic territory. Left segmental colectomy removed a more restrictive segment of the colon and left the origin of the inferior mesenteric artery unmolested. Both groups were similar with regard to preoperative risk factors. The number of early postoperative abdominal and extra-abdominal complications was similar in both groups. Overall, early postoperative mortality was 4% higher, in left hemicolectomy (6%) than in the left segmental colectomy (2%). Median survival was 10 years, and nearly equivalent in both groups. The two actuarial survival curves were similar. Bowel movement frequency was significantly increased after left hemicolectomy during the first postoperative year. Their results suggest that survival after left segmental colectomy is equivalent to that of left hemicolectomy.

Inadvertent perforation of the bowel during curative resection for colon carcinoma has a definite adverse effect. Slanetz (745) reported a drop in 5-year survival rates from 29% to 14% when disruption occurred during dissection. Local recurrence developed in 75% of cases involving spillage of malignant cells.

Colorectal Specialization and Surgical Volume

In an audit from a Scottish series of 646 anastomoses, the overall anastomotic leak rate was 4.8% (3.2% for colonic carcinoma and 8.9% after resection for rectal carcinoma) (300). Intersurgeon variation was scrutinized. When the anastomosis was performed by five of the 28 surgeons responsible for 50% of the patients, the leak rate was 4.2% vs. 14.3% for the others. The authors support the concept of specialized units.

The impact of the variability in surgical skill among surgeons has also been reported in a multicenter study by Reinbach et al. (897) There was a significant difference between colorectal surgeons with regard to postoperative mortality rates, which varied from 8% to 30%, anastomotic leakage rates, which ranged from 0% to 25%, wound sepsis rates, which ranged from 6% to 35%, and local recurrence rates, which ranged from 0% to 29%. The 10-year survival rate varied from 0% to 63%. There are many studies that now stress the point that we cannot ignore the fact that there exists a variability of skill among surgeons.

Volume

Meyerhardt et al. (923) studied a nested cohort of 1330 patients with stage II and stage III rectal carcinoma participating in a multicenter adjuvant chemotherapy trial. They analyzed differences in rates of sphincter-preserving operations, overall survival, and carcinoma recurrence by hospital surgical volume. They observed a significant difference in the rates of abdominoperineal resections across tertiles of hospital procedure volume (46.3% for patients resected at low-volume, 41.3% at medium-volume, and 31.8% at high-volume hospitals). This higher rate of sphincter-sparing operation at high-volume centers was not accompanied by any increase in recurrence rates. Hospital surgical volume did not predict overall disease free, or local recurrence-free survival. Patients who did not complete the planned adjuvant chemotherapy, those who underwent operation at low-volume hospitals had a significant increase in carcinoma recurrence (hazard ratio 1.94) and a nonsignificant trend toward increased overall mortality and local recurrence. In contrast, no significant volume-outcome relation was noted among patients who did complete postoperative therapy.

Shrag et al. (901) conducted a retrospective population-based cohort study utilizing the Surveillance, Epidemiology and End Results-Medicare linked database identified 2815 rectal carcinoma patients aged 65 and older. They found surgeon volume was better than hospital procedure volume as predicting long-term survival and can have a significant impact on survival for patients with rectal carcinoma. From the same database Shrag et al. (924) identified 24,166 colon carcinoma patients aged 65 and older. As opposed to their findings with rectal carcinoma, high-hospital procedure remained a strong predictor of low postoperative mortality rates for each outcome with and without adjustment for surgeon procedure volume. Surgeon-specific procedure volume was also an important predictor of surgical outcomes for 30-day mortality, and for 2-year mortality, although this effect was attenuated after adjusting for hospital volume. Hospital volume and surgeon volume were each an important predictor of the ostomy rate. Among high-volume institutions and surgeons, individual providers with unusually high ostomy rates could be identified. Both hospital and surgeon-specific procedure volumes predict outcomes following colon carcinoma resection; but hospital volume may exert a stronger effect. In an analysis of 600 patients undergoing resections for rectal carcinoma, Hermanek and Hohenberger (903) reported that the patients of low-volume surgeons experienced an increased risk of local recurrence. Borowski et al. (925) examined surgeon-volume and specialization as defined as membership of the Association of Coloproctology of Great Britain and Ireland as independent prognostic factors for operative morbidity and mortality for patients undergoing operations for colorectal carcinoma. A total of 5948 patients in a regional center in the United Kingdom underwent operations with an operative mortality of 7.9%. Mortality risk was significantly reduced for surgeons who performed more than 20 operations per year while ACPGBI membership was not significant. Although membership demonstrated an interest, it did not necessarily represent specialty training. Surgeons with a high-case volume or specialized interest were more likely to achieve bowel continuity than low-volume surgeons and nonspecialists following rectal resection. There was no significant difference in anastomotic leak rate (5.1%).

Martling et al. (902) compared outcomes in patients being operated upon by high-volume surgeons (more than 12 operations per year) with low-volume surgeons (12 operations or fewer per year). Forty-six surgeons operated on 652 patients. Five high-volume surgeons operated on 48% of the patients. In these, outcome was significantly better than in patients treated by low-volume surgeons (local recurrence rate 4% vs. 10%; rate of rectal carcinoma death 11% vs. 18%).

Wibe (926) examined the influence of caseload on long-term outcome following standardization of rectal carcinoma surgery at a national level. Data relating to all 3388 Norwegian patients with rectal carcinoma treated for cure were recorded in a national database. Treating hospitals were divided into four groups according to their annual caseload: hospitals in group 1 carried out 30 or more procedures, those in group 2 performed 20 to 29 procedures, group 3 10 to 19 procedures, and group 4 fewer than 10 procedures. The 5-year local recurrence rates were 9.2%, 14.7%, 12.5%, and 17.5% and 5-year overall survival rates were 64.4%, 64.0%, 60.8%, and 57.8%, respectively, in the four hospital caseload groups. An annual hospital caseload of fewer than 10 procedures increased the risk of local recurrence compared with that in hospitals where 30 or more procedures were performed each year (hazard ratio 1.9). Overall survival was lower for patients treated at hospitals with an annual caseload of fewer than 10 versus hospital for 30 or more (hazard ratio 1.2).

Colorectal Specialization

Callahan et al. (904) examined the relationship of surgeon subspecialty training and interests to in-hospital mortality while controlling for both hospital and surgeon volume. A large Statewide Planning and Research Cooperative System was used to identify 48,582 in patients who underwent colectomy. Surgical subspecialty training and interests was defined as surgeons who were members of the Society of Surgical Oncology (training/interest $n=68$) or the American Society of Colon and Rectal Surgeons (training/interest $n=61$). Overall mortality for colectomy patients was 4.6%; the adjusted mortality rate for subspecialty versus nonspecialty-trained surgeons was 2.4% versus 4.8%, respectively. For colectomies, risk-adjusted mortality is substantially lower when performed by subspecialty interested and trained surgeons, even after accounting for hospital and surgeon volume and patient characteristics. These findings may have implications for surgical training programs and for regionalization of complex surgical procedures.

Rosen et al. (905) examined variations in operative mortality among surgical specialists who perform colorectal surgery. Mortality rates were compared between six board-certified colorectal surgeons and 33 other institutional surgeons using comparable colorectal procedure codes and a validated database indicating patient severity of illness. Thirty-five ICD-9-CM procedure codes were used to identify 2805 patients who underwent colorectal surgery. Atlas, a state-legislated outcome database, was used by the hospital's Quality Assurance Department to rank the Admission Severity Group of 1753 patients (higher ASG, 0–4, indicates increasing medical instability). Colorectal surgeons had an eight-year mean in-hospital mortality rate of 1.4% compared with 7.3% by other institutional surgeons. There was a significantly lower mortality rate for colorectal surgeons compared with other institutional surgeons in ASG2 (0.8% vs. 3.8%, respectively) and ASG3 (5.7% and 16.4%, respectively). Board-certified colorectal surgeons had a lower in-hospital mortality rate than other institutional surgeons as patients' severity of illness increased.

Platell et al. (906) reviewed patients with colorectal carcinoma managed in general surgery units versus a colorectal unit. These results were compared to a historical control group treated within general surgical units at the same hospital. There were 974 patients involved in the study with no significant differences in the demographic details for the three groups. Patients in the colorectal group were more likely to have rectal carcinoma and stage I carcinomas and less likely to have stage II carcinomas. Patients treated in the colorectal group had a significantly higher overall 5-year survival when compared with the general surgical group and the historical control group (56% vs. 45% vs. 40%, respectively). Survival regression analysis identified age, ASA scores, disease stage, adjuvant chemotherapy, and treatment in a colorectal unit (hazards ratio 0.67) as significant independent predictors of survival. The results suggest that there may be a survival advantage for patients with colon and rectal carcinoma being treated within a specialist colorectal unit.

Read et al. (907) determined the effect of surgeon specialty on disease-free survival and local control in patients with carcinoma of the rectum. The records of 384 consecutive patients treated by colorectal surgeons ($n = 251$) and noncolorectal surgeons ($n = 133$) were reviewed independently by physicians in the Division of Radiation Oncology. Local recurrence was defined as pelvic recurrence occurring in the presence or absence of distant metastatic disease. Actuarial disease-free survival and local control rates at five years were 77% and 99% for colorectal surgeons versus 68% and 84% for noncolorectal surgeons. Multivariate analysis revealed that pathologic stage and background of the surgeon were the only independent predictors of disease-free survival and that pathologic stage, background of the surgeon, and proximal location of the carcinoma were independent predictors of local control. Sphincter preservation was more common by colorectal surgeons (52%) than noncolorectal surgeons (30%). They concluded good outcome for patients with carcinoma of the rectum is associated with subspecialty training in colon and rectal surgery.

Dorrance et al. (908) examined the effect of the surgeon's specialty on patient outcome after potentially curative colorectal carcinoma surgery and to identify factors that may help explain differences in outcome among specialty groups. In a large teaching hospital, 378 patients underwent potentially curative operation for colorectal carcinoma by surgeons with specialty interests, vascular or transplant, general, and colorectal surgeons. At a median follow-up of 45 months the only factors associated with a significant reduced local recurrence rate were the length of the resection specimen (odds ratio, 0.56) and colorectal specialty. Patients operated on by a general surgeon were 3.42 times more likely to develop a local recurrence than those operated on by a colorectal surgeon. For overall recurrence, early stage disease, absence of vascular invasion, and colorectal specialty were the only factors associated with significantly improved outcome at multivariate analysis. These data show that surgeons with an interest in colorectal carcinoma achieve lower local and overall recurrence rates compared with vascular, transplant, or general surgeons.

Martling et al. (927) evaluated the effects of an initiative to teach the TME technique on outcomes at five years after surgery. The study population comprised all 447 patients who underwent abdominal operations for rectal carcinoma in Stockholm County. Outcomes were compared with those in the Stockholm I (790 patients) and Stockholm II (542 patients) radiotherapy trials. The permanent stoma rate was reduced from 60.3% and 55.3% in the Stockholm I and II trials respectively to 26.5% in the TME project. Five-year local recurrence rates decreased from 21.9% and 19.1% to 8.2%, respectively. Five-year carcinoma-specific survival rates increased from 66.0% and 65.7% in the Stockholm trials to 77.3% in the TME project (hazard ratio 0.62). They concluded, a surgical teaching program had a major impact on rectal carcinoma outcome.

McArdle and Hole (871) conducted a study to determine whether differences in survival following surgery for colorectal carcinoma were due to differences in caseload or degree of specialization. The outcome in 3200 patients who underwent resection for colorectal carcinoma was analyzed on the basis of caseload and degree of specialization of individual surgeons. Carcinoma-specific survival at five years following curative resection varied among surgeons from 53.4% to 84.6%; the adjusted hazard ratios varied from 0.48 to 1.55. Carcinoma-specific survival rate at five years following curative resection was 70.2%, 62.0%, and 65.9% for surgeons with a high, medium, and low case volume, respectively. There were no consistent differences in the adjusted hazard ratios by volume. Carcinoma-specific survival rate at five years following curative resection was 72.7% for those treated by specialists and 63.8% for those treated by nonspecialists; the adjusted hazard ratio for nonspecialists was 1.35. They concluded the differences in outcome following apparently curative resection for colorectal carcinoma among surgeons appear to reflect the degree of specialization rather than case volume. It is likely that increase specialization will lead to further improvements in survival.

Perioperative Blood Transfusion

Clinical and experimental studies indicate that transfusion of blood has immunomodulating properties and that the behavior of some neoplasms may be influenced by the immune system of the host. It has been suggested that blood transfusion in the perioperative period adversely affects the rate of carcinoma recurrence and is even associated with increased mortality (758,759). Leite et al. (760) noted a 5-year survival rate of 37% for patients who were transfused compared with 60% for nontransfused patients. Furthermore, it has been suggested that the number of units blood transfused perioperatively in patients operated on for colon carcinoma has a progressively strong negative influence on survival (761). It has been reported that the incidence of recurrence is higher in those patients who receive transfusion during the operation than in those who receive transfusion either before or after operation; however, the study indicated that factors influencing the need for blood transfusion during the operation had a greater bearing on prognosis than the receipt of the blood per se (762). As with other prognosis discriminants, various authors have presented conflicting views (872,873). To resolve some of the controversy of the degree of immunomodulation by perioperative blood transfusion and its effect on oncologic surgery, Chung, Steinmetz, and Gordon (762) reviewed all studies published between 1982 and 1990 using the statistical method of Mantel-Haentszel-Peto to determine a cumulative estimate of the direction and magnitude of this association. Some 20 papers were included in the analysis, representing 5236 patients. The cuumulative odds ratios (95% confidence interval) of disease recurrence, death from carcinoma, and death from any cause were 1.80 (1.30 to 2.51), 1.76 (1.15 to 2.66), and 1.63 (1.12 to 2.38), respectively. These results support the hypothesis that perioperative blood transfusion is associated with an increased risk of recurrence of colorectal carcinoma and death from this malignancy.

Splenectomy has been considered a possible factor in the survival of patients operated on for colorectal carcinoma (928). The mechanism responseible for this adverse impact is undefined, but it may fall into the category of modulation of the immune response. Others disagree (929).

Previous Appendectomy

Armstrong et al. (765) studied a series of 519 patients presenting with carcinoma of the cecum in relation to a history with or without previous appendectomy. Previous appendectomy was associated with a higher incidence of local fixity, invasion of the abdominal wall, metastatic spread, and poor differentiation. These differences were reflected in a significantly lower resection rate for carcinomas in patients who had undergone appendectomy. The survival of patients who had previously had appendectomy was significantly reduced. Local recurrence was more common and often was noted to be in the old appendectomy wound itself. In this study appendectomy did not increase the risk of carcinogenesis in the cecum but worsened the prognosis for patients who subsequently developed carcinoma of the cecum.

■ PATHOLOGIC FEATURES

Numerous pathologic features have been studied in an effort to define and refine the prognosis of a given patient. In a very meticulous and thorough study Newland et al. (732) analyzed data from 579 patients collected prospectively during a follow-up ranging between 6 months and 21.5 years. Six variables showed significant independent effects on survival on multivariate analysis. In diminishing potency, these variables were apical lymph node involvement, spread involving a free serosal surface, invasion beyond the muscularis propria, location in the rectum, venous invasion, and high-grade malignancy. Significant independent effects also were shown for patient age and gender. The number of involved lymph nodes added no significant independent prognostic information. The authors recommend that all six independent variables be included in any future protocol for stratifying this prognostically diverse group of patients. Many of the individual discriminants are discussed below.

Location

Most reports suggest that rectal carcinoma has a poorer prognosis than colon carcinoma (732,740,742). In the report by Polissar, Sim, and Francis (735) colon carcinoma resulted in a significantly worse prognosis than rectal carcinoma. Newland et al. (732) reported a hazard ratio of 1.53. In contrast, the study by Martin et al. (876) found no difference in 5-year survival rates on the basis of site of the carcinoma. In patients with colon carcinoma, opinion has differed as to whether a right-sided lesion has a better prognosis (740), a left-sided lesion has a better prognosis (674), or the prognoses are equal. Several authors believe that right-sided lesions carry a poorer prognosis (768).

Size

In contrast to other malignancies, it has been reported that the size of a carcinoma of the colon bears little relationship to prognosis (732,877). Other authors have expressed the opposite opinion (769,770).

Configuration

The macroscopic features of a colon carcinoma appear to reflect its biologic activity. Polypoid lesions tend not to deeply invade the bowel wall, whereas ulcerating lesions more often penetrate the wall and are associated with a poorer prognosis. Lumen encirclement is a strong prognostic discriminant (742). Rate of survival with full circumferential involvement was found to be 29.7% at 5 years, whereas when less than half of the lumen was involved, the 5-year survival rate was 53.9% (740).

Survival and local recurrence are significantly better for patients with exophytic (polypoid and sessile) carcinomas than for those with nonexophytic (ulcerated and flat raised lesions) (912). Exophytic lesions include significantly more stage T1 and fewer T2 and T3 carcinomas, and a significantly smaller proportion of carcinomas that show venous and lymphatic invasion than the nonexophytic lesions.

Microscopy

Although histologic grading is valuable in assessing prognosis, no uniform system of grading exists. Broders' grade 1 carries a relatively good prognosis, while grades 3 and 4 have a poor prognosis. Approximately one half of patients fall into the grade 2 category, which makes this grading system of limited help. Furthermore, there is frequently a discrepancy between the preoperative and postoperative assessments. In their review, Sugarbaker, Gunderson, and Wittes (422) summarized the findings of many studies and concluded that malignancies of higher grades have less chance for cure than those of lower grades. Other microscopic features associated with a diminished chance for cure include more advanced primary lesions, cases involving increased frequency of venous invasion, increased frequency of distant metastases, increased frequency of perineural invasion, and increased frequency of metastases to lymph nodes. Preoperative biopsy is of limited prognostic value unless a poorly differentiated lesion is present, in which case the likelihood of lymphatic metastases is greater. Newland et al. (732) estimated that the hazard ratio for survival for patients with a high-grade carcinoma was 1.48.

Carcinomas that secrete large amounts of mucus are associated with reduced survival. Yamamoto et al. (777) compared the clinicopathologic features of patients with a mucinous carcinoma (6.6% of their patients) to a nonmucinous carcinoma. They found that mucinous carcinomas were more likely to invade adjacent viscera (29% vs. 10%), show lymph node involvement beyond the pericolic region (50% vs. 26%), have a reduced rate of curative resection (34% vs. 69%), have a higher recurrence rate (27% vs. 19%), and result in a poorer 5-year survival rate (33% vs. 53%). Green et al. (878) found that stage for stage, the 5-year overall survival rate was the same for mucinous and nonmucinous carcinomas. However, the 5-year survival rate for mucinous carcinoma of the rectum was decidedly more poor than nonmucinous carcinoma (11% vs. 57%). In a review of 352 patients with colorectal carcinoma followed for a minimum of 5 years, Secco et al. (776) found that mucinous adenocarcinomas represented 11.1% and signet-ring cell carcinomas represented 1.1% of cases. Mucinous carcinomas were most frequently located in the rectum (61.5%) and in the sigmoid colon (15.3%). Patients presented with Dukes' C and metastatic disease in 41% and 15% of cases, respectively. Disease recurrence was more frequently observed in patients with mucinous (51.7%) or signet-ring lesions (100%) compared with adenocarcinomas. Five-year survival rates were 45%, 28%, and 0% in patients with adenocarcinoma, mucinous adenocarcinoma, or signet-ring cell carcinomas, respectively.

Signet-ring cell adenocardnomas (i.e., cells with abundant intracellular mucus) have a particularly poor prognosis. Chen et al. (789) identified 61 signet ring cell carcinoma patients and compared their clinical data and outcomes to those of 144 consecutive patients with nonsignet ring cell mucinous rectal carcinomas and 2414 consecutive patients with nonmucinous rectal carcinomas. The incidence of signet ring cell carcinomas was 1.39% of rectal carcinomas. Mean patient age at onset of signet-ring cell carcinomas (48.1 years) was significantly lower than that for nonsignet ring cell mucinous carcinomas (57.4 years) and nonmucinous carcinomas (62.6 years). The proportion of late stage (TNM III and IV) carcinomas was significantly higher in signet ring cell carcinomas (90%) than in nonsignet-ring mucinous carcinomas (69%) and nonmucinous carcinomas (48%). There were more carcinomas located in the lower rectum in signet ring cell carcinomas (46%) than in nonsignet-ring mucinous carcinomas (34%) and nonmucinous carcinomas (29%). Signet ring cell carcinomas were significantly larger (5.7 cm) than nonsignet cell mucinous carcinoma (4.3 cm) and nonmucinous lesions (3.8 cm). A higher% of patients with signet ring cell carcinoma (42.6%) received abdominoperineal resection for treatment. In carcinomas with TNM stage IV the rate of spread via hematogenous route was significantly lower in signet ring cell carcinomas (18.5%) than in nonsignet cell mucin (43.5%) and in nonmucinous carcinomas (69%). The rate of spread via seeding to the peritoneum was lower in signet cell carcinomas (22.2%) than in nonsignet cell mucin carcinomas (43.5%) but higher than in nonmucinous carcinomas (2.7%). The rate of spread via the lymphatic route was higher in signet cell ring carcinomas (44.4%) than in nonsignet cell mucinous carcinomas (26.1%) and significantly higher than in nonmucinous carcinomas (12.3%). The 1-, 2-, and 5-year overall signet cell carcinoma survival rates were 73.9%, 36.3%, and 23.3%, respectively, which were significantly poorer than those of nonsignet cell mucin carcinomas and nonmucinous carcinomas. For the signet cell carcinomas, the 1-, 2-, and 5-year disease-free survival rates of signet cell carcinoma were 84%, 44.2%, and 30.3%, respectively which are comparable with general data of stage III rectal carcinoma in the world. They concluded diffuse infiltration of signet ring cells enhances the tendency of mucinous carcinomas of the rectum in more local extension and easier lymphatic spreading but not at peritoneal seeding.

Nissan et al. (790) compared 46 patients with signet ring cell carcinomas with 3371 patients with primary nonsignet ring cell carcinomas. Lymphatic and peritoneal spread was more common among the signet cell ring carcinoma group. Approximately one-third of signet ring cell carcinoma patients presented with metastatic disease. Mean survival time of signet ring cell carcinoma group was 45.4 months compared with 78.5 months for the control patients group. The cumulative survival curve of patients with signet ring cell carcinoma resembles that of patients with poorly differentiated rectal carcinomas.

The pathologic diagnosis of scirrhous carcinoma of the large bowel carries a very poor prognosis. Extent of penetration of the bowel wall is associated with a reduced prognosis. Greater extramural spread is associated with an increased incidence of nodal involvement (877). Hase et al. (786) examined 663 specimens from patients who underwent curative resection for colorectal carcinoma and identified small clusters of undifferentiated malignant cells ahead of the invasive front of the lesion, which they labeled "tumor budding." The presence of this feature resulted in a diminished 5-year survival rate (22% vs. 71%). In a study of 138 patients, Tanaka et al. (787) reported recurrence in 48% of patients with "tumor budding" compared with 4.5% without this histologic feature. Cumulative disease-specific survivals at five years were 74% and 98%, respectively. In a review of 196 resected stage II and III colon carcinomas, Okuyama et al. (788) found budding detected significantly more frequently in lesions with lymph node metastases (stage III) than in lesions without it. Patients with budding-positive lesions had worse outcome than those with budding-negative lesions with 50.6% with budding-positive lesions and 8.1% with budding-negative lesions developing recurrence. Patients with budding-positive lesions had a worse prognosis than patients without it. Moreover, no significant difference in survival curves was observed between patients with budding-positive stage II lesions and those with stage III lesions.

An additional histologic feature that may correlate with prognosis is the presence or absence of an inflammatory infiltrate. For patients whose resected specimens demonstrated infiltration of lymphocytes around blood vessels, together with hyperplasia of paracortical regions in lymph nodes, Pihl et al. (671) found a 5-year recurrence-free interval of 85%, while patients who lacked these characteristics exhibited a survival rate of 69%.

Gagliardi et al. (785) studied the relationship between acinar growth patterns in 138 patients with rectal carcinoma and survival. Lesions were classified according to size, 28 microacinar and 110 macroacinar. Patients with microacinar (small regular tubules) had a significantly reduced 5-year survival rate compared with those with macroacinar (large irregular tubules) lesions (43% vs. 68%).

Residual Disease

Local residual disease predicts poor patient survival after resection for colorectal carcinoma. Chan et al. (792) determined the prevalence of residual carcinoma in a line of resection in a large prospective series and identified other pathology variables that may influence survival in the absence of distant metastases. The overall prevalence of residual carcinoma in a line of resection was 5.9%. Of 12 pathology variables examined, only high grade and apical node metastases were independently associated with survival in the subset of 120 patients with residual disease in a line of resection but without distant metastases. The 2-year survival rate for patients with neither of these adverse features was 46.4% as compared with only 7.7% in those who had both.

Dukes' Staging

The numerous eponymous modifications of the Dukes classification have not allowed any meaningful comparison to be made from one report to another. However, within each of these modifications a more advanced stage represents a poorer prognosis. If a staging system of local, regional, and distant categories were adopted, it might permit comparison and agreement on survival of a given category of patient.

Histologic activity offers a means of estimating biologic behavior, and this association has been reflected in the Dukes classification. The effect of Dukes' staging on survivorship was reported from the Lahey Clinic in Boston in a study of 344 patients treated for colorectal carcinoma. The uncorrected 5-year survivorship for Dukes' A, B, and C patients was 85%, 65%, and 46%, respectively, while the corresponding corrected values were 100%, 78%, and 54% (740).

Newland et al. (732) conducted a multivariate survival analysis on the depth of invasion. For spread beyond the muscularis propria, the authors found a hazard ratio of 1.68, and for spread involving the free serosal surface, the hazard ratio was 1.71. In another report, the same authors found that the survival rates of patients with clinicopathologic stages A or B closely matched their expected survival as predicted from the general population (930). Males with stage B carcinomas were the only exception and their reduced survival rates were due to four clinical variables (cardiovascular complications, permanent stoma, urgent operation, or respiratory complications) and one pathologic variable (direct spread involving a free serosal surface).

Greene et al. (751) proposed a new TNM staging strategy for node positive colon and rectal carcinoma because the current stage III designation of colon carcinoma excludes prognostic subgroups stratified for mural penetration (T1-4) or nodal involvement (N1 vs. N2). They analyzed 50,042 patients with stage III colon carcinoma reported to the National Cancer Data Base. Three distinct subcategories with a traditional stage III cohort of colon carcinoma were identified—IIIA: T1/2, N1; IIIB: T3/4, N1; and IIIC: any T, N2. Five-year observed survival rates for these three subcategories were 59.8%, IIIA; 42.0%, IIIB; and 27.3%, IIIC. Analysis of this large data set supports stratification into three subsets, confirming the benefit of adjuvant chemotherapy in each subgroup. They subsequently analyzed data entered in the National Cancer Data Base for 5987 stage III patients with rectal carcinoma (931). Five-year observed survival rates for stage III subcategories were 55.3% in IIIA; 35.3% in IIIB; and 24.5% in IIIC. Stratifying for treatment outcome, stage IIIA patients having operation alone had poorer observed 5-year survival (39%) than patients treated with operation and adjuvant chemotherapy or radiation therapy (60%). Similar outcomes occurred in IIIB (operation alone 21.7% and chemo/radiotherapy 40.9%) and in IIIC (operation alone 12.2% and chemo/radiotherapy 28.9%). The effect of postoperative adjuvant therapy was beneficial in all subsets.

Lymph Node Status

The most important prognostic variable in colon carcinoma is the presence or absence of lymph node metastases. Patients with colorectal carcinoma found to have regional lymph node metastases after curative resection form a large and prognostically diverse group. In studies focusing on the level of lymph node involvement and the number of affected lymph nodes, the number of lymph nodes involved correlates with survival in some reports. In a report by Corman, Veidenheimer, and Coller (7), if more than three lymph nodes were positive, the overall survival rate was 18%, but with one to three nodes involved, the survival rate was 45% to 50%. At St. Mark's Hospital in London, the 5-year survival rate is approximately 60% when one node is affected, 35% when two to five nodes are involved, and 20% when six or more nodes are affected (230). An analysis of the NSABP clinical trials by Wolmark, Fischer, and Wieand (784) revealed a relative risk of death of 1.9 and 3.4 for patients with one to four and five to nine positive lymph nodes, respectively. Gardner et al. (792) also found that prognosis worsened with an increased number of involved lymph nodes. Patients who had six or more involved nodes were 4.6 times as likely to die from the disease as patients with only one involved node. Cohen et al. (771) reported that when one to three nodes were involved, the 5-year survival rate was 66%, but was reduced to 37% when four or more nodes were positive. Similarly, Tang et al. (795) found that the number of lymph nodes involved had an impact on survival. In a retrospective study of 538 patients, the 5-year survival rate for patients with one to three positive nodes was 69%, 44% for four to nine positive nodes, and 29% for 10 or more positive nodes. On the other hand, Newland et al. (733) reported that the number of involved lymph nodes added no significant independent prognostic information. Most potent in their analysis was apical node involvement, which they calculated to have a hazard ratio of 1.79 in their multivariate survival analysis. Such involvement was present in 9% of their node-positive patients. Malassagne et al. (794) found that both the number of lymph nodes involved as well as apical node involvement were prognosticators. The 5-year survival rates were 17% and 45% for patients with and without apical lymph node involvement, respectively, and 44% and 6% for those with four or fewer nodes involved compared with those with more than four positive nodes, respectively.

Swanson et al. (932) examined data from the National Cancer Data Base to determine whether the number of examined lymph nodes is prognostic for T3N0 colon carcinoma. A total of 35,787 prospectively collected cases of T3N0 colon carcinomas that were surgically treated and pathologically reported as T3N0M0 were analyzed. The 5-year relative survival rate for T3N0M0 colon carcinoma varied from 64% if one or two lymph nodes were examined to 86% if >25 lymph nodes were examined. Three strata of lymph nodes (1–7, 8–12, and ≥ 13) distinguished significantly different observed 5-year survival rates. These results demonstrate that the prognosis of T3N0 colon carcinoma is dependent on the number of lymph nodes examined. A minimum of 13 lymph nodes should be examined to label a T3 colon carcinoma as node negative.

Fisher et al. (933) examined the presumably negative nodes of a larger cohort of patients for what they designated nodal mini micrometastases on parameters of survival. Mini micrometastases were detected by immunohistochemical staining of the original lymph node sections with anticytokeratin A1/A3 in a total of 241 Dukes' A and B patients with rectal and 158 with colonic carcinoma. Nodal mini micrometastases were detected in 18% of patients in this cohort but this additional finding failed to exhibit any significant relationship to overall recurrence free survival. Other reports have recorded mini micrometastases in 19% to 39% of cases and this probably relates to the number of sections taken at the time of study. Sakuragi et al. (934) sought predictive markers of lymph node metastases to assist in management of 278 T1 colorectal carcinomas. Depth of submucosal invasion and lymphatic channel invasion were accurate predictive factors for lymph node metastases. The authors believe these two factors could be used in selecting appropriate cases for operation after endoscopic resection.

Tepper et al. (935) analyzed data from 1664 patients with T3, T4, or node positive rectal carcinoma treated in a National intergroup trial of adjuvant therapy with chemotherapy and radiation therapy to assess the association between the number of lymph nodes found by the pathologist in the surgical specimen and the time to relapse and survival outcomes. No significant differences were found by quartiles among patients determined to be node positive. Approximately 14 nodes need to be studied to define nodal status accurately. Examining greater number of nodes increases the likelihood of proper staging.

Venous Invasion

In a personal study of more than 1000 operative specimens, Morson and Dawson (230) found regional venous involvement in 35% of cases. Submucosal venous spread occurred in 10%, and in 25% there was evidence of permeation of extramural vessels. In the former cases, there was little or no effect on prognosis, but extramural venous involvement reduced 5-year survival rates from 55% to approximately 30%. In the report by Corman, Veidenheimer, and Coller (7), patients with Dukes' C lesions and blood vessel invasion had a 31% 5-year survival rate compared with 43% without blood vessel invasion. Comparable figures for Dukes' B lesions were 55% and 70%, respectively. The former% is not significant, but the latter reached statistical significance. A subsequent report from the Lahey Clinic found a difference with and without blood vessel invasion (740). Minsky et al. (803) reviewed a series of 168 patients who underwent potentially curative resection. The authors found that patients who had extramural blood vessel invasion had a significantly decreased 5-year survival rate compared with patients who had intramural blood vessel invasion or no vascular invasion at all. When extramural and intramural invasion were combined, the difference disappeared. Krasna et al. (804) found that the 3-year survival rate decreased from 62.2% in patients without vascular invasion to 29.7% in patients demonstrating vascular invasion. In 128 operative specimens, Horn, Dahl, and Morild (800) identified venous invasion in 22%. The 5-year survival rate in those with venous invasion was 32.9% vs. 84.3% for those without venous invasion. Newland et al. (732) identified venous invasion in 28.8% of their series, and in 81% of those patients extramural veins were involved. The authors calculated a hazard ratio of 1.49 in the multivariate survival analysis.

In a very thorough study Sternberg et al. (801) investigated venous invasion as a predictor of prognosis in colorectal carcinoma. The reported incidence of venous invasion in colorectal carcinoma specimens varies between 10% and 89.9%, mainly as a result of the interobserver variability and differences in specimen processing. Their study goal was to assess and compare the incidence of venous invasion diagnosed on H&E-stained tissue versus tissue stained with both H&E and an elastic fiber stain. Venous invasion was assessed on sections from 81 colorectal carcinomas resected from patients with synchronous distant metastases. Only stage IV carcinomas were studied for the following reasons: (1) it can be assumed that in all patients with distant hematogenous metastases venous invasion had occurred, thus enabling the false negative rate to be calculated; (2) there can be no dispute about the clinical relevance of the various characteristics of venous invasion identified in the carcinomas of patients with synchronous distant hematogenous metastases; and (3) to eliminate the effect of variance in carcinoma staging on the incidence of venous invasion. Initially, H&E-stained sections were studied for venous invasion. Sections that were negative or questionable with regard to venous invasion were then stained with an elastic fiber stain and a second final search for venous invasion was carried out. Venous invasion was identified in 51.9% on H&E-stained sections. The addition of the elastic fiber stain enabled the diagnosis of venous invasion in 38.5% of the remaining specimens, increasing the overall incidence to 70.4%. Of the 57 positive specimens, venous invasion was minimal in 47.4%, intermediate in 8.8%, and massive in 43.9%. Only intramural veins were involved in 31.6%, only extramural veins in 45.6%, and both intramural and extramural veins in 22.8% of the positive specimens. The filling type of venous invasion was found in 71.9%, the floating type in 49.1%, and the infiltrating type in 10.5% of the positive specimens. There was no significant difference between the incidence of venous invasion in the colon (70%) versus rectal and rectosigmoid carcinomas (71.4%) nor in the incidence of venous invasion in patients with hepatic (70%) versus nonhepatic (72.7%) metastases. Only minimal venous invasion is required for the seeding of clinically relevant hematogenous metastases, and emphasizes the careful dedicated search for venous invasion that is required from the pathologist. Although extramural venous invasion was predominant in stage IV colorectal carcinomas, in a third of lesions only intramural venous invasion was found. This suggests that intramural venous invasion may also seed clinically relevant hematogenous metastases, and should therefore also be considered as an indicator of poor prognosis.

Perineural Invasion

Perineural invasion has been shown to have a detrimental effect on prognosis. Its presence may be part of the overall penetration of the bowel wall. The association of disseminated disease has been reported (799). Krasna et al. (804) found that the 3-year survival rate decreased from 57.7% in patients without neural invasion to 29.6% in patients with neural invasion. Of 128 operative specimens examined by Horn, Dahl, and Morild (800), neural invasion was demonstrated in 32%. The 5-year survival rate in patients with neural invasion was 64.3% compared with 81.1% when neural invasion was not demonstrated.

Ueno et al. (807) investigated perineural invasion in 364 patients who underwent curative resection for rectal carcinoma penetrating the muscular layer. A grading system was established based on the "intensity" (number of perineural invasion foci in a 20-power field) and "depth" (distance from the muscularis propria). PNI-0 was defined as without perineural invasion, PNI-1 as intensity of less than five foci and depth less than 10 mm, and PNI-2 as five or more foci or 10 mm or greater depth of invasion. Perineural invasion was observed in 14% and strongly correlated with pathological lymph node metastases. Five-year survival was related to the perineural invasion (74% in PNI-0, 50% in PNI-1, and 22% in PNI-2). The rate of local recurrence was also related to PNI stage: 43% in PNI-2 and 9% in PNI-0 and PNI-1. The PNI grading system may be useful in prognosis and may allow case selection for intensive postoperative adjuvant therapy.

■ BIOCHEMICAL AND SPECIAL INVESTIGATIONS

Preoperative CEA Levels

An analysis of data from 945 patients entered into the NSABP revealed a strong correlation between preoperative CEA levels and the Dukes' classes (813). The mean CEA level progressively increased with each Dukes' category, and the mean value for each of the four classes was significantly different. Mean values (± SE) for Dukes' A, B, C, and D (metastatic or contiguous disease) were 3.9 ± 0.6, 9.3 ± 1.4, 32.1 ± 8.9, 251 ± 84, respectively. The prognostic function was independent of the number of positive histologic lymph nodes and unrelated to the presence or absence of obstruction. Preoperative levels correlated with the degree of lumen encirclement by the carcinoma, with lesions involving more than one half the circumference being associated with significantly lower preoperative CEA levels. The relative risk of developing a treatment failure was associated with preoperative CEA in both Dukes' B and C patients. For patients with Dukes' B lesions, those with a CEA of 2.5 to 10 had 1.2 times the likelihood of developing a recurrence as those with less than 2.5, while those with a CEA level greater than 10 had 3.24 times the likelihood. For patients with Dukes' C lesions the respective risks were 1.77 and 1.76. Although some authors have come to the same conclusion (813), others have found the correlation true only for patients with Dukes' C lesions (812). An important caveat to note is that poorly differentiated carcinomas produce little CEA, and therefore a normal preoperative CEA in a patient with a poorly differentiated carcinoma does not suggest a favorable prognosis (817). Several authors have found CEA determinations to be of little prognostic significance (881). However, a clearer relationship has been demonstrated between persistently elevated levels of CEA in the postoperative period and early recurrence (936).

Liver Function Tests

Abnormal results of liver function tests have been associated with a poor prognosis (818), but not uniformly so (747).

Other Blood Tests

Low serum protein levels have been reported to be associated with a poor prognosis. Factors found to have no effect on prognosis include hemoglobin level, white blood count, and erythrocyte sedimentation rate (747).

DNA Distribution

Several studies have reported that patients who exhibit an abnormal DNA pattern, that is, other than the normal diploid pattern, suffer a higher recurrence rate (819,822,937,744). Giaretti et al. (938) found DNA aneuploidy present in 31% of adenomas and 74% of adenocarcinomas. DNA ploidy correlated with the size and the degree of dysplasia but not with histologic type. From the same center, it was determined that fresh-frozen material gave a higher incidence of DNA aneuploidy than paraffin-embedded material (79% vs. 41%) (938) Armitage et al. (819) found that 55% of their patients had cells with abnormal DNA (aneuploid). Of this group, only 19% of patients survived 5 years, compared with 43% of patients with diploid neoplasms. In contrast, Jones, Moore, and Schofield (882) found that after the surgeon's assessment of operability, the pathologic classification, and the patient's age were considered, the DNA ploidy status conferred no independent survival value. Halvorsen and Johannesen (939) reported a significant survival advantage in patients with diploid lesions compared to those with nondiploid lesions but no difference between carcinoma of the rectum and colon. The authors concluded that ploidy does not contribute to the explanation of why patients with rectal carcinoma had a poorer prognosis than those with colon carcinoma. Venkatesh, Weingart, and Ramanujam (823) compared two parameters in DNA analysis and found that the odds of survival were 3.7 times greater in patients with aneuploidy rather than aneuploidy plus an S-phase fraction >20%.

Genetic Alteration

Among the most recent factors considered in the galaxy of prognostic discriminants are molecular genetic alterations (826). Fractional allelic loss, a measure of allelic deletions, has provided independent prognostic information. Distant metastases were significantly associated with high fractional allelic loss and with deletions of 17p and 18q. Further associations were found between allelic losses and a family history of carcinoma, left-sided location of a carcinoma, and absence of extracellular mucin.

Jen et al. (827) reported that patients with stage II disease have a 5-year survival rate of 93% when the carcinoma has no evidence of allelic loss of chromosome 18q, but only 54% when there was an allelic loss. In patients with stage III disease, 5-year survival is 52% without allelic loss and 38% with loss. An overall hazard ratio for death in patients with allelic loss of chromosome 18q is 2.83. It has also been reported that patients with CD44 v6-positive carcinomas have a poorer prognosis than those with negative lesions (839). Overexpression of *ras* p21 was reportedly associated with an increased incidence of lymphatic invasion, depth of invasion, incidence of liver metastases, and decreased operative curability and long-term survival (840).

Overall expression of *p53* has been found to be an independent predictor of recurrence in Dukes' B and C carcinomas by some authors (832,833) and not a predictor by others (890). Auvinen et al. (829) reported patients with *p53* overexpression had a corrected 5-year survival rate of 37% compared with that of 58% in patients with normal expression. Corresponding 10-year rates were 34% and 54%, respectively. *TP53* gene mutations (topographic genotyping) have been associated with decreased survival (831).

Shibata et al. (828) found that in patients with stage II disease whose carcinoma expressed *DCC*, the 5-year survival rate was 94.3%, whereas in patients with *DCC*-negative lesions, the survival rate was 61.6%. In patients with stage III disease, the survival rates were 59.3% and 33.2%, respectively.

Wang et al. (841) used DNA chip technology to systematically identify new prognostic markers for relapse in Dukes' B carcinoma patients. Gene expression profiling identified a 23-gene signature that predicts recurrence in Dukes' B patients. The overall performance accuracy was 78%. Thirteen of 18 relapse patients and 15 of 18 disease-free patients were predicted correctly, giving an odds ratio of 13. The clinical value of these markers is that the patients at a high predictive risk of relapse (13-fold risk) could be upstaged to receive adjuvant therapy, similar to Dukes' C patients. A series of other genetic alterations proposed as prognostic factors in colorectal carcinoma have been cited (230).

Lim et al. (917) analyzed the association between MSI status and clinicopathological features and prognosis in 248 sporadic colorectal carcinoma patients of which 9.3% had MSI+ carcinomas. MSI+ sporadic colorectal carcinomas were found predominantly in the proximal colon and were associated with poor differentiation, a lower preoperative serum CEA level, and less frequent systemic metastases than MSI− carcinomas. Low grade, low T-stage, no lymph node metastases, no systemic metastases, adjuvant chemotherapy, and MSI+ status were independent favorable prognostic factors for survival in sporadic colorectal carcinoma patients.

Kohen-Corish et al. (940) undertook a detailed analysis of the prognostic significance of MSI-L and loss of MGMT protein expression in colon carcinoma in 183 patients with clinicopathologic stage C colon carcinoma who had not received adjuvant therapy. They showed that MSI-L defines a group of patients with poorer survival than MSS patients and that MSI-L was an independent prognostic indicator in stage III colon carcinoma. Loss of MGMT protein expression was associated with the MSI-L phenotype but was not a prognostic factor for overall survival in colon carcinoma. p-16 methylation was significantly less frequent in MSI-L than in MSI-H and MSS carcinomas and was not associated with survival.

To derive a more precise estimate of the prognostic significance of MSI, Popat et al. (918) reviewed and pooled data from 32 eligible studies that reported survival in a total of 7642 cases, including 1277 with MSI. There was no evidence of publication bias. The combined hazard ratio estimate for overall survival associated with MSI was 0.65. This benefit was maintained restricting analyses to clinical trial patients (HR = 0.69) and patients with locally advanced colorectal carcinoma (HR = 0.67).

Sialomucin Staining

Oncogenic transformation of colonic epithelium is accompanied by increased secretion of sialomucin at the expense of the normally predominant sulfomucins. For patients who exhibit a sialomucin-predominant pattern, there is an increased incidence for local recurrence and a predicted diminution of 5-year survival (850).

Nuclear Morphometry

In search of a reliable prognostic discriminant, Mitmaker, Bégin, and Gordon (853) used nuclear morphometry to assess 100 cases of colorectal carcinoma in which patients who underwent curative resection were followed for at least 5 years. Each case was staged according to the Dukes' classification and graded histologically. The nuclear shape factor was defined as the degree of circularity of the nucleus, with a perfect circle recorded as 1.0. A nuclear shape factor >0.84 was associated with a poor outcome. This variable proved to be a highly significant predictor of survival and independent of the variables of sex, age, histologic grade, and Dukes' classification.

Plasminogen Activity

Studies of tissue plasminogen activity have revealed that overall survival curves are related to the ratio of urokinase-type plasminogen activators to tissue-type plasminogen activators (854). A ratio >0.22 in normal mucosa of patients with Dukes' B and C carcinoma has a decreased probability of survival with a Cox's hazard ratio of 2.8.

Sialyl Lewis^x Antigen Expression (Sle^x)

Based on data of 114 patients who underwent curative resections, sialyl Lewis^x antigen–positive patients had a higher incidence of recurrence in distant organs, especially in the liver, than that of sialyl Lewis^x–negative patients (845). The 5-year disease-free survival rates of sialyl Lewis^x–positive and –negative patients were 57.7% and 89.1%, respectively.

PCNA Labeling Findings

Proliferating cell nuclear antigen expressions of the invasive margin of a carcinoma was shown to be significantly higher in patients who were noted to have venous invasions, a higher potential for metastases to lymph nodes and liver, and less differentiated lesions (848).

An effort has been made to tabulate the various prognostic discriminants that have been considered important (see Table 15). At a glance, the reader will recognize the controversy engendered in the efforts to sort out the important factors.

RECURRENT DISEASE

■ FOLLOW-UP

The most appropriate follow-up for patients who have been operated on for carcinoma of the colon has not been determined. Any follow-up program should focus on the detection of resectable anastomotic and locoregional failure, liver and lung metastases, and metachronous lesions. In a retrospective analysis of 5476 patients with colon or rectal carcinoma, Cali et al. (941) calculated the annual incidence for metachronous carcinomas to be 0.35%. Current recommendations for follow-up are described in Chapter 25. However, the wisdom of any type of follow-up has been questioned. The rationale for such a stance is the belief that little effective therapy is available when recurrences develop. Opponents argue that intensive follow-up is not worth the effort and expense, since as many as 62% of new lesions are detected when the patient presents with symptoms between scheduled follow-up sessions (936,942–944). Proponents of intensive follow-up state that if a recurrent or metachronous lesion is detected when a patient is asymptomatic, the probability of cure by repeat resection will be increased, since the newly detected lesion will be at a more favorable stage than if the patient were symptomatic (945,946). In support of the latter argument, Buhler et al. (945) reported on a series in which patients with asymptomatic anastomotic recurrence had a re-resection rate of 66%, with a survival rate of 12 to 72 months, whereas none of the patients who were symptomatic had a resection for cure and the survival rate in this group was 1 to 24 months. In a report in which 1293 patients were rigorously followed, 299 recurrences were detected in 168 patients (local recurrence, 40%; liver metastases, 29%; and other, 31%) (946). Of these patients, 51% with local recurrence and 47% with liver metastases were asymptomatic. Radical operation was performed in 50% of those with local recurrences and in 26% of those with liver metastases. The 3-year survival rate after reoperation was 35% in those with local recurrence and 33% in those with liver metastases. The 5-year survival rates were 23% and 15%, respectively. These results demonstrate the benefit of aggressive follow-up. Yamamoto et al. (947) reported the results of 974 patients who underwent a curative resection. Recurrence developed locally in 7.2%; liver, 4.8%; and lung, 3.6%. The%s of patients who underwent reoperation or curative resection were 77% and 24% of those with local recurrence, 34% and 38% of those with liver metastases, and 17% and 100% of those with pulmonary metastases, respectively. The 3- and 5-year survival rates were 13% and 9% after reoperation for local recurrence, 14% and 0% for liver metastases, and 53% and 53% after reoperation for pulmonary metastases, respectively.

In an extensive review by Wade et al. (578) of 22,715 patients who underwent colectomy for carcinoma, 12,150 presented with metastatic disease. The estimated surveillance costs averaged $1.3 million per life saved by resection, or $203,000 per year of added life. Despite the apparent high price tag for postoperative studies, the authors believe that surveillance should continue. The costs of eliminating surveillance after curative colectomy would be paid every year by the patients who would die annually with recurrent carcinoma of the colon and rectum, by those who would lose 20 to 28 months of added life gained on average with resection of their isolated colorectal metastases, and by the patients whose cure would be sacrificed. There is a need to determine which tests and regimens can best identify metastatic disease at an early enough stage to allow curative treatment for those who will benefit from it.

■ INCIDENCE

In an excellent review, Devesa, Morales, and Enriquez (688) found that the incidence of recurrence varied because of multiple biases of classification and treatment, different methods of determining recurrence, and statistical manipulation. From their study it was noted that all series quote the incidence of recurrence by Dukes' staging or by some modification of Dukes' staging (e.g., Dukes' A from 0% to 13%, Dukes' B from 11% to 61%, and Dukes' C from 32% to 88%). Although anastomotic recurrences are not uncommon with low anterior resection, such a development following a right hemicolectomy or intraperitoneal anastomosis is considered a rare entity.

■ CONTRIBUTING FACTORS

Sugarbaker, Gunderson, and Wittes (422) have suggested several possible reasons that "curative" resections fail: (1) metastases in the lymphatic channels or nodes may result in unrecognized residual carcinoma, (2) malignant cells may be exfoliated from the primary lesion into veins prior to or during the operation, (3) malignant cells may persist at the circumferential margins of resection, and (4) malignant cells may be disseminated at the time of resection. Implantation is more likely to result in the development of early recurrence at the suture line, whereas metachronous carcinogenesis provides a likely explanation for the development of late recurrences (948). Indeed, all four mechanisms may play a role to a lesser or greater extent.

■ PATTERNS

Depending on the location of the original resection, patterns of recurrence vary with respect to the development of local, anastomotic, regional, or distant failure as well as the time to recurrence (949,950). The definition of local recurrence generally includes recurrence in areas contiguous to the bed of the primary resection or recurrence at the site of anastomosis. Distant spread represents metastases to sites beyond the location of resection. Local pelvic failure is common in rectal carcinoma because of narrow radial margins defined by the anatomic limits of dissection. Colon carcinoma tends to fail in the peritoneal cavity, the liver, or distant sites, with a relatively small component of isolated local failure. This pattern explains the emphasis on radiotherapy as adjuvant therapy for rectal carcinoma and systemic chemotherapy for colonic carcinoma. In a review of several series, Devesa, Morales, and Enriquez (688) found that 30% to 50% of patients with recurrence of colon carcinoma manifested locoregional failure. Distant metastases are present in up to 80% of patients with recurrence. The liver is most often involved in 50% to 80% of autopsy studies, followed by lung, bone, and other sites. In a follow-up of 487 patients for a median of 48 months (range, 15 to 132 months) Bohm et al. (951) documented recurrence in 31%. Of those, distant metastases were found in 51%, only local recurrence in 31%, and both local and distant metastases in 18%. In the review by Obrand and Gordon (952) the reported recurrence rates after curative resection of large bowel adenocarcinoma varied widely from 3% to 50%.

The patterns of recurrence from several selected series are presented in Table 16. It is often difficult to separate series of colon carcinoma from those of rectal carcinoma because the reports often are combined.

Rodriguez-Bigas et al. (953) conducted a retrospective analysis of the prognostic significance of anastomotic recurrence in 50 patients with colorectal carcinoma. All carcinomas were located above 10 cm from the anal verge. Forty anastomotic recurrences (80%) followed resection of sigmoid or proximal rectal lesions. The overall disease-free interval was 13 months, with 90% of recurrences diagnosed within 24 months of the primary resection. Forty-five recurrences (90%) were associated with synchronous or metachronous metastases. The overall median survival rate following the recurrence was 16 months (37 months if the anastomosis was the only recurrence site). Of five patients alive without evidence of disease, all were asymptomatic, and recurrence was confined to the anastomosis. The authors concluded that anastomotic recurrence following resection of colorectal carcinoma frequently heralds disseminated disease but can be potentially resected for cure if it is the only site in an otherwise asymptomatic patient. Willett et al. (694) reported that in patients with obstructing lesions, local failure developed in 42%, approximately, one third of whom had local failure only. In patients with perforated carcinoma, 44% developed local failure. The incidence of local failure and distant metastases in their control group was 14% and 21%, respectively.

With respect to the time frame, Russell et al. (949) found that 70% of all recurrences of colon carcinoma were detected within 2 years of operation and 90% were detected within 4 years. A review of the literature by Devesa, Morales, and Enriquez (688) noted that 60% to 84% of recurrences became apparent within 2 years of the initial operation and 90% within 4 years (median, 22 months). With respect to location, Malcolm et al. (957) found overall recurrence rates of 24%, 10%, 11.5%, and 34%, respectively, for carcinoma of the right, transverse, left, and sigmoid colon.

In a study to determine the incidence and patterns of recurrence after curative resection of colorectal carcinoma, Obrand and Gordon (952) conducted a retrospective review of 524 patients, 448 operated on with curative intent. The overall recurrence rate was 27.9%. The anastomotic recurrence rate was 11.7%. Locoregional recurrence rates, including anastomotic recurrences, were higher in patients with rectal lesions than colon lesions (20.3% vs. 6.2%). Distant metastases developed in 14.4% of patients (13.9% for colon carcinoma and 15.5% for rectal carcinoma). The average time to recurrence was 21.3 months (median, 17 months; range, 2 to 100 months). The average time for anastomotic

TABLE 16 ■ Patterns of Recurrence Following Curative Resection for Colon Carcinoma

Author(s)	No. of Patients	Duration of Follow-Up (Yr)	Recurrence (%) Local	Distant	Local and Distant	Total	Time to Recurrence (Mo)	5-Year Survival (%)
Olson et al. (952) (1980)	214	5.0	7		16	23		49
Malcolm et al. (893) (1981)	191	5.0	1	22	5	28	1–102	21
Boey et al. (953) (1984)	146		10	15	10	35	4–40	
Russell et al. (948) (1984)	550	4.0	5	19	10	34	2–102	
Umpleby et al. (674) (1984)	329	5.0	18	22	7	47		27
Willett et al. (954) (1984)	533	5.0	6	12	13	31		63
Gunderson, Sosin, and Levitt (955) (1985)	91		19	20		39		
Galandiuk et al. (956) (1992)[a]	818	2.0–11.5	5	34	4	43	0.5–98 (median, 17)	
Obrand and Gordon (951) (1997)[a]	448	1–15 (median, 70 mo)	13	13	2	28	2–100 (median, 17)	47[b]

[a]Includes colon and rectal carcinoma.
[b]47% alive at average of 80 months.

recurrence was 16.2 months vs. 22.9 months for distant disease and 18.9 months for regional recurrence. Colon recurrences occurred at a median of 16 months vs. 17 months for rectal recurrences. Patients with Dukes' A lesions had a 17.6% recurrence rate, those with Dukes' B had a 23.4% rate, and those with Dukes' C had 43.7%. Patients who did not undergo any intervention after diagnosis of recurrence survived an average of 28 months. Those who received palliative treatment survived an average of 39 months. Of those patients who underwent reoperation, 24% had re-resection for cure. Anastomotic re-resections accounted for 20 of 30 resections. A majority of recurrences (69.4%) occurred within 24 months of the original operation and 95% recurred by 48 months. For those who received adjuvant therapy, the mean and median times to recurrence were 25.4 and 22.0 months, respectively. For those patients who did not receive any adjuvant treatment, the mean and median times to recurrence were 19.8 and 16.0 months, respectively. Neither of these reached statistical significance on multivariate analysis. Forty-seven percent of these patients were alive at a mean 8 months. Those who died of their disease did so at an average of 53 months. Positive predictive factors for recurrence included the site of the lesion (rectum vs. colon), stage, invasion of contiguous organs, and presence of perforation. Age, sex, degree of differentiation, mucin secretion, and gross morphology were not found to be predictive factors.

Risk factors previously associated with increased recurrence rates include patient's sex, age, Dukes' stage, site of primary carcinoma (colon vs. rectum), infiltration of adjacent organs, perforation, and histology and size of the carcinoma, among others. Adverse prognostic factors reported by Galandiuk et al. (957) include males doing worse than females, rectum worse than colon, Dukes' C worse than B, grades 3 and 4 worse than 1 and 2, adhesions and/or invasion worse than none, perforation worse than none, nondiploid worse than diploid.

The clinical relevance of seeking factors, capable of predicting recurrence is to permit the physician to focus on subsets of patients who might most appropriately be targeted for aggressive adjuvant therapy and postoperative surveillance programs that will expedite the diagnosis of recurrent disease at a time when potentially curative therapy can be instituted. This is true even for patients who develop metastatic disease such as liver or lung metastases where curative resections are still favorable in selected circumstances.

Disease recurrence in the abdominal wall from primary colorectal carcinoma has received renewed attention after the recognition of port site metastases in patients undergoing laparoscopic colorectal resections. Koea et al. (958) reviewed 31 patients presenting to Memorial Sloan-Kettering Cancer Center with recurrent disease in the abdominal wall between 7 and 183 months after operation. Primary carcinomas were located in the right colon in 17 patients, left colon in 2 patients, sigmoid colon in 7 patients, and rectum in 3 patients. Nineteen percent of primary carcinomas were perforated, 45% were poorly differentiated, 92% were transmural (T3 or T4), and 51% had lymph node metastases at presentation. Twenty-two patients presented with a symptomatic abdominal wall mass, whereas recurrence in the abdominal wall was found incidentally in nine patients undergoing laparotomy. Four patients had isolated abdominal wall disease whereas the remaining 27 were found to have associated intra-abdominal disease. Six patients who were left with residual intra-abdominal carcinoma after abdominal wall resection had a median survival of four months. Twenty-five patients underwent a histologically complete resection of recurrence restricted to the abdominal wall alone ($n=4$; median survival time, 18 months), abdominal wall and in continuity resection of adherent viscera ($n=15$; median survival time, 12.5 months), or resection of abdominal wall and intra-abdominal recurrence at a distant site ($n=6$, median survival time, 22 months, although only one patient remained alive with disease). The actual two-year and five-year survival rates were 16% and 3%, respectively. They concluded abdominal wall metastases are often indicators of recurrent intra-abdominal disease; aggressive resection in patients with disease restricted to the abdominal wall and associated adherent viscera can result in local disease control.

CLINICAL FEATURES

The first suspicion of recurrence may be the insidious failure of general health signaled by malaise, weight loss, and anorexia. Vague discomfort as well as occasional bowel symptoms may be present. General physical examination is usually unrewarding, but as the disease progresses, a mass in the abdominal wall or within the abdominal cavity as well as ascites may be present. Anastomotic recurrences may be detected by endoscopy.

INVESTIGATIONS

In the detection of local recurrence or peritoneal seeding, physical examination and radiologic tests are not sensitive. Barium enema examination may reveal the recurrence, but sometimes minor changes have been interpreted as a surgical tailoring defect and anastomotic recurrences are not likely to be detected early. Colonoscopy will more directly detect anastomotic recurrences, but mucosal disruption caused by locoregional recurrence is reported to occur in <3% of patients (936).

Barillari et al. (959) evaluated the effectiveness of routine colonoscopy in 481 patients who underwent curative resection. Approximately 10% of patients developed intraluminal recurrences, with more than half arising in the first 24 months. CT is not a reliable diagnostic test for low volume masses on peritoneal surfaces. Jacquet et al. (960) found an overall sensitivity of 79%. Sensitivity was 90% for nodules >0.5 cm but only 28% for nodules <0.5 cm. Sensitivity was lowest in the pelvis (60%).

The newest technology available to detect recurrent disease is ^{18}fluorodeoxyglucose (^{18}FDG) PET. Delbeke et al. (961) assessed the accuracy of ^{18}FDG-PET in patients with recurrent colorectal carcinoma in detecting liver metastases compared with CT and CT portography, detecting extrahepatic metastases compared with CT and evaluating the impact on patient management. Fifty-two patients previously treated for colorectal carcinoma presented on 61 occasions with suspected recurrence and underwent PET of the entire body. The final diagnosis was obtained by pathology ($n=44$) or clinical and radiological follow-up ($n=17$). A total of 166 suspicious lesions were identified. Of the 127 intrahepatic lesions, 104 were malignant and of the 39 extrahepatic lesions, 34 were malignant. PET was more accurate (92%) than CT and CT portography (78% and 80%, respectively) in detecting liver metastases and more accurate than CT for extrahepatic metastases (92% and 71%, respectively). PET detected unsuspected metastases in 17 patients and altered surgical management in 28% of patients. They concluded PET is the most accurate noninvasive method for staging patients for recurrent metastatic colorectal carcinoma and plays an important role in management decisions in this setting.

Libutti et al. (962) evaluated the PET scan and CEA scan as a means of localizing recurrent colorectal carcinoma. In 28 patients explored, disease was found at operation in 94%. Ten had unresectable disease. PET scan predicted unresectable disease in 90% of patients. CEA scans failed to predict unresectable disease in any patient. In 16 patients found to have resectable disease or disease that could be treated with regional therapy, PET scan predicted this in 81% and CEA scan in 13%.

Desai et al. (963) determined the effect of PET on surgical decision-making in patients with metastatic or recurrent colorectal carcinoma. A total of 114 patients with advanced colorectal carcinoma were imaged with CT and PET scans. Forty-two of the 114 patients deemed to have resectable disease on the basis of CT, PET altered therapy in 40% on the basis of extrahepatic disease, bilobar involvement, thoracic involvement, retroperitoneal lymphadenopathy, bone involvement, and supraclavicular disease. In 25 patients with liver metastases, only PET found additional disease in 72%, extrahepatic disease, chest disease, retroperitoneal lymphadenopathy, and bone disease. Both scans underestimated small-volume peritoneal metastases discovered at laparotomy.

Whiteford et al. (964) evaluated the records of 105 patients who underwent 101 CT and 109 PET scans for suspected metastatic colorectal carcinoma. Clinical correlation was confirmed at time of operation, histologically, or by clinical course. The overall sensitivity and specificity of PET scan in detection of clinically relevant carcinoma were higher (87% and 68%) than for CT plus other conventional diagnostic studies (66% and 59%). The sensitivity of PET scan in detecting mucous carcinoma was lower (58%) than for nonmucinous carcinoma (92%). The sensitivity of PET scanning in detecting locoregional recurrence was higher than for CT plus colonoscopy (90% vs. 71%, respectively). The sensitivity of PET in detecting hepatic metastases was higher than for CT (89% vs. 71%). The sensitivity of PET scanning in detecting extrahepatic metastases exclusive of locoregional recurrence was higher for CT plus other conventional diagnostic studies (94% vs. 67%). PET scanning altered clinical management in a beneficiary manner in 26% of cases when compared with evaluation of CT plus other conventional diagnostic studies.

Johnson et al. (965) compared CT scan with PET scan in clinical decision making. A retrospective review of 41 patients with metastatic colorectal carcinoma in patients who had both CT and PET scans before operative exploration was performed. All patients underwent reexploration. Findings were divided into hepatic, extrahepatic, and pelvic regions of the abdomen. PET scan was found to be more sensitive than CT scan when compared with operative findings in the liver (100% vs. 69%), extrahepatic region (90% vs. 52%), and abdomen as a whole (87% vs. 61%). Sensitivities of PET scan and CT scan were not significantly different in the pelvic region (87% vs. 61%). In each case specificity was not significantly different between the two examinations. However, PET scanning is more sensitive than CT scanning and more likely to give the correct result when actual metastatic disease is present.

■ ROLE OF CARCINOEMBRYONIC ANTIGEN

One area in which CEA may be of value is in the early detection of recurrence. However, this is not always the case, and when the CEA level is elevated, there is often other evidence of recurrence. In their review of the literature, Devesa, Morales, and Enriquez (688) found higher than normal blood CEA levels in $<50\%$ of patients with early or localized failure and in approximately 75% of patients with widely disseminated disease nearly always involving the liver. The percentage of patients with lung metastases or peritoneal seeding who show elevated CEA levels is very low. False positive results are found in 6% to 25% of cases. Transient elevations of CEA have been reported to occur in 7% to 36% of patients without demonstrable recurrent carcinoma.

In a remarkable series reported by Minton et al. (966) in which a CEA-directed second-look procedure was practiced on asymptomatic patients, approximately half of the patients were found to have a recurrence amenable to resection for cure. The 5-year survival rate for this group was 30%. In those patients with recurrences after a second-look procedure, a small select group was slated to undergo a third-look (and possibly a fourth-look) procedure in an attempt to make them disease-free. The authors justify this aggressive approach because of the unresponsiveness of colorectal carcinoma to other treatment modalities.

Careful preoperative assessment must be performed to exdude those patients with unresectable metastatic disease. The surgeon must be aware that CEA levels may be elevated in nonmalignant conditions. Several authors have reported the benefit of a CEA-directed second-look operation (954,967,968). However, most surgeons have not encountered such uniformly encouraging results. In a selected review of four series comprising 203 patients, Wanebo and Stevens (809) found 80% with recurrent carcinoma. Disease was localized in 46%, and 54% had distant metastases. CEA levels at exploration ranged from 6.5 ng/mL (Ohio State University) to 25 ng/mL (Memorial Sloan-Kettering Cancer Center); 36% of the entire group underwent resection for cure, but the range was 7% (Roswell Park Memorial Institute) to 72% (Ohio State University).

Hida et al. (968) reported on the usefulness of postoperative CEA monitoring for second-look operations. Seven hundred fifty-six patients with Dukes' B and C, who had undergone curative resection, were monitored postoperatively using CEA and imaging techniques. A second-look operation was performed on any patient with a potentially resectable recurrence and, in addition, a second-look operation was performed when a persistently rising CEA value was detected. Recurrence developed in 18.8% of patients and 90.8% of the recurrences were detected within the first 3 years following curative resection. When comparing carcinomas of the colon with those of the rectum, the former were associated with significantly more hepatic and intra-abdominal recurrences, whereas the latter had significantly more locoregional and pulmonary recurrences. Seventy-two patients underwent a second-look operation. Of those patients, 54.2% had all of their disease resected and 1.4% had no detectable disease at the second look. Among the 142 patients with recurrence, 50% of patients underwent a second-look operation. The resectable group carried a significantly better survival than the unresectable recurrence group (41.3% vs. 5.2%). The authors concluded that complete removal of colorectal carcinoma recurrences by second-look operations, on the basis of postoperative, follow-up CEA, and imaging technique findings, results in improved survival.

■ TREATMENT

Operative Treatment

Reluctance on the part of many surgeons to engage in the close follow-up of patients who previously have undergone resection for carcinoma of the colon and rectum lies in the pessimistic reports of the limited prospect for patients being amenable to reexcisional surgery. Bohm et al. (951) reported that 24% of patients could undergo further curative resection but only 25% of those (6% of all recurrences) were free of disease for more than 2 years. Nevertheless, some reports have been encouraging and it is well worthwhile to operate on some of these individuals (969). Follow-up is important for several reasons: (1) a second primary large bowel malignancy may be detected at an early stage of development, (2) patients who have had a colorectal carcinoma are at a higher risk of developing a primary malignancy in another organ (e.g., the breast or endometrium), and (3) recurrent disease may be diagnosed when it is localized and thus be amenable to curative therapy. Gwin, Hoffman, and Eisenberg (970) reviewed 28 patients with nonhepatic intra-abdominal recurrence of carcinoma of the colon and were able to report 15 patients who had a median actuarial survival of 25.5 months. Disease-free survival was prolonged for these patients when the time to recurrence was >16 months. Patients who underwent palliative resection did better than those who had a bypass. Using CEA-directed second-look operations, Minton et al. (966) reported a re-resection for cure in 60% of patients with a 5-year survival of 30%. In a review of several series published in the 1980s, Herfarth, Schlag, and Hohenberger (971) found reoperation rates ranging from 18% to 60%, with an average of 31%.

The value of operation for patients with incurable colorectal carcinoma is controversial. Law et al. (972) evaluated the outcomes of 180 patients undergoing operation for incurable colorectal carcinoma. Seventeen patients died in the postoperative period. Operative mortality was significantly higher in patients with nonresection procedures. Median survival of patients with resection was significantly longer than in those without resection (30 weeks vs. 17 weeks). Other independent factors that were significantly associated with poor survival were the presence of ascites, presence of bilobar liver metastases and absence of chemotherapy and/or radiation therapy. In the presence of these factors, the balance between the benefit and risk of operation should be carefully considered before decision for operative treatment.

Browne et al. (973) reported their experience with surgical resection for patients with locoregional recurrent colon carcinoma. A total of 744 patients with recurrent colon carcinoma were identified and 100 (13.4%) underwent exploration with curative intent for potentially resectable locoregional recurrence: 75 with isolated locoregional recurrence, and 25 with locoregional recurrence and resectable distant disease. The median follow-up for survivors was 27 months. Locoregional recurrence was classified into four categories: anastomotic; mesenteric/nodal; retroperitoneal; and peritoneal. Median survival for all patients was 30 months. Fifty-six patients had an R0 resection (including distant sites). Factors associated with prolonged disease-specific survival included R0 resection; age <60 years; early stage of primary disease; and no associated distant disease. Poor prognostic factors included more than one site of recurrence and involvement of the mesenteric/nodal basin. The ability to obtain an R0 resection was the strongest predictor of outcome, and these patients had a median survival of 66 months.

Intraoperative Radiotherapy

Because of the inadequacy of operation or radiation therapy alone to treat recurrent locally advanced disease, a multimodality approach of intraoperative electron beam radiotherapy (IORT) combined with operation has been advocated (974). Willett et al. (974) reported that 5-year actuarial local control and disease-free survival rates for 30 patients undergoing this treatment program were 26% and 19%, respectively.

Taylor et al. (975) reported on 100 colon carcinoma patients treated with combination therapy including surgical resection, chemotherapy, and external plus intraoperative radiotherapy. The 5-year survival was 24.7%. The 38 patients with recurrent disease whose disease was completely resected had a 37.4% 5-year survival.

Endoscopic Laser Therapy

For the recurrent lesion that is unresectable, relief of obstruction and control of bleeding or secretions may be obtained by the use of endoscopic laser therapy (976). This therapy offers no relief of pain nor would there be any expected improvement in survival. However, an important advantage of this mode of therapy is that it can be performed with little or no sedation, thus avoiding the risks of general anesthesia and major surgery. In addition, it can be performed on an outpatient basis in most cases and can be applied on a repetitive schedule because there is no limiting cumulative dose for laser energy. Finally, systemic side effects are few, and thus patient acceptance is good (977). The symptoms of obstruction or bleeding can be controlled in 80% to 90% of patients with a complication rate of <10% and a mortality rate of approximately 1% (504,978–985). (Laser therapy is described in detail in Chapter 7.) Not all reports support the palliative virtues of lasers. In one report, two thirds of patients with large lesions showed little improvement and required alternative operative management (986). Courtney et al. (987) reported their experience with high powered diode laser to palliate 57 patients with inoperable colorectal carcinoma with neodymium:yttrium-aluminum-garnet (Nd:YAG). The median number of treatments received by each patient was 3 (range, 1–16 treatments), with a median interval between treatments of 9.5 (range, 1–25) weeks. Lifelong palliation of symptoms occurred in 89% of patients. Major complications were two perforations and one hemorrhage, giving an overall complication rate of 5.3%. One of the patients who experienced perforation died, giving an overall mortality rate of 1.8% for the procedure. The median survival by laser therapy was 8.5 months with a probability of survival at 24 months of 15%. The role of metallic stenting has been described in detail on page 564. For the individual in whom laser therapy or stenting is unsuitable or unsuccessful and who ultimately presents with an obstruction secondary to recurrence, a stoma may be the last desperate effort at palliation.

Cytoreductive Surgery and Hyperthermic Intraperitoneal Chemotherapy

Hyperthermic intraoperative intraperitoneal chemotherapy has been recently proposed to treat peritoneal carcinomatosis arising from colon carcinoma, which is usually regarded as a lethal clinical entity. Pilati et al. (988) reviewed 46 patients treated for peritoneal carcinomatosis from colorectal carcinoma. Thirty-four patients were treated with complete cytoreductive surgery immediately followed by intraoperative hyperthermic intraperitoneal chemotherapy with mitomycin C and cisplatin. No operative deaths were reported. The postoperative morbidity rate was 35%. No severe locoregional or systemic toxicity was observed. The two-year overall survival was 31% and the median survival time and the median time to local disease progression were 18 and 13 months, respectively. Survival and local disease control in patients with well and moderately differentiated colon carcinoma were significantly better than in those with poorly differentiated lesions. Considering the dismal prognosis of this condition, hyperthermic intraoperative intraperitoneal chemotherapy seems to achieve encouraging results in a selected group of patients affected with resectable peritoneal carcinomatosis arising from colon carcinoma.

Verwaal et al. (990) evaluated the outcome after the treatment of peritoneal carcinomatosis of colorectal carcinoma by cytoreduction and hyperthermic intraperitoneal chemotherapy. Recurrence within the study period of 7.5 years was 65%. For patients who had undergone a gross incomplete initial cytoreduction, the median duration of survival after recurrence was 3.7 months. If a complete cytoreduction had been accomplished initially, the median duration of survival after recurrence was 11.1 months. After effective initial treatment, a second surgical debulking for recurrence disease resulted in a median survival duration of 10.3 months and after treatment with chemotherapy it was 8.5 months. The survival was 11.2 months for patients who received radiotherapy for recurrent disease. Patients who did not receive further therapy survived 1.9 months. They concluded treatment of recurrence after cytoreduction and hyperthermic intraperitoneal chemotherapy is often feasible and seems worthwhile in selected patients.

Management of Malignant Ureteral Obstruction

The patient who develops a malignant ureteral obstruction poses a special and difficult problem in the decision-making process. A thoughtful and reasoned approach to the subject was outlined by Smith and Bruera (991), from whom much of the following information has been obtained. The patient presents with an upper urinary tract obstruction with clinical manifestations including flank pain, hematuria, fever, sepsis, and pyuria. In cases of high-grade obstruction, oliguria, anuria, or uremia may be presenting features. The diagnosis may be suspected based on retroperitoneal lymphadenopathy seen on abdominal pelvic CT or hydronephrosis seen on abdominal ultrasonography. The imaging method of choice for proving ureteral obstruction is excretory urography.

It is in the management of these patients that the decision-making process is difficult. An important consideration in the decision to treat these patients is their performance status. Some patients are already bedridden, severely symptomatic, and may not require treatment of their obstruction. Other patients may still be active with expressed, clearly defined personal goals that they can achieve with a few more months of life. For those patients deemed appropriate for aggressive therapy, both pharmacologic and urologic interventions may prove beneficial. It has clearly been shown that resection is contraindicated (568).

Pharmacologic treatments include the use of agents with antineoplastic activity or agents capable of reducing edema. In the latter category, patients with acute or chronic renal failure are treated with intravenous rehydration and a trial of high-dose corticosteroids (intravenous dexamethasone, 10 mg every 6 hours for 48 hours).

The role of urologic intervention in the management of malignant ureteral obstruction in advanced disease is not well defined. Some authors contend that active intervention is unwarranted with long-term progression of an underlying malignancy. Keidan et al. (991) reviewed 20 patients with advanced pelvic malignancy and concluded that before recommending percutaneous nephrostomy, the factors of in-hospital mortality (35% never left the hospital), limited survival (an additional 35% spent <6 weeks at home before they died), significant morbidity (55% required multiple tube changes), and poor quality of life should be considered. Others argue that decision making should be guided by clinical indications and contraindications. Published indications for urinary diversion in malignant ureteral obstruction include bilateral hydronephrosis, unilateral ureteral obstruction with renal insufficiency, and unilateral pyelonephrosis. Contraindications include the evidence of rapid progression of underlying disease for which no further antineoplastic treatment is planned, other life-threatening medical problems for which no further treatment is planned, and asymptomatic unilateral malignant ureteral obstruction with normal stable renal function in patients whose previous ureteral stenting has failed. Endoscopic retrograde placement of double J (double pigtail)-type ureteral stents is generally considered the first-line urinary diversion procedure. Failing this, percutaneous nephrostomy tubes can be placed successfully in nearly all cases. Open nephrostomy, with its significant mortality and complication rates associated with prolonged hospitalization, makes this a less attractive option. Anterograde and bidirectional stenting, subcutaneous stenting, and cutaneous ureterostomy have a limited role. In the final analysis, the decision regarding the management of ureteral obstruction needs to be highly personalized and follow a careful discussion with the patient and/or his or her family.

Nonoperative Treatment

For the most part, radiotherapy has not been used in the treatment of recurrent carcinoma of the colon because of the effects of radiation on the remaining abdominal viscera. However, specific localized areas of known recurrence can be treated by radiotherapy.

Chemotherapy in the form of various drugs, dosage scheduling, and routes of administration has been used for the treatment of colon carcinoma. The most frequently used drug has been 5-FU, which offers expected response rates in the 15% range. In the past, drug combinations have not enjoyed major success when compared with 5-FU alone, but the combination of 5-FU and leucovorin has led several investigators to publish encouraging response rates in patients with advanced disease.

Douillard et al. (992) investigated the efficacy of irinotecan in patients whose disease was refractory to fluorouracil. In a series of 387 patients that compared irinotecan plus fluorouracil and leucovorin to fluorouracil and leucovorin in a multicenter randomized trial, the response rate was higher in the irinotecan group (49% vs. 31%). Time to progression was longer (6.7 months vs. 4.4 months), the overall survival higher (median 17.4 months vs. 14.1 months) but grade 3 and 4 toxic effects were more frequent in the irinotecan group. In another multicenter trial, Saltz (993) compared the same groups plus a third group receiving irinotecan alone. The combination group with irinotecan resulted in longer progression free survival (median 7.0 months vs. 4.3 months), a higher response rate (39% vs. 21%), and longer overall survival (median 14.8 months vs. 12.6 months). Grade 3 diarrhea was more common with irinotecan. de Gramont et al. (994) studied fluorouracil and leucovorin with or without oxaliplatin as first-line treatment in advanced colorectal carcinoma. Patients allocated to the group with oxaliplatin had longer progression-free survival (median 9.0 months vs. 6.2 months), better response rate (50.7% vs. 22.3%). The overall survival did not reach significance (median 16.2 months vs. 14.7 months). Patients receiving oxaliplatin experienced higher frequencies of grade 3/4 neutropenia (41.7% vs. 5.3%), grade 3/4 diarrhea (11.9% vs. 5.3%), and grade 3 neurosensory toxicity (18.2% vs. 0%).

In a multicenter phase II study, Sorbye et al. (995) evaluated the efficacy and safety of oxaliplatin combined with the Nordic bolus schedule of fluorouracil and folinic acid as first-line treatment in metastatic colorectal carcinoma. Eighty-five patients were treated with oxaliplatin (85 mg/m^2) as a two-hour infusion on day 1 followed by a three-minute bolus injection with 5-FU (500 mg/m^2) and 30 minutes later by a bolus injection of folinic acid (60 mg/m^2) every second week. The same dose of 5-FU and folinic acid were also given on day 2. Of the 51 assessable patients the response rate was 62%. The estimated median time to progression was 7 months and the medial overall survival was 16.1 months in the intent-to-treat population. Neutropenia was the main adverse event with Grade 3 to 4 toxicity in 58% of patients. Febrile neutropenia developed in 8% and neuropathy in 54%. Hospitalization for treatment-related toxicity was needed in 25% of patients. Nevertheless, they concluded oxaliplatin combined with bolus Nordic schedule of 5-FU/folic acid is a well tolerated, effective, and feasible bolus schedule as first-line treatment for metastatic colorectal carcinoma.

Three agents with differing mechanisms of action are available for treatment of advanced colorectal carcinoma: fluorouracil, irinotecan, and oxaliplatin. Goldberg et al. (996) compared the activity and toxicity and three different two-drug combinations in patients with metastatic colorectal carcinoma who had not been treated previously for advanced disease. A total of 795 patients were concurrently randomly assigned to receive irinotecan and bolus fluorouracil plus leucovorin (IFL), oxaliplatin and infused fluorouracil plus leucovorin (FOLFOX) or irinotecan and oxaliplatin (IROX). A median time to progression of 8.7 months, response rate of 45% and median survival time of 19.5 months were observed for FOLFOX. These results were significantly superior to those observed for IFL for all end points (6.9 months, 31%, and 15.0 months, respectively) or for IROX (6.5 months, 35%, and 17.4 months, respectively) for time to progression and response. The FOLFOX regimen had significantly lower rates of severe nausea, vomiting, diarrhea, febrile neutropenia, and dehydration. Sensory neuropathy and neutropenia were more common with the regimens containing oxaliplatin. They concluded the FOLFOX regimen should be considered as standard therapy for patients with advanced colorectal carcinoma.

Tournigard et al. (997) investigated folinic acid, 5-FU, and irinotecan (FOLFIRI) followed by folinic acid, 5-FU, and oxaliplatin (FOLFOX6), and FOLFOX6 followed by FOLFIRI in previously untreated patients. In first-line therapy, FOLFIRI achieved 56% response rate and 8.5 months median progression-free survival versus FOLFOX6 which achieved 54% response rate and 8 month median free survival. Second-line FOLFIRI achieved 4% response rate and 2.5-month median progression-free survival versus FOLFOX6 which achieved 15% response rate and a 4.2-month progression-free survival. In first-line therapy, National Cancer Institute Common Toxicity Criteria grade 3/4 mucositis, nausea/vomiting, and grade 2 alopecia were more frequent with FOLFIRI, and grade 3/4 neutropenia and neurosensory toxicity were more frequent with FOLFOX6. Both sequences achieved a prolonged survival and similar efficacy.

Collucci et al. (998) in a multicenter Italian trial compared the irinotecan, leucovorin, and fluorouracil regimen (FOLFIRI) versus the oxaliplatin, leucovorin, and fluorouracil regimen (FOLFOX4) in 360 previously untreated patients with advanced colorectal carcinoma. They found no difference in overall response rates, median time to progression, and overall survival for patients treated with the FOLFIRI or FOLFOX4 regimen. Both therapies seem effective as first-line treatment in these patients. The difference between these two combination therapies is mainly in the toxicity profile.

Ibrahim et al. (999) reported on a single multicenter randomized trial in 463 patients with metastatic colorectal carcinoma whose disease had recurred or progressed during or within six months of completion of therapy with a combination of bolus 5-FU, leucovorin, and irinotecan.

Study arms included infusional 5-FU/leucovorin alone, oxaliplatin alone, and the combination of oxaliplatin infusional 5-FU/leucovorin. There were no complete responders. The partial response rates were 0%, 1%, and 9% for the 5-FU/leucovorin, oxaliplatin, oxaliplatin plus 5-FU/leucovorin treatments, respectively. The median times to radiographic progression of disease were 2.7, 1.6, and 4.6 months, respectively. Common adverse events associated with combination treatment included peripheral neuropathy, fatigue, diarrhea, nausea, vomiting, stomatitis, and abdominal pain. Neutropenia was the major hematologic toxicity. A small but statistically significant improvement in response rate was observed in the combination arm of oxaliplatin and infusional 5-FU and leucovorin in a population that has no other treatment options. An interim analysis of radiographic time to progression, with approximately 50% of events, revealed that time to progression was longer in the combination arm. This improvement in response rate and the interim analysis showing a longer radiographic time to progression were the bases of approval for oxaliplatin. The trial results demonstrate that the efficacy of single agent oxaliplatin is similar to that of infusional 5-FU/leucovorin and that oxaliplatin should not be used alone in this patient population except in clinical trials. Caution should be exercised in choosing the regimen if bolus 5-FU is used together with oxaliplatin due to excessive toxicities.

Most recently Kohne et al. (1000) reported that adding irinotecan to a standard weekly scheduled of high dose infusional fluorouracil and leucovorin can prolong progression-free survival. The median progression-free survival increased to 8.5 months from 6.4 months. The median overall survival time was increased from 16.9 to 20.1 months. The objective response rate was 62.2% in the irinotecan group and 34.4% in the other group.

The limited response rates of current chemotherapeutic regimens underscore the need for newer modalities of therapy. Recognizing the role of the VEGF in promoting angiogenesis in neoplasms, Hurwitz et al. (1001) conducted a study using bevacizumab, a monoclonal antibody against vascular endothelial growth factor in combination with chemotherapy. Of 813 patients with previously untreated metastatic colorectal carcinoma, they randomly assigned 402 to receive irinotecan, bolus fluorouracil, and leucovorin (IFL) plus bevacizumab (5 mg/kg of body weight every two weeks) and 411 to receive IFL plus placebo. The median duration of survival was 20.3 months in the group given IFL plus bevacizumab as compared with 15.6 months in the group given IFL plus placebo, corresponding to a hazard ratio for death of 0.66. The median duration of progression-free survival was 10.6 months in the group with IFL plus bevacizumab as compared with 6.2 months in the group with IFL plus placebo (hazard ratio for progression 0.54); the corresponding rates of response were 44.6% and 34.8%. The median duration of the response was 10.4 months in the group given IFL plus bevacizumab as compared with 7.1 months in the group given IFL plus placebo (hazard ratio for progression 0.62). Grade 3 hypertension was more common during treatment with IFL plus bevacizumab than with IFL plus placebo (11.0% vs. 2.3%) but was easily managed. They concluded the addition of bevacizumab to fluorouracil-based combination chemotherapy results in statistically significant and clinically meaningful improvement in survival among patients with metastatic colorectal carcinoma.

Any recommendation for toxic regimens of chemotherapy should be made only after careful consideration of the high level of toxicity and the diminished quality of life for the patient.

There has been renewed enthusiasm for the direct intra-arterial infusion of chemotherapeutic agents, specifically delivery into the liver. In their review of the literature, Blumgart and Fong (555) found six trials in which hepatic artery response rates were 48% to 62% compared with 0% to 21% for intravenous therapy. However, it must be pointed out that this increase in response rate translated to an improved survival in only one study and then only in subset analysis. Furthermore, potential complications associated with arterial infusional therapy included skin breakdown (1.0%); catheter break, misplacement, migration, leak, or kink (5.3%); pump pocket infection (1.2%); pump pocket hematoma or seroma (6.3%); and catheter-artery thrombosis or aneurysm (5.0%) (566). Added to this should be the chemotherapy complications, which included chemical hepatitis and sclerosing cholangitis (10.6%); gastritis, nausea, or vomiting (24.9%); ulcer (9.3%); and diarrhea (10.6%) (566). In my opinion, improved survival with attendant quality of life should be a benchmark to which to aspire.

In their review of the literature on hepatic arterial therapy of hepatic metastases, Vauthey et al. (566) noted that although the progression of disease may best be controlled by hepatic artery chemotherapy, its clear-cut survival advantage has yet to be demonstrated. A meta-analysis of seven randomized trials evaluating the possible benefit of hepatic artery infusion using FUDR compared with intravenous chemotherapy showed a survival advantage only when untreated controls were included (1002).

Since those meta-analyses, two other randomized trials of hepatic artery infusion have been published. The German Cooperative Group randomized 168 patients with unresectable liver metastases from colorectal carcinoma to hepatic artery infusion of 5-FUDR, hepatic artery infusion of 5-FU/leucovorin or intravenous 5-FU/leucovorin (1003). Response rates were higher in the two hepatic artery infusion arms but with no significant differences in time to progression. The Medical Research Council and the European Organization for the Research and Treatment of Cancer groups compared hepatic artery infusion (5-FU/leucovorin) with intravenous 5-FU/leucovorin given as per the de Gramont regimen (1004). Response rates were assessed in 183 patients and were nearly identical (22% for hepatic artery infusion, 19% for intravenous 5-FU/leucovorin). No differences between the arms were noted for toxicity or progression-free or overall survival. Of note, both the above trials utilized subcutaneous ports rather than implantable pumps and had significant catheter-related problems (36% of hepatic artery patients in the MRC/EORTC trial). The Cancer and Leukemia Group B (CALGB) recently completed trial 9481 which compared systemic 5-FU/leucovorin with hepatic artery infusion of FUDR, leucovorin, and dexamethasone (1005). Unfortunately, only 135 patients out of an accrual goal of 340 were randomized. The response rate (48% vs. 25%) was higher in the hepatic artery infusion group, though time to progression was not significantly different (5.3 months vs. 6.8 months), with time to hepatic progression better in the hepatic artery infusion arm (9.8 months vs. 7.3 months) and time to extrahepatic progression better in systemic arm (7.8 months vs. 23.3 months). The median overall survival time was statistically significantly better in the hepatic artery infusion arm (22.7 months vs. 19.9 months). In absolute terms, this three month advantage would appear marginal considering the hepatic artery infusion group required an operation with its attendant complications. Furthermore, even enthusiasts of hepatic artery infusion concede with the improved rates of response and survival reported with irinotecan and oxaliplatin-based regimens, a new standard of care for first-line treatment of metastatic colorectal carcinoma will have to be used as control arms in the evaluation of hepatic artery infusion trials (619). On the basis of trials performed, hepatic artery infusion does not represent the standard treatment option for patients with hepatic metastases from colorectal carcinoma.

The most recent publication on the subject is by Keer et al. (1006) who conducted a randomized trial to compare an intrahepatic arterial fluorouracil and folinic acid regimen with the standard intravenous de Gramont fluorouracil and folinic acid regimen for patients with carcinoma of the colon or rectum, with metastases confined to the liver. They randomly allocated 290 patients from 16 centers to receive either intravenous chemotherapy (folinic acid 200 mg/m^2, fluorouracil bolus 400 mg/m^2 and 22-hour infusion (600 mg/m^2, day 1 and 2, repeated every 14 days) or intra-arterial hepatic chemotherapy designed to be equitoxic (folinic acid 200 mg/m^2, fluorouracil 400 mg/m^2 over 15 minutes and 22-hour infusion 1600 mg/m^2 day 1 and day 2, repeated every 14 days). For patients allocated to the intrahepatic arterial infusion, 37% did not start their treatment and another 29% had to stop before receiving six cycles of treatment because of catheter failure. The intrahepatic artery group received a median of two cycles (0–6), compared with 8.5 (6–12) for the intravenous group. Median overall survival was 14.7 months for the intrahepatic artery group and 14.8 months for the intravenous group. Their results showed no evidence of an advantage in progression-free survival or overall survival for the intrahepatic artery group. In a commentary on this article, Bonetti (1007) noted that since 1986, eight phase-3 trials have compared hepatic artery infusion with either intravenous chemotherapy or best supportive care in the treatment of unresectable hepatic metastases from colorectal carcinoma. The main conclusions of a meta-analysis of seven randomized trials were that hepatic artery infusion is associated with a higher response rate (41% vs. 14%) but similar median survival (16 months vs. 12.2 months).

Martin et al. (1008) examined the survival and toxicity of hepatic arterial infusion pump following resection and/or radiofrequency ablation of all liver metastases. Patients received FUDR via the hepatic artery infusion pump at standard doses. Complications were graded according to a standard five-point grading scale. Thirty-four of 86 patients underwent placement of hepatic artery infusion pump at the time of hepatic resection or ablation. The hepatic artery group demonstrated a significantly greater number (median 5 vs. 2) and size (median 5 cm vs. 3 cm) of hepatic lesions compared to the group without hepatic artery infusion pump. The hepatic artery infusion pump experienced a greater frequency of complications (53% vs. 33%), with 18% in the hepatic artery infusion pump group demonstrating biliary sclerosis. There were no deaths within 30 days of operation. Median survival was similar in both groups (hepatic artery infusion pump 20 months, no hepatic artery infusion pump 24 months). Adjuvant hepatic artery infusion chemotherapy was associated with significantly greater morbidity and given the availability of newer active systemic agents and regimens, the value of adjuvant hepatic artery infusion pump chemotherapy following hepatic resection or ablation remains controversial.

Isolated reports have shown the efficacy of chemotherapy for recurrent malignancy in the pelvis by administration through a catheter introduced via the axillary artery (1009). Other forms of therapy tried have included external or internal liver irradiation, immunotherapy, hyperthermic therapy, hepatic artery ligation, and hepatic artery embolizaton—all without convincing evidence of sustained therapeutic advantage. The most recent effort has been intraperitoneal hyperthermic perfusion with mitomycin C for peritoneal metastases with a median response duration of 6 months (1010).

For patients in whom no active treatment is available, it is imperative that the treating physician ensure that the patient is relieved of pain by the prescription of progressively strong analgesics as necessary. Chronic severe carcinoma pain often is not well controlled because of an inadequate understanding of the nature of pain.

Common causes of chronic pain in patients with carcinoma include (1011):

1. Peripheral neuropathies due to radiation, chemotherapy (typically platinum, paclitaxel, and vincristine), erosion by the malignancy
2. Radiation fibrosis
3. Chronic postsurgical incisional pain
4. Phantom pain
5. Arthopathies and musculoskeletal pain due to changes in posture or mobility
6. Visceral pain due to damage to viscera or blockage due to the malignancy

Most chronic pain in patients with carcinoma is neuropathic pain.

Physicians often unnecessarily limit the dosage of analgesia because they have the ill-founded fear that the patient will become addicted to the drug. The basis of rational management is an appropriate analgesic given regularly in dosages adequate to suppress pain continuously. The stable of drugs might include traditional analgesics such as acetylsalicylic acid, acetaminophen, and pentazocine; anti-inflammatory agents such as acetylsalicylic acid, indomethacin, and phenylbutazone, valuable in the management of painful bony metastases; psychotropic analgesics such as tricyclic antidepressants (e.g., amitriptyline) and phenothiazine tranquilizers; and, ultimately, narcotics such as meperidine, methadone, codeine, and morphine. Drug selection climbs the "analgesic ladder" from nonopioid for mild pain to opioid with or without adjuvant medication for severe pain from carcinoma

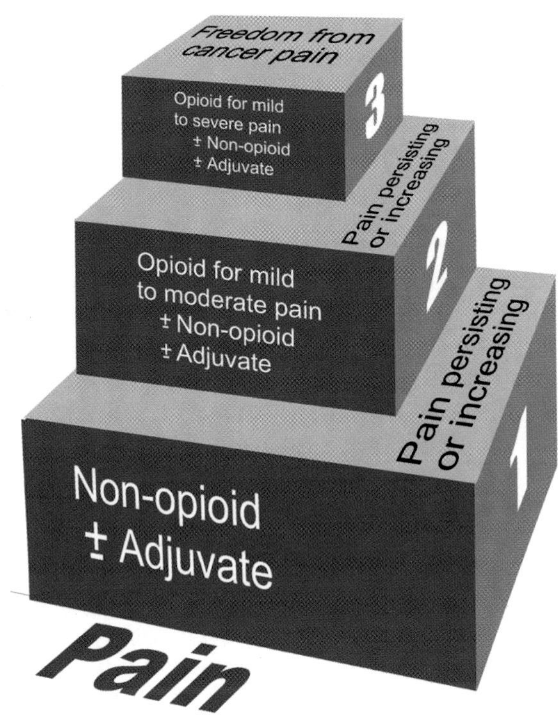

FIGURE 64 ■

(1012) (Fig. 64). A combination of agents is often useful. Since many of the narcotics result in constipation, patients should be prescribed laxatives at the same time (see Chapter 33). For patients in whom pain cannot be controlled by traditional oral and parenteral methods, Waterman, Hughes, and Foster (1013) have used epidural and intrathecal infusion with morphine. Excellent or good relief of pain was obtained in 70% of patients. It is a method of delivery that can be used in an outpatient setting. For patients in whom the pain is still not controlled, regional therapies should be considered, such as celiac plexus block or sympathetic blockade. Failing this, a neuroablative procedure should be offered, such as rhizotomy, neurolysis of primary afferent nerves or their ganglia, or cordotomy (1012).

An often neglected aspect of the care of patients with advanced carcinoma is the anorexia and associated weight loss suffered by these terminally ill patients. Foltz et al. (1014) determined that nutritional counseling produced a significant increase in caloric intake. The augmented regimen included a target caloric intake with 25% of total calories derived from protein sources as well as zinc and magnesium supplementation. Increases in intake were not associated with significant weight gain or increased percent protein intake, but they had some effect on minimizing weight loss or stabilizing weight, even in patients with advanced disease who were undergoing systemic chemotherapy.

■ RESULTS OF REOPERATION

The virtue of re-resection of local recurrence for cure has been questioned, but it is undeniable that some patients with local recurrence are amenable to cure. Reports of success for the resection of local recurrence for cure have varied widely, but 5-year survivals in the 30% range have been recorded (966).

Since many reports have documented that most recurrences occur within the first 2 years after resection of the primary lesion (942), it seems reasonable to concentrate follow-up efforts during that period. Those opposed to intensive follow-up state that the poor reoperation rate for cure, ranging from 7% to 20%, negates the cost and effort applied (936,942–944). However, Buhler et al. (945) noted that repeat resections for cure were possible in 66% of patients who were asymptomatic at the time that the recurrent lesion was detected, whereas in symptomatic patients, the lesion was usually unresectable. In a series of 30 patients with anastomotic recurrence, Vassilopoulos et al. (1015) found that the majority of patients were diagnosed within 2 years of initial operation, but in this series the diagnosis was usually based on persistent signs and symptoms. Nevertheless, resection for cure was still feasible in 50% of the cases, with a 5-year survival rate of 49% and only a 3% operative mortality rate. In the report by Pihl et al. (1016) an anastomotic recurrence rate of 2.7% was detected with a re-resection rate of 40%. Other authors also believe that re-resection offers the best outlook with regard to survival (1017). Barillari et al. (959) detected a 10% intraluminal recurrence rate in a series of 481 patients. Of the 29 patients who underwent a second operation, 17 had a radical procedure and, in this group, the 5-year survival rate was 70.6%. The authors concluded that asymptomatic patients more frequently underwent another operation for cure and thus had a better survival rate.

■ INTESTINAL OBSTRUCTION DUE TO RECURRENT CARCINOMA

A very difficult situation that challenges the clinical judgment of even the most experienced surgeon is the management of patients presenting with bowel obstruction after treatment of the primary malignancy when the feared cause is metastatic disease. Inappropriate operation does not improve outcome. Stellato and Shenk (1018) reviewed the literature on this subject and concluded that patients should be treated as any other patient manifesting intestinal obstruction, the rationale being that 26% to 38% of the bowel obstructions in patients with a history of malignancy are not secondary to recurrent or metastatic disease and that operative mortality rates for patients with carcinoma are comparable (9% to 15%) with those of patients presenting with obstruction without a history of malignancy. While 10% to 30% of patients obtain relief of obstruction by nasogastric decompression (two thirds within 3 days) 40% require operation. More than 35% of those with obstruction due to recurrent carcinoma obtain relief of their symptoms with operation. Predictors of poor outcome include the presence of shock, ascites, or an abdominal mass, with mortality rates of 100%, 70%, and 54%, respectively. Known carcinomatosis has a 40% 30-day mortality rate. Van Ooijen et al. (1019) reviewed the management of 59 patients with intestinal obstruction (38 patients with advanced carcinoma of the ovary and 21 patients with peritoneal carcinomatosis of other organs). The authors concluded that operative therapy for the relief of intestinal obstruction should only be considered in patients who do not present with manifest ascites or palpable masses and in patients with carcinoma of the ovary for whom effective chemotherapy is available. The rationale is simply that patients with masses or ascites had a median postoperative survival of only 36 days. Percutaneous gastrostomy should be the method of choice for other patients.

Although the overall prognosis is poor in patients with malignant obstruction, the median survival being 6 months, operation still offers the best hope for palliation (1018). Lau and Lorentz (1020) believe that a more aggressive approach is appropriate. In a review of 30 patients with unresectable intra-abdominal disease, 63% had bowel function restored. Obstruction recurred after a mean symptom-free interval of 120 days in eight of 19 patients initially relieved. Another operation was performed in three of these patients. The authors believe that their results, with a median survival of 192 days for those who benefitted from operation, justify a more positive approach toward this problem and when conservatism fails, laparotomy should be undertaken in patients who are not terminally ill.

Butler et al. (1021) also believe in an aggressive approach. The authors reviewed 54 patients with small bowel obstruction who had a previous diagnosis of carcinoma. Forty patients were initially treated nonoperatively, and 28% of those resolved after a mean 7 days of nasogastric suction. Five developed recurrent small bowel obstruction. Thirty-seven patients underwent laparotomy, at which time 68% were found to have obstruction due to recurrent carcinoma, with a mean survival of 5 months. Major postoperative complications occurred in 49% of patients, the most common being failure of resolution of the obstruction. The 30-day and in-hospital mortality rates of the 25 surgically treated patients were 24% and 28%, respectively. The authors concluded that (1) patients should be given an initial trial of nonoperative therapy, (2) patients with no known recurrence or a long interval to development of small bowel obstruction should be aggressively treated with early operation if nonoperative treatment fails, and (3) for patients with known abdominal recurrence in whom nonoperative therapy fails, the results of operative palliation are grim.

Miller et al. (1022) conducted a study to determine the efficacy and long-term prognosis for operative versus nonoperative treatment of small bowel obstruction secondary to malignant disease. There were 32 patients accounting for 74 admissions. Colorectal neoplasm was the principal primary malignant disease that led to small bowel obstruction. The median time between diagnosis of the malignant disease and small bowel obstruction was 1.1 years. At their initial presentation, 80% of patients were treated by operation but 47% of these patients had an initial trial of nonoperative treatment. Re-obstruction occurred in 57% of patients who were operated on compared with 72% of patients who were not. The median time to re-obstruction was 17 months for patients who underwent operation compared with 2.5 months for patients who did not. Also, 71% of patients were alive and symptom free 30 days after discharge from the operative treatment compared with 52% after nonoperative treatment. Postoperative morbidity was 67%. Mortality was 13%, and 94% of patients eventually died from complications of their primary disease. They concluded that small bowel obstruction secondary to malignant disease usually indicates a grim prognosis. Operative treatment has better outcome than nonoperative management in terms of symptom free interval and re-obstruction rates. However, it is marked by high postoperative morbidity. They recommend that after a short trial of nasogastric decompression, patients with obstruction secondary to malignant disease be operated on if clinical factors indicate they will survive the operation.

For patients with malignant large bowel obstruction, stent placement may successfully relieve obstruction and this subject has been described on page 562. Other methods to relieve malignant large bowel obstruction include NdYAG laser or balloon dilatation. Krouse et al. in their excellent review of palliative care of the patient with malignant obstruction detailed the wide ranged possible pharmacologic management (1023). It may include opioids for pain control, metoclopramide for nausea and vomiting; other antiemetics (prochloperazine, promethazine, and haloperidol to mention a few). Treatment of dehydration and nutritional depletion is controversial. Octreotide will be effective in the relief of symptoms of malignant bowel obstruction. Corticosteroids have been used in the hope of reducing edema around the malignancy.

August et al. (1024) reported on the use of home parenteral nutrition in patients with inoperable malignant bowel obstruction. In a review of 17 patients so treated, most patients and families (82%) perceived therapy as beneficial, with a median survival of 90 days. In most circumstances, members of the nutritional support team agreed in that home parenteral nutrition facilitates compassionate home care for carefully selected patients. Despite their encouraging report, one should be circumspect about embarking on such a program.

At times, because of diffuse involvement of the intestine by carcinomatosis, a percutaneous endoscopic gastroscopy may avoid the need for celiotomy. When used selectively, it can improve the quality of life of the carcinoma patient by relieving intractable vomiting and by providing an avenue for nutrition in a partially functioning gastrointestinal tract.

Parker and Baines (1025) questioned the philosophy of the compulsion to operate on the assumption that obstruction always demands operative intervention. The authors point out a mortality rate of 13% with a median survival of 10 months, but in malnourished patients the mortality rate can climb to 72%. Emergency operation increases the mortality rate threefold and, although survival may be increased by a few months, the relief of symptoms lasts only 2 months overall. To counteract these depressing data, good prognostic factors include an early stage or low-grade initial lesion, a long interval from first operation, a well-nourished patient, and the fact that in one third of patients with previous carcinoma, the obstruction is caused by benign disease. The decision to operate must be made with as much information as possible. Barium studies, CT, MRI, ultrasonography, or endoscopic evaluation may be beneficial. When the decision is made not to operate, adequate analgesia, antiemetics, and antisecretogogues should be administered.

COLORECTAL CARCINOMA COMPLICATING PREGNANCY

Colorectal carcinoma in pregnancy is a rare condition and has been estimated to occur in 0.001% to 0.100% of pregnancies (1026). As of 1993, 205 cases were reported in the literature. Colorectal carcinoma that presents in pregnancy usually does so at an advanced stage because the individuals are young and the diagnosis is usually not entertained, while any symptoms that do arise are often attributed to the pregnancy

(1027). The most common presenting complaint is abdominal pain followed by nausea and vomiting, constipation, abdominal distention, rectal bleeding, fever, and backache.

To better characterize the disease under this circumstance, Bernstein, Madoff, and Caushaj (1026) surveyed the membership of the American Society of Colon and Rectal Surgeons and identified 41 cases of large bowel carcinoma who presented during pregnancy or the immediate postpartum period. The mean age at presentation was 31 years (range, 16 to 41 years). Spatial distribution within the large bowel was as follows: right colon, 3; transverse colon, 2; left colon, 2; sigmoid colon, 8; and rectum, 26. Staging at presentation was Dukes' A, 0; B, 16; C, 17; and metastatic, 6. Two patients were unstaged. The average follow-up was 41 months. The stage-for-stage survival was similar to patients with colorectal carcinoma in the general population. For those with rectal lesions, the 5-year survival rate for Dukes' B was 83% and Dukes' C, 27% and for the colon, 75% and 33%, respectively. Noteworthy was the distal distribution, with 64% in their series and 86% in the literature located in the rectum, in contradistinction to the changing distribution in the general population where a migration to the right has been documented. Also, patients presented at an advanced stage (60% had Dukes' C or metastatic) and this probably accounts for the poor prognosis generally attributed to patients who develop colorectal carcinoma during pregnancy. A delay in diagnosis may in part account for the advanced stage of these lesions. It has been suggested that elevated levels of circulating estrogen and progesterone may stimulate growth of the carcinomas. The poor prognosis may in part be a reflection of the patient's age, as many believe that patients younger than 40 years of age are destined to a poor outcome.

Operative excision is the treatment of choice but, in pregnancy, operability, period of gestation, religious belief, and the patient's desire for children might be considered. In the first two trimesters, the appropriate operation should be recommended, leaving the pregnancy intact (1027). Total abdominal hysterectomy has been recommended if the uterus is found to be involved (1028). If the lesion is unre-sectable or is obstructing, a colostomy or "hidden" colostomy should be performed to help provide time for the fetus to reach viability. In the third trimester, it has been suggested that treatment be delayed until fetal pulmonary maturity is demonstrated. At that time, labor may be induced or a cesarean section performed, often without the lesion being removed. Simultaneous removal is not usually recommended because of increased vascularity in the pelvis. The definitive operation can be delayed for a few weeks after vaginal delivery. In the event the lesion is inoperable, the pregnancy can be allowed to proceed until viability is ensured, following which palliative measures can be undertaken.

Colorectal carcinoma coupled with pregnancy is a devastating combination yielding a poor prognosis. Whether this apparent poor prognosis reflects a delay in diagnosis, a biologically aggressive carcinoma in young women, or a hormonally driven carcinoma remains to be determined (1026).

OVARIAN CARCINOMA INVOLVING THE COLON

Involvement of the colon by advanced ovarian carcinoma is not uncommon. In these circumstances, the question arises as to the propriety of large bowel resection. Hertel et al. (1029) reported on 100 patients with FIGO stage IIIc ovarian carcinoma who underwent pelvic en bloc resection with excision of the rectosigmoid colon as part of the primary or secondary cytoreductive operation. Malignant involvement of the rectum was confirmed histopathologically: infiltration of the serosa in 28% of patients, infiltration of the muscularis in 31% of patients and infiltration of the mucosa in 14% of patients. Histopathologically confirmed pelvic R0 resection was achieved in 85% of patients. Pelvic recurrence occurred in 4.7% of 85 optimally debulked patients compared to 60% of 15 patients with suboptimal pelvic resection status. End colostomy could be prevented in 94% of patients. They concluded pelvic en bloc surgery with rectosigmoid resection was justified by histopathological outcome since deperitonealization with preservation of the rectosigmoid would have left malignancy in-situ in 73% of patients with suspected cul-de-sac involvement. This recommendation of course can only be made if there is no other evidence of metastatic disease as is the usual situation with ovarian carcinoma.

MALAKOPLAKIA AND COLORECTAL CARCINOMA

Malakoplakia is a characteristic inflammatory condition which is usually seen in the urogenital tract. Gastrointestinal malakoplakia is seen in association with a variety of conditions such as ulcerative colitis, diverticular disease, adenomatous polyps, and carcinoma. Pillay and Chetty (1030) reported four cases of colorectal carcinoma associated with malakoplakia. Three of the cases were encountered in males and the patients ranged in age from 55 to 64 years. One case each occurred in the cecum/ascending colon and descending colon while the remaining two were located in the rectum. All four cases were Dukes' stage B carcinoma. Furthermore, all four cases had spread to pericolonic fat and two had perforated. Microscopic examination showed the malakoplakia to be present at the infiltrating edge of the carcinoma. The draining lymph nodes were involved by malakoplakia to varying degrees in all cases. From their series and the literature review, malakoplakia associated with colorectal carcinoma tends to occur in elderly males in the rectum. The malakoplakia is found at the infiltrating front of the carcinoma and is not admixed with the neoplastic glands. Although lymph node involvement by malakoplakia has been reported only once previously, all four cases in this series showed evidence of involvement. The association does not appear to have any prognostic significance.

OTHER MALIGNANT LESIONS

CARCINOID

The carcinoid neoplasm is one member of a collection of neoplasms grouped together because of a common biochemical function. These neoplasms all incorporate and store large amounts of amine precursor (5-hydroxytryptophan) and have the ability to decarboxylate this substrate, leading to the production of several biologically active amines; thus is derived the acronym APUD (amine precursor uptake and decarboxylation) (1031).

■ INCIDENCE

Carcinoids arise from neuroectodermal derivatives. The gastrointestinal tract is the most common site and in decreasing order of frequency, the locations of carcinoids are the appendix, ileum, rectum, colon, and stomach (1032). Approximately 5% of all carcinoids are located in the colon (1032). The% of all gastrointestinal carcinoids has been reported to vary from 0.6% to 7.0% (1033). In the Connecticut Registry with 54 colonic carcinoids, 48% were in the cecum, 16% in the ascending colon, 6% in the transverse colon, 11% in the descending colon, 13% in the sigmoid colon, and 6% were not assigned (1034). The incidence of rectal carcinoids was 1.3% of noncarcinoid neoplasms of the rectum; for the colon, the incidence was 0.3% of noncarcinoid neoplasms of the colon (1035). In the Connecticut Registry, the age-adjusted incidence was 0.31 cases per 100,000 population/year (1034). Colonic involvement accounted for only 2.5% of all gastrointestinal carcinoids and 2.8% of all carcinoids (1036). Rectal carcinoids accounted for 12% to 15% of all carcinoids, and carcinoids of the remainder of the colon accounted for 7% of all carcinoids (1037).

■ CLINICAL FEATURES

Carcinoids most commonly occur in the seventh and eighth decades of life, with a female preponderance of 2:1 (1031,1036). Colonic carcinoids may present as a simple polyp or as a gross malignancy that is indistinguishable from carcinoma radiologically and has an "apple core" appearance. These carcinoids may be entirely asymptomatic, found in 0.014% of rectal examinations, or they may produce symptoms indistinguishable from those of carcinoma. Colonic carcinoids are usually symptomatic (1036). Once they have been diagnosed, a search for other neoplasms should be made because the incidence of synchronous and metachronous neoplasms has been reported as high as 42% (1036). Gastrointestinal carcinoid is associated with a high incidence of second primary malignancy. Gerstle, Kaufman, and Koltun (1038) reviewed their experience with 69 patients with carcinoids of the gastrointestinal tract and found that 42% had second synchronous neoplasms and 4% had a metachronous neoplasm. The gastrointestinal tract was the site of 43% of these additional neoplasms with half of these being carcinomas of the colon and rectum. Tichansky et al. (1039) conducted a search of the National Cancer Institute Surveillance, Epidemiology, and End Result database from 1973 to 1996 and found 2086 patients with colorectal carcinoids. Patients with colorectal carcinoids had an increased rate of carcinoma in the colon and rectum, small bowel, esophagus/stomach, lung/bronchus, urinary tract, and prostate, when compared with the control population. Most of the gastrointestinal carcinomas were synchronous carcinomas whereas lesions outside the gastrointestinal tract were mostly metachronous neoplasms. After the diagnosis of colorectal carcinoid neoplasms, patients should undergo appropriate screening and surveillance for carcinoma at these other sites.

Most gastrointestinal carcinoids are incidentally discovered at laparotomy or autopsy. The discovery of an asymptomatic gastrointestinal carcinoid during the operative treatment of another malignancy will usually only require resection and has little effect on the prognosis of the individual. Carcinoids may be associated with multiple endocrine neoplasia, especially of the parathyroid, but most of these are associated with carcinoids of foregut origin (1040). Carcinoids of midgut and hindgut origin occur more frequently and produce significant endocrine relationships other than serotonin production. The diagnosis may be established by demonstrating elevated blood levels of serotonin or elevated urinary levels of 5-hydroxyindoleacetic acid.

In the series reported by Rosenberg and Welch (1036), 44% of patients had signs of local spread, while 38% of patients had distant metastases. The liver was involved in 35.5% of the patients and the lung in 8%. In a review by Berardi (1041), 57% of patients with colonic carcinoids already had metastases, and of these, 42% had distant metastases. In the series reported by Gerstle, Kaufman, and Koltun (1038), the overall incidence of metastatic carcinoid at presentation was 32%. The most common sites of metastatic disease were lymph nodes in 82%, liver in 68%, satellite lesions to adjacent small bowel in 32%, peritoneum in 27%, and omentum in 18%. Only one of 18 appendiceal carcinoids metastasized and then only to the local lymph nodes. Four of nine colorectal carcinoids metastasized to the lymph nodes and liver. Other sites of metastatic disease included bone (1042).

■ PATHOLOGY

Macroscopically, carcinoids may vary in appearance from nodular thickening in the mucosa and submucosa to a sessile or pedunculated polypoid lesion, and they may have a yellowish tinge. Larger lesions may ulcerate and become annular, or they may obstruct and metastasize to regional lymph nodes or the liver (Fig. 65). The malignant character of these lesions correlates with size, location, and tissue invasion. Carcinoids of the appendix and rectum rarely metastasize (1037). Lesions <2 cm rarely metastasize, whereas 80% of lesions >2 cm in diameter do metastasize. Superficially invasive lesions have a better prognosis than do deeply penetrating ones. In his review Berardi (1041)

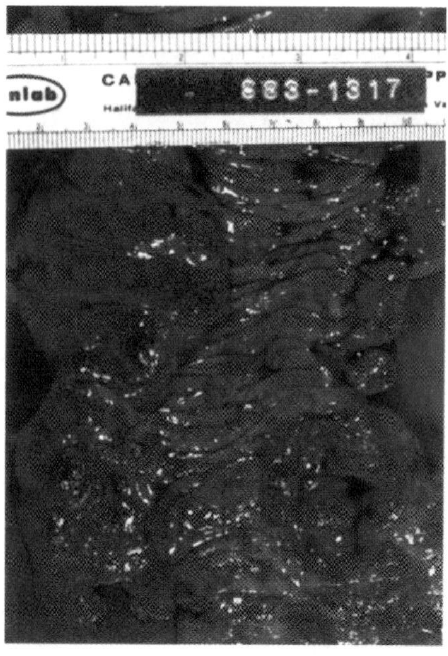

FIGURE 65 ■ Macroscopic features of a carcinoid of the large bowel. Lesion appears as a yellowish-tinged protruding mass.

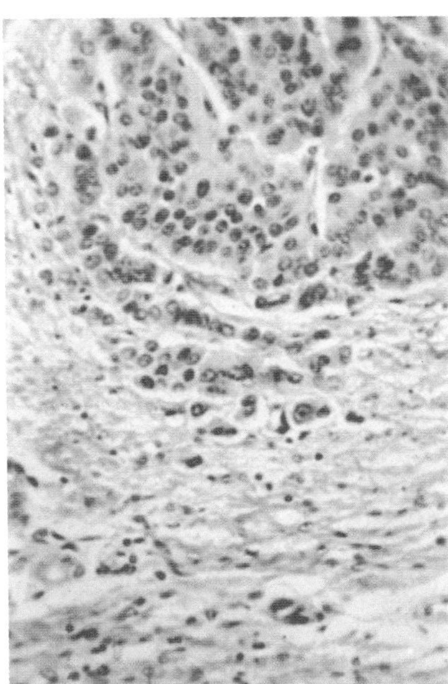

FIGURE 66 ■ Microscopic features of a carcinoid with uniform small cells in a trabecular anastomotic pattern. Although the lesion is not cytologically malignant, invasion into the muscle is evident. *Source*: Courtesy of H. Srolovitz, M.D., Montreal, Quebec.

found multiple carcinoids in 4.2% of patients with colonic carcinoids as compared with 30% of patients with ileal carcinoids. Associated malignancy of the colon was found in 2.5% of patients with colonic carcinoids as compared with 30% to 53% of patients with ileal carcinoids.

Microscopically, carcinoids consist of uniform, small, round or polygonal cells with prominent round nuclei and eosinophilic cytoplasmic granules (Fig. 66). They usually demonstrate one of five histologic patterns: insular, trabecular, glandular, undifferentiated, or mixed. In decreasing order of median survival time in years, the growth patterns ranked as follows: mixed insular plus glandular, 4.4; insular, 2.9; trabecular, 2.5; mixed insular plus trabecular 2.3; mixed growth pattern, 1.4; glandular, 0.9; and undifferentiated, 0.5 (1043).

■ IMAGING PROCEDURES

The hypervascular nature of carcinoids and their metastases allows an aggressive role by the radiologist in diagnosis and interventional management (1044). Double-contrast studies still best define the primary neoplasms. The "spoke wheel" configuration of the desmoplastic mesenteric masses and lymph node metastases are best seen by CT, whereas hepatic metastases can be demonstrated by CT, CT angioportography, ultrasonography, MRI, and octreotide scintigraphy. Superior mesenteric angiography of the small bowel and cecum is useful when scanning procedures are not revealing. Percutaneous needle biopsy with radiologic guidance may confirm the diagnosis.

Octreotide scintigraphy may have a fourfold impact on patient management (1045). It may detect resectable lesions that would be unrecognized with conventional imaging techniques, it may prevent operation in patients whose lesions have metastasized to a greater extent than can be detected with conventional imaging, it may direct the choice of therapy in patients with inoperable carcinoids, and in the future it may be used to select patients for radionuclide therapy.

■ CHEMICAL ACTIVITY

Carcinoids secrete serotonin, a substance with pronounced pharmacologic effects, including flushing of the face, neck, anterior chest wall, and hands; increased peristalsis leading to diarrhea; constriction of bronchi presenting as wheezing; and cardiac valvular lesions with right-sided heart failure (pulmonary stenosis). Other components of the syndrome include a rise in pulmonary arterial pressure, hypotension, edema, pellagra-like skin lesions, peptic ulcers, arthralgia, and weight loss (1046). This constellation of symptoms, known as the carcinoid syndrome, usually occurs with metastases to the liver. Other products such as bradykinins, histamine, vasoactive intestinal, peptide, adrenocorticotropic hormone (ACTH), 5-hydroxytryptophan, and prostaglandins produce part of the syndrome complex. The syndrome occurs primarily with carcinoids of the small bowel but not with those of the colon or rectum.

Foregut carcinoids, which are argentaffin negative and argyrophil positive, produce the serotonin precursor 5-hydroxytryptophan. Midgut carcinoids are usually both argyrophil positive and argentaffin positive, are frequently multicentric in origin, and may be associated with the carcinoid syndrome. Hindgut carcinoids are rarely argyrophil positive or argentaffin positive, are usually unicentric,

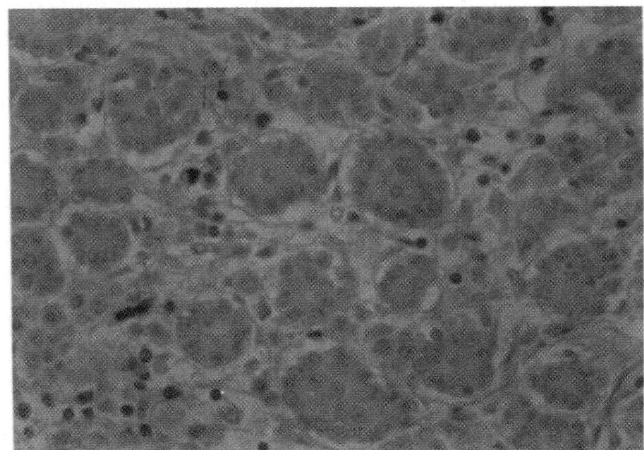

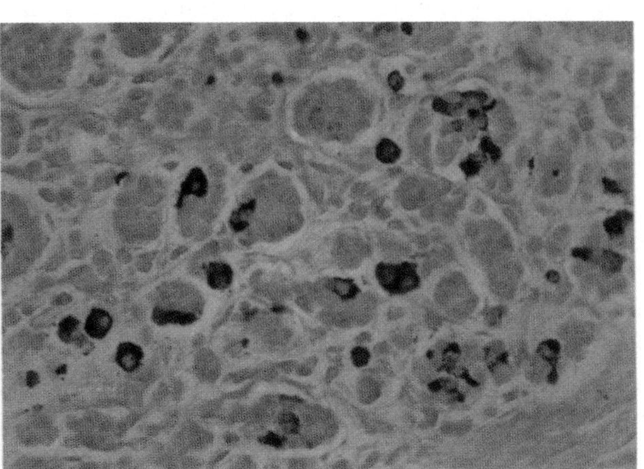

FIGURE 67 ■ (**A**) Microscopic appearance of a carcinoid with demonstration of argyrophilic granules by Fontana's stain. (**B**) Microscopic appearance of a carcinoid demonstrating argentaffin tissue. *Source*: Courtesy of L.R. Bégin, M.D., Montreal, Quebec.

and are not usually associated with the carcinoid syndrome (Fig. 67). The carcinoid syndrome is a rare clinical entity that occurs with a prevalence of 1.6% in patients with carcinoids and almost only if liver metastases are present (1047). Berardi (1041) estimated that <5% of colonic carcinoids cause the carcinoid syndrome. In a series by Rosenberg and Welch (1036), 4.2% of patients either had symptoms suggestive of the syndrome or elevated 5-hydroxyindoleacetic acid levels.

■ TREATMENT

Appendiceal carcinoids <1 cm in diameter can be treated adequately by appendectomy, but if they are ≥2 cm in diameter, a right hemicolectomy should be performed (1032). The rationale for the latter recommendation is that the average rate of metastases is 30% (1032). For lesions between 1 and 2 cm, in which the risk of metastases is between 0% and 1%, the decision-making process is more difficult. Appendectomy is probably sufficient but additional criteria may be considered, such as extension to the mesoappendix or subserosal lymphatic invasion (1048). A more aggressive approach may be advised for younger patients (1032). Gouzi et al. (1049) recommended that other than having a size >2 cm and base location, the presence of mucin production is a further indication for secondary right hemicolectomy.

The recommended treatment for small bowel carcinoids is wide segmental resection. Because the average lymph node involvement is 44% (1032), relevant lymph node drainage should be included. Meticulous intraoperative examination is indicated because 20% to 40% of small bowel carcinoids are multicentric and simultaneous adenocarcinomas of other parts of the gastrointestinal tract occur at a rate of 8% to 29% (1032).

For colonic carcinoids, the standard operation for adenocarcinoma should be performed.

Metastatic disease occurs more frequently with carcinoids of the colon. If there is distant disease, resection of the primary lesion is still recommended to alleviate symptoms because a long survival period is possible (1037). Partial hepatectomy should be considered if technically feasible (1046,1050). Beaton, Homan, and Dineen (1051) have shown the value of aggressive operative debulking in reducing and sometimes obliterating the manifestations of the syndrome. For patients with unresectable metastatic carcinoids to the liver, combining either operative hepatic dearterialization or hepatic intra-arterial embolization with chemotherapy has reportedly been effective in inducing regression of the liver metastases (1044,1050,1052). Chemotherapeutic agents used have included 5-FU, streptozotocin delivered via hepatic artery or portal vein catheters, or FUDR and doxorubicin administered systematically (1052). A number of other pharmacologic and cytotoxic agents have been used to control the carcinoid syndrome (1046). Each is aimed at neutralizing one of the pharmacologically active products released by the carcinoid. Vinik and Moattari (1053) have reported the successful use of somatostatin analog in the management of the carcinoid syndrome. The symptoms of diarrhea, flushing, and wheezing can be dramatically reduced or even abolished. Ahlman et al. (1050) pursued an aggressive policy in the management of patients with midgut carcinoid syndrome and bilobar disease. After primary operation to relieve symptoms of intestine obstruction and ischemia, the authors performed successful embolizations of hepatic arteries. Patients with remedial disease were treated by octreotide. In a series of 64 patients, the authors obtained a 70% 5-year survival rate.

■ RESULTS

Five-year survival rates for patients with colonic carcinoids are reported to be 52% (1035). Survival rates reported by Rosenberg and Welch (1036) were 51%, 25%, and 10% at 2, 5, and 10 years, respectively. In the Connecticut Registry, 2- and 5-year survival rates were 56% and 33%, respectively. The 5-year survival by Dukes' staging was A, 83%; B, 43%; C, 35%; and metastatic, 21%. In a 25-year population-based study of 36 colonic carcinoids, Spread et al. (1033) found a perioperative mortality of 22%. Actuarial survival rates at 2 and 5 years were 34% and 26%, respectively. In the authors' review, the size of the lesion and invasion into muscularis propria, the two major histopathologic prognostic factors for carcinoids, were not found to influence survival significantly. Stage, histologic pattern, differentiation, nuclear grade, and mitotic rate (>20 mitosis/10 hpf) proved to be prognostic factors. The 5-year survival rate in patients with appendiceal carcinoids was 90% to 100% (1032). The overall 5-year survival rate for small bowel carcinoids was 50% to 60% (1032). The 5-year survival rate decreases from 75% for local disease to 59% for patients with positive nodes to 20% to 35% if liver metastases are present.

LYMPHOMA

■ INCIDENCE

Lymphoma may occur as a primary lesion or as part of a generalized malignant process involving the gastrointestinal tract. As a primary lesion it constitutes only 0.5% of all cases of neoplastic disease of the colon, and yet it is the second most common malignant disease of the colon. Lymphoma comprises 6% to 20% of cases of primary gastrointestinal lymphoma (1037,1054–1057) and accounts for 5% to 10% of all non-Hodgkin's lymphoma (1055). It most commonly involves the cecum (70%), with the rectum and ascending colon next in order of frequency (1055,1057). A more recent publication cited distribution sites of primary large bowel lymphoma as cecum 37.5%, descending colon 25%, ascending colon 25%, and rectum 12.5% (1056). It can occur at any age from 3 years to 81 years, but the average age is 50 years. Men are affected twice as often as women but a recent publication cited the reverse (1056).

■ PATHOLOGY

Lymphomas represent a diverse group of neoplasms. At least six major classifications of non-Hodgkin's lymphoma are in use, but there is no consensus among them. Three macroscopic types are seen (230). Annular or plaquelike thickenings are the most common type, followed by bulky protuberant growths, and, rarely, thickened and aneurysmal dilatations of the bowel wall. The cut surface has a

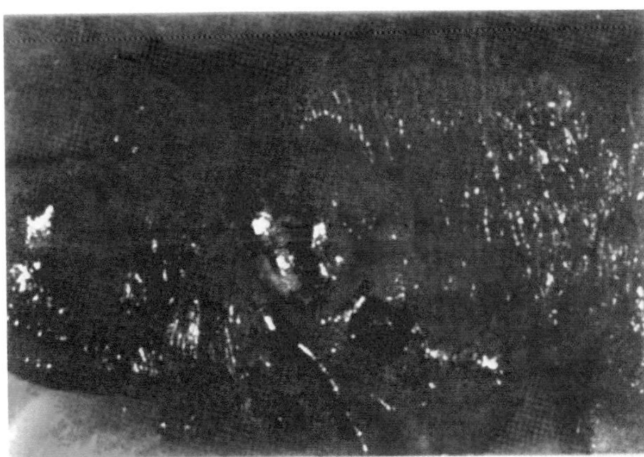

FIGURE 68 ■ Grayish fish-flesh appearance of a lymphoma of the large bowl. Note that the mucosa is intact.

uniform fleshy appearance (Fig. 68). Regional lymph nodes are involved in one half of all cases, but such involvement is not related to prognosis (230). Multiple primary foci are quite common. Malignant lymphomas may present as multiple polypoid protrusions of the entire colon and may mimic adenomatosis coli. Roentgenographically, 86% of colonic lymphomas are single lesions, 8% are multiple discrete lesions, and 6% show a diffuse colonic involvement (1037). Dawson, Cornes, and Morson (1059) presented these criteria for a primary lymphoma of the gastrointestinal tract: (1) no palpable peripheral lymphadenopathy, (2) normal roentgenographic findings except at the primary site, (3) normal white blood cell count and differential, (4) predominance of the alimentary tract lesion with only regional lymph node involvement, and (5) no involvement of the liver or spleen.

The large series of large bowel lymphomas reported by Jinnai, Iwasa, and Watanuki (1055) were classified histologically in order of frequency as follows: histiocytic, lymphocytic, mixed, and Hodgkin's disease. The incidence of each variety varies from series to series, but in the combined series it was as follows: histiocytic type, 43%; lymphocytic type, 29%; mixed type, 14%; Hodgkin's disease, 3.5% (Fig. 69) (1054).

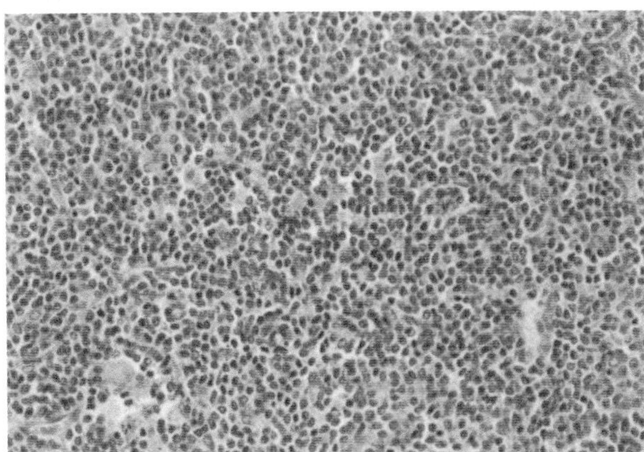

FIGURE 69 ■ Microscopic features of a poorly differentiated lymphoma of the colon demonstrating a somewhat nodular pattern, pleomorphism, and a degree of cellular necrosis. *Source*: Courtesy of L.R. Bégin, M.D., Monteral, Quebec.

In one series of 15 patients, histologically 40% were classified as high grade and 60% as intermediate-grade non-Hodgkin's lymphoma. The neoplasms usually presented at an advanced stage: in 87%, the lymphoma had spread to the adjacent mesentery, the regional lymph nodes, or both when first diagnosed (1057).

■ CLINICAL FEATURES

Lymphomas of the colon are characterized by abdominal pain in more than 90% of patients. Otherwise, the symptoms may be indistinguishable from those of carcinoma, with changes in bowel habits such as diarrhea or constipation, bleeding, weight loss, weakness, and possibly fever. Tender abdominal masses are present in 80% of patients on initial examination (1054). If ulceration supervenes, bleeding may be more prominent. Obstruction occurs in 20% to 25% of patients, but perforation is infrequent (1054). Multiple lesions constitute 8% of cases (1060).

The radiologic signs observed during barium enema studies for non-Hodgkin's lymphoma are as follows: a small nodular pattern frequently with multiple lesions (45.7%), a diffuse or infiltrating pattern (25.4%), a filling defect (22.9%), endoluminal and exoluminal images (17.8%), ulcerating patterns (3.4%), and a pure mesenteric form (0.8%) (1061). Lymphomas of the colon may produce the same radiologic appearance as carcinomas and similarly may be indistinguishable from carcinomas at laparotomy The colonoscopic appearance of a follicular lymphoma is seen in Fig. 70. Biopsy will clarify the diagnosis, but diagnosis still may be difficult because of the superficial nature of the biopsy.

Once the diagnosis is made, staging should be performed through an adequate history, physical examination, barium enema, complete blood count, liver function tests, chest x-ray films, bone marrow assay, CT scan of the abdomen, and lymphangiography (1037).

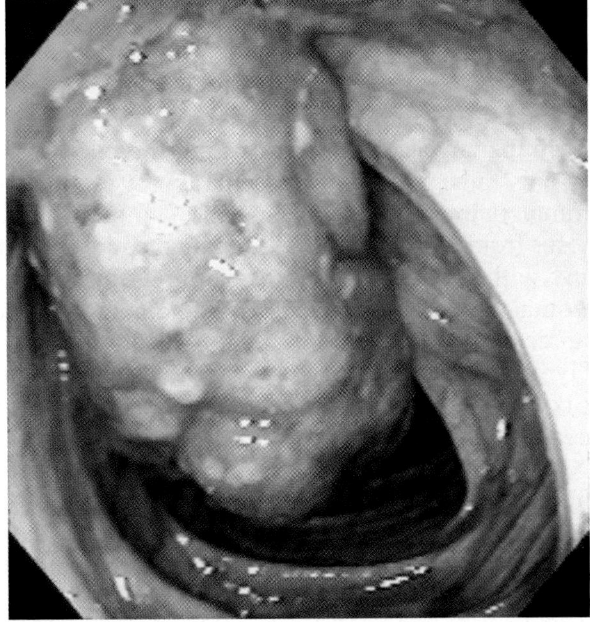

FIGURE 70 ■ Colonospic appearance of a colonic lymphoma.

■ TREATMENT

The treatment of primary lymphoma of the colon is resection. At laparotomy, appropriate staging with liver biopsy, lymph node biopsy, and splenectomy has been recommended (1037). Only one third of lymphomas are confined to the bowel wall at laparotomy (1060). For unresectable lesions, radiation is beneficial. Chemotherapy is recommended for systemic disease.

■ RESULTS

The overall 5-year survival rate is approximately 40% (range, 20% to 55%) (1054,1058).When regional lymph nodes are involved, 5-year survivals fall to 12%. There is a marked difference in survival rate between patients who undergo resection only and those who receive supplementary radiotherapy, 83% vs. 16% (1060).

In a series of 130 cases of primary lymphoma of the large intestine, Jinnai, Iwasa, and Watanuki (1055) reported a resection rate for cure of 55%, with most operations being abdominoperineal resections and others low anterior resections or hemicolectomies. Survival rates at 5 years and 10 years were 39.8% and 33.2%, respectively. Corresponding survival rates after curative resection were 44.2% and 40%. Prognosis was better when the lesion was $\leq$5 cm in diameter, intraluminal, and without lymph node metastases. When lymphomas were analyzed according to histologic type, 5-year and 10-year survival rates of curative resection were both 38.9% for histiocytic type, both 43% for lymphocytic type, 43.8% and 21.9% for the mixed type, and both 100% for Hodgkin's disease. Overall 5-year survival rates were 25.4%, 33.2%, 35.4%, and 40%, respectively. The growth pattern for the lesions was intraluminal for about 50%, extramural in 15%, intramural in 25%, and unknown in the remainder. Corresponding 5-year survival rates were 47%, 20%, and 12%. The 10-year survival rates were the same for intraluminal and extramural lesions, but no patients in the intramural group survived $>$7 years. The 5- and 10-year survival rates were 18.5% for patients with lymph node metastases, and 45.4% and 37.1%, respectively, for patients without metastases.

Doolabh et al. (1062) reported their experience with seven cases of primary colonic lymphoma which represented 1.4% of all non-Hodgkin's lymphoma, 14% of gastrointestinal non-Hodgkin's lymphoma and 0.9% of all colonic malignancies diagnosed during the period of their study. The most common presentation was nonspecific abdominal pain. The lack of specific symptoms delayed diagnoses from 1 to 12 months. All patients underwent laparotomy with resection. The most common location of the lymphoma was the cecum (71%). Regional lymph nodes were affected in all but one patient. All lymphomas were B-cell lymphomas (five small noncleaved cell and two large cell). Six of seven patients received adjuvant chemotherapy. Of the six patients available for follow-up, four remained alive (12, 19, 23, and 25 months after diagnosis). In both patients who died, the disease recurred diffusely.

Fan et al. (1063) identified 37 cases of primary colorectal lymphoma that comprised 0.48% of all cases of colon malignancies. The most common presenting sign and symptoms were abdominal pain (62%), abdominal mass (54%), and weight loss (43%). The most frequent site of involvement was the cecum (45%). Histologically, 78% were classified as high-grade and 22% as intermediate-grade to low-grade lymphoma. Fifty-seven percent of cases received adjuvant chemotherapy. The 5-year survival was 33% for all patients and 39% for patients treated with combination chemotherapy.

SARCOMA

There is a large variety of very uncommon neoplasms arising from mesenchymal tissues. The malignancies that fit into this category are classified as sarcomas. They include leiomyosarcoma, liposarcoma, hemangiosarcoma, fibrosarcoma, fibrous histiocytoma, neurofibrosarcoma, lymphangiosarcoma, and Kaposi's sarcoma.

Leiomyosarcoma of the colon is a rare pathologic entity, with only 58 recorded cases at the time of review of the literature by Suzuki et al. (1064) This type of sarcoma occurs two to six times more commonly in the rectum than in the colon in both sexes and most commonly appears in the fifth and sixth decades of life (1065). The lesion arises from the smooth muscle of the bowel. Macroscopically, it may range from a small nodule to a large mass, which is covered by mucosa in its early stages but eventually may become ulcerated (Fig. 71). The lesion may be intramural, endoenteric, exoenteric or dumbbell shaped (endoenteric and exoenteric) in position. It is usually a low-grade malignancy, and histologically it may be very difficult to differentiate from a benign leiomyoma (Fig. 72). Hematogenous spread results in metastases to the liver and the lung (1066). Regional lymph nodes are rarely involved. Early diagnosis is seldom accomplished before complications such as bleeding or obstruction occur (1066). Symptoms are similar to those of carcinoma: changes in bowel habit, rectal bleeding, passage of mucus, and, in the more advanced stage, weight loss. If the lesion is causing obstructive symptoms, abdominal pain may occur either as an ache or cramping. Rarely will an abdominal mass be palpable. Barium enema reveals a polypoid or constricting lesion that is usually indistinguishable from carcinoma. Colonoscopy and biopsy may be helpful if they are performed preoperatively. The treatment is resection as performed for carcinoma, and, in fact, the diagnosis will probably be made only after histiologic examination of the resected specimen. Curative resection has been reported in

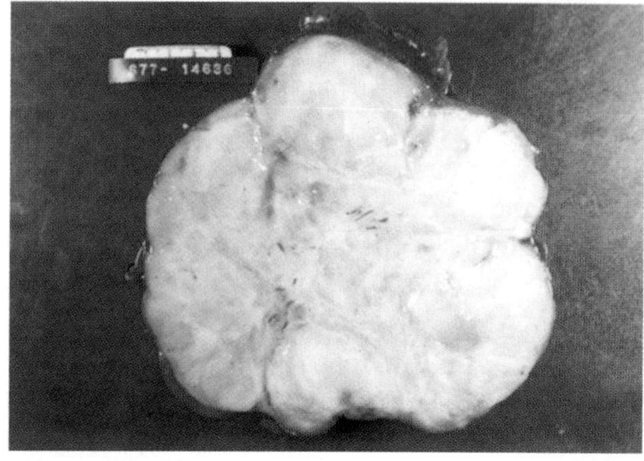

FIGURE 71 ■ Macroscopic appearance of a transected leiomyosarcoma of the descending colon.

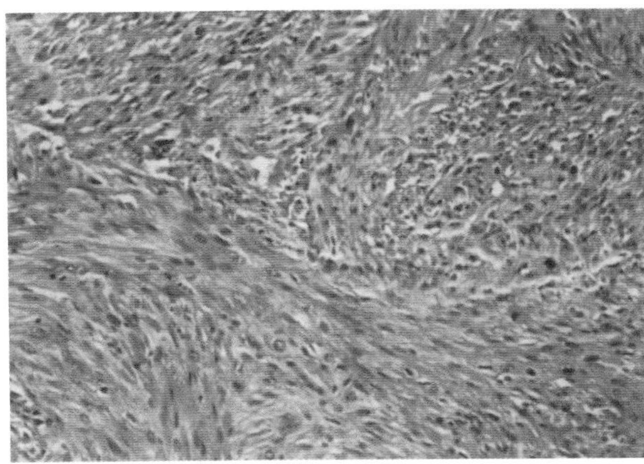

FIGURE 72 ■ Microscopic features of the leiomyosarcoma shown in Figure 71. Relatively well-differentiated cells may be difficult to distinguish from those of a benign leiomyoma. *Source*: Courtesy of L.R. Bégin, M.D., Monteral, Quebec.

45% of patients (1067). The 5-year survival rates are meaningless because of the paucity of cases. Pulmonary and hepatic metastases may occur many years later. The prognosis depends on the Broders grade, with grades 1 and 2 representing better prognoses than grades 3 and 4 (1067). Shiu et al. (1065) noted that endoenteric lesions carried a good prognosis and that exoenteric neoplasms invaded adjacent structures or perforated into the peritoneal cavity. Three clinicopathologic factors adversely affect prognosis: (1) lesions >5 cm in diameter, (2) extraintestinal invasion or perforation, and (3) high histopathologic grade of malignancy. Patients rarely survive 5 years after operation and almost two thirds die within 1 year (1069). Radiation or chemotherapy, alone or in combination, have not been found to be effective (1069).

For the most part, the other sarcomas in this group are pathologic curiosities, and their symptomatology and management are similar to those of leiomyosarcoma. For example a primary osteosarcoma arising in the colon has been reported (1070). The ultimate diagnosis of these conditions is probably also made from the resected specimen (1071).

SQUAMOUS CELL CARCINOMA

Primary squamous cell carcinoma of the large intestine is another exceedingly uncommon neoplasm. It is estimated that adenosquamous and squamous cell carcinoma of the large intestine comprise 0.05% to 0.10% of all large bowel malignancies (1072). Only 72 cases had been reported in the English-language literature until 1992 (1072). Subsequently, DiSario et al. (1) reported another 75 cases. In their review of the literature, Michelassi et al. (1073) found synchronous squamous cell carcinoma of the colon present in 3.2% of the collected cases; 10% had either antecedent, synchronous, or metachronous adenocarcinoma of the colon. The reported age range was 32 to 91 years. Mixed adenosquamous cell carcinoma occurs in men and women with equal frequency, but there are twice as many men in the squamous cell group. It has been suggested that a number of criteria must be satisfied before a diagnosis of primary squamous cell carcinoma of the large bowel is entertained (1074): (1) there must be no evidence in any other organ of a squamous cell carcinoma that might spread directly into the lower bowel or provide a source of intestinal metastases, (2) the affected bowel should not be involved in a fistulous tract lined with squamous cells (colocutaneous fistulas have been described in association with squamous cell carcinoma), and (3) when squamous cell carcinoma occurs in the rectum, care must be taken to exclude origin from the anal canal (i.e., there should be a lack of continuity between the lesion and the anal canal epithelium).

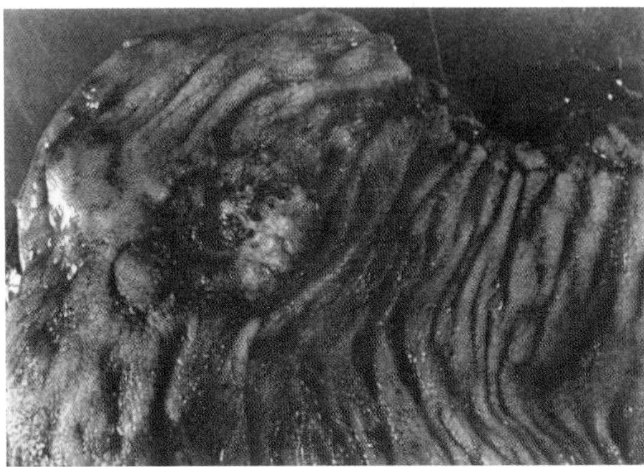

FIGURE 73 ■ Example of a squamous cell carcinoma of the large bowel, showing features similar to those of an adenocarcinoma.

Several mechanisms that have been proposed for the pathogenesis of this entity were reviewed by Vezeridis et al. (1075). They include (1) proliferation of uncommitted reserve or basal cells following mucosal injury, (2) squamous metaplasia of glandular epithelium, resulting from chronic irritation, (3) origin from embryonal nests of committed or uncommitted ectodermal cells remaining in an ectopic site after embryogenesis, (4) squamous metaplasia of an established colorectal adenocarcinoma, and (5) squamous differentiation arising in an adenoma. Associated conditions that have been described include ulcerative colitis, irradiated bowel, chronic colocutaneous fistulas, schistosomiasis, and colonic duplication (1073).

Symptoms, investigations, and assessment are similar to those of colon carcinoma. Lesions are distributed throughout the large bowel with 25% to 50% of all reported cases located in the rectum (1072,1076). Coexistent disease has been reported—schistosomiasis, ulcerative colitis,

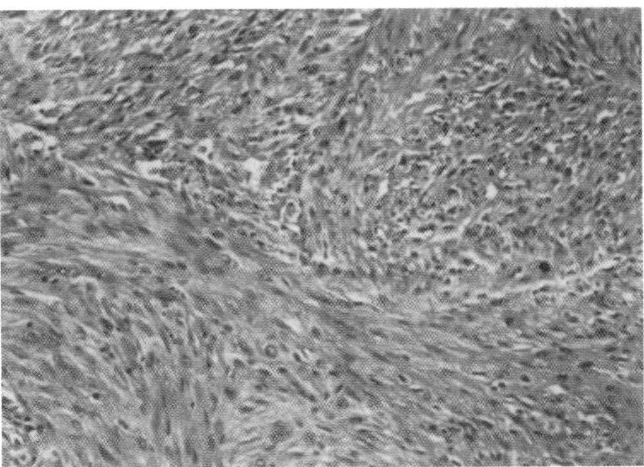

FIGURE 74 ■ Microscopic features of a squamous cell carcinoma with clusters of squamous cells in the stroma.

colonic duplication, amebiasis, ovarian carcinoma previously treated with radiation, prostatic carcinoma, and ovarian teratoma. Macroscopic features may not be dissimilar to those of adenocarcinoma (Fig. 73). Microscopic features are demonstrated in Fig. 74. Of the cases in the literature, approximately half were pure squamous cell carcinoma, and the other half were mixed adenosquamous cell carcinoma. Treatment consists of resection of the affected segment. For rectal lesions, it has been suggested that multimodality therapy, as described by Nigro, be the first line of treatment and that only when this therapy fails should extensive operative procedures be used (1074). On the other hand, the Nigro protocol may be used as adjuvant therapy. The 5-year survival rate was 50% for patients with Dukes' B lesions and 33% for those with Dukes' C lesions; no patients with metastatic disease survived (1073).

ADENOSQUAMOUS CARCINOMA

This malignancy contains both adenocarcinomatous and squamous carcinomatous elements that are separate although contiguous thus making a distinction from the common squamous metaplasia in an adenocarcinoma (230). It may be found in all parts of the large bowel but mostly in the right colon and rectum. They are very aggressive neoplasms that may have a worse prognosis than the more common form of colonic adenocarcinoma. Furthermore, the squamous component, in particular, may have a greater potential for metastasizing and can do so as an undifferentiated-appearing carcinoma (1077). Frizelle et al. (1078) searched the Mayo Clinic Tissue Registry for all primary cases of squamous and adenosquamous carcinoma of the colon and rectum. Cases were divided into pure squamous cell carcinoma ($n = 11$), mixed adenosquamous carcinoma ($n = 31$), and adenocarcinoma with benign-appearing squamous metaplasia (adenoacanthoma; $n = 2$). Right-sided lesions were the most common (43%). Metastatic disease was evident at presentation in 49% of patients, the most common sites in order being liver, peritoneal, and lung. The 5-year overall survival was 34%, stage I to III disease had a 65% 5-year survival rate, and stage IV mean survival time was 8.5 months. For node-positive and node-negative disease, 23% and 85%, respectively, survived five years.

PLASMACYTOMA

Primary plasmacytoma involving the colon is an exceedingly rare lesion (1079,1080). Presenting symptoms are nonspecific for gastrointestinal disease and may include abdominal pain, rectal bleeding, weight loss, nausea, vomiting, and anorexia. The lesion may be single or multiple and consists of polypoid or nodular protrusions. In the presence of intestinal involvement, appropriate scans and bone marrow biopsy should be obtained to rule out bone and marrow involvement. Microscopically, the plasmacytoma lesion is composed of many plasma cells. In most cases treatment has consisted of resection of the involved colon. An 80% 10-year survival can be expected (1037). However, if the diagnosis can be made by colonoscopic biopsy, treatment options include chemotherapy and radiotherapy (1081).

MELANOMA

Primary melanoma of the colon is a distinctly uncommon entity. Indeed, since melanoblasts are necessary for the development of melanoma and since they are found in tissues of ectodermal-origin (not in the large intestine above the mucocutaneous junction), it is questionable whether primary intestinal melanoma occurs at all. When the colon is involved, the disease is usually metastatic in origin.

Tessier et al. (1082) conducted a review of the literature in which they identified 88 cases of metastatic melanoma to the colon to which they added 24 patients. The mean age of their patients was 63.9 years. The interval time between diagnosis of the primary and metastatic disease to the colon was 7.5 years. Presenting symptoms included bleeding (51%), obstruction (29%), pain (20%), weight loss (11%), and perforation (7%). The frequency of these symptoms is comparable to those in the literature. Colonoscopy was the most commonly used diagnostic test (58%), followed by exploratory laparotomy (25%), autopsy (8%), and barium enema (8%). Resection was performed in 61% of patients with 39% having positive lymph nodes. The 1-year survival rate was 60% and the 5-year survival rate was 33%.

Much of the following information has been obtained from the review by Tessier et al. Radiologic studies of the gastrointestinal tract have shown a wide variation of abnormalities with the small intestine having the most diverse findings. A "bull's eye" or "target" sign on barium studies is a well-described finding in the small intestine, stomach, and duodenum. Findings of colonic involvement on barium studies may include multiple submucosal nodules, intussusception, large ulcerative lesions, and extrinsic masses compressing the colon. Macroscopically, the lesions are characteristically mucosal or submucosal, may be polypoid or infiltrative, single or multiple, melanotic or amelanotic.

On endoscopic examination these lesions may appear amelanotic but may have enough pigmentation to be easily recognizable on gross or microscopic examination. Intussusception of the colon, multiple colonic polyps, and fungating masses resembling colon carcinoma have been described on endoscopy. Colonoscopy is not only the most reliable study but also offers the benefit of obtaining tissue for diagnosis. Special stains such as nuclear S-100 and cytoplasmic HMB-45 may be necessary to secure the diagnosis.

There has been much debate as to the benefit of operation in patients with metastatic disease to the gastrointestinal tract from malignancy. Resection was performed in 75% of patients in the series of Tessier et al. and in 61% of patients from historic data. The average time until death after operation was 27.5 months. Nonoperative candidates died within 7.8 months after diagnosis. Patients with negative nodes had an average survival of 34.7 months whereas those with positive nodes lived an average of 20.4 months. In their group, 87.5% of patients had another organ involved at the time of presentation highlighting the rarity of isolated colonic metastases. From the literature review the long-term survival for isolated colonic metastases was 58.7 months. It would appear, therefore, that resection of isolated metastases to the colon is beneficial and negative nodal status is indicative of a favorable prognosis. Over 90% of patients who underwent operative resection of gastrointestinal metastases have also reported improvement in their symptoms further supporting a role for operative intervention in symptomatic patients. In the series of Tessier et al., patients presenting with obstruction or perforation had a dismal prognosis with no patient surviving longer than 10 months.

LEUKEMIC INFILTRATION

Although a solid neoplasm is not involved in leukemia of the colon, it might be appropriate to include this disease in this section.

The following account draws heavily from the work of Moir, Scudamore, and Benny (1083). The underlying pathology of leukemia of the colon is a neutropenic enterocolitis with primarily cecal involvement (typhlitis). The edema and hemorrhagic infarction may be seen elsewhere in the gastrointestinal tract. Neutropenic enterocolitis occurs particularly in patients with acute myelogenous leukemia undergoing high-dose cytosine arabinoside chemotherapy but also is seen in patients with other hematologic disorders (1084).

Four pathophysiologic mechanisms have been proposed: (1) enteric vascular ischemia caused by stasis or shock contributes to mucosal ulceration and subsequent invasion by pathogens, (2) mucosal necrosis caused by intramural neoplastic infiltrate alone or in combination with necrosis induced by chemotherapy allows entry of organisms into the bowel wall, (3) bleeding into the mucosa or submucosa secondary to thrombocytopenia causes mucosal disruption and subsequent invasion by colonic flora, and (4) focal fecal ulceration provides entry for pathogens (1085).

The clinical triad is comprised of neutropenia, sepsis, and abdominal pain (1086). The onset, which is heralded by prodromal fever, watery or bloody diarrhea, and abdominal distention, occurs during the phase of severe neutropenia. Symptoms may localize in the right lower quadrant with an associated increase in systemic toxicity. The diagnosis can be confirmed by several reexaminations, abdominal radiographs (showing partial small bowel obstruction, thickened and irregular mucosal folds, and air within the bowel wall), ultrasonography, or radionucleotide scans (gallium-labeled or indium-labeled white blood cells). CT findings include an edematous cecum and/or right colon, spiculation, and inflammation of the pericolic fat, and pneumatosis—all thought to be pathognomonic for neutropenic typhlitis (1086).

The mainstay of management is complete bowel rest with total parenteral nutrition, nasogastric suction, broad-spectrum antibiotics, and avoidance of laxatives or antidiarrheal agents. Granulocyte support may be helpful. Patients with a history of typhlitis should have prophylactic bowel rest and total parenteral nutrition instituted at the beginning of further chemotherapy. Patients with ongoing severe systemic sepsis who do not respond to chemotherapy and those with overt perforation, obstruction, massive hemorrhage, or abscess formation will require operative intervention. All necrotic material must be resected, usually by right hemicolectomy, ileostomy, and mucous fistula. Depending on the extent of bowel involvement, a more extensive resection may be required. Anastomosis is not advised. To prevent recurrence, elective right hemicolectomy has been suggested if additional courses of chemotherapy are required (1086).

NEUROENDOCRINE LESIONS OF THE COLORECTUM

In their review of the subject, Vilor et al. (1087) noted that neuroendocrine proliferations have been classified into three types: benign (glicentin, PP- or peptide YY-producing carcinoid), low-grade malignant (serotonin-producing carcinoid), and high-grade malignant (neuroendocrine carcinoma). Neuroendocrine carcinomas have further been subdivided into the oat cell type and intermediate cell type. The incidence in neuroendocrine carcinomas is $<0.1\%$ of all malignancies at this site. Thomas and Sobin (1088) noted that only 38 of 108,303 colonic and 18 of 46,618 rectal malignancies were small cell carcinomas. The preferred sites of occurrence are the cecum and rectum (1089). Microscopically, neuroendocrine neoplasms are recognized by their characteristically cytologic appearance with lack of tubule formation and submucosal growth pattern. They are argyrophilic and diffusely immunoreactive for neuron-specific enolase and synaptophysin. Most reported cases show metastases to the lymph nodes or distant organs at the time of diagnosis. Only approximately 10% of patients survive 1 year.

The most recent report on neuroendocrine carcinomas of the colon and rectum was by Bernick et al. (1090). They identified 38 patients with neuroendocrine carcinomas from a database comprising 6495 patients (0.6%). These endocrine carcinomas did not include carcinoids. Average patient age was 57 years—44.7% males and 55.3% females. Location of the carcinomas was as follows: 17 colon, 14 rectum, 6 anal canal, and 1 appendix. Pathology was reviewed and carcinomas were categorized as small cell carcinomas ($n=22$) or large cell neuroendocrine carcinoma ($n=16$). Eighty percent stained positive by means of immunohistochemistry for neuroendocrine markers, including chromogranin, synaptophysin, and/or neuron-specific enolase. Metastatic disease was detected at the time of diagnosis in 69.4% of patients. As a group, these carcinomas had a poor prognosis with a mean survival of 10.4 months. One, two, and three year survival was 46%, 26%, and 13%, respectively. There was no significant difference in survival based on pathological subtypes. Median follow-up time was 9.4 months.

MEDULLARY CARCINOMA OF THE COLON

Wick et al. (1091) studied 68 sporadic colorectal carcinomas with medullary features and compared them with 35 poorly differentiated purely "enteric" colorectal carcinomas and 15 purely neuroendocrine carcinomas of grades II and III, all in patients lacking a family history of colorectal carcinoma. Medullary carcinomas were significantly more common in the ascending colon than were enteric carcinomas, but there was no significant dissimilarity to neuroendocrine carcinomas. Purely enteric carcinomas occurred more often in the rectosigmoid than medullary carcinomas or neuroendocrine carcinomas. Medullary carcinomas arose in older patients and a marked sex difference also was noted. Despite an infiltrated growth pattern, medullary carcinoma was less likely than enteric carcinomas to manifest with stage III or IV disease, but there was no stage-related difference from neuroendocrine carcinomas. Although the histologic images of medullary carcinomas were evocative of neuroendocrine differentiation, chromogranin positivity and synaptophysin reactivity in that group did not differ meaningfully from enteric colorectal carcinomas but was dissimilar to the 100% labeling of neuroendocrine carcinomas. p53 immunolabelling was similar in the three groups of carcinomas. Follow-up data in the study cases showed that 5-year mortality was 40% for medullary carcinomas, 59% for enteric carcinomas, and 93% for neuroendocrine carcinomas. Medullary colorectal carcinoma seems to be a distinct clinicopathologic variant of colorectal carcinoma, which does not have a neuroendocrine lineage. The biologic behavior of medullary carcinoma was better than that for enteric carcinomas or neuroendocrine carcinomas.

CARCINOSARCOMA

A unique case of carcinosarcoma of the colon has been reported (1092). It invaded the bowel wall deeply, metastasized widely, resisted multiagent chemotherapy, and caused the patient's death four years later. It was composed of adenosquamous carcinoma admixed with sarcoma showing osseous, cartilaginous, and nonspecific spindle-cell differentiation.

SCHWANNOMA

Schwannomas of the colon and rectum are uncommon. Miettinen et al. (1093) identified 20 colorectal schwannomas from the files of the Armed Forces Institute of Pathology. The schwannomas occurred equally in men and women in a wide age range (18–87 years). The most common location was cecum, followed by sigmoid and rectosigmoid, transverse colon, descending colon and rectum. The lesions commonly presented as polypoid intraluminal protrusions often with mucosal ulceration. Rectal bleeding, colonic obstruction, and abdominal pain were the most common presenting symptoms. The most common histologic variant ($n=15$) was a spindle-cell schwannoma with a trabecular pattern and vague or no Verocay bodies. These neoplasms ranged from 0.5 to 5.5 cm in diameter. A lymphoid cuff with germinal centers typically surrounded these lesions and focal nuclear atypia was often present, but mitotic activity never exceeded 5 per 50 HPF. All lesions were strongly positive for S-100 protein and negative for CD117 (KIT), neurofilament proteins, smooth muscle actin, and desmin. Colorectal schwannomas behaved in a benign fashion with no evidence of aggressive behavior or connection with neurofibromatosis 1 or 2, based on follow-up information on 18 patients.

ANGIOSARCOMA

Colorectal sarcomas are rare, accounting for less than 0.001% of all colorectal malignancies. Brown et al. (1094) recently reviewed the literature on the subject and the following information has been extracted from that review. Thirteen cases of colonic angiosarcoma have been reported in the literature. The majority (61%) of the patients were female. The locations of the sarcoma were: sigmoid ($n=5$), cecum ($n=4$), rectum ($n=2$), descending colon ($n=1$), and multiple colonic sites ($n=1$). Most patients presented with rectal bleeding ($n=7$), abdominal pain ($n=6$), abdominal mass ($n=5$), and/or weight loss ($n=3$). Although chronic lymphedema, radiation, thorium dioxide (Thorotrast) exposure, and a number of syndromes have been cited as risk factors for angiosarcoma, none of these were noted in the cases of colonic angiosarcoma reported in the literature. The presence of a foreign body, a predisposing factor noted in other cases of angiosarcoma, were seen in only one patient with colonic angiosarcoma who had a surgical sponge left in the abdomen after previous operation.

The histomorphology revealed dissecting, atypical vascular channels with plump and layered endothelial cells and areas of solid and spindled cells with an infiltrative and destructive growth pattern typical of angiosarcoma. The differential diagnosis would include sarcomatoid carcinoma, metastatic melanoma, and other sarcomas. Size has been shown to be an independent prognostic factor in angiosarcoma. In this series, five of six patients with a colonic angiosarcoma <5 cm in largest diameter were alive at last follow-up (13–24 months postoperative). Conversely, only 1 of 6 patients with size ≥ 5 cm was alive at last follow-up.

Patient age ranged from 16 to 77 years. Six of seven patients older than aged 60 years had rapid progression of their disease leading to death, whereas four of six patients younger than aged 60 years were still alive at the last reported follow-up (13–36 months postoperatively).

A review of the current literature on colorectal angiosarcoma revealed that surgical excision is the only management shown to result in long-term survival. All survivors had surgical resection of the lesion and none received adjuvant radiotherapy or chemotherapy for the primary lesion. The patient with the longest recorded survival is a 16-year-old female who had multiple peritoneal metastases at the time of her original operation. Despite incomplete resection of the lesion and no adjuvant therapy, the patient was alive and well at 36 months follow-up. These early findings suggest that the patient's age at the time of diagnosis may influence the prognosis of the disease.

With so few reported cases of angiosarcoma of the colon and rectum, the role of adjuvant therapy is unclear. Generally, there seems to be little or no survival benefit with adjuvant chemotherapy in the treatment of sarcoma and limited experience in angiosarcoma has shown similarly disappointing results. However, doxorubicin-based regimens have shown response rates of 25% in subset analysis of a randomized controlled trial of chemotherapy in sarcoma. The role of adjuvant radiotherapy is unclear.

CHORIOCARCINOMA

Primary choriocarcinoma of the colon is a very rare neoplasm with only seven reported cases in the world literature, all but two of which was associated with an adjacent adenocarcinoma (1095). This has led to the suggestion that colonic choriocarcinomas may arise from the more typical adenocarcinoma a process of further de-differentiation. The overall poor prognosis may reflect the late diagnosis and the high volume of metastatic disease.

METASTASES FROM OTHER SOURCES

Patients who present with a suspected colonic neoplasm and a past history of another malignancy should be considered to have possible metastatic disease, especially if the constriction appears extramucosal and the lesion is at the splenic flexure. If the colonic lesion is a squamous carcinoma, an extracolonic source should be sought because primary squamous cell carcinoma of the colon is extremely rare. Metastases from carcinoma of the lung (1096) or breast (1097,1098) presenting as primary colonic neoplasms have been reported. In a review of the literature, Washington and McDonagh (1099) found the most common sources of metastases to the colon and rectum to be melanoma, lung, and breast. From their own series of surgical autopsy specimens, the authors added gynecologic, bladder, prostate, and pancreas. Survival after the development of gastrointestinal involvement is generally poor, with most patients surviving <1 year. However, long-term palliation may be achieved in a small subset of patients, chiefly with single small bowel deposits of melanoma or those with breast carcinoma responsive to tamoxifen.

For patients with locally advanced ovarian carcinoma with contiguous extension to or encasement of the reproductive organs, pelvic peritoneum, cul-de-sac, and sigmoid colon, Bristow et al. (1100) reported on 31 consecutive patients undergoing radical oophorectomy and en bloc rectosigmoid colectomy with primary stapled anastomosis. All patients had advanced stage epithelial ovarian carcinoma; International Federation of obstetrics and Gynecology (FIGO) stage III B (6.5%), stage III C (64.5%), and stage IV (29%). There was one anastomotic breakdown requiring reoperation and colostomy. Complete clearance of macroscopic pelvic disease was achieved in all cases. Overall, 87.1% of patients were left with optimal ($\leq$1 cm) residual disease and 61.3% were visibly disease free. There were no postoperative deaths but major and minor postoperative morbidity occurred in 12.9% and 35.5% of patients, respectively. They concluded resection of locally advanced ovarian carcinoma contributes significantly to a maximal cytoreductive effort.

REFERENCES

1. DiSairo JA, Burt RW, Kendrick ML et al. Colorectal cancers of rare histologic types compared with adenocarcinomas. Dis Colon Rectum 1994; 37:1277–1280.
2. Jemal A, Murray T, Ward E, et al. MS Cancer Statistics 2005, CA 55:10–30.
3. McLaughlin JR, Dryer D, Mao Y, et al. Canadian Cancer Statistics Toronoto, Canada: National Cancer Institute of Canada, 2005.
4. Surveillance, Epidemiology, and End Results (SEER). SEER Cancer Statistics Review 1975–2001. Seer.cancer.gov. Accessed July 4, 2004.
5. Hayne D, Brown RS, McCormack M, Quinn MJ, Payne HA, Babb P. Current trends in colorectal cancer: site, incidence, mortality and survival in England and Wales. Clin Oncol (R Coll Radiol) 2001; 13(6):448–52.
6. Correa P, Haenszel W. The epidemiology of large bowel cancer. Adv Cancer Res 1978; 26:1–141.
7. Corman ML, Veidenheimer MC, Coller JA. Colorectal carcinoma: a decade of experience at the Lahey Clinic. Dis Colon Rectum 1979; 22:477–479.
8. Axtell LM, Cutler SJ, Myers MH, eds. End results in cancer, report no. 4. National Institutes of Health. Pub. no. 73–272. Bethesda, Md.: US Department of Health, Education and Welfare, 1972:217.
9. Fuchs CS, Giovannucci EL, Colditz GA, et al. A prospective study of family history and the risk of colorectal cancer. N Engl J Med 1994; 331: 1669–1674.
10. Slattery ML, Mori M, Gao R, et al. Impact of family history of colon cancer on development of multiple primaries after diagnosis of colon cancer. Dis Colon Rectum 1995; 38:1053–1058.
11. Hall NR, Bishop DT, Stephenson BM, et al. Hereditary susceptibility to colorectal cancer. Relatives of early onset cases are particularly at risk. Dis Colon Rectum 1996; 39:739–743.
12. St. John DJB, McDermott FT, Hoppes JL, et al. Cancer risk in relatives of patients with common colorectal cancer. Ann Intern Med 1993; 118:785–790.
13. Genetics of colorectal cancer (PDQ^R), Nov 19, 2003. http://www.cancer.gov/cancerinfo/pdq/genetics/colorectal.
14. Mamazza J, Gordon PH. The changing distribution of large intestinal cancer. Dis Colon Rectum 1982; 25:558–562.
15. Obrand DI, Gordon PH. The continued change in the distribution of colorectal carcinoma. Br J Surg 1998; 85:246–248.
16. Qing SH, Rao KY, Jiang HY, Wexner SD. Racial differences in the anatomical distribution of colorectal cancer: a study of differences between American and Chinese patients. World J Gastroenterol 2003; 9(4):721–725.
17. Cucino C, Buchner AM, Sonnenberg A. Continued rightward shift of colorectal cancer. Dis Colon Rectum 2002; 45:1035–1040.
18. Takada H, Ohsawa T, Iwamoto S, et al. Changing site distribution of colorectal cancer in Japan. Dis Colon Rectum 2002; 45:1249–1254.
19. Bang KM, White JE, Gause BL, et al. Evaluation of recent trends in cancer mortality and incidence among Blacks. Cancer 1988; 61:1255–1261.
20. Lynch HT, Rubinstein WS, Locker GY. Cancer in Jews: introduction and overview. Fam Cancer 2004; 3(3–4):177–192.
21. Kune GA, Kune S, Watson LF. Perceived religiousness is protective for colorectal cancer: data from the Melbourne Colorectal Cancer Study. J R Soc Med 1993; 86:645–647.
22. Vobecky J, Devroede G, Caro J. Risk of large bowel cancer in synthetic fiber manufacture. Cancer 1984; 54:2537–2542.
23. de Verdier MG, Plato N, Steinbeck G, et al. Occupational exposures and cancer of the colon and rectum. Am J Ind Med 1992; 22:291–303.
24. Homa DM, Garabrand DH, Gillespie BW. A meta-analysis of colorectal cancer and asbestos exposure. Am J Epidemiol 1994; 139:1210–1212.
25. Demers RY, Burns PB, Swanson GM. Construction occupations, asbestos exposure, and cancer of the colon and rectum. J Occup Med 1994; 36:1027–1031.
26. Spiegelman D, Wegman DH. Occupational-related risks for colorectal cancer. J Natl Cancer Inst 1985; 75:813–821.
27. Avni A, Feuchtwanger MM. Juvenile versus adult colonic cancer: distinct different etiologic factors. Dis Colon Rectum 1984; 27:842.
28. Acquavella JF, Douglass TS, Philips SC. Evaluation of excess colorectal cancer incidence among workers involved in the manufacture of polypropylene. J Occup Med 1988; 30:438–442.
29. Lewis RJ, Schnatter AR, Lerman SE. Colorectal cancer incidence among polypropylene manufacturing workers. An update. J Occup Med 1994; 36:652–659.
30. Walker Am, Cohe AJ, Loughlin JE, et al. Mortality from cancer of the colon or rectum among workers exposed to ethyl acrylate and methyl methacrylate. Scand J Work Environ Health 1991; 17:7–19.
31. Lennard-Jones JE, Melville DM, Morson BC, et al. Precancer and cancer in extensive ulcerative colitis: findings among 401 patients over 22 years. Gut 1990; 31:800–806.
32. Greenstein AJ, Sachar DB, Smith H, et al. A comparison of cancer risk in Crohn's disease and ulcerative colitis. Cancer 1981; 48:2742–2745.
33. Ekbom A, Helmick C, Zack M, et al. Ulcerative colitis in colorectal cancer: a population based study. N Engl J Med 1990; 323:1228–1233.
34. Munkholm P. Review article: the incidence and prevalance of colorectal cancer in inflammatory bowel disease. Aliment Pharmacol Ther 2003; 18(Suppl 2):1–5.
35. Ekbom A, Helmick C, Zack M, et al. Increased risk of large bowel cancer in Crohn's disease with colonic involvement. Lancet 1990; 336:357–359.
36. Allen JI. Molecular biology of colorectal cancer: a clinician's view. Perspect Colon Rectal Surg 8:181–202, 195.
37. Knudson A. Hereditary cancer, oncogenes, and antioncogenes. Cancer Res 1985; 45:1437.
38. Lynch HT, Smyrk T. Hereditary non-polyposis colorectal cancer (Lynch syndrome): an updated review. Cancer 1996; 78:1149–1167.
39. Foulkes WD, Thiffault I, Gruber SB, et al. The founder mutation MSH2*1906G->C is an important cause of hereditary nonpolyposis colorectal cancer in the Ashkenazi Jewish population. Am J Hum Genet 2002; 71:1395–412.
40. Guillem JG, Rapaport BS, Kirchhoff T, et al. A636P is associated with early-onset colon cancer in Ashkenazi Jews. J Am Coll Surg 2003; 196: 222–225.
41. Nystrom-Lahti M, Kristo P, Nicolaides NC, et al. Founding mutations and alu-mediated recombination in hereditary colon cancer. Nature Med 1995; 1: 1203–1206.
42. Peltomaki P. Role of DNA mismatch repair defects in the pathogenesis of human cancer. J Clin Oncol 2003; 21:1174–1179.
43. Burt RW, Bishop T, Cannon LA, et al. Dominant inheritance of adenomatous polyps and colorectal cancer. N Engl J Med 1985; 312:1540–1544.
44. Solomon E, Voss R, Hall V. Chromosome 5 allele loss in human colorectal carcinomas. Nature 1987; 328:616–619.
45. Law DS, Olschwang S, Monpezat JP, et al. Concerted non-syntenic allelic loss in human colorectal carcinoma. Science 1988; 241:961–965.
46. Fearon ER, Vogelstein B. A genetic model for colorectal tumorigenesis. Cell 1990; 61:759–767.

47. Wang L, Patel U, Gosh L, et al. Mutation in the NM23 gene is associated with metastasis in colorectal cancer. Cancer Res 1993; 53:717–720.
48. Aaltonen LA, Peltomaki P, Leach FS, et al. Clues to the pathogenesis of familial colorectal cancer. Science 1993; 260:812–816.
49. Lu SL, Kawabata M, Imamura T, et al. HNPCC associated with germline mutation in the TGF-beta type II receptor gene. Nat Genet 1998; 19:17–18.
50. Liu B, Nicolaides NC, Markowitz S, et al. Mismatch repair gene defects in sporadic colorectal camcers with microsatellite instability. Nat Genet. 1995; 7:48–55..
51. DeFrancisco J, Grady WM. Diagnosis and management of hereditary non-polyposis colon cancer. Gastrointest Endosc 2003; 58:390–408.
52. Lawes DA, SenGupta S, Boulos PB. The clinical importance and prognostic implications of microsatellite instability in sporadic cancer. Eur J Surg Oncol 2003; 29:201–212.
53. Piepoli A, Santoro R, Cristofaro G, et al. Linkage analysis identifies gene carriers among members of families with hereditary non-polyposis colorectal cancer. Gastroenterology 1996; 110:1404–1409.
54. Vasen HFA, Mecklin JP, Khan PM, et al. The International Colaborative Group on Hereditary Non-Polyposis Colorectal Cancer (ICG-HNPCC). Dis Colon Rectum 1991; 34:424–425.
55. Aaltonen LA, Sankila R, Mecklin JP, et al. A novel approach to estimate the proportion of hereditary non-polyposis colorectal cancer of total colorectal cancer burden. Cancer Detect Prev 1994; 18:57–63.
56. Boland CR, Brown EF, Evans RM, Goldberg A, Short MP. Identifying and Managing Risk for Hereditary Nonpolyposis Colorectal Cancer and Endometrial Cancer (HNPCC) American Medical Association and America Gastroenterological Association Continuing Medical Edueda 2001; 1–21.
57. Umar A, Boland CR, Terdiman JP, et al. Revised Bethesda Guidelines for hereditary nonpolyposis colorectal cancer (Lynch syndrome) and microsatellite instability. J Natl Cancer Inst 2004; 96(4):261–268.
58. Pinol V, Castells A, Andreu M, et al. Gastrointestinal oncology group of the Spanish gastroenterological association. Accuracy of revised Bethesda guidelines, microsatellite instability, and Immunohistochemistry for identification of patients with hereditary non polyposis colorectal cancer. JAMA 2005; 293(16):1986–1994.
59. De Jong AE, Morreau H, Van Pujjenbroek M, et al. The role of mismatch repair gene defects in the development of adenomas in patients with HNPCC. Gastroenterology 2004; 126(1):42–48.
60. Cunningham C, Dunlop MG. Molecular genetic basis of colorectal cancer susceptibility. Br J Surg 1996; 83:321–329.
61. Mecklin JP, Jarvinen HJ. Tumor spectrum in Cancer Family Syndrome (hereditary non-polyposis colorectal cancer). Cancer 1991; 68:1109–1112.
62. Aarnio M, Mecklin JP, Aaltonen LA, Nystrom-Lahti M, Jarvinen HJ. Life-time risk of different cancers in hereditary non-polyposis colorectal cancer (HNPCC) syndrome. Int J Cancer 1995; 64:430–433.
63. Brezden-Masley C, Aronson MD, Bapat B, et al. Hereditary nonpolyposis colorectal cancer-molecular basis. Surgery 2003; 134:29–33.
64. Plaschke J, Engel C, Kruger S, et al. Lower incidence of colorectal and later age of disease onset in 27 families with pathogenic MSH6 germline mutations compared with familes with MLH1 or MSH2 mutations: the German Hereditary Nonpolyposis Colorectal Cancer Consortium. J Clin Oncol 2004; 22(22):4486–4494.
65. Lindor NM, Rabe K, Petersen GM, et al. Lower cancer incidence in Amsterdam-I criteria families without mismatch repair deficiency: familial colorectal cancer type X. JAMA 2005; 293(16):1979–1985.
66. Jass JR. Colorectal adenomas in surgical specimens from subjects with hereditary non-polyposis colorectal cancer. Histopathology 1995; 27:263–267.
67. Mecklin JP, Sipponen P, Jarvinen H. Histopathology of colorectal carcinomas and adenomas in cancer family syndrome. Dis Colon Rectum 1986; 29:849–853.
68. Sankila R, Aaltonen LA, Jarvinen HJ, et al. Better survival rates in patients with MLH1-associated hereditary colorectal cancer. Gastroenterology 1996; 110:682–687.
69. Tomoda H, Baba H, Oshiro T. Clinical manifestations in patients with hereditary non-polyposis colorectal cancer. J Surg Oncol 1996; 61:262–266.
70. Rodriguez-Bigas MA, Lee PHV, O'Malley L, et al. Establishment of a hereditary non-polyposis colorectal cancer registry. Dis Colon Rectum 1996; 39:649–653.
71. Hampel H, Frankel WL, Martin E, et al. Screening for the Lynch syndrome (hereditary nonpolyposis colorectal cancer). N Engl J Med 2005; 352(18): 1851–1860.
72. Lynch HT, Smyrk T, Lynch JF. Overview of natural history, pathology, molecular genetics, and management of HNPCC (Lynch syndrome). Int J Cancer (Pred Oncol) 1996; 36:38–43.
73. Jarvinen HJ, Aarnio M, Mustonen H, et al. Controlled 15-year trial on screening for colorectal cancer in families with hereditary nonpolyposis colorectal cancer. Gastroenterology 2000; 118:829–834.
74. de Vos tot Nederveen Cappel WH, Nagengast FM, Griffioen G, Menko FH, Taal BG, Kleibeuker JH, Vasen HF. Surveillance for hereditary nonpolyposis colorectal cancer: a long-term study on 114 families. Dis Colon Rectum 2002; 45(12):1588–1594.
75. Mecklin JP, Jarvinen H. Treatment and follow-up strategies in hereditary nonpolyposis colorectal carcinoma. Dis Colon Rectum 1993; 36:927–929.
76. Itoh H, Houlsten RS, Harocopos C, et al. Risk of cancer death in first-degree relatives of patients with hereditary non-polyposis cancer syndrome. (Lynch type II): a study of 130 kindreds in the United Kingdom. Br J Surg 1990; 77:1367–1370.
77. Brown GJ, St John DJ, Macrae FA, Aittomaki K. Cancer risk in young women at risk of hereditary nonpolyposis colorectal cancer: implications for gynecologic surveillance. Gynecol Oncol 2001; 80:346–349.
78. Watson P, Butzow R, Lynch HT, et al. International Collaborative Group on HNPCC. The clinical features of ovarian cancer in hereditary nonpolyposis colorectal cancer. Gynecol Oncol 2001; 82:223–228.
79. Meijers-Heijboer H, Wijnen J, Vasen H, ET AL. The CHEK2 1100delC mutation identifies families with a hereditary breast and colorectal cancer phenotype. Am J Hum Genet 2003; 72:1304–1314.
80. Wong N, Lasko D, Rabelo R, Pinsky L, Gordon PH, Foulkes W. Genetic counselling and interpretation of gentic tests in familial adenomatous polyposis and hereditary nonpolyposis colorectal cancer. Dis Colon Rectum 2001; 44:271–279.
81. Rabelo R, Foulkes W, Gordon PH, et al. Role of molecular diagnostic testing in familial adenomatous polyposis and hereditary nonpolyposis colorectal cancer families. Dis Colon Rectum 2001; 44:437–446.
82. Dunlop MG, Farrington SM, Carothers AD, et al. Cancer risk associated with germline DNA mismatch repair gene mutations. Hum Mol Genet 1997; 6:105–110.
83. Xia L, Shen W, Ritacca F, et al. A truncated hM SH2 transcript occurs as a common variant in the population: implications for genetic testing. Cancer Res 1996; 56:2289–2292.
84. Keller M, Jost R, Kadmon M, et al. Acceptance of and attitude toward genetic testing for hereditary nonpolyposia colorectal cancer: a comparison of participants and nonparticipants in genetic counseling. Dis Colon Rectum 2004; 47:153–162.
85. Gritz ER, Peterson SK, Vernon SW, et al. Psychological impact of genetic testing for hereditary nonpolyposis colorectal cancer. J Clin Oncol 2005; 23(9): 1902–1910.
86. ASHG Statement. Professional disclosure of familial genetic information. The American Society of Human Genetics Social Issues Subcommittee on Familial Disclosure. Am J Hum Genet 1998; 62:474–483.
87. Lerman C, Marshall J, Audrian J, et al. Genetic testing for colon cancer susceptibility: anticipated reactions of patients and challenges to providers. Int J Cancer (Pred Oncol) 1996; 69:58–61.
88. Hadley DW, Jenkins JF, Dimond E, de Carvalho M, Kirsch I, Plamer CGS. Colon cancer screening practices after genetic counseling and testing for hereditary nonpolyposis colorectal cancer. J Clini Oncol 2004; 22:39–44.
89. Offit K. Clinical Cancer Genetics. Risk counseling and management. 1st ed. New York: Wiley-Liss, 1998:301.
90. Jass JR, Whitehall VL, Young J, Leggett BA. Emerging concepts in colorectal neoplasia. Gastroenterology 2002; 123:862–876.
91. Lamprecht SA, Lipkin M. Chemoprevention of colon cancer by calcium, vitamin D and folate: molecular mechanisms. Nat Rev Cancer 2003; 3:601–614.
92. Nagao M, Sugimura T. Carcinogenic factors in food with relevance to colon cancer development. Mutat Res 1993; 290:43–51.
93. Miller AB, Howe GR, Jain M, et al. Food items and food groups as risk factors in a case-control study of diet and colo-rectal cancer. Int J Cancer 1983; 32: 155–161.
94. Willett WC, Stampfer MJ, Colditz GA, et al. Relation of meat, food, and fiber intake to the risk of colon cancer in a prospective study amongst women. N Engl J Med 1990; 323:164–172.
95. Nigro ND, Singh DV, et al. Effect of dietary beef fat on intestinal cancer formation in rats. J Natl Cancer Inst 1975; 54:439–442.
96. Reddy BS, Maruyana H. Effect of dietary fish oil on colon carcinogenesis in rats. Cancer Res 1986; 46:3367–3370.
97. Chao A, Thun MJ, Connell CJ. Meat consumption and risk of colorectal cancer. JAMA 2005; 293(2):233–234.
98. Larsson SC, Rafter J, Holmberg L, Bergvist L, Wolk A. Red meat consumption and risk of cancers of the proximal colon, distal colon and rectum: the Swedish Mammography Cohort. Int J Cancer 2005; 113(5):829–834.
99. Norat T, Bingham S, Ferrari P, et al. Meat, fish, and colorectal cancer risk: the European Prospective Investigation into cancer and nutrition. J Natl Cancer Inst 2005; 97:906–916.
100. Burkitt DP. Epidemiology of cancer of the colon and rectum. Cancer 1971; 28:3–13.
101. Fleiszer D, MacFarlane J, Murray D, et al. Protective effect of dietary fiber against chemically induced bowel tumours in rats. Lancet 1978; 2:552–553.
102. Nigro ND, Bull AW, Klopfer BA, et al. Effect of dietary fiber on intestinal carcinogenesis in rats. J Natl Cancer Inst 1979; 62:1097–1102.
103. Greenwald P, Lanza E, Eddy GA. Dietary fiber in the reduction of colon cancer. J AM Diet Assoc 1987; 87:1178–1188.
104. Trock B, Lanza E, Greenwald P. Dietary fiber, vegetables and colon cancer: critical review and meta-analysis of the epidemiological evidence. J Natl Cancer Inst 1990; 82:650–661.
105. Freudenheim JL, Graham S, Horvath PJ, et al. Risks associated with source of fibre and fibre components in cancer of the colon and rectum. Cancer Res 1990; 52:3295–3300.

106. Frentzel-Beyme R, Cheng-Claude J. Vegetarian diets and colon cancer: the German experience. Am J Clin Nutr 1994; 59(suppl):1143S–1152S.
107. Asano T, McLeod RS. Dietary fibre for the prevention of colorectal adenomas and carcinomas. Cochrane Database Syst Rev 2002(2):CD003430.
108. Fuchs CS, Giovannucci EL, Colditz GA, et al. Dietary fiber and the risk of colorectal cancer and adenoma in women. N Engl J Med 1999; 340:169–176.
109. Michels KB, Giovannucci, Joshipura KJ, et al. Prospective study of fruit and vegetable consumption and incidence of colon and rectal cancers. J Natl Cancer Inst 2000; 92:1740–1752.
110. Terry P, Giovannucci E, Michels KB, et al. Fruit, vegetables, dietary fiber, and risk of colorectal cancer. J Natl Cancer Inst 2001; 93:525–533.
111. Peters U, Sinha R, Chatterjee N, et al. Prostate, Lung, Colorectal, and Ovarian Cancer Screening Trial Project Team. Dietary fibre and colorectal adenoma in a colorectal cancer early detection programme. Lancet 2003, 361: 1491–1495.
112. Meyer F, White E. Alcohol and nutrients in relation to colon cancer in middle-aged adults. Am J Epidemiol 1993; 138(4):225–236.
113. Howe GR, Benito E, Castelleto R, et al. Dietary intake of fiber and decreased risk of cancers of the colon and rectum: evidence from the combined analysis of 13 case-control studies. J Natl Cancer Inst 1992; 84:1887–1896.
114. Bingham SA, Day NE, Luben R, et al. European Prospective Investigation into Cancer and Nutrition. Dietary fibre in food and protection against colorectal cancer in the European Prospective Investigation into Cancer and Nutrition (EPIC): an observational study. Lancet 2003 361:1496–1501.
115. Slattery ML, Sorenson AW, Ford MH. Dietary calcium intake as a mitigating factor in colon cancer. Am J Epidemiol 1988; 128:504–514.
116. Garland C, Shekelle RD, Barrett-Connor E, et al. Dietary vitamin D and calcium and risk of colorectal cancer: a 19 year prospective study in men. Lancet 1985; 1:307–309.
117. Rozen P, Fireman Z, Wax Y, et al. Oral calcium suppresses colonic mucosal proliferation of persons at risk for colorectal neoplasia. Gastroenterology 1987; 92:1603.
118. Wargovich MJ, Lynch PM, Levin B. Modulating effects of calcium in animal models of colon carcinogenesses and short-term studies in subjects at increased risk for colon cancer. Am J Clin Nutr 1991; 54:2025–2055.
119. Baron JA, Beach M, Mandel JS, et al. Calcium supplements for the prevention of colorectal adenomas, Calcium Polyp Prevention Study Group. N Engl J Med 1999; 340:101–117.
120. Wu K, Willett WC, Fuchs CS, Colditz GA, Giovannucci EL. Calcium intake and risk of colon cancer in women and men. J Natl Cancer Inst 2002; 94:437–446.
121. Wallace K, Baron JA, Cole BF, et al. Effect of calcium supplementation on the risk of large bowel polyps. J Natl Cancer Inst 2004; 96(12):921–925.
122. Larsson SC, Bergkvist L, Wolk A. Magnesium intake in relation to risk of colorectal cancer in women. JAMA 2005; 293(1):86–89.
123. Vernie LN. Selenium in carcinogenesis. Biochim Biophys Acta 1984; 738: 203–217.
124. Rumi G, Imre I, Sulle G, et al. Selenium in the blood of patients with colorectal cancer and neoplastic polyp. Acta Physiol Hung 1992; 80:275–279.
125. Finley JW. Reduction of cancer risk by consumption of selenium-enriched plants: enrichment of broccoli with selenium increases the anticarcinogenic properties of broccoli. J Med Food 2003; 6:19–26.
126. Nelson RL, Davis FG, Sutter E, et al. Serum selenium and colonic neoplastic risk. Dis Colon Rectum 1995; 38:1306–1310.
127. Jacobs ET, Jiang R, Alberts DS, et al. Selenium and colorectal adenoma: results of a pooled analysis. J Natl Cancer Inst 2004; 96(22):1669–1675.
128. Nigro ND, Bull AW. Prospects for the prevention of colorectal cancer. Dis Colon Rectum 1987; 30:751–754.
129. Wargovich MJ. New dietary anticarcinogens and prevention of gastrointestinal cancer. Dis Colon Rectum 1988; 31:72–75.
130. Wattenberg LW. Chemoprevention of cancer. Cancer Res 1985; 45:1–8.
131. Nigro ND, Bull AW, Wilson PS, et al. Combined inhibitors of carcinogenesis or intestinal cancer in rats. J Natl Cancer Inst 1982; 69:103–107.
132. Colacchio TA, Memoli VA. Chemoprevention of colorectal neoplasms. Arch Surg 1986; 121:1421–1424.
133. Lognecker MP. A case-control study of alcoholic beverage consumption in relation to risk of cancer of the right colon and rectum in men. Cancer Causes Control 1990; 1:5–14.
134. Pollack ES, Nomura AMY, Heilbrun LK, et al. Prospective study of alcohol consumption and cancer. N Engl J Med 1984; 310:617–621.
135. Newcomb PA, Storer BE, Marcus PM. Cancer of the large bowel in women in relation to alcohol consumption: a case-control study in Wisconsin (United States). Cancer Causes Control 1993; 4:405–411.
136. Kato I, Tominaga S, Ikari A. A case-control study of male colorectal cancer in Aichi Prefecture, Japan: with special reference to occupational activity level, drinking habits and family history. Jpn J Cancer Res 1990; 81:115–121.
137. Riboli E, Cornée J, Macquart-Moulin G, et al. Cancer and polyps of the colorectum and lifetime consumption of beer and other alcoholic beverages. Am J Epidemiol 1991; 133:157–166.
138. Serralva MS, Anjos J, Vilaca F. Colorectal carcinoma in patients older than 65 years: prognostic factors. Br J Surg 1995; 82(suppl 1):35–36.
139. Carstensen JM, Bygren LO, Hatscheck T. Cancer incidence among Swedish brewery workers. Int J Cancer 1990; 45:393–396.
140. Maekawa SJ, Aoyama N, Shirasaka D, et al. Excessive alcohol intake enhances the development of synchronous cancerous lesion in colorectal cancer patients. Int J Colorectal Dis 2004; 18:171–175.
141. Sharpe CR, Siemiatycki J, Rachet B. Effects of alcohol consumption on the risk of colorectal cancer among men by anatomical subsite (Canada). Cancer Causes Control 2002; 13:483–491.
142. Kikendall JW, Bowen PE, Burgess MB, et al. Cigarettes and alcohol as independent risk factors for colonic adenomas. Gastroenterology 1989; 97: 660–664.
143. Giovannucci E, Rimm EB, Stampfer MJ, et al. A prospective study of cigarette smoking and risk of colorectal adenoma and colorectal cancer in U.S. men. J Natl Cancer Inst 1994; 86:183–191.
144. Giovannucci E, Colditz GA, Stampfer MJ, et al. A prospective study of cigarette smoking and risk of colorectal adenoma and colorectal cancer in U.S. women. J Natl Cancer Inst 1994; 86:192–199.
145. Chao A, Thun MJ, Jacobs EJ, Henley SJ, Rodriguez C, Calle EE. Cigarette smoking and colorectal cancer mortality in the cancer prevention study II. J Natl Cancer Inst 2000; 92:1888–1896.
146. Jain M, Cook GM, Davis FG, et al. A case-control study of diet and colorectal cancer. Int J Cancer 1980; 26:757–768.
147. Potter JD, McMichael AJ. Diet and cancer of the colon and rectum: a case-control study. J Natl Cancer Inst 1986; 76:557–569.
148. Kritchevsky D. Epidemiology of fibre, resistant starch and colorectal cancer. Eur J Cancer Prev 1995; 4:345–352.
149. Phillips RL, Snowdon DA. Dietary relationships with fatal colorectal cancer among Seventh-Day Adventists. J Natl Cancer Inst 1985; 74:307–317.
150. Stemmerman GN, Nomura MY, Heilbrun LK. Dietary fat and the risk of colorectal cancer. Cancer Res 1984; 44:4633–4637.
151. Berry EM, Zimmerman J, Ligumsky M. The nature of dietary fat and plasma lipids in relation to the development of polyps and carcinoma of the colon. Gastroenterology 1985; 88:1323.
152. Freudenheim JL, Graham S, Marshall JR, et al. A case-control study of diet and rectal cancer in western New York. Am J Epidemiol 1990; 131: 612–624.
153. Giovannucci E, Stampfer MJ, Colditz GA, et al. Multivitamin use, folate, and colon cancer in women in the Nurses' Health Study. Ann Intern Med 1998; 129:517–524.
154. Fernandez E, Chatenoud L, La Vecchia C, Negri E, Franceschi S. Fish consumption and cancer risk. Am J Clin Nutr 1999; 70:85–90.
155. Jao SW, Beart RW Jr., Reiman HM, et al. Colon and anorectal cancer after pelvic irradiation. Dis Colon Rectum 1987; 30:953–958.
156. Matsuo T, Ito M, Sekine I, et al. Mucosal de novo cancer of the rectum following radiation therapy for uterine cancer. Intern Med 1993; 32:427–429.
157. Tamai O, Nozato E, Miyazato H, et al. Radiation-associated rectal cancer: report of four cases. Dig Surg 1999; 16(3):238–243.
158. Martins A, Sternberg SS, Attiyeh FF. Radiation-induced carcinoma of the rectum. Dis Colon Rectum 1980; 23:572–575.
159. Shirouzu K, Isomoto H, Morodomi T, et al. Clinicopathologic characterisitics of large bowel cancer developing after radiotherapy for uterine cervical cancer. Dis Colon Rectum 1994; 37:1245–1249.
160. Hareyama M, Okubo O, Oouchi A, et al. A case of carcinoma of the rectum after radiotherapy for carcinoma of the cervix. Radiat Med 1989; 7:197–200.
161. Baxter NN, Tepper JE, Durham SB, Rothenberger DA, Virnig BA. Increased risk of rectal cancer after prostate radiation: a population-based study. Gastroenterology 2005; 128(4):819–824.
162. Labow SB, Hoexter B, Walrath DC. Colonic adenocarcinomas in patients with ureterosigmoidostomies. Dis Colon Rectum 1979; 22:157–158.
163. Sheldon CA, McKinley CR, Hartig PR, et al. Carcinoma at the site of ureterosigmoidostomy. Dis Colon Rectum 1983; 26:55–58.
164. Van Driel MF, Zwiers W, Grand S, et al. Juvenile polyps at the site of a ureterosigmoidostomy. Report of 5 cases. Dis Colon Rectum 1988; 31: 553–557.
165. Guy RJ, Handa A, Traill Z, Mortensen NJ, et al. Rectosigmoid carcinoma at previous ureterosigmoidostomy site in a renal transplant recipient: report of a case. Dis Colon Rectum 2001; 44(10):1534–1539.
166. Kalble T, Tricker AR, Friedl P, et al. Ureterosigmoidostomy: long-term results, risk of carcinoma, and etiological factors for carcinogenesis. J Urol 1990; 144:1110–1114.
167. Kliment J, Luptak J, Lofaj M, et al. Carcinoma of the colon after ureterosigmoidostomy and trigonosigmoidostomy for extrophy of the bladder. Int Urol Nephrol 1993; 25:339–343.
168. Husmann DA, Spence HM. Current status of tumor of the bowel following ureterosigmoidostomy. A review. J Urol 1990; 144:607–610.
169. Zaridze DG. Environmental etiology of large-bowel cancer. J Natl Cancer Inst 1983; 70:389–400.
170. Hill MJ. Mechanism of colorectal carcinogenesis. Joosens JV, Hill MJ, Geboers J, eds. Diet and Human Carcinogenesis. Amsterdam: Elsevier Science, 1986:149–164.
171. Jorgensen T, Rafaelsen S. Gallstones and colorectal cancer—There is a relationship, but it is hardly due to cholecystectomy. Dis Colon Rectum 1992; 35:24–28.

172. Schernhammer ES, Leitzmann MF, Michaud DS et al. Cholecystectomy and the risk for developing colorectal cancer and distal colorectal adenomas. Br J Cancer 2003; 88:78–83.
173. Legergren J, Ye W, Ekbom A. Intestinal cancer after cholecystectomy: is bile involved in carcinogenesis? Gastroentelogy 2001; 121(3):542–547.
174. Wynder El, Reddy BS. Metabolic epidemiology of colorectal cancer. Cancer 1974; 34:801–806.
175. Moorehead RJ, McKelvey STD. Cholecystectomy and colorectal cancer. Br J Surg 1989; 76:250–253.
176. Gafa M, Sarli L, Sansebastiano G, et al. Prevention of colorectal cancer. Role of association between gallstones and colorectal cancer. Dis Colon Rectum 1987; 30:692–696.
177. Hickman MS, Salinas HC, Schwesinger WH. Does cholecystectomy affect colonic tumorigenesis? Arch Surg 1987; 12:334–336.
178. McMichael A, Potter JD. Host factors in carcinogenesis: certain bile acid metabolic profiles that selectively increase the risk of colon cancer. J Natl Cancer Inst 1985; 75:185–191.
179. Nielsen GB, Theodoro A, Tulinius A, et al. Cholecystectomy and colorectal carcinoma: a total-population historical prospective study. Am J Gastroenterol 1991; 88:1486–1490.
180. McFarlane MJ, Welch KE. Gallstones, cholecystectomy, and colorectal cancer. Am J Gastroenterol 1993; 88:1994–1999.
181. Abrams JS, Anton JR, Dreyfuss DC. The absence of a relationship between cholecystectomy and the subsequent occurrence of cancer of the proximal colon. Dis Colon Rectum 1983; 26:141–144.
182. Kune GA, Kune S, Watson LF. Large bowel cancer after cholecystectomy. Am J Surg 1988; 156:359–362.
183. Kaibara N, Wakatsuki T, Mizusawa K, et al. Negative correlation between cholecystectomy and the subsequent development of large bowel carcinoma in a low risk Japanese population. Dis Colon Rectum 1986; 29:644–646.
184. Ekbom A, Yuen J, Adami HO, et al. Cholecystectomy and colorectal cancer. Gastroenterology 1993; 105:142–147.
185. Neugent AI, Murray TI, Garbowski GC, et al. Cholecystectomy as a risk factor for colorectal adenomatous polypoid carcinoma. Cancer 1991; 68: 1644–1647.
186. Boulos PB, Cowin AP, Karamanolis DG, et al. Diverticula, neoplasia, or both? Early detection of carcinoma in sigmoid diverticular disease. Ann Surg 1985; 202:607–609.
187. Morini S, Angelis P, Manurita L, et al. Association of colonic diverticula with adenomas and carcinomas. A colonoscopic experience. Dis Colon Rectum 1988; 31:793–796.
188. Persky V, Andrianopoulos G. The etiology of cancer of the colon. It it all in the diet? Nelson RL, ed. Problems in Current Surgery. Controversies in Colon Cancer. Philadelphia: JB Lippincott, 1987:11–23.
189. Thune I, Lund E. Physical activity and risk of colorectal cancer in men and women. Br J Cancer 1996; 73:1134–1140.
190. Slattery ML, Edwards S, Curtin K, et al. Physical activity and colorectal cancer. Am J Epidemiol 2003; 158:214–224.
191. Terry MB, Neugut AI, Bostick RM, et al. Risk factors for advanced colorectal adenomas: a pooled analysis. Cancer Epidemiol Biomarkers Prev 2002; 11:622–629.
192. Colbert LH, Hartman TJ, Malila N, et al. Physical activity in relation to cancer of the colon and rectum in a cohort of male smokers. Cancer Epidemiol Biomakers Prev 2001; 10:265–268.
193. Longnecker MP, de Verdier MG, Frumkin H, et al. A case-control study of physical activity in relation to risk of cancer of the right colon and rectum in men. Int J Epidemiol 1995; 24:42–50.
194. White E, Jacobs EJ, Daling JR. Physical activity in relation to colon cancer in middle-aged men and women. Am J Epidemiol 1996; 144:42–50.
195. Quadrilatero J, Hoffman-Geotz L. Physical activity and colon cancer. A systematic review of potential mechanisms. J Sports Med Phys Fitness 2003; 43(2):121–138.
196. Neugent AI, Santos J. The association between cancers of the small bowel and large bowel cancers. Epidemiol Biomarkers Prev 1993; 2:551–553.
197. Sonnenberg A, Müller AD. Constipation and cathartics as risk factors of colorectal cancer: a meta-analysis. Pharmacology 1993; 47(suppl 1):224–233.
198. Singh S, Morgan BF, Broughton M, et al. A 10 year prospective audit of outcome of surgical treatment for colorectal carcinoma. Br J Surg 1995; 82: 1486–1490.
199. Brodeurs MJM, Lambe M, Bacon JA, et al. History of child-bearing and colorectal cancer risk in women aged less than 60: an analysis of Swedish routine registry data 1960–1984. Int J Cancer 1996; 66:170–175.
200. Newcomb PA, Storer BE. Postmenopausal hormone use and risk of large bowel cancer. J Natl Cancer Inst 1995; 87:1067–1071.
201. Calle EE, Miracle-McMahill HL, Thun MJ, et al. Estrogen replacement therapy and risk of fatal colon cancer in a prospective cohort of postmenopausal women. J Natl Cancer Inst 1995; 87:517–523.
202. Jacobs EJ, White E, Weiss NS. Exogeneous hormone reproductive history, and colon cancer (Seattle, Washington, U.S.). Cancer Causes Control 1994; 5: 359–366.
203. Marcus PM, Newcomb PA, Young T, et al. The association of reproductive and menstrual characteristics, and colon and rectal cancer risk in Wisconsin women. Ann Epidemiol 1995; 5:303–309.
204. Grodstein F, Newcomb PA, Stampfer MJ. Postmenopausal hormone therapy and the risk of colorectal cancer: a review and meta-analysis. Am J Med 1999; 106:574–582.
205. Baris D, Gridley G, Ron E, et al. Acromegaly and cancer risk: a cohort study in Sweden and Denmark. Cancer Causes Control 2002; 13:395–400.
206. Mullen PJ, Wilson HK, Majury CW, et al. Bile acids and the increased risk of colorectal tumors after truncal vagotomy. Br J Surg 1990; 77:1085–1090.
207. Fisher SG, Davis F, Nelson R, et al. Large bowel cancer following gastric surgery for benign disease: a cohort study. Am. J. Epidemiol. 1994; 139:684–92.
208. Little J, Owen RW, Fernandez F, et al. Asymptomatic colorectal neoplasia and fecal characteristics: a case-control study of subjects participating in the Nottingham fecal occult blood screening trial. Dis Colon Rectum 2002; 45: 1233–1241.
209. Babbs CF. Free radicals and the etiology of colon cancer. Free Radic Biol Med 1990; 8:191–200.
210. Gorbach SL, Goldin BL. The intestinal microflora and the colon cancer connection. Rev Infect Dis 1990; 12:S252.
211. Knekt P, Reunanen A, Takkunen H, et al. Body iron stores and risk of cancer. Int J Cancer 1994; 56:379–382.
212. Vesterinen E, Pukkala E, Timonen T, et al. Cancer incidence among 78,000 asthmatic patients. Int J Epidemiol 1993; 22:976–982.
213. Howden CW, Hornung CA. A systematic review of the association between Barrett's esophagus and colon neoplasm. Am J Gastoenterol 1995; 90: 1814–1819.
214. Vaughan TL, Kiemeney LALM, McKnight B. Colorectal cancer in patients with esophageal adenocarcinoma cancer. Epidemiol Biomar Prev 1995; 4:93–97.
215. Seigers CP, von Hertzberg-Lottin E, Otte M, et al. Anthanoid laxative abuse—A risk for colorectal cancer? Gut 1993; 34:1099–1101.
216. Younes M, Katikaneni RR, Lechago J. Association between mucosal hyperplasia of the appendix and adenocarcinoma of the colon. Histopathology 1995; 26:33–37.
217. Erlinger TP, Platz EA, Rifai N, Helzlsouer KJ. C-reactive protein and the risk of incident colorectal cancer. JAMA 2004; 291:585–590.
218. Woolcott CG, King WD, Marrett LD. Coffee and tea consumption and cancers of the bladder, colon and rectum. Eur J Cancer Prev 2002; 11:137–145.
219. Kavan MG, Engdahl BE, Kay S. Colon cancer: personality factors predictive of onset and stage of presentation. J Psychosom Res 1995; 39:1031–1039.
220. Galloway DJ, Indran M, Carr K, et al. Dietary manipulation during experimental carcinogenesis: a morphological study in the rat. Int J Colorectal Dis 1987; 2:193–200.
221. Shatzkin A, Kelloff G. Chemo-and dietary prevention of colorectal cancer. Eur J Cancer 1995; 31A:1198–1204.
222. Cassidy A, Bingham SA, Cummings JH. Starch intake and colorectal cancer risk; an international comparison. Br J Cancer 1994; 69:937–942.
223. Thun MJ, Namboodiri MM, Heath CW. Aspirin use and reduced risk of fatal colon cancer. N Engl J Med 1991; 325:1593–1596.
224. Rosenberg L, Palmer JR, Zauber AG, et al. A hypothesis: non-steroidal anti-inflammatory drugs reduce the incidence of large bowel cancer. J Natl Cancer Inst 1991; 83:355–358.
225. Smalley W, Ray WA, Daugherty J, Griffin MR. Use of nonsteroidal anti-inflammatory drugs and incidence of colorectal cancer: a population-based study. Arch Intern Med 1999; 159:161–166.
226. Baron JA, Cole BF, Sandler RS, et al. A randomized trial of aspirin to prevent colrectal adenomas. N Engl J Med 2003; 348:891–899.
227. Sturmer T, Glynn RJ, Lee IM, Manson JE, Buring JE, Hennekens CH. Aspirin use and colorectal cancer: post-trial follow-up data from the Physicians' Health Study. Ann Intern Med 1998; 128:713–720.
228. Burke CA, Bauer WM, Lashner B. Chemoprevention of colorectal cancer: slow, steady progress. Cleve Clin J Med 2003; 70:346–350.
229. Greenwald P, Kellofff G, Burch-WhitmanC, et al. Chemoprevention. CA Cancer J Clin 1995; 45:31–49.
230. Morson BC, Dawson IMP. Gastrointestinal Pathology. Day DW, Jass JR, Price AB, Shepherd NA, Sloan JM, Talbot JC, Warren BF, Williams GT. 4th Ed. Malden Oxford: Blackwell Science 2003.
231. Papp JP, Levine EJ, Thomas FB. Primary linitis plastica carcinoma of the colon and rectum. Am J Gastroenterol 1995; 90:141–145.
232. Broders AC. Grading of carcinoma. Minn Med 1925; 8:726–730.
233. Dukes CE. The classification of cancer of the rectum. J Pathol Bacteriol 1932; 35:323–332.
234. Jass JR, Atkin WS, Cuzick J, et al. The grading of rectal cancer: historical perspectives and multivariate analysis of 447 cases. Histopathology 1986; 10: 437–459.
235. Gibbs NM. Undifferentiated carcinoma of the large intestine. Histopathology 1977; 1:77–84.
236. Sundblad AS, Paz RA. Mucinous carcinomas of the colon and rectum and their relation to polyps. Cancer 1982; 50:2504–2509.

237. Bonello JC, Sternberg SS, Quan SHQ. The significance of signet cell variety of adenocarcinoma of the rectum. Dis Colon Rectum 1980; 23:180–183.
238. Umpleby HC, Ranson DL, Williamson RCN. Peculiarities of mucinous colorectal carcinoma. Br J Surg 1985; 72:715–718.
239. Okuno M, Ikehara T, Nagayama M, et al. Mucinous colorectal carcinoma: clinical pathology and prognosis. Ann Sure 1988; 54:681–685.
240. Anthony T, George R, Rodriguez-Bigas M, et al. Primary signet-ring cell carcinoma of the colon and rectum. Ann Surg Oncol 1996; 3:344–348.
241. Shirouza K, Isomoto H, Morodomi T, et al. Primary linitis plastica carcinoma of the colon and rectum. Cancer 1994; 74:1863–1868.
242. Hase K, Shatney CH, Mochizuki H, et al. Long-term results of curative resection of "minimally invasive" colorectal cancer. Dis Colon Rectum 1995; 38:19–26.
243. Novello P, Duvillard P, Goandjouan S, et al. Carcinomas of the colon with multidirectional differentiation. Report of two cases and review of fhe literature. Dig Dis Sci 1995; 40:100–106.
244. Begin LR, Gordon PH, Alpert LC. Endophytic malignant transformation within flat adenoma of the colon: a potential diagnostic pitfall. Virchows Arch A Pathol Anat 1993; 442:415–418.
245. Kudo S, Tamura S, Nakajima T, et al. Depressed type of colorectal cancer. Endoscopy 1995; 27:54–57.
246. Kubota O, Kino I, Kimura T, et al. Nonpolypoid adenomas and adenocarcinomas found in background mucosa of surgically resected colons. Cancer 1996; 77:621–626.
247. Minamoto T, Sawaguchi K, Ohta T, et al. Superficial-type adenomas and adenocarcinomas of the colon and rectum: a comparative morphological study. Gastroenterology 1994; 106:1436–1443.
248. Tada S, Yao T, Iida M, et al. A clinicopathologic study of flat colorectal carcinoma. Cancer 1994; 74:2430–2435.
249. Iishi H, Kitamura S, Nakaizumi A, et al. Clinicopathologic features and endoscopic diagnosis of superficial early adenocarcinomas of the large intestine. Dig Dis Sci 1993; 38:1333–1337.
250. Togashi K, Konishi F, Koinuma K, et al. Flat and depressed lesions of the colon and rectum: pathogenesis and clinical management. Ann Acad Med Singapore 2003; 32:152–158.
251. Nivatvongs S. Surgical management of early colorectal cancer. World J Surg 2000; 24:1052–1055.
252. Mulsow J, Winter DC, O'Keane JC, O'Connell PR. Sentinel lymph node mapping in colorectal cancer. Br J Surg 2003; 90(6):659–667.
253. Bilchik AJ, Nora DT, Sobin LH, et al. Effect of lymphatic mapping on the new tumor-node-metastasis classification for colorectal cancer. J Clin Oncol 2003; 21:668–672.
254. Saha S, Dan AG, Berman B, et al. Lymphazurin 1% versus 99 mTc sulfur colloid for lymphatic mapping in colorectal tumors: a comparative analysis. Ann Surg Oncol 2004; 11:21–26.
255. Bembenek A, Rau B, Moesta T, et al. Sentinel lymph node biopsy in rectal cancer—not yet ready for routine clinical use. Surgery 2004; 135: 498–505.
256. Bertagnoli M, Redston M, Miedma B, et al. Sentinel node staging of resectable colon cancer: results of CALG B 80001. Proc Am Soc Clin Oncol 2004; 22:2465 (abstr. 3506; suppl).
257. Read TE, Fleshman JW, Caushaj PF. Sentinel lymph node mapping for adenocarcinoma of the colon does not improve staging accuracy. Dis Colon Rectum 2005; 48:80–85.
258. Stojadinovic A, Allen PJ, Protic M, et al. Colon sentinel lymph node mapping: practical surgical applications. J Am Coll Surg 2005; 201(2):297–313.
259. Cimmino VM, Brown AC, Szocik JF, et al. Allergic reactions to isosulfan blue during sentinel node biopsy-a common event. Surgery 2001; 130(5): 439–442.
260. Gutman M, Fidler IJ. Biology of human colon cancer metastases. World J Surg 1995; 19:226–234.
261. Griffiths JD, McKinna JA, Rowbotham HD, et al. Carcinoma of the colon and rectum: circulating malignant cells and five-year survival. Cancer 1973; 31:226–236.
262. Weiss L, Grundmann E,.Torhorst J, et al. Hematogenous metastatic patterns in colonic carcinoma: an analysis of 1541 necropsies. J Pathol 1986; 150:195–203.
263. Taylor I. Liver metastases from colorectal cancer: lessons from the past and present clinical studies. Br J Surg 1996; 83:456–460.
264. Killingback M, Wilson E, Hughes ESR. Anal metastases from carcinoma of the rectum and colon. Aust N Z J Surg 1965; 34:178–187.
265. Norgren J, Svensson JD. Anal implantation metastases from carcinoma of the sigmoid colon and rectum. A risk when performing anterior resection with the EEA stapler. Br J Surg 1985; 72:602.
266. Rollinson PD, Dundas SAC. Adenocarcinoma of the sigmoid colon seeding into preexisting fistula-in-ano. Br J Surg 1984; 71:664–665.
267. Rosenberg IL. The etiology of colonic suture-line recurrence. Ann R Coll Surg Engl 1979; 61:251–257.
268. Scott NA, Taylor BA, Wolff BG, et al. Perianal metastases from a sigmoid carcinoma—objective evidence of a clonal origin. Report of a case. Dis Colon Rectum 1988; 31:68–70.
269. Thomas DJ, Thompson MR. Implantation metastasis from adenocarcinoma of sigmoid colon into fistula-in-ano. J R Soc Med 1992; 85:361.
270. Murakami S, Terakado M, Hashimoto T, Tsuji Y, Okubo K, Hirayama R. Adrenal metastasis from rectal cancer: report of a case. Surg Today 2003:126–130.
271. Conti JA, Kemeny N, Klimstra D, et al. Colon carcinoma metastatic to the trachea. Report of a case and a review of the literature. Am J Clin Oncol 1994; 17:227–229.
272. Araki K, Kobayashi M, Ogata T, et al. Colorectal; carcinoma metastatic to skeletal muscle. Hepatogastroenterology 1994; 41:405–408.
273. Kupfer HWEM, Theunissen P, Delaere KPJ. Urethral metastasis from a rectal carcinoma. Acta Urol Belg 1995; 63:31–32.
274. Bhutani MS, Pacheco J. Metastatic colon carcinoma to oral soft tissues. Spec Care Dentist 1992; 12:172–173.
275. Vasilevsky CA, Alou-Khalel A, Rochon L, et al. Carcinoma of the colon presenting as tonsillar metastases. J Otolaryngol 1997; 26:325–326.
276. Gabriel WB, Dukes CE, Bussey HJR. Lymphatic spread in cancer of the rectum. Br J Surg 1935; 23:395–413.
277. Turnbull RB, Kyle K, Watson FR, et al. Cancer of the colon: the influence of the no-touch isolation technique on survival rates. Ann Surg 1967; 166:420–427.
278. Wong JH, Severino R, Honnebier MB, Tom P, Namiki TS. Number of nodes examined and staging accuracy in colorectal carcinoma. J Clin Oncol 1999; 17(9):2896–2900.
279. Jass JR, Chapuis PH, Dixon MF, et al. Symposium on staging of colorectal cancer. Int J Colorectal Dis 1987; 2:123.
280. Greene FL, Page DL, Floming ID, et al. American Joint Committee for Cancer. Cancer Staging Handbook. 6th ed. New York: Springer-Verlag, 2002:127–138.
281. Astler VB, Coller FA. The prognostic significance of direct extension of carcinoma of the colon and rectum. Ann Surg 1954; 139:846–852.
282. Chapuis PH, Dent MF, Newland RC, et al. An evaluation of the American Joint Committee pTNM staging method for cancer of the colon and rectum. Dis Colon Rectum 1986; 29:6–10.
283. Chapuis PH, Dixon MF, Fielding LP, et al. Staging of colorectal cancer (Symposium). Int J Colorectal Dis 1987; 2:123–138.
284. Davis NC, Newland RC. Terminology and classification of colorectal adenpearcinoma. The Australian clinicopathological staging system. Aust N Z J Surg 1983; 53:211–221.
285. Gastrointestinal Tumor Study Group. Adjuvant therapy of colon cancer. Results of a prospectively randomized trial. N Engl J Med 1984; 310:737–743.
286. Terrazas JM, Val-Bernal JF, Buelta L. Staging of carcinoma of the colon and rectum. Surg Gynecol Obstet 1987; 165:255–259.
287. Goligher JC. The Dukes' A, B, and C categorization of the extent of spread of carcinomas of the rectum. Surg Gynecol Obstet 1976; 146:793–794.
288. Kirklin JW, Dockerty MB, Waugh JM. The role of the peritoneal reflection in the prognosis of carcinoma of the rectum and sigmoid colon. Surg Gynecol Obstet 1949; 88:326–331.
289. Zinkin LD. A critical review of the classifications and staging of colorectal cancer. Dis Colon Rectum 1983; 26:37–43.
290. Newland RC, Chapuis PH, Smyth EJ. The prognostic value of substaging colorectal carcinoma. A prospective study of 1117 cases with standardized pathology. Cancer 1987; 60:852–857.
291. Spratt JS Jr. Gross rates of growth of colonic neoplasms and other variables affecting medical decisions and prognosis. In: Burdette WJ, ed. Carcinoma of the Colon and Antecedent Epithelium. Springfield, III.: Charles C Thomas, 1970:66–77.
292. Finlay IG, Brunton GF, Meek D, et al. Rate of growth of hepatic metastases in colorectal carcinoma. Br J Surg 1982; 69:689.
293. Havelaar I, Sugarbaker PH. Rate of growth of intraabdominal metastases from colon and rectal cancer followed by serial EOE CT. Cancer 1984; 54:163–171.
294. Bolin S, Nilsson E, Sjodahl R. Carcinoma of the colon and rectum—growth rate. Ann Surg 1983; 198:151–158.
295. Burnett KR, Greenbaum El. Rapidly growing carcinoma of the colon. Dis Colon Rectum 1981; 24:282–286.
296. Matsui T, Tsuda S, Yao K, Iwashita A, Sakurai T, Yao T. Natural history of early colorectal cancer: evolution of a growth curve. Dis Colon Rectum 2000; 43(suppl 10):S18–S22.
297. Aldridge MC, Phillips RKS, Hittinger R, et al. Influence of tumour site on presentation, management and subsequent outcome in large bowel cancer. Br J Surg 1986; 73:663–670.
298. Mandava N, Kumar S, Pizzi WF, et al. Perforated colorectal carcinomas. Am J Surg 1996; 172:236–238.
299. Runkel NS, Schlag P, Schwarz V, et al. Outcome after emergency surgery for cancer of the large intestine. Br J Surg 1991; 78:183–188.
300. The consultant surgeons and pathologists of the Lothian and Borders health boards. Lothian and Borders large bowel cancer project: immediate outcome after surgery. Br J Surg 1995; 82:888–890.

301. Beart RW Jr., Melton LJ, Maruta M, et al. Trends in right and left sided colon cancer. Dis Colon Rectum 1983; 26:393–398.
302. Farrands PA, Hardcastle JD. Colorectal screening by a self-completion questionnaire. Gut 1984; 25:445–447.
303. Ramsay JA, Rose TH, Ross T. Colonic carcinoma presenting as an appendiceal abscess in a young woman. Can J Surg 1996; 39:53–56.
304. Beart RW, Steele GD Jr., Menck HR, et al. Management and survival of patients with adenocarcinoma of the colon and rectum: a national survey of the commission on cancer. J Am Coll Surg 1995; 181:225–236.
305. Acher PL, Al-Mishlab T, Rahman M, Bates T. Iron-deficiency anaemia and delay in the diagnosis of colorectal cancer. Colorectal Dis 2003; 5:145–148.
306. Church J, McGannon E. Family history of colorectal cancer: how often and how accurately is it recorded? Dis Colon Rectum 2000; 43:1540–1544.
307. Rosato FE, Shelly WB, Fitts WT Jr., et al. Non-metastatic cutaneous manifestations of cancer of the colon. Am J Surg 1969; 117:277–281.
308. Halak M, Hazzan D, Kovacs Z, Shiloni E. Synchronous colorectal and renal carcinomas: a noteworthy clinical entity. Report of five cases. Dis Colon Rectum 2000; 43:1314–1315.
309. Vasilevsky CA, Gordon PH. Colonoscopy in the follow-up of patients with colorectal carcinoma. Can J Surg 1988; 31:188–190.
310. Evers BM, Mullins RJ, Mathews TH. Multiple adenocarrinomas of the colon and rectum: an analysis of incidences and current trends. Dis Colon Rectum 1988; 31:518–522.
311. Pinol V, Andreu M, Castells A, et al. Synchronous colorectal neoplasms in patients with colorectal cancer: predisposing individual and familial factors. Dis Colon Rectum 2004; 47:1192–1200.
312. Adloff M, Arnaud JP, Bergamaschi R, et al. Synchronous carcinoma of the colon and rectum: prognostic and therapeutic implications. Am J Surg 1989; 157:299–302.
313. Langevin JM, Nivatvongs S. The true incidence of synchronous cancer of the large bowel: a prospective study. Am J Surg 1984; 147:330–333.
314. Rider JA, Kirsner JB, Moeller HC, et al. Polyps of the colon and rectum. JAMA 1959; 170:633.
315. Slater G, Fleshner P, Aufses AH. Colorectal cancer location and synchronous adenomas. Am J Gastroenterol 1988; 83:832–836.
316. Chu DZ, Giacoo G, Martin RG, Guinee VF. The significance of synchronous carcinoma and polyps in the colon and rectum. Cancer 1986; 57:445–450.
317. Lee TK, Barringer M, Myers RT, et al. Multiple primary carcinoma of the colon and associated extracolonic primary malignant tumors. Ann Surg 1982; 195:501–507.
318. Tanaka H, Hiyama T, Hanai A, et al. Second primary cancers following colon and rectal cancer in Osaka Japan. Jpn J Cancer Res 1991; 82:1356–1365.
319. Schoen RE, Weissfeld JL, Kuller LH. Are women with breast, endometrial, or ovarian cancer at increased risk for colorectal cancer? Am J Gastroenterol 1994; 89:835–842.
320. De Dombal FT, Matharu SS, Staniland JR, et al. Presentation of cancer to hospital as "acute abdominal pain." Br J Surg 1980; 67:413–416.
321. Ohman U. Prognosis in patients with obstructing colorectal carcinoma. Am J Surg 1982; 143:742–747.
322. Wolloch Y, Zer M, Lurie M, et al. Ischemic colitis proximal to obstructing carcinoma of the colon. Am J Proctol 1979; 30:17–22.
323. Saegesser F, Sandblom P. Ischemic lesions of the distended colon. A complication of obstructive colorectal cancer. Am J Surg 1975; 129:309–315.
324. Ueyama T, Yao T, Nakamura K, et al. Obstructing carcinoma of the colon and rectum: clinicopathologic analysis of 40 cases. Jpn J Clin Oncol 1991; 21: 100–109.
325. Seow-Choen F, Chua TL, Goh HS. Ischemic colitis and colorectal cancer: some problems and pitfalls. Int J Colorectal Dis 1993; 8:210–212.
326. Wolmark N, NSABP Investigators. The prognostic significance of tumour location and bowel obstruction in Dukes' B and C colorectal cancer. Ann Surg 1983; 198:743–750.
327. Umpleby HC, Williamson RCN. Survival in acute obstructing colorectal carcinoma. Dis Colon Rectum 1984; 27:299–304.
328. Panwalker AP. Unusual infections associated with colorectal carcinoma. Rev Infect Dis 1988; 10:347–364.
329. Lam S, Greenberg R, Bank S. An unusual presentation of colon cancer: purulent pericarditis and cardiac tamponade due to Bacteroides fragilis. Am J Gastroenterol 1995; 90:1518–1520.
330. Belinkie SA, Narayanan NC, Russell JC, et al. Splenic abscess associated with streptococcus bovis septicemia and neoplastic lesions of the colon. Dis Colon Rectum 1983; 26:823–824.
331. Silver SC. Streptococcus bovis endocarditis and its association with colonic carcinoma. Dis Colon Rectum 1984; 27:613–614.
332. Legier J. Streptococcus salivarius meningitis and colonic carcinoma. South Med J 1991; 84:1058–1059.
333. Lonardo A, Grisendi A, Pulvirenti M, et al. Right colon adenocarcinoma presenting as bacteroides liver abscesses. J Clin Gastroenterol 1992; 14:335–338.
334. Teitz S, Guidetti-Sharon A, Monro H, et al. Pyeogenic liver abscess: warning indicator of silent colonic cancer. Dis Colon Rectum 1995; 58:1220–1223.
335. Kudsk KA. Occult gastrointestinal malignancies producing metastatic clostridium septicum infections in diabetic patients. Surgery 1992; 112:765–772.
336. Lorimer JW, Eldus LB. Invasive *clostridium septicum* infection in association with colorectal carcinoma. Can J Surg 1994; 37:245–249.
337. Poleski MH, Gordon PH. Screening for carcinoma of the colon: pitfalls of the hemoccult test. In: Nelson RL, ed. Problems in Current Surgery. Controversies in Colon Cancer. Philadelphia: JB Lippincott, 1987:1–10.
338. Nivatvongs S, Fryd DS. How far does the proctosigmoidoscope reach? N Engl J Med 1980; 303:380–382.
339. Marks G, Gathright JB, Boggs HW, et al. Guidelines for use of the flexible fiberoptic sigmoidoscope in the management of the surgical patient. Dis Colon Rectum 1982; 23:187–190.
340. Traul DG, Davis CB, Pollock JC, et al. Flexible fiberoptic sigmoidoseopy—the Monroe Clinic experience. A prospective study of 5,000 examinations. Dis Colon Rectum 1983; 26:161–166.
341. Bernard D, Tasse D, Morgan S, et al. Is preoperative colonoscopy in carcinoma a realistic and valuable proposition? Can J Surg 1987; 30:87–89.
342. Isler JT, Brown PC, Lewis FG, et al. The role of preoperative colonoscopy in colorectal cancer. Dis Colon Rectum 1987; 30:435–439.
343. Finan PJ, Ritchie JK, Hawley PR. Synchronous and early metachronous carcinomas of the colon and rectum. Br J Surg 1987; 74:945–947.
344. Reilly JC, Rusin LC, Theuerkauf FJ Jr. Colonoscopy: its role in cancer of the colon and rectum. Dis Colon Rectum 1982; 25:532–538.
345. Sollenberger LL, Eisenstat TE, Rubin RJ, et al. Is preoperative colonoscopy necessary in carcinoma of the colon and rectum. Am Surg 1988; 54: 113–115.
346. Thomas RD, Fairhurst JJ, Frost RA. Wessex regional radiology audit: barium enema in colorectal carcinoma. Clin Radiol 1995; 50:647–650.
347. Peel AL, Benyon L, Grace RH. The value of routine preoperative urological assessment in patients undergoing elective surgery for diverticular disease or carcinoma of the large bowel. Br J Surg 1980; 67:42–47.
348. Vezeridis MP, Petrelli NJ, Mittelman A. The value of routine preoperative urologic evaluation in patients with colorectal carcinoma. Dis Colon Rectum 1987; 30:758–760.
349. Phillips R, Hittinger R, Saunders V, et al. Pre-operative urography in large bowel cancer: a useless investigation? Br J Surg 1983; 70:425–427.
350. Tartter PI, Steinberg BM. The role of preoperative intravenous pyelogram in operations performed for carcinoma of the colon and rectum. Surg Gynecol Obstet 1986; 163:65–69.
351. Grace RH, Hale M, Mackie G, et al. Role of ultrasound in the diagnosis of liver metastases before surgery for large bowel cancer. Br J Surg 1987; 74:480–481.
352. Rafaelsen SR, Kronborg O, Larsen C, et al. Intraoperative ultrasonography in detection of hepatic metastases from colorectal cancer. Dis Colon Rectum 1995; 38:355–360.
353. Meijer S, Pavel MA, Cuesta MA, et al. Intra-operativc ultrasound in detection of liver metastases. Eur J Cancer 1995; 31A:1210–1211.
354. Machi J, Isomoto H, Kurohiji T, et al. Accuracy of intraoperative ultrasonography in diagnosing liver metastases from colorectal cancer: evaluation with postoperative follow up results. World J Surg 1991; 15: 551–557.
355. Takeuchi N, Ramirez JM, Mortensen NJM, et al. Intraoperative ultrasonography in the diagnosis of hepatic metastases during surgery for colorectal cancer. Int J Colorectal Dis 1996; 11:92–95.
356. Kerner BA, Oliver GC, Eisenstat TE, et al. Is preoperative computerized tomography useful in assessing patients with colorectal carcinoma? Dis Colon Rectum 1993; 36:1050–1053.
357. Theoni RF, Rogalla P. CT for the evaluation of carcinomas in the colon and rectum. Semin Ultrasound CT MR 1995; 16:112–126.
358. Mauchley DC, Lynge DC, Langdale LA, Stelzner MG, Mock CN, Billingsley KG. Clinical utility and cost-effectiveness of routine preoperative computed tomography scanning in patients with colon cancer. Am J Surg 2005; 189(5):512–517.
359. Tempero M, Brand R, Holderman K, et al. New imaging techniques in colorectal cancer. Semin Oncol 1995; 22:448–471.
360. Zerhouni EA, Rntter C, Hamilton SR, et al. CT and MR imaging in the staging of colorectal carcinoma: report of the Radiology Diagnostic Oncology Group II. Radiology 1996; 200:443–451.
361. Johnson K, Bakhsh A, Young D, Martin TE Jr., Arnold M. Correlating computed tomography and positron emission tomography scan with operative findings in metastatic colorectal cancer. Dis Colon Rectum 2001; 44: 354–357.
362. Bertsch DJ, Burak WE, Young DC, et al. Radioimmunoguided surgery for colorectal cancer. Ann Surg Oncol 1996; 3:310–316.
363. Arnold MW, Hitchcock CL, Young DC, et al. Intra-abdominal patterns of disease dissemination in colorectal cancer identified using radioimmunoguided surgery. Dis Colon Rectum 1996; 39:509–513.
364. Dominguez JM, Wolff BE, Nelson H, et al. ^{111}In-CYT-103 scanning in recurrent colorectal cancer—does it affect standard management? Dis Colon Rectum 1996; 39:514–519.

365. Moffat FL, Pinsky CM, Hammershaimb L, et al. Clinical utility of external immunoscintigraphy with the IMMU-4 technetium-99m Fab' antibody fragment in patients undergoing surgery for carcinoma of the colon and rectum: results of a pivotal, phase III trial. J Clin Oncol 1996; 14: 2295–2305.
366. Corman ML, Galandiuk S, Block GE, et al. Immunoscintigraphy with ^{111}In-satumomab pendetide in patients with colorectal adenocarcinoma: performance and impact on clinical management. Dis Colon Rectum 1994; 37: 129–137.
367. Galandiuk S. Immunoscintigraphy in the surgical management of colorectal cancer. J Nucl Med 1993; 34:541–544.
368. Limberg B. Diagnosis and staging of colonic tumors by conventional abdominal sonography as compared with hydrocolonic sonography. N Engl J Med 1992; 327:65–69.
369. Leveson SH, Wiggins PA, Giles GR, et al. Deranged liver blood flow patterns in the detection of liver metastases. Br J Surg 1985; 72:128–130.
370. Dian-Yuan Z, Fu-cai F, Ya-li Z, et al. Comparison of Sham's test for rectal mucus to an immunological test for fecal occult blood in large intestinal carcinoma screening. Analysis of a checkup of 6480 asymptomatic patients. Chin Med J 1993; 106:739–742.
371. Sakamoto K, Muranti M, Ogawa T, et al. Evaluation of a new test for colorectal neoplasms: a prospective study of a symptomatic population. Cancer Biother 1993; 81:49–54.
372. Chen YL. The diagnosis of colorectal cancer with cytologic brushings under direct vision at fiberoptic colonoscopy. A report of 59 cases. Dis Colon Rectum 1987; 30:342–344.
373. Rosman AS, Federman O, Feinman L. Diagnosis of colonic cancer by lavage cytology with an orally administered balanced electrolyte solution. Am J Gastroenterol 1994; 89:51–56.
374. Gold P, Freedman SO. Demonstration of tumor-specific antigens in human colonic cardnomata by immunological tolerance and absorption techniques. J Exp Med 1965; 121:439–462.
375. Gold P. The carcinoembryonic antigen (CEA): discovery and three decades of study. Perspect Colon Rectal Surg 1996; 9(2):1–47.
376. Kyzer S, Mitmaker B, Gordon PH, et al. Proliferative activity of colonic mucosa at different distances from primary adenocarcinoma as determined by the presence of statin: a non proliferation-specific nuclear protein. Dis Colon Rectum 1992; 35:879–883.
377. Stein R, Juweid M, Mattes MJ, Goldbenberg DM. Carcinoembryonic antigen as a target for radioimmunotherapy of human medullary thyroid carcinoma: antibody processing, targeting, and experimental therapy with 131I and 90Y labeled MAbs. Cancer Biother Radiopharm 1999; 14(1):37–47.
378. Bockhorn M, Frilling A, Rewerk S, et al. Lack of elevated serum carcinoembryonic antigen and calcitonin in medullary thyroid carcinoma. Thyroid 2004; 14: 468–470.
379. Moorehead RJ, Hoper M, McKelvey STD. Assessment of ornithine decarboxylase activity in rectal mucosa as a marker for colorectal adenomas and carcinoma. Br J Surg 1987; 74:364–365.
380. Narisawa T, Takahashi M, Niwa M, et al. Increased mucosal ornithine decarboxylase activity in large bowel with multiple tumors, adenocarcinoma and adenomas. Cancer 1989; 63:1572–1576.
381. Gelister JSK, Jass RJ, Mahmoud M, et al. Role of urokinase in colorectal neoplasia. Br J Surg 1987; 74:460–463.
382. Fazio VW, Tekkis PP, Remzi F, Lavery IC. Assessment of operative risk in colorectal cancer surgery: the Cleveland Clinic Foundation colorectal cancer model. Dis Colon Rectum 2004; 47(12):2015–2024.
383. Portnoy J, Kagan E, Gordon PH, et al. Prophylactic antibiotics in elective colorectal surgery. Dis Colon Rectum 1983; 26:310–313.
384. Rubin RJ, White RA, Eisenstat TE, et al. Left subcostal transverse incision combined with the right lateral position for excising the splenic flexure: a reintroduction. Perspect Colon Rectal Surg 1988; l(2):41–47.
385. Thomas WM, Morris DL, Hardcastle JD. Contact ultrasonography in the detection of liver metastases from colorectal cancer: an in vitro study. Br J Surg 1987; 74:955–956.
386. Busuttil RW, Foglia RP, Longmire WP. Treatment of carcinoma of the sigmoid colon and upper rectum. A comparison of local segmental resection and left hemicolectomy. Arch Surg 1977; 112:920–923.
387. Dwight RW, Higgins GA, Keehn RJ. Factors influencing survival after resection in cancer of the colon and rectum. Am J Surg 1969; 117:512–522.
388. Grinnell RS. Results of ligation of inferior mesenteric artery at the aorta in resections of carcinoma of the descending and sigmoid colon and rectum. Surg Gynecol Obstet 1965; 170:1031–1046.
389. Pezim ME, Nicholls RJ. Survival after high or low ligation of the inferior mesenteric artery during curative surgery for rectal cancer. Ann Surg 1984; 200:729–733.
390. Enker WE, Laffer VT, Black GE. Enhanced survival of patients with colon and rectal cancer is based upon wide anatomic resection. Ann Surg 1979; 190:350–360.
391. Brief DK, Brener BJ, Goldenkrantz R, et al. Defining the role of subtotal colectomy in the treatment of carcinoma of the colon. Ann Surg 1991; 213:248–252.
392. Fisher ER, Turnbull RB Jr. The cytologic demonstration and significance of tumor cells in the mesenteric venous blood in patients with colorectal carcinoma. Surg Gynecol Obstet 1955; 100:102–108.
393. Cole WH, Packard D, Southwick HW. Carcinoma of the colon with special reference to the prevention of recurrence. JAMA 1954; 155:1549–1553.
394. Turnbull RB Jr., Kyle K, Watson FR, et al. Cancer of the colon: the influence of the no-touch technique on survival rates. Ann Surg 1967; 166:420–427.
395. Cohn I Jr., Floyd CE, Atik M. Control of tumor implantation during operations of the colon. Ann Surg 1963; 157:825–838.
396. Long RTL, Edwards RH. Implantation metastases as a cause of local recurrence of colorectal carcinoma. Am J Surg 1989; 157:194–201.
397. Wiggers T, Jeekel J, Arends JW. No-touch isolation technique in colon cancer: a controlled prospective trial. Br J Surg 1988; 75:409–415.
398. Gordon PH, Dalrymple S. The use of staples for reconstruction after colonic and rectal surgery. In: Ravitch MM, Steichen FM, eds. Principles and Practice of Surgical Stapling. Chicago: Year Book Medical Publishers, 1987:402–431.
399. Welter R, Charlier A, Psalmon F. Personal communication. In: Steichen FM, Ravitch MM, eds. Stapling in Surgery. Chicago: Year Book Medical Publishers, 1988:271.
400. Chassin JL, Rifkind KM, Turner JW. Errors and pitfalls in stapling gastrointestinal anastomoses. Surg Clin North Am 1984; 64:441–459.
401. Kyzer S, Gordon PH. The stapled functional end-to-end anastomoses following colonic resection. Int J Colorectal Dis 1992; 7:125–131.
402. Chassin JL, Rifkind KM, Sussman B, et al. The stapled gastrointestinal anastomosis: incidence of postoperative complications compared with the sutured anastomosis. Ann Surg 1978; 188:689–696.
403. Fortin CL, Poulin EC, Leclerc V. Evaluation de utilisation des appareils d'autosuture en chirurgie digestive. Can J Surg 1979; 22:580–582.
404. Brodman RF, Brodman HR. Staple suturing of the colon above the peritoneal reflection. Arch Surg 1981; 116:191–192.
405. Reuter MJP. Les sutures mécaniques en chirurgie digestive et pulmonaire. Thesis. Univérsity Louis Pasteur, Faculté de Médecine de Strasbourg, France, 1982.
406. Scher KS, Scott-Conner C, Jones CW, et al. A comparison of stapled and sutured anastomoses in colonic operations. Surg Gynecol Obstet 1982; 155: 489–493.
407. Steichen FM, Ravitch MM. Stapling in Surgery. Chicago: Year Book Medical Publishers, 1984:271.
408. Tuchmann A, Dinstl K, Strasser K, et al. Stapling devices in gastrointestinal surgery. Int Surg 1985; 70:23–27.
409. Kracht M, Hay JM, Fagniez PL, et al. Ileocolonic anastomosis after right hemicolectomy for carcinoma: stapled or hand-sewn? A prospective, multicenter, randomized trial. Int J Colorectal Dis 1993; 8:29–33.
410. Corman ML. Colon and Rectal Surgery. 2nd ed Philadelphia: JB Lippincott, 1989:417.
411. Abcarian H, Pearl RK. Simple technique for high ligation of the inferior mesenteric artery and vein. Dis Colon Rectum 1991; 34:1138.
412. Heald RJ. Anterior resection of the rectum. In: Fielding LP, Goldberg SM, eds. Rob and Smith's Operative Surgery. Surgery of the Colon, Rectum, and Anus. 5th ed. London: Butterworth-Heinemann Ltd, 1993:456–471.
413. Birnkrant A, Sampson J, Sugarbaker PH. Ovarian metastases from colorectal cancer. Dis Colon Rectum 1986; 29:767–771.
414. Graffner HOL, Aim POA, Oscarson JEA. Prophylactic oophorectomy in colorectal carcinoma. Am J Surg 1983; 146:233–235.
415. Sielezneff I, Salle E, Antoine K, Thirion X, Brunet C, Sastre B. Simultaneous bilateral oophorectomy does not improve prognosis of postmenopausal women undergoing colorectal resection for cancer. Dis Colon Rectum 1997; 40(11):1299–1302.
416. Young-Fadok TM, Wolff B, Nivatvongs S, et al. Prophylactic oophorectomy in colorectal carcinoma: preliminary results. Dis Colon Rectum 1998; 41: 277–285.
417. Cutait R, Lesser ML, Enker WE. Prophylactic oophorectomy in surgery for large bowel cancer. Dis Colon Rectum 1983; 26:6–11.
418. O'Brien PH, Newton PB, Metcalf JS, et al. Oophorectomy in women with carcinoma of the colon and rectum. Surg Gynecol Obstet 1981; 153:827–830.
419. MacKeigan JM, Ferguson JA. Prophylactic oophorectomy and colorectal cancer in premenopausal patients. Dis Colon Rectum 1979; 22:401–405.
420. Blamey S, McDermott F, Pihl E, et al. Ovarian involvement in adenocarcinoma of the colon and rectum. Surg Gynecol Obstet 1981; 153:42–44.
421. Steele G, Augenlicht L, Begg C, et al. National Institutes of Helth consensus development conference statement—adjuvant therapy for patients with colon and rectal cancer. JAMA 1990; 264:1444.
422. Sugarbaker PH, Gunderson LL, Wittes RE. Colorectal cancer. In: DeVita VT Jr., Hellman S, Rosenberg SA, eds. Cancer Principles and Practices of Oncology. 2nd ed. Philadelphia: JB Lippincott, 1985:795–884.
423. Duttenhaver JR, Hoskins RB, Gunderson LL, et al. Adjuvant postoperative radiation therapy in the management of adenocarcinoma of the colon. Cancer 1986; 57:955–963.
424. Ghossein NA, Samala EC, Alpert S, et al. Elective postoperative radiotherapy after incomplete resection of a colorectal cancer. Dis Colon Rectum 1981; 24:252–256.

425. Wong CS, Harwood AR, Cummings BJ, et al. Postoperative local abdominal irradiation for cancer of the colon above the peritoneal reflection. Int J Radiat Oncol Biol Phys 1985; 11:2067–2071.
426. Kopelson G. Adjuvant postoperative radiation therapy for colorectal carcinoma above the peritoneal reflection. I. Sigmotd colon. Cancer 1983; 51:1593–1598.
427. Kopelson G. Adjuvant postoperative radiation therapy for colorectal carcinoma above the peritoneal reflection. II. Antimesenteric wall, ascending and descending colon and cecum. Cancer 1983; 52:633–636.
428. Minsky BD. Adjuvant radiation therapy for colon cancer. Cancer Treat Rev 1995; 2:407–414.
429. Schabel FM Jr. Rationale for perioperative anticanccr treatment. Recent Results Cancer Res 1985; 98:1–10.
430. Gastrointestinal Tumor Study Group. Adjuvant therapy of colon cancer: results of a prospectively randomized trial. N Engl J Med 1984; 310:737–743.
431. Gilbert JM, Hellman K, Evans M, et al. Randomized trial of oral adjuvant ražoxane (ICRF 159) in resectable colorectal cancer: five year follow-up. Br J Surg 1986; 73:446–450.
432. Grage TB, Moss SE. Adjuvant chemotherapy in cancer of the colon and rectum: demonstration of effectiveness of prolonged 5-FU chemotherapy in a prospectively controlled randomized trial. Surg Clin North Am 1981; 61:1321–1329.
433. Higgins GA Jr., Amadeo JH, McElhinney J, et al. Efficacy of prolonged intermittent therapy with combined 5-fluorouracil and methyl CCNU following resection for carcinoma of the large bowel. A Veterans Administration Surgical Oncology Group report. Cancer 1984; 53:1–8.
434. Laurie J, Moertel C, Fleming T, et al. Surgical adjuvant therapy of poor prognostic colorectal cancèr with levamisole alone or combined levamisole and 5-fluorouracil. A North Central Cancer Treatment Group and Mayo Clinic study. Proc Am Soc Clin Oncol 1986; 5:316.
435. Panettiere FJ, Rogers AR. SWOG large bowel post-operative program. Proceedings of the Fourth International Conference on the Adjuvant Therapy of Cancer [abstr T7]. 1984:94.
436. Buyse M, Zelenuick-Jacquolte A, Chalmers TC. Adjuvant therapy for colorectal cancer, why we still don't know. JAMA 1988; 259:3571–3578.
437. Windle A, Bell PRF, Shaw D. Five year results of a randomized trial of adjuvant 5-fluorouracil and levamisole in colorectal cancer. Br J Surg 1987; 74:569–572.
438. Laurie J, Moertel C, Fleming T, et al. Surgical adjuvant therapy of large bowel carcinoma: an evaluation of levamisole and the combination of levamisole and 5-fluorouracil. A study of the North Central Cancer Treatment Group and Mayo Clinic. J Clin Oncol 1989; 7:1447–1456.
439. Moertel C, Fleming TR, Macdonald JS, et al. Levamisole and fluorouracil for adjuvant therapy of resected colon carcinoma. N Engl J Med 1990; 322:352–358.
440. Wolmark N, Rocketter H, Mamounas E, et al., Clinical trial to assess the relative efficacy of fluorouracil and leucovorin, fluorouracil and levamisole, and fluorouracil, leucovorin and levamisole in patients with Dukes B and C carcinoma of the colon: Results from National Surgical Adjuvant Breast and Bowel Project C-04. J. Clin. Oncol. 1999; 17: 3553–9.
441. Le Voyer TE, Sigurdson ER, Hanlon AL, et al. Colon cancer survival is associated with increasing number of lymph nodes analyzed: a secondary survey of intergroup trial INT-0089. J Clin Oncol 2003; 21:2912–2119.
442. Poplin EA, Benedetti JK, Estes NC, et al. Phase III Southwest oncology group 6415/Intergroup 0153 randomized trial of fluorouracil, leucovorin, and levamisole versus fluorouracil continuous infusion and lovamisole for adjuvant treatment of stage III and high-risk stage II colon cancer. J Clin Oncol 2005; 23(9):1819–1825.
443. Thirion P, Michiels S, Pignon JP,et al. Modulation of fluorouracil by leucovorin in patients with advance colorectal cancer: an updated meta-analysis. J Clin Oncol 2004; 22(18):3766–3775.
444. Moertel CG, Flaming TR, Macdonald JS, et al. Fluorouracil plus levamisole as effective adjuvant therapy after resection of stage III colon carcinoma: a final report. Ann Intern Med 1995; 122:321–326.
445. Wolmark N, Fisher B, Rockette H, et al. Postoperative adjuvant chemotherapy or BCG for colon cancer. Results from NSABP protocol C-01. J Natl Cancer Inst 1988; 80:30–36.
446. Wolmark N, Rockette H, Fisher B, et al. The benefit of leucovorin-modulated fluorouracil as postoperative adjuvant therapy for primary colon cancer: results from National Surgical Adjuvant Breast and Bowel Project Protocol C-03. J Clin Oncol 1993; 11:1879–1887.
447. Piedbois P, Buyse M, Rustum Y, et al. Modulation of fluorouracil by leucovorin in patients with advanced colorectal cancer: evidence in terms of response rate. J Clin Oncol 1992; 10:896–903.
448. Wolmark N, Bryant J, Smith R, et al. Adjuvant 5-fluorouracil and leucovorin with or without interferon alfa-2a in colon carcinoma: National Surgical Adjuvant Breast and Bowel Project protocol C-05. J Natl Cancer Inst 1998; 90: 1810–1816.
449. Mamounas EP, Wieand S, Wolmark N, et al. Comparative efficacy of adjuvant chemotherapy in patients with Dukes' B versus Dukes' C colon cancer: results for four National Surgical Adjuvant Breast and Bowel Project adjuvant studies (C-01, C-02, C-03, and C-04). J Clin Oncol 1999; 17: 1349–1355.
450. International Multicentre Pooled Analysis of B2 Colon Cancer Trials (IMPACT B2) investigators. Efficacy of adjuvant fluorouracil and folinic acid in B2 colon cancer. J Clin Oncol 1999; 17:1356.
451. International Multicentre Pooled Analysis of Colon Cancer Trials (IMPACT} investigators. Efficacy of adjuvant fluorouracil and folinic acid in colon cancer. Lancet 1995; 345:939–944.
452. Dubé S, Heyen F, Jenicek M. Adjuvant chemotherapy in colorectal carcinoma. Results of a meta-analysis. Dis Colon Rectum 1997; 40:35–41.
453. Sakamoto J, Ohashi Y, Hamada C, Buyse M, Burzykowski T, Piedbois P, Meta-Analysis Group of the Japanese Society for Cancer of the colon and Rectum; Meta-Analysis Group in Cancer. Efficacy of oral adjuvant therapy after resection of colorectal cancer: 5-year results from three randomized trials. J Clin Oncol 2004; 22:484–492.
454. Andre T, Boni C, Mounedji-Boudiaf L, et al. Multicenter International Study of Oxaliplatin/5-Fluorouracil/Leucovorin in the Adjuvant Treatment of Colon Cancer (MOSAIC) Investigators. Oxaliplatin, fluorouracil, and leucovorin as adjuvant treatment for colon cancer. N Engl J Med 2004; 350:2343–2351.
455. Martenson JA Jr., Willett CG, Sargent DJ, et al. Phase III study of adjuvant chemotherapy and radiation therapy compared with chemotherapy alone in the surgical adjuvant treatment of colon cancer: results of intergroup protocol 0130. J Clin Oncol 2004; 22:3277–3283.
456. Weiss L, Grundmann E, Torhost J, et al. Hematogenous metastatic patterns in colonic carcinoma: an analysis of 1,541 necropsies. J Pathol 1986; 150:195–203.
457. Taylor L, Machin D, Mullee M, et al. A randomized control trial of adjuvant portal vein cytotoxic perfusion in colorectal cancer. Br J Surg 1985; 72:359–363.
458. Swiss Group for Clinical Cancer Research (SAKK). Long-term results of a single course of adjuvant intraportal chemotherapy for colorectal cancer. Lancet 1995; 345:349–353.
459. Wolmark N, Bockette H, Wickerham DL, et al. Adjuvant therapy for Dukes' A, B, and C adenocarcinoma of the colon with portal vein. Fluorouracil hepatic infusion: preliminary results of National Surgical Adjuvant Breast and Bowel Project Protocol C-02. J Clin Oncol 1990; 8:1466–1475.
460. Wereldsma J, Bruggink E, Meijer W, et al. Adjuvant portal liver infusion in colorectal cancer with 5-fluorouracil/heparin vs. urokinase vs. control. Results of a prospective randomized clinical trial (colorectal adenocarcinoma trial). Cancer 1990; 65:425.
461. Piedbois P, Buyse M, Gray R, et al. Portal vein infusion is an effective adjuvant treatment for patients with colorectal cancer. Proc Am Soc Clin Oncol 1995; 14:192.
462. Chau I, Chan S, Cunninghan D. Overview of preoperative and postoperative therapy for colorectal cancer: the European and United States perspectives. Clin Colorectal Cancer 2003; 3(1):19–33.
463. Haydon A. Adjuvant chemotherapy in colon cancer: what is the evidence? Intern Med J 2003; 33:119–124.
464. Chapuis PH, Dent OF, Bokey EL, Newland RC, Sinclair G. Adverse histopathological findings as a guide to patient management after curative resection of node-positive colonic cancer. Br J Surg 2004; 91:349–354.
465. Figueredo A, Charette ML, Maroun J, Brouwers MC, Zuraw L. Adjuvant therapy for stage II colon cancer: a systematic review from the Cancer Care Ontario Program in evidence-based care's gastrointestinal cancer disease site group. J Clin Oncol 2004; 22:3395–3407.
466. Benson AB 3rd, Schrag D, Somerfield MR, et al. American Society of Clinical Oncology recommendations on adjuvant chemotherapy for stage II colon cancer. J Clin Oncol 2004; 22:3408–3419.
467. Ribic CM, Sargent DJ, Moore MJ, et al. Tumor microsatellite-instability status as a predictor of benefit from fluorouracil-based adjuvant chemotherapy for colon cancer. N Engl J Med 2003; 349:247–257.
468. Culakova E, Khorama A, Kuderer M, Crawford J, Dale DC, Lyman GH. For the ANC study group. Hospitalization with febrile neutropenia in colorectal cancer patients. J Clin Oncol 2004; 22:145; 295.
469. Arora A, Potter J. Older patients with colon cancer: is adjuvant chemotherapy safe and effective? J Am Geriatr Soc 2003; 51:567–569.
470. Rothenberg ML, Meropol NJ, Poplin EA, Van Custem E, Wadler S. Morality associated with irinotecan plus bolus fluorouracil/leucovorin: summary findings of an independent panel. J Clin Oncol 2001; 19:3801–3807.
471. Colorectal Cancer Chemotherapy Study Group of Japan–The 2nd Trial. Results of a randomized trial with or without 5-FU-based preoperative chemotherapy followed by postoperative chemotherapy in resected colon and rectal carcinoma. Jpn J Clin Oncol 2003; 33:288–296.
472. Douillard JY, Hoff PM, Skillings JR, et al. Multicenter phase III study of uracil/tegafur and oral leucovorin versus fluorouracil and leucovorin in patients with previously untreated metastatic colorectal cancer. J Clin Oncol 2002; 20:3605–3616.
473. Kabbinavar FF, Hambleton J, Mass RD, Hurwitz HI, Bergsland E, Sarkar S. Combined analysis of efficacy: the addition of bevacizumab to fluorouracil/ leucovorin improves survival for patients with metastatic colorectal cancer. J Clin Oncol 2005; 23(16):3706–3712.
474. Hurwitz HI, Fehrenbacher L, Hainsworth JD, et al. Bevacisumab in combination with fluorouracil and leucovorin: an active regimen for first-line metastatic colorectal cancer. J Clin Oncol 2005; 23(15):3502–3508.

475. Lise M, Gerard A, Nitti D, et al. Adjuvant therapy for colorectal cancer. The EORTC experience and a review of the literature. Dis Colon Rectum 1987; 30:847–854.
476. Gray BN, Walker C, Andrewartha L, et al. Melbourne trial of adjuvant immunotherapy in operable large bowel cancer. Aust N Z J Surg 1988; 58:43–46.
477. Wiesenfeld M, O'Connell MJ, Wieand HS, et al. Controlled clinical trial of interferon-α vs. postoperative surgical adjuvant therapy for colon cancer. J Clin Oncol 1995; 13:2324–2329.
478. Reithmulller G, Schnieder-Godicke E, Schlimok G, et al. Randomized trial of monoclonal antibody for adjuvant therapy of resected Dukes' C colorectal carcinoma. Lancet 1994; 343:1177–1183.
479. Guillou PJ. Potential impact of immunobiotechnology on cancer therapy. Br J Surg 1987; 74:705–710.
480. McArdle CS, Hole DJ. Emergency presentation of colorectal cancer is associated with poor 5-year survival. Br J Surg 2004; 91:605–609.
481. Jestin P, Nilsson J, Heurgren M, Pahlman L, Glimelius B, Gunnarsson U. Emergency surgery for colonic cancer in a defined population. Br J Surg 2005; 92:94–100.
482. Amsterdam E, Krispin M. Primary resection with colostomy for obstructive carcinoma of the left side of the colon. Am J Surg 1985; 150:558–560.
483. White CM, Macfie J. Immediate colectomy and primary anastomoses for acute obstruction due to carcinoma of the left colon and rectum. Dis Colon Rectum 1985; 28:155–157.
484. Sjodahl R, Franzen T, Nystrom PO. Primary versus staged resection for acute obstructing colorectal carcinoma. Br J Surg 1992; 79:685–688.
485. Nozoe T, Yasuda M, Honda M, Inutsuka S, Korenaga D. Obstructing carcinomas of the colon and rectum have a smaller size compared with those of non-obstructing carcinomas. Oncol Rep 2001; 8:1313–1315.
486. Smithers BM, Theile DE, Cohen JR, et al. Emergency right hemicolectomy in colon carcinoma: a prospective study. Aust N Z J Surg 1986; 56:749–752.
487. Lee YM, Law WL, Chu KW, Poon RT. Emergency surgery for obstructing colorectal cancers: a comparison between right-sided and left-sided lesions. J Am Coll Surg 2001; 192(6):719–725.
488. Deans GT, Krukowski ZH, Irwin ST. Malignant obstruction of the left colon. Br J Surg 1994; 81:1270–1276.
489. Porter JA, Salvati EP, Rubin RJ, et al. Complications of coiostomies. Dis Colon Rectum 1989; 32:299–303.
490. Wong SK, Eu KW, Lim SL, et al. Total colectomy removes undetected proximal synchronous lesions in acute left-sided colonic obstruction. Tech Coloproctol 1996; 4:87–88.
491. Stephenson BM, Shandall AA, Farouk R, et al. Malignant left-sided bowel obstruction managed by subtotal/total colectomy. Br J Surg 1990; 77:1098–1102.
492. Perez MD, de Fuenmayor ML, Calvo N, et al. Morbidity of emergency subtotal colectomy in obstructing carcinoma of the left colon. Br J Surg 1995; 82(Suppl):33.
493. Lau PW, Lo CY, Law WL. The role of one stage surgery in acute left-sided colonic obstruction. Am J Surg 1995; 169:406–409.
494. Chrysos E, Athanasakis E, Vassilakis JS, Zoras O, Xynos E. Total colectomy and J-pouch ileorectal anastomosis for obstructed tumors of the rectosigmoid junction. ANZ J Surg 2002; 72:92–94.
495. Tan SG, Nambiar R. Resection and anastomosis of obstructed left colonic cancer: primary or staged? Aust N Z J Surg 1995; 65:728–731.
496. Stewart J, Diament RH, Brennan TG. Management of obstructing lesions of the left colon by resection on table lavage and primary anastomosis. Surgery 1993; 114:502–505.
497. Kressner U, Antonsson J, Ejerblad S, et al. Intraoperative colonic lavage and primary anastomosis—an alternative to the Hartmann procedure in emergency surgery of the left colon. Eur J Surg 1994; 160:287–292.
498. Scotia Study Group. Single-stage treatment for malignant left-sided colonic obstruction: a prospective randomized clinical trial comparing subtotal colectomy with segmental resection following intraoperative irrigation. Br J Surg 1995; 82:1622–1627.
499. Chiappa A, Zbar A, Biella F, Staudacher C. One-stage resection and primary anastomosis following acute obstruction of the left colon for cancer. Am Surg 2000; 66:619–622.
500. Goodall RG, Park M. Primary resection and anastomosis of lesions obstructing the left colon. Can J Surg 1988; 31:167–168.
501. Ravo B. Colorectal anastomotic healing and intracolonic bypass procedure. Surg Clin North Am 1988; 68:1267–1294.
502. Kronborg O. The missing randomized trial of two surgical treatments for acute obstruction due to carcinoma of the left colon and rectum. Int J Colorectal Dis 1986; 1:162–166.
503. Fielding LP, Stewart-Brown S, Blesovsky L. Large bowel obstruction caused by cancer. A prospective study. Br Med J 1979; 2:515–517.
504. Eckhauser ML, Mansour EG. Endoscopic laser therapy for obstructing and/or bleeding colorectal carcinoma. Am Surg 1992; 58:358–362.
505. Dohmoto M. New method-endosopic implantation of rectal stent in palliative treatment of malignant stenosis. Digestiva 1991; 3:1507–1512.
506. Tejero E, Mainar A, Fernandez L, Tobio R, De Gregorio MA. New procedure for the treatment of colorectal neoplastic obstructions. Dis Colon Rectum 1994; 37:1158–1159.
507. Dauphine CE, Tan P, Beart W Jr., Vukasin P, Cohen H, Corman ML. Placement of self-expanding metal stents for acute malignant large-bowel obstruction: a collective review. Ann Surg Oncol 2002; 9:574–579.
508. Khot UP, Lang AW, Murali K, Parker MC. Systematic review of the efficacy and safety of colorectal stents. Br J Surg 2002; 89:1096–1102.
509. Law WL, Choi HK, Lee YM, Chu KW. Palliation for advanced malignant colorectal obstruction by self-expanding metallic stents: prospective evaluation of outcomes. Dis Colon Rectum 2004; 47:39–43.
510. Saida Y, Sumiyama Y, Nagao J, Uramatsu M. Long-term prognosis of pre-operative "bridge to surgery" expandable metallic stent insertion for obstructive colorectal cancer: comparison with emergency operation. Dis Colon Rectum 2003; 46(suppl 10):S44–S49.
511. Martinez-Santos C, Lobato RF, Fradejas JM, Pinto I, Ortega-Deballon P, Moreno-Azcoita M. Self-expandable stent before elective surgery versus. emergency surgery for the treatment of malignant colorectal obstructions: comparison of primary anastomosis and morbidity rates. Dis Colon Rectum 2002; 45: 401–406.
512. Johnson R, Marsh R, Corson J, Seymour K. A comprison of two methods of palliation of large bowel obstruction due to irremovable colon cancer. Ann R Coll Surg Engl 2004; 86:99–103.
513. Meisner S, Hensler M, Knop FK, West F, Wille-Jorgensen P. Self-expanding metal stents for colonic obstruction: experiences from 104 procedures in a single center. Dis Colon Rectum 2004; 47:444–450.
514. Suzuki N, Saunders BP, Thomas-Gibson S, Akle C, Marshall M, Halligan S. Colorectal stenting for malignant and benign disease: outcomes in colorectal stenting. Dis Colon Rectum 2004; 47:1207–1207.
515. Tomiki Y, Watanabe T, Ishibiki Y, et al. Comparison of stent placement and colostomy as palliative treatment for inoperatble malignant colorectal obstruction. Surg Endosc 2004; 18:1572–1977.
516. Sebastian S, Johnston S, Geoghegan T, Torreggiani W, Buckley M. Pooled Analysis of the efficacy and safety of self-expanding metal stenting in malignant colorectal obstruction. Am J Gastroenterol 2004; 99(10):2051–2057.
517. Carne PW, Frye JN, Robertson GM, Frizelle FA. Stents or open operation for palliation of colorectal cancer: a retrospective, cohort study of perioperative outcome and long-term survival. Dis Colon Rectum 2004; 47(9): 1455–1461.
518. Tsai MA, Yang YC, Leu FJ. Obstructive colitis proximal to partially obstructive colonic carcinoma: a case report and review of the literature. Int J Colorectal Dis 2004; 19:268–272.
519. Rowe VL, Frost DB, Huang S. Extended resection for locally advanced colorectal carcinoma. Ann Surg Oncol 1997; 4:131–136.
520. Glass RE, Fazio VW, Jagelman DG, et al. The results of surgical treatment of cancer of the colon at the Cleveland Clinic from 1965–1975. A classification of the spread of colon cancer and long term survival. Int J Colorectal Dis 1986; 1:33–39.
521. Gall FP, Tonak J, Altendorf A. Multivisceral resections in colorectal cancer. Dis Colon Rectum 1987; 30:337–341.
522. Hunter JA, Ryan JA, Schultz P. En bloc resection of coln cancer adherent to other organs. Am J Surg 1987; 154:67–71.
523. Orkin BA, Dozois RR, Beart RW Jr., Patterson DE, Gunderson LL, Ilstrup DM. Extended resection for locally advanced primary adenocarcinoma of the rectum. Dis Colon Rectum 1989; 32:286–292.
524. Eisenberg SB, Kraybill WG, Lopez MJ. Long-term results of surgical resection of locally advanced coiorectal carcinoma. Surgery 1990; 108:779–786.
525. Montesani C, Ribotta G, DeMilito R, et al. Extended resection in the treatment of colorectal cancer. Int J Colorectal Dis 1991; 6:161–164.
526. Curley SA, Carlson GW, Shumato CR, et al. Extended resection for locally advanced colorectal carcinoma. Am J Surg 1992; 163:553–559.
527. Izbicki JR, Hosch SB, Knoefel WT, et al. Extended resections are beneficial for patients with locally advanced colorectal cancer. Dis Colon Rectum 1995; 38:1251–1256.
528. Carne PW, Frye JN, Kennedy-Smith A, et al. Local invasion of the bladder with colorectal cancers: surgical management and patterns of local recurrence. Dis Colon Rectum 2004; 47:44–47.
529. Nakafusa Y, Tanaka T, Tanaka M, Kitajima Y, Sato S, Miyazaki K. Comparison of multivisceral resection and standard operation for locally advanced colorectal cancer: analysis of prognostic factors for short-term and long-term outcome. Dis Colon Rectum 2004; 47(12):2055–2063.
530. Curley SA, Evans DB, Ames FC. Resection for cure of carcinoma of the colon directly involving the duodenum or pancreatic head. J Am Coll Surg 1994; 179:587–592.
531. Koea JB, Conlon K, Paty PB, Guillem JG, Cohen AM. Pancreatic or duodenal resection or both for advanced carcinoma of the right colon: is it justified? Dis Colon Rectum 2000; 43:460–465.
532. Talamonti MS, Shumate CR, Carlson GW, et al. Locally advanced carcinoma of the colon and rectum involving the urinary bladder. Surg Gynecol Obstet 1993; 177:481–487.
533. Kroneman H, Castelein A, Jeekel J. En bloc resection of colon carcinoma adherent to other organs: an efficacious treatment? Dis Colon Rectum 1991; 34:780–783.
534. Poeze M, Houbiers JGA, van de Velde CJH, et al. Radical resection of locally advanced colorectal cancer. Br J Surg 1995; 82:1386–1390.

535. Landercasper J, Stolee RT, Steenlage E, et al. Treatment and outcome of right colon cancers adherent to adjacent organs or the abdominal wall. Arch Surg 1992; 127:841–846.
536. Yamada K, Ishizawa T, Niwa K, Chuman Y, Aikou T. Pelvic exenteration and sacral resection for locally advanced primary and recurrent rectal cancer. Dis Colon Rectum 2002; 45:1078–1084.
537. Lopez MJ, Monafo WW. Role of extended resection in the initial treatment of locally advanced colorectal carcinoma. Surgery 1993; 113:365–372.
538. Campbell SC, Church JM, Fazio VW, et al. Combined radical retropubic prostatectomy and proctosigmoidectomy for en bloc removal of locally invasive carcinoma of the rectum. Surg Gynecol Obstet 1993; 176:605–608.
539. McNamara DA, Fitzpatrick JM, O'Comnnell PR. Urinary tract involvement by colorectal cancer. Dis cancer Rectum 2003; 46:1266–1276.
540. Cady B, Monson DO, Swinton NW Sr. Survival of patients after colonic resection for carcinoma with simultaneous liver mects-tases. Surg Gynecol Obstet 1970; 131:697–700.
541. Joffe J, Gordon PH. Palliative resection for colorectal carcinoma. Dis Colon Rectum 1981; 24:355–360.
542. Liu SEM, Church JM, Lavery IC, et al. Operation in patients with incurable colon cancer—is it worthwhile? Dis Colon Rectum 1997; 40:11–14.
543. Takaki HS, Ujiki GT, Shields TS. Palliative resection in the treatment of primary colorectal cancer. Am J Surg 1977; 133:548–550.
544. Goslin R, Steele G, Zamcheck N, et al. Factors influencing survival in patients with hepatic metastases from adenocardnoma of the colon or rectum. Dis Colon Rectum 1982; 25:749–754.
545. Makela J, Haukipuro K, Laitinen S, et al. Palliative operations for colorectal cancer. Dis Colon Rectum 1990; 33:846–850.
546. Feqiz G, Ramacciato G, Indinnimeo M, et al. Synchronous large bowel cancer: a series of 47 cases. Ital J Surg Sci 1989; 19:23–28.
547. Bussey HJR, Wallace MH, Morson BC. Metachronous carcinomas of the large intestine and intestinal polyps. Proc R Soc Med 1967; 60:208–210.
548. Chu DZJ, Giacco G, Martin RG, et al. The significance of synchronous carcinoma and polyps in the colon and rectum. Cancer 1986; 57:445–450.
549. Passman MA, Pommier RF, Vetto JT. Synchronous colon primaries have the same prognosis as solitary colon cancers. Dis Colon Cancer 1996; 39:329–334.
550. Fogler R, Weiner E. Multiple foci of colorectal carcinoma. Argument for subtotal colectomy. N Y State J Med 1980; 80:47–51.
551. Gervaz P, Bucher P, Neyroud-Caspar I, Soravia C, Morel P. Proximal location of colon cancer is a risk factor for development of metachronous colorectal cancer: a population-based study. Dis Colon Rectum 2005; 48:227–232.
552. Shitoh K, Konishi F, Miyakura Y, Togashi K, Okamoto T, Nagai H. Microsatellite instability as a marker in predicting metachronous multiple colorectal carcinomas after surgery: a cohort-like study. Dis Colon Rectum 2002; 45:329–333.
553. Finlay IG, McArdle CS. Occult hepatic metastases in colorectal carcinoma. Br J Surg 1986; 73:732–735.
554. Machi J, Isomoto H, Kurohiji T, et al. Detection of unrecognized liver metastases from colorectal cancer by routine use of operative ultrasonography. Dis Colon Rectum 1986; 29:405–409.
555. Blumgart LH, Fong Y. Surgical options in the treatment of hepatic metastases from colorectal cancer. Curr Probl Surg 1995; 32:335–421.
556. Finlay IG, Meek D, Branton F, et al. Growth rate of hepatic metastases in colorectal carcinoma. Br J Surg 1998; 75:641–644.
557. Wigmore SJ, Madhavan K, Redhead DN, Currie EJ, Garden OJ. Distribution of colorectal liver metastases in patients referred for hepatic resection. Cancer 2000; 89:285–287.
558. Van Ooijen B, Oudkerk M, Schmitz PIM, et al. Detection of liver metastases from colorectal carcinoma: is there a place for routine computed tomography arteriography. Surgery 1996; 119:511–516.
559. Strasberg SM, Dehdashti F, Siegel BA, Drebin JA, Linehan D. Survival of patients evaluated by FDG-PET before hepatic resection for metastatic colorectal carcinoma: a prospective database study. Ann Surg 2001; 233:293–299.
560. Rodgers MS, Collinson R, Desai S, Stubbs RS, McCall JL. Risk of dissemination with biopsy of colorectal liver metastases. Dis Colon Rectum 2003; 46:454–458.
561. Fuhrman GM, Curley SA, Hohn DC, et al. Improved survival after resection of colorectal liver metastases. Ann Surg Oncol 1995; 2:537–541.
562. Bengtsson G, Carlsson G, Hafstrom L, et al. Natural history of patients with treated liver metastases from colorectal cancer. Am J Surg 1981; 141:586–589.
563. Nagorney DM. Hepatic resection for metastases from colorectal cancer. Nelson RL, ed. Problems in Current Surgery. Controversies in Colon Cancer. Philadelphia: JB Lippincott, 1987:83–92.
564. Palmer M, Petrelli NJ, Herrera L. No treatment option for liver metastases for colorectal adenocarcinoma. Dis Colon Rectum 1989; 32:698–701.
565. Stangl R, Altendorf-Hofmann A, Charnley RM, et al. Factors influencing the natural history of colorectal liver metastases. Lancet 1994; 343:1405–1410.
566. Vauthey JN, Marsch R, de W, et al. Arterial therapy of hepatic colorectal metastases. Br J Surg 1996; 83:447–445.
567. Hughes KS, Scheele J, Sugarbaker PH. Surgery for colorectal cancer metastatic to the liver. Optimizing the results of treatment. Surg Clin North Am 1989; 69:339–359.
568. Schlag P, Hohenberger P, Herforth C. Resection of liver metastases in colorectal cancer—competitive analysis of treatment results in synchronous versus metachrounous metastases. Eur J Surg Oncol 1990; 16:360–365.
569. Petrelli N, Gupta B, Piedmonte M, et al. Morbidity and survival of liver resection for colorectal adenocarcinoma. Dis Colon Rectum 1991; 34: 889–904.
570. Doci R, Gennari L, Bignami P, et al. One hundred patients with hepatic metastases from colorectal cancer treated by resection: analysis of prognostic determinants. Br J Surg 1991; 78:797–801.
571. Rosen CB, Nagorney DM, Taswell HF, et al. Perioperative blood transfusion and determinants of survival after liver resection for metastatic colorectal carcinoma. Ann Surg 1992; 216:492–505.
572. Nakamura S, Yokoi Y, Suzuki S, et al. Results of extensive surgery for liver metastasis in colorectal carcinoma. Br J Surg 1992; 79:35–38.
573. Van Ooijen B, Wiggers T, Meijer S, et al. Hepatic resections for colorectal cancer metastases in the Netherlands. A multi-institutional 10-years study. Cancer 1992; 70:28–34.
574. Grayowski TJ, Iwatsuki S, Madariaga JR, et al. Experience in resection for metastatic colorectal cancer: analysis of clinical and pathologic risk factors. Surgery 1994; 116:703–711.
575. Scheele J, Stang R, Altendorf-Hofmann A, et al. Resection of colorectal liver metastases. World J Surg 1995; 19:59–71.
576. Hananel N, Garzon J, Gordon PH. Hepatic resection for colorectal livery metastases. Am Surg 1995; 61:444–447.
577. Rougier PH, Milan C, Lazorthes F, et al. Prospective study of prognostic factors in patients with unresected hepativ metastases from colorectal cancer. Br J Surg 1995; 82:1397–1400.
578. Wade TP, Virgo KS, Li MJ, et al. Outcomes after detection of metastatic carcinoma of the colon and rectum in a national hospital system. J Am Coll Surg 1996; 182:353–361.
579. Wanebo HJ, Chu QD, Vezeridis MP, et al. Patient selection for hepatic resection of colorectal metastases. Arch Surg 1996; 131:322–329.
580. Ohlsson B, Stenram U, Tranberg KG. Resection of colorectal liver metastases: 25-year experience. World J Surg 1998; 22:268–276.
581. Fong Y, Fortner J, Sun RL, Brennan MF, Blumgart LH. Clinical score for predicting recurrence after hepatic resection for metastatic colorectal cancer: analysis of 1001 consecutive cases. Ann Surg 1999; 230:309–318.
582. Buell JF, Rosen S, Yoshida A, et al. Hepatic resection: effective treatment for primary and secondary tumors. Surgery 2000; 128:686–693.
583. Elias D, Ouellet JF, Bellon N, Pignon JP, Pocard M, Lasser P. Extrahepatic disease does not contraindicate hepatectomy for colorectal liver metastases. Br J Surg 2003; 90:567–574.
584. Kato T, Yasui K, Hirai T, et al. Therapeutic results for hepatic metastasis of colorectal cancer with special reference to effectiveness of hepatectomy: analysis of prognostic factors for 763 cases recorded at 18 institutions. Dis Colon Rectum 2003; 46(suppl):S22–S31.
585. Teh CS, Ooi LL. Hepatic resection for colorectal metastases to the liver: The National Cancer Centre/Singapore General Hospital experience. Ann Acad Med Singapore 2003; 32:196–204.
586. Weber JC, Bachellier P, Oussoultzoglou E, Jaeck D. Simultaneous resection of colorectal primary tumour and synchronous liver metastases. Br J Surg 2003; 90:956–962.
587. Lefor AT, Hughes KS, Shiloni E, et al. Intra-abdominal extrahepatic disease in patients with colorectal hepatic metastases. Dis Colon Rectum 1988; 31: 100–103.
588. Wagner JS, Adson MA, VanHeerden JA, et al. The natural history of hepatic metastases from colorectal cancer. Ann Surg 1984; 199:502–508.
589. Luna-Perez P, Rodriguez-Coria DF, Arroyo B, Gonzalez-Macouzet J. The natural history of liver metastases from colorectal cancer. Arch Med Res 1998; 29(1):319–324.
590. Ruo L, Gougoutas C, Paty PB, Guillem JG,Cohen AM, Wong WD. Elective bowel resection for incurable stage IV colorectal cancer: prognostic variables for asymptomatic patients. J Am Coll Surg 2003; 196:722–728.
591. Kuo LJ, Leu SY, Liu MC, Jian JJM, Cheng SH, Chen CM. How aggressive should we be in patients with stage IV colorectal cancer? Dis Colon Rectum 2003; 46:1646–1652.
592. de Santibanes E, Lassalle FB, McCormack L, et al. Simultaneous colorectal and hepatic resections for colorectal cancer: postoperative and long term outcomes. J Am Coll Surg 2002; 195:196–202.
593. Chua HK, Sondenna K, Tsiotos GG, Larson DR, Wolff BG, Nagorney DM. Concurrent vs. staged colectomy and hepatectomy for primary colorectal cancer with synchronous hepatic metastases. Dis Colon Rectum 2004; 47:1310–1316.
594. Tocchi A, Mazzoni G, Brozzetti S, Miccini M, Cassini D, Bettelli E. Hepatic resection in stage IV colorectal cancer: prognostic predictors of outcome. Int J Colorectal Dis 2004 19: 580–5.
595. Tanaka K, Shimada H, Matsuo K, et al. Outcome after simultaneous colorectal and hepatic resection for colorectal cancer with synchronous metastases. Surgery 2004; 136:650–659.
596. Attiyeh FF, Wichern WA. Hepatic resection for primary metastatic tumours. Am J Surg 1988; 156:368–373.

597. Adson MA. Resection of liver metastases – when is it worthwhile? World J Surg 1987; 11:511–520.
598. Bozzetti F, Doci R, Bignami P, et al. Patterns of failure following surgical resection of colorectal cancer, liver metastases. Rationale for a multimodal approach. Ann Surg 1987; 205:264–270.
599. Tanaka K, Adam R, Shimada H, Azoulay D, Levi F, Bismuth H. Role of neoadjuvant chemotherapy in the treatment of multiple colorectal metastases to the liver. Br J Surg 2003; 90:963–969.
600. Allen PJ, Kemeny N, Jarnagin W, Dematteo R, Blumgart L, Fong Y. Importance of response to neoadjuvant chemotherapy in patients undergoing resection of synchronous colorectal liver metastases. J Gastrointest Surg 2003; 7:109–115.
601. Iwatsuki S, Dvorchik I, Madariaga JR, et al. Hepatic resection for metastatic colorectal adenocarcinoma: a proposal of a prognostic scoring system. J Am Coll Surg 1999; 189:291–299.
602. Smith DL, Soria JC, Morat L, et al. Human telomerase reverse transcriptase (hTERT) and Ki-67 are better predictors of survival than established clinical indicators in patients undergoing curative hepatic resection for colorectal metastases. Ann Surg Oncol 2004; 11:45–51.
603. Imamura H, Seyama Y, Kokudo N, et al. Single and multiple resections of multiple hepatic metastases of colorectal origin. Surgery 2004; 135:508–517.
604. Jaeck D. The significance of hepatic pedicle lymph nodes metastases in surgical management of colorectal liver metastases and of other liver malignancies. Ann Surg Oncol 2003; 10:1007–1011.
605. Elias D, Sideris L, Pocard M, et al. Results of R0 resection for colorectal liver metastases associated with extrahepatic disease. Ann Surg Oncol 2004; 11:274–280.
606. Martin R, Paty P, Fong Y, et al. Simultaneous liver and colorectal resections are safe for synchronous colorectal liver metastasis. J Am Coll Surg 2003; 197:223–241.
607. Nelson RL, Freels S. A systematic review of hepatic artery chemotherapy after hepatic resection of colorectal cancer metastatic to the liver. Dis Colon Rectum 2004; 47:739–745.
608. Clancy TE, Dixon E, Perlis R, Sutherland FR, Zinner MJ. Hepatic arterial infusion after curative resection of colorectal cancer metastases: a meta-analysis of prospective clinical trials. J Gastrointest Surg 2005; 9:198–206.
609. Bines SD, Doolas A, Jenkins L, et al. Survival after repeat hepatic resection for recurrent colorectal hepatic metastases. Surgery 1996; 120:591–596.
610. Wanebo HJ, Chu QD, Avradopoulos KA, et al. Current perspectives on repeat hepatic resection for colorectal carcinoma: a review. Surgery 1996; 119: 361–371.
611. Pinson CW, Wright JK, Chapman WC, et al. Repeat hepatic surgery for colorectal cancer metastases to the liver. Am Surg 1996; 223:765–776.
612. Fernandez-Trigo V, Shamsa F, Sugarbaker PH. Repeat liver resections from colorectal metastasis. Surgery 1995; 117:296–304.
613. Oue FG, Nagorney DM. Resection of "recurrent" colorectal metastases to the liver. Br J Surg 1994; 81:255–258.
614. Takahashi S, Inoue K, Konishi M, Nakagouri T, Kinoshita T. Prognostic factors for poor survival after repeat hepatectomy in patients with colorectal liver metastases. Surgery 2003; 133:627–634.
615. Suzuki S, Sakaguchi T, Yokoi Y, et al. Impact of repeat hepatectomy on recurrent colorectal liver metastases. Surgery 2001; 129:421–428.
616. Oshowo A, Gillams A, Harrison E, Lees WR, Taylor I. Comparison of resection and radiofrequency ablation for treatment of solitary colorectal liver metastases. Br J Surg 2003; 90:1240–1243.
617. Berber E, Pelley R, Siperstein AE. Predictors of survival after radiofrequency thermal ablation of colorectal cancer metastases to the liver: a prospective study. J Clin Oncol 2005; 23(7):1358–1364.
618. Ueno H, Mochizuki H, Hashiguchi Y, Hastsuse K, Fujimoto H, Hase K. Predictors of extrahepatic recurrence after resection of colorectal liver metastases. Br J Surg 2004; 91:327–333.
619. Cohen DA, Kemeny EN. An update on hepatic arterial infusion chemotherapy for colorectal cancer. The Oncologist 2003; 8:553–556.
620. Gray BN, Anderson JE, Burton MA, et al. Regression of liver metastases following treatment with yttrium-90 microspheres. Aust N Z J Surg 1992; 62:105–110.
621. Stubbs RS, Cannan RJ, Mitchell AW. Selective internal radiation therapy with 90yttrium microspheres for extensive colorectal liver metastases. J Gastrointest Surg 2001; 5(3):294–302.
622. Lang EK, Brown CL. Colorectal metastases to the liver: selective chemoembolization. Radiology 1993; 189:417–422.
623. Stuart K. Chemoembolization in the manangement of liver tumors. The Oncologist 2003; 8:425–437.
624. Weaver ML, Atkinson D, Zemel R. Hepatic cryosurgery in the treatment of unresectable metastases. Surg Oncol 1995; 4:231–236.
625. Ruers TJ, Joosten J, Jager GJ, Wobbes T. Long-term results of treating hepatic colorectal metastases with cryosurgery. Br J Surg 2001; 88:844–849.
626. Scheele J, Altendorf-Hofmann A, Stangl R, et al. Pulmonary resection for metastatic colon and upper rectum cancer: is it useful? Dis Colon Rectum 1990; 33:745–752.
627. Saclarides TJ, Krueger BL, Szeluga DJ, et al. Thoracotomy for colon and rectal cancer metastases. Dis Colon Rectum 1993; 36:425–429.
628. Brister SJ, de Varennes B, Gordon PH, et al. Contemporary operative management of pulmonary metastases of colorectal origin. Dis Colon Rectum 1988; 31:786–792.
629. Kanemitsu Y, Kato T, Hirai T, Yasui K. Preoperative probability model for predicting overall survival after resection of pulmonary metastases from colorectal cancer. Br J Surg 2004; 91:112–120.
630. Watanabe I, Arai T, Ono M, et al. Prognostic factors in resection of pulmonary metastasis from colorectal cancer. Br J Surg 2003; 90(11):1436–1440.
631. Negri F, Musolino A, Normon AR, Landos G, Pastorino U, Chong E, Cunningham D. The development for preoperative chemotherapy strategy for patients selected to undergo pulmonary metastectomy from colorectal cancer. J Clin Oncol 2004; 145:202S.
632. King J, Glenn D, Clark W, et al. Percutaneous radiofrequency ablation of pulmonary metastases in patients with colorectal cancer. Br J Surg 2004; 91: 217–223.
633. Ike H, Shimada H, Ohki S, Togo S, Yamaguchi S, Ichikawa Y. Results of aggressive resection of lung metastases from colorectal carcinoma detected by intensive follow-up. Dis Colon Rectum 2002; 45:468–473.
634. Ishikawa K, Hashiguchi Y, Mochizuki H, Ozeki Y, Ueno H. Extranodal cancer deposit at the primary tumor site and the number of pulmonary lesions are useful prognostic factors after surgery for colorectal lung metastases. Dis Colon Rectum 2003; 46:629–636.
635. Zink S, Kayser G, Gabius HJ, Kayser K. Survival, disease-free interval, and associated tumor features in patients with colon/rectal carcinomas and their resected intra-pulmonary metastases. Eur J Cardiothorac Surg 2001; 19:908–913.
636. Irshad K, Ahmad F, Morin JE, Mulder DS. Pulmonary metastases from colorectal cancer: 25 years of experience. Can J Surg 2001; 44:217–221.
637. Vogelsang H, Haas S, Hierhoizer C, Berger U, Siewert JR, Prauer H. Factors influencing survival after resection of pulmonary metastases from colorectal cancer. Br J Surg 2004; 91:1066–1071.
638. Mineo TC, Ambrogi V, Tonini G, et al. Longterm results after resection of simultaneous and sequential lung and liver metastases from colorectal carcinoma. J Am Coll Surg 2003; 197:386–391.
639. Ike H, Shimada H, Togo S, Yamaguchi S, Ichikawa Y, Tanaka K. Sequential resection of lung metastasis following partial hepatectomy for colorectal cancer. Br J Surg 2002; 89:1164–1168.
640. Nagakura S, Shirai Y, Yamato Y, Yokoyama N, Suda T, Hatakeyama K. Simultaneous detection of colorectal carcinoma liver and lung metastases does not warrant resection. J Am Coll Surg 2001; 193:153–160.
641. Traina TA, Loonard GD, Tang L, Paty PB, Maki RG. Problems in colon cancer and a child with Renal Lymphoma: CASE 1. Metastatic colon cancer to the ovaries in a Krukenberg-like pattern. J Clin Oncol 2005; 23(22): 5255–5256.
642. Herrera-Ornelas L, Natarajan N, Tsukada Y, et al. Adenocarcinoma of the colon masquerading as primary ovarian neoplasia. An analysis of ten cases. Dis Colon Rectum 1983; 26:377–380.
643. Morrow M, Enker WE. Late ovarian metastases in carcinoma of the colon and rectum. Arch Surg 1984; 119:1385–1388.
644. Huang PP, Weber TK, Mendoza C, Rodriguez-Bigas MA, Petrelli NJ. Long-term survival in patients with ovarian metastases from colorectal carcinoma. Ann Surg Oncol 1998; 5(8):695–698.
645. Besbeas S, Stearns MW Jr. Osseous metastases from carcinomas of the colon and rectum. Dis Colon Rectum 1978; 21:266–268.
646. Bonnheim DC, Petrelli NJ, Herrera L, et al. Osseous metastases from colorectal carcinoma. Am J Surg 1986; 151:457–459.
647. Scuderi G, Macri A, Sfuncia G, et al. Sternal metastasis as initial presentation of a unknown rectal cancer. Int J Colorectal Dis 2004; 19:292–293.
648. Wong ET, Berkenblit A. The role of topotecan in the treatment of brain metastases. The Oncologist 2004; 9:68–79.
649. Alden TD, Gianino JW, Saclarides TJ. Brain metastases from colorectal cancer. Dis Colon Rectum 1996; 39:541–545.
650. Hammond MA, McCutcheon IE, Elsouki R, et al. Colorectal carcinoma and brain metastases: distribution, treatment and survival. Ann Surg Oncol 1996; 3:453–463.
651. Farnell GF, Buckner JC, Cascino TL, et al. Brain metastases from colorectal carcinoma. The long-term survivors. Cancer 1996; 78:74–76.
652. Knorr C, Reingruber B, Meyer T, Hohenberger W, Stremmel C. Peritoneal carcinomatosis of colorectal cancer: incidence, prognosis, and treatment modalities. Int J Colorectal Dis 2004; 19:181–187.
653. Glehen O, Kwiatkowski F, Sugarbaker PH, et al. Cytoreductive surgery combined with perioperative intraperitoneal chemotherapy for the management of peritoneal carcinomatosis from colorectal cancer: a multi-institutional study. J Clin Oncol 2004; 22:3284–3292.
654. Culliford AT 4th, Brooks AD, Sharma S, et al. Surgical debulking and intraperitoneal chemotherapy for established peritoneal metastases from colon and appendix cancer. Ann Surg Oncol 2001; 8(10):787–795.
655. Verwaal VJ, van Ruth S, de Bree E, et al. Randomized trial of cytoreduction and hyperthermic intraperitoneal chemotherapy versus systemic chemotherapy and palliative surgery in patients with peritoneal carcinomatosis of colorectal cancer. J Clin Oncol 2003; 21:3737–3743.

656. Verwaal VJ, van Ruth S, Witkamp A, Boot H, van Slooten G, Zoetmulder FA. Long-term survival of peritoneal carcinomatosis of colorectal origin. Ann Surg Oncol 2005; 12:65–71.
657. Shen P, Hawksworth J, Lovato J, et al. Cytoreductive surgery and intraperitoneal hyperthermic chemotherapy with mitomycin C for peritoneal carcinomatosis from nonappendiceal colorectal carcinoma. Ann Surg Oncol 2004; 11:178–186.
658. Elias D, Delperro JR, Sideris L, et al. Treatment of peritoneal carcinomatosis from colorectal cancer: impact of complete cytoreductive surgery and difficulties in conducting randomized trials. Ann Surg Oncol 2004; 11(5):518–521.
659. Mainprize KS, Berry AR. Solitary splenic metastasis from colorectal carcinoma. Br J Surg 1997; 84:70.
660. Rendi MH, Dhar AD. Cutaneous metastasis of rectal adenocarcinoma. Dermatol Nurs 2003; 15:131–132.
661. Tsai HL, Huang YS, Hsieh JS, Huang TJ, TSai KB. Signet-ring cell carcinoma of the rectum with diffuse and multiple skin metastases–a case report. Kaohsiung J Med Sci 2002; 18:359–362.
662. Gabriele R, Borghese M, Conte M, Bosso L. Sister Mary Joseph's nodule as a first sign of cancer of the cecum: report of a case. Dis Colon Rectum 2004; 47:115–117.
663. Yan BK, Nyam DC, Ho YH. Carcinoma of the rectum with a single penile metastasis. Singapore Med J 2002; 43:39–40.
664. Tutton MG, George M, Hill ME, Abulafi AM. Solitary pancreatic metastasis from a primary colonic tumor detected by PET scan: report of a case. Dis Colon Rectum 2001; 44:288–290.
665. Chagpar A, Kanthan SC. Vaginal metastasis of colon cancer. Am Surg 2001; 67:171–172.
666. Charles W, Joseph G, Hunis B, Rankin L. Problems in colon cancer and a child with renal lymphoma: CASE 2. metastatic colon cancer to the testicle presenting as testicular hydrocele. J Clin Oncol 2005; 23(22):5256–5257.
667. Tiong HY, Kew CY, Tan KB, Salto-Tellez M, Leong AF. Metastatic testicular carcinoma from the colon with clinical, immunophenotypical, and molecular characterization: report of a case. Dis Colon Rectum 2005; 48:582–585.
668. Radhakrishnan CN, Bruce J. Colorectal cancers in children without any predisposing factors. A report of eight cases and review of the literature. Eur J Pediatr Surg 2003; 13:66–68.
669. Killingback M, Barron P, Dent O. Elective resection and anastomosis for colorectal cancer: a prospective audit of mortality and morbidity 1976–1998. ANZ J Surg 2002; 72:689–698.
670. Platell CF, Semmens JB. Review of survival curves for colorectal cancer. Dis Colon Rectum 2004; 47(12):2070–2075.
671. Pihl E, Hughes ESR, McDermott FT, et al. Carcinomas of the colon—cancer specific long-term survival. A series of 615 patients treated by one surgeon. Ann Surg 1980; 192:114–117.
672. Stefanini P, Castrini G, Pappalardo G. Surgical treatment of cancer of the colon. Int Surg 1981; 66:125–131.
673. Zhou YG, Yu BM, Shen YX. Surgical treatment and late results in 1226 cases of colorectal cancer. Dis Colon Rectum 1983; 26:250–256.
674. Umpleby HC, Bristol JB, Rainey JB, et al. Survival of 727 patients with single carcinoma of the large bowel. Dis Colon Rectum 1984; 27:803–810.
675. Isbister WH, Fraser J. Survival following resection for colorectal cancer. A New Zealand national study. Dis Colon Rectum 1985; 28:725–727.
676. Wied U, Nilsson T, Knudson JB, et al. Postoperative survival of patients with potentially curable cancer of the colon. Dis Colon Rectum 1985; 28:233–235.
677. Davis NC, Evans EB, Cohen JR. Colorectal cancer: a large unselected Australian series. Aust N Z J Surg 1987; 57:153–159.
678. Moreaux J, Catala M. Carcinoma of the colon: long term survival and prognosis after surgical treatment in a series of 798 patients. World J Surg 1987; 11:804–809.
679. Brown SGW, Walsh S, Sykes PA. Operative mortality rate and surgery for colorectal cancer. Br J Surg 1988; 75:645–647.
680. Enblad P, Adami HO, Bergstrom R, et al. Improved survival of patients with cancers of the colon and rectum. J Natl Cancer Inst 1988; 80:586–591.
681. Jatzko G, Lisborg P, Wette V. Improving survival rates for patients with colorectal cancer. Br J Surg 1992; 79:588–591.
682. Clemmensen T, Sprechler M. Recording of patients with colorectal cancer on a database: results and advantages. Eur J Surg 1994; 160:175–178.
683. Carraro PG, Segala M, Cesana BM, Tiberio G. Obstructing colonic cancer: failure and survival patterns over a ten-year follow-up after one-stage curative surgery. Dis Colon Rectum 2001; 44:243–250.
684. Read TE, Mutch MG, Chang BW, et al. Locoregional recurrence and survival after curative resection of adenocarcinoma of the colon. J Am Coll Surg 2002; 195:33–40.
685. Morin NA, Obrand DF, Shrier I, Gordon PH (unpublished data). 2006.
686. Eisenberg B, Decosse JJ, Harford F, et al. Carcinoma of the colon and rectum: the natural history reviewed in 1704 patients. Cancer 1982; 49:1131–1134.
687. Staib L, Link KH, Blatz A, Beger HG. Surgery of colorectal cancer: surgical morbidity and five- and ten-year results in 2400 patients–monoinstitutional experience. World J Surg 2002; 26:59–66.
688. Devesa JM, Morales V, Enriquez JM, et al. Colorectal cancer. The bases for a comprehensive follow-up. Dis Colon Rectum 1988,31: 636–52.
689. The National Cancer Data Base Report on colon cancer, Nov 23, 2004. www.facs.org.
690. Kelley WE, Brown PW, Lawrence W Jr., et al. Penetrating, obstructing, and perforating carcinomas of the colon and rectum. Arch Surg 1981; 116: 381–384.
691. Brief DK, Brener BJ, Goldenkranz R, et al. An argument for increased use of subtotal colectomy in the management of carcinoma of the colon. Am Surg 1983; 49:66–72.
692. Crooms JW, Kovalcik PJ. Obstructing left-sided colon carcinoma. Appraisal of surgical options. Ann Surg 1984; 50:15–19.
693. Phillips RKS, Hittinger R, Fry JS, et al. Malignant large bowel obstruction. Br J Surg 1985; 72:296–302.
694. Willett C, Tepper JE, Cohen A, et al. Obstructive and perforative colonic carcinoma: patterns of failure. J Clin Oncol 1985; 3:379–384.
695. Serpell JW, McDermott FT, Katrivessis H, et al. Obstructing carcinomas of the colon. Br J Surg 1989; 76:965–969.
696. Mulcahy HE, Skelly MM, Husain A, et al. Long-term outcome following curative surgery for malignant large bowel obstruction. Br J Surg 1996; 83:46–50.
697. Chen HS, Sheen-Chen SM. Obstruction and perforation in colorectal adenocarcinoma: an analysis of prognosis and current trends. Surgery 2000; 127:370–376.
698. Hughes ESR, McDermott FT, Polglasse A, et al. Total and subtotal colectomy for colonic obstruction. Dis Colon Rectum 1985; 28:162–163.
699. Morgan WP, Jenkins N, Lewis P, et al. Management of obstructing carcinoma of the left colon by extended right hemicolectomy. Am J Surg 1985; 149:327–329.
700. Feng YS, Hsu H, Chen SS. One-stage operation for obstructing carcinomas of the left colon and rectum. Dis Colon Rectum 1987; 30:29–32.
701. Halevy A, Levi J, Orda R. Emergency subtotal colectomy. A new trend for treatment of obstructing carcinoma of the left colon. Ann Surg 1989; 210:220–223.
702. Slors JFM, Taat CW, Mallonga ET, et al. One-stage colectomy and ileorectal anastomosis for complete left-sided obstruction of the colon. Neth J Surg 1989; 41:1–4.
703. Stephenson BM, Shandall AA, Farouk R, et al. Malignant left-sided large bowel obstruction managed by subtotal/total colectomy. Br J Surg 1990; 77:1098–1102.
704. Antal SC, Kovacs ZG, Feigenbaum V, et al. Obstructing carcinoma of the left colon: treatment by extended right hemicolectomy. Int Surg 1991; 76: 161–163.
705. Tan SG, Nambiar B, Rauff A, et al. Primary resection and anastomosis in obstructed descending colon due to cancer. Arch Surg 1991; 126:748–751.
706. Murray J, Schoetz DJ Jr., Coller JA, et al. Intraoperative colonic lavage and primary anastomosis in non-elective colon resection. Dis Colon Rectum 1991; 34:527–531.
707. Stewart J, Diament RH, Brennan TG. Management of obstructing lesions of the left colon by resection, on table lavage, and primary anastomosis. Surgery 1993; 114:502–505.
708. Arnaud JP, Bergamaschi R. Emergency subtotal/total colectomy with anastomosis for acutely obstructed carcinoma of the left colon. Dis Colon Rectum 1994; 37:685–688.
709. Michowitz M, Avnieli D, Lazarovici J, et al. Perforation complicating carcinoma of the colon. J Surg Oncol 1982; 19:18–21.
710. Badia JM, Sitges-Serra A, Pia J. Perforation of colonic neoplasms. Review of 36 cases. Int J Colorectal Dis 1987; 2:187–189.
711. Carraro PG, Segala M, Orlotti C, Tiberio G. Outcome of large-bowel perforation in patients with colorectal cancer. Dis Colon Rectum 1998; 41(11): 1421–1426.
712. Khan S, Pawlak SE, Eggenberger JC, Lee CS, Szilagy EJ, Margolin DA. Acute colonic perforation associated with colorectal cancer. Am Surg 2001; 67: 261–264.
713. Scott NA, Jeacock J, Kingston RD. Risk factors in patients presenting as an emergency with colorectal cancer. Br J Surg 1995; 82:321–323.
714. Anderson JH, Hale D, McArdle CS. Elective versus emergency surgery for patients with colorectal cancer. Br J Surg 1992; 79:706–709.
715. Fitzgerald SD, Longo WE, Daniel GL, et al. Advanced colorectal neoplasia in the high-risk elderly patient: is surgical resection justified? Dis Colon Rectum 1993; 36:161–166.
716. Gervaz P, Pakart R, Nivatvongs S, Wolff BG, Larson D, Ringel S. Colorectal adenocarcinoma in cirrhotic patients. J Am Coll Surg 2003; 196:874–879.
717. Kotake K, Honjo S, Sugihara K. Changes in colorectal cancer during a 20-year period: an extended report from the multi-institutional registry of large bowel cancer, Japan. Dis Colon Rectum 2003; 46(suppl 10):S32–S43.
718. Wang HZ, Huang XF, Wang Y, Ji JF, Gu J. Clinical features, diagnosis, treatment and prognosis of multiple primary colorectal carcinoma. World J Gastroenterol 2004; 10(14):2136–2139.
719. Papaconstantinou HT, Sklow B, Hanaway MJ, et al. Characteristics and survival patterns of solid organ transplant patients developing de novo colon and rectal cancer. Dis Colon Rectum 2004; 47(11):1898–1903.

720. Phillips RKS, Hittinger R, Blesovsky L, et al. Large bowel cancer and surgical pathology and its relationship to survival. Br J Surg 1984; 71:604–610.
721. Jass JR. Pathologists' perspective on colorectal cancer. Perspect Colon Rectal Surg 1991; 4:327–332.
722. Adkins RB, Delozier JB, McKnight WG, et al. Carcinoma of the colon in patients 35 years of age and younger. Ann Surg 1987; 53:141–145.
723. Behbehani A, Sakwa M, Erlichman R, et al. Colorectal carcinoma in patients under age 40. Ann Surg 1985; 202:610–614.
724. Koh SJ, Johnson WW. Cancer of the large bowel in children. South Med J 1986; 79:931–935.
725. Rao BN, Pratt CB, Fleming ID, et al. Colon carcinoma in children and adolescents. Cancer 1985; 55:1322–1326.
726. Okuno M, Ikehara T, Nagayama M, et al. Colorectal carcinoma in young adults. Am J Surg 1987; 154:265–268.
727. Phillips RK, Hittinger R, Blesovsky L, et al. Local recurrence following curative resection for large bowel cancer. I. The overall picture. Br J Surg 1984; 71:12–16.
728. Cusack JC, Giacco GG, Cleary K, et al. Survival factors in 186 patients younger than 40-years old with colorectal adenocarcinoma. J Am Coll Surg 1996; 183:105–112.
729. Palmer ML, Herrera L, Petrelli NJ. Colorectal adenocarcinoma in patients less than 40 years of age. Dis Colon Rectum 1991; 34:343–345.
730. O'Connell JB, Maggard MA, Livingston EH, Yo CK. Colorectal cancer in the young. Am J Surg 2004; 187:343–348.
731. Chapuis PH, Dent OF, Fisher R, et al. A multivariate analysis of clinical and pathological variables in prognosis of resection of large bowel cancer. Br J Surg 1985; 72:698–702.
732. Newland RC, Dent OF, Lyttle MNB, et al. Pathologic determinants of survival associated with colorectal cancer with lymph node metastases. Cancer 1994; 73:2076–2082.
733. de Mello J, Struthers L, Turner R, et al. Multivariate analysis as aid to diagnosis and assessment of prognosis in gastrointestinal cancer. Br J Surg 1983; 48:341–348.
734. McArdle CS, McMillan DC, Hole DJ. Male gender adversely affects survival following surgery for colorectal cancer. Br J Surg 2003; 90:711–715.
735. Polissar L, Sim D, Francis A. Survival of colorectal cancer patients in relation to duration of symptoms and other prognostic factors. Dis Colon Rectum 1981; 24:364–369.
736. Mzabi R, Himal HS, Demers R, et al. A multiparametric computer analysis of carcinoma of the colon. Surg Gynecol Obstet 1976; 143:959–964.
737. Adam IJ, Mohamdee MO, Martin IG, et al. Role of circumferential margin involvement in the local recurrence of rectal cancer. Lancet 1994; 344: 707–711.
738. Griffin MR, Bergstralh EJ, Coffey RJ, et al. Predictors of survival after curative resection of carcinoma of the colon. Cancer 1987; 60:2318–2324.
739. Steinberg SM, Barkin JS, Kaplan RS, et al. Prognostic indicators of colon tumors: the Gastrointestinal Tumour Study Group experience. Cancer 1986; 57:1866–1870.
740. de Leon ML. Schoetz DJ, Coller JA, et al. Colorectal cancer. Lahey Clinic experience, 1972–1976. An analysis of prognostic indicators. Dis Colon Rectum 1987; 30:237–242.
741. Fielding LP, Phillips RKS, Frye JS, et al. The prediction of outcome after curative for large bowel cancer. Lancet 1986; 2:904–907.
742. Wolmark N, Wieand HS, Rockette HE, et al. The prognostic significance of tumour location and bowel obstruction in Dukes' B and C colorectal cancer: findings from the NSABP clinical trials. Ann Surg 1983; 198:743–752.
743. McArdle CS, Hole DJ. Emergency presentation of colorectal cancer is associated with poor 5-year survival. Br J Surg 2004; 91:605–609.
744. Venkatesh KS, Weingart DJ, Ramanujam PJ. Comparison of double and single parameters in DNA analysis for staging and as a prognostic indicator in patients with colon and rectal carcinoma. Dis Colon Rectum 1994; 37:1142–1147.
745. Slanetz CA Jr. The effect of inadvertent intraoperative perforation on survival and recurrence in colorectal cancer. Dis Colon Rectum 1984; 27:792–797.
746. James RD, Donaldson D, Gray R, Northover JM, Stenning SP, Taylor I. AXIS collaborators. Randomized clinical trial of adjuvant radiotherapy and 5-fluorouracil infusion in colorectal cancer (AXIS). Br J Surg 2003; 90: 1200–1212.
747. Wiggers T, Arends JW, Volovics A. Regression analysis of prognostic factors in colorectal cancer after curative resection. Dis Colon Rectum 1988; 31:33–41.
748. Bonfanti G, Bonzetti F, Doci E, et al. Results of extended surgery for cancer of the rectum and sigmoid. Br J Surg 1982; 69:305–307.
749. Habib NA, Peck MA, Sawyer CN, et al. An analysis of the outcome of 301 malignant colorectal tumors. Dis Colon Rectum 1983; 26:601–605.
750. Wood CB, Gills CR, Hole D, et al. Local tumour invasion as a prognostic factor in colorectal cancer. Br J Surg 68:326–328.
751. Greene FL, Stewart AK, Norton HJ. A new TNM staging strategy for node-positive (stage III) colon cancer: an analysis of 50,042 patients. Ann Surg 2002; 236:416–421.
752. Sugarbaker PH, Corlew S. Influence of surgical techniques in patients with colorectal cancer: a review. Dis Colon Rectum 1982; 25:545–557.
753. Zirngibl H, Husemann B, Hemanek P. Intraoperative spillage ot tumor cells in surgery for rectal cancer. Dis Colon Rectum 1990; 33:610–614.
754. Porter GA, Soskolne CL, Yakimets WW, Newman SC. Surgeon related factors and outcome in rectal cancer. Ann Surg 1998; 227:157–167.
755. Akyol AM, Mcgregor JR, Galloway DJ, et al. Anastomotic leaks in colorectal cancer surgery: a risk factor for recurrence? Int J Colorectal Dis 1991; 6: 179–183.
756. Fujita S, Teramoto T, Watanabe M, et al. Anastomotic leakage after colorectal cancer surgery: a risk factor for recurrence and poor prognosis. Jpn J Clin Oncol 1993; 23:299–302.
757. Bell SW, Walker KG, Rickard MJ, et al. Anastomotic leakage after curative anterior resection results in a higher prevalence of local recurrence. Br J Surg 2003; 90:1261–1266.
758. Parrott NR, Lennard TWJ, Taylor RMR. Effect of perioperative blood transfusion on recurrence of colorectal cancer. Br J Surg 1986; 73:970–973.
759. Wobbes T, Joosen KHG, Kuypers HHC, et al. The effect of packed cells and whole blood transfusion on survival after curative resection for colorectal carcinoma. Dis Colon Rectum 1989; 32:743–748.
760. Leite JPM, Granjo MEM, Martins MI, et al. Effect of perioperative blood transfusions on survival of patients after radical surgery for colorectal cancer. Int J Colorectal Dis 1993; 8:1129–1133.
761. Arnoux R, Corman J, Peloquin A, et al. Adverse effect of blood transfusions on patient survival after resection of rectal cancer. Can J Surg 1998; 31:121–126.
762. Francis DMA, Judson RT. Blood transfusion and recurrence of cancer of the colon and rectum. Br J Surg 1987; 74:26–30.
763. Chung M, Steinmetz OK, Gordon PH. Perioperative blood transfusion and outcome after resection for colorectal carcinoma. Br J Surg 1993; 80:927–932.
764. Nowacki MP, Szymandera JJ. The strongest prognostic factors in colorectal carcinoma. Surgicopathologic stage of disease and postoperative fever. Dis Colon Rectum 1985; 26:263–268.
765. Armstrong CP, Ahsan Z, Hinchley G, et al. Appendicectomy and carcinoma of the caecum. Br J Surg 1989; 76:1049–1053.
766. Meyerhardt JA, Tepper JE, Niedzwieki D, et al. Impact of body mass index on outcomes and treatment-related toxicity in a patients with stage II and III rectal cancer: findings from Intergroup Trial 0114. J Clin Oncol 2004; 22:648–657.
767. Halvorsen TB, Seim E. Tumor site: a prognostic factor in colorectal cancer? a multivariate analysis. Scand J Gastoenterol 1987; 22:124–128.
768. Alley PG, McNee RK. Age and sex differences in right colon cancer. Dis Colon Rectum 1986; 29:227–229.
769. Bjerkeset T, Morild J, Mark S, et al. Tumor characteristics of colorectal cancer and their relationship to treatment and prognosis. Dis Colon Rectum 1987; 30:934–938.
770. Steinberg SM, Barwick KW, Stablein DM. Importance of tumour pathology and morphology in patients with surgically resected colon cancer. Findings from the Gastrointestinal Tumor Study Group. Cancer 1986; 58:1340–1345.
771. Cohen AM, Tremiterra S, Candeh F, et al. Prognosis of node-positive colon cancer. Cancer 1991; 67:1859–1861.
772. Ogiwara H, Nakamura T, Baba S. Variables related to risk of recurrence in rectal cancer without lymph node metastases. Ann Surg Oncol 1994; 1:199–104.
773. Schmitz-Moormann P, Himmelmann GW, Baum U, et al. Morphological predictors of survival in colorectal carcinoma: Univariate and multivariate analysis. J Cancer Res Clin Oncol 1987; 113:586–592.
774. McDermott FT, Hughes ESR, Pihl E, et al. Prognosis in relation to symptom duration in colon cancer. Br J Surg 1981; 68:846–849.
775. Lindmark G, Gerdin B, Pahlman L, et al. Prognostic predictors in colorectal cancer. Dis Colon Rectum 1994; 37:1219–1227.
776. Secco GB, Pardelli B, Campora E, et al. Primary mucinous adenocarcinomas and signet-ring cell carcinomas of colon and rectum. Oncology 1994; 51: 30–34.
777. Yamamoto S, Mochizuki H, Hase K, et al. Assessment of clinicopathologic features of colorectal mucinous adenocarcinoma. Am J Surg 1993; 166: 257–261.
778. Sadahiro S, Ohumura T, Saito T, et al. An assessment of the mucous component in carcinoma of the colon and rectum. Cancer 1989; 64:1113–1116.
779. Nozoe T, Anai H, Nasu S, Sugimachi K. Clinicopathological characteristics of mucinous carcinoma of the colon and rectum. J Surg Oncol 2000; 75: 103–107.
780. Consorti F, Lorenzotti A, Midiri G, Di Paola M. Prognostic significance of mucinous carcinoma of colon and rectum: a prospective case-control study. J Surg Oncol 2000; 73:70–74.
781. Kanemitsu Y, Kato T, Hirai T, et al. Survival after curative resection for mucinous adenocarcinoma of the colorectum. Dis Colon Rectum 2003; 46: 160–167.
782. Halvorsen TB, Seim E. Association between invasiveness, inflammatory reaction, desmoplasia and survival in colorectal cancer. J Clin Pathol 1989; 42:162–166.
783. Nadel L, Mori K, Shinya H. Primary linitis plastica of the colon and rectum. Report of two cases. Dis Colon Rectum 1983; 26:738–742.
784. Wolmark N, Fischer B, Wieand HS. The prognostic value of the modifications of the Dukes' C classification of colorectal cancer. An analysis of the NSABP clinical trials. Ann Surg 1986; 203:115–122.
785. Gagliardi G, Stepniewska KA, Hershman MJ, et al. New grade related prognostic variable in rectal cancer. Br J Surg 1995; 82:599–602.

786. Hase K, Shatney C, Johnson D, et al. Prognostic value of tumor "budding" in patients with colorectal cancer. Dis Colon Rectum 1993; 36:627–635.
787. Tanaka M, Hashiguchi Y, Ueno H, Hase K, Mochizuki H. Tumor budding at the invasive margin can predict patients at high risk of recurrence after curative surgery for stage II, T3 colon cancer. Dis Colon Rectum 2003; 46:1054–1059.
788. Okuyama T, Nakamura T, Yamaguchi M. Budding is useful to select high-risk patients in stage II well-differentiated or moderately colon adenocarcinoma. Dis Colon Rectum 2003; 46:1400–1406.
789. Chen JS, Hsieh PS, Hung SY, et al. Clinical significance of signet ring cell rectal carcinoma. Int J Colorectal Dis 2004; 19:102–107.
790. Nissan A, Guillem JG, Paty PB, Wong WD, Cohen AM. Signet-ring cell carcinoma of the colon and rectum: a matched control study. Dis Colon Rectum 1999; 42:1176–1180.
791. Kang H, O'Connell JB, Maggard MA, Sack J, Ko CY. A 10-year outcomes evaluation of mucinous and signet-ring cell carcinoma of the colon and rectum. Dis Colon Rectum 2005; 46:1161–1168.
792. Chan CL, Chafai N, Rickard MJ, Dent OF, Chapuis PH, Bokey EL. What pathologic features influence survival in patients with local residual tumor after resection of colorectal cancer? J Am Coll Surg 2004; 199:680–686.
793. Gardner B, Feldman J, Spivak Y, et al. Investigations and factors influencing the prognosis of colon cancer. Am J Surg 1987; 153:541–544.
794. Malassagne B, Valleur P, Serra J, et al. Relationship of apical lymph node involvement to survival in resected colon carcinoma. Dis Colon Rectum 1993; 36:645–653.
795. Tang R, Wang JY, Chen JS, et al. Survival impact of lymph node metastases in TNM stage III carcinoma of the colon and rectum. J Am Coll Surg 1995; 180:705–712.
796. Khubchandani M. Relationship of symptom duration and survival in patients with carcinoma of the colon and rectum. Dis Colon Rectum 1985; 28:585–587.
797. Wong JH, Steinemann S, Tom P, Morita S, Tauchi-Nishi P. Volume of lymphatic metastases does not independently influence prognosis in colorectal cancer. J Clin Oncol 2002; 20:1506–1511.
798. Rothenberg KH. Genetic information and health insurance: state legislative approaches. J Law Med Ethics 1995; 23:312–319.
799. Martin EW, Joyce S, Lucas J, et al. Colorectal carcinoma in patients less than 40 years of age. Pathology and prognosis. Dis Colon Rectum 1981; 24:25–28.
800. Horn A, Dahl O, Morild I. Venous and neural invasion as predictors of recurrence in rectal adenocarcinoma. Dis Colon Rectum 1991; 34:798–804.
801. Sternberg A, Amar M, Alfici R, Groisman G. Conclusions from a study of venous invasion in stage IV colorectal adenocarcinoma. J Clin Pathol 2002; 55:17–21.
802. Horn A, Dahl O, Morild I. The role of venous and neural invasion on survival in rectal adenocarcinoma. Dis Colon Rectum 1990; 33:598–601.
803. Minsky BD, Mies C, Recht A, et al. Resectable adenocarcinoma of the rectosigmoid and rectum. II. The influence of blood vessel invasion. Cancer 1988; 61:1417–1424.
804. Krasna MJ, Flanebaum L, Cody RP, et al. Vascular and neural invasion in colorectal carcinoma. Incidence and prognostic significance. Cancer 1988; 61:1018–1023.
805. Tissot E, Naouri A, Naouri C, et al. Potentially curative surgery of colon carcinoma: influence of blood vessel invasion. Br J Surg 1995; 82(suppl 1):36.
806. Shirouzu K, Isomoto H, Kakegana T. Prognostic evaluation of perinueral invasion in rectal cancer. Am J Surg 1993; 165:233–237.
807. Ueno H, Hase K, Mochizuki H. Criteria for extramural perineural invasion as a prognostic factor in rectal cancer. Br J Surg 2001; 88:994–1000.
808. Bosch B, Guller U, Schnider A, et al. Perioperative detection of disseminated tumour cells is an independent prognostic factor in patients with colorectal cancer. Br J Surg 2003; 90(7):882–888.
809. Meyerhard JA, Catalano PJ, Haller DG, et al. Impact of diabetes mellitus on outcomes in patients with colon cancer. J Clin Oncol 2003; 21:433–440.
810. Hojo K, Koyama Y. Postoperative follow-up studies on cancer of the colon and rectum. Am J Surg 1982; 143:293–295.
811. Lewi H, Blumgart LH, Carter DC, et al. Preoperative carcinoembryonic antigen and survival in patients with colorectal cancer. Br J Surg 1984; 71: 206–208.
812. Wanebo HJ, Stevens W. Surgical treatment of locally recurrent colorectal cancer. In: Nelson RL, ed. Problems in Current Surgery. Controversies in Colon Cancer. Philadelphia: JB Lippincott, 1987:115–129.
813. Wolmark N, Fisher B, Wieand HS, et al. The prognostic significance of preoperative carcinoembryonic antigen levels in colorectal cancer. Results from NASBP clinical trials. Ann Surg 1984; 199:375–382.
814. Wang JY, Tang R, Chiag JM. Value of carcinoembryonic antigen in the management of colorectal cancer. Dis Colon Rectum 1994; 37:272–277.
815. Wiratkapun S, Kraemer M, Seow-Choen F, Ho YH, Eu KW. High preoperative serum carcinoembryonic antigen predicts metastatic recurrence in potentially curative colonic cancer: results of a five-year study. Dis Colon Rectum 2001; 44:231–235.
816. Wang WS, Lin JK, Chiou TJ, et al. Preoperative carcinoembryonic antigen level as an independent prognostic factor in colorectal cancer: Taiwan experience. Jpn J Clin Oncol 2000; 30:12–16.
817. Steele G, Zamcheck N. The use of carcinoembryonic antigen in the clinical management of patients with colorectal cancer. Cancer Detect Prev 1985; 8:421–427.
818. Lahr CJ, Soong SJ, Cloud G, et al. A multifactoria analysis of prognostic factors in patients with liver metastases from colorectal carcinoma. J Clin Concol 1983; 1:720–726.
819. Armitage NC, Robins RA, Evans DF, et al. The influence of tumour DNA abnormalities on survival in colorectal cancer. Br J Surg 1985; 72: 828–830.
820. Banner BF, Tomas-de la Vega JE, Roseman DL, et al. Should flow cytometric DNA analysis precede definitive surgery for colon carcinoma. Ann Surg 1986; 202:740–744.
821. Emdin SO, Stenling R, Roos G. Prognostic value of DNA content in colorectal carcinoma. A flow cytometric study with some methodologic aspects. Cancer 1987; 60:1282–1287.
822. Kokal W, Sheibani, K, Terz J, et al. Tumor DNA content in the prognosis of colorectal carcinoma. JAMA 1986; 255:3123–3127.
823. Giaretti W, Danova M, Geido G, et al. Flow cytometric DNA index in the progress of colorectal cancer. Cancer 1991; 67:1921–1927.
824. Garrity MM, Burgart LJ, Mahoney MR, et al. North Central Cancer Treatment Group Study. Prognostic value of proliferation apoptosis, defective DNA mismatch repair, and p53 overexpression in patients with resected Dukes' B2 or C colon cancer: a North Central Cancer Treatment Group Study. J Clin Oncol 2004; 22:1572–1582.
825. Diep CB, Thorstensen L, Meling GI, Skovlund E, Rognum TO, Lothe RA. Genetic tumor markers with prognostic impact in Dukes' stages B and C colorectal cancer patients. J Clin Oncol 2003; 21:820–829.
826. Kern SE, Fearon ER, Tersmette KWF, et al. Allelic loss in colorectal carcinoma. JAMA 1989; 261:3099–3103.
827. Jen J, Kim H, Piantadosi S, et al. Allelic loss of chromosome 18q and prognosis in colorectal cancer. N Engl J Med 1994; 331:213–221.
828. Shibata D, Reale MA, Lavin P, et al. The DCC protein and prognosis in colorectal cancer. N Engl J Med 1996; 335:1727–1732.
829. Jernvall P, Makinen MJ, Karttunen TJ, Makela J, Vihko P. Morphological and genetic abnormalities in prediction of recurrence in radically operated colorectal cancer. Anticancer Res 1999; 19:1357–1362.
830. Sarli L, Bottarelli L, Bader G, et al. Associated between recurrence of sporadic colorectal cancer, high level of microsatellite instability, and loss heterozygosity at chromosome 18q. Dis Colon Rectum 2004; 47(9): 1467–1482.
831. Pricolo VE, Finkelstein SD, Wu TT, et al. Prognostic value of TP53 and K-ras-2 mutational analysis in stage III carcinoma of the colon. Am J Surg 1996; 171:41–46.
832. Diez M, Gonzalez A, Enriquez JM, et al. Prediction of recurrence in B-C stages of colorectal cancer by p-53 expression. Br J Surg 1995; 82(Suppl 1):26.
833. Auvinen A, Isola J, Visakorpi T, et al. Overexpression of p53 and long-term survival in colon carcinoma. Br J Cancer 1994; 70:293–296.
834. Sun XF, Carstensen JM, Stall O, et al. Prognostic significance of p53 expression in relation to DNA ploidy in colorectal adenocarcinoma. Virchows Arch A Pathol Anat 1993; 423:443–448.
835. Yamaguchi A, Nakagawara G, Kurosake Y, et al. p53 immunoreaction in endoscopic biopsy specimens of colorectal cancer, and its prognostic significance. Br J Cancer 1993; 68:399–402.
836. Allegra CJ, Paik S, Colangelo LH, et al. Prognostic value of thymidylate synthase, Ki-67, and p53 in patients with Dukes' B and C colon cancer: a National Cancer Intitute-National Surgical Adjuvant Breast and Bowel Project collaborative study. J Clin Oncol 2003; 21:241–250.
837. Petersen S, Thames HD, Nieder C, Petersen C, Baumann M. The results of colorectal cancer treatment by p53 status: treatment-specific overview. Dis Colon Rectum 2001; 44:322–333.
838. Gervaz P, Bouzourene H, Cerottini JP, et al. Colorectal cancer: distinct genetic categories and clinical outcome based on proximal or distal tumor location. Dis Colon Rectum 2001; 44:364–372.
839. Herrlich P, Pals S, Ponta H. CD 44 in colon cancer. Eur J Cancer 1995; 31A:1116–1122.
840. Miyahara M, Saito T, Kaketani K, et al. Clinical significance of ras p21 over expression for patients with an advanced colorectal cancer. Dis Colon Rectum 1991; 34:1097–1102.
841. Wang Y, Jatkoe T, Zhang Y, et al. Gene expression profiles and molecular markers to predict recurrence of Dukes' B colon cancer. J Clin Oncol 2004; 22: 1564–1571.
842. Gonen M, Hunmer A, Zervoudakis A, et al. Thymidylate synthase expression in hepatic tumors is a predictor of survival and progression in patients with resectable metastatic colorectal cancer. J Clin Oncol 2003; 21:406–412.
843. Broll R, Busch P, Duchrow M, et al. Influence of thymidylate synthase and p53 protein expression on clinical outcome in patients with colorectal cancer. Int J Colorectal Dis 2005; 20(2):94–102.
844. Kopp R, Rothbauer E, Mueller E, Schildberg FW, Jauch KW, Pfeiffer A. Reduced survival of rectal cancer patients with increased tumor epidermal growth factor receptor levels. Dis Colon Rectum 2003; 46:1391–1399.

845. Nakmori S, Kameyama M, Imaoka S, et al. Increased expression of sialyl Lewis[x] antigen correlates with poor survival in patients with colorectal carcinoma: clinicopathological and immunohistochemical study. Cancer Res 1993; 53:3632–3637.
846. Nakayama T, Watanabe M, Katsumata J, et al. Expression of Sialyl Lewis[x] as a new prognostic factor for patients with advanced colorectal carcinoma. Cancer 1995; 75:2051–2052.
847. Nakagoe T, Fukushima K, Hirota M, et al. Immunohistochemical expression of sialyl Le[x] antigen in relation to survival of patients with colorectal carcinoma. Cancer 1993; 72:2323–2330.
848. Teixeira CR, Tanaka S, Haruma K, et al. Proliferating cell nuclear antigen expression at the invasive tumor margin predicts malignant potential of colorectal carcinomas. Cancer 1994; 73:575–579.
849. Al-Sheneber IF, Shibata HR, Sampalis J, et al. Prognostic significance of proliferating cell nuclear antigen expression in colorectal cancer. Cancer 1993; 71:1954–1959.
850. Habib NA, Dawson PM, Bradfield JWB, et al. Sialomucins at resection margin and likelihood of recurrence in colorectal carcinoma. Br Med J 1986; 293:521–523.
851. Villias K, Markidis P, Simatus G, et al. Mucin production and survival in colorectal carcinoma. Br J Surg 1995; 82 (Suppl 1):37.
852. Bonatsos G, Velmahos GC, Davaris P, et al. The role of sialomucin of resection margins on local recurrence and survival of patients radically operated on for colorectal carcinoma. Res Surg 1992; 4:68–70.
853. Mitmaker B, Begin LR, Gordon PH. Nuclear shape as a prognostic discriminant in colorectal carcinoma. Dis Colon Rectum 1991; 34:249–259.
854. Verspaget HW, Sier CPM, Ganesh S, et al. Prognostic value of plasminogen activities and their inhibitors in colorectal cancer. Eur J Cancer 1995; 31A: 1105–1109.
855. Hole DJ, McArdle CS. Impact of socioeconomic deprivation on outcome after surgery for colorectal cancer. Br J Surg 2002; 89(5):586–590.
856. Adloff M, Arnaud JP, Schloegel M, et al. Colorectal cancers in patients under 40 years of age. Dis Colon Rectum 1986; 29:322–325.
857. Enblad G, Enblad P, Adami HO, et al. Relationship between age and survival in cancer of the colon and rectum with special reference to patients less than 40 years of age. Br J Surg 1990; 77:611–616.
858. Lee PY, Fletcher WS, Sullivan ES, et al. Colorectal cancer in young patients: characteristics and outcome. Am Surg 1994; 60:607–612.
859. Liang JT, Huang KC, Cheng AL, Jeng YM, Wu MS, Wang SM. Clinicopathological and molecular biological features of colorectal cancer in patients less than 40 years of age. Br J Surg 2003; 90:205–214.
860. Turkiewicz D, Miller B, Schache D, Cohen J, Theile D. Young patients with colorectal cancer: how do they fare? ANZ J Surg 2001; 71:707–710.
861. Chung YF, Eu KW, Machin D, et al. Young age is not a poor prognostic marker in colorectal cancer. Br J Surg 1998; 85(2):1255–1259.
862. O'Connell JB, Maggard MA, Liu JH, Etzioni DA, Ko CY. Are survival rates different for young and older patients with rectal cancer? Dis Colon Rectum 2004; 47(12):2064–2069.
863. Paraf F, Jothy S. Colorectal cancer before the age of 40: a case-control study. Dis Colon Rectum 2000; 43:1222–1226.
864. Irvin TT. Prognosis of colorectal carcinoma in the elderly. Br J Surg 1988; 75:419–421.
865. Arnaud JP, Schloegel M, Ollier JC, et al. Colorectal cancer in patients over 80 years of age. Dis Colon Rectum 1991; 34:896–898.
866. Mulcahy HE, Patchett SE, Daly L, et al. Prognosis of elderly patients with large bowel cancer. Br J Surg 1994; 81:736–738.
867. Barrier A, Ferro L, Houry S, Lacaine F, Huguier M. Rectal cancer surgery in patients more than 80 years of age. Am J Surg 2003; 185:54–57.
868. Schillaci A, Cavallora A, Nicolanti V. The importance of symptom duration in relation of prognosis of carinoma of the large intestine. Surg Obstet Gynecol 1984; 158:423–426.
869. Goodman D, Irvin TT. Delay in diagnosis and prognosis of carcinoma of the right colon. Br J Surg 1993; 80:1327–1329.
870. Rouffet F, Hay JM, Vacher B, et al. Curative resection for left colonic carcinoma: hemicolectomy vs. segmental colectomy. A prospective, controlled, multicenter trial. French Association for Surgical Research. Dis Colon Rectum 1994; 37:651–659.
871. McArdle CS, Hole DJ. Influence of volume and specialization on survival following surgery for colorectal cancer. Br J Surg 2004; 91:610–617.
872. Crowson MC, Hallissey MT, Kiff RS. Blood transfusion in colorectal cancer. Br J Surg 1989; 76:522–523.
873. Weiden PL, Bean MA, Schultz P. Perioperative blood transfusion does not increase the risk of colorectal cancer recurrence. Cancer 1987; 60:870–874.
874. Sibbering DM, Locker AP, Hardcastle JD, et al. Blood transfusion and survival in colorectal cancer. Dis Colon Rectum 1994; 37:358–363.
875. Fucini C, Bandettini L, D'Elia M, et al. Are postoperative fever and/or septic complications prognostic factors in colorectal cancer resected for cure. Dis Colon Rectum 1985; 28:94–95.
876. Martin MB, Frontier T, Jarman W, et al. Colon and rectal carcinoma. Forty years and 1400 cases. Am Surg 1987; 53:146–148.
877. Wolmark N, Fisher B, Wieand HS, et al. The relationship of depth of penetration and tumour size to number of positive nodes in Dukes' C colorectal carcinoma. Cancer 1984; 53:2707–2712.
878. Green JB, Timmcke AE, Mitchell WT, et al. Mucinous carcinoma—just another colon cancer? Dis Colon Rectum 1993; 36:47–54.
879. Minsky B. Clinicopathologic impact in colorectal carcinoma. Dis Colon Rectum 1990; 33:714–719.
880. Bessa X, Pinol V, Castellvi-Bel S, et al. Prognostic value of postoperative detection of blood circulating tumor cells in patients with colorectal cancer operated on for cure. Ann Surg 2003; 237:368–375.
881. Moertel CG, O'Fallon JR, Go VL, et al. The preoperative carcinoembryonic antigen test in the diagnosis, staging, and prognosis of colorectal cancer. Cancer 1986; 58:603–611.
882. Jones DJ, Moore M, Schofield PF. Prognostic significance of DNA ploidy in colorectal cancer. A prospective flow cytometric study. Br J Surg 1988; 75:28–33.
883. Enker WE. Flow cytometric determination of tumor cell DNA content and proliferative index as prognostic variables in colorectal cancer. Perspect Colon Rectal Surg 1990; 3:1–28.
884. Michelassi F, Ewing CH, Montag A, et al. Prognostic significance of polidy determination in rectal cancer. Hepatogastroenterology 1992; 39:222–225.
885. Deans GT, Williamson K, Heatley M, et al. The role of flow cytometry in carcinoma of the colon and rectum. Surg Gynecol Obstet 1993; 177: 377–382.
886. Morgan M, Koorey D, Painter D, et al. p53 and DCC immunohistochemistry in curative rectal cancer surgery. Int J Colorectal Dis 2003; 18:188–195.
887. Iacopetta B. TP53 mutation in colorectal cancer. Hum Mutat 2003; 21:271–276.
888. Allega CJ, Parr Al, Wold LE, et al. Investigation of the prognostic and predictive value of thymidylate synthase, p53, and Ki-67 in patients with locally advanced colon cancer. J Clin Oncol 2002; 20:1735–1743.
889. Gallego MG, Acenero MJ, Ortega S, Delgado AA, Cantero JL. Prognostic influence of p53 nuclear overexpression in colorectal carcinoma. Dis Colon Rectum 2000; 43:971–975.
890. Grewal H, Guillem JG, Klimstra DS, et al. p53 Nuclear over-expression may not be an independent prognostic market in early colorectal cancer. Dis Colon Rectum 1995; 38:1176–1181.
891. Mulder JWR, Baas IO, Polak MM, et al. Evaluation of p53 protein expression as a marker for long-term prognosis in colorectal carcinoma. Br J Cancer 1995; 71:1257–1262.
892. Suzuki H, Matsumoto K, Koide A, et al. Correlation of p53 with the clinicopathologic features and prognosis of colorectal carcinoma. Jpn J Surg 1994; 24:85–87.
893. Johnston PG, Benson AB 3rd, Catalano P, Rao MS, O'Dwyer PJ, Allegra CJ. Thymidylate synthase protein expression in primary colorectal cancer: lack of correlation with outcome and response to fluorouracil in metastatic disease sites. J Clin Oncol 2003; 21:815–819.
894. Malcolm AW, Perencevich NP, Olson RM, et al. Analysis of recurrence patterns following curative resection for carcinoma of the colon and rectum. Surg Gynecol Obstet 1981; 152:131–136.
895. Pescatori M, Maria G, Betrani B, et al. Site, emergency, and duration of symptoms in prognosis of colorectal cancer. Dis Colon Rectum 1982; 25:33–40.
896. Sanfelippo PM, Beahrs OH. Factors in the prognosis of adenocarcinoma of the colon and rectum. Arch Surg 1972; 104:401–406.
897. Reinbach DH, McGregor JR. Murray GD, et al. Effect of surgeon's speciality interest on the type of resection performance for colorectal cancer. Dis Colon Rectum 1994; 37:1020–1023.
898. Myerson RJ, Michalski JM, King ML, et al. Adjuvant radiation therapy for rectal carcinoma: predictors of outcome. Int J Radiat Oncol Biol Phys 1995; 32:41–50.
899. Harmon JW, Tang DG, Gordon TA, et al. Hospital volume can serve as a surrogate for surgeon volume for achieving excellent outcomes in colorectal resection. Ann Surg 1999; 230(3):404.
900. Ko Cy, Chang JT, Chaudhry S, Kominski G. Are high-volume surgeons and hospitals the most important predictors of in-hospital outcome for colon cancer resection? Surgery 2002; 132:268–273.
901. Schrag D, Panageas KS, Riedel E, et al. Hospital and surgeon procedure volume as predictors of outcome following rectal cancer resection. Ann Surg 2002; 236:583–592.
902. Martling A, Cedermark B, Johansson H, Rutqvist LE, Holm T. The surgeon as a prognostic factor after the introduction of total mesorectal excision in the treament of rectal cancer. Br J Surg 2002; 89:1008–1013.
903. Hermanek P, Hohenberger W. The importance of volume in colorectal cancer surgery. Eur J Surg Oncol 1996; 22:213–215.
904. Callahan MA, Christos PJ, Gold HT, Mushlin AI, Dally JM. Influence of surgical subspecialty training on in-hospital mortality for gastrectomy and colectomy patients. Ann Surg 2003; 238:629–636.
905. Rosen L, Stasik JJ Jr., Reed JF 3rd, Olenwine JA, Aronoff JS, Sherman D. Variations in colon and rectal surgical mortality. Comparison of specialties with a state-legislated database. Dis Colon Rectum 1996; 39:129–135.
906. Platell C, Lim D, Tajudeen N, Tan JL, Wong K. Does surgical sub-specialization influence survival in patients with colorectal cancer? World J Gastroenterol 2003; 9:961–964.
907. Read TE, Myerson RJ, Fleshman JW, Fry RD, Birnbaum EH, Walz BJ, Kodner IJ. Surgeon speciality is associated with outcome in rectal cancer treatment. Dis Colon Rectum 2002; 45:904–914.

908. Dorrance HR, Docherty GM, O'Dwyer PJ. Effect of surgeon speciality interest on patient outcome after potentially curative colorectal cancer surgery. Dis Colon Rectum 2000; 43:492–498.
909. Smith JAE, King PM, Lane RHS, Thompson MR. Evidence of the effect of 'specialization' on the management, surgical outcome and survival from colorectal cancer in Wessex. Br J Surg 2003; 90:583–592.
910. Hafstrom L, Holmin T. Relationship between postoperative temperature and survival in patients resected for colorectal cancer. Am J Surg 1978; 135: 312–314.
911. Michelassi F, Vannucci L, Montag A, et al. Importance of tumor morphology for the long term prognosis of rectal adenocarcinoma. Am Surg 1988; 54: 376–379.
912. Chambers WM, Khan U, Gagliano A, Smith RD, Sheffield J, Nicholls RJ. Tumor morphology as a predictor of outcome after local excision of rectal cancer. Br J Surg 2004; 91:457–459.
913. Jass JR, Love SB, Northover JMA. A new prognostic classification of rectal cancer. Lancet 1987; 1:1303–1306.
914. Fulmes M, Setrakian S, Raj PK, Bogard BM. Cancer biology and necrotic changes in metastatic lymph nodes and survival of colon cancer patients. Am J Surg 2005; 189:364–368.
915. Smyth EF, Sharma A, Sivarajasingham N, Hartley J, Manson JR, Cawkwell L. Prognostic implications of hMLH1 and p53 immunohistochemical status in right-sided colon cancer. Dis Colon Rectum 2004; 47(12):2086–2091.
916. Hemminki A, Mecklin JP, Jarvinen H, Aaltonen LA, Joensuu H. Microsatellite instability is a favorable prognostic indicator in patients with colorectal cancer receiving chemotherapy. Gastroenterology 2000; 119:921–928.
917. Lim SB, Jeong SY, Lee MR, et al. Prognostic significance of microsatellite instability in sporadic colorectal cancer. Int J Colorectal Dis 2004; 19(6): 533–537.
918. Popat S, Hubner R, Houlston RS. Systematic review of microsatellite instability and colorectal cancer prognosis. J Clin Oncol 2005; 23(3):609–618.
919. Svendson LB, Sorensen C, Kjersgaard P, et al. The influence of age upon the survival of curative operation for colorectal cancer. Int J Colorectal Dis 1989; 4:123–127.
920. Coburn MC, Pricolo VE, Soderberg CH. Factors affecting the prognosis and management of carcinoma of the colon and rectum on patients more than eighty years of age. J Am Coll Surg 1994; 179:65–69.
921. Nilsson E, Bolin S, Sjodeh R. Carcinoma of the colon and rectum. Delay in diagnosis. Acta Chir Scand 1982; 148:617–622.
922. Wang SH, Lin JK, Moul YC, et al. Long-term prognosis of patients with obstructing carcinoma of the right colon. Am J Surg 2004; 187:497–500.
923. Meyerhardt JA, Tepper JE, Niedzwiecki D, et al. Impact of hospital procedure volume on surgical operation and long-term outcomes in high-risk curatively resected rectal cancer: findings from the Intergroup 0114 study. J Clin Oncol 2004; 22:166–174.
924. Schrag D, Panageas KS, Riedel E, et al. Surgeon volume compared to hospital volume as a predictor of outcome following primary colon cancer resection. J Surg Oncol 2003; 83:68–78.
925. Borowski DW, Kelly SB, Ratcliffe AA, et al. Small caseload in colorectal cancer surgery is associated with adverse outcome. Br J Surg 2004; 91(suppl 1):73.
926. Wibe A, Eriksen MT, Syse A, Tretli S, Myrvold HE, Soreide O. Norwegian rectal cancer group. Effect of hospital caseload on long-term outcome after standardization of rectal cancer surgery at a national level. Br J Surg 2005; 92:217–224.
927. Martling A, Holm T, Rutqvist LE, et al. Impact of a surgical training programme on rectal cancer outcomes in Stockholm. Br J Surg 2005; 92(2):225–229.
928. Davis CJ, Ilstrup DM, Pemberton JH. Influence of splenectomy on survival rate of patients with colorectal cacner. Am J Surg 1988; 155:173–179.
929. Varty PP, Linehan IP, Boulos PB. Does concurrent splenectomy at colorectal cancer resection influence survival? Dis Colon Rectum 1993; 36:602–606.
930. Newland RC, Dent OF, Chapuis PH, et al. Survival after curative resection of lymph node negative colorectal carcinoma. Cancer 1995; 76:564–571.
931. Greene FL, Stewart AK, Norton HJ. New tumor-node-metastasis staging strategy for node-positive (stage III) rectal cancer: an analysis. J Clin Oncol 2004; 22:1778–1784.
932. Swanson RS, Compton CC, Stewart AK, Bland KI. The prognosis of T3N0 colon cancer is dependent on the number of lymph nodes examined. Ann Surg Oncol 2003; 10:65–71.
933. Fisher ER, Colangeio L, Wieand S, Fisher B, Wolmark N. Lack of influence of cytokeratin-positive mini micrometastases in "Negative Node" patients with colorectal cancer: findings from the national surgical adjuvant breast and bowel projects protocols R-01 and C-01. Dis Colon Rectum 2003; 46: 1021–1025.
934. Sakuragi M, Togashi K, Konishi F, et al. Predictive factor for lymph node metastasis in T1 stage colorectal carcinomas. Dis Colon Rectum 2003; 46: 1626–1632.
935. Tepper JE, O'Connell MJ, Niedzwiecki D, et al. Impact of number of nodes retrieved on outcome in patients with rectal cancer. J Clin Oncol 2001; 19:157–163.
936. Beart RW Jr., O'Connell MJ. Postoperative follow-up of patients with carcinoma of the colon. Mayo Clin Proc 1983; 58:361–363.
937. Araki Y, Isomoto H, Morodomi T, et al. Survival of rectal carcinoma patients studied with flow cytometric DNA analysis. Kurume Med J 1990; 37:277–283.
938. Giaretti W, Sciallero S, Bruno S, et al. DNA flow cytometry of endoscopically examined colorectal adenomas and adenocarcinomas. Cytometry 1988; 9:238–244.
939. Halvorsen TB, Johannesen E. DNA ploidy, tumour site, and prognosis in colorectal cancer. A flow cytometric study of paraffin-embedded tissue. Scand J Gastroenterol 1990; 25:141–148.
940. Kohen-Corish MR, Daniel JJ, Chan C, et al. Low microsatellite instability is associated with poor prognosis in stage C colon cancer. J Clin Oncol 2005; 23(11):2318–2324.
941. Cali RL, Pitsch RM, Thorson AG, et al. Cumulative incidence of metachronous colorectal cancer. Dis Colon Rectum 1993; 36:388–393.
942. Tornqvist A, Ekelund G, Leandoer L. The value of intensive follow-up after curative resection for colorectal carcinoma. Br J Surg 1982; 69:725–728.
943. Cochrane JP, Williams JT, Faber RG, et al. Value of outpatient follow-up after curative surgery for carcinoma of the large bowl. Br Med J 1980; 280: 593–595.
944. Ekman CA, Gustavson J, Henning A. Value of a follow-up study of recurrent carcinoma of the colon and rectum. Surg Gynecol Obstet 1977; 145:895–897.
945. Buhler H, Seefeld U, Deyhle P, et al. Endoscopic follow-up after colorectal cancer surgery. Early detection of local recurrence? Cancer 1984; 54:791–793.
946. Wenzl E, Wunderlich M, Herbst F. Results of a rigorous follow-up system in colorectal cancer. Int J Colorectal Dis 1988; 3:176–180.
947. Yamamoto Y, Imai H, Iwamoto S, et al. Surgical treatment of the recurrence of colorectal cancer. Jpn J Surg 1996; 26:164–168.
948. Umpleby HC, Williamson RCN. Anastomotic recurrence in large bowel cancer. Br J Surg 1987; 74:873–878.
949. Russell A, Tong D, Dawson LE, et al. Adenocarcinoma of the proximal colon: Sites of initial dissemination and patterns of recurrence following surgery alone. Cancer 1984; 53:360–367.
950. Gunderson LL, Tepper JE, Dosoretz DE, et al. Patterns of failure after treatment of gastrointestinal cancer. In: Cox JD, ed. Proceedings of CROS-NCI Conference on Patterns of Failure after Treatment of Cancer. Vol. 2. Cancer Treatment Symposium, 1983.
951. Bohm B, Schwenk W, Hucke HP, et al. Does methodic long-term follow-up affect survival after curative resection of colorectal carcinoma? Dis Colon Rectum 1993; 36:280–286.
952. Obrand DI, Gordon PH. Incidence and patterns of recurrence following curative resection for colorectal carcinoma. Dis Colon Rectum 1997; 40:15–24.
953. Rodriguez-Bigas MA, Stulc JP, Davidson B, et al. Prognostic significance of anastomotic recurrence from colorectal adenocarcinoma. Dis Colon Rectum 1992; 35:838–842.
954. Boey J, Cheung HC, Lai CK, et al. A prospective evaluation of serum carcinoembryonic antigen (CEA) levels in the management of colorectal carcinoma. World J Surg 1984; 8:279–286.
955. Willett CG, Tepper JE, Cohen AM, et al. Failure patterns following curative resection of colonic carcinoma. Ann Surg 1984; 200:685–690.
956. Gunderson LL, Sosin H, Levitt S. Extrapelvic colon–Areas of failure in reoperation series: implications for adjuvant therapy. Int J Radiat Oncol Biol Phys 1985; 11:731–741.
957. Galandiuk S, Wieand HS, Moertel CG, et al. Patterns of recurrence after curative resection of carcinoma of the colon and rectum. Surg Gynecol Obstet 1992; 174:27–32.
958. Koea JB, Lanouette N, Paty PB, Guilem JG, Cohen AM. Abdominal wall recurrence after colorectal resection for cancer. Dis Colon Rectum 2000; 43:628–632.
959. Barillari P, Ramacciato G, Manetti G, et al. Surveillance of colorectal cancer. Effectiveness of early detection of intraluminal recurrences on prognosis and survival of patients treated for cure. Dis Colon Rectum 1996; 38:388–393.
960. Jacquet P, Jelinek JS, Stenes MA, et al. Evaluation of computed tomography in patients with peritoneal carcinomatosis. Cancer 1993; 72: 1631–1636.
961. Delbeke D, Vitola JV, Sandler MP, et al. Staging recurrent metastatic colorectal carcinoma with PET. J Nucl Med 1997; 38:1196–1201.
962. Libutti SK, Alexander HR Jr., Choyke P, et al. A prospective study of 2-[18F] fluoro-2-deoxy-D-glucose/positron emission tomography scan 99mTc-labeled arcitumomab (CEA-scan), and blind second-look laparotomy for detecting colon cancer recurrence in patients with increasing carcinoembryonic antigen levels. Ann Surg Oncol 2001; 8(10):779–786.
963. Desai DC, Zervos EE, Arnold MW, Burak WE Jr., Mantil J, Martin EW Jr. Positron emission tomography affects surgical management in recurrent colorectal cancer patients. Ann Surg Oncol 2003; 10:59–64.
964. Whiteford MH, Whiteford HM, Yee LF, et al. Usefulness of FDG-PET scan in the assessment of suspected inetastatic or recurrent adenocarcinoma of the colon and rectum. Dis Colon Rectum 2000; 43:759–767.
965. Johnson K, Bakhsh A, Young D, Martin TE Jr, Arnold M. Correlating computed tomography and positron emission tomography scan with operative findings in metastatic colorectal cancer. Dis Colon Rectum 2001; 44: 354–357.

966. Minton JP, Hoehn JL, Gerber DM, et al. Results of a 400 patient carcino-embryonic antigen second-look colorectal cancer study. Cancer 1985; 55: 1284–1290.
967. Staab HJ, Anderer FA, Stumpf E. Eighty-four potential second-look operations based on sequential carcino-embryonic antigen determinations and clinical investigations in patients with recurrent gastrointestinal cancer. Am J Surg 1985; 149:198–204.
968. Hida J, Yasutomi M, Shindoh K, et al. Second-look operation for recurrent colorectal cancer based on carcino-embryonic antigen and imaging techniques. Dis Colon Rectum 1996; 39:74–79.
969. Waldron RP, Donovam JA. Clinical follow-up and treatment of locally recurrent colorectal cancer. Dis Colon rectum 1987; 30:428–430.
970. Gwin JL, Hoffman JP, Eisenberg BL. Surgical management of nonhepatic intra-abdominal recurrence of carcinoma of the colon. Dis Colon Rectum 1993; 36:540–544.
971. Herfarth C, Schlag P, Hohenberger P. Surgical strategies in locoregional recurrences of gastrointestinal carcinoma. World J Surg 1987; 11:504–510.
972. Law NL, Chan WF, Lee YM, Chu KW. Non-curative surgery for colorectal cancer: critical appraisal of outcomes. Colorectal Dis 2004; 19:197–202.
973. Bowne WB, Lee B, Wong WD, et al. Operative salvage for locoregional recurrent colon cancer after curative resection: an analysis of 100 cases. Dis Colon Rectum 2005; 48:897–909.
974. Willett CG, Shelleto PC, Teppa JE, et al. Intraoperative electron beam radiation therapy for recurrent locally advanced rectal or rectosigmoid carcinoma. Cancer 1991; 67:1504–1508.
975. Taylor WE, Donohue JH, Gunderson LL, et al. The Mayo clinic experience with multimodality treatment of locally advanced or recurrent colon cancer. Ann Surg Oncol 2002; 9:177–185.
976. Wodnicki H, Goldeberg RI, Kaplan SR, et al. The laser. An alternative for palliative treatment of obstructing intraluminal lesions. Am Surg 1988; 54: 227–230.
977. Buchi KN. Endoscopic laser surgery in the colon and rectum. Dis Colon Rectum 1958; 31:739–748.
978. Bown SG, Barr H, Mathewson K, et al. Endoscopic treatment of inoperable colorectal cancers with the Nd:YAG laser. Br J Surg 1986; 73:949–952.
979. Faintuch JS. Endoscopic laser therapy in colorectal carcinoma. Hematol Oncol Clin North Am 1989; 3:155–170.
980. Krasner N. Lasers in the treatment of colorectal disease. Symposium. Int J Colorectal Dis 1989; 4:1–29.
981. Tan CC, Ifeikhar SY, Allan A, et al. Local effects of colorectal cancer are well palliated by endoscopic laser therapy. Eur J Surg Oncol 1995; 21:648–652.
982. Mandava N, Petrelli N, Herrera L, et al. Laser palliation for colorectal carcinoma. Am J Surg 1991; 162:212–215.
983. Chia YC, Ngoi SS, Goh PMY. Endoscopic Nd:YAG laser in the palliative treatment of advanced low rectal carcinoma in Singapore. Dis Colon Rectum 1991; 34:1093–1096.
984. Arrigoni A, Pernazio M, Spandre M, et al. Emergency endoscopy: recanalization of intestinal obstruction caused by colorectal cancer. Gastrointest Endosc 1994; 40:576–580.
985. Dittrich K, Armbruster C, Hoffer F, et al. Nd:YAG laser treatment of colorectal maliganancies: an experience of $4\frac{1}{2}$ years. Lasers Surg Med 1992; 12:199–203.
986. Bright N, Hale P, Mason R. Poor palliation of colorectal malignancy with the neodymium yttrium-aluminum-garnet laser. Br J Surg 1992; 79:308–309.
987. Courtney ED, Raja A, Leicester RJ. Eight-years experience of high-powered endoscopic diode laser therapy for palliation of colorectal carcinoma. Dis Colon Rectum 2005; 48:845–850.
988. Pilati P, Mocellin S, Rossi CR, et al. Cytoreductive surgery combined with hyperthermic intraperitoneal intraoperative chemotherapy for peritoneal carcinomatosis arising from colon adenocarcinoma. Ann Surg Oncol 2003; 10:508–513.
989. Verwaal VJ, Boot H, Aleman BM, van Tinteren H, Zoetmulder FA. Recurrences after peritoneal carcinomatosis of colorectal origin treated by cytoreduction and hyperthermic intraperitoneal chemotherapy: location, treatment, and outcome. Ann Surg Oncol 2004; 11:375–379.
990. Smith P, Bruera E. Management of malignant ureteral obstruction in the palliative care setting. J Pain Symptom Manage 1995; 10:481–486.
991. Keidan RD, Greenberg RE, Hoffman JP, et al. Is precutaneous nephrostomy for hydronephrosis appropriate in patients with advanced cancer? Am J Surg 1988; 156:206–208.
992. Douillard JY, Cunningham D, Roth AD, et al. Irinotecan combined with fluorouracil compared with fluorouracil alone as first-line treatment for metastatic colorectal cancer: a multicentre randomised trial. Lancet 2000; 355: 1041–1047.
993. Saltz LB,.Cox JV, Blanke C, et al. Irinotecan plus fluorouracil and leucovorin for metastatic colorectal cancer. Irinotecan Study Group. N Engl J Med 2000; 343: 905–914.
994. de Gramont A, Figer A, Seymour M, et al. Leucovorin and fluorouracil with or without oxaliplatin as first-line treatment in advanced colorectal cancer. J Clin Oncol 2000; 18:2938–2947.
995. Sorbye H, Glimelius B, Berglund A, et al. Multicenter phase II study of Nordic fluorouracil and folinic acid bolus schedule combined with oxaliplatin as first-line treatment of metastatic colorectal cancer. J Clin Oncol 2004; 22:31–38.
996. Goldberg RM, Sargent DJ, Morton RF, et al. A randomized controlled trial of fluorouracil plus leucovorin, irinotecan, and oxaliplatin combinations in patients with previously untreated metastatic colorectal cancer. J Clin Oncol 2004; 22:22–30.
997. Tournigand C, Andre T, Achille E, et al. FOLFIRI followed by FOLFOX6 or the reverse sequence in advanced colorectal cancer: a randomized GERCOR study. J Clin Oncol 2004; 22:229–237.
998. Colucci G, Gebbia V, Paoletti G, et al. Phase III randomized trial of FOLFIRI vs FOLFOX4 in the treatment of advanced colorectal cancer: A multicenter study of the gruppo Oncologico Dell'italia Meridionale. J Clin Oncol 2005; 23:4866–4875.
999. Ibrahim A, Hirschfeld S, Cohen MH, Griebel DJ, Williams GA, Pazdur R. FDA drug approval summaries: Oxaliplatin. The Oncologist 2004; 9:8–12.
1000. Kohne CH, van Custem E, Wils J, et al. Phase III study of weekly high-dose infusional fluorouracil plus folinic acid with or without irinotecan in patients with metastatic colorectal cancer: European Organization for Research and Treatment of Cancer Gastrointestinal Group (GI) study 40986. J Clin Oncol 2005; 23(22):4856–4865.
1001. Hurwitz H, Fehrenbacher L, Novotny W, et al. Bevacizumab plus irinotecan, fluorouracil, and leucovorin for metastatic colorectal cancer. N Engl J Med 2004; 350:2335–2342.
1002. Meta-analysis Group in Cancer. Reappraisal of hepatic arterial infusion in the treatment of nonresectable liver metastases from colorectal cancer. J Natl Cancer Inst 1996; 88:252–258.
1003. Lorenz M, Muller HH. Randomized, multicenter trial of fluorouracil plus leucovorin administered either via hepatic arterial or intravenous infusion versus fluorodeoxyuridine administered via hepatic arterial arterial infusion in patients with nonresectable liver metastases from colorectal carcinoma. J Clin Oncol 2000; 18:243–254.
1004. Kerr DJ, McArdle CS, Ledermann J, et al. Intrahepatic arterial versus intravenous fluorouracil and folinic acid for coloreactal cancer liver metastases: a multicentre randomised trial. Lancet 2003; 361:368–373.
1005. Kemeny N, Neidwiecki D, Hollis D, et al. Hepatic arterial infusion (HAI) versus systemic therapy for hepatic metastases from colorectal cancer: a CALGB randomized trial of efficacy, quality of life (QOL), cost effectiveness, and molecular markers. Proc Am Soc Clin Oncol 2003; 22:252a.
1006. Keer DJ, McArdle CS, Ledermann J, et al. Medical Research Council's colorectal cancer study group; European Organisation for Research and Treatment of Cancer colorectal cancer study group. Intrahepatic arterial versus intravenous fluorouracil and folinic acid for colorectal cancer liver metastases: a multicentre randomized trial. Lancet 2003; 361:368–73.
1007. Bonetti A. Hepatic artery infusion for liver metastases from colorectal cancer. Lancet 2003; 361:358–359.
1008. Martin RC, Edwards MJ, McMasters KM. Morbidity of adjuvant hepatic arterial infusion pump chemotherapy in the management of colorectal cancer metastatic to the liver. Am J Surg 2004; 188(6):714–721.
1009. Duprat G, Chalaoui J, Sylvestre J, et al. Intra-arterial infusion chemotherapy in rectal cancer. Can J Surg 1984; 27:57–59.
1010. Schneebaum S, Arnold MW, Staubus A, et al. Intraperitoneal hyperthermic perfusion with mitomycin C for colorectal cancer with peritoneal metastases. Ann Surg Oncol 1996; 3:44–50.
1011. Ballantyne JC. Chronic pain following treatment for cancer: the role of opioids. The Oncologist 2003; 8:567–575.
1012. Cherny NI, Portenoy RK. The management of cancer pain. CA Cancer J Clin 1994; 44:262–303.
1013. Waterman NG, Hughes S, Foster WS. Control of cancer pain by epidural infusion of morphine. Surgery 1991; 110:612–616.
1014. Foltz A, Besser P, Ellenberg S, et al. Effectiveness of nutritional counseling on caloric intake, weight change and percent protein intake in patients with advanced colorectal and lung cancer. Nutrition 1987; 3:263–271.
1015. Vassilopoulos PP, Yoon JM, Ledesma EJ, et al. Treatment of recurrence of adenocarcinoma of the colon and rectum at the anastomotic site. Surg Gynecol Obstet 1981; 152:777–780.
1016. Pihl E, Hughes ESR, McDermott FT, et al. Recurrence of carcinoma of the colon and rectum at the anastomotic suture line. Surg Gynecol Obstet 1981; 53:495–496.
1017. Makela J, Kairaluoma MI. Reoperation for colorectal cancer. Acta Chir Scand 1986; 152:151–155.
1018. Stellato TA, Shenk RR. Gastrointestinal emergencies in the oncologic patient. Semin Oncol 1989; 16:521–531.
1019. Van Ooijen B, van der Burg MEL, Planting ASTH, et al. Surgical treatment of gastric drainage only for intestinal obstruction in patients with carcinoma of the ovary or peritoneal carcinomatosis of other origin. Surg Gynecol Obstet 1993; 176:469–474.
1020. Lau PWK, Lorentz TG. Results of surgery for malignant bowel obstruction in advanced unresectable, recurrent colorectal cancer. Dis Colon Rectum 1993; 36:61–64.
1021. Butler JA, Cameron BL, Morrow M, et al. Small bowel obstruction in patients with a prior history of cancer. Am J Surg 1991; 162:624–628.

1022. Miller G, Boman J, Shrier I, Gordon PH. Small-bowel obstruction secondary to malignant disease: an 11-year audit. Can J Surg 2000; 43:353–358.
1023. Krouse RS, McCahill LE, Easson AM, Dunn GP. When the sun can set on an unoperated bowel obstruction: management of malignant bowel obstruction. J Am Surg 2002; 195:117–128.
1024. August DA, Thorn D, Fisher RL, et al. Home parenteral nutrition for patients with inoperable malignant bowel obstruction. J Parenter Enteral Nutr 1991; 15:323–327.
1025. Parker MC, Baines MJ. Intestinal obstruction in patients with advanced malignant disease. Br J Surg 1996; 83:1–2.
1026. Bernstein MA, Madoff RD, Caushaj PF. Colon and rectal cancer in pregnancy. Dis Colon Rectum 1993; 36:172–178.
1027. Van Voorhis B, Cruikshank DP. Colon carcinoma complicating pregnancy. A report of two cases. J Reprod Med 1989; 34:923–927.
1028. Nesbitt JC, Moise KJ, Sawyers JL. Colorectal carcinoma in pregnancy. Arch Surg 1985; 120:636–639.
1029. Hertel H, Diebolder H, Herrmann J, Kohler C, Kuhne-Heid R, Possover M, Schneider A. Is the decision for colorectal resection justified by histopathologic finding: a prospective study of 100 patients with advanced ovarian cancer. Gynecol Oncol 2001; 83:481–484.
1030. Pillay K, Chetty R. Malakoplakia in association with colorectal carcinoma: a series of four cases. Pathology 2002; 34(4):332–335.
1031. Nakano PH, Bloom RR, Brown BC, et al. Apudomas. Am Surg 1987; 53: 505–509.
1032. Stinner B, Kisker O, Zielke A, et al. Surgical management for carcinoid tumors of small bowel, appendix, colon and rectum. World J Surg 1996; 20:183–188.
1033. Spread C, Berkel H, Jewell L, et al. Colonic cacinoid tumors. A population-based study. Dis Colon Rectum 1994; 37:482–491.
1034. Ballantyne GH, Savoca PE, Flannery JT, et al. Incidence and mortality of carcinoids of the colon. Cancer 1992; 69:2400–2405.
1035. Godwin JD II. Carcinoid tumors. An analysis of 2837 cases. Cancer 1975; 36:560–569.
1036. Rosenberg JM, Welch JP. Carcinoids of the colon: a study of 72 patients. Am J Surg 1985; 149:775–779.
1037. Walker MJ. Rare tumours of the colon and rectum. In: Nelson RL, ed. Problems in Current Surgery. Controversies in Colon Cancer. Philadelphia: JB Lippincott1987:99:141–153.
1038. Gerstle JT, Kaufman GL, Koltun WA. The incidence, management, and outcome of patients with gastrointestinal carcinoids and secondary primary malignancies. J Am Coll Surg 1995; 180:427–432.
1039. Tichansky DS, Cagir B, Borrazzo E, et al. Risk of second cancers in patients with colorectal carcinoids. Dis Colon Rectum 2002; 45:91–97.
1040. Duh QY, Hybarger CP, Geist R. Carcinoids associated with multiple endocrine neoplasia syndromes. Am J Surg 1987; 154:142–148.
1041. Berardi RS. Carcinoid tumors of the colon (exclusive of the rectum): review of the literature. Dis Colon Rectum 1972; 15:383–391.
1042. Jolles PR. Rectal carcinoid metastatic to the skeleton. Scintigraphic and radiographic correlation. Clin Nucl Med 1994; 19:108–111.
1043. Johnson LA, Lavin P, Moertel CG, et al. Carcinoids: the association of histologic growth pattern and survival. Cancer 1983; 51:882–889.
1044. Wallace S, Ajani JA, Charn Sangavej C, et al. Carcinoid tumors: imaging procedures and interventional radiology. World J Surg 1996; 20:147–156.
1045. Kwekkeboom DJ, Krenning EP. Somatostatin receptor scintigraphy in patients with carcinoid tumors. World J Surg 1996; 20:157–161.
1046. Wood HF, Bax NDS, Smith JAR. Small bowel carcinoid tumors. World J Surg 1985; 9:921–929.
1047. Creutzfeldt N. Carcinoid tumors: development of our knowledge. World J Surg 1996; 20:126–131.
1048. Bowman GA, Rosenthal D. Carcinoid tumors of the appendix. Am J Surg 1983; 146:700–703.
1049. Gouzi JL, Laigneau P, Delalonde JP, et al. Indications for right hemicolectomy in carcinoid tumors of the appendix. Surg Gynecol Obstet 1993; 176: 543–547.
1050. Ahlman H, Westberg G, Wangberg B, et al. Treatment of liver metastases of carcinoid tumors. World J Surg 1996; 20:196–202.
1051. Beaton H, Homan W, Dineen P. Gastrointestinal carcinoids and the malignant carcinoid syndrome. Surg Genecol Obstet 1981; 152:268–272.
1052. Azizkhan RG, Tegtmeyer CJ, Wanebo HJ. Malignant rectal carcinoid: a sequential multidisciplinary approach for successful treatment of hepatic metastases. Am J Surg 1985; 149:210–214.
1053. Vinik A, Moattari AR. Use of somatostatin analog in the management of carcinoid syndrome. Dig Dis Sci 1989; 34(Suppl):14S–27S.
1054. Henry CA, Berry RE. Primary lymphoma of the large intestine. Am Surg 1988; 54:262–266.
1055. Jinnai D, Isawa Z, Watanuki T. Malignant lymphoma of the large intestine—operative results in Japan. Jpn J Surg 1983; 13:331–336.
1056. Pandey M, Kothari KC, Wadhwa MK, Patel HP, Patel SM, Patel DD. Primary malignant large bowel lymphoma. Am Surg 2002; 68:121–126.
1057. Zighelboim J, Larson MV. Primary colonic lymphoma. Clinic presentation, histopathologic features, and outcome with combination chemotherapy. J Clin Gastroenterol 1994; 18:291–297.
1058. Zinzani PL, Magagnoli M, Pagliani G, et al. Primary intestinal lymphoma: clinical and therapeutic features of 32 patients. Haematologica 1997; 82: 305–308.
1059. Dawson IMP, Cornes JS, Morson BC. Primary malignant lymphoid tumours of the intestinal tract. Report of 37 cases with study of factors influencing prognosis. Br J Surg 1961; 49:80–89.
1060. Contreary K, Nance FC, Becker WF. Primary lymphoma of the gastrointestinal tract. Ann Surg 1990; 191:593–598.
1061. Bruneton JN, Thyss A, Bourry J, et al. Colonic and rectal lymphoma. A report of 6 cases and review of the literature. Fortschr Rontgenstr 1983; 138:283–287.
1062. Doolabh N, Anthony T, Simmang C, et al. Primary colonic lymphoma. J Surg Oncol 2000; 74:257–262.
1063. Fan CW, Changchien CR, Wang JY, Chen JS, Hsu KC, Tang R, Chiang JM. Primary colorectal lymphoma. Dis Colon Rectum 2000; 43:1277–1282.
1064. Suzuki A, Fukuda S, Tomita S, et al. An unusual case of colonic leiomyosarcoma presenting with fever. Significant uptake of radioactivity of gallium-67 in the tumor. Gastroenterol Jpn 1984; 19:486–492.
1065. Shiu MH, Farr GH, Egeli RA, et al. Myosarcomas of the small and large intestine: a clinicopathologic study. J Surg Oncol 1983; 24:67–72.
1066. Stavorovsky M, Jaffa AJ, Papo J, et al. Leiomyosarcoma of the colon and rectum. Dis Colon Rectum 1980; 23:249–254.
1067. Akwari OE, Dozois RR, Weiland LN, et al. Leimyosarcoma of the small and large intestine. Cancer 1978; 42:1375–1384.
1068. Berkley KM. Leiomyosarcoma of the large intestine, excluding the rectum. Int Surg 1981; 66:177–179.
1069. Nuessle WR, Magill TR III. Leiomyosarcoma of the transverse colon. Report of a case with discussion. Dis Colon Rectum 1990; 33:323–326.
1070. Shimazu K, Funata N, Yamamoto Y, Mori T. Primary osteosarcoma arising in the colon: report of a case. Dis Colon Rectum 2001; 44:1367–1370.
1071. Smith JA, Bhathal PS, Cuthbertson AM. Angiosarcoma of the colon. A report of a case with long-term survival. Dis Colon Rectum 1990; 33: 330–333.
1072. Schneider TA, Birkett DH, Vernava AM. Primary adenosquamous and squamous cell carcinoma of the colon and rectum. Int J Colorectal Dis 1992; 7: 144–147.
1073. Michelassi F, Mishlove LA, Stipa F, et al. Squamous cell carcinoma of the colon. Experience of the University of Chicago. Review of the literature, report of two cases. Dis Colon Rectum 1988; 31:228–235.
1074. Lafreniere R, Ketcham AS. Primary squamous carcinoma of the rectum. Report of a case and review of the literature. Dis Colon Rectum 1985; 25:967–972.
1075. Vezeridis M, Herrera LO, Lopez GE, et al. Squamous cell carcinoma of the colon and rectum. Dis Colon Rectum 1983; 26:188–191.
1076. Juturi JV, Francis B, Koontz PW, Wilkes JD. Squamous-cell carcinoma of the colon responsive to chemotherapy. Dis Colon Rectum 1999; 42:102–109.
1077. Cerezo L, Alvarez M, Edwards O, Price G. Adenosquamous carcinoma of the colon. Dis Colon Rectum 1985; 28:597–603.
1078. Frizelle FA, Hobday KS, Batts KP, Nelson H. Adenosquamous and squamous carcinoma of the colon and upper rectum: a clinical and histopathologic study. Dis Colon Rectum 2001; 44:341–346.
1079. Sidani MS, Campos MM, Joseph JI. Primary plasmacytomas of the colon. Dis Colon Rectum 1983; 26:182–187.
1080. Lattuneddu A, Farneti F, Lucci E, Garcea D, Ronconi S, Saragoni L. A case of primary extramedullary plasmacytoma of the colon. Int J Colorectal Dis 2004; 19:289–291.
1081. Sperling RI, Fromowitz FB, Castellano TJ. Anaplastic solitary extramedullary plasmacytoma of the cecum. Report of a case confirmed by immunoperoxidase staining. Dis Colon Rectum 1987; 30:894–898.
1082. Tessier DJ, McConnell EJ, Young-Fadok T, Wolff BG. Melanoma metastatic to the colon: case series and review of the literature with outcome analysis. Dis Colon Rectum 2003; 46:441–447.
1083. Moir CR, Scudamore CH, Benny WB. Typhlitis: selective surgical management. Am J Surg 1986; 151:563–566.
1084. Taylor AJ, Dodds WJ, Gonyu JE, et al. Typhlitis in adults. Gastrointest Radiol 1985; 10:363–369.
1085. McClenathan JA. Metastatic melanoma involving the colon. Report of a care. Dis Colon Rectum 1989; 32:70–72.
1086. Keidan RD, Fanning J, Gatenby RA, et al. Recurrent typhlitis. A disease resulting from aggressive chemotherapy. Dis Colon Rectum 1989; 32:206–209.
1087. Vilor M, Tsutsumi Y, Osamura RY, et al. Small cell neuroendocrine carcinoma of the rectum. Case report. Pathol Int 1995; 45:605–608.
1088. Thomas R, Sobin L. Gastrointestinal cancer. Cancer 1995; 75(Suppl): 154–169.
1089. Saclarides TJ, Szeluga D, Staren ED. Neuroendocrine cancers of the colon and rectum: results of 10 year experience. Dis Colon Rectum 1994; 37:635–642.
1090. Bernick PE, Klimstra DS, Shia J, et al. Neuroendocrine carcinomas of the colon and rectum. Dis Colon Rectum 2004; 47:163–169.
1091. Wick MR, Vitsky JL, Ritter JH, et al. Sporadic medullary carcinoma of the colon: A clinicopathologic comparison with nonhereditary poorly differentiated enteric-type adenocarcinoma and neuroendocrine colorectal carcinoma. Am J Clin Pathol 2005; 123(11):56–65.

1092. Weidner N, Zekan P, Carcinosarcoma of the colon. Report of a unique case with light and immunohistochemical studies. Cancer 1986; 58: 1126–1130.
1093. Miettinen M, Shekitka KM, Sobin LH. Schwannomas in the colon and rectum: a clinicopathologic and immunohistochemical study of 20 cases. Am J Surg Pathol 2001; 25:846–855.
1094. Brown CJ, Falck VG, MacLean A. Angiosarcoma of the colon and rectum: report of a case and review of the literature. Dis Colon Rectum 2004; 47(12): 2202–2207.
1095. Le DT, Austin RC, Payne SN, Dworkin MJ, Chappell ME. Choriocarcinoma of the colon: report of a case and review of the literature. Dis Colon Rectum 2003; 46:264–266.
1096. Carr CS, Boulos DB. Two cases of solitary metastases from carcinoma of the lung presenting as primary colonic tumours. Br J Surg 1996; 83:647.
1097. Voravud N, El-Naggai AK, Balch CM, et al. Metastatic lobular breast carcinoma simulating primary colon cancer. Am J Clin Oncol 1992; 15:365–369.
1098. Law WL, Chu KW. Scirrhous colonic metastasis from ductal carcinoma of the breast: report of a case. Dis Colon Rectum 2003; 46:1424–1427.
1099. Washingtom K, McDonagh D. Secondary tumors of the gastrointestinal tract: surgical pathologic findings and comparison with autopsy survey. Mod Pathol 1995; 8:427–433.
1100. Bristow RE, del Carmen MG, Kaufman HS, Montz FJ. Radical oophorectomy with primary stapled colorectal anastomosis for resection of locally advanced epithelial ovarian cancer. J Am Coll Surg 2003; 197:565–574.

24 Malignant Neoplasms of the Rectum

Philip H. Gordon

ADENOCARCINOMA

It has become customary in textbooks on colon and rectal surgery to divide malignant neoplasms of the colon and rectum into separate chapters. We have continued this tradition but recognize that the division is purely arbitrary. Consequently, this chapter will omit topics that the two subjects have in common—epidemiology, etiology, pathogenesis, and much of the pathology except those features that are characteristic of the rectum. These topics are discussed in detail in Chapter 23. General assessment of the patient is similar, but certain items will be highlighted. Therapeutic options in specific circumstances will differ and consequently will be discussed in detail.

MECHANISMS OF SPREAD OF RECTAL CARCINOMA

The general mechanisms of spread for carcinoma of the rectum are similar to those of the colon, but because of the rectum's location within the pelvis, it is appropriate to elaborate on these mechanisms, especially as they may pertain to treatment.

DIRECT EXTENSION

Carcinoma of the rectum originates in the mucosa. Eventually it penetrates the thickness of the rectal wall rather than growing in the longitudinal axis. Untreated, it finally involves the full thickness of the rectum and may invade adjacent tissues.

TRANSPERITONEAL SPREAD

Peritoneal involvement by carcinoma of the rectum probably starts from local extension, continues through the peritoneum, and is disseminated within the peritoneal cavity. Once the carcinoma has spread throughout the peritoneal cavity, it is beyond hope of operative cure.

IMPLANTATION

It has been postulated that desquamated malignant cells from carcinoma of the colon or rectum may implant on anal wounds after hemorrhoidectomy, fistulectomy, fissurectomy, and the cut ends of bowel. This subject is discussed in Chapter 23.

LYMPHATIC SPREAD

Miles (1) believed that the draining lymphatic pathways of carcinoma of the rectum followed three directions: upward along the superior rectal glands, laterally along the middle rectal nodes, and downward to the inguinal nodes. His belief was based on an autopsy study in which most patients died from advanced disease with proximal blockade of the lymph nodes. Later studies revealed that lesions of the upper and middle thirds of the rectum drain upward along the superior rectal vessels; lesions in the lower third drain both upward along the superior mesenteric vessels and laterally along the middle rectal vessels and frequently along the internal iliac glands (2). More recent studies, employing lymphoscintigraphy, have demonstrated lymphatic drainage proximally along the inferior mesenteric vessels (3,4). Retrograde drainage of carcinoma is unusual unless the proximal lymph nodes are blocked or the carcinoma is poorly differentiated (5). Spread to inguinal nodes generally does not occur unless the carcinoma has invaded the dentate line.

Retrograde Intramural Metastases

With the present trend of performing a low anterior resection for carcinoma of the middle and upper rectum, the surgeon must select a site that compromises neither the adequacy of the resection nor the ability to perform a sphincter-saving procedure. It therefore becomes necessary to define an adequate distal margin. A comprehensive prospective study of this subject was conducted by Quer et al. (6). Examinations included 91 specimens obtained directly from the operating room. To obviate shrinkage, the specimens were stretched to conform to the preoperative or operative length measurements and were then immediately fixed for 48 hours in 10% formalin. If the two patients who had clinically obvious metastatic deposits were excluded, only one of 89 patients had retrograde spread beyond 1.5 cm, and 86 had no retrograde intramural spread. To decrease the chance of error, they recommended a margin of 2.5 cm below the lowest grossly palpable or visible edge of the carcinoma. This margin is adequate from the standpoint of retrograde intramural spread when the lesions were of low-grade malignancy. For high-grade malignancy, they advised against performing low anterior resections unless a margin of 6 cm or more could be obtained.

Grinnell (7) carried out a similar study. Of 76 patients with carcinoma of the rectum who had resection for cure, 67 patients had no retrograde intramural spread. Of the nine patients with retrograde spread, only three had spread beyond 1 cm from the lower margin of the carcinoma. Two had a poorly differentiated carcinoma, whereas the other one had retrograde subserosal venous spread. More recent studies have confirmed the limited nature of distal intramural spread in that it is within 2 cm in 95% of cases (8–11). It has been reported that even poorly differentiated carcinomas derive no significant benefit from a longer distal margin (12).

Retrograde Extramural Metastases

Spread of malignant cells in lymphatics is normally embolic from the primary lesion to regional nodes and then from node to node, with occasional bypassing of a node or a group of nodes. However, if lymph node metastases have developed, lymph flow may become blocked and be forced to seek alternate routes. As lymph pressure increases, lymphatic valves become incompetent, and retrograde flow and metastases may occur. Metastases retrograde to pararectal nodes occurred in only 1.6% of 309 cleared specimens of rectal carcinoma. All appeared to be the result of proximal lymphatic blockage from metastases (13).

VENOUS SPREAD

The development of distant metastases from primary carcinoma can result only from dissemination of malignant cells into the bloodstream. Circulating malignant cells are found infrequently in the peripheral blood of patients with carcinoma of the colon and rectum. However, the incidence rises during induction of anesthesia (28%), and such cells have been identified in the peripheral blood of 50% of patients during the operation (14). Surprisingly, follow-up studies of patients who had malignant cells in the peripheral blood during the operation have not shown any adverse effect on the ultimate prognosis (14). Unfortunately, little is known about the factors that favor the implantation of circulating malignant cells and subsequent metastases. The incidence of vascular spread correlates with the depth of invasion and histologic grade (15). The most common site of distant metastases for carcinoma of the rectum is the liver, followed by the lungs. The significance of venous involvement is described in Chapter 23.

CLINICAL FEATURES

SYMPTOMS

Many carcinomas of the rectum produce no symptoms initially and are discovered only as part of a routine proctosigmoidoscopy. Bleeding is the most common symptom of rectal carcinoma and is all too often incorrectly attributed by the patients to hemorrhoids. Profuse bleeding is unusual, and anemia is found only in the late stage. Occasionally considerable mucus may appear in the stool. As the disease progresses, the patient will notice a change in caliber of the stool because of partial obstruction. Complete obstruction is rare with carcinoma of the rectum because of the organ's large lumen and frequent sloughing of the lesion. If located low in the rectum, a carcinoma may cause a feeling of incomplete evacuation after a bowel movement or an urge to defecate, which is also known as tenesmus. Mild abdominal symptoms such as bloating or cramps may occur. Severe rectal or low back pain occurs only when local fixation is extensive and the major nerve trunks are involved by pressure or by invasion. If the carcinoma has invaded the bladder, signs of cystitis or a fistula may become apparent.

In the report of the commission on cancer (16) in which 5696 patients with carcinoma of the rectum were diagnosed, the presenting symptoms in order of frequency were rectal bleeding (60.4%), change in bowel habits (43.3%), occult bleeding (25.8%), abdominal pain (20.9%), malaise (9.1%), bowel obstruction (9%), pelvic pain (5%), emergency presentation (3.4%), and jaundice (0.8%).

GENERAL AND ABDOMINAL EXAMINATION

The general physical examination is essential for determining the extent of local disease, disclosing distant metastases, and appraising the operative risk of the patient with regard to nutritional, cardiovascular, pulmonary, and renal status. Particular attention should be directed to the liver, inguinal and supraclavicular lymph nodes, and the presence of jaundice. The development of inguinal lymph node metastases augurs poorly for the patient as median survival following discovery is approximately one year if the diagnosis is made at the same time or within one year of the primary and about 16 months if made more than one year after the primary lesion (17).

Digital Rectal Examination

Despite the sophisticated imaging technology available, useful and important information can be obtained from the digital rectal examination. A hard protuberant mass with a central ulceration is characteristic of a rectal carcinoma. The lesion may occupy a varying degree of the circumference of the rectum or may even be annular. Evaluation of the carcinoma should be made with respect to location and extent, mobility or fixity, size and gross configuration, and involvement in relation to extension to adjacent viscera or fixation to the sacrum. These are all helpful in establishing the true nature of the problem and hence direct appropriate therapy. The all-important digital rectal examination is such an age-old examination that studies have not been considered necessary. One exception is the report by Nicholls et al. (18) who assessed the depth and invasion of rectal carcinomas prior to operation and found colorectal specialists had an accuracy of 67% to 83% whereas the accuracy for trainees for 44% to 78% thus highlighting the need for experience. Others have reported similar accuracy for T-staging (67–84%) (19,20).

INVESTIGATIONS

ENDOSCOPY

The crucial nature of the endoscopic assessment, including sigmoidoscopy and colonoscopy, is fully explained in Chapter 23. This is especially true for rigid sigmoidoscopy, during which it is of utmost importance to carefully record the lesion's size, lower margin distance from the anal verge, and gross appearance. The flexible sigmoidoscope does not provide the examiner with an accurate measurement of the distance from the distal margin of the carcinoma to the anal verge. Multiple biopsies always should be done to confirm the diagnosis and establish the grade of the carcinoma. All patients with carcinoma of the rectum should have the remaining colon assessed for the presence of synchronous neoplastic lesions. The preferred method of examination is colonoscopy performed preoperatively if possible or at least at some reasonable time within the first year of operation.

ROUTINE LABORATORY BLOOD WORK

A complete blood count may reveal the presence of anemia. Abnormal liver function tests may suggest the presence of metastatic disease. A carcino-embryonic antigen determination is obtained as a baseline against which subsequent values may be compared. In addition, urinalysis, coagulation studies, and renal function tests are obtained.

RADIOLOGY

Chest X-Ray Examination

A chest X-ray examination is required for all patients with carcinoma of the rectum. It is the most practical and noninvasive method to detect pulmonary metastases. It is also a rough guide to evaluate pulmonary status.

Barium Enema

For patients in whom a total colonoscopy has not been performed or is not available, a barium enema, preferably an air-contrast study, should be obtained to rule out a synchronous carcinoma or polyp unless a high-grade obstruction is present. In a review of 545 patients with carcinoma of the rectum, of the 118 patients who underwent barium enema, synchronous carcinomas were detected in 9.3% and polyps in 14.7% (21). The investigators noted that 29% of the synchronous carcinomas and 11% of the polyps were beyond the reach of the flexible sigmoidoscope.

Intravenous Pyelography and Cystoscopy

An intravenous pyelogram (IVP) is still advised by some surgeons in patients with carcinoma of the rectum to outline the anatomy of the ureters, detect anomalies, evaluate renal function, and reveal obstructive uropathy. Cystoscopy is indicated when bladder symptoms suggest invasion by the rectal carcinoma or when the IVP suggests bladder involvement. Many surgeons do not obtain an IVP unless the lesion is large and fixed or the computed tomography (CT) scan demonstrates invasion into adjacent organs.

Imaging Techniques

The role of the various imaging techniques is discussed in Chapters 3 and 23. Of specific relevance to carcinoma of the rectum is the use of the CT scan in assessing the extent of pelvic disease. A recent review of the literature cited a meta analysis of 78 studies including 4897 patients that found an accuracy for T staging of 73% (22). Cance et al. (23) reported that a negative CT scan will fail to detect 10% of patients with small liver metastases or positive periaortic lymph nodes. Lupo et al. (24) compared water enema CT in 57 patients with standard CT in 64 patients and found the former to be more accurate in the preoperative staging of rectal carcinoma (84.2% vs. 62.5%). The diagnostic gain was mainly evident in the identification of rectal wall invasion within or beyond the muscle layer (94.7% vs. 61%). Tada and Endo (25) used abdominal ultrasonography to detect lateral pelvic lymph node involvement and reported an accuracy rate of 92.5%.

Ultrasonographic images of the normal colon and rectum identify five distinct layers: (i) mucosa, (ii) mucosa and muscularis mucosae, (iii) submucosa plus interface between submucosa and muscularis propria, (iv) muscularis propria minus the interface between the submucosa and muscularis propria, and (v) serosa and perirectal fascia (26). The first, third, and fifth layers are hyperechoic, whereas the second and fourth layers are hypo-echoic (Fig. 1). A Tl lesion is confined to the first three layers, a T2 lesion infiltrates the fourth layer, a T3 lesion involves all layers into perirectal tissues, and a T4 lesion extends into adjacent organs (Fig. 2).

The development of intrarectal ultrasonography has introduced a new dimension in the treatment of patients with rectal carcinoma. This diagnostic modality has proven to be a useful tool in the preoperative assessment of patients who might be candidates for local forms of therapy. The layers of the rectal wall can be identified and

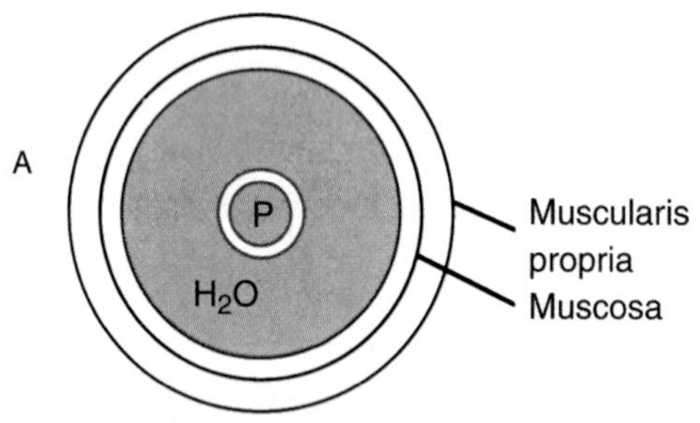

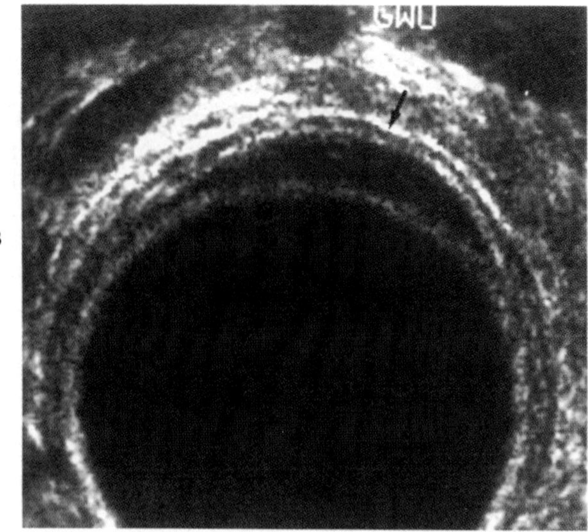

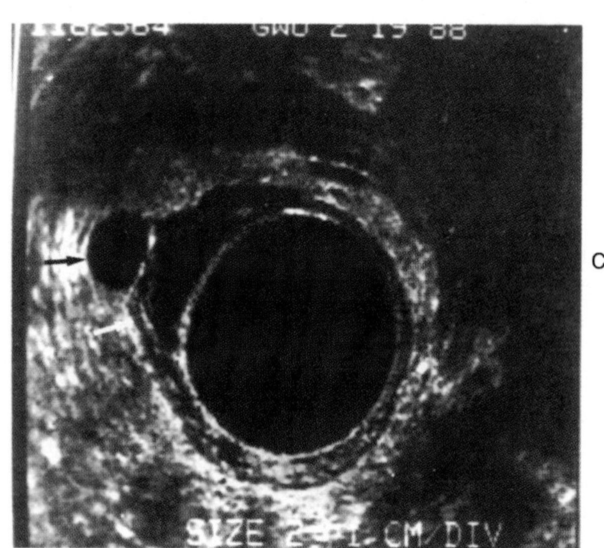

FIGURE 1 ■ (**A**) Five ultrasonographic layers of rectum. Layers of rectal wall are seen as rings, which represent interfaces between tissues of different density. Critical ring is outer dark ring, which represents muscularis propria. Penetration of this ring by carcinoma denotes Dukes' stage B. (**B**) Carcinoma of rectum. Outer dark interface (*arrow*) is intact adjacent to thicker dark layer that represents carcinoma. (**C**) Carcinoma of rectum with regional lymph node involvement. White arrow marks outer dark interface that disappears into adjacent thickening of carcinoma. Irregular surface of carcinoma where muscularis propria ring is not discernible denotes full bowel wall penetration. Black arrow points out large lymph node. *Source*: Courtesy of Lee E. Smith, M.D., Washington, D.C., U.S.A.

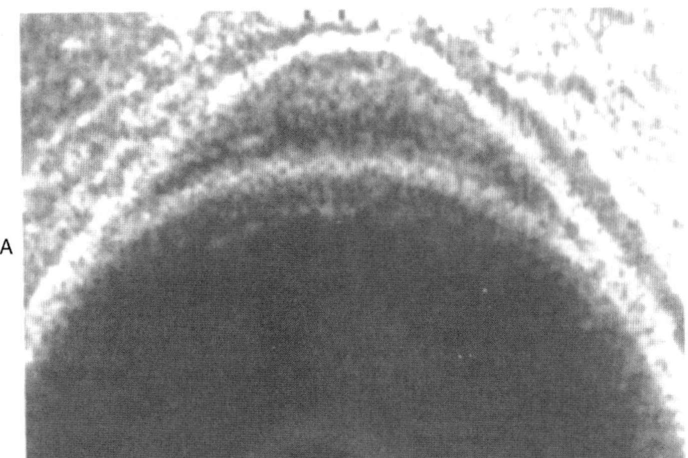

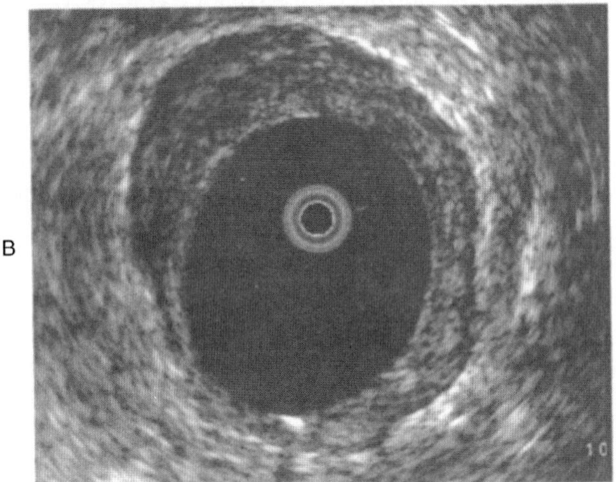

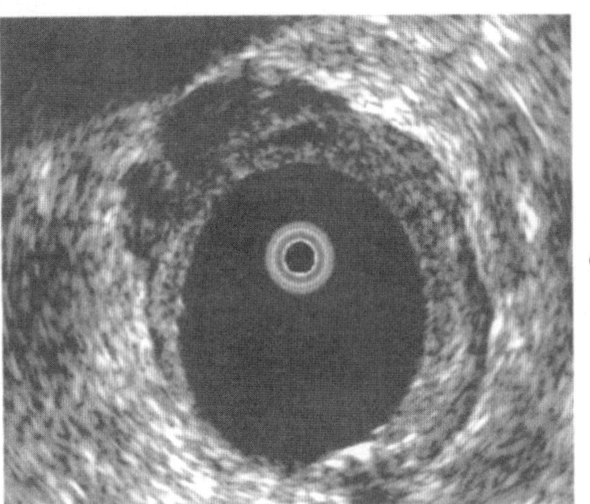

FIGURE 2 ■ (**A**) Tl carcinoma. Thickening of mucosa and submucosa layer. (**B**) T2 carcinoma. Expansion of mucosa and submucosa into muscularis propria. (**C**) T3 carcinoma. Extension through full thickness of rectal wall. *Source*: Courtesy of Michael Hill, M.D., George Washington University, Washington, D.C., U.S.A.

the depth of penetration determined. The status of lymph nodes also can be assessed. Marohn (27) reviewed the literature on the subject of endorectal ultrasonographic staging for rectal carcinoma. From 26 reports, which included 1966 patients, the average accuracy for staging was 88% (range, 75–96%). Sensitivity ranged from 55% to 100%, specificity from 24% to 100%, positive predictive value from 55% to 100%, negative predictive value from 85% to 100%, percent overstaging from 10% to 40%, and percent understaging from 1% to 30%. Values tend to vary with depth of penetration.

Garcia-Aguilar et al. (28) evaluated the accuracy of endorectal ultrasonography in preoperative staging of 1184 patients with rectal carcinoma or villous adenoma. They compared the endorectal ultrasonographic staging with the pathology findings based on the surgical specimens in 545 patients who had surgery (307 by transanal excision, 238 by radical proctectomy) without adjuvant preoperative chemoradiation. Overall accuracy in assessing the level of rectal wall invasion was 69%, with 18% of the neoplasms overstaged and 13% understaged. Accuracy depended on the stage and on the ultrasonographer. Overall accuracy in assessing nodal involvement in the 238 patients treated with radical surgery was 64%, with 25% overstaged and 11% understaged. In this study, the accuracy of endorectal ultrasonography in assessing the depth of invasion, particularly for early carcinomas was lower than previously reported. Differences in imaging interpretation may in part explain the discrepancies in accuracy between studies.

Kauer et al. (29) determined the accuracy of endosonography in the local staging of 458 rectal carcinomas. The overall rate for correctly classified patients was 69% with respect to the T category and 68% with respect to the N category. There was no difference between the 7.5-MHz and the 10-MHz scanners. In terms of accuracy, the T3 category carcinomas were the most (86%) and the T4 carcinomas the least (36%) accurately classified. Overstaging of carcinomas (19%) was much more frequent than understaging (12%). A high interobserver variability of 61% to 77% was noted. For pT1 carcinomas, the 10-MHz scanner was almost two times more accurate than the 7.5-MHz scanner (71% vs. 36%). The accuracy of endosonographic staging of rectal carcinoma very much depends on the T category.

A review of this subject found almost identical values with accuracy for T-staging varying between 69% and 97% (22). The latter review found higher accuracy for superficial lesions but more limited for deeply penetrating carcinomas. Yet, another review of 16 publications cited similar data with an overall accuracy rate of 83% for T-stage and 75% for N-stage (30). Approximately 14% of rectal carcinomas cannot be staged accurately because stenosis prevents insertion of the ultrasound probe (30).

Endorectal ultrasonography's ability to detect metastatic lymph nodes lags behind its ability to assess depth of invasion. Lymph node status can be predicted with an accuracy ranging from 73% to 85% (31–35). It is feasible and safe to perform biopsy of pararectal lymph nodes under direct ultrasonographic guidance. Ultrasonography-directed lymph node biopsy has a sensitivity of 71%, specificity of 89%, a positive predictive value of 92%, and a negative predictive value of 62%.

When endorectal ultrasonography staging is incorrect for depth of penetration, it is usually because of overstaging rather than understaging. Overstaging is presumably due to the related inflammatory cell infiltration around the carcinoma, which can have the same ultrasonographic characteristic as malignancy. Other potential explanations include an inflammatory response to a previous biopsy or compression of the rectal wall by the water-filled balloon leading to obliteration of the five-layer echo structure. It may also occur when a carcinoma is located on a haustral fold or sharp angulation that can result in tangential imaging. Overstaging most commonly occurs with T2 lesions that appear as T3 lesion (30). Understaging can be caused by microscopic infiltration, which is not detectable by the resolution obtained by the current ultrasonography instruments. Preoperative radiation therapy can influence the accuracy of staging by causing thickening of the rectal wall with loss of its five sonographic layers secondary to inflammation and/or fibrosis. Another variable is operator experience.

Williamson et al. (36) assessed the ability and accuracy of endorectal ultrasonography to predict changes in the stage of rectal carcinoma after preoperative chemoradiation. Of 15 patients studied, sonographic evidence of level of invasion and nodal status were each downstaged in 38% of patients. Pathologic evaluation revealed that the level of invasion was downstaged in 47% and nodal status in 88% compared with the initial endorectal ultrasonography staging. The authors concluded that although the method demonstrated shrinkage, it did not closely predict pathologic results. Bernini et al. (37) found downstaging in 53% with wall invasion and in 72% with lymph node involvement. The authors found endorectal ultrasonography of limited value in this setting because of overstaging. Fleshman et al. (38) reported that preoperative radiation therapy makes transrectal ultrasonography and CT scan less effective as staging techniques. A recent review suggested that the T-stage accuracy after radiation is 50% with a 40% overstaging rate (30). Lymph node staging accuracy is also decreased.

The introduction of magnetic resonance imaging (MRI) providing a high contrast soft tissue resolution without the need for imaging radiation was promising. However, in a recent review, the overall accuracy reported for body coil MRI ranges from 59% to 88% and is not better than CT (22). With the introduction of endoluminal coils reported T-stage accuracies varied from 71% to 91% (22). Further improvement was expected with the phased array coil but most reports record T-stage accuracy rates from 65% to 86% (22). The latter technique may be accurate and reliable for the prediction of circumferential resection margin with accuracy rates reported as high as 93% to 97% (22). Preoperative MRI may be of prognostic value in rectal carcinoma and may be helpful in selecting patients for neoadjuvant radio/chemotherapy. This idea is supported by the study of Martling et al. (39) who found five-year overall survival to be 77% when radial margins were not involved but only 43% when they were involved. Bisset et al. (40) reported the MRI detected penetration of carcinoma through the fascia propria with a sensitivity of 67%, specificity of 100%, and accuracy of 95%. This method of assessment may offer a new way to select those patients who require preoperative neoadjuvant therapy.

A number of comparative studies of different imaging techniques have been conducted. Leite et al. (41) compared water enema CT and transrectal ultrasonography in 40 patients with rectal carcinoma. The authors believe the former improves local staging without the difficulties associated with transrectal ultrasonography as in cases with stenoses and lesions located at a high level. Endorectal ultrasonography has been used in the evaluation of recurrence. CT is reported to be more accurate than intrarectal ultrasonography in the detection of recurrent carcinoma (42).

Tempero et al. (26) collated four series comprising 258 patients in which endorectal ultrasonography was compared to CT. Endorectal ultrasonography was superior in T stage (82% vs. 68%) and in N stage (83% vs. 66%). With respect to lymph node evaluation: (i) the likelihood of lymph node metastases is very low if lymph nodes are not identified, (ii) hyperechoic lymph nodes suggest nonspecific inflammatory changes, (iii) hypoechoic lymph nodes suggest metastases, and (iv) lymph nodes with mixed echoic patterns cannot be accurately classified and should be considered malignant. Overall accuracy of lymph node assessment in seven combined series comprising 566 patients was 80% (range, 70–83%) (26).

A more recent review of comparative studies supported these findings of superiority of US over CT with accuracy of 87% versus 76% for T stage, and 78% versus 62% for N-stage (30). Nevertheless, CT scanning provides excellent definition of distant and locoregional spread.

Meyenberger et al. (43) compared endoscopic ultrasonography to MRI with an endorectal coil in 21 patients. The results of preoperative examination were compared to histopathologic findings with a special focus on transmural invasion. Endoscopic ultrasonography identified all carcinomas, whereas MRI missed one carcinoma. Endoscopic ultrasonography was superior to MRI (accuracy, 83% vs. 40%). The MRI could not differentiate between T1 and T2 lesions. The accuracy of MRI in assessing perirectal infiltration was 80% compared to 100% with ultrasonography. Local recurrence was found in six patients all detected by endorectal ultrasonography and one missed by the MRI. In this study, endoscopic ultrasonography was more useful. MRI was found to be more operator-dependent (44). A more recent review suggested similar accuracy for MRI and US for staging rectal carcinoma (30).

Katsura et al. (45) using a radial scanner for endo-rectal ultrasonography in 120 patients with rectal carcinoma, found an accuracy rate of 92% in assessing wall penetration. No swollen lymph nodes were found in 35 of 98 cases but metastatic disease was found in five of these 35 cases (14.3%). Metastatic disease was observed more frequently in lymph nodes with a diameter greater than 5 mm (53.8%) and with an uneven and markedly hypoechoic pattern (72.3%).

In a study of 20 patients with rectal carcinoma, McNicholas et al. (46) evaluated MRI and found it accurate in all but one case with respect to transmural invasion and it diagnosed metastatic deposits in lymph nodes in 12 patients. It overstaged one patient with enlarged lymph nodes but the nodes were found to be histologically negative.

Kim et al. (47) studied the accuracy rates and clinical usefulness of MRI in preoperative staging of rectal carcinoma in 217 patients with histologically proven rectal carcinoma who had surgical resections performed. The MRI criteria for determining the depth of invasion was the degree of disruption of the rectal wall. Metastatic perirectal lymph nodes were considered to be present if they showed heterogeneous texture, irregular margin, and enlargement (greater than 10 mm). The accuracy of the MRI for determining depth of invasion was 81% and regional lymph node invasion was 63%. In the T-stage, accuracy rate of T1 was 75%, T2 was 54%, T3 was 87%, and T4 was 86%. The specificity of lymph node invasion was 41% and the sensitivity was 85%. The accuracy rate of regional lymph node involvement was 63%. T1 and T2 were overstaged in 25% and 46%, respectively, and T3 was understaged in 9.2%. The accuracy rate to detect metastatic lateral pelvic lymph node was 29% after lateral pelvic lymph node dissection was done. The accuracy rate in assessing levator ani malignant involvement was 72%. The accuracy of three dimensional endorectal ultrasound and endorectal MRI in the assessment of the infiltration depth of rectal carcinoma is comparable to conventional endorectal ultrasound (44).

Brown et al. (48) determined the accuracy of preoperative MRI in the evaluation of pathological prognostic factors that influence local recurrence and survival in 98 patients undergoing total mesorectal excision (TME) for biopsy-proven rectal carcinoma. There was 94% agreement between MRI and pathology assessment of T-stage. Agreement between MRI and histological assessment of nodal status was 85%. Although involvement of small veins by carcinoma was not discernible using MRI, large (caliber greater than 3 mm) extramural venous invasion was identified correctly in 15 of 18 patients. MRI predicted circumferential resection margin involvement with 92% agreement. Seven of nine patients with peritoneal perforation of the carcinoma (stage T4) were identified correctly using MRI. It may allow both better selection and assessment of patients undergoing preoperative therapy.

Branagan et al. (49) assessed whether preoperative MRI scans were able to predict (i) pathologic carcinoma and node stage, and (ii) those patients with pathologically clear circumferential resection margin. From a total of 40 patients, MRI correctly staged the carcinoma in 20 patients, understaged in 12, and overstaged in eight. Statistically, there was poor correlation between pathologic and radiologic staging of the carcinoma. MRI correctly staged node status in 27 patients, overstaged in nine, and understaged in four. Statistically, there was poor correlation between pathologic and radiologic node staging. MRI correctly reported the status of circumferential resection margin in 39 patients and understaged one patient. Statistically, there was good correlation between pathologic and radiologic reporting the circumferential resection margin involvement.

In a comparative study, Thaler et al. (50) found preoperative endoluminal ultrasonography to be accurate in 60% and MRI in 48% for preoperative staging of rectal carcinoma, but the differences were not significant. Others have found an MRI sensitivity of 84% and specificity of 93% in deter mining extramural extension (51). Billingham (52) reviewed seven series from the literature that encompassed 306 patients and found the accuracy of CT and MRI for detecting depth of invasion to be 76% and 83%, respectively.

Staging of colonic neoplasms by endoscopic ultrasonography has not gained importance because to date preoperative staging is without any clinical consequences. This may change with the introduction of minimally invasive surgical procedures and endoscopic resection techniques as an alternative to conventional open operation. Stergiou et al. (53) performed endorectal ultrasound with a miniprobe in 54 consecutive patients with colonic neoplasms who had been referred for endoscopic resection or for laparoscopic resection of their lesions. A sufficient endorectal ultrasound evaluation of the colonic lesion was possible in 93% of patients. The infiltration depth was correctly classified in 17 adenomas, 16 T1, 8 T2, 5 T3, and 1 T4 carcinoma (accuracy for T-staging 94%). Two T2 and one T3 carcinomas were overstaged by endorectal ultrasound while no understaging was recorded. The lymph node status was correctly classified in 84% of patients and a false-negative lymph node status was found in 8%. The overall accuracy of endorectal ultrasound was 80%. Miniprobe endorectal ultrasound is not optimal accuracy for staging of colonic neoplasms but with refinement may find a role in the future.

Heriot et al. (54) prospectively assessed the impact of PET scanning on the management of 46 primary rectal carcinomas. The operative management of 78% was unchanged as a result of the PET scan even though PET scan upstaged disease in 8% and downstaged disease in 14%. In 17%, management was altered because of the PET scan findings including 13% in which operation was cancelled and 4% in which the radiotherapy field was changed. Where available, follow-up confirmed the appropriateness of the PET scan induced management change in each case. Overall stage of disease was changed following PET scanning in 39% of patients. In view of this, they suggest that PET scanning be considered part of the standard investigation for such patients.

PREOPERATIVE PREPARATION

With growing fiscal constraints, same-day admission has come into vogue and indeed is being mandated by a growing number of health centers and insuring agencies unless the patient suffers from severe comorbid disease—in which case patients should be admitted to the hospital in sufficient time to allow measures designed to establish the optimum physical condition. In addition to laboratory studies, an electrocardiogram, especially in patients over 40 years old, always should be obtained and pulmonary function tests performed if indicated. A vigorous mechanical and antibiotic bowel preparation such as one of those described in Chapters 4 and 23 should be undertaken. For otherwise healthy patients, outpatient preparation has become increasingly utilized with patients arriving at the hospital on the morning of operation.

Potential complications such as impotence in males should be discussed with patients preoperatively. If abdominoperineal resection is anticipated, patients ideally should be visited by an enterostomal therapist who shall discuss and give information regarding life with a colostomy. Successful stomal management usually begins with preoperative education, and this greatly facilitates adjustment to the colostomy, which most patients find difficult. The ideal site for the colostomy is marked preoperatively.

RADICAL EXTIRPATIVE OPERATIONS

■ ASSESSMENT OF RESECTABILITY

Cases classified as operable are those in which the surgeon considers the conditions favorable for removal of the disease by operation. Inoperability is determined either by an unsatisfactory general condition that renders the patient unsuitable for operation or by an advanced disease state that is beyond hope for cure. In most cases it is only at exploratory laparotomy that an accurate assessment of the resectability of a rectal carcinoma can be made. Clinical examination alone gives no reliable information as to venous or lymphatic spread unless the spread is extensive or obvious distant metastases are present. Fixation of the primary growth as determined by rectal examination is unreliable in estimating the resectability. Preoperative CT scanning of the pelvis adds further information, but the ultimate decision is made at the time of laparotomy. The decision to resect is determined by the degree of fixation of the growth, the presence and extent of hepatic metastases, and the presence and extent of other metastases or peritoneal seedings.

Although fixation of a rectal carcinoma to an adjacent organ or the pelvis does not necessarily indicate contiguous spread, such appears to be the case more often with rectal carcinoma than with colon carcinoma. In a study of 625 patients who had undergone rectal excision, Durdey and Williams (55) noted that 27% of the patients had fixation—by malignant invasion (20%) and by inflammatory tissue (7%). Inflammatory attachment does not increase the risk of recurrence or decrease survival. Even for an incurable situation, palliative resection may relieve the patient of symptoms such as bleeding, tenesmus, and obstruction. In an unresectable case, the patient may benefit by an operation in which an obstructing lesion may be "bypassed" with a "hidden" colostomy (56).

■ SELECTION OF APPROPRIATE OPERATION

A host of factors influence the choice of operation for a given patient. Probably the most important factor is the level of the lesion. For practical purposes the rectum is divided into thirds (Fig. 3). The lower third extends from the anorectal ring (3–4 cm from the anal verge) to 7 cm from the anal verge, the middle third is 7 to 11 cm from the anal verge, and the upper third is 11 to 15 cm from the anal verge.

With the present knowledge of the usual lymphatic pathways at different levels of the rectum, it is generally accepted that low anterior resection is the treatment of choice for carcinoma of the upper third of the rectum. Abdominoperineal resection is the treatment of choice for many patients with carcinoma of the lower third of the rectum. However, with growing expertise, surgeons have become increasingly confident in offering an extended low anterior resection to a select number of patients whose

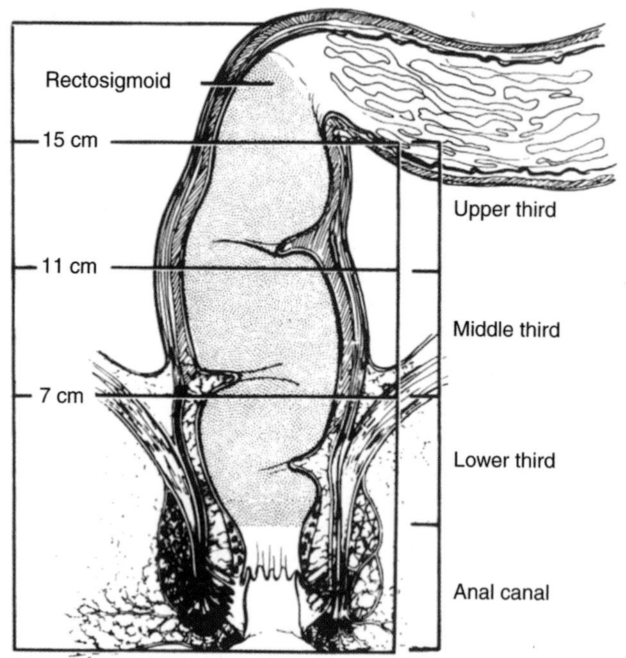

FIGURE 3 ■ Three levels of rectum.

carcinoma lie in the lower third of the rectum. The move toward sphincter-preserving operations began when technical expertise improved and anorectal physiology studies demonstrated that the distal 1 to 2 cm of rectum and upper internal anal sphincter were not absolutely necessary for continence. It has been suggested that it is now technically possible to remove rectal carcinoma that is extending into the anal canal with preservation of the anal sphincter mechanism and with a satisfactory oncologic outcome (57). However, enthusiasm for sphincter saving operations must be tempered by concern over incontinence and recurrence in suboptimally selected patients. Ultra-low colorectal and coloanal anastomosis together with a colonic pouch or coloplasty, produces acceptable function in many patients. There is still controversy about the risk of implantation of malignant cells, the place of downsizing neoadjuvant therapy, and true long-term functional outcome. Despite these concerns, surgeons should strive to perform rectal resection with sphincter preservation for low-lying rectal carcinoma whenever possible. The rationale is the same as noted in the following discussion on middle third lesions.

Controversy exists on the best curative resection for carcinoma of the middle third of the rectum. The technical difficulties in performing the low anastomosis and the high morbidity from anastomotic leaks and sepsis are well known. Another concern to the surgeon is what constitutes an adequate distal margin for resection. Studies of operative specimens have shown that a distal margin of 2 cm from the lower border of the carcinoma is adequate to contain both intramural and retrograde lymphatic spread (6,7,13). Indeed, one study showed that three quarters of rectal carcinomas exhibited no intramural spread (58). The exception to this generalization is the poorly differentiated carcinoma; for this lesion a distal margin of at least 6 cm has been suggested (6). The clinical studies by Wilson and Beahrs (59) noted no difference in suture line recurrence, pelvic recurrence, or five-year survival rates whether the distal margin was less than 2 cm or more than

5 cm from the lesion. Anastomoses as low as the levator ani muscle have been performed with complete maintenance of anal continence. Other factors influencing the choice between a sphincter-saving operation and abdominoperineal resection for carcinoma of the middle third of the rectum include body build, sex, obesity, lesion level, local spread, perforation or abscess, size and fixation of lesion, histologic grade of carcinoma (particularly undifferentiated carcinoma), presence of obstruction, adequacy of bowel preparation, and general medical condition. However, most patients with carcinoma of the middle third of the rectum can undergo a sphincter-saving operation.

From a Nationwide Inpatient Sample database, Purves et al. (60) reported that rectal carcinoma patients treated by high-volume surgeons are five times more likely to undergo sphincter-sparing procedures than those treated by low-volume surgeons. This has significant implications for those seeking a sphincter-preserving option for the treatment of their rectal carcinoma.

A comparison of the amount of tissue excised with a low anterior resection and an abdominoperineal resection is best described pictorially (Fig. 4). From the point of view of the proximal extent of dissection, the two operations are identical. The amount of tissue removed laterally is the same in both procedures. With respect to the distal line of resection, a margin as long as a 2 cm can be obtained, and there appears to be no benefit from sacrifice of the sphincter. Distal dissection of the vessels, mesorectum, and lymphatics are otherwise identical. Consequently, over the past 20 years, abdominoperineal resection has increasingly been displaced by low anterior resection (61).

Numerous reports have shown that sphincter-saving operations for carcinoma of the middle third of the rectum give comparable morbidity, mortality, and five-year survival rates to abdominOperineal resection (62–68). Although these reports were not controlled trials and are therefore not comparable, they do support the concept that in properly selected cases, a sphincter-saving operation is a good alternative for carcinoma of the middle third of the rectum. Sphincter-saving procedures currently in use include low anterior resection and the pull-through operations.

To determine the procedure of choice for rectal carcinoma, particularly low rectal carcinoma, Di Betta et al. (69) completed a search according to evidence based methods of comparative studies and national surveys published since 1990. Comparative studies between abdominoperineal resection and sphincter saving operations with a minimum of 50 patients presenting with carcinoma in the lower one-third of the rectum were analyzed including 6570 patients. Postoperative morbidity after abdominoperineal resection and sphincter saving operation is comparable and postoperative mortality decreased to 2% or less. The type of operation was not identified as a prognostic factor in terms of local disease control and survival. Quality of life is significantly inferior after abdominoperineal resection. National data reveal an abdominoperineal resection rate for carcinoma of the whole rectum (up to 16 cm) at 50% or higher and sphincter saving operations still would represent only 32% of the radical resections for low rectal carcinoma. All available evidence indicates that sphincter saving operations should be the procedure of choice for rectal carcinoma, even in the lower one-third. An abdominoperineal resection should only be performed when the carcinoma invades the anal sphincters and negative resection margins cannot be achieved by a sphincter saving operation.

Still other considerations may enter the decision in selecting the appropriate operation. Preexisting anal incontinence may impede against a sphincter-saving operation

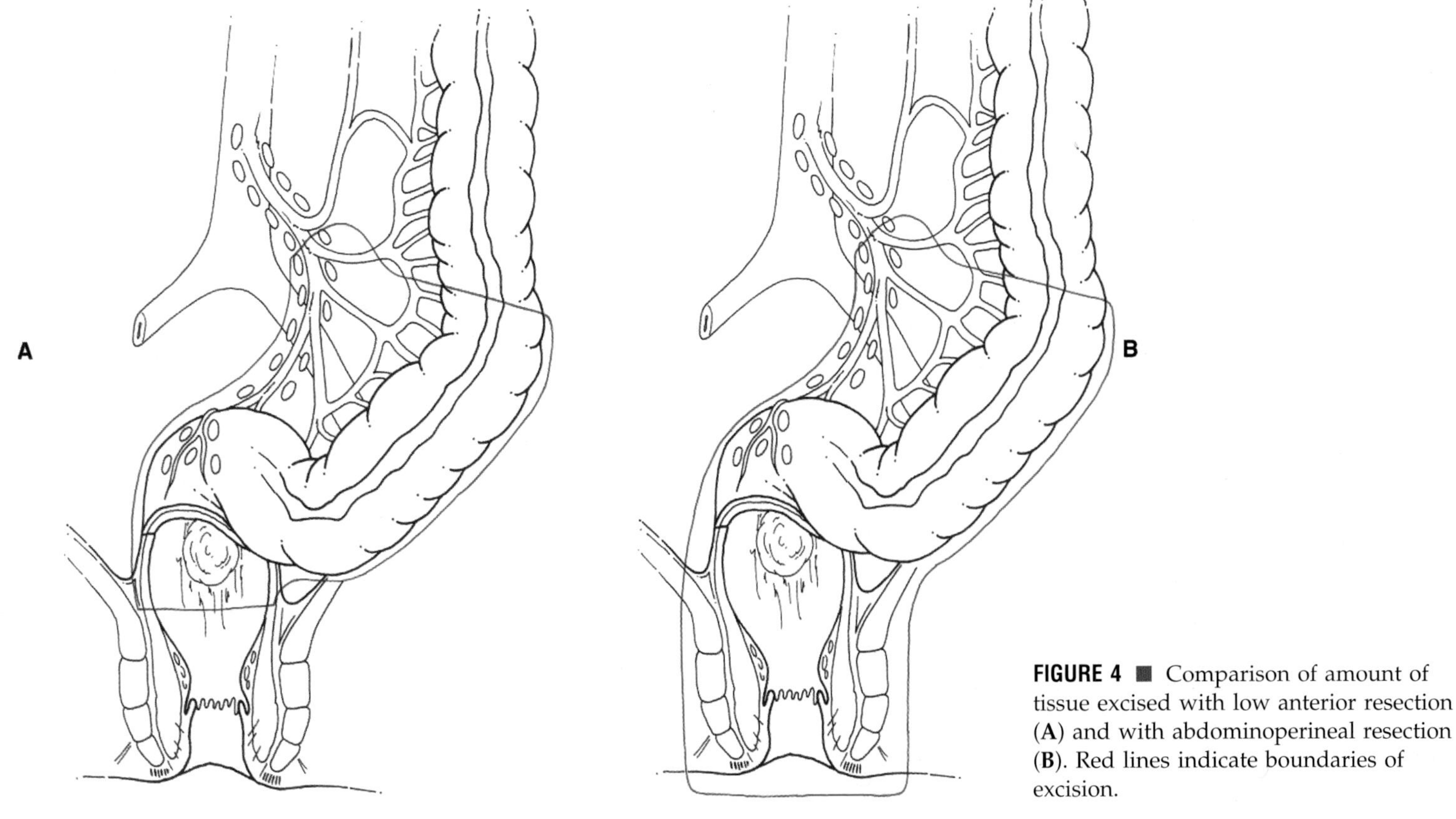

FIGURE 4 ■ Comparison of amount of tissue excised with low anterior resection (**A**) and with abdominoperineal resection (**B**). Red lines indicate boundaries of excision.

because rectal resection removes the reservoir function, and both the frequency of bowel movements and incontinence may be increased. An allied consideration is advanced age where decreased continence may prove problematic. However, this should not be an overriding consideration. The presence of extensive pelvic disease, which may ultimately obstruct the bowel, may be a relative contraindication to restoring intestinal continuity.

By the same token, patients with disseminated disease may not live long enough to benefit from establishment of intestinal continuity such as a coloanal anastomosis and later closure of an ileostomy. These patients would benefit from a permanent stoma. It should be noted that in the past operations for rectal carcinoma have focused mainly on avoidance of local recurrence and preservation of the anal sphincter. These goals were and still are very important. However, a patient who suffers from stool incontinence, straining and frequent bowel movements after sphincter saving rectal resection might have done better with a stoma. The time has now come to take more account of the postoperative quality of life of the patient and to modify our therapeutic options accordingly.

OPERATIVE PROCEDURES

Low Anterior Resection

Precise definitions of extent of resection have varied from author to author. The term "anterior resection" is a recollection from the days when posterior proctectomy was in vogue and the term anterior resection differentiated the abdominal approach from the posterior approach. The operation, which entails removal of the sigmoid colon and anastomosis of the proximal sigmoid or descending colon to the proximal rectum, is probably better-called a sigmoid resection.

The term "low anterior resection" is applied when the operation necessitates full mobilization of the rectum and transection of both lateral ligaments. The anastomosis is performed below the anterior peritoneal reflection. The term "extended low anterior resection" refers to a resection in which the anastomosis is constructed at or just above the levator ani muscles.

Because of the lateral curves of the rectum, it is possible that a carcinoma at the 7 cm level may be at the 12 cm level after full rectal mobilization. This is especially true with a posterior lesion. The feasibility of low anterior resection is decided on only after the rectum has been completely mobilized posteriorly, anteriorly, and laterally. If low anterior resection is to be done, the distal clearance should be at least 2 cm from the lower margin of the carcinoma. The splenic flexure must be taken down if there is any question of tension at the anastomosis. At the completion of the anastomosis the pelvic peritoneum is left open so that the hollow of the sacrum freely communicates with the peritoneal cavity to allow drainage of the accumulated fluid. Drains are generally not used. Closed suction drainage may be used in selected cases when the pelvis is not completely dry. A proximal ileostomy or colostomy is rarely performed. However, when the integrity of the anastomosis is in question, the surgeon should not hesitate to perform a complementary diverting stoma, either a transverse colostomy or an ileostomy.

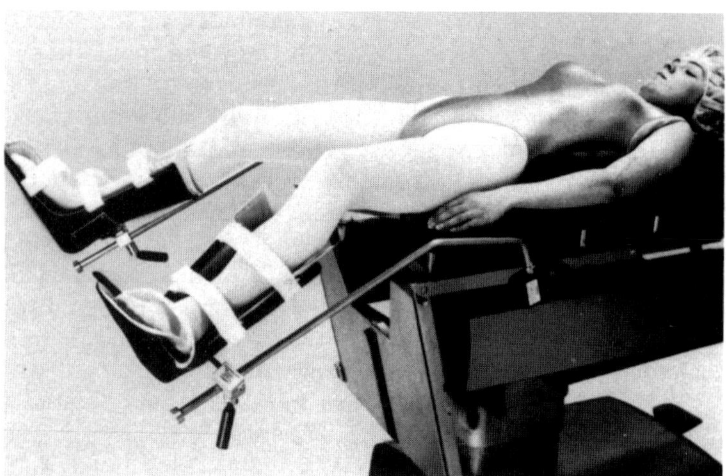

FIGURE 5 ■ Allen stirrups. With simple padding, stirrups minimize risk of pressure on calf and eliminate pressure on peroneal nerve. Thighs are slightly abducted and hips and knees slightly flexed. *Source*: Courtesy Allen Medical Systems, Bedford Heights, Ohio, U.S.A.

Position

The patient is placed supine and in a slight Trendelenburg position for better exposure of pelvic structures and to aid in venous return from the lower extremities. The lower extremities are placed in Yellow Fin or Allen stirrups, with the buttocks slightly elevated and near the edge of the table. With the knees flexed and the hips minimally flexed and abducted simultaneously, access to the abdomen and perineum is obtained (Fig. 5). Care should be taken to avoid excess abduction lest excessive traction be placed on the sciatic nerve. The lower extremities are best placed in a neutral position with only enough abduction to permit access to the perineum. Pressure over the fibular head has the potential to cause peroneal nerve palsy, and undue calf pressure may result in a compartment syndrome (70). Therefore adequate padding should be employed. The second assistant can be positioned between the patient's legs. A No. 16 Foley catheter is inserted into the bladder, and the urine output is monitored continuously throughout the operation.

Incision

Depending on the body habitus, both a transverse incision at a level between the pubis and umbilicus and a lower midline incision provide satisfactory exposure (Fig. 6A). If the proposed transverse incision interferes with the ideal location of a possible stoma, a midline incision should be used. A self-retaining retractor aids exposure.

Mobilization of Sigmoid Colon

After packing the small bowel into the upper abdomen, the sigmoid colon is mobilized by incising the lateral peritoneal reflection (white line of Toldt). The incision is carried cephalad to the distal descending colon and caudad parallel to the rectum until the cul-de-sac is reached. The extent of proximal mobilization depends on the redundancy of the sigmoid colon. If the sigmoid colon is short, the splenic flexure may require mobilization. This can be accomplished conveniently with a cautery or a scissors. The intersigmoid fossa acts as a useful guide to the ureter located just behind it (Fig. 6B). The retroperitoneal areolar tissue is pushed aside with a stick sponge so that a fan-shaped flap of

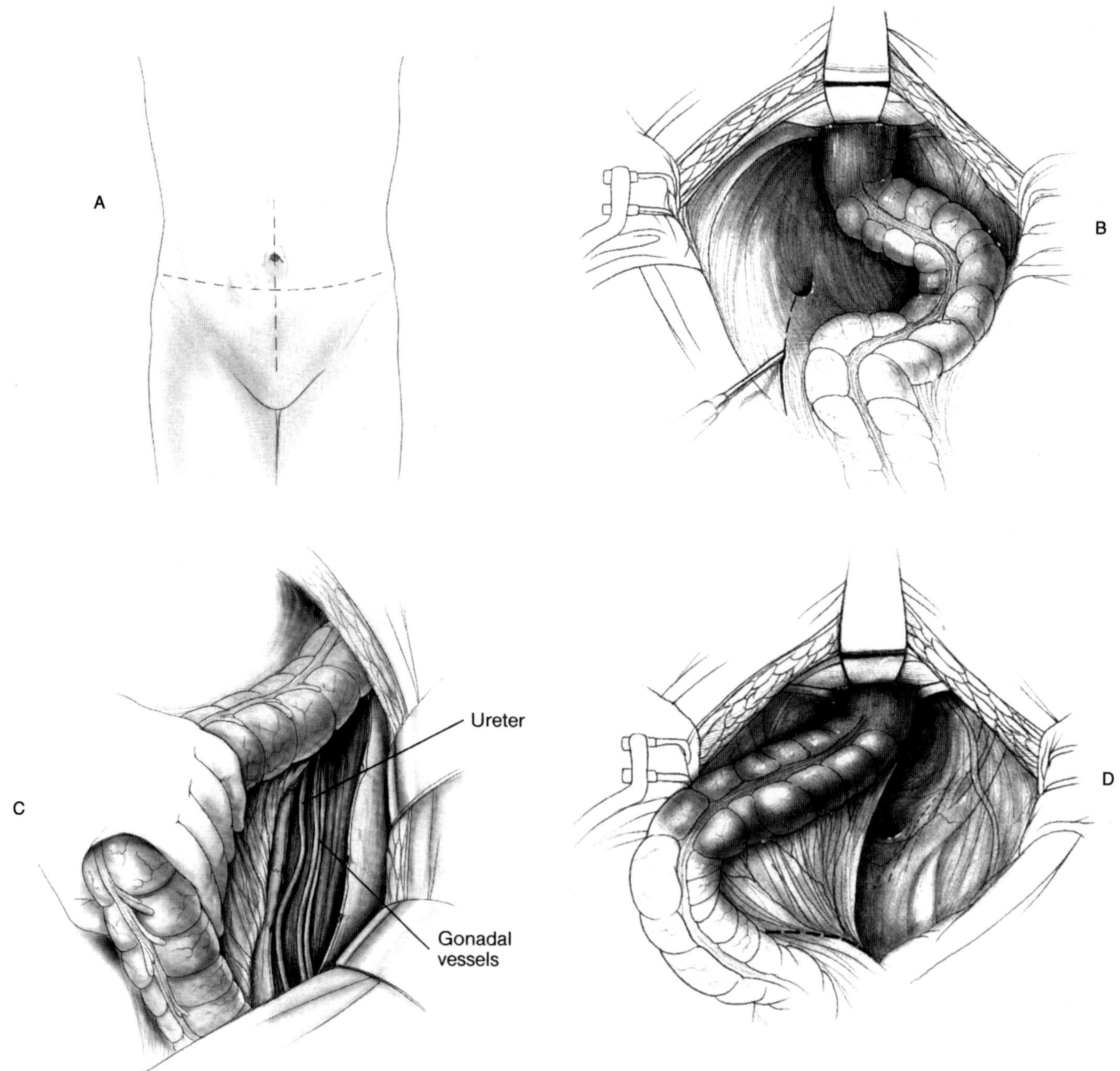

FIGURE 6 ■ Low anterior resection. (**A**) Incision selection. (**B**) Intersigmoid fossa is a marker of the underlying ureter. (**C**) Mobilization of sigmoid colon. Ureter is just medial to left spermatic or left ovarian vein. (**D**) T-shaped incision from colon toward inferior mesenteric artery and then toward the cul-de-sac. (*E to M on next pages*)

sigmoid mesentery is created. The left spermatic or left ovarian vein can be identified. At the level of the iliac crest, the ureter is just medial to this vein (Fig. 6C). Next the peritoneum on the right side of the sigmoid and rectum is incised, starting near the sigmoid vessels and continuing toward the origin of the inferior mesenteric artery. A T-shaped incision is made in the peritoneum, again parallel to the rectum, and carried down to the pelvis until the cul-de-sac is reached (Fig. 6D). Unless invasion or inflammation of the pelvis is encountered, the right ureter is not routinely identified although some surgeons believe it should be. The inferior mesenteric artery is identified and doubly clamped, divided, and doubly ligated just distal to the take-off of the left colic artery (Fig. 6E,F). Before the inferior mesenteric artery is clamped, care should be taken to ensure that the ureter is out of harm's way. The inferior mesenteric vein is ligated at the corresponding level.

Posterior Mobilization of Rectum

By drawing the rectum taut, a plane of areolar tissue behind the rectum at the level just above the promontory of the sacrum can be identified. With sharp dissection, the retrorectal space can usually be entered easily with minimal bleeding. Care must be taken at this point to develop the plane *anterior* to the presacral nerves. At the level just below the promontory, these nerves bifurcate (Fig. 6G,H).

There are four key zones where nerve damage may occur: (i) the inferior mesenteric artery origin (sympathetic

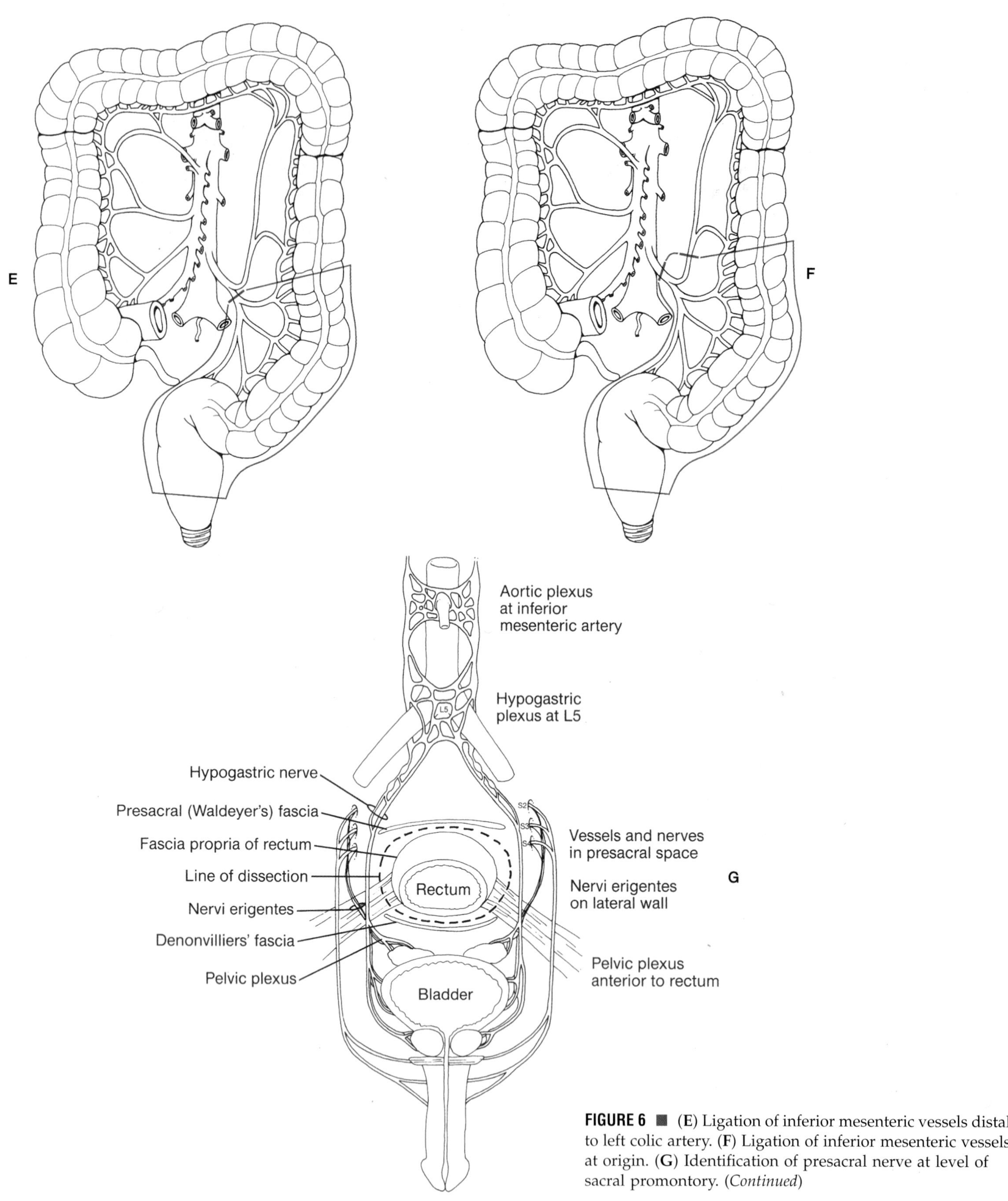

FIGURE 6 ■ (**E**) Ligation of inferior mesenteric vessels distal to left colic artery. (**F**) Ligation of inferior mesenteric vessels at origin. (**G**) Identification of presacral nerve at level of sacral promontory. (*Continued*)

hypogastric nerves), (ii) posterior rectal dissection (sympathetic hypogastric nerves), (iii) lateral dissection (mixed sympathetic and parasympathetic), and (iv) anterior dissection (cavernous nerves) (57).

Further cautery dissection in a semicircular manner readily mobilizes the rectum until the lateral stalks become prominent (Fig. 6I). The plane is developed by sharp dissection. At the S3 or S4 level, the rectosacral fascia, which varies from a thin fibrous band to a thick ligament, is encountered. The fascia is cut with a long heavy scissors or electrocautery (Fig. 6J). Failure to do so risks tearing the presacral venous plexus, which may then bleed

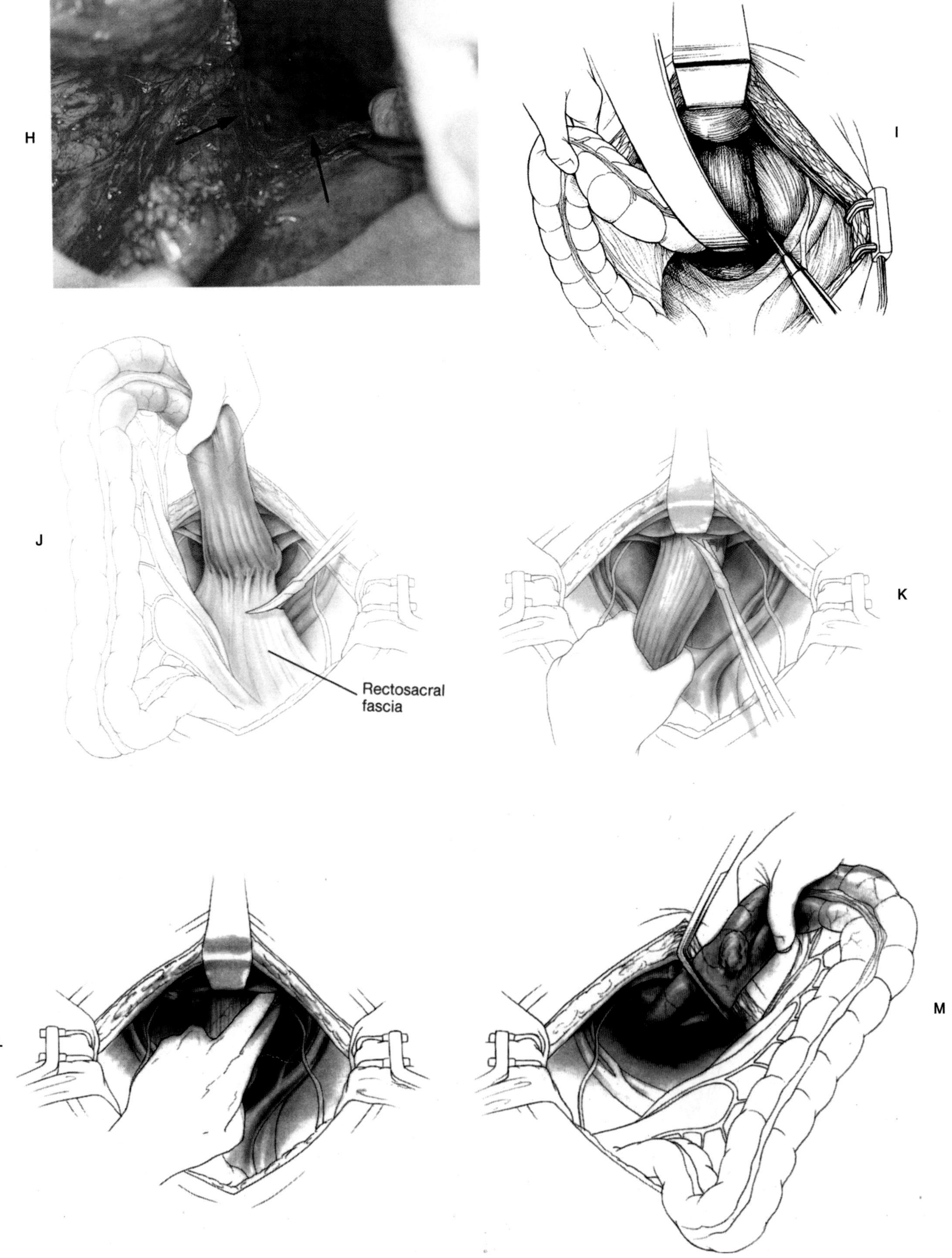

FIGURE 6 ■ (**H**) Presacral nerves (*arrows*) passing over sacral promontory into the pelvis. (**I**) At level of sacral promontory, presacral space is entered and developed. Cautery mobilization of posterior rectal wall and development of lateral stalks are done. (**J**) Division of rectosacral fascia by cautery or scissors. (**K**) Anterior mobilization of rectum by cautery or scissors. (**L**) Division of lateral stalks. (**M**) Right-angle bowel clamp placed distal to carcinoma.

profusely and can be difficult to control. Once this fascia is cut, the level of the coccyx is reached. Prior to posterior mobilization, some surgeons have found it easier to transect the proximal colon initially and reflect it anteriorly to facilitate exposure of the mesorectum. The use of a lighted pelvic retractor may dramatically facilitate pelvic exposure both posteriorly and anteriorly.

Although massive presacral bleeding during rectal mobilization is uncommon, it can rapidly destabilize a patient. Harrison et al. (71) described the anatomic basis of injury and summarized their experience with muscle fragment welding for control of massive presacral bleeding during rectal mobilization. Rectus abdominis muscle welding for the control of presacral bleeding was first described by Xu and Lin (72) in 1994. Harrison et al. (71) found this method to be an easy, rapid, extremely effective means of controlling a potentially life-threatening complication. The technique involves direct pressure held over the bleeding site with a finger or sponge stick while the patient is resuscitated. Once the patient is hemodynamically stable, a 1.5 to 2 cm^2 segment of rectus abdominis muscle is harvested from the incision and held in place with a forceps over the bleeding area while vigorous suctioning is implemented to expose the presacral operative field. Electrocautery at a high setting (100 Hz) is then applied to the forceps and transmitted to the muscle fragment, literally welding the bleeding site (Fig. 7). The muscle fragment or coagulum may actually fall free from the site, but the source of bleeding is welded closed.

Advantages of the muscle welding method include its efficacy (all eight patients in whom it was used by Harrison et al. (71) had prompt cessation of their hemorrhage); applicability with multiple bleeding sites; ready availability of the equipment required is already on the operative field; and the lack of foreign bodies left in the patient that require removal with the risk of secondary hemorrhage or anastomotic disruption. The anatomic basis for bleeding is the sacral-basivertebral veins that traverse the body of the sacrum to connect the internal vertebral venous system with the presacral venous plexus in at least 16% of patients (73). Because the adventitia of these veins blends with the sacral periosteum at the edge of the foramen, lifting or disrupting the presacral fascia during pelvic dissection can lacerate the veins, causing the ruptured ends to retract into the sacral foramina (73). The presacral venous plexus is composed of contributions from the two lateral sacral veins and the middle sacral vein (Fig. 8). Because this entire pelvic venous system lacks valves, it has been estimated that with the patient in the lithotomy position, the hydrostatic pressure in the presacral plexus is up the three times that of the inferior vena cava. Bleeding from small vessels in this area can be torrential and extremely difficult to control. Surgeons have traditionally relied upon direct pressure or electro-coagulation to contain the hemorrhage. Nivatvongs and Fang (74) have described the use of a titanium thumbtack for bleeding arising from bone. In very rare circumstances, prolonged packing for several days can be employed (75,76). Another described procedure involves the use of cyanoacrylate adhesive-coated hemostatic gelatin sponge placed over the bleeding vessel.

Anterior Mobilization of Rectum

In men the peritoneum at the rectovesical reflection is incised; mobilization is continued in the plane between

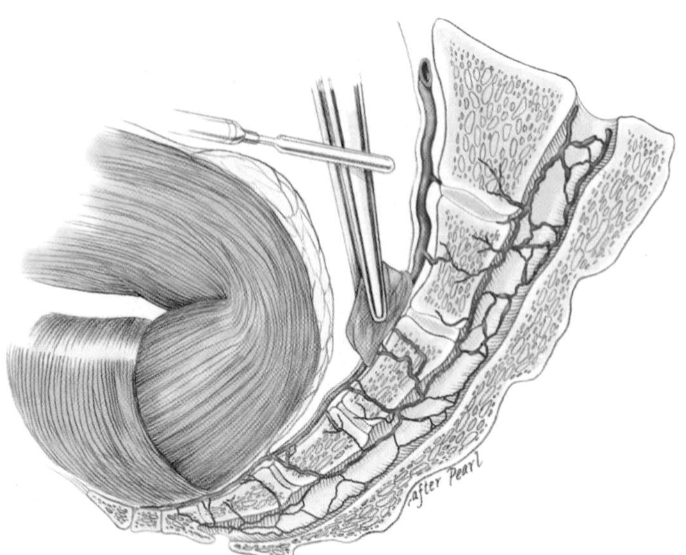

FIGURE 7 ■ Muscle welding with patch of rectus muscle on the bleeding site.

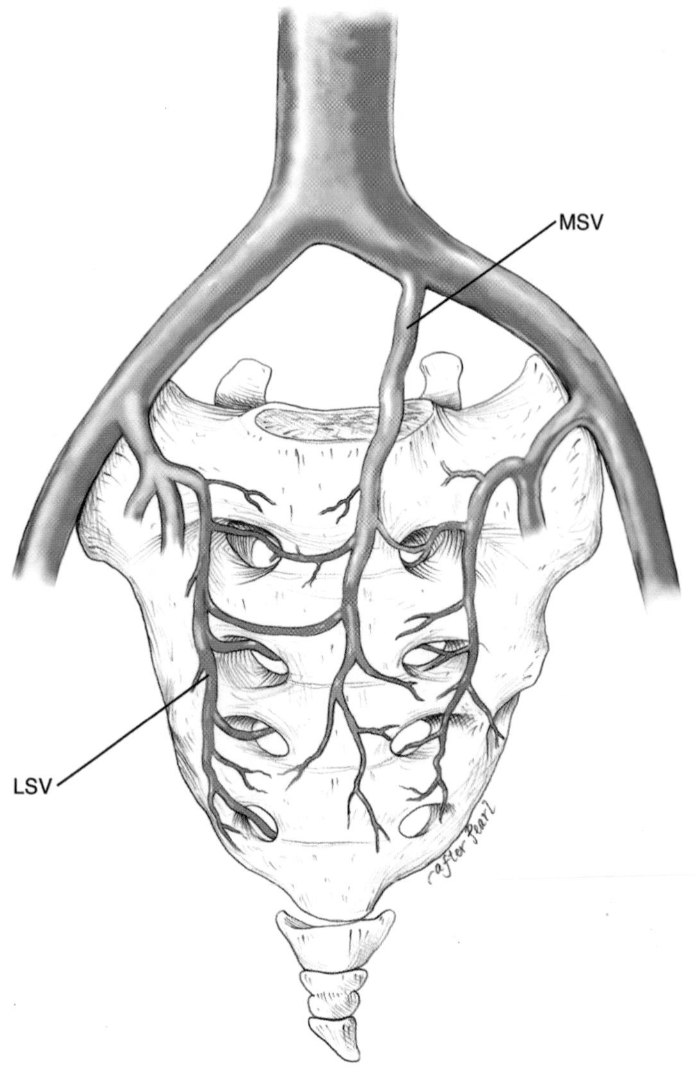

FIGURE 8 ■ Presacral venous plexus with communication with basivertebral veins.

the seminal vesicles and Denonvilliers' fascia. For posterior lesions, the plane posterior to Denonvilliers' fascia is pursued to diminish the risk of nerve damage. Most parasympathetic nerve damage probably occurs with anterior dissection. The cavernous nerves lie anteriorly to Denonvilliers' fascia, at the posterolateral border of the apex and base of the prostate. At this point, they lie closely related to the rectum. Controversy exists about the best anterior plane of excision; some recommend taking Denonvilliers' fascia whereas others believe it important to stay posterior to this fascia. The actual dissection performed should probably be tailored to the specific surgical situation, with emphasis on the position of the carcinoma (57). Dissection is extended distally until the rectum is separated from the seminal vesicles and is continued distal to the prostate (Fig. 6K). Bleeding is controlled with electrocoagulation.

Junginger et al. (77) conducted a study to determine the frequency of identification and preservation of the pelvic autonomic nerves and to identify a possible link between postoperative micturition disturbances and the extent of the radical resection in 150 patients with carcinoma of the rectum. The pelvis autonomic nerves were identified completely in 72%, partially in 10.7%, and not at all in 17.3%. Multivariate analysis showed gender, T stage, blood loss, curative operation, previous operation, learning curve, and depth of penetration of the rectal wall (T1/T2 vs. T3/T4) exerted an independent influence on achievement of complete pelvic nerve identification. Discharge from hospital with a urinary catheter occurred in 10.7% of patients. Identification and preservation of pelvic autonomic nerves was associated with low bladder dysfunction rates (4.5% vs. 38.5%).

In women the rectovaginal reflection is incised and the plane is developed between the rectum and the vagina until the pubis can be felt anteriorly. Exposure may be facilitated by passage of a suture around each fallopian tube, with elevation and retraction of the uterus anteriorly by attaching the sutures to the self-retaining retractor.

Dividing Lateral Ligaments (Stalks)

At this stage the rectum has been mobilized posteriorly to the tip of the coccyx and anteriorly to the level of the pubis. The rectum remains attached laterally on each side by the pelvic fascia or lateral ligaments (containing the accessory middle rectal vessels). The rectum is pulled taut with the left hand, and the right hand is placed behind the rectum and swept laterally on each side of the ligament, with care taken to avoid the ureters. The ligaments then can be divided by electrocautery. Alternatively, the ligaments are clamped, divided, and ligated (Fig. 6L).

Based on the recommendation by Heald et al. (78), an effort is made to excise the mesorectum rather than following the tendency to cone down through the mesorectum to the proposed distal line of resection. The latter technique leaves mesorectum in the pelvis, and Heald cautions that this is the main reason for local recurrence (78,79). For lesions located higher in the rectum, the distal portion of mesorectum may be left undisturbed but given an adequate distal margin; transection of the mesorectum is performed perpendicular to the rectal wall and not in a cone fashion. When adequate mobilization has been achieved, a right-angle bowel clamp is placed across the rectum distal to the carcinoma (Fig. 6M). At this point some surgeons irrigate the rectal stump with a cancericidal agent. Greater emphasis had been placed on this measure by European surgeons than by North American surgeons. This maneuver may disqualify patients who are otherwise eligible for clinical trials of adjuvant therapy.

Agaba (80) evaluated the effectiveness of cytocidal rectal washout in reducing the incidence of local recurrence. Of 141 patients who underwent curative anterior resection for carcinoma of the rectum and rectosigmoid, 90 patients underwent rectal washout using cetrimide before anastomosis while 51 patients did not have rectal washout before anastomosis. Among the washout group, the local recurrence rate was 4.4% compared with 5.9% among the no washout group. Because of the size of this study they were unable to demonstrate the benefit or lack thereof of this cytocidal agent in reducing local recurrence.

Inadvertent Rectal Perforation

An embarrassing but nevertheless real case scenario is the occasional inadvertent rectal perforation during the mobilization of a carcinoma of the rectum. It has been reported that the spillage of malignant cells in this situation results in a higher incidence of local recurrence (81). The question arises as to "what exactly should the surgeon do in such situations?" Several suggestions have been made. Irrigation with sterile water has been recommended with the hope that the hypo-osmolar nature of this solution will lyse any released malignant cells. Irrigation with povi-done-iodine (Betadine) has been used, also in the hope of killing malignant cells. If radiation has not been given preoperatively, a course of postoperative radiotherapy should be considered.

Anastomosis with Circular Stapler

The introduction of staplers into operative use in North America has markedly facilitated intestinal anastomoses. The advent of the circular stapler has extended the limits of low anterior resection by enabling surgeons to perform highly reliable anastomoses at a lower level than was technically possible with a traditional hand-sewn anastomosis, thus sparing a considerable number of patients from abdominoperineal resection and a permanent colostomy. The general principles of anastomoses must be maintained; generally, tissues not fit to sew should not be stapled. Conditions that are unfavorable for a hand-sewn anastomosis are also unfavorable for staples. Staples are only one method, albeit a convenient one, to establish intestinal continuity. Considerations of adequate blood supply, absence of tension, accurate apposition of tissue, and absence of sepsis apply equally to both stapled and hand-sutured anastomoses. A variety of staplers are commercially available (Fig. 9).

The technique and pitfalls with the use of the circular stapler have been described previously in detail (82). Having determined that a low anterior resection with a circular stapler is feasible, the surgeon prepares the proximal bowel by clearing 1 to 1.5 cm from the proposed proximal resection margin. A pursestring suture may be applied using the specially designed fenestrated clamp (Fig. 10A). The

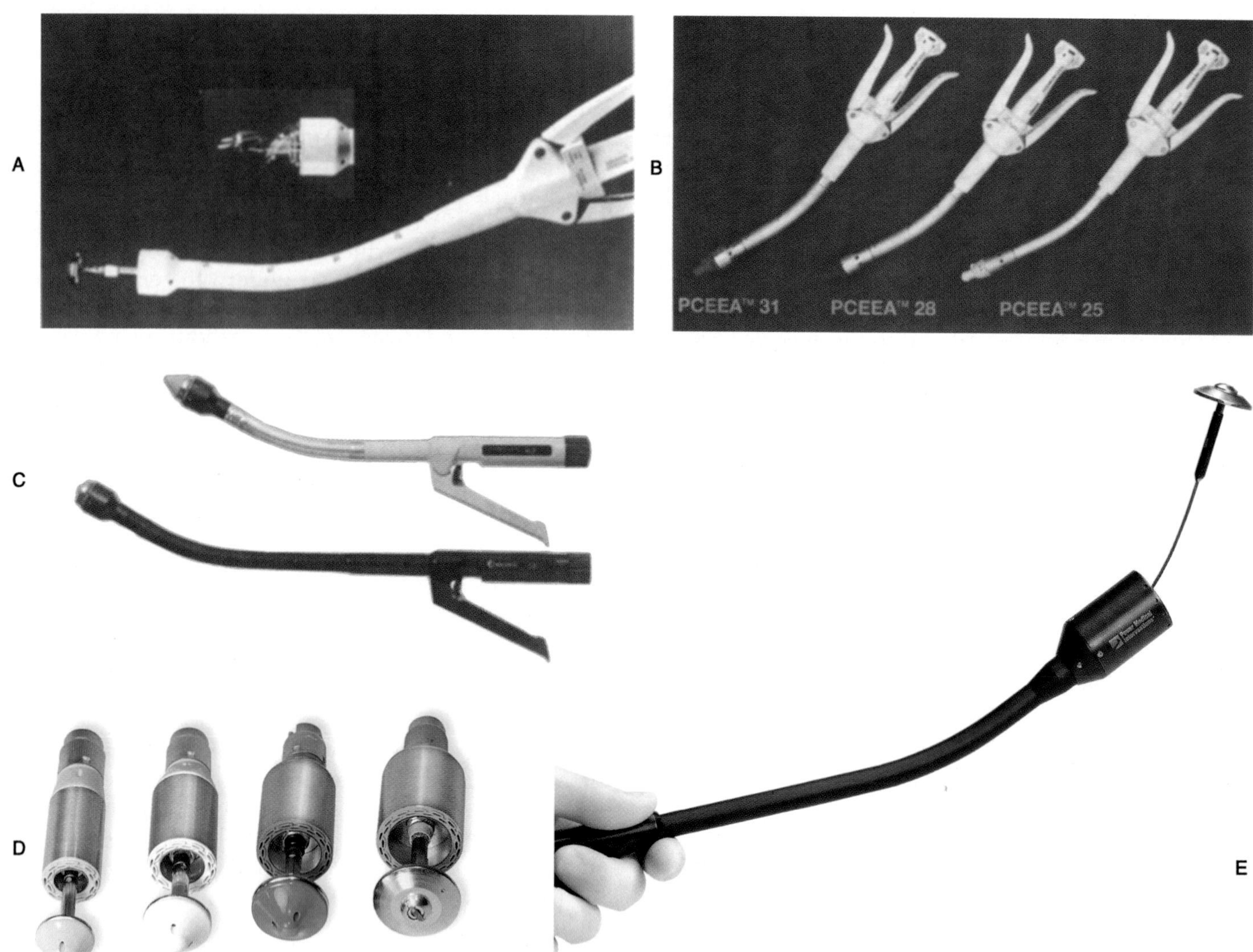

FIGURE 9 ■ Circular staplers. (**A**) United States Surgical disposable EEA stapler. (**B**) Curved CEEA staplers. (**C**) Ethicon ILS disposable staplers. (**D**) Circular staplers which connect to a long flexible drivenshaft: 21, 25, 29, and 33mm size. (**E**) Transanal 29mm circular stapler with flexible wire trocar. *Source*: (**A**) and (**B**) Courtesy of United States Surgical Corp., Norwalk, Connecticut, U.S.A. (**C**) Courtesy of Ethicon, Inc., Somerville, New Jersey, U.S.A. (**D** and **E**) Courtesy of Power Medical Interventions, Langhorne, Pennsylvania, U.S.A.

anvil is detached from the instrument and inserted into the proximal bowel after its transection (Fig. 10B). The proximal pursestring suture is tied to avoid contamination from the proximal bowel. Attention is then directed to the distal stump. The rectum is prepared in a similar manner, except that for low anastomoses, the width of the pelvis is not adequate to permit application of the instrument and a Keith needle. A right-angle clamp is placed distal to the carcinoma and the bowel is transected. A whipstitch of 2–0 Prolene is placed on the rectal stump, with evenly spaced bites taken 4 to 5 mm from the cut edge (Fig. 10A). Sizers are used to determine the appropriate diameter of the stapler cartridge.

Before insertion of the circular stapler, the operator must confirm the presence of the staples, circular knife, and Teflon ring. The appropriate size instrument is selected, lubricated, and inserted through the anus in the closed position with the handle up. The instrument is advanced until the cartridge is visualized through the rectal lumen, the central shaft is extruded, and the distal pursestring suture is tied (Fig. 10B). The anvil is then engaged into the central shaft (Fig. 10C). Turning the wing nut clockwise closes the stapler, while the abdominal operator ensures that the gap is free of sponges, mesentery, bladder, and other tissues, especially vaginal (Fig. 10D). Care must be taken to ensure adequate dissection to separate the rectum from the vaginal wall. Failure to do so runs the risk of entrapment of a portion of the posterior vaginal wall, which will probably lead to the development of a rectovaginal fistula. As the stapler is being closed, the perineal operator can check with a digital examination of the vagina that the vaginal wall is not being incorporated. When the stapler is fully closed, the safety is released and the stapler is activated by squeezing the handle firmly. This action places a double, staggered, circular row of stainless steel staples that join the two ends of the bowel, while a circular knife simultaneously cuts two rings of tissue inside the staple line, thus creating an inverted end-to-end anastomosis (Fig. 10E).

To remove the instrument, the stapler is opened by turning the wing-nut counterclockwise one and a half completed turns. The stapler is rotated in an arc and should

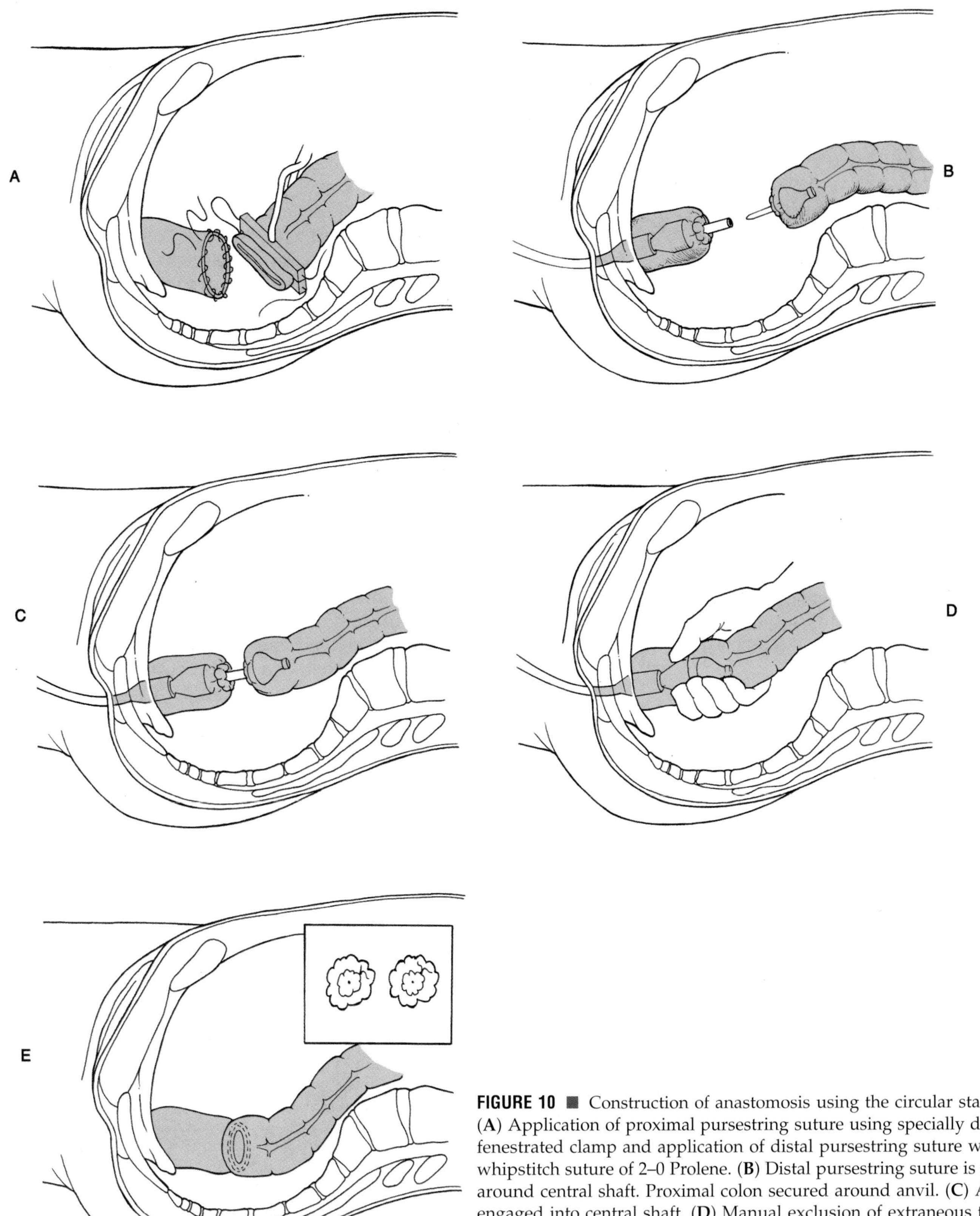

FIGURE 10 ■ Construction of anastomosis using the circular stapler. (**A**) Application of proximal pursestring suture using specially designed fenestrated clamp and application of distal pursestring suture with a whipstitch suture of 2–0 Prolene. (**B**) Distal pursestring suture is secured around central shaft. Proximal colon secured around anvil. (**C**) Anvil engaged into central shaft. (**D**) Manual exclusion of extraneous tissue during approximation of bowel ends. (**E**) Completed anastomosis with "rings of confidence." *Source*: Adapted from Ref. 83.

move independently of the bowel. The instrument is then removed in the direction of the curve of the instrument by a simple, gentle, simultaneous withdrawing and back-and-forth rotational motion. When difficulty is encountered in extraction of the instrument, guide sutures are placed through the anastomosis to help lift the anastomosis over the anvil (Fig. 11). A check is made to ensure that the rings of tissue excised are intact. Anastomoses may be inspected directly with a sigmoidoscope, looking for bleeding or obvious disruption. The integrity of the anastomosis is further tested by insufflating air into the bowel via the sigmoidoscope with saline in the pelvis. The abdominal operator checks for bubbles arising from the anastomosis. If an air leak is present, sutures can be placed to correct the defect. These sutures may be placed by the abdominal operator, but in the case of a very low anastomosis, per anal

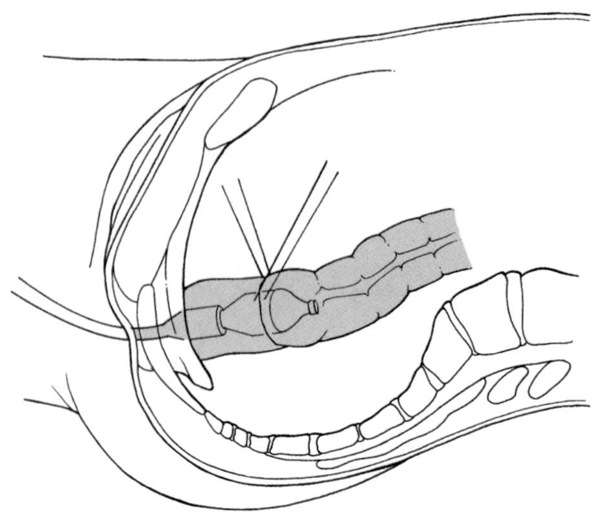

FIGURE 11 ■ Suture placement through anastomosis to help lift anastomosis over anvil. *Source*: Adapted from Ref. 83.

access may be more appropriate. A diverting stoma is not required unless the surgeon is unable to accomplish the closure or is in some way unhappy about the integrity of the anastomosis.

If excess laxity exists in the bowel, the peritoneum on the right side of the pelvis is closed. One side is left open to freely communicate with the generalized peritoneal cavity so that any fluid will be readily absorbed. More recently, the peritoneum has not been closed at all, and no adverse effects have appeared. It is unlikely that a loop of small bowel will pass around the colon that was led to the pelvis.

A technical problem that is not infrequently encountered is the discrepancy in the diameter of the bowel ends to be anastomosed. Probably the simplest way to enlarge the bowel lumen is by insertion of progressively larger sizers (e.g., sizers by United States Surgical Corp., Norwalk, Connecticut, U.S.A.). A second option is the use of a sponge forceps to stretch the bowel. Yet another technique is the very slow expansion of a 30 mL Foley balloon catheter with saline after it is positioned in the bowel lumen (84). All these methods of dilation may result in tearing of the bowel wall. Simple techniques of enlarging the diameter of the bowel lumen for performing end-to-end anastomoses using the EEA stapler were described by Tchervenkov and Gordon (85). If the transected bowel end cannot be dilated to accept a staple cartridge of appropriate size and the pursestring suture has already been applied, an incision can be made along the anti-mesenteric border of the colon. Ideally, the purse-string suture will have been placed so that the free ends are at the antimesenteric position of the circumference of the bowel (Fig. 12A). It is a simple matter to incise the bowel between the two ends of the suture (Fig. 12B) and then continue the suture along the newly created border past the apex of the incision to meet the other end of the suture (Fig. 12C). The new configuration of the circumference will be egg shaped (Fig. 12D).

If it is apparent from the outset that the bowel caliber is definitely too small and will not be successfully dilated by the previously described methods, the oblique application of the pursestring clamp will result in a larger diameter of the bowel end (Fig. 13).

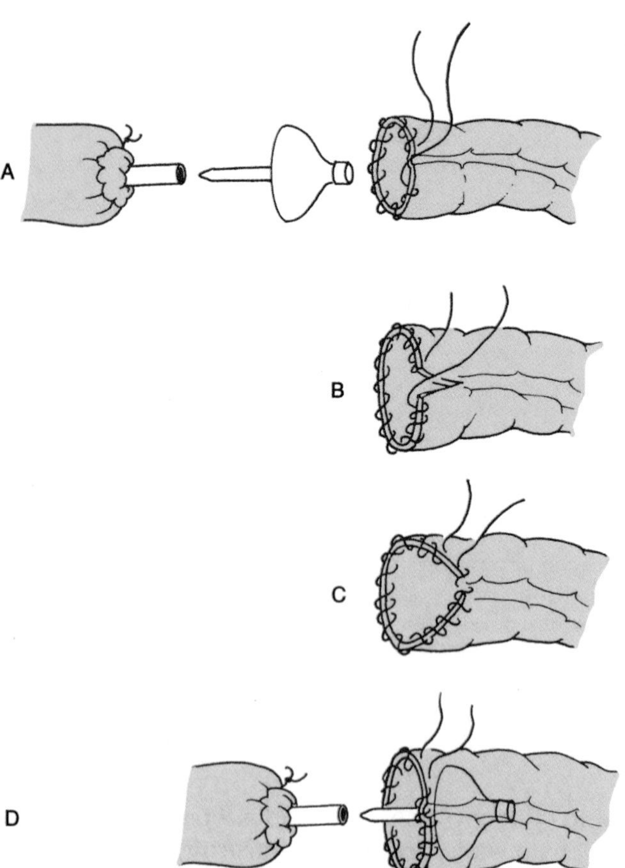

FIGURE 12 ■ (**A**) Application of pursestring clamp such that one end is on antimesenteric border. (**B**) Incision of bowel along taenia between sutures. (**C**) Continuation of suture along newly created border. (**D**) Completed application of pursestring suture. *Source*: Adapted from Ref. 85.

Double-Stapling Technique

Knight and Griffin (86) introduced the double-stapling technique (Fig. 14). The cited advantage of this technique is the elimination of the need for a distal pursestring suture. A Roticulator or regular linear stapler is placed on the rectum distal to the carcinoma. The instrument is fired, a right-angle bowel clamp is applied distal to the carcinoma, and the rectum is transected just proximal to the stapler. Depending upon the variety of circular stapler used, the technique varies slightly. With the CEEA instrument

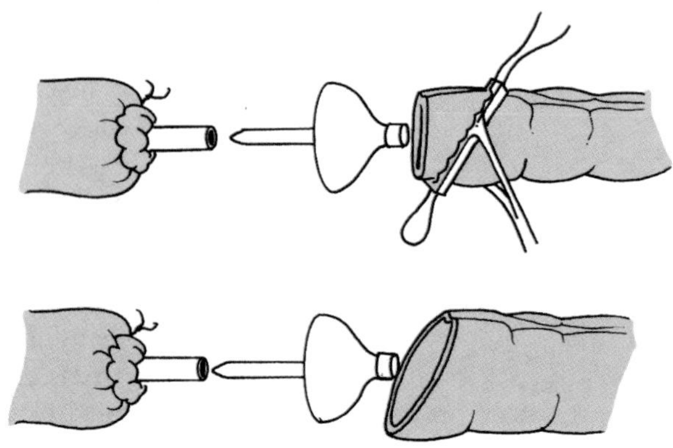

FIGURE 13 ■ Oblique application of pursestring clamp. *Source*: Adapted from Ref. 85.

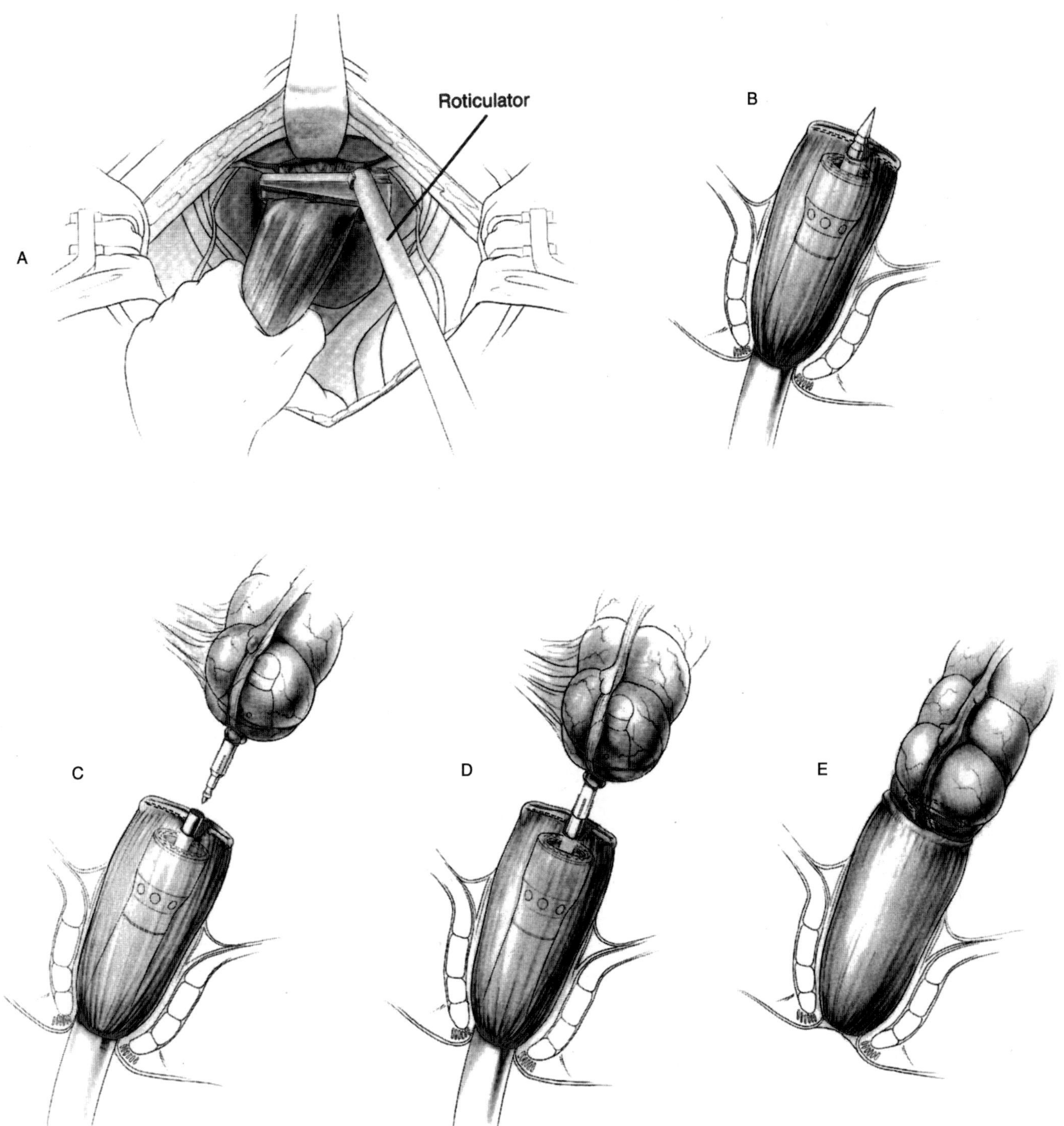

FIGURE 14 ■ Double-stapling technique. (**A**) Roticulator applied to distal rectum and pursestring clamp applied to proximal colon. (**B**) CEEA introduced with trocar piercing at level of anastomosis. (**C**) Trocar removed and detachable anvil inserted into proximal bowel. (**D**) Anvil engaged in central shaft. (**E**) Anastomosis completed.

the detachable anvil is removed and a trocar is placed in the central shaft, which is then retracted within the cartridge. The instrument is introduced through the anus and advanced to the staple line. The trocar is extruded through the staple line and removed; the anvil previously inserted into and secured on the proximal bowel is engaged into the central shaft. The anvil is approximated to the cartridge and the instrument is activated. The instrument is withdrawn and the anastomosis is inspected. The Ethicon circular stapler has the trocar built into the central shaft and hence one step is removed. When using a circular instrument care should be exercised to ensure that the trocar penetrates the suture line or the area immediately adjacent to it. If a rim of tissue between the stapled rectum and the ring of tissue excised remains, it may become ischemic and result in a leak.

Griffin et al. (87) reviewed 75 patients and found an anastomotic leak rate of 2.7% and a 2.7% incidence of stenosis that required treatment. No deaths were reported. Moran et al. (88) encountered a clinical leak rate of 9% and a stricture rate of 5% in a series of 55 patients. Laxamana et al. (89) reported on the long-term follow-up of 189 patients who underwent a double-stapling technique. The postoperative mortality was 1.6% and the clinical leak rate

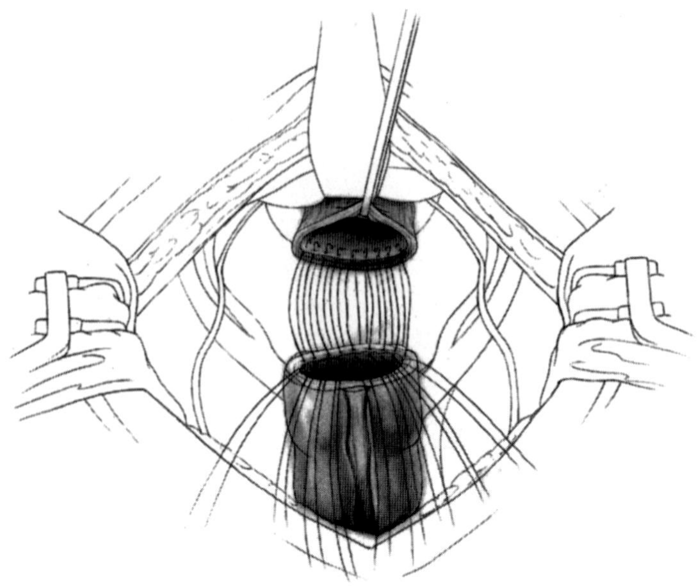

FIGURE 15 ■ Single-layer hand-sutured anastomosis. Alignment of posterior wall and placement of sutures before tying.

7.3%, significantly higher at 20% for the lower one-third of the rectum. Other surgeons have evaluated the safety of this technique (90).

Hand-Sutured Anastomoses

Many surgeons still prefer hand-sutured anastomoses. Although two-layered anastomoses were once considered standard technique, the trend is now toward single-layer anastomoses. The open technique, with no clamping of the bowel ends, prevents injury to the bowel wall. For approximation of the posterior wall, vertical mattress sutures are used. The first bite is full thickness on each side, but on the return bite only mucosa and submucosa are included (Fig. 15). Popularly used suture materials are 4–0 polypropylene, 4–0 polyglycolic acid, or poly-glactin. All knots are tied inside the lumen. An interrupted full-thickness suture with only mucosal inversion as described by Gambee is used for the anterior wall (Fig. 44 in Chapter 23). Many surgeons prefer a two-layer anastomosis: an outer seromuscular layer of 4–0 nonabsorbable or absorbable suture and a continuous inner layer of 4–0 absorbable suture. Details of suture techniques are described in Chapter 23 and illustrated in Figs. 46 and 47 of that chapter.

Abdominoperineal Resection

Proctectomy for carcinoma has evolved from a procedure that originally consisted primarily of a perineal excision to the classic Miles procedure. In the latter procedure, the rectum is mobilized via the abdominal route and buried below the reconstructed pelvic peritoneum; it is removed via a perineal route. The two-team, or synchronous combined excision gained popularity and remains my preference, as well as the technique of choice of many surgeons today. The Miles method permits a simultaneous approach to the rectum and shortens the operating time.

Abdominal Part of Operation

The initial dissection in an abdominoperineal resection is almost identical to that described for a low anterior resection. The one exception is that a conservative incision is made in the peritoneum on each side of the rectum. A flap of peritoneum is elevated on each side. Conserving the peritoneum facilitates closure at the end of the operation. Once the decision is made that an abdominoperineal resection is required, the perineal phase of the operation begins.

COMPLETION OF ABDOMINAL PORTION IN SYNCHRONOUS COMBINED EXCISION OF RECTUM

PREPARING COLOSTOMY AND RECONSTRUCTION OF PELVIC FLOOR ■ The site in the proximal sigmoid or distal descending colon chosen for the colostomy is cleaned and transected, an act easily accomplished with a stapler (Fig. 16A). With blunt finger dissection, an extraperitoneal tunnel is created from the left flank toward the site of the colostomy (Fig. 16B). A 2 cm disk of skin and subcutaneous tissue is excised at the premarked colostomy site. The anterior fascia is incised in a cruciate manner, the rectus muscle is split, and the posterior fascia and peritoneum are incised in a cruciate manner. The opening should admit two fingers loosely. The colon is then brought through the extraperitoneal tunnel to the colostomy aperture (Fig. 16C). It should be matured at the completion of the abdominal part of the procedure. Details of colostomy construction are described in Chapter 32.

With the synchronous combined excision, the rectum is passed to the perineal operator when that portion of the dissection is complete. If the patient is to be repositioned, the stapled end of the rectal stump is dropped into the pelvis. The pelvic peritoneum is closed with continuous 4–0 absorbable suture (Fig. 16D). It is at this point that preservation of the peritoneal flaps is appreciated. The abdominal cavity is copiously irrigated with saline and closed in layers.

INTRAPERITONEAL COLOSTOMY ■ If the extraperitoneal colostomy cannot be performed conveniently, the colon is brought out through the colostomy aperture, and the projecting limb is attached to the lateral abdominal wall using interrupted 4–0 absorbable sutures to prevent herniation of the small bowel. Nevertheless, the extraperitoneal technique is much preferred because of fewer complications related to peristomal herniation, prolapse, retraction, and internal herniation.

MATURATION OF COLOSTOMY ■ The staples at the end of the colostomy are excised. The colostomy limb may be sutured to the anterior fascia. It is preferable to evert the stoma 1 cm rather than making it flush with the skin. The stoma is immediately matured with interrupted 3–0 or 4–0 chromic catgut (Fig. 16E). A temporary colostomy bag is then applied.

PERINEAL PORTION WHEN SYNCHRONOUS COMBINED EXCISION OF RECTUM IS USED ■ During the original positioning of the patient, 2-in. tape is placed on each buttock to retract it laterally and permit better exposure of the perineum. In the male, the external genitalia also are taped to keep them out of the way of the perineal operator. The dissection is not begun until the abdominal operator has confirmed that the rectum is resectable.

The perineal phase of the operation is begun by placing a heavy, silk pursestring suture around the anus. An

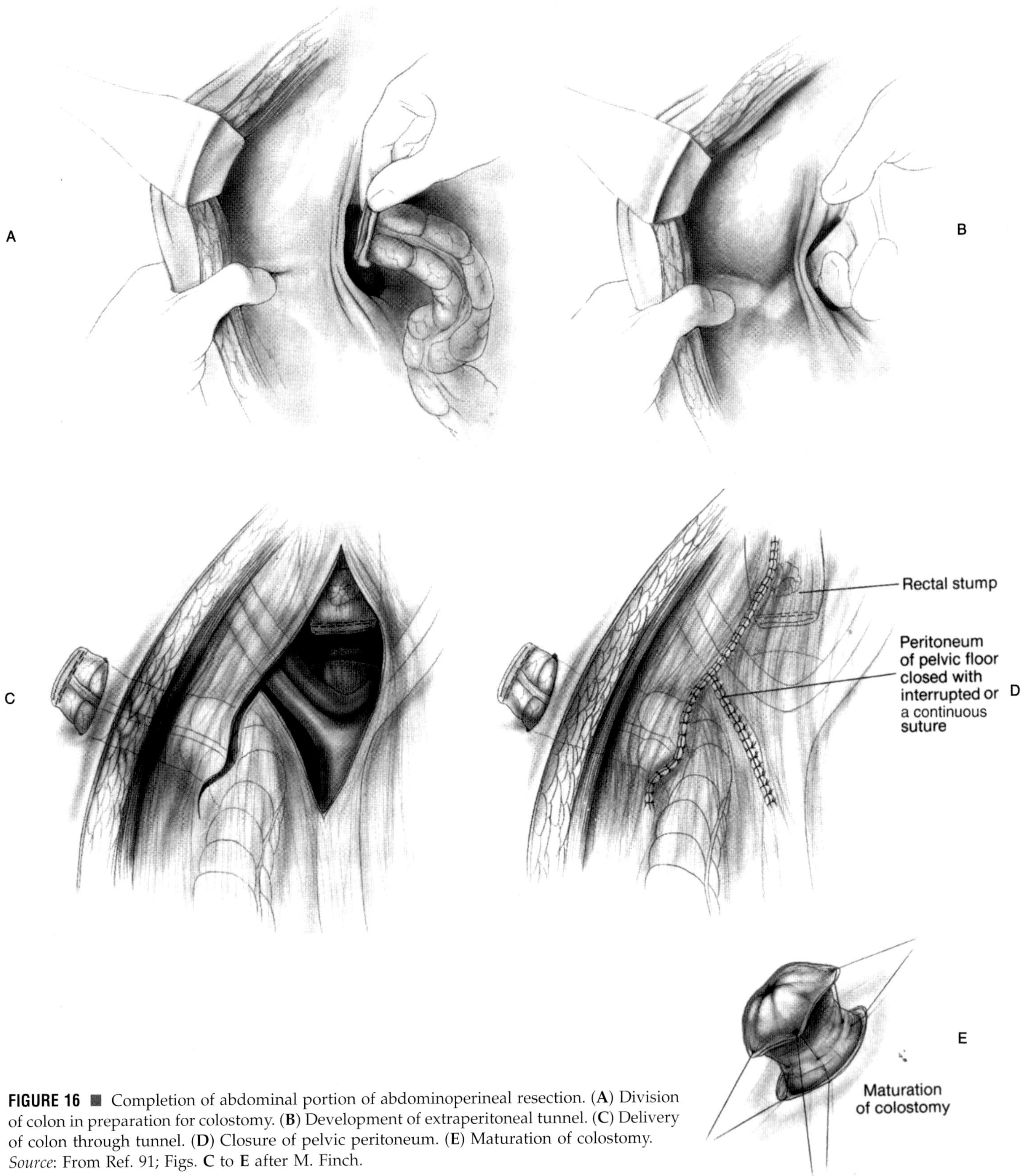

FIGURE 16 ■ Completion of abdominal portion of abdominoperineal resection. (**A**) Division of colon in preparation for colostomy. (**B**) Development of extraperitoneal tunnel. (**C**) Delivery of colon through tunnel. (**D**) Closure of pelvic peritoneum. (**E**) Maturation of colostomy. *Source*: From Ref. 91; Figs. **C** to **E** after M. Finch.

elliptical incision is made to encompass an adequate margin of tissue (Fig. 17A). A wider margin is obtained for low-lying lesions than for more proximal ones. The skin edges are then grasped with baby Kocher clamps. Spring retractors will aid exposure (Fig. 17B). Dissection is continued with a cautery or scissors to incise the fat in the ischioanal fossa. Cautery dissection results in less bleeding. The inferior rectal vessels on each side may require ligation. Deeper dissection is started posteriorly where the anococcygeal ligament is divided. Care should be taken to remain anterior to the coccyx because of the tendency to migrate to a superficial plane. Anteriorly dissection is

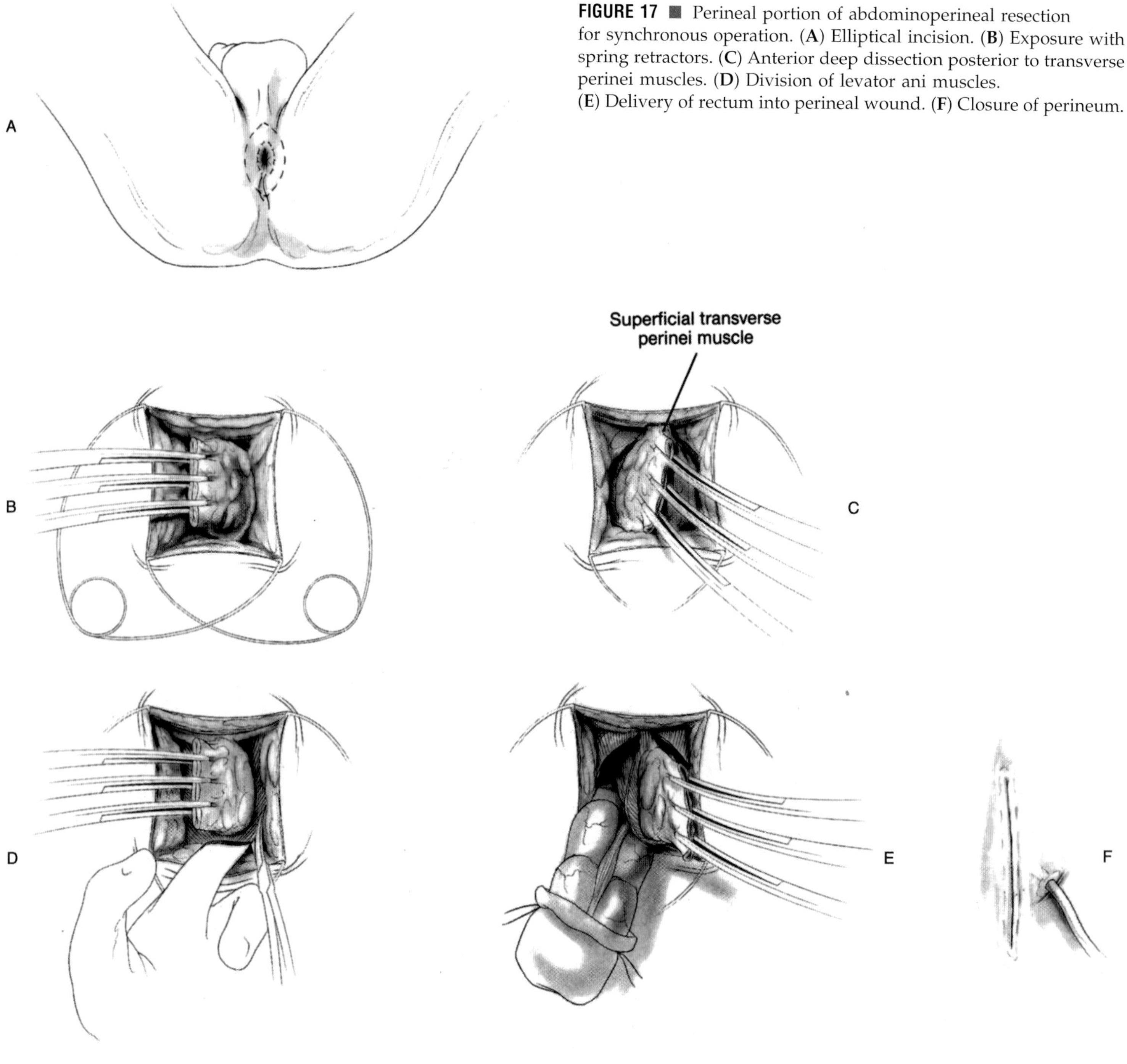

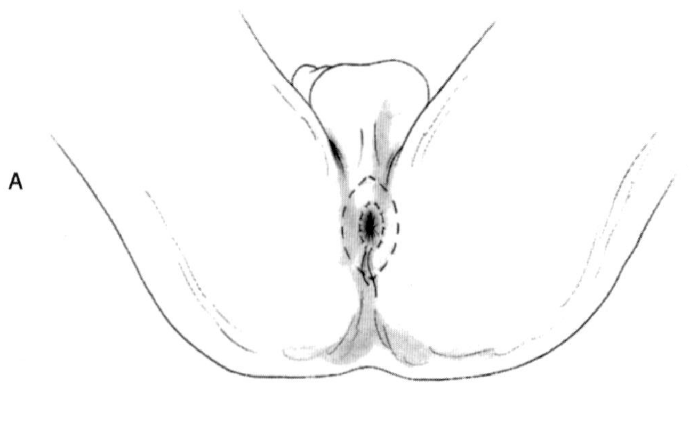

FIGURE 17 ■ Perineal portion of abdominoperineal resection for synchronous operation. (**A**) Elliptical incision. (**B**) Exposure with spring retractors. (**C**) Anterior deep dissection posterior to transverse perinei muscles. (**D**) Division of levator ani muscles. (**E**) Delivery of rectum into perineal wound. (**F**) Closure of perineum.

continued posterior to the transverse perinei muscles (Fig. 17C). Attention is once again directed posterior to the rectum, where a finger can pierce through the levator ani muscles just anterior to the coccyx to enter the presacral plane where the abdominal dissection has led (Fig. 17D). The muscle is divided between clamps and ligated or can often simply be divided with cautery. This is continued laterally on each side. At this point, the rectum can be delivered into the perineal wound posteriorly (Fig. 17E). This maneuver facilitates the anterior dissection. In the female, the rectum can easily be dissected from the vaginal wall. For lesions located on the anterior wall, it may be advisable to excise the posterior vaginal wall in continuity with the rectal wall. Reconstructing the vaginal wall and introitus is not a difficult task. In men, caution must be exercised to avoid injury to the urethra. This is the most difficult part of the operation. Misjudgment of tissue incision might result in entry into the rectum or membranous urethra. Palpation of the Foley catheter will help ascertain the appropriate plane. As muscle is divided on each side of the midline, the plane between the prostate and rectum is developed. By alternating displacement of the rectum from one side to the other and using cautious scissor or cautery dissection, the rectum is eventually separated from the prostate and urethra. Once this dissection is complete, the diseased rectum can be removed. The pelvis and perineal wound then are copiously irrigated with saline. After hemostasis has been ensured, a suction catheter is placed in the pelvis and brought out through a separate stab wound in the perineum. Alternatively, some surgeons prefer transabdominal drainage in the belief that this is easier for the patient in the postoperative period. The tapes placed on the buttocks at the beginning of the operation are now released. The ischioanal fat is approximated with absorbable sutures and the skin is closed with subcutaneous 3–0 Vicryl (Fig. 17F). In the extraordinary situation in which satisfactory control of bleeding has not been obtained, the pelvic wound can be packed with gauze rather than closed primarily. This may be accomplished via the perineum or through an abdominal route and brought out through the lower end of the wound (76). Wounds should be inspected regularly because of the possibility of perineal sepsis. If an abscess were to develop, it would be necessary to open the wound promptly.

PERINEAL PORTION OF ABDOMINOPERINEAL RESECTION WHEN PATIENT IS REPOSITIONED ■ With the recognized advantages of the synchronous combined excision of the rectum, there is seldom, if ever, a need for this technique. When employed, the patient is turned to the prone position with a 6-in. roll placed under the pubis (Fig. 18A). The buttocks are spread apart with 2-in. tape. The perineal area is prepared and draped. A purse-string suture of No. 1 silk is placed around the anus to avoid fecal spillage. An elliptical incision is made around the anus, just lateral to the boundary of the external sphincter muscle (Fig. 18B). Bleeding points are electrocoagulated. The incision is deepened circumferentially. Posteriorly, the anococcygeal ligament and the anococcygeal raphe are incised close to the tip of the coccyx. Once this is completed, the pelvic cavity is entered and the rectal stump can be delivered (Fig. 18C). The levator ani muscles on each side of the rectum are clamped, cut, and tied. Alternatively, they can be divided by cautery. At this point the remaining rectum is only attached to the prostate in men or the vagina in women (Fig. 18D). An incision is made to include Denonvilliers' fascia on the anterior wall of the rectum. Again for posterior lesions dissection posterior to Denonvillier's fascia would appear appropriate. Through this plane the rectum is sharply dissected from the prostate gland or vagina. Usually a moderate amount of bleeding occurs over the prostatic capsule or vagina, requiring electrocoagulation or a stick-tie.

CLOSURE OF PERINEAL SPACE ■ The perineal space is copiously irrigated with saline. Complete hemostasis must be obtained. A closed suction drain is placed in the perineal space and brought out through a small stab wound more anteriorly so that the patient will not sit on it. The subcutaneous tissue is closed with interrupted absorbable sutures (Fig. 18E). The skin is closed with subcuticular absorbable sutures. The drain is connected to continuous suction and left in place until the drainage is less than 10 mL per eight-hour shift on two or three consecutive shifts, which usually takes about five days (Fig. 18F).

PACKING OF PERINEAL WOUND ■ Closure of the perineal space should not be done if the wound continuously oozes or if gross fecal spillage has occurred. Instead, the wound should

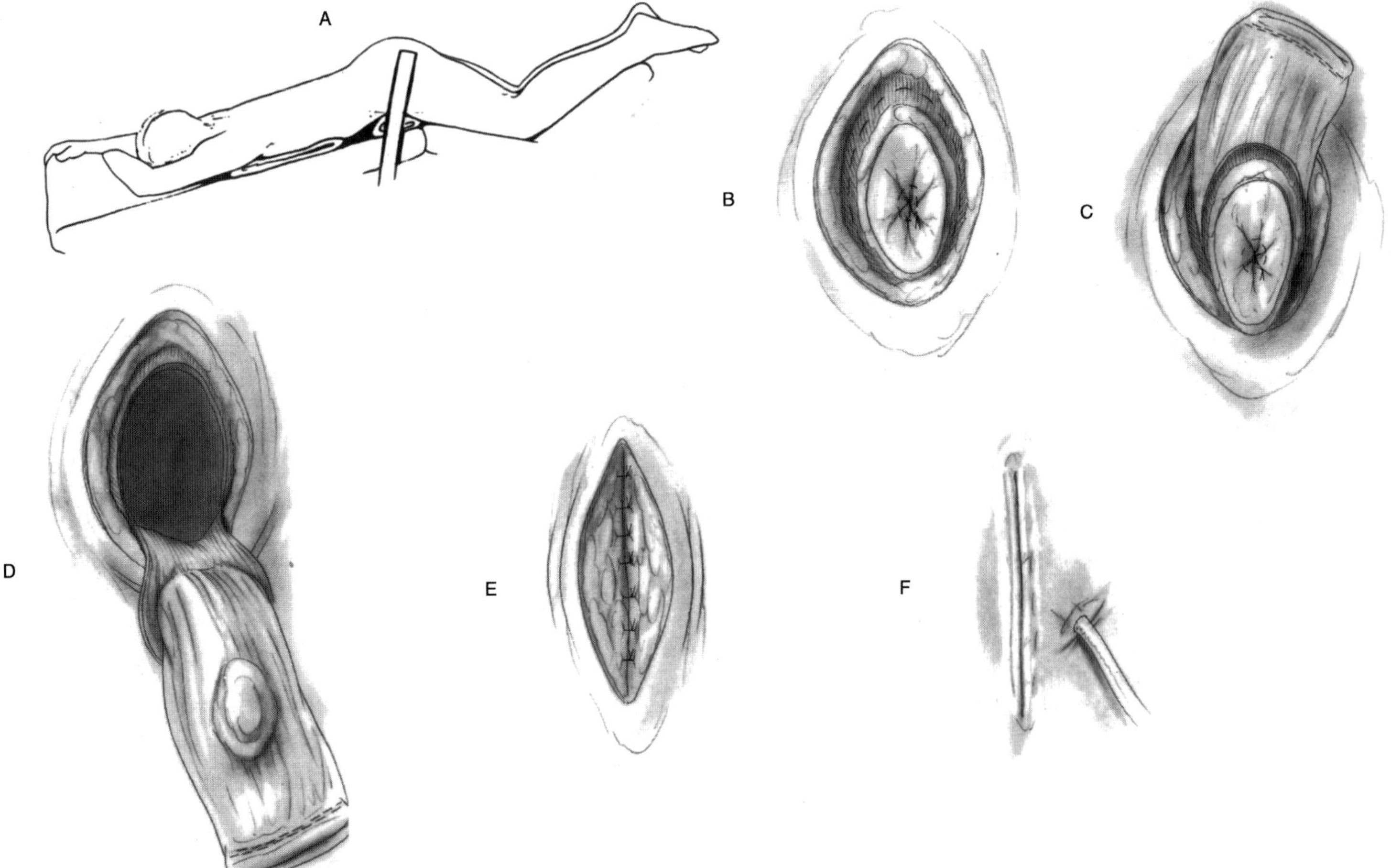

FIGURE 18 ■ Perineal portion when patient is repositioned. (**A**) Position. (**B**) Elliptical incision after placement of pursestring suture. (**C**) Delivery of rectal stump. (**D**) Remaining rectal attachment. (**E**) Closure of perineum. (**F**) Completed operation.

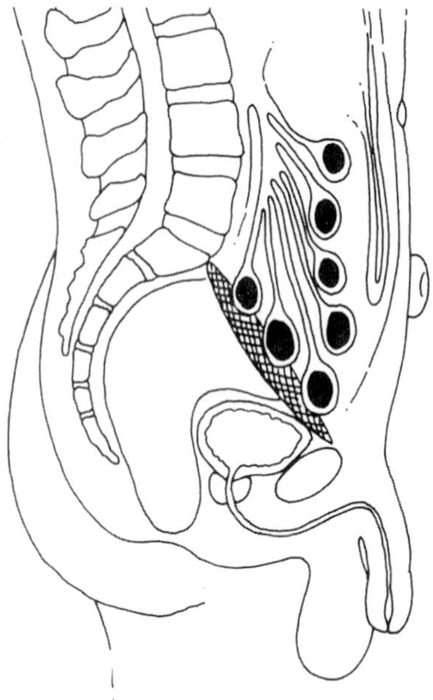

FIGURE 19 ■ Placement of sling from sacral promontory to anterior abdominal wall.

be packed with a rubber dam over Kerlex gauze. This packing should be removed in 48 hours. The rubber dam permits removal without the gauze adhering to adjacent tissue.

For patients in whom postoperative radiotherapy is anticipated, elimination of the small bowel from the pelvis diminishes the chance of radiation enteritis. To this end it has been recommended that a mesh be sutured to the pelvic brim. Devereux et al. (92) have successfully adopted the use of an absorbable polyglycolic acid mesh sling to protect against radiation enteritis (Fig. 19). In addition, a silicone rubber prosthesis can be used to fill the pelvic cavity (93). The Silastic material is of water density and does not interfere with radiation therapy.

Restoration of Continuity after Sphincter Preserving Operations

Reconstructive options following a sphincter-sparing resection for rectal carcinoma include straight colorectal anastomosis, straight coloanal anatomosis, colonic pouch-anal anastomosis, and coloplasty. Several factors must be considered in the selection of an appropriate technique for restoration of continuity if the postoperative neo-rectal function is to be optimized. Very low anterior resection and anastomosis can result in less than perfect function, the so-called anterior resection syndrome which is characterized by frequency, urgency, and soiling (94) and is thought to be due to the loss of the reservoir function as well as diminished compliance (95). The lower the level of the anastomosis, the more adverse the functional outcome. This is supported by reports that patients undergoing very low anterior resection have poorer quality of life scores than those undergoing high anterior resection (96) or even abdominoperineal resection (97). Postoperative function is also impaired in patients who have a straight colorectal anastomosis and receive postoperative radiotherapy or in those who have preoperative radiotherapy followed by anastomosis of colon to an irradiated rectal remnant (98). Direct coloanal anastomosis may be associated with patients experiencing increased frequency of defecation, increased nocturnal defecation, fecal urgency, and incontinence (95).

Coloanal Anastomosis

Parks (99) described a technique in which the rectum is transected just above the anorectal ring (Fig. 20A). The anal mucosa above the dentate line is removed through the anal orifice (Fig. 20B). The proximal colon is drawn down into the anorectal remnant and sutured to the level of the dentate line (Fig. 20C,D). A proximal ileostomy or colostomy is constructed to protect the anastomosis.

Coloanal anastomoses have historically been associated with a price to be paid for the restoration of intestinal continuity. Apart from the anastomotic leakage, functional outcome has been affected with varying degrees of urgency and alteration in continence. Miller et al. (100) assessed the anorectal factors with manometric studies of 30 patents who underwent rectal excision and stapled coloanal anastomosis. Only 11 patients experienced perfect continence. Those with poor continence had lower resting and squeeze pressures. Poor function was more common in women. The authors raised the possibility that occult damage may have arisen before low anterior resection and such damage might be detected with preoperative manometry and endoanal ultrasonography.

Patey et al. (101) reported on their experience in 140 patients with resection and coloanal anastomosis. There were no deaths and the five-year actuarial survival was 73%. Pelvic recurrence was documented at an actuarial rate of 11% at five years.

Braun et al. (102) compared 63 patients who underwent intersphincteric resection with direct coloanal anastomosis and 77 who had an abdominoperineal resection. During the mean follow-up period of 6.7 years, of those patients with curative resection, 11% presented with pelvic recurrence, and 33% with distant metastases after coloanal anastomosis; the rates of recurrence and distant metastases after abdominoperineal resection were 17% and 35%, respectively. The corrected five-year survival rates were 62% following coloanal anastomosis and 53% following abdominoperineal resection. Eighty-five percent of the patients with coloanal anastomosis reported good functional results regarding anal continence. This study demonstrates that the intersphincteric resection with coloanal anastomosis is a valuable surgical technique for rectal carcinoma with the benefit of preservation of continence.

Leo et al. (103) reported on 141 consecutive patients treated for a primary carcinoma of the distal rectum from 3.5 to 8 cm from the anal verge. Patient stratification, included 31 Dukes' stage A (T2N0), 44 stage B (T3N0), and 66 stage C (T2N+ to T3N+). Overall recurrence rate was 9.2%. Perfect continence was documented in 61% of cases. The only pathological factor related to local recurrence was lymphocytic reaction inside and around the carcinoma.

Saito et al. (104) extended their indication for sphincter saving operation. They investigated the curability and functional results of intersphincteric resection and additional partial external sphincter resection for carcinoma of the anorectal junction. Thirty-five patients with carcinoma located between 0 and 2 cm above the dentate line underwent abdominotransanal rectal resection with TME. All patients underwent diverting colostomy. Twenty patients received preoperative radio/chemotherapy. All patients had curative intent with microscopic safety margins. No postoperative mortality was encountered. Morbidity was identified in 13 patients and included peri-anastomotic

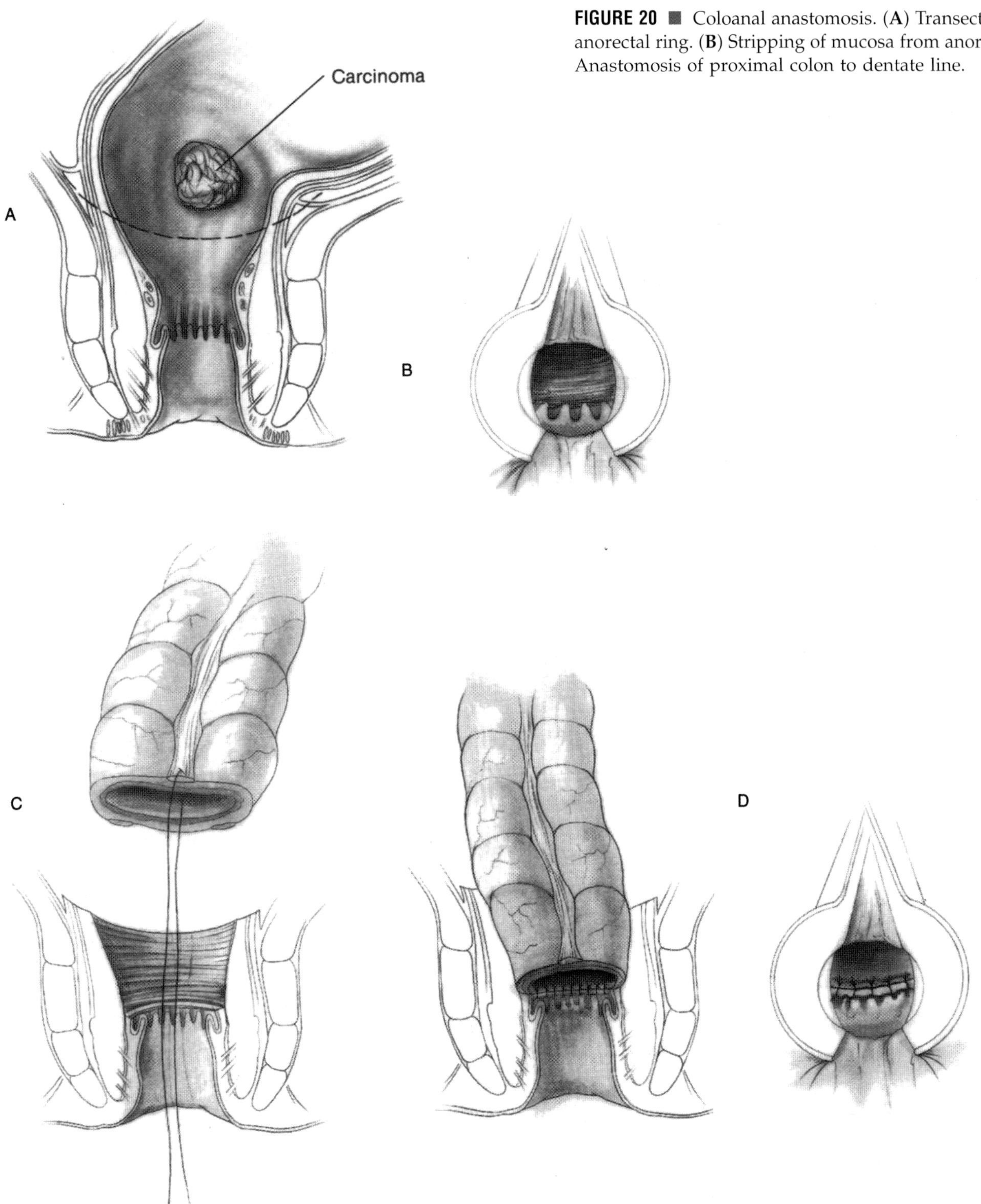

FIGURE 20 ■ Coloanal anastomosis. (**A**) Transection of rectum at level of anorectal ring. (**B**) Stripping of mucosa from anorectal stump. (**C**) and (**D**) Anastomosis of proximal colon to dentate line.

abscess, anastomotic leakage and fistula; postoperative bleeding, infection, peri-anastomotic stenosis, and anovaginal fistula. One of these patients required a permanent colostomy. Five patients developed recurrence during the median observation period of 23 months. Two of these patients underwent curative resection of liver or lung metastases. Twenty-one patients had undergone stoma closure and although continence was satisfactory in all, five displayed occasional minor soiling 12 months after stoma closure. Anal canal manometry demonstrated significant reduction in maximum resting pressure but acceptable functional results were obtained. They believe these procedures can be recommended for low rectal carcinoma patients who are candidates for abdominoperineal resection.

Gamagami et al. (105) assessed the influence of partial excision of the superior portion of the anal canal when necessary for margin clearance in distant rectal carcinoma on fecal continence after coloanal anastomosis. The 209 patients were categorized into three groups according to their level of anastomosis from the anal verge: 43 group 1 patients with anastomosis 0.5 to less than 2 cm from the anal verge, 75 group 2 patients with anastomosis 2 cm to less than 3 cm from the anal verge, and 73 group 3 patients with anastomosis 3 to 2.5 cm from the anal verge. In the first year, there was progressive improvement in anal continence in all three groups. At two years, 50% in group 1, 73% in group 2, and 62% in group 3 were fully continent. The proportion of all patients fully continent in group 1 remained unchanged as compared to continued improvement in groups 2 and 3 following the first year. At four years, 50% in group 1, 80% in group 2, 68% in group 3 were completely continent.

Nathanson et al. (106) reported that straight (nonreservoir) coloanal anastomoses with postoperative pelvic radiotherapy had significant adverse effects on anorectal function, with higher rates of clustering and frequency of defecation than with preoperative radiotherapy. No differences in continence rates were demonstrated. They attribute the adverse effects of postoperative radiotherapy to irradiation of the neorectum, which is spared when treatment is given preoperatively.

Olagne et al. (107) assessed the functional outcome of patients who had delayed coloanal anastomosis for a lower third rectal carcinoma after preoperative radiotherapy in 35 patients. Colorectal resection was performed about 32 days after the end of the radiotherapy. The distal colon stump was pulled through the anal canal. On postoperative day 5, the colonic stump was resected and a direct coloanal anastomosis performed without colostomy diversion. There was no mortality. There was no leakage. One patient had a pelvic abscess. One patient had necrosis of the left colon requiring reoperation. Another delayed coloanal anastomosis could be performed. Median follow-up was 43 months. Function was considered good in 59% and 70% at one and two years, respectively. They concluded this procedure is a safe and effective sphincter preserving operation that avoids a diverting stoma for patients with rectal carcinoma of the lower third of the rectum.

Most recently, Rullier et al. (108) assessed the oncologic outcome of patients treated by conservative radical surgery for carcinomas below 5 cm from the anal verge. Ninety-two patients with a nonfixed rectal carcinoma at 1.5 to 4.5 cm from the anal verge and without external sphincter infiltration underwent TME with intersphincteric resection, that is, removal of the internal sphincter to achieve adequate distal margin. Patients with T3 disease or internal sphincter infiltration received preoperative radiotherapy. There was no mortality and morbidity was 27%. The rate of complete microscopic resection (R0) was 89% with 98% negative distal margin and 89% negative circumferential margin. In 58 patients with a follow-up of more than 24 months, the rate of local recurrence was 2% and the five-year overall and disease free survival were 81% and 70%, respectively. They concluded, the technique of intersphincter resection permits us to achieve conservative surgery in patients with a carcinoma close to or in the anal canal without compromising local control and survival.

J Pouch

Establishment of a colonic reservoir analogous to the J-shaped ileal pouch was originally described by Lazorthes et al. (109,110) and has gained favor with a growing number of surgeons (111–114). Advocates of the procedure believe that adding capacity in the form of a colonic reservoir can substantially reduce dysfunction and greatly improve quality of life. Urgency is diminished and continence is improved. Technically, it is simple to make the reservoir in many cases, but in patients with obesity or a foreshortened mesentery, construction may prove difficult or impossible. The anastomosis itself is no more difficult than that of the straight coloanal reconstruction. Some patients may develop difficulty with evacuation and it is important to use no more than 12 to 16 cm of colon for the two-loop construction (115).

The operative technique of dissection follows the general oncologic principles previously enunciated. The splenic flexure will most likely require mobilization unless there is considerable redundancy of the colon. The proximal sigmoid or distal descending colon is used for reconstruction. An anastomosing instrument is applied at the line of transection to both divide the bowel and close the end (Fig. 21A). A colonic J pouch is made with 7 to 8 cm of bowel by folding the colon and creating a side-to-side anastomosis with a stapler introduced through the apex of the pouch (Fig. 21B,C). A double-stapling technique can be used to establish intestinal continuity. A temporary ileostomy is created. A sutured anastomosis can be constructed (Fig. 22).

Hallböök et al. (116) measured blood flow by laser Doppler fiowmetry before construction of a straight or J-pouch anastomosis. In the straight group (end-to-end anastomosis), blood flow levels at the site intended for anastomosis were significantly decreased following dissection of bowel. In the pouch group (side to end), blood levels at the site of the anastomosis were similar following dissection of the bowel and pouch construction. They concluded unaffected blood flow at the side of the anastomosis of the pouch might be a favorable factor for anastomotic healing.

Mortensen et al. (117) reported on a consecutive series of 23 patients with colonic J pouch-anal anastomosis for low rectal carcinoma. The mean distance from the pouch-anal anastomosis to the anal verge was 3.5 cm (range, 2.0–4.5 cm). In 19 surviving patients a mean of seven months after ileostomy closure, mean bowel frequency was 2.1 (range, one to four) per day, five patients had urgency, four had mild fecal seepage up to three times per week, and seven patients had some degree of incomplete evacuation. In 13 patients, there were no manometric differences before and after operation with respect to maximum tolerated volume or maximum resting pressure, but maximum squeeze pressure was significantly lower after operation (mean, 189 vs. 132 cm H_2O before and after operation, respectively). The authors believe that colonic pouch reconstruction should be considered as an alternative to straight coloanal anastomosis in patients undergoing very low anterior resection.

The physiologic deficiency in patients undergoing a low anterior resection for rectal carcinoma was highlighted in a study by Lewis et al. (118). In a series of 34 patients that were divided into three groups on the basis of residual rectum (none, less than 4 cm, greater than 4 cm) and a control group of 10 patients in whom the rectum was left intact, resting anal pressure was lower and the capacity of the neorectum was less after coloanal than after colorectal anastomosis. The greater the length of the residual rectum, the greater was the capacity of the neorectum. Their findings support the use of a colonic pouch when the entire rectum or almost the entire rectum has been removed.

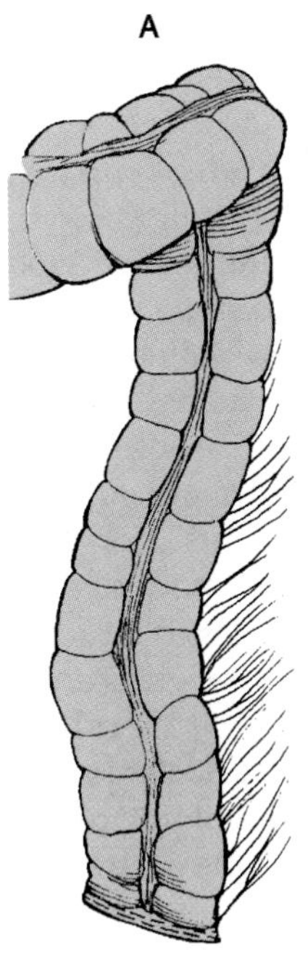

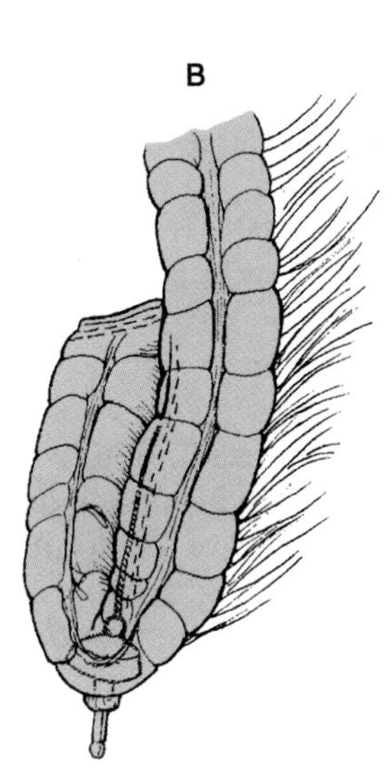

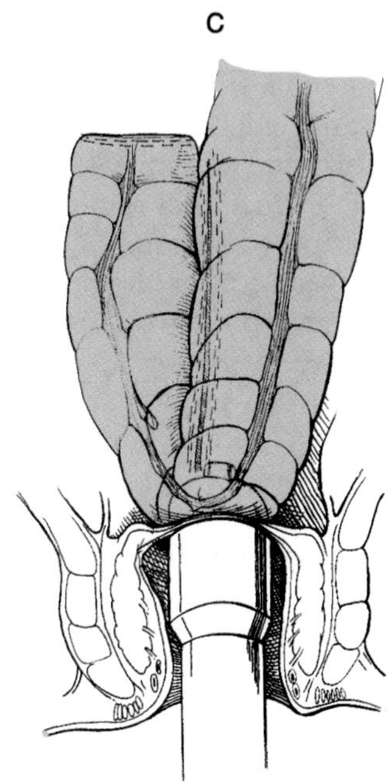

FIGURE 21 ■ (**A**) Transected proximal bowel. (**B**) Completed colonic J pouch with anvil secured by pursestring suture in apex of pouch. (**C**) Double-stapling technique used to construct side-to-end coloanal anastomosis.

A remarkable case of a patient developing a carcinoma in a colonic J pouch after a low anterior resection for villous adenoma was reported (119).

In a review of the literature, McNamara and Parc (95) found that up to 20% of patients suffer evacuation problems and require the use of enemas or suppositories to evacuate the pouch. This has been attributed to the use of excessively large reservoirs with pouches as large as 12 cm. They compared the number of bowel movements for 24 hours in eight series that compared coloanal anastomosis and the colonic J-pouch and with a follow-up of six weeks to two years found with the former a range of 2.0 to 6.4 (range 6–20) and with the latter 1.4 to 3.1 (range 4–10), statistically significant in most series. Hida et al. (120) conducted a prospective randomized study to determine optimum pouch size. They found that a 5-cm pouch was significantly superior to a 10-cm pouch with respect to evacuation function. Dehni and Parc (121) reviewed the different aspects of colonic J-pouch reconstruction with special focus on functional results and complications. They cited five randomized controlled trials comparing colon pouch anal anastomosis and straight coloanal anastomosis. According to the current literature, local recurrence rate and survival are comparable after either a low anterior resection, a coloanal anastomosis or an abdominoperineal resection for rectal carcinoma. In terms of functional outcome, there is mounting evidence supporting the superiority of the colonic J-pouch reconstruction over a straight anastomosis. The advantage of the pouch is most marked in the early postoperative period but may persist up to two years. Comparative studies have shown better results with pouch reconstruction in terms of stool frequency, urgency, nocturnal movements, and continence one year after operation. However, problems with evacuation of stools from the pouch are reported by 20% to 30% of patients in the long-term follow-up. Smaller pouches may reduce this difficulty. Overall, the use of a colonic J-pouch is compatible with curative operation and has the additive benefit of optimizing the postoperative quality of life of patients after total rectal resection for carcinoma.

Laurent et al. (122) compared handsewn or stapled colonic J-pouch-anal anastomosis performed after complete proctectomy and TME for carcinoma of the rectum. They found stapled coloanal anastomosis to be significantly faster than handsewn coloanal anastomosis and it had similar functional results.

Machado et al. (123) randomized 150 patients with rectal carcinoma undergoing TME and coloanal anastomosis to receive either a colonic pouch or a side-to-side anastomosis using the descending colon. A large proportion of the patients received short-term preoperative radiotherapy (78%). There was no significant difference in surgical outcome between the two techniques with respect to anastomotic height (4 cm), perioperative blood loss (500 mL), hospital stay (11 days), postoperative complications, reoperations, or pelvic sepsis rates. Comparing

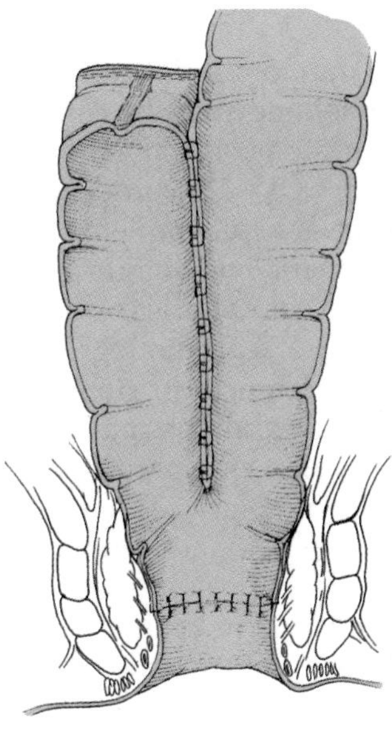

FIGURE 22 ■ Hand-sutured coloanal anastomosis for colonic J pouch.

functional results in the two study groups, only the ability to evacuate the bowel in less than 15 minutes at 16 months reached a significant difference in favor of the pouch. They concluded that either a colonic J-pouch or a side-to-end anastomosis performed on the descending colon in low anterior resection with total mesorecal excision are methods that can be used with similar expected functional and surgical results. Machado et al. (124) compared the functional and physiologic outcome two years after low anterior resection and TME with a colonic J-pouch or a side-to-end anastomosis in 35 patients. There was no statistical difference in functional outcome between groups at two years. Maximum neorectal volume increased in both groups but was approximately 40% greater at two years in pouches compared with the side-to-side anastomosis. Anal sphincter pressure volumes were halved postoperatively and did not recover during follow-up of two years. Male gender, low anastomotic level, pelvic sepsis, and the postoperative decrease of sphincter pressures were independent factors for more incontinence symptoms.

Dehni et al. (125) compared long-term bowel habits in 28 patients receiving preoperative radiation for rectal carcinoma followed by colonic J-pouch-anal anastomosis with those of 97 patients having similar rectal carcinoma surgery without radiation. The number of bowel movements per 24 hours in patients with or without radiation was 1.8. In the irradiated group, diarrhea (39% vs. 13%) and nocturnal defecation (36% vs. 15%) were more frequent than in the nonirradiated group. No other significant difference existed between groups with regard to stool clustering, use of protective pads, ability to defer evacuation more than 15 minutes, ability to evacuate the bowel within 30 minutes, incontinence score, use of medications, or dietary restriction.

Sailer et al. (126) reported that patients with a pouch reconstruction had a significantly better quality of life, particularly in the early postoperative period. Patients undergoing low anterior rectal resection and coloanal J-pouch reconstruction may expect not only better functional results but also an improved quality of life in the early months after operation compared with patients who receive a straight coloanal anastomosis.

In a detailed study Heah et al. (127) reported that pouches made from sigmoid or descending colon give similar bowel function after ultra-low anterior resection for rectal carcinoma.

Ho et al. (128) conducted a randomized controlled study to compare functional outcome following the colonic J-pouch and the straight coloanal anastomosis immediately after ultra-low anterior resection. Of 42 consecutive patients recruited, 19 of the straight group completed the study. At six months, the pouch patients had significantly less frequent stools (32.9 vs. 49 per week) and less soiling at passing flatus (38% vs. 73.7%). At two years, both groups had improved with no longer any differences in stool frequency (7.3 vs. 8 per week) and soiling and passing flatus (38% vs. 53%). Anal squeeze pressures were significantly impaired in both groups up to two years. The rectal maximum tolerable volume and compliance were not different between groups. Rectal sensory testing on the barostat phasic program showed impairment at six months and recovery at two years suggesting that postoperative recovery of residual afferent sympathetic nerves may play a role in functional recovery.

Wang et al. (129) reported the outcome of 30 consecutive patients with colonic J-pouch-anal anastomosis without a diverting stoma. All patients had carcinoma of the lower two-thirds of the rectum. Functional results were compared with those of 21 rectal carcinoma patients with straight coloanal anastomosis who underwent operation in the same period and 20 normal patients. There were two anastomotic leakages and one postoperative death. After one year, patients with pouch anastomosis had significantly less frequency of defecation and rectal urgency compared with those with straight anastomosis; 48% of patients with straight anastomosis had more than five bowel movements per day whereas all patients with pouch anastomosis had five or fewer bowel movements per day. Manometric studies showed that the maximum tolerable volume was significantly higher in patients with pouch anastomosis (81 vs. 152 mL).

If construction of a colonic J-pouch is not possible due to lack of colonic length, especially after prior colonic resections, the ileocecal interpositional reservoir may offer an alternative to rectal replacement. Hamel et al. (130) studied the functional results of the long-term follow-up of patients after TME and ileocecal interposition as rectal replacement. At five years, 78% of the patients were continent; mean stool frequency was 2.5 per day.

Da Silva et al. (131) assessed the impact of diverticular disease on function and on postoperative complications of the colonic J-pouch with pouch-anal anastomosis. The presence of diverticular disease in the colonic J-pouch was assessed on pouchogram prior to ileostomy closure. The median follow-up period was 22 months. Twenty-four patients comprised the diverticular group and 42 were in the nondiverticular group. The total evacuation score and total incontinence score did not significantly differ between the two groups. Furthermore, there was no significant difference in the total incidence of pouch complications between the two groups. The presence of diverticular disease in a colonic J-pouch does not seem to have an impact on pouch function or the postoperative complication rate.

Good function of the colonic-J-pouch reconstruction in the elderly would obviate the need for colostomy that is sometimes performed because of concern about fecal incontinence which increases with age. Hida et al. (132) compared functional outcome in 20 patients age 75 years or older (older group), and 27 patients age 60 to 74 years (old group) and 60 patients age 59 or younger (young group), three years after colonic J-pouch reconstruction, using a functional scoring system with a 17-item questionnaire [score range, 0 (overall good) to 26 (overall poor)]. The functional scores in the three age groups were satisfactory and similar. Among patients with anastomoses 1 to 4 cm from the anal verge, all 17 categories on the questionnaire in the three age groups were similar. Among patients with anastomoses 5 to 8 cm from the anal verge, only the use of laxatives or glycerine enemas was more common in the older group than in the old and young group (90% vs. 38.5% and 43.3%). They concluded that low anterior resection with colonic J-pouch reconstruction provides excellent functional outcome, including continence, for elderly patients.

Gervaz et al. (133) evaluated the impact of adjuvant chemoradiation therapy on pouch function in 74 patients with midrectal or low rectal carcinomas (less than 10 cm from the anal verge) who underwent a proctectomy with coloanal anastomosis with colonic J-pouch reconstruction.

The mean age of patients was 68.9 years and the mean duration of follow-up was 28.8 months. There were 28 patients in the surgery alone group and 17 patients who received either preoperative (13) or postoperative (4) adjuvant chemoradiation therapy. Patients in the surgery along group had a significantly better continence score: 18.1 versus 13.3 and were less likely to experience evacuatory problems (evacuation score 21.3 vs. 16.4). Use of pad was more frequent in the chemoradiation therapy than in the surgery alone group (53% vs. 18%). The incidence of functional disorders was also more frequent in the irradiated group of patients: incontinence to gas (76% vs. 43%) to liquid stool (64% vs. 25%) and to solid stool (47% vs. 11%). Moreover, irradiated patients reported more frequent pouch-related specific problems such as clustering (82% vs. 32%) and sensation of incomplete evacuation (82% vs. 32%). Finally, regression analysis demonstrated that radiation-induced sphincter dysfunction was progressive over time. Both preoperative and postoperative chemoradiation adversely affects continence and evacuation in patients with colonic J-pouch.

Harris et al. (134) identified seven reasons for failure to be able to construct a colonic J-pouch. These reasons were: (i) technical (narrow pelvis, bulky anal sphincters or need for mucosectomy, diverticulosis, insufficient colon length or pregnancy), and (ii) nontechnical (complex surgery or distant metastases present). Failure to construct a neorectal reservoir occurred in 30.7% of patients. This was reduced to 5.3% of patients in the latter period of the study.

Coloplasty

To overcome poor bowel function after resection of the distal rectum with a straight reanastomosis, a neo-reservoir using a colonic J-pouch has been advocated. However, difficulties in reach, inability to fit the pouch into a narrow pelvis, and postoperative evacuation problems can make the colonic J-pouch problematic. Furst et al. (135) randomized 40 consecutive patients with distal rectal carcinoma (less than 12 cm from the anal verge) into the J-pouch or coloplasty group. A low rectal resection and coloanal anastomosis was performed in all patients. The construction of a coloplasty pouch was feasible in all cases for the coloplasty group but not in 25% of patients of the J-pouch group because of colonic adipose tissue (Fig. 23). Six months after operation or stoma closure the stool frequency was 2.75 +/− 1 per day in the J-pouch group and 2 +/− 2 per day in the coloplasty group, respectively. There was no significant difference in resting and squeeze pressure and neo-rectal volume between the two groups. They found similar functional results in the coloplasty group compared to the J-pouch group. The neo-rectal sensitivity was increased in the coloplasty group. Therefore the colonic coloplasty seems to be an attractive pouch design because of its feasibility, simplicity, and effectiveness. They speculate that the advantage of the colonic J-pouch is not in creating a larger neo-rectal reservoir but is rather related to decreased motility. Mantyh et al. (136) compared the functional results after a low colorectal anastomosis among patients receiving a coloplasty (20), colonic J-pouch (16), or straight anastomosis (17). Maximum tolerated volume was significantly favorable in the coloplasty and colonic J-pouch group versus the straight anastomosis group. The compliance was also significantly favorable for the coloplasty and the colonic J-pouch group versus the straight anastmosis group. The coloplasty and colonic J-pouch had significantly fewer bowel movements per day than the straight anastomosis group. Similar complications rates were noted in the three groups. Patients with a coloplasty and low colorectal anastomosis seem to have similar functional outcome along with similar pouch compliance compared with patients with colonic J-pouch and low colorectal anastomosis. However, the coloplasty may provide an alternative method to the colonic J-pouch for a neo-rectal reservoir construction when reach or narrow pelvis prohibits its formation. Technically, it may also be easier to construct.

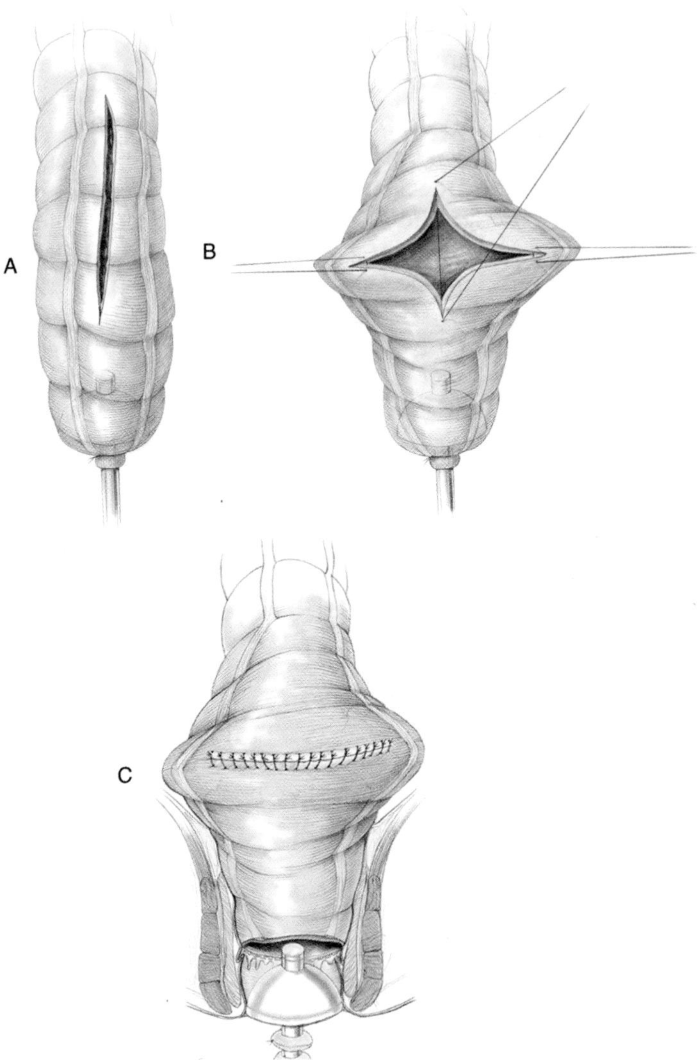

FIGURE 23 ■ Coloplasty construction. (**A**) An 8 to 10 cm longitudinal incision is made between the tenia 4 to 6 cm from the cut edge of the colon. (**B**) The longitudinal opening is closed in a transverse manner with interrupted 2-0 polyglycolic sutures starting with stay sutures in the middle and at each end. (**C**) Completed coloplasty and withdrawal of circular stapler after completion of the coloanal anastomosis.

Z'graggen et al. (137) reported on 41 patients who underwent low anterior rectal resection with continuity restored by a transverse coloplasty pouch anastomosis and the colon was defunctionalized for three months. Intraoperative complications occurred in 7%, none related to the transverse coloplasty pouch. There were no hospital deaths and the total complication rate was 27%; an anastomotic leakage rate of 7% was recorded. The stool frequency was 3.4 per 24-hours at two months follow-up and gradually decreased to 2.1 per 24-hours at eight months. Stool dysfunctions such as stool urgency, fragmentation, and incontinence were regularly observed until six months; the incidence significantly decreased thereafter. None of the patients had difficulty in pouch evacuation.

The most recent report by Remzi et al. (138) compared the quality of life, functional outcome, and complications among 162 patients undergoing coloplasty (69) colonic J-pouch (43) or straight anastomosis (50). Usually coloplasty or straight anastomosis was favored in male patients with a narrow pelvis or when a handsewn anatomosis was used. Quality of life assessment with the short form-36 questionnaire revealed better scores in coloplasty and colonic J-pouch groups. The coloplasty (1.0) and colonic J-pouch (1.0) groups had fewer night bowel movements than the straight anastomosis (1.5). The coloplasty group also had fewer bowel movements per day than the straight anastomosis group (3.8 vs. 4.8); also, less clustering and less anti-diarrheal medication use were observed than in the straight anastomosis group. Colonic J-pouch patients with hand-sewn anastomosis had a higher anastomotic leak rate (44%) than the patients in the coloplasty with hand-sewn anastomosis group (3.6%). They concluded, coloplasty seems to be a safe, effective technique for improving the outcome of low colorectal or coloanal anastomosis. It is especially applicable when a colonic J-pouch anastomosis is technically difficult.

Other Procedures

A variety of pull-through operations have been described. Their operative morbidity and functional outcome have often left a lot to be desired. Because other operations have supplanted them, none of the pull-through operations will be described here.

Kraske's approach, or the parasacral approach to rectal resection, commanded some popularity in the early part of the century but because of the associated problems of sepsis, anastomotic leaks, and fecal fistulas, it fell into disrepute. Kraske's operation is seldom used for the treatment of rectal carcinoma.

The abdominosacral resection championed by Localio et al. (139) enjoyed the favor of some surgeons, but enthusiasm has waned with the introduction of the circular stapler.

In an effort to create a sutureless anastomosis, analogous to Murphy's button, Hardy et al. (140) developed a biofragmentable ring composed of polyglycolic acid and barium sulfate. A multicenter trial compared the biofragmentable ring anastomosis to the stapled and sutured anastomoses. No statistical differences emerged with respect to the complication rate, in particular, of the anastomotic leaks (141). The biofragmentable ring has not been adapted for low anastomoses and indeed has not garnered great enthusiasm among surgeons.

Extended resections will be described in more detail under the operative treatment of recurrent disease but may also be applied to patients who initially present with locally advanced disease. Moriya et al. (142) described en bloc excision of the lower ureter and internal iliac vessels for locally advanced upper rectal and rectosigmoid carcinomas. Excellent prognoses were noted with respect to local control and functional results in eight patients.

Double Dynamic Graciloplasty

In patients with a very low rectal carcinoma, an abdominoperineal resection with creation of a permanent colostomy is the operative treatment of choice. Creation of a colostomy can be avoided without compromise of oncologic principles by delivering the distal colon to the perineum and wrapping it with both gracilis muscles, creating a new sphincter and pelvic floor. These muscles are electrically stimulated by an implanted neurostimulator. The details of the dynamic graciloplasty were described in Chapter 15. In a series of 11 patients so treated by Geerdes et al. (143) with a follow-up of 1.3 years, continence was achieved in seven patients, and two patients were awaiting completion of therapy. In two patients, necrosis of the distal colon led to failure of the technique. There were no local recurrences but two patients had distant metastases.

■ POSTOPERATIVE CARE

Postoperative management of the patient is discussed at length in Chapter 4.

■ RESULTS

The same difficulty encountered in determining the survival, morbidity, and mortality rates of colon carcinoma has been encountered with rectal carcinoma. Martling et al. (144) analyzed the prognostic value of surgeons' and pathologists' assessment of clearance in 1550 patients with primary rectal carcinoma who underwent resection. In patients assessed as having a complete surgical clearance, recurrence developed in 33.3%. For patients with an uncertain or incomplete clearance, recurrence rate was 59.5% and 61%, respectively. The relative risk of recurrence was twice as high when the surgeon or pathologist disagreed than when they both agreed on the complete clearance. Survival in patients with a complete, uncertain, or incomplete surgical clearance was 55.3%, 23.0%, and 10%, respectively. An effort was made to present representative data in Tables 1–4.

A frequently debated point is the virtue of sphincter-saving operations. Proponents of abdominoperineal resection believe anything less than the radical operation might jeopardize the patient's chance of cure. However, evidence suggests that this is not the case. From a multicenter trial, Wolmark and Fisher (68) found no survival advantage of abdominoperineal resection over low anterior resection. A review of several series from the literature concurred (63,66,67,178–182).

The general acceptance of the circular stapler method mandates a detailed discussion of the technique, with its inherent advantages and disadvantages as they relate to results. We reviewed a series of 215 anastomoses that I constructed with the circular stapler following resection (183). The operative mortality was 0.47%, with the one death being unrelated to the anastomosis. Intraoperative complications included bleeding, difficult extraction, instrument failure, incomplete "doughnuts," and deficient anastomoses. Early postoperative complications included one leak and a number of complications unrelated to the anastomoses. Anastomotic stenosis developed in 27 patients,

TABLE 1 ■ Operative Mortality, Five-Year Survival Rate, and Local Recurrence of Carcinoma of Rectum

Author(s)	No. of Potentially Curable Patients	Operative Mortality (%)	Five-Year Survival Rate: Crude (%)	Five-Year Survival Rate: Corrected (%)	Local Recurrence Rate (%)
Pählman et al. (145) (1985)	161	5	60		
Davis et al. (146) (1987)	235	3	42	55	
Enblad et al. (147) (1988)	23,603		42		
Michelassi et al. (148) (1988)	154	3	53	53	12
Amato et al. (149) (1991)	147	4–2[a]			11–12[a]
Tagliacozzo and Accordino (150) (1992)	274	3	59		17
MacFarlane et al. (79) (1993)	135	2	78		4
Fandrich et al. (151) (1994)	331		80, 40, 30[b]		14
Adam et al. (152) (1994)	141	6	62		23
Clemmesen and Sprechler (153) (1994)	196		50		6, 11, 22[b]
Enker et al. (154) (1995)	246	1	74		7
Hermanek et al. (155) (1995)	887		55		
Laxamana et al. (89) (1995)	189	2	78		9
Singh et al. (156) (1995)	251				8
Zaheer et al. (157) (1998)	514	2	80, 83, 78[c]		4, 6, 7[c]
Killingback et al. (158) (2001)	549	3	73		7
Staib et al. (159) (2002)	1099	1			16
Croxford et al. (160) (2004)	683				4
Wibe et al. (161) (2004)[a]	2136	3	63 overall 69, 62, 59[d]	–	12 overall, 9, 13, 15[a]
Law et al. (162) (2005)	224[e]	2	71	81	6
Gordon et al. (163) (2006) (unpublished data)	184	2	64		18

[a]Abdominoperineal plus anterior resection.
[b]According to Dukes' classification.
[c]Abdominoperineal resection, coloanal anastomosis, low anterior resection.
[d]Upper middle lower third of rectum.
[e]Stage II.

but only eight were permanent and only three of these were symptomatic. Two of these patients were treated with balloon dilatation. Anastomotic recurrences developed in 13.1% of patients. The time to recurrence ranged from 5 to 39 months. The overall follow-up time ranged from 4 to 124 months. Our experience and that of many other surgeons has shown the circular stapling device to be a reliable method for performing anastomoses to the rectum in a safe and expeditious manner.

One concern with the circular stapler is the high incidence of narrowing of the anastomoses. Others who have recorded complications after use of the EEA stapler in rectal anastomoses have reported narrowings ranging from 0% to 30% (Table 5). Few authors have given their definition of stenosis. Leff et al. (191) and Fazio (199) have defined a stricture as narrowing that does not allow passage of a 15 mm sigmoidoscope. I have considered as stenotic any anastomosis that did not accept the 19 mm sigmoidoscope.

TABLE 2 ■ Results of Curative Low Anterior Resection for Carcinoma of Rectum

Author(s)	No. of Patients	Operative Mortality (%)	Five-Year Survival Rate: Crude (%)
Fedorov and Odarjuk (164) (1983)	356	4	62
Zhou et al. (165) (1983)	158	1	63
Williams et al. (66) (1985)	100	7	74
Malmberg et al. (166) (1986)	83	5	71
Davis et al. (146) (1987)	111	5	39
Heberer et al. (167) (1987)	354	4	76
Belli et al. (168) (1988)	74	3	67
Amato et al. (149) (1991)	78	2	
Jatzko et al. (169) (1992)	175	3	77
Isenberg et al. (170) (1995)	89		45
Singh et al. (156) (1995)	135	4	
Enker et al. (154) (1995)	170	1	81
Laxamana et al. (89) (1995)	186	2	78
Zaheer et al. (157) (1998)	272	2	78
Killingback (158) (2001)	468	3	—
Wibe et al. (171) (2004)	1315	3	68
Law and Chu (164) (2004)	419	2	74 (disease specific)
Law et al. (162) (2005)	224[a]	2	71
Gordon et al. (163) (2006) (unpublished data)	129	2	63

[a]Stage II.

TABLE 3 ■ Results of Curative Abdominoperineal Resection for Carcinoma of Rectum

Author(s)	No. of Patients	Operative Mortality (%)	Five-Year Survival Rate: Crude (%)
Fedorov and Odarjuk (165) (1983)	829	8	53
Zhou et al. (166) (1983)	251	1	48
Elliot et al. (172) (1984)	196	2	39
Williams et al. (67) (1985)	33	4	68
Davis et al. (146) (1987)	104	1	56
Heberer et al. (168) (1987)	317	7	73
Huguier et al. (173) (1990)	100	1	45
Amato et al. (149) (1991)	69	4	
Jatzko et al. (170) (1992)	72	1	49
Isenberg et al. (171) (1995)	53		56
Singh et al. (156) (1995)	45	4	
Enker et al. (154) (1995)	76	1	60
Zaheer et al. (157) (1998)	169	2	80
Killingback et al. (158) (2001)	58	3	
Dehni et al. (174) (2003)	91[a]	1	76
Law and Chu (164) (2004)	69	2	60 disease specific
Wibe et al. (161) (2004)	821	3	55
Gordon et al. (163) (2006) (unpublished data)	21	0	57

[a]Some patients received preoperative radiology, some postoperative radiotherapy, some chemotherapy.

The problem of stenosis is probably an ischemic one, and in the enthusiasm to clear the bowel for application of the pursestring instrument, excess blood supply is stripped from the edge. By decreasing the amount of bowel that is prepared for the anastomosis, I have noted a decrease in the incidence of stenosis from 20% in my early experience to 13% in subsequent patients. In the last 72 cases, the incidence of stenosis was further reduced to 4.2%.

From the point of view of anastomotic security, reported clinical rates of leakage have ranged from 0% to 16% (Table 5). Those who have studied patients with meglumine diatrizoate (Gastrografin) enemas have found radiologic leakage rates ranging from 3% to 36% and even higher if only very low anterior resections were considered (211). Several authors have compared stapled with hand-sewn anastomoses (212–214). In two of these series stapled anastomoses fared better than hand-sewn anastomoses. In the report by Beart and Kelly (212) the two techniques were equal, but it must be noted that in 12% of the patients in that series, the rectum was preserved as a result of the stapling procedure. Other authors have reported that the use of a circular stapling device has diminished the need for abdominoperineal resection (63,187,188,215–218), and I certainly support this view. In the report by McGinn et al. (203) stapled anastomoses suffered a 12% clinical leak, whereas hand-sutured anastomoses experienced only a 3% clinical leak. These results are clearly at variance with other reports.

Concern has been expressed that the introduction of the circular stapling devices might result in a higher incidence of anastomotic or local recurrence (Table 6) (194,219–221). The concern is that surgeons might compromise on the distal margin of resection. It might also be argued that since a lower anastomosis can be created with a circular stapling device, a greater distal margin might be achieved in a given case while still preserving the anal sphincter.

TABLE 4 ■ Five-Year Survival Rate According to Stage Following Curative Resection of Carcinoma of Rectum

		Dukes' A			Dukes' B			Dukes' C		
Author(s)	No. of Patients	No.	Crude (%)	Corrected (%)	No.	Crude (%)	Corrected (%)	No.	Crude (%)	Corrected (%)
Rosen et al. (175) (1982)	180	45	86		75	65		60	33	
Hojo (176) (1986)	273		93			73			49	
Malmberg et al. (167) (1986)	83	26	96		32	72		25	45	
Davis et al. (146) (1987)	235		75	98		55	72		31	40
Michelassi et al. (148) (1988)	154					60	61		43	43
Fandrich et al. (151) (1994)	371		70–80[a]			45			30	
Hermanek et al. (155) (1995)	864	257	74		257	62		350	40	
Enker et al. (154) (1995)	246				99	87		147	64	
Sugihara et al. (177) (1996)	214	55	96		72	84		87	67	
Staib et al. (159) (2002)		259	91		269	73		215	38	
Dehni et al. (174) (2003)	91	34	88		26	84		31	54	
Gordon et al. (163) (2006) (unpublished data)	186	59	63		63	73		54	46	

[a]Submucosa or muscularis propria.
[b]Some patients received preoperative radiotherapy, some postoperative radiotherapy, some chemotherapy.

TABLE 5 ■ Complications with Circular Stapler

Author(s)	No. of Cases	Leaks (%)[a]		Stenosis (%)
		Clinical	Radiologic	
Cutait et al. (184) (1981)	49	12	b	6
Killingback (185) (1981)	64	9	b	14
Dorricott et al. (186) (1982)	50	6	20	b
Friis, Hjortrup, and Nielson (187) (1982)	38	11	b	b
Goligher (188) (1982)	101	3	9	5
Hamelmann et al. (189) (1982)	54	11	28	17
Helm and Rowe (190) (1982)	78	9	b	5
Leff et al. (191) (1982)	106	8	b	11
Polglase et al. (192) (1982)	19	16	36	30
Vezeridis et al. (193) (1982)	58	0	b	3
Anderberg et al. (194) (1983)	34	12	b	b
Fegiz, Angelini, and Bezzi (195) (1983)	134	16	30	b
Isbister, Beasley, and Dowle (196) (1983)	88	15	b	1
Kennedy et al. (197) (1983)	236	3	b	b
Resnick, Burstein, and Viner (198) (1983)	61	3	b	b
Fazio (199) (1984)	183	3	6	1
Hedberg and Helmy (200) (1984)	63	3	b	10
Steichen and Ravitch (201) (1984)	33	6	b	b
Fazio (202) (1984)	85	1	4	b
McGinn et al. (203) (1985)	58	12	24	b
Gillen and Peel (180) (1986)	55	6	24	b
Malmberg et al. (166) (1986)	96	14	b	b
Antonsen and Kronberg (204) (1987)	178	15	b	8
Zannini et al. (205) (1987)	209	9	b	9
Belli et al. (168) (1988)	74	4	b	3
Dehong et al. (206) (1991)	84	5	b	b
Steegmuller and Brown (207) (1991)	133	3	b	b
Kyzer and Gordon (183) (1992)	215	0.4	b	13
Moran et al. (88) (1992)	55	9	b	5
Karanjia et al. (208) (1994)	219	11	6	b
Fingerhut et al. (209) (1995)[c]	54	4	7	16
Fingerhut et al. (209) (1995)[d]	85	0	b	5
Detry et al. (210) (1995)	1000	4	b	0.5

[a]Percentages have been rounded to the closest whole number.
[b]Not addressed.
[c]Infraperitoneal anastomoses.
[d]Supraperitoneal anastomoses.

Several reports have shown that five-year survival rates for patients with carcinoma of the middle third of the rectum are at least as good or better with the use of a low anterior resection than with abdominoperineal resection (62,63,66–68) It also has been reported that local recurrences are higher after abdominoperineal resections than after low anterior resections (66,227). Since anastomoses are being created at a lower level than possible before the introduction of the stapler, if the incidence of local recurrence after the use of the EEA stapler is shown to be higher than with the conventional hand-sutured anastomoses, it might be appropriate to compare at least some of these recurrences to recurrences in patients who have had abdominoperineal resection. In an effort to shed light on this controversy, Wolmark et al. (226) compared the incidence of local recurrence in patients undergoing stapled or hand-sewn anastomoses following curative resection of Dukes' B and C colorectal carcinoma. There were 99 patients in the sutured group and 82 in the stapled group. The patients' average time in the study was 41 months. Analyses of the distal resection margins were made in the two groups. For anterior resections the length of distal margin was 2.7 ± 0.2 cm for hand-sewn anastomoses and 2.8 ± 0.2 cm for those effected by the EEA instruments. No significant difference emerged in the development of local recurrences as a first site of treatment failure when hand-sewn and stapled anastomoses were compared. If any trend was in evidence, it was in favor of the patient cohort with stapled anastomoses, in which the local recurrence was 12% compared with 19% for the hand-sewn group. The authors concluded that the use of stapled anastomoses does not compromise the patient.

In their review of the literature (18 reports), Enker et al. (154) reported that conventional operations are associated with a worldwide incidence of pelvic recurrence of 30% and disseminated disease in 60% to 65%. Local recurrence has been reported to be related to depth of penetration of the bowel wall. Willett et al. (230) reviewed the clinical course of 64 such patients undergoing abdominoperineal resection. Follow-up revealed that all 12 patients with disease limited to the submucosa were free of recurrence. Recurrence developed in eight of the 52 patients with muscularis propria involvement. The six-year actuarial disease-free survival, local control, and freedom from distant metastases rates for these patients were 80%, 84%, and 85%, respectively.

Croxford et al. (160) reported that the recurrence rate following TME is influenced by the level of the carcinoma.

TABLE 6 ■ Local Recurrence with Circular Stapler

Author(s)	No. of Cases	Follow-Up Mean or Range (mo)	Local Recurrence Rate (%)
Heald and Leicester (222) (1981)	40	16	3
Hurst et al. (219) (1982)	32	7–25	32
Anderberg et al. (194) (1983)	34	5	21
Fegiz et al. (195) (1983)	102	9–38	9
Isbister et al. (196) (1983)	63	?	14
Luke et al. (223) (1983)	79	24	22
Kennedy et al. (224) (1985)	63	44	36
Leff et al. (225) (1985)	70	36	11
Rosen et al. (221) (1985)	76	24	21
Gillen and Peel (180) (1986)	55	>24	15
Malmberg et al. (166) (1986)	96	65	18
Wolmark et al. (226) (1986)	82	41	12
Carlsson et al. (227) (1987)	40	78	35
Colombo et al. (179) (1987)	61	6–52	10
Neville et al. (228) (1987)	76	43	24
Zannini et al. (205) (1987)	108	>24	18
Belli et al. (168) (1988)	74	37	4
Akyol et al. (229) (1991)	152	24	19
Amato et al. (149) (1991)	40	24	13
Dehong et al. (206) (1991)	84	?	4
Kyzer and Gordon (183) (1992)	215	4–124	13
Moran et al. (88) (1992)	55	24–84	7

Overall recurrence rate was 4% in a series of 480 patients with upper, middle, and lower third rates being 0%, 2%, and 7%, respectively.

With the growing number of publications reporting results of TME or partial mesorectal excision, it might be appropriate to report their results separately and these are listed in Table 7. A caveat in interpreting these results is that in many of these publications there are a large number of exclusions which would make their survival rates artificially enhanced and local recurrence diminished over potentially previous reports of survival and local recurrence rates so that results are not necessarily comparable to the historical controls. For example, in the report by Heald et al. (232) exclusions resulted in a 50% decrease in local recurrence (6 to 3%) and a five-year survival improvement from 68% to 80%. With the usual emphasis on technical expertise, Cecil et al. (239) reported that following TME the local recurrence rate was 2% for Dukes' A cases, 4% for Dukes' B, and 7.5% for Dukes' C. The systemic recurrence rate was 8% for Dukes' A, 18% for Dukes' B, and 37% for Dukes' C. They believe if surgical priority is given to the difficult task of excision of the whole mesorectum, anterior resection with TME in node positive rectal carcinoma, recurrence rates of less than 10% can be achieved. Once again, case exclusion may have favorably biased results. Kockerling et al. (240), monitored 1581 consecutive patients who underwent curative resection (R0) for rectal carcinoma, for recurrence and survival. No patient received adjuvant radiotherapy or chemotherapy. The median follow-up time was greater than 13 years. The local recurrence rate decreased from 39.4% to 9.8% during the study period. The observed five-year survival rate improved from 50% to 71%. Three hundred and six patients with local recurrence had a significantly lower observed five-year survival rate. A total of 1285 patients had no local recurrence but 275 of them developed distant metastases

TABLE 7 ■ Operative Mortality, Survival and Local Recurrence Following Curative Mesorectal Excision for Carcinoma of Rectum

Author(s)	No. of Potentially Curative Patients	Operative Mortality	Overall Survival (%)	Local Recurrence (%)
Arbman et al. (231) (1996)	129	2	68 (4 yr)	4 (4 yr)
Heald et al. (232) (1998)	405	3	80 (5 yr)	3 (5 yr)
Hall et al. (233) (1998)	152	3	68 (5 yr)	11 (41 months)
Dahlberg et al. (234) (1999)	83	2	75 (5 yr)[a]	12
	119[b]	–	–	3[b]
Martling et al. (235) (2000)	381	3	91 (2 yr)	6 (2 yr)
Kapiteijn et al. (236) (2001)	937	3	82 (2 yr)	8 (2 yr)
	924[b]		82 (2 yr)	3
Nesbakken et al. (237) (2002)	161	3	66	11 (5 yr)
Bulow et al. (238) (2003)	311	7	77 (3 yr)	11 (3 yr)
Wibe et al. (161) (2004)	2136	3	63	12 (5 yr)

[a]Carcinoma-specific survival.
[b]Received preoperative radiotherapy.

(stage I 8%; stage II 16%; stage III 40%). Better quality operation had no effect on the incidence of initial distant metastases that remained constant.

Local recurrence continues to be a major problem following surgical treatment for rectal carcinoma and proposed ways of reducing this remain controversial. McCall et al. (241), reviewed published surgical series in which adjuvant therapies were not used and follow-up on at least 50 patients was available. Fifty-one papers reported follow-up on 10,465 patients with a median local recurrence rate of 18.5%. Local recurrence was 8.5%, 16.3%, and 28.6% in Dukes' A, B, and C patients, respectively, 16.2% following anterior resection, and 19.3% following abdomino-perineal resection. Nine papers (1176 patients) reported local recurrence rates of 10% or less. Local recurrence was 7.1% in 1333 patients having TME and 12.4% in 476 patients having extended pelvic lymphadenopathy. In 52% of cases, local recurrence was reported to have occurred with no evidence of disseminated disease. Surgical technique is an important determinant of local recurrence risk.

Some reports include all patients with carcinoma of the rectum including those treated by abdomino-perineal resection or low anterior resection. Further difficulty in comparison of local recurrence rates is the very definition of local recurrence—local recurrence alone, or local recurrence combined with distant spread. The varying observation times also plays a role. In some series, the rate is calculated on the basis of all patients and others report curative resection only. Also, the stage of the disease should be considered as pointed out as in the study of Bulow where a higher proportion of patients with Dukes' C carcinomas were in the control group (238). Another point to note is that leak rates of 8% to 16% are higher than should be expected following such operations. In the Hall report 73% of patients had a diverting stoma and mortality rates up to 7% were reported (233). What these reports do clearly emphasize is that careful oncologic operations can and should be performed by those specifically trained in the conduct of these procedures in a specialized unit and this should result in a reduction in the frequency in abdominoperineal resection, postoperative complications, mortality, local recurrence, and improved survival (233,234). The importance was further emphasized by the report of Nagtegaal (242). They reviewed the pathology reports of all patients entered into a Dutch multicenter randomized trial. A three-tiered classification was applied to assess completeness of the TME. Prognostic value of this classification was tested using the data of all patients who did not receive any adjuvant treatment. In 24% of 180 patients, the mesorectum was incomplete. Patients in this group had an increased risk of local and distant recurrence 36.1% versus 20.3% recurrence in the group with complete mesorectum.

In their very comprehensive study, Wibe et al. (161) examined the outcome of carcinoma of the lower rectum, particularly the rates of local recurrence and survival for carcinoma located in this area that have been treated by anterior or abdominoperineal resections. The prospective observational national cohort study that is part of the Norwegian Rectal Cancer Project, included all patients undergoing TME in 47 hospitals. A total of 2136 patients with rectal carcinoma within 12 cm of the anal verge were analyzed; 62% anterior resection and 38% abdomino-perineal resections. The lower edge of the carcinoma was located 0 to 5 cm from the anal verge in 791 patients, 6 to 8 cm in 558 patients, and 9 to 12 cm in 787 patients. According to the TNM classification, there were 33% stage I, 35% stage II, and 32% stage III. The five-year local recurrence rate was 15% in the lower level, 13% in the intermediate level, and 9% in the upper level. It was 10% local recurrence after anterior resection and 15% after abdomino-perineal resection. Fifty percent of recurrences occurred within 19 months and 90% within 40 months. The five-year survival rate was 59% in the lower level, 62% in the intermediate level, and 69% in the upper level, respectively, and it was 68% in the anterior resection group and 55% in the abdominoperineal resection group. Overall survival declined with increasing age with mortality rate of those greater than 79 years, six times those less than 50 years. Females survived better than males. The level of the carcinoma influenced the risk of local recurrence but the operative procedure anterior resection versus abdomino perineal resection did not. On the contrary, operative procedure influenced survival but level of the carcinoma did not. In addition to patient and carcinoma characteristics (T4 lesions), intraoperative bowel perforation that occurred in 9% of patients (16% APR, 4% anterior resection) and positive circumferential margins that occurred in 8% of patients (12% after APR, 5% after anterior resection), five-year survival negative circumferential margins (66% vs. 31% with positive margin) were identified as significant prognostic factors which were more common in the lower rectum explaining the inferior prognosis for carcinoma in this region. At 44 months follow-up, the observed local recurrence rate was 23% after perforation and 9% in patients with no perforation. They concluded that T4, R1 resections and/or intraoperative perforation of the carcinoma of bowel wall are main features of low rectal carcinoma causing inferior oncologic outcomes for malignancies in this area. If the operation is optimized preventing intraoperative perforation and involvement of the circumferential margin, the prognosis for carcinoma of the lower rectum seems not to be different from that of carcinomas at higher levels. In that case, the level of the carcinoma or the type of resection will not be indicators for selecting patients for radiotherapy.

Optimizing surgical techniques (TME) for rectal carcinoma can reduce the rate of local recurrence and increase overall survival. This was clearly exemplified by the results of the Norwegian Registry (243). In a national audit for the period of 1986 to 1988, 28% of patients developed local recurrence following treatment with a curative intent. Five-year overall survival was 55% for patients younger than 75 years. In 1994, the Norwegian Rectal Cancer Group was founded with the aim to improve the surgical standard by implementing TME on a national level. A rectal carcinoma registry recorded 5382 patients with a carcinoma located within 16 cm of the anal verge and 3432 patients underwent rectal resection with a curative intent. Of these, 9% had adjuvant radiotherapy and 2% were given chemotherapy. There was a rapid implementation of the new technique as 78% underwent TME in 1994 increasing to 96% in 1998. After 39 months mean follow-up, the rate of local recurrence was 8% and five-year survival was 71% for patients younger than 75 years. Specialization of surgeons, feedback of results, and a separate rectal carcinoma registry are thought to be major contributors to the improved treatment.

Ike et al. (244) reviewed the medical records of 71 patients with T3 or T4 primary rectal carcinomas who underwent a curative pelvic exenteration. The postoperative mortality, hospital death, and morbidity rates were 1.4%, 4.2%, and 66.2%, respectively. The overall five-year survival rate after total pelvic exenteration was 54.1%. The five-year survival rate was 65.7% for patients with T3 lesions and 39% for patients with T4 lesions. Postoperative survival was affected by age, stage of disease, and lymph node metastases. They concluded total pelvic exenteration might enable long-term survival in young patients with stage T3 and T4 primary rectal carcinomas and little or no lymph node metastases.

Manfredi et al. (245) determined factors influencing local recurrences from the cancer registry of the Cote d'Or (France). The five-year cumulative recurrence rate was 22.7%. The two variables significantly associated with local recurrence risk were stage at diagnosis and the macroscopic type of growth. There was a nonsignificant decrease in the local recurrence rate in patients treated by preoperative radiotherapy compared with that in the patients treated by operation alone. The proportion of patients re-resected for cure was 25.2%, an increase from 13% in 1976 to 1985 to 37.9% in 1986 to 1995.

Killingback et al. (158) examined local recurrence after curative resection for carcinoma of the rectum in which operative technique of TME was not performed. Total excision of the distal mesorectum was not performed in the upper third or mid rectum. Curative resections were performed in 549 patients of whom 17 died postoperatively (3%). Sphincter saving resection was performed in 88% and abdominoperineal resection in 11%. The pathology stages (Dukes') were A, 29.7%, B, 34.7%, C, 35.7%. Follow-up for a minimum of five years was recorded in 97.2% of patients. The median period of follow-up was 82 months. Local recurrence confined to the pelvis occurred in 3.2% of patients, and local recurrences associated with distant metastases occurred in 4.5% of patients. The total five-year local recurrence rate was 7.6%. Local recurrence was increased in stage C carcinomas. Diathermy dissection in the pelvis was associated with a decreased local recurrence rate. The five-year survival rate in curative resection was 72.5%.

Bonadeo et al. (246) assessed the local recurrence rate and prognostic factors for local recurrence in patients undergoing curative anterior or abdomino perineal resections without radiotherapy in 514 consecutive patients. In 417 patients, postoperative chemotherapy was limited to patients with stage III lesions. The five-year local recurrence rate was 9.7% with a median time to diagnosis of 15 months. Local recurrence rates in stage I, II, and III were 3.1%, 4.1%, and 24.1%, respectively. In relation to node status, local recurrence rates were N0, 4.1%; N1, 12.6%; N2, 32.1%; and N3, 59.3%. Lower third carcinomas had a higher local recurrence rate than middle and upper third lesions 17.9%, 7.1%, 5.1%, respectively.

Zaheer et al. (157) reported on the outcome of patients undergoing resection of rectal carcinoma achieved by abdominoperineal resection, coloanal anastomosis, anterior resection without adjuvant therapy. Among 514 patients who underwent operation alone, abdominoperineal resection was performed in 169 patients, coloanal anastomosis in 19, anterior resection in 272, and other procedures in 54. Eighty-seven percent of patients were operated on with curative intent. The mean follow-up was 5.6 years; follow-up was complete in 92%. Abdominoperineal resection and coloanal anastomosis were performed excising the envelope of rectal mesentery posteriorly and the supporting tissues laterally from the sacral promontory to the pelvic floor. Anterior resection was performed using an appropriately wide rectal mesentery resection technique if the carcinoma was high; if the carcinoma was in the middle or low rectum, all mesentery was resected. The mean distal margin achieved by anterior resection was 3 +/- 2 cm. Mortality was 2%. Anastomotic leaks after anterior resection occurred in 5% and overall transient urinary retention in 15%. Eleven percent of patients had a wound infection. The local recurrence and five-year disease free survival rates were 7% and 78%, respectively, after anterior resection; 6% and 83%, respectively, after coloanal anastomosis; 4% and 80%, respectively, after abdominoperineal resection. Patients with stage III disease had a 60% disease-free survival. The overall failure rate of 40% in stage III disease means that surgical approaches alone are not sufficient to achieve better long-term survival rates.

Vironen et al. (247) conducted a study to find out whether TME technique alone or combined with preoperative radiotherapy reduces local recurrence rate and improves survival. A conventional surgical technique was used during the first period (144 patients) and TME alone or combined with preoperative radiotherapy during the second period (61). After anterior resection (5%) during the first period, and 9% during the second period developed anastomotic leaks. Operative 30-day mortality was 1% and 0%, respectively. Actuarial local recurrence rate was 17% in the first period and 9% in the second period. Actuarial crude five-year-survival improved from 55% to 78% and carcinoma-specific survival improved from 67% to 86% between the two study periods.

Parks (248) reported on 76 patients who underwent a resection with coloanal anastomoses. Pelvic sepsis following colonic necrosis and anastomotic breakdown developed in two patients. Pelvic sepsis without anastomotic breakdown developed in another eight patients. Local recurrence developed in 8%. Survival at the three-year follow-up examination was 66% and at five years was 63%. Good functional results were reported in 69 of the 70 patients. In a report from St. Mark's Hospital in London, Sweeney et al. (249) reviewed 84 patients who underwent this operation. They found a low mortality of 2.4%, but a high complication rate with pelvic sepsis in 40.5% and anastomotic dehiscence in 47.6%. The crude five-year survival rate was 56%; local recurrence developed in 9.2% and was associated with systemic recurrence in another 9.2%. Functional results were deemed satisfactory in 92%. The authors concluded that for patients in whom the only alternative was abdominoperineal resection, their results showed no disadvantage in terms of potential cure, and functional results are acceptable. Enker et al. (250) reported on 41 patients in whom this technique was used. At 31 months,

75% were disease free. Functional results were reported to be good in 80% of patients. Similar encouraging results have been reported by others (251–255).

Kohler et al. (256) reported the results of 31 patients with a very low localization of the carcinoma (distal margin 1.3 cm above the dentate line) who underwent a low anterior rectal resection with coloanal anastomosis. If the function of the sphincter was acceptable and they could exclude infiltration of the carcinoma into the sphincter through endosonography, they relocated the resection plane distally into the intersphincteric region to obtain an acceptable margin of safety. After intersphincteric rectal dissection, the anastomosis was hand sewn, using interrupted sutures from the perineal approach, 2.5 to 3 cm above the anal verge, implementing Parks' retractor. A protective stoma was performed in all cases. Postoperative mortality was 0%. The leakage rate was 48%. Only 16% later needed additional operation for anastomotic strictures or for rectovaginal fistulas. Long-term observation showed that the anastomosis healed well in 87.1%. During the follow-up period of 6.8 years, 19.4% developed progression of their carcinoma (9.7% local recurrence and 12.9% distant spread). The five-year survival rate was 79% (Dukes' A 100%, Dukes' B, 67%, and Dukes' C, 44%). Anorectal incontinence for liquid stool developed in 29.6% and for solid stool in 3.7% of patients. Average stool frequency was 3.3 times per day. Resting pressure decreased significantly by 29% whereas squeeze pressure did not change. They concluded, in selected patients with carcinomas close to the dentate line, and intersphincteric resection of the rectum may help to avoid an abdominoperineal excision of the rectum with a terminal stoma, without any curtailment of oncologic standards.

Ho et al. (257) investigated the functional outcome in elderly patients following low anterior resection for carcinoma of the rectum. The study included 87 patients with carcinoma of the middle and lower rectum who underwent curative low anterior resection with TME and remained alive without recurrence for at least six months following the resection or closure of stoma. Anorectal manometry and questionnaire survey of the patients' bowel function were performed during follow-up (median 24.1 months). The median number of bowel motions was 2.5 per day in both elderly and young patients. Complete continence was achieved in 71.3% of patients, with both elderly and young patients performing similarly. The most common symptoms were clustering of bowel motions and urgency, which occurred in 30.3% and 34.9% of patients, respectively, regardless of age. Manometric findings were also similar between the elderly and the younger patients.

An elderly patient undergoing anterior resection for rectal carcinoma has a reasonably good expectation of acceptable continence. Phillips et al. (258) reviewed functional results one year after restorative operation in patients older than age 75 years. A total of 133 patients who had restorative anterior resection were alive at one year. Significant problems with bowel function or continence were denied by 85% of patients. One patient had already reported severe difficulty and had been given a definitive stoma for incontinence. The remaining 14%, although experiencing some problems with continence, did not consider the situation serious enough to contemplate a stoma.

Rengan et al. (259) conducted a trial to determine whether preoperative external-beam radiation therapy can increase the rate of sphincter preservation for patients with distal cT2N0 carcinoma of the rectum who refused an abdominoperineal resection. There were 27 patients with distal rectal carcinomas stage T2 by clinical and/or endorectal ultrasound who were judged by the operating surgeon to require an abdominoperineal resection and were treated with preoperative pelvic radiation alone (50.4 Gy). Operation was performed four to seven weeks later. The median follow-up was 55 months. The pathologic complete response rate was 15% and 78% of patients who underwent a sphincter-sparing procedure. The crude incidence of local failure for patients undergoing a sphincter sparing procedure was 10% and the five-year actuarial incidence was 13%. The actuarial five-year survival for patients undergoing sphincter preservation was as follows: disease-free, 77%; colostomy-free, 100%; and overall, 85%. Their data suggest that for patients with cT2N0 distal rectal carcinoma who required abdominoperineal resection, preoperative pelvic radiation improves sphincter preservation without an apparent compromise in local control or survival.

Engel et al. (260) assessed rectal carcinoma patients' quality of life by using the European Organization for Research and Treatment of Cancer QLQ-30 and CR38 questionnaires in 329 patients. Overall, anterior resection patients had better quality of life scores than abdominoperineal extirpation patients. High-anterior resection patients had significantly better scores than both low-anterior resection and abdominoperineal extirpation patients. Low-anterior resection patients, however, overall had a better quality of life than abdominoperineal extirpation patients, especially after four years. Abdominoperineal extirpation patients' quality of life scores did not improve over time. Stoma patients had significantly worse quality of life scores than nonstoma patients. Quality of life improved greatly for patients whose stoma was reversed. Anterior resection and nonstoma patients, despite suffering micturation and defecation problems, had better quality of life scores than abdominoperineal extirpation and stoma patients.

Schmidt et al. (261) assessed the differences in perceived quality of life over time among patients treated with anterior resection or abdominoperineal resection for rectal carcinoma. In a prospective study, the European Organization for Research and Treatment of Cancer (EORTC) Quality of Life Questionnaire C30 and a disease-specific module were administered to patients with rectal carcinoma before operation, at discharge, and 3, 6, and 12 months after the operation. Comparisons were made between patients receiving an anterior resection and those receiving an abdominoperineal resection. Data were available for 212 patients of whom 112 were female and 100 male. No differences in the distribution of age, sex, or disease stage were observed between groups. EORTC function scales showed no significant differences, including body image scales, between patients receiving an anterior resection and those receiving an abdominoperineal resection. In symptom scores, anterior resection patients had more difficulty with diarrhea and constipation, whereas patients with abdominoperineal resection experienced more impaired sexuality and pain in the anoperineal region. At discharge, patients receiving an anterior resection were more confident about their future.

Ranbarger et al. (81) reported on the prognostic significance of intraoperative perforation of the rectum during abdominoperineal resection. In their review of 250 patients, they found that 25.6% sustained an intraoperative perforation. Perforation did not affect the long-term outcome in patients with Dukes' A carcinoma or those with metastatic disease, but patients with Dukes' B and Dukes'C carcinomas experienced an increased recurrence (57% vs. 34%), most dramatically with Dukes' B lesions (25.9% vs. 8.1%), and a decreased five-year survival rate (31% vs. 46%). Porter et al. (262) reviewed 178 patients who underwent an abdominoperineal resection, 42 (24%) of whom had an inadvertent perforation. Local recurrence was significantly higher in the perforated group than the nonperforated group (54% vs. 17%). Similarly, five-year survival was significantly decreased with inadvertent perforation (29% vs. 59%). The detrimental implications of inadvertent perforation mandate meticulous avoidance.

Malignant fixation of carcinoma of the rectum is associated with a poor prognosis. Durdey and Williams (55) studied 625 patients who had undergone rectal excision and found that fixation was present in 27% (20% by malignant extension and 7% by inflammatory attachment). Corrected five-year survival rates were 28.5% in patients with malignant fixation, 68.9% in those with mobile lesions, and 64.6% when the carcinoma was tethered by inflammation. The incidence of local recurrence in the three groups was 41.3%, 15.1%, and 20%, respectively.

Phang et al. (263) conducted a retrospective population-based study to determine the influence of emergent presentation (obstruction, perforation, massive hemorrhage) on outcomes. There were 452 invasive carcinomas of the rectum of which 45 were emergent and 407 nonemergent. Disease-specific survival at four years for emergent and nonemergent stage II carcinomas were 66% versus 80%, respectively, and for stage III carcinomas 60% versus 73%, respectively. Local recurrence rates at four years for emergent and nonemergent stage II carcinomas were 20% versus 15%, respectively, and for stage III carcinomas 70% versus 20%, respectively. Resection more frequently involved a stoma for emergent (60%) than for nonemergent (35%) cases. Percent of patients having complete staging investigations were similar between emergent (42%) and nonemergent patients (39%). Adjuvant radiation was given in similar proportion to emergent (61%) and nonemergent (55%) patients. Adjuvant chemotherapy was given to a slightly higher proportion of emergent patients (63%) than nonemergent patients (43%).

Vironen et al. (264) compared perioperative morbidity, mortality, and survival after operation for rectal carcinoma in patients younger than and aged 75 years or older. Of 294 patients, 32% were aged 75 or older and comprised the elderly group. Major curative operation was possible in 62% of patients in the elderly group and in 74% of patients in the younger group. Among those operated on with curative intent, 34% of the older age group and 27% in the younger age group had complications. Thirty-day mortality was 2% and 0%, respectively. Although five-year crude survival was significantly lower in the older age group (43% vs. 65%), five-year carcinoma-specific survival (60% vs. 70%) and disease-free five-year survival (60% vs. 69%) were similar in both groups. The 17 patients treated with local excision had a carcinoma-specific survival of 81% and 83% in younger and older groups, respectively. After palliative resection, the two-year survival was similar (20% vs. 25%) in both groups. They concluded that major curative rectal carcinoma surgery in selected elderly patients can be performed with similar indications, perioperative morbidity, and mortality, as well as five-year carcinoma-specific and disease-free survival as in younger patients.

A very important aspect relates to careful operative technique. Eriksen et al. (265) reviewed the outcome of inadvertent perforation of the bowel during resection of rectal carcinoma. The study included a prospective national cohort of 2873 patients undergoing major resection for rectal carcinoma at 54 Norwegian hospitals. The overall perforation rate was 8.1%. The risk of perforation was significantly greater in patients undergoing abdominoperineal resection (odds ratio 5.6) and in those aged 80 years or more (odds ratio 2.0). The five-year local recurrence rate was 28.8% following perforation compared with 9.9% in patients with no perforation. Survival rates were 41.5% and 67.1%, respectively. The high local recurrence rates and reduced survival following perforation called for increased attention to avoid this complication.

A recent review by Leong (266) of multiple studies has shown that specialization in rectal carcinoma surgery results in lower postoperative morbidity and mortality, local and distant recurrence, and higher rates of sphincter saving resections.

Kressner et al. (267) investigated whether an abdominal or perineal septic complication was associated with rectal carcinoma recurrence in 228 patients. There was no clear difference in the overall incidence of recurrence between the infection group (36%) and the noninfection group (26%). The incidence of local recurrence was higher in the infection group (23%) than the noninfection group (9%). This increased risk was restricted to patients with a perineal infection (33% vs. the noninfection group), whereas patients with an abdominal infection (13%) did not differ from the noninfection group.

Sexual dysfunction is a recognized complication in men undergoing pelvic surgery for rectal carcinoma but there is little information on the influence of such surgery on sexual health in women. Platell et al. (268) evaluated sexual health in 50 women undergoing pelvic surgery for rectal carcinoma. A control group comprised women who had undergone operation for colonic carcinoma during the same interval. Of the 50 women in the study group who were contacted, 22 completed questionnaires. Sixty-two women in the control group were contacted and 19 completed questionnaires. Women in the study group were significantly younger than those in the control group. Compared with those of the control group, women who had undergone pelvic surgery were significantly more likely to feel less attractive, feel that the vagina was either too short or less elastic during intercourse, experience superficial pain during intercourse, and complain of fecal soiling during intercourse. Women in the study group were concerned that these limitations would persist for the rest of their lives. There were no differences between the two groups in relationship to sexual arousal or libido. They concluded that pelvic surgery for rectal carcinoma has a significant influence on sexual health of women.

Schmidt et al. (269) investigated how sexuality and quality of life are affected by age, gender, and type of operation in 516 patients who had undergone operation for rectal carcinoma. Quality of life data was received from 261 patients. For patients receiving abdominoperineal resection, sexuality was most impaired. Females reported more distress from the medical treatment: insomnia, fatigue, and constipation. Both genders had impaired sexual life; however, males had significantly higher values and felt more distressed by this impairment. Younger females felt more distress through impaired sexuality. In males sexuality was impaired independent of age. Adjuvant therapy had no influence on sexuality but on quality of life one year after operation.

LOCAL FORMS OF THERAPY

RATIONALE

The advantage of a purely local form of treatment for an early lesion is self-evident. Elimination of the necessity to recommend a major resectional operation, with its attendant morbidity and mortality, is most attractive. The theoretical disadvantage of a local form of therapy for carcinoma of the rectum is the failure to remove nodes along the inferior mesenteric vessels. However, not all these patients have lymph node involvement. With the high morbidity of abdominoperineal resection and low anterior resection, clinicians continue the search for a lesser procedure that would still be adequate for long-term survival. The goal is to identify patients with carcinoma that is still confined to the bowel wall without lymph node metastases (Dukes' A). This accounts for about 15% of carcinomas of the rectum. The advent of intrarectal ultrasonography has gone a long way to accurately identify these patients. In their review of the literature, Sharma et al. (270) noted that depth of invasion provides the best estimate of the probability of lymph node spread this occurring in 0% to 12% of T_1, 12% to 28% of T_2 and 36% to 79% of T_3 lesions. Additional factors considered important predictors of lymph node spread are histologic grade, lymphovascular invasion of the rectal wall, mucinous histology, and ulceration of the carcinomas. Proponents of local forms of therapy agree that even when local therapy fails, salvage by abdominoperineal resection can be expected with the same hope for cure as if it had been the initial form of therapy. For patients who are deemed unfit to withstand a major rectal excision or for patients who refuse an operation that necessitates a colostomy, a number of purely local forms of treatment have been used.

PROCEDURES

Local Excision

For a select small group of patients, perhaps 3% to 5% of all patients with carcinoma of the rectum, per anal local excision of the carcinoma may prove to be the treatment of choice (271,272). Criteria for the selection of patients for a local excision are not well defined. Ideally lesions should be in the distal third of the rectum, mobile, not deeply penetrating the wall, less than a third of the circumference of the rectal wall, preferably polypoid rather than ulcerated, and well or moderately well differentiated, with no suggestion of anal sphincter involvement. Furthermore, there should be no palpable or radiologic evidence of regional lymph node involvement. Consideration is given to a local form of treatment because it has been estimated that the risk of regional lymph node involvement is only 10% in selected cases (273). In an effort to determine selection criteria for local excision, Minsky et al. (274) studied 168 patients who had undergone curative resection for carcinoma of the rectum (low anterior resection or abdominoperineal resection). Patients with T1 lesions (submucosal invasion) had a zero incidence of positive lymph nodes regardless of size, grade, histology, and vessel or lymphatic invasion. All other categories had a 19% incidence of lymph node positivity. Huddy et al. (275) investigated the incidence of lymph node involvement in 454 rectal excision specimens. For lesions that were confined to the bowel wall, lymph node metastases were identified in 20% although two-thirds had only one or two involved nodes. For lesions confined to the submucosa, lymph node involvement occurred in 11%. The availability of intrarectal ultrasonography should help to define the status of these lesions and hence provide a comfort level that the disease is confined to the bowel wall. Billingham (52) reviewed five series from the literature that encompassed 761 patients. The percentages of lymph node involvement were related to depth of invasion and were as follows: submucosa (12%), muscularis propria (35%), subserosa (44%), and serosa (58%).

To determine the frequency of lymph node metastases, Blumberg et al. (276) reviewed 318 patients with T1 and T2 rectal carcinomas who underwent radical resection. Of these, 159 (48 T1 and 111 T2) were potentially eligible for curative local excision (less than or equal to 4 cm in size, less than or equal to 10 cm from the anal verge, no synchronous metastases). The overall frequency of lymph node metastases was 15% (T1, 10%; T2, 17%). Differentiation (well-differentiated or moderately differentiated, 14%; and poorly differentiated, 30%), and lymphatic vessel invasion (lymphatic vessel invasion-negative, 14%; and lymphatic vessel invasion-positive, 33%) influenced the risk of lymph node metastases. However, only blood vessel invasion (blood vessel invasion-negative 13% and blood vessel invasion-positive 33%) reached statistical significance as a single predictive factor. Carcinomas with no adverse pathologic features (low risk group) had a lower overall frequency of lymph node metastases (11%) compared with the remaining carcinomas (high risk groups 31%). However, even in the most favorable group (T1 carcinomas with no adverse pathologic features), lymph node metastases were present in 7% of patients.

Nascimbeni et al. (277) reviewed the clinical records of 7543 patients who underwent operative treatment for carcinoma of the colon to determine the risk factors for lymph node metastases. For the depth, the submucosa was divided into upper third (sm1), middle third (sm2), and lower third (sm3). The incidence of T1 lesions was 8.6% (353 patients). The lymph node metastasis rate was 13%. Significant predictors of lymph node metastasis were sm3, lymphovascular invasion, and lesions in the lower third of the rectum. They concluded T1 colorectal carcinomas with lymphovascular invasion, sm3 depth of invasion and location in the lower third of the rectum have a higher risk of lymph node metastases. These lesions should have an oncologic resection. In a case of the lesion in the lower third of the rectum, local excision plus adjuvant chemotherapy may be an alternative.

Sakuragi et al. (278) retrospectively analyzed 278 consecutive cases of T1 stage colorectal carcinoma resected using endoscopic resection or bowel surgery to seek predictive markers of lymph node metastasis to assist patient management. Twenty-one had lymph node metastasis. Depth of submucosal invasion (greater than or equal to 2000 μm) and lymphatic channel invasion significantly predicted risk of lymph node metastasis. When these two factors were adopted for the prediction of lymph node metastasis, sensitivity, specificity, positive predictive value, and negative predictive value were 100%, 55.6%, 15.6%, and 100%, respectively. They concluded, these two factors could be used in selecting appropriate cases for operation after endoscopic resection.

Okabe et al. (279) evaluated the clinical significance of location as a risk factor for lymph node metastasis in 428 T1 adenocarcinomas of the colon and rectum treated by radical resection. Location was assigned as right colon (cecum to transverse), left colon (splenic flexure to sigmoid), or rectum (0–18 cm from the anal verge). The overall rate of lymph node metastasis was 10%. On univariate analysis, lymph node metastasis was significantly more common in the rectum (15%) compared to the left colon (8%), or right colon (3%). However, on multivariate analysis, deep submucosal invasion and lymphovascular invasion were independent and significant risk factors, whereas location was not. T1 colorectal carcinomas have a progressively higher risk of lymph node metastasis as their location becomes more distal. However, the increasing rate of lymph node metastasis observed in carcinomas of the left colon and rectum is explained by a higher prevalence of high-risk pathologic features. In early colorectal carcinomas, morphology of the carcinoma is the strongest clinical predictor of metastatic behavior.

In a review of the literature, an enormously wide range of the incidence of lymph node involvement was cited: T1, 6% to 11%; T2, 10% to 35%, and T3, 25% to 65% (30). T1 lesions are usually amenable to local excision if they satisfy the above selection criteria. T3 lesions are clearly unsuitable because of the high incidence of lymph node metastases. There is considerable controversy about the suitability of T2 lesions and this will be elaborated upon below.

The advantage of local excision over other forms of local treatment is that it provides the opportunity to assess the diseased tissue histologically. Local excision also may be used for palliation in patients with overt disseminated malignant disease or in patients who are too old or too ill to withstand a major operation or who are unwilling to accept a colostomy.

The technique of local excision is similar to that described in Chapter 19 for benign lesions. The major difference, of course, is that the full thickness of the rectal wall is excised. The patient is placed in the prone or supine position, depending on the location of the lesion. Exposure is obtained through a Parks or Pratt retractor. A full-thickness excision is made around the lesion, leaving a 1 cm rim of normal rectal wall. The defect is closed transversely with full-thickness mattress sutures of 4–0 polyglycolic acid or polyglactin (Fig. 24).

Some surgeons prefer to leave the wound open (280). The excised specimen is pinned on a board to facilitate the histologic interpretation by the pathologist.

Gopaul et al. (281) reviewed 64 patients treated with local excision for rectal carcinoma. The median follow-up was 37 months. There were 15 local failures with a median time to local failure of 12 months. Seven patients were salvaged with further operation (four by repeat local excision, four by abdominoperineal resection, and one by low anterior resection). The incidence of local recurrence increased with advancing stage of the carcinoma (T1, 13%; T2, 24%; T3, 71%), histologic grade of differentiation (well, 12%; moderately, 24%; poorly, 44%), and margin status [negative, 16%; close (within 2 mm), 33%; positive, 50%]. Sixteen percent of carcinomas less than or equal to 3 cm failed compared with 47% for carcinomas greater than 3 cm. Nine percent of T2 patients treated with adjuvant radiotherapy recurred locally compared with 36% without radiation therapy. Three of four T3 patients who received radiation therapy failed locally compared with two of three who did not. The overall survival at five years was 71%, and disease-free survival was 83%. Actuarial local failure was 27% and freedom from distant metastasis was 86%. The sphincter preservation rate was 90% at five years. They concluded, local excision alone is an acceptable option for well differentiated, T1 carcinomas less than or equal to 3 cm. Adjuvant radiation is recommended for T2 lesions. The high local recurrence rate in patients after local

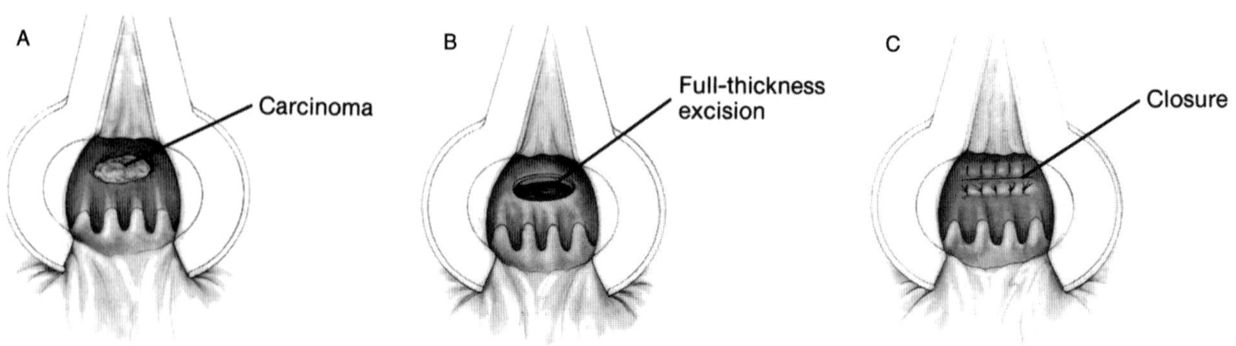

FIGURE 24 ■ Local excision of carcinoma of rectum. (**A**) Exposure of carcinoma. (**B**) Full-thickness disk excision with perirectal fat exposed. (**C**) Completed closure.

excision of T3 lesions with or without adjuvant radiotherapy would mandate a radical resection.

Nascimbeni et al. (282) identified 114 patients who had T1 sessile adenocarcinoma in the lower third or middle third of the rectum to compare the long-term recurrence rate, long-term survival and risk factors for patients treated with local excision or oncologic resection. Patients who received adjuvant therapy or who had pedunculated lesions were excluded. The mean follow-up was 9.2 years; median follow-up was 8.1 years. They compared 70 patients who underwent local excision with 74 patients who underwent oncologic resection. Among patients with lesions in the middle or lower third of the rectum (i) the five-year and 10-year outcomes were significantly better for overall survival (90.4% vs. 72%) and disease-free survival (83.6% vs. 69.8%) in the oncologic resection group compared with 72.4% and 44.3% overall survival and 66.6% and 39.6 disease-free survival for local excision. There were no significant differences in local recurrence or distant metastasis; (ii) multivariate risk factors for long-term carcinoma-free survival were invasion into the lower third of the submucosa, local excision, and older than age 68 years; and (iii) for lesions with invasion into the lower third of the submucosa, the oncologic resection group had lower rates of distant metastasis and better survival. Among patients with lesions in the lower third of the rectum (i) the five-year and ten-year outcome showed no significant differences in survival, local recurrence, or distant metastasis between the two groups; and (ii) for lesions with invasion into the lower third of the submucosa, the oncologic resection showed a trend of improved survival which was not statistically significant, possibly because of the lower statistical power from the small sample size. They concluded, patients who undergo local excision or oncologic resection for T1 carcinoma in the lower two-thirds of the rectum have a high incidence of local recurrence and distant metastasis.

A meta-analysis indicates that local recurrence occurs in 9.7% of patients (range 0–24%) in patients with T1 carcinomas, 25% (range 0–67%) of those with T2 carcinomas and 38% (range 0–100%) of those with T3 carcinomas (283).

The overall results of local excision for carcinoma of the rectum are presented in Table 8. It is once again stressed that these series are not necessarily comparable because patient selection and degree of bowel wall penetration will differ. A general idea of possible results can be gleaned from these reports, however.

Graham et al. (299) reviewed 10 published series in which local excision was used as definitive treatment for patients with invasive rectal carcinoma located within 6 cm of the anal verge. The overall five-year crude survival rate was 69% (range, 55–100%) and the cancer-specific survival rate was 89% (range, 82–100%). Local recurrence developed in 19% (range, 0–27%), but 56% (range, 22–100%) of these patients were cured with additional operations. The pathologic features of positive surgical margins, poorly differentiated histology, and increased depth of invasion were associated with increased local recurrence and decreased survival.

Lock et al. (287) assessed the outcome of 152 patients who underwent local excision of their carcinoma of the rectum at St. Mark's Hospital, London, England, between 1948 and 1984. The authors continued their institutional policy of local excision being justified if the carcinoma is well or moderately well differentiated and the lesion is judged completely excised. Following local excision, if the lesion is deemed incompletely removed, a radical operative procedure is indicated. In cases with high-risk lesions (e.g., those with deep penetration, poor differentiation but completely removed, or lymphatic involvement) adjuvant radiotherapy can be considered. Of 56 patients with low-grade malignancy, three underwent early reoperation (low anterior resection). There was one death from carcinoma. Of the 81 patients with average-grade malignancy, 10 died from carcinoma—two after early reoperation and eight following recurrence. Of the 15 patients with high-grade malignancy, six underwent early reoperation and three of these died from carcinoma. Among the nine patients who did not undergo early reoperation, there were three related deaths (two from carcinoma, one after rectal excision for recurrence). The authors concluded that local excision is a valid therapy for patients with low-grade lesions, not recommended for those with average-grade lesions, and they questioned the necessity for early reoperation in patients with high-grade lesions.

Green et al. (289) reviewed 104 patients who underwent diskectomy with intent to cure, representing 16% of patients with carcinoma of the rectum. Of the nine patients whose operation was converted to a more radical procedure because of failure to meet criteria for cure, five had no residual disease and two died from carcinoma. The remaining 95 patients were followed up from 1 to 152 months (mean 64.1 months). The overall recurrence rate was 22.4% (Tl, 10.6%; T2, 38.9%; and T3, 100%; well differentiated, 0%; moderately differentiated, 21.1%; and moderately to poorly differentiated, 58.3%). The authors concluded that transanal diskectomy remains an option for cure in selected patients.

Muto and Oya (300) reviewed colorectal T1 (submucosally invasive carcinoma) in terms of pathology, diagnosis, and treatment. The incidence of T1 carcinomas was approximately 10% and the percentage of node metastases was 10% to 11%, whereas hepatic metastases was less than 1%. Macroscopically, they were divided into three types: polypoid, ulcerating, and flat. The ulcerating type was divided into two subgroups: polypoid growth and nonpolypoid growth based on the histologic appearance of resected specimens. The tools for detecting T1 carcinomas were fecal occult blood test and colonoscopy, and magnifying colonoscopy and chromography facilitate more precise diagnosis. Ultrasonography also was useful for the correct diagnosis of the depth of carcinoma invasion. Most polypoid and some flat T1 carcinomas were safely treated by polypectomy or endoscopic mucosal resection alone; however, when resected specimens contained risk factors for metastasis such as deep invasion (sm-2, sm-3) and vessel invasion, additional surgery was necessary for cure. For rectal T1 carcinomas, the most appropriate procedure should be carefully selected from several therapeutic options to preserve anal function.

Chambers et al. (297) conducted a study to determine whether the morphology of 91 rectal carcinomas predicts outcome following treatment by local excision. Morphology was divided into four types: polypoid, sessile, ulcerated, and flat raised. Survival and local recurrence

TABLE 8 ■ **Results of Local Excision of Carcinoma of the Rectum**

Author(s)	No. of Patients	Mean Follow-Up (Yr)	Five-Year Survival Rate[a](%)	Local Recurrence (%)	Salvage Procedure Performed (%)
Biggers, Beart, and Ilstrup (284) (1986)	141	≥5.0	65	27	ND
Heberer et al. (168) (1987)	42	5.0	84	7	ND
Horn, Halvorsen, and Morild (285) (1989)	17[b]	4.3	100	0	
	14[c]	4.8	83	43	66
Killingback (286) (1992)	40	5.0	72	25	50
Billingham (52) (1992)	33		88	27	56
Lock, Ritchie, and Hawley (287) (1993)	126	>5.0	93	14	61
Willett et al. (288) (1994)	32[b] 22[c]		66	20	ND
Green et al. (289) (1994)	104	5.0	T1 93 T2 83 T3 0	11 39 100	ND
Faivre et al. (290) (1996)	126	7.3	85	28	69
Obrand and Gordon (291) (1996)	19	5.0	82	26	60
Taylor et al. (20) (1998)	24	4.3	52	46	70
Chakravarti et al. (292) (1999)	52	4.3	T1+T2 (66)[e] (74)[f]	28[e] 18[f]	78 84
Steele et al. (293) (1999)	59	4.0	T1 85 (78)[d]	7	50
Varma et al. (294) (1999)	37	6.0	T1 95 T2 83 T3 57	5 45 25	100
Mellgren et al. (295) (2000)	108	4.4	T1 72 T2 65	18[f] 47	89
Paty et al. (296) (2002)	125	6.7	T1 74 T2 72	17 26	82
Chambers et al. (297) (2004)	Δ56 □35	5.0 5.0	91 54	9 40	ND ND
Gopaul et al. (281) (2004)	53	30	71 (83%)[d]	27	67
Nascimbeni et al. (282) (2004)	70	9.2	T1 72.4 (66.6)[d]	7	
Madbouly et al. (298) (2005)	52	46	T1 75	29	93

Note: ND, no data;, overall survival; Δ, exophytic; □, nonexophytic. Survival and recurrence data are of 10 years.
25% regional radiotherapy one-half of which also received chemotherapy.
[a]Not certain which values are crude or corrected.
[b]Invasion of submucosa only.
[c]Invasion of muscularis propria.
[d]Survival (disease-free survival).
[e]Operation alone.
[f]Adjuvant chemoradiation.

were significantly better for patients with exophytic (polypoid and sessile) carcinomas than for those with nonexophytic (ulcerated and flat raised) lesions. The exophytic group included significantly more stage T1 and fewer T2 and T3 carcinomas, and a significantly smaller proportion of carcinomas that showed venous and lymphatic invasion than the nonexophytic. Nonexophytic carcinomas were associated with high-risk histopathological features that rendered carcinomas of this type unsuitable for local excision.

Paty et al. (296) reported on 125 patients with T1 and T2 carcinomas of the rectum treated by local excision as definitive operation. Thirty-one patients were selected to receive adjuvant radiation therapy. Fifteen of these 31 patients received adjuvant radiation in combination with 5 fluorouracil chemotherapy. Median follow-up was 6.7 years. Ten-year local recurrence and survival rates were 17% and 74% for T1 rectal carcinomas and 26% and 72% for T2 carcinomas. Median time to relapse was 1.4 years for local recurrence and 2.5 years for distant recurrence. In patients receiving radiotherapy, local recurrence was delayed (median 2.1 years vs. 1.1 years), but overall rates of local and overall recurrence and survival rates were similar to patients not receiving radiotherapy. Among 26 carcinoma deaths, 28% occurred more than five years after local excision. No clinical or pathologic features were predictive of local recurrence. Intra-lesional vascular invasion was the only significant predictor of survival. Among patients who developed recurrence, the pattern of first clinical recurrence was predominantly local: 50% local only, 18% local and distant, and 32% distant only. Among patients with isolated local recurrence, 82% underwent salvage resection. Actuarial survival among these salvaged patients was 30% at six years after salvage. They concluded the long-term risk of recurrence after local excision of T1 and T2 rectal carcinomas is substantial. Two-thirds of patients with recurrence have local failure implicating inadequate resection in treatment failure. In their study, neither adjuvant radiotherapy nor salvage operation was reliable in preventing or controlling local recurrence. The postoperative interval to death was as long as 10 years, raising concern that mortality may be higher than is generally appreciated. Additional treatment strategies are needed to improve the outcome of local excision.

To evaluate nationwide patterns of surgical treatment and survival of early stage rectal carcinoma using data from the National Cancer Database, Baxter et al. (301) examined rectal carcinoma cases reported to the National Cancer Database during three time periods; 1989 to 1991, 1994 to 1996, and 1999 to 2001. Patients had T1 or T2 carcinomas that were clinically and pathologically node negative and no neoadjuvant therapy was received. A total of 25,815 patients meeting selection criteria were identified; 28% in the first period, 36% in the second, and 36% in the third. T1 lesions were identified in 30%. Rates of local excision increased over time, both for T1 lesions (22–46%) and T2 lesions (6–17%). Local excision was more common in T1 lesions, the elderly (greater than 75 years), African Americans, and women. The five-year survival of patients with T1 lesions was similar to those treated with local excision and radical resection; 77% versus 80%, however, survival was worse with local excision for those with T2 lesions; 66% versus 73%. The use of local excision for stage I rectal carcinoma is increasing both for T1 and T2 lesions. This does not appear to have negative consequences for T1 lesions; however, local excisions for T2 lesions were associated with worse five-year survival. Although some of this effect may be due to inadequate staging for local excision, at the current time they believe local excision for T2 lesions should be used with great caution.

Sengupta and Tjandra (283) conducted a literature review of 41 studies on curative local excision of rectal carcinoma. Local excision preserves anorectal function and seems to have limited morbidity (0–22%). Local excision alone was associated with local recurrences in 9.7% (range 0–24%) of T1, 25% (range 0–67%) of T2, and 38% (range 0–100%) of T3 carcinomas. The addition of adjuvant chemoradiotherapy after local excision yields local recurrence rates of 9.5% (range 0–50%) for T1, 13.6% (range 0–24%) for T2, and 13.8% (range 0–50%) for T3 carcinomas. Factors other than T stage that lead to higher local recurrence rates after local excision include poor histologic grade, the presence of lymphovascular invasion, and positive margins. Local recurrences after local excision can be surgically salvaged 84 of 114 patients (74%) in 15 studies, with a disease-free survival rate between 40% and 100% at a follow-up of 0.1 to 13.5 years.

Madbouly et al. (298) reviewed their results of T1 low rectal carcinoma undergoing local excision alone. Patients with poorly differentiated carcinomas, perineural or lymphovascular invasion, or with mucinous component were excluded. Fifty-two patients underwent transanal excision during the study period. Five-year recurrence was estimated to be 29.4%, five-year carcinoma-specific and overall survival rates were 89% and 75%, respectively. Fourteen of 15 patients with recurrence underwent salvage treatment with 56.2% five-year survival. Gender, preoperative staging by endorectal ultrasound, distance from the anal verge, size of the carcinoma, location, and T1 status discovered after transanal excision of a villous adenoma did not influence local recurrence or carcinoma-specific survival. This high recurrence and low salvage rate raises the issue about the role of transanal excision alone for early rectal carcinoma and the possible need for adjuvant therapy or increased role of the resective procedures.

In a series of 19 patients on whom I performed a per anal local excision, there were no intraoperative complications and postoperative complications included urinary retention in one patient and bleeding in one patient (291). Local recurrence developed in 26% of patients but salvage operation was successful in 60% of these patients. The five-year corrected survival rate was 82%. In this review, neither size nor grade of the carcinoma correlated with recurrence. The recurrence rate was higher in patients with inadequate margins of excision and ulcerative lesions. Minsky (302) reported an increase from 6% to 56%. Killingback (286) reported increases from 23% to 36% if margins were positive for malignant cells. Of the 19 patients in our series, resection margins were involved in one patient, who died of other causes at 13 months without evidence of recurrence. Margins of normal tissue were noted to be small in four patients and unassessable in one. Recurrence occurred in three of these five patients.

Hahnloser et al. (303) determined the frequency and outcome of radical resection (within 30 days) after local excision of rectal carcinoma. Fifty-two locally excised rectal carcinomas (29 transanal and 23 polypectomies) were followed by radical operation (24 abdominoperineal resections and 28 low anterior resections) within seven days. Radical operation was performed because of a malignant polyp ($n=42$), positive margins ($n=5$), lymphovascular invasion (n=3), and T3 stage carcinoma ($n=2$). Twenty-three percent were found to have nodal involvement and 29% showed residual carcinoma in the resected specimen. The T2-3 N0-1 stage controls were well matched. No significant difference in location, size, adjuvant therapy, or length of follow-up was noted. Length of follow-up was not different. For T1, the controls were also comparable. Nodal involvement was 21% in T1 study cases and 15% in T1 primary radical-surgery controls, with a trend toward location in the lower third of the rectum in both groups (58% and 50%, respectively). Local recurrence rates were 3% in the study group, 5% for patients undergoing primary radical-operation, and 8% for local excision alone. Distant metastasis (11%, 12%, and 13%, respectively) and overall five-year survival were also not significantly different (78%, 89%, and 73%, respectively). They concluded, nodal involvement in attempted locally excised rectal carcinomas is not uncommon. Local excision of rectal carcinoma followed by radical operation within 30 days in carcinoma patients does not compromise outcome compared with primary radical-operation.

Conflicting reports regarding the results of salvage operations for local recurrence have been published. Cuthbertson and Simpson (304) achieved good salvage results by radical resection. On the other hand, Killingback (286) found that five of 10 patients with local recurrence were suitable for radical resection, and only one of these survived the malignant disease (dying of cardiac disease three years after resection).

Friel et al. (305) determined the outcome of 29 patients who underwent salvage radical operation for local recurrence after a full thickness local excision for stage I rectal carcinoma. Recurrence involved the rectal wall in 90% and was purely extrarectal in only 10%. Mean time between local excision and radical operation was 26 months. The resection was considered curative in 79%. At a mean follow-up of 39 (range 2–147) months after radical operation, 59% remained free of disease. The disease-free survival rate was 68% for patients with favorable histology versus 29% for patients with unfavorable histology.

Weiser et al. (306) examined surgical salvage of locally recurrent rectal carcinoma in 50 patients following initial transanal excision of T1 or T2 rectal carcinomas. Eight patients had resectable synchronous distant disease. Salvage procedures included abdominoperineal resection (31), low anterior resection (11), total pelvic exenteration (4), and transanal excision (3). One patient had unresectable disease at exploration, requiring diverting ostomy. Of the 49 patients who underwent successful salvage, 55% required an extended pelvic dissection with en bloc resection of one or more of the following structures: pelvic sidewall and autonomic nerves (18); coccyx or portion of sacrum (6); prostate (5); seminal vesicle (5); bladder (4); portion of the vagina (3); ureter (2); ovary (1); and uterus (1). Complete pathologic resection (R0) was accomplished in 47 of 49 patients. Of the eight patients with distant and local recurrence, two underwent synchronous resection and six had delayed metastasectomy. Five-year disease-specific survival was 53%. Factors predictive of survival included evidence of any mucosal recurrence on endoscopy, low presalvage carcinoembryonic antigen, and absence of poor pathologic features (lymphovascular and perineural invasion). Patients who required an extended pelvic resection had a worse survival rate. Other salvage rates are reported to be between 25% and 100% (291).

Baron et al. (307) compared the impact on survival of "immediate" resection for adverse features versus "salvage" resection for clinical recurrence. Of 155 patients who underwent some form of local therapy, 21 patients underwent abdominoperineal resection and/or low anterior resection, whereas another 21 patients underwent salvage operation for local recurrence. The disease-free survival rate was 94.1% for the former and 55.5% for the delayed group. The authors therefore recommended that immediate operation be performed when adverse pathologic features are present in the excised specimen.

Adjuvant therapy has been used in an effort to decrease the incidence of recurrence after local excision (308). Bennett et al. (309) reported a recurrence rate of 16% after the administration of 45 Gy to 19 patients who underwent local excision. Bailey et al. (19) reported on 53 patients who underwent local excision; 24 received full-dose radiotherapy postoperatively. With a follow-up ranging from 12 to 130 months, there was only an 8% recurrence rate. Minsky (302) reviewed the results from seven institutions, with series numbers ranging from 12 to 46 patients who underwent margin-negative local excision and postoperative pelvic radiotherapy. Some also received adjuvant chemotherapy. They found a local recurrence rate ranging from 6% to 18%. Of the three institutions that reported failure by stage, local recurrence developed in 3% of patients with T1 lesions, 10% of patients with T2 lesions, and 24% of patients with T3 lesions. Minsky therefore recommended that T3 lesions be treated by extended resection with preoperative or postoperative radiotherapy.

Wagman et al. (310) reported on 39 patients who underwent a local excision followed by postoperative radiation therapy + or − 5-FU based chemotherapy. The median follow-up was 41 months and 11 patients had positive margins. The five-year actuarial colostomy-free survival was 87% and overall survival was 70%. Crude local failure increase with T stage: 0% T1, 24% T2, and 25% T3. Of the eight patients (21%) who developed local failure, five underwent salvage abdominoperineal resection and were locally controlled. Actuarial local failure at five years was 31% for T2 disease and 27% for the total patient group. In the 32 patients with an intact sphincter, 94% had good to excellent sphincter function. They believe local excision and postoperative therapy remains a reasonable alternative to abdominoperineal resection in selected patients.

Lamont et al. (311) reviewed 27 T1 lesions treated with local excision, 10 of whom received postoperative chemoradiation, and no local recurrences were identified. Of 17 T1 patients who did not receive adjuvant treatment, local recurrence occurred in 24%. In all cases of local recurrence, lesions had been excised to negative margins, none were poorly differentiated, none exhibited vascular or lymphatic invasion. Their data suggested a trend toward improved local control with adjuvant therapy after local excision of T1 rectal carcinomas.

Coco et al. (312) reported that the addition of radiotherapy in the treatment of patients with T2 lesions provided equivalent survival to T1 who underwent local excision without adjuvant radiotherapy. In their series of 22 patients with T1 and 15 patients with T2 lesions overall survival was 75%, whereas the corrected survival rate was 90%.

Graham et al. (313) reported on the use of postoperative chemotherapy and radiotherapy, using 5-fluorouracil (5-FU) and leucovorin, with radiation in doses of 45 Gy plus a perineal boost of 9 Gy. Three of 14 patients so treated experienced grade 3 to 4 toxicity manifested by cystitis, proctitis, or perineal skin desquamation, but there were no local recurrences and only one case of distant metastases.

Russel et al. (314) assigned 65 eligible patients into one of three treatment groups following local excision: observation, or adjuvant treatment with 5-FU fluorouracil and one of two different dose levels of locoregional radiation. Minimum follow-up was five years and median follow-up was 6.1 years. Locoregional failure correlated with T-category revealed: T1, 4%; T2, 16%; T3, 23%. Locoregional failure escalated with percentage involvement of the rectal circumference; 6% among patients with carcinomas involving 20% or less of the rectal circumference, and 18% among patients with carcinomas involving 21% to 40% of the circumference. Distant dissemination rose with T-category with 4% T1, 12% T2, and 31% T3. Actuarial freedom from pelvic relapse at five years was 88% based on the entire study population and 86% for the less favorable patients treated with adjuvant radiation and 5-FU.

Chakravarti et al. (292) reported on 99 patients with T1 or T2 carcinomas, 52 patients treated by local excision alone, and 47 patients treated by local excision plus adjuvant irradiation. Twenty-six of these 47 patients were treated by irradiation in combination with 5 fluorouracil chemotherapy. The five-year actuarial local control and recurrence-free survival rates were 72% and 66%, respectively, for the local excision alone group and 90% and 74%, respectively for the adjuvant irradiation group. This improvement in outcome was evident despite the presence of a higher risk patient population in the adjuvant irradiation group. Adverse pathologic features such as poorly differentiated histology and lymphatic or blood vessel invasion decreased local control and recurrence free survival rates in the local excision only group. Adjuvant radiation significantly improved five-year outcomes in patients with high-risk pathologic features. Furthermore, adjuvant radiotherapy extended the time to recurrence from 13.5 months to 55 months. The authors recommend adjuvant chemoradiation for all patients undergoing local excision for T2 carcinomas and for T1 carcinomas with high-risk pathologic features. The four cases of late local failures beyond five years in the adjuvant irradiation group underlines the need for careful long-term follow-up in these patients. The authors reviewed five other studies with local excision plus postoperative radiotherapy that had reported local control from 76% to 86% and five-year survivals, 75% to 85%.

The Cancer and Leukemia Group B (CALGB) and collaborators (293) reviewed 177 patients who had T1/T2 carcinomas less than or equal to 4 cm in diameter, which encompassed less than or equal to 40% of the bowel circumference, and were less than or equal to 10 cm from the dentate line. Of the 177 patients, 59 patients who were eligible for the study had T1 carcinomas and received no further treatments; 51 eligible T2 patients received external beam irradiation (5400 cGY/30 fractions five days/week) and 5-FU after local excision. At 48 months median follow-up, six-year survival and failure-free survival rates of the eligible patients were 85% and 78%, respectively. Eight patients died of disease, four with distant recurrence only. One T1 patient is alive with distant disease. Two T1 and seven T2 patients experienced isolated local recurrences; all underwent salvage abdominoperineal resection. After APR, one T1 and four of the seven T2 patients were free of disease at the time of last visit (two to seven years). One T1 patient died of local and distant disease. Three of seven T2 patients died with distant disease. The authors concluded that sphincter preservation could be achieved with excellent carcinoma control without initial sacrifice of anal function in most patients.

Our own experience with 64 cases, 11 of which received adjuvant radiotherapy revealed the incidence of local recurrence increased with advancing stage: T1 13%, T2 24%, T3 71% (281). However, the addition of postoperative radiotherapy reduced the local recurrence rate of T2 lesions to 9%. Overall and disease-free survival at five years was 71% and 83%. Salvage operations were performed in 67% of patients with locoregional recurrence and the five-year sphincter preservation rate was 90%. Predictors of local failure in our study were size greater than 3 cm, transmural penetration (T3), and positive marginal status.

Taylor et al. (20) reported that the addition of adjuvant radiotherapy reduced their recurrence after local excision from 46% to 13% and the five-year disease-free survival increased from 52% to 81%. Varma et al. (294) reported that none of their 19 patients who received adjuvant therapy, either chemotherapy or radiotherapy developed a local recurrence. Steele et al. (293) conducted a prospective multi-institutional trial to determine whether survival of patients with T1 and T2 carcinomas of the rectum who were treated with local excision would be comparable to historical controls treated with radical operation (APR). T1 patients ($n = 59$) had no further treatment while T2 patients ($n = 51$) received postoperative radiation (5400 cGY/30 fractions) and 5-FU (500 mg/m^2 days 1–3 and 29–31). For T1 lesions, the six-year overall survival was 87% and disease-free survival 83% and the corresponding values for T2 lesions 85% and 71%. Patients who developed only local recurrence (T1 and T2) all underwent salvage APR. At 48 months comparison of their experiences with historical data from the National Cancer Database (American Joint Commission on Cancer) showed no significant therapeutic disadvantage in the sphincter-sparing approach. The follow-up was too short to determine whether patients who failed locoregional disease can be cured by salvage radical operation. At the end of their study, they believed their data allowed the following conclusions: (i) sphincter preservation is not easy to accomplish in a uniformly defined manner; (ii) sphincter preservation approaches are significantly less morbid than radical operations; (iii) predictors of outcome are not yet assessable because of relatively few recurrences; and (iv) salvage therapy effectiveness is not yet determined.

Schell et al. (315) believe that patients who have initially bulky (T3) lesions and experience significant downstaging after neoadjuvant chemoradiotherapy, peranal excision appears to be a safe and effective treatment preserving sphincter function and avoiding laparotomy. They reported 74 patients diagnosed with locally advanced T3 rectal carcinomas. After neoadjuvant therapy, 14.9% of patients who had significant downstaging of their carcinomas were selected to undergo peranal excision of their residual rectal carcinomas. Carcinomas were located between 1 and 7 cm from the anal verge and were located in lateral, anterior, and posterior positions. Mean follow-up was 55.2 months. There were no local recurrences, nodal metastases, or operative mortalities. Nine percent developed distant metastases (pulmonary nodules) and lived 30 months after peranal excision.

Ruo et al. (316) evaluated the clinical outcome of 10 selected patients with invasive distal rectal carcinoma (six T2 and four T3) treated with preoperative radiotherapy with or without 5-FU based chemotherapy. A full thickness local excision was performed four to six weeks after completion of radiotherapy, primarily because of co-morbid diseases or patient refusal or permanent colostomy. Median follow-up was 28.5 months. Only one positive microscopic margin was detected. Among three cases of complete pathological response, two remain without evidence of disease. All patients retained sphincter function and avoided creation of a stoma. Two patients developed recurrence, one with widespread disease including pelvic recurrence 26 months after operation and the other with distant disease only at 23 months. There were four deaths, two unrelated to carcinoma, one of undetermined cause after seven years and one after widespread recurrence at 26 months with death four months later. Two-year actuarial survival was 78%. This pilot study demonstrated that preoperative radiotherapy and full thickness local excision avoids major abdominal operation yet facilitates sphincter preservation, excision with negative margins and short-term local control in selected patients with distal rectal carcinoma.

Electrocoagulation

Many carcinomas of the lower and middle thirds of the rectum are treated locally for cure with electrocoagulation by some surgeons. Details and results of this technique are described in Chapter 19. The results have been encouraging.

Intracavitary Radiotherapy

In 1973, Papillon (317) of Lyons, France, introduced a method for delivering high-dose radiotherapy to a small area in a short period of time. The technique, known as the Papillon treatment of contact radiotherapy, or intracavitary radiotherapy, is attractive in that it requires no operation. It can be delivered in an outpatient setting and is reported to have good results in selected patients. The radiation is delivered through a special 3 cm-diameter proctoscope. At each visit 3000 rads can be delivered, and lesions usually respond after the delivery of 9 to 15 Gy. Selected lesions should be within 10 cm from the anal verge, preferably not larger than 3 cm and certainly not more than 3 × 5 cm, in which case overlapping fields can be delivered. The lesions should be polypoid, well differentiated, or moderately well differentiated and have no evidence of regional lymph node involvement. With these restrictions, less than 10% of rectal carcinomas are suitable for intracavitary radiotherapy (318).

In his most recent report of 310 patients, Papillon (318) noted a five-year survival rate of 76%, a local recurrence rate of 8.3%, and a death rate from carcinoma of 7.7%. The results of other investigators reviewed by Papillon reveal a local recurrence of 18% to 30%.

For elderly poor-risk patients with TNM classification T2 or T3 carcinomas of the lower third of the rectum, Papillon established a protocol of a short intensive course of external beam irradiation (30 Gy over 12 days) followed two months later by intracavitary radiation. In a series of 71 patients followed up for more than three years, the death rate from carcinoma was 11%, and the death rate from intercurrent disease was 27%. At five years, the death rate from carcinoma was 16%.

Sischy et al. (319) applied intracavitary radiotherapy successfully for a selected group of 192 patients and reported local control in 95% and five-year survival rates of 94%. They believe this form of treatment may be applicable in 15% to 20% of all rectal carcinomas. Hull et al. (320) reviewed 126 patients who received endocavitary radiotherapy with curative intent. With a mean time to recurrence of 16.1 (range 1–56) months, 29% of patients had a recurrence. Following additional treatments, 14 additional patients were rendered free of disease. They concluded endocavitary irradiation initially rendered 71% of patients free of disease. With additional treatment another 11% were rendered free of disease. In the subgroup of patients followed more than five years, 68% had no evidence of disease at follow-up after endocavitary irradiation, and 91% had no evidence of disease with additional treatment. The size of the lesion, differentiation, morphology, and distance from the anal verge did not influence recurrence. Debulking or operative excision before endocavitary irradiation did not increase recurrence.

Horiot et al. (321) reported on 200 patients treated with intracavitary radiotherapy. Local failure occurred in 4.4% of patients with T1 lesions and 19.5% in those with T2 lesions and nodal failure in 0.9% of T1 lesions and 9.2% of those with T2 lesions. Ultimate local control after salvage of failures was 94.5%. A functional sphincter was preserved in 95% of patients with local control. Reed et al. (322) reported 32 patients who received 75 to 120 Gy of endocavitary radiation (2–4 doses of 30 Gy at three-week intervals). The carcinomas were polypoid in 22 patients, sessile in five, and ulcerated in five. After a mean follow-up of 43 months (range, 6–103 months) four of five patients with ulcerated lesions developed recurrence (80%) compared to only 15% for sessile or polypoid lesions. Furthermore, time to recurrence was shorter in the group with ulcerated lesions. The authors recommended that these patients should be considered for operation initially. Schild et al. (323) evaluated the results of 20 patients treated with curative intent. Radiation doses ranged from 20 to 155 Gy and one to four fractions. In follow-up from 5 to 84 months (median, 55 months), local control was achieved in 18 of 20 patients (89%) and the five-year survival rate was 76%.

We reported the clinical outcome of 15 patients with low rectal adenocarcinoma treated with the long source–skin distance of endorectal irradiation technique (324). This method was designed at McGill University in 1986 as an alternative to the standard short source–skin distance rectal irradiation that was developed by Papillon. The only preparation required is two cleansing enemas prior to treatment. Fourteen patients were treated with curative intent and one for palliation. The median total dose was 85 Gy (range, 60–135 Gy) in a median of three fractions (range, 3–5) over a median treatment time of five weeks (range, 2–9.5 weeks). With a mean follow-up of 39 months and a median of 24 months (range, 3 months to 8.7 years), actuarial overall survival and disease-free survival rates were 50.8% and 71.4%, respectively, at 8.7 years. Subsequent to that report, one patient died of distant metastatic disease. One patient treated with curative intent required an abdominoperineal resection for progressive disease. Treatments were tolerated well by all patients. Four patients required steroid enemas for localized proctitis for a short period of time. They all responded well and had complete resolution of symptoms. Our results are comparable with those in other reports in the literature, and the complications are similar in type and frequency to other published series. The long source–skin distance technique may be an acceptable alternative to the standard short source–skin distance technique.

Winslow et al. (325) examined outcomes after salvage abdominoperineal resection for recurrence in 38 patients after endocavitary radiation. The mean time to recurrence after completion of endocavitary radiation was 21 months with 29% having persistent disease, 63% recurrent disease, and 8% a second primary. At abdominoperineal resection, 47% had transection of the carcinoma, specimen perforation, or injury to the genitourinary or gynecologic tract and 24% had positive radial margins. The mean time to perineal wound healing was 56 days postoperatively with 36.8% taking more than 60 days. Re-recurrence developed in 45% of patients at a mean of 21 months after salvage, with a local control rate of 26% at 45 months of follow-up. Median disease-specific survival from completion of endocavitary radiation was 115.5 months with a five-year disease-specific survival rate of 66%. Patients with recurrent disease after endocavitary radiation had significantly better disease-specific survival than those with persistent disease (median survival 115 vs. 25 months). Although technically difficult and associated with a high morbidity, abdominoperineal resection salvage was possible in 55% of patients failing endocavitary radiation in this study.

Cryotherapy

Cryotherapy is another form of local tissue destruction. However, the technique is associated with considerable malodorous discharge and post-treatment bleeding (326). It has not found general acceptance. A noted exception is the report by Heberer et al. (168), who treated 268 patients by cryotherapy as a primary procedure and 20 because of locoregional recurrence. Indications for palliative treatment were high operative risk in 67% and advanced incurable and unresectable disease in 21%. Fourteen patients refused a colostomy or radical operation, and 19 patients had multiple factors. Three deaths occurred during the treatment courses—all due to perforation. Two of the deaths resulted from necrosis of the carcinoma related to cryotherapy, and one was caused by perforation of the descending colon due to chronic obstruction by uncontrolled intrapelvic disease. Predictably, results were favorable for the early carcinomas, 77% of which disappeared with no evidence of disease. With respect to quality of life, cryotherapy enabled 80% of all patients to avoid a colostomy. For the 162 patients without evidence of metastatic disease, the five-year survival was about 35%.

Laser Therapy

Mathus-Vliegan (327) reported on the use of laser therapy for the management of carcinomas with endosonographic evidence of infiltration no deeper than the submucosa without evidence of lymph node involvement. Of the 15 patients who fulfilled these requirements, together with 15 patients treated in the presonographic era, complete eradication was achieved in 78 patients. No recurrence was seen in a median follow-up period of three years. Since the authors believe eradication is possible in greater than 90% of cases, they suggest that curative laser treatment be considered in highly selected cases. Its role in palliation was discussed in Chapter 23.

External Beam Radiotherapy

External beam radiation has been used as primary definitive therapy for selected cases of carcinoma of the rectum. Cummings (328) reported the use of 45 to 50 Gy in 144 patients. He reported an uncorrected five-year survival rate of 22%. The rates were 36% for patients with mobile lesions and 11% for those with fixed lesions. He suggested it is possible to offer initial high-dose radiation followed by a period of observation of up to six months (provided the carcinoma is regressing) before recommending operative intervention. Sischy (329) has reported a similar experience. Most physicians, however, do not consider external beam radiotherapy the first-line recommendation.

SPECIAL CONSIDERATIONS

DISTAL MARGINS

Controversy has long raged over what should be the ideal, necessary, or even acceptable distal margin of resection. The distal margin of resection is determined by the likelihood of downward lymphatic spread and intramural spread of the carcinoma. Based on a better understanding of distal intramural spread, it would appear unnecessary to demand the traditional 5 cm distal margin, especially when it may mean sacrifice of the anal sphincter. Wilson and Beahrs (59) demonstrated that a 2 cm distal margin is probably adequate to encompass any distal intramural lymphatic spread. From the same institution Beart (330) reported that no significant differences appeared in 5- and 10-year survival rates in patients whose length of distal margin ranged from less than or equal to 2 cm to greater than or equal to 5 cm for those who underwent a low anterior resection. Several reports have suggested that the 5 cm distal margin is too stringent a requirement (10,58,254,331). Pollet and Nicholls (10) found no significant difference in either local recurrence or survival when distal margins of less than 2 cm were compared to distal margins greater than 2 cm. Vernava et al. (254) found that a distal margin of even 0.8 cm in the fresh unpinned specimen provided adequate clearance for most rectal carcinomas. In a review of 273 patients with sphincter-saving operations, Hojo (176) concluded that a 2 cm distal margin is adequate. Madsen and Christiansen (9) found in their series of 43 specimens that all potentially curable carcinomas would have been adequately resected with a margin of only 1.5 cm. Heimann et al. (332) found that patients having anterior resection with distal margins of less than or equal to 1 cm had an extremely high recurrence rate (36%) but that the rates of pelvic recurrence did not continue to improve when the distal margins were greater than 2 cm.

In a labor-intensive study, Kirwan et al. (333) examined 7626 sections with a mean number of 381 per "doughnut" for 20 patients who underwent a low anterior resection. In 19 of the 20 patients, no malignant tissue was encountered. In the patient in whom carcinoma was identified, the perirectal lymphatics were involved, which the authors believed represented lymphatic rather than contiguous spread. The authors concluded that the classic 5 cm margin of resection is not necessary in low anterior resection for carcinoma.

To ascertain the optimal distal margin of resection of sphincter-saving surgery, Shirouzu et al. (334) examined 610 consecutive patients who underwent resection for carcinoma. Distal spread was found in 10% overall, but in only 3.8% of patients who underwent curative operation. Distal spread was not seen in stage I; however, it was seen 1.2% in stage II, and 5.1% in stage III, but this was confined to within a 1 cm length. Most patients with distal spread had a lower survival rate and died of distant metastases rather than local recurrence. The authors concluded that a distal margin of resection of 1 cm might be appropriate clearance for most rectal carcinomas. Vernava et al. (335) also reported that distal margins as short as 0.8 cm do not prejudice cure nor do they increase the risk of local recurrence. Measurements were made in the fresh, not pinned, resected specimens. In a series of 243 patients, anastomotic recurrence rates for margins less than 0.8 cm were 30% vs. 10.5% for greater than 0.8 cm. The five-year survival rate in patients with distal margins less than 0.8 cm was 49.3% vs. 67.5% in those with greater distal margins. In a study of 55 patients, Kwok et al. (336) found distal intramural spread of greater than 10 mm in only three patients, all of whom had advanced disease.

Although most authors agree that the 5 cm distal margin is not necessary, dissenting opinions exist. Enker et al. (337) reported that for patients with Dukes' B carcinoma with a resection margin of less than 5 cm, the recurrence rate was 20% compared to 7% if the margin was greater than 5 cm. For Dukes' C lesions with margins less than10 cm, the recurrence rate of 37% compared to 7% if the margin was greater than10 cm. Perhaps the patients with distal margins greater than10 cm had upper rectal lesions and the survival differences were due to greater mesorectal excision. Tonak et al. (338) noted a local recurrence rate of 33% for margins less than 3 cm and only 13% for margins greater than 3 cm. Despite these reports, for patients with a well-differentiated or moderately distinct carcinoma, a 2 cm distal margin seems adequate.

Review of previous studies reveals that 5% to 19% of rectal carcinomas will have intramural spread of greater than 1 cm (339). Moore et al. (340) determined the adequacy of a distal margin of less than or equal to 1 cm in 94 patients with locally advanced rectal carcinoma requiring preoperative combined modality therapy. Distal margin length ranged from 0.1 to 9.5 cm (median 2.0 cm) and did not correlate with local recurrence or recurrence free survival. Estimates of recurrence free survival and local recurrence at three years for the less than or equal to 1 cm versus greater than 1 cm and the less than or equal to 2 cm versus greater than 2 cm groups were not significantly different. Their data suggest that for patients with locally advanced rectal carcinoma undergoing resection and preoperative combined modality therapy distal margins less than or equal to 1 cm do not seem to compromise oncologic outcome.

Nakagoe et al. (341) examined microscopic distal intramural spread in 134 consecutive specimens of resected rectal carcinoma. Distal intramural spread was noted in 24.6% of patients. Patients with distal intramural spread had a shorter disease-specific or disease-free survival time after curative operation than those without distal intramural spread. Most patients with distal intramural spread developed distant reccurrence. Distal intramural spread was an independent risk factor for poor prognosis in patients with rectal carcinoma.

It has generally been reported that patients with poorly differentiated carcinoma exhibit a greater extent of distal intramural spread; hence a longer distal margin is required even if the resection entails an abdominoperineal resection. However, Elliot et al. (12) reviewed 42 patients with poorly differentiated carcinoma of the rectum and found no significant difference in the five-year survival rate or in local recurrence between those patients who underwent abdominoperineal resection and those who underwent low anterior resection, despite the fact that the average distal margin of those who had a sphincter-saving operation was only 2.7 cm.

■ CIRCUMFERENTIAL MARGINS

A long overlooked factor in the development of local recurrence following resection for rectal carcinoma is the circumferential margin. Although the literature is replete with discussion and heated debate as to appropriate distal margins, Quirke et al. (342) emphasized the importance of obtaining an adequate circumferential margin in order to secure a cure. In the most recent report from that institution, Hall et al. (233) examined the prognostic significance of circumferential margin involvement in resected specimens after potentially curative operations. Of 152 patients having curative resection, 13% had carcinomas within 1 mm of the circumferential margin. After follow-up until death or a median period of 41 months, recurrent disease was seen in 24% of patients with a negative margin and 50% with a positive margin. Local recurrence, however, was not significantly different in the two groups (11% and 15%, respectively). They concluded that when mesorectal excision is performed, circumferential margin involvement is more an indicator of advanced disease than inadequate local surgery. Patients with an involved margin may die from distant disease before local recurrence becomes apparent. Wibe et al. (343) examined the prognostic impact of the circumferential resection margin on local recurrence, distant metastasis, and survival rates. From the Norwegian national population-based rectal carcinoma registry, 686 patients underwent TME with a known circumferential margin. None of the patients had adjuvant radiotherapy. Following potential curative resection and after a median follow-up of 29 (range 14–60) months, the overall local recurrence rate was 7%: 22% among patients with a positive resection margin and 5% in those with a negative margin (greater than 1 mm). Forty percent of patients with a positive margin developed distant metastases, compared with 12% of those with a negative margin. Therefore, what is the value of extending the distal margin for 2 to 5 cm if the lateral margins of resection are involved? Information on circumferential margin is important in the selection of patients for postoperative adjuvant therapy.

■ TOTAL MESORECTAL EXCISION

In recent years the subject of TME has become increasingly discussed and promoted as the "gold standard" in operative technique when operating for cure upon patients with carcinoma of the rectum. A growing number of publications have raved as to the efficacy and indeed the necessity for religiously adhering to the principle of TME in each and every patient who is to undergo a curative resection. Many of these publications can be classified as testimonials and hence it may be appropriate to review the recommendation and at least try to place it in proper perspective. To broach the subject it is important to consider the definition of what TME is, to review the mechanism of spread of carcinoma of the rectum with particular focus on how it pertains to TME, to consider why TME has been deemed necessary in particular on how it relates to the incidence of local recurrence after radical resection, and finally, to weigh the available evidence to decide whether TME is really required in the operative management of each and every patient who suffers from carcinoma of the rectum (344).

TME may be defined as complete excision of all mesorectal tissue enveloped in an intact visceral layer of the pelvic fascia that has no carcinoma at the lateral or circumferential margins. The procedure has been popularized by Heald since he and his colleagues first advocated the technique in 1982 (78). In fact, details of the operation (not labeled TME at the time) were described a half century earlier by Abel in his address entitled "The Modern Treatment of Cancer of the Rectum" to the Interstate Postgraduate Medical Assembly of North America in Milwaukee, Wisconsin October 21, 1931 (345).

The salient components of the operation as recommended by Heald are as follows (Fig. 25). Meticulous dissection of the avascular plane between the mesorectum and parietes is completed under direct vision. Precise, sharp dissection is undertaken around the integral mesentery of the hindgut that envelops the entire midrectum. The excised specimen therefore includes the entire posterior, distal and lateral mesorectum out to the plane of the inferior hypogastric plexuses that have been carefully preserved. Anteriorly the specimen includes intact Denonvilliers' fascia and the peritoneal reflection. In their most recent publication, Heald et al. (346) stressed the importance of dissecting anterior to Denonvilliers' fascia until dissection is beyond the carcinoma in order to optimize outcomes in the technically challenging but rewarding operation. They describe the fascia as intimately adherent to the anterior mesorectal envelope. They describe a loose areolar tissue between Denonvilliers' fascia and the seminal vesicles. The desire to dissect posterior to the fascia is because it is perilously close to the neurovascular bundles and other authors believe this may be appropriate for posterior lesions (Fig. 26). The characteristic smooth, bilobed, encapsulated appearance posteriorly and distally reflects the contours of the pelvic floor and the midline anococcygeal raphe. This procedure adds to operative time and complications but is has been claimed that it eliminates virtually all locally recurrent disease after "curative" resection. By adopting this technique, the amount of the rectum with adequate blood supply above the levator is limited, and only 3 to 4 cm can safely be used for anastomosis. This may explain the high leak rate reported by Heald et al. (78,79) and their recommendation for diversion.

Hermanek et al. (347) stressed that the pathological examination of resected rectal carcinoma should always include a visual assessment of the mesorectal excision to ensure oncologic adequacy. The clinical practice guidelines of the German Cancer Society recommends reporting the distal extent of mesorectal excision (total or partial without coning) and excision in an inviolate fascia envelope. Macroscopic evaluation of the resection specimen is supplemented by stain marking after postoperative filling the inferior mesenteric or superior rectal artery with ink or methylene blue solution. They believe the pathological assessment of adequacy of mesorectal excision should be taken into account in selection for adjuvant radiotherapy. Sterk et al. (348) performed specimen angiography to confirm completeness of the removed mesorectum. The rectal blood supply comes almost exclusively through the superior rectal vessels. Thus the fascia covering the mesorectum forms, as far as the rectal vascularization is concerned, a closed compartment. The mesorectal vessels are enclosed in the fibrous avascular mesorectal fascia. They run close above the fascia. In the case of an incomplete mesorectal excision, the specimen angiography shows a stain leaking from the mesorectal fascia.

The rationale for proposing this operation is based on the observation that one of the mechanisms of spread of rectal carcinoma is retrograde extramural metastases. Pathologic assessment of resected specimens has been

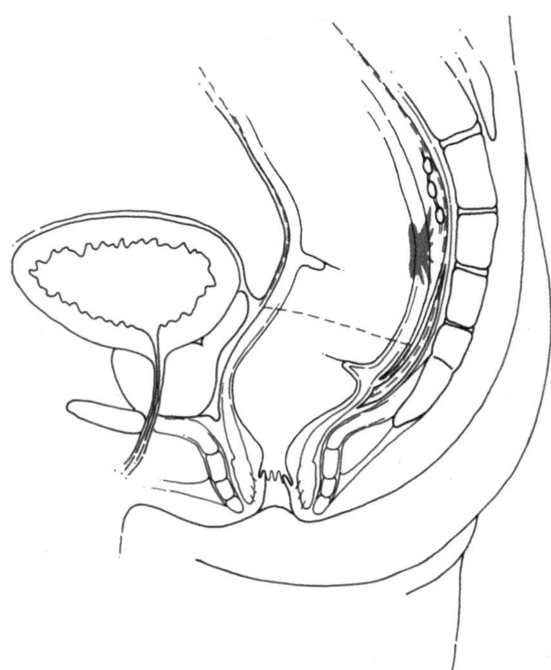

FIGURE 25 ■ Total excision of mesorectum.

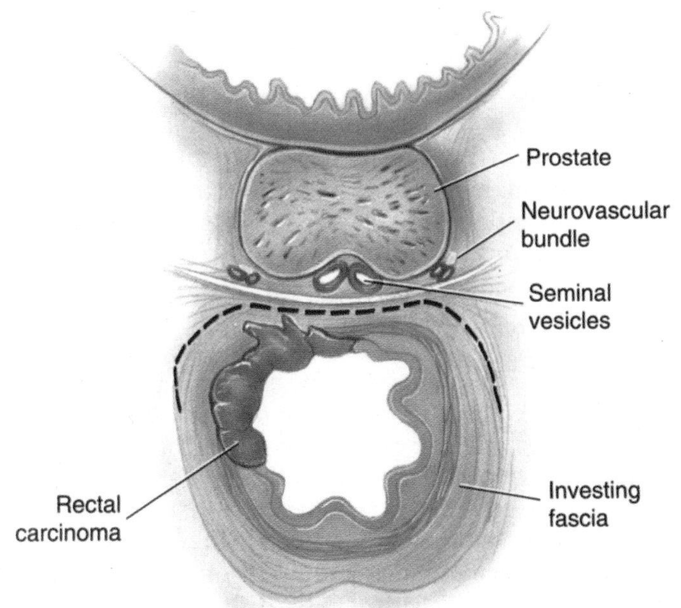

FIGURE 26 ■ The extent of resection for total mesorectal excision.

conducted by a number of investigators. In the study of 100 specimens, Heald et al. (78), found distal spread in five patients the furthest being 4 cm distal to the mural lesion. Cawthorn et al. (349), also related the extent of mesorectal spread as a prognostic factor after operation for rectal carcinoma. From a study of 167 consecutive patients, the authors noted that the five-year survival rate was significantly greater in patients with slight mesorectal spread (less than 4 mm) than in those with more extensive mesorectal spread (55% vs. 25%). Scott et al. (350), noted that distal mesorectal spread often exceeds intramural spread and found distal mesorectal spread in 4 of 20 patients who underwent TME. Patients with deposits in the distal mesorectum had a worse outcome at four-year follow-up, a greater risk of local recurrence, and an increased frequency of distant metastasis. Choi (351) found distal spread in 11 of 53 specimens studied but the furthest deposit was only 2 cm away.

Reynolds et al. (352) conducted a detailed pathologic evaluation of the mesorectum from 50 consecutive patients who underwent curative resection for rectal carcinoma. Of 21 patients with Duke's B lesions, five had discrete foci of adenocarcinoma with no evidence of lymph node metastases, as did 12 of 23 patients with Duke's C lesions. In 12 patients, the distal mesorectum was involved, and in one a mesorectal deposit 5 cm distal of the lower mural level of the carcinoma was retrieved. In five of these 12 cases, mesorectal involvement was greater than 2 cm below the mural level of the lesion. In five cases, overt mesorectal deposits were identified in the absence of mesorectal node involvement. It can thus be seen distal extramural retrograde spread has not been reported greater than 5 cm and rarely greater than 3 cm.

Prabhudesai et al. (353) studied the impact of extranodal deposits on the outcome of rectal carcinoma in 55 patients whose resected specimens for rectal carcinoma were staged as Dukes C or Dukes B. Distant metastases were diagnosed earlier in patients with extranodal deposits (mean 14 months) compared with controls (mean 37 months). On follow-up, 31% from the extranodal deposit group developed liver metastases compared with 11.5% of the control group. Local recurrence was seen in 17.2% of patients from the extranodal deposit group and 3.8% of the control group. Carcinoma-related mortality was higher in the extranodal deposit group (16 vs. 7 patients). The three-year actuarial survival was 48.3% in patients with extranodal deposits and 65.4% in those without. A significant association was noted between the number of extranodal deposits and intramural vascular invasion, extramural vascular invasion, perineural invasion, and lymph node involvement. These data suggest that extranodal deposit is a distinct form of metastatic disease in patients with rectal carcinoma. The association with vascular invasion and earlier development of metastases probably infers that a significant proportion of extranodal deposits may represent blood born spread. These foci of malignant cells should be considered as indicators of poor prognosis.

The rationale for advocating TME is that Heald believes local recurrence is the result of spread of carcinoma into the mesorectum. A very large range of local recurrences have been reported after radical resection for carcinoma of the rectum (3–36%) (Table 1, Table 6). McCall et al. (354) in a review of 52 articles in the literature in which at least 50 patients were included (10,465 patients) found a median local recurrence rate of 18.5% for operation alone. The true rates are probably higher because in their review, patients up to 20 cm from the anal verge were included and hence these would in most series be considered colon carcinoma. Local recurrence was 8.5%, 16.3%, and 28.6% in Dukes' A, B, and C patients, respectively, 16.2% following anterior resection and 19.3% following abdomino-perineal resection. Nine papers (1176 patients) reported local recurrence rates of 10% or less. Routine cytocidal stump washout in 1364 patients was associated with 12.2% local recurrence. Although not a comparative value in light of the other numbers, it did not appear to be very helpful.

Others also support the adoption of TME (355,356). Bokey et al. (357) have cited numerous reasons for the wide range of reported local recurrence rates. These include case mix, surgical expertise, definition of recurrence (pelvic only vs. pelvic and distant metastases), incomplete histopathology reporting, lack in clarity in definition of curative operation, variable length of follow-up, variability in data collection, and variability in calculation of local recurrence rate. Notwithstanding these difficulties, it is important to seek ways of decreasing the incidence of local recurrence.

In a 1993 report of patients of MacFarlane et al. (79) an independent analyst reviewed 135 patients with Dukes' B and C carcinomas of the rectum who underwent curative resection (126 anterior resections and nine abdominoperineal resection). With follow-up over a 13-year period, the actuarial recurrence rate at five years was 4% and the overall recurrence rate was 18%. Ten-year figures were 4% and 19%. The operative mortality was 2%. The five-year disease-free survival was 78% (Dukes' B, 85%; Dukes' C, 68%). Of nagging concern in the tabulation of their data was the 25% exclusion rate of what was considered to be incurable or believed to harbor residual disease on the sidewall of the pelvis. The authors further reported that the results from TME alone were substantially superior to the best results reported by the North Central Cancer Treatment Group (358) (NCCTG) with conventional operation plus radiotherapy or combination chemoradiotherapy: 5% local recurrence at five years compared with NCCTG 25% (radiotherapy) and 13% (chemoradiotherapy), respectively; and 22% overall recurrence compared with NCCTG 62.7% (radiotherapy) and 41.5% (chemoradiotherapy), respectively.

These large differences are somewhat hard to reconcile and may imply that residual disease remained more often in the NCCTG patients than those who underwent TME. Possibly some undefined reason may have contributed to the difference. I mention this because the pathologic studies conducted to determine the incidence of metastatic disease in the mesorectum distal to the mural lesion (i.e., the extramural retrograde metastases) reveal a relatively low incidence that would not account for the difference between the Heald and the NCCTG reported incidences of local recurrence. TME results are also superior to the National Surgical Adjuvant Breast and Bowel Project (NSABP), in which a five-year recurrence rate of 70% was seen in a similar group treated by operation alone (359).

Enker et al. (154) reported on 246 patients who underwent resection of rectal carcinoma according to the principles of TME (low anterior resection, 69%; abdominoperineal resection, 31%). The operative mortality rate was 0.8%. The overall five-year survival rate was 74.2% (86.7% for patients with Dukes' B and 64% for patients with Dukes' C lesions). Adjuvant radiotherapy with or without chemotherapy was administered to 70 patients. Pelvic recurrences were observed in 7.3%. They believe TME is compatible with both autonomic nerve and sphincter preservation, thus preserving sexual and urinary function in most patients. Furthermore, statistics revealed that adjuvant radiation therapy was of no benefit in preventing local recurrence. The investigators' results led them to question the current role of combined-modality adjuvant therapy in patients who have undergone resection in accordance with TME. They noted that various trials of adjuvant radiotherapy have reduced the incidence of local failure to approximately 15% but that such adjuvant treatment has no impact on survival. The results of chemoradiation following conventional resection do not approach the rates achieved by TME. Furthermore, the morbidity and mortality of adjuvant treatment are frequently ignored. Situations these authors believe appropriate for adjuvant treatment include (i) patients with marginally resectable or unresectable disease; (ii) patients with N2 disease, perineural invasion, or multiple adverse pathologic features in the mesorectum; and (iii) patients with T3, Nl, M0 disease.

A summary of local recurrence of other authors reporting on TME have ranged from 0% to 13% with most in the 6% to 9% range (344). Wibe (360) who reviewed 3516 patients in the Norwegian Cancer Registry, reported on the largest series of patients undergoing TME. After a mean follow-up period of 36 months, local recurrence rates were 6.4% for low anterior resection and 8.2% for abdominoperineal resection compared to 11% and 14.3%, respectively, after conventional operation. Noteworthy was the fact that local recurrence rates in 25 departments operating on more than 10 patients per year varied from 1.8% to 20.6%. Ridgway and Darzi (361) reviewed local recurrence rates following TME from selected series with more than 50 patients combining 13 studies with 6058 patients followed two to 10 years. The average local recurrence rate was 6.6%. In a recent review, the five-year survivals have ranged from 64% to 83% (95).

In an effort to even further decrease the incidence of local recurrence, several investigators have added adjuvant therapy to TME. Local recurrence rates in these reports have ranged from 0% to 4.0% (344), but the adjuvant therapy has varied from series to series and from patient to patient within any given series and follow-up has been relatively short. In their comprehensive most recent review of the literature, Colquhoun et al. (362) analyzed seven case series that employed TME and found that with a follow-up of one to seven years local recurrence rates varied from 5% to 9%. In one study in which postoperative radiotherapy was employed, the local recurrence rate was reduced to 1.5% with a follow-up of two years. No meaningful conclusion can be drawn from these reports only to say that there may be advantage to add adjuvant therapy to TME.

The cost of improved survival is not inconsequential. Procedures require more operating room time, transfusion requirements have increased, and anastomosotic leak rates have increased to 17.4% (11%, clinical: 6.4%, radiologic) to the point that MacFarlane et al. (79) now routinely fashion a protective colostomy. In their detailed analysis of these later complications, there were 11% of major anastomotic leaks associated with peritonitis or a pelvic collection and 6.4% minor leaks that were asymptomatic and detected by contrast enema. All major leaks occurred at an anastomotic height of less than 6 cm (208). Major leaks were associated with failure to function in 11 of 62 patients with a defunctioning colostomy in 13 of 157 patients. Of the 24 patients with major leaks, three died and only nine patients with major leakage and a temporary stoma have had these closed. Nesbakken et al. (363) evaluated the long-term functional outcome after anastomotic leakage in the treatment of rectal carcinoma in 92 patients who underwent low anterior resection with TME. Eighteen percent developed clinical anastomotic leakage. The functional outcome of 11 of 12 patients in whom a stoma was subsequently closed and bowel continuity was restored without stricture was compared with that of 11 matched patients who had undergone low anterior resection without leakage. Nine patients made an uneventful recovery after the initial treatment of anastomotic leakage. Eight developed serious septic complications, of whom, four had a pelvic abscess. Five patients had chronic complications that precluded closure of the stoma. Patients who had experienced leakage showed reduced neo-rectal capacity, more evacuation problems and a trend to more fecal urgency and incontinence than control patients. Nesbakken et al. (364) examined the frequency of urinary and sexual dysfunction following rectal excision for carcinoma. Spontaneous flowmetry, residual volume of urine measurement and urodynamic examinations including cystometry and simultaneous detrusor pressure and urinary flow recording, was carried out before and three months after curative rectal excision. Forty-nine consecutive patients, 39 of whom had a TME and 10 of partial mesorectal excision were examined before operation at 35 again after operation. In two patients, a weak detrusor was detected before operation. Two patients developed signs of bladder denervation after operation. Transitory moderate urinary incontinence appeared in four other women. Six of 24 men reported some reduction in erectile function and one became impotent. Two men reported retrograde ejaculation. All the complications were seen in the TME group.

Kim et al. (365) assessed the safety of TME with pelvic autonomic nerve preservation in terms of voiding and sexual function in males with rectal carcinoma. They performed urine flowmetry using Urodyn and a standard questionnaire using the International Index of Erectile Function and the International Prostate Symptom Score before and after surgery in 68 males with rectal carcinoma. Significant differences in mean maximal urinary flow rate and voided volume were seen before and after operation but no differences in residual volume before and after operation were apparent. The total International Prostate Symptom Score was increased after operation. Five International Index of Erectile Function domain scores (erectile function, intercourse satisfaction, orgasmic function, sexual desire, and overall satisfaction) were significantly decreased after operation. Erection was possible in 80.9%; penetration ability was possible in 75%. Complete inability for erection and intercourse was observed in 5.5%. Retrograde ejaculation was noted in 13.2%. International Index of Erectile Function domains such as sexual desire and overall satisfaction were greatly decreased in 57.4% and 63.2%, respectively.

Urinary dysfunction may occur after mesorectal excision and pelvic autonomic nerve preservation in patients with rectal carcinoma. Kneist et al. (366) identified factors predictive of long-term urinary catheterization in 210 patients without significant urologic problems who underwent resection of rectal carcinomas with mesorectal excision. Eight patients (3.8%) required long-term urinary catheterization: two after complete pelvic autonomic nerve preservation (2 of 168) and six in whom a pelvic autonomic nerve preservation was incomplete (6 of 42). Incomplete pelvic autonomic preservation (odds ratio 13.8) was a predictive factor for major urinary dysfunction.

Peeters et al. (367) investigated risk factors associated with symptomatic anastomotic leakage after TME. Patients with operable rectal carcinoma were randomized to receive short-term radiotherapy followed by TME or to undergo TME alone. Eligible Dutch patients who underwent an anterior resection (924 patients) were studied retrospectively. Symptomatic anastomotic leakage occurred in 11.6%. Pelvic drainage and the use of defunctioning stoma were significantly associated with a lower anastomotic failure rate. A significant correlation between the absence of a stoma and anastomotic dehiscence was observed in both men and women, for both distal and proximal rectal carcinomas. In patients with anastomotic failure, the presence of pelvic drains and a covering stoma were both related to a lower requirement for a surgical reintervention. They concluded, placement of one or more pelvic drains after TME might limit the consequences of anastomotic failure. The clinical decision to construct a defunctioning stoma is supported by this study.

A novel solution to the problem of increased stool frequency, urgency, and incontinence following TME was described by von Flüe et al. (368). An interpositional ileocecal graft based on its original blood supply was rotated counterclockwise and placed between the sigmoid colon and the anal canal. In 20 consecutive patients, at six-month follow-up, 16 patients showed excellent and four patients showed good defecation quality with maximal tolerable volumes, compliance, and mean colonic transit time comparable to age and gender matched healthy volunteers.

Before fully endorsing TME other information must be considered. Quirke (342) emphasized the importance of adequate circumferential margins to secure cure. In a review of 141 patients undergoing curative resection 25% of patients were found to have involved margins. The hazard of local recurrence was 12.2 and for survival 3.2. For patients with a positive margin at five-year follow-up local recurrence was 78% compared with 10% for patients with negative margins. In a more recent report (233) the same group reviewed 152 curative resections and at a median follow-up of 41 months found a local recurrence of 11% if margins were negative compared with 15% if margins were positive. Overall recurrence was 24% for those with negative margins and 50% for those with positive margins. The authors now concluded that circumferential involvement was more an indicator of advanced disease than inadequate local surgery. Patients with involved margins may die from distant disease before local recurrence becomes apparent.

Lopez-Kostner (369) and colleagues compared the outcomes of the treatment of upper rectal carcinoma ($n = 229$) in which TME was not performed with outcomes of sigmoid colon carcinoma ($n = 225$) and lower rectal carcinomas ($n = 437$). The risk of local recurrence alone, local and distant recurrence, death as a result of carcinoma or any recurrence or death as a result of carcinoma was 3.5, 2.7, 2.1, and 1.9 times higher for patients with lower rectal carcinoma than for patients with upper rectal carcinoma or sigmoid colon carcinoma. The outcome for upper rectal and sigmoid carcinomas was the same.

Another important contribution was that of Bokey and colleagues (357) who reviewed a series of 596 patients who had no adjuvant therapy and had a five-year actuarial recurrence rate of 11%. In their study independent predictive factors for local recurrence were: (i) positive nodes (hazard ratio 5.5); (ii) distal margin less than 1 cm (3.8); (iii) venous invasion (2.6); and (iv) total anatomic dissection (2.0). Pertinent to this discussion these authors noted no difference in the local recurrence between those patients in whom the mesorectum was divided or fully excised.

So in this morass of opinionated authors and plethora of often confusing data, what conclusions can the operating surgeon draw? It seems clear that from pathologic studies cited and the operative results obtained, that TME for the upper rectum and possibly even upper part of mid rectum is not necessary. For patients with carcinoma of the distal rectum, a "standard" dissection in the appropriate plane "automatically" includes a TME. The key would seem to be careful not to cone down through the mesentery but rather to proceed in the areolar plane outside the investing fascia of the rectum and when the appropriate distal margin is obtained a sharp incision is made perpendicular to the bowel thus including in the mesorectum any potential extramural retrograde spread. Indeed upon review of Heald's original publication on the subject (78), it can be observed that he had stated that "this technique was not necessary for some upper rectal carcinomas which mobilized up so well that they could be resected like sigmoid lesions, i.e., the mesorectum was transected at least 5 cm below the carcinoma." I certainly support Heald's contention that precise operative technique is fundamental to a sound oncologic resection, but do not concur that TME is necessary for all patients undergoing operation for a rectal carcinoma. This dissertation in no way is to be misinterpreted as casting any disparaging remarks on Heald's enthusiasm for the procedure. On the contrary, he is to be complimented for drawing our attention to the serious problem of local recurrence following operation for rectal carcinoma and suggesting a plan of action to diminish the problem.

■ RADICAL LYMPHADENECTOMY

The role of extended proximal lymphadenectomy will be considered in the discussion on high ligation of the inferior mesenteric artery. The role, if any, of radical pelvic lymphadenectomy is unclear. Advocates of the extended procedure claim improved survival. A report by Enker et al. (154), in which TME was adopted, resulted in an improved survival rate of 74% and so they no longer adopt extended lymphadenectomy as a standard operative approach. A report by Michelassi et al. (148) found no statistical reduction in pelvic recurrence by the addition of pelvic lymphadenectomy. Hojo et al. (370) reported on 437 patients who underwent curative resection for carcinoma of the middle and lower rectum. Abdominoperineal resections were performed in 262 patients and low anterior resections in 175 patients. The overall pelvic recurrence rate was 12.4%. In a comparison of wide ileopelvic and conventional lymphadenectomy, local recurrence rates according to Dukes' stage were 0% and 5.2% for Dukes' A, 21.9% and 6.3% for Dukes' B, and 32.8% and 23.6% for Dukes' C, respectively. Corresponding five-year survival rates were 94% and 91% for Dukes' A, 88% and 74% for Dukes' B, and 61% and 43% for Dukes' C patients.

The operation, however, is associated with significant morbidity, which may include impotence, urinary bladder difficulties, possible vascular injury with subsequent deep venous thrombosis, and sciatic nerve injury. Hojo et al. (370) noted that the extent of operation increased intraoperative bleeding from 1500 to 1900 ML, the anastomotic leak rate from 16.9% to 22.8%, the incidence of long-term neurogenic bladder from 8.8% to 39.4%, and the incidence of impotence from 37.5% to 76%. In order to decrease the urinary and sexual morbidity that follows radical pelvic lymphadenectomy for rectal carcinoma, Hojo et al. (371) began selective preservation of the pelvic autonomic nerves. One hundred and thirty-four patients with rectal carcinoma underwent a curative resection (52 abdominoperineal resections, 82 sphincter-saving resections) with extended pelvic lymphadenectomy and selective pelvic autonomic nerve preservation. Pelvic autonomic nerve preservation was classified into five degrees depending on the extent of pelvic dissection. First-degree indicated complete preservation of the nerves; second-degree indicated destruction of the hypogastric plexus; third-degree indicated partial preservation of the pelvic autonomic plexus; fourth-degree indicated bilateral or unilateral preservation of only the fourth pelvic parasympathetic nerve; and fifth-degree indicated complete destruction of the pelvic autonomic nerves. Most patients with first-degree preservation were able to void spontaneously 7 to 10 days following the operation. However, 28 of 36 patients (78%) with fifth-degree preservation had not regained bladder sensation by the third postoperative week and were discharged with an indwelling catheter; 21 of 36 (58%) had not regained bladder sensation by the sixtieth postoperative day. The cystometric data indicate a progressive decline in bladder sensation and function with increasingly extensive pelvic dissection. However, preservation of only the fourth parasympathetic nerve (fourth-degree preservation) resulted in partial sparing of bladder sensation and voiding function. Evaluation of sexual function in males below 60 years of age revealed that only 12 of 39 patients (31%) recovered erectile function and only six of 39 (19%) recovered normal ejaculatory function in the first postoperative year. In most of these patients, the pelvic autonomic plexus was preserved (i.e., first-degree preservation). Four patients with partial preservation recovered erectile function. Complete pelvic autonomic nerve preservation is the best way to prevent urinary and sexual morbidity after rectal resection. The opposing goals of maximizing the chance for cure and minimizing morbidity must be individualized and balanced in each patient.

By contrast, Glass et al. (372) analyzed the results of 75 patients who underwent extended pelvic lymphadenectomy in an attempt to improve the prognosis but found no improvement in survival. By comparing the results of current series to those of patients previously operated on in the hospital, the five-year survival rates of extended resection and conventional techniques by Dukes' stage were Dukes' A, 100% vs. 82.4%; Dukes' B, 78.3% vs. 65.6%; Dukes' C_1, 29.2% vs. 40.4%; and Dukes' C_2, 25% vs. 22.4%. The authors concluded that extension of the conventional operation is unlikely to improve results. Moreira et al. (373) also failed to demonstrate a benefit in terms of local recurrence and survival rates.

In contrast, Moriya et al. (374) reported promising results using nerve-sparing operations with lateral node dissection for advanced lower rectal carcinoma. With respect to technique, nerve-sparing procedures were distinguished as three types—total autonomic nerve preservation, complete preservation, and partial preservation of the pelvic nerve with lateral dissection. In the authors' opinion, total autonomic nerve preservation should be applied to patients with Dukes' A carcinoma, complete preservation should be used for patients with Dukes' B, and partial preservation of the pelvic nerve with lateral dissection is appropriate for patients with Dukes' C, on the basis of findings from endorectal ultrasonography. Cutting the lateral ligament of the rectum, which consists primarily of autonomic nerves, is the most intense phase during this nerve-sparing technique. The dissection should start along the internal iliac vessels and advance downward to the middle rectal artery, while removing the lymphatic tissue covering them. By meticulous sharp cuts of fascia on the piriform muscle, the surgeon can expose the root of the pelvic nerves. In 133 patients who underwent this nerve-sparing operation with lateral dissection for lower rectal carcinoma, the authors analyzed survival and functional results, operative burdens, and modes of recurrence. In 84% of patients, an acceptable level of urinary function was preserved. The five-year survival rate was 67% in all patients, 88% for Dukes' A, 74% for Dukes' B, and 59% for Dukes' C. According to the number of positive nodes, the five-year survival rate comprised 83% of patients with up to three involved nodes, and 34% of those with more than four nodes. Local recurrence rates were 2.7% in patients with Dukes' B and 13% with Dukes' C. The authors believe at present, a pelvic nerve-sparing procedure with lateral dissection is the most promising operation, guaranteeing both adequate lymphadenectomy and preservation of urinary function.

In the most recent review of the controversy, Morita et al. (375) continue to support the use of lateral node dissection and pelvic autonomic nerve preservation, but in a commentary following the article Moriya now believes that the number of patients who have suffered loss of function (impotence and bladder dysfunction) because of lateral node dissection is no match for the very rare patient who benefits from it. Hocht et al. (376) analyzed data to evaluate the pattern of recurrence in rectal carcinoma with special emphasis on lateral extension. Initially 54% of the evaluated patients were N0, and the others were distributed evenly between N1 and N2; initial T stage was T1 in 2%, T2 in 24%, T3 in 60%, and T4 in 13%. Recurrent carcinomas were situated mainly in the posterior part of the bony pelvis. The pelvic sidewall was a rare site of recurrence and involved in fewer than 5%. Because most recurrences arise in the central pelvis extending surgery to include dissecting the iliac vessels would probably offer only a moderate benefit, which must be balanced against potential side effects. Fujita et al. (377) investigated the oncologic outcome of patients who underwent curative operation for lower rectal carcinoma to clarify whether lateral pelvic node dissection conferred any benefit. A total of 246 patients who underwent curative operation for stage II and III lower rectal carcinoma were reviewed. Forty-two of these patients did not undergo lateral pelvic lymph node dissection. There was no difference in survival among patients with stage II and III disease between the two groups. However, in patients with pathological N1 lymph node metastases, the five-year disease free survival was 73% in patients who had lateral pelvic lymph node dissection compared with 35.3% among those who did not. They believe a randomized trial is needed to verify the benefit of lateral pelvic lymph node dissection.

Nagawa et al. (378) evaluated the effectiveness of preoperative radiation therapy for advanced lower rectal carcinoma to preserve the function of pelvic organs and reduce local recurrences in a prospective randomized, controlled study. The patients were randomly allocated to complete autonomic nerve preserving surgery without lateral node dissection, or surgery with dissection of the lateral lymph nodes including autonomic nerves followed by oral administration of carmofur for one year. No difference was observed in either survival or disease-free survival between groups. There was no difference between the two groups in terms of recurrence rate. A significant difference was observed in urinary and sexual function one year after surgery. Their study suggests that lateral node dissection is not necessary in terms of curability for patients with advanced carcinoma of the lower rectum who undergo preoperative radiotherapy.

Koda et al. (379) examined whether lateral lymph node dissection with or without preoperative chemoradiotherapy benefits patients with rectal carcinoma. A total of 452 consecutive cases of curatively resected pT2, pT3, and pT4 middle to lower rectal carcinomas were retrospectively analyzed. Of these, 265 patients underwent curative lateral lymph node dissection and 155 chemoradiotherapy. Lateral lymph node metastases were identified in 7.7% of patients. Of the pT3/pT4 extraperitoneal carcinoma patients, 13.5/18.8% had lateral lymph node metastases. In the treatment of middle rectal carcinomas and pT2 extraperitoneal carcinomas, lateral lymph node dissection either with or without chemoradiotherapy did not improve survival rate.

Other surgeons have conceded that when lymph nodes on the lateral pelvic wall are implicated, the condition is essentially incurable, since removal of all involved tissue will probably not be complete. Hida et al. (380) investigated the therapeutic efficacy of lateral lymph node dissection. They studied 198 patients with rectal carcinoma who underwent lateral lymph node dissection. The rate of metastases to lateral lymph nodes was 11.1% and metastases to the lateral lymph nodes occurred more frequently with lower rectal carcinoma classified as pT3 or pT4 in the TNM system. The rate of local recurrence was 12.5% and the five-year survival rate after curative resection was 70.1%. The five-year survival rate in patients with metastases to the lateral lymph nodes was 25.1% and this rate was significantly lower than the five-year survival of 74.3% in patients without metastases to the lateral lymph nodes. Urinary dysfunction was observed in 67.5% of patients, and male sexual dysfunction was found in 97.4% of men younger than 60 years of age with prior sexual ability. They concluded the prognosis for patients with metastases to the lateral lymph nodes is poor and the improvement in survival rate from lateral lymph node dissection is minimal.

Furthermore, the operation will be prolonged, and the extended dissection will undoubtedly be associated with more bleeding and ultimately a greater morbidity and mortality. No convincing evidence exists to support a significant survival advantage with the radical operation to compensate for the increased morbidity.

■ CONCOMITANT PELVIC ORGAN EXCISION

The incidence of occult ovarian metastases from carcinoma of rectum and colon is about 6%. For this reason bilateral salpingo-oophorectomy should be considered, especially when the carcinoma is in the lower part of the rectum where the lymphatics communicate directly to the ovaries and fallopian tubes. The risk of this added surgical procedure is small and the benefit to the patient may be significant. Most of these patients have passed menopause, thus minimizing the adverse physiologic effect.

Lymphatic drainage from the lower part of the rectum also communicates with the uterus, cervix, and broad ligament. Theoretically a total hysterectomy should be performed, along with abdominoperineal resection for carcinoma of the lower rectum. However, because a hysterectomy may add to the morbidity and mortality, such practice is usually limited to only those patients in whom associated pathology such as direct extension of the carcinoma or large fibroids exists.

A rich lymphatic system communicates between the lower rectum and the posterior vaginal wall. A concomitant partial vaginectomy may be required in women with locally advanced rectal carcinoma. Ruo et al. (381) identified 64 patients requiring a partial vaginectomy during resection of primary rectal carcinoma. Locally advanced disease was reflected by presentation with malignant rectovaginal fistula ($n=6$) or carcinomas described as bulky or adherent/tethered to the rectovaginal septum ($n=32$). Thirty-five patients received adjuvant radiation with or without chemotherapy. At a median follow-up of 22 months, 42% of patients developed recurrent disease, with most of these occurring at distant sites. The five-year overall survival was 46% with a median survival of 44 months. The two-year local recurrence-free survival was 84%. The crude local failure rate was 16% and local recurrence was more common in patients with a positive as opposed to a negative microscopic margin (50% vs. 13%, respectively).

Positive nodal status had a significant effect on overall survival. Excision of the posterior vaginal wall if attached should be included in abdominoperineal resection for carcinoma on the anterior wall of the lower rectum. This should not add significantly to the risk of the procedure.

The seminal vesicles and prostate usually are not removed along with abdominoperineal resection of the rectum unless there is direct extension of the carcinoma into them. Bladder wall not involving the trigone can be excised in continuity. In the rare situation in which the bladder and prostate are involved by the disease, they can be removed if the patient is an acceptable medical risk and agreeable to the operation. Consideration can be given to a cystoprostatectomy and ileal bladder resection in addition to the abdominoperineal resection, but it must be remembered that this is a formidable undertaking and is associated with significant morbidity and mortality. The role for a procedure of this magnitude is clearly limited. If this procedure is being considered, it would be wise to seek the counsel of a urologist.

Sokmen et al. (382) reported fixation of the locally advanced rectal carcinoma at the time of operation as an important prognostic variable. It may be difficult to determine whether fixation is caused by inflammatory adhesions or by direct extension tethering the carcinoma to the surrounding pelvic structures. Of 83 patients with rectal carcinoma, 24% had locally advanced lesions. Perioperative mortality was 5%. Only 24% showed histopathological confirmed carcinoma adhesion into adjacent structures. There was no significant difference between the patients with positive and negative histopathological confirmation of malignant spread in terms of survival rates. The presence of local extension does not necessarily mean incurability and sound surgical judgment should dictate that in the face of a tethered lesion, must one extend the surgical intervention radically to resect any malignancy en bloc.

Orkin et al. (383) reviewed 65 patients who underwent extended resection for locally advanced carcinoma of the rectum. Their study included 37 abdominoperineal resections, 20 low anterior resections, and eight Hartmann's procedures. Attached viscera most frequently resected were the uterus, 32; ovaries, 37; partial vagina, 25; and bladder, 26. Examination of these organs revealed carcinomatous involvement in 57%. This extended resection represented only 1.5% of patients who underwent operation for carcinoma of the rectum. No deaths occurred; the incidence of morbidity was 20%, and the five-year survival rate was 52%. A similar experience was reported by Federov et al. (384). When a carcinoma is fixed to the sacrum, Sugarbaker (385) has advocated partial sacrectomy and en bloc resection. He reported a survival time of more than three years in four of six patients so treated.

■ PALLIATIVE THERAPY FOR ADVANCED RECTAL CARCINOMA

Palliative therapy for advanced rectal carcinoma constitutes a major health care issue. A workshop was held on this challenging problem and much of the following information was derived from the summary of that undertaking (386). About three-quarters of the patients with rectal carcinoma are treated with curative intent. The remaining 25% of patients are treated for palliation and half of these will undergo abdominal operation as part of their palliative treatment. Of the patients treated with curative intent, approximately 40% will develop recurrences that cannot be treated with curative intent. It can thus be estimated that in the United States 20,000 to 30,000 patients per year will require palliative care for rectal carcinoma.

The primary goal of palliative therapy is to maximize the quality of remaining life. Palliative care is a complex undertaking and requires collaboration of a multidisciplinary team. The treatment plan should focus on pain and symptom management and treatment should be commensurate with the expected improved quality of life. Most patients with incurable rectal carcinoma fear the development of severe pain. Reassurance and good communication about all aspects of the disease process in combination with optimal pain control by modern pain management methods should play a pivotal role in the palliative treatment regimen.

Investigations, especially when clinical findings include malnutrition, ascites, extensive lymphadenopathy and palpable metastases should be minimized. If operative palliation appears feasible, resectability and extent of abdominal metastases should be assessed with CT of the abdomen and pelvis. Endorectal ultrasound and MRI should be used only if resectability is uncertain. If the primary lesion is resectable and abdominal metastases are absent, further imaging studies, e.g., PET scan may be indicated. Diagnostic laparoscopy is occasionally useful to determine if palliative resection would be beneficial.

Rectal carcinoma may be deemed incurable for several reasons. The patient may have advanced locoregional disease or distant metastases. There may be significant co-morbidities rendering the patient unfit for operation or the patient may simply decline an operation that consequently results in the construction of a permanent colostomy. For the most part, operative palliative therapy is generally indicated if the patient will tolerate the procedure and if the operation has a high likelihood of relieving symptoms related to the carcinoma and maintaining normal functions to maximize the quality of life. Operative intervention is only one of several options for palliation. The indication for surgical palliation depends on symptoms, extent of local disease, expected duration of life, and perioperative morbidity and mortality. Indications forcing the surgeon's hand include bowel obstruction, rectal perforation with localized sepsis or fistula formation, rectovesical, rectoprostatic, or rectovaginal fistula formation, or fecal incontinence. Resection should not be considered if there is extensive pelvic disease, lower extremity lymphedema, invasion of ileofemoral vessels, extensive lymphatic involvement, sciatic nerve pain, bilateral ureteral obstruction, neural or bony involvement at a higher than S1/S2 level, DVT, multiple peritoneal metastases, nonresectable distant metastases (liver, lung, etc.), or if life expectancy is less than three to six months. Anterior resection with anastomosis is considered if clearance allows the rectal reminant to be longer than 3 to 4 cm. Increased risk of anastomotic breakdown due to preoperative irradiation, the disadvantage of a temporary proximal stoma, and the time to achieve good anal function should be taken into account and indeed may negate the creation of an anastomosis. A Hartmann operation is often a better alternative if the patient is willing to accept a permanent colostomy when anal function is poor. Perineal wound healing is obviated. Whereas posterior vaginectomy and hysterectomy are not a deterrent to palliative rectal resection, more extensive pelvic exenterations are rarely performed because of their high morbidity and diminished quality of life. Surgical treatment for patients with unresectable carcinomas is frequently limited to construction of a sigmoid colostomy for fecal diversion; this is now often performed laparoscopically. Construction of an end stoma with an adjacent small mucous fistula (end loop) avoids the disadvantages of a loop colostomy. Loop stomas are useful in patients with short life expectancy and with significant obesity. With extensive local disease but not complete obstruction a hidden colostomy may be created and the patient may succumb from metastatic disease before complete obstruction occurs. In a number of patients, colostomies are being replaced by endorectal debulking and endorectal stenting particulary for mid and low rectal lesions. Seldom may these lesions be amenable to peranal excision.

In the minds of some surgeons, it seems hard to justify a low anterior resection or abdominoperineal resection in patients who obviously have no chance for long-term survival. Because of the high morbidity and mortality, some authors have advocated lesser procedures (387). On the other hand, most of these patients are symptomatic. If untreated, the symptoms invariably become worse with progression of the disease. A colostomy without excision of the primary lesion affords little palliation and only adds to the inconvenience of stoma care. Although a colostomy may overcome obstructive symptoms, it does nothing to relieve the incessant diarrhea with bleeding and mucus discharge or the sacral and sciatic nerve pain. The most reliable way to diminish these symptoms is excision of the carcinoma-bearing rectum.

In a series of 125 patients who underwent palliative operative treatment, Moran et al. (387) found a median survival of 6.4 months for those who underwent a diverting colostomy, 14.8 months for abdominal resection, and 14.7 months for per anal excision. Longo et al. (388) reviewed a series of 103 patients, 68 of whom underwent palliative resection and 55 of whom were treated without resection (colostomy or nonoperative treatment). The postoperative mortality was similar in both groups. The survival time was significantly better in patients who underwent resection, but this is probably a reflection of the more extensive disease in patients who did not undergo resection. Resection may also improve the quality of life.

The optimal use of radical surgery to palliate primary rectal carcinomas presenting with synchronous distant metastases is poorly defined. Nash et al. (389) reviewed 80 stage IV rectal carcinoma patients to evaluate the effectiveness of radical operation without radiation as local therapy. Seventy-six percent of patients received chemotherapy; response information was available for 34 patients. Radical resection was accomplished by low anterior resection ($n=65$), abdominoperineal resection ($n=11$), and Hartmann's resection ($n=4$). Surgical complications were seen in 15% with one death and four reoperations. The local recurrence rate was 6% with a median time to local recurrence of 14 months. Only one patient received pelvic radiotherapy as salvage treatment. One patient required subsequent diverting colostomy. Median survival was 25 months. The extent of metastases and response to chemotherapy were determinants of prolonged survival. They concluded that radical surgery without radiotherapy would be able to provide durable local control with acceptable morbidity.

The results of the largest series of palliative operations were reported by Johnson et al. (390). In a total of 338 patients, the operative mortality for patients undergoing resection was 11.7%; colostomy, 5.3%; and diagnostic laparotomy, 6.8%. The carcinoma-specific survival rate was longer in patients undergoing resection, but this only reflects a bias of patient selection toward more favorable cases. The five-year survival rate for the palliative operation was 4.5% with a median survival of 10 months.

In a symposium on advanced carcinoma of the rectum, Gordon et al. (391) discussed the subject of palliative resection in patients who have established metastatic disease. It was believed that palliative resection of the primary lesion is very important because it eliminates the constant urge for stool, the bleeding problem, and the pelvic pressure symptoms. In these patients, an anastomosis can be done and the usual margin for a curative resection is not required. A low anterior resection is an option, even with liver metastases. There is also a role for palliative abdominoperineal resection, and patients who survive the procedure may have palliation for up to two to three years. In the presence of ascites, there is concern about the ability of the anastomosis to heal. If there is extensive pelvic disease and concern that there might be residual carcinoma in the pelvis, perhaps an anatomosis will not work well, and the patient will be better served by a colostomy. If an extensive portion of the patient's liver has been replaced by malignancy, perhaps nothing should be done. Endocavitary radiation, local excision, fulguration, or some primary control of the rectal lesion can be considered, knowing that the patient has a limited life expectancy of less than six months. Electrocoagulation and/or laser or intraluminal stenting may be used to open a channel through an obstructing rectal malignancy for palliation. These patients have a limited lifespan, and it is preferable to make them comfortable without a major operation, if possible. Nevertheless, there are certain situations when Hartmann's procedure is appropriate for palliation. If the carcinoma is large and bulky, removal of the lesion can prevent tenesmus, pain, bleeding, and impending obstruction. At the same time, if the carcinoma is located so low that an anastomosis would result in a perineal colostomy, Hartmann's procedure is appropriate. It alleviates the patient's symptoms and offers better quality of life for the time remaining.

Heah et al. (392) analyzed the outcomes of 28 patients treated by Hartmann's procedure versus 26 patients by abdominoperineal resection. Postoperatively, Hartmann's procedure group started oral intake at a mean of 2.3 days, and stomas were functioning at a mean of 3.1 days compared with 2.6 days for oral intake and three days for stoma functioning in the abdominoperinreal resection group. Hartmann's procedure group was ambulant after a mean of 2.4 days versus a mean of 3.2 days in the abdominoperineal resection group. Postoperative abdominal wound infection occurred in 18% and 19%, respectively, in the Hartmann and abdominoperineal groups. Forty-six percent of patients had perineal wound sepsis, and 38% had perineal wound pain in the abdominoperineal resection group. These complications were absent in Hartmann's procedure group. Postoperative stay was similar in both groups. They concluded that Hartmann's procedure offers superior palliation compared with abdominoperineal resection because it provides good symptomatic control without any perineal wound complications and pain.

In patients with a large resectable carcinoma, significant palliation can be achieved in terms of pain, tenesmus, and obstruction with a palliative abdominoperineal resection recognizing that the operation will not necessarily allow the patient to live any longer but will certainly make the patient more comfortable for the time remaining. If the patient is otherwise a good risk, abdominoperineal resection may be the best palliative procedure.

The prognosis and role of operation in patients with incurable rectal carcinoma was studied by Mahteme et al. (393). The authors noted that resection of the primary lesion in patients with incurable carcinoma was followed by a median survival of 7.5 months, approximately four months longer than that after laparotomy without resection. Massive liver involvement, abnormal liver function tests, peritoneal growth, or abnormal lymph nodes correlated with a short survival. Local symptoms demanded active surgical treatment in approximately 15% of patients with a retained primary carcinoma. A colostomy was necessary for intestinal obstruction in 12% of patients. The authors believe their results support a selective approach to patients with incurable rectal carcinoma.

In light of these findings, I tend to favor resection of the rectum or a limited low anterior resection for patients with tenesmus, excessive bleeding, or perineal pain. Exceptions are patients whose general condition is considered too poor to withstand the operation or the presence of malignant disease that has disseminated extensively.

Self-expanding metal stents have become a useful addition to the palliative armamentorium in the past decade. Stent placement is indicated in patients with obstructing rectal carcinoma who have extensive disease, who are poor surgical candidates, and who have incurable recurrent disease after resection. Stent placement does not palliate rectal bleeding. In experienced centers, stents are successfully placed in approximately 90% of cases. Stenting has been discussed in detail in Chapter 23.

Laser ablation is still a useful therapy for some patients, particularly when the predominant symptom is rectal bleeding. In patients with obstructing rectal carcinoma, several repeated treatment sessions may be necessary to achieve initial luminal patency and further sessions will become necessary every few months or as symptoms recur. Palliation of obstructive symptoms is achieved after two to five laser sessions in 80% to 90% patients and lasts up to six months. Complications occur in 5% of 15% of patients that are mostly minor, although perforation, sepsis, and death have been reported. Laser therapy is an important adjunct in patients with recurrent obstruction after self-expanding metal stent placement. Laser ablation is not effective in treating painful infiltration of pelvic nerves by the malignancy. Argon plasma coagulation is a cost-effective alternative to laser treatment for control of bleeding but it is less useful for treating rectal obstruction. Injection therapy of rectal carcinoma using alcohol or sclerosing agents has a great advantage of being low cost and simple. Photo-dynamic therapy, endoscopic electrocoagulation, and cryotherapy are less suitable because of side effects or complications. Photo-dynamic therapy is limited by the cutaneous photo-toxicity of the systemically administered hematoporphyrin.

Chemotherapy and external beam radiotherapy play an important role in the palliation of the incurable carcinoma. Lesions that are asymptomatic or minimally symptomatic can be managed with chemotherapy or with chemotherapy and radiation. Combination regimens (especially with newer agents Irinotecan and oxaliplatin) may achieve responses in excess of 75% for chemotherapy-naïve rectal carcinoma and offer a considerable chance for palliation and may offer a survival benefit. The addition of pelvic radiation therapy should be made dependent on the extent of extrapelvic metastases and the size of the rectal carcinoma. A large rectal carcinoma might best be offered pelvic radiation.

Radiation alone has definite benefits in relieving symptoms. Pain and bleeding can be treated with success in 75% of patients with low doses of radiation. However, symptom relief is relatively short-lived and can be expected to last for three to nine months. It is most useful in patients with advanced disease and a short life expectancy. Radiation therapy does not offer a survival benefit. Addition of chemotherapy will generally increase survival. Attempts have been made to improve palliation in patients with locally recurrent carcinoma by combining surgery with external beam and intraoperative radiotherapy if available.

Nakfoor et al. (394) reported on 145 patients with locally advanced rectal carcinoma who underwent moderate to high dose preoperative irradiation followed by resection, 93 of whom received 5-FU. At operation, intraoperative electron beam irradiation was administered to the surgical bed of 73 patients with persistent malignancy or residual disease in the pelvis. No differences in sphincter preservation, pathological downstaging or resectability rates were observed by 5-FU use. However, there were statistically significant improvements in five-year actuarial local control and disease specific survival in patients receiving 5-FU during irradiation compared with patients undergoing irradiation without 5-FU. For the 73 patients selected to receive intraoperative electron beam irradiation, local control and disease-specific survival correlated with resection extent. For the 45 patients undergoing complete resection and intraoperative electron beam irradiation, the five-year actuarial local control and disease specific survival were 89% and 63%, respectively. These figures were 65%, 32% for the 28 patients undergoing intraoperative radiotherapy for residual disease. Treatment strategies using 5-FU during irradiation and intraoperative radiotherapy for patients with locally advanced rectal carcinoma are beneficial and well tolerated.

Patients should not be considered for operation, chemotherapy, or radiation therapy if they have significant pre-existing medical conditions, are unable to maintain alimentation because of metastatic disease, or are so debilitated in their performance status that they are limited to bed-to-chair existence. Parenteral administration of fluids may provide some additional comfort, however, total parenteral nutrition or tube feedings have not been shown to be of benefit in the nonsurgical carcinoma patient.

■ HARTMANN'S PROCEDURE

Occasionally one encounters a carcinoma of the middle third of the rectum that can be resected with an adequate lower margin of clearance, but it is technically difficult to safely perform a low anastomosis, or the likelihood of local recurrence is high. In such situations, closure of the distal rectal stump with establishment of an end sigmoid colostomy is an alternative to abdominoperineal resection. Likewise, in the presence of an obstructing carcinoma of the rectum, where one is faced with poorly prepared bowel, Hartmann's procedure might be considered. However, this procedure should be performed with caution since the complication rate of pelvic abscess as the principal cause of death is high.

ReMine and Dozois (395) reviewed 107 patients who underwent Hartmann's procedure for carcinoma of the rectum. In approximately half of these patients the operation was considered palliative. In only 10% of patients was intestinal continuity reestablished. Doci et al. (396) reported a consecutive series of 50 patients who underwent Hartmann's resection for palliation because of advanced disease (62%), poor risk conditions and advanced age (24%), and intraoperative complications or a difficult primary anastomosis (14%). The overall operative morbidity and mortality were 80% and 8%, respectively, with pelvic sepsis accounting for 37.5% of the complications. The overall five-year survival rate for patients undergoing operation for cure was 46%.

An extended Hartmann's procedure is occasionally useful in rectal resections, because anastomotic, perineal, and functional problems are eliminated. Tottrup and Frost (397) reported 163 patients undergoing rectal resection with colostomy and closure of the rectal remnant. Pelvic sepsis developed in 18.6%. When the rectum had been transected less than 2 cm above the pelvic floor, 32.9% developed an abscess in contrast to 7.8% after higher transection. Other risk factors were male gender and missing foot pulses. Only 61% of pelvic abscesses healed after a median of 59 days, leaving 39% unhealed after an observation period of 277 days.

■ UNRESECTABLE CARCINOMA OF THE RECTUM

When confronted with a carcinoma that is unresectable, the surgeon has a difficult decision. The spectre of a future colonic obstruction may motivate many surgeons to perform an immediate diverting colostomy despite the fact that the patient does not have an obstruction and the surgeon knows many patients will die of metastatic disease before they develop an obstruction. The "hidden" colostomy, in combination with nonoperative therapy, such as radiotherapy, electrocoagulation, and, more recently, the neodymium-yttrium-aluminum-garnet (Nd:YAG) laser, provides these patients a better quality of life.

The "hidden" colostomy is not a new procedure. It was initially described in 1967, but is a procedure that is seldom considered or remembered (398). The technique of construction of the hidden colostomy is not difficult (56,398). A short transverse incision is made in the right upper quadrant over the rectus muscle and deepened through the subcutaneous tissue, anterior rectus sheath, rectus muscle, posterior rectus sheath, and peritoneum.

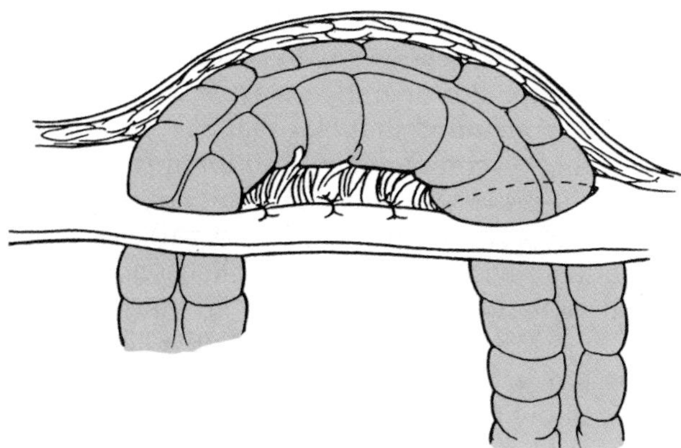

FIGURE 27 ■ Hidden colostomy.

The proximal transverse colon is mobile and generally easily delivered into the incision. The omentum is gently dissected off the right side of the transverse colon to facilitate delivery of the intestine. A small window, approximately 3 cm, is created adjacent to the portion of the intestine to be delivered. The purpose of the window is to allow the creation of a fascial bridge. The intestine is then delivered into the wound and three sutures of 0 Vicryl (polyglactin 910) are used to approximate the fascia through the mesenteric window (Fig. 27). Care must be taken to ensure adequate width of the bridge because, if a narrow bridge is created, the intestine may be acutely angulated and the patient may experience an obstruction at the level of the operative site during the early postoperative period (Fig. 28). A small subcutaneous pocket is created above and below the incision to allow better seating of the transposed colon. A few catgut sutures are used to approximate the subcutaneous tissue superficial to the colon and the skin is closed with 3–0 subcuticular Vicryl.

In the event that the distal part of the intestine becomes obstructed, it is a simple matter to open the colostomy. Using local infiltrative anesthesia, a short incision is made superficial to the transposed intestine. The colon is opened and immediately matured. The wound should be quarantined with drapes during the opening of the intestine and after aspiration of the initial flood of intestinal contents, a gauze can be inserted into each of the distal and proximal intestinal

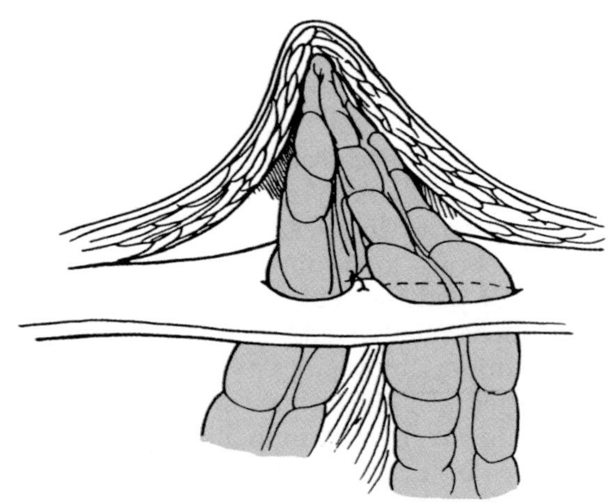

FIGURE 28 ■ Collapsed hidden colostomy due to inadequate length of fascial bridge.

loops while the colostomy is matured. The gauze is then removed and an appliance promptly applied.

Of six patients on whom I performed this procedure, two died without signs of obstruction. One patient with carcinoma of the ovary responded to chemotherapy and had no subsequent symptoms of obstruction. Two patients underwent opening of their colostomy eight and nine months later. After courses of chemotherapy and radiotherapy, one patient underwent a pelvic exenteration.

■ HIGH LIGATION OF INFERIOR MESENTERIC ARTERY

In performing abdominoperineal resections for carcinoma of the rectum, if the inferior mesenteric artery is ligated below the take-off of the left colic artery, a significant number of patients (7–11%) will have lymph node metastases at the origin of the inferior mesenteric artery. These metastases would not have been removed unless a high ligation had been performed (399). Based on this finding, many surgeons advocated ligation of the inferior mesenteric artery at the origin of the aorta, hoping to improve long-term survival rates. In a study of 179 specimens with high ligation by Grinnell (400), 19 (10.6%) had lymph node metastases between the point of ligation of the artery at the aorta and the level of its left colic branch. These were nodes that would not have been removed if ligation had been carried out at a point distal to the left colic artery. However, follow-up records of these 19 patients showed that none were salvaged by the radical procedure. This suggests that still higher aortocaval nodes were involved and were beyond the reach of operation. A study by Busuttil et al. (401) of treatment for carcinoma of the sigmoid colon and upper rectum also failed to show any benefit of ligating the inferior mesenteric artery at its origin. Indeed, the complication rate after segmental colectomy was a third as great as that for the radical left hemicolectomy. The hospital mortality rate was 1% after the former and 6.2% after the latter, whereas the five-year survival rate was 70.3% after the former and 56.3% after the latter.

Surtees et al. (402) reviewed the results of a series of 250 patients who underwent resection of carcinoma of the rectum at St. Mark's Hospital in London. For patients with Dukes' C carcinomas, survival rate did not improve if ligation of inferior mesenteric artery at its origin was performed instead of ligation distal to the left colic artery. Other authors have also reported the failure of high ligation to confer a survival benefit (403,404).

In a series of 198 patients with rectal carcinoma who underwent resection with high ligation of the inferior mesenteric artery, Hida et al. (405) found the incidence of metastases to lymph nodes surrounding the origin of the inferior mesenteric artery (root nodes) was 8.6%. Inferior mesenteric artery root nodal metastases occurred more frequently with pT3 and pT4 carcinomas. The five-year survival rate in patients with inferior mesenteric artery root nodal metastases was 38.5%; this rate was significantly lower than in those without inferior mesenteric root nodal metastases (73.4%), clearly an indicator of more advanced disease.

The only contrary publication on the subject was by Slanetz and Grimson (406). They reviewed a series of 2409 consecutive patients undergoing curative resection with detailed descriptions of the operative procedure and lymphatic drainage in the surgical specimens that provided a unique database to provide meaningful comparisons between high and intermediate level ligation. The probability of five-year survival rate increased with high ligation from 73.9% to 84% in patients with Dukes' B colon carcinomas and from 49% to 58% in patients with Dukes' C1 colon carcinomas. In patients with Dukes' A C (lymph node involvement but not penetration of the full thickness of the muscularis propria) carcinomas, high ligation increased five-year survival rate from 64.9% to 80.4%. In patients with Dukes' C carcinomas with involved middle level lymph nodes, the five-year survival rate increased from 20.5% to 33% and the death rate from recurrent carcinoma fell from 77% to 59% with high ligation. In patients with Dukes' A C carcinomas with four or fewer involved nodes, the five-year survival rate was increased by high ligation from 50% to 78.6% in the colon and from 40% to 71.4% in the rectum. When more than four lymph nodes were involved, the survival rate had been unaffected by the level of ligation. Although high ligation reduced distant recurrences, its greatest effect was observed in the incidence of local and suture line recurrence. The five-year local recurrence rate in patients with Dukes' B who were managed by high ligation was 11.4% compared with 18.7% with intermediate ligation. In patients with Dukes' C carcinoma the local recurrence rate was 20.8% five years following high ligation compared with 30.7% for intermediate ligation. In patients with Dukes' B carcinoma who were undergoing curative resections, the incidence of suture line recurrence was 3.9% following high ligation compared with 5.5% following intermediate ligation. In patients with Dukes' C carcinoma, the incidence of suture line recurrence was 6.9% with high ligation and 11.4% with intermediate ligation. They concluded in certain stages of colorectal carcinoma, the more extensive resection of mesenteric lymphatic drainage associated with high ligation appears to increase the survival rate and reduce the recurrence rate following curative resections.

High ligation is of no value in the treatment of Dukes' A and B lesions, nor is it of any value if metastases have occurred (407). High ligation is of potential benefit to the patient with a Dukes' C lesion only at the precise time when nodal metastases have spread to a level proximal to the left colic artery but have not spread to the origin of the inferior mesenteric artery (Fig. 29). This clearly constitutes only a small number of patients. The additional operative morbidity and mortality would probably negate any potential benefit.

■ MARKING THE RECTUM

When a polyp has been removed from the rectum and the pathologist reports the excised tissue to contain invasive adenocarcinoma, a low anterior resection may be recommended. At the time of operation it will be impossible to determine the level at which the lesion was located and the level at which the rectum is to be transected. To mark the site, the rectum can be injected with methylene blue at the commencement of the procedure. Injection of 0.25 ML usually turns the external surface blue at the time of laparotomy. If the injection is insufficient, the rectum will not be marked,

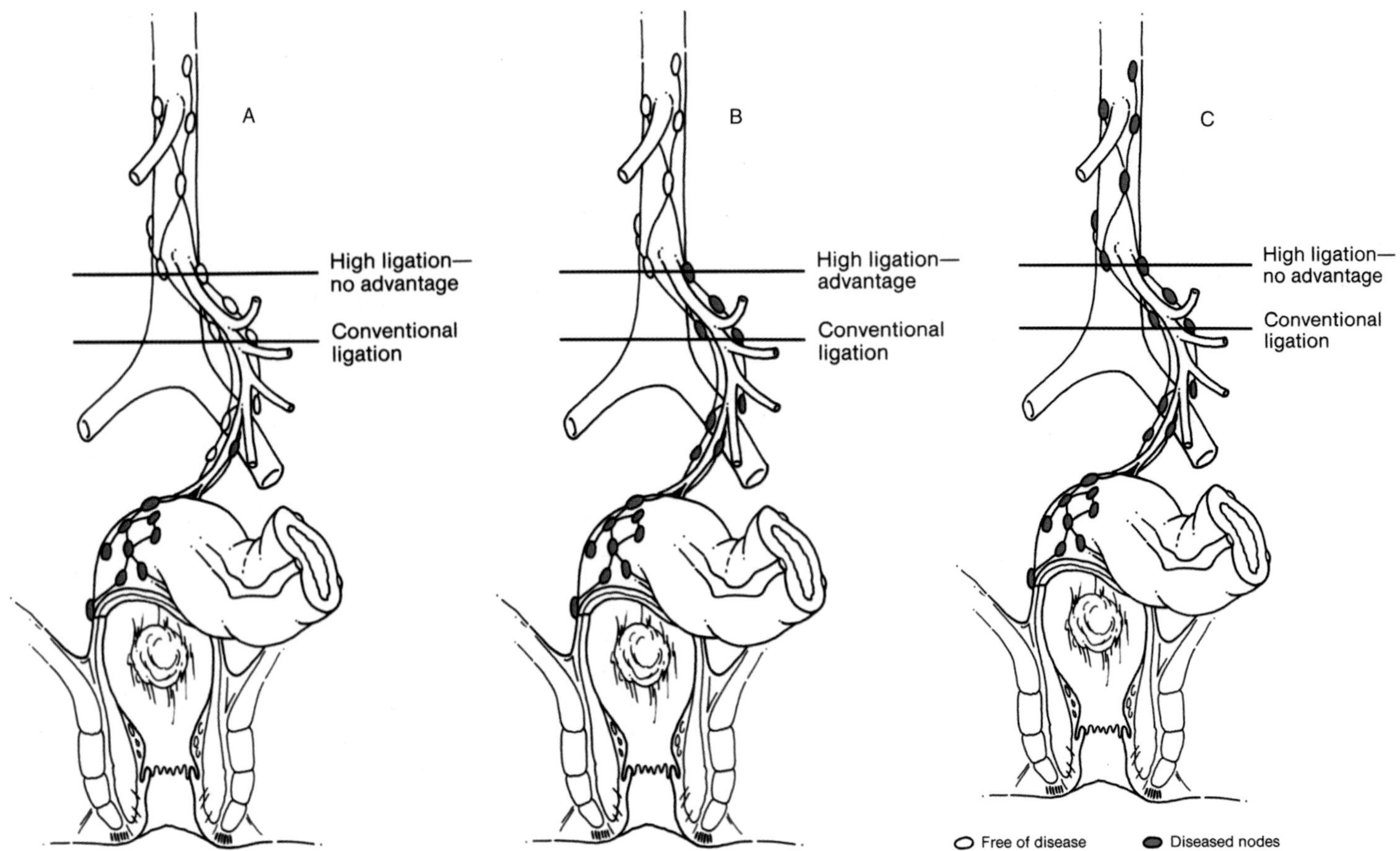

FIGURE 29 ■ Potential value of high ligation of inferior mesenteric artery. (**A**) Conventional low ligation would be sufficient. (**B**) High ligation provides potential benefit. (**C**) Proximal lymphatic spread is beyond confines of even high ligation. *Source*: Adapted from Ref. 407.

but if excess methylene blue is injected, the entire pelvis may be stained. Injecting the appropriate amount permits identification of the correct level for transection.

ADJUVANT THERAPY FOR CARCINOMA OF THE RECTUM

■ RADIOTHERAPY

Although the resectability of carcinoma of the rectum has remarkably increased during the past five decades, the five-year survival rate has not substantially improved. Radical operation remains the principal treatment for rectal carcinoma, but unfortunately failure, particularly local recurrence, is a common event (30–50%) (408). The symptoms of locally recurrent disease such as pelvic pain and altered bowel habit are often difficult to palliate and many patients die from locally recurrent disease. The search for additional treatment modalities to employ in conjunction with operative excision has been widespread during the past several decades. It has long been known that carcinoma of the rectum is relatively sensitive to irradiation. Both preoperative and postoperative adjuvant radiation therapy has been evaluated in randomized trials involving thousands of patients. Most studies have reported that both pre- and postoperative radiotherapy significantly reduce local recurrence but do not improve survival compared with results obtained from resection alone.

McLean and Duncan (408) published an excellent review of randomized trials of adjuvant radiotherapy and some of the following information has been derived from their article.

Preoperative Irradiation

Interpretation of results in the literature is difficult. Many of the reports are not controlled trials, the modes of treatment were different, and the dosages varied widely from a mere single dose of 500 cGy in the immediate preoperative period to multiple doses totaling 5000 cGy or more.

Preoperative adjuvant radiotherapy offers three potential advantages (408,409): (i) an increase in resectability and the probability of achieving a curative resection; (ii) "downstaging" of the resected carcinoma; and (iii) a reduction in the number of viable malignant cells, which may then reduce the probability of both local and distant relapses. Other potential advantages cited include decreased seeding of malignant cells, less acute toxicity, increased radiosensitivity because of more oxygenated cells, and enhanced sphincter preservation (410). The possible disadvantages include (408): (i) the loss of accurate surgical staging, which may confound the selection of patients for adjuvant chemotherapy; (ii) delay in performing the definitive curative procedure; and (iii) a potential increase in the risk of postoperative mortality and morbidity.

Furthermore, routine use of preoperative radiation will subject many patients to unnecessary therapy, because information from randomized trials suggests that 20% to 30% of patients have Tl or T2 lesions. These patients risk bowel, bladder, and systemic toxicity. Patients with unresectable disease or those found to have extensive liver metastases may be excluded from being given inappropriate additional therapy. Women in their childbearing years should be informed of the sacrifice of fertility and induction of premature menopause. The increasing availability of sophisticated imaging techniques such as the PET scan may decrease the number of patients who are overtreated.

The results of the European Organisation for Research and Treatment of Cancer (EORTC) were reported by Gerard et al. (411). The report included 466 patients who were randomized to groups of operation only or operation and 34.5 Gy preoperatively. High morbidity and mortality were noted in the irradiated group, although the values did not reach statistical significance. Both perineal wound healing and hospitalization was prolonged in irradiated patients. During a mean follow-up of 75 months, no improvement in the survival rate of irradiated patients was noted, but the rate of local recurrence decreased.

The Medical Research Council in the United Kingdom conducted a trial in which patients were randomly assigned into groups for no adjuvant treatment, a course of 2000 cGy in 10 fractions, or a single exposure of 500 cGy (412). With a minimum follow-up of four years neither form of adjuvant radiotherapy yielded a survival benefit, nor was the incidence of local recurrence reduced.

Other authors support the use of preoperative radiotherapy (413–416). Mendenhall et al. (417) reviewed a series of 132 patients with rectal carcinoma who underwent preoperative radiotherapy with a variety of doses. Compared with historical controls treated by operation alone, the local recurrence rate at five years was 8% versus 33%, and the five-year absolute survival rate was 66% versus 40%.

Some authors have reported improved survival rates (418). Preoperative radiotherapy has reportedly been beneficial in the treatment of unresectable carcinoma (415,419). It also has been suggested that no increase in morbidity or mortality occurs with preoperative radiotherapy (420).

A report on preoperative short-term radiation therapy in operable rectal carcinoma was provided by the Stockholm Rectal Cancer Study Group (421). The investigators randomized 849 patients in a controlled clinical trial (Stockholm I Trial) of radiation therapy (2500 cGy over five to seven days) before operation versus operation alone. At a median follow-up time of 107 months (range, 62–144 months) the incidence of pelvic recurrence was significantly lower (422). A reduction was observed in all Dukes' stages, but no differences with respect to frequency of distant metastases or overall survival were observed. The time to local recurrence or distant metastases and survival was significantly prolonged in the irradiation group. However, the postoperative morbidity was significantly higher among irradiated patients, and the postoperative mortality was 8% in the radiation therapy group compared to 2% in the operation alone group.

Pählman and Glimelius (423) reported on a multicenter trial in which patients with Astler-Goller stages B_2, C_1, C_2 were randomized to treatments of 25.5 Gy in five to seven days preoperatively (236 patients) and 60 Gy postoperatively (235 patients). No radiation-related complications or increased mortality were noted. The incidence of perineal wound sepsis was increased in the abdominoperineal resection group that received radiotherapy. Although the local recurrence was statistically lower after preoperative than postoperative radiotherapy (12% vs. 21%), with a minimum follow-up of three years and a mean follow-up of 6.3 years, the two groups had equal survival rates. From their review of randomized controlled radiotherapy trials, Pählman and Glimelius (424) believed that the reduction in local recurrence is higher if radiotherapy is given preoperatively rather than postoperatively. The effect of radiation is also dependent on the dose of each fraction and the total treatment time.

In an initial report from a Swedish multicenter study examining the role of preoperative irradiation in the treatment of patients with resectable rectal carcinoma, 1168 patients were recruited into a nationwide Swedish trial (425). Patients were randomly allocated to receive either preoperative irradiation (25 Gy in five fractions over one week) followed by operation within one week or operation alone. In each group, 454 patients underwent curative operation. The postoperative mortality rates did not differ, 4% after irradiation versus 3% after operation alone, but the postoperative mortality rate was significantly higher in patients treated with a two- rather than three- or four-portal technique (15% vs. 3%). Perineal wound infections were found more frequently in patients receiving irradiation (20% vs. 10%). No difference in the incidence of anastomotic dehiscence or other postoperative complication was found between the groups. In the most recent report on the Swedish Rectal Cancer Trial (426) it was stated that irradiation did not increase postoperative mortality. After five years follow-up, the rate of local recurrence was 11% in the group receiving preoperative radiotherapy and 27% in the group undergoing operation alone. The difference was found in all subgroups defined according to Dukes' stage. The overall five-year survival rate was 58% for those receiving preoperative radiotherapy and 48% for those undergoing operation alone. The cancer-specific survival rates at nine years among patients treated with curative resection were 74% and 65%, respectively.

The Stockholm Rectal Cancer Study Group initiated a second trial in March 1987 (Stockholm II Trial). The protocol was identical with that of the first trial, except that a four-portal technique was used, the target volume was reduced, and patients older than 80 years old were excluded. In both trials, the patients were treated with a fractionation dose of 5 Gy over five or seven days (treatment interruption occurred during the weekend). The Stockholm I Trial used a two-field technique to a large volume, including the anus, rectum, perirectal tissues, perineum, and regional lymph node stations (the inguinal lymph nodes, the obturator foramina, and the paravertebral lymph nodes) up to the level of the second lumbar vertebra. In the Stockholm II Trial, a four-field box technique was used and the treatment volume was reduced cranially. The latter technique is believed to reduce risk of radiation-related complications. The Stockholm II Trial closed when 557 patients had been included. In a preliminary report from this trial (427), the local recurrence rate was reduced, the length of survival improved after preoperative radiotherapy, and there was no significant increase in postoperative mortality in irradiated patients compared with nonirradiated patients (2% vs. 1%).

Holm et al. (428) assessed the outcome of abdominoperineal resection and anterior resection in the treatment of rectal carcinoma in relation to adjuvant preoperative radiotherapy in 1292 patients. Patients in the radiotherapy group received 25 Gy over five to seven days [776 patients (60%) had been treated with abdominoperineal resection and 516 (40%) with anterior resection]. The overall postoperative complication rate was 33% in the group who underwent abdominoperineal resection and 29% in those who had undergone anterior resection. In both groups, complications occurred more frequently in irradiated patients. The anastomotic leakage rate after anterior resection was similar in irradiated and nonirradiated patients (13% vs. 12%). The postoperative mortality rate was similar after abdominoperineal resection and anterior resection (4% vs. 3%). Postoperative mortality rate was increased in irradiated patients compared with nonirradiated and this was higher after abdominoperineal resection (7% vs. 1%) than after anterior resection (4% vs. 2%). There was no statistically significant difference in survival between the abdominoperineal resection and the anterior resection. Radiotherapy did not significantly influence the overall survival in either of the two surgical groups. There was no statistical difference in local recurrence between abdominoperineal resection and anterior resection groups, but radiotherapy significantly reduced local recurrence, regardless of the operative method. After abdominoperineal resection the local recurrence rate was 16% in irradiated patients and 28% in nonirradiated patients. Corresponding figures after anterior resection were 11% and 24%. The cumulative incidence of distant metastases was 27% after abdominoperineal resection and 26% after anterior resection. These investigators reviewed the causes of death after operation in an attempt to identify risk factors for postoperative mortality in patients treated with high doses of preoperative radiotherapy (429). The majority of deaths were from cardiovascular disease or infection. The authors noted that the risk of death was related to the preoperative radiotherapy technique, that is, patients irradiated with a two-portal technique and a relatively large volume compared with those radiated with a four-portal technique and a limited volume.

Holm et al. (430) reported on 1027 curatively operated patients included in two prospective randomized trials of preoperative radiotherapy for rectal carcinoma patients (Stockholm I and II trials). The goal was to assess whether long-term intercurrent morbidity and mortality were increased in patients allocated to the preoperative treatment. Preoperative radiotherapy significantly increased the incidence of venous thromboembolism (7.5% vs. 3.6%), femoral neck and pelvic fractures (5.3% vs. 2.4%), intestinal obstruction (13.5% vs. 8.5%), and postoperative fistulas (4.8% vs. 1.9%). For arterial disease and genitourinary tract diseases, no difference in risk was found between irradiated and nonirradiated patients. Radiotherapy significantly reduced rectal carcinoma deaths in both trials and also improved overall survival in the Stockholm II Trial.

Pelvic radiation-related complications are a direct function of the volume of the radiation-field, the overall treatment time, fraction size, radiation energy, total dose, and technique (431). Small bowel-related complications, a dreaded consequence, are directly proportional to the volume of small bowel in the radiation field. Surgical techniques employed to minimize toxicity to the small bowel from radiation therapy include reperitonealization of the pelvic floor, retroversion of the uterus, construction of an omental sling, placement of an absorbable mesh, placement of pelvic clips to delineate high-risk areas, and insertion of tissue expanders (431). Some radiation therapy techniques include using the prone position, multiple-field techniques (three-field preferred), computerized dosimetry, high-energy linear accelerator (greater than or equal to 6 mv) doses that do not exceed 5040 cGy to the small bowel, a standard fraction size (180 to 200 cGy/day), and bladder distention (431). The importance of technique was highlighted in the report from the Swedish Rectal Cancer Trial in which in-hospital mortality was similar in patients receiving preoperative therapy (4%) when compared with those who underwent operation alone (3%). However, in the group of patients irradiated with two beams, the rate of in-hospital mortality was considerably higher (15%) than in those irradiated with three or four beams (3%) (426). Sphincter function has also been a concern following pelvic radiation. A preliminary analysis of response to a questionnaire about anal function that was sent to all recurrence-free patients who had undergone a sphincter-saving procedure and were alive at least five years following treatment in the Swedish Rectal Cancer Trial indicated that patients who underwent irradiation had more problems with the number of bowel movements, incontinence, urgency, and soiling than those who underwent operation alone (426).

Dahlberg et al. (432) investigated the effect of preoperative high dose radiotherapy in long-term bowel function in patients treated with anterior resection in the Swedish Rectal Cancer Trial. Median bowel frequency per week was 20 in the irradiated group and 10 in the surgery alone group. Incontinence for loose stools, urgency, and emptying difficulties were all more common after irradiation. Sensory function such as discrimination between gas and stool and ability to safely release flatus did not however differ between groups. Thirty percent of the irradiated group stated that they had an impaired social life because of bowel dysfunction compared with 10% of the surgery alone group. The study indicates that high dose radiotherapy influences long-term bowel function thus emphasizing the need for finding predictive factors for local recurrence to exclude patients with very high probability for cure with surgery alone and to use optimized radiation techniques. The investigators now suggest that to minimize disturbance of bowel function, the routine inclusion of the anal canal in the irradiated volume in proximal carcinomas should probably be avoided.

Preoperative radiotherapy followed by proctectomy and colonic J-pouch anastomosis significantly increases nocturnal defecation frequency (36% vs. 15%) and diarrhea (39% vs. 13%) compared with similar nonirradiated patients but had no influence on the other bowel-habit parameters studied (98).

Goldberg et al. (433) reported a prospective randomized multicenter trial that compared preoperative radiotherapy followed by operation with operation alone for rectal carcinoma less than or equal to 12 cm from the anal verge (Imperial Cancer Research Fund). Of 468 patients, 228 were randomized to radiotherapy (3–5 Gy over five days within two days of operation) followed by operation and 239 to operation alone. Follow-up until either the patient's death or five years after the procedure was achieved in 97% of patients. The operative mortality rate for radiotherapy and operation was 9% compared with 4% for operation alone. Cardiovascular and thromboembolic complications were more common after radiotherapy and operation (13%) than after operation alone (3%). Of the 280 patients who had curative operation, 52% of those who had radiotherapy and operation and 56% of those who had operation alone survived five years. Local treatment failure was identified during follow-up in 17% of patients with radiotherapy and operation and 24% for operation alone. It occurred in 33 of 258 patients who had a curative resection (radiotherapy and operation, 9%; operation alone, 16%). Long-term survival was unaffected but long-term local recurrence was reduced by the addition of low-dose radiotherapy to the operation. Perioperative mortality, however, was increased.

Kerman et al. (409) reported an analysis of a 14-year experience of moderately high-dose (4500–5000 cGy) preoperative radiation as an adjuvant to low anterior resection of 95 cases of adenocarcinoma of the rectum. The treatment was well tolerated, without treatment-related mortality, and with a low incidence (5.2%) of severe complications. The local recurrence rate was 4.2% and the distant failure rate was 10.5%. At five years, the actuarial survival rate was 66% and the disease-free survival rate was 64%. At 10 years, the actuarial survival rate and disease-free survival rate were 52%. The authors concluded that moderately high-dose (4500–5000 cGy) neoadjuvant radiation in clinically resectable adenocarcinoma of the rectum in which one segment of the anastomosis is in the preoperative radiation field is a safe, effective adjuvant to low anterior resection and that it offers patients excellent local control, long-term survival, and sphincter preservation.

In an uncontrolled study, Bannon et al. (434) reported on sphincter-sparing procedures for patients with carcinoma of the distal 3 cm of the rectum following high-dose radiation. Following administration of 4500 to 7000 cGy, 65 patients underwent transanal abdominal radical proctosigmoidectomy and 44 patients underwent full-thickness local excision with a mean follow-up of 40 months. Local recurrence rates were 9% and 14%, respectively, and five-year actuarial survival rates were 85% and 90%, respectively.

Minsky et al. (435) reported 30 patients (two with T2 and 28 with T3) with rectal carcinoma 3 to 7 cm from the anal verge who underwent preoperative radiotherapy (46.8 to the pelvis and a 3.6 Gy boost) followed by a low anterior resection and coloanal anastomosis. The incidence of local failure was a crude rate of 12% and a four-year actuarial rate of 23%. The four-year actuarial survival rate was 75%. Function was good or excellent in 77% of patients, with median number of two bowel movements. The authors thought that this technique was an alternative to an abdominoperineal resection.

Myerson et al. (436) reported on 251 patients with carcinoma of the rectum who received 40 to 50 Gy followed by operation six to seven weeks later. The five-year rates for local control and freedom from disease were 90% and 73%, respectively.

Izar et al. (437) reported on 241 patients with rectal carcinoma who underwent preoperative radiotherapy with 36 Gy. The postoperative mortality rate was 2.9%. The most frequent complications were delayed healing of abdominal wounds, 18%; perineal wounds, 14%; and intestinal obstruction, 5%. Local failure occurred in 12% (Dukes' A, 10%; B, 12%; and C, 23%). Five- and 10-year actuarial survival rates were 70% and 50%, respectively.

Pacelli et al. (438) compared neoadjuvant treatment of preoperative radiotherapy (38 Gy) plus intraoperative radiotherapy (10 Gy: $n = 69$) to no preoperative treatment in a series of 113 patients with middle and lower T_3 rectal carcinomas consecutively submitted to TME. Overall, 68.2% of patients were downstaged by the preoperative regimens. Postoperative complications were comparable in the two groups. Five-year disease specific survival was 81.4% and 58.1% in preoperative radiotherapy plus intraoperative radiotherapy group and TME group, respectively. Corresponding figures for disease-free survival were 73.1% and 57.2% in the two groups, respectively. The rates of local recurrence at five years were 6.6% and 23.2% in preoperative radiotherapy plus intraoperative radiotherapy and TME groups, respectively.

Minsky reviewed 12 modern randomized trials of preoperative radiation therapy for clinically resectable rectal carcinomas. All used low to moderate doses of radiation. Overall, most of the trials showed a decrease in local recurrence and this difference reached statistical significance in six of the trials. Although in some trials, a subset analysis has shown a significant improvement in survival, the Swedish Rectal Cancer Trial is the only one that reported a survival advantage for the total treatment group (58% vs. 48%) (426). Given that the other 11 randomized trials of preoperative radiation therapy did not report a survival benefit, these data clearly need to be confirmed by additional studies (439). The most recent trial reported was the Dutch CKVO 95–04 study in which 1805 patients with clinically resectable (T_1 to T_3) disease were randomized to operation alone (with a TME or to extensive short course preoperative radiation therapy followed by operation with TME) (236). Although radiation significantly decreased the local recurrence rate (8% vs. 2%), there was no difference in two-year survival (82%). With longer follow-up, the five-year local recurrence rate was higher with operation alone (12%); however, it was significantly decreased (6%) with preoperative radiation followed by operation with TME (440). Second, even if future trials confirm a survival benefit, there are other equally important endpoints in rectal carcinoma that need to be addressed. These include acute toxicity, sphincter preservation and function, and quality of life. For example, acute toxicity in the Dutch CKVO 95–04 trial included 10% neurotoxicity, 29% perineal wound complications, and 12% postoperative leaks (441). In the patients who developed postoperative leaks, 80% required operation resulting in an 11% mortality rate. Hartley et al. (442) reported a 6% mortality with 5 Gy × 5 followed by TME.

Two meta-analyses reported conflicting results. While both reported a decrease in local recurrence, the analysis by Camma et al. (443) showed a survival advantage, whereas the analysis by the Colorectal Cancer Collaborative Group (439) did not.

The benefit of adjuvant radiotherapy for resectable rectal carcinoma has been extensively studied, but data on survival are still equivocal despite a reduction in the rate of local recurrence. At least 28 randomized controlled trials have compared outcomes of operation for rectal carcinoma combined with preoperative or postoperative radiotherapy with those of operation alone. The Colorectal Cancer Collaborative Group conducted a collaborative meta-analysis of these results to give a more balanced view of the evidence and to increase statistical precision. They analyzed individual patient data from 22 randomized comparisons between preoperative (6350 patients in 14 trials) or postoperative (2157 in eight trials) radiotherapy and no radiotherapy for rectal carcinoma. Overall survival was only marginally better in patients who were allocated to radiotherapy than those allocated to operation alone (45% vs. 42.4% at five years and 26.9% vs. 25.3% at 10 years). Rates of apparently curative resection were not improved by preoperative radiotherapy (85% radiotherapy vs. 86% control). Yearly risk of local recurrence was 46% lower in those who had preoperative radiotherapy than those who had operation alone and 37% lower in those who had postoperative treatment than those who had operation alone. Fewer patients who had preoperative radiotherapy died from rectal carcinoma than those who had operation alone (45% vs. 50%, respectively) but early (less than or equal to 1 year after treatment) deaths from other causes increased (8% vs. 4% died). Preoperative radiotherapy (at biologically effective doses greater than or equal to 30 Gy) reduces the risk of local recurrence and death from rectal carcinoma. Postoperative radiotherapy also reduces local recurrence but short preoperative radiation schedules seem to be at least as effective as longer schedules. In this systematic review of data from 8507 patients in 22 trials of adjuvant radiotherapy for rectal carcinoma, radiotherapy both before and after operation substantially reduced the risk of local recurrence in apparently curatively resected patients and moderately reduced deaths from rectal carcinoma. The largest reductions were in studies of preoperative radiotherapy with biologically effective doses of 30 Gy or more; no significant reductions were recorded in studies of radiotherapy schedules with low biologically effective doses.

One of the most important controversies with preoperative therapy is whether the degree of downstaging is adequate to enhance sphincter preservation. An analysis of 1316 patients treated on two previously published Scandinavian trials of intensive short course radiation showed the downstaging was most pronounced when the interval between the completion of radiation and operation was at least 10 days (444). In the Dutch CKVO 95–04 trial, where the interval was one week, there was no downstaging (445). Data from the Lyon R90–1 trial of preoperative radiation suggest that an interval of more than two weeks following the completion of radiation increases the chance of downstaging (446). Whether increasing interval between the end of intensive short-course radiation and surgery to greater than or equal to four weeks will increase downstaging is not known. This question is being addressed in an ongoing randomized trial from Sweden (Stockholm III trial). Even if preoperative radiation therapy were effective, I would not perform an anastomosis through a portion of bowel that several weeks earlier harboured a malignancy. Furthermore, sphincter preservation without good function is of questionable benefit. In a series of 73 patients who underwent operation, Grumann et al. (97) reported that 23 patients who underwent an abdominoperineal resection had a more favorable quality of life compared with the 50 who underwent a low anterior resection.

Guillem et al. (447) conducted a prospective analysis to determine the operating surgeon's ability to assess response to combined modality therapy (CMT) in 94 prospectively accrued patients with locally advanced rectal carcinoma. Clinical assessment using digital rectal examination (DRE) underestimated pathologic response in 78%. In addition, DRE was able to identify only 21% with a pathologic complete response. There were no clinical overestimates of response. None of the clinicopathologic characteristics of the carcinoma examined had a significant impact on DRE estimation of response. Given the inaccuracy of DRE following preoperative CMT, it should not be used a sole means of assessing efficacy of therapy nor for selecting patients following CMT for local therapies.

The timing of operation following neoadjuvant therapy for rectal carcinoma is not well defined. An interval of six to eight weeks between completion of preoperative chemo-radiation therapy and operative resection of advanced rectal carcinoma has been described. Stein et al. (448) studied whether a longer time interval between completion of therapy and resection increases disease downstaging and affects perioperative mortality. They enrolled 40 patients with advanced carcinoma of the rectum who underwent preoperative chemoradiation on a prospective trial with irinotecan (50 mg/m^2), 5-FU (225 mg/m^2), and concomitant external-beam radiation (45–54 Gy) followed by complete resection of the carcinoma with TME. The patients were divided into two groups with 33 eligible patients: Group A (four- to eight-week time interval) and Group B (10–14-week interval). There were no statistical differences in perioperative morbidity with three anastomotic leaks in Group A. The carcinomas were downstaged in 58% of patients in Group A and 43% of those in Group B. Nodal down staging occurred in 78% of Group A and 67% of Group B. The pathologic complete response rate was 21% in Group A and 14% in Group B and a residual microfocus of carcinoma was found in 33% of patients in Group A and 42% of those in Group B. These differences were not statistically significant. They concluded a longer interval between completion of neoadjuvant chemoradiation and operative resection did not increase the response of advanced rectal carcinoma in this cohort. Francois et al. (446) presented contrary data. They suggested that a long interval between preoperative irradiation and operation provides increased downstaging with no detrimental effect on toxicity and early clinical results. They randomized 20 patients with rectal carcinoma accessible to digital examination, staged T_2 to T_3, NX, MO before radiotherapy (39 Gy in 13 fractions) into two groups: in the short interval group, operation had to be performed within two weeks after completion of radiation therapy, compared with six to eight weeks in the long interval group. A long interval between preoperative radiotherapy and operation was associated with a significantly better clinical response (53.1% in the short group and 71.7% in the long group), and pathologic downstaging (10.3% in the short group and 26% in the long group). At a median follow-up of 33 months, there were no differences in morbidity, local relapse, and short-term survival between the two groups. Sphincter preserving operation was performed in 76% of cases in the long group and 68% in the short group. They believe that when sphincter preservation is questionable, a long interval may increase the chance of successful sphincter-saving operation. This issue continues to remain controversial.

Marijnen et al. (449) reported on the heath related quality of life and sexual functioning of 990 patients who underwent TME and were randomly assigned to short-term preoperative radiotherapy (5 × 5 Gy). Patients without a recurrence the first two years were analyzed ($n = 990$). Daily activities were significantly fewer for preoperative radiotherapy patients three months postoperatively. Irradiated patients recovered slower from defecation problems than TME-only patients. Preoperative radiotherapy had a negative effect on sexual functioning in males and females. Irradiated males had more ejaculation disorders and erectile functioning deteriorated over time. Preoperative radiotherapy had similar effects in patients who underwent a low anterior resection versus an abdominoperineal resection. Patients with an abdominoperineal resection scored better on the physical and psychologic dimension than low anterior resection patients, but worse on voiding.

With the information available at this time, the effect of preoperative irradiation on carcinoma of the rectum can be summarized as follows: the resectability may be improved in those patients with a fixed rectal carcinoma (450); malignant cells in the regional lymph nodes may be destroyed and thus may convert the disease to a more favorable stage; and local seeding of malignant cells, in addition to distant dissemination, may be decreased by altering the viability of shed malignant cells.

Currently, no unanimous agreement on the dose of radiation to be delivered exists. A frequently administered dosage is 40 to 45 Gy delivered over four to six weeks with a six-week interval before operation. For patients who have received radiotherapy, it has been customary to establish a protective ileostomy or colostomy, but some reports suggest that it is safe to perform an anastomosis if the radiation dose does not exceed 45 Gy (451,452).

A summary of recent published randomized trials is provided in Table 9. Caution should be exercised when data from different sources are cited, because each trial has different patient selection criteria, different radiotherapy schedules and fields, and different end points. As seen from the table, only the Swedish trials observed significant improvement in overall survival with preoperative radiotherapy. There is some overlap between the Swedish Rectal Cancer Trial and the so-called Stockholm II Trial in that 316 patients who were enrolled in Stockholm were also included in the Swedish Rectal Cancer Trial (426). The Sao Paulo study also demonstrated improvement, but only 68 patients were entered (454).

Postoperative Radiotherapy

Since most recurrent carcinoma of the rectum is localized in the pelvis and usually occurs in those patients with Dukes' B or C lesions, some authors believe that postoperative irradiation is more appropriate when details of the pathologic staging have been established. Gunderson and Sosin (457) cited the following advantages and disadvantages of postoperative irradiation.

TABLE 9 ■ **Results of Randomized Trials of Preoperative Radiotherapy**

Trial (Authors)	No. of Patients	Dose (Gy/Fractions)	Dukes' Stage C (%)	Local Recurrence (%)	Distant Metastases (%)	Overall Years Survival (%)
MRC 1 (412) (1984)	824	Control	46 No difference	No difference		38
		5/1	45			41
		20/10	36[a]			40
VASOG 2 (453) (Higgins, Humphrey, and Dweight, 1986)	361	Control	41			42
		34.5/18	35			43
EORTC (411) (Gerard et al., 1990)	466	Control	59	30	39	59
		34.5/15	55	15[a]	39	69
Sao Paulo (454) (Resis Neto, Guilici, and Reis Neto, 1989)	68	Control	47	47	32	34
		40/20	26[a]	15[a]	15[a]	80[a]
Norway (455) (Dahl et al., 1990)	309	Control	28	21	21	58
		32.5/18	18[a]	15	23	57
ICRF (433) (Goldberg et al., 1994)	468	Control	No difference	24		40
		15/3		17[a]		39
Northwest Region (456) (Marsh, James, and Schofield, 1994)	284	Control		37	36	70
		20/4		13[a]	43	70
Stockholm I (422) (Cedermark et al., 1995)	849	Control	28	28	37	36
		25/5-7	28	14[a]	30	36
Stockholm II (427) (Cedermark et al., 1996)	557	Control		21	26	56
		25/5		10[a]	19[a]	70[a]
SRCT (426) (1997)	1168	Control		27		48
		25/5		11		58[a]
Dutch (Kapiteijn et al., 2001) (236)	937	Preop 5/5	33	2 (2 yr)	15 (2 yr)	82 (2 yr)
	924	TME alone	36	8	17	82

[a]Statistically significant.
Abbreviations: MRC, Medical Research Council; VASOG, Veterans' Administration Surgical Oncology Group Trial II; EORTC, European Organisation for Research and Treatment of Cancer; ICRF, Imperial Cancer Research Foundation; SRCT, Swedish Rectal Cancer Trial.

Advantages

1. The total extent of the carcinoma is known and thus irradiation is unnecessary, particularly in those patients who have Dukes' A lesions.
2. Postoperative irradiation could be used in patients with either anterior resection or abdominoperineal resection and therefore would potentially benefit a larger number of patients. This treatment does not delay operation or alter pathologic staging.

Disadvantages

1. Postoperative irradiation has no effect on cells that may be spread at the time of operation.
2. Residual malignant cells in tissues rendered hypoxic as a result of operation may be more resistant to ionizing irradiation than those in a normal oxygenated environment.
3. A long delay in initiating postoperative irradiation could ensue if postoperative complications occur or perineal wound healing is delayed.

Hoskins et al. (458) reported on 97 patients who received postoperative radiotherapy. When compared with a historical control group of 103 patients, a statistically significant decrease in local recurrence at 3 years was noted in patients with Dukes' B_2 or C lesions. The Gastrointestinal Tumor Study Group (GITSG) trial consisted of a four-arm study in which patients were randomized to the following treatment groups: operation alone, chemotherapy, radiotherapy, or combination chemotherapy (459). After a median follow-up of more than 5 years, recurrence was seen in 55% of patients in the control group, in 46% who received chemotherapy or radiotherapy, and in only 30% of those who received combination treatment. Fisher et al. (359) reported on 555 patients entered into the multicenter NSABP Protocol R-01. Patients were randomized to receive operation alone; postoperative adjuvant chemotherapy with 5-FU, semustine, and vincristine; or postoperative radiotherapy (46 to 47 Gy). The postoperative radiotherapy group demonstrated an overall reduction in local and regional recurrence from 25% to 16%, but no significant benefit in overall disease-free survival or the survival rate was found. In summary, postoperative radiotherapy appears to decrease the risk of local recurrence but results in no significant improvement in survival rate.

Martijn et al. (460) reported a retrospective analysis of 178 patients receiving adjuvant postoperative radiotherapy (median total dosage, 50 Gy) after curative operation for adenocarcinoma of the rectum and rectosigmoid. The overall 5-year survival rate was 42% and the 5-year disease-free survival rate was 37%. The respective rates for the Gunderson-Sosin stage B_2 patients were 59% and 53% and 25% and 25% for stage C_2 patients. Five-year local relapse rates were 27% for stage B and 40% for stage C_2 carcinomas.

De Neve et al. (461) reviewed the results of postoperative radiotherapy given to 40 patients with gross or microscopically proven residual disease after resection of rectal or rectosigmoid carcinoma. Mean radiation dosage was 50 Gy. Survival for patients with microscopic residual disease was 40% at 5 years compared to 12% for those with gross residual disease.

Mak et al. (462) reported on the late complications of postoperative radiation therapy used to treat 224 patients with rectal carcinoma. The median dose was 54 Gy. Forty-seven patients received concomitant 5-FU. The small bowel obstruction rate was 30% for extended field radiotherapy, 21% for single pelvic field, and 9% for multiple pelvic fields with median time to obstruction of 7 months. Small bowel obstruction was correlated with post-surgical adhesions prior to radiotherapy and absence of reperitonealization at time of the initial operation.

Tang et al. (463) compared 127 patients with Astler-Coller stage B_2 or C rectal carcinoma who underwent operation and postoperative radiotherapy to 122 patients undergoing operation alone. Severe or life-threatening radiation-related complications were encountered in 8% of patients. Postoperative radiotherapy did not improve survival. Five-year survival rates for patients with Dukes' B_2 for operation alone and operation and radiotherapy were 80% and 64%, respectively, and for Dukes' C, 52% and 41%, respectively.

A summary of randomized trials of postoperative radiotherapy is presented in Table 10.

TABLE 10 ■ Results of Randomized Trials of Postoperative Radiotherapy

Trial (Authors)	No. of Patients	Dose (Gy/Fractions)	Dukes' Stage	Local Recurrence (%)	Distant Metastases (%)	Overall 5-Year Survival (%)
GITSG (459) (1985)	227	Operation alone	B_2 and C	24	34	43
		CT		27	27	57
		40–48 Gy/22–27		20	30	50
		CT + 40–44 Gy/22–24		11	26	59
Denmark (464) (Balsev et al., 1986)	494	Operation alone	B/C	18	14	Similar
		50 Gy/25		16	19	
NSABP (359) (Fisher et al., 1988)	555	Operation alone	B and C	25	27	43
		CT		21	24	53*
		46–47 Gy/26–27		16	31	50
Netherlands (465) (Treurniet-Donker et al., 1991)	172	Operation alone	B_2/C	33	26	57
		50 Gy/25		20	36	45
MRC3 (466) (Gates et al., 1995)	469	Operation alone	B/C	34	35	38
		40 Gy/20		213*	31	41

*Statistically significant.

Abbreviations: CT, Chemotherapy; GITSIG, Gastrointestinal Tumor Study Group; MRC, Medical Research Council; NSABP, National Surgical Adjuvant Breast and Bowel Project.

Preoperative vs. Postoperative Radiotherapy

Pählman and Glimelius (423) reported on a study that compared patients who received 2550 cGy preoperatively to those who received 6000 cGy postoperatively. The authors found no significant difference in the survival rate, but a local recurrence rate of 12% after preoperative radiotherapy was better than the 21% noted after postoperative radiotherapy.

Preoperative and Postoperative Irradiation (Sandwich Therapy)

The search continues to improve the survival rate in patients with carcinoma of the rectum and to reduce morbidity and unnecessary treatment. Using 500 cGy preoperatively is attractive since this amount of irradiation does not interface with wound healing or alter pathologic staging. The "sandwich technique" uses a single dose of 500 cGy preoperatively and 4500 cGy over 5 weeks postoperatively. The postoperative dose can be eliminated if the resected specimen does not warrant further radiotherapy. Sause et al. (467) used this protocol in 353 patients with carcinoma of the ascending and descending colon and rectum. Five-year follow-up estimates of no preoperative therapy vs. preoperative therapy were as follows: local recurrence, 29% vs. 26%; metastasis, 41% vs. 43%; and survival, 54% vs. 54%. No benefit was derived from preoperative treatment. Bayer et al. (468) proposed a different treatment regimen, with 3000 cGy administered preoperatively, and only patients with Dukes' B or C lesions received another 3000 cGy postoperatively. However, the follow-up time was too short to permit any conclusions. From a nonrandomized retrospective analysis Botti et al. (469) compared 124 patients who received preoperative and postoperative radiotherapy (40), postoperative radiotherapy (30), or operation alone (54). Operative mortality was 2% in the sandwich radiotherapy group vs. 7% in the operation alone group. After a median follow-up of 60 months, the actuarial locoregional recurrence rate at 5 years was 3% for the sandwich radiotherapy group compared with 18% and 30% for the postoperative radiotherapy and surgery group alone, respectively. The actuarial 5-year survival rates were 86%, 50%, and 28% in the sandwich radiotherapy group, postoperative radiotherapy group, and operation alone group, respectively.

Intraoperative Irradiation

For selected patients in whom a fixed carcinoma has responded to external beam radiation, Tepper et al. (470) suggest that the addition of intraoperative radiation therapy increases the regional and probably the overall disease-free survival rate beyond that found when external beam radiation alone is used. Encouraging preliminary results also have been reported by Sischy (471). Intraoperative radiotherapy has been recommended for patients with fixed, unresectable carcinomas. It is believed that direct delivery of the high-dose radiotherapy may enhance control of the disease. Valentini et al. (472) reported on 15 studies at the fifth IORT International Congress held in 1994; 700 patients with rectal carcinoma had undergone intraoperative radiation therapy. In primary carcinoma unresectable for cure and in local recurrence it is evidenced that external beam radiotherapy plus operation plus intraoperative radiation therapy enable an improvement in local control and survival compared to external radiotherapy alone. In the Mayo Clinic experience 50 patients treated with external beam radiotherapy (45–50 Gy) plus operation showed a 24% local control and 24% three-year survival, while 20 patients in the intraoperative radiation therapy group (10–20 Gy) showed 80% local control and 50% three-year survival. At the Massachusetts General Hospital 103 patients with rectal carcinoma unresectable for cure were given preoperative radiotherapy (50.4 Gy) and, if at operation frozen sections revealed residual disease or a disease-free margin less than 5 mm, intraoperative radiation therapy (15 Gy) was performed. Local control in the former was 67%, while it was 82% in the latter group. Five-year disease-free survival was similar (55% vs. 54%). Investigators of the Fox Chase Cancer Center in Philadelphia stated that in the presence of residual carcinoma intraoperative radiation therapy is ineffective. Significant intraoperative radiation therapy-induced perioperative and late toxicities have been reported—irradiation of ureters resulting in a 44% rate of obstruction requiring stents, peripheral neuropathies (32%), bone necrosis, fatal bleeding from a Hartmann pouch, and enteritis.

Gunderson et al. (473) evaluated 123 patients with previously unirradiated locally recurrent colorectal carcinomas who received intraoperative electron radiation therapy usually as a supplement to external beam irradiation and maximum resection. All received external beam radiation therapy with or without concomitant 5-FU-based chemotherapy (45 Gy in 25 fractions and a boost of 5.4 to 9 Gy in three to five fractions). Maximum resection was performed before or after external beam radiation. Intraoperative electron radiation therapy doses ranged from 10 to 20 Gy in 119 of 123 patients, Central failure (within the intraoperative electron field) was documented in 11%, with a five-year actuarial. rate of 26%. Local relapse (in the external beam field) occurred in 20%, with a five-year rate of 37%. Distant metastases occurred in 54%, with a five-year rate of 72%. Median survival was 28 months, with overall survival at two, three, and five years of 62%, 39%, and 20%, respectively. Although there was a trend for reduction in local relapse rates with gross total versus partial resection, this neither achieved statistical significance nor translated into improved survival. Disease control within the intraoperative electron and external fields is decreased when the surgeon is unable to accomplish a gross total resection. Therefore it is reasonable to consistently add 5-FU or other dose modifiers during external beam radiation therapy and to evaluate the use of dose modifiers in conjunction with intraoperative electron radiation therapy (sensitizers and hyperthermia). Even with locally recurrent lesions, the aggressive multimodality approaches, including intraoperative electron radiation therapy, have resulted in improved local control and long-term survival rates of 20% versus an expectecd 5% with conventional techniques. Sadahiro et al. (474) reported the efficacy of intraoperative radiotherapy for curatively resected rectal carcinoma in 62 patients who received preoperative radiotherapy with 20 Gy. Retrospective comparisons were made with 248 patients treated by operation alone. Survival, disease-free survival, and local recurrence-free survival in the intraoperative radiotherapy group were significantly more favorable than in the nonintraoperative radiotherapy group. Differences in survival were observed in stage II patients but not in stage I or stage III patients. The local failure rate was 2.6% in the intraoperative radiotherapy group and 11.3% in the nonintraoperative radiotherapy group. The distant metastasis rate was 18% in the intraoperative radiotherapy group and 19.5% in the nonintraoperative radiotherapy group. There was a significantly higher rate of wound infection in the intraoperative radiotherapy group. However, in reviewing a series of 71 patients who received intraoperative radiotherapy for locally advanced carcinoma, Fuchs and Bleday (475) noted high rates of complications, 78.9% averaging 2.83 complications per patient. One of the most severe complications observed was massive iliac artery bleeding or blowout. Two such cases were successfully treated with angiographic embolization, both patients presented to the hospital emergently with considerable blood loss requiring intensive care unit resuscitation in the range of 6 to 19 units of blood. The necessity for specialized expensive equipment, as well as the cooperation of the radiation oncologist, anesthesiologist, and surgeon, will limit the acceptance of this regimen unless dramatic results can be obtained.

■ CHEMOTHERAPY

Adjuvant chemotherapy involves the postoperative use of cancericidal drugs to eradicate microfoci of malignant cells. The most useful single agents for colorectal carcinoma have been 5-FU and 2′-deoxy-5-fluorouridine (5-FUDR). Most investigators use 5-FU because of its identical effectiveness to 5-FUDR and lower cost. 5-FU blocks the formation of thymidylic acid and therefore the biosynthesis of DNA.

The NSABP Protocol R-01 (359) used 5-FU, semustine, and vincristine and found an improved disease-free survival rate and overall survival rate. However, the observed advantage was restricted to males and was more advantageous in those younger than 65 years of age. The advantage continues to be significant at eight years (476).

The GITSG trial reported an overall survival benefit for patients treated with adjuvant postoperative radiation (4000–4800 cGy) and chemotherapy (5-FU and semustine) following low anterior resection or abdominoperineal resection for Dukes-Kirklin B_2, C_1, and C_2 carcinomas (459). The recurrence rate was 55% in control patients and 33% among patients receiving a combination of radiation therapy and chemotherapy. O'Connell et al. (477) studied 660 patients with TNM stage II and III rectal carcinoma to determine whether the efficacy of chemotherapy could be improved by administering 5-FU by protracted infusion throughout the course of radiotherapy and whether the omission of semustine would reduce the toxicity and delayed complications of chemotherapy without decreasing its efficacy. At a median follow-up of 46 months, patients who received a protracted infusion had a significantly increased time to relapse, 53% to 63% (a decrease of 27%), and improved survival, 60% to 70% (a decrease of 30% in their death rate). The addition of semustine provided no benefit. In a study of 141 patients with curative resection for colorectal carcinoma, approximately one-third of which were carcinoma of the rectum, patients were randomized to a control group (operation alone); resection and 5-FU group; or resection, 5-FU, and levamisole group (478). With a five-year follow-up, patients who had received levamisole had a survival advantage. Patients who died of recurrence of the carcinoma in the control group comprised 52%; in the group who underwent resection and 5-FU, 44%; and in the group receiving 5-FU and levamisole, 32%.

■ COMBINATION CHEMORADIOTHERAPY

Frustration with inadequate results has led to the recommendation of combined chemotherapy and radiotherapy. GITSG published encouraging results (459). In a four-arm study that compared operation alone, chemotherapy (5-FU and semustine), radiotherapy (4000–4800 cGy), and combined radiation (4400 cGy) and chemotherapy (5-FU and semustine), the results showed an advantage for combined treatment for time to recurrence and survival rate. It has been suggested that the preoperative irradiation combined with 5-FU suppositories can reduce the incidence of postoperative recurrence (479). In an effort to improve resectability and possibly survival, Sischy et al. (480) employed chemosensitizers (5-FU and mitomycin) combined with moderate-dose radiation for carcinomas larger than 5 cm requiring abdominoperineal resection. In a series of 60 patients, the size of the lesions at operation decreased by more than 50% in over 75% of patients. No residual carcinoma was found in 10%, and only microscopic foci were present in another 21%. Only 24% of resected specimens contained positive lymph nodes. Of the 33 patients followed up for five years, 60% were alive and well. As in the treatment of anal carcinoma, chemosensitizers may play a role in the treatment of rectal carcinoma in the future.

Krook et al. (358) reported on the NCCTG 794751 trial. Patients with T3, T4, N1, N2 (equivalent to Dukes' B and C) lesions were randomized to treatment with postoperative radiation alone (45 Gy delivered in 180 cGy fractions five days a week over five weeks plus a 5.4 Gy boost delivered in 180 cGy fractions to the carcinoma bed after acute radiation tolerance was demonstrated) or to radiation (similar dosage) plus concurrent 5-FU. The latter treatment was both preceded and followed by a cycle of systemic therapy with 5-FU plus methyl-CCNU (semustine). For the combined modality, chemotherapy was initiated with a single dose of methyl-CCNU at 130 mg/m^2 of body surface area. 5-FU was administered by rapid intravenous injection at 300 mg/m^2 on days 1 through 5. On day 36, a course of 5-FU was given at 400 mg/m^2 daily for five days. Four weeks later (on day 64), therapy of 5-FU and radiation was initiated. 5-FU was given by rapid intravenous injection at a dose of 500 mg/m^2 during the first three days of radiation and repeated during the first three days of the fifth week of radiation. One month after radiation, a single dose of methyl-CCNU was given (100 mg/m^2) plus 5-FU (300 mg/m^2) for five days. One month later, 5-FU was given at 400 mg/m^2 daily for five days. After a median follow-up time of more than seven years, the combined modality showed a relative reduction in recurrence of 34% (63% vs. 42%), with an initial 46% reduction in pelvic recurrence and a 37% reduction in distant metastases. In addition, the overall patient death rate was reduced by 29%, and carcinoma-related deaths dropped by 36%. The five-year disease-free survival rate increased from 42% to 63%, and the overall five-year survival rate increased from 47% to 58%.

In the NSABP R-02 trial, 694 eligible patients with Dukes' B or C carcinoma of the rectum were randomly assigned to receive either postoperative adjuvant chemotherapy alone ($n=348$) or chemotherapy with postoperative radiotherapy ($n=346$) (481). All female patients ($n=287$) received 5-FU plus LV chemotherapy; male patients received either MOF ($n=207$) or 5-FU plus LV ($n=200$). The average time on study for surviving patients was 93 months. Postoperative radiotherapy resulted in no beneficial effect on disease-free survival or overall survival regardless of which chemotherapy was utilized, although it reduced the cumulative incidence of locoregional relapse from 13% to 8% at five-year follow-up. Male patients who received 5-FU plus LV demonstrated a statistically significant benefit in disease-free survival at five-years compared with those who received MOF (55% vs. 47%) but not in five-year overall survival (65% vs. 62%). The addition of postoperative radiation therapy to chemotherapy in Dukes' B and C rectal carcinoma did not alter the subsequent incidence of distant disease, although there was a reduction in locoregional relapse when compared with chemotherapy alone.

While a logical argument may be made for the elimination of radiotherapy in the postoperative setting on the basis of the outcome from the study described here, enthusiasm for the approach must be tempered by the confirmed demonstration that radiotherapy is effective in reducing the incidence of locoregional recurrence, an event that can be associated with substantial morbidity and an attenuation in quality of life. Whether the 5% absolute decrease in the cumulative incidence of locoregional relapse is sufficient to justify the routine use of postoperative radiotherapy is a decision that must be made by the clinician. In a thoughtful and provocative editorial that followed this publication, Haller (482) noted that although it is accepted that a beneficial outcome of adjuvant treatment of rectal carcinoma is prevention of clinically relevant local recurrences, most clinicians and patients would agree that overall survival and quality of life are more pertinent end points of treatment. Since it is likely that most of the long-term morbidity of postoperative chemotherapy and radiation therapy is due to the late effects of the radiation therapy, it is reasonable to ask whether all patients should be exposed to this treatment and whether similar clinical outcomes could be achieved with improved surgical techniques or with systemic chemotherapy alone. If radiation therapy reduces local recurrence, then perhaps its use should be limited to those patients with particularly high-risk anatomic or biologic determinants for this pattern of failure, i.e., those with greater local extension (macroscopic T3 or T4) or multiple lymph node involvement.

Theodoropoulos et al. (483) evaluated the impact of response to preoperative and, specifically, of T-level downstaging, nodal downstaging, and complete pathologic response after chemoradiation therapy on oncologic outcome of 88 patients with locally advanced rectal carcinoma. T-level downstaging after neoadjuvant treatment was demonstrated in 41% and complete pathologic response was observed in 18%. Of the 42 patients with ultrasound-positive nodes, 27 had no evidence of nodal involvement on pathologic evaluation (64%). The overall response rate (T-level downstaging or nodal downstaging) was 51%. At a median follow-up of 33 months, 86.4% of patients were alive. The overall recurrence rate was 10.2% (three patients had local and six had metastatic recurrences). Patients with T-level downstaging and complete pathologic response were characterized by significantly better five-year survival and better overall survival. None of the patients with complete pathologic response developed recurrence or died during the follow-up period.

Burmeister et al. (484) conducted a phase 2 study to collect data prospectively on the toxicity of postoperative combined chemoradiation therapy. The prescribed radiation dose was 50.4 Gy in 28 fractions, and the 5-FU chemotherapy was 450 mg/m^2 given with fractions 1 to 3 and 26 to 28 ($n=80$). On completion of the radiation therapy, the patient was given a further four cycles of bolus 5-FU at monthly intervals. Acute toxicity of the therapy was significant with 16% of patients experiencing severe bowel morbidity. The other major side effects of the therapy were skin reactions, neutropenia and bladder problems. Late bowel toxicity was also severe. The local in field relapse rate was 10%. The majority of relapses were at distant sites, mostly in the liver and lungs. The actuarial survival at five years was 55%. They concluded that the combined adjuvant postoperative chemoradiation therapy using their protocol was effective but had significant acute and late morbidity. The optimum regimen for those patients requiring postoperative adjuvant therapy is yet to be determined.

Tepper et al. (485) published the final report of the gastrointestinal Intergroup 0114. All patients had a potentially curative resection and were treated with two cycles of chemotherapy followed by chemoradiation therapy and two additional cycles of chemotherapy. Chemotherapy regimens were bolus 5-FU, 5-FU and leucovorin, 5-FU and levamisole, and 5-FU leucovorin and levamisole. Pelvic irradiation was given to a dose of 45 Gy to the whole pelvis and a boost to 50.4 to 54 Gy. One thousand, six hundred and ninety-five patients were entered and fully assessable with a median follow-up of 7.4 years. There was no difference in overall survival or disease-free survival by drug regimen. Disease free survival and overall survival decreased between years five and seven (from 54% to 50% and 64% to 56%, respectively), although recurrence free rates had only a small decrease. The local recurrence rate was 14% [9% in low-risk (T1 to N2+) and 18% in high-risk patients (T3N+, T4N)]. Overall, seven-year survival rates were 70% and 45% for the low-risk and high-risk groups, respectively. Males had a poorer overall survival rate than females. There is no advantage to leucovorin or levamisole containing regimens over bolus 5-FU alone in the adjuvant treatment for rectal carcinoma when combined with irradiation. Local and distant recurrence rates are still high especially in T3N+ and T4 patients even with full adjuvant chemoradiation therapy.

The EORTC trial compared preoperative radiotherapy (34.5 Gy) to the same treatment and chemotherapy (5-FU) and found no difference in local recurrence, distant metastases, disease-free survival, or overall survival (486).

In an ongoing effort to improve survival, preoperative chemoradiation has been tried by several investigators. In a study by Meade et al. (487) patients underwent preoperative endorectal ultrasonography staging followed by high-dose radiotherapy combined with 5-FU. Following resection, the downstaging was recorded in 14 of 20 patients and no residual disease was present in eight patients. Local recurrence developed in two patients. Disease-free survival was noted in 17 patients with 9 to 51 month follow-up. Others have also reported encouraging results for preoperative chemoradiation (488).

In a nonrandomized trial, Stryker et al. (489) compared the results of chemoradiation (45–50 Gy plus 5-FU plus mitomycin, four to eight weeks prior to operation) in 30 patients with stage II and III rectal carcinoma with the results of treatment in 56 patients who did not undergo preoperative chemoradiation of which 24 patients received postoperative adjuvant chemoradiation. Five-year actuarial control rates were 96%, 83%, and 88%, respectively. Disease-free survival rates were 80%, 57%, and 47%, respectively. Overall survival rates were 85%, 48%, and 78%, respectively.

Kollmorgan et al. (490) studied the adverse effects of long-term bowel function following postoperative chemoradiotherapy for rectal carcinoma. The authors compared two similar groups of patients who underwent anterior resection. One group received postoperative radiation and chemotherapy, while the other did not. The chemoradiotherapy patients had more bowel movements per day (median seven vs. median two) and more of these patients had clustered bowel movements (42% vs. 3%), nighttime movements (46% vs. 14%), incontinence (occasional, 39% vs. 7%; frequent, 17% vs. 0%), and inability to differentiate stool from gas (39% vs. 15%). More patients in the chemoradiation group had to wear a pad (41% vs. 10%), were unable to defer defecation longer than 15 minutes (78% vs. 19%), had liquid stools sometimes or always (29% vs. 5%), regularly used Lomotil and/or Imodium (58% vs. 5%), and had perianal skin irritation (41% vs. 12%). Overall, 93% of the patients receiving chemoradiation reported that their bowel function was different than before operation versus 61% of the nonradiation group who so reported. Although it may improve survival, adjuvant postoperative chemoradiotherapy also results in significant long-term detrimental effects on bowel function. Physicians should inform patients of these effects before the treatment is initiated.

Picciocchi et al. (491) entered 64 patients with stage II or III rectal carcinoma into a study to receive preoperative radiotherapy, 37.8 Gy combined with continuous 5-FU and mitomycin C. Toxicity was recorded in 27% of patients with one patient dying from the effects of chemotherapy. Of the 61 patients operated on, 46 underwent low anterior resections and 15 underwent abdominoperineal resection. There were no postoperative mortalities but morbidity was recorded at 28%, 8.7% sustaining anastomotic dehiscences. Definitive histologic staging was downgraded from initial clinical staging (stage 0, 0–5; stage I, 0–19; stage II, 13–21; stage III, 48–15; and stage IV, 0–1). With a median follow-up of 23 months, the incidence of local recurrence was 5% and that of distant metastases was 8%.

Multidisciplinary treatment efforts continue to select patients who would benefit most from perioperative treatment while minimizing toxicity. Suggested criteria for the selection of neoadjuvant therapy include patients with carcinomas of the distal rectum that are locally advanced by either clinical or imaging criteria, poorly differentiated carcinomas, circumferential lesions, or carcinomas that are obstructing or perforated (492).

Garcia-Aguilar et al. (493) studied the prognostic value of pathologic complete response to preoperative chemoradiation in rectal carcinoma patients. They prospectively followed up 168 consecutive patients with ultrasound stages II (57) and III (122) rectal carcinoma treated by preoperative chemoradiation followed by radical resection with mesorectal excision; 161 had a curative resection. Average follow-up was 37 months. Downstaging occurred in 58% of patients, including 13% patients who had a pathologic complete response. The estimated five-year rate of local recurrence was 5%; of distant metastases, 14%. None of the patients with pathologic complete response has developed disease recurrence. They found no difference in survival among patients with pathologic stage I, stage II, or stage III carcinomas. They concluded a pathologic complete response to preoperative chemoradiation is associated with improved local control and patient survival.

Ruo et al. (494) found that a marked response to preoperative radiotherapy +/− chemotherapy may be associated with good long-term outcome but was not predictive of recurrence free survival. The presence of poor histopathologic features and positive nodal status are the most important prognostic indicators after neo-adjuvant therapy. Stipa et al. (495) evaluated the impact of preoperative radiation and chemotherapy on primary rectal carcinoma and mesorectal lymph nodes in 187 consecutive patients who underwent abdominoperineal resection or low anterior resection for locally advanced stage T3-4. Comparison of pre-combined modality therapy, endorectal ultrasound stage with pathologic stage revealed a decrease in T stage in 49% as well as a decrease in the percentage of individuals with positive mesorectal lymph nodes, from 54% to 27%. The incidence of residual mesorectal lymph node involvement remains significant and parallels increasing stage. They believe that locally advanced distal rectal carcinoma should continue to include formal resection. Rullier et al. (496) reported 43 patients who underwent preoperative radiochemotherapy (50 Gy range 40–54) and concomitant chemotherapy with 5-FU continuous infusion ($n=36$) or bolus ($n=7$) for rectal carcinoma located 2 to 6 cm from the anal verge. There were 40 T3 lesions, and three T4 lesions. Sphincter saving resection was performed six weeks after treatment in 25 patients by using intersphincteric resection. Coloanal anastomoses were associated with a colonic pouch in 86% of the patients, and all patients had a protecting stoma. There were no deaths related to the preoperative radiochemotherapy and operation. Acute toxicity was mainly due to diarrhea with 54% of grade 1 to 2. Four anastomotic fistulas and two pelvic hematomas occurred; all patients but one had closure of the stoma. Downstaging was observed in 42% of the patients and was associated with a greater radial margin. After a median follow-up of 30 months, the rate of local recurrence was 2%, and 10% had distal metastases. Overall and disease-free survival rates were both 85% at three years. Functional results were good (Kirwin continence I, II) in 79% of the available patients ($n=37$). They were slightly altered by intersphincteric resection (57% vs. 75%) for perfect continence; but were significantly improved by a colonic pouch (74% vs. 16%). They concluded these results suggested preoperative radiochemotherapy allowed sphincter saving resection to be performed with good local control and good functional results in patients with T3 low rectal carcinomas.

Read et al. (497) reviewed 191 consecutive patients undergoing abdominal surgical procedures for primary rectal carcinoma, 89% of whom were treated with preoperative external beam radiotherapy. Curative resection was performed in 80% including low anterior resection with coloproctostomy or coloanal anastomosis ($n=103$), abdominoperineal resection ($n=44$), Hartmann's procedure ($n=4$), and pelvic exenteration ($n=1$). Mean follow-up of patients undergoing curative resection was 96 months. Palliative procedures were performed in 20%. Perioperative mortality was 0.5%. Complications occurred in 34%. The anastomotic leak rate was 4%. Disease-free five-year survival rate by pathologic stage was as follows: stage I, 90%; stage II, 85%; stage III, 54%; stage IV, 0% and no residual carcinoma, 90%. Of the 152 patients treated with curative resection, disease-free survival rate was 80% at five years. The carcinoma recurred in 21% treated with curative resection. The predominant pattern of recurrence was distant failure only. Overall, local recurrence (local and local plus distant) at five years was 6.6%. The local recurrence rate paralleled stage: stage I, 0%; stage II, 6%; stage III, 20%; and no residual carcinoma, 0%.

The review of retrospective data by Minsky (410) suggests that preoperative combined modality therapy increases pathologic downstaging compared with preoperative radiation without chemotherapy, and is associated with a lower incidence of acute toxicity compared with postoperative combined-modality therapy. In general, the incidence of grade 3/4 acute toxicity during the combined-modality segment is 15% to 25%, the complete response rates are 10% to 30% pathologic, and 10% to 20% clinical, and the incidence of local recurrence is 2% to 10%. In his review of 5 oxaliplatin-based combined modality therapy studies in which 45 to 50.4 Gy were used in combination with 5-FU, leucovorin, and oxaliplatin (one study substituted ralitrexal for 5-FU) pathologic complete response rates varied from 14% to 37% (410). Volter et al. (498) combined irinotecan with hyperfractionated radiation (1.6 Gy twice daily to 41.6 Gy) and encountered a high incidence of anastomotic leak and/or abscess of 30%.

Despite a lack of randomized data demonstrating clinical benefit, preoperative chemoradiation has been increasingly used in patients with T_3 disease in North America (499). Luna-Perez et al. (500) evaluated the feasibility, morbidity, and functional results of anal sphincter preservation after preoperative chemoradiation therapy and coloanal anastomosis in 32 patients with rectal carcinoma located between 3 and 6 cm above the anal verge. Twenty-two patients underwent coloanal anastmosis with the J-pouch; ten underwent straight anastomosis. The mean distal surgical margin was 1.3 cm. Major complications included coloanal anastomotic leakage (3); pelvic abscess (3); and coloanal stenosis (2). Mean follow-up was 25 months. Recurrences occurred in four patients and were local and distant (1) and distant (3). Anal sphincter function was perfect (20), incontinent to gas (3), occasional minor leak (2), frequent major soiling (3), and colostomy ($n=2$). They concluded that in patients with locally advanced rectal carcinoma located 3 to 6 cm from the anal verge who are traditionally treated with abdominoperineal resection, preservation of anal sphincter after preoperative chemoradiation therapy plus complete rectal excision with coloanal anastomosis is feasible and is associated with acceptable morbidity and no mortality.

To determine whether patients downsized with preoperative chemoradiotherapy may be potential candidates for local excision, Bedrosian et al. (501) investigated residual disease patterns in 219 patients after neoadjuvant treatment. Preoperatively, 88% were staged as T3 and 47% had clinical N1 disease. The pathologic complete response rate was 20%. T stage was downsized in 64% of the patients and 69% of patients with clinical N1 disease were rendered node negative. Seventeen percent of patients downsized to less than or equal to T2 had residual disease in the mesentery. With a median follow-up of 40 months, 83% of patients remain alive and free of disease. Local recurrence developed in 4.1% of patients. Although response rates to preoperative chemoradiotherpay within the bowel wall and lymph node basin are similar, one in six patients with pT0-2 carcinomas will have residual disease in the rectal mesentery and nodes.

Stipa et al. (495) evaluated the impact of preoperative radiation and chemotherapy on primary mid and distal rectal carcinomas and mesorectal lymph nodes in 187 consecutive patients who underwent abdominoperineal resection or low anterior resection for locally advanced (T3-4) carcinoma. Comparison of pre-combined modality therapy, endorectal ultrasound stage with pathologic stage revealed a decrease in stage in 49% as well as a decrease in the percentage of individuals with positive mesorectal lymph nodes from 54% to 27%. They concluded following preoperative combined modality therapy, the incidence of residual mesorectal lymph node involvement remains significant and care for locally advanced distal rectal carcinoma should continue to include formal rectal resection.

Enker (502) noted that despite recent enthusiasm, neoadjuvant therapy in previous studies have indicated that from 10% to 30% of patients demonstrate objective regression of disease (i.e., a complete pathologic response) after neoadjuvant therapy. The corollary is that 70% to 90% of patients harbour residual mesorectal carcinoma despite their preoperative treatment requiring formal curative rectal and mesorectal resection. Furthermore, no proven correlation exists between the regression of the primary carcinoma and the regression of regional, mesorectal node disease. Whereas shrinkage of a bulky primary carcinoma situated within a narrow pelvis can offer the surgeon an easier opportunity to perform an adequate resection, shrinkage alone is not a sign of clinical downstaging in a disease that is overwhelmingly regional in its presentation (greater than or equal to T3, or N1–N2 in 65% to 80% of patients). Designing patient care around the aftereffects of response to chemoradiotherapy as opposed to determining treatment of the original stage of presentation has many pitfalls and hazards. Therefore, shrinkage of the primary carcinoma is not a sufficient foundation upon which to alter treatment from one's original intentional to perform a regional resection in such patients despite regression of the primary lesion after radiation and chemotherapy.

Onaitis et al. (503) reported up to 30% of patients with locally advanced rectal carcinoma have a complete clinical or pathologic response to neoadjuvant chemoradiation. They analyzed complete clinical and pathologic responders among 141 rectal carcinoma patients treated with neoadjuvant chemoradiation. Clinical restaging after treatment consisted of proctoscopic examination and often CT scan. Clinical complete responders had no advantage in local recurrence, disease-free survival, or overall survival rates when compared with clinical partial responders. Pathologic complete responders also had no recurrence or survival advantage when compared with pathologic partial responders. Of the 34 pathologic T0 lesions, 13% had lymph node metastases. They concluded clinical assessment of complete response to neoadjuvant chemoradiation is unreliable. Micrometastatic disease persists in a proportion of patients despite pathologic complete response.

Hofheinz et al. (504) evaluated the feasibility and efficacy of capecitabine in combination with weekly irinotecan (CAPIRI) with concurrent pelvic radiotherapy in 19 patients with locally advanced rectal carcinoma. All patients underwent operation and R0 resection was achieved in all patients. Pathologic complete remission was observed in four patients and another five patients had only microfoci of residual disease. They concluded preoperative chemoradioatherapy with CAPIRI is feasible and well tolerated.

It must be remembered that chemoradiation is not without its complications. Chessin et al. (505) reported on complications of 297 consecutive patients with locally advanced rectal carcinoma treated with preoperative combined modality therapy (radiation: 5040 cGy; chemotherapy: 5-FU-based) and then operation. Major complications were defined as those requiring medical or surgical treatment. Median follow-up was 43.9 months. There were no postoperative mortalities, but there were 145 major complications in 98 patients (33% of the study population). The most common complications were small bowel obstruction (11%) and wound infection (10%), anastomotic leaks (4%) and pelvic abscesses (4%) in patients treated with low anterior resection. Postoperative complications had no significant impact on oncologic outcomes. Although postoperative mortalities are rare, complications requiring treatment can be anticipated in one-third of patients undergoing preoperative combined modality therapy and TME. They recommend a policy of selective fecal diversion after preoperative combined modality therapy and TME for locally advanced rectal carcinoma to achieve low rates of pelvic sepsis but this may lead to an increased incidence of small bowel obstruction.

Most recently, Habr-Gama et al. (506) conducted a study to determine the correlation between final stage and survival in patients receiving neoadjuvant chemoradiation treatment regardless of initial disease stage. Two hundred and sixty patients with distal (0–7 cm from anal verge) rectal carcinoma considered resectable were treated by neoadjuvant chemoradiotheapy with 5-FU and leucovorin plus 5040 cGy. Patients with incomplete clinical response eight weeks after chemoradiotherapy completion were treated by radical resection. Patients with complete clinical response were managed by observation alone. Seventy-one patients (28%) showed complete clinical response (clinical stage 0). One hundred and sixty-nine patients showed incomplete clinical response and were treated with operation. In 22 of these patients (9%), pathologic examination revealed pT0 N0 M0 (stage p0), 59 patients (22%) had stage I, 68 patients (26%) had stage II, and 40 patients (50%) had stage III disease. Overall survival rates were significantly higher in stage c0 compared with stage p0. Disease-free survival rate showed better results in stage c0, but the results were not significant. Five year overall and disease-free survivals were 97.7% and 84% (stage 0); 94% and 74% (stage I); 83% and 50% (stage II); and 56% and 26% (stage III), respectively. Carcinoma-related overall and disease-free survival may be correlated to final pathologic staging following neoadjuvant chemoradiotherapy for distal carcinoma. Also stage 0 is significantly associated with improved outcome.

Moore et al. (507) conducted a review to determine whether prolongation of the interval between preoperative combined modality therapy and operation resulted in an increased pathologic complete response rate. They identified 155 rectal carcinoma patients undergoing preoperative pelvic external beam radiation and 5-FU chemo based therapy followed by rectal resection. A pathologic complete response occurred in 15% of patients. A pathologic complete response occurred in 19% of patients with an interval greater than 44 days versus 12% in those with an interval less than or equal to 44 days. The benefit of a prolonged interval between completion of preoperative combined modality therapy and operation remains unclear.

The German Rectal Cancer Group addressed the controversy of preoperative versus postoperative chemoradiotherapy (508). Patients with clinically staged T3/T4 N+ rectal carcinoma were randomly assigned to preoperative or postoperative chemoradiotherapy: 50.4 Gy in 28 fractions were applied to the carcinomas and the pelvic lymph nodes. 5-FU (1 g/m^2/day) was administered concomitantly during the first and fifth week of radiotherapy as 120 hours continuous infusion. Four additional cycles of 5-FU adjuvant chemotherapy (500 mg/m^2/day $\times$ 5 day, q four weeks) were delivered. Chemoradiotherapy was identical in both arms except for a small-volume boost of 5.4 Gy in the postop arm. The interval between chemoradiotherapy and operation was four to six weeks in both arms. Techniques of operation were standardized and included TME. Median follow-up was 43 months (range 4–89 months). Of 823 patients randomized in 26 participating institutions, 392 and 405 were evaluable in the postop and preop chemoradiotherapy arms, respectively. The five-year pelvic and distant recurrence rates were 11% versus 7% and 34% versus 30%, respectively. Fewer patients experienced chronic anastomotic stenosis following preoperative chemoradiotherapy versus postoperative chemoradiotherapy (2.7% vs. 8.5%). Following preoperative chemoradiotherapy, there was significant down staging of the carcinoma with a 8% pathologic complete response rate. The UICC-stages were I to IV: 18%, 28%, 39%, 7%, missing 8% in the postoperative chemoradiotherapy arm versus 24%, 28%, 27%, 6%, missing 7% in the preoperative chemoradiotherpy arm. In the subgroup of 188 patients with low lying carcinomas who were declared by the surgeon prior to randomization to require an abdominoperineal resection, 19% underwent a sphincter saving procedure in the postoperative chemotherapy arm. This was significantly increased to 39% following preoperative chemoradiotherapy.

In the most recent update of their data, Sauer et al. (509) reported 421 patients were randomly assigned to receive preoperative chemoradiotherapy and 402 patients to receive postoperative chemoradiotherapy. The overall survival rates were 76% and 74%, respectively. The five-year cumulative incidence of local relapse was 6% for patients assigned to preoperative chemoradiotherapy and13% to the postoperative treatment group. Grade 3 and 4 toxicity effects occurred in 27% of patients in the preoperative treatment group as compared with 40% of patients in the postoperative treatment group. The corresponding rates of long-term toxic effects were 14% and 24%, respectively. They concluded preoperative chemoradiotherapy as compared to postoperative chemoradiotherapy improved local control and was associated with reduced toxicity but did not improve overall survival.

Ravasco et al. (510) investigated the impact of dietary counseling or nutritional supplements on outcomes in carcinoma patients: nutritional, morbidity, and quality of life during and three months after radiotherapy. A total of 111 colorectal carcinoma patients referred for radiotherapy, stratified by stage, were randomly assigned: group 1 ($n = 37$), dietary counseling (regular foods); group 2 ($n = 37$), protein supplements; group 3 ($n = 37$), ad libitum intake. Nutritional intake (dietary history), status (Ottery's Subjective Global Assessment), and quality of life (European Organization for Research and Treatment of Cancer Quality of Life Questionnaire version 3.0) were evaluated at baseline, at the end, and three months after radiotherapy. At radiotherapy completion, energy intake increased in groups 1 and 2, group 1 more than group 2, and decreased in group 3. Protein intake increased in groups 1 and 2, group 1 less than group 2, and decreased in group 3. At three months, group 1 maintained nutritional intake and group 2 and 3 returned to baseline. After radiotherapy and at three months, rates of anorexia, nausea, vomiting, and diarrhea were higher in group 3. At radiotherapy completion, in group 1, all quality of life function scores improved proportionally to adequate intake or nutritional status; whereas in group 2 only three of six function scores improved proportionally to protein intake, and in group 3 all scores worsened. At three months, group 1 patients maintained/improved function, symptoms, and single-item scores; in group 2, only few function and symptoms scores improved; in group 3, quality of life remained as poor as after radiotherapy.

The results of the randomized trials of combined chemoradiation is presented in Table 11.

IMMUNOTHERAPY

Malignant cells have repeatedly been found in the systemic venous blood in a high percentage of patients undergoing colonic or rectal excision for carcinoma (14). Their presence or absence in the peripheral blood during the operation in no way correlates with survival, suggesting that host factors are important in preventing the growth of these circulating cells (513). Many other observations support the premise of a close relationship between immunologic competency and the growth of human carcinomas (513).

The rationale of using immunotherapy for carcinoma assumes patients have potential antineoplastic immunity that is either blocked or at a low level, but that can be effectively stimulated to destroy malignant cells (514) A variety of modalities have been used to increase immunocompetence. Specific methods include the use of living carrier cells, neuraminidase, and purified tumor antigen (515). Nonspecific immunologic adjuvants have been shown to

TABLE 11 ■ Results of Randomized Trials of Combined Chemoradiation

Trial (Author)	No. of Patients	Dose (Gy/Fraction)	Local Recurrence (%)	Distant Metastases (%)	Overall Five-year Survival (%)
EORTC (486)	247	Preop 34.5 Gy/15.0	15	30	59
(Boulis-Wassif et al., 1984)		Preop 34.5 Gy/15.0 + 5-FU	15	30	46
GITSG (459) (1985)	227	Operation alone	24	34	43
		CT	27	27	57
		Postop 40–48 Gy/22–27	20	30	50
		CT + 40–44 Gy/22–21	11	26	59
NCCTG (358)	209	Postop 45 Gy/25 + 5.4 Gy boost	23	46	38
(Krook et al., 1991)		Postop 45 Gy/25 + 5-FU	14[a]	29[a]	53[a]
GITSG (511) (1992)	210	Postop 44.4 Gy/23 + 5-FU	15	25	44
		Postop 41.4 Gy/23 + 5-FU + Semustine	11	33	46
Intergroup (477)	660	50.4/28 Gy + CT bolus	11	40	60
(O'Connell et al., 1994)		54 Gy/30 + CT continuous	8	31	70[a]
NARCPG (512)	144	Operation alone	30	-	46
(Tveit et al., 1997)		Postop 46 Gy + 5-FU	12[a]	-	64
NSABP R-02 (481)	694	MOF 5-FU-leucovorin	}13	}29	}66
(Wolmark et al., 2000)		5-FU + postop 46 Gy (26/5) 5-FU-leucovorin + postop 46 Gy	} 8[a]	}31	}68
CAO/ARO/A10–94	405	Preop 50.4/28	7%[a]	30%	78%
Sauer (508) (2003)	392	Postop 50.4/28 + 5.4 Gy	11%	34%	73%

[a]Statistically significant.

Abbreviations: CT, chemotherapy; EORTC, European Organisation for Research and Treatment of Cancer; GITSG, Gastrointestinal Tumor Study Group; MOF, methyl CCNU, vincristine sulfate (Oncovin), 5-FU; NCCTG, North Central Cancer Treatment Group; NSABP, National Surgical Adjuvant Breast and Bowel Project. NARCPG Norwegian Adjuvant Rectal Cancer Project Group.

be effective in eliciting an immune response against a wide range of neoplasms, including colorectal carcinoma. The most widely used immunoadjuvants are bacillus Calmette. Guerin (BGG), *Corynebacterium parvum* (*C. parvam*), and methanol-extracted residue of BCG (MER). Only nonspecific adjuvants have been used in colorectal carcinoma.

Another approach is combination immunotherapy and chemotherapy Chemoimmunotherapy aims at combining the "debulking" capacity of chemotherapy with the potential of immunotherapy for controlling microscopic disease and therefore producing long-term disease-free survival.

Reed et al. (516) noted that patients given *C. parvum* had less immunosuppression secondary to chemotherapy than the control group and were able to receive chemotherapy twice as frequently. It may be that *C. parvum* exhibited no immunotherapeutic value in these patients but merely allowed the more aggressive utilization of chemotherapy.

Immunotherapy is most effective when the bulk of the carcinoma is small, either from surgical removal or in response to chemotherapy or radiation therapy. Immunotherapy can only be effective in an immunocompetent host. Immunotherapy at the M.D. Anderson Hospital in Houston using BCG showed improvement in survival rates (517). Unfortunately, the results were not compared to a control group, making interpretation difficult. In the NSABP study, BCG was used but did not result in improved survival rates (359).

■ SUMMARY

Despite a lack of randomized data demonstrating clinical benefit, preoperative chemoradiation has been increasingly used in patients with T3 disease in North America (499).

The phlethora of information from the published data and the controversies amongst the various experts makes it very difficult to mandate a course of action for each clinical situation. Even the magnitude of the different problems encountered in the treatment of rectal carcinoma varies tremendously. In their comprehensive review of the literature, Colquhoun et al. (362) analyzed nine randomized clinical trials designed to determine the effects of neoadjuvant therapy in the treatment of rectal carcinoma with a follow-up that varied from two to seven years. The recurrence rates following operation alone ranged from 8% to 30%. With the addition of adjuvant therapy, rates ranged from 2.4% to 27%. The death rate was reduced by 25% to 29% in two studies in which postoperative chemoradiotherapy was given and by 21% in one study in which preoperative chemoradiotherapy was given. In the remaining six trials, no survival benefit was derived from adjuvant therapy. In a meta-analysis of 36 randomized clinical trials using neoadjuvant and adjuvant therapy, Ooi et al. (518) demonstrated the morbidity of such treatments to be frequent but tolerable. Short-term (acute) complications of preoperative radiotherapy include lethargy, nausea, diarrhea, and skin erythema or desquamation. These acute effects develop to some degree in most patients during treatment but are usually self-limiting. With preoperative radiotherapy the incidence of perineal wound infection increases from 10% to 20%. The acute toxicities after postoperative radiotherapy for rectal carcinoma occur in 4% to 48% of cases, and serious toxicities requiring hospitalization or operative intervention occur in 3% to 10% of cases. The main problems with postoperative radiotherapy are small bowel obstruction (5–10%), delay in starting radiotherapy caused by delayed wound healing (6%), postoperative fatigue (14%), and toxicities precluding completion of adjuvant therapy (49–97%). The morbidity and mortality of both preoperative and postoperative radiotherapy are higher in elderly patients and when two-portal rather than three-portal or four-portal radiation technique is used. After combined adjuvant chemotherapy and radiotherapy, acute hematologic and gastrointestinal toxic effects are frequent (5–50%). Delayed radiation toxicities include radiation enteritis (4%), small bowel obstruction (5%), and rectal stricture (5%). Nevertheless, Colquhoun et al. (362) concluded in their review that adjuvant treatment remains indicated for patients with T3-4N0 and T1-4N1-2 carcinomas. Careful consideration should be given to those patients greater than 80 years who are less likely to experience recurrence based on age alone and who appear less tolerant of the toxicity associated with adjuvant therapy of any sort.

Despite many randomized trials of adjuvant therapy for rectal carcinoma, no consensus currently exists. Although the early trials of postoperative radiation and/or chemotherapy led to the 1991 NIH Consensus Statement, subsequent protocols of preoperative therapy challenged the consensus. Given the variation in timing and amount of radiation therapy used in existing trials, and given the lack of consensus on this topic, decision analysis provides a means to determine optimal adjuvant therapy. Kent et al. (519) conducted a literature search. Baseline values and ranges were determined from reference sources restricted to randomized controlled trials. Model variables included adverse effects and overall survival. They found postoperative combination therapy (expected value = 0.68) is the preferred treatment in terms of overall survival, in comparison to postoperative radiation alone, preoperative combination therapy, and preoperative radiation alone. Their decision analysis demonstrated a preference for postoperative combination therapy for stage II and III rectal carcinoma in terms of overall survival.

POSTOPERATIVE COMPLICATIONS

The complications associated with rectal surgery are discussed in detail in Chapter 36.

RECURRENT DISEASE

■ FOLLOW-UP

The rationale and policy for the follow-up of patients with carcinoma of the large bowel is detailed in Chapter 25. Most anastomotic recurrences will be detected within two years of operation.

■ INCIDENCE

A wide range of recurrence rates has been reported. As might be expected, the incidence of recurrence increases with the duration of follow-up. Long-term follow-up and an intensive search for recurrence, including a high autopsy rate, are factors that yield an increase in both total and local recurrence rates (227). One series of 101 patients followed up for five years turned up a recurrence rate of 39%, whereas a series of 231 patients followed up for 18 years yielded an incidence of 54% (227). In a thorough review of the literature, Sagar and Pemberton (520) found that the incidence of local recurrence after curative resection of rectal carcinoma ranged from 3% to 32%. Values varied, depending on the Dukes' stage of the disease and the portion of the rectum involved, that is, the upper, middle, or lower third. Lower values were seen with Dukes' A and proximal rectal lesions, whereas high values were seen with Dukes' C and distal rectal lesions. Abdominoperineal resections often have been recommended over low anterior resections because of the fear of local recurrence. However, when compared for the same degree of differentiation and stage of the carcinoma, local recurrence rates following low anterior resection are reportedly the same as rates for abdominoperineal resection (66,68,520,521). Other prognostic discriminants were fully discussed in Chapter 23.

In a review of 1008 patients undergoing potentially curative resection, McDermott et al. (331) reported that local recurrence developed in 14% of patients after resection of the upper third of the rectum compared with 21% for the middle third and 26% for the lower third. No relationship between local recurrence and the type of curative resection performed was documented. In a study that supported an intensive follow-up program to detect early local recurrence of colorectal carcinoma, Schiessel et al. (522) found that 22% of patients developed recurrence. Most of the recurrences (76%) developed after operation for rectal carcinoma. The rate of local recurrence was similar after a sphincter-saving operation (14.4%) as for an abdominoperineal resection (16.7%). An overall recurrence rate for rectal carcinoma was 14.7% as opposed to 4.4% after colonic carcinoma. Local recurrence only developed in 74.6% of patients, whereas disseminated disease was manifest in the other 25.4%. Castro-Sousa et al. (523) reported on 84 patients with carcinoma of the rectum who underwent radical excision. There was no significant difference in the incidence of recurrence between the group with sphincter preservation (17%) and abdominoperineal resection (13%). Rullier et al. (524) also found no difference in local recurrence between sphincter preservation (27.8%) and abdominoperineal resection (30.8%), but these rates are appreciably higher.

Following low anterior resection, Pilipshen (525) found that local recurrence rates varied from 14% to 43%. Local recurrence rates following low anterior resection with the use of the circular stapler are noted in Table 6 (3–36%). Quirke et al. (342) reported that in different hands, the incidence of local recurrence after resection of rectal carcinoma varies from 4% to 40%. In a dramatic departure from the generally high rates of recurrence, Heald (526) noted a remarkably low local recurrence rate of only 2.6%. He attributed this favorable outcome to complete excision of the mesorectum. It has been reported that wide pelvic lymphadenectomy can reduce the incidence of recurrence to 6% to 8%. Pihl et al. (527) also reported the amazing low anastomotic recurrence rate of 3% after resection of carcinoma of the rectum.

■ FACTORS CONTRIBUTING TO RECURRENCE

A number of local factors may contribute to the development of local recurrence following a low anterior resection of the rectum: (i) incomplete excision of the primary lesion, either inadequate distal or lateral margins of resection, or incomplete removal of the mesorectum; (ii) implantation of exfoliated neoplastic cells on the anastomosis or other raw surface; and (iii) development of metachronous lesions at the site of the anastomosis. General prognostic discriminants were described in great detail in Chapter 23. In their local recurrence rate of 20%, Feil et al. (528) reported that local recurrence depended on Dukes' stage, grading, gross appearance, lymphatic stroma reaction, venous invasion, perineural invasion, and margin of clearance. In a review of factors that influence local recurrence, Twomey et al. (529) conducted a meta-analysis of the English language literature through 1988 and found that adjuvant radiotherapy with doses of 3000 cGy or more resulted in a reduction of up to 40% in local recurrence in all but the lowest risk patient.

■ PATTERNS OF RECURRENCE

Pilipshen (525) has classified local recurrence with a view toward possible further treatment. He defined the five categories as follows:

- *Anastomotic.* Recurrence arising in and contained to bowel wall.
- *Perianastomotic.* Recurrence in proximity or involving the anastomosis by extensive disease with inward invasion.
- *Perineal.* Recurrence in the perineal scar following abdominoperineal resection. If minimal, the scar may be amenable to resection.
- *Pelvic wall.* Recurrence fixed to bone, major blood vessels, and/or nerves, usually precluding resection.
- *Anterior genitourinary.* Recurrence that, if amenable to resection, involves pelvic exenteration.

In most instances, however, recurrences overlap these categories at the time of diagnosis.

Gunderson and Sosin (457) reported that in patients who develop recurrent disease, local recurrence alone was noted in 50% of patients and in 92% with distant metastases. In an autopsy series, Welch and Donaldson (530) found that 25% of the patients died of only local disease, 25% of distant disease, and 50% of combined regional and distant metastases. Among patients who develop recurrent disease, Pilipshen et al. (531) found that the pelvis was the single site of recurrence in 53% or was combined with other sites in 63%. They suggested that resection of local recurrent disease would be feasible in 20% of patients who underwent low anterior resection and in 10% of patients who underwent abdominoperineal resection.

In a review of the patterns of recurrence following curative abdominoperineal resection, Rosen et al. (175) found that 43% of patients developed recurrence, 10% developed local recurrence, and the other 33% manifest with distant metastases. They noted that local recurrence appears much earlier in patients with Dukes' C lesions than in those with Dukes' B lesions (6 months vs. 21.5 months). However, once recurrence appears, differences in survival time from recurrence to death were not significant (10.5 months vs. 17 months), regardless of whether the initial presentation of recurrence was local or distant.

In a review of 1008 patients who underwent curative resection, McDermott et al. (331) found that 11% of patients developed local recurrence without evidence of systemic spread, whereas 9% developed both local and systemic recurrence. Of the patients who developed metastases, the recurrence was evident within two years in 60%. Of the patients who died from recurrence, 27% had evidence of local recurrence only, 24% had combined local and systemic recurrence, and 48% had evidence of systemic spread only. The corresponding median survival times were 35, 34, and 39 months, respectively.

Luna-Perez et al. (532) reported on the patterns of recurrence in a group of 49 patients treated with pelvic exenteration and radiotherapy. Thirty-one received preoperative radiotherapy, 4500 cGy. Six weeks later they performed posterior pelvic exenteration in 21 patients and total pelvic exenteration in 10. Nine patients received postoperative radiotherapy, 5000 cGy, after a posterior pelvic exenteration. Of nine patients who had surgery, only seven had posterior pelvic exenteration and two had total pelvic exenteration. Surgical mortality occurred in 16% of those patients who received preoperative radiotherapy. The median follow-up was 52 months. Recurrences occurred in 23% of those patients who received preoperative radiotherapy (local, one patient; local/distant, one; distant, four); in 88% of those patients treated with surgery only (local/distant, four; distant, four); and in 11% of those treated with postoperative radiotherapy (distant, one). The five-year survival rate for patients who received radiotherapy was 66% vs. 44% for those treated with surgery only. The authors concluded that local control of locally advanced primary rectal adenocarcinoma requiring a pelvic exenteration is improved by the addition of radiotherapy. When recurrences do occur, they are predominantly at extrapelvic sites. The extensive review of the patterns of recurrence reported by Obrand and Gordon was described in Chapter 23.

■ CLINICAL FEATURES

With anastomotic recurrence, the patient may be asymptomatic, but an irregularity may be found upon follow-up rectal, digital, or vaginal examination, or recurrence may be seen during sigmoidoscopy. Symptoms, when present, may include bleeding, narrowed stools, or pain. A biopsy confirms the diagnosis.

Following abdominoperineal resection with perineal recurrence, a mass may be seen. Pelvic recurrence may be asymptomatic or may manifest with pain or pressure in the abdomen, pelvis, or perineum (Fig. 30). The pain may also radiate to the back, buttocks, or lower extremities. Urinary tract symptoms may develop, or vaginal bleeding may occur. As many as half the patients with recurrence are symptom free at the time of diagnosis (522).

■ INVESTIGATIONS

A barium enema is not necessary for diagnosing an anastomotic recurrence following low anterior resection but may show a narrow-caliber lumen and rule out a synchronous

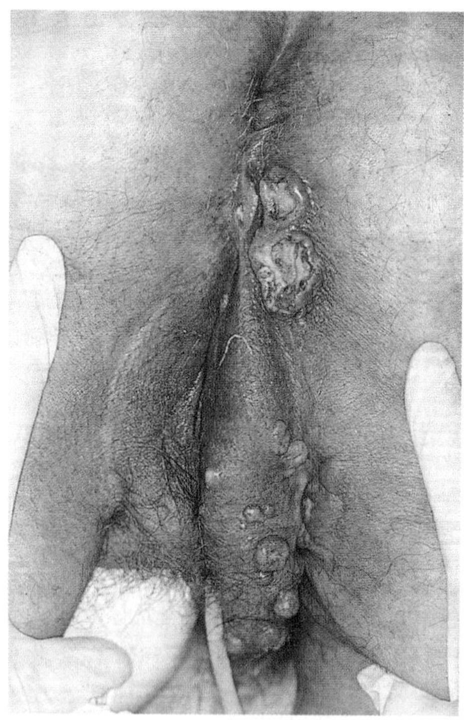

FIGURE 30 ■ Perineal recurrence with ulcerating masses and numerous metastatic nodules along vulva and groin.

neoplastic lesion if a colonoscopy is not planned or unable to to performed. Investigations should include a search for the extent of disease using an IVP, which may show ureteral displacement or compression although this information can usually be obtained from a CT scan. The carcinoembryonic antigen (CEA) level may or may not be elevated in patients with a pelvic recurrence. A search for disseminated disease also should be made. CT scanning is probably the most useful test to determine a recurrence. Postoperative changes, especially after abdominoperineal excision of the rectum, mimic recurrent disease and serial scans may be of benefit especially if a postoperative baseline scan had been obtained. Following abdominoperineal resection, percutaneous biopsy under CT guidance will confirm the diagnosis (533). MRI may also demonstrate the extent of a pelvic recurrence and/or guide percutaneous biopsy. Intrarectal ultrasonography may detect early intramural or extrarectal recurrences before there is evidence of intraluminal recurrence (534). Lohnert et al. (535) conducted a prospective study to assess the diagnostic potential of endorectal and endovaginal ultrasound to detect asymptomatic resectable local recurrence. In 338 patients, 721 endoluminal ultrasound examinations were added to routine follow-up of rectal and left colonic carcinoma. A total of 116 patients (34.3%) were shown to have local recurrence, which was suggested by endoluminal ultrasound and proven by endoluminal ultrasound guided needle biopsy in all cases of unclear pararectal structures that could not be verified by endoscopic biopsy. Digital examination failed to detect local recurrence in 91 patients, endoscopy failed to detect local recurrence in 80 patients, and the levels of markers for carcinoma were normal in 25 patients with confirmed local recurrence. In 33 cases of local recurrence, both digital examination and endoscopy results were normal. Twenty-five patients in whom carcinoembryonic antigen levels, digital examinations, and endoscopy results were normal, underwent potential curative reoperation, with total resection of the local recurrence. All 25 patients were still alive at the end of the study period, and 21 were free from disease. On the other hand, only 6 of 67 patients with local recurrence detectable by conventional follow-up could be operated on with curative intention. Detecting radiolabeled monoclonal antibodies with a hand-held gamma-counter probe appears to be of some help in intraoperative decision making at the time of second-look operation. Unnecessary operation can be avoided and the extent of potentially curative resections may be expanded (536). Moore et al. (537) found that PET scanning is an accurate modality for detecting pelvic recurrence of rectal carcinoma after full dose external beam radiotherapy. It correctly identified 16 of 19 recurrences for a sensitivity of 84% and specificity of 88%. Overall accuracy was 87%.

■ TREATMENT OF RECURRENT DISEASE

Effective therapy for pelvic or perineal recurrence is limited. It appears, however, that to adopt a totally therapeutic nihilistic attitude is not entirely warranted. Resectional therapy has proven curative in some, albeit a limited number, patients [estimated by some to be up to one-third of patients (520)] and palliative care can lessen the discomfort of many of these patients.

Yamada et al. (538) studied 83 patients with locally recurrent rectal carcinoma for survival benefit by re-resection. Sixty patients underwent resection for recurrent carcinoma including total pelvic exenteration in 30 patients and sacrectomy in 23 patients. The extent of locally recurrent carcinoma classified by the pattern of pelvic invasion was: localized, sacral invasion, and lateral invasion. This simple classification proved to be helpful to the surgeon making a recommendation for treatment as the pattern of pelvic invasion was a significant prognostic factor that independently influenced survival after resection of recurrent carcinoma. The five-year survival rates were 38% in the localized type (recurrent carcinoma localized to adjacent pelvic organs or connective tissue), 10% in the sacral invasion type (recurrent carcinoma invading the lower sacrum S3-4–5, coccyx, or periostium) and 0% in the lateral invasive type (recurrent carcinoma invading the sciatic nerve, greater sciatic foramen, lateral pelvic wall or upper sacrum S1/2). Hence resection for locally recurrent rectal carcinoma is potentially curative in patients with localized or sacral invasion patterns of recurrence, but alternatives should be explored in patients with recurrence involving the lateral pelvic wall.

Operative Treatment

In selected circumstances when technically possible, the best chance for cure following a recurrence is re-resection. Failing that, radical surgery may offer good palliation and a better quality of life (520). More than 50% of these patients have disease amenable to operative resection (520). In a review of seven reports from the literature, Herefarth et al. (539) deemed that 31% of patients with locoregional recurrence may be suitable for curative reintervention. This was a paltry increase of only 6% over reports two and three decades earlier, despite the advanced technology used in the postoperative follow-up.

In the case of a previous low anterior resection, occasionally it may be feasible to effect a re-resection with an extended low anterior resection, but more likely an abdominoperineal resection will be necessary. In preparation for operation, insertion of ureteral catheters may be helpful to identify the ureters. Segall et al. (540) reviewed 12 patients who underwent abdominoperineal resection for recurrence subsequent to low anterior resection. These procedures were technically more difficult, but no death occurred. Although no long-term cures resulted, significant palliation was achieved, and one patient survived more than eight years. In the series reviewed by Schiessel et al. (522) the treatment of local recurrence was operative in 86.5% of patients (48.6% of the patients underwent radical resection and 51.4% underwent palliative operation). The type of operative intervention depended on the localization of the recurrence and included abdominoperineal resection, sacral excision, or pelvic exenteration. Hojo (176) performed re-resection in 22 of 30 patients with anastomotic recurrence; 11 had curative resections.

Suzuki et al. (541) reported on 65 patients who underwent re-resection for recurrent rectal carcinoma. Procedures included abdominoperineal resection, wide local resection, Hartmann's procedure, low anterior resection, and abdominosacral resection along with an en bloc resection of adherent organs, including vagina, uterus, bladder, prostate, seminal vesicles, and sacrum when appropriate. There were no deaths, but 17 severe complications occurred. Three-year, five-year, and median survivals were 57, 34, and 45 months, respectively. The cumulative probability of failure was 24%, 41%, and 47% at one, three, and five years, respectively. Cumulative risk of distant metastases was 30%, 51%, and 62% at one, three, and five years, respectively. The authors concluded that complete excision of locally recurrent carcinoma would be able to provide a significant number of patients with long-term survival.

Wiggers et al. (542) reviewed 163 patients with local recurrence of rectal carcinoma after previous "curative" resection and of the 35 patients who underwent exploratory laparotomy, 27 were amenable to re-resection. There was no operative mortality but, with a median follow-up of 42 months, local re-recurrence developed in 59% of patients. The estimated five-year survival rate was 20%.

Saito et al. (543) reviewed 58 consecutive patients with local recurrence of rectal carcinoma after previous "curative" resection. Of the 58 patients, 27 underwent re-resection, nine had palliative resection, and 22 were treated by conservative therapy. Among the 27 patients with curative resections, 17 received preoperative radiotherapy (40 Gy) plus operation, and 10 operation alone. No patients were lost to follow-up; median follow-up time was 36.3 months. The overall rate of curative resection was 46.6%. With regard to surgical procedure, abdominoperineal resection with or without sacral resection was standard following previous low anterior resection and total pelvic exenteration with or without sacral resection was common after abdominoperineal resection. There was a high incidence of morbidity (71.4%) after total pelvic exenteration. Re-recurrence was observed in 44.4% after curative re-resection. There was local re-recurrence in 22.2%. The local re-recurrence rate was 11.8% with radiotherapy plus operation and 40% with operation alone. The estimated five-year survival following curative re-resection was 45.6% (61.2% with radiotherapy plus operation, 29.6% with operation alone). Huguier et al. (544) reported that of 80 patients having local recurrence, 48% underwent a re-resection combined in 10 cases with resection of metastases. The incidence of asymptomatic detected recurrence was higher after anterior resection (39%) than after abdominoperineal resection (18%). Re-resection was performed more often in the past two decades after anterior or Hartmann first procedure than after abdominoperineal resection (67% vs. 21%) and more often in asymptomatic patients than in symptomatic patients (71% vs. 38%). The actuarial five-year survival rate after re-resection was 20%. They concluded early detection of local recurrence with PET scan leads to an improved re-resection rate.

Boyle et al. (545) assessed the outcome of a series of 64 patients who underwent resection of locally recurrent rectal carcinoma with curative intent. The median time interval between resection of primary carcinoma and surgery for locally recurrent disease was 31 months. Twenty-three patients had central disease, 10 patients had sacral involvement, 21 patients had pelvic sidewall involvement, and 10 patients had both sacral and sidewall involvement. Fifty-seven patients underwent resection of the carcinoma. Thirty-nine out of 57 patients underwent wide resection (abdominoperineal excision of rectum, anterior resection, or Hartmann's procedure) whereas 18 patients (31.6%) required radical resection, pelvic exenteration, or sacrectomy. Curative, negative resection margins were obtained in 36.8% of patients who had excision. Perioperative mortality was 1.6%. Significant postoperative morbidity occurred in 40% of patients.

Vermaas et al. (546), compared the results of preoperative radiotherapy followed by operation with operation alone for recurrent rectal carcinoma. With 92 patients suitable for resection with curative intent, preoperative radiation with a median dosage of 50 Gy was performed in 59 patients; 33 patients did not receive preoperative radiotherapy. The median follow-up of patients alive for the total group was 16 months. Complete resections were performed in 64% of the patients who received preoperative radiation and 45% of the nonirradiated patients. A complete response with radiotherapy was found in 10% of the preoperative irradiated patients. There were no differences in morbidity and reintervention rate between the two groups. Local control after preoperative radiotherapy was statistically significantly higher after three and five years. Overall survival and metastasis-free survival were not different in both groups. Complete response to preoperative radiotherapy was predictive for an improved survival.

Garcia-Aguilar et al. (547) analyzed the outcome of patients with isolated local recurrence after radical treatment for rectal carcinoma in 87 patients. Symptomatic treatment alone or chemotherapy and/or radiation therapy was provided in 23 patients (26%) and surgical exploration was performed in 64 patients. In 22 patients (25%), the carcinoma was considered unresectable at operation ($n = 13$) or was resected for palliation with gross or microscopic-positive margins ($n = 9$). In 48% curative intent resection was performed. The only independent predictors of resectability were younger age at diagnosis, earlier stage of the primary carcinoma, and initial treatment by sphincter-saving procedure. There was no difference in survival between patients who had no operation and those who had palliative operation. The estimated five-year survival rate for patients who had curative intent resection was better than for those who had no operation or palliative operation (35% vs. 7%). Of the 42 patients who underwent curative intent resection, 33% developed a second recurrence at a mean of 15 months after reoperation. Twenty-five percent of patients developed major complications.

Hahnloser et al. (548) assessed the results of multimodality therapy for patients with recurrent rectal carcinoma and analyzed factors predictive of curative resection and prognostic for overall survival. A total of 394 patients underwent surgical exploration for recurrent rectal carcinoma. Ninety were found to have unresectable local or extrapelvic disease and 304 underwent resection of the recurrence. Overall five-year survival was 25%. Curative, negative resection margins were obtained in 45% of patients; in these patients a five-year survival of 37% was achieved compared to 16% in patients with either microscopic or gross residual disease. Overall survival was significantly decreased for symptomatic pain and more than one fixation. Survival following extended resection of adjacent organs was not different from limited resection (28% vs. 21%). Perioperative mortality was only 0.3% but significant morbidity occurred in 26% of patients with pelvic abscess being the most common complication. They concluded long-term survival can be achieved especially for patients with no symptoms and minimal fixation of the recurrence in the pelvis provided no gross residual disease remains. Lopez-Kostner et al. (549) determined whether salvage operation in appropriate selected patients could significantly lengthen disease-free survival after a previously curative resection for rectal carcinoma. Of 937 patients who underwent operation with curative intent, 8.6% experienced local recurrence. Thirty-six patients with locally current rectal carcinoma were referred from other institutions. Of 117 patients with locally recurrent rectal carcinoma, 36.7% underwent salvage operation. Factors associated with higher chance of receiving salvage operation were female gender, the first operation performed at outside institutions, and transanal local excision as the initial operation. For 43 patients who underwent salvage operation, five-year carcinoma-specific and disease-free survival rates were 49.7% and 32.2%, respectively. A trend for poor prognosis was observed in patients with recurrence diameter greater than 3 cm and fixation of the carcinoma.

Mannaerts et al. (550) compared three treatment modalities for patients with locally recurrent rectal carcinoma. Ninety-four patients were treated with electron-beam radiation therapy only, 19 with combined preoperative electron-beam radiation therapy and operation and 33 with intraoperative radiation therapy-multimodality treatment. The three-year survival, disease-free survival and local control rates were 14%, 8%, and 10%, respectively, in the electron-beam radiation therapy only group and 11%, 0%, and 14%, respectively, in the combined electron-beam radiation therapy surgery group. The overall intraoperative radiation therapy multimodality treatment group showed significant better three-year survival, disease-free survival, and local control rates of 60%, 43%, and 73%, respectively compared with the historical control groups.

Isolated perineal recurrence after abdominoperineal resection of the rectum may be suitable for wide local excision. Cure is rare as perineal deposits are usually associated with disease deeper in the pelvis. Local excision results in some palliation but may also result in nonhealing wounds and even enterocutaneous fistulas.

To determine the value of total pelvic exenteration, Lopez et al. (551) reviewed the results of 24 patients undergoing the procedure, which involved removal of the distal colon and rectum along with the lower ureters, bladder, internal reproductive organs, perineum, draining lymph nodes, and pelvic peritoneum. The operative mortality was 20% (9% during the past decade) with an overall survival rate of 42%.

Falk et al. (552) reported on 45 patients who underwent pelvic exenteration for advanced primary or recurrent adenocarcinoma. Many patients had previous radiotherapy. The operative mortality was 15.5%. Of the 16 patients who had palliative exenteration, nine died, seven of progressive malignancy (median survival, five months). Exenteration was deemed curative in 22 patients, but six died of the disease (median survival, 15.5 months). At the time of reporting, four patients were alive at 11,17, 21, and 23 months. After operation the remaining 12 patients were disease free at 4 to 21 months postoperatively (median, 10.5 months).

Sugarbaker (385) reported on six patients who underwent en bloc resection for rectal carcinoma with sacrectomy for lesions fixed posteriorly. Voiding occurred spontaneously, but the men were impotent. Four of six such patients survived more than three years. Temple and Ketcham (553) performed five en bloc resections and one sacral resection only. The operative mortality was 9% with an 18% five-year survival. Pearlman et al. (554) reported on 19 patients. Four underwent extended proctectomy, four underwent a standard pelvic exenteration, and 12 had sacropelvic exenterations. One operative death occurred, two died free of disease, four died of disease, two are alive with disease, and eight are living free of disease at the time of publication. The authors believe that radiation is not as effective as radical operation.

Wanebo et al. (555) have used abdominosacral resection with or without pelvic exenteration for pelvic recurrence in 53 patients, 47 with curative intent. Almost all the patients had been irradiated previously (4000–5900 cGy). Organs resected included the rectum, 18; bladder, 25; partial bladder, two; prostate and/or seminal vesicles, 19; vagina, two; total abdominal hysterectomy, eight; segmental bowel resection, eight; and other, eight. The level of sacral resection was L5-S1, one; high SI or Sl-2, 26; mid-S2 or mid-S3, 14; and low S4-5, six. Added resection included sidewall pelvic vessels in two patients and pelvic lymph node dissection in 46. The operative mortality rate was 8.5% and postoperative morbidity was encountered in most patients. Survivors had relief of sacral root pain and good motor function. The division of SI, S2, S3 roots compromises bladder function, resulting in bladder denervation. Although this can be managed by Crede's method of voiding and the use of α-agonists or self-catheterization, it requires careful attention and care by the attending physician. The actuarial five-year survival rate was 33% and the median survival was 39 months. Temple and Ketcham (556) described a unique palliative approach of radical debridement for recurrent carcinoma ulcerating through the perineum that cannot be controlled by other means. Seven patients were treated with resection of the recurrence along with portions of the sacrum. Coverage was obtained with myocutaneous flaps. Temple and Ketcham believe that the duration and quality of life are improved with this method.

Tepper et al. (557) reported on the prevalence and influence of salvage therapy among patients with recurrent disease following curative resection of T3, T4 rectal carcinomas in the intergroup study 0114. A total of 1792 patients were entered into the study and 1696 were assessable. After a median of 8.9 years of follow-up, 715 patients (42%) had disease recurrence, and an additional 10% died without evidence of disease. Five hundred patients with follow-up information available had a single organ or single site of first recurrence (73.5% of all recurrences). A total of 171 patients (34% of those with a single organ or single site of recurrence) had a potentially curative resection of the metastatic or locally recurrent disease. Single-site first recurrences in the liver, lung, or pelvis occurred in 448 patients (90% of the single-site recurrences), with 159 (35%) of these undergoing surgical resection for attempted cure. Overall survival differed significantly between the resected and nonresected groups with overall five-year probabilities of 0.27 and 0.06, respectively. From their data, the chance of a long-term cure for surgical salvage of rectal carcinoma recurrence is approximately 27%.

Jimenez et al. (558) reviewed 55 patients undergoing total pelvic exenteration for locally advanced or recurrent colorectal carcinoma. Indications for operation were recurrent colorectal carcinoma in 71% and primary rectal carcinoma in 29%. Of 39 patients with recurrent colorectal carcinoma, 85% had previous radiotherapy and 64% had previous abdominoperineal resection. At the time of pelvic exenteration, 49% of patients receiving intraoperative radiation and 20% required sacrectomy. Complete resection with negative margins was achieved in 73%. Perioperative mortality after pelvic exenteration was 5.5% and complications including perineal wound infection (40%), pelvic abscess (20%), abdominal wound infection (18%), and cardiopulmonary events (18%). Median disease-specific survival for all patients was 48.9 (range, 3.2–105.6) months. Less satisfactory outcomes are observed in patients whose indication for pelvic exenteration is recurrent colorectal carcinoma after abdomoniperineal resection.

Ike et al. (559) reviewed charts of 45 patients with rectal carcinoma who underwent curative total pelvic exenteration for local recurrence. Post-operative morbidity was 77.8% and in-hospital death occurred in 13.3% of patients. The overall five-year survival rate was 14.1%. The five-year survival rates stratified according to the expectation of curability were 31.6% for absolutely curative resection, 7.8% for relatively curative resection, and 0% for noncurative resection. The disease-free interval was the only independent prognostic factor. There was no benefit from perioperative radiation or intraoperative continuous pelvic peritoneal perfusion of the pelvis. They concluded total pelvic exenteration for local recurrence of rectal carcinoma would be able to achieve long-term survival when curative resection is possible and the disease-free interval would be long.

Bakx et al. (560) reported on the results of 26 patients who underwent sacral resection for both primary and recurrent rectal carcinoma as well as recurrent anal carcinoma. Sacral resection alone was performed in five patients, with abdominoperineal resection in six patients and exenteration in 13 patients. Median operating time was six hours (range 2.5–10 hours) with median blood loss of 3600 ML (range 420–11,500 ML). A transpelvic rectus abdominis musculocutaneous flap was used in 50% and an omental transposition in 65% of procedures. There was only one death. Estimated two and five-year survivals were 82% and 51%, respectively. There were 27 major complications (five requiring re-laparotomy). They believe their results support the use of sacral resection in patients with nonmetastatic malignant disease.

Mannaerts et al. (561) reported their results in patients with locally advanced primary (13) or locally recurrent rectal (37) carcinoma with dorsolateral fixation who underwent abdominosacral resection as part of a multimodality treatment, i.e., preoperative irradiation, operation, and intraoperative irradiation. Margins were microscopically negative in 52%, microscopically positive in 36%, and positive with gross residual disease in 12%. Operation time ranged from 210 to 590 minutes and blood loss ranged from 400 to 10,000 ML. No operative or hospital deaths occurred. Postoperative complications occurred in 82%; most notably were perineal wound infections or dehiscence (48%). Other complications were postoperative urinary retention or incontinence (18%), peritonitis, grade II neuropathy, and fistula formation. The three-year overall survival, disease-free survival, and local control rates were respectively 41%, 31%, and 61%. Completeness of the resection (negative vs. positive margins was a significant factor influencing survival, disease-free survival, and local control.

Moriya et al. (562) evaluated the effectiveness or total pelvic exenteration with distal sacrectomy for fixed recurrent carcinoma that developed from primary rectal carcinoma in 57 patients. Negative margins were present in 84%. Two hospital deaths were observed in the early period and none in the later period. The most common sacral amputation level was the S3 superior margin, followed by the S4 inferior margin and the S2 margin. The most frequent complication was sacral wound dehiscence in 51%, followed by pelvic sepsis in 39%. The incidence of pelvic sepsis in the latter period was significantly decreased to 23% compared with 72% in the earlier period. Negative margins and negative CEA predicted improved survival. In 48 patients with negative margins, three-year and five-year disease-specific survivals were 62% and 42%, respectively.

Shirouzu et al. (563) reported on 26 patients who underwent total pelvic exenteration for locally advanced colorectal carcinoma with an 8% mortality rate. In patients with stage II primary disease the five year survival rate was 71% (mean survival, 58 months). In patients with stage III, the mean survival was 14 months and in stage IV, the mean survival was five months. In patients who underwent curative operation for recurrent disease, the five-year survival rate was 25% (mean survival, 33 months). In their review of the literature, Sagar and Pemberton (520) noted that if patients are selected carefully, pelvic exenteration is associated with a median survival of 21 to 30 months and a five-year survival rate of ≤50%.

In their review of pelvic exenteration for recurrent colorectal carcinoma, Yeung et al. (564) noted that after they combined a series of 13 reports in the literature, the incidence of pelvic recurrence by Dukes' staging was 11%, 23%, and 35% for Dukes' A, B, and C, respectively, with an overall recurrence rate of 25%. It is very clear that the incidence of recurrence is dependent on the length of follow-up, but approximately 70% of failures occur within two years of treatment. A significant portion of patients with local recurrence have disease confined to the pelvis without distant metastases. Faced with the problem of isolated pelvic recurrence, complete extirpation may have a chance of cure or at least good palliation. Elements of the procedure consist of a composite that in women are radical hysterectomy, total cystectomy, and abdominoperineal resection; and in men total cystectomy, radical prostatectomy, and abdominoperineal resection. More radical resection may include sacrectomy. In their series of 43 patients ranging in age from 31 to 77 years, the median duration from the time of the initial operation to exenteration was 39.7 months. Of the patients studied, 60% had received radiotherapy. Internal iliac vessels were ligated, but involvement of common and external iliac vessels implied inoperability. The most popular form of urinary diversion was the ileal conduit. In their series of 43 patients, 26 had ileal conduits, six had colonic conduits, and 11 had wet colostomies. Among the different constructions of a continent reservoir, the ileal colonic (Indiana) pouch was attractive because it utilized the least amount of ileum along with the ascending colon, which has the greatest likelihood of not being exposed to pelvic radiation. The learning curve for this procedure is steep with high postoperative morbidity and mortality rates. Cited operative mortality rates fell from 13% to 20% to from 2% to 7% as experience accumulated. Complication rates range from 30% to 75%. Types of complications included enteric fistula, conduit leak and/or fistula, bowel obstruction, pelvic hemorrhage/abscess, urosepsis, renal failure, wound infection, deep venous thromboses/pulmonary embolus, myocardial infarction/cardiac arrest, cerebrovascular accident, sepsis (nonpelvic), gastrointestinal hemorrhage, prolonged ileus, and hernia. The reoperation rate was high among this group of patients in whom the complication rate was even higher. These sobering statistics mandate that a careful patient selection process was undertaken prior to embarking on this procedure. Survival rates following this procedure have not been overly encouraging. Reported rates of recurrence range from 40% to 70% and overall five-year survival rates from 10% to 20%. However, this should be compared to a 2% to 3% five-year survival rate for untreated disease. Even in a palliative setting, symptomatic improvement is often prompt and long-standing. Up to 89% of patients with curative intent have significant palliation from pain. Moreover, some of these patients achieve remarkable psychological improvement and an enhanced quality of life.

Since it was first reported in 1948, pelvic exenteration has been used in the treatment of advanced pelvic malignancy. The original procedure has been modified in an attempt to preserve urinary or fecal continence. Rodriguez-Bigas and Petrelli (565) conducted a literature review on selected series of total pelvic exenterations and modified pelvic exenterations in order to assess and discuss the different types of pelvic exenterations and the indications, contraindications, morbidity, mortality, and results of these procedures. According to the series reviewed, morbidity after pelvic exenteration ranges between 32% and 84%, postoperative mortality ranges from 0% to 14%, and five-year survival varies from 23% to 68%. These numbers indicate that total pelvic exenteration and its modifications are a complex group of surgical procedures with significant early and late postoperative morbidity and mortality. While the authors think that these findings indicate that pelvic exenteration should only be undertaken by experienced surgeons at specialized centers, they also caution that, above all, their findings indicate that the potential curability of a patient with adjacent organ involvement should not be compromised by doing less than an en bloc resection.

Kakuda et al. (566) reviewed 22 patients who underwent pelvic exenteration for recurrent rectal carcinoma. Seventeen underwent potentially curative resection, five were for palliation only. There was one operative death. Fifteen suffered at least one complication; nine suffered multiple complications. Ten patients required re-admission to the hospital. The overall disease-free interval was 11 months. Potentially curative and palliative resections resulted in median survivals of 20.4 and 8.4 months, respectively. While patients may derive oncologic and palliative benefits from exenteration, the price in terms of operative morbidity remains high.

Although resection of locally recurrent rectal carcinoma has been associated with improved survival, symptomatic relief has been incompletely characterized. Miner et al. (567) reviewed 105 consecutive patients requiring repeat operation for locally recurrent rectal carcinoma. They were observed for a minimum of two years or until death. An operation was performed with palliative intent in 23% of patients. Before repeat operation, 79% of the palliative intent patients had symptoms: 21% bleeding, 42% obstruction, and 21% pain. After repeat operation with palliative intent, improvement was noted in 40% with bleeding, 70% with obstruction, and 20% with pain. Additional or recurrent symptoms were noted in 87% during follow-up. Seventy-seven percent of patients had an operation with nonpalliative intent. Before repeat operations, 57% of nonpalliative patients had symptoms, with 32% experiencing bleeding, 11% obstruction, and 19% pain. After repeat operation with nonpalliative intent, initial improvement was noted in 88% with bleeding, 78% with obstruction, and 40% with pain. During follow-up, symptoms arose in 37% of the initially asymptomatic patients and additional or recurrent symptoms were seen in 63% of those previously symptomatic. They noted, the recurrence or development of new symptoms makes a complete asymptomatic clinical course uncommon.

Shoup et al. (568) reported survival after operation and intraoperative radiotherapy for recurrent rectal carcinoma. Of 634 patients undergoing resection for recurrent rectal carcinoma, 111 received intraoperative radiotherapy with curative intent and 100 were available for follow-up. With a median follow-up of 23.2 months, 60% recurred: 33% locally and 45% distantly and 22% at both sites. Of all variables analyzed, only complete resection with microscopically negative margins and the absence of vascular invasion in the recurrent specimen predicted improved disease-free and disease-specific survival. Median disease-free survival and median disease-specific survival were 31.2 and 66.1 months, respectively, for complete resection compared with 7.9 and 22.8 months for resection for microscopic or grossly positive margins. Median disease-free survival and median disease-specific survival were 6.4 and 16.1 months, respectively, in the presence of vascular invasion in the recurrent specimen compared with 23.3 and 57.3 months in the absence of vascular invasion. Complete resection and the absence of vascular invasion were the only predictors of improved local control.

Kuehne et al. (569) evaluated the use of fractionated perioperative high-dose-rate brachytherapy in association with wide surgical excision (debulking). All patients had abdominal exploration, aggressive debulking of the carcinoma, and placement of afterloading brachytherapy catheters. Patients underwent simulation on postoperative day 3 and received 1200 to 2500 cGy of fractionated high-dose-rate brachytherapy between postoperative days 3 and 5. All patients had involvement of the lateral pelvic sidewall and/or the sacrum. Follow-up ranged from 18 to 93 months and was available in 27 patients of which 37% were alive at the time of the report. Nine patients were without evidence of disease. Eighteen percent died of noncarcinoma related causes without evidence of recurrent disease. Five complications potentially related to treatment (three abscesses, two fistulas) occurred in five patients.

Cheng et al. (570) conducted a retrospective chart review of 142 patients with recurrent rectal carcinoma, 27 of whom had unilateral or bilateral hydronephrosis. Distant metastatic disease was present in 55% of these patients. Twelve patients (45%) with hydronephrosis and local recurrent disease on evaluation were analyzed. Six of the 12 patients underwent exploratory laparotomy with none found to have resectable disease. Their mean survival after diagnosis of recurrent disease was 14 months. Based on their results, the presence of hydronephrosis (unilateral or bilateral) in recurrent rectal carcinoma portends a survival equivalent to the presence of distant metastases. Therefore, they do not believe potentially curative resection has a role for patients with locally recurrent rectal carcinoma in the presence of hydronephrosis.

Kelly and Nugent (571) described the use of intrarectal formalin instillation to control intractable rectal bleeding from advanced pelvic malignancy. The technique involves insertion of a foley catheter to the top of the rectum and inflating the balloon to 30 cc. Paraffin gauze and gel are applied to the anal skin following which 40 ML of 4% formalin is infused into the rectum for two minutes and then removed. The rectum is irrigated with normal saline for five minutes. They found formalin instillation into the rectum is an option when one is faced with rectal hemorrhage from inoperable pelvic malignancies.

To provide local control and palliation of pain, a multimodality approach that includes external beam radiation therapy, surgical resection, and intraoperative electron irradiation has been used at the Mayo Clinic for patients with locally advanced anal or recurrent rectal carcinomas involving the sacrum (572). Sixteen consecutive patients underwent surgical exploration, sacrectomy, and intraoperative electron radiation therapy. Proximal extent of resection was S2-3 in four patients, S3-4 in five, and S4-5 in five. Two patients underwent resection of the anterior table of the sacrum. Margins were clear in 11, close in three, and microscopically involved in two patients. Operative times ranged from 6 to 17 hours (median, 12.5 hours), and blood loss ranged from 300 to 12,600 ML (median, 3350 ML). No operative deaths resulted. Major postoperative complications occurred in eight patients (50%): posterior wound infections and dehiscence, urinary leak, and ileal fistula. Five patients (31%) developed no complications, and three patients (19%) developed minor complications. The survival rate was 68% at one year and 48% at two years. Rodriguez-Bigas et al. (573) found that both unilateral and bilateral hydro nephrosis are contraindications for potentially curative resection for recurrent rectal carcinoma. Wanebo et al. (555) also identified lateral pelvic node and marrow involvement as contraindications for resection in patients with advanced or recurrent disease.

Management of Sacral and Perineal Defects

The management of sacral and perineal defects following abdominoperineal resection and radiation can prove very difficult. Loessin et al. (574) presented their experience with treating persistent sacral and perineal defects secondary to radiation and abdominoperineal resection with or without sacrectomy. Fifteen consecutive patients were treated with an inferiorly based transpelvic rectus abdominis muscle or musculocutaneous flap. The technique as described by the authors is performed with the patient in the lithotomy position using two teams. The abdomen is opened in the midline, and the pelvis is cleared of all adhesions and bowel. The urologists place ureteral stents preoperatively in all patients to help avoid ureteral injury. After the pelvis has been cleared, very aggressive debridement of the perineal wound is performed so that fresh bleeding tissue and healthy bone are encountered. Leaving behind a nidus for infection or dead bone will result in failure. At this point, the rectus abdominis muscle or musculocutaneous flap is elevated. The flap is raised as an island flap connected only to the inferior epigastric pedicle (Fig. 31A). The entire muscle and skin unit is then passed into the pelvis via a 5 cm incision placed in the posterior sheath/peritoneum, starting at the point of the inferior epigastric vessels and running superiorly (Fig. 31B). The skin muscle unit is now carefully checked so that no twisting or kinking of the vascular leash is encountered. To "fit" the muscle and/or skin into the perineal wound, blunt dissection with the fingers must be performed "gingerly" so that a four-finger-breadth passage is created in the perineal wound (Fig. 31C). It is during this maneuver that bleeding or ureter or bladder injury may occur. Once this is accomplished, the pelvic cavity is copiously irrigated, bleeding observed and controlled, and the urinary tract checked for injury. At this point, the skin, muscle unit may be pulled and pushed into the defect. The perineal skin (Fig. 31D) and the abdomen can be closed.

Postoperatively, the patient is maintained on an air flotation mattress for five days. Patients are allowed to ambulate on day 7. Drains in the pelvis and abdomen are removed on day 10. Fourteen of the 15 patients healed, and seven patients had no complications. The remaining eight patients required one or more operative debridements and/or prolonged wound care to accomplish a healed wound. The authors concluded that difficult post-irradiated perineal and sacral wounds would be healed with persistent surgical attention to adequate debridement, control of infections, and a well-vascularized muscle flap. The most satisfying aspects for patients are elimination of a foul-smelling discharge, discontinuation of multiple daily dressing changes, and reduction in the degree of chronic pain. Others have found this technique useful (575). Yeh et al. (576) used a variety of myocutaneous flaps to accomplish the same goal. Jain et al. (577) reported on the use of the transpelvic placement of the rectus abdominis muscle in a series of patients, 87% of whom received radiation therapy (muscle only was used in four patients, muscle with skin grafting in eight, and a musculocutaneous flap in three). Healing was complete in 12 of 15 patients at discharge.

Yeh et al. (576) reported on nine patients who underwent 10 myocutaneous flap reconstructions for large perineal or pelvic defects following surgical extirpation of recurrent rectal carcinoma at Fox Chase Cancer Center. All nine patients had been previously treated with radiation therapy. Resection was determined by the extent of recurrence and included perineal resection, pelvic exenteration, cystectomy, sacrectomy, or coccygectomy. Extent of disease necessitated intraoperative radiation therapy in one case and placement of brachy-therapy catheters in four. Bilateral gracilis flaps were used in four, unilateral in three, gluteus maxi-mus in two, and combined gluteal and gracilis flaps in one patient. Six perineal and four combined perineal and vaginal defects were reconstructed. The length of hospitalization averaged 17.5 days. Acute surgical flap-related complications included three cases of minor wound infection or separation. Chronic flap complications consisted of one fistula from a ureterocolostomy, five persistent sinuses that ultimately healed, and one incidence of delayed minimal wound separation. One late abscess necessitated reoperation for drainage. Perioperative mortality was zero. There was a single case of delayed flap loss at two years in the setting of malnutrition and neglect. The median actuarial survival rate following reconstruction is 32 months. A single patient had local failure, two had distant disease, and two were disease free. Patients indicated that to a large extent they were able to pursue normal activities. Pain was nonexistent or minimal in all patients surveyed. Patients with pain, bleeding, or infection from locally recurrent rectal carcinoma may survive many months.

Chessin et al. (578) cited a major source of morbidity after abdominoperineal resection after external beam pelvic radiation to be perineal wound complications, seen in up to 66% of cases. They determined the effect of rectus abdominus myocutaneous flap reconstruction on perineal wound morbidity in 19 patients with anorectal carcinoma treated with external beam pelvic radiation followed by abdominoperineal resection and rectus abdominus myocutaneous flap reconstruction of the perineum. A control group of

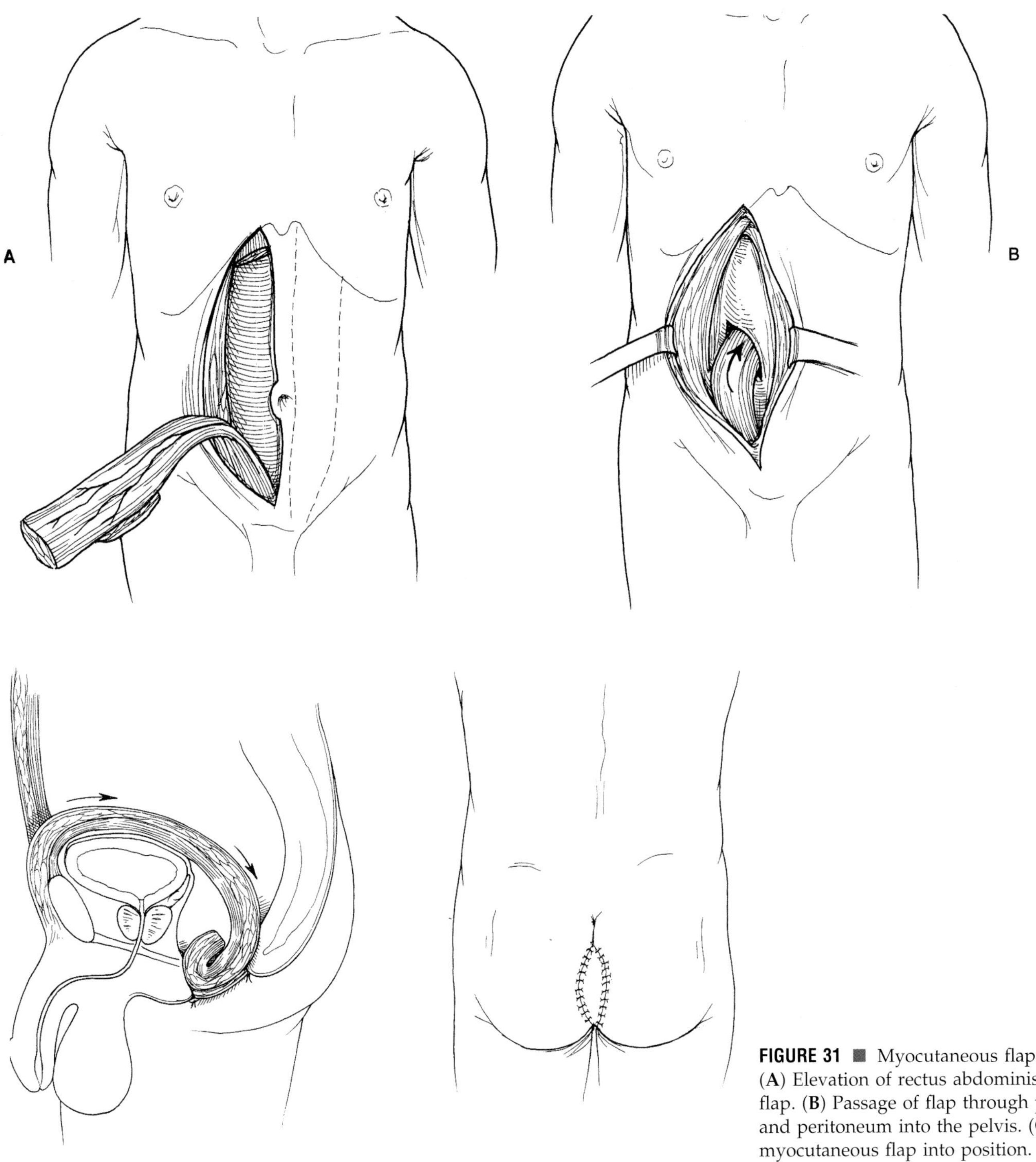

FIGURE 31 ■ Myocutaneous flap reconstruction. (**A**) Elevation of rectus abdominis myocutaneous flap. (**B**) Passage of flap through posterior sheath and peritoneum into the pelvis. (**C**) Securing myocutaneous flap into position. (**D**) Completed perineal closure.

59 patients with anorectal carcinoma treated with similar radiation doses that subsequently underwent an abdominoperineal resection without a rectus abdominus myocutaneous flap during the same time period was used. Perineal wound complications occurred in 15.8% of the flap patients and 44% of the control patients. The incidence of other complications was not different between groups (42.1% vs. 42.4%). They believe because other complications are not increased, flap closure of the perineal wound should be strongly considered in this patient population. The advantages of musculocutaneous flap reconstruction of the irradiated pelvis and perineal wound include reduction of dead space, interposition of well-vascularized, nonirradiated tissue, and replacement of resected skin. The disadvantages of these flaps include the added time for the surgical procedure, the added costs, and the potential morbidity (such as infections, flap loss, seroma, ventral and perineal hernia, and abdominal bulge) of such procedures. These disadvantages are usually offset by lower rates of perineal wound complications (579).

Local Ablation

The use of laser treatment for palliation in patients with unresectable recurrent carcinoma of the rectum has been described in some length in Chapter 23. Electrocoagulation has also been employed under these circumstances to avoid a colostomy (580). Of 15 patients so treated, nine were alive at 8 to 16 months without colostomy. Salvati and Rubin

(581) reported that 16 of 19 patients so treated were spared a colostomy. Good palliation of obstruction, bleeding, and pain have been reported with the use of the urologic resectoscope, a procedure that required no anesthetic or long operative time. In one series a colostomy was avoided in 14 of 15 patients (582).

The most common application of cryotherapy is treatment of recurrent, unresectable carcinomas of the rectum. The goal is the avoidance of a stoma. In a report of 219 patients so treated, Fritsch et al. (583) noted that local eradication of recurrent disease was achieved in 30% and symptoms were relieved in a further 24%. However, complications were not inconsequential, with bleeding in 14%, stenoses in 26%, and other complications, including peritonitis, in another 8%. Furthermore, the malodorous discharge was distressing. Heberer et al. (168) also reported avoidance of a stoma in 80% of 268 patients treated with cryotherapy.

Nonoperative Treatment

Radiotherapy

Radiotherapy is probably the most frequently adopted modality for the treatment of recurrent disease. It is reasonably effective in the control of pain and may shrink the mass and diminish drainage from ulcerated lesions. The ability to deliver radiation depends on whether the patient received adjuvant radiotherapy following the operation. In a series of 85 patients who developed pelvic recurrence after abdominoperineal resection, Villalon and Green (584) reported a 92% response to pain and an 80% response to mass (shrinkage). In a series of 143 patients, Pacini et al. (585) reported control of symptoms in 80% of patients. Dobrowsky and Schmid (586) obtained a 90% response rate. The crude survival time is 19.8 months following palliative radiotherapy (525,586).

Chemotherapy

Systemic chemotherapy has not demonstrated dramatic or long-term effects. Some palliation has been reported with the use of intraarterial 5-FU and mitomycin (587). The combination of hyperthermia and chemotherapy has been reported to offer better pain control (588). 5-FU and folinic acid (Leucovorin) is a frequently used combination at the present time (589).

Hyperthermia and Chemoradiotherapy

Nishimura et al. (590) reported on the addition of hyperthermia to radiation therapy for primarily unresectable as well as recurrent colorectal carcinoma. The authors found a response rate of 54% compared to 36% for radiotherapy alone.

In a nonrandomized trial, Ichikawa et al. (591) compared the results of postoperative combined radiation plus 5-FU suppositories plus hyperthermia (35 patients) to no pretreatment (41 patients). In the pretreatment group, local recurrence was lower (10.4% vs. 27.1%), and survival was improved (81.8% vs. 67.6%). The authors believe that this is a promising modality for advanced carcinoma of the lower rectum.

Gonzalez et al. (592) reported on 72 patients with either unresectable or recurrent colorectal carcinoma who were treated with combined radiotherapy (50 Gy) and hyperthermia (administered within 30 minutes of radiation intending to reach temperatures of 41°C over 30 minutes). Toxicity consisted of local pain (33%) and general discomfort (17%). Hyperthermia was prematurely stopped in 17% of patients. Palliation was achieved in 75% of patients with a mean duration of 12 months. Objective (CT scan) remission was obtained in 15%. Median survival was four months, and 17% of the patients were alive at three years after treatment.

Korenga et al. (593) retrospectively compared 23 patients treated with preoperative hyperthermia, chemotherapy, and radiotherapy with 48 patients treated by operation alone and operation and chemotherapy. The incidence of local recurrence was zero in the first group, but 15% and 10%, respectively, in the second group. The authors concluded that preoperative treatment decreased the frequency of local recurrence and the likelihood of spread during operation.

Pain Control

The principles of pain control and general comfort of the patient are described in Chapter 23. Narcotics should be prescribed liberally. For patients with intractable pain, neurosurgical procedures such as a chordotomy or rhizotomy are effective for pain control.

■ RESULTS OF REOPERATION

Controversy exists regarding the value of reoperation for recurrent carcinoma, and reported cure rates vary considerably. Pilipshen (525) reviewed a number of reports in the literature in which recurrences were re-resected by extended low anterior resection, abdominoperineal resection, or pelvic exenteration, even with partial sacrectomy. The overall "cure" was approximately 25%, but local repeat recurrence ranged from 25% to 50%.

Schiessel et al. (522) reported on 109 patients treated by operation with a radical procedure in 53 cases. The operative mortality was 4.6%, with a 50% survival rate at 17 months. Gagliardi et al. (594) reported on 55 patients who had resection of locally recurrent rectal carcinoma. The five-year survival rate was 18% with a median survival of 24 months. At a median follow-up of 28 months, 53% of patients developed a second local recurrence and 24% metastases only. Operative mortality was 5% and complications occurred in 22%. The authors' review of the literature revealed a probability of survival at one year to range from 30% to 98% and after three years, 0% to 62%. Williams et al. (595), in their review of the English literature, have suggested that the operative mortality rate should be less than 10% and can be less than 5% in primary cases of total pelvic exenteration. In their review of the literature regarding exenterative surgery for recurrent disease, Sagar and Pemberton (520) found an operative mortality rate ranging from 0% to 8.5%, a morbidity rate of 10% to 44%, survival rate of 18% to 49% at five years, and a local recurrence rate of 18% to 69%.

OTHER MALIGNANT LESIONS OF THE RECTUM

■ CARCINOID

Only those features specifically relevant to rectal as opposed to colonic carcinoids or carcinoids in general are discussed here. Derivation and histochemical characteristics have been discussed in the section on colonic carcinoids (Chapter 23). When the embryologically derived divisions of foregut, midgut, and hindgut are considered, the carcinoid neoplasm arising in each area has a characteristic chemicopathologic manifestation (596). Hindgut carcinoids, which include rectal carcinoids, do not produce serotonin and they are not considered to give rise to the carcinoid syndrome (596).

■ CLINICAL PRESENTATION

Rectal carcinoids comprise only 0.1% of all rectal neoplasms (597). They occur with no sex predominance and are most commonly found in the sixth and seventh decades of life. Carcinoids will be discovered in 0.05% of all patients who undergo sigmoidoscopy (598). In sigmoidoscopic examination of 21,522 asymptomatic adults, Matsui et al. (599) found 16 carcinoids (prevalence, 0.07%). In Chapter 23 it was stated that the appendix is the most common location for gastrointestinal carcinoids but in a review of 175 patients with gastrointestinal carcinoids from the Ochsner Clinic in New Orleans, Jetmore et al. (600) found that the rectum represents the most common primary site. The authors found that the distribution of carcinoids was rectum, 55%; ileum, 12%; appendix, 12%; colon, 6%; stomach, 6%; jejunum, 2%; pancreas, 2%; and other, 5%. The typical finding during rectal examination is a solitary mobile submucosal nodule with an intact overlying mucosa. Its color varies from yellow-gray to tan-pink. Its size is usually from 1 to 1.5 cm. An erythematous change or a depression may be seen (599). In only 2% to 4% of cases do multiple nodules occur. Symptoms are encountered in 50% of patients and include bleeding, change in bowel habits, pain, pruritus, or weight loss (601). None of the 86 patients with rectal carcinoids removed by Fitzgerald et al. (601) developed a carcinoid syndrome, a finding noted by others (597).

Malignancy has been reported in 39% of cases, and in these the significant findings related to a size greater than 2 cm in diameter with invasion through the muscularis propria. The malignant variety is frequently ulcerated, with bleeding being part of the clinical presentation. The incidence of metastatic disease is less in hindgut carcinoids (rectum, 18%) than in either midgut (jejunoileal, 34%; colon, 60%) or foregut (stomach, 23%; bronchus, 21%) (602). An association with long-standing chronic inflammatory bowel disease such as ulcerative colitis has been suggested (603). A secondary malignancy was found in eight of 43 patients with rectal carcinoids reported by Sauven et al. (603).

■ INVESTIGATION

As with carcinoma of the rectum, intrarectal ultrasonography has been useful in the evaluation of carcinoids. Yoshikane et al. (604) found an overall accuracy of 75% in determining the depth of invasion as well as lymph node metastases.

Kobayashi et al. (605) evaluated the diagnostic value of endoscopic ultrasonography in 66 rectal carcinoids to determine whether a lesion is indicated for endoscopic polypectomy. They concluded rectal carcinoids that satisfy the following three conditions are indicated for local resection, including endoscopic polypectomy: a maximum diameter of less than or equal to 10 mm, no invasion of the muscularis propria, and no depression or ulceration in the lesion. Endoscopic ultrasonography also is useful for estimating the depth of invasion of rectal carcinoids.

■ PATHOLOGY

Macroscopically, carcinoids may have a yellow appearance, but in most cases this is not a striking feature. Microscopically, they consist of rosettes, ribbons, or masses of uniform small, round, or polygonal cells with prominent nuclei and acidophilic cytoplasmic granules. Immunohistochemically, carcinoids show focal or diffuse positivities for chromagranin A and/or neuron-specific enolase and often to pancreatic polypeptide (599).

No absolute histologic difference exists between benign and malignant rectal carcinoids. Size and histologic evidence of invasion into the muscularis propria are helpful in distinguishing benign from malignant lesions. Indeed, the only consistent microscopic feature of malignancy is invasion of the muscularis propria (597). In a review of 24 rectal carcinoids, Shirouzu et al. (606) found that all lesions less than 2 cm in diameter had neither muscle-layer invasion nor lymph node metastases except for atypical carcinoids. In patients with metastatic carcinoid Gerstle et al. (607) found 77% of patients had invasion through the muscularis propria. Of 86 patients with carcinoids less than 2 cm reported by Fitzgerald et al. (601) only one with a 1.5 cm ulcerated lesion developed liver metastases. In the review by Spread et al. (608), 64% of patients already had metastatic disease at time of presentation and another 22% were Dukes' C.

■ TREATMENT

The pathologic data of these neoplasms indicate that those greater than 2 cm in diameter should, in general, be treated by abdominoperineal resection or low anterior resection, if feasible (609,610). Carcinoids less than 2 cm in diameter with an atypical histologic appearance also indicate the need for abdominoperineal resection because of the risk of lymphatic involvement (606). For small lesions, treatment consists of total excisional biopsy, leaving a margin of normal tissue. This treatment permits assessment of the depth of penetration. If there is invasion of the muscularis propria, a resection appropriate for carcinoma should be performed, because 47% of these lesions have been shown to have metastases (609).

■ RESULTS

Nauneim et al. (609) reported on the results of treatment of 595 patients with rectal carcinoids. The five-year survival rate for patients with no metastases was 92%; for patients with regional lymph node involvement, 44%; and for patients with distant metastases, 7%. Tsioulias et al. (611) found that the nuclear DNA pattern was a factor of significant prognostic value. In a study of 22 patients with rectal carcinoids, three patients with synchronous or metachronous metastases had an aneuploid DNA pattern, whereas 19 patients without metastases showed a diploid DNA pattern. No other single clinical or pathologic feature could predict more accurately the malignant potential and subsequent course of the rectal carcinoid. On the other hand, Fitzgerald et al. (601) found DNA ploidy of no useful prognostic value. In a review of 35 patients with rectal carcinoids, only four lesions were malignant and all patients died despite radical operative treatment (597). Because radical treatment was largely unsuccessful, the authors of this review advocated a flexible operative approach.

Sauven et al. (603) also questioned whether aggressive operation is warranted. In their management of 43 patients with anorectal carcinoids, no recurrence developed in the 18 patients who underwent local excision. Lesions that were more advanced than T2 or greater than 2 cm in diameter were always fatal. All 13 patients with involved lymph nodes died of metastatic disease with a median survival of 10 months. The authors concluded that if local excision permits complete resection, radical extirpation would provide little benefit.

Matsui et al. (599) treated 16 small polypoid carcinoids by local excision and at an average 79 months follow-up, all were alive and disease free. Fitzgerald et al. (601) found that radical resection of rectal carcinoids with ulceration or greater than or equal to 2 cm is associated with a poor prognosis. However, survival may be long term, even in the presence of metastatic disease. Others have also reported that patients with carcinoids greater than 2 cm or invading beyond the muscularis propria die of metastatic disease despite radical resection (597,603). In a review of 85 patients with rectal carcinoids less than 2 cm, Jetmore et al. (600) found that treatment by local excision or fulguration resulted in no recurrences with an average five-year follow-up. Ten patients with metastasizing carcinoids fared poorly despite radical operation, with only one surviving five years.

LYMPHOMA

CLINICAL PRESENTATION

These lesions are less common than the rectal carcinoid. The disease is more common in women (2:1) and is usually seen beyond the age of 50. The incidence is reported to be 0.19% to 1.3% of all rectal neoplasms (602). The rectum is the site of 21.7% of lymphomas of the large intestine (612). In homosexual men with AIDS, non-Hodgkin's lymphoma is one of the two most common malignancies but is nevertheless a rare neoplasm (613).

The patient usually seeks treatment because of rectal bleeding or an alteration in bowel habits. However, a significant proportion may present with nothing more than generalized malaise and vague abdominal pain.

The lesion is detected on rectal examination and through sigmoidoscopy. The macroscopic appearance bears no relationship to the histologic structure. The growth patterns seen in the rectum vary. The growth may be bulky and protuberant with ulceration, it may appear as annular or plaquelike thickenings of the bowel wall, or it may manifest as multiple malignant lymphomatous polyposis.

The histologic varieties were described under the colonic lymphomas (Chapter 23). The aggressive nature of the AIDS-related lymphoma usually results in disseminated disease at the time of diagnosis. The extent of the disease should be assessed with CT scans, chest X-ray films, and a bone marrow biopsy.

TREATMENT AND RESULTS

The treatment of local or even regional disease is resection whenever possible (614). Devine et al. (615) reported on 61 patients with lymphoma involving the rectum; 49 had extensive lymphoma with secondary involvement of the rectum and 12 had lymphoma confined to the rectum. Those with widespread lymphoma were treated with chemotherapy, radiotherapy, or both. Five of the 12 patients with localized disease underwent resection. The overall five-year survival rate was 20%; the rate decreased to 15% with widespread disease and jumped to 50% when disease was confined to the rectum. Patients who underwent excision did better than those treated nonoperatively. Jinnai et al. (616) noted that the best prognosis occurred in patients with intraluminal lymphomas that were less than or equal to 5 cm and without lymph node metastases. For patients with widespread disease, those in whom the rectum is secondarily involved, or patients with AIDS, operation would seem inappropriate. These patients may benefit from chemotherapy and radiotherapy.

Radiotherapy has a limited place in the primary treatment of rectal lymphoma and is not a substitute for operation. Radiotherapy is useful in the palliation of inoperable cases and as an adjunct to operation when resection is considered incomplete, either in relation to the primary lesion or the associated lymph node metastases. Adjuvant chemotherapy plays an important role in the treatment of these malignancies.

It is important to realize that long-term survivors have been reported following incomplete removal of gastrointestinal malignant lymphomas, including patients with lymph node involvement. With advances in cytotoxic drug therapy and, to a lesser extent, in radiotherapy, resection has a prominent place even when the surgeon is doubtful as to the completeness of the resection and thus the ultimate success.

Lymphosarcoma has been associated with chronic ulcerative colitis (617). Caution is emphasized when reviewing rectal biopsies for staging of colitis, because in some of the cases confusion has arisen between chronic inflammatory infiltrate and lymphosarcoma. In such cases radical excision of the colon is clearly required.

Perry et al. (618) reported on 22 patients with primary lymphoma of the rectum. Twelve of the 22 died, three-quarters within two years of diagnosis with a follow-up of 10 months to 10 years. In a review of the Mayo Clinic experience, Devine et al. (615) found a five-year survival rate of 50% for lymphomas confined to the rectum, but only 15% when disease was widespread. Postoperative radiotherapy has been reported to enhance survival (615,619).

SARCOMA

As with the colon, a large variety of very uncommon neoplasms of mesenchymal origin may be found in the rectum. These have more recently been described as mural-based stromal neoplasms (620). The benign lesions tend to be submucosal, range in size from 1 to 7 cm (mean, 2.1 cm), lack nuclear atypia, and display a mitotic activity not exceeding one mitosis per 50 high-power microscopic fields. In contrast lesions exhibiting a malignant behavior are located in the muscularis propria, range in size from

1.6 to 11 cm (mean, 4.5 cm), manifest necrosis in 67% of patients, demonstrate moderate atypia, and display a mitotic count ranging from 5 to 58 mitoses per 50 high-power microscopic fields.

The most common of these neoplasms is the leiomyosarcoma. Leiomyosarcoma of the rectum occurs at all ages and in both sexes, but it is more common beyond the sixth decade of life and represents approximately 0.07% to 0.1% of all malignancies (621,622). In a review of 81,000 cases of malignancy entered into the Armed Forces Central Medical Registry, Feldtman et al. (623) found seven cases of leiomyosarcoma of the rectum. This neoplasm accounted for 0.06% of all gastrointestinal malignancies and 0.3% of all rectal malignancies.

Bleeding, constipation, and rectal pain are the most common symptoms. In addition, the patient may complain of a pressure sensation, diarrhea, dysuria, or difficult defecation (621).

The majority of lesions are palpable on digital examination. They vary in size from 1 to 20 cm, are predominantly endorectal lesions, and in the more malignant forms have extensive perirectal invasion (621,624). Most lesions appear as submucosal masses and approximately 44% are ulcerated. The consistency may be firm, soft, or hard (621).

Histologically, interlacing bands of distinct, spindle-shaped cells are seen. The criterion of malignancy is simple in the high-grade forms. It is based upon the number of mitoses per high-power field (625). It is on this definition that the decision for a more definitive operation is based. Leiomyosarcoma of the rectum grows slowly and metastasizes late. Spread is by direct extension into contiguous structures and by bloodstream to liver, lungs, brain, and bone. Lymphatic metastases are rare. Blood-borne metastases to liver and lung are the most common cause of death (622).

Attempts have been made to modify the treatment according to the histologic classification of the neoplasm. Because of the difficulty in determining malignancy, supposedly benign lesions treated by local excision have a high recurrence rate. When local recurrence develops and in lesions diagnosed primarily as malignant, the treatment of choice is wide local excision rather than lymphatic clearance, but abdominoperineal resection may be necessary. In a review of the literature, Labow and Hoexter (624) calculated a 20% five-year survival rate. Survival is generally poor, with a five-year survival rate between 20% and 40% and local recurrence rates as high as 20% to 86% (626). Randleman et al. (627) reported on 22 patients with leiomyosarcoma. Treatment consisted of wide local excision in 10 patients and radical excision in 11. One lesion was unresectable. None of the patients had lymph node involvement. The 5-year and 10-year survival rates were 62% and 40%, respectively. Adjuvant therapy had no effect on survival. The authors concluded that lesions less than 2.5 cm in size can be treated by wide local excision, whereas larger lesions require radical resection.

In a review of the literature involving 135 cases, Khalifa et al. (621) found the same 5- and 10-year survival figures whether the patient was treated by radical or local excision. Survival at 5 and 10 years was 38.9% and 9.7%, respectively. The patient survival rate was related to the degree of differentiation of the neoplasm; poorly differentiated lesions had a poor prognosis. However, local excision was followed by 67.5% recurrence. They concluded that abdominoperineal resection is still the procedure of choice. Local excision might be considered for small lesions of low-grade malignancy in poor-risk patients. Radiotherapy is of limited benefit. Chemotherapy [doxorubicin (formerly adriamycin)] may prove effective in one-third of cases (621).

Yeh et al. (628) presented the prognosis after resection of 40 patients with rectal leiomyosarcoma. The mean age was 58.7 years. Anal bleeding and perianal pain were the two most common symptoms at initial diagnosis. Twenty-nine patients received a radical surgical resection, such as abdominoperineal resection and low anterior resection; the other 11 patients received a wide local excision, such as transrectal excision or Kraske's operation. Sixteen lesions were classified as high-grade leiomyosarcoma, and 23 as low-grade. With a median follow-up of 35 months, 48% developed recurrence or metastasis postoperatively. The overall and disease-free (one year, three years, and five years) survival rates were 97%, 90%, and 75% and 90%, 59%, and 46%, respectively. Patients less than 50 years ($n=9$) and high-grade leiomyosarcoma, showed poor prognosis in the disease-free survival curve. There was a strong trend toward higher local recurrence rates for the wide local excision group than for the radical resection (55% vs. 24%). There was no difference in the incidence of distant metastasis between the two groups with different operation types. The metastasis rates of the wide local excision and radical excision groups were 27% and 38%, respectively.

GASTROINTESTINAL STROMAL TUMOR (GIST)

Changchien et al. (629) reported the outcome of curative resection of rectal GIST. Diagnostic immunohistochemical staining with CD34, CD117, S-100, desmin, and muscle-specific actin was performed in 46 consecutive patients with previously diagnosed rectal leiomyosarcoma who underwent curative resection. CD44, Bcl-2, P53, and Ki-67 staining were performed on neoplasms rediagnosed as GIST for the prognostic evaluation. There were 91.3% of patients with rectal GIST (18 females and 24 males; mean age 58.4 years). Twenty-nine patients underwent radical surgical resections, such as abdominoperineal resection or low anterior resection whereas the other 13 patients underwent wide local excision, such as transrectal excision or Kraske's operation. Sixteen neoplasms were classified as high-grade GIST and 26 as low-grade. No neoplasms had a positive P53 stain. Recurrence or metastasis developed in 64.3% of patients postoperatively (median follow-up 52 months). The one-year, two-year, and five-year disease-free survival rates were 90.2%, 76.7%, and 43.9%, respectively. Of these patients with recurrence, subsequent resections in 12 patients with local recurrence, transarterial embolization of the neoplasm or STI-571 chemotherapies in three patients with distant metastasis were performed. The one-year, two-year and five-year overall survival rates were 97.4%, 94.3%, and 83.7%, respectively. The group with wide local excision had a higher local recurrence rate than that of the radical resection group (77% vs. 31%) despite smaller size (4.5 vs. 7.2 cm). There was no difference in the incidence of distant metastasis between the two groups. Younger age (less than 50 years), higher histologic grade, positive Bcl-2 status, and larger neoplasms (greater than 5 cm) were factors associated with significantly poor prognosis for rectal GIST. Radical resection was superior to wide local excision in the prevention of local recurrence, but not that of distant metastases.

Lo et al. (630) described a case of GIST of the rectum who declined abdominoperineal resection. Neoadjuvant treatment with imatinib decreased the size of the lesion permitting sphincter-sparing transanal excision. The patient had no evidence of disease for 24 months postoperatively until she recurred with lung metastases. Microdissection genotyping of the recurrent lesion revealed a deletion in exon 11.

SECONDARY CARCINOMA

It is unusual for the rectum to be invaded secondarily by carcinoma. The most common malignancies to do so are large bowel carcinomas, usually of the sigmoid colon, which may involve pelvic structures, including the rectum. It is rare for prostatic carcinomas to invade Denonvilliers' fascia and present as a rectal neoplasm. It is more common for prostatic carcinoma to grow in a circumferential fashion around the rectum, giving the appearance of an annular carcinoma without a break in mucosal continuity. This malignancy has the appearance of a bulky, infiltrating rectal carcinoma. The diagnosis can only be made following a biopsy (631).

The pouch of Douglas is a common site for metastatic implantation following transperitoneal spread from carcinoma of any of the intra-abdominal organs. The most common sites of origin are the stomach and ovary. Any metastatic neoplasm can present in this site; the breast is a typical site for such a malignancy (632). Carcinoma of the cervix rarely involves the rectum (633).

Metastatic renal cell carcinoma involving the rectum has been reported (634).

MISCELLANEOUS NEOPLASMS

Extraordinarily rare neoplasms such as granular cell neoplasms of the rectum have been reported (635,636).

Primary teratoma of the rectum is exceedingly rare. Takao et al. (637) reported the 48th case in the world literature and provided the following information on the subject. It is thought rectal teratoma may arise from an aberrant germ cell in the embryonic digestive tract. Most cases are women with a wide range age range 8 to 80 years (mean 42.5 years). Initial symptoms may include prolapse of the lesion or hair, or bloody stool. On examination, it is often located on the anterior wall of the rectum. The diagnosis is easy if hair is found on the surface. Endorectal ultrasound demonstrates a heterogeneous echo pattern different from that of submucosal neoplasms. The treatment of choice is endoscopic excision as most teratomas are pedunculated. All primary rectal teratomas are pathologically benign.

Primary rectal malignant melanoma is an exceptionally rare neoplasm associated with an extremely poor prognosis despite aggressive treatment. Hazzan et al. (638) presented two patients with bulky lesions of the lower rectum above the squamocolumnar junction. Both patients underwent abdominoperineal resection and postoperatively were treated with autologous melanoma cell vaccine. One patient was considered disease free for months after operation; the second one developed supraclavicular lymph nodes and right lung metastasis after seven months.

REFERENCES

1. Miles WE. Pathology of spread of cancer of rectum and its bearing upon surgery of cancerous rectum. Surg Gynecol Obstet 1931; 52:350–359.
2. Block IR, Enquist IF. Lymphatic studies pertaining to local spread of carcinoma of the rectum in female. Surg Gynecol Obstet 1961; 112:41–46.
3. Bucci L, Saifi R, Meraviglia F, et al. Rectal lymphoscintigraphy. Dis Colon Rectum 1984; 27:370–375.
4. Miscusi G, Masori L, Dell'Anna A, et al. Normal lymphatic drainage of the rectum and anal canal revealed by lymphoscintigraphy. Coloproctology 1987; 9:171–174.
5. Hermanek P. Evolution and pathology of rectal cancer. World J Surg 1982; 6:502–509.
6. Quer EA, Dahlin DC, Mayo CW. Retrograde intramural spread of carcinoma of the rectum and rectosigmoid. Surg Gynecol Obstet 1953; 96:24–30.
7. Grinnell RS. Distal intramural spread of carcinoma of the rectum and rectosigmoid. Surg Gynecol Obstet 1954; 99:421–430.
8. Hughes TG, Jenevein EP, Poulos E. Intramural spread of colon carcinoma. Am J Surg 1983; 146:697–699.
9. Madsen PM, Christiansen J. Distal intramural spread of rectal carcinoma. Dis Colon Rectum 1986; 29:279–282.
10. Pollet WG, Nicholls RJ. The relationship between the extent of distal clearance and survival and local recurrence rates after curative anterior resection for carcinoma of the rectum. Ann Surg 1984; 198:159–163.
11. Williams NS. The rationale of preservation of the anal sphincter in patients with low rectal cancer. Br J Surg 1984; 71:575–581.
12. Elliot MS, Todd IP, Nicholls RJ. Radical restorative surgery for poorly differentiated carcinoma of the mid-rectum. Br J Surg 1982; 69:564–568.
13. Grinnell RS. Lymphatic block with atypical and retrograde lymphatic metastasis and spread in carcinoma of the colon and rectum. Ann Surg 1966; 163:272–280.
14. Griffiths JD, McKinna JA, Rowbotham HD, et al. Carcinoma of the colon and rectum: circulating malignant cells and five-year survival. Cancer 1973; 31:226–236.
15. Dukes CE, Bussey HJR. The spread of rectal cancer and its effect on prognosis. Br J Cancer 1958; 12:309–320.
16. Beart RW, Steele GD Jr, Menck HR, et al. Management and survival of patients with adenocarcinoma of the colon and rectum: a national survey of the commission on cancer. J Am Coll Surg 1995; 181:225–236.
17. Mesko TW, Rodriguez-Bigas MA, Petrelli NJ. Inguinal lymph node metastases from adenocarcinoma of the rectum. Am J Surg 1994; 168:285–287.
18. Nicholls RJ, Mason AY, Morson BC, Dixon AK, Fry IK. The clinical staging of rectal cancer. Br J Surg 1982; 69:404–409.
19. Bailey HR, Huval WV, Max E, et al. Local excision of carcinoma of the rectum for cure. Surgery 1992; 111:555–561.
20. Taylor RH, Hay JH, Larsson SN. Transanal Local Excision of Selected Low Rectal Cancers. Am J Surg 1998; 175:360–363.
21. Isabel-Martinez L, Chapman AH, Hall RI. The value of barium enema in the investigation of patients with rectal carcinoma. Clin Radiol 1988; 39:531–533.
22. Beets-Tan RG, Beets GL. Rectal cancer: how accurate can imaging predict the T stage and the circumferential resection margin? Int J Colorectal Dis 2003; 18:385–391.
23. Cance WG, Cohen AM, Enker WE, et al. Predictive value of a negative computed tomographic scan in 100 patients with rectal carcinoma. Dis Colon Rectum 1991; 34:748–751.
24. Lupo L, Angelelli G, Pennarale O, et al. Improved accuracy of computed tomography in local staging of rectal cancer using water enema. Int J Colorectal Dis 1996; 11:60–64.
25. Tada M, Endo M. Ultrasonographic examination for lateral lymphatic spread and local recurrence of rectal cancer. Preoperative detection and evaluation. Dis Colon Rectum 1995; 38:1047–1052.
26. Tempero M, Brand R, Holderman K, et al. New imaging techniques in colorectal cancer. Semin Oncol 1995; 22:448–471.
27. Marohn MR. Endorectal ultrasound. Postgraduate course syllabus. SAGES 1997:126–153.
28. Garcia-Aguilar J, Pollack J, Lee SH, et al. Accuracy of endorectal ultrasonography in preoperative staging of rectal tumors. Dis Colon Rectum 2002; 45:10–15.
29. Kauer WK, Prantl L, Dittler HJ, Siewert JR. The value of endosonographic rectal carcinoma staging in routine diagnostics: a 10-year analysis. Surg Endosc 2004; 18:1075–1078.
30. Savides JJ, Master SS. Endoractal ultra sound in rectal cancer. Gastrointest Endosc 2002; 56(suppl):512–518.
31. Wong WD, Orrom WJ, Jensen LL. Preoperative staging of rectal cancer with endorectal ultrasonography. Perspect Colon Rectal Surg 1990; 3:315–334.

32. Glaser F, Schlag P, Herfarth C. Endorectal sonography for the assessment of invasion of rectal tumors and lymph node involvement. Br J Surg 1990; 77:883–887.
33. Sentovich SM, Blatchford GJ, Falk PM, et al. Transrectal ultrasound of rectal tumors. Am J Surg 1993; 166:638–642.
34. Hunerbein M, Below C, Schlag PM. Three-dimensional endorectal ultrasonography for staging of obstructing rectal cancer. Dis Colon Rectum 1996; 39:636–642.
35. Herzog U, von Flue M, Tondelli P, et al. How accurate is endorectal ultrasound in the preoperative staging of rectal cancer? Dis Colon Rectum 1993; 36: 127–134.
36. Williamson PR, Hellinger MD, Larach SW, et al. Endorectal ultrasound of T3 and T4 rectal cancers after preoperative chemo-radiation. Dis Colon Rectum 1996; 39:45–49.
37. Bernini A, Deen KI, Madoff RD, et al. Preoperative adjuvant radiation with chemotherapy for rectal cancer: its impact on stage of disease and the role of endorectal ultrasound. Ann Surg Oncol 1996; 3:131–135.
38. Fleshman JW, Myerson RJ, Fry RD, et al. Accuracy of transrectal ultrasound in predicting pathologic stage of rectal cancer before and after preoperative radiation therapy. Dis Colon Rectum 1992; 35:823–829.
39. Martling A, Holm T, Bremmer S, Lindholm J, Cedermark B, Blomqvist L. Prognostic value of preoperative magnetic resonance imaging of the pelvis in rectal cancer. Br J Surg 2003; 90:1422–1428.
40. Bissett IP, Fernando CC, Hough DM, et al. Identification of the fascia propria by magnetic resonance imaging and its relevance to preoperative assessment of rectal cancer. Dis Colon Rectum 2001; 44:259–265.
41. Leite JS, Castro-Sousa F, Tralhao G, et al. Preoperative staging of rectal carcinoma: water enema CT vs. transrectal ultrasound. Br J Surg 1995; 82(suppl l):2–3.
42. Romano G, Esercizio L, Santangelo M, et al. Impact of computed tomography vs. intrarectal ultrasound on the diagnosis, resectability, and prognosis of locally recurrent rectal cancer. Dis Colon Rectum 1993; 36:261–265.
43. Meyenberger C, Boni RAH, Bertschinger P, et al. Endoscopic ultrasound and endorectal magnetic resonance imaging: a prospective, comparative study for preoperative staging and follow-up of rectal cancer. Endoscopy 1995; 27:469–479.
44. Hunerhein M, Pegios W, Rau B, Vagi TJ, Felix R, Schlag PM. Prospective comparison of endorectal ultrasound, three-dimensional endorectal ultrasound, and endorectal MRI in the preoperative evaluation of rectal tumors. Preliminary results. Surg Endosc 2000; 14:1005–1009.
45. Katsura Y, Yamada K, Ishizawa T, et al. Endorectal ultrasonography for the assessment of wall invasion and lymph node metastasis in rectal cancer. Dis Colon Rectum 1992; 35:362–368.
46. McNicholas MMJ, Joyce WP, Dolan J, et al. Magnetic resonance imaging of rectal carcinoma: a prospective study. Br J Surg 1994; 81:911–914.
47. Kim NK, Kim MJ, Park JK, Park SJ, Min JS. Preoperative staging of rectal cancer with MRI: accuracy and clinical usefulness. Ann Surg Oncol 2000; 7:732–737.
48. Brown G, Radcliflfe AG, Newcombe RG, DallimoreNS, Bourne MW, Williams GT. Preoperative assessment of prognostic factors in rectal cancer using high-resolution magnetic resonance imaging. Br J Surg 2003; 90:355–364.
49. Branagan G, Chave H, Fuller C, McGee S, Finnis D. Can magnetic resonance imaging predict circumferential margins and TNM stage in rectal cancer? Dis Colon Rectum 2004; 47:1317–1322.
50. Thaler W, Watzka S, Martin F, et al. Preoperative staging of rectal cancer by endoluminal ultrasound vs. magnetic resonance imaging. Preliminary results of a prospective comparative study. Dis Colon Rectum 1994; 37:1189–1193.
51. Kasunoki M, Yanagi H, Kamikonya N, et al. Preoperative detection of local extension of carcinoma of the rectum using magnetic resonance imaging. J Am Coll Surg 1994; 179:653–656.
52. Billingham RP. Conservative treatment of rectal cancer. Extending the indications. Cancer 1992; 70:1355–1363.
53. Stergiou N, Haji-Kermani N, Schneider C, et al. Staging of colonic neoplasms by colonoscopic microprobe ultrasonography. Int J Colorectal Dis 2003; 18: 445–449.
54. Heriot AG, Hicks RJ, Drummond EG, et al. Does positron emission tomography change management in primary rectal cancer? A prospective assessment. Dis Colon Rectum 2004; 47:451–458.
55. Durdey P, Williams NS. The effect of malignant and inflammatory fixation of rectal carcinoma as prognosis after rectal excision. Br J Surg 1984; 71:787–790.
56. Kyzer S, Gordon PH. Hidden colostomy. SurgGynecol Obstet 1993; 177: 181–182.
57. Tytherleigh MG, McC Mortensen NJ. Options for sphincter preservation in surgery for low rectal cancer. Br J Surg 2003; 90:922–933.
58. Williams NS, Dixon ME, Johnson D. Reappraisal of the 5 cm rule of distal excision for carcinoma of the rectum: a study of distal intramural spread and of patients' survival. Br J Surg 1983; 70:150–154.
59. Wilson SM, Beahrs OH. The curative treatment of carcinoma of the sigmoid, rectosigmoid, and rectum. Ann Surg 1976; 183:556–565.
60. Purves H, Pietrobon R, Hervey S, Guller U, Miller W, Ludwig K. Relationship between surgeon caseload and sphincter preservation in patients with rectal cancer. Dis Colon Rectum 2005; 48:195–202.
61. Mettlin C, Mittelman A, Natarajan N, et al. Trends in the United States for the management of adenocarcinoma of the rectum. SurgGynecol Obstet 1981; 153:701–706.
62. Jarvinen HJ, Ovaska J, Mecklin JP. Improvements in the treatment and prognosis of colorectal carcinoma. Br J Surg 1988; 75:25–27.
63. Nicholls RJ, Ritchie JR, Wadsworth J, et al. Total excision or restorative resection for carcinoma of the middle third of the rectum. Br J Surg 1979; 66:625–627.
64. Slanetz CA, Herter FP, Grinnell RS. Anterior resection versus abdominoperineal resection for cancer of the rectum and rectosigmoid. Am J Surg 1972; 123:110–117.
65. Stearns MW Jr. The choice among anterior resection, the pull-through and abdominoperineal resection of the rectum. Cancer 1974; 34:969–971.
66. Williams NS, Durdey P, Johnston D. The outcome following sphincter saving resection and abdominoperineal resection for low rectal cancer. Br J Surg 1985; 72:595–598.
67. Williams NS, Johnston D. Survival and recurrence after sphincter saving resection and abdominoperineal resection for recurrence of the middle third of the rectum. Br J Surg 1984; 71:278–282.
68. Wolmark N, Fisher B. An analysis of survival and treatment failure following abdominoperineal resection and sphincter-saving resection in Dukes'; B and C rectal carcinoma. Ann Surg 1986; 204:480–487.
69. Di Betta E, D'Hoore A, Filez L, Penninckx F. Sphincter saving rectum resection is the standard procedure for low rectal cancer. Int J Colorectal Dis 2003; 18:463–469.
70. Bergqvist D, Bohe M, Ekelund G. Compartment syndrome after prolonged surgery with leg supports. Int J Colorectal Dis 1990; 5:1–5.
71. Harrison JL, Hooks VH, Pearl RK, et al. Muscle fragment welding for control of massive presacral bleeding during rectal mobilization: a review of eight cases. Dis Colon Rectum 2003; 49:1115–1117.
72. Xu J, Lin J. Control of presacral hemorrhage with electrocautery through a muscle fragment pressed on the bleeding vein. J Am Coll Surg 1994; 179:351–352.
73. Qinyao W, Weijun S, Youren Z, et al. New concepts in severe hemorrhage during proctectomy. Arch Surg 1985; 12:1013–1020.
74. Nivatvongs S, Fang DT. The use of thumb tacks to stop massive presacral hemorrhage. Dis Colon Rectum 1986; 29:589–590.
75. Metzger PP. Modified packing technique for control of presacral pelvic bleeding. Dis Colon Rectum 1988; 31:981–982.
76. Zama N, Fazio VW, Jagelman DG, et al. Efficacy of pelvic packing in maintaining hemostasis after rectal excision for cancer. Dis Colon Rectum 1988; 31:923–928.
77. Junginger T, Kneist W, Heintz A. Influence of identification and preservation of pelvic autonomic nerves in rectal cancer surgery on bladder dysfunction after total mesorectal excision. Dis Colon Rectum 2003; 46:621–628.
78. Heald RJ, Husband EM, Ryall ROH. The mesorectum in rectal cancer surgery: The clue to pelvic recurrence. Br J Surg 1982; 69:613–616.
79. MacFarlane JK, Ryall RDH, Heald RJ. Mesorectal excision for rectal cancer. Lancet 1993; 341:457–460.
80. Agaba EA. Does rectal washout during anterior resection prevent local tumor recurrence? Dis Colon Rectum 2004; 47:291–296.
81. Ranbarger KR, Johnston WD, Chang JC. Prognostic significance of surgical perforation of the rectum during abdominoperineal resection for rectal carcinoma. Am J Surg 1982; 143:186–188.
82. Gordon PH, Dalrymple S. The use of staples for reconstruction after colonic and rectal surgery. In: Ravitch MM, Steichen FM, eds. Principles and Practice of Surgical Stapling. Chicago: Year Book Medical Publishers, 1987:402–431.
83. Gordon PH, Vasilevsky CA. Experience with stapling in rectal surgery. Surg Clin North Am 1984; 64:555–566.
84. Minichan DP. Enlarging the bowel lumen for the EEA stapler. Dis Colon Rectum 1982; 25:61.
85. Tchervenkov CI, Gordon PH. Simple techniques of enlarging the diameter of the bowel lumen for the performance of end-to-end anastomoses using the EEA stapler. Dis Colon Rectum 1984; 27:630–631.
86. Knight CD, Griffin FD. Techniques of low rectal reconstruction. Curr Probl Surg 1983; 20:391–456.
87. Griffin FD, Knight CD, Whitaker JM. The double stapling technique for low anterior resection. Ann Surg 1990; 211:745–752.
88. Moran BJ, Blenkinsop J, Finnis D. Local recurrence after anterior resection for rectal cancer using a double stapling technique. Br J Surg 1992; 79: 836–838.
89. Laxamana A, Solomon MJ, Cohen Z, et al. Long-term results of anterior resection using the double-stapling technique. Dis Colon Rectum 1995; 38: 1246–1250.
90. Julian TB, Ravitch MM. Evaluation of the safety of end-to-end (EEA) stapling anastomosis across linear stapled closures. Surg Clin North Am 1984; 64: 567–577.
91. Goldberg SM, Gordon PH, Nivatvongs S. Essentials of Anorectal Surgery. Philadelphia: JB Lippincott 1980; Chpt. 16, p. 182.
92. Devereux DF, Eisenstat T, Zinkin L. The safe and effective use of postoperative radiation therapy in modified Astler-Coller stage C3 rectal cancer. Cancer 1989; 63:2393–2396.
93. Sugarbaker PH. Intrapelvic prosthesis to prevent injury of the small intestine with high dosage pelvic irradiation. SurgGynecol Obstet 1983; 157:269–271.

94. Mcdonald PJ, Heald RJ. A survey of postoperative function after rectal anastomosis with circular stapling devices. Br J Surg 1983; 70:727–729.
95. McNamara DA, Parc R. Methods and results of sphincter-preserving surgery for rectal cancer. Cancer Control 2003; 10:212–218.
96. Renner K, Rosen HR, Novi G, Hobleng N, Schiessel R. Quality of life after surgery for rectal cancer: do we still need a permanent colostomy? Dis Colon Rectum 1999; 42:1160–1167.
97. Grumann MM, Noack EM, Hoffman IA, et al. Comparison of quality of life in patients undergoing abdominoperineal extirpation or anterior resection for cancer. Ann Surg 2001; 233:149–156.
98. Dehni N, McNamara DA, Schlegel RD, et al. Clinical effects of preoperative radiation therapy on anorectal function after proctectomy and colonic J-pouch-anal anastomosis. Dis Colon Rectum 2002; 45:1635–1640.
99. Parks AG. Transanal technique in low rectal anastomosis. Proc R Soc Med 1972; 65:975–976.
100. Miller AS, Lewis WG, Williamson MER, et al. Factors that influence functional outcome after coloanal anastomosis for carcinoma of the rectum. Br J Surg 1995; 82:1327–1330.
101. Patey PB, Enker WE, Cohen AM, et al. Treatment of rectal cancer by low anterior resection with coloanal anastomosis. Ann Surg 1994; 219:365–373.
102. Braun J, Treutner KH, Winketan G, et al. Results of inter-sphincteric resection of the rectum with direct coloanal anastomosis for rectal carcinoma. Am J Surg 1992; 163:407–412.
103. Leo E, Belli F, Andreola S, et al. Total rectal resection and complete mesorectum excision followed by coloendoanal anastomosis as the optimal treatment for low rectal cancer: the experience of the National Cancer Institute of Milano. Ann Surg Oncol 2000; 7:125–132.
104. Saito N, Ono M, Sugito M, et al. Early results of intersphincteric resection for patients with very low rectal cancer: an active approach to avoid a permanent colostomy. Dis Colon Rectum 2004; 47:459–466.
105. Gamagami R, Istvan G, Cabarrot P, Liagre A, Chiotasso P, Lazorthes F. Fecal continence following partial resection of the anal canal in distal rectal cancer: long-term results after coloanal anastomoses. Surgery 2000; 127:291–295.
106. Nathanson DR, Espat NJ, Nash GM, et al. Evaluation of preoperative and postoperative radiotherapy on long-term functional results of straight coloanal anastomosis. Dis Colon Rectum 2003; 46:888–894.
107. Olagne E, Baulieux J, de la Roche E, et al. Functional results of delayed coloanal anastomosis after preoperative radiotherapy for lower third rectal cancer. J Am Coll Surg 2000; 191:643–649.
108. Rullier E, Laurent C, Bretagnol F, Rullier A, Vendrely V, Zerbib F. Sphinctersavhig resection for all rectal carcinomas: the end of the 2-cm distal rule. Ann Surg 2005; 241:465–469.
109. Lazorthes F, Fages P, Chiotasso P, et al. Resection of the rectum with construction of a colonic reservoir and colo-anal anastomosis for carcinoma of the rectum. Br J Surg 1986; 73:136–138.
110. Lazorthes F, Chiotasso P, Gamagami RA, et al. Late clinical outcome in a randomised prospective comparison of colonic J pouch and straight coloanal anastomosis. Br J Surg 1997; 84:1449–1451.
111. Nicholls RJ, Lubowski DZ, Donaldson DR. Comparison of colonic reservoir and straight colo-anal reconstruction after rectal excision. Br J Surg 1988; 75:318–323.
112. Dehni N, Tiret E, Singland JD, et al. Long-term functional outcome after low anterior resection: comparison of low colorectal anastomosis and colonic J-pouch-anal anastomosis. Dis Colon Rectum 1998; 41:817–823.
113. Hallbook O, Pahlman L, Krog M, et al. Randomized comparison of straight and colonic J pouch anastomosis after low anterior resection. Ann Surg 1996; 224:58–65.
114. Harris GJ, Lavery IC, Fazio VW. Function of a colonic J pouch continues to improve with time. Br J Surg 2001; 88:1623–1627.
115. Nicholls J, Hall C. Treatment of cancer of the lower rectum. Br J Surg 1996; 83:15–18.
116. Hallböök O, Johansson K, Sjodahl R. Laser Doppler blood-flow measurement in rectal resection for carcinoma—Comparison between the straight and colonic J pouch reconstruction. Br J Surg 1996; 83:389–392.
117. Mortensen NJM, Ramirez JM, Tekeuchi N, et al. Colonic J pouch-anal anastomosis after rectal excision for carcinoma: Functional outcome Br J Surg 1995; 82:611–613.
118. Lewis WG, Holdsworth PJ, Stephenson BM, et al. Role of the rectum in the physiological and clinical results of coloanal and colorectal anastomosis after anterior resection for rectal carcinoma. Br J Surg 1992; 79:1082–1086.
119. Stebbing JF, Mortensen NJ McC. Carcinoma in a colon J pouch reservoir after low anterior resection for villous adenoma. Br J Surg 1995; 82:172.
120. Hida J, Yasutomi M, Fujimoto K, et al. Functional outcome after low anterior resection with low anastomosis for rectal cancer using the colonic J-pouch. Prospective randomized study for determination of optimum pouch size. Dis Colon Rectum 1996; 39:986–991.
121. Dehni N, Parc R. Colonic J-pouch-anal anastomosis for rectal cancer. Dis Colon Rectum 2003; 46:667–675.
122. Laurent A, Parc Y, McNamara D, Parc R, Tiret E. Colonic J-pouch-anal anastomosis for rectal cancer: a prospective, randomized study comparing handsewn vs. stapled anastomosis. Dis Colon Rectum 2005; 48:729–734.
123. Machado M, Nygren J, Goldman S, Ljungqvist O. Similar outcome after colonic pouch and side-to-end anastomosis in low anterior resection for rectal cancer: a prospective randomized trial. Ann Surg 2003; 238:214–220.
124. Machado M, Nygren J, Goldman S, Ljungqvist O. Functional and physiologic assessment of the colonic reservoir or side-to-end anastomosis after low anterior resection for rectal cancer: a two-year follow-up. Dis Colon Rectum 2005; 48:29–36.
125. Dehni N, McNamara DA, Schlegel RD, Guiguet M, Tiret E, Parc R. Clinical effects of preoperative radiation therapy on anorectal function after proctectomy and colonic J-pouch-anal anastomosis. Dis Colon Rectum 2002; 45: 1635–1640.
126. Sailer M, Fuchs KH, Fein M, Thiede A. Randomized clinical trial comparing quality of life after straight and pouch coloanal reconstruction. Br J Surg 2002; 89:1108–1117.
127. Heah SM, Seow-Choen F, Eu KW, Ho YH, Tang CL. Prospective, randomized trial comparing sigmoid vs. descending colonic J-pouch after total rectal excision. Dis Colon Rectum 2002; 45:322–328.
128. Ho YH, Seow-Choen F, Tan M. Colonic J-pouch function at six months versus straight coloanal anastomosis at two years: randomized controlled trial. World J Surg 2001; 25:876–881.
129. Wang JY, You YT, Chen HH, Chiang JM, Yeh CY, Tang R. Stapled colonic J-pouch-anal anastomosis without a diverting colostomy for rectal carcinoma. Dis Colon Rectum 1997; 40:30–34.
130. Hamel CT, Metzger J, Curti G, Degen L, Harder F, von Flue MO. Ileocecal reservoir reconstruction after total mesorectal excision: functional results of the long-term follow-up. Int J Colorectal Dis 2004; 19:574–579.
131. da Silva GM, Kaiser R, Borjesson L, et al. The effect of diverticular disease on the colonic J pouch. Colorectal Dis 2004; 6:171–175.
132. Hida J, Yoshifuji T, Tokoro T, et al. Long-term functional outcome of low anterior resection with colonic J-pouch reconstruction for rectal cancer in the elderly. Dis Colon Rectum 2004; 47:1448–1454.
133. Gervaz P, Rotholtz N, Wexner SD, et al. Colonic J-pouch function in rectal cancer patients: impact of adjuvant chemoradiotherapy. Dis Colon Rectum 2001; 44:1667–1675.
134. Harris GJ, Lavery IC, Fazio VW. Reasons for failure to construct the colonic J-poiich. What can be done to improve the size of the neorectal reservoir should it occur? Dis Colon Rectum 2002; 45:1304–1308.
135. Furst A, Suttner S, Agha A, Beham A, Jauch KW. Colonic J-pouch vs. coloplasty following resection of distal rectal cancer: early results of a prospective, randomized, pilot study. Dis Colon Rectum 2003; 46:1161–1166.
136. Mantyh CR, Hull TL, Fazio VW. Coloplasty in low colorectal anastomosis: manometric and functional comparis with straight and colonic J-pouch anastomosis. Dis Colon Rectum 2001; 44:37–42.
137. Z'graggen K, Maurer CA, Birrer S, Giachino D, Kern B, Buchler MW. A new surgical concept for rectal replacement after low anterior resection: the transverse coloplasty pouch. Ann Surg 2001; 234:780–785.
138. Remzi FH, Fazio VW, Gorgun E, et al. Quality of life, functional outcome, and complications of coloplasty pouch after low anterior resection. Dis Colon Rectum 2005; 48:735–743.
139. Localio SA, Eng K, Coopa GF. Abdominosacral resection for midrectal cancer: a 15 year experience. Ann Surg 1983; 198:320–324.
140. Hardy TG, Pace WC, Maney JW, et al. A bioffagmentable ring for sutureless bowel anastomosis. An experimental study. Dis Colon Rectum 1985; 28: 484–490.
141. Corman ML, Prager ED, Hardy TG, et al. Comparison of the Valtrac biofragmentable anastomosis ring with conventional suture and stapled anastomosis in colon surgery. Results of a prospective randomized clinical trial. Dis Colon Rectum 1989; 32:183–187.
142. Moriya Y, Hojo K, Sawada T. En bloc excision of lower ureter and internal iliac vessels for locally advanced upper rectal and rectosigmoid cancers. Use of ileal segment for ureteral repair. Dis Colon Rectum 1988; 31:872–878.
143. Geerdes BP, Zoetmulder FAN, Baeten CGMI. Double dynamic graciloplasty and coloperineal pull-through after abdominoperineal resection. Eur J Cancer 1995; 31A:1248–1252.
144. Martling A, Singnomklao T, Holm T, Rutqvist LE, Cedermark B. Prognostic significance of both surgical and pathological assessment of curative resection for rectal cancer. Br J Surg 2004; 91:1040–1045.
145. Pählman L, Glimelius B, Enblad P. Clinical characteristics and their relation to surgical curability in adenocarcinoma of the rectum and rectosigmoid. A population-based study on 279 consecutive patients. Acta Chir Scand 1985; 151:685–693.
146. Davis NE, Evans EB, Cohen JR, et al. Colorectal cancer: a large unselected Australian series. Aust N Z J Surg 1987; 57:153–159.
147. Enblad P, Adami HO, Bergstrom R, et al. Improved survival of patients with cancers of the colon and rectum. J Natl Cancer Inst 1988; 80:586–591.
148. Michelassi F, Block GE, Vannucci L, et al. A 5 to 21 year follow-up and analysis of 250 patients with rectal adenocarcinoma. Ann Surg 1988; 208: 379–386.
149. Amato A, Pescatori M, Butti A. Local recurrence following abdominoperineal excision and anterior resection for rectal carcinoma. Dis Colon Rectum 1991; 34:317–322.

150. Tagliacozzo S, Accordino M. Pelvic recurrence after surgical treatment of rectal and sigmoid cancer. A prospective clinical trial in 274 patients. Int J Colorectal Dis 1992; 7:135–140.
151. Fandrich F, Schroder DW, Saliveros E. Long-term survival after curative resection for carcinoma of the rectum. J Am Coll Surg 1994; 178:271–275.
152. Adam IJ, Mohamdee MD, Martin IG, et al. Role of circumferential margin involvement in the local recurrence of rectal cancer. Lancet 1994; 344:707–711.
153. Clemmesen T, Sprechler M. Recording of patients with colorectal cancer on a database: Results and advantages. Eur J Surg 1994; 160:175–178.
154. Enker WE, Thaler HT, Craner ML, et al. Total mesorectal excision in the operative treatment of carcinoma of the rectum. J Am Coll Surg 1995; 181:335–346.
155. Hermanek P, Wiebelt H, Staimmer D, et al. Prognostic factors of rectum carcinoma—Experience of the German multicentre study SGCPC. Tumori 1995; 81(suppl):60–64.
156. Singh S, Morgan BF, Broughton M, et al. A 10-year prospective audit of outcome of surgical treatment for colorectal carcinoma. Br J Surg 1995; 82: 1486–1490.
157. Zaheer S, Pemberton JH, FaroukR, Dozois RR, Wolff BG, Ilstrup D. Surgical treatment of adenocarcinoma of the rectum. Ann Surg 1998; 227:800–811.
158. Killingback M, Barron P, Dent OF. Local recurrence after curative resection of cancer of the rectum without total mesorectal excision. Dis Colon Rectum 2001; 44:473–483.
159. Staib L, Link KH, Blatz A, Beger HG. Surgery of colorectal cancer: surgical morbidity and five- and ten-year results in 2400 patients—monoinstitutional experience. World J Surg 2002; 26:59–66.
160. Croxford M, Salerno G, Walson M, Sexton R, Heald RJ, Moran BJ. Does the height of the tumour influence the local recurrence rate in low rectal cancer treatment by total mesorectal resection? Br J Surg 2001; 91(suppl 1):1.
161. Wibe A, Syse A, Andersen E, TretH S, Myrvold HE, Soreide O. Norwegian Rectal Cancer Group. Oncological outcomes after total mesorectal excision for cure for cancer of the lower rectum: anterior vs. abdominoperineal resection. Dis Colon Rectum 2004; 47:48–58.
162. Law WL, Ho JW, Chan R, Auj G, Chu KW. Outcome of anterior resection for stage II rectal cancer without radiation: the role of adjuvant chemotherapy. Dis Colon Rectum 2005; 48:218–226.
163. Gordon PH, Shrier J, Obrand DI, Unpublished 2006.
164. Fedorov VD, Odarjuk TS. Sphincter saving operation for cancer of the rectum. Coloproctology 1983; 6:336–338.
165. Zhou XG, Yu BM, Shen YX. Surgical treatment and late results in 1226 cases of colorectal cancer. Dis Colon Rectum 1983; 26:250–256.
166. Malmberg M, Graffner H, Ling L, et al. Recurrence and survival after anterior resection of the rectum using the end to end anastomotic stapler. Surg Gynecol Obstet 1986; 163:231–234.
167. Heberer C, Denecke H, Demmel N, et al. Local procedures in the management of rectal cancer. World J Surg 1987; 11:499–503.
168. Belli L, Beati CA, Frangi M, et al. Outcome of patients with rectal cancer treated by stapled anterior resection. Br J Surg 1988; 75:422–424.
169. Jatzko G, Lisborg P, Wette V. Improving survival rates for patients with colorectal cancer. Br J Surg 1992; 79:588–591.
170. Isenberg J, Keller HW, Pichlmaier H. Middle and lower third rectum carcinoma: Sphincter saving or abdominoperineal resection? Eur J Surg Oncol 1995; 21:265–268.
171. Law WL, Chu KW. Abdominoperineal resection is associated with poor oncological outcome. Br J Sur 2004; 91:1493–499.
172. Elliot MS, Steven DM, Terblanche J. Abdominoperineal resection of the rectum for carcinoma at Groote Schuur Hospital, Cape Town, 1971–1982. S Afr Med J 1984; 65:411–413.
173. Huguier M, Depoux F, Houry S, et al. Adenocarcinoma of the rectum treated by abdominoperineal excision: Multivariate analysis of prognostic factors. Int J Colorectal Dis 1990; 5:144–147.
174. Dehni N, McFadden N, McNamara DA, Guiguet M, Tiret E, Pargj R. Oncologic results following abdominoperineal resection for adenocarcinoma of the low rectum. Dis Colon Rectum 2003; 46:867–874.
175. Rosen L, Veidenheimer MC, Coller JA, et al. Mortality, morbidity, and patterns of recurrence after abdominoperineal resection for cancer of the rectum. Dis Colon Rectum 1982; 25:202–208.
176. Hojo K. Anastomotic recurrence after sphincter saving resection for rectal cancer. Length of distal clearance of the bowel. Dis Colon Rectum 1986; 29: 11–14.
177. Sugihara K, Moriya Y, Akasu T, et al. Pelvic autonomic nerve preservation for patients with rectal carcinoma. Oncologic and functional outcome. Cancer 1996; 78:1871–1880.
178. Christiansen J. Place of abdominoperineal resection in rectal cancer. J R Soc Med 1988; 81:143–145.
179. Colombo PL, Foglieni CLS, Morone C. Analysis of recurrence following curative low anterior resection and stapled anastomosis for carcinoma of the middle third and lower rectum. Dis Colon Rectum 1987; 30:457–464.
180. Gillen P, Peel ALG. Comparison of the mortality, morbidity and incidence of local recurrence in patients with rectal cancer treated by either stapled anterior resection or abdominoperineal resection. Br J Surg 1986; 73:339–341.
181. Pescatori M, Mattana C, Maria G, et al. Outcome of colorectal cancer. Br J Surg 1987; 74:370–372.
182. Yeatman TJ, Bland KI. Sphincter saving procedures for distal carcinoma of the rectum. Ann Surg 1989; 209:1–18.
183. Kyzer S, Gordon PH. Experience with the use of the circular stapler in rectal surgery. Dis Colon Rectum 1992; 35:696–706.
184. Cutait DE, Cutait R, Da Silva JH, et al. Stapled anastomosis in colorectal surgery. Dis Colon Rectum 1981; 24:155–160.
185. Killingback M. Intrapelvic restorative resection for carcinoma of the large bowel, Hunterian Lecture. Royal College of Surgeons of England, April 1, 1981.
186. Dorricott NJ, Braddley RM, Keighley MRB, et al. Complications of rectal anastomoses with end-to-end anastomosis (EEA) stapling instrument. Ann R Coll Surg Engl 1982; 64:171–174.
187. Friis J, Hjortrup A, Nielson OV. Sphincter-saving resection of the rectum using the EEA auto staples. Acta Chir Scand 1982; 148:379–381.
188. Goligher JC. The use of circular staplers for the construction of colorectal anastomoses after anterior resection. In: Heberer G, Denecke H, eds. Colorectal Surgery. Berlin: Springer-Verlag, 1982:107–113.
189. Hamelmann H, Thiede A, Jostarndt L, et al. Stapler anastomoses in the low rectal third. In: Heberer G, Denecke H, eds. Colorectal Surgery. Berlin: Springer-Verlag, 1982:115–119.
190. Helm W, Rowe PH. Rectal anastomosis with the EEA stapling instrument. Ann R Coll Surg Engl 1982; 64:356–357.
191. Leff EI, Hoexter B, Labow SB, et al. The EEA stapler in low colorectal anastomoses: initial experience. Dis Colon Rectum1982; 162(235):704–707.
192. Polglase AL, Cunningham GE, Hughes ESR, et al. Initial clinical experience with the EEA stapler. Aust N Z J Surg 1982; 52:71–75.
193. Vezeridis M, Evans TJ, Mittelman A, et al. EEA stapler in low anterior anastomosis. Dis Colon Rectum 1982; 35:364–367.
194. Anderberg B, Enblad P, Sjodahl R, et al. The EEA stapling device in anterior resection for carcinoma of the rectum. Br J Surg 1983; 149:99–103.
195. Fegiz G, Angelini L, Bezzi M. Rectal cancer: Restorative surgery with the EEA stapling device. Int Surg 1983; 68:13–18.
196. Isbister WH, Beasley SW, Dowle CS. The EEA stapler—A Wellington experience. Coloproctology 1983; 6:323–326.
197. Kennedy HL, Rothenberger DA, Goldberg SM, et al. Colo-colostomy and coloproctostomy utilizing the circular intraluminal stapling devices. Dis Colon Rectum 1983; 26:145–148.
198. Resnick SD, Burstein AE, Viner YL. Use of the stapler in anterior resection for cancer of the rectosigmoid. Isr J Med Sci 1983; 19:128–133.
199. Fazio VW. Advances in the surgery of rectal carcinoma utilizing the circular stapler. Spratt JS, ed. In: Neoplasms of the Colon, Rectum and Anus. Philadelphia: WB Saunders, 1984:268–288.
200. Hedberg SE, Helmy AH. Experience with gastrointestinal stapling at the Massachusetts General Hospital. Surg Clin North Am 1984; 64:511–528.
201. Steichen FM, Ravitch MM. Stapling in Surgery. Chicago: Year Book Medical Publishers, 1984:271.
202. Fazio VW, Jagelman DG, Lavery IC, McGonale BA. Evaluation of the proximate-ILS circular stapler. Ann Surg 1985; 201:108–114.
203. McGinn FP, Gartell PC, Clifford PC, et al. Staples or sutures for low colorectal anastomoses: a prospective randomized trial. Br J Surg 1985; 73:603–605.
204. Antonsen HK, Kronborg O. Early complications after low anterior resection for rectal cancer using the EEA stapling device: a prospective trial. Dis Colon Rectum 1987; 30:579–583.
205. Zannini G, Renda A, Lepore R, et al. Mechanical anterior resection for carcinoma of the midrectum: long-term results. Int Surg 1987; 72:18–19.
206. Dehong Y, Yue T, Qinglan C, et al. Anterior resection with EEA stapler and manual sutures: comparison of two patient groups. In: Ravitch MM, Steichen FM, Welter R, eds. Current Practice of Surgical Stapling. Philadelphia: Lea & Febiger, 1991:101–103.
207. Steegmuller KW, Brown S. Experience with 140 stapled colorectal anastomoses. Ravitch MM, Steichen FM, Welter R, eds. Current Practice of Surgical Stapling. Philadelphia: Lea & Febiger, 1991:269–271.
208. Karanjia ND, Corder AP, Beam P, et al. Leakage from stapled low anastomosis after total mesorectal excision for carcinoma of the rectum. Br J Surg 1994; 81:1224–1226.
209. Fingerhut A, Hay JM, Elhadad A, et al. Supraperitoneal colorectal anastomosis: hand-sewn versu circular staples—a controlled clinical trial. Surgery 1995; 118:479–485.
210. Detry RJ, Kartheuser A, Delriviere L, et al. Use of the circular staples in 1000 consecutive colorectal anastomoses: experience of one surgical team. Surgery 1995; 117:140–145.
211. Goligher JC, Lee PWR, Lintott DJ. Experience with the Russian model 249 suture gun for anastomosis of the rectum. Surg Gynecol Obstet 1979; 148:517–524.
212. Beart RW Jr, Kelly KA. Randomized prospective evaluation of the EEA stapler for colorectal anastomosis. Am J Surg 1981; 141:143–147.
213. Adloff M, Arnaud JP, Beehary S. Stapled vs sutured colorectal anastomosis. Arch Surg 1980; 115:1436–1438.
214. Scher KR, Scott-Conner C, Jones CW, et al. A comparison of stapled and sutured anastomoses in colonic operations. Surg Gynecol Obstet 1982; 155:489–493.
215. Brown AA, Gasson JE, Brown RA. Experience with the EEA stapler in carcinoma of the lower rectum. S Afr Med J 1981; 21:258–261.

216. Goligher JC. The use of stapling devices for the construction of low rectal anastomoses. Ann Chir Gynaecol 1980; 69:125–131.
217. Heald RJ. Towards fewer colostomies—The impact of circular stapling devices on the surgery of rectal cancer in the district hospital. Br J Surg 1980; 67: 198–200.
218. Odou MW, O'Connell TX. Changes in the treatment of rectal carcinoma and effects on local recurrence. Arch Surg 1986; 121:1114–1116.
219. Hurst PR, Prout WG, Kelly JM, et al. Local recurrence after low anterior resection using the staple gun. Br J Surg 1982; 69:275–276.
220. Heald RJ, Husband EM, Ryall RDH. The mesorectum in rectal cancer surgery: the clue to pelvic recurrence? Br J Surg 1982; 69:13–16.
221. Rosen CB, Beart RW, Duane M, et al. Local recurrence of rectal carcinoma after hand sewn and stapled anastomoses. Dis Colon Rectum 1985; 28:305–309.
222. Heald RJ, Leicester RJ. The low stapled anastomoses. Br J Surg 1981; 68:333–337.
223. Luke M, Kirkegaard P, Lendorf A, et al. Pelvic recurrence rate after abdominoperineal resection and low anterior resection for rectal cancer before and after introduction of the stapling technique. World J Surg 1983; 7:616–619.
224. Kennedy HL, Langevin JM, Goldberg SM, et al. Recurrence following stapled coloproctostomy for carcinomas of the mid portion of the rectum. Surg Gynecol Obstet 1985; 160:513–516.
225. Leff EI, Shaver JO, Hoexter B, et al. Anastomotic recurrences after low anterior resection: stapled vs hand sewn. Dis Colon Rectum 1985; 28:164–167.
226. Wolmark N, Gordon PH, Fisher B, et al. A comparison of stapled and hand sewn anastomoses in patients undergoing resection for Dukes' B and C colorectal cancer: an analysis of disease free survival and survival from NSABP randomized clinical trials. Dis Colon Rectum 1986; 29:344–350.
227. Carlsson V, Lasson A, Ekelund G. Recurrence rates after curative surgery for rectal carcinoma, with special reference to their accuracy. Dis Colon Rectum 1987; 30:431–434.
228. Neville R, Fielding LP, Amendola C. Local tumor recurrence after curative resection for rectal cancer: a ten year hospital review. Dis Colon Rectum 1987; 30:12–17.
229. Akyol AM, McGregor JR, Galloway DJ, et al. Recurrence of colorectal cancer after sutured and stapled large bowel anastomoses. Br J Surg 1991; 78: 1297–1300.
230. Willett CG, Lewandrowski K, Donnelly S, et al. Are there patients with stage I rectal carcinoma at risk for failure after abdominoperineal resection? Cancer 1992; 69:1651–1655.
231. Arbman G, NilsSon E, HallbookO, Sjodahl R. Local recurrence following total mesorectal excision for rectal cancer. Br J Surg 1996; 83:375–379.
232. Heald RJ, Moran BJ, Ryall RD, Sexton R, MacFarlane JK. Rectal cancer: the Basingstoke experience of total mesorectal excision, 1978–1997. Arch Surg 1998; 133:894–899.
233. Hall NR, Finan PJ, Al-Jaberi T, et al. Circumferential margin involvement after mesorectal excision of rectal cancer with curative intent: predictors of survival but not local recurrence. Dis Colon Rectum 1998; 41:979–983.
234. Dahlberg M, Glimelius B, Pahlman L. Changing strategy for rectal cancer is associated with improved outcome. Br J Surg 1999; 86:379–384.
235. Martling AL, Holm T, Rutqvist LE, Moran BJ, Heald RJ, Cedemark B. Effect of a surgical training programme on outcome of rectal cancer in the County of Stockholm. Stockholm Colorectal Cancer Study Group, Basingstoke Bowel Cancer Research Project. Lancet 2000; 356:93–96.
236. Kapiteijn, Marijnen CA, Nagtegaal ID, et al. Preoperative radiotherapy combined with total mesorectal excision for resectable rectal cancer. N Engl J Med 2001; 345:638–646.
237. Nesbakken A, Nygaard K, Westerheim O, Mala T, Lunde OC. Local recurrence after mesorectal excision for rectal cancer. Eur J Oncol 2002; 28:126–134.
238. Bulow S, Christensen IJ, Harling H, Kronborg O, Fenger C, Nielsen HJ; Danish TME Study Group; RANX05 Colorectal Cancer Study Group. Recurrence and survival after mesorectal excision for rectal cancer. Br J Surg 2003; 90: 974–980.
239. Cecil TD, Sexton R, Moran BJ, Heald RJ. Total mesorectal excision results in low local recurrence rates in lymph node-positive rectal cancer. Dis Colon Rectum 2004; 47:1145–1149.
240. Kockerling F, Reymond MA, Altendorf-Hofmann A, Dworak O, Hohenberger W. Influence of surgery on metachronous distant metastases and survival in rectal cancer. J Clin Oncol 1998; l6:324–329.
241. McCall JL, Cox MR, Wattchow DA. Analysis of local recurrence rates after surgery alone for rectal cancer. Int J Colorectal Dis 1995; 10:126–132.
242. Nagtegaal ID, van de Velde CJ, van der Worp E, Kapiteijn E, Quirke P, van Krieken JH. Cooperative Clinical Investigators of the Dutch Colorectal Cancer Group. Macroscopic evaluation of rectal cancer resection specimen: clinical significance of the pathologist in quality control. J Clin Oncol 2002; 4(20):1729–1734.
243. Wibe A, Eriksen MT, Syse A, Myrvold HE, Soreide O. Norwegian Rectal Cancer Group. Total mesorectal excision for rectal cancer-what can be achieved by a national audit? Colorectal Dis 2003; 5:471–477.
244. Ike H, Shimada H, Yamaguchi S, Ichikawa Y, Fujii S, Ohki S. Outcome of total pelvic exenteration for primary rectal cancer. Dis Colon Rectum 2003:474–480.
245. Manfredi S, Benhamiche AM, Meny B, Cheynel N, Rat P, Faivre J. Population-based study of factors influencing occurrence and prognosis of local recurrence after surgery for rectal cancer. Br J Surg 2001; 88:1221–1227.
246. Bonadeo FA, Vaccaro CA, Benati ML, Quintana GM, Garione XE, Telenta MT. Rectal cancer: local recurrence after surgery without radiotherapy. Dis Colon Rectum 2001; 44:374–379.
247. Vironen JH, Halme L, Sainio P, et al. New approaches in the management of rectal carcinoma result in reduced local recurrence rate and improved survival. Eur J Surg 2002; 168:158–164.
248. Parks AG. Per anal anastomosis. World J Surg 1982; 6:531–538.
249. Sweeney JL, Ritchie JK, Hawley PR. Resection and sutured per anal anastomosis for carcinoma of the rectum. Dis Colon Rectum 1989; 32:103–106.
250. Enker WE, Stearns MW Jr, Janov AJ. Per anal coloanal anastomosis following low anterior resection for rectal carcinoma. Dis Colon Rectum 1985; 28: 576–581.
251. Cohen AM, Enker WE, Minsky BD. Proctectomy and coloanal reconstruction for rectal cancer. Dis Colon Rectum 1990; 33:40–43.
252. Drake DB, Pemberton JH, Beart RW, et al. Coloanal anastomosis in the management of benign and malignant rectal disease. Ann Surg 1987; 206:600–605.
253. Hautefeuille P, Valleus P, Perniceni T, et al. Functional and oncologic results after coloanal anastomoses for low rectal carcinoma. Ann Surg 1988; 207:61–64.
254. Vernava AM III, Robbins PL, Brabbee GW. Restorative resection: Coloanal anastomosis for benign and malignant disease. Dis Colon Rectum 1989; 32:690–693.
255. Wunderlich M, Hansuch JK, Schiessel R. Results of coloanal anastomosis. A prospective study. Int J Colorectal Dis 1986; 1:157–161.
256. Kohler A, Athanasiadis S, Ommer A, Psarakis E. Long-term results of low anterior resection with intersphincteric anastomosis in carcinoma of the lower one-third of the rectum: analysis of 31 patients. Dis Colon Rectum 2000; 43:843–850.
257. Ho P, Law WL, Chan SC, Lam CK, Chu KW. Functional outcome following low anterior resection with total mesorectal excision in the elderly. Int J Colorectal Dis 2003; 18:230–233.
258. Phillips PS, Farquharson SM, Sexton R, Heald RJ, Moran BJ. Rectal cancer in the elderly: patients' perception of bowel control after restorative surgery. Dis Colon Rectum 2004; 47:287–290.
259. Rengan R, Paty JP, Wong WD, et al. Distal cT2N0 Rectal Cancer: Is There an Alternative to Abdominoperineal Resection? J Clin Oncol 2005; 23:4905–4912.
260. Engel J, Kerr J, Schlesinger-Raab A, Eckel R, Sauer H, Holzel D. Quality of life in rectal cancer patients: a four-year prospective study. Ann Surg 2003; 238:203–213.
261. Schmidt CE, Bestmann B, Kuchler T, Longo WE, Kremer B. Prospective evaluation of quality of life of patients receiving either abdominoperineal resection or sphincter-preserving procedure for rectal cancer. Ann Surg Oncol 2005; 12:117–123.
262. Porter GA, O'Keefe GE, Yakimets WW. Inadvertent perforation of the rectum during abdominoperineal resection. Am J Surg 1996; 172:324–327.
263. Phang PT, MacFarlane JK, Taylor RH, et al. Effect of emergent presentation on outcome from rectal cancer management. Am J Surg 2003; 185:450–454.
264. Vironen JH, Sainio P, Husa AI, Kellokumpu IH. Complications and survival after surgery for rectal cancer in patients younger than and aged 75 years or older. Dis Colon Rectum 2004; 47:1225–1231.
265. Eriksen MT, Wibe A, Syse A, Haffner J, Wiig JN. Norwegian Rectal Cancer Group Norwegian Gastrointestinal Cancer Group. Inadvertent perforation during rectal cancer resection in Norway. Br J Surg 2004; 91:210–216.
266. Leong AF. Total mesorectal excision (TME)—twenty years on. Ann Acad Med Singapore 2003; 32:159–162.
267. Kressner U, Graf W, Mahteme H, PahJman L, Glimelius B. Septic complications and prognosis after surgery for rectal cancer. Dis Colon Rectum 2002; 45:316–321.
268. Platell CF, Thompson PJ, Makin GB. Sexual health in women following pelvic surgery for rectal cancer. Br J Surg 2004; 91:465–468.
269. Schmidt CE, Bestmann B, Kuchler T, Longo WE, Kremer B. Ten-year historic cohort of quality of life and sexuality in patients with rectal cancer. Dis Colon Rectum 2005; 480:483–492.
270. Sharma A, Hartley J, Monson JR. Local excision of rectal tumors. Surg Oncol 2003; 12:51–61.
271. Killingback MJ. Indications for local excision of rectal cancer. Br J Surg 1985; 72(suppl):S54–S56.
272. Whiteway J, Nicholls RJ, Morson BC. The role of surgical local excision in the treatment of rectal cancer. Br J Surg 1985; 72:694–697.
273. Morson BC. Histological criteria for local excision. Br J Surg 1985; 72(suppl):S53–S54.
274. Minsky BD, Rich T, Recht A, et al. Selection criteria for local excision with or without adjuvant radiation therapy for rectal cancer. Cancer 1989; 63:1421.
275. Huddy SPJ, Hasband EM, Cook MG, et al. Lymph node metastases in early rectal cancer. Br J Surg 1993; 80:1457–1458.
276. Blumberg D, Paty PB, Guillem JG, et al. All patients with small intramural rectal cancers are at risk for lymph node metastasis. Dis Colon Rectum 1999; 42:881–885.
277. Nascimbeni R, Burgart LJ, Nivatvongs S, Larson DR. Risk of lymph node metastasis hi Tl carcinoma of the colon and rectum. Dis Colon Rectum 2002; 45:200–206.
278. Sakuragi M, Togashi K, Konishi F, et al. Predictive factors for lymph node metastasis in Tl stage colorectal carcinomas. Dis Colon Rectum 2003; 46: 1626–1632.

279. Okabe S, Shia J, Nash G, et al. Lymph node metastasis in Tl adenocarcinoma of the colon and rectum. J Gastrointest Surg 2004; 8:1032–1039.
280. Lavery IC, Jones IT, Weakley FL, et al. Definitive management of rectal cancer by contact (endocavitary) irradiation. Dis Colon Rectum 1987; 30:835–838.
281. Gopaul D, Belliveau P, Vuong T, et al. Outcome of local excision of rectal carcinoma. Dis Colon Rectum 2004; 47:1780–1788.
282. Nascimbeni R, Nivatvongs S, Larson PR, Burgart LJ. Long-term survival after local excision for Tl carcinoma of the rectum. Dis Colon Rectum 2004; 47: 1773–1779.
283. Sengupta S, Tjandra JJ. Local excision of rectal cancer: what is the evidence? Dis Colon Rectum 2001; 44:1345–1361.
284. Biggers OR, Beart RW Jr, Ilstrup DM. Local excision of rectal cancer. Dis Colon Rectum 1986; 29:374–377.
285. Horn A, Halvorsen JF, Morild I. Transanal extirpation for early rectal cancer. Dis Colon Rectum 1989; 32:769–772.
286. Killingback MJ. Local excision of carcinoma of the rectum. World J Surg 1992; 16:437–446.
287. Lock MR, Ritchie JK, Hawley PR. Reappraisal of radical local excision for carcinoma of the rectum. Br J Surg 1993; 80:928–929.
288. Willett CG, Compton CC, Shellito PC, et al. Selection factors for local excision or abdominoperineal resection of early stage rectal cancer. Cancer 1994; 73:2716–2720.
289. Green JD, Riether RD, Rosen L, et al. Transanal diskectomy for cure of rectal adenocarcinoma: is clinical judgment accurate? [abstract]. Dis Colon Rectum 1994; 37:5.
290. Faivre J, Chaume JC, Pigot F, et al. Transanal electro resection of small rectal cancer: a sole treatment. Dis Colon Rectum 1996; 39: 270–278.
291. Obrand DI, Gordon PH. Results of local excision for rectal carcinoma. Can J Surg 1996; 39:463–468.
292. Chakravarti A, Compton CC, Shellito PC, et al. Long-term follow-up of patients with rectal cancer managed by local excision with and without adjuvant irradiation. Ann Surg 1999; 230:49–54.
293. Steele GD Jr, Herndon JE, Bleday R, et al. Sphincter-sparing treatment for distal rectal adenocarcinoma. Ann Surg Oncol 1999; 6:433–441.
294. Varma MG, Rogers SJ, Schrock TR, Welton ML. Local excision of rectal carcinoma. Arch Surg 1999; 134:863–867.
295. Mellgren A, Sirivongs P, Rothenberger DA, Madoff RD, Garcia-Aguilar J. Is local excision adequate therapy for early rectal cancer? Dis Colon Rectum 2000; 43:1064–1071.
296. Paty PB, Nash GM, Baron P, et al. Long-term results of local excision for rectal cancer. Ann Surg 2002; 236:522–529.
297. Chambers WM, Khan U, Gagliano A, Smith RD, Sheffield J, Nicholls RJ. Tumour morphology as a predictor of outcome after local excision of rectal cancer. Br J Surg 2004; 91:457–459.
298. Madbouly KM, Remzi FH, Erkek BA, et al. Recurrence after transanal excision of Tl rectal cancer: should we be concerned? Dis Colon Rectum 2005; 48: 711–719.
299. Graham RA, Garnsey L, Jessup JM. Local excision of rectal carcinoma. Am J Surg 1990; 160:306–312.
300. Muto T, Oya M. Recent advances in diagnosis and treatment of colorectal T1 carcinoma. Dis Colon Rectum 2003; 46(suppl):S89–S93.
301. Baxter NN, Stewart AR, Nelson H. Local Excision for rectal cancer. J Clin Oncol 2004; 22:145–273.
302. Minsky BD. Clinical experience with local excision and postoperative radiotherapy for rectal-cancer. Dis Colon Rectum 1993; 36:405–409.
303. Hanloser D, Wolff BG, Larson DW, Ping J, Nivatvongs S. Immediate radical resection after local excision of rectal cancer: an oncologic compromise? Dis Colon Rectum 2005; 48:429–437.
304. Cuthbertson AM, Simpson R. Curative local excision of rectal adenocarcinoma. Aust N Z J Surg 1986; 56:229–231.
305. Friel CM, Cromwell JW, Marra C, Madoff RD, Rothen berger DA, Garcia-Aguilar J. Salvage radical surgery after failed local excision for early rectal cancer. Dis Colon Rectum 2002; 45:875–879.
306. Weiser MR, Landmann RG, Wong WD, et al. Surgical salvage of recurrent rectal cancer after transanal excision. Dis Colon Rectum 2005; 48:1169–1175.
307. Baron PL, Enker WE, Zakowski MF, et al. Immediate vs. salvage resection after local treatment for early rectal cancer. Dis Colon Rectum 1995; 38: 177–181.
308. Rouanet P, Saint Aubert B, Fabre JM, et al. Conservative treatment for low rectal carcinoma by local excision with or without radiotherapy. Br J Surg 1993; 80:1452–1456.
309. Bennett CJ Jr, Sombeck MD, Mendanhall WM, et al. Conservative alternatives in the management of early carcinoma of the rectum. South Med J 1993; 86:409–413.
310. Wagman R, Minsky BD, Cohen AM, Safe L, Paty PB, Guillem JG. Conservative management of rectal cancer with local excision and postoperative adjuvant therapy. Int J Radiat Oncol Biol Phys 1999; 44:841–846.
311. Lamont JP, McCarty TM, Digan RD, Jacobson R, Tulanon P, Lichliter WE. Should locally excised T1 rectal cancer receive adjuvant chemoradiation? Am J Surg 2000; 80:402–405.
312. Coco C, Magistrelli P, Netri G, et al. Combined modality therapy in low risk (T2 NO) rectal cancer. Rays 1995; 20:156–164.
313. Graham RA, Atkins MB, Karp DD, et al. Local excision of rectal carcinoma. Early results with combined chemoradiation therapy using 5-fluorouracil and leucovorin. Dis Colon Rectum 1994; 37:308–312.
314. Russell AH, Harris J, Rosenberg PJ, et al. Anal sphincter conservation for patients with adenocarcinoma of the distal rectum: long-term results of radiation therapy oncology group protocol 89–02. Int J Radiat Oncol Biol Phys 2000; 46:313–322.
315. Schell SR, Zlotecki RA, Mendenhali WM, Marsh RW, Vauthey JN, Copeland EM III. Transanal excision of locally advanced rectal cancers downstaged using neoadjuvant chemoradiotherapy. J Am Coll Surg 2002; 194:584–590.
316. Ruo L, Guillem JG, Minsky BD, Quan SH, Paty PB, Cohen AM. Preoperative radiation with or without chemotherapy and full-thickness transanal excision for selected T2 and T3 distal rectal cancers. Int J Colorectal Dis 2002; 17:54–58.
317. Papillon J. Endocavitary irradiation of early rectal cancer for cure: a series of 123 cases. Proc R Soc Med 1973; 66:1179–1181.
318. Papillon J. Present status of radiation therapy in the conservative management of rectal cancer. Radiother Oncol 1990; 17:275–283.
319. Sischy B, Hinson EJ, Wilkinson DR. Definitive radiation therapy for selected cancer of the rectum. Br J Surg 1988; 75:901–903.
320. Hull TL, Lavery IC, Saxton JP. Endocavitary irradiation: an option in select patients with rectal cancer. Dis Colon Rectum 1994; 37:1266–1270.
321. Horiot JC, Gerard JP, Maingen P. Conservative and curative management of rectal adenocarcinomas by local radiotherapy alone. Eur J Cancer 1995; 31A:1340–1342.
322. Reed NP, Cataldo PA, Garb JL, et al. The influence of local tumor ulceration on the effectiveness of endocautery radiation for patients with early rectal carcinoma. Cancer 1995; 76:967–971.
323. Schild SE, Martenson JA, Gunderson LL. Endocavitary radiotherapy of rectal cancer. Int J Radiat Oncol Biol Phys 1996; 34:677–682.
324. Mahajan A, Shenouda G, Gordon PH, et al. Long source-skin distance rectal irradiation technique: a review of results. Radiother Oncol 1996; 40:63–67.
325. Winslow ER, Kodner IJ, Mutch MG, Birnbaum EB, Fleshman JW, Dietz DW. Outcome of salvage abdominoperincal resection after failed endocavitary radiation in patients with rectal cancer. Dis Colon Rectum 2004; 47:2039–2046.
326. Lambrianidas HL, Ghilchick MG. Cryosurgery in the treatment of rectal carcinoma. Postgrad Med J 1983; 59:244–245.
327. Mathus-Vliegan EMH. Laser ablation of early colorectal malignancy. Endoscopy 1993; 25:462–468.
328. Cummings BJ. Radiation therapy and rectal carcinoma. The Princess Margaret Hospital experience. Br J Surg 1985; 72(suppl):S64–S66.
329. Sischy B. The role of radiation therapy in the management of carcinoma of the rectum. Contemp Surg 1987; 30:13–26.
330. Beart RW Jr. Rectal and anal cancers. In: Steele G Jr, Osteen RT, eds. Colorectal Cancer. New York: Marcel Dekker, 1986:170.
331. McDermott FT, Hughes ESR, Pihl E, et al. Local recurrence after potentially curative resection for rectal cancer in a series of 1008 patients. Br J Surg 1985; 72:34–37.
332. Heimann TM, Szporn A, Bolnick K, et al. Local recurrence following surgical treatment of rectal cancer. Comparison of anterior and abdominoperineal resection. Dis Colon Rectum 1986; 29:862–864.
333. Kirwan WO, Drumm J, Hogan JM, et al. Determining safe margin of resection in low anterior resection for rectal cancer. Br J Surg 1988; 75:720.
334. Shirouzu K, Isomoto H, Kakegawa T. Distal spread of rectal cancer and optimal distal margin of resection for sphincter-preserving surgery. Cancer 1995; 76:388–392.
335. Vernava AM, Moran M, Rothenberger DA, et al. A prospective evaluation of distal margins in carcinoma of the rectum. Surg Gynecol Obstet 1992; 175:333–336.
336. Kwok SPY, Lau WY, Leung KL, et al. Prospective analysis of the distal margin of clearance in anterior resection for rectal carcinoma. Br J Surg 1996; 83:969–972.
337. Enker WE, Laffer UT, Block GE. Enhanced survival of patients with colon and rectal cancer is based upon wide anatomic resection. Ann Surg 1979; 190: 350–360.
338. Tonak J, Gall FP, Hermanek P, et al. Incidence of local recurrence after curative operations for cancer of the rectum. Aust N Z J Surg 1982; 52:23–27.
339. Gibbs P, Chao MW, Tjandra JJ. Optimizing the outcome for patients with rectal cancer. Dis Colon Rectum 2003; 46:389–402.
340. Moore HG, Riedel E, Minsky BD, et al. Adequacy of 1-cm distal margin after restorative rectal cancer resection with sharp mesorectal excision and preoperative combined-modality therapy. Ann Surg Oncol 2003; 10:80–85.
341. Nakagoe T, Yamaguchi E, Tanaka K, et al. Distal intramural spread is an independent prognostic factor for distant metastasis and poor outcome in patients with rectal cancer: a multivariate analysis. Ann Surg Oncol 2003; 10:163–170.
342. Quirke P, Durdey P, Dixon MF, et al. Local recurrence of rectal adenocarcinoma due to inadequate surgical resection: Histologic study of lateral tumour spread and surgical excision. Lancet 1986; 2:996–999.
343. Wibe A, Rendedal PR, Svensson E, et al. Prognostic significance of the circumferential resection margin following total mesorectal excision for rectal cancer. Br J Surg 2002; 89:327–334.
344. Gordon PH. Is total mesorectal excision really important? J Surg Oncol 2000; 74:177–180.

345. Abel AL. The modern treatment of cancer of the rectum. Milwaukee Proc 1931:296–300.
346. Heald RJ, Moran G, Brown G, Daniels IR. Optimal total mesorectal excision for rectal cancer is by dissection in fromt of Denonvilliers fascia. Br J Surg 2004; 91:121–123.
347. Hermanek P, Hermanek P, Hohenberger W, Klimpfinger M, Kockerling F, Papadopoulos T. The pathological assessment of mesorectal excision: implications for further treatment and quality management. Int J Colorectal Dis 2003; 18:335–341.
348. Sterk P, Kasperk R, Opitz T, Schubert F, Klein P. Vascular organization in the mesorectum: angiography of rectal resection specimens. Int J Colorectal Dis 2000; 15:225–228.
349. Cawthorn SJ, Parums DV, Gibbs NM, et al. Extent of mesorectal spread and involvement of lateral resection margin as prognostic factors after surgery for rectal cancer. Lancet 1990; 35:1055–1059.
350. Scott N, Jackson P, Al-Jaberi T, et al. Total mesorectal excision and local recurrence: a study of tumour spread in the mesorectum distal to rectal cancer. Br J Surg 1995; 82:1031–1033.
351. Choi JS, Kim SJ. Kim YI, et al. Nodal metastasis in the distal mesorecturn: need for total mesorectal excision of rectal cancer. Yonsei Med J 1996; 37:243–250.
352. Reynolds JV, Joyce WP, Dolan J, et al. Pathological evidence in support of total mesorectal excision in the management of rectal cancer. Br J Surg 1996; 83: 112–115.
353. Prabhudesai A, Arif S, Finlayson CJ, Kumar D. Impact of microscopic extranodal tumor deposits on the outcome of patients with rectal cancer. Dis Colon Rectum 2003; 46:1531–1537.
354. McCall JL, Cox MR, Wattchaw DA. Analysis of local recurrence rates after surgery alone for rectal cancer. Int J Colorectal Dis 1995; 10:126–132.
355. Leo E, Belli F, Andreola S, et al. Total rectal resection, mesorectal excision, and coloendoanal anastomosis: a therapeutic option for the treatment of low rectal cancer. Ann Surg Oncol 1996; 3:336–343.
356. Heald RJ. Rectal cancer: The surgical options. Eur J Cancer 1995; 31A:1189–1192.
357. Bokey EL, Ojerskog B, Chapuis PH, et al. Local recurrence after curative resection of the rectum for cancer withour adjuvant therapy: role of total anatomical resection. Br J Surg 1999; 86:1164–1170.
358. Krook JE, Moertel CG, Gunderson LL, et al. Effective surgical adjuvant therapy for high risk rectal carcinoma. N Engl J Med 1991; 324:709–715.
359. Fisher B, Wolmark N, Rockette H, et al. Postoperative adjuvant chemotherapy or radiation therapy for rectal cancer: results from NSABP protocol R-01. J Natl Cancer Inst 1988; 80:21–29.
360. Wibe A. On behalf of the Norwegian Recta Cancer Group and the Norwegian Cancer Registry presented at the ASCRS Annual Meeting. Washington. DC. May 1–6, 1999.
361. Ridgway PF, Darzi AW. The role of total mesorectal excision in the managment of rectal cancer. Cancer Control 2003; 10:205–211.
362. Colquhoun P, Wexner SD, Cohen A. Adjuvant therapy is valuable in the treatment of rectal cancer despite total mesorectal excision. J Surg Qncol 2003; 83:133–139.
363. Nesbakken A, Nygaard K, Lunde OC. Outcome and late functional results after anastomotic leakage following mesorectal excision for rectal cancer. Br J Surg 2001; 88:400–404.
364. Nesbakken A, Nygaard K, Bull-Njaa T, Carlsen E, Eri LM. Bladder and sexual dysfunction after mesorectal excision for rectal cancer. Br J Surg 2000; 87: 206–210.
365. Kim NK, AahnTW, Park JK, et al. Assessment of sexual and voiding function after total mesorectal excision with pelvic autonomic nerve preservation in males with rectal cancer. Dis Colon Rectum 2002; 45:1178–1185.
366. Kneist W, Heintz A, Junginger T. Major urinary dysfunction after mesorectal excision for rectal carcinoma. Br J Surg 2005; 92:230–234.
367. Peeters KC, Tollenaar RA, Marijnen CA, et al. Risk factors for anastomotic failure after total mesorectal excision of rectal cancer. Br J Surg 2005; 92:211–216.
368. von Flüe MO, Degen LP, Beglinger C, et al. Ileocecal reservoir reconstruction with physiologic function after total mesorectal cancer excision. Ann Surg 1996; 224:204–212.
369. Lopez-Kostner F, Lavery IC, Hool GP, et al. Total mesorectal excision is not necessary for cancer of the upper rectum. Surgery 1998; 124:612–618.
370. Hojo K, Sawada T, Moriya Y. An analysis of survival and voiding, sexual function after wide ileopelvic lymphadenectomy in patients with carcinoma of the rectum compared with conventional lymphadenectomy. Dis Colon Rectum 1989; 32:128–133.
371. Hojo K, Vernava AM III, Sugihara K, et al. Preservation of urine voiding and sexual function after rectal cancer surgery. Dis Colon Rectum 1991; 34: 532–539.
372. Glass RE, Ritchie JK, Thompson HR, et al. The results of surgical treatment of cancer of the rectum by radical resection and extended abdominosacral lymphadenectomy. Br J Surg 1985; 72:599–601.
373. Moreira LF, Hizuta A, Iwagaki H, et al. Lateral lymph node dissection for rectal carcinoma below the peritoneal reflection. Br J Surg 1994; 81:293–296.
374. Moriya Y, Sugihara K, Akasu T, et al. Nerve-sparing surgery with lateral node dissection for advanced lower rectal cancer. Eur J Cancer 1995; 31A: 1229–1232.
375. Morita T, Murata A, Koyama M, Totsuka E, Sasaki M. Current status of autonomic nerve-preserving surgery for mid and lower rectal cancers: Japanese experience with lateral node dissection. Dis Colon Rectum 2003; 46(suppl): S78–S87.
376. Hocht S, Mann B, Germer CT, et al. Pelvic sidewall involvement in recurrent rectal cancer. Int J Colorectal Dis 2004; 19:108–113.
377. Fujita S, Yamamoto S, Akasu T, Moriya Y. Lateral pelvic lymph node dissection for advanced lower rectal cancer. Br J Surg 2003; 90:1580–1585.
378. Nagawa H, Muto T, Sunouchi K, et al. Randomized, controlled trial of lateral node dissection vs. nerve-preserving resection in patients with rectal cancer after preoperative radiotherapy. Dis Colon Rectum 2001; 44:1274–1280.
379. Koda K, Saito N, Oda K, Takiguchi N, Sarashina H, Miyazaki M. Evaluation of lateral lymph node dissection with preoperative chemo-radiotherapy for the treatment of advanced middle to lower rectal cancers. Int J Colorectal Dis 2004:188–194.
380. Hida J, Yasutomi M, Fujimoto K, Maruyama T, Okuno K, Shindo K. Does lateral lymph node dissection improve survival in rectal carcinoma? Examination of node metastases by the clearing method. J Am Coll Surg 1997; 184:475–480.
381. Ruo L, Paty PB, Minsky BD, Wong WD, Cohen AM, Guillem JG. Results after rectal cancer resection with in-continuity partial vaginectomy and total mesorectal excision. Ann Surg Oncol 2003; 10:664–668.
382. Sokmen S, Terzi C, Unek T, Alanyali H, Fuzun M. Multivisceral resections for primary advanced rectal cancer. Int J Colorectal Dis 1999; 14:282–285.
383. Orkin BA, Dozois RR, Beart RW, et al. Extended resection for locally advanced primary adenocarcinoma of the rectum. Dis Colon Rectum 1989; 32:286–292.
384. Fedorov VD, Odaryuk TS, Shelygin YA. Results of radical surgery for advanced rectal cancer. Dis Colon Rectum 1989; 32:567–571.
385. Sugarbaker PH. Partial sacrectomy for en bloc excision of rectal cancer with posterior fixation. Dis Colon Rectum 1982; 25:208–211.
386. Stelzer M. Summary statement 2003 SSAT-AGA-ASGE Workshop on Palliative Therapy of Rectal Cancer Gastrointestinal Surg 2004; 8:253–258.
387. Moran MR, Rothenberger DA, Lahr CJ, et al. Palliation for rectal cancer. Resection? Anastomosis? Arch Surg 1987; 122:640–643,.
388. Longo WE, Ballantyne GH, Bilchik HJ, et al. Advanced rectal cancer: what is the best palliation? Dis Colon Rectum 1988; 31:842–847.
389. Nash GM, Salte LB, Kemeny NE, et al. Radical resection of rectal cancer primary tumor provides effective local therapv m patients with stage IV disease. Ann Surg Oncol 2002; 9:954–960.
390. Johnson WR, McDermott FT, Pihl E, et al. Palliative operative management in rectal carcinoma. Dis Colon Rectum 1981; 24:606–609.
391. Gordon PH, Fry RD, Segall MM, et al. Advanced carcinoma of the rectum. Perspect Colon Rectal Surg 1994; 7:235–244.
392. Heah SM, Eu KW, Ho VH, Leong AF, Seow-Choen F. Hartmann's procedure vs. abdominoperineal resection for palliation of advanced low rectal cancer. Dis Colon Rectum 1997; 40:1313–1317.
393. Mahteme H, Pählman L, Gimelius B, et al. Prognosis after surgery in patients with incurable rectal cancer: a population-based study. Br J Surg 1996; 83: 1116–1120.
394. Nakfoor BM, Willett CG, Shellito PC, Kaufman DS, Daly WJ. The impact of 5-fluorouracil and intraoperative electron beam rradiation therapy on the outcome of patients with locally advanced primary rectal and rectosigmoid cancer. Ann Surg 1998; 228:194–200.
395. ReMine SG, Dozois RR. Hartmann's procedure: Its use with complicated carcinomas of sigmoid colon and rectum. Arch Surg 1981; 116:630–633.
396. Doci R, Audisio RA, Bozzetti F, et al. Actual role of Hartmann's resection in elective surgical treatment for carcinoma of rectum and sigmoid colon. Surg Gynecol Obstet 1986; 163:49–53.
397. Tottrup A, Frost L. Pelvic sepsis after extended Hartmann's procedure. Dis Colon Rectum 2005; 48:251–255.
398. Turnbull RB, Weakley FL Jr. Atlas of Intestinal Stomas. St. Louis: CVMosby, 1967:161–165.
399. Grinnell RS, Hiatt RB. Ligation of the inferior mesenteric artery at the aorta in resections for carcinoma of the sigmoid and rectum. Surg Gynecol Obstet 1952; 94:526–534.
400. Grinnell RS. Results of ligation of inferior mesenteric artery at the aorta in resections of carcinoma of the descending and sigmoid colon and rectum. Surg Gynecol Obstet 1965; 120:1031–1036.
401. Busuttil RW, Foglia RP, Longmire WP Jr. Treatment of carcinoma of the sigmoid colon and upper rectum. Arch Surg 1977; 112:920–923.
402. Surtees P, Ritchie JK, Phillips RKS. High versus low ligation of the inferior mesenteric artery in rectal cancer. Br J Surg 1990; 77:618–621.
403. Bland KI, Polk HC. Therapeutic measures applied for the curative and palliative control of colorectal carcinoma. Surg Annu 1983; 15:123–161.
404. Corder AP, Karanjia ND, Williams JD, et al. Flush aortic tie versus selective preservation of the ascending left colic artery in low anterior resection for rectal carcinoma. Br J Surg 1992; 79:650–652.
405. Hida J, Yasutomi M, Maruyama T, et al. Indication for using high ligation of the inferior mesenteric artery in rectal cancer surgery. Examination of nodal metastases by the clearing method. Dis Colon Rectum 1998; 41: 984–987.

406. Slanetz CA Jr, Grimson R. Effect of high and intermediate ligation on survival and recurrence rates following curative resection of colorectal cancer. Dis Colon Rectum 1997; 40:1205–1218.
407. Rothenberger DA, Wong WD. Rectal cancer—Adequacy of surgical management. Surg Annu 1985; 17:309–336.
408. McLean CM, Duncan W. Rectal cancer: a review of randomized trials of adjuvant radiotherapy. Clin Oncol 1995; 7:349–358.
409. Kerman HD, Roberson SH, Bloom TS, et al. Rectal carcinoma. Long-term experience with moderately high doses preoperative radiation and low anterior resection. Cancer 1992; 69:2813–2819.
410. Minsky BD. Oxaliplatin-based combined-modality therapy for rectal cancer. Semin Oncol 2003; 30(4 suppl 15):26–33.
411. Gerard A, Buyse M, Nordlinger B, et al. Preoperative radiotherapy as adjuvant treatment of rectal cancer. Ann Surg 1988; 308:606–612.
412. Medical Research Council. The evaluation of low-dose preoperative x-ray therapy in the management of operable rectal cancer; Results of a randomly controlled trial. Br J Surg 1984; 71:21–25.
413. Cummings BJ, Rider WD, Harwood AR, et al. Radical external beam radiation therapy for adenocarcinoma of the rectum. Dis Colon Rectum 1983; 26:30–36.
414. Fortier GA, Constable WC. Preoperative radiation therapy for rectal cancer. Arch Surg 1986; 121:1380–1385.
415. James RD, Schofield PF. Resection of "inoperable" rectal cancer following radiotherapy. Br J Surg 1985; 72:279–281.
416. Papillon J. The future of external beam irradiation as initial treatment of rectal cancer. Br J Surg 1987; 74:449–454.
417. Mendenhall WM, Bland KI, Copeland EM, et al. Does preoperative radiation therapy enhance the probability of local control and survival in high-risk distal rectal cancer. Ann Surg 1992; 215:696–706.
418. Friedmann P, Garb JL, Pare WC, et al. Survival following moderate dose preoperative radiation therapy for carcinoma of the rectum. Cancer 1985; 55: 967–973.
419. Cummings BJ. A critical review of adjuvant preoperative radiation therapy for adenocarcinoma of the rectum. Br J Surg 1986; 73:332–338.
420. Duncan W. Adjuvant radiotherapy and rectal cancer: the MRC trials. Br J Surg 1985; 72(suppl):S59–S62.
421. Stockholm Rectal Cancer Study Group. Preoperative short-term radiation therapy in operable rectal carcinoma. A prospective randomized trial. Cancer 1990; 66:49–55.
422. Cedermark B, Johansson H, Rutqvist L, et al. The Stockholm I Trial of preoperative short term radiotherapy in operable rectal carcinoma. Cancer 1995; 75:2269–2275.
423. Påhlman L, Glimelius B. Pre- or postoperative radiotherapy in rectal and rectosigmoid carcinoma. Report from a randomized multicenter trial. Ann Surg 1990; 211:187–195.
424. Påhlman L, Glimelius B. The value of adjuvant radio(chemo)-therapy for rectal cancer. Eur J Cancer 1995; 31A:1347–1350.
425. Påhlman L. Initial report from a Swedish multicentre study examining the role of preoperative irradiation in the treatment of patients with resectable rectal carcinoma. Br J Surg 1993; 80:1333–1336.
426. Swedish Rectal Cancer Trial. Improved survival with preoperative radiotherapy in resectable rectal cancer. N Engl J Med 1997; 336:980–987.
427. Cedermark B, SRCS Group. Randomized study on preoperative radiation therapy in rectal carcinoma. Ann Surg Oncol 1996; 3:423–430.
428. Holm T, Rutqvist LE, Johansson H, et al. Abdominoperineal resection and anterior resection in the treatment of rectal cancer: results in relation to adjuvant preoperative radiotherapy. Br J Surg 1995; 182:1213–1216.
429. Holm T, Rutqvist LE, Johansson H, et al. Postoperative mortality in rectal cancer treated with or without preoperative radiotherapy: causes and risk factors. Br J Surg 1996; 83:964–968.
430. Holm T, Singnomklao T, Rutqvist LE, et al. Adjuvant preoperative radiotherapy in patients with rectal carcinoma. Adverse effects during long-term follow up of two randomized trials. Cancer 1996; 78:968–976.
431. Cohen AM, Minsky BD, Schilsky RL. Cancer of the rectum. In: deVita VT Jr, Hellman S, Rosenberg SA, eds. Cancer Principles and Practice of Oncology. Philadelphia: Lippincott-Raven, 1997:1197–1251.
432. Dahlberg M, Glimelius B, Graf W, Pahlman L. Preoperative irradiation affects functional results after surgery for rectal cancer: results from a randomized study. Dis Colon Rectum 1998; 41:543–549.
433. Goldberg P, Nicholls RJ, Porter N, et al. Long-term results of a randomised trial of short-course low-dose adjuvant preoperative radiotherapy for rectal cancer: reduction in local treatment failure. Eur J Cancer 1994; 30A:1602–1606.
434. Bannon JB, Marks GJ, Modiuddin M, et al. Radical and local excisional methods of sphincter-sparing surgery after high-dose radiation for cancer of the distal 3 cm of the rectum. Ann Surg Oncol 1995; 2:221–227.
435. Minsky BD, Cohen AM, Enker WE, et al. Sphincter preservation with preoperative radiation therapy and coloanal anastomosis. Int J Radiat Oncol Biol Phys 1995; 31:553–559.
436. Myerson RS, Michalski JM, King ML, et al. Adjuvant radiation therapy for rectal carcinoma: predictors of outcome. Int J Radiat Oncol Biol Phys 1995; 32: 41–50.
437. Izar F, Fourtanier G, Pradere B, et al. Preoperation radiotherapy as adjuvant treatment in rectal cancer. World J Surg 1992; 16:106–111.
438. Pacelli F, Di Giorgio A, Papa V, et al. Preoperative Radiotherapy Combined With Intraoperative Radiotherapy Improve Results of Total Mesorectal Excision in Patients with T_3 Rectal Cancer. Dis Colon Rectum 2004; 47: 170–179.
439. Colorectal Cancer Collaborative Group. Adjuvant radiotherapy for rectal cancer: asystematic overview of 8507 patients from 22 randomised trials. Lancet 2001; 358:1291–1304.
440. van de Velde CJH. Preoperative radiotherapy and TME-surgery for rectal cancer. Detailed analyses in relation to quality control in a randomized trial. Proc Am Soc Clin Oncol 2002; 21:127a (abstract 506).
441. Marijnen CA, Kapiteijn E, van de Velde CJ, et al. Acute side effects and complications after short-term preoperative radiotherapy combined with total mesorectal excision in primary rectal cancer: report of a multicenter randomized trial. J Clin Oncol 2002; 20:817–825.
442. Hartley A, Giridharan S, Gray L, et al. Retrospective study of acute toxicity following short-course preoperative radiotherapy. Br J Surg 2002; 89:889–895.
443. Camma C, Giunta M, Fiorica F et al. Preoperative radiotherapy for resectable rectal cancer: a metaanalysis. JAMA 2000; 284:1008–1015.
444. Graf W, Dahlberg M, Osman MM, et al. Short-term preoperative radiotherapy results in down-staging of rectal cancer: a study of 1316 patients. Radiother Oncol 1997; 43:133–137.
445. Marijnen CA, Nagtegaal ID, Klein Kranenbarg E, et al. No downstaging after short-term preoperative radiotherapy in rectal cancer patients. J Clin Oncol 2001; 19:1976–1984.
446. Francois Y, Nemoz CJ, Baulieux J, et al. Influence of the interval between preoperative radiation therapy and surgery on downstaging and on the rate of sphincter-sparing surgery for rectal cancer: The Lyon R90–01 randomized trial. J Clin Oncol 1999; 17:2396–2402.
447. Guillem JG, Chessin DB, Shia J, et al. Clinical examination following preoperative chemoradiation for rectal cancer is not a reliable surrogate end point. J Clin Oncol 2005; 23:3475–3479.
448. Stein DE, Mahmoud NN, Anne PR, et al. Longer time interval between completion of neoadjuvant chemoradiation and surgical resection does not improve downstaging of rectal carcinoma. Dis Colon Rectum 2003; 46: 448–453.
449. Marijnen CA, van de Velde CJ, Putter H, et al. Impact of short-term preoperative radiotherapy on health-related quality of life and sexual functioning in primary rectal cancer: report of a multicenter randomized trial. J Clin Oncol 2005; 23:1847–1858.
450. Mella O, Dahl O, Horn A, et al. Radiotherapy and resection for apparently inoperable rectal adenocarcinoma. Dis Colon Rectum 1984; 27:663–668.
451. Friedmann P, Garb JL, McCabe DP, et al. Intestinal anastomosis after preoperative radiotherapy for carcinoma of the rectum. Surg Gynecol Obstet 1987; 164:257–260.
452. Roberson SH, Heron HC, Kerman HD, et al. Is anterior resection of the rectosigmoid safe after preoperative radiation? Dis Colon Rectum 1985; 28: 254–259.
453. Higgins GA, Humphrey EW, Dweight RW. Preoperative radiation and surgery for cancer of the rectum: Veterans' Administration Surgical Oncology Group Trial II. Cancer 1986; 58:352–359.
454. Reis Neto JA, Guilici FA, Reis Neto JA Jr. A comparison of non-operative vs preoperative radiotherapy in rectal carcinoma. A 10-year randomized trial. Dis Colon Rectum 1989; 32:702–710.
455. Dahl O, Horn A, Morild I, et al. Low dose preoperative radiation postpones recurrences in operable rectal cancer. Results of a randomized multicenter trial in Western Norway. Cancer 1990; 66:2286–2294.
456. Marsh P, James R, Schofield P. Adjuvant preoperative radiotherapy for locally advanced rectal carcinoma. Dis Colon Rectum 1994; 37:1205–1214.
457. Gunderson LL, Sosin H. Areas of failure found at reoperation (second or symptomatic look) following "curative surgery" for adenocarcinoma of the rectum. Cancer 1974; 34:1278–1292.
458. Hoskins RB, Gunderson IX, Dosoretz DE, et al. Adjuvant postoperative radiation therapy in carcinoma of the rectum and rectosigmoid. Cancer 1985; 55:61–71.
459. GITSG. Prolongation of the disease-free interval in surgically treated rectal carcinoma. N Engl J Med 1985; 312:1465–1472.
460. Martijn H, de Neve W, Lybeert ML, et al. Adjuvant postoperative radiotherapy for adenocarcinoma of the rectum and rectosigmoid. A retrospective analysis of locoregional control, survival, and prognostic factors on 178 patients. Am J Clin Oncol 1995; 18:277–281.
461. De Neve W, Martijn H, Lybeert MM, et al. Incompletely resected rectum, rectosigmoid or sigmoid carcinoma: results of postoperative radiotherapy and prognostic factors. Int J Radiat Oncol Biol Phys 1991; 21:1297–1302.
462. Mak AC, Rich TA, Schultheiss JE, et al. Late complications of postoperative radiation therapy for cancer of the rectum and rectosigmoid. Int J Radiat Oncol Biol Phys 1994; 28:597–603.
463. Tang R, Wang J-Y, Chen JS, et al. Postoperative adjuvant radiotherapy in Astler-Coller Stage B2 and C rectal cancer. Dis Colon Rectum 1992; 35: 1057–1065.
464. Balsev I, Pedersen M, Teglbjaerg PS, et al. Postoperative radiotherapy in Dukes B and C carcinoma of the rectum and rectosigmoid. a randomized multicentre study. Cancer 1986; 58:22–28

465. Treurniet-Donker AD, van Putten WL, Wereldsma JC, et al. Postoperative radiation therapy for rectal cancer: An interim analysis of a prospective randomized multicentre trial in The Netherlands. Cancer 1991; 67:2042–2048.
466. Gates G. On the behalf of the MRC Rectal Cancer Working Party. Results of the MRC trial of postoperative radiotherapy for operable rectal cancer. UKCCR Meeting on Colorectal Cancer Oxford, U.K.: March 20, 1995.
467. Sause WT, Pajak JF, Noyes RD, et al. Evaluation of preoperative radiation therapy in operable colorectal cancer. Ann Surg 1994; 220:668–675.
468. Bayer I, Turani H, Lurie H, et al. The Sandwich approach: irradiation-surgery-irradiation in rectal cancer. Four years experience. Dis Colon Rectum 1988; 28:222–224.
469. Botti C, Cosimelli M, Impiombata FA, et al. Improved local control and survival with the "sandwich" technique of pelvic radiotherapy for resectable rectal cancer. A retrospective multivariate analysis. Dis Colon Rectum 1994; 37(suppl 2):S6–S15.
470. Tepper JE, Cohen AM, Wood WC, et al. Intraoperative electron beam radiotherapy in treatment of unresectable rectal cancer. Arch Surg 1986; 121: 421–423.
471. Sischy B. Intraoperative electron beam radiation therapy with particular reference to treatment of rectal carcinoma—primary and recurrent. Dis Colon Rectum 1986; 29:714–718.
472. Valentini V, de Santis M, Morganti AG, et al. Intraoperative radiation therapy (IORT) in rectal cancer: Methodology and indications. Rays 1995; 20:73–89.
473. Gunderson LL, Nelson H, Martenson JA, et al. Intraoperative electron and external beam irradiation with or without 5-fluorouracil and maximum surgical resection for previously unirradiated, locally recurrent colorectal cancer. Dis Colon Rectum 1996; 39:1379–1395.
474. Sadahiro S, Suzuki T, Ishikawa K, et al. Intraoperative radiation therapy for curatively resected rectal cancer. Dis Colon Rectum 2001; 44:1689–1695.
475. Fuchs JR, Bleday R. Massive iliac artery bleeding in patients receiving intraoperative radiation therapy for advanced rectal cancer: report of two cases. Dis Colon Rectum 2004; 47:383–386.
476. Wolmark N, Rockette H, Fisher B, et al. The benefit of leukovorin-modulated fluorouracil as postoperative adjuvant therapy for primary colon cancer: results from National Surgical Adjuvant Breast and Bowel Project Protocol C-03. J Clin Oncol 1993; 11:1879–1887.
477. O'Connell MJ, Martensen JA, Wieand HS, et al. Improving adjuvant therapy for rectal cancer by combining protracted infusion fluorouracil with radiation therapy after curative surgery. N Engl J Med 1994; 331:502–507.
478. Windle R, Bell PRF, Shaw D. Five year results of a randomized trial of adjuvant 5-fluorouracil and levamisole in colorectal cancer. Br J Surg 1987; 74:569–572.
479. Takahashi T, Mizusawa H, Kato T, et al. Preoperative irradiation and 5-fluorouracil suppository for carcinoma of the rectum. Am J Surg 1988; 156:58–62.
480. Sischy B, Graney MJ, Hinson J, et al. Preoperative radiation therapy with sensitizers in the management of carcinoma of the rectum. Dis Colon Rectum 1985; 28:56–57.
481. Wolmark N, Wieand HS, Hyams DM, et al. Randomized trial of postoperative adjuvant chemotherapy with or without radiotherapy for carcinoma of the rectum: National Surgical Adjuvant Breast and Bowel Project Protocol R-02. J Natl Cancer Inst 2000; 92:388–396.
482. Haller DG. Defining the optimal therapy for rectal cancer. JNCI 2000; 92: 361–362.
483. Theodoropoulos G, Wise WE, Padmanabhan A, et al. T-level downstaging and complete pathologic response after preoperative chemoradiation for advanced rectal cancer result in decreased recurrence and improved disease-free survival. Dis Colon Rectum 2002; 45:895–903.
484. Burmeister BH, Schache D, Burmeister EA, et al. Synchronous postoperative adjuvant chemoradiation therapy for locally advanced carcinoma of the rectum. Int J Colorectal Dis 2004; 19:55–59.
485. Tepper JE, O'Connell M, Niedzwiecki D, et al. Adjuvant therapy in rectal cancer:analysis of stage, sex and local control-final report of intergroup 0114. J Clin Oncol 2002; 20:1744–1750.
486. Boulis-Wassis, Ferard A, Loygue J, et al. Final results of a randomized trial on the treatment of rectal cancer with preoperative radiotherapy alone or in combination with 5-fluorouracil followed by radical surgery; Trial of the European Organization for Research and Treatment of Cancer. Gastrointestinal Tract Cancer Cooperative Group. Cancer 1984; 53:1811–1818.
487. Meade PG, Blatchford GJ, Thorson AG, et al. Preoperative chemoradiation downstages locally advanced ultrasound-staged rectal cancer. Am J Surg 1995; 170:609–613.
488. Chari RS, Tyler DS, Anscher MS, et al. Preoperative radiation and chemotherapy in the treatment of adenocarcinoma of the rectum. Ann Surg 1995; 221:778–787.
489. Stryker SJ, Kiel KD, Rodemaker A, et al. Preoperative "chemoradiation" for stages II and III rectal carcinoma. Arch Surg 1996; 231:514–519.
490. Kollmorgan CF, Meagher AP, Wolff BG, et al. The long-term effect of adjuvant postoperative chemoradiotherapy for rectal carcinoma on bowel function. Ann Surg 1994; 220:676–682.
491. Picciocchi A, Coco C, Magistrelli P, et al. Combined modality therapy of resectable high risk rectal cancer. Rays 1995; 20:182–189.
492. Enker WE. The elusive goal of preoperative staging in rectal cancer. Ann Surg Oncol 2004; 11:245–246.
493. Garcia-Aguilar J, Hernandez de Anda E, Sirivongs P, Lee SH, Madoff RD, Rothenberger DA. A pathologic complete response to preoperative chemoradiation is associated with lower local recurrence and improved survival in rectal cancer patients treated by mesorectal excision. Dis Colon Rectum 2003; 46:298–304.
494. Ruo L, Tickoo S, Klimstra DS, et al. Long-term prognostic significance of extent of rectal cancer response to preoperative radiation and chemotherapy. Ann Surg 2002; 236:75–81.
495. Stipa F, Zernecke A, Moore HG, et al. Residual mesorectal lymph node involvement following neoadjuvant combined-modality therapy: rationale for radical resection? Ann Surg Oncol 2004; 11:187–191.
496. Rullier E, Goffre B, Bonnel C, Zerbib F, Caudry M, Saric J. Preoperative radiochemotherapy and sphincter-saving resection for T3 carcinomas of the lower third of the rectum. Ann Surg 2001; 234:633–640.
497. Read TE, Ogunbiyi OA, Fleshman JW, et al. Neoadjuvant external beam radiation and proctectomy for adenocarcinoma of the rectum. Dis Colon Rectum 2001; 44:1778–1790.
498. Volter V, Stupp R, Matter M, et al. Preoperative hyperfractionated accelerated radiotherapy (HART) and concomitant CPT-11 in rectal carcinoma. A phase I/II study. Proc Am Soc Clin Oncol 2001; 20:126b (abstr 2254).
499. Chau I, Chan S, Cunningham D. Overview of preoperative and postoperative therapy for colorectal cancer: the European and United States perspectives. Clin Colorectal Cancer 2003; 3:19–33.
500. Luna-Perez P, Rodriguez-Ramirez S, Hernandez-Pacheco F, Gutierrez De La Barrera M, Fernandez R, Labastida S. Anal sphincter preservation in locally advanced low rectal adenocarcinoma after preoperative chemoradiation therapy and coloanal anastomosis. J Surg Oncol 2003; 82:3–9.
501. Bedrosian I, Rodriguez-Bigas MA, Feig B, et al. Predicting the node-negative mesorectum after preoperative chemoradiation for locally advanced rectal carcinoma. J Gastrointest Surg 2004; 8:56–63.
502. Enker WE. The elusive goal of preoperative staging in rectal cancer. Ann Surg Oncol 2004; 11:245–246.
503. Onaitis MW, Noone RB, Fields R, et al. Complete response to neoadjuvant chemoradiation for rectal cancer does not influence survival. Ann Surg Oncol 2001; 8:801–806.
504. Hofheinz RD, von Gerstenberg-Helldorf B, Wenz F, et al. Phase I trial of capecitabine and weekly irinotecan in combination with radiotherapy for neoadjuvant therapy of rectal cancer. J Clin Oncol 2005; 23:1350–1357.
505. Chessin DB, Enker W, Cohen AM, et al. Complications after preoperative combined modality therapy and radical resection of locally advanced rectal cancer: a 14-year experience from a specialty service. J Am Coll Surg 2005; 200:876–882.
506. Habr-Gama A, Perez RQ, Nadalin W, et al. Long-term results of preoperative chemoradiation for distal rectal cancer correlation between final stage and survival. J Gastrointest Surg 2005; 9:90–99.
507. Moore HG, Gittleman AE, Minsky BD, et al. Rate of pathologic complete response with increased interval between preoperative combined modality therapy and rectal cancer resection. Dis Colon Rectum 2004; 47:279–286.
508. Sauer R. Adjuvant versus neoadjuvant combined modality treatment for locally advanced rectal cancer: first results of the German rectal cancer study (CAO/ARO/AIO-91). Int J Radiat Oncol Biol Phys 2003; 57(suppl 2):S124–S125.
509. Sauer R, Becker H, Hohenberger W, et al. Preoperative versus postoperative chemoradiotherapy for rectal cancer. N Eng J Med 2004; 351:1731–1740.
510. Ravasco R Monteiro-Grillo T. Vidal PM, Camilo ME. Dietary counseling improves patient outcomes: a prospective, randomized, controlled trial in colorectal cancer patients undergoing radiotherapy. J Clin Oncol 2005; 23: 1431–1438.
511. Gastrointestinal Tumor Study Group. Radiation therapy with fluorouracil with or without semustine for the treatment of patients with surgical adjuvant adenocarcinoma of the rectum. J Clin Oncol 1992; 10:549–557.
512. Tviet KM, Guldvog I, Hagen S, et al. Randomized controlled trial of postoperative radiotherapy and short-term time-scheduled 5-fluorouracil against surgery alone in the treatment of Dukes B and C rectal cancer. Norwegian Adjuvant Rectal Cancer Project Group. Br J Surg 1997; 84:1130–1135.
513. Holmes EC, Eilber FR, Morton DL. Immunotherapy of malignancy in humans. Current status. JAMA 1975; 232:1052–1055.
514. MacDonald JS. The immunobiology of colorectal cancer. Semin Oncol 1976; 2:421–431.
515. Martin DS. The necessity for combined modalities in cancer therapy. Hosp Pract 1973:129–136.
516. Reed RC, Gutterman JW, Mavligit GM, et al. Phase I trial of intravenous (IV) and subcutaneous (SC) *Corynebacterium parvum* (Cp). Am J Clin Oncol 1975; 16:228.
517. Mavligit GM, Gutterman JV, Burgess MA, et al. Adjuvant immunotherapy and chemo immunotherapy in colorectal cancer of the Dukes' C classification: preliminary clinical results. Cancer 1975; 36(suppl):2421–2427.
518. Ooi B, Tjandra JJ, Green MD. Morbidities of adjuvant chemotherapy and radiotherapy for resectable rectal cancer. Dis Colon Rectum 1999; 42:403–418.

519. Kent TS, Miller A, Bennett A, Weber T. Decision analysis for adjuvant therapy of rectal cancer. J Am Coll Surg 2003; 197:571.
520. Sagar PM, Pemberton JH. Surgical management of locally recurrent rectal cancer. Br J Surg 1996; 83:293–304.
521. Fick ThE, Baeten CGMI, von Meyenfeldt MF, et al. Recurrence and survival after abdominoperineal and low anterior resection for rectal cancer without adjuvant therapy. Eur J Surg Oncol 1990; 16:105–108.
522. Schiessel R, Wunderlich M, Herbst F. Local recurrence of colorectal cancer: effect of early detection and aggressive surgery. Br J Surg 1986; 73:342–344.
523. Castro-Sousa F, Leite JS, Alves FC, et al. Results of sphincter saving resection in rectal carcinoma: morbidity and local recurrence. Br J Surg 1995; 82(suppl 1):1.
524. Rullier E, Laurent C, Carles J, et al. Sphincter saving resection and local recurrence in the treatment of low rectal cancer stage B and C. Br J Surg 1995; 82(suppl 1):3–4.
525. Pilipshen S. Cancer of the rectum: local recurrence. In: Fazio VW, ed. Current Therapy in Colon and Rectal Surgery. Toronto: Brian C. Decker, 1990:137–149.
526. Heald RJ. Rectal cancer: anterior resection and local recurrence—a personal review. Perspect Colon Rectal Surg 1988; 1:1–26.
527. Pihl E, Hughes ESR, McDermott FT, et al. Recurrence of carcinoma of the colon and rectum at the anastomotic suture line. Surg Gynecol Obstet 1981; 153:495–496.
528. Feil W, Wunderlich M, Kovatz E, et al. Rectal cancer: factors influencing the development of local recurrence after radical anterior resection. Int J Colorectal Dis 1988; 3:195–200.
529. Twomey P, Burchell M, Strawn D, et al. Local control in rectal cancer. A clinical review and meta-analysis. Arch Surg 1989; 124:1174–1179.
530. Welch JP, Donaldson GA. Detection and treatment of recurrent cancer of the colon and rectum. Am J Surg 1978; 135:505–511.
531. Pilipshen SJ, Heilweil M, Quan SHQ, et al. Patterns of pelvic recurrence following definitive resection of rectal cancer. Cancer 1984; 53:1354–1362.
532. Luna-Perez P, Delgado S, Labastida S, et al. Patterns of recurrence following pelvic exenteration and external radiotherapy for locally advanced primary adenocarcinoma. Ann Surg Oncol 1996; 3:526–533.
533. Butch RJ, Wittenberg J, Mueller PR, et al. Presacral masses after abdominoperineal resection for colorectal carcinoma. The need for needle biopsy. AJR 1985; 144:309–312.
534. Ramirez JM, Mortensen NJ McC, Takeuchi N, et al. Endoluminal ultrasonography in the follow up of patients with rectal cancer. Br J Surg 1994; 81:692–694.
535. Lohnert MS, Doniec JM, Henne-Bruns D. Effective of endoluminal sonography in the identification of occult local rectal cancer recurrences. Dis Colon Rectum 2000; 43:483–491.
536. Cohen AM, Martin EW Jr, Lavery I. Radioimmunoguided surgery using iodine 125 B72.3 in patients with colorectal cancer. Arch Surg 1991; 126: 349–352.
537. Moore HG, Akhurst T, Larson SM, Minsky BD, Mazumdar M, Guillem JG. A case-controlled study of 18-fluorodeoxyglucose positron emission tomography in the detection of pelvic recurrence in previously irradiated rectal cancer patients. J Am Coll Surg 2003; 197:22–28.
538. Yamada K, Ishizawa T, Niwa K, Chumarn Y, Akiba T. Patterns of pelvic invasion are prognostic in the treatment of locally recurrent rectal cancer. Br J Surg 2001; 88:988–993.
539. Herefarth C, Schlag P, Hohenberger P. Surgical strategies in locoregional recurrences of gastrointestinal carcinoma. World J Surg 1987; 11:504–510.
540. Segall MM, Goldberg SM, Nivatvongs S, et al. Abdominoperineal resection for recurrent cancer following low anterior resection. Dis Colon Rectum 1981; 24:80–84.
541. Suzuki K, Dozois RR, Devine RM, et al. Curative reoperations for locally recurrent rectal cancer. Dis Colon Rectum 1996; 39:730–736.
542. Wiggers T, de Vries MR, Veeze-Kuypers B. Surgery for local recurrence of rectal carcinoma. Dis Colon Rectum 1996; 39:323–328.
543. Saito N, Koda K, Takiguchi N, et al. Surgery for local pelvic recurrence after resection of rectal cancer. Int J Colorectal Dis 1998; 13:32–38.
544. Huguier M, Houry S, Barrier A. Local recurrence of cancer of the rectum. Am J Surg 2001; 182:437–439.
545. Boyle KM, Sagar PM, Chalmers AG, Sebag-Montefiore D, Cairns A, Eardley I. Surgery for locally recurrent rectal cancer. Dis Colon Rectum 2005; 48:929–937.
546. Vermaas M, Ferenschild FT, Nuyttens JJ, et al. Preoperative radiotherapy improves outcome in recurrent rectal cancer. Dis Colon Rectum 2005; 48: 918–928.
547. Garcia-Aguilar J, Cromwell JW, Marra C, Lee SH, Madoff RD, Rothenberger DA. Treatment of locally recurrent rectal cancer. Dis Colon Rectum 2001; 44:1743–1748.
548. Hahnloser D, Nelson H, Giinderson LL, et al. Curative potential of multimodality therapy for locally recurrent rectal cancer. Ann Surg 2003; 237:502–508.
549. Lopez-Kostner F, Fazio VW, Vignali A, Rybicki LA, Lavery IC. Locally recurrent rectal cancer: predictors and success of salvage surgery. Dis Colon Rectum 2001; 44:173–178.
550. Mannaerts GH, Rutten HJ, Martijn H, Hanssens PE, Wiggers T. Comparison of intraoperative radiation therapy-containing multimodality treatment with historical treatment modalities for locally recurrent rectal cancer. Dis Colon Rectum 2001; 44:1749–1758.
551. Lopez MJ, Kraybill WG, Downey RS, et al. Exenterative Surgery for locally advanced rectosigmoid cancers. Is it worthwhile? Surgery 1987; 102:644–651.
552. Falk RE, Moffat FL, Makowka L, et al. Pelvic exenteration for advanced primary and recurrent adenocarcinoma. Can J Surg 1985; 28:539–541.
553. Temple WJ, Ketcham AS. Sacral resection for control of pelvic tumors. Am J Surg 1992; 163:370–374.
554. Pearlman NW, Steigmann GV, Donohue RE. Extended resection of fixed rectal cancer. Cancer 1989; 63:2438–2441.
555. Wanebo HJ, Koness RJ, Vezeridis MP, et al. Pelvic resection of recurrent rectal cancer. Ann Surg 1994; 220:586–597.
556. Temple WJ, Ketcham AS. Surgical palliation for recurrent rectal cancers ulcerating in the perineum. Cancer 1990; 65:1111–1114.
557. Tepper JE, O'Connell M, Hollis D, Niedzwiecki D, Cooke E, Mayer RJ. Intergroup Study 0114. Analysis of surgical salvage after failure of primary therapy in rectal results from Intergroup Study 0114. J Clin Oncol 2003; 21:3623–3628.
558. Jimenez RE, Shoup M, Cohen AM, Paty PB, Guillem J, Wong WD. Contemporary outcomes of total pelvic exenteration in the treatment of colorectal cancer. Dis Colon Rectum 2003; 46:1619–1625.
559. Ike H, Shimada H, Ohki S, Yamaguchi S, Ichikawa Y, Fujii S. Outcome of total pelvic exenteration for locally recurrent rectal cancer. Hepatogastroenterology 2003; 50:700–703.
560. Bakx R, van Lanschot JJ, Zoetmulder FA. Sacral resection in cancer surgery: surgical technique and experience in 26 procedures. J Am Coll Surg 2004; 198:846–851.
561. Mannaerts GH, Rutten HJ, Martijn H, Groen GJ, Hanssens PE, Wiggers T. Abdominosacral resection for primary irresectable and locally recurrent rectal cancer. Dis Colon Rectum 2001; 44:806–814.
562. Moriya Y, Akasu T, Fujita S, Yamamoto S. Total pelvic exenteration with distal sacretomy for fixed recurrent rectal cancer in the pelvis. Dis Colon Rectum 2004; 47:2047–2053.
563. Shirouzu K, Isomoto H, Kakegawa T. Total pelvic exenteration for locally advanced colorectal carcinoma. Br J Surg 1996; 83:32–35.
564. Yeung RS, Moffat FL, Falk RE. Pelvic exenteration for recurrent colorectal carcinoma: a review. Cancer Invest 1994; 12:176–188.
565. Rodriguez-Bigas MA, Petrelli NJ. Pelvic exenteration and its modifications. Am J Surg 1996; 171:293–301.
566. Kakuda JT, Lamont JP, Chu DZ, Paz IB. The role of pelvic exenteration in the management of recurrent rectal cancer. Am J Surg 2003; 186:660–664.
567. Miner TJ, Jaques DP, Paty PB, Guillem JG, Wong WD. Symptom control in patients with locally recurrent rectal cancer. Ann Surg Oncol 2003; 10:72–79.
568. Shoup M, Guiliem JG, Alektiar KM, et al. Predictors of survival in recurrent rectal cancer after resection and intraoperative radiotherapy. Dis Colon Rectum 2002; 45:585–592.
569. Kuehne J, Kleisli T, Biernacki P, et al. Use of high-dose-rate brachytherapy in the management of locally recurrent rectal cancer. Dis Colon Rectum 2003; 46:895–899.
570. Cheng C, Rodnguez-Bigas MA, Petrelli N. Is there a role for curative surgery for pelvic recurrence from rectal carcinoma in the presence of hydronephrosis? Am J Surg 2003; 182:274–277.
571. Kelly SR, Nugent KP. Formalin instillation for control of rectal hemorrhage in advanced pelvic malignancy: report of two cases. Dis Colon Rectum 2002; 45:121–122.
572. Magrini S, Nelson H, Gunderson LL, et al. Sacropelvic resection and intraoperative electron irradiation in the management of recurrent anorectal cancer. Dis Colon Rectum 1996; 39:1–9.
573. Rodriguez-Bigas MA, Herrera L, Petrelli NJ. Surgery for recurrent rectal adenocarcinoma in the presence of hydronephrosis. Am J Surg 1992; 164:18–21.
574. Loessin SJ, Moland NB, Devine RM, et al. Management of sacral and perineal defects following abdominoperineal resection and reduction with transpelvic muscle flaps. Dis Colon Rectum 1995; 38:940–945.
575. McAllister E, Wells K, Chaet M, et al. Perineal reconstruction after surgical extirpation of pelvic malignancies using the trans-pelvic transverse rectus abdominal myocutaneous flap. Ann Surg Oncol 1994; 1:164–168.
576. Yeh KA, Hoffman JP, Kusiak JE, et al. Reconstruction with myocutaneous flaps following resection of locally recurrent rectal cancer. Am Surg 1995; 61:581–589.
577. Jain AK, De Franzo AJ, Marks MW, et al. Reconstruction of pelvic exenterative wounds with transpelvic rectus abdominis flaps: a case series. Ann Plast Surg 1997; 38:115–123.
578. Chessin DB. Hartley J, Cohen AM, et al. Rectus flap reconstruction decreases perineal wound complications after pelvic chemoradiation and surgery: a cohort study. Ann Surg Oncol 2005; 12:104–110.
579. Butler CE, Rodriguez-Bjgas MA. Pelvic reconstruction after abdominoperineal resection: is it worthwhile? Ann Surg Oncol 2005; 12:91–94.
580. Christiansen J, Kirkegaard P. Treatment of recurrent rectal cancer by electroresection/coagulation after low anterior resection. Dis Colon Rectum 1983; 12:41–44.
581. Salvati EP, Rubin RJ. Electrocoagulation as primary therapy for rectal carcinoma. Am J Surg 1976; 132:583–586.
582. Kurz KR, Pitts WR, Speer D, et al. Palliation of carcinoma of the rectum and pararectum using the urologic resectoscope. Surg Gynecol Obstet 1988; 166:60–62.

583. Fritsch A, Seidl W, Walzel C, et al. Palliative and adjunctive measures in rectal cancer. World J Surg 1982; 6:569–577.
584. Villalon AH, Green D. The use of radiotherapy for pelvic recurrence following abdominoperineal resection for carcinoma of the rectum. A ten year experience. Aust N Z J Surg 1981; 51:149–151.
585. Pacini P, Cionini L, Pirtoli L, et al. Symptomatic recurrences of carcinoma of the rectum and sigmoid. The influence of radiotherapy on the quality of life. Dis Colon Rectum 1986; 29:865–868.
586. Dobrowsky W, Schmid AP. Radiotherapy of presacral recurrence following radical surgery for rectal carcinoma. Dis Colon Rectum 1985; 28:917–919.
587. Patt YZ, Peters RE, Chuang VP, et al. Palliation of pelvic recurrence of colorectal cancer with intra-arterial 5-fluorouracil and mitomycin. Cancer 1985; 56:2175–2180.
588. Estes NG, Morphis JG, Hornback NB, et al. Intraarterial chemotherapy and hyperthermia for pain control in patients with recurrent rectal cancer. Am J Surg 1986; 152:597–601.
589. Machover D, Timus M, Schwartenberg L, et al. Treatment of advanced colorectal and gastric adenocarcinoma with 5-fluorouracil combined with high dose leucovorin. An update. In: Bruckner HW, Rustum YM, eds. Advances in Cancer Chemotherapy. The Current Status of 5-Fluorouracil, Leucovorin, Calcium Combination. New York: Park Row Publishers, 1984:55–64.
590. Nishimura Y, Hiraoka M, Akuta K, et al. Hyperthermia combined with radiation therapy for primarily unresectable and recurrent colorectal cancer. Int J Radiat Oncol Biol Phys 1992; 23:759–768.
591. Ichikawa D, Yamaguchi T, Yoshioka Y, et al. Prognostic evaluation of preoperative combined treatment for advanced cancer in the lower rectum with radiation, intraluminal hyperthermia, and 5-Fluorouracil suppository. Am J Surg 1996; 171:346–350.
592. Gonzales DG, van Dijk JDP, Blank LECM. Radiotherapy and hyperthermia. Eur J Cancer 1995; 31A:1351–1355.
593. Korenga D, Matsushima T, Adachi Y, et al. Preoperative hyperthermia combined with chemotherapy and radiotherapy for patients with rectal carcinoma may prevent early local pelvic recurrence. Int J Colorectal Dis 1992; 7:206–209.
594. Gagliardi G, Hawley PR, Hershman MJ, et al. Prognostic factors in surgery for local recurrence of rectal cancer. Br J Surg 1995; 82:1401–1405.
595. Williams LF, Huddleston CB, Sawyers JL, et al. Is total pelvic exenteration reasonable primary treatment for rectal carcinoma. Ann Surg 1988; 207:670–678.
596. Creutzfeldt W. Carcinoid tumors: Development of our knowledge. World J Surg 1996; 20:126–131.
597. Burke M, Shepherd N, Mann CV. Carcinoid tumors of the rectum and anus. Br J Surg 1987; 74:358–361.
598. Pronay G, Nagy G, Vjszaszy L, et al. Carcinoid tumors of the rectum. Ann Gastroenterol Hepatol 1982; 18:313–315.
599. Matsui K, Iwase T, Kitagawa M. Small, polypoid-appearing carcinoid tumors of the rectum: clinicopathologic study of 16 cases and effectiveness of endoscopic treatment. Am J Gastroenterol 1993; 88:1949–1953.
600. Jetmore AB, Ray JE, Gathright JB, et al. Rectal carcinoids: The most frequent carcinoid tumors. Dis Colon Rectum 1992; 35:717–725.
601. Fitzgerald SD, Meagher AP, Moniz-Pereira P, et al. Carcinoid tumor of the rectum. DNA ploidy is not a prognostic factor. Dis Colon Rectum 1996; 39:643–648.
602. Godwin JD II. Carcinoid tumors. An analysis of 2837 cases. Cancer 1975; 36:560–569.
603. Sauven P, Ridge JA, Quan SH, et al. Anorectal carcinoid tumors. Is aggressive surgery warranted? Ann Surg 1990; 21:67–71.
604. Yoshikane H, Tsukamoto Y, Niwa Y, et al. Carcinoid tumors of the gastrointestinal tract: evaluation with endoscopic ultrasonography. Gastrointest Endosc 1993; 39:375–383.
605. Kobayashi K, Katsumata T, Yoshizawa S, et al. Indications of endoscopic polypectomy for rectal carcinoid tumors and clinical usefulness of endoscopic ultrasonography. Dis Colon Rectum 2005; 48:285–291.
606. Shirouzu K, Isomoto H, Kakegawa T, et al. Treatment of rectal carcinoid tumors. Am J Surg 1990; 160:262–265.
607. Gerstle JT, Kaufman GL, Koltun WA. The incidence, management, and outcome of patients with gastrointestinal carcinoids and secondary primary malignancies. I Am Coll Surg 1995; 180:427–432.
608. Spread C, Berkel H, Jewell L, et al. Colonic carcinoid tumors. A population-based study. Dis Colon Rectum 1994 37:482–491.
609. Nauneim KS, Zeitels J, Kaplan EL, et al. Rectal carcinoid tumors—Treatment and prognosis. Surgery 1983; 94:670–676.
610. Stinner B, Kisker O, Zielke A, et al. Surgical management for carcinoid tumors of small bowel, appendix, colon and rectum. World J Surg 1996; 20: 183–188.
611. Tsioulias G, Muto T, Kubota Y, et al. DNA ploidy pattern in rectal carcinoids. Dis Colon Rectum 1991; 34:31–36.
612. Bruneton JN, Thyss A, Bourry J, et al. Colonic and rectal lymphomas. A report of six cases and review of the literature. Fortschr Röntgenstr 1983; 138:283–287.
613. Lee MH, Waxman M, Gillooley JF. Primary malignant lymphoma of the anorectum in homosexual men. Dis Colon Rectum 1986; 29:413–416.
614. Onhi SK, Keane PF, Sackier JM, et al. Primary rectal lymphoma and malignant lymphomatous polyposis. Two cases illustrating current methods in diagnosis and management. Dis Colon Rectum 1989; 32:1071–1074.
615. Devine RM, Beart RW Jr, Wolff BG. Malignant lymphoma of the rectum. Dis Colon Rectum 1986; 29:821–824.
616. Jinnai D, Iwasa Z, Watanuko T. Malignant lymphoma of the large intestine—Operative results in Japan. Jpn J Surg 1983; 13:331–336.
617. Vieta JO, Delgado GE. Chronic ulcerative colitis complicated by—colonic lymphoma: report of a case. Dis Colon Rectum 1976; 19:56–62.
618. Perry PM, Cross RM, Morson BC. Primary malignant lymphoma of the rectum (22 cases). Proc R Soc Med 1972; 65:72.
619. Shepherd NA, Hall PA, Coates PJ, et al. Primary malignant lymphoma of the colon and rectum: a histopathological and immunohistochemical analysis of 45 cases with clinicopathologi-cal correlations. Histopathology 1988; 12:235–252.
620. Hague S, Dean PJ. Stromal neoplasms of the rectum and anal canal. Hum Pathol 1992; 23:762–767.
621. Khalifa AA, Bong WL, Rao VK, et al. Leiomyosarcoma of the rectum. Report of a case and review of the literature. Dis Colon Rectum 1986; 29:427–432.
622. Moore DO, Hilbun BM. Leiomyosarcoma of the rectum. A case report and review of the literature. Contemp Surg 1986; 29:132–137.
623. Feldtman RW, Oram-Smith JC, Teers RJ, et al. Leiomyosarcoma of the rectum: the military experience. Dis Colon Rectum 1981; 24:402–403.
624. Labow SB, Hoexter B. Leiomyosarcoma of the rectum: Radical vs conservative therapy and report of three cases. Dis Colon Rectum 1977; 20:603–605.
625. Akawri OE, Dozois RR, Weiland LH, et al. Leiomyosarcoma of the small and large bowel. Cancer 1978; 42:1375–1384.
626. Kessler KJ, Kerlakian GM, Welling RE. Perineal and perirectal sarcomas. Report of two cases. Dis Colon Rectum 1996; 39:468–472.
627. Randleman CD, Wolff BG, Dozois RR, et al. Leiomyosarcoma of the rectum and anus. Int J Colorectal Dis 1989; 4:91–96.
628. Yeh CY, Chen HH, Tang R, Tasi WS, Lin PY, Wang JY. Surgical outcome after curative resection of rectal leiomyosarcoma. Dis Colon Rectum 2000; 43: 1517–1521.
629. Changchien CR, Wu MC, Tasi WS, et al. Evaluation of prognosis for malignant rectal gastrointestinal stromal tumor by clinical parameters and immunohistochemical staining. Dis Colon Rectum 2004; 47:1922–1929.
630. Lo SS, Papachristou GL, Finkelstein SD, Conroy WP, Schraut WE, Ramanathan RK. Neoadjuvant imatinib in gastrointestinal stromal tumor of the rectum: report of a case. Dis Colon Rectum 2005; 48:1316–1319.
631. Lasser A. Adenocarcinoma of the prostate involving the rectum. Dis Colon Rectum 1978; 21:23–25.
632. Cervi G, Vettoretto N, Vinco A, et al. Rectal localization of metastatic lobular breast cancer: report of a case. Dis Colon Rectum 2001; 44:453–455.
633. Christodoulopoulos JB, Papaionnou AN, Drakopoulou EP, et al. Carcinoma of the cervix presenting with rectal symptomatology: Report of three cases. Dis Colon Rectum 1972; 15:373–376.
634. Rosito MA, Damin DC, Lazzaron AR, et al. Metastatic renal cell carcinoma involving the rectum. Int J Colorectal Dis 2002; 17:359–361.
635. Okano A, TakaKuwa H, Nishi A. Granular cell tumor of the rectum Gastrointest. Endosc 2001; 54:624.
636. Nakachi A, Miyazato H, Oshiro T, Shimoji H, Shiraishi M, Muto Y. Granular cell tumor of the rectum: a case report and review of the literature. J Gastroenterol 2000; 35:631–634.
637. Takao Y, Shimamoto C, Hazama K, et al. Primary rectal teratoma: EUS features and review of the literature. Gastrointest Endosc 2000; 51:353–355.
638. Hazzan D, Reissmann P, Halak M, Resnick MB, Lotem M, Shiloni E. Primary rectal malignant melanoma: report of two cases. Tech Coloproctol 2001; 5:51–54.

25 Large Bowel Carcinoma: Screening, Surveillance, and Follow-Up

Santhat Nivatvongs

DETECTION OF EARLY COLORECTAL CARCINOMA

Data in 2005 showed that there were 145,290 estimated new cases of colon and rectal carcinomas in the United States, and of these, 40,340 (28%) were carcinomas of the rectum. Of this 56,290 (combined colon and rectum) will die, a death rate of 39%. In the United States, between 1991 and 2001, the death rate from carcinoma of colon and rectum has improved by 5% in men, and 4% in women (1).

Survival for colon and rectal carcinoma is closely related to the clinical and pathologic stage of the disease at diagnosis. Data from the German Multicenter Study in colorectal carcinoma showed five-year survival rates in stages I, II, III, and IV as 76%, 65%, 42%, and 16%, respectively (surgical mortality not excluded) (2).

A good starting point for an analysis of the pattern of colorectal carcinoma can be seen in data from the National Cancer Data Base (NCDB) (3) (Table 1). It shows the stages at diagnosis in different age groups and ethnicity. These data show the better stage in patients over 70 years for both carcinoma of colon and rectum. Ethnicity is another significant factor. African-Americans are less likely to present with stage I or II than are non-Hispanic whites. Hispanics are also slightly less likely to be diagnosed with stage I or II colorectal carcinoma than non-Hispanic whites. However, Asians have a pattern of stage and diagnosis similar to that of non-Hispanic whites (data not shown), and the sample of native Americans is too small to draw any conclusion about the stage at presentation. The data from NCDB suggest that age and ethnicity are important factors to consider in the diagnosis of colorectal carcinoma (3).

It has become clear that if the disease can be detected at an early stage, the overall prognosis can be improved, with another benefit that some colorectal carcinomas can even be prevented. Most colorectal carcinomas are asymptomatic until a late stage, when some partial obstruction occurs, causing abdominal pain or change in bowel habits. Although carcinoma of the colon and rectum bleeds occasionally and unpredictably, it may be possible to diagnose it in an early stage by examining for occult blood in the stool. Through many observations and studies, including current knowledge of molecular genetics of colorectal carcinoma, the natural history of colorectal carcinoma starts with one crypt. The numerous mutations of genes slowly give rise to a small polyp and then progresses to an invasive carcinoma that eventually metastasizes. The National Polyp Study (NPS) showed that it takes about 10 years for the development of an invasive carcinoma from a "clean" colon (4). This lengthy, stepwise natural history provides a window of opportunity for detecting early carcinoma and

TABLE 1 ■ Distribution of Adenocarcinoma of the Colon and Rectum by American Joint Commitee on Cancer (AJCC) Stage, Age at Diagnosis, and Ethnicity of Patients Diagnosed in 1993 at Hospitals Participating in the National Cancer Data Base

Category and Site	Distribution by Stage (%)				No. of Cases
	I–II	III	IV	Total (%)	
Age					
Colon					
< 50	44	27	29	100	2503
50–59	47	27	26	100	4130
60–69	53	26	21	100	9112
70–79	57	25	19	100	12,871
≥80	59	25	16	100	8661
Subtotal					37,277
Rectum					
< 50	50	33	17	100	1338
50–59	53	30	17	100	2406
60–69	58	27	15	100	4273
70–79	59	26	15	100	4579
≥80	62	22	16	100	2238
Subtotal					14,834
Ethnicity					
Colon					
Non-Hispanic white	55	25	20	100	32,463
Hispanic	51	29	20	100	680
African-American	48	27	25	100	3087
Subtotal					36,230
Rectum					
Non-Hispanic white	58	27	15	100	11,731
Hispanic	53	27	20	100	372
African-American	54	25	21	100	950
Subtotal					13,053

Source: From Ref. 3.

removing malignant polyps (Fig. 1). Thus screening strategy can be directed toward detecting early carcinoma to reduce morbidity and mortality as well as removing premalignant polyps to reduce the incidence of colorectal carcinoma.

EARLY DIAGNOSIS OF COLORECTAL CARCINOMA

Colorectal carcinoma fulfills all the criteria for justified screening. First, it is common and serious: it is the second leading cause of death from carcinoma in the United States, affecting men and women equally. Treatment of patients with advanced colorectal carcinoma is largely unsuccessful. In 2005 the overall survival rate was 61% (1). Second, various screening tests have been shown to achieve accurate detection of early-stage colorectal carcinomas (5–9). Third, evidence from controlled trials and case-control studies suggests varying degrees of persuasiveness that removing adenomatous polyps reduces the incidence of colorectal carcinoma and detecting early-stage carcinomas reduces mortality from the disease. Finally, screening benefits outweigh its harms. The various ways of screening for colorectal carcinoma all have cost-effectiveness ratios comparable to those of other generally accepted screening tests (10).

WHAT IS SCREENING?

Screening identifies individuals who are more likely to have colorectal carcinoma or adenomatous polyps from among those without signs or symptoms of disease (10). It is the use of simple, affordable, and acceptable tests to identify a subgroup of the at-risk population more likely to have a clinically significant lesion or abnormality (11). Screening, which refers primarily to a population approach, has been used interchangeably with early detection. Case finding refers to early detection on an individual basis. These terms refer to the identification of individuals with an increased probability of having colorectal neoplasia (4). The goal of screening for colorectal carcinoma is to reduce mortality from the disease.

It is important to note that once the screening results are positive, a complete investigation of the entire colon and rectum is mandated, preferably by CT colonography, total colonoscopy, or with flexible sigmoidoscopy and barium enema, to identify colorectal polyps or carcinomas.

Screening should be accompanied by efforts to optimize the participation of patients and healthcare providers, and to remind patients and providers about the need for rescreening at recommended intervals (12).

WHO SHOULD BE SCREENED?

Most people in the United States are not currently screened for colorectal carcinoma. Seeff et al. (13) analyzed data from the National Health Interview Survey which demonstrated that less than half of the U.S. population age ≥50 years reported undergoing hemoccult occult blood test (FOBT) and endoscopy (sigmoidoscopy, colonoscopy, or proctoscopy) within recommended time intervals. A lack of awareness by the respondent of the need for the test and a lack of recommendation by the physician for the test to be performed were found to be the most commonly reported barriers to undergoing the test. Lack of physician recommendation clearly was an important barrier; among persons who reported undergoing no colorectal carcinoma testing or none recently, only 5% reported that a physician had recommended colorectal carcinoma testing.

Approximately 75% of all new cases of colorectal carcinoma occur in people with no known predisposing factors for the disease. Incidence increases with age, beginning around 40 years (14). People with no predisposing factors are considered to be at average risk for colorectal

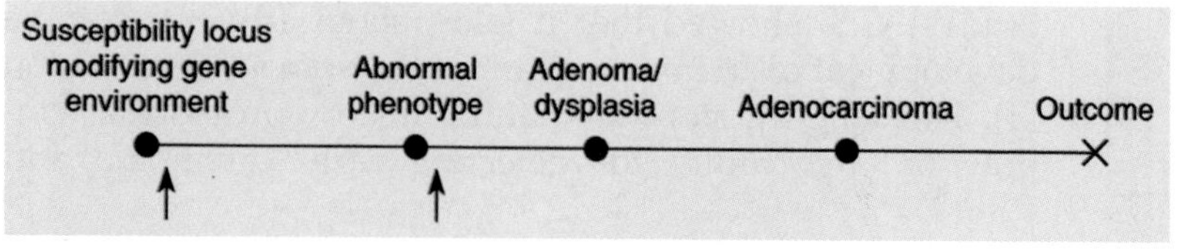

FIGURE 1 ■ The natural history of colorectal carcinoma. *Source*: From Ref. 4.

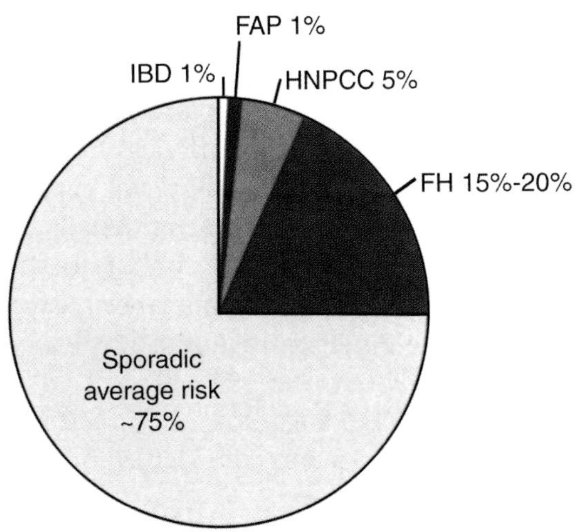

FIGURE 2 ■ Annual new cases of colorectal carcinoma in men and women ≥ 50 years of age with no special risk factors. *Abbreviations*: FAP, familial adenomatous polyposis; FH, family history; HNPCC, hereditary nonpolyposis colon cancer; IBD, inflammatory bowel disease. *Source*: From Ref. 10.

carcinoma. People with a family history of colorectal carcinoma (i.e., one or more parents, siblings, or children with the disease) but without any apparent defined genetic syndrome account for most of those at high risk (15%–20%). Hereditary nonpolyposis colon cancer (HNPCC) accounts for 4–7% of all cases and familial adenomatous polyposis (FAP) about 1%. The remainder, about 1%, are attributed to a variety of uncommon conditions: chronic ulcerative colitis, Crohn's colitis, Peutz-Jeghers syndrome, and familial juvenile polyposis, in which the colorectal carcinoma risk is elevated but is not as high as in HNPCC and FAP (Fig. 2) (10). Other risk factors that should be kept in mind include older age, a diet high in saturated fats and low in fiber, excessive alcohol consumption, and sedentary lifestyle (15).

Screening people at average risk for colorectal carcinoma is different from screening people at high risk. Clinicians should determine an individual patient's risk status well before the earliest potential initiation of screening. The individual's risk status determines when screening should be initiated, and what tests and frequency are appropriate (Fig. 3) (12).

Risk stratification can be accomplished by asking several questions aimed at uncovering the risk factors for colorectal cancer (12). They are as follows:

1. Has the patient had colorectal carcinoma or an adenomatous polyp?
2. Does the patient have an illness (e.g., inflammatory bowel disease) that predisposes him or her to colorectal carcinoma?
3. Has a family member had colorectal carcinoma or an adenomatous polyp? If so, how many, was it a first-degree relative (parent, sibling, or child) and at what age was the carcinoma or polyp first diagnosed?

A positive response to any of these questions should prompt further efforts to identify and define the specific condition associated with increased risk.

SCREENING PEOPLE AT AVERAGE RISK FOR COLORECTAL CARCINOMA

Men and women at average risk should be offered screening with one of the following options beginning at 50 years. A study of a screening colonoscopy in 40–49 years old people confirmed that colorectal carcinomas are uncommon at this age group, supporting the recommendation that screening in average risk people begin at age 50 years (16).

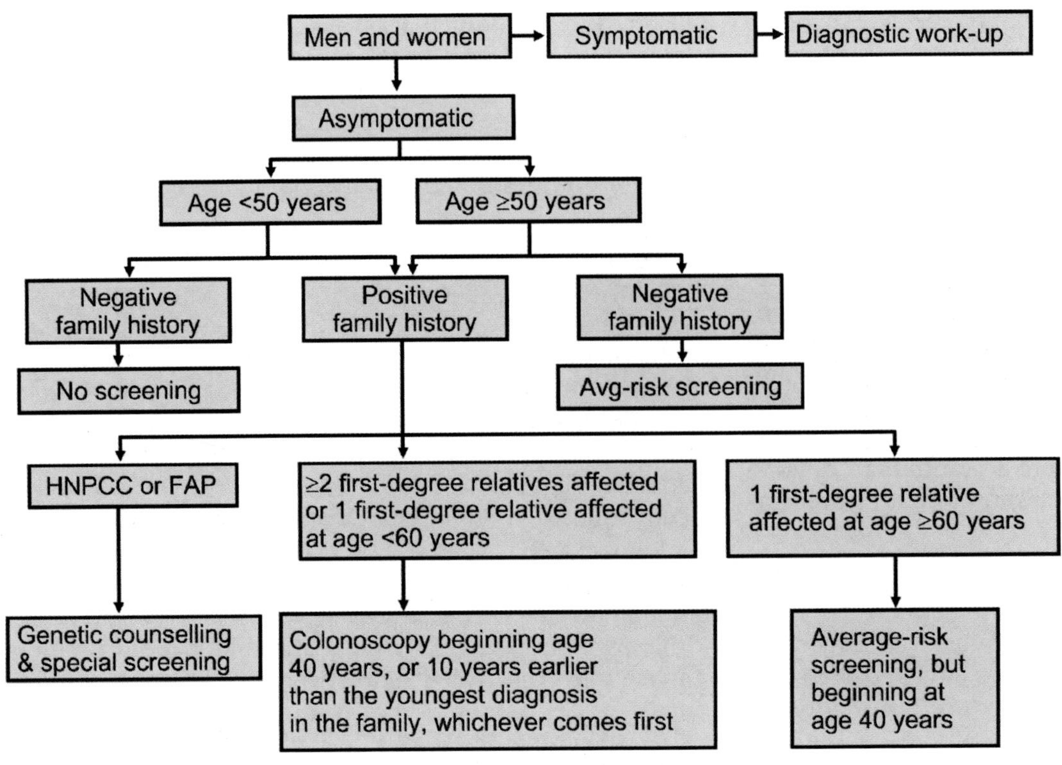

FIGURE 3 ■ The algorithm for colorectal carcinoma screening. *Abbreviations*: AVG, average; HNPCC, hereditary nonpolyposis colorectal cancer; FAP, familial adenomatous polyposis. *Source*: From Ref. 12.

The rationale for presenting multiple options is that no single test has unequivocal superiority, and that giving patients a choice allows them to apply personal preferences and may increase the likelihood that screening will occur. The strategies are not equal with regard to evidence of effectiveness, magnitude of effectiveness, risk, or up-front costs. Reviewing the rationale section for each screening test below will provide clinicians with information that they can use in presenting the relative effectiveness of each test to patients. These tests are recommended by the American Gastroenterological Association (12) as well as the American Cancer Society guidelines (17).

The following excerpts are heavily taken from the American Gastroenterological Association, presented by Winawer et al. (12).

■ FECAL OCCULT BLOOD TEST

This test offers yearly screening with fecal occult blood test (FOBT) using Guaiac-based test with dietary restriction (confined to red meat alone by waiting three days before developing the test) or an immunochemical test without dietary restriction. Two samples from each of three consecutive stools should be examined without rehydration. The patients with a positive test on any specimen should be followed up with colonoscopy (12). The American Gastroenterological Society recommend yearly testing because it is more effective than screening every two years. Rehydration is not recommended. Newer Guaiac-based and immunochemical tests are available that have improved sensitivity and appear to maintain acceptable specificity. Dietary restrictions during testing are commonly recommended to reduce the false-positive rate for the more sensitive Guaiac-based tests but are not necessary for the immunochemical and less sensitive Guaiac-based tests.

With longer (18 years) follow-up in the Minnesota trial, FOBT screening every other year was found to reduce colorectal cancer mortality by 21% (18), a rate consistent with the results of the biennial screening in the two European trials (7,8). The incidence of colorectal carcinoma was also reduced in the screened group (19). A systematic review of three clinical trials (5–7,19) has shown that a restricted diet does not reduce the positivity rate for the older, less-sensitive Guaiac-based tests and that very restricted diets may reduce compliance rates (20).

Disadvantages of FOBT are that currently available tests for occult blood fail to detect many polyps and some carcinomas. Also, most people who test positive will not have colorectal neoplasia (have a false-positive test result) and, thus, will undergo the discomfort, cost, and risk of colonoscopy without benefit. Colonoscopy is recommended for all those with a positive FOBT because it was a diagnostic procedure used throughout most of the trials, and because it is substantially more accurate than double-contrast barium enema for the detection of both small carcinomas and adenomas (21).

■ FLEXIBLE SIGMOIDOSCOPY

Screening with flexible sigmoidoscopy is recommended every five years. Case-controlled studies have reported that sigmoidoscopy was associated with reduced mortality for colorectal carcinoma (22–24). Colon carcinoma risk in the area beyond the reach of the sigmoidoscope was not reduced. A five-year interval between screening examinations is a conservative choice. It is supported by the observation that a reduction in colorectal carcinoma deaths related to screening sigmoidoscopy was present up to 10 years from the last screening examination (22), and that repeat colonoscopy five years after a negative colonoscopy found few instances of advanced neoplasia (25), and follow-up of a cohort of patients after polyp excision showed that development of advanced neoplasia was rare up to five years after a negative colonoscopy (26). The interval is shorter than for colonoscopy because flexible sigmoidoscopy is less sensitive than colonoscopy.

Several studies have shown that the prevalence of proximal advanced adenomas in patients without distal adenomas is in the 2–5% range (27–30). A flexible sigmoidoscopy followed by colonoscopy if a polyp was found would have identified 70–80% of patients with advanced proximal neoplasia (28). In one randomized controlled trial, screening sigmoidoscopy followed by colonoscopy when polyps were detected was associated with an 80% reduction in colorectal carcinoma incidence (31).

■ COMBINED FOBT AND FLEXIBLE SIGMOIDOSCOPY

FOBT is done every year combined with flexible sigmoidoscopy every five years. When both tests are performed, the FOBT should be done first because a positive result is an indication for colonoscopy, obviating the need for the sigmoidoscopy examination. The effectiveness of this combined screening strategy in reducing mortality has never been studied directly in a randomized trial. It is likely that the combination of both screening methods is more effective than either method of screening alone for several reasons: FOBT may be less sensitive for distal colon lesions (32), case-controlled studies report screening FOBT and sigmoidoscopy each are associated with reduced colorectal carcinoma mortality after controlling for the other (22,33), and a nonrandomized controlled trial reported a 43% reduction (which was not statistically significant) in colorectal carcinoma deaths in people screened with FOBT and sigmoidoscopy relative to sigmoidoscopy alone (6). The disadvantage of the FOBT/sigmoidoscopy strategy is that people incur the inconvenience, cost, and complications of both tests with an uncertain gain in effectiveness.

■ COLONOSCOPY

Colonoscopy is offered every 10 years. Although there are no studies evaluating whether screening colonoscopy alone reduces the incidence or mortality from colorectal carcinoma in people at average risk, several lines of evidence support the effectiveness of screening colonoscopy (12). There is direct evidence that screening sigmoidoscopy reduces colorectal carcinoma mortality (22,23), and colonoscopy allows more of the large bowel to be examined. Colonoscopy has been shown to reduce the incidence of colorectal carcinoma in two cohort studies of people with adenomatous polyps (26,34). Colonoscopy permits detection and removal of polyps and biopsy of carcinoma throughout the colon. However, colonoscopy involves greater cost, risk, and inconvenience to the patient than other screening tests, and not all examinations visualize the entire colon. The added value of colonoscopy over sigmoidoscopy screening, therefore, involves a tradeoff of incremental benefits and harms (12).

Choice of a 10-year interval between screening examinations for average-risk people (if the preceding examination is negative) is based on estimates of the sensitivity of colonoscopy and the rate at which advanced adenomas develop. The dwell time from the development of adenomatous polyps to transformation into carcinoma is estimated to be at least 10 years on average (26,35).

In two large prospective studies of screening colonoscopy, about half of patients with advanced proximal neoplasms had no distal colonic neoplasms (28,29). Similarly, a prospective study of distal colon findings in a cohort of average-risk persons with carcinoma proximal to the splenic flexure found that 65% had no neoplasm distal to the splenic flexure (36). A randomized controlled trial of sigmoidoscopy with follow-up colonoscopy for all patients with polyps compared with no screening demonstrated a significant reduction in colorectal carcinoma incidence in the screened patients (31). A cohort of 154 asymptomatic average-risk persons with negative screening colonoscopies had < 1% incidence of advanced neoplasms at a second colonoscopy five years later (25), lending support to the recommended interval of 10 years. Two colonoscopy studies suggested that flat and depressed adenomas account for 22% and 30% of adenomas (37,38), and one report suggests that dye spraying is necessary to not miss these lesions (37). However, the precise prevalence and clinical significance of flat adenomas is uncertain.

By the end of 2000, the U.S. Medicare had decided to reimburse for colonoscopy screening. Colonoscopy as the best primary screening test began to be discussed and to be advocated by some gastroenterology organizations (39).

■ DOUBLE-CONTRAST BARIUM ENEMA (DCBE)

This test is recommended every five years. There are no randomized trials evaluating whether screening DCBE reduces the incidence or mortality from colorectal carcinoma in people at average risk of the disease. The sensitivity of DCBE for large polyps and carcinomas is substantially less than with colonoscopy, the procedure does not permit removal of polyps or biopsy of the carcinomas, and DCBE is more likely than colonoscopy to identify artifacts and other findings (such as stool) as polyps. Patients with an abnormal barium enema need a subsequent colonoscopy.

DCBE is included as an option because it offers an alternative (albeit less sensitive) means to examine the entire colon, it is widely available, and it detects about half of large polyps, which are most likely to be clinically important. Adding flexible sigmoidoscopy to DCBE is not recommended in the screening setting. A five-year interval between DCBE examinations is recommended because DCBE is less sensitive than colonoscopy in detecting colonic neoplasms.

In a prospective study of DCBE in a surveillance population with a spectrum and prevalence of disease similar to a screened population, DCBE detected 53% of adenomatous polyps 6–10 mm in size, and 48% of those >1 cm in size compared with colonoscopy (21). In a nonrandomized study of 2193 consecutive colorectal carcinoma cases in community practice, the sensitivity for carcinoma was 85% with DCBE and 95% with colonoscopy (40).

SCREENING PEOPLE AT INCREASED RISK FOR COLORECTAL CARCINOMA

Screening high-risk people can take several forms. Patients can begin screening at an earlier age if polyps and carcinomas arise at an earlier age, they can be screened more frequently if the evolution from small polyps to carcinoma is more rapid, they can be screened by tests that reach the right colon if the carcinoma occurs more proximally, or they can be screened with more sensitive methods, such as colonoscopy or DCBE rather than FOBT or sigmoidoscopy. Patients already found to have adenomatous polyps are at increased risk for colorectal carcinoma and are candidates for surveillance rather than screening (10).

■ FAMILY HISTORY OF COLORECTAL CARCINOMA OR ADENOMATOUS POLYP

This group consists of individuals having one or more first-degree relatives (parent, sibling, or child) with colorectal carcinoma or adenomatous polyps diagnosed at age < 60 years. There is significant evidence that carcinomas arise at an earlier age in these people than in average-risk persons. In effect, the risk of a 40-year-old person with a family history of colorectal carcinoma is comparable to that of an average-risk 50-year-old person (41) Screening colonoscopy should be started at age 40 years or 10 years younger than the earliest diagnosis in their family, whichever comes first, and repeated every five years (12). Colorectal carcinoma screening recommendations for people with familial or inherited risk is in Table 2.

The lifetime risk of colon carcinoma in people with family history of colon carcinoma is in Table 3.

■ GENETIC SYNDROMES

See Chapter 22 for screening of familial adenomatous polyposist (FAP) and Chapter 23 for screening of HNPCC.

■ DETECTION OF SECOND MALIGNANCIES

Some patients have a higher incidence of a second malignancy than the normal population. Analysis of the Utah Cancer Registry, which documented more than 35,000 carcinomas, revealed that Utah men with one carcinoma have a 1.2 times greater likelihood of developing another carcinoma and Utah women have a 1.5 times greater likelihood than did other persons in the Utah population of the same race, sex, and age who have not had a previous malignancy. In particular, men with primary carcinoma of the colon and rectum have a higher incidence of developing a second carcinoma in the colon, rectum, prostate, or bladder (42). A complete colonic examination with colonoscopy or flexible sigmoidoscopy combined with barium enema to check metachronous lesions should be performed every five years.

At present, the glycoprotein, prostate-specific antigen (PSA) is the most useful marker available for the diagnosis and management of prostate carcinoma. However, PSA is prostate specific but is not sufficiently specific to be used alone as a screening test for prostate carcinoma. PSA is also produced by normal prostatic tissue and can indicate the presence of benign prostatic hyperplasia (BPH).

TABLE 2 ■ **Colon Carcinoma Screening Recommendations for People with Familial or Inherited Risk**

Familial Risk Category	Screening Recommendation
First-degree relative affected with colorectal carcinoma or an adenomatous polyp at age ≥ 60 years, or two second-degree relatives affected with colorectal carcinoma	Same as average risk but starting at age 40 years
Two or more first-degree relatives[a] with colon carcinoma, or a single first-degree relative with colon carcinoma or adenomatous polyps diagnosed at an age < 60 years,	Colonoscopy every five years, beginning at age 40 years or 10 years younger than the earliest diagnosis in the family, whichever comes first
One second-degree or any third-degree relative[b,c] with colorectal carcinoma	Same as average risk
Gene carrier or at risk for familial adenomatous polyposis[d]	Sigmoidoscopy annually, beginning at age 10–12 years[e]
Gene carrier or at risk for HNPCC	Colonoscopy, every 1–2 years, beginning at age 20–25 years or 10 years younger than the earliest case in the family, whichever comes first

[a]First-degree relatives include parents, siblings, and children.
[b]Second-degree relatives include grandparents, aunts, and uncles.
[c]Third-degree relatives include great-grandparents and cousins.
[d]Includes the subcategories of familial adenomatous polyposis, Gardner syndrome, some Turcot syndrome families, and AAPC.
[e]In AAPC, colonoscopy should be used instead of sigmoidoscopy because of the preponderance of proximal colonic adenomas. Colonoscopy screening in AAPC should probably begin in the late teens or early 20s.
Abbreviations: HNPCC, hereditary nonpolyposis colon cancer; AAPC, attenuated adenomatous polyposis coli.
Source: From Ref. 12.

The combination of the PSA test and digital rectal examination provides reliable early detection of prostatic carcinoma. These should be performed annually (43).

For a 55-year-old man presenting to a physician's office, it is prudent to obtain a serum PSA concentration and perform a digital rectal examination. If both are normal, the patient should be followed with an annual evaluation. If the results of the digital rectal examination are unremarkable but the serum PSA level is mildly elevated (range, 4.1–10.0 µg/L), transrectal ultrasonography should be performed (44). Cytologic examination of urine for exfoliated cells should be performed annually, if indicated.

In women, a second carcinoma is more likely to occur in the colon, rectum, cervix, uterus, or ovary (44). Thus a complete large bowel examination should be performed every five years. Mammograpny, pelvic examination, and a Papanicolaou smear test should be performed as part of a routine annual checkup as appropriate.

TABLE 3 ■ **Familial Risk**

Familial Setting	Approximate Lifetime Risk of Colon Carcinoma
General population risk in the U.S.	6%
One first-degree relative with colon carcinoma[a]	2–3-fold increased
Two first-degree relatives with colon carcinoma[a]	3–4-fold increased
First-degree relative with colon carcinoma diagnosed at ≤50 years	3–4-fold increased
One second- or third-degree relative with colon carcinoma[b,c]	About 1.5-fold increased
Two second-degree relatives with colon carcinoma[b]	About 2–3-fold increased
One first-degree relative with an adenomatous polyp[a]	About 2-fold increased

[a]First-degree relatives include parents, siblings, and children.
[b]Second-degree relatives include grandparents, aunts, and uncles.
[c]Third-degree relatives include great-grandparents and cousins.
Source: From Ref. 12.

NEW SCREENING TESTS

There are a couple emerging screening tests that are not yet ready for mass screening but have promising potential.

COMPUTED TOMOGRAPHY COLONOGRAPHY (CTC, VIRTUAL COLONOSCOPY)

At the time of this writing, computed tomography colonography (CTC) is not yet ready for a mass screening test for colorectal carcinoma. It is used as a backup for an incomplete colonoscopy, or for patients who are not suitable for a colonoscopy. However, the advances in technology, techniques, and clinical studies have progressed rapidly. It will be just a matter of time that CTC will become another option for colorectal carcinoma screening (see Chapter 3).

FECAL DNA TESTING

Fecal DNA testing is based on the idea that, because carcinoma is a disease of mutations that occur as tissue evolves from normal to adenoma to carcinoma, those mutations should be detectable in stool (39). Preliminary reports that persons with advanced carcinoma have detectable DNA mutations in stool (45) provided the basis for a large study, using a panel of 21 mutations, in more than 4000 asymptomatic persons who received screening colonoscopy, fecal DNA testing, and FOBT with Hemoccult II (46). The DNA marker panel, including mutations in APC, *K-ras*, and p53, showed a sensitivity of 52% for colorectal carcinoma and specificity of 94% (40).

Such stool-based testing is appealing because it is noninvasive, requires no special colonic preparation, and has the capability of detecting neoplasia throughout the entire length of the colon (47). Because the DNA alterations in colorectal carcinoma are heterogeneous, future assays will need to detect mutations in the number of genes in addition to what we have known at this time. The future of such an approach would seem promising if sensitivity could be increased by additional markers such as methylation and if cost could be reduced (39,47).

WHEN TO STOP SCREENING

There is no direct evidence as to when screening should stop, but indirect evidence supports stopping screening in people nearing the end of life. Polyps take at least 10 years to progress to carcinoma, and screening to detect polyps may not be in the patient's best interest if he or she is not expected to live at least that long. Also, screening and diagnostic tests are, in general, less well tolerated by elderly people. Therefore there will come a time in most peoples' lives when the rigors of screening and diagnostic evaluation of positive tests are no longer justified by the potential to prolong life. The age at which to stop screening depends on the judgment of the individual patient and his or her clinician, taking into account the lead time between screening and its benefits and the patient's life expectancy (10).

SURVEILLANCE

Surveillance is the monitoring of people known to have colon or rectal disease.

AFTER REMOVAL OF ADENOMATOUS POLYPS

The main options for surveillance are colonoscopy and DCBE. The best evidence of the effectiveness of surveillance is from colonoscopy. In the National Polyp Study (NPS), a cohort of 1418 patients who had undergone complete colonoscopy and removal of one or more adenomatous polyps from the colon or rectum were followed up for an average of 5.9 years per patient with periodic colonoscopy. After adjusting for age, sex, and polyp size, rates of carcinoma were 76–90% lower than expected when compared with three reference groups (from published reports) who had not undergone surveillance. The study used reference groups as controls, with the assumption that patients undergoing polypectomy would have experienced the same incidence of carcinoma as the reference populations who have not undergone polypectomy (Fig. 4).

The optional frequency of surveillance was also studied in the NPS. All patients who had undergone prior polypectomy were randomized to undergo surveillance colonoscopy either one and three years or only three years after polypectomy. The two groups showed no difference in the proportion of detected adenomatous polyps with advanced pathology (3% in both groups) (48). This suggests that the first follow-up screening after polypectomy can be deferred for at least three years. The study also showed that if the results of the first surveillance colonoscopy are negative, subsequent examinations are highly unlikely to reveal further adenomatous polyps.

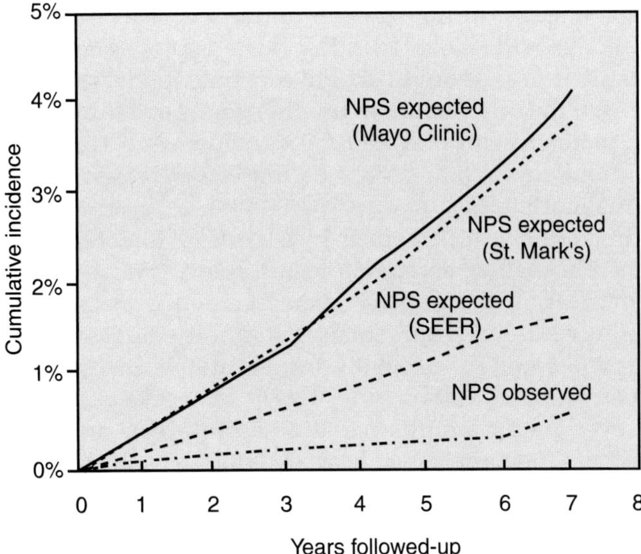

FIGURE 4 ■ The observed and expected incidences of colorectal carcinoma in a National Polyp Study cohort after having undergone colonoscopic polypectomy. *Abbreviations*: NPS, National Polyp Study; SEER, Surveillance, Epidemiology, and End Results (Program). *Source*: From Ref. 26.

There have been no reported studies of surveillance after polypectomy using barium enema and no reported studies comparing surveillance with barium enema versus colonoscopy (10).

New evidence supports the concept that colonoscopic polypectomy reduces subsequent colorectal carcinoma incidence (12). A study of postpolypectomy surveillance demonstrated a 66% reduction in colorectal carcinoma incidence, similar to the previous report of the NPS (34).

There is no direct evidence related to when to stop surveillance. As with screening, the age at which surveillance should stop depends on the judgment of patients and their clinicians, taking into account the patient's medical history and comorbidity. The characteristics of the polyps removed and the results of follow-up examinations should also be taken into account.

IN PEOPLE WITH INFLAMMATORY BOWEL DISEASE

The primary goal of surveillance for colorectal carcinoma in patients with inflammatory bowel disease is to detect moderate to severe dysplasia and early carcinoma rather than polyps. Surveillance should be performed in patients with a history of the disease for about eight years, after which time the risk of carcinoma starts to appear. It is debatable whether surveillance alone is a reliable indicator of prophylactic proctocolectomy (see details in Chapter 26).

IN PEOPLE WITH URETEROSIGMOIDOSTOMY

Ureterosigmoidostomy has been replaced for the most part by ileocystoplasty or the ileal conduit and therefore few patients have this condition. Recently it has been found that patients with ureterocystoplasty or ileal conduit have an equally high risk of developing carcinoma as patients with ureterosigmoidostomy. It takes an average 18 years (range, 5–29 years) for patients with ileocystoplasty or ileal conduit to develop malignancy. Most of the carcinomas or adenomas are at the anastomotic line. At one time in the experimental animal model (rats), it was believed that fecal matter was needed in the urinary stream to develop neoplasia. Later studies disputed this concept and the recent findings of malignancy in ileocystostomy or iteal conduit also confirm that urine alone can cause the malignancy. The pathogenesis is unclear but it appears in animal studies (rats) and the findings in humans that nitrosamines produced by gram negative bacteria are probably part of the mechanism in carcinogenesis (49). Patients with ureterosigmoidostomy should have a flexible sigmoidoscopy or colonoscopy. The examinations should begin on the 10th anniversary of the original operation and should be repeated annually (46). If a polyp is found at the anastomotic line, endoscopic removal is not advisable because most of them are situated at the site of the ureterosigmoidostomy (50,51). If possible, the patient should have an alternative of urinary diversion (51,52).

FOLLOW-UP AFTER CURATIVE RESECTION

Patients with a colorectal carcinoma should have a colonoscopy before the operation to rule out synchronous neoplasms. If the colon is obstructed preoperatively, colonoscopy should be performed approximately six months after operation. If this or a complete preoperative examination is normal, subsequent colonoscopy should be offered after three years; and then, if normal, every five years (12).

The goals of follow-up are to detect local recurrences, distant metastasis, metachronous carcinomas and adenomas, and detection of other primary carcinomas.

The rationale for postoperative follow-up of colorectal carcinoma is based on the assumption that detection of a recurrence in an asymptomatic patient indicates carcinoma at an earlier stage that can be more effectively treated than those detected at a more advanced symptomatic stage.

In general, the investigation includes history and physical examination, endoscopy, carcinoembryonic antigen (CEA), liver function tests, ultrasonography and/or computed tomography (CT) scan, and chest x-ray films.

Approximately 30–50% of patients who undergo curative resection for carcinoma of the colon and rectum have a recurrence (53). In the series by Sugarbaker et al. (54), 85% of patients who develop recurrence do so within 2.5 years, and all sites of recurrence develop at approximately the same period of time, with a median of 17 months. The series by Pihl et al. (55) revealed that 50% of liver metastases are clinically obvious within 21–22 months of treatment, compared with 22–34 months for pulmonary metastases. Recurrences within the abdominal cavity are noted in 84% of all recurrences; 15% have recurrences involving distant metastases only (54). Approximately 35% of patients have liver metastasis. Of these, the liver is the only site of metastasis in approximately 20%. Between 10% and 22% have pulmonary metastases and approximately 10% of these patients have metastasis isolated to the lungs (53).

INVESTIGATION TO DETECT RECURRENCES AND METASTASES

Careful history taking and physical examination provide an effective means of surveillance. Several prospective studies showed that patient symptoms and physical signs can provide the first indication of recurrent carcinoma in 21–48% of those with advanced disease (56,57). In a study by Beart et al. (58) 168 patients who had undergone colorectal resection for cure were followed at least every 15 weeks for up to four years. In 41 of 48 patients, symptoms developed before detection by physical examination or biochemical and radiologic investigations. The symptoms included coughing, abdominal and pelvic pain, change in bowel habit, rectal bleeding, and malaise. Physical examination is a frequent indicator of recurrence but is not as sensitive as the presence of symptoms. All patients with positive physical findings were found to have symptoms or a positive CEA test. Recurrent carcinoma that is symptomatic or that can be detected on physical examination is likely to be advanced and not curable (56).

Alkaline phosphatase seems to be the most sensitive liver function test (58). However, it also has a high false positive rate and, therefore, has little predictive value if used alone (56).

Because chest x-ray films are noninvasive and inexpensive, most clinicians order them annually. Any patient with a questionable or positive lesion should undergo a chest CT scan.

A CT scan of the abdomen is not performed routinely, because the results are somewhat unreliable. Its limitation in detecting early pelvic recurrence is compounded by the fact that postoperative artifacts in the pelvis may persist for as long as two years. However, a CT scan is invaluable for assessing symptomatic patients and for confirming the clinical impression of recurrences (59). A CT scan to detect liver metastases is more accurate, with 85–90% sensitivity; this is similar to ultrasonography and magnetic resonance imaging (MRI). When CT scan is doubtful, positron emission tomography (PET) can be helpful (60).

A systemic review and meta-analysis of randomized trials suggests a survival benefit associated with performing CT (every 3–12 months) (61). However, others have reported that CT scan did not increase the number of curative hepatectomies (62). The track record for detecting curable pelvic or local relapse is also disappointing (63–65). When adjuvant radiation therapy is used, related posttreatment changes further complicate the interpretation of such imaging (66).

CEA is a sensitive marker for identifying recurrence or metastases. CEA level is elevated most commonly in patients with hepatic metastases; 95% of these patients have increased plasma CEA levels. On the other hand, in patients with local abdominal or pelvic recurrences, 17–25% have normal CEA levels. Of the 70 patients with recurrences, 89% have elevated plasma CEA levels before the recurrences are detected by any other means. However, CEA does not always detect recurrences or metastases at a resectable stage. In the series reported by Beart et al. (58), 48 patients with elevated CEA were explored and only one patient was thought to have a potentially resectable lesion. On the other hand, in another series of 146 asymptomatic patients with elevated CEA, evidence of recurrence was found in 95%, and 58% of these were resectable for potential cure (67).

In an uncontrolled study by Moertel et al. (68), using a patient population entered into a large National Surgical Adjuvant Trial, the patients were accrued from a variety of settings ranging from small community clinics to large universities and are probably representative of carcinoma in most practices nationwide. Every 12 weeks of the first year, every four months for the second year, and every six months thereafter, they have evaluations supplemented by hemoglobin and chemical analysis of the blood and chest radiographs. At 24 and 48 weeks and then annually, they underwent either proctoscopy, colon radiography, or total colonoscopy. Performance of the CEA test was optional, according to the usual practice of the responsible physician. Of a total of 1216 patients with resected carcinoma of the colon, 1017 (84%) had CEA monitoring. Among 417 monitored patients with recurrence, 59% had a preceding elevation of CEA concentration. Of 600 patients without recurrence, 16% showed a false positive result. CEA testing is most sensitive for detecting hepatic or retroperitoneal metastases and relatively insensitive for local, pulmonary, or peritoneal involvement. Surgical explorations were performed in 115 patients with CEA elevations, and 47 recurrences, usually hepatic, were resected with curative intent. On the other hand, 38 patients with normal CEA concentrations and 23 patients not monitored also underwent such resection—usually for a pulmonary or local recurrence. Of all CEA-monitored patients, 2.3% were alive and disease free more than one year after the salvage operation (2.9% of those with CEA elevations and 1.9% of those with no elevations). Of patients with no CEA monitoring, 2% were also alive and disease free more than one year after the salvage operation. The authors concluded that carcinoma cures attributable to CEA monitoring are, at best, infrequent. It is questionable whether this small gain justifies the substantial cost in dollars and the physical and emotional stress that this intervention may cause patients.

Although intensive postoperative follow-up programs, including CEA evaluation, do identify recurrence earlier and thus result in higher resectable rates, they do not translate into a higher survival. Ohlsson et al. (63) of Sweden conducted a prospective randomized study investigating the value of intense postoperative follow-up compared with no follow-up in 107 patients followed up from 5.5–8.8 years. The study showed no difference in survival. A similar but larger prospective randomized study was conducted by Kjeldsen et al. (64) of Denmark. It consisted of 597 patients who also showed no improvement in overall survival or in disease-related survival.

Richard and McLeod (53) critically examined the literature on postoperative follow-up of patients with colorectal carcinoma through a Medline search for articles published from 1966 through February 1996. The report included randomized controlled clinical trials, cohort studies, and descriptive studies. From the findings of their review, the authors believe that there is inconclusive evidence either to support or refute the value of follow-up surveillance programs to detect recurrent colorectal carcinoma. The authors pointed out many flaws in most of the studies, including small sample sizes, patient bias, and variations in follow-up protocols. The authors estimated that even if postoperative surveillance were effective, the survival benefit would not be $>10\%$. On the other hand, in a meta-analysis of 3283 patients in seven nonrandomized studies, Bruinvels et al. (69) found a 9% better overall survival rate in intensively followed patients, including more asymptomatic recurrences and more operations for recurrence.

Surgeons and patients should understand the limitations of an intensive postoperative follow-up to detect recurrences and metastases. The follow-up regimen should be discussed and individualized to fit each patient's needs.

METACHRONOUS CARCINOMAS AND POLYPS

The goal of surveillance after colorectal resection for carcinoma is to clear the adenomas if this has not been done preoperatively and to detect metachronous carcinoma. The incidence of metachronous carcinoma of the large bowel is approximately 2%–4% within 3–20 years (70–72). Periodic examination of the large bowel with colonoscopy every three to five years provides the most accurate results. An alternative is to use flexible sigmoidoscopy combined with DCBE, possible CT colography in the near future.

There are no controlled studies of the effectiveness of surveillance strategies in this situation. Available information suggests that the metachronous carcinomas have biological behavior that is not different from initial carcinomas except in increased frequency of occurrence.

OTHER PRIMARY MALIGNANCIES

The detection of other primary carcinomas is not important until the patient has achieved long-term survival. This fact has usually been ignored, unrealized, or forgotten. Enblad et al. (42) analyzed the occurrence of a second primary malignant disease in 38,166 patients with carcinoma of the colon and in 23,603 patients with carcinoma of the rectum, as reported to the Swedish Cancer Registry between 1960 and 1981. The overall relative risk (RR) of developing a second primary malignant disease was significantly increased both after carcinoma of the colon (women, RR = 1.4; men, RR = 1.3) and rectum (women, RR = 1.4; men, RR = 1.3). The increased risk of secondary primary diseases occurs in the stomach, small intestine, ovary, endometrium, cervix, breast, kidney, bladder, and prostate (Table 4).

SUMMARY

Despite the plethora of publications on the subject of follow-up strategies for patients who have undergone curative resection for colorectal carcinoma, there is no general agreement on the optimal follow-up program. The efficacy of aggressive and intensive surveillance remains

TABLE 4 ■ The Relative Risk of Secondary Primary Malignancy

Site of Second Malignancy	Sex	Primary Lesions of Colon (RR)	Primary Lesion of Rectum (RR)
Stomach	M	1.3	1.0
	F	1.0	1.3
Small intestine (carcinoid, adenocarcinoma)	M	10.2	3.8
	F	5.1	2.0
Kidney	M	1.5	1.2
	F	1.5	1.3
Bladder	M	1.5	1.3
	F	2.0	1.7
Prostate	M	1.3	1.3
Ovary	F	3.0	1.5
Endometrium	F	1.7	1.7
Cervix	F	1.1	1.4
Breast	F	1.3	1.3

Abbreviation: RR, relative risk.
Source: From Ref. 42.

TABLE 5 ■ Summary of Guideline for Colorectal Surveillance after Primary Surgery with Curative Intent

Test or Procedure	ESMO (73)	ASCO (74)	ASCRS (75)	ONTARIO'S (76)
History and physical examination	History is taken. Clinical exam only in patients with suspicious symptoms	Every 3–6 months for first 3 years; annually thereafter	Three times per year for 2 years	For Stage IIB and III, every 6 months for 3 years; annually for an additional 3 years
Fecal occult-blood test	Restricted to patients with suspicious symptoms	No routine testing	Not recommended	Not addressed
Liver function tests	Restricted to patients with suspicious symptoms	No routine testing	No routine testing	Not addressed
CEA	Restricted to patients with suspicious symptoms	Every 2–3 months for Stage II or III for 2 years or longer. Only in patients who can undergo liver resection	Three times per year for 2 years	For Stage IIB and III, every 6 months for 3 years; annually for additional 3 years
Chest X-ray	Restricted to patients with suspicious symptoms	No routine testing. Order when CEA is elevated or symptoms suggestive of pulmonary metastasis	No routine testing	For Stage IIB and III, every 6 months for 3 years; annually for additional 3 years
Flexible sigmoidoscopy and endoscopic ultrasound	Every 6 months for 2 years in carcinoma distal sigmoid or rectum. Endorectal ultrasound	For patients who have not received pelvic irradiation. Direct imaging of rectum periodically. For patients who have received pelvic irradiation, direct imaging is not suggested	Periodic anastomotic examination	Not addressed
Colonoscopy and barium enema	Every 5 years	Every 3–5 years	Every 3 years	Annually if there is a polyp; 3–5 years if no polyp
CT abdomen	Restricted to patients with suspicious symptoms	Not routine	Not routine	For Stage IIB and III, every 6 months for 3 years; annually for additional 3 years
Ultrasonography of the abdomen	Of liver every year for 3 years	Not addressed	Not addressed	For Stage IIB and III, every 6 months for 3 years; annually for additional 3 years

Abbreviations: ASCO; American Society Clinical Oncology; ASCRS, American Society of Colon and Rectal Surgeons; CEA, carcinoembryonic antigen; CT, computed tomography; ESMO, European Society for Medical Oncology.

a topic of intense debate. Some data support the contention that surveillance leads to increased rates of early detection and resection of recurrence but this has not necessarily always translated into improved survival. What constitutes the ideal or even preferred follow-up program remains controversial, and this is clearly reflected by the lack of uniformity among practicing clinicians.

It is important that patients understand the limitations of the postoperative follow-up no matter how minimal or extensive it is. They should actively participate in the decision-making of the follow-up plan.

Guidelines from some major societies are helpful on this issue. See Table 5 (73–76).

REFERENCES

1. Jemal A, Murray T, Warel B, et al. Cancer Statistic 2005. CA Cancer J Clin 2005; 55:10–30.
2. Hermanek P, Sobin LH. Colorectal carcinoma. Hermanek P, Gaspodarowicz MK, Henson DE, Hutter RVP, Sobin LH, eds. Prognostic Factors in Cancer. HCII. International Union Against Cancer. Berlin: Springer-Verlag, 1995:64–79.
3. Jessup JM, Menck HR, Fremgen A, Winchester DP. Diagnosing colorectal carcinoma: Clinical and molecular approaches. CA Cancer J Clin 1997; 47:70–92.
4. Winawer SW, Zauber AG, Stewart E, O'Brien MJ. The natural history of colorectal cancer. Opportunities for intervention. Cancer 1991; 67:1143–1149.
5. Mandel JS, Bond JH, Church TR, et al. Reducing mortality from colorectal cancer by screening for fecal occult blood. N Engl J Med 1993; 328:1365–1371.
6. Winawer SJ, Flehinger BJ, Schottenfeld D, Miller DG. Screening for colorectal cancer with fecal occult blood testing and sigmoidoscopy. J Natl Cancer Inst 1993; 85:1311–1318.
7. Kronborg O, Fenger C, Olsen J, Jorgensen OD, Sondergaard O. Randomized study of screening for colorectal cancer with fecal-occult blood test. Lancet 1996; 348:1467–1471.
8. Hardcastle JD, Chamberlain JO, Robinson MHE, et al. Randomized controlled trial of fecal-occult-blood screening for colorectal cancer. Lancet 1996; 348: 1472–1477.
9. Kewenter J, Brevinge H, Engaras B, Haglind E, Ahren C. Results of screening, rescreening and follow up in a prospective randomized study for detection of colorectal cancer by fecal occult blood testing. Results for 68,308 subjects. Scand J Gastroenterol 1994; 29:468–473.
10. Winawer SJ, Fletcher H, Miller L, et al. Colorectal cancer screening: Clinical guidelines and rationale. Gastroenterol 1997; 112:594–642.
11. Bond JH. Screening for colorectal cancer: Confuting the refuters. Gastrointest Endosc 1997; 45:105–109.
12. Winawer S, Fletcher R, Rex D, et al. Colorectal cancer screening and surveillance: Clinical guidelines and rationale—update based on new evidence. Gastroenterol 2003; 124:544–560.
13. Seeff LC, Nadel MR, Klabunde CN, Thompson T, Shapiro JA, Vernon SW, Coates RJ. Patterns and predictors of colorectal cancer test use in the adult U.S. population. Cancer 2004; 100:2093–2103.
14. Surveillance, epidemiology and results (SEER) program, 1973–1992. Bethesda, Maryland: National Cancer Institute.
15. Potter JD, Slattery ML, Bostick RM, Gapstur SM. Colon cancer: A review of the epidemiology. Epidemiol Rev 1993; 15:499–545.
16. Imperiale TF, Wagner MS, Liney, Larkin GN, Rogge JD, Ransohoff DF. Results of screening colonoscopy among persons 40 to 49 years of age. N Engl J Mech 2002; 346:1781–1785.

17. Smith RA, Cokkinides V, Eyre H. American cancer society guidelines for early detection of cancer, 2005 CA cancer J Clin 2005; 55:31–44.
18. Mandel JS, Church TR, Ederer F, Bond JH. Colorectal cancer mortality: effectiveness of biennial screening for fecal occult blood. J Nah Cancer Inst 1999; 91:434–437.
19. Mandel JS, Church TR, Bond JH, et al. The effect of fecal occult-blood screening on the incidence of colorectal cancer. N Engl J Med 2000; 343:1603–1607.
20. Pignone M, Campbell MK, Carr C, Phillipe C. Meta-analysis of dietary restriction during fecal occult blood testing. Eff Clin Pract 2001; 4:150–156.
21. Winower SJ, Stewart ET, Zauber AG, et al. For the National Polyp Study Work Group: A comparison of colonoscopy and double contrast barium enema for surveillance after polypectomy National Polyp Study Work Group. N Engl J Med 2000; 342:1766–1772.
22. Selby JV, Friedman GO, Quesenberry CP Jr, Weiss NS. A case-control study of screening sigmoidoscopy and mortality from colorectal cancer. N Engl J Med 1992; 326:653–657.
23. Newcomb PA, Norfleet RG, Storer BE, Surawicz T, Marcus PM. Screening sigmoidoscopy and colorectal cancer mortality. J Natl Cancer Inst 1992; 84: 1572–1575.
24. Muller AD, Sonnenberg A. Protection by endoscopy against death from colorectal cancer. Arch Intern Med 1995; 155:1741–1748.
25. Rex DK Cummings OW, Helper DJ, et al. Five year incidence of adenomatous adenomas after negative colonoscopy in asymptomatic average-risk persons. Gastroenterol 1996; 111:1178–1181.
26. Winawer SJ, Zauber AG, Ho MN, et al. Prevention of colorectal cancer by colonoscopic polypectomy. The National Polyp Study Work Group. N Engl J Med 1993; 329:1977–1981.
27. Levin TR, Palitz A, Grossman S, et al. Predicting advanced proximal colonic neoplasia with screen sigmoidoscopy. JAMA 1999; 2818:1611–1617.
28. Lieberman DA, Weiss DG, Bond JH, Ahnen DJ, Garewal H, Chejfec G. Use of colonoscopy to screen symptomatic adults for colorectal cancer. Veterans Affair Cooperative Group. N Engl J Med 2000; 343:162–168.
29. Imperiale TF, Wagner DR, Lin CY, Larkin GN, Rogge JD, Ransohoff DF. Risk of advanced proximal neoplasms in asymptomatic adults according to the distal colorectal findings. N Engl J Med 2000; 343:169–174.
30. Farraye FA, Wallace M. Clinical significance of small polyps found during screening with flexible sigmoidoscopy. Gastrointest Endorc Clin NAM 2002; 12:41–51.
31. Thiis-Evensen E, Hoft GS, Sauer J, Langmark F, Majak BM, Vatn MH. Population-based surveillance by colonoscopy: Effect on the incidence of colorectal cancer. Scand J Gastroenternal 1999; 34:414–420.
32. Jorgensen OD, Kronborg O, Fenger C. A randomized study of screening for colorectal cancer using fecal occult blood testing: Results after 13 years and seven biennial screening rounds. Gut 2002; 50:29–32.
33. Selby JV, Friedman GD, Quesenberry CP Jr., Weiss NS. Effect of fecal occult blood testing on mortality from colorectal cancer. A case-control study. Ann Intern 1993; 118:1–6.
34. Citarda F, Tomaselli G, Capocaccia R, Barcherini S, Crespi M. Efficacy in standard clinical practice of colonoscopic polypectomy in reducing colorectal cancer incidence. Gut 2001; 48:812–815.
35. Hofstad B, Vatri M. Growth rate of colon polyps and cancer. Gastrointest Endosc Clin N Anm 1997; 7:345–363.
36. Rex DK, Chak A, Vasudeva R, et al. Prospective determination of distal colon findings in average-risk patients with proximal colon cancer. Gastrointest Endosc 1999; 49:727–730.
37. Rembacken BJ, Fujii T, Cairus A, et al. Flat and depressed colonic neoplasms: A prospective study of 1000 colonoscopies in the UK. Lancet 2000; 355:1211–1214.
38. Saitohy, Waxman I, West AB, et al. Prevalence and distinctive biologic features of flat colorectal adenomas in a North American population. Gastroentrol 2001; 120:1657–1665.
39. Ransohoff DF. Colon cancer screening in 2005: status and challenges. Gastroenterol 2005; 128:1685–1695.
40. Rex DK, Rahmani EY, Haseman JH, Lemmei GT, Kaster S, Buckley JS. Relative sensitivity of colonoscopy and barium enema for detection of colorectal cancer in clinical practice. Gastroenterol 1997; 112:17–23.
41. Fuchs CS, Giovannucci EL, Colditz GA, Hunter DJ, Speizer FE, Willet NC. A prospective study of family history and risk of colorectal cancer. N Engl J Med 1994; 331:1669–1674.
42. Enblad P, Adami HO, Glimelius B, Krusemo W, Pahlman L. The risk of subsequent primary malignant diseases after cancers of the colon and rectum. Cancer 1990; 65:2091–2100.
43. Barry MJ. Prostate-specific-antigen testing for early diagnosis of prostate cancer. N Engl J Med 2001; 344:1373–1377.
44. Oesterling JE. Prostate-specific antigen. Improving its ability to diagnose early prostate cancer. JAMA 1992; 264:2236–2238.
45. Ahlquist DA, Skoletsky JE, Boynton KA, et al. Colorectal cancer screening by detection of altered human DNA in stool: Feasibility of a multitarget assay panel. Gastroenterol 2000; 119:1219–1227.
46. Imperiale TF, Ransohoff DF, Itz Kowitz SH, Turnbull BA, Ross ME. Fecal DNA versus fecal occult blood for colorectal-cancer screening in an average-risk population. N Engl J Med 2004; 351:2704–2714.
47. Walsh JME, Terdiman JP. Colorectal cancer screening. Scientific Review. JAMA 2003; 289:1288–1296.
48. Winawer SJ, Zauber AG, O'Brien MJ, et al. Randomized comparison of surveillance intervals after colonoscopic removal of newly diagnosed adenomatous polyps. N Engl J Med 1993; 328:901–906.
49. Filmer RB, Spencer JR. Malignancies in bladder augmentations and intestinal conduits. J Urol 1990; 143:671–678.
50. Woodhouse CRJ. Guidelines for monitoring of patients with ureterosigmoidostomy. Gut 2002; 51(suppl V):V15–V16.
51. Hurlstone DP, Wells JM, Bhala N, McAlindon ME. Ureterosigmoid anastomosis: risk of colorectal cancer and implications for colonoscopists. Gastrointest Endosc 2004; 59:248–254.
52. Azimuddin K, Khubchandani IT, Stasik JJ, Rosen L, Riether RD. Neoplasia after ureterosigmoidostomy. Dis Colon Rectum 1999; 42:1632–1638.
53. Richard CS, McLeod RS. Follow-up of patients after resection for colorectal cancer: A position paper of the Canadian Society of Surgical Oncology and the Canadian Society of Colon and Rectal Surgeons. Can J Surg 1997; 40:90–100.
54. Sugarbaker PH, Gianola FJ, Dwyer A, Neuman NR. A simplified plan for follow-up of patients with colon and rectal cancer supported by prospective studies of laboratory and radiologic test results. Surgery 1987; 102:79–87.
55. Pihl E, Hughes ESR, McDermott FT. Lung recurrence after curative surgery for colorectal cancer. Dis Colon Rectum 1987; 30:417–419.
56. Kelly CJ, Daly JM. Colorectal cancer. Principles of postoperative follow-up Cancer 1992; 70:1397–1408.
57. Goldberg RM, Fleming TR, Tangen CM, et al. Strategies for identifying resectable recurrence and success rates after resection. Ann Intern Med 1998; 129:27–35.
58. Beart RW Jr, Metzger PP, O'Connell MJ, Schutt AJ. Postoperative screening of patients with carcinoma of the colon. Dis Colon Rectum 1981; 24:585–588.
59. Zheng G, Eddleston B, Schofield PF, Johnson RJ, James RD. Computed tomographic scanning in rectal carcinoma. J R Soc Med 1984; 877:915–920.
60. Tzimas GN, Koumanis DJ, Meterissian S. Positron emission tomography and colorectal carcinoma: An update. JACS 2004; 198:645–652.
61. Renchan AG, Egger M, Saunders Mp, O'Dwyer ST. Impact on survival of intensive follow up after curative resection for colorectal cancer: Systematic review and meta-analysis of randomized trials. BMJ 2002; 384:813–818.
62. Schoemaker D, Black R, Giles L, Toouli J. Yearly colonoscopy, liver CT, and chest radiography do not influence 5-year survival of colorectal cancer patients. Gastroenterol 1998; 114:7–14.
63. Ohlsson B, Breland W, Ekberg H, Graffner H, Tranberg KG. Follow-up after curative surgery for colorectal carcinoma: Randomized comparison with no follow-up Dis Colon rectum 1995; 38:619–626.
64. Kjeldsen BJ, Kronborg O, Fenger C, Jorgensen OD. A prospective randomized study of follow-up after radical surgery for colorectal cancer. Br J Surg 1997; 84:666–669.
65. Pietra N, Sarli L, Costi R, Ouchemi C, Grattarola M, Peracchia A. Role of follow-up in management of local recurrences of colorectal cancer: A prospective randomized trial. Dis Colon Rectum 1998; 41:1127–1133.
66. Pfister DG, Benson III Al B, Somerfield MR. Surveillance strategies after curative treatment of colorectal cancer. N Engl J Med 2004; 350:2375–2382.
67. Martin EW Jr., Minton JP, Carey LC. CEA-directed second look surgery in the asymptomatic patient after primary resection of colorectal carcinoma. Ann Surg 1985; 202:310–317.
68. Moertel CG, Fleming TR, Macdonald JS, Haller DG, Laurie JA, Tangen C. An evaluation of the carcinoembryonic antigen (CEA) test for monitoring patients with resected colon cancer. JAMA 1993; 270:943–947.
69. Bruinvels DJ, Stiggelbous AM, Kievit J, van Houwelingen HC, Habberna JDF, van de Velde CJH. Follow-up of patients with colorectal cancer. A meta-analysis. Ann Surg 1994; 219:174–182.
70. Tornqvist A, Ekelund G, Leandoer, L. Early diagnosis of metachronous colorectal carcinoma. Aust N Z J Surg 1981; 51:442–445.
71. Luchtefeld MA, Ross DS, Zander JD, Folse JR. Late development of metachronous colorectal cancer. Dis Colon Rectum 1987; 30:180–184.
72. Herald RJ, Bussey HJR. Clinical experiences at St. Mark's Hospital with multiple synchronous cancers of the colon and rectum. Dis Colon Rectum 1975; 18:6–10.
73. ESMO minimum clinical recommendations for diagnosis, adjuvant treatment and follow-up of colon cancer. Ann Oncol 2001; 12:1053–1054.
74. Benson III Al B, Desch CE, Flynn PJ, et al. 2000 update of American Society of Clinical Oncology Colorectal Cancer Surveillance guidelines. J Clin Onc 2000; 18:3586–3588.
75. The Standards Practice Task Force. The American Society of Colon and Rectal Surgeons. Practice parameters for the surveillance and follow-up of patients with colon and rectal cancer. Dis Colon Rectum 2004; 47:807–817.
76. Figueredo A, Rumble RB, Maroun J, et al. Follow-up of patients with curatively resected colorectal cancer: a practice guideline. BMC Cancer 2003; 3:26–38.

26 Ulcerative Colitis

Santhat Nivatvongs

INTRODUCTION

Ulcerative colitis is a nonspecific inflammatory bowel disease (IBD) that affects both sexes and occurs at all ages, with maximal onset between the second and fourth decades. The etiology is unknown, and no epidemiologic studies to date suggest that a transmissible causative agent is responsible for the disease.

EPIDEMIOLOGY AND ETIOLOGY

Epidemiology is the study of the distribution and the factors important in determining the nature of disease. At present, the understanding of the epidemiology in patients with ulcerative colitis is limited. Little is known about the distribution, and even less about the nature of the disease. Studies on ulcerative colitis are difficult because mild cases may be overlooked and not recorded, whereas severe cases often are referred to major medical centers. The disease is uncommon and has marked geographic differences in incidence rates. Most of the reported series are from developed countries in North America and Europe. Ulcerative colitis is less common in Asia, Africa, and South America. Garland et al. (1) studied 15 regions in the United States and found the incidence was 5.48 to 5.87 per 100,000 in the white population. A study from Rochester, Minnesota, is unique in that the population is stable and access to comprehensive medical record linkage and indexing system are complete (2). The incidence in the years between 1960 and 1979 was 15 per 100,000 people. Age-specific incidence was roughly bimodal in appearance (Fig. 1). A similar stable population from Denmark showed a similar pattern, with an annual incidence of 8.1 per 100,000 inhabitants (3). Most authors report that the incidence of ulcerative colitis has remained constant during the past two decades or that it has declined recently (4). In Japan, the incidence rate of

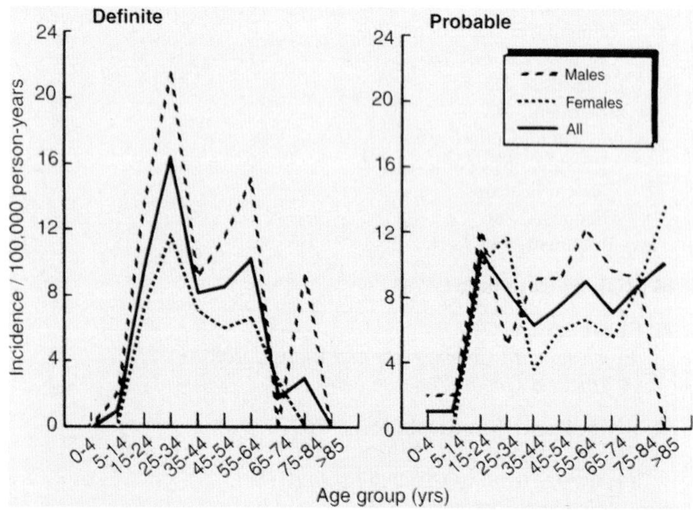

FIGURE 1 ■ Age-specific incidence of "definite" and "probable" chronic ulcerative colitis among Rochester, Minnesota, residents. The "definite" category requires radiologic or endoscopic documentation of ulcerative colitis at least twice, six months apart. "Probable" is only one observation or the observation spanned for a period of less than six months. *Source*: From Ref. 2.

ulcerative colitis increased to 0.25 per 100,000 population and to a peak of 0.49 in 1974. There has been a tendency to remain at the same level since 1975 (5).

It has been suggested that IBD may either be environmental in origin or involve a genetic predisposition that can be triggered by an environmental stimulus (1). The nature of these factors is unknown. Speculation has included increased sugar consumption, a low-fiber diet, food allergies, food additives, infectious agents, and shortened breastfeeding time as some of the many environmental influences that may contribute to the etiology of IBD (4). Although Crohn's disease is associated with smoking and smoking has detrimental effects on the clinical course of the disease, ulcerative colitis is largely a disease of nonsmokers and former smokers. Furthermore, cigarette smoking may even result in a beneficial influence on the course of ulcerative colitis (6). In addition, Mormons and nonsmokers have a high incidence of ulcerative colitis. In contrast, smokers have approximately a two-fold increased risk of developing Crohn's disease than nonsmokers, often 5 to 15 years after smoking begins (7). Cigarette smoking is protective against developing ulcerative colitis at any age, particularly at younger ages (8).

Familial aggregation of ulcerative colitis has been recognized for many years (9,10). Substantial evidence indicates genetic factors play a role in the predisposition of IBD. However, these conditions are not inherited in a Mendelian pattern. Any genetic predisposition to ulcerative colitis probably is influenced by social factors such as diet, smoking habits, or use of oral contraceptives (11,12). In fact, among the risk factors for IBD, family history is the most consistent. Farmer et al. (13) investigated the family history of 838 patients with IBD onset before 21 years of age. Of 316 patients with ulcerative colitis, 29% had a positive family history. In a study reported by Lashner et al. (14), 22% of all probands had family members with IBD. Of the 10,819 patients with ulcerative colitis registered in Japan, 197 (1.8%) had a positive history of ulcerative colitis. Parent–child and sibling relationships are much more common than relationships involving more distant relatives (5). Ulcerative colitis probands tend to have more relatives diagnosed with ulcerative colitis, and Crohn's disease probands have more relatives with Crohn's disease. The two diseases are distinct and follow separate inheritance patterns (14).

During acute episodes of IBD, neutrophils flood the lamina propria. Once present in tissues, neutrophils actively bind bacteria opsonized by antibodies and C36 component of complement by virtue of specific receptors. Once bound, neutrophil metabolism increases dramatically and the bacteria or the coated particles are ingested (15). Seventy-five percent of ulcerative colitis patients exhibit perinuclear antineutrophil cytoplasmic antibodies (p-ANCA). However, the presence of p-ANCA does not correlate with the activity or extent of colitis and is thought to be an epiphenomenon (7,15,16).

Extensive immunologic reviews by Strober and James (17) stressed that ulcerative colitis is not an autoimmune disease and that no evidence establishes any immunologic disorder as the primary cause of ulcerative colitis. However, the immune system is an important mediator of the pathology of chronic ulcerative colitis (CUC). Clinically it has been observed that the severity of the disease correlates with the presence of immune cells in the intestinal lesions, that the extraintestinal manifestations of disease resemble immune-complex disorders, and that immunosuppressive drugs that inhibit the release of soluble activation factors are effective in controlling the disease (18).

An enormous amount of work has been done to understand the etiology of ulcerative colitis but without success; as Ekbom put it, "a lot of data but little knowledge" (19).

CLINICAL COURSE

Ulcerative colitis is a dynamic disease characterized by remissions and exacerbations. The clinical spectrum ranges from an inactive or quiescent phase to a low-grade active disease and finally to a fulminant disease. The rectum almost invariably is involved. The disease is homogenous, with involvement ranging from the rectum (proctitis) to the rectum and sigmoid (proctosigmoiditis) to typical full-blown proctocolitis involving the entire colon and rectum. Ulcerative colitis does not involve the small bowel; however, the distal few inches of the terminal ileum frequently are inflamed because of reflux of the diarrheal stool from the cecum. This inflammation is called "backwash ileitis" and is reversible. It must not be confused with the ileitis of Crohn's disease.

CLINICAL MANIFESTATIONS

The basic symptoms of ulcerative colitis are diarrhea and bleeding from the rectum. Massive hemorrhage is encountered infrequently. The severity of diffuse, oozing of blood from the diseased mucosa is directly related to the stage, extent, and intensity of the inflammatory process. The onset of ulcerative colitis may be insidious, with minimal bloody stools and/or diarrhea, or there may be explosive severe diarrhea, bleeding, tenesmus, crampy abdominal pain, and fever. The diarrhea may occur as often as once every one to two hours. Patients with ulcerative colitis commonly report cramping prior to and relieved by a bowel movement, often localized to the left lower quadrant, reminiscent of altered defecation reported in irritable bowel syndrome. Persistent pain is an uncommon feature except in severe active disease, when inflammation extends to the serosa (20). Nocturnal diarrhea is a sign of an organic problem. The stool is usually small in amount, and often only blood and mucus are passed. Loss of weight and development of malaise and anemia depend entirely on severity and duration of the disease. Physical findings are nonspecific and depend on severity of the disease. Abdominal distention in association with the toxic signs of fever, tachycardia, and an elevated white blood cell count is an ominous sign of toxic megacolon. When constipation occurs, it most often is associated with disease limited to the rectum and sigmoid colon, most likely resulting from spasm.

DIAGNOSIS

The diagnosis of ulcerative colitis must be made by endoscopy. Since the rectum almost invariably is involved, proctoscopy or flexible sigmoidoscopy is regarded as essential and sufficient, especially in very ill patients. A complete evaluation with total colonoscopy is contraindicated during the acute attack because of the risk of perforation. After patients have recovered from the acute stage, total colonoscopy should be performed to determine the extent of the disease.

The mucosa in a patient with ulcerative colitis ranges from granular, with minimal edema and friability in the milder stage to frank ulceration with marked edema and bleeding from the mucosa in the acute stage. Multiple random biopsies of the mucosa should be done to check for any mucosal dysplasia, particularly when the disease has been present for more than 10 years and is not an acute stage.

If possible, both barium enema examination and colonoscopy should be done to complement the findings. Use of a barium enema, however, is contraindicated when the disease is in an acute stage. In a patient with long-standing ulcerative colitis, the colon is foreshortened and has lost normal haustration (Fig. 2). Tiny ulcers are seen as fine marginal irregularities. Deep ulcers are seen as "collar buttons" or a linear collection of barium parallel to the bowel lumen. Benign stricture of the colon in long-standing ulcerative colitis is uncommon and usually is from spasm or hypertrophy of the muscularis mucosa. Stricture in a patient with ulcerative colitis must be presumed malignant until proven otherwise.

The important part of the initial diagnosis of ulcerative colitis is to exclude infectious causes of colitis, and to differentiate it from Crohn's colitis (see Chapter 27).

ASSESSMENT OF SEVERITY

Attacks of ulcerative colitis vary widely in severity, and management must be tailored accordingly. Assessment of the extent and severity of the disease is essential at the time of diagnosis and during recurrence and for determining the effect of medical treatment (21). A simple classification of the severity of an attack was devised many years ago Truelove and Witts (22). It is a useful, objective set of criteria for therapeutic trials and in day-to-day clinical practice (23,24). In this classification, the degree of severity is based on six simple clinical signs (Table 1) (25).

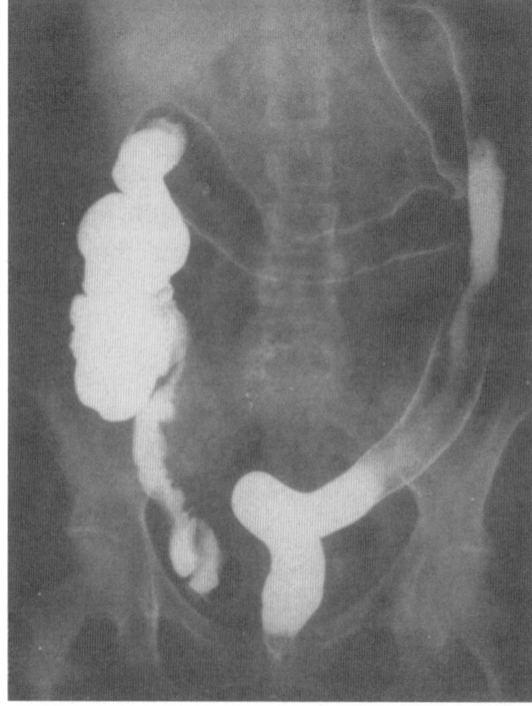

FIGURE 2 ■ Foreshortening and loss of normal haustration in colon with long-standing ulcerative colitis.

Another useful method was devised by Schroeder of the Mayo Clinic to assess ulcerative colitis activity (Box 1). This can be easily applied to a study group of patients.

Roseth et al. (27) found that fecal calprotectin is useful to assess disease activity in ulcerative colitis. Although other parameters such as fecal excretion of indium 1110-labeled granulocyte have been found to be an excellent correlation with both the histological and endoscopic evaluation of disease activity of IBD, it is an expensive test (27,28).

Calprotectin is a 36-kD calcium-binding protein with antimicrobial properties. This protein is located in the cytosol fraction of both PMN and monocytes/macrophages. Calprotectin can accurately be assessed in plasma and stools by enzyme-linked immunosorbent assay (ELISA) (29).

Roseth et al. (27) evaluated 62 consecutive patients with ulcerative colitis who came for colonoscopic surveillance. Fecal samples were collected two days before the colonoscopy and was stored at less than 20°C until further analysis. The endoscopic mucosal inflammation was graded (0–3) as well as biopsy for microscopic inflammation grading (0–3). The fecal concentrations of calprotectin were determined by ELISA.

The result showed that the correlation between the endoscopic and histological grading of inflammation activity was significant. There was a significant correlation between the histological grading of disease activity and that of fecal calprotectin. Patients with active disease (Grade 2 or 3) had higher fecal calprotectin concentrations than patients with no/low activity (Grade 1 or 2). There was also a significant difference between patients with no/low activity and those with normal colonoscopy.

In 39 patients with pancolitis, there was a significant correlation between the histological grading of inflammation and the fecal calprotectin levels. A similar pattern was found in 25 patients with left-sided colitis and proctitis.

Finally, when disease activity was assessed by different hematological parameters (hemoglobin, erythrocyte sedimentation rate, C-reactive protein, platelets, and serum albumin), no correlation was found between these and the

TABLE 1 ■ **Definition of Severity of Attack of Ulcerative Colitis**

	Severity of Attack[a]	
Symptoms	**Severe**	**Mild**
Diarrhea	Six or more stools daily	Four or fewer stools daily
Blood in stool	Large amount	Small amount
Fever	99.5°F or higher (evening)	None
Tachycardia	90/min or more	None
Anemia	75% hemoglobin or less	None
Elevated erythrocyte sedimentation rate	30 mm/hr or more	Normal

[a]Moderate = Intermediate between severe and mild.
Source: From Ref. 25.

BOX 1 ■ Scoring System for Assessment of Ulcerative Colitis Activity[a]

Stool frequency	Findings of flexible proctosigmoidoscopy
0 = normal number of stools for the patient 1 = one to two stools more than normal 2 = three to four stools more than normal 3 = five or more stools more than normal	0 = normal or inactive disease 1 = mild disease (erythema, decreased vascular pattern, and mild friability) 2 = moderate disease (marked erythema, absent vascular pattern, friability, and erosions) 3 = severe disease (spontaneous bleeding, ulceration)
Rectal bleeding	**Physician's global assessment**
0 = no blood seen	0 = normal
1 = streaks of blood with stool less than half the time	1 = mild disease
2 = obvious blood with stool most of the time	2 = moderate disease
3 = blood alone passed	3 = severe disease

Scoring:
0=No symptoms of colitis, the patient felt well, and the scoping score is 0.
1=Mild symptoms and scope findings that are mildly abnormal.
2=More serious abnormalities, scoping, and symptoms, score of 1 to 2.
3=Scoping and symptoms scores are 2 to 3, and the patient probably requires corticosteroid therapy and possibly hospitalization.
[a]The score reflects the patient's recorded symptoms, the flexible sigmoidoscopic appearance of rectum and sigmoid mucosa, and other pertinent indexes, such as physical findings and the patients' performance status.
Source: From Ref. 26.

endoscopic or histological grading of disease activity nor the fecal calprotectin levels. The authors concluded that fecal calprotectin assessment is a useful parameter of disease activity in ulcerative colitis; it reflects the degree of inflammation rather than the extent of the disease.

PATHOLOGIC FEATURES

GROSS APPEARANCE

The inflammation in patients with ulcerative colitis is confined to the mucosa and submucosa. The bowel is foreshortened in long-standing cases, but the bowel wall on the outside is neither thickened nor inflamed. The disease starts in the rectum and is more severe there than in more proximal parts of the colon unless the rectum is treated locally with steroid enemas, in which case the rectum may appear less severely affected or even grossly normal. The appearance of the mucosa varies according to severity of the disease. Typically, the mucosa is granular, swollen, and friable (Fig. 3). In severe cases, there are patchy full-thickness ulcerations of the mucosa (Fig. 4). In long-standing ulcerative colitis, most of the mucosa may be lost and "burned out." The mucosa may show multiple polyps, which are regenerations of inflamed mucosa resulting from previous ulcerations. They are referred to as "pseudopolyps" or "inflammatory polyps."

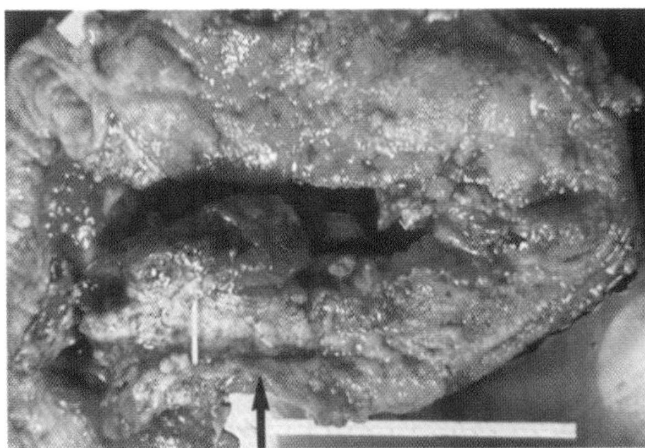

FIGURE 3 ■ Granular appearance of mucosa in chronic ulcerative colitis. Also note narrowing of sigmoid colon caused by carcinoma (*arrow*).

The distribution of disease can be a very useful feature in distinguishing between ulcerative colitis and Crohn's disease. Ulcerative colitis is a contiguous process that nearly always involves the rectum. There is proximal extension from the rectum to a varying degree. In some cases, initial rectum involvement is followed by more proximal extension over time. In other cases, the disease remains localized to the rectum that is called "ulcerative proctitis." In a minority of cases, the entire colon is involved at the initial presentation. The transition from involved to uninvolved mucosa usually occurs gradually, is occasionally abrupt, and is never characterized by intervening uninvolved mucosa. The presence of uninvolved mucosa distal to a diseased segment is known as a "skip lesion" and strongly suggests Crohn's disease rather than ulcerative colitis (30).

The gross appearance of the colon and rectum depends on the severity of the disease. In acute or fulminant disease, the serosa is hyperemic but is soft and otherwise appears quite normal. Shortening of the colon is best seen on barium study and is difficult to appreciate on celiotomy.

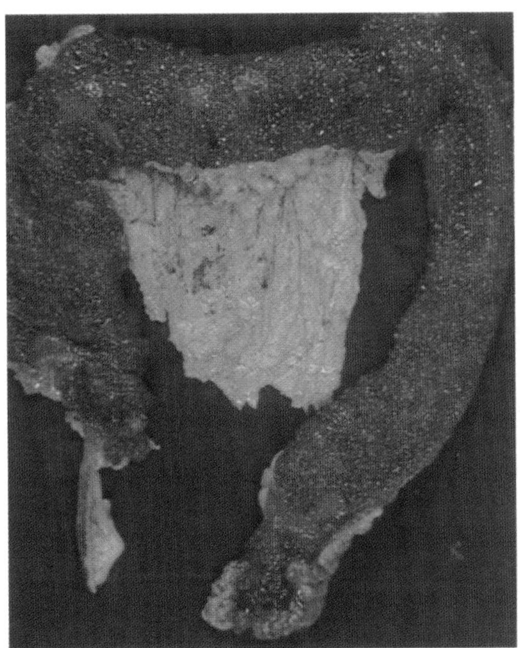

FIGURE 4 ■ Deep ulcerations in severe ulcerative colitis.

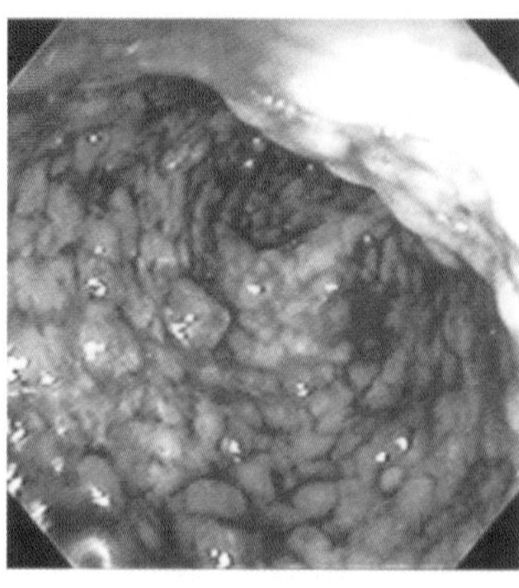

FIGURE 5 ■ Pseudopolyposis associated with ulcerative colitis.

Stricture formation occurs in 5% to 12% of patients. In a series reported by Gumaste et al. (31) including 1156 patients with ulcerative colitis, 59 (5%) had 70 separate strictures in the colon and rectum. Twenty-four percent of the strictures proved to be malignant. Three striking features of malignant strictures are apparent as compared to benign strictures: (i) appearance late in the course of the disease (61% after 20 years of disease vs. 0% before 10 years), (ii) location proximal to splenic flexure (86%), and (iii) symptomatic large bowel obstruction (100% vs. 14% in benign strictures). Benign strictures are caused by hypertrophy of muscularis mucosa and are reversible (32).

Endoscopically, the granularity and friability and congested, velvety appearance of the mucosa can be easily recognized. There may be full-thickness ulceration of the mucosal layer, generally patchy but never separated by intervening normal mucosa. The degree of ulceration varies from small punctate lesions to broad areas with undermining of adjacent mucosa. Occasionally, linear ulcers referred to as "tram-line ulcers" may occur in ulcerative colitis along the taenia coli, although the presence of deep linear ulcers ("rake ulcers") suggests Crohn's disease (30).

Pseudopolyps, or better referred to as inflammatory polyps, are actually islands of intact mucosa that become relatively elevated through the ulceration of adjacent mucosa (Fig. 5). Quiescent disease is usually characterized by a smooth, uniform, atrophic, and nonfriable mucosa but may have granular mucosal surface. Absence of normal haustral folds is the rule. In some cases, the mucosa may appear perfectly normal endoscopically, but biopsies from these ostensibly normal areas almost always contain histologic evidence of chronic disease (30).

■ MICROSCOPY

The hallmark of active ulcerative colitis is the presence of polymorphonuclear (PMN) leukocytosis within the lamina propria, crypt, and surface epithelium and crypt lumina. As a rule, the PMN leukocytosis within the lamina propria is a relatively lesser component when compared with the active inflammation in the crypts. PMN leukocytosis will also be characteristically present within the epithelium of the crypts, a finding termed "cryptitis," in addition to forming aggregates within the crypt lumina, known as "crypt abscess." The crypt abscess may rupture into adjacent tissue forming a foreign body granuloma in response to exposed mucin, a finding that can be confused with epithelioid granulomas of Crohn's disease (30).

It should be emphasized that although PMN leukocytes are seen in the lamina propria, crypt epithelium, and crypt lumina in active IBD, they are also seen in infectious colitis. This underscores the importance of ruling out infectious disease. In general, extensive crypt abscesses and cryptitis will favor ulcerative colitis or Crohn's disease over an infectious colitis; however, there is extensive overlap histologically. Secondarily thrombosed vessels may be seen and should not be taken as an indication of a primary ischemic event. The histologic features of these ulcer-based biopsies are not specific, and sampling from the edge of the ulcers or adjacent mucosa is more likely to be informative (30).

The epithelium in actively inflamed mucosa shows varying degrees of regenerative change in response to the inflammation. The characteristic features of regenerative epithelium include loss of mucin, prominent basophilic cytoplasm with plump hyperchromatic nuclei, and increased numbers of mitoses that involve the superficial portion of the crypts. Mucin depletion is a characteristic feature of CUC but is nonspecific since an adenomatous polyp, as well as dysplastic epithelium, also has mucin depletion (30).

While the acute changes above are seen, there are also nearly always underlying features of chronicity even when the clinical history is quite short. From a diagnostic standpoint, the presence of these features of chronicity is often more important than the acute inflammatory component since in an acute inflammatory background, evidence of chronicity suggests an active IBD rather than an infectious colitis. Typical features of chronicity include irregular spacing of glands with crypt distortion, loss of parallelism, size variation, and crypt branching (Fig. 6). Branched glands are rarely seen in conditions other than chronic IBD. Other features of chronicity include foreshortening of the glands and mucosal atrophy, Paneth's cell metaplasia, enteroendocrine cell hyperplasia, and thickening of the muscularis mucosa. A thickened muscularis mucosa is usually more prominent distally and is thought to account partially for the gross shortening of the bowel. In some cases of CUC, a prominent hyperplasia of lymphoid follicles is present. This

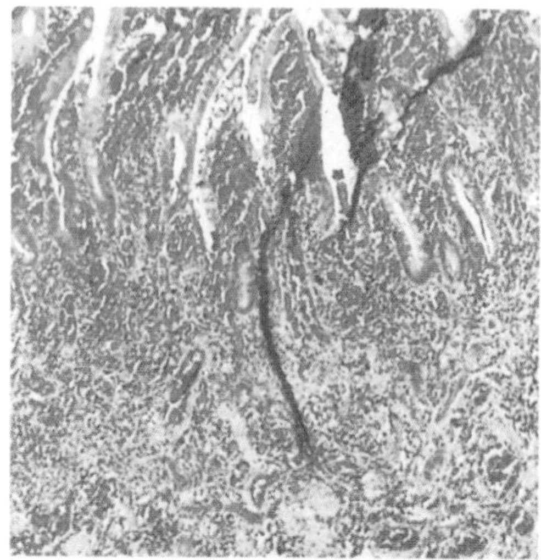

FIGURE 6 ■ Infiltrations of acute and chronic inflammatory cells in mucosa and submucosa in active ulcerative colitis.

generally occurs in the rectum, and has been referred to as "lymphoid follicular proctitis." The lymphoid follicles in ulcerative colitis are present in the lamina propria adjacent to the muscularis mucosa and in the superficial submucosa, as opposed to those in Crohn's disease, which are found in the deeper submucosa, muscularis propria, and subserosal adipose tissue (30).

Ulcerative colitis has been divided into three major disease phases: active colitis, resolving colitis, and quiescent colitis. These phases nearly always have the above-described features of chronicity. As active disease abates, either spontaneously or as a result of treatment, the phase of resolution takes place and is characterized by a decrease in acute inflammation, prominent epithelium regeneration, and a progressive restoration of the goblet cell population. Fulminant ulcerative colitis refers to a severe form of active ulcerative colitis in which the deep submucosa and muscularis propria are involved. This takes the form of deep V-shaped ulcers that may extend deep into the muscularis propria and may be associated with muscle necrosis (myocytolysis). The degree of disease activity in the adjacent mucosa is usually severe, and extensive superficial ulceration and mucosal denudation are common (30).

Instances of overlap between ulcerative colitis and Crohn's disease are rare, which suggests major fundamental differences in the evolution of these diseases, although in the early stages, it is common to have a mix of clinical and pathologic features that made a precise diagnosis difficult and often subjective (33). In their opinion, Finkelstein et al. (33) believe ulcerative colitis and Crohn's disease do represent two separate and unique diseases and failure to arrive at a clear distinction often is due to deficiencies in clinicopathologic correlation or inadequate tissue sampling.

DIFFERENTIAL DIAGNOSIS

Many conditions cause diarrhea and bleeding that mimic ulcerative colitis. It is essential to differentiate these diseases since their natural history, course, and management are different. Part of the investigation in patients with the clinical diagnosis of ulcerative colitis should include examination of stool for pathogenic bacteria, ova, and parasites and biopsy of large bowel mucosa, even though it appears grossly normal.

■ CROHN'S DISEASE

Crohn's disease is another nonspecific or idiopathic IBD that has features both similar and in contrast to ulcerative colitis (Chapter 27).

■ *CLOSTRIDIUM DIFFICILE* COLITIS

General Considerations

C. difficile is a gram-positive, spore-forming, anaerobic microorganism. Up to 40% of newborns may harbor *C. difficile* and its toxin without harm, yet severe and even lethal enterocolitis is well recognized in association with antibiotic administration in older children and adults (34). About 3% of healthy adults and 20% to 40% of hospitalized patients are colonized with *C. difficile*, which in healthy persons is metabolically inactive in the spore form (35,36). The disease is the consequence of overgrowth of *C. difficile* and its toxin (37). In the past it was believed that lincomycin and clindamycin caused the infection (38,39), but it is known now that any antibiotic can give rise to the colitis. The disease can even occur without prior use of an antibiotic (40).

C. difficile is an important nosocomial pathogen, and some hospitals and long-term care facilities have reported epidemics of diarrhea caused by this agent (41).

Clinical Features

The *C. difficile* toxin affects the mucosa of the large bowel, causing watery diarrhea, fever, and leukocytosis. Bleeding per rectum is generally not a feature. The signs and symptoms vary according to the severity of the condition. Patients with more severe disease may present with or without diarrhea. In the absence of diarrhea, the only clues to diagnosis may be a high fever, a moderate or marked PMN leukocytosis, lower or diffuse abdominal pain, tenderness and distension (42). In extreme cases, toxic megacolon can develop. The diarrhea may develop during the course of the antibiotic treatment or several weeks after its discontinuation.

Diagnosis

Since it takes a few days to obtain the results, the cytotoxin assay that uses tissue culture has been the gold standard for diagnosis. It is the most sensitive test. However, most laboratories do not offer tissue-culture assays, and the results of the assay are not available for 24 to 48 hours. The most practical tests are the enzyme immunoassays and the toxin-culture assays of the stool. Enzyme immunoassays are offered by most laboratories and have good specificity, but a high enough toxin A or toxin B must be present for the test to be positive. Therefore, there is a false-negative rate of 10% to 20%. Commercially available reagents will detect the toxin A or toxin A and toxin B. Those that detect both toxin A and toxin B are preferred, because 1% to 2% of cases involve strains of *C. difficile* that produce only toxin B. The results of this test should be available within hours or within one day (41).

The diagnosis can also be made by culturing stool on selected medium, including the toxin-culture assay, with broth cultures of isolates to identify toxigenic strains. The advantage of this approach, if it is done correctly, is the high degree of sensitivity. Limitations are the lack of specificity, the delay of three to four days before results are available, and the small number of laboratories that offer this test (41).

It may be useful to test more than one stool specimen for *C. difficile* toxin. Performing enzyme immunoassays on two or three specimens, rather than one, not only increases the diagnostic yield by 5% to 10%, but also increases the cost (41).

If the diagnosis is in doubt, a proctoscopy or flexible sigmoidoscopy should be next. Grossly, the mucosa appears normal or demonstrates mild inflammation similar to that with mild proctocolitis or has typical yellowish, plaque-like membranes on the inflamed mucosa—thus use of the term "pseudomembranous colitis" in the past. There is no membrane formation on the large bowel mucosa in at least 50% of the cases of antibiotic-induced colitis. If pseudomembranes are seen, it is specific, because nearly all cases are attributed to *C. difficile* infection (41). Involvement of the large bowel also can be patchy or segmental; thus proctoscopy and flexible sigmoidoscopy may not detect the disease, and colonoscopy may become necessary. A retrospective study by Bergstein et al. (43) showed that there is no apparent difference in the rate of detection of pseudomembranes between rigid sigmoidoscopy (57%), flexible sigmoidoscopy (50%), and colonoscopy (50%).

Treatment

The most important step in the treatment is stopping the antibiotics. In most patients, the diarrhea improves within a few days. To avoid retention of the toxin in the large bowel, antidiarrheal drugs should not be prescribed. Specific treatment is indicated if the diarrhea continues or if the patient must continue the implicated antibiotics.

Vancomycin, metronidazole, and bacitracin are effective. With the lower cost of metronidazole (250 times cheaper than vancomycin), it should become the first-line treatment. If this fails, then vancomycin or bacitracin should be instituted. Regardless of therapy, relapse or asymptomatic carriage can occur and may be the result of reacquisition of *C. difficile* from the environment or sporulation. When treatment is discontinued, the spores revert to a vegetative form, and the disease may relapse within days.

Metronidazole is given orally at a dose of 500 mg three times daily or 250 mg four times daily for 7 to 14 days. Vancomycin is administered orally at a dose of 125 mg four times a day for 7 to 14 days. Bacitracin is given orally at a dose of 25,000 U four times a day for 7 to 14 days (41,44,45). In prospective randomized trials, metronidazole and vancomycin showed equivalent efficacy; bacitracin is less effective than vancomycin in clearing *C. difficile* from the stool. Cholestyramine, which has been recommended as primary therapy for mild cases, binds *C. difficile* toxin but cannot be used with vancomycin because it also binds this drug (44).

Relapse occurs in 20% to 25% of cases (41). Recurrent disease may reflect relapse of infection due to the original infecting organism or infection by a new strain (46). Tapering doses of vancomycin as described by Tedesco et al. (47), may be used: 125 mg four times a day for one week, 125 mg twice a day for one week, and 125 mg every third day for two weeks. The rationale for pulsed doses of vancomycin is that the spored forms will germinate to the vegetative plate during the vancomycin-free period and then will be treated by the next pulse of vancomycin. Tapering doses of metronidazole may be more cost effective (44).

Others have proposed the administration of anion-exchange resins to absorb *C. difficile* toxin (such as 4 g of cholestyramine three times daily), or the use of agents to antagonize *C. difficile* (such as *Saccharomyces boulardii* or *Lactobacillus* strain GG). Enemas with human stool or stool flora obtained from broth cultures have also been suggested as a means of reconstituting normal flora. Response rates are good, but this solution is usually unnecessary and carries a potential risk of transmission of retroviruses or other agents (41).

Severely ill patients who show no response to an adequate medical treatment, require a colectomy, in rare instances (41).

Dallal et al. (48) reviewed 2334 hospitalized patients with *C. difficile* colitis from January 1989 to December 2000. Sixty-four patients died or underwent colectomy for fulminant colitis. In 2000, the incidence of *C. difficile* colitis in hospitalized patients increased from a baseline of 0.68% to 1.2% and the incidence of patients with *C. difficile* colitis in whom life-threatening symptoms developed increased from 1.6% to 3.2%. Forty-four patients required a colectomy and 20 patients died directly from *C. difficile* colitis. A recent surgical procedure and immunosuppression were common predisposing conditions. Lung transplant patients were 46 times more likely to have *C. difficile* colitis and eight times more likely to have severe disease. Abdominal computed tomography scan correctly diagnosed all patients, whereas 12.5% of toxin assays and 10% of endoscopies were falsely negative. Patients undergoing colectomy (89% underwent a total abdominal colectomy and ileostomy) for *C. difficile* colitis had an overall death rate of 57%. Significant predictors of death after colectomy were preoperative vasopressor requirements and age.

Longo et al. (49) used the computer-based search, the Veterans Administration Data Processing Center, for patients with *C. difficile* colitis who subsequently underwent colectomy from fiscal year 1997 to 2000 (total number of patients with *C. difficile* during this period of time was not known). Sixty-seven patients with mean age of 69 (range 40–86 years), 99% of them males, were identified. All 67 patients had *C. difficile* verified in the colectomy specimens. Thirty six of 67 patients (54%) developed *C. difficile* colitis during hospitalization for an unrelated illness and 30 of 36 patients (87%) after a surgical procedure. Thirty one of 67 patients (46%) developed *C. difficile* colitis at home. There was no history of diarrhea in 25 of 67 patients (37%). Forty three of 67 patients (64%) presented with an acute surgical abdomen. Abdominal computed tomography correctly diagnosed 45 or 46 patients (98%) who were imaged. Twenty six of 67 patients (39%) underwent colonoscopy; all 26 were found to have severe inflammation or pseudomembranes. Fifty three of 67 patients (80%) underwent a total colectomy; 14 of 67 underwent segmental colonic resection. Perforation and infarction were found in 59 of 67 patients (58%) at surgery. Overall mortality was 48%. Mean hospitalization was 36 (range 2–297) days.

Patients with fulminant *C. difficile* colitis often present with an unexplained abdominal illness with a marked leukocytosis that rapidly progresses to shock and peritonitis. Although frequently developed during a hospitalization and often after a surgical procedure, it may develop outside of a hospital setting or even at home. Diarrhea may be absent and stool cytology may be negative for *C. difficile* toxin. Perforation and infarction are frequently found at surgery. Mortality from fulminant *C. difficile* colitis remains high despite surgical intervention (49).

Clostridium difficile: The Recent Outbreak in Quebec Hospitals

In March 2003, several hospitals in Quebec, Canada, noted a marked increase in the incidence of *C. difficile*-associated diarrhea. Because of this problem, Loo et al. (50) conducted a prospective study at 12 Quebec hospitals to determine the incidence of nosocomial *C. difficile*-associated diarrhea and its complication and a case-controlled study to identify risk factors for the disease. Isolates of *C. difficile* were typed by pulsed-field gel electrophoresis and analyzed for binary toxin genes and partial deletions in the toxin A and B repressor gene tcdC.

The results showed that a total of 1703 patients with 1719 episodes of nosocomial *C. difficile*-associated diarrhea were identified. The incidence was 22.5 per 1000 admissions. The 30-day attributable mortality rate was 6.9%. Case patients were more likely than matched controls to have received fluoroquinolones [odds ratio (OR), 3.9] or cephalosporins (OR, 3.8). A predominant strain, resistant to fluoroquinolones, was found in 129 of 157 isolates (82%), and binary toxin genes and partial deletions in the tcdC gene were present in 132 isolates (84%). The authors concluded that a strain of *C. difficile* that was resistant to fluoroquinolones and had binary toxin and a partial deletion of tcdC gene was responsible for this outbreak of *C. difficile*-associated diarrhea. Exposure to fluoroquinolones or cephalosporins was a risk factor.

This study supports the concept that a more vigorous strain of *C. difficile* is causing epidemic disease at selected locations and is associated with more frequent and more severe disease, as indicated by higher rates of toxic megacolon, leukemoid reaction, shock, requirement of colectomy, and death (51). What should we do? Bartlett and Perl (51) suggested that control hinges on prevention, recognition of cases, and optimal management of disease. Physicians and infection-control personnel need to monitor for an increasing incidence of *C. difficile*-associated disease on the basis of some classic features: the administration of antibiotics complicated by diarrhea, fever, leukocytosis, sometimes with a leukemoid reaction, and hypoalbuminemia or toxic megacolon, or both. Standard stool assays available in most laboratories will not identify this epidemic strain, but the strain might be suspected on the basis of the number of severity of cases. Treatment consists of the prompt discontinuation of the implicated antimicrobial agent and the administration of oral metronidazole; for severely ill patients and those who do not have a prompt response to metronidazole, oral vancomycin should be considered.

Prevention efforts should include fastidious use of barrier precautions, isolation of the patient, careful cleaning of the environment with sporicidal agents active against *C. difficile*, and fastidious use of hand hygiene. This last requirement should include washing hands with soap and water as a supplement to the use of alcohol-based sanitizers, because such sanitizers do not eradicate *C. difficile*.

Particularly important is antibiotic stewardship with restraint in the use of epidemiologically implicated antimicrobial agents, usually second- and third-generation cephalosporins, clindamycin, fluoroquinolones, or a combination of the three (51,52).

■ *CAMPYLOBACTER* GASTROENTERITIS

General Considerations

Campylobacter is a microaerophilic, gram-negative, rapidly mobile bacillus. It formerly was unknown as a human pathogen because of lack of culture techniques in the past to isolate it from the stool. Since the report by Skirrow (53) in 1977, *Campylobacter jejuni* has been recognized as one of the most common worldwide causes of acute bacterial infection of the gastrointestinal tract. *Campylobacter* enteritis is a zoonosis (i.e., its main source is animals), and is transmitted to humans by consumption of contaminated food, including water, milk, and meat. Poultry is the primary source because of the high rates of colonization of commercially available chickens in which culture positivity is around 88% (54).

Clinical Features

Campylobacter infection can affect both the large and small intestine. It may present as acute colitis that mimics IBD. The incubation period is two to five days (range, 1–10 days). The clinical picture resembles other acute infectious diarrheas. Patients often have headaches, myalgia, and fever before the onset of diarrhea. Colicky abdominal pain usually is severe and may mimic that of acute appendicitis if it is localized to the right lower quadrant.

Diagnosis

Direct microscopic examination of fecal specimens by dark-field or phase-contrast microscopy may provide a presumptive diagnosis of campylobacteriosis because this organism exhibits a typical darting motility (55). A definitive diagnosis requires a stool culture, which must be delivered rapidly to the laboratory. A special medium is required for culture, and the laboratory must be instructed to look for this organism. Endoscopic findings in the rectum and colon range from mild nonspecific colitis to frank ulcerations. Biopsy of the colonic mucosa shows nonspecific inflammation and is not diagnostic.

Treatment

Campylobacter colitis is self-limited and generally does not require specific treatment. For patients in whom treatment is indicated, some authors recommend erythromycin as the drug of choice because of its low cost and low levels of resistance. It must be started early, on the first day of illness, or possibly as late as the second or the third day (56). The dosage is 500 mg administered orally twice daily for five days (57). Another effective treatment is quinolone antibiotics such as Ciprofloxacin. Patients respond rapidly to either a single 750 mg dose of Ciprofloxacin or 500 mg twice daily for three days. The most significant problem in using Ciprofloxacin has been the rapid rise in antimicrobial resistance. Most quinolone resistances against *Campylobacter* have come from the United States because of the use of this antibiotic in poultry (56).

■ SALMONELLA ENTEROCOLITIS

General Considerations

Nontyphoidal salmonellosis is the leading cause of bacterial food poisoning. The pathogen is *Salmonella enteritidis*, which is transmitted by eating contaminated food, particularly raw eggs (58). *S. enteritidis* invades the bowel mucosa and multiplies in the lamina propria of the large bowel. Sometimes it enters the bloodstream, causing septicemia. Diarrhea is caused by its enterotoxin.

Clinical Features

The incubation period is within 24 hours. The onset of illness is abrupt, with headache, nausea, vomiting, fever, abdominal cramps, and diarrhea. The diarrhea is watery with a large volume. The course of the disease is usually 48 hours.

Diagnosis

S. enteritidis is easy to isolate from stool. The 4-methylumbelliferyl-caprilate (MUCAP) test is used for rapid identification of *Salmonella* strains from agar plates (55). Endoscopic examination of the rectum and the colon reveals edema and hyperemic mucosa, signs that are usually not confused with those of ulcerative colitis.

Treatment

Specific treatment with antibiotics is not indicated. In fact, antibiotics may prolong excretion of the bacteria (59). Ciprofloxacin 500 mg twice a day for three to five days is an appropriate empirical antibiotic of choice for patients who are moderately to severely ill with signs of an invasive pathogen, such as fever, blood in stool, fecal leukocytes, or prolonged duration of diarrhea (56).

■ *ESCHERICHIA COLI* 0157:H7

Escherichia coli 0157:H7 (*E. coli* 0157:H7) is an important virulence human pathogen. North American gastroenterologists probably encounter one or more patients every year who are infected with this organism (60). *E. coli* expressing somatic antigen 157 and flagellar (H) antigen 7 was first recognized as a pathogen in two nearly simultaneous reports in 1983 by Karmali et al. (61) at the Hospital for Sick Children in Toronto, and Riley et al. (62) at the Centers for Disease Control. There was an epidemiologic association between the consumption of hamburgers and the development of hemorrhagic colitis. Microbiologic investigation showed the presence of a previously unknown pathogen, *E. coli* 0157:H7, in the stools of most of the infected patients whose microbiologic cultures were performed early in illness (60).

The basic microbiologic characteristics of *E. coli* 0157:H7 do not differ from those of other *E. coli*. The cardinal virulence trait of *E. coli* 0157:H7 has been considered to be its ability to produce Stx1, Stx2, or both. Almost all strains from North America have a gene that encodes Stx2; approximately two-thirds have a gene that encodes Stx1. *E. coli* 0157:H7 may infect persons of any age, but children less than age 10 and the elderly have the highest frequency of extraintestinal complications and death. Large epidemics and clustered infections in North America, Europe, and Japan give the impression that most cases of *E. coli* 0157:H7 infection are associated with outbreaks.

Clinical Features

Patients infected with *E. coli* 0157:H7 are in considerable abdominal pain and present a compelling picture for relief of symptoms. In severe cases, the patients have bloody diarrhea. Some patients infected with *E. coli* 0157:H7 have mild gastrointestinal symptoms. Particularly in children, the patients may develop hemolytic-uremic syndrome (HUS) (61). Most notably, *E. coli* 0157:H7 infections present abruptly, usually in previously healthy hosts, with symptoms that have lasted no more than a week. Prediarrheal herald signs of *E. coli* 0157:H7 include a self-limited fever, abdominal pain, irritability, fatigue, headache, myalgias, and confusion. Vomiting can occur at any stage of the illness. Abdominal pain frequently is intense and is disproportionate to findings on physical examination. The pain usually is spasmodic and intermittent in nature. Fever is reported by about one-third of the patients, usually soon after the diarrhea becomes bloody. The absence of a fever at the time of presentation tends to distinguish *E. coli* 0157:H7 infections from other bacterial diarrheas (60).

Diagnosis

Acute bloody diarrhea is an urgent medical problem. The timely performance of a complete stool culture is the most important component of diagnostic evaluation of this disorder. Unless it is known that the laboratory routinely includes a sorbitol MacConkey agar plate to screen all stools, the physician should order a stool culture—and should include *E. coli* 0157:H7 when considering this pathogen.

At the time of presentation of a patient with bloody diarrhea and on learning that a patient has a positive *E. coli* 0157:H7 culture, it is important to obtain a complete blood count, electrolytes, blood urea nitrogen (BUN), and creatinine determinations. These values become the baseline determinations in monitoring the patients for the development of extraintestinal complications of *E. coli* 0157:H7 infection, such as HUS. Urinalysis is not particularly helpful at this stage. Blood cultures almost never are positive in *E. coli* 0157:H7 infections. Sigmoidoscope examination and biopsy rarely are necessary (60).

Treatment

Antimotility agents, anticholinergic agents, or opioid narcotics should not be used. Patients with bloody diarrhea or patients with intense pain should be admitted to the hospital. The most important medical complication of *E. coli* 0157:H7 infection is HUS, which is a process that has prominent components of thrombotic and renal tubular injury. Adequate hydration counteracts microvascular thrombi to maintain organ profusion and to maintain glomerular filtration rate and renal tubular flow is the principle measure (60).

It is easy to underestimate the degree of hydration in patients infected with the *E. coli* 0157:H7. The volume of the stools produced by infected patients is not large, but evacuations are frequent. Many patients probably have some degree of vascular injury and capillary leakage, without or in advance of HUS, and such patients might not manifest the cutaneous signs of dehydration. Vomiting and poor oral intake compound the problem. Normal saline or normal saline with 5% dextrose, or lactated Ringer's solution must be adequately instituted. Potassium can be added as needed. Patients who are receiving the aforementioned fluid regimen should be monitored in the hospital by following the complete blood count closely, usually on a daily basis. A falling platelet count is the initial manifestation of microangiopathy, and a rising platelet count heralds the end of this process and can be used to stop the aggressive infusion. Urine output should be monitored closely. Referral to a specialist experienced in managing HUS should be made at the earliest suggestion of renal insufficiency (60).

Consideration for *C. difficile* arises in the setting of *E. coli* 0157:H7 infections in two situations. The first is at the time of presentation of a patient with bloody diarrhea, in whom the physician considers the possibility that acute *C. difficile* infection is the cause. In Tarr et al. (60) experience, *E. coli* 0157:H7 infections have a more fulminant onset than those caused by *C. difficile*. In the second situation, both *E. coli* 0157:H7 and *C. difficile* may occur in the same patient (60). Even in this situation, antimicrobial therapy aimed, such as metronidazole or vancomycin, at eradicating or suppressing any diagnosed *C. difficile* infection should be discouraged. Such therapy could increase the risk of developing HUS (60).

Complications

There are two important complications of *E. coli* 0157:H7 and HUS that usually become apparent in the post-HUS phase. The first is biliary lithiasis, which can occur in 10% of the children with HUS. Presumably the pigment load during the acute episode of hemolysis causes biliary sludging that progresses to gallstones. The second complication, colonic structures, may present itself after HUS as abdominal pain and bloating. Colonic structures may become apparent during the convalescent phase of HUS or within several weeks of discharge from the hospital (60).

■ AMEBIASIS

General Considerations

Amebiasis is a water-borne disease caused by the protozoan *Entamoeba histolytica*. It is transmitted by feces-oral spread. Infection with *E. histolytica* is worldwide, with the incidence as high as 50% in endemic areas (63).

E. histolytica exists in two forms: the mobile trophozoite and the cyst. The trophozoite is the parasitic form that dwells in the lumen or wall of the colon. When diarrhea occurs, the trophozoites are passed unchanged in the liquid stool. In the absence of diarrhea, the trophozoites usually encyst before leaving the gut. The cysts are highly resistant to environmental change and are responsible for transmission of the disease. The infective stage of the disease is the cyst, which gains entry to humans in food or drink contaminated by feces. Trophozoites released from the cysts in the small bowel are carried to the large bowel, where they multiply and live commensally.

The pathogenesis of invasive amebiasis requires the adherence of *E. histolytica* to colonic mucosa. *E. histolytica* contains numerous proteolytic enzymes that cause damage to the mucosa, giving rise to inflammation (64).

Clinical Features

Amebic colitis can affect all age groups, and stool tests of virtually all infected patients are positive for *E. histolytica* (65). Most patients are asymptomatic but are cyst passers and carriers. Some patients manifest with a chronic nondysenteric syndrome consisting of intermittent diarrhea, abdominal pain, flatulence, and weight loss (66). During an acute or chronic attack there is frequently some degree of liver tenderness and hepatomegaly. Diarrhea, a hallmark of disease, is caused by damage to the colonic mucosa and stimulation of intestinal secretion (67). Fulminant colitis is infrequent and has high morbidity and mortality rates. Such patients are gravely ill with fever, leukocytosis, abdominal pain, profuse bleeding, diarrhea, and occasionally gangrene and perforation of the colon. Fulminant colitis often is associated with a liver abscess.

Diagnosis

Identification of *E. histolytica* in stool, as either trophozoites or cysts, confirms the diagnosis. Proctoscopy or flexible sigmoidoscopy is useful in diagnosing asymptomatic patients. The spectrum of rectal and colonic abnormalities ranges from nonspecific thickening of the mucosa to classic flask-shaped ulcers (67). In most patients, the inflammation of the mucosa is diffuse, granular, and friable and is indistinguishable from that of ulcerative colitis. Biopsy reveals severe inflammation and numerous trophozoites (68).

The new assay using polymerase chain reaction (PCR) has been designed to detect *E. histolytica*-specific DNA. PCR has proved to be as specific as antigen detection and isoenzyme analysis for the identification of *E. histolytica* in fresh stool. Overall, PCR appears to be specific, rapid, and technically simple. Serology can be used to diagnose amebic abscess as well as amebic colitis. The indirect hemagglutination assay is 99% sensitive for amebic liver abscess (may be negative early in the disease process) and 88% sensitive for amebic colitis. Serology can be positive for years after infection (possibly secondary to colonization), which limits its specificity as a diagnostic test, especially in endemic areas (67).

Treatment

It is controversial whether asymptomatic intestinal amebiasis should be treated. Development of a liver abscess is unlikely (69). For symptomatic intestinal amebiasis, metronidazole is the drug of choice, 750 mg orally three times a day for 10 days (70). Even in such doses, metronidazole is less effective in the intestinal form than in the hepatic form of the disease. Tetracycline, 500 mg orally four times a day for 10 days, may be added.

Fulminant amebic colitis is a life-threatening disease. Once the diagnosis of fulminant amebic colitis is made, the patient must be urgently taken to the operating room. In patients with extensive involvement of the colon, a subtotal colectomy with ileostomy and the Hartmann procedure is the procedure of choice. In a series of 55 patients with fulminant or necrotizing amebic colitis, the overall mortality was 89%. Of 25 patients who required surgery, the mortality rate was 76% (71).

■ COLLAGENOUS COLITIS

General Considerations

Collagenous colitis was first described by Lindstrom (72) in 1976. It is a "new" IBD that should be suspected in older patients with watery diarrhea who have radiographically and endoscopically normal findings. It bears no known relationship to Crohn's disease or ulcerative colitis, and its pathogenesis remains unknown. More than 80% of patients with this disorder have been women, with a mean age of 60 years (73). Association with various gastrointestinal, autoimmune, and rheumatologic conditions has been observed in some patients (74).

Clinical Features

Watery diarrhea can be intermittent or continuous, from a mean of eight stools per day and up to 30, and may last for months or years. The diarrhea can be "secretory" in that it is large in volume and may not abate despite fasting. Only rarely is the diarrhea severe and acute enough to cause dehydration.

A study on the mechanism of diarrhea in collagenous colitis by Burgel et al. (75) revealed that reduced net Na^+ and Cl^- absorption is the prominent diarrheal mechanism accompanied by a secretory component of active electrogenic chloride secretion. The subepithelial collagenous band as a significant diffusion barrier is a cofactor. Down-regulation of tight junction molecules but not epithelial apoptosis is a structural correlate of barrier dysfunction contributing to diarrhea by a leak flux mechanism.

Colicky abdominal pain is often present and nausea, vomiting, weight loss, and fecal incontinence may be the accompanying features (74). Collagenous colitis is typically a chronic disease that follows a benign and sometimes remitting and relapsing course. There is only one report in the literature in which collagenous colitis may have played a role in an ultimately fatal outcome. Surgical therapy is rarely needed, with only two cases requiring colectomy for refractory disease in an extensive review of the literature by Zins et al. (74).

Diagnosis

Biopsy of colonic mucosa is essential for the diagnosis of collagenous colitis. The hallmark for the diagnosis is the subepithelial collagen layer of eosinophilic band immediately subjacent to the surface epithelium, with mild chronic inflammatory infiltrate in the lamina propria (Fig. 7) (76,77). The collagen band varies in thickness and bears no relationship to severity of the disease. A study from the Mayo Clinic included 172 patients with collagenous colitis (78). In 113 of 123 rectal biopsy specimens, 116 of 121 sigmoid specimens, and 68 of 70 descending colon biopsy specimens, the findings were diagnostic of collagenous colitis. This suggests that initial colonoscopy and procurement of proximal biopsy specimens are infrequently necessary to establish a diagnosis of collagenous colitis, and that flexible sigmoidoscopy in conjunction with biopsies is sufficient in most patients. However, 5 of 97 patients with collagenous colitis had nondiagnostic biopsies and required biopsy of the more proximal colon to establish the diagnosis. Most of these patients were treated with anti-inflammatory medication. Thus for patients in whom the diagnosis of collagenous colitis is strongly suggested, but in whom biopsy specimens obtained at flexible sigmoidoscopy are nondiagnostic, colonoscopy should be considered. The study of small bowel biopsy specimens rarely shows changes consistent with celiac sprue, and therefore small bowel biopsies to search for celiac disease seem unwarranted unless other findings suggest the presence of intestinal malabsorption.

Stool examinations in 116 patients with collagenous colitis were positive for fecal leukocytosis in 55%. This frequent finding helps to establish the inflammatory nature of collagenous colitis. However, it is not sufficiently sensitive to be used clinically in making the diagnosis (78).

Lymphocytic colitis is a condition that has many clinical similarities to those of collagenous colitis. It differs from collagenous colitis histologically only by the absence of the abnormal subepithelial collagen band in biopsy specimens (Fig. 8). The exact association between lymphocytic and collagenous colitis is unclear. Only two well-documented examples of conversion from lymphocytic to collagenous colitis are known (79).

Varghese et al. (80) reported a case of a patient with severe diarrhea caused by lymphocytic colitis and concurrent celiac sprue who did not respond to maximal medical therapy. A proctocolectomy with ideal pouch–anal anastomosis (IPAA) was performed with patient's satisfaction at eight months follow-up.

Treatment

Agents that could potentially cause diarrhea (e.g., excess caffeine, alcohol, and dairy products) should be discontinued. Nonsteroidal anti-inflammatory drugs (NSAID) use should be decreased or eliminated if possible. Antidiarrhea therapy (e.g., loperamide or diphenoxylate) is effective in many patients and is usually well tolerated. If patients do not

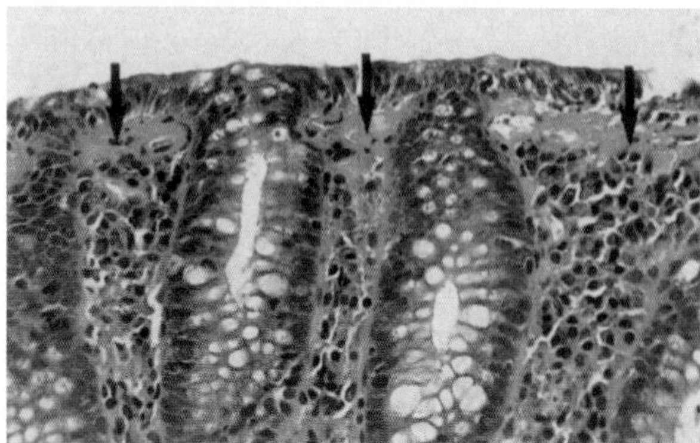

FIGURE 7 ■ Subepithelial collagen layer of eosinophilic band and inflammatory infiltrate in lamina propria in collagenous colitis (*arrows*). *Source*: Courtesy of Herschel A. Carpenter, M.D. Mayo Clinic, Rochester, MN, U.S.A.

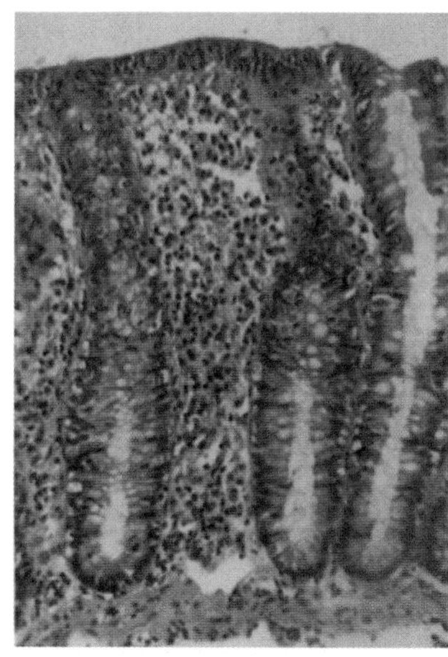

FIGURE 8 ■ Lymphocytic colitis lymphocytic infiltration in lamina propria. Note the absence of a subepithelial collagen band.

respond to these agents, treatment with bismuth subsalicylate (eight 262-mg tablets/day in divided doses) is beneficial in many patients, often with long-lasting benefit (81).

Many patients with microscopic colitis (collagenous colitis or lymphocytic colitis) are treated with mesalamine or sulfasalazine, either as first-line therapy or for those not responding to the therapy discussed above. Although these drugs were reported to be effective in the majority of patients, several large series have reported a benefit in fewer than 50% of patients. Cholestyramine therapy may be more effective, but many patients do not tolerate it due to its texture or side effects (82).

Patients refractory to medications outlined above may respond to corticosteroids. Corticosteroids have been among the most effective drugs used for therapy in large uncontrolled series. However, relapse after steroid withdrawal is common with many patients becoming steroid-dependent. Thus, before beginning corticosteroid therapy, the diagnosis should be reconsidered an alternative diagnosis, such as coexistent celiac sprue or infection, should be excluded (81).

Budesonide, a potent synthetic steroid with high first-pass hepatic metabolism, resulting in low systemic bioavailability and less risk of side effects, has been effective in three placebo-controlled trials (82–84). The response rate in those treated with budesonide ranges from 57% to 100% which was superior to response to placebo in each study. In these controlled trials, there was little or no toxicity, but relapse was common after stopping treatment.

For steroid-refractory or steroid-dependent patients, immunomodulation therapy with azathioprine or six-mercaptopurine can be used, although side effects are common (81).

RISK OF CARCINOMA

One of the most serious complications of ulcerative colitis is the development of colon and rectal carcinoma. The most important risk factors are total involvement of the large bowel and long duration (85,86). Young age at the onset of colitis is probably not an independent risk factor; however, since younger patients have an early onset of risk, the duration of risk is longer, leading to a relatively high cumulative incidence of carcinoma (85). Duration and extent of the disease are the most important risk factors for development of carcinoma (87,88). Patients may develop carcinoma after 5 to 10 years of the disease, but the risk is only approximately 3%, and some authors have not found any carcinoma during the first decade. The risk becomes obvious after 10 years and rises to 50% and 75% after 30 and 40 years of disease, respectively (Fig. 9) (86).

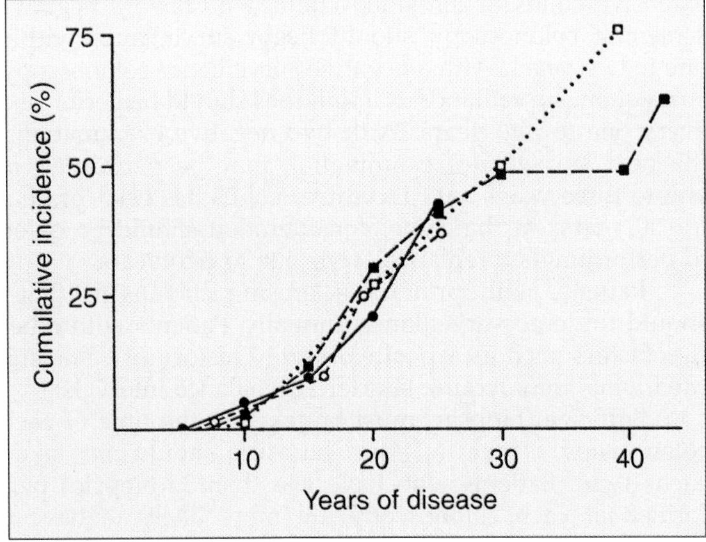

FIGURE 9 ■ Risk of carcinoma in extensive ulcerative colitis. Note the identical risk in four different series. *Source*: From Ref. 86.

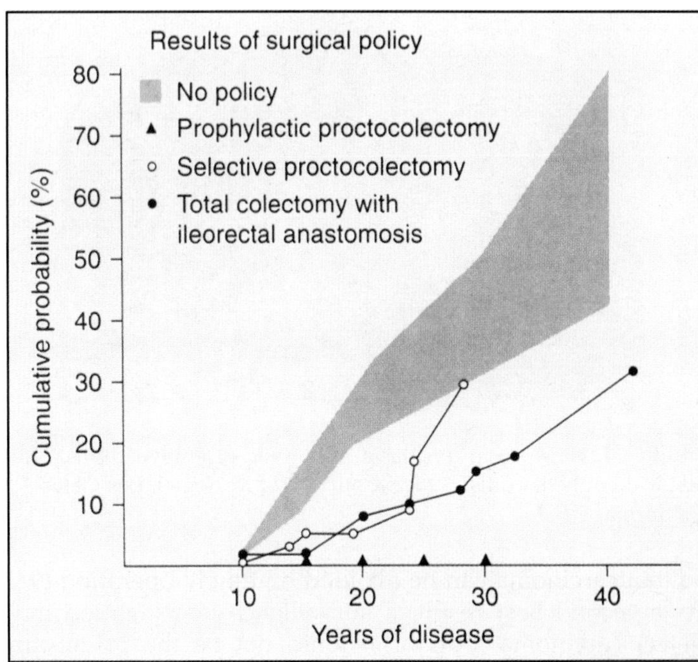

FIGURE 10 ■ Surgical treatment reduces incidence of carcinoma in ulcerative colitis. *Source*: From Ref. 86.

In long-standing extensive ulcerative colitis, the severity of colonic inflammation, as detected by colonoscopic biopsy histologic examination, is an important determinant of the risk of colorectal neoplasia. There have been a few reports of large-bowel carcinoma in patients with ulcerative colitis that was limited to the rectum and/or left colon (85,89,90).

There is an increased risk of colorectal carcinoma among patients with left-sided ulcerative colitis, but this risk is substantially lower compared to the risk among patients with pancolitis. Moreover, the latency period is 10 to 15 years longer compared to pancolitis before patients with left-sided colitis are at risk of colorectal carcinoma (87,88).

The only effective way to prevent carcinoma of the large bowel in ulcerative colitis is a total proctocolectomy (TPC). Preserving the rectum with colectomy and ileorectal anastomosis does not protect completely against the development of rectal carcinoma. Again, the risk increases with time (Fig. 10) (86).

SURVEILLANCE

Periodic follow-up of patients with long-standing ulcerative colitis with endoscopy, particularly colonoscopy and biopsy, has been a common practice. The goal of surveillance or "watch-over" is to detect premalignant changes

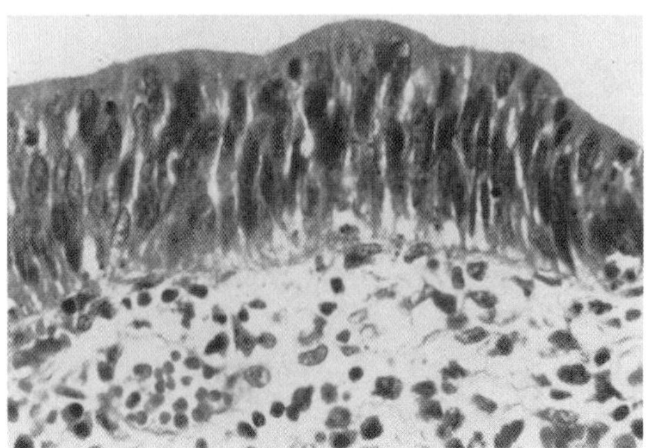

FIGURE 11 ■ Mucosal dysplasia in chronic ulcerative colitis. Note atypical epithelial cells. *Source*: Courtesy of M. Segall, Los Gatos, California, U.S.A.

so that carcinoma can be avoided by timely operation (91). As a second best result, a surveillance investigation may detect carcinoma, but this should not be the prime aim because invasive malignancy is always dangerous. This strategy is based on the assumption that a dysplastic lesion (Fig. 11) can be detected before invasive carcinoma has developed. So far there has been no valid epidemiologic evidence that carcinoma surveillance in ulcerative colitis saves lives. However, circumstantial evidence suggests that it does (91).

Lennard-Jones (91) reviewed the reports of four series, each from a hospital serving a local region (92–95). A total of 423 patients, most of whom had extensive ulcerative colitis, were investigated regularly by colonoscopy (1844 examinations) over a period of 12 to 15 years between 1973 and 1991. A small number of patients with dysplasia or carcinoma were seen over a relatively long period of time. No death from carcinoma occurred during surveillance in any series, but 11 (2.6%) of 425 patients were operated upon for premalignant lesions and three (0.6%) for curable Dukes' stage A carcinoma. Only two deaths from carcinoma occurred outside the program. The importance of initial screening colonoscopy was demonstrated.

Encouraging results from the surgical treatment for carcinoma found as a result of a surveillance program have been observed. These hospitals reported five-year survival rates of 77%, 88%, and 87%, respectively, after surgical treatment of patients with carcinoma detected as the results of a surveillance program. In each hospital, these figures exceeded the survival rates of 37%, 15%, and 55%, respectively, observed among other patients surgically treated for colorectal carcinoma–complicating ulcerative colitis (96,97). Although these comparisons do not constitute proof that surveillance allows treatment of carcinoma at an earlier stage than among patients outside the program, the results are suggestive and encouraging (91).

■ PROBLEMS WITH COLONOSCOPY AND BIOPSY

Colonoscopy has several limitations. First, neoplastic mucosa may appear endoscopically normal, making it impossible to identify suspicious areas that should be biopsied. Second, when random biopsies are performed, only a very small portion of the colon is sampled, and the potential for sampling error is great. Third, colonoscopy with biopsy carries a risk of misinterpretation by the pathologist. Expert pathologists estimate that up to 48% of patients with low-grade dysplasia (LGD) may be misdiagnosed as having only ulcerative colitis. Such errors are due to combination of sampling and interpretive difficulties with colonoscopic biopsies. Likewise, the false-negative rates for high-grade dysplasia (HGD) and carcinoma are estimated at 40% and 10%, respectively. False-positive rates range from 2% (for LGD diagnosed as HGD) to 15% (for ulcerative colitis diagnosed as LGD). Thus, the accuracy of surveillance is somewhat limited (98,99). Since it is well accepted that the risk of colorectal carcinoma in ulcerative colitis is greater than that of the general population, colonoscopic surveillance of patients with ulcerative colitis should be supported. In most studies, the compliance of patients in surveillance programs is excellent, in the neighborhood of 85% to 91% (98).

Physicians and surgeons should also recognize the limited nature of the existing data on dysplasia surveillance and shakiness of the premise on which such a costly practice is based. An analysis of 10 prospective studies of dysplasia surveillance with a total of 1225 patients has shown that when colectomy is performed for HGD, carcinoma is already present in 30% to 40% of the patients (100). Of particular concern is that approximately half of these carcinomas are advanced (Dukes' stage C or D). If the practice of surveillance is to wait for HGD to develop before recommending colectomy, it would be too late. The probability of finding carcinoma in patients undergoing colectomy with low grade or indefinite dysplasia is also worrisome (8–9%), although the data in this category are insufficient to be conclusive (100).

■ A PRACTICAL GUIDE

In the absence of randomized prospective trials, it is not possible to determine the full impact of dysplasia surveillance in patients with ulcerative colitis. The following is a practical guide (101,102).

Colonoscopy should be performed in ulcerative colitis patients eight to ten years after the onset of ulcerative colitis symptoms. At the time of this examination, the extent of disease should also be evaluated. Patients with extensive colitis or left-sided colitis who have a negative screening colonoscopy should begin surveillance within one to two years. With a negative surveillance colonoscopy, subsequent surveillance examinations should be performed every one to two years. With two negative examinations, the next surveillance examination may be performed in one to three years until ulcerative colitis has been present for 20 years. At that time, consideration should be given to performing surveillance every one to two years.

Patients with primary sclerosing cholangitis (PSC) should undergo surveillance annually. Patients with other risk factors such as a positive family history of colorectal carcinoma, may require shorter surveillance intervals.

Sufficient biopsies must be taken at the time of each colonoscopy. Three to four biopsies should be taken each 10 cm. Patients who have less than 33 biopsies performed at each colonoscopy are more likely to have a missed diagnosis for dysplasia.

One or more biopsies reported "indefinite for dysplasia" should be reviewed by an experienced gastrointestinal pathologist. If the diagnosis is confirmed, a follow-up surveillance examination should be performed within three to six months.

Any biopsies reported "positive for low-grade dysplasia (LGD)" should be confirmed by an experienced gastrintestinal pathologist. Controversy exists about the management of LGD because the natural history is unknown at this time. There is evidence showing that LGD may progress to HGD or even colorectal carcinoma. An unrecognized synchronous colorectal carcinoma may already be present in up to 20% of individuals who undergo surgery shortly thereafter.

A patient confirmed to have multifocal flat LGD (two or more biopsies with LGD from a single screening or surveillance examination) or repetitive flat LGD (two or more examinations with at least a single focus on LGD) should be strongly encouraged to undergo prophylactic total proctocolectomy. Recent evidence indicates that the five-year rate of progression to HGD or colorectal carcinoma for patients with confirmed unifocal LGD (only one biopsy positive for LGD) seems to be similar to that of multifocal LGD. Therefore, such a patient should also be offered the option of undergoing prophylactic proctocolectomy.

If an operative strategy is deferred and the patient elects to continue with surveillance, a repeat examination should be performed within three months or no later than six months from the discovery of LGD. Repeat examinations should include sufficient samplings so that there is no error in the histologic diagnosis. It must be stressed that for patients who elect to pursue a nonoperative strategy for LGD, subsequent negative examinations (i.e., no dysplasia) is not sufficiently reassuring to return to routine surveillance. Therefore, continued more frequent examinations (less than or equal to six months) should be pursued.

As with LGD, finding of HGD should be confirmed by a pathologist from an expert center. If confirmed total proctocolectomy should be performed, given the high rate of synchronous and metachronous adenocarcinoma.

Raised lesions encountered within areas of colitis may include one or more polyps that visually resemble sporadic adenomas and may be amenable to complete polypectomy. If polypectomy is complete and biopsies of surrounding mucosa (four biopsies taken immediately adjacent to the raised lesion and submitted separately) are negative for dysplasia, and, in addition, there is no dysplasia elsewhere in the colon, a follow-up examination should be performed within six months, with regular surveillance resumed if no dysplosia is found. However, if dysplasia is present in the surrounding mucosa, or if dysplastic polypoid lesion is nonresectable or does not resemble a typical adenoma, a high risk of associated synchronous colorectal carcinoma would justify recommending a complete proctocolectomy. The alternative option of segmental colectomy has not been evaluated in the literature and should be restricted to carefully selected patients with serious mitigating circumstances. Marking a raised lesion with India ink at the time of colonoscopy is advisable.

Adenoma-like polyps encountered in areas of the colon that are endoscopically and microscopically free of disease involvement may be managed according to standard recommendations for postpolypectomy follow-up of sporadic adenomas.

In special circumstances, prophylactic proctocolectomy may be recommended in the absence of LGD or HGD. Such special situations include the persistence of symptomatic ulcerative colitis requiring intermittent or persistent steroid therapy for 15 to 20 years or the presence of multiple pseudopolyps that may hide dysplastic lesions or make it difficult to obtain suitable biopsies.

The need for molecular screening of patients with long-standing extensive ulcerative colitis is well recognized. Detection p55 and K-*ras* mutations in patients with ulcerative colitis have been detected. Although promising, this technique is not yet ready for practical use (103–105).

EXTRACOLONIC MANIFESTATIONS

There are many extracolonic manifestations of IBD. The most serious are the hepatobiliary disorders

HEPATIC DYSFUNCTION

Asymptomatic parenchymal liver disease with liver function test abnormalities is the most common manifestation (106). Fatty infiltration of the liver is present in as many as 50% of patients with ulcerative colitis, and cirrhosis is present in 3% to 4% (107,108). Control of the primary disease medically or surgically will reverse or improve the fatty infiltration of the liver, but once cirrhosis has developed, it is irreversible. Pericholangitis frequently is associated with IBD. It may not be clinically apparent, but liver function tests may reveal elevated aspartate transaminase (AST), or serum glutamic oxaloacetic transaminase (SGOT). The diagnosis is confirmed by a liver biopsy that shows intensive infiltration of the portal triads.

PRIMARY SCLEROSING CHOLANGITIS AND BILE DUCT CARCINOMA

PSC is a chronic cholestatic syndrome of unknown cause characterized by fibrosis of the intrahepatic and extrahepatic bile ducts (109,110). It is associated almost specifically with CUC and is uncommon with Crohn's disease (111). PSC is diagnosed best by endoscopic retrograde cholangiopancreatography, which shows characteristic bead-like extrahepatic and intrahepatic bile ducts (112) (Fig. 12).

The frequency of PSC in patients with IBD has been reported to be between 7.4% and 7.5%. This probably underestimates the true number of cases because no systematic cholangiographic studies have been performed in asymptomatic IBD patients. Most IBD patients who develop PSC are younger than 40 years of age, and 70% of the patients are men. PSC may manifest preceding development of IBD for as long as seven years (113). Some investigators suggest that nearly all patients with PSC have developed or will subsequently develop IBD (114).

Whether total proctocolectomy will reverse or improve the condition has been a subject of debate for some time. Cangemi et al. (109) prospectively studied the progression of clinical, biochemical, cholangiographic, and hepatic histologic features in 45 patients with PSC associated with ulcerative colitis. Twenty patients who had undergone proctocolectomy were compared with 25

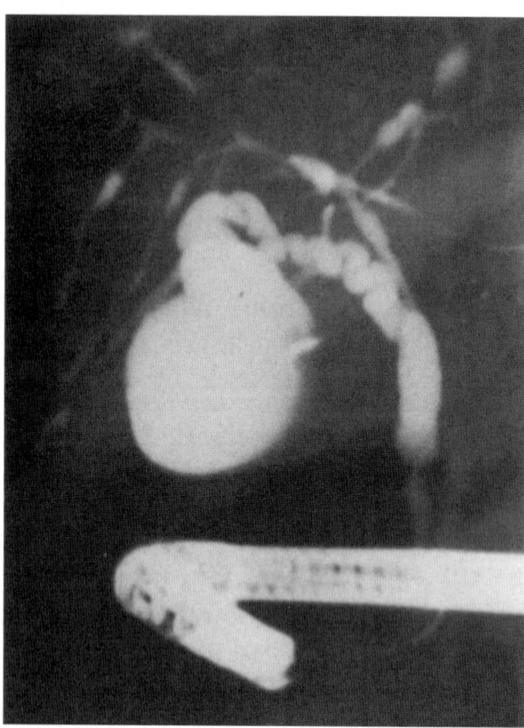

FIGURE 12 ■ Endoscopic retrograde cholangiopancreatography shows characteristic beadlike bile ducts in primary sclerosing cholangitis. *Source*: From Ref. 112.

patients who had not. All patients were followed up for a minimum of one year, and the overall duration of follow-up was similar in both groups (4.1 vs. 3.9 years). The results revealed that proctocolectomy for ulcerative colitis has no beneficial effect on PSC.

Substantial evidence suggests that genetic susceptibility and immunologic factors play a pivotal role in the development of PSC. The HLA-B8 haplotype and the HIA-DR3 haplotype are found in the majority of patients with ulcerative colitis and PSC. Patients with ulcerative colitis and the HLA-B8 and HLA-DR3 haplotypes have been estimated to have a 10-fold increase in the relative risk of developing PSC (115). A number of humoral abnormalities have been documented in PSC. Hypergammaglobulinemia, high titers of smooth muscle antibody (SMA) and antinuclear antibody (ANA), neutrophil-specific nuclear antibody (ANNA), and antineutrophil cytoplasmic antibody (ANCA) have been reported (114). Various cellular immune abnormalities have also been observed in patients with PSC. There is a significant decrease in the total number of circulatory T-cells because of a large decrease in the suppressor and/or cytotoxic T-cell component (116,117).

Many patients with PSC are asymptomatic and are diagnosed because of a cholestatic biochemical profile identified during a routine examination. Among symptomatic patients, the most common complaints are the insidious onset of fatigue and pruritus and jaundice. Other symptoms include abdominal pain, fever, and weight loss as well as the complications of severe liver disease such as bleeding varices, ascites, and encephalopathy. Patients may exhibit manifestations of other immune diseases such as thyroiditis and chronic active hepatitis as well as symptoms of chronic pancreatitis. The differential diagnosis of PSC includes secondary sclerosing cholangitis, primary biliary cirrhosis, extrahepatic obstruction, chronic active hepatitis, and idiopathic adulthood ductopenia (114).

The natural history of PSC is important to define because it allows assessment of prognosis in individual patients and helps identify at what juncture medical or surgical intervention should be undertaken. In general, PSC is a progressive disease that can lead to liver failure and death. A median survival time of 9 to 12 years appears to be independent of geographic and environmental influences. In asymptomatic patients, the 8-year survival is 80%; in symptomatic patients the 8-year survival is 50% (118).

Treatment of PSA is often palliative. Only liver transplantation is curative. Some medications have been used with minimal success to slow the progress of the disease.

Antibiotics are often used to treat cholangitis. Cholestyramine is also used to treat pruritus (114). Corticosteroids combined with colchicine showed no benefit (119). Azathioprine and 6-MP have not been shown to help (120). A double-blind, placebo-controlled prospective trial of d-penicillamine showed no beneficial effects (121).

High doses of ursodeoxycholic acid [(UDCA) 25 to 30 mg/kg/day] have been shown to substantially improve in biochemical, cholangiographic, and histologic parameters. UCDA is associated with immunomodulatory effect and is approved for the treatment of primary biliary cirrhosis (122). UDCA has also shown to significantly decrease the risk for developing colorectal dysplasia or carcinoma in patients with ulcerative colitis and PSC (123).

In a meta-analysis using MEDLINE search by Soetikno et al. (124), comparing the risk of colorectal neoplasia (dysplasia and carcinoma) in patients with ulcerative colitis with and without PSC, 11 studies met all the eligibility criteria for the meta-analysis. Patients with ulcerative colitis and PSC are at increased risk of colorectal dysplasia and carcinoma compared with patients with ulcerative colitis alone; OR 4.79 with the Mantel-Haenszel method. This increased risk is present even when the risk of colorectal carcinoma alone is considered; OR 4.09 using Mantel-Haenszel method. Patients with ulcerative colitis associated with PSC should have more intensive colonoscopic surveillance.

In patients who require proctocolectomy because of intractable ulcerative colitis, or because of colorectal mucosal dysplasia or carcinoma, an ileoanal pouch can be done if there is no contraindication such as carcinoma of low rectum (125). Unless orthotopic liver transplantation (OLT) is planned, every effort should be made to avoid a permanent ileostomy because peri-ileostomy varices may develop if the patient's condition progresses to portal hypertension.

OLT is the only known curative treatment for PSC (126). Prophylactic proctocolectomy before OLT is not necessary (127). Among 57 patients who underwent OLT for PSC and ulcerative colitis performed at Mayo Clinic, none of the patients had their colon or rectum removed. Three patients developed colorectal carcinoma, with a mean follow-up of 4.2 years, an incidence approximately 1% per person per year. The cumulative incidence of dysplasia was 15% at five years and 21% at eight years after OLT. However, this risk of colorectal neoplasia (dysplasia and carcinoma) had no impact on patient survival (127). The Birmingham group reported by Vera et al. (128) found that the incidence of colorectal carcinoma after OLT was 5.3% (8 of 152 patients with PSC), compared with 0.6% (7 of 1184) in non-PSC cases. All colorectal carcinomas in the PSC group were in patients with ulcerative colitis and an intact colon, with the cumulative risk 14% and 17% after 5 and 10 years, respectively. The risk factors for colorectal carcinoma were colonic dysplasia after OLT, duration of colitis longer than 10 years, and pancolitis. Patients with colorectal carcinoma had a reduced five-year survival of 55% versus 75%.

ARTHRITIS

An extensive study in patients with ulcerative colitis by Orchard et al. (129) showed that peripheral arthropathies Type I occurred in 3.6% of patients and Type II occurred in 2.5%. Type I (pauciarticular) is defined as less than five joints involved. In this type, the condition is acute, self-limited attacks (less than 10 weeks). It often coincides with relapses of the colitis. It is strongly associated with extraintestinal manifestations of IBD. Type II (polyarticular) is defined as five or more joints involved. In this type, the symptoms usually persist for months to years. It runs a course independent of the colitis. It is associated with uveitis but not with other extraintestinal manifestations.

The pathophysiology of joint pain in IBD is now better understood. Mucosal inflammation can absorb specific bacterial products, dietary antigens, and digestive enzymes. There are reports of detectable levels of serum bacterial lipopolysaccharides, formulated oligopeptides, and antibodies to bacteria lipid A and peptidoglycan (130). Such absorption is germane to the production of distant inflammation because these microbial products can activate immunoregulatory cells, complement, and the kallikrein system and forward the production of proinflammatory cytokines (131).

Synovitis may occur without obvious clinical disease, a picture most frequently described in infancy. Synovitis has a sudden joint pain with frequent effusion and tenderness. Acute synovitis occurs in approximately 20% of patients, and most commonly in association with increased activity of the disease. The patterns of joint involvement are consistent with large joints, particularly knees, ankles, hips, and shoulders. This typical abrupt, self-limiting, and nondeforming arthritis mirrors only a transient exposure to peptidoglycan and is improved by medical therapies that alter bacterial flora or restore a degree of mucosal integrity through the reduction of inflammation (131). Arthritis alone is not an indication for bowel resection.

ANKYLOSING SPONDYLITIS AND SACROILIITIS

In IBD, the majority of sacroiliitis patients are clinically asymptomatic, yet 65% of patients have abnormal magnetic resonance imaging (MRI) results. Progressive joint sclerosis may occur in patients who exhibit continuing infection (131).

Ankylosing spondylitis occurs in 3–5% of patients with IBD. Those at highest risk are HLA-B27 positive and have a family member with either idiopathic ankylosing spondylitis or another spondyloarthropathic syndrome (131).

It is important to remember that sacroiliac joints are uniformly involved in ankylosing spondylitis and that this axial progression occurs without an apparent contemporaneous relationship to clinically active inflammatory bowel disease. Physical examination reveals tenderness of the sacroiliac joint, global loss of truncal motion, flattening of the lumbar lordosis, and in cases of advanced disease, decreased chest expansion and cervical fusion in forward flexion. In long-standing ankylosing spondylitis, spinal pain in the lumbar or thoracic region may eventually disappear as the spinal ligaments or the apophyseal joints ossify. In general, any recurrence of lumbar pain or a change in the character of cervical pain signifies a spinal neurologic complication such as cervical atlantoaxial subluxation (131).

Medical or surgical treatment has little or no effect on sacroiliitis or ankylosing spondylitis. The goal of treatment is the retardation of disability and the limiting of deformity. Exercise programs emphasizing deep breathing, swimming, and erect posture should be considered, especially for those who are HLA-B27 positive who may have a more aggressive course. Although few clinical symptoms may appear, cortical and trabecular bone loss may approach 1% to 2.5% of bone mass per year (131).

ERYTHEMA NODOSUM

The most common cutaneous manifestation of IBD is erythema nodosum, arising in at least 10% to 15% of patients with ulcerative colitis and Crohn's disease. It appears early in the course of IBD, and, in almost 80% of cases, in conjunction with some form of peripheral arthropathy. The clinical appearance of tender, symmetric, distributed, subcutaneous red and raised nodules is a reflection of the critical pathologic feature of a septal panniculitis composed primarily of a lymphohistiocytic infiltrate. The probable cause is a bacterial antigen or inflammatory cell products (131).

Of all the extraintestinal manifestations, erythema nodosum is the most responsive to treatment of the bowel, and persistence of the lesions indicates inadequate control of the IBD (132). Treatment with prednisone 40 mg/day as a simple morning dose is recommended (133). For steroid-refractory patients with mild to moderate gut symptoms, azathioprine should be used, and if not tolerated, methotrexate. For severely active, steroid-refractory disease, proctocolectomy should be considered (132).

PYODERMA GANGRENOSUM

An uncommon but serious condition, pyoderma gangrenosum occurs almost exclusively in patients with IBD. The lesion begins as an erythematous plaque, papule, or bleb, usually situated on the pretibial region but occasionally elsewhere. Lesions soon progress into an ulcerated, necrotizing, and painful wound with ragged, purple–red margins. They are multiple in 71% of patients and over half are situated below the knees. In the series from St. Mark's Hospital (134), ulcerative colitis was active in 50% and Crohn's disease was active in 75% of patients when pyoderma gangrenosum was diagnosed. The cause is most likely immunologic in origin.

Pyoderma gangrenosum may or may not parallel activity of IBD. The treatment is to control activity of IBD with steroids and to use topical agents, such as an antibiotic cream. Intravenous cyclosporine may be helpful in healing persistent lesions (135). Pyoderma adjacent to an ileostomy is best treated medically and with modifications of the appliance under the supervision of an enterostomal therapist. Surgical relocation of the stoma to an uninvolved site is the last resort, because the lesions may recur at the new stoma (132).

ULCERS OF MOUTH

Aphthous ulcerations of the buccal mucosa, soft palate, gums, lips, tongue, and uvula are frequent complications of IBD. They do not parallel the activity of the bowel disease (132). Treatment is symptomatic. Control of the active bowel disease helps resolve these oral lesions. In addition, a variety of local therapeutic measures are helpful, including topical anesthetic or the use of triamcinolone in Orabase (135).

EYE DISEASES

Ocular complications in IBD include episcleritis, uveitis, iritis, and conjunctivitis. It occurs in less than 10% of cases, but can be associated with significant morbidity, including blindness (136). Episcleritis is the most common abnormality and is characterized by a rapid development of eye redness but without loss of vision. Iritis and uveitis are uncommon but are much more serious complications with acute onset of painful eyes associated with blurred vision and headache. These complications may precede the development of IBD (131,137).

The basic treatment is to treat the underlying IBD.

A high index of suspicion is vital to detect and properly manage the pleomorphic spectrum of eye disease associated with IBD. The patient with a red eye associated with a visual defect or severe eye pain requires immediate referral to a specialist. Vomiting in the context of a unilateral red eye must be managed as acute angle closure glaucoma until an alternative diagnosis is secure. Infectious complications such as viral conjunctivitis are very contagious and easily transmitted to health personnel and other patients. Clinicians must be aware of the diverse spectrum of eye involvement in IBD and include routine ocular evaluation in the care of these multisystem diseases (138).

ULCERATIVE COLITIS AND PREGNANCY

A review of 10 series comprising more than 1300 pregnancies reported by Miller (139) revealed that the average patient with ulcerative colitis has a very good chance of a normal full-term delivery. Data from Korelitz (140) showed that 83% of mothers with ulcerative colitis delivered healthy newborns. Premature delivery was noted in 2.5% and spontaneous abortion in 12%, but no stillbirths or congenital abnormalities were observed. Babies born to mothers with ulcerative colitis exhibit lower-than-normal birth weights, but these results do not achieve statistical significance. Ulcerative colitis does not affect the mode of delivery or the incidence of preeclampsia or eclampsia during the gestational period (141).

If ulcerative colitis is quiescent at the onset of pregnancy, the odds favor that it will remain quiescent throughout. If, on the other hand, the disease is active, it will likely continue to be active or worsen during pregnancy. However, if the patient with active ulcerative colitis is brought into remission with drug therapy, the course of the disease is similar to that of the patient whose disease is quiescent at the onset of pregnancy. Exacerbation or worsening of the disease during pregnancy most likely occurs during the first trimester. The postpartum course of the disease is based on the continuation of the disease during the last month of pregnancy (140).

Most drugs used in the treatment of the pregnant IBD patient are the same as those used in patients who are not pregnant. These drugs include corticosteroids, sulfasalazine, 5-aminosalicylic acid (5-ASA), antibiotics, and immunosuppressive medications, all of which might be already established when pregnancy is recognized. Sulfonamides have generally been considered safe medications during all stages of pregnancy and lactation. Sulfasalazine reaches the breast milk at a level equal to 45% of that in the maternal serum. These medications can cross the placenta and displace unconjugated bilirubin from albumin, introducing a theoretical risk of drug-induced neonatal jaundice and kernicterus. The amount of sulfasalazine in breast milk is negligible. Neither sulfasalazine nor 5-ASA has been shown to cause harm to the neonate (140).

Steroids are well tolerated by the fetus. This is probably because the concentration of steroids in the fetus is one-eighth that in the mother (140). Experimental studies have implicated azathioprine and 6-MP in low fetal birth weights and congenital abnormalities. Seven of 103 neonates born to human renal transplant recipients who took azathioprine at a higher dose than that used to treat IBD, demonstrated birth defects (140,141). However, Alstead et al. (142) showed no complications in the fetus when azathioprine had been continued throughout pregnancy.

DRUGS FOR ULCERATIVE COLITIS

Medications have remained the primary treatment for ulcerative colitis. There are several drugs that are effective in the treatment of ulcerative colitis. The surgeons should be familiar with them.

SULFASALAZINE (AZULFIDINE)

Sulfasalazine has been a mainstay of treatment for CUC since the 1950s. It consists of 5-ASA linked by an azo bond to sulfapyridine. 5-ASA is the therapeutic component. When ingested orally, sulfasalazine is largely unabsorbed from the small intestine and delivered intact to the colon, where the azo bond is split by bacteria to release 5-ASA, which exerts a topical action on inflamed colonic mucosa. The sulfapyridine component, which is largely absorbed, systemically accounts for much of the toxicity of sulfasalazine. The precise mechanism of action of 5-ASA in IBD is unknown but may involve the inhibition of leukotriene synthesis, inhibition of granulocyte activation, or scavenging of oxygen-derived free radicals. Up to 50% of patients taking sulfasalazine experience at least one side effect produced by the drug. However, most side effects are not serious and are reversible. Dose-related side effects are most common and include anorexia, nausea, vomiting, epigastric discomfort, and headache. Rarely, a dose-related hemolytic anemia is clinically evident. More rare idiosyncratic reactions to sulfasalazine include fever, rash, exfoliative dermatitis, neutropenia, agranulocytosis, pancreatitis, hepatitis, pneumonitis, polyarteritis, pulmonary infiltration, and lupus erythematosus. Reversible decreases in sperm number or function are common in men taking sulfasalazine, and infertility may result. Most toxicity resulting from sulfasalazine is thought to relate to sulfapyridine moiety rather than the 5-ASA component. In patients who experience fever or skin rashes, desensitization has permitted the reintroduction of the drug in selected cases at a very low initial dose, after which the dose is increased gradually in small increments. However, sulfasalazine should not be resumed after a serious or life-threatening reaction (143).

■ AMINOSALICYLATES

The anti-inflammatory properties of 5-ASA are apparently related to its topical effects on the inflamed colonic mucosa. If administered orally, 5-ASA (mesalamine) is rapidly absorbed in the small intestine and excreted in the urine. Thus, it does not reach the colon in amounts sufficient to be therapeutically effective. In some delayed-release forms, such as Asacol (Procter & Gamble, Cincinnati, Ohio, U.S.A.) and Rowasa (Solvay Pharmaceuticals, Marietta, Georgia, U.S.A.), 5-ASA is coated with an acrylic resin that dissolves only at an intraluminal pH > 6 (Asacol) or 7, thus allowing delivery of 5-ASA to the distal ileum and colon where the intraluminal pH approaches 6 to 7. In another slow-release formulation of 5-ASA, Pentasa (Merion Merrell Dow, Kansas City, Missouri, U.S.A.) capsules dissolve in the stomach to release microgranules of 5-ASA coated with a semi-permeable membrane of ethylcellulose. This mechanism allows release of 5-ASA throughout the gastrointestinal tract, including the small intestine. Pentasa was, in fact, developed for the treatment of small bowel Crohn's disease and preliminary trials suggested that it might be effective. Pentasa has also been known to be effective in maintaining remission of ulcerative colitis (143).

In a second type of oral 5-ASA preparation, 5-ASA is linked to a carrier less toxic or less absorbent systemically than sulfapyridine. The prototype of such azo bond components is olsalazine (Dipentum, Kabi Pharmacia, Piscatawai, New Jersey, U.S.), which consists of two 5-ASA molecules linked by an azo bond (143).

Like sulfasalazine, olsalazine must undergo bacterial cleavage in the colon to allow release of the 5-ASA. One common side effect of olsalazine not seen as often with other 5-ASA compounds is diarrhea, which occurs in up to 20% of patients who receive the drug. The diarrhea is thought to result from olsalazine-induced stimulation of ileal secretion of fluid and electrolytes and often subsides despite continuation of the drug, which should be taken with meals (143).

Renal function should be monitored in all patients receiving 5-ASA preparations because of the known nephrotoxic effects in rats and rare reports of nephrotoxicity in humans. However, long-term 5-ASA therapy has been proven to be as safe with regard to nephrotoxicity as maintenance sulfasalazine therapy (143).

In the treatment of severe ulcerative pancolitis, there is no evidence that high-dose oral 5-ASA is better than or even comparable to systemic corticosteroids. In patients with inactive to moderately active ulcerative colitis, who are established on and tolerating sulfasalazine therapy, there appears to be no benefit in switching to an oral 5-ASA preparation. 5-ASA enemas have been shown to be at least as effective as hydrocortisone enemas as initial therapy or for relapses of distal ulcerative colitis and effective for maintenance of remission as well. A response is often seen in three to six weeks but occasionally may take as long as four to six months. In the treatment of distal ulcerative colitis, 5-ASA enemas are probably more effective than oral 5-ASA combinations. Enema preparations have the limitation generally of reaching only the splenic flexure of the colon. They are also inconvenient for long-term maintenance therapy and are quite expensive. Suppositories containing 500 mg of 5-ASA have shown benefits in the treatment of proctitis when administered two or three times a day (143).

■ CORTICOSTEROIDS

Corticosteroids are effective drugs for the treatment of ulcerative colitis because of their broad spectrum of anti-inflammatory and immunosuppressive actions. They suppress inflammatory mediators, inhibit neutrophil and macrophage chemotaxis, and depress cellular immunity. In ulcerative colitis, steroids act primarily to alter the immune function of leukocytes in the gut wall. Alternative immunosuppressive drugs are for the most part less potent, have a slower onset of action, and are toxic. Thus, therapy with prednisone or prednisolone is a mainstay of treatment for patients with moderate to severe exacerbations of ulcerative colitis who do not respond to 5-ASAs (144). Although response rates to steroids are high, efficacy comes at a significant cost. Unpleasant cosmetic effects caused by glucocorticoids are almost universal. Further, more serious metabolic consequences, such as hypertension, diabetes mellitus, osteoporosis, and an increased susceptibility to infection, are frequent. In the absence of safe, effective alternatives to long-term corticosteroid therapy, many patients opt for colectomy to treat their disease. There is no evidence that corticosteroids maintain remission in ulcerative colitis or Crohn's disease (144).

■ BUDESONIDE

Budesonide is a second generation corticosteroid. Taken orally, it has greater than 100 times higher affinity for the steroid receptor than hydrocortisone and has a rapid first-pass metabolism through the liver, thereby reducing systemic exposure (145,146). When administered as an enema, only 10% to 15% of the active drug reaches the systemic circulation. An enema preparation of budesonide has been effective for distal ulcerative colitis (147). However, the reduction of systemic side effects of budesonide as compared with prednisone is relative. At high doses, the full spectrum of glucocorticoid-associated side effects can be observed. Budesonide is much more expensive than prednisone (145).

■ ANTIBIOTICS

Although metronidazole has become an important drug in the treatment of colonic and perineal Crohn's disease, it does not appear to be effective in treating ulcerative colitis.

■ IMMUNOSUPPRESSIVE DRUGS

The immunosuppressant azathioprine and its metabolite 6-mercaptopurine, used in association with corticosteroids, may be useful in treating ulcerative colitis unresponsive to standard therapy alone. The mechanism of action is unknown but may involve an inhibitory effect on T-cell production. Azathioprine and 6-mercaptopurine also appear to prevent relapses in patients with ulcerative colitis, although long-term maintenance therapy with these drugs is often avoided because of the concern about the increased risk of malignancy. The adverse effects of azathioprine and 6-mercaptopurine include acute pancreatitis in approximately 3% and fever and rash in 2% of those given the drugs (148). Nausea is common, and in some patients drug-induced diarrhea may be confused with a flare-up of bowel disease. Concerns about lymphoma and bone marrow suppression have been raised, but these complications appear with a standard drug dose of 50 mg per day. The patient's peripheral blood counts should be monitored during therapy (143).

Cyclosporine, an immunosuppressant used to prevent rejection of transplanted organs, has been used in the treatment of refractory IBD. Cyclosporine is a peptide originally derived from soil fungi that causes a depression of helper T-cell function and inhibits interleukin-2. It appears to have a more rapid onset of action than either azathioprine or 6-mercaptopurine, and benefit is often seen within two weeks. The first multicenter controlled trial using cyclosporine, 4 mg/kg/day by continuous infusion, improves 82% of patients with severe ulcerative colitis compared to 0% of patients receiving placebo (149). Cyclosporine may prove useful in preventing, or at least in delaying, the need for urgent surgery. Cyclosporine has also shown promise when administered as enemas to patients with refractory distal ulcerative colitis. By this route of administration, cyclosporine is thought to act locally, because it undergoes first-pass intestinal metabolism (150). Oral cyclosporine therapy is complicated by slow, incomplete, and variable intestinal absorption (147).

The major drawbacks of cyclosporine are its expense and side effects, including hypertension, renal dysfunction, gingival hypertrophy, anorexia, nausea and vomiting, tremor, and paresthesias. The aim is to use it for a short time as a "bridge" to the use of other agents that are safer for long-term use but are initially limited by a slow onset of action (6-mercaptopurine, azathioprine) or lower efficacy in patients with refractory active disease (mesalamine) (151).

MEDICAL MANAGEMENT

The medical therapy of ulcerative colitis depends on extent of involvement and severity of the disease at presentation.

PROCTITIS

Proctitis refers to an ulcerative process involving the rectum. Rectal bleeding, urgency, and tenesmus are frequent symptoms. In contrast to more extensive forms of colitis, patients may sometimes present with constipation rather than diarrhea. The mainstay of therapy is the use of topical treatments in the form of 5-ASA suppositories or steroid foams. The former is preferred, given its proven efficacy as a long-term maintenance therapy (152,153). In a patient with mild to moderate proctitis, treatment can be initiated with one 5-ASA suppository twice a day. A response should be seen within two to three weeks. The same dose can be continued until the patient is symptom free and can then be tapered gradually to a dose of one suppository every three nights. Maintenance therapy is not recommended (152).

Occasionally, because of discomfort or anal irritationtation, a patient does not tolerate suppositories, in which case oral medications are an alternative. Sulfasalazine or oral 5-ASA are effective. Their beneficial effect should be seen within two weeks. Once remission has been achieved, these agents can be tapered gradually to maintenance doses. The use of prednisone is rarely warranted in patients with severe refractory proctitis.

PROCTOSIGMOIDITIS

Proctosigmoiditis or distal colitis refers to involvement of the distal 30 to 40 cm of colonic mucosa. Similar to proctitis, this form of colitis is often amenable to therapy solely with topical agents. Most patients with proctosigmoiditis present with mild to moderate disease manifested by bloody diarrhea and absent or mild systemic symptoms.

Therapy for mild to moderate proctosigmoiditis can be initiated with 5-ASA enemas or hydrocortisone enemas. The former is preferred because of its proven efficacy in maintaining remission in ulcerative colitis (154). Therapy can be started with a single nightly 4 g 5-ASA enema and then waiting three to four weeks to assess the therapeutic response. If symptoms persist, an early morning 5-ASA or hydrocortisone enema can be added to the therapy. This treatment can then be tapered to a maintenance frequency of a single 5-ASA enema every third night. A randomized, controlled, multicenter trial (155) demonstrated that budesonide and hydrocartisone foam had similar efficacy and safety for patients with proctosigmoiditis; the remission rates were 53% and 52%, respectively. Foams are more acceptable to patients than enemas. For the patient who does not respond to topical therapy or poorly tolerates it, oral 5-ASA preparations are an effective alternative. In this situation, oral 5-ASA is often used in combination with topical agents. Sulfasalazine (Azulfidine), mesalamine (Pentasa, Asacol), and olsalazine (Dipentum) have proven to be equally effective in the treatment of active ulcerative colitis (152).

Sulfasalazine, 1 g/day, mesalamine, 1 to 1.2 g/day, or olsalazine, 500 mg/day, can be started, and if tolerated, can be increased every few days. Sulfasalazine is preferred because of its low cost. One common error in management is accepting a therapeutic failure when these medications have not been pushed to the maximum dose. Generally, for active disease, sulfasalazine can be increased to a maximum of 4 to 6 g/day (156), mesalamine to 4.8 g/day (26), and olsalazine to 3 g/day (157). At these doses, the latter two agents may be better tolerated. These drugs may require three to four weeks to exert the maximal therapeutic effect. Once the patient is in remission, these agents can be tapered to maintenance doses of sulfasalazine, 2 g/day; mesalamine, 1.2 to 2.4 g/day; oralsalazine, 1 g/day. Folate, 1 mg/day, is recommended for patients on long-term sulfasalazine (152).

Prednisone, at a dose of 40 to 60 mg, is indicated for the patient with severe distal colitis or with moderate colitis who has not improved with 5-ASA. This dose can be continued for a 10-day period before it is slowly tapered. Patients who respond to steroid therapy begin to feel a marked improvement within 24 to 48 hours.

■ LEFT-SIDED COLITIS AND PANCOLITIS

Left-sided colitis refers to inflammation up to the level of the splenic flexure. Pancolitis is defined as inflammation of the colonic mucosa diffusely up to and beyond the hepatic flexure. In these more extensive forms of colitis, the combination of oral 5-ASA medications and enemas is often used from the onset of exacerbation. These patients may have symptoms of rectal involvement (urgency, tenesmus) that predominate, justifying the concomitant use of topical therapy.

In a randomized double-blind study (158), combined oral and enema treatment with mesalamine (Pentasa®) is superior to oral therapy alone in patients with mild to moderate extensive ulcerative colitis. The oral dosage was 2 g of mesalamine twice daily and an enema at bedtime containing 1 g of mesalamine. Once the patient is in remission, one can attempt to taper and discontinue the enemas followed by reduction of oral mesalamine to a maintenance dose (152). Antidiarrheal medications may also be effective for symptomatic relief (152). Loperamide, an opiate, is the preferred drug because of its safety and efficacy (159). It is contraindicated in the acutely ill patient because of the risk of precipitating toxic megacolon.

For patients with moderate to severe colitis from the onset or moderate colitis that has not improved after adequate 5-ASA therapy, corticosteroids and immunosuppressive agents are then used, respectively, in a stepwise fashion (160).

■ ANEMIA IN INFLAMMATORY BOWEL DISEASE

The topic of anemia in IBD receives little attention. At a random point in time, one-third of the IBD population suffers from anemia (161). Anemia in IBD is still a frequent complication, affecting cognitive function, ability to work, and general well-being, and can be effectively prevented or treated. Anemia of chronic diseases such as IBD, rheumatoid arthritis, chronic infection, or malignancy has a similar mechanism. Both ineffective erythropoiesis and reduced red blood cell life span contribute to the anemia (161).

In general, enteric-coated formulations should be avoided, because they may release their iron content beyond the intestinal side of maximal iron absorption. Because of more side effects and less efficacy, the intramuscular or subcutaneous route of parenteral iron administration is obsolete (161).

Nonenteric coated oral iron might work for patients with moderate anemia (hemoglobin > 10.5 g/dL). The projected total iron requirement for a 70 kg patient with hemoglobin 8.0 g/dL and a ferritin of 15 mcg/L would be approximately 1995 mg. Presuming a high iron absorption (10% of 200 mg/day), perfect compliance, and no continuous blood loss, oral iron therapy may need 100 days to replace such an iron deficit. Most patients, however, are continuously losing blood, have less daily absorption, and do not tolerate this amount of oral iron. To overcome the obstacles of oral iron therapy in severe anemia, an intravenous iron therapy is needed.

Because of the concern over the risk of anaphylactic reactions to iron dextran, iron sucrose, which is tolerated well, should be used. A 10 mL iron sucrose (corresponding to 200 mg Fe) diluted in 250 mL of normal saline solution and given intravenously over 60 minutes. Iron sucrose infusion is given twice during the first two weeks and once a week thereafter. This regime can correct anemia in 80% of IBD patients. The remaining 20% can be correctable by the addition of recombinant human erythropoietin (rHu EPO) (161).

■ SEVERE OR FULMINANT COLITIS

Severe colitis is characterized by bloody diarrhea associated with weight loss, volume deplection, fever, and severe anemia. Fulminant colitis refers to patients with severe disease who appear toxic. These patients are at risk of progressing to toxic megacolon and possible bowel perforation. Patients with severe and fulminant disease require immediate hospital admission. The mainstays of therapy are bowel rest and parenteral steroids (152).

Hydrocortisone, 100 mg intravenously every eight hours, prednisolone, 30 mg intravenously every 12 hours, or methylprednisolone, 16 to 20 mg intravenously every eight hours, can be used. The latter two may be preferred because they have less sodium-retaining and potassium-wasting properties. Some physicians prefer prednisolone because the parenteral dose is equal to the oral dose. All three standard steroid preparations may also be given as a 24-hour continuous infusion (152). In patients who have not received steroids within the previous 30 days, intravenous adrenocorticotropic hormone (ACTH), 120 U per 24 hours, may be superior to standard parenteral steroids (162). Patients should feel significant improvement within 48 hours of intravenous therapy.

Often the addition of 5-ASA enemas or hydrocortisone enemas twice a day may be helpful, particularly if the predominant symptoms are lower abdominal pain, tenesmus, and urgency. There have been no randomized-controlled trials that have compared the effectiveness of parenteral steroids alone to the combination of steroids and mesalamine (5-ASA) in severe colitis. If a patient's flare-up coincides with the recent increase or addition of a 5-ASA agent, the medication should be withheld during the patient's hospital stay. Some 5-ASA compounds have been found to cause flare-ups of colitis (163).

The role of antibiotics in severe ulcerative colitis is unclear. The limited data available do not seem to support their use in this situation. Controlled trials assessing the addition of intravenous metronidazole (164) and/or metronidazole and tobramycin (165) to parenteral steroids in severe ulcerative colitis did not demonstrate their superiority to steroids alone (165). However, there may be a subgroup of patients with nontoxic severe ulcerative colitis and an incomplete response to corticosteroids who manifest low-grade fever and leukocytosis with bands who will respond to a course of broad-spectrum antibiotics (166). In patients with high fevers, leukocytosis and bands, and peritoneal signs or megacolon, broad-spectrum antibiotics are clearly indicated. Patients with dilated colon who undergo decompression with a nasogastric tube are asked to roll supine to prone every two hours to help redistribute gas (167).

Patients with toxic megacolon should respond to therapy within 72 hours; if not, colectomy is indicated. Less severely ill patients should respond to intensive parenteral steroids within seven days. Those who do not respond are candidates for surgery or intravenous cyclosporine. Based on a recent placebo-controlled study in patients with severe ulcerative colitis who were treated with a high dose of steroid, mesalamine-based medications, and loperamide or codeine, Lichtiger et al. (149) showed that cyclosporine, 4 mg/kg/day, given by intravenous infusion, showed a dramatic response rate of 82% compared to the placebo group of 0%. The mean response time was seven days (range, 3–14 days). The adverse effects included a single case of grand mal seizure, paresthesia (36%), and diastolic hypertension (36%). No notable nephrotoxicity was found. In a randomized, double-blind control study conducted by van Assche et al. (168) comparing intravenous cyclosporine 4 mg/kg (38 patients) to 2 mg/kg (35 patients). The results showed that there was no difference in clinical response rate (84.2% versus 85.7%, median time to response was four days), colectomy rates (13.1% vs. 8.6%), and adverse events.

In patients who have a history of chronic and frequently relapsing ulcerative colitis, surgery is preferred because it is curable. Cyclosporine may be suitable in the patient with new-onset ulcerative colitis presenting as severe or fulminant disease and who may not feel adequately prepared for surgery. The long-term outcome of patients who have had their bowel salvaged with cyclosporine is undetermined (152).

Those individuals in whom cyclosporine therapy is contemplated must have the physical and emotional ability to undergo the weeks to months of intensive therapy, undertake timely blood draws, frequent office visits, and be willing and able to take maintenance therapy with 6-MP or azathioprine. Contraindications include patients with active or chronic infections, seizures, hypertension, renal insufficiency, electrolyte abnormalities, or other serious medical or psychologic problems (169).

Infliximab (Remicade®) is a monoclonal antibody against tumor necrosis factor. It has been known to be effective in the treatment of active Crohn's disease. Its role for the treatment of ulcerative colitis has not been established. Jarnerot et al. (170) conducted a randomized double-blind trial of infliximab or placebo in severe to moderately severe ulcerative colitis not responding to conventional treatment with corticosteroid. The primary end point was colectomy or death three months after randomization. Forty-five patients were included (24 Infliximab and 21 placebo). The dosage of infliximab was 4 to 5 mg given as a slow infusion. The results showed that no patient died. Seven patients in the infliximab group and 14 in the placebo group had a colectomy (odds ratio of 4.9) within three months after randomization. No serious side effects occurred. The authors concluded that infliximab is an effective and safe rescue therapy in patients experiencing an acute severe or moderately severe attack of ulcerative colitis not responding to conventional treatment.

Two multicenters randomized, double-blind, placebo-controlled studies—the Active Ulcerative Colitis Trials 1 and 2 (ACT 1 and ACT 2, respectively) conducted globally between March 2002 and March 2005 were to evaluate the efficacy of infliximab for induction and maintenance therapy in adults with ulcerative colitis (171). In each study, 364 patients with moderate-to-severe active ulcerative colitis despite treatment with concurrent medications received placebo or Infliximab (5 or 10 mg/kg of body weight) intravenously at weeks 0, 2, and 6 and then every eight weeks through week 46 (in ACT 1) or week 22 (in ACT 2). Patients were followed for 54 weeks in ACT 1 and 30 weeks in ACT 2.

The results showed that in ACT 1, 69% of patients who received 5 mg of Infliximab and 61% of those who received 10 mg had a clinical response at week 8, as compared with 37% of those who received placebo ($p < 0.001$ for both comparisons with placebo). The response was defined as a decrease in the Mayo score of at least three points and at least 30%, with an accompanying decrease in the subscore for rectal bleeding of at least one point or an absolute rectal-bleeding subscore of 0 or 1. In ACT 2, 64% of patients who received 5 mg of infliximab and 69% of those who received 10 mg had a clinical response at week 8, as compared with 29% of those who received placebo ($p < 0.001$ for both comparisons with placebo). In both studies, patients who received infliximab were more likely to have a clinical response at week 30 ($p \leq 0.002$ for all comparisons). In ACT 1, more patients who received 5 mg or 10 mg of infliximab had a clinical response at week 54 (45% and 44%, respectively) than did those who received placebo (20%, $p < 0.001$ for both comparisons).

The authors concluded that patients with moderate-to-severe active ulcerative colitis treated with infliximab at weeks 0, 2, and 6 and every eight weeks thereafter were more likely to have a clinical response at weeks 8, 30, and 54 than were those receiving placebo.

Similar to Crohn's disease, maintenance treatment with repeated infliximab infusions will probably be necessary in ulcerative colitis as well, which seems particularly important in patients who escape a colectomy to avoid further hospitalization and risk of later surgery. It can be expected that the majority of patients will suffer from another ulcerative colitis attack once the biologic effect of infliximab has disappeared. For this reason, it is unlikely that the way in which infliximab was used in these studies represents the ideal approach to severe ulcerative colitis. However, the event of infliximab in the therapeutic armamentarium of ulcerative colitis means a significant step forward in the management of this disease (172).

Drugs best avoided or used with great caution during an acute attack include antidiarrheal drugs, such as codeine, diphenoxylate, and loperamide, because there is fairly strong circumstantial evidence that they may predispose to toxic megacolon. Heavy doses of sedatives should be avoided but can be given in moderation if the patient is unable to sleep because of apprehension. Iron therapy for anemia is contraindicated during an acute attack, but a course of a well-absorbed iron preparation, such as ferrous fumarate, is often indicated when the attack has been checked. Appreciable anemia during an acute attack requires treatment by blood transfusion.

■ STEROID-REFRACTORY ULCERATIVE COLITIS

Regardless of the extent of colonic involvement, some patients receive corticosteroid therapy but remain symptomatic with active disease. Therapeutic considerations in this group with steroid-refractory colitis include operation and further medical treatment. Before considering any other therapeutic agents, one must make certain that the patients have received maximum oral and topical 5-ASA therapy. There is no evidence that substituting one form of 5-ASA with another has any benefit.

Immunosuppressants, such as azathioprine or its metabolite 6-MP, are effective in patients with chronic active ulcerative colitis that is unresponsive to steroids. Because operation in ulcerative colitis is curative, many physicians are hesitant about using these medications and risking the development of potential serious side effects. Patients who do not desire operation or who are at high surgical risk are candidates for this therapy. Patients with resistant proctosigmoiditis or left-sided colitis are also suitable candidates for immunomodulators. They are effective in 60% to 70% patients who have refractory disease (152).

The therapy is initiated with a dose of 50 mg/day. Because a full therapeutic response may not occur for three to six months, patients should be maintained on prednisone therapy for at least two months before attempting to reduce the dose. The 6-MP or azathioprine is increased gradually, if necessary, to a maximum dose of 2 to 2.5 mg/kg/day. Blood counts should be monitored. New onset abdominal pain should be assessed promptly to rule out pancreatitis. The medications are discontinued and are contraindicated if pancreatitis occurs. Up to 10% of patients have to stop using immunosuppressants because of toxicity that includes leukopenia, pancreatitis, and infection. If, after six months of 6-MP or azathioprine, the patient has not improved, operation should be strongly considered (152).

Although the preliminary clinical trial by Kozarek et al. (173) showed that 75% of patients with intractable ulcerative colitis improved with oral methotrexate, a recent double-blind, randomized Israeli multicenter trial showed that methotrexate at a weekly oral dose of 12.5 mg is not found to be better than placebo in the induction or maintenance of remission in patients with refractory chronic active ulcerative colitis (174).

Continuation or resumption of smoking has been shown to have a beneficial effect on the clinical course of ulcerative colitis patients, with a reduction in symptoms and fewer hospitalizations. Nicotine may be responsible for the potentially beneficial effect of smoking on ulcerative colitis. Transdermal nicotine may be efficacious for the induction of remission in mild to moderately active ulcerative colitis, but is ineffective for maintenance. It may be reasonable to consider transdermal nicotine patches in carefully selected patients with mild to moderate refractory ulcerative colitis that has not responded to 5-ASA and steroids, especially in former smokers. Given the substantial negative impact on overall health, cigarette smoking should never be recommended (175).

■ STEROID-DEPENDENT ULCERATIVE COLITIS

Some patients with CUC remain well on oral corticosteroids but become symptomatic when these medications are tapered. The major concern in these patients is the potential toxicity associated with long-term steroid administration. Azathioprine and 6-MP have proven effective as steroid-sparing and long-term remitting agents.

How long should patients in remission remain on these medications? A retrospective analysis reviewed the outcome of patients who have been on long-term administration of 6-MP for ulcerative colitis. This study suggested that despite a remission of up to 1.5 years, patients who discontinued 6-MP have a significant risk of relapse (176). Bitton and Peppercorn (152) recommended tapering the 6-MP and azathioprine after 1.5 to 2 years of clinical remission.

NATURAL HISTORY OF TREATED ULCERATIVE COLITIS

The outcome of ulcerative colitis is difficult to predict. The presentation and the treatment of the disease vary greatly. Current medical management has changed greatly from the past and, thus, modifies the course of the disease. A couple of studies have looked at the natural history of patients with ulcerative colitis who obtained adequate treatment.

■ COURSE OF SEVERE ULCERATIVE COLITIS

Simple criteria are needed to predict which patients with severe ulcerative colitis will respond poorly to intensive medical treatment and require colectomy. Travis et al. (24), of Oxford, U.K., conducted a prospective study in patients with severe ulcerative colitis admitted to the hospital. All patients received aggressive and intensive management. Patients who did not respond had the opportunity to receive cyclosporine. The study involved 51 consecutive episodes of severe colitis affecting 49 patients. All of the severe episodes were treated with intravenous and rectal hydrocortisone and 14 of 51 with cyclosporine. The study monitored 36 clinical, laboratory, and radiographic variables. The follow-up was one year. The criteria for severe colitis were defined by Truelove (Table 1) (25).

It could be predicted on day 3 that 85% of patients with more than eight stools on that day, or a stool frequency between three and eight, together with a C-reactive protein greater than 45 mg/L, would require colectomy. For patients given cyclosporine, 4 of 14 avoided colectomy but two continued to have symptoms. Complete responders remained in remission for a median of nine months and had a 5% chance of colectomy. After seven days of treatment, patients with more than three stools per day or visible blood had a 60% chance of continued symptoms and a 40% chance of colectomy in the following months.

The criteria for a complete response were stringent (stool frequency of fewer than three without visible blood after seven days). Only 42% of episodes responded completely to intensive medical treatment. Seventy-three percent of the incomplete responders still had stool frequency of more than three per day or visible blood, and 43% ultimately required colectomy.

Cyclosporine (5 mg/kg/day) is effective in 50% of patients who have not responded to intravenous corticosteroids. Forty-three percent of these responders require colectomy within three months. The 50% of patients who do not respond require a colectomy. The role of cyclosporine for treatment of severe ulcerative colitis is yet to be defined. Only bowel frequency and C-reactive protein evaluation are the most useful inflammatory markers.

■ COURSE OF ACTIVE AND CHRONIC ULCERATIVE COLITIS

Langholz et al. (177) studied a population base of patients with ulcerative colitis in Copenhagen, Denmark, over a period of 25 years 1962–1987. The study analyzed the course of the disease regarding short- and long-term disease activity, predicting the pattern of disease course, and impact of the disease on work, hospital admissions, and frequency of visits to outpatient clinics. These patients were treated according to the severity of their disease with sulfasalazine or mesalamine, glucocorticoids (topical and systemic), and colectomy.

There were 1161 patients with ulcerative colitis with a mean follow-up of 11.7 years. The follow-up was 99.9%. The colectomy rate was 9% in the year of diagnosis, 3% per year in the following four years, and then approximately 1% per year. The cumulative colectomy rate was 24%, 30%, and 32% at 10, 15, and 25 years after diagnosis, respectively. The probability of undergoing colectomy was correlated to the extent of disease at diagnosis, with a cumulative probability of 35% in patients with pancolitis, 19% in patients with substantial colitis, and 9% in patients with proctosigmoiditis initially after five years. High disease activity at diagnosis, manifested as systemic symptoms such as weight loss and fever, had a high chance of requiring colectomy.

Twenty-three percent of patients had only one disease episode (median observation, 3 years; range, 1–25 years), whereas 77% had continuous or relapsing disease after the initial episode (mean observation, 10 years; range, 1–25 years).

The cumulative probability of being completely relapse-free decreased rapidly with time, 18.4% after five years and 10.6% after 25 years. The patients without relapse after 25 years did not differ in clinical appearance at diagnosis from those with intermittent disease.

About half of patients with ulcerative colitis will be in remission at any time, although 90% have an intermittent course. Relapses are unpredictable, except that disease activity in previous years indicates with 70% to 80% probability that the disease will continue the following year. The cumulative probability of a continuous active course is very low, 1% after five years and 0.1% after 25 years. However, the probability of an intermittent course with remission and relapses increases with time, 90% 25 years after the diagnosis.

Contrary to expectation that those with systemic symptoms and extensive involvement at diagnosis would probably have a course with several flare-ups, a higher proportion of patients with systemic symptoms are in continuous remission up to seven years after the diagnosis.

Only 6 of 1161 patients developed a colorectal carcinoma during the observation period. This does not differ from the general population calculated from the Danish National Cancer Registry. This result reflects presumably the active surgical policy that removes patients with highly active disease with a course of continuous activity (178).

There is a risk of death in the first year, but the mortality due to colitis is low (less than 0.8%), reflecting a small number of patients with severe active pancolitis.

Although ulcerative colitis is troublesome, the probability of maintaining working capacity after 10 years is 92.8%.

INDICATIONS FOR OPERATION

■ INTRACTABILITY

It is not uncommon for patients with long-standing ulcerative colitis to become dependent on corticosteroids to function adequately. They may have diarrhea several times a day, anemia, and weakness. They continue to function and are not totally incapacitated. In this situation, although an operation is usually recommended, the patient should enter the decision-making process. Since the introduction of the ileoanal pouch procedures, many patients feel more comfortable in accepting an operation earlier; at present, intractability to medical treatment has become the most common indication for an operation in patients with ulcerative colitis.

■ FULMINANT COLITIS

Currently it is generally accepted that severe attacks of ulcerative colitis should be resuscitated vigorously with medical treatment and operated on within 24 hours if the patient's condition deteriorates and within five days if there is no significant improvement. With adoption of this early operative approach, the mortality rate has fallen to less than 3% (179,180).

■ TOXIC MEGACOLON

Toxic megacolon is an emergency, life-threatening complication of ulcerative colitis, Crohn's colitis, and other forms of colitides such as salmonellosis, ischemic colitis, and *C. difficile* colitis (181,182). Toxic megacolon may occur as an acute exacerbation of the disease, but in more than 60% of patients it develops as an initial manifestation (183). Nevertheless, it is a rare complication, which probably reflects better management of the patient medically and the earlier referral of patients for an operation.

"Toxic megacolon" is a clinical term for acute colitis with segmental or total dilatation of the colon (Fig. 13). Usually these patients are very ill with high fever, abdominal pain and tenderness, tachycardia, and leukocytosis. Patients may develop toxicity without megacolon or megacolon without severe toxic signs. The etiology of megacolon is unclear, but there are known factors that precipitate the condition: antidiarrheal agents, opiates, belladonna alkaloids, and barium enema.

Patients with toxic megacolon require vigorous resuscitation to maintain homeostasis. Antibiotics to treat colonic bacterial flora are given as soon as possible. To prevent adrenal dysfunction, administration of intravenous hydrocortisone is mandatory for patients who have been taking, or recently have been treated with, corticosteroids. If the patient never has taken corticosteroids and a decision has been made to try medical measures, hydrocortisone should be started. Properly managed, more than half of

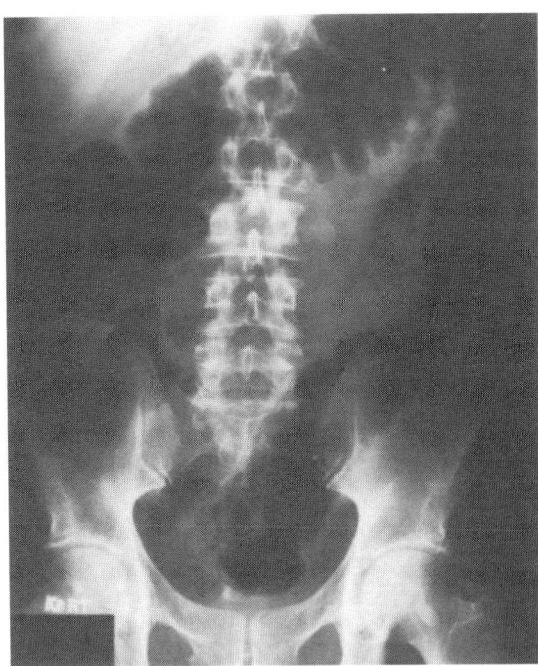

FIGURE 13 ■ Acute ulcerative colitis complicated by toxic megacolon.

these patients respond to medical treatment, and the operation can be postponed to an elective procedure.

Transient toxic dilatation of the colon is itself not an indication for operation, but if there is any deterioration, an operation may be indicated within 24 hours. This approach minimizes the incidence of colonic perforation, which is associated with a 20% mortality rate compared with a 4% rate if there is no perforation (181). Grant and Dozois (184) studied the clinical course of 38 patients with toxic megacolon who were treated successfully nonoperatively (32 patients had ulcerative colitis and six had Crohn's colitis). The follow-up ranged from 3 to 22 years (average, 13 years). Eleven patients (29%) suffered second episodes of fulminant colitis or recurrent toxic megacolon. Ultimately, 18 patients (47%) underwent colon resection, which was performed on an emergency or urgent basis in 15. The authors believed that medical management of toxic megacolon should be regarded almost exclusively as preparation for imminent operation. Controversy exists as to whether TPC or subtotal colectomy with the rectum left behind should be done. The TPC has the advantage that the entire disease is eliminated. In expert hands it can be done with low morbidity and mortality (185). On the other hand, a subtotal colectomy without removal of the rectum is a significantly lesser operation for the very ill patient, but part of the diseased bowel is left behind, risking continued complications. Since the introduction of the ileoanal pouch procedure, the trend is to preserve the rectum if feasible, particularly in young patients, hoping that the ileoanal pouch procedure can be performed at a later date. Approximately 50% of patients with Crohn's colitis have minimal involvement of the rectum, making it logical not to remove the rectum at this critical time. In selected patients, an ileorectal anastomosis can be done as a second stage.

■ MASSIVE BLEEDING

Massive bleeding caused by ulcerative colitis is rare. Nevertheless, it occasionally represents the principal indication for an emergency operation. The frequency of severe hemorrhage reported in the literature ranges from 0% to 4.5%. However, this relatively rare complication accounts for approximately 10% of all urgent colectomies for ulcerative colitis (186).

■ PROPHYLAXIS FOR CARCINOMA

Although TPC is the only way to prevent the development of carcinoma in patients with long-standing ulcerative colitis, it is difficult to justify an operation in patients who are asymptomatic or who have minimal symptoms and do not require any medication. Nevertheless, many patients decide to have an operation performed as prophylaxis.

■ CARCINOMA

A study of ulcerative colitis and colorectal carcinoma, using a population-based chart of 3117 patients, was conducted by Ekbom et al. (187). It confirmed the existence of an increased risk of colorectal carcinoma, with the relative risk of 14.8 for patients with pancolitis as compared with the general population. The extent of disease at diagnosis and the age at diagnosis, especially if 15 years older or younger, were strong and independent determinants of this increase in relative risk.

Carcinoma in patients with ulcerative colitis apparently does not develop from the ordinary adenoma–carcinoma sequence but arises directly from the flat mucosa. The carcinoma also usually is of the infiltrating type rather than the polypoid type or is found in the submucosa, making it difficult to detect even with colonoscopy and biopsy (Fig. 14). Approximately 20% of carcinomas in patients with ulcerative colitis are incurable at the time of diagnosis. It is not unusual to find multiple carcinomas of the colon and rectum in these patients. The five-year survival rate for patients with carcinoma complicating ulcerative colitis is generally poor and ranges from

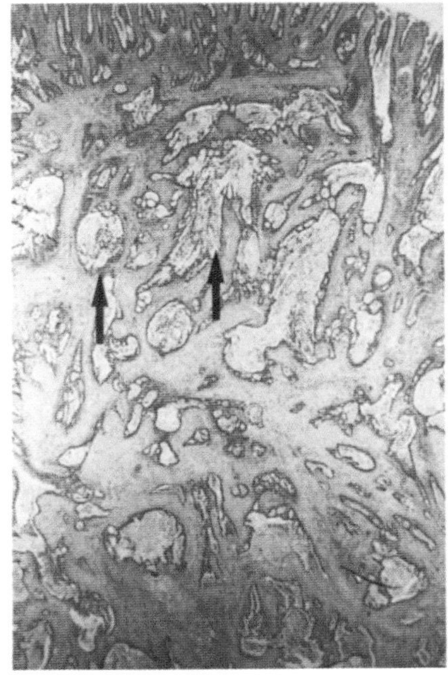

FIGURE 14 ■ Infiltrating carcinoma of colon in a patient with chronic ulcerative colitis (*arrows*). Note normal mucosa overlying the carcinoma.

19% to 55% (188). The poor prognosis is attributed to the late stage of the disease by the time carcinomas are detected. However, when matched with a similar stage in noncolitic patients, there is no statistically significant difference in the five-year survival rate (188,189).

■ CUTANEOUS AND SYSTEMIC COMPLICATIONS

Most extracolonic manifestations except PSC, cirrhosis, and ankylosing spondylitis improve after the disease is removed. If the colitis is severe and the complications are significant, an operation should be considered strongly.

OPERATIVE OPTIONS

■ TOTAL PROCTOCOLECTOMY AND ILEOSTOMY

TPC and ileostomy removes the entire disease and has been considered the "gold standard" against which other procedures must be compared. The advantages of this procedure include its relatively low-morbidity rate and freedom from functional problems when compared with other sphincter-saving procedures. The main disadvantage is the need for a permanent ileostomy, which many patients have difficulty adapting to or accepting psychologically.

Technique of Mobilizing Rectum

The patient is placed in the combined position with both legs in stirrups. The technique for performing the colectomy for ulcerative colitis is similar to colectomy for carcinoma (see Chapter 23). However, the mobilization of the rectum and its removal are performed differently to avoid damage to the pelvic nerves that supply the bladder and also to maintain sexual function in men.

The distal sigmoid colon is dissected from the mesentery close to its wall. The superior rectal vessels are ligated at the promontory of the sacrum. The avascular presacral space is entered at the promontory of sacrum. A St. Mark's retractor with a lip is placed behind the posterior rectum retracting the rectum forward. Any adherent fibers are cut with electrocautery. The retractor is constantly adjusted. Once the rectosacral fascia is cut, the supralevator space is entered and the levator ani muscle is visualized, indicating completion of the posterior mobilization. With this technique, the presacral sympathetic plexuses are not disturbed. The peritoneum and endopelvic fascia on each side of the rectum are incised with electrocautery close to the rectal wall. The anterior peritoneal reflection is incised with electrocautery, starting at the midline in the avascular plane just posterior to the seminal vesicle or vagina. This incision should be carried laterally to the edge of the seminal vesicle or vagina and then curved down posterolaterally to avoid damage to the pelvic nerves and blood vessels that enter anterolaterally. The entire rectum then can be mobilized, using mostly sharp dissection with electrocautery all the way down to the levator ani muscle. The rest of the anorectum is removed through the perineal phase.

Intersphincteric Proctectomy

Intersphincteric proctectomy is the removal of the anorectum with preservation of the entire external sphincter muscles and the levator ani muscle (Fig. 15A). After making an elliptic skin incision, electrocautery is used to develop the intersphincteric plane (Fig. 15B). In this plane, the anal canal, along with the internal sphincter, can be separated easily from the external sphincter muscles. With electrocautery the dissection is usually easy, and blood loss is minimal. The dissection is carried proximally in a circumferential manner to the level of the levator ani muscle, where the dissection will meet with the mobilized rectum from above (Fig. 15C). The entire specimen then is removed. The perineal wound is closed with two layers of interrupted 2–0 or 3–0 monofilament synthetic sutures, starting at the levator ani muscle. The skin is closed with subcuticular suture of 3–0 monofilament synthetic absorbable suture, or left open.

If available, the greater omentium is mobilized and filled in the pelvis. After the abdomen is washed thoroughly with normal saline solution, a closed suction drain is placed in the presacral space and is brought out through a separate stab wound in the left lower abdomen. It is left for five days or until the output is approximately 20 mL/day. The pelvic peritoneum is not closed. The ileostomy is constructed in the right lower quadrant and is matured.

■ COLECTOMY WITH ILEOSTOMY AND HARTMANN'S PROCEDURE

Colectomy with ileostomy and Hartmann's procedure is a much less extensive operation for very ill patients with fulminant colitis or toxic megacolon. The risk of damaging the pelvic nerves also is eliminated during the acute inflammation of the rectum and the pelvis. Another important aspect is the preservation of the anorectum for the future construction of an ileoanal pouch. In an emergency situation, colectomy with ileostomy and Hartmann's procedure has become the operation of choice for most patients, particularly young patients.

With this operation, after the abdominal colectomy has been performed, the terminal ileum is brought out as an ileostomy in the right lower quadrant. The lower sigmoid colon just above the promontory of sacrum is divided with a stapler. It is important to leave a rectal tube or a Foley catheter in the rectum for a few days to avoid perforation of the rectal stump. Large amounts of gas can be formed by bacteria. One of the major disadvantages of leaving the diseased rectum behind is the continuation of active disease that may require a subsequent urgent proctectomy. However, this problem is uncommon. It occurred in only three instances at St. Mark's Hospital, London, in 18 years (179). When urgent proctectomy is mandatory because of acute bleeding, the rectum can be stapled and divided just above the levator ani muscle. The anal sphincter is not disturbed, and an ileoanal pouch procedure can still be performed in the future.

■ COLECTOMY WITH ILEORECTAL ANASTOMOSIS

In properly selected patients, particularly young patients with good anal continence and good rectal compliance, in the presence of mild or moderately inflamed mucosa, colectomy with ileorectal anastomosis works well. The advantage of preserving the rectum is obvious. The patients continue to have bowel movements naturally. Because the rectum is

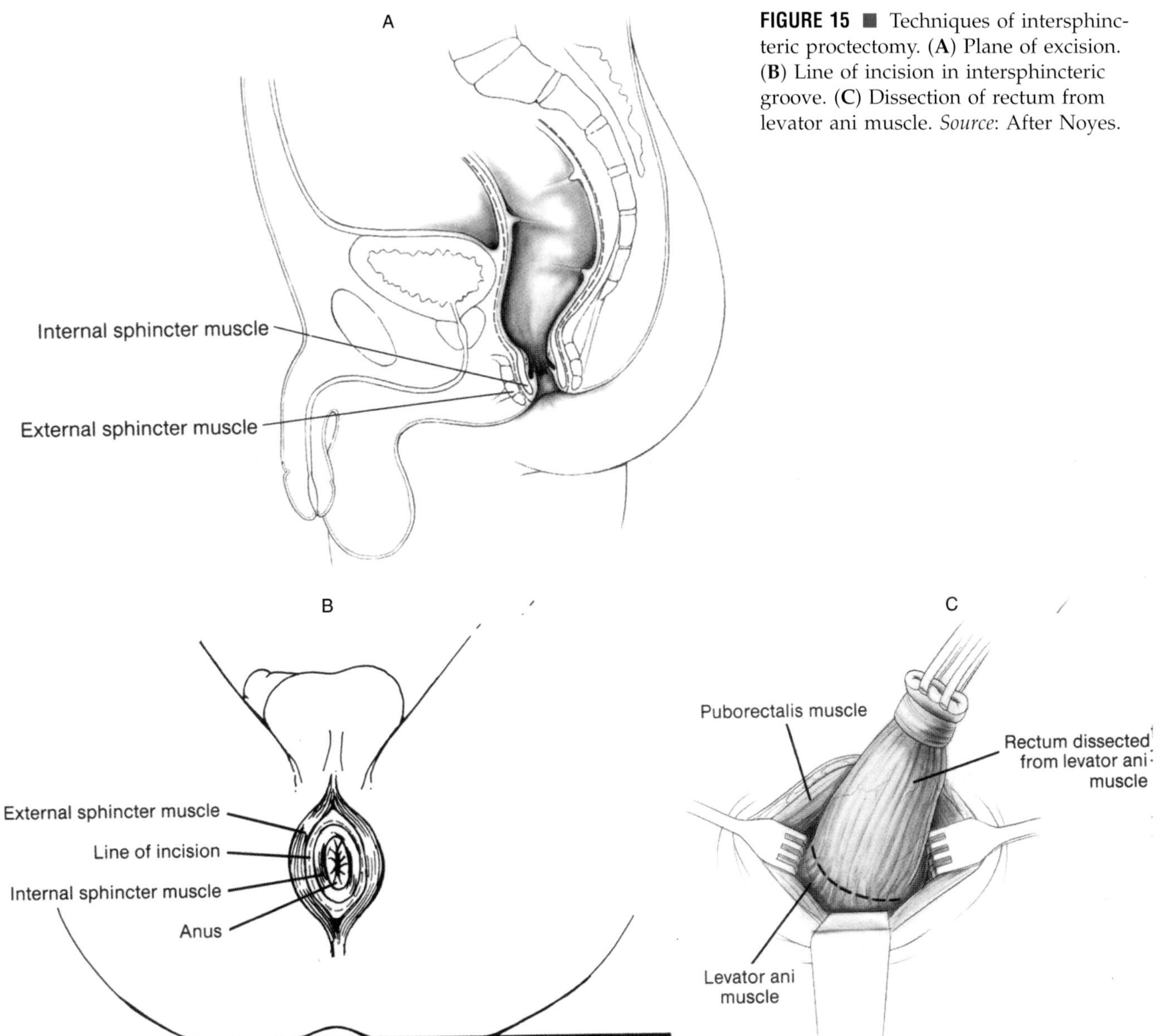

FIGURE 15 ■ Techniques of intersphincteric proctectomy. (**A**) Plane of excision. (**B**) Line of incision in intersphincteric groove. (**C**) Dissection of rectum from levator ani muscle. *Source*: After Noyes.

not disturbed, the chance of impotence from mobilization of the rectum during the operation is completely eliminated. This is particularly important for young male patients.

This operation has several disadvantages. Bowel movements may occur as often as 6 to 10 times per day; there is a risk of incontinence if the patients are not properly selected. The disease in the rectum may exacerbate. The segment of rectum is still at risk for the development of carcinoma. This risk, however, is relatively low—approximately 5% at 15 to 20 years (190). Patients must return for a periodic biopsy examination to check for mucosal dysplasia. Patients also should understand that they might require another operation to remove the rectum when indicated.

The reported success rate for ileorectal anastomosis varies from series to series. The series from the Cleveland Clinic showed a success rate of 75% in 109 patients with ileorectal anastomosis followed from 1 to 22 years (mean 8.2 years) (191). The series from Stockholm showed a 43% success rate in 60 patients, with a mean time of observation of 13 years (192). The series from Mayo Clinic showed acceptable functional results in 87.5% and 91% reported an improvement in their quality of life, in 42 patients. The follow-up was 6.5 ± 4.8 years (193). These differences probably reflect the selection of patients for the procedure and the duration of the follow-up. The most common reasons for failure are persistence of disease in the rectum and severe diarrhea (190,192). The positive preoperative prognostic factor is mild rectal disease (192). Approximately 10% of cases are considered suitable for ileorectal anastomosis (192). This number likely will be lower since the acceptance of the ileoanal pouch procedure.

■ TOTAL PROCTOCOLECTOMY WITH CONTINENT ILEOSTOMY (KOCK'S POUCH)

The continent ileostomy was pioneered by Kock (194) of Sweden in 1969. It was introduced to serve those patients who do not desire to wear an ileostomy appliance for the conventional Brooke ileostomy. The vast experience with Kock's pouch was centered in a few medical centers in Europe and the United States throughout the 1970s. The procedure, however, has never been used widely in private practice. The reason is obvious: it is plagued with complications. The incidence of early postoperative complications, including intra-abdominal abscess, peritonitis, suture line leakage, fistulas, small bowel obstruction, and stomal necrosis, is 23%. The incidence of late complications, particularly valve dysfunction requiring revisional operations, is as high as 54% (195).

Technique

During the 1970s the technique for constructing a Kock's pouch was changed and modified several times. The latest improvement is securing the nipple valve with rows of staples placed longitudinally (196). The technique for proctocolectomy is the same as that for conventional ileostomy. Depending on the thickness of the abdominal wall, the terminal 5 to 10 cm of terminal ileum is used for the outlet. Proximal to the outlet, 10 cm of ileum is reserved for construction of the valve and the adjacent 30 cm for the pouch (Fig. 16A). The mesentery supplying the segment of the ileum for the valve is cleared of peritoneum and fat in a triangular shape, taking care to preserve the main blood vessels. The purpose of fat clearance is to make the tissue less bulky when it later is intussuscepted to secure the valve in the pouch.

The reservoir construction is begun by opening the 30 cm segment of bowel along its antimesenteric border. The segment is folded into a U shape, with the terminal segment positioned cranially and the bottom of the U to the left-hand side of the patient. The two 15 cm limbs of the U are sutured with continuous 3–0 synthetic absorbable sutures (Fig. 16B). The incision on the afferent loop extends approximately 2 cm beyond the connecting point. This maneuver avoids later kinking of the afferent loop when the reservoir is attached to the abdominal wall. The valve then is constructed by grasping the bowel wall through the open lumen and intussuscepting the intestine into the future reservoir (Fig. 16C). The valve should be 5 cm long. The intussuscepted position is maintained by staples, which are applied with a linear stapler or an anastomosing stapler without a knife. The full length of the arms of the instrument should be used when applying the staples (Fig. 16D). Four rows of staples are used, one on each side of the mesentery and the remainder in the other two quadrants. The tip of the valve is anchored to the wall of the reservoir by the application of a fifth row of staples to prevent eversion of the valve (Fig. 16E). Before this row of staples is applied, the opposing areas of the valve tip and the reservoir wall are electrocoagulated to denude the muscularis layer and, promote firm attachment. The intestinal plate then is folded, and the reservoir is closed with continuous inverted 3–0 synthetic absorbable sutures (Fig. 16F). The corners of the reservoir are pushed downward between the mesenteric leaves so that the former posterior aspect of the reservoir is brought up anteriorly (Fig. 16G). At this time, the reservoir is tested for valve incompetence by injecting air through a catheter. The reservoir is attached to the anterior abdominal wall at the site of the ileostomy in the right lower quadrant (Fig. 16H and I). The ileostomy is made flush with the skin level.

Postoperative Management

The reservoir continuously is drained with a specially designed bullet-tipped catheter (197). It is left in the pouch for two weeks. After this time the catheter is clamped intermittently for one-hour periods during the day but is connected to the bag for drainage at night. Three weeks after the operation, the catheter is clamped for two-hour periods. The pouch is irrigated with water. After four weeks, the catheter is removed, and the patient is trained to empty the reservoir every three hours and gradually to decrease the frequency of intubation to three to four times per day and not during the night. The patient is encouraged to irrigate the pouch once a day or more often if the consistency of the discharge is thick (196).

Valve Malfunction

Nipple valve malfunction causing obstruction and incontinence is the most common late complication of Kock's pouch. Malfunction includes valve extrusion, eversion, stomal hernia, and fistula formation (196–198). The use of multiple longitudinal rows of staples to anchor the valve and the prolonged use of a catheter to drain the pouch during the first month after operation decrease the frequency of these complications markedly.

The extruded nipple valve can be repaired with the existing desusscepted segment. The stoma is taken down, and the pouch is dissected free from its attachments. An enterotomy is made in the pouch for exposure. The nipple valve is reconstructed in the same manner as described earlier and the pouch replaced to its original position (Fig. 17).

More often the valve requires reconstruction. The stoma and the pouch are freed. The stoma and the damaged valve are excised from the pouch (Fig. 18A). The afferent limb is divided 15 cm from the pouch. An enterotomy is made on the pouch for exposure, and a nipple valve is reconstructed in the same manner as previously described (Fig. 18B). The reservoir is rotated so that the stoma is passed through the anterior abdominal wall for the ileostomy (Fig. 18C). The proximal cut end of the ileum is attached to the opening at the previously excised valve or is reattached at a new appropriate site (Fig. 18D).

Results

The improvement in constructing the continent ileostomy appears to have matured. A review by Vernava and Goldberg (195) showed that the complication rate has been reduced to an acceptable level (Table 2). Construction of a continent ileostomy provided a group of patients who were not satisfied with their conventional ileostomy with great satisfaction and improved their quality of life in several aspects, including improvement in working capacity, leisure activities, and sexual life (200). Other studies also showed a positive effect in 90% of patients (195).

Current Use of Continent Ileostomy

The continent ileostomy largely has been replaced by the ileoanal pouch procedure. At present, its main place is for patients who previously have had a TPC and Brooke ileostomy and strongly desire to have a continent stoma and for

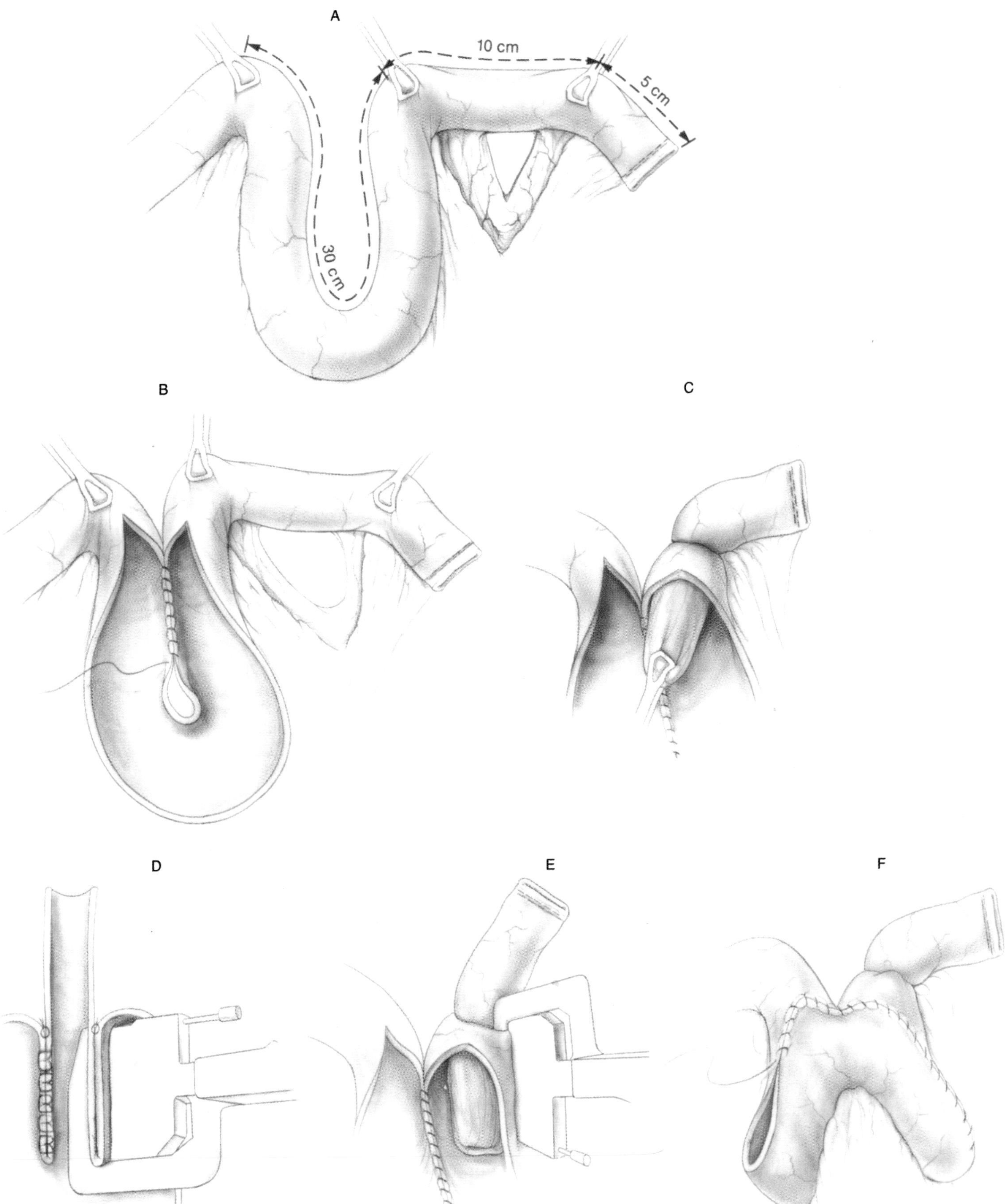

FIGURE 16 ■ Construction of Kock's pouch. (**A**) 45 cm of terminal ileum is used: 30 cm for pouch, 10 cm for valve, and 5 cm for ileostomy. Mesentery on segment for valve is cleared from fat in a triangular shape. (**B**) A segment of terminal ileum is folded into a U with a 15 cm limb. Antimesenteric border is incised, and inner wall is sutured with 3–0 absorbable continuous suture. Note incision on afferent loop extended 2 cm beyond connecting point. (**C**) Segment for valve is intussuscepted into future reservoir. (**D**) With a linear stapler, valve is anchored in four quadrants. (**E**) Fifth row of staples is applied between valve and wall of reservoir. (**F**) Intestinal plate of reservoir is folded and closed with 3–0 absorbable continuous sutures. (*G–I on next page*)

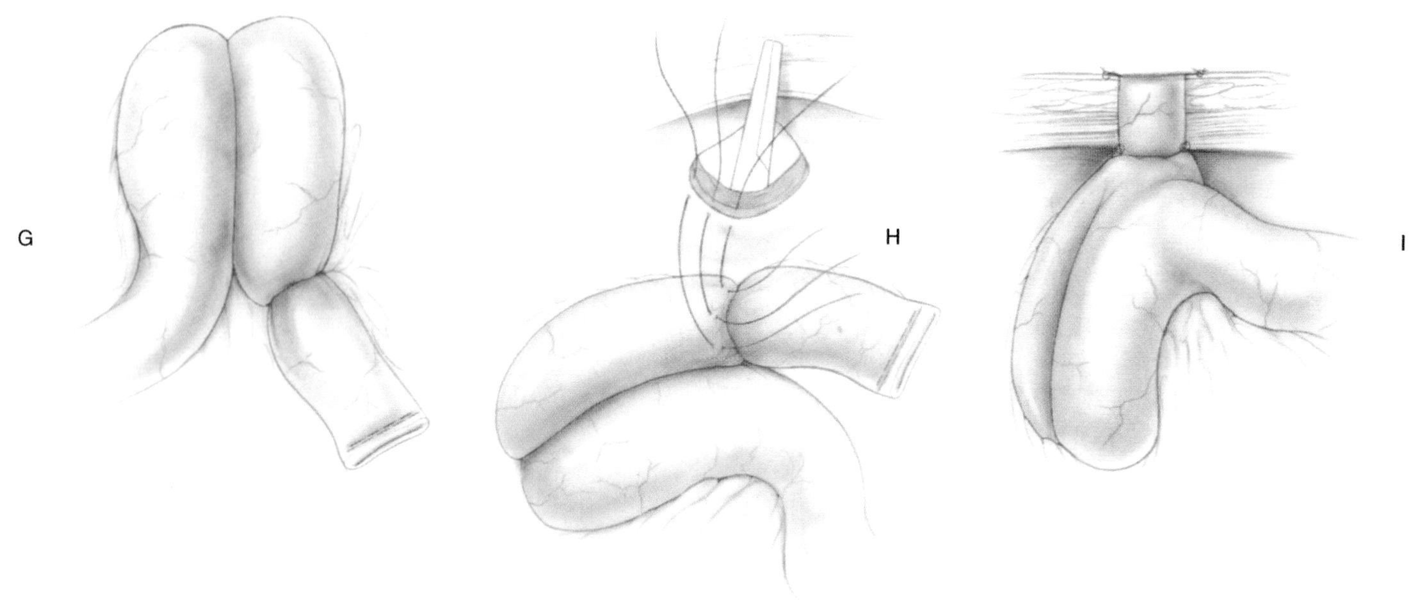

FIGURE 16 ■ (*Continued*) (**G**) Pouch is pushed downward between mesenteric leaves. (**H**) Reservoir is fixed to anterior abdominal wall. (**I**) Ileostomy limb is brought through abdominal wall and sutures are placed. *Source*: From Ref. 196.

patients who are denied an ileoanal pouch procedure because of anal incontinence. Patients who have problems with their conventional ileostomy and patients with a failed ileoanal pouch can be considered candidates for a continent ileostomy (197,201,202).

A follow-up report from Göteborg, Sweden (203) is important first-hand information. This is the institution where continent ileostomy was pioneered by Professor Kock. The study consisted of 68 patients who had had a continent ileostomy performed between 1967 and 1974; and these 68 patients were available for long-term follow-up. The median age at follow-up was 60 (range, 40–89) years. The results showed that 65% of the patients had at least one operation and 50% of the patients had undergone three or more reoperations. Most were revision procedures related to nipple valve dysfunction and/or fistula. Patients evacuate their pouch a median of four times every 24 hours. Minor peristomal skin irritation occurred in 10%. Episodes of pouchitis were reported by a third of the patients. Seventy-eight percent of the patients rated that overall health as good, very good, or excellent. The authors concluded that although revisional operations may be needed to restore continence, continent ileostomy has a good durability. They agreed with other authors that conversion of the failed ideal pouch-anal anastomosis to a continent ileostomy may be a reasonable alternative and gratifying results have been reported. They speculated, "the next decade may well see a great revival of interest in the continent ileostomy, thus some surgical teams should be conversant with the technique and be prepared to offer patients this operation as a second alternative."

■ TOTAL PROCTOCOLECTOMY WITH ILEAL POUCH–ANAL ANASTOMOSIS

Although continent ileostomy can be regarded as the procedure of the 1970s, TPC with ileal pouch-anal anastomosis (IPAA) has been the procedure of the 1980s, was marching through the 1990s, and continues on into the 21st century. For many patients with ulcerative colitis, IPAA has become the procedure of choice. TPC with IPAA not only eliminates the disease, but also preserves the anal sphincter.

Evolution of Proctocolectomy with Sphincter Preservation

The concept of preserving the anal sphincter and maintaining bowel continuity after excision of the colon and rectum is not new. In 1888, Julius Von Hochenegg of Vienna devised his pull-through method of coloanal anastomosis whereby the distal anorectal mucosa was stripped through the anus and the proximal gut pulled through the sphincter apparatus. In 1910, Vignolo of Pisa interposed an isolated segment of ileum to bridge the gap between the sigmoid colon and the anus after abdominosacral resection of a rectal malignancy. He clearly described a sutured anastomosis between the ileal segment and the stripped upper anal canal (204). The first ileoanal anastomosis is attributed to Rudolph Nissen of Berlin, who in 1933 performed a total colectomy with ileoanal anastomosis in a 10-year-old child with polyposis. The early postoperative results were gratifying (204). Ravitch and Sabiston (205) experimented with TPC, anorectal mucosectomy, and ileoanal anastomosis in 28 dogs. They found the technique was feasible and the anal function reasonable. In 1948, Ravitch (206) reported on two patients with long-standing ulcerative colitis who underwent colectomy, anorectal mucosectomy, and ileoanal anastomosis. Both patients withstood the operation well and had excellent fecal continence. Both patients had two formed stools a day and none at night.

In 1952, Best (207) reviewed the literature on patients undergoing colectomy with ileoanal anastomosis. There were 12 patients with ulcerative colitis and 17 with polyposis. The overall satisfactory results were approximately 50%, but there were numerous complications, particularly sepsis and anastomotic leaks. He was pessimistic about

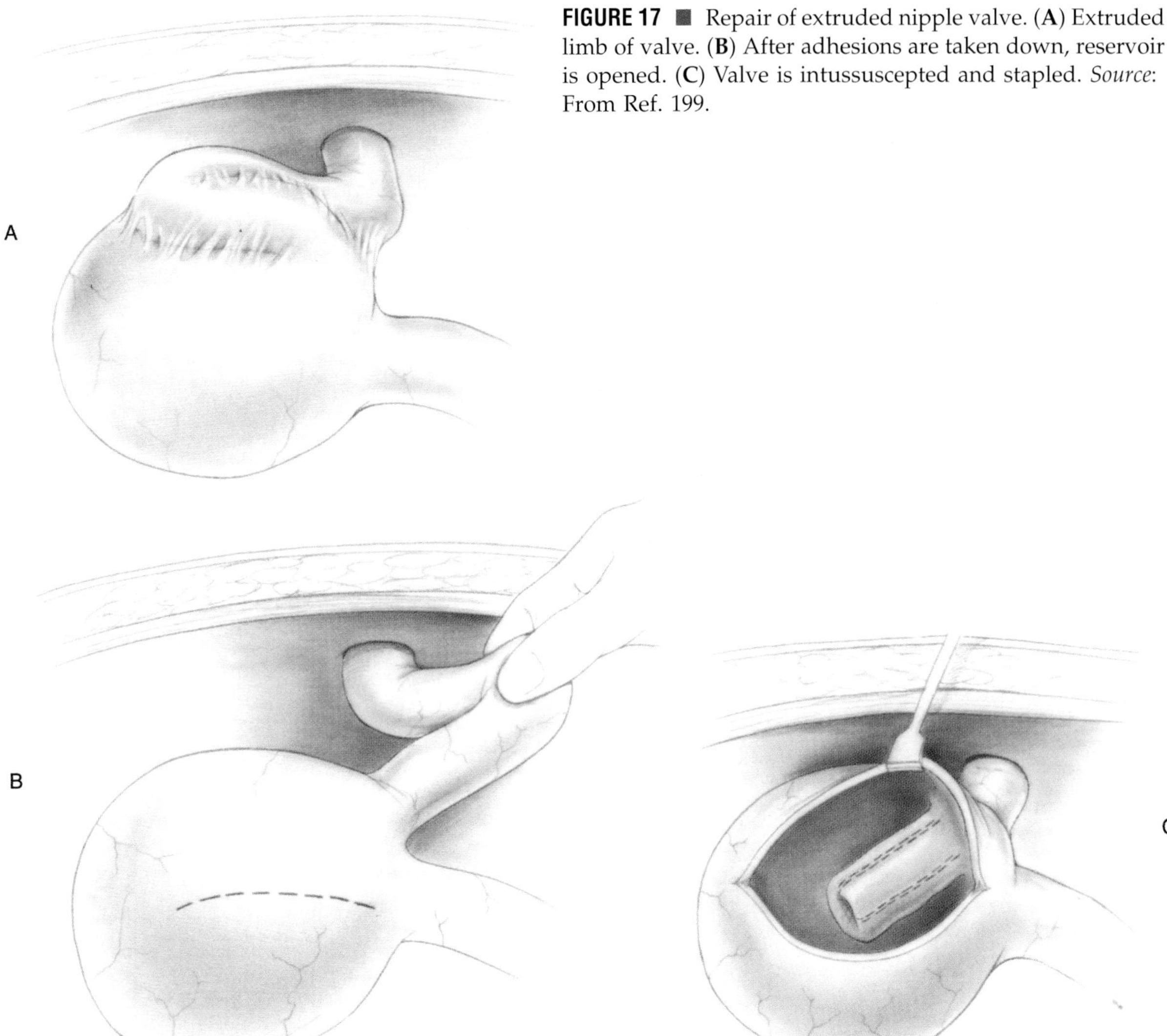

FIGURE 17 ■ Repair of extruded nipple valve. (**A**) Extruded limb of valve. (**B**) After adhesions are taken down, reservoir is opened. (**C**) Valve is intussuscepted and stapled. *Source*: From Ref. 199.

the operation and stated, "I have difficulty in convincing myself that facing the issues described is worth the sweat and tears of both patient and surgeon." However, Best was convinced that ileoanal anastomosis was a feasible procedure. In 1951, Goligher (208) performed two proctocolectomies with ileoanal anastomosis and gave his opinion: "I certainly would not presume to condemn an operation on such a limited experience, but these results as they stand are discouraging and indicate quite clearly that the functional condition after this operation is not always satisfactory. Nevertheless, I propose to experiment further with this procedure."

Because of the problem with frequent bowel movements, fluid and electrolyte imbalance, fistulas and abscesses, Valiente and Bacon (209) reasoned that if the rate of bowel movements could be diminished to a reasonable level, the bulk of these problems would be solved. To solve the frequency problem, they believed that creating a reservoir would obviate the almost constant need to evacuate. They wrote, "The pouch is constructed in a similar manner as the technique used in the so-called *pantaloon* operation for cases of total gastrectomy. It is our belief that if an adequate pouch can be obtained and the sphincter mechanism can be preserved intact, it would be possible for these patients to retain the ileal contents enough so that only three to four bowel movements take place every day" (Fig. 19).

Valiente and Bacon applied their concept to seven dogs. Although five of them died, the authors concluded from the two remaining dogs, "... a satisfactory and adequate pouch was established, the sphincter control was preserved in its entirety, the number of stools decreased and their consistency became mushy to formed, the perineal irritation was minimal. The capacity of the pouch to empty has been demonstrated by X-ray studies." In discussing Valiente and Bacon's paper, Rupert Turnbull stated, "I think this is in the dream stage, however, at the present time; ... I believe that somewhere in the future someone may perhaps solve this problem" (209).

In 1977, Martin et al. (210) reported on a proctocolectomy with anorectal mucosectomy to 1 cm above the mucocutaneous junction. The terminal ileum was anastomosed to the anal canal. A complementary loop ileostomy also was performed. Seventeen patients with ulcerative colitis who were between the ages of 11 and 20 years underwent this procedure. The results in 15 patients were successful, with good fecal continence. Overall complications were significant, particularly pelvic infection and cuff abscess.

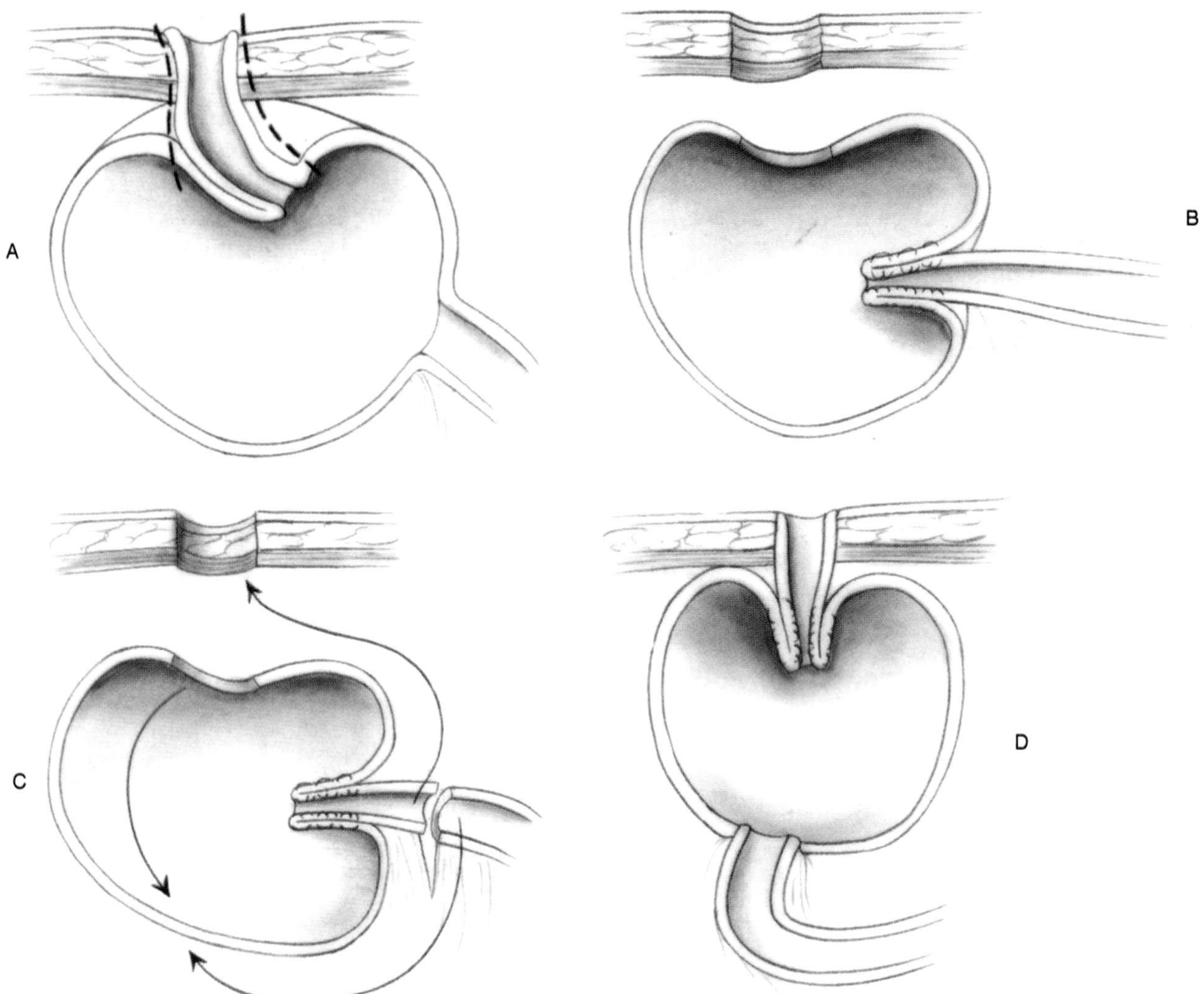

FIGURE 18 ■ Reconstruction of a new nipple valve. (**A**) Entire pouch and ileostomy are taken down. (**B**) Entire efferent limb of reservoir is excised and defect is closed. (**C**) Afferent limb 15 cm from reservoir is transected for reconstruction of valve. An enterotomy is made on the pouch. Nipple valve is intussuscepted into pouch and stapled in four quadrants. (**D**) Pouch is rotated. Newly constructed nipple valve, along with ileostomy limb, is brought through previous ileostomy site and anchored. Proximal cut end of ileum is anastomosed to reservoir as new afferent limb. *Source*: From Ref. 196.

Ileoanal anastomosis enjoyed its place briefly in the late 1970s and early 1980s (211,212). It was soon obvious that some kind of reservoir was needed to reduce the intolerable number of bowel movements in most patients, particularly in adults (213).

In 1978, Parks and Nicholls (214) were the first to show that proctocolectomy, stripping of the anorectal mucosa, and a pouch–anal anastomosis were feasible in patients with ulcerative colitis. They subsequently reported their experience with this operation in 21 patients (17 with ulcerative colitis, four with polyposis). Continence was good, and the average number of bowel movements was four per day (215). This report convinced others that a breakthrough in the operative treatment of ulcerative colitis had been achieved.

TABLE 2 ■ **Complications after Continent Ileostomy**

Complication	%
Pouch ileitis	15–30
Nipple valve slippage	3–25
Fistulas	0–10
Stomal stricture	10
Nipple prolapse	4–6
Complications requiring revisional operation	12–25
Stomal necrosis	?

Source: From Ref. 195.

■ SELECTION OF PATIENTS

TPC with IPAA is a major operation with a potentially high complication rate if not performed properly. The functional results are not perfect, particularly if the patients are not properly selected physically and mentally. The stool in the pouch is watery or at best semisolid, and good anal sphincter control is required to achieve reasonable continence. Patients with known poor anal continence should not be considered for IPAA. Although patients older than the age of 50 years have more frequent bowel movements and have less satisfactory sphincter control (216), age per se should not necessarily be the determining factor. If the patient is fit, understands the less-than-perfect outcome, and still desires to have the procedure, it should be considered.

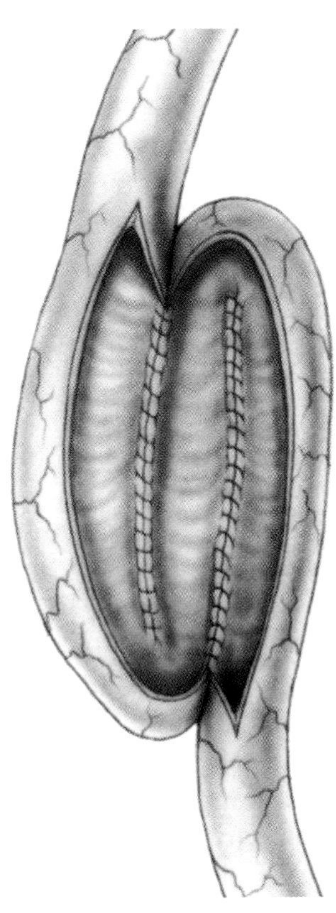

FIGURE 19 ■ "Pantaloon" pouch, comprising three segments of bowel. *Source*: From Ref. 209.

Patients with fulminant colitis and those with colitis and toxic megacolon should not have a simultaneous IPAA because of the high risk of intra-abdominal sepsis. Instead, a colectomy with a Hartmann procedure and an ileostomy should be done first. It will not compromise the results of later IPAA in any way (217,218). Hayvaert et al. (219) found that morbidity after elective IPAA was 27% compared with 66% for fulminant colitis. Pouch–anal leak occurred in 11% versus 41%, respectively. Although the differences do not reach statistical significance, it probably is due to the small number of patients. When properly selected in patients with fulminant ulcerative colitis who are hemodynamically stable, characterized by absence of tachycardia and hypotension, IPAA with ileostomy can be safely performed without major complication (220). Only 12 of 737 patients with IPAA were elected for the procedure. Harms et al. (221) also reported excellent results. Their successes involved the correction of anemia and severe hypoproteinemia via prolonged postoperative hyperalimentation, rapid steroid tapering, and an awareness of problem-related adrenal insufficiency (221). A prospective study comparing two- and three-stage procedures by Nicholls et al. (222) showed that the incidence of pelvic sepsis (18% and 17%, respectively) and small-bowel obstruction (19% and 15%, respectively) do not differ.

Overweight males have a higher risk of anastomotic stricture, reflecting the difficulty of the operation. This in turn may result in tension in the anastomosis, with disruption, ischemia, and stricture complications (223). Preoperative counseling for IPAA should include discussion of the risk of intraoperative abandonment. Browning and Nivatvongs (224) retrospectively reviewed 1789 IPAA attempts at the Mayo Clinic. Intraoperative abandonment occurred in 74 patients (4.1%). Patients in whom the operation was abandoned were older than patients in whom it was not (38 years vs. 33 years; $p < 0.01$), with age older than 40 years conferring a relative risk of 1.87 versus age younger than 40 years. IPAA was abandoned for technical reasons in 32 patients (43%), intraoperative diagnosis of Crohn's disease in 27 patients (36%), colorectal carcinoma in 10 patients (14%), mesenteric desmoid in three patients (4%), and miscellaneous reasons in two patients (3%). Among the abandonment of IPAA for technical reasons (1.8% of total series), a body mass index greater than or equal to 25 kg/m^2, male gender, and age greater than or equal to 40 years significantly increased the risk (224).

Happy patients are those who are highly motivated to have the procedure. The surgeon should keep in mind that the Brooke ileostomy remains the benchmark against which other options must be compared.

Various Methods of Pouch Construction

The single most important function of an ileal pouch is as a reservoir to hold the gastrointestinal contents. Whether it is an isoperistaltic or an antiperistaltic pouch does not seem to matter significantly. The pouch should be large enough to hold ileal contents but small enough to fit in the pelvis. The original type of reservoir reported by Parks and Nicholls in 1978 (214) is called an S pouch, and it used three segments of the terminal ileum. In 1980, Utsunomiya et al. (225) described a two-loop segment called a J pouch. In 1980, Fonkalsrud (226) introduced a side-to-side pouch. In 1985, Nicholls and Pezim (227) modified a double J pouch to expand the capacity; the result is called a W pouch. It soon was learned that the configuration of the pouch is not the determining factor in predicting functional outcome (228–230). At the present time, the J pouch is the reservoir that almost all surgeons use.

Technique of J-Pouch Construction

Abdominal Proctocolectomy

The patient is positioned to allow access to the abdomen and perineum. Mobilization of the colon and rectum is exactly the same as that described for TPC and ileostomy for ulcerative colitis.

The terminal ileum is transected flush with the cecum, using a linear stapler. The ileal branch of the ileocolic vessels must be preserved at this point but may need to be sacrificed later. The rectum is transected just above the levator ani muscle, using a linear stapler. The root of the small bowel mesentery is mobilized to the level of the ligament of Treitz.

Preparation of Terminal Ileum and Its Mesentery

A site 15 to 20 cm proximal to the stapled cut end of the terminal ileum is chosen and folded for the J-pouch construction. It will reach the anus if this point extends 6 cm beyond the top of the symphysis pubis (231). The most important part of the pouch procedure is to obtain adequate length of the mesentery. It is usually necessary to release tension by transversely incising the peritoneum of the stretched mesentery of the small bowel.

The mesentery is transilluminated to delineate the arcade of the blood vessels formed by the ileocolic artery and the terminal ileal branch of the superior mesenteric artery. Because traction is placed on the small bowel at the predetermined site for the pouch, either the ileocolic or the superior mesenteric vessel has the most tension and needs to be sacrificed to obtain the maximal length for the pouch to reach. Only one of the two vessels can be taken. If the ileocolic vessel has to be sacrificed, the procedure is performed near its origin. If the superior mesenteric vessel has to be taken, the procedure is performed at a site in the distal one-third. Transillumination is necessary to visualize the arcades of blood supply. It is important that an arcade of blood vessels connects between the ileocolic and the superior mesenteric vessels (Fig. 20). In fresh cadaver, the increase in mesenteric length is greater after superior mesenteric vessels divisions than after ileocolic vessels division (232).

Goes et al. (233) reported a technique of preserving the middle colic vessels along with the marginal vascular arcade from the middle colic artery to the ileal branch of the ileocolic artery. In this way, both the ileocolic vessels and the distal third of the superior mesenteric vessels can be sacrificed. In cadaver dissection, this technique adds a mean 3.6 cm (range, 2.5–5 cm) over the conventional technique of taking out one vessel. This technique may prove to be very useful, pending further study.

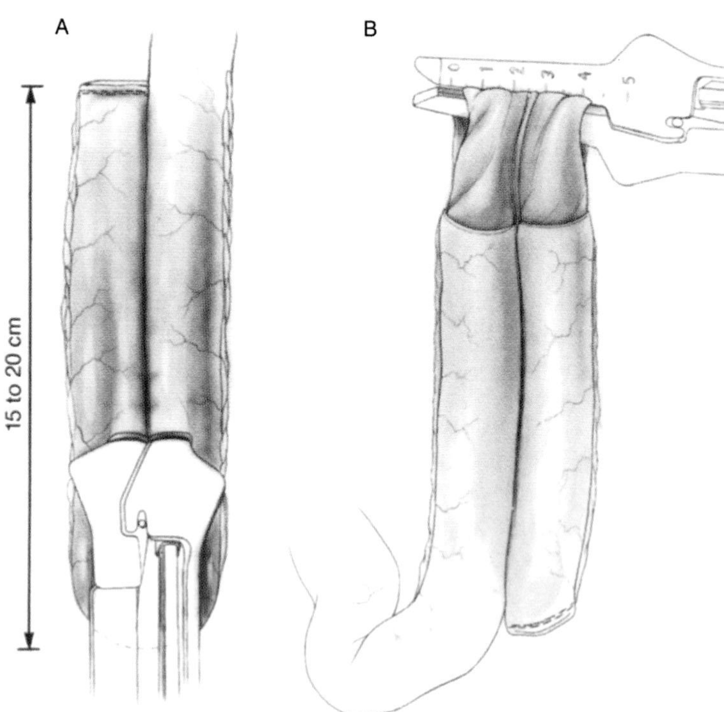

FIGURE 21 ■ Construction of J pouch. (**A**) A 15 to 20 cm segment of terminal ileum is folded into shape of a J. An enterotomy is made 6 to 7 cm from base of J. Anastomosing stapler is activated in both directions. Multiple firings are required. (**B**) Septum at base of pouch is everted and divided.

Construction of Pouch

The J pouch is made from the distal 30 to 40 cm of ileum folded in half. Two small enterotomies are made approximately 5 cm from the base of the future reservoir. An anastomosing stapler is introduced and activated in the direction of the base, then in the opposite direction (Fig. 21A). Multiple firings of the stapler are needed, depending on the length of the stapler chosen. With this technique, the ridge at the base of the pouch is everted through the enterotomies and transected with the stapler to prevent obstruction of the outlet of the pouch (Fig. 21B). The enterotomies are closed transversely or longitudinally with one closed transversely or longitudinally with one layer of running 3–0 braided synthetic absorbable suture. This kind of construction is for anorectal mucosectomy technique through its base (frequently called the apex). A pursestring suture is placed at the base to prevent excessive stretching, and an enterotomy is made within the pursestring suture. Multiple firings of the stapler are needed to complete the entire length of the pouch (Fig. 22). In this way, no bridge is created, and the opening at the base is used later in an anastomosis with the anus. This technique is preferred by some surgeons because it eliminates the need for the enterotomy and the distal bridge is eliminated automatically. However, in the former technique, when the pouch is brought down to the anus, the anastomosis can be performed at the most distal part of the pouch, which is usually the site of the base (apex). I prefer this technique because I can get about 1 cm better reach (for the hand-sewn anastomosis).

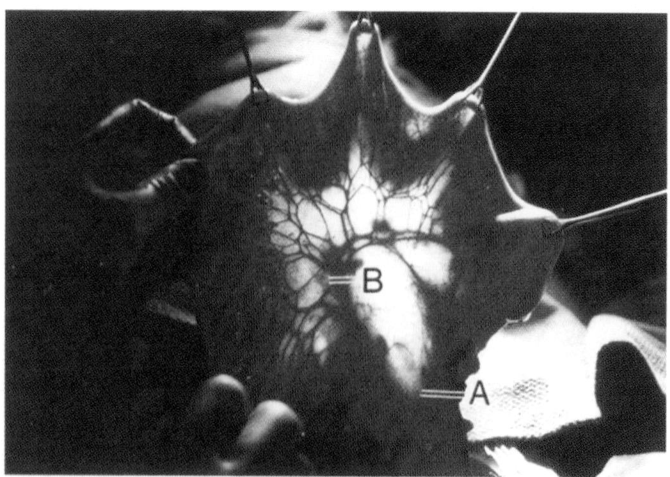

FIGURE 20 ■ Technique of lengthening mesentery in J-pouch construction. Arterial supply of terminal ileum. Note site of taking ileocolic vessels (**A**) and site of taking superior mesenteric vessels (**B**). It is important to note that only one of the two vessels can be sacrificed.

Technique of S-Pouch Construction

Parks and Nicholls (214) were the first to construct the S pouch as a reservoir and to anastomose it to the anus.

Preparation of Terminal Ileum and Its Mesentery

Unlike the J pouch, the S-pouch reservoir reaches the anal canal with its efferent limb, the end of the terminal ileum. The ileal branch of the ileocolic artery is ligated and divided near its origin. The last vascular arcade near the tip of the terminal ileum must not be injured (Fig. 23). Additional incisions on the peritoneum of the mesentery usually provide extra length.

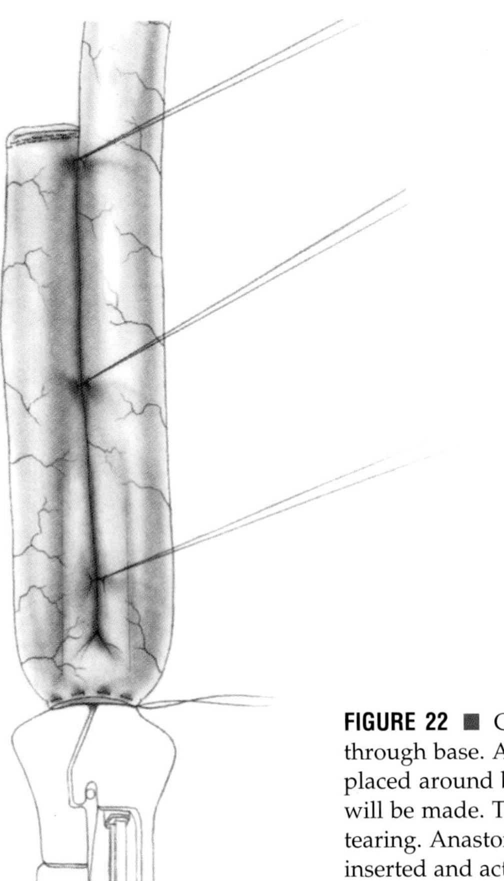

FIGURE 22 ■ Construction of J pouch through base. A pursestring suture is placed around base where enterotomy will be made. This suture will prevent tearing. Anastomosing stapler is inserted and activated. Multiple firings may be needed.

Construction of Pouch

The terminal ileum, with 10 to 12 cm in each limb, is folded twice with a 2 cm projection that will be an outlet of the pouch for anastomosis to the anus (Fig. 24A). Originally, Parks et al. (215) used 15 cm for each limb and a 5 cm projection. However, a pouch that size with a long efferent limb resulted in an incidence of evacuation difficulties as high as 50%. The ileum is opened on its antimesenteric border, and the posterior walls are sutured using one continuous layer of 3–0 braided synthetic absorbable sutures (Fig. 24B). Finally, the anterior wall of the pouch is approximated using one continuous layer of 3–0 braided synthetic absorbable sutures (Fig. 24C).

Other Types of Pouch

Fonkalsrud (226) preferred to use a lateral reservoir. The reach by this type of pouch to the anus is similar to that of the S pouch. It is constructed by forming a side-to-side anastomosis between two 15 cm limbs of terminal ileum, with a 2 cm projection for the pouch–anal anastomosis (Fig. 25).

To increase the capacity of the pouch, hoping to improve the functional results, Nicholls and Lubowski (235) developed a four-loop reservoir (W pouch). The terminal ileum is folded into two U-shaped configurations, with each limb 12 cm long. The antimesenteric border in each limb is incised. The posterior wall is sewn together with one running layer of 3–0 braided synthetic absorbable sutures. The cut edges in the anterior wall are approximated using one layer of continuous 3–0 braided synthetic absorbable sutures (Fig. 26).

Anorectal Mucosectomy

The technique and the concept of mucosectomy have changed. It is now known that the rectum can be transected down to the level of the levator ani muscle without compromising anal sphincter function. The shorter stripping procedure reduces the time of operation, bleeding, contamination, and the risk of infection, and it favors better expansion of the neorectum (236).

From the abdominal part, the rectum is transected at just above the levator ani muscle using TA 30 stapler. Mucosectomy is performed per anum. Two Gelpi retractors are placed at right angles at the anoderm to efface the anus. Normal saline solution is injected in the submucosal plane around the anal canal. Using electrocautery or scissors, the mucosa is stripped from the underlying internal sphincter, starting at the dentate line and carried up to the stapled rectum, where it is removed en bloc with the submucosal tube. Using this technique, the entire length of the internal sphincter muscle is preserved. The disposable Lone Star self-retaining retractor (Lone Star Medical Products, Houston, Texas, U.S.A.) is used, which further facilitates the dissection (237). The anus is effaced circumferentially by eight elastic adjustable stays (Fig. 27). This technique is helpful when the cheeks of the buttocks are deep. However, the stays pulling the dentate line move distally, hampering the reach of the pouch for the anastomosis. If this is the case, Gelpi retractors should be used at the time of anastomosis.

My preference in anorectal mucosectomy is to remove in four separate strips. From the abdominal phase, the rectum is transected at about 6 cm from the anal verge (measured by digital examination) using electrocautery. This leaves approximately 4 cm of anorectal mucosa from the dentate line. The anorectum is exposed with a Pratt anal speculum. The mucosa is injected with normal saline solution to raise it from the underlying internal sphincter muscle. Using scissors, the submucosa at the dentate line in that quadrant is dissected to cut end of the rectum. The posterior quadrant is started first and ended in the anterior quadrant. I do not believe that mild to moderate stretching with the Pratt speculum for 1 to 2 minutes in each quadrant damages the sphincter muscles. The advantage of this technique is that it is consistently easy to perform.

Ileal Pouch–Anal Anastomosis

The pouch is delivered to the denuded anorectal cuff using a Babcock clamp. The base of the pouch is anastomosed to the anus at the dentate line using interrupted 3–0 braided synthetic absorbable sutures (Fig. 28).

A closed suction drain is placed in the presacral space behind the pouch and is brought out through a separate stab wound in the left lower quadrant. A No. 20 Malecot catheter or a Penrose drain is placed in the pouch for four to five days. This helps avoid retention of fluid in the event of hypersecretion from the pouch.

Stapled Pouch–Anal Anastomosis Without Mucosectomy

Because of the consistently low resting pressure in patients after mucosectomy and IPAA, particularly in those with fecal soiling (238,239) it was speculated that injury to the anal canal or internal sphincter might be the cause. In a

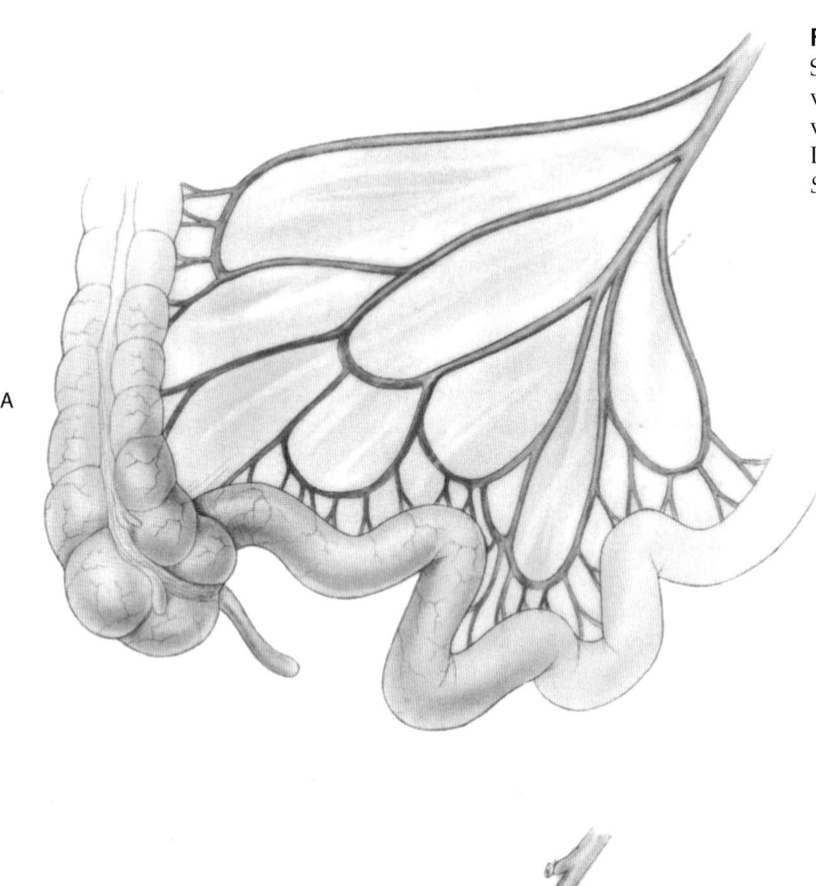

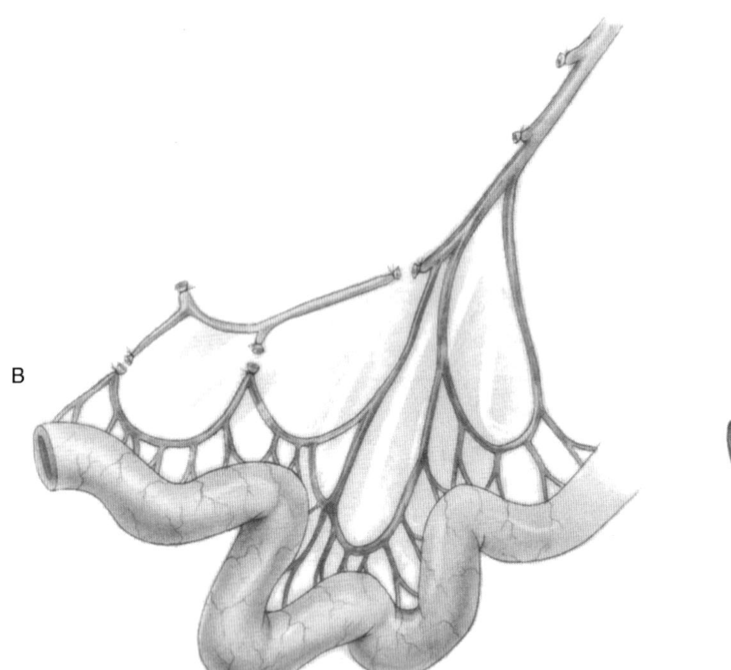

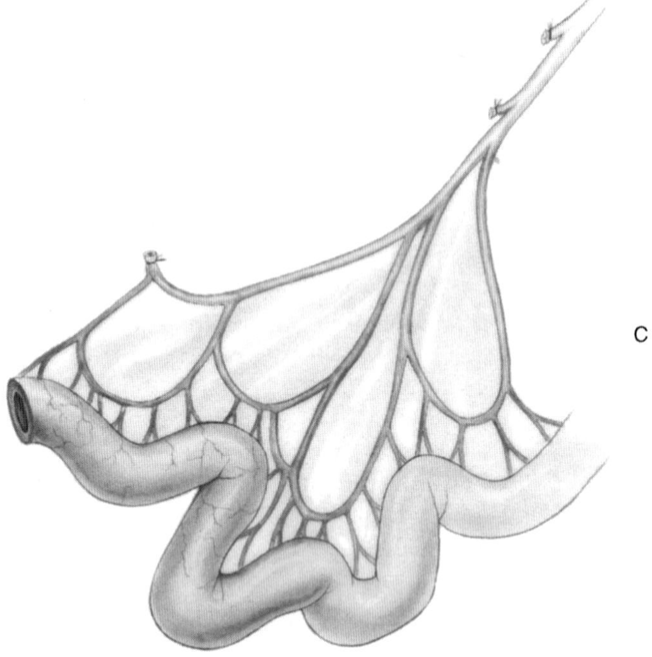

FIGURE 23 ■ Technique of lengthening mesentery in S pouch. (**A**) Identification of right colic and ileocolic vessels. (**B**) Right colic artery is divided. (**C**) Ileocolic vessels are ligated and divided near their origin. Last arterial arcade to terminal ileum must be preserved. *Source*: From Ref. 234.

small series of patients reported by Keighley (240) the resting pressure was lower in the group of patients after endoanal mucosectomy than after abdominal mucosectomy and the incidence of leakage was also higher in the endoanal mucosectomy group. This was not a randomized trial, and the duration of follow-up was short; but it suggested that endoanal mucosectomy causes damage, possibly from prolonged stretching of the anal canal during the procedure. To improve continence, many authors have advocated a pouch–anal anastomosis without mucosectomy, leaving 1 to 2 cm of transitional zone epithelium above the dentate line, using double-stapled technique.

Technique

The abdominal colectomy is performed in the same manner as for IPAA with mucosectomy. The rectum is transected 4 cm proximal to the dentate line using a linear stapler 30 or 50 mm in width (Fig. 29A). The level of transection must be verified precisely by checking (with a finger through the anus) the level of the stapler before preparing the anorectal stump.

The J pouch is constructed using an anastomosing stapler through the base of the pouch (see Fig. 22). A medium-size circular stapler with the trocar retracted into the cartridge is inserted into the anal canal, and the trocar

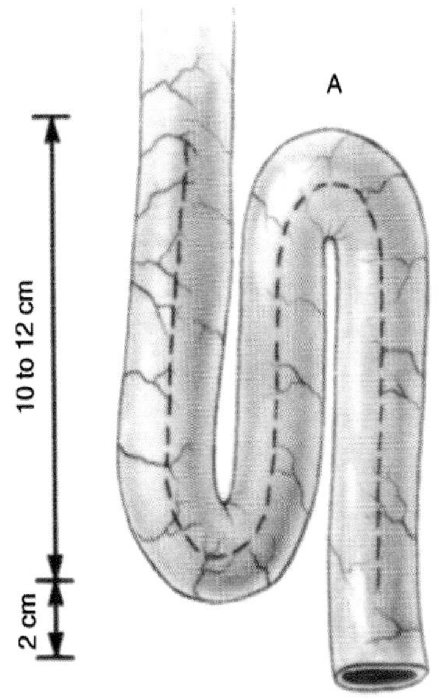

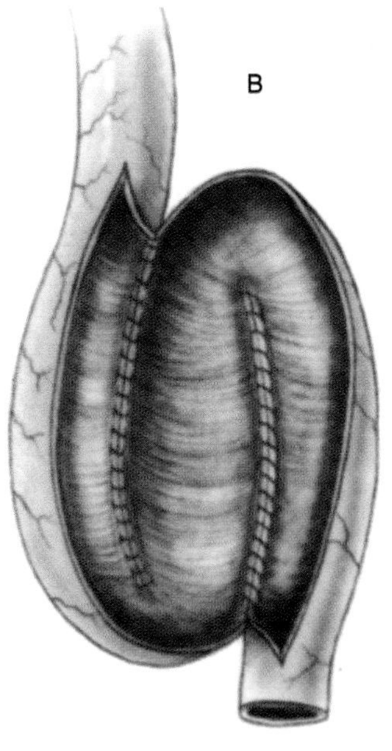

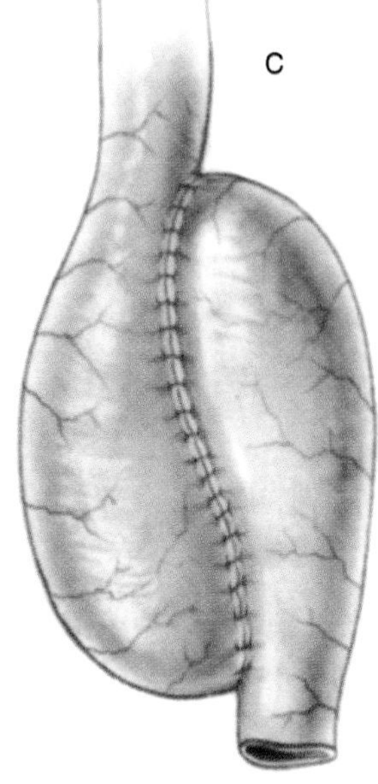

FIGURE 24 ■ Construction of S pouch. (**A**) Terminal ileum is folded (10–12 cm for each limb) to make three segments, with a 2 cm projection remaining. (**B**) Incision is made on antimesenteric border of bowel. Posterior walls are closed with one continuous layer of 3–0 absorbable sutures. (**C**) Pouch is completed with one-layer closure of anterior wall using one continuous layer of absorbable sutures. Note the short projection of only 1 to 1.5 cm. *Source*: From Ref. 215.

is projected through the staple line and then removed (Fig. 29B). The anvil of the stapler is inserted into the base of the J pouch, and a pursestring suture of 2–0 Prolene is tied around the shaft. The anvil pin is engaged into the central shaft where the trocar was removed. The anvil is approximated to the cartridge, and the instrument is activated, after which it is disengaged and removed from the anal canal (Fig. 29C). The two donut rings should be checked for their completeness, because an incomplete donut ring may indicate an incomplete anastomosis. The anastomosis should be 2 cm proximal to the dentate line and should be palpated with the index finger through the anus to detect any defect. The pelvis is then filled with saline solution. The ileum above the pouch is clamped, and a small amount of air is introduced via the anal canal to check for an air leak. A closed-suction drain is placed in the presacral space behind the pouch. A number 22 Malecot catheter is left in the pouch for drainage of any hypersecretion of fluid. It is left in as dependent drainage for 4 or 5 days.

The stapled pouch–anal anastomosis is easier and quicker to perform than IPAA with mucosectomy. Some authors do not routinely use a diverting loop ileostomy.

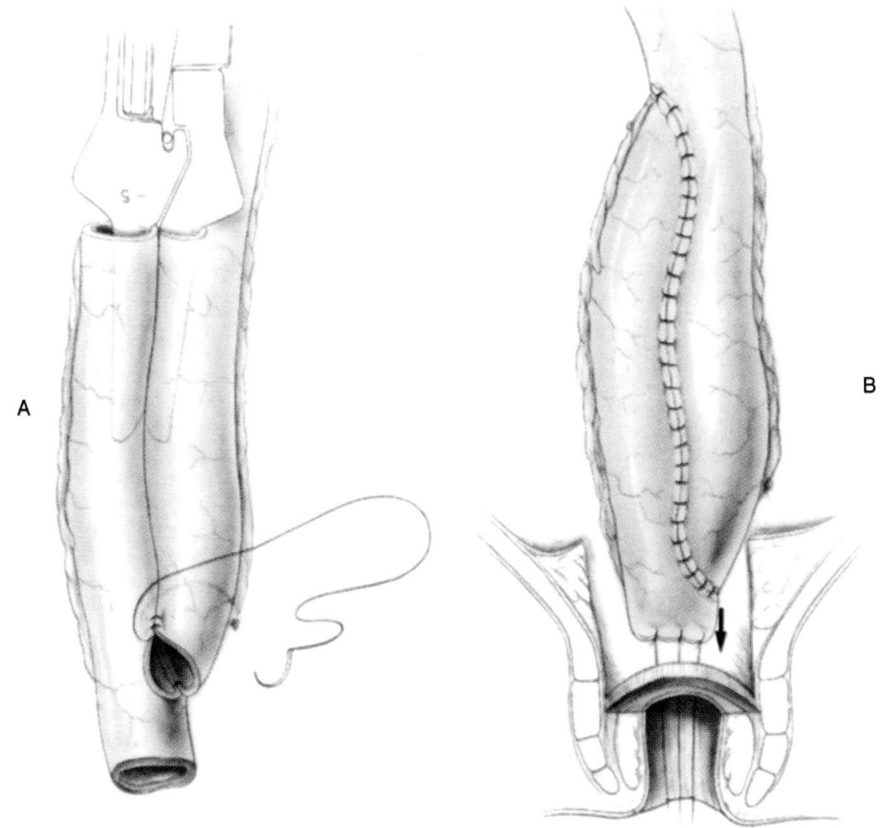

FIGURE 25 ■ Lateral reservoir. (**A**) A 15 cm segment of terminal ileum is divided. With an anastomosing stapler, segment is anastomosed side to side with proximal part of ileum. (**B**) Enterotomies for stapler are closed with continuous sutures. Entire reservoir anastomosis is sewn over with a second layer of continuous absorbable sutures.

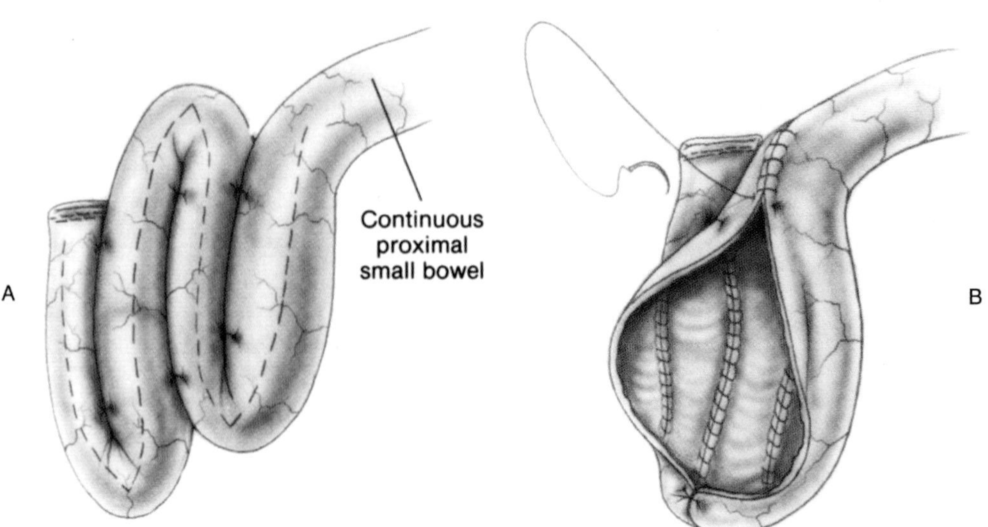

FIGURE 26 ■ Construction of W pouch. (**A**) Four segments of terminal ileum are folded in two U configurations. Antimesenteric border is incised. (**B**) Posterior walls are closed with one layer of continuous 3–0 absorbable sutures. Anterior wall is closed with one layer of continuous 3–0 absorbable sutures.

The Issue of Leaving Anal Transitional Zone Behind

Proponents of stapled pouch–anal anastomosis showed that without mucosectomy, incontinence, particularly seepage, seldom occurs. They believed that the transitional zone is not true mucosa and therefore acute inflammation or flare-ups of colitis are unlikely and the risk of developing carcinoma is extremely low (241–245). However, in the presence of dysplasia of the colon or rectum, synchronous colorectal carcinoma, or active disease in the area, preservation of the transitional zone of the anal canal is not recommended (246,247).

Objections to preserving the anal mucosa include the risk of carcinoma and persisting or recurring inflammation causing symptoms, A study by Curran et al. (248) of anal mucosa in 24 specimens from patients with ulcerative colitis showed that the anal mucosa was inflamed in each patient and no significant difference could be demonstrated between the degrees of inflammation in their rectal and anal mucosa. In 21% the inflammatory changes were most severe in the anal canal. Tsunoda et al. (249) studied the stripped anorectal mucosa in patients with IPAA to determine the incidence of dysplasia in 118 patients with ulcerative colitis. Although the overall rate of dysplasia was 2.5%, dysplasia was present in three specimens of stripped anorectal mucosa out of 12 patients with dysplasia of the colonic resection specimens (25%). Dysplasia also was present in 8% of the stripped anorectal mucosa when the disease was more than 12 years old and 0% when the disease was less than 10 years old.

In an effort to determine whether the anal transitional zone (ATZ) should be removed with the IPAA procedure, Ambroze et al. (250) studied 50 proctocolectomy specimens from 50 ulcerative colitis patients and from 50 patients with rectal carcinoma who served as controls. The authors found that the columnar epithelium of the rectal mucosa formed

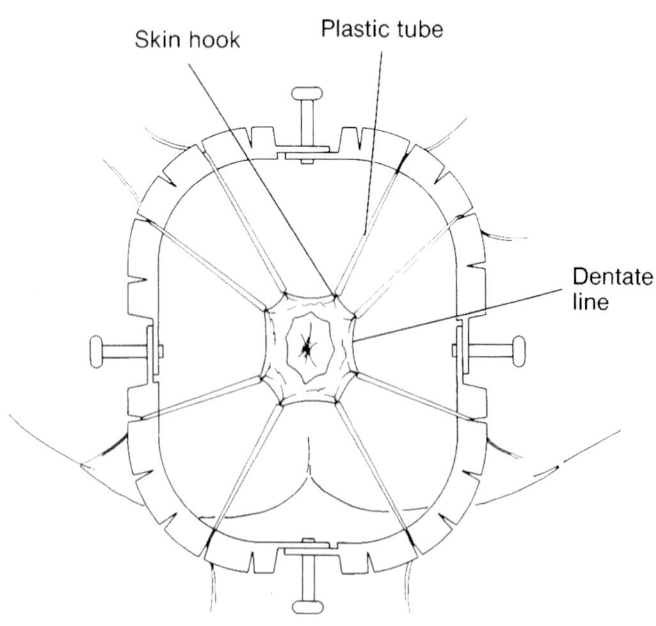

FIGURE 27 ■ Technique of anorectal mucosectomy with patient in lithotomy position in stirrups. The Lone Star, a self-retaining retractor, is used to efface anal canal. Its eight elastic stays can be adjusted to facilitate mucosectomy and anastomosis of the pouch to dentate line. *Source*: From Ref. 237.

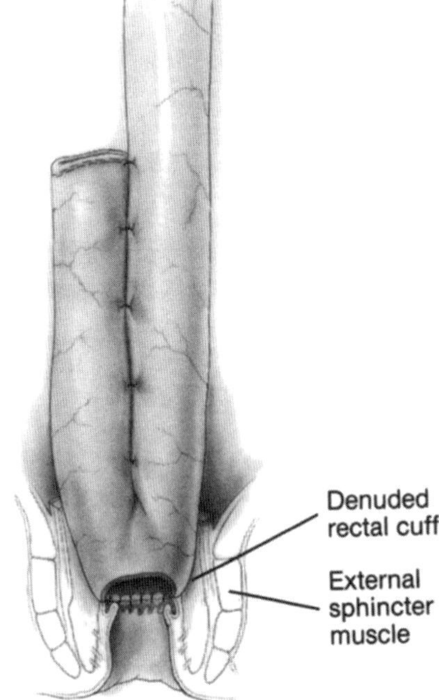

FIGURE 28 ■ Pouch–anal anastomosis. Pouch is delivered through denuded anorectum and is anastomosed to dentate line with one layer of interrupted 3–0 synthetic absorbable suture.

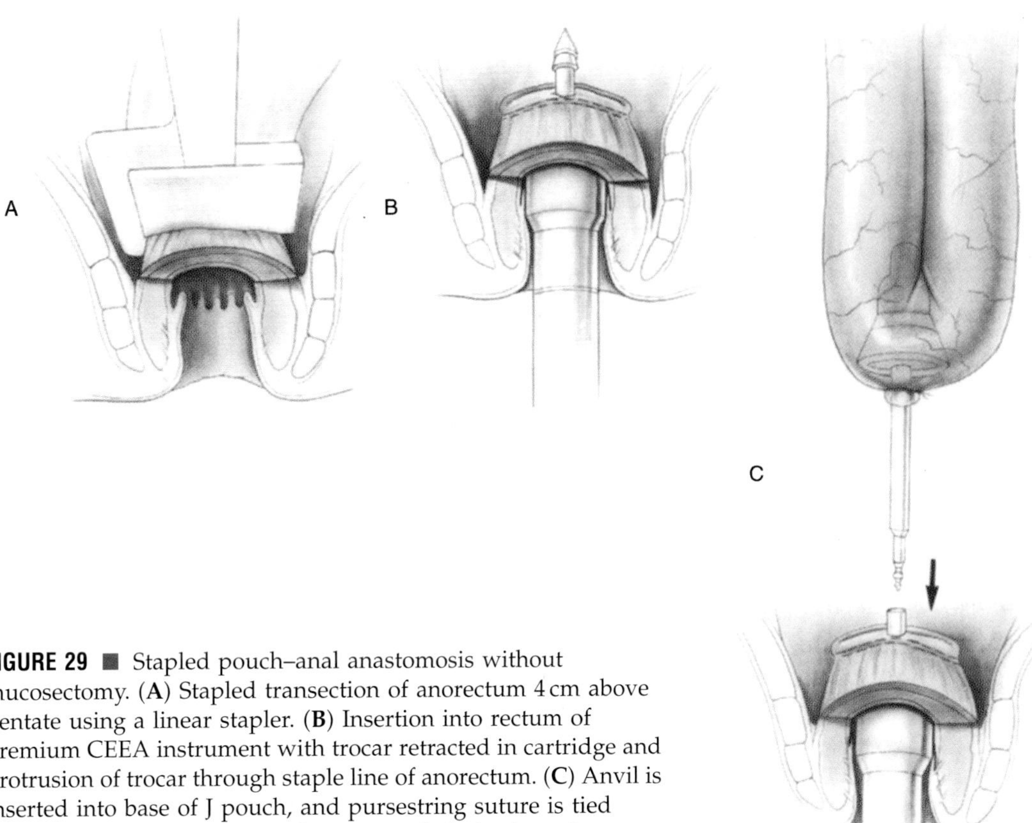

FIGURE 29 ■ Stapled pouch–anal anastomosis without mucosectomy. (**A**) Stapled transection of anorectum 4 cm above dentate using a linear stapler. (**B**) Insertion into rectum of premium CEEA instrument with trocar retracted in cartridge and protrusion of trocar through staple line of anorectum. (**C**) Anvil is inserted into base of J pouch, and pursestring suture is tied around shaft. Anvil is engaged into central shaft where the trocar was removed and approximated to cartridge. Instrument is activated and anastomosis is completed. *Source*: From Ref. 240.

digitations within 1 cm of the dentate line in 89% of the specimens. Although the transitional epithelium does not become inflamed in ulcerative colitis, the columnar epithelium that extends past the transitional epithelium causes inflammation of the anal canal.

In a study of ATZ in 113 patients who had stapled pouch–anal anastomosis for ulcerative colitis, Thompson-Fawcett et al. (251) found that inflammatory activity in the ATZ was very low, and if present, it was usually associated with inflammatory activity in the columnar epithelium of the cuff. The amount of columnar epithelium within the ATZ was small. It seemed unlikely the ATZ would be primarily involved in the inflammatory process of ulcerative colitis. The authors believe that routine follow-up biopsies of the ATZ is indicated.

Even mucosectomy is not without risk. O'Connell et al. (252) found small islets of residual rectal mucosa in 21% of the patients who underwent IPAA with mucosectomy. However, the remnants of the rectal mucosa do not regenerate (253). Stripping the mucosa starting at the dentate line does not always remove the entire ATZ. In 9% of the specimens studied by Ambroze et al. (250), the columnar epithelium was in direct apposition to the dentate line. The study by Fenger (254) showed that ATZ extends 3 to 6 mm below the dentate line. Adenocarcinoma has been reported in patients who underwent IPAA with mucosectomy, presumably arising from a remnant of the rectal mucosa (255,256). Long-term periodic examination of the anal canal and the pouch is recommended. Despite leaving the entire ATZ behind in stapled IPAA, most authors believe that the risk of the inflammation or dysplasia in this small area is low (257). However, long-term annual examinations with biopsies of the anorectal mucosa are advisable (247). If mucosa dysplasia is found, a transanal mucosectomy, or if necessary, an abdominal approach is recommended (258).

Another controversy involves the functional results between the two techniques, particularly fecal incontinence, especially during the night. The reports from most series show that the stapled technique without mucosectomy has less fecal incontinence (244,259–261). These comparisons do not take into account the proper technique of mucosectomy and the excessive time spent overstretching the anal canal. Becker et al. (262) have shown that in 66 of 79 patients, mucosectomy specimens contain smooth muscle. The degree of smooth muscle loss is associated with reduced anal sphincter pressure, increased stool frequency, and more frequent nocturnal leakage of stool. This study suggests that performing the technique of mucosectomy properly is crucial for the best results.

The high incidence of nocturnal incontinence [up to 55% (263,264)] in mucosectomy IPPA has been thought to be from damage of the internal sphincter muscle, coupled with losing the ATZ, which may be essential for sensation and discrimination. The resting pressure drops 42% to 54% after mucosectomy for IPAA (264–266). Most studies on stapled anastomosis without mucosectomy showed the incidence of nocturnal incontinence to be approximately 8% to 18% (267,268). Tuckson et al. (261) found that the stapled anastomosis without mucosectomy has a higher mean anal resting pressure (64.6 ± 5.3 mm Hg) than IPAA mucosectomy with hand-sewn anastomosis

(47.9 ± 33 mm Hg). Others have reported similar findings (269). Miller et al. (270) found anal sensation is better but resting pressure does not differ between nonmucosectomy and mucosectomy patients.

Prospective randomized trials comparing anal function (continence, urgency, frequency, etc.) between mucosectomy and nonmucosectomy patients were conducted by Seow-Choen et al. (271) and Luukkonen and Jarvinen (272). Both trials showed no advantages between the two. A case-control study by McIntyre et al. (273) also showed no statistical difference between the two groups. An uncontrolled study by Guzzetti et al. (274) showed more fecal incontinence in patients who had undergone mucosectomy.

It appears that both proponents for mucosectomy IPPA (275) and nonmucosectomy stapled anastomosis (259) have good reasons. It is important, if mucosectomy is performed, not to take or injure the internal sphincter muscle. It is a common finding that the muscle is included in the specimen (262). The surgeon should develop techniques to strip off the anorectal mucosa quickly to avoid prolonged stretching of the anal canal. The denuded anorectum must be reexamined for any residual mucosa. Similarly, the nonmucosectomy stapled technique should also be performed properly. The anastomosis should be 1 to 2 cm above the dentate line. It is not advisable to anastomose the pouch to the dentate line as the functional result has been shown to be inferior (276). An anastomosis 4 cm above the dentate line is likely a pouch–rectal anastomosis and should be avoided.

Loop Ileostomy

A loop ileostomy is recommended for IPAA in patients with ulcerative colitis. It allows the reservoir and the anastomosis to heal and regain their function. IPAA without a diverting ileostomy, however, has been performed successfully in a few carefully selected patients, but should be used with caution (277). The results in a group of 50 patients who underwent IPAA (stapled technique) without diverting ileostomy at the Cleveland Clinic (278) were compared to 50 patients who underwent a diverting ileostomy during the same period of time. Anastomotic leak and pelvic abscess were more common in patients without ileostomy (7 of 50, 14% vs. 2 of 50, 4%). Eight of these nine patients were taking greater than or equal to 20 mg of prednisone per day.

Septic complications requiring reoperation (6% vs. 0%), prolonged ileus and fever of unknown origin (10% vs. 4%) were also more common in patients without ileostomy. Despite similar functional results at six weeks and at 12 months, patients without ileostomy have a poorer quality-of-life index (5 vs. 8, 10 being best) in the early period (0–6 weeks) of pouch function. Overall, IPAA with a loop ileostomy was safer than without in this series, especially in patients taking greater than or equal to 20 mg prednisone per day. At the Mayo Clinic, 96% of IPAAs (with anorectal mucosectomy) are performed with a loop ileostomy. In properly selected patients, a one-stage IPAA without ileostomy is performed with excellent results. Strict criteria are applied: no tension at the anastomosis, good blood supply of terminal ileum, good general health, and no steroid intake (279). Gorfine et al. (280) performed IPAA with anorectal mucosectomy, without ileostomy, if the patients did not take immunosuppressive drugs and were taking less than 20 mg of prednisone daily in the month preceding surgery. When compared to a similar group with ileostomy, the rates of septic complications and functional results were similar. A randomized trial was conducted on IPAA with and without ileostomy in a small number of patients by Grabler et al. (281). The results showed no difference in morbidity and mortality. Several other authors have performed IPAA without ileostomy almost exclusively (282–286).

At the Mayo Clinic, we continue to perform loop ileostomy for IPAA and to reserve IPAA without ileostomy for selected criteria as alluded to previously by Galandiuk et al. (279). However, an increasing number of IPAA procedures can be performed without ileostomy.

The loop ileostomy is closed approximately two to three months after the operation, provided the pouchogram shows no leak or pelvic abscess. Approximately 80% to 98% of loop ileostomy closures can be performed with an incision around the ileostomy without the need to open the abdomen (263,287).

A loop of ileum as close to the pouch as possible (usually 45–60 cm from the apex of the pouch) is brought out through the aperture, which was premarked in the right lower quadrant. This loop of bowel should not be turned or twisted. Both the functional and nonfunctional stomas are matured with 3–0 monofilament synthetic absorbable sutures. No rod is needed to support the ileostomy.

Creation of a loop ileostomy is not without problems, particularly small bowel obstruction and wound infection. Some authors avoid a loop ileostomy because of complications reported as high as 52% (281). However, in the large series of 1504 patients reported by Wong et al. (288) showed an overall complication rate of 11.4%. The complications included small bowel obstruction (6.4%), wound infection (1.4%), abdominal septic complication (1%), and enterocutaneous fistulas (0.6%). There were no significant differences in complication rates and length of hospitalization between hand sewn and stapled closure techniques. Closure of the loop ileostomy also has significant complications. Small bowel obstruction is the most common finding, accounting for approximately 10% (287,289–291). Exploratory celiotomy for peritonitis after ileostomy closure occurs 1% to 7% (287,289–291).

In patients with complications of the ileal pouch or concomitant medical problems, the loop ileostomy should not be closed for an extended period of time. Delaying ileostomy closure for more than six months has no deleterious effect on pouch function (292).

Which Type of Pouch to Use?

Which type of pouch to use is a matter of personal preference. Most surgeons favor the J pouch but may switch to an S pouch if the J pouch cannot reach the anus with ease. It always is wise not to construct the pouch until it is determined that the pouch will reach the anus. This can be done by simulating the pouch configuration and drawing it down to the pelvis.

What to Do When the Pouch Won't Reach?

Proper dissection of the small-bowel mesentery and division of the ileocolic vessels or distal one-third of the superior mesenteric vessels as described earlier, will give an adequate length for the J-pouch or S-pouch to the upper anal canal in almost all the cases. However, in certain situations, the pouch does not reach. Chick et al. (293) reported a case of using saphenous vein grafts after division of the superior mesenteric vessels (the ileocolic vessels had been divided) to extend the length of the small-bowel mesentery. A 15-cm saphenous vein was harvested from the upper thigh and interposed end-to-end between the stump of the superior mesenteric vessels to the distal artery and vein of the devascularized segment. Microvascular technique and the operative microscope were used. The added length had allowed the correction of a 6 cm deficit, a successful J-pouch anal anastomosis. There were no operative or postoperative complications except for a minor wound infection.

We had such a situation in a case of a young and thin patient who underwent an urgent total abdominal colectomy with retention of the rectum. The ileocolic vessels were divided at the time of construction of an end-ileostomy. The patient was readmitted to the hospital six weeks later for a small-bowel obstruction, not relieved by conservative management. Exploratory celiotomy was performed; a small-bowel volvulus was found, about one foot proximal to the ileostomy. This was successfully corrected with a derotation.

Six months later, an ileal pouch was performed. The small-bowel mesentery was foreshortened because of the previous volvulus. The only way to make the pouch reach was to divide the superior mesenteric vessels. A vascular surgeon was consulted. The superior mesenteric vessels were divided at a convenient area well below the duodenum. A 10-cm saphenous vein was harvested from the left inner thigh (patient was already in combined position). This was interposed to the superior mesenteric artery. Microvascular technique using a microscope was not necessary and it was not necessary to reconnect the superior mesenteric vein. We obtained a strong pulsation of the graft and the entire small bowel had an excellent blood flow, confirmed by a Doppler. We achieved about 5 cm extra length. The J pouch reached the upper anal canal without tension, using double-staple technique. The patient did well and the loop ileostomy was closed two and a half months later (*Disease Colon and Rectum*, in press).

I believe this is an important technique to know, keeping in mind that complications of the graft can occur especially blood clots. It is essential to have a competent vascular surgeon to perform the procedure, and it should be used only as the last option.

SPECIAL SITUATIONS

■ INDETERMINATE COLITIS

All patients who plan to undergo IPAA should have a preliminary diagnosis of ulcerative colitis based on clinical diagnosis, including history, physical examination, endoscopy, and often a biopsy. In some patients, the diagnosis cannot be ascertained even at the time of proctocolectomy, after frozen section of the specimen, because of the unusual distribution of inflammation, deep linear ulcers, neural proliferation, transmural inflammation, fissures, creeping fat, and retention of the goblet-cell population. This "indeterminate" colitis (294) accounted for 5% of 1519 patients who underwent IPAA for CUC at the Mayo Clinic (295).

In a prospective study of 499 patients with preoperative diagnosis of ulcerative colitis at the Cleveland Clinic Florida (296), 20 patients or 4% had the diagnostic changes after the proctocolectomy: 2.6% as indeterminate colitis, and 1.4% as Crohn's colitis.

In a review of an IPAA registry at the Mayo Clinic (295), 1437 patients with CUC and 82 patients with indeterminate colitis who underwent IPAA were compared. Patients with indeterminate colitis and CUC were comparable in terms of gender and duration of follow-up. The mean follow-up was 83 (range, 1–192) months. The mean age of CUC was higher (34 vs. 31). At 10 years, patients with indeterminate colitis had significantly more episodes of pelvic sepsis (17% indeterminate colitis vs. 7% CUC), pouch fistula (31% vs. 9%), and pouch failure (27% vs. 11%). Importantly, during follow-up, fully 15% of patients with indeterminate colitis, but only 2% of patients with CUC, had their original diagnosis changed to Crohn's disease. When the outcomes of these patients newly diagnosed with Crohn's disease were considered separately, the rate of complications for the remaining patients with indeterminate colitis was identical to that of patients with CUC. Functional outcomes were comparable among all three groups. The authors concluded that after IPAA, patients with indeterminate colitis who did not develop Crohn's disease subsequently experienced long-term outcomes nearly identical to patients with CUC. Crohn's disease, whether it develops after surgery or CUC or indeterminate colitis, is associated with poor long-term outcome.

Similar results have been reported by others (296,297). It appears that if the final diagnosis is not obvious Crohn's disease, IPAA can be performed with reasonable confidence (298–301). This approach should be made with caution. The series from the Lahey Clinic (302) indicated perineal complication rate of 50% in indeterminate patients with IPAA compared with 3% in patients with CUC. It is comparable to the perineal complication rate in Crohn's disease of 66%. The pouch failure rate was 28% compared with 17% in patients with CUC. If in doubt during the operation, it is reasonable to withhold the IPAA by performing a colectomy and a Hartmann procedure and an ileostomy. This will provide time to re-evaluate the specimen and a long-term follow-up before the final diagnosis.

The diagnosis of IBD is based on a combination of clinical, histologic, endoscopic, and radiologic data. The distinction between ulcerative colitis and Crohn's disease can be difficult to observe because of the lack of a gold standard to differentiate between the two. There are no reliable immunohistochemical markers, but the combined application of serologic markers, p-ANCA, and anti-saccharomyces cerevisiae antibodies (ASCA) increases the diagnostic accuracy for Crohn's disease and ulcerative colitis. Evaluation of the upper gastrointestinal tract can also increase the sensitivity and specificity for the diagnosis of IBD, because Crohn's disease may involve the upper gastrointestinal tract, while ulcerative colitis leaves the upper gastrointestinal tract unaffected. Currently, a diagnosis of indeterminate colitis is considered only when the disorder is confined to the colon. Whether any involvement of the upper gastrointestinal tract can occur is not known. During follow-up, patients with indeterminate colitis can be categorized as having Crohn's disease when upper gastrointestinal tract involvement, small bowel involvement, or fistula formation develops or when granulomas and/or transmural lymphoid hyperplasia are found. However, it is currently unknown whether the occurrence of fistulas is typical of Crohn's disease and excludes indeterminate colitis. Indeterminate colitis is generally considered to be a temporary diagnosis. Indeterminate colitis patients with negative serology for p-ANCA and ASCA are more likely to remain indeterminate colitis patients. Therefore, the possibility that indeterminate colitis could be a separate entity needs to be confirmed (303).

■ INADVERTENT CROHN'S DISEASE

Crohn's disease of the colon and rectum and/or the small bowel is contraindicated for IPAA because of the likelihood of recurrent Crohn's disease in the pouch or in the rest of the small bowel. Despite the best attempts to make the preoperative and intraoperative diagnosis of ulcerative colitis, approximately 2% of patients subsequently proven to have Crohn's disease after the IPAA has already been made (295). What should be done next in this situation is one of the most important decisions for any patient.

Detecting the differentiation between ulcerative colitis and Crohn's disease and making a perfect diagnosis can be difficult or inaccurate in up to 15% of patients (304). The only absolute difference that can be used to distinguish the two conditions is the presence of small bowel disease in Crohn's disease, because all other features are only relatively discriminatory. Macroscopic fat wrapping and the presence of skip lesions are helpful when present in the colon (305). Granulomas, although a classic feature of Crohn's disease, do not occur in every patient and may be present in ulcerative colitis and infective enteritis, particularly *Campylobacter* spp. (304,305). Granulomas may also be seen following diversion of the fecal stream in patients with ulcerative proctitis in the three-stage IPAA, particularly in association with ruptured crypts (305–307). High-dose systemic steroids, 5-ASA, and azathioprine may modify the histologic appearance of mucosal biopsy specimens and thereby alter the diagnostic features normally seen in the disease (305).

A retrospective review of the prospectively maintained IPAA database was undertaken at the Cleveland Clinic (308) to identify patients with a diagnosis of Crohn's disease after IPAA. Sixty patients (32 females; median age 33) (range, 55–74 years) who underwent IPAA for ulcerative colitis subsequently had that diagnosis revised to Crohn's disease. Median follow-up of all patients was 46 (range, 4–158) months. Twenty-one of the 60 patients with Crohn's disease developed active Crohn's disease. In this group, the follow-up was 63 (range, 0–132) months from the time of diagnosis. Six of them underwent pouch removal, and one had permanent dysfunction (two-thirds still had the pouch intact). There was no pouch loss in those with asymptomatic Crohn's disease.

The results showed that for the patients who still had the pouch intact, the median daily bowel movement was seven (range, 3–20); 50% of the patients rarely or never experienced urgency, and 59% reported perfect or near perfect continence. Median quality of life, health, and happiness scores were 9.9 and 10 out of 10. The authors concluded that with the low-pouch–loss rate and good functional outcome in patients with Crohn's disease, it might be possible to perform ileoanal pouch procedure in a certain group of colonic Crohn's disease.

In a series from Mayo Clinic (295), 38 patients had the diagnosis changed to Crohn's disease after a successful IPAA for CUC. In the median follow-up of 83 (range, 1–192) months, this group of patients did not experience complications until developing Crohn's disease. The probability of pouchitis, small-bowel obstruction, and stricture were not different when compared to the ulcerative colitis group. However, the complications were higher in other parameters. The overall probability of remaining free of complications was less than 5% for Crohn's disease at five years versus 50% for ulcerative colitis; the probability of a pouch fistula was 65% versus 9%; the probability of a pelvic sepsis was 25% versus less than 5% at seven years; the probability of pouch failure was 50% versus 10% at 10 years.

In spite of the high rate of complications, the functional outcomes (fecal incontinence, number of bowel movements) in those patients with Crohn's disease who had an intact pouch, it was similar to those patients with ulcerative colitis. This is likely because of the fact that patients with complex Crohn's disease had lost their pouch during the follow-up period, leaving only patients with Crohn's disease with reasonable functioning pouches intact available for follow-up. These findings support those from the Cleveland Clinic who found that the functional results and quality of life of the patients undergoing IPAA were similar to that of the patients with ulcerative colitis (308).

Because of the acceptable outcome in Crohn's disease developed after IPAA, some surgeons are optimistic about the possibility of offering IPAA in selected group of patients with Crohn's disease such as those who have no involvement of the small bowel and no perianal diseases, and patients who are highly motivated to have IPAA (308,309). The hurdle at present is an inability to properly select the patients before the IPAA (308). However, most surgeons are against IPAA in known Crohn's disease of the colon because of the high complications (295,302,310). Once the diagnosis of Crohn's disease has been made after IPAA, there is no reason to remove the pouch. Removal of the pouch is advisable only when medical treatment has failed.

The issue of Crohn's disease of the IPAA may have some answers in the near future. Colombel et al. (311) showed for the first time that Infliximab might significantly contribute to the salvage of pouch in patients developing Crohn's disease-related complications after IPAA. The study was performed on 26 patients with IPAA and Crohn's disease-related complications at the Mayo Clinic. The median time between IPAA and the diagnosis of Crohn's disease was 4.5 years (range, 0.6–16 years). The main reasons for changing the original ulcerative colitis diagnosis to Crohn's disease were complex perianal or pouch fistulizing disease in 14 patients (54%), prepouch ileitis in 5 (19%), and both prepouch ileitis and complex fistula in seven (27%). Patients received one to three doses of Infliximab over eight weeks as induction therapy. Subsequently, the patients received a variable number of maintenance infusions.

The results at a short-term follow-up, 16 of 26 patients (62%) had a complete response, 6 of 26 (23%) had a partial response, and 4 of 26 (15%) had no response. Information regarding long-term follow-up was available in 24 patients. After a median follow-up of 21.5 months (range, 3–44 months), eight patients (33%) either had their pouch resected or had a persistent diverting ileostomy. The pouch was functional in 16 of 24 (67%) patients, with either good ($n = 7$) or acceptable ($n = 7$) clinical results in 14 of 24 (58%). Of those 14 patients, 11 were under long-term, on demand, or systemic maintenance treatment with Infliximab. In the study, the authors were not able to identify predictors of response to Infliximab. Administration of infliximab in this group of patients was demonstrated to be safe. Infusion reaction and serum sickness-like disease was observed in 2 of 26 patients, which was in accordance with their short- and long-term safety experience observed in a consecutive series of 500 patients with Crohn's disease treated with Infliximab at the Mayo Clinic.

The authors concluded that Infliximab proved to be beneficial and safe in both the short- and long-term treatment of patients with an IPAA performed for a presumed diagnosis of ulcerative colitis who subsequently developed Crohn's disease-related complications. Maintenance therapy with Infliximab was required to maintain symptomatic remission in most of the patients. Although it is generally accepted that IPAA is contraindicated in patients with Crohn's disease, their results lend further support to some surgeons in performing IPAA in selected patients with no history of anal manifestations and no evidence of small bowel involvement (311).

ULCERATIVE COLITIS WITH CARCINOMA

Occasionally, the surgeon encounters a patient who is a candidate for TPC with IPAA but who also has associated carcinoma of the colon or rectum. A review of several series in the literature revealed that a surprisingly high proportion of carcinoma is unsuspected (312). TPC with IPAA can be performed provided the operation does not compromise curative resection and the predicted prognosis is good (313). IPAA should be avoided in patients with carcinoma of the middle and lower rectum because the proctectomy for IPAA is not an adequate operation for the carcinoma and the possible need for chemoradiation therapy is likely to damage the ileoanal pouch. An alternative consideration is to perform resection and have the IPAA done later after a period of observation and appropriate adjuvant therapy because of the difficulty in intraoperative staging (314).

In a series of 1616 patients who underwent IPAA at the Mayo Clinic from January 1981 to December 1994 inclusive, 82 patients (5%) had a coexisting colorectal neoplasm (315). Seventy-seven patients had adenocarcinoma, four patients had a carcinoid, and one had a sarcoma. Fifty-nine patients (72%) had CUC and 23 (28%) had familial adenomatous polyposis (FAP). The mean age at operation was 32 years (range, 13–60 years) for FAP patients and 38 years (range, 15–56 years) for CUC patients. The mean duration of disease was 13.7 years for patients with CUC. The report was restricted to 77 patients with adenocarcinoma. A preoperative diagnosis of colorectal carcinoma was made in 79% of patients. The distribution of 95 carcinomas in 77 patients was identified as follows: sigmoid, 25 patients; rectum, 21; cecum, 12; ascending colon, 11; transverse colon, 10; descending colon, 8; splenic flexure, 6; and hepatic flexure, 2. Among the 21 rectal carcinomas, four were in the proximal rectum, five in the mid-rectum, and three in the distal rectum. The stages of the carcinomas are shown in Table 3.

TABLE 3 ■ Stage and Location of Colon and Rectal Cancers

Stage	Colon	Rectal	Total
0 (T0 N0 M0)	6	3	9
I (Tl, 2 N0 M0)	19	12	31
II (T3, 4 N0 M0)	14	1	15
III (Any T N + M0)	17	5	22
All	56	21	77

Source: From Ref. 315.

The functional results in patients with carcinoma were compared with those in patients without carcinoma. There were no differences. However, pouch failure was more common in patients with carcinoma than in patients without carcinoma (16% vs. 7%). This was attributable to radiation injury in patients with carcinoma of the rectum and to progression of disease. The overall long-term survival rate was 84%. The recurrence rate was 32%, which is comparable to the rate reported for non-IPAA patients of 43% (316) (Table 4). This study shows that IPAA can be performed after CUC with carcinoma provided an oncologic resection is not compromised and the patients can enter an appropriate adjuvant therapy. Other authors also arrived at the same conclusion (317,318).

TABLE 4 ■ Recurrence of All Colon and Rectal Cancers According to TNM Stage

Stage	Number	Local (%)	Systemic (%)	Overall (%)
0 (T0 N0 M0)	9	0 (0)	0 (0)	0 (0)
I (T1, 2 N0 M0)	31	0 (0)	0 (0)	0 (0)
II (T3, 4 N0 M0)	15	3 (20)	1 (7)	4 (27)
III (Any T N + M0)	22	5 (23)	3 (14)	8 (36)
All	77	8 (10)	4 (5)	12 (16)

Source: From Ref. 315.

ADENOCARCINOMA IN ILEAL POUCH–ANAL ANASTOMOSIS

Proctocolectomy plus IPAA is frequently performed in long-standing ulcerative colitis. Many of these patients are young and may live another 50 or more years. This operation still leaves at-risk tissues behind: the columnar rectal mucosal remnant at the site of the anastomosis and the ATZ. Even in the mucosectomy technique, some islands of mucosa may be left behind (252). The ATZ in itself also has some columnar epithelium that frequently extends below the dentate line (254). There are two sites that the carcinoma may occur: the anorectal cuff (ATZ plus remnants of rectal mucosa at the anastomosis), and the ileal pouch itself.

To evaluate the long-term risk of dysplasia of the ATZ, O'Riodain et al. (245) performed serial ATZ biopsies in 210 patients who had IPAA for ulcerative colitis or indeterminate colitis. None of the patients had the preoperative diagnosis of carcinoma of the rectum or of dysplasia within 8 cm of the anal verge. Biopsies of the ATZ every six months to two years for at least five years postoperatively, the median follow-up was 77 (range, 60–124) months. The results showed ATZ dysplasia developed in seven patients 4 to 51 (median, 11) months postoperatively. There was no association with gender, age, preoperative disease duration or extent of colitis, but the risk of ATZ dysplasia was significantly increased in patients with prior carcinoma or dysplasia in the colon or rectum. The authors concluded that ATZ dysplasia after IPAA is infrequent, is most common in the first two to three years postoperatively, and may apparently disappear on repeated biopsy. ATZ preservation did not lead to the development of cancer in the ATZ after five to ten years of follow-up. This is in agreement with the results of the studies done by others (319,320). The authors recommend a long-term surveillance to monitor dysplasia. If repeated biopsy confirms persistent dysplasia, ATZ excision with neo-IPAA is recommended. A similar study was performed by Coull et al. (321) in 135 patients who underwent IPAA for ulcerative colitis. The median follow-up was 56 (range, 12–145) months. The median time since diagnosis of ulcerative colitis was 8.8 (range, 2–32) years. The cuff biopsies showed no dysplasia or carcinoma, although chronic inflammation was present in 94% of the cuff biopsies. The authors concluded that since there was no evidence of either dysplasia or carcinoma in the columnar cuff mucosa up to 12 years after the pouch formation, the cuff surveillance in the first decade after IPAA may be unnecessary unless there is a HGD or carcinoma in the original resection specimen.

The study by Thompson-Fawcett and Mortensen showed that if carcinoma is present in a colon that has been removed for ulcerative colitis, there is a 25% incidence of dysplasia in the columnar cuff in the short term. They have the opinion that those who are spared from carcinoma by colectomy are likely to have a similar risk of developing dysplastic change in the columnar cuff with longer follow-up (322).

What about the risk of carcinoma of the pouch itself? Herline et al. (323) performed biopsies in 160 patients with IPAA for ulcerative colitis. The average length of follow-up from pouch construction to time of surveillance and biopsy was 8.4 ± 4.6 years. There were 52% of patients whose pouches were older than 10 years (mean, 12.7 ± 2) at the time of surveillance. The results showed that only 1% had focal, LGD in the pouch. The authors concluded that even with long-term follow-up of IPAA patients, there is little evidence to support routine biopsy of the ileal mucosa in ulcerative colitis patients. The same conclusions were made by Borjesson et al. (324), and Thompson-Fawcett et al. (325).

Case reports of adenocarcinoma in the ileoanal pouch–anal anastomosis are summarized on Table 5 (255,256,326–338). It is striking to see the preponderance in males. Almost all the patients have long history of ulcerative colitis. About half of the carcinomas develop in the anorectal cuff and another half in the pouch itself. There are several patients who have carcinoma of the colon or rectum at the time of the IPAA (255,332,336,337). The treatment of carcinoma in IPAA is the same as for carcinoma of the low rectum.

The a first case of squamous cell carcinoma at the anorectal cuff was reported by Schaffzin and Smith (339). This occurred in a 47-year-old woman who underwent proctocolectomy and IPAA after 16 years of ulcerative colitis. Twenty-five years after the IPAA, she underwent a pouchoscopy for fever and poor pouch function. A 3×3

TABLE 5 ■ Adenocarcinoma in Ileal Pouch–Anal Anastomosis

Author/Year/Ref.	Age at Dx of CA	Gender	Hx of CUC (Year)	Duration After IPAA (Year)	Technique		Site	
					Stapled	Mucosectomy	A–R Cuff	Pouch
Hassan, 2003 (326)	38	M	10	22 mo		x		x
Bell, 2003 (327)	24	M	15	12	x		x	
Bentram, 2003 (328)	63	M	44	13		x		x
Nagi, 2003 (329)	28	M	NS	5		x	x	
Baratsis, 2002 (330)	49	M	24	2	x		x	
Hyman, 2002 (331)	41	M	13	5	x		x	
[a]Laureti, 2002 (332)	46	M	20	2		x	x	
Rotholtz, 2001 (333)	72	M	6	7	x		x	
Heuschen, 2001 (334)	48	M	23	3		x		x
Iwama, 2000 (335)	50	M	NS	15		x		x
[a]Vieth, 1998 (336)	35	F	18	2		x		x
[a]Sequens, 1997 (337)	54	F	9	1	x		x	
Rodriguez-Sanjuan, 1995 (338)	52	F	18	20 mo		x		x
Puthu, 1992 (256)	51	M	17	6	NS	NS	x	
[a]Stern, 1990 (255)	59	M	35	3		x		x

[a]Patient had adenocarcinoma of colon or rectum at the time of IPAA

Abbreviations: A–R Cuff, Anorectal cuff, including anal transitional zone plus rectal mucosa remnant; CA, adenocarcinoma; CUC, chronic ulcerative colitis; Hx, history; M, male; F, female; mo, month; NS, not stated.

mass was found at the level of the anastomosis, at the anorectal ring. Biopsies proved to be an invasive squamous cell carcinoma in the background of normal intestinal mucosa. The patient underwent chemoradiation and responded well. There was no long-term follow-up.

■ PREGNANCY

Most women who have IPAA are relatively young and are of reproductive age. Problems occasionally arise when they become pregnant. What is the effect of IPAA on fertility? Can the patient carry the pregnancy to full-term without jeopardizing the function? Is vaginal delivery safe, or is it wise to perform a cesarean section?

The effect of IPAA on fertility has been studied by Oresland et al. (340). Hysterosalpingography disclosed abnormalities in the majority of patients. The fallopian tubes adhered to the pelvic floor in half of the patients, and occlusion of one or both tubes was demonstrated in 50% of patients. Two-thirds of the women who attempted to become pregnant failed to do so during a five-year follow-up, indicating a high incidence of infertility. Other authors also found reduced fertility after proctocolectomy and ileal pouch procedure (341,342). Dyspareunia occurs in 7% to 33% of patients after IPAA. The reason may be related to anatomic changes in the pelvis and perineum, such as deformity of the vaginal vault, dilatation of the dorsal fornix, and displacement of the vagina toward the coccyx, as found in women after a proctectomy (343).

A study was conducted by Hahnloser et al. at the Mayo Clinic (344) to evaluate pregnancy, delivery, and functional outcome in females before and after IPAA for CUC. The study consisted of patients aged 40 years or younger at the time of IPAA with a mean follow-up after the operation of 13 years. A total of 141 females were pregnant after the CUC diagnosis, but before the IPAA (236 pregnancies; mean, 1.7) and 87% delivered vaginally. A mean of five (range, 1–16) years after IPAA, 135 females were pregnant (232 pregnancies; mean, 1.7). There was no difference in birth weight, duration of labor, delivery complications, vaginal delivery rates (59% before vs. 54% after IPAA), and unplanned cesarean section (19% vs. 14%). Planned cesareans occurred only after IPAA and were prompted by obstetrical concerns in only one of eight. Pouch function at first follow-up after delivery (mean, seven months) was similar to pregravida function. After IPAA, daytime stool frequency was the same after delivery as pregravida (5.4 vs. 5.4) but was increased at the time of last follow-up (68 months after delivery; 5.4 vs. 6.4). The rate of occasional fecal incontinence also was higher (20% after IPAA and 21% pregravida vs. 36% at last follow-up). No difference in functional outcome was noted compared with females who were never pregnant after IPAA ($n = 307$). Age and becoming pregnancy did not affect the probability of pouch-related complications such as stricture, pouchitis, and obstruction. The authors concluded that successful pregnancy and vaginal delivery occur routinely in females with CUC before and after IPAA. The method of delivery should be dictated by obstetrical considerations. Ravid et al. of University of Toronto (345) also reported a similar favorable outcome. In contrast, the study by Remzi et al. of Cleveland Clinic (346) showed that the risk of sphincter injury and quality of life were significantly worse after vaginal delivery when compared with cesarean section in patients with IPAA. However, in the short term, this did not seem to substantially influence pouch function or quality of life; however, the long-term effects remain unknown. In their study, 82 women who had at least one live birth after IPAA participated in the study. Sixty-two patients had cesarean section after IPAA and 20 had vaginal delivery. The mean follow-up was 4.9 years. The vaginal delivery group had significantly higher incidence of anterior sphincter defect by anal endosonography (50% vs. cesarean section delivery group 13%). The mean squeeze anal pressure was significantly higher in the patients who had cesarean section delivery than that of vaginal delivery. Quality of life evaluated by time trade-off method also was significantly better in the cesarean section delivery group (1 vs. vaginal delivery group 0.9). The authors suggested that a planned cesarean section might eliminate these potential and factual concerns in IPAA patients.

There was a report by Aouthmany and Horattas (347) in an unusual case of ileal pouch perforation in pregnancy. It is a rare case that a colorectal surgeon may encounter some day. The case was a 30-year-old multigravida with an uncomplicated pregnancy at 27 weeks gestation. The patient was admitted to the perinatal ward for preterm labor. The patient had a proctocolectomy and IPAA for ulcerative colitis previously. Forty-eight hours after admission, she developed acute generalized abdominal pain with associated dyspnea. A spiral computed tomography (CT) of the chest to rule out pulmonary embolus revealed free intra-abdominal air. An emergency cesarean section was performed which resulted in a viable female infant. At surgery, a 3-mm perforation at the end of the J-limb of the pouch was identified. The cause for the perforation was related to its adhesion to the back of the uterus. The adhesions were taken down and the perforation was primarily repaired. Her postpartum course was uncomplicated.

■ OLDER PATIENTS

Two questions often arise: How do IPAA patients do when they get older? Can IPAA be successful in older patients?

Among 1400 IPAA patients at the Mayo Clinic, 75 consecutive subjects were identified as having had the operation for at least 10 years (348). Sixty-one patients were available for study. Functional results were evaluated at 1 year and at 10 years after the IPAA in each patient. Stool frequency (7 ± 3, mean $\pm$ SD) remained unchanged at 1 and 10 years. Excellent daytime continence at one year was achieved in 82% of patients; 10 years later it dropped to 71%. Frequent incontinence was 2% and 8%, respectively, and nighttime incontinence slightly deteriorated at 10 years but was not statistically significant. It appears that sphincter function deteriorates slightly 10 years after the procedure, and most patients remain quite happy. A longer follow-up for 15 years in 409 patients at the same institution showed that the function of the pouch and the quality of life remain intact (349). Others have reported similar results and complications in patients 50 years of age or older versus younger patients (350–352).

Keighley (353) reported the outcome of 30 patients over the age of 50 years from 154 individuals having IPAA for ulcerative colitis. Of this group, seven were in their sixties and five were in their seventies. The eventual outcome in terms of pouch excision and complications for these patients did not differ from younger patients. The functional results were marginally inferior to those under 50 years of age but the incidence of soiling was almost exactly the same. Reissman et al. (354) compared the outcome of 14 patients 60 years of age or older to 126 patients under the age of 60. The morbidity rate (21% vs. 21%) and mortality rate (0% vs. 0.8%) and functional and physiologic results were not different. These patients had a double-stapled ileoanal reservoir. Good to excellent outcomes are also reported in patients 70 years old and older (355). It appears that IPAA can be offered to older patients with an expectation of good outcome.

Older patients live a more sedentary life and are more philosophical about lifestyle choices; therefore, few would choose a stoma when first presented with a choice. But when given the facts about the risk of Crohn's disease, reoperation, pouch failure, pouchitis, and numerous defecation and seepage problems, many elderly patients choose a permanent ileostomy. This is not to say that pouch surgery has no place in the treatment of the elderly. Patients with minimal symptoms from colitis may prefer to avoid a stoma, but, if that is their inclination, they must be informed of the true outcome of IPAA (353).

COMPLICATIONS

TPC with IPAA for ulcerative colitis has been performed since the first report by Parks and Nicholls (214) in 1978. Vast experience has been accumulated in terms of understanding the function of the pouch, patient preparation, patient selection, and particularly operative techniques. The use of a short mucosectomy and rectal cuff has made the operation much easier and consequently decreased the number of pelvic complications. The shortening of the outflow projection of the S pouch to 1 to 1.5 cm has eliminated the problem of the outflow obstruction (234,356).

Despite being a major and technically demanding surgery in frequently sick patients, proctocolectomy and IPAA has a low mortality. The main reasons are that most of the patients are typically young, in the early to mid-thirties, and most of the operations are performed in major medical centers. In a series of 1603 patients with IPAA from the Mayo Clinic (1407 for CUC, 187 for FAP, 9 for other diagnoses), three deaths (0.2%) occurred postoperatively because of pulmonary embolism perforated gastric ulcer, and subarachnoid hemorrhage (357). Late deaths occurred in 29 patients (1.8%), 10 months to 10.4 years after the operation. The most common cause of death was malignancy, including colon and rectal carcinoma (10 patients), hematologic malignancies (four patients), cholangiocarcinoma (three patients), and germ-cell carcinoma (one patient). The rest died from other causes, but none was directly attributable to the IPAA procedure. In a series of 1005 patients from the Cleveland Clinic, four patients (0.41%) died during the early postoperative period (358).

SMALL BOWEL OBSTRUCTION

A survey of the literature reveals an overall frequency of intestinal obstruction after IPAA ranging from 15% to as high as 44%, and the incidence of obstruction requiring operative intervention hovers between 5% and 20% (359). In a recent series from the Cleveland Clinic, of 1005 patients undergoing IPAA from 1983 to 1993 (including ulcerative colitis, Crohn's disease, and FAP) 254 patients (25.3%) had small bowel obstruction (7.5% early and 17.8% later), and 70 patients (27.6%) required reoperation (358). Two-thirds of the patients with small bowel obstructions—stomal stenosis, volvulus or internal hernia, and adhesive bands—had the temporary loop ileostomy as their cause. The leading cause was stomal rotation, a common technique of placing the functioning side inferiorly to facilitate the outflow (360). This technique is totally unnecessary and should be abandoned. After closure of the ileostomy, most obstructions are due to adhesions and anastomotic strictures (359).

In a long-term follow-up of 202 patients with IPAA for ulcerative colitis at the Mayo Clinic (361) the cumulative probability of developing small bowel obstruction 5 years after ileostomy closure was 14%, whereas at 10 years it was 22%.

PELVIC ABSCESS

Most recent series cite the incidence of pelvic abscess as 4% to 6% (358,362–364). A pelvic abscess most probably results from contamination of the presacral space, either during the operation or postoperatively if there is partial disruption of the pouch–anal anastomosis, which may or may not be apparent radiologically. On occasion, a pelvic abscess will become evident clinically only after the ileostomy has been closed and intestinal continuity restored. The patient usually has a fever, pelvic or low back pain sometimes radiating into the lower extremities, and leukocytosis. A pouchogram or CT scan may demonstrate a leak communicating with an abscess cavity or distortion and anterior displacement of the ileal reservoir. A CT scan of the pelvic area often not only is diagnostic but also may help determine the operative approach or may be used to guide treatment (365). However, not all pelvic abscesses are catastrophic or require major abdominal operations. In the initial series of 188 patients who had an ileoanal anastomosis at the Mayo Clinic (366), 9 of the 21 patients in whom a pelvic abscess developed, could be treated by local drainage and antibiotics. In some situations CT-guided drainage also has been successful. In approximately half of the patients transabdominal exploration with evacuation of the purulent collection and placement of drains was required to overcome the septic process. If the ileostomy had been closed, it was reestablished. In some instances the ileal reservoir must be excised because of the insurmountable pelvic sepsis despite one or even multiple revisional operations. In the series at the Mayo Clinic, pelvic sepsis was responsible for half of the reservoirs that required excision.

■ LEAKAGE OF POUCH AND POUCH–ANAL ANASTOMOSIS

Leakage of the pouch and of the pouch–anal anastomosis occurs in 2% to 10% (216,263,358,363). Asymptomatic leaks revealed by X-ray studies most often are diagnosed when the patient returns to have the ileostomy closed and intestinal continuity restored. Such leaks represent incomplete healing of the anastomosis or the ileal reservoir, and the only treatment needed is to defer closure of the ileostomy, usually for a few months, after which the patient is restudied. In most instances, the leak will have disappeared by then, and the ileostomy can be closed. In a few cases, a perianastomotic leak persists for 9 or even 12 months without causing any symptoms. If the leak is small and asymptomatic, the ileostomy can be closed without adverse sequelae (365). Patients with symptomatic leaks may present with low-grade fever, perineal or low-back (sacral) pain, and intermittent perianal purulent discharge. A preoperative pouchogram may show a small sinus tract starting in the vicinity of the anastomosis and extending for a variable length, most often behind the pouch. The pouch should be examined with the patient under anesthesia, the tract curetted, and the patient placed on an antibiotic such as metronidazole. Usually the symptoms will resolve rapidly, and the sinus tract heals. The temporary ileostomy may be closed in the presence of an asymptomatic persistent sinus tract. Failure to heal a symptomatic or large sinus tract should suggest Crohn's disease, and the ileostomy should be left in place (365).

■ VAGINAL FISTULA

Ileal pouch–vaginal fistula occurs in about 6% of patients with IPAA. Sepsis and technical factors (e.g., length of cuff) are the most common contributors (367). Its incidence varies from 4% to 12% (358,368–372). About one-fourth to one-third of the fistulas occur before closure of the ileostomy, and about two-thirds to three-fourths appear after the ileostomy has been closed with the mean of five to seven months (range, 10 days to 9 months) (369–372). Vaginal fistula occurs in both mucosectomy with hand-sewn pouch–anal anastomosis and double-stapled anastomosis without mucosectomy with equal frequency (372). Most fistulas are at the anastomosis and low in the vagina. In a small number of cases, the origin of the fistula is the suture line of the pouch. Similarly, fistula high in the vagina has also been reported (370).

Approximately 75% of patients with ileal pouch–vaginal fistula undergo colectomy for acute fulminant ulcerative colitis, and the pouch is constructed either simultaneously or later as a three-stage procedure (369). Another high-risk group includes patients in whom IPAA is performed in one stage without a temporary diverting ileostomy. Tekkis et al. (373) identified factors associated with pouch fistula: female, perianal abscess, fistula-in-ano, Crohn's disease, abnormal anal manometry, and pelvic sepsis.

Ninety-two percent of the fistulas are recognized clinically (369). Tests that are helpful to diagnose and assess the origin and direction of the fistulous tract include pouchography, ultrasonography, CT, contrast enemas, fistulography, MRI, and examination under general or regional anesthesia (370).

The basic principle in the management of the pouch–vaginal fistula is delaying closure of the diverting ileostomy from a few to several months. It is important to treat sepsis with antibiotics and drainage of any pelvic or perineal abscesses. This strategy alone has healed three of five patients reported by Groom et al. (372). If the ileostomy has been closed, it should be re-established but the success rate for the fistula to heal is poor (374). Experience has shown that pouch–vaginal fistulas that occur after closure of the ileostomy are much more difficult to manage (370–372).

Because the intra-anal procedures for ileoanal pouch–vaginal fistula have been disappointing, resulting in healing at best, approximately 50%, Burke et al. (375) used a transvaginal approach to achieve direct access to the internal opening, enabling closure without damage to the anal sphincter. Fourteen patients were treated, all had IPAA for ulcerative colitis and all were defunctioned. The median age was 40 (range, 25–52) years. Median follow-up was 18 (range, 6–60) months. The operation was successful in 11 of the 14 patients, after one attempt in six patients, after two attempts in four, and after three attempts in one patient. The operation failed in three patients, who had a permanent ileostomy. There was no fecal incontinence in those successful patients.

The technique consisted of an inverted T-shaped incision made along the midline longitudinal access of the posterior vaginal wall with the horizontal limb at the junction of the perineal skin with the posterior vaginal wall. The vagina was dissected from the anal canal and ileal pouch on each side, creating two lateral flaps to expose the anterior wall of the pouch and the ileoanal anastomosis. The internal opening in the bowel was then excised and the defect closed transversely using interrupted 2–0 synthetic absorbable sutures. The vaginal flaps were then replaced and approximated with the same type of interrupted sutures leaving a closed wound. A mechanical bowel preparation was not performed as the patients were defunctioned. All were given intravenous antibiotics.

Johnson et al. (376) studied 24 of 619 (4%) women who had IPAA complicated by pouch–vaginal fistula. An additional five women had the IPAA performed at another institution and were referred for management of their pouch–vaginal fistula. An additional five women had the IPAA performed at another institution and were referred for management of their pouch–vaginal. In additional five women had the IPAA performed at another institution and were referred for management of their pouch-reginal fistula. Local and/or combined abdominoperineal repairs were performed in 22 of 29 patients. Combined abdominoperineal repairs were associated with a higher success rate than that of local perineal repairs (53% vs. 8%, respectively, at 10 years after repair). Overall, 50% (11 of 22) of patients who underwent surgical repair of a pouch–vaginal fistula had a successful result with a functioning pouch and no recurrence of the fistula, and 21% (6 of 29) of patients required pouch excision.

Shah et al. (377) studied 60 females (mean age, 33.3 ± 1.3 years) who had IPAA complicated with pouch–vaginal fistulas. Preoperative diagnosis was ulcerative colitis in 88%, indeterminate colitis 10%, and FAP 2%. The average time to pouch–vaginal fistula was 21 months (range, 1–132 months). Primary treatment modalities included the following: local repairs ($n=46$, 77%), the majority of which were ileal advancement flaps; redo restorative proctocolectomy ($n=6$, 10%); and pouch excision ($n=5$, 8%). Initial healing was achieved in 20 patients. An additional 11 patients with recurrences healed after repeat procedures. The overall healing rate was 52% at 49.4 ± 3.8 months follow-up. Pouch failure was the eventual outcome in 13 (22%) patients and 16(27%) patients had persistent pouch–vaginal fistula. A delayed diagnosis of Crohn's disease was made in 24 patients. Crohn's disease patients had lower success rate following ileal advancement flaps compared with the non-Crohn's (25% vs. 48%, respectively), much lower overall healing rates of their pouch–vaginal fistulas (17% vs. 75%, respectively), and a higher incidence of pouch failure (33% vs. 14%, respectively).

Pouch–vaginal fistulas can persist and recur indefinitely, even after repeated repairs. Repair in those patients with Crohn's disease uniformly failed within five years from primary repair. Patients with recurrent pouch–vaginal fistulas and ulcerative colitis should be offered salvage surgery because successful closure following initial failure occurs in approximately 50% (378).

■ ANAL STRICTURE

Some degree of narrowing of the anal canal at the anastomosis is common and presents no problem. A lumen that admits the distal interphalangeal joint of the index finger (312) or admits a 1-cm diameter proctoscope is satisfactory. Anastomotic strictures can occur after pelvic sepsis. Other factors such as undue tension on the IPAA, inadequate blood supply, and poor technique may be play important roles (365).

In a study of strictures in 213 patients (out of 1884 IPAA, 11.2%; 11% for CUC, and 12% for FAP) with IPAA at the Mayo Clinic (379), there were two kinds of strictures: nonfibrotic and fibrotic, on the basis of the presence or absence of a fibrotic segment in the anal canal anastomosis that was responsible for pouch-outlet obstruction requiring at least one dilatation. Strictures were nonfibrotic in 86% of patients and fibrotic in 14%. A greater number of strictures were observed after a hand-sewn anastomosis ($p=0.03$). Intraoperative technical difficulties were associated with 13% of all strictures regardless of the type of stricture. Treatment with dilatation was successful in 95% of nonfibrotic strictures but only 45% of fibrotic strictures ($p=0.0001$). Surgical treatment was required in 25 strictures (12%), including excision of the strictured segment with mucosal advancement flap (five patients), excision of the pouch with permanent ileostomy (nine patients), or redo pouch (three patients).

Significant stricture of the pouch–anal anastomosis occurs in 5% to 16% of patients. The stricture is usually apparent on postoperative examination before closure of the ileostomy. Mild strictures can be dilated with a finger or Hegar dilators in the office or clinic, preferably gradually graduating from a No. 13 to No. 18 Hegar dilator. A tight stricture (5 mm or smaller) should be dilated with the patient under anesthesia, and repeated dilatation will be required. Occasionally a tight band in the anoderm or internal sphincter muscle requires incision.

Anal stenosis occurred in 14.2% of the hand-sewn and 39.6% of the stapled anastomoses in a series from St. Mark's Hospital (380). Although sepsis, ischemia, and tension at the anastomosis are well-known predisposing factors to the development of anastomotic stenosis, there is no evidence that these play any part in the patients who develop a stenosis in this series. In the series from Lewis et al. (381) of Leeds, U.K., 16% of patients with IPAA developed severe and persistent anal stricture. Factors that significantly predisposed the patient to the development of an ileoanal anastomotic stricture were (i) use of the small (25 mm) diameter stapling gun, (ii) use of a W pouch, (iii) use of a defunctioning ileostomy, and (iv) anastomotic dehiscence and pelvic abscess (381). The functional outcome after dilatation of a stricture was as good as the outcome in patients who did not have a stricture (381).

In a long and tight anal stricture, dilatation is not possible, or the stricture rapidly recurs. Fazio and Tjandra (382) described a transanal technique using pouch advancement and neo-ileoanal anastomosis.

Before operation, the pathology of the original specimen was re-examined to exclude Crohn's disease; if necessary, further biopsies of the ileal pouch were taken. Bowel preparation with polyethylene glycol electrolyte lavages and antibiotic prophylaxis were used. A Foley catheter was inserted to empty the bladder. The operation was performed with the patient in the prone jackknife position under general anesthesia using muscle relaxants.

The anus was everted using radially placed 1–0 Dexon sutures through the anal verge, including the superficial portion of the internal anal sphincter and the perineum. Effacement of the lower anal canal helped to bring the strictured anastomosis into the operative field. The distance of the stricture from the dentate line was carefully noted. A lighted Ferguson anal retractor was gently inserted into the anorectal canal to enhance exposure. Isotonic saline (10 mL) was injected circumferentially into the submucosa of the anal canal at and below the stricture to improve the accuracy of the depth of incision.

An incision was made at or just above the dentate line and below the strictured anastomosis. The incision was continued around the circumference of the anal canal using cautery (Fig. 30A). Using sharp, pointed scissors, the stricture ring and ileal loop immediately above the anastomosis were radially dissected and raised as a circumferential flap to expose the underlying internal anal sphincter (Fig. 30B). Bleeding points were controlled using electrocautery. Taking care not to damage the sphincter complex, cephalad dissection in this plane led to the pelvis (supralevator space) outside the ileal pouch and superior to any preserved rectal muscular cuff. Using a combination of sharp and blunt dissection, the ileal pouch was mobilized circumferentially for a distance of 12 cm from the anal verge. Tissue forceps (Babcocks) or stay sutures were applied to the edge of the stricture allowing for manipulation of the pouch, facilitating the freeing from the pouch of adhesions in the pelvis. This mobilization allowed delivery of the structured segment and normal distal pouch beyond the anal verge (Fig. 30C). The stricture and a margin of the pouch were excised, leaving a fresh edge of ileum level with the dentate line. The mobilized ileal pouch was then anastomosed to the anal canal at the level of the dentate line without

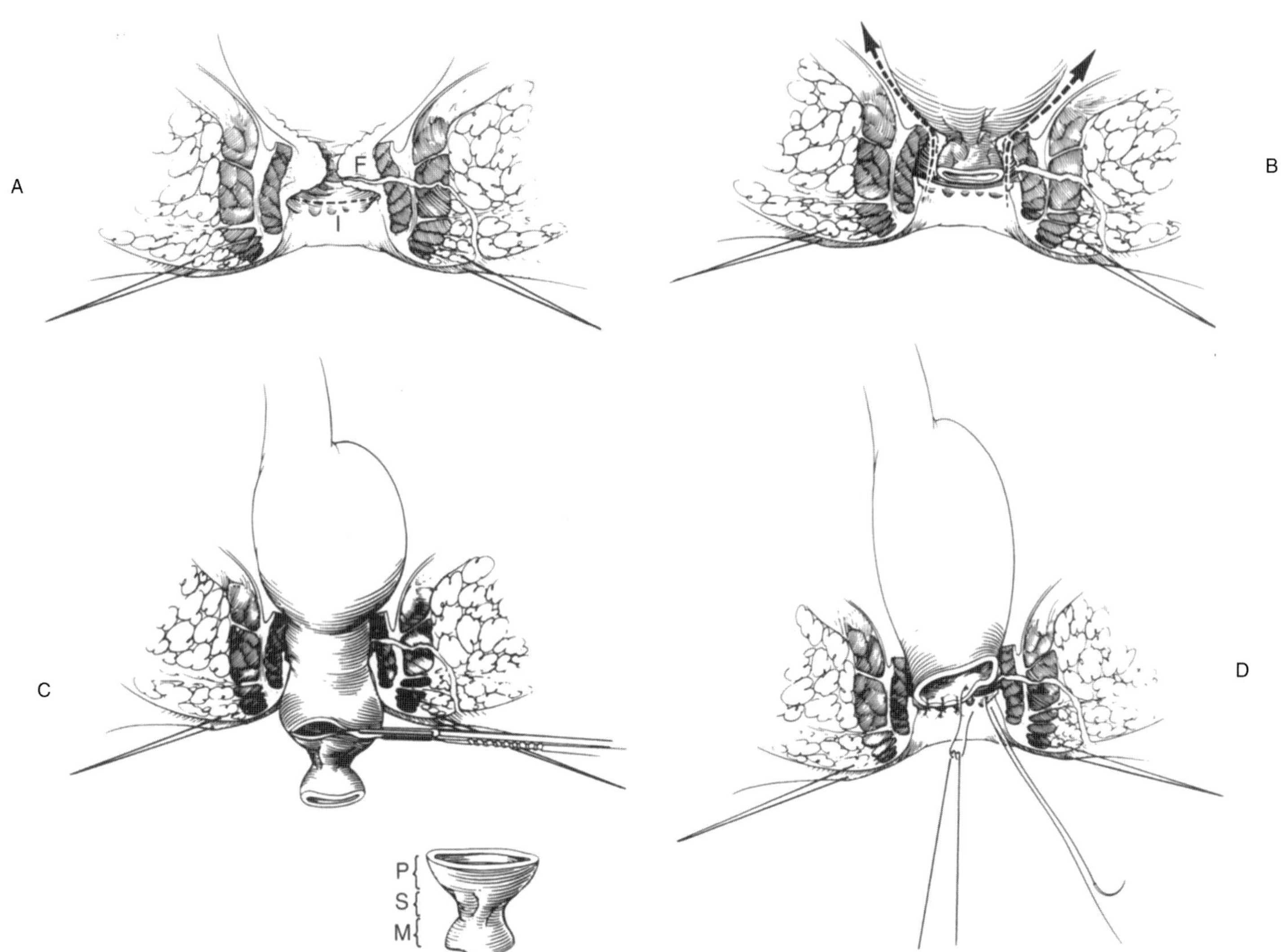

FIGURE 30 ■ A transanal technique using pouch advancement and neo-ileoanal anastomosis. (**A**) A circumferential incision (*I*) is made at or just above the dentate line and below the stricture. A fistula tract (*F*) associated with ileal pouch–anal anastomosis may be present. (**B**) Plane of dissection between the ileal pouch and the underlying sphincter muscles. (**C**) The mobilized pouch with the strictured segment is advanced beyond the anal verge. The stricture (*S*) and a cuff of the pouch (*P*) are excised to leave a freshened edge of the ileal pouch. (*M*) Anal mucosa (if any is left). (**D**) Anastomosis of the freshened edge of ileal pouch with the anal canal. If a fistula is present, the external component of the tract should be separately drained with a mushroom catheter. *Source*: From Ref. 382.

tension using interrupted 2–0 braided synthetic absorbable sutures (Fig. 30D). In one case, tension on the anastomosis was relieved by placing six radial sutures between the seromuscular layer of the pouch and the lower part of the internal sphincter. A diverting stoma was not used.

This technique can be extended to repair anovaginal or anoperineal fistula associated with strictured ileoanal anastomosis, as occurred in two of the patients in this study. Similarly, it may be performed for certain complex fistulas without associated stricture. The tract was identified and marked with a nylon loop. The internal opening of the tract through the internal sphincter was exposed, excised in an elliptical fashion, and then closed transversely with 2–0 braided synthetic absorbable sutures. The mobilized ileal pouch was then advanced to cover the closed end of the tract and anastomosed to the anal canal as described. The external component of the fistula tract was managed by drainage using a mushroom catheter for six weeks, by which time the drainage had ceased. The catheter was removed at a follow-up consultation.

After operation, the patients were allowed sips of fluid for two days, followed by a liquid diet. A normal diet was given after five days. Prophylactic antibiotics were continued for 48 hours.

Although the technique described here has been used successfully in only three patients, it is useful and should be included in the armamentarium of the pouch surgeon. In cases where the stricture is so long (for example, >5 cm) that mobilization from the perineum alone is unlikely to be successful, an abdominoperineal approach is recommended as the primary procedure.

■ DIFFICULT EVACUATION

Anal stricture is the leading cause of difficult evacuation and can be easily diagnosed. Another group of patients has severe difficulty evacuating the pouch but without mechanical obstruction. These patients require catheterization. Herbst et al. (383) reported 11 patients (excluding mechanical anal stricture) who had difficult bowel movements three to 24 times per 24 hours.

There are two basic causes for the outflow obstruction. The first is a long efferent ileal limb, which occurs especially in S pouches. This type of limb is seen only rarely owing to a trend away from this form of pouch. The second is a long anorectal stump. This is becoming more frequent owing to the increase in stapled pouch–anal anastomosis. While stapling techniques have been described as ensuring an anastomosis within the anal canal, use of the doubling stapling technique may result in high anastomosis (383).

Major salvage surgery is indicated in patients who would otherwise require a permanent ileostomy. The patient must be prepared for failure and must also be made aware that a good functional result cannot be guaranteed. Salvage surgery requires abdominal reoperation and a temporary ileostomy. At operation, the pouch is fully mobilized abdominally to the level of the pouch–anal or pouch-rectal anastomosis, and the part of pouch or anorectal stump that causes the obstruction resected. The pouch is then sewn back to the anal canal at the level of the dentate line. In the series reported by Herbst et al. (383), all but one patient had a decrease in the 24-hour frequency of stools, but four out of 11 patients continued to refuse catheterization. Satisfaction was achieved in 8 of the 11 patients.

■ PORTAL VEIN THROMBOSIS

Portal vein thrombosis (PVT) is rare under any circumstances. However, Remzi et al. (384) found it to be a common incidental finding when CT scan of the abdomen is performed for various condition after IPAA for ulcerative colitis.

In a review of 94 patients who had a CT abdomen performed after IPAA, a median of 20 days (range, 3–70) after the operation at the Cleveland Clinic. The reasons for CT scan were because of abdominal pain, fever, leukocytosis, and delayed bowel function. PVT was diagnosed in 42 of 94 patients (45%). PVT was diagnosed at initial reading of the scan in 11 patients, and on review in 31. Septic complications of IPAA caused these symptoms and signs in 45 patients, 20 of whom had PVT. Twenty-two patients were found to have had PVT without evidence of any septic source. There is no specific treatment for PVT. However the authors treat these patients initially with heparin followed by coumadin for 3 to 6 months. All but one patient with PVT recovered without any sequelae or recurrence of the symptoms. The good news is that if this PVT goes undiagnosed, no serious emergences occur, even when not treated (384).

■ POUCHITIS

Pouchitis is an acute and/or chronic inflammation of the ileal reservoir, a common complication in patients with ulcerative colitis who undergo IPAA. It is not related to the type of pouch constructed (385). The prevalence varies widely from less than 7% to as high as 59% (386–389). This large variation reflects differences in diagnostic criteria and duration of follow-up and is responsible for much of the confusion surrounding pouchitis (386,387). The risk of developing pouchitis is highest during the initial six-month period. The cumulative risk levels off after two years. Fewer than 10% of patients have severe, chronic pouchitis, and only 1% to 3% need pouch removal (388).

Symptoms of pouchitis include increased stool frequency, urgency, bright red bleeding, fecal incontinence, abdominal pain, malaise, fever, and the extraintestinal manifestations of IBD. The most common symptoms are bloody effluent, nausea and vomiting, and fever (390). Symptoms alone, however, are not sufficient to diagnose pouchitis. Other conditions produce similar symptoms, for instance, outlet obstruction, bacterial or parasitic infections, recurrent Crohn's disease, and functional bowel syndrome (386).

The accurate diagnosis of pouchitis should include clinical, endoscopic (Fig. 31), and microscopic criteria (391). The pouchitis disease activity index (PDAI) developed by Sandborn et al. (392) provides a useful guide to abnormal findings (Table 6). It is simple and objective, and its score gives a quantitation severity of the disease. Pouchitis is defined as a total score of greater than or equal to seven points (Table 6). Using PDAI as the guide, only 10% of patients with previously diagnosed pouchitis met the diagnostic criteria. No asymptomatic patient qualified for a diagnosis of pouchitis by PDAI criteria (392).

The cause of pouchitis is unknown. The condition is disease-related in that colitis patients have a much greater incidence of pouchitis than do patients undergoing the operation for FAP. Also, colitis patients who have extraintestinal manifestations of the disease are more likely to get pouchitis than those without extraintestinal manifestations (393). In contrast, patients with backwash ileitis are not predisposed to the condition (394). Although mechanical causes, such as anastomotic stricture and excessively large pouches that empty poorly, sometimes cause pouchitis, in most patients a mechanical problem cannot be identified. Pouchitis seems to be related to stasis in the pouch, with subsequent proliferation of bacteria in the lumen of the pouch, especially anaerobic bacteria (395,396). The bacteria or their exotoxins appear to damage the mucosa of the pouch. Erosions, ulcerations, and an acute inflammatory response then appear. One supporting fact of the stasis-bacterial overgrowth theory is that metronidazole, an antibiotic directed primarily at anaerobic bacteria, decreases bacterial counts and improves inflammation and symptoms. However, this theory does not explain why colitis patients are more susceptible to pouchitis than polyposis patients. A study of tissue biopsy samples from patients with pouchitis compared to findings in patients with normal pouches, conventional ileostomies, and normal ileum, using electron microscopy and bacteriologic culture was undertaken by McLeod et al. (397). Intramural bacteria

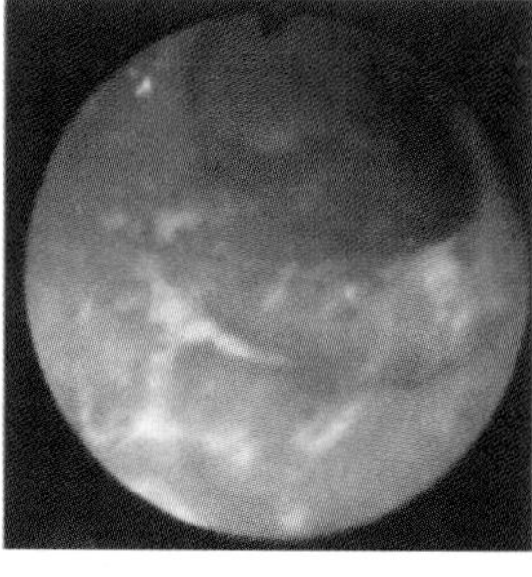

FIGURE 31 ■ Inflammation with the superficial ulcerations of mucosa in a patient with pouchitis.

TABLE 6 ■ Elements of the Pouchitis Disease Activity Index[a]

Criteria	Score
Clinical	
Stool frequency	
Usual postoperative stool frequency	0
One to two stools/day greater than postoperative usual	1
Three or more stools/day greater than postoperative usual	2
Rectal bleeding	
None or rare	0
Present daily	1
Fecal urgency or abdominal cramps	
None	0
Occasional	1
Usual	2
Fever (temperature < 37.8°C)	
Absent	0
Present	1
Endoscopic inflammation	
Edema	1
Granularity	1
Friability	1
Loss of vascular pattern	1
Mucous exudates	1
Ulceration	1
Acute histologic inflammation	
Polymorphonuclear leukocyte infiltration	
Mild	1
Moderate with crypt abscess	2
Severe with crypt abscess	3
Ulceration per low-power field (mean)	
< 25%	1
25% to 50%	2
> 50%	3

[a]Pouchitis is defined as a total score of ≥ 7 points.
Source: From Ref. 392.

were present more frequently in tissue samples of both normal and inflamed pouches, but they were also observed in biopsy samples from conventional ileostomies and in normal ileum. Aerobic bacterial counts were increased in biopsy samples from patients with endoscopic and histologic evidence of pouchitis compared with those with normal pouches, whereas anaerobic counts did not differ significantly. Although the significance of these findings is unknown, they suggest that aerobic bacteria may play a role in the pathogenesis of pouchitis.

The ileal pouch develops an altered mucosal anatomy when compared with the anatomy of a healthy ileum. The pouch mucosa has shortened, blunted villi and elongated crypts that show an increased rate of crypt cell production. Mucous cells of the colonic type appear in the mucosa. In fact, the mucosal histology of the ileal pouch resembles the mucosal histology of the colon.

Total fecal concentrations of short-chain fatty acids in patients with pouchitis were significantly lower than those in asymptomatic control patients. Specifically, acetic acid and butyric acid concentrations were significantly decreased, whereas those of propionate were not (398). This finding has led to the hypothesis that pouchitis may be caused by a deficiency of nutrients for the ileal or colonic epithelium (398,399). Accordingly, a deficiency of butyric acid (a primary nutrient of colonocytes) or of glutamine (a major nutrient of enterocytes) may contribute to the syndrome of pouchitis, similar to the pathophysiologic basis for diversion colitis. Treatment of pouchitis with butyrate suppositories was disappointing. Only three of nine patients responded favorably. Treatment with glutamine suppositories yielded encouraging results. Six of ten patients so treated developed no recurrent symptoms. Given the lack of a placebo control, it is unclear whether these two therapies are similarly effective or similarly ineffective (400).

Another possibility is that the mucosal ischemia that results in the production of oxygen free radicals, which in turn incite inflammation, may have a role in the development of pouchitis. Allopurinol, a xanthine oxidase inhibitor, fails to prevent pouchitis in a randomized-controlled trial (401).

Broad-spectrum antibiotics are the mainstay of treatment for pouchitis. The most commonly used antibiotic is metronidazole. Most patients with pouchitis have an initial response to metronidazole. The usual dose is 250 to 500 mg three times a day for 7 to 10 days. Clinical improvement usually occurs within 24 to 48 hours. Patients with frequent relapses of pouchitis may require long-term suppressive metronidazole therapy with doses ranging from 250 mg every third day to 250 mg three times a day. Side effects of metronidazole that may limit long-term administration include nausea and peripheral neuropathy. In a small, randomized clinical trial (402), 16 patients were randomized to a two-week course of ciprofloxacin 1000 mg/day ($n = 7$) or metronidazole 20 mg/kg/day ($n = 9$). Both medications significantly reduced the PDAI score. Ciprofloxacin had a greater reduction in overall PDAI (6.9 ± 1.2 vs. 3.8 ± 1.7), symptom score (2.4 ± 0.9 vs. 1.3 ± 0.9), and endoscopic score (3.6 ± 1.3 vs. 1.9 ± 1.5). None of the patients in the ciprofloxacin group experienced adverse effects, whereas three patients in the metronidazole group (33%) developed vomiting, unpleasant taste, or transient peripheral neuropathy. The authors recommended ciprofloxacin as one of the first-line therapies for acute pouchitis.

Gosselink et al. (403) conducted a study comparing the effect of ciprofloxacin and metronidazole on the microbial flora of patients with pouchitis. Patients treated with ciprofloxacin had significantly larger reductions in PDAI score compared with patients treated with metronidazole. During pouchitis-free periods, the patients had flora characterized by high numbers of anaerobes and no or low numbers of pathogens. This flora resembles normal colon flora. During pouchitis episodes, they formed a significant decrease of anaerobes, a significant increase of aerobic bacteria and significantly more numbers of pathogens, such as *Clostridium perfringens* (in 95% of samples) and hemolytic strains of *Escherichia coli* (in 57% of the samples). Treatment with metronidazole resulted in a complete eradication of the anerobic flora, including *C. perfringens*. However, no changes in the numbers of *E. coli* were found. In contrast, when the patient was treated with ciprofloxacin, not only *C. perfringens*, but also all coliforms including hemolytic strains of *E. coli* disappeared. The larger part of the anaerobic flora was left undisturbed. This study strongly suggests a role of pathogenic bacteria (*C. perfringens* and/or hemolytic strains of *E. coli*) in pouchitis. Treatment with ciprofloxacin is superior because it eradicates both pothogens and results in an optimal restoration of normal pouch flora; of note, ciprofloxacin does not disturb the majority of anerobic bacteria. Alternatives to metronidazole include, amoxicilin/clavulanic acid, erythromycin, and tetracycline (393).

The first step in the treatment of pouchitis is to confirm the diagnosis using pouch endoscopy and biopsy specimens in patients with compatible symptoms. Once the diagnosis is confirmed, treatment is initiated with metronidazole or ciprofloxacin. For patients whose symptoms fail to respond, treatment with other types of broad-spectrum antibiotics often is the next step. When patients requiring suppressive antibiotic therapy develop bacterial resistance after prolonged treatment, cycling three or four antibiotics in one-week intervals is sometimes helpful. Those patients who do not respond to metronidazole, ciprofloxacin or other antibiotics should be treated with anti-inflammatory or immunosuppressive agents. Initial local pouch treatment often includes mesalamine enemas or suppositories or steroid enemas. In more refractory cases, sulfasalazine, oral mesalamine, and oral steroids may be useful. Some patients may require combination therapy with multiple agents similar to the treatment for patients with IBD. A small number of cases are refractory to all forms of medical therapy, and these patients should be referred to a surgeon for consideration of pouch reconstruction or excision (396).

Patients who have chronic pouchitis should be considered for probiotic therapy. Probiotics are live organisms, typically bacteria, found as commensals in the human gastrointestinal tract. The mechanism of action of probiotics in pouchitis is unclear (400).

Gionchetti et al. (404) evaluated the efficacy of a probiotic preparation (VSL3) containing 5×10^{11}/g of viable lyophilized bacteria of four strains of lactobacilli, three strains of bifidobacteria, and one strain of *Streptococcus salivarius* subsp. *thermophilus* compared with placebo in maintenance of remission of chronic pouchitis. Forty patients in clinical and endoscopic remission were randomized to receive either VSL3, 6 g/day, or an identical placebo for nine months. Patients were assessed clinically every month and endoscopically and histologically every two months or in the case of a relapse. The results showed that three patients (15%) in the VSL3 group had relapses within the nine months follow-up period, compared with 20 (100%) in the placebo group. Fecal concentration of lactobacilli, bifidobacteria, and *S. thermophilus* increased significantly from baseline levels only in the VSL3-treated group. The authors concluded that oral administration of this probiotic preparation is effective in preventing flare-ups of chronic pouchitis.

Gosselink et al. (405) investigated the efficacy of probiotic *Lactobacillus rhamnosus* GG in long-term delaying the first onset of pouchitis. Thirty-nine patients who underwent an IPAA between 1996 and 2001, started immediately after the operation with daily intake of *L. rhamnosus* GG in a fermented product. Seventy-eight patients, in whom an IPAA was performed between 1989 and 1996, received no *L. rhamnosus* GG. The results showed that the first episodes of pouchitis were observed less frequently in patients with a daily intake of *L. rhamnosus* GG (cumulative risk at three years: 7% vs. 29%). The authors concluded that daily intake of fermented products containing *L. rhamnosus* GG provides significant clinical benefit, without side effects. The authors recommended a daily intake of *L. rhamnosus* GG (dose $1–2 \times 10^{11}$ bacteria) to delay the first onset of pouchitis. This single strain as a part of a fermented product is less expensive than the lyophilized mixture, VSL3.

The frequency of refractory pouchitis ranges from 4.5% to 5.5%, with severe intractable pouchitis leading to excision of the pouch in 0.3% to 1.3% of patients (400). In a study of the clinical outcome of 100 patients at the Mayo Clinic who underwent IPAA for ulcerative colitis, 32 patients developed pouchitis, 21 had recurrent pouchitis, and 11 had one to two episodes of acute pouchitis. Of the recurrent pouchitis, 16 had frequent relapses of acute pouchitis, and five had chronic pouchitis. Of the five with chronic pouchitis, three required maintenance suppressive therapy and two required pouch excision (400).

Finally, it is important to review the clinical course and natural history of patients with pouchitis to gain some perspective on the seriousness of this problem and to determine whether the increasing incidence of pouchitis should lead to reconsideration of the use of proctocolectomy with ileal reservoir creation in patients with ulcerative colitis. At the Mayo Clinic, the cumulative percentage of patients with ulcerative colitis with IPAAs who have developed at least one episode of pouchitis is 32% (406). Of patients with pouchitis, 39% have a single acute episode that responds to treatment with antibiotics (393). The remaining 61% of patients with pouchitis have at least one recurrence, and many of these patients believe that pouchitis recurs often enough to constitute a chronic problem (393). Fifteen percent of patients with pouchitis (5% of all patients with IPAA) require maintenance suppressive therapy and have been labeled as having "chronic pouchitis" (393,406). Almost half of these patients with chronic pouchitis (2% of all patients with IPAA) require pouch excision because of pouchitis. The benefit of surgery compared with the risk of pouchitis assessment is still favorable for the IPAA operation in appropriately selected patients with ulcerative colitis, given the natural history of pouchitis reported to date. The cumulative probability of pouchitis increases from 28% at five years to 38% at 10 years and to 47% at 15 years (349).

A useful treatment algorithm for pouchitis is given in Figure 32 (400).

■ REOPERATION FOR POUCH-RELATED COMPLICATIONS

Pouch-related complications occur in from 12% to 22% of patients. They include anastomotic stricture, perianal fistula or abscess, intra-abdominal fistula or abscess, residual septum in a J pouch, a long efferent limb in an S pouch, and unsatisfactory pouch function (363,407). What is the outcome for these patients? Galandiuk et al. (407) reviewed their experience with 114 patients at the Mayo Clinic. Complications prevented initial ileostomy closure in 25% of the patients. The salvage procedures performed included anal dilatation for stricture with the patient under anesthesia, placement of a seton and/or fistulotomy for perianal fistula, unroofing anastomotic sinuses, simple drainage and antibiotic administration for perianal abscess, abdominal exploration with drainage of intra-abdominal abscess with or without establishment of ileostomy, and complete or partial reconstruction of the reservoir for

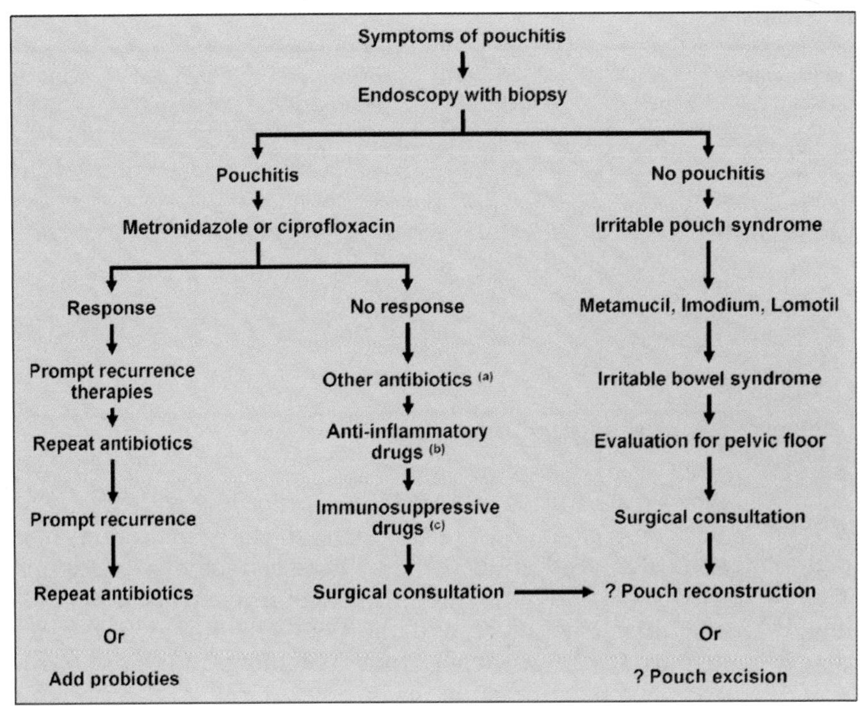

FIGURE 32 ■ Treatment algorithm for pouchitis. (**a**) Other antibiotics indicates: rifaximin; amoxicillin/clavulanate; erythromycin; tetracycline; and cycling of multiple antibiotics. (**b**) Anti-inflammatory drugs indicates: bismuth subsalicylate, mesalamine enemas, sulfasalazine, and oral mesalamine. (**c**) Immunosuppressive drugs indicates: budesonide, steroid enemas, oral steroids, azathioprine. *Source*: From Ref. 400.

patients with inadequate emptying. None of the reoperated patients died, and reoperation led to restoration of pouch function in two-thirds of the patients. However, 20% of the 114 pouches required excision. Excision was especially common among patients who had pelvic sepsis.

Satisfactory results have been reported in a subgroup of patients who required disconnection of the pouch, pouch revision, and reconnection of the pouch (408,409). The series from the Mayo Clinic included 23 patients with various problems (Table 7) (408). At a median follow-up of five years (range, 1–10 years), 11 patients reported good-to-excellent function, 5 reported fair function, 1 reported recurrent pouchitis, and 6 were unsuccessful (three had gross incontinence, two had excessive bowel movement, and one had Crohn's disease). The operative technique consisted of mobilizing and disconnecting the pouch from the anal anastomosis. The pouch was delivered out of the pelvis and revised according to the nature of the problem. In this series problems included excision of a long efferent spout with or without excision of the original pouch, excision of the original pouch with construction of a new pouch, excision of a long blind end of a J pouch, rotation of the pouch on its long axis, and excision of fistulous tracts with repair of pouch. After the repair, the pouch was anastomosed to the anal canal at the dentate line. A covering loop ileostomy was performed in each case.

Similarly, Hulten et al. (410) disconnected and revised failing pouches but converted them to continent ileostomies. The procedures were successfully performed in five patients with various problems: high evacuation frequency and urgency, perianastomotic abscess, incontinence, a pouch–vaginal fistula, and persistent pelvic pain. However, follow-up was not reported.

The Cleveland Clinic group reported 59 patients with a fistula from the pouch to various sites: 24 vaginal, 11 cutaneous, 16 perineal, and 8 presacral (411). Among these patients, 111 operations (range, 1–7) were performed. Pouch excision was required in 32%. Overall, 68% were successful.

Salvage surgery for major complications following IPAA is worthwhile (412). One significant finding is that, in general, significant pelvic sepsis precludes successful pouch salvage (413,414).

TABLE 7 ■ **Indication for Reoperation and Outcome in 23 Patients**

Problem	Number of Patients	Treatment	Outcome
Long efferent spout	9	New pouch (5) Revised pouch (4)	Success (7)
Sepsis and/or fistula	4	Revised pouch	Success (2)
Blind limb	3	Revised pouch	Success (1)
Twisted pouch	3	New pouch (1) Old pouch retained (2)	Success (3)
Ileal pouch–anal anastomosis	3	Old pouch retained	Success (3)
No pouch, (only folded J)	1	New pouch	Success (1)

Source: From Ref. 408.

■ SEXUAL DYSFUNCTION

The impact of restorative proctocolectomy on sexual function is important because patients are generally young and in their reproductive years. Despite using an operative technique that spares presacral nerves and preserves the pelvic floor and anal canal, sexual dysfunction still occurs. In the series from the Mayo Clinic in which 670 IPAAs were performed for ulcerative colitis, impotence occurred in 1% and retrograde ejaculation in 3% (415). In females dyspareunia occurred in 7%. A prospective study of 100 male patients with IPAA from Göteborg, Sweden, revealed impotence in 2% (excluding preoperative impotence) and retrograde ejaculation in 2% (416). Damgaard et al. (417) from Denmark also reported a similar incidence. The sexual dysfunction in females was greater: dyspareunia in

TABLE 8 ■ Causes of Complete Failure of Ileal Pouch–Anal Anastomosis

	Number of Patients	Number of Failures	Incontinence/ Diarrhea (%)	Fistula/ Sepsis (%)	Intractable Pouchitis (%)	Crohn's Disease (%)	Perianal Disease (%)	Others (%)
Tulchinsky et al. (420)	631 (only UC)	61 (9.7%)	30	52	11	–		7
Lepisto (421)	486 (includes FAP)	26 (5.3%)	19	35	12	15		19
MacRae et al. (418)	551 (includes FAP)	58 (10.5%)	21	41	10	19	4	5
Foley et al. (419)	460 (includes FAP)	16 (3.5%)	24	33	–	33	–	10
Wexner et al. (364)	180 (includes FAP)	14 (8%)	36	7	14	36	–	7
Dozois et al. (415)	670(only UC)	25 (4%)	44	–	–	12	–	44

Abbreviations: UC, ulcerative colitis; FAP, familial adenomatous polyposis.

7% (excluding preoperative dyspareunia) and fecal leaks during intercourse in 2% (excluding preoperative leaks).

■ COMPLETE FAILURE OF ILEAL POUCH–ANAL ANASTOMOSIS

Despite a complex operation and the relatively high complication rate after TPC with IPAA, the incidence of total failure requiring excision of the pouch or the establishment of a permanent ileostomy is relatively low—3.5% to 10.5% (Table 8) (364,415,418–421).

Pouch excision, even in specialist hands, is a major undertaking with a low but significant risk of postoperative death (1.5%) and a high rate of early and late morbidity (62%). The most frequent complication is small bowel obstruction (16%), requiring a reexploration in 4%. Of the local complications, in the immediate postoperative period, pelvis sepsis (6%) is the most frequent, requiring drainage but without a celiotomy.

The most common late complication is related to the perineal wound, particularly persistent perineal sinus, which require further surgery in 40% (420,422).

MacLean et al. (423) reconstructed ileal pouch in 57 patients with failed IPAA for ulcerative colitis (included, FAP). Basically, the failed pouch was fully immobilized and divided at the level of anorectal ring. If possible, the pouch was preserved (70%). If not, the pouch was excised and a new reservoir was constructed from the distal terminal item (30%). Then a mucosectomy or excision of the remaining outlet of the pouch was performed via the perineal approach. In all cases, handsewn pouch-anal anastamosis was performed. The pelvis was drained with a closed suction drain. A diverting ileostomy was constructed in all cases. Intestinal continuity was usually restored three months later.

The causes for the pouch failure were: pouch-vaginal fistula in 21 patients, pelvic sepsis in 14, long outlet with obstructed defecaction in 14, anastomotic stricture in 5, pouch-perineal fistula in 2, and chronic pouchitis in 1. The mean age of the patients was 33.9 (±10.4) years. There were 14 males. There was no perioperative deaths.

Postoperative complications occured in 51%. Pouch leak/pelvic sepsis was the most common complication, occurring in 12 patients (21%), followed by pouch-vaginal fistula, which occurred in 9 (16%). Other complications include small bowel obstruction in 5 (9), wound infection in 3 (5%), pouch-perineal fistula in 1 (2%), and retrograde ejaculation in 1 (2%)

Twenty-two percent of patients failed and required pouch excision. The functional results and the quality of life were considered good.

■ FUNCTIONAL RESULTS

Anorectal function after the IPAA procedure is the result of the complex interaction of many factors, including anal sphincter and puborectalis muscle activity, reservoir capacity, compliance, motility and emptying, anorectal pelvic floor sensation and innervation, upper intestinal activity, stool consistency, content, volume, and transit (424). The functional results most important in determining patient satisfaction are frequency of bowel movements per day and fecal continence. Both stool frequency and fecal soiling improve during the first two years, particularly in the first 12 months (425).

■ STOOL FREQUENCY

The reported frequency of bowel movements varies from series to series. Regardless of the type of pouch, the number of bowel movements ranges from three to nine (average, six) during the day and zero to one (average, one) during the night (216,263,426,427). As a rule, the frequency is greater immediately after the operation and gradually decreases to its minimum within a year. Frequent stools are related to the increased fecal output after IPAA. Healthy persons produce about 150 g of stool per day that is passed with a frequency that ranges from three motions per day to one motion every three days. In contrast, IPAA patients who have lost their colons expel a mean of 650 g of stool per day passed as five semisolid motions per 24 hours. The fourfold increase in fecal output probably accounts for the fourfold increase in frequency of defecation (238). The greater the fecal output, the greater the number of stools per day (Fig. 33).

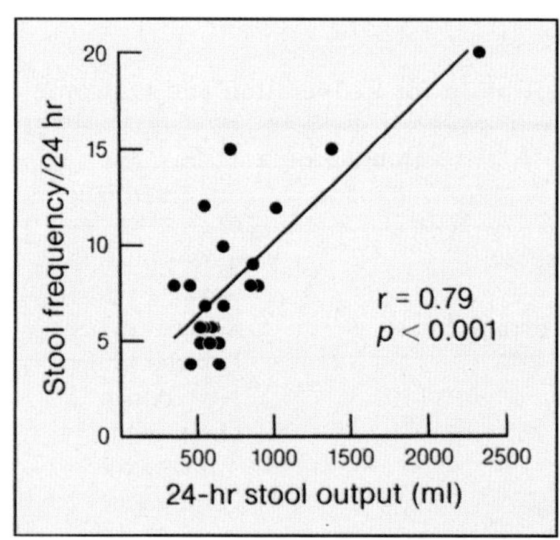

FIGURE 33 ■ Graph of 24-hour stool frequency compared with stool output per 24 hours after ileal pouch–anal anastomosis. *Source*: From Ref. 238.

Decreasing the fecal volume could be of great benefit to IPAA patients. A small volume of thicker stool would decrease the frequency of stools and probably also improve continence. The volume of fecal output can be decreased by about one-third by the use of loperamide hydrochloride (428), but the chronic use of this medication is expensive and unattractive to many patients. Bulking agents have also been used to thicken the stool but, unfortunately, do not decrease fecal output.

Efforts are being made to develop new methods of decreasing enteric output. A somatostatin analogue might diminish fecal output in IPAA patients, because it has done so in patients with conventional ileostomies (429). A careful trial in IPAA patients has not yet been reported. Calcium taken orally may also have a role (430). Slowing small intestinal transit to allow more time for absorption is an attractive hypothesis, but reversing intestinal segments in an attempt to do so has not been successful, at least not in dogs (431). Electrical pacing of the small intestine backward to slow transit and improve absorption has achieved more success in dogs with jejunal loops (432) but not in dogs with ileostomy (433). The human small intestine has also been paced, but the human small bowel absorption with pacing has not yet been achieved. In fact, decreasing fecal output below a minimal volume may not be desirable. It may be that fecal output, like urinary output, must maintain a certain minimal volume each day in order to assume that digestion and absorption from the small intestine can proceed normally. Reducing fecal volume below minimal level may impair digestion and absorption.

■ FECAL INCONTINENCE

The incidence of fecal incontinence varies from series to series, depending on the method of study and the definition of incontinence. The long-term results of 409 patients (218 men, 191 women) with IPAA at the Mayo Clinic who were followed annually for 15 years gives a more accurate reflection of long-term outcome than has been previously reported (349).

At one year 81% of patients never experienced any daytime fecal incontinence; by 10 years that percentage had dropped to 55% and remained at 55% until 15 years.

This decrease in perfect continence was accompanied by an increase in only occasional and not frequent episodes of daytime fecal incontinence.

Fecal incontinence at night also worsened over time; whereas 47% of patients never had incontinence at one year, this decreased to only 24% by 15 years. Unlike daytime incontinence, however, this decrease in perfect continence was accompanied by an increase in frequent fecal incontinence. Interestingly, the percentage of patients recording their stools as being liquid doubled over the 15-year period (6–13%), while the percentage who described their stool as solid decreased from 34% to 18%.

Despite these changes, the use of medications to alter transit (stool bulking agents, loperamide, diphenoxylate, and cholestyramine) remained stable at about 50% of patients throughout the follow-up. Importantly, the ability of the patients to discriminate stool from gas remained constant.

The functional outcome in 409 patients at 1, 5, 10, and 15 years of follow-up is given in Table 9.

TABLE 9 ■ Functional Outcome in 409 Patients at 1, 5, 10, and 15 Years of Follow-Up

	1-yr	5-yr	10-yr	15-yr	P
Mean age at follow-up, y	33.6	38	42.9	49.2	
Stool frequency, No.					
Mean Stools/day	5.5	5.6	5.6	6.2	< 0.001
Mean Stools/night	1.1	1.3	1.5	2.0	< 0.001
Stool consistency					
Liquid	6%	6%	5%	13%	< 0.001
Semiliquid (porridge)	60%	64%	75%	69%	
Solid	34%	30%	20%	18%	
Can differ gas from stool	75%	83%	80%	72%	< 0.001
Pad usage	33%	30%	22%	24%	< 0.005
Medication usage	53%	45%	47%	44%	0.01

Source: From Ref. 349.

Two major prerequisites must be present to achieve fecal continence: a compliant, receptive fecal reservoir of adequate size that empties well and a competent barricade to fecal outflow provided by an intact pelvic floor and a strong anal sphincter.

The ileal J-pouch provides a compliant reservoir of adequate volume that empties well. Measurements of J-pouches have shown a rate of distensibility of 15 mL/mm Hg of intrapouch pressure, a maximum tolerable volume of 320 mL, and a voluntary emptying rate of 11 mL of stool per minute (238,434,435). The patients emptied 84% of pouch content spontaneously at will (436). These values are similar to those of the healthy rectum.

Other motor features of the pouch, however, do not mimic the motility of the healthy rectum. The healthy rectum exhibits few if any contractions when distended to 350 mL. In contrast, large amplitude phasic contractions appear in most ileal pouches at a threshold of distention of approximately 100 mL (Fig. 34). The contractions increase intrapouch pressure to a value near anal sphincter pressure. The increases in pouch pressure are usually accompanied by increases in anal sphincter pressure (437), but sometimes pouch contractile strength exceeds anal sphincter strength. When this happens, leakage may result (438).

A method of decreasing the strength of pouch contractions as the pouch fills has not yet been devised. Anticholinergics have been used with anecdotal success, but large enough doses to inhibit pouch contraction have undesirable side effects, secondary to the inhibition of contraction in smooth muscle elsewhere. The contractile response of most pouches seems to depend mainly on the size of the pouch, rather than the particular style of pouch. Excessively large pouches, however, are not recommended because they do not empty well and may predispose the patient to pouchitis. A method of preventing or markedly reducing the strength of ileal pouch contractions as the pouch fills is yet to be devised.

The anal sphincters are reasonably well but not perfectly preserved by the operation. Resting analsphincteric strength, largely a function of the internal anal, sphincter, is decreased approximately 15% after the procedure (Fig. 35) (439). Among 50 IPAA patients we studied, resting sphincter pressure was 56 mm Hg, while resting pressure in healthy controls was 65 mm Hg (440). Moreover, anal

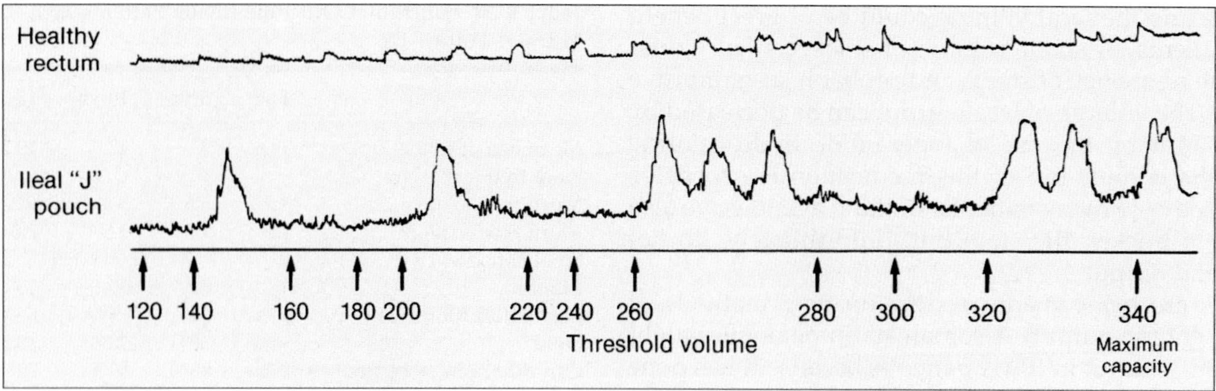

FIGURE 34 ■ Manometric tracing showing intraluminal pressure response of healthy rectum (*top*) and to distention of ileal pouch (*bottom*). Note appearance of large pressure waves at threshold volume of 140 mL distention in pouch. *Source*: From Ref. 238.

small waves superimposed on the resting pressure had a slower frequency and a larger amplitude in pouch patients than in controls. The resting pressure in some patients decreased more at night as sleep deepened than it did in healthy controls (441). There were periods during which pressures in patients decreased to near zero during rapid eye movement sleep.

The decrease in resting anal sphincter pressure may be due to mechanical damage from dilatation of the sphincter during the anal mucosal stripping or from direct injury to the sphincter during the stripping. It is also possible that partial extrinsic denervation of the sphincter occurs when the distal rectal wall and its adjacent vasculature are transected. Adrenergic fibers that accompany the vessels are known to augment anal sphincter strength, at least in the dog (442). Clearly, careful mucosal dissection, minimal dilatation of the sphincter during operation, and the protection of sphincter innervation are keys to maintaining a well-functioning anal sphincter postoperatively.

New methods of augmenting resting anal sphincter strength after surgery would be welcome. Anal sphincter resting pressure can be increased by loperamide hydrochloride (428) and sodium valproate (443) and perhaps by biofeedback. Whether that strength can be further augmented with adrenergic drugs is unknown.

In contrast to anal sphincter resting pressure, anal sphincter squeeze pressure, a function of the external anal sphincter, is usually well maintained after IPAA (Fig. 36) (439,440). While damage to the striated muscle of the external sphincter or its innervation in some patients who have episodic fecal leakage has been documented (444), overall anal squeeze pressure after mucosectomy IPAA is similar to healthy controls (439,440,444,445). Also, the anorectal angle and pelvic floor dynamics are well maintained (446).

METABOLIC FUNCTION

Whether creation of the ileal pouch changes absorption of fluid, electrolytes, and other substances has been of concern to clinicians. Much of the accumulated knowledge has been gained from studies of patients with Kock's pouch, which has a similar construction and surface area.

The plasma level of electrolytes, calcium, and phosphorus showed no changes. The ileal reservoir is capable of absorbing vitamin B_{12} instilled with intrinsic factor. Most studies show normal serum vitamin B_{12}, but some show borderline or low vitamin B_{12} absorption. It was not known whether this decrease is due to decreased ileal absorptive capacity secondary to morphologic mucosal changes or to altered absorption caused by overgrowth of bacterial flora. Serum folate levels were normal in patients with Kock's pouch, and no folate deficiency anemia has been noted.

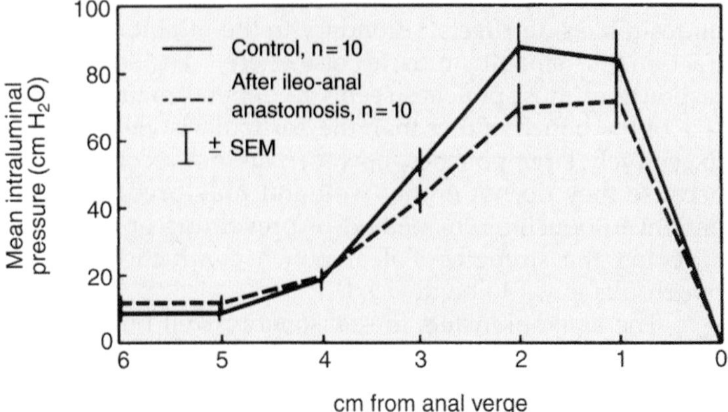

FIGURE 35 ■ Anal sphincter resting pressure profile of 10 patients with ileal pouch anal anastomosis and those of 10 healthy nonoperated controls. *Source*: From Ref. 439.

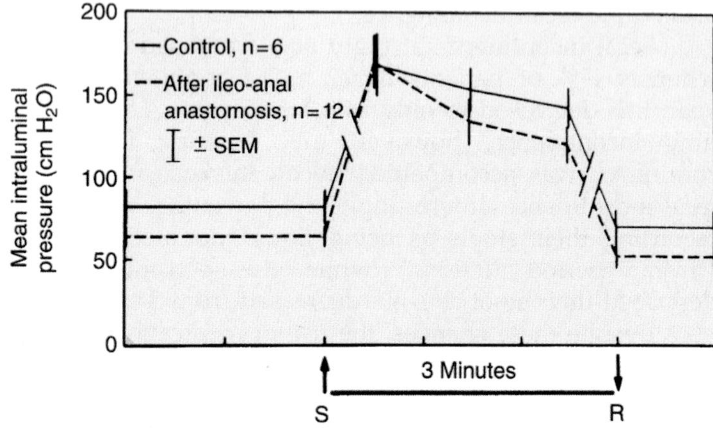

FIGURE 36 ■ Anal sphincter squeeze pressure from 12 patients with ileal pouch anal anostomosis and six healthy nonoperated controls. *Source*: From Ref. 439.

Serum iron and total iron-binding capacity levels are normal in patients with Kock's pouch. However, serum iron levels have been reported as low in a few patients with IPAA. Whether this is related to iron malabsorption has not been substantiated.

Most reports found no evidence of fat malabsorption in ileal reservoir patients, although some have detected steatorrhea in patients with Kock's pouch. Since the steatorrhea improved with administration of oral antibiotics, it was likely the result of stasis in the pouch. Bile salts absorbed primarily in the terminal ileum, therefore, are an important metabolic consideration in long-term follow-up of ileal reservoir patients. Several investigators have demonstrated an increased fecal loss of bile acids, presumably caused by excessive deconjugation of bile acids by bacterial overgrowth. However, structural mucosal changes, specifically shortening of villi, may account for some of the bile salt malabsorption (234).

PATIENT SATISFACTION WITH ILEAL POUCH–ANAL ANASTOMOSIS

When patients with ulcerative colitis require an operation, most if not all, discuss the options and the suitability of each option for their particular needs with their surgeon. The options include TPC and ileostomy, TPC with mucous fistula, colectomy with ileorectal anastomosis, TPC and Kock's pouch, and TPC and IPAA. The advantages and disadvantages, including the risk of morbidity and mortality, are discussed fully. As a rule, the patients participate in the decision making and are the ones who make the final decision, unless their choice is contraindicated or is not suitable.

Despite an imperfect functional result, including an average of six bowel movements per day and some seepage of feces in 20% of the patients during the day and 52% during the night (263), most patients with the IPAA procedure are happy with the results and are glad of their choice. Most large series reported a satisfaction rate of 94% to 95% (356,427,447). This result must be interpreted with caution. Most patients go to such referral centers mainly because they want to have the IPAA. They are the patients who hate a permanent ileostomy. They are also the patients who do not have contraindications to the procedure. Nevertheless, in properly selected patients with ulcerative colitis, TPC with IPAA provides much satisfaction.

To assess whether the improvement with IPAA is due to the absence of a stoma or the preservation of fecal continence, functional and performance activity were assessed in 406 patients with Brooke ileostomies, 313 with Kock's pouches, and 298 with IPAA (448). Patients with IPAA had fewer restrictions in sports participation and sexual activity than those with Kock's pouch, but those with Kock's pouches had fewer restrictions in those activities but more restrictions in travel than those with Brooke ileostomy. In contrast, performance in the categories of social life, recreation, work, and family were similar between the groups. Another retiospective study was conducted by Kohler et al. (449) comparing 160 patients undergoing cholecystectomy as controls and 240 patients with IPAA during an eight-year period from 1982 to 1989. Cholecystectomy was chosen as the comparative procedure because it is an intra-abdominal operation thought to result in few long-term adverse sequelae. No difference was found with regard to patient assessment of quality of life, health, status, and satisfaction. Scores for the quality-of-life dimension of family life, social life, recreational activities, sex life, occupational work, housework, sports, and travel were similar. These results have remained stable over an eight-year period.

Hahnloser et al. (349) prospectively assessed quality of life in a cohort of 409 patients followed annually for 15 years after IPAA for ulcerative colitis. They found that social activities, sports, traveling, recreational activities, family relationship, work around home, and other activities did not deteriorate with time. Sexual activities were not restricted at 5 years, but by 10 and 15 years after IPAA, mild restrictions were reported by 15% and 17% and severe restrictions by 2% and 4%, respectively. Grouped by gender, no difference was noted at 5 and 10 years, but at 15 years of follow-up, more men than women reported severe sexual restrictions (6% men vs. 2% women), whereas more women were only mildly restricted (14% men vs. 20% women. At 5, 10, and 15 years, 100%, 95%, and 91%, respectively, of patients had kept the same job, and work was not affected by surgery in 85%, 91%, and 83%, respectively. Diet was unchanged in 61% of patients or slightly more restricted in 39% at 15 year follow-up.

McLeod et al. (450) found no difference in satisfaction and quality of life among patients who have had a Brooke ileostomy, Kock's pouch, and IPAA for ulcerative colitis. The quality of life was improved after surgery and was high regardless of the surgical procedure used.

Proctocolectomy with a well-constructed Brooke ileostomy should remain the gold standard treatment for ulcerative colitis against which IPAA must be compared. Notwithstanding the fact that TPC and ileostomy has proven to be a durable, reliable operation with few complications and hence has stood the test of time, patients, given a choice, usually prefer an IPAA with its higher complication rate so as to be able to maintain a normal route of evacuation. Bamberger and Otchy (451) showed that, barring other disqualifying illness, active duty soldiers can anticipate continuation of their military career (not combat) following IPAA.

REFERENCES

1. Garland CF, Lilienfeld AM, Mendeloff AI, Markowitz JA, Terrell KB, Garland FC. Incidence rates of ulcerative colitis and Crohn's disease in fifteen areas of the United States. Gastroenterology 1981; 81:1115–1124.
2. Stonnington CM, Phillips SF, Melton LJ III, Zinsmeister AR. Chronic ulcerative colitis: Incidence arid prevalence in a community. Gut 1987; 28: 402–409.
3. Langholz B, Munkholm P, Nielsen GH, Kreiner S, Binder V. Incidence and prevalence of ulcerative colitis in Copenhagen County from 1962 to 1987. Scand J Gastroenterol 1991; 26:1247–1256.
4. Sonnenberg A. Geographic variation in the incidence of and mortality from inflammatory bowel disease. Dis Colon Rectum 1986; 29:854–861.
5. Kitahora T, Ulsunomiya T, Yokota A. Epidemiological study of ulcerative colitis in Japan: Incidence and familial occurrence. J Gastroenterol 1995; 30(suppl 8):5–8.
6. Birrenbach T, Bocker U. Inflammatory bowel disease and smoking. A review of epidemiology, pathophysiology, and therapeutic implications. Inflamm Bowel Dis 2004; 10:848–859.

7. Lashner BA. Epidemiology of inflammatory bowel disease. Gastroenterol Clin North Am 1995; 24:467–474.
8. Regueiro M, Kip KE, Cheung O, Hegazi RA, Plevy S. Cigarette smoking and age at diagnosis of inflammatory bowel disease. Inflamm Bowel Dis 2005; 11:42–47.
9. Kirsner JB. Genetic aspects of inflammatory bowel disease. Clin Gastroenterol 1973; 2:557–575.
10. Monsen W, Brastrom O, Nordenvall B, Sorstad J, Hellers G. Prevalence of inflammatory bowel disease among relatives of patients with ulcerative colitis. Scand J Gastroenterol 1987; 22:214–218.
11. Mayberry JF. Recent epidemiology of ulcerative colitis and Crohn's disease. Int J Colorectal Dis 1989; 4:59–66.
12. Loftus EV. Clinical epidemiology of inflammatory bowel disease: incidence, prevalence, and environmental influences. Gastroenterology 2004; 126:1504–1517.
13. Farmer RG, Michener WM, Mortimer EA. Studies of family history among patients with inflammatory bowel disease. Clin Gastroenterol 1980; 9:271–278.
14. Lashner BA, Evans AA, Kirsner JB, Hanauer SB. Prevalence and incidence of inflammatory bowel disease in family members. Gastroenterology 1986; 91:1396–1400.
15. Reumaux D, Colombel JF, Masy E. Anti-neutrophil cytoplasmic auto-antibodies (ANCA) in ulcerative colitis (LIC): no relationship with disease activity. Inflamm Bowel Dis 2000; 6:270–274.
16. Steven C. Pathogenesis. Semin Colon Rectal Surg 1993; 4:2–13.
17. Strober W, James SP. The immunologic basis of inflammatory bowel disease. J Clin Immunol 1986; 6:415–432.
18. Nelson H. Immunology of chronic ulcerative colitis. Semin Colon Rectal Surg 1990; 1:147–157.
19. Ekbom A. The epidemiology of IBD. A lot of data but little knowledge. How shall we proceed? Inflamm Bowel Dis 2004; 10(suppl):532–534.
20. Sands BE. From symptom to diagnosis: clinical distinction among various forms of intestinal inflammation. Gastroenterology 2004; 126: 1518–1532.
21. Camilheri M, Proano M. Advances in the assessment of disease activity in inflammatory bowel disease. Mayo Clin Proc 1989; 64:800–807.
22. Truelove SC, Witts LJ. Cortisone in ulcerative colitis. Final report on a therapeutic trial. Br Med J 1955; 29(4947):1041–1048.
23. Seo M, Okada M, Yao T, Ueki M, Arima S, Okumura M. An index of disease activity in patients with ulcerative colitis. Am J Gastroenterol 1992; 87:971–976.
24. Travis SPL, Farrant JM, Ricketts C, et al. Predicting outcome in severe ulcerative colitis. Gut 1996; 38:905–910.
25. Truelove SC. Medical management of ulcerative colitis and indications for colectomy. World J Surg 1988; 12:142–147.
26. Schroeder KW, Tremaine WJ, Ilstrup DM. Coated oral 5-aminosalicylic acid therapy for mildly to moderately active ulcerative colitis: a randomized study. N Engl J Med 1987; 317:1625–1629.
27. Roseth AG, Aadland E, Johnson J, Raknerud N. Assessment of disease activity in ulcerative colitis by fecal calprotectin, a novel granulocyte marker protein. Digestion 1997; 58:176–180.
28. Saverymuttu SH, Camilleri M, Rees H, Lavender JP, Hodgson HJE, Chadwick VS. Indium-III-granulocyte scanning in the assessment of disease activity in inflammatory bowel disease. Gastroenterology 1986; 90: 1121–1128.
29. Roseth AG, Fagerhol MK, Aadland E, Schjonsby H. Assessment of the neutrophil dominating protein calprotectin feces: a methodological study. Scand J Gastroenterol 1992; 27:793–798.
30. Batts KP, Weiland L. Pathology of ulcerative colitis. Semin Colon Rectal Surg 1990; 1:132–146.
31. Gumaste V, Sachar DB, Greenstein AJ. Benign and malignant colorectal strictures in ulcerative colitis. Gut 1992; 33:938–941.
32. Goulson SJM, McGovern VJ. The nature of benign strictures in ulcerative colitis. N Engl J Med 1969; 281:290–295.
33. Finkelstein SD, Sasatomi E, Regueiro M. Pathologic features of early inflammatory bowel disease. Gastroenterol Clin N Am 2002; 31: 133–145.
34. Seaver RL. Screening for Clostridium difficile in chronic inflammatory bowel disease in relapse. Is it helpful? Is it cost efficient? J Clin Gastroenterol 1986; 8:397–400.
35. Viscidi R, Willey S, Bartlett JG. Isolation rates and toxigenic potential of Clostridum difficile isolates from patient populations. Gastroenterology 1981; 81:5–9.
36. McFarland LV, Mulligan ME, Kwok RY, Stamm WE. Nosocomial acquisition of Clostridium difficile infection. N Eng J Med 1989; 320:204–210.
37. Bardhett JG, Chang TW, Gurwith M, Gorbach SL, Onderdonk AB. Antibiotic-associated pseudomembranous colitis due to toxin-producing Clostridia. N Engl J Med 1978; 298:531–534.
38. Scott AJ, Nicholson GI, Kerr AR. Lincomycin as a cause of pseudomembranous colitis. Lancet 1973; 2:1232–1234.
39. Tedesco FJ, Barton RW, Alpers DH. Clindamycin associated colitis. Ann Intern Med 1974; 81:429–433.
40. Wold A, Mendelow H, Bartlett JG. Non-antibiotic-associated pseudo-membranous colitis due to toxin-producing clostridia. Ann Intern Med 1980; 92:798–799.
41. Bartlett JG. Antibiotic-associated diarrhea. N Engl J Med 2002; 346: 334–339.
42. Kyne L, Farrell RJ, Kelly CP. Clostridium difficile. Gastroenterol Cl N Am 2001; 30:753–777.
43. Bergstein JM, Kramer A, Wittman DH, Aprahamian C, Queb-beman EJ. Pseudomembranous colitis: How useful is endoscopy? Surg Endosc 1990; 4:217–219.
44. Rosen L. Antibiotic-associated colitis. Perspect Colon Rectal Surg 1991; 4: 205–217.
45. Marts BC, Longo WE, Vernava AM III, Kennedy DJ, Daniel GL, Jones I. Patterns and prognosis of Clostridial difficile colitis. Dis Colon Rectum 1994; 37:837–845.
46. Aslam S, Hamill RJ, Musher DM. Treatment of Clostridium difficile-associated disease: old therapies and new strategies. Lancet Infect Dis 2005; 5:549–557.
47. Tedesco FJ, Gordon D, Fortson WC. Approach to patients with multiple relapses of antibiotic-associated pseudomembranous colitis. Am J Gastroenterol 1985; 80:867–868.
48. Dallal RM, Harbrecht BG, Boujoukas AJ, et al. Fuluinant Clostridium difficile: An under appreciated and increasing cause of death and complications. Ann Surg 2002; 3:363–372.
49. Longo WE, Mazuski JE, Virgo KS, Lee P, Bahadursingh AN, Johnson FE. Outcome colectomy for Clostridium difficile colitis. Dis Colon Rectum 2004; 47:1620–1626.
50. Loo VG, Poirier L, Miller MA, et al. A predominantly clonal multi-institutional outbreak of Clostridium difficile—associated diarrhea with high morbidity and mortality. N Engl J Med ; 353:2442–2449.
51. Bartlett JG, Perl TM. The new clostridium difficile—What does it mean?. Engl J Med 2005; 353:2503–2505.
52. Muto CA, Pokrywka M, Shutt K, et al. A large outbreak of Clostridium difficile-associated disease with an unexpected proportion of deaths and colectomies at a teaching hospital following increased fluoroquinolone use. Infect Control Hosp Epidemiol 2005; 26:273–280.
53. Skirrow MB. Campylobacter enteritis: A "new" disease. Br Med J 1977; 2:9–11.
54. Smith K, Besser J, Hedberg C, et al. Quinolone-resistent Campylobacter jejuni infections in Minnesota, 1992–1998, N Engl J Med 1999; 344:1525–1532.
55. Turgeon DK, Fritoche TR. Laboratory approaches to infections diarrhea. Gastroenterol Clin N Am 2001; 30:693–707.
56. Oldfield III EC, Wallace MR. The role of antibiotics in the treatment of infections diarrhea. Gastroenterol Clin N Am 2001; 30:817–836.
57. McNuety CAM. The treatment of Campylobacter infections in man. J Antimkrob Chemother 1987; 19:281–284.
58. Update: Salmonella enteritidis infections in the Northeastern United States. mmWR 1987; 36:204–205.
59. Nye FJ. Do antibiotics really prolong salmonella excretion? Antimicrob Chemother 1981; 7:215–216.
60. Tarr PI, Neill MA. Escherichia coli 0157:H7. Gastroenterol Clin N Am. 2001; 30:735–751.
61. Karmali M, Steele B, Petric M, Lim C. Sporadic cases of hemolytic-uremic syndrome associated with fecal cytotoxin and cytotoxin-producing Escherichia coli in stools. Lancet 1983; 1:619–620.
62. Riley L, Remis R, Helgerson S, et al. Hemorrhagic Colitis associated with a rare Escherichia coli serotype. N Engl J Med 1983; 308:681–685.
63. Hossain MM, Ljungstrom I, Glass RI, Lundin L, Stoll BJ, Huldt G. Amoebiasis and giardiasis in Bangladesh: Parasitological and serological studies. Trans R Soc Trop Med Hyg 1983; 77:552–554.
64. Ravdin JI. Pathogenesis of disease with Entamoeba histolytica. Studies of adherence toxins and contact-dependent cytolysis. Rev Infect Dis 1986; 8:247–260.
65. Adams EB, MacLeod IN. Invasive amebiasis. I. Amebic dysentery and its complications. Medicine 1977; 56:315–323.
66. Haider Z, Rasul A. Chronic non-dysenteric intestinal amebiasis. A review of 159 cases. J Pakistan Med Assoc 1975; 25:75–78.
67. Katz DE, Taylor DN. Parasitic infections of the gastrointestinal tract. Gastroenterol Clin N Am 2001; 30:797–815.
68. Blumencranz H, Kasen L, Romen J, Way J, LeLeiko NS. The role of endoscopy in suspected amebiasis. Am J Gastroenterol 1983; 78:15–18.
69. Kean BH. The treatment of amebiasis. A recurrent agony. Commentary. JAMA 1976; 235:501.
70. Drugs for parasitic infections. Med Lett 1984; 26:27–34.
71. Takahashi T, Gambon-Dominguez A, Gonnez-Mendez TJM, et al. Fulminant ametic colitis. Analysis of 55 cases. Dis Colon Rectum 1997; 40:1362–1367.
72. Lindstrom CG. "Collagenous colitis" with watery diarrhea—A new entity?. Pathol Eur 1976; 11:87–89.
73. Bayless TM, Giardiello FM, Lazenby A, Yardley JH. Collagenous colitis [editorial]. Mayo Clin Proc 1987; 62:740–741.
74. Zins BJ, Sandborn WJ, Tremaine WJ. Collagenous and lymphocytic colitis: Subject review and therapeutic alternatives. Am J Gastroenterol 1995; 90:1394–1400.
75. Burgel N, Bojarshi C, Mankertz J, Zeitg M, Fromm M, Schulzhe JD. Mechanisms of diarrhea in collagenous colitis. Gastroenterology 2002; 123:433–443.
76. Wang KK, Carpenter HA, Schroeder KW, Tremaine WJ. Collagenous colitis: A clinicopathologic correlation. Mayo Clin Proc 1987; 62:665–671.
77. Case records of the Massachusetts General Hospital. Case 29–1988. N Engl J Med 1988; 319:162–168.

78. Zins BJ, Tremaine WJ, Carpenter HA. Collagenous colitis: Mucosal biopsies and association with fecal leukocytes. Mayo Clin Proc 1995; 70: 430–433.
79. Cruz-Correa M, Giardiello FM, Bagoless TM. A typical forms of inflammatory bowel disease: microscopic colitis and pouchitis. Curr opin Gastroenterol 2000; 16:343–348.
80. Varghese L, Galandiuk S, Tremaine WI, Burgart LJ. Lymphocytic colitis treated with proctocolectomy and ileal J-pouch and amastomosis. Dis Colon Rectum 2002; 45:123–126.
81. Pardi DS. Microscopic colitis. An update. Inflamm Bowel Dis 2004; 10:860–870.
82. Baert F, Schmit A, D'haens G, etal. The Belgian 1BD Research and Codali Brussels, Belgium. Budesonide is collagenous colitis: A double-blind plauto-controlled trial with histologic follow-up. Gastroenterology 2002; 122:20–25.
83. Miehche S, Heymer P, Bethke B et al. Budiaonide treatment for collagenous colitis: A randomized, double-blind, plauto-controlled, multicenter trial. Gastroenterology 2002; 123:978–984.
84. Bonderup OK, Hansen JB, Birket-Smith L, Vestergaard V, Teglbjaerg PS, Fallingborg J. Budesonide treatment of collagenouos colitis: a randomized, double fluid, placebo-controlled trial with morphometric analysis. Gut 2003; 52:248–251.
85. Gillen CD, Walmsley RS, Prior P, Andrews HA, Allan RN. Ulcerative colitis and Crohn's disease: a comparison of the colo-rectal cancer risk in extensive colitis. Gut 1994; 35:1590–1592.
86. Devroede G. Risk of cancer in inflammatory bowel disease. In: Winawer SJ, Schottenfeld D, Sherlock P, eds. Colorectal Cancer: Prevention, Epidemiology and Screening. New York: Raven Press, 1980:325–334.
87. Ekbom A, Helmick C, Zack M, Adami HO. Ulcerative colitis and colorectal cancer. A population-based study. N Engl J Med 1990; 323:1228–1233.
88. Ekbom A. Rick of cancer in ulcerative colitis. J gastrointest Surg 1998; 2:312–313.
89. Farmer RG, Hawk WA, Turnbull RB Jr. Carcinoma associated with mucosal ulcerative colitis and with transmural colitis and enteritis (Crohn's disease). Cancer 1971; 28:289–292.
90. Cook MG, Goligher JC. Carcinoma and epithelial dysplasia complicating ulcerative colitis. Gastroenterology 1975; 68:1127–1136.
91. Lennard-Jones JE. Surveillance in ulcerative colitis: Is it worthwhile? Does it save lives? Inflam Bowel Dis 1995; 1:76–79.
92. Johnson B, Ahsgren L, Anderson LO, Sterling R, Rutegard J. Colorectal cancer surveillance in patients with ulcerative colitis. Br J Surg 1994; 81:689–691.
93. Lynch DAF, Lobo AJ, Sobala GM, Dixon MF, Axon ATR. Failure of colonoscopic surveillance in ulcerative colitis. Gut 1993; 34:1075–1080.
94. Leidenius M, Kellokumper I, Husa A, Riihelu M, Sipponen P. Dysplasia and carcinoma in longstanding ulcerative colitis: an endoscopic and histological surveillance programme. Gut 1991; 32:1521–1525.
95. Lofberg R, Brostrom O, Karlen P, Tribukait B, Ost A. Colonoscopic surveillance in long-standing total ulcerative colitis: A 15-year follow-up study. Gastroenterology 1990; 99:1021–1031.
96. Connell WR, Talbot IC,HarpazN. Clinicopathological characteristics of colorectal carcinoma complicating ulcerative colitis. Gut 1994; 35:1419–1423.
97. Choi PM, Nugent FW, Schoetz DJ Jr, Silverman ML, Haggit RC. Colonoscopic surveillance reduces mortality from colorectal cancer in ulcerative colitis. Gastroenterology 1993; 105:418–424.
98. Provenzale D, Onken J. Surveillance issues in inflammatory bowel disease. J Clin Gastroenterol 2001; 32:99–105.
99. Provenzale D, Knowdley KV, Arora S, Wong JB. Prophylactic colectomy or surveillance for chronic ulcerative colitis? A decision analysis. Gastroenterology 1995; 109:1188–1196.
100. Bernstein CN, Shanahan F, Weinstein WM. Are we telling patients the truth about surveillance colonoscopy in ulcerative colitis? Lancet 1994; 343:71–74.
101. Itzknoitz SH, Present DH. Consensus conference: Colorectal cancer screening and surveillance in inflammatory bowel disease. Inflam Bowel Dis 2005; 3:314–321.
102. Banks PA, Present DH. Surveillance in ulcerative colitis: Is it worthwhile? Does it save lives? Or does it just give discontent? Inflam Bowel Dis 1995; 1:84–85.
103. Rosman-Urbach M, Niv Y, Birk Y, e al. A high degree of aneuploidy, loss of b 53 gene, and low soluble p53 protein serum levels are detected in ulcerative colitis patients. Dis Coloo Rectum 2004; 47:304–313.
104. Hussain SP, Amstad P, Raja K, et al. Increased p53 mutation load in noncancerous colon tissue from ulcerative colitis: a cancer-prone chronic inflammatory disease. Cancer Res 2000; 60:3333–3337.
105. Lang SM, Stratais DF, Heinzlmann M, Heldwein W, Wiebecke B, Loeschke K. Molecular screening of patients with long standing extensive ulcerative colitis: detection of p53 and K-ras mutation by single strand confirmation polymorphism analysis and differential hybridization in colonic lavage fluid. Gut 1999; 44:822–825.
106. Lupinetti M, Mehigan D, Cameron JL. Hepatobiliary complications of ulcerative colitis. Am J Surg 1980; 139:113–118.
107. Eade MN, Cooke WT. Hepatobiliary disease associated with ulcerative colitis. Postgrad Med 1973; 53:112–118.
108. Bush A, Mitchison H, Walt R, Baron JH, Boylston AW, Summerfield JA. Primary biliary cirrhosis and ulcerative colitis. Gastroenterology 1987; 92:2009–2018.
109. Cangemi JR, Wiesner RH, Beaver SJ, et al. Effect of proctocolectomy for chronic ulcerative colitis on the natural history of primary sclerosing cholangitis. Gastroenterology 1989; 96:790–794.
110. Talwackar J, Lindor KD. Primary sclerossing cholangitis. Inflamm Bowel Dis 2005; 11:62–72.
111. Lavery IC. Nonenteric complications of inflammatory bowel disease. Semin Colon Rectal Surg 1990; 1:183–185.
112. Nivatvongs S. Colon, rectum, and anal canal. James EC, Corry RJ, Perry JF Jr, eds. Basic Surgical Practice. Philadelphia: Hanley & Belfus, 1987:323.
113. Broome W, Lofberg R, Lundgvist K, Veress B. Subclinical time span of inflammatory bowel disease in patients with primary sclerosing cholangitis. Dis Colon Rectum 1995; 38:1301–1305.
114. Flamm SL, Chopra G. Hepatobiliary manifestations. Semin Colon Rectal Surg 1993; 4:62–74.
115. Chapman RW. Role of immune factors in the pathogenesis of primary sclerosing cholangitis. Semin Liver Dis 1991; 11:1–4.
116. Lindor KD, Wiesner RH, Katzmann JA, LaRusso NF, Beaver SJ. Lymphocyte subsets in primary sclerosing cholangitis. Dig Dis Sci 1987; 32:720–725.
117. Snook JA, Chapman RW, Sachdev GK, et al. Peripheral blood and portal tract lymphocyte populations in primary sclerosing cholangitis. J Hepatol 1989; 9:36–41.
118. Talwalker JA, Lindor KD. Primary sclerosing cholangitis. Inflam Bowel Dis 2005; 11:62–72.
119. Lindor KD, Wiesner RH, Colwell LJ, Steiner B, Beaver S, LaRusso NF. The combination of prednisone and colchicine in patients with primary sclerosing cholangitis. Am J Gastroenterol 1991; 86:57–61.
120. Kaplan MM. Medical approaches to primary sclerosing cholangitis. Semin Liver Dis 1991; 11:56–63.
121. La Russo NF, Wiesner RH, Ludwig J, MacCarthy RL, Beaver SJ, Zinsmeister AR. Prospective trial of penicillanine in primary sclerosing cholangitis. Gastroenterology 1988; 95:1036–1042.
122. Pardi DS, Loftus EV Ja, Kremers WK, Keach J, Linder KD. Ursodeoxycholic acid as a chemopreventive agent in patients with ulcerative colitis and primary sclerosing cholangitis. Gastroenterology 2003; 124:889–893.
123. Brentnall TA. Ursodiol: Good drug makes good. Editorial. Gastroenterology 2003; 124:1139.
124. Soetikno RM, Otto SI, Heidenreich PA, Young HS, Blackstone MO. Internal risk of colorectal neoplasia in patients with primary sclerosing cholangitis and ulcerative colitis is a meta-analysis. Gastrointestinal Endroc 2002; 56:48–54.
125. Poritz LS, Koltun WA. Surgical management of ulcerative colitis in the presence of primary sclerosing cholangitis. Dis Colon Rectum 2003; 46:173–178.
126. MacLean AR, Lilly L, Cohen Z, O'Connor B, McLeod RS. Outcome of patients undergoing his transplantation for primary sclerosing cholangitis. Dis Colon Rectum 2003; 46:112–118.
127. Loftus LV, Aguilar KZ, Sandborn WJ, et al. Risk of colorectal neoplasia in patients with primary sclerosing cholangitis and ulcerative colitis following orthotopic liver transplantation. Hepatalogy 1998; 27:685–690.
128. Vera A, Gunson BK, Ussatoff V, Nightugale P, etal. Colorectal cancer in patients with inflammatory bowel disease after liver transplantation for sclerosing cholangitis. Transplantation 2003; 75:1983–1988.
129. Orchard TR, Woodsworth BP, Jewell. Peripheral arthropathies in inflammatory bowel disease: their articular distribution and natural history. Gut 1998; 42:387–391.
130. Sartor RB, Cleland DR, Cartalano CG, Schwab JH. Serum antibody response indicates intestinal absorption of bacterial cell wall pepticloglycan in inflammatory bowel disease patients. Gastroenterology 1985; 88:1571A.
131. Levine JB, Lukawski-Trubish D. Gastrointestinal considerations in inflammatory bowel disease. Gastroenterol Clin North Am 1995; 34:633–646.
132. Tremaine WJ. Treatment of erythema nodosum, aphthous stomatitis, and pyoderma gangrenosum in patients with IBD. Inflamm Bowel Dis 1998; 4:68–69.
133. Grand RJ. Treatment of extraintestinal manifestations of inflammatory bowel disease. Inflamm Bowel Dis 1998; 4:72.
134. Levitt MD, Ritchie JK, Lennard-Jones JE, Phillips RKS. Pyoderma gangrenosum in inflammatory bowel disease. Br J Surg 1991; 78:676–678.
135. Banks PA, Present DH. Treatment of erythema nodosum, aphthous stomatitis, and pyoderma gangrenosum in patients with IBD. Inflamm Bowel Dis 1998; 4:73.
136. Orchard TR, Chua CN, Ahmad T, et al. Uveitis and erythema nodosun in inflammatory bowel disease: clinical features and the role of HLA genes. Gastroenterology 2002; 123:714–718.
137. Lavery I. Nonenteric complications of inflammatory bowel disease. Semin Colon Rectal Surg 1990; 1:183–185.
138. Mintz R, Feller ER, Bahr RL, Shah SA. Ocular manifestations of inflammatory bowel disease. Inflamm Bowel Dis 2004; 10:135–139.
139. Miller JP. Inflammatory bowel disease in pregnancy: a review. J R Soc Med 1986; 79:221–225.
140. Korelitz BI. Pregnancy. Semin Colon Rectal Surg 1993; 4:48–54.
141. Davidson JM, Lindheimer MD. Pregnancy in women with renal allographs. Semin Nephrol 1984; 4:240–251.
142. Alstead EM, Lennard-Jones JE, Farthing MJG, Clark ML. Safety of azathioprine in pregnancy in inflammatory bowel disease. Gastroenterology 1990; 99:443–446.

143. Friedman LS. New medical therapies. Semin Colon Rectal Surg 1993; 4:14–24.
144. Feagan BG. Oral budesonide therapy for ulcerative colitis: a topical tale [editorial]. Gastroenterology 1996; 110:2000–2002.
145. van Deventer SJH. Is budesonide an advance in the treatment of Crohn's disease?. Inflamm Bowel Dis 2001; 7:62–63.
146. Peppercorn MA. Advances in drug-therapy for inflammatory bowel disease. Ann Intern Med 1990; 112:50–60.
147. Hanauer SB, Schulman MI. New therapeutic approaches. Gastroenterol Clin North Am 1995; 24:523–540.
148. Present DH, Meltzer JJ, Krumholz MP, Wolke A, Korelitz BI. 6-Mercaptopurine in the management of inflammatory bowel disease: Short- and long-term toxicity. Ann Intern Med 1989; 111:641–649.
149. Lichtiger S, Present DH, Kornbluth A, et al. Cyclosporine in severe ulcerative colitis refractory to steroid therapy. N Engl J Med 1994; 330:1841–1845.
150. Kolars JC, Awni WM, Merion RM, Watkins PB. First-pass metabolism of cyclosporine by the gut. Lancet 1991; 338:1488–1490.
151. Sandborn WJ. A critical review of cyclosporine therapy in inflammatory bowel disease. Inflam Bowel Dis 1995; 1:48–63.
152. Bitton A, Peppercorn MA. Medical management of specific clinical presentations. Gastroenterol Clin North Am 1995; 24:541–558.
153. Campieri M, Gionchetti P, Belluzzi A, et al. Topical treatment with 5-aminosalicylic in distal ulcerative colitis by using a new suppository preparation. A double-blind placebo-controlled trial. Int J Colorectal Dis 1990; 5:79–81.
154. Sutherland LR, Martin FP, Greer S, et al. 5-aminosalicylic acid enemas in the treatment of distal ulcerative colitis, proctosigmoiditis, and proctitis. Gastroenterology 1987; 92:1894–1898.
155. Bar-Meir S, Fidder HH, Faszczgls M, et al. The International Budesonide study group. Dis Colon Rectum 2003; 46:929–936.
156. Dick AP, Grayson MJ, Carpenter RG, Petrie A. Controlled trial of sulphasalazine in the treatment of ulcerative colitis. Gut 1964; 5:437–442.
157. Zinberg J, Molinas S, Das KM. Double-blind placebo-controlled study of olsalazine in the treatment of ulcerative colitis. Am J Gastroenterol 1990; 85: 562–566.
158. Marteau P, Probert CS, Lindgren S, et al. Combined oral and enema treatment with pentasa (mesalazine) is superior to oral therapy alone in patients with extensive mild/moderate active ulcerative colitis: a randomized, double blind, placebo controlled study. Gut 2005; 54:960–965.
159. Barrett KE, Dharmathaption K. Pharmacological aspects of therapy in inflammatory bowel disease: antidiarrheal agents. J Clin Gastroenterol 1988; 10:57–63.
160. Haghighi DB, Lashner BA. Left-sided Ulcerative colitis. Gasterentrol Clin N Am 2004; 33:271–284.
161. Gasche C. Anemia in IBD: The overlooked villain. Inflamm Bowel Dis 2000; 6:142–150.
162. Meyers S, Sachar DB, Goldberg JG, Janowitz HD. Corticotropin versus hydrocortisone in the intravenous treatment of ulcerative colitis. A prospective, randomized, double-blind clinical trial. Gastroenterology 1983; 85:351–357.
163. Schwartz AG, Targan SR, Saxon A. Sulfasalazine induced exacerbation of ulcerative colitis. N Engl J Med 1982; 306:409–412.
164. Chapman RW, Selby WS, Jewell DP. Controlled trial of intravenous metronidazole as an adjunct to corticosteroids in severe ulcerative colitis. Gut 1986; 27:1210–1212.
165. Mantzaris GJ, Hatzis A, Kontogiannis P, Triadaphyllon G. Intravenous tobramycin and metronidazole as an adjunct to corticosteroids in acute severe ulcerative colitis. Am J Gastroenterol 1994; 89:43–46.
166. Peppercorn MA. Are antibiotics useful in the management of nontoxic severe ulcerative colitis. J Clin Gastroenterol 1993; 17:14.
167. Present DH, Wolfson D, Gelernt IM. Medical decompression of toxic megacolon by rolling—a new technique with favorable long-term follow-up. J Clin Gastroenterol 1985; 10:485–490.
168. van Assche G, D'Heans G, Noman M, et al. Randomized, double-blind comparison of 4 mg/kg versus 2 mg/kg intravenous cycloporine in severe ulcerative colitis. Gastroenterology 2003; 125:1025–1031.
169. Chang JC, Cohan RD. Medical management of severe ulcerative colitis. Gastroentrol Clin N Am 2004; 33:235–250.
170. Jarnerot G, Hertervig E, Friis-Lidy Z, et al. Infliximab as rescue therapy in severe to moderately severe ulcerative colitis: a randomized, placeb-controlled study. Gastroentrology 2005; 128:1805–1811.
171. Rutgeerts P, Sandborn WJ, Feagan BG, et al. Infliximab for induction and maintenance therapy for ulcerative colitis. N Eng J Med 2005; 353:2462–2476.
172. D'Haens G. Infliximab for ulcerative colitis: Finally same answers Editorial. Gastroenterology 2005; 128:2161–2166.
173. Kozarek RA, Patterson DJ, Gelfand MD, Botoman VA, Ball TJ, Wilske KR. Methotrexate induces clinical and histologic remission in patients with refractory inflammatory bowel disease. Ann Intern Med 1989; 110:353–356.
174. Oren R, Arber N, Odes S, et al. Methotrexate in chronic active ulcerative colitis: a double-blind, randomized Israeli multicenter trial. Gastroenterology 1996; 110:1416–1421.
175. Solern CA, Loftus EV Jr. Management of refractory inflammatory bowel disease. Gastroenterol Clin N Am 2004; 33:319–334.
176. George J, Pou R, Bodian C, Rubin P, Present D. 6-Mercaptopurine is effective in chronic ulcerative colitis but how long do you use it? Gastroenterology 1994; 106:A686.
177. Langholz E, Murikholm P, Davidsen M, Binder V. Course of ulcerative colitis: Analysis of changes in disease activity over years. Gastroenterology 1994; 107:3–11.
178. Hodgson HJF. The natural history of treated ulcerative colitis. Gastroenterology 1994; 107:300–308.
179. Hawley PR. Emergency surgery for ulcerative colitis. World J Surg 1988; 12:169–173.
180. Albrechtsen D, Bergan A, Nygaard K, Gjone E, Flatmark A. Urgent surgery for ulcerative colitis: Early colectomy in 132 patients. World J Surg 1981; 5:607–615.
181. Heppell J, Farkough E, Dube S, Peloquin A, Morgan S, Bernard D. Toxic megacolon—an analysis of 70 cases. Dis Colon Rectum 1986; 29:789–792.
182. Greenstein AJ, Sachar DB, Gibas A, et al. Outcome of toxic dilatation in ulcerative and Crohn's colitis. J Clin Gastroenterol 1985; 7:137–144.
183. Campiesi M, Gionchetti P, Belluzzi A, et al. Efficiency of 5-aminosalicylic acid enemas versus hydrocortisone enemas in ulcerative colitis. Dig Dis Sci 1987; 32(suppl):S67–S70.
184. Grant CS, Dozois RR. Toxic megacolon: ultimate fate of patients after successful medical management. Am J Surg 1984; 147:106–110.
185. Lee ECG, Truelove SC. Proctocolectomy for ulcerative colitis. World J Surg 1980; 4:195–201.
186. Robert JH, Sachar DB, Aufses AH, Greenstein AJ. Management of severe hemorrhage in ulcerative colitis. Am J Surg 1990; 159:550–555.
187. Ekbom A, Helmick C, Zack M, Adami HO. Ulcerative colitis and colorectal cancer. A population-based study. N Engl J Med 1990; 323:1228–1233.
188. Lavery IC, Chiulli RA, Jagelman DG, Fazio VW, Weakley FL. Survival with carcinoma arising in mucosal ulcerative colitis. Ann Surg 1982; 195:508–512.
189. van Heerden JA, Beart RW Jr. Carcinoma of the colon and rectum complicating chronic ulcerative colitis. Dis Colon Rectum 1980; 23:155–159.
190. Hawley PR. Ileorectal anastomosis. Br J Surg 1985; 72(Suppl):S75–S82.
191. Oakley JR, Lavery IC, Fazio VW, Jagelman DG, Weakley FL, Easley K. The fate of the rectal stump after subtotal colectomy for ulcerative colitis. Dis Colon Rectum 1985; 28:394–396.
192. Leijonmarck CE, Lofberg R, Ost A, Hellers G. Long-term results of ileo-rectal anastomosis in ulcerative colitis in Stockholm County. Dis Colon Rectum 1990; 33:195–200.
193. Pastore RLO, Wolff BG, Hodege D. Total abdominal colectomy and ileorectal anastomosis for inflammatory bowel disease. Dis Colon Rectum 1997; 40:1455–1464.
194. Kock NG. Intra-abdominal "reservoir" in patients with permanent ileostomy. Preliminary observations on a procedure resulting in fecal continence in five ileostomy patients. Arch Surg 1969; 99:223–231.
195. Vernava AM, Goldberg SM. Is the Kock pouch still a viable option? Int J Colorectal Dis 1988; 3:135–138.
196. Kock NG, Brevinge H, Öjerskog B. Continent ileostomy. Perspect Colon Rectal Surg 1989; 2(2):71–84.
197. Dozois RR, Kelly KA, Beart RW Jr, Beahrs OH. Continent ileostomy: The Mayo Clinic experience. In: Dozois RR, ed. Alternatives to Conventional Ileostomy. Chicago: Year Book, 1985:180–191.
198. Fazio VW, Church JM. Complications and function of continent ileostomy at the Cleveland Clinic. World J Surg 1988; 12:148–154.
199. From Goligher JC. Surgery of the Anus, Rectum, and Colon. London: Bailliere Tindall, 1980, p. 810.
200. Öjerskog B, Hallstrom T, Kock NG, Myrvold HE. Quality of life in ileostomy patients before and after conversion to the continent ileostomy. Int J Colorectal Dis 1988; 3:166–170.
201. Hulten L. The continent ileostomy (Kock's pouch) versus the restorative proctocolectomy (pelvic pouch). World J Surg 1985; 9:952–959.
202. Castillo E, Thomassie LM, Whitlow CB, Margolin DA, Malcolm J, Beck DE. Continent Ileostomy: Current experience. Dis Colon Rectum 2005; 48: 1263–1268.
203. Berndtsson IEK, Lindholm E, Oresland T, Hulten L. Health-related quality of life and pouch function in continent ileostomy patients: a 30-year perspective. Dis Colon Rectum 2004; 47:2131–2137.
204. Stryker SJ, Dozois RR. The ileoanal anastomosis: Historical perspectives. In: Dozois RR, ed. Alternatives to Conventional Ileostomy. Chicago: Year Book, 1985:255–265.
205. Ravitch MM, Sabiston DC. Anal ileostomy with preservation of the sphincter. A proposed operation in patients requiring total colectomy for benign lesions. Surg Gynecol Obstet 1947; 84:1095–1099.
206. Ravitch MM. Anal ileostomy with sphincter preservation in patients requiring total colectomy for benign conditions. Surgery 1948; 24:170–187.
207. Best R. Evaluation of ileoproctostomy to avoid ileostomy in various colon lesions. JAMA 1952; 150:637–642.
208. Goligher JC. The functional results after sphincter-saving resections of the rectum. Ann R Coll Surg Engl 1951; 8:421–439.
209. Valiente MA, Bacon HE. Construction of pouch using "pantaloon" technique for pull-through of ileum following total colectomy. Am J Surg 1955; 90: 742–750.
210. Martin LW, LeCoultre C, Schubert WK. Total colectomy and mucosal proctectomy with preservation of continence in ulcerative colitis. Ann Surg 1977; 186:477–480.

211. Telander RL, Smith SL, Marcinek HM, O'Fallon WM, van Heerden JA, Perrault J. Surgical treatment of ulcerative colitis in children. Surgery 1981; 90:787–794.
212. Beart RW Jr, Dozois RR, Kelly KA. Ileoanal anastomosis in the adult. Surg Gynecol Obstet 1982; 154:826–828.
213. Beart RW Jr. Surgical management of chronic ulcerative colitis. Semin Colon Rectal Surg 1990; 1:186–194.
214. Parks AG, Nicholls RJ. Proctocolectomy without ileostomy for ulcerative colitis. Br Med J 1978; 2:85–88.
215. Parks AG, Nicholls RJ, Belliveau P. Proctocolectomy with ileal reservoir and anal anastomosis. Br J Surg 1980; 67:533–538.
216. Fleshman JW, Cohen Z, McLeod RS, Stern H, Blair J. The ileal reservoir and ileoanal anastomosis procedure. Factors affecting technical and functional outcome. Dis Colon Rectum 1988; 31:10–16.
217. Penna C, Daude F, Pare R, et al. Previous subtotal colectomy with ileostomy and sigmoidostomy improves the morbidity and early functional results after ileal pouch-anal anastomosis in ulcerative colitis. Dis Colon Rectum 1993; 36:343–348.
218. Galandiuk S, Pemberton JH, Tsao J, Ilstrup DM, Wolff BG. Delayed ileal pouch-anal anastomosis. Complications and functional results. Dis Colon Rectum 1991; 34:755–758.
219. Hayvaert G, Penninckx F, Filez L, Aerts R, Kerremans R, Rutgeerts P. Restorative proctocolectomy in elective emergency cases of ulcerative colitis. Int J Colorectal Dis 1994; 9:73–76.
220. Ziv Y, Fazio VW, Church JM, Milsom JW, Schroeder TK. Safety of urgent restorative proctocolectomy with ileal pouch-anal anastomosis for fulminant colitis. Dis Colon Rectum 1995; 38:345–349.
221. Harms BA, Myers GA, Rosenfeld DJ, Starling JR. Management of fulminant ulcerative colitis by primary restorative proctocolectomy. Dis Colon Rectum 1994; 37:971–978.
222. Nicholls RJ, Holt SD, Lubowski DZ. Restorative proctocolectomy with ileal reservoir: Comparison of two-stage vs three-stage procedures and analysis of factors that might affect outcome. Dis Colon Rectum 1989; 32:323–326.
223. Browning SM, Nivatvongs S. Intraoperative abandonment of ileal pouch-anal anastomosis: The Mayo Clinic experience. J Am Coll Surg 1998; 186:441–446.
224. Browning SM, Nivatvongs S. Intraoperative abandonment of ileal pouch-anal anastomosis for technical reasons [abstract]. Dis Colon Rectum 1998; 41:A27.
225. Utsunomiya J, Iwama T, Imajo M, et al. Total colectomy, mucosal proctectomy and ileoanal anastomosis. Dis Colon Rectum 1980; 23:459–466.
226. Fonkalsrud EW. Total colectomy and endorectal ileal pull-through with internal ileal reservoir for ulcerative colitis. Surg Gynecol Obstet 1980; 150:1–8.
227. Nicholls RJ, Pezim ME. Restorative proctocolectomy with ileal reservoir for ulcerative colitis and familial adenomatous polyposis: a comparison of three reservoir designs. Br J Surg 1985; 72:470–474.
228. Beck DE. The effect of different reservoir designs. Semin Colon Rectal Surg 1996; 17:109–113.
229. Hewett PJ, Stitz R, Hewett MK, Ng B. Comparison of the functional results of restorative proctocolectomy for ulcerative colitis between the J and W configuration ileal pouches with sutured ileoanal anastomosis. Dis Colon Rectum 1995; 38:567–572.
230. Pescatori M. The results of pouch surgery after ileo-anal anastomosis for inflammatory bowel disease: the manometric assessment of pouch continence and its reservoir function. World J Surg 1992; 16:872–879.
231. Smith L, Friend WG, Medwell SJ. The superior mesenteric artery The critical factor in the pouch pull-through procedure. Dis Colon Rectum 1984; 27:741–744.
232. Martel P, Blanc P, Bothereau H, Malafosse M, Gallot. Comparative anatomical study of division of the ileocolic pedicle or the superior mesenterial pedicle for ineseuteric lengthening. Br J Surg 2002; 89:775–778.
233. Goes RN, Nguyen P, Huang D, Beart RW Jr. Lengthening of the mesentery using the marginal vascular arcade of the right colon as the blood supply to the ileal pouch. Dis Colon Rectum 1995; 38:893–895.
234. Wong WD, Rothenberger DA, Goldberg SM. Ileoanal pouch procedures. Curr Probl Surg 1985; 23:9–18.
235. Nicholls RJ, Lubowski DZ. Restorative proctocolectomy: the four loop (W) reservoir. Br J Surg 1987; 74:564–566.
236. Dozois RR. Technique of ileal pouch-anal anastomosis. Perspect Colon Rectal Surg 1989; 2:85–94.
237. Roberts PL, Schoetz DJ Jr, Murray JJ, Coller JA, Veidenheimer MC. Use of new retractor to facilitate mucosal proctectomy. Dis Colon Rectum 1990; 33: 1063–1064.
238. O'Connell PR, Pemberton JH, Brown ML, Kelly KA. Determinants of stool frequency after ileal pouch-anal anastomosis. Am J Surg 1987; 153:157–164.
239. Oresland T, Fasth S, Nordgren S, Akervall S, Hulten L. Pouch size: The important functional determinant after restorative proctocolectomy. Br J Surg 1990; 77:265–269.
240. Keighley MRB. Abdominal mucosectomy reduces the incidence of soiling and sphincter damage after restorative proctocolectomy and J-pouch. Dis Colon Rectum 1987; 30:386–390.
241. Kmiot WA, Keighley MRB. Totally stapled abdominal restorative proctocolectomy. Br J Surg 1989; 76:961–964.
242. Heald RJ, Allen DR. Stapled ileo-anal anastomosis: a technique to avoid mucosal proctectomy in the ileal pouch operation. Br J Surg 1986; 73:571–572.
243. Johnston D, Holdsworth PJ, Nasmyth DG, et al. Preservation of the entire anal canal in conservative procto-colectomy for ulcerative colitis: a pilot study comparing end-to-end ileo-anal anastomosis without mucosal resection with mucosal proctectomy and endo-anal anastomosis. Br J Surg 1987; 74:940–944.
244. Sands LR, Wexner SD. The role of the double-stapled technique and the ileoanal pouch. Semin Colon Rectal Surg 1996; 7:77–83.
245. O'Riodain MG, Fazio VW, Lavery IC, et al. Incidence and natural history of dysplasia of the anal transitional zone after ileal pouch-anal anastomosis: results of a five-year to ten-year follow-up. Dis Colon Rectum 2000; 43:1660–1665.
246. Eu KW, Seow-Choen F. The role of mucosectomy and the ileoanal pouch. Semin Colon Rectal Surg 1996; 7:72–76.
247. Ziv Y, Fazio VW, Sirimarco MT, Lavery IC, Goldblum JR, Petras RE. Incidence, risk factors, and treatment of dysplasia in the anal transitional zone after ileal pouch-anal anastomosis. Dis Colon Rectum 1994; 37:1281–1285.
248. Curran FT, Sutton TD, Jass JR, Hill GL. Ulcerative colitis in the anal canal of patients undergoing restorative proctocolectomy [abstract]. Br J Surg 1990; 77:1420.
249. Tsunoda A, Talbot IC, Nicholls RJ. Incidence of dysplasia in the anorectal mucosa in patients having restorative proctocolectomy. Br J Surg 1990; 77:506–508.
250. Ambroze WL, Pemberton JH, Dozois RR, Carpenter HA. Does retaining the anal transitional zone (ATZ) fail to extirpate chronic ulcerative colitis (CUC) after ileal pouch-anal anastomosis (IPAA)? [abstract]. Dis Colon Rectum 1991; 34:20.
251. Thompson-Fawcett MW, Mortensen NJM, Warren BF. "Cuffitis" and inflammatory changes in the columnar cuff, anal transitional zone, and ileal reservoir after stapled pouch-anal anastomosis. Dis Colon Rectum 1999; 42:348–355.
252. O'Connell PR, Pemberton JH, Weiland LH, et al. Does rectal mucosa regenerate after ileo-anal anastomosis? Dis Colon Rectum 1987; 30:1–5.
253. Heppell J, Weiland LH, Perrault J, Pemberton JH, Telander RL, Beart RW Jr. Fate of the rectal mucosa after rectal mucosectomy and ileoanal anastomosis. Dis Colon Rectum 1983; 26:768–771.
254. Fenger C. The anal transitional zone. Acta Pathol Microbiol Immunol-Scand 1987; 85(suppl 289):1–42.
255. Stern H, Walfisch S, Mullen B, McLeod R, Cohen Z. Cancer in an ileo-anal reservoir: a new late complication? Gut 1990; 31:473–475.
256. Puthu D, Rajan N, Rao R, Rao L, Venugopal P. Carcinoma of the rectal pouch following restorative proctocolectomy. Report of a case. Dis Colon Rectum 1992; 35:257–260.
257. Lavery IC, Sirimarco MT, Ziv Y, Fazio VW. Anal canal inflammation after ileal pouch-anal anastomosis. The need for treatment. Dis Colon Rectum 1995; 38:803–806.
258. Fazio VW, Tjandra JJ. Transanal mucosectomy. Ileal pouch advancement for anorectal dysplasia or inflammation after restorative proctocolectomy. Dis Colon Rectum 1994; 37:1008–1011.
259. Cohen Z. Ileoanal pouches—Is mucosectomy unnecessary? Can J Gastroenterol 1993; 7:263–265.
260. Gemlo BT, Belmonte C, Wiltz O, Madoff RD. Functional assessment of ileal pouch-anal anastomotic techniques. Am J Surg 1995; 169:137–142.
261. Tuckson W, Lavery IC, Fazio V, Oakley J, Church J, Milsom J. Manometric and functional comparison of ileal pouch anal anastomosis with and without anal manipulation. Am J Surg 1991; 161:90–96.
262. Becker JM, LaMorte W, Marie GST, Ferzoco S. Extent of smooth muscle resection during mucosectomy and ileal pouch-anal anastomosis affects anorectal physiology and functional outcome. Dis Colon Rectum 1997; 40:653–660.
263. Pemberton JH, Kelly KA, Beart RW Jr, Dozois RR, Wolff BG, Ilstrup DM. Ileal pouch-anal anastomosis for chronic ulcerative colitis. Long-term results. Ann Surg 1987; 206:504–513.
264. Becker JM, McGrath KM, Meagher MP. Later functional adaptation after colectomy, mucosal proctectomy, and ileal pouch-anal anastomosis. Surgery 1991; 110:718–725.
265. Lindquist K. Anal manometry with microtransducer technique before and after restorative proctocolectomy. Dis Colon Rectum 1990; 33:91–98.
266. Luukkonen P. Manometric follow-up of anal sphincter function after an ileo-anal pouch procedure. Int J Colorectal Dis 1988; 3:43–46.
267. Johnston D, Holdsworth DJ, Nasymth DG, et al. Preservation of the entire anal canal in conservative proctocolectomy for ulcerative colitis: a pilot study comparing end-to-end ileo-anal anastomosis without mucosal resection with mucosal proctectomy and endo-anal anastomosis. Br J Surg 1987; 74: 940–944.
268. Lavery IC, Tuckson WB, Easley KA. Internal anal sphincter function after total abdominal colectomy and stapled ileal pouch-anal anastomosis without mucosal proctectomy. Dis Colon Rectum 1989; 32:950–953.
269. Sugarman HJ, Newsome HF, DeCosta G, Zfass AM. Stapled ileoanal anastomosis for ulcerative colitis and familial polyposis without a temporary diverting ileostomy. Ann Surg 1991; 213:606–619.
270. Miller R, Bartolo DCC, Orrom WJ, Mortensen NJM, Roe AM, Cervero F. Improvement of anal sensation with preservation of the anal transition zone after ileoanal anastomosis for ulcerative colitis. Dis Colon Rectum 1990; 33:414–418.

271. Seow-Choen S, Tsunoda A, Nicholl S. Prospective randomized trial comparing anal function after hand-sewn ileoanal anastomosis with mucosectomy versus stapled ileoanal anastomosis without mucosectomy in restorative proctocolectomy. Br J Surg 1991; 78:430–434.
272. Luukkonen P, Jarvinen H. Stapled vs hand-sutured ileoanal anastomosis in restorative proctocolectomy. A prospective randomized study. Arch Surg 1993; 128:437–440.
273. McIntyre PB, Pemberton JH, Beart RW Jr, Devine RM, Nivatvongs S. Double-stapled vs. hand-sewn ileal pouch-anal anastomosis in patients with chronic ulcerative colitis. Dis Colon Rectum 1994; 37:430–433.
274. Guzzetti G, Poggioli G, Marchetti F, et al. Functional outcome in handsewn versus stapled ileal pouch-anal anastomosis. Am J Surg 1994; 168:325–329.
275. Dozois RR, Juharz E. Ileoanal pouches—Is mucosectomy essential? Can J Gastroenterol 1993; 7:258–262.
276. Deen KI, Williams JG, Billingham GC, Keighley MRB. Randomized trial to determine the optimum level of pouch-anal anastomosis in stapled restorative proctocolectomy. Dis Colon Rectum 1995; 38:133–138.
277. Metcalf AM, Dozois RR, Kelly KA, Wolff BG. Ileal pouch-anal anastomosis without temporary diverting ileostomy. Dis Colon Rectum 1986; 29:33–35.
278. Hyman NH, Fazio VW, Tuckson WB, Lavery IC. Consequences of delayed ileostomy closure after ileal pouch-anal anastomosis. Dis Colon Rectum 1992; 35:870–873.
279. Galandiuk S, Wolff BG, Dozois RR, Beart RW Jr. Ileal pouch-anal anastomosis without ileostomy. Dis Colon Rectum 1991; 34:870–873.
280. Gorfine SR, Gelernt IM, Bauer JJ, Harris MT, Kreel I. Restorative proctocolectomy without diverting ileostomy. Dis Colon Rectum 1995; 38:188–194.
281. Grabler SP, Hosie KB, Keighley MRB. Randomized trial of loop ileostomy in restorative proctocolectomy. Br J Surg 1992; 79:903–906.
282. Mowschenson PM, Critchlow JF. Outcome of early surgical complications following ileoanal pouch operation without diverting ileostomy. Am J Surg 1995; 169:143–146.
283. Sugarman HJ, Newsome HH. Stapled ileoanal anastomosis without a temporary ileostomy. Am J Surg 1994; 167:58–66.
284. Sagar PM, Lewis W, Holdsworth PJ, Johnston D. One-stage restorative proctocolectomy without temporary defunctioning ileostomy. Dis Colon Rectum 1992; 35:582–588.
285. Jarvinen HJ, Luukkonen P. Comparison of restorative proctocolectomy with and without covering ileostomy in ulcerative colitis. Br J Surg 1991; 78: 199–201.
286. Hainsworth PJ, Bartolo DCC. Selective omission of loop ileostomy in restorative proctocolectomy. Int J Colorect Dis 1998; 13:119–123.
287. Senapati A, Nicholls RJ, Ritchie JK, Tibbs CJ, Hawley PR. Temporary loop ileostomy for restorative proctocolectomy. Br J Surg 1993; 80:628–630.
288. Wong KS, Remzi, Gorgun E, et al. Loop ileostomy closure after restorative proctocolectomy: Outcome in 1504 patients. Dis Colon Rectum 2005; 48: 243–250.
289. Lewis P, Bartolo DCC. Closure of loop ileostomy after restorative proctocolectomy. Ann R Coll Surg Engl 1990; 72:263–265.
290. Fineberg SM, McLeod RS, Cohen Z. Complications of loop ileostomy. Am J Surg 1987; 153:102–107.
291. Metcalf AM, Dozois RR, Beart RW, Kelly KA, Wolff BG. Temporary ileostomy for ileal pouch-anal anastomosis. Function and complications. Dis Colon Rectum 1986; 29:300–303.
292. Hyman NH, Fazio VW, Tuckson WB, Lavery IC. Consequences of ileal pouch-anal anastomosis for Crohn's disease. Dis Colon Rectum 1991; 34:653–657.
293. Chick LR, Brown RE, Walton RL. Microvascular reconstruction of a devascularized ileal segment during ileo-anal anastomosis. J Reconstructr Microsurg 1988; 4:359–361.
294. Price AB. Overlap in the spectrum of non-specific inflammatory bowel disease—Colitis indeterminate. J Clin Pathol 1978; 31:567–577.
295. Yu CS, Pemberton JH, Larson D. Ileal pouch-anal anastomosis in patients, with indeterminate colitis. Long-term results. Dis Colon Rectum 2000; 43:1487–1496.
296. Pishori T, Dinnewitzer A, Zmora O, et al. Outcome of patients with indeterminate colitis undergoing double-stapled ileal pouch-anal anastomosis. Dis Colon Rectum 2004; 47:717–721.
297. Delaney CP, Remzi FH, Gramlich T, Dadvand B, Fazio VW. Equivalent function, quality of life and pouch survival rates after ileal pouch-anal anastomosis for indeterminate and ulcerative colitis. Ann Surg 2002; 236:43–48.
298. Brown CJ, MacLean AR, Cohen Z, Machae HM, O'Connor BI, McLeod RS. Crohn's disease and indeterminate colitis and the ileal pouch-anal anastomosis: Outcomes and patterns of failure. Dis Colon Rectum 2005; 48:1542–1549.
299. Rudolph WG, Uthoff SMS, McAuliffe TL, Goode ET, Petras RE, Galandiuk S. Indeterminate colitis. The real story. Dis Colon Rectum 2002; 45:1528–1534.
300. Dozois RR. Indeterminate colitis and its relationship to Crohn's disease. Colorectal Dis 2001; 3(suppl):54–57.
301. Tekkis PP, Heriot AG, Smith O, et al. Long-term outcomes of restorative proctocolectomy for Crohn's disease and indeterminate colitis. Colorect Dis 2005; 7:218–223.
302. Kolton WA, Schoetz DS Jr, Roberts PL, Murray JJ, Coller JA, Veidenheimer MC. Indeterminate colitis predisposes to perineal complications after ileal pouch-anal anastomosis. Dis Colon Rectum 1991; 34:857–860.
303. Geboes K, De Hertogh G. Indeterminate colitis. Inflamm Bowel Dis 2003; 9:324–331.
304. Price AB, Jewkes J, Sanderson PJ. Acute diarrhea: Campylobacter colitis and the role of the rectal biopsy. J Clin Pathol 1979; 32:990–997.
305. Lucarotti ME, Freeman BJC, Warren BF, Durdey P. Synchronous proctocolectomy and pouch formation and the risk of Crohn's disease. Br J Surg 1995; 82:755–756.
306. Warren BF, Shepherd NA. The role of pathology in pelvic ileal reservoir surgery. Int J Colorectal Dis 1992; 7:68–75.
307. Warren BF, Shepherd NA, Bartolo DCC, Bradfield JWB. Pathology of the defunctioned rectum in ulcerative colitis. Gut 1993; 34:514–516.
308. Hartley JE, Fazio VW, Remzi FH, et al. Analysis of the outcome of ileal pouch-anal anastomosis in patients with Crohn's disease. Dis Colon Rectum 2004; 47:1808–1815.
309. Regimbeau JM, Panisy Pocard M, Bouhniky Y, et al. Long-term results of ileal pouch-anal anastomosis for colorectal Crohn's disease. Dis Colon Rectum 2001; 44:769–778.
310. Braveman JM, Schoetz DJ, Marcello PW, et al. The fate of the ileal pouch in patients developing Crohn's disease. Dis Colon Rectum 2004; 47:1613–1619.
311. Colombel JF, Ricart E, Loftus EV Jr, et al. Management of Crohn's disease of the ileal pouch with Infliximab. Am J Gastroenterol 2003; 98:2240–2244.
312. Church JM. The ileal pouch-anal anastomosis in patients with cancer of the colon and rectum. Semin Colon Rectal Surg 1996; 7:93–97.
313. Taylor BA, Wolff BG, Dozois RR, Kelly KA, Pemberton JH, Beart RW Jr. Ileal pouch-anal anastomosis for chronic ulcerative colitis and familial polyposis coli complicated by adenocarcinoma. Dis Colon Rectum 1988; 31:358–362.
314. Wiltz O, Hashmi HF, Schoetz DJ Jr, et al. Carcinoma and the ileal pouch-anal anastomosis. Dis Colon Rectum 1991; 34:805–809.
315. Radice E, Nelson H, Devine RM, et al. Ileal pouch anal anastomosis in patients with colorectal cancer: Long-term functional and oncologic outcomes. Dis Colon Rectum 1998; 41:11–17.
316. Galandiuk S, Wieand HS, Moertel CG, et al. Patterns of recurrence after curative resection of carcinoma of the colon and rectum. Surg Gynecol Obstet 1992; 174:27–32.
317. Gorfine SR, Harris HT, Buf DS. Restorative proctocolectomy for ulcerative colitis complicated by colorectal cancer. Dis Colon Rectum 2004; 47:1377–1385.
318. Remzi FH, Preen M. Rectal cancer and ulcerative colitis: does it change the therapeutic approach? Colorectal Dis 2003; 5:483–485.
319. Remzi FH, Fazio VW, Delaney CP, et al. Dysplasia of the anal transitional zone after ileal pouch-anal anastomosis. Results of prospective evaluation after a minimum of ten years. Dis Colon Rectum 2003; 46:6–13.
320. Thompson-Fawcett MW, Rest NA, Warren BF, Mortensen NJ. Aneuploidy and columnar cuff surveillance after stapled ileal pouch-anal anastomosis in ulcerative colitis. Dis Colon Rectum 2000; 43:408–413.
321. Coull DB, Lee FD, Henderson AP, Anderson JH, Mc Kee RF, Finlay FG. Risk of dysplasia in the columnar cuff after stapled restorative proctocolectomy. Br J Surg 2003; 90:72–75.
322. Thompson-Fawcett MW, Mortensen NJ Mc C. Anal transitional zone and columnar cuff in restorative proctocolectomy. Br J Surg 1996; 83: 1047–1055.
323. Herline AJ, Meisinger LL, Rusin LC, et al. Its routine pouch surveillance for dysplasia indicated for ileoanal pouches? Dis Colon Rectum 2003; 46: 156–159.
324. Borjesson L, Willen R, Haboubi N, Duffs SB, Hulten L. The risk of dysplasia and cancer in the ileal pouch mucosa after restorative proctocolectomy for ulcerative proctocolitis is low: a long-term follow-up study. Colorectal Dis 2004; 6:494–498.
325. Thompson-Fawcett MW, Marcus V, Redston M, Cohen Z, Mc Leod RS. Risk of dysplasia in long-term ileal pouches and pouches with chronic pouchitis. Gastroenterology 2001; 121:275–281.
326. Hassan C, Zullo A, Speziale G, Stella F, Lorenzetti R, Morini S. Adenocarcinoma of the ileoanal pouch anastomosis: an emerging complication? Int J Colorectal Dis 2003; 18:276–278.
327. Bell SW, Parry B, Neill M. Adenocarcinoma in the anal transitional zone after ileal pouch for ulcerative colitis. Report of a case. Dis Colon Rectum 2003; 46:1134–1137.
328. Bentrem DJ, Wang KL, Stryler SJ. Adenocarcinoma in an ileal pouch occurring 14 years after restorative proctocolectomy. Report of a case. Dis Colon Rectum 2003; 46:544–546.
329. Nagi SS, Chaudhary A, Gondal R. Carcinoma of pelvic pouch following restorative proctocolectomy: report of a case and review of the literature. Dig Surg 2003; 20:63–65.
330. Baratsis S, Hadjidimitriou F, Christodoulou M, Lariou K. Adenocarcinoma in the anal canal after ileal pouch-anal anastomosis for ulcerative colitis using a double stapling technique. Dis Colon Rectum 2002; 45:687–692.
331. Hyman N. Rectal cancer as a complication of stapled IPAA. Inflamm Bowel Dis 2002; 8:43–45.
332. Laureti S, Ligolini F, D'Errico A, Rago S, Poggioli G. Adenocarcinoma below ileoanal anastomosis for ulcerative colitis. Report of a case and review of the literature. Dis Colon Rectum 2002; 45:418–421.
333. Rotholtz NA, Pikarsky AJ, Singh JJ, Wexner SD. Adenocarcinoma arising from along the rectal stump after double-stapled ileorectal J-pouch in a patient with

ulcerative colitis: the need to perform a distal anastomosis. Report of a case. Dis Colon Rectum 2001; 44:1214–1217.
334. Heuschen WA, Heuschen G, Autochbach F, Allemeyer EH, Herfarth C. Adenocarcinoma in the ileal pouch: late risk of cancer after restorative proctocolectomy. Int J Colorectal Dis 2001; 16:126–130.
335. Iwama T, Kamikawa J, Higachi T, et al. Development of invasive adenocarcinoma in long-standing diverted Ileal J-Pouch for ulcerative colitis. Dis Colon Rectum 2000; 43:101–104.
336. Vieth M, Grunaweld M, Niemeyer C, Stolte M. Adenocarcinoma in an ileal pouch after prior proctocolectomy for carcinoma in a patient with ulcerative pancolitis. Virchows Arch 1998; 433:281–284.
337. Sequens R. Cancer in the anal canal (transitional zone) after restorative proctocolectomy with stapled ileal pouch-anal anastomosis. Int J Colorectal Dis 1997; 12:254–255.
338. Rodrignez-Sanjuan JC, Polavieja MG, Naranjo A, Castillo J. Adenocarcinoma in an ileal pouch-for ulcerative colitis. Letter Dis Colon Rectum 1995; 38:779–780.
339. Schaffzin DM, Smith LE. Squamous-cell carcinoma developing after an ileoanal pouch procedure: Report of a case. Dis Colon Rectum 2005; 48:1086–1089.
340. Oresland T, Palmblad S, Ellstrom M, Berndtsson I, Crona N, Hulten L. Gynecological and sexual function related to anatomical changes in the female pelvis after restorative proctocolectomy. Int J Colorectal Dis 1994; 9:77–81.
341. Gorgun E, Remzi FH, Goldberg JM, et al. Fertility is reduced after restorative proctocolectomy with ileal pouch anal anastomosis: A study of 300 patients. Surgery 2004; 136:795–803.
342. Olsen KO, Juelsson M, Laurberg S, Oresland T. Fertility after ileal pouch- and anastomosis in women with ulcerative colitis. Br J Surg 1999; 86:493–495.
343. Counihan TC, Roberts PL, Schoetz DJ Jr, Coller JA, Murray JJ, Veidenheimer MC. Fertility and sexual and gynecologic function after ileal pouch-anal anastomosis. Dis Colon Rectum 1994; 37:1126–1129.
344. Hahnloser D, Pemberton JH, Wolff BG, et al. Pregnancy and delivery before and after ileal pouch-anal anastomosis for inflammatory bowel disease: immediate and long-term consequences and outcomes. Dis Colon Rectum 2004; 47:1127–1135.
345. Ravid A, Richard CS, Spencer LM, et al. Pregnancy, delivery and pouch function after ileal pouch-anal anastomosis for ulcerative colitis. Dis Colon Rectum 2002; 45:1283–1288.
346. Remzi FH, Gorgun E, Bast J, et al. Vaginal delivery after ileal pouch-anal anastomosis: a Word of Caution. Dis Colon Rectum 2005; 48:1691–1699.
347. Aouthmany A, Horattas MC. Ileal pouch perforation in pregnancy: Report of a case and review of the literature. Dis Colon Rectum 2004; 47:243–245.
348. McIntyre PB, Pemberton JH, Wolff BG, Beart RW, Dozois RR. Comparing functional results one year and 10 years after ileal pouch anal anastomosis for chronic ulcerative colitis. Dis Colon Rectum 1994; 37:303–307.
349. Hahnloser D, Pemberton JH, Wolff BG, Larson DR, Crownhart BS, Dozois RR. The effect of ageing on function and quality of life in ileal pouch patients A single cohort experience of 40% patients with chronic ulcerative colitis. Ann Surg 2004; 240:615–623.
350. Bauer JJ, Gorfine SR, Gelernt IM, Harris MT, Kreel I. Restorative proctocolectomy in patients older than fifty years. Dis Colon Rectum 1997; 40:562–565.
351. Lewis WG, Sagar PM, Holdswroth PJ. Restorative proctocolectomy with end to end pouch-anal anastomosis in patients over age of fifty. Gut 1993; 34:948–952.
352. Chapman JR, Larson DW, Wolff BG, et al. Ileal pouch-anal anastomosis Does age at the time of surgery affect outcome? Arch Surg 2005; 140:534–540.
353. Keighley MRB. The role of pouch-anal anastomosis in the elderly. Semin Colon Rectal Surg 1996; 7:98–101.
354. Reissman P, Tesh TA, Weiss EG, Nogueras JJ, Wexner SD. Functional outcome of the double stapled ileoanal reservoir in patients more than 60 years of age. Am Surg 1996; 62:178–183.
355. Delaney CP, Dadvand B, Ramzi FH, Church JM, Fazio VW. Functional outcome quality of life, and complication after ileal pouch-anal anastomosis in selected septuagenarians. Dis Colon Rectum 2002; 45:890–894.
356. Cohen Z, McLeod RS. Proctocolectomy and ileoanal anastomosis with J-shaped or S-shaped ileal pouch. World J Surg 1988; 12:164–168.
357. Kollmorgen CF, Nivatvongs S, Dean PA, Dozois RR. Long-term deaths following ileal pouch-anal anastomosis. Dis Colon Rectum 1996; 39:525–528.
358. Fazio VW, Ziv Y, Church JM, et al. Ileal pouch-anal anastomoses complications and function in 1005 patients. Ann Surg 1995; 222:120–127.
359. Francois Y, Dozois RR, Kelly KA, et al. Small intestinal obstruction complicating ileal pouch-anal anastomosis. Ann Surg 1989; 209:46–50.
360. Marcello PW, Roberts PL, Schoetz DJ Jr, Coller JA, Murray JJ, Veidenheimer MC. Obstruction after ileal pouch-anal anastomosis: a preventable complication. Dis Colon Rectum 1993; 36:1105–1111.
361. Meagher AP, Farouk R, Dozois RR, Kelly KA, Pemberton JH. Ileal pouch-anal anastomosis for chronic ulcerative colitis: complications and long-term outcome in 1310 patients. Br J Surg 1998; 85:800–803.
362. Scott NA, Dozois RR, Beart RW Jr, Pemberton JH, Wolff BG, Ilstrup DM. Postoperative intra-abdominal and pelvic sepsis complicating ileal pouch-anal anastomosis. Int J Colorectal Dis 1988; 3:149–152.
363. Schoetz DJ Jr, Coller JA, Veidenheimer MC. Can the pouch be saved? Dis Colon Rectum 1988; 31:671–675.
364. Wexner SD, Wong WD, Rothenberger DA, Goldberg SM. The ileoanal reservoir. Am J Surg 1990; 159:178–185.
365. Dozois RR. Pelvic and perianastomotic complications after ileoanal anastomosis. Perspect Colon Rectal Surg 1988; 1:113–121.
366. MetcalfAM, Dozois RR, Kelly KA, Beart RW Jr, Wolff BG. Ileal "J" pouch–anal anastomosis: Clinical outcome. Ann Surg 1985; 202:735–739.
367. Lolohea S, Lynch AC, Robertson GB, Frizelle FA. Ileal pouch-anal anastomosis–vaginal fistula: a review. Dis Colon Rectum 2005; 48:1802–1810.
368. Lee PY, Fazio VW, Church JM, Hull TL, Eu KW, Lavery IC. Vaginal fistula following restorative proctocoletomy. Dis Colon Rectum 1997; 40:752–759.
369. Wexner SD, Rothenberger DA, Jensen L, et al. Ileal pouch vaginal fistulas: Incidence, etiology, and management. Dis Colon Rectum 1989; 32:460–465.
370. Paye F, Penna C, Chiche L, Tiret E, Frileux P, Parc R. Pouch-related fistula following restorative proctocolectomy. Br J Surg 1996; 83:1574–1577.
371. O'Kelly TJ, Merrett M, Mortensen NJ, Dehn TCB, Kettlewell M. Pouch-vaginal fistula after restorative proctocolectomy: Etiology and management. Br J Surg 1994; 81:1374–1375.
372. Groom JS, Nicholls RJ, Hawley Pr, Phillips RKS. Pouch-vaginal fistula. Br J Surg 1993; 80:936–940.
373. Tekkis PP, Fazio VW, Remzi F, Heriot AG, Manilich E, Strong SA. Risk factors associated with ileal pouch-related fistula following restorative proctocoletomy. Br J Surg 2005; 92:1270–1276.
374. Korsgen S, Keighley MRB. Poor outcome of a defunctioning stoma after pouch construction for ulcerative colitis. Dig Surg 2000; 17:147–149.
375. Burke D, van Laarhoven JHM, Herbst F, Nicholls RJ. Trans vaginal repair of pouch-vaginal fistula. Br J Surg 2001; 88:241–245.
376. Johnson PM, O'Connor BI, Cohen Z, McLeod RS. Pouch-Vaginal fistula after ileal pouch-anal anastomosis: treatment and outcome. Dis Colon Rectum 2005; 48:1249–1253.
377. Shah NS, Remzi F, Massmann A, et al. Management and treatment outcome of pouch-vaginal fistulas following restorative proctocolectomy. Dis Colon Rectum 2003; 46:911–917.
378. Herist AG, Tekkis PP, Smith JJ, Bona R, Cohen RG, Nicholls RJ. Management and outcome of pouch-vaginal fistulas following restorative proctocolectomy. Dis Colon Rectum 2005; 48:451–458.
379. Prudhomme M, Dozois RR, Godlewski G. Mathison S, Fabbro-Peray P. Anal canal structures after ileal pouch-anal anastomosis. Dis Colon Rectum 2003; 46:20–23.
380. Senapati A, Tibbs CJ, Ritchie JK, Nicholls RJ, Hawley PR. Stenosis of the pouch anal anastomosis following restorative proctocolectomy. Int J Colorectal Dis 1996; 11:57–59.
381. Lewis WG, Kuzu A, Sagar PM, Holdsworth PJ, Johnston D. Stricture at the pouch-anal anastomosis after restorative proctocolectomy. Dis Colon Rectum 1994; 37:120–125.
382. Fazio VW, Tjandra JJ. Pouch advancement and neo ileoanal anastomosis for anastomotic stricture and anovaginal fistula complicating restorative proctocolectomy. Br J Surg 1992; 79:694–696.
383. Herbst F, Sielezneff I, Nicholls RJ. Salvage surgery for ileal pouch outlet obstruction. Br J Surg 1996; 83:368–371.
384. Remzi FH, Fazio VW, Oncel M, et al. Portal vein thrombi after restorative proctocolectomy. Surgery 2002; 132:655–662.
385. Pescatori M, Mattana C. Factors affecting anal continence after restorative proctocolectomy. Int J Colorectal Dis 1990; 5:213–218.
386. Mignon M, Steitler C, Phillips SF. Pouchitis—a poorly understood entity. Dis Colon Rectum 1995; 38:100–103.
387. Shouten WR. Pouchitis. Perspect Colon Rectal Surg 1993; 6:225–240.
388. Stahlberg D, Gullberg K, Liljeqvist L, Hellers G, Lofberg R. Pouchitis following pelvic pouch operation for ulcerative colitis. Incidence, cumulative risk, and risk factors. Dis Colon Rectum 1996; 39:1012–1018.
389. Macafee DAL, Abercrombie JF, Maxwell-Armstrong C. Pouchitis. Coloreetal Dis 2004; 8:142–152.
390. Fleshman JW. Pouchitis. Semin Colon Rectal Surg 1996; 7:102–108.
391. Moskowitz RL, Shepherd NA, Nicholls RJ. An assessment of inflammation in the reservoir after restorative proctocolectomy with ileoanal ileal reservoir. Int J Colorectal Dis 1986; 1:167–174.
392. Sandborn WJ, Tremaine WJ, Batts KP, Pemberton JH, Phillips SF. Pouchitis after ileal pouch-anal anastomosis: a pouchitis disease activity index. Mayo Clin Proc 1994; 69:409–415.
393. Lohmuller JL, Pemberton JH, Dozois RR, Ilstrup D, van Heerden J. Pouchitis and extraintestinal manifestations of inflammatory bowel disease after ileal pouch-anal anastomosis. Ann Surg 1990; 211:622–629.
394. Gustavsson S, Weiland LH, Kelly KA. Relationship of backwash ileitis to ileal pouchitis after ilea pouch-ana anastomosis. Dis Colon Rectum 1987; 30:25–28.
395. Fozard BJ, Pemberton JH. Results of pouch surgery after ileo-anal anastomosis: The implications of pouchitis. World J Surg 1992; 16:880–884.
396. Sandborn WJ. Pouchitis following ileal pouch-anal anastomosis: Definition, pathogenesis, and treatment. Gastroenterology 1994; 107:1856–1860.
397. McLeod RS, Antonioli D, Cullen J, et al. Histologic and microbiology features of biopsy samples from patients with normal and inflamed pouches. Dis Colon Rectum 1994; 37:26–31.
398. Wischmeyer P, Pemberton JH, Phillips SF. Chronic pouchitis after ileal pouch-anal anastomosis: Responses to butyrate and glutamine suppositories in the pilot study. Mayo Clin Proc 1993; 68:978–981.

399. Sagar PM, Taylor BA, Godwin P, et al. Acute pouchitis and deficiencies of fuel. Dis Colon Rectum 1995; 38:488–493.
400. Mahadevan U, Sandborn WJ. Diagnosis and management of pouchitis. Gastroenterology 2003; 124:1636–1650.
401. Joelsson M, Andersson M, Bark T, et al. Allopurinol as prophylaxis against pouchitis following ileal pouch-anal anastomosis for ulcerative colitis.A randomized placebo-controlled double-blind study. Scand J Gastroenterol 2001; 36:1179–1184.
402. Shen B, Achkar JP, Lashner BA, et al. A randomized clinical treat of eiprofloxacin and metronidazole to treat acute pouchitis. Inflann Bowel Dis 2001; 7: 301–305.
403. Gosselink MP, Shouten WR, van Lieshout LMC, Hop WCJ, Laman JD, Embden JGH. Eradication of pathogenic bacteria and restoration of normal pouch flora: Comparison of metronidazole and eiprofloxacin in the treatment of pouchitis. Dis Colon Rectum 2004; 47:1519–1525.
404. Gionchetti P, Rizzello F, Venturi A, et al. Oral bacteriotherapy as maintenance treatment in patients with chronic pouchitis: a double-blind, placebo-controlled trial. Gastrointerology 2000; 119:305–309.
405. Gosselink MP, Schouten WR, van Lieshout LMC, Hop WC, Laman JD, Embden JGHR. Delay of the first onset of pouchitis by oral intake of the probiotic strain Lactobacillus rhamnosus GG. Dis Colon Rectum 2004; 47:876–884.
406. Penna C, Dozois RR, LaRusso NF, Tremaine WJ. Pouchitis after ileal pouch anal anastomosis for chronic ulcerative colitis occurs with increased frequency in patients with associated primary sclerosing cholangitis [abstract]. Gastroenterology 1994; 106:A751.
407. Galandiuk S, Scott NA, Dozois RR, et al. Ileal pouch-anal anastomosis. Reoperation for pouch-related complications. Ann Surg 1990; 212:446–454.
408. Sagar PM, Dozois RR, Wolff BG, Kelly KA. Disconnection, pouch revision and reconnection of the ileal pouch-anal anastomosis. Br J Surg 1996; 83:1401–1405.
409. Korsgen S, Nikiteas N, Ogunbiyi OA, Keighley MRB. Results from pouch salvage. Br J Surg 1996; 83:372–374.
410. Hulten L, Farth S, Hallgren T, Oresland T. The failing pelvic pouch conversion to continent ileostomy. Int J Colorectal Dis 1992; 7:119–121.
411. Ozuner G, Hull T, Lee P, Fazio VW. What happens to a pelvic pouch when a fistula develops? Dis Colon Rectum 1997; 40:543–547.
412. Saltzberg SS, DiEdwardo C, Scott TE, La Morte WW, Stucchi AF, Becker JM. Ileal pouch salvage following failed ileal pouch-anal anastomosis. J Gastrointest Surg 1999; 3:633–641.
413. Ogunbiyi OA, Korsgen S, Keighley MRB. Pouch salvage. Longterm outcome. Dis Colon Rectum 1997; 40:548–552.
414. Farouk R, Dozois RR, Pemberton JH. Incidence and subsequent impact of pelvic abscesses after ileal pouch-anal anastomosis for chronic ulcerative colitis. Dis Colon Rectum 1998; 41:1239–1243.
415. Dozois RR, Kelly KA, Welling DR, et al. Ileal pouch-anal anastomosis: Comparison of results in familial adenomatous polyposis and chronic ulcerative colitis. Ann Surg 1989; 210:268–273.
416. Oresland T, Fasth S, Nordgren S, Hulten L. The clinical and functional outcome after restorative proctocolectomy. A prospective study in 100 patients. Int J Colorectal Dis 1989; 4:50–56.
417. Damgaard B, Wettergren A, Kirkegaard, P. Social and sexual function following ileal pouch-anal anastomosis. Dis Colon Rectum 1995; 38: 286–289.
418. MacRae HM, McLeod RS, Cohen Z, O'Connor BI, Ton ENC. Risk factors for pelvic pouch failure. Dis Colon Rectum 1997; 40:257–262.
419. Foley EF, Schoetz DJ Jr, Roberts PL, Marcello PW, Murray JJ, Coller JA, Veidenheimer MC. Rediversion after ileal pouch-anal anastomosis. Causes of failures and predictors of subsequent pouch salvage. Dis Colon Rectum 1995; 38:793–798.
420. Tulchinsky H, Hawley PR, Nicholls J. Long-term failure after restorative proctocolectory for ulcerative colitis. Ann Surg 2003; 238:229–234.
421. Lepisto A, Luukkonen P, Jarvinen HJ. Cumulative failure rate of ileal pouch-anal anastomosis and quality of life after failure. Dis Colon Rectum 2002; 45:1289–1294.
422. Karoui M, Cohan Richard, Nicholls J. Results of surgical removal of the pouch after failed restorative proctoclectory. Dis Colon Rectum 2004; 47:869–875.
423. MacLean AR, O'Connor B, Parkes R, Cohen Z, McLeod RS. Reconstructive surgery for failed ileal pouch-anal anastomosis. A viable surgical option with acceptable results. Dis Colon Rectum 2002; 45:880–886.
424. Smith LE, Orkin BA. Physiology of the ileo-anal anastomosis. Semin Colon Rectal Surg 1990; 1:118–127.
425. Young-Fedok TM, Wolff BG. Long-term functional outcome with ileal pouch-anal anastomosis. Semin Colon Rectal Surg 1996; 7:114–120.
426. Becker JM, Raymond JL. Ileal pouch-anal anastomosis. A single surgeon's experience with 100 consecutive cases. Ann Surg 1986; 204:375–383.
427. Wexner SD, Jensen L, Rothenberger DA, Wong WD, Goldberg SM. Long-term functional analysis of the ileo-anal reservoir. Dis Colon Rectum 1989; 32: 275–281.
428. Emblem R, Stien R, Morkrid L. The effect of loperamide on bowel habits and anal sphincter function in patients with ileo-anal anastomosis. Scand J Gastroenterol 1989; 24:1019–1024.
429. Williams NS, Cooper JC, Axon ATR, King RFGJ, Barker M. Use of a long acting somatostatin analogue in controlling life threatening ileostomy diarrhea. BMJ 1984; 289:1027–1028.
430. Barsoum G, Winslet M, Kappas A, Keighley MRB. Influence of dietary calcium supplementation on ileo-anal pouch function [abstract]. Gut 1990; 31: A1170–A1177.
431. Williams NS, King RFGJ. The effect of a reversed ileal segment and artificial valve on intestinal transit and absorption following colectomy and low ileorectal anastomosis in the dog. Br J Surg 1985; 72:169–174.
432. Collin J, Kelly KA, Phillips SF. Enhancement of absorption from the intact and transected canine small intestine by electrical pacing. Gastroenterology 1979; 76:1422–1428.
433. Connell PR, Kelly KA. Enteric transit and absorption after canine ileostomy: Effect of pacing. Arch Surg 1987; 122:1011–1018.
434. Taylor BM, Cranley B, Kelly KA, Phillips SF, Beart RW Jr, Dozois RR. A clinical physiologic comparison of ileal pouch-anal and straight ileoanal anastomosis. Ann Surg 1983; 198:462–468.
435. O'Connell PR, Kelly KA, Brown ML. Scintigraphic assessment of neorectal function. J Nucl Med 1986; 27:422–427.
436. Soper NJ, Chapman NJ, Kelly KA, Brown ML, Phillips SF, Go VLW. The ileal brake after ileal pouch-anal anastomosis. Gastroenterology 1990; 98:111–116.
437. Ferrara A, Pemberton JH, Hanson RB. Preservation of continence after ileoanal anastomosis by the coordination of ileal pouch and anal canal motor activity. Am J Surg 1992; 163:83–89.
438. Stryker SJ, Kelly KA, Phillips SF, Dozois RR, Beart RW Jr. Anal and neorectal function after ileal pouch-anal anastomosis. Ann Surg 1986; 203:55–61.
439. Heppell J, Kelly KA, Phillips SF, Beart RW Jr, Telander RL, Perrault J. Physiologic aspects of continence after colectomy, mucosal proctectomy and endorectal ileo-anal anastomosis. Ann Surg 1982; 195:435–443.
440. O'Connell PR, Stryker SJ, Metcalf AM, et al. Anal canal pressure and motility after ileoanal anastomosis. Surg Gynecol Obstet 1988; 166:47–54.
441. Orkin BA, Soper NJ, Kelly KA, Dent J. The influence of sleep on anal sphincteric pressure in health and after ileal pouch-anal anastomosis. Dis Colon Rectum 1992; 35:137–144.
442. Kubota M, Szurszewski JH. Innervation of the canine internal anal sphincter [abstract]. Gastroenterology 1984; 86:1146.
443. Shoji Y, Kusunoki M, Sakanoue Y, Utsunomiya J. Effects of sodium valproate on various intestinal motor functions after ileal J pouch-anal anastomosis. Surgery 1993; 113:560–563.
444. Stryker SJ, Daube JR, Kelly KA, Telander RL, Phillips SF, Beart RW Jr, Dozois RR. Anal sphincter electromyography after colectomy, mucosal rectectomy, and ileoanal anastomosis. Arch Surg 1985; 20:713–716.
445. Hallgren T, Fasth S, Nordgren S, Oresland T, Hulten L. The stapled ileal pouch-anal anastomosis: a randomized study comparing two different pouch designs. Scand J Gastroenterol 1990; 25:1161–1168.
446. Barkel DC, Pemberton JH, Pezim ME, Phillips SF, Kelly KA, Brown ML. Scintigraphic assessment of the anorectal angle in health and after ileal pouch-anal anastomosis. Ann Surg 1988; 208:42–49.
447. Pemberton JH, Phillips SF, Ready RR, Zinsmeister AR, Beahrs OH. Quality of life after Brooke ileostomy and ileal pouch–anal anastomosis. Ann Surg 1989; 209:620–628.
448. Kohler LW, Pemberton JH, Zinsmeister AR, Kelly KA. Quality of life after proctocolectomy. A comparison of Brooke ileostomy, Kock pouch, and ileal pouch-anal anastomosis. Gastroenterology 1991; 101:679–684.
449. Kohler LW, Pemberton JH, Hodge DO, Zinsmeister AR, Kelly KA. Long-term functional results and quality of life after ileal pouch-anal anastomosis and cholecystectomy. World J Surg 1992; 16:1126–1132.
450. McLeod RS, Churchill DN, Lock AM, Vanderburgh S, Cohen Z. Quality of life of patients with ulcerative colitis preoperatively and postoperatively. Gastroenterology 1991; 101:1307–1313.
451. Bamberger PK, Otchy DP. Ileoanal pouch in the active duty population. Dis Colon Rectum 1997; 40:60–66.

27 Crohn's Disease

Santhat Nivatvongs and Philip H. Gordon

INTRODUCTION

Crohn's disease is a nonspecific inflammatory bowel disease of the gastrointestinal tract. Reviewing the proceedings of the Pathological Society of London from 1850 through 1899, Fielding (1) found 31 cases with features of Crohn's disease and 25 cases of possible Crohn's disease. It is of interest that the great majority of cases involved the large bowel. Originally the diseases were diagnosed as obstruction, stricture, and ulcerative colitis.

In 1932 Crohn et al. (2) described "a disease of the terminal ileum, affecting mainly young adults, characterized by a subacute or chronic necrotizing and cicatrizing inflammation." They noted that the disease process frequently led to stenosis of the lumen of the intestine associated with formation of multiple fistulas. These authors called the disease "regional ileitis" and believed that it involved only the terminal ileum. The disease entity was recognized rapidly and the eponym "Crohn's disease" became widely used.

In 1960 Lockhart-Mummery and Morson (3) were the first to report Crohn's disease of the large intestine. Their clinical and pathologic study made it clear that Crohn's disease is different from ulcerative colitis and that the two entities do not occur together in the same patient. It is now recognized that Crohn's disease can occur anywhere in the gastrointestinal tract from the mouth to the anus (4), usually in association with Crohn's disease of the bowel, but that it may precede the intestinal manifestations by many years.

EPIDEMIOLOGY

Russell and Stockbrügger (5) updated the epidemiology of inflammatory bowel disease and much of the following information has been obtained from their comprehensive review. There has been a time trend in incidence, with a rapid increase in frequency of Crohn's disease occurring between 1965 and 1980 and after a slower increase reached a plateau. This is in contrast to ulcerative colitis where the incidence leveled off. The precise incidence of Crohn's disease is difficult to determine. The noted increase is partly due to the improved recognition of the disease and to better diagnostic methods, but these advances cannot completely explain the marked increase in incidence (6). Furthermore, there are considerable geographic variations that range from 1 to 10 per 100,000 population (Table 1) (5). The highest rates are reported in Scandinavian countries and Scotland followed by England and North America, but are lower in Central and Southern Europe. One study from Denmark showed the incidence of Crohn's disease to be 2.7 per 100,000 population compared to 8.1 per 100,000 for ulcerative colitis. This prevalence was 34 per 100,000 population for Crohn's disease compared to 117 per 100,000 for ulcerative colitis (8). Garland et al. (7) found the incidence to range from 3.40 to 4.95 per 100,000 white population in 15 areas in the United States. The authors found a tri-modal age distribution with peaks at ages 20 to 29, 50 to 59, and 70 to 79 in white males (Fig. 1) and 20 to 29, 50 to 59, and 70 to 79 in white females (Fig. 2).

Anseline (15) found an incidence of 2.1 per 100,000 population in the Hunter Valley region of Australia. The prevalence for patients requiring operation was 34 per

TABLE 1 ■ Incidence and Prevalence of Crohn's Disease in Various Geographic Regions

Author(s)	Country	Annual Incidence/ 100,000	Prevalence/ 100,000
Garland et al. (7) (1981)	United States (15 areas)	3.4–4.95	
Binder et al. (8) (1982)	Denmark	2.70	34.0
Haug et al. (9) (1989)	Western Norway	5.30	
Stowe et al.(10) (1990)	Rochester, NY, U.S.A.	5.00	
Probert et al. (11) (1993)	England		
	Europeans		75.8
	South Asians		33.2
Maté-Jimenez et al. (12) (1994)	Spain	1.61	19.8
	Urban	1.87	
	Rural	0.86	
Odes et al. (13) (1994)	Israel	4.20	50.6
	Asian-African-born Jews	4.60	55.0
	European-American-born Jews	3.90	58.7
	Bedouin Arabs		8.2
Tsianos et al. (14) (1994)	Greece	0.30	
Anseline (15) (1995)	Australia	2.10	34.0
Lindgren et al. (16) (1996)	Sweden		94.0
Manousos et al. (17) (1996)	Crete, Greece	3.00	
Moum et al. (18) (1996)	Southeastern Norway	5.80	
Tragnone et al. (19) (1996)	Italy	2.30	
Hanauer and Meyers (20) (1997)	United States		50.0
Lapidus et al. (21) (1997)	Sweden	4.6	
Loftus et al. (22) (1998)	Olmsted County, U.S.A.	5.8	144
Yao et al. (23) (2000)	Japan	1.2	13.5
Loftus et al. (24) (2002)	North America	3.1–14.6	26.0–198.5

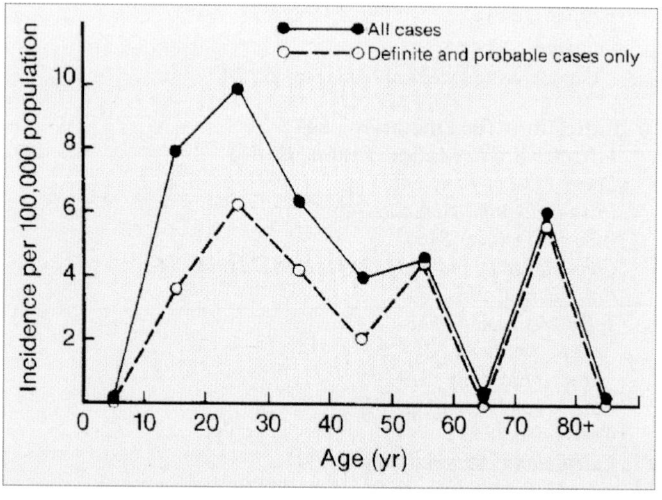

FIGURE 1 ■ Age-specific incidence rate of Crohn's disease per 100,000 population: white males. *Source*: From Ref. 7.

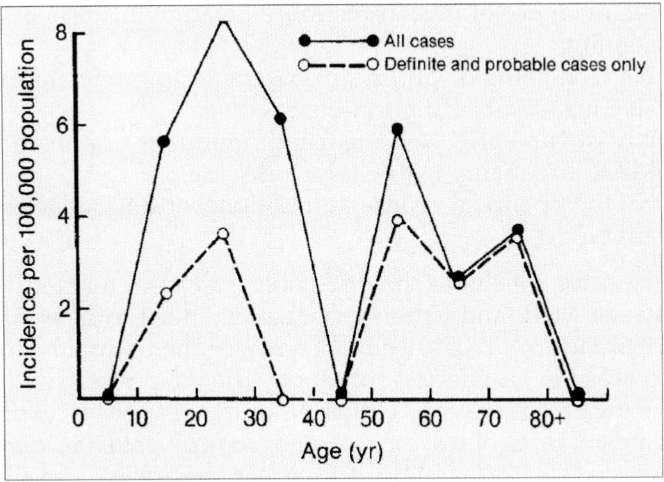

FIGURE 2 ■ Age-specific incidence rate of Crohn's disease per 100,000 population: white females. *Source*: From Ref. 7.

100,000. There was a slight female preponderance, with a peak incidence in the third decade of life. In a community-based study of 225 patients in Norway, the annual incidence was 5.8 per 100,000, with a peak of 11.2 per 100,000 for those 15 to 24 years old (5). There was no gender difference.

Lapidus et al. (21) evaluated the incidence of Crohn's disease in Stockholm County between 1955 and 1989 in a cohort of 1936 patients with Crohn's disease. The mean increase in incidence was 15% per five-year period with a mean annual incidence of 4.6 per 100,000 during the last two decades. The mean incidence for the entire study period was similar for men and women. The mean age at diagnosis increased from 25 years in 1960 to 1964 to 32 years in 1985 to 1989, partly because of an increasing proportion of patients aged at least 60 years at diagnosis. The proportion of patients with colonic Crohn's disease at the time of diagnosis increased from 15% to 32%, whereas the proportion of patients with ileocecal disease decreased from 58% to 41% during the study period. Elderly patients had a higher proportion of small bowel disease and a lower proportion of ileocolic disease compared with younger patients.

In Japan, the number of patients with Crohn's disease has increased remarkably (23). The prevalence and the annual incidence of patients with Crohn's disease in Japan were estimated to be approximately 2.9 and 0.6 per 100,000 population in 1986 and 13.5 and 1.2 per 100,000 population in 1998, respectively. Characteristic features of Crohn's disease in Japan are that the male:female ratio exceeds two, and there is no second peak of incidence in the age group of 55 to 65 years. Clinically, Crohn's disease with only multiple small aphthous ulcerations, which is the earliest stage of disease that is diagnosable, was found in 5% of patients.

Crohn's disease exhibits a bimodal age distribution, with a peak onset between 15 and 30 years and a second smaller peak between 55 and 80 years. Women are, in general, at a 20% to 30% greater risk than men of developing Crohn's disease. Ethnicity has long been described to play a role, with a remarkable predominance of Jewish patients in the North American and South African series. The incidence rates of Crohn's disease in Israel is higher among those born in Europe or America than in those born in Israel. In England, Hindus and Sikhs have a lower incidence of Crohn's disease than the general population. American black and Indian populations are at a low risk of inflammatory bowel disease.

ETIOLOGY AND PATHOGENESIS

The true etiology of Crohn's disease is yet to be determined. Sartor (25) reviewed the three most recent theories for the etiology of Crohn's disease as (i) a specific infectious agent; (ii) a defective mucosal barrier resulting in increased exposure to antigens; and (iii) an abnormal host response to ubiquitous agents, such as luminal constituents or dietary antigens. Much of the following information has been gleaned from that review.

The infectious agents currently postulated as etiologic bases in Crohn's disease are *Mycobacterium paratuberculosis*, the paramyxovirus or measles virus, and most recently under investigation, *Listeria monocytogenes*. The rationale underlying the theory that *M. paratuberculosis* may be a causative agent in Crohn's disease is based on its remarkable resemblance to ileocecal tuberculosis caused by *M. tuberculosis*. *M. tuberculosis* has been detected in up to 65% of patients with Crohn's disease based on results of biopsies of resected tissue with the highly sensitive polymerase chain reaction (PCR) test and has not yet been cultured in any patient without Crohn's disease. A general lack of epidemiologic evidence linking *M. paratuberculosis* to Crohn's disease is the first of several reasons why this etiologic theory creates controversy. According to Sartor (25), no increased incidence of Crohn's disease among farmers and their families, or among veterinarians, has been found. Furthermore, Crohn's disease does not respond to antimycobacterial agents; however, it does respond to steroids, which would presumably activate a mycobacterial infection.

A number of recent papers have rekindled the debate of a specific association between *Mycobacterium avium paratuberculosis* (MAP) and Crohn's disease. The strength of association between MAP and Crohn's disease in a study depends on (i) showing MAP in Crohn's disease patients and (ii) showing its absence in persons without Crohn's disease. Naser and colleagues found MAP DNA in 46% of individuals with Crohn's disease but also in 20% of healthy controls (26). Viable MAP was cultured from the blood of 50% of patients with Crohn's disease and none of the individuals without inflammatory bowel disease—data contributing to the evidence that MAP might be a cause of Crohn's disease. Sechi et al. (27) determined what proportion of people in Sardinia, a community where *Mycobacterium avium* subspecies *paratuberculosis* infection is endemic, attending for ileocolonoscopy with or without Crohn's disease was infected with this pathogen. Twenty-five patients (83.3%) with Crohn's disease and three control patients (10.3%) were positive (odds ratio 43.3). *Mycobacterium avium* subspecies *paratuberculosis* grew in cultures from 63.3% of Crohn's patients and from 10.3% of control patients (odds ratio 14.9). *Mycobacterium avium* subspecies *paratuberculosis* was detected in the majority of Sardinian Crohn's disease patients. The finding of the organism colonizing a proportion of people without Crohn's disease is consistent with what occurs in other conditions caused by a primary bacterial pathogen in susceptible hosts.

An argument against a MAP Crohn's disease link has been that the pathogenesis of these conditions is considered to be different. Histologic and immunologic studies of Crohn's disease have resulted in three somewhat different overlapping models of Crohn's disease etiology; (i) a primary dysfunction of intestinal integrity, (ii) an excess immune reactivity in the intestinal tract, or (iii) an immune-deficiency to a component of the intestinal flora (28). This latter immune-deficiency model has gained increasing attention since the discovery of the two first Crohn's disease susceptible genes NOD2/CARD15 (29) mapped to chromosome 16 and OCTN (30). Behr et al. (31) suggested that NOD2 mutations may confer susceptibility to mycobacterial infection when they reported a case where Crohn's disease, MAP-NOD2 mutations were documented together in the same patient.

Conflicting results exist about the presence of MAP-specific IS900 DNA in Crohn's disease tissues. Autschbach et al. (32) examined IS900 in a large number of gut samples from patients with Crohn's disease ($n = 100$) and ulcerative colitis ($n = 100$), and noninflamed control tissues ($n = 100$). IS900 PCR detection rate was significantly higher in Crohn's disease tissues samples (52%) than in ulcerative colitis (2%) or in non-inflammatory bowel disease (5%) specimens. In Crohn's disease patients, IS900 DNA was detected in samples from both diseased small bowel (47%) as well as from the colon (61%). No firm association between MAP-specific IS900 detection rates and clinical phenotypic characteristics in Crohn's disease could be established. However, corticosteroid medication constituted a factor which tended to have a negative influence on IS900 DNA detection rates in Crohn's disease.

In a commentary on the above paper, Sartor (33) summarized the arguments for and against MAP causation of Crohn's disease. Factors in favor of the hypothesis include:

1. Clinical and pathological similarities between Johne's and Crohn's disease;
2. Presence in food chain (milk, meat) and water supplies;
3. Increased detection of MAP in Crohn's disease tissues by culture, polymerase chain reaction (PCR); fluorescent in situ hybridization;
4. Positive blood cultures of MAP in Crohn's disease patients;
5. Increased serological responses to MAP in Crohn's disease patients;
6. Detection of MAP in human breast milk by culture and PCR;
7. Progression of cervical lymphadenopathy to distal ileitis in a patient with MAP infection;
8. Therapeutic responses to combination antituberculosis therapy that include macrolide antibiotics.

Factors that speak against the hypothesis include:

1. Differences in clinical and pathological responses in Johne's and Crohn's disease;
2. Lack of epidemiological support of transmissible infection;
3. No evidence of transmission to humans in contact with animals infected with MAP;
4. Genotypes of Crohn's and bovine MAP isolates not similar;
5. Variability in detection of MAP by PCR (0–100% in Crohn's disease and ulcerative colitis tissues) and serologic testing;
6. No evidence of mycobacterial cell wall by histochemical staining;
7. No worsening of Crohn's disease with immunosuppressive agents or HIV infection;
8. No documented cell-mediated immune responses to MAP in patients with Crohn's disease;
9. No therapeutic response to traditional antimycobacterial antibiotics.

Sartor concludes that to establish a causal relationship between MAP and Crohn's disease, we need to determine if clearance of MAP selectively changes the natural history of disease in an infected subset of patients, perform definitive investigations of cellular immune responses to this organism in Crohn's disease and control patients, determine if NOD2/CARD15 and other microbial signaling pathways influence intracellular MAP infection and clearance, and review results of ongoing large multi-institutional studies to detect MAP in shared coded tissues by various molecular and culture methods. If MAP is responsible for a subset of Crohn's disease, public health measures must be implemented to eliminate the source of infection in our food chain and food processing practices must be modified. In addition, the medical community must develop ways to efficiently and cost effectively screen for MAP infection and develop methods to efficiently clear this organism from infected tissues, possibly through a combination of effective antibiotics and immunostimulants that enhance innate clearance responses.

The theory that Crohn's disease may be the result of a persistent measles infection is based on a number of factors. Analysis of resected tissue by electron microscopy has confirmed the presence of paramyxovirus-like particles in intestinal epithelial cells and endothelial lesions. Furthermore, elevated antimeasles serum antibodies have been found in a high number of patients with Crohn's disease. Wakefield et al. (34) believe that Crohn's disease may be a chronic granulomatous vasculitis in reaction to a persistent infection with measles virus within the vascular epithelium. This granulomatous inflammation, perhaps aggravated by a hypercoagulable state or mechanical stress, results in the clinical features of Crohn's disease. Although controversial, the incidence of Crohn's disease does not appear to be altered by measles vaccination.

Most recently, *L. monocytogenes* has come under investigation as a possible factor in the pathogenesis of Crohn's disease. Immunohistochemical staining of tissue samples and positive serology has been noted. Enteric pathogens may not only play a role in the etiology of Crohn's disease, but may also contribute to the exacerbation or reactivation of both ulcerative colitis and Crohn's disease. Prospective studies have documented that 25% of inflammatory bowel disease recurrences have been stimulated by viral or bacterial respiratory infections.

The second theory in the infectious etiology of Crohn's disease involves a defective mucosal barrier leading to increased exposure to luminal antigens and proinflammatory molecules. There is an abundance of viable bacteria, particularly anaerobes, in the luminal distal ileum and in the colon that can stimulate an inflammatory response. An intrinsically leaky epithelium could result in continuous stimulation of the underlying lamina propria cells that not only initiates but also perpetuates intestinal inflammation.

Confirmed data indicate that enhanced permeability of the mucosa has been found in 10% of asymptomatic relatives of patients with Crohn's disease. Relatives of patients with Crohn's disease also demonstrate increased mucosal permeability when exposed to nonsteroidal anti-inflammatory drugs. Further investigation is needed to determine whether this breach in the mucosal barrier is a primary defect or merely the consequence of on-going inflammation.

It is quite possible that Crohn's disease may be caused by an abnormal host immune response to ubiquitous agents such as luminal bacterial constituents and dietary antigens. Several factors help support this theory. Disease is found in areas of highest bacterial concentrations; inflammation improves when luminal bacteria are decreased by antibiotics, bowel rest, or bypass; serum and secreted antibodies increase in response to ubiquitous bacteria, anaerobes in particular; and luminal bacteria invade mucosal ulcers and translocate to the mesenteric lymph nodes. It is also possible that the high bacterial load facilitates a secondary invasion of fistulas and ulceration by viable bacteria, exacerbating inflammation. Furthermore, the uptake of proinflammatory bacterial constituents into the portal circulation and lymph nodes may perpetuate inflammation and cause systemic manifestations.

Sartor (35) proposes the following sequence of events in the etiology and pathogenesis of Crohn's disease. Nonspecific intestinal inflammation can be induced by a wide variety of enteric infections or ingested toxins. Resultant increased mucosal permeability leads to enhanced uptake of toxic luminal bacterial products, which potentiates local injury. The vast majority of hosts respond to these injurious events by promptly downregulating the inflammatory response and rapidly healing the mucosal damage without residual scarring. The genetically susceptible host, however, who lacks the ability to suppress the inflammatory response efficiently, has inappropriate amplification of the immune cascade. In response to constant exposure to phlogistic luminal constituents, these patients develop an unrestrained inflammatory response, leading to tissue destruction, chronic inflammation, and fibrosis. Thus inflammatory bowel disease is caused by a genetically determined defective downregulation of inflammation driven by ubiquitous antigens. Luminal anaerobic bacterial antigens are the stimuli in Crohn's disease. Spontaneous or therapy-induced remissions can be achieved, but the risk of reactivation of inflammation is high because of the frequent exposure to triggering episodes that can reignite the inflammatory cascade. This theory suggests that the intestine is in a constant state of controlled inflammation, mediated by a balance between aggressive luminal forces and host-protective mechanisms. This delicate balance can be deranged by any number of environmental triggering events and is in disequilibrium in inflammatory bowel disease.

A host of other etiologic or pathogenetic factors play greater or lesser roles in the genesis of Crohn's disease. There is an increased frequency of positive family history of Crohn's disease compared with controls (10–20%) (5). Studies of familial incidence of Crohn's disease among close relatives confirmed an increased risk ranging from 17 to 35 times that of the general population (36). A positive family history is present more often in patients with Crohn's disease than in those with ulcerative colitis, which suggests that genetic factors may be either relatively more important or more penetrant in the pathogenesis of Crohn's disease (37). There is a pronounced concordance in the site of the disease for family members with Crohn's disease, and the familial occurrence in Crohn's disease is less frequent when the disease is located in the colon rather than elsewhere (38). The age-adjusted risk of relatives is highest for siblings and offsprings (8–9%) followed by parents (3–4%), whereas the risk for second-degree relatives seems not to be increased. Probert et al. (11) found that the comparative risk of developing Crohn's disease among first-degree relatives of patients with Crohn's disease was increased by up to 35 times. The higher concordance rates of Crohn's disease in monozygotic twins than in dizygotic twins support the argument that genetic factors are an important component in the development of Crohn's disease. The term "genetic anticipation" is used to describe earlier onset, of disease, increased severity or both in succeeding generations of families affected by a particular disease. Polito et al. (39) studied 27 pairs of two-generation first-degree relatives. The authors found evidence of a lower age at diagnosis and a greater extent of disease in the younger member of two-generation pairs affected by Crohn's disease, as well as the association with paternal transmission, suggesting that genetic anticipation does occur in Crohn's disease.

Three major variants of the CARD15 gene confer susceptibility to Crohn's disease. Annese et al. (40) investigated the possible association of CARD15 variants with specific clinical characteristics including the occurrence of anti-Saccharomyces cerevisiae antibodies (ASCA) and anti-neutrophil cytoplasmic antibodies (ANCA), in a large cohort of inflammatory bowel disease patients and their unaffected relatives. Patients studied included 316 Crohn's disease patients (156 with positive family history), 408 ulcerative colitis patients (206 with positive family history), 588 unaffected relatives, and 205 unrelated healthy controls. Single nucleotide polymorphisms (SNPs) R702W, G908R, and L1007finsC of the CARD15 gene were investigated. Compared to healthy controls, the frequency of all three variants in Crohn's disease was significantly increased: 8.7% versus 4.1% for R702W, 7.3% versus 2.7% for G908R, 9.3% versus 0.7% for L1007finsC. At least one risk allele was found in 38.2%, 13.7%, and 15.1% of Crohn's disease, ulcerative colitis, and healthy controls, respectively. The L1007finsC risk allele was also significantly increased in unaffected relatives of familial (9.5%) and sporadic (9%) Crohn's disease compared to 0.7% for healthy controls. Carriers of two risk alleles in 16 healthy relatives were asymptomatic after five to eight years of follow-up. Crohn's disease carriers of at least one variant were younger, more likely to have ileal localization, stenosing pattern, previous resective surgery, and presence of ASCA. No difference in SNPs frequency between familial and sporadic cases of Crohn's disease was found. In their population, both familial and sporadic Crohn's disease patients carrying at least one major variant of CARD15 had an aggressive clinical course.

Freeman (41) reported the unusual occurrence of very late phenotypical expression of familial ileocolic Crohn's

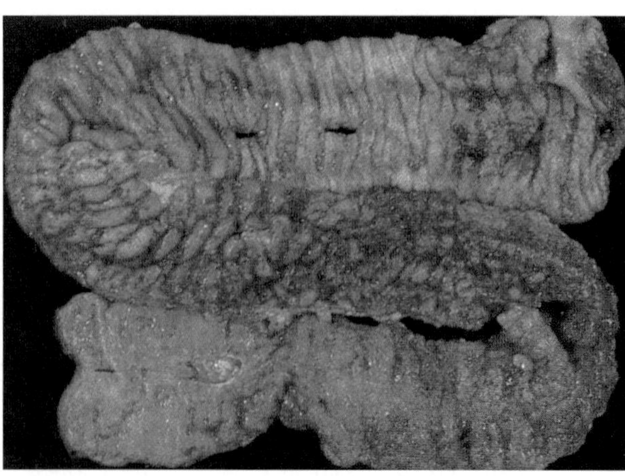

FIGURE 3 ■ Cobblestone appearance of Crohn's colitis.

disease in three elderly sisters. The observations reflect a possible gene-based predisposition to Crohn's disease or alternatively, disease clustering related to a commonly shared environmental factor. He also noted in the literature the initial diagnosis of Crohn's disease reported in a 92-year-old patient.

Freeman (42) evaluated 1000 patients with Crohn's disease for a family history. There were 140 patients who reported a relative with Crohn's disease. Of these, all 87 first-degree relatives were confirmed to have Crohn's disease (37 men and 51 women). Siblings, particularly women, were most commonly affected in comparison with parents or children. There were 65 with a single-affected first-degree relative and 22 with multiple-affected first-degree relatives. In this series, the tendency to have a female sibling with Crohn's disease was further increased in those with multiple-affected first-degree relatives. Although the age of diagnosis of children was less than the age of diagnosis in the respective parents, there were almost identical numbers of mother–child and father–child pairs. Patients with multiple first-degree relatives were older with more extensive disease in both ileal and colonic sites compared with those with only a single first-degree relative and more frequent colonic disease.

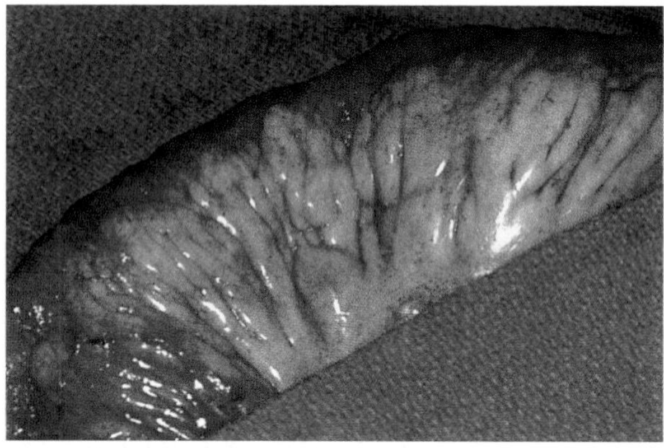

FIGURE 4 ■ Creeping of fat on small bowel wall in Crohn's disease.

Kugathasan et al. (43) investigated the effect of CARD15 mutations on disease manifestation, disease progression, and the risk of early surgery in childhood-onset Crohn's disease. Genotyping for three CARD15 mutations: R702W, G908R, and 3020insC, was performed in 186 children with Crohn's disease from a prospective cohort. The mean age of Crohn's disease was 12.4 years. The frequency of allelic mutations observed was 6.6% for R702W, 6% for G908R, and 13.1% for 3020insC. Of Caucasian Crohn's disease children, 42% had at least one CARD15 mutation. None of the non-Caucasian children with Crohn's disease had any CARD15 mutation. A significant association was detected for 3020insC. Ileal location (odds ratio 4.3) and stricturing disease (odds ratio 6.6) was more frequent and the risk of surgery was higher (hazard ratio = 5.8) and surgery occurred earlier (hazard ratio = 2.2) in those children with 3020insC mutation compared with those without 3020insC. Genetic testing may identify children with Crohn's disease who are at risk of early surgery.

Helio et al. (44) evaluated the allele frequencies of the CARD15 variants R702W, G908R, and 1007fs in Finnish inflammatory bowel disease patients and searched for possible associations between CARD15 variants and occurrence of familial forms of inflammatory bowel disease or complicated forms of Crohn's disease. The frequency of NOD2 gene variants was lower in genetically homogenous Finns than in other populations. The 1007fs variant was associated with Crohn's disease. The occurrence of

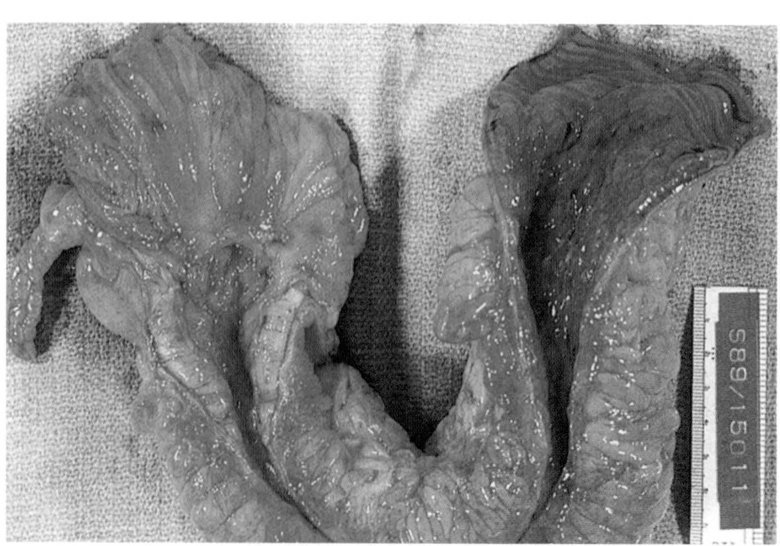

FIGURE 5 ■ Terminal ileum and cecum. Marked thickening of terminal ileum, severely compromised lumen and sharp cutoff of disease of ileocecal valve.

CARD15 variants predicted ileal location as well as stricturing and penetrating forms of Crohn's disease.

A number of other contributing factors have been implicated. Dietary factors have been implicated with a high intake of refined sugar and starch and low intake of fresh fruit associated with Crohn's disease. Conflicting reports have been related to the intake of dietary fiber and no consensus has emerged regarding dietary fat. Dietary studies are made difficult by uncooperative patients, by the fact that the relevant diet may have occurred many years in the past, and because clinical or subclinical disease may alter the diet. Smoking appears to be directly associated with the development of Crohn's disease. The risk factor in the Oxford study was 3.4 (36). Others have found a similar relative risk of 3.0 (45). Smokers have more symptoms and following resection the risks of clinical, endoscopic, and operative recurrence are increased compared with nonsmokers (5).

Several studies have shown a link between taking oral contraceptives and developing Crohn's disease. One study reported relative risk for use for one to three years, and greater than three years at 2.5 and 4.3, respectively (45). It appears that the risk increases after oral contraceptives have been used for five years or longer and it diminishes after discontinuation, disappearing after approximately five years. The mechanism by which oral contraceptives might lead to Crohn's disease is unclear (36). A meta-analysis of 16 studies found the use of oral contraceptives associated with a modest increase in the development of Crohn's disease (relative risk, 1.44). Most studies report a higher incidence of inflammatory bowel disease in higher socioeconomic class. Controversy continues regarding any possible relationship to psychopathology. Despite the tremendous amount of research done on Crohn's disease, at the present time "we know neither its cause nor its cure" (4).

PATHOLOGY

Crohn's disease is a transmural, predominantly submucosal inflammation having a cobblestone appearance on colonoscopy or on inspection of the gross specimen (Fig. 3). In severe and chronic disease the bowel wall becomes thickened and rigid, with creeping of fat on the bowel wall, which may progress until the affected bowel may appear to be encased in mesenteric fat (Figs. 4 and 5). Characteristic "cork-screwing" of vessels on the serosal surface is noted along with obliteration of the gut mesenteric angle and enlargement of mesenteric lymph nodes. Single or multiple strictures may be present in both the colon and small bowel. Inflamed bowel may become adherent to adjacent viscera and form fistulas. Deep linear ulcers are also characteristic of Crohn's disease (Fig. 6), but the earliest recognizable mucosal change is the aphthoid ulcer, which may enlarge into discontinuous serpiginous ulcers (46). The long linear ulcers may subsequently become "railroad track" scars. Inflammatory polyps may occur. Microscopic features include submucosal edema, lymphoid aggregation (Fig. 7), lymphoplasmacytic infiltrate, and ultimately, fibrosis. The histologic hallmark of the disease is sarcoid-type epitheloid granuloma (Fig. 8). In resected specimens, granulomas are present in 50% to 60% of cases and in regional lymph nodes in 20% to 38% of cases. The incidence of granulomas in biopsies varies from 15% to 36% (46).

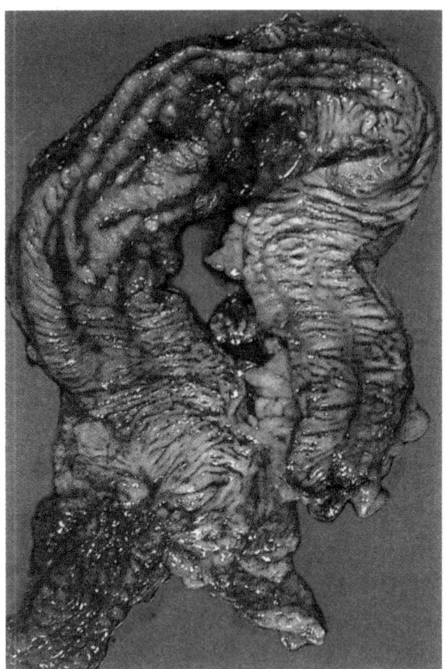

FIGURE 6 ■ Deep linear ulcers of transverse and ascending colon in Crohn's disease.

Epithelioid granuloma is one of the best histological criterion for distinguishing Crohn's disease from other inflammatory bowel diseases. Heresbach et al. (47) evaluated epithelioid granuloma occurrence in incident Crohn's disease cases and examined the associations between epithelioid granulomas and outcome. They reviewed the histological reports of endoscopic and surgical specimens in a cohort of 188 consecutive incident Crohn's disease cases and recorded the occurrence of epithelioid granulomas, isolated giant cells, and microgranulomas. Follow-up was at least five years. Granulomas were found in 37% of patients including 25% at presentation. Median time from Crohn's disease diagnosis to epithelioid granuloma detection was 0.16 months overall and 9.6 months in patients who became epithelioid granuloma positive during follow-up. Isolated giant cells were found in 6% of patients and

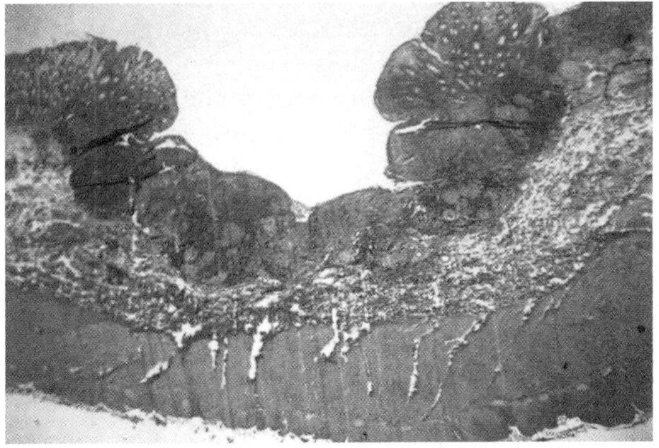

FIGURE 7 ■ Mucosal ulcerations with submucosal edema and lymphoid aggregations.

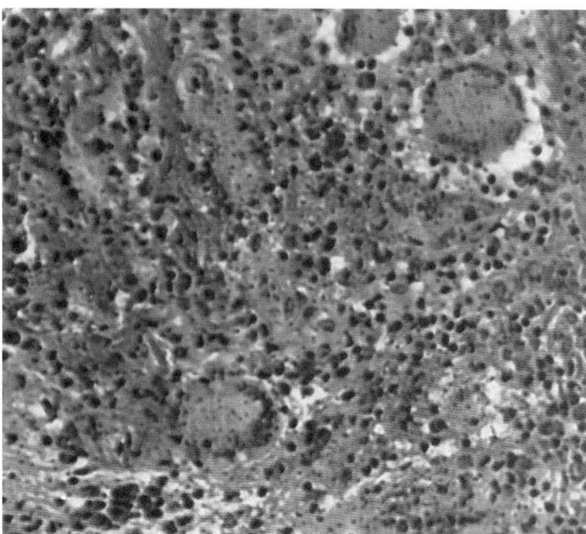

FIGURE 8 ■ Sarcoid-type epitheloid granulomas.

microgranulomas in 12%. Epithelioid granuloma detection increased with the number of endoscopic sampling procedures; sampling site had no influence. Epithelioid granulomas were associated with surgical resection but not immunosuppressive therapy. Thus, epithelioid granulomas may separate Crohn's disease into two pathological subsets and may indicate aggressive disease.

CLINICAL MANIFESTATIONS

Crohn's disease has been described as a panenteric disease. The onset of Crohn's disease is insidious. Symptoms are subtle and manifestations are protean, depending on which part of the bowel is involved. Abdominal pain is a typical symptom of ileocolitis, whereas diarrhea and bleeding per rectum are the signs and symptoms of Crohn's colitis. Weight loss associated with anemia and hypoproteinemia is common in active Crohn's disease. The characteristic triad of symptoms is abdominal pain, diarrhea, and weight loss. Other symptoms include anorexia, fever, and recurrent oral aphthous ulcerations. Signs of pallor, cachexia, clubbing, an abdominal mass or tenderness, or evidence of obstruction should be sought (20). A history of perianal disease, extraintestinal manifestations, evidence of retarded growth, or failure of the development of secondary sex characteristics in children raises suspicion. Occasionally there may be a fulminant onset.

Factors recognized to exacerbate Crohn's disease include intercurrent infections (upper respiratory and enteric), cigarette smoking, and nonsteroidal anti-inflammatory drugs (NSAIDs) (20). Stress and psychologic predisposition are unproven factors. Narcotic analgesia should be avoided outside the perioperative setting because of the potential for tolerance and abuse in the setting of chronic disease (48). Patients with familial Crohn's disease are characterized by an early age of onset and more extensive disease (49).

The distribution of Crohn's disease in the gastrointestinal tract has varied from report-to-report and is summarized in Table 2. Of those with a large bowel pattern, two-thirds have total involvement. Only half of the patients with Crohn's colitis have rectal involvement.

TABLE 2 ■ Anatomic Distribution of Crohn's Disease

		Area of Involvement			
Author(s)	No. of Patients	Small Bowel (%)	Ileocolic (%)	Colon (%)	Perianal (%)
Farmer et al. (50)	615	27	41	29	3
Greenstein (51)	1124	39	45	16	
Ritchie (52)	332	23	33	44	
Anseline (15)	130	35	32	28	5
Platell et al. (53)	306	21	32	42	5

One of the uncommon but potentially dramatic complications is the psoas abscess. Fever, abdominal tenderness, limb pain, and hip contracture are typical signs but are only present in half of the cases (54). The diagnosis is made by computed tomography (CT) scan. Initial therapy consists of CT-guided percutaneous drainage under cover of broad-spectrum antibiotics. This should be followed by resection of the affected bowel.

Deveaux et al. (55) compared multiple variables among black patients with Crohn's disease requiring operation to those of white patients in 345 patients requiring operation for Crohn's disease. The mean age at diagnosis was 28 years for white males, 20 years for black males, and 30 years for white females, 28 years for black females. Thirty-seven percent of white females presented with obstructive symptoms versus 12% of black females. Sixty-five percent of black females presented with inflammatory symptoms compared with 28% of white females. Of females presenting with fistulas, 15% of black patients had a rectovaginal fistula compared with 5% of white patients. Seventeen percent of black males and 21% of white males had intra-abdominal fistulas. None of these differences were statistically significant. The incidence of fistulas at presentation, mean number of fistulas, total numbers of operations, and family history of inflammatory bowel disease did not differ. Crohn's disease does not seem to be more severe among black patients who had an early diagnosis.

In patients with rapidly deteriorating inflammatory bowel disease, cytomegalovirus (CMV) infection should be kept in mind as one of the differential diagnoses (56). We have also witnessed this clinical situation in which multiple spontaneous colonic perforations have developed.

DIAGNOSIS

The diagnosis of Crohn's disease is confirmed by a variety or combination of endoscopic, radiographic, or pathologic studies that document the typical focal, asymmetric, transmural, and occasional granulomatous features (20). A high index of suspicion is required for patients with chronic diarrhea. Stools should be examined for the presence of enteric pathogens, ova, and parasites, and *Clostridium difficile* toxin (20).

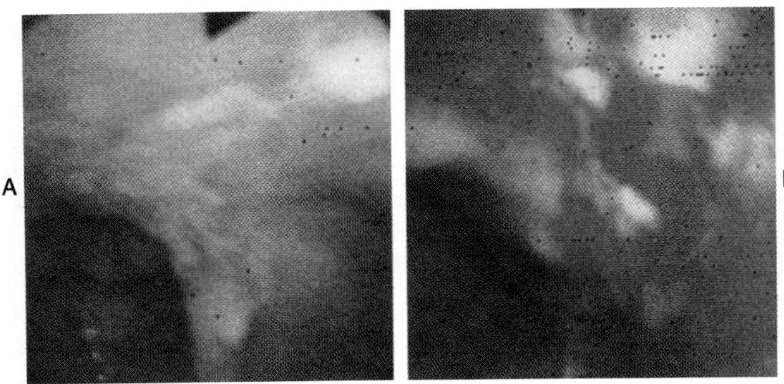

FIGURE 9 ■ (**A**) Mild Crohn's disease. (**B**) Severe Crohn's disease.

■ ENDOSCOPY

Since only half of the patients with Crohn's colitis have rectal involvement, proctosigmoidoscopy does not constitute adequate examination. Colonoscopy is the most sensitive tool for diagnosis of Crohn's colitis, particularly in mild and early disease, which is not seen on barium enema studies. Typically, the disease is patchy in distribution. Edema of the mucosa and aphthous ulcers is features of early Crohn's disease. Deep linear ulcers and fibrotic strictures are also typical. However, some patients have granular and friable mucosa with continuous and homogeneous involvement of the entire colon and rectum (Fig. 9). In such a situation it is impossible to differentiate Crohn's disease from ulcerative colitis. Biopsies of the mucosa are rarely definitive unless a sarcoid-type giant cell granuloma is seen.

Although radiographic contrast studies are superior to endoscopy for diagnosing fistulas, endoscopic procedures have a definite role in the evaluation and management of fistulizing Crohn's disease (57). Endoscopy allows for tissue sampling, and provides information regarding the extent and severity of gastrointestinal inflammation, and the presence of such complications as strictures and carcinoma. Preoperative colonoscopy has particular value in assessing an enterocolonic fistula, and has important implications regarding the type of operation performed.

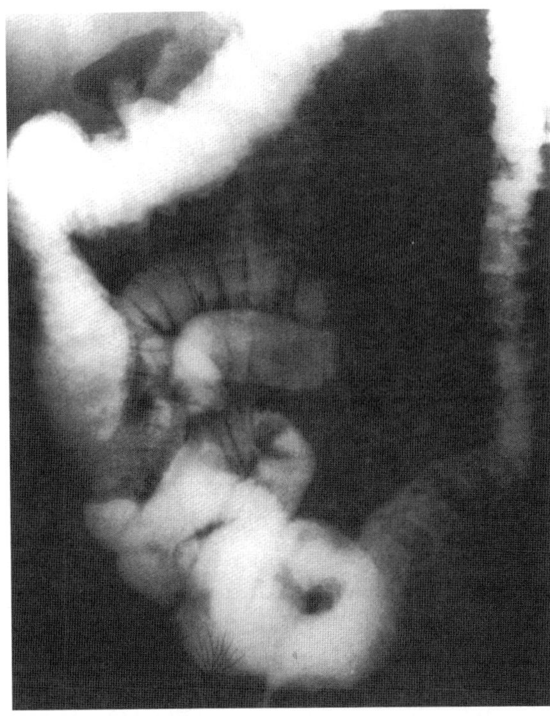

FIGURE 10 ■ Barium enema study in Crohn's colitis shows irregular nodular defects of the left colon and transverse colon.

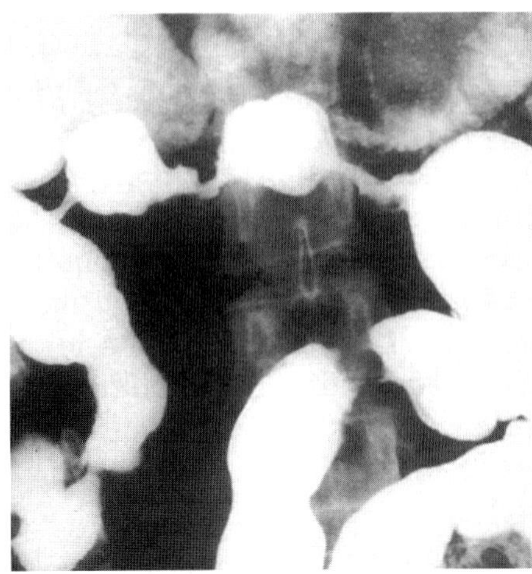

FIGURE 11 ■ Upper gastrointestinal and small bowel follow-through demonstrating multiple strictures of the small bowel.

■ CONTRAST STUDIES

It is important that not only the diagnosis but also the extent of Crohn's disease be established. Upper intestinal and small bowel follow-through barium studies should always be performed. One of the striking radiologic features of Crohn's disease of the colon is frequency of concomitant involvement of the small bowel. The characteristic radiographic features of Crohn's colitis are skip lesions, contour defects, longitudinal and transverse ulcers, cobblestone-like mucosal pattern, narrowing or stricture, thickening of the haustral margin, irregular nodular defects, and involvement of the terminal ileum as seen on barium enema studies (Fig. 10). Small bowel enteroclysis is a more sensitive means of evaluating jejunal and ileal findings. Examples of radiologic findings are seen in Figures 11 and 12.

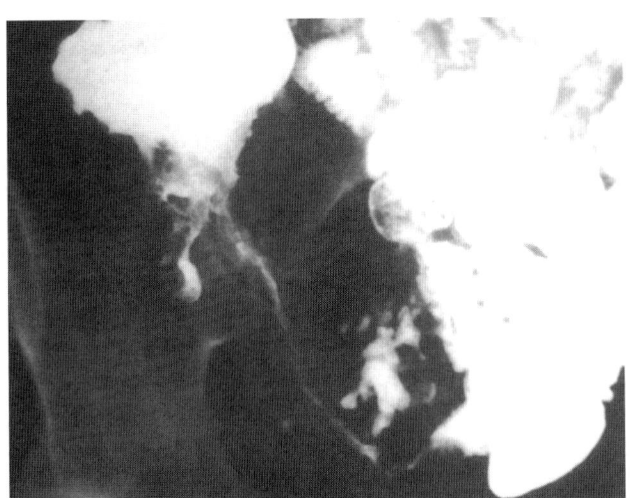

FIGURE 12 ■ Upper gastrointestinal and small bowel follow-through demonstrating 12 cm stenotic distorted segment of terminal ileum contracted cecum.

Otterson et al. (58) conducted a study to determine the accuracy of barium radiography compared with intraoperative evaluation with passage of a balloon catheter for assessment of stricturing Crohn's disease. In 118 patients, 230 strictures were identified by barium examination; 365 strictures were identified using the balloon catheter technique. Barium examination overestimated or underestimated the number of strictures in 36% of patients. Overall, barium radiography was least accurate in patients with strictures amenable to strictureplasty. Failure to be able to wean from steroids may suggest a missed stricture. Their data suggests that careful exploration and intraoperative, intraluminal testing of intestinal patency identify additional strictures compared with barium radiographs in a significant number of patients with Crohn's disease.

■ NUCLEAR SCANS

A report on the use of indium-111-labeled granulocyte scan has shown that this nuclear medicine technique is extremely accurate in delineating the anatomic extent of disease both in the large and the small intestine. This test is well tolerated by patients and requires no bowel preparation. It is dependent on the normal function of the patient's granulocytes for its imaging and can be used to differentiate patients with diarrhea caused by obstructive symptoms from those with symptoms arising from acute inflammation. The latter group are best treated medically, whereas those patients having scirrhous obstruction without inflammation can be treated only by operation (59).

Li et al. (60) analyzed the ability of 99mTc-HMPAO leukocyte scintigraphy to distinguish Crohn's disease from ulcerative colitis. The diagnostic criteria were established by reviewing 99mTc-HMPAO leukocyte scintigrams in 123 patients with histologically proven Crohn's disease (83) or ulcerative colitis (40). Uptake in the right iliac fossa, with or without other segments of colon, irregular bowel uptake, small bowel uptake, or colonic activity with rectal sparing was all strongly suggestive of Crohn's disease. Left-sided colitis was found to indicate ulcerative colitis. Total colitis occurred in both ulcerative colitis and Crohn's disease. The criteria were later tested in an additional 62 patients with excellent results (accuracy, 98%). In 63 patients in whom the results of barium radiology were also available, the accuracy of scintigraphy was higher (93% and 83%, respectively).

■ ASCA TEST

Kaila et al. (61) determined the utility of the anti-saccharomyces cerevisiae antibodies (ASCA) test [enzyme-linked immunosorbent assay (ELISA) test] in their investigation of patients with gastrointestinal symptoms. The study population included Crohn's disease ($n = 114$), ulcerative colitis ($n = 74$), indeterminate colitis ($n = 31$), celiac disease ($n = 9$), irritable bowel syndrome ($n = 75$), other diagnoses ($n = 33$), and no disease ($n = 45$). ASCA had a sensitivity of 37% and specificity of 97% for diagnosing Crohn's disease and an odds ratio for a diagnosis of Crohn's disease of 18.4. The 47 ASCA-positive patients included the following diagnoses: Crohn's disease = 39, ulcerative colitis = 3, indeterminate colitis = 1, celiac disease = 3, and no disease = 1. The likelihood of having an inflammatory disease if ASCA is positive was nearly 40-fold. A positive ASCA test using this assay nearly clinches a diagnosis of some form of inflammatory intestinal disease, which is highly likely to be Crohn's disease. Klebl et al. (62) also reported that the combined detection of ASCA immunoglobulin IgA and ASCA IgG by indirect immunofluorescence as well as ELISA may optimize the discrimination of Crohn's disease from ulcerative colitis.

■ ULTRASONOGRAPHY

The spectrum of enteric and perienteric changes associated with Crohn's disease can be evaluated with ultrasonography (63). Classic features include gut wall thickening, stricture, creeping fat, hyperemia, mesenteric nodes, and mucosal abnormalities. Complications include inflammatory masses, fistula, obstruction, perforation, and appendicitis. Although barium enema examination and endoscopy remain the major investigative tools for evaluation of mucosal disease, ultrasonography is excellent for evaluation of both mural and extraintestinal disease (63). Its advantages include lack of radiation, which makes it a valuable tool for initial evaluation of patients with abdominal pain or an abdominal mass. This is especially true if perforation or obstruction is suspected or if the patient is pregnant or refuses other means of investigation. In many cases, ultrasonography can effectively replace modalities that use ionizing radiation for the diagnosis and serial evaluation of extraluminal complications. In addition, ultrasonography can be used to assess the response to treatment and to detect postoperative recurrence. Ultrasonography allows accurate identification of patients in whom the possibility of operation or percutaneous intervention would justify other means of investigation, particularly CT. During the ultrasound examination, unsuspected extraintestinal complications, such as gallstones, renal calculi, hydronephrosis, fatty liver, and sclerosing cholangitis, can be detected. Diseases other than Crohn's disease that might be responsible for the patient's symptoms, such as a ruptured ovarian cyst or appendicitis, can also be diagnosed with ultrasonography.

Parente et al. (64) prospectively investigated the accuracy of ultrasound compared with X-ray procedures and intraoperative findings in detecting small bowel strictures complicating Crohn's disease as well as its reliability in assessing disease extent and location within the bowel in a series of 296 consecutive patients with proven Crohn's disease. Overall, sensitivity and specificity of ultrasound in assessing the anatomical distribution of Crohn's disease were 93% and 97%, respectively. The extent of ileal disease measured at ultrasound correlated well with that determined by X-ray ($r = 0.52$) in medically treated patients as well as with that measured intraoperatively in surgical patients ($r = 0.64$). One or more stenoses were detected in 35.5% of patients at small bowel enteroclysis in the non-operative Crohn's disease group compared with 82% in the operative Crohn's disease series. Sensitivity, specificity, and positive predictive values of bowel ultrasound in the detection of strictures were 79%, 98%, and 95% in nonoperative Crohn's disease patients and 90%, 100%, and 100% in operative Crohn's disease cases, respectively.

■ COMPUTED TOMOGRAPHY

CT has been described as the premier imaging procedure for evaluating the mural and extraintestinal manifestations of inflammatory bowel disease (65). It plays a critical role in detecting abscesses, in differentiating various causes of mesenteric abnormalities, and in discovering extraintestinal complications.

Schratter-Sehn et al. (65) compared transrectal or transvaginal endoscopic ultrasonography with CT in the diagnosis of perirectal fistulas, abscesses, and diffuse inflammatory changes in the lower pelvis in 25 patients with Crohn's disease. Results were verified by operation in eight patients and by correlation with findings on endoscopy, barium radiography, and fistulography, and the clinical course in all other patients. Endoscopic ultrasonography was superior to CT in diagnosing fistulas (14 vs. 4 correct diagnoses) and inflammatory infiltration of the lower pelvic muscles (11 vs. 2 correct diagnoses). The methods were equivalent in diagnosing anorectal abscesses. CT was superior in the detection of inflammatory changes in the pararectal fasciae and fatty tissue, which could not be detected by endoscopic ultrasonography.

Hassan et al. (66) compared the accuracy of CT enteroclysis to that of endoscopy in detecting bowel wall alteration of the terminal or neoterminal ileum in 39 patients with Crohn's disease. Diagnoses used ileocolonoscopy with histology; clinical activity was measured by Crohn's Disease Activity Index (CDAI). Contrast-enhanced spiral CT of the abdomen was performed after distention of the small bowel with an enema of methylcellulose. Retrograde ileocolonoscopy diagnosed 30 patients with Crohn's disease of the ileum, while nine patients served as controls. CT enteroclysis detected Crohn's disease in 86.7% and in none of the control group. Three of four patients with false-negative findings on CT enteroclysis had postsurgical Crohn's disease recurrence. The overall sensitivity and specificity of CT enteroclysis for ileal Crohn's disease detection were 86.7% and 100% (PPV = 100%; NPV = 69.2%) and 94.1% and 100% (PPV = 100%; NPV = 90%), respectively.

■ MAGNETIC RESONANCE IMAGING

Haggett et al. (67) evaluated the role of magnetic resonance imaging (MRI) in the demonstration of the pelvic and perianal complications of Crohn's disease. Twenty-five patients with active Crohn's disease were studied. The MRI results were correlated with operative and clinical findings. In 16 patients, cutaneous, deep perineal, or enterovesical fistulas or abscesses were diagnosed at MRI, which showed close correlation with findings at examination under anesthesia. In eight patients no fistulas or abscesses were seen at MRI nor was there any evidence of complications on clinical examination and flexible sigmoidoscopy. There was one false negative examination in a patient who had a colovesical fistula.

Horsthuis et al. (68) recently reviewed the potential of MRI to evaluate disease activity in Crohn's disease. MRI has intrinsic advantage over other techniques, including noninvasiveness and the absence of ionizing radiation. For perianal fistulizing disease MRI has become a mainstay in evaluation of disease, as localization and extent of disease can be very well appreciated using both T2-weighted and T1-weighted sequences, fat suppression, and intravenous contrast medium. Imaging of the small bowel and colon in Crohn's disease is more complicated due to bowel peristalsis and respiratory movement. However, using fast breath-hold sequences and intravenous spasmolytic medication, images of good diagnostic quality can be acquired. To obtain sufficiently distended bowel, MR enteroclysis can be performed. Abdominal MRI is a valuable imaging technique for evaluation of luminal, transmural, and extraintestinal manifestations of Crohn's disease as degree of disease activity, presence of luminal pathology (e.g., stenosis) and extraintestinal manifestations of disease (e.g., abscesses, fistulas) can be accurately assessed.

Koh et al. (69) evaluated the sensitivity and specificity of MRI in assessing the activity of Crohn's disease in 30 symptomatic patients. Twenty-three patients had active disease and seven patients had inactive disease. One hundred and twenty-four of a total of 168 bowel segments were examined with both MRI and endoscopy or surgery. On a per patient basis, MRI had an overall sensitivity of 91% and a specificity of 71% for active disease. The Crohn's disease activity index had a sensitivity of 92% and a specificity of 28%. On a per segment basis, MRI had a sensitivity of 59% and a specificity of 93%. Bowel wall thickening of greater than 4 mm, bowel wall enhancement, and increased mesenteric vascularity were useful in identifying active disease.

■ CAPSULE ENDOSCOPY

In their review of the literature, Legnani and Kornbluth (70) noted a number of recently published studies report diagnostic yields for Crohn's disease from capsule endoscopy of over 70% in patients with negative or inconclusive findings on prior small bowel series and ileocolonoscopy. Capsule endoscopy is a more sensitive examination than traditional radiography. Most series report a positive influence on patient outcome based on capsule findings. "Mucosal breaks" are seen in 14% of normal volunteers, even in the absence of recent NSAIDs. Capsule retention occurs in less than 1% of patients with suspected Crohn's disease, but retention rates of 4% to 6% are reported in patients with established Crohn's disease.

Dubcenco et al. (71) studied the accuracy of capsule endoscopy in the evaluation of small bowel Crohn's disease. Capsule endoscopy yielded a sensitivity and a specificity of 89.6% and 100%, respectively, and a positive predictive value and a negative predictive value of 100% and 76.9%, respectively, whereas small bowel series were 27.6%/100% and 100%/32%.

■ VIRTUAL COLONOSCOPY

Biancone et al. (72) compared findings from virtual colonoscopy versus conventional colonoscopy for assessing the postoperative recurrence of Crohn's disease. Conventional colonoscopy showed perianastomotic recurrence in 15 of 16 patients. Perianastomotic narrowing or stenosis was detected by virtual colonoscopy in 11 of these 15 patients. There were 11 true-positive, one true-negative, and zero false-positive and four false-negative findings (73% sensitivity, 100% specificity, 100% positive predictive value, 20% negative predictive value, 75% accuracy). Among the eight patients showing a rigid stenosis of the anastomosis not allowing passage of the colonoscope, virtual colonoscopy detected narrowing or stenosis in seven patients. The current findings suggest that although the widespread use of virtual colonoscopy in Crohn's disease is currently not indicated because of possible false-negative findings, this technique may represent an alterative to conventional colonoscopy in noncompliant postsurgical patients with a rigid stenosis not allowing passage of the endoscope.

■ NEW DIAGNOSTIC CRITERIA

New diagnostic criteria for Crohn's disease were established by the Research Committee of Inflammatory Bowel Disease, set up by the Japanese Ministry of Health and Welfare. For a definitive diagnosis, one of the following three conditions is required: (i) longitudinal ulcer or luminal deformity induced by longitudinal ulcer or cobblestone pattern, (ii) intestinal small aphthous ulcerations arranged in a longitudinal fashion for at least three months plus noncaseating granulomas, and (iii) multiple small aphthous ulcerations in both the upper and lower digestive tract not necessarily with longitudinal arrangement, for at least three months, plus noncaseating granulomas. Moreover, ulcerative colitis, ischemic enterocolitis, and acute infectious enterocolitis should be excluded (22).

■ DIFFERENTIAL DIAGNOSIS

Depending upon the mode of presentation, a number of entities may be included in the differential diagnosis. In the acute phase, acute appendicitis or processes, such as infection caused by *Yersinia, Campylobacter, Shigella,* and *Salmonella,* might be considered. Tuberculosis might also be considered. In a more insidious onset, lymphoma and chronic mesenteric ischemia can produce a similar picture.

One particular infection, *Escherichia coli* 0157:H7, may closely mimic right-sided colonic Crohn's disease (73). CT scans show cecal thickening and mass effects with multiple mesenteric lymph nodes and sparing of the rest of the colon. Colonoscopy reveals a mucosal pattern consistent with Crohn's disease. Therefore, patients presenting with acute bleeding, diarrhea, and displaying CT features of right-sided Crohn's disease might best have *E. coli* 0157:H7 infection excluded before therapy for Crohn's disease is initiated.

NATURAL HISTORY

The natural history of Crohn's disease in any individual patient is not entirely predictable. Generally, the course of the disease is one of remission and exacerbation, but, nevertheless, tends to be slowly progressive and frequently leads to the eventual development of complications that require operation. Unlike ulcerative colitis, Crohn's disease can involve both the small and large bowel with characteristic segmental involvement. If the pattern were known, treating physicians might be able to intercept the development of many of the well-recognized complications. However, numerous investigators have provided us with relevant information regarding progression, treatment, long-term outcome, and quality of life.

Freeman (74) reviewed data on the natural history of long-standing Crohn's disease from a clinical database of over 1000 patients and found eight patients (5 women, 3 men) who had disease documented for over 50 years. In spite of complex histories with either stricturing or penetrating complications, all currently have either no symptoms or minimal disease activity, often without the need for ongoing pharmacologic treatment. Most significantly, their clinical courses were all characterized by prolonged asymptomatic periods, often for more than a decade, before the recurrence of symptomatic disease. Pathological findings in all patients revealed granulomatous inflammatory disease, often recurring intermittently over many decades. Moreover, the location of the findings implied that the disease has a tendency to evolve, not only in a temporal dimension, but also extending geographically within the gastrointestinal tract. These clinical and pathological features in long-standing Crohn's disease suggest that recurring or multiple discrete initiating events, rather than a single initiating event, could be involved in the etiology and pathogenesis of Crohn's disease.

Crohn's disease tends to run a clinical course with seasonal exacerbations. The highest relapse rates are found in the autumn and winter, whereas the lowest are in the summer (75). This observation suggests that exogenous factors may be involved in the relapse of Crohn's disease.

Sachar (76) reported 70% of patients with Crohn's disease undergo at least one operation. This group is almost evenly divided between those with fibro-stenotic obstruction and those with other complications—ulceration, fistulization, or abscess. Unfortunately, operation only resets the clock. The recurrence rate is 8% to 10% per year.

Of patients with Crohn's disease who have not previously undergone operative treatment and who are in symptomatic remission, 25% to 50% experience symptomatic recurrence after one year and 40% to 65% have recurrence by two years (77). Of patients who have undergone resection, 30% to 50% have symptomatic recurrence during the first five postoperative years and 50% to 80% have symptomatic recurrence by 10 years postoperative (77).

Makowiec et al. (78) evaluated the disease progress and the long-term outcome in 323 patients with Crohn's colitis followed up for a mean of 9.8 years. The probabilities of having pancolitis or rectal disease were 77.1% and 78.8% after 15 years, respectively, and higher in patients with initially left-sided or segmental colitis compared with right-sided colitis. The chance of having perianal fistulas was 43.3% after 15 years. The risk of undergoing colonic resection was 62.2% after 15 years and higher in the presence of right-sided colitis. The cumulative risk of colectomy was 18.2% after 15 years and higher in patients with pancolitis, left-sided colitis, or in the presence of perianal fistulas. The 15-year probabilities of having a proctectomy

(12%) and having a temporary stoma (21%) were only influenced by the presence of perianal fistulas but not by rectal disease or pattern of colitis. Most patients with colonic Crohn's disease will eventually have pancolitis but only 20% of them will lose the colon. The proctectomy rate is low despite a high frequency of rectal disease. Perianal fistulas and the presence of total or left-sided colonic involvement are adverse risk factors with regard to preservation of colonic length.

Agrez et al. (79) studied the natural history of Crohn's disease in a well-defined population. They identified 42 of 103 residents of Olmsted County, Minnesota, U.S.A., as having Crohn's disease who had undergone one or more operative procedures. Follow-up extended to 32 years, with a median of 8.5 years. Thirty-six patients underwent at least one definitive resection; eight of these patients subsequently underwent a second definitive operation. The likelihood that any patient would undergo operation was greatest within the first year of diagnosis. The percentages of patients in whom recurrent disease developed after the first and second definitive resections were 50% and 37%, respectively. Approximately half the patients who experienced a recurrence underwent further operation. The site of diseased bowel and sex were not factors specifically influencing recurrence rates. Patients 40 years of age and older who underwent operation appeared to fare better with respect to recurrent disease than younger patients. Although the authors' findings suggest cumulative risks of recurrent disease after definitive resection similar to those reported from larger population groups or major referral centers, the proportion of patients who underwent operation during the natural history of their Crohn's disease was much less than generally reported. The authors concluded that operation for Crohn's disease is not inevitable and that evidence to the contrary may imply both a treatment and a referral bias.

Munkholm et al. (80) followed up a cohort of 373 patients with Crohn's disease to estimate the probability for remission and relapse with time and working capacity. The clinical course of Crohn's disease differs markedly over time, from ever-relapsing cases to a quiescent course with remission for several years, interrupted by years with relapse. No predictive factors have been found for the subsequent course with regard to age, sex, extent of disease at diagnosis, and treatment in the year of diagnosis. The relapse rate within the year of diagnosis and the following two years, however, does correlate positively with the relapse rate in the following five years. Furthermore, the relapse rate for one year during the disease course influences the relapse rate the following year, indicating a disease pattern over time with waves of at least two years' duration. A slight tendency toward burning out was found. The disease course, reflected in working capacity for patients, showed that a minor portion—up to 15% after 15 years—become incapable and obtain a disability pension, while 75% of patients each year are fully capable of work. Within 10 years 50% of the patients will not have experienced any year with impaired capacity for work.

Loftus et al. (24) quantified through systemic review, the epidemiology and natural history of Crohn's disease in North America. The prevalence of Crohn's disease in North America ranges from 26.0 to 198.5 cases per 100,000 persons. The incidence rates range from 3.1 to 14.6 cases per 100,000 person-years. Most patients have a chronic intermittent disease course, while 13% have an unremitting disease course and 10% have a prolonged remission. Less than half require corticosteroids at any point. During any given year, approximately 10% are treated with corticosteroids and 30% are treated with 5-aminosalicylates. Up to 57% of patients require at least one operative resection.

Mendelsohn et al. (81) traced 1000 patients hospitalized with Crohn's disease to identify those who died, the events preceding death, and their relationship to Crohn's disease. The authors considered any management early in the disease that might have influenced outcome. They introduced the term "virulent" Crohn's disease to describe those patients with most or all of the following criteria: young age at onset, multiple operative procedures, short bowel/malabsorption, chronic steroid therapy, narcotic addiction, and sepsis. Twenty-five patients (2.6%) had died. Major events preceding 18 deaths related to Crohn's disease were virulent Crohn's disease (six), gastrointestinal neoplasms (six), complications in the elderly (five), and complications of drug therapy (one). Seven deaths probably unrelated to Crohn's disease were attributed to extraintestinal neoplasms (four) and myocardial infarction (three). Death was related to Crohn's disease or its treatment in 72% and perhaps in all. Ten of the 25 died at age 46 or younger (mean, 36 years; range, 25–46 years). Twenty-two (88%) who died had undergone operation for Crohn's disease (mean, 3.3 procedures), including eight who died postoperatively (six elderly), attributable to sepsis in seven and pulmonary embolism in one. The events preceding death suggest that early aggressive nonoperative therapy for severe Crohn's disease warrants a careful controlled evaluation.

Cottone et al. (82) reviewed a series of 531 patients with Crohn's disease and found that there was an excess of deaths from neoplasms of the digestive organs (1 observed, 0.37 expected). The mortality from Crohn's disease was not increased.

Goldberg et al. (83) reviewed 152 of 399 Crohn's patients (38%) diagnosed over 20 years, who lived within a geographically defined area at the time of diagnosis and who had undergone at least one operation. One hundred seventy-one resections were performed in 160 operations during a mean follow-up of 60 months. Forty-eight percent of patients had undergone their first resection within 10 years of diagnosis, and 39% of those had undergone a second resection within 10 years of the first.

The typical site of recurrent disease following restorative resection is the neoterminal ileum. Following total proctocolectomy (TPC) and ileostomy, recurrent disease develops in the prestomal ileum. Approximately 30% to 40% of patients having restorative operation develop a symptomatic recurrence within five years, 50% to 60% by 10 years, and 70% to 75% within 15 years (84). Only 15% to 20% of patients requiring total proctocolectomy and ileostomy can be expected to develop recurrence over the course of 15 to 20 years.

Polito et al. (85) examined the influence of age at diagnosis of Crohn's disease on disease site, type, and course. Younger age at diagnosis (less than 20 years) compared with an older age (greater than or equal to 40 years) was associated with a greater prevalence of family history of Crohn's disease (29.9% vs. 13.6%), greater small bowel involvement (88.7% vs. 57.5%), more stricturing disease (45.8% vs. 28.8%), and a higher frequency of operation (70.6% vs. 55.3%). Older age at diagnosis was associated with a greater prevalence of colonic disease (84.8% vs. 71.2%) and the inflammatory subtype (54.5% vs. 34.4%).

In a long-term follow-up study (4.4 ± 3.2 years, mean ± SD) of 203 patients with Crohn's disease in Japan, Iida et al. (86) evaluated the prognoses relative to life span and operation. Cumulative survival rates 5 and 10 years after diagnosis were 98.9% and 98.9%, respectively. These figures were not different from the expected survival rates in the sex- and age-matched general population. Cumulative operation rates 5 and 10 years after the onset of symptoms were 16.2% and 39.1%, respectively. In a second study, the authors investigated 419 patients with Crohn's disease diagnosed at nine institutions. The follow-up period was 6.3 ± 3.9 years. Cumulative survival rates 5 and 10 years after diagnosis were 99.2% and 96.9%, respectively. Cumulative operation rates 5 and 10 years after the onset of symptoms were 30.3% and 70.8%, respectively. These results indicate that the prognosis of Japanese patients with Crohn's disease may be superior to those in Western countries.

Specific segments of the population have been studied. Sedgwick et al. (87) studied the natural history of a cohort of 68 children with Crohn's disease. Fifty-four of the 68 patients were treated surgically, with a total of 135 operations. Fifty percent of the cohort had a major operation within five years of onset of symptoms, and median time to a second operation was four years. The types of major operation performed in juvenile onset patients differed significantly from those recorded in adults, with a higher rate of exploratory laparotomy in younger patients. With a mean follow-up of seven years, 18% had a permanent stoma. There were five deaths, of which three were postoperative. This study highlights the frequency of surgical intervention in young people with Crohn's disease.

Nwokolo et al. (88) reviewed the influence of pregnancy on the natural history of Crohn's disease. The authors found patients with distal ileal and colonic Crohn's disease who had been pregnant in the past subsequently needed fewer resections. Pregnancy could influence the natural history of Crohn's disease, either by decreasing immune responsiveness or by retarding fibrous stricture formation, which is the most common indication for operative intervention.

Roberts et al. (89) reviewed the clinical course of Crohn's disease in older patients. The records of 50 patients whose initial diagnosis of Crohn's disease was made after the age of 50 years with a median age of 60 years (range, 50–78 years) followed for a median of 95.5 months (range, 81.1–236.6 months). The most common presenting signs and symptoms were abdominal pain (82%), diarrhea (70%), weight loss (56%), bleeding from the gastrointestinal tract (26%), abdominal mass (16%), and fistula (14%). Initial operations performed were ileocolic resection (38%), proctocolectomy (16%), small bowel resection (10%), colostomy (2%), and a variety of segmental resections' of the colon (34%). The overall recurrence rate of disease in patients, in whom all obvious disease was resected, based on distribution of disease, was 80% (ileocolitis), 38% (ileitis), and 35% (colitis). Crohn's disease more often affects the distal gastrointestinal tract in older age groups. After resection, however, the clinical course is similar to that in the younger population. The high recurrence rate of Crohn's colitis is probably a result of the large number of initial segmental resections.

Lapidus et al. (90) assessed the features and clinical course of 507 patients with colorectal Crohn's disease. Colonic distribution was segmental in 40%, total in 31%, and left-sided in 26%. Perianal/rectal fistulas occurred in 37%. In patients who obtained clinical remission, the five-year cumulative relapse rate after diagnosis was 67%. At the initial presentation of Crohn's disease, the frequency of major surgery decreased from 24% to 14% over time. Still, the overall long-term probability of major surgery after 10 years was unaltered (49% vs. 47%). The presence of fistulas increased the probability of surgical resection (relative risk = 1.7), whereas left-sided disease was associated with a decrease (relative risk = 0.6). Twenty-four percent of patients developed inflammation in the small bowel. The cumulative risk for permanent ileostomy was 25%, 10 years after diagnosis.

To compare the time course of clinical recurrences and reoperations following primary resection for fistulization versus fibrostenotic obstruction and ileal Crohn's disease, Sachar et al. (91) performed a retrospective cohort study of 71 patients undergoing their first resection. Among these 71 patients, 35 were classified as fistulizing and 36 as fibrostenotic. With a mean follow-up of 73 months to reoperation, the fistulizing and fibrostenotic patients experienced virtually identical numbers of clinical recurrences: 25 from the former group and 24 from the latter. The recurrences appeared very slightly earlier among the fistulizing than among the fibrostenotic group, but the difference did not approach statistical significance. Only 18 patients came to reoperation during follow-up: 12 from the fistulizing and 6 from the fibrostenotic group. The earliest reoperation in the fistulizing group occurred at 14 months and in the fibrostenotic group at 44 months. There was a trend for earlier reoperation in the fistulizing group but the difference was not statistically significant.

Schwartz et al. (92) studied the cumulative incidence and natural history of fistulas in Crohn's disease in the community. At least one fistula occurred in 35% of patients, including 20% who developed perianal fistulas. A fistula developed in 46% of patients before or at the time of formal diagnosis. The cumulative risk of any fistula was 33% after 10 years and was 50% after 20 years (perianal, 21% after 10 years and 26% after 20 years). At least one recurrent fistula occurred in 34% of patients. Most fistulizing episodes (83%) required operations. Perianal fistulizing episodes resulted in bowel resection in 23% of patients.

Louis et al. (93) assessed the association between rapid development of a penetrating or stricturing pattern of Crohn's disease and demographic and clinical characteristics as well as NOD2/CARD15 genotype in 163 patients with a firm diagnosis of Crohn's disease and who had nonpenetrating nonstricturing disease at diagnosis. Five years after diagnosis, there were 67.5% of patients with nonstricturing nonpenetrating disease, 11% with stricturing disease, and 21.5% with penetrating disease. Only disease location and number of flares per year were significantly discriminant between the three subgroups. Ileal location of the disease was associated with a stricturing pattern while a high number of flares were associated with a penetrating pattern. Active smoking was also associated with a penetrating pattern compared with a nonstricturing nonpenetrating pattern only. They concluded that early development of stricturing or penetrating behaviour in Crohn's disease is influenced by disease location, clinical activity of the disease, and smoking habit, but not by NOD2/CARD15 genotype.

Freeman (94) assessed mortality, intestinal malignancy, and the need for resection in 224 patients with early onset disease. Mean follow-up was 12.2 years. Most patients were diagnosed from ages 13 to 19 years. Ileocolonic disease was most common (57.1%), while upper intestinal involvement (18.8%) was frequent. Complex disease with strictures (28.6%) or penetrating complications (46.6%) were common. One patient with early onset disease died from a drug overdose and one developed rectal carcinoma. One or more intestinal resections were required in 56.3% of patients. More than one resection was needed in 23.2% of patients. The mean time from diagnosis to first resection was 4.2 years and from first to second resection was 6.6 years with most resections required in the first two years. Most patients who needed one or more resections had ileocolonic disease and had complex stricturing or penetrating disease.

Allez et al. (95) conducted a study to determine whether the presence of severe endoscopic lesions may predict a higher risk of colectomy and penetrating complications. Severe endoscopic lesions were defined as extensive and deep ulcerations covering more than 10% of the mucosal area of at least one segment of the colon. Among the 102 patients included, 53 had severe endoscopic lesions at index colonoscopy. During the follow-up (median = 52 months), 37 patients underwent colonic resection. Probabilities of colectomy at one, three, and eight years were 20%, 26%, and 42%, respectively. Risk of colectomy was independently affected by the presence of severe endoscopic lesions at index colonoscopy (relative risk = 5.4), a Crohn's disease activity index level greater than 288 (relative risk = 2.2), and the absence of immunosuppressive therapy during the follow-up (relative risk = 2.4). Probabilities of colectomy were 31% and 6% at one year, 42% and 8% at three years, and 62% and 18% at eight years in patients with and without severe endoscopic lesions, respectively. All six patients with penetrating complications during the follow-up had severe endoscopic lesions at index colonoscopy. They concluded that patients with Crohn's disease exhibiting deep and extensive ulcerations at colonoscopy have a more aggressive clinical course with an increased rate of penetrating complications and surgery.

CLASSIFICATION

A number of classifications of Crohn's disease have been suggested but none has been generally accepted. An international working party commissioned for the 1998 World Congress of Gastroenterology in Vienna developed a classification of Crohn's disease based on objective variables and this has become known as the Vienna Classification (96). Eight outcome-related variables relevant to Crohn's disease were identified and stepwise evaluated in 413 consecutive cases, a database survey, and by clinical considerations. Allocation of variables was conducted with well-defined Crohn's disease populations from Europe and North America. Three variables were finally selected: Age at diagnosis [below 40 years (A1), equal to or above 40 years (A2)], Location [terminal ileum (L1), colon (L2), ileocolon (L3), upper gastrointestinal (L4)], and Behavior [nonstricturing nonpenetrating (B1), stricturing (B2), penetrating (B3)]. Analyses revealed associations between age at diagnosis and location, and between behavior and location. The Vienna classification of Crohn's disease provides distinct definitions to categorize Crohn's patients into 24 groups. A number of investigators have applied this classification to a variety of databases to determine its clinical relevance.

Freeman (97) applied this classification to a single clinician database of 877 patients comprised of 56.1% women and 43.9% men. Of these patients, 84.4% were diagnosed before 40 years of age and 15.6% were diagnosed by 40 years of age or older. Disease was located in the terminal ileum in 25.3% of patients, colon alone in 27.2% of patients, and ileocolon in 34.6% of patients. Another 113 (13.1%) of patients had disease in the upper gastrointestinal tract, usually with disease also in the terminal ileum (23 patients), colon (12 patients), or ileocolon (71 patients). Only 7 of the 877 patients had disease located in the upper gastrointestinal alone with no distal disease. Disease behavior could be classified as nonstricturing and nonpenetrating in 29.2% of patients, stricturing in 33.6% of patients and penetrating in 37.2% of patients. Of the 877 patients with Crohn's disease, 837 were white, 38 were Asian and 2 were black. In this Canadian teaching hospital at the University of British Columbia, Crohn's disease predominantly affects women, and young adults with a high rate of stricturing and penetrating complications. Freeman (98) used a modified Vienna classification schema to explore the specific role of age at diagnosis on both disease location and disease behavior. There were 1015 consecutively evaluated patients, including 449 males and 566 females. Disease was most often located in the ileocolon and could be most often classified as complex disease (i.e., in greater than 70%) with strictures or penetrating complications. For both male and females, with increasing age at diagnosis, disease became less extensive, more often localized in the colon alone, and disease behavior could be characterized as more complex, especially with penetrating disease complications. Freeman (99) further reported patients with longstanding Crohn's disease including 81 females and 69 males who were seen continuously by a single clinician for at least 20 years to learn more about the natural history of the disease. Additional retrospective data were available extending for more than 40 years and 13 had died usually with an advanced malignancy. To evaluate disease expression, phenotypic clinical characteristics defined by the 1998 Vienna classification for Crohn's disease were used and included age at diagnosis, location of disease, and disease behavior at the time of diagnosis or 10 years or 20 years after diagnosis. Most patients were initially diagnosed before the age of 40 years (94%) and had ileocolonic disease (65.3%). At diagnosis, both females and males were most often classified with inflammatory disease (nonstenosing, nonpenetrating); however, over the course of the disease, particularly in the first decade, decreased numbers of patients with inflammatory disease and increased numbers with penetrating disease were seen. In addition, some with stenosing disease eventually developed penetrating disease. Disease localized to ileum alone was most often complicated by stricture formation, whereas ileocolonic disease was usually complicated by a penetrating complication. This shift in disease behavior indicates that Crohn's disease is a dynamic process that phenotypically evolves and progresses with time.

Cosnes et al. (100) assessed the long-term evolution of the disease behavior of Crohn's disease according to the Vienna classification and determined the predictive factors and prognostic implications of this evolution in 2002 patients. They found 60% developed a stricturing ($n = 254$) or a penetrating ($n = 945$) complication. Twenty-year actuarial rates of inflammatory, stricturing, and penetrating disease were 12%, 18%, and 70%, respectively.

Louis et al. (101) assessed the stability over the course of the disease of its location and behavior as determined according to the Vienna classification in 297 Crohn's disease patients. The location of the disease remained relatively stable over the course of the disease. Although the proportion of patients who had a change in disease location became statistically significant after five years, over 10 years only 15.9% of patients had a change in location. They observed a more rapid and prominent change in disease behavior, which was already statistically significant after one year. Over 10 years, 45.9% of patients had a change in disease behavior. The most prominent change was from nonstricturing nonpenetrating disease to either stricturing (27.1%) or penetrating (29.4%) disease. Age at diagnosis had no influence on either location or behavior of disease. Ileal Crohn's disease was more often stricturing, and colonic or ileocolonic Crohn's disease was more often penetrating: this was already the case at diagnosis and became more prominent after 10 years. They concluded that behavior of Crohn's disease according to the Vienna classification varies dramatically over the course of the disease and cannot be used in phenotype-genotype analyses.

Veloso et al. (102) described the clinical course of Crohn's disease in a well-defined homogeneous group of 480 patients followed up from diagnosis to 20 years. Definitions of patient subgroups were made according to the Vienna classification. Patients with ileal disease had a greater need for surgical and a lesser need for immunosuppressive treatment; patients with ileocolonic disease were diagnosed at an earlier age and showed a lower probability of remaining in remission during the disease course; patients with colonic disease needed less surgical or steroid treatment; patients with intestinal penetrating disease were frequently submitted to abdominal surgery, whereas those with anal-penetrating disease often needed immunosuppressive treatment. Approximately 40% of the patients were in clinical remission at any time but only about 10% maintained a long-term remission free of steroids after their initial presentation. A more benign clinical course could be predicted in patients who stayed in remission in the year after diagnosis. They believe the grouping of patients with Crohn's disease according to the Vienna classification and/or the clinical activity in the year after diagnosis is useful in predicting the subsequent course of disease.

The discovery of a series of genetic and serological markers associated with disease susceptibility and phenotype in inflammatory bowel disease has led to the prospect of an integrated classification system involving clinical, serological, and genetic parameters. Another working party assembled for the Montreal 2005 World Congress of Gastroenterology reviewed current clinical classification systems in Crohn's disease and while an integrated system is not proposed for clinical use at present, the introduction of a widely accepted clinical subclassification is strongly advocated. They recommended a modification of the Vienna classification as follows:

- Introduction of an early age of onset category (diagnosis at 16 years or younger)
- Allow for the coclassification of location L4 (upper gastrointestinal involvement with L1 to L3
- Inclusion of a modifier for perianal disease

A summary of the revised Montreal classification is as follows:

Age at diagnosis (A)	
A1 16 years or younger	
A2 17–40 years	
A3 Over 40 years	
Location (L)	*Upper GI Modifier (L4)*
L1 Terminal ileum	L1 + L4
L2 Colon	L2 + L4
L3 Ileocolon	L3 + L4
L4 Upper GI	–
Behavior (B)	*Perianal Disease Modifier (p)*
B1 Nonstricturing Nonpenetrating	B1p
B2 Stricturing	B2p
B3 Penetrating	B3p

Although an enormous amount of work has gone into the effort at classification by world expert gastroenterologists, the exact value of the classification to clinical relevance is yet to be determined.

MEDICAL MANAGEMENT

As with ulcerative colitis, there is no specific medical therapy for Crohn's disease. The aims of treatment are to reduce bowel inflammation, promote symptomatic relief for intestinal and extraintestinal manifestations, and correct nutritional disturbances. Control, rather than cure of the disease, is the expectation of treatment. The goal is to eliminate symptoms to maintain general well being with as few side effects and long-term sequelae as possible. Mild and moderately severe disease can be treated on an outpatient basis. For severe attacks the patient should be admitted to the hospital for bowel rest and vigorous therapy.

SULFASALAZINE AND 5-AMINOSALICYLIC ACID

Sulfasalazine has two molecular components, sulfapyridine and 5-aminosalicylic acid (5-ASA). 5-ASA inhibits both cyclooxygenase and 5-lipoxy-genase, which in turn inhibit prostaglandin and leukotriene synthesis. There is some evidence that 5-ASA can directly consume and detoxify the oxygen radicals released during respiratory bursts of granulocytes (59). Sulfasalazine has no effect on small intestinal and perianal disease. The National Cooperative Crohn's Disease (NCCD) study showed that when given alone sulfasalazine is effective in the control of active disease. It is not a useful adjunct to prednisone in active Crohn's disease. Furthermore, sulfasalazine provides no prednisone-sparing effect to allow more rapid or complete withdrawal of the prednisone (103).

Review of available information reveals that mesalamine preparations remain the mainstay of therapy for mild to moderately active Crohn's colitis (104). Pentasa (Marion-Merrell Dow, Kansas City, Missouri, U.S.A.) is effective only at doses of 4 g/day. Singleton et al. (105) conducted a double-blind randomized prospective-controlled trial comparing placebo with three daily doses of mesalamine in 310 patients. Mesalamine (Pentasa), 4 g/day, resulted in a remission rate of 43% in the treatment of acute Crohn's disease compared with 18% in the placebo group. Asacol (Proctor & Gamble, Cincinnati, Ohio, U.S.A.), at a dose of 3.2 g/day, has been shown to be effective in the treatment of mild to moderately active Crohn's colitis or ileocolitis (106). For the treatment of Crohn's disease, higher doses than physicians are used to prescribing may be necessary. For example, 4.8 to 6.0 g/day of Asacol may be required (12–15 tablets), whereas 24 tablets of Pentasa or 30 tablets of sulfasalazine may be needed to accomplish the same goal.

ANTIBIOTICS

In the management of patients with acute exacerbations of Crohn's disease, antibiotics are often recommended on the premise that the inflammation is transmural. The rationale for using antibiotics is based on their effect in decreasing luminal bacterial concentration, secondary tissue invasion, and micro abscesses that complicate Crohn's disease, as well as bacterial translocation and dissemination, an effect that, in turn, reduces systemic complications (25).

More recently, Sartor reviewed the subject of therapeutic manipulation of the enteric microflora in inflammatory bowel disease (107). Clinical and experimental studies suggest that the relative balance of aggressive and protective bacterial species is altered in these disorders. Antibiotics can selectively decrease tissue invasion and eliminate aggressive bacterial species or globally decrease luminal and mucosal bacteria concentrations depending on their spectrum of activity. Alternatively, administration of beneficial bacterial species (probiotics), poorly absorbed dietary oligosaccharides (prebiotics), or combined probiotics and prebiotics (synbiotics) can restore a predominance of beneficial *Lactobacillus* and *Bifidobacterium* species. Current clinical trials do not fulfill evidence-based criteria for using these agents in inflammatory bowel diseases, but multiple nonrigorous studies and widespread clinical experience suggest that metronidazole and/or ciprofloxacin can treat Crohn's colitis and ileocolitis (but not isolated ileal disease), perianal fistulas, and pouchitis.

There is evidence, based on controlled trials, that metronidazole is effective as primary therapy in Crohn's disease. Its mechanism of action includes suppression of anaerobes and possible immunosuppression, although this is questionable, and there is some evidence that it may block adhesion molecules. The indications for use of metronidazole according to Sartor (25) are as primary therapy for Crohn's colitis and enterocolitis, perianal disease, and possibly prevention of postoperative recurrence of Crohn's disease.

Regarding metronidazole dosing, Sartor (25) emphasized a low dose of 10 mg/kg/day as needed to avoid intolerance is appropriate for colitis and ileocolitis. A high dose of 20 mg/kg/day is required for chronic administration in perianal disease. Response of perianal fistulas may require three months of treatment, which is associated with a high risk of peripheral neuropathy. It has been shown that 10% to 50% of patients who received a high dose of the drug for more than six months experience adverse effects. This rate drops to less than 5% with the lower dose, 10 mg/kg/day, which is effective therapy for intestinal Crohn's disease.

Prantera et al. (108) investigated the efficacy and the safety of a combination of metronidazole and ciprofloxacin compared with methylprednisolone in treating 41 consecutive patients with active Crohn's disease. Patients were randomly allocated to receive, for 12 weeks, ciprofloxacin, 500 mg twice daily, plus metronidazole, 250 mg four times daily, or methylprednisolone, 0.7 to 1 mg/kg/day, with variable tapering to 40 mg, followed by tapering of 4 mg weekly. Ten of the 22 antibiotic patients (45.5%) and 12 of the 19 steroid patients (63%) obtained clinical remission at the end of the 12-week study. The authors suggested that metronidazole and ciprofloxacin could be an alternative to steroids in treating the acute phase of Crohn's disease.

CORTICOSTEROIDS

Corticosteroids are the mainstay for treatment of active symptomatic Crohn's disease in both the colon and the small intestine. The anti-inflammatory activity of steroids is mediated by their inhibition of cellular lipids, which stabilizes cellular membranes and prevents release of free arachidonic acid (59). Another characteristic of steroids is immunosuppressive activity. Good initial symptomatic response can be expected in 75% to 90% of patients, although this response is not necessarily associated with improved radiologic appearance.

For active disease, prednisone, 40 to 60 mg orally, given in three to four divided doses, is maintained for 10 to 14 days. The dosage is then tapered at the rate of 5 mg a week. The dose of prednisone is increased if there is any sign of relapse.

In very ill patients, prednisolone, 60 mg intravenously, is given as a continuous infusion or hydrocortisone, 100 mg every eight hours, and tapered as patient improves until the patient is ready for oral prednisone. Rectal administration of hydrocortisone is useful in treating distal colonic and rectal disease. There has been no evidence to support the use of prophylactic steroid therapy in both quiescent disease and after operative treatment (109).

Budesonide is a corticosteroid analog. Because of its rapid first-pass metabolism by the liver, its systemic bioavailability is low and it should have little suppression of adrenal function and few side effects. Greenberg et al. (110) compared daily doses of 3, 9, and 15 mg of oral controlled-release budesonide with placebo in an 8-week trial of 258 patients. The optimal efficacy was seen at the 9 mg dose (51% remission vs. 20% with placebo). Rutgeerts et al. (111) reported on a European trial of 176 patients comparing a 9 mg dose of budesonide to prednisolone, 40 mg daily on a tapering schedule over an 8-week interval. At 10 weeks, 53% of budesonide-treated patients were in remission compared with 66% of those treated with prednisolone, but side effects were less common with budesonide.

Fedorak and Bistritz (112) recently reviewed the use of budesonide in the treatment of Crohn's disease. Two commercially available enteric-coated pH-dependent release formulations (Entocort EC and Budenofalk) deliver budesonide to the ileum and proximal colon regions most commonly affected in Crohn's disease. The drug's effectiveness in this disease has been proven in multiple, placebo-controlled trials, where it has been shown to be superior to mesalamine and placebo, and equivalent to prednisolone for the control of mild to moderate active right-sided Crohn's disease. This beneficial therapeutic effect comes with less adrenal suppression and a small improvement in the clinical adverse effect profile, as compared with prednisolone. However, budesonide provides no benefit over the conventional therapy for left-sided colonic disease, and it is less effective for the treatment of more severe disease activity and more distal colonic disease. Continuous budesonide does not prolong remission and is, therefore, best used in an intermittent fashion to treat acute exacerbations. Kane et al. (113) reviewed randomized controlled trials comparing budesonide to corticosteroids, 5-ASA products or placebo to assess the effectiveness and safety for inducing remission of active Crohn's disease and for maintaining remission. Trials had to report on the effectiveness of treatment (defined as decreasing or maintaining Crohn's disease activity index scores ≤150) or adverse events. Budesonide was more likely to induce remission than placebo (relative risk = 1.8) or 5-ASA (relative risk = 1.7) although only one trial compared budesonide to 5-ASA products. Although budesonide induced remission less frequently than conventional corticosteroids (relative risk = 0.9) there was no significant difference between conventional corticosteroids and budesonide for inducing remission among patients with a low disease activity (initial CDAI = 200–300). Budesonide was significantly less likely to cause corticosteroid-associated adverse events than conventional corticosteroids (relative risk = 0.7). No significant difference in total adverse events or corticosteroid-associated adverse events was demonstrated between budesonide and 5-ASA or placebo. Although budesonide is 13% less effective for the induction of remission in active Crohn's disease than conventional corticosteroids, it is less likely to cause corticosteroid-related adverse effects. Budesonide is ineffective in maintaining remission.

Akerkar et al. (114) reported that the relative risk for developing corticosteroid-associated complications in elderly Crohn's disease patients is 7.64 for mental status changes, 1.46 for hypertension, 1.53 for hyperglycemia, 1.59 for hypokalemia, 1.09 for nosocomial infections, and 1.09 for congestive heart failure.

■ IMMUNOSUPPRESSIVE AGENTS

6-Mercaptopurine and Azathioprine

Immunosuppressive agents, such as 6-mercaptopurine (6-MP) and azathioprine, are frequently used agents in the management of patients with Crohn's disease, but the benefit is often not realized for several months. A long-term randomized double-blind study of 6-MP by Present et al. (115) demonstrated that 67% of subjects with Crohn's disease who were taking 6-MP improved in comparison with only 8% for those receiving placebo. In this study the mean time for response to 6-MP was 3.1 months, and 20% of the subjects required more than four months of treatment before improving. The authors also reported that 75% of the subjects receiving 6-MP were able to decrease or eliminate concomitant corticosteroid therapy.

A study by Markowitz et al. (116) included 36 adolescents with Crohn's disease who were treated with 6-MP for at least six months. Seventeen patients had ileocolonic disease and nine had pancolonic disease; seven had disease of the small intestine and three of the partial colon. All patients had received corticosteroids, sulfasalazine, antibiotics, and nutritional support for 5.0 ± 3 years before 6-MP was administered. However, intractable symptoms persisted. The results showed that during the first six months of 6-MP use, 50% of patients were able to completely discontinue the use of prednisone. At the end of a full year of 6-MP therapy, 80% of patients no longer required corticosteroids. While nearly 40% of subjects had perianal fistulas or abscesses before starting 6-MP treatment, only 14% had them during the therapy. Accordingly, the subjects with no signs of perianal disease increased from 22% to 53% while undergoing 6-MP therapy. In general, subjects with extensive colonic involvement seemed to have the best response, but differences were not significant because of the small sample size of each subgroup (116). O'Brien and Bayless (117) suggested that immunosuppressive agents also may be effective in the treatment of ileitis.

Present (118) recommended the following protocol for the administration of 6-MP: 50 mg 6-MP daily; check white blood cell count weekly for the first four to six weeks, thereafter every other week, and after many years every three to four months. Patients are told to discontinue the drug immediately if they develop a sore throat or fever. After four weeks, the dosage of 6-MP can be raised gradually to 75 to 100 mg daily. The vast majority of patients will require 50 to 75 mg to respond.

Korelitz et al. (119) reported observations after 20 years of clinical experience with 6-MP in 148 patients with Crohn's disease who had not satisfactorily responded to steroids and other drugs. Defined therapeutic goals were achieved in 68%. Major successes included (i) elimination of steroids (66%), (ii) healing of internal fistulas and abscesses or improvement by elimination of discharge and tenderness (64%), and (iii) healing or improvement by elimination of pain, tenderness, and discharge of perirectal fistulas and abscesses (87%). Other therapeutic goals that achieved 100% success were healing or marked improvement of Crohn's disease in the stomach and duodenum, and permitting operation to be performed electively after 6-MP allowed margins for resection to be delineated. 6-MP was less effective in achieving therapeutic goals of preventing recurrent small bowel obstruction (43%) and elimination of abdominal masses (55%). Seventy-eight percent of patients showed a reduction in the activity index with a mean of 43%. In the review 6-MP was demonstrated to be effective in achieving major therapeutic goals in two of three patients with severe Crohn's disease.

D'Haens et al. (120) treated 19 patients with recurrent ileitis following right hemicolectomy for Crohn's disease with azathioprine. Therapy resulted in induction of maintenance of clinical remission in all 15 evaluable patients.

Pearson et al. (121) conducted a meta-analysis of nine randomized placebo-controlled trials. The authors found that azathioprine and 6-MP benefits those with active disease but steroids should be maintained and tapered while waiting for these agents to take effect. Therapy should be continued for at least 17 weeks and preferably for 26 to 52 weeks. Benefit was accrued to patients with quiescent and fistulous disease and steroid-sparing effect was confirmed. The incidence of adverse side effects is near 10%. The dose of azathioprine ranged from 2 to 3 mg/kg/day for active disease and 1 to 2.5 mg/kg/day for maintenance therapy. Azathioprine and 6-MP remain the second-line immunosuppressive drugs (104).

The greatest negative factor in the use of immunosuppressive has been the fear of toxicity and neoplasia, particularly lymphoma, which has been well known in transplant patients. In patients with Crohn's disease, the risk of treatment with 6-MP is unknown and is probably small, but study of more patients with longer follow-up will be needed before the incidence can be determined. In the experience of Present (122), 8% of patients manifested some form of hypersensitivity to 6-MP. This includes fever, joint pain, and pancreatitis. The pancreatitis associated with 6-MP appears to be in the form of allergy or hypersensitivity in that it occurs within the first three to four weeks of therapy, recurs on challenge, and produces no long-term sequelae. If pancreatitis symptoms begin, blood amylases should be drawn and the drug promptly withdrawn (123).

Present (122) pointed out that about 5% of patients with Crohn's disease might require 6-MP and suggested that the drug be used earlier in the course of disease instead of waiting until operation is required. The indications for 6-MP are (i) steroid toxicity, steroid dependence; (ii) fistulization (perianal, enterocutaneous, internal fistula); and (iii) recurrent Crohn's disease with previous multiple small bowel resections with the goal to avoid operation, which may result in short bowel syndrome.

Methotrexate

Lemann et al. (123) reported the results of the use of methotrexate in 39 patients with Crohn's disease refractory to conventional treatment, including azathioprine. The probability of remission was 72% at three months. The probability of remission and steroid withdrawal was 42% at 12 months. In patients in clinical remission, the probability of relapse on methotrexate was 58% at 12 months. Although toxicity was acceptable, the long-term benefit was more limited.

In a subsequent report Lemann et al. (124) reported on the long-term efficacy and safety in 49 patients with Crohn's disease who were treated with methotrexate for greater than or equal to six months. In all, 41 patients achieved complete remission and were maintained on methotrexate for a median of 18 months (range 7–59 months). In these patients, the probabilities of relapse were 29%, 41%, and 48% at one, two, and three years, respectively. A higher rate of relapse was observed in women and in patients with ileocolitis. Adverse reactions were recorded in 24 patients, requiring discontinuation of methotrexate in five. A liver biopsy was performed in 11 patients; a mild steatosis was found in five, a slight dilation of the sinusoids in one, a granulomatous hepatitis with a mild portal fibrosis in one, and a slight periportal fibrosis in one patient. They concluded that the long-term benefit of maintenance therapy with methotrexate in patients with chronically active Crohn's disease demonstrated only moderate side effects.

The North American Crohn's Study Group investigators (125) studied the efficacy of 25 mg of intramuscular methotrexate weekly for 16 weeks and a tapering dose of prednisone or placebo on 141 steroid-dependent Crohn's disease patients (approximately 75% with colonic involvement). Remission was defined by the Crohn's disease activity index and the ability to discontinue steroid treatment. By these criteria, methotrexate was significantly superior to placebo. Side effects of methotrexate included nausea, anorexia, stomatitis, diarrhea, hematologic toxicity, interstitial pneumonitis, and hepatic toxicity.

Alfadhli et al. (126) conducted a systemic Cochrane review of the evidence for the effectiveness of methotrexate for induction of remission in patients with active Crohn's disease in the presence and absence of concomitant steroid therapy. Selected criteria included randomized controlled trials involving patients of age greater than 17 years with refractory Crohn's disease defined by conventional clinical, radiological, and endoscopic criteria, which was categorized as being active (Crohn's disease activity index >150). The outcome measure was the rate of induction of remission and complete withdrawal from steroids in the treatment and control groups after more than 16 weeks of treatment. A secondary outcome was induction of remission with reduction in steroid dose of at least 50%. Three small studies, which employed low doses of methotrexate orally, showed no statistically significant difference between methotrexate and placebo/control medication-treated patients. One small study, which used a higher dose of intravenous/oral methotrexate, showed no statistically significant difference between methotrexate and azathioprine. A larger study, which employed a higher dose of methotrexate intramuscularly, showed substantial benefit. Adverse effects were more common with high-dose intramuscular methotrexate therapy than with placebo. They concluded that there is evidence from a single large randomized trial on which to recommend the use of methotrexate 25 mg intramuscularly weekly for induction of remission and complete withdrawal from steroids in patients with refractory Crohn's disease. There is no evidence on which to base a recommendation for use of lower dose of oral methotrexate.

Cyclosporine

Mixed reports of the efficacy of cyclosporine in the clinical response of patients with Crohn's disease have been published. In a European trial of 182 patients, the long-term treatment of chronic active Crohn's disease with cyclosporine plus low-dose steroids did not offer an advantage compared with low-dose steroids alone (127). In a study of eight patients with acute refractory Crohn's disease, intravenous cyclosporine was administered but, although there was improvement in six patients after discontinuation of treatment, relapse is to be expected (128).

Sandborn et al. (129) reviewed the literature and found clinical response rates of active Crohn's disease to high-dose cyclosporine in uncontrolled pilot studies to range from 0% to 100%, with an overall mean response of 63%. Three large multicenter controlled trials of low-dose oral cyclosporine (lesser than or equal to 5 mg/kg/day) for treatment of chronically active Crohn's disease and Crohn's disease remission maintenance failed to show a beneficial effect compared with placebo. The clinical response rates in the only controlled trial of high-dose cyclosporine (7.6 mg/kg/day) for active Crohn's disease was 59% compared with 32% for placebo, although the benefit did not persist after cyclosporine was discontinued. Sandborn et al. (129) conducted a study to determine whether high-dose oral cyclosporine (greater than or equal to 5 mg/kg/day) would be more effective than low-dose cyclosporine (lesser than or equal to 5 mg/kg/day). They found that with a 6-week course of oral cyclosporine (8 mg/kg/day), the clinical response did not correlate with intestinal or blood cyclosporine concentrations. However, cyclosporine side effects, including nephrotoxicity, gingival hyperplasia, hypertrichosis, hypertension, paresthesias, tremor, headache, and peroneal nerve palsy, were common.

McDonald et al. (130) conducted a Cochrane review to evaluate the effectiveness of oral cyclosporine for induction of remission in patients with active Crohn's disease in the presence and absence of concomitant steroid therapy. Prospective, randomized, double-blinded, placebo-controlled trials of parallel design, with treatment duration of a minimum of 12 weeks, comparing oral cyclosporine therapy with placebo for treatment of patients with active Crohn's disease were eligible for inclusion of which there were four. All data were analyzed on an intention-to-treat basis. The results of this review demonstrate that low-dose (5 mg/kg/day) oral cyclosporine is not effective for the induction of remission in Crohn's disease. Patients treated with low-dose oral cyclosporine are more likely than placebo-treated patients to experience adverse events including renal dysfunction. The use of low-dose oral cyclosporine for the treatment of chronic active Crohn's disease does not appear to be justified. Higher doses of cyclosporine are not likely to be useful for the long-term management of Crohn's disease because of the risk of nephrotoxicity and the availability of other proven interventions.

Tacrolimus

Ierardi et al. (131) reported the results of a prospective, open-label, uncontrolled study in 13 patients affected by Crohn's disease with resistance to steroids treated with long-term oral tacrolimus. Tacrolimus was administered at the doses 0.1 to 0.2 mg per day/kg and adjusted in order to achieve levels of 5–10 ng/mL; only mesalazine was continued concomitantly. Steroids and total parental nutrition were tapered when appropriate. Median treatment was 27.3 months. Only one patient dropped out due to adverse events. Crohn's disease activity index score significantly decreased after six months in 11 patients; for one year in nine of them, and seven years in two of them. The inflammatory bowel disease life quality questionnaire score significantly increased over the same periods. In three out of six patients, complete closure of fistulas occurred. Tacrolimus allowed total parenteral nutrition to be withdrawn in three out of five patients. Supplementation with low-dose steroids was required in five patients. Two patients underwent operation. They concluded that tacrolimus therapy may represent a therapeutic option in Crohn's disease when conventional therapies fail.

Although some encouraging reports have been published with the use of immunosuppressive agents, the unbridled enthusiasm for their use should be tempered by the recognition of the frequent failures and the side effects suffered by even those in whom response is obtained. Furthermore, response is often slow to achieve and dissipates when treatment is discontinued. They may have a role for patients who do not respond to 5-ASA preparations and steroids but should not be continued indefinitely to the detriment of the patient when an anatomically defined area of affected bowel can wisely be resected.

Although immunosuppressants have been used more frequently over the last 25 years, there is no significant decrease of the need for operation or of intestinal complications of Crohn's disease (132).

■ BIOLOGIC MODIFIERS

Infliximab (Remicade) a chimeric monoclonal antibody against TNF-alpha has evolved as a promising therapeutic option in the treatment of Crohn's disease.

Wenzl et al. (133) reported the nationwide experience with infliximab for the treatment of Crohn's disease in Austria. A total of 748 infusions were administered to 153 patients. After the first treatment course an excellent or good response occurred in 83% of patient with luminal disease, and 71% of patients with fistulous disease. After the first treatment course, 71% of patients received further infliximab therapy. At a mean follow-up of 29 months, 50% of patients had improved since baseline without requiring operation for Crohn's disease. Steroid withdrawal was achieved in 25% of patients. Surgery had been performed in one-third of patients and was associated with lacking response to the first treatment course and with fistulous disease. Comedication with azathioprine favored the initial response and steroid withdrawal. One patient died from myocarditis.

Miehsler et al. (134) presented their experience with infliximab in the treatment of four patients with internal fistulas in Crohn's disease—entero-enteral and entero-abdominal, parastomal, entero-vesical. Each was treated with three infusions of infliximab (5 mg/kg body weight) with intervals of two and four weeks. In addition, three patients had strictures and two patients had perianal fistulas. After the three infusions of infliximab, internal fistulas remained unchanged in all patients. The perianal fistulas present in two cases were healed. The concluded treatment with three infusions of infliximab (5 mg/kg body weight) led to healing of only the perianal fistulas, whereas the internal fistulas were not influenced and was no alternative for operation. Poritz et al. (135) evaluated the role of infliximab in supplanting operation for fistulizing Crohn's disease. They reviewed 26 patients (14 males; mean age, 38 years; range, 19–80 years) who received a mean of three (range, one to six) doses of infliximab (5 mg/kg) with the intent to cure fistulizing Crohn's disease. Nine patients (35%) had perianal, six (23%) enterocutaneous, three (12%) rectovaginal, four (15%) peristomal, and four (15%) intra-abdominal fistulas. Nineteen (73%) of the patients had prior operation for Crohn's disease. Six patients (23%) had a complete response to infliximab with fistula closure, 12 (46%) with a partial response, and eight (31%) had no response to infliximab. Fourteen (54%) of the patients still required operation for their fistulizing Crohn's disease after infliximab therapy (10 bowel resections, four perianal procedures), whereas half (6/12) of the patients treated with infliximab who still had open fistulas after treatment declined operative intervention. Five of six patients with fistula closure on infliximab had perianal or rectovaginal fistulas. None of the patients with either enterocutaneous or peristomal fistulas were healed with infliximab. Although it was associated with a 61% complete or partial response rate, infliximab therapy did not supplant the need for operative intervention in the majority of patients with fistulizing Crohn's disease.

Mendoza et al. (136) reported their experience with infliximab treatment with 28 patients treated (7 with inflammatory and 21 with fistulizing disease). Patients received a total of 116 infusions of infliximab: 57.1% (4 of 7) of patients with luminal disease had complete response within a median of 17.5 days (range, 15–28 days), and 62% (13 of 21) of patients with fistulizing disease had complete response within a median of nine days (range, 6–51 days). All patients (5) without relapse received concomitant treatment with immune modifiers. The group of patients with previous resection or perianal fistula repair had complete response more frequently (odds ratio = 30).

In their review Panaccione et al. (137) noted in randomized, placebo-controlled clinical trials, 33% of patients treated with infliximab 5 mg/kg achieved remission (Crohn's disease activity score < 150), compared with only 4% of those receiving placebo. Additionally, infliximab is the only drug therapy shown to be effective for the treatment of fistulizing Crohn's disease. The ACCENT I trial found that 58% of 573 patients responded to an initial infusion of infliximab 5 mg/kg but there was no placebo arm (138).

Grange et al. (139) reported the use of infliximab 5 mg/kg given at weeks 0, 5, and 9 for a patient with Crohn's disease who had a severe and rapidly extensive corticosteroid-resistant pyoderma gangrenosum of the leg. A dramatic response was observed within 72 hours with a favorable effect persisting for four weeks after each infliximab infusion. Complete healing was achieved at week 11.

The Canadian Association of Gastroenterology published the following clinical guidelines for the use of infliximab in Crohn's disease (140). Indications include as follows:

1. Moderate to severe Crohn's disease: infliximab is indicated for patients who demonstrate continuing symptoms, despite the optimal use of conventional therapies with glucocorticoids and an adequate trial of immunosuppressive therapy (6-MP, azathioprine, or methotrexate), and for patients who are unable to tolerate conventional therapy including glucocorticoids and immunosuppressive therapy
2. Fistulizing Crohn's disease: (infliximab is indicated for patients with symptomatic enterocutaneous and perianal fistula)

With regard to initial dosing, there is evidence to suggest that initial dosing with three infusions at weeks 0, 2, and 6 results in higher remission and response (by approximately 15%) at 14 weeks than dosing at 0 and 14. They further state that there is sufficient evidence to suggest that patients receiving infliximab should receive concomitant immunosuppressant therapy to reduce the formation of antibodies to infliximab, decrease the likelihood of infusion reactions and possibly increased overall response. Patients with Crohn's disease who require therapy with infliximab should receive concomitant immunosuppressive therapy (e.g., 6-MP, azathioprine or methotrexate) if no contraindications exist, even if the patient has failed to respond to these medications in the past. Administration of hydrocortisone intravenously 30 minutes before infusion of infliximab reduces the incidence of antibodies to infliximab and increases measurable infliximab levels in the serum. Corticosteroids should be tapered and discontinued. For patients who are unable to discontinue corticosteroids the role of infliximab in long-term management should be reassessed.

With regard to maintenance dosing in moderate to severe Crohn's disease, regular repeat dosing every eight weeks is effective in maintaining clinical response after an induction regimen. In patients with recurrence of symptoms following an initial infliximab-induced response or remission, therapy with infliximab (5 mg/kg) intravenously is effective in reestablishing and maintaining remission. Patients who have lost response during the maintenance dosing with 5 mg/kg may regain response if the dosing is increased to 10 mg/kg or the infusion intervals are shortened. For patients with fistulizing Crohn's disease, regular repeat dosing every eight weeks is effective in maintaining clinical response after an induction regimen. In patients with recurrence of symptoms following initial infliximab-induced response or remission, therapy with infliximab (5 mg/kg) intravenously may be effective in reestablishing and maintaining remission. Patients who have lost response during maintenance dosing (5 mg/kg) may regain response if the dosing is increased to 10 mg/kg or if the infusion intervals are shortened.

Akobeng and Zachos (141) conducted a systemic Cochrane review to evaluate the effectiveness of TNF-alpha blocking agents in inducing remission in patients with active Crohn's disease. They included only randomized controlled trials in which patients with active Crohn's disease (defined by a validated Crohn's disease activity index) were randomly allocated to receive a TNF-alpha blocking agent in the treatment arm, or to receive placebo or another treatment in the comparison arm. Outcome measures reported in the primary studies included clinical remission, clinical response, and changes in disease activity index. Ten studies were identified of which four met the inclusion criteria. There is evidence from one randomized controlled trial that suggests that a single intravenous infusion of the monoclonal antibodies cA2, infliximab, may be effective for induction of remission in Crohn's disease. There was no difference in the response rates among infliximab doses of 5, 10, or 20 mg/kg. The results of two other trials suggested that CDP571, the genetically engineered TNF monoclonal antibody, might also be effective in reducing disease activity index at two weeks after an infusion. They did not find any evidence to support the use of etanercept in Crohn's disease. The reviewer's conclusions were that there is evidence from one randomized controlled trial suggesting that a single infusion of infliximab may be effective for induction of remission in Crohn's disease. Based on this review, they recommend a dose of 5 mg/kg.

Infliximab has been advocated for patients with various anorectal complications associated with Crohn's disease. Van der Hagen et al. (142) assessed the healing rate of complex perianal fistulas in Crohn's disease after a multistep strategy, including induction treatment with infliximab in case of active proctitis, followed by definitive operation. Patients with complex fistulas in Crohn's disease underwent pretreatment with noncutting setons, and in cases of severe recurrent fistulas or abscesses, a diverting stoma. Infliximab was added in cases of active proctitis. Seventeen patients were included of which seven patients were treated by operation only, and in 10 patients infliximab was added. After a median follow-up of 19 (range, 8–40) months, fistula healing was observed in 17 patients (100%). One patient of the infliximab group developed a recurrent fistula (10%) after 24 months, and in one patient (10%) soiling occurred. Two patients of the surgical group developed a recurrent fistula (29%) and soiling occurred in two patients (29%).

Poggioli et al. (143) conducted a pilot study to determine the feasibility and safety of the local injection of infliximab in selected patients with severe perianal Crohn's disease. The study included 15 patients with complex perianal Crohn's disease in which sepsis was not controlled using surgical and medical therapy. Among them, four had previously undergone intravenous infusion of infliximab with no significant response, nine had contraindications for intravenous infusion, and two had associated stenosing ileitis and severe coloproctitis. The injection of 15 to 21 mg of infliximab, associated with operative treatment, was performed at the internal and external orifices and along the fistula tract. No major adverse effects were reported. Ten of 15 patients healed after 3 to 12 infusions. A controlled randomized trial is required to prove the value.

Rubenstein et al. (144) reported that operations account for one half, and hospitalizations for one-third, of overall costs for patients with Crohn's disease. Infliximab induces remission and heals fistulas in Crohn's disease but is more costly than traditional therapies. They reviewed the impact upon resource use in Crohn's disease for at least one full year both before and after initial infliximab infusion. There were 79 patients (59% female, mean age 38.6 years). A decrease was seen in the annual incidence of all operations (38%), gastrointestinal operations (18%), endoscopies (43%), emergency room visits (66%), all outpatient visits (16%), outpatient GI visits (20%), all radiologic examinations (12%), and nonplain films (13%). Fistula patients ($n = 37$) had decreases in hospitalizations (59%); GI operations (59%); all operations (66%); all, GI and surgical outpatient visits (27%, 26%, 70%, respectively); emergency room visits (64%); all radiologic examinations (40%); and nonplain films (61%). Patients with luminal disease ($n = 42$) had decreases in endoscopies (52%), and emergency room visits (69%). Patients of both genders and all ages experienced decreases in resource use. They concluded that this decrease in the use of healthcare resources raises the potential of overall cost savings in Crohn's disease receiving this drug.

Having reviewed the potential benefits of infliximab, the purported advantages must be balanced with the numerous and sometimes lethal side effects reported with this agent. Colombel et al. (145) evaluated the short- and long-term safety in 500 patients with Crohn's disease treated with infliximab at the Mayo Clinic. The 500 patients received a median of three infusions and had a median follow-up of 17 months. Forty-three patients (8.6%) experienced a serious adverse event of which 30 (6%) were related to the infliximab. Acute infusion reactions occurred in 19 of 500 patients (3.8%). Serum sickness-like disease occurred in 19 of 500 patients and was attributed to infliximab in 14 (2.8%). Three patients developed drug-induced lupus. One patient developed a new demyelination disorder. Forty-eight patients had an infectious event, of which 41 (8.2%) were attributed to infliximab. Twenty patients had a serious infection: two had fatal sepsis, eight had pneumonia (of which two cases were fatal), six had viral infections, two had abdominal abscesses requiring surgery, one had arm cellulitis, and one had histoplasmosis. Nine patients had a malignant disorder, three of which were possibly related to infliximab. A total of 10 deaths were observed. For five of these patients (1%), the events leading to death were possibly related to the infliximab. They concluded that clinicians must be vigilant for the occurrence of infrequent but serious events.

Reported adverse reactions to infliximab include respiratory tract infections, including cough, sinusitis, pharyngitis, and bronchitis; nervous system effects, including headache, dizziness, and pain; musculoskeletal effects, including arthralgias and back pain; abdominal pain, including nausea and diarrhea, and chills and fever (146). Hypersensitivity reactions consisting of dyspnea, urticaria, and hypotension occur in approximately 10% of patients. Following treatment with infliximab serious opportunistic infections including reactivation of latent tuberculosis has occurred. By decreasing the immune response, tuberculosis can become symptomatic. Williams (147) reported a case of meningitis caused by *L. monocytogenes* six days after the second infusion of infliximab and reviewed eight other such cases reported in the literature. Singh et al. (148) presented a case of cutaneous Nocardia infection in a patient who was taking infliximab for Crohn's disease. A demyelination-like syndrome in Crohn's disease after infliximab therapy has been reported (149). Infliximab infusion should be terminated if demyelination is suspected. Other reported side effects include congestive heart failure, lupus-like syndrome, induction of autoantibodies and injection site reactions (150). It is important for clinicians to be aware of these side effects when prescribing therapy. Phelan and Wooltorton (151) reported that the U.S. Food and Drug Administration (FDA) has recently advised of serious hematologic events including leukopenia, neutropenia, thrombocytopenia, and pancytopenia in some patients taking infliximab. A potential side effect of an immune-modifying medication is the possibility of initiating a malignancy. The most commonly reported malignancy is lymphoproliferative disorder. In a report evaluating infliximab, nine patients reportedly developed a lymphoproliferative disorder, eight of which were lymphomas. It is unclear whether infliximab contributes to malignancy or whether the patient's disease condition itself leads to malignancy. A few studies have indicated a possible association between infliximab therapy for Crohn's disease and the onset of lymphoma (146). The FDA warned that in controlled studies of all TNF-alpha blocking agents, including Remicade, more cases of lymphoma have been observed among patients receiving the agents than among control group patients. Malignancies have also been observed in open-label, uncontrolled clinical studies at a rate several-fold higher than expected in the general population. Patients with Crohn's disease or rheumatoid arthritis, particularly patients with highly active disease and/or chronic exposure to immunosuppressant therapies, may be at a higher risk (up to several-fold) than the general population for the development of lymphoma. FDA has recommended a warning concerning malignancy be added to the labeling for all therapeutic agents that block TNF (152). Nicholson et al. (146) reported two patients who developed newly diagnosed metastatic colonic carcinoma during the treatment with infliximab. Both patients developed their carcinoma within one year of therapy with infliximab for Crohn's disease and both patients were receiving surveillance colonoscopy.

There has been a question as to whether these agents might increase the postoperative complication rate. Colombel et al. (153) conducted a study to determine whether the use of steroids, immunosuppressive agents, or infliximab prior to abdominal surgery for Crohn's disease is associated with an increased rate of early postoperative complications. Documented information included the use of infliximab within eight weeks before and four weeks after operation and dose and duration of corticosteroids, azathioprine/6-MP, and methotrexate. Septic complications included wound sepsis, intra-abdominal and extra-abdominal infections. Nonseptic complications included Crohn's disease recurrence, small bowel obstruction, gastrointestinal bleeding, and thromboembolism. Two hundred and seventy patients were operated upon including 107 patients who received steroids, 105 patients who received immunosuppressants (64 azathioprine, 38 6-MP, 4 methotrexate) and 52 who received infliximab. Forty-eight patients underwent urgent or emergency operation and 222 underwent elective operation. Septic complications occurred in 19% of patients including wound sepsis in 10%, anastomotic leak in 3%, and intra-abdominal abscess in 2%, and extra-abdominal infections in 7%. Nonseptic complications occurred in 7% of patients. Preoperative use of high- or moderate-dose steroids, immunosuppressives, or infliximab was not associated with greater complication rates. No deaths occurred. Marchal et al. (154) also conducted a study to determine whether the preoperative use of infliximab may increase the risk of perioperative complications. There were 40 patients who received one or more infusions prior to intestinal resection (31 of 40 within 12 weeks). The incidence of early minor (15% vs. 12.8%) and major (12.5% vs. 7.7%) and late minor (2.5% vs. 5.1%) and major (17.5% vs. 12.8%) complications and the mean hospital stay after operation (10.3 vs. 9.9 days) were similar in both groups. A trend toward an increased early infection rate was found in infliximab pretreated patients (6 vs. 1) but more patients in this group received corticosteroids and/or immunosuppressives (29 vs. 16 patients). They concluded that the use of infliximab before intestinal resection does not prolong the hospital stay and does not increase the rate of postoperative complications.

Other monoclonal antibodies have been used in the treatment of Crohn's disease. Schreiber et al. (155) investigated the efficacy and safety of certolizumab pegol (a polyethylene-glycolated Fab fragment of antitumor necrosis factor, CDP870) in Crohn's disease. In a placebo-controlled, phase II study, 292 patients with moderate to severe Crohn's disease received subcutaneous certolizumab 100, 200, or 400 mg or placebo at weeks 0, 4, and 8. At all time points, the clinical response rates were highest for certolizumab 400 mg, greatest at week 10 (certolizumab 400 mg 52.8%; placebo 30.1%) but not significant at week 12 (certolizumab 400 mg, 44.4%; placebo 35.6%). They concluded that certolizumab 400 mg may be effective and is well tolerated in patients with active Crohn's disease.

Sandborn et al. (156) reported on the use of natalizumab, a humanized monoclonal antibody against alpha 4-integrin. Induction therapy with natalizumab for Crohn's disease resulted in small, nonsignificant improvements in response (56% and 49%) and remission rates (37% and 30%). Patients who had a response had significantly increased rates of sustained response (61% vs. 28%) and remission (44% vs. 26%) if natalizumab was continued every four weeks. The benefit of natalizumab will need to be weighed against the risk of serious adverse effects including progressive multifocal leukoencephalopathy.

■ ANALGESICS

Cross et al. (157) characterized the prevalence of narcotic use and contributing factors in Crohn's disease patients. Narcotic use was identified in 13.1% of patients. Narcotic users were more likely to be female (72% vs. 49%), had higher rates of disability (15.4% vs. 3.6%), and a longer duration of disease (17 vs. 12.9 years). In addition, they took more medication (6.97 vs. 4.7) and had a higher prevalence of neuropsychiatric drug use (37% vs. 19%). Crohn's disease patients receiving narcotics had worse disease activity (HBI 9.1 vs. 5.0) and diminished quality of life (Sinflammatory bowel diseaseQ 44.2 vs. 51.6). Active disease [HBI score $\geq$ 4 (odds ratio 3.9)], polypharmacy [use of greater than or equal to five drugs (odds ratio 5.5)], and smoking (odds ratio 2.8) were associated with narcotic use. Narcotic use may be an indicator of more severe disease because it is associated with increased disease activity and decreased quality of life.

■ NUTRITION

The pathogenesis of malnutrition in Crohn's disease was well described by Stokes (158). Patients may have a reduced food intake because of anorexia or fear of abdominal pain after eating. Increased requirements and decreased synthesis may result from active inflammation or sepsis. One reason for diet therapy is an interruption in the inflammatory cascade through a change in dietary fatty acid sources. Specifically, this entails the substitution of omega-6 fatty acids, such as arachidonate, for omega-3 fatty acids, found principally in fish oils and certain vegetable oils. These fatty acids can diminish synthesis of those inflammatory mediators by competitive inhibition of the enzymes involved and substitution for the omega-6 fatty acids in the cell wall (59). An enteric loss of nutrients may be due to exudation of the intestinal mucosa or an interrupted enterohepatic circulation. Malabsorption may be caused by loss of absorptive surface from disease or operation, stagnant loop syndrome from strictures, fistula or surgical blind loops, mucosal cell disease, or lymphangiectasia. Miscellaneous causes of malnutrition include a rapid gastrointestinal transit, effects of medical therapy, or effects of parenteral nutrition without trace element supplements.

For these and other reasons, a dietary therapy has been suggested for treating Crohn's disease. The concept of the use of an elemental diet or total parenteral nutrition as primary therapy has at best been controversial. Potential uses of elemental diets in Crohn's disease include induction of remission, treatment of steroid-dependent/resistant patients, growth failure, malnutrition, preoperative preparation, and maintenance of remission. Clinical experience indicates that patients with distal colonic or perianal disease respond poorly to therapy with elemental diets compared to those with small bowel or ileocecal disease. In the acute phase, total parenteral nutrition has often been recommended as primary therapy but blind and excessive reliance on total parenteral nutrition is not appropriate because bowel rest does not stop the disease process. Nutritional replenishment for the malnourished patient with acutely active Crohn's disease is self-evident (159). A meta-analysis of eight randomized trials totaling 413 patients found that enteral nutrition, as a sole therapy, was inferior to corticosteroids (160). In a separate analysis of five trials, including 134 patients, there appeared to be no difference in the efficacy of elemental versus nonelemental formulas. In a review article, Wu and Craig (161) concluded that drug therapy plays the primary role in the induction and maintenance of remission in Crohn's disease, but that total parenteral nutrition may have an adjunctive role in achieving remission in steroid-refractory patients.

Total parenteral nutrition may support the severely nutritionally depleted patient but should not take the place of more definitive treatment.

Evans et al. (162) examined the safety and feasibility of providing short-term, in-home total parenteral nutrition (TPN) for patients with inflammatory bowel disease for whom the alternative is prolonged hospitalization or early operation. A quality-of-life phone interview was conducted at the time of review. Fifteen patients were identified whose average age was 35 years. The underlying diagnosis was Crohn's disease in 10 and ulcerative colitis in five. The indications for home TPN were complex internal fistulas, and resolving sepsis in two, postoperative septic complications (anastomotic leak/enterocutaneous fistula) in five, high output proximal stomas in four, prolonged ileus/partial obstruction in three, and spontaneous enterocutaneous fistula in one. The average duration of home TPN was 75 days (range, 7–240 days). Two patients (13%) failed home TPN (one with uncontrolled sepsis; one with dehydration) and were readmitted to hospital. Home TPN was discontinued in one patient whose enterocutaneous fistula failed to heal with nonoperative treatment. Home TPN was successful in 12 patients (80%): eight (53%) who underwent planned definitive operation and four (27%) whose conditions resolved without operation. Complications of home TPN were line sepsis and pulmonary aspergillosis in one patient. All patients preferred home TPN to further hospitalization and reported good or excellent qualify of life at home.

■ SMOKING CESSATION

Yamamoto and Keighley (163) reviewed the impact of smoking on disease recurrence after operation for Crohn's disease from 10 studies that examined the relationship between smoking and disease recurrence after operation. Approximately half of the patients were smokers at the time of operation. In most studies, smoking significantly increased the risk of postoperative disease recurrence. Smokers had an approximately twofold increased risk of recurrence compared with nonsmokers and the effect of smoking was dose-dependent. The increased risk of recurrence among smokers was more prominent in women than in men, and longer duration of smoking increased the risk of recurrence. Ex-smokers had a similar recurrence rate to nonsmokers and giving up smoking soon after operation was associated with a lower probability of recurrence. Encouraging patients to stop smoking is an important part of the management of Crohn's disease.

Ryan et al. (164) examined the impact of smoking, quitting smoking, and other factors on reoperation for recurrent Crohn's disease in 584 patients who had undergone an operation for ileocecal Crohn's disease. Smokers were more likely to have undergone one, two, and three reoperations for recurrence at any site [relative incidence risk (RIR): RIR 1.32; RIR 1.55; and RIR 1.77, respectively] and were more likely to have undergone one reoperation for recurrent ileocecal Crohn's disease (RIR 1.48). Patients who quit smoking were less likely to have undergone one, two, and three reoperations for recurrence at any site (RIR 0.25, RIR 0.30, and RIR 0.25, respectively) and were less likely to have undergone one reoperation for recurrent ileocecal Crohn's disease (RIR 0.27). This study also indicates that patients with ileocecal Crohn's disease who stop smoking reduce the risk of reoperation for recurrent Crohn's disease.

Johnson et al. (165) offered an updated review of the effects of smoking on Crohn's disease. Smokers with

Crohn's disease have a more aggressive disease requiring more therapeutic intervention. Smoking cessation is associated with a 65% reduction in the risk of relapse as compared with continued smokers, a similar magnitude to that obtained with immunosuppressive therapy. Although difficult to achieve, smoking cessation can best be encouraged by accessing appropriate counseling services, nicotine replacement therapy, and bupropion. Using a combination of these treatments there is an improved chance of success of up to 20% compared with an unassisted quit attempt. Smoking cessation unequivocally improves the course of Crohn's disease and should be a primary therapeutic aim in smokers with Crohn's disease.

■ PROBIOTICS

Antibiotics are often employed in the treatment of Crohn's disease. However, indiscriminate suppression of intestinal bacterial may be harmful and long-term use of antibiotics is burdened by side effects and by the risk of developing bacterial resistance. Manipulation of enteric flora with probiotic compounds would be a possible and appealing alternative. Prantera and Scribano (166) investigated the efficacy of probiotics in reducing the endoscopic recurrence rate or in reducing the severity of recurrent lesions at one year after operation. Forty-five patients were randomized to receive *Lactobacillus rhamnosus* strain GG or placebo for 12 months. The results showed no difference in endoscopic and clinical remission between the two groups.

Intestinal bacteria play a key role in inflammatory bowel disease. Probiotics attempt to modify disease by favorably altering bacterial composition, immune status, and inflammation. Some data exist that possibly show an efficacy of probiotics as maintenance therapy in chronic relapsing pouchitis. Obstacles to providing probiotic therapy include selection of appropriate strains, poor regulated probiotic quality standardization, processing and human biologic factors which impair probiotic viability, difficulty in maintaining new bacterial populations in the gut, and local product unavailability (167).

■ SUMMARY

Bebb and Scott (168) reviewed all placebo-controlled trials of the commonly used drugs in Crohn's disease for both the induction and maintenance of remission to determine the efficacy. Prednisolone/prednisone is the most effective drug to achieve remission with a remission rate of 60%. Aminosalicylates are only moderately effective in achieving remission, but more effective in high dose (e.g., Pentassa 4 g/day) and less effective in maintaining remission. Both azathioprine and infliximab are associated with remission induction and maintenance rates of 40% to 66%. Methotrexate intramuscularly has a remission induction rate of 39%.

In a review of article, Kamm (169) recently summarized the clinical management of Crohn's disease in relation to the treatment of acute disease and the maintenance of remission. The medication used to achieve these two goals may or may not be the same. Some patients with mildly active disease may respond to high-dose (4 g/day) mesalazine (mesalamine), and 5-ASA may also be helpful in weaning a patient off steroids after treatment for a flare up. However, the value of 5-ASA in maintaining remission in Crohn's disease remains controversial. Subgroups of patients may be helped, for example, patients with Crohn's disease who have experienced a relapse within the last two years may benefit. Steroids form the first-line therapy for acute episodes of inflammation but do not maintain remission. Azathioprine and mercaptopurine are the first-line drugs for the maintenance of remission in moderate to severe Crohn's disease, and by titrating the dose up from 2 mg/kg daily, some previously resistant patients will be brought into remission. One half of patients who do not tolerate azathioprine will tolerate mercaptopurine. Methotrexate is effective in inducing and maintaining remission, and is useful for patients who fail azathioprine treatment. Thalidomide is not proven in controlled studies, but two open studies have demonstrated its efficacy. The optimal dose, however, remains to be defined. Purified liquid diets with food exclusion can induce remission in patients with active disease, but food exclusion is difficult to maintain long-term. Infliximab can induce and maintain remission in patients resistant to other therapies, with two-thirds of patients initially responding to treatment. One-third go into remission and of those who respond to a single treatment approximately half maintain remission when treated regularly for a year. Infliximab is, however, associated with an increased risk of infection and its effect on carcinoma incidence is uncertain. The development of antibodies against the drug is associated with a loss of effect and allergic infusion reactions.

Guidelines for Medical Management

With the variety of agents available, no fixed regimen or algorithm can be constructed in the management of patients with Crohn's disease. Oftentimes, 5-ASA products are initially used for Crohn's colitis or ileocolitis. If no response, antibiotics may be added, usually metronidazole but also ciprofloxacin or tetracycline. Failing this, steroids are introduced and failing steroids, immunosuppressive agents are offered.

Hanauer and Meyers (20) reviewed the practice guidelines developed under the auspices of The American College of Gastroenterology. The following information has been extracted from their excellent review. Therapeutic recommendations depend on the disease location, severity, and complications. Therapeutic approaches are individualized according to the symptomatic response and tolerance to medical intervention. Therapy is divided into acute and maintenance phases. Operation is advocated for obstructing stenoses, suppurative complications, or medically intractable disease.

Mild to Moderate Active Crohn's Disease

This category applies to ambulatory patients able to tolerate oral alimentation without manifestations of dehydration, toxicity (high fevers, rigors), abdominal tenderness, painful mass, or obstruction. Ileal, ileocolonic, or colonic disease is treated with an oral aminosalicylate (sulfasalazine, 3 to 6 g/day, or mesalamine, 3.2 to 4.8 g/day in divided doses). Alternatively, metronidazole, 10 to 20 mg/kg/day, can be administered and may be effective in a proportion of patients not responding to sulfasalazine.

Moderate to Severe Disease

This category applies to patients who have failed to respond to treatment for mild to moderate disease or those with more prominent symptoms of fevers, significant weight loss (more than 10%), abdominal pain and tenderness (without rebound), intermittent nausea or vomiting (without obstructive findings), or significant anemia. After infection or abscess is excluded, patients with moderate to severe presentation are treated with prednisone, 40 to 60 mg/day, administered until resolution of symptoms and resumption of weight gain (generally 7 to 28 days). Infection or abscess requires appropriate antibiotic therapy or drainage (percutaneous or operative). Elemental diets may be an alternative to steroid therapy.

Severe to Fulminant Disease

This category refers to patients with persisting symptoms despite the introduction of steroids as an outpatient or individuals presenting with high fever, persistent vomiting, evidence of intestinal obstruction, rebound tenderness, cachexia, or evidence of an abscess. These patients should be hospitalized. Surgical consultation is indicated for patients with obstruction or tender abdominal mass. An abdominal mass should be evaluated via ultrasonography or CT to exclude an abscess. Abscesses require percutaneous or operative drainage. Once an abscess has been excluded or the patient has been receiving oral steroids, parenteral corticosteroids equivalent to 40 to 60 mg of prednisone are administered in divided doses or as a continuous infusion. There is no specific role for total parenteral nutrition in addition to steroids but nutritional support via elemental feeding or parenteral hyperalimentation is indicated for patients unable to tolerate an oral diet for more than five to seven days.

Remission

This category refers to patients who are asymptomatic or without inflammatory sequelae and includes patients who have responded to acute medical intervention or have undergone resections without gross residual disease. Patients requiring systemic steroids are usually not considered to be "in remission." Corticosteroids should not be used as long-term agents to prevent relapse of Crohn's disease. Mesalamine or azathioprine/6-MP do provide maintenance benefits and should be considered for patients responding to acute medical intervention. Mesalamine should also be considered to reduce the likelihood of recurrence after resection.

INDICATIONS FOR OPERATION

It is currently accepted that Crohn's disease is a pangastrointestinal disease and that recurrence can develop in any segment of the gastrointestinal tract. Therefore, the objectives of operative treatment are relief of symptoms, correction of complications, restoration of health and function when medical treatment has failed, prevention of development of carcinoma, and withdrawal of medications (steroids and immunosuppressive agents) or, succinctly stated, establishment of a normal quality of life.

When to operate on a patient with Crohn's disease has been a subject of controversy. Those who favor early operation argue that there is no benefit in prolonging the patient's suffering if medical treatment has shown no significant improvement and there is no virtue in waiting until serious complications develop. They claim good or fair results in approximately 90% of patients, with an overall 50% recurrence rate during the first 15 years of follow-up (170). Studies by Hulten (171) also showed that the disease itself was a more important factor in malnutrition than the loss of diseased bowel. Arguments against early operation relate to the fact that because recurrence and reoperation rates are high, postponing the operation or regarding operation as a last resort will result in fewer resections and thus the chance of developing short bowel syndrome becomes less likely.

Edna et al. (172) analyzed the annual incidence of laparotomy for Crohn's disease in a defined population in Middle Norway in a retrospective study of 102 consecutive abdominal operations for Crohn's disease in 74 patients. The median follow-up after the primary operation was 6.2 years. The number of operations increased for every five-year period: the corresponding annual incidence rates for primary operations from 1975 were 0.2, 1.9, 3.3, 4.7, and 5.4 per 100,000 inhabitants. The Vienna classification divided this purely surgical material into meaningful groups.

Sands et al. (173) aimed to define the rate of early operation for Crohn's disease and to identify risk factors associated with early operation. Of 345 eligible patients, 69 (20.1%) required operation within three years of diagnosis excluding the 14 patients (4.1%) who had major operations at the time of diagnosis. Overall, the interval between diagnosis and operation was short; one half of all patients who required operation underwent their operation within six months of diagnosis. Risk factors identified as significantly associated with early operation included the following: smoking; disease of small bowel without colonic involvement; nausea and vomiting or abdominal pain on presentation; neutrophil count; and steroid use in the first six months. Disease localized to the colon only, blood in the stool, use of 5-ASA and lymphocyte count were inversely associated with risk of early operation.

The timing of the decision for operation in Crohn's disease is based on an evaluation of the symptom severity of the disease, medical treatment failure or side effects, and perceptions of operative risk. Optimal evaluation of these competing factors should result in operation timed to the patient's best advantage, achieving maximal relief of symptoms with minimal operative disadvantage. The timing of the decision to perform intestinal resection for Crohn's disease is strongly influenced by the patient's medical advisers. A factor probably not considered often enough is the patient's view with these variables in mind. Scott and Hughes (174) asked 80 patients if they would have preferred their ileocolonic resection and anastomosis for Crohn's disease to be carried out sooner, later, or at the same time that it was done. Seventy of the patients replied (88%). No patient preferred their operation to have been later, while 74% thought it should have been earlier. A preferred operation time was given to 69 resections, between zero months, that is, at the same time, and 15 years earlier. The median preferred operation time was 12 months earlier (7 to 18 months earlier). The remaining 18 patients were satisfied with the timing of their operation. Reasons given for earlier operation in 58 resections included the severity of Crohn's symptoms preoperatively (97%), the ability to eat normally after resection (86%), feeling of well-being after the resection (62%), and abolishing the need for drugs (43%). Patients preferring an earlier operation time were less likely to have had a previous resection than patients in the "same time" group.

Regardless of one's philosophy, it is inappropriate to proceed to operation before an adequate trial of medical management has been given enough time to work. Similarly, it is a mistake to delay operation until serious complications have developed. Unfortunately, it is these complications that comprise many of the indications for operation.

■ INTRACTABILITY TO MEDICAL TREATMENT

As with ulcerative colitis, intractability is the most common indication for the operative treatment of Crohn's disease at the present time. Of course, the definition of intractability is clearly not the same for all treating physicians or indeed for patients.

■ BOWEL OBSTRUCTION

Obstruction, particularly of the small bowel, can be caused by the inflammatory process of active Crohn's disease, a fibrotic stricture from chronic disease, or an abscess or phlegmon causing a mass effect. In the absence of an obvious abscess, the initial management should be medical, but if there is no response to treatment, urgent or emergent operation may become necessary.

The initial treatment of acute obstruction should be bowel rest, intravenous fluids, and steroids. The rationale of the latter is that obstruction is due, at least in part, to inflammation and edema. With repeated obstruction, chronic fibrosis may result and operative relief will be required, although emergency operation is rarely necessary. Other causes of obstruction might include an impacted food bolus or an unrecognized malignancy. If the patients have had a previous laparotomy, adhesions may be the causative factor.

The operative indication for patients with obstruction may be modified by the possibility of balloon dilatation. Intestinal strictures associated with Crohn's disease may occur in "virgin" bowel or as an anastomotic stricture. Efforts to treat this problem without an operation have included balloon dilatation, which has met with mixed results. Lavy (175) treated 10 patients (five with strictures of the left colon and five anastomotic strictures after ileotransversostomy) with dilatation followed by injection of 40 mg of triamcinolone with a sclerotherapy needle. With a follow-up of 1.5 to 3 years, two patients required additional dilatation and injection one year later, while the other eight patients remained well. This treatment may diminish the need for operative procedures.

In Crohn's disease, multiple areas of small bowel stenosis are relatively common, but there are only 11 reported cases with stenosis complicated by enterolithiasis. Yuan et al. (176) described three patients with multiple strictures, enterolithiasis, and refractory iron-deficiency anemia. The chronic anemia was severe, requiring multiple transfusions in two patients. One patient developed a perforation and a second had carcinoma within one of the saccular dilatations between strictures. Management of this stricture-enterolith-anemia triad requires removal of the enteroliths and correction of the strictures by strictureplasty and/or resection. If the operation of choice is strictureplasty, however, meticulous inspection and biopsy of each proposed site of enteroplasty is essential to rule out carcinoma. Others have also described enterolothic intestinal obstruction in Crohn's disease (177).

■ INTRA-ABDOMINAL ABSCESS

An intra-abdominal abscess associated with Crohn's disease is usually the result of a sealed perforation of the bowel. At present, most patients with this condition do not require exploratory celiotomy because CT-guided percutaneous drainage is highly successful in combination with the administration of antibiotics. If percutaneous drainage is not feasible, or if the sepsis cannot be controlled and the patient's condition deteriorates, an exploratory celiotomy and bowel resection should be performed.

Procaccino et al. (178) conducted a retrospective analysis in an effort to determine optimal operative therapy for psoas abscess. Forty patients were cured with one operation. Twenty-one patients required two operations, four patients required three operations, and two patients required more than three operations. The reason for failure of treatment was failure to resect the diseased bowel or to drain the psoas abscess adequately. The most common etiologies were Crohn's disease in 49 patients, postoperative sepsis in eight patients, and complications of renal disease in four patients. There were two deaths. Failure to recognize and treat psoas abscess results in considerable morbidity.

Garcia et al. (179) compared the long-term outcome of medical, percutaneous, and surgical treatment of abdominal and pelvic abscesses complicating Crohn's disease. Fifty-one subjects were identified with a mean follow-up of 3.8 years. Fewer patients developed recurrent abscesses after initial surgical drainage and bowel resection (12%) than patients treated with medical therapy only or percutaneous drainage (56%). One half of the patients treated nonoperatively ultimately required operation, whereas only 12% of those treated with initial operation required reoperation during the follow-up period. Most failures of nonoperative therapy occurred within three months. In this series operative management of abscesses in Crohn's disease was more effective than medical treatment or percutaneous drainage for prevention of abscess recurrence.

Yamaguchi et al. (180) elucidated the incidence and natural course of abdominal abscess complicating Crohn's disease. Of 352 patients with Crohn's disease, 35 patients (9.9%) had abscesses. The cumulative incidence of complication with an abscess was 9% and 25%, respectively, 10 and 20 years after Crohn's disease onset. Of the 35 Crohn's disease patients with abscess, 60% had an operation prior to the present study. The age when the abscess developed was 30.1 years and the duration of illness from the onset of Crohn's disease until development of an abscess was 10.8 years (range, 0–29 years). The location of involvement was: abdominal wall (40%); peritoneal cavity (29%); retroperitoneal or ileopsoas (26%); and subphrenic region (6%). In terms of location of abscess, it occurred most often on the right side (65.7%). Almost all abscesses occurred near the site of an anastomosis. Diseased segments of the bowel responsible for the abscess formation were categorized radiographically as showing mild stenosis (6.5%), intermediate stenosis and/or simple fistula (41.9%), and severe stenosis and/or multiple fistulas (51.6%). Conservative treatment (including drainage of abscess alone was effective in seven patients (20%) and operation was needed in 28 patients (80%). During the 5.3 year follow-up after treatment for the abdominal abscess, 26% of patients had recurrence of an abscess mostly within three years.

■ INTERNAL FISTULA

Because of its transmural nature, Crohn's disease of the small bowel and the large bowel frequently adheres to adjacent organs, such as urinary bladder, bowel, uterus, vagina, and stomach. With progression of active disease, subsequent erosion into these organs may give rise to a fistula. Approximately 32% to 35% of patients with Crohn's disease have developed an internal fistula, and most of these patients have Crohn's disease, of the small intestine (181). Uncomplicated enteroenteric fistulas require no operation. Ileosigmoid fistulas generally arise due to diseased terminal ileum. Management depends on symptoms and whether there is primary involvement of the sigmoid colon. Asymptomatic patients require no operation. Symptomatic patients should undergo a terminal ileal resection and closure of sigmoid if it is secondarily involved or sigmoid resection if it is primarily involved. Enterovesical fistulas are treated by resection of diseased bowel (usually terminal ileum) with closure of bladder and interposition of omentum between bladder repair and enteric suture line. Gastric fistulas in Crohn's disease are very rare. Greenstein et al. (182) found six cases of cologastric fistula among 907 patients with Crohn's disease (0.6%) and one case of ileogastric fistula among 1211 patients with ileal disease (0.08%). Recommended therapy is colon or ileal resection with wedge excision of the stomach.

Sachar et al. (183) sought to determine the association between perianal and intestinal fistulization by analyzing the cases of Crohn's disease recorded in databases from six international centers totaling 5491 cases of Crohn's disease in the United States, France, Italy, and The Netherlands. Among the 1686 cases with isolated ileal disease, the evidence of an association between perianal disease and internal fistulization was not consistent across centers, with relative risks ranging from 0.8 to 2.2. For patients with Crohn's colitis ($n = 1655$), the association was much stronger and more consistent with an estimated common relative risk of 3.4.

Lavy and Yasin (184) treated enterocutaneous fistulas using somatostatin. Five patients with Crohn's disease were treated with four daily injections of 300 μg octreotide. The total period of treatment was eight weeks. Closure of fistulas was achieved in four of the five patients. They believe somatostatin may have a role in treating Crohn's disease enterocutaneous fistulas and may prevent operation or prolonged immunosuppressive therapy.

Solem et al. (185) described the clinical features and outcomes of patients with fistulas to the urinary system in Crohn's disease. A total of 78 patients (56% men) were identified. Patients presented with pneumaturia (68%), dysuria (64%), recurrent urinary tract infections (32%), and fecaluria (28%). Cystoscopy and CT of the abdomen/pelvis had the highest diagnostic yield (74% and 52%, respectively). Fistulas originated from the ileum (64%), colon (21%), rectum (8%), and multiple sites (7%). Urinary tract sites included bladder (88%), urethra (6%), urachus (3%), ureter (1%), and other (1%). Median follow-up was 1.1 year (0–22.3 years). A total of 70 patients (90%) had operation, with medical treatment first attempted in four patients with antibiotics and/or immunosuppressants. One patient had adequate symptom relief without operation on antibiotic suppression alone. Six patients required a partial cystectomy but no patient had a cystectomy or nephrectomy. Only three surgical patients had recurrent urinary system fistulas.

Of 213 patients undergoing surgical treatment for Crohn's disease, Ikeuchi et al. (186) found 55 patients (25.8%) to have 81 intra-abdominal fistulas. The most common indication for operation was intestinal obstruction. A fistula represented a single indication for operative treatment in nine patients (15.5%). All patients with intra-abdominal fistulas underwent resection of the diseased intestinal segment. Only one patient died postoperatively from multiple organ failure because of anastomotic breakdown.

Khanna and Gordon (187) reported a case of a patient who had a gastro-colic fistula secondary to Crohn's disease and it is from their review of the literature that the following information has been obtained. Development of a gastro-colic fistula secondary to Crohn's disease is thought to be a result of colitis in the transverse colon with deep ulceration and subsequent fibrosis and fistula formation to the adjacent stomach. Hence, it has been suggested that the correct term for the fistula would be "colonogastric" fistula. The classic triad of symptoms in patients with colonogastric fistulas secondary to Crohn's disease comprises diarrhea, weight loss, and fecal halitosis or vomiting, but is only present in 30% of cases. Diarrhea, weight loss, and abdominal pain are seen in approximately 50% of patients with Crohn's-related colonogastric fistulas but these symptoms can easily be attributed to an uncomplicated exacerbation of the underlying disease process. Hence, it is very difficult to determine the presence of a colonogastric fistula based on history alone. The presence of feculent vomiting or fecal halitosis, which is pathognomonic of a colonogastric fistula, may help in the diagnosis. The symptoms associated with Crohn's-related colonogastric fistulas are thought to be secondary to reflux of the colonic contents through the fistulous tract with secondary injury to the upper gastrointestinal tract. This retrograde flow of fecal material may result in bacterial overgrowth and be responsible for the debilitating diarrhea and malnutrition that occur with a colonogastric fistula. Vitamin B_{12} malabsorption may occur. Physical findings in a patient with a colonogastric fistula usually include malnourishment and dehydration. Abdominal findings are often nonspecific and minimal; findings may be limited to diffuse abdominal tenderness and distention. Laboratory indices are also nonspecific and also limited to electrolyte abnormalities related to vomiting and diarrhea plus anemia, hypoproteinemia and avitaminoses secondary to the patient's malnourished state. Plain films of the abdomen are usually nonspecific. The diagnosis of a colonogastric fistula is usually confirmed by a barium enema, which is reported to have close to 100% diagnostic accuracy in revealing the fistula. Upper gastrointestinal barium study is only effective in disclosing colonogastric fistulas in approximately one quarter to one-third of the cases; this is likely because the fistulous opening is usually so small that contrast material preferentially passes through the pyloric channel as the stomach empties by antral contraction. Although esophogastroduodenoscopy and colonoscopy do not demonstrate the fistula well, these examinations are essential preoperatively because they delineate the extent and severity of the disease and hence provide useful information on which the surgeon can base a decision as to the type of resection required. Medical therapy may play a role in managing Crohn's-related colonogastric fistulas. Greenstein and associates (188) reported that two patients in their series became asymptomatic and showed radiologic closure of the fistulas with prolonged courses of 6-MP. In light of today's enthusiasm for infliximab in the treatment of fistulous disease, there may be a role for this agent. However, it is generally accepted that operation is the definitive treatment for colonogastric fistula. In the severely debilitated patient, a two-stage procedure with a proximal diverting stoma has been advised but a preoperative course of intravenous hyperalimentation for the severely malnourished patient may obviate this. In terms of the type of operation, a variety of procedures have been recommended, depending on the extent of the disease. Most authors advocate resection of the diseased colon and excision and primary repair of the fistulous opening. In some cases, because of the size of the fistula or significant involvement of the stomach, gastric wedge resection of the fistula or a partial gastrectomy may be required.

■ COLOCUTANEOUS AND ENTEROCUTANEOUS FISTULA

The process of colocutaneous or enterocutaneous fistula is similar to that of internal fistula in which the diseased bowel adheres to the abdominal wall and invades through the skin or an abscess breaks through the skin. Most spontaneous fistulas are due to ileal rather than colonic disease. Enterocutaneous fistulas commonly follow operation and generally represent recurrent disease. Bowel rest and antibiotics are often the initial therapy. Once the fistula has developed, urgent operation is seldom required unless associated with sepsis, but the fistula rarely heals without resection. Nevertheless, in some cases it is worthwhile to try treatment with hyperalimentation or immunosuppressants.

Hill et al. (189) meticulously defined the principles of surgical and metabolic management of patients with external small bowel fistulas in association with Crohn's disease. A consecutive series of 85 patients (26 with Crohn's disease) was studied. In 69 of the 85 patients (82%), successful closure of the fistula was achieved (36 spontaneously and 33 operatively), and the mortality rate was 16%. The overall results were similar for Crohn's patients, except that spontaneous closure occurred significantly less often (in 4 of 26 patients). Two distinct types of Crohn's fistula were observed. In 10 patients, the fistula arose in the early postoperative period and was not associated with residual Crohn's disease. The pattern of behavior and overall results of treatment of these patients were the same as for non-Crohn's patients. In 16 patients whose fistula arose from an area of Crohn's disease (six postoperatively and 10 spontaneously after discharge of an abscess), spontaneous closure was not observed. Operation was undertaken in 15 of these patients and was successful in 14. One patient died. Studies of body stores of protein showed that massive losses (2% per day) occurred in patients in whom sepsis was uncontrolled, despite intravenous nutrition. Although the total energy expenditure of Crohn's patients was no different from that of non-Crohn's patients (45 kcal/kg/day), studies of total body protein while the patients were being given intravenous nutrition showed that, when active Crohn's disease remained in situ, the expected increase in body protein stores of approximately 1 kg did not occur. The authors concluded that fistulas unassociated with residual Crohn's disease should be managed along conventional lines. Those fistulas arising from diseased small intestine also require operation. This is performed after sepsis has been drained, metabolic deficits (but not necessarily deficits of body protein) have been corrected, and the anatomy of the fistula has been defined. The operative procedure involves resection of the bowel involved and performance of a primary anastomosis.

Poritz et al. (190) presented the results of surgical management of entero- and colocutaneous fistulas associated with Crohn's disease in 51 patients (56 operative procedures). Previous operation for Crohn's disease had been carried out in 84% of patients. The fistula site was enterocutaneous in 64% of patients, colocutaneous in 21% and anastomotic in 14%; another 16% had associated enteroenteric fistulas. The onset of the fistula followed abscess drainage in 27% and occurred at the site of recurrent disease in 73%. Initially 71% of patients underwent conservative management prior to operation; 28% underwent operation directly. Surgical procedures were: 25 ileocolic resections, eight stoma revisions with resection, eight small bowel resections, seven subtotal colectomies, four partial colectomies, three proctocolectomies, and one fistula tract excision. Postoperative complications occurred in 11% of patients. Mean follow-up was 48.6 months. Recurrence as defined by either clinical examination or reoperation was documented in 16% of patients, with a mean time to recurrence of 27 months. They concluded that entero- and colocutaneous fistulas usually occur from a site of active disease. Operative management with bowel resection, including the fistula, is the preferred method of treatment.

■ FULMINANT COLITIS

Similar to ulcerative colitis, fulminant colitis is treated vigorously with intravenous fluids and electrolytes, high doses of intravenous corticosteroids, and broad-spectrum antibiotics. Urgent operation should be performed within 24 hours if the patient's condition deteriorates and within five days if there is no significant improvement.

Olsen and Gilbert (191) reviewed the subject of cytomegaloviras (CMV) infection and Crohn's colitis and the following information was taken from their review. CMV infection can complicate both ulcerative colitis and Crohn's disease. The virus belongs to the herpes family and 40% to 100% of the adult population has been infected. Most infections are subclinical and lead to lifelong latency. However, in immunocompromised individuals such as transplant recipients and AIDS patients, the virus can cause severe disease. The prevalence of CMV complicated colitis in patients with inflammatory bowel disease has been estimated at 0.53% to 4% but in patients presenting with severe steroid refractive Crohn's disease, it is thought to be much higher at 11% to 36%. Clinical pointers to viral complication include persistent severe hypokalemia, high spiking pyrexia, lymphadenopathy, and bone marrow suppression but such features are also seen in patients with uncomplicated severe steroid-resistant Crohn's colitis. The recommendation means of diagnosis is histologic examination of biopsies from the affected mucosa and ulcer beds. Serological tests and virus isolation from blood or feces do not prove colonic infection. With early diagnosis, some patients with CMV infection superimposed on colonic disease might be spared operation. When CMV infection is found to be complicating Crohn's colitis, steroid treatment should be reduced, other immunomodulatory treatments stopped, and ganciclovir 10 to 15 mg/kg daily in divided doses given for two to three weeks. Such treatment has reduced emergency colectomy rates from 80% to 33% and case fatality from 33% to 5% in patients with severe steroid-refractory inflammatory bowel disease complicated by CMV. However, about one-fifth of patients so treated need colectomy within three months because the underlying bowel disease has become reactivated or the viral infection has persisted.

■ TOXIC MEGACOLON

This condition can occur in both ulcerative colitis and Crohn's disease. The reader is referred to the discussion of toxic megacolon in Chapter 26.

■ FREE PERFORATION

Free perforation of small bowel Crohn's disease occurs in 1% of cases but some reports are higher because of incorporation of ruptured abscess and colonic perforation (192). A similar incidence of 1% to 3% occurs in Crohn's disease of the large bowel (193,194). Once this condition has been diagnosed, emergency operation must be performed and the perforated bowel resected, usually a small bowel resection or subtotal colectomy and ileostomy with peritoneal lavage. Greenstein et al. (195) noted a 3.8% mortality following resection and anastomosis in 52 patients. Survival of 100% was reported in 18 patients treated by resection and exteriorization. Primary anastomosis may be appropriate for small bowel but the clinical decision will depend on the degree of contamination, the state of the bowel ends, general nutritional status, and the absence of distal obstruction.

Veroux et al. (196) evaluated the incidence of free peritoneal perforation among 208 patients with Crohn's disease surgically treated. Five patients (2.4%) suffered from free peritoneal perforation. In one patient, free peritoneal perforation was the first symptom of Crohn's disease. In three cases, the perforation was in the small bowel and in two in the large bowel. All cases had a resection of the involved bowel and in two cases an ileostomy was performed in order to prevent severe peritonitis. There was neither mortality nor major complications. In their review, they found 100 cases of free peritoneal perforation. No correlation seemed to exist with previous corticosteroid treatment. The most appropriate treatment is resection of the involved bowel with immediate or in case of severe sepsis delayed anastomosis.

Werbin et al. (197) evaluated the incidence and treatment results of free perforation in 160 patients with Crohn's disease and followed for a mean period of five years. Of the 83 patients (52%) requiring operative intervention, 13 (15.6%) were operated due to free perforation. The mean age of the perforated Crohn's disease was 33 years and the mean duration of symptoms prior to operation was six years. The location of the free perforation was the terminal ileum in 10 patients, the mid ileum in two patients, and the left colon in one patient. Operative treatment included 10 ileocecectomies, two segmental resections of small bowel, and resection of left colon with transverse colostomy and mucus fistula in one patient. There was no operative mortality and mean postoperative hospital stay was 21 days. All patients were followed for a mean of 58 months. Six patients (42%) required a second operation during the follow-up period.

Ikeuchi et al. (198) investigated the characteristics of free perforation in Japanese patients with Crohn's disease. They reviewed the data for 104 patients with free perforation in Crohn's disease reported in the Japanese literature, in addition to 22 patients from their hospital. There were 89 men and 37 women with ages ranging from 16 to 92 years. Free perforation was the presenting sign of the disease in 72 patients. The perforation sites were the jejunum in seven, the ileum in 102, and the colon in 17. Multiple perforations occurred in 13 patients. Steroid therapy was administered in 25 patients, but the relationship between steroid therapy and free perforation had not been well established. The incidence of free perforation in Crohn's disease in Japan was between 2.9% and 10.5%. This incidence was higher than that in Western countries. Ninety-eight patients were treated with resection and drainage, and 22 patients with resection and diversion (details not known in six patients). There were no patients with simple closure of the perforation site. Anastomotic rupture occurred in 13 patients. Five patients died after the operation. Four of the five patients had multiple perforations.

Freeman (199) reported 15 new cases of spontaneous free perforation of the small intestine—nine female patients and six male patients—in a series of 1000 consecutively evaluated patients with Crohn's disease seen during the period spanning 20 years, for an estimated frequency of 1.5%. Spontaneous free perforation was the presenting clinical feature of Crohn's disease in nine (60%) of the newly discovered cases. Most perforations were located in the ileum rather than in the jejunum, and there were no duodenal perforations. One patient with extensive intestinal disease presented with concomitant free perforations of the jejunum and ileum, while a second patient had two free ileal perforations that developed independently, separated by about six years. No perforations were the result of a superimposed malignant process, i.e., adenocarcinoma or lymphoma. There have been no mortalities, and the subsequent clinical course of these patients has been limited to a minority requiring corticosteroid or immunosuppressive medications, or further resections.

■ MASSIVE BLEEDING

Massive bleeding caused by Crohn's disease has been reported to occur in 1% to 13% of patients (200). The site of the bleeding should be established and may require the investigations described in Chapter 35.

Cirocco et al. (201) identified four patients of 631 admissions (0.6%) for Crohn's disease with life-threatening gastrointestinal hemorrhage. These and 34 similar cases from the medical literature were reviewed to provide a composite of those at risk and elucidate appropriate diagnostic and therapeutic maneuvers. The study revealed a preponderance of young men (2:1) with an average age of 35 years (range, 14–89 years), the majority of whom (60%) had had Crohn's disease for an average of 4.6 years (range, 0–18 years). The site of bleeding resembled the general distribution for Crohn's disease, with small bowel disease predominating (66% involved the ileum). The five cases of exsanguination (13% of the total) were all men with known Crohn's disease (average, 5.8 years) involving the ileum alone or in part. Mesenteric arteriography was positive in 17 patients, providing precise preoperative localization resulting in no mortality in this group. Excluding those who presented with exsanguination, operation was necessary to cease hemorrhage in 91% of patients (30 of 33). Ileocolectomy was the most frequently performed procedure (53%). In follow-up, only one patient (3.5%) required further resection for recurrent bleeding, and two other patients (7%) required further therapy for nonhemorrhagic recurrence.

Kostka and Lukas (202) reported on the clinical features and course of bleeding in six of 156 patients with Crohn's disease. The six patients consisted of three males and three females, ranging in age from 17 to 42 years. Three patients were known to have Crohn's disease, whereas three presented with acute bleeding as the initial symptoms of Crohn's disease. There were 11 separate episodes of severe hemorrhage: three patients bled only once, two bled twice, and one bled four times. The precise bleeding site was correctly identified in four of eleven episodes: twice by colonoscopy and twice by angiography. Primary bleeding episodes subsided without operation in four of six patients, but three of these four patients rebled massively, and operation followed in two of these cases. An emergency operation was necessary to stop hemorrhage in four patients; two of them underwent operation during their first hemorrhagic episode, and two patients underwent operation during a repeated episode of hemorrhage. As a consequence, one ileectomy and three ileocolectomies had to be performed. During the follow-up of the resected patients, no recurrence of hemorrhagic or nonhemorrhagic Crohn's disease was observed in three patients, two, five, and six years after operation and only one patient required further therapy three years after operation for recurrent bleeding. For this, super selective embolization of a peripheral branch of the superior mesenteric artery was used. Two nonresected patients are doing well in a course of remission. They concluded that a conservative approach may be suggested as the first-line therapy, but operation is inevitable in patients suffering from massive bleeding and in patients with recurrent bleeding.

Veroux et al. (203) characterized the clinical features and course of acute gastrointestinal bleeding in Crohn's disease at their institution. Five patients had gastrointestinal bleeding with a mean duration of the Crohn's disease of six years. The source of bleeding was identified in four patients (80%). Endoscopy was, in all patients, the first diagnostic procedure. A Hartmann total colectomy with closure of the rectal stump and ileostomy was performed in three patients, while two patients with ileal massive bleeding were treated conservatively. One patient had a recurrence of bleeding from the small bowel one week later but didn't require operative treatment. One patient with pancolonic Crohn's disease died on the 10th postoperative day because of multiorgan failure and septic complications. Recurrent hemorrhage should be an appropriate indication for operation.

Belaiche et al. (204) defined epidemiological characteristics and therapeutic options of hemorrhagic forms of Crohn's disease in 34 cases. Acute lower gastrointestinal hemorrhage defined as acute rectal bleeding originating in diseased bowel and requiring a transfusion of at least two units of red blood cells within 24 hours. Upper gastrointestinal tract hemorrhage or anal lesions and postoperative bleeding were excluded. Mean age at time of hemorrhage was 34.2 years. Mean duration of disease before the hemorrhage was 5.6 years. The hemorrhage occurred during a flare up of the disease in 35% of cases. The hemorrhage was more frequent in colonic disease (85%) than in isolated small bowel disease (15%). The origin of bleeding was identified in 65% of cases, by colonoscopy (60%), by angiography (three patients) or at operation (one patient). The bleeding lesion was an ulcer in 95% of cases, most often in the left colon. The treatment was surgical in 20.5% (colectomy in 36%), endoscopical (seven patients, including five successes), or medical. Hemorrhage recurred in 12 patients (35%) within a mean time of three years (four days to eight years) requiring operation in three cases. No deaths were observed.

Gastrointestinal bleeding in patients with Crohn's disease presents both a diagnostic and therapeutic challenge. The bleeding site may be difficult to localize preoperatively and multiple segments of gross disease can lead to uncertainty as to the precise source at the time of laparotomy. Remzi et al. (205) described the combined use of provocative angiography and highly selective methylene blue injection preoperatively to accurately identify the site of hemorrhage and direct bowel resection. Methylene blue, injected distally into the bleeding vessel during angiography stains the bowel at the bleeding site. This allows the bleeding lesion to be removed with a limited resection thus preserving bowel length.

■ CARCINOMA PREVENTION

The risk of carcinoma in long-standing Crohn's disease is well established but prophylactic operation does not appear warranted. Patients with chronic and active Crohn's colitis require periodic surveillance through colonoscopy and biopsy. Dysplasia is frequently seen when a malignancy is present, both in remote and adjacent mucosa. In small bowel Crohn's disease, upper gastrointestinal and small bowel follow-through barium studies should be obtained. A stricture in long-standing Crohn's disease should be considered a possible sign of carcinoma. A bypassed segment of Crohn's disease should be resected if possible.

CARCINOMA

Similar to carcinoma associated with ulcerative colitis, carcinoma occurring with Crohn's disease tends to demonstrate aggressive histologic features (206). The prognosis is directly related to the stage of the disease at the time of operative treatment.

EXTRACOLONIC MANIFESTATIONS

Most extracolonic manifestations—except primary sclerosing cholangitis, which is rare with Crohn's disease, cirrhosis, and ankylosing spondylitis—improve after the diseased bowel has been removed. If medical treatment fails to improve the symptoms, operation should be considered.

GROWTH RETARDATION

Severe growth retardation is an important indication for operation. Timing of the operation is of the essence because operation must be conducted prior to puberty and closure of the epiphyses. Otherwise, catch-up growth will not occur.

OVERVIEW

The frequency of indications for operation for Crohn's disease varies from center-to-center depending on the referral patterns of that particular institution. In a report by Anseline (15), indications for operation were chronic obstruction, 43%; phlegmon/abscess, 12%; fistula, 3%; bleeding, 1%; fulminant colitis, 22%; and chronic colitis, 29%. For patients with Crohn's colitis, the primary indication for the initial operation in a series of 166 patients at the Cleveland Clinic was internal fistulas and abscesses, 25%; perianal disease, 23%; chronic ill health, 21%; toxic megacolon, 19%; and intestinal obstruction, 12% (207).

INTERVENTIONAL OPTIONS AND THEIR RESULTS

ILEOCECAL RESECTION

Hulten (171) summarized the concerns regarding the operative treatment of Crohn's disease of the small bowel or ileocecum. He cited three disadvantages. They are as follows:

1. It often causes a fair amount of operative morbidity and mortality, especially when performed in the presence of septic complications. To reduce these immediate hazards, a strong case can certainly be made for an earlier resort to operation before the onset of such complications.
2. It is followed by a high incidence of recurrence of the disease, amounting to about 50% by 10 years. Claims that the risk of recurrence can be reduced by using a more radical type of resection have not been substantiated. Fortunately, recurrences can usually be excised with no increased likelihood of further recurrence, and by a combination of resection and re-resection as required, many patients can be afforded prolonged periods of symptomatic relief.
3. Normal intestinal absorption is impaired, especially after major or repeated resections of the small bowel. The consequences are diarrhea and possible hematologic and nutritional disturbances and a predisposition to the formation of biliary and urinary calculi. But even a loss of up to 50% of the entire small intestine is often compatible with a reasonably good state of general health, particularly if most of the colon has been preserved. Fortunately, such extensive intestinal losses are rare, even after two or three resections.

Traditional therapy for patients with terminal ileitis found at laparotomy for appendicitis has been to perform appendectomy when the cecum is normal and to leave the diseased ileum in place. Weston et al. (208) assessed the role of ileocolic resection in the setting of acute ileitis by reviewing the records of 1421 patients with Crohn's disease. Crohn's disease was found at laparotomy for presumed appendicitis in 36 patients (2.5%). Ten patients underwent ileocolic resection, 23 had appendectomy, and three had exploratory laparotomy alone. After initial ileocolic resection, five patients (50%) required no further resection, with a mean follow-up time of 12.4 years (range, 4–19 years). Of 26 patients treated traditionally, 24 (92%) required ileocolic resection for intractability or complications of Crohn's disease. Thirty-eight percent required resection within one year and 65% within three years (intractability in eight, obstruction in three, fistula in four, and perforation in two). Of 24 patients who subsequently underwent resection, only six (25%) required further small bowel resection for Crohn's disease with a mean follow-up time of 13 years (range, 0.1–34 years). The authors concluded that the majority of patients found to have Crohn's disease at laparotomy for appendicitis required early ileocolic resection. Therefore, the traditional dictum of nonoperative therapy for these patients may not be in their best long-term interest and merits reevaluation.

Andersen and Kehlet (209) assessed the outcome with multimodal rehabilitation in 32 consecutive ileocolic resections for Crohn's disease in 29 patients who received epidural analgesia and enforced postoperative oral nutrition and mobilization with a scheduled stay of two days. Median time to defecation was 2.5 days and postoperative hospital stay was three days. During a 30-day postoperative follow-up, there were two readmissions, one for mechanical bowel obstruction and one because of fever and vomiting. Complications included one wound abscess, one cystitis, and one pneumonia.

Resegotti et al. (210) conducted a study to determine whether a side-to-side stapled ileocolonic anastomosis produces fewer anastomotic leaks than those with a hand-sewn end-to-end ileocolonic anastomosis in 122 consecutive patients undergoing elective ileocecal or ileocolonic resection for Crohn's disease: 71 had hand-sewn end-to-end anastomosis and 51 had side-to-side stapled anastomosis. The choice between the two anastomoses was left to the surgeon's preference. In the hand-sewn group, there were 14.1% anastomotic leaks and in the stapled group there was a 2% anastomotic leak. Mortality was 1.4% in the hand-sewn group and 0% in the stapled group. Complications other than anastomotic leak developed in 11 patients in the hand-sewn and in six patients in the stapled group. Mean postoperative hospital stay was 12.3 days in the hand-sewn group and 9.7 days in the stapled group. Although confirmation from randomized controlled trials is required, side-to-side anastomosis seems to substantially decrease anastomotic leaks in surgical patients with Crohn's disease compared with hand-sewn end-to-end anastomosis.

■ TOTAL PROCTOCOLECTOMY AND ILEOSTOMY

Total proctocolectomy and ileostomy remains the "gold standard" operative treatment when Crohn's disease involves the entire colon and rectum or if fecal incontinence is too severe to preserve the rectum. This operation eliminates the large bowel disease completely. It is not indicated in the acutely ill patient except for the very rare occurrence of a rectal perforation or profuse hemorrhage. Operative mortality for this procedure has ranged from 1.5% to 4% (211). However, recurrence still can develop in the small bowel. In a series reported by Goligher (212), 162 patients with Crohn's disease were followed up for a mean period of 15 years (range, 7–25 years) after this operation, and recurrence was detected in 15%. The frequency of recurrence has reportedly ranged from 3.3% to 46% (211). A most important factor influencing the incidence of recurrence is the length of follow-up, with a cumulative recurrence rate of 5% at 1 year after operation to roughly 20% at 12 years (211). Approximately 90% of recurrences develop in the distal ileum within 25 cm of the ileostomy (213).

Another relatively common problem with this operation is the perineal wound. In a survey of 144 patients who underwent total proctocolectomy for Crohn's disease, Goligher (212) found perineal wound healing to be straightforward in 62% of patients, delayed but eventually complete in 28%, and very troublesome in 10%. The technique of total proctocolectomy and ileostomy is the same as for ulcerative colitis (see Chapter 26).

Goligher (211) stressed the important point that an ileostomy constructed in association with a total proctocolectomy or subtotal colectomy for Crohn's disease is quite different from that performed in conjunction with the same operation for ulcerative colitis in that it is frequently sited at a higher level in the small bowel due to the necessity to resect a variable amount of terminal ileum implicated in the disease process. Several consequences may arise. First, absorption of fluid and electrolytes from the lower ileum may be less efficient with a tendency to electrolyte depletion. The replacement of fluid, electrolytes, and nutrition may be required. Second, the major site of vitamin B12 absorption is the lower ileum and resection may require need for replacement. Finally, the lower ileum is also the site of bile acid reabsorption and resection may predispose to cholesterol gallstone formation.

■ SUBTOTAL COLECTOMY WITH CLOSURE OF RECTAL OR SIGMOID STUMP OR MUCOUS FISTULA AND ILEOSTOMY

This operation removes most of the colonic disease, but the part of the disease found in the rectum or sigmoid colon remains. It is suitable for severe colonic disease in very ill patients who require urgent operation, in patients with toxic dilatation or fulminant colitis, in patients who might be candidates for an ileorectal anastomosis but with whom there is some doubt as to whether the rectum is absolutely normal, in those whose debilitated general condition might not permit a safe anastomosis, and in patients who normally would be considered for a total proctocolectomy but because of severe sepsis from very gross perianal fistulization or ulceration may appear likely to be more safely managed by a two-stage procedure (211). It is also appropriate for patients in whom the exact nature of the inflammatory bowel disease is uncertain, thus avoiding the risk of performing a restorative proctocolectomy in patients with Crohn's disease. In the urgent setting, it is the favored operation because of its simplicity and safety with no pelvic dissection or anastomosis.

Hyman et al. (214) assessed the safety and outcomes in 74 patients undergoing subtotal colectomy with ileostomy for ulcerative colitis or Crohn's colitis. The mean age was 35.9 years. Median duration of disease was 36 months, but 28 patients had colitis for less than one year, whereas 10 patients had disease of greater than 10 years duration at the time of colectomy. Median preoperative hospital stay was seven days and median postoperative length of stay was 6.5 days. Sixty-six patients underwent operation for refractory exacerbation, five for free perforation, two for abscess, and one patient for hemorrhage. After operation, 36.5% of patients had a change in diagnosis. Complications occurred in 23% of patients. In the ulcerative colitis patients, 31 of 52 ultimately underwent ileal pouch-anal anastomosis (IPAA) but 39% chose either completion proctectomy or no further operation. They concluded that subtotal colectomy with ileostomy remains a safe and effective treatment for patients requiring urgent operation for severe inflammatory bowel disease. Because of the substantial incidence of change in diagnosis and satisfaction in many patients with an ileostomy, subtotal colectomy with ileostomy may be preferable to primary ileal pouch-anal anastomosis even when a pouch is considered safe.

In these often critically ill patients, controversy exists as to the best management of the distal bowel. Options include a Hartmann stump, a mucous fistula, or placement of the bowel end in the subcutaneous layer. For severely inflamed bowel, Hartmann's procedure may be appropriate as it affords the opportunity to remove more diseased bowel. The distal end may also be transected with staples (or closed with suture) and be buried in the subcutaneous layer. Should this end dehisce, a mucous fistula develops rather than a pelvic abscess. A mucous fistula may be created initially but imposes upon the patient the management of a second opening.

Subtotal colectomy with a retained rectum or sigmoid colon was performed by Goligher (211) in 15% to 20% of patients with large bowel Crohn's disease. This operation permits other options. For example, if the rectum or sigmoid colon has minimal disease, an ileorectal anastomosis can be constructed at a later date. On the other hand, if the disease continues to be troublesome a proctectomy can be performed in the future. With the present evidence of a definite risk of development of carcinoma, the retained rectum or sigmoid colon should not be left in place indefinitely. Poppen et al. (215) reported on intersphincteric and perimuscular perineal excision of the rectum. They noted laparotomy was avoided in 28 of 29 patients who had closure of the rectal stump with ileostomy. Of course, this can be performed only if the rectal stump is short.

■ FATE OF RECTAL STUMP

To determine prognostic factors relating to the fate of the retained rectal segment after operation for Crohn's colitis, Guillem et al. (216) studied the records of 47 patients who underwent creation of an excluded rectal stump. Disease developed in 70% in the excluded rectal segment by five years, 51% had completion proctectomy by 2.4 years, and 19% retained a rectum with disease at a median follow-up period of five years (range, 2–13 years). At a median follow-up time of six years (range, 2–21 years), 30% were without clinical disease. Neither initial involvement of the terminal ileum nor endoscopic inflammatory changes seen in the rectum predicted eventual disease of the excluded rectal segment. However, initial perianal disease complicating Crohn's colitis was predictive of persistent excluded rectal segment disease and often required proctectomy. Primary total proctocolectomy (TPC) of early completion proctectomy may be indicated in this subgroup of patients.

Lock et al. (217) reported the late results of 127 patients undergoing colonic excision and ileostomy with a mean follow-up of 11.5 years. Of 101 patients who had a subtotal colectomy with rectal preservation, 58 subsequently underwent either rectal excision (46 patients) or ileorectal anastomosis (six patients), or both of these operations (six patients). The most common indication for removal of the rectum was persistent severe anorectal disease, although hemorrhage, perforation, and carcinoma were also seen. Whenever a portion of the bowel affected by Crohn's disease cannot be kept under endoscopic or radiologic surveillance, such as in an anal stricture with a preserved rectal stump, resection is generally indicated (207). The fate of the rectum after colectomy and ileostomy was also examined by Harling et al. (218). The authors reviewed 84 patients who had colectomy with ileostomy and oversewing of the rectum. The operative mortality was 6%. After a median 7.7 years of follow-up, 25 ileorectal anastomoses had been undertaken, 16 of which were successful. Twenty-nine proctectomies were performed. The resulting 10-year cumulative risk of proctectomy was 50%. While the risk of proctectomy was significantly less among patients with a normal rectum at colectomy compared with patients with proctitis, the initial macroscopic degree of proctitis did not correlate with the risk of subsequent proctectomy. The five-year cumulative ileal resection rate in 29 patients with a rectum in situ but out of circuit was 29%.

Cirincione et al. (219) presented a review of the literature and three cases of carcinoma developing in the defunctioned rectal stump despite surveillance proctoscopy. One patient developed squamous cell carcinoma of the anal canal and two patients developed adenocarcinoma of the rectum. One patient died and the other developed recurrence. The authors recommend interval perineal proctectomy in all patients undergoing low Hartmann's procedure for severe anorectal Crohn's disease in whom rectal preservation is not possible. Regularly scheduled interim surveillance proctoscopy performed every two years with biopsies of macroscopically normal-appearing and abnormal-appearing rectal mucosa and curetting of fistulous tracts is also recommended to decrease the possibility of missing occult malignancies.

■ COLECTOMY WITH ILEORECTAL ANASTOMOSIS

In 25% to 50% of patients with Crohn's disease of the large bowel, the rectum and the distal sigmoid colon are spared, so colectomy with ileorectal anastomosis seems to be ideally suited (211,220). Although some surgeons are prepared to perform a primary or secondary ileorectal anastomosis even when some degree of Crohn's proctitis is present, Goligher (211) advised ileorectal anastomosis only for patients with an absolutely normal rectal mucosa and, at most, only minimal anal complications. Even so, he found the recurrence rate to be 71%, with a mean follow-up of 15 years (range, 7–25 years). Eighty percent of these patients required conversion to ileostomy (211). These high recurrence rates also were experienced by other authors (213,221). In the series reported by Ambrose et al. (220) involving 63 consecutive patients with Crohn's colitis treated through colectomy and ileorectal anastomosis, the cumulative recurrence rate at 10 years was 64% and the cumulative reoperation rate was 48%. Serious postoperative complications occurred in 10 patients, particularly postoperative intra-abdominal abscesses; nearly all of the patients with such complications had major precipitating factors, the most common of which was urgent colectomy for either bleeding or severe colitis.

Chevalier et al. (222) reported on 83 patients who underwent colectomy and ileorectal anastomosis for Crohn's disease of the large bowel. There were two postoperative deaths and seven anastomotic leaks. Fifty-two patients retained a functioning anastomosis with a mean follow-up of eight years. Forty had an excellent or good functional result. The cumulative proportion of patients with a functioning ileorectal anastomosis was 77% and 63% at 5 and 10 years, respectively. Patients presenting with perforating Crohn's disease had a significantly increased risk of failure of the anastomosis. Perianal Crohn's disease following ileorectal anastomosis was significantly related to the need to defunction or excise the rectum.

Longo et al. (223) reviewed 121 patients who underwent ileorectal anastomosis for Crohn's colitis. Preoperatively 63% were found to have mild or moderate proctitis and 37% had rectal sparing. Small bowel disease was associated in 52%, while perianal disease was present in 15%. Sixty-five ileorectal anastomoses were performed at the time of subtotal colectomy, while 56 were done after previous operation. Anastomotic leaks occurred in 3%. There were no operative deaths. Ten percent with protecting stomas never underwent closure. Among the remaining 118 patients with functioning ileorectal anastomoses, 23% required later proctectomy and 13% required proximal diversion, with the mean period with a functioning ileorectal anastomosis in these 46 patients being 4.1 years. An additional 13 patients required preanastomotic resection and neoileorectal anastomoses and 11 required proximal small bowel resection. The mean duration of function of all 118 ileorectal anastomosis was 9.2 years. At the time of review, after a mean follow-up of 9.5 years, 72 patients (61%) retained a functioning ileorectal anastomosis with 44 being free of disease while 28 were being treated with steroids or antidiarrheal medication. The mean stool frequency was 4.7 per day. In patients with Crohn's colitis, ileorectal anastomosis should be considered as an alternative to proctocolectomy if the rectum is not severely diseased and sphincter function is not compromised.

Total colectomy for Crohn's disease of the colon may be restorative with ileorectal anastomosis or with an ileostomy and rectal stump. Rieger et al. (224) retrospectively audited the results of total colectomy and in particular assessed the number of patients who had a permanent ileostomy and whether this was related to disease in the rectum at the time of the original operation. Thirty-eight patients were identified (mean 35 years; range, 17–65 years). One patient died perioperatively from an anastomotic leak. Median follow-up for the remaining patients was seven years (range, 1–29 years). Ileorectal anastomosis was performed in 17 patients and total colectomy and ileostomy in 20 patients. Indications for operation were failure of medical treatment (61%), toxic colitis (18%), abscess (8%), perforation (5%), large bowel obstruction (5%), and colovesical fistula (3%). Subsequent proctectomy (14 patients, 38%) was more likely with subtotal colectomy and ileostomy (nine patients, 45%) than ileorectal anastomosis (five patients, 29%). Additionally, seven patients had diversion of the rectum making 21 with an ileostomy (57%). Rectal involvement at the time of the original procedure significantly increased the likelihood of permanent ileostomy. The presence of anal disease did not increase the prospect of ileostomy. One patient died with advanced adenocarcinoma in a defunctioned rectum.

■ ILEOSTOMY

The use of fecal diversion has been advocated in Crohn's colitis to achieve colonic healing, to minimize morbidity during colonic resection in debilitated patients, to facilitate limited resection in the presence of diffuse disease, and in the face of failure of medical treatment, symptomatic perianal disease, and prevention or delay of proctocolectomy in young patients (225). Winslet et al. (225) evaluated the long-term results of fecal diversion alone for Crohn's disease predominantly confined to the colon. The clinical course of 44 patients undergoing elective proximal fecal diversion for Crohn's disease of the colon was reviewed. Sustained disease remission was obtained in 70%. Diversion was associated with a significant reduction in steroid requirements and a significant improvement in hemoglobin, erythrocyte sedimentation rate, and albumin. Sixteen patients (36.4%) required a proctocolectomy, 19 patients (43.2%) remained defunctioned, and four patients (9%) died. Five patients had intestinal continuity restored, which remained intact in four patients for a mean follow-up of 99 months (range, 21–153 months). Fecal diversion for Crohn's disease of the colon produces a high incidence of sustained disease remission, but for the majority of patients the prospect of future restoration of intestinal continuity is limited.

The hope that a temporary defunctioning ileostomy to permit diseased bowel to rest and recover has not been realized and has been abandoned. As an urgent procedure, with a view to later resection, Zelas and Jagelman (226) used diversion as a temporary measure in poor-risk patients to enable them to proceed more safely with resection at a later date. The authors believe that loop ileostomy to establish fecal diversion has a definite role in the initial operative management of the severely ill patients with Crohn's colitis. They used it in 79 patients as the initial procedure in severe, debilitating Crohn's colitis or ileocolitis. Clinical improvement, as measured by subjective and objective criteria and length of hospitalization, occurred in 91% of patients. Definitive operation was undertaken at a later stage under more ideal circumstances without mortality. The late relapse rate of 33% in this series led them to recommend definitive operation electively at an earlier stage after initial clinical improvement. The mortality was 5.1%. Goligher (211) has not found this two-stage approach necessary.

Edwards et al. (227) assessed the effect of fecal diversion on the natural history of a refractory Crohn's colitis and severe perianal disease. Some 73 patients underwent a defunctioning stoma (55 for refractory Crohn's colitis and 18 for perianal disease). Acute remission was achieved in 63 patients (48 for refractory Crohn's colitis and 15 for perianal disease). Twenty-nine patients had subsequent closure of the defunctioning stoma (25 of 48 acute responders with refractory Crohn's colitis and 4 of 15 acute responders with perianal disease). Eleven patients with a refractory Crohn's colitis and two with perianal disease achieved good long-term function without disease relapse (median follow-up 36 months). Overall, 52 patients have undergone proctocolectomy or remain with a defunctioning stoma (37 with refractory Crohn's colitis and 15 with perianal disease). They concluded that fecal diversion is associated with acute clinical remission in the majority of patients with refractory Crohn's colitis and perianal disease, but sustained benefit occurs less often. For selected patients, diversion alone offers a realistic alternative to major bowel resection.

■ SEGMENTAL COLON RESECTION

Occasionally, the surgeon finds Crohn's disease limited to a short segment of the colon. Goligher (211) found segmental disease occurred in approximately 6% of patients with Crohn's colitis. In such cases, a segmental resection with anastomosis appears to work well. The propriety of segmental resection has been questioned because of the high recurrence rates reported, up to 62% at 5.5 years (228). total proctocolectomy and ileostomy for Crohn's colitis offers a low recurrence rate but commits patients to a permanent ileostomy. In contrast, segmental resection may predispose patients to recurrence and further operation but may delay or avoid a stoma in select individuals. It appears logical that preservation of the remaining portion of the colon would result in better bowel function and thus may prove, especially, important in the elderly. Segmental resection or even abdominoperineal resection may rid patients of debilitating symptoms. There have been a few reports of this situation in the literature, typically in small series (228–231). Of 12 patients treated by Goligher (211) over a period of 10 to 25 years, three eventually underwent further resection but the nine others were trouble-free.

Prabhakar et al. (232) reported on 53 patients who had a segmental colon resection without a permanent stoma. Of 49 patients available for a mean follow-up of 14 years, Crohn's disease of the colon involved the right, left, and both sides of the colon in 12, 31, and 6 patients, respectively, and involved less than one-third, one- to two-thirds, and more than two-thirds of the colon in 23, 25, and 1 patient, respectively. In 22 of 49 patients (45%) no further therapy was required. Of the 55% of patients who required further therapy, 22% were managed medically and 33% were managed operatively. Three recurrences developed in the small bowel. The remaining 24 developed in the colon. For the 16 patients with recurrence requiring operation, mean time to recurrence was 51 ± 14 months; in all cases, recurrent disease involved the colon, with four anastomotic recurrences. At first recurrence, 10 patients underwent another limited colon resection and six patients underwent completion proctectomy with permanent ileostomy. Five patients required a third procedure, only one of which resulted in a permanent ileostomy. Therefore, 86% of patients remained stoma-free and 14% ultimately required permanent ileostomy, with a mean stoma-free interval of 23 ± 4 months. The authors concluded that colon resection without proctectomy in select patients with limited colonic Crohn's disease can delay or avoid the necessity of a permanent stoma.

Polle et al. (233) evaluated the outcome after segmental colonic resection in 91 patients with a median follow-up of 8.3 years. Thirty patients (33%) had at least one re-resection, of whom 20 finally underwent total proctocolectomy. Female sex and a history of perianal disease were identified as independent risk factors for resection: odds ratio 12.5 and 13.9, respectively. Forty (44%) of the 91 patients had a stoma at the end of the study period. Of 30 patients who had re-resection, 24 finally had a stoma.

Compared with subtotal colectomy, segmental resection is reported to be associated with a higher rate of re-resection. Andersson et al. (234) compared segmental resection (31) to subtotal colectomy with anastomosis (20) with regard to re-resection, postoperative symptoms, and anorectal function. The re-resection rate did not differ between groups in either the entire study population or the subgroup of patients with comparable colonic involvement. Segmentally resected patients had fewer symptoms, fewer loose stools, and better anorectal function. Multivariate analysis revealed the number of colonic segments removed to be the strongest predictive factor for postoperative symptoms and anorectal function. They concluded that segmental resection should be considered in limited Crohn's colitis.

Martel et al. (235) analyzed the outcome of patients treated by segmental colectomy for colonic Crohn's disease. Among 413 patients undergoing operations for Crohn's disease, 84 had a segmental colectomy (cases of terminal ileitis with limited cecal involvement were not included). In the 84 patients, operations included right segmental colectomy, 55%; left segmental colectomy, 40%; associated right and left colectomy, 5%. A stoma was established in 32% of patients. Operative mortality was zero. Twelve patients (14%) had postoperative complications (including six cases of anastomotic leakage). Reoperation was required in 44% of patients and the mean time to operation was 4.5 years. Twenty-six of these patients suffered colonic recurrence and were treated by total colectomy ($n = 9$) or new segmental resection ($n = 17$). The only factor that correlated with risk recurrence was youth. At the end of the study, 13 patients still had a stoma. Eighty percent were fully satisfied or satisfied. There was no evidence of a high risk of postoperative complications, surgical recurrence, or the requirement of a permanent stoma in patients suffering from colonic Crohn's disease who are treated according to a "bowel-sparing policy."

■ OPERATIONS FOR INTESTINAL FISTULA

Crohn's disease is complicated by internal fistulas in 30% to 40% of patients (236). The general principle is resection of the primarily affected diseased segment (e.g., terminal ileum) and closure of the defect in the secondarily involved organ (e.g., bladder, stomach, or duodenum). In the ileosigmoid fistula, the ileum is almost always the perpetrator and the sigmoid innocent and the ileum must, therefore, be removed. By contrast, in colojejunal fistulas, the colon is the perpetrator; therefore, the affected portion of colon must be resected (76). Young-Fadok et al. (237) reviewed the medical records of 90 patients with ileosigmoid fistula and Crohn's disease. A preoperative diagnosis of ileosigmoid fistula was made in 77% of patients. Sigmoid repair was performed in 47.8%, sigmoid resection in 35.6%, a more extensive procedure in 13.3%, and 3.3% either had operation elsewhere or were observed. The repair and resection groups were similar with respect to age, length of Crohn's disease, and preoperative symptoms. There was no significant difference between groups in the incidence of postoperative complications. There were no postoperative deaths. Average length of stay was 8.3 days following repair and 9.9 days after resection. Reasons for resection included significant purulence or inflammation, a large fistula defect, a defect on the mesenteric border of the sigmoid, and active sigmoid Crohn's disease. Surgeon's assessment of the presence of Crohn's disease in the sigmoid correlated with pathologic examination and was aided by knowledge of recent endoscopic appearance and biopsy results. Intraoperative frozen section and colonoscopy were helpful in distinguishing serosal inflammation from active Crohn's disease.

Saint-Marc et al. (238) reviewed their experience with 30 patients with ileosigmoid fistulas who underwent operation. Among them, 15 had a preoperative colonoscopy. The sigmoid was thought to be affected by Crohn's disease in seven patients or stricture in two patients and was resected. In 21 patients in whom the sigmoid was thought to be affected by proximity, simple suture was performed in 15 and a wedge resection in six. Eleven patients had a temporary stoma (37%). One had coloproctectomy. One patient died postoperatively. One patient had postoperative sigmoidocutaneous fistula after conservative treatment. Histology of the sigmoid specimen showed Crohn's disease in eight patients (27%), including five of nine resected specimens and three of 21 conservative procedures. All patients with Crohn's misdiagnosis did not have preoperative colonoscopy. Nine of 11 stomas were closed in a median delay of four months. With a median delay of nine years, four patients again underwent operation for recurrent colonic Crohn's disease, and all of them underwent operation initially without preoperative colonoscopy. The authors concluded that preoperative endoscopic assessment of the colon is a reliable guide to use when choosing between sigmoid resection or a conservative approach and can result in reduced morbidity and improved long-term results.

McNamara et al. (181) reviewed the operative treatment of 63 patients with enterovesical fistula in Crohn's disease to evaluate its effectiveness and long-term results. Distribution of anatomic pattern was 34.9% ileal, 7.9% colonic, and 57.2% ileocolic. Nineteen patients (30.1%) had previous abdominal operation for Crohn's disease. Presenting symptoms included frequency and dysuria in 93.6%, pneumaturia in 79.3%, and fecaluria in 63.4%; 60.3% of patients had all three features. Enterovesical fistula was confirmed preoperatively in 43 patients, suspected clinically in 15 patients, and diagnosed intraoperatively in five patients. Sixty-one of 63 patients underwent operation with resection of the phlegmon or abscess with the diseased bowel and curettage or resection of the fistula. After curettage of the bladder defect, pelvic and bladder drainage was instituted. Coexistent fistulas, most commonly ileosigmoid, occurred in 31 patients. Intra-abdominal abscesses were found in 21 patients, 15 of whom required two-stage procedures. One patient died (mortality, 1.6%), urine leak occurred in 3.2%, and wound infection occurred in 1.6%. Follow-up (mean, 106 months) identified one recurrence of enterovesical fistula due to Crohn's disease. Enterocutaneous fistulas developed in 6.4% and 17.4% required further resections for Crohn's disease.

Yamamoto et al. (239) examined clinicopathological features and management of enterovesical fistula complicating Crohn's disease in 30 patients. Urological symptoms were present in 22 patients; pneumaturia in 18, urinary tract infection in seven, and hematuria in two. In five patients clinical symptoms were successfully managed by conservative treatment and they required no operative treatment for enterovesical fistula. Twenty-five patients required operation. All the patients were treated by resection of disease bowel and pinched off the dome of the bladder. No patient required resection of the bladder. The foley catheter was left in situ for an average of two weeks after operation. Three patients developed early postoperative complications; two bowel anastomotic leaks, and one intra-abdominal abscess. All these complications were associated with sepsis and multiple fistulas at the time of laparotomy. After a median follow-up of 13 years, three patients having postoperative sepsis (anastomotic leak or abscess) developed a recurrent fistula from the ileocolonic anastomosis to the bladder, which required further operation. In the other 22 patients without postoperative complications, there has been no fistula recurrence.

Michelassi et al. (248) reviewed 639 patients who underwent operative treatment for complications of Crohn's disease. Of those, 222 patients (34.7%) were found to have 290 intra-abdominal fistulas. A fistula was diagnosed preoperatively in 69.4% of patients, intraoperatively in 27%, and only after examination of the specimen in 3.6%. The fistula represented the primary or single indication for operative treatment in 6.3% and one of several indications in the remaining patients. Of 165 patients with an abdominal mass or abscess, 41.8% had a fistula. All patients underwent resection of the diseased intestinal segment, 73.1% with primary anastomosis and the remaining with a temporary or permanent stoma. The fistula was directly responsible for a stoma in only 7.2% of patients and was never responsible for a permanent stoma. Resection of the diseased bowel achieved en bloc removal of the fistula in 145 cases. Removal of 93 additional fistulas required resection of the diseased bowel segment along with closure of a fistulous opening on the stomach or duodenum in 14, bladder in 35, or rectosigmoid in 44. When the fistula drained through a vaginal cuff in four patients, the opening was left to close by secondary intention. When the fistula opened through the abdominal wall in 46, the fistulous tract was debrided. In the remaining two enterosalpingeal fistulas, en bloc resection of the involved salpinx accomplished complete removal of the fistula. There was a dehiscence of one duodenal and one bladder repair, 6% of patients experienced postoperative septic complications, and one patient died.

Duodenocolic fistulas deserve special attention. They are very uncommon. Murray et al. (241) found only three duodenocolic fistulas in 70 patients with Crohn's disease. They are thought to arise from primarily involved colon, often strictured with or without an abscess. Formation of a fistula may decompress the bowel and relieve pain but is followed by ascending bacterial growth. Patients may be asymptomatic. The diagnosis may be made by colonoscopy or confirmed with an upper gastrointestinal tract study and small bowel follow-through or barium enema. Treatment consists of segmental resection of the colon (right hemicolectomy) and closure of the duodenal defect. Should severe disease involve the duodenum with stricturing, consideration for a gastroenterostomy would be appropriate (236).

■ BYPASS OPERATION

An example of this operation is a side-to-side ileo-transverse colostomy for inflammatory or obstructive Crohn's disease of the terminal ileum. Because of the high mortality with bowel resection, bypass operation was the standard approach in the past. However, this approach was plagued with complications related to disease activity in the retained segment, abscess, fistula, perforation, and carcinoma.

In a review of their experience at the General Hospital in Birmingham, U.K., in 1972, Alexander-Williams and Haynes (242) concluded that because of the high complication rate with bypass operation, excision should be advocated. Also, by that time the mortality rate for excision had fallen much lower than 10%. Bypass operation for Crohn's disease has no place in present-day practice. An exception can be made when the inflammatory mass firmly adheres to other organs, thus preventing a safe excision. Bypass operations are also used for gastroduodenal Crohn's disease.

■ SMALL BOWEL RESECTION

The justification for operation on the small intestine follows similar principles to operation on the large bowel. Indications for operation include failure of medical treatment, the need to alleviate symptoms of obstruction, or eliminate septic complications. These patients are not infrequently malnourished and have low serum albumin concentrations. Ideally, operation should be advised before complications arise. Once a decision to operate is made, it must be decided what length of the intestine is to be resected. Extensive resections do not reduce the risk of recurrence; therefore, only macroscopically affected bowel should be resected. The proposed anastomotic margin might best be inspected and if the mucosal surface is severely ulcerated, an additional portion of intestine should be removed. Anastomosis can be constructed with staples or hand-sewn, as described in Chapter 23.

■ STRICTUREPLASTY

The concept of a minimal operation for Crohn's disease, particularly of the small intestine, is based on the rationale that it is impossible to cure Crohn's disease by excision because it is a panintestinal disease that eventually can recur in any part of the remaining intestine. The surgeon is required only to treat the complications and to conserve as much intestine as possible. In the case of stricture, excision is not necessary if the narrowing can be corrected (242). The purpose of strictureplasty is to correct the small bowel obstruction and to preserve the length of the small intestine. It is not intended to replace small bowel resection. In patients with diffuse jejunoileitis, multiple strictureplasties rather than resection may be particularly appropriate.

Review of the records at the General Hospital in Birmingham, U.K., revealed that strictureplasty for Crohn's disease was first performed there in 1961 by Bryan Booke (242). The patient had both Crohn's disease and radiation enteritis with stricture at the site of a previous ileotransverse anastomosis. The stricture was divided longitudinally and sewn transversely, providing relief of the patient's obstructive symptoms. The strictureplasty remained patent without ulceration for 10 years. Encouragement for the concept of strictureplasty came initially in the late 1970s, when reports from India showed that tuberculous enteric strictures could be treated as effectively by strictureplasty as by excision (243). A pioneer in the concept of treating Crohn's stricture through strictureplasty was the late Emmanuel Lee (244) of Oxford, who operated on patients with intestinal obstruction and malnutrition in whom resection had previously been thought to be contraindicated, either because of diffuse small bowel involvement or fear of development of a "short bowel" due to a previous excision.

Strictureplasty is ideal for short strictures of small intestine in quiescent disease (Fig. 13). Patients with multiple short strictures are also good candidates. If there is shortage of small intestine because of previous excision, preservation of the intestine through strictureplasty also should be considered. However, when operation is performed for the first time, a simple bowel resection with anastomosis is preferred because it eliminates the diseased bowel. Strictureplasty is used mainly for the small intestine. Of 106 strictureplasties performed in 37 patients, the ileum accounted for 54% of the sites (242) (Table 3).

Tjandra and Fazio (245) reviewed the indications and contraindications for strictureplasty. Situations in which

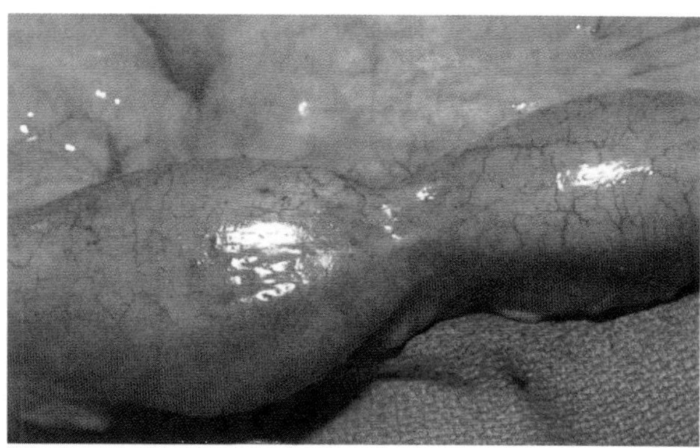

FIGURE 13 ■ A short stricture in Crohn's disease of the ileum.

strictureplasty should be considered include (i) diffuse changes with symptomatic strictures, especially if dilatation of proximal bowel is present; (ii) previous extensive (longer than 100 cm) resection of small bowel; (iii) rapid symptomatic recurrence within 12 months of previous resection; (iv) evidence of short bowel syndrome; and (v) presence of fibrotic strictures. Presence of macroscopically active disease in the stricture alone is not a contraindication. The authors went on to cite some indications in which strictureplasty is contraindicated: (i) presence of overt perforation, (ii) presence of fistula or inflammatory phlegmon at the intended site, (iii) multiple strictures within a short segment, (iv) likelihood of excessive tension at strictureplasty closure, and (v) serum albumin level less than 20 g/L. Circumstances in which strictureplasty requires cautious assessment include (i) strictures longer than 30 cm (a very long stricture is best dealt with by resection), (ii) serious comorbid medical illness, and (iii) serum albumin level between 20 and 30 g/L.

Futami and Arima (246) reviewed their early and late results of strictureplasty in 103 patients with obstructive Crohn's disease undergoing 293 strictureplasties (Heineke-Minkulicz, 234; Finney, 22; Jaboulay, 35; side-to-side isoperistaltic strictureplasty, 1). Mean age at operation was 31.4 years. Forty-four patients had at least one previous operation and synchronous other operative procedures were performed in 62 patients. For 41 patients with strictureplasty alone, 154 strictureplasties were done. The site and number of strictures treated by strictureplasty was as follows: duodenum, 2; small intestine, 265; ileocecal region, 6; colon, 4; recurrence at previous anastomosis, 11; and recurrence at previous strictureplasty, 5. The mean number of strictureplasties per patient was 2.8. There was no operative mortality. Septic complications related to strictureplasty

TABLE 3 ■ **Sites of 106 Strictureplasties (37 Patients)**

Site	%
Ileum	54
Jejunum	34
Ileocecal	5
Duodenum	5
Ileorectal	2
TOTAL	100

Source: Modified from Ref. 242.

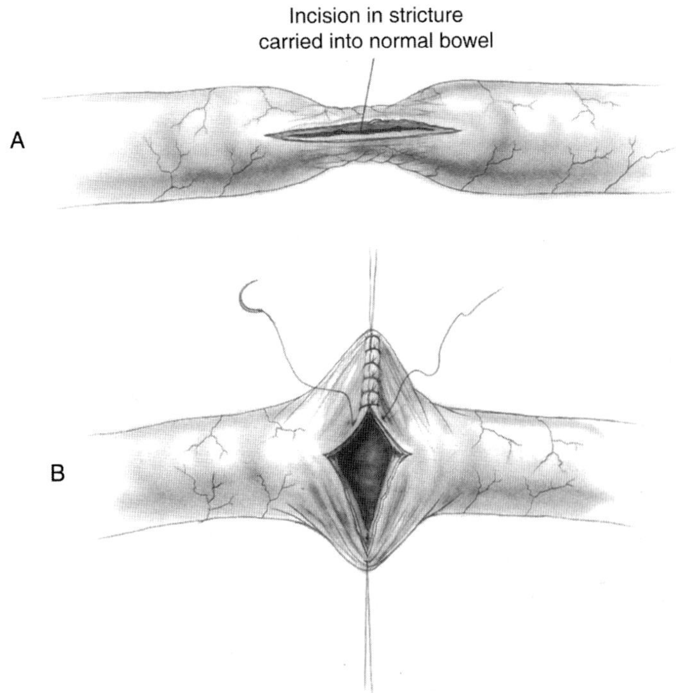

FIGURE 14 ■ **(A)** Stricture is opened along anterior bowel wall. **(B)** Enterotomy is closed transversely. *Source*: Modified from Ref. 247.

developed in four patients and reoperation was needed in two patients (1.9%). Mean duration of follow-up was 80 months. For all patients, the 5- and 10-year reoperation rate was 45% and 62%, respectively. Further operation was required in 44% of patients for recurrence of whom 20% of patients had recurrence at the site of the strictureplasty, which was restrictured in 14 patients and perforating disease in seven patients. Perforating disease for recurrence was more frequent at the site treated by the Finney or Jaboulay procedure compared with Heineke-Mikulicz.

Technique and Results

A short stricture is treated the same way as a Heineke-Mikulicz pyloroplasty for peptic ulcer disease. A longitudinal incision is made over the stricture and carried approximately 2 cm beyond the thickened bowel proximally and distally with a scalpel or by electrocautery. The bowel lumen is carefully examined because bands of scar are frequently present and must be excised. A stay suture is placed at the middle of the incision on each side (Fig. 14A). The enterotomy is then closed transversely with one layer of 4–0 absorbable suture (Fig. 14B). A Gambee suture works well for this closure. Strictureplasty can be performed in as many places as necessary in the individual patient. For a long stricture the incision is made over the entire length with 2 cm beyond the thickened area on each side (Fig. 15A). This segment of bowel is then folded into an inverted U (Fig. 15B), and a Finney-type anastomosis is performed with one layer of sutures of 4–0 absorbable material (Fig. 15C). An alternative is to use an intestinal stapling device (Fig. 16).

Michelassi et al. (248) reported the results of a prospective longitudinal study of a new bowel-sparing procedure (side-to-side isoperistaltic strictureplasty) in patients with extensive Crohn's disease. Of 469 consecutive patients with Crohn's disease of the small bowel, 71 patients (15.1%) underwent at least one strictureplasty; of these, 21 (4.5%) underwent a side-to-side isoperistaltic strictureplasty. Fourteen of the latter procedures were constructed in the jejunum, four in the ileum, and three with ileum overlapping colon. The average length of the strictureplasty was 24 cm. Performance of this strictureplasty instead of a resection resulted in preservation of an average

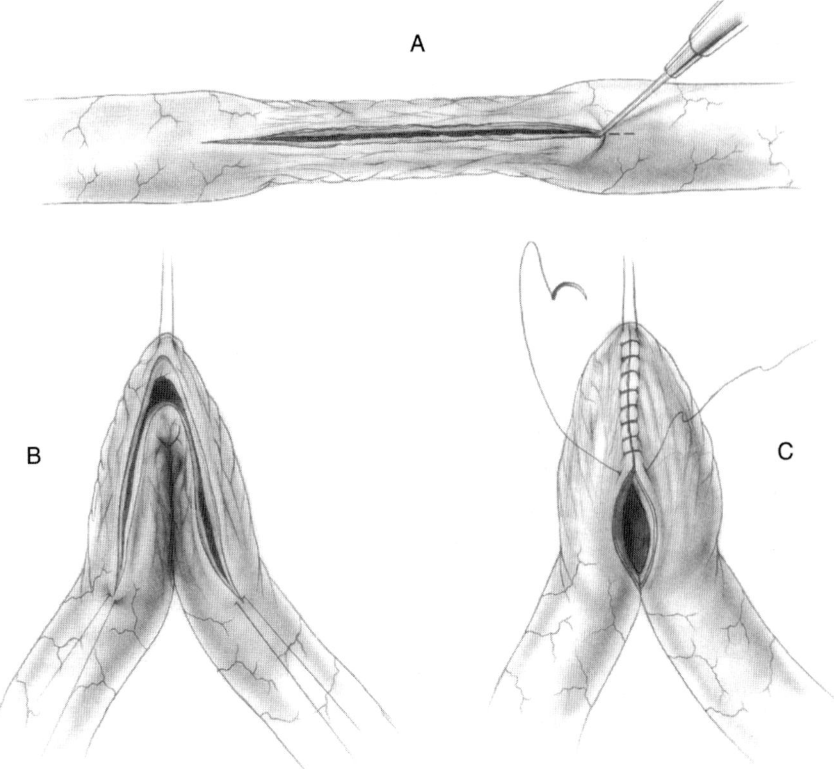

FIGURE 15 ■ **(A)** Long segment of stricture is opened. **(B)** Bowel is folded into an inverted U. **(C)** Side-to-side anastomosis is made. *Source*: Modified from Ref. 247.

of 17% of small bowel length. One patient suffered a postoperative gastrointestinal hemorrhage. All patients were discharged on oral feedings after a mean of 8 days. With follow-up extending to 7.5 years in 20 patients (one patient died of unrelated cause), radiographic, endoscopic, and histopathologic examination of this strictureplasty suggests regression of previously active Crohn's disease.

Tonelli et al. (249) reported results obtained with a side-to-side isoperistaltic strictureplasty for single or multiple strictures that affected long bowel tracts in 31 patients. Indications for operation included subocclusion in 22 patients, malnutrition in 9 patients, and fistula or abscess in 6 patients. Two side-to-side isoperistaltic strictureplasties were performed in the jejunum, 6 in the jejunum-ileum, 16 in the proximal ileum, 1 in the terminal ileum, and 6 in the ileo-cecal tract. The average length of side-to-side isoperistaltic strictureplasty was 32 cm (range, 10-54). Sixteen patients also underwent concomitant bowel resection and 17 patients have received additional strictureplasty. There was no perioperative mortality, nor were there any postoperative complications requiring reoperation. In all patients, intestinal occlusion and malnutrition were resolved. At an average follow-up of 26.4 months, 6 patients required reoperation, but in only one of them did the recurrence involve a previous strictureplasty site. They concluded side-to-side isoperistaltic strictureplasty seems to provide a technical solution leading to improvement when long intestinal inflamed tract is treated.

Since a stricture of the small bowel may not be obvious, it can be missed easily when the serosal surface is examined. It is important that the entire small bowel be examined to rule out other areas of stricture. Through an enterotomy, a standard No. 16 Foley catheter or, preferably, a Baker's long intestinal tube is passed throughout the

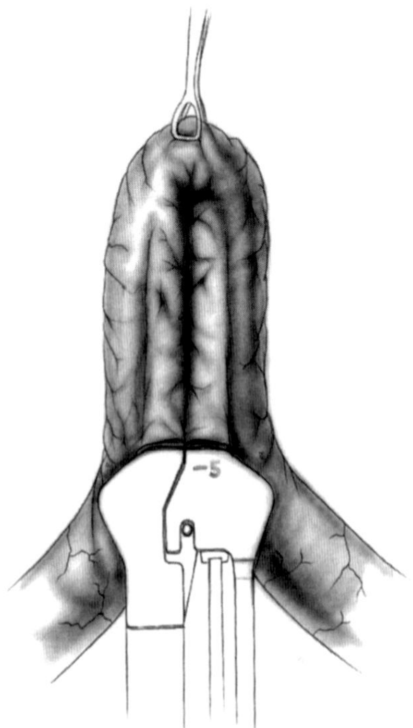

FIGURE 16 ■ With a stapling device, a side-to-side anastomosis is made for a long stricture.

length of the small bowel by intussuscepting the bowel over the tube. The balloon is inflated with water to give it a diameter of 2 cm. This is the size below which obstructive symptoms are unlikely to occur (250). The areas of stricture are noted and strictureplasty is performed at each area as indicated.

The technique can be applied to small bowel strictures as well as ileocolic anastomotic strictures following a previous resection (251). The results of strictureplasty from reported series of a sizable number are collated in Table 4. Nivatvongs (263) also reviewed the status of strictureplasty in Western countries. From cumulative series of patients he collated a mortality of 0%, perioperative hemorrhage (≥3 units) in 2% to 4%, fistula/abscess in 6% to 8%, reoperation for septic complications in 2% to 5%, and nonstrictureplasty-related complications in 1% to 2%. With respect to outcome, with a follow-up ranging from six months to seven years, symptomatic recurrence developed in 24% to 36% (15% reoperative and 9% to 22% medical/nonoperative). Symptomatic restricture of stricture site occurred in 2.5% to 57%.

Tichansky et al. (264) conducted a meta-analysis of multiple variables for outcome on 506 patients who underwent 1825 strictureplasties for Crohn's disease. There was minimal morbidity and zero mortality. Ninety percent of strictures were less than 10 cm in length. Approximately 85% used the Heineke-Mikulcz technique and 13% used the Finney strictureplasty. Forty-four percent of procedures included concurrent bowel resection. The recurrence rate of Crohn's disease and the proportion of patients requiring additional operations after strictureplasty was increased in patients with longer study duration after operation who showed symptoms of active disease, who experienced preoperative weight loss, or who received the Heineke-Mikulicz procedure. The proportion of patients requiring additional operation was decreased when a Finney strictureplasty was used as compared with those treated by the Heineke-Mikulcz procedure.

More recently, Roy and Kumar (265) undertook a literature review of long-term studies on strictureplasty to evaluate its safety and efficacy. They collected the information from seven studies since the meta-analysis of Tichansky et al. (264). There were 461 patients who underwent 1408 strictureplasties with a mean or median follow-up of 69 months. They calculated a hemorrhage rate of 3.3%, obstruction 1.5%, fistula 2.4%, abscess 0.7%, and anastomotic leak at 0.9%

Despite residual disease, relief of symptoms and return to general well-being have occurred in more than 90% of patients (250).

In a study attempting to define whether there is an increased need for reoperation in patients with Crohn's disease of the small bowel treated by strictureplasty compared to those treated by small bowel resection, 41 patients who underwent strictureplasty were compared with 41 patients treated with small bowel resection. The need for reoperation at the original site of operation was similar in both groups at similar intervals (266).

Ozuner et al. (267) conducted a study to determine reoperative rates for Crohn's disease following strictureplasty in 162 patients who underwent 698 strictureplasties. The cumulative five-year incidence of reoperative

TABLE 4 ■ Results of Strictureplasty

Author(s)	No. of Patients	No. of Procedures	Mortality	Complications				Follow-up (mo)	Further Operation (%)
				Overall (%)	Fistula/ Leak (%)	Sepsis/ Abscess (%)	Bleeding (%)		
Alexander-Williams (250) (1986)	57	146	0		8			36	14
Spencer et al. (252) (1994)	35	71	0	14				36	17
Quandalle et al. (253) (1994)	22	107	0			5	5	36	22
Baba and Nakai (254) (1995)	69		0		0		0	37	17
Serra et al. (255) (1995)	43	154	0		2			54	33
Stebbing et al. (256) (1995)	52	241	0			4		50	36
Hurst et al. (257) (1998)	57	109		12	2 (Fistula/Leak and Sepsis/Abscess combined)		2	38	12
Yamamoto et al. (258) (1999)	87	245	0	–	8 (Fistula/Leak and Sepsis/Abscess combined)		–	104	44
Sampietro et al. (259) (2000)	104		0	6	3	3	–	60	25
Tonelli et al. (260) (2000)	44	174	0	–	0	–	–	48	23
Dietz et al. (261) (2001)	314	1124	–	18	4	5	11	90	34
Laurent et al. (262) (2002)	18	68	0	–	6	6	–	63	6

recurrence was 28%. The authors further found no difference between the cumulative reoperative rate at five years for patients who underwent strictureplasty alone and those who underwent strictureplasty plus resection. Operative recurrence was managed by new strictureplasty, restrictureplasty, or bowel resection. Tonelli et al. (249) reported restrictures of previous strictureplasty sites requiring operation occurred in 8.8% of cases. Hurst and Michelassi (257) reported an identical 8.8% reoccurrence of the site of a previous strictureplasty.

Stebbing et al. (256) found that most symptomatic recurrence was caused by new segments of stricturing or perforating disease, and recurrence of Crohn's disease at a strictureplasty site was noted in only 3.7%. A third operation was required in 13% of patients. The authors also found that patients undergoing strictureplasty alone were no more likely to require reoperation than those who had a concomitant resection at the first procedure.

Multiple strictureplasties are prone to collectively ooze and cause the hemoglobin and hematocrit levels to drop in the postoperative period. Ozuner and Fazio (268) conducted a retrospective analysis of 139 patients with Crohn's disease who underwent a total of 523 strictureplasties. Poststrictureplasty hemorrhage occurred in 9.3%. The average drop in hemoglobin and hematocrit levels in these patients was 5.8 g/dL and 0.174 g/dL, respectively. Initially, management of these patients includes close observation, evaluation of vital signs, fluid replacement, and study for coagulation disorders to rule out other possible sources of bleeding. If hemoglobin and hematocrit levels drop substantially or if a patient becomes symptomatic, prompt blood transfusion is recommended. Most patients respond promptly to transfusion alone. Bleeding usually occurs at the suture site, is temporary, ceases early, and requires no further intervention. Hematologic abnormalities, if present, should be corrected rapidly with platelets and fresh frozen plasma and, for the long term, with iron, folate, vitamin B_{12}, or appropriate trace elements. If bleeding continues or patients require multiple blood transfusions, they should have a red blood cell nuclear scan or an angiogram. If clips were applied intraoperatively, the bleeding site and strictureplasty sites can be precisely located. There are no strict guidelines as to when to proceed with the red blood cell scan or angiogram. Vasopressin infusion (0.2 U/min) through the bleeding vessel is most effective in controlling the bleeding. Also Gelfoam (The Upjohn Co., Kalamazoo, Michigan, U.S.A.), coils, or other techniques can be used to embolize the bleeding vessel feeding the strictureplasty site. It is suggested that the angiography catheter be left in the vessel for 24 hours or until it is certain that bleeding has been effectively controlled. Other sources of hemorrhage can also be identified during angiography as well (e.g., anastomotic bleeds, iatrogenic injury to mesenteric vessels, or. omental vessels). If the patient shows signs and symptoms of shock, celiotomy should be performed. Usually this kind of bleeding is not from a strictureplasty site. Poor intraoperative hemostasis is the most common cause.

Yamamoto and Keighley (269) examined the outcome of strictureplasty for recurrence at the ileocolonic anastomosis after resection in Crohn's disease in 42 patients. The method of ileocolic strictureplasty was Heineke-Mikulicz reconstruction for a short stricture (< 6 cm) in 41 patients and Finney construction for a long stricture (20 cm) in one. Synchronous operations were performed for co-existing small bowel Crohn's disease in 17 patients: strictureplasty in 8, resection in 2, and both in 7. Postoperatively, there were two intra-abdominal abscesses, which were treated conservatively. There were no deaths. All except 2 patients had complete relief of symptoms after operation. Most of the patients who had preoperative weight loss gained weight (median gain, +2.6 kg). After a median follow-up of 99 months, 57% of patients had a symptomatic recurrence. Three patients were successfully managed by medical treatment. The other 21 patients (50%) required operation for recurrence (recurrence at the previous ileocolic stricture site). They concluded, strictureplasty is a safe and efficacious procedure for ileocolonic anastomotic recurrence in Crohn's disease.

Yamamoto et al. (270) assessed the outcome of strictureplasty for duodenal Crohn's disease in 13 patients.

Ten patients underwent strictureplasty as the primary procedure and in three, strictureplasty was used as the revision procedure after previous bypass operation. Two patients developed anastomotic breakdown and were treated either by Roux-en-Y duodenojejunostomy or partial gastrectomy. Symptoms of obstruction persisted in four patients after strictureplasty; three eventually resolved after prolonged nasogastric aspiration, but the other required gastrojejunostomy. In the long-term, six patients developed restricture at the previous strictureplasty site. Five required repeat strictureplasty and the other patient underwent duodeno-jejunostomy. One patient who had repeat strictureplasty required a further strictureplasty because of restricture at the previous strictureplasty site. Overall, 9 of 13 patients required further operation because of early postoperative complications or restricture at the strictureplasty site. They concluded strictureplasty for duodenal Crohn's disease is associated with a high incidence of postoperative complications and restricture.

Dietz et al. (271) reported their experience with strictureplasty for diffuce Crohn's jejunoileitis in 123 patients. Nineteen patients (15%) were receiving TPN for short-bowel syndrome, and 81 (66%) were taking chronic steroids. Total number of strictureplasties performed was 701 (median, 5/patient). Seventy percent of patients underwent a synchronous bowel resection. Recurrence was defined as the need for reoperation. Patients with diffuse jejunoileitis were also compared with 219 patients with limited small bowel Crohn's disease undergoing strictureplasty. The overall morbidity rate was 20%, with septic complications occurring in 6%. The surgical recurrence rate was 29% with a median follow-up period of 6.7 years. The recurrence rate in diffuse jejunoileitis patients did not differ from that seen in patients with limited small bowel Crohn's disease. Short duration of disease and short interval since last operation were significant predictors of accelerated recurrence.

Broering et al. (272) defined the efficacy of strictureplasty and resection in patients with obstructive Crohn's disease of the colon. Quality of life was evaluated in follow-up examinations using the Inflammatory Bowel Disease Questionnaire. The incidence of postoperative surgical recurrence was 36% in those treated by strictureplasty and 24% in those treated by resection. Postoperative morbidity was 16.1% in the former and 22.3% in the latter. There was no significant difference between the groups in quality of life measures (177 vs. 182 points). They concluded, strictureplasty in Crohn's colitis is a valuable surgical technique which results in low recurrence rates and in surgical outcome comparable to that in resection without sacrificing functional large bowel length.

A novel indication for strictureplasty was reported by Matzke et al. (273) in a patient who developed an isolated stricture of the mid portion of her ileal pouch nine years after proctocolectomy and J-ileal pouch-anal anastomosis for ulcerative colitis. With repeated episodes of pouchitis and reevaluation her diagnosis was changed to Crohn's disease. A mid pouch strictureplasty alleviated her obstructive symptoms and is an alternative to pouch excision in the management of patients with Crohn's disease.

Broering et al. (274) defined the results of strictureplasty and resection in terms of quality of life, surgical recurrence, and postoperative complications in 67 patients with Crohn's disease of the small bowel. Quality of life was evaluated in follow-up examinations using the Inflammatory Bowel Disease Questionnaire. Postoperative morbidity was 14.8% after strictureplasty and 17% after resection. Fifty percent of the patients treated by strictureplasty and 37% treated by resection developed recurrent disease. Quality of life measurement revealed no significant difference between patients treated by strictureplasty or resection.

Jaskowiak and Michelassi (275) reported a case of small bowel adenocarcinoma developing at the site of a prior strictureplasty in a patient seven years postoperatively in the absence of any other preneoplastic disease of the small bowel. Presenting symptoms were progressive obstruction after a long period of quiescent disease.

Of occasional concern during the performance of a strictureplasty is the presence of a carcinoma at the stricture site. Partridge and Hodin (276) presented such a case and their review of the literature found a 15% increased incidence of carcinoma in patients with Crohn's disease compared with the general population. The incidence of small bowel carcinoma has been reported to be 3-fold to 100-fold increased compared with the general population. There may be no masses nor distension of the bowel segment apart from the stricture. Whenever there is mucosal ulceration or any other suspicion of malignancy an intraoperative biopsy would be recommended.

■ PERCUTANEOUS DRAINAGE OF INTRA-ABDOMINAL ABSCESS

Sahai et al. (277) reviewed 27 percutaneous drainage procedures performed in 24 patients with intra-abdominal abscesses associated with Crohn's disease. They were classified as successes (56%) or failures (44%) on the basis of the need for an operative procedure within 30 days of catheter removal. Patients whose abscesses were successfully drained had significantly fewer associated fistulas (46.6% vs. 92%), and their abscesses tended more often to be first (rather than recurrent), spontaneous (rather than postoperative), located in the right lower quadrant, and smaller. Patients whose abscesses were successfully drained also tended to spend more time with the catheter in place and required more imaging procedures. Complications were noted in four cases (15%), enterocutaneous fistula at the site of catheter insertion in three cases, and postprocedure fever in one case. Hospital stay was significantly shorter after successful drainage (16.3 ± 6.9 vs. 31.7 ± 22.1 days). After a total of 543.5 patient-months of follow-up, subsequent intra-abdominal Crohn's-related operation was required in only two of the successes and one failure. The authors concluded that (i) percutaneous drainage of Crohn's abscess successfully obviates the need for early operation in approximately 50% of cases, and this benefit is maintained on long-term follow-up; (ii) percutaneous drainage shortens hospital stay; (iii) Crohn's abscesses in various locations, single or multiple, with or without an associated fistula, may be successfully drained percutaneously; and (iv) the presence of an associated fistula may be a risk factor for failure.

■ STRICTURE DILATATION

Couckuyt et al. (278) reported their experience with hydrostatic balloon dilation of Crohn's strictures of the colon in 55 patients followed for a mean 33.6 months. Patients ranged in age from 17 to 74 years (mean, 39.5 years). All participating patients had symptoms of obstruction (intermittent severe abdominal cramps, abdominal distention, and altered bowel habits) and radiographically demonstrated "narrow" strictures. The patients' symptoms were resistant to medical therapy. Dilation was performed using Microvasive Rigiflex balloon catheters (Watertown, Massachusetts, U.S.A.) passed through a standard 2.8 mm colonoscope instrument channel under direct visualization. An 18 mm balloon was used first, followed by either 20 or 25 mm balloons. The balloons were inflated to recommended pressures for two minutes. Two to six inflations were performed per session. Light general anesthesia was used. Prophylactic antibiotics were not administered and all patients were observed overnight after the procedure. Successful dilation was achieved in 90% and after successful dilation the passage of a 13.8 mm diameter colonoscope was possible in 51 of the 70 procedures. In eight patients, dilation was not successful secondary to the length or angulation of the stricture. Procedure time was an average of one hour. Complications occurred in six patients (8%), including two localized perforations and two retroperitoneal perforations, which were managed conservatively with intravenous antibiotics. Two intraperitoneal perforations occurred, which were treated successfully with one-stage resection. Complete long-term relief of obstructive symptoms was reported in 20 of 55 patients after one procedure. Eighteen patients required a second dilation at a mean interval of 1.5 years. Successful long-term results were achieved in 13 of these 18 patients, resulting in a total long-term success in 34 of 55 patients (62%). Nineteen patients (34%) required operation for persistent or recurrent obstructive symptoms.

In general, fibrous strictures respond well to mechanical dilation, whereas inflammatory strictures may not, over the long term, because the inflammatory process itself accounts for the observed luminal compromise. Medical therapy should represent the mainstay of treatment in these patients. While the authors' results are encouraging, some technical aspects are worth considering in regard to the role they may play in the relatively high rate of complications (8% of procedures) and eventual requirement for operation (32% of patients). The choice of an 18 F balloon to begin may be too large and could potentially result in excessive numbers of perforations. The use of smaller-caliber balloons with more gradual progression to larger size might reduce the frequency of perforations.

Ramboer et al. (279) reported on the use of endoscopic balloon dilation combined with local corticosteroid injection in the treatment of stenoses in recurrent Crohn's disease. Of 13 patients, 11 of whom previously had right hemicolectomy, treated with a Microvasive Rigiflex balloon with a pressure of 35 psi maintained for two minutes followed by injection of betamethasone, 5 mg circumferentially, no operations were required. The mean follow-up was 47 months. There were 52 treatment sessions without perforation and with relief of symptoms. Kelly and Hunter (280) described endoscopic balloon dilatation in three patients with obstructive symptoms from duodenal strictures due to Crohn's disease. The use of hydrostatic balloon dilatation of colonic strictures in Crohn's disease represents a potentially valuable technique in the management of these problematic complications.

Singh et al. (281) evaluated the safety and efficacy of endoscopic balloon dilatation with or without intralesional steroid injection, of symptomatic upper gastrointestinal and lower gastrointestinal Crohn's disease strictures. Technical success was defined as the ability of the scope to traverse the stricture postdilatation. Long-term success rate was claimed if a patient remained asymptomatic and did not require operation or further endoscopic dilatation. Over four years they performed 29 stricture dilatations on 17 patients with 20 strictures. The mean follow-up period was 18.8 months. Stricture locations were as follows: rectal, 5; sigmoid, 2; colocolonic anastomosis, 3; ileocolonic anastomosis, 4; ileum, 1; descending colon, 1; cecum, 1; and distal duodenal bulb, 3 patients. Technical success was achieved in 96.5% of stricture dilatations. Ten strictures (34.5%) were dilated to <15 mm and 19 (65.5%) to ≥ 15 mm. Long-term success rate in the <15 mm group was 70% and in the ≥ 15 mm group was 68.4%. Four quadrant steroid injections were done on 11 strictures. The recurrence rate in this group was 10% and that in the non-steroid group 31.3%. The overall long-term success was 76.5% by intent-to-treat analysis. Three perforations occurred (all colonic) during 29 stricture dilatations, a complication rate of 10% with no mortalities.

For a patient with longstanding Crohn's disease with radiographic evidence of small bowel obstruction caused by ileal stricture and poor nutritional status, Bickston et al. (282) described the use of a metallic enteral stent as a bridge to resection. Two Wallstents were placed; luminal patency was subsequently confirmed by a fluoroscopic study. The patient tolerated a regular diet.

Morini et al. (283) evaluated the long-term clinical outcome in 43 Crohn's patients after endoscopic dilatation for ileal or neoileal strictures. Endoscopic dilatation was technically successful in 79% of Crohn's disease patients with a mean number of dilatations per patient of 3. During a mean follow-up of 63.7 months, a positive long-term outcome was observed in 52.9% of patients, whereas operation was necessary in the remaining 16 cases. The risk of operation was distinctly higher within 2 years post dilatation than in the next two years (26.4% vs. 8.3% respectively). No clear clinical, endoscopic or radiologic predictive factors for successful outcome were identified.

Sabate et al. (284) evaluated the safety and long-term efficacy of per-endoscopic hydrostatic balloon dilatation in 38 patients with Crohn's disease. Strictures were located as follows: ileocolonic (26) or colo-colonic (2) anastomosis, colon (4), ileum (3), proximal jejunum (1), and ileo-cecal valve (5); three patients had two strictures accessible to dilatation. The mean length of the strictures was 2.1 cm. Thirty-two of the 38 patients were successfully dilated and followed for a mean of 22.8 months until operation or last news. The probabilities of obstructive symptom recurrence were 36% at one year and 60% at 5 years. Twelve patients had a second dilatation and 3 a third. The probabilities of operation for stricture were 26% at one year and 43% at five years. Results were not influenced by age, sex, activity of disease, passage of the stricture by the colonoscope or concomitant medical therapies. Complications occurred in 9.4% of the 53 dilatation sessions, with only one perforation.

Brooker et al. (285) conducted a review to determine whether long-acting steroid injection into strictures after dilatation may decrease the need for further stricture dilatation and improve the outcome in symptomatic patients. There were 14 patients who underwent a total of 26 dilatations with triamcinolone injected (median dose 20 mg, 10-40 mg) in 20 of the procedures. Seven patients (50%) had sustained remission after a single dilatation and steroid injection, with a median follow-up period of 16.4 months. Four patients (28.5%) required more than one dilatation (median 3 dilatations, range 2-4) to control their symptoms, with a median follow-up period of 27.8 months. Endoscopic management failed in 3 patients (21.4%) who were referred for operation. There were no complications due to dilatation or triamcinolone injection.

Dear and Hunter (286) reported 16 of 22 patients had resolution of their obstructive symptoms after balloon dilatation although one third of patients required more than 2 dilatations over the follow-up period. Six of 22 patients had persisting symptoms after endoscopic treatment, requiring operation. There were no complications noted after any of the 71 dilatations that were performed.

■ LIKELIHOOD OF STOMA NECESSITY

Post et al. (287) reviewed 746 patients with Crohn's disease treated operatively within a 13-year interval in whom 227 stomas (159 primary and 68 secondary) were created. The main indication (64%) for primary stoma was severe perianal or genital fistulous disease. Revisional operation for stomal complications was more common following colostomy than ileostomy (31% vs. 5%). Twenty years after the first symptoms of Crohn's disease, the cumulative risks of receiving any stoma or a permanent stoma were 41% and 14%, respectively. Four parameters were shown to be independently associated with the risk for any stoma as well as a permanent one. First, increased risk coincided with rectal inflammation, perianal fistula, or abscess, and absence of small intestinal involvement. Second, long-standing symptomatic disease before the first operative intervention reduced the risks of a permanent stoma. Third, the long-term chances of closure following temporary stoma were 75% when used for anastomotic protection or avoidance, 79% after postoperative complications, and 40% for perianal or genital fistulas or for rectal inflammation or stenosis. Finally, rectal disease and perianal fistula were the only independent predictors of a low possibility of stoma closure during follow-up. In their review, Singh et al. (288) noted that for patients with Crohn's colitis and perianal disease the reported rate of proctectomy is 12–20%.

■ FATE OF ILEAL POUCH-ANAL ANASTOMOSIS IN UNSUSPECTED CROHN'S DISEASE

Because the distinction between ulcerative colitis and Crohn's disease can be difficult, some patients with Crohn's disease inadvertently undergo an IPAA. Sagar et al. (289) reviewed the long-term outcome of patients with Crohn's disease who had undergone mucosectomy with hand-sewn IPAA (J pouch in 35, S pouch in one, and W pouch in one). All patients underwent preoperative colonoscopy and biopsy. Histologic examination of the resected specimen at the time of IPAA showed features of ulcerative colitis in 22, indeterminate colitis in nine, or Crohn's disease in six. The stoma was closed in all patients. A total of 11 of 37 patients developed complex fistulas (pouch-cutaneous in six, pouch-vaginal in four, or pouch-vesical in one). Crohn's disease recurred in the pouch in 20, anal canal in four, pouch and anal canal in 10, and elsewhere in three. After 10 years (range, 3–14 years), the pouch remained in situ in 20 patients in whom frequency of bowel movement was seven times (3–10) per 24 hours in situ but defunctioned in seven patients and excised in 10 patients (failure rate, 45%). The authors concluded that inadvertent IPAA for Crohn's disease is associated with a high rate of failure (45%) but an acceptable long-term functional result if the pouch can be kept in situ. These data are not to be misconstrued as advocating an IPAA in patients with Crohn's disease, but rather to point out the complication and failure rates.

Grobler et al. (290) reported on 20 of 81 patients treated by restorative proctocolectomy for presumed ulcerative colitis who had some features of Crohn's disease. Ten were classified as definite Crohn's disease and 10 as indeterminate colitis. These pathologic features were first apparent during synchronous colectomy and pouch construction in 10 of 11 cases. In the remainder, histologic features of possible Crohn's disease were first identified during rectal excision in six, preliminary subtotal colectomy in two, and after pouch excision in two. Complications were marginally more common in patients with features of possible Crohn's disease: pelvic sepsis, 30% versus 20%; fistulas, 45% versus 16%; ileal stenosis, 40% versus 21%; pouchitis, 50% versus 26%; and small bowel obstruction, 25% versus 13%. Pouch excision or a persistent proximal stoma has been necessary in six patients with possible Crohn's disease (30%) compared with nine (15%) of the remainder. Median hospital stay, however, was the same and stool frequency in those with a functioning pouch was comparable. These results show that there is a higher complication rate if there are features of Crohn's disease but that the medium-term functional results are acceptable if the pouch can be retained.

Brown et al. (291) determined the outcome of patients with Crohn's disease and indeterminate colitis who have an ileal pouch-anal anastomosis. From a total of 1,270 patients who underwent restorative proctocolectomy, 36 had Crohn's disease and 21 had indeterminate colitis. Pouch complications were significantly more common in patients with Crohn's disease (64%) and indeterminate colitis (43%) compared with patients with ulcerative colitis (22%). Similarly, 56% of patients with Crohn's disease had their pouch excised or defunctioned, compared with 10% of patients with indertiminate colitis and 6% with ulcerative colitis. The functional results in patients with Crohn's disease with a successful pouch were not significantly different from those with indeterminate colitis or ulcerative colitis. Although complication rates may be higher in patients with indeterminate colitis compared with ulcerative colitis, the overall pouch failure rate is similar.

They believe Crohn's disease should remain a relative contraindication to restorative proctocolectomy, whereas ileal pouch-anal anastomosis is an acceptable alternative for patients with indeterminate colitis.

Tekkis et al. (292) evaluated the short-term and long-term outcomes of patients undergoing restorative proctocolectomy for Crohn's disease and indeterminate colitis. There were 52 patients with Crohn's disease or indeterminate colitis from a total of 1,652 patients undergoing restorative proctocolectomy. Patients with indeterminate colitis or indeterminate colitis favoring ulcerative colitis (group 1, n = 26) had a pouch failure rate of 11.5% versus 57.5% for patients with Crohn's disease or indeterminate colitis favoring Crohn's disease (group 2, n = 26). Pouch salvage was undertaken in 15 patients with a 13.3% failure rate and patients in group 2 were 2.6 times more likely. No significant differences were evident between Crohn's disease and indeterminate colitis with regards to pelvic sepsis (19.2% vs. 15.4%), anastomotic stricture (23.1% vs. 21.7%), small bowel obstruction (26.9% vs. 26.9%) or pouchitis (15.4% vs. 11.5%). The 24 hour bowel frequency (7.5 vs. 8), fecal urgency, daytime or nighttime incontinence were similar between patients with Crohn's disease or indeterminate colitis. Patients in group 2 were more likely to develop a pouch-related fistula than in patients in group 1. They conclude that patients with indeterminate colitis should remain candidates for restorative proctocolectomy but careful preoperative assessment is advised to exclude clinical signs favoring the diagnosis of Crohn's disease. The complications associated with failure are extensive and the option of reconstructive surgery in patients with Crohn's disease should be questioned. Heriot et al (293) further reported that repair of pouch vaginal fistulas in patients with Crohn's disease uniformly failed within 5 years from primary repair.

Braveman et al. (294) reviewed their experience with patients receiving an ileal pouch-anal anastomosis for cure but subsequently found to have Crohn's disease. There were 32 such patients (4.1%) identified from a registry of 790 ileal pouch-anal anastomosis patients. The preoperative diagnosis was ulcerative colitis in 24 patients and indeterminate colitis in 8 patients. Median follow-up was 153 (range 13-231 months). The median time from ileal pouch-anal anastomosis to diagnosis of Crohn's disease was 19 (range 0-188 months). Complications occurred in 93%, including perineal abscess/fistula (63%), pouchitis (50%), anal stricture (38%). Pouch failure (excision or current diversion) occurred in 9 patients (29%) at a median of 66 (range 6-187) months. Two of these 9 patients had preoperative anal disease. Comparing patients with failed pouches (n = 9) to patients with functioning pouches (n = 23), post ileal pouch-anal anastomosis perineal abscess (67 v.26%) and pouch fistula (89% vs. 30%) were more commonly associated with pouch failure. Preoperative clinical, endoscopic, and pathologic features were not predictive of pouch failure or patient outcome. For those with a functional pouch, 50% have been or are currently on medication to treat active Crohn's disease. This group had 6 bowel movements in 24 (range 3-10) hours, with leakage in 60% and pad usage in 45%. They concluded patients who undergo ileal pouch-anal anastomosis and are subsequently found to have Crohn's disease experience significant morbidity. They choose not to recommend the routine application of ileal pouch-anal anastomosis in any subset of patients with known Crohn's disease.

Hartley et al. (295) reviewed their experience with patients with ileal pouch-anal anastomosis for apparent mucosal ulcerative colitis who were subsequently found to have Crohn's disease to determine whether selected patients with Crohn's disease may be candidates for ileal pouch-anal anastomosis. There were 60 patients (32 females; median age 33 years) who underwent ileal pouch-anal anastomosis for mucosal ulcerative colitis who subsequently had that diagnosis revised to Crohn's disease. Median follow-up of all patients was 46 months. No pre-ileal pouch-anal anastomosis factors examined were predictors of the development of recrudescent Crohn's disease. The overall pouch loss rate for the entire cohort was 12% and 33% for those with recrudescent Crohn's disease. Median daily bowel movements in those with ileal pouch-anal anastomosis in-situ at the time of collective data was 7, with 50% of patients rarely or never experiencing urgency and 59% reporting perfect or near perfect continence. Median quality of life, health, and happiness scores were 9.9 and 10 of 10. They concluded the secondary diagnosis of Crohn's disease after ileal pouch-anal anastomosis is associated with protracted freedom from clinically evident Crohn's disease, low pouch loss rate, and good functional outcome. Such results can only be improved by the continued development of medical strategies for the long-term suppression of Crohn's disease. They believe these data support a prospective evaluation of ileal pouch-anal anastomosis in selected patients with Crohn's disease.

Regimbeau et al. (296) reported ten-year results of ileal pouch-anal anastomosis in selected patients with colorectal Crohn's disease for whom coloprotectomy and definitive end ileostomy was the only alternative. There were 41 patients (22 females/19 males) with a mean age of 36 years who underwent ileal pouch-anal anastomosis for colorectal Crohn's disease. None had passed or present history of anal manifestations or evidence of small bowel involvement. Diagnosis of Crohn's disease was established preoperatively in 26 patients on the resected specimen after ileal pouch-anal anastomosis, or after occurrence of Crohn's disease-related complication in 15 patients. Follow-up was 113 months. There was no postoperative death. Eleven (27%) patients experienced Crohn's disease-related complications, 47 months after ileal pouch-anal anastmosis: 2 had persistent anal ulcerations with pouchitis and granulomas on pouch biopsy and were treated medically; 2 experienced extrasphincteric abscesses and 7 presented pouch-perineal fistulas which were treated surgically. Among them, 3 patients with persistent perineal fistula despite operation required definitive end ileostomy. Of the 20 patients followed for more than 10 years, 7 (35%) experienced Crohn's disease-related complications which required pouch excision in 2 (10%). These good results justify the use of ileal pouch-anal anastomosis in selected patients with colorectal Crohn's disease, (i.e. no past or present history of anal manifestations and no evidence of small bowel involvement), for whom the only alternative is definitive end ileostomy.

HOW MUCH BOWEL TO RESECT

The early theory of Crohn and associates was that all affected bowel with a reasonable margin of 30 cm on each side and all draining lymph nodes should be excised (2). Support of wide resection also was favored by Wolff et al. (297). In a series of 710 patients with Crohn's disease, recurrence was 89% when the anastomotic margins contained microscopic disease. This compared to 55% recurrence in patients with clear margins. However, other studies showed that a limited resection of gross disease was adequate, and the recurrence did not appear higher despite microscopic disease at the site of anastomosis (298–302). The conservative preference is based on the principle that Crohn's disease is a truly pan intestinal disease with multifocal potential and an operative cure is impossible to obtain. Hence, some surgeons perform resection only to correct the complications and not to try to eliminate the entire disease. This philosophy should diminish the risk of disability associated with short bowel syndrome. Following this principle, Alexander-Williams and Haynes (242) were prepared to perform anastomoses to bowel afflicted by minor degrees of ulceration. They found that there was no higher incidence of anastomotic leak when diseased bowel was used in comparison with the results when the ends of the bowel were normal on microscopy.

Fazio et al. (303) conducted a randomized controlled trial to determine the effect of resection margins on the recurrence of Crohn's disease in the small bowel. A total of 152 patients undergoing ileocolic resection for Crohn's disease were randomly assigned to two groups in which the proximal line of resection was 2 cm (limited resection) or 12 cm (extended resection) from the macroscopically involved area. Patients also were classified by whether the margin of resection was microscopically normal (category 1), contained nonspecific changes (category 2), were suggestive but not diagnostic for Crohn's disease (category 3), or were diagnostic for Crohn's disease (category 4). Recurrence was defined as reoperation for recurrent preanastomotic disease. Median follow-up time was 55.7 months. Disease recurred in 25% of patients in the limited resection group and 18% of patients in the extended resection group. In the 90 patients in category 1 with normal tissue, recurrence occurred in 16, whereas in the 41 patients with some degree of microscopic involvement, recurrence occurred in 13. Recurrence rates were 36% in category 2, 39% in category 3, and 21% in category 4. The authors concluded that recurrence of Crohn's disease is unaffected by the width of the margin of resection from macroscopically involved bowel.

With all of these controversies, it seems logical to stay in the middle ground, that is, to resect the grossly diseased bowel without concern for microscopic disease.

OVERVIEW OF RESULTS

The long-term prognosis, including operation rates, the incidence of recurrent disease, morbidity and mortality and current status, has been analyzed by a number of investigators. Andrews et al. (304) reported on a group of 360 patients with Crohn's colitis followed for a mean period of 14.9 years. The overall operation rate was 76%. Prolonged spontaneous or drug-induced remission occurred at all sites: right-sided disease (11%), extensive colonic disease (21%), and left-sided disease (38%). The cumulative reoperation rates at 5 and 10 years after right hemicolectomy were 26% and 46%, after colectomy and ileorectal anastomosis were 46% and 60%, and after panproctocolectomy were 10% and 21%, respectively. There was a two-fold excess mortality rate from related Crohn's disease deaths during the period of review, but the mortality rate has fallen with time. There have only been 11 related deaths in the last decade, of which eight were probably unavoidable. At review the status of most patients was good, although treatment had included a permanent stoma in less than half (41%) the patients still under review. All but 14 patients were well and symptom-free and only 16 were receiving specific medical treatment.

In a series of 130 patients operated on for Crohn's disease in Australia, there were seven postoperative deaths, all the result of septic complications following operation for large bowel disease (15) Thirty-six patients required a subsequent operation with a mean time to recurrence of 3.7 years. The cumulative recurrence rates were 24% at five years, 28% at 10 years, and 31% at 15 years.

In their review of the subject, Tjandra and Fazio (305) found the operative mortality for Crohn's colitis to be 2%. Late related mortality (2–5%) may be due to complications of operation, particularly small bowel obstruction or after operation for complications of recurrent disease. The operative mortality after emergency operation is higher, 7.8% in toxic megacolon and 29.4% in the presence of free perforation of the colon.

Tjandra and Fazio (305) also studied the matter of recurrence rates following operation for Crohn's disease and the following data have been extracted from their review. It must be acknowledged that the definition of recurrence rates varies from report-to-report and at least in part accounts for the variation in rates. Some have defined recurrence as those with clinically symptomatic disease, others reported those who require reoperation, and still others have followed patients closely and have recognized endoscopic evidence of disease. Furthermore, recurrence rates have varied with anatomic distribution of disease, operation performed, and more important, are related to length of follow-up. Notwithstanding these confounding factors, some results follow. At 14 years after initial operation, the cumulative risk of recurrence of patients with ileocolic disease is 50%, for terminal ileum disease alone 38%, and for large bowel disease alone 32%. Total proctocolectomy is associated with a lower probability of a recurrence than colectomy and ileorectal anastomosis (15–20% versus 50–70%) over a median follow-up of 15 years. The ileal recurrence rates after total proctocolectomy are significantly less than those following colectomy and ileorectal anastomosis. Segmental colectomy had even higher recurrence rates that approached 62% at five years. The cumulative probability after total proctocolectomy is estimated at 7% at five years, 11% at 10 years, and 22% at 20 years (52). The cumulative recurrence rates for ileorectal anastomosis is 34% at five years, 49% at 10 years, 55% at 20 years, and 73% at 30 years (52).

There is a predilection of recurrence for specific sites after a certain operative procedure (305). For patients with Crohn's colitis, the current operation performed at the

Cleveland Clinic is total proctocolectomy in one or more stages (76%), followed by colectomy with or without anastomosis (21%). Much less commonly, ileostomy alone or a bypass (3%) is performed (305). The most common site of recurrence for total proctocolectomy and ileostomy is the terminal ileum, immediately above the ileostomy; after ileorectal anastomosis, in the rectum or ileum; and after segmental colectomy, in the remaining large bowel. Recurrences that occur late (>10 years) are more often successfully managed medically than those that occur early. At the Cleveland Clinic the cumulative recurrence rate at 11 years in patients without terminal ileum disease is 23% compared with 46% for patients with terminal ileal disease (305).

Lock et al. (217) studied the fate of the rectum following colectomy and ileostomy. Of 101 patients who had subtotal colectomy with rectal preservation, 58 subsequently underwent either rectal excision (46 patients), ileorectal anastomosis (6 patients) or both of these operations (6 patients).

Nordgren et al. (306) analyzed the long-term results of an aggressive approach to the operative treatment of 136 patients after first resection for primary Crohn's disease. Mean follow-up was 16.6 years; 18 patients died (three of Crohn's disease). The cumulative risk for a second resection was 0.40 at 10 years and 0.45 at 15 years. Cumulative risk for a third and fourth resection was 0.5 at 10 years. The authors concluded that an aggressive surgical approach in Crohn's disease is associated with low operative mortality and morbidity and good functional results and offers good symptomatic relief.

Platell et al. (307) reported the results of treatment of 360 patients with Crohn's disease. The mean age at diagnosis was 33.4 years. The distribution of the disease was small bowel (32.3%), small bowel and colon (26.5%), colon (39.9%), and anal disease alone (1.6%). A total of 416 abdominal operations were performed on 204 patients. The most common indications for operation were failed medical therapy (21.9%), small bowel obstruction (15.9%), enteric fistula (10.1%), and intra-abdominal abscess (10.1%). The most frequently performed procedures were ileocolic resection with anastomosis (28.8%), small bowel resection (9.4%), and total colectomy and ileostomy (7%). Postoperative complications included anastomotic leaks (4%), intra-abdominal abscess formation (3.6%), and enterocutaneous fistulas (6%). Three patients died during the review period. During the mean follow-up of 84.4 months, 30% of patients developed recurrence requiring further operation at a mean 72.7 months postoperatively. The most frequent site for a recurrence was the preanastomotic terminal ileum (61.7%). Platell et al. (307) concluded that the majority of patients with Crohn's disease would require resection at some stage. This can be performed with a low mortality and morbidity and a recurrence rate of around 5% a year.

Leung and Jones (308) reported a consecutive series of 92 patients with Crohn's disease who underwent operation. The mean length of follow-up was 46 months. Forty patients had disease in more than one site, compared with 52 patients with single site disease. In total, 184 procedures were performed. Patients with the combination of colonic and anorectal disease required more operative interventions than patients with other disease distributions. At follow-up, all patients with disease confined to the small intestine or ileocecal region were free of symptoms with only 9 taking medication. No patients presenting with colonic disease had symptomatic disease or were taking any anti-inflammatory medication at time of follow-up. However, in the group of patients with anorectal or the combination of colonic and anorectal disease, 42% had ongoing symptoms (predominantly anorectal). Fifteen patients had a stoma at some point during their surgical course. Those with small bowel or colonic disease had better outcomes following operation compared to those with anorectal disease.

Fichera et al. (309) prospectively evaluated the long-term outcomes of patients with isolated Crohn's disease to identify patients that may benefit from initial more aggressive resection. They identified 179 patients with Crohn's disease operated on for primary colonic disease: 55 patients underwent segmental colectomy, 49 total abdominal colectomies, and 75 total proctocolectomies. Patients with diffuse colonic involvement were significantly less likely to undergo segmental colectomy than total abdominal colectomy or total proctocolectomy. Patients with distal involvement or pancolitis were significantly less likely to undergo segmental colectomy than total abdominal colectomy or total proctocolectomy. Overall, there were 24.4% with surgical Crohn's recurrences during follow-up: 38.8% in the segmental colectomy, 22.9% in the total abdominal colectomy and 9.3% in the total proctocolectomy group. There was a significant difference in time to recurrence between the 3 groups. Segmental colectomy patients had a significantly shorter time to first recurrence than total proctocolectomy patients. After adjusting for extent of disease, the segmental colecotomy group had a significantly greater risk of surgical recurrence than the total proctocolectomy group. Total proctocolectomy patients were significantly less likely to be still taking medications one year after the index operation than total abdominal colectomy patients and segmental colectomy patients. During follow-up, patients with isolated distal disease were significantly more likely to require a permanent stoma than patients with isolated proximal disease. They concluded a more aggressive approach should be considered in patients with diffuse and distal Crohn's colitis. Total proctolectomy and the properly selected patients is associated with low morbidity, lower risk of recurrence, and longer time to recurrence. Patients after total proctocolectomy are more likely to be weaned off all Crohn's-related medications. Long-term rate of permanent fecal diversion is significantly higher in patients with distal disease.

Delaney et al. (310) assessed the effect of surgery for Crohn's disease on quality of life in the early postoperative period. Preoperative and 30-day postoperative quality of life were determined in 82 patients using Cleveland Global Qualify of Life scores (range from 0[worst] to 10 [best possible] quality of life). The incidence of complications was 23% (11% were major). There was a significant improvement in quality of life 30 days after surgery. Female patients and those who did not develop complications within 30 days of operation had a significantly greater improvement in quality of life after operation than other groups.

To determine whether reoperation at the ileostomy in Crohn's disease reflects recurrence of disease or a complication of stoma construction, Ecker et al. (311) reviewed 92 patients who underwent colectomy followed up for 5.4 years. In 28 patients (30.4%) a total of 42 operations were necessary. The clinical indication was prestomal recurrence in 5 reoperations (11.9%) and stoma complications in 37 (88.1%). In contrast, ileal recurrence was demonstrated histologically in 28 specimens (66.7%) and healthy ileum in the rest. There was a statistically significant association between fibrotic recurrence and stoma stenosis/retraction and a trend for association between penetrating recurrence and peristomal ulceration. The cumulative risk for first reoperation due to clinical recurrence was calculated at 3.3% and 14.0% at 5 and 10 years postoperatively, whereas the corresponding figures for stomal complications were 25.7% and 40.0%. In contrast, the cumulative risk that a recurrence was found histologically on the occasion of the reoperation was 23.0% and 35.0% while the probability that the ileum was healthy in the case of a stoma complication remained low. In conclusion, most reoperations after ileostomy construction in Crohn's disease are associated histologically with recurrent inflammation.

Norris et al. (312) conducted a retrospective review of all patients with histologically proven Crohn's disease to assess whether an older cohort was at an increased risk. A total of 156 patients had 298 laparotomies for histopathologically proven Crohn's disease. The frequency distribution of age at last laparotomy was bimodal, and the statistically determined cut-off age between younger and older cohorts was 55 years. Thirty-three patients were old than 55 years. There was no difference in duration of symptoms before first diagnosis (older, 17 months vs. younger, 25 months), previous number of Crohn's operations (42.4% vs. 39.8%), or duration of known Crohn's disease. Isolated large bowel disease was more common in the elderly cohort (42.4% vs. 18.7%). Small bowel and ileocecal resections were more common in the younger cohort (72.4% vs. 51.6%). There was one death in each cohort (overall mortality 1.3%) and anastomotic leak rates were 4.3% (older) versus 5.3% (younger) despite frank sepsis present in 21.2% of all subjects at the time of operation. The older group had more cardiac (18.3% vs. 0.8%) and respiratory complications (18.2% vs. 2.4%) and a longer mean but not median postoperative hospital admission. They concluded, clinical features and presentation are similar in the older and younger Crohn's patients having a laparotomy. However, in the older patient there is a greater likelihood of large bowel disease, ileocecal resection is done less commonly, there is a higher risk of minor cardiopulmonary postoperative complications, but with similar mortality and anastomotic leak rates to the younger patient.

Krupnick and Morris reviewed the long-term results of resection for Crohn's disease (313). They noted 70% to 90% of patients will require operative intervention. Operations for small bowel Crohn's disease is usually necessary for unrelenting stenotic complications of the disease. Fistula, abscess, and perforation can also necessitate operative intervention. Most patients benefit from resection or strictureplasty with an improved quality of life and remission of disease, but recurrence is common and 33% to 82% of patients will need a second operation, and 22% to 33% will require more than two resections. Short-bowel syndrome is unavoidable in a small percentage of Crohn's patients because of recurrent resection of affected small bowel and inflammatory destruction of the remaining mucosa. Although previously a lethal and unrelenting disease with death caused by malnutrition, patients with short-bowel syndrome today can lead productive lives with maintenance on TPN. This lifestyle, however, does not come without a price. Severe TPN complications such as sepsis of indwelling central venous catheters and liver failure do occur.

Hurst et al. (314) elucidated the features, indications, and surgical treatment in patients affected by complications of Crohn's disease in 513 consecutive patients who were operated on for 542 occurrences of Crohn's disease. Indications for abdominal surgery were often multiple but included failure of medical management (n = 220), obstruction (n = 94), intestinal fistula (n = 68), mass (n = 56), abdominal abscess (n = 33), hemorrhage (n = 7), and peritonitis (n = 9). Four hundred sixty-four abdominal procedures were performed, necessitating 425 intestinal resections and 97 strictureplasties. The use of a strictureplasty was more common in the second half of the study (16% vs 7.3%, second half versus first half). Perioperative complications occurred in 75 of the 464 abdominal operations (16%). There were no deaths. One hundred and thirty patients (25%) required operation for perineal complications of Crohn's disease. The presence of Crohn's disease in the rectal mucosa was associated with a higher risk for permanent stomas in patients requiring operation for treatment of perianal Crohn's (67% vs. 11%). They concluded, patterns of surgical treatment in Crohn's disease are changing with more emphasis on non-resectional options. The presence of rectal involvement significantly increases the need for an permanent stoma in patients with perianal Crohn's disease.

Tay et al. (315) analyzed the impact of immunomodulator therapy on the rate of intra-abdominal septic complications in Crohn's disease patients undergoing bowel reanastomosis or strictureplasty. Immunomodulator agents included azathioprine, 6-MP, methotrexate, and infliximab. Intra-abdominal septic complications developed in 11% of operations. Immunodomulator use was associated with fewer (5.6%) compared with 25% of patients not on therapy. Intra-abdominal septic complications were not influenced by steroid use, smoking status, preoperative abscess, or fistula or albumin levels.

Uno et al. (316) estimated the mortality and cause of death by Crohn's disease in Japan in nine affiliated hospitals and followed up for 8.4 years. Death occurred in 6 of 544 patients. Cumultative survival rates for patients with Crohn's disease were 99.7% at 5 years, 99.3% at 10 years, and 96.8% at 15 years; there was no significant difference between genders or the age-matched expected survival rate of the Japanese population.

Bernell et al. (317) conducted a study to account for recurrence rates, present risk factors for recurrence after primary colectomy, and account for the ultimate risk of having a stoma after colectomy with ileorectal anastomosis in a population-based cohort of 833 patients with Crohn's colitis. The cumulative 10-year risk of a symptomatic recurrence was 58% and 47% respectively after colectomy with ileorectal anastomosis and segmental colonic resection. In colectomy with ileostomy, lower rates were found with respectively 24% and 37% after subtotal colectomy and proctocolectomy with ileostomy. The multivariate analysis showed that perianal disease, ileorectal anastomosis, and segmental resection were independent risk factors for postoperative recurrence. In 76% of patients with ileorectal anastomosis, a stoma-free function could be retained during a median follow-up of 12.5 years.

Bernell et al. (318) assessed the risk for resection and postoperative recurrence in the treatment in a population-based cohort of 907 patients with primary ileocecal Crohn's disease. Resection rates were 61%, 77%, and 83% at 1, 5, and 10 years respectively after the diagnosis. Relapse rates were 28% and 36% 5 and 10 years after the first resection. A younger age at diagnosis resulted in a low resection rate. The presence of perianal Crohn's and long resection segments increased the incidence of recurrence, and resection for a palpable mass and/or abscess decreased the recurrence rate.

Bernell et al. (319) assessed the impact of possible risk factors on intestinal resection and postoperative recurrence of Crohn's disease in a population-based cohort of 1,936 patients. The cumulative rate of intestinal resection was 44%, 61%, and 71% at 1, 5, and 10 years after diagnosis. Postoperative recurrences occurred in 33% and 44% at 5 and 10 years after resection. The relative risk of surgery was increased in patients with Crohn's disease involving any part of the small bowel, in those having perianal fistulas, and those who were 45 to 59 years of age at diagnosis. Female gender and perianal fistulas as well as small bowel and continuous ileocolic disease, increased the relative risk of recurrence. The frequency of operation has decreased over time, but the postoperative relapse rate remains unchanged.

Yamamoto et al. (320) reviewed their overall experience of single-stage proctocolectomy for Crohn's disease in 103 patients. Principal indications for proctocolectomy were chronic colitis (49%), acute colitis (37%), and anorectal disease (14%). The commonest postoperative complication was delayed perineal wound healing (35%) followed by intra-abdominal sepsis (17%) and stomal complications (15%). In 23 patients, the perineal wound healed between 3 and 6 months after proctocolectomy, whereas in 13 patients the wound remained unhealed for more than 6 months. There were 2 hospital deaths (2%) caused by sepsis. The 5-year, 10-year and 15-year cumultative reoperation rates for small bowel recurrence were 13%, 17%, and 25% respectively after a median follow-up of 18.6 years. Factors affecting reoperation rate for recurrence were gender (male; hazard ratio 2.4 vs. female) and age at operation ($\leq$ 30 years: hazard ratio 2.6 vs. $>$ 30 years). The following factors did not affect the reoperation rate: duration of symptoms, smoking habits, associated perforating disease, coexisting small-bowel disease, postoperative complications, and medical treatment.

Yamamoto et al. (321) examined risk factors for intra-abdominal sepsis after operation in 343 patients who underwent 1008 intestinal anastomosis during 566 operations for primary or recurrent Crohn's disease. Intra-abdominal septic complications, defined as anastomotic leak, intra-abdominal abscess, or enterocutaneous fistula, developed after 76 operations (13%). Intra-abdominal septic complications were significantly associated with preoperative low albumin levels ($<$ 30g/l), preoperative steroid use, abscess at the time of laparotomy, and fistula at the time of laparotomy. The intra-abdominal septic complication rate was 50% in patients with all these four risk factors, 29% of patients with three risk factors, 14% of patients with two risk factors, 16% in patients with only one risk factor and 5% in patients with none of these risk factors. The following factors did not affect the incidence of septic complications: age, duration of symptoms, number of previous bowel resections, site of disease, type of operation (resection, strictureplasty, or bypass), covering stoma, and number, site, or method (sutured or stapled) of anastomoses.

CHALLENGING ANATOMIC LOCATIONS OF CROHN'S DISEASE

OROPHARYNX

Crohn's disease occasionally involves mucosal membranes of the oropharynx, usually in conjunction with disease elsewhere. Rarely, the respiratory tract may be involved. Patients may complain of painful oral ulcers, glossitis dysphagia, or odynophagia (and result in reduced food intake), malnutrition, and weight loss (322). Lip fissuring, gingival hyperplasia, angular cheilitis, mucosal tags, cobblestoning plaques, polypoid lesions, perioral erythema; and pyostomatitis vegetans may be present (323). Most patients with oral lesions require no specific oral treatment. Mild analgesics and Orabase (Squibb) may be useful (322). For very symptomatic lesions, the gamut of medical agents described in this chapter has been tried.

Clark et al. (324) reported a case of a 24 year old lady who presented with cervical lymphadenopathy, the subsequent investigation of which resulted in the identification of the disease both in this node and in the tonsils. It is noted that these lesions may precede the classical intestinal manifestations.

ESOPHAGUS

Esophageal Crohn's disease is a rare finding. The presumptive diagnosis is based on esophageal inflammation aphthous ulcers occurring in the presence of Crohn's involvement in other areas of the gastrointestinal tract. The average age at diagnosis is 40 years with no gender predominance. Symptoms include progressive dysphagia, weight loss odynophagia, epigastric pain, and chest discomfort. Nausea and heartburn are uncommon. Hoarseness due to involvement of the larynx or tracheobronchial tree is rare (325). Pulmonary symptoms may predominate if there is significant regurgitation and aspiration or a fistulous communication with a bronchus. Radiologic findings include esophageal stricture, fistulous tracts, thickened folds, asymmetric esophagitis, and cobblestoning of the mucosa, and ulcerations. Endoscopic findings include hyperemia, inflammation, friability, nodular thickening, inflammatory mass, cobblestoning, ulceration, and stricturing. Biopsies are usually too superficial to make a definitive diagnosis. Aminosalicylates and immunosuppressives have produced equivocal results, but response has occurred with the use of steroids. Complete healing of lesions has been reported in two-thirds of patients after a two- to four-week course of steroids (326). Esophagectomy is required in 40% to 50% of patients. Indications for operation are extensive stricture and fistula formation (325). Complications have included reflux esophagitis, late stricture, empyema with esophagocutaneous fistula formation, pneumonia, respiratory insufficiency, sepsis, and gastric retention (in patients who do not have a pyloroplasty) (325). Mortality has been 8%.

Decker et al. (327) reviewed the clinical features and outcome of patients with esophageal Crohn's disease at the Mayo Clinic. Twenty patients (0.2%), with esophageal involvement were identified. Median age at diagnosis was 31 years (range, 7 to 77 years). Eleven patients (55%), were female. Extraesophageal Crohn's disease preceded or was found at the same time as the diagnosis of esophageal Crohn's in all cases. Sixteen patients (80%) had symptoms referable to the esophagus. Endoscopic findings included ulcers in 17 (85%), erythema or erosions in 8 (40%), and strictures in 4 patients (20%). One patient had a fistula. The most common histologic finding were active chronic inflammation (75%) and ulcer (30%). No granulomata were identified. Approximately one half of their patients improved with first-line therapy. Eleven patients (55%) received immune modifier therapy. Six showed significant improvement on azothioprine, 6-mercaptopurine, or cyclosporine. Esophageal dilatation was required in 6 patients, and 3 patients required operation.

Rudolph et al. (328) reviewed the literature and in addition to their three cases found 72 additional cases of esophageal Crohn's disease. Among these, 75 patients who were on average 34 years old, esophageal disease was the presenting symptom in 41 patients (55%). The diagnosis was difficult in 13 patients, in whom no distal bowel disease was detected at the time of initial esophageal presentation. The most common presentation was dysphagia associated with aphthous or deep ulcerations (52 patients). In 11 of these patients, oral aphthous ulcerations were also present. Esophageal stenosis or fistulas to surrounding structures were present in 27 patients and led to operation in 17 patients. Most of the unfavourable outcomes were in this group of 27 patients with esophageal complications including 5 deaths. Fourteen additional patients required operation for Crohn's disease of other areas. Responses of uncomplicated ulcerative disease of the esophagus tended to be favourable if the medical regimen included prednisone. Clinical patterns of esophageal Crohn's disease were divided into three categories: ulcerative, stenosing, and asymptomatic.

■ GASTRODUODENUM

Duodenal involvement by Crohn's disease is a rare condition. The reported incidence has ranged from 0.5% to 4% (329). The gastric antrum and pylorus may be involved in up to 60% of cases (330,241). In one series, distal disease was previously known in 51.7% of patients and an additional 30.3% were found, to have unsuspected disease discovered during the investigation of duodenal complications. Of patients with seemingly isolated disease, distal involvement developed in 56% of patients and only 7.9% did not have disease after an 11.7-year follow-up (331).

Primary Crohn's disease characteristically affects young persons (average age, 26 years) with no gender predilection (331). Isolated involvement may be late to diagnose because symptoms are usually attributed to peptic ulcer disease. Symptoms related to the upper gastrointestinal tract may be limited or overshadowed by diarrhea or other symptoms from disease in the more distal portion of the intestine. Symptoms include epigastric pain, nausea, vomiting, loss of weight, hematemesis, or melena. Contrast studies remain the most useful for diagnosis. Radiographic investigations may reveal thickened folds, nodular changes, aphthous ulcers, fissuring, cobblestoning, or stenosis (Fig. 17).

Endoscopic features may include gastric and duodenal ulceration, especially linear or serpiginous (323). The antrum may be poorly distensible, and a rigid pyloric

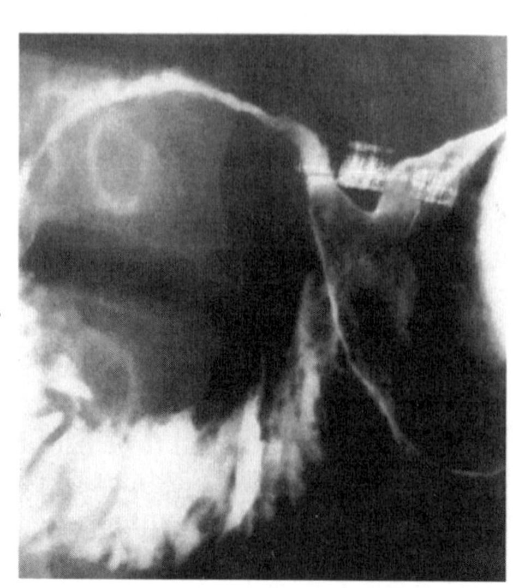
A

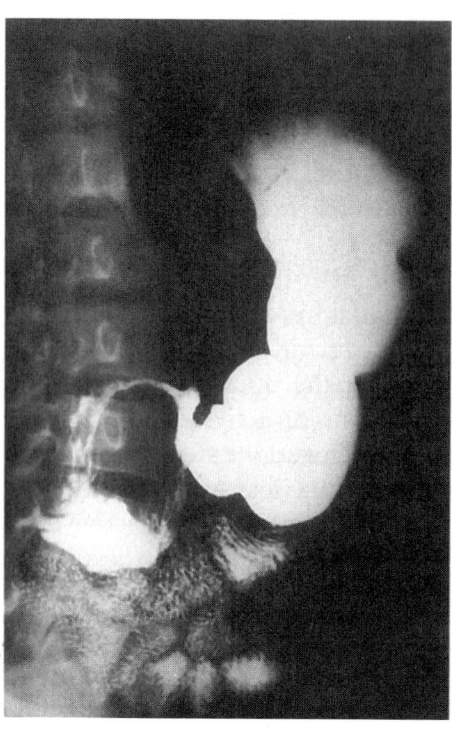
B

FIGURE 17 ■ (**A** and **B**) Radiographs showing duodenal Crohn's disease.

or pyloroduodenal stenosis may be observed. Patchy or diffuse nodules and aphthous ulcers with cobblestoning may be present. Strictures and fistula from the stomach or duodenum into nearby intestinal loops or the pancreaticobiliary tree may be appreciated (e.g., greater curvature of the stomach to splenic flexure or ileocolic anastomosis, duodenum). Alcantara et al. (332) conducted a prospective study of 41 patients diagnosed as having Crohn's disease to evaluate the degree of upper gastrointestinal tract involvement. In 56%, endoscopic alterations were found most frequently affecting the antrum and duodenum. Lesions encountered were aphthoid erosions, ulcers, thickening of folds, nodules, erythema, and stenosis. Granulomas were found in biopsies in 19.5% the patients. They were more frequent in those demonstrating endoscopic alterations (26%) than in those with normal endoscopic findings (11%).

Clinically, the condition may present in one of two ways, either as an intrinsic lesion or as secondary involvement (usually from right colonic disease or from an ileocolic anastomosis in the case of recurrence).

Operation is required in about one-third of patients generally for gastric outlet obstruction (192,331,333). Bleeding is a rare indication because now effective H_2 blockers are available. In this anatomically difficult area, bypass procedures (gastro-jejunostomy and/or duodenal jejunostomy) are generally recommended (333). If gastroenterostomy is performed, the patient is subject to marginal ulceration and, hence, a vagotomy is often recommended. However, the role of vagotomy remains controversial. The debate focuses on the risk of postvagotomy diarrhea vs. risk of marginal ulceration. How the availability of powerful H_2 blockers might modify the latter recommendation is unknown. For short segment duodenal strictures, strictureplasty may be the appropriate solution. Fistulas between regions of active disease in the terminal ileum and colon and the stomach or duodenum may occur. Weight loss and diarrhea are the most common complaints. There is active disease in the stomach and duodenum in less than 10% of cases. Barium enema demonstrates retrograde flow of barium into the duodenum. Resection of the involved bowel and primary closure of the stomach or duodenum with serosal patch and interposition of omentum are important principles of management. A large duodenal defect may be treated by duodenojejunal anastomosis, serosal onlay patch, or drained into a Roux-en-Y limb.

Murray et al. (241) reviewed 70 patients with primary Crohn's disease of the duodenum. Of these, 27 (38.5%) required an operation. Of the 22 patients treated by the authors, four (18%) had only gastroduodenal disease and 13 (59%) had associated gastric involvement. Sukhabote and Freeman (334) examined the clinical features of 22 patients with Crohn's disease of the upper gastrointestinal tract. In most cases, a benign clinical course was observed with only one patient coming to operation. Upper abdominal pain (90%), weight loss (>50%), and nausea and vomiting (>30%) were the common symptoms. Endoscopic features included mucosal erosions, thickening of mucosal folds, ulceration, granularity, nodularity, and cobblestoning. Patients were treated with pharmacologic agents for Crohn's disease as well as ranitidine and sucralfate.

Poggioli et al. (329) reviewed 12 patients with duodenal Crohn's disease, an incidence of 3.6%. The male to female ratio was 2:1 with a mean age of 44.8 years (range, 24 to 71 years). A duodenal fistula was present in three patients while the other nine had an intrinsic lesion. Five of the nine patients had stenotic lesions and they presented with typical symptoms of "high" obstruction with postprandial pain, vomiting, and weight loss. All patients were diagnosed preoperatively with endoscopic and histologic evidence of Crohn's disease and were treated operatively. The four patients with duodenal lesions with morphologic appearance of peptic ulcer disease had diffuse jejunoileal disease. Their symptoms were also ulcer-like, with pain, heartburn, and dyspepsia. Three of four also had recurrent episodes of bleeding. The diagnosis was established by the presence of aphthoid ulcers with a coexisting jejunoileal or ileocolic location of Crohn's disease. Treatment of patients with duodenal fistula consisted of resection of source and primary closure of the duodenal breach. Duodenal stenosis was treated with strictureplasty in three patients and duodenojejunostomy in two patients. Patients with ulcer-like symptoms were treated nonoperatively. Medical treatment consisted of H_2 blockers and omeprazole but two patients required steroids. Following strictureplasty in one patient, gastric inertia developed and led to subtotal gastrectomy with a Billroth II gastrojejunostomy. Strictureplasty can be considered the treatment of choice for duodenal stenosis up to the third portion. For stenoses extending from the third portion of the duodenum to the ligament of Treitz, duodenojejunostomy is advocated because of technical difficulties of strictureplasty.

Yamamoto et al. (335) assessed the clinical features and management of 14 patients with gastroduodenal fistulas in patients with Crohn's disease. In 6 patients, a gastroduodenal fistula was diagnosed before operation whereas 8 gastroduodenal fistulas were discovered during operation for distal Crohn's disease. In 6 patients, the fistula originated from Crohn's disease in the transverse colon, and in 6 patients it originated from recurrent disease at an ileocolic anastomosis; these patients had no gross evidence of gastroduodenal Crohn's disease. In one patient, the ileocolonic-duodenal fistula closed on medical treatment. The other 11 patients underwent resection of the diseased bowel and closure of the gastric or duodenal fistulas. The two remaining fistulas were from the duodenum to the abdominal wall; both had primary Crohn's duodenitis. One duodenocutaneous fistula was treated by debridement of the duodenal fistula and simple closure of the defect; the other was treated by limited duodenal excision around the fistula and by duodenojejunostomy. In all patients, gastroduodenal fistulas were cured, and there have been no fistula recurrences. Simple closure of the gastroduodenal component of the fistula is generally advised for gastroduodenal fistulas.

In their recent review Mottet et al. (336) noted that symptomatic gastroduodenal manifestations of Crohn's disease are rare with less than 4% of patients being clinically symptomatic. Gastroduodenal involvement may, however, be found endoscopically in 20% and in up to 40% of cases histologically, most frequently as Helicobacter pylori-negative focal gastritis, usually in patients with concomitant distal ileal disease. In practice, the activity of concomitant distal Crohn's disease usually determines the indication for therapy, except in the presence of obstructive gastroduodenal symptoms. With the few data available, it seems correct to say that localized gastroduodenal disease should be treated with standard medical therapy used for more distal disease, with the exception of sulfasalazine and mesalamine with pH-dependent release. Presence of symptoms of obstruction needs aggressive therapy. If medical therapy with steroids and immunomodulatory drugs does not alleviate the symptoms, balloon dilatation and operative intervention are options to consider.

■ DIFFUSE JEJUNOILEITIS

Diffuse jejunoileitis is an uncommon, but important manifestation of Crohn's disease because of the associated high morbidity and challenges in medical management. It has been reported in 3% to 10% of all cases (337). Tan and Allan (337) analyzed the outcome in 34 patients with diffuse jejunoileitis. It presents in younger patients (mean age at diagnosis, 26.4 years) than those with distal ileal Crohn's disease (mean age at diagnosis, 33.3 years). Nearly all presented with clear-cut abdominal symptoms, including a combination of colicky abdominal pain (91%), weight loss (62%), and diarrhea (53%). Other symptoms include malnutrition, growth arrest, hypoalbuminemia, and peripheral edema. Most patients had severe symptoms reflected by the fact that 77% had been treated with corticosteroids for periods of more than 6 months at some stage during their follow-up. The mean follow-up from diagnosis was 16 years. Twenty eight patients (82%) had at least one operation for diffuse jejunoileitis and two thirds of the patients (21) required two or more operations. The frequency of operative intervention was particularly high in the younger patients ($r = 0.71$). The proportion of patients requiring operation was highest in the first year after diagnosis. The annual operative rate was 15% for the first 10 years, and then it fell to 5.2% in years 11 to 15, and 2.6% in years 16 to 20. The data suggest that the disease burns itself out over time. The increasing use of strictureplasty for short strictures and the minimal use of resection have eliminated problems associated with the short small bowel syndrome. The long-term prognosis of these patients is good. In the study by Tan and Allan (337), only two patients died (one of perforation of the jejunum and another of an unrelated bronchogenic carcinoma). After a mean interval from diagnosis of 16 years, 24 of 32 living patients were well and symptom free. Only eight had abdominal symptoms, of whom three were receiving corticosteroid treatment, and one was being given azathioprine. The combination of anti-inflammatory drugs with the relief of recurrent obstructive symptoms by strictureplasty can together produce a good long-term prognosis in most parents with diffuse jejunoileitis.

Keh et al. (338) compared the outcome of patients who were surgically treated for jejunal Crohn's disease to those whose disease was confined to the ileocecal region from a database of 724 surgically treated Crohn's disease patients. Twenty-eight patients with jejunal Crohn's disease at their first operation (12 jejunal alone, 16 also involving other sites) were identified. The median age in both groups was 21 years with a median follow-up period of 19 years. The 3, 5, and 10 years reooperation rates for the groups with jejunal disease were 43%, 50%, and 61% compared to 22%, 30%, and 51% with ileocecal disease respectively.

Freeman (339) reported 39 patients with jejunoileal Crohn's disease followed for a mean duration of over 16 years. Over 80% of patients had concomitant colonic and/or gastroduodenal involvement with Crohn's disease, suggesting that this entity may represent a specific clinical phenotype of extensive disease localization. Classification of Crohn's disease behaviour using the Vienna classification schema revealed that virtually all patients in this study suffered from intestinal stricture formation or penetrating disease complications. Moreover, pharmacological therapies with corticosteroids and immunosuppressant drugs were rarely successful, with virtually all patients requiring at least one and usually multiple intestinal resections. Finally, most patients required long-term nutritional support, often with home parenteral nutrition.

Higuero et al. (340) evaluated the clinical characteristics, therapeutic modalities and long-term outcome in 18 patients with jejunoileitis and compared them to 36 matched controls without jejunoileitis. Mean follow-up was 7.6 years in both groups. At time of Crohn's disease jejunoileitis diagnosis, the following signs were significantly more frequent in patients with jejunoileal Crohn's disease than in controls: malnutrition (39% vs.3%), pain suggesting obstruction (33% vs. 8%), vomiting (28% vs. 5%). Patients with Crohn's disease jejunoileitis were more frequently male: male/female ration = 2.0/1.1. Upper digestive involvement (esophagus, stomach, and duodenum) (67% vs. 36%) and small intestine strictures (61% vs. 19%) were more frequent in Crohn's disease jejunoileitis. Initial management was more "aggressive" in Crohn's disease jejunoileitis than in controls: steroids in 62% vs. 30%, azathioprine in 39% vs. 3%, total parenteral nutrition in 28% vs. 8% and operation in 33% vs. 17%. During follow-up, the need for azathioprine therapy and operation were more frequent in Crohn's disease jejunoileitis than in controls (extensive small bowel resection in 2 patients). In 10 of 18 patients, jejunoileitis involvement was diagnosed with a median delay of 3.6 years (range 0.5 to 14.5) after Crohn's disease diagnosis and at time of Crohn's disease diagnosis in the 8 others; outcome after Crohn's disease jejunoileitis diagnosis was similar in these two groups. In their experience, the main revealing signs of jejunoileitis are obstruction and malnutrition. Patients with Crohn's disease jejunoileitis required more often azathioprine and operation than patients without jejunoileitis. Jejunoileitis is a severe form of Crohn's disease more frequently complicated by extensive small bowel resection.

Yamamoto et al. (341) reviewed the long-term outcome of surgical treatment for diffuse jejunoileal Crohn's disease in 46 patients who required operation. Strictureplasty was used for short strictures without perforating disease (perforation, abscess, fistula). Long strictures (< 20 cm) or perforating disease were treated with resection. During an initial operation, strictureplasty was used on 63 strictures in 18 patients (39%). After a median follow-up of 15 years, there were 3 deaths: 1 from postoperative sepsis, 1 from small-bowel carcinoma, and 1 from bronchogenic carcinoma. Thirty-nine patients required 113 reoperations for jejunoileal recurrence. During 75 of the 113 reoperations (66%), strictureplasty was used in 315 strictures. Only 2 patients experienced the development of short-bowel syndrome and required home parenteral nutrition. At publication, 4 patients were symptomatic and required medical treatment. All other patients were asymptomatic and required neither medical treatment nor nutritional support. Most patients with diffuse jejunal Crohn's disease can be restored to good health with minimal symptoms by surgical treatment that includes strictureplasty.

■ APPENDIX

Prieto-Nieto et al. (342) found Crohn's disease confined to the vermiform appendix is rare. The incidence was 0.2% of all patients diagnosed with Crohn's disease at La Paz University Hospital, Madrid, Spain, in 20 years. They reviewed the clinical records of 10 patients with isolated appendiceal Crohn's disease. The preoperative diagnosis was acute appendicitis in all 10 cases, and all patients underwent appendectomy. Postoperative complications were limited to an enterocutaneous fistula in one patient. There was no evidence of recurrence during a mean follow-up period of 14.5 years (range 2–25 years). They concluded, that Crohn's disease when confined to the appendix is less aggressive than in other sections of the intestine, with a low recurrence rate and incidence of postoperative fistula.

■ PERIANAL AND ANAL CANAL CROHN'S DISEASE

Perianal and anal canal disease, a frequent manifestation of Crohn's disease, may be the first sign of the disease and sometimes precedes the onset of intestinal symptoms by many years. The incidence of anal problems in Crohn's disease varies greatly among reported series as low as 3.8% and as high as 61% to 80% (288). Different distributions of the disease also have different incidences of perianal disease. Generally, patients with large bowel Crohn's disease have a higher incidence of perianal manifestations than those with small bowel involvement. The incidence of perianal disease from several reports is cited in Table 5.

The diagnosis of perianal and anal Crohn's disease is easy if the surgeon knows the patient's history of Crohn's disease. However, if the anal and perianal disease is the first manifestation, an accurate diagnosis can be difficult or missed altogether. There are some features of anal and perianal disease that are suggestive of Crohn's disease, for example, multiplicity of lesions, lateral location fissures, deep ulceration of perianal skin and anal canal, anal stricture, and multiple fistulas. Most lesions are less painful than they appear. Complete colonic examinations with colonoscopy or flexible sigmoidoscopy with barium enema should be performed to rule out associated colorectal Crohn's disease. Upper gastrointestinal studies with small bowel follow-through are also part of the investigation. Endoanal ultrasonography may be useful in evaluating fistulous tracks and the presence of sepsis but is limited if the patient has severe pain or an underlying stricture (288). MRI may be useful for evaluating the integrity of the internal and external sphincter as well as identifying complex fistulas and abscesses (288). For patients with a great deal of pain, examination under anesthesia may detect and provide an opportunity to drain sepsis. Biopsies of perianal lesions usually yield only nonspecific inflammation (331) but may permit exclusion of a malignancy in a long-standing fistula or stricture.

Efforts to classify perianal disease associated with Crohn's disease have been made but because of the diversity of the pathologic processes, obvious difficulties are encountered. Hughes (354) proposed a classification based on type and severity of pathologic process. This clinical classification of perianal Crohn's disease (Box 1) is based on the presence of certain structural abnormalities: ulceration, fistula/abscess, and strictures. Each of these three structural abnormalities is graded on a scale from zero to two depending on severity (zero not present, two severe). There is an associated subsidiary classification covering associated conditions, proximal disease, and disease activity (APD) (Box 2). These provide useful comparative checklists that allow intergroup comparison by giving a concise score instead of a subjective, confusing, and lengthy description.

Francois et al. (355) assessed the value of Hughes' pathogenic classification. Patients with primary specific lesions (condyloma, cavitating ulcer, fissure) underwent more abdominal interventions (68% vs. 31%) as well as proctologic interventions (2.9 vs. 1.35 operations patient). Perfect continence was recorded ultimately in 31.8% of patients in the first group compared to 62.5% in the second group. This study showed the very poor prognosis of anal perineal fistulas in Crohn's disease.

There is no question that the perianal disease associated with Crohn's disease results in morbidity for the patient. A number of available indices have been used

TABLE 5 ■ Incidence of Perianal Disease in Crohn's Disease

Author(s)	Small Bowel (%)	Large Bowel (%)	Small and Large Bowels (%)	Overall (%)
Rankin et al. (NCCS) (343)	26	47	41	36
Williams et al. (344)	14	52	–	22
Hobbiss and Schofield (345)	11	40	53	33
Hughes et a1. (346)	–	–	–	78
Markowitz et al. (347)	41	36	54	49
Lockhart-Mummery (348)	34	58	58	55
Goebell (349)	10	43 R100[a]	26	26
Kangas (350)	–	–	–	42
Palder et al. (351)	67	51	60	62
McKee and Keenan (352)	–	–	–	31
Platell et al. (53)	21	48	32	42
Sangwan et al. (353)	18	48	33	–

[a]R, With rectal disease.

BOX 1 ■ Cardiff Classification of Perianal Crohn's Disease (UFS)

U (Ulceration)	F (Fistula/Abscess)	S (Stricture)
0. Not present	0. Not present	0. Not present
1. Superficial fissures	1. Low/superficial.	1. Reversible stricture
(a) Posterior and/or anterior	(a) Perianal	(a) Anal canal-spasm
(b) Lateral	(b) Anovulval, anoscrotal	(b) Low rectum-membrane
(c) With gross skin tags	(c) Intersphincteric	(c) Spasm with severe pain, no sepsis
2. Cavitating ulcers	(d) Anovaginal	2. Irreversible
(a) Anal canal	2. High	(a) Anal stenosis
(b) Lower rectum	(a) Blind supralevator	(b) Extrarectal stricture
(c) With extension toperineal skin (aggressive ulceration)	(b) High direct (anorectal)	
	(d) High complex	
	(e) Rectovaginal	
	(c) Ileoperineal	

Source: From Ref. 354.

to assess the extent to which patients are troubled, or indeed incapacitated by the various perianal and anal disorders. These include the Crohn's Disease Activity Index (CDAI), the simple Harvey-Bradshaw index (HBDAI), the Physician Global Assessment (MDGA), the Patient Global Assessment (PGA), and the most recently described Perianal Disease Activity Index (PDAI). The latter index was described and reported by Irvine (356) to be simple and clinically useful when administered twice to clinically stable patients. The author conducted a study to assess the degree of impairment and response to therapy in 37 patients. Each of five elements was graded on a 5-point Likert scale in these patients at 124 visits (Box 3). The CDAI, HBDAI, PDAI, and treatment were recorded and the indices validated against MDGA and PGA. There was strong correlation of PDAI with MDGA and PGA, but poor correlation of PDAI with CDAI and HBDAI. It was found that physicians prescribed more aggressive treatment for patients with higher PDAI scores.

There is evidence that perianal Crohn's disease may heal if active Crohn's disease elsewhere in the gut is treated successfully. Such treatment may include bowel resection. The healing rate has been reported between 47% and 80% (357). These results must be interpreted with caution because many anorectal lesions also heal spontaneously.

The management of perianal Crohn's disease can be considered either medical or surgical. In the medical management, a large number of agents have been tried. These include steroids, sulfasalazine, a host of 5-ASA products now available, antibiotics (metronidazole, ciprofloxacin, clarithromycin, and others), immunosuppressive agents (6-MP, azathioprine, methotrexate, and cyclosporine), and bowel rest with total parenteral nutrition, the latter not to be discussed as there is no evidence of its value in definitive resolution of symptoms. Although there is some evidence of efficacy reported by enthusiasts for each of the above modalities, overall results of treatment have been mixed. Neither the initial response rate nor the recurrent symptoms following cessation of treatment is ideal.

There is little evidence to suggest a benefit from steroids and aminosalicylates in the treatment of perianal disease. Present et al. (115) reported a 31% fistula-in-ano closure with 6-MP compared with 6% for placebo. An added benefit was the ability to decrease steroid dose in 75% of patients compared with 36% in the placebo group. Lecomte et al. (358) reported that one third of patients with perianal lesions of Crohn's disease demonstrated a clear improvement during azathioprine or 6-mercaptopurine therapy. Patients aged 40 years or older with recent perianal disease and without fistula were the best responders.

Brandt et al. (359) reported a beneficial response of metronidazole for perineal Crohn's disease. However, in the 26 patients reviewed in follow-up it was noted that when the dosage was decreased, there was a 100% exacerbation of symptoms. The cessation of medication was successful in only 28% patients. Healing could be achieved with drug introduction but long-term therapy (12 to 36 months) was necessary. In the recommended dose of 20 mg/kg/day, complications arose such as paresthesias (50%), which resulted in cessation of treatment. Other annoying side effects included a metallic taste, dark urine, anorexia, nausea, vomiting, and vertigo.

West et al. (360) reported that perianal fistulas in Crohn's disease are predominantly colonized by skin flora (gram-positive microorganisms). Therefore, antimicrobial treatment should be directed toward these microorganisms. Ciprofloxicin is a commonly used antibiotic.

BOX 2 ■ Subsidiary Classification (APD)

A (Associated Anal Conditions)	P (Proximal Intestinal Disease)	D (Disease Activity—In Anal Lesions)
0. None	0. No proximal disease	1. Active
1. Hemorrhoids	1. Contiguous rectal disease	2. Inactive
2. Malignancy	2. Colon (rectum spared)	3. Inconclusive
3. Other (specify)	3. Investigation incomplete	

Source: From Ref. 354.

BOX 3 ■ Perianal Crohn's Disease Activity Index

Discharge
0. No discharge
1. Minimal mucous discharge
2. Moderate mucous or purulent discharge
3. Substantial discharge
4. Gross fecal soiling

Pain/Restriction of Activities
0. No activity restriction
1. Mild discomfort, no restriction
2. Moderate discomfort, some limitation
3. Marked discomfort, marked limitation
4. Severe pain, severe limitation

Restriction of Sexual Activity
0. No restriction
1. Slight restriction
2. Moderate limitation
3. Marked limitation
4. Unable to engage in

Type of Perianal Disease
0. No perianal disease/skin tags
1. Anal fissure or mucosal tear
2. <3 Perianal fistulas
3. ≥3 Perianal fistulas
4. Anal sphincter ulceration or fistulas with significant undermining of skin

Degree of Induration
0. No induration
1. Minimal induration
2. Moderate induration
3. Substantial induration
4. Gross fluctuance/abscess

Total Score__________

Source: From Ref. 356.

Present and Lichtiger (361) touted the virtues of cyclosporine. In a report of 16 patients (10 perirectal, four enterocutaneous, and two rectovaginal fistulas), cyclosporine was administered intravenously, 4 mg/kg/day, and then switched to oral 6 to 8 mg/kg/day. Despite only seven closures (44%) and a 36% relapse rate, the regimen was labeled effective. Complications included paresthesias (75%), hirsutism (19%), hypertension (25%), and nephrotoxicity (6%).

Azathioprine and 6-MP have been found to result in a closure of fistula-in-ano in 31% to 75% of cases (288). Methotrexate has reportedly been effective in up to 50% of cases. Relapse following cessation of treatment is not uncommon. Mycophenolate mofetil and tacrolimus have shown some promise but relapse is common when treatment is terminated.

In his review of literature Rutgeerts (362) noted the management of perianal fistulizing disease resistant to standard treatment has greatly improved with the introduction of the anti-tumor necrosis factor-alpha antibody, infliximab. Complete arrest of the drainage of fistula is obtained in 46% of patients 10 weeks after the administration of 5–10 mg/kg of infliximab at weeks 0, 2, and 6 and, on average, lasts for 12 weeks. He believes a treatment algorithm for fistulizing Crohn's disease should involve the early and optimal use of immunosuppressives and/or infliximab.

McNamara et al. (363) performed a literature search of the use of infliximab for perianal disease. They found the use of infliximab at a dose of 5 mg/kg at intervals of 0, 2, and 6 weeks results in significant improvement in disease in approximately 70% of patients with fistulas. Prior examination under anesthesia with placement of non-cutting seton sutures in fistula tracts is a useful adjunct in many patients. Preliminary results show a benefit from maintenance infliximab therapy and from concomitant use of immunosuppressants such as azathioprine.

Lavy et al. (364) proposed the use of hyperbaric oxygen in the management of patients with perianal Crohn's disease. The authors noted that the indolent nature of Crohn's disease is compatible with ischemia and secondary bacterial invasion. The rationale for hyperbaric oxygen is that it improves tissue oxygenation and can restore a favorable cellular milieu in which the wound-healing process and host antibacterial mechanisms (especially against anaerobes) are enhanced. They treated 10 patients who were previously nonresponders to salicylates, steroids, metronidazole, and 6-MP with the hyperbaric chamber. Each patient received 20 treatments of 90 min/day, six days/wk of 100% oxygen at 2.5 atmospheres absolute. Repeat courses of 20 sessions were given to nonresponders. Complete healing resulted after one course in three patients, two courses in two patients, three courses in two patients, and improved in one and no improvement in two. Healing was maintained in the 18-month follow-up. Colombel et al. (365) evaluated hyperbaric oxygen in 10 consecutive patients with severe perineal Crohn's disease. There were four superficial fissures, four cavitating ulcers, six low or superficial fistulas, two high fistulas, and one irreversible anal stenosis. All patients had received one or more medical treatments without healing the perineal lesions, and all had had previous operations for perineal lesions. Two patients did not complete treatment. Eight patients completed at least 30 hyperbaric oxygenation sessions and were evaluable. Six of eight patients treated were healed, three completely and three partially. All patients who healed completely received hyperbaric oxygen as an additional treatment to a local perineal operation. The authors concluded that hyperbaric oxygen might be useful as a last resort treatment of chronic perineal Crohn's disease resistant to other treatments or as a complement to operation.

Yamamoto et al (366) assessed the role of fecal diversion in 31 patients with perianal Crohn's disease. The principal indications for fecal diversion were severe perianal sepsis in 13 patients, recurrent deep anal ulcer in 3, complex anorectal fistula in 9, and rectovaginal fistula in 6. Twenty-five patients (81%) went into early remission and 6 (19%) failed to respond. Of the 25 early responders, 17 relapsed at a median duration of 23 months after fecal diversion. By contrast, 8 patients (26%) went into complete remission and required no further operation at a median duration of 81 months after diversion. Altogether, 22 patients required operation at a median duration of 20 months after fecal diversion: proctectomy in 21 and repeated drainage of anal sepsis in 1. At time of publication, intestinal continuity had been restored in only

3 patients (10%). There were no parameters to identify in whom a successful outcome is likely.

Egan and Sandborn (138) recently summarized the medical treatment of perianal Crohn's disease as follows: physicians caring for Crohn's disease today have a great array of therapeutic options to choose from. Traditionally, antibiotics such as metronidazole are used for perianal fistulas, although no controlled evidence supports this practice. Infliximab 5 mg/kg administered at weeks 0, 2, and 6 and azathioprine 2–2.5 mg/kg or 6-mercaptopurine 1.5 mg/kg are the drugs with the best established roles for the medical treatment of active fistulizing disease. A recent placebo-controlled trial evaluated tacrolimus for the treatment of perianal Crohn's disease. Although rates of complete fistula closure were not better in the active treatment group, more fistulas improved with tacrolimus than with placebo. Thus, in patients with active perianal fistula who do not respond to infliximab along with azathioprine or 6-mercaptopurine, tacrolimus is a potential alternative therapy. The value of continued infliximab infusions in patients with fistula who had an initial response to 3 doses of infliximab 5 mg/kg was evaluated in the ACCENT II trial. Sixty-nine percent of patients responded to the initial induction course of infliximab (defined as > 50% reduction in number of draining fistulas) and were then randomized to maintenance infliximab every 8 weeks or placebo. The median time to loss of response was 14 weeks in placebo-treated patients versus > 40 weeks in infliximab-treated patients, a highly significant difference. Therefore, Crohn's disease patients with persistent or recurrent perianal fistula after initial response to 3 dose infliximab induction therapy along with azathioprine or 6-mercaptopurine, should be treated with 8 weekly infliximab infusions.

Because of the diversity of pathologic processes it seems appropriate to deal with the surgical management of the different lesions separately.

Excoriation

Excoriation, superficial abrasions, and maceration of the perianal skin and perineum are not the disease itself but usually occur as the result of diarrhea and secondary infection by bacteria and fungi.

Anal Skin Tags

Skin tags are the most common finding among patients with anal Crohn's disease. Typically, they are edematous thickened skin 1 to 2 cm in size. The tags frequently cause pain on sitting and make the anal region difficult to clean. Most skin tags persist after 10 years of follow-up (367). Management is expectant with warm baths and cleansing. Operation is not usually indicated. For patients where tags interfere with perianal hygiene, fibrous tags may be removed.

Hemorrhoids

In 1977, Jeffrey et al. (368) reported on 20 patients with Crohn's disease who underwent 26 courses of treatment. This represented about 0.04% of about 50,000 patients with hemorrhoids. Hemorrhoidectomy was followed by 11 complications (10 fistula-in-ano) and six patients who ultimately required proctectomy were attributed to the previous hemorrhoidectomy. The authors, therefore, strongly cautioned against hemorrhoidectomy in this setting. However, more recently, Wolkomir and Luchtefeld (369) reported on 17 patients who underwent nemorrhoidectomy with uncomplicated healing in 15 patients. With a mean follow-up of 11.5 years, only one patient required proctectomy for an unrelated cause.

Perineal Ulceration

Bizarre ulcerations and undermining of subcutaneous tissue may occur in patients with Crohn's disease. They occur with an incidence of 1.9% to 5.1% and seem to predict future intestinal disease (288). Swelling, pain, and pocketing of pus may be a prominent clinical manifestation. Treatment is nonspecific with warm baths, curettage of ulceration, and unroofing of undermined tissue. For painful ulcers, Hughes (354) used direct injection of local depot methylprednisolone and reported pain relief in five of seven patients.

Skin lesions are the most common extraintestinal manifestation of Crohn's disease. Lesions that develop at sites remote from the gastrointestinal tract and have granulomas on histologic examination are termed "metastatic cutaneous" Crohn's disease. Management is difficult as medical treatment is often ineffective. Williams et al. (370) described the use of operative debridement of areas of perineal metastatic cutaneous Crohn's disease in five patients, all of whom had failed to improve after a variety of medical treatments. One patient had a poor result with continuing mild perineal discharge and four had a good outcome with complete resolution of symptoms and satisfactory cosmetic results.

Fissure-in-Ano

Anal fissure is a common manifestation and constitutes 21–35% of anal complications in Crohn's disease (288). Unlike the ordinary anal fissure, which occurs in the posterior or anterior midline of the anus, fissures in Crohn's disease can occur at any location around the anus. They are most commonly located posteriorly (41%), lateral (9%–20%), and multiple (32–33%) (288). They are often bluish in appearance, deep, and have undermined edges. The pain is relatively mild compared to the appearance. In a long-term follow-up of 53 patients with fissures, only 10 (19%) still had fissures 10 years later and none had new fissures. Approximately 50% of these patients developed anal stenosis, but fecal incontinence was not a problem in these patients (367). An abscess or fistula can subsequently develop in 26% of patients (288).

For the most part, management is nonoperative. If patients are experiencing severe pain, an examination under anesthesia is indicated to rule out sepsis. For unresponsive patients, judicious use of lateral internal sphincterotomy is recommended. Wolkomir and Luchtefeld (369) reported on 25 patients who underwent 27 operations. Uncomplicated healing within two months occurred in 22 patients. With a mean follow-up of 7.5 years, two patients underwent proctectomy, neither related to the fissure operation. Fleshner et al. (371) reviewed 56 patients with fissure-in-ano associated with Crohn's disease and found that 84% of them were symptomatic. Sixty-six percent of the fissures were in the midline and 32% were multiple. Medical treatment healed 50% of patients. Predictive factors for healing included male gender, painless fissures, and acute fissures. Of 56 patients with follow-up, 26% developed an abscess with fistula in the base of the fissure. The authors concluded that medical treatment alone is more ominous and recommended a more liberal use of lateral internal sphincterotomy. However, it would still seem wise to give the patient an opportunity to heal without the benefit of an operation. All nine patients who underwent lateral internal sphincterotomy by Platell et al. (53) healed.

Anal Stenosis

The development of narrowing of the anal canal is not uncommon in patients suffering from Crohn's disease. Hughes (354) described two types of stricture: (i) a spasmodic stricture dependent on smooth muscle contraction and absent when patients are examined under anesthesia, and (ii) stricture secondary to infection manifesting either as an intraluminal membrane or extramucosal fibrotic tissue. A bulk-forming agent and a periodic one-finger dilatation will usually maintain an adequate-sized orifice to permit satisfactory defecation. Dilatation can also be achieved with progressively larger Hagar dilators. In very selected circumstances, a lateral internal sphincterotomy might be indicated. Long anorectal strictures are usually accompanied by severe proctitis, which may ultimately lead the patient to a proctectomy.

Anorectal Abscesses

Anorectal abscesses occur relatively commonly in the natural history of Crohn's disease (23–62% of patients) (288). Ischioanal abscesses account for 39–43% and approximately 70% are associated with fistula-in-ano (288). The trans-sphincteric is the commonest type of fistula with an incidence of 29–47% (288). About the only noncontroversial aspect of the management of patients with anorectal suppuration is that incision and drainage are indicated. Incisions should be small and close to the anus in the event of the development of a fistula-in-ano. In a series of 38 patients with anorectal abscesses, associated with Crohn's disease reported by Pritchard et al. (372), 30 abscesses were simple and eight were complex horseshoe abscesses. After incision and drainage, 45% to 56% of patients developed recurrent abscesses and 31% to 44% subsequently required proctectomy, depending on whether a mushroom catheter was inserted at the time of drainage. Why catheter insertion should cause this difference is unclear. In the report by Platell et al. (53), the incision and drainage of anorectal sepsis were followed by a 13% recurrence rate.

Rectovaginal Fistula

Spontaneous vaginal fistulas, mostly rectovaginal ones, were reported in 3.5% to 23% of patients with Crohn's disease (288,373). Management of these fistulas always has been difficult and depends on the severity of rectal disease and the symptomatology. When no rectal disease is present, a local repair should prove satisfactory. In the presence of rectal disease with minimal symptoms, if the patient is not excessively disturbed, no treatment may be recommended. With severe rectal disease, with large and high fistulas in markedly symptomatic patients, proctectomy is generally required. For moderate disease, Irvine and Keighley (357) have suggested a local repair under cover of a stoma.

Heyen et al. (373) reviewed 28 patients with vaginal fistulas in complicated Crohn's disease. Twelve required early operation, including local closure and small bowel resection, and five patients underwent total proctocolectomy. Conservative management was used in 16 patients, but in none of these did the fistula close spontaneously. Subsequent proctocolectomy was required in seven patients; although two patients with high vaginal fistulas were managed by total colectomy, end ileostomy, and over-sewing of the rectal stump. Only two high fistulas resulting from ileal Crohn's disease resolved with resection and anastomosis of the diseased segment alone. Local repair was unsuccessful despite repeated operations in two of five patients. Two patients died of malignancy arising within a chronic vaginal fistula. Although some vaginal fistulas complicating Crohn's disease cause little disability and can be managed symptomatically, they do not heal by conservative therapy or by a proximal defunctioning stoma alone. In time, severe bowel symptoms develop in the majority of patients and necessitate proctectomy.

Morrison et al. (374) reviewed 12 patients with rectovaginal fistula associated with Crohn's disease. Primary fistula repair was performed in four patients and four others had staged repair with preliminary fecal diversion. Four patients with severe colonic and anorectal disease had total proctocolectomy performed as the first procedure. Of the eight patients who underwent repair, complete healing occurred in six patients. One patient had a persistent fistula, while the other underwent total proctocolectomy after three unsuccessful repairs. Success of operation correlated with quiescent intestinal disease and absence of rectal involvement.

Scott et al. (375) reviewed 67 women with anorectal Crohn's disease with a goal of determining the prognostic effect of the presence of a vaginal fistula. Eighteen of 29 patients with anorectal/vaginal fistula underwent local operation, defunctioning stoma, or proctectomy, whereas only 13 of 38 patients without rectovaginal fistula did so. The authors, therefore, concluded that a vaginal fistula forbade an adverse effect, not a surprising finding.

Successful closure of rectovaginal fistula associated with Crohn's disease has been reported using a rectal advancement flap (376) or a vaginal approach (377). Of course, rectal inflammation must be controlled before a repair is attempted as the presence of intense proctitis is almost certainly a formula for failure (378).

Fistula-in-Ano

The incidence of fistula-in-ano associated with Crohn's disease reported by various authors is listed in Table 6. In the series by Keighley and Allan (379), fistula-in-ano was second only to skin tags in frequency of perianal Crohn's disease. In a study of the natural history of perianal Crohn's disease, Buchmann et al. (367) reported that in approximately one-third of patients with low fistulas, spontaneous healing occurred, in one-third healing took place

TABLE 6 ■ Fistula-in-Ano in Crohn's Disease

Author(s)	Incidence (%)
Kodner and Fry (380)	14–38
Markowitz et al. (347)	11
Lockhart-Mummery (348)	10
Wolff et al. (381)	14
Bernard et al. (382)	24
Van Dongen and Lubbers (383)	28
Radcliffe et al. (384)	9
Goebell (349)	30
Kangas (350)	11
Palder et al. (351)	14
Nordgren et al. (385)	20
Halme and Sainio (386)	31 (17–49)
Sugita et al. (387)	56
Platell et al. (53)	31

after fistulotomy, and in one-third fistulas persisted after 10 years of follow-up. In the series reported by Allan and Keighley (357), 14 of 40 patients with low-lying fistula-in-ano had spontaneous healing. In 13 patients the fistulas persisted and in 10 patients proctectomy was required. Low anal fistulas in perianal Crohn's disease often are asymptomatic and may heal spontaneously.

A major controversy concerns the management of patients with an anal fistula in the presence of Crohn's disease. Such a fistula may be very complex and may involve varying degrees of the sphincter mechanism. Extensive procedures expose these patients to the risk of not healing and inducing or worsening anal incontinence. However, other patients with Crohn's disease have fairly simple fistulas but are nonetheless severely troubled with them. In these cases, a fistulotomy for relief of symptoms is indicated. If no rectal disease exists, the risk of worsening the situation is minimal. Simple intersphincteric fistulas may be handled easily, and transsphincteric fistulas may be treated with or without the use of a seton. Extrasphincteric fistulas, however, invariably indicate active rectal involvement, and proctectomy is usually the only chance for control. If anorectal suppuration is present, establishing adequate drainage to allow the sepsis to subside before proceeding to proctectomy is beneficial.

Sloots et al. (388) studied the fistulous tracts in 41 patients with Crohn's disease by physical examination, sondage of the fistula, proctoscopy, and hydrogen peroxide enhanced transanal ultrasound. The main tract and ramification of the fistula were classified according to the anatomical Parks' classification. Only nine (22%) patients had a single inter- or transsphincteric fistula. In 12% of patients, a single supra- or extrasphincteric fistula was found, in 34% more than one fistula tract, and in 32% an anovaginal fistula was present. Thus, 78% of patients had a surgically difficult to treat fistula. In the ramified fistula, the main tract follows the Parks' classification, but ramifications may have a bizarre pattern which is not in agreement with this classification.

Although operations on the anal canal of patients with Crohn's disease have been considered a relative contraindication, we do not always believe this to be the case. A review by Bayer and Gordon was conducted of 28 patients with fistula-in-ano associated with Crohn's disease (389). An effort was made to classify the fistula-in-ano according to Parks' classification, but many fistulas were complicated and did not neatly fit into one of the described categories (9 intersphincteric, 10 transsphincteric, and 9 complex). Patients underwent fistulotomy (three with a seton). Complete healing was achieved in 71.4% of cases with an average healing time of 3.5 months. With an average follow-up of 71 months, postoperative function was good in 20 patients (71.5%). Of the remaining eight patients, five ultimately underwent total proctocolectomy because of the severity of their colorectal disease. One patient developed alteration of continence and two patients developed stenosis. There were two recurrences.

In a report by Levien et al. (390), 29 of 46 patients undergoing operative treatment of a fistula-in-ano accomplished primary healing (63%), but 10% of these patients (22%) developed a recurrence. Of the 27 patients who required more than one operation, 18 ultimately achieved a stage of minimal disability, whereas four required proctectomy (11%) and five had continuing disability. The most favorable group of patients comprised those with an internal opening and normal rectum (18 out of 21 healed). Morrison et al. (391) reported on 32 patients, 19 of whom underwent fistulotomy, eight partial fistulotomy, and five fistulotomy preceded by diversion. Seven patients required more than one operation. Healing was ultimately accomplished in 94%, and only two patients developed a recurrence. In that series, success of the operation correlated with the absence of rectal disease and quiescent disease elsewhere in the gastrointestinal tract.

In a review from St. Mark's Hospital, London, by Marks et al. (392), of 125 fistulas associated with Crohn's disease, one-third were classified as low (superficial, intersphincteric, and low transsphincteric) and 33 as rectovaginal; of the remaining ones, seven were extrasphincteric, 24 had intersphincteric and transsphincteric extensions, and four were unclassified. A series by Hobbiss and Schofield (345) revealed 21 of 26 patients had low fistulas. Twenty of 22 patients in the latter series underwent a definitive operation with no significant prolongation of healing time and four recurrences. In the former series, 32 of the 46 patients with low fistulas underwent fistulotomy, with 25 healing successfully. Five patients with transsphincteric fistulas so treated healed successfully.

Hesterberg et al. (393) reported on the use of an anocutaneous flap to treat patients with anovaginal fistulas with Crohn's disease. Following excision of the fistulous tract, the sphincter is sutured, and an anocutaneous flap created with a wide base at the perineum is anastomosed to the rectal mucosa covering the internal opening of the fistula. Seven of 10 patients so treated suffered from Crohn's proctitis and in these patients a protective enterostomy was constructed before the operative closure of the fistula. All fistulas healed primarily. With a median follow-up of 18 months, a relapse occurred in three patients. Makowiec et al. (394) reported 36 rectal advancement flap repairs performed in 32 patients with perianal Crohn's disease. There were 12 anovaginal and 20 transsphincteric fistulas. Patients were followed prospectively for a mean 19.5 months. The prognostic influence of fistula type, rectal disease, intestinal disease, and fecal diversion on recurrence was assessed. Four of 36 repairs showed primary failure, the operated fistula recurred in 11 patients after a median of seven months, and a new fistula developed in six patients. The fistula recurrence rate was higher in patients with anovaginal fistula or Crohn's colitis but did not correlate with disease activity. Transitory mild incontinence of stool was observed in one patient only. Although rectal advancement flap repair does not cure perianal fistulas in most patients with Crohn's disease, those without Crohn's colitis may have long-term benefit. The authors concluded that short-term improvement of symptoms justifies this simple procedure even in patients with anovaginal fistula.

Complex fistulas should be approached with more caution. White et al. (395) recommend treating patients with complex fistulas with long-term indwelling setons placed through the fistulous tract and tied loosely to maintain the patency of the fistula without cutting through the sphincters. At the time of insertion, although abscesses are incised and drained, no attempt is made to divide the superficial tissues or the sphincter overlying the fistulous tract. In 10 patients 18 fistulas were so treated, and the patients were followed for four months to seven years. Excellent palliation was obtained despite severe proctitis in six of the patients, and none required proctectomy. Some patients required multiple seton insertion. This technique is aimed at delaying or preventing the need for proctectomy and sparing the patient's having a permanent stoma for as long as possible.

Koganei et al. (396) evaluated the efficacy of long-term seton drainage in the management of 13 patients with Crohn's fistulas—five intersphincteric and eight transsphincteric. With a mean follow-up of 12.1 months, perianal pain disappeared or improved in all patients, as did pyrexia. Discharge and tenderness disappeared or diminished in 77% and induration disappeared or improved in 69%. Overall good results were achieved in 10 patients but three required redrainage. The authors concluded that seton management was worthwhile.

Thornton et al. (397) reviewed the results of long-term indwelling seton or depezzar catheter in the management of perianal Crohn's disease. All patients underwent an intraoperative endorectal ultrasound to identify the extent of the fistulas and to assess anal wall thickness. Fistulas were classified by Parks' criteria. All patients then underwent insertion of a seton or depezzar catheter under ultrasound guidance. All patients were followed clinically and with endorectal ultrasound. Twenty-eight patients with 43 complex perianal Crohn's fistulas were identified. Median follow-up was 13 months. Twenty-one percent of patients developed recurrent or new perianal symptoms while the seton was in situ. Eleven percent of patients required further operative intervention. The median anal wall thickness at the time of diagnosis was 18.5 mm reducing to a median of 14 mm after seton insertion and symptom control. No patient reported deterioration in fecal continence after seton insertion. Patient age, reduction in anal wall thickness after seton insertion, and length of follow-up were significant predictors of long-term symptom control. They concluded that long-term indwelling seton is an effective management modality for complex perianal Crohn's fistulas.

Shinozaki et al. (398) conducted a study to clarify the current status of operation for anal fistula in Crohn's disease with simultaneous intestinal resection. There were 39 of 239 Crohn's patients who underwent long-term seton drainage. The patients were divided into two groups: patients who received simultaneous bowel and anus operation ($n = 11$) and a control group ($n = 28$). There were 74% of patients who received two seton drains or more with a mean of 2.7. Two or more operations were performed on 54% of the patients. The rate of seton drain removal was 52% at 12 months after operation and 86% at 24 months. The cumulative rate of seton drains remaining at 12 months after the first operation was 10% in the simultaneous group and 37.7% in the control group. After total removal of seton drains, 33% of patients recurred. All the patients who had recurrences belonged to the control group. Continence did not deteriorate after seton drainage. Enterostomy was required in 26% of patients and no patient received proctectomy. They concluded that healing of Crohn's anal fistula was significantly better in the simultaneous group than in the control group, and the recurrence rate was lower in the simultaneous group.

Topstad et al. (399) evaluated the efficacy of infliximab combined with selective seton drainage in the healing of fistulizing anorectal Crohn's disease. Twenty-nine patients received a mean of three (range, 1–5) doses of infliximab 5 mg/kg. Twenty-one patients had perianal fistula; eight had rectovaginal fistulas, four with combined rectovaginal/perianal fistula. A complete response rate occurred in 67% of patients with perianal fistula (mean follow-up nine months), with 4 of the 14 patients relapsing (mean six months), but all had a complete response to retreatment (mean nine months). A partial response occurred in four patients (19%), defined by decreasing drainage (two patients) or infliximab dependence (two patients) requiring repeated dosing every six to eight weeks. Three patients (14%) had no response. Seton drainage was used before infusion in 13 perianal patients with perianal infection and 17 were treated with maintenance azathioprine or methotrexate. Of eight patients with rectovaginal fistula, complete response occurred in one, partial response in five, and no response in two. Total partial responders became infliximab-dependent. A complete response was observed in one patient with isolated rectovaginal fistula, a partial response in five. No patient with a combined rectovaginal/perianal fistula had a complete response. Concomitant rectovaginal fistula was a poor prognostic indicator for successful infliximab therapy.

Van Bodegraven et al. (400) reported that short-term treatment of Crohn's disease-associated fistulas with infliximab does not induce disappearance of fistulous tracts, irrespective of therapeutic response. In all patients, remainders of fistulous tracts were demonstrated by endosonographic techniques.

A growing number of surgeons have adopted an operative policy and their results are presented in Table 7. Notwithstanding the good results reported in these studies plus gratifying, results in patients whom we have treated, a general word of caution must be issued to counsel against the radical treatment of a fistulous abscess in a patient with Crohn's disease, for healing in some patients tends to be prolonged; therefore, removal of large amounts of tissue may result in inordinate healing times. On the other hand,

TABLE 7 ■ Results of Operation for Crohn's Fistula-in-Ano

Author(s)	No. of Patients	Treatment	Healed (%)
Hellers et al. (401) (1980)			
Small bowel	22	Local	62
Ileocolic	21	Local	57
Large bowel	56	Local	17
Sohn et al. (402) (1981)	100	Parks' fistulectomy	85
Marks et al. (392) (1981)	46	Lay open	80
Hobbiss and Schofield (345) (1982)	20	Lay open	100
Bernard et al. (382) (1986)	27	Lay open	63
Van Dongen and Lubbers (383) (1986)	28	Local	79
Fuhrman and Larach (403) (1989),	19	Lay open	95
Levien et al. (390) (1989),	46	Lay open	63
Morrison et al. (391) (1989),	32		
	19	Lay open	94
	8	Seton	
	5	Division and lay open	
Fry et al. (404) (1989)	13	Lay open	100
	3	Sliding flap	100
Williams et al. (405) (1991)	33	Lay open	93
Nordgren et al. (385) (1992),	23		
Ileocolic	12	Lay open	83
Large bowel	11	Lay open	36
Francois et al. (355) (1993),	35	Lay open	86
Bayer and Gordon (389) (1994),	28	Lay open	71
Williamson et al. (406) (1995),	35	Lay open ± seton	74
McKee and Keenan (352) (1996)			
Low	34	Lay open	62
High	19	Lay open seton, flap	42
Platell et al. (53) (1996)	44	Lay open	91
Scott and Northover (407) (1996)	27	Lay open	81
	27	seton	85

failure to perform an early fistulotomy may permit a relatively simple fistula to blossom into a more difficult management problem.

We believe that early definitive operation will reduce the progression of a simple and uncomplicated fistula to a complex one. Our results along with the results of several other authors support this course of action. The fear of poor wound healing has not been realized. Of course, care must be taken of the musculature. Setons should be judiciously employed. The poor results occur in those patients who have associated rectal disease in combination with complex bizarre fistulization. Principles of operative management include (i) not to operate if asymptomatic, (ii) ideally to operate if disease is quiescent, (iii) to treat active disease (aggressive medical treatment is required to control bowel disease preoperatively), (iv) to minimize tissue excision, and (v) to be conservative. Patients with a high fistula in perianal Crohn's disease may require a proctectomy (357).

A carcinoma arising in an anal fistula in the absence of Crohn's disease occurs rarely. Carcinoma arising in an anorectal fistula of Crohn's disease is likewise rare.

Because of the difficulty in treating these fistulas, they may be chronic. Due to the chronicity of the perianal inflammation, these patients may be predisposed to malignant transformation. This is complicated further by the delay in diagnosis because these symptoms usually are attributed to the fistula and biopsy examination usually is performed late. The development of carcinoma in chronic perineal sinuses is rare and only 14 cases have been described in the literature, of which half were squamous cell carcinoma. It has been postulated that the environment of chronic injury and repair leads to this neoplastic change (408). One report cites an incidence of malignant transformation in 0.7% of Crohn's disease patients (409).

Ky et al. (409) encountered seven such patients, four of which were squamous cell carcinoma and three adenocarcinomas. Two deaths in the patients with squamous cell carcinoma and one in the patients with adenocarcinomas suggests a poorer prognosis in both types of malignancy than when these lesions occur without Crohn's disease. Carcinoma arising in a Crohn's fistula can be very difficult to diagnosis. Examination may be limited by pain, stricture, or induration of the perianal tissues. Examination under anesthesia can also overlook the lesion. Diagnostic examination under anesthesia yields increases with biopsies or curettage of the fistulous tracts.

Sivarajasingham et al. (410) presented a case of perianal Hodgkin's lymphoma in a patient with Crohn's disease who was on long-term immunosuppression and whose symptoms would normally be attributed to Crohn's disease. Diagnosis was based on the morphological appearance of atypical cells in the lamina propria and the immunohistochemical profile of Reed Sternberg and Hodgkin's cells showing a coexpression of CD15 and CD30. This is a reminder that perianal complaints in patients with inflammatory bowel disease may be a manifestation of other pathology.

Rectourethral Fistula

Rectourethral fistula in Crohn's disease is a rare occurrence and as of 1995 only 13 cases had been reported (411). Consequently, definitive management has been individualized. Successful medical treatment has included metronidazole. Immunosuppressive agents have not reportedly been helpful. Diversion alone has met with mixed results. In the absence of rectal disease, the rectal flap has proved successful (412). With severe rectal disease, proctectomy may be the most appropriate solution.

Perineal Wound

The perineal wound after proctectomy has always been a concern to surgeons. The presence of perianal disease has a marked effect on healing of proctectomy wounds after rectal excision. Of 27 proctectomies performed in patients with perianal Crohn's disease, 19 were followed up for persistent perineal sinus (70%). Complete perineal healing occurred in all nine patients who had had a rectal excision, in the absence of perianal disease (379). Similar poor perineal healing also was reported in a small series by Williams and Hughes (413). In a series of 144 patients undergoing total proctocolectomy and ileostomy for Crohn's disease by Goligher (211), healing of the perineal wound was straight forward in 62%, delayed but eventually complete in 28%, and very troublesome in 10% (3% were left with persistent sinus).

A number of factors have been shown to influence healing (414): severity of perianal disease, severity of rectal disease, high preoperative fistula, rectovaginal fistula, fecal contamination at time of operation, postoperative perineal sepsis, antibiotic coverage, gender, age, and use of steroids.

Management of the established unhealed perineal sinus has proved problematic and frustrating (211). The wound should be carefully examined to rule out the presence of an enterovaginal fistula. A sinogram or small bowel follow-through should exclude this possibility. The simplest maneuver is to curette and revise the wound, a procedure that can be repeated. The wound may not collapse because of the fibrotic nature of the cavity wall. More aggressive approaches include saucerization with split-thickness skin graft, wide excision, including the coccyx and skin flap rotation, or muscle or musculocutaneous flaps using gracilis, gluteus maximus, or rectus abdominis muscle to obliterate the unhealed wound.

Combined Perianal Disease

A number of surgeons report on the overall management of patients with perianal Crohn's disease. One such example is a report by Sangwan et al. (353). They reviewed the records of 66 patients, 3.8% of 1735 patients with Crohn's disease with symptomatic perianal Crohn's disease treated by local operations. All patients had intestinal disease that was limited to the colon in 32 patients (48%), ileocolonic region in 22 patients (33%), and ileum in 12 patients (18%). Types of perianal disease encountered included 57 with perianal suppuration, 47 with anal fistula, 21 with anal fissure, five with anal stenosis, three with gluteal abscess, two with scrotal abscess, and two with anovaginal fistula. A total of 321 episodes of anal complications necessitated 256 local interventions. Local anorectal operations performed included simple incision and drainage of abscess (57), fistulotomy (35), incision and drainage of complex anorectal abscesses and fistulas and insertion of seton (24), internal sphincterotomy (6), fissurectomy (1), and anal dilation (3). Of 24 patients with horseshoe abscesses and fistulas managed with insertion of a seton and 35 patients who underwent fistulotomy as a primary procedure or in conjunction with drainage of an abscess, none experienced fecal incontinence as a direct result of the operation. Thirteen patients required proctectomy to control perianal disease, and a similar number underwent total proctocolectomy for extensive intestinal disease. Forty patients (61%) continue to retain a functional anus. The authors concluded that patients with symptomatic low anal fistula involving minimum sphincter musculature could be treated safely with fistulotomy. In treatment of patients with horseshoe abscesses and high fistulas, aggressive local operative intervention using a seton permits preservation of the sphincter and good postoperative function.

McKee and Keenan (352) reviewed the outcome of treatment of 127 of 415 patients with Crohn's disease who had perianal involvement. In 56 patients, perianal disease was the presenting complaint. Ninety-nine of the 127 patients had colonic involvement. Thirty-two were treated with metronidazole and 41 were treated with azathioprine, with at least temporary improvement in 91% and 68%, respectively. Seventy patients had treatment for fistula-in-ano and, in 50% of patients, permanent healing was achieved. In general, treatment and outcome were largely related to the extent and severity of gut involvement. Proctectomy was performed in 32 patients (11 because of ongoing colonic disease). Only seven patients had proctectomy solely because of perianal disease. Proctectomy was necessary in 32 of 99 patients with colitis and perianal disease but in none of the 28 patients without colonic involvement. Primary healing of the perineal wound was obtained in 17 patients and only one patient had an unhealed perineal wound at the time of reporting. The authors concluded that perianal Crohn's disease does not inevitably lead to panproctocolectomy. Cautious operation for fistula when rectal inflammation is quiescent is worthwhile. Loss of bowel continuity is more likely when colitis coexists with perianal disease. Panproctocolectomy is often indicated because of the combination of colitis and perianal disease rather than for perianal disease alone.

Traditionally, proctectomy has been the treatment for severe complex fistula-in-ano from Crohn's disease. Marchesa et al. (415) reported on 13 patients (12 women) with severe perianal Crohn's disease and multiple fistulas who underwent a circumferential transanal sleeve advancement flap procedure. There were no postoperative deaths or major morbidity. One year after operation, the fistula had healed in 8 of 13 patients (with three requiring additional operations before healing). Of patients in whom the procedure failed, three underwent proctectomy for progression of disease and the other two had recurrence of a rectovaginal fistula six and eight months after operation. Of six variables evaluated (previous procedure, steroid use, steroid dosage, associated Crohn's disease, associated procedures, and diverting stoma), only associated procedures were significantly related to a successful outcome.

Joo et al. (416) evaluated the outcome of patients undergoing endorectal advancement flap repair for perianal Crohn's disease in 31 procedures performed on 26 patients. The mean patient age was 40.2 years. Type of fistulas included: rectovaginal (64.5%), fistula-in-ano (25.9%), rectourethral (3.2%), and others (6.5%). The mean length of follow-up was 17.3 months. The mean length of hospitalization was 3.7 days. A temporary diverting stoma was created in six patients with a 66.7% surgical success rate. Twenty-one of the 26 patients had previous procedures consisting of 38.7% bowel resections, 19.4% seton placements, 12.9% drainages, and 19.4% diverting ileostomies. Eleven patients had multiple procedures. Ultimately fistulas were eradicated in 71% of cases including 75% with rectovaginal fistulas and 63.6% with other fistulas. There was no mortality; morbidity included flap retraction in one patient who required antibiotics for five days and bleeding in one patient who required reoperation. Success was noted in 25% of patients with small bowel Crohn's disease as compared to 87% without small bowel Crohn's disease. They concluded that endorectal advancement flap is an effective surgical modality for the treatment of fistulas due to perianal Crohn's disease but is less apt to succeed in patients with concomitant small bowel Crohn's disease.

Michelassi et al. (417) elucidated features, surgical procedures, and long-term results in 224 patients with anorectal complications of Crohn's disease. Presenting complications included abscesses ($n = 36$), fistula-in-ano

($n = 51$), rectovaginal fistula ($n = 20$), anal stenosis ($n = 40$), anal incontinence ($n = 11$), or a combination of features ($n = 66$). Twenty-four patients did not undergo operative treatment; the remaining 200 patients underwent 284 procedures. Ultimately, 139 patients (62%) retained anorectal function; reasons for proctectomy in the remaining 85 patients included disease ($n = 66$), extensive fistular disease ($n = 15$), fecal incontinence ($n = 2$), and tight anal stenosis ($n = 1$). Patients with rectal disease had a significantly higher rate of proctectomy than patients with rectal sparing (77.6% vs. 13.6%). In the absence of rectal involvement, patients with multiple complications have a significantly higher rate of proctectomy than patients with single complications (23% vs. 10%). Complete healing and control of sepsis can be achieved in the majority of patients. Active rectal disease and multiple complications significantly increase the need for proctectomy.

In summary, perianal Crohn's disease pursues a relatively benign course. Perianal and anal areas should be kept clean and operation should be aimed at relieving symptoms, such as through incision and drainage of perianal abscess, gentle dilatation of anal stricture, and curettage or unroofing of infected fistulous tracts. The need for proctectomy is uncommon. It is useful to remember that "incontinence in Crohn's disease is due to aggressive surgeons and not to progressive disease." (418).

SPECIAL CONSIDERATIONS

EXTRACOLONIC MANIFESTATIONS

Involvement of other organ systems in Crohn's disease is similar to involvement in ulcerative colitis. Extraintestinal manifestations recorded in one series included peptic ulcer, arthritis, skin lesions (pyoderma gangrenosa or erythema nodosa), cholelithiasis, renal calculi, and eye lesions (uveitis). Most reports have grouped them as inflammatory bowel disease (see Chapter 26).

Freeman (419) reviewed 50 patients with erythema nodosum and pyoderma gangrenosum associated with Crohn's disease. Forty-one of 566 women (7.2%) and nine of 449 men (2.0%) were affected. Of these (4.4%) had erythema nodosum and (0.7%) had pyoderma gangrenosum including 0.2% with both dermatologic disorders at different times during their clinical courses. Recurrent erythema nodosum was detected in nine patients (20%) including eight women, while recurrent pyoderma gangrenosum was seen in two patients (28.6%). There was an age-dependent effect on the appearance of erythema nodosum with the highest percentage seen in those younger than 20 years of age. Detection rates for erythema nodosum in women approached the low men's rates in Crohn's disease at older than 40 years of age. Most patients with these dermatologic disorders had colonic disease with or without ileal involvement as well as complex disease, usually with penetrating complications. The study documents a sex-based and age-dependent effect on the clinical expression of erythema nodosum in Crohn's disease. This suggests that some components of the inflammatory process in Crohn's disease may be modulated by estrogen-mediated events, particularly in adolescents and young adults.

Metastatic Crohn's disease is a rare complication of Crohn's disease that has been infrequently reported in the literature. Sams et al. (420) reported a patient with chronic ulceration of the penis who ultimately was diagnosed with Crohn's disease following an initial misdiagnosis of pyoderma gangrenosum. Both pyoderma gangrenosum and cutaneous (metastatic) Crohn's disease may occur in the setting of inflammatory bowel disease. Clinical distinction between pyoderma gangrenosum and cutaneous Crohn's disease may be difficult because clinical and pathologic features often are similar. Although surgical debridement is therapeutic in cutaneous Crohn's disease, it may lead to increased tissue loss and disease progression (pathergy) in pyoderma gangrenosum. Thus, it is important to determine a definitive diagnosis before surgical debridement, especially, in tissue-sensitive sites. Guest and Fink (421) reported a case where submammary, inguinal, and perineal disease was observed in a patient many years after proctocolectomy. The patient had severe cutaneous metastatic Crohn's disease in the absence of active gastrointestinal disease. Biancone et al. (422) described the development of an unusual granulomatous skin lesion of the forehead in a patient with established Crohn's disease showing no postoperative recurrence.

Although not a true extraintestinal manifestation of Crohn's disease, kidney stones are increased in patients with bowel disease, particularly those who have had resection of part of their gastrointestinal tract. Worcester (423) reviewed the subject and the following information has been extracted from that review. These stones are usually calcium oxalate, but there is a marked increase in the tendency to form uric acid stones, as well, particularly in patients with colon resection. These patients all share a tendency to chronic volume contraction due to loss of water and salt in diarrheal stool, which leads to decreased urine volumes. They also have decreased absorption; therefore, diminishing urinary excretion, of citrate and magnesium, which normally act as inhibitors of calcium oxalate crystallization. Patients with colon resection and ileostomy form uric acid stones, as loss of bicarbonate in the ileostomy effluent leads to formation of acid urine. This, coupled with low urine volume, decreases the solubility of uric acid, causing crystallization and stone formation. Prevention of stones requires treatment with alkalinizing agents to raise urine pH to about 6.5, and attempts to increase urine volume, which increases the solubility of uric acid and prevents crystallization. Patients with small bowel resection may develop steatorrhea; if the colon is present, they are at risk of hyperoxaluria due to increased permeability of the colon to oxalate in the presence of fatty acids, and increased concentrations of free oxalate in the bowel lumen due to fatty acid binding of the luminal calcium. Therapy involves a low-fat, low-oxalate diet, attempts to increase urine volume, and agents such as calcium given to bind oxalate in the gut lumen. Correction of hypocitraturia and hypomagnesuria are also helpful.

Urinary tract complications in Crohn's disease are common. Ben-Ami et al. (424) determined the incidence of urinary tract complications in patients with Crohn's disease and reported their experience over 15 years. Clinical and radiological findings of 312 patients with Crohn's disease were reviewed. Simple cystitis was the most common problem, occurring in 51 patients. There were 22 patients with urinary tract complications that required hospitalization. Six patients had ileovesical fistulas. All six patients were treated surgically. Four patients had ureteral obstruction and hydronephrosis, three of whom responded well to conservative treatment. In one patient, the affected ileal segment was resected. Four patients suffered from retroperitoneal abscess accompanied by urinary symptoms. Twelve patients developed right kidney stones. All of the patients suffered from longstanding Crohn's disease with bowel obstruction. Surprisingly, most of the severe complications occurred in men, although 70% of the patients were women.

Gumbo et al. (425) reported the case of a patient with Crohn's disease and recurrent pneumonia secondary to occult ileopulmonary fistula and reviewed five other cases in the literature. Patients often present with chronic cough productive of feculent sputum, pleuritic chest pain, and signs of pulmonary consolidation that fail to respond completely to antibiotic therapy. Mixed enteric flora is cultured from sputum and bronchial washings in most cases. Bronchoscopy findings range from chronic bronchial inflammation to feculent material in the airways. Barium enema is often diagnostic. Surgery and Crohn's-specific therapy are key components of curative therapy.

Omori et al. (426) reported a case of pulmonary involvement of Crohn's disease in a patient with known Crohn's disease. Lung biopsy through thoracoscopy was performed and revealed signs of chronic inflammation with multiple subepithelial noncaseating and epithelioid granulomas on pathologic examination. Intravenous steroids were required in the initial management of life-threatening pulmonary dysfunction. Oral steroid dosage had slowly been tapered over one month. After 36 months, the patient's condition was stable on continued treatment with prednisone and mesalazine.

Granulomatous bronchiolitis and necrobiotic nodules may be a manifestation of Crohn's disease in the absence of microbial agents (427). While a multiplicity of complex pulmonary changes may occur in Crohn's disease, their clinical recognition and precise pathological definition may be particularly important if treatment with a biological agent, such as infliximab, is being considered.

Freeman and Freeman (428) conducted a study to determine the rate of avascular necrosis (osteonecrosis) in patients with Crohn's disease. Over 20 years, 877 patients with Crohn's disease, 56% women and 43% men were evaluated with patient follow-up data available for a mean of 7.8 years. In this group, four men were seen with osteonecrosis. No woman was affected. Patient ages ranged from 19 to 36 years at the time of diagnosis of their Crohn's disease and all were white. In one patient, disease was confined to the colon while three patients had disease involving the terminal ileum and colon. Two patients received corticosteroids as well as parenteral nutrition during the course of their disease. Two patients did not receive corticosteroids or parenteral nutrition. Of 877 patients with Crohn's disease, 55.5% received corticosteroids during the course of the disease, 22.4% received at least one course of parenteral nutrition, and 14.3% received both corticosteroids and parenteral nutrition. A total of 35.5% had at least one small intestinal resection. The overall rate of avascular necrosis in Crohn's disease was less than 0.5% but for men with Crohn's disease was about 1%. In this series, risk of osteonecrosis could not be attributed to corticosteroid use, parenteral nutrition, or both forms of therapy administered together. Small intestinal resection with loss of small intestinal absorptive area was not a risk factor for the development of osteonecrosis.

Mesenteric arterial thrombosis has been described as a complication of Crohn's disease (429).

■ HEPATOBILIARY MANIFESTATIONS

Hepatobiliary manifestations occur quite frequently in patients suffering from chronic ulcerative colitis and Crohn's disease and carry with them considerable morbidity and mortality. Although the true incidence is difficult to determine, clinically significant hepatobiliary disease occurs in 5% to 10% of patients (430). For those hepatobiliary manifestations that respond to therapy of the underlying bowel disease, medical and/or surgical therapy must be aggressively pursued.

Multiple hepatobiliary complications have been described in patients with Crohn's disease, including hepatitis, cholangitis, steatosis, and amyloidosis. Gallbladder involvement has been frequently reported in such patients. Rettally et al. (431) reviewed the association of Crohn's disease and gallbladder disease. The incidence of gallstones has been reported to be two-fold greater than in the general population, this being especially likely when the ileum is involved or after its resection. Additionally, acalculous cholecystitis has been described in severely ill patients. A search of the literature provided only three cases of acute cholecystitis and histopathological evidence of active Crohn's disease of the gallbladder (431). The predominant clinical picture was common in all three cases was that of upper gastrointestinal symptoms, with abdominal pain more often localized to the right upper quadrant in an ill-appearing patient prompting investigations or interventions for biliary disease. Small bowel involvement was concomitantly identified in all cases. Furthermore, the pathological findings in the gallbladder were similar to those seen in the bowel such as transmural inflammation, granulomatous change, and lymphatic channel dilatation. Isolated involvement of the gallbladder with Crohn's disease manifesting as acute cholecystitis has also been reported (432).

Lapidus et al. (433) evaluated the prevalence of gallstone disease in a defined cohort of Crohn's disease patients, the possible risk factors, and the relative risk compared with the general population. The prevalence of gallstone disease was related to disease extent, previous intestinal resection, age and gender. They found that 26.4% had gallstone disease ($RR = 1.8$). The number of previous intestinal resections was the only significant risk factor. There was no significant difference in gallstone disease between gender (28.2% vs. 24.1%) or age (34% vs. 21.8%). The lack of association between disease extent and the site of previous intestinal resection, together with a previous finding of normal cholesterol saturation of the bile in patients with Crohn's disease, indicate that these patients may develop pigment stones rather cholesterol stones.

Gallstone disease is reported to be higher in patients with Crohn's disease than in the general population. Chew et al. (434) studied the prevalence of cholecystectomy in patients with Crohn's ileitis and attempted to identify any associated risk factors and determine whether it is justified to perform prophylactic cholecystectomy during ileocolic resection. A total of 191 patients with Crohn's ileitis who were treated medically or who had an ileocolic resection were reviewed. They concluded that the prevalence of gallstone disease in Crohn's ileitis requiring cholecystectomy is similar to that of the general population with a female predominance. In addition, the number of patients requiring cholecystectomy after ileal resection is low. Thus, synchronous prophylactic cholecystectomy during ileocolic resection for Crohn's ileitis is not justified.

Kreuzpaintner et al. (435) reviewed the literature on the subject of liver abscesses complicating Crohn's disease and the following information has been gleaned from their review. There were 59 cases with Crohn's disease and liver abscesses reported. In 72.9% men are affected; 62.2% of the patients suffered from active and 37.8% from inactive Crohn's disease. In 52.9% of inactive patients and 7.1% of patients with active Crohn's disease, the liver abscess presented as the initial manifestation of Crohn's disease. Implicated in the development of liver abscesses were the following: 29.8% received cortisone, 20% antibiotics, 21.6% had an intra-abdominal intervention for Crohn's disease in the previous 12 months, 28% exhibited intra-abdominal abscesses except one perianal, 15% showed intra-abdominal perforations (one was walled-off, in one patient the gallbladder was perforated) and in 18% intra-abdominal fistula existed. Clinically, the diagnosis of liver abscess often is difficult because there are only nonspecific symptoms. These include fever, chills, pain, and tenderness in the right upper quadrant. A leucocytosis is always present and in some patients the serum alkaline phosphatase is elevated. In the presence of underlying Crohn's disease the diagnosis of liver abscess is difficult to establish because leucocytosis and other symptoms present may be attributed to the inflammatory bowel disease. In 47.2% of patients abscesses were solitary, in 9.4% double abscesses and in 43.4% multiple abscesses were found. Pathogens were cultured in 83.8% from aspirates of the abscesses. Together with the results of one positive blood culture, streptococcus milleri was the dominating pathogen with 19.6%. Other prevalent pathogens in abscesses were streptococci, anaerobes, and enterobacteriaceae. There were 3.9% of cultures that remained sterile. Different mechanisms can lead to the development of a liver abscess: direct extension from an intra-abdominal abscess, concomitant biliary sepsis, pylephlebitis, and portal bacteremia. The assumption that pylephlebitis and portal bacteremia can cause liver abscesses is supported by the following investigations: from patients with Crohn's disease during surgery, mesenteric lymph nodes were removed which showed bacterial growth in 19.8% as compared to 5.6% and 0% in ulcerative colitis and other controls, respectively. From these data it may be considered that in Crohn's disease bacteria invade lymph vessels and the vascular system, leading to portal bacteremia and pylephlebitis, respectively. During colonoscopy in patients with active inflammatory bowel disease, bacteremia with obligate anaerobes could be detected in 40% as compared to 0% in patients with inactive inflammatory bowel disease and controls. The clinical and statistical observation of a cluster of bacterial endocarditis in patients with active inflammatory bowel disease is in line with these pathogenetic considerations. In the reviewed cases, 43 patients received antibiotics. Another eight patients (15.7%) were treated with antibiotics only, four of them with success; their abscesses were described as large, multiple, multiple small, or solitary. In four patients the diagnosis of the liver abscess was made only at autopsy and they were described as multiple or multiple small. In four patients (7.8%) a percutaneous aspiration was performed, in 21 patients (41.2%) a percutaneous catheter drainage, and in 15 patients (29.4%) a surgical catheter drainage. In each patient either an open aspiration, percutaneously and surgically inserted catheter drainage and a lobectomy were required. Altogether seven patients (13.7%) died. The fatalities occurred from the period of 1947 to 1983. Subsequently, no fatalities by liver abscesses were reported. This was attributed to the newly established imaging techniques like ultrasound and computerized tomography. To date the most clinically efficacious therapy of pyogenic liver abscesses has been the percutaneous catheter drainage combined with appropriate antibiotics. A surgical drainage is to be considered if the primary disorder requires an intra-abdominal intervention at the same time or if a percutaneous drainage technically is not feasible. In principle, exclusive antibiotic therapy is to be avoided because antibiotics alone lead to an unacceptably high mortality; the reports vary between 67% and 100%.

■ RISK OF CARCINOMA

Itzkowitz and Yio (436) reviewed the role of inflammation in the pathogenesis of carcinoma in patients with inflammatory bowel disease. Chronic inflammation as a cause of carcinoma is supported by the fact that colon carcinoma risk increases with longer duration of colitis, greater anatomic extent of colitis, the concomitant presence of other inflammatory manifestations such as primary sclerosing cholangitis, and the fact that certain drugs used to treat inflammation, such as 5-aminosalicylates and steroids, may prevent the development of colorectal carcinoma. The major carcinogenic pathways that lead to sporadic colorectal carcinoma, namely chromosomal instability, microsatellite instability, and hypermethylation, also occur in colitis-asssociated colorectal carcinoma. Unlike normal colonic mucosa, however, inflamed colonic mucosa demonstrates abnormalities in these molecular pathways even before any histological evidence of dysplasia or carcinoma. Whereas the reasons for this are unknown, oxidative stress likely plays a role. Reactive oxygen and nitrogen species produced by inflammatory cells can interact with key genes involved in carcinogenic pathways such as p53, DNA mismatch repair genes, and even DNA base excision repair genes. Other factors such as NF-kappaB and cyclooxygenases may also contribute. These observations offer compelling support for the role of inflammation in colon carcinogenesis.

Greenstein (437) reviewed the subject of malignancy in Crohn's disease and much of the following material is drawn from his comprehensive review. Carcinomas developing in patients with inflammatory bowel disease differ from those that arise from the adenoma–carcinoma sequence in that they develop at a young age, their anatomic distribution is different, they are influenced by sites of disease, and they are more frequently multiple and mucinous. Noteworthy is the fact that dysplasia precedes the carcinoma, which allows for surveillance. Crohn's disease carcinomas have a more proximal distribution, may occur throughout the gastrointestinal tract, and may occur in association with fistulas or excluded loops. Colorectal carcinoma in Crohn's disease may occur in normal-appearing bowel.

In a subsequent review, Greenstein (438) noted Crohn's disease carcinomas are more proximally distributed than Ulcerative Colitis carcinomas. Both tend to occur at the site of the overt disease and both develop at earlier ages (47 yrs UC, 50 yrs CD) than in the de novo colorectal carcinoma (70 years). The absolute cumulative colon carcinoma frequencies (8% UC, 7% CD) are identical after 20 years, emphasizing the importance of regular surveillance in both types of inflammatory bowel disease. Moreover, the increased risk of colon carcinoma exists in patients with Crohn's disease even when Crohn's disease is confined to the small bowel, and patients with inflammatory bowel disease have increased risks of developing extraintestinal and reticuloendothelial neoplasms in both Crohn's disease and Ulcerative Colitis, as well as ano–vulval and malignant melanoma in Crohn's disease. Colitic colorectal carcinomas are often diffuse, extensive, multiple, and right-sided with insidious presentation. The prognosis is no worse after operation than that of de novo colorectal carcinoma. Most small bowel carcinomas in Crohn's disease are adenocarcinomas rather than sarcomas, and present at a younger age, more diffusely and more distally than de novo carcinomas, usually making them undiagnosable at a curable early stage; indeed, two-thirds present with intestinal obstruction. Strictures of the colon are common in patients with inflammatory bowel disease, and they have a 10-fold risk for colon carcinoma, 30-fold for Ulcerative Colitis, and six-fold for Crohn's disease. The risk increases with disease duration. The indications for operation are absolute, relative and incidental, and the procedures include segmental resection, total proctocolectomy, subtotal colectomy, and palliative procedures.

Controversy continues regarding the incidence of colorectal carcinoma in patients with Crohn's disease. Reports range from 2% to 5% of patients with Crohn's colitis. While incidence estimates of 7 to 20 times more than expected have been suggested, some authors dispute any association between the two diseases. Person et al. (439) conducted a population-based study of 1251 subjects with Crohn's disease. The authors failed to demonstrate an increased occurrence of colorectal carcinoma. Munkholm et al. (440) followed up a cohort of 373 patients and found that the overall mortality and lifetime risk of carcinoma in patients with Crohn's disease were not increased, although the risk of rare small bowel carcinoma was significantly increased.

A review of the literature by Shorter (441) found that long-standing disease (greater than seven years) and extensive Crohn's colitis, regardless of age of onset, were associated with a twenty-fold increased risk of colonic carcinoma. In Uppsala, Sweden, a cohort of 1655 patients with Crohn's disease was studied during follow-up from 1958 to 1984 (442). There was an increased overall risk of 2.5. The relative risk was similar for males and females. Duration of follow-up did not affect risk. Relative risk for disease of the terminal ileum was one; for terminal ileum and parts of the colon, 3.2; and for colon alone, 5.6. Patients in whom colonic involvement by Crohn's disease was diagnosed before 30 years of age had a higher relative risk (20.9) than those diagnosed at older ages (2.2). The study reported by Savoca et al. (206) also showed that the risk of carcinoma with long-standing Crohn's colitis is significant and that the risk is highest in areas of active disease (Fig. 18).

Gillen et al. (443) reported that the relative risk of 4.9 for colorectal carcinoma increased to 13.3 for patients less than 25 years old at onset of Crohn's disease and to 18.2 if corrected for extensive colitis. If both factors are present, the risk rises to 57.2.

The association of colorectal carcinoma with small bowel Crohn's disease remains unresolved but is probably real. These carcinomas differ from de novo carcinomas of the small bowel in that there is a lower average age at diagnosis (45 years vs. 60 years), the site is more distal (76% vs. 20%), the mean postoperative survival is less (8 months vs. 32 months), and there is an increase in the proportion of multifocal or diffuse carcinomas. The incidence of carcinoma increases with long-standing duration of Crohn's disease. The prognosis of carcinoma of the small bowel in patients with Crohn's disease is poor (5% five-year survival compared with 20% to 30% five-year survival for de novo small bowel carcinomas).

Colorectal strictures develop in 5% to 17% of patients with colonic Crohn's disease. The frequency of carcinoma in patients with stricture (6.8%) is higher than in those without strictures (0.7%) (437). There is no difference in symptoms between patients with benign and malignant strictures. The mean age of patients with malignant

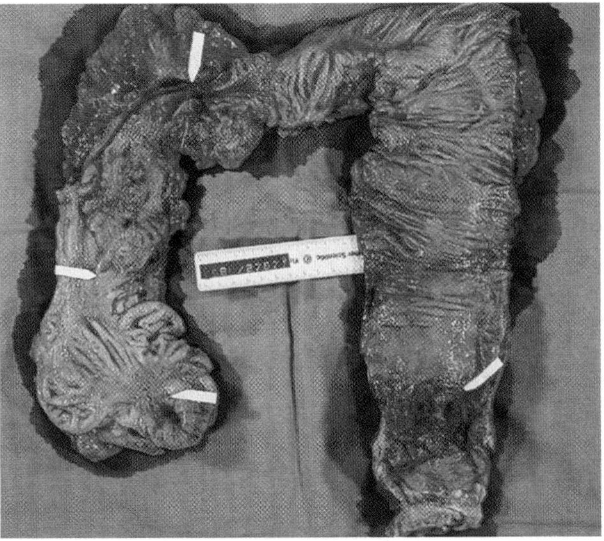

FIGURE 18 ■ Carcinoma of the rectum (80% circumference) in an area of mild inflammation. Stricture hepatic flexure secondary to fibrosis of Crohn's disease. Mild right-sided Crohn's disease with incidental diverticular disease descending colon.

strictures is higher than with benign stricture (57 years vs. 41 years). In view of the high rate of malignancy, colonoscopy with biopsy is essential in patients with Crohn's disease with colonic stricture, and operation is mandatory when the stricture cannot be fully assessed during colonoscopy.

Unlike ulcerative colitis, a segmental resection may be the appropriate treatment, in patients with segmental disease. Subtotal colectomy may be more appropriate depending on the extent of the Crohn's disease. Total proctocolectomy is reserved for those with extensive or universal colitis, especially those with perianal disease in whom reconstruction of intestinal continuity is inadvisable. Segmental resection is the preferred treatment for Crohn's enteritis. Palliative procedures for very advanced disease may include diversionary stoma.

The five-year survival for colorectal carcinoma in patients with Crohn's disease is 45%, which increases to 56% if excluded loops are omitted (437). Survival for small bowel carcinoma is 23% at three years. Mortality for carcinoma in excluded bowel has been reported as high as 100% (437). The most recent report of carcinomas developing in a small bowel Crohn's stricture found only nine such cases (444). All patients had Crohn's disease for more than 10 years. The average age of patients was 48 years compared to 65 years for de novo carcinomas. In patients with Crohn's disease, carcinoma affects the duodenum twice as commonly as jejunum, and four times as commonly as ileum. The two-year disease-free survival is 9% compared with 15% to 25% for de novo carcinomas. Fifty-nine percent of all carcinomas complicating Crohn's disease were discovered incidentally during pathologic examination of resected specimens. If small bowel alone is considered, this figure rises to 70%.

Nikias et al. (445) reviewed the medical records of 16 patients with the simultaneous diagnosis of Crohn's disease and colorectal carcinoma to identify risk factors that may account for Crohn's disease-associated colorectal carcinoma being cited with increasing frequency. There were 18 carcinomas: four in the right colon, four in the transverse colon, two in the descending colon, and eight rectal lesions. Median age at presentation was 48 years. The mean duration of Crohn's disease before presentation of carcinoma was 19.7 years. Two lesions were discovered in strictured bowel segments. Two patients had multiple carcinomas. One had simultaneous cecal and left colon adenocarcinomas. The other underwent resection of a right colon lesion and five years later presented with a transverse colon carcinoma. Eight patients had rectal carcinoma; all were diagnosed preoperatively. Six of these patients had a history of severe perianal Crohn's disease. Six had undergone multiple incision and drainage procedures for anorectal abscesses and fistulas. Two developed malignancies in defunctionalized rectal stumps. One of these patients presented with simultaneous squamous rectal carcinoma and papillary bile duct cholangiocarcinoma. Symptoms of chronic inflammatory disease may obscure clinical manifestations of occult malignancy and thereby delay diagnosis. Crohn's patients with long-standing anorectal or perianal disease and stricture may well warrant surveillance endoscopy and biopsy of involved areas with the hope of earlier detection and treatment of these rectal carcinomas.

The development of malignancy in patients with Crohn's disease may apply particularly to those with chronic complicated anorectal disease. Of some 2500 patients with Crohn's disease seen at St. Mark's Hospital in London, 15 are known to have developed carcinoma of the lower gastrointestinal tract. Malignancy occurred in the colon in two patients, in the upper two-thirds of the rectum in one, in the lower third of the rectum in seven, and in the anus in five. The 12 patients with carcinoma arising in the anus or lower rectum had long-standing severe anorectal Crohn's disease, which included a stricture (four), fistula (four), proctitis (one), abscess (two), and enlarged anal skin tags (one).

Michelassi et al. (446) reported 14 cases of intestinal adenocarcinoma complicating Crohn's disease, seven occurring in the small bowel and seven in the large bowel. In both locations, two-thirds of patients were male. The average ages at the time of diagnosis of Crohn's disease and of carcinoma were similar between the two groups of patients, 28 and 48 years, respectively. The diagnosis of carcinoma was suspected or obtained preoperatively in only four cases of large bowel carcinoma. In two patients with large bowel carcinoma and five with small bowel carcinoma, the diagnosis was made at laparotomy. In the remaining cases, only careful histologic examination revealed the carcinoma. Six small bowel carcinomas were located in the ileum, and five colonic carcinomas were distal to the splenic flexure. Two small bowel and one large bowel carcinomas were multifocal and had surrounding mucosal dysplasia. All carcinomas except one small bowel carcinoma underwent resection. Survival correlated with stage of carcinoma at resection; no patient with regional or distant metastasis survived five years, in comparison with an 83% five-year actuarial survival rate of patients with carcinoma confined to the intestinal wall. Mean survival was six months for patients with small bowel carcinoma in comparison with 65 months for patients with large bowel carcinoma, reflecting a tendency toward more advanced lesions in the small bowel group.

It has been reported that Crohn's disease that has an equivalent anatomic extent of disease in the colon and duration of disease is associated with an identical risk for colorectal carcinoma as chronic ulcerative colitis (447). Choi and Zelig (448) reported on the similarity of colorectal carcinoma in Crohn's disease and ulcerative colitis. The authors reviewed 80 patients with colorectal carcinoma complicating Crohn's disease or ulcerative colitis with median ages at diagnosis of colorectal carcinoma of 54.5 years and 43 years, respectively. The median duration of disease to the diagnosis of carcinoma was long (Crohn's disease, 15 years; ulcerative colitis, 18 years). Most carcinomas developed after more than eight years of disease (Crohn's disease, 75%; ulcerative colitis, 90%). Patients with multiple carcinomas at diagnosis were equally common (Crohn's disease, 11%; ulcerative colitis, 12%). Carcinoma occurred in the area of macroscopic disease in most patients (Crohn's disease, 85%; ulcerative colitis, 100%). Mucinous and signet ring histologic features were equally common (Crohn's disease, 29%; ulcerative colitis, 21%). Dysplasia was present with similar frequency in both diseases (Crohn's disease, 73%; ulcerative colitis, 79%). The overall five-year survival rates were also similar (Crohn's disease, 46%; ulcerative colitis, 50%). These findings show that carcinomas complicating Crohn's disease and ulcerative colitis have strikingly similar clinicopathologic features. It is suggested that patients with extensive Crohn's disease of long duration without prior resection would benefit from a surveillance program that emphasizes biopsies in areas of macroscopic disease.

Stahl et al. (449) reviewed the records of 25 patients with Crohn's disease and colorectal carcinoma to help clarify the nature of this association. Only 22 patients were available for complete retrospective analysis. The median age at diagnosis of Crohn's disease was 37 years (range, 15–67 years), and the median age at diagnosis of carcinoma was 54.5 years (range, 32–76 years). The median duration of symptoms preceding the discovery of colorectal carcinoma was 18.5 years (range, 0–32 years). Carcinoma arose in colonic segments with known Crohn's disease in 77% of patients, and six patients (27%) had associated colonic mucosal dysplasia. One lesion was classified as Dukes' stage A, nine lesions were Dukes' stage B, five lesions were Dukes' stage C, and seven lesions were metastatic. Patients with an onset of Crohn's disease before the age of 40 years had primarily Dukes' stage C or metastatic disease and consequently poor survival. Most patients presented with nonspecific signs and symptoms, with nothing to distinguish the activity of the Crohn's disease from the presence of the colorectal neoplasm. The authors concluded that younger patients with long-standing Crohn's disease should be considered for colonic surveillance to permit earlier diagnosis and treatment of potential colorectal carcinoma.

Ribeiro et al. (450) reviewed the clinical features and estimated the long-term survival of 30 patients with colorectal carcinoma complicating Crohn's disease. All patients were operated on and follow-up was complete for all patients to 10 years after operation, to the time of death, or to the closing date of the study. The 30 patients in the series had 33 colorectal adenocarcinomas; 10% presented with two synchronous carcinomas. The patients were relatively young (mean age 53 years) and had longstanding Crohn's disease (duration greater than 20 years in 87%). The five-year actuarial survival was 44% for the overall series: 100% for stage A, 86% for stage B, 60% for stage C. All five patients with excluded bowel carcinoma died of large bowel carcinoma within 2.4 years; by contrast, the actuarial five-year survival for patients with in-continuity carcinomas was 56%. They concluded that the incidence, characteristics, and prognosis of colorectal carcinoma complicating Crohn's disease are similar to the features of carcinoma in ulcerative colitis including age, multiple neoplasms, long duration of disease and greater than 50% five-year survival rate (without excluded loops). These observations suggest the advisability of surveillance programs for Crohn's disease of the colon similar to those for ulcerative colitis of comparable duration and extent.

Lynch et al. (451) recently reviewed the association inflammatory bowel disease in Ashkenazi Jews and the relationship to familial colorectal carcinoma. They noted that the NOD2 mutation shows a significant increased frequency in Jews when compared to non-Jews. While there is an increased incidence of colorectal carcinoma in patients with inflammatory bowel disease, it nevertheless is important to realize that inflammatory bowel disease likely accounts for no more than 1% to 3% of all cases of colorectal carcinoma in Ashkenazi Jews. Importantly, however, awareness of the increased colorectal carcinoma risk in inflammatory bowel disease may aid immeasurably in preventive interventions. The molecular pathway leading to colorectal carcinoma in inflammatory bowel disease appears to be different from the well-known adenoma–carcinoma sequence, given the fact that these carcinomas appear to arise from either flat, dysplastic tissue or dysplasia-associated lesions or masses. An important model, but by no means an absolute one, for colon carcinogenesis in inflammatory bowel disease follows progression from an absence of dysplasia, to indefinite dysplasia, to low-grade dysplasia, on to high-grade dysplasia, and ultimately to invasive carcinoma. This carcinogenetic process relates to the disease duration with respect to the extent of colonic involvement and may also involve primary sclerosing cholangitis. Given this knowledge of an increased risk for colorectal carcinoma, surveillance colonoscopy should initially be performed 8 to 10 years after onset of symptoms as opposed to diagnosis, and it should be performed one to two years after eight years of disease in patients with pancolitis or after 15 years in those with left-sided colitis. A search for dysplasia of colonic mucosa with biopsies performed in all four quadrants every 10 cm throughout the colon is important. Additional biopsies should be taken of any flat lesions, masses, or strictures. Prophylactic colectomy may be indicated when dysplasia is confirmed by knowledgeable pathologists.

Jess et al. (452) studied a population-based cohort of 374 patients with Crohn's disease in order to determine the long-term risk of intestinal and extraintestinal malignancies. The risk of small bowel adenocarcinoma was significantly increased, independent of age and gender (standardized morbidity ratio, 66.7). The risk of colorectal carcinoma was not increased either in the total group of patients or in patients with colonic Crohn's disease exclusively (standardized morbidity ratio, 1.64). Extraintestinal carcinoma did not occur more frequently than expected. This population-based study of patients with Crohn's disease revealed no increase in colorectal carcinoma risk possibly due to maintenance of treatment with 5-ASA preparations and operation in treatment failure. In contrast, the risk of small bowel carcinoma was increased more than 60-fold. The risk of extraintestinal carcinoma was not increased and no lymphomas were observed.

Solem et al. (453) described the clinical features, outcomes, and risk factors of small bowel adenocarcinoma in Crohn's disease. Two controls with Crohn's disease were selected for each case, matched by gender and age. Nine cases (four males) were identified. The patients presented with abdominal pain (89%), obstruction (89%), and weight loss (78%). The carcinoma was located in the ileum in eight patients (89%) and jejunum in one patient (11%). All cases but one had advanced disease with either lymph node involvement or metastases. All cases had operation with one receiving adjuvant chemotherapy. No significant risk factors were found. The mortality rates at one and two years were 42% and 61%.

Sjodahl et al. (454) studied the risk of Crohn's disease-associated colorectal carcinoma in 335 patients with rectal or anal carcinoma. Approximately three Crohn's patients per million inhabitants were diagnosed with rectal or anal carcinoma every year, which is 1% of the total number of cases. At diagnosis of carcinoma, 36% were aged below 50 years and 58% below 60 years. Corresponding figures for all cases of anal and rectal carcinoma were 5% and 18%, respectively. Present knowledge from the literature implies that there is an increased risk of rectal and anal carcinoma only in Crohn's disease patients with severe proctitis or severe chronic perianal disease. However, the rectal remnant must also be considered a risk factor. The outcome is the same as in sporadic carcinoma at a corresponding stage but the prognosis is often poor due to the advanced stage of carcinoma at diagnosis. They suggest that six high-risk groups should be recommended annual surveillance after a duration of Crohn's disease of 15 years including extensive colitis, chronic severe anorectal disease, rectal remnant, strictures, bypassed segments and sclerosing cholangitis.

Freeman (455) reviewed his database of 877 patients with Crohn's disease and found six patients with colorectal carcinoma (i.e., overall rate of 0.7%). All of these patients were men with an initial diagnosis of Crohn's disease established at a mean age of approximately 28 years, with either ileocolic disease or colonic disease alone, but not with ileal disease alone. Although there was a predominance of women in the overall study population (56.1%), no women developed colorectal carcinoma. The clinical behavior of Crohn's disease was classified as nonstricturing in all six patients with colorectal carcinoma, but in two patients Crohn's disease was complicated by a perirectal abscess or fistula. All carcinomas were located in the rectum and were diagnosed 30 years, 22 years, 7 years, 18 years, 20 years, and 40 years after Crohn's disease was initially diagnosed. In three patients the carcinoma was detected in a residual stump after partial colon resection at least 10 years earlier. In five patients, localized extension of disease through the serosa, nodal or distant metastases (liver and lung) was found at the time of diagnosis.

Freeman (456) tabulated myeloid and lymphoid malignancies compared with intestinal carcinomas in 1000 consecutive evaluated patients with Crohn's disease. Myeloid and lymphoid neoplasms were present in 0.5% of patients while carcinoma in the intestinal tract was detected in 1%. Most of the patients with a malignancy had Crohn's disease for a prolonged period of more than 20 years and had negative outcomes, including death or presentations with advanced disease. In this cohort, lymphoma was not detected in a single patient after diagnosis of Crohn's disease, possibly reflecting the limited use of immunosuppressives or infused biological agents in that clinical practice. Bypassed rectal stumps were associated with subsequent colorectal carcinoma in half of all males with colon carcinoma suggesting an important risk factor following colectomy in Crohn's disease. Epithelial dysplasia was detected in only a single male patient before colorectal carcinoma implying that this histopathological marker may be a poor predictor of subsequent colon carcinoma development in Crohn's disease, an inflammatory bowel process that is typically patchy or focal in distribution in the intestinal tract.

Sigel et al. (457) determined the prevalence, grade, and type of dysplasia found adjacent to and distant from 30 Crohn's-related adenocarcinomas. Most of the patients were male (70%). The median ages at diagnosis of Crohn's disease and adenocarcinoma were 34 and 49 years, respectively. The extent of Crohn's disease included ileocolitis in 21 patients, only colonic disease in six patients, and only small bowel disease in three. In most cases (67%), carcinoma was found incidentally at operation. All carcinomas arose in areas involved by Crohn's disease. Eight (27%) adenocarcinomas arose in small bowel and 22 (73%) arose in the colon, including two in out-of-circuit rectums. Most carcinomas (63%) were poorly differentiated. Dysplasia was found adjacent to the carcinoma in 87% of cases. Of the colorectal carcinomas, 86% had adjacent dysplasia, and 41% had distant dysplasia. They concluded that most cases of Crohn's-related intestinal adenocarcinoma have dysplasia in adjacent mucosa, and 41% of those arising in the colorectum have distant dysplasia, supporting a dysplasia–carcinoma sequence in Crohn's disease.

The recommendation for the follow-up of patients with Crohn's disease has changed in light of the recognition of the risk of developing carcinoma. If one were to extrapolate results from a review of 10 prospective studies (1225 patients) of surveillance colonoscopy in ulcerative colitis patients by Bernstein et al. (458), immediate colectomy would be recommended for all patients diagnosed with high-grade or low-grade dysplasia. These authors found that 43% of patients with a dysplasia-associated lesion or mass already had carcinoma at immediate colectomy. The risks of carcinoma at immediate colectomy were 42% for high-grade and 19% for low-grade dysplasia. Of patients found to have high-grade dysplasia after the initial colonoscopy, 32% had carcinoma. Of patients with untreated low-grade dysplasia, 16% to 29% progressed to a dysplasia-associated lesion or mass, high-grade dysplasia, or carcinoma. Of patients with indefinitive results, 28% progressed to high-grade dysplasia and 9% to carcinoma. The risk of progression to dysplasia was only 2.4% for patients whose initial result was negative.

Eaden (459) recently reviewed the subject of colorectal carcinoma and inflammatory bowel disease. The risk of colorectal carcinoma for any patient with ulcerative colitis is estimated to be 2% after 10 years, 8% after 20 years, and 18% after 30 years of disease. The relative risk of colorectal carcinoma in Crohn's colitis is approximately 5.6% and should raise the same concerns as an ulcerative colitis. Risk factors for colorectal carcinoma include disease duration, early onset, extensive disease, primary sclerosing cholangitis and a family history of sporadic colorectal carcinoma. All patients should have a review colonoscopy 8 to 10 years after diagnosis to establish the extent of disease. Surveillance should begin 8 to 10 years after disease onset for pancolitis and 15 to 20 years after disease onset for left-sided disease. Regular surveillance is recommended with a screening interval every three years in the second decade of disease and annually by the fourth decade. Random biopsies should be taken at regular intervals with the attention paid to dysplasia-associated lesions or masses, irregular plaques, villiform elevations, ulcers and strictures. Dysplasia is recognized as a premalignant condition, but the likelihood of progression to carcinoma is difficult to predict. High-grade dysplasia, confirmed by two expert gastrointestinal pathologists, is a strong indication for colectomy, as is low-grade dysplasia, although the diagnosis of low-grade dysplasia is unreliable. Surveillance programs indicate that overall five-year survival rate is higher in surveyed patients, although patients still present with Dukes' stage C carcinoma or disseminated malignancy. Surveillance has huge socioeconomic implications. As surveillance is not 100% effective, alternative ways of reducing the carcinoma risk with chemopreventive agents, such as aminosalicylates, are being considered.

Mpofu et al. (460) conducted a Cochrane review to assess the evidence that endoscopic surveillance may prolong life by allowing earlier detection of colon carcinoma or its precursor lesion, dysplasia in patients with inflammatory bowel disease. In one study, 2/40 of the patients dying of colorectal carcinoma had undergone surveillance colonoscopy on at least one occasion compared with 18/102 of the control (*RR* 0.28). One of the 40 patients who died from colorectal carcinoma had undergone surveillance colonoscopies on two or more occasions compared with 12/102 controls (*RR* 0.22) in contrast to a more modest effect observed for patients who had only one colonoscopy (*RR* 0.43). In another study, carcinoma was detected in a significantly earlier stage in the surveillance group; 15/19 had Dukes' stage A or B carcinoma in the surveilled group compared to 9/22 in the nonsurveilled group. The five-year survival rate was 77.2% for carcinomas occurring in the surveillance group and 36.3% for the nonsurveillance group. Four of 19 patients in the surveillance group died from colorectal carcinoma compared to 11/22 patients in the nonsurveillance group (*RR* 0.42). A third study found that 4 of 91 patients in the surveillance group died from colorectal carcinoma compared to 2 of 95 patients in the nonsurveilled group (*RR* 2.09). Colectomy was less common in the surveillance group, 33 compared to 51 and was performed four years later (after 10 years of disease) in the surveillance group. For the pooled data analysis, 8/110 patients in the surveillance group died from colorectal carcinoma compared to 13/117 patients in the nonsurveillance group (*RR* 0.81). These reviewers concluded that there is no clear evidence that surveillance colonoscopy prolongs survival in patients with extensive colitis. There is evidence that carcinomas tend to be detected at an earlier stage in patients who are undergoing surveillance and these patients have a correspondingly better prognosis but lead-time bias could contribute substantially to this apparent benefit. There is indirect evidence that surveillance is likely to be effective at reducing the risk of death from inflammatory bowel disease-associated colorectal carcinoma and indirect evidence that it is acceptably cost effective.

The most recent screening recommendations are derived from a panel of international experts assembled to develop consensus recommendations for the performance of surveillance (461). The following recommendations are taken from their deliberations. Patients who have only had small intestinal Crohn's disease without colonic involvement are not considered to be at high risk for colorectal carcinoma but should be managed according to general population colorectal carcinoma screening guidelines. For patients with Crohn's colitis, the Committee endorses the notion that the risk of colorectal carcinoma is similar to that of ulcerative colitis if there is comparable surface area involvement and disease duration. Carcinoma risk in Crohn's colitis occurs after 8 to 10 years of disease, and screening should start at this time. All patients with primary sclerosing cholangitis not previously known to have inflammatory bowel disease should undergo a colonoscopy to determine their status. This procedure should include biopsies from normal appearing mucosa, because microscopic evidence of colitis may not be visually apparent. For those patients shown to have inflammatory bowel disease, screening and subsequent surveillance should begin at the time of primary sclerosing cholangitis onset. Patients with major colonic involvement (at least one-third of the colon involved with disease as determined endoscopically) who have harbored disease for 8 to 10 years from onset of symptoms should undergo a screening colonoscopy. If no dysplasia or carcinoma is found, a surveillance examination protocol should be started within two years. After a negative surveillance colonoscopy, subsequent surveillance should be performed every one to two years. With two negative examinations, the next surveillance examination may be performed in one to three years until Crohn's colitis has been present for 20 years. At that time surveillance should be performed every one to two years. The recommendations for management after an abnormal finding in Crohn's colitis are identical to those for ulcerative colitis. For patients with segmental Crohn's colitis, if a dysplastic or malignant lesion is detected and operation is planned, it is not known whether a segmental resection alone is sufficient or whether an ulcerative colitis-based approach for total proctocolectomy should be considered. If the endoscopist is unable to pass a stricture and perform surveillance with a standard pediatric endoscope, a barium enema or computerized tomographic colonography should be considered to evaluate the proximal colon. If there is more than 20 years of disease, the approximately 12% rate of concomitant carcinoma warrants consideration for operation (total colectomy or segmental resection).

■ CHEMOPREVENTION OF COLORECTAL CARCINOMA

Patients with inflammatory bowel disease have increased risk for colorectal carcinoma and hence prevention has been increasingly important. The two adopted methods to prevent the development of colon carcinoma in clinical practice include prophylactic colectomy and colonoscopic surveillance. Patients and physicians seldom accept colectomy as a routine preventive method and most patients do not undergo appropriate colonoscopic surveillance. Chemoprevention refers to the use of natural or synthetic chemical agents to reverse, suppress, or to delay the process of carcinogenesis. Prevention of colorectal carcinoma by administration of chemopreventive agents is one of the most promising options for inflammatory bowel disease patients who are at increased risk of the disease. The chemopreventive efficacy of nonsteroidal anti-inflammatory drugs against intestinal neoplasms has been well established. But with reports that NSAIDs aggravate the symptoms of colitis, their sustained use for the purpose of carcinoma chemoprevention has been relatively contraindicated in inflammatory bowel disease patients. Another hopeful candidate chemoprevention drug for inflammatory bowel disease patients is 5-ASA, which is well tolerated by patients and has limited systemic adverse effects, and no gastrointestinal toxicity. 5-ASA lacks the well-known side effects of long-term NSAIDs use. Retrospective correlative studies have suggested that the long-term use of 5-ASA in inflammatory bowel disease patients may significantly reduce the risk of the development of colorectal carcinoma (462). According to the literature, this agent might well satisfy clinical expectations with respect to a safe and effective chemopreventive agent.

■ CROHN'S DISEASE AND PREGNANCY

In the seminal publication by Crohn et al. in 1956, the disease in relation to pregnancy was divided into four categories (463). Category 1 consists of patients with previously diagnosed disease, quiescent at conception. Category 2 consists of patients with active disease at conception. Category 3 consists of patients with onset of disease during pregnancy. Category 4 consists of patients with the onset of Crohn's disease in the postpartum period. In the review of the literature by Goettler and Stellato (464), they reported studies that indicate the activity of Crohn's disease is unaffected by pregnancy and that fetal mortality and morbidity are not significantly increased. When relapses of Crohn's disease do occur during pregnancy, they usually present during the first trimester. In approximately 25% of patients, worsening of the baseline Crohn's disease activity occurs during the postpartum period attributed to the sudden decrease in endogenous corticosteroids after delivery. Overall, 70% to 90% of pregnancies in Crohn's patients resulted in live births. This is, however, affected by disease activity. Abortion, prematurity, or low birth weight occurred in 50% of patients with active disease, but occurred in only 21% of patients with quiescent disease at conception. Diagnosis of Crohn's flair or complications during pregnancy may be made more difficult by the pregnancy, but the diagnosis is considered when the patient carries a preexisting diagnosis of Crohn's disease.

In the literature, values for infertility in inflammatory bowel disease are almost certainly overestimates because longer follow-up can only increase the number of pregnancies, and in most series it is not certain that all eligible patients were trying to conceive (465,466). Factors suggested as underlying subfertility in patients with Crohn's disease include dyspareunia, tubal occlusion, nutritional deficiencies, and presence of active disease with associated general ill health and medical advice against pregnancy. Indeed, patients who underwent resection had higher pregnancy rates (465).

Lindhagen et al. (467) reviewed the fertility and outcome of pregnancy in 78 women younger than 40 years of age treated with resection. The median follow-up time after the primary operation was 12.8 years. During the observation time there were 87 pregnancies in 44 patients. Neither the number of live births, nor the frequency of abortions, differed from that expected in the general population. There was no stillbirth. The localization of the disease was not significant. From the authors' study, operative intervention had no deleterious effects on fertility or outcome of pregnancy.

A review of the literature by Miller (465), including 748 pregnancies in patients with Crohn's disease, showed that the overall chance of delivery of a normal infant was similar to that in the general population. However, the coexistence of severe disease may lead to an increase in the risk of spontaneous abortion, stillbirth, or premature delivery. A study by Baird et al. (466), including 177 women with Crohn's disease, showed no evidence of increased risk of pregnancy loss, but the risk of preterm birth was significantly elevated in patients with Crohn's disease.

Woolfson et al. (468) reviewed 78 pregnancies in 50 patients to evaluate the effects of Crohn's disease on the outcome of pregnancy and the influence of the pregnancy on the course of Crohn's disease. Overall, 21 pregnancies (27%) had abnormal outcomes, including nine spontaneous abortions, six infants small for gestational age, five premature infants, and an infant who developed respiratory distress. Eight patients (50%) with active disease compared with 13 patients (21%) with inactive disease at conception had abnormal outcomes. During pregnancy 15 (55%) with active disease and six (12%) with inactive disease had an abnormal outcome. Neither medical nor surgical treatment, independent of disease activity, appeared to affect the outcome adversely. Eighteen of 73 patients (25%) with quiescent or mild disease relapsed, and seven of 16 patients with some disease activity improved (44%). Of 34 patients on medication, nine relapsed (27%), and of 39 patients not on medication, nine relapsed (24%). These results suggest that the outcome of pregnancy is not adversely affected by Crohn's disease. However, patients with active disease at conception and/or during the pregnancy have poorer outcomes independent of the use of medication or requirement of operation. Neither pregnancy nor medications taken affect the course of the disease.

Nielsen et al. (469) also studied pregnancy in Crohn's disease. The course of 109 pregnancies in 68 women with Crohn's disease was studied. A total of 76 children were delivered. There were no gemellary deliveries, and none of the children had congenital malformations. Pregnancy entailed no increased risk of an exacerbation of the bowel disease. As compared with the reference population and with women with ulcerative colitis, the total material showed an increased risk of premature delivery and spontaneous abortion, but a further analysis showed that this was due only to an increased risk in women with active disease at the time of conception and in women who had undergone bowel resection during pregnancy. Birth weight and birth length corresponded to those in the reference population. Treatment with sulfasalazine and corticosteroids did not influence the course of pregnancy or the frequency of neonatal jaundice or malformations. The authors concluded that in Crohn's disease a pregnant woman should be given the same medical treatment as when not pregnant. Generally, the women should be advised preferably to conceive at a time when their bowel disease is inactive.

Approximately 25% of patients with Crohn's disease develop a relapse during pregnancy or the puerperium. This figure may not differ from that of nonpregnant patients with Crohn's disease, but it suggests that the first trimester and the puerperium are the most likely times for relapse. Review of the literature also revealed that approximately one-third of patients improved, one-third-remain unchanged, and one-third deteriorated during the course of gestation and the puerperium. Thus two-thirds of such patients are likely to contend with active disease during pregnancy (465).

Rogers and Katz (470) conducted a review of the course of Crohn's disease during pregnancy and its effect on pregnancy outcome. The authors found that active disease at the onset of pregnancy tends to remain active and quiescent disease tends to remain quiescent. Stillbirths and spontaneous abortions occur at a rate similar to the general population, but preterm delivery occurs two to three times the general population. A history of perianal disease is not a reason for abdominal delivery. Disease activity is the best predictor of pregnancy outcome.

Bush et al. (471) conducted a study to determine whether inflammatory bowel disease is associated with increased risk of adverse perinatal outcome. It was a case-controlled study of 116 singleton pregnancies with inflammatory bowel disease compared to 56,398 singleton controls. Patients with inflammatory bowel disease were slightly older (32.8 vs. 30.6 years), more likely to be Caucasian or Asian than Black or Latino (92% vs. 57%), and have private health insurance (32% vs. 3%). inflammatory bowel disease was associated with an increased risk of labor induction (32% vs. 24%), chorioamnionitis (7% vs. 3%), and Cesarean section (32% vs. 22%), but there were no differences in neonatal outcomes. Subgroup analysis demonstrated an increased risk of low birth weight in the ulcerative colitis group versus the Crohn's group (19% vs. 0%). Patients with prior operation for inflammatory bowel disease had a lower incidence of low birth weight (0% vs. 12%). Flares during pregnancy were associated with an increased risk of preterm delivery (27% vs. 8%) and low birth weight (32% vs. 3%). They concluded that inflammatory bowel disease was an independent risk factor for Cesarian section but there was no increase in adverse perinatal outcome. Crohn's disease prior to inflammatory bowel disease operation and quiescent disease were associated with a lower risk of low birth weight.

Crohn's disease commonly affects women of childbearing age. In the most recent review by Mottet et al. (472), available data on Crohn's disease and pregnancy show that women with Crohn's disease can expect to conceive successfully, carry to term, and deliver a healthy baby. Control of disease activity before conception and during pregnancy is critical, to optimize both maternal and fetal health. Generally speaking, pharmacological therapy for Crohn's disease during pregnancy is similar to pharmacological therapy for nonpregnant patients. Patients maintained in remission by way of pharmacological therapy should continue it through their pregnancy. Most drugs including sulfasalazine, mesalazine, corticosteroids, and immunosuppressors such as azathioprine and 6-MP, are safe, whereas methotrexate is contraindicated.

The diagnosis of Crohn's disease developing for the first time during pregnancy is very rare but may pose a diagnostic challenge because symptoms typical of Crohn's disease—colicky abdominal pain, distention, nausea, and vomiting—are all frequently experienced during pregnancy. Standard radiologic investigations are contraindicated because of radiation exposure. Rigid and flexible sigmoidoscopy can be performed safely. Ultrasonography scanning may identify thickened terminal ileum or an intra-abdominal abscess. MRI is a safe noninvasive investigation and has been useful in establishing the diagnosis of Crohn's disease (473).

Goettler and Stellato (464) reviewed the English language literature for all reported cases of Crohn's disease presenting in pregnancy. Their review found a maternal mortality of 4% and morbidity of 40% and a fetal mortality of 38%, with 24% normal outcome of pregnancy. Abscess and perforation are commonly the initial manifestation of Crohn's disease because of delay in diagnosis and decreased physiologic ability to control intra-abdominal infections during pregnancy (464).

The medical treatment for Crohn's disease is similar to that of ulcerative colitis. (For the effects of medications on pregnancy, see Chapter 26.) Oral 5-ASA appears to be safe for the management of inflammatory bowel disease during pregnancy (474). Operation for colitis during pregnancy is rare. If the acute attack becomes intractable to aggressive medical management with obvious deterioration of the patient's condition, operation is indicated despite the pregnant state. Hill et al. (475) reported six patients who developed acute intraperitoneal sepsis during pregnancy. All the women recovered and five had healthy babies. The other had a miscarriage when a colonic anastomosis dehisced. Indications for operation are the same as for nonpregnant patients. For acute sepsis, Hill et al. (475) recommend removal of the source of the sepsis and exteriorization of the bowel ends.

Operations performed during the first trimester are associated with an increased risk of miscarriage. For planned procedures during the second trimester, the risk is lower. In the third trimester, laparotomy may be complicated by premature delivery and technical difficulties.

Goettler and Stellato (464) reviewed the surgical management of Crohn's disease during pregnancy. Patients presenting with peritoneal signs should undergo operation without delay. Free perforation is not unexpected because abscesses are typically less well controlled in pregnancy. Because the omentum is separated from the intestines by the bulk of the uterus, the abscess may be adjacent to the uterus and decompress into the peritoneal cavity with the onset of labor. Maternal and fetal mortality of negative laparotomy is significantly less than the delay in treating abscess or perforation. In most of the major studies presenting Crohn's disease in pregnancy, active disease was successfully controlled with medical therapy. Operation was required in only 2% of those patients. When operation was required, the inflammatory bowel disease is usually advanced with perforation or abscess. Prognosis for both mother and fetus is poor. Isolated reports have recommended that when diffuse peritonitis is encountered in the pregnant abdomen, that a stoma be constructed rather than performing an anastomosis. In the collected case reports by Goettler and Stellato (464), 11 patients had operative intervention described; eight of these had primary anastomosis rather than an ileostomy. Of these patients, two had intestinal anastomotic dehiscence. It seems reasonable to avoid anastomosis in a grossly contaminated field, as with nonpregnant patients, keeping in mind that anastomotic leak places pregnant patients at higher risk of generalized peritonitis rather than localized abscess, and this places both the mother and fetus at increased risk.

RECURRENCE

FACTORS INFLUENCING RECURRENCE

Many factors have been considered that may affect recurrence but there is no general agreement that age, sex, perioperative blood transfusion, duration of disease, the length of bowel resected, or the presence of ileal disease have any effect. Disease at resection margins appears also not to be implicated. The presence of perianal disease is associated with a greater risk of recurrence. Excision of the rectum has a lower recurrence rate but operation with anastomosis has a higher recurrence rate.

To determine the recurrence rate that requires reoperation, Whelan et al. (476) studied 438 patients who had undergone operation and were followed up for a mean of 13 years. Those patients with ileocolic disease had a slightly higher recurrence: 53% compared with 45% for colonic and 44% for small intestinal patterns. Second recurrences were from the ileocolic pattern (35%), colonic (34%), and small intestine (38%). The estimated median time of recurrence was similar among these three groups. The presence of an internal fistula or perianal disease as an indication for operation was associated with a higher likelihood of recurrence and a shortened estimated median time to recurrence.

Sachar et al. (477) studied 93 patients who underwent first resection at Mount Sinai Hospital in New York. In the entire series recurrence rates were lowest in patients with the longest preoperative duration. The same tendency was especially marked among the 68 patients without ileostomy. Likewise, among the 38 patients with ileitis, the relative risk of recurrence was significantly lower for those with disease duration exceeding 10 years. The recurrence rates among patients with ileitis, ileocolitis, and colitis were similar. Sex and age did not have an influence on recurrence rates in this series.

In a prospective cohort follow-up of 89 patients who had ileal resection for Crohn's disease, colonoscopy was performed within the first year of resection along with other clinical and laboratory examinations at six-month intervals (478). The most important predictor of recurrence was preoperative severity of Crohn's disease as determined by colonoscopy. In 19 patients who had normal neoterminal ileum at the time of resection macroscopically and microscopically all showed inflammation endoscopically six months after operation. This suggested that the recurrence was not from residual disease at the resected terminal ileum.

Raab et al. (479) investigated the factors that influenced the risk of symptomatic recurrence in patients with Crohn's disease who were treated with primary resection. Data regarding age, gender, time from diagnosis to operation, medication, preoperative infectious complications, laboratory values, emergency and/or elective procedures, location and extent of disease, and resection margins were analyzed in relation to recurrence in 353 patients who were undergoing a "curative" resection. Univariate analyses showed a higher risk of recurrence in women with ileal and ileocolonic disease than in men, in patients with ileocolonic disease compared with those with isolated ileal disease, and in ileal disease patients with an increased disease extent. In a multivariate analysis performed on patients with ileal disease, increased disease extent, limited resection on the colonic side, and referral from other hospitals were three independent variables that indicated an increased risk of recurrence. Length of disease-free resection margins did not influence the risk of recurrence. These results favor a conservative approach, particularly in patients with extensive disease.

Aeberhard et al. (480) conducted a study of the long-term course of surgically treated Crohn's disease designed to identify prognostic factors predictive of the time course and probability of recurrence. In their series of 101 patients with a median follow-up of 13 years, there was a 96% follow-up. The only variable that had a statistically significant effect on the time to reoperation was characterization of disease at the time of operation as perforating as opposed to nonperforating. Median interval between the first and second intestinal operation was 1.7 years for the perforating group and 13 years for the nonperforating group and the median time between any two operations during the study period was two years for the perforating group and 9.9 years for the nonperforating group. The risk of having to undergo reoperation for recurrence was greatest during the first two years after an operation, and this was mainly because of a short time to recurrence in the perforating group of indications. Thereafter, the yearly hazard of requiring further operation was maintained at approximately 5%.

Anseline et al. (481) studied eight factors that might predict recurrence in 130 patients operated on for Crohn's disease. There was a highly significant relationship between the presence of granulomas and subsequent recurrence. There was a trend to increased recurrence in patients with ileocolic disease and segmental colectomy. Age, sex, length of history, indication for operation, and affected lines of transection were not associated with recurrence.

Scott et al. (482) reviewed 92 patients who had undergone 102 ileocolonic anastomoses constructed after resection of intestinal Crohn's disease. The authors noted no influence of the anastomotic configuration (i.e., end-to-side, or side-to-side) on the incidence of symptomatic recurrence.

Scarpa et al. (483) compared recurrence rate after stapled side-to-side ileocolonic anastomosis to those after stapled end-to-side or hand-sewn side-to-side anastomosis to distinguish the role of suture technique and anastomotic configuration in the prevention of Crohn's disease recurrence. Twelve of them had stapled side-to-side anastomosis, 36 stapled end-to-side anastomosis, and 36 hand-sewn side-to-side anastomosis. No statistically significant difference between the three groups was observed in early postoperative follow-up. The stapled side-to-side anastomosis group obtained a better symptom-free survival than the stapled end-to-side group. In the stapled and hand-sewn side-to-side groups, reoperation were significantly lower than in the stapled end-to-side group.

Ikeuchi et al. (484) compared the outcome of patients undergoing stapled anastomosis with that of patients having hand-sewn anastomosis in 63 patients undergoing intestinal resection for Crohn's disease. The group undergoing stapling comprised 30 patients and 37 anastomoses. The group with a hand-sewn anastomosis comprised 33 patients and 45 anastomoses. The median follow-up period was 87 months. There was a significant difference in cumulative recurrences between the groups. They found stapled anastomoses after resection for Crohn's disease may delay reoperation in patients with symptomatic recurrence.

Munoz-Juarez et al. (485) conducted a case-control comparative analysis of patients with Crohn's disease treated with wide-lumen stapled anastomosis (side-to-side, functional end-to-end) and a matched (age and gender) group treated with conventional sutured end-to-end anastomosis. A total of 138 patients with Crohn's disease were treated, 69 with wide-lumen stapled anastomosis and 69 with conventional sutured end-to-end anastomosis. Fewer complications occurred after the wide-lumen stapled anastomosis. A total of 55 patients developed recurrent Crohn's disease symptoms, 57% in the conventional sutured end-to-end anastomosis, and 24% in the wide-lumen stapled anastomosis group. Median follow-up was 70 and 46 months, respectively. After conventional sutured end-to-end anastomosis, 18 reoperations were required, 15 for anastomotic stricture, and three for fistulization. After wide-lumen stapled anastomosis, three reoperations were necessary, two for stricture, and one for fistulization. The cumulative reoperation rate for anastomotic recurrence was significantly lower for the wide-lumen stapled anastomosis group.

Among the many factors studied by Poggioli et al. (486), the only risk factor identified was duration of disease before the initial operation. D'Haens, Gasparaitis, and Hanauer (487) found a close correlation between the duration of postoperative recurrence with the extent of preoperative disease. Holzheimer et al. (488) reviewed six variables (age, sex, site of diseased bowel, histologic evidence of Crohn's disease, indication for operation and incidence of postoperative complications), and incidence and time of recurrence in 104 surviving patients of 106 who underwent a first resection for Crohn's disease. Patients were followed up for a mean 4.5 years. Presentation with acute perforation was associated with a higher incidence of recurrence (10 of 14 compared with 26 of 90), and more than doubled the risk of that recurrence developing within six years. The same was true for development of a postoperative complication. The corresponding figures were 14 of 26 compared with 22 of 78. The development of postoperative complications is a previously unrecognized risk factor for early recurrence in Crohn's disease.

Silvis et al. (489) studied the effect of blood transfusion on postoperative recurrence of Crohn's disease. Overall, perioperative blood transfusion showed no effect on recurrence but has a beneficial effect on the postoperative recurrence of Crohn's disease in parous women. Klein et al. (490) demonstrated that 65% of patients operated on for Crohn's disease had lesions of the small bowel at perioperative endoscopy. However, endoscopic lesions left in place after "curative" operation, have no influence on early endoscopic anastomotic recurrences in Crohn's disease. Heimann et al. (491) reviewed 164 patients undergoing intestinal resection for Crohn's disease to identify clinical criteria that may help recognize patients with Crohn's disease who are at high risk for early symptomatic postoperative recurrence. Patients with symptomatic recurrent disease within 36 months were defined as having an early recurrence. Multivariate analysis revealed that the number of anastomoses was the most important prognostic indicator, followed by inflammation at the resection margins. Patients requiring an ileostomy had a significantly lower early recurrence rate than those having single or multiple anastomoses. There was no significant correlation between inflammation at the margins and early recurrence in patients requiring an ileostomy or a single anastomosis. When the margins were examined in patients with two or more anastomoses, 91% with inflammation at either margin experienced early recurrence. Patients having multiple anastomoses with normal margins had the same recurrence rate as patients with single anastomosis (42%).

There has been considerable debate on the importance of surgical margins in the treatment of Crohn's disease. Krause et al. (492) reported a study of 186 patients divided retrospectively into two groups, one with radical resection of 10 cm or more of disease-free margins included in the resection specimen and the other with specimens with less than 10 cm of uninvolved bowel. Follow-up of more than 14 years showed that the group with the wider margins had a recurrence of 31% and a better quality of life than with the nonradical resection group, which had a recurrence rate of 83%. Softley et al. reported a similar result in patients with a margin of normal tissue of less than 4 cm (including those with histologically positive margins) had a recurrence rate that was 10 times higher than that of a control group (493). A contrary report by Raab et al. based on 353 patients undergoing curative resection suggested that the length of the disease-free margin did not influence recurrence rates (494). A prospective study examining this issue of length of uninvolved bowel was carried out by Fazio et al. (495). Patients undergoing ileocolic resection were assigned randomly to have a proximal margin of either 2 cm of grossly uninvolved bowel or 12 cm of uninvolved bowel. No significant difference in recurrence rate was found in the 56 patients undergoing extended resection in comparison to that of the 75 patients undergoing more limited resection although the recurrence rate in the extended margin group was lower (18% vs. 25%). The length of proximal margin was examined in another prospective randomized study; patients with a length of 5 cm or more and less than 5 cm of uninvolved mucosa were compared with no significant difference (496). Wolff (497) noted several papers have suggested a benefit from a microscopically disease-free clearance at the margin of the anastomosis while an equal number have shown no difference in terms of relapse rates (498–500). The prospective randomized controlled trial by McLeod et al. (496) showed no difference between groups with and without marginal microscopic involvement.

Glehen et al. (501) conducted a prospective study comparing jejunoileal length in patients with Crohn's disease and the general population to determine whether this parameter can be related to outcome and management of Crohn's disease complications. Small bowel length was measured during abdominal operation prior to bowel resection in 93 patients with Crohn's disease and 92 patients without inflammatory or small bowel disease. Small bowel length was shown to be shorter in patients with Crohn's disease (462 cm vs. 657 cm) and was correlated to sex and height. There was no correlation of small bowel length to clinical expression (perforating or nonperforating), site, or outcome. Small bowel length is not a prognostic factor of postoperative relapse. The presence of perineal disease and systemic abnormalities seem to be the only prognostic factors in surgical recurrence. Sex, age at onset, time of first surgery, site of disease, and mode of onset are not predictive of surgical recurrence. They recommend minimal intestinal resection or strictureplasty or leaving asymptomatic intestinal lesions when surgically treating Crohn's disease complications in patients at high risk of surgical relapse and initial short bowel.

Morpurgo et al. (502) studied 92 patients with Crohn's disease affecting the colon to characterize disease behavior and to determine whether such patients might be candidates for sphincter-sparing surgery. Mean follow-up after diagnosis was 82 months. There were 39 patients with granulomatous colitis and 53 patients without granulomas. There was no statistical difference in the age at diagnosis or presence of small bowel (23% vs. 27%), ileocolic (34% vs. 30%), or perineal (36% vs.22%) disease in these patients. At initial presentation, 88% of patients with pancolitis had colitis alone without other sites of intestinal disease compared with only 37% of patients with segmental colitis. Patients with granulomas and patients with segmental colitis at presentation have a significantly higher recurrence when compared with patients without granulomas and patients with pancolitis. Thirteen patients without granulomatous disease and eight with granuloma underwent ileal pouch-anal anastomosis. Seven patients (three with granuloma and four without granuloma) had recurrence of Crohn's disease in the ileal pouch; two required pouch removal and a permanent diversion for fistulizing disease in the ileal pouch and five were successfully treated conservatively without operation. The presence of granulomas and segmental involvement of the colon in patients with Crohn's colitis may reflect a more virulent clinical course. Ileal pouch-anal anastomosis may be considered as an option in select patients with Crohn's colitis without small bowel or perianal disease. Based on their data, patients with nongranulomatous pancolitis may be better candidates for sphincter-sparing operations.

Scarpa et al. (503) reviewed the records of 120 patients treated for stenosing Crohn's disease and reported the risk factors for recurrence of stenosis to be younger age, acute obstruction, emergency conditions, postoperative complications, small bowel disease, ileo-ileal anastomosis, and type of suture.

Borley et al. (504) investigated the hypothesis that there is an aggressive subtype of Crohn's disease characterized by early recurrence and that disease location and surgical procedures are associated with differing patterns of recurrence. They analyzed 280 patient records totaling 482 major abdominal operations. There was a significantly higher recurrence rate for ileal disease than for ileocolic or colic disease (median reoperation free-survival 37.8 vs. 47.8% and 54.7 months, respectively) and there was a significantly shorter reoperation-free–survival for those patients treated by strictureplasty alone or strictureplasty combined with resection than for those treated by resection alone (41.7 and 48.6 vs. 51 months, respectively) but only disease site was confirmed as an independent risk factor for recurrence. These data suggest that there is no evidence for the existence of a separate early recurring, aggressive disease type.

Maconi et al. (505) evaluated patients with Crohn's disease, using transabdominal ultrasound, the morphologic characteristics of the diseased bowel wall before and after conservative operation and assessed whether these characteristics and their behavior in the postoperative follow-up are useful and reliable prognostic factors of clinical and surgical recurrence. In 85 consecutive patients treated with strictureplasty and miniresections for Crohn's disease, clinical and ultrasonographic evaluations were performed before and six months after operation. Assessed before operation were the maximum bowel wall thickness, the length of the bowel wall thickening, the bowel wall echo pattern (homogeneous, stratified, and mixed), and the postoperative bowel wall behavior, classified as normalized, improved, unchanged, or worsened. A significant correlation was found between a long preoperative bowel wall thickening and surgical recurrence. Bowel wall thickness after operation was unchanged or worsened in 43.3% of patients; in these patients, there was a high frequency of previous operation. Patients with unchanged or worsened bowel wall thickness had a higher risk of clinical and surgical recurrence compared with those with normalized or improved bowel wall thickness.

Hofer et al. (506) reviewed patients who had undergone abdominal surgery for Crohn's disease to determine risk factors for recurrence. Mean follow-up was 4.4 years. Patients with fistulizing type of symptoms, extraintestinal manifestations, corticosteroid treatment or male gender experienced significant earlier reoperation. Recurrent disease, histologic evidence of inflamed resection margins, patient's age at the time of primary diagnosis and operation, and the presence of epitheloid granulomas did not show significant influence on recurrence-free intervals.

Bernell et al. (507) assessed the risk for resection and postoperative recurrence in the treatment of ileocecal Crohn's in a population-based cohort of 907 patients. Resection rates were 61%, 77%, and 83% at 1, 5 and 10 years, respectively after the diagnosis. Relapse rates were 28% and 36%, 5 and 10 years after the first resection. A younger age at diagnosis resulted in a low resection rate. The presence of perianal Crohn's disease and long resection segments increased the incidence of recurrence, and resection for a palpable mass and/or abscess decreased the recurrence rate.

Bernell et al. (508) assessed the impact of possible risk factors on intestinal resection and postoperative recurrence in Crohn's disease. Data on initial intestinal resection and postoperative recurrence were evaluated retrospectively in a population-based cohort of 1936 patients. The cumulative rate of intestinal resection was 44%, 61%, and 71% at 1, 5, and 10 years, respectively, after diagnosis. Postoperative recurrences occurred in 33% and 44% at 5 and 10 years, respectively, after resection. The relative risk of operation was increased in patients with Crohn's disease involving any part of the small bowel, in those having perianal fistulas, in those who were 45 to 59 years of age at diagnosis. Female gender and perianal fistulas as well as small bowel and continuous ileocolonic disease, increase the relative risk of recurrence. They found three-fourths of patients with Crohn's disease will undergo an intestinal resection and half of them will ultimately relapse. The frequency of operation is decreased over time but the postoperative relapse rate remains unchanged.

Lifestyle factors have been shown to influence prognosis in Crohn's disease. Timmer et al. (509) assessed the effects of smoking and oral contraceptive use on clinical relapse rates. Of 152 patients, 40% had a relapse. Analysis showed unfavorable outcomes for women, current smokers, and use of oral contraceptives. Recent operation was associated with a decreased risk of relapse. The Cox model retained current smoking versus never smoking (hazard ratio = 2.1), oral contraceptive use (hazard ratio = 3.0) and medical compared with operative induction of remission (hazard ratio = 2.1) as predictors of relapse. Ex-smokers did not have an increased risk. Finally, sex, age, time in remission, disease location, and disease duration were not significant predictors.

Froehlich et al. (510) recently reviewed the treatment of postoperative Crohn's disease. At one year after first resection, up to 80% of patients showed an endoscopic recurrence, 10% to 20% have clinical relapse, and 5% have surgical recurrence. Smoking is one of the most important risk factors for postoperative recurrence. Preoperative disease activity and the severity of endoscopic lesions in the neo-terminal ileum within the first postoperative year are predictors of symptomatic recurrence. Mesalamine is generally the first-line treatment used in the postoperative setting but still provokes considerable controversy as to its efficacy, in spite of the results of a meta-analysis. Immunosuppressive treatment (azathioprine, 6-MP) is based on scant evidence but is currently used as a second-line treatment in postoperative patients at high risk for recurrence, with symptoms or with early endoscopic lesions in the neo-terminal ileum. Nitroimidazole antibiotics (metronidazole, ornidazole) are also effective in the control of active Crohn's disease in the postoperative setting. Given their unknown toxicity, they may be used as a third-line treatment as initial short-term prevention therapy rather than for long-term use. Conventional corticosteroids, budesonide, or probiotics have no proven role in postoperative prophylaxis. Infliximab has not as yet been studied for use in the prevention of relapse after surgery.

Yamamoto (511) recently combined an extensive study to examine factors affecting postoperative recurrence of Crohn's disease by a Medline-based literature review. Smoking significantly increases the risk of recurrence (risk is approximately twice as high), especially in women and heavy smokers. Quitting smoking reduces the postoperative recurrence rate. A number of studies have shown a higher risk when the duration of disease before operation was short. There were, however, different definitions of short among the studies. Prophylactic corticosteroids are not effective in reducing the postoperative recurrence. A number of randomized controlled trials offer evidence of the efficacy of 5-ASA (mesalazine) in reducing postoperative recurrence. Recently, the therapeutic efficacy of the immunosuppressive drugs (azathioprine and 6-MP) in the prevention of postoperative recurrence has been investigated in several studies and reported that these drugs might help prevent the recurrence. Further clinical trials would be necessary to evaluate the prophylactic efficacy of immunosuppression. Several studies showed a higher recurrence rate in patients with perforating disease than those with nonperforating disease. However, evidence for differing recurrence rates and perforating and nonperforating disease is inconclusive. A number of prospective studies reported that a stapled functional end-to-end anastomosis was associated with a lower recurrence rate compared with other types of anastomosis. However, prospective randomized studies would be necessary to draw a definite conclusion. Many studies found no difference in the recurrence rates between patients with radical resection and nonradical resection. Therefore, minimal operative procedures including strictureplasty have been justified in the management of Crohn's disease. In this review the following factors do not seem to be predictive of postoperative recurrence: age at onset of disease, sex, family history of Crohn's disease, anatomical site of disease, length of resected bowel, presence of granuloma in the specimen, blood transfusions, and postoperative complications. The most significant factor affecting postoperative recurrence of Crohn's disease is smoking. Smoking significantly increases the risk of recurrence. A short disease duration before operation seems albeit to be a very minor degree to be associated with a higher recurrence rate. 5-ASA has been shown with some degree of confidence to lead to a lower recurrence rate. The prophylactic efficacy of immunosuppressive drugs should be assessed in the future. A wide anastomotic technique for resection may reduce postoperative recurrence rate though this should be investigative with prospective randomized trials.

■ MAINTAINING REMISSION IN CROHN'S DISEASE

One of the greatest challenges in managing Crohn's disease is to maintain remission. Within two years of establishing medical remission an estimated 35% to 80% of patients relapse (478). It has long been recognized that the long-term use of sulfasalazine has proven beneficial in the reduction of exacerbations in ulcerative colitis. Much effort has been directed at studies attempting to maintain remission and prevent or at least reduce the development of recurrence following either medical treatment or resection of diseased intestine.

Feagen (512) reviewed the subject of maintenance of remission in patients treated for Crohn's disease from which much of the following information has been obtained. The proportion of individuals who experience a symptomatic relapse after the induction of medical remission has been estimated at 35% to 80% over two years. The variability of this estimate likely reflects diversity in definitions of relapse and the heterogeneic patient populations studied. Endoscopic recurrence occurs, almost uniformly, within a three-year period after an operation in which all visible disease has been resected. Clinical recurrence rates are considerably lower than those reported in endoscopic studies and range between 23% and 37% at one year increasing to 40% to 55% at five years. With respect to risk factors for postoperative recurrence, involvement of multiple segments of intestine is associated with increased risk. Patients with multiple anastomoses or those with inflammation at the surgical margins are also more likely to relapse but this it not universally agreed upon. The length of small bowel involved in a postoperative recurrence correlated with the length of diseased intestine before operation. Surgical recurrence rates are significantly higher in female smokers compared with nonsmokers. Smoking is a risk factor for clinical, surgical, and endoscopic recurrence. Operations for inflammatory complications of Crohn's disease (i.e., abscess) or previous operation for Crohn's disease increase the risk of recurrence.

Stark and Tremaine (77) reported the results of a meta-analysis of more than 30 clinical trials on maintenance therapy in Crohn's disease. At least four trials demonstrated statistically significant results using 5-ASA compared with placebo. A summary of the review is shown in Table 8. Oral 5-ASA preparations reduce recurrence rates by about 40% when administered to patients with quiescent Crohn's disease. Messori et al. (520) also performed a meta-analysis of five clinical trials conducted to determine the value of 5-ASA in maintaining remission in Crohn's disease. The pooled relapse-free rates in the treatment group were 91% at six months, 84% at 12 months, and 72% at 24 months. The corresponding rates in the control group were 77%, 60%, and 52%, respectively. The cost for preventing each relapse can be between $4000 and $10,000, which compares favorably with the average cost of treating a relapse. A subsequent report by McLeod et al. (521) revealed that in a randomized controlled trial of 163 patients 3 g of mesalamine (Rowasa or Salofalk) daily reduced symptomatic recurrence rates to 31% from 41 % in the control group.

Caprilli et al. (522) conducted a double-blind randomized multicenter prospective controlled trial to evaluate whether 4 g/day of mesalazine may offer therapeutic advantages over 2.4 g/day in the prevention of both endoscopic and clinical postoperative recurrence of Crohn's disease. Two hundred and six patients submitted to the first or second intestinal resection for Crohn's disease limited to the terminal ileum with or without the involvement of the cecum/ascending colon were enrolled. Of these, 101 were randomly allocated to receive 4 g/day of mesalazine (Asacol) and 104 to receive 2.4 g/day starting two weeks after operation. Eighty-four patients in the 4 g/day group and 81 patients in the 2.4 g/day group were evaluated by endoscopy. They concluded that the 4 g/day regimen of mesalazine does not offer a clinically significant advantage over a 2.4 g/day regimen in the prevention of postoperative endoscopic and clinical recurrence of Crohn's disease at one-year follow-up.

Salomon et al. (523) reported on a meta-analysis of 12 placebo-controlled trials evaluating the efficacy of single-drug therapy for the induction and maintenance of remission in Crohn's disease. The authors noted nearly identical rates of relapse with sulfasalazine, prednisolone, or azathioprine, demonstrating a 90% maintenance of remission rate at three months that decreased to 25% at 36 months. A meta-analysis of 10 randomized controlled trials (1022 patients) of sulfasalazine or mesalamine in the prevention of symptomatic relapse in quiescent disease revealed that the risk of clinical relapse at one year was reduced by the use of these drugs, but subgroup analysis found that the observed benefit was seen with only the mesalamine preparation (524). Efficacy was noted with ileal and ileocolic disease and not with colonic disease alone. This, together with another meta-analysis (520), suggests that mesalamine at higher doses is an effective agent to maintain remission in Crohn's disease. A more recent report on this subject is a double-blind, placebo-controlled study of mesalamine, 750 mg four times a day for 48 weeks, in maintaining remission in 293 patients with Crohn's disease (525). Patients were stratified according to the method of induction of remission (medical or surgical). Twenty-five percent who received mesalamine had a relapse compared with 36% receiving placebo. Of mesalamine-treated patients, 25% had relapsed by 249 days of follow-up compared with 154 days for placebo-treated patients. Subgroup analysis showed that patients with ileocecal-colonic disease or female patients had fewer relapses on mesalamine therapy than placebo-treated patients (21% vs. 41% and 19% vs. 41%, respectively). In this study, mesalamine treatment reduced relapse compared with placebo treatment, although conventional statistical significance was not achieved.

Ardizzone et al. (526) compared the efficacy and safety of azathioprine and mesalamine in the prevention of clinical and surgical relapse in patients who have undergone operations for Crohn's disease. In a prospective, open-label, randomized study, 142 patients received azathioprine (2 mg/kg/day) or mesalamine (3 g/day) for 24 months. Clinical relapse was defined as the presence of symptoms with a Crohn's disease activity index score greater than 200 and surgical relapse as the presence of symptoms refractory to medical treatment or complications requiring operation. After 24 months, the risk of clinical relapse was comparable in the azathioprine and mesalamine groups. No difference was observed with respect to

TABLE 8 ■ Placebo-Controlled Trials of Preparations of 5-Aminosalicylic Acid to Prevent Recurrent Crohn's Disease

Author(s)	Agent (dosage)	No. of Patients	Type of Remission	Site of Prior Disease	Relapse (definition)	Duration of Trial (mo)	Relapse Rate 5-ASA vs. Placebo (p value)
Positive Results							
Thomson (513)	Claversal (1.5 g/day)	209	S, M	I, IC, C	Clinical	12	12 mo, 22.4% vs. 36.2% (0.0395)
Prantera et al. (514)	Asacol (2.4 g/day)	125	M	I, IC, C	Clinical	12	12 mo, 34% vs. 55% (0.02)
Caprilli et al. (515)	Asacol (2.4 g/day)	83	S	I, IC	Endoscopic	12	12 mo, 7.34% vs. 38.70% (<0.01)
Gendre et al. (516)	Pentasa (2 g/day)	161	S, M	SB, SB + C, C	Clinical	24	12 mo, 28% vs. 68% (<0.05) 24 mo, 55% vs. 71% (<0.05)
Negative results							
Fiasse et al. (517)	Claversal (1.5 g/day)	62	S	I, IC	Clinical	12	12 mo, 54% vs. 37% (ns)
Brignola et al. (518)	Pentasa (2 g/day)	44	M	I, IC, C	Clinical	4	4 mo, 42.4% vs. 59% (ns)
Florent et al. (519)	Claversal (1.5 g/day)	126	S	I, IC, C	Endoscopic	3	3 mo, 50% vs. 63% (ns)

Abbreviations: 5-ASA, 5-Aminosalicylic acid; C, colon; I, ileum; M, medical remission; ns, not significant; S, postsurgical remission; SB, small bowel.
Source: From Ref. 77.

surgical relapse at 24 months between the two groups. In a subgroup analysis, azathioprine was more effective than mesalamine in preventing clinical relapse in patients with previous intestinal resections (OR, 4.83). More patients receiving azathioprine withdrew from treatment due to adverse events than those receiving mesalamine (22% vs. 8%).

Akobeng and Gardener (527) conducted a systemic Cochrane review to evaluate the efficacy of oral 5-ASA agents for the maintenance of medically reduced remission in Crohn's disease. They included randomized control trials, which compared oral 5-ASA agents with either placebo or sulphasalazine, with treatment durations of at least six months. The main outcome measure was the occurrence of relapse as defined by the primary studies. They assumed the participants who dropped out of the study and on whom there was no postwithdrawal information, had relapse during the study period. The odds ratio for six studies where participants were followed up for 12 months was 1.0. They found no evidence in this review to suggest that 5-ASA preparations are superior to placebo to the maintenance of medically induced remission in patients in Crohn's disease.

Stark and Tremaine (77) reviewed four controlled trials studying long-term low-dose steroid therapy (7.5–15 mg) and concluded that the weight of evidence is that corticosteroids do not have a major benefit in the prevention of recurrence of Crohn's disease. Lofberg et al. (528) evaluated the efficacy and safety of budesonide, a corticosteroid analog, given in an oral controlled-release formulation for maintenance of remission in patients with ileal and ileocecal Crohn's disease. Of 176 patients with active Crohn's disease who had achieved remission (Crohn's disease activity index score ≤ 150) after 10 weeks of treatment with either budesonide or prednisolone, 90 were randomized to continue with once-daily treatment of 6 mg of budesonide, 3 mg of budesonide, or placebo for up to 12 months in a double-blind, multicenter trial. After three months, 19% of the patients in the 6 mg group had relapsed compared with 45% in the 3 mg group and 44% in the placebo group. The corresponding results after 12 months were 59% in the 6 mg budesonide group, 74% in the 3 mg group, and 63% in the placebo group. The authors concluded that 6 mg budesonide once daily is significantly more efficacious than placebo in prolonging time to relapse in Crohn's disease and causes only minor systemic side effects. Rutgeerts et al. (529) reported that budesonide is only slightly less effective than prednisolone in inducing remission but had fewer side effects and caused less suppression of pituitary–adrenal function. In a double-blind multicenter trial, Greenberg et al. (530) studied the value of oral controlled-release budesonide as maintenance treatment for Crohn's disease. It was well tolerated and prolonged remission in Crohn's disease of ileum and proximal colon but this effect was not sustained at one-year follow-up.

Sandborn et al. (531) evaluated the efficacy and safety of oral budesonide for maintenance of remission in patients with mild to moderately active Crohn's disease of the ileum and/or ascending colon. Four double-blind placebo-controlled trials with identical protocols were combined and comprised 380 patients with Crohn's disease in medically induced remission (288). Patients were randomized to receive oral budesonide 3 mg, 6 mg, or placebo daily for 12 months. The median time to relapse was 268, 170, and 154 days for budesonide 6 mg, budesonide 3 mg and placebo groups, respectively. They concluded that budesonide 6 mg a day is effective for prolonging time to relapse and for significantly reducing relapse rates at three and six months but not 12 months.

Steinhart et al. (532) evaluated the effectiveness and safety of conventional systemic steroid therapy in maintaining clinical remission in Crohn's disease in a Cochrane review. Selection criteria included randomized double-blind placebo-controlled trials involving patients of any age with Crohn's disease in clinical remission as defined by a CDAI less than 150 or by the presence of no symptoms or only mild symptoms at the time of entry into the trial. The experimental treatment consisted of oral conventional corticosteroid therapy (excluding budesonide, fluticasone, etc.). Clinical disease relapse was used as the outcome measure of interest. Three studies were judged as eligible for inclusion for a total number of subjects included in the analysis at the time points of 6, 12, and 24 months being 142, 131, and 95 for the corticosteroid group and 161, 138, and 87 for the control group. The odds ratio for relapse on active treatment was 0.71, 0.82, and 0.72 at 6, 12, and 24 months, respectively. The reviewer's conclusions were that the use of conventional systemic corticosteroids in patients with clinically quiescent Crohn's disease does not appear to reduce the risk of relapse over a 24-month period of follow-up.

Rutgeerts et al. (533) reported a double-blind controlled trial in which metronidazole, 20 mg/kg divided three times daily for three months, was used to prevent recurrence of ileal disease after curative resection of the ileum and partial right colonic resection. This regimen reduced the incidence of recurrent lesions in the neoterminal ileum (52% vs. 75%) and significantly reduced the incidence of severe ileal disease (13% vs. 43%) compared with placebo. Metronidazole also significantly reduced symptomatic recurrence rates at one year (4% vs. 25%) and showed a trend toward improvement at two and three years.

Bouhnik et al. (534) assessed the value of azathioprine or 6-MP in patients who were in a prolonged clinical remission (greater than six months without steroids). In patients on therapy, the cumulative probabilities of relapse at one and five years were 11% and 32%, respectively. In patients who stopped therapy, the probabilities of relapse at one and five years were 38% and 75%, respectively. However, after four years of remission, the risk of relapse was similar; therefore, the usefulness of continued therapy is questionable. Azathioprine and 6-MP effectively suppress chronic disease activity and maintain medication-induced remission, but the potential risks of side effects may outweigh the benefit of continuous treatment to prevent relapse in asymptomatic patients (77).

Orally administered corticosteroids, sulfasalazine, metronidazole, azathioprine, and cyclosporine have not proved of benefit in the prevention of recurrence in Crohn's disease. Nonetheless, corticosteroids, metronidazole, and azathioprine can control chronically active disease.

Hanauer et al. (535) conducted a randomized controlled trial to assess the benefit of maintenance infliximab therapy in patients with active Crohn's disease who respond to a single infusion of infliximab. The 573 patients with a score of at least 220 on the CDAI received a 5 mg/kg intravenous infusion of infliximab at week 0. After assessment response at week 2, patients were randomly assigned to repeat infusions of placebo at weeks 2 and 6 and then every eight weeks thereafter until week 46 (group I), repeat infusions of 5 mg/kg of infliximab at the same time points (group II), or 5 mg/kg of infliximab at weeks 2 and 6 followed by 10 mg/kg (group III). There were 58% of patients who responded to a single dose of infliximab within two weeks. At week 30, 21% of group I patients were in remission compared with 39% of group II and 45% of group III patients. Thus, patients in groups II and III combined were more likely to sustain clinical remission than patients in group I (OR 2.7). Patients with Crohn's disease who respond to an initial dose of infliximab are more likely to be in remission at weeks 30 and 54, to discontinue corticosteroids, and to maintain their response for a longer period of time, if infliximab treatment is maintained every eight weeks.

Sands et al. (536) performed a multicenter, double-blind, randomized, placebo-controlled trial to evaluate the efficacy of infliximab maintenance therapy in 306 adult patients with Crohn's disease and one or more draining abdominal or perianal fistulas of at least three months duration. Patients received 5 mg of infliximab per kilogram of body weight intravenously on weeks 0, 2, and 6. A total of 195 patients who had a response at weeks 10 and 14, and 87 patients who had no response were then randomly assigned to receive placebo or 5 mg of infliximab per kilogram every eight weeks and to be followed to week 54. The time to loss of response was significantly longer for patients who received infliximab maintenance therapy than for those who received placebo maintenance (more than 40 weeks vs. 14 weeks). At week 54, 19% of patients in the placebo maintenance group had a complete absence of draining fistulas, as compared with 36% of patients in the infliximab maintenance group.

Hanauer et al. (537) presented the following balanced view for the lifetime channeling of infliximab for Crohn's disease. It is clear that when treatment with infliximab is introduced, induction therapy alone does not alter the natural history of Crohn's disease. Rutgeerts demonstrated that after a single infusion of infliximab, approximately 80% of responders would relapse within a year unless retreatment is provided (538). The French study group GETAID, has recently demonstrated that discontinuing azathioprine maintenance therapy after four years leads to an increased risk of clinical recurrence within one year that amounts to a 60% risk of relapse at five years (539). The real issue is where to position the introduction of infliximab for the treatment of Crohn's disease. Given the safety risks and the risk of immunogenicity (development of antibodies to infliximab and eventual infusion reactions and loss of response), and the recognition that once on infliximab, always on infliximab, it will be important to define which patients should be started on infliximab therapy. Hanauer currently recommends infliximab, primarily, for patients failing other medications, administers the three-dose regimen plus azathioprine or methotrexate for all patients, and anticipates the requisite for indefinite therapy. In the absence of data demonstrating long-term superiority of infliximab plus azathioprine compared to corticosteroids plus azathioprine, he fears administration of infliximab as a bridge therapy to an alternate immune modifier. This concern is due to the recognition that retreatment after a hiatus can lead to the development of antibodies to infliximab and ultimately loss of response to this highly efficacious therapy from which there is no current rescue aside from operation.

Borgaonkar et al. (540) conducted a Cochrane review to evaluate the effects of antituberculous therapy for the maintenance of remission in patients with Crohn's disease. They identified a total of seven randomized trials, which included 355 patients. The analysis of all seven trials yielded an odd ratio for maintenance of remission of 1.36. The reviewer's conclusion was that antituberculous therapy might be effective at maintaining remission in patients with Crohn's disease when remission has been induced with corticosteroids combined with antituberculous therapy. However, the results, which support this conclusion come from a subgroup of only two trials with small numbers of patients and should be interpreted with caution. Use of this therapy cannot be recommended on the basis of this evidence.

In a less than encouraging review of the strategies to prevent postoperative recurrence in Crohn's disease, Rutgeerts (541) provided the following summary. The majority of patients with Crohn's disease require resection in the course of their disease. Most of them will suffer symptomatic recurrence in the years after their operation leading to new complications and sometimes repeated operation. Smoking, perforating behavior of the disease, and ileal or ileocolonic locations seem to predispose to early and aggressive recurrence. No clear prophylactic drug regime has been identified. Sulfasalazine and 5-ASA are only mildly protective and meta-analysis of all studies does not show superiority over placebo. Glucocorticosteroids are not efficacious. Nitroimidazole antibiotics, metronidazole and ornidazole prevent early endoscopic recurrence and postpone symptomatic relapse but are not well tolerated. Immunosuppression with azathioprine or 6-MP is attractive but hard data concerning their efficacy are still lacking. No data are available on the use of biologicals for the prevention of postoperative Crohn's disease.

Diminished bone mineral density is a recognized complication of Crohn's disease. Maintenance treatment with infliximab improves bone mineral density in patients with Crohn's disease (542).

SUMMARY

Egan and Sandborn (138) recently reviewed the subject of the treatment of Crohn's disease and remission and their results are summarized as follows: 6-MP and azathioprine are the benchmark drugs for the maintenance of long-term symptomatic remission in Crohn's disease. Although the benefit of these drugs is well established, a recent noninferiority (equivalence) study addressed the question of when to discontinue 6-MP or azathioprine in patients who experience years-long remission. Among Crohn's disease patients in remission for at least 42 months, withdrawal of azathioprine leads to an 18-month relapse rate of 21% compared with 8% among the group randomized to continue active treatment with statistical analysis indicating that azathioprine withdrawal was not equivalent to continued azathioprine. Thus, both in induction followed by long-term treatment studies and in a withdrawal of treatment trial, azathioprine and 6-MP have been found to be superior to placebo for maintenance of remission in Crohn's disease.

5-ASA drugs have been extensively studied for the prevention of Crohn's disease flares. The results of some of these studies suggested that mesalamine was efficacious for the maintenance of medically or surgically induced remission of Crohn's disease, but more studies showed no benefit over placebo. Meta-analysis showed no significant benefit over placebo in medically induced remission or a marginal benefit in surgically induced remission. Similarly, sulfasalazine and olsalazine were found to be not superior to placebo for remission maintenance. For these reasons, 5-ASA drugs should not be prescribed to Crohn's disease patients for maintenance of remission.

Conventional corticosteroids are not effective in maintaining Crohn's disease remission at doses low enough to avoid obvious adverse effects with long-term use. However, controlled ileal release budesonide 6 mg/day was found to be effective for prolongation of time to relapse and maintenance of remission at six months but not one year in patients with Crohn's disease in medically induced remission. Budesonide 6 mg/day is more effective than placebo or mesalamine 3 g/day for maintenance of remission in patients with steroid-dependent Crohn's disease.

Metronidazole at a dose of 20 mg/kg per day in divided doses delays the recurrence of the severe endoscopic lesions of Crohn's disease after ileal resection when administered for three months after surgery. However, side effects are problematic and clinical recurrence rates at one, two, and three years in the intention-to-treat population were not significantly lower by three months of metronidazole therapy. Thus, the role of metronidazole for postoperative maintenance of remission and clinical remission remains uncertain.

Methotrexate maintenance therapy was studied in patients who had entered symptomatic remission with Methotrexate 25 mg once weekly. At a dose of 15 mg weekly, methotrexate was superior to placebo in this 40-week trial, with long-term remission rates of 65% versus 39% in placebo-treated patients. Furthermore, 55% of patients who relapsed and were retreated with methotrexate 25 mg a week entered symptomatic remission at 40 weeks.

The benefit of eight weekly infusions of infliximab in Crohn's disease patients who experienced clinical benefit from a single infusion of this agent was studied in a large clinical trial involving 573 patients. The ACCENT I trial reported that of 58% patients who responded to an initial infusion of infliximab 5 mg/kg, remission rates after 30 weeks were 21%, 39%, and 45% in the groups randomized to eight weekly maintenance treatments with placebo, 5 or 10 mg/kg infliximab, respectively. Dose escalation from 5 to 10 mg/kg or dose interval shortening from every eight weeks to every six weeks or even every four weeks appears to increase the number of patients successfully maintained.

These data, along with the results of older studies, support the following management approach for the treatment of Crohn's disease in remission. Azathioprine or 6-MP, methotrexate, and infliximab have been proven efficacious for maintaining medically induced remission in Crohn's disease. Although budesonide prolongs the time to relapse, it does not meet the conventional definition of efficacy (maintenance of remission for one year). Most patients who enter remission with drug therapy will relapse without maintenance treatment. Therefore, azathioprine, 6-MP, methotrexate, or infliximab, and in some cases budesonide, should be administered to avoid symptomatic relapse. Because of the expense and the need for concomitant immunosuppressive therapy to prevent immunogenicity, infliximab should be reserved for patients unable to take or refractory to these other drugs. Budesonide should only be administered to patients with distal small intestine and right colon disease, and most studies suggest that the duration of benefit with maintenance budesonide is less than one year. This is considerably shorter than the benefit reported in the studies of azathioprine, 6-MP, and methotrexate for remission maintenance. Therefore, azathioprine, 6-MP, and methotrexate should be prescribed for most Crohn's disease patients in medically induced remission. Symptomatic relapse tends to occur after azathioprine and 6-MP are stopped so therapy with these agents should be continued indefinitely in most patients in the absence of a contraindication to continuation. Patients who require infliximab to enter remission but relapse despite the use of azathioprine, 6-MP, or methotrexate should receive eight weekly infusion of infliximab. Whether all patients require the immediate institution of maintenance therapy with one of these agents is unclear. Data indicate that 56% to 68% of Crohn's patients who are treated with corticosteroids are not in remission one year later, so most patients will require maintenance therapy, and practitioners should have a low threshold for beginning immunosuppressive maintenance therapy.

The time to symptomatic relapse after intestinal resection in Crohn's disease is highly variable. Because many patients with a short segment of stricturing Crohn's disease at the terminal ileum do not experience recurrent symptoms soon after operation, they do not necessarily treat all postoperative patients. Natural history studies have shown that symptomatic recurrence is preceded by endoscopic recurrence and the severity of endoscopic changes predicts future disease activity. Therefore, an alternative to treating all patients with azathioprine or 6-MP is to stratify postoperative patients by the presence or absence of neoterminal ulcers 6 to 12 months after operation and to treat only those with severe ulcers. However, immediate postoperative maintenance therapy may be indicated in those patients with residual unresected disease, a prior history of aggressive disease (including internal fistula or abscess), a short clinical course before operation, or multiple prior resections. Metronidazole has been shown to reduce the frequency of severe ulcers after terminal ileum and right colon resection, but the utility of this agent in the prevention of symptomatic relapse has not been established. Although postoperative remission maintenance

BOX 4 ■ **Comparison of Ulcerative Colitis and Crohn's Colitis**

Manifestation	Ulcerative Colitis	Crohn's Colitis
Clinical Features		
Bleeding per rectum	3+	1+
Diarrhea	3+	3+
Abdominal pain	1+	3+ Especially with involvement of ileum
Vomiting	R	3+
Fever	R	2+
Palpable abdominal mass	R	2+
Weight loss	+	3+
Clubbing	R	1+
Rectal involvement	4+	1+
Small bowel involvement	0	4+
Anal and perianal involvement	R	4+
Risk of carcinoma	1+	1+
Clinical course	Relapses/remission	Slowly progressive
Radiologic		
Thumb printing sign on barium enema	R	1+
Endoscopic		
Distribution	Symmetric	Asymmetric
Continuous involvement	4+	1+
Rectal	4+	1+
Vascular architecture	Absent	1+
Friability	4+	1+
Erythema	3+	1+
Spontaneous petechiae	2+	R
Profuse bleeding	1+	R
Aphthous ulcer	0	4+
Serpiginous ulcer	R	4+
Deep longitudinal ulcer	0	4+
Cobblestoning	0	4+
Mucosa surrounding ulcer	Abnormal	±Normal
Pseudopolyps	2+	2+
Bridging	R	1 +
Gross Appearance		
Thickened bowel wall	0	4+
Shortening of bowel	2+	R
Fat creeping onto serosa	0	4+
Segmental involvement	0	4+
Aphthous ulcer	R	4+
Linear ulcer	0	4+
Microscopic Picture		
Depth of involvement	Mucosa and submucosa	Full thickness
Lymphoid aggregation	0	4+
Sarcoid-type granuloma	0	4+
Fissuring	0	2+
Goblet cell mucin depletion	4+	1+
Intramural sinuses	0	1+
Operative Treatment		
Total proctocolectomy	Excellent option in selected patients	Indicated in total large bowel involvement
Segmental resection	R	Frequent
Ileal pouch procedure	"Gold standard"	Contraindicated
Prognosis		
Recurrence after total proctocolectomy	0	3+
Complications		
Internal fistula	R	4+
Intestinal obstruction (stricture or infection)	0	4+
Hemorrhage	1+	1+
Sclerosing cholangitis	1+	R
Cholelithiasis	0	2+
Nephrolithiasis	0	2+

Abbreviations: R, Rare; 0, not found; 1+, may be present; 2+, common; 3+, usual finding; 4+, characteristic (not necessarily common).
Source: From Refs. 546, 547.

studies are mostly lacking, they frequently prescribe azathioprine or 6-MP in this patient population.

An enteric-coated preparation of fish oil has been shown to be effective in reducing the rate of relapse in patients with Crohn's disease in remission who are at high risk of relapse (543). Belluzzi et al. (544) performed a one-year, double-blind, placebo-controlled study to investigate the effects of a new fish oil preparation in the maintenance of remission in 78 patients with Crohn's disease who had a high risk of relapse. The patients received either nine fish oil capsules containing a total of 2.7 g of omega-3 fatty acids or nine placebo capsules daily. Among patients in the fish oil group, 28% had relapses and among the patients in the placebo group, 69% had relapses. After one year, 59% in the fish oil group remained in remission compared with 26% in the placebo group. They concluded that in patients with Crohn's disease in remission, a novel enteric-coated fish oil preparation is effective in reducing the rate of relapse. Because of minimal side effects, fish oil might be an ideal maintenance agent in Crohn's disease. However, fish oil supplementation cannot be recommended as the sole maintenance agent at present. It does, however, seem prudent to promote a diet rich in fish oil in patients with Crohn's disease.

Hirakawa et al. (545) examined the effect of an elemental diet in the maintenance of remission of 84 patients. Follow-up revealed that the cumulative continuous remission rates after one, two, and four years were 94%, 63%, and 63%, respectively, in the group receiving home elemental enteral hyperalimentation; 75%, 66%, and 66%, respectively, in the group receiving home elemental enteral hyperalimentation and drugs; 63%, 42%, and 0%, respectively, in the group receiving drugs; and 50%, 33%, and 0%, respectively, in the group receiving no maintenance therapy. The authors believe that elemental diet therapy is effective, not only for the induction of remission but also for the maintenance of remission in Crohn's disease.

REFERENCES

1. Fielding JF. Crohn's disease in London in the latter half of the nineteenth century. Ir J Med Sci 1984; 153:214–220.
2. Crohn BB, Ginzburg L, Oppenheimer GD. Regionalileitis. JAMA 1932; 99: 1323–1329.
3. Lockhart-Mummery HE, Morson BC. Crohn's disease (regional enteritis) of the large intestine and its distinction from ulcerative colitis. Gut 1960; 1:87–105.
4. Janowitz HD. Crohn's disease—50 years later. N Engl J Med 1981; 304: 1600–1602.
5. Russell MGVM, Stockbrügger RW. Epidemiology of inflammatory bowel disease: an update. Scand J Gastroenterol 1996; 31:417–427.
6. Rose JDR, Roberts GM, Mayberry JF, et al. Cardiff Crohn's jubilee: The incidence over 50 years. Gut 1988; 29:346–351.
7. Garland CF, Lilienfeld AM, Mendeloff AI, et al. Incidence rates of ulcerative colitis and Crohn's disease in fifteen areas of the United States. Gastroenterology 1981; 81:1115–1124.
8. Binder V, Both H, Hansen PK, et al. Incidence and prevalence of ulcerative colitis and Crohn's disease in the county of Copenhagen, 1962 to 1978. Gastroenterology 1982; 83:563–568.
9. Haug K, Schrumpf E, Halvorsen JF, et al. Epidemiology of Crohn's disease in Western Norway. Scand J Gastroenterol 1989; 24:1271–1275.
10. Stowe SP, Redmond SR, Stormont JM, et al. An epidemiologic study of inflammatory bowel disease in Rochester, New York. Hospital incidence. Gastroenterology 1990; 98:104–110.
11. Probert CSJ, Jayanthi V, Hughes AO, et al. Prevalence and family risk of ulcerative colitis and Crohn's disease: An epidemiologic study among Europeans and South Asians in Leicestershire. Gut 1993; 34:1547–1551.
12. Maté-Jimenez J, Munoz S, Vicent D, et al. Incidence and prevalence of ulcerative colitis and Crohn's disease in urban and rural areas of Spain from 1981 to 1988. J Clin Gastroenterol 1994; 18:27–31.
13. Odes HS, Locker C, Neumann L, et al. Epidemiology of Crohn's disease in Southern Israel. Am J Gastroenterol 1994; 89:1859–1862.
14. Tsianos EV, Masalas CN, Merkouropoulos M, et al. Incidence of inflammatory bowel disease in northwest Greece: rarity of Crohn's disease in an area where ulcerative colitis is common. Gut 1994; 35:369–372.
15. Anseline P. Crohn's disease in the Hunter Valley Region of Australia. Aust N Z J Surg 1995; 65:564–569.
16. Lindgren A, Wallerstedt S, Olsson R. Prevalence of Crohn's disease and simultaneous occurrence of extraintestinal complications and cancer. An epidemiologic study in adults. Scand J Gastroenterol 1996; 31:74–78.
17. Manousos ON, Koutroubakis I, Potamianos S, et al. A prospective epidemiologic study of Crohn's disease in Heraklion, Crete. Incidence over a 5-year period. Scand J Gastroenterol 1996; 31:599–603.
18. Moum B, Vatn MH, Ekbom A, et al. Incidence of Crohn's disease in four countries in southeastern Norway, 1990–1993. A prospective population-based study. Scand J Gastroenterol 1996; 31:355–361.
19. Tragnone A, Corrao G, Miglio F, et al. Incidence of inflammatory bowel disease in Italy: A nationwide population-based study. 1996.
20. Hanauer SB, Meyers S. Management of Crohn's disease in adults. Am J Gastroenterol 1997; 92:559–566.
21. Lapidus A, Bernell O, Hellers G, Persson PG, Lofberg R. Incidence of Crohn's disease in Stockholm county 1955–1989. Gut 1997; 41:480–486.
22. Loftus EV Jr., Silverstein MD, Sandborn WJ, Tremaine WJ, Harmsen WS, Zinsmeister AR. Crohn's disease in Olmsted County, Minnesota, 1940–1993: incidence, prevalence, and survival. Gastroenterology 1998; 114:1161–1168.
23. Yao T, Matsui T, Hiwatashi N. Crohn's disease in Japan: diagnostic criteria and epidemiology. Dis Colon Rectum 2000; 43(10 suppl):S85–S93.
24. Loftus EV Jr., Schoenfeld P, Sandborn WJ. The epidemiology and natural history of Crohn's disease in population-based patient cohorts from North America: a systematic review. Aliment Pharmacol Ther 2002; 16:51–60.
25. Sartor RB. Current theories in the etiology of Crohn's disease. Mt Sinai Newslett 1995; 2:2–6.
26. Naser SA, Ghobrial G, Romero C, Valentine JF. Culture of *mycobacterium avium* subspecies paratuberculosis from the blood of patients with Crohn's disease. Lancet 2004; 364(9439):1039–1044.
27. Sechi LA, Scanu AM, Molicotti P, et al. Detection and isolation of *mycobacterium avium* subspecies paratuberculosis from intestinal mucosal biopsies of patients with and without Crohn's disease in Sardinia. Am J Gastroenterol 2005; 100:1529–1536.
28. Koresnik JR. Past and current theories of etiology of IBD: toothpaste, worms, and refrigerators. J Clin Gastroenterol 2005; 39(4 Suppl 2):S59–S65.
29. Hugot JP, Chamaillard M, Zouali H, et al. Association of NOD2 leucine-rich repeat variants with susceptibility to Crohn's disease. Nature 2001; 411(6837):599–603.
30. Peltekova VD, Wintle RF, Rubin LA, et al. Functional variants of OCTN cation transporter genes are associated with Crohn disease. Nat Genet 2004; 36(5): 471–475.
31. Behr MA, Semret M, Poon A, Schurr E. Crohn's disease, mycobacteria, and NOD2. Lancet Infect Dis 2004(3):136–137.
32. Autschbach F, Eisold S, Hinz U, et al. High prevalence of *Mycobacterium avium* subspecies paratuberculosis IS900 DNA in gut tissues from individuals with Crohn's disease Gut 2005; 54:944–949.
33. Sartor RB. Does *mycobacterium avium* subspecies paratuberculosis cause Crohn's disease? Gut 2005; 54:896–898.
34. Wakefield AJ, Ekbom A, Dhillon AP, et al. Crohn's disease: pathogenesis and persistent measles virus infection. Gastroenterology 1995; 108:911–916.
35. Sartor RB. Current concepts of the etiology and pathogenesis of ulcerative colitis and Crohn's disease. Gastroenterol Clin North Am 1995; 24:475–507.
36. Mayberry JF. Recent epidemiology of ulcerative colitis and Crohn's disease. Int J Colored Dis 1989; 4:59–66.
37. Shohat T, Rotter J. Genetics of IBD. IBD News. National Foundation for Ileitis and Colitis. 1989; 10:4–5.
38. Cottone M, Brignola C, Rosselli M, et al. Relationship between site of disease and familial occurrence in Crohn's disease. Dig Dis Sci 1997; 41: 129–132.
39. Polito JM, Rees RC, Childs B, et al. Preliminary evidence of genetic anticipation in Crohn's disease. Lancet 1996; 347:798–800.
40. Annese V, Lombardi G, Perri F, et al. Variants of CARD15 are associated with an aggressive clinical course of Crohn's disease—an IG-IBD study. Am J Gastroenterol 2005; 100:84–92.
41. Freeman HJ. Crohn's disease defined in three elderly sisters. Can J Gastroenterol 2005; 19:251–252.
42. Freeman HJ. Familial Crohn's disease in single or multiple first-degree relatives. J Clin Gastroenterol 2002; 35:9–13.
43. Kugathasan S, Collins N, Maresso K, et al. CARD15 gene mutations and risk for early surgery in pediatric-onset Crohn's disease. Clin Gastroenterol Hepatol 2004; 2:1003–1009.
44. Helio T, Halme L, Lappalainen M, et al. CARDIS/NOD2 gene variants are associated with familially occuring and complicated forms of Crohn's disease. Gut 2003; 52:558–562.
45. Katschinski B, Fingerle D, Scherbaum B, et al. Oral contraceptive use and cigarette smoking in Crohn's disease. Dig Dis Sci 1993; 38:1596–1600.

46. Tanaka M, Riddell RH. The pathological diagnosis and differential diagnosis of Crohn's disease. Hepato-gastroenterol 1990; 37:18–31.
47. Heresbach D, Alexandre JL, Branger B, et al. ABERMAD (Association Bretonne d'Etude et de Recherche sur les Maladies de I'Appareil Digestif). Frequency and significance of granulomas in a cohort of incident cases of Crohn's disease. Gut 2005; 54:215–222.
48. Kaplan MA, Korelitz BI. Narcotic dependence in inflammatory bowel disease. J Clin Gastroenterol 1988; 10:275–278.
49. Colombel JF, Grandbostien B, Gower-Rousseau C, et al. Clinical characteristics of Crohn's disease in 72 families. Gastroenterology 1996; 111:604–607.
50. Farmer RG, Hawk WA, Turnbull RB. Clinical patterns in Crohn's disease: a statistical study of 615 cases. Gastroenterology 1975; 68:627–635.
51. Greenstein AJ. The surgery of Crohn's disease. Surg Clin North Am 1987; 67:573–596.
52. Ritchie JK. The results of surgery for large bowel Crohn's disease. Ann R Coll Surg Engl 1990; 72:155–157.
53. Platell C, Mackay J, Collopy B, et al. Anal pathology in patients with Crohn's disease. Aust N Z J Surg 1996; 66:5–9.
54. Cools D, Bosmans E. Psoas abscess. A rare complication of Crohn's disease. Acta Chir Belg 1996; 96:165–167.
55. Deveaux PG, Kimberling J, Galandiuk S. Crohn's disease: presentation and severity compared between black patients and white patients. Dis Colon Rectum 2005; 48:1404–1409.
56. Coban S, Ensari A, Kuzu MA, Yalcin S, Palabiyikoglu M, Ormeci N. Cytomegalovirus infection in a patient with Crohn's ileocolitis. J Gastroenterol 2005; 19:109–111.
57. Regueiro M. The role of endoscopy in the evaluation of fistulizing Crohn's disease. Gastrointest Endosc Clin N Am 2002; 12:621–633.
58. Otterson MF, Lundeen SJ, Spinelli KS, et al. Radiographic underestimation of small bowel stricturing Crohn's disease: a comparison with surgical findings. Surgery 2004; 136: 854–860.
59. Nelson RL. New medications for inflammatory bowel disease. Semin Colon Rectal Surg 1990; 3:168–175.
60. Li DJ, Freeman A, Miles KA, et al. Can $^{99}Tc^{m}$ HMPAO leucocyte scintigraphy distinguish between Crohn's disease and ulcerative colitis? Br J Radiol 1994; 67:472–477.
61. Kaila B, Orr K, Bernstein CN. The anti-Saccharomyces cerevisiae antibody assay in a province-wide practice: accurate in identifying cases of Crohn's disease and predicting inflammatory disease. Can J Gastroenterol 2005; 19:717–721.
62. Klebl FH, Bataille F, Hofstadter F, Herfarth H, Scholmerich J, Rogler G. Optimising the diagnostic value of anti-Saccharomyces cerevisiae-antibodies (ASCA) in Crohn's disease. Int J Colorectal Dis 2004; 19:319–324.
63. Sarvrazin J, Wilson SR. Manifestations of Crohn disease at US. Radiographics 1996; 16:499–520.
64. Parente F, Maconi G, Bollani S, et al. Bowel ultrasound in assessment of Crohn's disease and detection of related small bowel strictures: a prospective comparative study versus x ray and intraoperative findings. Gut 2002; 50:490–495.
65. Schratter-Sehn AU, Lochs H, Vogelsang H, et al. Endoscope ultrasonography versus computed tomography in the differential diagnosis of perianorectal complications in Crohn's disease. Endoscopy 1993; 35:582–586.
66. Hassan C, Cerro P, Zullo A, Spina C, Morini S. Computed tomography enteroclysis in comparison with ileoscopy in patients with Crohn's disease. Int J Colorectal Dis 2003; 18:121–125.
67. Haggett PJ, Moore NR, Shearman JD, et al. Pelvic and perineal complications of Crohn's disease: assessment using magnetic resonance imaging. Gut 1995; 36:407–410.
68. Horsthuis K, Lavini Mphill C, Stoker J. MRI in Crohn's disease. J Magn Reson Imaging 2005; 22:1–12.
69. Koh DM, Miao Y, Chinn RJ, et al. MR imaging evaluation of the activity of Crohn's disease. AJR Am J Roentgenol 2001; 177:1325–1332.
70. Legnani P, Kornbluth A. Video capsule endoscopy in inflammatory bowel disease 2005. Curr Opin Gastroenterol 2005; 21:438–442.
71. Dubcenco E, Jeejeebhoy KN, Petroniene R, et al. Capsule endoscopy findings in patients with established and suspected small-bowel Crohn's disease: correlation with radiologic, endoscopic, and histologic findings. Gastrointest Endosc 2005; 62:538–544.
72. Biancone L, Fiori R, Tosti C, et al. Virtual colonoscopy compared with conventional colonoscopy for stricturing postoperative recurrence in Crohn's disease. Inflamm Bowel Dis 2003; 9:343–350.
73. Ilnyckyj A, Greenberg H, Bernstein CN. Escherichia coli 0157:H7 infection mimicking Crohn's disease. Gastroenterology 1997; 112:995–999.
74. Freeman HJ. Temporal and geographic evolution of longstanding Crohn's disease over more than 50 years. Can J Gastroenterol 2003; 17:696–700.
75. Zang L, Anderson FH. Seasonal change in the exacerbations of Crohn's disease. Scand J Gastroenterol 1996; 31:79–82.
76. Sachar DB. Maintenance strategies in Crohn's disease. Hosp Pract 1996; 15: 99–106.
77. Stark ME, Tremaine WJ. Maintenance of symptomatic remission in patients with Crohn's disease. Mayo Clin Proc 1993; 68:1183–1190.
78. Makowiec F, Schmidtke C, Paczalla D, et al. Progression and prognosis of Crohn's colitis. Zeitschrift fur Gastroenterologic 1997; 35:7–14.
79. Agrez MV, Valente RM, Pierce N, et al. Surgical history of Crohn's disease in a well-defined population. Mayo Clin Proc 1982; 57:747–752.
80. Munkholm P, Langholz E, Davidson M, et al. Disease activity courses in a regional cohort of Crohn's disease patients. Scand J Gastroenterol 1995; 30:699–706.
81. Mendelsohn RR, Korelitz BI, Gleim GW. Death from Crohn's disease. Lessons from a personal experience. J Clin Gastroenterol 1995; 20:22–26.
82. Cottone M, Magliocco A, Rosselli M, et al. Mortality in patients with Crohn's disease. Scand J Gastroenterol 1996; 31:372–375.
83. Goldberg PA, Wright JP, Gerber M, et al. Incidence of surgical resection for Crohn's disease. Dis Colon Rectum 1993; 36:736–739.
84. Glotzer DJ. Surgical therapy for Crohn's disease. Gastroenterol Clin North Am 1995; 24:577–596.
85. Polito JM, Childs B, Mellits ED, et al. Crohn's disease: Influence of age and diagnosis on site and clinical type of disease. Gastroenterology 1996; 111: 580–586.
86. Iida M, Yaov T, Okada M. Long-term follow-up study of Crohn's disease in Japan. The Research Committee of Inflammatory Bowel Disease in Japan. J Gastroenterol 1995; 30(suppl 8):17–19.
87. Sedgwick M, Barton R, Hamer-Hodges W, et al. Population based study of surgery in juvenile onset Crohn's disease. Br J Surg 1991; 78:171–175.
88. Nwokolo CU, Tan WC, Andrews HA, et al. Surgical resections in parous patients with distal ileal and colonic Crohn's disease. Gut 1994; 35: 220–223.
89. Roberts PL, Schoetz DJ Jr., Pricolo R, et al. Clinical course of Crohn's disease in older patients: A retrospective study. Dis Colon Rectum 1990; 33:458–462.
90. Lapidus A, Bernell O, Hellers G, Lofberg R. Clinical course of colorectal Crohn's disease: a 35-year follow-up study of 507 patients. Gastroenterology 1998; 114:1151–1160.
91. Sachar DB, Subramani K, Mauer K, et al. Patterns of postoperative recurrence in fistulizing and stenotic Crohn's disease, a retrospective cohort study of 71 patients. J Clin Gastroenterol 1996; 22(2):114–116.
92. Schwartz DA, Loftus EV Jr., Tremaine WJ, et al. The natural history of fistulizing Crohn's disease in Olmsted County Minnesota. Gastroenterology 2002; 122:875–80.
93. Louis E, Michel V, Hugot JP, et al. Early development of stricturing or penetrating pattern in Crohn's disease is influenced by disease location, number of flares, and smoking but not by NOD2/CARD15 genotype. Gut 2003; 52:552–557.
94. Freeman HJ. Long-term prognosis of early-onset Crohn's disease diagnosed in childhood or adolescence. Can J Gastroenterol 2004; 18:661–665.
95. Allez M, Lemann M, Bonnet J, Cattan P, Jian R, Modigliani R. Long term outcome of patients with active Crohn's disease exhibiting extensive and deep ulcerations at colonoscopy. Am J Gastroenterol 2002; 97:947–953.
96. Gasche C, Scholmerich J, Brynskov J, et al. A simple classification of Crohn's disease: report of the Working Party for the World Congress of Gastroenterology, Vienna 1998. Inflamm Bowel Dis 2000; 6(1):8–15.
97. Freeman HJ. Application of the Vienna Classification for Crohn's disease to a single clinician database of 877 patients. Can J Gastroenterol 2001; 15:89–93.
98. Freeman HJ. Age-dependent phenotypic clinical expression of Crohn's disease. Clin Gastroenterol 2005; 39:774–777.
99. Freeman HJ. Natural history and clinical behavior of Crohn's disease extending beyond two decades. J Clin Gastroenterol 2003; 37:216–219.
100. Cosnes J, Cattan S, Blain a, Beaugerie L, Carbonnel F, Pare R, Gendre, JP. Long-term evolution of disease behavior of Crohn's disease. Inflamm Bowel Dis 2002; 8:244–250.
101. Louis E, Collard A, Oger AF, Degroote E, Aboul Nasr El Yafi FA, Belaiche J. Behaviour of Crohn's disease according to the Vienna classification: changing pattern over the course of the disease. Gut 2001; 49:777–82.
102. Veloso FT, Ferreira JT, Barros L, Almeida S. Clinical outcome of Crohn's disease: analysis according to the Vienna classification and clinical activity. Inflamm Bowel Dis 2001; 7:306–313.
103. Singleton JW, Summers RW, Kern F Jr., et al. A trial of sulfasalazine as adjunctive therapy in Crohn's disease. Gastroenterology 1979; 77:887–897.
104. Barnett JL. Medical management of colorectal Crohn's disease. Current opinion. Gastroenterology 1996; 12:26–31.
105. Singleton JW, Hanauer SB, Gutnick GL, et al. Mesalamine capsules for the treatment of active Crohn's disease: results of a 16-week trial. Gastroenterology 1993; 104:1293–1301.
106. Tremaine WJ, Schroeder KW, Harrison JM, et al. A randomized, double-blind, placebo-controlled trial of the oral mesalamine (5-ASA) preparation, Asacol, in the treatment of symptomatic Crohn's colitis and ileocolitis. J Clin Gastroenterol 1994; 19:278–282.
107. Sartor RB. Therapeutic manipulation of the enteric microflora in inflammatory bowel diseases: antibiotics, probiotics, and prebiotics. Gastroenterology 2004; 126:1620–1633.
108. Prantera C, Zannoni F, Schribano ML, et al. An antibiotic regimen for the treatment of active Crohn's disease: a randomized, controlled trial of metronidazole plus ciprofloxacin. Am J Gastroenterol 1996; 91:328–332.
109. Summers RW, Switz DM, Sessions JT Jr., et al. National cooperative Crohn's disease study: results of drug treatment. Gastroenterology 1979; 77:847–869.

110. Greenberg GR, Feagan BG, Martin F, et al. The Canadian inflammatory bowel disease study group: oral budesonide for active Crohn's disease. N Engl J Med 1994; 331:836–841.
111. Rutgeerts P, Lofberg R, Malchow H, et al. A comparison of budesonide with prednisolone for active Crohn's disease. N Engl J Med 1994; 331:842–845.
112. Fedorak RN, Bistritz L. Targeted delivery, safety, and efficacy of oral enteric-coated formulations of budesonide. Adv Drug Deliv Rev 2005; 57:303–316.
113. Kane SV, Schoenfeld P, Sandborn WJ, Tremaine W, Hofer T, Feagan BG. The effectiveness of budesonide therapy for Crohn's disease. Aliment Pharmacol Ther 2002; 16(8):1509–1517.
114. Akerkar GA, Peppercorn MA, Hamel MB, et al. Corticosteroid-associated complications in elderly Crohn's disease patients. Am J Gastroenterol 1997; 92:461–464.
115. Present DH, Korelitz BI, Wisch N, et al. Treatment of Crohn's disease with 6-Mercaptopurine. A long-term, randomized, double-blind study. N Engl J Med 1980; 302:981–987.
116. Markowitz J, Rosa J, Grancher K, et al. Long-term 6-Mercaptopurine treatment in adolescents with Crohn's disease. Gastroenterology 1990; 99:1347–1351.
117. O'Brien J, Bayless T. Immunosuppressive agents in the treatment of Crohn's disease including ileitis and ileocolitis (abstract). Gastroenterology 1989; 96:A370.
118. Present DH. 6-Mercaptopurine and other immunosuppressive agents in the treatment of Crohn's disease and ulcerative colitis. Gastroenterol Clin North Am 1989; 18:57–71.
119. Korelitz BI, Adler DJ, Mendelsohn RA, et al. Long-term experience with 6-mercaptopurine in the treatment of Crohn's disease. Am J Gastroenterol 1993; 88:1198–1205.
120. D'Haens G, Geboes K, Ponette E, et al. Healing of severe recurrent ileitis with azathioprine therapy in patients with Crohn's disease. Gastroenterology 1997; 112:1475–1481.
121. Pearson DC, May GR, Fick GH, et al. Azathioprine and 6-mercaptopurine in Crohn's disease: a meta-analysis. Am Int Med 1995; 122:132–142.
122. Present DH. Current concepts in treating inflammatory bowel disease with immunosuppressive agents. IBD News. National Foundation for Ileitis and Colitis 1985; 6:1–3.
123. Lemann M, Chamiot-Prieuo C, Mesnard B, et al. Methotrexate for the treatment of refractory Crohn's disease. Alment Pharmacial Ther 1996; 10:309–314.
124. Lemann M, Zenjari T, Bouhnik Y, et al. Methotrexate in Crohn's disease: long-term efficacy and toxicity. Am J Gastroenterol 2000; 95:1730–1734.
125. Feagan BG, Rochon J, Fedorak RN, et al. Methotrexate for the treatment of Crohn's disease. N Engl J Med 1995; 332:292–297.
126. Alfadhli AA, McDonald JW, Feagan BG. Methotrexate for induction of remission in refractory Crohn's disease. Cochrane Database Syst Rev 2005; Jan 25(1):CD003459.
127. Stange EF, Modigliani R, Pena AS, et al. European Trial of cyclosporine in chronic active Crohn's disease: a 12-month study. Gastroenterology 1995; 109:774–782.
128. Santos JV, Baudet JA, Casellas FJ, et al. Intravenous cyclosporin for steroid-refractory attacks of Crohn's disease. Short- and long-term results. J Clin Gastroenterol 1995; 20:207–210.
129. Sandborn WJ, Tremaine WJ, Lawson GM. Clinical response does not correlate with intestinal or blood cyclosporine concentrations in patients with Crohn's disease treated with high dose oral cyclosporine. Am J Gastroenterol 1996; 91:37–43.
130. McDonald JW, Feagan BG, Jewell D, Brynskov J, Stange EF, Macdonald JK. Cyclosporine for induction of remission in Crohn's disease. Database Syst Rev 2005; Apr 18(2):CD000297.
131. Ierardi E, Principi M. Francavilla R, et al. Oral tacrolimus long-term therapy in patients with Crohn's disease and steroid resistance. Aliment Pharmacol Ther 2001; 15:371–377.
132. Cosnes J, Nion-Larmurier I, Beaugerie L, Afchain P, Tiret E, Gendre JP. Impact of the increasing use of immunosuppressants in Crohn's disease on the need for intestinal surgery. 2005; 54:237–241.
133. Wenzl HH, Reinisch W, Jahnel J, Stockenhuber F, Tilg H, Krichgatterer A, Petritsch W. Austrian infliximab experience in Crohn's disease: a nationwide cooperative study with long-term follow-up. Eur J Gastroenterol Hepatol 2004; 16:767–773.
134. Miehsler W, Reinisch W, Kazemi-Shirazi L, et al. Infliximab: lack of efficacy on perforating complications in Crohn's disease. Inflamm Bowel Dis 2004; 10(1):36–40.
135. Poritz LS, Rowe WA, Koltun WA. Remicade does not abolish the need for sugery in fistulizing Crohn's disease. Dis Colon Rectum 2002; 45(6):771–775.
136. Mendoza JL, Garcia-Paredes J, Cruz Santamaria DM, et al. Infliximab treatment and prognostic factors for response in patients with Crohn's disease. Rev Esp Enferm Dig 2002; 94:269–279.
137. Panaccione R. Canadian Consencus Group on the use of infliximab in Crohn's disease. Infliximab for the treatment of Crohn's disease: review and indications for clinical use in Canada Can J Gastroenterol 2001; 15:371–375.
138. Egan LJ, Sandborn WJ. Advances in the treatment of Crohn's disease. Gastroenterol 2004; 126:1574–1581.
139. Grange F, Djilali-Bouzina F, Weiss AM, Polette A, Guillaime JC. Corticosteriod-resistant pyoderma gangrenousm associated with Crohn's disease: rapid cure with infliximab. Dermatology 2002; 205:278–280.
140. Panaccione R, Fedorak RN, Aumais G, et al. Canadian Association of Gastroenterology. Canadian Association of Gastroenterology Clinical Practice Guidelines: the use of infliximab in Crohn's Disease. Can J Gastroenterol 2004; 18(8):503–508.
141. Akobeng AK, Zachos M. Tumor necrosis factor-alpha antibody for induction of remission in Crohn's disease. Cochrane Database Syst Rev 2004; 1:CD003574.
142. van der Hagen SJ, Baeten CG, Soeters PB, Russel MG, Beets-Tan RG, van Gemert WG. Anti-TNF-alpha (infliximab) used as induction treatment in case of active proctitis in a multistep strategy followed by definitive surgery of complex anal fistulas in Crohn's disease: a preliminary report. Dis Colon Rectum 2005; 48:758–767.
143. Poggioli G, Laureti S, Pierangeli F, et al. Local injection of Infliximab for the treatment of perianal Crohn's disease. Dis Colon Rectum 2005; 48:768–774.
144. Rubenstein JH, Chong RY, Cohen RD. Infliximab decreases resource use among patients with Crohn's disease. J Clin Gastroenterol 2002; 35:151–156.
145. Colombel Jf, Loftus EV Jr., Tremaine WJ, et al. The safety profile of inflixamab in patients with Crohn's disease: the Mayo clinic experience in 500 patients. Gastroenterology 2004; 126:19–31.
146. Nicholson T, Orangio GR, Brandenburg D, Wolf DC, Pennington EE. Crohn's colitis presenting with node-negative colon cancer and liver metastasis after therapy with infliximab: report of two cases. Dis Colon Rectum 2005; 48:1651–1655.
147. Williams G, Khan AA, Schweiger F. Listeria meningitis complicating infliximab treatment for Crohn's disease. Can J Infect Dis Med Microbiol 2005; 16:289–292.
148. Singh SM, Rau NV, Cohen LB, Harris H. Cutaneous nocardiosis complicating management of Crohn's disease with infliximab and prednisone. CMAJ 2004; 171:1063–1064.
149. Freeman HJ, Flak B. Demyelination-like syndrome in Crohn's disease after infliximab therapy. Can J Gastroenterol 2005; 19:313–316.
150. Scheinfeld N. A comprehensive review and evaluation of the side effects of the tumor necrosis factor alpha blockers etanercept, infliximab and adalimumab. J Dermatolog Treat 2004; 15:280–294.
151. Phelan C, Wooltorton E. Infliximab and serious hematologic events. CMAJ 2004; 171:1045.
152. http://www.fda.gov/medwatch/SAFETY/2004/safety04.htm.
153. Colombel JF, Loftus EV Jr., Tremaine WJ et al. Early postoperative complications are not increased in patients with Crohn's disease treated perioperatively with infliximab or immunosuppressive therapy. Am J Gastroenterol 2004; 99:878–883.
154. Marchal L, D'Haens G, Van Assche G, et al. The risk of post-operative complications associated with infliximab therapy for Crohn's disease: a controlled cohort study. Aliment Pharmacol Ther 2004; 19(7):749–754.
155. Schreiber S, Rutgeerts P, Fedorak RN, et al. CDP870 Crohn's Disease Study Group. A randomized, placebo-controlled trial of certolizumab pegol (CDP870) for treatment of Crohn's disease. Gastrenterology. 2005; 129:807–818.
156. Sanborn WJ, Colombel JF, Enns R, et al. International Efficacy of Natalizumab as Active Crohn's Therapy (ENACT-1) Trial Group; Evaluation of Natalizumab as Continuous Therapy (ENACT-2) Trial Group. Natalizumab induction and maintenance therapy for Crohn's disease. N Engl J Med 2005; 353:1912–125.
157. Cross RK, Wilson KT, Binion DG. Narcotic use in patients with Crohn's disease. Am J Gastroenterol 2005; 100:2225–2229.
158. Stokes MA. Crohn's disease and nutrition. Br J Surg 1992; 79:391–394.
159. Bernstein CN, Shanahan F. Critical appraisal of enteral nutrition as primary therapy in adults with Crohn's disease. J Gastroenterol 1996; 91:2075–2079.
160. Griffiths AM, Ohlsson A, Sherman PM, et al. Meta-analysis of enteral nutrition as a primary treatment of active Crohn's disease. Gastroenterology 1995; 108:1056–1067.
161. Wu S, Craig RM. Intense nutritional support in inflammatory bowel disease. Dig Dis Sci 1995; 40:843–852.
162. Evans JP, Steinhart AH, Cohen Z, McLeod RS. Home total parenteral nutrition: an alternative to early surgery for complicated inflammatory bowel disease. J Gastrointest Surg 2003; 7:562–566.
163. Yamamoto T, Keighley MR. Smoking and disease recurrence after operation for Crohn's disease. Br J Surg 2000; 87:398–404.
164. Ryan WR, Allan RN, Yamamoto T, Keighley MR. Crohn's disease patients who quit smoking have a reduced risk of reoperation for recurrence. Am J Surg 2004; 187:219–225.
165. Johnson GJ, Cosnes J, Mansfield JC. Review article: smoking cessation as primary therapy to modify the course of Crohn's disease. Aliment Pharmacol Ther 2005; 21:921–931.
166. Prantera C, Scribano ML. Probiotics and Crohn's disease. Dig Liver Dis 2002; 34(suppl 2):S66–S67.
167. Tamboli CP, Caucheteux C, Cortot A, Colombel JF, Desreumaux P. Probiotics in inflammatory bowel disease: a critical review. Best Pract Res clin Gastroenterol 2003; 17:805–820.

168. Bebb JR, Scott BB. How effective are the usual treatments for Crohn's disease? Aliment Pharmacol Ther 2004; 20:151–159.
169. Kamm MA. Review article: chronic active disease and maintaining remission in Crohn's disease. Aliment Pharmacol Ther 2004; 20(suppl 4):102–105.
170. Ekelund GR, Lindhagen T. Controversies in the surgical management of Crohn's disease. Perspect Colon Rectal Surg 1989; 2:1–18.
171. Hulten L. Surgical treatment of Crohn's disease of the small bowel or ileocecum. World J Surg 1988; 12:180–185.
172. Edna TH, Bjerkeset T, Skreden K. Abdominal sugery for Crohn's disease during 30 years in Middle Norway. Hepatogastroenterology 2004; 51: 481–484.
173. Sands BE, Arsenault JE, Rosen MJ, et al. Risk of early surgery for Crohn's disease: implications for early treatment strategies. Am J Gastroenterol 2003; 98:2712–2718.
174. Scott NA, Hughes LE. Timing of ileocolonic resection for symptomatic Crohn's disease—The patient's view. Gut 1994; 35:656–657.
175. Lavy A. Triamcinolene improves outcome in Crohn's disease strictures. Dis Colon Rectum 1997; 40:184–186.
176. Yuan JG, Sachar DB, Koganei K, et al. Enterolithiasis, refractory anemia, and strictures of Crohn's disease. J Clin Gastroenterol 1994; 18:105–108.
177. Khare DK, Bansal R, Doraisamy S, Gupta S. Crohn's disease presenting as enterolithic intestinal obstruction. Am J Surg 2004; 187:408–409.
178. Procaccino JA, Lavery IC, Fazio VW, et al. Psoas abscess: difficulties encountered. Dis Colon Rectum 1991; 34:784–789.
179. Garcia JC, Persky SE, Bonis PA, Topazian M. Abscesses in Crohn's disease: outcome of medical versus surgical treatment. J Clin Gastroenterol 2001; 32:409–412.
180. Yamaguchi A, Matsui T, Sakurai T, et al. The clinical characteristics and outcome of intraabdominal abscess in Crohn's disease. J Gastroenterol 2004; 39:441–448.
181. McNamara MJ, Fazio VW, Lavery IC, et al. Surgical treatment of enterovesical fistulas in Crohn's disease. Dis Colon Rectum 1990; 33:271–276.
182. Greenstein AJ, Present DH, Sachar DB, et al. Gastric fistulas in Crohn's disease. Report of cases. Dis Colon Rectum 1989; 32:888–892.
183. Sachar DB, Bodian CA, Goldstein ES, et al. Task Force on Clinical Phenotyping of the IOIBD. Is perianal Crohn's disease associated with intestinal fistulization? Am J Gastroenterol 2005; 100:1547–1549.
184. Lavy A, Yasin K. Octreotide for enterocutaneous fistulas of Crohn's disease. Can J Gastroenterol 2003; 17:555–558.
185. Solem CA, Loftus EV Jr., Tremaine WJ, Pemberton JH, Wolff BG, Sandborn WJ. Fistulas to the urinary system in Crohn's disease: clinical features and outcomes. Am J Gastroenterol 2002; 97:2300–2305.
186. Ikeuchi H, Shoji Y, Yamamura T. Management of fistulas in Crohn's disease. Dig Surg 2002; 19:36–39.
187. Khanna MP, Gordon PH. Gastrocolic fistulization in Crohn's disease: a case report and a review of the literature. Can J Surg 2000; 43:53–56.
188. Greenstein AJ, Present DH, Sachar DB, et al. Gastric fistulas in Crohn's disease. Report of cases. Dis Colon Rectum 1989; 32(10):888–892.
189. Hill GL, Bourchier RG, Witney GB. Surgical and metabolic management of patients with external fistulas of the small intestine associated with Crohn's disease. World J Surg 1988; 12:191–197.
190. Portiz LS, Gagliano GA, Mcleod RS, MacRae H, Cohen Z. Surgical management of entero and colocutaneous fistulae in Crohn's disease: 17 years experience. Int J Colorectal Dis 2004; 19:481–485.
191. Olsen S, Gilbert J. Cytomegalovirus infection in Crohn's colitis. J R Soc Med 2004; 97:335–336.
192. Mowatt JI, Burnstein MJ. Free perforation of small bowel Crohn's disease: A case report and review. Can J Gastroenterol 1993; 7:300–302.
193. Softley A, Clamp SE, Bouchier IAD, et al. Perforation of the intestine in inflammatory bowel disease. An OMGE survey. Scand J Gastroenterol 1988; 23(suppl 144):24–26.
194. Bundred NJ, Dixon JM, Lumsden AB, et al. Free perforation in Crohn's colitis. A ten-year review. Dis Colon Rectum 1985; 28:35–37.
195. Greenstein AJ, Mann D, Sachar DB, et al. Free perforation in Crohn's disease. I. A survey of 99 cases. Am J Gastroenterol 1985; 80: 682–689.
196. Veroux M, Angriman I, Ruffolo C, et al. A rare surgical complication of Crohn's disease: free peritoneal perforation. Minerva Chir 2003; 58: 351–354.
197. Werbin N, Haddad R, Greenberg R, Karin E, Skornick Y. Free perforation in Crohn's disease. Isr Med Assoc J 2003; 5:175–177.
198. Ikeuchi H, Yamamura T. Free perforation in Crohn's disease: review of the Japanese literature. J Gastroenterol 2002; 37:1020–1027.
199. Freeman HJ. Spontaneous free perforation of the small intestine in Crohn's disease. Can J Gastroenterol 2002; 16:23–27.
200. Renison DM, Forouhar FA, Levine JB, et al. Filiform polyposis of the colon presenting as massive hemorrhage. An uncommon complication of Crohn's disease. Am J Gastroenterol 1983; 78:413–416.
201. Cirocco WC, Reilly JC, Rusin LC. Life-threatening hemorrhage and exsanguination from Crohn's disease: report of four cases. Dis Colon Rectum 1995; 38:85–95.
202. Kostka R, Lukas M. Massive, life-threatening bleeding in Crohn's disease. Chir Belg 2005; 105:168–174.
203. Veroux M, Angriman I, Ruffol C, et al. Severe gastrointestinal bleeding in Crohn's disease. Ann Ital Chir 2003; 74(2):213–215.
204. Belaiche J, Louis E, D'Haens G, et al. Acute lower gastrointestinal bleeding in Crohn's disease: characteristics of a unique series of 34 patients. Belgian IBD Research Group. Am J Gastroenterol 1999; 94(8):2177–2181.
205. Remzi FH, Dietz DW, Unal E, Levitin A, Sands MJ, Fazio VW. Combined use of preoperative provocative angiography and highly selective methylene blue injection to localize an occult samll-bowel bleeding site in a patient with Crohn's disease: report of a case. Dis Colon Rectum 2003; 46:260–263.
206. Savoca PE, Ballantyne GH, Cahow CE. Gastrointestinal malignancies in Crohn's disease. A 20-year experience. Dis Colon Rectum 1990; 33:7–11.
207. Fazio VW, Wu JS. Surgical therapy for Crohn's disease of the colon and rectum. Surg Clin North Am 1997; 77:197–210.
208. Weston LA, Roberts PL, Schoetz DJ Jr., et al. Ileocolic resection for acute presentation of Crohn's disease of the ileum. Dis Colon Rectum 1996; 39: 841–846.
209. Anderson J, Kehlet H. Fast track open ileo-colic resections for Crohn's disease. Colorectal Dis 2005; 7:394–397.
210. Resegotti A, Astegiano M, Farina EC, et al. Side-to-side stapled anastomosis strongly reduces anastomotic leak rates in Crohn's disease surgery. Colon Rectum 2005; 48:464–468.
211. Goligher JC. Surgical treatment of Crohn's disease affecting mainly or entirely the large bowel. World J Surg 1988; 12:186–190.
212. Goligher JC. The long-term results of excisional surgery for primary and recurrent Crohn's disease of the large bowel. Dis Colon Rectum 1985; 28: 51–55.
213. Scammell BE, Andrews H, Allan RN, et al. Results of proctocolectomy for Crohn's disease. Br J Surg 1987; 74:671–674.
214. Hyman NH, Cataldo P, Osler T. Urgent subtotal colectomy for severe inflammatory bowel disease. Dis Colon Rectum 2005; 48:70–73.
215. Poppen B, Svenberg T, Bark T. Perineal excision of the rectum. Br J Surg 1996; 83:366–367.
216. Guillem JG, Roberts PL, Murray JJ, et al. Factors predictive of persistent or recurrent Crohn's disease in excluded rectal segments. Dis Colon Rectum 1992; 35:768–772.
217. Lock MR, Fazio VW, Farmer RG, et al. Proximal recurrence and the fate of the rectum following excisional surgery for Crohn's disease of the large bowel. Ann Surg 1981; 194:754–760.
218. Harling H, Hegnhoj J, Rasmussen TN, et al. Fate of the rectum after colectomy and ileostomy for Crohn's colitis. Dis Colon Rectum 1991; 34:931–935.
219. Cirincione E, Gorfine SR, Bauer JJ. Is Hartmann's procedure safe in Crohn's disease? Report of three cases. Dis Colon Rectum 2000; 43:544–547.
220. Ambrose NS, Keighley MRB, Alexander-Williams J, et al. Clinical impact of colectomy and ileorectal anastomosis in the management of Crohn's disease. Gut 1984; 25:223–227.
221. Krause W, Ejerblad S, Bergman JA. Crohn's disease. A long-term study of the clinical course in 186 patients. Scand J Gastroenterol 1985; 20:516–524.
222. Chevalier JM, Jones DJ, Ratelle R, et al. Colectomy and ileorectal anastomosis in patients with Crohn's disease. Br J Surg 1994; 81:1379–1381.
223. Longo WE, Oakley JR, Lavery IC, et al. Outcome of ileorectal anastomosis for Crohn's colitis. Dis Colon Rectum 1992; 35:1066–1071.
224. Rieger N, Collopy B, Fink R, Mackay J, Woods R, Keck J. Total colectomy for Crohn's disease. Aust N Z J Surg 1999; 69:28–30.
225. Winslet MC, Andrews H, Allan RN, et al. Fecal diversion in the management of Crohn's disease of the colon. Dis Colon Rectum 1993; 36:757–762.
226. Zelas P, Jagelman DG. Loop ileostomy in the management of Crohn's colitis in the debilitated patient. Ann Surg 1980; 191:164–168.
227. Edwards CM, George BD, Jewell DP, Warren BF, Mortensen NJ, Kettlewell MG. Role of a defunctioning stoma in the management of large bowel Crohn's disease. Br J Surg 2000; 87:1063–1066.
228. Longo WE, Ballantyne GH, Cahow E. Treatment of Crohn's colitis. Segmental or total colectomy? Arch Surg 1988; 123:588–590.
229. Sanfey H, Bayless TM, Cameron JL. Crohn's disease of the colon. Is there a role for limited resection? Am J Surg 1984; 147:38–42.
230. Stern HS, Goldberg SM, Rothenberger DA, et al. Segmental versus total colectomy for large bowel Crohn's disease. World J Surg 1984; 8:118–122.
231. Allan A, Andrews MB, Hilton CJ, et al. Segmental colonic resection is an appropriate operation for short skip lesions due to Crohn's disease in the colon. World J Surg 1989; 13:611–616.
232. Prabhakar LP, Laramee C, Nelson H, et al. Avoiding a stoma: role for segmental or abdominal colectomy in Crohn's colitis. Dis Colon Rectum 1997; 40: 71–78.
233. Polle SW, Slors JF, Weverling GJ, Gouma DJ, Hommes DW, Bemelman WA. Recurrence after segmental resection for colonic Crohn's disease. Br J Surg 2005; 92:1143–1149.
234. Andersson P, Olaison G, Hallbook O, Sjodahl R. Segmental resection or subtotal colectomy in Crohn's colitis? Dis Colon Rectum 2002; 45(1):47–53.
235. Martel P, Betton PO, Gallot D, Malafosse M. Crohn's colitis experience with segmental resections; results in a series of 84 patients. J Am Coll Surg 2002; 194:448–453.
236. Ilijevski NS, Petrovic MJ, Rabrenovic LB, et al. Duodenocolic fistula in Crohn's disease. Eur J Surg 1997; 163:223–226.

237. Young-Fadok TM, Wolff BG, Meagher A, et al. Surgical management of ileosigmoid fistulas in Crohn's disease. Dis Colon Rectum 1997; 40:558–561.
238. Saint-Marc O, Vaillant J-C, Frileux P, et al. Surgical management of ileosigmoid fistulas in Crohn's disease: role of preoperative colonoscopy. Dis Colon Rectum 1995; 38:1084–1087.
239. Yamamoto T, Keighley MR. Enterovesical fistulas complicating Crohn's disease: clinicopathological features and management. Int J Colorectal Dis 2000; 15:211–215.
240. Michelassi F, Stella M, Balestracci T, et al. Incidence, diagnosis, and treatment of enteric and colorectal fistulae in patients with Crohn's disease. Ann Surg 1993; 218:660–666.
241. Murray JJ, Schoetz DJ Jr., Nugent FW, et al. Surgical management of Crohn's disease involving the duodenum. Am J Surg 1984; 147:58–65.
242. Alexander-Williams J, Haynes IG. Conservative operations for Crohn's disease of the small bowel. World J Surg 1985; 9:945–951.
243. Katariya RN, Sood S, Rao DG, et al. Strictureplasty for tubercular stricture of the gastrointestinal tract. Br J Surg 1977; 64:496–498.
244. Lee ECG, Papaioannou N. Minimal surgery for chronic obstruction in patients with extensive or universal Crohn's disease. Ann R Coll Surg Engl 1982; 64:229–233.
245. Tjandra JJ, Fazio VW. Techniques of strictureplasty. Perspect Colon Rectal Surg 1992; 5:189–198.
246. Futami K, Arima S. Role of strictureplasty in surgical treatment of Crohn's disease. J Gastroenterol 2005; 40(suppl 16):35–39.
247. Corman ML. Colon and Rectal Surgery. 2nd ed Philadelphia: JB Lippincott, 1989:831.
248. Michelassi F, Hurst RD, Melis M, et al. Side-to-side isoperistaltic strictureplasty in extensive Crohn's disease: a prospective longitudinal study. Ann Surg 2000; 232:401–408.
249. Tonelli F, Fedi M, Paroli GM, Fazi M. Indications and results of side-to-side isoperistaltic strictureplasty in Crohn's disease. Dis Colon Rectum 2004; 47:494–501.
250. Alexander-Williams J. The technique of intestinal strictureplasty. Int J Colorect Dis 1986; 1:54–57.
251. Sharif H, Alexander-Williams J. Strictureplasty for ileo-cloic anastomic strictures in Crohn's disease. Int J Colorectol Dis 1991; 6:214–216.
252. Spencer MP, Nelson H, Wolff BG, et al. Strictureplasty for obstructive Crohn's disease: The Mayo experience. Mayo Clin Proc 1994; 69:33–36.
253. Quandalle P, Gambiez L, Colombel JF, et al. Long-term follow up of strictureplasty in Crohn's disease. Acta Gastroenterol Belg 1994; 57:314–319.
254. Baba S, Nakai K. Strictureplasty for Crohn's disease in Japan. J Gastroenterol 1995; 30(suppl 8):135–138.
255. Serra J, Cohen Z, McLeod RS. Natural history of strictureplasty in Crohn's disease: 9-year experience. Am J Surg 1995; 38:481–485.
256. Stebbing JF, Jewell DP, Kettlewell MGW, et al. Long-term results of recurrence and reoperation after strictureplasty for obstructive Crohn's disease. Br J Surg 1995; 82:1471–1474.
257. Hurst RD, Michelassi F. Strictureplasty for Crohn's disease: techniques and long-term results. World J Surg 1998; 22:359–363.
258. Yamamoto T, Keighley MR. Factors affecting the incidence of postoperative septic complications and recurrence after strictureplasty for jejunoileal Crohn's disease. Am J Surg 1999; 178:240–245.
259. Sampietro GM, Cristaldi M, Poretta T, Montecamozzo G, Danelli P, Taschieri AM. Dis Colon Rectum 2000; 17:261–267.
260. Tonelli F, Ficari F. Strictureplasty in Crohn's disease: surgical option. Dis Colon Rectum 2000; 43:920–926.
261. Dietz DW, Laureti S, Strong SA, et al. Safety and longterm efficacy of strictureplasty in 314 patients with obstructing small bowel Crohn's disease. J Am Coll Surg 2001; 192:330–337.
262. Laurent S, Detry O, Detroz B, et al. Strictureplasty in Crohn's disease: short- and long-term follow-up. Acta Chir Belg 2002; 102:253–255.
263. Nivatvongs S. Strictureplasty for Crohn's disease of small intestine. Present status in Western Countries. J Gastroenterol 1995; 30(suppl 8):139–142.
264. Tichansky D, Cagir B, Yoo E, Marcus SM, Fry RD. Strictureplasty in Crohn's disease: meta-analysis. Dis Colon Rectum 2000; 43:911–919.
265. Roy P, Kumar D. Strictureplasty. Br J Surg 2004; 91:1428–1437.
266. Sayfan J, Wilson DAL, Allan A, et al. Recurrence after strictureplasty or resection for Crohn's disease. Br J Surg 1989; 76:335–338.
267. Ozuner G, Fazio VW, Lavery FC, et al. Reoperative rates for Crohn's disease following strictureplasty. Dis Colon Rectum 1996; 39:1191–1203.
268. Ozuner G, Fazio VW. Management of gastrointestinal bleeding after strictureplasty for Crohn's disease. Dis Colon Rectum 1995; 38:297–300.
269. Yamamoto T, Keighley MR. Long-term results of strictureplasty for ileocolonic anastomotic recurrence in Crohn's disease. J Gastrointest Surg 1999; 3:555–560.
270. Yamamoto T, Bain IM, Connolly AB, Allan RN, Keighley MR. Outcome of strictureplasty for duodenal Crohn's disease. Br J Surg 1999; 86:259–262.
271. Dietz DW, Fazio VW, Laureti S, Strong SA, Hull TL, Church J, Remzi FH, Lauvery IC, Senagore AJ. Stricturplasty in diffuse Crohn's jejunoileitis: safe and durable. Dis Colon Rectum 2002; 45:764–770.
272. Broering DC, Eisenberger CF, Koch A, et al. Strictureplasty for large bowel stenosis in Crohn's disease: quality of life after surgical therapy. Int J Colorectal Dis 2001; 16: 81–87.
273. Matzke GM, Kang AS, Dozois EJ, Sandborn WJ. Mid pouch strictureplasty for Crohn's disease after ileal pouch-anal anastomosis: an alternative to pouch excision. Dis Colon Rectum 2004; 47:782–786.
274. Broering DC, Eisneberger CF, Koch A, Bloechle C, Knoefel WT, Izbicki JR. Quality of life after surgical therapy of small bowel stenosis in Crohn's disease. Dig Surg 2001; 18:124–130.
275. Jaskowiak NT, Michelassi F. Adenocarcinoma at a strictureplasty site in Crohn's disease: report of a case. Dis Colon Rectum 2001; 44:284–287.
276. Partridge SK, Hodin RA. Small bowel adenocarcinoma at a strictureplasty site in a patient with Crohn's disease: report of a case. Dis Colon Rectum 2004; 47:778–781.
277. Sahai A, Belair M, Gianfelice D, et al. Percutaneous drainage of intra-abdominal abscesses in Crohn's disease: short- and long-term outcome. Am J Gastroenterol 1997; 92:275–278.
278. Couckuyt H, Gevers AM, Coremans G, et al. Efficacy and safety of hydrostatic balloon dilatation of ileocolonic Crohn's studies: a prospective long-term analysis. Gut 1995; 36:577–580.
279. Ramboer C, Verhamme M, Dhondt E, et al. Endoscopic treatment of stenosis in recurrent Crohn's disease with balloon dilatation combined with local corticosteroid injection. Gastroenterol Endosc 1995; 42:252–255.
280. Kelly SM, Hunter JO. Endoscopic balloon dilatation of duodenal strictures in Crohn's disease. Postgrad Med J 1995; 71:623–624.
281. Singh VV, Draganov P, Valentine J. Efficacy and safety of endoscopic balloon dilation of symptomatic upper and lower gastrointestinal Crohn's disease strictures. J Clin Gastroenterol 2005; 39:284–290.
282. Bickston SJ, Foley E, Lawrence C, Rockoff T, Shaffer HA Jr., Yeaton P. Terminal ileal stricture in Crohn's disease: treatment using a metallic enteral endoprosthesis. Dis Colon Rectum 2005; 48:1081–1085.
283. Morini S, Hassan C, Lorenzetti R, et al. Long-term outcome of endoscopic pneumatic dilatation in Crohn's disease. Dig Liver Dis 2003; 35:893–897.
284. Sabate JM, Villarejo J, Bouhnik Y, et al. Hydrostatic balloon dilatation of Crohn's strictures. Aliment Pharmacol Ther 2003; 18:409–413.
285. Brooker JC, Beckett CG, Saunders BP, Benson MJ. Long-acting steroid injection after endoscopic dilation of anastomotic Crohn's strictures may improve the outcome: a retrospective case series. Endoscopy 2003; 35:333–337.
286. Dear KL, Hunter JO. Colonoscopic hydrostatic ballon dilation of Crohn's strictures. J Clin Gastroenterol 2001; 33:315–318.
287. Post S, Herfarth CH, Schumacher H, et al. Experience with ileostomy and colostomy in Crohn's disease. Br J Surg 1995; 82:1629–1633.
288. Singh B, McC Mortensen NJ, Jewell DP, George B. Perianal Crohn's disease. Br J Surg 2004; 91(7):801–814.
289. Sagar PM, Dozois RR, Wolff BG. Long-term results of ileal pouch-anal anastomosis in patients with Crohn's disease. Dis Colon Rectum 1996; 39:893–898.
290. Grobler SP, Hosie KB, Affie E, et al. Outcome of restorative proctocolectomy when the diagnosis is suggestive of Crohn's disease. Gut 1993; 34:1384–1388.
291. Brown CJ, Maclean A, Cohen Z, et al. Crohn's disease and indeterminate colitis and ileal pouch-anal anastomosis: outcomes and patterns. Dis Colon Rectum. 2005; 48(8):1542–1549.
292. Tekkis PP, Heriot AG, Smith O, Smith JJ, Windsor AC, Nicholls RJ. Long-term outcomes of restorative proctocolectomy for Crohn's disease and indeterminate colitis. Colorectal Dis 2005; 7:218–223.
293. Heriot AG, Tekkis PP, Smith JJ, Bona R, Cohen RG, Nicholls RJ. Management and outcome of pouch-vaginal fistulas following restorative proctocolectomy. Colon Rectum 2005; 48:451–458.
294. Braveman JM, Schoetz DJ Jr., Marcello PW, et al. The fate of the ileal pouch in patients developing Crohn's disease. Dis Colon Rectum 2004; 47:1613–1619.
295. Hartley JE, Fazio VW, Remzi FH, et al. Analysis of the outcome of ileal pouch-anal anastomosis in patients with Crohn's disease. Dis Colon Rectum 2004; 47:1808–1815.
296. Regimbeau JM, Panis Y, Pocard M, et al. Long-term results of ileal pouch-anal anastomosis for colorectal Crohn's disease. Dis Colon Rectum 2001; 44: 769–778.
297. Wolff BG, Beart RW Jr., Frydenberg HB, et al. The importance of disease-free margins in resections for Crohn's disease. Dis Colon Rectum 1983; 26:239–243.
298. Hamilton SR, Reese J, Pennington L, et al. The role of resection margin frozen section in the surgical management of Crohn's disease. Surg Gynecol Obstet 1985; 160:57–62.
299. Rico DJ, Manunta A, Bergamaschi R, et al. Surgical management of Crohn's disease: how much to resect? Digitale Bild-diagn 1987; 4:41–44.
300. Cooper JC, Williams NS. The influence of microscopic disease at the margin of resection on the recurrence rates in Crohn's disease. Ann R Coll Surg Engl 1986; 68:23–26.
301. Wettergren A, Christensen J. Risk of recurrence and reoperation after resection for ileocolic Crohn's disease. Scand J Gastroenterol 1991; 26:1319–1322.
302. Funayama Y, Sasaki I, Naito H, et al. Surgical results in Crohn's disease: An analysis in review of cumulative risk of recurrence and reoperation. Jpn J Gastroenterol 1991; 88:33–39.
303. Fazio VW, Marchetti F, Church JM, et al. Effect of resection margins on the recurrence of Crohn's disease in the small bowel. A randomized controlled trial. Ann Surg 1996; 224:563–573.
304. Andrews HA, Lewis P, Allan RN. Prognosis after surgery for colonic Crohn's disease. Br J Surg 1989; 76:1184–1190.

305. Tjandra JJ, Fazio VW. Surgery for Crohn's colitis. Int Surg 1992; 77:9–14.
306. Nordgren SR, Fasth SB, Oresland TO, et al. Long-term follow-up in Crohn's disease. Mortality, morbidity, and functional status. Scand J Gastroenterol 1994; 29:1122–1128.
307. Platell C, Mackay J, Callopy B, et al. Crohn's disease: A colon and rectal department experience. Aust N Z J Surg 1995; 65:570–575.
308. Leung R, Jones IT. Clinical experience with Crohn's disease. ANZ J Surg 2005; 75:471–474.
309. Fichera A, McCormack R, Rubin MA, Hurst RD, Michelassi F. Long-term outcome of surgically treated Crohn's colitis: a prospective study. Dis Colon Rectum 2005; 48:963–969.
310. Delaney CP, Kiran RP, Senagore AJ, et al. Quality of life improves within 30 days of surgery for Crohn's disease. J Am Coll Surg 2003; 196:714–721.
311. Ecker KW, Gierend M, Kreissler-Haag D, Feifel G. Reoperations at the ileostomy in Crohn's disease reflect inflammatory activity rather than surgical stoma complications alone. Int J Colorectal Dis 2001; 16:76–80.
312. Norris B, Solomon MJ, Eyers AA, West RH, Glenn DC, Morgan BP. Abdominal surgery in the older Crohn's population. Aust N Z J Surg 1999; 69:199–204.
313. Krupnick AS, Morris JB, The long-term results of resection and multiple resections in Crohn's disease. Semin Gastrointest Dis 2000; 11(1):41–51.
314. Hurst RD, Molinari M, Chung TP, Rubin M, Michelassi F. Prospective study of the features, indications, and surgical treatment in 513 consecutive patients affected by Crohn's disease. Surgery 1997; 122:661–667.
315. Tay GS, Binion DG, Eastwood D, Otterson MF. Multivariate analysis suggests improved perioperative outcome in Crohn's disease patients receiving immunomodulator therapy after segmental resection and/or strictureplasty. Surgery 2003; 134:565–572.
316. Uno H, Yao T, Matsui T, et al. Mortality and cause of death in Japanese patient with Crohn's disease. Dis Colon Rectum 2003; 46(10 suppl):S15–S21.
317. Bernell O, Lapidus A, Hellers G. Recurrence after colectomy in Crohn's colitis. Dis Colon Rectum 2001; 44:647–654.
318. Bernell O, Lapidus A, Hellers G. Risk factors for surgery and postoperative recurrence in 907 patients with primary ileocaecal Crohn's disease. Br J Surg 2000; 87:1697–1701.
319. Bernell O, Lapidus A, Hellers G. Risk factors for surgery and postoperative recurrence in Crohn's disease. Ann Surg 2000; 23:38–45.
320. Yamamoto T, Allan RN, Keighley MR. Audit of single-stage proctocolectomy for Crohn's disease: postoperative complications and recurrence. Dis Colon Rectum 2000; 43:249–256.
321. Yamamoto T, Allan RN, Keighley MR. Risk factors for intra-abdominal sepsis after surgery for Crohn's disease. Dis Colon Rectum 2000; 43:1141–1145.
322. Freeman HJ. Upper gastrointestinal tract Crohn's disease. Can J Gastroenterol 1990; 4:26–32.
323. Ficarra G, Cicchi P, Amorosi A, et al. Oral Crohn's disease and pyostomatitis vegetans. An unusual association. Oral Surg Oral Med Oral Pathol 1993; 75:220–224.
324. Clark MP, Benjamin E, Alusi G. A rare case of Crohn's disease in head and neck surgery. J Laryngol Otol 2003; 117(2):146–147.
325. Howden FM, Mills LR, Rubin JW. Crohn's disease of the esophagus. Am Surg 1994; 60:656–660.
326. D'Haens G, Rutgeerts P, Geboes K, et al. The natural history of esophageal Crohn's disease: three patterns of evaluation. Gastrointest endosc 1994; 40:296–300.
327. Decker GA, Loftus EV Jr., Pasha TM, Tremaine WJ, Sandborn WJ. Crohn's disease of the esophagus: clinical features and outcomes. Inflamm Bowel Dis 2001; 7:113–119.
328. Rudolph I, Goldstein F, DiMarino AJ Jr. Crohn's disease of the esophagus: Three cases and a literature revies. Can J Gastroenterol 2001; 15:117–122.
329. Poggioli G, Stocchi L, Laureti S, et al. Duodenal involvement of Crohn's disease. Three different clinicopathologic patterns. Dis Colon Rectum 1997; 40:179–183.
330. Nugent FW, Roy MA. Duodenal Crohn's disease: an analysis of 89 cases. Am J Gastroenterol 1989; 84:249.
331. Schoetz DJ Jr. Gastroduodenal Crohn's disease. Perspect Colon Rectal Surg 1992; 5:145–152.
332. Alcantara M, Rodrigues R, Potenciano JLM, et al. Endoscopic and bioptic findings in the upper gastrointestinal tract in patients with Crohn's disease. Endoscopy 1993; 25:282–286.
333. Michelassi F, Block GE. Surgical management of Crohn's disease. Adv Surg 1993; 26:307–322.
334. Sukhabote J, Freeman HJ. Granulomatous (Crohn's) disease of the upper gastrointestinal tract: A study of 22 patient with mucosal granulomas. Can J Gastroenterol 1993; 7:605–609.
335. Yamamoto T, Bain IM, Connolly AB, Keighley MR. Gastroduodenal fistulas in Crohn's disease: clinical features and management. Dis Colon Rectum 1998; 41:1287–1292.
336. Mottet C, Juillerat P, Gonvers JJ, et al. Treatment of gastroduodenal Crohn's disease. Digestion 2005; 71:37–40 (Epub 2005 Feb 4, 2005).
337. Tan WC, Allan RN. Diffuse jejunoileitis of Crohn's disease. Gut 1993; 34:1374.
338. Keh C, Shatari T, Yamamoto T, Menon A, Clark MA, Keighley MR. Jejunal Crohn's disease is associated with a higher postoperative recurrence rate than ileocaecal Crohn's disease. Colorectal Dis 2005; 7:366–368.
339. Freeman HJ. Long-term clinical behavior of jejunoileal involvement in Crohn's disease. Can J Gastroenterol 2005; 19:575–578.
340. Higuero T, Merle C, Thiefin G, et al. Jejunoileal Crohn's disease: a case-control study. Gastroenterol Clin Biol 2004; 28:160–166.
341. Yamamoto T, Allan RN, Keighley MR. Long-term outcome of surgical management for diffuse jejunoileal Crohn's diease. Surgery 2001; 129:96–102.
342. Prieto-Nieto et al. Crohn's disease limited to the appendix. Am J Surg 2001; 182:531–533.
343. Rankin GB, Watts HD, Clifford S, et al. National cooperative Crohn's disease study: extraintestinal manifestations and perianal complications. Gastroenterology 1979; 4:914–920.
344. Williams DR, Coller JA, Corman ML, et al. Anal complications in Crohn's disease. Dis Colon Rectum 1981; 24:22–24.
345. Hobbiss JH, Schofield PF. Management of perianal Crohn's disease. J R Soc Med 1982; 75:414–417.
346. Hughes LE, Donaldson DR, Williams JG, et al. Local depot methyl prednisolone injection for painful anal Crohn's disease. Gastroenterology 1983; 94: 709–711.
347. Markowitz J, Daum F, Aiges H, et al. Perianal disease in children and adolescents with Crohn's disease. Gastroenterology 1984; 86:829–833.
348. Lockhart-Mummery HE. Anal lesions in Crohn's disease. Br J Surg 1985; 75(suppl):S95–S96.
349. Goebell H. Perianal complications in Crohn's disease. Neth J Med 1990; 32:S47–S51.
350. Kangas E. Anal lesions complicating Crohn's disease. Ann Chir Gynecol 1991; 80:336–339.
351. Palder SB, Shandling B, Bilik R, et al. Perianal complications of pediatric Crohn's disease. J Pediatr Surg 1991; 26:513–515.
352. McKee RF, Keenan RA. Perianal Crohn's disease—Is it all bad news? Dis Colon Rectum 1996; 39:136–142..
353. Sangwan YP, Schoetz DJ Jr., Murray JJ, et al. Perianal Crohn's disease: Results of local surgical treatment. Dis Colon Rectum 1996; 39:529–535.
354. Hughes LE. Clinical classification of perianal Crohn's disease. Dis Colon Rectum 1992; 35:928–932.
355. Francois Y, Vignal J, Descos L. Outcome of perianal fistulae in Crohn's disease—value of Hughes pathogenic classification. Int J Colorectal Dis 1993; 8:39–41.
356. Irvine EJ. Usual therapy improves perianal Crohn's disease as measured by a new disease activity index. J Clin Gastroenterol 1995; 70:27–32.
357. Irvine A, Keighley MRB. Management of perianal Crohn's disease. World J Surg 1988; 12:198–202.
358. Lecomte T, Contou JF, Beaugerie L, et al. Predictive factors of response of perianal Crohn's disease to azathioprine or 6-mercaptopurine. Dis Colon Rectum 2003; 46:1469–1475.
359. Brandt LJ, Bernstein LH, Boley SJ, et al. Metronidazole therapy for perineal Crohn's disease: a follow up study. Gastroenterology 1982; 83:383–387.
360. West RL, Van der Woude CJ, Endtz HP, Hansen BE, Ouwedijk M, Boelens HA, Kusters JG, Kuipers EJ. Perianal fistulas in Crohn's disease are predominantly colonized by skin flora: implications for antibiotic treatment? Dig Dis Sci 2005; 50:1260–1263.
361. Present DH, Lichtiger S. Efficacy of cyclosporine in the treatment of fistula of Crohn's disease. Dig Dis Sci 1994; 39:374–380.
362. Rutgeerts P. Review article: treatment of perianal fistulizing Crohn's disease. Aliment Pharmacol Ther 2004; 20(suppl 4):106–110.
363. McNamara DA, Brophy S, Hyland JM. Perianal Crohn's disease and infliximab therapy. Surgeon 2004; 2:258–263.
364. Lavy A, Weisz G, Adir Y, et al. Hyperbaric oxygen for perianal Crohn's disease. J Clin Gastroenterol 1994; 19:202–205.
365. Colombel JF, Mathieu D, Bouault JM, et al. Hyperbaric oxygenation in severe perineal Crohn's disease. Dis Colon Rectum 1995, 38:609–614.
366. Yamamoto T, Allan RN, Keighley MR. Effect of fecal diversion alone on perianal Crohn's disease. World J Surg 2000; 24:1258–1262.
367. Buchmann P, Keighley MRB, Allan RN, et al. Natural history of perianal Crohn's disease. Ten-year follow-up: a plea for conservation. Am J Surg 1980: 140:642–644.
368. Jeffrey PJ, Parks AG, Ritchie JK. Treatment of hemorrhoids in patients with inflammatory bowel disease. Lancet 1977; 1:1084–1088.
369. Wolkomir AF, Luchtefeld M. Surgery for symptomatic hemorrhoids and anal fissures in Crohn's disease. Dis Colon Rectum 1993; 36:545–547.
370. Williams N, Scott NA, Watson JS, et al. Surgical management of perineal and metastatic cutaneous Crohn's disease. Br J Surg 1993; 80:1596–1598.
371. Fleshner PR, Schoetz DJ Jr., Roberts PL, et al. Anal fissure in Crohn's disease. A plea for aggressive management. Dis Colon Rectum 1995; 38:1137–1143.
372. Pritchard TJ, Schoetz DJ, Caushaj FP, et al. Strictureplasty of the small bowel in patients with Crohn's disease. An effective surgical option. Arch Surg 1990; 125:715–717.
373. Heyen F, Winslet MC, Andrews H, et al. Vaginal fistulas in Crohn's disease. Dis Colon Rectum 1989; 32:379–383.
374. Morrison JG, Gathright JB, Ray JE, et al. Results of operation for rectovaginal fistula in Crohn's disease. Dis Colon Rectum 1989; 32:497–499.
375. Scott NA, Nair A, Hughes LE. Anovaginal and rectovaginal fistula in patients with Crohn's disease. Br J Surg 1992; 79:1379–1380.

376. Jones JF, Fazio VW, Jagelman DG. The use of transanal rectal advancement flaps in the management of fistulas involving the anorectum. Dis Colon Rectum 1987; 30:919–923.
377. Sher ME, Bauer JJ, Gelernt I. Surgical repair of the rectovaginal fistulas in patients with Crohn's disease: Transvaginal approach. Dis Colon Rectum 1991; 34:641–648.
378. Cohen JL, Strieker JW, Schoetz DJ Jr., et al. Rectovaginal fistula in Crohn's disease. Dis Colon Rectum 1989; 32:825–828.
379. Keighley MRB, Allan RN. Current status and influence of operation on perianal Crohn's disease. Int J Colored Dis 1986; 1:104–107.
380. Kodner IJ, Fry RD. Inflammatory bowel disease. Clin Symp 1982; 34:27–29.
381. Wolff GB, Culp CE, Beart RW Jr., et al. Anorectal Crohn's disease: a long-term perspective. Dis Colon Rectum 1985; 28:709–711.
382. Bernard D, Morgan S, Tasse D. Selective surgical management of Crohn's disease of the anus. Can J Surg 1986; 29:318–321.
383. Van Dongen LM, Lubbers ESC. Perianal fistulas in patients with Crohn's disease. Arch Surg 1986; 121:1187–1190.
384. Radcliffe AG, Ritchie JK, Hawley PR, et al. Anovaginal and rectovaginal fistulas in Crohn's disease. Dis Colon Rectum 1988; 31:94–99.
385. Nordgren S, Fasth S, Hulten L. Anal fistulas in Crohn's disease: Incidence and outcomes of surgical treatment. Int J Colored Dis 1992; 7:214–218.
386. Halme L, Sainio AP. Factors related to frequency, type, and outcome of anal fistulas in Crohn's disease. Dis Colon Rectum 1995; 38:55–59.
387. Sugita A, Koganei K, Harada H, et al. Surgery for Crohn's anal-fistulas. J Gastroenterol 1995; 30(suppl 8):143–146.
388. Sloots CE, Felt-Bersma RJ, Poen AC, Cuesta MA, Meuwissen SG. Assessment and classification of fistula-in-ano in patient with Crohn's disease by hydrogen peroxide enhanced transanal ultrasound. Int J colorectal Dis 2001; 16:292–297.
389. Bayer I, Gordon PH. The selected operative management of fistula-in-ano in Crohn's disease. Dis Colon Rectum 1994; 37:760–765.
390. Levien DH, Surrell J, Mazier P. Surgical treatment of anorectal fistulas in patients with Crohn's disease. Surg Gynecol Obstet 1989; 169:133–136.
391. Morrison JG, Gathright JB Jr., Ray JE, et al. Surgical management of anorectal fistulas in Crohn's disease. Dis Colon Rectum 1989; 32:492–496.
392. Marks CG, Ritchie JK, Lockhart-Mummery HE. Anal fistulas in Crohn's disease. Br J Surg 1981; 68:525–527.
393. Hesterberg R, Schmidt WO, Muller F, et al. Treatment of anovaginal fistulas with an anocutaneous flap in patients with Crohn's disease. Int J Colorectal Dis 1993; 8:51–54.
394. Makowiec F, Jehle C, Becker HD, et al. Clinical course after transanal advancement flap repair of perianal fistula in patients with Crohn's disease. Br J Surg 1995; 82:602–606.
395. White RA, Eisenstat TE, Rubin RJ, et al. Seton management of complex anorectal fistulas in patients with Crohn's disease. Dis Colon Rectum 1990; 33: 587–589.
396. Koganei K, Sugita A, Harada H, et al. Seton treatment of perianal Crohn's fistulas. Jpn J Surg 1995; 35:32–36.
397. Thornton M, Solomon MJ. Long-term indwelling seton for complex anal fistulas in Crohn's disease. Colon Rectum 2005; 48:459–463.
398. Shinozaki M, Koganei K, Fukushima T. Simultaneous anus and bowel operation is preferable for anal fistula in Crohn's disease. J Gastroenterol 2002; 37:611–616.
399. Topstad DR, Panaccione R, Heine JA, Johnson DR, Maclean AR, Buie WD. Combined seton placement, infliximab infusion, and maintenance immunosuppressive improve healing rate in fistulizing anorectal Crohn's disease: a single center experience. Dis Colon Rectum 2003; 46:577–583.
400. van Bodegraven AA, Sloots CE, Felt-Bersma RJ, Meuwissen SG. Endosonographic evidence of persistence of Crohn's disease-associated fistulas after infliximab treatment, irrespective of clinical response. Dis Colon Rectum 2002; 45:39–45.
401. Hellers G, Bergstrand O, Ewerth S, et al. Occurrence and outcome after primary treatment of anal fistulae in Crohn's disease. Gut 1980; 21: 525–527.
402. Sohn N, Korelitz BI, Weinstein MA. Anorectal Crohn's disease: definitive surgery for fistulas and recurrent abscesses. Am J Surg 1980; 139:394–397.
403. Fuhrman G, Larach SW. Experience with perirectal fistulas in patients with Crohn's disease. Dis Colon Rectum 1989; 32:847–848.
404. Fry RD, Shemesh EI, Kodner IJ, et al. Techniques and results in the management of anal and perianal Crohn's disease. Surg Gynecol Obstet 1989; 168:42–48.
405. Williams JG, Rothenberger DA, Nemer FG, et al. Fistula-in-ano in Crohn's disease. Results of aggressive surgical treatment. Dis Colon Rectum 1991; 34:378–384.
406. Williamson PR, Hellinger MD, Larach SW, et al. Twenty-year review of the surgical management of perianal Crohn's disease. Dis Colon Rectum 1995; 38:389–392.
407. Scott HJ, Northover JM. Evaluation of surgery for perianal Crohn's fistulas. Dis Colon Rectum 1996; 39:1039–1043.
408. Bahadursingh AM, Longo WE. Malignant transformation of chronic perianal Crohn's fistula. Am J Surg 2005; 189:61–62.
409. Ky A, Sohn N, Weinstein MA, Korelitz BI. Carcinoma arising in anorectal fistulas of Crohn's disease. Dis Colon Rectum 1998; 41:992–996.
410. Sivarajasingham N, Adams SA, Smith ME, Hosie KB. Perianal Hodgkin's lymphoma complicating Crohn's disease. Int J Colorectal Dis 2003; 18:174–176.
411. Santoro GA, Bucci L, Frizelle FA. Management of rectourethral fistulas in Crohn's disease. Int J Colored Dis 1995; 10:183–188.
412. Fazio VW, Jones IT, Jagelman DG, et al. Rectourethral fistulas in Crohn's disease. Surg Gynecol Obstet 1987; 164:148–150.
413. Williams JG, Hughes LE. Abdominoperineal resection for severe perianal Crohn's disease. Dis Colon Rectum 1990; 33:402–407.
414. Scammell BE, Keighley MRB. Delayed perineal wound healing after proctectomy for Crohn's disease. Br J Surg 1986; 73:150–152.
415. Marchesa P, Hull TL, Fazio VW. Advancement sleeve flaps for treatment of severe perianal Crohn's disease. Br J Surg 1998; 85:1695–1698.
416. Joo JS, Weiss EG, Nogueras JJ, Wexner SD. Endorectal advancement flap in perianal Crohn's disease. Am Surg 1998; 64:147–150.
417. Michelassi F, Melis M, Rubin M. Hurst RD. Surgical treatment of anorectal complications in Crohn's disease. Surgery 2000; 128:597–603.
418. Alexander-Williams J, Buchmann P. Perianal Crohn's disease. World J Surg 1980; 4:203–208.
419. Freeman HJ. Erythema nodosum and pyoderma gangrenosum in 50 patients with Crohn's disease. Can J Gastroenterol. 2005; 19:603–606.
420. Sams HH, Kiripolsky MG, Boyd AS, King LE Jr. Crohn's disease of the penis masquerading as pyoderma gangrenosum: a case report and review of the literatrure. Cutis 2003; 72:432–437.
421. Guest GD, Fink RL. Metastatic Crohn's disease: case report of an unusual variant and review of the literature. Dis Colon Rectum 2000; 43:1764–1766.
422. Biancone L, Geboes K, Spagnoli LG, et al. Metastatic Crohn's disease of the forehead. Inflamm Bowel Dis 2002; 8(2):101–105.
423. Worcester EM. Stones from bowel disease. Endocrinol Metab Clin North Am 2002; 31:979–999.
424. Ben-Ami H, Ginesin Y, Behar DM, Fischer D, Edoute Y, Lavy A. Diagnosis and treatment of urinary tract complications in Crohn's disease: an experience over 15 years. Can J Gastroenterol 2002; 16:225–229.
425. Gumbo T, Rice TW, Mawhorter S. Recurrent pneumonia from an ileobronchial fistula complicating Crohn's disease. J Clin Gastroenterol 2001; 32:365–367.
426. Omori H, Asahi H, Inoue Y, Irinoda T, Saito K. Pulmonary involvement in Crohn's disease report of a case and review of the literature. Inflamm Bowel Dis 2004; 10:129–134.
427. Freeman HJ, Davis JE, Prest ME, Lawson EJ. Granulomatous bronchiolitis with necrobiotic pulmonary nodules in Crohn's disease. Can J Gastroenterol 2004; 18:687–690.
428. Freeman HJ, Freeman KJ. Prevalence rates and an evaluation of reported risk factors for osteonecrosis (avascular necrosis) in Crohn's disease. Can J Gastroenteroal 2000; 14:138–143.
429. Sanghavi P, Paramesh A, Dwivedi A, Markova T, Phan T. Mesenteric arterial thrombosis as a complication of Crohn's disease. Dig Dis Sci 2001; 46: 2344–2346.
430. Memon MI, Memon B, Memon MA. Hepatobiliary manifestations of inflammatory bowel disease. HPB Surg 2000; 11:363–371.
431. Retally CA, Trevino HH, Molina K, Kane SV. Crohn's disease involving the gallbladder. case report and review of the literature. Am J Gastroenterol 2003; 98:509–511.
432. Sharma AK, Nawroz IM, Evgenikos N, Daniel T. Isolated involvement of the gallbladder by Crohn's disease manifesting as acute cholecystitis. J Gastrointest Surg 2005; 9:357–359.
433. Lapidus A, Bangstad M, Astrom M, Muhrbeck O. The prevalence of gallstone disease in a defined cohort of patients with Crohn's disease. Am J Gastroenterol 1999; 94:1261–1266.
434. Chew SS, Ngo TQ, Douglas PR, Newstead GL, Selby W, Solomon MJ. Cholecystectomy in patients with Crohn's ileitis. Colon Rectum 2003; 46: 1484–1488.
435. Kreuzpaintner G, Schmidt WU, West TB, Tischendorf FW. Two large liver abscesses complicating Crohn's disease. Z Gastroenterol 2000; 38:837–840.
436. Itzkowitz SH, Yio X. Inflammation and cancer IV. Colorectal cancer in inflammatory bowel disease: the role of inflammation. Am J Physiol Gastrointest Liver Physiol 2004; 287:G7–G17.
437. Greenstein AJ. Malignancy in Crohn's disease. Perspect Colon Rectal Surg 1995; 8:137–159.
438. Greenstein AJ. Cancer in inflammatory bowel disease. Mt Sinai J Med 2000; 67:227–240.
439. Person PG, Karlen P, Bernell O, et al. Crohn's disease and cancer: A population-based cohort study. Gastroenterology 1994; 107:1675–1679.
440. Munkholm P, Langholz E, Davidson M, et al. Intestinal cancer risk and mortality in patients with Crohn's disease. Gastroenterology 1993; 105:1716–1723.
441. Shorter RG. Risk of intestinal cancer in Crohn's disease. Dis Colon Rectum 1983; 26:686–689.
442. Ekbom A, Helmick C, Zack M, et al. Increased risk of large bowel cancer in Crohn's disease with colonic involvement. Lancet 1990; 336:357–359.
443. Gillen CD, Andrews HA, Prior P, et al. Crohn's disease and colorectal cancer. Gut 1994; 35:651–656.

444. Balaji V, Thompson MR, Marley NJE, et al. Occult small bowel adenocarcinoma in a Crohn's stricture. J R Soc Med 1997; 90:45.
445. Nikias G, Eisner T, Katz S, et al. Crohn's disease and colorectal carcinoma: Rectal cancer complicating long-standing active perianal disease. Am J Gastroenterol 1995; 90:216–219.
446. Michelassi F, Testa G, Pomidor WJ, et al. Adenocarcinoma complicating Crohn's disease. Dis Colon Rectum 1993; 36:654–661.
447. Gillen CD, Walmsley RS, Prior P, et al. Ulcerative colitis and Crohn's disease: A comparison of the colorectal cancer risk in extensive colitis. Gut 1994; 35:1590–1592.
448. Choi PM, Zelig MP. Similarity of colorectal cancer in Crohn's disease and ulcerative colitis: implications for carcinogenesis and prevention. Gut 1994; 35:950–954.
449. Stahl TJ, Schoetz DJ Jr., Roberts PL, et al. Crohn's disease and carcinoma: Increasing justification for surveillance?. Dis Colon Rectum 1992; 35:850–856.
450. Ribeiro MB, Greenstein AJ, Sachar DB, et al. Colorectal adenocarcinoma in Crohn's disease. Ann Surg 1996; 223:186–193.
451. Lynch HT, Brand RE, Locker GY. Inflammatory bowel disease in Ashkenazi Jews: implications for familial colorectal cancer. Fam Cancer 2004; 3:229–232.
452. Jess T, Winther KV, Munkholm P, Langholz E, Binder V. Intestinal and extra-intestinal cancer in Crohn's disease: follow-up of a population-based cohort in Copenhagen Country, Denmark. Aliment Pharmacol Ther 2004; 19:287–293.
453. Solem CA, Harmsen WS, Zinsmeister AR, Lostus EV Jr. Small intestinal adenocarcinoma in Crohn's disease: a case-control study. Inflamm Bowel Dis 2004; 10(1):32–35.
454. Sjodahl RI, Myrelid P, Soderholm JD. Anal and rectal cancer in Crohn's disease. Colorectal Dis 2003; 5:490–495.
455. Freeman HJ. Colorectal cancer complicating Crohn's disease. Can J Gastroenterol 2001; 15:231–236.
456. Freeman HJ. Tabulation of myeloid, lymphoid and intestinal malignancies in Crohn's disease. Can J Gastroenterol 2002; 16:779–784.
457. Sigel JE, Petras RE, Lashner BA, Fazio VW, Goldblum JR. Intestinal adenocarcinoma in Crohn's disease: a report of 30 cases with a focus on coexixting dysplaisa. Am J Surg Pathol 1999; 23:651–655.
458. Bernstein CN, Shanahan F, Weinstein WM. Are we telling patients the truth about surveillance colonoscopy in ulcerative colitis? Lancet 1994; 343:71–74.
459. Eaden J. Review article: colorectal carcinoma and inflammatory bowel disease. Aliment Pharmacol Ther 2004 20(suppl 4):24–30.
460. Mpofu C, Watson AJ, Rhodes JM. Strategies for detecting colon cancer and/or dysplasia in patients with inflammatory bowel disease. Cochrane Database Syst Rev 2004; (2):CD000279.
461. Itzkowitz SH, Present DH; Crohn's and Colitis Foundation of America Colon Cancer in IBD Study Group. Consensus conference: Colorectal cancer screening and surveillance in inflammatory bowel disease. Bowel Dis 2005; 11:314–321.
462. Cheng Y, Desreumaux P. 5-aminosalicylic acid is an attractive candidate agent for chemoprevention of colon cancer in patients with inflammatory bowel disease. World J Gastroenterol 2005; 21(11):309–314.
463. Crohn BB, Korelitz BI, Yarnis H. Regional ileitis complicating pregnancy. Gastroenterology 1956; 31:615–624.
464. Goettler CE, Stellato TA. Initial presentation of Crohn's disease in pregnancy: report of a case. Dis Colon Rectum 2003; 46:406–410.
465. Miller JP. Inflammatory bowel disease in pregnancy: a review. J Roy Soc Med 1986; 79:221–225.
466. Baird DD, Narendranathan M, Sandler RS. Increased risk of preterm birth for women with inflammatory bowel disease. Gastroenterology 1990; 99: 987–994.
467. Lindhagen T, Bohe M, Ekelund G, et al. Fertility and outcome of pregnancy in patients operated on for Crohn's disease. Int J Colorectal Dis 1996; 1:25–27.
468. Woolfson K, Cohen Z, McLeod RS. Crohn's disease and pregnancy. Dis Colon Rectum 1990; 33:869–873.
469. Nielsen OH, Andreasson B, Bondesen S, et al, Pregnancy in Crohn's disease. Scand J Gastroenterol 1984; 19:724–732.
470. Rogers RG, Katz VL. Course of Crohn's disease during pregnancy and its effect on pregnancy outcome: a retrospective review. Am J Perinatal 1995; 12:262–264.
471. Bush MC, Patel S, Lapinski RH, Stone JL. Perinatal outcomes in inflammatory bowel disease. J Matern Fetal Neonatal Med 2004; 15:237–241.
472. Mottet C, Juillerat P, Gonvers JJ, et al. Pregnancy and Crohn's disease. Digestion 2005; 71:54–61 (Epub 2005 Feb 4, 2005).
473. Shoenut JP, Semelka RC, Silverman R, et al. MRI in the diagnosis of Crohn's disease in two pregnant women. J Clin Gastroenterol 1993; 17:244–247.
474. Habal FM, Hui G, Greenberg GR. Oral 5-aminosalicylic acid for inflammatory bowel disease in pregnancy: Safety and clinical course. Gastroenterology 1993; 105:1057–1060.
475. Hill J, Clark A, Scott MA. Surgical treatment of acute manifestations of Crohn's disease during pregnancy. J R Soc Med 1997; 90:64–66.
476. Whelan G, Farmer RG, Fazio VW, et al. Recurrence after surgery in Crohn's disease. Relationship to location of disease (clinical pattern) and surgical indication. Gastroenterology 1985; 88:1826–1833.
477. Sachar DB, Wolfson DM, Greenstein AJ, et al. Risk factors for postoperative recurrence of Crohn's disease. Gastroenterology 1983; 85:917–921.
478. Rutgeerts P, Geboes K, Vantrappen G, et al. Predictability of the postoperative course of Crohn's disease. Gastroenterology 1990; 99:956–963.
479. Raab Y, Bergstrom R, Ejerblad S, et al. Factors influencing recurrence in Crohn's disease: an analysis of a consecutive series of 353 patients treated with primary surgery. Dis Colon Rectum 1996; 39:918–925.
480. Aeberhard P, Berchtold W, Riedtmann H-J, et al. Surgical recurrence of perforating and nonperforating Crohn's disease: a study of 101 surgically treated patients. Dis Colon Rectum 1996; 39:80–87.
481. Anseline PF, Wlodarczyk J, Murugasu R. Presence of granulomas is associated with recurrence after surgery for Crohn's disease: experience of a surgical unit. Br J Surg 1997; 84:78–82.
482. Scott NA, Sue-Ling HM, Hughes LE. Anastomotic configuration does not affect recurrence of Crohn's disease after the ileo-colonic resection. Int J Colorectal Dis 1995; 10:67–69.
483. Scarpa M, Angriman I, Barollo M, et al. Role of stapled and hand-sewn anastomoses in recurrence of Crohn's disease. Hepatogastroenterology 2004; 51:1053–1057.
484. Ikeuchi H, Kusunoki M, Yamamura T. Long-term results of stapled and hand-sewn anastomoses in patients with Crohn's disease. Dig Surg 2000; 17:493–496.
485. Munoz-Juarez M, Yamamoto T, Wolff BG, Keighley MR. Wide-lumen stapled anastomosis vs. conventional end-to-end anastomosis in the treatment of Crohn's disease. Dis Colon Rectum 2001; 44:20–25.
486. Poggioli G, Laureti S, Seller! S, et al. Factors affecting, recurrence in Crohn's disease. Results of a prospective audit. Int J Colorectal Dis 1996; 11:294–298.
487. D'Haens GR, Gasparaitis AE, Hanauer SB. Duration of recurrent ileitis after ileocolonic resection correlates with presurgical extent of Crohn's disease. Gut 1995; 36:715–717.
488. Holzheimer RG, Molloy RG, Whittmann DH. Postoperative complications predict recurrence of Crohn's disease. Eur J Surg 1995; 161:129–135.
489. Silvis R, Steup WH, Brand A, et al. Protective effect of blood transfusion on postoperative recurrence of Crohn's disease in parous woman. Transfusion 1994; 34:242–247.
490. Klein O, Colombel JF, Lescut D, et al. Remaining small bowel endoscopic lesions at surgery have no influence on early anastomotic recurrence in Crohn's disease. Am J Gastroenterol 1995; 90:1949–1952.
491. Heimann TM, Greenstein AJ, Lewis B, et al. Prediction of early symptomatic recurrence after intestinal resection in Crohn's disease. Ann Surg 1993; 218:294–299.
492. Krause U, Ejerblad S, Bergman L. Crohn's disease. A long-term study of the clinical course in 186 patients. Scand J Gastroenterol 1985; 20:516–524.
493. Softley A, Myren J, Clamp SE, Bouchier IAD, Watkinson G, de Dombal FT. Factors affecting recurrence after surgery for Crohn's disease. Scand J Gastroenterol 1988; 23(suppl 144):31–34.
494. Raab Y, Bergstrom R, Ejerblad S, Graf W, Pahlman L. Factors influencing recurrence in Crohn's disease. An analysis of a consecutive series of 353 patients treated with primary surgery. Dis Colon Rectum 1996; 39:918–25.
495. Fazio VW, Marchetti F, Church JM, et al. Effect of resection margins on the recurrence of Crohn's disease in the small bowel. A randomized controlled trial. Ann Surg 1996; 224:563–573.
496. McLeod RS, Wolff BG, Steinhart AH, et al. Prophylactic mesalamine treatment decreases postoperative recurrence of Crohn's disease. Gastroenterology 1995; 109:404–413.
497. Wolff BG. Resection margins in Crohn's disease. Br J Surg 2001; 88:771–772.
498. Pennington L, Hamilton SR, Bayless TM, Cameron JL. Surgical management of Crohn's disease. Influence of disease at margin of resection. Ann Surg 1980; 192:311–318.
499. Wolff BG, Beart RW Jr, Frydenberg HB, Weiland LH, Agrez MW, Ilstrup DM. The importance of disease-free margins in resections for Crohn's disease. Dis Colon Rectum 1983; 26:239–243.
500. Kontanagi H, Kramer K, Fazio VW, Petras RE. Do microscopic abnormalities at resection margins correlate with increased anastomotic recurrence in Crohn's disease?. Retrospective analysis of 100 cases. Dis Colon Rectum 1991; 34:909–916.
501. Glehen O, Lifante JC, Viganl J, et al. Small bowel length in Crohn's disease. Int J Colorectal Dis 2003; 18:423–427.
502. Morpurgo E, Petras R, Kimberling J, Ziegler C, Galandiuk S. Characterization and clinical behavior of Crohn's diseases initially presenting predominantly as colitis. Dis Colon Rectum 2003; 46:918–924.
503. Scarpa M, Angriman I, Barollo M, et al. Risk factors for recurrence of stenosis in Crohn's disease. Acta Biomed Ateneo Parmense 2003; 74(suppl 2):80–83.
504. Borley NR, Mortensen NJ, Chaudry MA, et al. Recurrence after abdominal surgery for Crohn's disease: relationship to disease site and surgical procedure. Dis Colon Rectum 2002; 45:377–383.
505. Maconi G, Sampietro GM, Cristaldi M, et al. Preoperative characteristics and postoperative behavior of bowel wall on risk of recurrence after conservative surgery in Crohn's disease: a prospective study. Ann Surg 2001; 233:345–352.
506. Hofer B, Bottger T, Hernandez-Richter T, Seifert JK, Junginger T. The impact of clinical types of disease manifestation on the risk of early postoperative recurrence in Crohn's disease. Hepatogastroenterology 2001; 48:152–155.
507. Bernell O, Lapidus A, Hellers G. Risk factors for surgery and postoperative recurrence in 907 patients with primary ileocecal Crohn's disease. Br J Surg 2000; 87:1697–1701.

508. Bernell O, Lapidus A, Hellers G. Risk factors for surgery and postoperative recurrence in Crohn's disease. Ann Surg 2000; 23:38–45.
509. Timmer A, Sutherland LR, Martin F. Oral contraceptive use and smoking are risk factors for relapse in Crohn's disease. The Canadian Mesalamine for Remission of Crohn's disease Study Group. Gastroenterology 1998; 114:1143–1150.
510. Froehlich F, Juillerat P, Felley C, et al. Treatment of postoperative Crohn's disease. Digestion 2005; 71:49–53 (Epub 2005 Feb 4, 2005).
511. Yamamoto T. Factors affecting recurrence after surgery for Crohn's disease. World J Gastroenterol 2005; 11:3971–3979.
512. Feagan BG. Maintenance therapy for inflammatory bowel disease. Am J Gastroenterol 2003; 98(12 suppl):S6–S17.
513. Thomson ABR. International Mesalamine Study Group. Coated oral 5-aminosalicylic acid versus placebo in maintaining remission of inactive Crohn's disease. Aliment Pharmacol Ther 1990; 4:55–64.
514. Prantera C, Pallone F, Brunetti G, et al. Italian IBD study group. Oral 5-aminosalicylic acid (Asacol) in the maintenance treatment of Crohn's disease. Gastroenterology 1992; 103:363–368.
515. Caprilli R, Andreoli A, Capurso Z, et al. 5-ASA in the prevention of Crohn's disease postoperative recurrence: an intensive report of the Italian Study Group of the Colon (GISC)(abstract). Gastroenterology 1992; 102:A601.
516. Gendre JP, Mary SY, Florent C, et al. Oral mesalamine (Pen-tasa) as maintenance treatment in Crohn's disease: a multi center placebo-controlled study. Gastroenterology 1993; 104:435–439.
517. Fiasse R, Fontaine F, Vanheuverzwyn R. Prevention of Crohn's disease recurrences after intestinal resection with Eudraqid-L-coated 5-aminosalicylic acid: preliminary results of a one year double-blind placebo controlled study (abstract). Gastroenterology 1991; 100:A208.
518. Brignola C, Iapnone P, Pasquali S, et al. Placebo-controlled trial of oral 5-ASA in relapse prevention of Crohn's disease. Dig Dis Sci 1992; 37:29–32.
519. Florent C, Cortot A, Quandale P, et al. Placebo-controlled trial of Claversal (C) in the prevention of early endoscopic relapse after "curative" resection for Crohn's disease (CD). Gastroenterology 1992; 102:A623.
520. Messori A, Brignola C, Trallori G, et al. Effectiveness of 5-aminosalicylic acid for maintaining remission in patients with Crohn's disease: a meta analysis. Am J Gastroenterol 1994; 89:692–698.
521. McLeod RS, Wolff BG, Steinhart AH, et al. Prophylactic mesalamine treatment decreases postoperative recurrence of Crohn's disease. Gastroenterology 1995; 109:404–413.
522. Caprilli R, Cottone M, Tonelli F, et al. Two nesalazine regimens in the prevention of the post-operative recurrence of Crohn's disease: a pragmatic, double-blind, randomized controlled trial. Aliment Pharmacol Ther 2003; 17:517–523.
523. Salomon P, Kornbluth A, Aisenberg J, et al. How effective are current drugs for Crohn's disease? A meta-analysis. J Clin Gastroenterol 1992; 14:212–215.
524. Steinhart AH, Hemphill D, Greenberg GR. Sulfasalazine and mesalamine for the maintenance therapy of Crohn's disease: A meta analysis. Am J Gastroenterol 1994; 89:2116–2124.
525. Sutherland LR, Martin F, Bailey RJ, et al. A randomized placebo-controlled, double-blind trial of mesalamine in the maintenance of remission of Crohn's disease. Gastroenterology 1997; 112:1069–1077.
526. Ardizzone S, Maconi G, Sampietro GM, et al. Azathioprine and Mesalamine for prevention of relapse after conservative surgery for Crohn's disease. Gastroenterology 2004; 127:730–740.
527. Akobeng AK, Gardener E. Oral 5-aminosalicylic acid for maintenance of medically-induced remission in Crohn's Disease. Cochrane Database Syst Rev 2005; Jan 25(1):CD003715.
528. Lofberg R, Rutgeerts P, Malchow H, et al. Budesonide prolongs time to relapse in ileal and ileocecal Crohn's disease. A placebo controlled one-year study. Gut 1996; 39:82–86.
529. Rutgeerts P, Lofberg R, Malchow H, et al. A comparison of budesonide with prednisolone for active Crohn's disease. N Engl J Med 1994; 331:873–874.
530. Greenberg GR, Feagan BG, Martin F, et al. Oral budesonide as maintenance treatment for Crohn's disease: a placebo-controlled, dose-ranging study. Gastroenterology 1996; 110:45–51.
531. Sandborn WJ, Lofberg R, Feagan BG, Hanauer SB, Campieri M, Greenberg Gr. Budesonide for maintanance of remission in patients with Crohn's disease in medically induced remission: a predetermined pooled analysis of four randomized, double-blind, placebo-controlled trials. Am J Gastroenterol 2005; 100:1780–1787.
532. Steinhart AH, Ewe K, Griffiths AM, Modigliani R, Thomsen OO. Corticosteroids for maintenance of remission in Crohn's disease. Cochrane Database Syst Rev 2003; 4:CD000301.
533. Rutgeerts P, Hiele M, Geboes K, et al. Controlled trial of metronidazole treatment for prevention of Crohn's recurrence after ileal resection. Gastroenterology 1995; 108:1617–1621.
534. Bouhnik Y, Lémann M, Mary JY, et al. Long-term follow up of patients with Crohn's disease treated with azathioprine or 6-mercaptopurine. Lancet 1996; 347:215–219.
535. Hanauer SB, Feagan BG, Lichtenstein GR, et al. ACCENT I Study Group. Maintenance infliximab for Crohn's disease: the ACCENT I randomised trial. Lancet 2002; 359(9317):1541–1549.
536. Sands BE, Anderson FH, Bernstein CN, et al. Infliximab maintenance therapy for fistulizing Crohn's disease. N Eng J Med 2004; 350:876–885.
537. Hanauer SB. Infliximab: lifetime use for maintenance is appropriate in Crohn's Disease. A balancing View: lifetime channelling of infliximab for Crohn's disease. Am J Gastroenterol 2005; 100:1438–1439.
538. Rutgeerts P, D'Haens G, Targan S, et al. Efficacy and safety of retreatment with anti-tumor necrosis factor antibody (infliximab) to maintain remission in Crohn's disease. Gastroenterology 1999; 117:761–769.
539. Treton X, Bouhnik Y, Mary JY, et al. Azathioprine withdrawal in patients with Crohn's disease maintained on prolonged remission under treatment is associated with a high risk of relapse. Gastroenterology 2004; 126(Suppl 2):A113.
540. Borgaonkar M, MacIntosh D, Fardy J, Simms L. Anti-tuberculous therapy for maintaing remission of Crohn's disease. Cochrane Database Syst Rev 2000; 2:CD000299.
541. Rutgeerts P. Strategies in the prevention of post-operative recurrence in Crohn's disease. Best Pract Res Clin Gastroenterol 2003; 17:63–73.
542. Bernstein M, Irwin S, Greenberg GR. Maintenance infliximab treatment is associated with improved bone improved bone mineral density in Crohn's disease. Am J Gastroenterol 2005; 100:2031–2035.
543. Kim Y. Can fish oil maintain Crohn's disease in remission? Nutr Rev 1996; 54:248–252.
544. Belluzzi A, Brignola C, Campieri M, et al. Effect of an enteric-coated fish-oil preparation on relapses in Crohn's disease. N Engl J Med 1996; 334: 1557–1560.
545. Hirakawa H, Fukuda Y, Tanida N, et al. Home elemental enteral hyper-alimentation (HEEH) for the maintenance of remission in patients with Crohn's disease. Gastroenterol Japanica 1993; 28:379–384.
546. Nivatvongs S. The colon, rectum, and anal canal. In James EC, Corry RJ, Perry JF Jr., eds. Basic Surgical Practice. Philadelphia: Hanley & Belfus, 1987:p. 325.
547. Ogorek CP, Fisher RS. Differentiation between Crohn's disease and ulcerative colitis. Med Clin North Am 1994; 78:1249–1258.

28 Diverticular Disease of the Colon

Philip H. Gordon

INTRODUCTION

The term "diverticulum" indicates an abnormal pouch or sac, opening from a hollow organ such as the intestine. It is derived from the Latin verb *divertere*, which means "to turn aside." Credit for the first description of diverticular disease has been given to Cruveilhier (1), who in 1849 described a series of small, pear-shaped, hernial protrusions of mucosa through the muscle coat of the sigmoid colon. From a historical perspective, diverticula were initially regarded as nothing more than a pathologic curiosity, but with time it was realized that they could be associated with inflammation, perforation, adhesions, fistulas, and stenosis. After World War I, contrast radiology revealed a growing prevalence of this disease. When finally recognized as clinically important, diverticula were treated medically unless complications supervened. More recently, physicians have shown a willingness to refer patients with diverticula for elective operation.

The presence of protrusions of the mucosa through the muscular wall of the bowel, commonly but not invariably associated with a muscular abnormality of the sigmoid colon, has been termed as "diverticulosis." When inflammation is superimposed, the term "diverticulitis" is used. Because many patients with this condition exhibit no evidence of inflammation, the encompassing term "diverticular disease" is used for the entire spectrum of the clinical consequences of the presence of diverticula of the colon.

PATHOLOGIC ANATOMY

In a detailed study of the anatomy and pathology of diverticular disease, Slack (2) examined the large intestine of 141 cadavers in which consecutive autopsies were performed and 36 consecutive operative specimens were removed because of diverticulitis. Diverticula had broken through the circular muscle in four main positions (Fig. 1). In approximately 40% of the cases, protrusions were also noted between the antimesenteric teniae. A large blood vessel coursed around the bowel on each side outside the muscular coat to penetrate through the mesenteric side of the antimesenteric teniae. In some cases, this vessel appeared to divide on the mesenteric side of the antimesenteric teniae into deep and superficial branches, with the deeper one piercing the circular muscle coat and the more superficial one passing external to or directly through the teniae. Small vessels arose from the main circumferential vessels and penetrated the circular muscle coat and the mesenteric teniae. The main circumferential vessel passed superficial to the diverticulum; in each case, small vessels passed along the neck of the diverticulum toward the lumen of the bowel.

INCIDENCE

Almy and Howell (3) noted that diverticulosis affects 30 million Americans annually, bringing 200,000 to the hospital and incurring health care costs in excess of one-third of a billion dollars in 1980. It is estimated that 30% of the population over the age of 60 and perhaps 60% of the population over the age of 80 may be affected (4). Connell (5) estimated the probable risk of the aged population developing diverticular disease to be at nearly 50%.

In fact, it is impossible to estimate the precise incidence of diverticular disease in the general population. Data on the incidence and prevalence of diverticular disease of the colon represent a crude overall blend of numbers derived from radiologic, surgical, and autopsy reports on both hospitalized and ambulatory populations. In any review of statistics, autopsy studies will underestimate the incidence of diverticulosis because of the care needed to demonstrate all diverticula. Radiologic studies will overestimate the occurrence because people have barium enemas for various symptoms. What is evident is that the incidence has gradually increased over the past several decades. For example, in 1930, Rankin and Brown (6) reported that barium enema examinations revealed that 5.7% of 24,620 cases had diverticulosis, as did 5.2% of 1925 autopsy cases at the Mayo Clinic. Heller and Hackler (7) reported that between 1909 and 1975, the autopsy incidence of diverticulosis had risen from 5% to 50%.

In a cross-sectional study, Hart et al. (8) identified 58 cases of perforated large-bowel diverticula living in a defined area with a population of 531,241. The incidence was 4.0 cases per 100,000 per year, it increased with age, and it was higher in men than women (5.8 vs. 3.1). The most frequently used drugs were nonsteroidal anti-inflammatory drugs (29%) and opiate analgesics (26%).

The incidence of diverticular disease steadily increases with age, from approximately 5% in the fifth decade to about 50% in the ninth decade, with a maximal incidence in the sixth, seventh, and eighth decades (4). Colcock (9) estimated that 10% to 20% of patients above the age of 40 have diverticula of the colon. Rodkey and Welch (10) found that the average age for men to have diverticula was 59 years and for women was 67 years, and that 75% of people over the age of 80 years have diverticulosis. Morson (11) noted that diverticular disease is uncommon in individuals under the age of 40, and estimated that one-third of persons over 60 years have diverticula, and that the incidence steadily increases with age. Painter and Burkitt (12) reported that up to two-thirds of individuals are affected by the age of 70. In the United Kingdom, 33% of individuals over the age of 45 have radiologic evidence of colonic diverticula (13). The incidence according to sex also varies from report to report. In an autopsy series, Parks (4) recorded the incidence of diverticular disease as 33% in men and 42% in women. However, in a similar study, Hughes (14) found the incidence of diverticular disease to be 45% in men and 40% in women. In a series of 280 unselected autopsies in Norway, Eide and Stalsberg (15) found the incidence of diverticular disease to be 25% in males and 43% in females. In a series of clinical cases of diverticular disease, Parks (4) found a male-to-female ratio of 2:3, and Rodkey and Welch (10) noted that 59% of cases were female and 41%, male. Morson (11) reported that diverticular disease was more common in men than women.

Geographic location is also important, for it appears that diverticulosis is a disease of Western man. A close relationship exists between the prevalence of diverticular disease and economic development and adoption of Western eating habits. Diverticula are common in Europe,

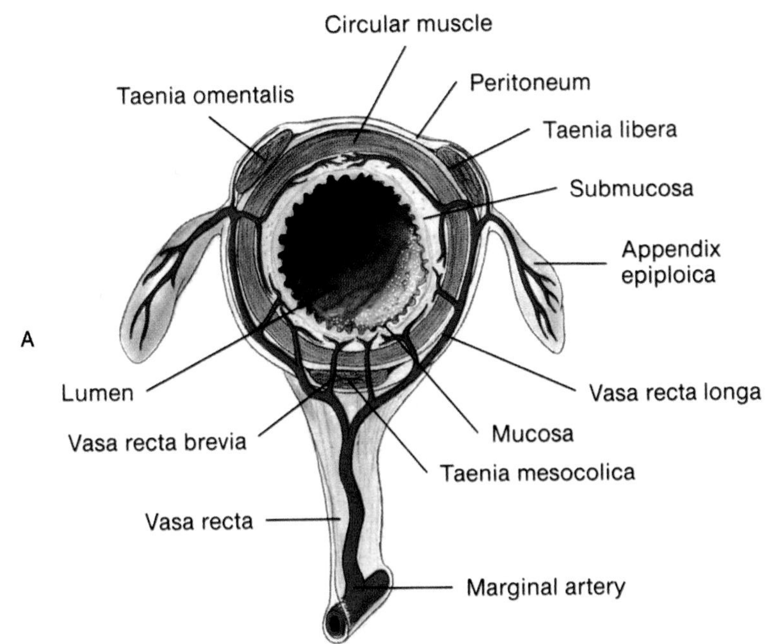

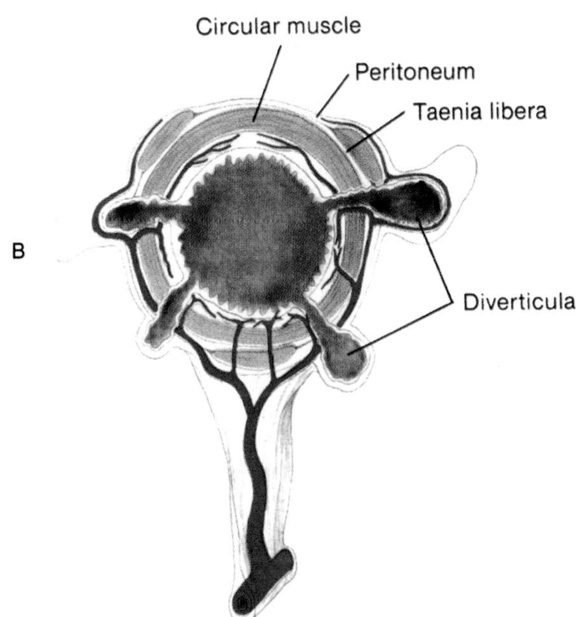

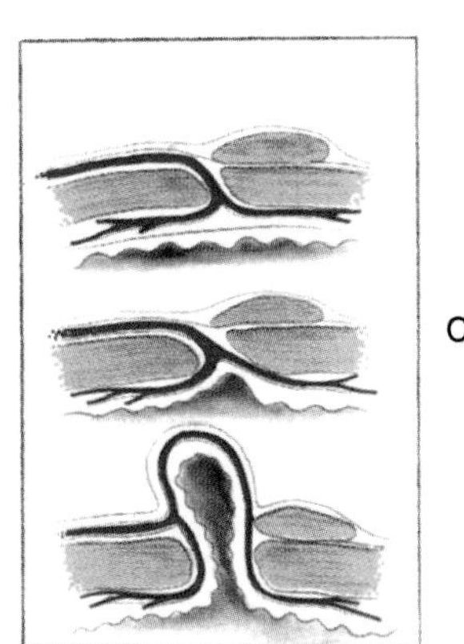

FIGURE 1 ■ (**A**) Cross section of the usual anatomic layers of colonic wall with special attention to the course of vessels. (**B**) Cross section demonstrating the location of diverticula as determined by Slack. (**C**) Relationship of the vessels to the diverticulum.

North America, and Australia, less common in South America, and rare in Africa and Oriental countries. In stark contrast to Western reports, Pan et al. (16) reviewed a 60-year experience in a hospital in China and found only 18 cases of colonic diverticula. The incidence as judged by autopsy cases and colonoscopic cases was 0.12% and 0.33% to 1.2%, respectively. In an autopsy study of 200 patients, Coode et al. (17) found diverticula in 5%, and most of these were situated in the cecum. The prevalence of diverticular disease is low in Iran, with only 2.4% of individuals over the age of 50 having this condition (18). In a study of the changing epidemiology of diverticular disease in Israel, Levy et al. (19) evaluated the findings from 1244 consecutive barium enemas and found colonic diverticula in 14.2%. The prevalence among Ashkenazic Jews was 19.7%, among Sephardic and Oriental Jews, 16%, and among Arabs, 9.5%. When compared to a similar study a decade earlier, results for the Ashkenazic group remained the same, whereas there was a threefold increase among the Sephardic and Oriental Jews and a sevenfold increase among Arabs.

Kang et al. (20) studied the frequency of colonic diverticular disease in British patients of Indian-subcontinent Asian origin compared with other ethnic groups by colonoscopic examination. Colonic diverticular disease was identified in 4% of the Indian-subcontinent Asian males and in 5% of the females compared with 22% and 23% in other ethnic groups, respectively.

Left-sided diverticula are predominant in the United States, Canada, the United Kingdom, Europe, Australia, Israel, Iran, Jordan, and Brazil. Right-sided diverticulosis is almost exclusively an Oriental condition and is more common than left-sided diverticula in Japan, Hawaii (among Japanese and Chinese individuals), China, Korea, Thailand, and Singapore (11). Kubo et al. (21) found that 76% of Japanese patients with diverticula had right-sided disease. To better understand the changing nature of diverticular disease of the colon in Japan, Nakada et al. (22) reviewed 6849 patients undergoing barium enema examination during an eight-year period from 1985 to 1992. Diverticular disease was found in 1074 patients (15.7%), including 702 males (65.4%) and 372 females (34.6%). During this eight-year period, there was an increase in frequency from 10.7% in 1985 to 17.8% in 1992. The percentage of patients with right-sided, bilateral, and left-sided diverticular disease was 69.2%, 17.5%, and 13.3%, respectively. The right-sided diverticular disease was more common in the younger age group and was predominant in male patients, whereas the left-sided diverticular disease increased with age, especially in female patients. Of the 1074 patients, 11 (1.0%) underwent operation in the same period. Regarding right-sided diverticular disease, only 2 of 743 patients received operation (0.3%). On the other hand, of the 143 patients with left-sided diverticular disease, nine patients (6.3%) underwent some form of operation. Nearly all patients diagnosed as having diverticula had either no symptoms or only mild symptoms, and only about 1% required operation. Right-sided diverticular disease of the colon seems to produce no serious clinical problems compared with left-sided diverticular disease. Miura et al. (23) also studied the spatial distribution of diverticular disease in the Japanese population. In 7543 double-contrast barium enemas, diverticula that were classified into right-sided, left-sided, and bilateral types, and the relationship of the frequency (detection rate) and numbers of diverticula to age were examined for the earlier (1982–1987) and later (1988–1992) periods. Diverticular disease was found in 22.2% of the male and 15.5% of the female examinees. The right-sided type predominated among the subjects. Frequency distribution by age of the bilateral type was similar to that of the left-sided type. Bilateral diverticular disease increased in frequency with advancing years in the sixth and seventh decades, the right-sided type increased in middle-aged subjects, and the left-sided type did not. The bilateral type was composed of diverticula in the right colon, where numbers were greater than in the pure right-sided type, but remained unchanged with increasing age, and diverticula in the left colon, where numbers were similar to the pure left-sided type, but did not increase with age. Increase in the prevalence of bilateral and not the pure left-sided form has contributed to the recent increase in diverticula in the left colon among the Japanese, and might have been preceded by an increase in the right-sided type.

Chan et al. (24) conducted a retrospective study to determine the prevalence of diverticulosis in Hong Kong Chinese adults. They analyzed 858 consecutive barium enema examinations over a period of 18 months. The prevalence of diverticulosis in their community was 25.1%, with no significant difference in the prevalence in male and female adults. The prevalence is lower than that in the Western countries, but higher than that in Asia. Moreover, the peak prevalence is at the 50 to 79 years age group, with lower prevalence in the older age groups. This may be explained by the rapid rise in prevalence in the younger age groups so that the age-related increase in prevalence becomes obscured. They postulate that this may be due to the Western cultural influence in their diet and lifestyle. There was no significant difference in the symptomatology of patients with and without diverticulosis, supporting the idea that diverticulosis alone is usually asymptomatic. There was predominance of right-hemicolon involvement in their subjects, in contrast to the left-hemicolon predominance in the Caucasian population. In patients with diverticulosis, 55.3% had only right-sided involvement, 32.6% had bilateral involvement, and only 12.1% had exclusively left-hemicolon involvement. Cecal and ascending colon diverticula were found in 6.4% and 17.6% of all adults under study, respectively.

Segal and Leibowitz (25) have described the emergence of diverticular disease in black South Africans. Diverticula in this population occur predominantly in the descending colon. The authors suggest that the variable anatomic distribution of diverticula in different ethnic groups implies that fiber deficiency is not the only factor responsible for the condition. Diverticular disease may comprise several entities with different causes.

Mendeloff (26) summarized data gathered by Painter and added information from newer publications. Information from the past few decades is presented in Tables 1 and 2. The incidence of diverticular disease increases as populations adopt Western lifestyles. Nevertheless, the right-sided colonic diverticulosis seen in Japanese and other Oriental peoples persists in spite of the markedly increased frequency of all diverticular disease.

ETIOLOGY

It is generally agreed that colonic diverticula are acquired. They are considered pulsion diverticula, which, under the influence of increased intraluminal pressure, are mucosal herniations that protrude through points of the bowel wall weakened by entry of blood vessels. Recognition of the segmentation mechanism of pressure production and its role in the localization of high intracolonic pressures has led

TABLE 1 ■ Frequency of Diverticulosis in Various Countries as Revealed by Barium Enema

Author(s)	Country	No. of Patients	%
Manousos et al. (27)	United Kingdom	109	7.6 (<60 yr) 34.9 (>60 yr)
Havia (28)	Finland	1,215	12.0
Vajrabukka et al. (29)	Thailand (1978–1979)	289	4.2
Dabestani et al. (18)	Iran (1972–1976)	556	1.6
Kubo et al. (21)	Japan (1965–1980)	12,505	7.8
Fatayer et al. (30)	Japan (1979–1981)	274	4.0
Levy et al. (19)	Israel (1979–1984)		
	Ashkenazim		17.3
	Sephardim-Orientals		12.3
	Arabs		5.4
Segal and Leibowitz (25)	South Africa		
	Blacks	440	2.7
	Whites	221	20.8

TABLE 2 ■ Frequency of Diverticulosis in Various Countries as Revealed by Autopsy

Author(s)	Country	No. of Patients	%
Cleland (31)	Australia (1940–1948)	3000	2.6
Hughes (14)	United Kingdom	200	45.0
Parks (4)	United Kingdom	300	37.0
Pan et al. (16)	China (1949–1982)	6896	0.1
Coode et al. (17)	China (1980, Hong Kong)	200	5.0
Paspatis et al. (32)	Crete	502	22.9

to some understanding of the pathogenesis of diverticular disease, but the etiology of the disease to a great degree remains a mystery. Painter (33) hypothesized that it is a deficiency disease caused by inadequacy of fiber brought about by the refining of carbohydrates.

In the past half century, the amount of cereal fiber consumed by individuals in the Western world has declined dramatically. Painter (33) believes that this dietary change is the most probable cause of the emergence of diverticular disease in Westernized populations in the twentieth century. A colon with a wide lumen is less able to form segments efficiently, and large-bore colons are found wherever individuals eat a diet containing plenty of roughage. By contrast, consuming the overrefined, fiber-deficient diet of the industrial countries produces small hard stools that pass through a narrower colon that can segment more easily. Higher pressures are needed to transport these stiff stools, and because the fecal stream is more viscous by the time it reaches the distal colon, it causes the sigmoid to segment excessively. Thus segmentation is the mechanism responsible for the pathogenesis of diverticula, and a fiber-deficient diet is the cause of the disease.

Burkitt et al. (34) studied the fiber intake of African natives and compared it to that of British subjects. They found that the Africans had a higher stool weight and a shorter transit time. They attributed the low incidence of diverticular disease to this high fiber intake. Bingham (35) provided an excellent summary of the dietary fiber intake of general populations and found that Africans consume 60 to 150 g/day; Europeans, 15 to 25 g/day; Japanese, 20 g/day; Canadian vegetarians, 30 g/day; and people in the United States, 13 to 20 g/day. In a study of barium enema examinations in vegetarians and non-vegetarians, Gear et al. (13) found a 12% incidence of diverticular disease in vegetarians, compared with a 33% incidence among non-vegetarians. Manousos et al. (36) found that patients with diverticula consumed significantly less brown bread and vegetables but more meat than controls.

Nakaji et al. (37) compared the etiology of right-sided diverticula in Japan with that of left-sided diverticula in the West. Diverticula occur predominantly in the right-sided colon (over 70%) in Japanese patients, and even among Japanese who emigrate, in contrast with the diverticula in Western patients. Incidence rates of colon diverticula have rapidly increased in Japan since World War II with the increased dietary fiber intake. The increased detection rate over time is higher in urban areas than in rural areas, and it corresponds to the distribution of dietary fiber intake. Furthermore, the significant relationship with right-sided diverticula with intraluminal pressure in Japan is similar to that of left-sided diverticula in the West, and the pathological feature of these diverticula are similar. The etiology of right-sided diverticula in Japan (and perhaps other Mongolian peoples) is very similar to that of left-sided diverticula in the West. The location may represent a difference in morphology of the large intestine between Mongolians (including Japanese) and Westerners, rather than environmental differences.

In a prospective study of 47,678 American men, Aldoori et al. (38) found that physical activity was inversely associated with the risk of symptomatic diverticular disease, with a relative risk of 0.60 for individuals engaged in vigorous activity. Jogging and running were the activities cited. From the same cohort of men, Aldoori et al. (39) found that smoking, caffeine, and alcohol intake are not associated with any substantial increased risk of symptomatic diverticular disease. Aldoori et al. (40) further examined prospectively dietary fiber calculated from food composition values from a prospective cohort of 43,881 U.S. male health professionals in the 40 to 75 years age group. Their findings suggest that the insoluble component of fiber was significantly associated with a decreased risk of diverticular disease (RR = 0.63), and this inverse association was particularly strong for cellulose (RR = 0.52).

Development of colonic diverticulosis is a function of age and declining colonic wall mechanical strength. The latter is partly a consequence of changes in the collagen structure. Wess et al. (41) measured collagen from unaffected human colons and those with colonic diverticulosis obtained at necropsy. The colonic total collagen content was constant with age. The acid solubility of the collagen, however, increased after the age of 40. At over 60 years, colonic diverticulosis was associated with an increased acid solubility ratio compared with values in unaffected colons (15:3 compared with 9:2). Stumpf et al. (42) reported that in patients with diverticulitis, there were decreased levels of mature collagen type I and increased levels of collagen type III, with a resulting lower collagen ratio I/III. The expression of matrix metalloproteinase-I was reduced significantly in the diverticulitis group, while the expression of matrix metalloproteinase-13 did not differ significantly between the two groups. Their findings support the theory of structural changes in the colonic wall as one of the major pathogenic factors in the development of diverticular disease.

Bode et al. (43) reported the contents of type I and III collagen telopeptides and total collagen were similar in diverticulosis and healthy tissue, whereas in malignant tissue, type III collagen was scarce. The rate of type I collagen synthesis was clearly increased in malignancy but not significantly in diverticulosis. However, type III collagen synthesis was increased in diverticulosis but not in malignancy. These changes may be a factor in the etiology of colonic diverticulosis.

PATHOGENESIS

PATHOPHYSIOLOGIC FINDINGS

Several investigators have conducted studies in patients with diverticular disease to determine whether their responses to various stimuli differ from those of individuals who do not harbor colonic diverticula. Painter found no difference in the resting pressure patterns in the sigmoid colon in healthy individuals vs. those with diverticulosis (44). By contrast Arfwidsson noted a higher mean resting pressure in patients with diverticulosis than in normal individuals (44). Using a neostigmine-stimulated motility index, Weinreich and Andersen (45) discovered that asymptomatic patients with diverticular disease had manometric tracings indistinguishable from those of healthy individuals, whereas those with abdominal pain had sigmoid motility similar to those with irritable bowel syndrome. Asymptomatic patients and those with diarrhea who had diverticular disease had colonic myoelectric activity similar to that of healthy individuals (46). Therapeutic doses of morphine cause the normal colon to generate increased pressure, with an even greater response evoked in segments of the colon containing diverticula (44). Neostigmine (prostigmin) also elicits an exaggerated response in diverticular segments compared with normal segments of colon. Food intake induces a marked increase in intraluminal pressure, and emotion also increases the motility of the colon. Patients with symptomatic diverticular disease have abnormal myoelectric activity, with an abnormal slow wave pattern with a predominant frequency of 12 to 18 cycles/min (47). The pattern changes toward normal when bran is given. Connell (48), in his study of patients with diverticular disease, found an exaggerated response to pharmacologic stimuli, an increased intraluminal pressure, and faster frequency waves and rapid contractions.

Painter and Burkitt (12) summarized their work and that of other investigators with regard to pressure in the human sigmoid colon. Under resting conditions, the normal human sigmoid colon harbors a basal pressure within a few millimeters of mercury of the atmospheric pressure. Superimposed on this basal pressure at irregular intervals are small waves of positive pressure, which last 10 to 20 seconds, are usually less than 10 mmHg in amplitude, and do not progress along the colonic lumen. The sigmoid colon beset with diverticula behaves the same way when at rest. Morphine causes the normal colon to generate waves of pressure that double in number but are usually less than 20 mmHg in amplitude. Segments of sigmoid that bear diverticula respond with pressures that sometimes exceed 90 mmHg, an observation believed to favor progression of the disease once established.

According to Painter and Burkitt (12), cineradiography has shown that the high pressures evoked by morphine and transmitted to the diverticula may inflate them like balloons; hence, the use of morphine as an analgesic is contraindicated in patients with acute diverticular disease because it may cause perforation. Instead, meperidine (Demerol) should be given because it lowers the intracolonic pressures, with reduced height and number of pressure waves, and it lessens the muscular activity of the colon, thus resting the bowel. Cineradiography also has revealed high-localized intraluminal pressures that are produced by segmentation of the colon, regardless of the stimulus that evokes them. Segmentation causes the colon to act not as a tube, but as a series of "little bladders," each of which has its outflow narrowed (Fig. 2) (12). High pressures can develop in these segments or bladders, and force the mucosa through the muscle wall of the colon. Segmentation, concerned in the transportation of colonic contents, normally plays a part in colonic physiology. Frequently, these contents are shunted back and forth in the sigmoid colon, presumably to aid in the absorption of water from the fecal stream. Thus Painter and Burkitt believe that diverticula are the outward visible sign of an inward disturbance of colonic motility. The cause of this abnormal behavior must be environmental and is probably due to changes in diet, which alter the consistency of the colon's contents.

Rees et al. (49) compared the response rate of circular and longitudinal muscle strips from the sigmoid colon of patients with diverticular disease to those of individuals with carcinoma. Longitudinal muscle strips from diverticular

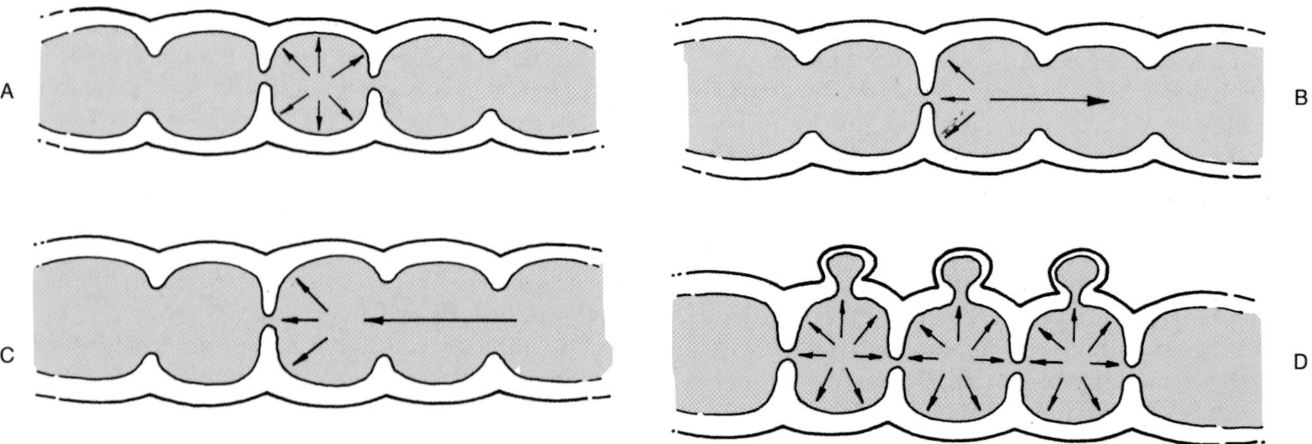

FIGURE 2 ■ Segmentation is concerned with the transportation and halting of feces in sigmoid colon. (**A**) Segmented colon. One segment has produced pressure by contracting. (**B**) Relaxation of contraction ring on one side of this segment allows contents to move into next segment, which harbors lower pressure. This is a mechanism by which contents are moved. (**C**) Feces are halted. Contraction rings act as baffles that slow and finally halt contents, and a pressure change results. Segmentation is seen in sigmoid as feces are shunted back and forth. (**D**) Segmented colon acting as a series of "little bladders" whose outflow is obstructed at both ends and which extrude diverticula by generating high-localized intrasegmental pressures. Segmentation is essential to pathogenesis of diverticula. Any factor that causes segmentation to occur more frequently or more efficiently favors causation of diverticula disease. *Source*: Modified from Ref. 12.

disease specimens were less responsive to acetylcholine, histamine, or adrenaline than those of controls. The response of diverticular circular muscle strips showed a small decrease to acetylcholine, a small increase to noradrenaline, and no change to histamine as compared to controls.

Clemens et al. (50) studied 10 asymptomatic diverticular disease patients, 11 symptomatic uncomplicated diverticular disease patients, and nine healthy controls to assess whether altered visceral perception or abnormal compliance of the colorectal wall plays a role in these clinical entities. Using a dual barostat device, sensations were scored and compliance curves obtained using stepwise intermittent isobaric distensions of the rectum and sigmoid, before and after a liquid meal. In the rectum, perception was increased in the symptomatic uncomplicated diverticular disease group compared with controls and the asymptomatic diverticular disease group. Rectal compliance curves were not different between the groups. In the sigmoid colon, perception in the pre- and postprandial periods was increased in symptomatic uncomplicated diverticular disease compared with controls, but not when compared with asymptomatic diverticular disease patients. Sigmoid volume–pressure curves had comparable slopes (compliance) in all groups but were shifted downward in symptomatic uncomplicated diverticular disease patients compared with asymptomatic diverticular disease patients in the preprandial period. They concluded symptomatic but not asymptomatic uncomplicated diverticular disease is associated with heightened perception of distension, not only in the diverticular bearing sigmoid, but also in the unaffected rectum.

Bassotti et al. (51) investigated basal and stimulated (postprandial) colonic motility in patients with diverticular disease, together with the detection of high-amplitude propagated contractions (mass movements). Motility data from patients were compared with those obtained in healthy control subjects. Ten patients and 16 control subjects of both sexes were recruited; colonic motility was recorded for a 24-hour period by a colonoscopically positioned manometric catheter. Two 1000-kcal mixed meals were served during the study. Compared with control subjects, patients with diverticular disease displayed significantly increased amounts of motility in the affected segments; the response to a physiologic stimulus (meal) was also abnormal in the patients' group. Diverticular disease patients also had a significant increase of forceful propulsive activity compared with control subjects (average $= 10.3 \pm 2.7$/subject/day high-amplitude propagated contractions for patients and 5.5 ± 0.8/subject/day for control subjects); interestingly, about 20% of such activity was abnormal, being propagated in a retrograde fashion. They concluded that patients with diverticular disease of the colon have abnormal motor and propulsive activities of the large bowel, which are confined to the affected segments. These findings are somewhat different than those of Clemens and the reason is unclear.

■ TRADITIONAL CONCEPT

The traditional belief is that diverticula develop as a result of elevated intraluminal pressures that arise because of segmentation of the colon. Bowel shortening might be explained by contracture of the teniae coli, which could cause thickening and hypersegmentation of the circular muscle layer.

Painter (44) summarized his extensive studies of the role of segmentation as the cause of diverticular disease and its symptoms as follows: Segmentation of the colon is the mechanism by which the colon propels its contents or halts material moving through its lumen. It involves the production of increased intraluminal pressures and has been demonstrated by recording the intracolonic pressures with open-ended tubes, while simultaneous cineradiography recorded the behavior of the colon. The intracolonic pressures produced by segmentation may exceed 90 mmHg. Fig. 3 shows three longitudinal sections of colon, each containing three leads recording from different levels of the colon. In the top section, the open lumen allows the colonic contents to move freely so that small movements of the colonic wall will result in no significant change of pressure. In the middle section, the center segment is demarcated from the others by two contraction rings that narrow the lumen on each side of it. Further contraction of this segment is resisted by its contents, which cannot flow freely into the neighboring bowel. A pressure change will be recorded by lead 2, but this pressure will not affect the adjacent segments. The bottom section shows the center segment contracted so that the lumen on each side of it is almost occluded. Further contraction of this segment would cause development of a very high pressure, which would be recorded by lead 2; leads 1 and 3, which lie in open bowel, would be unaffected. This center segment behaves like a "little bladder" whose outflow is obstructed, thus generating very high pressures. These pressures cause herniation of the mucosa.

Painter and Burkitt (12) further postulate that an unrefined diet containing adequate fiber may prevent diverticulosis for the following reasons:

1. The colon that copes with a large volume of feces has a wide diameter, will generate a lower intraluminal pressure, and is less prone to produce diverticula.
2. Patients with a diet high in fiber have a shorter colonic transit time, so the colon absorbs water for less time and has to propel a less viscous fecal stream. Hence, the colon probably produces less pressure and is less apt to become trabeculated and to bear diverticula.
3. Suppression of the call to stool favors drying of the feces and increasing generation of pressure. The swiftly passed soft stool subjects the sigmoid colon to less strain and does not favor the development of diverticula.

■ CHANGING CONCEPTS

Departing from conventional teaching, Ryan (52) suggested that there are two kinds of diverticular disease. The more common variety has the classic muscle abnormality, is chiefly confined to the left colon, and is characterized by bowel symptoms with pain, inflammation, and perforative and fistula complications. Older patients are generally affected. The other one has no muscle abnormality but does have extensive densely packed diverticula throughout the colon in which bleeding is common, perhaps caused by a connective tissue abnormality that, on the one hand, allows

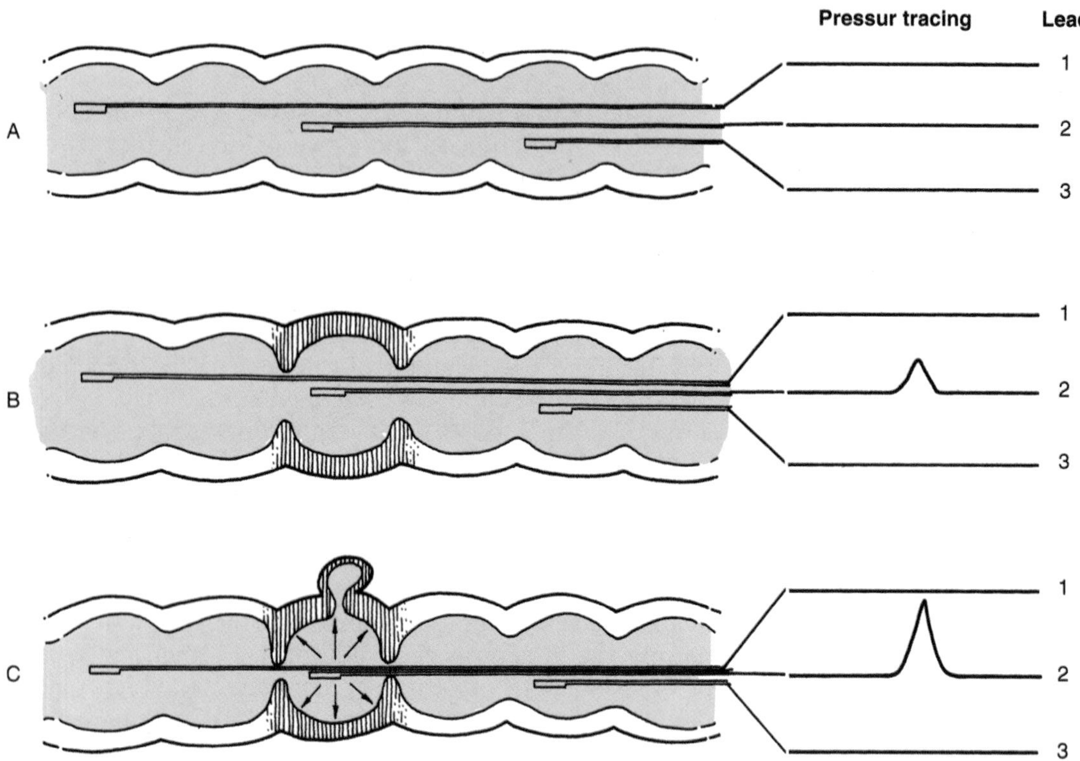

FIGURE 3 ■ Segmentation causing high pressures and pulsion force responsible for diverticulosis. *Source*: From Ref. 12.

development of diverticula in the absence of abnormal intraluminal pressures and, on the other hand, provides inadequate support for vessels in the diverticular wall or for vascular malformations, which are therefore likely to bleed. Ryan's clinical evidence suggests that both acute and chronic pain may be caused by either inflammation or muscle spasm. Ryan further proposed that perforation may be due to abnormal intraluminal pressures rather than diverticular inflammation. In a series of 100 consecutive hospital admissions, Ryan (52) found the reasons to be acute diverticulitis, 36%; bleeding, 18%; free perforation and peritonitis, 10%; perforation and local abscess, 6%; fistula, 14%; stricture, 6%; and chronic diverticulitis, 10%.

Mann (53) also departed from the traditional concept and postulated that the underlying defect was related to the smooth muscle of the bowel at the level of the rectosigmoid. He observed that the smooth muscle of the rectosigmoid junction behaved differently from the sigmoid colon above or the rectum below. Manometric studies of this zone showed that in response to a stimulus causing contraction of the colon above and the rectum beneath, the smooth muscle of the rectosigmoid junction relaxed. Based on this observation, Mann hypothesized that if in response to aging processes, dietary faults, and constipation, the rectosigmoid loses its ability to relax sufficiently in advance of a peristaltic wave of contraction, a zone of low-grade resistance will build. To overcome this resistance, muscle hypertrophy would take place, and abnormal pressures would develop in the sigmoid colon. With repeated peristalsis, high pressure would be distributed to the entire pelvic colon. Mann believed that this theory would explain the progression of disease better, and he stated that the rectosigmoid must be resected during definitive treatment.

In his review and assessment of available information, Manousos (54) concluded that the clinical spectrum of diverticular disease results from the interaction of two factors: intraluminal pressure and weakness of the colonic wall in different proportions. When the tensile strength of the wall is high, no diverticula can develop, regardless of the long-standing presence of increased intracolonic pressures; however, when the colonic wall is weak, even smaller degrees of colonic hypermotility can lead to the development of multiple diverticula of the colon. In their review of the literature regarding the origin of symptoms in diverticula disease, Simpson et al. (55) concluded that it would seem likely that several interrelated processes such as muscular dysfunction, visceral hypersensitivity, and inflammation are involved in symptom generation. The foregoing discussions reinforce the fact that neither the etiology nor pathogenesis of diverticular disease is well understood.

PATHOLOGY

In a patient with uncomplicated diverticular disease, the sigmoid colon appears shortened and its wall thickened compared with that of a healthy person. Characteristically, diverticula are of the pulsion type and were described by Whiteway and Morson (56) as occurring in two rows between the mesenteric and antimesenteric teniae. Occasionally, protrusions may be situated in the antimesenteric intertenial area. Meyers et al. (57) described four rows of diverticula, all related to penetrating vasa recta. The row of diverticula closest to the mesenteric teniae is related to vasa recta brevia, whereas those proximal to the antimesenteric teniae protrude along the course of the vasa recta longa. Slack (2) also described the diverticula as being present in four rows. From the external surface, diverticula are frequently not apparent because they project into the appendices epiploicae (Fig. 1B).

The muscle abnormality is the most consistent and important feature in diverticular disease of the sigmoid colon (11). When the colonic wall is sectioned, the interior aspect reveals round or slit-like openings, which may at times be inconspicuous and detected only when fecal matter is in the orifice. The muscular coat is thickened, and the mucosal layer is heaped into transverse folds that project into the lumen. The luminal diameter is reduced in size. The thickened longitudinal and circular muscle layers have been considered responsible for shortening the sigmoid colon and pleating the mucosa, with the creation of a saccular appearance (Fig. 4). Narrowing of the lumen may be due to these redundant folds but in part may be secondary to pericolic fibrosis (11).

Microscopically, diverticula possess two coats: an inner mucosal layer and an outer serosal layer. An artery, vein, and attenuated muscle may be seen close to the neck of the diverticulum (Fig. 5). Antimesenteric diverticula do not entirely herniate through the circular muscle fibers, but they have a thinned layer of circular muscle in their wall.

In patients with diverticular disease, both muscle layers are greatly increased in thickness. There has been much conjecture about whether the muscle thickening is due to hypertrophy or hyperplasia. In their study of the thickened bowel, Whiteway and Morson (56) failed to reveal evidence of cellular hypertrophy or hyperplasia. Instead, they attributed the thickening to the presence of elastic tissue, specifically in the teniae (58). This progressive elastosis causes longitudinal foreshortening of the colon, accentuating the semicircular corrugations of the shortened circular muscle. The source of the elastosis is uncertain, but this muscle abnormality precedes the development of diverticulosis. It is characteristic of diverticular disease in that it is never seen in other segmental or diffuse inflammatory conditions of the colon. Why the muscle abnormality occurs predominantly in the sigmoid colon is unclear. It is postulated that the muscle of the sigmoid colon is different from that of the more proximal colon because it appears thicker and shows an increased capacity for muscular spasm.

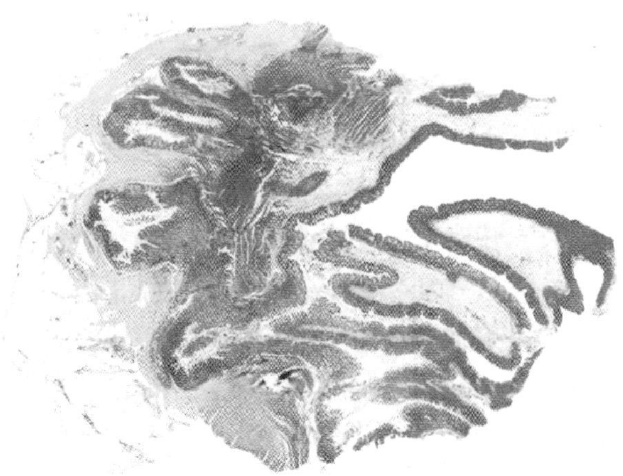

FIGURE 5 ■ Photomicrograph of several diverticula penetrating the colonic wall. *Source*: Courtesy of Esther Lamoureux, M.D., Montreal, Quebec, Canada.

A

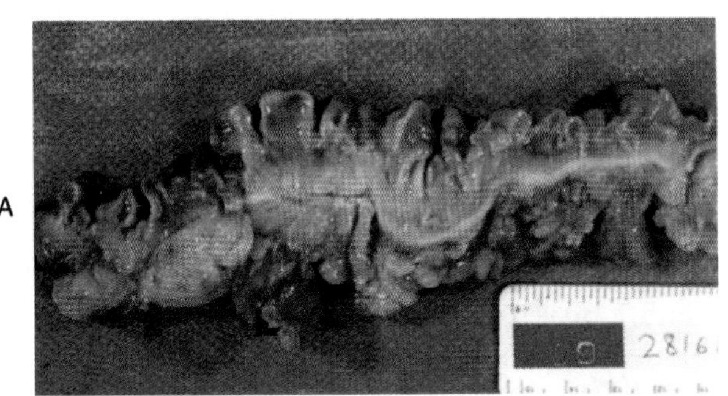

B

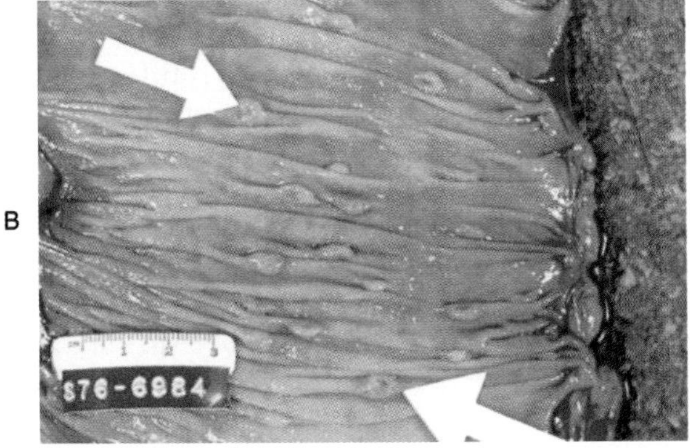

FIGURE 4 ■ (**A**) Resected sigmoid colon demonstrating muscle thickening, mucosal pleating, and narrowed lumen. (**B**) Example of right-sided diverticula in thin-walled colon. *Source*: Courtesy of Esther Lamoureux, M.D., Montreal, Quebec, Canada.

Evidence of inflammatory change is not shown in approximately a quarter to one-third of all specimens resected for diverticular disease (11,59). When inflammation does occur, it is noted in the extramural pericolic tissues. The pericolitis may be due to micro-perforation or macro-perforation of a diverticulum.

Killingback et al. (60) proposed the need for a better classification of the surgical pathology of diverticular disease treated by elective resection. They conducted a prospective audit over a 25-year period on 206 patients managed by elective resection, with a postoperative mortality of 1.0% and a total morbidity of 51.5%. The surgical pathology was classified as noninflammatory, 12.6%; localized diverticulitis, 43.7%; and extracolonic diverticulitis, 44.2%. They believe this classification is useful in relating to the technical requirements of the operation. Post-operative morbidity is associated with the presence and severity of inflammatory pathology, and therefore the case mix of any series will have a significant impact on this aspect.

PATTERNS OF DISEASE

The most frequent site of diverticular disease is the sigmoid colon. According to the law of Laplace, the tension in the wall of a hollow cylinder is inversely proportional to its radius multiplied by the pressure within the cylinder. This implies that the intraluminal pressure is greater where the lumen is narrowed—in this case in the sigmoid colon, thus explaining the increased likelihood that pulsion diverticula will develop in this particular area (48).

Even as far back as 1930, Rankin and Brown (6) reported on 24,620 cases with barium enema examination and 1225 cases involving autopsy at the Mayo Clinic and found diverticulosis to be located only in the sigmoid colon in 29%, in the sigmoid colon and other areas in 68%, and in other areas but not the sigmoid colon in 3%. In a series of 521 clinical cases of diverticular disease, Parks (4) found the sigmoid colon alone to be involved in 65.5% and in combination with other regions in 96%; 6.7% had total colonic involvement. Rodkey and Welch (10) found the sigmoid colon to be involved in 94% of cases. Only sporadic cases of rectal diverticulosis have been reported (61).

An entirely different pattern of diverticular disease was reported from Japan. Of 615 patients with diverticular disease of the colon reviewed by Sugihara et al. (62), 429 had diverticula in the cecum and ascending colon (70%), 98 in the sigmoid and descending colon (16%), and 88 in both the right and the left colon (14%). The right-sided type was more common in younger patients and more predominant in men, whereas the left-sided type was more common in the elderly and showed no sexual predilection. More than 50% of patients were asymptomatic, and 25% complained of disturbed bowel function. The frequency of diverticulitis was not related to location but to the number of diverticula. Acute inflammation was a complication in 61 patients (14%) with right-sided diverticula and in 16 patients (16%) with left-sided diverticula. Many patients with right-sided diverticula improved with medical treatment. When indicated, the operative treatment of choice was drainage and supplemental appendectomy. In a small series of cases reported from China, right-sided diverticula comprised approximately 60% of the cases (16).

NATURAL HISTORY

Despite the prevalence of diverticulosis of the colon estimated to be 15% to 37% (4,15), it is an asymptomatic condition in most patients. Why some patients develop symptoms and others do not is unknown. It is estimated that 10% to 25% of patients with diverticulosis will develop diverticulitis (4,5,63). Of patients with diverticulitis of the colon, 10% to 33% eventually require operative intervention (4,64,65). From his extensive personal studies and thorough review of the literature, Parks (4) summarized the following features of diverticular disease. The incidence increases with advancing years, and there is an increased risk of hemorrhage in the elderly. In young patients, the disease often pursues an aggressive course. There seems to be a change in the incidence according to sex, with more recent reports recording a higher incidence in females. Progression of disease relative to number and size of diverticula does not occur in 70% of patients, and it is doubtful that the frequency of attacks of diverticulitis is related to the number of diverticula present. In the majority of patients with diverticula localized to the distal colon, the disorder will not necessarily progress relentlessly and involve additional segments. Progression more often occurs within the segment of bowel initially affected. On an average, patients with extensive involvement are not older, and may indeed be younger than those with localized disease.

Parks (4) also noted severe complications to occur as commonly in patients with distal disease as in those with total colonic involvement. Indeed, after an operation to eradicate distal disease, it was unusual for inflammatory complications to develop in the proximal bowel. However, hemorrhage occurred more readily from the proximal bowel, but this bleeding may not necessarily be of diverticular origin and may be due to vascular ectasias which are known to be more common in the right colon. Parks estimated that 10% to 25% of patients with diverticular disease will develop an inflammatory complication, which can cause major difficulties. In a study of 294 asymptomatic patients followed up for an average of 15 years, clinical diverticulitis developed in 25%, obstruction in 5%, clinical perforation in 5%, and significant hemorrhage in 5% (66). In another study of 503 patients with diverticular disease followed up for 18 years, only two required operation (67). The author suggests that at least 10% of patients will become symptomatic within five years, 25% in 6 to 10 years, and 37% by 11 to 18 years after diagnosis.

In terms of duration of symptoms, one-half of the patients with diverticular disease are in good health until approximately 1 month before presentation, and three-quarters have symptoms for less than 1 year. Patients who present with serious complications may be asymptomatic until hours before admission. The correlation between symptoms and pathologic findings is poor, for one-third of resected specimens fail to show evidence of inflammation. Analysis of the prognosis relative to symptoms reveals that pain confined to the left lower quadrant is associated with a better prognosis than widespread pain. There is no correlation between the site of pain and the number or location of diverticula. Cases involving disturbance of bowel habit have an immediate and a long-term prognosis that are less favorable. Nausea, vomiting, persistent urinary symptoms, and a palpable mass are associated with a high complication rate and a less favorable prognosis.

The initial attack in many patients with inflammatory diverticular disease will respond to bowel rest and broad-spectrum antibiotics. One-third to two-thirds of patients will have recurrent attacks or continue to have symptoms. Approximately one-fourth of patients whose attack resolves after conservative treatment will require further hospital admission for recurrent episodes of inflammation. More than 70% will continue to have intermittent symptoms, and only 10% will remain symptom free after a second hospital admission for diverticulitis. Approximately half of the patients who require readmission because of a second attack do so within 1 year of the first attack, and 90% are admitted within 5 years.

The outcome of recurrent attacks is different. Medical treatment of recurrent disease is less effective than treatment of the presenting attack. The complication rate increases with subsequent attacks: 23% for one attack and 58% for more than one attack. Although the addition of unprocessed bran to the diet of patients with diverticular disease will reduce pain in approximately 80% of patients, it has not been shown that such a diet reduces the incidence of inflammatory attacks.

Farmakis et al. (68) reported on the natural history of complicated diverticular disease based on details of 300 patients entered into a national audit. Questionnaires were sent to the general practitioners of 176 patients with this condition, 5 years after hospital admission; 120 responded. Of these 120 patients, 10 died from recurrent complicated diverticular disease, 29 died from other disorders, and 81 remained alive. Forty of 110 patients (excluding those who died from recurrence) were still symptomatic or were so at the time of unrelated death. Thirty-nine patients developed a severe complication after the index admission, 14 of who had the same complication initially. Of the 77 patients initially managed by sigmoid resection, only two developed recurrent complications compared with 37 of 43 managed conservatively. Of the 10 patients who died from recurrent diverticular disease, nine had not undergone sigmoid colectomy at or after the original admission. These data argue for interval sigmoid colectomy in most patients who initially present to hospital with complicated diverticular disease to prevent the later development of potentially lethal complications.

Makela et al. (69) reviewed the outcome of 366 patients admitted with acute diverticulitis. There were significantly more males than females in the age group less than 50 years, and young males underwent operative treatment during the first treatment period more frequently than the others. Young patients were operated on without mortality and all their temporary colostomies were closed. Older patients died more often of diseases unrelated to the diverticular disease during the years after the first episode of acute diverticulitis. Recurrences of diverticular diseases developed in 22% of patients and they were significantly more common in patients less than 50 years than in the older age groups. Males less than 50 years often developed complications of diverticular disease after two hospital admissions. Based on their data, they recommend resection for all patients after two episodes of acute diverticulitis that resolves after conservative treatment with antibiotics.

Of all patients with diverticula, approximately 1% will require operative treatment (70). An estimated 15% to 30% of patients needing hospital admission require operation (3). Ryan reported this number to be 25% (52). Follow-up studies reveal that 2% to 10% of these patients will have troublesome symptoms or a major recurrence and that up to 25% will have minor symptoms. Of the patients who have residual diverticula, more than 80% will be asymptomatic, only rarely will such patients require further resection. Development of diverticula after resection of the affected segment does not often occur if there has been an adequate resection of the distal bowel with the thickened muscle. The establishment of a colostomy, although a potentially helpful measure in the resolution of inflammation, in no way eliminates the possibility of acute exacerbation of the disease. Closure of a colostomy without resection is associated with an inordinately high recrudescence rate (approximately 65–75%) and is seldom justified today. The immediate risk to life for the elective operation is 2% to 3% and in an emergency situation is 10% to 12%.

Ambrosetti et al. (71) evaluated immediate and late outcomes of acute left colonic diverticulitis and correlated them with age. Diagnosis relied on results of operation, computed tomography (CT), and Gastrografin enema. Two hundred twenty-six patients were urgently hospitalized for acute left colonic diverticulitis. Twenty-one percent were younger than 50 years. Twenty-nine percent were operated on during their first hospitalization. The remaining patients treated conservatively underwent CT and an enema within 72 hours of admission. Thirty-three percent of patients older than 50 years required operation during their first attack, compared with 15% younger than 50 years, although on CT severe diverticulitis was found in 26% of patients older than 50 years and in 37% of patients younger than 50 years. Of the patients treated conservatively, 28% younger than 50 years experienced recurrences or complications after their first discharge compared with 13% older than 50 years. The authors concluded patients younger than 50 years were significantly more prone to recurrences and complications after conservative treatment of their diverticulitis, whereas older patients required operation significantly more often during their first hospitalization. However, recurrences are not more severe than first attacks and respond favorably to conservative measures.

Chautems et al. (72) evaluated the long-term natural history of sigmoid diverticulitis in 118 patients treated non-operatively after a first acute episode. Patients had a poor outcome if they had persisting or recurring diverticulitis diagnosed by CT. Diverticulitis was graded mild or severe on CT according to Ambrosetti's criteria. They investigated whether young age ($\leq$50 years old) and severe diverticulitis were risk factors for a poor outcome. With a median follow-up of 9.5 years, 80 patients had no complications and 38 had remote complications. The incidence of remote complications was the highest (54% at five years) for young patients with severe diverticulitis on CT and the lowest (19% at five years) for older patients with mild disease. Young age and severe diverticulitis taken separately were both statistically significant factors of poor outcome. They proposed that after a first acute episode of diverticulitis treated non-operatively, elective colectomy should be offered to young patients ($\leq$50 years old) with severe diverticulitis on CT.

Using a statewide administrative database and identifying all patients hospitalized non-electively for diverticulitis, Anaya and Flum (73) determined the lifetime risk of emergency colectomy/colostomy for patients with diverticulitis. A total of 25,058 patients (mean age 69 years, 60% females) were hospitalized for an initial episode of diverticulitis. Of the 20,136 patients treated without initial operation, 19% had recurrences, with younger patients (< 50 years) more likely to have a recurrence than older patients (27% vs. 17%). While only 5.5% of patients had recurrent hospitalizations during which an emergency colectomy/colostomy was performed, it occurred more commonly in younger patients (7.5% vs. 5%). The adjusted hazard ratio for emergency colectomy/colostomy in younger patients was 39% higher than in older patients (hazard ratio 1.39). Among all patients, the adjusted hazard ratio for emergency colectomy/colostomy was 2.2 times higher than each subsequent admission (hazard ratio 2.2). The predicted probability of emergency colectomy/colostomy was highest in younger patients with multiple rehospitalizations. They concluded that age and number of recurrent events were associated with the risk of emergency colectomy/colostomy after successful nonoperative management in patients with diverticulitis and individualization of recommendations regarding elective colectomy based on these factors may be appropriate.

The association of hiatal hernia, cholelithiasis, and diverticular disease of the colon (Saint's triad) has been

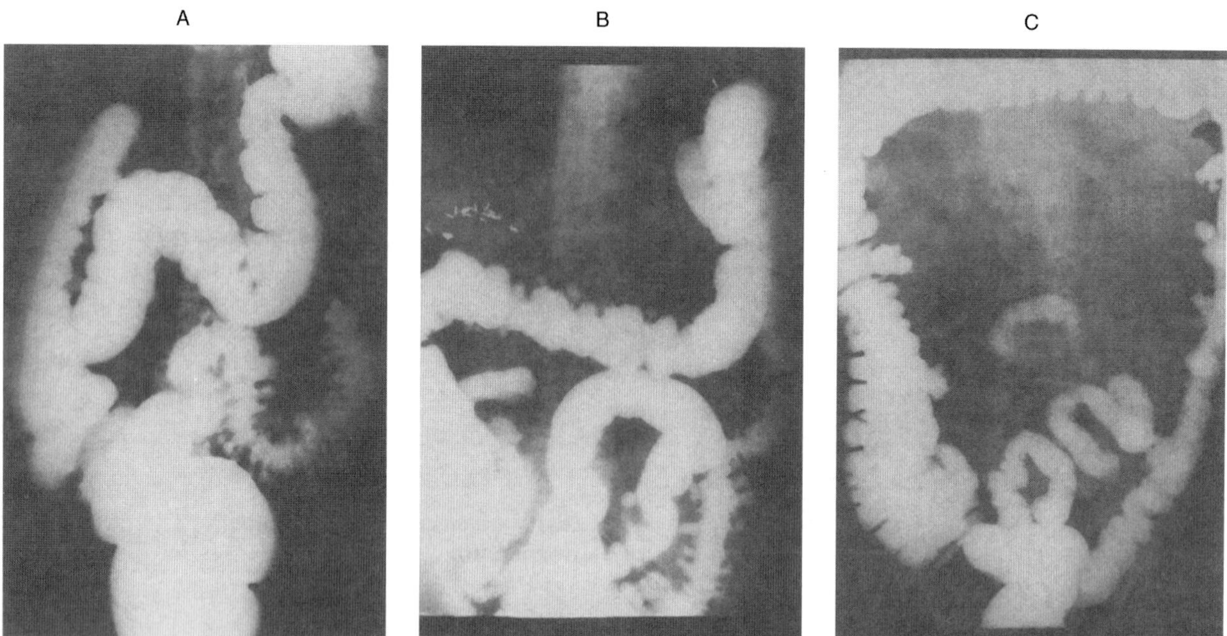

FIGURE 6 ■ (**A**) Barium enema demonstrating extensive sigmoid diverticular disease. (**B**) Barium enema showing diverticular disease involving entire colon. (**C**) Barium enema indicating wide-mouth diverticula.

estimated to be 3% to 6%. It has been suggested that irritable bowel syndrome is related to diverticular disease of the colon and may, indeed, be a prodromal phase of the disease, but reports have failed to demonstrate a clear association. Although diverticular disease and carcinoma of the colon are seen in the same patient population, no causal relationship has been found between the two.

CLINICAL MANIFESTATIONS

SYMPTOMS

Most often, uncomplicated diverticular disease is asymptomatic, and it may be discovered incidentally during a barium enema examination. Some patients may experience ill-defined left-sided abdominal discomfort located most often in the left lower quadrant. Associated symptoms of anorexia, flatulence, nausea, and alteration in bowel habits may occur. The patient's history may reveal passage of "rabbit-ball" stools or attacks of diarrhea. The diagnosis is often made during the investigation of patients with irritable bowel syndrome. Rectal bleeding is uncommon in patients with uncomplicated diverticular disease (74). Patients with a history of rectal bleeding in whom a barium study has shown only diverticular disease should be investigated further as though the diverticula were not present. Some patients will present with a history of narrow-caliber stools, which suggests a neoplasm, but subsequent investigation reveals diverticular disease.

PHYSICAL EXAMINATION

In patients with diverticulosis, no abnormal physical signs will be found during an abdominal examination. Similarly, digital rectal examination is unrevealing. A rigid sigmoidoscopic examination also usually is not revealing, because examination beyond the rectosigmoid junction often is impossible. Only rarely can the mouths of diverticula be seen.

DIAGNOSIS

In the absence of specific symptoms and signs, the diagnosis is most often established through a barium enema examination, which is also the best way to determine the extent and severity of the diverticulosis. Diverticula may be distributed throughout the entire colon, but it is the left colon, particularly the sigmoid, that is most often affected (Fig. 6). The size and shape of the diverticula vary greatly. A common radiologic finding is some degree of colonic spasm, that in its grossest form may produce a characteristic zigzag appearance (Fig. 7). In the chronic state, the lumen may become stenotic and the bowel will be more

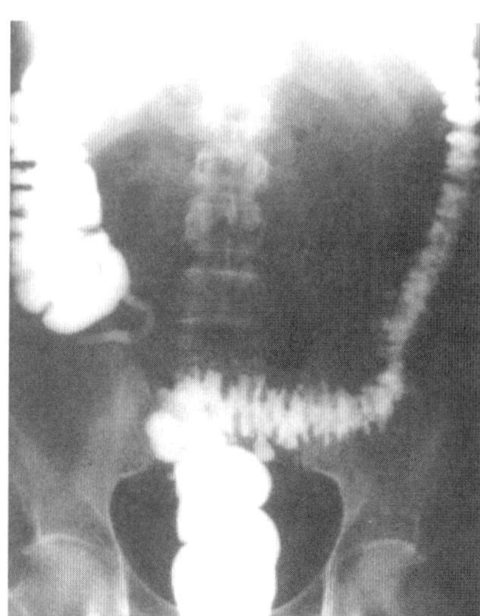

FIGURE 7 ■ Area of spasm with a zigzag appearance in sigmoid colon.

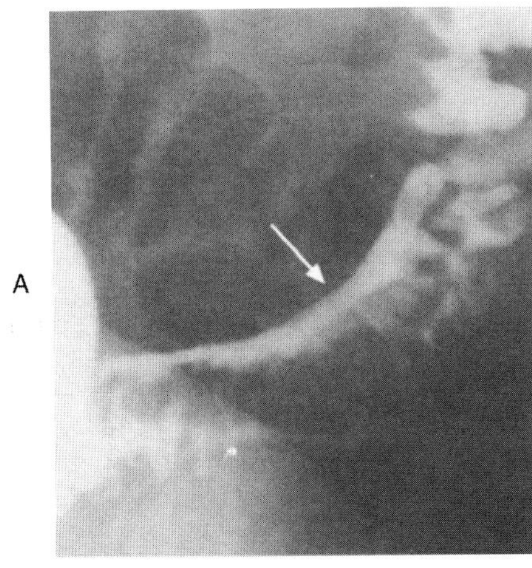

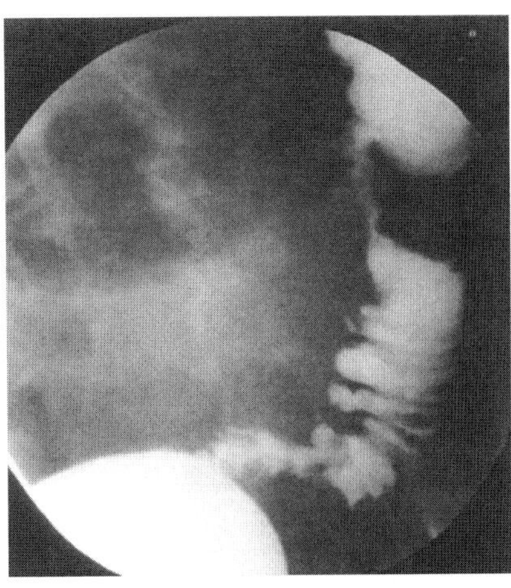

FIGURE 8 ■ (**A**) Extended area of stenosis with a long intramural sinus tract. (**B**) Two areas of narrowing: one in the sigmoid and one in the mid-descending colon, each representing strictures secondary to diverticulitis.

rigid (Fig. 8A) (75). Simultaneous sites of narrowing may occur (Fig. 8B). Fistulas to adjacent viscera such as the bladder may be seen (Fig. 9). The use of the flexible sigmoidoscope may allow identification of the presence of sigmoid diverticular disease. Patients who present with symptoms suggestive of bowel disease may undergo colonoscopic examination at which time the diagnosis also may be made but colonoscopy may overlook minor degrees of diverticulosis (Fig. 10). Colonoscopy has proved to be a useful tool in differentiating diverticular disease from carcinoma. However, the endoscopist must be certain that the area of narrowing has been traversed to rule out a malignancy.

A review of the literature by Hunt (76) showed that carcinoma was identified in 17% of 125 patients with complicated diverticular disease, and additional diagnosis was made in 32%. The cecum was reached in 61%. The presence of bleeding strongly suggested the presence of a concomitant lesion. In a group of 135 patients with persistent bleeding, in whom barium enema examination showed only diverticular disease, 11% had carcinoma, and an additional diagnosis was made in 37%.

Boulos et al. (77) carried out colonoscopy in 65 patients in whom a double-contrast barium enema for bowel symptoms had shown sigmoid diverticular disease. In 19 patients, the barium enema examination had shown neoplastic lesions (polyps in 17 and carcinoma in two), but colonoscopy showed no polyp in 9 of the 17 patients. In one, a carcinoma, not a polyp, was found, and of the two carcinomas, only one was confirmed. In 46 patients, the barium enema showed diverticular disease only, but colonoscopy revealed polyps in 8 patients and carcinoma in 3. Thus in 35% of patients, conclusions based on the barium enema examination were inaccurate. Colonoscopy revealed neoplastic lesions in 31%, an incidence that the authors believe to be great enough to recommend the use of routine colonoscopy in patients with symptomatic diverticular disease, especially those with rectal bleeding.

Kewenter et al. (74) found that minor rectal bleeding was uncommon in patients with uncomplicated diverticular disease, and reported that patients with a history of rectal bleeding in whom a barium enema showed diverticular disease should be investigated as though the diverticula were not present.

Schreyer et al. (78) evaluated the feasibility of magnetic resonance imaging (MRI)-based colonography to assess 14 consecutive patients with clinically suspected diverticulitis. All patients underwent abdominal CT as gold standard. Inflammation as judged by CT was identically assessed on an MRI; additionally, the 3-D models gave a comprehensive image for surgical planning. This comprehensive 3-D model could replace presurgical planning barium enema, with concurrent assessment of the residual colon.

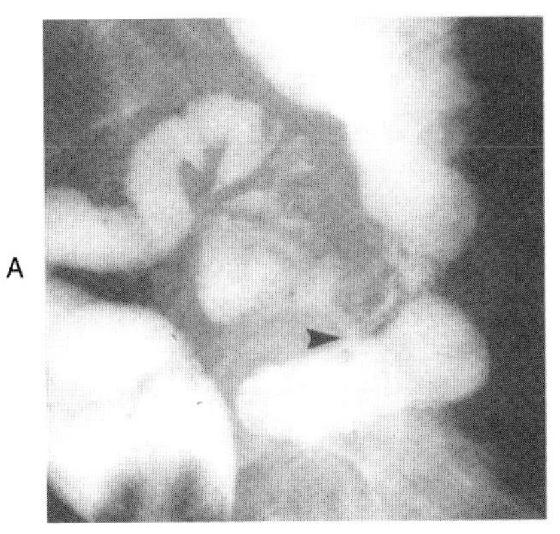

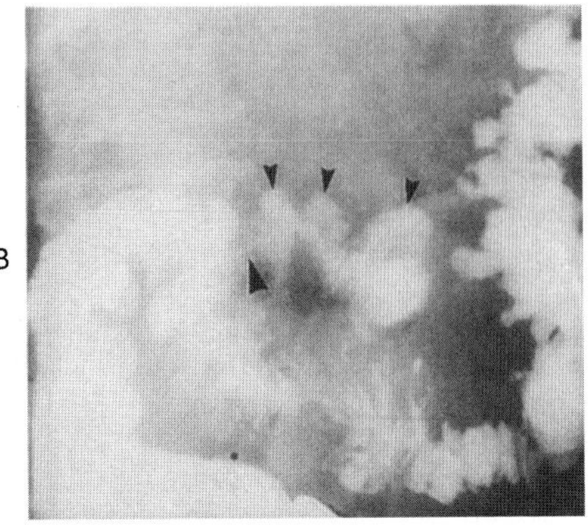

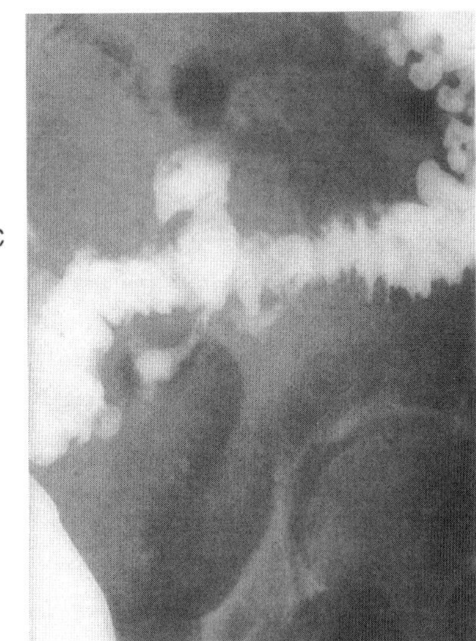

FIGURE 9 ■ (**A**) Colovesical fistula (communication denoted by arrow). (**B**) Coloenteric fistula (communication denoted by arrows). (**C**) Walled-off pericolic abscess with colovaginal fistula.

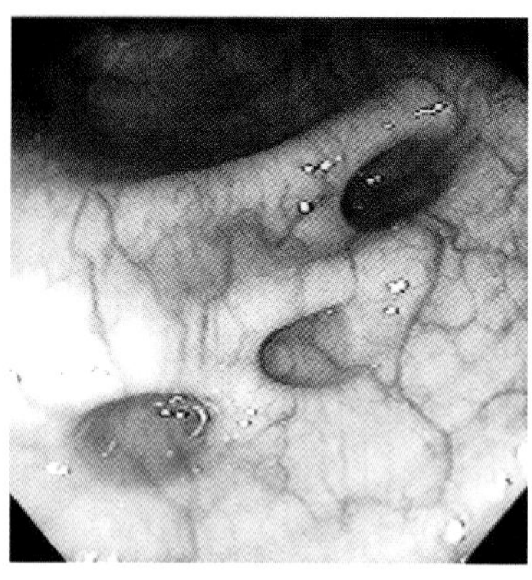

FIGURE 10 ■ Colonoscopic appearance of a diverticulum.

■ DIFFERENTIAL DIAGNOSIS

Depending on the presenting symptom complex, the differential diagnosis of diverticular disease may be quite lengthy. Clearly, the most important entity is carcinoma. A number of radiologic features have been considered in establishing the differential diagnosis. For example, in a patient with diverticular disease, the affected segment of bowel is often longer than in one with carcinoma. The transition from normal to diseased bowel with diverticular disease is more gradual than with carcinoma, in which it is usually abrupt. With diverticular disease, the mucosa is preserved, but it is destroyed in carcinoma. The presence of diverticula in an area of colonic narrowing favors the diagnosis of diverticular disease but in no way rules out the presence of a concomitant carcinoma. Despite these points of differentiation, radiologic distinction between diverticular disease and carcinoma may be impossible (Figs. 11 and 12). In a review of barium enema studies of 73 patients with diverticular disease of the colon, with and without neoplasms, Schnyder et al. (79) concluded that radiologic recognition of an associated neoplasm in a colon with diverticular disease can be made correctly only approximately half the time. Even during laparotomy, it may be difficult to differentiate the two entities.

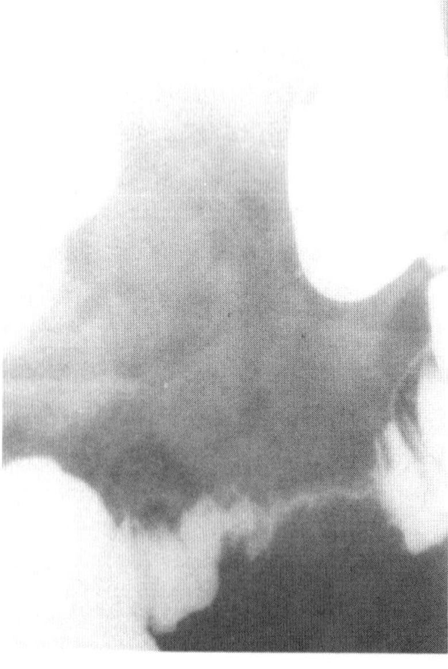

FIGURE 11 ■ Stricture at junction of sigmoid and descending colon. Mucosa is intact. Only a single diverticulum is seen. Patient had only diverticular disease.

Patients with irritable bowel syndrome present with intestinal symptoms, but investigations fail to reveal any anatomic abnormalities. It has been suggested that irritable bowel syndrome may precede the development of diverticular disease and represents one end of the spectrum of a motility disorder, but no evidence has been found for a causal relationship between the two conditions. The symptoms in some patients with localized Crohn's disease may mimic those of diverticulitis. Associated symptoms of diarrhea, rectal bleeding, weight loss, and perianal disease would suggest Crohn's disease. Sigmoidoscopic examination may not be helpful because the rectum may be spared in Crohn's disease. Indeed, the two conditions may coexist. Berman et al. (80) found that patients who required a second colonic resection for diverticulitis had Crohn's disease and diverticulitis.

Patients with ischemic colitis usually present with bloody diarrhea and abdominal pain. A barium enema will demonstrate thumbprinting to establish the diagnosis.

The distinction between colonic diverticula and polyps is usually readily apparent on an air-contrast examination. On rare occasions, a diverticulum may be responsible for an intraluminal projection on barium enema, resulting in diagnostic confusion. One such abnormality is an inverted diverticulum. In one study, inverted diverticula appeared as broad-based, smooth, sessile polyps measuring 1.5 to 2.0 cm with a characteristic central umbilication and/or evidence of barium within the polyp (81). This phenomenon may also be observed at endoscopy and inadvertent diverticulectomy has been performed (82,83) with its potential for perforation and bleeding.

Depending on the modes of presentation, other entities that may be included in the differential diagnosis are ulcerative colitis, appendicitis, pelvic inflammatory disease, ureteral colic, small bowel obstruction, and endometriosis. With respect to age, the differential diagnosis in the elderly might include ischemia, carcinoma, volvulus, obstruction, penetrating ulcer, and nephrolithiasis/urosepsis. In young and middle-aged individuals, diagnoses to entertain include appendicitis, salpingitis, inflammatory bowel disease, penetrating ulcer, and urosepsis.

■ TREATMENT

■ DIET

Because patients with diverticular disease have increased intraluminal pressures, a high-fiber diet has been recommended for them. A high-bulk diet reduces colonic pressure and removes the presumed underlying disorder in diverticular disease. Thompson and Patel (84) reviewed the results of seven placebo-controlled trials of bran and bulking agents in the treatment of diverticular disease. From these studies, it was apparent that ingestion of 20 to 30 g of bran is necessary to achieve a therapeutic effect. Taylor and Duthie (47) found that bran tablets were effective in producing a significant increase in stool weight, a decrease in transit time, and reversion of an abnormal rapid electric rhythm in colonic smooth muscle from 80% to 40%. The dose as well as the length of time the substance is

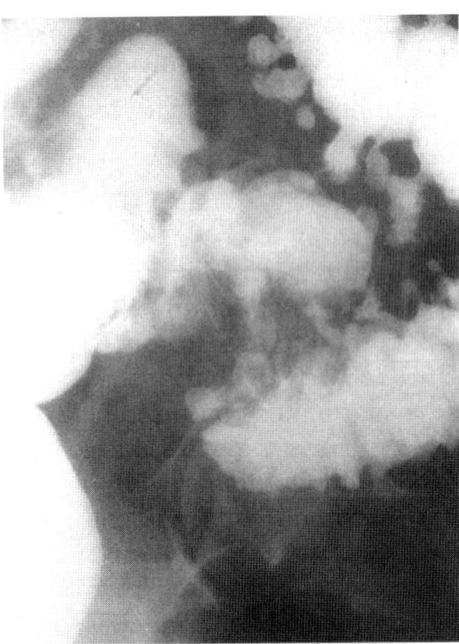

FIGURE 12 ■ Narrowed mid-sigmoid colon with question of overhanging edges and destroyed mucosa suspicious of carcinoma. Patient proved to have diverticular disease.

administered seems to be important. Although the trials failed to show a clear-cut benefit in every case, it is logical to advise the use of bran in patients with symptomatic uncomplicated diverticular disease. Coarse bran has a more significant effect on stool-weight, speeds transit time, and reduces intraluminal pressure in the colon when compared to fine bran (85).

Although epidemiologic evidence suggests that a high-fiber diet prevents the formation of diverticula, there is little evidence that once diverticula are formed the use of bran and bulking agents will prevent the complications of diverticular disease. An exception to this belief is the study by Hyland and Taylor (86), suggesting that among those who already have diverticula complications and recurrences of diverticulitis are reduced with a high-fiber diet. Although advocated by some, the elimination of foods with seeds is of questionable value.

■ MEDICATION

Bulk-Forming Agents

Diets high in fiber may control the symptoms of diverticular disease effectively. Examples of high-fiber foods are listed in Table 9 of Chapter 33. Because many patients find a high-fiber diet unpalatable, the addition of bulk-forming agents provides a suitable substitute. Many proprietary preparations contain psyllium, and their addition to the diet can provide an effective supplement.

Analgesics

Analgesics, when prescribed, should be non-constipating. Pentazocine reduces the motility of the sigmoid colon in patients with diverticular disease while relieving pain (87). However, meperidine (Demerol) is probably the agent of choice because it decreases intraluminal pressure and is less likely to produce disorientation (3). Morphine should not be used because it increases intracolonic pressure (44).

Anticholinergics

The recommendation for using anticholinergic agents is based on the observed hypermotility of the sigmoid colon in many symptomatic patients with diverticular disease; however, their value has never been documented clearly.

Antibiotics

Papi et al. (88) conducted a double-blind, placebo-controlled trial to determine the efficacy of long-term intermittent administration of a poorly absorbed antibiotic in obtaining symptomatic relief in uncomplicated diverticular disease of the colon. A series of 168 patients received either a fiber supplement (glucomannan, 2 g/day) plus rifaximin, 400 mg twice a day (a rifamycin derivate with broad-spectrum bacterial activity including anaerobes), for seven days every month (84 patients), or glucomannan, 2 g/day, plus placebo, two tablets twice a day for seven days every month (84 patients). After 12 months, 70% of patients treated with rifaximin were symptom free or mildly symptomatic compared to 40% in the placebo group. Symptoms such as bloating and abdominal pain or discomfort were primarily affected by the antibiotic treatment. No advantage was accrued in preventing diverticulitis. Latella et al. (89) examined the efficacy of cyclic long-term administration of rifaximin, in obtaining symptom relief in patients with uncomplicated diverticular disease, and compared the incidence of episodes of diverticulitis in the group treated with rifaximin to that in a group receiving fiber supplementation alone. In a multicenter prospective open trial, 968 outpatients with uncomplicated symptomatic diverticular disease were randomized to either fiber supplementation with 4 g/day glucomannan plus 400 mg rifaximin twice daily for seven days every month ($n = 558$) or 4 g/day glucomannan alone ($n = 346$). After 12 months, the group treated with glucomannan and rifaximin showed fewer symptoms (abdominal pain/discomfort, bloating, tenesmus, diarrhea, abdominal tenderness) and a lower global symptomatic score. Overall, 56.5% of the patients treated with glucomannan and rifaximin and 29.2% of those treated with glucomannan alone were asymptomatic at 12 months. The rate of complications (diverticulitis and rectal bleeding) was 1.34% in the rifaximin and glucomannan group and 3.22% in the glucomannan alone group.

Brandimarte and Tursi (90) investigated the effectiveness of the combination of rifaximin/mesalazine (Asacol, Mesasal, Pentasa, Salofalk) followed by mesalazine alone to evaluate tolerability and effectiveness in symptomatic remission in 90 consecutive patients with symptomatic uncomplicated diverticular disease. Symptoms assessed, scoring them on a quantitative scale, included constipation, diarrhea, abdominal pain, rectal bleeding, and mucus with stool. All patients were treated with 800 mg/day rifaximin plus 2.4 g a day mesalazine for 10 days, followed by 1.6 g / day mesalazine for 8 weeks. This study was completed by 95.6% of patients. The total score decreased from 1439 to 44. After the eighth week of treatment, 81% of patients were completely asymptomatic with mesalazine alone (total symptomatic score: 0), while 18.6% showed only slight symptoms (total score: 44). After 4 and 6 weeks of treatment, 2% of patients showed recurrence of diverticulitis with mesalazine alone and 2% were withdrawn from the study for diarrhea after starting mesalazine. Their results showed that rifaximin/mesalazine followed by mesalazine alone is effective in resolving symptoms in patients with symptomatic uncomplicated diverticular disease. Further confirmation of this finding will be necessary before general recommendations can be made for its adoption.

■ OPERATION

Indications

At one time, operation for diverticular disease was reserved solely for treating the complications of the disease: perforation, development of an abscess, fistula formation, obstruction, and massive hemorrhage. Because operations for complicated diverticular disease have higher operative morbidity and mortality rates, some surgeons recommend a more aggressive attitude toward elective operations.

Certain valid indications for elective resection have evolved. Factors affecting the decision of whether to recommend a resection include the patient's age, general health, and life expectancy; the severity of the episode (or episodes); and the matter of urinary tract involvement. Patients who suffer repeated attacks of diverticulitis (two or more) are candidates for operation, but the absolute number is not the sole criterion. The severity of the attack (did it require hospitalization?), the interval between attacks (e.g., every 9 months or 9 years?), the association of urinary symptoms, and the bona fide nature of the attack (or was it simply transient left lower quadrant pain?) must be considered. Patients with a persistent tender mass are candidates for operation. Patients with persistent symptoms attributed to colonic dysfunction associated with left lower quadrant discomfort are possible candidates for resection; however, caution must be exercised in recommending resection for this group of patients because the surgeon should feel confident that these symptoms are attributable to the diverticular disease. Patients with a previous attack of diverticulitis and residual radiologic evidence of a perforation or abscess that had successfully been treated nonoperatively are candidates for resection. A narrowed or marked deformity of the sigmoid colon on barium enema examination along with the inability to exclude coexisting carcinoma is another valid criterion that is less frequently applicable today with the availability of colonoscopic assessment. Patients with persistent urinary symptoms suggestive of an impending colovesical fistula are also candidates. Elective resection has been advised after only one attack of diverticulitis, especially if the patient is less than 55 years or if there is radiologic evidence of a leak or obstruction (91,92). However, one must be circumspect about advising operation after only one episode of acute diverticulitis, even for the young patient.

Patients who have undergone transplantation are subject to a variety of colonic complications, including perforated diverticulitis (93). A higher percentage of renal transplant patients develop free perforation as opposed to walled-off perforation because of the use of immunosuppressive agents and steroids. Therefore, it is recommended that such patients with only one attack but who require chronic immunosuppressive therapy undergo early operative treatment, and it has even been suggested that patients with extensive diverticular disease undergo elective resection before transplantation.

Dominguez Fernandez et al. (94) noted that the incidence of diverticulosis is especially high among patients with autosomal dominant polycystic kidney disease. They evaluated the prevalence of diverticulosis in these patients awaiting renal transplantation and the incidence of bowel perforation following allogenic kidney transplantation due to polycystic kidney disease. There were 46 patients who underwent transplantation for this disease. There was one patient who developed a sigmoid perforation under postoperative immunosuppression. Surgical treatment was a Hartmann's procedure. A sigmoid resection was necessary in one patient due to diverticulitis without perforation. They did not find a higher prevalence of diverticulosis with autosomal polycystic kidney disease nor did they see a higher incidence of sigmoid perforation during post-transplant immunosuppression in their study.

Although much has been written on the subject, absolute indications for elective resection in diverticular disease are lacking. For the most part, a consensus does exist regarding patients who have sustained two attacks of diverticulitis. Practice parameters for the treatment of sigmoid diverticulitis published by the American Society of Colon and Rectal Surgeons recommend resection after two attacks of uncomplicated diverticulitis (95). For patients with complicated diverticulitis defined as the development of an abscess or a fistula, resection is recommended after one attack. The Practice Parameters Committee of the American College of Gastroenterology recommend that elective (prophylactic) surgery may be reasonable in patients with recurrent attacks of diverticulitis, patients with complicated disease (e.g., fistulas and abscess), or in young or immunosuppressed patients (96). They further state that as diverticulitis may recur in as few as one of four patients, surgery is not generally indicated after a single uncomplicated episode. The Scientific Committee of the European Association for Endoscopic Surgery held a consensus development conference on the diagnosis and treatment of diverticular disease and recommended that after two attacks of diverticular disease, elective resection should be considered. The Committee also recommended surgery for patients in whom concomitant carcinoma cannot be excluded and those with chronic complications (fistula, stenosis, or bleeding).

Janes et al. (97) performed a medline literature search on surgery for diverticular disease. They found most people with diverticulosis to be asymptomatic. Diverticular disease occurs in over 25% of the population, increasing with age. After one episode of diverticulitis, one-third of patients have recurrent symptoms; after a second episode, a further third have a subsequent episode. Perforation is commonest during the first episode of acute diverticulitis. After recovering from an episode of diverticulitis, the risk of an individual requiring an urgent Hartmann's procedure is 1 in 2000 patient-years of follow-up. Surgery for diverticular disease has a high complication rate and 25% of patients have ongoing symptoms after bowel resection. Based on these findings, they concluded there is no evidence to support the idea that elective surgery should follow two attacks of diverticulitis.

An even less aggressive approach has been recommended. Richards and Hammitt (98) used a Markov model to compare the costs and outcomes of performing surgery after one, two, or three uncomplicated attacks of uncomplicated diverticulitis. The optimum timing of surgery in terms of cost effectiveness is unknown. They found that surgery after the third attack is cost saving, yielding more years of life and quality-adjusted life years at a lower cost than the other two strategies, and hence recommend prophylactic resection after the third attack of diverticulitis.

Determining the optimal strategy for elective colectomy in patients with diverticular disease involves a balance of the morbidity, mortality, cost, and quality of life associated with both elective and expectant management. Salem et al. (99) used decision and cost analysis to simulate the clinical and economic outcomes after recovery from an episode of nonsurgically treated diverticulitis to determine the preferable management strategy. A Markov model was constructed to evaluate lifetime risks of death and colostomy, care costs, and quality of life associated with elective colectomy after subsequent episodes of diverticulitis. Performing colectomy after the fourth rather than the second episode in patients older than 50 years resulted in 0.5% fewer deaths, 0.7% fewer colostomies, and saved US $1035 per patient. In younger patients, performing colectomy after the fourth episode, when compared with after the first episode, resulted in 0.1% fewer deaths and 2% fewer colostomies, and saved US $5429 per patient. Expectant management through three recurrent episodes with elective colectomy after the fourth episode was the dominant strategy across the full range of variables tested.

Chapman et al. (100) also thought it is time to rethink the "rules." They conducted a study to update our understanding of morbidity, mortality, characteristics, and outcomes of 337 patients with complicated diverticular disease. The mean age of patients was 65 years and 70% had one or more comorbidities. A total of 46.6% had a history of at least one prior diverticulitis episode, whereas 53.4% presented with complicated diverticular disease as their first episode. Overall mortality was 6.5% (86.4% associated with perforation, 9.5% anastomotic leak, 4.5% patient managed nonoperatively). A total of 89.5% of the perforation patients who died had no history of diverticulitis. Steroid use was significantly associated with perforation rates as well as mortality. Comorbidities such as diabetes, collagen-vascular disease, and immune system compromise were also highly associated with death. Overall morbidity was 41.4%. Older age, gender, steroids, comorbidities, and perforation were significantly associated with morbidity. They concluded that the fact that the majority of patients presenting with complicated diverticular disease as their first episode calls into question the current practice of elective resection as a stratagem for reducing mortality. Immunocompromised patients may benefit from early resection.

The exact timing for elective operation has been clouded with more recent publications, and it would appear that sound clinical judgment plays a key role in the decision-making process.

Preparation of Patient

The general preparation and bowel preparation, both mechanical and antibiotic, are discussed in Chapter 4.

Principles of Resection

Changing Management

Rodkey and Welch (10) reviewed the changing patterns in the operative treatment of 1244 cases of diverticular disease at the Massachusetts General Hospital in Boston from 1911 to 1983. The major trends they noted included (i) a decrease in hospital admissions but a sustained number of operations; (ii) the increased severity of disease in hospitalized patients as manifested by an increased percentage of patients with immunosuppression and other diseases and by an increased number of patients with sepsis and generalized peritonitis; (iii) an increased percentage of cases with one-stage resection and anastomosis; and (iv) the finding that in patients with generalized peritonitis resection of the perforated segment at the time of the original operation resulted in the lowest mortality rate.

Over the most recent 20-year period of the study, 17.7% of 362 patients diagnosed with diverticulitis underwent operation. The trend toward a one-stage procedure was evident, regardless of the indication for operation. The authors compared operative procedures for various indications in the two most recent decades, 1964 to 1973 and 1974 to 1983. For example, in cases of a pericolic abscess, a one-stage resection and anastomosis were performed in 92% of cases, but in the preceding decade, it was used in only 64% of the cases. For patients with a perforation and pelvic abscess, a one-stage resection and anastomosis were performed in 47% of cases but in only 11% in the previous decade. Among patients operated on for generalized peritonitis, the primary focus of disease was excised at the primary operation in 69% of cases but in only 6% in the previous decade. The mortality rate was reduced from 35% in the first decade to 22% in the second. In patients with sepsis, who had the primary focus excised during the initial operation, the average hospitalization was 30 days, and morbidity was 57 days; when the primary focus was not excised during the initial operation, the figures were 56 days and 232 days, respectively. When colonic obstruction was the indication for operation, a one-stage resection and anastomosis were performed in 72% of cases, but these procedures were performed in only 30% during the prior decade. Eleven percent of patients with a fistula had a one-stage operation in the first decade and 35% in the second decade. When massive colonic bleeding was the main indication for operation, segmental resection was performed when the bleeding point was identified, and subtotal colectomy was performed when it was not identified. For patients in whom chronic pain was the indication for operation, only 75% of patients underwent a one-stage resection in the first decade, whereas in the most recent decade, 98% were treated by a single-stage operation.

Extent of Resection

For patients with a sound indication for operation, few surgeons would object to the concept of performing resection and primary anastomosis for uncomplicated diverticular disease.

The exact extent of the resection has varied from surgeon to surgeon, however. Certain principles should be adopted. Ideally, the entire thickened contracted segment, not just the part involved in the inflammatory process, should be resected, and an anastomosis should not be performed in thickened bowel. It also is generally agreed that every diverticulum does not require resection. Distally, diverticular disease does not usually involve the rectum, so the proximal rectum is the distal extent. Follow-up of patients with previous resection has revealed that recurrent diverticulitis in diverticula proximal to the sigmoid is uncommon.

A review by Benn et al. (101) included 501 patients who underwent elective resection for sigmoid diverticular disease and allowed the establishment of principles to determine the extent of resection (102). As revealed in the literature, overall recurrent diverticulitis develops in 7% of patients, and 20% of these patients require reoperation. In these studies, symptoms and signs of recurrent diverticulitis developed in 10.4% of patients; in 12.5% of them, the sigmoid colon had been used for the distal margin of anastomosis, and in 6.7% of them the rectum had been used. Barium enema studies performed in 61 of these patients 5 to 9 years after resection revealed progression of diverticula in 14.7%. The lowest incidence of recurrence was found when the descending colon was anastomosed to the upper rectum. Reoperation was required in 3.4% of patients in whom the sigmoid colon was used as the distal anastomotic site and in 2.2% of those in whom the rectum was used. The authors therefore concluded that the entire distal sigmoid colon should be removed during resection for diverticular disease. Barium enemas performed in 43% of the patients after resection revealed diverticula in 71% of that group.

From a purely technical point of view, if the descending colon is riddled with diverticula, common sense dictates that the anastomosis should be created through the distal transverse colon to avoid a difficult or hazardous anastomosis. The presence of an occasional diverticulum may be a nuisance but should not create a significant problem. In patients with abundant pericolic fat, it may be difficult to identify the extent of the diverticular disease, so caution should be exercised in the selection of the proximal line of resection.

Another technical point regarding the blood supply appears to be important. Tocchi et al. (103) recommend presentation of the inferior mesenteric artery in colorectal resections for complicated diverticular disease in order to reduce the risk of leakage of a colorectal anastomosis. They randomized 86 patients in a group in which the integrity of the inferior mesenteric artery was preserved and a group of 77 patients in which the inferior mesenteric artery was divided at its origin. Operative time was superior in the inferior mesenteric artery preserved group. Morbidity and mortality were similar in both groups, being 17.4% and 1.1% in the group with preservation of the inferior mesenteric artery compared with 19.5% and 1.3% in the group in which the mesentery artery was divided, respectively. However, a significant difference was noted when determining the incidence of radiologic dehiscence and clinical dehiscence, which was 18.1% and 10.4%, respectively, in the group in which the inferior mesenteric artery was divided, compared to 7% and 2%, respectively, in the group in which the inferior mesenteric artery was preserved. Furthermore, no strictures were noted in follow-up of patients in the group in which the inferior mesenteric artery was preserved but two strictures were detected in patients in whom the inferior mesenteric artery was divided.

Preoperative Ureteral Status and Ureteral Catheters

In the past, surgeons would usually obtain a preoperative intravenous pyelogram (IVP) to determine any obvious involvement of the ureter. This has mostly been supplanted by CT scanning; even if the ureter does not appear to be involved, it is wise to insert a left ureteral catheter before operation. Although placement of the catheter does not eliminate intraoperative injury to the ureter, it may prove helpful during the dissection. Kyzer and Gordon (104) studied the necessity for preoperative ureteral catheter insertion for colorectal operations. To determine what complications might be associated with ureteral catheter use, the charts of all patients undergoing ureteral catheterization in combination with colorectal procedures were reviewed. The indications for operation, the presence or absence of urinary tract symptoms, and IVP findings (if performed) were recorded. The length of time for the procedure, size and number of catheters, and complications were noted. From the operative report, a retrospective grading of necessity for ureteral catheterization was assessed according to a scale from A to D. There were 120 ureteral catheterizations performed, bilaterally in 60% of cases. Complications included renal colic (1) oliguria (1), and anuria (2). Intraoperatively, one ureter was cut and one ureter tied, but this was recognized through palpation, and the ligature was removed. Retrospective grading deemed ureteral catheterization necessary in 27.5% of cases. The authors concluded that catheters are helpful in selected cases.

For patients with bilateral catheter insertion, complications can be reduced by ensuring urine output prior to removal of the second catheter.

Operative Options for Elective Situations

In unusual circumstances, the surgeon may choose an operation usually meant for a patient with complicated diverticular disease, but almost invariably, the selection for elective operation is resection and primary anastomosis.

Resection

On entry into the abdomen, the sigmoid colon may be found to be adherent to a variety of viscera and to the posterior and lateral walls. One of the first decisions to be made by the surgeon is whether or not the lesion is a carcinoma, because carcinoma would mandate a wider resection. The determination may be impossible, but when the surgeon is in doubt, the disease is probably inflammatory in nature. Careful and often tedious dissection is necessary to separate attached viscera. A "pinching" maneuver may be helpful to achieve separation. In doing so, it is not uncommon to enter a pericolic abscess, but this should not inhibit continued dissection. With adjacent viscera retracted, the sigmoid colon is then freed from the abdominal wall, with special care taken to protect the left ureter. In the event of dense fibrosis, the prior insertion of ureteral catheters, which can be palpated, may be most helpful. The inflammatory process rarely extends toward the rectum; consequently, a soft, pliable portion of proximal rectum can be prepared for the distal anastomosis. Proximally the anastomosis should be extended at least to the descending colon. Some surgeons recommend routine mobilization of the splenic flexure, which is not necessary in all cases. The surgeon's choice determines the technique for reestablishing intestinal continuity, and the options are those described in Chapter 23 for resection of colon carcinoma.

Some specific difficulties related to diverticular operations may be encountered. If the sigmoid colon cannot be readily mobilized because of dense adhesions, dissection may be resorted to by transecting the colon early in the operation and retracting the sigmoid colon forward to expose the posterior abdominal wall. By dissecting along the wall of the sigmoid colon, the vital structures of the ureter and iliac vessels may be avoided. The colon is foreshortened; therefore, the surgeon must be certain that there is no tension on the anastomosis. The mesentery is shortened and thickened; thus extra caution may be required in securing the blood supply. The appendices epiploicae tend to be very fatty and must be cleared in preparation for anastomosis. In addition, because the diverticula enter the base of the fatty appendages, they must be considered. In many patients who undergo resection for diverticular disease, the muscle wall is considerably thickened and it is unwise to create an anastomosis through this thickened wall. If such thickening is identified at the level of transection, further excision is indicated. Occasionally the descending colon may contain such extensive diverticular disease that there is not a satisfactory portion through which an anastomosis can be performed. Under these circumstances, the surgeon should not hesitate to extend the resection proximally and anastomose the transverse colon to the upper rectum.

Results

Breen et al. (59) reported that 94% of 82 patients operated on for diverticular disease improved. Individuals from whom specimens with no histologic evidence of inflammatory changes were found were less likely to have favorable results. Preoperative factors that might help predict the likelihood of a less successful outcome include the presence of bowel management problems for more than one year and abdominal pain not localized to the left lower quadrant. Munson et al. (105) reported that a surprising 27% of patients who underwent resection continued to have symptoms. Moreaux and Vons (106) reviewed 177 consecutive patients operated on electively for diverticular disease of the sigmoid colon. The indications for operation were: colovesical fistula (12), suspicion of residual abscess (39), two or more previous attacks of acute inflammation (52), chronic symptoms (72), and suspicion of carcinoma (2). An abscess was found at operation in 76 patients (43%), and this was extracolic with local peritonitis in 52 patients (29%). An unsuspected abscess was found in 25 of the 72 patients operated on for chronic symptoms. Colonic resection with primary anastomosis was performed in 95% of the 177 patients, and in 94% of those 52 patients with an extracolic abscess. There were no postoperative deaths and no clinical anastomotic leakages. Long-term results were very good in 85% of the 177 patients and in 82% of the 72 patients operated on for chronic symptoms. The results of this series suggest that a one-stage procedure can be safely performed with some technical precautions in most patients operated on electively for diverticular disease, even if an extracolic abscess is found. The good long-term results in patients operated on for chronic symptoms suggest that such symptoms should be taken into account with respect to surgical indications.

Pessaux et al. (107) studied a total of 46 potential preoperative and intraoperative risk factors for mortality and morbidity in 582 patients who underwent elective sigmoid resection for diverticulitis. The operative mortality was 1.2% and the overall morbidity was 24.9%. Analysis revealed two statistically significant independent risk factors of mortality: age>75 years [odds ratio (OR)= 7.9] and obesity (OR = 5.2). The abdominal morbidity was 6.5%. The absence of antimicrobial prophylaxis administration with ceftriaxone was the only significant risk factor for abdominal morbidity. The extra-abdominal morbidity was 18.4%. Both chronic pulmonary disease (OR = 2.9) and cirrhosis (OR = 12) proved to be significant risk factors for extra-abdominal morbidity. Weight control prior to operation, routine administration of prophylactic preoperative antibiotics, and preoperative optimization of respiratory status of patients with chronic pulmonary disease could decrease the postoperative mortality and morbidity associated with elective sigmoid resection for diverticulitis.

Thaler et al. (108) evaluated variables on recurrence rates after sigmoid resection for diverticulitis. Recurrence after operation was defined as left lower quadrant pain, fever, and leucocytosis, with consistent CT and/or contrast enema findings on admission and after 6 weeks. Anastomosis level was based on muscle layer configuration (teniae coli) at the distal resection margin. There were 236 patients (105 females) with a mean age of 60.4 years available for follow-up at a mean of 67 months. The median duration of preoperative symptoms was 18 months. All but one patient (99%) had at least one admission before operation. Laparoscopic resection was performed on 59% of patients while open resection was performed on 41% of patients. The conversion rate was 13% and the 30-day complication rate was 23% with 0.4% 30-day mortality and a 2.1% reoperation rate. The splenic flexure was mobilized in 47% of patients. Anastomoses were fashioned by a stapler in 73% of patients and were anastomosed to the rectum in 72% of patients. Specimen length was 17.9 ± 5.9 cm with inflammation at the proximal margin in 14%. Recurrence developed in 5% of patients at a mean of 78 months, with reoperation in only one patient. The level of anastomosis was the only predictor recurrence. Patients with colosigmoid anastomoses had a four times higher risk of having a recurrence compared with patients with colorectal anastomoses.

Thorn et al. (65) reviewed the functional results after elective colonic resection in 75 consecutive patients. Major complications included anastomotic leakage, bleeding, and bowel obstruction in 13% of patients with a total complication rate of 33%. Recurrent diverticulitis developed in 8% of patients. Fifty patients classified their result as excellent or good. Functional symptoms or symptoms suggestive of irritable bowel syndrome before the operation, predicted a less successful result. Diverticular disease operations were hampered by postoperative complications but resulted, in most cases, in good functional outcome and a low rate of recurrent disease.

Horgan et al. (109) reported that patients with diverticular disease might present with chronic symptoms but never develop diverticulitis. They reviewed the outcome of surgical intervention in this subgroup of patients with atypical (smoldering) diverticular disease. Of 930 patients who underwent sigmoid resection for diverticular disease, 47 (5%) fit the inclusion criteria for smoldering diverticular disease and underwent sigmoid colectomy with primary anastomosis. A minimum of 12 months of follow-up was completed in 68% of these patients. Evidence of acute or chronic inflammatory changes was present in 76% of resected specimens. Complete resolution of symptoms occurred in 76.5% with 88% being pain free. They concluded that the diagnosis and presentation of atypical smoldering diverticular disease is an uncommon and poorly defined entity. However, sigmoid resection in this subgroup of patients is safe and is associated with resolution of symptoms in the majority of cases. The results of elective resection and primary anastomosis for a selected series of patients are tabulated in Table 3.

COMPLICATIONS

The frequency with which complications occur in patients with diverticular disease is impossible to determine. To use operative intervention as an index to the incidence would underestimate the frequency of complications because many of these patients do not undergo operation for a variety of reasons. To determine the relative frequency of the various complications, the indications for operation were gleaned from the comprehensive report by Rodkey and Welch (10): pericolic abscess, 10.9%; perforation with local peritonitis or pelvic abscess, 32.3%; generalized peritonitis, 14.6%; obstruction, 10.9%; bleeding, 8.2%; fistula, 9.7%; and pain, 13.4%. McConnell et al. (117) characterized the gender and age differences in 934 patients with clinically symptomatic sigmoid diverticular disease requiring operation. There are 443 men and 491 women with an average age of 64. Forty-nine patients presented with massive rectal bleeding (males 3.6%, females 1.6%), 329 with chronic diverticulitis (males 15.8%, females 19.3%), 61 with obstructive symptoms (males 2.7%, females 3.9%), 148 with fistulas (males 8%, females 7.8%), 170 with perforation (males 8.7%, females 9.4%), 79 with abscess (males 4.0%, females 4.5%), 59 with stricture (males 2.2%, females 4%), and 39 with acute diverticulitis (males 2.2%, females 1.9%). Overall, patients younger than 50 years presented more often with chronic or recurrent diverticulitis. They noted that female patients present, on average, five years later than males with complications requiring operation. Overall, men had a high incidence of bleeding, whereas women present more often with stricture and obstruction. Young males present more with fistula, whereas older males present with bleeding. Young females present with perforation, and older females present with chronic diverticulitis and stricture.

Retrospective studies have suggested an association between consumption of nonsteroidal anti-inflammatory drugs (NSAIDs) and the complications of diverticular disease. Wilson et al. (118) entered 92 patients into a prospective study of the complications of diverticular disease over a three-year period; 31 were taking NSAIDs compared with only four age- and sex-matched controls from a representative general practice. A second control group comprised 306 patients with carcinoma of the colon in whom NSAID consumption was again significantly lower than in patients with diverticular disease (22 of 306 vs. 31 of 92). Of the 31 patients taking NSAIDs, 19 presented with a perforation or peritonitis. By contrast, only eight of the 61 patients not taking NSAIDs had such complications. Eleven patients presented with bleeding of whom five were taking NSAIDs and six were not. Patients admitted with complications of diverticular disease have a high incidence of NSAID intake, and it appears that NSAID consumption is associated with a more severe form of the disease. Aldoori et al. (119) prospectively examined the relationship between self-reported use of NSAIDs and acetaminophen and the risk of symptomatic diverticular disease. A total of 35,615 male health professionals, at baseline and free of diagnosed diverticular disease, in the age group of 40 to 75 years, residing in 50 U.S. states were sent follow-up questionnaires about use of NSAIDs and acetaminophen. During four years of follow-up, they documented 310 newly diagnosed cases of symptomatic diverticular disease. Regular and consistent use of NSAIDs and acetaminophen were positively

TABLE 3 ■ **Results of Elective Resection and Primary Anastomosis for Diverticular Disease**

Author(s)	No. of Patients	Operative Mortality (%)	Complication Rate (%)	One-Stage (%)	Two-Stage (%)	Three-Stage (%)
Bokey et al. (110) (1981)	47	4.3	21	64	36	
Eisenstat et al. (111) (1983)	135	2.2		100		
Hackford et al. (112) (1985)	86	1	18			
Benn et al. (101) (1986)	501	1.6		81	11	8
Levien et al. (113) (1989)	46	0	60	89	7	
Killingback (114) (1990)	146	1.4		75	12	12
Moreaux and Vons (106) (1990)	177	0	6	95	5	
Netri et al. (115) (2000)	44	2	16	89		
Vinas-Salas et al. (116) (2001)	38	2.6	16	100		
Thorn et al. (65) (2002)	75	0	33	100		
Pessaux et al. (107) (2004)	582	1.2	25			

associated with the overall risk of symptomatic diverticular disease (RR for NSAIDs = 2.24 and for acetaminophen 1.81). Most of this positive association was attributable to cases associated with bleeding, particularly for acetaminophen (RR for NSAIDs = 4.64 and for acetaminophen 13.63).

Wilcox et al. (120) evaluated the association between NSAID use in a prospective case control study evaluating 105 patients with lower gastrointestinal (GI) bleeding. The age-, race-, and gender-adjusted risks for lower GI bleeding associated with NSAID use were significant (OR = 2.6). The risk associated with diverticular bleeding (OR = 3.4). Goh et al. (121) conducted a retrospective review of 20 patients admitted with colonic perforation in diverticular disease. Of the 20 patients with perforation, 45% were taking NSAIDs for four weeks or longer compared with 15% of the control group of sex-matched patients diagnosed with diverticular disease not complicated by perforation (RR = 2.9). Nineteen percent of all patients with diverticular disease were taking NSAIDs compared with 10% of the second control group, which consisted of 600 age- and sex-matched randomly selected patients with no known diverticular disease admitted as emergencies in the same period (RR = 1.8). The findings indicate a strong association between the use of NSAIDs and the perforation of colonic diverticula.

Morris et al. (122) tested the hypothesis that three classes of drugs namely NSAIDs, opioid analgesics, and corticosteroids are risk factors for perforated diverticular disease. With ophthalmology and dental controls, opioid analgesics (RR = 1.8 and 3.1, respectively), NSAIDs (RR = 4.0 and 3.7, respectively) and for corticosteroids (RR = 5.7 and 7.8, respectively) were all positively associated with perforated colonic diverticular disease.

Mpofu et al. (123) studied sigmoid diverticular abscess perforation in 64 patients with rheumatic conditions and 320 controls from a similar geographic area. The results showed that independent of rheumatic diagnosis, corticosteroid treatment is strongly associated with sigmoid diverticular abscess perforation (OR = 31.9) and nonsteroidal anti-inflammatory drugs only weakly associated (OR = 1.8). A rheumatic diagnosis is strongly associated with the development of sigmoid diverticular abscess perforation (OR = 3.5).

■ ACUTE DIVERTICULITIS

Definition

When a segment of diverticula-bearing colon becomes acutely inflamed, the entity is referred to as acute diverticulitis, which is associated with fever, leukocytosis, and sometimes a mass. It differs from the clinical situation of "painful diverticular disease" described by Painter (33), in which the patient experiences left lower quadrant pain and possibly waves of pain down the left side of the abdomen without fever or elevated white blood cell count. However, the sigmoid colon may be palpable in the latter category of patients.

Incidence

Approximately 10% to 25% of patients with known diverticulosis will develop one or more bouts of diverticulitis (4,5,63,66,67). Diverticulitis developed in approximately 15% of more than 26,000 cases of diverticulosis seen at the Mayo Clinic (6). In a small series of patients from China, the incidence of diverticulitis was 16.7% in patients with diverticulosis (16). A report from Japan noted that in 1124 cases of diverticular disease of the colon seen over a 15-year period, diverticulitis occurred in 2.4% (124). Among patients who require hospitalization, 10% to 20% require an emergency operation (125,126); during the operation, generalized or fecal peritonitis is found in 20% to 60% (64,127).

Pathogenesis

The reason as to why a diverticulum becomes infected by bacteria that are normally found in the colon is unknown. Mechanical trauma caused by fecaliths has been suggested as a cause, but high intracolonic pressures may be responsible. Morson (11) stated that diverticula become inflamed because fecal matter is not discharged through the narrow neck, becomes inspissated to produce a fecalith, and abrades the mucosal lining of the sac to produce low-grade chronic inflammation. Commonly only one diverticulum becomes inflamed, and it is unusual for more than three or four to be affected. Because of the thin wall of the diverticulum, local peritonitis is common. Perforation, which often is contained locally, may then ensue and may become adherent to adjacent viscera. Free perforation is uncommon. Resolution might result in later fibrosis around the colon. Pericolic abscesses usually become walled-off, and, with repeated episodes of inflammation, the colon may become enshrouded by fibrous tissue.

Clinical Features

Patients with acute diverticulitis usually present with steady left lower quadrant pain, which varies in intensity, depending on the degree of the inflammation. The pain may radiate to the suprapubic region, the back, or the left groin. It commonly persists for several days and then may disappear entirely until further exacerbation of the diverticulitis occurs. Alteration in bowel habit, with constipation or diarrhea, may occur. If an element of obstruction is present, abdominal distention may develop. Occasionally anorexia, nausea, and vomiting may supervene. Rectal bleeding is distinctly uncommon during the acute episode, but slight bleeding may be noted. If the inflammatory process involves the bladder, symptoms of dysuria, urgency, and frequency may develop. A low-grade fever usually is present.

Physical findings depend on the severity of the inflammatory process. In milder cases, left lower quadrant tenderness and rebound can be demonstrated, and a tender mass may be palpable. In more severe cases, abdominal distention may develop, either secondary to an ileus or to partial obstruction. A digital rectal examination reveals some tenderness in the pelvis, or a mass may be felt. Use of rigid sigmoidoscopy may be limited because of pain.

A number of unusual extraperitoneal presentations of diverticulitis have been reviewed by Ravo et al. (128) Tracking may occur along fascial planes or paths of least resistance, and the disease may be manifested along various anatomic pathways of the abdomen, retroperitoneum, and pelvis and reach such diverse places as the abdominal wall, flank, perineum, scrotum, buttocks, vagina, hip

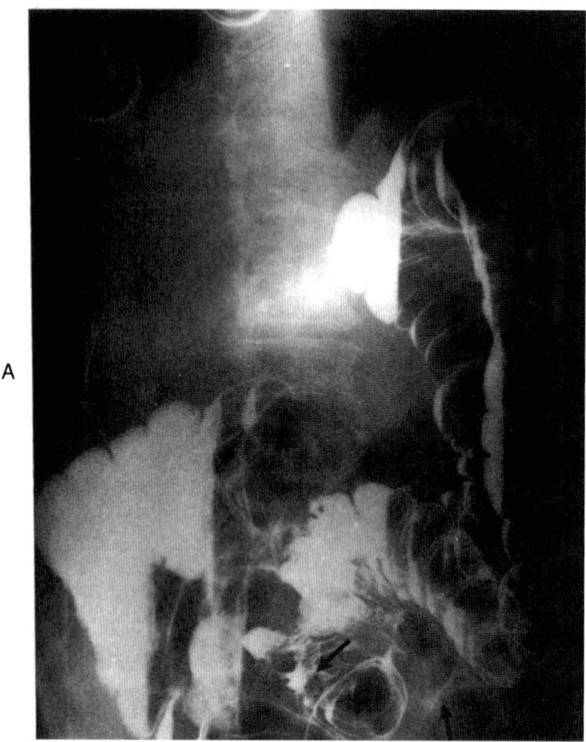

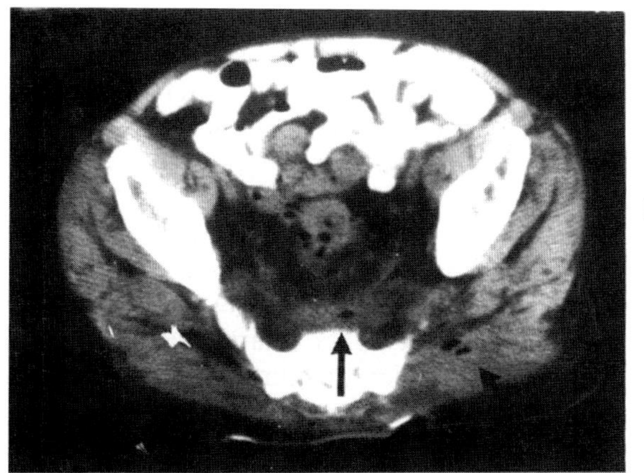

FIGURE 13 ■ (**A**) Barium enema showing severe diverticular disease of sigmoid colon with diverticulitis, perforation, and a tract leading to gluteal region. (**B**) Computed tomography showing gas and streaking in prevertebral tissue and gas in soft tissue in gluteal region. *Source*: Courtesy of David A. Rothenberger, M.D., St. Paul, Minnesota, U.S.A.

joints, thigh, lower extremities, mediastinum, and neck. The clinical manifestations vary tremendously, depending on the direction of spread (Fig. 13).

Diagnosis

In many cases, the clinical manifestations of the disease will allow the physician to arrive at the diagnosis with reasonable confidence. Associated constitutional disturbances (i.e., pyrexia, tachycardia, nausea, and vomiting) may be present. In severe cases, the diagnosis may be confused with other causes of an acute abdomen. The leukocyte count is not especially helpful and has been found to be normal in two-thirds of patients with acute complications of diverticular disease (112).

An abdominal series rarely offers any specific diagnostic information. When the diagnosis is entertained but not certain, or for the patient with left lower quadrant peritonitis of uncertain cause, the use of ultrasonography, a CT scan of the abdomen, or a water-soluble contrast enema can be considered (129). The small bowel is involved in 7% of cases, with manifestations including coloenteric fistula, small bowel obstruction, or inflammatory changes secondary to an associated mass (130). A contrast study may identify perforation of a diverticulum. Spreading cellulitis and an abscess adjacent to the diverticula produce radiographic alterations consisting of spasm, irritability, shortening, narrowing, rigidity, distention, and thickening of the folds (75). Hiltunen et al. (131) studied 53 patients with clinically suspected diverticulitis with water-soluble contrast enema. The diagnosis was confirmed in only 47% of cases. Normal contrast studies were seen in a quarter of patients, whereas one had ischemic colitis, three had colon carcinoma, and the remainder had nondiverticular causes of their symptoms. The authors believe the water-soluble contrast enema is safe and useful in investigating patients with suspected diverticulitis. If the findings are normal, investigations can be directed elsewhere without undue delay.

Yacoe and Jeffrey (132) reviewed the sonographic findings of colonic diverticulitis. An abnormal colonic segment at the point of maximum tenderness is the most common sonographic feature of diverticulitis occurring in approximately 85% of cases. Inflamed diverticula are demonstrated in 70% to 85% of cases as echogenic shadowing outpouchings of the thickened colon. Shadowing fecaliths occasionally may be demonstrated. The presence of a hypoechoic region of marked mural thickening suggests a mural abscess. Hyperechoic foci within the collection indicate the presence of gas bubbles. Peridiverticular inflammation is demonstrated sonographically as regional increased echogenicity in the pericolic fat. The presence of an extraluminal hypoechoic collection is evidence of peridiverticular abscess. Extraluminal hyperechoic foci are evidence of mesenteric gas. Linear echogenic foci are suggestive of fistulous tracts. Additional findings may include focal thickening of the bladder, gas within the bladder, hydronephrosis, and liver abscess. In a prospective study of 123 patients with clinical signs of acute intestinal inflammation, Verbanck et al. (133) found that the sensitivity of ultrasonography in diagnosing acute colonic diverticulitis was 84.6% and the specificity 80.3%. The predictive values of positive and negative sonograms were 76.0% and 87.7%, respectively. Of the 52 patients with subsequently proven acute colonic diverticulitis (radiologic, colonoscopic, or surgical), 44 presented sonographically with a thickened (>4 mm) hypoechoic bowel wall. In 15 patients, enlarged fluid-filled bowel loops were also present. Air-containing diverticula were demonstrated in three patients, abscesses in eight patients, and colovesical fistulas in two patients. Eight large abscesses were successfully treated without emergency surgery by percutaneous sonographically guided evacuation. The diagnoses of patients who initially presented with clinical signs of acute diverticulitis, but who were misdiagnosed included Crohn's disease, ischemic colitis, lymphoma, left-sided appendicitis, and *Yersinia* ileitis.

Schwerk et al. (134) prospectively studied the clinical value of high-resolution real-time sonography for the diagnosis of acute and complicated colonic diverticulitis in 130 consecutive patients with abdominal complaints. The results of ultrasonographic investigation were compared with those of clinical examination on admission. Regarding history and initial clinical evaluation, diverticulitis was graded as "highly suspected" in 19 (36.5%) out of a total of 52 patients with later proven colonic diverticulitis (prevalence, 40%), as "possible but equivocal" in 24 (46.2%), and as "very unlikely" in the remaining nine (17.3%) patients. Ultrasonography enabled the diagnosis of diverticulitis with an overall accuracy of 97.7%, a sensitivity of 98.1%, and a specificity of 97.5%. The predictive values of positive and negative ultrasonographic examinations were 96.2% and 98.5%, respectively. The echomorphologic features of acute diverticulitis include visualization of a colon segment presenting with local tenderness on gradual compression, which shows hypoechogenic thickening of the wall and a target-like appearance in the transverse view due to inflammatory changes and muscular thickening. Sonographic signs of peridiverticulitis (hyperechoic halo) were found in 96% of patients and echogenic diverticula in 86%. Of the 13 abdominal abscesses, 12 (92%) were detected on initial ultrasonographic examination and could be treated by percutaneous drainage in seven cases, while six required operative intervention.

Ripolles et al. (135) evaluated the role of ultrasound in the diagnosis and management of acute diverticulitis in 208 hospitalized patients. Diverticulitis was retrospectively classified as either simple or complicated, the latter being defined by the presence of extraluminal air and/or abscesses. Diverticulitis was finally diagnosed in 203 patients. Ultrasound exhibited a sensitivity of 86% in 77 cases who underwent operation and of 94% in the global 203 patients. Of the 34 patients with diverticulitis and emergency operation, 10 had false negative ultrasound exams. Of patients with signs of complicated diverticulitis in the initial ultrasound study, 27% required emergency operation compared with only 3% with ultrasound evidence of simple diverticulitis. Of the patients with diverticulitis undergoing conservative management, 32% developed complications during follow-up period. The patients under the age of 50 with signs of complicated diverticulitis suffered more complications (65%) than the patients in the other group. In 26% of subjects with recurrences, these were either similar to or less than the first episode in 84% of cases.

Hollerweger et al. (136) investigated the sonographic appearance and detectability of inflamed diverticula in 175 consecutive patients with clinically suspected diverticulitis. Outpouchings from the colonic wall centered in the pericolic inflammation were considered inflamed diverticula. They were divided into four groups. Sonography showed inflamed diverticula in 77% of 102 patients with diverticulitis. Inflamed diverticula were hypoechoic in 37%, predominantly hyperechoic in 4%, hyperechoic with surrounding hypoechoic rim in 41%, and hyperechoic with acoustic shadowing in 18% of patients. In 23% of patients, no inflamed diverticulum was demonstrable. This group included 17 patients with complicated diverticulitis and six false-negative cases. An inflamed diverticulum as a sign of diverticulitis yielded an overall sensitivity of 77% and a specificity of 99%. Sensitivity in uncomplicated disease was 96%. In patients with complicated diverticulitis, an inflamed diverticulum is often not detectable.

Hulnick et al. (137) performed CT scans on 43 patients with diverticulitis. Their findings in decreasing order of frequency included inflammation of the pericolic fat, 98%; diverticula, 84%; thickening of the colonic wall, 70%; pericolic abscess, 35%; peritonitis, 16%; fistula, 14%; colonic obstruction, 12%; and intramural sinus tracts, 9%. Secondary findings included distant abscess (12%) and ureteral obstruction (7%). With the contrast enema, the extent of pericolic inflammation was underestimated in 41% of examinations.

Hachigian et al. (138) used CT in place of contrast enemas as the initial imaging study to evaluate 59 patients with the clinical diagnosis of acute sigmoid diverticulitis. CT established that three patients (5%) were hospitalized with an incorrect clinical diagnosis. Thirty-seven patients (62.7%) were identified as having uncomplicated acute diverticulitis. These patients were all treated successfully with nonsurgical therapies and were discharged in an average of 6.8 days. In the remaining 19 patients (32.2%), CT revealed complicated acute diverticulitis by helping to identify abscess, fistula, peritonitis, or obstruction. Of these 19 patients, 11 required urgent operation or CT-guided percutaneous drainage of an abscess. The four patients whose abscesses were drained percutaneously responded favorably and underwent an elective single-stage resection. The average hospital stay for patients with complicated diverticulitis was 13.6 days. CT has the advantage of providing information about extracolonic pathology and anatomic variation useful for surgical planning. Additionally, early CT-guided needle drainage allowed downstaging of complicated diverticulitis, avoided emergent operation, and permitted single-stage elective resection.

Werner et al. (139) evaluated the use of multislice CT for detection of clinically suspected left-sided colonic diverticulitis in 120 patients. Acute diverticulitis was proven in 55.8% of patients with an accuracy of 98%. Contained perforation or abscess formation was detected with an accuracy of 96% and 98%, respectively. In 25.8% of patients, diagnoses other than diverticulitis caused abdominal pain, which was correctly diagnosed by CT in 71%. The CT as well as other concurrently performed diagnostic methods showed normal findings and no causes for the patient symptoms in 18.4% of patients.

Poletti et al. (140) explored CT and demographic predictors for unfavorable outcome of nonoperative treatment in patients with a first event of left colonic diverticulitis. The admission CT scans of 168 consecutive patients with a diagnosis of left colonic diverticulitis who underwent nonoperative treatment and had an 18-month follow-up were reassessed by three radiologists unaware of the clinical findings. Unfavorable outcome was defined as a failure of nonoperative treatment 18 months after admission, which required either operation or rehospitalization for antibiotic treatment. Among these 168 patients, 68% had an uneventful outcome, but nonoperative treatment failed in 32%. The presence of an abscess (OR = 6.18) or extraintestinal gas pocket ≥ 5 mm (OR = 4.26) was the only CT finding significantly associated with failure of nonoperative treatment.

Both CT scanning and contrast enemas are reasonably reliable methods of detecting diverticulitis. Neither a negative CT scan nor a negative contrast enema study excludes the diagnosis of diverticulitis. In a comparison of barium enema and CT scanning in the diagnosis of acute diverticulitis, Johnson et al. (141) studied 102 patients to determine the sensitivity of the two techniques. The contrast enema was correct in 77% of patients, falsely negative in 15%, and indeterminate in 7%. The CT examination was diagnostic in 41%, consistent with the diagnosis of diverticulitis in 38%, and falsely negative in 21% of patients. Although the CT scan portrayed the extraluminal extent of disease better, it provided significant information altering therapy in only one of 28 patients. No complications occurred in any patient as a result of using a contrast enema or CT scan. Johnson et al. believe that the contrast enema should remain the initial routine examination for the evaluation of patients with suspected diverticulitis. CT scanning should be reserved for patients who are unable to have an adequate contrast enema, those with suspected distant or diffuse abdominal abscesses, those who are unresponsive to medical therapy, and those who are candidates for percutaneous drainage.

Smith et al. (142) analyzed 31 patients with diverticulitis who underwent CT scanning as well as a contrast enema. There was almost equal sensitivity to abnormality of approximately 90%. Contrast enema produced a specific diagnosis of diverticulitis in 61%, using stringent positive criteria, and an additional 29% with suggestive findings. Comparative CT-specific diagnoses in those 31 cases were made in 65%, and suggestive in 23%. CT was particularly useful diagnostically in cases of retrograde obstruction on contrast enema. The authors conclude that contrast enema should be the primary mode of approach, while CT can be a valuable follow-up when the diagnosis is still in doubt, or if it is possible that patient management might be altered by additional information.

Ambrosetti et al. (143) compared the performance between water soluble contrast enema and CT. Diverticulitis was considered moderate when CT showed localized thickening of the colonic wall (5 mm or more) and inflammation of pericolic fat, and contrast enema showed segmental luminal narrowing and tethered mucosa; it was considered severe when abscess, extraluminal air, or contrast, or all three were observed on CT, and when one or both of the last two signs were seen on contrast enema. Both CT and contrast enema were performed on 420 patients. The performance of CT was significantly superior to contrast enema in terms of sensitivity (98% vs. 92%), which was calculated from patients who had their colon removed and whose diverticulitis was histologically proven, and in the evaluation of the severity of inflammation (26% vs. 9%). Moreover, of 69 patients who had an associated abscess seen on CT, only 29% had indirect signs of this complication on contrast enema. They concluded that in the diagnostic evaluation of acute left colonic diverticulitis, CT should be preferred to contrast enema as the initial radiologic examination.

Labs et al. (144) also evaluated the role of CT scanning in 42 patients with complications of diverticular disease. Diverticular abscesses were diagnosed preoperatively by CT scanning in 10 patients through the triad of diverticula, a segmentally thickened colon, and extravisceral fluid collections with or without associated gas. Contrast enemas suggested the presence of a diverticular abscess in only two of eight patients studied. Colovesical fistula was diagnosed by CT scanning preoperatively in 11 of 12 patients with a triad of air in the bladder, thickened colon adjacent to an area of thickened bladder, and colonic diverticula. Contrast enemas demonstrated a fistula in only three of eight patients studied. The remaining 20 patients had uncomplicated acute diverticulitis, and CT findings included segmentally thickened colon with diverticula. In total, CT scanning correctly visualized acute complications in 21 of 22 patients, and it excluded an abscess or fistula in all 20 patients with uncomplicated acute diverticulitis. The authors concluded that CT scanning is the most sensitive and specific test for diagnosing complications of acute diverticulitis.

Ambrosetti et al. (145) conducted a prospective study to examine factors that may predict a poor outcome (complications and recurrences) after a first attack of diverticulitis, which has been successfully managed conservatively. Twenty-four of 107 patients who entered the study had a poor outcome: persistent diverticulitis (nine cases), recurrence (seven cases), colonic stenosis (six cases), residual parasigmoid abscess (one case), and colovesical fistula (one case). Of the 18 men aged 50 or younger, eight had a poor outcome compared with 16 of the remaining 89 patients. Of 76 patients with mild findings on CT (localized thickening of colonic wall and inflammation of pericolic fat), 12 (16%) had a poor outcome compared with 11 of 23 patients (48%) whose CT was estimated as severe (abscess and/or extraluminal air and/or extraluminal Gastrografin). These results suggest that elective colectomy can be proposed after a first attack of acute left diverticulitis in men up to the age of 50 years and/or in patients whose initial CT reveals findings of severe diverticulitis.

In the evaluation of a patient with left lower quadrant pain in whom the suspected diagnosis is acute diverticulitis, controversy exists as to whether barium enema or CT scan should be used for initial evaluation. It should be noted that the misdiagnosis rate of diverticulitis based on clinical criteria alone might be as high as 34% to 67% (129). This underscores the need for a reliable imaging technique. Diverticulitis can be diagnosed reliably and safely with either a contrast enema or a CT scan. If peritonitis is suspected, water-soluble contrast should be used. Support is growing for the use of CT because it defines the extent of disease better than does contrast enema and also shows the entire abdomen and pelvis, allowing a greater likelihood of making an alternative diagnosis if diverticulitis is not present. The contrast enema has the advantage of more accurately depicting the luminal diameter, better defining the size and location of fistulas, more accurately detecting colon carcinoma, and being less expensive. In many instances, both CT and contrast enema may be needed to fully evaluate the patient with suspected diverticulitis. The studies should be considered complementary, but CT scan is probably the best initial test (146).

Fiberoptic endoscopy yields little, if any, useful information, and its use risks perforating an acutely inflamed bowel. It would therefore be an unwise maneuver.

Management

Patients who present with a mild case of diverticulitis may be treated on an outpatient basis. Clear liquids by mouth and a broad-spectrum antibiotic for a week to 10 days are prescribed. Anticholinergics have been used for patients with pain attributed to colonic spasm but are of doubtful value. As symptoms subside, solid food can be reintroduced into the diet. For patients with a more severe inflammatory process, hospitalization is necessary. The mainstay of therapy is bowel rest, intravenous fluids, and broad-spectrum antibiotics.

Antibiotic therapy for diverticulitis is not a well-studied subject, and hence prescribed antibiotics are often related to the whims of the prescribing physician. Coverage ideally is aimed at both gram-negative aerobes and anaerobes and gram-positive organisms. The following are suggested regimens in the Sanford Guide to Antimicrobial Therapy 2004 (147). For patients with mild diverticulitis, recommended outpatient treatment includes trimethoprim-sulfamethoxazole double strength (480 mg) b.i.d. or ciprofloxacin 500 mg b.i.d. plus metronidazole 500 mg q6h PO for 7 to 10 days. An alternative is amoxicillin/clavulanate (Augmentin) 500 mg/125 mg t.i.d.) PO × 7 to 10 days. For mild to moderate disease, which includes peridiverticular abscess (inpatients), the primary suggested regimen includes pipercillin/tazobactam 3.375 g IV q6h, or 4.5 g IV q8h, or ampicillin/sulbactam (Unasyn) 3 g IV q6h, or ticarcillin clavulanate (Timentin) 3.1 g IV q6h, or ertapenem 1 g IV q day. Alternative regimens include ciprofloxacin 400 mg IV q12h or levofloxacin 750 mg IV q24h plus metronidazole 500 mg IV q6h or 1 g IV q12h. For severe life-threatening disease, primary regimens include imipenem cilastatin (Primaxin) 500 mg IV q6h or meropenem 1 g IV q8h. Alternative regimens may include ampicillin plus metronidazole and (ciprofloxacin 400 mg IV ql2h or levofloxacin 750 mg TV q24h) or ampicillin 2 g IV q6h and metronidazole 500 mg IV q6h plus antipseudomonal aminoglycosidic antibiotics. Ertapenem is less active against pseudomonas aeruginosa/Acinetobacter species than imipenem or meropenem. This role of enterococci remains debatable but drugs active against enterococci should probably be included in patients with valvular heart disease. For patients with severe penicillin/cephalosporin allergy, aztreonam 2 g q6h and metronidazole 500 mg IV q6h, or 1 g IV q12h, or ciprofloxacin 400 mg IV q12h, or levofloxacin 750 mg IV qd plus metronidazole are prescribed. For patients with renal impairment, treatment with combination antibiotics such as sulbactam-ampicillin, imipenem-cilastatin, or ticarcillin-clavulanate acid may be considered. Based on in-vitro data, one could substitute gatifloxacin/moxifloxacin for ciprofloxacin/levofloxacin but insufficient clinical data is available. Optimal duration for antibiotic therapy for acute diverticulitis is unclear but recommendations have varied from 7 to 14 days. The ever-popular cephalosporins have fallen into disfavor because of the increased incidence of *Clostridium difficile* following their use. Antibiotics, which have been considered high risk for the development of *C. difficile* have, included ampicillin and amoxicillin, amoxicillin clavulanate, second and third generation cephalosporins, and clindamycin. Moderate-risk antibiotics have included the penicillins except amoxicillin and ampicillin, quinolones, tetracyclines, carbapenems, first generation cephalosporins, trimethoprim-sulfamethoxazole, and macrolides. Low-risk antibiotics that have been considered are aminoglycosides, metronidazole, vancomycin, ticarcillin-clavulanate, and rifampin.

Cephalosporins, in particular third-generation cephalosporins, appear to disproportionately predispose to *C. difficile* diarrhea compared to other commonly prescribed antibiotics (148). Other publications have also reported the association of *C. difficile*–associated diarrhea with the use of cephalosporins (149–152). In one study with 60 patients with *C. difficile* enterotoxin in their stool, 85% of patients had been on ceftriaxone +/or ceftazidime in the proceeding six weeks. No patient on ticarcillin/clavulanate developed *C. difficile*–associated diarrhea (153). In our institution, Miller et al. (154) noted antibiotic utilization (reflected in decreased second and third generation cephalosporin use, along with increased ticarcillin/clavulanate and fluoroquin dose use) resulted in a temporally related marked decrease in the hospital-wide nosocomial *C. difficile*–associated diarrhea incidence rate from 15 per 100 admissions (148 per 100,000 patient days) to 5 per 100 admissions (58 per 100,000 patient days).

Nasogastric suctioning may not be necessary unless there is evidence of obstruction or the patient develops nausea or vomiting. The efficacy of anticholinergic drugs in the acute setting is unsubstantiated. The use of morphine is contraindicated because of the well-documented increase in intraluminal pressure after its administration. The patient's symptoms should begin to subside within 48 hours, and, if resolution continues, the patient is investigated approximately three weeks later. If medical therapy should fail, an urgent operation may be required. If the patient should present with an acute abdomen with evidence of a spreading peritonitis, immediate operation would be mandatory. Approximately one-third of patients admitted to the hospital with diverticulitis will require operation during the first admission (10).

Results and Prognosis

For the patient with an initial uncomplicated episode of diverticulitis, medical management is indicated because 70% to 85% of patients recovering from the attack will have no further recurrences (3,4,155). In an extensive study by Parks (4), 297 patients admitted to the hospital for only medical treatment were followed up for 2 to 16 years. Of all patients in the study, 2% died from diverticular disease, 4% were alive and had had severe symptoms of this condition, 26% were alive and had had mild symptoms of diverticulitis, and 40% were alive and entirely free of complaints about the bowel. Of the original 297 patients, 25% had to reenter the hospital for a second admission (half of them within one year), 4% for a third time, and 2% for a fourth time. Of the patients who were readmitted, 6.7% underwent operative treatment, and 2% died. Munson et al. (105) found that of 32 medically treated patients, 62.5% continued to have symptoms.

The risk of recurrent symptoms after an attack of acute diverticulitis has variously been reported to range from as low as 7% to as high as 62%, with most authors accepting an approximation of one-third to one-quarter as a reasonable estimate of recurrence (3,4,95,105,126). The chance of the need for a second hospitalization varies from 11% to 25% (71,156). Recurrent attacks are less likely to respond to medical therapy and have a higher mortality rate (3,4,95); therefore most authorities agree that elective resection is indicated after two attacks of uncomplicated diverticulitis, although this recommendation has been questioned (157).

Parks (4) reported that the complication rate increases with subsequent attacks, with a 23% rate after one attack and a 58% rate after more than one attack. In stark contrast, Haglund et al. (64) analyzed the short- and long-term outcome in 392 patients admitted to the hospital with an initial attack of acute diverticulitis. Emergency operation was required in 25% of patients after the first attack, with an operative mortality rate of 20%. Of the 295 patients treated medically and followed up for 2 to 12 years, 25% developed recurrent attacks, almost one-half within 1 year after the first attack had subsided, with a risk of an attack in the first year of approximately 10%. Once the initial attack had subsided, the yearly risk of suffering another attack was calculated at approximately 3%. No perforations occurred, and medical treatment was uneventful in all cases. All perforations and the vast majority of other complications occurred in association with the initial attack. After the first attack, the disease appeared to run a benign course, and the risk of dying from unrelated diseases was greater than the risk of dying from acute diverticulitis or its complications. In view of their findings, the authors concluded that the increased risk of elective "prophylactic" sigmoid resection in patients who are in the early stages of diverticular disease or who have recovered from acute diverticulitis could hardly be justified. Operation may be considered in patients with persistent incapacitating symptoms and for patients with complications.

Nylamo (158) reviewed 57 patients who were treated nonoperatively for colonic diverticulitis and were followed up for at least 10 years. Of the 24 patients who experienced two or more episodes of diverticulitis, only 3 had resection for recurrent attacks. None of the patients had any serious complications during follow-up.

Tudor et al. (159) reported on a prospective national audit of 300 patients with complicated diverticular disease from 30 hospitals. Complications present on admission included acute phlegmon (104), pericolic abscess (34), purulent peritonitis (40), large bowel obstruction (31), fecal peritonitis (23), pericolic abscess complicated by fistula (28), and lower GI bleeding (40). The overall mortality rate was 11.3% (acute phlegmon, 4%; purulent peritonitis, 27%; pericolic abscess, 12%; fecal peritonitis, 48%; large bowel obstruction, 6%; bleeding, 2%; and fistula, 4%). Acute phlegmon was treated without operation in 75% and by resection in 23.1%. Management of purulent peritonitis generally involved Hartmann's procedure (62%) or resection and primary anastomosis (15%). Similarly, patients with pericolic abscess usually underwent Hartmann's procedure (38%) or resection and primary anastomosis (35%). The principal operation for fecal peritonitis was Hartmann's resection (83%). Large bowel obstruction was managed conservatively in four patients (13%), by Hartmann's procedure in nine (29%), and by resection and primary anastomosis with or without a proximal stoma in 13 (42%). Most patients (82%) with fistula associated with an abscess were managed by resection and primary anastomosis; 90% with acute GI bleeding were treated without operation.

Detry et al. (160) studied two groups of patients with diverticulitis to determine optimum management and outcome. A "phlegmonous" diverticulitis (no pericolic abscess) was diagnosed in 78 cases (group 1). A pericolic abscess was identified in 42 cases (group 2). The medical treatment was successful in 97% of the patients of group 1. Only 15 patients required a delayed elective resection for recurrence or chronic complications within the next 24 months. There were no operative deaths. All the other patients were doing well after a mean follow-up of five years, without any disease-related death. Patients presenting with a localized pericolic abscess (group 2, 42) were initially treated either conservatively (22) or by a more or less extensive drainage (20). There were two deaths in the "conservative" group. Primary or delayed colonic resection was indicated in 34 cases because of uncontrolled sepsis, recurrence, or secondary chronic complications. The authors concluded that accurate classification of the disease is essential. If no peritonitis has developed, the presence of an abscess is the main determinant in both prognosis and treatment. Most patients who develop an acute phlegmonous diverticulitis do well with conservative treatment, and prophylactic resection is not indicated. Curative colectomy is reserved for patients developing persistent complications over the next few months. On the other hand, high rates of recurrence and complication are observed among the patients with a pericolic abscess. Drainage of the abscess, possibly followed by a secondary elective colectomy, could be the appropriate treatment.

Larson et al. (155) reviewed 99 patients treated medically for acute diverticulitis and followed up for an average of 9.2 years; 73% had no further symptoms or hospital admissions once they recovered from their episode of acute diverticulitis. In light of these findings, it is somewhat difficult to justify performing an operation after only one attack of diverticulitis.

Similarly, Sarin and Boulos (161) reviewed 164 patients who presented with acute complications of diverticular disease and were prospectively followed up for a median of 48 months. Medical treatment of acute diverticulitis was effective in 85% of 86 patients, with a mortality of 1.3% and a recurrence rate of 2% per patient year follow-up. All 37 patients presenting with bleeding responded to conservative management without mortality and a readmission rate, with further bleeding of 5% per patient year. Patients who required colonic resection had a mortality of 12% but with no further admissions with complications of diverticular disease. They believe that the low risk of readmission with recurrent disease after successful conservative treatment of the acute complications of diverticular disease does not justify elective operation in this group of patients.

Follow-Up Care and Advice

After complete resolution of an attack of acute diverticulitis, patients are customarily advised to follow a high-fiber diet.

Although the addition of unprocessed bran is helpful in controlling the symptoms of pain, there is no evidence to support the claim that it reduces the frequency of inflammatory attacks.

Indications for Operation

An operation is indicated for the patient who fails to respond to medical measures or for the patient who presents with generalized peritonitis. Failure of nonoperative therapy may be apparent within hours or may take 3 to 5 days. The decision to operate depends on the severity of peritoneal contamination as judged by the degree and extent of tenderness and systemic disturbance. If signs are confined to the left lower quadrant, performing an operation is not urgent. Urgent operation was required in less than one-third of all emergency admissions with acute diverticulitis (64), in 25% of the series of 224 patients reported by Wedell et al. (162).

The matter of when to resect after an acute episode of diverticulitis resolves is controversial. No set time interval must elapse before performing an elective resection. The inflammatory process usually resolves within a few weeks, but it may take longer if the initial process was extensive.

Operative Options

The following sections discuss operative options available in the treatment of patients with complicated diverticular disease. The advantages and disadvantages of each option are highlighted and provide reasons why certain trends in operative therapy have developed. Although comparisons of different procedures are necessary to arrive at a recommendation, reported series are almost never comparable for a number of reasons. Not all the patients being treated in each series are similar, for some series include patients with only localized diverticulitis and some will include patients with a perforation; however, more often than not both types of patients have been inappropriately assigned to one category to supplement the small numbers collected. Many studies fail to define precisely the type and extent of peritonitis at the time of operation. It is not always clear whether patients have a purulent or fecal peritonitis or whether there is a localized abscess or a fistula. For example, Nagorney et al. (163) reported that the operative mortality rate was 9% for patients with spreading purulent peritonitis, 6% for those with diffuse purulent peritonitis, and 35% for those with fecal peritonitis. Series are frequently compared from different eras when different support facilities and different antibiotics were being used. Because the reports are not of randomized trials, the potential for selection biases arises. Nonetheless, certain trends have emerged. With cognizance of the above limitations, an effort has been made to present a summary of current trends of operative therapy.

Transverse Colostomy and Drainage (Three-Stage Procedure)

The traditional recommendation for patients who suffer from perforated sigmoid diverticulitis with abscess formation has been a staged operation with an initial diversionary colostomy and drainage, a subsequent resection, and finally closure of the colostomy. A transverse loop colostomy is constructed, and the infected area is drained (Fig. 14). The advantage of the procedure is that it is a relatively easy operation. However, Killingback (114) states that this approach to acute diverticulitis, with or without pericolic abscess, is tenable only if the surgeon has decided that no free or indirect perforation exists. Several disadvantages of the operation include the necessity for a colostomy for some time, and in some cases the stoma remains permanently. Experience has shown that with this regimen, the combined morbidity and mortality rates of the three stages are high, and the procedure is associated with long periods of hospitalization (Table 4). The presence of the perforated sigmoid colon and a column of stool in the left colon predictably permits a continuing focus of sepsis. Simple defunctionalizing of a segment of colon does not necessarily ensure resolution of the inflammatory process. In fact, progressive disease may persist, and fistulization may occur in spite of an adequate diverting colostomy.

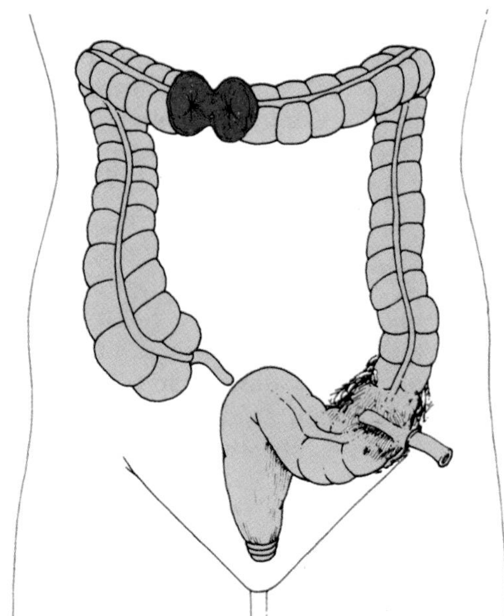

FIGURE 14 ■ Drainage of pericolic abscess and establishment of diverting transverse colostomy.

TABLE 4 ■ **Results of Drainage and Proximal Colostomy for Perforated Diverticulitis**

Author(s)	No. of Patients	Operative Mortality (%)
Greif et al. ROL (164)	306	12[a]
	505	29[b]
Edelmann (127)	25	36
Sakai et al. (165)	11	64
Wara et al. (166)	50	26
Killingback (167)	59	12
Ryan (168)	23	30
Cullen and Ferguson (169)	25	58
Nagorney et al. (163)	31	26
Lambert et al. (170)	16	38
Finlay and Carter (171)	37	24
Hold et al. (172)	46	13
Wedell et al. (162)	10	40

[a]Localized peritonitis.
[b]Generalized peritonitis.
Abbreviation: ROL, review of the literature.

Finally, the patient is faced with at least two further procedures. The question of how long to allow the inflammation to "cool off" is a debatable issue. The recommendations have ranged from 6 weeks to 6 months.

In general, this option is not recommended unless the surgeon believes that he or she is unable to mobilize the colon. In an elective setting, the three-stage procedure was used in 22 patients by Hackford et al. (112) The cumulative operative mortality rate was 14% and the morbidity rate was 24%, with a completion of operative therapy of 76%.

Greif et al. (164) collected information on patients with perforated sigmoid diverticulitis from a review of 19 references in the world literature. In the group of 510 patients with localized peritonitis, those who were initially resected had a 2% operative mortality rate, whereas those who underwent a proximal diversion had a 12% operative mortality rate. Of 833 patients with perforated diverticulitis and generalized peritonitis who underwent an emergency operation, the operative mortality rate was 12% for patients who underwent initial resection, compared with 29% who underwent colostomy and drainage. Classen et al. (173) have presented the best results for the three-stage operation. In a review of more than 200 patients, the combined operative mortality rate reported was 11%: 8.5% for first stage, 0.7% for second stage, and 4% for third stage.

In a study of 83 patients by Wara et al. (166), the outcome was unacceptable. Of 25 patients with generalized peritonitis who managed only by proximal colostomy and drainage, 11 died. Only 58% subsequently underwent a resection of the diseased segment, and even fewer (46%) eventually had their intestinal continuity restored.

The use of drainage alone has been associated with a mortality rate of 24% to 89% (170,174).

Drumm and Clain (175) have proposed that all patients with purulent peritonitis secondary to perforating diverticulitis be managed by a defunctioning transverse colostomy and drainage. They further recommend that subsequent management consist of simple closure of the colostomy after a check barium enema. They substantiate their recommendation with 20 cases, but their recommendation is generally not accepted. Indeed, it is considered inappropriate. Krukowski and Matheson (174) reported previous experience that indicated that symptoms would recur in 50% to 70% of patients managed in this fashion. This is certainly not a good option for patients with a perforation. In all likelihood, many of the patients with acute diverticulitis without evidence of an overt perforation who have undergone a diverting colostomy and drainage procedure very well may have resolved the inflammatory process without an operation.

In conclusion, transverse colostomy and drainage are rarely, if ever, indicated, especially for patients with generalized peritonitis and overt perforation. A possible reasonable indication for this operation is the elderly debilitated patient with intestinal obstruction caused by diverticulitis, or the situation in which the surgeon believes that he or she cannot mobilize the colon.

Exteriorization and Resection with Colostomy and Mucous Fistula (Mikulicz Operation)

This operation entails the exteriorization of the perforated segment of bowel with the establishment of a proximal colostomy and mucous fistula side by side (Fig. 15). Advantages of this procedure over simple diversion include the removal of the perforated segment of bowel from the peritoneal cavity, the establishment of a sigmoid colostomy, which is easier to manage than a transverse colostomy, and the necessity to use only two stages to effect intestinal continuity. It results in a single stoma, but appliance placement is difficult.

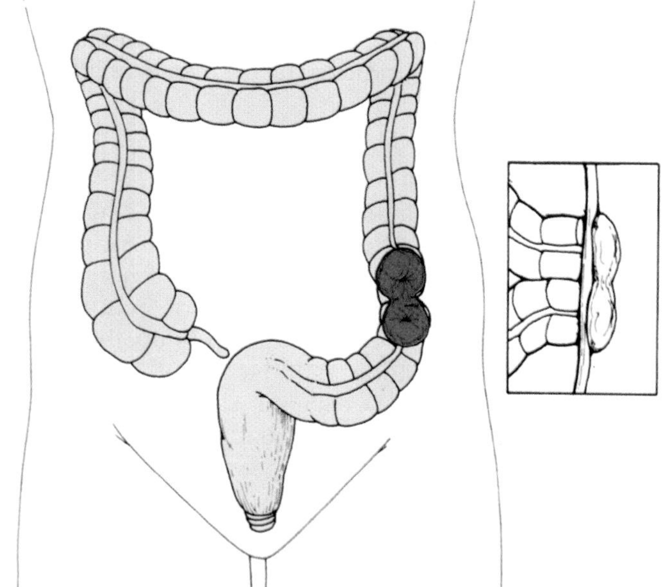

FIGURE 15 ■ Mikulicz operation.

Advocates of this procedure are few (176). Watkins and Oliver (177) used this procedure in 12 consecutive patients, without any mortality. Sakai et al. (165) exteriorized the perforation either as a loop or a "blow hole" in 14 patients. They considered it an ideal treatment, because it was effective, fast, and opened few tissue planes. There were no deaths in their series, nor was there recurrent intra-abdominal infection.

The disadvantage of the operation is that with the foreshortened inflamed mesentery and the distal extent of the disease, there seldom is a distal length of bowel adequate for the mucous fistula to reach skin level. In conjoining the two loops of bowel, the ideal stoma site most likely is compromised. The operation has a poor reputation for retraction of distal bowel. Killingback (114) described the method as too tentative and uncertain.

In conclusion, this procedure is seldom applicable and apparently has no advantage over resection with colostomy and mucous fistula.

Resection with Sigmoid Colostomy and Closure of Rectal Stump (Hartmann's Procedure)

This operation was originally performed for removal of a rectal carcinoma (178). It entails the resection of the perforated segment of sigmoid colon along with closure of the rectal stump and the establishment of an end sigmoid colostomy (Fig. 16A). When technically feasible, most surgeons recommend that the distal bowel be brought out as a mucous fistula (Fig. 16B). In most circumstances, Hartmann's operation is almost certainly the procedure of choice for patients suffering from a free perforation and

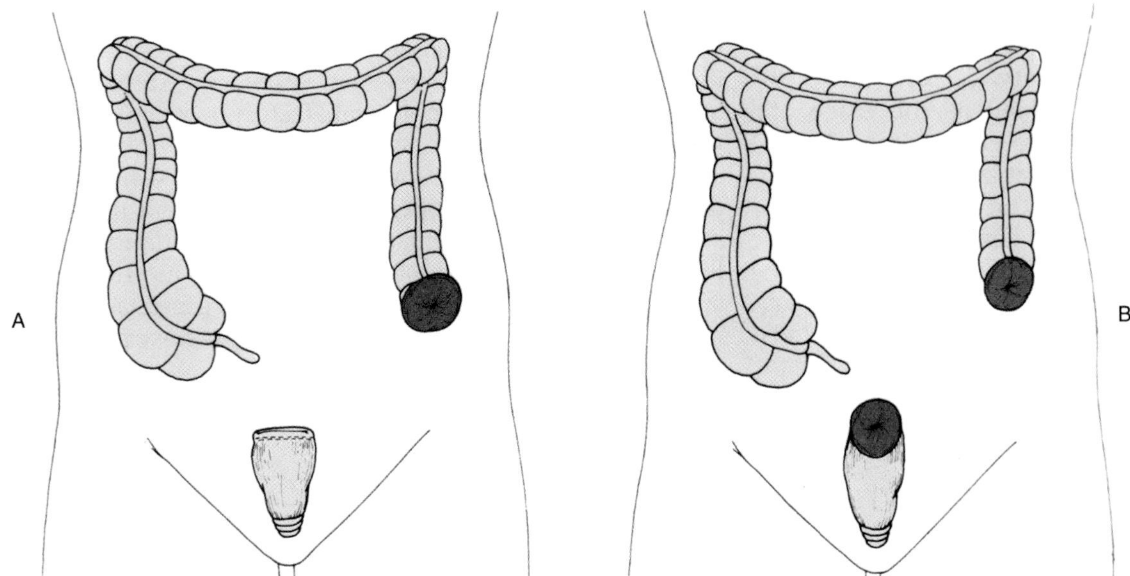

FIGURE 16 ■ (**A**) Classic Hartmann's procedure. (**B**) Sigmoid resection with mucous fistula.

generalized peritonitis. The advantage of this procedure is that the septic focus is removed by the primary operation, thus eliminating the continued source of contamination. Resection requiring some dissection of tissue planes does not appear to spread the infective process. The preventable mortality of this disease is due to immediate or delayed effects of sepsis.

The mortality related to cardiovascular or pulmonary disease may be more difficult to reduce. Anastomosis in the presence of a perforated obstructed colon can be avoided in the presence of an acutely inflamed intestine, fecal contamination, free pus, and an emergency situation. The patient is more inclined to accept a satisfactory single-barrel left-sided colostomy than a transverse loop colostomy, which is more difficult to manage. Disadvantages include the fact that the second stage of the operation requires a major abdominal procedure. This objection may be overcome with the advent of laparoscopic closure of the colostomy.

When the abdomen is opened, the surgeon may be intimidated by the large phlegmonous mass. However, the acute inflammatory nature of the disease often permits blunt dissection to proceed without injury to adjacent structures, in particular, the small bowel and left ureter. Little in the way of sharp dissection is necessary, but it is invariably needed for resection at a later stage. It is wise to begin dissection in normal tissues proximal and distal to the mass. Division of peritoneal attachments will permit entry into the appropriate plane (i.e., just posterior to the colon wall and anterior to the ureter and left gonadal vessels). Attachments to abdominal wall, bladder, ureter, and pelvis are systematically divided until the affected colon is mobilized. Difficult dissections can be facilitated by division of the colon at the proposed proximal line of resection, and reflecting the colon anteriorly provides more working room (179). The mesocolon is opened to allow insertion of the surgeon's hand. Using a proximal-to-distal dissection, the colon is lifted away from the retroperitoneal structures including the ureter, gonadal, and iliac vessels. Mesenteric vessels are ligated and divided as identified. Approaching the most adherent area from all sides eventually results in release of the fixed bowel. The bowel distal to the inflammatory mass, usually at approximately the level of the sacral promontory, can be closed with a stapling device. The retrorectal space should not be dissected unless necessary for the drainage of an abscess. The bowel proximal to the inflamed mass is then transected (if not already done) and an end sigmoid colostomy is constructed. Mobilizing the splenic flexure is undesirable in the presence of gross contamination. Fowler et al. (180) reported on a patient who presented with a perforated diverticulitis in the Hartmann's pouch. They therefore recommend that, especially for steroid-dependent patients known to be at a high risk for complications and recurrent disease, all distal diseased bowel be resected during the initial procedure.

A devastating complication following the Hartmann's procedure is leakage from the rectal stump. Schein et al. (181) reported their experience with 11 patients who encountered this problem. Nine of the rectal stumps were manually sutured and two were created with the use of a linear stapler. In 10 patients, the diagnosis was made during a laparotomy that was undertaken for persistent intra-abdominal infection. In two patients, the stump was debrided and refashioned with a linear stapler placed distal to the diseased bowel. Nine patients were managed with a "washout system." A large tube was secured in the open rectum with a pursestring suture and a second tube inserted via the anus to the rectum and secured to the perianal skin. A third sump drain was placed in the pelvis. Postoperatively, 4 L of normal saline was infused daily for five to seven days. Subsequently the pelvic, proximal, and distal rectal tubes were removed in that order. The mortality rate was 27%. The authors recommend that during emergency resection when local and systemic circumstances are not favorable, it may be prudent to irrigate the rectum and leave its stump open with an adequate drainage system. When the stump is closed, it is advisable to decompress the stump via sigmoidoscopy or even irrigate the rectum to minimize abdominal contamination should leakage subsequently occur. If stump closure appears tenuous, a wide bore catheter might wisely be placed via the anus into the rectal stump for several days.

One of the major criticisms of this procedure is the considerable difficulty encountered when an attempt is made to reestablish intestinal continuity. Certain principles should be considered when embarking on this stage of therapy. First, timing of the second procedure is important. The more severe the initial contamination, the longer will be the period required for resolution. In most cases, three months is a reasonable convalescent period for achieving normalcy. Second, the remaining colon must be assessed for residual diverticular disease. Any residual diverticular disease in the distal segment of bowel should be resected to allow distal anastomosis to the proximal rectum. Resecting every diverticula-bearing portion of colon proximal to the anastomosis is not essential unless the disease is so extensive that there is not a satisfactory segment of colon in which to construct an anastomosis.

A number of intraoperative techniques have been described to assist the operation. The advent of the CEEA stapler has dramatically facilitated the operation (Fig. 17). First, the colostomy is mobilized, the edges are freshened, and a purse-string suture is placed. The anvil is detached and inserted in the proximal bowel, and the purse-string suture

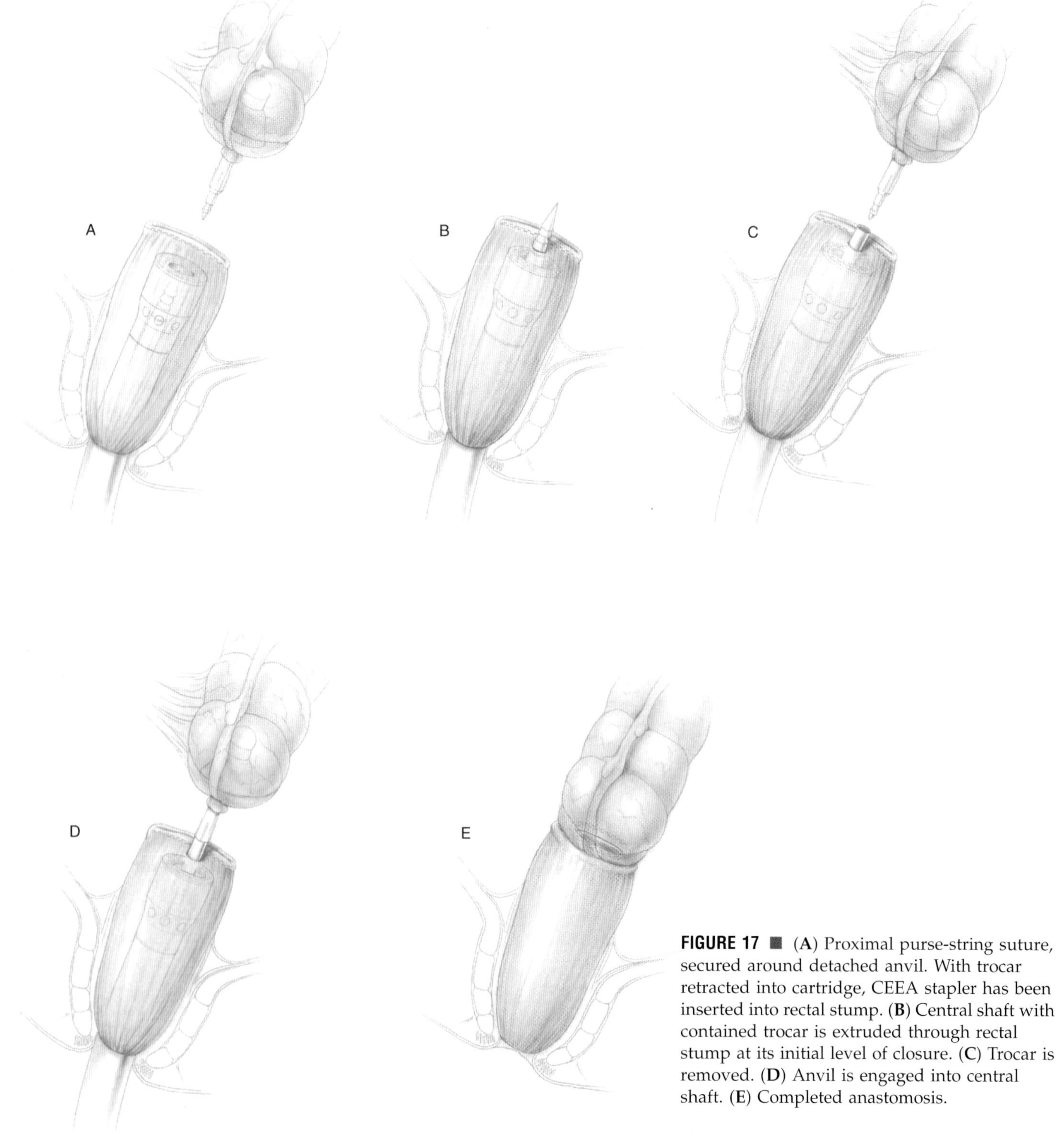

FIGURE 17 ■ (**A**) Proximal purse-string suture, secured around detached anvil. With trocar retracted into cartridge, CEEA stapler has been inserted into rectal stump. (**B**) Central shaft with contained trocar is extruded through rectal stump at its initial level of closure. (**C**) Trocar is removed. (**D**) Anvil is engaged into central shaft. (**E**) Completed anastomosis.

is tied. If the distal bowel was resected to the level of the proximal rectum during the initial operation, no further resection is required. The CEEA instrument with a piercing tip is applied to the central shaft and is retracted in the cartridge. The instrument is then inserted through the anus and advanced to the apex of the rectum. The only part of the rectal stump that must be dissected is an area just large enough for the cartridge of the stapler. If the wing nut is turned, the piercing tip and central shaft are protruded through the rectal stump, the piercing tip is removed, and the anvil is reunited with the central shaft. No purse-string suture is required on the distal bowel. The anvil is approximated to the cartridge and the instrument is activated, thus creating the anastomosis. If a lesser distal resection was performed during the initial operation, removal of the distal sigmoid colon is indicated to allow anastomosis to the proximal rectum. Under these circumstances, the usual technique for establishing continuity with the EEA stapler is used. The ILA can be used with equal efficacy (Ethicon Endosurgical).

Salem et al. (182) assessed the costs and outcomes of colostomy and colostomy reversal in patients with diverticulitis using a Washington state administrative database. There were 5420 patients who underwent colostomy for diverticulitis and its related complications. The rate of colostomy reversal was 56.3% (80% in patients less than 50 years, and 30% in patients over 77 years). (In their review of 33 studies, the average reversal rate was 72%.) The in-hospital mortality rate after colostomy reversal was 0.36% and was 2.6% in those over the age of 77. The length of time from colostomy to its reversal was approximately five months. They concluded that the impact of colostomy and reversal operations of both the patients and the healthcare system is significant.

Numerous reports on perforated diverticulitis have shown decreased morbidity and mortality rates after primary resection of the diseased segment compared to those for staged procedures. The largest series was reported by Wigmore et al. (183) but included patients with diagnoses other than only diverticulitis. A total of 178 patients, under the care of seven different surgical units, underwent reversal of Hartmann's procedure during a five-year period. The mortality rate of the study group was 0.6%, the anastomotic leak rate was 3.9%, and the incidence of anastomotic stricture was 6.7%. The median time interval between resection and reversal was 92 days and no relation was found between timing and complications. Anastomotic strictures occurred significantly more commonly in stapled than in sutured anastomoses; however, leaks were equally common in both types. The mean age of the patients who developed major complications was not statistically different from that of the rest of the study group and there was no difference in premorbid state. The authors believe that the low complication rates reported in this series may be attributable to the high level of operator experience in performing this technically difficult procedure, which was done by a consultant in 66% of cases and by a senior registrar in 33%.

Primary resection with colostomy has been widely adopted during the past decade for the treatment of patients with severe complications of diverticulitis. Because of this, Peoples et al. (184) conducted a retrospective review of all patients undergoing operation for colonic diverticular disease during the two time periods 1974 to 1978 (196) and 1982 to 1986 (230). Forty-three patients had abscess or peritonitis from 1974 to 1978, whereas 52 had these complications from 1982 to 1986. Colostomy and drainage alone were used for 31 of 43 patients (72%) from 1974 to 1978, while primary resection with colostomy was used for 39 of 52 patients (75%) from 1982 to 1986. Despite this shift in the treatment method, mortality increased from 14% in 1974 to 1978 to 19% in 1982 to 1986. Patients with peritonitis had identical mortalities (22%) during both periods. Patients with abscess experienced an increase in mortality from 8% in 1974 to 1978 to 15% in 1982 to 1986. In the authors' review, the widespread use of primary resection for patients with severe complications of diverticulitis appears not to have altered mortality for those with diffuse peritonitis and may have worsened the outcome for those with abscess. The reasons are unclear for the apparent discrepancy between their findings and other reports.

Kronberg (185) conducted a prospective randomized trial on 62 patients with diffuse peritonitis from perforated diverticulitis of the left colon, comparing acute transverse colostomy, suture, and omental covering of a visible perforation, with acute resection without primary anastomosis. For purulent peritonitis, the postoperative mortality rate was significantly higher after acute resection (6 of 25) than after colostomy (none of 21). In those treated by acute resection, the mortality rate age was not significantly higher after Hartmann's procedure (5 of 15) than after exteriorization of both lumens (1 of 10). The postoperative mortality rate in patients with fecal peritonitis did not differ significantly between colostomy (6 of 10) and acute resection (two of six). Stomas became permanent in 4 of 25 patients with diverticulitis surviving acute colostomy and in 7 of 22 surviving acute resection. The author concluded that the suture and transverse colostomy is superior to resection for purulent peritonitis because of the lower postoperative mortality rate and despite the shorter hospital stay in those surviving acute resection. However the operative mortality rate for resection in his trial is considerably higher than that reported by most other authors.

Celicout and Zeitoun (186) reported the results of a multicenter randomized trial comparing Hartmann's procedure with perforation suture and colostomy for patients with generalized peritonitis due to perforated sigmoid diverticulitis. Both procedures exhibited an equally high operative mortality rate of 22% but the authors favored Hartmann's procedure because of the significantly lower reintervention rate (5% vs. 20%) due to persistent peritonitis.

A tabulation of operative morbidity and mortality rates is provided in Table 5. Some patients in certain series had a modified Hartmann's procedure with creation of a mucous fistula. Factors associated with increased risk of death included persistent sepsis, fecal peritonitis, preoperative hypotension, and prolonged duration of symptoms (163). The results of restoration of intestinal continuity are provided in Table 6. Haas and Fox reviewed the fate of the forgotten rectal pouch after a Hartmann's procedure without any reconstruction (200). They examined 45 patients at least one year after an operation for a variety of indications and found that 25 patients were asymptomatic. The others reported pain, mucus, discharge,

TABLE 5 ■ Results of Hartmann's Procedure for Perforated Diverticulitis

Author(s)	No. of Patients	Operative Mortality (%)	Complication Rate (%)
Greif et al. ROL (164)	204[a]	2	
	316[b]	12	
Auguste et al. (187)	65	12	95
Hackford et al. (112)	19	16	35
Nagorney et al. (163)	84	7	41
Lambert et al. (170)	30	17	
Mallonga et al. (188)	38	5	13
Finlay and Carter (171)	38	21	
Marien (189)	36	11	42
Alanis et al. (190)	26	15	23
Berry et al. (191)	29	28	69
Hold et al. (172)	76	12	21
Kerner et al. (192)	66	2	39
Hiltunen and Matikaainen (193)	41	15	60
Kronberg (185)	15	33	
Ambrosetti et al. (71)	51	4	
Keck et al. (194)	53	9	57
Wigmore et al. (183)	124	6	
Celicout and Zeitoun (186)	53	22	
Thaler et al. (195)	63	32	24
Wedell et al. (162)	31	23	–
Khosraviani et al. (196)	72	10	43
Gooszen et al. (197)	28	25	46
Schilling et al. (198)	42	10	46

[a]Localized peritonitis.
[b]Generalized peritonitis.
Abbreviation: ROL, review of the literature.

bleeding, or passage of bowel contents. Of the 24 patients operated on for diverticulitis, 12 had proctitis, and 2 had polyps. The proctitis should be treated with reanastomosis.

In conclusion, notwithstanding the prospective randomized trial on the subject by Kronberg (185), Hartmann's procedure has evolved as the treatment of choice for patients with purulent or fecal peritonitis. However, because of the very high operative morbidity and mortality, some surgeons have questioned the wisdom of this procedure (185,191,195). It is no longer the treatment of choice for a patient with an abscess, which should be treated primarily by percutaneous drainage; if this drainage should be unsuccessful, Hartmann's procedure then can be considered or, according to Kronberg, suture and transverse colostomy.

Resection with Primary Anastomosis and Proximal Colostomy

Using resection and primary anastomosis with a proximal diverting transverse colostomy has the advantage of the diseased segment being resected, an anastomosis being created, and there being no need to establish continuity in the area of the inflammatory process (Fig. 18). Alternatively, a diverting ileostomy can be created.

The disadvantage is that another operation is required to close the colostomy, an operation that has its own attendant complications. The timing of the closure of the colostomy is debatable, and recommendations have ranged from 6 weeks to 3 months. Before closure, the anastomosis should be examined by sigmoidoscopy and barium enema to ensure that healing has occurred and that the lumen is patent. In 13 patients who were treated in this manner, Hackford et al. (112) encountered no mortality and a cumulative morbidity rate of 22%. In a series of 29 patients so treated, Hold et al. (172) reported a 7% mortality and a 38% complication rate.

Landen and Nafteux (201) conducted a prospective study on 20 patients to determine whether primary anastomosis with diverting colostomy constitutes a valid alternative to the Hartmann's procedure for patients with diffuse peritonitis due to perforated diverticulitis of sigmoid origin. Restoration of colonic continuity was programmed six weeks later, after verification of the anastomosis by Gastrografin enema. Operative mortality and morbidity was 15% and 50%, respectively. No patients showed signs of suture disruption. Mean length of hospitalization was 20 days. Closure of the colostomy using a small

TABLE 6 ■ Results Following Restoration of Intestinal Continuity After Hartmann's Procedure

Author(s)	No. of Patients	Operative Mortality (%)	Complication Rate (%)	Restoration (%)
Hackford et al. (112)	10	0	0	63
Nagorney et al. (163)	73	1	17	75
Lambert et al. (170)	25	0		94
Mallonga et al. (188)	30	0	3	83
Marien (189)	22	0	46	69
Alanis et al. (190)	14			64
Kerner et al. (192)	58	0	39	88
Hiltunen and Matikaainen (193)	27	0	26	77
Keck et al. (194)	48	2	26	83
Le Neel et al. (199)	64	0	18	70
Wigmore et al. (183)	102	1	29	52
Thaler et al. (195)	34	6	29	54
Wedell et al. (162)	31	–	–	31
Khosraviani et al. (196)	72	0	–	70
Gooszen et al. (197)	28	4	–	57
Schilling et al. (198)	42	3	–	76

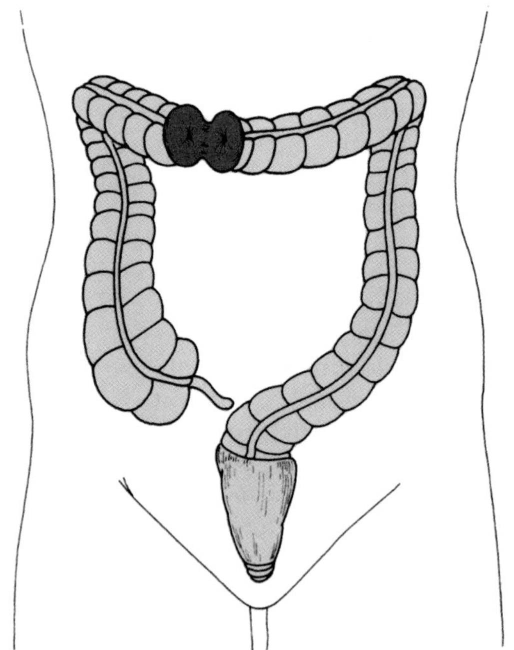

FIGURE 18 ■ Resection with primary anastomosis and proximal diverting transverse colostomy.

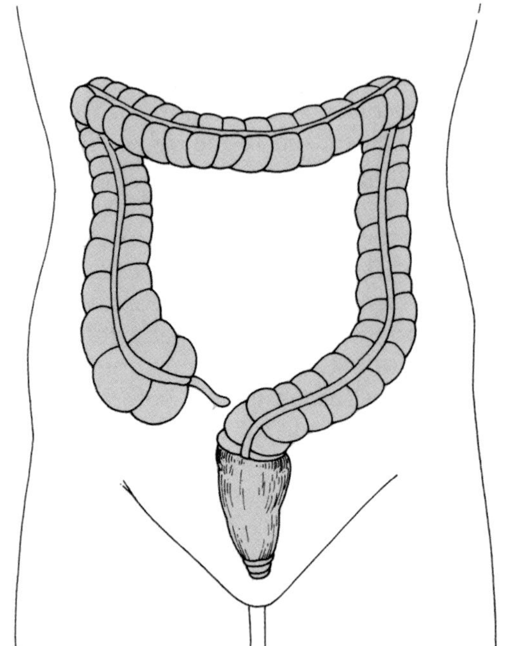

FIGURE 19 ■ Resection and primary anastomosis.

peristomal incision was performed in all surviving patients after a mean delay of 45 days. Mean length of hospitalization for colostomy closure was seven days without mortality. Primary anastomosis was found to be as safe as Hartmann's procedure but appears to be superior in terms of total length of hospital stay, interval of stomal closure, and rates of stomal closure.

Gooszen et al. (197) reported 32 patients who underwent resection, primary anastomosis, and defunctioning stoma with an operative mortality of 16%, with 16% requiring reoperation for abscess or infection. When they compared their results to a similar group of patients who underwent a Hartmann's procedure, a greater incidence of morbidity was noted with the Hartmann's procedure and they therefore prefer primary anastomosis with covering stoma.

Wedell et al. (162) reported 148 patients who underwent primary resection and primary anastomosis with a stomal closure rate of 89% dramatically better than their stomal closure rate of 23% following a Hartmann's operation.

In conclusion, this operation is a viable option, but it is not popular today.

Resection and Primary Anastomosis

A number of authors have adopted the operation of primary resection and anastomosis without a protecting colostomy (Fig. 19). Most surgeons believe that this operation is far too dangerous for general application. Anastomoses created after resection of inflamed, unprepared bowel suffer clinical leakage rates as high as 17% to 30%, a complication that proves fatal in a substantial proportion of patients (174). In addition, mortality rates of 28% to 50% have been reported after primary resection and immediate anastomosis (174). Results of some series with highly selected patients and encouraging results are presented in Table 7. Farkouh et al. (202) reported on 15 patients with perforated diverticulitis and diffuse peritonitis on whom an immediate anastomosis was constructed. Their criteria for operation were that (i) the bowel must not be distended, (ii) the bowel should be empty of feces, (iii) edema of the bowel wall at the resection site should be minimal, (iv) the distal segment of colon should be above the peritoneal reflection, (v) there should be no fecal contamination, and (vi) the patient's general condition should be reasonably good. When these criteria were met, the procedure was found to be safe, with results including one anastomotic leak, an average hospital stay of 11 days, and one death from acute pulmonary edema. The authors reviewed nine series,

TABLE 7 ■ **Results Following Resection and Primary Anastomosis for Acute or Perforated Diverticulitis**

Author(s)	No. of Patients	Mortality Rate (%)	Complication Rate (%)
Farkouh et al. (202)	15	7	
Ryan (168) ROL	73	8	
	12	0	
Rodkey and Welch (10)	63[a]	0	
	62[b]	5	
	32[c]	3	
Hackford et al. (112)	86	1	18
Alanis et al. (190)	29	3	50
Hold et al. (172)	70	3	16
Wedell et al. (162)	148	1	–
Hoemke et al. (157)	113	2	–
Gooszen et al. (203)	45	7	d
Schilling et al. (198)	13	8	33
Blair and Germann (204)	28	9	24

[a]Localized perforation (pericolic abscess).
[b]Pelvic abscess.
[c]Obstruction.
[d]48 complications in 45 patients.
Abbreviation: ROL, review of the literature.

including their own, with a total of 73 patients so treated. The operative mortality rate was 8.2%.

Auguste et al. (187) suggest that a colostomy is not necessary if a pericolic abscess is confined to the mesentery or if the abscess is localized to the pelvis. Ravo et al. (205) described a technique in which a soft, pliable tube is attached above the anastomotic site and passed through the anastomosis to protect the latter in the presence of maximal fecal loading, gross dehiscences, or fecal peritonitis. This one-stage intracolonic bypass was used in 28 patients, with no deaths and no anastomotic leakages. Intracolonic bypass may facilitate this operation, but more experience must be accumulated before a general recommendation can be made for its use.

Hackford and Veidenheimer (63) believe that the ability to achieve bowel preparation is pertinent to the decision to perform an anastomosis. This was accomplished in 96% of their patients who underwent primary resection but in only 30% to 40% of patients who underwent Hartmann's procedure.

Blair and Germann (204) reported 33 cases of resection and primary anastomosis. Five of these cases were protected with a proximal diverting stoma giving an incidence of 85% unprotected primary anastomosis in a group of patients undergoing emergency operation for acute sigmoid diverticulitis. There was one anastomotic leak, seven wound infections, and three deaths with an average length of stay of nine days. They concluded the practice of resection and primary anastomosis for acute sigmoid diverticulitis has an acceptable morbidity and mortality.

Gooszen et al. (203) reported a series of 45 patients to evaluate the feasibility of a primary anastomosis for acute complicated diverticular disease. Acute Physiology and Health Evaluation (APACHE) II score, Mannheim Peritonitis Index (MPI), and Hughes' peritonitis classification were used to classify patients and to detect factors predictive of postoperative outcome. The MPI includes different weights according to whether peritonitis is purulent (six points) or feculent (12 points), as well as other factors such as age over 50 (five points), female sex (five points), preoperative duration of peritonitis greater than 24 hours (four points), diffuse generalized peritonitis (six points), and organ failure (seven points) involving either kidney or lung, shock, or intestinal obstruction (206).

Neither anastomotic leakage (8.8%) nor death (6.6%) was related to a higher MPI, APACHE II, or Hughes' score. More postoperative septic complications were seen in patients with MPI over 16. Death, anastomotic leakage, reintervention, and wound infection were observed more frequently in patients who presented with colonic obstruction than in those with abscess or perforation.

Lee et al. (207) reported on 33 patients with complications of diverticulitis who underwent intraoperative colonic lavage in an attempt to perform primary anastomosis. In five patients, the operation included creation of a colostomy. The indication for operation was obstruction in 39%, persistent abscess or phlegmon in 39%, perforation in 18%, and hemorrhage in 3%. According to Hinchey's classification system, 18 patients had stage I disease, 10 had stage II, five patients had stage III, and none had stage IV. The single anastomotic complication in the series was responsible for the sole operative mortality. The morbidity rate of 42%, included three intraoperative complications (two splenic injuries and one ureteral laceration), two intra-abdominal abscesses (6%), and six wound infections (18%). In their experience, intraoperative colonic lavage has proven to be a safe method for accomplishing single-stage resection of the colon in selected patients with diverticulitis who require an urgent operation. When there is no evidence of diffuse purulent or feculent peritonitis, they believe this is the preferred method for treating patients who are hemodynamically stable.

Salem and Flum (208) conducted a systematic literature review, and identified 98 published series dealing with surgical management of perforated diverticulitis with peritonitis, either with primary resection and anastomosis or with the Hartmann's procedure. Operative mortality data from patients with diverticular peritonitis undergoing Hartmann's procedure ($n = 1051$) were derived from 54 studies. Considering the Hartmann's procedure and its reversal procedures together, the mortality rate was 19.6% (18.8% for the Hartmann's procedure and 0.8% for its reversal), the wound infection rate was 29.1% (24.2% for the Hartmann's procedure and 4.9% for its reversal), and stoma complications and anastomotic leaks (in the reversal operation) occurred in 10.3% and 4.3%, respectively. Of 569 reported cases of primary anastomosis from 50 studies, the aggregated mortality rate was 9.9% (range, 0–75) with an anastomotic rate of 13.9% (range, 0–60), and a wound infection rate of 9.6% (range, 0–26). They concluded reported mortality and morbidity in patients with diverticular peritonitis who underwent primary anastomosis were not higher than those in patients undergoing Hartmann's procedure. This suggests that primary anastomosis is a safe operative alternative in certain patients with peritonitis.

A Hartmann's procedure may continue to be a sound strategy in patients with septic shock secondary to peritonitis as the resulting hypotension, desaturation, and acidosis may indeed lead to injured anastomotic healing. However, recent clinical reports have suggested that in the absence of septic shock, a primary anastomosis may be performed safely during bacterial peritonitis (162,198, 203). Constructing an anastomosis relieves the patient from the burden of a colostomy and obviates a need for an additional operation to restore intestinal continuity.

In summary, the introduction of on-table lavage has modified the thinking of some surgeons. Details of the technique are fully described in Chapter 23. In selected cases, resection and primary anastomosis might be considered a suitable, safe operation (174). Despite encouragement for greater use of this operation by some surgeons, at present its use seems inappropriate in patients with generalized peritonitis.

Laparoscopic Management of Generalized Peritonitis Due to Perforated Colonic Diverticula

A novel but as yet not generally accepted method is the use of laparoscopic peritoneal lavage in conjunction with parenteral fluids and antibiotic therapy in the management of generalized peritonitis secondary to perforated diverticular disease of the colon (209). O'Sullivan et al. (209) assessed a cohort of eight patients with generalized peritonitis secondary to perforated diverticular disease of the left colon that was diagnosed laparoscopically. All the patients had purulent peritonitis but no fecal contamination. They were treated with laparoscopic peritoneal lavage and intravenous fluids and antibiotics.

All patients made a complete recovery, with resumption of normal diet within 5 to 8 days. No patient required surgical intervention during a 12- to 48-month follow-up. This approach merits further assessment as an alternative to the traditional open surgical management.

Percutaneous Drainage of Diverticular Abscesses

Ever-expanding technology has introduced a more palatable method for managing patients in whom progression of their diverticulitis has resulted in a pericolic or pelvic abscess. In instances in which the abscess is confined, the most appropriate method of treatment is CT-guided or ultrasonography-guided percutaneous drainage, with the patient receiving broad-spectrum antibiotics (210,211). Catheters connected to dependent drainage are left in place until drainage ceases and there is resolution of pain and fever. Periodic flushing is performed to ensure patency. A repeat CT scan can be performed at the time of catheter removal. Sinography may help confirm closure of the fistula or collapse of the abscess cavity before catheter removal. With this method, patients can be discharged from the hospital; then after a period of approximately 4 to 6 weeks, which allows resolution of the inflammatory process, the patient can return for an elective resection, thus converting a multiple-stage operation to a single-stage one. The optimal time to wait before elective resection has not been determined, with some surgeons recommending only 10 to 28 days.

In a report of 19 patients followed up for an average of 17.4 months after percutaneous drainage, 15 required drainage for fewer than three weeks, and three patients developed gross fecal fistulas (212). The treatment plan of preoperative drainage followed by resection and primary anastomosis was completed in 74% of patients in a safe and effective manner. Three patients (16%) required urgent operation because of persistent infection. One death resulted from poorly controlled sepsis in a patient who refused operation. Once drainage has been established, these authors offer the following important principles of successful treatment: (i) maintenance of catheter patency by routine saline solution irrigation, (ii) immediate replacement of nonfunctioning catheters, (iii) sinography once or twice weekly to assess abscess shrinkage and fistula patency, (iv) administration of appropriate broad-spectrum antibiotics and bowel rest or low-residue diet, (v) intravenous nutritional support when appropriate, and (vi) catheter removal only when drainage ceases and the abscess is completely collapsed.

Kaiser et al. (213) analyzed 511 patients admitted for acute diverticulitis and found an abscess in 19.4% of patients (74 pericolic, 25 pelvic). CT-guided drainage was performed in 16 patients, one failure requiring a two-stage operation. Whereas conservative treatment failed in 6.8% in patients without abscess or perforation, 22.2% of patients with an abscess required an urgent resection (68.2%, one stage; 31.8%, two stage). Recurrence rates were 13% for mild cases, as compared to 41.2% in patients with a pelvic abscess treated conservatively with/without CT-guided drainage. Of all surgical cases, resection/primary anastomosis was achieved in 73.6% with perioperative mortality of 1.1% and leak rate of 2.1%. They concluded CT evidence of diverticular abscess has a high risk of failure from nonoperative management regardless of the patient's age. They believe after treatment of diverticulitis with CT evidence of an abscess, physicians should strongly consider elective operation in order to prevent recurrent diverticulitis.

Ambrosetti et al. (214) proposed a more selective management for the treatment of patients with abscess associated with diverticular disease. In their long-term follow-up of 73 patients with diverticular abscess (median of 43 months) following successful conservative treatment of their abscesses, elective colectomy was not deemed mandatory. They noted that of the 45 patients with a mesocolic abscess, 15% required operation during their first hospitalization versus 39% of the 28 patients with a pelvic abscess. At the end of follow-up, 58% of the 38 patients with a mesocolic abscess who had successful conservative treatment during their first hospitalization did not need operative treatment versus 47% of the 17 who had a pelvic abscess. However, 51% of the patients with a mesocolic abscess had surgical treatment versus 71% of those with a pelvic abscess. They concluded that, considering the poor outcome of a pelvic abscess associated with acute left-sided colonic diverticulitis, percutaneous drainage followed by secondary colectomy seems justified. Mesocolic abscess has a better outcome and at least some of them do not need to be drained or operated upon. Drainage, which was undertaken only if a favorable response was not observed 48 hours after parenteral antibiotics, was mostly done for large abscesses with a statistically significant cut-off size of 5 cm. Mesocolic abscess by itself is not an absolute indication for colectomy for two reasons: first because half do not require operation and second, no patient had complications that required emergency operation.

The only limitation to this procedure is the inability to find a safe access route (e.g., when an abscess is covered by bowel). Potential complications include perforation of a viscus, fistula formation, injury to a major blood vessel with hemorrhage, pneumothorax, spread of sepsis to adjacent tissue, and septicemia. There is also the possibility of inadequate drainage and recurrent sepsis. Results of CT-guided percutaneous drainage of diverticular abscesses are listed in Table 8.

Laparotomy and Incision with Drainage of Abscess

This treatment option, although once considered appropriate, is probably no longer a viable consideration. An

TABLE 8 ■ Results of Computed Tomography-Guided Percutaneous Drainage of Diverticular Abscesses

Author(s)	No. of Patients	Success Rate (%)[a]	Catheter-Related Complications
Mueller et al. (215)	21	76	0
Neff et al. (216)	16	94	0
Stabile et al. (212)	19	74	0
Kaiser et al. (213)	16	94	–

[a]Resolution of symptoms, multistage operation not required.

exception to this statement is the situation in which the radiologist is unable to gain safe percutaneous access to the abscess; under this circumstance an operative approach would be indicated. Most surgeons would perform Hartmann's procedure with drainage of the abscess, but in exceptional circumstances, drainage alone might be considered. Even then, a complementary colostomy would probably be established.

PARADIGM SHIFT IN THE MANAGEMENT OF DIVERTICULITIS ■ Salem et al. (217) evaluated temporal trends in the use of operative and nonoperative interventions in the management of diverticulitis using the state of Washington administrative database. Of the 25,058 patients hospitalized nonelectively with diverticulitis (mean age 69 years, 60% female), there were only minimal changes in the frequency of admission over time (0.006% increase per year). The odds of an emergency colectomy at initial hospitalization decreased by 2% each year whereas the odds of percutaneous abscess drainage increased 7% per year. Among patients undergoing percutaneous drainage, the odds of operative interventions decreased by 9% compared to patients who did not have a percutaneous intervention. The proportion of patients undergoing colostomy during emergency operations remained essentially stable over time (range, 49–61%), as did the proportion of patients undergoing prophylactic colectomy after initial nonsurgical management (approximately 10%).

Extended Colectomy

The extended colectomy has been recommended for treating massive bleeding of undetermined origin in patients with diverticular disease. It has also been proposed for men under age 50 who harbor extensive disease (218). Crowson and McCaughan (219) reported on 45 patients who underwent total abdominal colectomy for management of their diverticular disease. The authors suggested three absolute indications for performing this operation in complicated diverticular disease: (i) massive hemorrhage, (ii) fistula formation, and (iii) extensive involvement of the entire colon. The morbidity rate compared favorably with that for segmental resection. More than one-half of the procedures were performed as a second-stage curative procedure. Although this procedure is an option to keep in mind in the unusual circumstance in which difficulty is encountered in creating an anastomosis without tension, it is seldom used in the management of patients with complications of acute diverticulitis.

■ MALIGNANT DIVERTICULITIS

Morganstern et al. (220) described a form of severe diverticulitis characterized by (i) phlegmonous inflammation of the sigmoid and rectosigmoid colon, often extending below the peritoneal reflection; (ii) frequent fistulization to the skin, urinary bladder, and small intestine; (iii) frequent colonic obstruction; and (iv) high postoperative morbidity, including wound infection, anastomotic leaks, pelvic abscesses, overwhelming sepsis, and a high postoperative mortality rate of 18% (3 out of 17 patients). This form was termed "malignant" diverticulitis because of the progressive nature of the disease process and the frequency of severe morbidity associated with it. It represents approximately 7% of patients undergoing operation for diverticular disease. For this fulminant variant of diverticulitis, the authors favor the three-stage resection. A multistaged procedure would not seem to be required with the current understanding of the disease.

■ MANAGEMENT OF YOUNG PATIENTS

Patients aged below 40 years account for 2% to 6% of those with diverticular disease (92,221) and include a preponderance of men (221,222). It has often been suggested that diverticular disease in the young patient is associated with a more virulent course and is characterized by recurrent inflammatory episodes and a propensity for serious complications (4,91,92,222,223). The severity of diverticulitis in younger patients is not easy to define because criteria to judge it are mostly based on the rate of emergency operation, which varies from 17% to 88% (224). This is a poor indication of severity because of the difficulty of diagnosing diverticulitis in young patients with an accuracy of 12% to 59% on admission (224).

Ambrosetti et al. (224) conducted a prospective study to compare acute left-sided colonic diverticulitis in patients aged 50 years or younger and in patients older than 50 years for severity of disease and immediate and late outcome. Of the 265 patients studied, 61 were aged 50 years or younger; of these, 49 were men. In all instances, diagnosis was confirmed radiologically or histologically. Fewer operations were performed on younger patients than on older patients (15% vs. 33%). Severe diverticulitis was found more often in younger men than older men (39% vs. 23%). After successful conservative treatment during the first hospitalization period, younger men had a statistically greater risk of poor outcome than older men (29% vs. 5%). The authors concluded that although younger men have severe acute diverticulitis more often than older men, operative treatment during the first episode is less often needed in younger men. On the other hand, after conservative treatment, younger men have a statistically greater chance of poor secondary outcome than older men.

Ouriel and Schwartz (92) reviewed the records of 15 patients under the age of 40 years with documented diverticular disease and found that 92 patients presented with acute diverticulitis, five presented with bleeding, and 18 were asymptomatic. An urgent operation was necessary in 16 patients, and another nine underwent resection during the initial hospitalization. Of the remaining 67 patients managed medically, 55% required readmission, with 23% having a serious complication and 45% undergoing a subsequent operation. The authors therefore recommend that patients have an elective resection after a "cooling-off" period to minimize morbidity and hospitalization.

In a review of the natural history of diverticular disease in patients under age 40 years. Chodak et al. (91) obtained a follow-up history in 14 of 17 patients initially treated medically. Mild symptoms were reported in seven, and the other seven required operation. Over a 14-year period, 27 of 37 patients had undergone operation.

Konvolinka (225) reviewed the records of 248 patients hospitalized for acute diverticulitis and found 11.7% of them to be under the age of 40 years, 76% male and 24% female. Operative intervention was required in 76% of cases compared to 17% of elderly cases. Obesity is the major comorbid condition. Early operative intervention is recommended following the first documented attack to avoid the potential for serious septic complications.

In a series of 58 patients with diverticulitis reviewed by Freischlag et al. (222), 17 (29%) were younger than 40 years. Fifteen of the 17 (88%) required urgent or emergent surgery for complications of diverticular disease, a significantly larger proportion than for patients over age 40 years (42%). In 13 patients, the operation was required during the first attack.

Schauer et al. (226) reviewed their experience in which 61 of 238 patients treated for acute diverticulitis were 40 years of age or younger. Younger patients more frequently required an operation on an urgent basis for complications of diverticulitis during the initial hospitalization. The most common indication for operation in young patients was perforation compared with recurrent disease for the older age group. The younger group had a sevenfold incidence of enteric fistulas complicating their acute episode of diverticulitis.

Cunningham et al. (223) compared the medical versus surgical management of diverticulitis for complications and outcomes in patients under the age of 40 years. Complications included readmission, recurrent symptoms after antibiotic therapy, and postoperative problems. A radiographic or surgical diagnosis of diverticulitis was made in 29 patients (18 surgical, 11 medical). Medically managed patients had significantly more emergency department visits (4.7 ± 6.6 vs. 0.3 ± 0.6) and readmissions (7 vs. 4). Three surgical patients (17%) had a total of six complications as compared with six medical patients (55%) with 25 complications. All medically treated patients had recurrent symptoms and six required operation. They believe operation is the indicated treatment for the first episode of diverticulitis in patients under the age of 40 years.

Minardi et al. (227) reviewed 22 patients with diverticulitis, aged 40 years and younger. Inclusion criteria were either a diagnosis of diverticulitis confirmed at operation, or positive CT findings and/or a positive contrast enema. The mean age in this study was 32.1 years. All 22 patients presented with abdominal pain. The next most common symptom was nausea and/or vomiting in 45% followed by fever and chills in 36%. Eighteen patients underwent an operation. Four patients were treated nonoperatively. Nineteen patients had diverticulitis of the sigmoid colon. The remaining three had right-sided diverticulitis. Two patients underwent right hemicolectomy and one underwent cecectomy. Of the 15 patients with sigmoid diverticulitis, 80% underwent a two-stage procedure of sigmoid colectomy and colostomy and Hartmann's pouch. Twenty percent of patients underwent a one-stage procedure of sigmoid colectomy and primary anastomosis. Two of three patients undergoing a one-stage procedure required reoperation. Postoperative complications occurred in 56% of patients. Two of these patients had septic complications. There was one death in the series. Colostomy closure was performed successfully in 75% of patients. The overall mortality was 4.5%. They believe, although rare, diverticulitis in a young patient is often a fulminant illness requiring operation early in the disease process.

The experience of others does not support the "virulent" label for diverticulitis in the young (228). Acosta et al. (221), in their review of 285 patients with acute diverticulitis, concluded that the behavior of the disease in patients 40 years or younger is probably not more virulent than in older patients. Similarly Vignati et al. (229) studied the natural history of documented diverticulitis that resolves after treatment with intravenous antibiotics and bowel rest in patients under the age of 50 years. Of the total of 40 patients, 25% required operation during the initial admission. Of the remaining 30 patients followed up for five to nine years, one-third required operation—all elective with single-stage resections. Based on their data, the authors do not recommend operation after a single episode of diverticulitis.

West et al. (230) in a series of 46 patients under the age of 50 years found that diverticulitis did not appear to take a more aggressive course than the same disease in older patients. Biondo et al. (231) reported on 327 patients treated for left colonic diverticulitis. Patients were divided into two groups: those aged 50 years or less (group 1, 72 patients) and those older than 50 years (group 2, 255 patients). The diagnosis was confirmed histologically or radiologically in all patients. During the first hospital stay, 69.1% of patients had successful conservative treatment, 23.9% needed emergency operation, and 7% had a semielective operation. The recurrence rate was 25.5% in group 1 and 22.3% in group 2. Overall, a mortality rate in patients who underwent an operation was 16.3%. The mortality rate was 0 in group 1 and 2.2% in group 2 after elective or semielective operation, and 0 in group 1 and 34.9% in group 2 after emergency operation. They concluded diverticulitis in young patients does not have a particularly progressive course and the risk of recurrence is similar to that of older patients. Similarly, Guzzo and Hyman (156) conducted a retrospective chart review of 762 patients admitted with sigmoid diverticulitis. During the study period, 31% of patients underwent operation. The outcomes in patients aged 50 years or younger (group 1), which represented 34% of the total population studied were compared with patients older than 50 years (group 2). The risk of requiring operation on initial hospital presentation was similar between the two groups (24% vs. 22%, respectively); however, group 1 patients were more likely to be treated operatively at some point during the study period (40% vs 26%) because of an increase in elective resections. Of the 196 patients in group 1 who had an initially medically managed admission, only one presented at a later date with perforation (0.5%). They concluded the risk of subsequent diverticular perforation in medically managed young patients with sigmoid diverticulitis is very low and hence these patients did not necessarily merit an operation.

Notwithstanding the enthusiasm for performing operation in the young patient, it must be remembered that Haglund et al. (64) found few serious complications in patients with subsequent attacks of diverticulitis. In light of these findings, the frequently espoused policy of recommending operation after a single attack of diverticulitis in young patients may not be warranted.

RECTAL DIVERTICULA

Diverticula of the rectum are extremely rare. The presence of uncomplicated rectal diverticulosis is probably of little clinical significance. They are considered to be true diverticula and are often solitary (61). Affected patients may experience rectal pain. A high-fiber diet and sitz baths have proven effective (232). When diverticulitis supervenes, inflammation and ulceration have been reported. Resolution of symptoms has been achieved through the use of antibiotics and evacuation of a mass. The condition should not be confused with carcinoma. If an abscess should develop, it can be drained through the rectum. For repeated inflammation, segmental resection should be considered.

CHRONIC DIVERTICULITIS

Chronic diverticulitis is an ill-defined entity possibly characterized by a low-grade inflammation caused by a past local perforation. Some patients have the muscle abnormality of left-sided diverticular disease with bowel symptoms. In some cases, the patients may have irritable bowel syndrome. Indications for elective operation already have been described.

PERFORATION

Patients with diverticulitis with perforation may have a variety of conditions, ranging from a small abscess between the leaves of the mesocolon to full-blown fecal peritonitis. There is little uniformity in the classification of the pathology, the indications for operation, or the operative management. Full credit for the introduction of some semblance of organization of the severity of the disease goes to Hughes et al. (233), who proposed a practical clinical classification based on operative findings to group patients according to the severity of their peritoneal contamination. They divided clinically acute diverticulitis into the following four main groups, according to patients with

1. Local peritonitis
2. Local pericolic or pelvic abscess
3. General peritonitis due to ruptured pericolic or pelvic abscess
4. General peritonitis due to free perforation of the colon.

Subsequent authors have proposed their own classifications. Localio and Stahl (234) called attention to the problem of terminology and underscored the observation that acute perforated diverticulitis may present as a free perforation with diffuse peritonitis or as a confined perforation with pericolic or mesocolic abscess formation. This classification provided a useful distinction in terms of clinical manifestations and appropriate operative management. In their classification of perforated diverticulitis, Miller and Wichern (235) made the distinction between patients with pericolic abscess, mesocolic abscess, or free perforation with diffuse peritonitis. Hinchey et al. (236) in a classification almost identical to that of Hughes et al. (233), divided their patients into four stages:

- Stage I: Pericolic or mesenteric abscess
- Stage II: Walled-off pelvic abscess
- Stage III: Generalized purulent peritonitis
- Stage IV: Generalized fecal peritonitis

Killingback (167) proposed the following more complicated classification:

1. Abscess
   a. Peridiverticular
   b. Mesenteric
   c. Pericolic (pelvic)
2. Perforation
   a. Free
   b. Concealed (indirect)
3. Gangrenous sigmoiditis
4. Peritonitis
   a. (i) serous, (ii) purulent, or (iii) fecal
   b. (i) local, (ii) pelvic, or (iii) generalized (diffuse)

The treatment recommended depends on which one of these entities is present. The need to define the extent of the inflammatory process is illustrated by the report of Haglund et al. (64), who noted that of 97 patients who underwent emergency operation, the operative mortality rate was 33% when a perforation was present and only 3% when only acute inflammation was present. Authors who are more liberal in their indications for operation (i.e., include a higher percentage of patients with only inflammation in their series) will report a lower operative mortality rate. The mortality rate for patients with localized peritonitis or an abscess is less than that associated with diffuse or fecal contamination (64,164,235,236).

The percentage of cases in each category varies greatly according to the aggressiveness of the surgeon in operating on patients with nonresponding acute diverticulitis. The surgeon who operates early and frequently will have a much larger percentage of patients in category I (Hinchey classification), whereas the conservative surgeon who is willing to "ride it out" will have a higher percentage in categories III and IV. Obviously all surgeons will operate promptly on patients with generalized peritonitis. Although the authors have not used the same classification, the type of perforation that can be expected (as determined from information in the articles) as described in the Hinchey classification is outlined in Table 9. It will be noted that the percentages vary greatly.

Localized (Pericolic Intramesenteric) Abscess

A walled-off perforation or abscess is the most common complication of sigmoid diverticulitis. It may occur in the pericolic region or may involve the mesentery.

TABLE 9 ■ Expected Frequency of Severity of Perforations of Diverticulitis

Author(s)	No. of Patients	Stage I (%)	Stage II (%)	Stage III (%)	Stage IV (%)
Hinchey et al. (236)	95	31	40	22	7
Killingback (167)	248	14	33	42	11
Auguste et al. (187)	116	21	35	35	9
Mallonga et al. (188)	38	21	18	40	21
Silvis and Keeman (237)	29	3	10	62	24
Alanis et al. (190)	65	18	63	17	2
Lee et al. (207)	33	55	30	15	0

The clinical manifestations of this type of abscess are confined to the left lower quadrant, with varying degrees of pain and tenderness occurring. Constitutional symptoms of tachycardia and leukocytosis are commensurate with the degree of inflammation.

A number of radiologic features have been described through the barium enema study, but recent advances in technology have facilitated the diagnosis. Barium should not be used in the presence of acute inflammation; when the diagnosis is in doubt, any contrast study should include a water-soluble contrast medium. Dye may be seen tracking in the immediate pericolic region or toward the pelvis. Less commonly, the mass may increase in size to involve the abdominal wall and on very rare occasions, may even track toward the perineum through the ischioanal fossa. An abscess may be differentiated from a phlegmon with the use of ultrasonography. CT scanning may prove very valuable, from both a diagnostic and a therapeutic point of view. Initial management consists of broad-spectrum antibiotic therapy and bowel rest. If symptoms worsen or do not improve, the presence of an undrained abscess should be suspected. In the past, at this point operative intervention was considered indicated, and a large number of operations have been recommended for these circumstances. The options have been outlined in the discussion of treatment of acute diverticulitis.

However, the development of the ability to drain these abscesses percutaneously under CT control has revolutionized the management of patients. The tremendous advantage is that what was formerly treated as a two- or three-stage procedure can now be converted into a one-stage elective, or at least a semielective, operation. After resolution of the acute inflammatory process, the patient can receive mechanical and antibiotic bowel preparation and proceed to an elective resection and primary anastomosis.

Pelvic Abscess

If a patient treated for acute diverticulitis fails to improve after three to five days of adequate medical therapy, a pericolic or pelvic abscess should be suspected. The signs and symptoms have already been described, but "protection" by contiguous structures may initially mask the presence of a pelvic abscess. Rectal or vaginal examination may reveal a tender bulging mass. Hypovolemia and gram-negative sepsis may occur. Once suspected, the diagnosis can be confirmed with ultrasonography or a CT scan. The patient should be treated with intravenous fluids, broad-spectrum antibiotics, and CT- or ultrasound-directed percutaneous drainage.

Purulent Peritonitis

Purulent peritonitis may arise from a persistently leaking diverticulitis or from the sudden rupture of a previously walled-off pericolic or pelvic abscess. The site of perforation is often not identified (95 of 248 times) (114). This situation demands immediate appropriate administration of fluids and electrolytes, correction of cardiopulmonary abnormalities, administration of parenteral antibiotics, and prompt operative treatment using the choices outlined under the options for treating acute diverticulitis. Probably the single most significant advance in the treatment of perforation associated with diverticulitis is primary resection of the perforated segment. No longer can the patient be considered too ill to withstand a major operative procedure; he or she must be considered too ill to withstand anything other than primary resection. In a patient with perforation during acute diverticulitis, it is the disease, not the operation that causes death.

Fazio (238) has offered a number of guidelines for conducting emergency operations on patients with generalized peritonitis secondary to perforated diverticulitis:

1. Resect the perforated segment.
2. Do not do more than you need to do. Definitive operation is a more extensive procedure.
3. Do not open further avenues of sepsis by performing extensive peritoneal dissection, either by mobilizing the splenic flexure or by entering the presacral space.
4. Do not make a mucous fistula. The distal sigmoid can be stapled and delivered to the lower end of the abdominal wound to avoid the need for a second appliance.
5. Examine the open specimen before closure of the abdomen. If a malignancy is found, a wider resection can be entertained if the patient's general status is satisfactory.

Following resection, copious irrigation with warm saline solution is helpful to dilute the bacterial inoculum. Opinion is divided on two matters: whether using an antibiotic irrigation is more efficacious than using saline and the use of drains. The general peritoneal cavity cannot be drained, but if an abscess cavity is present, the use of suction catheters might be appropriate. At the time of the definitive operation, the principles concerning the extent of the operation as described for elective procedures should be adopted.

Fear of anastomotic leakage has long dominated surgical practice when confronted with the presence of peritonitis during laparotomy, as in the case of perforated diverticulitis. This has led to the common practice of resection of the inflamed bowel followed by end-colostomy (Hartmann's procedure) to avoid the construction of a primary anastomosis. This may be a sound strategy in patients with septic shock secondary to peritonitis as the resulting hypotension, desaturation, and acidosis may indeed lead to impaired anastomotic healing. However, recent clinical studies suggest that, in the absence of septic shock, a primary anastomosis may be performed safely during bacterial peritonitis (162,198,203). Constructing a primary anastomosis releases the patient from the burden of a colostomy and the need for an additional operation to restore continuity. In spite of this, many surgeons including the author are still reluctant to perform a primary anastomosis in the presence of peritonitis and the Hartmann's procedure remains popular.

Fecal Peritonitis

The least common but potentially most devastating type of perforation is a free perforation in which the patient rapidly develops a generalized fecal peritonitis. This situation is associated with the greatest mortality rate (163,174,236,239). The patient presents with a rather sudden onset of abdominal pain and distention. Examination may reveal a septic patient with constitutional signs of fever, tachycardia, and even hypotension in the advanced stage. Abdominal examination may reveal distention, tenderness, guarding, or rigidity. Leukocytosis of varying degrees will be present. In elderly patients and those being treated with steroid drugs, symptoms and signs of peritonitis may be minimal or absent. An abdominal series will usually reveal free air.

Patients with fecal peritonitis demand immediate treatment with fluid replacement, blood volume restoration, broad-spectrum, antibiotics, and immediate operation. Emergency resection of the sigmoid colon is the best treatment for these patients (174). The general principles discussed in the previous section also pertain to this condition.

Results

Outcome depends, for the most part, on the severity of the disease (type of peritonitis) and the type of operation performed. For example, Nagorney et al. (163) found a 6% mortality rate for patients with diffuse purulent peritonitis and a 35% rate for those with fecal peritonitis. The difference in operative mortality according to the type of operation is clearly depicted in Tables 4 and 5. Factors identified as having an increased risk of death include persistent sepsis, fecal peritonitis, preoperative hypotension, and prolonged duration of symptoms. In the report by Elliott et al. (240), 28% of 463 patients admitted with acute diverticulitis required an operation and in this group the mortality rate was 18%. All deaths occurred in patients who had on operation for septic complications or bowel obstruction.

In an excellent review of the world literature on emergency surgery for diverticular disease complicated by generalized and fecal peritonitis, Krukowski and Matheson (174) showed a clear advantage in terms of both immediate morbidity and mortality in performing primary resection instead of operations in which the colon was retained. In a painstakingly detailed analysis, they tabulated data on the mortality rate of the first emergency operation in a total of 1282 patients described in 57 publications between 1957 and 1984. The collective mortality rate relative to the various operations was as follows: drainage with or without suture, 28.1%; colostomy with or without suture, with or without drainage, 25.7%; exteriorization, 13.1%; resection without anastomosis, 12.2%; resection with anastomosis, 9%; and resection with anastomosis with colostomy, 6.1%. Those who have attempted to quantify morbidity unanimously agree that intraperitoneal and wound sepsis, length of hospital stay, and failure to complete the proposed course of treatment are very much higher in the group of patients treated with a lesser operation. They concluded that when an operation is necessary for treatment of generalized peritonitis or failed medical management, the affected sigmoid loop should be resected and the operation should be completed as Hartmann's procedure. Only in the most favorable circumstances should a primary anastomosis be considered after on-table irrigation of the colon.

Silvis and Keeman (237) attempted to determine outcome relative to the stage of the disease and the type of operation performed. The lack of uniform classification of the severity of perforation is one of the main problems in comparing results of emergency operations in patients with complicated diverticulitis. In their review of several studies, including their own, the patient mortality rate was low with either a staged resection (approximately 5%) or a primary resection (no mortality recorded) for stage I disease. For stage II disease, the mortality rates were also similar, approximately 8% and 5%, respectively. Some series combined stages III and IV. For stage III disease, the operative mortality rate was approximately 17% for staged resection and 8% for primary resection. For stage IV disease, the operative mortality rate was 64% for staged resection and 28% for primary resection. The present trend is to preserve the use of primary sigmoid resection and anastomosis for perforations in stages I and II, and to perform Hartmann's procedure for stages III and IV.

An exception to this statement is the report by Regenet et al. (241), who compared primary resection with intraoperative colonic lavage and Hartmann's procedure. Of the 60 patients who underwent emergency laparotomy for diverticular peritonitis (Hinchey stages III, IV), primary resection and anastomosis with intraoperative colonic lavage was performed on 27 patients and Hartmann's procedure in 33. Mortality with intraoperative colonic lavage was 11% and with Hartmann's procedure was 12%. The incidence of postoperative complication was significantly higher and the mean hospital stay was significantly longer after Hartmann's procedure than after primary resection with intraoperative colonic lavage. They concluded that primary resection with intraoperative colonic lavage should be an alternative to Hartmann's procedure for diffuse purulent and stercoral peritonitis.

Makela et al. (242) reviewed 133 patients admitted to a university hospital for diverticular perforation. They noted that the annual prevalence of perforated sigmoid diverticulitis in Finland is increasing. It was 2.4 per 100,000 in the year 1986 and 3.8 per 100,000 in the year 2000. The resection rate was 90%; after resection, 45 primary anastomoses, 75 Hartmann's colostomies, and one covering colostomy were performed. The overall complication rate was 32%, without any significant difference between the procedures. Overall mortality was 9% without significant difference between the procedures. Forty-five percent of the colostomies have been closed. The Mannheim Peritonitis Index (MPI) score can be used in predicting the outcome of patients admitted for perforated sigmoid diverticulitis. More recently, Makela et al. (243) reviewed 172 patients with diverticular perforation and evaluated prognostic indicators of postoperative complications and mortality. The resection rate was 91%; 64 primary anastomoses, 93 Hartmann's procedures, and 2 covering colostomies were performed. The overall complication rate was 33%. In patients under 70 years, the MPI and the American Society of Anesthesiologists (ASA) score were independent prognostic factors. None of the factors predicted morbidity in patients over 70 years. Overall mortality rate was 8%, without any significant difference between the procedures. All patients who died presented with ASA scores of III to IV. Only the MPI score seemed to be an independent predictor of mortality. Age alone was not an independent predictor of mortality.

Zeitoun et al. (206) conducted a multicenter randomized clinical trial involving a comparison of primary resection and suture, drainage with proximal colostomy followed by secondary resection for patients with generalized peritonitis complicating sigmoid diverticulitis. A total of 105 patients were randomized to undergo primary or secondary resection. The main end point was occurrence of generalized or localized peritonitis. The Mannheim peritonitis index score was calculated for each patient to check for comparability of groups. Patients were then analyzed according to whether the MPI score was less than 21 (good prognosis), 21, or greater (poor prognosis). Postoperative peritonitis occurred less often after primary than secondary resection, whether considering the first procedure only (1 of 55 patients vs. 10 of 48 patients) or all procedures (1 of 55 vs. 12 of 48). Likewise, early reoperation was performed less often following primary resection than secondary resection (2 of 55 vs. 9 of 48 and 2 vs. 11), leading to a shorter median hospital stay for patients having primary resection (15 days) than those undergoing secondary resection (24 days). The mortality did not differ significantly with regard to operative policy (primary resection 24% vs. secondary resection 19%) or type of peritonitis (fecal in 27% vs. purulent 19%). No patients died following a second or third procedure. They concluded that primary resection is superior to secondary resection in the treatment of generalized peritonitis complicating sigmoid diverticulitis because of significantly less postoperative, fewer reoperations and shorter hospital stay.

■ FISTULA

Incidence

Fistula formation is believed to evolve from a localized perforation to which an adjacent viscus becomes adherent. Ultimately the abscess or feces begin to drain through that viscus. It is not entirely clear as to how often fistula development occurs in patients with diverticular disease. Hool et al. (244) reviewed more than 2300 patients with diverticular disease, 80 of whom required operation, and only four fistulas were noted, for an incidence of 5%. On the other hand, Corman (245) found that 33% of 155 patients who underwent resection had a fistula. However, in a review of the literature, Colcock and Stahmann (246) found that 19% of 1555 patients who underwent resection had a colonic fistula. Other reported series are listed in Table 10. It is not surprising to find that there is a discrepancy in the incidence of fistula because series from large referral centers can be expected to contain a larger percentage of fistulas.

TABLE 10 ■ Incidence of Fistula Formation in Patients with Diverticular Disease Requiring Operation

Author(s)	No. Requiring Operation	No. of Fistulas	Incidence (%)
Colcock and Stahmann ROL (246)	1555	296	19
Orebaugh et al. (247)	144	14	10
Hool et al. (244)	80	4	5
Pheils et al. (248)	80	20	25
Corman (245)	155	51	33
Rodkey and Welch (10)	350	39	11
Woods et al. (249)	412	92	22
Bahadursingh et al. (250)	192	9	6

Abbreviation: ROL, review of the literature.

Types and Frequency

A large variety of fistulas have been described in patients with diverticular disease. The relative frequency of the different types is difficult to ascertain because authors often report on only one type or only certain types of fistulas, so representative series are seldom, if ever, available. The most common variety is the colovesical fistula, followed by colocutaneous, colovaginal, and coloenteric fistulas. Other distinctly uncommon fistulas that have been described include coloureteral (246,251), colouterine (111,246,249,252), colosalpingeal (246,253,254), coloperineal (10,246), sigmoid-appendiceal (255), colovenous (256), and colocholecystic (257) ones. The frequency of each of these fistulas as reported by their authors is described in Table 11.

Clinical Manifestations

Much of the following information has been obtained from a review of internal fistulas associated with diverticular disease conducted by Woods et al. (249). The clinical manifestations depend on the type of fistula present. The mean age of patients ranges from 55 to 65, with an overall range of 38 to 84. Patients with a colovesical fistula are preponderantly male, with ratios ranging from 2:1 to 6:1 (249,260). Presumably the uterus, which interposes itself between the bladder and the colon in the female, acts as a protective shield. Approximately 50% of the female patients had had a hysterectomy (249). It is of interest to note that in a series of 48 fistulas of all types associated with diverticular disease, there was a female predominance with a 3:1 ratio (259). Looking specifically at colovesical fistula, the female preponderance was maintained with a 2:1 ratio but 60% of these women had undergone a hysterectomy. In many cases, the symptoms are preceded by the symptoms of diverticulitis, and a pericolic abscess may burst into an adjacent viscus. With a colovesical fistula, the symptoms may include those of cystitis (70–80%), namely dysuria, frequency, and hematuria; lower abdominal pain (30–90%); pneumaturia (60%); and fecaluria (40–70%). Bowel symptoms may be absent in up to 36% of patients (261), and the presenting symptoms are those of a urinary tract infection. Very rarely, the patient may pass urine from the rectum (10%). Systemic toxicity may occur in 20% to 50% of patients, and a mass is present in less than 30% of cases.

Fazio et al. (262) reviewed the records of 93 patients with colocutaneous fistulas associated with diverticulitis. Ninety-five percent of fistulas developed after an operation, whereas only 5% developed spontaneously. The presence of a diverting stoma did not prevent fistula formation but did decrease morbidity. Twenty-eight patients had a fistula to other organs, 20 involving the small bowel. Clinical manifestations in addition to stool passing through the fistula include fever, a mass, obstruction, skin excoriation, rectal bleeding, or peritonitis. Incidence of recent weight loss (40%) and hypoalbuminemia (47%) was high. Factors leading to persistence of fistulas included sepsis (42 patients), distal obstruction caused by residual sigmoid colon (38 patients), and presence of Crohn's disease or carcinoma.

Patients with a colovaginal fistula may present with abdominal pain and discharge of pus, stool, or flatus through the vagina. Vaginal examination will reveal an

TABLE 11 ■ Types of Fistula Formation Reported for Patients with Diverticular Disease

	Author(s)						
Type	Colcock and Stahmann (246)		Eisenstat et al. (111)	Wassef et al. (258)	Rodkey and Welch (10)	Woods et al. (249)	Vasilevsky et al. (259)
Colovesical	21 (33%)	131 (53%)	12 (67%)	16 (55%)	16 (41%)	60 (65%)	23 (48%)
Colocutaneous	22 (34%)	77 (31%)	4 (22%)	5 (17%)	6 (15%)		2 (4%)
Colovaginal	7 (11%)	4 (2%)		7 (24%)	7 (18%)	23 (25%)	21 (44%)
Coloenteric	6 (9%)	25 (10%)	1	4 (14%)	8 (21%)	6 (6.5%)	1
Colouterine	1	2	1			3 (3%)	
Colosalpingeal	1						1
Coloureteral	1	1					
Coloperineal	1	1			1		
Colocolic	1	3			1		
Miscellaneous	3	2					
Total	64	246 (ROL)	18	32	39	92	48

Abbreviation: ROL, review of the literature.

opening, usually at the apex of the vaginal vault (75%), or a mass may be detected during a pelvic or abdominal examination. Many of these patients have previously undergone a hysterectomy. For example, in the series by Woods et al. (249), 83% of such patients had had a previous hysterectomy. In the series reported by Vasilevsky et al. (259), 95% of the women had undergone a previous hysterectomy. In a review of 69 patients from the literature by Grissom and Snyder (263), 71% had a history of hysterectomy. Although the thick-walled uterus is usually resistant to fistula formation, occasionally fistulization may occur. Some patients may develop a purulent or fecal vaginal discharge.

Patients with coloenteric fistulas also may have abdominal pain and develop diarrhea, depending on the portion of small bowel affected. Rarely an abscess may burrow through the levator ani muscle and the ischioanal fossa, and present in the perineum as an ischioanal abscess. Only five cases of coloureteric fistula have been reported in the literature up to 1994 (264).

Diagnosis

Diagnosis of a colovesical fistula may be either rather simple or difficult. Passage of stool through the urethra is diagnostic but uncommon. Unexplained recurrent urinary tract infections that fail to respond to appropriate antimicrobial therapy should alert the physician to the possible diagnosis. Pneumaturia that occurs at the end of voiding is strongly suggestive of colovesical fistula, but gas-producing organisms in the bladder might simulate the condition, particularly in patients with diabetes.

The reliability of various investigative modalities has varied. Flexible sigmoidoscopy and colonoscopy may rule out inflammatory bowel disease or malignancy but will usually fail to demonstrate the fistula. An abdominal series may demonstrate an air–fluid level in the bladder. A barium enema may demonstrate the communication in 5% to 80% of the cases but will show the diverticular disease. It is probably the most common way in which the diagnosis is made. Cystoscopy may reveal cystitis, and the opening may be seen (46%) (249). Some abnormality was found in 92% of patients with bullous edema or localized cystitis (249). An intravenous pyelogram may help in assessing renal function and in verifying the presence of two functioning kidneys or other abnormalities. Passage in the urine of ingested dyes or charcoal is diagnostic. Cystograms have demonstrated the fistula in up to 30% of cases. The Bourne test, consisting of radiography of the centrifuged urine samples obtained immediately after a barium enema, was positive in 9 of 10 patients, and it was the only positive evidence of an otherwise occult colovesical fistula in 7 of them (265). CT scanning has reliably detected the presence of a colovesical fistula, and it may be useful in assessing the extent and degree of pericolonic inflammation, thus playing a role in both the preoperative surgical planning and the diagnosis (266). Radiographic abnormalities include intravesical gas, focal bladder wall thickening, extraluminal mass, and sometimes the fistulous tract (Fig. 20). Some now regard this to be the most sensitive diagnostic study (266).

A barium enema will demonstrate the communication of a colovaginal fistula in 34% to 49% of the cases (259,263). The opening in the vaginal vault was found at or near the

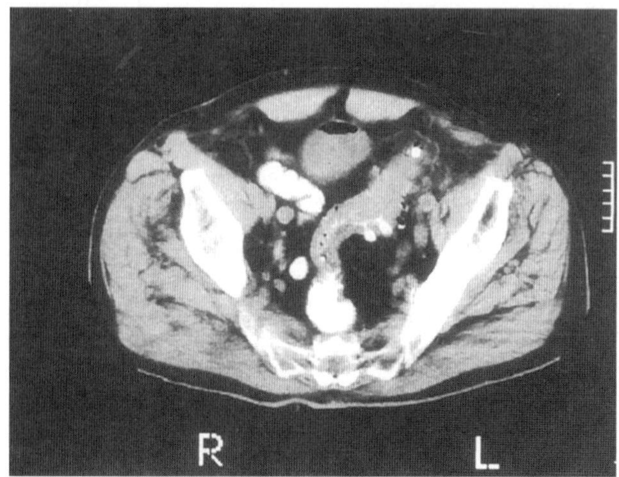

FIGURE 20 ■ Computed tomography demonstrating thickened bowel wall in area of sigmoid diverticular disease. Air in the bladder is demonstrated.

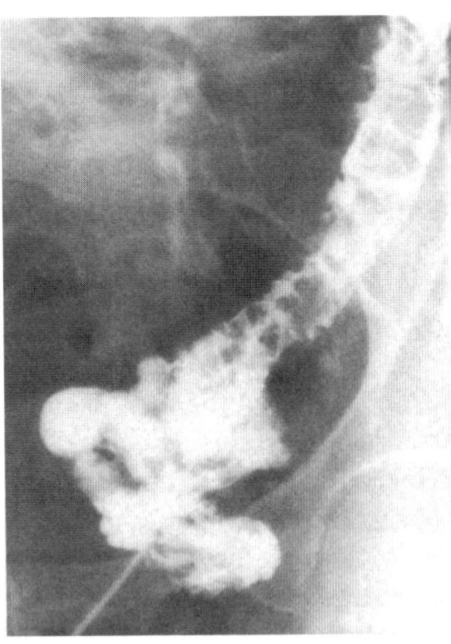

FIGURE 21 ■ Fistulogram demonstrating communication between vaginal vault and colon. A previous barium enema did not demonstrate the fistula.

apex of the vagina by vaginoscopy in 29% to 90% of cases (259,263). If the fistula is strongly suspected and unproven, a fistulogram can be used as demonstrated in Fig. 21. Vaginography has been described as the investigation of choice for clinically suspected vaginal fistulas (267). The technique employs a Foley catheter with a 30 cc balloon that is inserted into the vagina and inflated to obtain a good seal. The injection of water-soluble contrast will usually visualize the fistula (Fig. 22). In a series of 24 patients, Giordano et al. (267) reported that vaginography successfully identified 19 fistulas with a sensitivity of 79%, but not all were of diverticular origin. Other methods that tried to identify fistulas include oral charcoal challenge, tandem colovaginoscopy, flexible vaginoscopy, CT, and in more recent years, MRI. Coloenteric fistulas usually can be demonstrated by a barium enema, whereas a hysterogram may demonstrate a colouterine fistula or colotubal fistula. A purulent vaginal discharge is usually present. The charcoal challenge test has been repeated to confirm the diagnosis of a colouterine fistula (268). Charcoal seen flowing from the cervical os during pelvic examination the day after ingestion of activated charcoal will confirm the diagnosis. The diagnosis of colocutaneous fistulas is usually quite apparent. External drainage of feces makes the diagnosis obvious. They usually occur in the clinical setting as a complication of a previous resection for diverticulitis or in a patient with a complicated diverticulitis who had a previous laparotomy or as a result of a percutaneous drainage of a diverticular abscess. Signs and symptoms other than external drainage of feces are absent in over half of patients.

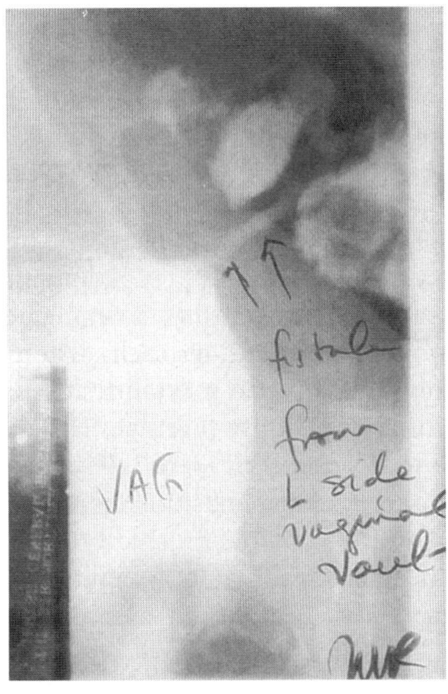

FIGURE 22 ■ Vaginogram demonstrating fistulous communication between left side of vaginal vault and the colon.

Principles of Treatment

The general principle of treating fistulas is to excise the offending organ of origin. A preliminary colostomy is generally not required. Although resective procedures comprise the treatment of choice, in highly selected patients nonoperative therapy has been reported as a viable option (269). Four patients with severe associated illnesses who were followed up for 3 to 14 years encountered little inconvenience and were without significant complications. Urinary contamination was treated with repeated courses of antibacterial therapy. Vasilevsky et al. (259) also reported on three patients (two colovesical and one colovaginal) treated nonoperatively. They were deemed poor operative candidates because of life-threatening cardiac or respiratory conditions.

Management

The operative management of patients with fistulas secondary to diverticular disease has changed dramatically over the years. Options include those already described, but the trend is toward a one-stage resection adopting the principles already outlined. The sigmoid colon is by definition adherent to the viscus in question.

With a colovesical fistula, adherence to both the bladder and the left ureter may be present. In the initial approach, it is probably best to mobilize the colon proximal and distal to the fistula. The colon may be pinched off the bladder by blunt dissection, but careful and often very tedious sharp dissection, with caution exercised not to injure the left ureter, usually is necessary to remove the colon from the bladder. Oftentimes, when the colon is freed from the bladder, an actual opening in the bladder is not seen. If an opening is present, it can be closed in two layers. Interrupted absorbable sutures should be used. Despite the fact that there is induration in this portion of the bladder, excising this portion is unnecessary because the induration will resolve after the colon has been excised.

The diseased bowel is resected, and a primary anastomosis usually is created. If suitable omentum is available, it is advantageous to place it between the bladder and bowel and tack it in place. Bladder drainage for at least 7 to 10 days is required, depending on the amount of bladder manipulation. In the series reported by Woods et al. (249), the bladder was managed by doing nothing (58%), by closure (20%), and by excision closure (22%), and omental interposition was used in 16 cases (27%).

For colovaginal fistulas, one-stage resection is advocated (270). Closure of the vagina is unnecessary in a patient with colovaginal fistula when the colon is freed from the vaginal vault. Similarly, a colouterine fistula requires no treatment of the uterine connection, but a hysterectomy may be performed as an elective procedure, as was done in two out of three cases reported by Woods et al. (249). Enteric openings require closure or may necessitate performing a small bowel resection. For a colotubal fistula, a salpingo-oophorectomy concomitant with the sigmoid resection is in order.

Results

In a series of patients in whom operations were performed for a variety of internal fistulas (mostly colovesical), Woods et al. (249) encountered a 3.5% operative mortality rate and a complication rate of 27%. The series included a variety of operative procedures, but the authors believe that a primary anastomosis can be performed with acceptable morbidity and mortality rates and is the procedure of choice, leaving staged procedures for use in highly selected patients.

Fazio et al. (262) reported that, in a series of patients with colocutaneous fistulas, 92 patients underwent operation, with 80% having one- or two-stage resection and anastomosis. One patient died postoperatively, and complications occurred in 48%. The operation was successful in that 77% of the patients had no stoma or fistula. The authors emphasized the role of diversion of the fecal stream in reducing morbidity from colonic fistulas. They further concluded that it is important to perform a true colorectal anastomosis and that patients with a complicated clinical course should be suspected of having Crohn's disease.

Vasilevsky et al. (259) conducted a study to assess the appropriate management of patients with diverticulitis complicated by fistula formation. There were 42 patients—32 women (76%) and 10 men (24%), who ranged in age from 46 to 89. Six of them had multiple fistulas. The types of fistulas included colovesical (48%), colovaginal (44%), colocutaneous (4%), colotubal (2%), and coloenteric (2%). Operative procedures consisted of resection and primary anastomosis in 38 patients (91%) and Hartmann's procedure in one patient because of a large phlegmon found at time of operation for a colovaginal fistula. Three patients were managed with antibiotics (two due to poor performance status, the third due to resolution of symptoms). There were no operative mortalities. The postoperative course was uncomplicated in 69%, while 12 patients (31%) experienced 19 complications (40%). These consisted of urinary tract infection (9.5%), atelectasis (7.1%), prolonged ileus (4.8%), arrhythmias (4.8%), renal failure, myocardial infarction, pseudomembranous colitis, peroneal nerve palsy, unexplained fever, and pulmonary edema (2.4% each). There were no anastomotic leaks and no mortalities. Hospital stay ranged from 6 to 31 days (average, 11.5 days). Fistulas due to diverticulitis were safely managed by resection and primary anastomosis without mortality and with acceptable morbidity in this series. Patients deemed to be poor operative risks can be managed with a course of nonoperative treatment.

Many health care institutions and providers have frequently challenged the value of specialization. Di Carlo et al. (271) conducted a review to determine whether there were any outcome differences in the management of fistulas complicating diverticulitis. There were 122 patients with 37 under the care of fully trained colorectal surgeons and 85 under the care of general surgeons. There were no significant differences in patient demographics, preoperative comorbidities, or the number of preoperative diagnostic investigations between the two groups. The colorectal surgeons performed more intraoperative ureteral stenting (55.5% vs. 24.4%). The general surgeons performed more initial diverting Hartmann's and colostomy procedures (27% vs. 5.4%). The patients in the general surgery group had longer postoperative lengths of stay (14 days vs. 11 days), and longer total lengths of stay (24 days vs. 14 days). The patients in the general surgery group experienced a higher rate of wound infections (12.9% vs. 5.4%), and a larger proportion of them experienced complications (41.2% vs. 27%). They concluded that specialization in colon and rectal surgery contributed to an improved outcome, with a lower rate of diverting procedures, a shorter hospital stay, and a lower rate of complications.

■ HEMORRHAGE

Incidence

Over the past four decades, what was believed to be the most common cause of massive lower intestinal hemorrhage has changed. In the 1960s, massive bleeding was attributed to carcinoma; in the 1970s, to diverticular disease; and in the 1980s, to vascular ectasias. These are not mutually exclusive diagnoses. In fact, the bleeding in many patients with known left-sided diverticular disease is attributed to vascular ectasias (272). Casarella et al. (273) compiled findings from 60 patients with acute rectal bleeding. The bleeding in one-half of the patients in whom a site was identified resulted from diverticulosis. Ninety-five percent of the bleeding sites were located to the right of the splenic flexure. The advent of angiography has changed the recognition of the cause of the bleeding. Kubo et al. (124) reported diverticular hemorrhage in 3.9% of 1124 cases, an incidence considerably lower than that in Western countries (3–27%) (274–277).

Pathogenesis

It was originally believed that bleeding associated with diverticular disease was due to inflammation. Subsequent evaluation of resected specimens has failed to demonstrate the implicated inflammatory process. Baer (278) attributed massive diverticular bleeding to chronic injury to the vasa recta, which lie in the submucosa of the diverticulum from the apex to the antimesenteric orifice. In a review of collected cases from the literature, she found a pathologically proved ruptured vasa recta within a diverticulum in 20 of 22 patients studied. The rupture can occur at the apex of the diverticulum or at the neck of the sac.

Clinical Manifestations

The characteristic presentation of the patient with diverticular bleeding is that of an otherwise healthy individual who gets the urge to move his or her bowels and suddenly passes a large amount of bright red– or maroon-colored stool. Bleeding stops spontaneously in an estimated 70% of cases, but 30% will continue to bleed and require emergency operative treatment (276). Approximately, 25% of patients who initially present with bleeding that has stopped, will present with rebleeding (279). If the bleeding is massive, tachycardia and hypotension may occur. Physical examination is usually unrewarding, as is abdominal examination. Sigmoidoscopy will reveal large amounts of blood and blood clots but usually no source of the bleeding.

Diagnosis and Investigation

A number of algorithms have been suggested for the management of patients with massive lower GI hemorrhage (see Chapter 35). The relative value of and appropriate order in which investigations such as barium enema, colonoscopy, nuclear scans, and angiography should be used have been hotly debated. In practice, the type of investigation and the order in which investigations are performed often depend on the preference of the surgeon, the availability of ancillary services, and the time of day when the patient is being assessed.

In the initial assessment, the upper GI tract should be ruled out as a bleeding source by gastric aspiration and possible gastroscopy. Sigmoidoscopy should be performed on all patients with lower GI hemorrhage, despite the fact that it is usually not a fruitful examination; however, mucosal changes associated with neoplastic or inflammatory diseases may be seen. Furthermore, the rectum is relatively inaccessible to inspection and palpation during laparotomy.

For many years, the barium enema was considered the appropriate initial study for determining the source of bleeding. It has even been suggested that a barium enema may be therapeutic in stopping the bleeding (280). However, if a barium enema is the initial study, the contrast material will preclude the possibility of other investigations; thus, this method is no longer favored. The demonstration of diverticula on a barium enema does not mean that they are the source of the bleeding, nor does it tell the examiner which diverticulum is the source (if, in fact, one is).

When confronted with a patient with massive rectal bleeding and after a sigmoidoscopic examination has been completed, it is probably wise to perform a nuclear scan. Two radionuclide techniques can be used to detect active GI bleeding. Technetium sulfur colloid scintigraphy uses a radiopharmaceutical that is rapidly cleared ($T_{\frac{1}{2}} = 3$ minutes in healthy individuals) from the intravascular space (281). The sensitivity is excellent, but a significant disadvantage is that patients must be bleeding actively during the few minutes in which the radiopharmaceutical is in the blood. An additional disadvantage of using sulfur colloid is that this agent normally accumulates in the liver and spleen, making it difficult to identify bleeding sites near these organs (Fig. 23).

An alternative technique is to use an intravascular tracer such as technetium-99m–labeled red blood cells or albumin. To localize the bleeding site, 5 to 70 mL of blood is needed. The advantage of this technique is that the patient can be monitored for active GI bleeding for as long

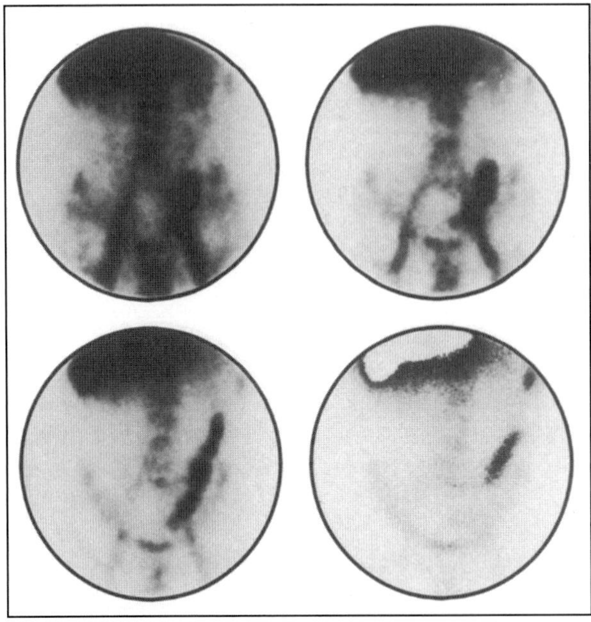

FIGURE 23 ■ Sulfur colloid study with consecutive two-minute images after injection. Dramatic extravasation noted in the left lower quadrant in a patient with diverticular disease. *Source*: Courtesy of G. Stern, M.D., Montreal, Quebec, Canada.

as 24 hours after a single injection. Using this technique, Markisz et al. (281) studied 39 patients and found that of the 22 patients with negative scans, eight underwent arteriography, with an active bleeding site identified in none. In 21 of the 22 patients, only medical treatment was required. Of the 17 patients with positive scans, the average age was older, the number of transfusions greater, the length of hospitalization longer, the number of patients requiring invasive therapy greater, and the number of deaths larger (six). The authors believe that red blood cell scintigraphy can be used effectively to screen patients for arteriography; and if an operation is required, the surgeon can use the results to plan it. The disadvantage with the blood pool agent is that if imaging is not done precisely at the time of active bleeding (i.e., at the time of extravasation), the radioactive agent may be propelled in the lumen and because of peristalsis, an erroneous localization may be made during delayed imaging (Fig. 24).

Hunter and Pezim (282) were less optimistic about the value of ^{99m}Tc-labeled red blood cell scintigraphy in localization of lower GI bleeding. In a review of 203 patients who underwent a scan and in whom the true site of bleeding was determined by other methods, including angiography and surgical pathology, the results of only 26% of the scans were positive and indicated a specific site of bleeding. A definitive bleeding site was identified in 22 patients by other means and correlated with a scan in only nine cases. The scan was incorrect in the remaining 13 cases, implying a localization error in 25% of the patients. A subgroup of 19 patients with a positive scan underwent a surgical procedure directed by the nuclear scan, and eight patients had an incorrect operation, for a surgical error of 42%. The authors therefore concluded that the value of the scan in localizing lower GI bleeding accurately is limited.

The use of colonoscopy in a patient with massive hemorrhage is debatable. Some authors have found the

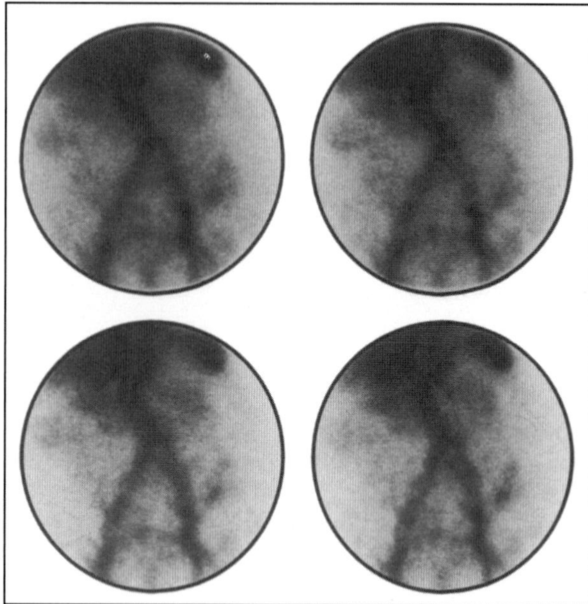

FIGURE 24 ■ Tagged red blood cell scan with films taken 0 to 30 minutes after injection. Extravasation is demonstrated in left lower quadrant. *Source*: Courtesy of G. Stern, M.D., Montreal, Quebec, Canada.

experience frustrating because of the amount of blood present and the failure to identify a source (Fig. 25). Other authors have found the examination fruitful. Forde (283) has been able to identify a bleeding source in up to 80% of patients. In the presence of massive bleeding, colonoscopy would seem to have limited application. Foutch (284) performed a retrospective study to determine if certain endoscopic features of a bleeding diverticulum predict outcome for patients and to assess the role of NSAIDs as a risk factor for hemorrhage. Over a 28-month period, colonoscopy was performed on 13 patients in whom a specific diverticulum was unequivocally identified as a cause for bleeding. Three patients had a visible vessel located inside a diverticulum, and one subject had an adherent clot with active bleeding. These colonoscopic findings were classified as stigmata of significant hemorrhage (SSH). In the remaining nine patients, the diverticula were ulcerated. This endoscopic finding was classified as stigmata of insignificant hemorrhage (SIH). Compared with patients with SIH, individuals with SSH experienced a greater number of bleeding episodes (3.5 vs. 1.3), had a lower initial hemoglobin concentration (8.2 g% vs. 12.5 g%), and required more transfusions (3.3 vs. 0) and invasive treatments (75% with SSH were managed by endoscopy or surgery vs. 0% for those with SIH). Seventy-five percent of subjects with SSH compared with 0% of patients with SIH had a combined exposure to NSAIDs and ASA. The author concluded the presence of a visible vessel or an adherent clot with active bleeding is a reliable marker for significant hemorrhage. Ulcerated diverticula are the cause of trivial bleeding, and presence of this endoscopic finding accurately predicts a benign clinical course. Furthermore, NSAIDs may be an important risk factor for diverticular bleeding. It is possible that combined exposure to NSAIDs and ASA results in more severe bleeding compared with the use of NSAIDs alone.

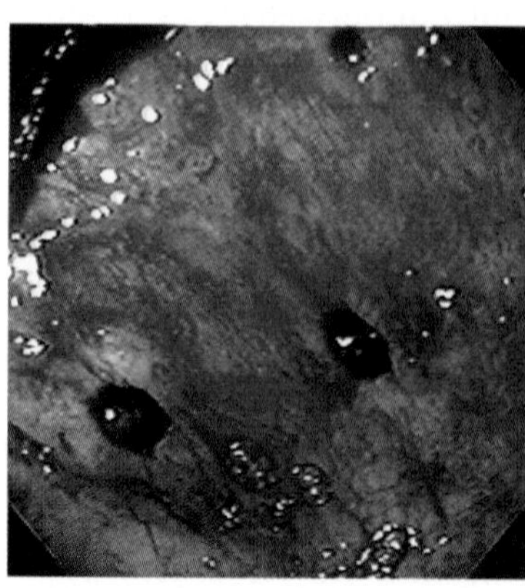

FIGURE 25 ■ Blood seen in ostia of diverticula but it cannot be definitely stated this is the source of bleeding or whether blood is just collecting in diverticula.

Jensen et al. (279) reported their evolving 10-year experience using urgent colonoscopy for the diagnosis and treatment of severe diverticular hemorrhage. They studied 121 patients with severe hematochezia from colonic diverticulosis. A diagnosis was made by urgent colonoscopy performed within 6 to 12 hours following admission. Colonic lavage, which required 3 to 4 hours consisted of 5 to 6 L of sulfate purge given orally in two-thirds of the cases and by nasogastric tube in remainder (279). Diverticular bleeding was defined as definite when active bleeding, a nonbleeding visible vessel, or an adherent clot was present and presumptive when diverticulosis was present in the absence of another bleeding source.

The authors performed diagnostic colonoscopy in 73 patients with severe lower GI bleeding and found a definitive diverticular source in 23%. Despite medical treatment (transfusion, correction of coagulopathy when present, cessation of anticoagulants, NSAIDs, and aspirin), 53% continued to bleed or had another episode of bleeding. Six such patients ultimately required partial colectomy to control the bleeding. They subsequently delivered endoscopic therapy to 21% with definite diverticular hemorrhage and achieved 100% permanent hemostasis during the median 30-month follow-up. Endoscopic therapy consisted of 1 to 2 mm aliquot injections of dilute epinephrine (1:20,000) into the four quadrants around the bleeding point. Nonbleeding visible vessels received bipolar electrocoagulation. Dilute epinephrine was injected into the adherent clot, which was then shaved off with a cold snare and the underlying vessel was treated with bipolar coagulation. The authors tattooed each treatment site.

Colonoscopy showed active bleeding in 50%, nonbleeding visible vessel in 20%, and an adherent clot in 30% of patients with definite diverticular bleeding seen during their most recent experience. The authors diagnosed a nondiverticular source more often in the initial phase of the study compared to the latter phase.

Selective angiography may prove helpful in identifying the bleeding source but positive results have varied widely (13–86%), the complication rate is about 10%, and it is expensive (285). If the radionuclide scan is negative, arteriography is probably not needed. If the study is positive, arteriography may not only confirm the finding but may also prove therapeutic. The logical order of cannulation should be the superior mesenteric artery, inferior mesenteric artery, and finally the celiac artery if no source has yet been found. Angiographic abnormalities include extravasation of dye or filling of a diverticulum. If a bleeding source is identified, it may be controlled by the use of vasopressin infusion, but rebleeding may occur in 30% of patients after initial control is obtained with vasopressin. The treating physicians must be cognizant of the side effects of this agent (decreased cardiac output, hypertension, erythema, and an antidiuretic effect). Local problems related to the catheter insertion include embolism, bleeding around the puncture site, hematoma, and limitation of activity. Efficacy of this treatment is in the range of 85% to 90% (286). Another therapeutic use of angiography is embolization of Gelfoam strips or an autologous blood clot (287–289). Patients, however, must be observed closely for potential necrosis of the bowel. For patients in whom angiography has failed to identify a bleeding site or in whom a site was identified but not controlled with vasopressin, a barium enema might next be considered as a therapeutic tool.

Management

Despite the (sometimes) alarming nature of the bleeding, replacement of blood is usually followed by spontaneous cessation of bleeding. How much blood should be administered before recommending an operation is controversial. Replacement of four units should alert the surgeon to the possible need for operation. Nahrwold (290) has offered the following indications for operative intervention: (i) administering 1500 mL of blood is necessary to accomplish resuscitation and bleeding continues, (ii) administering 2000 mL of blood is necessary to maintain vital signs during a 24-hour period, (iii) bleeding, no matter how much, continues for 72 hours, and (iv) rebleeding occurs within one week of cessation of significant hemorrhage. The elderly tolerate blood loss less well than young individuals; therefore, early operative intervention is mandatory in elderly patients. Anywhere from 10% to 25% of patients continue to bleed and require operative intervention (291).

Considerable controversy has centered on determining the most appropriate operation. In an effort to identify the source of the bleeding and perform a lesser operation, historically a number of techniques were used, including multiple colotomies, divided colostomy, intraoperative sigmoidoscopy, blind left hemicolectomy, and, more recently, right hemicolectomy. However, with the numerous modalities of investigation currently available, these techniques should be abandoned.

If a previous diagnostic investigation has revealed the source of the bleeding, the appropriate segmental resection should be performed. If no source has been identified, intraoperative colonoscopy may be used to identify a source. If there is still no evidence of a specific bleeding site, total abdominal colectomy and ileorectal anastomosis should be performed. The rationale for the extended resection is based on the 30% rebleeding rate in cases having blind segmental resection (276,292).

Renzulli et al. (293) reviewed the data on 42 consecutive patients with acute colonic diverticular bleeding with a mean follow-up of 4.1 years. Preoperative localization of the bleeding site was possible in six patients (14%)—by colonoscopy in two and by angiography in four. Ten patients underwent segmental colectomy with primary anastomosis and 32 subtotal colectomies with primary ileorectostomy. Subtotal colectomy is the more extensive operative procedure (longer resected bowel, greater blood loss), and although it was performed in older patients, there were no significant differences between segmental and subtotal colectomy with respect to operation time, morbidity, mortality, hospital stay, number of bowel movements, continence scores, rebleeding rate, or patient satisfaction. They concluded that subtotal colectomy with primary ileorectostomy for colonic diverticular bleeding that was not localized is a safe and effective procedure providing complete bleeding control and preserving continence.

There are a variety of options for endoscopic therapy in patients with acute lower GI bleeding (294). Only about 20% of patients with lower GI bleeding have a lesion that can be treated through the endoscope (294).

Ramirez et al. (295) described the use of endoscopic injection of epinephrine 1:10,000 (2–10 mL) into the neck of the bleeding diverticulum as an effective, simple, and safe endoscopic maneuver. In four cases, they arrested active hemorrhage and prevented early rebleeding. They believe that such a therapeutic modality should not only be added to the endoscopist's armamentarium, but should also be considered as a first-line approach for such patients. Others have also advocated this technique (182,296).

Bloomfeld et al. (297) identified 13 patients who underwent colonoscopic hemostatic management for the treatment of acute diverticular bleeding. Therapy consisted of epinephrine injection and/or multi-polar electrocoagulation. Five patients (38%) experienced rebleeding within 30 days of the index bleed, four of whom required operation and three patients (23%) had late bleeding. There were no complications of endoscopic therapy.

A number of other endoscopic methods to obtain hemostasis have been described. The endoscopic approach is useful when the source of bleeding can be visualized endoscopically (279). Coagulation therapy can be administered with any of the available monopolar, bipolar, or electronically heated (Heater) catheter probes (294). Argon plasma coagulation is also feasible (298), but the walls of the diverticula are thin and can be easily perforated. The use of endoclips in the treatment of massive colonic diverticular bleeding has been described with placement of hemoclips on and around the visible vessel (99,299). Endoscopic band ligation of bleeding colonic diverticula has also been described (300). The use of a fibrin sealant has been described (301).

The successful use of barium impaction therapy was reported in which barium sulfate solution was prepared by mixing 220 g of water, 800 g of barium sulfate powder, and 1 mg of epinephrine (302). The solution was administered using a double balloon enema tip. An additional 400 mL of barium was administered. After confirming that the ascending colon and cecum were filled with barium, the enema tip was clamped and the patient's position was changed every 5 minutes (prone, left lateral, supine, and right lateral positions) for 2 hours. The patient remained in the radiology department the entire time. After this procedure, hematochezia stopped. Several barium-impacted diverticula were visible in an abdominal radiograph 6 days later. Oral feeding was resumed eight days after the impaction therapy and rebleeding did not occur 13 months after the barium impaction therapy. Koperna et al. (303)

evaluated the efficacy of barium as a treatment option for severe diverticular bleeding in 102 patients who needed transfusion of two or more units of blood. They compared the clinical efficacy of surgical resection, conservative treatment, and therapeutic barium enema. Conservative treatment led to a rebleeding rate of 43.3%, which differed significantly from a 15.9% rebleeding rate after therapeutic barium enema. No rebleeding was registered in surgically treated patients. Sixty percent of patients in whom therapeutic barium enema failed were treated by colonic resection without mortality, while 77% of patients who had rebleeding after conservative treatment were successfully treated with barium enema. Overall, barium enema was the most frequently applied second-line treatment (56.5%). The mortality after operation was significantly higher than that after other treatment modalities (33% vs. 1%). They concluded that therapeutic barium enema is the treatment of choice for the first bleeding episode, whereas operative resection should be performed if rebleeding occurs.

In patients with a minor degree of persistent rectal bleeding in whom contrast studies have revealed diverticular disease, the bleeding should not be attributed solely to that disease, for Teague et al. (304) found that 20% of 40 patients with diverticular disease and persistent rectal bleeding had carcinoma of the colon.

Results

Bleeding of diverticular origin ceases spontaneously in 70% of cases, but 30% will continue to bleed and require emergency operation (276). The frequency of delayed or recurrent bleeding is uncertain but is estimated at 10% to 25% of patients (276). The frequency of bleeding recurrence ranges from 0% to 25% (275). Within the first 24 hours, it occurs in 20% of patients, whereas late recurrence occurs in 12% (276). The incidence of rebleeding depends on the amount of bowel resected, but the exact incidence is unknown. If subtotal colectomy and ileorectal anastomosis have been performed, the incidence approaches zero.

Of considerable controversy is the recommendation for elective interval resection. The recommendation is made because of the estimated rebleeding rate of up to 25%. Some authors recommend the resection after two episodes of bleeding attributable to diverticular disease, but most physicians favor a conservative approach. The indications for elective resection to avoid further bleeding have not been well defined.

■ OBSTRUCTION

Obstruction secondary to diverticular disease is uncommon. It is usually a consequence of perforation, or it may result from repeated episodes of inflammation with an acute episode on chronic presentation (305). It also may be caused by a loop of small bowel becoming adherent to a diverticular mass. When obstruction supervenes, abdominal pain, distention, and constipation are present. These symptoms may be associated with the already described symptoms of diverticulitis. Because of the obstruction's presumed association with perforation, the condition is confirmed by using plain films of the abdomen and water-soluble contrast enemas. Barium is withheld when there is any hint of peritoneal signs of leakage. The most specific finding is deformed and spiculated, inflamed diverticula. The majority of patients have radiologic findings of incomplete obstruction and possibly localized signs of sepsis.

Most patients with obstruction caused by diverticular disease will respond to nonoperative management. Repeated bouts of obstruction or marked areas of narrowing require resection on an elective basis. Very rarely will a preliminary colostomy be required. In most circumstances in which an operation is necessary for a patient who has obstruction secondary to diverticulitis, a resection (if this is technically feasible) is the treatment of choice. Usually Hartmann's procedure is performed.

■ MISCELLANEOUS

Pneumopylephlebitis and Hepatic Abscess

Pylephlebitis, or septic thrombophlebitis of the portal vein, is a rare but often fatal condition (306). It may progress to hepatic abscess formation. The two are distinct pathologic entities that may arise from a common source of suppuration. In their review, Waxman et al. (306) found only 56 cases of diverticulitis as the source of pylephlebitis and/or hepatic abscess. The combination occurred in only 10% of cases, with the majority of patients presenting with a solitary hepatic abscess. In his series of 22 patients, Lin (307) found evidence of diverticulitis as the source of sepsis in only 30% of the patients.

Treatment consists of drainage of the abscess and administration of appropriate antibiotics. Resection of the diseased sigmoid is advocated (308–310). The occurrence of hepatic portal venous gas has also been reported in patients with diverticulitis (311,312). It is believed to be uniquely associated with intramesocolic perforation (312). Hepatic portal venous gas may prove difficult to diagnose because abdominal signs and symptoms may be vague or absent. Despite reports of the successful nonoperative treatment of septic thrombophlebitis of the inferior mesenteric vein from sigmoid diverticulitis (313,314) once the diagnosis is established, operative treatment seems more appropriate. It appears though that portal and mesenteric gas is not associated with the grave prognosis of necrotic bowel.

Ureteral Involvement

Ureteral involvement in diverticulitis is unusual. The left ureter is more commonly involved but right-sided and bilateral instances have been reported (315). The three types of involvement are fistula, stricture, and compression, with compression being the most frequent. Ney et al. (315) reported three instances of hydronephrosis and hydroureter and were able to find only 31 documented cases of these complications in the literature. These complications resolve after definitive treatment of the diverticulitis, and the initial plan for managing the intestinal disease does not need alteration except with the proviso that the retroperitoneum be examined for the presence of a fibrotic inflammatory reaction (316). If such a reaction is present, performing ureterolysis is suggested. The wisdom of ureterolysis could be questioned because in the analogous situation where the right ureter is obstructed in

Crohn's disease, ureterolysis is not recommended. Siminovitch and Fazio (316) recommend obtaining urograms preoperatively in patients scheduled to undergo intestinal surgery. The proximity of the sigmoid colon to the left ureter should cause more instances of this complication than are reported.

Subcutaneous Emphysema

Subcutaneous emphysema in association with GI perforations occurs mainly in the elderly, most likely in those with diverticulitis. Abdominal wall emphysema develops because of mechanical factors, with direct communication through a colocutaneous fistula (317), high intraintestinal pressures, or infection with gas-producing organisms, or it originates in the respiratory tract. Subcutaneous emphysema as distant as the cervical region has been associated with diverticular perforation of the sigmoid colon (318). Localized signs of perforation may be absent in patients receiving corticosteroids. The time at which subcutaneous emphysema appears in relationship to symptoms can be used to predict whether inflammation is associated with the process. Thus if subcutaneous emphysema is detected within 48 hours after the onset of the illness, infection is unlikely to be a major contributing factor. If it appears after a 48 hour interval, infection invariably is associated with the disease. The presence of air per se in the soft tissues has no damaging effect. Subcutaneous emphysema will regress when another route of passage is found from the bowel.

Necrotizing Fasciitis

Harrison and Ellis reported the unusual complication of abdominal wall necrotizing fasciitis secondary to perforated sigmoid diverticular disease (319). Necrotizing fasciitis, a variant of acute nonclostridial dermal gangrene, is usually initiated by an operative procedure or by spontaneous trauma. Associated with perforated diverticulitis, it requires radical excision of the necrotic abdominal wall and resection of the offending segment of bowel.

Pyoderma Gangrenosum

Pyoderma gangrenosum with its erythematous papule or pustule that progresses rapidly to an ulceration with a violaceous overhanging border has been associated with a ruptured diverticulum with retroperitoneal abscess formation and bacterial sepsis (320). Resection of the affected colon leads to complete resolution of the cutaneous disease.

Orthopedic Manifestations

Leg pain was the sole mode of presentation for five cases of diverticulitis in one series (321). In the 15 cases of thigh abscesses and emphysema reported due to diverticular disease, 70% died (321,322). The mortality is, in part, due to delayed recognition and treatment. The diagnosis of retroperitoneal perforation might be entertained in patients with unexplained symptoms of the leg, especially if accompanied by fever and leukocytosis. Once diagnosed, broad-spectrum antibiotic coverage and immediate operation are mandatory. An unusual case of a right thigh and leg abscess secondary to a perforated sigmoid diverticulitis was reported (323). An urgent Hartmann's procedure was required following which 1.5 L of purulent material was evacuated via a thigh incision and multiple distal counterincisions were needed to obtain adequate drainage.

RESULTS AND PROGNOSIS

The number of persons with diverticular disease in the United States between 1983 and 1987 was estimated at 1.9 million (324). The percentage of persons with diverticular disease who had any limitation in activity was estimated to be 6% and those with limitation in major activity 15%. The annual number of physician contacts for diverticular disease was 2,237,000.

Mortality from diverticular disease before the age of 65 was less than one per 100,000 population in 1985 (324). For those aged 85 and above, the mortality rate was nearly 10 times that of persons aged 65 to 74.

Making a precise assessment of the morbidity and mortality related to the treatment of patients with diverticular disease is difficult. Many authors pool data from elective and emergency operations or separate results according to the indications for operation or the type of operation performed. Therefore it may be inappropriate to apply such an assessment based on combined data to a given patient with a particular complication who is about to undergo a specific operation. One such review of morbidity and mortality rates in relation to indication for operation was reported by Corman (247, p. 684) and is summarized in Table 12.

An overview of complications that occurred in the large series of patients reported by Rodkey and Welch (10) is presented in Table 13. A total of 569 operations were performed on 350 patients. The mortality rate for one-stage resection and anastomosis was 1.5% (3 of 195 patients); of two-stage procedures, 13.9% (10 of 72 patients); and of three-stage procedures, 15.2% (9 of 59 patients). Sepsis was the leading cause of death, and generalized peritonitis carried with it a 25% overall mortality rate. From their thorough review, the authors concluded that (i) in patients with generalized peritonitis, excision of the primary focus of disease during the initial operation was associated with a lower mortality rate than that for operations in which the primary site was not excised, and (ii) in patients with localized peritonitis or pelvic abscess there was no significant difference in mortality between operations in which the

TABLE 12 ■ Surgery for Diverticular Disease: Morbidity and Mortality

Presentation	No of. Patients	No. of Complications[a]	No. of Deaths	Mortality (%)
Phlegmon	99	56	7	7
Fistula	51	44	3	6
Abscess	33	31	2	6
Obstruction	9	6	1	10
Perforation	7	9	1	14
Total	199	146	14	9 (average %)

[a]Some patients had more than one complication.
Source: From Ref. 245.

TABLE 13 ■ Complications with 569 Operations Performed on 350 Patients

Operative	No. of Patients	Postoperative	No. of Patients
Splenic injury (splenectomy)	7	Respiratory failure	20
Hemorrhage	6	Wound abscess	14
Colonoscopic perforation	3	Anastomotic leak	12
Ureteral injury	2	Renal failure	12
		Peritonitis	10
		Incisional hernia	10
		Hemorrhagic shock	8
		Ileus	8
		Thrombocytopenia	8
		Miscellaneous	47

Source: From Ref. 10.

primary site was excised and those in which it was not. Mortality rates varied with the urgency of the situation. The operative mortality rate for emergency operations (<24 hours) was 10.2%, for urgent operations (1–30 days), 9.7%, and for elective operations, 2.4%. The major lessons learned include the need for (i) performing the operations without delay on immunosuppressed patients with perforation, (ii) resecting the primary site of perforation during the initial operation in patients with generalized peritonitis, (iii) applying and elaborating the indications for elective resections to prevent the necessity for an emergency operation, (iv) using selected arteriography more frequently in cases of massive hemorrhage, and (v) taking care to avoid injury to the spleen during the operation because such an injury carries with it an increased mortality rate.

In a series of 38 patients reported by Smirniotis et al. (325), four of the five deaths occurred in patients in whom the perforated segment was not resected. Therefore resection is strongly recommended. Stefansson et al. (326) identified 130 patients who underwent emergency operation for sigmoid diverticulitis during a 20-year period. They analyzed the postoperative mortality according to age, gender, concomitant disease, number of diverticulitis attacks, and operation (79 not resected, 51 resected) and compared the outcome in patients subjected to resection to those not resected. Operative findings included phlegmon, abscess, generalized purulent peritonitis, and local or generalized fecal peritonitis. After the first emergency operation, 20 patients (15%) died and after a subsequent colostomy closure, two patients died. Overall mortality was 17%. Fifty-five percent of the patients who died had been operated on for phlegmonous diverticulitis or an abscess. Age and concomitant diseases were the most prominent risk factors for death. In a multivariate analysis, patients not resected had a threefold postoperative mortality compared with those resected (13% vs. 4%). Postoperative complications were observed in 26% of patients. Among those not resected, significantly more patients had permanent colostomies compared to those resected. Therefore when sigmoid diverticulitis is revealed during an exploratory laparotomy, a resection should be attempted.

Bahadursingh et al. (250) reviewed the outcome of 192 patients with complicated diverticular disease. A previous attack of diverticulitis was documented in 61% of patients. Of the investigations performed, 66.7% had a CT scan of the abdomen and pelvis, 20% underwent contrast enema, 32% underwent colonoscopy and 1% underwent a small bowel series. The abnormal findings on the CT scan were as follows: diverticular abscess (16%), diverticulitis (37%), diverticulosis without inflammation (15%), free air (10%), and fistula (1%). The locations of the diverticular abscesses were pelvic (36%), pericolic sigmoid (36%), and "other," which included interloop (28%). Preoperative abscess drainage occurred in 5%, which were either percutaneous (3%) or transrectal (2%). A fistula occurred in 6% of patients: colovesical (3%), colocutaneous (1%), enterocolic (1%), or colovaginal (1%). Overall, 38% underwent operation. All patients undergoing operation had a resection of their colon. The operative findings were localized abscess in 22%, purulent/fecal peritonitis in 17%, and phlegmon in 14%. A primary resection with anastomosis was performed in 92% of patients with 56% having a protecting stoma. An unsuspected carcinoma was found in 7% of patients. Overall, 15% developed a complication related to diverticulitis. Morbidity was 15.1% at which 34% were infection related. The symptoms were present for an average of 14 days, most patients were female (59%), and most had a previous attack of diverticulitis. They concluded the practice of resection and primary anastomosis for acute diverticulitis has an acceptable morbidity and mortality. For high-risk anastomoses, a covering loop ileostomy and not a Hartmann's procedure is preferred.

Although the probability that diverticular disease is the cause of death is extremely low, the incidence of diverticular disease increases with age, and the mortality rate from complications of diverticular disease also increases with advancing age. In addition, people are living to an older age; hence more patients might be expected to have the complications of diverticular disease. Mendeloff (26) determined that diverticulitis ranked very low as a cause of death: 0.5 deaths per 100,000 for the population aged less than 64 years; 6.2 for white females and males and 2.7 and 4.4 for nonwhites, respectively, for ages 65 to 74 years; 12.9 for white males, 16.8 for white females, 7.3 for nonwhite males, and 4.2 for nonwhite females ages 75 to 84 years; and 24.1 for white males, 30.2 for white females, 9.6 for nonwhite males, and 11.6 for nonwhite females ages 85 years and over.

The wide variation in geographic distribution of the disorder has led investigators to implicate diet as an etiologic or at least contributing factor. Experimental studies using dietary manipulation have suggested that diverticular disease may be a fiber-deficiency disease. If it is, a simple lifestyle change during early adult life may produce a reduction in the absolute risk of the development of diverticular disease. However, with the current conflicting views about the pathogenesis of diverticular formation, it may be necessary to know more about the other ingredients of the diet that may be contributing factors (26).

RIGHT-SIDED DIVERTICULA

INCIDENCE

Right-sided diverticula may be seen in conjunction with universal, diverticular disease, or may be isolated to the right side only. Diverticula of the cecum and ascending colon occur at a younger age than diverticula of the left colon and are associated with an equal sex distribution. They are more common in Orientals than in Whites and rarely occur in the West, where the incidence is 0.9% to 3.6% (327). In a review of 780 patients with colonic diverticulitis, Fischer and Farkas (328) found 12 patients with acute diverticulitis of the cecum or ascending colon for an incidence of 1.5%. From Hong Kong, Lo and Chu (329) reported right-sided diverticulitis to account for 17% of all colonic diverticulitis in their population. In Singapore, Tan et al. (330) noted a 10% incidence of diverticular disease through barium enema study, and in two-thirds of these patients, the diverticula were on the right side. In the same republic, Lee (331) conducted an autopsy survey of diverticular disease of the large bowel. Of 1014 colons examined, diverticula were present in 19%. The lesion appeared earlier in life and was more common in men, and there was a predominance of right colon involvement. Tan et al. (330) and Lee (331) believe that although adoption of the Western diet may influence the prevalence of diverticular disease, the site of predilection is determined more by racial or genetic predisposition. All diverticula examined histologically were false, including the 20% that were solitary diverticula. The distribution of solitary diverticula was similar to that of multiple diverticulosis.

To evaluate the relationship between long-term dietary habits and the prevalence of right-sided diverticulosis in the general population, Lin et al. (332) performed a retrospective case control study. They reviewed the records of 3105 screening colonoscopies performed on healthy asymptomatic adults. A single-blinded nurse interviewed all case and control subjects in order to establish their dietary habits during the previous decade. A total of 86 cases of right-sided diverticulosis were included whereas 106 controls were randomly selected. There was a marked association between meat consumption frequency and right-sided diverticulosis with an OR of 24.8 between the most and least frequent consumers of meat products. There was no association with vegetable or fruit consumption frequency, laxative use, supplemental fibre intake, smoking, or family history.

Miura et al. (333) conducted a study to determine whether the incidence of solitary diverticula (defined as 1 or 2 diverticula in this study) and multiple (3 or more) diverticula of the right colon is increased in Japan. A total of 13,947 consecutive barium enema examinations performed in the period from 1982 to 1997 were reviewed. Right-sided and bilateral diverticula have increased in frequency across time; however, left-sided diverticula have not. Patients with one or two diverticula in the right colon of right-sided disease unexpectedly had increased across time in both genders, and patients with three or more diverticula in the right colon of right-sided disease have shown an increase in males. The number of diverticula of the right colon showed no increase across time or with aging. Diverticula of the right colon might be an acquired disease and self-limiting in development, because the frequency did not increase substantially in the elderly and because the number changed little across time and with aging.

■ PATHOLOGY

Right-sided diverticula are thought by some authors to be congenital, and most are true diverticula (i.e., contain all layers of the intestine); however, other authors believe that most right-sided diverticula are false diverticula (330). Lo and Chu (329) found 18 of 21 specimens resected for right-sided diverticulitis to contain false diverticula. Markham and Li (334) found 30 of 35 resected specimens to have false diverticula. Murayama et al. (335) measured the thickness of right colonic muscle and suggested that these diverticula are of the same etiology as left-sided diverticula. Morson (11) described a muscular abnormality expressed by an increase in the number of haustral folds and hypertrophy of lymphoid tissue at the mouths of the diverticula.

Sugihara et al. (336), using a catheter-tipped transducer, found that after intravenous injection of neostigmine, high-pressure waves were more frequently observed and the colonic motility index was greater in patients with diverticular disease than in controls. They suggested that high intraluminal pressure and abnormal motility in the ascending colon play important roles in the pathogenesis of right-sided diverticular disease.

The solitary diverticulum has a shorter and wider neck than that of the multiple varieties (337). Its location is most commonly anteromedial, followed by its occurrence on the anterolateral wall of the cecum (330). Cecal diverticula are solitary in 77% to 81% of cases, and they are multiple in 19% to 23% of cases (338).

■ CLINICAL MANIFESTATIONS

A solitary diverticulum may exist unsuspected until diverticulitis supervenes. The majority of patients with right-sided diverticula are asymptomatic, and the diagnosis is made at the time of radiologic investigation. Some patients may experience vague right-sided abdominal pain. The average age of patients with right-sided diverticula is 10 to 15 years less than that for patients with diverticula of the left colon (339).

Right-sided diverticular disease differs from left-sided disease in that it occurs in patients at a younger age, has an equal sex distribution, runs a self-limiting course, and does not seem to become more severe or extensive with increasing age.

Pieterse et al. (340) identified four distinct morphologic groups of patients with right-sided diverticular disease, each with a distinct clinical presentation. One group had solitary false diverticula mimicking acute appendicitis and at operation was found to have inflamed cecal masses. A second group had diverticula formed on the basis of defects in the muscularis propria, had a mean age 30 years older than the previous group, and presented with hemorrhage, and at laparotomy the appearance of the bowel was unremarkable. A third group had diverticula similar to that seen on the left side of the colon, and the last group had the true congenital cecal diverticula.

Right-sided diverticulitis mimics acute appendicitis but occurs at an average age of 40 (338). The patient presents with symptoms of pain (usually in the right lower quadrant, but the pain may be epigastric or in the right flank), pyrexia, nausea, or vomiting. During examination, the patient may have varying degrees of tenderness, guarding, and rebound tenderness or a right lower quadrant mass. Leukocytosis is usually present.

■ RADIOLOGIC FINDINGS

Plain films of the abdomen are generally not helpful. A nonspecific ileus or sentinel loop, a mass, or a fecalith may be seen, but these signs also occur with patients with appendicitis. The major sonographic finding in patients with uncomplicated acute diverticulitis of the right colon is a hypoechoic round or oval focus protruding from a segmentally thickened colonic wall (341). CT scanning may be useful in making the early diagnosis of diverticulitis of the cecum and ascending colon (342). It may show a thickened colonic wall, an extraluminal mass, haziness, and linear strands in the adjacent pericolic fat and thickened nearby fascial planes. Differentiation from appendicitis may be impossible unless CT demonstrates an intramural abscess or cecal diverticula in association with an inflammatory process that is located cephalad to a normal appearing cecal caput and periappendiceal region (343). A perforated cecal carcinoma should be suspected if the constellation of CT findings is dominated by soft-tissue components and not by pericecal inflammatory reaction.

Chou et al. (344) described the sonographic findings of right-sided colonic diverticulitis. Sonography detected 21 inflamed diverticula with one false positive and two false negative results. The most typical sonographic feature of an inflamed diverticulum of the right colon was a rounded or oval-shaped hypoechoic or nearly anechoic structure (52%) protruding out from the segmentally thickened colonic wall. Some of them might contain strong echoes representing gas or feces (43%), or stone in the lumen (5%). Regional pericolic of peridiverticular fat thickening was noted in 57% of patients and segmental colon wall thickening in 38%. Ultrasound examination yielded an overall accuracy of 99.5%. A positive sonogram made the likelihood of acute right-sided diverticulitis 456.5 times greater compared with the pretest clinical impression. Ultrasonography differentiated acute right-sided colonic diverticulitis from acute appendicitis with 100% accuracy.

MRI can be useful in the diagnosis of right colonic diverticulitis, which may be seen as an outpouching of the right colon (345). An inflamed diverticulum with adjacent colonic wall thickening and surrounding inflamed fat are characteristic MR signs. MRI can be a valuable alternative to CT in young or pregnant patients who have suspected appendicitis and an equivocal ultrasound result.

However, the correct diagnosis is generally not made because the patient is usually operated on for acute appendicitis and the diagnosis is made at the time of laparotomy. In a review of the literature, Sardi et al. (327) found that the correct diagnosis was made 7% of the time, and acute appendicitis was the most common preoperative diagnosis (68%). Features that may help distinguish between the two diseases include the facts that (i) cecal diverticulitis tends to be more prolonged and less acute in presentation; (ii) fever, anorexia, nausea, and vomiting occur less often with diverticulitis; (iii) a mass is more commonly present; and (iv) patients tend to be older (338). Patients also may present with varying degrees of bleeding.

■ MANAGEMENT

Even at the time of laparotomy, the precise diagnosis may not be made because the inflamed mass may be mistaken for carcinoma. In their review of the literature, Graham and Ballantyne (338) found that among 367 cases, the surgeon correctly identified cecal diverticulitis in 58% of instances and believed the diagnosis was a neoplasm in 40% of instances. If there is a circumscribed area of inflammation and the diagnosis is certain, such as occurs in two-thirds of the cases, diverticulectomy (local excision) is the preferred method of treatment (327,330,338). If a large mass is present and there is a concern about the possibility of malignancy, such as occurs in the other one-third of the cases, performing a right hemicolectomy is indicated (327,329,338,346). Intraoperative colonoscopy may help differentiate a benign condition from a malignant one (347).

The infrequent occurrence of right colon diverticulitis in the developed West has led to a controversy in the management of this disease. In Singapore, Ngoi et al. (348) continued to avoid colectomy whenever possible because this disease is usually nonprogressive. They reviewed 68 patients treated by conservative operation to evaluate the effectiveness of this treatment policy. Almost 70% of their patients were younger than 40 years, and the clinical presentation was indistinguishable from acute appendicitis. Diverticulectomy was performed only for inflamed and perforated diverticula (25 cases), while the nonperforated diverticulum was left alone (40 cases). The inflammation invariably responded to antibiotic therapy. Only three patients had colonic resection because a malignant neoplasm could not be excluded. There were no adverse sequelae over a mean follow-up period of 3.5 years, except for one patient who had recurrent attacks of right colon diverticulitis necessitating colectomy. With this policy of management they encountered no mortality, and morbidity was 19%, mostly wound infections.

Papaziogas et al. (349) presented their experience of the surgical management of eight cases of cecal diverticulitis over a 25-year period. The mean age of the patients was 54.2 years. Five patients underwent diverticulectomy, two patients underwent ileocecal resection, and one patient underwent suture of the perforated diverticulum. The postoperative course was uneventful. At long-term follow-up (mean 14.6 years), none of the patients who underwent diverticulectomy mentioned any symptom or complication. They concluded that diverticulectomy if technically feasible could be considered as an adequate therapy for cecal diverticulitis. Aggressive resection should be considered in cases of extensive inflammatory changes. On the other hand, Fang et al. (350) propose aggressive resection for cecal diverticulitis. This is based on a study of 85 patients. Nonoperative management was applied to 18 patients initially. Three patients had recurrent diverticulitis during follow-up. These patients responded satisfactorily to another course of medical treatment. Laparotomy was performed in 67 patients. Acute appendicitis was the preoperative diagnosis in 70% of patients. Of the other patients, six received operation because of repeated attacks of diverticulitis, seven had preoperative CT diagnosis of cecal diverticulitis with perforation, five had preoperative diagnosis of cecal neoplasm, and two had medical treatment failure. All these patients received right hemicolectomy. In the 47 patients with a preoperative diagnosis of acute appendicitis, 24 received appendectomy, 9 received diverticulectomy, and 14 received right hemicolectomy. Overall, 34 patients received right hemicolectomy, 9 received diverticulectomy, and 24 received appendectomy only. In the right hemicolectomy group, there were two deaths with underlying diseases and five complications. In the appendectomy group, there was no postoperative mortality but in seven patients recurrent diverticulitis developed. Three of them required right hemicolectomy. They concluded the natural history of cecal diverticulitis varies from benign and self-limiting to fulminant in the oriental population. Less than 40% of patients were successfully treated initially with conservative methods and none developed recurrence during the follow-up period. They therefore recommend aggressive surgical resection for patients with a definite diagnosis.

In the less acute case in which the diagnosis of cecal diverticulitis is made before the operation and the patient may present with a mass, radiologic examination may suggest the correct diagnosis. Under these circumstances, nonoperative management with antibiotics and fluids may result in resolution of the symptoms.

Komuta et al. (351) reviewed the records of patients with acute right colonic diverticulitis with the goal of establishing therapeutic guidelines. The 80 patients who were suffering a first attack were successfully were treated with bowel rest and antibiotics. Two of these 80 patients underwent an elective operation at the surgeon's discretion during the original hospitalization and one needed an urgent operation. Of the 78 patients who responded to medical therapy, 20.5% developed recurrent right colonic diverticulitis. All 16 patients who had a second attack were successfully treated with medical therapy. Three of the 16 patients underwent an elective operation during this rehospitalization period. Of the 13 patients who had a second attack and had responded to medical therapy, there was a third attack in two patients (15.4%). Both of these patients were again successfully treated with medical therapy. There was no morbidity and mortality related to recurrence with an average time from the first attack to study contact of 35.2 months. Unlike acute uncomplicated left colonic diverticulitis, their findings indicated that after two documented episodes, medical treatment alone rather than elective surgery might be considered as an effective guideline for the treatment of acute uncomplicated right colonic diverticulitis.

So et al. (352) reported a series of 25 cases of bleeding right colonic diverticulosis selected from the colonoscopic reports of 190 patients who presented with acute lower GI bleeding. Bleeding diverticulosis was present in 30% of patients of which 44% suffered from right-sided disease. A history of hypertension was present in 64% of patients. Patients presented with either fresh blood in stools or melena. Blood transfusions were required in 60% of patients. Colonoscopy showed blood clots in the right colon in 60% and active bleeding from the right colon diverticula in 12%. The bleeding stopped spontaneously in 64%. The other patients required operation because of continuous or recurrent bleeding. All had a right hemicolectomy performed. There were no deaths. No patients had further bleeding during the median seven-month follow-up period.

In the event of massive hemorrhage from right-sided diverticula, the principles outlined above are invoked; if the bleeding does not stop and the bleeding site is identified, a right hemicolectomy is the appropriate treatment.

■ RESULTS

Kovalcik and Surtarsic (353) reported on 11 patients, most of who underwent a resection and primary anastomosis with no deaths or anastomotic leaks. Gouge et al. (354) also reported on 14 patients who underwent resection and anastomosis without any resulting deaths or leakage. In a report by McFee et al. (339), of 18 patients, all but one underwent resection with one leak and no deaths resulting. Arrington and Judd (355) reported on 33 patients with cecal diverticulitis. None had a free perforation. One patient required repeated drainage of a pericecal abscess before a definitive procedure. Of the remaining 32 patients with an inflammatory mass, 26 underwent right hemicolectomy, five had a cecectomy or partial colectomy, and two had simple excision of the diverticulum. No deaths and only one postoperative complication, an intra-abdominal abscess that required drainage, occurred. Lo and Chu (329) conducted a retrospective review on 22 surgically treated Chinese patients with documented right colon diverticulitis. Only one diagnosis subsequently proved correct. The pathology was easily recognized in four patients during operation, while examination of the resected specimen confirmed the intraoperative suspicion in 13 patients. The right colon was resected and an ileocolonic anastomosis performed in 21 patients; the remaining patients underwent diverticulectomy and drainage of a pericolic abscess. There was no postoperative mortality, and four patients developed wound infection. In a series of 35 patients reported by Markham and Li (334), five patient underwent diverticulectomy and the remaining patients right hemicolectomy. Harada and Whelan (356) reported on a conservative management of 90 cases of cecal diverticulitis at the University of Hawaii hospitals. The most common preoperative diagnosis was acute appendicitis, occurring in 73% of patients. A right colectomy or cecectomy was performed in 49 patients, an appendectomy in 29, and a diverticulectomy in 10. Seventeen complications occurred, only one of which was in the appendectomy group. Follow-up of up to 10 years was successful in 27 of 29 appendectomy patients, only four of whom had recurrent pain. There were no instances of a missed cecal carcinoma. The authors concluded that in those patients in whom carcinoma can be ruled out and in whom there is no evidence of abscess formation, appendectomy combined with postoperative antibiotics is a safe and effective method for the treatment of cecal diverticulitis. Fischer and Farkas (328) treated 12 patients with right-sided diverticulitis. Of the 11 patients who underwent laparotomy, seven had a right hemicolectomy, three had an appendectomy, and only one had a laparotomy. There was no mortality and only one complication occurred. The authors compiled the treatment and operative mortality rate of 279 cases collected from the literature. Resectional therapy had an operative mortality rate of 1.7%. More recent reviews of the literature report a mortality rate of 1.4% to 2.5% (327,338).

Law et al. (357) compared the results of emergency operation for patients with right-sided and left-sided diverticulitis (37 right-sided, 23 left-sided). Patients with right-sided disease were significantly younger (mean age 41.9 vs. 74.2 years) and there was a tendency for male predominance (78.4% vs. 56.5%). All patients with right-sided disease had localized peritonitis while 74% of patients with perforated left-sided diverticulitis had generalized fecal or purulent peritonitis. Mortality rates for right-sided disease and left-sided disease were 0% and 13%, respectively, and morbidity rates were 14.2% and 61%, respectively. Longer hospital stay was also found in patients with left-sided diverticulitis.

Diverticulitis of the transverse colon is exceedingly rare. In their review of the literature, Jasper et al. (358) disclosed 31 cases of transverse colon diverticulitis. Medical therapy with bowel rest and antibiotics is appropriate for transverse colon diverticulitis when free perforation and peritoneal signs are absent and the inflammation is contained as shown by CT. Operative exploration should be reserved for patients with diffuse peritonitis. The recommended treatment is extended right hemicolectomy. If perforation should supervene, performing a segmental resection with colostomy and mucous fistula has been recommended (359). For acute solitary diverticulitis of the transverse colon with a mass, resection and primary anastomosis are usually advocated (360).

GIANT COLONIC DIVERTICULUM

A giant colonic diverticulum is a rare clinical entity (361–364). Up to 1995, only 70 cases had been reported—40 males and 30 females with an age range of 32 to 90 (365). It is most commonly located in the sigmoid colon, arises from the antimesenteric border, and ranges in size from 4 to 30 cm (365,366). They are usually single but may be multiple. McNutt et al. (363) reviewed the three types of giant colonic diverticula described in the literature. One type is the pseudogiant colonic diverticulum, which results when a diverticulum increases in size without evidence of perforation. Remnants of muscularis mucosa or muscularis propria may be found in the wall, but the lining is usually granulation tissue interspersed with colonic mucosa. The second type results from perforation of the diverticulum and subsequent development of an abscess that remains in communication with the bowel lumen. This is an inflammatory giant colonic diverticulum because the wall of the diverticulum comprises no portion of the bowel wall except scar tissue. The third type contains all the layers of the bowel wall and is a true giant colonic diverticulum. Its pathogenesis is uncertain but is believed to represent a complication of diverticulosis. Other theories include distention of the diverticulum from a gas-forming organism or a ball-valve mechanism causing gas entrapment.

Patients may suffer vague abdominal pain, constipation, or diarrhea, and nausea and vomiting or may note a mass in the abdomen. Three types of complications have been described: infection and perforation, volvulus of the cyst, and obstruction of the small bowel resulting from adhesions (366). During physical examination, a large tender hypertympanitic mass may be found in the lower abdomen.

A plain film of the abdomen may reveal a gas-filled mass, but the diagnosis is usually made by barium enema examination. The differential diagnosis of abdominal gas-filled cysts included pneumatosis cystoides intestinalis, Meckel's diverticulum, giant duodenal diverticulum, duplication of the bowel, emphysematous cystitis, emphysematous cholecystitis, volvulus of the large bowel, pseudocyst of the pancreas, and tubo-ovarian abscess. Early operative treatment is necessary because the complication rate is high (17%) and includes perforation, volvulus, obstruction, and carcinoma (365). Treatment involves resection of the sigmoid colon in continuity with the diverticulum.

COEXISTING DISORDERS

CROHN'S DISEASE

Schmidt et al. reported the association of Crohn's disease and diverticulitis.(367). The involvement of diverticula by Crohn's disease may cause an increased incidence of diverticulitis (368). Of 21 patients with Crohn's disease and associated diverticulitis who underwent resection, diverticulitis could be pathologically confirmed in 48%. The clinical or radiologic recognition of the coexistence of the two diseases is often difficult, but this coexistence can be confirmed by microscopic examination (11).

Berman et al. (80) reported on 25 patients who had Crohn's disease in a colonic specimen resected for presumed diverticulitis. They presented a syndrome of combined diverticulitis and Crohn's disease heralded by anorectal disease, rectal bleeding, and fistulas. The illness is characterized by multiple operations, failure of diversionary procedures to control distal disease, and a high incidence of lethal pelvic sepsis. In patients whose disease persists after colonic resection, and recurs distally after diversion or forms fistulas late after resection for diverticulitis or who require multiple resections for clinical diverticulitis, Crohn's disease should be suspected.

Gledhill and Dixon (369) reviewed the histological specimens of 11 consecutive individuals having a colonic resection showing histologic features of both Crohn's disease and diverticulitis. In nine patients, the Crohn's-like reaction was confined to the segment bearing the diverticula. They had no clinical evidence of Crohn's disease. They concluded a Crohn's-like inflammatory response can be a localized reaction to diverticulitis and does not necessarily indicate chronic inflammatory bowel disease.

Burroughs et al. (370) noted that histologic appearances indistinguishable from Crohn's disease have been described in patients undergoing sigmoid colectomy for complicated diverticular disease. They investigated whether this finding represents coincidental dual pathology or merely a granulomatous colitis confined to the diverticular segment. Eight patients whose sigmoid colectomy specimens showed acute diverticulitis and granulomatous inflammation were identified. All had a preoperative diagnosis of diverticular disease and no previous evidence of Crohn's disease. Noncaseating epithelioid granulomas unrelated to foreign material and usually unrelated to inflamed diverticula, were present in the bowel wall of seven cases and in the regional lymph nodes of five. Three had granulomatous vasculitis and two had granulomas in "background" mucosa. Mural lymphoid aggregates were identified in all cases. However, fissuring ulcers distinct from inflamed diverticula were not identified. On median follow-up of 51 months, none of the patients developed evidence of chronic inflammatory bowel disease. They concluded that caution should be exercised to avoid an inappropriate diagnosis of Crohn's disease.

■ ADENOMAS AND CARCINOMAS

De Masi et al. (371) assessed the value of colonoscopy in the diagnosis of neoplasms associated with diverticular disease. In their review of 149 patients, examination could not be completed in 16% because of an impassable stricture in the left colon. Concurrent lesions were diagnosed in 69%, and carcinoma was found in 6%. They concluded that colonoscopy is indicated for patients with diverticulosis with symptoms because a precise differential diagnosis can be obtained. When colonoscopy is prevented because of a stricture, an operation is indicated. Rodkey and Welch (10) found polyps in 7% of patients operated on for diverticular disease. In 60 patients in whom a barium enema examination showed diverticular disease alone, colonoscopy revealed 13 polyps and one carcinoma, for a 23% incidence of neoplasia associated with diverticular disease (372). Therefore patients with persistent large bowel symptoms in whom a barium enema shows diverticular disease should undergo colonoscopic examination to unveil undetected neoplasia.

A review by Boulos et al. (373) included 105 patients with symptomatic sigmoid diverticular disease, in whom colonoscopy revealed an associated carcinoma in 7% and adenoma in 28%. The authors therefore recommend colonoscopy in patients with diverticular disease, particularly in those over the age of 60 years.

Stefansson et al. (374) compared the sensitivity between double-contrast barium enema and sigmoidoscopy in diagnosing neoplastic lesions in the sigmoid colon in patients with diverticulosis. In 52 patients with severe diverticulosis ($\geq$15 diverticula), the double-contrast barium enema detected one out of four polyps found by sigmoidoscopy. In 54 patients with mild diverticulosis ($<$15 diverticula), double-contrast barium enema detected 7 of 10 polyps found by sigmoidoscopy. Successful bowel preparation did not influence the outcome of the double-contrast barium enema. Sigmoidoscopy was incomplete in 17 (16%) of the patients; females were more difficult to examine, as were those with a previous pelvic operation. The authors concluded that neither double-contrast barium enema nor sigmoidoscopy alone is sufficient to detect all neoplastic lesions in the sigmoid colon in patients with sigmoid diverticulosis of the colon.

Carcinoma or an adenoma may occur simultaneously with diverticular disease. In a review of 385 patients with colonic carcinoma, coexisting diverticular disease was found in 25% (375). Furthermore, approximately half of the patients had evidence of associated diverticulitis. The authors suggested that carcinoma of the colon may even contribute to the development of diverticulosis and diverticulitis because of an elevation of intraluminal pressure. In a series of 351 patients undergoing resection for diverticulitis, Bacon et al. (376) found a coexisting carcinoma in 7.7%. When the sigmoid colon is resected as an emergency procedure for presumed diverticular disease, coincidental carcinoma is found in 20% to 25% of the patients (377,378). This impressive statistic underscores the fact that when resection is avoided with less florid inflammatory changes, the presence of a malignancy must be eliminated once the acute episode has resolved.

Stefansson et al. (379) noted that certain similar epidemiologic characteristics suggest a common etiology for colon carcinoma and diverticulosis of the colon. The hypothesis that patients with diverticulosis are at an increased risk of developing colon carcinoma was tested in a retrospective, population-based, cohort study in Sweden. A total of 7159 patients who had been given a hospital discharge, diagnosis of diverticulosis or diverticulitis of the colon between 1965 and 1983, were followed up during 1985 by means of record linkage procedures. After excluding the first two years of follow-up, there was not a significant increase in risk (SIR) overall for colon carcinoma (SIR = 1.2) or for rectal carcinoma (SIR = 1.1). The observed number of right-sided colon carcinomas was as expected (SIR = 0.9). In contrast, an increased risk of left-sided colon carcinoma was found, both overall (SIR = 1.8) and consistently in men and women as well as in different age groups. This risk increased, the longer the follow-up. These results do not support the hypothesis of a common etiology in diverticular disease and colonic carcinoma but suggest a causal relationship between diverticular disease and carcinoma of the left colon. This excess risk is not great enough to justify any screening procedures for carcinoma in patients with known diverticular disease but patients with diverticular disease and a change in symptoms should have malignant disease excluded. Stefansson also found that there is a causal association between sigmoid diverticulitis and long-term risk of left-sided colon carcinoma (OR = 4.2) (380).

Paspatis et al. (32) conducted an autopsy study to determine the prevalence of large bowel polyps and diverticulosis in the population on Crete. Data were collected from a total of 502 autopsies (320 men, 182 women; median age 65 years). Polyps were found in 21.1% of cases. These were adenomas in 14.5%, hyperplastic polyps in 4.9%, and mucosal tags in 1.5%. Diverticulosis of the large bowel was found in 22.9%. The prevalence of adenomas and diverticulosis increased with advanced age. The prevalence of colonic diverticulosis in Crete is slightly lower than that which has been reported in most other studies in economically developed countries. The prevalence of colorectal adenomas in Crete is one of the lowest rates reported in Europe and is compatible with the known low incidence of colorectal carcinoma in Crete.

Kieff et al. (381) also tried to determine the relationship between distal diverticulosis and risk of colorectal neoplasia. Patients undergoing first time colonoscopy for any indication were eligible if they had no prior polypectomy, colonic resection, or inflammatory bowel disease. The 502 participants were 67% male with a mean age of 58.6 years. Twenty-three percent had extensive diverticulosis, 36% had one or more than one adenoma, and 14% had advanced neoplasia. Overall, comparison of those with extensive distal diverticulosis versus few or no diverticula revealed no differences in the risks of any neoplasia or advanced neoplasia, either distally (26.7% vs. 25.4%; 12.9% vs. 8.8%, respectively) or proximally (25% vs. 18.4%; 6% vs. 4.9%). Compared to women with few or no distal diverticula, however, women with extensive distal diverticulosis were more likely to have any neoplasia and advanced neoplasia, both distally (34.6% vs. 16.3%; 23.1% vs. 5.7%) and proximally (30.8% vs. 14.9%; 11% vs. 4.3%).

Morini et al. (382) also evaluated the possible association between diverticular disease and both adenomas and colorectal carcinoma in 630 patients undergoing colonoscopy. Inclusion criteria were age above 45 years and performance of total colonoscopy. Adenomas were defined as advanced when they were greater than 1 cm in diameter and/or the percentage of the villous component was more than 30% and/or high-grade dysplasia was present. At endoscopy, 47% presented evidence of diverticular disease. Adenomas were found in 31.9% of patients with diverticular disease and in 28.9% of patients without. The prevalence of adenomas located in the sigmoid colon was significantly higher in patients with diverticula than in controls (64.1% vs. 41.8%). Similarly, the detection of advanced adenomas located in the sigmoid colon was more likely in patients with diverticula than in controls (59.9% vs. 37.5%). Colorectal carcinoma prevalence was similar in patients with and without diverticula (8.3% vs. 7.1%).

■ ULCERATIVE COLITIS

Ulcerative colitis and diverticulitis can coexist, but the association is much less common than Crohn's disease and diverticulitis (11). Ulcerative colitis is most likely to be apparent by associated clinical symptoms and sigmoidoscopic findings.

■ SAINT'S TRIAD

Burkitt and Walker stressed the association of colonic diverticulosis with cholelithiasis plus hiatal hernia (383). The association is found in an estimated 3% to 6% of the general population (66).

■ ARTHRITIS

A causal association between acute diverticulitis of the sigmoid colon and arthritis has rarely been reported. Alba et al. (384) reported the case of a 60-year-old patient who developed migrating arthritis of the knee ankle during the recurring episode of acute diverticulitis of the sigmoid colon. Treatment with NSAIDs and antibiotics had little effect on joint disease. Arthritis promptly improved after resection of the sigmoid colon, and 30 months later the patient was free of symptoms in the previously affected joints.

Five previous cases of diverticulitis-associated arthritis have been reported. Lower limbs are affected with knees and ankles being the most commonly involved joints. Pyoderma gangrenosum has also been reported in four patients with diverticulitis and arthritis. Colon resection is recommended for patients with diverticulitis-associated arthritis, which does not respond properly to antibiotic therapy.

SPECIAL PROBLEMS

■ SIMILARITY TO GYNECOLOGIC DISEASE

Patients with diverticulitis may present with symptoms that suggest a gynecologic problem. The management of such patients is discussed in Chapter 37.

■ IMMUNOCOMPROMISED PATIENT

Immunocompromised patients include those receiving organ transplants, patients taking steroids, patients with carcinoma undergoing chemotherapy, patients with acquired immunodeficiency syndrome, patients who have diabetes mellitus, and patients who are chronic alcoholics (70).

The immunocompromised patient presents a special problem, because the clinical course is often one of minimal or no symptoms and findings. The patients may fail medical treatment and require operative intervention. The morbidity and mortality of these patients is high. To make the diagnosis, a high index of suspicion must be maintained. Furthermore, these patients should be treated aggressively. For example, in a comparison of immunocompromised vs. nonimmunocompromised patients, with acute diverticulitis, Perkins et al. (385) found that medical treatment was successful in 76% of 45 nonimmunocompromised patients, whereas there was 100% failure in 10 immunocompromised patients, with every patient requiring an operation. The immunocompromised patients had a higher incidence of sepsis, peritonitis, and perforation. The authors found that performing a colostomy and resection resulted in fewer complications in these patients than did performing colostomy and drainage.

Starnes et al. (386) reported on the results of performing an operation for diverticulitis in patients with renal failure. The overall morbidity rate was 88% and the mortality rate was 28%, with sepsis being the major cause of morbidity and mortality.

Tyau et al. (387) reviewed the records of 209 patients with acute diverticulitis (40 immunocompromised patients and 169 nonimmunocompromised patients). Free perforation into the peritoneal cavity occurred in 43% (17 of 40) of immunocompromised patients and 14% (24 of 169) of nonimmunocompromised patients. Operations were performed in 58% (23 of 40) of immunocompromised patients and 33% (55 of 169) of nonimmunocompromised patients. Postoperative morbidity was 65% (15 of 23) in immunocompromised patients and 24% (13 of 55) in nonimmunocompromised patients; postoperative mortality was 39% (9 of 23) and 2% (1 of 55), respectively. The authors conclude that acute diverticulitis in the immunocompromised patient carries a greater risk of free perforation and need for operation than in the nonimmunocompromised patient. Furthermore, the prognosis for immunocompromised patients who undergo operation is worse than that for nonimmunocompromised patients.

REFERENCES

1. Cruveilhier J. Traité d'Anatomie Pathologique. Paris: Baillière, 1849.
2. Slack WW. The anatomy, pathology, and some clinical features of diverticulitis of the colon. Br J Surg 1962; 50:185–190.
3. Almy TP, Howell DA. Diverticula of the colon. N Engl J Med 1980; 302: 324–331.
4. Parks TG. Natural history of diverticular disease of the colon. Clin Gastroenterol 1975; 4:53–69.
5. Connell AM. Pathogenesis of diverticular disease of the colon. Adv Intern Med 1977; 22:377–395.
6. Rankin FW, Brown PW. Diverticulitis of the colon. Surg Gynecol Obstet 1930; 50:836–847.
7. Heller SN, Hackler LR. Changes in the crude fiber content of the American diet. Am J Clin Nutr 1978; 31:1510–1514.
8. Hart AR, Kennedy HJ, Stebbings WS, Day NE. How frequently do large bowel diverticula perforate? An incidence and cross-sectional study. Eur J Gastroenterol Hepatol 2000; 12:661–665.
9. Colcock BF. Diverticular Disease of the Colon. Philadelphia: WB Saunders, 1971.
10. Rodkey GV, Welch CE. Changing patterns in the surgical treatment of diverticular disease. Ann Surg 1984; 200:466–478.
11. Morson BC. Pathology of diverticular disease of the colon. Clin Gastroenterol 1975; 4:37–52.
12. Painter NS, Burkitt DP. Diverticular disease of the colon. A 20th century problem. Clin Gastroenterol 1975; 4:3–21.
13. Gear JSS, Ware A, Fursdon P, et al. Symptomless diverticular disease and intake of dietary fiber. Lancet 1979; 1:511–514.
14. Hughes LE. Postmortem survey of diverticular disease of the colon. Gut 1969; 10:336–351.
15. Eide TJ, Stalsberg H. Diverticular disease of the large intestine in Northern Norway. Gut 1979; 20:609–615.
16. Pan GZ, Liu TH, Chen MZ, Chang HC. Diverticular disease of the colon in China. A 60 year retrospective study. Chin Med J 1984; 97:391–394.
17. Coode PE, Chan KW, Chan YT. Polyps and diverticulosis of the large intestine. A necropsy survey in Hong Kong. Gut 1985; 26:1045–1048.
18. Dabestani A, Aliabadi P, Shah-Rookh FD, et al. Prevalence of colonic diverticular disease in Southern Iran. Dis Colon Rectum 1981; 24: 385–387.
19. Levy N, Stermer E, Simon J. The changing epidemiology of diverticular disease in Israel. Dis Colon Rectum 1985; 28:416–418.
20. Kang JY, Dhar A, Pollok R, et al. Diverticular disease of the colon: ethnic differences in frequency. Aliment Pharmacol Ther 2004; 19:765–769.
21. Kubo A, Ishiwata J, Maeda Y, et al. Clinical studies on diverticular disease of the colon. Jpn J Med 1983; 22:185–189.
22. Nakada I, Ubukata H, Goto Y, et al. Diverticular disease of the colon at a regional general hospital in Japan. Dis Colon Rectum 1995; 38: 755–759.
23. Miura S, Kodaira S, Aoki H, et al. Bilateral type diverticular disease of the colon. Int J Colorectal Dis 1996; 11:71–75.
24. Chan CC, Lo KK, Chung EC, Lo SS, Hon TY. Colonic diverticulosis in Hong Kong: distribution pattern and clinical significance. Clin Radiol 1998; 53:842–844.
25. Segal I, Leibowitz B. The distributional pattern of diverticular disease. Dis Colon Rectum 1989; 32:227–229.
26. Mendeloff AI. Thoughts on the epidemiology of diverticular disease. Clin Gastroenterol 1986; 15:855–877.
27. Manousos ON, Truelove SC, Lumsden K. Transit times of food in patients with diverticulosis or irritable colon syndrome and normal subjects. Br Med J 1967; 3:760–763.
28. Havia T. The irritable bowel syndrome. A follow-up study with special reference to the development of diverticula. Acta Chir Scand 1971; 137: 569–572.
29. Vajrabukka T, Saksornchai K, Jimakorn P. Diverticular disease of the colon in a Far Eastern community. Dis Colon Rectum 1980; 23:151–154.
30. Fatayer WT, A-Khalef MM, Shalam KA, et al. Diverticular disease of the colon in Jordan. Dis Colon Rectum 1983; 26:247–249.
31. Cleland JB. Incidence of diverticulosis. Br Med J 1968; 1:579.
32. Paspatis GA, Papanikolaou N, Zois E, Michalodimitrakis E. Prevalence of polyps and diverticulosis of the large bowel in the Cretan population. An autopsy study. Int J Colorectal Dis 2001; 16:257–261.
33. Painter NS. Diverticular disease of the colon: the first of the Western diseases shown to be due to a deficiency of dietary fibre. S Afr Med J 1982; 61: 1016–1020.
34. Burkitt DP, Walker ARP, Painter NS. Dietary fiber and disease. JAMA 1974; 229:1068–1074.
35. Bingham S. Dietary fiber intake: intake studies, problems, methods and results. In: Trowell H, Burkitt DP, Heaton K, eds. Dietary Fiber; Fiber Depleted Foods and Disease. New York: Academic Press, 1985.
36. Manousos ON, Day E, Jhonou A, et al. Diet and other factors in the etiology of diverticulosis: an epidemiological study in Greece. Gut 1985; 26: 544–549.
37. Nakaji S, Danjo K, Munakata A, et al. Comparison of etiology of right-sided diverticula in Japan with that of left-sided diverticula in the West. Int J Colorectal Dis 2002; 17:365–373.
38. Aldoori WH, Giovannucci EL, Rimm EB, et al. Prospective study of physical activity and the risk of symptomatic diverticular disease in man. Gut 1995; 36:276–282.
39. Aldoori WH, Giovannucci EL, Rimm EB, et al. A prospective study of alcohol, smoking, caffeine, and the risk of symptomatic diverticular disease in men. Ann Epidemiol 1995; 5:221–228.
40. Aldoori WH, Giovannucci EL, Rockett HR, Sampson L, Rimm EB, Willett WC. A prospective study of dietary fiber types and symptomatic diverticular disease in men. J Nutr 1998; 128:714–719.
41. Wess L, Eastwood MA, Weso TJ, et al. Cross linking of collagen is increased in colonic diverticulosis. Gut 1995; 37:91–94.
42. Stumpf M, Cao W, Klinge U, Klosterhalfen B, Kasperk R, Schumpelick V. Increased distribution of collagen type III and reduced expression of matrix metalloproteinase 1 in patients with diverticular disease. Int J Colorectal Dis 2001; 16:271–275.
43. Bode MK, Karttunen TJ, Makela J, Risteli L, Risteli J. Type I and III collagens in human colon cancer and diverticulosis. Scand J Gastroenterol 2000; 35: 747–752.
44. Painter NS. The cause of diverticular disease of the colon; its symptoms and its complications. J R Coll Surg Edinb 1985; 30:118–122.
45. Weinreich J, Andersen D. Intraluminal pressure in sigmoid colon. II. Patients with sigmoid diverticula and related conditions. Scand J Gastroenterol 1976; 11:581–586.
46. Hyland JMP, Darby CF, Hammond P, et al. Myoelectric activity of the sigmoid colon in patients with diverticular disease and the irritable colon syndrome suffering from diarrhea. Digestion 1980; 20:293–299.
47. Taylor I, Duthie HL. Bran tablets and diverticular disease. Br Med J 1976; 1:988–990.
48. Connell AM. Applied physiology of the colon. Factors relevant to diverticular disease. Clin Gastroenterol 1975; 4:23–36.
49. Rees BI, Bond J, Spriggs TLB, et al. Observations on the muscle abnormality of the human sigmoid colon in diverticular disease. Br J Clin Pharmacol 1980; 9:229–232.
50. Clemens CH, Samsom M, Roelofs J, van Berge Henegouwen GP, Smout AJ. Colorectal visceral perception in diverticular disease. Gut 2004; 53: 717–722.
51. Bassotti G, Battaglia E, Spinozzi F, Pelli MA, Tonini M. Twenty-four hour recordings of colonic motility in patients with diverticular disease: evidence for abnormal motility and propulsive activity. Dis Colon Rectum 2001; 44:1814–1820.
52. Ryan P. Two kinds of diverticular disease. Ann R Coll Surg Engl 1991; 73: 73–79.
53. Mann CV. Problems in diverticular disease. Proctology 1979; 1:20–25.
54. Manousos ON. Diverticular disease of the colon. Dig Dis 1989; 7:86–103.
55. Simpson J, Scholefield JH, Spiller RC. Origin of symptoms in diverticular disease. Br J Surg 2003; 90:899–908.
56. Whiteway J, Morson BC. Pathology of the aging—diverticular disease. Clin Gastroenterol 1985; 14:829–846.
57. Meyers MA, Volberg F, Katzen B. The angioarchitecture of colonic diverticula—significance in bleeding diverticulosis. Radiology 1973; 108: 249–262.
58. Whiteway J, Morson BC. Elastosis in diverticular disease of the sigmoid colon. Gut 1985; 26:158–166.
59. Breen RE, Corman ML, Robertson WG, et al. Are we really operating on diverticulitis? Dis Colon Rectum 1986; 29:174–176.
60. Killingback M, Barron PE, Dent OF. Elective surgery for diverticular disease: an audit of surgical pathology and treatment. ANZ J Surg 2004; 74: 530–536.
61. Halpert RO, Crnkovich FM, Schreiberg MH. Rectal diverticulosis: a case report and review of the literature. Gastrointest Radiol 1989; 14:274–276.
62. Sugihara K, Muto T, Morioka Y. Diverticular disease of the colon in Japan. A review of 615 cases. Dis Colon Rectum 1984; 27:531–537.
63. Hackford AW, Veidenheimer MC. Diverticular disease of the colon. Current concepts and management. Surg Clin North Am 1985; 65:347–363.
64. Haglund U, Hellberg R, Johnsen C, et al. Complicated diverticular disease of the sigmoid colon. An analysis of short- and long-term outcome in 392 patients. Ann Chir Gynecol 1979; 68:41–46.

65. Thorn M, Graf W, Stefansson T, Pahlman L. Clinical and functional results after elective colonic resection in 75 consecutive patients with diverticular disease. Am J Surg 2002; 183:7–11.
66. Boles RS, Jordan SM. The clinical significance of diverticulosis. Gastroenterology 1958; 35:579–581.
67. Horner JL. Natural history of diverticulosis of the colon. Am J Dig Dis 1958; 3:343–350.
68. Farmakis N, Tudor RG, Keighley MRB. The 5-year natural history of complicated diverticular disease. Br J Surg 1994; 81:733–735.
69. Makela J, Vulolio S, Kiviniemi H, Laitinen S. Natural history of diverticular disease: when to operate?. Dis Colon Rectum 1998; 41:1523–1528.
70. Roberts PL, Veidenheimer MC. Current management of diverticulitis. Adv Surg 1994; 27:189–208.
71. Ambrosetti P, Robert JH, Witzig JA, et al. Acute left colonic diverticulitis: a prospective analysis of 226 consecutive cases. Surgery 1994; 115: 546–550.
72. Chautems RC, Ambrosetti P, Ludwig A, Mermillod B, Morel P, Soravia C. Long-term follow-up after first acute episode of sigmoid diverticulitis: is surgery mandatory? A prospective study of 118 patients. Dis Colon Rectum 2002; 45:962–966.
73. Anaya DA, Flum DR. Risk of emergency colectomy and colostomy in patients with diverticular disease. Arch Surg 2005; 140:681–685.
74. Kewenter J, Hellzen-Ingemarsson A, Kewenter G, et al. Diverticular disease and minor rectal bleeding. Scand J Gastroenterol 1985; 20: 922–924.
75. Marshak RH, Lindner AE, Maklansky D. Diverticulosis and diverticulitis of the colon. Mt Sinai J Med 1979; 46:261–276.
76. Hunt RH. The role of colonoscopy in complicated diverticular disease: a review. Acta Chir Belg 1979; 78:349–353.
77. Boulos PB, Salmon PR, Karamanolis DG, et al. Is colonoscopy necessary in diverticular disease? Lancet 1984; 1:95–96.
78. Schreyer AG, Furst A, Agha A, et al. Magnetic resonance imaging based colonography for diagnosis and assessment of diverticulosis and diverticulitis. Int J Colorectal Dis 2004; 19:474–480.
79. Schnyder P, Moss AA, Theoni RF, et al. A double blind study of radiologic accuracy in diverticulitis, diverticulosis and carcinoma of the sigmoid colon. J Clin Gastroenterol 1979; 1:55–66.
80. Berman IR, Corman ML, Coller JA, et al. Late onset Crohn's disease in patients with colonic diverticulitis. Dis Colon Rectum 1979; 22:524–529.
81. Glick SN. Inverted colonic diverticulum: air contrast barium enema findings in six cases. AJR 1991; 156:961–964.
82. Ladas SD, Prigouris SP, Pontelidaki C, et al. Endoscopic removal of inverted sigmoid diverticulum—Is it a dangerous procedure? Endoscopy 1989; 21:243–244.
83. Schuman BM. Endoscopic diverticulectomy in the sigmoid colon. Gastrointest Endosc 1982; 28:189–190.
84. Thompson WG, Patel DG. Clinical picture of diverticular disease of the colon. Clin Gastroenterol 1986; 15:903–916.
85. Smith AN, Drummond E, Eastwood MA. The effect of course and fine Canadian Red Spring wheat and French soft wheat bran on colonic motility in patients with diverticular disease. Am J Clin Nutr 1981; 34: 2460–2463.
86. Hyland JMP, Taylor I. Does a high fiber diet prevent the complications of diverticular disease?. Br J Surg 1980; 67:771–779.
87. Stanciu C, Bennett JR. Colonic response to pentazocine. Br Med J 1974; 1: 312–313.
88. Papi C, Ciaco A, Koch M, et al. Efficacy of rifaximin in the treatment of symptomatic diverticular disease of the colon: a multicentre double-blind placebo-controlled trial. Aliment Pharmacol Ther 1995; 9:33–39.
89. Latella G, Pimpo MT, Sottili S, et al. Rifaximin improves symptoms of acquired uncomplicated diverticular disease of the colon. Int J Colorectal Dis 2003; 18:55–62.
90. Brandimarte G, Tursi A. Rifaximin plus mesalazine followed by mesalazine alone is highly effective in obtaining remission of symptomatic uncomplicated diverticular disease. Med Sci Monit 2004; 10(5):PI70–PI73.
91. Chodak GW, Rangel DM, Passaro E Jr. Colonic diverticulitis in patients under age 40: need for earlier diagnosis. Am J Surg 1981; 141:699–702.
92. Ouriel K, Schwartz SI. Diverticular disease in the young patient. Surg Gynecol Obstet 1983; 156:1–5.
93. Bernstein WC, Nivatvongs S, Tallent MB. Colonic and rectal complications of kidney transplant in man. Dis Colon Rectum 1973; 16:255–263.
94. Dominguez Fernandez E, Albrecht KH, Heemann U, et al. Prevalence of diverticulosis and incidence of bowel perforation after kidney transplantation in patients with polycystic kidney disease. Transpl Int 1998; 11:28–31.
95. Wong WD, Wexner SD, Lowry A, et al. Practice parameters for the treatment of sigmoid diverticulitis-supporting documentation. The standards Task Force. The American Society of Colon and Rectal Surgeons. Dis Colon Rectum 2000; 43:290–297.
96. Stollman NH, Raskin JB. Diagnosis and management of diverticular disease of the colon in adults. Ad Hoc Practice Parameters Committee of the American College of Gastroenterology. Am J Gastroenterol 1999; 94: 3110–3121.
97. Janes S, Meagher A, Frizelle FA. Elective surgery after acute diverticulitis. Br J Surg 2005; 92:133–142.
98. Richards RJ, Hammitt JK. Timing of prophylactic surgery in prevention of diverticulitis recurrence: a const-effectiveness analysis. Dig Dis Sci 2002; 47:1903–1908.
99. Salem L, Veenstra DL, Sullivan SD, Flum DR. The timing of elective colectomy in diverticulitis: a decision analysis. J Am Coll Surg 2004; 199: 904–912.
100. Chapman J, Davies M, Wolff B, et al. Complicated diverticulitis: is it time to rethink the rules? Ann Surg 2005; 242:576–581.
101. Benn PL, Wolff BG, Ilstrup DM. Level of anastomosis and recurrent colonic diverticulitis. Am J Surg 1986; 151:269–271.
102. Wolff BG, Ready RL, MacCarty RL, et al. Influence of sigmoid resection on progression of diverticular disease of the colon. Dis Colon Rectum 1984; 27:645–647.
103. Tocchi A, Mazzoni G, Fornasari V, Miccini M, Daddi G, Tagliacozzo S. Preservation of the inferior mesenteric artery in colorectal resection for complicated diverticular disease. Am J Surg 2001; 182:162–167.
104. Kyzer S, Gordon PH. The prophylactic use of ureteral catheters during colorectal operations. Am Surg 1994; 60:212–216.
105. Munson KD, Hensien MA, Jacob LN, et al. Diverticulitis: a comprehensive follow-up. Dis Colon Rectum 1996; 39:318–322.
106. Moreaux J, Vons C. Elective resection for diverticular disease of the sigmoid colon. Br J Surg 1990; 77:1036–1038.
107. Pessaux P, Muscari F, Ouellet JF, et al. Risk factors for mortality and morbidity after elective sigmoid resection for diverticulitis: prospective multicenter multivariate analysis of 582 patients. World J Surg 2004; 28: 92–96.
108. Thaler K, Baig MK, Berho M, et al. Determinants of recurrence after sigmoid resection for uncomplicated diverticulitis. Dis Colon Rectum 2003; 46: 385–388.
109. Horgan AF, McConnell EJ, Wolff BG, The S, Paterson C. Atypical diverticular disease: surgical results. Dis Colon Rectum 2001; 44:1315–1318.
110. Bokey EL, Chapuis PH, Pheils MT, et al. Elective resection for diverticular disease and carcinoma. Comparison of postoperative morbidity and mortality. Dis Colon Rectum 1981; 24:181–182.
111. Eisenstat TE, Rubin RJ, Salvati EP. Surgical management of diverticulitis. The role of the Hartmann procedure. Dis Colon Rectum 1983; 26: 429–432.
112. Hackford AW, Schoetz DJ Jr, Coller JA, et al. Surgical management of complicated diverticulitis. Dis Colon Rectum 1985; 28:317–321.
113. Levien DH, Mazier WP, Surrell JA, et al. Safe resection for diverticular disease of the colon. Dis Colon Rectum 1989; 32:30–32.
114. Killingback M. Diverticulitis of the colon. In: Fazio VW, ed. Current Therapy in Colon and Rectal Surgery. Toronto: BC Decker, 1990: 222–231.
115. Netri G, Verbo A, Coco C, et al. The role of surgical treatment in colon diverticulitis: indications and results. Ann Ital Chir 2000; 71:209–214.
116. Vinas-Salas J, Villalba-Acosta J, Scaramucci M, et al. Complications of colonic diverticular disease. Comparative study of two series. Rev Esp Enferm Dig 2001; 93:649–658.
117. McConnell EJ, Tessier DJ, Wolff BG. Population-based incidence of complicated diverticular disease of the sigmoid colon based on gender and age. Dis Colon Rectum 2003; 46:1110–1114.
118. Wilson RG, Smith AN, MacIntyre IMC. Complications of diverticular disease and non-steroidal anti-inflammatory drugs: a prospective study. Br J Surg 1990; 77:1103–1104.
119. Aldoori WH, Giovannucci EL, Rimm EB, et al. Use of acetaminophen and nonsteroidal anti-inflammatory drugs: a prospective study and the risk of symptomatic diverticular disease in men. Arch Fam Med 1998; 7:255–260.
120. Wilcox CM, Alexander LN, Cotsonis GA, Clark WS. Nonsteroidal anti-inflammatory drugs are associated with both upper and lower gastrointestinal bleeding. Dig Dis Sci 1997; 42:990–997.
121. Goh H, Bourne R. Non-steroidal anti-inflammatory drugs and perforated diverticular disease: a case-control study. Ann R Coll Surg Engl 2002; 84: 93–96.
122. Morris CR, Harvey IM, Stebbings WS, Speakman CT, Kennedy HJ, Hart AR. Epidemiology of perforated colonic diverticular disease. Postgrad Med J 2002; 78(925):654–658.
123. Mpofu S, Mpofu CM, Hutchinson D, Maier AE, Dodd SR, Moots RJ. Steroids, non-steroidal anti-inflammatory drugs, and sigmoid diverticular abscess perforation in rheumatic conditions. Ann Rheum Dis 2004; 63: 588–590.
124. Kubo A, Kagaya T, Nakagawa H. Studies on complications of diverticular disease of the colon. Jpn J Med 1985; 24:39–43.
125. Kyle J, Davidson AI. The changing pattern of hospital admissions for diverticular disease of the colon. Br J Surg 1975; 62:537–541.
126. Parks TG, Connell AM. The outcome of 455 patients admitted for treatment of diverticular disease of the colon. Br J Surg 1970; 57:775–778.
127. Edelmann G. Surgical treatment of colonic diverticulitis: report of 205 cases. Int Surg 1981; 66:119–124.

128. Ravo B, Khan SA, Ger R, et al. Unusual extraperitoneal presentations of diverticulitis. Am J Gastroenterol 1985; 80:346–351.
129. Wexner SD, Daily TH. The initial management of left lower quadrant peritonitis. Dis Colon Rectum 1986; 29:635–638.
130. Frager E, Wolf EL, Frager JD, et al. Small intestinal complications of diverticulitis of the sigmoid colon. JAMA 1986; 256:3258–3261.
131. Hiltunen KM, Kolehmainen H, Vuorinen T, et al. Early water-soluble contrast enema in the diagnosis of acute colonic diverticulitis. Int J Colorectal Dis 1991; 6:190–192.
132. Yacoe ME, Jeffrey RB. Sonography of appendicitis and diverticulitis. Radiol Clin North Am 1994; 32:899–912.
133. Verbanck J, Lambrecht S, Rutgeerts L, et al. Can sonography diagnose acute colonic diverticulitis in patients with acute intestinal inflammation? A prospective study. J Clin Ultrasound 1989; 17:661–666.
134. Schwerk WB, Schwarz S, Rothmund M. Sonography in acute colonic diverticulitis: a prospective study. Dis Colon Rectum 1992; 35:1077–1084.
135. Ripolles T, Agramunt M, Martinez MJ, Costa S, Gomez-Abril SA, Richart J. The role of ultrasound in the diagnosis, management and evolutive prognosis of acute left-sided colonic diverticulitis: a review of 208 patients. Eur Radiol 2003; 13:2587–2595.
136. Hollerweger A, Macheiner P, Rettenbacher T, Brunner W, Gritzmann N. Colonic diverticulitis: diagnostic value and appearance of inflamed diverticula-sonographic evaluation. Eur Radiol 2001; 11:1956–1963.
137. Hulnick DH, Megibow AJ, Balthazar EJ, et al. Computed tomography in the evaluation of diverticulitis. Radiology 1984; 152:491–495.
138. Hachigian MP, Honickman S, Eisenstat TE, et al. Computed tomography in the initial management of acute left-sided diverticulitis. Dis Colon Rectum 1992; 35:1123–1129.
139. Werner A, Diehl SJ, Farag-Soliman M, Duber C. Multi-slice spiral CT in routine diagnosis of suspected acute left-sided colonic diverticulitis: a prospective study of 120 patients. Eur Radiol 2003; 13:2596–2603.
140. Poletti PA, Platon A, Rutschmann O, et al. Acute left colonic diverticulitis: can CT findings be used to predict recurrence? AJR Am J Roentgenol 2004; 182:1159–1165.
141. Johnson CD, Baker ME, Rice RP, et al. Diagnosis of acute colonic diverticulitis: comparison of barium enema and CT. Am J Roentgenol 1987; 148:541–546.
142. Smith TR, Cho KC, Morehouse HT, et al. Comparison of computed tomography and contrast enema evaluation of diverticulitis. Dis Colon Rectum 1990; 33:1–6.
143. Ambrosetti P, Jenny A, Becker C, Terrier TF, Morel P. Acute left colonic diverticulitis—compared performance of computed tomography and water-soluble contrast enema: prospective evaluation of 420 patients. Dis Colon Rectum 2000; 43:1363–1367.
144. Labs JD, Sarr MG, Fishman EK, et al. Complications of acute diverticulitis of the colon: improved early diagnosis with computerized tomography. Am J Surg 1988; 155:331–356.
145. Ambrosetti P, Robert J, Witzig JA, et al. Prognostic factors from computed tomography in acute left colonic diverticulitis. Br J Surg 1992; 179: 117–119.
146. Trenkner S, Thompson WM. Questions and answers. AJR 1995; 165:733.
147. Gilbert DN, Moellering RC, Eliopoulos GM, Sande MA, eds. The Sanford Guide to Antimicrobial Therapy 2004. 34th edition Hyde Park, Vt: Antimicrobial Therapy, Inc, 2004.
148. Starr JM, Impallomeni M. Risk of diarrhoea, Clostridium difficile and cefotaxime in the elderly. Biomed Pharmacother 1997; 51:63–67.
149. Werth B, Kobler E, Reinhart WH, Ciorciaro C, Hartmann K, Kuhn M. Clostridium difficile associated diarrhea in cephalosporin administration: experiences of the Swiss Adverse Drug Reaction Reporting System 1981–1995. Schweizeriche Medizinische Wocherschritt Suppl 1997; 89:55–89.
150. Spencer RC. The role of antimicrobial agents in the aetiology of Clostridium difficile-associated disease. J Antimicrob Chemother 1998; 41(suppl C): 21–27.
151. Ludlam H, Brown N, Sule O, Redpath C, Coni N, Owen G. An Antibiotic Policy associated with reduced risk of clostridium difficile associated diarrhea. Age Aging 1999; 28:578–580.
152. Thomas C, Riley TV. Restriction of third generation cephalosporin use reduces the incidence of clostridium difficile associated diarrhea in hospitalized patients. Commun Dis Intell 2003; 27(suppl):528–531.
153. Anand A, Bashey B, Mir T, Glatt AE. Epidemiology, clinical manifestations and outcome of clostridium difficile associated diarrhea. Am J Gastroenterol 1994; 89:519–523.
154. Miller MA, Cohen E, Consolacion N, Orenstein P, Amihod B. Control of hyper endemic nosocomial clostridium difficile associated diarrhea by substitution of second/third generation cephalosporin utilization with ticarcillin/clavunalate fluoroquinolone. Presented at 42nd ICAAC, San Diego, California, September 2002. p. 331.
155. Larson DM, Master SS, Spiro HM. Medical and surgical therapy in diverticular disease. A comparative study. Gastroenterology 1976; 71: 734–737.
156. Guzzo J, Hyman N. Diverticulitis in young patients: is resection after a single attack always warranted?. Dis Colon Rectum 2004; 47:1187–1190.
157. Hoemke M, Treckmann J, Schmitz R, Shah S. Complicated diverticulitis of the sigmoid: a prospective study concerning primary resection with secure primary anastomosis. Dig Surg 1999; 16:420–424.
158. Nylamo E. Diverticulitis of the colon: role of surgery in preventing complications. Ann Chir Gynaecol 1990; 79:139–142.
159. Tudor RG, Farmakis N, Keighley MRB. National audit of complicated diverticular disease: analysis of index cases. Br J Surg 1994; 81:730–732.
160. Detry R, Jamez J, Karthensen A, et al. Acute localized diverticulitis: optimum management requires accurate staging. Int J Colorectal Dis 1992; 7:38–42.
161. Sarin S, Boulos PB. Long-term outcome of patients presenting with acute complications of diverticular disease. Am R Coll Surg Engl 1994; 76(2): 117–120.
162. Wedell J, Banzhaf G, Chaoui R, Fischer R, Reichmann J. Surgical management of complicated colonic diverticulitis. Br J Surg 1997; 84:380–383.
163. Nagorney DM, Adson MA, Pemberton JH. Sigmoid diverticulitis with perforation-and generalized peritonitis. Dis Colon Rectum 1985; 28:71–75.
164. Greif JM, Fried G, McSherry CK. Surgical treatment of perforated diverticulitis of the sigmoid colon. Dis Colon Rectum 1980; 23:483–487.
165. Sakai L, Daake J, Kaminski DL. Acute perforations of sigmoid diverticula. Am J Surg 1981; 142:712–716.
166. Wara P, Sorensen K, Berg V, et al. The outcome of staged management of complicated diverticular disease of the sigmoid colon. Acta Chir Scand 1981; 147:209–214.
167. Killingback M. Management-of perforative diverticulitis. Surg Clin North Am 1983; 63:97–115.
168. Ryan P. Changing concepts in diverticular disease. Dis Colon Rectum 1983; 26:12–18.
169. Cullen KW, Ferguson JC. Diverticular disease as a surgical emergency. Br J Clin Pract 1984; 38:20–24.
170. Lambert ME, Knox RA, Schofield PF, et al. Management of septic complications of diverticular disease. Br J Surg 1986; 73:576–579.
171. Finlay IG, Carter DC. A comparison of emergency resection and staged management in perforated diverticular disease. Dis Colon Rectum 1987; 30:929–933.
172. Hold M, Denck H, Bull P. Surgical management of perforating diverticular disease in Austria. Int J Colorectal Dis 1990; 5:195–199.
173. Classen JN, Bonardi R, O'Mara CS, et al. Surgical treatment of acute diverticulitis by stage procedure. Ann Surg 1976; 184:582–586.
174. Krukowski ZH, Matheson NA. Emergency surgery for diverticular disease complicated by generalized and fecal peritonitis: a review. Br J Surg 1984; 71:921–927.
175. Drumm J, Clain A. The management of acute colonic diverticulitis with suppurative peritonitis. Ann R Coll Surg Engl 1984; 66:90–91.
176. Weckesser EC. Functional exteriorized colon for perforations due to diverticulitis. Am J Surg 1980; 139:298–300.
177. Watkins GL, Oliver GA. Surgical treatment of acute perforative sigmoid diverticulitis. Surgery 1971; 69:215–219.
178. Hartmann H. Nouveau procédé d'ablation des cancers de la partie terminale du colon pelvien. Congres Fr Chir 1923; 30:2241.
179. Abcarian H, Pearl RK. A safe technique for resection of perforated diverticulitis. Dis Colon Rectum 1990; 33:905–906.
180. Fowler C, Aaland M, Johnson L, et al. Perforated diverticulitis in a Hartmann pouch. Dis Colon Rectum 1986; 29:662–664.
181. Schein M, Kopelman D, Nitecki G, et al. Management of the leaking rectal stump after Hartmann's procedure. Am J Surg 1993; 165:285–287.
182. Salem L, Anaya DA, Roberts KE, Flum DR. Hartmann's colectomy and reversal in diverticulitis: a population-level assessment. Dis Colon Rectum 2005; 48:988–995.
183. Wigmore SJ, Duthie GS, Young IE, et al. Restoration of intestinal continuity following Hartmann's procedure: the Lothian experience 1987–1992. Br J Surg 1995; 82:27–30.
184. Peoples JB, Vilk DR, Macguire JP, et al. Reassessment of primary resection of the perforated segment for colonic diverticulitis. Am J Surg 1990; 159:291–294.
185. Kronberg O. Treatment of perforated sigmoid diverticulitis: a prospective randomized trial. Br J Surg 1993; 80:505–507.
186. Celicout B, Zeitoun G. Generalized peritonitis in sigmoid acute diverticulitis: surgical treatment—a randomized study of French Research Associations. Br J Surg 1996; 83(suppl 2):24.
187. Auguste L, Borrero E, Wise L. Surgical management of perforated diverticulitis. Arch Surg 1985; 120:450–452.
188. Mallonga ET, Brummelkamp WH, van Gulik TM, et al. The Hartmann procedure: its role in acute complicated diverticulitis. Neth J Surg 1986; 38:171–174.
189. Marien B. The Hartmann procedure. Can J Surg 1987; 30:30–31.
190. Alanis A, Papanicolou GK, Tadros RR, et al. Primary resection and anastomosis for treatment of diverticulitis. Dis Colon Rectum 1989; 32:933–939.
191. Berry AR, Turner WH, Mortensen NJM, et al. Emergency surgery for complicated diverticular disease. A five-year experience. Dis Colon Rectum 1989; 32:849–854.

192. Kerner B, Oliver GC, Eisenstat TE, et al. Use of the Hartmann procedure in the treatment of complicated acute diverticulitis. Semin Colon Rectal Surg 1990; 1:87–92.
193. Hiltunen KM, Matikaainen M. The Hartmann procedure in the treatment of complicated sigmoid diverticulitis. Res Surg 1991; 3:222–225.
194. Keck JO, Collopy BT, Ryan PJ, et al. Reversal of Hartmann's procedure: effect of timing and technique on ease and safety. Dis Colon Rectum 1994; 37: 243–248.
195. Thaler K, Gero S, Ball PG, et al. Surgical management of perforating sigmoid diverticular disease with general peritonitis. Br J Surg 1996; 83(suppl 2):36.
196. Khosraviani K, Campbell WJ, Parks TG, Irwin ST. Hartmann procedure revisited. Eur J Surg 2000; 166:878–881.
197. Gooszen AW, Gooszen HG, Veerman W, van Dongen VM, Hermans J, Klien Kranenbarg E. Operative treatment of acute complications of diverticular disease: primary or secondary anastomosis after sigmoid resection. Eur J Surg 2001; 167:35–39.
198. Schilling MK, Maurer CA, Kollmar O, Buchier MW. Primary vs. secondary anastomosis after sigmoid colon resection for perforated diverticulitis (Hinchey stage III and IV): a prospective outcome and cost analysis. Dis Colon Rectum 2001; 44:699–703.
199. Le Neel JC, Letessier E, Grenier F, et al. Restoration of colorectal continuity after Hartmann's procedure: a report of 150 cases. Br J Surg 1995; 82(suppl 1):32.
200. Haas PA, Fox TA. The fate of the forgotten rectal pouch after Hartmann's procedure without reconstruction. Am J Surg 1990; 159:106–111.
201. Landen S, Nafteux P. Primary anastomosis and diverting colostomy in diffuse diverticular peritonitis. Acta Chir Belg 2002; 102:24–29.
202. Farkouh E, Hellou G, Allard M, et al. Resection and primary anastomosis for diverticulitis with perforation and peritonitis. Can J Surg 1982; 25:314–316.
203. Gooszen AW, Tollenaar RA, Geelkerken RH, Smeets HJ, Bemelman WA, van Schaardenburgh P. Prospective study of primary anastomosis following sigmoid resection for suspected acute complicated diverticular disease. Br J Surg 2001; 88:693–697.
204. Blair NP, Germann E. Surgical management of acute sigmoid diverticulitis. Am J Surg 2002; 183:525–528.
205. Ravo B, Mishrick A, Addei K, et al. The treatment of perforated diverticulitis by one-stage intracolonic bypass procedure. Surgery 1987; 102:771–775.
206. Zeitoun G, Laurent A, Rouffet F, et al. Multicentre, randomized clinical trial of primary versus secondary sigmoid resection in generalized peritonitis complicating sigmoid diverticulitis. Br J Surg 2000; 87: 1366–1374.
207. Lee EC, Murray JJ, Coller JA, Roberts PL, Schoetz DJ Jr. Intraoperative colonic lavage in nonelective surgery for diverticular disease. Dis Colon Rectum 1997; 40:669–674.
208. Salem L, Flum DR. Primary anastomosis or Hartmann's procedure for patients wiht diverticular peritonitis? A systematic review. Dis Colon Rectum 2004; 47:1953–1964.
209. O'Sullivan GC, Murphy D, O'Brien MG, et al. Laparoscopic management of generalized peritonitis due to perforated colonic diverticulitis. Am J Surg 1996; 171:432–434.
210. Gerzof SC, Johnson WC. Radiologic aspects of diagnosis and treatment of abdominal abscesses. Surg Clin North Am 1984; 64:53–66.
211. Greco RS, Kamath C, Nosher JL. Percutaneous drainage of peridiverticular abscess followed by primary sigmoidectomy. Dis Colon Rectum 1982; 25: 53–55.
212. Stabile BE, Puccio E, van Sonnenberg E, et al. Preoperative percutaneous drainage of diverticular abscesses. Am J Surg 1990; 159:99–105.
213. Kaiser AM, Jiang JK, Lake JP, et al. The management of complicated diverticulitis and the role of computed tomography. Am J Gastroenterol 2005; 100: 910–917.
214. Ambrosetti P, Chautems R, Soravia C, Peiris-Waser N, Terrier F. Long-term outcome of mesocolic and pelvic diverticular abscesses of the left colon: a prospective study of 73 cases. Dis Colon Rectum 2005; 48:787–791.
215. Mueller PR, Saini S, Wittenburg J, et al. Sigmoid diverticular abscesses: percutaneous drainage as an adjunct to surgical resection in 24 cases. Radiology 1987; 164:321–325.
216. Neff CC, van Sonnenberg E, Casola G, et al. Diverticular abscesses: percutaneous drainage. Radiology 1987; 163:15–18.
217. Salem L, Anaya DA, Flum DR. Temporal changes in the management of diverticulitis. J Surg Res 2005; 124:318–323.
218. Gallagher DM, Russel TR. Surgical management of diverticular disease. Surg Clin North Am 1978; 58:563–572.
219. Crowson WN, McCaughan JJ. Total abdominal colectomy in the surgical management of diverticular disease of the colon. Twenty years experience. South Med J 1972; 65:1443–1447.
220. Morganstern L, Weiner R, Michel SL. "Malignant" diverticulitis. A clinical entity. Arch Surg 1979; 114:1112–1116.
221. Acosta JA, Grebenc ML, Doberneck RC, et al. Colonic diverticular disease in patients 40 years old or younger. Am Surg 1992; 58:605–607.
222. Freischlag J, Bennion RS, Thompson JE. Complications of diverticular disease of the colon in young people. Dis Colon Rectum 1986; 29:639–643.
223. Cunningham MA, Davis JW, Kaups KL. Medical versus surgical management of diverticulitis in patients under age 40. Am J Surg 1997; 174: 733–735.
224. Ambrosetti P, Robert JH, Witzig JA, et al. Acute left colonic diverticulitis in young patients. J Am Coll Surg 1994; 179:156–160.
225. Konvolinka CW. Acute diverticulitis under age forty. Am J Surg 1994; 167: 562–565.
226. Schauer PR, Ramos R, Ghiatas AA, et al. Virulent diverticular disease in obese men. Am J Surg 1992; 164:443–448.
227. Minardi AJ Jr, Johnson LW, Sehon JK, Zibari GB, McDonald JC. Diverticulitis in the young patient. Am Surg 2001; 67:458–461.
228. Schweitzer J, Casillas RA, Collins JC. Acute diverticulitis in the young adult in not "virulent." Am Surg 2002; 68(12):1044–1047.
229. Vignati PV, Welch JP, Cohen JL. Long-term management of diverticulitis in young patients. Dis Colon Rectum 1995; 38:627–629.
230. West D, Robinson EK, Delu AN, Ligon RE, Kao S, Mercer DW. Diverticulitis in the younger patient. Am J Surg 2003; 186:743–746.
231. Biondo S, Pares D, Marti Rague J, Kreisler E, Fraccalvieri D, Jaurrieta E. Acute colonic diverticulitis in patients under 50 years of age. Br J Surg 2002; 89: 1137–1141.
232. Chiu TCT, Bailey HR, Hernandez AJ. Diverticulitis of the mid rectum. Dis Colon Rectum 1983; 26:59–60.
233. Hughes ESR, Cuthbertson AM, Carden ABG. The surgical management of acute diverticulitis. Med J Aust 1963; 1:780–782.
234. Localio SA, Stahl WM. Diverticular disease of the alimentary tract. I. The colon. Curr Probl Surg 1967; 29:1–78.
235. Miller DW, Wichern WA. Perforated diverticulitis. Appraisal of primary versus delayed resection. Am J Surg 1971; 121:536–540.
236. Hinchey EJ, Schaal PGH, Richards GK. Treatment of perforated disease of the colon. Adv Surg 1978; 12:86–109.
237. Silvis R, Keeman JN. Complicated diverticulitis in acute surgery. Neth J Surg 1988; 40:117–120.
238. Fazio VW. Acute perforated diverticulitis. In: Fischer JE, ed. Common Problems in Gastrointestinal Surgery. Chicago: Year Book, 1989:386–393.
239. Hollender LF, Meyer CH, Alexiou D, et al. Therapeutic principles in emergency colonic surgery. Int Surg 1981; 66:307–310.
240. Elliott TB, Yego S, Irvin TT. Five-year audit of the acute complications of diverticular disease. Br J Surg 1997; 84:535–539.
241. Regenet N, Pessaux P, Hennekinne S, et al. Primary anastomosis after intraoperative colonic lavage vs. Hartmann's procedure in generalized peritonitis complicating diverticular disease of the colon. Int J Colorectal Dis 2003; 18:503–507.
242. Makela J, Kiviniemi H, Laitinen S. Prevalence of perforated sigmoid diverticulitis is increasing. Dis Colon Rectum 2002; 45:955–961.
243. Makela JT, Kiviniemi H, Laitinen S. Prognostic factors of perforated sigmoid diverticulitis in the elderly. Dig Surg 2005; 22:100–106.
244. Hool GJ, Bokey EL, Pheils MT. Diverticular coloenteric fistulae. Aust NZ J Surg 1981; 51:358–359.
245. Corman ML. Colon and Rectal Surgery, 2nd ed. Philadelphia: JB Lippincott, 1989:505, 684.
246. Colcock BP, Stahmann FD. Fistulas complicating diverticular disease of the sigmoid colon. Ann Surg 1972; 175:838–846.
247. Orebaugh JE, McCris JA, Lee JF. Surgical treatment of diverticular disease of the colon. Am Surg 1978; 44:712–715.
248. Pheils MT, Chapuis PH, Bokey EL. Diverticular disease: a retrospective study of surgical management, 1970–1980. Aust NZ J Surg 1982; 52:53–56.
249. Woods RJ, Lavery JC, Fazio VW, et al. Internal fistulas in diverticular disease. Dis Colon Rectum 1988; 31:591–596.
250. Bahadursingh AM, Virgo KS, Kaminski DL, Longo WE. Spectrum of disease and outcome of complicated diverticular disease. Am J Surg 2003; 186:696–701.
251. Maeda Y, Nakashima S, Misaki T. Ureterocolic fistula secondary to colonic diverticulitis. Int J Urol 1998; 5:610–612.
252. Senthilhes L, Foulatier O, Verspyck E, Roman H, Scotte M, Marpeau L. Colouterine fistula complicating diverticulitis: a case report and review of the literature. Eur J Obstet Gynecol Reprod Biol 2003; 110:107–110.
253. Williams SM, Nolan DJ. Colosalpingeal fistula: a rare complication of colonic diverticular disease. Eur Radiol 1999; 9:1432–1433.
254. Parikh VA. Colosalpingeal fistula: a rare complication of diverticular disease of the colon. J Clin Gastroenterol 1997; 24:187–188.
255. Libson E, Bloom RA, Verstandig A, et al. Sigmoido-appendiceal fistula in diverticular disease. Diagn Imaging Clin Med 1984; 53:262–264.
256. Sonnenshein MA, Cone LA, Alexander RM. Diverticulitis with colovenous fistula and portal venous gas. J Clin Gastroenterol 1986; 8:195–198.
257. Goenka P, Iqbal M, Manalo G, Youngberg GA, Thomas E. Colo-cholecystic fistula: an unusual complication of colonic diverticular disease. Am J Gastroenterol 1999; 94:2558–2560.
258. Wassef R, Morgan S, Tasse D, et al. Les fistules dans la maladie diverticulaire du colon: Etude de 29 cas. Can J Surg 1983; 26:546–549.
259. Vasilevsky CA, Belliveau P, Trudel J, Stein BL, Gordon PH. Fistulas complicating diverticulitis. Int J Colorectal Dis 1998; 13:57–60.
260. Krompier A, Howard R, Macewen A, et al. Vesicocolonic fistulas in diverticulitis. J Urol 1976; 115:664–666.

261. Pheils MT. Vesico-colic fistula due to diverticulitis. Aust NZ J Surg 1972; 41:237–240.
262. Fazio VW, Church JM, Jagelman DG, et al. Colocutaneous fistulas complicating diverticulitis. Dis Colon Rectum 1987; 30:89–94.
263. Grissom R, Snyder TE. Colovaginal fistula secondary to diverticular disease. Dis Colon Rectum 1991; 34:1043–1049.
264. Cirocco WC, Priolo SR, Golub RW. Spontaneous ureterocolic fistula: a rare complication of colonic diverticular disease. Am Surg 1994; 60:832–835.
265. Amendola MA, Agha FP, Dent TL, et al. Detection of occult colovesical fistula by the Bourne Test. Am J Roentgenol 1984; 142:715–717.
266. Jarrett TW, Vaughan ED. Accuracy of computerized tomography in the diagnosis of colovesical fistula secondary to diverticular disease. J Urol 1995; 153:44–46.
267. Giordano P, Drew PJ, Taylor D, et al. Vaginography—investigation of choice for clinically suspected vaginal fistulas. Dis Colon Rectum 1996; 39:568–572.
268. Huettner PC, Flakier NJ, Welch WR. Colouterine fistula complicating diverticulitis: charcoal challenge test aids in diagnosis. Obstet Gynecol 1992; 80:550–552.
269. Amin M, Nallinger R, Polk HC. Conservative treatment of selected patients with colovesical fistula due to diverticulitis. Surg Gynecol Obstet 1984; 159:442–444.
270. Colonma JO, Kang J, Giuliano AE, Hiatt JR. One-stage repair of colovaginal fistula complicating acute diverticulitis. Am Surg 1990; 56:788–791.
271. Di Carlo A, Andtbacka RH, Shrier I, et al. The value of specialization—is there an outcome difference in the management of fistulas complicating diverticulitis. Dis Colon Rectum 2001; 44:1456–1463.
272. Baum S, Athanasoulis CA, Waltman AC, et al. Angiodysplasia of the right colon: a cause of gastrointestinal bleeding. Am J Roentgenol 1977; 129:789–794.
273. Casarella WJ, Galloway SJ, Taxin RN, et al. "Lower" gastrointestinal tract hemorrhage: new concepts based on arteriography. Am J Roentgenol 1974; 121:357–368.
274. Gennaro AR, Rosemond GP. Colonic diverticula and hemorrhage. Dis Colon Rectum 1973; 16:409–415.
275. Knutson OH, Wahlby L. Colonic haemorrhage in diverticular disease—diagnosis and treatment. Acta Chir Scand 1984; 150:259–264.
276. McGuire HH, Haynes BW. Massive hemorrhage from diverticulosis of the colon: guidelines for therapy based on bleeding patterns observed in fifty cases. Ann Surg 1972; 175:847–855.
277. Williams RA, Wilson SE. Current management of massive lower gastrointestinal bleeding. Int Surg 1980; 2:157–163.
278. Baer JW. Pathogenesis of bleeding colonic diverticulosis: new concepts. Crit Rev Diagn Imaging 1978; 11:1–20.
279. Jensen DM, Machicado GA, Jutabha R, Kovacs TO. Urgent colonoscopy for the diagnosis and treatment of severe diverticular hemorrhage. N Engl J Med 2000; 342:78–82.
280. Adams JT. The barium enema as treatment for massive diverticular bleeding. Dis Colon Rectum 1974; 17:439–441.
281. Markisz JA, Front D, Royal HD, et al. An evaluation of ^{99m}Tc-labelled red blood cell scintigraphy for the detection and localization of gastrointestinal bleeding sites. Gastroenterology 1982; 83:394–398.
282. Hunter JM, Pezim ME. Limited value of technetium-^{99m}-labelled red cell scintigraphy in localization of lower gastro-intestinal bleeding. Am J Surg 1990; 159:504–506.
283. Forde KA. Colonoscopy in acute rectal bleeding. Gastrointest Endosc 1981; 27:219–220.
284. Foutch PG. Diverticular bleeding: Are nonsteroidal anti-inflammatory drugs risk factors for hemorrhage and can colonoscopy predict outcome for patients? Am J Gastroenterol 1995; 90:1779–1784.
285. Buttenschoen K, Buttenschoen DC, Odermath R, Beger HG. Diverticular disease-associated hemorrhage in the elderly. Langenbecks Arch Surg 2001; 386:8–16.
286. Athanasoulis CA. Angiography in the management of patients with gastrointestinal bleeding. Adv Surg 1983; 16:1–23.
287. Goldberger LE, Bookstein JJ. Transcatheter embolization for treatment of diverticular hemorrhage. Radiology 1977; 122:613–617.
288. Matolo NM, Link DP. Selective embolization for control of gastrointestinal hemorrhage. Am J Surg 1979; 138:840–844.
289. Miller MD, Johnsrude IS, Jackson DC. Improved technique for transcatheter embolization of arteries. Am J Roentgenol 1978; 130:183–184.
290. Nahrwold DL. Diverticular bleeding. In: Fischer JE, ed. Common Problems in Gastrointestinal Surgery. Chicago: Year Book, 1989:363–370.
291. Parsa F, Gordon HE, Wilson SE. Bleeding diverticulosis of the colon: a review of 83 cases. Dis Colon Rectum 1975; 18:37–41.
292. Drapanas T, Pennington DG, Kappelman M, et al. Emergency subtotal colectomy: preferred approach to management of massive bleeding diverticular disease. Ann Surg 1973; 177:519–526.
293. Renzulli P, Maurer CA, Netzer P, Dinkel HP, Buchler MW. Subtotal colectomy with primary ileorectostomy is effective for unlocalized, diverticular hemorrhage. Langenbecks Arch Surg 2002; 387:67–71.
294. Gostout CJ. The role of endoscopy in managing acute lower gastrointestinal bleeding. NEJM 2000; 342:125–127.
295. Ramirez FC, Johnson DA, Zierer ST, et al. Successful endoscopic hemostasis of bleeding colonic diverticula with epinephrine ingestion. Gastrointest Endosc 1996; 43:167–170.
296. Kim YI, Marcon NE. Injection therapy for colonic diverticular bleeding. A case study. J Clin Gastroenterol 1993; 17:46–48.
297. Bloomfeld RS, Rockey DC, Shetzline MA. Endoscopic therapy of acute diverticular hemorrhage. Am J Gastroenterol 2001; 96:2367–2372.
298. Mauldin JL. Therapeutic use of colonoscopy in active diverticular bleeding. Gastrointest Endosc 1985; 31:290–291.
299. Simpson PW, Nguyen MH, Lim JK, Soetikno RM. Use of endoclips in the treatment of massive colonic diverticular bleeding. Gastrointest Endosc 2004; 59:433–437.
300. Farrell JJ, Graeme-Cook F, Kelsey PB. Treatment of bleeding colonic diverticula by endoscopic band ligation: an in-vivo and ex-vivo pilot study. Endoscopy 2003; 35:823–829.
301. Andress HJ, Mewes A, Lange V. Endoscopic hemostatis of a bleeding diverticulum of the sigma with fibrin sealant (letter). Endoscopy 1993; 25:193.
302. Matsuhashi N, Akahane M, Nakajima A. Barium impaction therapy for refractory colonic diverticular bleeding. AJR 2003; 180:490–492.
303. Koperna T, Kisser M, Reiner G, Schulz F. Diagnosis and treatment of bleeding colonic diverticula. Hepatogastroenterology 2001; 48:702–705.
304. Teague RH, Thornton JR, Manning AP, et al. Colonoscopy for investigation of unexplained rectal bleeding. Lancet 1978; 1:1350–1351.
305. Jackson BR. The diagnosis of colonic obstruction. Dis Colon Rectum 1982; 25:603–609.
306. Waxman BP, Cavanagh LL, Nayman J. Suppurative pylephlebitis and multiple hepatic abscesses with silent colonic diverticulitis. Med J Aust 1979; 2:376–378.
307. Lin C. Suppurative pylephlebitis and liver abscess complicating chronic diverticulitis. Mt Sinai J Med 1973; 40:48–55.
308. Liebert CW. Hepatic abscess resulting from asymptomatic diverticulitis of the sigmoid colon. South Med J 1981; 74:71–73.
309. Wallack MK, Brown AS, Austrian R, et al. Pyogenic liver abscesses secondary to asymptomatic sigmoid diverticulitis. Ann Surg 1976; 184:241–243.
310. Perez-Cruet MJ, Grable E, Dropkin MS, et al. Pylephlebitis associated with diverticulitis. South Med J 1993; 86:578–580.
311. Cambria RP, Margolies MN. Hepatic portal venous gas in diverticulitis. Survival in steroid-treated patient. Arch Surg 1982; 117:834–835.
312. Jensen JA, Tsang D, Minnis JF, et al. Pneumopylephlebitis and intramesocolic diverticular perforation. Am J Surg 1985; 150:284–287.
313. Sywak M, Romano C, Raber E, Pasieka JL. Septic thrombophlebitis of the inferior mesenteric vein from sigmoid diverticulitis. J Am Coll Surg 2003; 196:326–327.
314. Draghetti MJ, Salvo AF. Gas in the mesenteric veins as a nonfatal complication of diverticulitis: report of a case. Dis Colon Rectum 1999; 42:1497–1498.
315. Ney C, Cruz FS, Carvajal S, et al. Ureteral involvement secondary to diverticulitis of the colon. Surg Gynecol Obstet 1986; 163:215–218.
316. Siminovitch JMP, Fazio VW. Obstructive uropathy secondary to sigmoid diverticulitis. Dis Colon Rectum 1980; 23:504–507.
317. Lipsit ER, Lewicki AM. Subcutaneous emphysema of the abdominal wall from diverticulitis with necrotizing fasciitis. Gastrointest Radiol 1979; 4:89–92.
318. Cappell MS, Marks M. Acute colonic diverticular perforation presenting as left ear pain and facial swelling due to cervical subcutaneous emphysema in a patient administered corticosteroids. Am J Gastroenterol 1992; 87:899–902.
319. Harrison BJ, Ellis H. Perforated sigmoid diverticulum with necrotizing fasciitis of the abdominal wall. J R Soc Med 1981; 74:625–626.
320. Kurgansky D, Foxwell MM. Pyoderma gangrenosum as a cutaneous/manifestation of diverticular disease. South Med J 1993; 86:581–584.
321. Haiart DC, Stevenson P, Hartley RC. Leg pain: an uncommon presentation of perforated diverticular disease. J R Coll Surg Edinb 1989; 34:17–20.
322. Terry JH. Unusual cases of perforated diverticulitis of the colon. J Fla Med Assoc 1990; 77:814–816.
323. Chankowsky J, Dupuis P, Gordon PH. Sigmoid diverticulitis presenting as a lower extremity abscess: report of a case. Dis Colon Rectum 2001; 44: 1711–1713.
324. Mendeloff AJ, Everhart JE. Diverticular Disease of the Colon. Pub. No. 94–1447. Bethesda, MD: US Department of Health and Human Services, National Institutes of Health, 1994:553–565.
325. Smirniotis V, Tsoutsos D, Fotopoulos A, et al. Perforated diverticulitis: a surgical dilemma. Int Surg 1991; 76:44–47.
326. Stefansson T, Pahhnan L, Ekbom A, et al. Surgery in acute diverticulitis, a retrospective population based study. 130 patients operated in the University Hospital in Uppsala Sweden, 1969–1989. Acta Univ Uppsala 1994.
327. Sardi A, Gokli A, Singer JA. Diverticular disease of the cecum and ascending colon. A review of 881 cases. Am Surg 1987; 53:41–45.
328. Fischer MG, Farkas AM. Diverticulitis of the cecum and ascending colon. Dis Colon Rectum 1984; 27:454–458.
329. Lo CY, Chu KN. Acute diverticulitis of the right colon. Am J Surg 1996; 171:244–246.
330. Tan EC, Tung KH, Tan L, et al. Diverticulitis of cecum and ascending colon in Singapore. J R Coll Surg Edinb 1984; 29:373–376.
331. Lee YS. Diverticular disease of the large bowel in Singapore. An autopsy survey. Dis Colon Rectum 1986; 29:330–335.

332. Lin OS, Soon MS, Wu SS, Chen YY, Hwang KL, Triadafilopoulos G. Dietary habits and right-sided colonic diverticulosis. Dis Colon Rectum 2000; 43:1412–1418.
333. Miura S, Kodaira S, Shatari T, Nishioka M, Hosoda Y, Hisa TK. Recent trends in diverticulosis of the right colon in Japan: retrospective review in a regional hospital. Dis Colon Rectum 2000; 43:1383–1389.
334. Markham NI, Li AKC. Diverticulitis of the right colon—experience from Hong Kong. Gut 1992; 33:547–549.
335. Murayama N, Baba S, Susumm K, et al. An aetiological study of diverticulosis of the right colon. Aust NZ J Surg 1981; 51:420–425.
336. Sugihara K, Muto T, Morioka Y. Motility study in right-sided diverticular disease of the colon. Gut 1983; 24:1130–1134.
337. Langdon A. Solitary diverticulitis of the right colon. Can J Surg 1982; 25: 579–581.
338. Graham SM, Ballantyne GH. Cecal diverticulitis. Review of the American experience. Dis Colon Rectum 1987; 30:821–826.
339. McFee AS, Sutton PG, Ramos R. Diverticulitis of the right colon. Dis Colon Rectum 1982; 25:254–256.
340. Pieterse AS, Rowland R, Miliauskas JR, et al. Right-sided diverticular disease of the colon: a morphological analysis of 16 cases. Aust NZ J Surg 1986; 56:471–475.
341. Wada M, Kikuchi Y, Doy M. Uncomplicated acute diverticulitis of the cecum and ascending colon: sonographic findings in 18 patients. AJR 1990; 155:283–287.
342. Crist DW, Fishman EK, Scatarige JC, et al. Acute diverticulitis of the cecum and ascending colon diagnosed by computed tomography. Surg Gynecol Obstet 1988; 166:99–102.
343. Birnbaum BA, Balthazar EJ. CT of appendicitis and diverticulitis. Radiol Clin North Am 1994; 32:885–898.
344. Chou YH, Chiou HJ, Tiu CM, et al. Sonography of acute right side colonic diverticulitis. Am J Surg 2001; 181:122–127.
345. Cobben LP, Groot I, Blickman JG, Puylaert JB. Right colonic diverticulitis: MR appearance. Abdom Imaging 2003; 28:794–798.
346. Schuler JG, Bayley J. Diverticulitis of the cecum. Surg Gynecol Obstet 1983; 156:743–748.
347. Mariani G, Tedoli M, Dina R, et al. Solitary diverticulum of the cecum and right colon: report of six cases. Dis Colon Rectum 1987; 30:626–629.
348. Ngoi SS, Chia J, Goh MY, Sim E, Rauff A. Surgical management of right colon diverticulitis. Dis Colon Rectum 1992; 35:799–802.
349. Papaziogas B, Makris J, Koutelidakis I, Paraskevas G, Oikonomou B, Atmatzidis K. Surgical management of cecal diverticulitis: is diverticulectomy enough? Int J Colorectal Dis 2005; 20:24–27.
350. Fang JF, Chen RJ, Lin BC, Hsu YB, Kao JL, Chen MF. Aggressive resection is indicated for cecal diverticulitis. Am J Surg 2003; 185:135–140.
351. Komuta K, Yamanaka S, Okada K, et al. Toward therapeutic guidelines for patients with acute right colonic diverticulitis. Am J Surg 2004; 187: 233–237.
352. So JB, Kok K, Ngoi SS. Right-sided colonic diverticular disease as a source of lower gastrointestinal bleeding. Am Surg 1999; 65:299–302.
353. Kovalcik PJ, Surtarsic DL. Cecal diverticulitis. Am Surg 1981; 47: 72–73.
354. Gouge TH, Coppa GF, Eng K, et al. Management of diverticulitis of the ascending colon. Am J Surg 1983; 145:387–391.
355. Arrington P, Judd CS. Cecal diverticulitis. Am J Surg 1981; 142:56–59.
356. Harada RN, Whelan TJ. Surgical management of cecal diverticulitis. Am J Surg 1993; 166:666–671.
357. Law WL, Lo CY, Chu KW. Emergency surgery for colonic diverticulitis: differences between right-sided and left-sided lesions. Int J Colorectal Dis 2001; 16:280–284.
358. Jasper DR, Weinstock LB, Balfe DM, Heiken J, Lyss CA, Silvermintz SD. Transverse colon diverticulitis: successful nonoperative management in four patients. Report of four cases. Dis Colon Rectum 1999; 42:955–958.
359. Shperber Y, Halevy A, Oland J, Orda R. Perorated diverticulitis of the transverse colon. Dis Colon Rectum 1986; 29:466–468.
360. Wilkinson S. Acute-solitary diverticulitis of the transverse colon in a child: report of a case. Dis Colon Rectum 1988; 31:574–576.
361. Heimann T, Aufses AH Jr. Giant sigmoid diverticula. Dis Colon Rectum 1981; 24:468–470.
362. Maresca L, Maresca C, Erickson E. Giant sigmoid diverticulum: report of a case. Dis Colon Rectum 1981; 24:191–195.
363. McNutt R, Schmitt D, Schulte W. Giant colonic diverticula—three distinct entities. Report of a case. Dis Colon Rectum 1988; 31:624–628.
364. Muhletaler CA, Berger JL, Robinette CL Jr. Pathogenesis of giant colonic diverticula. Gastrointest Radiol 1981; 6:217–222.
365. Naber A, Sliutz AM, Foeitas H. Giant diverticulum of the sigmoid colon. Int J Colorectal Dis 1995; 10:169–172.
366. Van Vugt AB, Sleeboom C, Dekker LA, et al. Giant cysts in diverticular disease of the sigmoid colon. Neth J Surg 1985; 37:183–186.
367. Schmidt GT, Lennard-Jones JE, Morson BC, et al. Crohn's disease of the colon and its distinction from diverticulitis. Gut 1968; 9:7–16.
368. Myers MR, Alonso DR, Morson BC, et al. Pathogenesis of diverticulitis complicating granulomatous colitis. Gastroenterology 1978; 74:24–31.
369. Gledhill A, Dixon MF. Crohn's-like reaction in diverticular disease. Gut 1998; 42:392–395.
370. Burroughs SH, Bowrey DJ, Morris-Stiff GJ, Williams GT. Granulomatous inflammation in sigmoid diverticulitis: two diseases or one? Histopathology 1998; 33:349–353.
371. De Masi E, Bertolotti A, Fegiz GF. The importance of endoscopy in the diagnosis of neoplasms associated with diverticular disease of the colon and its effect on surgical treatment. Ital J Surg Sci 1984; 14:195–199.
372. Aldridge MC, Sim AJW. Colonoscopy findings in symptomatic patients without x-ray evidence of colonic neoplasms. Lancet 1986; 2:833–834.
373. Boulos PB, Cowin AP, Karamanolis DG, et al. Diverticula, neoplasia or both? Early detection of carcinoma in sigmoid diverticular disease. Ann Surg 1985; 202:607–609.
374. Stefansson T, Bergman A, Ekbom A, et al. Accuracy of double contrast barium enema and sigmoidoscopy in the detection of polyps in patients with diverticulosis. Acta Radiol 1994; 85:442–446.
375. Stavbrovsky M, Finkelstein T. Colonic cancer and associated diverticulitis. Int Surg 1979; 64:49–53.
376. Bacon HE, Tse GN, Herabat T. Co-existing carcinoma with peridiverticulitis of the colon. Dis Colon Rectum 1973; 16:500–503.
377. Krukowski ZH, Koruth NM, Matheson NA. Evolving practice in acute diverticulitis. Br J Surg 1985; 72:684–686.
378. Smallwood JA. Diverticular disease: emergency surgical problems. Hosp Update 1982; 8:1554–1561.
379. Stefansson T, Ekbom A, Sparen P, Pahlman L. Increased risk of left sided colon cancer in patients with diverticular disease. Gut 1993; 34:499–502.
380. Stefansson T, Ekbom A, Sparen P, Pahlman L. Association between sigmoid diverticulitis and left-sided colon cancer: a nested, population-based, case control study. Scand Gastroenterol 2004; 39:743–747.
381. Kieff BJ, Eckert GJ, Imperiale TF. Is diverticulosis associated with colorectal neoplasia? A cross-sectional colonoscopic study. Am J Gastroenterol 2004; 99:2007–2011.
382. Morini S, Hassan C, Zullo A, et al. Diverticular disease as a risk factor for sigmoid colon adenomas. Dig Liver Dis 2002; 34:635–639.
383. Burkitt DP, Walker ARP. Saint's triad. Confirmation and explanation. South Afr Med J 1976; 50:2136–2138.
384. Alba S, Nascimbeni R, Di Betta E, Villanacci V, Salerni B. Arthritis as a rare extra-intestinal manifestation of acute sigmoid diverticulitis. Dig Surg 2001; 18:233–234.
385. Perkins JD, Shield CF, Chang FC, et al. Acute diverticulitis. Comparison of treatment in immunocompromised and non-immunocompromised patients. Am J Surg 1984; 148:745–748.
386. Starnes HF, Lazarus JM, Vineyard G. Surgery for diverticulitis in renal failure. Dis Colon Rectum 1985; 28:827–831.
387. Tyau ES, Prystowsky JB, Joehl RJ, et al. Acute diverticulitis. A complicated problem in the immunocompromised patient. Arch Surg 1991; 126:855–859.

29 Volvulus of the Colon

Santhat Nivatvongs

INTRODUCTION

Volvulus refers to a torsion or twist of an organ on a pedicle. It can involve the stomach, spleen, gallbladder, small bowel, right colon, transverse colon, splenic flexure, or sigmoid colon (1). Volvulus of the large bowel results from the colon's twisting on its mesentery, producing symptoms either by narrowing of the bowel lumen, strangulation of the blood vessels, or both.

Widespread differences based on geographic and epidemiologic factors are seen in the distribution of volvulus. Overall in the United States, the sigmoid colon accounts for 43% to 71% of the cases of colonic volvulus. Most of the remaining cases involve the cecum and the right colon; volvulus of the transverse colon or splenic flexure is relatively rare, accounting for only 2% to 5% and 0% to 2%, respectively (2). In Olmstead County, Minnesota, during the period 1960 through 1980, the age-adjusted incidence of sigmoid volvulus and cecal volvulus was 1.67 and 1.20 per 100,000 population per year, respectively (3). In an unusual report from the high-altitude area of the Bolivian and Peruvian Andes at 13,000 feet above sea level, sigmoid volvulus accounted for 79% of all intestinal obstruction. The reason is not clear but may be related to the increased gas volume in the bowel because of high altitude (4).

SIGMOID VOLVULUS

INCIDENCE AND EPIDEMIOLOGY

In the United States sigmoid volvulus is an infrequent cause of intestinal obstruction and occurs much less often than carcinoma or diverticulitis as a cause of colonic obstruction. In an extensive review Ballantyne (5) found that only 3.4% of 4766 cases of intestinal obstruction and 9.6% of 1206 cases of colonic obstruction in the United States were caused by sigmoid volvulus. The highest reported worldwide incidence appeared in a study from northern Iran by Scott (6), who found that sigmoid volvulus was the cause of 85% of colonic obstructions. Johnson (7) reported 13 cases of sigmoid volvulus in a series of 24 bowel obstructions from Ethiopia (7). Increased frequency of sigmoid volvulus in Pakistan, India, Brazil, and Eastern Europe also has been reported (5). Although volvulus does occur with increased frequency in the Soviet Union (5), the previously reported data from the 1920s (8), in which more than 50% of cases of bowel obstruction were caused by volvulus, may not be accurate today because of changing epidemiologic and dietary factors.

Among reported cases of sigmoid volvulus from the United States, Ballantyne (5) has isolated the following epidemiologic factors:

1. *Sex.* Sigmoid volvulus is more common in men, occurring in 63.7% of men in a collected review of 571 patients. Bruusgaard (9) had previously attributed this finding to the wider female pelvis and more relaxed abdominal musculature, which afford an early volvulus a better chance of spontaneous reduction.
2. *Age.* Analysis of data from 43 studies reveals that the average age at which sigmoid volvulus occurs in English-speaking countries is 60 to 65 years, although it tends to occur 15 to 20 years earlier in other parts of the world. Other data suggest a trend toward earlier onset in English-speaking countries as well (10).
3. *Race.* Racial differences have been noted in many U.S. studies on sigmoid volvulus. Review of 221 patients in 10 series revealed that two-thirds 146 were black, one-third 74 were white, and one was Hispanic.
4. *Residence.* Review of nine U.S. studies revealed that 45.1% of 244 patients were admitted to the hospital from another institution. Of all patients, 54.9% came from private homes, 32.4% from mental institutions, and 12.7% from nursing homes.

Typically, then, the sigmoid volvulus patient in the United States is male, black, elderly, and may be institutionalized. In other parts of the world the typical patient is also male but is younger and living at home, probably in a rural area.

■ ETIOLOGY

In order for it to twist on itself, the sigmoid colon must be long and floppy, with a narrow mesenteric root. It can be congenital or acquired, particularly after previous abdominal surgery causing scar at the root of the sigmoid mesentery.

The concept of the etiology of intestinal volvulus is based on the fact that bowel when distended becomes elongated. By direct measurement, the antimesenteric border of the bowel increased its length by 30% whereas the mesenteric border increased by only 10% (11). As the bowel distends, it rotates in response to the need to accommadate this disproportionate increase in the length of its antimesenteric border. Perry (11) created a model using thin latex rubber tubing gathered up on its "mesenteric" border by a stiffer adhesive rubber strip to limit the elongation of this border. A latex rubber sheet was used to produce a deep "mesentery" (Fig. 1). Inflation of the "bowel" produced a 180° volvulus (Fig. 2). The same result follows the inflation of an isolated segment of cadaver ileum in which the mesentery has been refashioned and sutured to make it deep with a narrow base (Fig. 3). An example of this concept in vivo can be observed. In Afghanistan, for example, during the feast of Ramadan, the incidence of this type of volvulus rises sharply from bloated intestine (12). "Red gut," a disease of sheep grazing alfalfa (lucerne), is thought to be the result of volvulus associated with bowel gas distention (13).

It becomes clear that in order to have a volvulus, the bowel has to be distended with air to float. Colon that is full of stool cannot float and twist but by its weight may twist on itself and is not a true volvulus. In fact, the gush-out of "stool" on reducing the sigmoid volvulus is an exudate from obstruction, not the loaded stool from constipation.

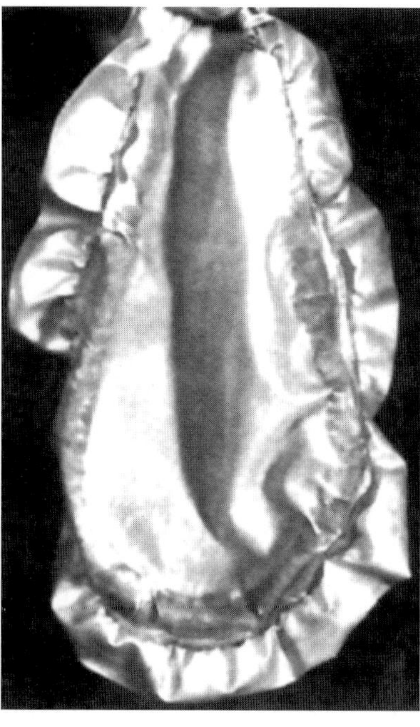

FIGURE 1 ■ Latex rubber model in flaccid state suspended from its base. *Source*: From Ref. 11.

A large number of precipitating or associated factors have been implicated in the genesis of sigmoid volvulus, including lead poisoning (14), vitamin B deficiency (14), adhesions (15), gout (15), Hirschsprung's disease (16), megacolon and diabetes (17), Parkinson's disease and other neurologic disorders (17), Chagas' disease (18), stroke (19), sprue (20), ischemic colitis (21), peptic ulcer (22), tuberculosis (22), cardiovascular disease (23), hypokalemia (24), pregnancy (25), and excessive enemas (26).

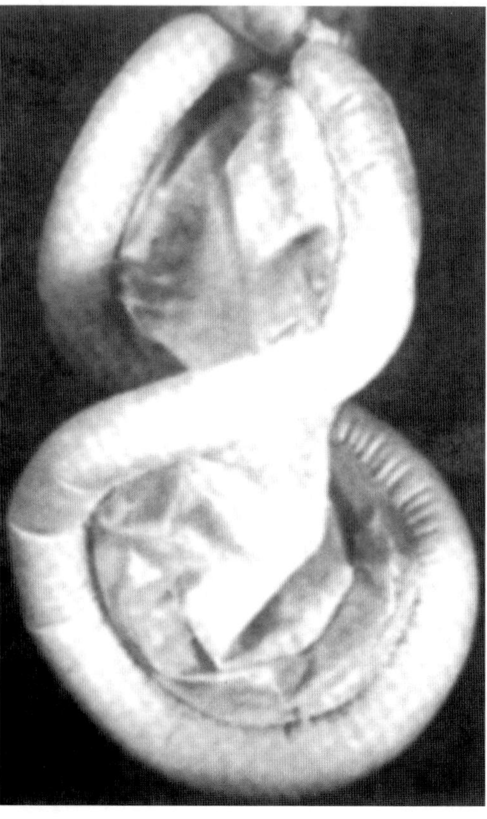

FIGURE 2 ■ The same model inflated with compressed air to 50 mm Hg. Note the rotation, which could be induced in either a clockwise or counterclockwise direction. *Source*: From Ref. 11.

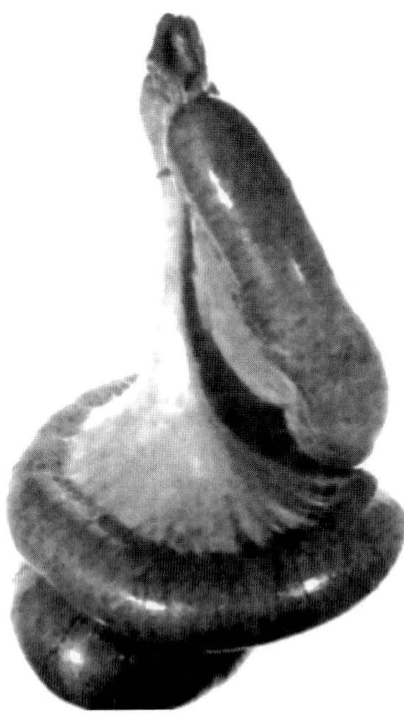

FIGURE 3 ■ The same model using cadaver ileum. Either clockwise or counterclockwise rotation could be induced on inflation. *Source*: From Ref. 11.

■ PATHOGENESIS

In a patient with a sigmoid volvulus, the twist of the sigmoid may be in a clockwise or counterclockwise direction, but it is usually counterclockwise around the axis of the mesocolon with varying degrees of rotation (Fig. 4). For significant obstruction to occur the torsion must be at least 180°. Torsion less than this is generally asymptomatic and can be considered physiologic.

The obstruction produced is a closed-loop type of mechanical obstruction that may be simple or strangulated. In the early stages of obstruction, peristalsis forces gas and fluid into the closed loop to remain trapped as the twist acts as a check valve to prevent release. Occasionally, some trapped air and gas are forced from the loop so that the diarrheal stools may occur.

With simple obstruction the bowel wall generally remains viable for a few days, largely because the sigmoid colon can tolerate more intraluminal pressure than other parts of the intestinal tract before signs of vascular compromise appear. Eventually strangulation will occur, with occlusion of the veins developing first, followed by occlusion of the arteries, mesocolic thrombosis, and infarction. Necrosis usually occurs first at the site of torsion but may include the entire loop.

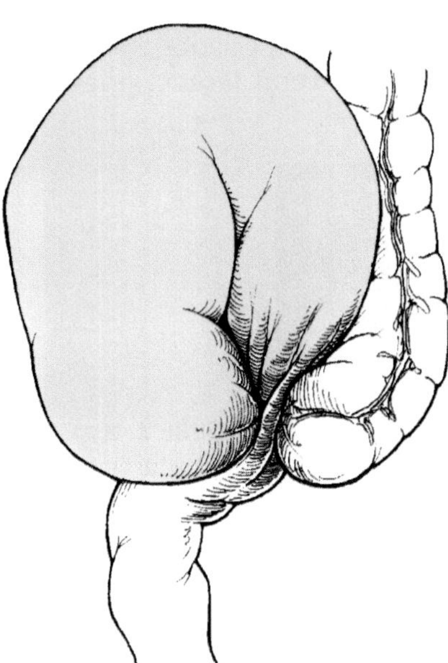

FIGURE 4 ■ Sigmoid volvulus twisted in counterclockwise direction.

In the acute fulminating variant of this disease, gangrene may occur much more rapidly because of a sudden, tight compression of the mesenteric vessels compounded by a rapid distention of the bowel lumen.

■ CLINICAL PRESENTATION

Although a chronic, painless variant of sigmoid volvulus has been described (27), the condition should be viewed as an acute disease. Hinshaw and Carter (28) have distinguished between two distinct clinical presentations of acute sigmoid volvulus depending on the rapidity of the twisting mesentery.

In the "acute fulminating type" the patient is generally younger, the onset of symptoms is sudden, and the course is rapid. Generally, there is little history of previous episodes, and symptoms include early vomiting, diffuse abdominal pain and tenderness, marked prostration, and the early appearance of gangrene. Distention may be minimal, and findings often are not distinctive. In its classic form the acute fulminating variety of sigmoid volvulus produces no distinctive diagnostic signs except for the clinical picture of an acute abdominal catastrophe; the actual diagnosis is made at celiotomy.

The second type, or "subacute progressive type," is the more common presentation. The patient is generally older, the onset more gradual, and the early course more benign. There is often a history of previous attacks and chronic constipation. Vomiting occurs late, pain is minimal, and signs of peritonitis are usually not present. Abdominal distention is generally extreme in this form, and radiographic findings are usually diagnostic.

■ DIAGNOSIS

In the acute fulminating type, the diagnosis of acute peritonitis is evident, immediate celiotomy is mandatory, and specific diagnostic measures are generally not indicated.

In the more common subacute progressive type, the diagnosis can be strongly suspected by the history and physical examination. In addition to a history of chronic constipation and possibly previous episodes, there is a recent history of gradual onset of cramping, lower abdominal pain, and progressive distention. Usually there is obstipation and absence of flatus, although there may be occasional diarrheal stools. Vomiting is uncommon as an early symptom. Marked abdominal distention and tympany are the most striking physical findings. Bowel sounds may be hyperactive or hypo-active but generally are not absent.

The diagnosis is usually confirmed by X-ray examination. A plain film of the abdomen classically shows a massively distended single loop of bowel on the right or left side of the abdomen with both ends in the pelvis and the bow near the diaphragm ("bent inner tube sign") (Fig. 5). Fluid levels may be seen in the sigmoid loop with little difference of levels in the upright position. The degree of distention of the proximal colon and small bowel on the right side of the abdomen varies. A Gastrografin enema

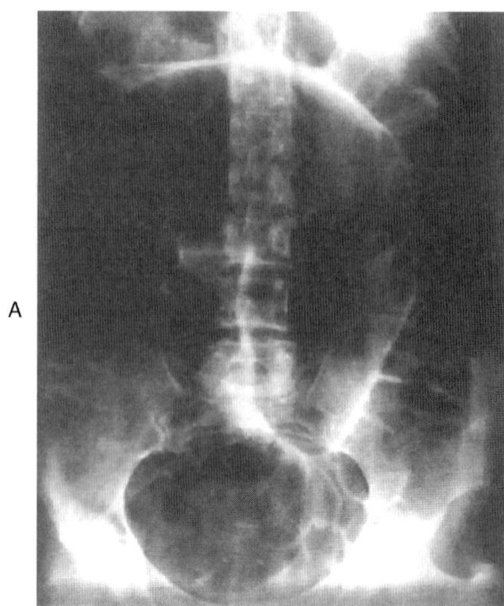

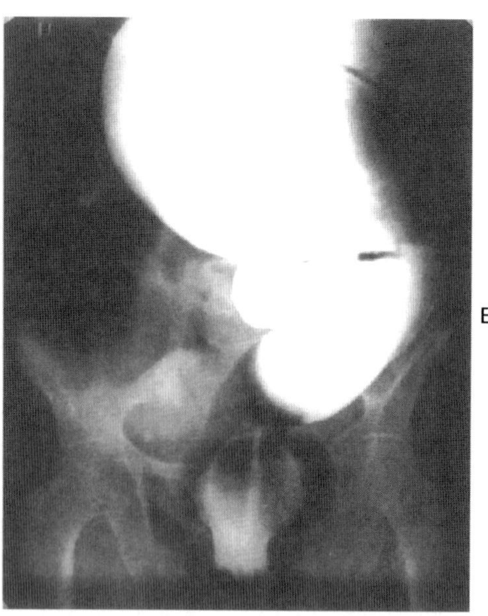

FIGURE 5 ■ Plain film (**A**) and contrast study (**B**) showing massively dilated sigmoid loop.

study reveals a pathognomonic finding of the Gastrografin column, ending sharply at the level of the site of torsion ("bird's beak" or "ace of spades" deformity) (Fig. 6). Burrell et al. (29) evaluated the plain abdominal radiographs in patients with sigmoid volvulus. Three signs, the apex of the loop under the left hemi-diaphragm, inferior convergence on the left, and the left flank overlap sign, are 100% specific as well as being highly sensitive. The sign that is least specific is a distended ahaustral sigmoid loop and an air:fluid ratio >2:1.

In approximately 30% to 40% of the cases, plain films can be equivocal. The transverse colon or small bowel distention can superimpose on the sigmoid loops; the two limbs may overlap, deviate laterally, or be oriented in an anteroposterior plane; the sigmoid can be fluid filled; or a dilated, redundant transverse colon or a closed-loop small bowel obstruction may mimic sigmoid volvulus (30,31). In these cases computed tomography (CT) may be helpful. The sigmoid afferent and efferent loops have a radial distribution around a low-attenuating adipose area (the twisted mesocolon) with a soft tissue center (the point of torsion). Engorged and stretched vessels converge toward the center. This feature is described as the "whirl sign" (Fig. 7). CT scan can also identify signs of strangulation (32).

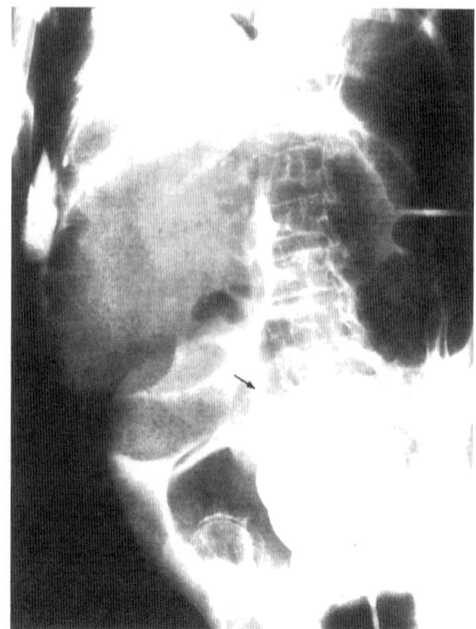

FIGURE 6 ■ "Bird's beak" deformity at the site of volvulus (*arrow*).

■ TREATMENT

Management of Nonstrangulated Sigmoid Volvulus

The goals of therapy in nonstrangulated sigmoid volvulus are directed at relief of acute torsion and prevention of recurrences. Ideally, the volvulus should be derotated and the colon decompressed. A few days later, after a full colonic preparation, sigmoid resection is performed. However, there are other lesser procedures to prevent recurrences such as tube sigmoid colostomy (33), mesosigmoidoplasty (34), and sigmoid colopexy (35).

Rigid Sigmoidoscopic Decompression

In 1947 Bruusgaard (9) described his experience with nonoperative reduction by sigmoidoscopy and passage of a rectal tube into the obstructed loop. The procedure was performed on 136 cases and was successful 123 times for a 90% success rate; four deaths occurred, with a mortality rate of 2.9%.

In the 1950s and 1960s greater experience was gained with the nonoperative method. Several larger series with

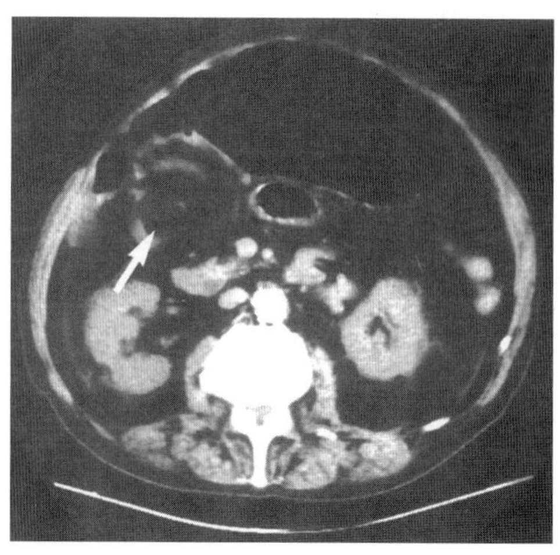

FIGURE 7 ■ A typical "whirl sign" of cecal volvulus (*arrow*). *Source*: Courtesy Richard Devine, M.D., Mayo Clinic, Rochester, Minnesota, U.S.A.

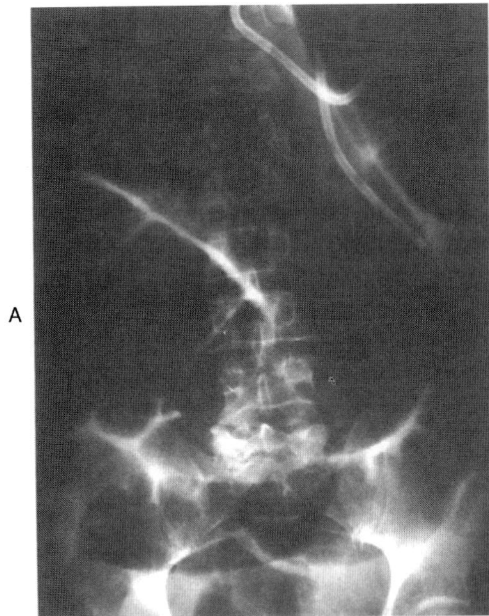

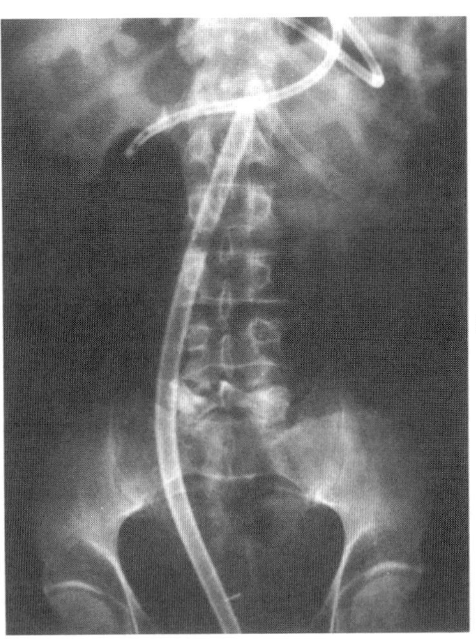

FIGURE 8 ■ (**A**) Abdominal film of patient with sigmoid volvulus. (**B**) Abdominal film of same patient after sigmoidoscopic decompression with a rectal tube in place.

equally impressive results were reported. Drapanas and Stewart (36) reported successful decompression with rectal intubation in 82 of 98 cases (84% success) with a 1.2% mortality rate; Wuepper et al. (19) were successful with this method in 44 of 54 cases, and had a mortality rate of 5.5%; and Shepherd (37) was successful in 78 of 89 cases, with a 3.4% mortality rate. In addition, in 1973 Arnold and Nance (23) had a 77% success rate in 114 cases.

Comparative figures for survival with operative detorsion have consistently yielded higher mortality rates than nonoperative reduction. Hinshaw and Carter (28) reported a 22% mortality rate for operative detorsion in 18 patients. Shepherd (37) reported a 16% mortality rate for 49 patients, and Sutcliffe (38) reported two deaths in 19 patients (11% mortality rate). Habr-Gama et al. (18) and Sharpton and Cheek (39) have reported mortality rates as low as 5% and 8%, respectively, and Gulati et al. (40) have reported a 35% mortality rate for 34 patients.

Nonoperative decompression thus has become the preferred initial treatment for nonstrangulated sigmoid volvulus. This approach, however, should not be used in three situations: (i) when there are clinical signs of nonviable bowel, (ii) if a trial of sigmoidoscopy has failed to achieve immediate reduction, and (iii) when volvulus repeatedly recurs. In these situations it is safest to proceed with immediate celiotomy.

The technique of sigmoidoscopic decompression is as follows. Preparation of the patient for surgery is begun so that if the nonoperative technique fails, operative intervention will not be delayed. Preferably the patient is placed in the prone jackknife position because this position facilitates the decompression by allowing the colon to fall away. The lateral decubitus position is acceptable if the patient cannot tolerate the jackknife position. The rigid sigmoidoscope is carefully inserted until the site of torsion is seen, and the mucosa is inspected carefully for signs of ischemia or necrosis. If the mucosa appears intact, a soft, well-lubricated 40 to 60 cm rectal tube is passed gently beyond the site of torsion until there is an immediate return of gas and stool from the obstructed loop. The rectal tube can be passed through the sigmoidoscope or along the side of the sigmoidoscope. The tube is then secured to the perianal skin and is left in place for at least 48 hours (Fig. 8). Recent reports showed a wide range of success rates in sigmoidoscopic decompression between 38% and 100% (2,35,41–44). When decompression is unsuccesful, strangulation of the sigmoid volvulus must be suspected, or the volvulus is beyond reach of the sigmoidoscope. Flexible sigmoidoscopy and colonoscopy are now widely used and have largely replaced the rigid sigmoidoscope.

Colonoscopic and Flexible Sigmoidoscopic Decompression

Despite the fact that many failures of sigmoidoscopic decompression of a sigmoid volvulus are related to gangrenous changes at the site of torsion, a significant number of failures occur because the rigid 25 cm sigmoidoscope does not reach the site of obstruction.

In 1976, Ghazi et al. (45) presented the first case of colonoscopic decompression of sigmoid volvulus with the site of obstruction measured at 105 cm from the insertion of the colonoscope. Subsequent favorable reports with both the full-length colonoscope (46–48) and the flexible sigmoidoscope (49) have appeared. A review of 25 cases of sigmoid volvulus revealed that 24 of the cases were safely decompressed colonoscopically, with the only failure occurring when the colonoscope was deliberately withdrawn when cyanotic mucosa was/identified 80 cm from the anus (47). Renzulli et al. (50) reported a success rate of only 58% in a small series of 12 patients. In a review of 189 patients with sigmoid volvulus from Veterans Affairs hospitals, using endoscopy (rigid sigmoidoscopy, flexible sigmoidoscopy, or endoscopy), the success rate was 81% (51).

Colonoscopic and flexible sigmoidoscopic decompression differs from rigid sigmoidoscopic decompression in that the colonoscope itself is passed through the site of torsion, often with gentle air insufflation as the scope is passed beyond the obstruction. Some authors have attached an external suction device to the biopsy portion of the colonoscope to facilitate removal of liquid, stool, and debris from the unprepared colon (52). Others have attached to the colonoscope a jejunostomy-type tube that is left as a decompressing stent that can be passed as far proximally as the cecum (53). A rectal tube can be passed after the volvulus has been reduced by passing the tube alongside with the flexible scope in place or after it has been withdrawn.

The precautions taken for rigid sigmoidoscopic decompression also apply to colonoscopic and flexible sigmoidoscopic decompression. If reduction does not occur promptly, the procedure should be terminated in favor of surgery. The procedure should also be abandoned in the presence of bloody drainage or cyanotic mucosa.

Flexible endoscopy is a sensitive means of diagnosing both acute sigmoid volvulus and intermittent sigmoid volvulus. Twisting spirals of mucosa are seen if the volvulus is still present. Even if the volvulus has spontaneously reduced, the mucosa at the site of volvulus demonstrates discrete and localized signs of inflammation. In addition the vascular markings are obscured and the mucosal folds are thickened. There may also be some granularity or friability. These findings are limited only to short segments of approximately 4 to 5 cm at both the rectosigmoid and the descending sigmoid junctions (54).

Surgical Management

Although the mortality rate of sigmoidoscopic deflation without further treatment is relatively low, at 5% to 8%, most deaths are the result of coexisting disease rather than a direct result of the procedure itself or complications related to the procedure (55). The recurrence from sigmoidoscopic deflation alone is high, 40% to 70% (2,37,42). With this high recurrence, it is obvious that further management is desirable. The mortality of surgery for sigmoid volvulus depends on whether the colon is gangrenous, and on the severity of intercurrent disease. Elective colon resection for sigmoid volvulus is most efficient. When properly performed, recurrence should not occur, although this complication has been reported (37,44).

Most authors have emphasized the need for elective resection in all patients who had an episode of sigmoid volvulus, although some have reserved elective resection for selected lower-risk patients. Shepherd (37) reported on 74 elective resections performed five to eight days after conservative treatment, with a mortality rate of 2.8%. Even in patients who have been classified as higher risk, the elective mortality rate should be lower than the risk of death from complications of recurrent volvulus.

Sigmoid Colon Resection

For a nonstrangulated colon, sigmoid colon resection can be performed as an elective procedure a few days later, after a bowel preparation. If an urgent exploratory celiotomy is necessary, the left colon and rectum can be irrigated with providone–iodine via a rectal tube. The mortality rate for sigmoid colon resection with primary anastomosis has been reported to be between 0% and 12.5% (37,41,56–58). For gangrenous bowel, sigmoid resection with a colostomy and Hartmann's procedure is the safest, although some authors perform an anastomosis. The operative mortality is between 0% and 38% (37,41,56–59). Even without gangrenous colon, emergency sigmoid resection with primary anastomosis has a high anastomotic leak rate (60).

Much of the mortality associated with elective sigmoid resection after volvulus can be reduced by taking advantage of the unique anatomic features of the sigmoid in these patients. Because the sigmoid is long and freely movable, the mesosigmoid is also long, and the points of peritoneal fixation are close together, the redundant loop usually can be delivered out of the abdominal cavity through a limited incision (Fig. 9). The peritoneum is

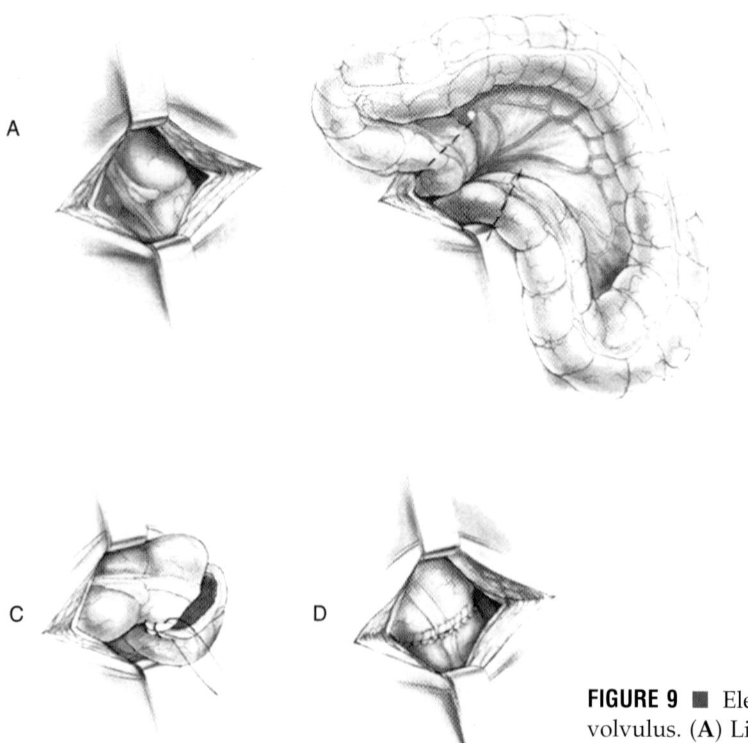

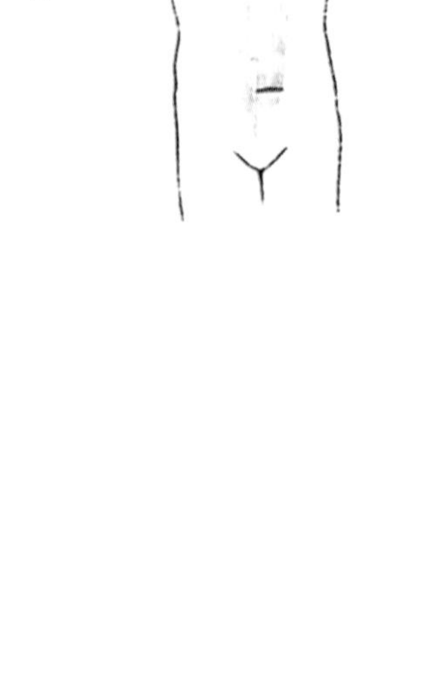

FIGURE 9 ■ Elective sigmoid resection after nonoperative decompression for volvulus. (**A**) Limited left lower quadrant incision. (**B**) Delivery of redundant sigmoid. (**C**) Anastomosis at level of abdominal wall after resection of redundant sigmoid. (**D**) Anastomotic segment dropped back into abdominal cavity.

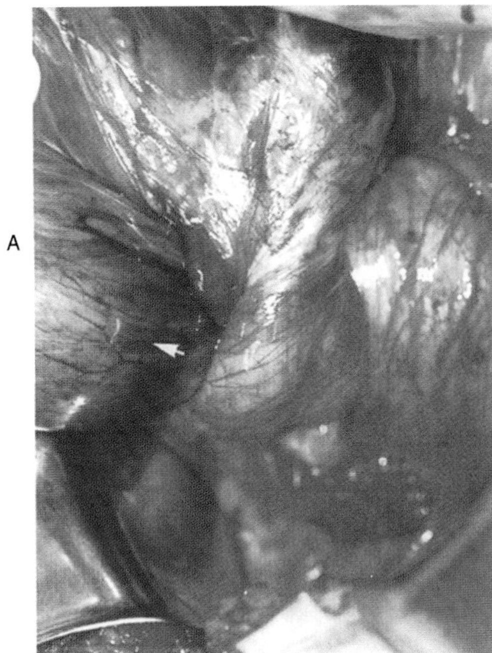

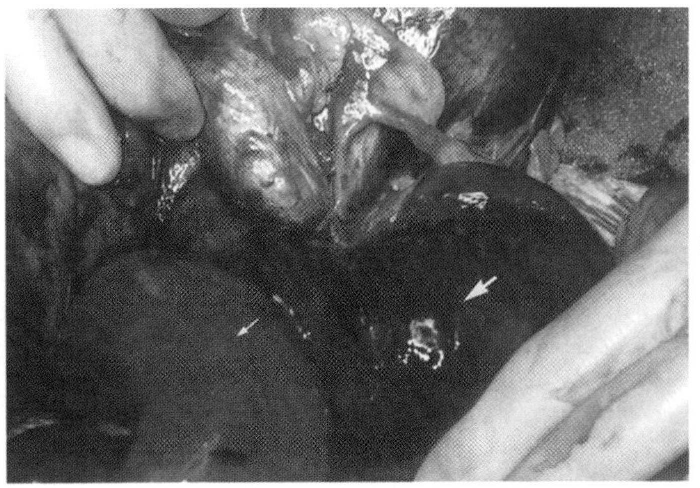

FIGURE 10 ■ Simultaneous sigmoid and cecal volvulus. (**A**) Sigmoid volvulus with gangrene (*arrow*). (**B**) Cecal volvulus with gangrene (*large arrow*). Note the inflamed terminal ileum (*small arrow*).

entered through a short transverse incision made in the left lower quadrant, dividing through the left rectus muscle. The redundant loop is delivered, the mesocolon is divided to free a proximal and a distal end, and the anastomosis is made on the surface of the abdomen. The bowel is then dropped back into the peritoneal cavity and the incision is closed. In elderly debilitated patients this procedure often can be performed with local anesthesia.

At operation, it is important to examine the entire abdomen to make certain that there is no volvulus at any other part. Simultaneous sigmoid and cecal volvulus is rare but has been reported (61). An example of this condition can be seen in Figure 10.

In the series reported by Grossmann et al. (51), 178 of 228 (78%) patients underwent a colostomy, with 44% considered to be urgent. Evidence of ischemia was present in 86 of 178 cases (48%), frank necrosis of the colon was observed in 59 of 178 cases (33%). Sigmoid resection was performed in 173 of 178 patients (97%): 107 of 173 patients (62%) had resection with colostomy; 66 of 173 patients (38%) had primary anastomosis; colostomy without sigmoid resection was performed in 2 of 178 patients (1%), and 3 of 178 patients (2%) underwent sigmoidopexy. There were no operative deaths. Twenty-five of 178 patients (14%) died within 30 days of surgery.

Nonresective Procedures

Even elective sigmoid colon resection has significant morbidity and mortality. In very ill patients a resection should be avoided, unless the bowel is gangrenous. Surgeons should know other effective but less radical procedures to prevent a recurrence.

Sigmoid Decompression and Colopexy

This is a unique procedure claimed to produce no recurrence and no death in 20 patients with nongangrenous sigmoid volvulus. The only complication was one wound infection (35). The author first deflated the sigmoid volvulus with an 18-gauge needle. With the collapsed sigmoid colon his success in sigmoidoscopic insertion of a rectal tube was 100%, and there was no incidence of stool leakage from the needle. Four to five days later, the patient was explored and a sigmoid colopexy performed.

The sigmoid colon is placed against the lateral and anterior abdominal wall at the left iliac fossa to determine the site of colopexy. Strips of Gore-Tex band are cut from a bifurcated vascular graft with the size and length suitable to encircling the colon and suturing to the abdominal wall without obstructing the bowel lumen. Usually six to eight strips are sutured at one end to the abdominal wall with interrupted 2–0 Prolene sutures. An arterial forceps is pushed through the mesocolon. The bands are then pulled through, wrapped around half the colonic circumference, and sutured with interrupted 2–0 Prolene to the abdominal wall (Fig. 11). Prolene or vicryl mesh is more practical.

This is a new technique that deserves attention. I believe decompression of the volvulus should be attempted with a rigid or a flexible sigmoidoscope first. If this is not successful, a percutaneous needle deflation should then be performed followed by placement of a rectal tube.

Mesosigmoidoplasty

The concept of this technique is to reduce the length of the mesosigmoid and broaden its attachment. It can be used in an elective or emergency situation but without gangrene. The sigmoid colon must be decompressed.

The peritoneum over the mesosigmoid is incised vertically in the midline starting from the base up to 2.5 cm from the mesenteric border of the sigmoid colon (Fig. 12). The flaps of peritoneum on each side are raised laterally. The flaps are then approximated transversely with continuous suture using synthetic absorbable sutures. The procedure is repeated over the other side of the meso-sigmoid.

Subrahmanyam (34) performed this technique in 126 patients (48 elective, 78 emergency). There was one death from aspiration pneumonia and two recurrences after two and six

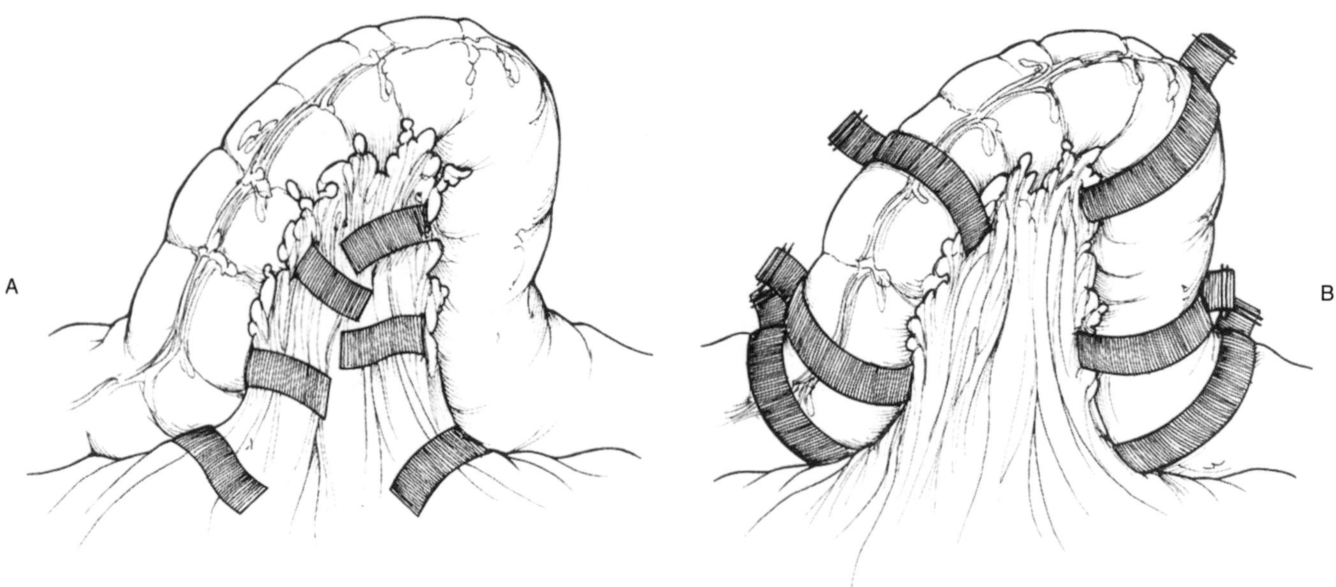

FIGURE 11 ■ (**A**) Strips of Gore-Tex band are sutured to the intra-abdominal wall and the loose ends are delivered through the sigmoid mesentery. (**B**) Gore-Tex bands sutured around the sigmoid colon.

months. The mean follow-up was 8.2 years. This technique may not be feasible in obese patients with fatty mesocolon.

Bach et al. (62) modified this technique by cutting the sigmoid mesentery in its full thickness longitudinally. The key to this modified technique is to preserve the first branch of the sigmoid vessel at the base of the mesentery, and the last vascular arcade near the colonic wall. Following the principles of mesosigmoidoplasty, the longitudinal slot of the mesosigmoid was sutured horizontally, using absorbable sutures on each aspect of the mesosigmoid (medial and lateral), taking only the peritoneal layer. Twelve patients were successfully performed. A short-term follow-up in eight patients from four to eight months showed no problems with recurrence, abdominal discomfort, or change in bowel habits.

Foley Catheter Sigmoidostomy

The aim of this technique is to fix the redundant sigmoid colon to the anterior abdominal wall. The Foley catheter is removed two weeks later.

Tanga (33) reported favorable results in 10 patients with a one-stage procedure consisting of detorsion and Foley catheter sigmoidostomy analogous to detorsion and cecostomy performed to treat cecal volvulus.

T-Fasteners Sigmoidopexy

This innovated technique was devised by Brown et al. (63) to endoscopically tag the stomach wall to the anterior abdominal wall for the percutaneous gastrostomy to prevent leaking around the tube. Gallagher et al. (64,65) applied this technique to fix the sigmoid colon to the anterior abdominal wall with the aid of colonoscopy, for sigmoid volvulus. The procedure is used exclusively for patients with sigmoid volvulus who are not candidates for general anesthetic.

The instruments consist of a T-fastener with cotton pledget, a washer to hold the pledget to the skin, a needle with slot to house the T-fastener, and a stylet for ejecting the fastener (Ross Laboratories, Columbus, Ohio, U.S.A.).

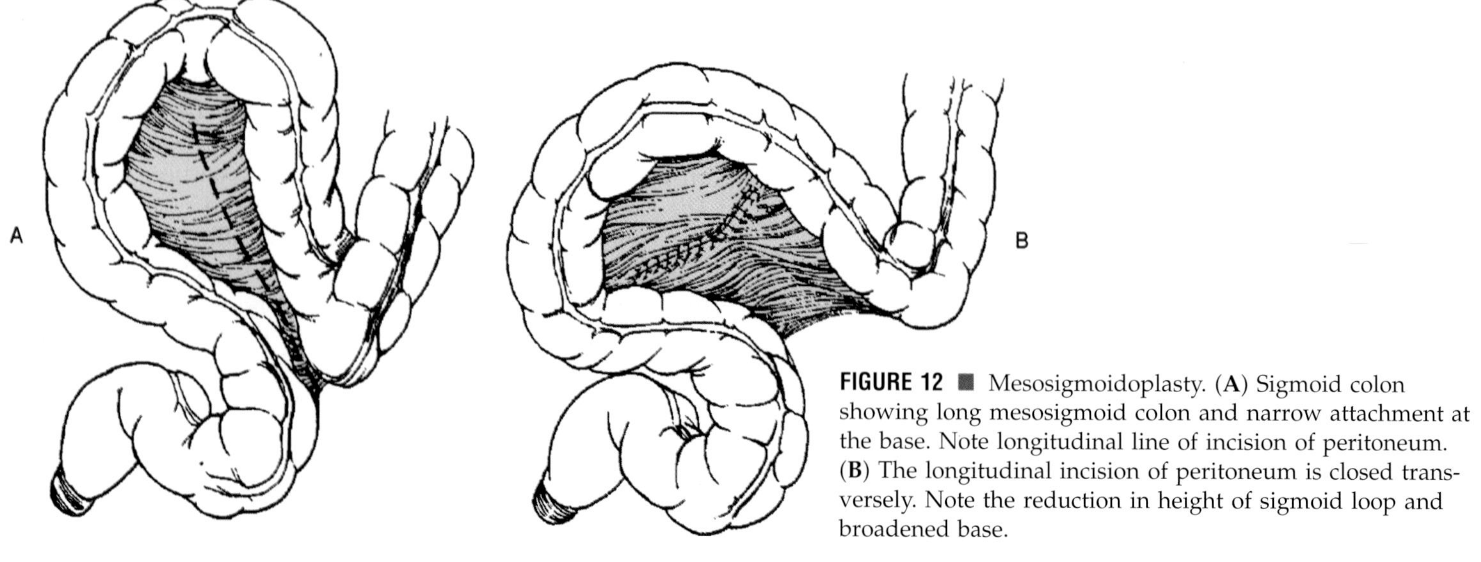

FIGURE 12 ■ Mesosigmoidoplasty. (**A**) Sigmoid colon showing long mesosigmoid colon and narrow attachment at the base. Note longitudinal line of incision of peritoneum. (**B**) The longitudinal incision of peritoneum is closed transversely. Note the reduction in height of sigmoid loop and broadened base.

The technique requires a successful detorsion and decompression of the viable sigmoid colon using a colonoscope. With the colonoscope as a guide, the T-fastener is deployed via the needle. The T-fastener then pulls the sigmoid colon up against the abdominal wall and is tightened on the skin over the cotton pledget (Fig. 13). Three to four T-fasteners are placed 4–5 cm apart, in a triangular disposition (65,66). These fasteners are cut at the skin level after 28 days (66). They will eventually pass through with stool. By this time, the sigmoid colon should adhere to the anterior abdominal wall. The procedure is performed under mild sedation.

Pinedo et al. (66) successfully performed this technique in two patients with a follow-up of 7 to 18 months. Gallagher et al. (65) reported six patients: one patient died of peritonitis, one patient developed a small bowel obstruction that resolved with conservative management, one patient had a recurrent volvulus of more proximal sigmoid colon at eight months—successfully treated with a repeated procedure.

Obviously, this appealing technique requires an improvement.

Comment: Nonresective procedures for sigmoid volvulus may not appear to be attractive but sometimes we have no choice because of the patient's extremely poor condition that cannot tolerate a major undertaking. Knowing other alternatives may be life-saving. A nonresective technique such as mesosigmoidopexy is valuable because it works well.

From time to time surgeons encounter a very old and frail nursing home patient with multiple recurrent sigmoid volvulus that could be successfully reduced, only to recur hours or days later. Such a case may benefit from using the T-fasteners. Although most surgeons are not familiar with this technique, endoscopists who have experience with the percutaneous gastroscopy may be able to help.

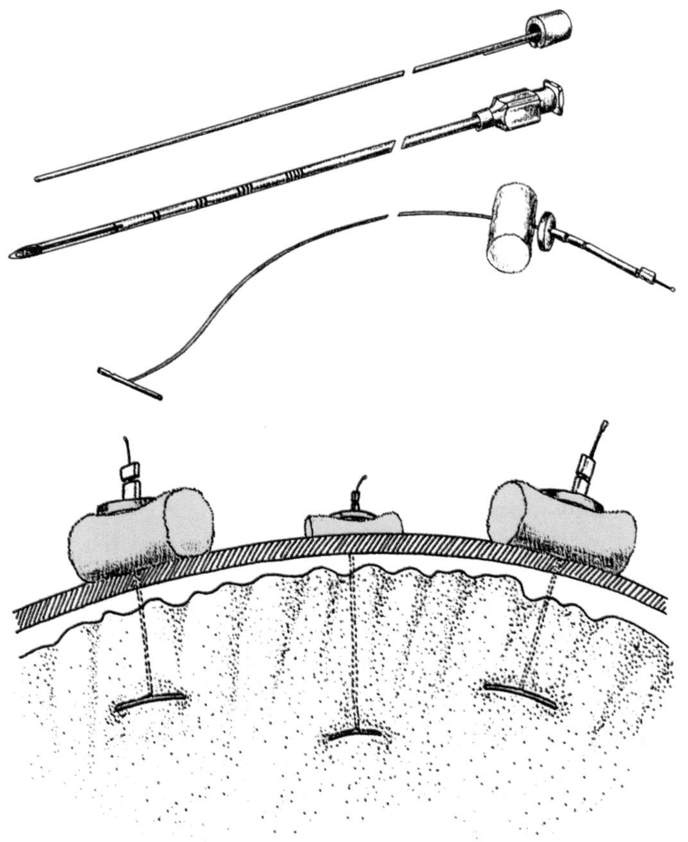

FIGURE 13 ■ T-fasteners. See details in text. *Source*: From Ref. 66.

ILEOSIGMOID KNOTTING

Ileosigmoid knotting is a unique entity in which a loop of ileum and the sigmoid colon wrap around each other. It was once called "double volvulus" but this term has been abandoned. It is rare in the Western world but is not uncommon in Africa, Asia, and the Middle East (67). Ileosigmoid knotting accounted for 8.8% of 773 cases of sigmoid volvulus and 1.7% of 4005 cases of all mechanical obstruction in the series from Turkey reported by Alver et al. (67). Other series dealing with this condition had a higher incidence, between 18% and 27% of all cases of volvulus.

Ironically, review of the world literature in 1932 showed that out of 161 cases, all but seven came from Russia or Scandinavia (37). At that time no cases had been reported from America or from Africa. The first case reports from the southern hemisphere appear to be from Sri Lanka in 1940 and India in 1953. From Africa, the first account was in 1952 from Uganda (37).

MECHANISM

Experience suggests that the knot is not initiated by the colon but by a hyperactive ileum that winds itself around the pedicle of a passive sigmoid loop. Bulk may be an important factor in stimulating small bowel activity. In the volvulus-belt region, it is customary to eat most of the day's food in one large evening meal. Several pounds of food are washed down with large quantities of liquid. The most common intestinal knotting occurs in the early hours of the morning (37). Alver et al. (67) summarize the different patterns of knotting (Fig. 14).

CLINICAL FEATURES

There are many differences between the clinical features of knotting and those of volvulus. Sigmoid volvulus is seen five times as often as intestinal knotting in males, whereas in females intestinal knotting is seen nearly twice as often as sigmoid volvulus in the series from Uganda (37). The age of patients with ileosigmoid knotting is also younger than patients with volvulus, 42 years versus 53 years. The absence of previous attacks is also striking, in contrast with sigmoid volvulus in which over 30% of the patients give a history of recurrent attacks of volvulus. Pain is the main complaint in every case. The onset is acute and occurs most commonly in the early hours of the morning, awakening the patient from sleep. Initial central colic gives way to constant agonizing generalized pain. Almost 75% of patients from Uganda arrive at the hospital on the day of onset compared with 25% of patients with volvulus of the sigmoid colon who arrive at the hospital in the first 24 hours (37).

Vomiting usually occurs at the onset of pain. In sigmoid volvulus, vomiting is a late feature and is often absent. Another striking feature of ileosigmoid knotting is that distention is not a common complaint by the patient, in contrast to sigmoid volvulus in which distention is obvious. The patient usually arrives at the hospital in shock,

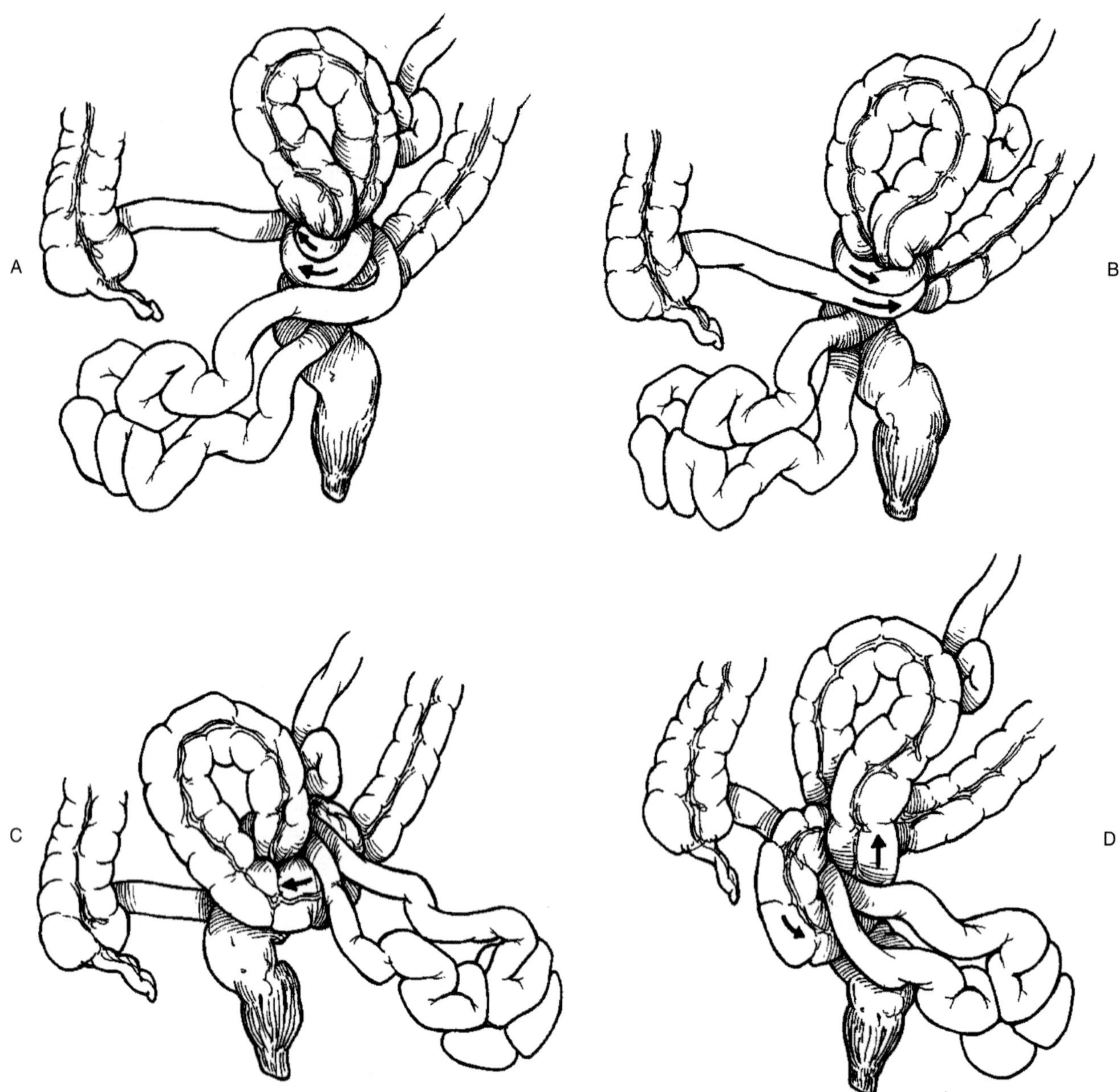

FIGURE 14 ■ Schematic diagrams showing the types of ileosigmoid knotting. The ileum (active component) wraps itself around the sigmoid colon (passive component) in a clockwise (**A**) and counterclockwise (**B**) direction. The sigmoid colon (active component) wraps itself around a loop of ileum (passive component) in a clockwise (**C**) and counterclockwise (**D**) direction.

with pale, cold, clammy skin. In the majority of cases, gangrene is present and a generalized peritonitis is found. It is usually abundantly obvious that a grave abdominal catastrophe has occurred. In regions where this condition is not uncommon, the diagnosis can be made with confidence from the clinical picture.

■ SURGICAL TREATMENT

Ileosigmoid knotting requires an emergency operation, because it cannot be reduced via an endoscope. The mortality of this condition is exceedingly high, 67% (67). With no other operation is death on the operating table seen so often. The abdominal cavity usually contains several liters of heavily bloodstained fluid. The bowel wall and the lumen are also full of blood, and there is little doubt that most deaths are due to hemorrhagic shock (37).

If the bowels are viable, the knot can be safely untied. After the bowel is decompressed, both the small bowel and the colon are resected with or without anastomosis, depending on the patient's condition and the condition of the bowel. The operating mortality for nongangrenous bowel is 28% in the series by Alver et al. (67).

Untying the knot in gangrenous bowel is difficult and time-consuming and carries the hazard of rupturing the gangrenous loop even after deflation. It also risks bacterial toxins and breakdown products escaping into the general circulation, causing irreversible septic shock (37). The gangrenous bowel should be removed en bloc with its mesentery. Anastomosis of the bowel should be avoided. The operative mortality in this situation is 40% to 50% (37,67,68).

Alver et al. (69) reported 12 cases of internal herniation concurrent with ileosigmoid knotting or sigmoid volvulus. Only cases of internal herniation through a congenital defect, mostly the mesentery, were included. The age of the patients ranged from 25 years to 72 years. Of note was the findings of gangrene of the small bowel or sigmoid colon in all of the patients at the time of the operation that required an en bloc resection. Postoperative morbidity and mortality were 33.3% in both.

SIGMOID VOLVULUS IN PREGNANCY

Sigmoid volvulus in pregnancy is a rare occurrence; there have been only 73 cases reported in a review by Alshawi (70). It is a potentially serious condition and should be recognized as a surgical emergency. Prompt management is necessary to minimize maternal and fetal morbidity and mortality (70). Alshawi (70) proposed that in the first trimester, a nonoperative procedure using colonoscopic detorsion and rectal tube decompression be recommended until the second trimester when sigmoid resection is performed for recurrent cases. In the third trimester, the treatment is nonoperative until fetal maturity and delivery when sigmoid resection can be performed.

CECAL VOLVULUS

INCIDENCE AND EPIDEMIOLOGY

Cecal volvulus occurs less commonly than sigmoid volvulus and accounts for approximately 1% of all cases of intestinal obstruction (71). Most reported cases have involved patients younger than those having sigmoid volvulus, with ages ranging from 30 to 70 years (72–74), although some authors have noted the occurrence of cecal volvulus in older patients as well (75,76). Most patients having recurrent or intermittent forms of cecal volvulus are younger, with 92% less than age 36 in one study (77). A clear predominance of women over men has been reported by most authors (75).

ETIOLOGY AND PATHOGENESIS

Unlike the acquired anatomic features of sigmoid volvulus, a distinct congenital anatomic variant is present in cecal volvulus patients, involving incomplete peritoneal fixation of the right colon and resulting in an abnormal ascending colon. Cadaver studies have reported that this variant is present in 10% to 22% or more of the population (78,79).

Given the anatomic prerequisite of a mobile cecum, a number of associated or precipitating factors have been implicated in the development of cecal volvulus. Among the frequently cited factors are congenital bands (78), adhesions from previous surgery (48,80), and trauma and manipulation from a recent abdominal operation (81). Coarse high-fiber diet have been implicated in the development of cecal volvulus in eastern Europe (78), although they have not been described as a factor elsewhere. Increased peristalsis caused by diarrhea or cathartics has been suggested as a predisposing factor (82), as has overeating (83). Distention related to obstruction has been implicated (84), as has pregnancy or space-occupying pelvic lesions (85). Rare congenital factors include nonrotation of the midgut (86) and torsion around a vitelline duct remnant (87). Clinically, the most important precipitating factor may be the presence of distal colonic obstruction. This obstruction reportedly can occur in as many as one-third (84) to one-half (88) of the cases of cecal volvulus.

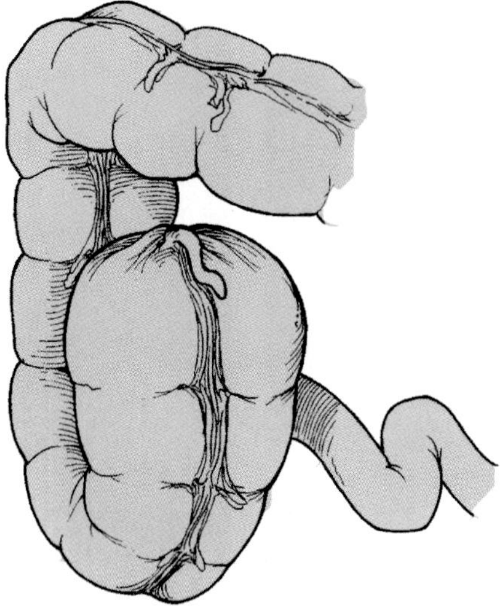

FIGURE 15 ■ Cecal bascule type of cecal volvulus.

A cecal volvulus tends to twist in a clockwise fashion, in contrast to the counterclockwise twist of a sigmoid volvulus. The resulting obstruction, however, is similarly of the closed loop and complete type.

A cecal bascule is an anterior and superior folding of the mobile cecum over the fixed distal ascending colon (Fig. 15). Although tension gangrene may develop, there is no major vessel obstruction. Some authors exclude this condition from being a cecal volvulus because it is not a true volvulus (75).

CLINICAL PRESENTATION

The clinical presentation of cecal volvulus may be divided into three major types: acute fulminating, acute obstructive, and intermittent or recurrent (73,77). In the acute fulminating type vascular obstruction occurs early, and the clinical picture is that of an acute surgical abdomen, with the need for immediate surgical intervention apparent. The acute obstructive type is more indolent and progressive, with findings related to the development of a closed loop cecal obstruction and distal small bowel obstruction. In this variant the patient generally presents with vague cramping, abdominal pain, nausea with or without vomiting, and slowly increasing abdominal distention. Abdominal X-ray films and a gastrografin enema study often are needed to confirm the diagnosis.

In the intermittent form the symptoms may vary from mild indigestion to severe cramping pains, but the symptoms last for only short periods and subside spontaneously, making the diagnosis difficult.

DIAGNOSIS

The diagnosis of cecal volvulus should be suspected from the history and usually can be confirmed by X-ray studies. Abdominal plain films may be confusing, because the lack of lateral fixation allows visualization of the mobile cecum anywhere in the abdomen. Closed loop filled with fluid may obscure in the image on the radiograph. Regardless of location, however, the most important single finding is the presence of a large dilated cecum. The loop often may be ovoid and midabdominal, or it may occupy the left upper quadrant, with its convex surface facing the left lower quadrant (due to its clockwise rotation). Distended loops

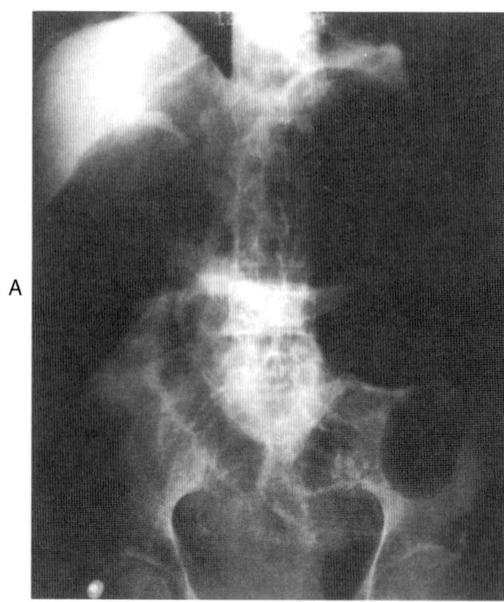

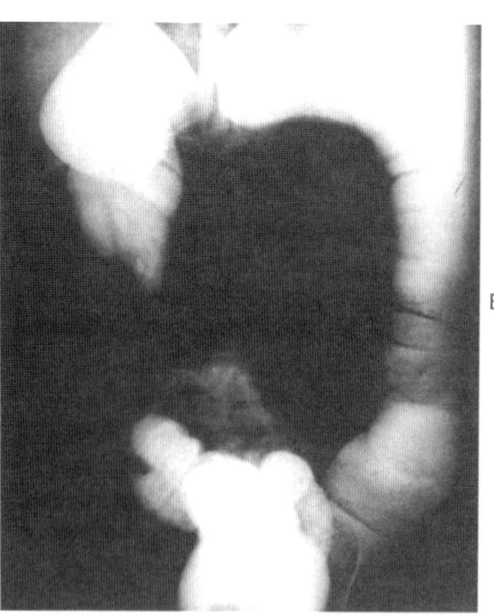

FIGURE 16 ■ (**A**) Abdominal film of patient with cecal volvulus showing dilated, abnormally positioned cecum with dilated distal small bowel loops. (**B**) Contrast study of same patient showing the site of torsion.

of small bowel are usually present (Fig. 16A). As in sigmoid volvulus, contrast studies are pathognomonic, with a characteristic "ace of spades" or "bird's beak" deformity seen at the site of torsion (Fig. 16B). CT of the abdomen reveals a typical "whirl sign" in the right abdomen with marked distention of the colon (Fig. 7).

CT abdomen gives the presence and location of the volvulus and gives the added benefit of allowing early identification of ischemia and perforation. Three-dimensional (3D) reconstruction may further improve diagnostic capabilities by allowing visualization of the entire small bowel in a single image (89).

■ TREATMENT

Nonoperative Reduction

Radiographic attempts at reduction of right-sided colonic volvulus are generally unsuccessful and potentially hazardous (90). Although success in colonoscopic decompression of cecal volvulus has been sporadically reported (47,71), the chance of success is slim. It only introduces more air into the colon and delays the operation. More appealing is the percutaneous decompression of the cecal volvulus (91). CT-guided percutaneous decompression of the acute massive dilatation of the cecum has been reported, using a No. 22 Chiba needle (92) or a trocar with insertion of a 12 Fr suprapubic cystostomy catheter (93). This approach should only be used as a last resort.

Operative Treatment

Most patients with cecal volvulus require urgent or emergency operation. Seventeen of 20 patients with cecal volvulus in the series reported by Geer et al. (94) required emergency operative intervention.

Little argument exists over the need for resectional therapy for gangrenous cecal volvulus or that the operation should consist of a right hemicolectomy. In most circumstances, an anastomosis should be avoided. The ileum is brought out as an ileostomy and the colon closed or brought out as mucous fistula. The mortality of ileocolectomy for gangrenous cecal volvulus is 22% to 40% (95,96).

Several options are available for the viable bowel. Ileocolectomy will cure the problem and eliminate a recurrence. However, the mortality rate is significant, 0% to 22% (95–98). The high mortality rate in some series has discouraged some surgeons from performing a resection. I believe the decision should be individualized. If the bowel is markedly edematous or does not have good color, an anastomosis should not be performed. The proximal end should be brought out as an ileostomy and the distal end closed. In the majority of cases, an ileocolectomy with a primary anastomosis can be performed.

Cecostomy is appealing in its simplicity and fixation to the abdominal wall to prevent a recurrence. It has become the procedure of choice for many surgeons (96,99). On the other hand, the high infection rate, the significant recurrence of 13% in one series, and the nuisance of postoperative care have made it not as popular as it should be.

Cecopexy has its advocates. The relatively high recurrent rate of 13% to 28.5% (75,95,100) has prompted some surgeons to perform a simultaneous cecopexy and tube

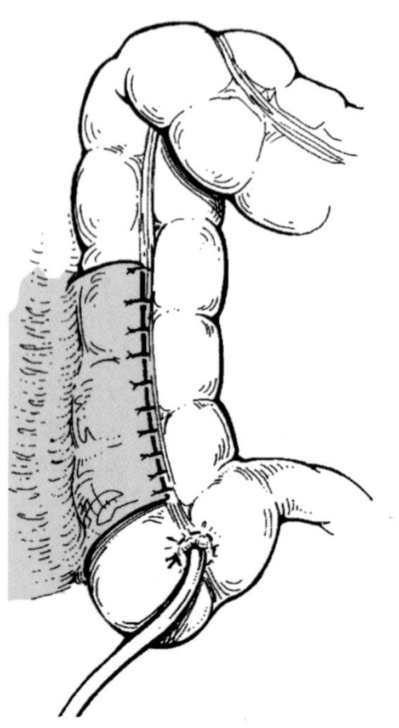

FIGURE 17 ■ Cecostomy and colopexy with a peritoneal flap.

cecostomy (75). Simple cecopexy involves suture of the peritoneum to the taenia of the right colon, using interrupted 3–0 or 4–0 nonabsorbable sutures. The peritoneal flap, if used, is made at the level of the ileocecal valve and is extended to cover the ascending colon up to but not including the hepatic flexure. After the flap has been tailored to cover half the circumference of the right colonic segment, it is sutured in place with interrupted nonabsorbable sutures (Fig. 17).

Detorsion of the cecal volvulus without any kind of colonic fixation is unreliable and should not be used alone.

Cecal volvulus in pregnancy is rare (101,102). Unlike sigmoid volvulus in which a nonsurgical correction with endoscopic detorsion is reasonably successful, most if not all cecal volvulus require surgical intervention. For a second and third trimester, a celiostomy can be performed under general anesthesia, and proceeds with an ileocolonic resection, or nonresection procedure as appropriate. Cecal volvulus in the first trimester will have to be done under spinal anesthesia. Unless it is gangrenous, a nonresective procedure such as a tube cecostomy or a colopexy seems to be a good option for the situation.

VOLVULUS OF TRANSVERSE COLON

■ INCIDENCE AND EPIDEMIOLOGY

Volvulus of the transverse colon is rare. Only 69 cases were reported in the literature before 1983 (103). A review of 306 cases of colonic volvulus from the 1960s revealed that only 4% of the cases involved the transverse colon (104). Age and sex distribution tend to parallel that for cecal volvulus rather than sigmoid volvulus, because patients with transverse colonic volvulus tend to be younger and more often are female (105,106).

■ ETIOLOGY AND PATHOGENESIS

A short transverse mesocolon and wide points of fixation of the hepatic and splenic flexures normally prevent the transverse colon from twisting. For transverse colonic volvulus to occur, certain congenital, physiologic, or mechanical factors must alter these relationships. Congenital factors include a freely movable right colon, a long meso-transverse colon, close proximity of fixation (106,107), or other visceral abnormalities, including the Chilaiditi syndrome (108,109) (hepatodiaphragmatic inter-position of the colon). Physiologic factors include chronic constipation from a variety of causes, high-fiber diet (106), and megacolon from Hirschsprung's disease (110) or scleroderma (111). Mechanical factors generally include some form of distal colonic obstruction, either from adhesion, neoplasm, stricture, or sigmoid volvulus (1,106,107).

■ CLINICAL PRESENTATION AND DIAGNOSIS

Eisenstat et al. (1) have described an acute fulminating and a subacute progressive variant of transverse colonic volvulus similar to types previously described for cecal volvulus and sigmoid volvulus. Patients with the acute type present with sudden severe pain, minimal distention, and rapid deterioration. The course of patients with the subacute type mimics the development of a distal small bowel obstruction, with gradual onset of pain, vomiting, and distention.

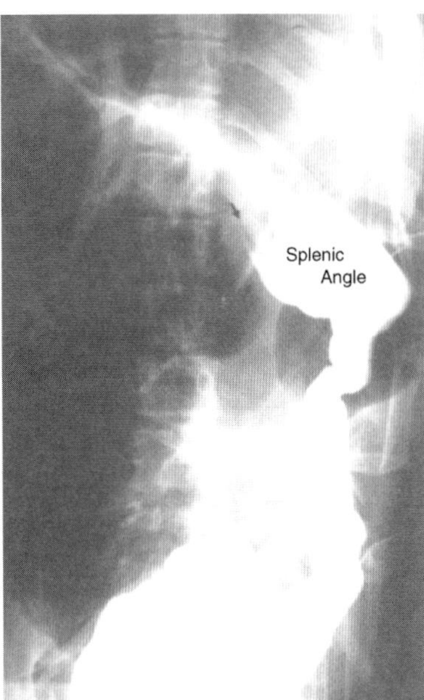

FIGURE 18 ■ Bird's beak deformity of transverse colonic volvulus. *Source*: Alain Ouimet, M.D., Montreal, Quebec.

Diagnosis is made on clinical grounds and is confirmed by radiographic evaluation of middle colonic obstruction, particularly the presence of distention of the proximal colon, with an empty distal bowel and two air-fluid levels seen in the upright and lateral decubitus positions (112). The two air-fluid levels represent proximal and distal transverse colonic limbs analogous to those seen with a sigmoid volvulus but distinct from the single air-fluid level seen with a cecal volvulus. Contrast studies will demonstrate the characteristic bird's beak deformity at the site of torsion (Fig. 18).

■ TREATMENT

Colonoscopic decompression and detorsion of transverse colonic volvulus has been reported (113,114) and may be the preferred initial procedure for the high-risk patient who has no evidence of nonviable bowel. The tendency for the volvulus to recur is documented by Anderson et al. (115), who found recurrent transverse colonic volvulus in three of four patients treated by operative detorsion, with or without simple colopexy. Many authors recommend resection as definitive treatment, either as a segmental colectomy or extended right hemicolectomy (1,105,106,113,114).

A number of colopexy procedures have been attempted previously, including suturing of the greater omentum or mesocolon to the anterior abdominal wall, right cecopexy with or without a peritoneal flap, and cecostomy (103). Mortensen and Hoffman (116) have described a parallel colopexy in which the redundant U-loop of transverse colon is sutured to the adjacent ascending and descending limbs of the colon with a continuous absorbable seromuscular suture (Fig. 19). This procedure may prove to be a useful alternative to resection in select cases. However, until more experience is available with this procedure or the other colopexy methods, segmental resection or extended right hemicolectomy should be considered the preferred treatment for nonstrangulated transverse colonic volvulus.

Cases involving gangrene or perforation should be managed by resection with colostomy and closure of the distal end or mucous fistula, or by extended right

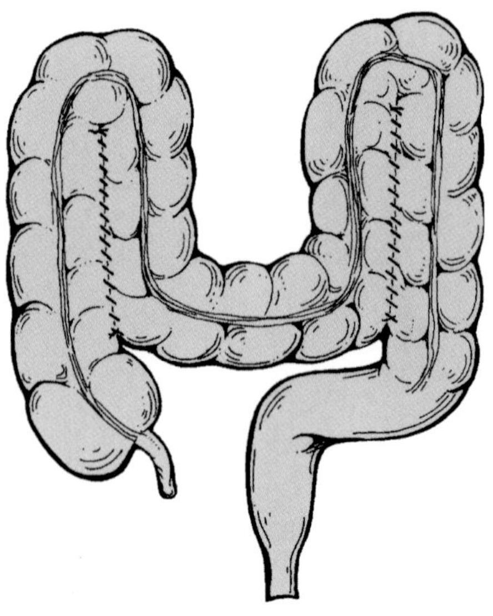

FIGURE 19 ■ Parallel colopexy. Redundant transverse colonic loop is sutured to the adjacent ascending and descending ends of the colon.

hemicolectomy and ileocolonic anastomosis. Mortality can be significant, as reported by Kerry and Ransom (104), who noted a 33% mortality rate among their cases of transverse colonic volvulus. Early diagnosis and aggressive therapy should dramatically lessen this figure.

SPLENIC FLEXURE VOLVULUS

INCIDENCE AND EPIDEMIOLOGY

Fewer than 25 cases of splenic flexure volvulus have been reported, including one case of "traveling volvulus," involving the sigmoid and splenic flexure (117). The average patient age among 22 reported cases was 50.5 years, and women outnumbered men by two to one (118,119).

ETIOLOGY, PATHOGENESIS, AND CLINICAL PRESENTATION

Splenic flexure volvulus normally is prevented by the limited mobility of this point of the colon because of the phrenocolic, gastrocolic, and splenocolic ligaments, along with the retroperitoneal position of the descending colon. For splenic flexure volvulus to occur, the normal anatomic arrangements must be altered, either by congenital deficiency or surgery, making the splenic flexure more mobile. Sixteen of 22 reported patients in a review by Naraynsingh and Raju (120) had had previous abdominal surgery. Congenital bands or adhesions also have been implicated in the etiology (119,120). Associated factors have included constipation and neuropsychiatric disorders (121). The clinical presentation of splenic flexure volvulus is similar to that seen with transverse colonic or cecal volvulus (Fig. 20).

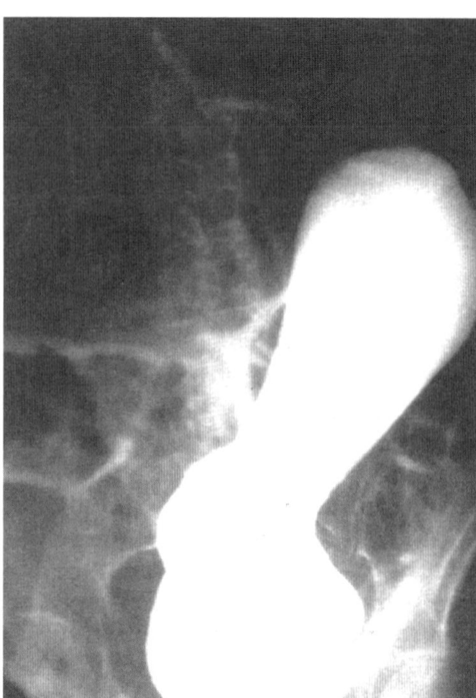

FIGURE 20 ■ Barium enema demonstrating obstruction of splenic flexure volvulus. *Source*: John Keyserlingk, M.D., Montreal, Quebec.

Radiographic diagnosis of a splenic flexure volvulus is suggested when the following are seen: (i) a markedly dilated, air-filled colon with an abrupt termination at the anatomic splenic flexure, (ii) two widely separated air-fluid levels, one in the transverse colon and the other in the cecum, (iii) an empty descending and sigmoid colon, and (iv) a characteristic bird's beak deformity at the anatomic splenic flexure indicated by contrast enema examination (122).

TREATMENT

Treatment is surgical and has consisted of either resection or detorsion with lysis of adhesions and/or fixation of the splenic flexure. One recurrence has been reported after simple colopexy (118). The only death occurred in an untreated patient. The low mortality rate may relate to the fact that strangulation of the splenic flexure occurs infrequently (117). Although experience with simple colopexy for sigmoid volvulus and transverse colonic volvulus suggests that recurrence may be a problem, the limited experience to date suggests that either resection or detorsion and fixation are acceptable alternative procedures (117,119,120).

REFERENCES

1. Eisenstat TE, Raneri AJ, Mason GR. Volvulus of the transverse colon. Am J Surg 1977; 134:396–399.
2. Brothers TE, Strodel WE, Ekhauser FE. Endoscopy in colonic volvulus. Ann Surg 1977; 206:1–4.
3. Ballantyne GH. Volvulus of the large intestine [Expert Commentary]. Perspect Colon Rectal Surg 1990; 3:56–60.
4. Asbun HJ, Castellanos H, Balderrama B, et al. Sigmoid volvulus in the high altitude of the Andes. Review of 230 cases. Dis Colon Rectum 1982; 35:350–353.
5. Ballantyne GH. Review of sigmoid volvulus. Clinical patterns and pathogenesis. Dis Colon Rectum 1982; 25:823–830.
6. Scott GW. Volvulus of the sigmoid flexure. Dis Colon Rectum 1965; 8:30–34.
7. Johnson LP. Recent experience with sigmoid volvulus in Ethiopia; its incidence and management by primary resection. Ethiop Med J 1965; 4:197–204.
8. Perlmann J. Klinische Beiträge zur Pathologie und chirurgischen Behandlung des Darmverschlusses. Arch Klin Chir 1925; 137:245–264.
9. Bruusgaard C. Volvulus of the sigmoid colon and its treatment. Surgery 1947; 22:466–478.
10. Northeast ADR, Dennison AR, Lee EG. Sigmoid volvulus: New thoughts on the epidemiology. Dis Colon Rectum 1984; 27:260–261.
11. Perry EG. Intestinal volvulus: A new concept. Aust N Z J Surg 1983; 53: 483–486.
12. Duke JH, Yar MS. Primary small bowel volvulus. Arch Surg 1967; 112:685–678.
13. Gumbrell RC, Jagusch KT. "Red gut" syndrome in lambs grazing lucerne. N Z Med J 1973; 21:178–179.
14. Berger KE, Lundberg EZ. Intestinal volvulus precipitated by lead poisoning. JAMA 1951; 147:13–16.
15. String ST, DeCosse JJ. Sigmoid volvulus: an examination of the mortality. Am J Surg 1971; 121:293–297.
16. Shepherd JJ. The epidemiology and clinical presentation of sigmoid volvulus. Br J Surg 1969; 56:353–359.

17. Berenyl MR, Schwartz GS. Megasigmoid syndrome in diabetes and neurologic disease; Review of 13 cases. Am J Gastroenterol 1967; 47:310–320.
18. Habr-Gama A, Haddad J, Simonsen O, et al. Volvulus of the sigmoid colon in Brazil: A report of 230 cases. Dis Colon Rectum 1976; 19:314–320.
19. Wuepper KD, Otteman MG, Stahlgren LH. An appraisal of the operative and non-operative treatment of sigmoid volvulus. Surg Gynecol Obstet 1966; 122: 84–88.
20. Glazer IM, Aldersberg D. Volvulus of the colon: a complication of sprue. Gastroenterology 1953; 24:159–172.
21. Meyers MS, Ghahremani GG, Govone AF. Ischemic colitis associated with sigmoid volvulus: new observations. AJR 1977; 128:591–595.
22. Friedlaender E. The surgical treatment of acute volvulus of the megasigmoid by primary resection. J Int Coll Surg 1961; 35:296–301.
23. Arnold GJ, Nance FC. Volvulus of the sigmoid colon. Ann Surg 1973; 177: 527–531.
24. Forward AD. Hypokalemia associated with sigmoid volvulus. Surg Gynecol Obstet 1966; 123:35–42.
25. Lord SA, Boswell WC, Hungerpiller JC. Sigmoid volvulus in pregnancy. Am Surg 1995; 62:380–382.
26. Schagen van Leeuwen JH. Sigmoid volvulus in a West African population. Dis Colon Rectum 1985; 28:712–716.
27. Verheyden CN, Newcomer AD, Beart RW Jr. Painless chronic sigmoid volvulus. JAMA 1978; 240:464–465.
28. Hinshaw DB, Carter R. Surgical management of acute volvulus of the sigmoid colon. A study of 55 cases. Ann Surg 1957; 146:52–60.
29. Burrell HC, Baker DM, Wardrop P, Evans AJ. Significant plain film findings in sigmoid volvulus. Clin Radiol 1993; 49:317–319.
30. Ott DJ, Chen MYM. Specific acute colonic disorders. Radiol Clin North Am 1994; 32:871–874.
31. Young WS, Engelbrecht HE, Stacker A. Plain film analysis in sigmoid volvulus. Clin Radiol 1978; 29:553–560.
32. Catalano O. Computed tomographic appearance of sigmoid volvulus. Abdom Imag 1996; 21:314–317.
33. Tanga MR. Sigmoid volvulus: a new concept in treatment. Am J Surg 1974; 128:119–121.
34. Subrahmanyam M. Mesosigmoplasty as definitive operation for sigmoid volvulus. Br J Surg 1991; 79:683–684.
35. Salim AS. Management of acute volvulus of the sigmoid colon: a new approach by percutaneous deflation and colopexy. World J Surg 1991; 15:68–73.
36. Drapanas T, Stewart JD. Acute sigmoid volvulus: concepts in surgical treatment. Am J Surg 1961; 101:70–77.
37. Shepherd JJ. Treatment of volvulus of sigmoid colon: a review of 425 cases. Br Med J 1968; 1:280–283.
38. Sutcliffe MML. Volvulus of the sigmoid colon. Br J Surg 1968; 55:903–910.
39. Sharpton B, Cheek RC. Volvulus of the sigmoid colon. Am surg 1976; 42: 436–440.
40. Gulati SM, Grover NK, Tagore NK, Taneja OP. Volvulus of the sigmoid in Delhi, India. Dis Colon Rectum 1974; 17:219–225.
41. Ballantyne GH, Bradner MD, Beart RW Jr., Ilstrup DM. Volvulus of the colon. Incidence and mortality. Ann Surg 1985; 202:83–92.
42. Mangiante EC, Croce MA, Fabian TC, Moore OF III, Britt LG. Sigmoid volvulus. A four-decade experience. Am Surg 1989; 55:41–44.
43. Keller A, Aeberhard P. Emergency resection and primary anastomosis for sigmoid volvulus in an African population. Int J Colorectal Dis 1989; 5:209–212.
44. Jacobs DM, Bubrick MP. Volvulus of the large intestines. Perspect colon Rectal Surg 1990; 3:34–55.
45. Ghazi A, Shinya H, Wolff WI. Treatment of volvulus of the colon by colonoscopy. Ann Surg 1976; 183:263–265.
46. Biery DL, Hoffman SMJ. Colonoscopic reduction of sigmoid volvulus. J Am Osteopath Assoc 1978; 77:543–545.
47. Orchard JL, Mehta R, Khan AH. The use of colonoscopy in the treatment of colonic volvulus: Three cases and review of the literature. Am J Gastroenterol 1984; 79:864–867.
48. Wertkin MG, Aufses AH Jr. Management of volvulus of the colon. Dis Colon Rectum 1978; 21:40–45.
49. Priuiti FW, Holt RW. Detorsion of sigmoid volvulus by flexible fiberoptic sigmoidoscopy. J Med Soc NJ 1984; 78:289–290.
50. Renzulli P, Maurer CA, Netzer P, Buchler MW. Preoperative colonoscopic derotation is beneficial in a acute colonic volvulus. Dig Surg 2002; 19:223–229.
51. Grossmann EM, Longo WE, Stratton MD, Virgo KS, Johnson FE. Sigmoid Volvulus in department of Veteran Affairs Medical Centers. Dis Colon Rectum 2000; 43:414–418.
52. Wissler DW, Morrissey JF. Use of an external suction-irrigation device in endoscopy. Gastrointest Endosc 1980; 26:11–12.
53. Bernton E, Meyers R, Reyna T. Pseudo-obstruction of the colon: Case report including a new endoscopic treatment. Gastrointest Endosc 1982; 28:90–92.
54. Ballantyne GH. Volvulus of the large intestine [Expert commentary]. Perspect Colon Rectal Surg 1990; 3:56–60.
55. Gibney EJ. Volvulus of the sigmoid colon. Surg Gynecol Obstet 1990; 173:243–255.
56. Begarani M, Conde AS, Longo R, Ilaliano A, Terenzi A, Venuto G. Sigmoid volvulus in West Africa: a prospective study on surgical treatments. Dis Colon Rectum 1993; 36:186–190.
57. Naaeder SB, Archampong EQ. One-stage resection of acute sigmoid volvulus. Br J Surg 1994; 82:1635–1636.
58. Degiannis E, Levy RD, Silwa K, Hale MJ, Saadia R. Volvulus of the sigmoid colon at Baragwanath hospital. South Afr J Surg 1996; 34:25–28.
59. Isbister WH. Large bowel volvulus. Int J Colorectal Dis 1996; 11:96–98.
60. Raveenthiran V. Restorative resection of unprepared left colon in gangrenous vs. viable sigmoid volvulus. Int J Colorectal Dis 2004; 19:258–263.
61. Moore JH, Cintron JR, Duarte B, Espinosa G, Abcarian H. Synchronous cecal and sigmoid volvulus. Report of a case. Dis Colon Rectum 1992; 35:803–805.
62. Bach O, Rudloff W, Post S. Modification of mesosigmoidoplasty for nongangueonus sigmoid volvulus. World J Surg 2003; 27:1329–1332.
63. Brown AS, Mueller PR, Ferricci JT. Controlled percutaneous gastrostomy: nylon T-fasteners for fixation of the anterior gastric wall. Radiology 1986; 158:543–544.
64. Gallagher HJ, Aitken D, Chapman A, Ambrose NS. Endoscopic T-bar sigmoidopexy. A novel and effective treatment of sigmoid volvulus. Colorectal Dis 2000; 2(suppl):68.
65. Gallagher HJ, Aitken D, Chapman A, Ambrose NS. Additional experience of endoscopic T-bar sigmoidopexy [Letter to Editor]. Dis Colon Rectum 2002; 45:1565–1566.
66. Pinedo G, Kirberg A. Percutaneous endoscopic sigmoidopexy in sigmoid volvulus with T-fasteners. Report of two cases. Dis Colon Rectum 2001; 44:1867–1870.
67. Alver O, Oren D, Tireli M, Kazabasi B, Akdemir D. Ileosigmoid knotting in Turkey. Review of 68 cases. Dis Colon Rectum 1993; 36:1139–1147.
68. Mallick IH, Winslet MC. Ileosigmoid knotting. Colorectal Dis 2004; 6:220–225.
69. Alver O, Oren D, Apaydin B, Yigitbasi R, Ersan Y. Internal hermiation concurrent with ileosigmoid knotting or sigmoid volvulus: Presentation of 12 patients. Survey 2005; 137:372–377.
70. Alshawi JS. Recurrent sigmoid volvulus in pregnancy: report of a case and review of the literature. Dis Colon Rectum 2005; 48:1811–1813.
71. Anderson MJ Sr., Okike N, Spencer RJ. The colonoscope in cecal volvulus: Report of three cases. Dis Colon Rectum 1978; 21:71–74.
72. Hendrick JW. Treatment of volvulus of the cecum and right colon. Arch Surg 1964; 88:364–373.
73. Hindshaw DB, Carter R, Joergenson EJ. Volvulus of the cecum or right colon. Am J Surg 1959; 98:175–183.
74. Jeck HS. Volvulus of the cecum with a review of the recent literature and report of a case occurring as a postoperative complication. Am J Surg 1958; 96:411–414.
75. Anderson JR, Welch GH. Acute volvulus of the right colon: an analysis of 69 patients. World J Surg 1986; 10:336–342.
76. Wolf RY, Wilson H. Emergency operation for volvulus of the cecum. Review of 22 cases. Am Surg 1966; 32:96–102.
77. Barss JA, Coury JJ, Koch DA, Sites EC, Hazledine HJ. Intermittent volvulus of the right colon. Am J Surg 1959; 97:316–320.
78. Wolfer JA, Beaton LE, Anson BJ. Volvulus of the cecum: anatomic factors in its etiology. Report of a case. Surg Gynecol Obstet 1942; 74:882–893.
79. Donhauser JL, Atwell S. Volvulus of the cecum. Arch Surg 1949; 58:129–148.
80. Burke JB, Ballantyne GH. Cecal volvulus: low mortality at a city hospital. Dis Colon Rectum 1984; 27:737–740.
81. Jordon GL Jr, Beahrs OH. Volvulus of the cecum as a post-operative complication. Report of six cases. Ann Surg 1953; 137:245–249.
82. Grover NK, Gulati SM, Tagore NK, Taneja OP. Volvulus of the cecum and ascending colon. Am J Surg 1973; 125:672–675.
83. Rehbar A, Easley GW, Mendoza CB Jr. Volvulus of the cecum. Am Surg 1973; 39:325–330.
84. Krippaehne WW, Vetto RM, Jenkins CC. Volvulus of the ascending colon: a report of twenty-two cases. Am J Surg 1967; 114:323–332.
85. Sorg J, Whitaker WG Jr., Richmond L. Volvulus of the right colon in the postpartum and postoperative period. JMA Ga 1977; 66:519–523.
86. Berger RB, Hillemeier AC, Stahl RS, Markowitz RI. Volvulus of the ascending colon: an unusual complication of non-rotation of the midget. Pediatr Radiol 1982; 12:298–300.
87. Bedard CK, Ramirez A, Holsinger D. Ascending colon volvulus due to a vitelline duct remnant in an elderly patient. Am J Gastroenterol 1979; 71:617–620.
88. Ritvo M, Farrell GE Jr., Shauffer IA. The association of volvulus of the cecum and ascending colon with other obstructive colonic lesions. Am J Roentgenol 1957; 78:587–598.
89. Moore CJ, Corl FM, Fishman EK. CT of cecal volvulus: unraveling the image. AJR 2001; 177:95–98.
90. Nay HR, West JP. Treatment of volvulus of the sigmoid colon and cecum. Arch Surg 1967; 94:11–13.
91. Patel D, Ansari E, Berman MD. Percutaneous decompression of cecal volvulus. Am J Radiol 1987; 148:747.
92. Crass JR, Simmons RL, Frick MP, Maile CW. Percutaneous decompression of the colon using CT guidance in Ogilvie syndrome. Am J Roentgenol 1985; 144:475–476.
93. Casola G, Withers C, van Sonnenberg E, Herba MJ, Saba RM, Brown RA. Percutaneous cecostomy for decompression of the massively distended cecum. Radiology 1986; 158:793–794.
94. Geer DA, Arnaud G, Beitter A, et al. Colonic volvulus. The Army Medical Center experience 1983–1987. Am Surg 1991; 57:295–300.

95. Todd GJ, Forde KA. Volvulus of the cecum: choice of operation. Am J Surg 1979; 138:632–634.
96. Rabinovich R, Simansky DA, Kaplan O, Mavor E, Manny J. Ceical volvulus. Dis Colon Rectum 1990; 33:765–769.
97. Burke JB, Ballantyne GH. Cecal volvulus. Low mortality at a city hospital. Dis Colon Rectum 1984; 27:737–740.
98. Madiba TE, Thomson SR. The management of cecal volvulus Dis Colon Rectum, 2002; 45:264–267.
99. Benacci JC, Wolff BG. Cecostomy: therapeutic indications and results. Dis Colon Rectum 1995; 38:530–534.
100. Tejler G, Jiborn H. Volvulus of the cecum. Report of 26 cases and review of the literature. Dis Colon Rectum 1988; 31:445–449.
101. John H, Gyr T, Giudici G, Martinoli S, Marx A. Cecal volvulus in pregnancy. Case report and review of literature. Arch Gynecol Obstet 1996; 258:161–164.
102. Montes H, Wolf J. Cecal volvulus in Pregancy. Gastroenterol 1999; 94: 2554–2556.
103. Gumbs MA, Kashan F, Shumofsky F, Yerubandi SR. Volvulus of the transverse colon: report of cases and review of the literature. Dis Colon Rectum 1983; 26:825–828.
104. Kerry R, Ransom HK. Volvulus of the colon: etiology, diagnosis and treatment. Arch Surg 1969; 29:78–85.
105. Fishman EK, Goldman SM, Patt PG, Berlanstein B, Bohlman ME. Transverse colon volvulus: diagnosis and treatment. South Med J 1983; 176:185–189.
106. Zinkin LD, Katz LD, Rosin JD. Volvulus of the transverse colon: report of a case and review of the literature. Dis Colon Rectum 1979; 22:492–496.
107. Boley SJ. Volvulus of the transverse colon. Am J Surg 1958; 96:122–125.
108. Orangio GR, Fazio VW, Winkelman E, McGonagle BA. The Chilaiditi syndrome and associated volvulus of the transverse colon: an indication for surgical therapy. Dis Colon Rectum 1986; 29:653–656.
109. Plorde JJ, Raker EJ. Transverse colon volvulus and associated Chilaiditis syndrome: case report and literature review. Am J Gastroenterol 1996; 91: 2613–2616.
110. Martin JD Jr., Ward CS. Megacolon associated with volvulus of transverse colon. Am J Surg 1944; 64:412–416.
111. Budd DC, Nirdlinger EL, Sturtz DL, Fouty WJ Jr. Transverse colon volvulus associated with scleroderma. Am J Surg 1977; 133:370–372.
112. Newton NA, Reines HD. Transverse colon volvulus: case reports and review. Am J Roentgenol 1977; 128:69–72.
113. Chang TH. Acute volvulus of the transverse colon: report of an unusual case. W Va Med J 1985; 81:95–98.
114. Joergensen K, Kronborg O. The colonoscope in volvulus of the transverse colon. Dis Colon Rectum 1980; 23:357–358.
115. Anderson R, Lee D, Taylor RV, Ross HM. Volvulus of the transverse colon. Br J Surg 1981; 68:179–181.
116. Mortensen NJM, Hoffman G. Volvulus of the transverse colon. Postgrad Med J 1979; 55:54–57.
117. Anderson MF, Pinckney L. The traveling volvulus. Dis Colon Rectum 1979; 22:276–278.
118. Goldberg M, Lernau OZ, Mogle P, Dermer R, Nissan S. Volvulus of the splenic flexure of the colon. Am J Gastroenterol 1984; 79:693–695.
119. Welch GH, Anderson JR. Volvulus of the splenic flexure of the colon. Dis Colon Rectum 1985; 28:592–593.
120. Naraynsingh V, Raju GC. Splenic flexure volvulus. Postgrad Med J 1985; 61:1007–1009.
121. Ballantyne GH. Volvulus of the splenic flexure: report of a case and review of the literature. Dis Colon Rectum 1981; 24:630–632.
122. Mindelzun RE, Stone JM. Volvulus of the splenic flexure: radiographic features. Radiology 1991; 181:221–223.

30 Mesenteric Vascular Diseases

Philip H. Gordon

Mesenteric vascular disease encompasses a family of diseases of which the end result is injury to the small or large bowel resulting from diminished blood flow or inadequate oxygen and nutrient delivery. Mesenteric disease is present in 18% of patients older than 65 years of age and in 70% of those undergoing aortofemoral bypass (1). The diseases vary from anatomically definable and clinically reproducible symptom complexes, such as those seen in superior mesenteric artery embolism, to more erratic and unpredictable patterns, such as those of ischemic colitis. The estimated frequency of causes of acute mesenteric ischemia are arterial occlusion 50%, nonocclusive mesenteric ischemia 20% to 30%, venous occlusion 5% to 15%, as well as extravascular sources such as incarcerated hernia, volvulus, intussusception, and adhesive bands (2). Although it is important to view these diseases clinically as individual entities often requiring different clinical approaches, it is equally important to recognize the common anatomic and physiologic principles involved in each syndrome.

VASCULAR ANATOMY

The intestinal tract has a generous overlapping blood supply, with blood flow averaging 1500 to 1800 mL/min. Wide variations in blood flow are possible in response to meals or exercise. The three main vessels supplying circulation to the bowel include the celiac axis, the superior mesenteric artery (SMA), and the inferior mesenteric artery (IMA). Because of the important collateral blood flow emanating from the hypogastric arteries at the level of the sigmoid colon, the hypogastrics also should be considered to be part of this system.

The celiac artery consists of three main trunks, which are the splenic, common hepatic, and left gastric arteries. The main collateral communication between the celiac and the SMA system is via the pancreaticoduodenal loop and to a lesser extent from the dorsal pancreatic artery. The pancreaticoduodenal artery originates as anterior and posterior superior pancreaticoduodenal branches that arise from the gastroduodenal artery, which is itself a branch of the common hepatic artery. This loop communicates around the duodenal sweep between the pancreatic border of the duodenum and the pancreas and unites with inferior pancreaticoduodenal vessels coming from the SMA. The pancreaticoduodenal loop can dilate considerably in the presence of ischemic disease. Another collateral vessel, the dorsal pancreatic artery, is a branch that traverses the pancreas, coming from either the splenic artery or the

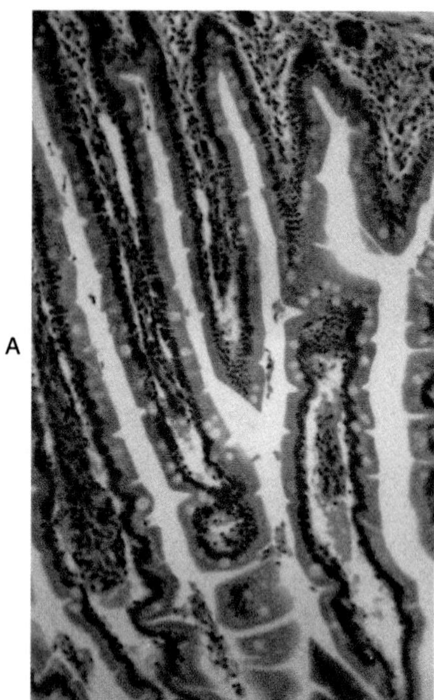

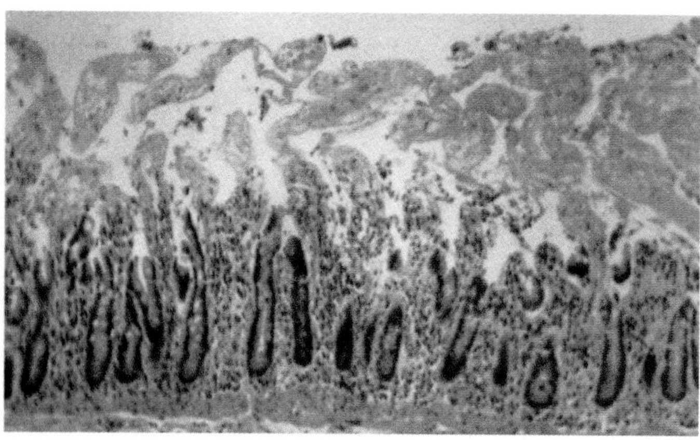

FIGURE 1 ■ (**A**) Microscopic section of normal small bowel villus pattern. (**B**) Section of small bowel having sustained ischemic injury, showing sloughing and loss of villus tips with preservation of cellular elements of villus at the base.

'common hepatic artery to join and collateralize with the SMA system below via the middle colic artery.

The SMA gives off the inferior pancreaticoduodenal artery as its first branch, and it then supplies virtually the entire blood supply to the jejunum and ileum via individual mesenteric arteries. At the level of the distal ileum a large ileocolic artery nourishes the terminal ileum and cecum. The ascending colon and transverse colon receive blood from branches that arise from the SMA more proximally. The right colic artery arises from the mid-portion of the SMA to supply the ascending colon. The middle colic artery frequently is spared from SMA embolism because it originates from the most proximal portion of the SMA before dividing into right and left branches.

The left branch of the middle colic artery traverses the mesocolon along the left side of the transverse colon, the splenic flexure, and the descending colon to ultimately collateralize with the IMA at the level of the mid-portion of the descending colon. The IMA communication between the left colic artery and the SMA circulation has been variously called the marginal artery, the arc of Riolan, the central anastomotic artery, and the meandering mesenteric artery. Two or more anastomotic arteries may be present (3). Discussion of the anatomy and varying nomenclature is elaborated in Chapter 1. The IMA also gives off sigmoidal branches and superior rectal branches; the latter branches communicate with the hypogastric system by means of middle and inferior rectal vessels (see Chap. 1).

In general, acute occlusion of any of the three main mesenteric vessels, either celiac, SMA, or IMA, is capable of causing varying degrees of acute infarction, whereas gradual occlusion of any one, two, or even three of these vessels can occur without injury, depending largely on the extent of the collateral circulation.

The arcade system and overlapping circulation within the small bowel end at the level of the villus, where the arterioles effectively become end vessels. A single arteriole, designated the main arteriole, enters through the core of the villus. This vessel arborizes into a tuft arrangement of capillaries at the tip of the villus and subsequently drains into venules that converge at the villus base to form the collecting venule (4). There is evidence for a countercurrent exchange mechanism similar to that seen in the renal nephron; in the villus the mechanism involves the central arteriole and the venules lying in close proximity at the base of the villus (5). During low-flow states, oxygen is shunted by diffusion from arteriole to venule, and this renders the villus tip vulnerable to ischemic injury (6). The high metabolic rate of the villus and the oxygen shunting make the villus the first part of the intestine to feel the impact of ischemic injury (Fig. 1).

PATHOPHYSIOLOGY OF INTESTINAL ISCHEMIA

The gut receives 20% of resting and 35% of postprandial cardiac output. Of this, 70% supplies the mucosa (1). Kaleya and Boley (7) summarized the microcirculation and collateral flow within the intestinal wall. An extensive network of vessels within the bowel wall arises from the vasa recta and vasa brevia on the mesenteric border of the bowel. These vessels give rise, sequentially, to the external muscular vascular plexus, then penetrate the muscular coat and form a rich submucosal plexus. The submucosal plexus is more extensive in the small bowel than in the colon and may make the small intestine more resistant to ischemia than the colon. A central arteriole originates from the submucosal plexus, loses its muscular coat, and arborizes into an extremely rich subepithelial capillary network within each individual villus. The flow through this redundant system is controlled by a network of resistance and capillary vessels, which, in turn, are affected by many functional, humoral, local, and neural influences. There are two primary mechanisms for the control of splanchnic vascular resistance. The first is neural. The sympathetic nervous system is important for the maintenance of resting splanchnic arteriolar tone and the primary mechanism of sympathetic control is neural. The second is humoral, consisting of a variety of circulating hormones, including catecholamines, vasoactive peptides, and inflammatory mediators such as histamine and the arachidonic acid metabolites. The important vasoconstrictor peptides include angiotensin II and vasopressin. Local factors play a role in intestinal blood flow. Prostaglandins, leukotrienes, and some thromboxane analogs produce splanchnic vasoconstriction. Local factors that accompany ischemia have potent vasodilatory effects on intestinal vessels. Hyperkalemia, hyperosmolarity, decreased local oxygen tension, adenosine, and high concentrations of carbon dioxide, causing local acidosis, dilate resistance vessels and produce local hyperemia. Exogenously administered vasodilators (e.g., papaverine) prevent and reverse the persistent vasoconstriction that follows a drop in SMA blood flow.

Inadequate intestinal perfusion is a consequence of either focal vascular occlusions or a low-flow state. Within 15 minutes of absolute ischemia, structural damage to the villi of the small bowel can be demonstrated; within three hours mucosal sloughing occurs. At six hours transmural necrosis is complete (1). The nature and rapidity of these processes are affected by two other factors: collateral circulation and disorders of splanchnic autoregulation. Despite the variety of conditions that predispose to ischemia, the histopathology and sequence of events remain consistent and predictable. Intestinal ischemia induces a spectrum of injury, from subtle changes in capillary permeability to transmural necrosis, and the final outcome depends on local as well as systemic factors (7). There basically are two separate factors responsible for the subsequent damage—tissue hypoxia and reperfusion injury. Hypoxia occurs during the period of ischemia and reperfusion injury when some flow is re-established. The early phase of acute intestinal ischemia involves mechanisms that ultimately cause volume loss and acidosis. Reversal of the ischemic injury is possible early in the process. Later in the course, bacterial invasion with endotoxic release, septicemia, and shock becomes more prominent and indicates full-thickness irreversible injury.

Following an episode of intestinal ischemia, the first event involves loss of circulatory blood volume with intense outpouring of fluid and protein through the injured villus. The most tenable explanation for this early extravasation of fluid is that the ischemic villus tip loses its absorptive function, while the crypt cells are relatively spared of injury and can continue their secretory functions (8). Loss of circulating blood volume and distention caused by intraluminal exudation contribute to a further decrease in perfusion. As submucosal layers are rendered ischemic, bowel edema develops, and this is followed by transudation of fluid into the peritoneal cavity, complicating the already serious hypovolemia. The intense volume loss alone can lead to profound hypovolemia, with the metabolic sequelae of hypoxia at the tissue level and lactic acidosis.

The changes that occur when intestine is deprived of an adequate blood supply are both metabolic and morphologic (7). Ultrastructural changes occur within 10 minutes and, by 30 minutes, extensive changes, including accumulation of fluid between cells and the basement membranes, are present. The tips of the villi then begin to slough, and a membrane of necrotic epithelium, fibrin, inflammatory cells, and bacteria accumulates. Later, edema appears, followed by bleeding into the submucosa. Cellular death progresses from the lumen outward until transmural necrosis of the bowel wall occurs.

Vasoactive substances released in response to intestinal ischemia act to further diminish perfusion. Release of myocardial depressant factor probably contributes to worsening the already diminished cardiac output. Other mediators such as cytokines, platelet-activating factor, and tumor necrosis factor are also released (1). Histamine release during ischemic reperfusion appears to play an important role in the progression of the shock state. Diamine oxidase, an enzyme that acts to inactivate histamine, has been shown to have a protective effect in intestinal ischemia (9). Also implicated in circulatory collapse following intestinal infarction is the vasoactive intestinal polypeptide (VIP), which acts as a potent vasodilator and contributes to the intense outpouring of intraluminal fluids (10,11).

Bacterial invasion does not occur until 24 hours or more into the course of the ischemic episode. In studies with an isolated colonic ischemia model, Bennion et al. (12,13) showed that by 72 hours the total number of anaerobic bacteria had increased, while aerobic bacteria counts had decreased. All anaerobe species were found to be increased, especially *Bacteroides*, as well as a variety of clostridial species, including *Clostridium difficile*. In the same animal model, cultures of portal venous blood and liver became infected with a mixed anaerobic flora by 24 hours. Systemic bacteremia followed portal venous bacteremia at 48 hours when aortic and peritoneal cultures grew mixed anaerobes. This suggests that ischemia-induced mucosal injury first causes portal vein bacteremia, followed by systemic bacteremia once the hepatic reticuloendothelial system becomes overwhelmed. These findings precede perforation, which causes more widespread bacterial dissemination within the peritoneal cavity from gross spillage of bowel contents.

Recent attention has been directed at the role of oxygen free radicals in the pathogenesis of reperfusion injury. Partial reduction of molecular oxygen results in the production of oxygen free radicals. These superoxide radicals mark the beginning of a metabolic cascade that results in the formation of highly toxic hydroxyl free radicals. The enzymes, superoxide dismutase and catalase, provide a defense against superoxide radicals by converting the radicals to peroxide and water. Cytotoxic effects of oxygen-derived free radicals result from peroxidation of the lipid components of cellular membranes and the degradation of the hyaluronic acid and collagen components of basement membranes and extracellular matrices (14,15). The resulting increased vascular permeability and mucosal membrane injury lead to enhanced transcapillary fluid transudation and interstitial edema. Studies by Granger et al. (16) have provided evidence that free radical scavenger enzymes substantially block the increased vascular permeability induced by ischemia, while antihistamines, indomethacin, and methylprednisone do not.

Parks et al. (17) subsequently have shown that experimentally generated oxygen free radicals cause increased vascular permeability in nonischemic bowel comparable to that seen with ischemia.

The source of superoxide production in intestinal ischemia appears to be the enzyme xanthine oxidase. Xanthine oxidase is abundant in small bowel mucosa, where it is most heavily concentrated in the villus tip. Substrates for the reaction include hypoxanthine, which is a catabolic product of adenosine triphosphate, and molecular oxygen available with reperfusion. The tissue damage occurs during reperfusion and not during the period of ischemia (1).

Andrei et al. (18) documented a fatal case of small bowel ischemia following laparoscopic cholecystectomy. Their literature review revealed at least six cases of small bowel ischemia following laparoscopic cholecystectomy. It is postulated this was due to the physiological adverse effects of pneumoperitoneum-associated intra-abdominal hypertension, compromising the mesenteric circulation.

DIAGNOSTIC STUDIES

Improved results in the treatment of most types of mesenteric vascular disease must come from earlier diagnosis. Diagnostic laboratory studies for mesenteric ischemia are based on measurements of physiologic derangements. Specific radiographic studies and other diagnostic procedures will be covered in the discussion of each disease process.

The white blood cell count generally is a reliable indicator of ischemic injury and often can be used to monitor the progress or the worsening of the disease. However, some studies have shown that as many as 25% of patients will have significant ischemic injury without elevation of the white blood cell count (7), emphasizing the need to consider other subjective and objective findings. Hematocrit may be a helpful guide to the status of ischemic disease because it can reflect the intense hypovolemia seen with significant small bowel injuries. Hematocrit levels as high as 60% can be seen in some patients, and this hemoconcentration may further contribute to the ischemic process by causing sludging and microvascular thrombosis.

Arterial blood gases show a metabolic acidosis pattern associated with intestinal infarction. The acidosis may precede the development of shock and may be of diagnostic significance (19). Some studies have shown a disproportionately high elevation of serum phosphate levels in the presence of intestinal ischemia, suggesting that serum phosphate may serve as a marker for the disease. Serum phosphate elevation, while not specific for bowel ischemia, is useful because it is so readily determined, and the phosphate elevation may precede irreversible ischemic injury (20).

A number of enzyme levels have been studied, but many are nonspecific and others are not readily available. Amylase, lactic dehydrogenase, and serum glutamate oxaloacetate transaminase levels often are elevated, but these elevations are nonspecific and generally are not reliable. Animal studies have shown that serum intestinal alkaline phosphatase (SIAP) levels are elevated in the presence of mesenteric ischemia disease but not in the presence of inflammatory disease or perforation (21). This could make SIAP levels a useful and specific marker in the future, although the test is not available for clinical use at this time. Creatine phosphokinase (CPK) isoenzyme levels also have been shown to be elevated in the presence of ischemic bowel disease (22,23), and assays for these enzymes are readily available. Animal studies have shown that fractionating the CPK into BB and MB bands can be especially helpful in the first 24 hours (23). The CPK-BB isoenzyme tends to be elevated in the first 12 hours, whereas the CPK-MB band becomes elevated in the second 12 hours, making these potentially useful diagnostic markers for early intestinal ischemia.

The level of diamine oxidase, a histamine catabolizing enzyme, has been shown to be elevated early in the face of intestinal ischemia, probably in response to the intensive release of histamine by the ischemic process (24). If this enzyme assay becomes available in the future, it may be helpful in differentiating ischemic injury from other inflammatory processes. The level of VIP also has been shown to be elevated, particularly early in ischemic disease (10), but an assay for VIP is not yet available in most medical centers.

Acosta et al. (25) assessed the value of the fibrinolytic marker D-dimer testing to diagnose SMA occlusion by means of likelihood ratios. Nine of 101 patients included had acute SMA occlusion. The median D-dimer concentration was 1.6 mg/L, which was higher than that in 25 patients with inflammatory disease or in 14 patients with intestinal obstruction. The combination of a D-dimer level greater than 1.5 mg/L, atrial fibrillation and female sex resulted in a likelihood ratio for acute SMA occlusion of 17.5, whereas no patient with a D-dimer concentration of 0.3 mg/L or less had acute SMA occlusion.

Scholz (26) described the following radiologic findings that may be expected in acute bowel ischemia with any modality that images the intestine: gasless abdomen, rapid transit, slow transit, ileus, bowel obstruction, unchanging loop of small bowel, blood blister formation, thumbprinting, thick folds, "stack of coins," thickening of bowel wall, persisting enhancement of thick bowel wall on computed tomography (CT), and prompt reversal of these findings if ischemia is reversed. The following findings indicate that bowel infarction is present or was present and that fibrotic healing has occurred: focal ulcer, shaggy mucosa, "collar button" ulcers, mesenteric or portal vein gas, intramural fistula, intraluminal mucosal cast, intraperitoneal air, stricture, and pseudodiverticulum. Wiesner et al. (27) published an extensive review of CT findings in acute bowel ischemia. These may consist of various morphologic changes, including homogeneous or heterogeneous hypoattenuating or hyerattenuating wall thickening, dilatation, abnormal or absent wall enhancement, mesenteric stranding, vascular engorgement, ascites, pneumatosis, and portal venous gas. Acute bowel ischemia may affect the small and/or large bowel and may be diffuse or localized, segmental or focal, and superficial or transmural; therefore, it can mimic various intestinal diseases. Acute bowel ischemia may involve more typical regions such as the left-sided colon; under such circumstances or if there are more specific CT findings such as pneumatosis or portal venous gas, the correct diagnosis will usually be suspected by the radiologist in an appropriate clinical setting. The CT appearance of acute bowel ischemic will depend on its cause, severity, localization, extent, and distribution, as well as the presence and degree of submucosal or intramural hemorrhage, superimposed bowel wall infection, and/or bowel wall perforation. Therefore, the CT findings in acute bowel ischemia may be as heterogeneous and nonspecific in these patients as their clinical and laboratory findings are. Klein et al. (28) reviewed the value of all diagnostic imaging of 54 patients with mesenteric infarction. The authors found CT (82%) and angiography (87.5%) to be highly sensitive but favored CT because it can also be used to rule out other causes of the acute abdomen. Chou et al. (29) evaluated the CT features of small bowel ischemia and necrosis and correlated the findings with clinical outcome or patient prognosis in 68 surgically or angiographically proved cases of small bowel ischemia. The CT features of intestinal ischemia were divided into three groups: (A) thinned bowel wall with poor enhancement, intramural gas, or portal venous gas; (B) thickened small bowel wall without superior mesenteric vein thrombosis; and (C) thickened small bowel wall with superior mesenteric vein thrombosis or intussusception. The evaluated factors include small bowel wall or mucosal enhancement pattern, small bowel dilatation, mesenteric edema, and CT evidence of narrowing or occlusion of the superior mesenteric artery or vein. Oral contrast material was not administered. Intramural gas and small bowel dilatation were associated with a higher bowel necrosis rate (eight of eight and 17 of 21, respectively) in group A. Poor mucosal enhancement of the thickened bowel wall indicated a higher bowel necrosis rate in groups B (six of seven) and C (12 of 12) than did normal mucosal enhancement. Only intramural gas was accompanied by a higher mortality (six of eight).

Sreenarasimhaiah (2) has recently summarized the value of imaging studies. CT imaging has evolved over several years into a very useful modality for diagnosis of mesenteric ischemia and is the test of choice in the diagnosis of acute mesenteric ischemia. Findings include focal or segmental bowel wall thickening, submucosal edema or hemorrhage, pneumatosis, and portal venous gas. Contrast-enhanced CT detects acute mesenteric ischemia with sensitivity rates exceeding 90%. CT has been able to detect nonvascular visceral abnormalities. CT angiography is also available. MRI with angiography is another noninvasive modality that rivals conventional angiography. In mesenteric venous disease, excellent visualization of the vascular anatomy is possible in addition to assessment of portal venous patency, flow direction, splanchnic thrombosis, and changes suggestive of portal hypertension. Three-dimensional gadolinium-enhanced reconstruction of vascular anatomy with a single breath hold and ultrafast scanning with digital subtraction angiography are also available. MRI with angiography has high sensitivity and specificity similar to those of CT angiography with the advantage of safer gadolinium agents and lack of ionizing radiation. Although MRI with angiography is an excellent tool for the evaluation of chronic mesenteric ischemia, it should not be the first technique used in the diagnosis of acute mesenteric ischemia, because of its potentially insufficient resolution to adequately identify nonocclusive low flow states or distal emboli. Burkart et al. (30) studied magnetic resonance (MR) measurements of mesenteric venous flow and found the imaging technique promising as a noninvasive screening test for chronic mesenteric ischemia. Duplex scanning may be of value in identifying major vessel occlusion (7). Laparoscopy may also be useful in the diagnosis but is limited by its inability to assess mucosal necrosis.

CLINICAL SYNDROMES

■ SUPERIOR MESENTERIC ARTERY EMBOLISM

SMA embolism is the most dramatic of the mesenteric vascular diseases and accounts for 33% to 50% of acute mesenteric ischemia (1,7,31). Most commonly, this originates as a consequence of atrial fibrillation. It affords the potential for complete reversal and resolution if diagnosis and treatment are carried out promptly.

Acosta et al. (32) assessed the incidence of acute thromboembolic occlusion of the superior mesenteric artery in a population-based study in those autopsies coded for bowel ischemia (997/23,446 clinical and 9/7569 forensic autopsies). Two forensic and 211 clinical autopsies demonstrated acute thromboembolic occlusion of the superior mensenteric artery with intestinal gangrene. Previous suspicion of intestinal ischemia was noted in only 33%. Sixteen patients were operated. The cause-specific mortality was 6/1000 deaths, the incidence of 8.6/100,000 person-years increasing exponentially with age. Mortality was 93%.

The disease is characterized by a sudden onset of severe abdominal pain that generally is out of proportion to the physical examination. Associated findings include forceful gastric emptying with vomiting in approximately one-half of the patients and diarrhea in one-third. The white blood cell count usually is elevated, and frequently a history of cardiac disease and/or previous embolic phenomena is present. Plain radiography may show dilated thickened bowel loops, a ground-glass appearance due to ascites, thumbprinting, and toxic dilatation or gas in the bowel wall, portal vein, or peritoneum. All these features indicate infarction, but one-fourth of patients with infarction have a normal plain abdominal radiograph (1). CT may show ascites, intestinal wall thickening, mucosal thumbprints, pneumatosis, and portal vein gas but may be normal in 30% of patients with proven mesenteric ischemia (1). Diagnosis is made by arteriogram. Characteristically, a sharp cutoff or meniscus sign is present at the site of the embolus several centimeters from the takeoff of the SMA. The most proximal branches supplying the proximal jejunum and the right transverse colon usually are not affected. This differentiates SMA embolism from SMA thrombosis, where the occlusion occurs at the origin of the vessel (Fig. 2).

Boley et al. (33) have reported good results with papaverine used as part of a nonoperative protocol; mortality rates have been $<59\%$ in papaverine-treated patients. Some favorable early results also have been seen with thrombolytic therapy (34–36). However, most patients with SMA embolism will need surgery, particularly when progression of the ischemic injury is suspected. The characteristic finding at surgery is a normal proximal jejunum with pulses present,

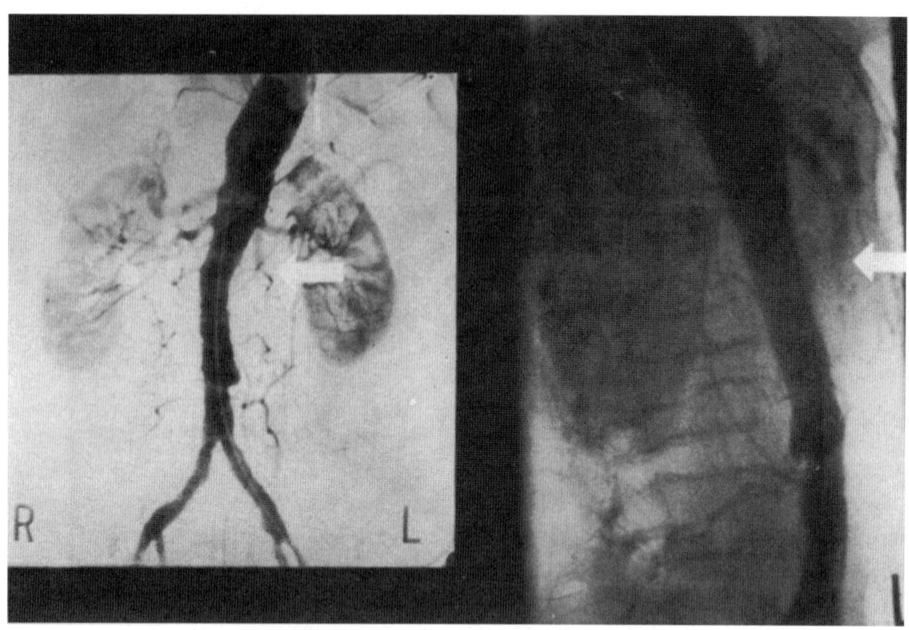

FIGURE 2 ■ Arteriogram showing SMA embolism with arrow pointing to site of occlusion forming a meniscus sign.

reflecting the more distal placement of the embolus beyond the origin of the SMA. The ischemic changes are seen from the level of the mid-portion of the jejunum to the transverse colon, and no pulses are found in any of the vessels to this large section of the small and large bowel. This differs from SMA thrombosis, which is accompanied by ischemic changes involving the entire jejunum, the ileum, and the right colon.

When diagnosed, a papaverine infusion 30 to 60 μg/hr through the indwelling SMA catheter has been advised (31). Treatment of SMA embolism includes embolectomy or arterial reconstruction. Resection should be limited to those cases in which intestinal segments are frankly infarcted (Fig. 3) (1,31). Early embolectomy alone usually is sufficient to restore perfusion (Fig. 4). Care must be taken to evacuate all distally propagated thrombi, and narrowing must be avoided when closing the arteriotomy site. The need for small bowel resection often may be avoided by re-evaluating the viability of the bowel 15 to 30 minutes after restoration of blood flow.

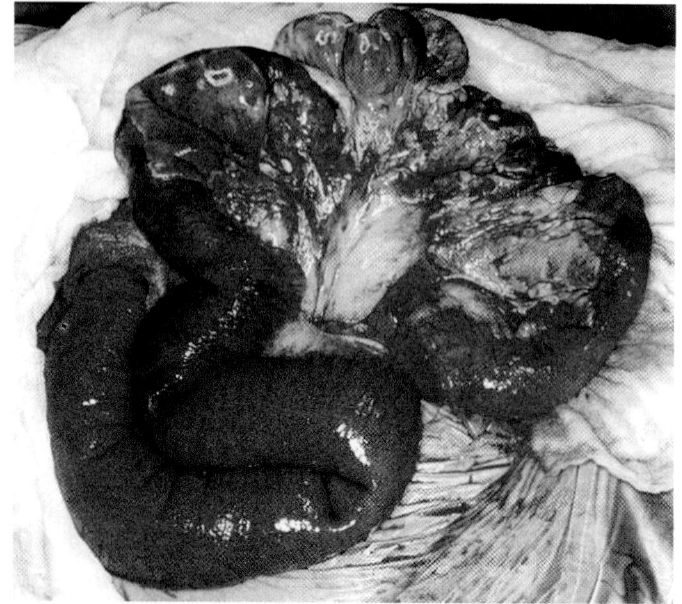

FIGURE 3 ■ Well-delineated necrotic small bowel.

Traditional methods of determining bowel viability following reperfusion are inaccurate. Reliance on the return of normal color, the presence of mesenteric pulsations, and peristalsis promotes unnecessary bowel resection in up to 50% of cases (37). It is much more accurate to determine viability by fluorescein dye injection or by Doppler ultrasonography. Both techniques are relatively simple and allow for more precise delineation of nonperfused and nonviable bowel (31,37,38). The use of surface oximetry to assess the adequacy of intestinal tissue oxygenation is especially promising. Sheridan et al. (39) have used a modified Clark oxygen electrode to measure tissue oxygen tension (PtO_2) and have established a reference range for intraoperative PtO_2 for the entire gastrointestinal tract. The papaverine infusion may be continued for 12 to 24 hours, and repeat angiograms may be obtained to ascertain that the vasoconstriction has been abolished (31). Heparin is controversial because gastrointestinal hemorrhage is a significant risk. Thrombolytic therapy with streptokinase, urokinase, or recombinant tissue plasminogen activators in cases of acute and subacute SMA embolism or thrombosis has been described (1).

The use of second-look laparotomy may maximize intestinal salvage for those cases in which viability is uncertain. The decision to perform a second-look procedure should be made at the time of the original operation. Re-exploration has been advocated 12 to 48 hours later, regardless of apparent clinical improvement or stabilization of the patient's overall condition. To avoid a formal second-look operation following massive resection for bowel infarction Sluttzki et al. (40) used laparoscopic inspection to assess the integrity of the anastomosis and viability of the remaining bowel. At the primary operation, two 10/12 mm laparoscopic trocars were inserted in the lower quadrants, and 48 to 72 hours later the abdominal contents were inspected laparoscopically in five consecutive patients. The authors found the technique safe and reliable in all patients. Because of concern about decreasing mesenteric blood flow, care was taken to limit the pressure to 15 mmHg during the procedure.

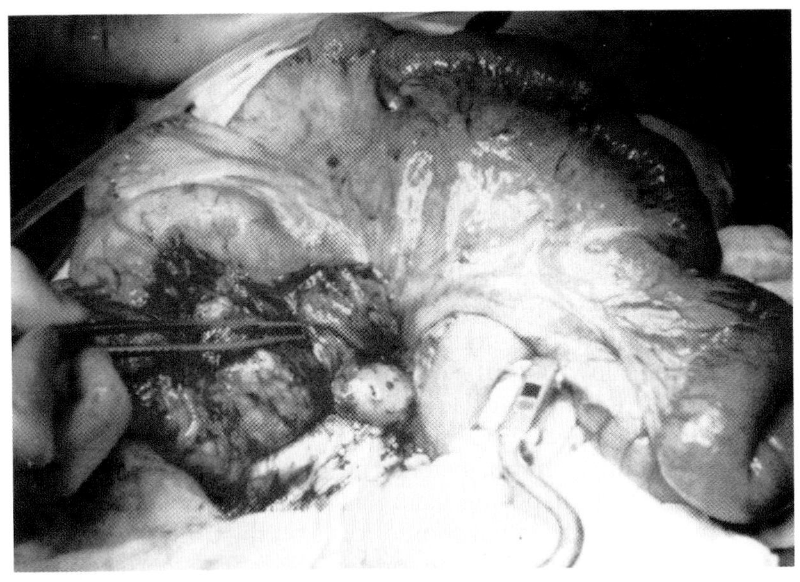

FIGURE 4 ■ Operative photo of SMA embolectomy site following restoration of blood flow. Ischemic sites are prominent at center of field indicating areas of small bowel that needed resection.

Anadol et al. (41) compared open and laparoscopic "second-look" procedures in patients with mesenteric ischemia. In the open group (41 patients), the abdomen was closed and a second-look laparotomy was performed in 23 patients. In the laparoscopic group (36 patients), a 10 mm trocar was inserted before closing the abdomen and second-look intervention was performed by a laparoscope in 23 patients. Sixteen of re-laparotomies in the open group (70%) revealed nothing and were unnecessary. Two patients (8%) in the laparoscopic group needed re-resection while 20 patients (87%) were rescued from unnecessary laparotomies.

Some authors are comfortable enough with Doppler assessment of bowel viability that they no longer recommend second-look procedures (42). In a review of the literature, Bergan (43) demonstrated that second-look operations are useful only for select patients. Of 49 patients who had survived SMA embolectomy, a second-look operation was not performed in 42 of these survivors. Among those seven patients in whom the second-look procedure was performed, resection was necessary in only two, suggesting that the yield from this operation is modest when it is not performed on an individualized basis. The use of a second-look operation is clearly indicated whenever bowel of questionable viability has been left behind (31). Sales et al. (44) reported on a series of 29 patients who underwent small bowel resection primarily for mesenteric artery occlusive disease. All patients were given an ostomy, and the authors believe that this policy decreased the mortality rate (34%) in their series. All the surviving patients had intestinal continuity restored.

Bingol et al. (45) reported 24 patients who underwent SMA embolectomy. The patients were divided into three groups according to the onset of symptoms and operation time. Group I ($n = 12$) patients were operated on in the first six hours after onset of symptoms; group II ($n = 9$) patients were operated on between six and 12 hours after onset of symptoms; and group III ($n = 3$) patients underwent embolectomy after 12 hours. Low dose (5–10 mg) local tissue-type plasminogen activator (t-PA) administration directly into the SMA was an additional procedure with the embolectomy in all patients. The macroscopic view of the intestine was normal in 15 patients (12 patients in group I and three patients in group II) 30 minutes after the administration of local t-PA. Segmental resection was necessary in four patients in group II. Extended resection was necessary in two patients in group II and three patients in group III and all the patients died during the early postoperative period. They suggest that exploratory laparotomy should be done in patients with sudden abdominal pain, nausea, vomiting, mild leucocytosis, and metabolic acidosis who have previous valvular heart disease or atrial fibrillation. Ultimately, selective low-dose t-PA (5–10 mg) administration reduces the length of intestinal portion to be resected.

Savassi-Rocha and Veloso (46) reported a case of SMA embolism in which arterial flow was re-established by selective intra-arterial infusion of streptokinase. They found 18 similar cases in the literature. This procedure could be an alterative to embolectomy in selected patients, i.e. patients with an early diagnosis, no evidence of intestinal necrosis and with partial occlusion and/or occlusion of secondary branches of the SMA. Frequent arteriographies and intensive care are necessary in this approach. The patient should be continuously monitored because of the possibility of treatment failure and the need for embolectomy.

■ SUPERIOR MESENTERIC ARTERY THROMBOSIS

SMA thrombosis is distinguishable from embolism because of the more insidious onset of symptoms and the prominence of hypovolemic signs initially and cardiovascular collapse later. It accounts for 5% to 50% of acute mesenteric ischemia (1,7,31). The usual presentation involves the gradual onset of abdominal pain associated with progressive distention and clinical signs of dehydration. Frequently there is anorexia, nausea and vomiting, and diarrhea with occult or gross blood. Leukocytosis is usually present. Often there is a history compatible with chronic intestinal insufficiency (1,47). Although a diagnosis can be made by arteriogram, most patients are so acutely ill at the time of presentation that surgery is inevitable, and often the definitive diagnosis is made at the time of operation. Arteriography usually shows a cutoff of SMA blood flow at its origin. When advanced disease is present, plain abdominal X-ray films may show air in the portal vein and the liver (Fig. 5).

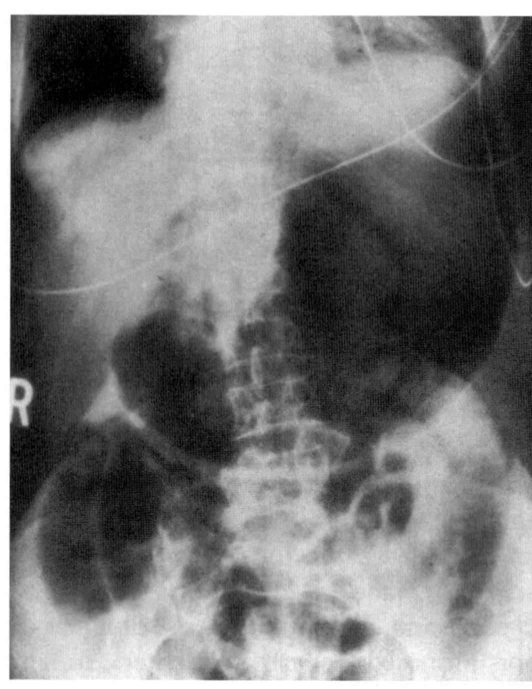

FIGURE 5 ■ Abdominal X-ray film of patient with massive small bowel infarction showing a dilated stomach and gas in the portal vein.

As with SMA embolism, initial operative management for arterial thrombosis must include revascularization of any extensive segment of ischemic bowel. Thromboendarterectomy for acute mesenteric arterial thrombosis has been associated with a high failure rate. Aortomesenteric bypass may be beneficial even if viability is not completely restored and resection becomes necessary (31). The graft may salvage marginally viable proximal jejunum, which ultimately may allow the patient to be maintained on oral alimentation. In addition, the graft may lessen the risk of anastomotic leak, since healing may be impaired if an anastomosis is performed in a potentially compromised but still viable small bowel. It has been argued that emergency bypass is doomed to failure because the gut has already infarcted, early graft thrombosis is almost universal, and the patient is likely to succumb from the systemic effects of reperfusion (1). For these reasons, extensive resection is probably preferable to time-consuming attempts at revascularization. Johnson et al. (48) reported on nine patients who underwent a bypass graft because of acute mesenteric thrombosis with an operative mortality of 22%. Survival at one year was 65% and at five years, 52%.

■ NONOCCLUSIVE MESENTERIC ISCHEMIA AND INFARCTION

Nonocclusive mesenteric infarction has been diagnosed with increasing frequency in intensive care unit settings among patients critically ill from other unrelated diseases. It accounts for 20% to 30% of cases of mesenteric ischemia (1,7,31). The signs and symptoms of nonocclusive mesenteric ischemia or infarction are similar to those of thrombotic infarction, except that nonocclusive disease tends to occur in a specific group of vulnerable patients. The disease should be suspected in any patient with cardiovascular disease and abdominal pain. Although the diagnosis is difficult to make, it is important to differentiate from other causes of ischemia because therapy is primarily nonoperative. Arteriography in these patients generally does not reveal an occlusion but shows reduced blood flow secondary to severe mesenteric vasospasm. Newer studies show that the renin–angiotensin axis, not catecholamines, may be the primary mediator of the splanchnic vasoconstriction seen in response to the severe physiologic stress associated with this condition (49,50).

Predisposing factors to nonocclusive ischemia include (1) patients with congestive heart failure who are taking digitalis and diuretics, (2) patients with valvular heart disease and low-output syndromes, (3) patients with digitalis intoxication and cardiac arrhythmia, (4) patients in shock or with prolonged hypovolemia, and (5) patients experiencing postoperative hypotension. The common denominator for all these predisposing factors is the low-flow state.

Initial treatment should focus on the underlying problem contributing to the presentation. The correction of hypovolemia, treatment of arrhythmias, and relief of congestive heart failure are crucial beginnings. Antibiotics may be helpful since the ischemia may result in a loss of the mucosal barrier to bacteria. A number of vasodilator drugs have been tried, but the one most frequently used is papaverine (30–60 mg/hr), usually given by angiographic catheter infusion until clinical and radiologic resolution, for up to five days (51,52). Epidural block and intraoperative splanchnic block also have been used to relieve the reflex component of the vasospasm. In many patients, nonthrombotic ischemia cannot be differentiated from infarction, and laparotomy is necessary for this distinction to be made. At laparotomy, all necrotic bowel should be resected; splanchnic block or epidural block may be added at that time. The prognosis for non-occlusive mesenteric ischemia tends to be poor largely because of the severity of the underlying illness that precipitates the ischemic event.

Ward et al. (53) adopted an aggressive approach to the management of these patients. In a review of 34 patients with nonocclusive mesenteric ischemia, seven patients underwent visceral arteriography, two of whom required operation and both died. Of the 29 patients who were explored, 21 had segmental injury and eight had massive injury. Of the 21 with segmental injury, 12 (57%) had a primary anastomosis, five of whom died (42%). Nine of 21 patients (43%) underwent delayed anastomosis, and two of them died (22%). None with massive injury underwent primary anastomosis. A second-look operation was performed on 22 of 29 patients (76%). Eleven of the 22 (50%) underwent further bowel resection. Overall, 55% survived.

Schuler and Hudlin (54) described the presentation and management of five cases of nonocclusive ischemic cecal necrosis. Four of the patients presented with right-sided abdominal pain, tenderness, and leucocytosis. The preoperative diagnosis was incorrect in all patients. Two patients were thought to have appendicitis, two were though to have carcinoma, and one was thought to have a perforated viscus. Each patient underwent a right hemicolectomy and four survived. Each of the patients had ischemic necrosis without evidence of emboli or vasculitis or hypotension. Ischemic necrosis of the cecum is an infrequent variant of ischemic colitis that should be considered in the differential diagnosis of the elderly patient presenting with right lower quadrant pain.

Neri et al. (55) reviewed the diagnostic and treatment methods that emerged from their experience in 371 patients with a diagnosis of aortic dissection. Mesenteric ischemia was present in 19% of patients. In 9% of patients, bowel ischemia was not associated with a false lumen anatomy or an extension of the dissection process. The mortality rate in patients with nonocclusive mesenteric ischemia was 86%; sepsis and multiple organ failure were the cause of death in all nonsurvivors. Surgical treatment was beneficial only in the early phases of the disease. In patients who underwent operation, the significant risk factors were severe coagulation disorders, postoperative cerebral ischemia, maximal oxygen extraction rate of more than 0.40, aortic calcinosis, chronic obstructive pulmonary disease, thrombosis of the false lumen, inotropic support, and chronic renal insufficiency. In suspected cases, an aggressive surgical attitude may represent the only means of reducing mortality.

■ MESENTERIC VENOUS THROMBOSIS

Mesenteric venous thrombosis accounts for 5% to 30% of all cases of gut ischemia (7,31). Bradbury et al. (1) classified the causes of mesenteric venous thrombosis (Table 1). To this list, Flaherty et al. (56) added a previously unrecognized cause of ischemia characterized by a vasculitis of mesenteric veins and their intramural tributaries. The authors proposed the term "mesenteric inflammatory veno-occlusive disease" to describe the entity.

Mesenteric venous thrombosis is characterized by the insidious onset of abdominal discomfort. The subacute nature of the symptoms may persist for 1 to 4 weeks. Progression of the disease is accompanied by more severe symptoms of crampy or diffuse abdominal pain, distention, or vomiting. The chief symptom of colicky pain is usually universal, nonlocalizing, and out of proportion to the meager findings of the physical examination. Mesenteric venous occlusion can often be differentiated from the previously described arterial occlusive syndromes by one of several commonly associated diseases that are present in most of the patients (Table 1). Between 15% and 44% of patients with primary venous thrombosis will have suffered previous thromboembolic disease (1). The physical examination is so nonspecific that it belies the seriousness of the situation. Physical findings vary with the stage of disease and may manifest as abdominal tenderness, distention, decreased bowel sounds, guarding, rebound tenderness, a temperature >38°C, and clinical signs of shock in 25% of patients.

TABLE 1 ■ Classification of the Causes of Mesenteric Venous Thrombosis

Primary (30%)	Secondary (60%)
Splenectomy	Portal hypertension; prehepatic, hepatic, and posthepatic
Polycythemia rubra vera	Injection sclerotherapy of esophageal varices
Sickle-cell disease	Portosystemic shunt insertion
Antithrombin III deficiency	Intra-abdominal sepsis; appendicitis, diverticulitis, pelvic abscess, visceral perforation, cholangitis
Protein C deficiency	Acute and chronic pancreatitis
Protein S deficiency	Intra-abdominal neoplasia
Dysfibrinogenemia	Gastroenteritis; bacterial, viral, and parasitic
Platelet disorders	Inflammatory bowel disease
Myeloproliferative disease	Abdominal trauma
Heparin cofactor II deficiency	Malignancy
Pregnancy	
Puerperium	**Idiopathic (10%)**
Contraceptive pill use	
Carcinomatosis	

Source: From Ref. 1.

In general, diagnostic laboratory studies are disappointing, the exception being diagnostic peritoneal lavage, which uniformly returns serosan-guinous fluid (57,58). A leukocytosis of 10,000 to 30,000/mm^3 with a leftward shift is often present. Evaluation for a hypercoagulable state should be made if the diagnosis is suspected. Radiographs, whether plain or with contrast, rarely assist in the diagnostic process. CT has established the diagnosis in 90% of cases by demonstrating thrombus directly (1). Small bowel follow-through findings may include marked thickening of the bowel wall and valvulae conniventes because of congestion and edema, separation of loops caused by mesenteric thickening, a long transition zone between involved and uninvolved bowel with progressive narrowing of the lumen by thickened wall, and thumbprints. Angiographic findings may include the demonstration of a thrombus in the superior mesenteric vein with partial or complete occlusion, failure to visualize the superior mesenteric or portal vein, slow or absent filling of mesenteric veins, arterial spasm, failure of arterial arcades to empty, and a prolonged blush in the involved segment (7). Diagnosis frequently is made at the time of operation.

Treatment of mesenteric venous thrombosis includes fluid resuscitation, antibiotics, and prompt heparinization (1). The development of an acute abdomen requires operative intervention. Operative findings include the presence of congested, cyanotic, bluish-black, edematous bowel with arterial pulsations present in the mesentery. Thrombosed veins may be clearly visible, and sectioning across the mesentery shows thrombus extruding from the mesenteric veins and brisk arterial bleeding. Occasionally a venous thrombectomy is helpful. If a long segment of bowel is involved and there is complete thrombosis of the superior mesenteric vein with possible extension to the portal vein, venous thrombectomy is indicated. A second-look operation should be performed, at which time a better assessment of the extent of nonviable bowel is made. Heparin therapy is instituted (7). For short segments of bowel involvement, thrombectomy would not appear to be indicated. A wide resection of involved bowel is recommended with a primary end-to-end anastomosis. If there is doubt regarding the wisdom of restoring intestinal continuity, the bowel can be brought to the surface as a stoma or re-examined at a "second look." Anticoagulant therapy with heparin is indicated and should be initiated during or immediately after operation (1,59,60), and anticoagulation therapy should be continued for several months postoperatively unless specifically contraindicated by other associated diseases. Following resection, about half of the patients experience recurrence if anticoagulants are not administered, and of those with recurrence, approximately 50% are found to have an associated deep venous thrombosis or pulmonary embolus (61). In the study cited, treatment with anticoagulants dramatically decreased mortality; without operation and without anticoagulant therapy, the natural history of mesenteric venous thrombosis resulted in a 95% mortality rate; with operation but without anticoagulant therapy, the mortality rate was 65%; and with operation followed by immediate anticoagulant therapy, the mortality rate was 35% (61).

Rhee et al. (62) evaluated the outcome of 72 patients with mesenteric venous thrombosis—53 acute and 19 chronic. A laparotomy was performed in 34 patients, 31 undergoing bowel resection and one an unsuccessful mesenteric venous thrombectomy. Mesenteric venous thrombosis recurred in 36%. The 30-day mortality rate was 27%. The long-term survival of patients with acute mesenteric venous thrombosis was worse than for chronic disease (36% vs. 83% at three years).

Divino et al. (63) analyzed nine patients treated surgically for mesenteric venous thrombosis. The most common presenting symptom was abdominal pain with bloody diarrhea in three patients; preoperative diagnosis of mesenteric vein thrombosis was suspected in two. Radiologic tests included plain X rays, CT, and ultrasound. The time to operation ranged from three hours to seven days after admission. All patients underwent resection of infarcted bowel with primary anastomosis and immediate postoperative anticoagulation. No patient underwent a second-look operation. The postoperative morbidity and mortality rates were 55% and 11%, respectively.

An algorithm outlining a possible approach to the management of mesenteric ischemia was published by Bradbury et al. (Fig. 6) (1).

■ CHRONIC MESENTERIC VASCULAR DISEASE

A detailed account of chronic mesenteric vascular disease or "intestinal angina" is beyond the scope of this text, and the reader is referred to textbooks of vascular surgery. However, any discussion of acute mesenteric vascular disease would be incomplete without a brief overview of the salient points of chronic mesenteric vascular disease.

Mesenteric angina is poorly understood partly due to problems involved in diagnosing and defining the disease as a clinical syndrome. The disease is difficult to induce experimentally because the rich mesenteric collateral circulation has made it difficult to develop a satisfactory animal model. Diagnosis is further complicated by the lack of correlation between arteriographic findings and clinical symptoms. Finally, clinical studies on this disease are remarkably limited, particularly when compared with the wealth of material available on vascular disease involving other organs or organ systems.

Croft et al. (64) reviewed autopsy material on 203 patients and tried to correlate arteriographic findings with clinical symptoms and autopsy findings. Critical stenosis on two of three vessels was seen in only four of their patients, and correlation with symptoms was not found. Other researchers have reported that complaints of intestinal angina precede acute intestinal infarction in a sizable percentage of cases. Kwoan and Connolly (47) noted that they found conspicuous warning signs present for several months in all 25 patients operated on for acute intestinal infarction.

The classic triad of symptoms is postprandial pain, fear of eating, and involuntary weight loss. The most consistent symptom complex involves the presence of postprandial pain in association with weight loss and malabsorption. The postprandial pain often is associated with "food fear," causing the patient to refuse to eat because of the fear of subsequent pain. The pain, which is directly related to eating, is experienced soon after a meal and lasts for several hours. Because patients with chronic mesenteric vascular disease frequently are cachectic in appearance, they sometimes are evaluated for the presence of widespread malignancy rather than vascular disease. Color flow duplex scanning is increasingly used as the first-line investigation of patients suspected of having mesenteric ischemia. When an arteriogram is performed, high-grade stenosis or complete occlusion of three mesenteric vessels suggests that significant ischemic disease may be present. No relationship has been found between the loss of intestinal absorptive function and the degree of reduced flow seen on angiography (65). Because of the prevalence of asymptomatic arterial stenosis, the diagnosis is difficult and the indications for surgery are unclear. In general, surgery should be considered when a patient has a clinical presentation that is compatible with intestinal ischemia, arteriographic evidence of critical stenosis in two of three vessels, and no plausible explanation for the abdominal pain.

A patient with intestinal angina and weight loss, in whom other causes have been excluded, and in whom angiography shows occlusive disease of at least two of three major visceral arteries, should be considered for revascularization. Few patients meet these criteria. Surgical options for reconstruction include bypass grafting, endarterectomy, and reimplantation. Bypass grafting has been the preferred procedure (48,66), with most authors recommending prosthetic grafts over autogenous vein grafts. Prosthetic grafts have less tendency for kinking when used between the aorta and the mobile SMA. They also are more readily available than vein grafts. Total revascularization of all affected vessels is preferred to single-vessel revascularization, since this may decrease the incidence of late recurrence (48,67,68). Because of the presence of significant atherosclerotic disease in the adjacent aorta, reimplantation is seldom performed.

Illuminati et al. (69) reported on 11 patients who underwent revascularization of 11 digestive arteries for symptomatic chronic mesenteric occlusive disease. Eleven superior mesenteric arteries and one celiac axis were revascularized. The revascularization techniques included retrograde bypass grafting in seven cases, antegrade bypass grafting in two, percutaneous arterial angioplasty in one, and arterial reimplantation in one case. There was no operative mortality. Cumulative survival rate was 88.9% at 36 months. Primary patency rate was 90% at 36 months. The symptom-free rate was 90% at 36 months. They found direct reimplantation, antegrade and retrograde bypass grafting, all allowed good mid-term results: the choice of the optimal method depends on the anatomic and general patient's status. Angioplasty alone yields poor results and should be limited to patients at poor risk for operation.

Leke et al. (70) reported their experience with a tailored surgical approach of 16 patients operated on for

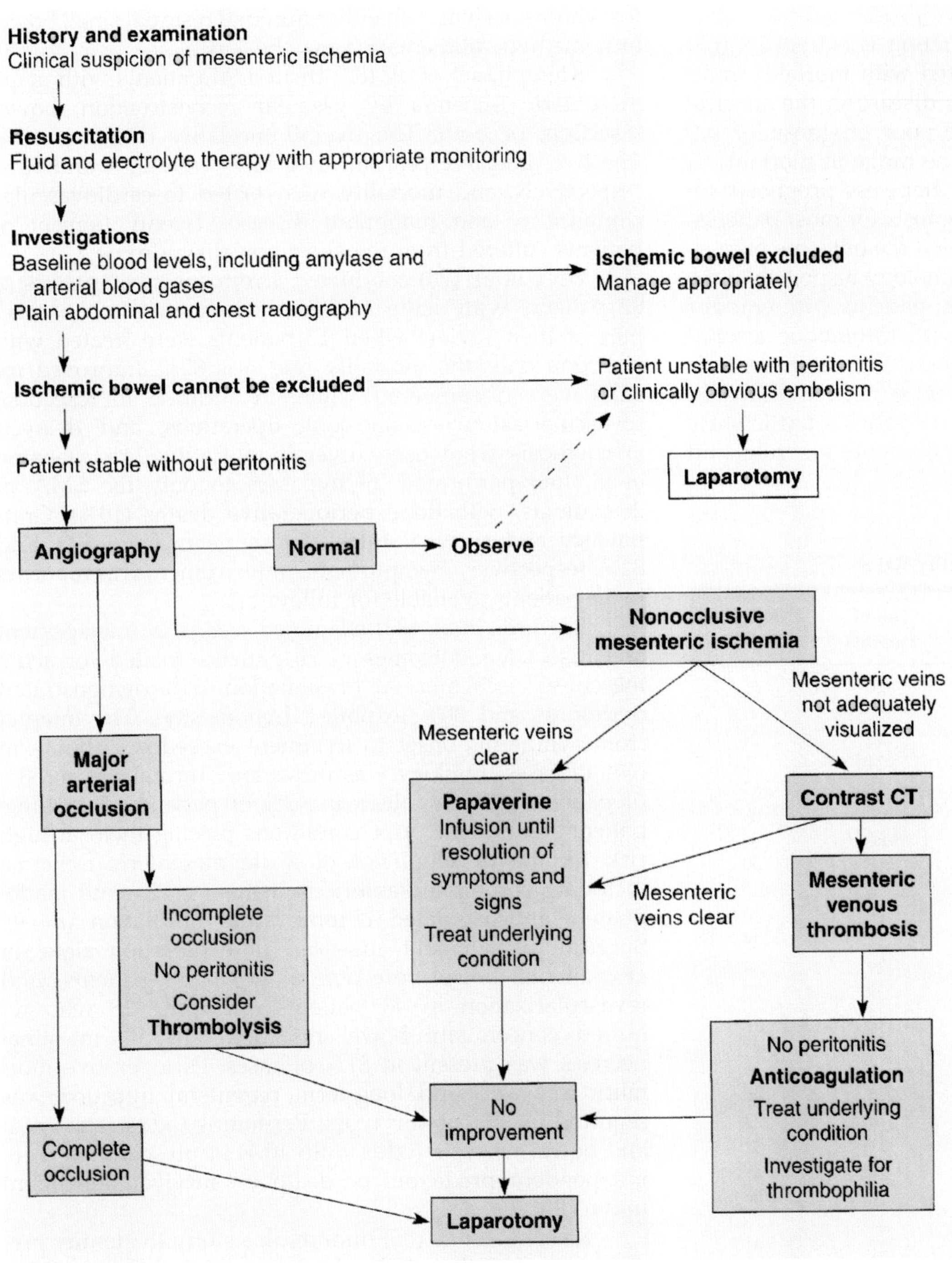

FIGURE 6 ■ Algorithm outlining possible approach to management of mesenteric ischemia. *Source*: From Ref. 1.

chronic mesenteric ischemia. The patients ranged in age from 32 to 80 years and 75% of patients were female. The most common preoperative complaints were postprandial abdominal pain and weight loss. Revascularization was tailored to the arterial anatomy and included bypass to the SMA alone (eight), bypass to the celiac artery and SMA (six), SMA reimplantation onto the aorta (one), SMA/IMA reimplantation (one), and transaortic endarterectomy of the celiac artery/SMA (one). There was one perioperative death (mortality 5.6%). Follow-up duplex scans at a mean of 34 months showed no graft thromboses.

Some early success has been reported following angioplasty for chronic mesenteric vascular disease (71–73). Success rates of 70% to 100% have been reported with recurrence rates of 10% to 50% within 4 to 28 months (1). If the patient's symptoms later recur following angioplasty, the history of having undergone successful angioplasty suggests that the patient may expect a favorable result from surgical reconstruction.

Kasirajan et al. (74) evaluated the efficacy of percutaneous angioplasty and stenting in comparison with traditional open surgical revascularization for the treatment of chronic mesenteric ischemia. Although the results of percutaneous angioplasty and stenting and open surgery were similar with respect to morbidity, death, and recurrent stenosis, percutaneous angioplasty and stenting was associated with a significantly higher incidence of recurrent symptoms and thus their suggestion that open surgery should be preferentially offered to patients deemed fit for open revascularization.

Results of Therapy

The prognosis for mesenteric infarction is extraordinarily grave, and this disease is associated with mortality rates that are among the highest of any disease in the surgical literature. Table 2 summarizes the poor prognosis of patients with mesenteric infarction; the range in mortality is from 24% to 90%. The seemingly hopeless prognosis reflects the late presentation and diagnosis for most patients.

Inderbitzi et al. (79) reported that the outcome of mesenteric ischemia varies with the pathology responsible; the mortality rate is reported as 50% in patients with embolic arterial occlusion, 95% in those with thrombotic arterial occlusion, 67% in those with nonocclusive mesenteric ischemia, and 30% in those with mesenteric thrombosis. Despite this, salvage is possible in some patients, particularly those who are younger and potentially more vigorous and for whom survival with either minimal residual small bowel or home hyperalimentation may be feasible.

TABLE 2 ■ Mesenteric Infarction Mortality Rates

Author(s)	Type of Ischemia	No. of Patients	Mortality Rate (%)
Guttormson and Bubrick (75)	IC	20	65
Levy et al. (76)	All	45	24
Brewster et al.[a] (77)	All	24	25
Parish et al. (78)	IC	16	62
Inderbitzi et al. (79)	All	100	68
	SMA e	60	50
	SMA t	15	90
	NOMI	6	67
	MVT	19	30
Longo et al. (80)	NOMI, IC	31	29
Sales et al. (44)	All	29	34
Rhee et al. (62)	MVT	31	27
Kaleya and Boley (7)	All	65	45
	SMA e	23	39
	SMA t	6	33
	NOMI	26	46
	MVT	6	33
Ward et al. (53)	NOMI	29	31
Longo et al.[a] (81)	IC	19	89
Klempnauer et al. (82)	All	90	66
	SMA e	21	76
	SMA t	27	81
	NOMI	12	83
	MVT	30	27
Divino et al. (63)	MVT	9	11
Neri et al. (55)	NOMI	73	86
Edwards et al. (83)	SMA e + t	76	62
Scharff et al. (84)	IC	129	29
Kasirajan et al. (85)	SAM e	20	60
	SAM t	55	56
	NOMI	6	38
	MVT	6	33
	Volvulus	3	33
	Hernia	8	13
Schoots et al.[b] (86)	SMA e	705	70
	SMA t	980	83
	MVT	394	45
	NOMI	556	78

[a]All patients following aortic reconstruction.
[b]Review of literature.
Abbreviations: IC, ischemic colitis; MVT, mesenteric venous thrombosis; NOMI, nonocclusive mesenteric insufficiency; SMA e, superior mesenteric artery embolus; SMA t, superior mesenteric artery thrombosis.

Klempnauer et al. (82) treated 90 patients with acute mesenteric ischemia by vascular reconstruction, bowel resection, or both. The overall mortality rate was 66%. The two- and five-year survival rates were 70% and 90%, respectively, and mortality was related to cardiovascular comorbidity and malignant disease. Twenty percent of patients suffered from the short bowel syndrome.

Levy et al. (76) conducted a retrospective analysis of 92 patients with acute mesenteric ischemia. In the early part of their review when 17 patients were treated with resection only, the mortality rate was 82%. Improved results were documented when, in addition to resection, revascularization, second-look operations, and delayed anastomosis were used (overall mortality, 24%). Gentile et al. (66) performed 29 bypasses to only the SMA in 26 patients, with three perioperative deaths (10%). Graft patency and survival rates at four years were 89% and 82%, respectively. Symptomatic improvement was reported in all patients available for follow-up.

Edwards et al. (83) examined trends in management and associated outcomes in 76 patients treated for acute mesenteric ischemia. At presentation, 64% demonstrated peritonitis and 30% exhibited hypotension. The interval from symptoms onset to treatment exceeded 24 hours in 63% of cases. Etiology was mesenteric thrombosis in 58% of patients and embolism in 42% of patients. Thirty-five patients (46%) had prior conditions placing them at high risk for the development of acute mesenteric ischemia including chronic mesenteric ischemia ($n = 26$) and inadequately anticoagulated chronic atrial fibrillation ($n = 9$). Surgical management consisted of exploration alone in 16 patients, bowel resection alone in 18 patients, and revascularization in 43 patients, including 28 who required concomitant bowel resection. Overall, intestinal necrosis was present in 81% of cases. Perioperative mortality was 62% and long-term parenteral nutrition was required in 31% of survivors. Peritonitis (odds ratio = 9.4) and bowel necrosis (odds ratio 10.4) at presentation were independent predictors of death or survival dependent upon TPN.

Kasirajan et al. (85) undertook a study to identify predictors of in-hospital death and length of stay in 107 patients diagnosed with acute bowel gangrene. Among the baseline factors that had a significant univariable association with mortality (51%) were age, symptom duration, preoperative and postoperative pH and lactic acid, history of hypertension, and renal failure. Symptom duration and history of hypertension were independent risk factors for mortality. Longer length of stay was invariably associated with symptom duration, systemic acidosis, vascular etiology, amount of resected bowel, and need for second-look procedures. The presence of multiple risk factors predictive of a high mortality rate may aid more realistic decision making for physicians, patients, and family members.

There are large differences in prognosis after acute mesenteric ischemia depending on etiology. Schoots et al. (86) analyzed the published data on survival following acute mesenteric ischemia over the past four decades in relation to disease etiology and mode of treatment. They conducted a systematic review of the available literature from 1966 to 2002 and performed quantitative analysis of data derived from 45 observational studies containing 3692 patients with acute mesenteric ischemia. They showed that the prognosis after acute mesenteric venous thrombosis is better than that following acute arterial mesenteric ischemia, the prognosis after mesenteric arterial embolism is better than that after arterial thrombosis or nonocclusive ischemia, the mortality rate following surgical treatment of arterial embolism and venous thrombosis (54.1% and 32.1%, respectively) is less than that after surgery for arterial thrombosis and nonocclusive ischemia (77.4% and 72.7%, respectively), and the overall survival after acute mesenteric ischemia has improved over the past four decades but overall is still only 28.4%. Surgical treatment of arterial embolism has improved outcome whereas the mortality rate following surgery for arterial thrombosis and nonocclusive ischemia remains poor.

Johnson et al. (48) reviewed the results of 21 patients who underwent arterial bypass grafts for the treatment of chronic ischemia. There were no intraoperative deaths. Survival at one year was 100%, 86% at three years, and 79% at five years. During follow-up, graft thrombosis occurred in three patients. Of the patients who underwent only a single SMA or celiac bypass, two of five died of bowel infarction; only one of 16 patients who underwent both celiac and SMA bypass had to undergo a repeat procedure because of graft occlusion. The authors' review of the literature, which encompassed eight other reports, revealed operative mortality rates ranging from 0% to 12%. In a series of 58 patients, McAfee et al. (68) reported a five-year survival rate of 73% for three-vessel repairs, 57% for two-vessel repairs, and 0% for one-vessel repair.

■ ISCHEMIC COLITIS

Colonic ischemia is the most common form of ischemic injury to the gut. It is usually focal, nonocclusive, and commonly involves a "watershed" area, typically the splenic flexure. A precipitating cause is found in fewer than 20% of patients. The syndrome of ischemic colitis has been defined only relatively recently. In 1963, Boley et al. (87) described a reversible component to colonic ischemia, and three years later Marston et al. (88) reported on the three stages of ischemic colitis and described the natural history of the disease. The incidence of ischemic colitis in general populations ranged from 4.5 to 44 cases per 100,000 person-years (89). The risk was increased two- to four-fold by either prevalent irritable bowel syndrome or chronic obstructive pulmonary disease. Most cases occur between the sixth and ninth decade of life, with men slightly more prone to this disease than women (90). However, other investigators found no significant sex predilection, while still others found the risk increased in females and in persons 65 years and older (7,89).

Etiology

Ischemic colitis is usually not associated with major vascular occlusion. The colon has a generous overlapping blood supply, with contributions from the SMA, IMA, and hypogastric arteries. Two regions that are believed to be anatomically vulnerable to ischemic disease are "Griffith's point," at the splenic flexure corresponding to the junction of the SMA (left branch of middle colic) and the IMA (ascending branch of left colon), and "Sudeck's critical point," corresponding to the junction of the IMA (last sigmoid branch) and hypogastric systems. A watershed phenomenon has been described to explain the vulnerability of these points, since perfusion between the overlapping circulations may be inadequate during periods of hemodynamic insult. Because of the vulnerability of the colon at the sigmoid and splenic flexure, these areas have historically been considered to be the most frequent sites of clinical ischemic colitis. The sigmoid site is probably not a clinically significant factor.

Occlusive events and low-flow states both have been associated with ischemic injury to the colon. The severity of ischemic colitis is influenced by several factors, including the duration of the decrease in blood flow, the caliber of occluded vessel, the rapidity of onset of ischemia, the metabolic requirements of the affected bowel, the presence of associated conditions such as colonic distention, the adequacy of collateral circulation, and the concentration and virulence of colonic bacteria (91). Colonic bacteria become a factor in the severity of the disease once the mucosal barrier has been compromised. For this reason, colonic ischemia may be less severe when it occurs postoperatively in patients who have undergone preoperative mechanical and antibiotic bowel cleansing. Lastly, distention of the involved colon segment is of importance because distention of the colonic lumen will compromise the transmural blood flow to that segment (92).

A number of predisposing factors that are associated with the development of ischemic colitis have been defined (Table 3) (93). In the largest series of patients with ischemic colitis studied for coagulation defects in the United States, the prevalence of clotting disorders was 28%; higher than that in the general population (8.4%) (94). Koutroubakis et al. (95) investigated the role of acquired and hereditary thrombotic risk factors in patients with a definite diagnosis of colon ischemia. The prevalence of antiphospholipid antibodies was significantly higher in patients with colon ischemia compared with inflammatory and healthy controls (19.4% vs. 0% and 1.9%). Among genetic factors only factor V Leiden was significantly associated with colon ischemia (22.2% vs. 0% and 3.8%). A combination of thrombophilic disorders was found in 25% of the cases. A comprehensive thrombophilic screening in colon ischemia revealed a congenital or acquired thrombophilic state in 72% of patients. This may represent evidence supporting the possible role of acquired and hereditary thrombotic risk factors in the pathogenesis of ischemic colitis (95). Low plasma protein Z levels may play a role in the disease development in some cases with ischemic colitis. Protein Z deficiency was found in patients' cases with ischemic colitis (18.2%) compared to diverticulitis (7.7%) and controls (3.0%) (96).

A host of drugs have reportedly been responsible for the development of ischemic colitis. Acute ischemic colitis has also been caused by an allergy to amoxicillin (97). The damage to the gut seemed to occur as a result of the hypotension suffered during an anaphylactic episode. A case of ischemic colitis possibly linked to the use of a

TABLE 3 ■ Colonic Ischemia: Etiologic Factors

Idiopathic (spontaneous)	Small vessel disease—*continued*	Medications—*continued*
Major vascular occlusion	Systemic vasculitis disorders	Gold
Trauma	Systemic lupus erythematosus	Nonsteroidal anti-inflammatory drugs
Thrombosis, embolization of mesenteric arteries	Polyarteritis nodosa	Neuroleptics
Arterial embolus	Allergic granulomatosis	Colonic obstruction
Cholesterol embolus	Scleroderma	Colon carcinoma
Aortography	Behçet's syndrome	Adhesions
Colectomy with inferior mesenteric artery ligation	Takayasu's arteritis	Stricture
Midgut ischemia	Thromboangiitis obliterans	Diverticular disease
Postabdominal aortic reconstruction	Buerger's disease	Rectal prolapse
Mesenteric venous thrombosis	Shock	Fecal impaction
Hypercoagulable states	Cardiac failure	Volvulus
Portal hypertension	Hypovolemia	Strangulated hernia
Pancreatitis	Sepsis	Pseudo-obstruction
Small vessel disease	Neurogenic insult	Hematologic disorders
Diabetes mellitus	Anaphylaxis	Sickle-cell disease
Rheumatoid arthritis	Medications	Protein C deficiency
Amyloidosis	Digitalis preparations	Protein S deficiency
Radiation injury	Diuretics	Antithrombin III deficiency
	Catecholamines	Cocaine abuse
	Estrogens	Long distance running
	Danazol	

Source: From Ref. 93.

weight loss drug Phentermine has been reported (98). Ischemic colitis has reportedly been associated with paclitaxel and carboplatin chemotherapy (99,100).

The FDA MedWatch system received 20 spontaneous reports of ischemic colitis associated with the use of tegaserod (Zelnorm) an agent used for the short-term treatment of constipation-predominant irritable bowel syndrome in women (101). The manufacturer of the drug states that in over 11,600 patients using tegaserod with a total of 3456 patient-years of exposure, no case of ischemic colitis was reported. They further note that patients with irritable bowel syndrome are approximately 3 to 4 times as likely to receive a diagnosis of ischemic colitis as are patients without irritable bowel syndrome. They also report that during postmarketing surveillance, 21 cases of ischemic colitis were reported worldwide. On the basis of worldwide use of Tegaserod, a postmarketing incidence of seven cases of ischemic colitis for 100,000 patient-years can be calculated. This approximates the incidence of ischemic colitis in the general population (7–47 cases per 100,000 patient-years) and significantly lower than that in the population of patients with irritable bowel syndrome (43–179 cases per 100,000 patient-years). Tegaserod therapy should be reserved for specific patients (women with irritable bowel syndrome and constipation) who have more moderate to severe symptoms (102). The duration of treatment should not exceed 12 weeks and therapy should be stopped after four weeks if there has been no response. Patients should be warned that they may experience potentially serious diarrhea or rarely intestinal ischemia. They should be advised to seek prompt medical attention if serious diarrhea, lightheadedness, or postural symptoms develop during treatment. The drug should be immediately stopped if rectal bleeding or new or worsening abdominal pain develops.

Frossard et al. (103) reported two cases of ischemic colitis in young women attributed to a high level of circulating estrogens due to pregnancy in the first case and the second due to oral contraceptive medication. Ischemic colitis has been reported with alosetron, a potent and selective serotonin antagonist that is used to treat diarrhea-predominant IBS (104). Meloxicam used to treat osteoarthritis has reportedly been a cause of ischemic colitis (105).

Cocaine use can result in visceral infarction, intestinal ischemia, and gastrointestinal tract perforation. Linder et al. (106) reported cocaine-associated colonic ischemia in three patients, and including theirs, 28 cases have been reported in the literature. Cocaine is a potentially life-threatening cause of ischemic colitis.

Dowd et al. (107) reported four cases linking ischemic colitis and orally administered nasal decongestants containing pseudoephedrine. On colonoscopy, all four patients had colitis primarily affecting the splenic flexure in the anatomical watershed area. Colonoscopic biopsies were consistent with ischemic injury. All cases responded to abstinence from pseudoephedrine and medical supportive therapy. None had a relapse since discontinuing the pseudoephedrine (8–12 months). The vasoconstrictive action of pseudoephedrine may predispose susceptible patients to develop ischemic colitis in the watershed area of the splenic flexure. Knudsen et al. (108) reported on the development of eight serious cases of ischemic colitis in patients with migraine treated with Sumatriptan.

To the already long list of conditions that predispose to intestinal ischemia, operative procedures such as cardiac bypass and gynecologic operations as well as colonoscopy and barium enema should be added (2). Mesenteric colitis following colonoscopy has been reported (109). Transient ischemic colitis following an airplane flight as the only predisposing factor has been reported (110). Ischemic colitis has been reported in patients with strict dieting (111). Ischemic colitis has been associated with herbal product ingestion (112).

Dee et al. (113) found that 3.1% of patients developed ischemia of the small and large bowel or both within 20 days after renal transplantation and 54.5% died as a result. The most prominent segment involved was the terminal ileum and ascending colon. Right colon involvement is associated with severe forms of ischemic colitis and occurs frequently in patients with chronic renal failure requiring hemodialysis (114).

A case of ischemic colitis associated with pheochromocytoma has been reported (115). Mesenteric inflammatory veno-occlusive disease is a rare cause of mesenteric ischemia that is diagnosed by histologic examination of the operative specimen. Complete resolution of the process following resection confirms a relative benign course of this disease (116).

Ischemic colitis is a rare but serious consequence of long-distance running (117). Physiologic shunting due to splanchnic vasoconstriction, intravascular volume depletion due to chronic dehydration, and possibly some element of hypercoaguability due to secondary polycythemia may have been causative factors. Ischemic colitis associated with the use of electrical muscle stimulation device exercise equipment has been reported (118). Ischemic colitis has been reported after flexible endoscopy in patients with connective tissue disorders (119,120), and the hemolytic uremic syndrome (121).

Walker et al. (122) sought predictors of colon ischemia in a group of 700 persons at least 20 years old with presumed colon ischemia and 6440 controls. Patients with colon ischemia were nearly three times as likely to have IBS than controls. A history of nonspecific colitis, lower gastrointestinal hemorrhage, systemic rheumatologic disorders, ischemic heart disease in the preceding six months, and abdominal surgery in the past month were also much more common in colon ischemia cases than controls. Use of a drug to treat diarrhea was strongly associated with risk. The most prevalent risk factor for colon ischemia was the use of drugs with the side effect of constipation, found in one-third of cases and one in nine controls. Cases had seen physicians, particularly gastroenterologists, much more commonly in the preceding six months than had controls. They concluded that clinically evident colon ischemia arose preferentially in persons with prior abdominal symptoms, many of whom carried a diagnosis of IBS. Drugs that reduce bowel motility may constitute a widespread and potentially avoidable risk factor. The frequency of a preceding doctor visit, without a specific diagnosis, suggested that colon ischemia might have a prolonged subacute presentation.

Classification

The three degrees of severity of ischemic colitis as classified by Marston et al. (88) include transient ischemia, ischemic stricture as a late sequela of a partial-thickness injury, and the gangrenous form. Gangrenous injury is seen in 15% to 20% of cases. Of the 80% to 85% of nongangrenous cases, most are transient and reversible. Chronic damage in the form of persistent segmental colitis occurs in 20% to 25% and strictures in 10% to 15% of cases (93).

The transient form is characterized by its reversibility and is associated with mucosal edema, congestion, superficial ulcerations, and petechiae (Fig. 7). Histologically, the

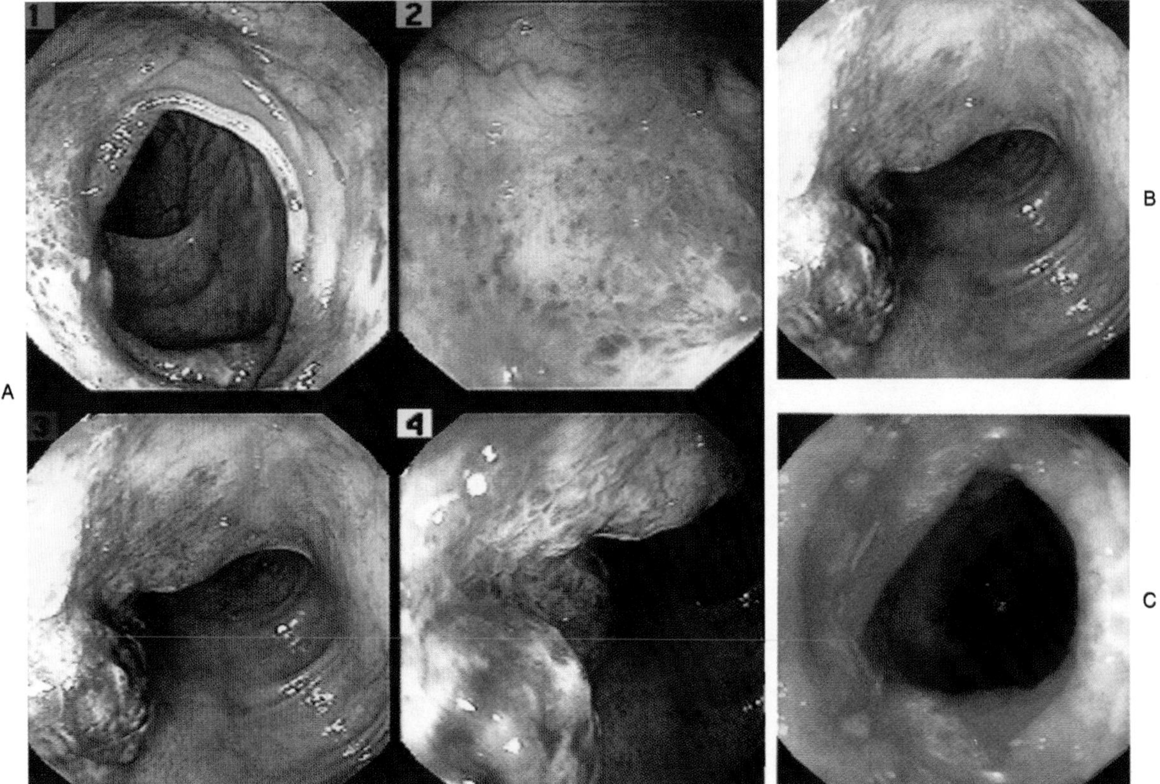

FIGURE 7 ■ (**A**) Acute, mild stage characterized by hyperemia, edema, and petechiae. 1 = mass, mid-transverse colon; 2 = mass, mid-transverse colon; 3 = mass, mid-ascending colon; 4 = mass, mid-ascending colon. (**B**) Acute stage with edema and submucosal hemorrhage. (**C**) Subacute stage consisting of edema, exudation, and ulceration. *Source*: Courtesy of David Morowitz, M.D., Washington, D.C.

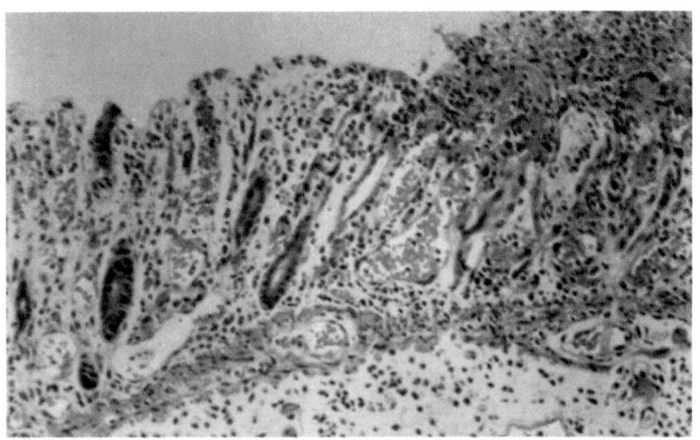

FIGURE 8 ■ Microscopic section of transient ischemic colitis showing sloughing and infiltration of the mucosa.

changes are confined predominantly to the mucosa and submucosa and consist of an intense inflammatory reaction with superficial sloughing of the mucosa, submucosal hemorrhage, and edema (Fig. 8). Multiple superficial ulcerations may develop. Gradually the blood is resorbed, and the edema resolves with complete structural and functional recovery in 1 to 2 weeks. Characteristic radiographic findings are either thumbprinting caused by submucosal hemorrhage or pseudotumors that reflect distortion of the bowel lumen by the same process (Fig. 9). Reoperative processes can return these changes to normal if perfusion is restored at this stage. On occasion patchy areas of acute ischemic colitis may be found on screening colonoscopy on many asymptomatic patients (Fig. 10A,B,C).

The ischemic stricture represents a partial-thickness injury that involves the mucosa and muscular layers and results in fibrosis and narrowing of the lumen over a period of weeks to months. Endoscopically, the stricture is characterized by fixed narrowing of the lumen and a mucosa that is replaced by granulation tissue (Fig. 11). Histologically, marked fibrosis is seen within the muscularis, the mucosa is replaced by granulation tissue, and hemosiderin-laden macrophages are prevalent (Fig. 12). On barium enema the stricture appears as an area of irreversible narrowing of the lumen. Dilatation proximal to the stricture suggests that the stricture may be significant, while the presence of a simple asymptomatic stricture may not be of clinical importance (Fig. 13).

Gangrenous ischemic colitis is characterized by full-thickness necrosis and infarction. Gross examination reveals the segment to be dilated with patchy or confluent gray-green or black discoloration (Fig. 14). Histologic sections reveal intense inflammation with transmural necrosis (Fig. 15). Contrast studies should be avoided in the presence of suspected gangrenous changes. Patients with gangrenous change will go on to perforation, sepsis, and death unless surgical intervention is undertaken promptly.

Despite similarities in the initial presentation of most episodes of colonic ischemia, the outcome of any single event cannot be predicted at its onset unless the initial physical findings indicate an intra-abdominal catastrophe. The clinical spectrum of colonic ischemia along with the relative frequencies of each type as reported by Brandt and Boley (123) is shown in Figure 16.

Patterns of Involvement

The reported anatomic site of involvement of ischemic colitis has varied considerably from series to series. Historically, ischemic colitis has been described as usually involving, or at least being most severe, near the splenic flexure where the arterial supply is a watershed area between the territories of the SMA and IMA. Numerous reports support this pattern of involvement (124–126). In a review of 1024 patients in the literature, Reeders et al. (90) found the incidence to be as follows: right colon, 8%;

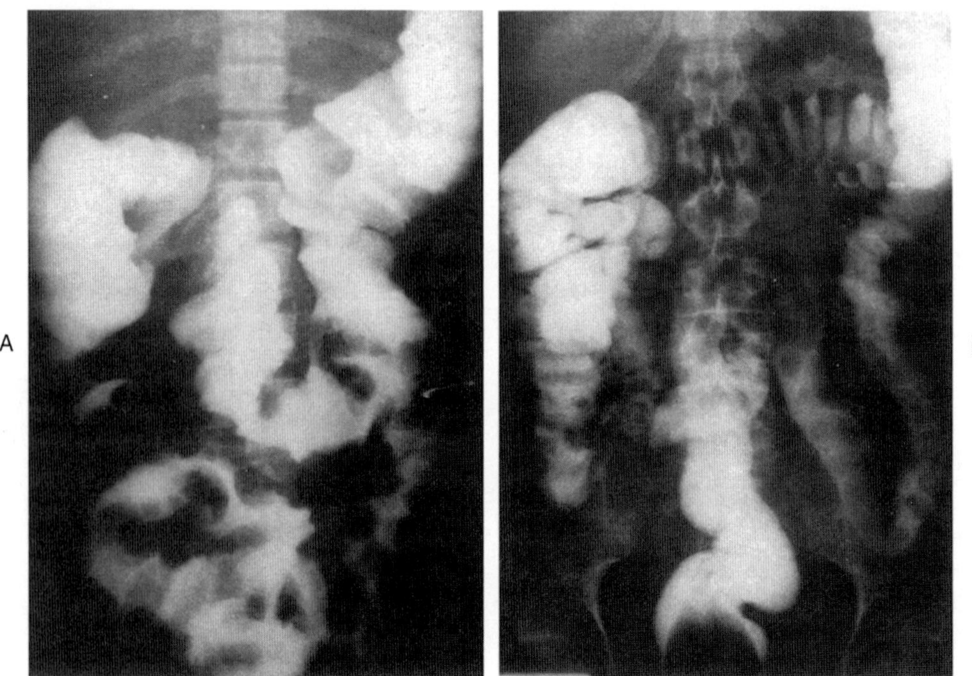

FIGURE 9 ■ (**A**) X-ray film of patient with ischemic colitis with thumbprinting seen in sigmoid colon. (**B**) X-ray film of patient with ischemic colitis segment showing pseudotumor formation in descending colon and sigmoid.

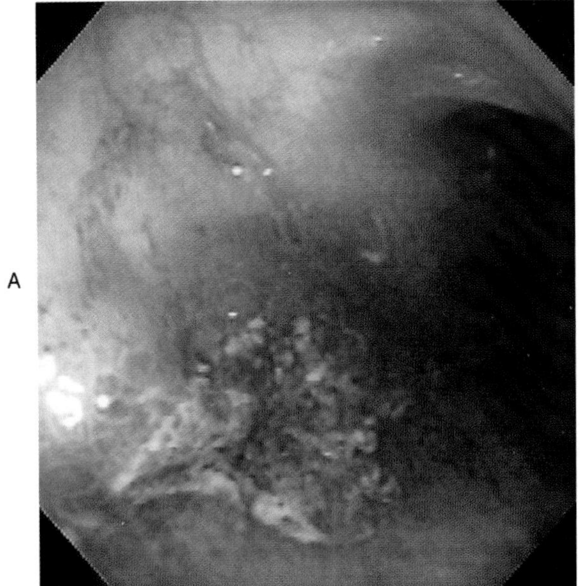

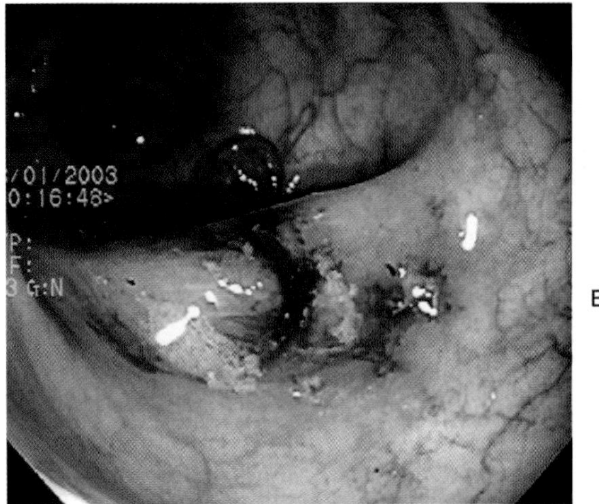

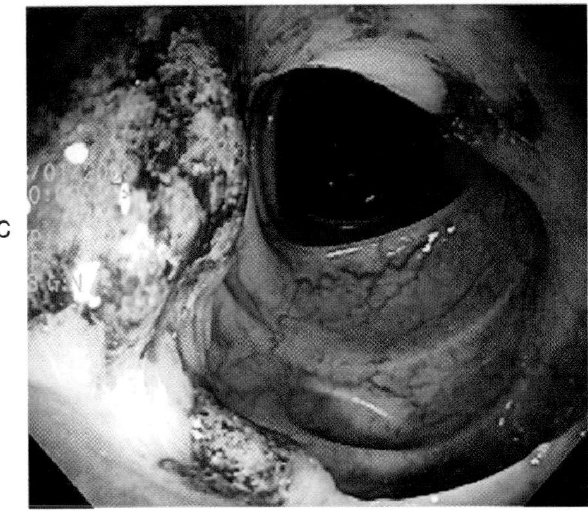

FIGURE 10 ■ (**A**) Mild ischemic colopathy; (**B**) isolated ischemic patch; (**C**) more dramatic patchy acute ischemic colitis.

transverse colon, 15%; splenic flexure, 23%; descending colon, 27%; and sigmoid colon, 23%. Rectal ischemia has been described in 4% of the cases in the above review, and only rarely does it progress to gangrene (127). A different pattern was found by Guttormson and Bubrick (75), who noted that ischemic disease can occur on the right side with equal or greater frequency, despite the richer blood supply to this segment of colon. Longo et al. (80) also reported in their series that the anatomic distribution of disease was different than that usually reported with ischemic colitis: right colon, 46%; splenic flexure, 4%; descending colon, 7%; rectosigmoid, 40%; and pancolitis, 8%. Others have also found a predilection for the right side of the colon (128).

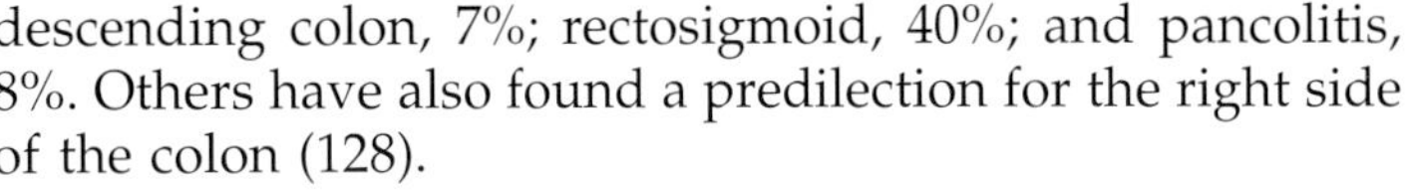

Clinical Manifestations

The presentation of this disease is variable. It frequently occurs in the elderly and debilitated patient, often in

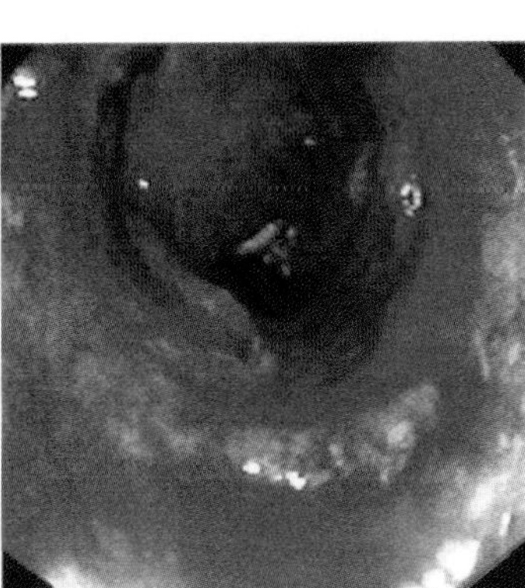

FIGURE 11 ■ Chronic stage with mucosal granularity, decreased haustration, and stricture.

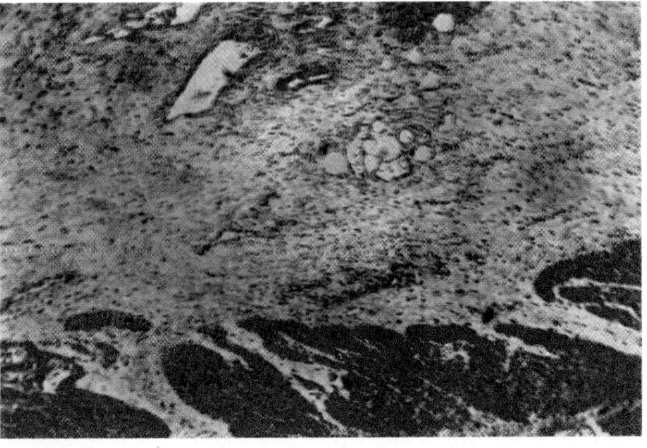

FIGURE 12 ■ Histologic section of ischemic stricture showing intense fibrosis.

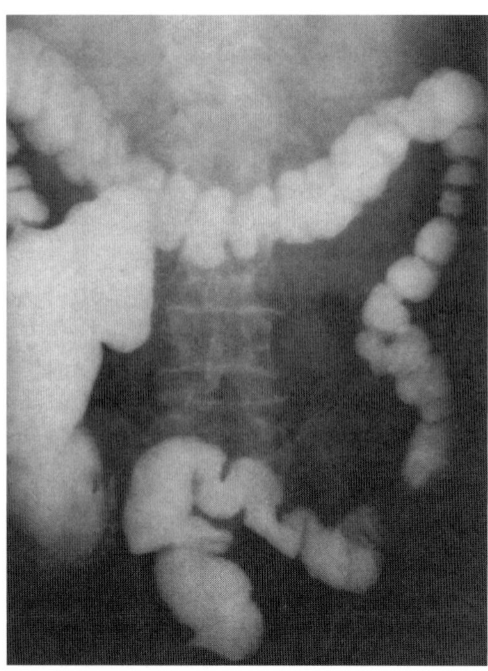

FIGURE 13 ■ X-ray film showing ischemic stricture of junction of descending and sigmoid colon.

association with severe comorbid disease. The medical diseases found most frequently by Longo et al. (80) were cardiovascular, 55%; diabetes mellitus, 23%; pulmonary, 21%; renal failure, 6%; and hematologic, 6%. The precipitating factors may not be evident. The outcome rests on numerous factors, including severity, extent, and rapidity of the ischemic insult in addition to the therapy given (93).

The symptoms of ischemic colitis include the sudden onset of crampy abdominal pain, usually on the left side if the disease involves the left side of the colon. There may be bloody diarrhea and often fever and abdominal distention. Blood loss is usually minimal. An urge to defecate may accompany the pain. Anorexia, nausea, and vomiting secondary to associated ileus may be present.

Newman and Cooper (129) compared the incidence and clinical characteristics of lower gastrointestinal bleeding due to ischemic colitis with those of lower gastrointestinal bleeding of other causes. Of 124 patients with lower GI bleeding, 24 cases were due to ischemic colitis, 62 to diverticulosis, 11 to inflammatory bowel disease, and 27 to other causes. The average age of patients

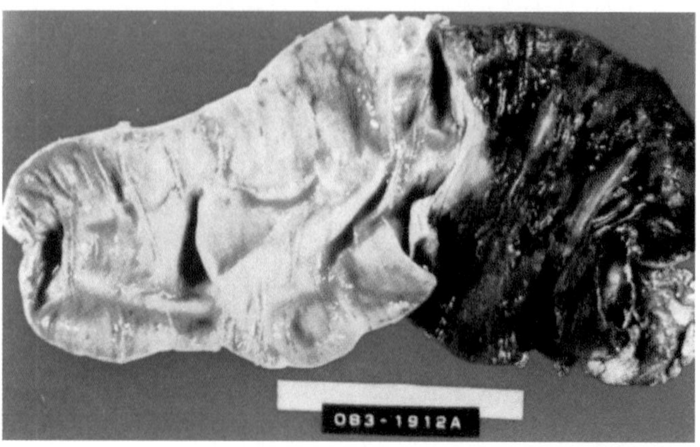

FIGURE 14 ■ Gross specimen of infarcted colonic segment.

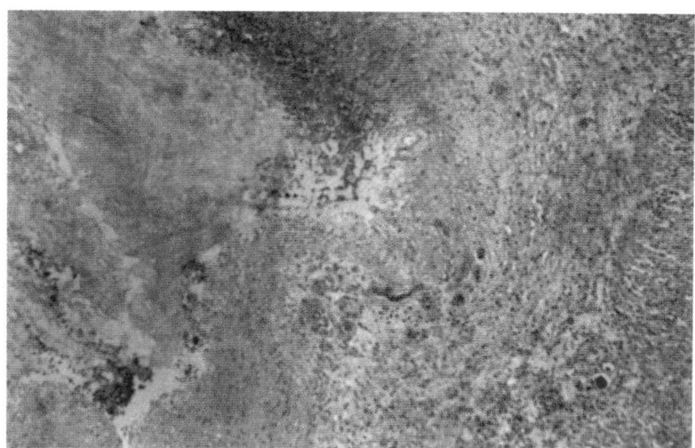

FIGURE 15 ■ Histologic section of infarcted segment of colon showing intense full-thickness inflammatory changes and necrosis.

in each group was 65.5, 76.5, 40.5, and 77.5 years, respectively. Patients with ischemic colitis were statistically younger than those with diverticular bleeding and others. The three patients with ischemic colitis underwent blood transfusion, while 23 with diverticulosis, 15 others, and none with IBD received blood. Three patients with ischemic colitis and one patient from the others group died. More women (75) than men (49) had lower GI bleeding—in total and within each group. Of women with lower GI bleeding, many more with ischemic colitis (44.4%) than with diverticulosis (3.0%), IBD (0%), or others (5.6%) were taking estrogen. In their series, ischemic colitis was the second most common cause of lower GI bleeding.

Ardigo et al. (130) reported two cases of spontaneous anal passage of a large bowel "cast" caused by acute ischemic injury. Their literature review revealed six cases of passage of a large bowel cast. In the eight total patients, infarcted muscularis propria was found in seven patients, five patients had a diversion procedure, and seven survived.

Abdominal examination may reveal mild distention and varying degrees of tenderness that usually correspond to the site of the ischemic colon. Rectal examination reveals stools positive for occult blood. Patients with the gangrenous variety may exhibit the picture of an abdominal catastrophe with signs of sepsis and shock. For patients hospitalized with another critical illness, a nonresolving ileus might raise the suspicion of an ischemic colitis.

Ullery et al. (131) reviewed charts of 100 patients with an ICD-9 code for mesenteric or intestinal ischemia. Compared to patients with mesenteric ischemia, those with colonic ischemia were older (61 vs. 77 years), were more likely to present with gastrointestinal bleeding (11% vs. 90%), and were less likely to report abdominal pain as their primary complaint (89% vs. 10%), or to receive a correct emergency department diagnosis (75% vs. 9%). Preventza et al. (132) investigated the demographics, etiology, clinical features, and prognosis of ischemic colitis in 39 young adults (<50 years of age). The mean age at diagnosis was 38 years; the female to male ratio was 1.8. Fifty-two percent of women were using oral contraceptives at the time of diagnosis. Other potential associations identified were vascular thromboembolism (four of 39), vasoactive drugs (four of 39), hypovolemia (four of 39), and vasculitis (two of 39); 19 patients (49%) had no identifiable predisposing factors.

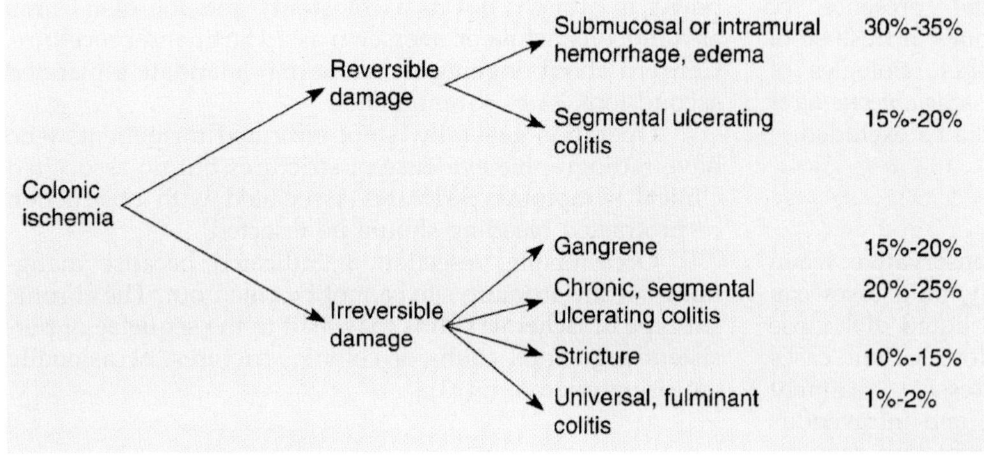

FIGURE 16 ■ Clinical spectrum of colonic ischemia. Relative frequencies of each type as reported by Brandt and Boley. *Source*: From Ref. 123.

Dominant presenting symptoms were abdominal pain (77%), bloody diarrhea (54%), and hematochezia (51%). Most patients were diagnosed at colonoscopy, and most disease was left-sided. Twenty-nine patients were successfully managed with intravenous fluids, broad-spectrum antibiotics, and bowel rest; 10 patients required operation. There was one disease-related death in the operative group.

Diagnosis

Unfortunately, there are no specific diagnostic tests. Patients usually exhibit leukocytosis. Abdominal series may reveal thickened bowel, suggest thumbprinting, or exhibit a distended colon. In a rare circumstance, toxic megacolon may supervene (133). A plain radiograph that demonstrates free air secondary to perforation, air within the bowel wall, or portal venous gas signifies colonic infarction and mandates emergency laparotomy. CT demonstrates only nonspecific findings, such as a thickened bowel wall (134). Ultrasonography has been reported to aid in the diagnosis but is not widely used (135).

There are no reliable serum markers of intestinal viability. Lange and Jackel (136) reported that a raised serum lactate concentration is the best marker for mesenteric ischemia. In a study of 85 patients with acute abdominal symptoms, the authors found that a raised plasma lactate concentration was always a sign of a life-threatening condition and usually indicated the need for an emergency operation. As a marker of mesenteric ischemia, its sensitivity was 100% and its specificity was 42%.

In the past, diagnosis was made by barium enema or exploratory laparotomy, but in recent years colonoscopy has been used with increased accuracy (75,137). Hemorrhagic nodules seen at colonoscopy represent bleeding into the submucosa. Sequential colonoscopies may confirm the diagnosis of colonic ischemia and help ascertain the outcome of the ischemic injury. The initial examination should be performed early because thumbprinting dissipates within days as the submucosal hemorrhages are either absorbed or evacuated into the colon lumen when the overlying mucosa ulcerates and sloughs. If ischemic colitis is not demonstrated, colonoscopy can help identify other forms of inflammatory bowel disease or rule out a malignancy. Areas of gray and green or black mucosa and submucosa are seen in patients with transmural infarction. Biopsy may be helpful in differentiating the disease from inflammatory processes, such as granulomatous colitis or atypical ulcerative colitis. Histologic evidence of mucosal infarction or ghost cells is pathognomonic of ischemia but is rare (93). Biopsies usually display nonspecific inflammatory changes. Other changes include vascular congestion, damage in the superficial half of the mucosa, loss of mucin and surface epithelial cells, and degeneration of normal crypt architecture. In the stricture phase, fibrosis dominates the biopsy picture.

The diagnosis of ischemic colitis depends on the recognition of clinical features (2). In patients in whom colonic ischemia is suspected but no signs of peritonitis are present, a sigmoidoscopy should be performed to identify mucosal changes. Computed tomography imaging is usually nonspecific and may only show thickening of the bowel wall. Mesenteric angiography usually has no role in the diagnosis of colon ischemia, because the mesenteric vessels and arcades are usually patent.

An excellent discussion of the differential diagnosis was presented by Gandhi et al. (93). According to their following description, *acute mesenteric arterial insufficiency* is characterized by significant abdominal pain. Patients also often have a history of previous distal emboli, dysrhythmias, or atherosclerotic heart disease. The diagnosis is established by arteriography. *Mesenteric venous occlusion* is characterized by the insidious onset of abdominal discomfort. Progression of disease is accompanied by more severe symptoms of crampy or diffuse abdominal pain, distention, or vomiting. Approximately 20% of cases are idiopathic, but the remainder is associated with liver disease, inflammatory bowel disease, hematologic disease, or hypercoagulable states, particularly malignancy. Ultrasonographic or CT scanning may reveal a lack of patency of the mesenteric veins, and venous filling will not be seen on arteriography. In the younger population, the possibility of *inflammatory bowel disease* should be entertained.

Patients with *acute diverticulitis* usually present with abdominal pain that is localized to the left lower quadrant; it may be related to a recent bowel movement. Up to 25% of patients will have had a previous attack. Physical examination reveals localized peritonitis in the left lower quadrant. Contrast enemas and a CT scan may reveal the diagnosis. *Infectious colitis* may also be mistaken for the ischemic variety. Watery diarrhea, fever, leukocytosis, and recent antibiotic usage characterize *pseudomembranous colitis*. Proctosigmoidoscopic examination may illustrate diffuse edema, multiple ulcerations, and the presence of pseudomembranes. Evidence of trophozoites in fresh stool specimens documents *amebic colitis.* Other etiologies of acute abdominal pain, such as *bowel obstruction, peptic ulcer disease, volvulus,* and *pancreatitis,* must also be excluded.

Treatment

Treatment of ischemic colitis can be conservative when the diagnosis is made early. Occasionally, mild cases can be managed on an outpatient basis with liquid diet, close observation, and possibly antibiotics. More serious cases require hospitalization, and more aggressive treatment includes bowel rest, nasogastric suction, and intravenous fluid replacement. Parenteral hyperalimentation may be helpful when a protracted course is suspected or the disease has been associated with underlying nutritional deficiencies. Antibiotics that are effective against both aerobic and anaerobic bacteria should be started. Cardiac function and oxygen delivery are optimized, and medications that may contribute to colonic ischemia are withdrawn if possible. Agents such as papaverine and dextran have been used to improve flow, but their value has not been proved. Patients who fail to improve on a conservative regimen should be treated surgically.

Patients with chronic segmental colitis should be treated symptomatically. Local steroid enemas may be of some benefit (93). The successful treatment of a patient with chronic segmental ischemic colitis suffering from persistent fever and diarrhea with 1500 mg mesalamine/day has been reported (138). Colonoscopy revealed multiple ulcers including a broad longitudinal one and erosions on friable and edematous mucosa of the sigmoid colon and rectum. A follow-up colonoscopy revealed a healing mucosa. Recurrent episodes of sepsis in otherwise asymptomatic patients with unhealed areas of segmental colitis may be an indication for resection.

Specific indications for operation include peritonitis, perforation, recurrent fever or sepsis, clinical deterioration in patients refractory to medical management with continuation of symptoms beyond 2 to 3 weeks, and gangrene visualized endoscopically. Other indications include fulminant colitis, massive hemorrhage, chronic protein losing colopathy, and symptomatic ischemic stricture (2). At operation, a wide resection of nonviable bowel should be performed. Intraoperative assessment of colonic viability may prove difficult. A palpable pulse in the SMA will rule out a correctable cause of midgut ischemia. With a normal-appearing serosa, determination of viability may be achieved with colonoscopy, evaluation of the antimesenteric serosal surface by hand-held continuous wave Doppler, tonometric measurement of intramural pH, pulse oximetry of transcolonic oxygen saturation, or intravenous fluorescein (93). It is still wise to open the resected specimen to inspect for mucosal injury. This is especially critical if an anastomosis is being considered. The surgeon should not be fooled by the dark appearance of mucosa secondary to melanosis coli, in which case the blood supply is normal and extended resection because of "black" mucosa is not necessary.

Primary anastomosis is usually unsafe in this setting, because postoperative progression of the ischemia can compromise the anastomotic site. The proximal limb of bowel is brought out as a colostomy and the distal limb as a mucous fistula or oversewn as a Hartmann procedure. Concern about ongoing ischemia may mandate a planned second look 24 to 48 hours later.

Operation generally is not indicated for patients who have radiographic evidence of strictures but no associated clinical symptoms. Strictures associated with obstruction or protracted bleeding should be resected.

Occasionally, resection is indicated because malignancy at the stricture site cannot be ruled out. The chronic subtype of ischemic colitis may lead to the sequelae of persistent segmental colitis or colonic strictures, occasionally requiring operation (93).

Results

The prognosis on the outcome for ischemic colitis varies considerably.

Abel and Russell (139) reported the management of 18 patients with ischemic colitis, nine of whom were treated conservatively with a mortality rate of 45% and nine of whom required an operation with a mortality rate of 55%. Reeders et al. (90) reported the results of treatment of 199 patients with ischemic colitis. Thirty-five patients underwent immediate operation for peritonitis, and all died. The remaining 164 patients were initially managed nonoperatively. Ninety-eight patients continued conservative treatment throughout their hospitalization, 57% of whom died. Among the remaining 66 patients initially treated nonoperatively who ultimately required an operation for progression of the disease, 51% died.

Longo et al. (80) identified 47 patients with nonocclusive ischemia of the large intestine. Overall, 15 of 16 patients were successfully treated nonoperatively with bowel rest and antibiotics, one of whom died. Among the 31 patients requiring resection, intestinal continuity was re-established in 14. Second-look laparotomies in eight patients revealed further ischemia in two (20%). The mortality rate in the operative group was 29%. No patient developed recurrent ischemia in a mean follow-up of 5.3 years. The authors found that while the course may be self-limited, elderly and diabetic patients as well as those developing ischemia following aortic surgery or hypotension continued to have a poor prognosis.

Parish et al. (78) reported on 38 patients identified with ischemic colitis. Among patients with spontaneous disease, the mortality rate was 24% compared with 54% in postoperative patients. Of the 16 patients requiring operative intervention, the mortality rate was 62%. In patients who required reoperation, the operative mortality rate was 88%. The mortality rate for nonoperative treatment was 14%. Guttormson and Bubrick (75) reviewed 39 patients with ischemic colitis and found an overall mortality rate of 53% (42% nonoperative treatment and 65% operative treatment). The authors' data showed a close association between ischemic colitis and a number of serious systemic diseases, including renal failure, arteriosclerotic heart disease, vascular disease, and hematologic, vasculitic, and connective tissue disorders.

Longo et al. (140) studied the outcome of 43 patients with ischemic colitis. Diagnosis was established by colonoscopy in 72%, whereas in the remainder diagnosis was made in the operating room. Ischemic colitis developed in the hospital in 40% of patients during admission for an unrelated illness. Segmental colitis was present in 72% of patients and 35% of these patients were successfully managed nonoperatively. In the patients with segmental colitis who required operation, the 30-day mortality rate was 22%. Among 17 patients with segmental ischemia treated by resection and stoma, 75% underwent eventual stoma closure.

Guivarc'h et al. (141) reported their experience in 88 cases of ischemic colitis including 76 cases of gangrene with 17 perforations, six cases with stenosis, and six cases that regressed. The left colon was involved in 59 cases with extension to the transverse colon in 20, the right colon in 10, and global involvement in 18. Abdominal pain, diarrhea, and abdominal distention occurred in 81%, 62%, and 78% of the cases, respectively. Colonoscopy was performed in 61 cases, a barium enema in 27. A colectomy was required in 77 patients: 50 left colectomies with 16 extensions to the transverse colon, 17 total colectomies, and 10 right colectomies. Morbidity was 53% in cases with perforated gangrene and 28% without perforation. There was no morbidity in stenosis and regressive forms. Intestinal continuity was conserved or re-established in 51 of the 62 survivors.

Scharff et al. (84) studied the outcome of 129 patients with colon ischemia. The mean age was 66 years; 47% were male. Risk factors included chronic renal failure (33%), receiving vasoactive drugs (57%), and atherosclerosis (56%). Of 43% with melena, 88% of patients survived. Of 33% with an acute abdomen, 51% died. Initially, 54% were treated nonoperatively of which 24% required operation. Of 76 patients who were treated operatively, 41% died. Eleven patients at operation had ischemia without colon infarction or perforation; 45% died. The overall mortality was 29%. Mortality rates remained high, despite treatment.

Medina et al. (142) reviewed the clinical characteristics of patients and analyzed predictive factors of poor outcome in 53 cases of ischemic colitis. Hypertension (51%) was the main risk factor associated with ischemic colitis. Peritonitis was present only in the severe group. Colonoscopy and histologic studies were the most used diagnostic procedures. Peripheral vasculopathy and right colonic involvement were risk factors for severe outcome. Five patients died during admission and among these the right colon was affected in four.

Colonic "Cast" Slough

The spontaneous passage per rectum of a full-thickness colon "cast" is a rare consequence of acute colonic ischemia. Foley et al. (143) reported a patient who had undergone a Hartmann's procedure for a perforated diverticular abscess, which was reversed six months later. On the first postoperative night after reversal the patient had a brief hypotensive episode, and three weeks later passed a 21 cm full-thickness infarcted piece of colon. The patient did not develop peritonitis and for 11 months experienced only mild symptoms. Under colonoscopic surveillance, the granulation tissue conduit connecting the remaining viable bowel became increasingly stenosed proximally and difficult to dilate. After three rapidly consecutive episodes of large-bowel obstruction, the patient required a laparotomy to resect the stricture and restore bowel continuity. From a literature review, this was the eighth case of its kind and the first in which such prolonged conservative management has been possible.

Idiopathic Mesenteric Phlebosclerosis

A new clinicopathologic disease was described by Iwashita et al. (144) and they proposed the term "idiopathic mesenteric phlebosclerosis." In fact, the entity was originally described by Koyama et al. (145) and later reviewed by Yoshinaga et al. (146) who found 18 cases. Iwashita et al. identified seven patients with calcifications in the small mesenteric veins and their intramural branches. Clinical findings included abdominal pain and diarrhea of a gradual onset and chronic course. A positive fecal occult blood test and mild anemia were often found. Patients had linear calcifications and stenosis in the right colon, which were discovered by plain abdominal radiography and barium enema, respectively. Endoscopic findings included edematous, dark-colored mucosa and ulcerations. Four patients underwent a subtotal colectomy because of persistent abdominal pain or ileus. The histopathologic findings were macroscopically characterized by a dark purple- or dark brown-colored colonic surface, the swelling and disappearance of plicae semilunares coli, and marked thickening of the colonic wall, while they were microscopically characterized by marked fibrous thickening of the venous walls with calcifications, marked submucosal fibrosis, deposition of collagen in the mucosa, and foamy macrophages within the vessel walls.

■ ISCHEMIC COLITIS AND AORTOILIAC SURGERY

Ischemic colitis is an infrequent but highly lethal complication following aortic surgery. It is unique because in part it may be a direct consequence of an anatomic change in blood flow resulting from ligation of the IMA (see Chap. 1). Ernst et al. (147) and Hagihara et al. (148) have evaluated patients endoscopically following abdominal aortic aneurysm resection and have found that the incidence of clinical ischemic disease was 1–2% and that the incidence of endoscopic disease was 6.8%. Endoscopic evidence of ischemic colitis was found in 60% of patients following emergency repair of abdominal aortic aneurysm, reflecting in part the hypovolemia, shock, and also the absence of mechanical or antibiotic bowel preparation prior to emergency operation. In a review of 2137 patients undergoing aortic reconstructive operations, Brewster et al. (77) found a 1.1% incidence of intestinal ischemia. Bjorck et al. (149) studied the incidence and clinical presentation of intestinal ischemia after 2930 aortoiliac/femoral operations. The estimated incidence of bowel ischemia was 2.8%. Among patients operated on for a ruptured aneurysm in shock, the estimated incidence of bowel ischemia was 7.3%. Of the 63 patients with intestinal ischemia, only 15 patients presented with early passage of bloody stools. In 60 patients (95%), the lesion affected the left colon within the reach of the sigmoidoscope. Champagne et al. (150) reviewed 88 patients who underwent emergent aortic reconstruction because of ruptured abdominal aortic aneurysms. Operative mortality was 42%. Colonoscopy was performed in 62 of 72 patients who survived more than 24 hours. Bowel ischemia was documented in 36% of patients. Of these, 62% had grade I or grade II ischemia at both initial and repeat endoscopy. Exploratory laparotomy with bowel resection was undertaken in 35% because of grade III ischemia. Two procedures were performed because of worsening ischemia discovered at repeat colonoscopy. In patients with colonoscopic findings of bowel ischemia, the mortality rate was 50%. In those with grade III necrosis who underwent resection the mortality rate was 55%. Elevated lactate levels, immature white blood cells, and increased fluid sequestration were all variables associated with the occurrence of colon ischemia. When the cardinal symptoms are not present, the surgeon may be alerted to the diagnosis by general signs of deterioration, such as oliguria, circulatory instability, septicemia, and coagulopathy.

In a review by Longo et al. (81) of 4957 patients who underwent operation of the abdominal aorta for abdominal aortic aneurysm, 58 (1.2%) had subsequent ischemic colitis. The mean time to diagnosis of ischemic colitis was 5.5 days after aortic surgery (range, 1–21 days). Of 17 patients initially treated nonoperatively, only one required a sigmoid resection. One of these patients required a resection for stricture 14 months later. Bowel resection with fecal diversion was required in 32 of 49 patients (65%)—13 for ischemia without infarction and 19 with infarction. The overall mortality rate was 54%, but that rate was 89% if bowel resection for bowel infarction was required (19 patients). Only two of 12 (16%) of those who required fecal diversion and survived underwent eventual stoma closure. Among seven patients who received second-look laparotomy for ischemic colitis, additional bowel resection was required in six. No patient had aortic graft infection diagnosed during the index hospitalization. The overall mean hospitalization duration after the diagnosis of ischemic colitis was 38 days (range, 1–164 days). The high overall mortality rate is almost identical to that of previous reports (151). In view of high mortality rates, routine postoperative colonoscopy, could be justified on high-risk patients (those with multiple risk factors and/or ruptured aneurysms) to enable timely reoperative intervention in patients suspected of full-thickness necrosis. Caution is advised in patients with ischemic colitis undergoing colonoscopy in that distention of the bowel with air may diminish colonic blood flow and further exacerbate the ischemia (152).

Brandt et al. (153) suggested that flexible sigmoidoscopy reliably predicts full thickness colonic ischemia following repair of ruptured aortic aneurysms. They believe patients with nonconfluent ischemia limited to the mucosa can be safely followed by serial endoscopic examinations. However, in contrast, Houe et al. (154) reviewed seven prospective nonrandomized reports on routine colonoscopy after abdominal aortic surgery. Endoscopy may disclose ischemic colitis but cannot separate transmural from clinically less important mucosal ischemia. Endoscopy had no impact on mortality in any of the prospective series.

For patients developing clinical ischemic colitis following aortic surgery, the mortality rate has been reported to be high after elective aneurysm resection and significantly higher after emergency operation, even as high as 60% to 100% (155). Brewster et al. (77) reported an overall mortality rate of 25% that rose to 50% if reoperation for bowel resection was required. Maupin, Rimar, and Villalba (156) reviewed 103 patients who underwent operation for a ruptured abdominal aortic aneurysm. Of the 71 survivors, ischemic colitis developed in 27%. For those who required bowel resection, the mortality rate was 58%, and hence the authors recommended flexible fiberoptic sigmoidoscopy in the early postoperative period to detect ischemic colitis prior to the onset of clinical sepsis. Bast et al. (157) conducted a prospective study of the incidence and risk factors for ischemic disease of the colon and rectum following operation for abdominal aortic aneurysm. In their series of 100 patients, routine postoperative colonoscopy revealed ischemic colonic disease, defined as ulceration or necrosis in 4.5% of patients undergoing elective operation and 17.6% of patients undergoing operation for ruptured aneurysms. Ligation of a patent IMA was not in this study related to the development of ischemic disease, nor was a prolonged (>1 hour) cross-damping of the aorta. Zelenock et al. (155) conducted a prospective study of 100 patients undergoing aortic reconstructive surgery in which patients underwent colonoscopy within 24 to 48 hours. Only three patients developed endoscopic evidence of ischemia, and no patient required bowel resection. The authors attributed their good results to utilization of adjunctive procedures to enhance colonic perfusion in 12 patients (IMA reimplantation, bypass to internal iliac artery, and anastomosis of aortofemoral bypass limb to adjacent common iliac artery).

Piotrowski et al. (158) conducted a retrospective review of 101 patients who were treated for abdominal aortic aneurysm, 71 (70%) of whom survived for longer than 24 hours postoperatively. Colonic ischemia, primarily left sided, was a perioperative complication in 24 patients (35%) and required colectomy in 11 patients (44%). Colectomy carried a 44% mortality rate compared to 20% in patients without this complication. Colonic ischemia occurred more frequently in patients with preoperative shock and a greater intraoperative blood loss, but showed no correlation with patient age, comorbid medical conditions, laboratory values, time to operation, or treatment of the IMA. Most patients with postoperative bowel ischemia, including eight of the 11 patients who required colectomy, were found to have chronic IMA occlusion. Revascularization of patent IMAs had little effect on outcome. Of the 17 patent IMAs, nine were reimplanted, and five patients (55%) developed bowel ischemia, two of whom required colectomy. Eight were ligated and three (39%) developed bowel ischemia, one of whom required colectomy. The authors concluded that preoperative shock was the most important factor predicting the development of colonic ischemia following ruptured abdominal aortic aneurysm.

Lane and Bentley (159) described two cases of rectal stricture formation following aortic aneurysm repair. A combination of hypotension, compromised internal iliac circulation, and poor collateral supply following inferior mesenteric artery ligation can result in acute ischemic proctitis—an infrequently described clinical entity. Ulceration and necrosis are the sequelae of prolonged ischemia and fibrous stricture formation may result. One patient responded to dilatation and posterior mid-rectal myotomy; the other failed to respond to conservative measures and eventually had an end colostomy fashioned following intractable symptoms.

Jarvinen et al. (160) defined the incidence and attendant mortality of intestinal infarction of 1752 patients who underwent abdominal aortic reconstruction as recorded in the Finnish National Vascular Registry. Among the 1752 operations, 27 patients had intestinal ischemia for an incidence of bowel infarction of 1.2%. Among patients operated on for a ruptured aneurysm it was 3.1%, whereas 1% for patients with nonruptured aneurysm and 0.6% of those operated on for aortoiliac occlusive disease developed intestinal infarction. In 14 patients (67%), the lesion affected the left colon. The overall 30-day mortality rate was 13% but reached 67% among those with intestinal infarction.

The frequency of ischemic colitis following aortoiliac surgery varies from 7% after repair of ruptured aortic aneurysm to 0.6% after bypass for aortoiliac occlusive disease (161). In order to analyze the predisposing factors and outcome of ischemic colitis, Van Damme et al. (161) reviewed their clinical experience of 28 cases (16 ruptured aortic aneurysms, seven elective aortic aneurysms, and five aortoiliac occlusive disease) of clinically evident colonic ischemia. Transmural necrosis was observed in 21 patients, 15 of which underwent Hartmann procedure with a mortality of 66%. All nonoperated grade III patients died. Overall, 16 of the 28 patients died at hospital (57% mortality rate). Associated colon revascularization could not avoid the evolution of colon necrosis in four patients. Reimplantation of a patent inferior mesenteric artery or internal iliac artery was performed in only 4.8% of all aortic reconstructions and did not influence the development of ischemic colitis. The authors conclude that a more liberal use of postoperative sigmoidoscopy could allow detecting colonic ischemia at an earlier stage and reduce ensuing mortality.

Colonic necrosis can complicate endovascular abdominal aortic aneurysm repair even when both internal iliac arteries are preserved (162). Advantageously, the clinical signs of severe colonic ischemia in endograft patients are not obscured by aftereffects of a laparotomy.

Although the most likely etiology of colonic ischemia following aortic surgery appears to be a sudden loss of blood flow from a patent IMA, a number of other factors have been described. These factors include failure to resume hypogastric flow, absence or injury to the collateral circulation, operative trauma to the colon, cholesterol emboli, or an aortoiliac steal syndrome in which blood flow is shunted from the colon to the extremities through the newly revascularized iliac or femoral vessels (163,164). Klok et al. (165) noted that all patients undergoing aortic reconstructive operations develop a significant drop in sigmoidal intramucosal pH. Return to a normal baseline within 6 to 12 hours after declamping probably predicts a postoperative course without ischemic colitis. Bjorck and Hedberg (166) also found that sigmoid intramucosal pH could be used to monitor patients undergoing aortic operations. In a study of 34 patients, eight patients developed major complications, four of whom had ischemic colitis and five of whom died. Sigmoid acidosis (pH $<$ 7.1) served as an early warning. If acidosis was reversed within 24 hours, no major complications developed; if prolonged, it was predictive of major morbidity.

Risk factors to the development of ischemia include prolonged cross-clamp time, rupture of the aortic aneurysm, hypotension, hypoxemia, arrhythmia, retroperitoneal hematoma with compression of the viscera and its blood supply, inadequacy of colonic collaterals, intraoperative injury or interruption of the marginal artery of Drummond or meandering mesenteric arcade, operative trauma to the colon, bowel distention, lack of preoperative bowel preparation (93), and ligation of a patent IMA. Ligation of the IMA was the most important feature in one series (74%) (77). Decisions on whether or not to reimplant the IMA should be based on Doppler ultrasonography, fluorescein dye injections, or IMA stump pressure (37,167).

Prevention of ischemic colitis can result from IMA reimplantation. Criteria for reimplantation of a patent IMA recommended by Brewster et al. (77) include severe SMA disease, an enlarged IMA or meandering mesenteric artery, exclusion of hypogastric circulation, loss of Doppler signal in sigmoid mesentery, poor IMA back-bleeding (stump pressure $<$40 mmHg), and a history of prior colon resection. Mechanical and antibiotic bowel preparation should also be considered in the preoperative preparation for elective aortic reconstruction. Intraoperative methods used to diminish the likelihood of colonic ischemia include preservation of the meandering mesenteric artery, avoidance of distal embolization of atherosclerotic debris, gentle handling of the colon, and intraoperative anticoagulation (93).

IMA reimplantation does not ensure colon viability in aortic surgery. Mitchell and Valentine (168) identified 10 patients with aortic surgery, five of whom underwent successful IMA reimplantation for inadequate Doppler signals on the antimesenteric border of the sigmoid colon. The other five patients did not undergo IMA reimplantation because they were deemed to have adequate blood perfusion. Transmural colon necrosis occurred in six of the 10 study patients, four of whom had IMA reimplantation. Three of the four patients with colon ischemia presenting less than 24 hours after aortic revascularization survived but both patients with late colon ischemia died of multisystem organ failure. Although transmural necrosis is a highly morbid complication after aortic surgery, timely colectomy may lead to survival in some patients.

Signs and symptoms may be difficult to detect in a patient who has just undergone a major reconstructive aortic operation. Bloody diarrhea during the first day or two after an aortic operation should alert the clinician of the diagnosis of ischemic colitis. Metabolic acidosis, leukocytosis, oliguria, tachycardia, and hypotension may develop with aggressive disease. Treatment follows the recommendation above with nonoperative treatment for mild forms of the disease and resection for severe irreversible transmural disease. In the latter case, primary anastomosis is contraindicated because of the potential for leakage and contamination of the aortic prosthesis.

Controversy exists as to the cause of ischemic colitis complicating endosvascular aneurysm repair. Occlusion of the hypogastric arteries during endovascular repair of aortoiliac aneurysm results in a significant incidence of buttock claudication, and has been suggested as a causative factor in the development of postprocedural colonic ischemia, in addition to factors such as systemic hypotension, embolization of atheromatous debris, and interruption of IMA inflow. To analyze the relationship between perioperative hypogastric artery occlusion and postoperative ischemic colitis, Geraghty et al. (169) reviewed their experience with bifurcated endovascular grafts in 233 patients. Unilateral perioperative hypogastric artery occlusion during the course of endovascular aortoiliac aneurysm repair occurred in 18.9% and 0.4% underwent bilateral hypogastric artery occlusion. In 1.7% signs and symptoms of ischemic colitis developed 2 ± 1.4 days postoperatively. In all patients, the diagnosis was confirmed at sigmoidoscopy, and initial treatment included bowel rest, hydration, and intravenous antibiotic agents. Three patients with bilateral patent hypogastric arteries required colonic resection 14.7 ± 9.7 days after the initial diagnosis and two of these three patients died in the postoperative period. Pathologic findings confirmed the presence of atheroemboli in the colonic vasculature in all three patients who underwent colonic resection. The fourth patient had undergone multiple manipulations of the left hypogastric artery in an unsuccessful attempt to preserve patency of this vessel during aortoiliac aneurysm repair. This patient recovered completely with nonoperative management. Perioperative unilateral hypogastric artery occlusion was not associated with a significantly higher incidence of postoperative ischemic colitis. Their extensive experience suggests that embolization of atheromatous debris to the hypogastric artery tissue beds during endovascular manipulations, rather than proximal hypogastric artery occlusion, is the primary cause of clinically significant ischemic colitis after endovascular aneurysm repair.

Ischemic Colitis Following Cardiopulmonary Bypass

Colonic ischemia following cardiopulmonary bypass is a rare development (0.06–0.2%), but when it occurs carries a high mortality rate (76%) (93). The clinical picture is subtle. Contributing factors of systemic hypovolemia, hypotension, and hypothermia result in reduction of blood flow through the intestinal microcirculation. Other insults may include long bypass times, use of inotropes that may induce splanchnic vasoconstriction, and the intra-aortic pump. The combination of these factors may result in sepsis and multiple organ failure. Timely operative intervention may be lifesaving.

Ischemic Colitis Proximal to Obstructing Carcinoma

An acute colitic process believed to be ischemic in nature may develop proximal to an obstructing carcinoma of the colon. Symptoms are usually attributed to the carcinoma. The major importance for recognition of this entity is that an anastomosis constructed in an unrecognized ischemic colon is in jeopardy of failure. When that condition is suspected, a biopsy may aid in the diagnosis. Other obstructing processes such as diverticulitis, volvulus, fecal impaction, or strictures from previous ischemic insults, operations, or radiation therapy may cause diminished colonic blood flow by the effects of sustained increased intraluminal pressure (93).

■ TOTAL COLONIC ISCHEMIA

A fulminating form of colonic ischemia involving all or most of the colon and rectum has been identified (124,170). These patients manifest a sudden onset of universal colitis with bloody diarrhea, fever, abdominal pain, and tenderness, often with signs of peritonitis. Contributing factors include large and small vessel arterial disease, decreased perfusion pressure, inadequacy of collateral circulation, and plasma viscosity (124). These patients are systemically ill, and management necessitates total abdominal colectomy and ileostomy. Ischemic pancolitis is rare with only a limited number of documented cases (140,141,170). All 12 cases reported by Longo et al. (140) required operation and 75% died. Both patients reported by Al-Saleh et al. (170) survived. In a surgical series of 88 cases of ischemic colitis reported by Guivarc'h et al. (141), 17 of the 18 patients with global involvement required total colectomy. Although indications for operation do not differ from those with segmental ischemia, Al-Saleh et al. (170) recommend vigilant examination of the entire colon at laparotomy as well as pre- or intraoperative colonoscopy in order to recognize the diffuse nature of the disease and institute appropriate management.

■ ISCHEMIC PROCTITIS

Ischemic proctitis is a rare condition that affects elderly patients with arteriosclerosis. It is most commonly seen following aortic operations in which hypotension develops secondary to blood loss. It has been reported to occur as a result of hypovolemic shock sustained through trauma (171). Ischemic proctitis has also been reported in association with adventitial fibromuscular dysplasia (172). Ischemic necrosis has complicated systemic lupus erythematosus (173). Up to 1992, 37 cases had been reported (174). In a review of 328 patients with ischemic colitis, Bharucha et al. (175) identified 10 patients with isolated proctosigmoiditis defined as involvement extending to no more than 30 cm above the dentate line. In the six patients with acute rectal ischemia (symptoms <4 weeks), clearly identifiable precipitating factors such as a major illness or hemodynamic disturbance were identified in four patients but in only one of four patients with chronic ischemic proctosigmoiditis (symptoms ≥ 4 weeks). Bloody diarrhea is the most common symptom. The diagnosis of ischemia is made by the mucosal appearance of the sigmoid and is differentiated from infectious proctitis by stool culture. Plain radiographic signs of ischemic proctitis are unlikely to be recognized until necrosis is established and extramural air is visible adjacent to the rectal wall (176). CT may reveal rectal wall thickening and/or perirectal stranding (175). Angiography may demonstrate atheromatous disease of the aortoiliac vessels. Biopsy and histopathologic changes may help differentiate this entity from idiopathic inflammatory bowel disease, especially if the hallmark feature of superficial epithelial necrosis is present. Mild ischemic proctitis may be treated with antibiotics and intravenous fluids, but full-thickness ischemia requires a Hartmann resection with low division of the rectum. Cataldo and Zarka (177) reported the use of topical instillation of 4% formalin in the treatment of refractory hemorrhagic ischemic proctitis. Complete proctectomy or abdominoperineal resection should not be necessary. Kishikawa et al. (178) reported a case of chronic ischemic proctitis that occurred spontaneously, and the following information was extracted from their review of the literature on this subject. Symptoms include diarrhea, fecal incontinence, abdominal pain, rectal pain, and bloody diarrhea. The endoscopic findings of chronic ischemic proctitis include atrophic mucosa with scattered white scars reflecting repeated episodes of ischemia and healing. Chronic ischemic proctitis should be suspected whenever ulcer formation or erosion is observed endoscopically in the context of atrophic mucosa and multiple whitish scars in the rectosigmoid colon with mucosal crypt atrophy or fibrosis evident in biopsy specimens. On CT, ischemic proctitis should be considered when mural thickening confined to the rectum and sigmoid colon is associated with perirectal fat stranding especially in elderly patients with known cardiovascular risk factors. Patients with ischemic proctitis fall into two groups: (1) those with atherosclerotic disease who have been hospitalized for some other disorder (myocardial infarction, pneumonia, and heart failure), and (2) those with mesenteric venous occlusion. Cocaine is the only agent that induces focal rectal ischemia and this effect of the drug demonstrates the importance of vasoconstriction in the pathogenesis of ischemic proctitis. Ischemic proctitis has been associated with mesenteric venous occlusion. Treatment of ischemic proctitis, acute or chronic, depends on the level of ischemia. Superficial mucosa ischemia should be treated conservatively with close monitoring for signs of sepsis or perforation. Operation is required for necrosis of the bowel wall. Nelson et al. (174) performed resection in four of six cases of acute ischemic proctitis.

REFERENCES

1. Bradbury AW, Brittendon J, McBride K, et al. Mesenteric ischemia: a multidisciplinary approach. Br J Surg 1995; 82:1446–1459.
2. Sreenarasimhaiah J. Diagnosis and management of intestinal ischaemic disorders. BMJ 2003; 326:1372–1376.
3. Moskowitz M, Zimmerman H, Felson B. The meandering mesenteric artery of the colon. Am J Roentgenol 1964; 92:1088–1099.
4. Jacobson LF, Noer RJ. The vascular pattern of the intestinal villi in various laboratory animals and man. Anat Rec 1952; 114:85–101.
5. Hallback DA, Hulten L, Jodal M, et al. Evidence for the existence of a countercurrent exchange in the small intestine in man. Gastroenterology 1978; 74: 683–690.
6. Lundgreh O. The circulation of the small bowel mucosa. Gut 1974; 15: 1005–1013.
7. Kaleya RN, Boley SJ. Acute mesenteric ischemia. Crit Care Clin 1995; 11: 479–512.
8. Robinson JWL, Winistorfer B, Mirtovitch V. Source of net water and electrolyte loss following intestinal ischemia. Res Exp Med 1980; 176:263–275.
9. Kusche J, Lorenz W. Stahlknecht CD, et al. Intestinal diamine oxidase and histamine release in rabbit mesenteric ischemia. Gastroenterology 1981; 80: 980–987.
10. Bateson PG, Buchanan KD, Stewart DM, et al. The release of vasoactive intestinal peptide during altered midgut blood flow. Br J Surg 1980; 67:131–134.
11. Modlin IM, Blood SR, Mitchell SC. Vasoactive intestinal plasma polypeptide (VIP) levels and intestinal ischemia. Esperienta 1978; 34:535–536.
12. Bennion RS, Wilson SE, Serota AI, et al. The role of gastrointestinal microflora in the pathogenesis of complications of mesenteric ischemia. Rev Infect Dis 1984; 6(suppl 1):S132–S138.
13. Bennion RS, Wilson SE, Williams RA. Early portal anaerobic bacteremia in mesenteric ischemia. Arch Surg 1984; 119:151–155.
14. Brawn K, Fridovich I. Superoxide radical and superoxide dismutases: threat and defense. Acta Physiol Scand 1980; 492:9–18.
15. Parks DA, Bulkley GB, Granger DN. Role of oxygen-derived free radicals in digestive tract disease. Surgery 1983; 94:415–422.
16. Granger DN, Rutili G, McCord JM. Superoxide radicals in feline intestinal ischemia. Gastroenterology 1981; 91:27–29.
17. Parks DA, Granger DN, Bulkley GB. Superoxide radicals and mucosal lesions in the ischemic small intestine. Fed Proc 1982; 44:1742.
18. Andrei VE, Schein M, Wise L. Small bowel ischemia following laparoscopic cholecystectomy. Dig Surg 1999; 16:522–524.
19. Brookes DH, Carey LC. Base deficit in superior mesenteric artery occlusion, an aid to early diagnosis. Ann Surg 1973; 177:352–356.
20. Jamieson WG, Marchuk S, Ronsom J, et al. The early diagnosis of massive intestinal ischemia. Br J Surg 1982; 69(suppl 5):S52–S53.
21. Barnett SM, Davidson ED, Bradley EL. Intestinal alkaline phosphatase and base deficit in mesenteric occlusion. J Surg Res 1976; 20:243–246.
22. Lamor W, Woodard L, Statland BE. Clinical implications of creatine kinase BB isoenzyme. N Engl J Med 1978; 299:834–853.
23. Graeber GM, Cafferty PJ, Reardon MI, et al. Changes in the serum total creatine phosphokinase (CPK) and its isoenzymes caused by experimental ligation of the superior mesenteric artery. Ann Surg 1981; 193:499–505.
24. Wollin A, Navert H, Bounous G. Effects of intestinal ischemia on diamine oxidase activity in rat intestinal tissue and blood. Gastroenterology 1981; 80: 349–355.
25. Acosta S, Nilsson TK, Bjorck M. D-Dimer testing in patients with suspected acute thromboembolic occlusion of the superior mesenteric artery. Br J Surg 2004; 91:991–994.
26. Scholz FJ. Ischemic bowel disease. Radiol Clin North Am 1993; 31:1197–1218.
27. Wiesner W, Khurana B, Ji H, Ros PR. CT of acute bowel ischemia. Radiology 2003; 226:635–650.
28. Klein HM, Lensing R, Klosterhalfen B, et al. Diagnostic imaging of mesenteric infarction. Radiology 1995; 197:79–82.
29. Chou CK, Mak CW, Tzeng WS, Chang JM. CT of small bowel ischemia. Abdomin Imaging 2004; 29:18–22.
30. Burkart DJ, Johnson CD, Reading CC, et al. MR measurements of mesenteric venous flow: prospective evaluation in healthy volunteers and patients with suspected chronic mesenteric ischemia. Radiology 1995; 194:801–806.
31. Stoney RJ, Cunningham CG. Acute mesenteric ischemia. Surgery 1993; 114:489–490.
32. Acosta S, Ogren M, Sternby NH, Bergqvist D, Bjorck M. Incidence of acute thrombo-embolic occlusion of the superior mesenteric artery—a population-based study. Eur J Vasc Endovasc Surg 2004; 27:145–150.
33. Boley SJ, Feinstein FR, Sammartano R, et al. New concepts in the management of emboli of the superior mesenteric artery. Surg Gynecol Obstet 1981; 153: 561–569.
34. Vujic I, Stanley J, Gobien R. Treatment of acute embolus of the superior mesenteric artery by topical infusion of streptokinase. Cardiovasc Intervent Radiol 1984; 7:94–96.
35. Pillari G, Doscher W, Fierstein J, et al. Low-dose streptokinase in the treatment of celiac and superior mesenteric artery occlusion. Arch Surg 1983; 118: 1340–1342.
36. Jamieson AC, Thomas RJS, Cade JF. Lysis of a superior mesenteric artery embolus following local infusion of streptokinase and heparin. Aust N Z J Surg 1979; 49:355–356.
37. Bulkley GB, Zuidema GD, Hamilton SR, et al. Intraoperative determination of small bowel viability following ischemic injury. Ann Surg 1981; 193: 628–637.
38. O'Donell JA, Hobson RW. Operative confirmation in evaluation of intestinal ischemia. Surgery 1980; 87:109–112.
39. Sheridan WG, Lowndes RH, Young HL. Intraoperative tissue oximetry in the human gastrointestinal tract. Am J Surg 1990; 159:314–319.
40. Sluttzki S, Halpern Z, Negri M, et al. The laparoscopic second look for ischemic bowel disease. Surg Endosc 1996; 10:729–731.
41. Anadol AZ, Ersoy E, Taneri F, Tekin EH. Laparoscopic "second-look" in the management of mesenteric ischemia. Surg Laparosc Endosc Percutan Tech 2004; 14:191–193.
42. Cooperman M. Intestinal ischemia. Mount Kisco, New York: Futura Publishing, 1983:147.
43. Bergan JJ. Acute intestinal infarction. Rutherford R, ed. Vascular surgery. 2nd ed. Philadelphia: WS Saunders, 1984:955.
44. Sales JP, Frileux P, Cugnenc PH, et al. Mesenteric infarction: improved survival after temporary enterostomy. Br J Surg 1993; 80:1029.
45. Bingol H, Zeybek N, Cingoz F, Yilmaz AT, Tatar H, Sen D. Surgical therapy for acute superior mesenteric artery embolism. Am J Surg 2004; 188:68–70.
46. Savassi-Rocha PR, Veloso LF. Treatment of superior mesenteric artery embolism with a fibrinolytic agent: case report and literature review. Hepatogastroenterology 2002; 49:1307–1310.
47. Kwoan JH, Connolly JE. Prevention of intestinal infarction resulting from mesenteric arterial occlusive disease. Surg Gynecol Obstet 1983; 157: 321–324.
48. Johnson KW, Lindsay TF, Walker PM, et al. Mesenteric arterial bypass grafts: early and late results and suggested surgical approach for chronic and acute mesenteric ischemia. Surgery 1995; 118:1–7.
49. Bailey RW, Bulkley GB, Hamilton SR, et al. Protection of the small intestine from non-occlusive mesenteric ischemic injury due to cardiogenic shock. Am J Surg 1987; 153:108–116.
50. Bailey RW, Bulkley GB, Hamilton SR, et al. Pathogenesis of non-occlusive ischemic colitis. Ann Surg 1986; 203:590–599.
51. Clark RA, Gallant TE. Acute mesenteric ischemia: Angiographic spectrum. AJR 1984; 142:555–562.
52. Kaleya RN, Sammartano RJ, Boley SJ. Aggressive approach to acute mesenteric ischemia. Surg Clin North Am 1992; 72:157–182.

53. Ward D, Vernava AM, Kammski DL, et al. Improved outcome by identification of high-risk non-occlusive mesenteric ischemia, aggressive reexploration, and delayed anastomosis. Am J Surg 1995; 170:577–581.
54. Schuler JG, Hudlin MM. Cecal necrosis: infrequent variant of ischemic colitis. Report of five cases. Dis Colon Rectum 2000; 43:708–712.
55. Neri E, Sassi C, Massetti M, et al. Nonocclusive intestinal ischemia in patients with acute aortic dissection. J Vasc Surg 2002; 36:738–745.
56. Flaherty MJ, Lie JT, Haggitt RC. Mesenteric inflammatory veno-occlusive disease. A seldom recognized cause of intestinal ischemia. Am J Surg Pathol 1994; 18:779–784.
57. Grendell JH, Ockner RK. Mesenteric venous thrombosis. Gastroenterology 1982; 82:358–372.
58. Benjamin E, Oropello JM, Iberti TJ. Acute mesenteric ischemia: pathophysiology, diagnosis and treatment. Dis Mon 1993; 39:131–210.
59. Khodadadi J, Rozencwajg J, Nacasch N, et al. Mesenteric vein thrombosis. Arch Surg 1980; 115:315–317.
60. Sack J, Aldrete JS. Primary mesenteric venous thrombosis. Surg Gynecol Obstet 1982; 154:205–208.
61. Kitchens CS. Evolution of our understanding of the pathophysiology of primary mesenteric venous thrombosis. Am J Surg 1992; 163:346–348.
62. Rhee RY, Gloviczki P, Mendonca CT. Mesenteric venous thrombosis: still a lethal disease in the 1990s. J Vasc Surg 1994; 20:688–697.
63. Divino CM, Park IS, Angel LP, Ellozy S, Spiegel R, Kim U. A retrospective study of diagnosis and management of mesenteric vein thrombosis. Am J Surg 2001; 181:20–23.
64. Croft RJ, Menon GP, Marston A. "Does intestinal angina exist?" A critical study of obstructed visceral arteries. Br J Surg 1981; 68:316–318.
65. Marston A, Clark JMF, Garcia JG, et al. Intestinal function and intestinal blood supply: a 20-year surgical study. Gut 1985; 26:656–666.
66. Gentile AT, Moneta GL, Taylor LM, et al. Isolated bypass to the superior mesenteric artery for intestinal ischemia. Arch Surg 1994; 129:926–932.
67. Hollier LH, Bernatz PE, Pairolaro PC, et al. Surgical management of chronic intestinal ischemia: a reappraisal. Surgery 1981; 90:940–946.
68. McAfee MK, Cherry KF, Naessens JM, et al. Influence of complete revascularization on chronic mesenteric ischemia. Am J Surg 1992; 164: 220–224.
69. Illuminati G, Calio FG, D'Urso A, Papaspiropoulos V, Mancini P, Ceccanei G. The surgical treatment of chronic intestinal ischemia: results of a recent series. Acta Chir Belg 2004; 104:175–183.
70. Leke MA, Hood DB, Rowe VL, Katz SG, Kohl RD, Weaver FA. Technical consideration in the management of chronic mesenteric ischemia. Am Surg 2002; 68:1088–1092.
71. Furrer J, Gruntzig A, Kugelmeier J, et al. Treatment of abdominal angina with percutaneous dilation of an arteria mesenterica superior stenosis. Cardiovasc Intervent Radiol 1980; 3:43–44.
72. Golden DA, Ring EJ, McLean GK, et al. Percutaneous transluminal angioplasty in the treatment of abdominal angina. AJR 1982; 139:247–249.
73. Birch SJ, Colapinto RF. Transluminal dilation in the management of mesenteric angina. Journal de l'Association Canadienne des Radtologistes 1982; 33:46–47.
74. Kasirajan K, O'Hara PJ, Gray BH, et al. Chronic mesenteric ischemia: open surgery versus percutaneous angioplasty and stenting. J Vasc Surg 2001; 33:63–71.
75. Guttormson NL, Bubrick MP. Mortality from ischemic colitis. Dis Colon Rectum 1989; 32:469–472.
76. Levy PJ, Krausz MM, Manny J. Acute mesenteric ischemia: improved results. A retrospective analysis of ninety-two patients. Surgery 1990; 107:372–380.
77. Brewster DC, Franklin DP, Cambria RP, et al. Intestinal ischemia following abdominal aortic surgery. Surgery 1991; 109:447–454.
78. Parish KL, Chapman WC, William LF. Ischemic colitis. An ever changing spectrum? Am Surg 1991; 57:118–121.
79. Inderbitzi R, Wagner HE, Seiler C, et al. Acute mesenteric ischemia. Eur J Surg 1992; 158:123–126.
80. Longo WE, Ballantyne GH, Gusberg RJ. Ischemic colitis. Patterns and prognosis. Dis Colon Rectum 1992; 35:726–730.
81. Longo WE, Lee TG, Barrett MG, et al. Ischemic colitis complicating abdominal aortic aneurysm surgery in the U.S. veteran. J Surg Res 1996; 60:351–354.
82. Klempnauer J, Grothues F, Bektas H, et al. Long-term results after surgery for acute mesenteric ischemia. Surgery 1997; 121:239–243.
83. Edwards MS, Cherr GS, Craven TE, et al. Acute occlusive mesenteric ischemia: surgical management and outcomes. Ann Vasc Surg 2003; 17:72–79.
84. Scharff JR, Longo WE, Vartanian SM, Jacobs DL, Bahadursingh AN, Kaminiski DL. Ischemic colitis: spectrum of disease and outcome. Surgery 2003; 134: 624–629.
85. Kasirajan K, Mascha EJ, Heffernan D, Sifuentes J III. Determinants of in-hospital mortality and length of stay for acute intestinal gangrene. Am J Surg 2004; 187:482–485.
86. Schoots IG, Koffeman GI, Legemate DA, Levi M, van Gulik TM. Systematic review of survival after acute mesenteric ischaemia according to disease aetiology. Br J Surg 2004; 91:17–27.
87. Boley SJ, Schwartz S, Lash J, et al. Reversible vascular occlusion of the colon. Surg Gynecol Obstet 1963; 116:53–60.
88. Marston A, Pheils MT, Thomas ML, et al. Ischemic colitis. Gut 1966; 7:1–15.
89. Higgins PD, Davis KJ, Laine L. Systematic review: the epidemiology of ischaemic colitis. Alimnet Pharmacol Ther 2004; 19:729–738.
90. Reeders JWAJ, Tytgat GNJ, Rosenbusch G, et al. Ischemic colitis. Dordrecht, The Netherlands: Martinus Nijhoff, 1984:30, 157.
91. Kaleya RN, Boley SJ. Colonic ischemia. Perspect Colon Rectal Surg 1990; 3: 62–81.
92. Saegesser F, Sandblom P. Ischemic lesion of the distended colon: a complication of obstructive colorectal cancer. Am J Surg 1975; 129:309–315.
93. Gandhi SK, Hanson MM, Vernava AM, et al. Ischemic colitis. Dis Colon Rectum 1996; 39:88–100.
94. Midian-Singh R, Polen A, Durishin C, Crock RD, Whittier FC, Fahmy N. Ischemic colitis revisited: a prospective study identifying hypercoagulability as a risk factor. South Med J 2004; 97:120–123.
95. Koutroubakis IE, Sfiridaki A, Theodoropoulou A, Kouroumalis EA. Role of acquired and hereditary thrombotic risk factors in colon ischemia of ambulatory patients. Gastroenterology 2001; 121:561–565.
96. Koutroubakis IE, Theodoropoulou A, Sfiridaki A, Kouroumalis EA. Low plasma protein Z levels in patients with ischemic colitis. Dig Dis Sci 2003; 48:1673–1676.
97. Perez-Carral C, Carreira J, Vidal C. Acute ischaemic colitis due to hypotension and amoxicillin allergy. Postgrad Med J. 2004; 80:298–299.
98. Comay D, Ramsay J, Irvine EJ. Ischemic colitis after weight-loss medication. Can J Gastroenterol 2003; 17:719–721.
99. Tashiro M, Yoshikawa I, Kume K, Otsuki M. Ischemic colitis associated with paclitaxel and carboplatin chemotherapy. Am J Gastroenterol 2003; 98:231–232.
100. Daniele B, Rossi GB, Losito S, Gridelli C, de Bellis M. Ischemic colitis associated with paclitaxel. J Clin Gastroenterol 2001; 33:159–160.
101. Brinker AD, Mackey AC, Prizont R. Tegaserod and ischemic colitis. N Engl J Med 2004; 351:1361–1364; discussion 1361–1364.
102. Wooltorton E. Tegaserod (Zelnorm) for irritable bowel syndrome: reports of serious diarrhea and intestinal ischemia. CMAJ 2004; 170:1908.
103. Frossard JL, Spahr L, Queneau PE, Armenian B, Brundler MA, Hadengue A. Ischemic colitis during pregnancy and contraceptive medication. Digestion 2001; 64:125–127.
104. Friedel D, Thomas R, Fisher RS. Ischemic colitis during treatment with alosetron. Gastroenterology 2001; 120:557–560.
105. Garcia B, Ramaholimihaso F, Diebold MD, Cadiot G, Thiefin G. Ischaemic colitis in a patient taking meloxicam. Lancet 2001; 357(9257):690.
106. Linder JD, Monkemuller KE, Raijman I, Johnson L, Lazenby AJ, Wilcox CM. Cocaine-associated ischemic colitis. South Med J 2000; 93: 909–913.
107. Dowd J, Bailey D, Moussa K, Nair S, Doyle R, Culpepper-Morgan JA. Ischemic colitis associated with pseudoephedrine: four cases. Am J Gastroenterol 1999; 94:2430–2434.
108. Knudsen JF, Friedman B, Chen M, Goldwaser, JE. Ischemic colitis and sumatriptan use. Arch Intern Med 1998; 158:1946–1948.
109. Rice E, DiBaise JK, Quigley EM. Superior mesenteric artery thrombosis after colonoscopy. Gastrointest Endosc 1999; 50:706–707.
110. Butcher JH, Davis AJM, Page A, Green B, Shepherd HA. Transient ischaemic colitis following an aeroplane flight: two case reports and review of the literature. Gut 2002; 51:746–747.
111. Shibata M, Nakamuta H, Abe S, et al. Ischemic colitis caused by strict dieting in an 18-year-old female: report of a case. Dis Colon Rectum 2002; 45:425–428.
112. Ryan CK, Reamy B, Rochester JA. Ischemic colitis associated with herbal product use in a young woman. J Am Board Fam Pract 2002; 15(4):309–312.
113. Dee SL, Butt K, Ramaswamy G. Intestinal ischemia. Arch Pathol Lab Med 2002; 126:1201–1204.
114. Flobert C, Cellier C, Berger A, et al. Right colonic involvement is associated with severe forms of ischemic colitis and occurs frequently in patients with chronic renal failure requiring hemodialysis. Am J Gasroenterol 2000; 95:195–198.
115. Sohn CI, Kim JJ, Lim YH, et al. A case of ischemic colitis associated with pheochromocytoma. Am J Gastroenterol 1998; 93:124–126.
116. Bao P, Welch DC, Washington MK, Herline AJ. Resection of mesenteric inflammatory veno-occlusive disease causing ischemic colitis. J Gastrointest Surg 2005; 9:812–817.
117. Lucas W, Schroy PC III. Reversible ischemic colitis in a high endurance athlete. Am J Gastroenterol 1998; 93:2231–2234.
118. Tsujimoto T, Takano M, Ishikawa M, et al. Onset of ischemic colitis following use of electrical muscle stimulation (EMS) exercise equipment. Intern Med 2004; 43:693–695.
119. Church JM. Ischemic colitis complicating flexible endoscopy in a patient with connective tissue disease. Gastrointest Endosc 1995; 41:181–182.
120. Versaci A, Macri A, Scuderi G, et al. Ischemic colitis following colonoscopy in a systemic lupus erythematosus patient: report of a case. Dis Colon Rectum 2005; 48:866–869.
121. Schwarz DA, Stork M, Wright J. Segmental colonic gangrene: a previously unreported complication of adult hemolytic uremic syndrome. Surgery 1994; 116:107–110.
122. Walker AM, Bohn RL, Cali C, Cook SF, Ajene AN, Sands BE. Risk factors for colon ischemia. Am J Gastroenterol 2004; 99:1333–1337.

123. Brandt LJ, Boley SJ. Colonic ischemia. Surg Clin North Am 1992; 72:203–229.
124. Welch GH, Shearer MG, Imrie CW, et al. Total colonic ischemia. Dis Colon Rectum 1986; 29:410–412.
125. West BR, Ray JE, Gathright JB. Comparison of transient ischemic colitis with that requiring surgical treatment. Surg Gynecol Obstet 1980; 151:366–368.
126. Sakai L, Keltner R, Kaminski D. Spontaneous and shock-associated ischemic colitis. Am J Surg 1980; 140:755–760.
127. Boley SJ, Corman M, Moosa AR, et al. Symposium. Management of colonic ischemia. Contemp Surg 1989; 34:73–104.
128. Landreneau RJ, Fry WJ. The right colon as a target organ of non-occlusive mesenteric ischemia. Arch Surg 1990; 125:591–594.
129. Newman JR, Cooper MA. Lower gastrointestinal bleeding and ischemic colitis. Can J Gastroenterol 2002; 16:597–600.
130. Ardigo GJ, Longstreth GF, Weston LA, Walker FD. Passage of a large bowel cast caused by acute ischemia: report of two cases. Dis Colon Rectum 1998; 41:793–796.
131. Ullery BS, Boyko AT, Banet GA, Lewis LM. Colonic ischemia: an under-recognized cause of lower gastrointestinal bleeding. J Emerg Med 2004; 27:1–5.
132. Preventza OA, Lazarides K, Sawyer MD. Ischemic colitis in young adults: a single-institution experience. J Gastrointest Surg 2001; 5:388–392.
133. Markoglou C, Avgerinos A, Mitrakan M, et al. Toxic megacolon secondary to acute ischemic colitis. Hepatogastroenterology 1993; 40:188–190.
134. Philpotts LE, Hecken JP, Westcott MA, et al. Colitis: use of CT findings in differential diagnosis. Radiology 1994; 190:445–449.
135. Ranschaert E, Verbille R, Marchal G, et al. Sonographic diagnosis of ischemic colitis. J Belge Radiol 1994; 77:166–168.
136. Lange H, Jackel R. Usefulness of plasma lactate concentration in the diagnosis of acute abdominal disease. Eur J Surg 1994; 160:381–384.
137. Tada M, Misaka F, Kawai K. Analysis of the clinical features of ischemic colitis. Gastroenterol Jpn 1983; 18:204–209.
138. Sano S, Nishimori I, Miyao M, et al. Successful use of mesalamine in the treatment of chronic segmental lesion in a case of ischemic colitis. J Gastroenterol Hepatol 2003; 18:882–883.
139. Abel ME, Russell TR. Ischemic colitis: comparison of surgical and nonoperative management. Dis Colon Rectum 1983; 26:113–115.
140. Longo WE, Ward D, Vernava AM III, Kaminski DL. Outcome of patients with total colonic ischemia. Dis Colon Rectum 1997; 40:1448–1454.
141. Guivarc'h M, Roullet-Audy JC, Mosnier H, Boche O. Ischemic colitis. A surgical series of 88 cases. J Chir (Paris) 1997; 134:103–108.
142. Medina C, Vilaseca J, Vitiela S, Fabra R, Armengol-Miro JR, Malagelada JR. Outcome of patients with ischemic colitis: review of fifty-three cases. Dis Colon Rectum 2004; 47:180–184.
143. Foley CL, Taylor CJ, Aslam M, Reddy KP, Birch HA, Owen ER. Failure of conservative management after the passage of a distal colonic "cast": report of a case. Dis Colon Rectum 2005; 48:1090–1093.
144. Iwashita A, Yao T, Schlemper RJ, et al. Mesenteric phlebosclerosis: a new disease entity causing ischemic colitis. Dis Colon Rectum 2003; 46:209–220.
145. Koyama N, Koyama H, Hanajima T, et al. Chronic ischemic colitis causing stenosis. Report of a case [in Japanese with English abstract]. Stomach Intestine (Tokyo) 1991; 26:455–460.
146. Yoshinaga S, Harada N, Araki Y, et al. Chronic ischemic colonic lesion caused by phlebosclerosis: a case report. Gastrointest Endosc 2001; 53:107–111.
147. Ernst CB, Hagihara PF, Daugherty ME, et al. Ischemic colitis incidence following abdominal aortic reconstruction: a prospective study. Surgery 1976; 80:417–421.
148. Hagihara PF, Ernst CB, Griffen WO Jr. Incidence of ischemic colitis following abdominal aortic reconstruction. Surg Gynecol Obstet 1979; 149:571–573.
149. Bjorck M, Bergqvist D, Troeng T. Incidence and clinical presentation of bowel ischemia after aortoiliac surgery—2930 operations from a population-based registry in Sweden. Eur J Vasc Endovasc Surg 1996; 12:139–144.
150. Champagne BJ, Darling RC III, Daneshmand M, et al. Outcome of aggressive surveillance colonoscopy in ruptured abdominal aortic aneurysm. J Vasc Surg. 2004; 39:792–796.
151. Schroder J, Christofferson JK, Anderson J, et al. Ischemic colitis complicating reconstruction of the abdominal aorta. Surg Gynecol Obstet 1985; 160:299–303.
152. Kozarek RA, Ernest DL, Silverman ME. Air pressure induced colon injury during diagnostic colonoscopy. Gastroenterology 1980; 78:7–14.
153. Brandt CP, Piotrowski JJ, Alexander JJ. Flexible sigmoidoscopy. A reliable determinant of colonic ischemia following ruptured abdominal aortic aneurysm. Surg Endosc 1997; 11(2):113–115.
154. Houe T, Thorboll E, Sigil U, Liisberg-Larsen O, Schroeder TV. Can colonoscopy diagnose transmural ischaemic colitis after abdominal aortic surgery? An evidence-based approach. Eur J Vasc Endovasc Surg 2000; 19:304–307.
155. Zelenock GB, Strodel WE, Knol JA, et al. A prospective study of clinically and endoscopically documented colonic ischemia in 100 patients undergoing aortic reconstructive surgery with aggressive colonic and direct pelvic revascularization compared with historic controls. Surgery 1989; 106: 771–780.
156. Maupin G-E, Rimar SD, Villalba M. Ischemic colitis following abdominal aortic reconstruction for ruptured aneurysm. A 10 year experience. Am Surg 1989; 55:378–380.
157. Bast TJ, van der Biezen JJ, Scherpenisse J, et al. Ischemic disease of the colon and rectum after surgery for abdominal aortic aneurysm: a prospective study of the incidence and risk factors. Eur J Vasc Surg 1990; 4:253–257.
158. Piotrowski JJ, Ripepi AJ, Yuhas JP, et al. Colonic ischemia: the Achilles heel of ruptured aortic aneurysm repair. Am Surg 1996; 62:557–560.
159. Lane TM, Bentley PG. Rectal strictures following abdominal aortic aneurysm surgery. Ann R Coll Surg Engl 2000; 82:421–423.
160. Jarvinen O, Laurikka J, Salenius JP, Lepantalo M. Mesenteric infarction after aortoiliac surgery on the basis of 1752 operations from the National Vascular Registry. World J Surg 1999; 23:243–247.
161. Van Damme H, Creemers E, Limet R. Ischaemic colitis following aortoiliac surgery. Acta Chir Belg 2000; 100:21–27.
162. Hinchliffe RJ, Armon MP, Tse CC, Wenham PW, Hopkinson BR. Colonic infarction following endovascular AAA repair: a multifactorial complication. J Endovasc Ther 2002; 9:554–558.
163. Connolly JE, Stammer EA. Intestinal gangrene as the result of mesenteric arterial steal. Am J Surg 1973; 126:197–204.
164. Cordorba A, Gordillo O. Mesenteric arterial steal syndrome secondary to bilateral lumbar sympathectomy. Int Surg 1979; 64:67–69.
165. Klok T, Moll FL, Leusink JA, et al. The relationship between sigmoidal intramucosal pH and intestinal arterial occlusion during aortic reconstructive surgery. Eur J Vasc Endovasc Surg 1996; 1:304–307.
166. Bjorck M, Hedberg B. Early detection of major complications after abdominal aortic surgery: predictive value of sigmoid colon and gastric intramucosal pH monitoring. Br J Surg 1994; 81:25–30.
167. Ernst CB, Hagihara PF, Daugherty ME, et al. Inferior mesenteric artery stump pressure: a reliable index for safe IMA ligation during abdominal aortic aneurysmectomy. Ann Surg 1978; 187:641–646.
168. Mitchell KM, Valentine RJ. Inferior mesenteric artery reimplantation does not guarantee colon viability in aortic surgery. J Am Coll Surg 2002; 194: 151–155.
169. Geraghty PJ, Sanchez LA, Rubin BG, et al. Overt ischemic colitis after endovascular repair of aortoiliac aneurysms. J Vasc Surg 2004; 40:413–418.
170. Al-Saleh N, Wehrli BM, Driman DK, Taylor BM. Ischemic pancolitis: recognizing a rare form of acute ischemic colitis. Can J Surg 2004; 47:382–383.
171. Ahmed I, Kerwat R, Morgan AR, et al. Rectal ischemia following hypovolemic shock. Br J Surg 1996; 83:508.
172. Quirke P, Campbell I, Talbot IC. Ischemic proctitis and adventitial fibromuscular dysplasia of the superior rectal artery. Br J Surg 1984; 71: 33–38.
173. Lazaris ACh, Papanikolaou IS, Theodoropoulos GE, Petraki K, Davaris PS. Ischaemic necrosis of the rectum and sigmoid colon complicating systemic lupus erythematosus. Acta Gastroenterol Belg 2003; 66:191–194.
174. Nelson RL, Briley S, Schuler JJ, et al. Acute ischemic proctitis: report of 6 cases. Dis Colon Rectum 1992; 35:375–380.
175. Bharucha AE, Tremaine WJ, Johnson CD, et al. Ischemic proctosigmoiditis. Am J Gastroenterol 1996; 91:2305–2309.
176. MacKay C, Murphy P, Rosenberg IL, et al. Case report: rectal infarction after abdominal aortic surgery. Br J Radiol 1994; 67:497–498.
177. Cataldo PA, Zarka MA. Formalin instillation for ischemic proctitis with unrelenting hemorrhage: report of a case. Dis Colon Rectum 2000; 43: 261–263.
178. Kishikawa H, Nishida J, Hirano E, et al. Chronic ischemic proctitis: case report and review. Gastrointest Endosc 2004; 60:304–308.

31

Radiation Injuries to the Small and Large Intestine

Santhat Nivatvongs

INTRODUCTION

Radiation therapy is an important means of control in patients with carcinoma of the cervix, uterus, prostate, testicles, bladder, and rectum. However, its role in the treatment of ovarian carcinoma has diminished over the past 20 years (1), but its role in the treatment of rectal carcinoma is strong (2–4). The injurious effects of X-rays on normal intestine were noted only two years after Roentgen's discovery of X-rays, when Walsh (5) described the case of a coworker who developed bowel dysfunction while exposed to X-rays. The man's symptoms cleared when he was kept from further exposure. Since that time, much has been written about the pathology and clinical symptomatology of radiation injury to individual organ systems. Some of the most serious injuries occur in the gastrointestinal tract, with damage to the small bowel, colon, and rectum. Despite improved technology and a better understanding of the effects of radiation on normal tissues, radiation injury is still a formidable problem. Many patients who are cured of carcinoma still suffer considerable morbidity and occasional mortality from the radiation itself.

INCIDENCE AND CLINICAL MANIFESTATIONS

The true incidence of radiation injury is difficult to assess accurately. Most large series estimate the incidence of chronic radiation injury to be between 5% and 11%, with approximately 20% of these requiring an operation (6). Krook et al. (7) reported a 6.7% incidence of bowel complications in patients who received postoperative chemoradiation for rectal adenocarcinoma.

Although the acute effects of radiation begin within hours of the commencement of radiation therapy, most patients will not experience the symptoms of acute radiation injury until 3000 to 4000 cGy have been delivered. Acute colitis and proctitis are manifested by abdominal pain, diarrhea, tenesmus, and rectal bleeding. There is little value in pursuing an aggressive diagnostic evaluation in this clinical setting. Approximately 50% to 70% of all patients undergoing therapeutic pelvic irradiation will develop these symptoms. A decrease of the daily dosage of the radiation is usually successful, and it is distinctly uncommon to have to discontinue the therapy (6).

Late complications can lead to a multitude of clinical problems. Patients may present with bowel obstruction, stricture, fistula formation, perforation, hemorrhage, and malabsorption. They may also experience fecal incontinence, either because of direct radiation damage to the anal sphincter or as a consequence of late radiation effects on pelvic nerves (8). One must keep in mind that patients who survive five or more years after their first malignancy may be at risk for the development of subsequent malignancies within the radiation fields (6).

Eighty-five percent of all patients who develop radiation injury present between 6 and 24 months after completion of radiation therapy (9–11). The remaining 15% of patients may develop complications years or even decades after treatment (12). In general, patients with rectal ulceration or proctitis present somewhat earlier in their course than with strictures and fistulas (13,14).

Damage to the small intestine is more serious and constitutes 30% to 50% of the radiation injuries severe enough to require operation (15,16). Urinary tract complications, including ureteral obstruction secondary to fibrosis, cystitis, and fibrotic changes in the bladder (with bladder dysfunction and fistula formation), occur in up to 28% of patients having late gastrointestinal complications (17,18).

Late complications can appear clinically as anorexia, malnourishment, colicky abdominal pain, bowel dysfunction (including diarrhea, obstipation, fecal urgency, and frequency of defecation with or without incontinence), rectal pain, rectal bleeding, dysuria, hematuria, chronic urinary tract infections, sepsis, and shock. Since many of these symptom complexes may be also seen in patients with recurrent malignancy, it is often difficult to distinguish late radiation injury from recurrent carcinoma.

MECHANISMS OF RADIATION INJURY

Ionizing radiation injures cells by the transfer of energy to critical biologic macromolecules, including DNA, proteins, and membrane lipids. Some damage occurs directly from absorption of energy by the target molecules. Indirect damage is caused by diffusible oxygen free radicals, highly reactive intermediates generated from the absorption of radiant energy by low-molecular-weight compounds. Water is, by far, the most abundant component of the cell, and the radiologic products of water are responsible largely for indirect free radical damage. When target macromolecules are irradiated directly or react with high-energy free radical intermediates, the targets themselves become ionized or transformed into free radicals. Although radiation can exert its damaging effects by these two different mechanisms, the end result is the same (19).

Damage to lipid membranes results, in part, from lipid peroxidation. Functionally, these changes are expressed as altered membrane fluidity and increased permeability, which can trigger the release of potent physiologic mediators that enhance the damage (19).

PATHOLOGY

The gastrointestinal tract is second only to the kidneys in radiosensitivity, and gastrointestinal tract injury is the major limiting factor affecting tolerance to radiation of the abdomen and pelvis (20,21). Although the small intestine is more radiosensitive than the large intestine, it is injured less frequently because of its mobility within the abdominal cavity. The sites of most severe injury after pelvic irradiation are in the lower sigmoid colon and upper rectum, probably because of their proximity to the field of radiation. Overt injury to the small intestine is less common but, when it occurs, is usually situated 6 to 10 cm from the ileocecal valve. These areas show the most severe derangement of vascular architecture and maximum reduction in microvascular volume (22).

At the cellular level, the injurious effect of radiation is still not fully understood. Ionizing radiation generates free radicals from intracellular water; they, in turn, can interact with DNA to block transcription and replication. Cells with a high proliferation rate such as those in the intestinal mucosa are more susceptible to such disruptions (23,24). More latent effects can occur in the vascular connective tissue, giving rise to complications later (23).

Grossly, early radiation injuries result in an edematous, thickened, and hyperemic mucosa. Areas of superficial ulceration or necrosis also may be present (Fig. 1) (25). In the small bowel, the villi become blunted, and in both the small and large bowels, the crypts become shortened, and cryptal microabscesses can form. Microscopically, the microvilli of the surface epithelium are shortened, prominent large nuclei are present, and the mitochondria and endoplasmic reticulum are dilated (15). The submucosa may show some cytologic atypia with bizarre, enlarged fibroblasts that could be mistaken for malignant cells (Fig. 2). A loss of the normal fibrillar pattern of collagen and the deposition of large amounts of hyalin also may be present in the submucosa (26). A hyalin-type substance thickens artery walls as well (21,27). Spasm and thrombosis may occur in the arterioles (Fig. 3), and vascular ectasias may develop (21,27). Infiltration by leukocytes can be seen throughout the full thickness of the bowel wall.

Late injuries are characterized by a severe degree of fibrosis. Grossly, the bowel appears pale and opaque, and is usually shortened. The mesentery becomes thickened and may be also shortened (15). Gross radiation changes may be indistinguishable from those of Crohn's disease, but the fat does not generally extend over the surface of the bowel as it does in Crohn's disease (Fig. 4) (28). Loops of small intestine may be fused with fibrous adhesions and

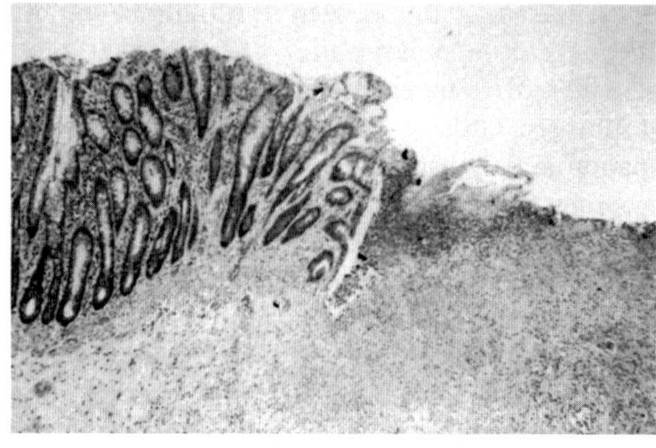

FIGURE 1 ■ Superficial ulceration showing loss of mucosa and inflammatory reaction in an acute radiation injury.

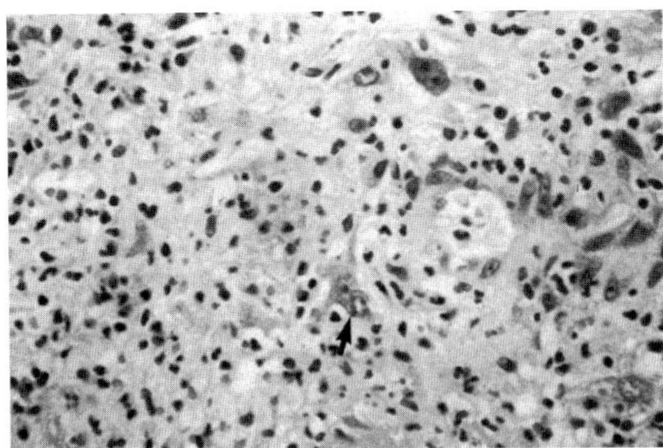

FIGURE 2 ■ Enlarged bizarre-shaped fibroblast (*arrow*) seen in tissue from an acute radiation injury.

normal tissue planes obliterated, giving rise to a "frozen pelvis" comparable to that seen with recurrent malignancy (15,28). Strictures, generally long and tapered, may appear; ulcers may develop and can be deep and progress to a fistula or perforation (28,29).

Histologically, the villi show thickening and flattening, with areas of atrophy and degeneration. There is a marked submucosal fibrosis with hyalinization (14). Telangiectasias may be prominent in the submucosa but may also occur throughout the bowel wall (Fig. 5). The arterioles show hyaline thickening of the media with intimal proliferation (26). Areas of venous and lymphatic sclerosis are noted, and venous and lymphatic ectasias can appear in the submucosa (14). The smooth muscle of both the small and large intestines may become hypertrophic, and the ganglion cells in the rectum also may undergo hypertrophy and degenerate; the latter change can affect function (8,16). The serosa and perirectal connective tissue usually show fibrosis with arterial hyalinization and intimal fibrosis (28).

A microradiography study using barium sulfate infusion by Carr et al. (22) showed that in radiation-injured bowel that requires resection, alterations in microvascular architecture are present in all sections, but these appearances vary with the type of lesion. At the site of fully developed strictures, a reduction in vascularity affects all layers of the intestinal wall. Histologically, these areas show pronounced fibrosis in the submucosa and muscularis propria together with severe vascular changes that

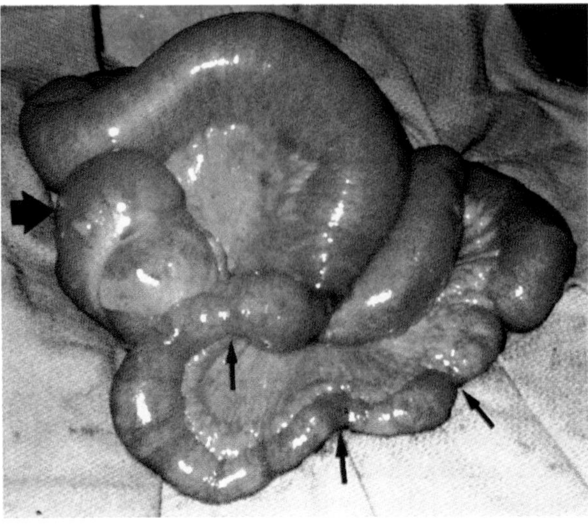

FIGURE 4 ■ Specimen from ileocolic resection for chronic radiation enteritis. Small arrows point to areas of stricture without fat wrapping in the ileum. Large arrow points to cecum. Note dilatation of the proximal nonstrictured small bowel.

consist of occlusive fibrin thrombi in capillaries and sometimes-occlusive intimal fibrosis in the small intramural arterial vessels. In sections taken from sites adjacent to perforations, avascularity zones are apparent. The mucosa vascular pattern is abnormal, and the severity of change parallels the reduction in vascularity in the remainder of the section. Capillary microthrombi are present in these mucosal vessels with or without accompanying mucosal necrosis.

PATHOGENESIS

Malabsorption with intractable diarrhea is one of the most serious consequences of radiation injury to the intestine. Several factors may be involved in the genesis of this problem, including increased bowel motility (30). The change in motility may stem from increased prostaglandin release, which can stimulate the smooth muscle of the small bowel (30,31). Loss of the brush border and its digestive enzymes may occur, causing a decrease in carbohydrate absorption arid osmotic diarrhea (27). Bacterial overgrowth in the

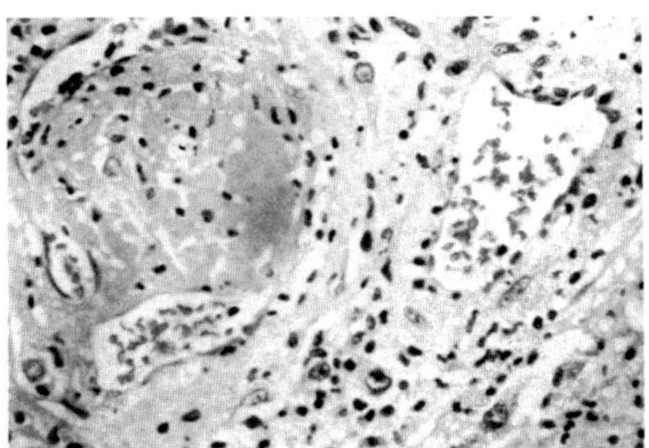

FIGURE 3 ■ Thrombosis and recanalization changes in arteriole in irradiated tissue.

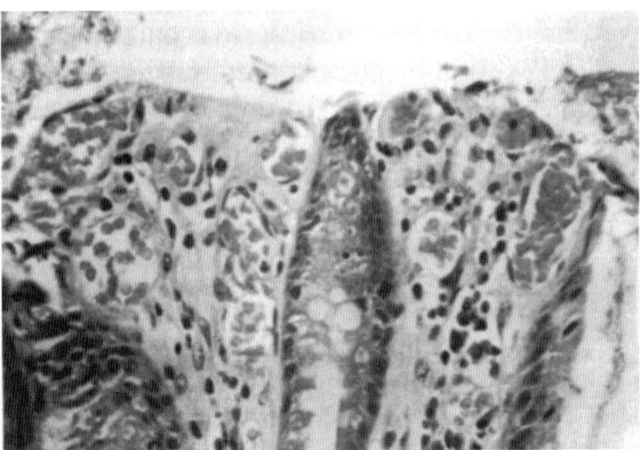

FIGURE 5 ■ Mucosal telangiectasias seen in a chronic radiation injury.

intestine can also cause malabsorption and subsequent diarrhea (32). Injury to the terminal ileum can cause a decrease in the absorption of bile salts, which has a dual effect. An increased bile salt load to the colon causes intraluminal sodium retention with an increase in intraluminal water retention. In addition, the bile salt pool decreases in size, with a decrease in the absorption of fats and the development of steatorrhea (32).

Although injury to the small intestine is chiefly responsible for malabsorption and diarrhea, injury to the rectum is responsible for the development of incontinence and the frequency and urgency of defecation. Stenosis of the rectosigmoid area sometimes is severe enough to cause these symptoms (26). Anal manometric study in patients with radiation proctitis showed a decrease in rectal volume and compliance. The physiologic length of the internal sphincter decreased while the squeeze pressure and external sphincter muscle function were normal. Rectosphincteric reflex was abnormal in several patients (8,16). Correlating these findings with histologic studies showed hypertrophy of smooth muscle and abnormalities in the myenteric plexus, including hypertrophy of the nerve fibers and a decrease in the number of ganglion cells within the plexus of Auerbach (33). A similarity between these findings and those of Hirschsprung's disease was apparent.

Another complication of intestinal radiation is the development of a primary carcinoma in the radiated tissue. This was first noted by Slaughter and Southwick (34) in 1957. In 1965, Black and Ackerman (35) developed criteria for the diagnosis of radiation-induced carcinoma. These criteria include a 10-year latency period from the time of radiation therapy and severe radiation changes in the adjacent tissues. Sandler and Sandler (36) demonstrated that patients who have had radiation therapy have a relative risk for developing a primary carcinoma in the radiated field 2.0 to 3.6 times that of the normal population. Patients who have undergone radiation in the pelvic region have careful surveillance beginning 10 years after completion of radiation therapy. Most of these neoplasms are likely to arise in the rectum and, therefore, should be within reach of a rigid or flexible sigmoidoscope.

Although one would expect high-dose radiation to be essential for the induction of colorectal carcinoma, in fact, the opposite may be true. Palmer and Spratt (37) found that patients who received low-dose radiation for benign gynecologic conditions had a greater chance (3.32%) of developing rectal carcinoma than those who received high-dose radiation (1.42%) to treat carcinoma of the cervix. Radiation-induced colorectal carcinomas were more often of mucinous histologic type (25% to 60% of cases) than carcinomas in nonradiated patients (10% of cases) (6). The fact that these carcinomas are of a different histologic type and that all colon carcinomas induced by radiation in rats are mucinous adenocarcinomas (38), lends further support to the concept that these carcinomas are radiation-induced.

Another pathologic process that can be confused with adenocarcinoma is colitis cystica profunda, which has been noted to occur in irradiated tissue. It is a rare condition characterized by the presence of epithelial mucous cysts that are generally deep to the mucosa (39,40). Although the glandular elements in the submucosa and muscularis propria may appear as adenocarcinoma, cytologic evidence of malignancy must he present before the lesions may be called adenocarcinoma.

PREDISPOSING FACTORS

The cumulative total dosage of radiation delivered to the tissues is an important determinant of any subsequent radiation damage. Strockbine et al. (41) in a review of 831 patients, noted no intestinal injuries when the total radiation dose was less than 3000 rads but found an injury rate of 36% among patients receiving 7000 rads. Assessment of the minimal and maximal tolerance doses for the gastrointestinal tract has shown that the small bowel is the most radiosensitive area.

Although total dosage is an important etiologic factor in the development of radiation injuries, patients receiving low-dose radiation can still suffer radiation damage to normal tissues (11,26). This damage can occur because cell injury is also dependent on the rate at which the radiation is delivered. Malignant cells do not self-repair as well as normal cells between doses of radiation; so malignant cells do not repopulate between doses as well as normal cells. Consequently, the normal cell population is better able to tolerate radiation that is given more frequently, especially when smaller doses are used (24,42). Doses of less than 200 rads per day comprise the regimen usually given for external beam radiation. Dosage rates are especially important when intracavitary radiation is used. Lee et al. (43) have shown that dosage rates greater than 60 rads per hour are associated with a higher incidence of bladder and rectal injuries.

It has long been known that some patients tolerate radiotherapy better than others. One important predisposing factor is, existing vascular damage from hypertension, diabetes mellitus, collagen vascular disease, and atherosclerosis (1,10,19,27,44–48). Second is a previous abdominal or pelvic operation that led to adhesions that immobilize the small bowel such that the same segment receives radiation with each treatment (19,49). A thin habitus has also been associated with a greater frequency of chronic radiation damage (47).

A strong correlation has also been made between radiation injury and various chemotherapeutic agents. Doxorubicin (Adriamycin), acti-mycin, bleomycin, and 5-fluorouracil (5-FU) enhance cell injury in the gastrointestinal tract; this necessitates reduction in radiation dosage when these agents are being used (50,51). Olsalazine is contraindicated during pelvis radiation therapy because it increases the risk of proctitis (52). Animal studies have shown that intraluminal contents, including pancreatic secretions, can predispose the patient to radiation injuries (53).

SMALL INTESTINE INJURIES

DIAGNOSIS

Injuries to the small bowel are not readily identified since it is the most difficult part of the gastrointestinal tract to study radiographically and it cannot be reached readily endoscopically. Small bowel studies are notoriously inexact; extensive narrowing may be present with normal

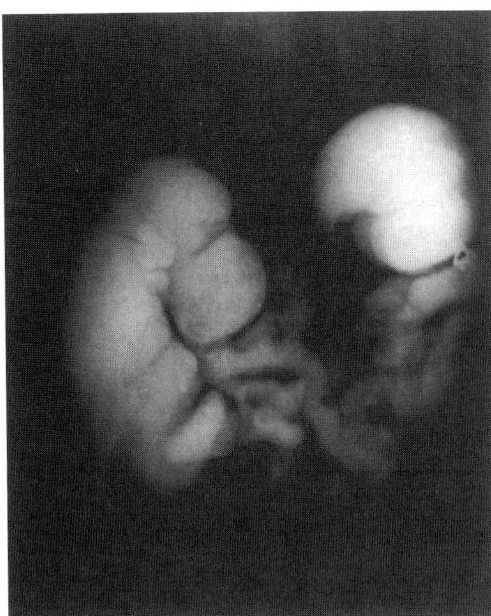

FIGURE 6 ■ Small bowel study in a patient with radiation enteritis showing "thumbprinting," submucosal edema, and fluid between small bowel loops.

radiologic findings. Positive findings, when present, are generally those of ischemia with "thumbprinting," nodular filling defects, and separation of loops secondary to edema and/or fibrosis (54) (Fig. 6). Strictures and fistulas also can be seen, but fistulograms are often necessary to localize enterocutaneous fistulas.

The recent progress in CT enterography will replace other radiologic tests for evaluating the small intestine (55,56).

Radiation-induced lesions may be especially difficult to distinguish from neoplastic invasion on X-ray studies. Most lesions secondary to radiation appear in the terminal ileum, whereas 58% of those caused by malignancy occur in the duodenum or jejunum (57). Angiography can help distinguish the two entities. Characteristic findings of radiation injury include arterial stenosis, decreased vascularity, luminal irregularities, and stenosis in the veins, with a decrease in the capillary phase in the bowel wall. In contrast, arteries supplying a malignancy tend to be dilated and are associated with a large number of tiny "tumor" vessels within the carcinoma during the capillary phase (58). The recent progress of technology using integrated PET-CT imaging is valuable for the differentiation of posttreatment changes from recurrent carcinoma (59).

The clinical manifestation of radiation damage to the small bowel can be divided into two groups according to the time of appearance. Acute enteral complications of radiation therapy occur either during or immediately following a course of radiation therapy. Nausea, vomiting, cramps, and intermittent diarrhea are all symptoms of acute radiation enteritis. Such symptoms are probably caused by a breakdown in the intestinal mucosa that is no longer able to absorb the usual fluids and nutrients. The mucosa is also unable to prevent the efflux of fluids from the underlying supporting stroma. These changes in the intestinal epithelium result in disorders of motility and transport of fluid and solutes (23,60).

Long-term complications of radiation therapy are usually manifestations of progressive vasculitis and interstitial fibrosis initiated by radiation therapy, often delivered many years before clinical signs develop. Partial or complete intestinal obstruction due to strictures or decreased motility, intestinal perforation, gastrointestinal bleeding, malabsorption, etc., and enteric fistulas are all long-term enteral complications of patients treated with abdominal or pelvic radiation therapy (23,60).

■ MEDICAL MANAGEMENT

No effective medical treatment is available. Conservative therapy can control many of the symptoms of radiation enteropathy. Antispasmodics, anticholinergics, opiates, a low-residue diet, and a diet low in fats and lactose can improve symptoms of abdominal pain and diarrhea (61,62). Lactose deficiency from villus blunting with emergent lactose intolerance is seen in 20% of consequent patients (63,64). Malabsorption studies should be done on patients who do not respond to the above measures. If a study reveals that a patient has abnormal bile salt absorption, the specific bile salt–binding resin, cholestyramine, can often decrease the diarrhea significantly (62,65,66). Cholestyramine is usually well tolerated although it blinds oral medications and should not be given concomitantly with other drugs (65). Oral antibiotics can help patients who have suspected bacterial overgrowth of the small bowel from intestinal stasis. 5-ASA and steroids are effective (67,68).

In some patients, elemental diets have been shown to decrease stool output while maintaining nutrition (69). For other patients either short-term or long-term total parenteral nutrition (TPN) may be needed. Some patients, in whom both medical and surgical therapies have failed, have done well with home TPN (70,71). TPN is often the initial treatment of choice for an enterocutaneous fistula, especially in the malnourished patient, although spontaneous closure is uncommon (72). TPN is invaluable for preparing the malnourished patient for operation.

■ SURGICAL MANAGEMENT

Selection of appropriate procedures should consider general as well as local aspects. Literature data indicate that over 40% of patients with radiation enteritis will not survive 2 years following operation, and over 60% of the deceased succumb to their primary malignancy (73). Operation is clearly indicated for obstruction, perforation, fistula that is unresponsive to TPN, abscess, and intractable bleeding or diarrhea. Although the number of patients requiring operation is small, the morbidity rate has been reported to be as high as 65% (72) and the mortality rate as high as 45% (74). Decisions concerning timing of operation and type of operation can be critical.

Often it is impossible to distinguish radiation injury from recurrent malignancy, thus influencing surgical decision-making. Walsh and Schofield (75) reported on 53 patients with small bowel obstruction who underwent exploratory laparotomy and found that 17 of the 53 patients had recurrent malignancy, whereas the others had obstruction from other causes. Most of the patients with malignancy received good palliation from the operation, and the authors concluded that operation should not be denied solely because of concern about recurrent carcinoma.

The most controversial issue relating to the surgical management of patients with small bowel radiation injury is whether to bypass or resect the abnormal bowel. The argument against resection with primary anastomosis is that dividing the mesenteric vessels will further jeopardize an already compromised bowel and that dissection around adhesions increases the risk of subsequent fistula formation (72). On the other hand, bypassing an irradiated segment leaves behind a diseased portion of bowel with the potential for fistula formation and the development of a blind-loop syndrome (76).

Surgical decision-making was proformaly influenced by a retrospective multicenter study with literature meta-analysis published in 1976 (71), which rather indiscriminately compared the surgical outcome of resection versus bypass, i.e., without consideration of the intestinal segment involved. The conclusion that bypass was superior to resection in terms of surgical complication and operative mortality had substantial impact for more than a decade (73).

Overall, an individualized approach selectively using bypass and resection is probably the safest course. For those cases in which most of the small bowel is involved and dense adhesions have formed in the pelvis, dissection should be avoided and a bypass procedure performed instead. On the other hand, resection is preferable if disease is confined to a short segment of small intestine or if wide resection and ileocolic anastomosis to the colon can be done. In the latter cases, frozen-section biopsy of the grossly normal colon segment can be helpful to rule out fibrosis, obliteration of vessels, or other evidence of significant radiation injury (27,61,78).

Strictureplasty is not recommended as a primary procedure for radiation strictures. However, in patients with limited intestinal reserve where strictures are located within long segments of diseased bowel which, if resected or bypassed, would have significant nutritional or metabolic consequences, strictureplasty may be an effective and safe tool to conserve intestinal length (79).

Despite high initial mortality and morbidity rates, life expectancy in patients with chronic radiation enteritis without recurrence of their primary neoplastic disease is good. Resection seems to provide a lower reoperative rate and a better 5-year survival and better quality of life than by-pass procedure (80,81).

Regardless of the procedure, special mention must be made of enterolysis. A high incidence of fistula formation and perforation has been reported after enterolysis because of either ischemia or small enterotomies made during the procedure (1,10). Enterolysis should be undertaken with great caution and generally only if the surgeon is willing to resect the involved bowel if necessary.

The management of small bowel fistulas can be particularly difficult. The fistula may be due to recurrent malignancy as well as radiation injury. It is useful to divide the management of patients with enteric fistulas into three phases: (i) stabilization, (ii) definition of the fistula, and (iii) definitive therapy (82). Stabilization of the patient includes fluid and electrolyte resuscitation, control of fistula output, and nutritional repletion of the chronically debilitated patient. To define the extent of the fistula, contrast studies, including large and small bowel X-ray films, as well as fistulograms are employed. Every effort is made to ascertain the full extent of the often-complex small bowel fistulas encountered. Despite prolonged TPN, no radiation-induced small bowel fistula has ever closed with conservative management alone. However, TPN with gut rest may be a valuable initial treatment. Poor results have been obtained with attempts at resection of the fistula or partial bypass; the best results have followed total exclusion of the involved segment of bowel (72,82,83). Smith et al. (82) reported a 92% success rate of total exclusion, bringing out one end of the excluded segment as a mucous fistula (Fig. 7). This compares favorably with a 67% success rate with resection and a 69% success rate with partial bypass.

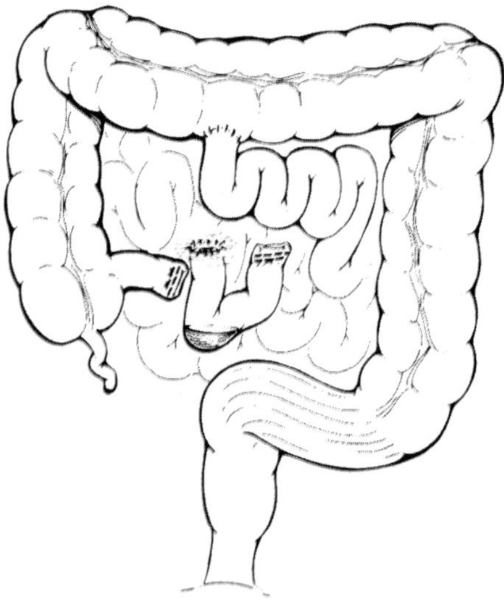

FIGURE 7 ■ Management of radiation-induced small bowel fistula by total exclusion of the involved segment, bringing out one end as a mucous fistula.

COLON AND RECTAL INJURIES

DIAGNOSIS

Injuries of the colon and rectum are more easily diagnosed and more readily denned than small bowel injuries. A digital examination alone can define areas of anorectal stenosis, and a bimanual examination can detect a frozen pelvis. Sometimes these examinations are painful, in which case they should be performed with the patient under general or regional anesthesia.

Proctoscopy or colonoscopy is essential to diagnosis, but each must be performed with caution because fixation of the bowel may make it vulnerable to perforation. The rectal mucosa can undergo a wide range of changes, with varying degrees of edema, increased friability, petechial hemorrhages, and diffuse oozing (26,31,84). Ulcerations may be present, usually on the anterior wall. The ulcers tend to have a sloughing gray base with flat edges (18). Biopsy may be required to rule out malignancy, but care must be taken in performing these biopsies, or a rectal fistula can result.

Proctitis associated with radiation therapy has been divided into three stages by Dean and Taylor (85). Stage I

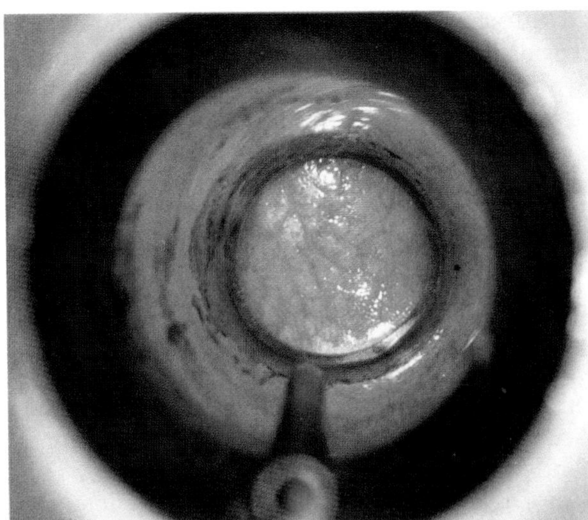

FIGURE 8 ■ Proctoscopic view of stage I radiation-induced proctitis with vascular congestion, edema, and friability.

consists of vascular congestion and friability of the rectal mucosa. The areas of severe injury are usually located on the anterior wall at the level of the cervix. Often there is a circumscribed area of thickening with a mucoid exudate present (Fig. 8). This stage is clinically accompanied by rectal bleeding, diarrhea, tenesmus, sphincter irritability, and mucoid discharge. Stage II is an ulcerative stage resulting from thrombosis of the small mucosal vessels. The mucosa is thickened and generally is covered with an exudate, but ischemia is more marked in this stage. Rectal pain is more severe and is associated with more bleeding and diarrhea. Stage III is characterized by progression of the ischemia with endarteritis, necrosis, and, sometimes, fistula formation. Rectal strictures are found in this stage (Fig. 9). Clinically, erosions can lead to massive hemorrhage, and the strictures can cause diarrhea with urgency, incomplete evacuation, and fecal or purulent drainage. Dean and Taylor (85) consider stages I and II amenable to medical therapy, whereas stage III generally requires surgical intervention.

DeCosse et al. (10) have divided patients with radiation-induced rectal injury into two groups. Group I consists of those with proctitis, rectal ulceration, or stenosis. In these patients, symptoms of bleeding, tenesmus, and rectal pain do not correlate with the degree of injury. When present, rectal stenosis is generally located proximal to the ulcers, usually 8 to 12 cm from the anal verge. The process is often reversible in these patients. Group II injuries consist of rectovaginal fistulas. These injuries are irreversible and require surgical intervention.

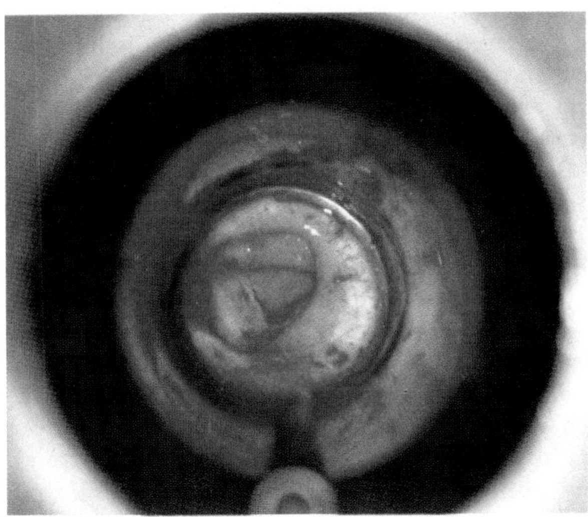

FIGURE 9 ■ Proctoscopic view of stage III radiation-induced proctitis with severe fibrosis and stricture.

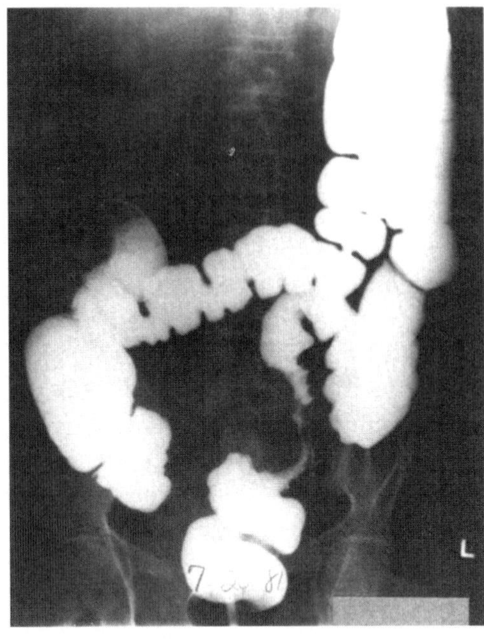

FIGURE 10 ■ Barium enema examination in a patient with radiation proctocolitis showing long rectosigmoid stricture.

Radiation injuries to the colon proximal to the rectosigmoid can be diagnosed by flexible colonoscopy and barium enema. Colonoscopy reveals a pale arid opaque mucosa at the injury site, suggesting fibrosis and submucosal edema. The surrounding tissue may appear more normal, but prominent submucosal telangiectasias may be present. The mucosa may be erythematous, granular, and friable when more active and acute distress is present (72,86). Barium enema studies reveal shortening and narrowing of the rectosigmoid region with loss of the normal curvature (9,15). The presacral space may increase secondary to thickening of the rectal wall and the perirectal tissues. These changes are best seen on lateral and oblique projections (11,54). The examination may reveal rigidity and lack of distensibility of the rectum. Atrophy of the mucosa may give a pipe stem appearance (9). When active disease is present, the mucosa may show a granular irregularity similar to that seen in other inflammatory bowel diseases with pseudopolypoid protrusions (9). Multiple areas of stricture may be present, and they can be difficult to distinguish from recurrent carcinoma (Fig. 10) (33).

■ MEDICAL MANAGEMENT

Antispasmodic agents, anticholinergics, and opiates can be helpful in treating patients with large bowel injuries. Use of a low-residue diet and stool softeners is beneficial because of the friability of the rectal mucosa and its vulnerability to damage from the fecal stream.

Sucralfate enema, given twice daily, has been shown to help (87). Aminosalicylic acid (ASA) derivatives, given rectally or orally, have not been shown to be of benefit (88).

Vitamin A stimulates various aspects of wound repair and wound healing. Levitsky et al. (89) reported a case of a patient with HIV infection who developed a symptomatic anal ulcer after receiving radiotherapy for anal squamous cell carcinoma. Vitamin A 8000 IU was given orally twice daily. Within 7 weeks his anorectal symptoms and anal ulcer were completely resolved.

In a prospective, randomized, double-blind, placebo-controlled trial of retinol palmitate (Vitamin A) for chronic radiation proctopathy with symptoms of diarrhea, rectal pain, rectal urgency, rectal bleeding, and fecal incontinence was reported (90). Nineteen patients were randomized: 10 to retinal palmitate 10,000 IU by mouth daily for 90 days, 9 to placebo. The results showed that the retinol palmitate group had significantly reduced symptoms. This series is small but may serve as the basis for a larger, multicenter trial for the future (90).

One of the mechanisms of radiation injury to the gastrointestinal tract is the indirect damage of the cell caused by diffusible oxygen free radicals (19). Antioxidants, which have a scavenging property for reactive oxygen metabolites (91), have been found to prevent tissue damage in radiation injury and ischemia-reperfusion injury (92).

Kennedy et al. (92) conducted a prospective study using Vitamins E and C in patients suffering from radiation injury of the rectum. Twenty patients (10 prostate carcinoma, 10 gynecological malignancies) who had received previous radiation treatment were referred for treatment with symptoms of rectal pain, bleeding, or diarrhea with and without urgency. Symptoms had been present for at least 6 months. The radiation exposure ranged from 1 to 36 years (average, 4 years). All of these patients had received some form of therapy for their symptoms and had failed to respond. In this study, the treatment was initiated with Vitamin E 400 IU, taken orally three times a day, and Vitamin C 500 mg taken orally three times a day. Other medications were discontinued.

The results showed that at 4–6 weeks of follow-up, there was a significant improvement in the bleeding, diarrhea, and urgency. However there was no significant improvement of rectal pain. All 10 patients who underwent a second follow-up interview reported sustained improvement in their symptoms 1 year later. The favorable results of Vitamin E and Vitamin C need to be confirmed by a double-blind placebo-controlled trial (92).

SURGICAL MANAGEMENT

Most colorectal radiation injuries do not require surgery, and operation on the previously irradiated colon has been associated with substantially high morbidity and mortality rates. However, if obstruction, perforation, fistula, persistent bleeding, intractable pain, or severe fecal incontinence develops, operative intervention is required.

For patients having proctocolitis with severe bleeding or intractable pain despite conservative treatment, a diverting colostomy should be performed. It will allow edema and infection to subside and will usually give immediate symptomatic relief. Preliminary experience with endoscopic laser coagulation of abnormal rectal vessels and bleeding, suggests that it can be useful in controlling bleeding when used either alone or with colostomy. Jao et al. (94) reviewed their experience with 62 patients treated surgically for radiation injury to the colon and rectum; 27 of the patients had colostomy alone as the initial treatment. Of the 24 patients who survived for follow-up, five had no further operation, 15 had the colostomy closed after a mean interval of 9.6 months, and nine required resection.

In patients requiring colostomy for radiation proctitis, the stoma itself has been associated with high incidence of complications, including peristomal fistula, stomal retraction, and necrosis. Mobilization of healthy proximal bowel and exteriorization of a significant length should minimize the occurrence of these problems (72,74). An ileostomy is easier to manage, and its construction does not interfere with the blood supply to the colon if a coloanal procedure is performed in the future.

Takedown of the colostomy or an ileostomy should not be attempted for at least six months and only after the rectal area has healed. Radiographic and endoscopic studies should be performed on the distal segment to rule out the interim development of stricture or fistula. Careful consideration must be always given to the possible progression of the disease (with recurrence of its symptoms) after colostomy takedown.

Although a permanent colostomy may be preferable for some patients with refractory disease, it will not control symptoms satisfactorily in some patients and will not be well accepted by others. Such patients should be considered for resection and anastomosis. Clinical studies have shown that colorectal anastomosis can be performed safely in the presence of moderate, acute, or chronic radiation change; anastomosis is clearly more hazardous when performed for clinically demonstrable radiation colitis or proctitis. Conventional anterior resection with low anastomosis in cases of radiation injury has been associated with complication rates as high as 71% (94). Although setting absolute guidelines for safe anastomosis after radiation therapy is not possible because of differences in radiation techniques and differences in individual responses, the following general guidelines are reasonable: (i) an anastomosis can be usually performed safely if the colon and rectum have received less than 4000 to 4500 rads; (ii) constructing a protective loop ileostomy is advised if anastomosis will be performed after radiation in the range of 4000 to 5500 rads; and (iii) anastomosis is generally unsafe after administration of 5500 to 6000 rads or more even if a protective loop ileostomy is added.

In 1978, Parks et al. (95) reported on five patients having an ultralow anterior resection and coloanal sleeve anastomosis. Four of the patients had rectovaginal fistulas and one had intractable pain from a radiation ulcer. All five patients had satisfactory result. The operation is performed with the patient in the lithotomy position, although the mucosal dissection can be accomplished initially with the patient in the prone jackknife position. In the abdominal phase, the colon is mobilized to include the splenic flexure, and the rectum is dissected close to the bowel. Dissection is continued beyond the necrotic rectal

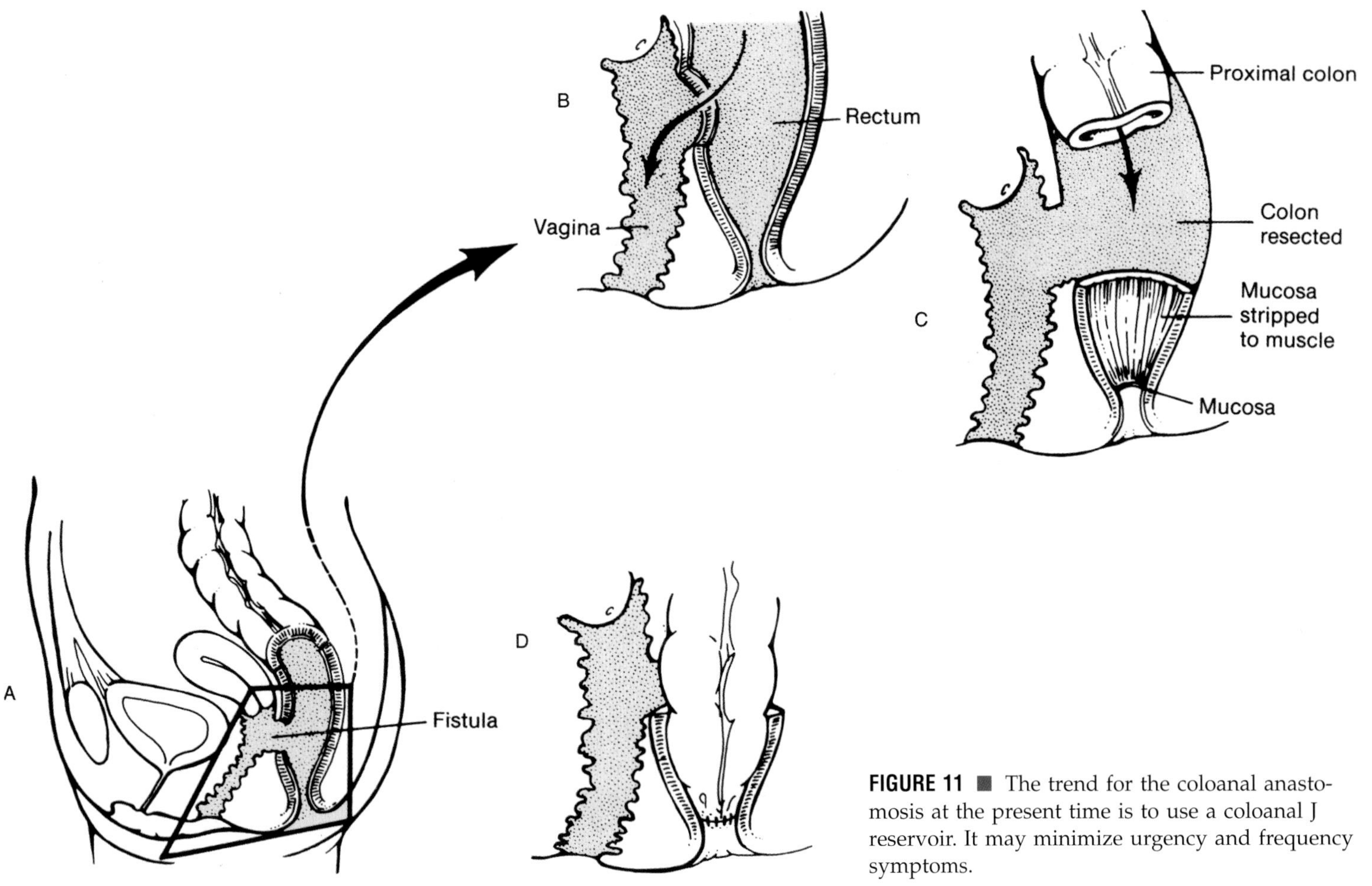

FIGURE 11 ■ The trend for the coloanal anastomosis at the present time is to use a coloanal J reservoir. It may minimize urgency and frequency symptoms.

tissue, stricture, ulcer, or fistula. The rectum is divided at this level. The colon is divided proximally at a nonirradiated site, and the rectosigmoid is removed. From the perineal approach, the submucosa of the distal rectum is infiltrated with an epinephrine solution, and the mucosa is dissected circumferentially with a scissors up to the point of proximal dissection. The proximal colon is then pulled through the denuded region with stay sutures, and a coloanal anastomosis is performed at the dentate line, with the use of interrupted 3–0 braided synthetic absorbable sutures. A temporary loop ileostomy is performed, to protect the anastomosis (Fig. 11).

Since the description by Parks et al. (95), other authors have reported similarly good results with this technique (96–100). Cooke and De Moor (98) reported good continence in the follow-up of 21 of 28 patients at one year. They did note that liquid stool with variable degrees of incontinence persisted in 79% of the patients who had an anastomosis at the dentate line for low-lying fistulas. This was not a problem for patients having anastomosis at a higher level. Cooke and De Moor (98) were also concerned about ischemia when the blood supply to the distal colon was based on the left colic artery. They had better results with the blood supply based on the left branch of the middle colic artery. Several authors have noted that the anorectum can form a narrow rigid tunnel just below the pelvic peritoneum in patients having a frozen pelvis (98,100). This tunnel can be enlarged by sharp dissection of the fibrous tissue anteriorly in the midline. Nowacki et al. (100) also noted that sometimes mucosectomy cannot be performed by the dissection method described by Parks; in these situations curettes may be used to remove the mucosa.

Radiation-induced rectovaginal fistulas generally require operation for closure. Local repair of the fistulas inevitably fails. Boronow (101) described five points to follow when treating rectovaginal fistulas: (i) recurrent carcinoma should be ruled out; (ii) the fecal stream must be diverted; (iii) acute radiation injuries should be allowed to subside; (iv) a new blood supply must be brought into the fistula repair area; and (v) the fistula itself should be closed. Based on these principles, various techniques for bringing new blood supply to the area have been tried. These sources of blood supply include gracilis muscle, adductor muscle, rectus muscle, omentum, and labial fat pads. Most repairs are performed through an episiotomy-type incision, with transverse repair of the colonic fistula. The new tissue with its blood supply is brought in and positioned in the rectovaginal septal region at the site of the fistula, and the vaginal mucosa is closed. Although these methods have had some success, the Parks coloanal sleeve anastomosis is especially well suited for this problem and should be considered the procedure of choice.

For low rectal strictures unresponsive to medical management, a diverting colostomy may be acceptable as definitive therapy for many patients. For patients wanting to maintain continuity, resection with the Parks sleeve anastomosis is usually the best choice. The Bricker-type fold-over anastomosis (102) and the Duhamel procedure (103) have now been outdated.

RADIATION PROCTITIS

Injury to the rectum is unavoidable when the patients receive pelvic irradiation. Acute radiation proctitis occurs during, or soon after, completing the course of radiotherapy. It is characterized histologically by epithelial meganucleosis, lack of mitotic activity, and patchy fibroblastic proliferation in the lamina propria with normal blood vessels.

Chronic radiation proctitis is characterized histologically by narrowing of the arterioles from subintimal fibrosis, telangiectasia of capillaries and postcapillary venules, endothelial degeneration, and platelet thrombi formation associated with severe fibrosis of the lamina propria and crypt distortion. These changes correspond to the progressive ischemia and resulting symptoms are managed by patients with chronic radiation proctitis (104).

CLINICAL MANIFESTATIONS

The incidence of both acute and chronic radiation proctitis correlates with the dose of the radiation. Smit et al. (105) reported an incidence of 20% when the total dose to the anterior rectal wall was 7500 cGy or below compared with 60% when the dose was above 7500 cGy.

Patients may present with symptoms of radiation proctitis from as early as the first week of therapy to as late as 30 years posttreatment. Patients who present during or soon after therapy may complain of diarrhea (with or without blood), nausea, abdominal cramping, tenesmus, sphincter irritability, mucoid discharge, and, less commonly, constipation. Hematuria and dysuria may be present because of concurrent radiation injury of urinary tract. In general, these patients do well in the short term, with conservative medical therapy, typically resolving over two to six months. Approximately 20% of the patients with acute radiation proctitis require temporary cessation of radiation treatments and the majority of these symptoms within 1 to 2 weeks. Once the acute radiation proctitis has resolved, many patients remain asymptomatic and suffer no further manifestation of radiation injury (106).

Approximately 1% to 20% of patients who receive radiation therapy develop chronic radiation proctitis. The clinical presentation is determined by the location and severity of the radiation injury. These include rectal bleeding, most commonly from mucosal telangiectasias, intense fibrosis causing frozen pelvis, major tissue destruction resulting in vaginal, enteric, or cutaneous fistulas, or severe stricture formation presenting as partial to complete obstruction of the rectum. Patient complaints vary widely from severe pain to no pain and from constipation to diarrhea with or without incontinence. A rectum that appears severely affected by radiation damage on endoscopic examination but does not bother the patient, does not warrant treatment (106).

SURGICAL MANAGEMENT

The safest operation for treatment of severe and intractable radiation proctitis is fecal diversion via a stoma. Fecal diversion, in most cases, allows the rectal mucosal edema and secondary infection to subside: Bleeding usually ceases and pain is typically relieved. Surgical therapy is indicated for obstruction, stricture, perforation of rectal vaginal fistula, fecal incontinence, intractable pain, and persistent bleeding. If the patient is young, with good fecal continence, the Parks' coloanal anastomosis, preferably a colonic J pouch, should be considered. Patients with severe disease should have a proctectomy.

Low rectal complications from radiation for carcinoma of the prostate present a difficult problem. Larson et al. (107) conducted a retrospective study on 5719 patients who underwent radiation therapy at the Mayo Clinic for carcinoma of the prostate, between 1990 and 2003. Fourteen patients developed rectal complications: 10 patients (71%) had documented rectourethral fistulas; four patients (29%) had either transfusion-dependent, persistent rectal bleeding, or fecal incontinence. The treatment included fecal diversion alone (20%), urinary and fecal diversion alone (50%), and primary repair with or without a tissue flap and fecal diversion (29%) in the 14 affected patients. Symptomatic improvement and resolution of these three complications occurred in 12 (85%) of the patients. However, only 2 (15%) were able to retain their intestinal continuity to achieve this outcome.

TREATMENT FOR HEMORRHAGIC RADIATION PROCTITIS

Minor bleeding from radiation proctitis can be improved by treating the constipation or diarrhea. A 5-ASA enema has not been found to be helpful. Sucralfate, 2 g suspended in 20 mL tap water delivered as an enema twice a day, has been reported to promote healing (108).

Persistent and severe bleeding radiation proctitis is uncommon but can be a challenge. Currently, there are nonoperative techniques that should be tried first before considering a colostomy or a proctectomy.

Argon plasma coagulation (APC) is highly effective in controlling hemorrhagic radiation proctitis (109–112). Villaciencio et al. (109) performed this on an outpatient via a flexible endoscope. The Argon gas flow rate used ranged from 1.2 to 2 L/min, the electrical power setting from 45 to 50 W, and the probe size from 2.7 to 3.2 mm diameter. An effort was made to treat individual telangiectasias, and whenever possible to avoid "painting" the rectal mucosa so as to minimize ulceration. The pulse duration was usually less than one second unless telangiectasias were virtually confluent, in which case longer pulse durations are used. All lesions were treated in a single session whenever possible. Telangiectasias in the skin of the anal canal are not treated but the area coagulated was extended to the dentate line when necessary. The authors have treated 12 patients, all of whom were anemic, and 4 had received blood transfusions. The mean number of treatment sessions was 1.7, and 10 patients were successfully treated in a single session. Rectal bleeding resolved within one month of the last treatment in 19 patients, usually on the day of the last procedure. Short-term side effects occurred in three (14%) patients (rectal pain, tenesmus, and/or abdominal distention); long-term complications (rectal pain, tenesmus, diarrhea) developed in four patients (19%).

Topical application of diluted formalin has been found to stop active bleeding from radiation proctitis. Saclarides et al. (113) reported success in stopping bleeding in 75% of the patients with a single treatment. The rest of the patients improved but continued to have bleeding. The 4% formalin solution is prepared by mixing 200 mL of 10% buffered formalin with 300 mL water. The patient was prepared with cleansing enemas before the procedure. The procedure was performed in the operating room under local, caudal, or general anesthesia. Approximately 400 to 500 mL was instilled in 30 to 50 mL aliquots via a rigid sigmoidoscope. Each aliquot is kept in contact with rectal mucosa for 30 seconds. Saline should be used liberally to irrigate the rectum between formalin aliquots and to wash the perineum in the event that the formalin has escaped externally. The authors used this technique only in severe cases. In the milder case, they used a formalin-soaked cotton-tip applicator. This is a technique favored by Seow-Choen et al. (114). They performed this procedure under caudal anesthesia in lithotomy position. Gauze sponges soaked in 4% formalin were held in direct contact with bleeding sites through a rigid sigmoidoscope until the bleeding site ceased to bleed, which usually took 2 to 3 minutes. The process was repeated at other sites until all the bleeding had stopped. Seven of the eight patients had cessation of bleeding in one session and had not rebled through 1 to 6 months of follow-up. The eighth patient required a second session for mild recurrent bleeding two weeks later. Other authors also found this method of treatment to be effective (115–118).

The histologic study of the rectal mucosa after formalin application was studied by Chautems et al. (117). Endoscopic biopsies were performed at three different occasions: for four patients, immediately before 4% formaldehyde application; for four patients, immediately after the application; and for three patients, 1 month later and at 1 year. The results showed that unspecified radiation-induced reactions were found on the baseline-biopsies. The rectal mucosa was erythematous and friable. It contained edematous granulation tissue with a mild acute inflammation, small neovessels, bizarre atypical radiation fibroblast and mild fibrosis. On the biopsies performed after the application of 4% formaldehyde, multiple fresh thromboses appeared in the areas of neovascularization. This occurred only in the superficial mucosa. On the biopsies of the rectum performed one month or 12 months later, there were signs of chronic changes related to the radiotherapy, and there were no signs of acute inflammation or thrombosed vessels. This was characterized by mild fibrosis of the lamina propria, hyalinized vessel wall and muscular degeneration of the muscularis mucosa.

INCREASED RISK OF RECTAL CARCINOMA AFTER PROSTATE RADIATION

Radiation therapy for prostate carcinoma has been associated with an increased rate of pelvic malignancies, particularly bladder carcinoma. The association between radiation therapy and colorectal carcinoma yield conflicting results (119). In a study by Brenner et al. (120), a 105% increase in the incidence of rectal carcinoma was found in prostate carcinoma patients following radiation (vs. surgery) after more than 10 years of follow-up; in addition, a 24% (nonsignificant) increase in the incidence of colon carcinoma was found after radiation. In the other study by Neugut et al. (121), no increased incidence of rectal carcinoma was found in prostate carcinoma patients after radiation (vs. no radiation), even in those with long-term follow-up. Both of these studies have limitations that may explain the discrepant result. Most important, the mean years of follow-up are limited in both studies. The Brenner et al. study (120); included patients diagnosed from 1973 through 1993, but the mean survival time after prostate carcinoma diagnosis was only four years. The mean follow-up time was not presented in the Neugut et al. study (121); however, it included patients diagnosed from 1973 through 1990 and was published 4 years earlier than the Brenner et al. study; so follow-up would be even shorter. Given that biologically, the latency period between radiation exposure and radiation-induced malignancy is at least 5 years, neither study had sufficient follow-up time to determine the true effect of radiation. Similarly, both studies included cases of rectal carcinoma discovered at two months (120) and six months (121) after prostate diagnosis; yet such early rectal carcinomas could not have resulted from radiation exposure, rather they may have been missed. Neither study excluded patients with prior history of colorectal carcinoma (119).

Baxter et al. (119) conducted a retrospective cohort study using Surveillance, Epidemiology, and End Results (SEER) registry data from 1973 to 1994. The study focused on men with prostate carcinoma, but with no previous history of colorectal carcinoma, treated with either surgery or radiation who survived at least five years: The authors evaluated the effect of radiation on development of carcinoma for three sites: definitely irradiated sites (rectum), potentially irradiated sites (rectosigmoid, sigmoid, and cecum), and nonirradiated sites (the rest of the colon). Using a proportional hazards model, they evaluated the effect of radiation on the development of colorectal carcinoma over time.

The result showed that a total of 30,552 men received radiation, and 55,263 underwent surgery only. Colorectal carcinomas developed in 1437 patients: 267 in irradiated sites, 686 in potentially irradiated sites, and 484 in nonirradiated sites. Radiation was independently associated with development of carcinoma over time in irradiated sites but not in the remainder of the colon. The adjusted hazard ratio for development of rectal carcinoma was 1.7 for the radiated group, compared with surgery-only group. The authors concluded that there was a significant increase in development of rectal carcinoma after radiation for prostate cancer. Radiation had no effect on development of carcinoma in the remainder of the colon, indicating that the effect is specific to directly irradiated tissue.

This study represents a significant improvement over prior analysis of the secondary consequences of radiation for prostate carcinoma. First, their study is based on a large number of men with prostate carcinoma, all of whom had their prostate disease confirmed microscopically, underwent treatment for their disease, and had long-term follow-up; the mean follow-up time was 9 years in the radiation group and 9.5 years in the surgery-only group. The authors included only men who survived at least 5 years; thus, biologically, all radiated patients were at risk for radiation-induced rectal carcinoma. They excluded men with previous colorectal carcinoma as well as men who developed a colorectal carcinoma in the first five years after prostate carcinoma treatment. Allowing for this lag time serves two purposes: (i) it excludes men diagnosed with colorectal carcinoma only because of more intense evaluation associated with complications of their prostate carcinoma treatment, and (ii) it is consistent with the hypothesis that radiation-induced carcinogenesis takes at least five years to manifest. The authors found no increase in the incidence of colon carcinoma in potentially irradiated sites and nonirradiated sites; by using other parts of the colon as control measures, they reduced the likelihood that any observed radiation effect in the rectum was merely because of confounding and demonstrated that carcinogenic effect of radiation is specific to irradiated sites (119).

PREVENTION

RADIATION TECHNIQUE

Because of the high morbidity and mortality associated with late radiation complications, prevention of these injuries has received increasing attention. Fractionating radiation doses and other refinements in radiotherapy techniques have helped decrease radiation complications. However, by identifying those patients most at risk, further precautions can be taken. Green (122,123) has successfully developed a program for minimizing small bowel injury in high-risk patients. He initially identified high-risk patients by doing small bowel contrast studies. When small intestine adhesions were identified in the pelvis, Green modified the total dose, altered the size of the radiated field, and used various positioning techniques such as the prone position and bladder distention to minimize small bowel exposure.

Use of the hyperfractionation technique has been suggested for other patients with increased risk factors. This involves giving the patient less than the usual 180 to 200 rads per day and spreading the dose across several daily treatments (1). The use of barium-soaked vaginal packing around the radium source has also been recommended as a way to displace the bladder anteriorly and the rectum posteriorly away from the radium source (85).

Emptying the rectum before insertion of intracavitary radiation has also been recommended as a way to protect it from radiation (72).

A number of other methods for minimizing injury have been tried or are being considered. Hypoxia renders tissue less susceptible to radial injury, but it has not been useful since it also makes the carcinoma less radiosensitive (15). Elemental diets, TPN, and protease have been suggested as beneficial by decreasing pancreatic secretions or altering function (1).

RADIOPROTECTIVE AGENTS

There have been reports that have addressed pharmacologic manipulations of the luminal environment of the animal intestine. An alkaline lumen provides some reduction in radiation mucosal damage. Alterations in osmolarity have little influence. Absence of either bile salts or proteolytic enzymes at the time of radiation delivery leads to significantly diminished damage. Studies on using 5-ASA-Type drugs to prevent radiation proctitis are largely unsuccessful (52,124,125).

Balsalazide is a new generation 5-ASA drug that yields a high concentration of active drug in the distal colon. Jahraus et al. (126) conducted a randomized, double-blind, placebo-controlled trial. Twenty-seven patients with carcinoma of the prostate received 2250 mg capsules of Balsalazide twice daily for 5 days before radiotherapy and continued for 2 weeks after completion of radiation treatment. The results showed that with the exception of nausea or vomiting seen in 3 patients on Balsalazide and 2 on placebo, all toxicities were appreciably lower in patients taking Balsalazide. Proctitis was prevented most significantly with a mean proctitis index of 35 in Balsalazide patients and 74 in placebo patients.

These results were encouraging but have not been confirmed in a cooperative group trial to assess its efficiency in a multi-institutional setting.

Glutamine and an elemental diet have been shown to protect the intestine from radiation damage (127,128). Oral luminal adrenocortical steroid, methyl prednisolone, provides some damage reduction (19).

From all these observations, it is possible that the small bowel lumen can be physiologically or pharmacologically perturbed at the time of radiation exposure to reduce mucosal damage. The small bowel, however, does not lend itself to such manipulations by oral route in the clinical situation. Absorption, secretion, peristalsis, and, perhaps, enzymatic activity combine to frustrate efforts to bathe the entire small bowel mucosa with a chosen concentration of any substance.

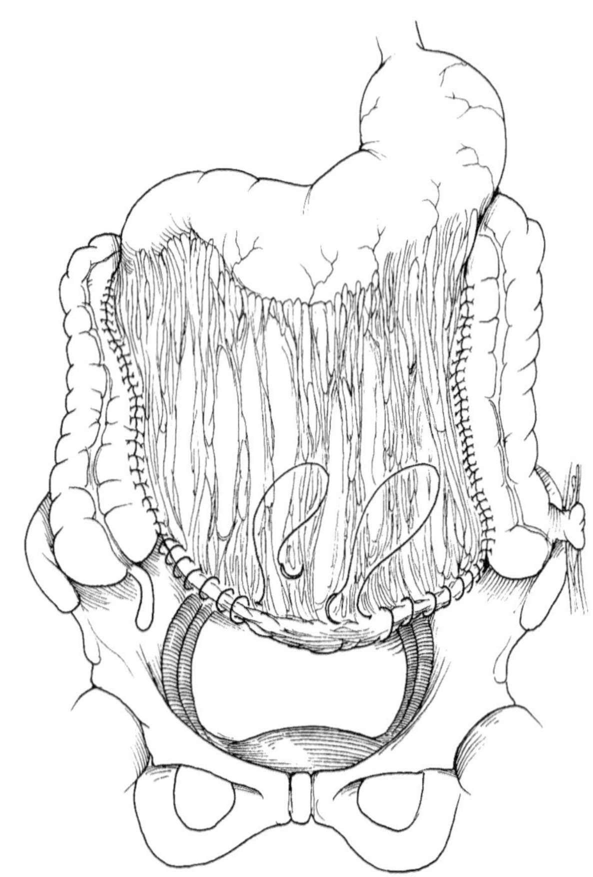

FIGURE 12 ■ Omental envelope. The apron of the greater ometum is sutured to the left and right colon and transversely, the pelvic brim and promontory of the sacrum.

■ SURGICAL TECHNIQUES

Three surgical techniques that are practical and useful to exclude the small intestine from the pelvis, and thus avoid or minimize radiation injury are the omental envelope (129–131) the absorbable mesh sling (132), and pelvic space tissue expander (133,134).

Omental Envelope

This technique can be accomplished only if the greater omentum has substantial size that can cover the upper to midabdominal cavity. The greater omentum is freed from any adhesion except at its pedicle to the greater curvature of the stomach. The cecum and terminal ileum are mobilized out of the pelvis. The entire small intestine is then covered with the entire greater omentum. The right free edge of the omentum is sutured to the anteromedial aspect of the ascending colon, beginning at the hepatic flexure and ending at the cecum (Fig. 12). This is accomplished with a continuous 3–0 braided or monofilament synthetic absorbable suture, taking full-thickness bites of the edge of the omentum to the seromuscular bites on the wall of the colon. Similarly, the left free edge of the omentum is sutured to the descending colon, beginning near the splenic flexure and ending at the level of descending sigmoid junction. The inferior free edge of the omentum begins at the previous suture at the cecum and continues transversely at the level of the pelvic brim, suturing the inferior free edge of the omentum to the posterior parietal peritoneum and ending in the midline on the sacral promontory where it meets the suture from the left side (Fig. 13).

If further descent of the omentum is required, it can be achieved by mobilizing the splenic and hepatic flexures of the colon and also by detaching the omentum from the greater curvature of the stomach. A final inspection is made to ascertain that no gaps exist in the suture lines so that herniation of the small intestine may be avoided (130). The series by Choi and Lee (131) compared 32 patients with omental envelope to 25 patients without. The former group was shown to protect the small bowel to radiation injury in both early and late follow-up. There has been no significant complication as the result of the omental hammock.

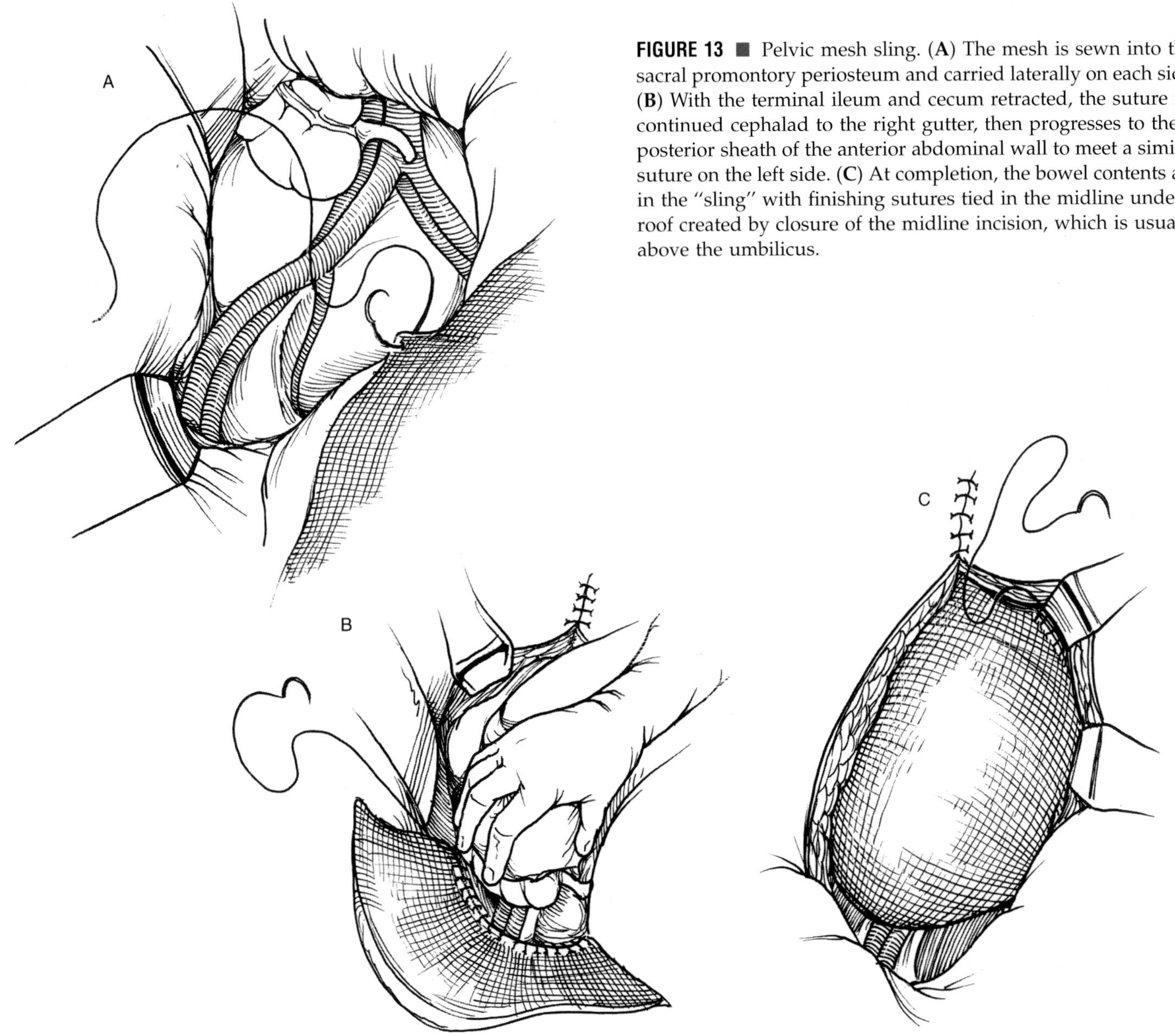

FIGURE 13 ■ Pelvic mesh sling. (**A**) The mesh is sewn into the sacral promontory periosteum and carried laterally on each side. (**B**) With the terminal ileum and cecum retracted, the suture is continued cephalad to the right gutter, then progresses to the posterior sheath of the anterior abdominal wall to meet a similar suture on the left side. (**C**) At completion, the bowel contents are in the "sling" with finishing sutures tied in the midline under a roof created by closure of the midline incision, which is usually above the umbilicus.

Pelvic Mesh Sling

A sheet of seven times 9 in. polyglycolic acid (Vicryl) mesh is sewn into the sacral promontory periosteum using two 2–0 monofilament synthetic absorbable sutures (Fig. 13A). The cecum and terminal ileum are mobilized to assure a more cephalad position. The suture on the right side incorporates the edge of the mesh to the sacral promontory and transversely to the posterior parietal peritoneum and continues cephalad to the right gutter on to the psoas and quadratus lumborum fascia (Fig. 13B). The suture then progresses to the posterior sheath of the anterior abdominal wall to meet the similar suture on the left side. The incision above the umbilicus is closed to allow suturing the mesh across the anterior abdominal wall. At completion, bowel contents are in the "sling" (Fig. 13C).

Devereux et al. (135) used this technique in 60 patients who received an average 5500 cGy in fractionated doses for rectal carcinoma and gynecologic malignancies. None has developed radiation enteritis with a mean follow-up of 28 months. Similar good results have also been obtained by Rodier et al. (136). In 60 patients with gynecologic malignancies who received irradiation between 4250 and 5800 cGy in fractions of 180 to 200 cGy per day, five days a week, 7% developed radiation enteritis, with a mean follow-up of 17.8 months (range, 1–57 months).

Tissue Expander in Pelvis

The concept of using tissue expander is to fill the pelvis cavity and exclude the small bowel from the radiation field. In the past, a saline-filled prosthesis for the breast augmentation was used. There are now available custom-designed pelvic tissue expanders with sewing straps (132). Sezeur et al. (134) used a silicone rubber molded balloon that can be filled with saline solution up to 600 mL, and has a spherical shape. A sheet of absorbable mesh is placed between the small bowel and the balloon. It is then fixed to the posterior and lateral pelvic walls to prevent small bowel herniation. The balloon is then filled with saline solution to the appropriate size, displacing the small bowel and ovary from the radiation field. They used this technique in 22 patients; one patient required its removal because of small bowel injury during the procedure. The rest of the patients showed no signs or symptoms of radiation enteritis, with the follow-up of 24.5 months (range, 10 to 73).

One disadvantage of using the tissue expander is that it must be removed at completion of the radiotherapy.

REFERENCES

1. Morgenstern L, Hart M, Lugo D, Friedman NB. Changing aspects of radiation enteropathy. Arch Surg 1985; 120:1225.
2. Andre N, Schmiegel W. Chemoradiotherapy for colorectal cancer. Gut 2005; 54:1194–1202.
3. Wheeler JMD, Dodds E, Warren BF, et al. Preoperative chemoradiotherapy and total urecorectal excisions surgery for locally advanced rectal cancer: Correlation with rectal cancer regression grade. Dis Colon Rectum 2004; 47:279–286.
4. Moore HG, Gittleman AE, Minsky BD, et al. Rate of pathologic complete response with increased interval between preoperative combined intrdality therapy and rectal cancer resection. Dis Colon Rectum 2004; 47:279–286.
5. Walsh D. Deep tissue traumatism from roentgen ray exposure. Br Med J 1897; 2:272.
6. Otchy DP, Nelson H. Radiation injuries of the colon and rectum. Surg Clin North Am 1993; 73:1017–1035.
7. Krook JE, Moertel CG, Gunderson LL, et al. Effective surgical adjuvant therapy for high-risk rectal carcinoma. N Engl J Med 1991; 324:709–715.
8. Kollmorgen CF, Meagher AP, Wolff BG, Pemberton JH, Martenson JA, Illstrup DM. The long-term effect of adjuvant postoperative chemoradiotherapy for rectal carcinoma on bowel function. Ann Surg 1994; 220:676–682.
9. Gilinsky NH, Bums DG, Barbezat GO, Levin W, Myers HS, Marks IN. The natural history of radiation-induced proctosigmoiditis: an analysis of 88 patients. Q J Med (New Series L11) 1983; 205:40.
10. DeCosse JJ, Rhodes RS, Wente WB, Reagan JW, Dworken HI, Holden WD. The natural history and management of radiation induced injury of the gastrointestinal tract. Ann Surg 1969; 170:369.
11. Palmer JA, Bush RS. Radiation injuries of the bowel associated with the treatment of carcinoma of the cervix. Surgery 1976; 80:458.
12. Harling H, Balsler I. Long-term prognosis of patients with severe radiation enteritis. Am J Surg 1988; 155:517–519.
13. Schofield PF, Holden D, Carr ND. Bowel disease after radiotherapy. J R Soc Med 1983; 76:463.
14. Wellwood JM, Jackson BT. The intestinal complications of radiotherapy. Br J Surg 1973; 60:814.
15. Kinsella TJ, Bloomer WD. Tolerance of the intestine to radiation therapy. Surg Gynecol Obstet 1980; 151:273.
16. Varma JS, Smith AN, Busuttil A. Correlation of clinical and manometric abnormalities of rectal function following chronic radiation injury. Br J Surg 1985; 72:875.
17. Cochrane JPS, Yarnold JR, Slack WW. The surgical treatment of radiation injuries after radiotherapy for uterine carcinoma. Br J Surg 1981; 68:25.
18. Kagan AR, Nussbaum H, Gilbert H, et al. A new staging system for irradiation injuries following treatment for cancer of the cervix uteri. Gynecol Oncol 1979; 7:166.
19. Delaney JP, Bonsack ME, Felemovicius I. Luminal route for intestinal radioprotection. Am J Surg 1993; 166:492–501.
20. Roswit B, Malsky SI, Reid CB. Severe radiation injuries of the stomach, small intestine, colon and rectum. Am J Roentgenol 1972; 114:460.
21. Girvin GW, Schnug GE, Cavanagh CR, McGonigle DJ. Complications of abdominal irradiation. Am J Surg 1971; 37:498.
22. Carr ND, Pullen BR, Hasleton PS, Schofield PF. Microvascular studies in human radiation bowel disease. Gut 1984; 25:448–454.
23. Smith DH, DeCosse JJ. Radiation damage to the small intestine. World J Surg 1986; 10:189.
24. Yeoh EK, Horowitz M. Radiation enteritis. Surg Gynecol Obstet 1987; 165:373.
25. Schmitz RL, Ghao JH, Bartolome JS. Intestinal injuries incidental to irradiation of carcinoma of the cervix of the uterus. Surg Gyhecol Obstet 1974; 138:29.
26. Villasanta U. Complications of radiotherapy for carcinoma the uterine cervix. Am J Obstet Gynecol 1972; 114:717.
27. Localio SA, Pachter HL, Gouge TH. The radiation-injury bowel. Surg Annu 1979; 11:181.
28. Berthrong M. Pathologic changes secondary to radiation. World J Surg 1986; 10:155.
29. Joelsson I, Raf L. Late injuries of the small intestine following radiotherapy for uterine carcinoma. Acta Chir Scand 1973; 139:1.
30. Yeoh EK, Lui D, Lee NY. The mechanism of diarrhea resulting from pelvic and abdominal radiotherapy: a prospective study using selenium-75 labelled conjugated bile acid and cobalt-labelled cyariocobalamin. Br J Radiol 1984; 57:1131.
31. Cunningham IGE. The management of radiation proctitis. Aust N Z J Surg 1980; 50:172.
32. Ludgate SM, Merrick MV. The pathogenesis of post-irradiation chronic diarrhea: measurement of SeHCAT and B_{12} absorption for differential diagnosis determines treatment. Clin Radiol 1985:275.
33. Varma JS, Smith AN. Anorectal function following coloanal sleeve anastomosis for chronic radiation injury of the rectum. Br J Surg 1986; 73:285.
34. Slaughter PD, Southwick HW. Mucosal carcinomas as a result of irradiation. Arch Surg 1957; 74:420.
35. Black WC, Ackerman LV. Carcinoma of the large intestine as a late complication of pelvic radiotherapy. Clin Radiol 1965; 16:2.
36. Sandler RS, Sandler DP. Radiation-induced cancers of the colon and rectum: assessing the risk. Gastroenterology 1983; 4:51.
37. Palmer JP, Spratt DW. Pelvic carcinoma following irradiation for benign gynecological diseases. Am J Obstet Gynecol 1956; 72:49–505.
38. Denman DL, Kirchner FR, Osborn JW. Induction of colon adenocarcinoma in the rat by x-irradiation. Cancer Res 1978; 3:1899–1905.
39. Gardiner GW, McAuliffe N, Murray D. Colitis cystica profunda occurring in a radiation-induced colonic stricture. Hum Path 1984; 15:295.
40. Valiulis AP, Gardiner GW, Mahoney LJ. Adenocarcinoma and colitis cystica profunda in a radiation-induced colonic stricture. Dis Colon Rectum 1985; 28:128.
41. Strockbine MF, Hancock JE, Fletcher GH. Complications in 83 patients with squamous cell carcinoma of die intact uterine cervix treated with 3000 rads or more whole pelvis irradiation. Am J Roentgenol 1970; 108:293.

42. Bourne RG, Kearsley JH, Grove WD, Roberts SJ. The relationship between early and late gastrointestinal complications of radiation therapy for carcinoma of the cervix. Int J Radiat Oncol Biol Phys 1983; 9:1445.
43. Lee KH, Kagan AR, Nussbaum H, Wollin M, Winkley JH, Norman A. Analysis of dose, dose-rate and treatment time in the production of injuries by radium treatment for cancer of the uterine cervix. Br J Radiol 1976; 49:430.
44. Yoonessi M, Romney S, Dayem H. Gastrointestinal tract complications following radiotherapy of uterine cervical cancer Past and present. J Surg Oncol 1981; 18:135.
45. Potish RA. Prediction of radiation-related small bowel damage. Radiology 1980; 135:219.
46. Potish RA, Jones TK Jr, Levitt SH. Factors predisposing to radiation-related small-bowel damage. Radiology 1979; 132:479.
47. Potish RA. Importance of predisposing factors in the development of enteric damage. Am J Clin Oncol 1982; 5:189.
48. Van Nagell JR, Maruyama Y, Parker JC Jr, Dalton WL. Small bowel injury following radiation therapy for cervical cancer. Am J Obstet Gynecol 1974; 118:163.
49. LoIudice T, Baxter D, Balint J. Effects of abdominal surgery on the development of radiation enteropathy. Gastroenterology 1977; 73:1093.
50. Danjoux CE, Catton GE. Delayed complications in colo-rectal carcinoma treated by combination radiotherapy and 5-Fluoro-uracil—Eastern Cooperative Oncology Group (ECOG) Pilot Study. Int J Radiat Oncol Biol Phys 1979; 5:311.
51. Phillips TL, Fu KK. Quantification of combined radiation therapy and chemotherapy effects on critical normal tissues. Cancer 1976; 37:1186.
52. Martenson JA, Hyland G, Moertel CG, et al. Olsasalazine is contraindicated during pelvic radiation therapy: results of a double-blind, randomized clinical trial. Int J Radiat Oncol Biol Phys 1996; 35:299–303.
53. Mulholland MW, Levitt SH, Song CW, Potish RA, Delaney JP. The role of luminal contents in radiation enteritis. Cancer 1984; 54:2396.
54. Rogers LF, Goldstein HM. Roentgen manifestations of radiation injury to the gastrointestinal tract. Gastrointest Radiol 1977; 2:281.
55. Hara AK, Leighton JA, Heigh RI, et al. Crohn disease of the small bowel: preliminary comparision among CT enterography, capsule endoscopy, small bowel follow-through, and ileoscopy. Radiology 2006; 233:128–134.
56. Boudiaf M, Jaff A, Soyer P, et al. Small-bowel disease: prospective evaluation of multi-detector row helical CT enteroclysis in 107 consecutive patients. Radiology 2004; 233:338–344.
57. Yuhasz M, Laufer I, Sutton G, Herlinger H, Caroline DF. Radiography of the small bowel in patients with gynecologic malignancies. Am J Roentgenol 1985; 144:303.
58. Dencker H, Holmdahl KH, Lunderquist A, Olivecrona H, Tylen U. Mesenteric angiography in patients with radiation injury of the bowel after pelvis irradiation. Am J Roentgenol 1972; 114:476.
59. Delbeke D. Integrated PET-CT imaging: implications for evaluation of patients with colorectal carcinoma. Seminars colon Rect Surg 2005; 16:69–81.
60. Scully RE, Mark FJ, McNeely WR, McNeely BW. Case records of the Massachusetts General hospital, case 9–1994. N Engl J Med 1994; 330: 627–630.
61. Morgenstern L, Thompson R, Friedman NB. The modern enigma of radiation enteropathy: Sequelae and solutions. Am J Surg 1977; 134:166.
62. McLaren JR. Sequelae of abdominal radiation and their medical management. Compr Ther 1977; 3:25.
63. Yeoh E, Horowrtz M, Antonietta R, Mueeke T, Maddox A, Chatterton B. Effect of pelvis: irradiation on gastrointestinal function: a prospective longitudinal study. Am I Med 1993; 95:397–406.
64. Nanielson A, Nyhlin H, Stendahl U, Stenling R, Suhr O. Chronic diarrhea after radiotherapy for gynecological cancer: occurrence and etiology. Gut 1991; 32:1180–1187.
65. Heusinkveld RS, Manning MR, Aristizabal SA. Control of radiation-induced diarrhea with cholestyramine. Int J Radiol Oncol Biol Phys 1978; 4:687.
66. Condon JR, Wolverson RL, South M, Brinkley D. Radiation diarrhea and cholestyramine. Postgrad Med J 1978; 54:838.
67. Baum CA, Biddle WL, Miner PB. Failure of 5-aminosalicylic acidenemas to improve chronic radiation proctitis. Dig Dis Sci 1989; 14:758–760.
68. Triantafillidis JK, Dadioti P, Nicolakis D, Mercias E. High dose of 5-aminosalicylic acid enemas in chronic radiation proctitis: comparison with betamethasone enemas. Am J Gastroenterol 1990; 85:1537–1538.
69. Beer WH, Fan A, Halsted CH. Clinical and nutritional implications of radiation enteritis. Am J Clin Nutr 1985; 41:85.
70. Miller DG, Ivey M, Young J. Home parenteral nutrition in treatment of severe radiation enteritis. Ann Intern Med 1979; 91:858.
71. Scolapio JS, Ukleja A, Burnes JU, Kelly DG. Outcome of patients with radiation enteritis treated with home parenteral nutrition. Am J Gastroenterol 2002; 97:662–666.
72. Russell JC, Wellch JP. Operative management of radiation injuries of the intestinal tract. Am J Surg 1979; 137:433.
73. Meissner K. Late radiogenic small bowel damage: guidelines for the general surgeon. Dig Surg 1999; 16:169–174.
74. Galland RB, Spencer J. Surgical aspects of radiation injury to the intestine. Br J Surg 1979; 66:135.
75. Walsh HPJ, Schofield PF. Is laparotomy for small bowel obstruction justified in patients with previously treated malignancy? Br J Surg 1984; 71:933.
76. Smith ST, Seski JC, Copeland LJ, Gershenson DM, Edwards CL, Herson J. Surgical management of irradiation-induced small bowel damage. Obstet Gynecol 1985; 65:563.
77. Swan RW, Fowler WC Jr, Boronow RC Surgical management of radiation injury to the small intestine. Surg Gynecol Obstet 1976; 142:325.
78. Dirksen PK, Matolo NM, Trelford JD. Complications following operation in the previously irradiated abdominopelvic cavity. Am Surg 1997; 43:234.
79. Dietz DW, Remzi FH, Fazio VW. Strictureplasty after obstructing small-bowel lesions in diffuse radiation enteritis—Successful outcome in fine patients. Dis Colon Rectum 2001; 44:1772–1777.
80. Onodera H, Nagayama S, Mori A, Fujimoto A, Tachibana T, Yonenaga Y. Reappraisal of surgical treatment for radiation enteritis. World J Surg 2005; 29:459–463.
81. Regimbeau JM, Panis Y, Gouzi JL, Fagniez PL, and the French University Association for Surgical Research. Operative and long-term results after surgery for chronic radiation enteritis Am J Surg 2001; 182:237–242.
82. Smith DH, Pierce VK, Lewis JL. Enteric fistulas encountered on a gynecologic oncology service from 1969 through 1980. Surg Gynecol Obstet 1984; 158:71.
83. Piver MS, Levitt SH. Enterovaginal and enterocutaneous fistulate in women with gynecologic malignancies. Obstet Gynecol 1976; 48:560.
84. Jackson BT. Bowel damage from radiation. Proc 1976; 69:683.
85. Dean RE, Taylor ES. Surgical treatment of complications resulting from irradiation therapy of cervical cancer. Am J Obstet Gynecol 1960; 79:34.
86. Reichelderfer M, Morrissey JF. Colonoscopy in radiation colitis. Gastrointest Endosc 1980; 26:41.
87. Kochhar R, Sriram PV, Sharma SC, Goel RC, Patel F. Natural history of late radiation procfusigmorditis treated with topical suspension. Dig Dis Sci 1999; 44:973–978.
88. Baum CA, Biddle WL, Miner PB Jr. Failure of 5-aminosalicyliz anol enemas to improve chronic radiation proctitis. Dig Dis Sci 1989; 34:758–760.
89. Levitsky J, Hong JJ, Jani AB, Ehrenpreis ED. Oral vitamin A therapy for a patient with a severely symptomatic postradiation anal ulceration. Report of a case. Dis Colon Rectum 2003; 46:679–682.
90. Ehrenpreis ED, Jani A, Levitsky J, Ahn J, Hong J. A prospective, randomized, double-blind, placebo-controlled trial of retinal palmitate (vitamin A) for symptomatic chronic radiation procfopathy. Dis Colon Rectum 2005; 48:1–8.
91. Niki E. Lipid antioxidants: how they may act in biological systems. Br J cancer 1987; 55:153–157.
92. Kennedy M, Bruninga K, Mutlu BA, Losurdo J, Choudhary S, Keshavarzian A. Successful and sustained treatment of chronic radiation proctitis with antioxidant Vitamins E and C. Am J Gastroenterol 2001; 96:1080–1084.
93. Borek C. Radiation and chemically induced transformation free radicals, antioxidants and cancer. Br J Cancer 1987; 55:74–86.
94. Jao SW, Beart RW, Gunderson LL. Surgical treatment of radiation injuries of the colon and rectum. Am J Surg 1986; 151:272.
95. Parks AG, Allen CLO, Frank JD, McPartlin JF. A method of treating post-irradiation rectovaginal fistulas. Br J Surg 1978; 65:417.
96. Allen-Mersh TG, Wilson EJ, Hope-Stone HF, Mann CV. The management of late radiation-induced rectal injury after treatment of carcinoma of the uterus. Surg Gynecol Obstet 1987; 164:521.
97. Browning GGP, Varma JS, Smith AN, Small WP, Duncan W. Late results of mucosal proctectomy and coloanal sleeve anastomosis for chronic irradiation rectal injury. Br J Surg 1987; 74:31.
98. Cooke SAR, De Moor NG. The surgical treatment of the radiation-damaged rectum. Br J Surg 1981; 68:488.
99. Gazet JC. Parks' coloanal pull-through anastomosis for severe, complicated radiation proctitis. Dis Colon Rectum 1985; 28:110.
100. Nowacki MP, Szawlowski AW, Borkowski A. Parks' coloanal sleeve anastomosis for treatment of post-radiation rectovaginal fistula. Dis Colon Rectum 1986; 29:817.
101. Boronow RC. Management of radiation-induced vaginal fistulas. Am J Obstet Gynecol 1971; 110:1.
102. Bricker EM, Johnston WD, Patwardhan RV. Repair of post-irradiation damage to colorectum. Ann Surg 1981; 193:555.
103. Starr DS, Lawrie GM, Morris GC Jr. Treatment of post-irradiation stricture of the rectum by the modified Duhamel procedure. Am J Surg 1979; 137:795.
104. Lisehora GB, Rothenberger DA. Radiation proctitis. Semin Colorect Surg 1993; 4:240–248.
105. Smit SGJM, Helle PA, Van Putten SJL. Late radiation damage in prostate cancer patients treated by high-dose external radiotherapy in relation to rectal dose. Int J Radiat Oncol Biol Phys 1990; 18:23–29.
106. Lisehora GB, Rothenberger DA. Radiation proctitis. Semin Colon Rectal Surg 1993; 4:240–248.
107. Larson DW, Chrouser K, Young-Fadok T, Nelson H. Rectal complications after modern radiation for prostates cancer: a colorectal surgical challenge. J Gastrointest Surg 2005; 9:461–466.
108. Kochhar R, Sharma SC, Gupta BB. Rectal sucralfate in radiation proctitis. Lancet 1988; 2:400.

109. Villaciencio RT, Rev DK, Rahmari E. Efficacy and complications of argon plasma coagulation for hematochezia related to radiation proctopathy. Gastrointest Endose 2002; 55:70–74.
110. Venkatesh KS, Ramanujam P. Endoscopic therapy for radiation proctitis-induced hemorrhage in patients with prostatic carcinoma using argon plasma coagulator application. Surg Endose 2002; 16:707–710.
111. Tjandra JJ, Serigupta S. Argon plasma coagulation is an effective treatment for refractory hemorrhagic radiation proctitis. Dis Colon Rectum 2001; 44:1759–1765.
112. Taief S, Rolachon A, Cerri JC, et al. Effective use of argon plasma coagulation in the treatment of severe radiation proctitis. Dis Colon Rectum 2001; 44:1766–1771.
113. Saclarides TJ, King DG, Franklin JL, Doolas A. Formalin instillation for refractory radiation-induced hemorrhagic proctitis. Dis Colon Rectum 1996; 39:196–199.
114. Seow-Choen F, Goh HS, Eu KW. A simple and effective treatment for hemorrhagic radiation proctitis using formalin. Dis Colon Rectum 1993; 36:135–138.
115. de Paradis V, Etienney I, Bauer P, et al. Formalin application in the treatment of chronic radiation-induced hemorrhagic proctitis—an effective but not risk-free procedure: A prospective study of 33 patients. Dis Colon Rectum 2005; 48:1535–1541.
116. Parikh S, Hughes C, Salvati EP, Eisenstad T, Oliver G, Chinn B, Notaro J. Treatment of Hemorrhagiz radiation proctitis with 4 percent formalin. Dis Colon Rectum 2003; 46: 596–600.
117. Chautems RC, Delgadillo X, Ruffia-Brandt L, Deleaval JP, Marti MCL, Roche B. Formaldehyde application for hemorrhagic radiation-induced proctitis: a clinical and histological study. Colorectal Dis 2003; 5:24–28.
118. Courter SF, Froese DP, Hart MJ. Prospective evaluation of formalin therapy for radiation proctitis. Am J Surg 1999; 177:396–398.
119. Baxter NN, Tepper JB, Durhan SB, Rothenberger DA, Virrig BA. Increased risk of rectal cancer after prostate radiation: A population-based study. Gastroenterology 2005; 128:819–824.
120. Brenner DJ, Curtis RE, Hall EJ, Ron E. Second malignancies in prostate carcinoma patients after radiotherapy compared with surgery. Cancer 2000; 88:398–406.
121. Neugut AI, Ahsan H, Robinson E, Ennis RD. Bladder carcinoma and other second malignancies after radiotherapy for prostate carcinoma. Cancer 1997; 79:1600–1604.
122. Green N. The avoidance of small intestine injury in gynecologic cancer. Int J Radiat Oncol Biol Phys 1983; 9:1385.
123. Green N, Melbye RW, Iba G, Kussin L. Radiation therapy for carcinoma of the prostate: The experience with small intestine injury. Int J Radiat Oncol Biol Phys 1978; 4:1049.
124. Resbent M, Marteau P, Cowen D, et al. A randomized double blind placebo controlled multicenter study of mesalazine for the prevention of acute radiation enteritis. Radiother Oncol 1997; 44:59–63.
125. Baughan CA, Canney PA, Bucharari RB, Piekering RM. A randomized trial to assess the efficiency of 5-aminosalicylic acid for the prevention of radiation enteritis. Clin Oncol 1993; 5:19–24.
126. Jahraus CD, Bettenhausen D, Malik W, Sellitti M, Stclair WH. Prevention of acute radiation-induced proctosigmoiditis by balsalazide: a randomized double-blind placebo controlled trial in prostate cancer patients. Int J Radiat Oncol Biol Phys 2005; 63:1483–1487.
127. Jensen JC, Schaefer R, Nwokedi E, et al. Prevention of chronic radiation enteropathy by dietary glutamine. Ann Surg Oncol 1994; 1:157–163.
128. McArdle AH, Reid EC, Laplante MP, Freeman CR. Prophylaxis against radiation injury. Arch Surg 1986; 121:879–885.
129. Lechner P, Cesnik H. Abdominopelvic omentopexy: preparatory procedure for radiotherapy in rectal cancer. Dis Colon Rectum 1992; 35:1157–1160.
130. De Luca FR, Ragins H. Construction of an omental envelope as a method of excluding the small intestine from the field of postoperative irradiation to the pelvis. Surg Gynecol Obstet 1985; 160:365.
131. Choi HJ, Lee HS. Effect of omental pedicle hammock in protection against radiation-induced enteropathy in patients with rectal cancer. Dis Colon Rectum 1995; 38:276–280.
132. Waddell BE, Lee RJ, Rodriguez-Bigas MA, Weber TK, Retrelli NJ. Absorbable must sling prevents radiation-induced bowel injury during "sandwich" chemoradiation for rectal cancer. Arch Surg 2000; 135:1212–1217.
133. Waddell BE, Radriguez MA, Lee RJ, Weber TK, Perrelli NJ. Prevention of chronic radiation enteritis. J Am Coll Surg 1999; 189:611–624.
134. Sezeur A, Marterla L, Abbou C, et al. Small intestine protecfim from radiation by means of a removable adapted prosthesis. Am J Surg 1999; 178:22–26.
135. Devereux DF, Chandler JJ, Eisenstat T, Zinkin L. Efficacy of an absorbable mesh in keeping the small bowel out of the human pelvis following surgery. Dis Colon Rectum 1988; 31:17–21.
136. Rodier JF, Janser JC, Rodier D, et al. Prevention of radiation enteritis by an absorbable polyglycolic acid mesh sling. A 60-case multi-centric study. Cancer 1991; 68:2545–2549.

32 Intestinal Stomas

Philip H. Gordon, Jean MacDonald, and Peter A. Cataldo

INTRODUCTION

Although the advent of restorative proctocolectomy and stapled low anterior anastomosis has lessened the need for permanent ileostomy and permanent end colostomy, the abdominal stoma still serves a critical function in the management of benign and malignant diseases. Currently, approximately 100,000 patients undergo stoma surgery in the United States, annually (1). Many of these patients will have major complications from the operation, and all of them will experience at least some problems as a result of the stoma. These problems are biopsychosocial in nature and may include surgical complications, peristomal skin complications, and problems with odor, noise, anxiety, depression, sexual dysfunction, and social isolation (2–4). The judicious assessment of the need for the stoma, careful surgical technique, and skilled enterostomal nursing are essential for a satisfactory outcome.

ILEOSTOMY

HISTORY

It was Baum who performed the first ever ileostomy in 1879 on a patient with an obstructing carcinoma of the ascending colon. The patient survived the ileostomy procedure but died from complications of a second operation that involved resecting the primary carcinoma and creating an ileocolic anastomosis. Kraussold, Billroth, Bergman, and Maydl were among the other 19th century surgeons who subsequently performed the ileostomy surgery. Maydl's patient is generally considered to be the first to survive and fully recover from an ileostomy performed in combination with resection for colon carcinoma (5).

In 1913, Brown (6) reported on 10 patients in whom he constructed an ileostomy. He made the stoma as an end ileostomy, closing off the distal end and bringing 2 inches of the proximal end out through the lower part of the incision. He inserted a catheter into the lumen and allowed it to separate as the surrounding tissue sloughed, and the bowel became granulated, contracted, and eventually formed a mucocutaneous junction with the abdominal wall skin. Brown achieved a favorable result in all of his patients.

The results of ileostomy surgery as reported by subsequent authors were uniformly disappointing. A variety of techniques were introduced, including the method of placing the terminal ileum through a separate right lower quadrant incision as an end ileostomy and various loop ileostomy techniques. The most significant achievement during this period, however, occurred in the late 1920s, when Dr. Alfred Strauss of Chicago performed an ileostomy and later a colectomy for ulcerative colitis on a young chemist named Koenig. Koenig subsequently designed an ileostomy appliance bag, commercially known as the Koenig-Rutzen bag. This appliance was used widely until the introduction of karaya in the 1950s.

In the following years, ileostomy-related fluid and electrolyte problems were identified and the need for earlier operation in patients with severe ulcerative colitis was recognized. The problem of high ileostomy output remained an obstacle to full rehabilitation for many patients until the, 1950s, when Warren and McKittrick (7) related the problem of ileostomy dysfunction to partial obstruction of the stoma at the level of the abdominal wall. A few years later Crile and Turnbull (8) showed that excessive ileostomy fluid loss in the early postoperative period resulted from serositis of the exposed ileal serosal surface. The authors subsequently showed that covering the exposed serosa with an everted layer of mucosa could prevent or minimize ileostomy dysfunction. The simplified full-thickness eversion technique described by Brooke (9) has since gained universal acceptance. Later technical developments include Goligher's description of the extraperitoneal ileostomy in 1958 (10) and the description by Kock et al. (11) of the continent ileostomy in the early 1970s.

Two events that were critical to the success of ileostomy surgery and the rehabilitation of the ileostomy patient were the formation of the first ileostomy club at Mount Sinai Hospital in New York in 1951 and the initiation of an educational program for enterostomal therapists [later to be known as enterostomal therapy (ET) nurses] by Rupert Turnbull at the Cleveland Clinic in 1961. Today the United Ostomy Association comprises 550 chapters and 34,000 members (personal communication, 1997). The speciality of ET nursing has matured and expanded as well, and in 1997, the number certified ET nurses exceeded 2300 (personal communication, 1997).

STOMAL PHYSIOLOGY

Physiologically left-sided colostomy output is very similar to that of normal bowel movements. There are essentially no significant physiologic abnormalities associated with left-sided colostomy; for that reason the physiology segment of this chapter will be dedicated to ileostomy output.

Ileostomy output clearly changes as the patient recovers from their operation and appears to have three distinct phases of adaptation. In the first three days, the output is bilious and liquid in nature and increases daily with the maximum output occurring on the third or fourth day. During the second phase, which occurs from the fourth to the sixth day following operation, the output stabilizes, thickens, and even decreases slightly. Phase III, adaptation, occurs from the first week to the eighth week following operation and is associated with a steady decrease in volume and thickening of the stoma output (12,13). After complete adaptation, the output from an end ileostomy created without significant ileal resection stabilizes between 200 and 700 cc/day.

Tang et al. (14) studied the ileostomy output of 60 patients who underwent restorative proctectomy with defunctioning ileostomy. By the fourth postoperative day, 65% of patients had a functioning ileostomy. Ileostomy output peaked at the fourth day with a median of 700 mL (range, 10–3250 mL) per 24-hour period. Output decreased after the 5th day, and by the 10th postoperative day, a median of 300 mL (range, 100–750 mL) per 24-hour period was reached despite normal intake. The authors noted that the critical period for acute dehydration was the third to eighth day and recommended aggressive fluid and electrolyte replacement. They therefore suggested that patients should not be discharged before 9 or 10 days after ileostomy construction.

Small bowel adaptation following ileostomy creation results in increased reabsorption of water and electrolytes.

In a normal individual, between 1500–2000 mL per day exit the terminal ileum into the colon. With ileostomy adaptation, 70% to 80% of this output is reabsorbed.

Historically, ileostomies were created without eversion and matured spontaneously in the first one to two weeks following operation. This was commonly associated with ileostomy dysfunction. In the 1950s, Warren and McKittrick related ileostomy dysfunction to partial obstruction due to stomal edema (7). This stomal edema was further clarified by Crile and Turnbull (8) when they showed that ileostomy effluent damaged the ileal serosa leading to serositis and subsequent edema and ileostomy obstruction. The primarily "matured" ileostomy described by Brooke has essentially eliminated ileostomy dysfunction (9).

Most patients are able to tolerate an unrestricted diet following postoperative recovery. Dietary changes have little effect on ileostomy output with the exception that fasting can decrease ileostomy output to between 50 and 100 mL/day. Studies have shown an elemental diet will decrease volume and concentration of digestive enzymes as well as bile acids (15). Diets high in fat, perhaps due to fat malabsorption and alternations in bile salt circulation, have been shown to increase stoma output to 20% above baseline (15,16). In addition, increases in oral fiber intake greater that 16 g/day have also been shown to increase output, stool frequency, and flatus (17).

Nutrition

Individuals with ileostomies associated with less than 100 cm of resected terminal ileum are able to maintain essentially normal nutrition. Although rare, fat malabsorption, from impaired bile salt absorption or reduced bile salt pool may cause osmotic diarrhea. Bile salt output may increase either by absorptive inhibition or perhaps by direct secretory stimulation on intestinal mucosa (15,18). Lactase deficiency and/or enterokinase deficiency may be more evident in individuals with an ileostomy. In the absence of significant terminal ileal resection, nutritional consequences of ileostomy are minimal and patients are able to maintain a normal weight and body composition. Resection of greater than 100 cm of terminal ileum or bacterial overgrowth may result in B12 malabsorption, and vitamin B supplementation may be necessary to prevent megaloblastic anemia.

Metabolic Changes

Normal individuals lose between 2 and 10 mEq of sodium in their stool on a daily basis, while the ileostomates lose approximately 60 mEq/day. In the review by Soybel (13), the daily steady-state of fecal losses following ileostomy compared to normal stool were: water, 100 to 150 mL vs. 650 mL; sodium, 1 to 5 mmol vs. 81 mmol; potassium, 5 to 15 mmol vs. 6 mmol; chloride, 1 to 2 mmol vs. 34 mmol. Symptomatic salt depletion, however, is rare due to renal compensation. Individuals with ileostomies have been shown to have chronically elevated mineralocorticoid levels that increase water and sodium reabsorption, compensating for the increased losses in the stool. Renal compensation combined with a normal diet make a chronic dehydration and salt depletion a rare circumstance in individuals with well-adapted ileostomies. Additionally, calcium, and magnesium levels are unaffected unless extensive terminal ileum has been resected.

Although the sodium concentration of ileostomy fluid rises and falls in relation to total body sodium levels, the usual sodium concentration is about 115 mEq/L. Others have reported the intestinal loss of sodium in patients with a conventional ileostomy to be 62 mmol/24 hours[a]. With dehydration, the sodium concentration falls and the potassium level rises; changes in the sodium/potassium ratio reflect the participation of the terminal ileum in sodium conservation during times of salt depletion. Normally the sodium/potassium ratio is about 12 and rarely rises above 15 (9). The pH is generally on the acidic side, just slightly below 7.

The bacteriologic composition of the ileostomy fluid is different from that of normal small or large intestine. Gorbach et al. (19) showed that the total number of bacteria in ileostomy effluent is approximately 80 times greater than that in the normal ileum. The ileostomy effluent contains a 100-fold increase in the number of aerobes, a 2500-fold increase in coliform bacteria, and increases in total anaerobes compared to the normal ileum.

The single most important factor influencing ileostomy output is the amount of uninjured intestine proximally (13). Increased body mass is associated with increased output. Water intake plays virtually no role. Elemental diets are associated with decreased volume while high fat content is associated with higher losses. Increases in fiber content increase ileostomy output by as much as 20% to 25% when dietary bran supplementation exceeds 16 g/day. Losses of nutrients such as carbohydrates and protein are also increased with diets high in fiber or fat. Overproduction of gastric acid contributes to the volume of ileostomy output. Ileostomy output decreases when patients receive antisecretory agents such as omeprazole, but such benefits are reaped only with patients with large ileostomy output ($\geq$2.61 L/day) or those who have had significant amounts of small bowel resected.

Intestinal transit does slow in individuals with end ileostomy. Using radioisotopes, Soper et al. demonstrated that gastric emptying was normal. However, oral stomal transit time was significantly increased compared to normal controls (348 min vs. 243 min) (20). Similar findings were observed in a study of transit times in individuals undergoing proctocolectomy and ileostomy (21). Similarly, Bruewer et al. demonstrated, by lactose breath test, that oral pouch transit time was prolonged in individuals undergoing proctocolectomy and IPAA (22). Adaptation occurs over a period greater than one year and the mechanism remains unknown. Theories include epithelial hypertrophy with an increased absorptive surface (23). In addition, an inverse relationship between nutrition and electrolyte absorption and intestinal transit time has been identified (24).

Bacterial flora in the ileostomy approaches that of the colon. Gorbach found an 80-fold increase in total number of organisms in the terminal ileum (19). Specifically coliforms were 2500 times more common than normal ileal fluid. However, ileostomy bacterial content was still considerably less than that or normal stool.

[a] For univalent molecules (e.g., Na^+, K^+) 1 mEq/L = 1 mmol/L.
For divalent molecules (e.g., Ca^{++}, Mg^{++}), 2 mEq/L = 1 mmol/L.

Bacteroides fragilis, a normal inhabitant of colonic stool, was rarely found in ileostomy output.

Individuals with inflammatory bowel disease, particularly associated with ileal resection and/or ileostomy, are at an increased risk for urinary stone formation. The incidence in these individuals' ranges from 3% to 13%, whereas it is 4% in the normal population (25). Uric acid stones are rare in the normal population, but comprise 60% of stones in individuals with an ileostomy (26). Low urinary volume and pH combined with increased concentrations of calcium and oxalate are thought to be responsible for this phenomenon (27). In addition, decreased urinary volume and decreased urinary pH facilitate stone precipitation (27). Prophylaxis and treatment consist of increasing daily fluid to increase urinary volume and urinary pH.

The association between ileostomies and gallstone formation has not been well established. Individuals with well-adapted ileostomies are found to have bile acid secretions similar to those with an intact colon (28,29). However, significant terminal ileal resection or extensive terminal ileal disease does affect the entero-hepatic circulation. Bile absorption and/or depletion may occur, resulting in increased saturation of bile that leads to bile salt precipitation and subsequent stone formation. Despite this, Ritchie found no increase in incidence in cholecystectomy rates in ileostomy patients compared with that in the normal population (30). However, Kurchin recommended prophylactic cholecystectomy in female individuals undergoing proctocolectomy or small intestinal resection for inflammatory bowel disease because of a threefold increase in asymptomatic gallstones (31).

Ileostomy Dysfunction

Significant diarrhea may occur in individuals with ileostomies for many reasons. It develops more rapidly and has greater physiologic consequences than when it occurs in individuals with a normal colon. Diarrhea may result from significant ileal resection, partial small obstruction, bacteria overgrowth, recurrent or persistent regional enteritis, or infections. In most cases, treatment is similar to those given to individuals with an intact colon. Specific attention must be paid to fluid and electrolyte repletion, however, because these individuals are at significant risk for dehydration and metabolic abnormalities.

Kusuhara et al. (32) found that the administration of a somatostatin analog, SMS 201–995 (100 μg thrice a day for five days), reduced the daily output of proximal ileostomies from 997 to 736 g along with a decrease in daily sodium and chloride excretion. The authors suggested a possible role for this agent in the management of a proximal ileostomy.

Bacterial overgrowth may develop when stasis occurs in the small bowel and can lead to deconjugation of bile salts and subsequent osmotic diarrhea as well as B12 malabsorption. Unconjugated bile salts impair sugar, water, sodium, and potassium reabsorption in the small intestine (33). In addition, anaerobic bacteria bind to the B12-intrinsic factor complex inhibiting reabsorption. Treatment is directed at eliminating the cause of stagnation in the small intestine and, if appropriate, antibiotics to decrease bacterial load.

■ TYPES OF ILEOSTOMIES

End Ileostomy

An end ileostomy is indicated after a total proctocolectomy for inflammatory bowel disease or familial polyposis, and in some cases after more limited resection for other colonic diseases. The procedure is rarely performed today without concomitant resection. It is potentially reversible when it has been performed with a partial or total colectomy (when the hazards of primary anastomosis between the ileum and colon or rectum were considered to be unacceptably high), such as in cases of ischemic infarction, peritonitis, or severe nutritional deficiency.

When the ileostomy is performed for benign inflammatory conditions, it is desirable to preserve as much ileum as possible; consequently the ileum should be divided within 1 to 2 cm of the ileocecal valve. If the resection is performed for benign conditions, it is possible to preserve the ileocolic artery, although collateral flow from the next proximal mesenteric vessel is sufficient to nourish the entire distal ileum.

Once the blood supply and mesentery have been taken, the ileum is divided between either staples or intestinal clamps. The small mesenteric vessels and fat are trimmed proximally for a distance of 5 to 6 cm. A 1-cm strip of mesentery is left attached to the terminal bowel in order to prevent ischemia. A 2.5- to 3-cm circumferential incision is made in the skin around the previously marked site in the right lower quadrant (Fig. 1A). Care should be exercised not to remove excess subcutaneous fat because its presence is beneficial in the support of the ileostomy appliance. Keating et al. (34) recommend the adoption of the use of a simple transverse incision 3 to 4 cm long on the apex of the skin fold. No skin or subcutaneous fat is excised so that on reversal of the stoma, the skin edges fall back together without tension. The ultimate wound is cosmetically better with less skin scarring. The fascia is exposed, and a cruciate incision is made through the fascia (Fig. 1B). The rectus muscle is spread apart with a hemostat, and the incision is carefully extended through the posterior rectus sheath and peritoneum, with a scissors or scalpel (Fig. 1C). The opening is extended to produce a defect of 3 to 4 cm that corresponds to the width of the tips of the index and middle fingers of a surgeon with average-size hands.

The ileum is drawn through the circular incision in the right lower quadrant so that the ileal mesentery is oriented cephalad, toward the diaphragm (Fig. 1D). Exteriorization of 5 to 6 cm of ileum should be accomplished (Fig. 1E). The mesenteric defect is closed by suturing the cut edge of the mesentery to the anterior abdominal wall 2 cm lateral to the midline incision from the ileostomy site to the ligamentum teres (Fig. 1F). The ileum may be secured to the peritoneum and posterior rectus fascia with interrupted or running absorbable sutures.

The extraperitoneal technique may be used as an alternative to closing the mesenteric defect, although this technique has the disadvantage of making ileostomy takedown more difficult. The technique may be better suited for colostomy construction following abdominoperineal resection.

The primary Brooke-type maturation of the ileostomy can either be performed at this point or after the abdominal

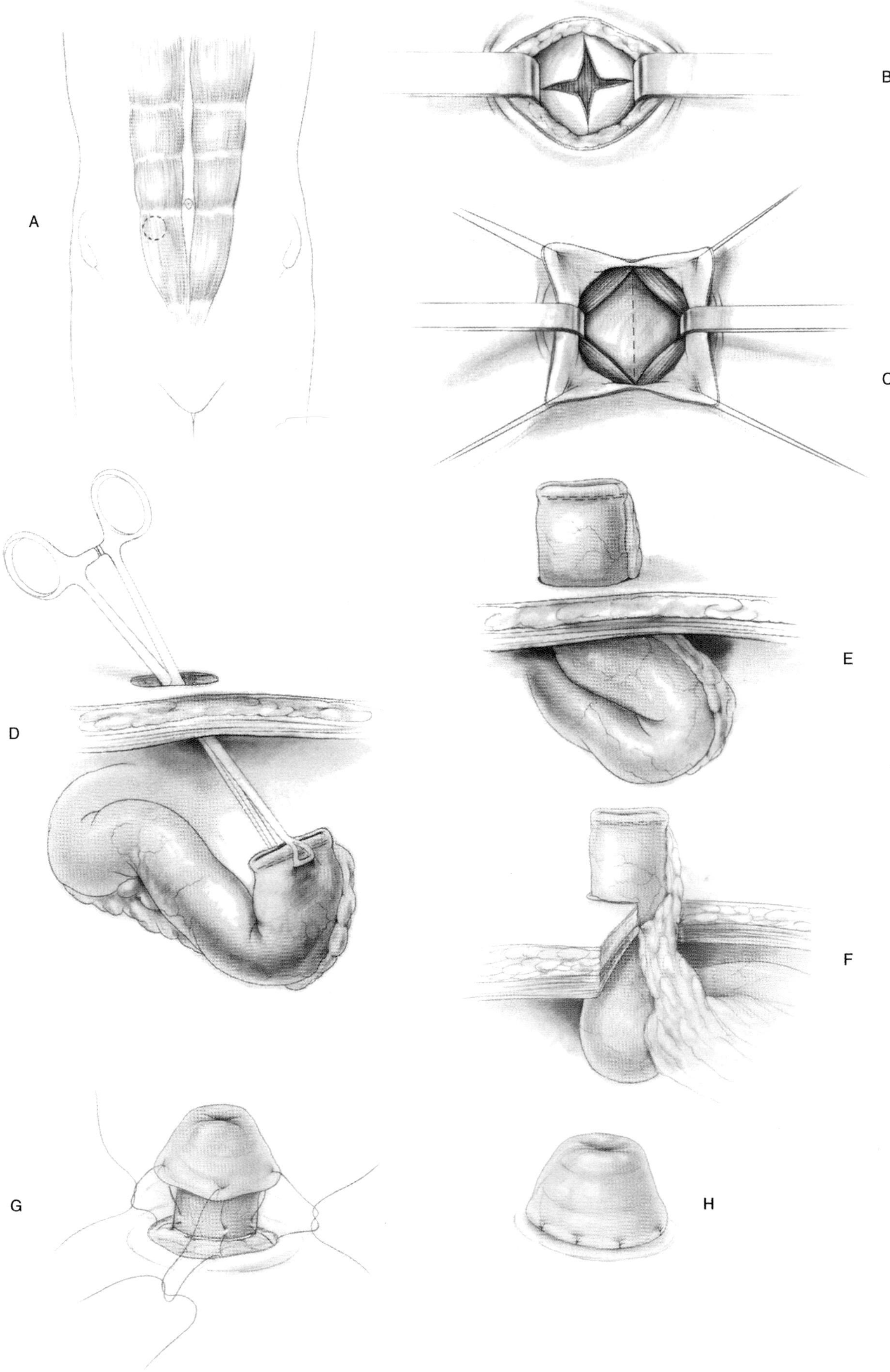

FIGURE 1 ■ Technique of Brooke end ileostomy construction (intraperitoneal method). (**A**) Skin and subcutaneous fat are resected over rectus muscle in preselected right lower qudrant site. (**B**) Cruciate incision is made in fascia. (**C**) Rectus muscle is retracted and peritoneal cavity is entered. (**D** and **E**) Ileum is delivered through ileostomy site. (**F**) Ileal mesentery is fixed to peritoneum from the ileostomy to the ligamentum teres. (**G** and **H**) Brooke maturation is done. (*I on next page*)

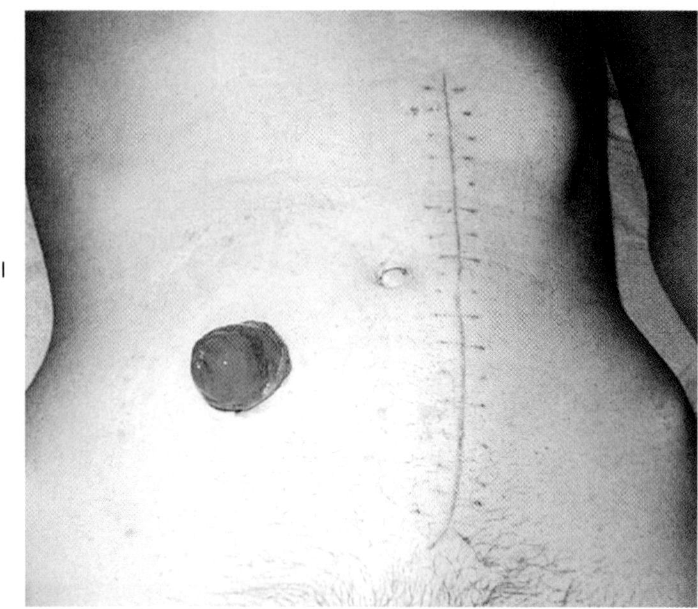

FIGURE 1 ■ (I) Well-constructed ileostomy showing satisfactory protrusion above skin level.

wall has been closed. The advantage of waiting until the abdomen is closed is that it prevents the spilling of ileostomy contents into the abdominal cavity and onto the wound. The advantage of maturing the stoma immediately is that it allows the surgeon to make adjustments as needed if inspection of the ileostomy suggests that its viability is tenuous. The mucosal surface should always be pink and should bleed freely at its edges. The primary maturation is performed by placing interrupted three-point buttressing sutures of absorbable suture between the tip of the ileum, the seromuscular layer of the ileum at the level of the fascia, and the skin (Fig. 1G). Interrupted sutures connecting the full-thickness bowel wall directly to the dermis of the skin are then added to secure the ileostomy (Fig. 1H). The ileostomy should protrude at least 2 cm beyond the abdominal wall (Fig. 1I). An appliance bag is fitted immediately in the operating room.

The Brooke ileostomy is now the most widely used technique for construction of an end ileostomy. In most patients it is relatively simple to perform and problems with retraction, serositis, or obstruction are uncommon. In some patients, however, the terminal ileal segment may be so edematous that full-thickness eversion using the Brooke technique is not possible. In these instances, the Turnbull technique may be useful (8). This involves resecting the distal serosa and muscularis and everting the mucosa over the proximal ileum.

The Guy rope suture technique is an alternative method of creating eversion in a thickened terminal ileum without the need for seromuscular resection. With this technique, three permanent 3–0 absorbable sutures are placed between the distal edge of the ileum and the full thickness of the skin. In addition, three temporary internal Guy traction sutures are placed 1.5 to 2 cm part inside the ileal lumen. Upward traction on the Guy sutures with simultaneous outward traction on the permanent external sutures helps to evert the thickened segment without damage or tearing of the mucosa (35).

Carlsen and Bergan (36) reviewed the complications of 358 end ileostomies: 224 were primary constructions, 96 were reconstructed by laparotomy, and 38 were local reconstruction. Only two ileostomies were primarily located on the left side. The mean length was 5 cm. The authors performed 11.6% reoperations after primary ileostomy and 7.3% and 7.9% reoperations after reconstruction by laparotomy and local approach, respectively. There were 12.9% and 8.7% reoperations after emergency and elective primary operations, respectively. Closing the lateral gutter or fixation of ileum to the rectus fascia did not significantly influence the number of reoperations. Postoperative discoloration of the ileostomy was not predictive of ileotomy dysfunction. Stenosis of the ileostomy, peristomal fistulas, and peristomal dermatitis were seen in 23 (10.3%), 21 (9.4%), and 18 (8%) of the patients after primary ileostomies, respectively. Patients with Crohn's disease had significantly more of these problems than patients with ulcerative colitis. Only a few patients had retraction of the ileostomy (2.7%), stomal prolapse (1.8%), or parastomal herniation (1.8%). Women had significantly more parastomal herniation than men; otherwise, there were no differences between the sexes.

Loop Ileostomy

The loop ileostomy is used to protect an ileoanal or high-risk colonic anastomosis. Although a loop transverse colostomy had traditionally been used to protect a low-lying colorectal anastomosis, Williams et al. (37) recommend the loop ileostomy whenever a stoma is needed to divert stool from the distal colorectum. The authors compared the loop ileostomy to the loop colostomy and found that the ileostomy had significantly less odor, required significantly fewer appliance changes, and had fewer overall problems than the colostomy. Others have advocated loop ileostomy as a superior method for diverting the bowel to cover a colonic or rectal anastomosis and found septic complications following ileostomy closure less frequent than those following colostomy closure. However, postoperative bowel obstruction and other serious complications such as severe dehydration requiring antidiarrheal medication and hospitalization, skin breakdown, and even cholelithiasis may occur, rarely (38).

Winslet et al. (39) assessed the defunctioning efficiency of the loop ileostomy using a radioisotope and dye technique. The median defunctioning capacity in patients without episodes of fecal discharge per rectum ($n = 18$) was 99% and was not affected by body position or the formation of a dependent stoma. In four patients who passed fecal material per rectum but who had no stomal retraction, the median defunctioning efficiency was 99%, and continued fecal discharge was considered to be due to mucopurulent secretion from active distal disease. In four patients who passed fecal material per rectum and also had a retracted stoma, the defunctioning efficiency was significantly reduced (median, 85%), owing to the overspill into the distal limb.

Chen and Stuart (40) reviewed the choice of a defunctioning stoma in restorative resection for colorectal carcinoma. The authors found the morbidity of stoma construction and closure comparable, but favored loop ileostomy because it is generally easier to manage.

Loop ileostomies are most commonly created at the time of laparotomy and bowel resection; therefore, exposure is generally through a midline incision. A segment of ileum several centimeters proximal to the ileocecal valve [which

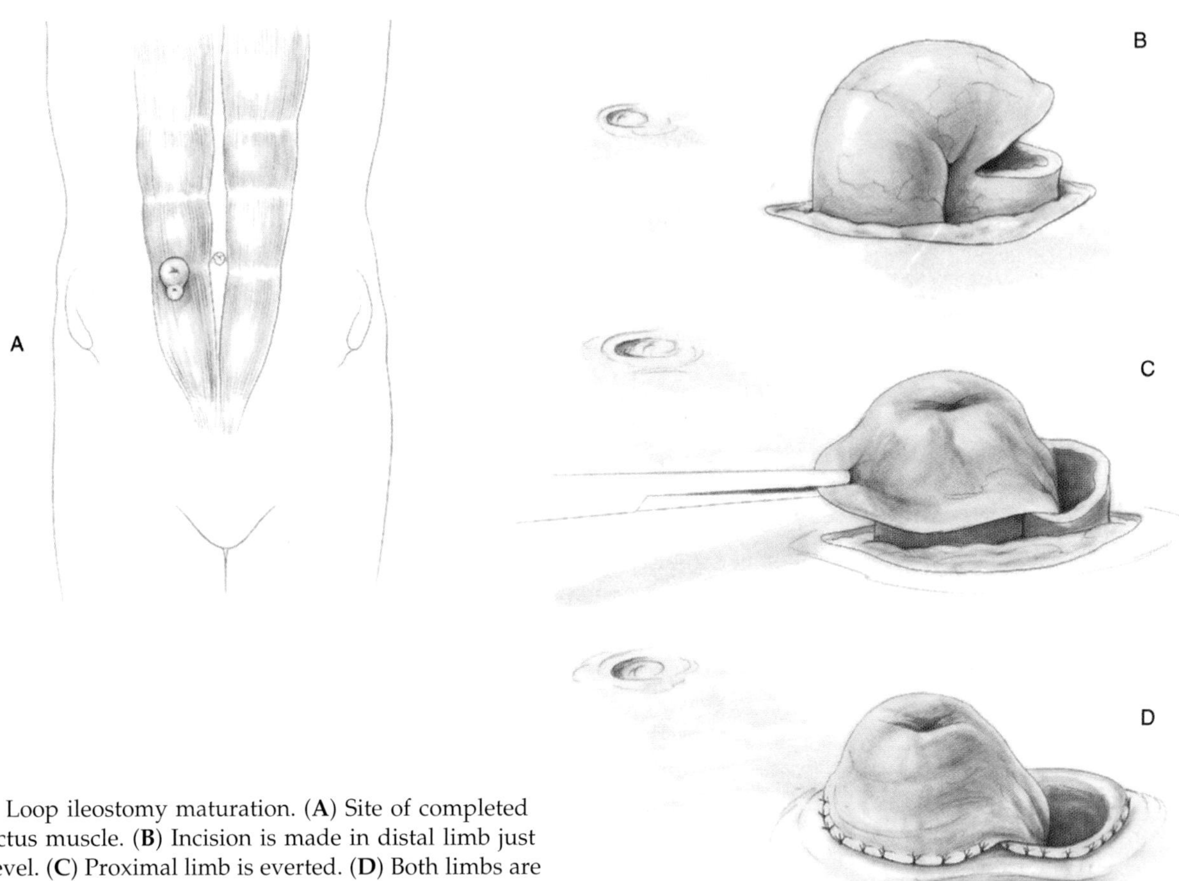

FIGURE 2 ■ Loop ileostomy maturation. (**A**) Site of completed loop over rectus muscle. (**B**) Incision is made in distal limb just above skin level. (**C**) Proximal limb is everted. (**D**) Both limbs are sutured to skin.

reaches the predetermined stoma site without tension (Fig. 2A)] is chosen and encircled with a penrose drain or grasped with a Babcock clamp. The distal limb is tagged with a suture or scored to insure correct orientation.

A disc of skin in excised and defect in the abdominal wall is created similar to or slightly larger than an of end ileostomy. The loop is then passed through the abdominal wall with care to avoid twisting. The suture marking the distal limb should be clearly visible.

The loop is matured by making an incision across the distal aspect of ileum from one mesenteric border to the other at skin level (Fig. 2B). This allows the functional limb to be the larger of the two stomas. The functional, or proximal limb will assume a cephalad position, and the defunctionalized loop will assume a caudad position. The distal loop is sutured to the dermis of the skin with 3–0 absorbable suture. The cephalad, proximal end is then everted to assume the appearance of an end ileostomy by placing three-point anchoring sutures through the ileostomy tip, the ileum at the fascia level, and the dermal layer of the skin (Fig. 2C). Interrupted sutures securing the remainder of the afferent opening to the skin level are placed to complete the stoma maturation (Fig. 2D). In most circumstances a stomal support rod is not necessary.

Some authors (37,41,42) prefer to rotate the loop 180° so that the afferent loop is in the caudad position and the defunctionalized efferent limb is cephalad to allow for maximal fecal diversion when the patient is upright. However, this increases the risk of bowel obstruction and does not improve diversion rates (43).

Prasad et al. (44) described a rodless end-loop ileostomy procedure in which the ileum is divided between surgical staples after only a short segment of mesentery has been taken and the stapled proximal end is brought out and matured as a Brooke ileostomy. The antimesenteric corner of the distal stapled end is brought out inferiorly, and a small distal ileostomy opening is created and matured primarily at the skin level (Fig. 3). Sitzmann (45) has described a similar technique in which the staple line of the distal limb is left closed and the limb is tacked to the afferent limb at the level of the fascia.

End-loop ileostomies may be created in any situation where a loop ileostomy is indicated. They may be particularly helpful in individuals with thick abdominal walls or short ileal mesenteries. In addition, if there is a significant likelihood that the "temporary" ileostomy may become permanent, an end-loop stoma may make long-term management easier for the ostomate. The end-loop ileostomy is constructed by dividing the ileum with staples and by elevating the ileum at a point where the bowel is redundant enough to permit elevation above the abdominal wall. This ileostomy is matured in the same way as a conventional incontinuity loop ileostomy (Fig. 4) (36).

■ LOOP ILEOSTOMY TAKEDOWN

Before closing a diverting ileostomy, it is important to ensure that there is no distal stricture as may be seen in patients with a diverting ileostomy constructed at the time of an ileal-pouch anal reservoir. Takedown of a loop ileostomy generally can be performed through a peristomal incision and usually does not necessitate a formal laparotomy. In some patients, particularly in those who are obese or have unusually dense adhesions, it may be necessary to open the previous abdominal incision and mobilize additional small bowel in order to safely perform the procedure.

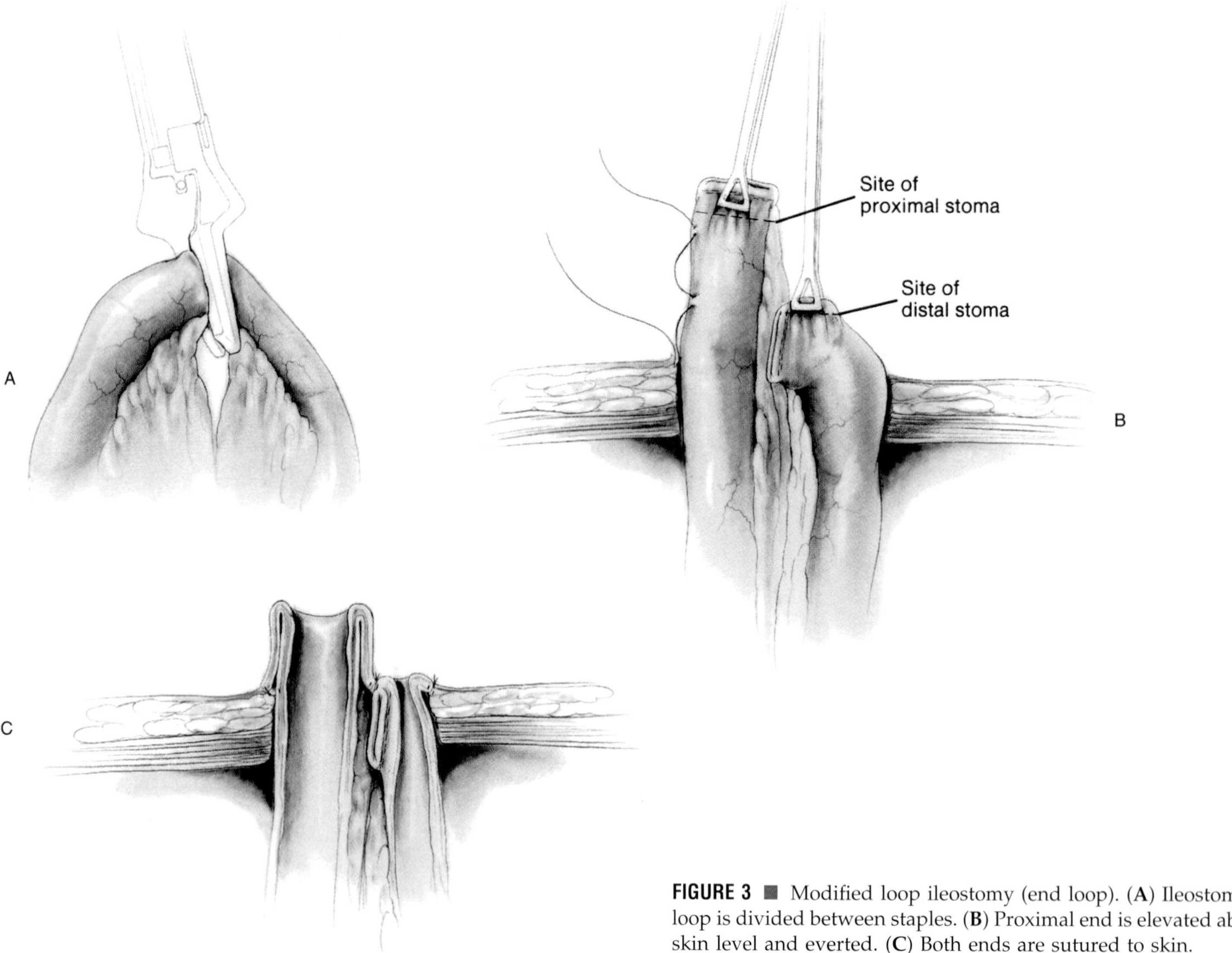

FIGURE 3 ■ Modified loop ileostomy (end loop). (**A**) Ileostomy loop is divided between staples. (**B**) Proximal end is elevated above skin level and everted. (**C**) Both ends are sutured to skin.

A smooth elliptical incision is made with 1 to 2 mm of skin taken above and below the ileostomy and extension of the incision approximately 1 cm from the medial and lateral edges of the stoma. The incision is extended down to the fascia and the peritoneum by sharp dissection, with meticulous care taken to avoid bowel injury. Once the proximal and distal limbs of the loop have been freed down to the peritoneal level, the remaining peritoneal attachments to the abdominal wall can be stripped away either by blunt or sharp dissection. The ileal segment has been adequately mobilized when it can be elevated from the incision and the wound edges are clear to the peritoneum (Fig. 5A and B). The surgeon then has three options of closure: anterior ileal wall closure, stomal resection with end-to-end anastomosis, and functional end-to-end stapled anastomosis.

The choice of anterior wall closure as opposed to resection and anastomosis is one that can be made at the time of surgery. It is often feasible to, simply resect the stomal margin and the attached rim of skin and then transversely close the bowel in either one or two layers or with staples (Fig. 5C and D). If induration or distortion of the lumen is present, however, it is safe to resect the edges of both limbs and perform a primary end-to-end anastomosis using healthy ileal tissue proximally and distally (Fig. 5E–I).

Kestenberg and Becker (46) proposed the technique of stapled functional end-to-end anastomosis because of the dissatisfaction they experienced with long operating times, anastomotic edema, stricture, and partial obstruction following end-to-end anastomosis. Their technique involves mobilizing both proximal and distal limbs of the ileostomy, then making a 1-cm enterotomy on each limb just below the ileostomy and firing the linear stapler through these enterotomies. The stoma is resected after a stapling device is fired just below the enterotomy segments (Fig. 6). A functional end-to-end anastomosis as depicted in Figure 40 in Chapter 23 can be used with equal efficacy.

van de Pavoordt et al. (47) reviewed their experience with closure of loop ileostomies. Ninety-three percent of the stoma closures were done through simple transverse incisions. The overall complication rate was 17%. Of the early postoperative complications (13%), the major complication was small bowel obstruction, commonly in patients in whom the stoma was protecting a pelvic ileal reservoir. Abdominal septic complications were 1%. The wound infection rate after healing by both secondary intention and primary skin closure was 3%. Only one incisional hernia was observed in the late postoperative period; in three patients, a posterior rectus sheath defect at the stoma site

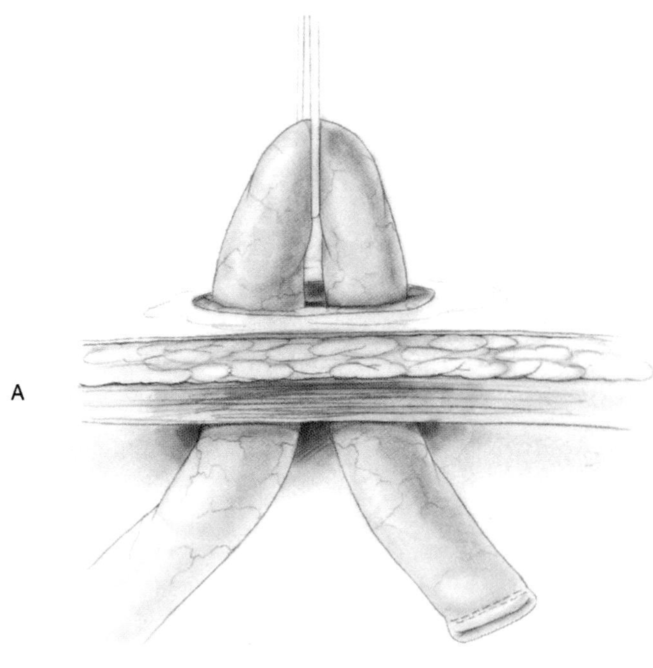

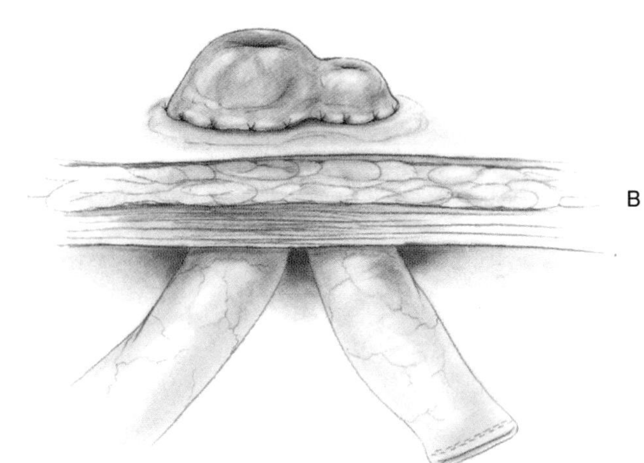

FIGURE 4 ■ An end-loop ileostomy. (**A**) Loop of ileum is elevated proximal to stapled end. (**B**) Completed maturation of loop.

was found incidentally at laparotomy, without clinical evidence of an incisional hernia.

COLOSTOMY

HISTORY

In 1776 Pillore, a French surgeon, created a cutaneous cecostomy for a wine merchant suffering from obstructing rectal carcinoma. Although the patient died two weeks later from a small bowel perforation induced by forced catharsis, the cecostomy was the first recorded instance of a successful colonic stoma being performed (48). At autopsy, the cecostomy was healthy. A number of sporadic reports of colostomies followed, and these generally involved construction of a loop colostomy for obstruction in adults or imperforate anus in infants. In 1793 Duret, a naval surgeon from Brent, performed the first successful left iliac colostomy for a case of imperforate anus in a child three-days old. The patient lived to the age of 45 years. In 1839 Ammusat, a Parisian surgeon, reported 29 cases of colostomy, with all of them sited in the lumbar area. Twenty-one of these cases involved infants with an imperforate anus; of these, four survived.

In 1884, Maydl introduced the technique of loop colostomy supported by a rod, when he suggested using a goose quill to support the loop against the abdominal wall. In 1881, Schitininger described the creation of an end sigmoid colostomy and an oversewn distal stump. This operation was the forerunner of the Hartmann procedure described in 1923, which consisted of sigmoid resection with end colostomy and an oversewn rectal stump (48). The operation of colostomy for obstruction came into widespread use in the 20th century.

Miles (49) has been credited for the 1908 description of the operation of end sigmoid colostomy and abdominoperineal resection. In fact, C.H. Mayo had previously described the technique in 1904. This operation, with the loop colostomy that preceded it, ushered in a new surgical era. The end sigmoid colostomy and loop diverting colostomy as described by Miles, Maydl, and others have now been performed by thousands of surgeons on hundreds of thousands of patients in this century with relatively few technical modifications. In the last two decades, the need for end sigmoid colostomy has diminished as surgical stapling techniques have made low anterior anastomosis more feasible (50). At the same time, there has been an increased interest in developing alternatives to permit continent function or control of colostomy output. These include magnetic stoma devices (51), the Conseal plug (Coloplast, Inc., Tampa, FL, U.S.A.) (52), and a silicone implantable ring (53). Although none of these products has enjoyed widespread acceptance, devices like these someday may become popular and important.

FECAL DIVERSION

Although the standard method of diverting the fecal stream away from the left colon has traditionally been the transverse loop colostomy, the indications for fecal diversion as well as the choice of a loop colostomy as the best means to achieve this have become controversial. The most common indications for diversion in the past have been obstruction or inflammation of the left colon, trauma to the colon, anterior resection of the rectum, and perineal sepsis. The increasing popularity of Hartmann's procedure with end colostomy for diverticulitis or obstructing carcinoma, the more aggressive use of primary resection and anastomosis in some of these cases, and the increasing reliance on primary closure for many colon injuries have no doubt decreased the popularity of loop colostomy in the emergency setting.

Fielding et al. (54) prospectively studied more than 2000 patients having elective colorectal anastomoses and found that 15.8% received a synchronous covering stoma to protect the anastomosis. No differences in mortality were

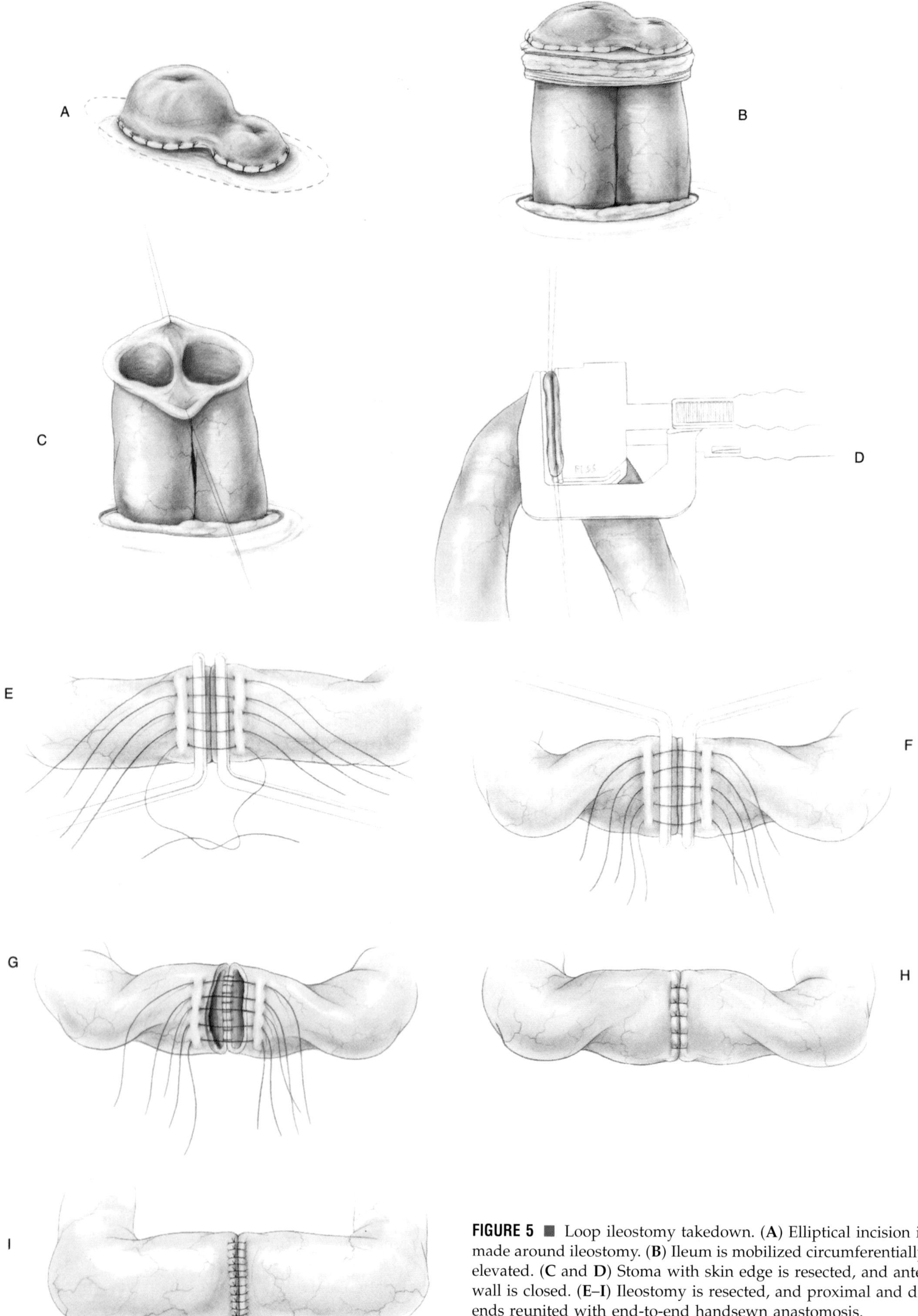

FIGURE 5 ■ Loop ileostomy takedown. (**A**) Elliptical incision is made around ileostomy. (**B**) Ileum is mobilized circumferentially and elevated. (**C** and **D**) Stoma with skin edge is resected, and anterior wall is closed. (**E–I**) Ileostomy is resected, and proximal and distal ends reunited with end-to-end handsewn anastomosis.

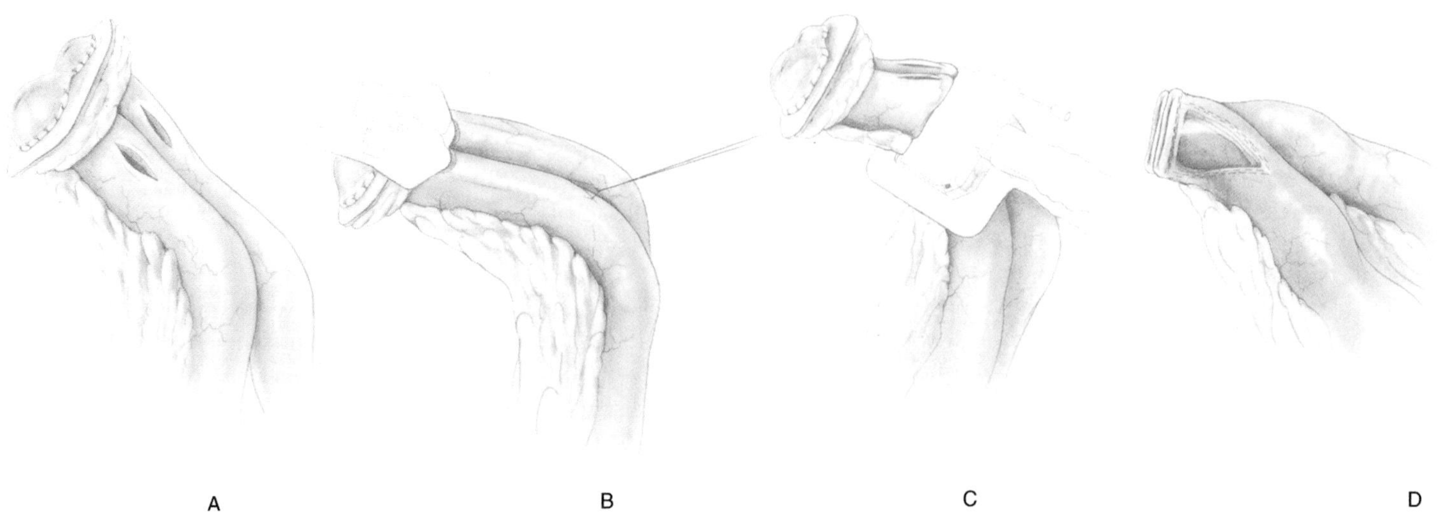

FIGURE 6 ■ Stapled ileostomy takedown. (**A**) Ileostomy is mobilized, and stab incisions are made on antimesenteric surface. (**B**) Stapler is positioned through stab wounds and fired. (**C**) Ileostomy is resected with linear stapler to include stab wounds in resection. (**D**) Functional end-to-end anastomosis.

observed between patients who had a covering stoma and those who did not, although significant differences in surgical practice were identified in different surgeons. The authors concluded that the covering diverting stoma was not necessary for surgeons who were able to keep their patients' leak rates at an acceptably low level.

Although many patients with colon and rectal injuries, particularly those with multiple abdominal injuries, need some type of fecal diversion, surgeons have increasingly recognized that the isolated and uncomplicated colonic injury treated promptly, can be managed successfully with primary closure (55).

The methods of diversion not involving resection include the "medical colostomy," ileostomy, cecostomy, and diverting colostomy. The concept of a "medical colostomy" using a chemically defined diet was recommended by Gordon for such anorectal procedures as sphincteroplasty, postanal repair, skin grafting following excision of a neoplasm or hidradenitis suppurativa, and repair of rectovaginal fistula (56). It puts the gastrointestinal tract at rest so that the repaired area does not have to be challenged with bowel movements. Today it would not appear necessary for most anal sphincter repairs nor for repairs of rectovaginal fistulas but would prove beneficial in the treatment of extrasphincteric fistulas. Robertson (57) achieved similar benefits with an elemental diet in 16 patients with inflammatory bowel disease, anorectal sphincter surgery, or wounds that had to be protected from fecal soiling. None of the patients on the elemental diet had bowel movements within three days of operation, and most had bowel movements only at five- to six-day intervals. Nutritional support, either by total parenteral nutrition or the elemental diet, is a useful alternative in select patients who need a brief period of gastrointestinal tract rest but do not otherwise need total prolonged fecal diversion.

The value of the loop ileostomy was discussed earlier and should be considered as an alternative to loop colostomy, in most patients. Both the loop ileostomy and loop colostomy, however, can pose management problems for the patient, and neither is an ideal stoma for long-term use. The comparative study by Williams et al. (37) showed that both loop ileostomy and loop transverse colostomy successfully defunctionalized the distal bowel. The ileostomy had fewer peristomal problems and fewer management problems than the colostomy, although dehydration from diarrhea or high ileostomy output could be a potential problem with the ileostomy, particularly in elderly patients.

Corman (58) has stated that "cecostomy could be removed from our surgical armamentarium with very little consequence to health care delivery." Others (59,60) have been more supportive of the cecostomy as a method of decompressing select patients without subjecting them to the morbidity of a loop colostomy. Attention has focused on less invasive ways of performing cecostomy, including the computed tomography CT-guided percutaneous method (61) and the percutaneous endoscopic method for nonobstructing colonic dilatation (62).

Winkler and Volpe (63) reviewed loop transverse colostomy among 29 patients in a community hospital and found that 5 patients died, 8 had complications, and only 18 patients underwent colostomy closure. The authors concluded that the first stage in the management of these patients should be resection of the diseased segment and that the colostomy should be end bearing and placed as close to the disease process as possible. Hopkins (64) supported the concept that temporary loop colostomy may not be "temporary" in many patients by reporting that colostomy closure was not performed in 19 of 45 patients (42%) having transverse colostomy for malignancy. Abrams et al. (65) similarly found that colostomy closure was not performed in 156 of 248 patients (63%) having transverse and left colostomies. The difficulties in managing a loop transverse colostomy compared to an end sigmoid colostomy are so substantial that the surgeon must always consider that the loop colostomy may ultimately subject the patients to a less-than-ideal colostomy for life.

Although much of the controversy on indications and methods for fecal diversion involves personal preferences on the part of individual authors, some general principle should be applicable for most patients. The principle of resecting primary disease and performing an end-bearing stoma in preference to a loop colostomy or other proximal diverting method is a sound principle that should be adhered to whenever possible. For other patients needing fecal diversion, the loop colostomy or loop ileostomy can be performed. In deciding whether to perform a fecal diversion for patients undergoing anterior resection or for patients with trauma, the surgeon must weigh the risks and consequences of anastomotic or colonic closure leakage against the morbidity and mortality of later colostomy takedown. These risks vary among patients and also among surgeons. The medical colostomy is a useful means of avoiding a surgical stoma in patients who need only short-term diversion to protect perineal wounds or perineal incisions. Tube cecostomy is of limited value and should be used only for decompression and not for fecal diversion.

Cecostomy

Since the turn of the century, tube cecostomy has been advocated mainly as a decompression procedure for acute colonic obstruction and as a safety valve for colonic resection. It has also been suggested for perforation or impending perforation of the cecum, for cecal volvulus, adynamic ileus of the colon and toxic dilatation in inflammatory bowel disease. The procedure is best performed as a tube cecostomy rather than a primary stoma. When a primary stoma is needed, it is better to perform a loop ileostomy or a loop transverse colostomy, since both are more diverting and are easier for the patients to manage.

The virtues of tube cecostomy, as cited by its proponents, are that it is easy to perform, can be carried out under local anesthesia, the cecum is the portion of colon most likely to perforate, it does not interfere with subsequent resection of the left side of the colon, and it may eventually close spontaneously. In cases of extreme obesity of the abdominal wall and when gross distention of the bowel has "used up" the leaves of the transverse mesocolon, transverse colostomy may be impossible. Under these circumstances, cecostomy may be the only method of relieving obstruction.

The use of cecostomy has frequently been criticized and has lost favor with many surgeons. Detractors point out that it provides less effective decompression than does a transverse colostomy and that it does not allow complete diversion.

Tube cecostomy can be performed as a primary operation through a right lower quadrant McBurney or right lateral transverse incision. Once the peritoneum is opened, the distended cecum is easily delivered through this incision. The serosal surface should be secured to the peritoneal surface with interrupted absorbable sutures. Two pursestring sutures of nonabsorbable material such as 3–0 silk are then placed around the apex of the cecum, and a No. 30-Fr Foley catheter or No. 36 to 40 DePessor catheter is inserted inside the pursestring sutures. The two pursestring sutures are tied, and the tube is secured in place. It is best to deliver the catheter through a stab wound either cephalad or caudad to this incision so that the incision can be closed primarily. The tube can be removed after 7 to 10 days, and the cecocutaneous fistula should close spontaneously.

Rosenberg and Gordon (66) conducted a retrospective review of 59 tube cecostomies to evaluate operative indications, outcome, and associated morbidity. Tube cecostomy was performed as a complementary procedure in 81.4% of cases; in the other 18.6%, it represented either the only operative intervention or the initial stage of a two-stage procedure. Complications included local infection in 32% of cases, pericatheter leak in 25%, skin excoriation in 24%, and pain in 12%. Catheters remained in place for an average of 14 days, but function was adequate in only 40% of cases. Cecal drainage persisted from 24 hours to 90 days after the tube was removed.

Two additional procedures were required to close persistent cecal fistulas. In addition, other reported complications included wound dehiscence, recurrence of a fistula after closure of the cecostomy, subcutaneous emphysema, prolapse of the omentum, stitch granuloma, evisceration, retraction, and hernia formation at the cecostomy site. Aseptic decompression of a distended cecum can be difficult and peritonitis and poor tube function after cecostomy have been responsible for a substantial number of deaths. Tube cecostomy fails to decompress the bowel adequately in as many as 50% of cases. The authors concluded that the high morbidity associated with this procedure militates against its use. Benacci and Wolff (60) were more encouraging about cecostomy. In a retrospective chart review of 67 patients who had catheter tube cecostomy placement, clinical indications for tube cecostomy were colonic pseudo-obstruction (39%), distal colonic obstruction (16%), cecal perforation (15%), cecal volvulus (13%), preanastomotic decompression (12%), and miscellaneous (5%). Operation was emergent in 64% of patients and elective in 36% of patients. Tube cecostomy was the primary procedure in 70% of patients and complementary in 36% of patients. Minor complications were seen in 45%, including pericatheter leak (15%), superficial wound infection (12%), tube occlusion (7%), skin excoriation (4%), premature tube dislodgement (4%), colocutaneous fistula (3%), and ventral hernia (12%). No patients required reoperation for tube-related morbidity. The authors concluded that catheter tube cecostomy is of therapeutic value in select clinical situations.

A protective diversionary cecostomy or transverse colostomy is now rarely warranted for left-sided colon procedures since this can be safely performed without diversion. A review of contemporary literature suggests that reasonable current indications for tube cecostomy include volvulus, pseudo-obstruction (if an attempt at colonoscopic decompression has failed), cecal perforation associated with an obstructed left-sided lesion, and to relieve obstruction in morbidly obese patients when transverse colostomy is technically impossible.

Loop Transverse Colostomy

In the past the loop transverse colostomy was a commonly used method to achieve temporary or short-term fecal diversion, whether necessitated by obstruction, inflammation, trauma, low colorectal anastomoses, or perineal wounds. Fontes et al. (67) studied the ability of the emergency loop colostomy to achieve total fecal diversion in 62 patients. The authors found that fecal diversion was virtually complete in all patients for the first three months but that the diversion became incomplete in about 15% of the patients in subsequent months, probably because of recession and retraction of the stoma. Schofield et al. (68) found that they could achieve total fecal diversion from a right transverse colostomy by rotating the stoma counterclockwise for 90° so that proximal limb was in the most dependent position caudad to the distal limb. Morris and Rayburn (69) studied 23 patients with loop colostomies by giving them barium by mouth. In no patient was barium found in the distal limb, indicating full diversion. At least 17 other individual techniques have been recorded in the literature to ensure complete fecal diversion from a loop colostomy (67). Most of these manipulations appear to be unnecessary, since a traditional loop colostomy should be able to achieve complete fecal diversion for a least a few months postoperatively. Complete diversions should rarely, if ever, be necessary for a longer period of time.

Loop Colostomy Construction

Although a seemingly endless number of techniques have been described for construction of a loop colostomy, three generic methods are used most often. The first involves construction of the loop colostomy over a fascial bridge without the use of a supporting rod or prosthetic bridge material. The second method involves the use of a rod or bridge, and the third method involves creating an end loop or divided type of colostomy. The dissatisfaction with the postoperative management problems caused by loops and bridges has no doubt led to the proliferation of techniques.

In addition to the three types of loop colostomies, a fourth type of diverting temporary colostomy has been described by Turnbull et al. (70) as part of an operation for the treatment of toxic megacolon complicating ulcerative colitis. That procedure consisted of a series of skin-level colostomies along with a loop ileostomy as the preliminary operative treatment of critically ill patients with toxic megacolon. This procedure is infrequently performed today, and a skin-level temporary colostomy with its attendant management problems is rarely, if ever, indicated.

Loop Colostomy Over Fascial Bridge

A transverse incision is made in the right upper quadrant at the previously marked stoma site. The incision is extended across the rectus fascia anteriorly and the rectus muscle fibers are separated. If the patient does not have a concomitant lower transverse incision, rectus can be divided between clamps and ligated to allow for a larger opening. If, however, a simultaneous lower transverse incision through the rectus muscle below the umbilicus has been made, then it is best not to devascularize rectus muscle in the right upper quadrant because of the risk of leaving an ischemic muscle segment between the two transverse incisions. The peritoneum is incised either sharply or with a fine hemostat, and the peritoneal cavity is entered.

The right transverse colon should be grasped with a Babcock forceps and elevated out of the incision, with care taken to identify the taeniae and confirm that the segment is colon. The incision may have to be enlarged if there is too much tension on the bowel as it leaves the abdominal wall. On occasion, it may be necessary to extend the incision and take down the hepatic flexure of the right colon to allow the right transverse colon enough mobility to be delivered through the incision, but this maneuver is usually not necessary.

Once the transverse colon has been elevated from the abdomen, the gastrocolic omentum adherent to the superior surface of the colon is cleaned away, and a short segment of mesocolon (<5 cm) is taken between clamps and ligated with sutures. The fascial bridge is defined by grasping the fascia and peritoneum together with either an Allis or Kocher clamp. Two or three sutures of heavy nonabsorbable material such as braided nylon or slowly absorbable material are placed through both the fascia and peritoneum of the superior lip of the incision, then through the window created between the colon and the mesocolon, and then through the fascia and peritoneum of the inferior lip on the opposite side. After all sutures have been placed, they are tied on the same side as the incision. The fascia should be felt carefully to make sure it is not constricting the lumen or blood supply of either loop. If the fascial or peritoneal openings are tight, they should be incised either medially or laterally but not along the fascial bridge. If the abdominal wall incision appears too large on either side, it can be partially closed with an interrupted nonabsorbable or slowly absorbable suture.

An incision is made across the apex of the colon. A primary maturation is performed with a 3–0 absorbable material such as vicryl or chromic catgut. The residual lateral or medial extension of the incision can be closed with a running subcuticular absorbable suture (Fig. 7).

Loop Transverse Colostomy Over Rod

This procedure is identical to that described for the fascial bridge technique, except that the colostomy is supported through the mesocolic defect by a grass rod, bridge, or other type of supporting material (Fig. 8). Regardless of type, the supporting structure is removed approximately 7 to 10 days after surgery, at which time the colostomy is adherent enough to the incision that it should not recede. Schofield et al. (68) described the operation of dependent proximal loop colostomy. This stoma avoids the complications of prolapse and paracolostomy hernia and is easy to close. It defunctions the distal colon as evidenced by the study of 10 patients given a radioactive tracer, chromium-51, by mouth and none spilled over into the distal loop.

End-Loop Colostomy

The end-loop colostomy is analogous to the end-loop ileostomy described by Prasad et al. (71). In this technique the transverse colon is divided between surgical staples. The proximal end is brought out as an end stoma through the incision, and the tip of the distal limb is brought out alongside the proximal stoma. The corner is opened and matured as a small distal stoma (Fig. 9). The end-loop colostomy eliminates the risk of distal segment prolapse and creates a stoma easier to care for postoperatively.

Unti et al. (72) conducted a retrospective review of their seven-year experience in 229 patients with end-loop-colostomies (136), ileocolostomies (71), and ileostomies (24). A total of 30 stoma-related complications were observed in 27 stomas, for an overall complication rate of 13.1%. The most common complications were skin excoriation secondary to leakage (3.5%), retraction (3.5%), partial necrosis (2.6%), and peristomal sepsis (1.8%). Mucocutaneous separation, prolapse, and stenosis were each seen in less than 1% of patients. No cases of stomal herniation, obstruction, or

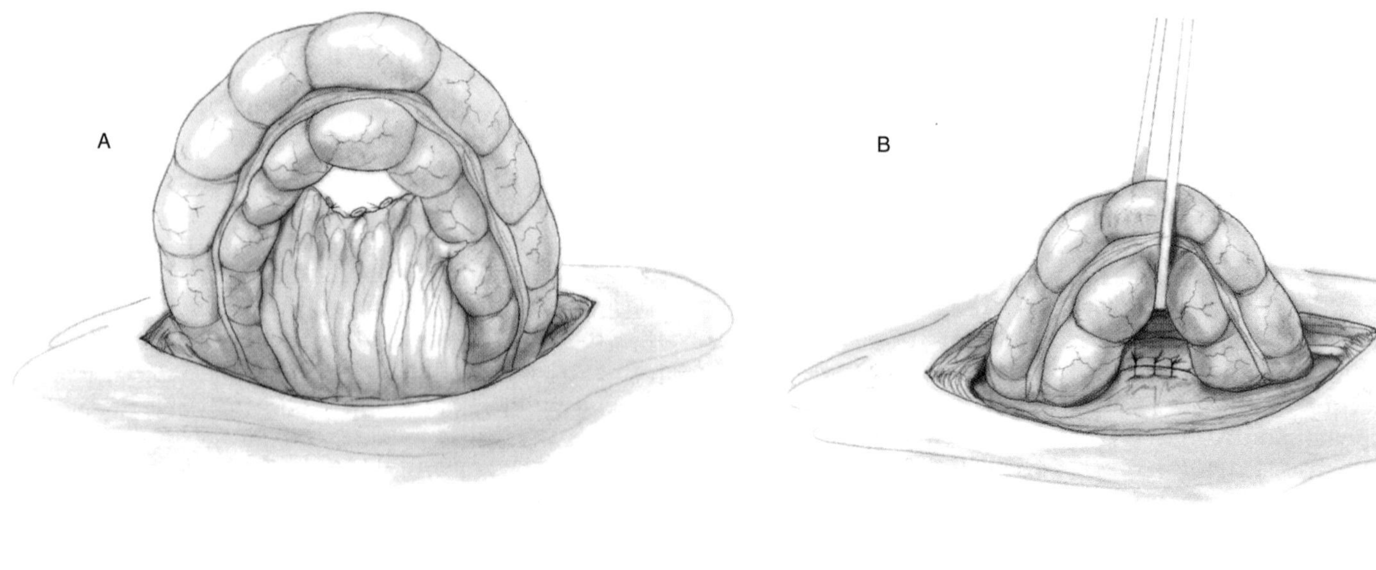

FIGURE 7 ■ Loop colostomy constructed over fascial bridge. (**A**) Window in mesocolon is formed and colon is elevated. (**B**) Fascial Bridge is created through mesocolic window with interrupted sutures. (**C**) Colon is opened and sutured to skin.

hemorrhage were encountered. Twelve deaths occurred, but none was attributed to stoma-related complications.

Hidden Colostomy

Sometimes a patient is found to have an unresectable carcinoma of the colon or rectum in association with extensive metastases or carcinomatosis. If the primary lesion is not causing complete or partial obstruction, the surgeon must decide between doing nothing and risking that the patient will need a second operation later for obstruction or creating a colostomy at the first operation, knowing that the patient may never need it. The hidden colostomy can be a useful technique in this setting.

The colostomy is performed as a loop over a fascial bridge proximal to the carcinoma, which is usually in the rectum. The colon is not elevated above the skin level but is instead buried in the subcutaneous fat where it can easily be identified later. Then if obstruction occurs, the colostomy can be opened at the bedside with the patient under local anesthesia. The resulting stoma is not anatomically ideal, but the patient is usually terminal or near terminal when it is performed, and overall it serves the patient well (see Chapter 24).

Loop Colostomy Closure

The decision to perform a temporary loop colostomy must always involve some consideration of the morbidity, the mortality, and the cost of colostomy closure. Parks and Hastings (73) reported that complications related to colostomy takedown decreased if colostomy closure was put off for 90 days or more. Williams et al. (74) analyzed the morbidity, mortality, and cost of colostomy closure in patients having a colostomy constructed for either trauma or nontraumatic diseases and found no significant differences in complication rates, although the authors noted that the colostomy was less likely to be closed if it was performed for nontraumatic disease. Thal and Yeary (75) reported no deaths and a relatively low complication rate of only 10.2% among 137 patients having a colostomy

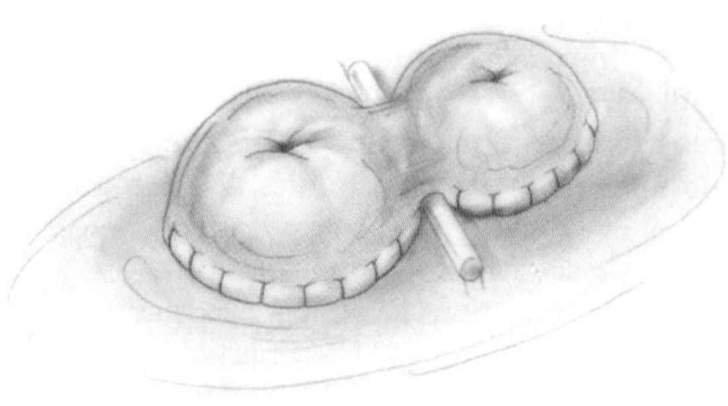

FIGURE 8 ■ Loop colostomy constructed over glass rod.

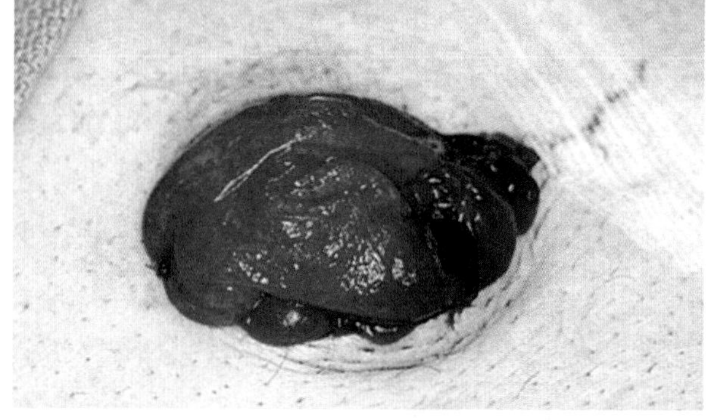

FIGURE 9 ■ End-loop colostomy with corner of distal limp incorporated into stoma. Overall appearance like an end colostomy.

closed following diverting colostomy for trauma. They emphasized the importance of meticulous surgical technique and attention to detail during the procedure.

Altomare et al. (38) reviewed the closure of 87 protective colostomies and identified hypoalbuminemia and interval to closure as risk factors. Operative mortality was 4.6%, major complications developed in 13% (fecal fistula, sepsis, intestinal obstruction, and myocardial insufficiency), and minor complications were recorded in 29% of patients. Colostomy closures within 30 days had a mortality rate of 12.5%, a major complication rate of 25%, and a minor complication rate of 50%. For closures performed between 31 and 90 days rates were 5.2%, 10.5%, and 36.8%, respectively. For closure after 90 days rates were 0%, 9.3%, and 9.3%, respectively. Their review of the literature, which included 26 reports, revealed a range of death rates from 0% to 4.6%, fecal fistula from 2% to 43%, and total complications from 5% to 61%. The authors emphasized that these data underscore the very significant morbidity and mortality associated with colostomy closure, and therefore the same skill and meticulous approach are required for this operation as for any major procedure performed on the colon.

Velmahos et al. (76) reported conflicting recommendations from a randomized trials of trauma patients in which they compared early (within 15 days of initial operation) and late (>90 days after initial operation) closure. The authors found no significant difference in morbidity between the two groups, with an overall complication rate of 26.3%. Technically, the early closure of colostomies was far easier than late closure, required significantly less operating time, and resulted in less intraoperative blood loss. The closure of end colostomies was more time consuming, both early and late, and caused more bleeding. Total hospitalization was marginally shorter overall for early closure, but late closure of end colostomies resulted in prolonged hospitalization. The authors recommend early closure of colostomies and the use of loop colostomies whenever possible as both safe and beneficial for patients with colonic injury after trauma. Contraindications to early closure include a nonhealing distal bowel, persistent would sepsis, and persistent postoperative instability.

The loop colostomy can be closed by any of three methods, including mobilization of the colostomy with closure of the anterior wall of the colon, mobilization with functional end-to-end surgical staple closure, and resection of the colostomy with primary end-to-end anastomosis. The three techniques are analogous to those used for loop ileostomy takedown. If the colon is satisfactorily mobilized proximally and distally, if the colon edges are satisfactorily debrided so that sutures or staples are placed only through healthy, noninflamed tissue, if the blood supply to both ends of the colon is satisfactory, and if there is no tension on the suture line, then all three methods should give comparably good results.

■ END SIGMOID COLOSTOMY

End sigmoid colostomy may be temporary or permanent. It is performed as a permanent procedure following abdominoperineal resection of the rectum for malignant disease, and it is also indicated as a definitive stoma for incontinent patients who are not suitable candidates for other procedures. End sigmoid colostomy may be performed as a temporary stoma following resection of the rectosigmoid for benign or malignant disease, and it may serve as a means of achieving temporary diversion for other conditions such as radiation proctitis. The end colostomy allows the patient to take advantage of the absorptive capacity of the proximal colon, making it the easiest type of intestinal stoma for the patient to manage.

A key technical consideration in end sigmoid colostomy construction involves deciding whether to fashion the colostomy as an extraperitoneal or intraperitoneal structure. Goligher (10) first described the extraperitoneal approach after observing that patients with both ileostomy and colostomy seemed especially predisposed to postoperative intestinal obstruction. The extraperitoneal colostomy was designed to prevent obstruction from occurring so frequently. Subsequently, Whittaker and Goligher (77) reviewed their experience with 251 patients and found that patients having an extraperitoneal iliac colostomy did not have a lower incidence of mechanical obstruction, but they did have a significantly lower incidence of pericolostomy herniation, prolapse, and recession compared to patients having an intraperitoneal colostomy.

The extraperitoneal colostomy is a good option for patients needing a permanent iliac colostomy. Extraperitoneal colostomy is also good for patients with ascites. The leaking of fluid is minimized or eliminated. For those patients needing only a temporary stoma, the intraperitoneal method is preferable, because takedown of the colostomy and subsequent reanastomosis are less difficult when the proximal colon has been left in an intraperitoneal position.

Technique of Extraperitoneal Colostomy Construction

The technique of extraperitoneal end sigmoid colostomy construction is the same whether it is performed as part of an abdominoperineal resection or as a permanent end colostomy for benign disease. Either a lower midline or transverse incision is suitable once it has been determined that the preselected stoma site will not be too close to either incision. A minimum of 3 cm and preferably 5 to 8 cm should separate the edge of the stoma from the abdominal incision.

Once the abdomen is opened, the sigmoid colon is mobilized by incising the lateral peritoneal reflection along the white line of Toldt, carefully identifying the left ureter as it crosses the left common iliac artery. The intraperitoneal rectosigmoid is then resected and the rectal stump, if retained, closed with staples. Otherwise, a complete proctectomy is performed as described in Chapter 24 for resection of rectal carcinoma. The colostomy site is then created by excising a disk of skin and separating subcutaneous fat down to the level of the fascia. It is important that a layer of fat be retained between the abdominal incision and the colostomy site so that the two wounds are not in direct communication at the subcutaneous level. This is easily averted by excising the skin disk and fat as an inverted cone or better still by not excising any subcutaneous fat. Goligher (10) originally recommended that the extraperitoneal colostomy be placed a little more laterally so that the rectus muscle is not included. Subsequent experience has shown that the extraperitoneal tunnel can be readily extended into the rectus sheath; this allows the stoma to be positioned medially through the rectus muscle. Although either method is acceptable, the more medial placement of the stoma is preferable because the rectus muscle adds extra support to the stoma. Sjödahl et al. (78) reported a dramatic reduction in parastomal hernia development when a permanent stoma was brought out through the rectus muscle. In a review of 130 patients, the prevalence of parastomal hernia was 2.8% when the stoma was constructed through the rectus muscle versus 21.6% when brought out lateral to the rectus muscle. In contrast, Ortiz et al. (79) found no correlation between the presence of parastomal hernia and the position of the stoma in the abdominal wall.

The left lateral peritoneal leaf is then grasped with a forceps, and an extraperitoneal tunnel is created by a combination of sharp and blunt dissection to connect with the colostomy wound in the abdominal wall. The tunnel is gently developed by finger dissection and the colon delivered through the tunnel so that 3 to 5 cm of colon comfortably protrudes above the skin level. The colon is then secured to the fascia with interrupted or running sutures of 3–0 polyglycolic acid. The pelvic peritoneum should be secured over the colon, and, if the procedure is performed as part of an abdominoperineal resection, the process of pelvic reperitonealization is completed at this time.

Primary maturation of the colostomy is performed using interrupted 3–0 absorbable sutures with the matured colostomy fashioned to protrude 1 to 2 cm above the abdominal wall. Maturation is accomplished by placing four anchoring stitches through the full thickness of the colon, then the colonic wall below the skin level, then the dermis. Interrupted simple sutures are placed between each of the four quadrants to complete the maturation (Fig. 10).

The intraperitoneal colostomy differs only in that the colon is delivered through the rectus muscle, and the defect in the left lateral peritoneal gutter is closed with interrupted slowly absorbable sutures.

Several techniques of end colostomy maturation using stapling devices have been described using either the linear skin stapler (80) or the circular stapling device (81). Both of these methods offer the simplicity and ease of stapling, but they might not allow the surgeon the same opportunity to optimize stomal contour and stomal protrusion for the individual abdominal wall.

Porter et al. (82) reported on 126 patients who underwent 130 end colostomies, 44 for benign, and 86 for malignant disease, and were followed for an average of 35 months. The left or sigmoid colon was used in 99 and the transverse colon in 31 patients. Stomas were made electively in 98 patients and urgently in 32. Seventy-six stomas were brought out through the incision and 54 from separate sites. There were 69 complications in 55 patients (44%), including 11 strictures, 9 wound infections, 14 hernias, 9 small bowel obstructions, 4 prolapses, 2 abscesses, 1 peristomal fistula, 17 skin erosions, and 2 poor stoma locations. Fifteen complications required reoperation. Five of these procedures included stoma revision. Total numbers of complications were not related to the stoma site, the disease process, the urgency of the procedure, or the segment of colon used. Wound infections, however, were increased in urgently made stomas. The incidence of hernia was equivalent in stomas brought out through the incision or at a separate site. Forty-one patients (30%) had 43 colostomies closed an average of 3.5 months after creation. Thirteen patients had 14 complications (five wound infections, six hernias, two small bowel obstructions, and one rectovaginal fistula). One patient died. Four patients required reoperation. There were no anastomotic leaks. Complications were equivalent in Hartmann closures and transverse colostomy closures. Complications were similar in stomas created for carcinoma and those created for diverticular disease.

■ CONTINENT COLOSTOMIES

Numerous devices have been introduced for uses with an end sigmoid colostomy to help the patient achieve greater control of both gas and stool output from the stoma. Interest in magnetic devices was stimulated by the work of Feustel and Hennig (83), who described a magnetic ring system in the early 1970s. The system consists of a magnetic ring that is implanted subcutaneously, and the colonic stoma is brought through the ring. An external magnetic cap fitted over the stoma mechanically prevents the expulsion of stool. A disposable charcoal filter disk on the undersurface of the cap permits gas to escape.

Khubchandani et al. (51), using careful patient selection methods, reported favorable results among 14 patients. Husemann and Hager (84) reported the results of 240 patients who underwent implantation of the Erlangen magnetic device. Forty-five rings were explored because of infection, pressure necrosis, parastomal hernia, invagination, prolapse, and stenosis. Although continence was obtained in 68% of patients, only 43% of surviving patients still use the system. Reasons given for not using the cap were pain and weight. Although the magnetic ring device has been successful in some patients, it has two main disadvantages. It requires a magnetic material to be permanently implanted in the abdominal wall and placement must be nearly perfect to allow for satisfactory function. For these reasons, the device has failed to gain widespread popularity.

In Prager's preliminary experience (53) with a two-part silicone device, three of five patients were able to achieve continence by inserting a specially designed inflatable plug into the stoma.

The Conseal colostomy system (Coloplast, Inc., Tampa, FL, U.S.A.) is composed of an open-cell polyurethane foam with a water-repellent cover. The cover contains a charcoal filter that enables intestinal gas to pass without odor while preventing the passage of fecal material. The Conseal plug expands to form a bell-shaped plug when it is inserted into the stoma (Fig. 11). Clague and Heald (52) evaluated the Conseal system in a multicenter trial of 100 patients and found that it was successful in approximately one-third of the patients. Patients who irrigated their colostomy tended to retain the plug longer than those who used the natural method. Cazador et al. (85) conducted another multicenter trial in which 43 patients were evaluated. No complications arose, and complete fecal continence was obtained in 71%. This continence device did not achieve its original promise.

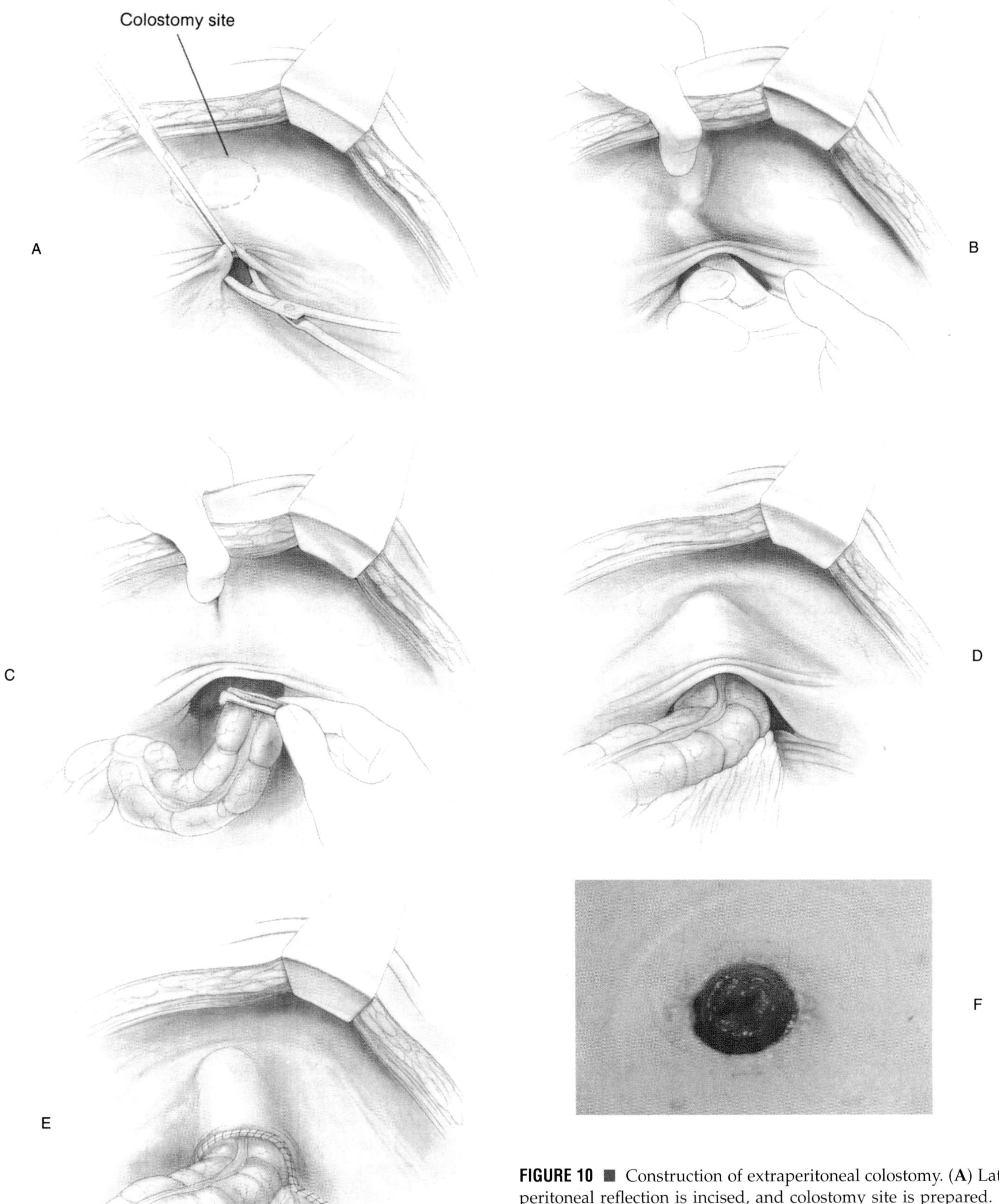

FIGURE 10 ■ Construction of extraperitoneal colostomy. (**A**) Lateral peritoneal reflection is incised, and colostomy site is prepared. (**B**) Extraperitoneal tunnel is dissected bluntly. (**C** and **D**) Colon is brought through tunnel. (**E**) Peritoneum is closed around colon, and pelvic floor reconstruction is completed. (**F**) Properly constructed colostomy with adequate protrusion above skin level.

A number of methods have been used to achieve continence without using external devices, the most promising being the intestinal smooth muscle graft. Schmidt (86) reported an 80% success rate with this procedure among 500 patients. The procedure consists of a free transplant of a 10 to 15 cm segment of colonic smooth muscle that is

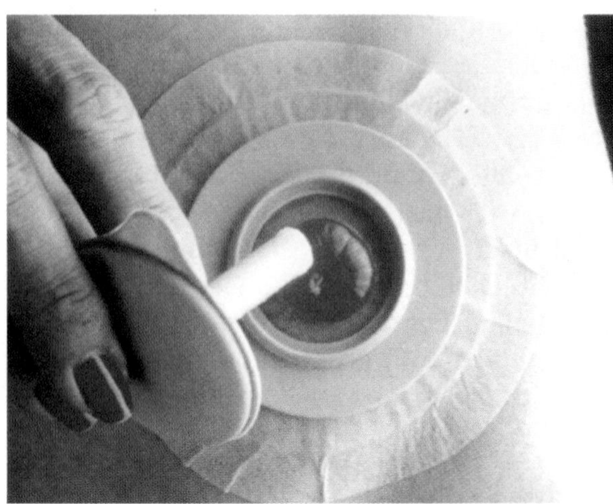

FIGURE 11 ■ Conseal system. Skin barrier is positioned around stoma, and plug is about to be inserted into stoma and snapped on to flange of skin barrier.

sutured to become ruffled into a muscle mass of about half that length. The graft is wrapped around the bowel and sutured to produce continence.

■ END COLOSTOMY TAKEDOWN

End colostomy takedown with intraperitoneal anastomosis involves mobilizing proximal and distal colonic segments and creating an end-to-end anastomosis using either staples or sutures. The previous abdominal incision, either vertical or transverse, needs to be reopened, and often, extensive adhesions need to be taken down. The colostomy is mobilized by making an elliptical incision around the skin and then dissecting down to the fascia and peritoneum until the colon is free. The mucous fistula or distal rectosigmoid is also mobilized, and the anastomosis can usually be performed without difficulty.

Before the advent of circular staplers, end sigmoid colostomy takedown with extraperitoneal anastomosis to a low-lying rectal stump was often an exceptionally difficult and hazardous procedure. This procedure has been greatly simplified by the introduction of the newer circular stapling devices. After the proximal sigmoid has been mobilized and prepared for anastomosis, the distal stump needs to be dissected only enough to define the apex and free the colon from adhesions that will inhibit smooth placement of the stapling device. The stapler is inserted per anum, and the device is opened so that the trocar can penetrate the apex of the rectal stump and bring the barrel of the device through that hole. A pursestring suture is placed on the proximal sigmoid and tied around the anvil shaft. This shaft is reengaged into the central shaft of the cartridge, and the anvil is approximated to the cartridge. The stapler is fired and then removed. The procedure should carry minimal morbidity as long as the apex of the rectal stump has been carefully defined and a clean circular anastomosis has been obtained (see Fig. 17 in Chapter 28). This particular operation lends itself well to a laparoscopic approach, which is described in detail in Chapter 38.

In the event that considerable residual sigmoid colon remains, the circular stapler may not reach the apex of the sigmoid stump. Also there may be kinking of rectum in the hollow of the sacrum. In either event, an additional portion of rectosigmoid will require resection.

The purported ease and safety of closure of loop colostomy are cited as reasons for avoiding end colostomy, with or without resection. Data comparing the complications of loop colostomy closure and end colostomy takedown and anastomosis are sparse. Mileski et al. (87) analyzed data from 93 consecutive colostomy closures, 62 of which were loop and 31 were end colostomies. The two groups were comparable with respect to age, underlying disease, and risk factors, such as coronary artery disease, diabetes, hypertension, steroid dependence, hypoalbuminemia, and smoking. Closure of end colostomies took longer and was associated with more blood loss than closure of loop colostomies. However, the mortality rates for closure of loop (4.8%) and end (3.2%) colostomies were not significantly different. The complication rates were identical (16%). Although none of the other risk factors was associated with increased rates of mortality or morbidity, the detrimental effects of steroid dependence and preoperative hypoalbuminemia were striking. The four deaths and 60% of the complications occurred in patients with steroid dependence or hypoalbuminemia, or both. The rates of wound infection after primary or secondary closure of the stoma site were not significantly different. The authors concluded that loop colostomy closure is not associated with fewer complications than closure of end colostomy, even though the latter takes longer to perform and is more difficult. Primary closure of the stomal site is safe and reduces the length of hospital stay.

Mosdell and Doberneck (88) reviewed the charts of 59 patients undergoing Hartmann's procedure and 43 patients undergoing ostomy closure after divided colostomy, loop colostomy, or divided ileostomy-colostomy. Ostomy closure after Hartmann's procedure was accomplished in 46 patients. These 46 patients (group I) were compared with the 43 patients having ostomy closure following divided colostomy, loop colostomy, or divided ileostomy-colostomy (group II). No deaths occurred in either group. The morbidity rate was 30% in group I and 19% in group II. Major complications involved wound, lung, small bowel, and colonic anastomoses. Anastomotic stricture rate was 9% in group I and 5% in group II. Small bowel and anastomotic complications in both groups occurred only when ostomy closure was performed after a delay of less than six months after ostomy construction. Stricture occurred only after end-to-end colocolostomy and coloproctostomy and did not occur after ileostomy or ileoproctostomy. All strictures were successfully treated by reoperation. Anastomotic leak and pelvic abscess did not occur in either group. The authors concluded that ostomy closure after Hartmann's procedure may be more difficult and time consuming than ostomy closure after loop colostomy, divided colostomy, or divided ileostomy-colostomy, but that ostomy closure after Hartmann's procedure does not result in a higher morbidity rate. The authors advise an interval of six months between ostomy construction and ostomy closure and submit that all patients whose general condition permits reoperation may safely undergo ostomy closure.

Pearce et al. (89) reviewed the outcome of 145 patients undergoing Hartmann's resection. The mortality rate of the primary procedure was 8%. Eighty patients also underwent reanastomosis. The interval between the primary and secondary procedures was found to be the most important risk factor. Six of 12 patients had clinical evidence of a leak when this interval was less than three months, compared with seven of 28 patients for three to six months, and none of 40 when the second operation was delayed for greater than six months. All deaths (three patients) and clinical septicemia (four patients) occurred in the two "early" groups. All colovaginal fistulas (three patients) and strictures (three patients) were associated with stapled anastomoses. No association was found between the complication rate following reanastomosis and the initial pathology or experience of the surgeon undertaking the secondary operation.

Keck et al. (90) reviewed the case records of 111 patients undergoing Hartmann's procedure mostly for advanced carcinoma and complicated diverticular disease. Of 96 patients who survived, 50 (52%) underwent reversal. Of those with diverticular disease, 40 of 48 (83%) underwent reversal. Mortality for Hartmann's reversal was 2%, anastomotic leak rate was 4%, and overall complication rate was 26%. Early reversal was performed in 13 patients and late reversal in 37 patients. There was no difference in these groups in mortality, morbidity, or anastomotic leakage. However, bed stay was longer in the early group and graded operative difficulty greater. In particular, cases in which adhesion density was most severe and in which accidental enterotomy occurred were more common in the early group.

Livingston et al. (91) questioned whether the risks after colostomy closure were exaggerated. The authors reviewed 121 patients who underwent colostomy closure for trauma. There was no mortality and a 4.9% incidence of major morbidity. Although there was no apparent relationship between the interval between colostomy creation and closure, three of the six major complications occurred in patients whose colostomies were closed soon after complicated initial injuries. The authors recommended that if the primary operation is complicated by intra-abdominal sepsis or major wound problems, six months should ensue before attempting closure. Long-term follow-up of these patients (mean, 39 months) disclosed a low incidence of late complications secondary to colostomy closure. Although the trend toward the increased use of primary repair of colon injuries in selected patients is supported, the authors' study indicates that the risk of colostomy closure has been exaggerated and should not be a factor in the decision to create a colostomy after colon trauma.

Khoury et al. (92) retrospectively reviewed the records of 46 patients who underwent colostomy closure. Patients ranged in age from 24 to 87 years, and 54% were women. Stomas had been created during emergency operations in 87%. Most operations (54%) were performed for complications of acute diverticulitis. Of the 46 procedures, 40 (87%) were end colostomies and six were loop colostomies. Stomas were closed at a range of 11 to 1357 days after creation (mean, 207 days; median, 116 days). Inpatient complications occurred in 15% of patients, including congestive heart failure (2%), cerebrovascular accident (4%), pneumonia (2%), enterocutaneous fistula (2%), and pulmonary embolus with death (2%). The most common long-term complication was midline wound hernia, which occurred in 10% of surviving patients. Overall complications occurred in 24%. The authors concluded that colostomy closure is a major operation.

■ COMPLICATIONS

Colostomy complications are similar to those associated with ileostomies. The most frequently encountered problems include ischemia, recession, prolapse, and parastomal hernia. Allen-Mersh and Thomson (93) reviewed 156 operations on 23 patients over a three-year period for correction of late colostomy complications and found that problems included stenosis in 65 patients, paracolostomy hernia 42, and prolapse in 16.

Leenen and Kuijpers (94) studied 266 patients with 345 stomas on the small and large bowel to determine possible etiologic factors for stomal complications. The overall complication rate for creating a stoma was 36%. No differences in overall complication rate were encountered when comparing acute and elective management; however, high-output stomas and necrosis were encountered more often in the acutely managed group. Preoperative contamination was followed more often by stomal retraction. Septic events, however, occurred less frequently than in the noncontaminated procedures. Moderate obesity had no significant influence on the outcome of the procedure. Adipose patients had a statistically significant greater number of necroses. The outcome of stoma surgery was greatly influenced by bowel quality. Crohn's disease and bowel ischemia were encountered in 50% of patients with stoma complications. In ischemic disease, significantly more necrosis was found. Retraction of the stoma occurred more often in patients with Crohn's disease. Patients with chronic ulcerative colitis did not have a higher complication rate.

Complications of ileostomy are common, although they can be minimized by careful surgical technique and good enterostomal nursing. Carlstedt et al. (95) reviewed the ileostomy complications in 203 patients operated on with proctocolectomy and ileostomy for ulcerative colitis and Crohn's disease. The crude rate of ileostomy complications necessitating reconstruction was 34% and was significantly higher in patients with Crohn's disease compared with patients with ulcerative colitis. The cumulative rate of surgical revision after eight years was 75% in the former group and 44% in the latter. Ileostomy stenosis and sliding recession were the two most common indications for reconstruction. Eighty-three percent of the revisions were performed as local procedures, making a formal laparotomy unnecessary. Causative factors such as surgical technique, length of concomitant ileal resection, and postoperative weight-gain were analyzed for possible influence on the rate of reconstruction, but no significant association was identified.

Khoo et al. (96) prospectively assessed the morbidity of creating and closing loop ileostomies in a consecutive series of 203 patients having an ileoanal pouch procedure. There was one death as a result of liver failure. One patient developed a persistent pouch-vaginal fistula that resulted in pouch excision. The remaining 201 patients had their ileostomy closed at a mean time of 10 weeks after the primary procedure. Only 7% needed reoperation to correct ileostomy-related problems. After ileostomy closure, complications were noted in only 2% of patients. Stothert et al. (97) reviewed the outcome of 49 high-risk patients having 51 stomas created as an emergency measure and found a morbidity of more than 50%. Feinberg et al. (98) found complications referable either to a temporary loop ileostomy or its closure in 69 of 117 patients undergoing loop ileostomy in association with the pelvic reservoir procedure and ileoanal anastomosis. Grobler et al. (99), in a randomized trial of loop ileostomy in restorative proctocolectomy, found that 52% of patients developed ileostomy-related complications. On the other hand, Wexner et al. (100) found that loop ileostomy was a safe option for fecal diversion in a study of 83 patients who required temporary fecal diversion after either ileoanal or low colorectal anastomosis (72 patients), for perianal Crohn's disease (5 patients), or for other reasons (6 patients). All loop ileostomies were supported with a rod, and fecal diversion was maintained for a mean of 10 weeks. Sixty-seven patients had re-establishment of intestinal continuity. Stoma closure was effected through a parastomal incision in 64 patients; in three, a laparotomy was required. The closure was stapled side to side in 49 patients, while a hand-sewn anastomosis was performed in the other 18 patients. All skin wounds were left open. Nine patients (10.8%) developed 10 complications. Four patients developed dehydration and electrolyte abnormalities secondary to high stoma output, two had anastomotic leaks that spontaneously healed following conservative management, one patient developed a superficial wound infection that spontaneously drained and one patient developed a partial small bowel obstruction that resolved without operation after a four-day hospitalization. One stoma retracted after supporting rod removal and prompted premature closure. There were no instances of stomal ischemia, hemorrhage, prolapse, or mortality in this series.

Leong et al. (101) conducted an actuarial analysis of complications of 150 permanent end ileostomies constructed over a 10-year period. By 20 years, the incidence of stomal complications approached 76% in patients operated on for ulcerative colitis and 59% in those with Crohn's disease. Revisional surgery rates were higher in patients with ulcerative colitis than in those with Crohn's disease (28% vs. 16%). Complications encountered were skin problems (cumulative probability, 34%), intestinal obstruction (23%), retraction (17%), parastomal herniation (16%), fistula or suppuration (12%), prolapse (11%), stenosis (5%), and necrosis (1%). Closure of the lateral space did not reduce the probability of developing intestinal obstruction (18% at 20 years in those with closure vs. 3% in those without). Fixation of the mesentery did not reduce the probability of developing prolapse of the ileostomy (11% in those with fixation vs. none in those without). The incidence of parastomal herniation was not reduced by siting through the rectus abdominis (21% in those sited through the body of the rectus abdominis vs. 7% in those sited through the oblique muscles). Some of the surgical dogmas relating to ileostomy construction are not supported by the results of this study.

In a review by Senapati et al. (102), of 310 patients who underwent restorative proctocolectomy, 296 had a covering ileostomy and 14 did not. The stoma had been closed in 88.9% at a median interval from formation of 12.0 weeks. Ileostomy-rated complications before closure occurred in 5.7%. Laparotomy for obstruction due to the ileostomy was required in 2.4%. Retraction requiring revision occurred in 1.0%, an abscess behind the stoma in 0.3%, and miscellaneous appliance problems in 2.4%. Following closure, 22.4% developed an ileostomy-related complication. There were 30 cases of small bowel obstruction, treated conservatively in 19 (7.2%) and by laparotomy in 11 (4.2%). Peritonitis requiring laparotomy occurred in 1.1%, and 0.8% developed an enterocutaneous fistula. There were 5.3% wound infections and 6.1% other miscellaneous problems. Significant complications associated with a temporary ileostomy were less frequent in this series than in some other reports. Obstruction was the most common complication and fistula was rare.

In the recent review of the complications of temporary loop ileostomy by Kaidar-Person et al. (103), factors suggested to predispose to stoma complications were high body mass index, inflammatory bowel disease, use of steroids and immunosuppressive therapy, diabetes, old age, emergency operation, operative technique, and surgeon experience. Preoperative evaluation and proper marking of the stoma site before an operation were associated with fewer adverse outcomes. In the review of 14 publications, the reported morbidity ranged from 3% to 100% (with many in the 35–45% range). Major complications included stenosis, small bowel obstruction, retraction, necrosis, prolapse, stricture, fistula, and parastomal hernia. Small bowel obstruction ranged from 0% to 17% (mostly in 3–8% range), high output 1% to 72% (mostly in the 3–5% range), appliances leakage 7% to 68% (mostly in 17–38% range) skin 2% to 41% (mostly in the 4–7% range), and reoperation rate 1% to 9%. Minor complications included dermatitis, electrolyte imbalance, and dehydration from high stoma output. The latter may often necessitate early closure of the stoma. Although not a complication, nonclosure of a temporary ileostomy ranged from 0% to 19%.

Bowel Obstruction

Small intestinal obstruction is a relatively common occurrence among ileostomy patients. It is usually caused by extrinsic compression from adhesions or an internal hernia, intraluminal compression from impacted boluses of food, or recurrent Crohn's disease.

Although food bolus obstruction is usually self-limited, it is clinically indistinguishable from complete extrinsic small intestinal obstruction. Food bolus obstructions tend to be complete and present as an impaction at a point of angulation or stricture at the fascial level. Since the impaction may occur after the ingestion of exotic or high-fiber foods, such as coconut, the patient often relates the onset of pain to a time just after eating these foods. The patient frequently has a history of similar episodes.

The onset of pain and obstructive symptoms tends to be sudden, and cessation of ileostomy output usually follows. With a partial high-grade obstruction, the patient describes passing a large volume of watery effluent from the stoma and may confuse this event with gastroenteritis. Whether the obstruction is complete or partial, significant dehydration can result from associated nausea and vomiting, as well as from the secretion of fluid into the dilated small bowel proximal to the obstruction. Toxicity is generally not present, and perforation and peritonitis are uncommon.

Management of food bolus obstruction should include fluid and electrolyte restoration, nasogastric suction, and close observation. Gentle irrigation of the ileostomy with a soft, well-lubricated rubber catheter, using 4 oz of either saline or liquid glycerine often dislodges the impaction and relieves the obstruction. Alternatively, lavage of the ileostomy with up to 500 mL of saline may be tried using an enema bag, a cone-tip irrigator, and an irrigation sleeve. Operation is rarely needed.

Mechanical extrinsic obstruction is less common but potentially more serious than intraluminal obstruction. Patients who have had operations for inflammatory bowel disease have a greater predilection for obstruction than those who have undergone abdominal operations and bowel resection for other disease. Hughes et al. (104) found a 9.1% incidence of small bowel obstruction requiring operation among 463 patients having resectional therapy for inflammatory bowel disease compared to a 2.3% incidence of operation among 2474 patients having resection for colon and rectal neoplasms. Two-thirds of the obstructions in this series were related to adhesions, and the other third was related to the stoma. Fasth and Hulten (42) noted a lower incidence of obstruction, approximately 3%, for patients with loop ileostomies.

Intestinal obstruction has been reported as an especially frequent complication following restorative proctocolectomy for inflammatory bowel disease. The obstructive events are related either to the temporary ileostomy or to the adhesions. Obstructive phenomena have been reported in up to 43.5% of patients having such restorative procedures (105). Francois et al. (106) reviewed the Mayo Clinic experience with small bowel obstruction complicating ileal pouch–anal anastomosis and found that 17% of their patients developed small bowel obstruction; 7.5% of these patients required operation. In this series, obstruction was more likely to occur in patients who had a temporary Brooke ileostomy (12.5%) than those who had a loop ileostomy (4.6%). Although the loop ileostomy with an open mesenteric defect laterally appears especially vulnerable to obstruction, it is clear that patients having either a Brooke end ileostomy or loop ileostomy are at risk.

Anderson et al. (107) described a simple technique to minimize the risk of volvulus following establishment of a loop ileostomy. A broad antimesenteric attachment of the seromuscular layer of ileum to the parietes at the stoma site is achieved with absorbable sutures, creating a broader fulcrum. After adopting this technique, no complications were noted in 30 patients followed up for a minimum of four years.

The patient with mechanical small bowel obstruction is often indistinguishable from the patient with food bolus obstruction. The initial management is the same, consisting of fluid and electrolyte resuscitation, nasogastric suction, and a brief trial of irrigation or lavage of the stoma. If pain persists despite nasogastric tube decompression and lavage of the stoma, then early operation is the safest course. If, however, the patient is comfortable with the nasogastric tube in place and if the abdomen is soft and free of signs of peritonitis, then the patient maybe observed for a period of 24 to 48 hours. Immediate operation must be considered if the patient develops increasing pain, increased distention, leukocytosis, or fever. For all patients with an uncertain obstruction and unsatisfactory course, early operation is often the safest approach. Although Francois et al. (106) emphasized that necrosis from small bowel obstruction complicating the loop or Brooke ileostomy was rare in their series, the consequences of additional small bowel loss from infarction in a patient who already has an ileostomy are significant and the need for resection must be avoided.

Stoma Ischemia

Stoma ischemia is present when a healthy stoma turns dark purple or black, usually within the first 24 hours after operation. Ischemia may be limited to the part of the stoma above the skin level, or it may extend deep to the fascial level, the peritoneal level, or the proximal intra-abdominal ileum. When a stoma becomes dark, the first priority is to assess the proximal extent of the ischemia. If the ischemia extends below the fascia and peritoneum, immediate revision is indicated to prevent perforation and peritonitis. Viability of the proximal mucosa can be assessed by inserting a test tube and illuminating it with a penlight. If the ischemia is limited to the level of the fascia or above, it is best to monitor this condition nonoperatively and revise the stoma at a later time if stenosis or other complications develop. A two-piece pouching system instead of a single appliance may be especially helpful in this case because it allows easy access to the stoma without removing the adhesive covering the peristomal skin. Another handy test in evaluating stoma ischemia is a pinprick test in which arterial bleeding may be seen from the muscle, even in the presence of mucosal necrosis. With ischemia limited to the mucosa, spontaneous resolution can usually be expected.

Ischemia following construction of a colostomy, especially an end sigmoid colostomy, is seen more frequently than ischemia following ileostomy construction. This occurs in part because the left colon is less mobile than the ileum and in part because the colon is often brought through a thickened abdominal wall under some tension. When an end sigmoid colostomy is performed for carcinoma, the left colic artery has usually been taken, often as part of a high ligation of the inferior mesenteric artery. In this case the blood supply through the marginal artery may be inadequate to nourish the stomal end.

A healthy stoma should be pink at all times. If the stoma is dusky or black in the first 24 hours, the extent of the ischemia must be evaluated (Fig. 12A). The technique of using a penlight inside a test tube described to evaluate ileostomy viability also works well for the colostomy. If uncertainty remains, 5 mL fluorescein dye can be injected intravenously for 10 minutes (108). A long-wave ultraviolet lamp is used to inspect the stoma after a test tube is inserted. If strong fluorescence of the mucosa is noted, viability is assured. A negative result is indeterminate. It might best be remembered that a dark or even black stoma postoperatively, especially a moist one, may not be a necrotic stoma or infarcted bowel, but perhaps melanosis coli (109). This should be considered as it requires no

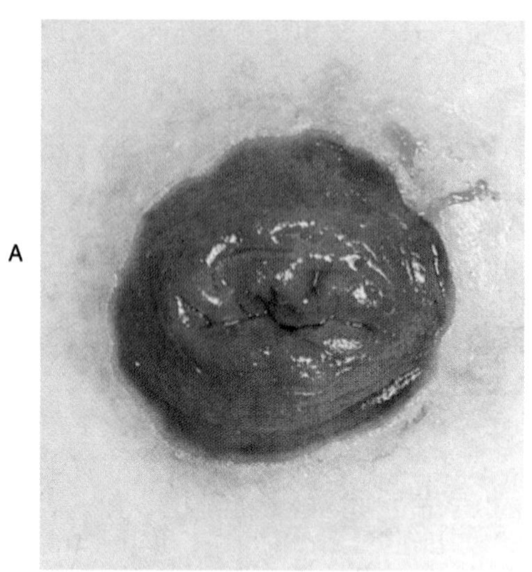

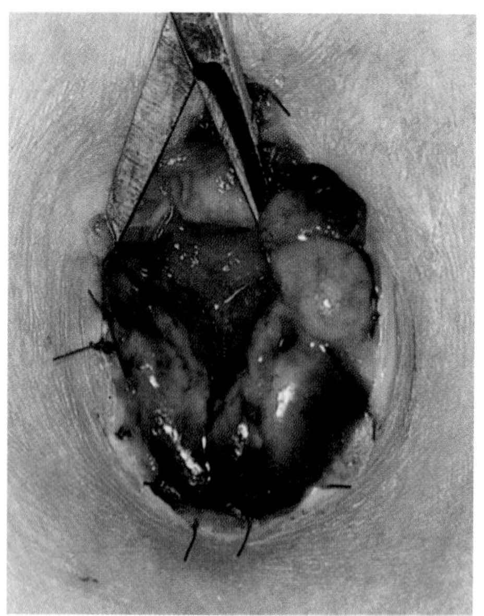

FIGURE 12 ■ (**A**) Ischemic colostomy. (**B**) Only distal-most portion of transverse colostomy is necrotic.

treatment and its recognition will obviate a needless operation. If in the early postoperative period, the cyanosis, ischemia, or necrosis is all above the fascial level, it is best to do nothing but manage the wound locally and let a mucocutaneous junction form by secondary intention (Fig. 12B). Stricture or recession is often the late consequence of ischemia, but such problems can be revised electively later. If necrosis extends below the level of the fascia and peritoneum, however, immediate laparotomy and colostomy revision should be undertaken to avoid perforation and peritonitis.

Mucocutaneous Separation

Mucocutaneous separation of the stoma from the skin may occur as a result of tension (i.e., creation of a skin opening too large for the exteriorized bowel). or superficial infection (Fig. 13). Good ET nursing is especially important when this problem occurs, and stenosis at the skin level is always possible as a late consequence. The subcutaneous tissue between the stoma and skin should be kept clean by packing the area with a paste material (e.g., Stomahesive) or absorptive powder until a new junction forms secondarily.

Stoma Stenosis

Stoma stenosis occurs as a consequence of ischemia or infection, although occasionally it can result from the opening in the skin or fascia being made too small at the time of stoma construction (Fig. 14). The stenosis can be managed initially with simple and gentle dilatation of the stoma in conjunction with a low-fiber diet. If the patient has recurrent obstructive episodes or pain, however, the stoma should be revised. Skin-level stenosis can be managed by detaching the skin from the mucosa, and by excising a small amount of skin to increase the trephine size. This incision can be extended down to the fascia, if necessary, where the fascial opening can be enlarged. The fascia and skin are resutured primarily and a new Brooke-type stoma fashioned. Malt et al. (110) described a technique for relieving stricture at the fascial level by performing a fasciotomy similar to those performed for compartment syndromes of the calf or forearm. With this technique, incisions are made above and below the ileostomy and away from the peristomal skin. A scissors is then slid through the grain of the anterior rectus sheath to the ileum and the stricture is relieved (Fig. 15).

Recession (Retraction)

Recession, or retraction, of an ileostomy or colostomy can occur in as many as 10% to 15% of patients (111). The recession can be intermittent or fixed. Intermittent recession, or telescoping, results from having too large a gap through the abdominal wall or from having inadequate fixation and adhesion formation between the stoma and the abdominal wall. With intermittent recession, the stoma length and protrusion are generally satisfactory when patients assume the upright position, but the stoma becomes flush with the skin or may recede below the skin level when patients lie supine and the abdominal muscles are relaxed. This often leads to soiling and leakage, since it is difficult to maintain a satisfactory appliance seal whenever the stoma does not protrude above the skin level. Fixed ostomy recession usually implies that the stoma was designed too short at the time of construction or that it became too short when the width of the abdominal wall increased after a period of postoperative weight gain (Fig. 16). Some patients with either fixed or intermittent ileostomy recession can be managed with skilled ET nursing. A convex faceplate placed firmly against the skin

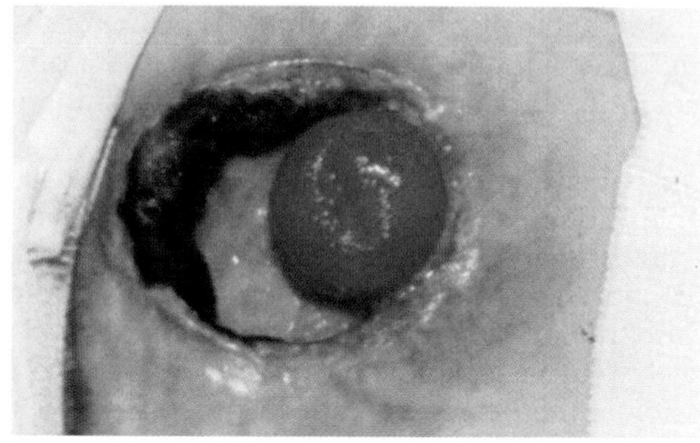

FIGURE 13 ■ Ileostomy with gaping mucocutaneous separation.

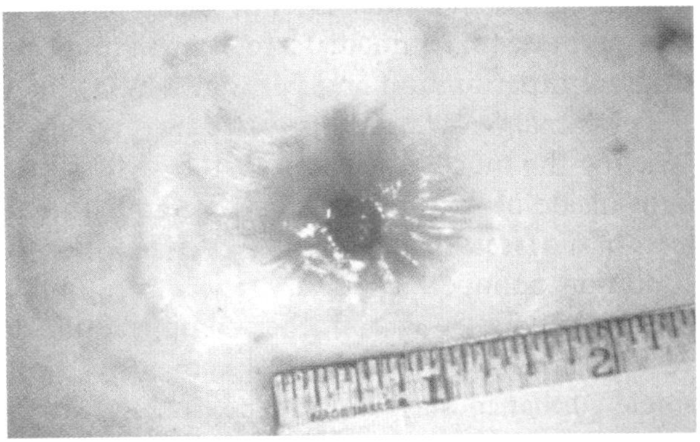

FIGURE 14 ■ Ileostomy stenosis with marked skin scarring.

sometimes allows patients to maintain a satisfactory seal and not need operative revision. If the patient continues to have leakage and soiling, then the ileostomy should be revised.

The simplest type of revision is performed locally by making a circumferential incision around the stoma at the mucocutaneous junction and extending the incision down to the level of fascia and peritoneum to free up the entire distal bowel that is then refixed to the peritoneum and fasci, and a new Brooke maturation is performed (Fig. 17).

Ostomy Prolapse

Introduction

Stomal prolapse may develop in any type of abdominal stoma. Rates are variable, but substantially lower than those of parastomal hernias. In a review of the *United Ostomy Association Registry*, Fleshman and Lewis found the rates as follows: ileostomy 3%, colostomy 2%, and urostomy less than 1% (112). Similarly, a Cook County Hospital registry including 1616 stomas found the overall incidence to be 2%. Age and lack of preoperative stoma site markings were predictive risk factors (113). However,

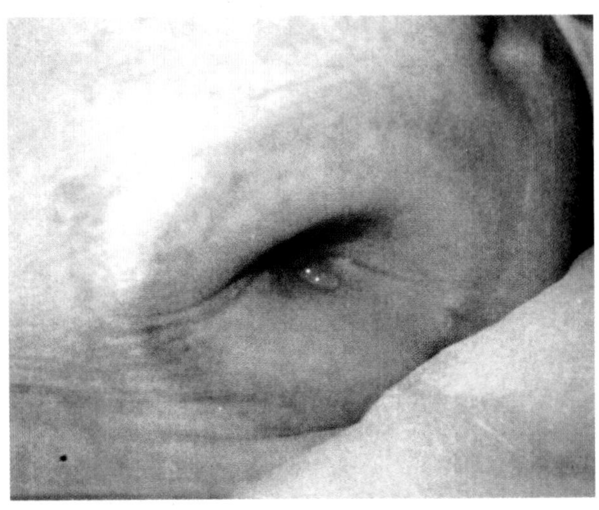

FIGURE 16 ■ Fixed recession of ileostomy.

registries tend to include predominantly individuals with permanent stomas, therefore, underestimate the risk of complications associated with temporary stomas.

The stoma at highest risk for prolapse has been the transverse loop colostomy and the distal defunctionalized limb is usually responsible. Reasons for this are unclear, but a large stoma aperture (particularly when stomas are created in an emergency setting), and a poorly fixed, redundant, distal transverse colon have been implicated. Incidence varies, but rates of prolapse as high as 47% have been found in association with loop colostomies (114).

Some authors divide prolapse into two types, fixed and sliding. Fixed prolapse is defined as permanent eversion of a greater than desired segment of bowel. This occurs because too much bowel has been everted at the time of stoma construction. It is uncommon and rarely requires treatment. The remainder of this segment will focus on sliding prolapse.

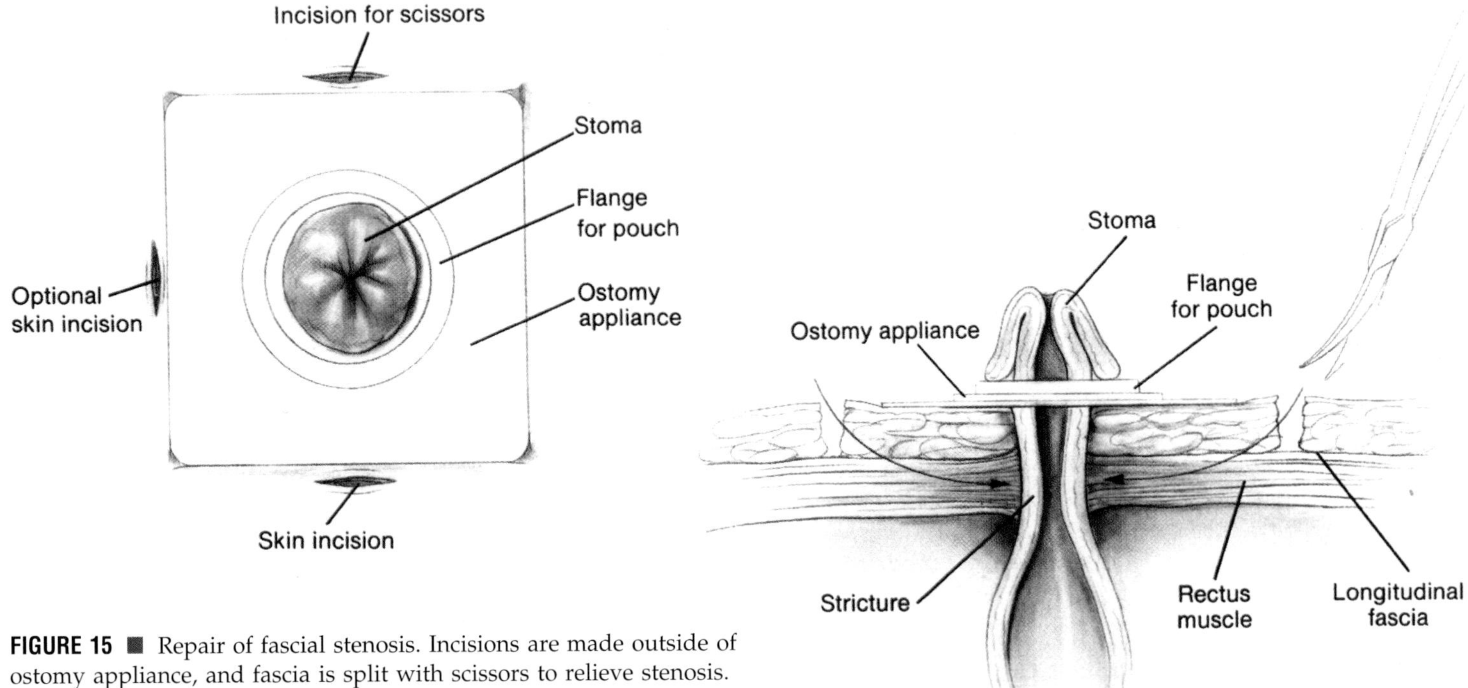

FIGURE 15 ■ Repair of fascial stenosis. Incisions are made outside of ostomy appliance, and fascia is split with scissors to relieve stenosis. *Source*: Modified from Ref. 110.

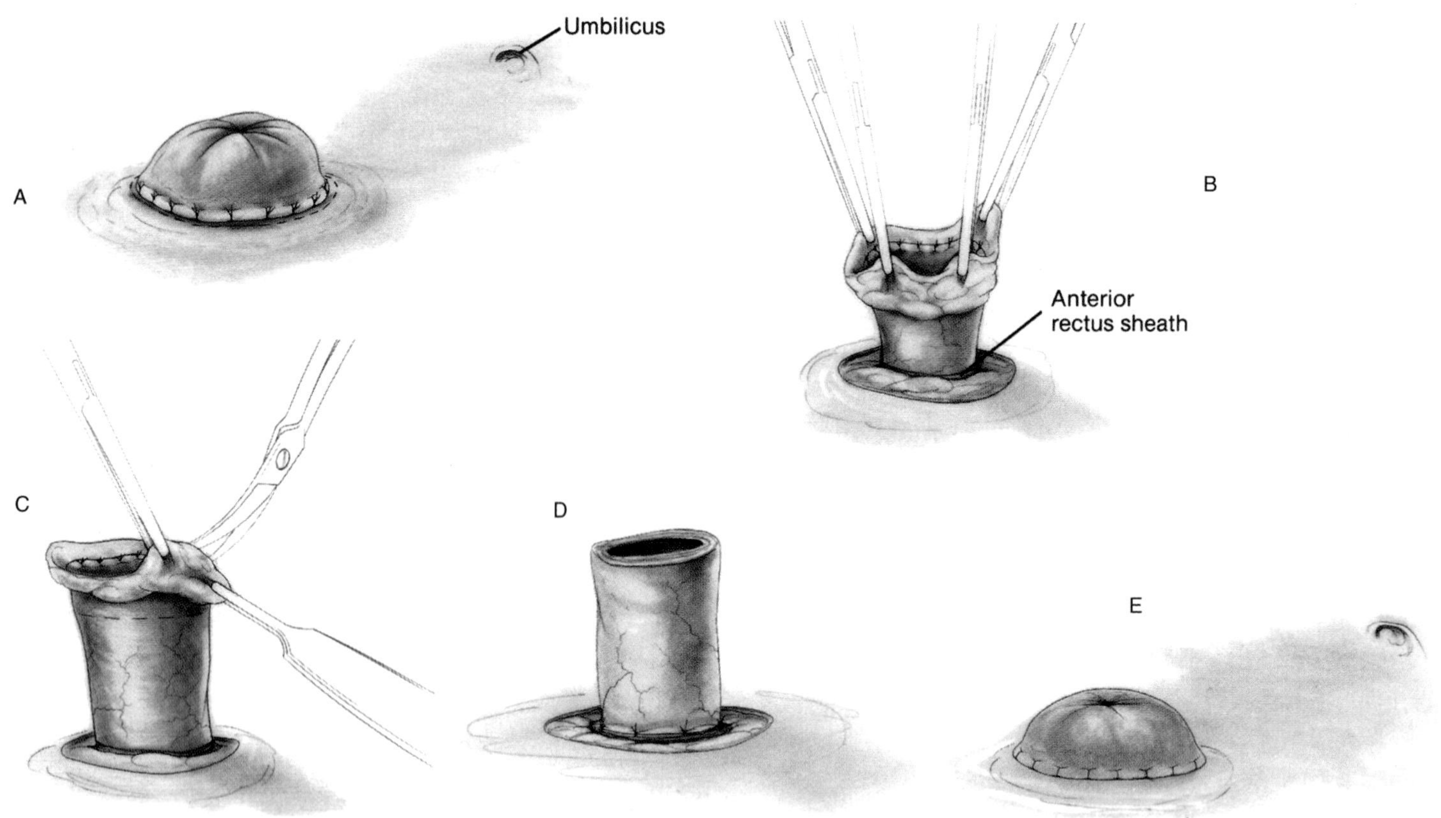

FIGURE 17 ■ Ileostomy revision. (**A**) Circumferential incision around stoma. (**B** and **C**) Stoma is mobilized to fascia and peritoneum, and tip is resected. (**D**) Ileum is fixed to fascia. (**E**) New Brooke maturation is done.

Sliding prolapse occurs when long segment of ileum or colon protrude through the stoma orifice intermittently, usually in response to Valsalva or increased abdominal pressure. Segments greater than 40 to 50 cm have been observed (Figs. 18 and 19).

Particularly when prolapse develops in colostomies, a parastomal hernia may also be present. It is essential that any concomitant hernia be identified prior to treatment, as the presence of a parastomal hernia will dictate the type of repair required. Allen-Mersh and Thomson identified a 50% incidence of hernia associated with colostomy prolapse, most commonly associated with end colostomies (93).

Symptoms

Stomal prolapse always presents as a stomal mass, but other symptoms include dislodgement of the appliance, bowel obstruction, and pain due to venous engorgement of the constricted, prolapsed segment. Diagnosis is ascertained by history and physical examination. The frequency and consequences of symptoms are important because minimally symptomatic, infrequent prolapse does not require repair.

When examining the abdomen, the prolapse should be reduced and a finger placed in the stomal orifice. Diligent inspection and palpation of the peristomal skin will determine the presence or absence of a hernia. If a hernia is present, its presence and symptoms should dictate the type of repair performed. The prolapse will, by necessity, be repaired during the process.

Treatment

Less than 10% of prolapse will be complicated by incarceration and/or strangulation. In these situations, treatment is urgent. In viable, incarcerated stomas table sugar may be sprinkled (large amounts) on the stoma to draw out water and decrease edema. This may allow for reduction of the prolapse with subsequent elective operation. If this is unsuccessful or if viability is in question, then it will be necessary to proceed with operation. If the bowel is nonviable, then an extra-abdominal resection and cutaneous recreation of the stoma is the preferred option. Otherwise any of the options mentioned in the ensuing sections may be applied.

When prolapse or any stoma complication develops, the surgeon should first determine if the stoma can be reversed and intestinal continuity can be reestablished. If this can be done safely, it should be the first surgical option even if earlier than previously planned. If this in not an option, then repair should be undertaken.

Regardless of the planned preoperative approach, all of the following should be accomplished prior to operation. A comprehensive history and physical must be performed not only to determine the patient's ability to tolerate an operation, but also to determine preoperative stoma related problems so that these can be addressed (i.e., odor, leakage, poorly fitting appliance, and poor stoma visualization). In addition, any disability or dysfunction that will limit stoma care, such as arthritis or poor vision, should be elicited. All patients should also be attended to by a trained stomatherapist and/or the surgeon preoperatively, in the event resiting of a stoma becomes necessary. Finally, at the time of operation, all patients need to be prepped and drapped for laparotomy and transabdominal repair even if preoperative plan dictates a parastomal approach.

Repair takes one of three forms: resection, revision, or resisting. Resection is most commonly employed for end

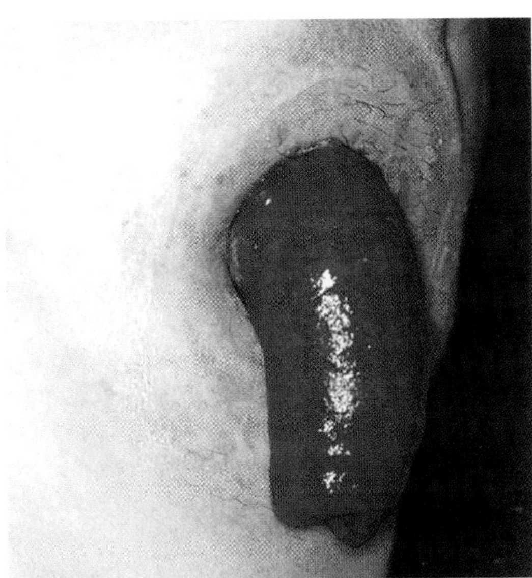

FIGURE 18 ■ Prolapsed ileostomy.

stomas. Resection simply involves mucocutaneous disconnection (care should be taken to prevent creating an oversized skin defect), eversion of the prolapsed segment, resection of any exteriorized bowel, and recreation of the stoma.

Simple prolapse can easily be repaired through a paracolostomy incision. The colon is mobilized in the same fashion as for local colostomy revision, with dissection down to the peritoneal cavity to free the colon circumferentially. The colon, with all its redundancy, is then delivered through the abdominal wall. The redundant sigmoid is resected, leaving a 5-cm protrusion above the abdominal wall. The sigmoid is fixed to the fascia with 3–0 nonabsorbable sutures, and a primary maturation is performed with 3–0 chromic catgut suture (Fig. 20).

Revision is most appropriate for prolapse of the distal limb of a transverse loop colostomy. In this case, through peristomal skin incision, the distal limb is dissected free and separated from the proximal limb. The open end is then closed and returned to the abdominal cavity. The fascial and skin defects are then tailored to an appropriate size and an end colostomy created. Care should be taken to insure proper orientation of the proximal and distal limbs as dropping the proximal, functional end of a transverse colostomy into the peritoneal cavity will have predictable, devastating consequences.

Prolapse is more common with a transverse colostomy than with an end colostomy, but transverse colostomy prolapse can be managed conservatively since the stoma is usually temporary (Fig. 21). When operation is indicated, several procedures have been proposed. Zinkin and Rosin (115) described a modification of an old procedure called "button colopexy" for patients who are not candidates for extensive revision. This procedure can be performed on an outpatient basis. It is performed by pressing the proximal and distal loop of bowel against the anterior abdominal wall by a finger inserted in the lumen, and then securing each loop against the abdominal wall with large nonabsorbable sutures tied over a button. Another option for the transverse colostomy prolapse in high-risk patients is dividing the loop colostomy into two limbs. The prolapsing proximal or distal colon limb is dissected free, the redundant tip is resected, and a new end colostomy is fashioned with a long Hartmann's pouch or a small mucous fistula.

Finally, resiting is best reserved for prolapsed stomas with other associated problems. As previously mentioned, this is an option for prolapse in association with hernia. However, resiting may be beneficial in other situations. If the stoma was originally poorly sited and this has lead to significant problems, then resiting may be appropriate. In addition, a transverse loop colostomy may be associated with other significant problems such as odor, leakage, or the need for an overly large unsightly appliance. Here, right colectomy and ileostomy may be the procedure of choice if reestablishment of continuity is not appropriate.

Parastomal Hernia

Parastomal hernias may develop around both ileostomies and colostomies (Fig. 22). The risk of parastomal hernia is increased with high intra-abdominal pressure, chronic cough, obesity, malnutrition, and use of immunosuppressive drugs and steroids. The probability of the occurrence of the risk of this complication may be reduced by locating the stoma through the rectus muscle. The incidence varies, but paraileostomy hernias are less frequent (0–28%) compared with colostomies (0–58%) (116). Advanced age of colostomates versus ileostomates, solid nature of feces, and larger size of colostomies versus ileostomies have all been implicated as causative factors (116).

A

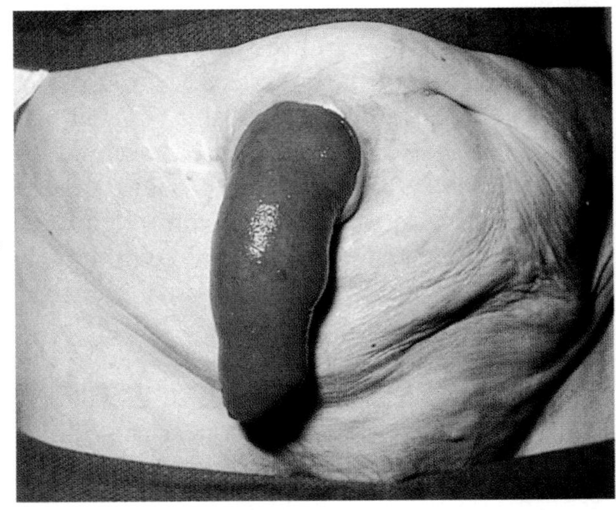

B

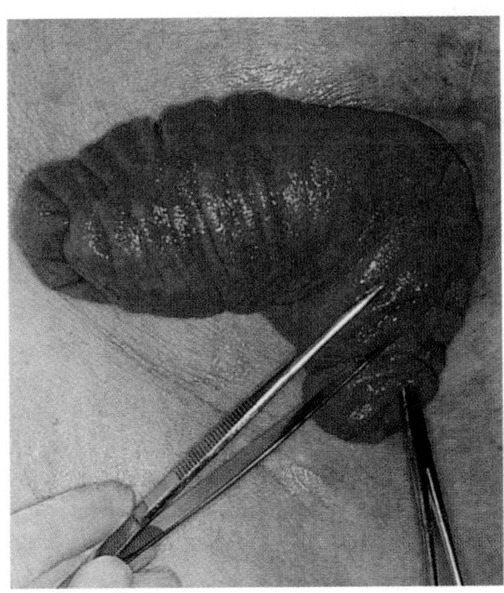

FIGURE 19 ■ (**A**) Dramatic end-colostomy prolapse. (**B**) End-transverse colostomy with prolapse of ascending colon and cecum. Forceps indicates the ileocecal valve and hemostat in appendiceal orifice.

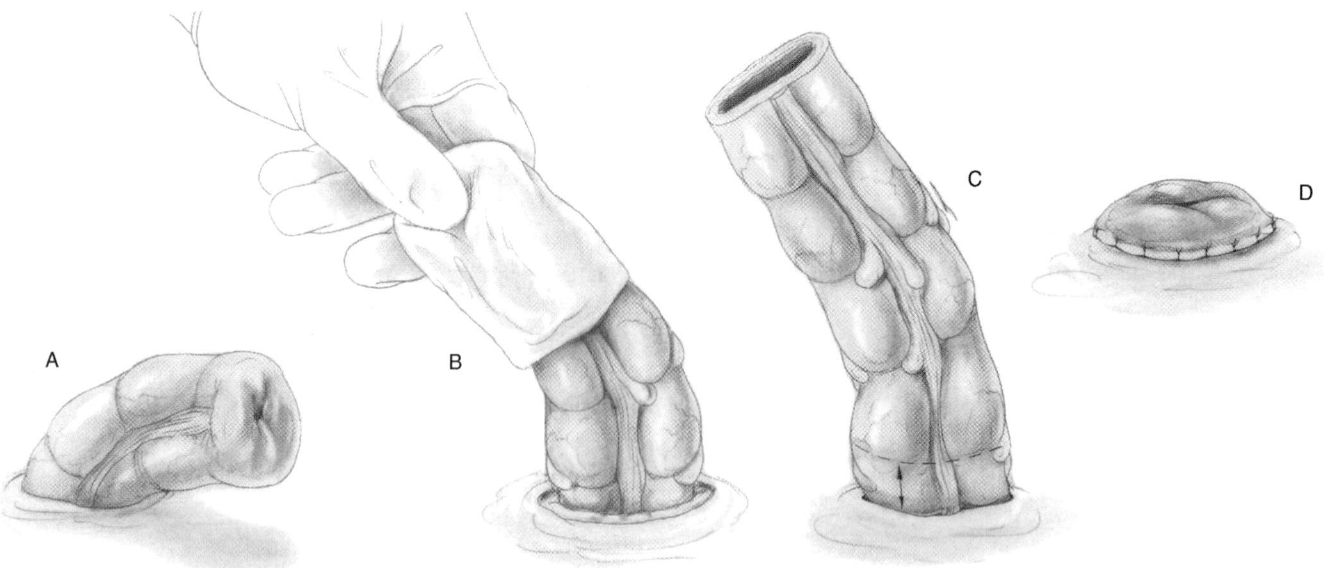

FIGURE 20 ■ Repair of prolapsed end colostomy. (**A** and **B**) Mucocutaneous junction of colostomy is incised and colon elevated. (**C**) Redundant colon is resected. (**D**) New colostomy is matured.

The most frequent complication of colostomy is parastomal hernia (Fig. 22). Parastomal hernia may be caused by poor operative technique, infection, incorrect location, too large a hole (early hernia), or by high intra-abdominal pressure due to obesity, constipation, prostatism, or chronic cough (late hernia) (117).

Carne et al. (118) reviewed the technical factors related to the construction of the stoma that may influence the incidence and success of the different methods of repair. They found parastomal hernia affects 1.8% to 28.3% of end ileostomies and 0% to 6.2% of loop ileostomies. Following colostomy formation, the rates are 4.0% to 48.1% and 0% to 30.8%, respectively. Site of stoma formation (through or lateral to rectus abdominus), trephine size, fascial fixation and closure of lateral space are not proven to affect the incidence of hernia. The role of extraperitoneal stoma construction is uncertain. Mesh repair gives a lower rate of recurrence (0–33%) than direct tissue repair (46–100%), or stoma relocation (0–76.2%).

FIGURE 21 ■ Prolapsed, partially ulcerated distal limb of transverse colostomy.

In addition, stoma placement lateral to the rectus muscle has been associated with increased risk of herniation. Birnbaum and Ferrier noted a fourfold increase in hernias when colostomies were placed through the oblique muscles (119). Similarly, Grier found a 10% risk in transrectus stomas compared with a 70% risk in those lateral to the rectus muscle (120). In contrast, several other series noted no significant differences (121–125). Regardless of whether hernias

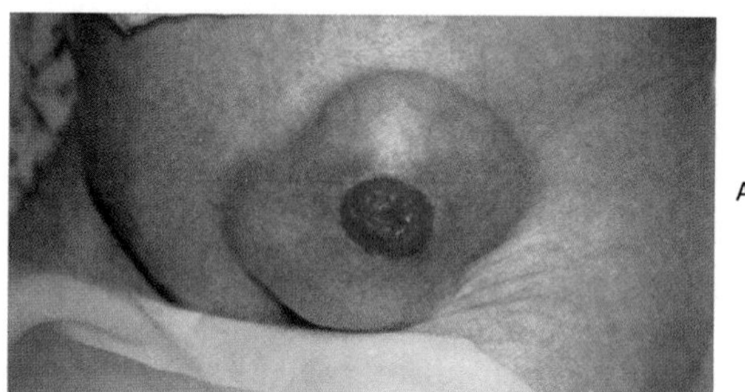

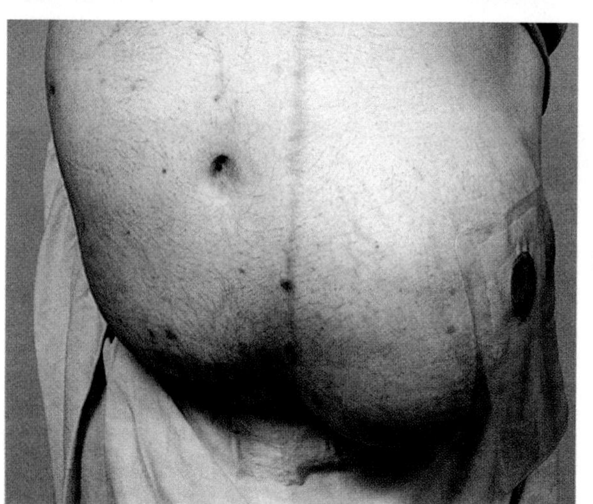

FIGURE 22 ■ (**A**) Large parastomal hernia around end sigmoid colostomy. (**B**) Huge paracolostomy hernia with laterally displaced ostomy opening.

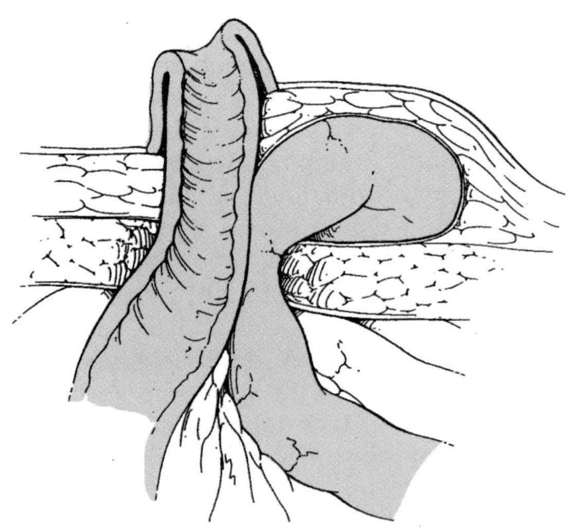

FIGURE 23 ■ True parastomal hernia. *Source*: From Ref. 126.

develop around ileostomies or colostomies, their presenting symptoms, evaluation, and treatment are similar.

Hernias commonly present as a mass in the peristomal skin or are discovered incidentally on physical examination. Additional symptoms include: difficulty maintaining an appliance seal, pain, small bowel obstruction, stoma outlet obstruction, skin excoriation, and difficulty with stoma irrigation.

A careful physical examination with a finger in the stoma is often all that is necessary to diagnose and characterize a parastomal hernia. Hernias have been divided into four types (116). Type I is a "true" parastomal hernia, where small bowel protrudes within a peritoneal sac through a fascial defect (Fig. 23). In Type II peritoneal contents protrude between the two layers of everted bowel in association with a prolapsed stoma (Fig. 24). Type III describes subcutaneous protrusion of the stoma between the fascia and the peristomal skin with no real fascial defect (Fig. 25). Type IV is a "pseudohernia" or a diffuse bulge due to weakness in the abdominal wall musculature and requires no treatment (Fig. 26).

As previously mentioned, a careful physical examination can distinguish between the four hernia types.

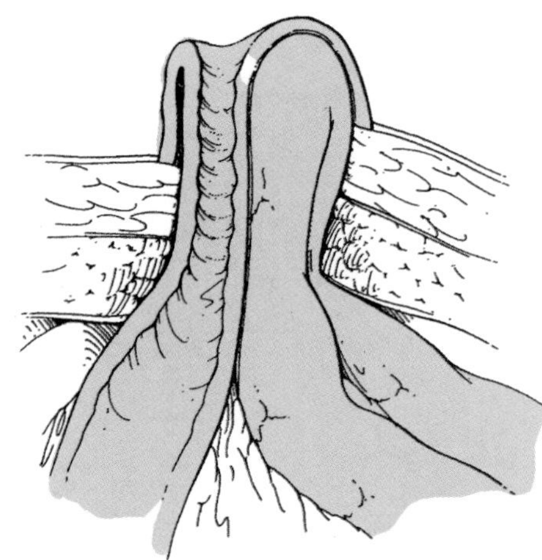

FIGURE 24 ■ Intrastomal hernia (may be associated with prolapse). *Source*: From Ref. 126.

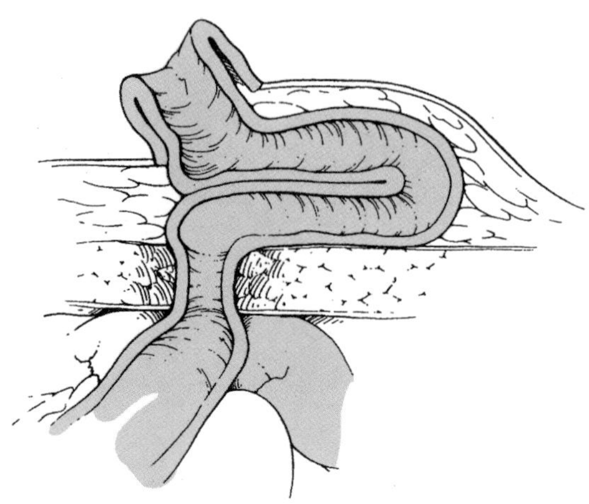

FIGURE 25 ■ Subcutaneuous prolapse (pseudohernia) with intact fascial ring. *Source*: From Ref. 126.

Occasionally an abdominal CT scan may be helpful if classification is difficult. It is essential to classify these hernias preoperatively as treatment will vary significantly.

Prior to recommending operation, it is important to note that stomal hernia repair may be associated with significant complications and success rates are variable. Consequently, not all parastomal hernias require repair. Asymptomatic patients may need no treatment. Minimally symptomatic patients can be treated with appliance modification with or with a support belt with the aid of a stoma therapist (Fig. 27).

If conservative measures fail, or if bowel obstruction or significant skin excoriation develops, operation is indicated. In several series, long term follow-up of stomas revealed between 15% and 32% of ostomates with hernias required operative repair (127,128).

Three surgical approaches are available for treatment of paraileostomy or paracolostomy hernias, local repair, transperitoneal repair, or stoma resiting (Fig. 28). Mesh can be used with any of the three techniques.

Regardless of the selected approach, all patients should be prepared for laparotomy and stoma resiting. Each patient should have one or two alternate stoma sites identified and marked by a stoma therapist or surgeon prior to operation. In cases where stoma placement is difficult or the abdominal wall has multiple scars and/or skin creases, patients may need to wear an appliance at the

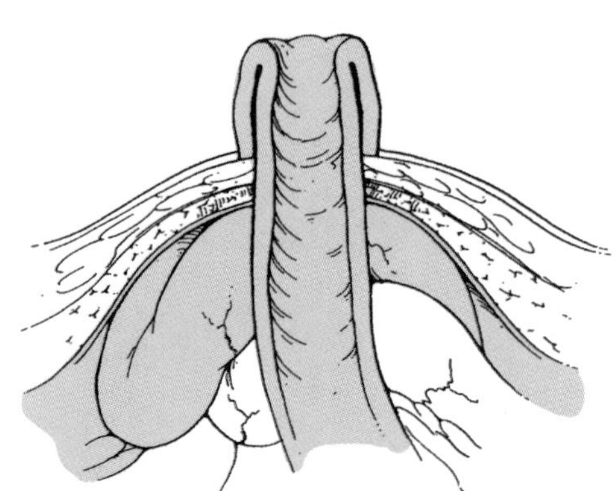

FIGURE 26 ■ Pseudohernia due to weakness of abdominal wall without fascial defect. *Source*: From Ref. 126.

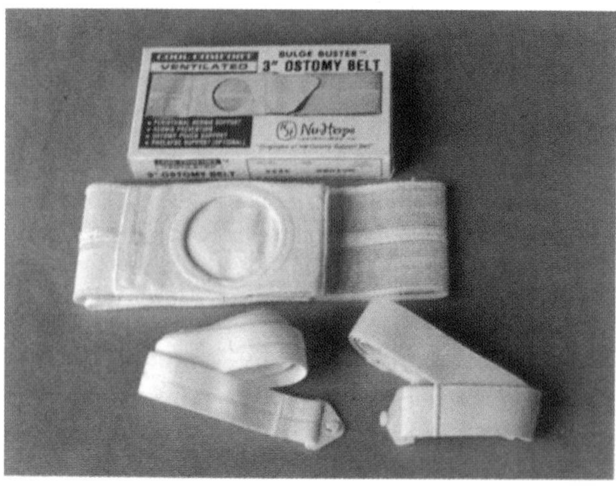

FIGURE 27 ■ Ostomy belts. Upper belt is designed to support parastomal hernia. Lower belts are attached to pouching systems.

prospective, new stoma sites for a day prior to operation to assess satisfaction.

Local approaches may vary, but all follow similar principles. An incision is made in the peristomal skin outside the footprint of the appliance; the hernia sac is separated from the surrounding, subcutaneous tissue, and reduced. Finally, the defect is repaired. Currently, mesh is used in nearly all the repairs as recurrence is almost inevitable without prosthetic material.

Although some parastomal hernias can be repaired by excision of the sac and local resuture of the fascia, recurrences are especially common if this method is used for larger hernias or hernias associated with weakened fascia. Repair of these hernias requires either the use of synthetic mesh or moving the stoma. Allen-Mersh and Thomson (93) found that relocating the stoma above and medial to the previous stoma tended to be less successful than resiting either to the right side of the abdomen or the umbilicus. Relocating is technically easier to do through the umbilicus, but stomal management is much easier from the patient's perspective if the stoma is on the right side. For some larger hernias, synthetic mesh (Marlex) can be used to close the hernia defect and the colon can be placed along either the medial or the lateral border of the mesh. Preferably the colon can be brought out through an opening created in the center of the mesh (Fig. 28). A number of modifications for the use of Marlex have been described (129,130).

Stephenson and Phillips (131) described an approach to the repair of a parastomal hernia that avoids laparotomy and maintains the existing stoma site. Under local anesthesia the stoma is mobilized about the mucocutaneous junction. The stoma is then brought out through a fresh adjacent area of abdominal wall and the defect repaired with a tension-free mesh. A drain is brought out at a distance not to interfere with appliance application. The stoma is then resited at its original position and anchored in place. Eight patients so treated had no recurrences at a mean follow-up of 15 months.

The transabdominal approach consists of the same steps performed through a midline laparotomy. The mesh may be placed intraperitoneally or in a supra-peritoneal position below the posterior rectus fascia. Geisler et al. (132) reported 11 patients undergoing parastomal hernia with an overall recurrence for mesh repair at a parastomal site of 63%. Wound infection occurred in sites of parastomal repair in 13% of parastomal hernia sites. Wound infection rates were statistically independent of type of hernia, variety of mesh, or operative approach.

Steele et al. (133) reviewed the rate of complications and outcomes with polypropylene mesh in parastomal hernia repairs in 58 patients. After closure of the fascia, the stoma was pulled through the center of the mesh, which was placed either above or below the fascia. There were 31 end colostomies, 24 end ileostomies, and 3 loop transverse colostomies. Mean follow-up was 51 months. Overall complications related to the polypropylene mesh were 36% (recurrence 26%, surgical bowel obstruction 9%, prolapse 3%, wound infection 3%, fistula 3%, and mesh erosion 2%). None of the patients had extirpation of their mesh. Complications were significantly associated with younger age (60 years vs. 67 years). Carcinoma patients with stomas had fewer complications. Inflammatory bowel disease, stomal type, mesh location, urgent procedures, steroid use, and surgical approaches were not significantly associated with an increased complication rate.

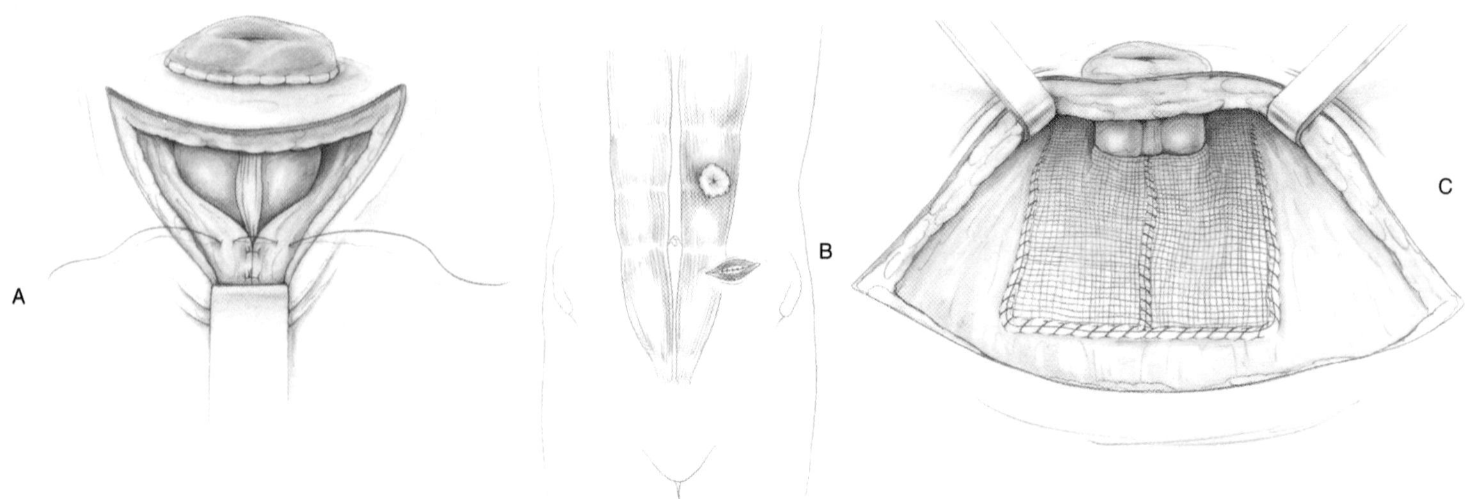

FIGURE 28 ■ Parastomal colostomy hernia. Types of repair: (**A**) Direct resuture of fascia after resecting hernia sac. (**B**) Repair of hernia after relocating stoma. (**C**) Repair with synthetic mesh.

Of the 15 patients with recurrence, 7 underwent successful repair for an overall success rate of 86%.

Janes et al. (134) determined the effect of stomal complications using a mesh at the primary operation. They randomized 27 patients to have a conventional stoma and 27 to have the mesh. No infection, fistula formation, or pain occurred (observation time, 2–28 months). At the 12-month follow-up, parastomal hernia was present in 8 of the 18 patients without a mesh and in none of the 16 patients in whom the mesh was used.

Finally, stoma resiting is a straight-forward approach and involves stoma takedown, necessary lysis of adhesions, and recreation of the stoma at a premarked, new location. The hernia and old stoma defect are closed appropriately, and may include mesh if a satisfactory repair cannot be otherwise obtained.

Success rates are variable, but local repair alone fails up to 64% patients (93), while success following prosthetic repair, either local or transabdominal, is associated with a greater than 80% success rate (135,136). Stomal resiting is associated with a 30% recurrence rate (128).

The risk of recurrence after parastomal hernia repair is considerable and is higher for fascial repair (76%) than for stoma relocation (33%) (137). However, complications are more common after stoma relocation (88%) than fascial repair (50%). This high rate reflects incisional hernia, which develops in 52% of patients. Botet et al. (117) reported their experience with a technique of stoma translocation without laparotomy. The original stoma was closed and dissected free from the abdominal wall. A disk of skin was excised 6 cm from the original site and a fascial opening created. The colon was drawn through the new site, the original colostomy opening sutured, and the colostomy matured. In 11 patients so treated, there were no recurrences with a follow-up ranging from 2 to 36 months.

Fistula

Although superficial fistulas can occur around a stoma because of stitch abscess, trauma, or other minor problems, a peristomal fistula is usually a serious problem. Fistulas can be especially troublesome when they occur after an ileostomy for Crohn's disease, since they almost invariably indicate recurrent disease. Many superficial fistulas heal spontaneously, but major fistulas below the skin level usually require formal stomal reconstruction, and the stoma often needs to be moved (111).

Greatorex (138) described a simple method of closing a fistula by debriding the fistula tract with a pipe cleaner soaked in 6% aqueous phenol solution. The procedure is based on the principle that many simple fistula tracts will close after careful debridement and the addition of a sclerosing agent. Fibrin glue can be used as an alternative to phenol.

Stomal Varices

Varices are abnormal portosystemic vascular connections and develop in response to increase in portal pressure. Sclerosing cholangitis, alcoholic cirrhosis, and extensive metastatic disease to the liver are the most common causes in ostomates. Other risk factors for the development of parastomal varices include splenomegaly, esophageal varices, advanced histologic stage at liver biopsy, low serum albumin, thrombocytopenia, and an increased prothrombin time (139). In individuals with ileostomies or colostomies, the surgical proximity of the portal (intestine) and systemic (skin) leads to the possibility of varices in individuals with liver disease. This should be kept in mind when chosing surgical options for the treatment of ulcerative colitis accompanied by sclerosing cholangitis. An ileal-pouch anal anastomosis, avoiding a permanent ileostomy, eliminates the risk of stomal varices in these individuals. The actual incidence of peristomal varices is unknown, but may be as high as 27% in patients with known hepatic dysfunction (140).

The management of bleeding from ileostomy varices poses a dilemma as recurrent bleeding is almost the rule following local treatment (43–100%) (141), and yet definitive control by portal decompression carries significant morbidity and mortality for most patients (142). Grundfest-Broniatowski and Fazio (143) have emphasized the hazards of portacaval shunting for bleeding stomal varices, particularly since shunting does not appear to improve overall survival in these patients. The authors recommend a conservative approach consisting of appliance refitting if the bleeding is related to trauma, local pressure, epinephrine compresses, and transfusions, if needed. Ligation of the varices with or without stoma revision generally stops hemorrhage in those patients who continue to bleed. Mucocutaneous disconnection interrupts the high-pressure portosystemic collaterals; only rarely is it necessary to resort to shunting. Stomal sclerotherapy with 3% sodium tetradecyl sulfate, ethanol, and saline in a 1:1:1 mixture (144), or 0.5% to 1% polidocanol (Ethoxysclerol), or almond oil containing 5% phenol (145) has been used with some success. Roberts et al. (141) recommended shunts after failure of local therapy. If decompressive shunt therapy is to be done, it is best to create a splenorenal shunt away from the right upper quadrant, since many of these patients ultimately become candidates for liver transplantation. For the occasional patient who continues to bleed despite conservative measures and is not a suitable candidate for portacaval shunting, percutaneous transhepatic embolization of varices has been reported successful and may be considered as an option (146).

Roberts et al. (141) reviewed their experience with 12 patients who had bleeding stomal varices. Stomal variceal bleeding occurred between 1 and 11 years (median, 5.5 years) after creation of the stoma. At the time of diagnosis, a typical caput medusae is seen around the stoma (Fig. 29). Control of bleeding initially consisted of direct pressure; recurrent bleeding occurred in one patient who died before definitive therapy could be performed. The remaining 11 patients underwent a total of 18 additional procedures to control bleeding stomal varices, including nine local procedures (suture ligation of the stoma in four, mucocutaneous disconnection in three, cauterization of the stoma in one, and transposition of the stoma in one), eight portosystemic shunts, and one liver transplantation. Seven patients died of hepatic failure a median of four years (range, one to nine years) after treatment. Recurrent bleeding occurred in three patients after local treatment and in one patient after a portosystemic shunt. Although local procedures may be effective for the initial control of bleeding, recurrent bleeding often occurs. Mortality is high because of the severity of the underlying liver disease.

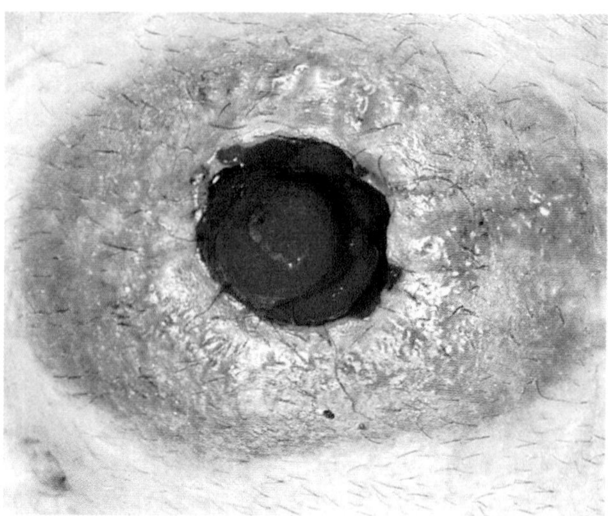

FIGURE 29 ■ Ileostomy with typical circumferential caput medusae. *Source*: Courtesy Pat Roberts, M.D., Burlington, Massachusetts, U.S.A.

In the last 10 years, the use of transjugular, intrahepatic, portosystemic shunting (TIPS) has increased substantially. It has been successfully applied to the treatment of variceal bleeding from many sites in individuals with portal hypertension, including stomal variceal hemorrhage (147,148). TIPS allows for treatment of the primary cause of variceal bleeding (portal hypertension) without the need for laparotomy. It has the additional advantage of not altering perihepatic anatomy in patients who are candidates for future liver transplantation.

In summary, the selection of treatment for individuals with bleeding stomal varices, whether from an ileostomy, urostomy, or colostomy should be based on the patients' underlying disease process and general medical condition. Simple, local measures are often a good first step to control hemorrhage, but bleeding will ultimately recur. They may be all that is necessary in individuals with end-stage liver disease who are not transplant candidates. Eliminating the underlying cause, however, is essential for long-term prevention of bleeding. Portosystemic shunting, either by TIPS in individuals who are transplant candidates, or by formal, surgical shunts in patients who are not, will ultimately be necessary.

Ulceration

Ulceration is either due to local trauma, infection, or recurrent Crohn's disease. Ulceration around the stoma implies recurrent Crohn's disease, whereas ulceration on the stoma itself may be the result of other causes. Ulcers should be treated symptomatically with good enterostomal care. Resection is not indicated unless ulcerations extend deep into the ileostomy or peristomal abdominal wall ulceration becomes unmanageable.

Diversion Colitis

Diversion colitis is an iatrogenic, nutritional complication following the creation of a diverting colostomy. It can occur regardless of whether the colostomy is performed as a loop colostomy or end colostomy with a defunctionalized Hartmann's pouch or mucous fistula. The colitis is a unique type of inflammatory process that can appear within weeks of fecal diversion and resolves rapidly once continuity has been reestablished. The histologic findings tend to be nonspecific and undistinguishable from ulcerative colitis. Diversion colitis develops due to the fact that the colon and rectum require luminal stool to meet the nutritional needs of the colonocytes. *N*-butyrate, a short chain fatty acid is the primary fuel source for colonic mucosal cells and is only available through luminal absorption from stool.

Korelitz et al. (149) proposed that short-chain fatty acids produced by anaerobic bacteria serve as a trophic factor for the distal colon and rectal mucosa. Harig et al. (150) administered short-chain fatty acids to the diverted segment of four patients with diversion colitis, and in each case the inflammation resolved. The best treatment for diversion colitis is to reestablish colonic continuity. If this is not possible, then short-chain fatty acid enemas may be of benefit. However, in most cases no treatment is necessary. Diversion colitis is often found incidentally on preoperative endoscopy of the defuntionalized limb. Patients occasionally suffer the minor inconvenience of mild tenesmus and small mucosy, bloody stools. Reassurance is usually all that is required.

The most important fact regarding diversion colitis or proctitis is to realize that it exists and that patients have not developed ulcerative proctitis precluding stoma takedown. The opposite is in fact true; stoma takedown and reestablishment of intestinal continuity will resupply the colon with *N*-butyrate and the diversion colitis will resolve.

OUTCOMES OF STOMAL CONSTRUCTION AND CLOSURE

The overall morbidity of closure of a temporary ileostomy ranges from 2% to 33% (103). In particular, small bowel obstruction occurs in 0% to 13% (mostly in the 6–10% range), wound infection 0% to 18% (mostly in the 3–7% range), and relaparotomy 0% to 13% (mostly in the 4–7% range). The incidence of incisional hernia at the previous stoma site varies from less than 1% to 12%.

Pokorny et al. (151) analyzed 533 patients with stoma closure. The overall stoma closure related mortality was 3%; the overall stomal closure related surgical complication rate was 20%. Wound infections (9%) and anastomotic leakage (5%) were the most common surgical complications. Age was the only significant risk factor for survival. Use of a soft silicone drain for intraperitoneal drainage (odds ratio 1.62) was the only risk factor for complications. In patients with carcinoma as the primary disease (odds ratio = 1.61) they observed significantly fewer complications. Stomal closure is so often considered a minor procedure but as clearly and appropriately pointed out in this article, it is associated with significant morbidity and mortality. This should not be unexpected because these patients are undergoing bowel operations and therefore should be accorded the same considerations and respect as any other patient undergoing bowel operation.

Moug et al. (152) reported on 100 consecutive patients undergoing elective closure of a loop ileostomy. The overall postoperative complication rate was 32% and mortality rate was 3%. Minor complications included wound infection, nausea and vomiting, and cardiac arrhythmia. Major complications were obstruction, ischemic bowel, sepsis, and anastomotic leak. The likelihood of postoperative complications increases significantly with increasing deprivation category scores. The overall complication rate in patients with low (1–2) intermediate (3–5), and high (6–7), scores were 0%, 26%, and 46%, respectively. Thus, high levels of socioeconomic deprivation significantly increased risk of postoperative complications after elective closure of loop ileostomies.

Bosshardt (153) reviewed his facility's experience with 383 fecal ostomies to determine the effect of advanced age on surgical outcome measures in a tertiary managed care medical center. There were 103 patients aged 70 years or older and 280 patients were younger than 70 years. There were 220 elective procedures and 163 emergency procedures. The diagnosis leading to creation of the ostomy was more often malignancy in older patients (75%) compared with younger patients (45%). Both age groups underwent a similar proportion of emergency procedures (older vs. younger patients, 44% vs. 42%); but more older patients were left with permanent stomas (59% vs. 41%). Older patients also had more preoperative comorbidities, higher American Society of Anesthesiologists score, longer hospital stays, and more postoperative complications. Thirty-day mortality was 6.8% in the older group versus 0.4% in the younger group. Fewer older patients were eligible for ostomy reversible (41% vs. 59%) and a smaller proportion of eligible older patients actually underwent the reversal procedure (78% vs. 95%). The complication rate associated with ostomy reversal was not significantly different in the two age groups. They concluded, patients aged 70 years and older undergo proportionally more permanent fecal ostomy procedures than younger patients. Furthermore, older patients tolerate ostomy reversal with minimal morbidity and should not be denied consideration based on age alone if they are eligible candidates.

Park et al. (113) analyzed 1616 patients with enteric stomas and found 34% of patients with complications. Among the total complications, 28% occurred early (<1 month postoperation) and 6% occurred late (>1 month). The most common early complications were skin irritations (12%), pain associated with poor stoma location (7%), and partial necrosis (5%). The most common late complications were skin irritation (6%), prolapse (2%), and stenosis (2%). The enteric stoma with the most complications was the loop ileostomy (75%). The enteric stoma with the least complications was the end transverse colostomy (6%). The general surgery service had the most complications (47%), followed by gynecology (44%), surgical oncology (37%), colorectal (32%), pediatric surgery (29%), and trauma (25%). Age, operating service, enteric stoma type and configuration, and preoperative enterostomal therapist marking were found to be variables that influenced stoma complications. They concluded, preoperative enterostomal site marking, especially in older patients, and avoiding the ileostomy, particularly in the loop configuration, can help minimize complications.

With respect to stoma-related complications and type of stoma, Edwards (154) presented a contrary view. For patients requiring defunctioning following anterior resection and total mesorectal excision, they conducted a randomized study to receive either loop ileostomy or loop transverse colostomy. Follow-up after stoma closure was a median of 36 months. There were 70 patients randomized (loop transverse colostomy 36 and loop ileostomy 34) of whom 63 underwent stoma closure (loop transverse colostomy 31 and loop ileostomy 32). There were no significant differences in the difficulty of formation or closure or in the postoperative recovery between the groups. However, there were 10 complications related directly to the stoma in the loop transverse colostomy group: fecal fistula (1), prolapse (2), parastomal hernia (2), incisional hernia during follow-up (5). None of these complications occurred in the loop ileostomy group. They concluded, the choice of diversion is loop ileostomy as a method of defunctioning a low anastomosis.

Kairaluoma et al. (155) examined the outcome of 349 intestinal stomas constructed in 342 patients. In 141 of these patients, the stoma could be considered as temporary. The 30-day mortality rate was 7%. The overall complication rate was 50%. Pure stoma related complications were observed in 12% of the patients. The final closure rate of temporary stomas was 67%. The closure rate was significantly higher if the temporary stomas were of the double-barrel type. There was no significant difference in the closure rate between patients with benign and malignant diseases, but the rate decreased significantly in age groups over 70 years. They concluded, 40% of stomas constructed are considered as temporary but only two-thirds of temporary stomas are closed subsequently.

Duchesne et al. (156) analyzed 164 ostomy patients to document the frequency and types of ostomy complications and the risk factors associated with them. Complications occurred in 25% of patients; 39% occurred within one month of the procedure. Complications included prolapse in 22%, necrosis in 22%, stenosis in 17%, irritation in 17%, infection in 15%, bleeding in 5%, and retraction in 5%. Gender, carcinoma, trauma, diverticulitis, emergency operation, ileostomy and ostomy location/type were not associated with a stoma complication. Significant predictors of ostomy malfunction included inflammatory bowel disease (odds ratio = 4.49) and obesity (odds ratio = 2.66). The care of an enterostomal nurse was found to prevent complications (odds ratio = 0.15).

ENTEROSTOMAL CARE AND REHABILITATION

The history of enterostomal therapy has been documented by Cataldo (157). He notes that the earliest stomas were not the artistry of pioneering surgeons but were created by acts of nature (i.e., the end results of strangulated hernia or penetrating trauma). Patients were left to their own devices to determine how to care for this new intrusion in their life. This, of course, is no longer true, and stoma care is an integral part of the overall management of these patients.

Whether the stoma is permanent or temporary, patients with abdominal stomas have multiple adjustment demands. Physical alterations resulting from construction of the stoma require immediate and long-term attention and will have an impact on the patient's biopsychosocial status for the duration of the stoma.

Rehabilitation of the person with an abdominal stoma begins preoperatively with a multidisciplinary health care team (158,159). The medical physician, surgeon, ET nurse specialist, and, most important, the patient and family offer unique contributions to the positive outcome of a well-rehabilitated person. In addition, individualized patient needs may necessitate a referral to a social worker, dietitian, home care nurse, counselor, or a well-rehabilitated ostomy patient visitor. Of particular importance within the team is the collaboration between the surgeon and ET nurse specialist.

Research addressing the unique rehabilitation issues of this patient group both preoperatively and postoperatively highlights the need for family support and pertinent information based on their learning needs (160). The following is a discussion of ostomy patient needs and interventions in the preoperative, postoperative, and long-term phases of rehabilitation.

■ PREOPERATIVE CONSIDERATIONS

Expected outcomes in the preoperative period include (i) well-informed patient and family, (ii) properly selected and marked stoma site, and (iii) manageable level of anxiety. Outcomes may not always be achievable during this phase because of acute illness. However, the plan of preoperative care is generally developed with these outcomes in mind (159,161,162).

Assessment and Planning

Preoperative assessment and planning are essential for successful rehabilitation of the ostomy patient. Ideally, education beings in the clinic setting prior to hospital admission when the patient is better able to absorb information provided by the ET nurse. When this is not possible, education provided at the bedside the day prior to or on the day of operation must take into account the heightened level of stress experienced by the patient and significant others. Family members are encouraged to attend preoperative teaching sessions since they not only provide much needed emotional support, but do also validate and reinforce information the patient may not have assimilated. The participation of family members in all phases of patient teaching also allows the ET nurse to address the needs and concerns of significant others which may not always reflect those of the ostomy patient. In addition, a study performed by Persson (163) showed that spouses of patients undergoing ostomy surgery for rectal carcinoma felt that when they were excluded from information sessions, they felt isolated and experienced greater fear. This situation can become a vicious cycle where the patient and significant others cease to communicate in an effort to protect each other from further stress and worry. In emergency situations, it may not be possible for the ET nurse to mark the stoma site or provide education and counseling. The surgeon must, therefore, select an appropriate stoma site.

Patient assessment in the preoperative period includes emotional and physical factors that will affect the individual's ability to manage routine ostomy care as well as the ability to adjust and return to a previous lifestyle. Any physical limitations such as manual dexterity or diminished eyesight must be noted to prepare for future teaching sessions. When communicating with a patient who has difficulty hearing, care must be taken to share delicate information while maintaining confidentiality in a busy hospital ward or clinic setting. The patient's previous contact with an individual who had an ostomy should be discussed to dispel any fear or misconception resulting from the experience.

Preoperative assessment of the patient's learning style and education assists the ET nurse in preparing to teach in all three domains required to master the care of an ostomy: cognitive, affective and psychomotor (164). Some patients will prefer to read as much information as possible while others will depend solely on demonstrations provided by the ET nurse. Patients who are illiterate may be reluctant to divulge this fact; therefore the ET nurse must be sensitive to behavior which indicates any learning disability. A patient's profession or hobby can contribute to the ability to master some of the technical components of ostomy care. An example of this would be that of a seamstress who would have little difficulty measuring and cutting a stoma opening in a pouch. In order to accurately gauge learning needs, both verbal and nonverbal cues must be observed while interacting with a patient. In some instances patients may indicate a need to limit information, particularly when they are feeling overwhelmed. Of utmost importance is the need to individualize teaching. A patient's religious background may present as an issue if the presence of a stoma restricts certain aspects of religious practice. The patient's emotional status, coping mechanisms, social support, financial concerns, and relationship issues should also be included in the preoperative assessment.

Knowledge of common concerns for the ostomy patient in the short and long term provides guidance for the physician and ET nurse. Numerous papers have been published on psychosocial issues of ostomy patients. Jeter (165) stressed the importance of preoperative teaching and counseling to fully recover and enjoy a satisfactory quality of life for patients undergoing operations for colorectal carcinoma resulting in a stoma. Common misconceptions about ostomies should be dispelled. An effort should be made to allay patients' fears associated with colorectal carcinoma and ostomy operations. Fears cited by Jeter (165) include those of the primary disease, long-term prognosis after operation, fear of operation, postoperative pain, inability to manage the appliance, rejection by family, inability to retain employment, and sexuality, and concern for social adjustment. Jeter lists certain concepts and facts that are considered essential for patients and family members to learn before hospital discharge. The list includes how to change appliances, where to buy ostomy supplies, signs and symptoms of early postoperative complications, person(s) to whom complications or ostomy problems should be reported, and sources of financial aid if necessary. Additional types of information that can be considered "nice to know" but not essential include Ostomy Association meeting dates, foods that cause gas and odor, travel information, details about operation, ostomy accessory items, and potential long-term complications.

A study examined the concerns of patients before and after discharge from the hospital and found eight common areas. They include, in order of importance, fear of stool leakage, odor, ability to participate in sports, necessity for further treatment, wearing a pouch, changing the pouch, change in body appearance, and participating in sexual love play and intercourse (166). Information related to these topics is included throughout this chapter.

Interventions

Much research has been performed in the area of adaptation to life with a stoma. Piwonka (160) found that regardless of time since operation, factors that remained the most influential on psychological adaptation were ostomy self-care, body image, and perceived social support. The importance of teaching technical skills must therefore be balanced with the need to explore psychosocial concerns. Information provided in the preoperative period is essential to patient understanding, decreased anxiety, and informed consent. Topics included are anatomy and physiology, terminology, disease process, planned operation changes in function, complications, and expected results. Not surprisingly, it is equally important to discuss what is to be removed as well as what is not to be removed during the operation. A discussion of ostomy function, diet, pouches, and general ostomy management is also provided (158,167).

Emotional concerns are addressed when the clinician seeks the patient's view of the coming operation and how it will affect the person's lifestyle and quality of life. Discussion of work, play, sexuality, and other patient-introduced concerns are also important. Diagrams, written pamphlets, and videotapes are useful and may be obtained from manufacturers at no charge. Educational materials are available from organizations such as the American Cancer Society and United Ostomy Association (see pp. 1068–1069). However, nothing replaces personal contact with the surgeon and ET nurse. The therapeutic relationship is intensely important at this most vulnerable time. Experienced clinicians know that a few well chosen, honest words of hope can arrest a great deal of anxiety, particularly during the preoperative period.

Stoma site selection and construction have a direct bearing on the quality of life for the person with a stoma. Leakage, odor, difficulty with pouch changes, increased equipment costs, and stoma revisions occur as a result of poor stoma location (168,169). Patients who experience recurrent leakage from poorly sealed pouches may become reclusive and limit their social contact for fear of an embarrassing incident (170). Therefore the primary technical intervention during this period is stoma site marking. Turnbull and Weakley (171) first emphasized the importance of stoma site selection and marking during the preoperative period. Recommendations of the past are the standards of today as experts agree that stoma sites are to be marked preoperatively, usually by the ET nurse specialist, and often in conjunction with the surgeon (168,172).

Primary requirements for the ideal stoma site include placement within the rectus muscle with approximately 6 to 7 cm of flat skin around the site. This will provide an anatomically stable area. The rectus muscle is palpated while the patient is supine, lifting his or her head off the pillow. The intraperitoneal stoma should pass through the rectus muscle to minimize future prolapse or parastomal hernia. Extraperitoneal stomas may be placed just lateral to the rectus muscle to facilitate making the extraperitoneal tunnel, although medial placement through the rectus muscle is preferable. The abdomen is assessed while the patient is supine, sitting, standing, and bending forward (Fig. 30). If the patient wears a brace or is in a wheelchair, the abdomen is assessed with these devices in use. When possible, trousers or skirts should be worn to establish the location of the beltline as this not only affects flange placement of the appliance but also the manner in which the pouch will be accommodated by clothing.

Abdominal topography is also evaluated. The area of the peristomal plane should ideally be free of incisions, sutures, drains, rods, bony prominences, umbilicus scars, and waistline and skin folds as they form defects in the abdominal contours that may result in pouch leakage (Figs. 31 and 32). The natural elevation of the infraumbilical area enables the patient to visualize the stoma well, which is critical to self-care (173). Therefore the site is usually marked at the apex of the infraumbilical bulge. Exceptions to this evaluation occur in the obese patient, younger child, or patient with a barrel-shaped abdomen. It is generally important to mark these stomas in the upper quadrants so that the patient is able to see, and therefore care for, the stoma independently (168).

Other challenges in stoma site selection include patients with multiple surgical scars. An adolescent patient

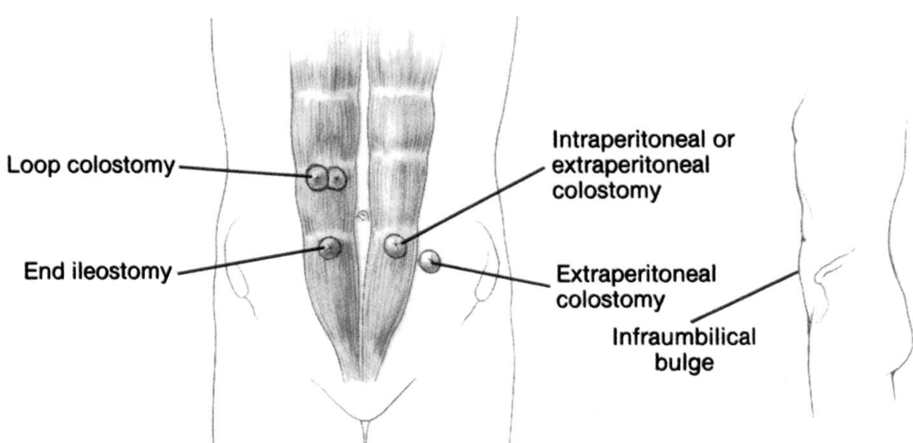

FIGURE 30 ■ Diagram of usual stoma sites for ileostomies and colostomies.

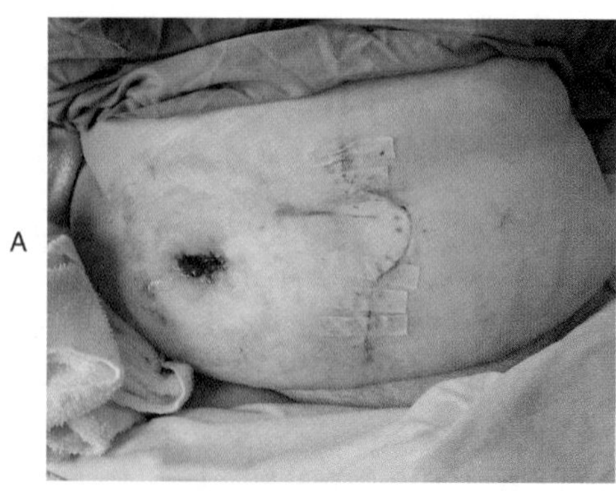
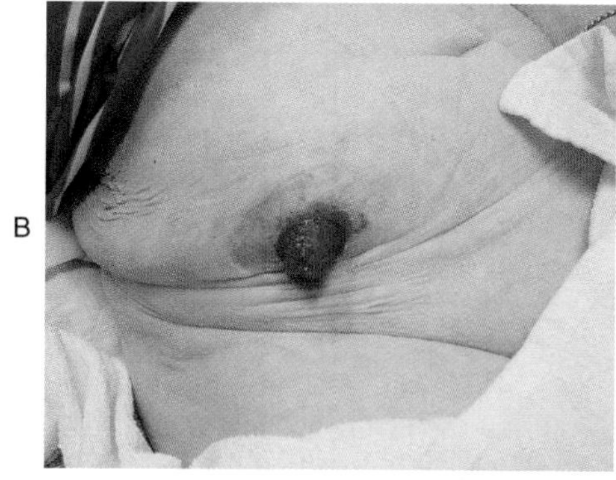
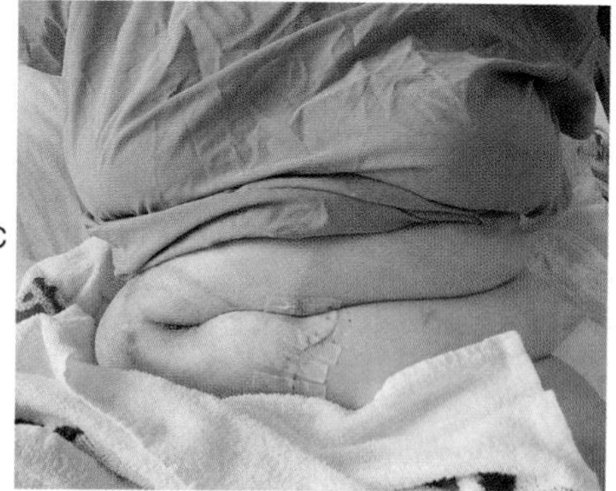

FIGURE 31 ■ (**A**) Poorly sited stoma in obese patient (supine). (**B**) Stoma difficult to visualize even with patient in semi Fowler's position (45°). (**C**) Stoma cannot be visualized when patient is seated upright (90°).

with Crohn's disease and multiple previous abdominal operations may have few good locations available (Fig. 33). When two stomas are planned, they should be located far enough apart so that each stoma may be pouched separately, if necessary. This holds true when one of the stomas is a mucous fistula since mucous discharge and odor may necessitate pouching (Fig. 34). For the patient undergoing pelvic exenteration, the colostomy should be placed lower than the urinary diversion to allow for clearance if an ostomy belt is used.

Site selection can be marked with a variety of methods but the most common and simplest would be to use indelible ink or silver nitrate. A waterproof clear film dressing can be used to protect the site if marking takes place well in advance of the operation.

■ POSTOPERATIVE ASPECTS OF CARE

Expected outcomes for the patient and family in the postoperative period include (i) mastery of basic ostomy care knowledge and skills, (ii) ability to express concerns and adaptive approaches toward resolution, and (iii) knowledge of resources needed for effective ostomy management in the home care and community settings (161,162).

Immediate Postoperative Care

Technical management of the patient postoperatively starts in the operating room with a properly fitted and applied pouching system. The pouch contains effluent, protects the peristomal skin and incision, and avoids soiling of monitoring leads and clothing in the area. Most pouching systems will maintain a seal for at least three to four days when used appropriately. Pouches applied early postoperatively are clear for later observation of mucosal vascularity. They are also drainable, which avoids frequent adhesive removal once the stoma begins to pass gas and stool. Presized systems are not recommended in the operating room since postoperative mucosal edema may occur that could result in stomal laceration and bleeding. Similarly, convex pouching systems are generally not used since the application of pressure to a newly sutured mucocutaneous suture line may result in separation (174). Rather, a sizable system is selected that will be cut to the size of the patient's stoma. Using this approach provides further benefits as inventory in the operating room is decreased and a standardized procedure reduces application errors.

Once the pouch has been selected, the stoma is measured. The correct size of the stoma is determined by using a measuring guide, and by selecting the size opening on the guide that will allow the pouch to cover peristomal

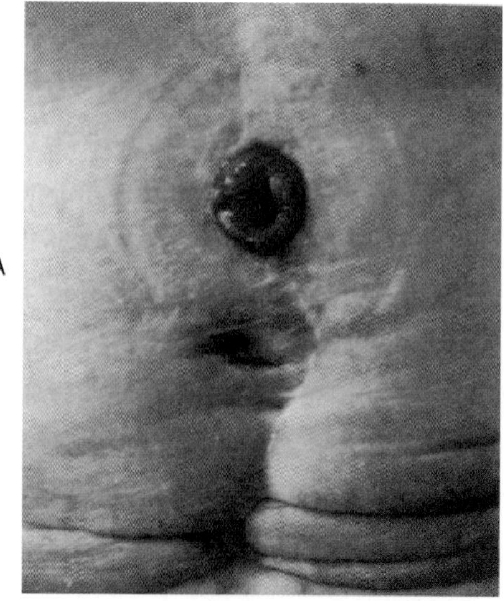
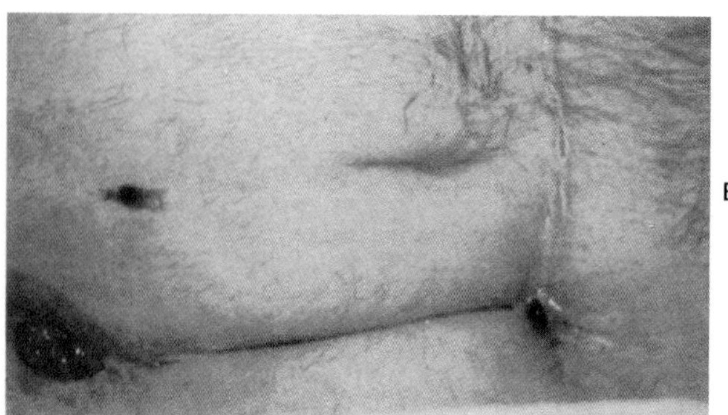

FIGURE 32 ■ Improperly placed stoma. (**A**) Improper placement of stoma above umpilicus and through midline incision will make it difficult to fit secure pouching system. (**B**) Unsuitable stoma because of placement that is too low, too lateral, and across transverse incision. Skin markings for suitable stoma sites on either right or left side are shown.

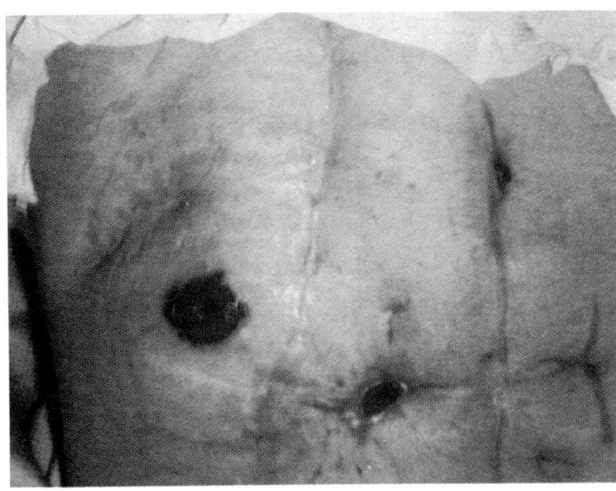

FIGURE 33 ■ Stoma placement must be individualized in patients with Crohn's disease and multiple previous scars and active fistula.

skin up to the mucocutaneous juncture (Fig. 35). The skin surrounding the stoma is cleansed with tap water or an appropriate commercial solution; then, allowed to completely dry prior to pouch application. For pouch application procedure, see specific procedures on pp. 1066–1067.

Rods and bridges used in stomal construction are obstacles to effective pouch adherence and delay routine patient teaching. They may also put tension on the stoma during pouching. When the rod is placed in a cephalad-to-caudad position or on the plane with the umbilicus, the patient may experience discomfort and limited mobility. Therefore a fascial bridge is recommended for loop stomas. However, if a rod or bridge is used, there are two options during pouch application. The device may be placed into the pouch, or the pouch may be applied over the device. The potential for leakage is less when the rod or bridge is placed into the pouch. During application of the pouch, the rod is guided into the aperture of the pouch first. Then the pouch is secured around the stoma, and the rod is adjusted to its original position. A label or notation is made directly on the front of the pouch as an indication to future caregivers that a supporting device is inside the pouch. The date for rod removal and the name of the person doing it must be established as part of the patient ostomy careplan to avoid unnecessary delay in teaching and promote patient comfort.

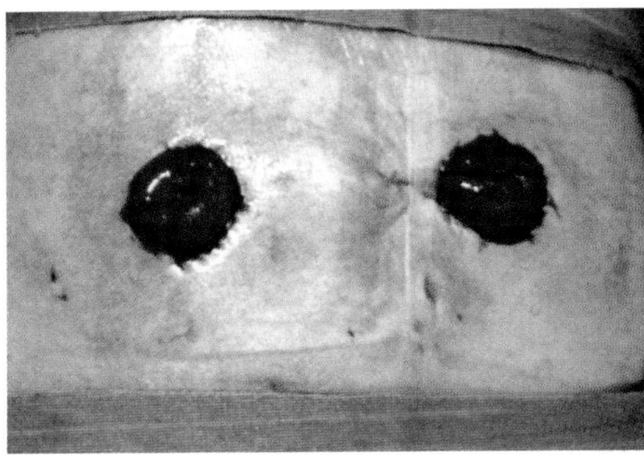

FIGURE 34 ■ Dual stomas in patients having colostomy and mucous fistula.

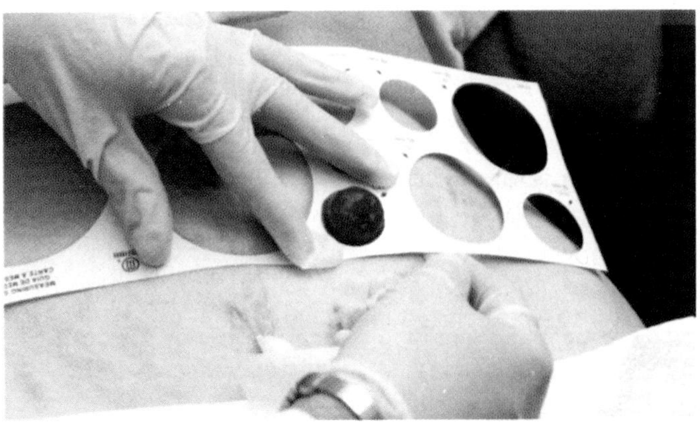

FIGURE 35 ■ Technique of measuring stoma (stoma-measuring guide).

Information and Emotional Support

Currently, the average hospital postoperative stay for patients undergoing abdominoperineal resection and sigmoid colostomy, total proctocolectomy and ileostomy, or restorative ileoanal reservoir is from 7 to 10 days. During this period, the patient experiences multiple educational and adjustment issues that will be ongoing in the posthospital period. However, basic skills to master in self-care are pouch emptying, pouch changing, skin care, and care of the incision. One technique used to begin teaching postoperatively is a "tour" of the abdomen. The ET nurse and patient embark on this "tour" by examining the stoma and peristomal skin. A discussion of normal values is initially undertaken. The color of the stoma and quality of the skin are discussed and, later, documented. The integrity of the mucocutaneous juncture and abdominal incision are assessed and documented. As the patient recovers, specific areas are included in postoperative teaching and support. A few are discussed here. However, Table 1 provides a comprehensive listing of topics to be included. Prioritizing patient needs is important, since hospital stays have

TABLE 1 ■ **Postoperative Components of the Rehabilitation Care Plan for Ostomates**

Technical Skills	Information	Emotion
Pouch emptying Pouch changing	Normal anatomy Function and appearance of the stoma	Individualized care Family inclusion
Peristomal skin cleansing	Diet	Time to discuss concerns
Stoma measurement	Odor and gas control	Role modeling support (i.e., caregivers and ostomy group members)
Ongoing stoma and peristomal skin assessment	Fluid and electrolyte needs Recognition of departures from normal Community resources (e.g., ostomy groups and suppliers)	Discussion of sexuality and return to previous lifestyle

become brief. Essential information, such as pouch emptying and changing, is completed prior to discharge.

Emotional care of the patient that promotes adaptation is important to be included in the care plan. One dimension of the ET nurse's role is supportive counseling. The patient is encouraged to explore the ostomy experience in discussion sessions with the ET nurse. The patient is allowed to identify concerns and to begin to resolve them. Focus is also on the concerns and fears of the family. By exploring these feelings and meanings for the patient, problems become more manageable, and the patient moves toward adaptation (159).

Unique Aspects of Care

Ileostomies may be temporary or permanent. Temporary ileostomies have been more frequently performed as a component of the restorative ileoanal reservoir. Issues unique to the patient with ileostomy include maintenance of peristomal skin integrity, fluid and electrolyte balance, prevention of small bowel obstruction, and psychosocial issues inherent to younger populations (i.e., childbearing, raising children, and professional and work situations). The expected function of a conventional ileostomy is 800 to 1000 mL per 24 hours or pouch emptying six to eight times in 24 hours. A drainable pouch is used and changed once every four to seven days (Table 2).

Transverse colostomies are generally intended to be temporary or palliative. They function similarly to ileostomies but with less fluid output. Stools may be malodorous. The pouch may be emptied four to six times in 24 hours. The change interval is also four to seven days.

Many of the operative procedures resulting in a transverse colostomy are performed on an emergency basis and present pouching challenges since these stomas are often exteriorized at the waistline or proximal to the ribcage. Changes in abdominal contour or contact with a rigid ribcage can cause stressors to the pouching system which will limit adhesion and cause subsequent leakage and skin irritation. The surgeon should consider these factors and construct a stoma in a lower quadrant whenever possible.

Descending and sigmoid colostomies are usually permanent and most frequently performed in older individuals. Concomitant health problems, such as arthritis, diabetes, or impaired vision, may provide additional challenges during rehabilitation. Descending and sigmoid colostomies begin to function three to seven days postoperatively. Therefore teaching in the hospital is shortened as the patient will have little experience with pouch emptying. Stools are not corrosive to the peristomal skin, yet protection is recommended to keep the skin clean and dry. Stool may be malodorous and a deodorizer required. As normal bowel function returns, there may be one to three stools a day. The question of whether to irrigate or use the natural method of colostomy control is usually discussed briefly preoperatively as management options. However, current thinking defers this decision to the outpatient clinic. Once the patient recovers from the operation and is able to provide self-care, discussion regarding colostomy irrigation is undertaken.

TABLE 2 ■ Stoma Management Quick Reference Guide

Type of Stoma	Output Characteristics	Management Approach
Ileostomy	Liquid to paste Active enzymes	Drainable pouch with skin barrier Change pouching system every 4 to 7 days Deodorizers: oral or pouch (powder, liquid, and tablet)
Transverse colostomy	Liquid to semiformed Low active enzymes	Drainable pouch with skin barrier Change pouching system every 4 to 7 days Deodorizers: oral or pouch (powder and liquid) No routine colostomy irrigations
Descending or sigmoid colostomy	Semiformed Minimal active enzymes	Natural method of control Drainable pouch with skin barrier Change pouching system every 4 to 7 days Deodorizer: oral or pouch (liquid) Colostomy irrigation method Irrigate every 1 to 2 days Closed or drainable pouch Skin barrier optional Stoma plug optional Diet to promote constipation

Peristomal Skin Care

Gold standard in peristomal skin care is that less is more. The goal is to prevent irritation and loss of skin integrity thus avoiding pain, infection and further pouching complications. The use of tap water, soft material, and gentle skin cleansing are recommended. The addition of soap is optional, but if used should be mild and free of perfumes, oil, and dye. Patients may need to be reminded that peristomal skin care is not a sterile procedure and therefore showering is an acceptable method of cleaning the skin. Careful hair removal of skin beneath the appliance is recommended to prevent folliculitis and will improve patient comfort with pouch removal. Coarse body hair can be clipped. The parastomal skin can be shaved with a safety razor using soap or with the use of a barrier powder on clean dry skin. Mechanical trauma is best avoided with careful removal of all the adhesive components of the appliance. Patients must be taught to gently pull the appliance away with one hand while the other hand anchors the adjacent skin. Reducing contact with chemicals will decrease the possibility of a local reaction and subsequent sensitization.

Diet, Gas, and Noise

Diet is a key to many postoperative concerns. Odor, gas, noise, diarrhea, bowel obstruction, and social activities may all be affected by fluid and food choices. Postoperatively, increased levels of gas and noise are expected as the surgical ileus resolves. However, complaints of excessive gas in the posthospital phase require assessment. They are frequently the result of eating habits and food choices (Box 1). Dietary restrictions are recommended in the literature, but few studies have been performed to substantiate these restrictions. Due to postoperative edema of the intestinal tract, patients with ileostomies are often

BOX 1 ■ Foods Affecting Bowel Function

Foods That Increase Odor	Foods That Increase Gas	Foods That May Help Control Odor or Gas	Foods That Thicken Stool (Decrease Output)	Foods That Loosen Stool (Increase Output)	High-Fiber Foods That May Cause Blockages
Asparagus	Beans	Fresh parsley	Applesauce	Green beans	Dried fruit
Broccoli	Beer/carbonated soda	Yogurt	Bananas	Beer, alcohol	Grapefruits, Apples
Brussels sprouts	Alcohol	Buttermilk	Cheese	Broccoli	Nuts
Cabbage	Broccoli		Boiled milk	Fresh fruits	Corn
Cauliflower	Brussels sprouts		Marshmallows	Grape juice	Raisins
Dried peas, beans and lentils	Cabbage		Pasta	Raw vegetables	Celery
Eggs	Cauliflower		Creamy peanut butter	Prunes/juice	Popcorn
Fish	Corn		Pretzels	Spicy foods	Coconut
Garlic, onions	Cucumbers		Rice	Fried foods	Seeds
Some spices	Pickles, sauerkraut		Bread	Chocolate	Coleslaw
Turnip	Mushrooms		Tapioca	Spinach	Oriental vegetables
Some strong chesses (e.g., Roquefort)	Dried peas, lentils		Toast	Leafy green vegetables	Meats with casings
Some medications	Radishes		Yogurt	Aspartame/ Nutrasweet®	Oranges
Some vitamin Preparations	Spinach		Bagels	Licorice	Mushrooms
	Dairy products		Soda crackers	Coffee	
	Onions		Potatoes	High-sugar foods	
	Turnips		Barley	Caffeinated beverages	
	Eggs		Oatmeal or oat bran		
	Melons				
	Peppers				
	Onions, chives				
	Chewing gum				

Source: From Ref. 166, 169.

advised to limit fiber intake for six to eight weeks following operation (175).

All ostomy patients are instructed to chew food very well, eat at regular intervals, drink eight 8-oz glasses (2 L) of fluid per day and to gradually return to a regular diet. The fact that most ostomates can return to a regular diet is supported by a survey of members of the United Ostomy Association which was performed to identify the dietary restrictions of patients with ileostomies (13%) colostomies (83%) and urostomies (4%). The findings indicated that 88% of respondents had resumed a regular diet following their ostomy surgery (175).

Small Bowel Obstruction

Small bowel obstruction is a complication of abdominal operations. In stoma patients, food bolus and adhesions are a frequent cause. Patients are instructed to recognize early the signs of obstruction (i.e., pain, decreased stomal output, stoma swelling, nausea, and vomiting). If obstruction occurs, a liquid diet is recommended with relaxation techniques (i.e., a warm bath). The pouch should be removed, if necessary, and the aperture cut larger to avoid laceration. The patient's physician should be contacted when the patient experiences prolonged obstruction, vomiting, or when pain is severe. An ileostomy lavage may be necessary (see the special procedure on pp. 1066–1067). Most commonly, the obstruction resolves with conservative management. Interestingly, the patient is usually able to identify the offending food. Patients are instructed to chew foods thoroughly and increase fluid intake when eating or eliminate offending foods from the diet (176).

Fluid and Electrolytes

Fluid and electrolyte balance is particularly important to patients with ileostomy or high-output transverse colostomy. Education includes information about dehydration as well as fluid and electrolyte balance. As previously stated, patients are encouraged to drink eight 8-oz glasses of fluids in a 24-hour period. If sodium depletion is in question, soups, bouillon, and Gatorade may be taken. Sources of potassium include orange juice, bananas, strong tea, and Gatorade.

Odor

Most pouching systems are odor proof. Therefore the only time a patient should experience odor is when the pouch is emptied. If this is offensive, pouch deodorizers, oral odor control tablets, or room deodorizers may be used. A liquid or powder deodorizer may be squirted into the bottom of the pouch following each emptying procedure. Oral deodorizers may also be effective, but should be manufactured specifically for the intended use. Room sprays are not always handy or effective, but are frequently used. If odor is detected under other circumstances, it is usually observed to be caused by leakage or an emptying spout that has not been properly cleaned. When a pouch leaks, it should be changed rather than taped for future attention. Pouch spouts may be kept clean by cuffing the spout back during emptying. Otherwise, spouts are cleaned with tissue and water after each emptying. Some patients attempt to manage odor by rinsing the pouch. However, rinsing with water is awkward and may result in decreased wear time.

Activities

Following abdominal operations, lifting restrictions serve to allow for healing and in avoiding abdominal hernia. Generally, heavy lifting (> 10 lbs) should be avoided during the first four to six weeks postoperatively. It is useful to give examples of lifting activities to be avoided (i.e., wet laundry, shoveling snow, lifting the garage door, carrying groceries). Following this period, however, patients may gradually return to previous physical activities involving lifting or heavy pushing and pulling. Sports, workouts, and other strenuous activities are generally permitted at that point.

There are no restrictions on sexuality following operation except that sexual intercourse is to be avoided until the patient has recovered. Abdominal tenderness, incision discomfort, and perineal pain may curtail sexual intercourse for a few weeks or more following discharge from the hospital.

Discharge Instructions

Most patients experience a degree of anxiety caring for their stomas without nursing assistance for the first time. Referral to a home care agency for short-term support is suggested to ease the transition from the hospital setting to the community. A referral to social services is initiated when planning for an interim or long-term care facility or to respond to questions regarding insurance coverage. Follow-up appointments with the physicians and ET nurse are also made. The ET nurse usually sees the patient in the clinic within two weeks of discharge. Depending on the institution, ostomy supplies may be provided or patients purchase supplies in amounts required for a short period, as adjustments will most likely be made at clinic appointments. The ostomy patient should be sent home with written instructions, a recent stoma pattern, a list of local suppliers, product codes, and reading material pertinent to their operative procedure.

Exercise and social contacts are important to physical and psychological recovery. Patients are encouraged to walk, see friends, and get out of the house as tolerated.

■ POSTHOSPITALIZATION MANAGEMENT

Expected outcomes in the long term include (i) prevention of complications, (ii) resumption of previous or desired lifestyle, and (iii) psychological adaptation to life with a stoma.

Generally, patients who avoid major complications with the stoma, peristomal skin, or pouching system are able to view the stoma as manageable sooner and move to resume previous lifestyles and psychological adaptation more easily. Therefore prevention and planning pre- and postoperatively are the keys to the outcomes seen during the posthospitalization phase. Lack of a properly constructed and sited stoma or effective enterostomal care results in complications, delayed patient adaptation, and additional expense (i.e., equipment, outpatient visits, or revision of the stoma) (168,174).

Technical and Educational Aspects

The recovering patient may be independent in care or require assistance with the stoma from a spouse or friend. In a long-term care facility, the nursing staff may be the caregivers. Whatever the circumstances, there is an ongoing need for refitting the pouching system as the stoma shrinks, abdominal contours change, and questions regarding peristomal skin care or treatment occur. This is also a particularly important time to educate the patient, as this is the time when the patient and the family express their questions and concerns are expressed by the patient and family.

Basic information should be reviewed. However, the goals of complication prevention and independence are primary in this period. Initially, patients in the hospital were taught to empty and change the pouching system. As the patient recovers and learning is increased, the standard for success is raised. When a problem occurs, patients are soon able to recognize and participate in technical problem solving. If pouch leakage occurs, the patient should assess the back of the appliance to determine where erosion took place. This can help establish what changes need to be made to the system to improve the seal. Leakage can take place if the pouch is not fitted properly or does not conform to the shape of the parastomal skin. The patient should also know that weight gain affects the peristomal plane and the abdominal contours, that also requires a refitting (174). Peristomal skin condition should be routinely checked by the patient at each pouch change. If a small area of erythema or denudation develops, the patient can independently intervene with an absorptive hydrocolloid powder. Under humid conditions, if an itchy, erythematous rash with satellite lesions develops, the patient should consider a candidiasis etiology and initiate use of an antifungal agent (177).

Colostomy Irrigation

Advanced knowledge for the patient with a descending or sigmoid colostomy includes discussion of management options: the natural method or colostomy irrigation. As the patient begins to resume his or her previous lifestyle, schedules, activities, sports, or other preferences may dictate how the stoma is managed. In the past, most patients were taught to irrigate as the acceptable means of management. However, today the pros and cons of irrigation are discussed, and the patient makes the final decision.

The natural method of colostomy control allows the colostomy to function normally with a pouching system in use. There is a wide variety of pouches available to patients with colostomies such as one or two piece systems as well as a drainable or closed pouch (with or without charcoal filter). The pouch may need to be emptied one to three times in a 24-hour period. The appliance is changed every five to seven days. Special instructions on diet are provided to avoid constipation. Many patients decide to continue with this method because it is simple and less time consuming. Although much has been written about the option of colostomy irrigation to "control" the bowel function, a technique that will permit many patients to be free of evacuations at unwanted times, we have observed that given the choice, most patients opt for the natural evacuation format. The availability of a variety of appliances permits patients to successfully manage their colostomy.

Alternatively, colostomy irrigation may be selected. The purpose of routine irrigation of a colostomy is to regulate the bowel and avoid stool discharges between irrigations. The procedure is intended as a convenience for patients. Those who have a high level of success are independent patients with previously predictable bowel function, good prognosis, absence of severe physical or mental limitations, good dietary habits, and absence of medications or current treatment that may result in loose stools. Contraindications for routine irrigation include diarrhea regardless of etiology, radiation enteritis, parastomal hernia, or the need for fluid restrictions due to renal failure. Precautions should be taken when there is a history of diverticulitis, angina, myocardial infarct, or spastic bowel (178). Patients considering routine irrigation are educated regarding the procedure, time requirements, and expected results. (See colostomy irrigation procedure on p. 1066.)

Since there is a possibility of stool leakage between irrigations, patients are instructed to use a pouching system. Discussion with the ostomate who chooses to irrigate include the need to consider long-term issues such as expected changes with aging that could interfere with the ability to irrigate independently. Individuals who select irrigation as a form of colostomy management must ensure that the medical nursing staff is advised of the need for continued irrigations in the event of hospitalization, or admission to a long-term care facility (179).

Jao et al. (180) retrospectively reviewed colostomy irrigation as a management option in 223 patients who had undergone abdominoperineal resection at the Mayo Clinic. Of that group, 134 (60%) of the patients irrigated and had good continence with only minor leakage of stool between irrigations. Of those who irrigated, 48 (22%) had regular stool leakage between irrigations and 41 (18%) patients discontinued irrigation for a number of reasons. Dini et al. (181) assessed 509 patients having a colostomy for rectal carcinoma as potential candidates for irrigation. Fifty-two patients were considered unsuitable and 40 refused to learn the technique. The remaining 417 patients (82%) adopted the irrigation method. Of these, 97% achieved full continence for periods of 24 to 48 hours. There was no case of colonic perforation; 31.6% had been irrigating from one to five years and 10.3% for more than five years. There was a reduction of more than 50% per 24-hour period in the number of appliances used by patients. The authors concluded that irrigation is a simple, safe, and cost-effective means of managing a colostomy and that with careful selection of patients, irrigation should be recommended as a routine part of rehabilitation. Sanada et al. (182) studied 214 ostomates to assess daily activities and psychosocial differences between patients who adopted natural evacuation compared to those who irrigated their colostomy. The authors found that colostomy irrigation imposes less distress on the patient, causes fewer skin problems, and is less of a financial burden. In daily activities, irrigation causes fewer difficulties compared to natural evacuation in the areas of bathing and sleeping. Furthermore, the authors found that the frequency of going outdoors remained the same as in preoperative days and that the patients were able to adjust to daily activities postoperatively. From a psychosocial standpoint, irrigation patients had a higher degree of self-esteem and had fewer anxieties and fewer worries than those using natural evacuation. The instruction of evacuation control, management of gas odor, and a great deal of psychosocial support must be given to natural evacuation patients (Fig. 36).

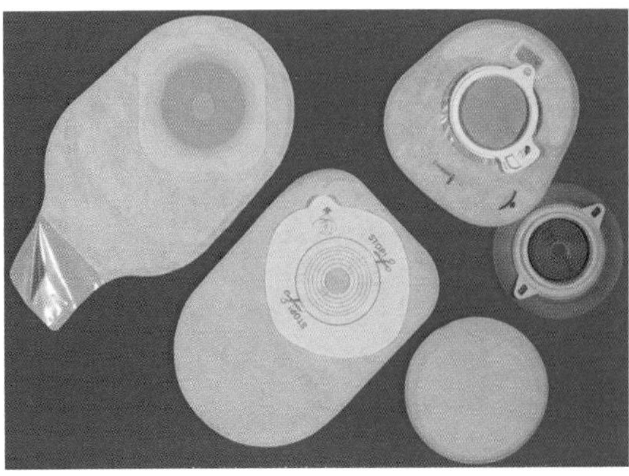

FIGURE 36 ■ Colostomy pouching options for patients using irrigation methods.

Surveillance

Over the long term, research has supported the need for outpatient follow-up. Follick et al. (183) reported that of 131 ostomy patients belonging to an ostomy support group, 84% reported problems in at least one aspect of ostomy management. Fifty-three percent experienced peristomal skin irritation, 38% identified leakage, 37% reported pouching problems, 37% experienced odor, and 34% complained of noise. In a survey from the Cleveland Clinic, ileostomy patients were surveyed to identify problems encountered. Forty-nine percent identified peristomal skin irritation, 42% stated noise and odor, and 29% had difficulty managing the pouching system (184). Based on this level of technical morbidity, outpatient services are required to intervene with proper treatment and attempt to prevent complications through routine preventive education and follow-up.

ET nurse specialists generally have routine surveillance programs. The intervals for follow-up may be within two weeks of discharge from the hospital, one month later, six weeks following that appointment, three months, six months, and annually. The condition of the stoma and peristomal skin is assessed as well as self-care techniques, activity levels, and intimacy concerns.

Follow-up education and reinforcement regarding dehydration and electrolyte replacement are also provided. This is particularly important in warm weather or during strenuous physical activities.

Ostomy equipment is expensive. In the United States, Medicare currently reimburses 80% of *medically necessary* equipment. However, "medically necessary" does not include all equipment available. Examples of currently reimbursable items under Medicare are cleansers, preparations, pouch covers, and additional closure clamps. Further, there is a guideline for the appropriate utilization of equipment. Organizations such as the United Ostomy Association and the Wound Ostomy Continence Nurse Society have lobbied to change some of the funding obstacles presented by Medicare (185). The maximum number of supplies allocated has been increased in some instances. For example, utilization of the number of drainable pouches which was initially limited to 10 per month, has been increased to 20. If there is a need for a greater number of supplies than allowed by Medicare, the patient's physician can provide a letter indicating the medical necessity for these additional items (186). In Canada, funding for ostomy supplies is a provincial mandate. There

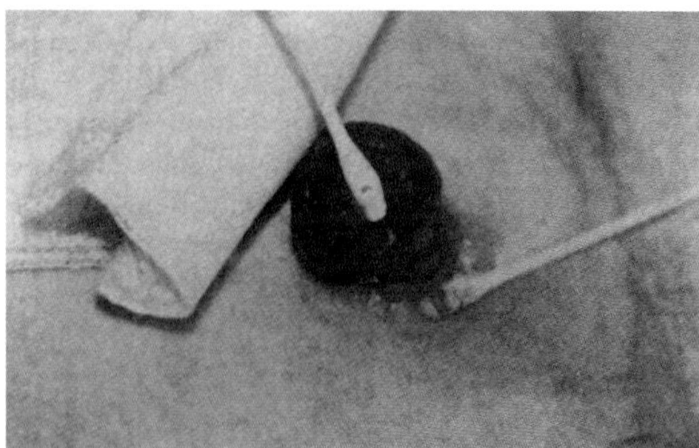

FIGURE 37 ■ Stoma laceration caused by pouching system.

are variations between provinces ranging from programs allocating 75% coverage to no provincial coverage whatsoever (187). The details required to determine whether private insurance will offer coverage is most frequently found under the prosthetic device or durable medical equipment portion of the policy.

■ LOCAL STOMA AND PERISTOMAL SKIN PROBLEMS

STOMA LACERATION ■ Stoma laceration can be caused by a pouching system that fits too closely, slides against the stoma or from an improperly fitted belt (Fig. 37). Patients with visual impairment can cause stoma trauma with improper application of the appliance. The most common site for laceration is inferolaterally. Correcting the stoma size opening and possibly discontinuing the use of a belt should alleviate further problems. When visual acuity is an issue, home health aid may be required to assist the patient with appliance change and prevent further trauma. Use of a hydrocolloid powder on lacerations will assist with healing.

CONTACT DERMATITIS ■ Contact dermatitis occurs in stoma patients as a response of the skin to contact with external agents. The etiology may be either an irritant or an allergic reaction (188). Irritant contact dermatitis—the most common type—is caused by mechanical injury to the skin from pouch removal, contact of the skin with stomal effluent, or irritation from solvents, cements, or other products acting alone or in combination (Fig. 38). Treatment of irritant contact dermatitis should include removal of the irritant chemicals, pouch refitting, and often patient education. Peristomal skin medications are usually not necessary, since the problem should resolve when the underlying cause has been removed. If the skin is erythematous and moist, applying the Stanley procedure will help to absorb moisture and provide an intact surface for adhesion of the appliance. This involves the application of three layers of a skin-barrier powder/and alcohol-free skin prep onto any denuded peristomal skin. Each layer is allowed to completely dry between applications.

Allergic contact dermatitis is an allergic reaction to a specific stomal product (Fig. 39). Because allergic contact dermatitis is relatively rare, it is important to search for an irritant cause first. If the condition is considered to be allergic, then patch testing should be performed to identify the causative agent and to confirm that the reaction is

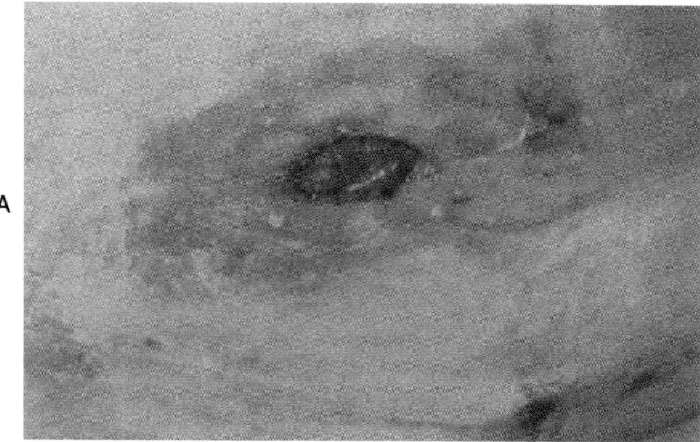

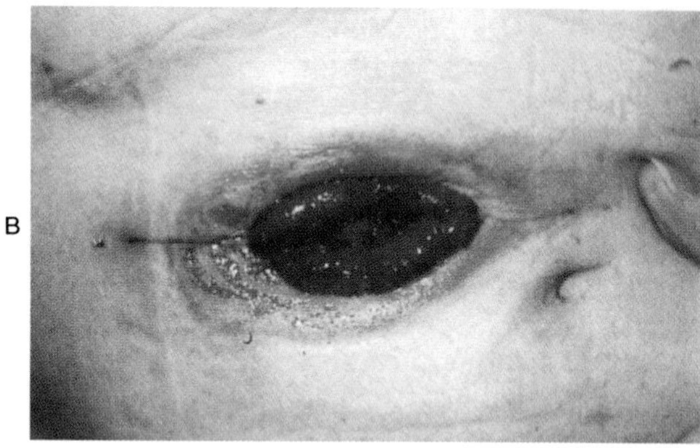

FIGURE 38 ■ Contact dermatitis. (**A**) Mechanical contact dermatitis caused by improper removal of pouching system. (**B**) Chemical contact dermatitis caused by irritation from fecal effluent.

allergic. It is important not to attribute what might be a simple irritant contact dermatitis to an allergic reaction, since this restricts the patient's ability to use the adhesive material that has been implicated in the allergic reaction, even though the material may otherwise have been useful for the patient.

YEAST INFECTION ■ Monilial yeast infections are frequent and commonly occur in the peristomal skin surrounding all types of stomas (Fig. 40). Although *Candida* infections tend to occur in the debilitated host, most peristomal monilial infections are due to local conditions such as pouch system leakage with proliferation of yeast under the pouch

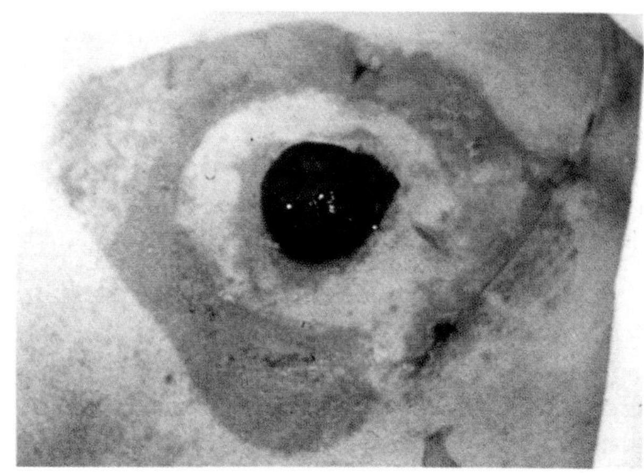

FIGURE 39 ■ Allergic contact dermatitis caused by reaction to pouch adhesive.

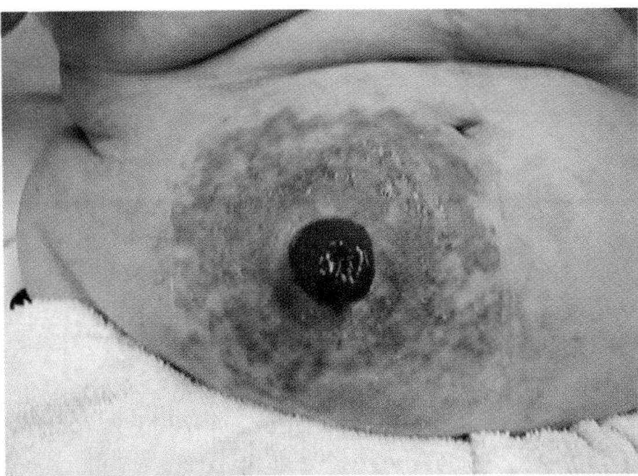

FIGURE 40 ■ Candidiases around ileostomy.

adhesive. Monilial yeast infection is characterized by bright red primary and satellite papular lesions. Usually the patient complains of itching and burning around the irritated skin. The condition is managed by applying nystatin powder (e.g., Mycostatin) at the time of routine pouch changing until the infection has resolved.

Pseudoepithelial Hyperplasia

Pseudoepithelial hyperplasia (PEH) presents as a wart-like thickening of epithelium that has been repeatedly exposed to highly liquid or corrosive effluent (Fig. 41). The affected area can be painful and bleed easily depending on the severity of PEH. The definitive treatment is to choose a pouching system that will protect the parastomal skin from contact with the offending effluent. Silver nitrate sticks or electrocautery can be used to control bleeding (189). More frequent appliance changes may be required initially to protect the affected area and provide comfort (189). In a suspicious situation biopsy may be appropriate to rule out carcinoma.

Psoriasis

Psoriasis may present on the peristomal skin as sharply demarcated, erythematous, weeping, papular lesions, or plaques with scales (Fig. 42). Treatment includes the use of a solid-form skin barrier such as a Hollister psoriasis dressing. Occasionally adjunctive treatment with corticosteroids may be indicated.

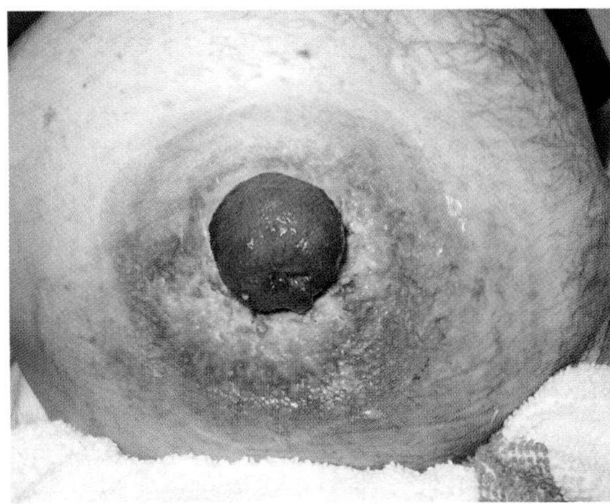

FIGURE 41 ■ Hyperplasia caused by chronic exposure of skin to effluent.

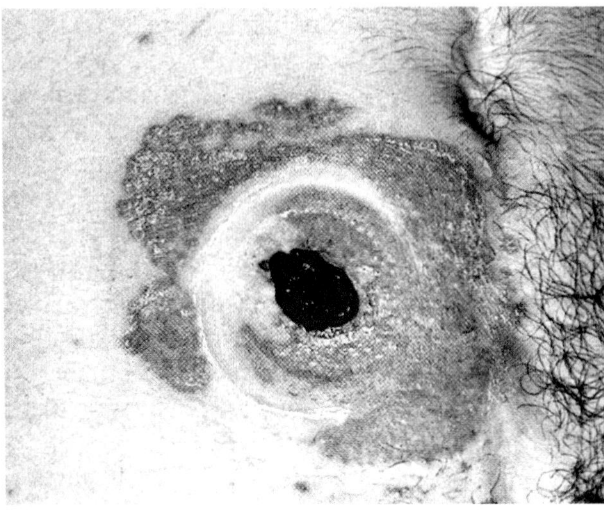

FIGURE 42 ■ Psoriasis surrounding umbilicus and peristomal skin.

PYODERMA GANGRENOSUM ■ Pyoderma gangrenosum may be associated with Crohn's disease, chronic ulcerative colitis, or a malignancy (Fig. 43). It was first described by Brunsting in 1930 and occurs in approximately 2% of patients whose Crohn's disease or ulcerative colitis results in the creation of a stoma (186,187,189,190). It presents clinically as an irregular ulcerated gangrenous area with ragged

A

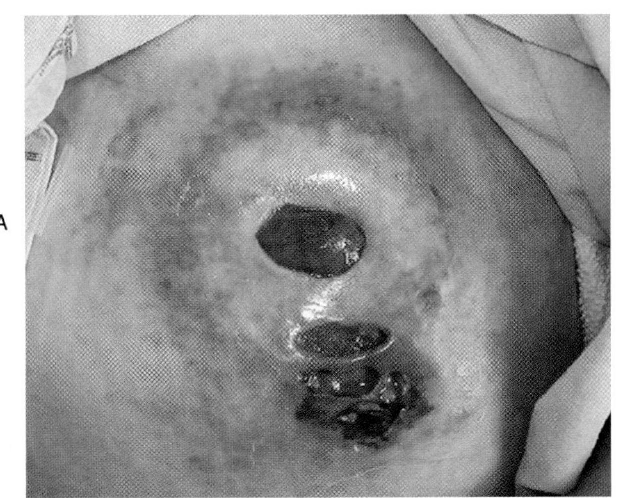

B

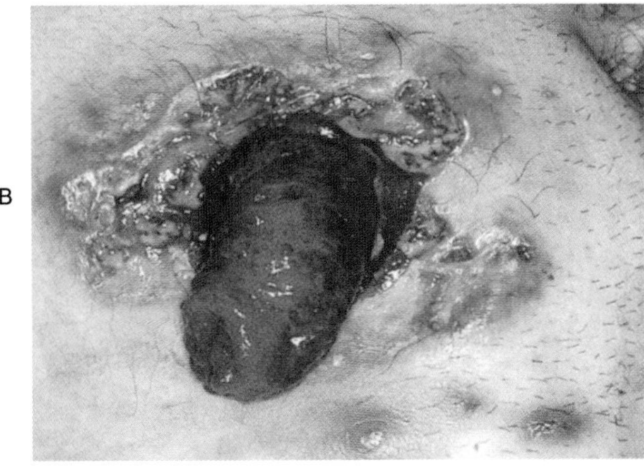

FIGURE 43 ■ (**A**) Pyoderma gangrenosum around sigmoid colostomy in patient with Crohn's disease. (**B**) Pyoderma gangrenosum around ileostomy in patient with Crohn's disease.

purple edges. Initially the skin may appear ecchymotic, and the patient complains of pain. Later the lesions undergo tunneling, resulting in increasingly large necrotic ulcers surrounded by a violaceous area. The treatment consists of administering a combination of corticosteroids (topical, systemic, and intralesional) and antibiotics. Topical management includes providing an adequate appliance seal, controlling wound pain and infection while applying principles of moist wound healing. In some cases the use of sodium cromoglycate spray in combination with betamethasone dipropionate ointment has been effective and does not interfere with the pouch seal. In accordance with wound care principles proper cleaning and an antimicrobial absorbent silver dressing (e.g., Aquacel Ag or Acticoat) can decrease the bacterial burden and promote healing (191). Further exudate control can be achieved by covering the primary dressing with a hydrocolloid such as Duoderm (Convatec) or Comfeel (Comfeel) prior to the application of the pouch. Intralesional injection of steroids (e.g., triamicinolone acetonide solution, 10 mg/mL administered at 2-week intervals on two or three occasions) may prove ideal because it is administered intermittently when the ostomy appliance is changed and it does not interfere with the adhesion of the divide.

Kiran et al. (192) reported on the outcome of peristomal pyoderma gangerenosum. Diagnosis was predominantly clinically based on a classic presentation of painful, undermined, peristomal ulceration. The underlying diagnosis was Crohn's disease in 11 patients, ulcerative colitis in 3 patients, indeterminate colitis in 1 patient, and posterior urethral valves in 1 patient. At the time of development of peristomal pyoderma gangrenosum the underlying disease was active in 69% of patients. Stoma care, ulcer debridement with unroofing of undermined edges, and intralesional corticosteroid injection was associated with 40% complete response rate and a further 40% partial response rate. Of five patients who received infliximab, four responded to therapy. Complete response after all forms of therapy, including stoma relocation in seven patients was 87%. They concluded local wound management and ET are extremely important for patients with peristomal pyoderma gangrenosum. Relocation of this stoma is reserved for persistent ulceration failing other therapies because peristomal pyoderma gangerenosum may occur at the new stoma site.

RECURRENT PERISTOMAL CARCINOMA ■ Recurrence of carcinoma in the peristomal field or on the stoma itself poses a serious management problem because pouch leakage odor and discomfort may be difficult to control (Fig. 44A). Frequent pouch refittings are often needed. Ideally, a recurrent malignancy should be managed by resection and relocation of the stoma, but this is not always feasible because recurrent stomal carcinoma is often a sign of widespread end-stage malignant metastatic disease.

Adenocarcinoma arising at the ileostomy stomacutaneous junction is exceedingly rare. The coexistence of ileal carcinoma and chronic ulcerative colitis is distinctly uncommon, and the development of ileal carcinoma in a patient following resection for chronic ulcerative colitis is exceptionally rare. Review of the literature until 1993 repealed only 12 such cases (194). Primary adenocarcinoma of a Brooke ileostomy has been reported in four cases of patients undergoing total proctocolectomy and ileostomy for familial adenomatous polyposis (194). A more recent review of the subject reported another case and noted there were now 35 other such cases (195). The most common presenting signs and symptoms include bleeding, ulceration, and the presence of a friable mass at the ileostomy (Fig. 44B). In addition, pain, intermittent ileostomy obstruction, stenosis, and retraction have been observed. These manifestations may occur decades following the initial operation for chronic ulcerative colitis (193).

Review of the literature until 2003 reveals one article that addresses the occurrence of metachronous adenocarcinoma occurring at a colostomy site. The authors found only seven other cases reported to the surgical association in Japan between 1983 and 1997 (196).

One cannot rely on biopsy of suspicious lesions, since in half the reported cases biopsies revealed only inflammation. Subsequent resections performed for ileostomy revision in these patients revealed adenocarcinoma in the resected specimens. It is therefore recommended that the presence of atypia within a biopsy specimen necessitates

A

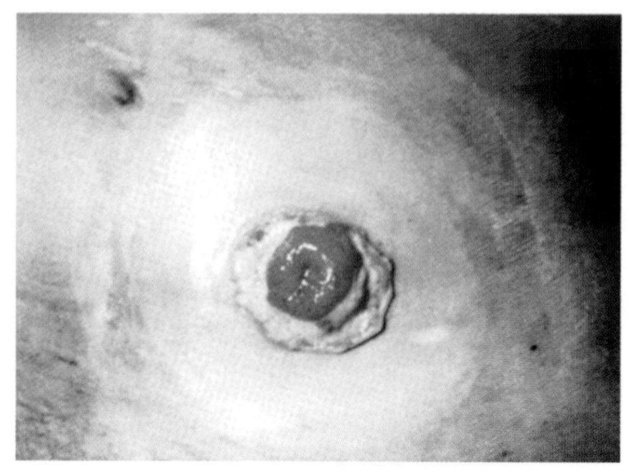

B

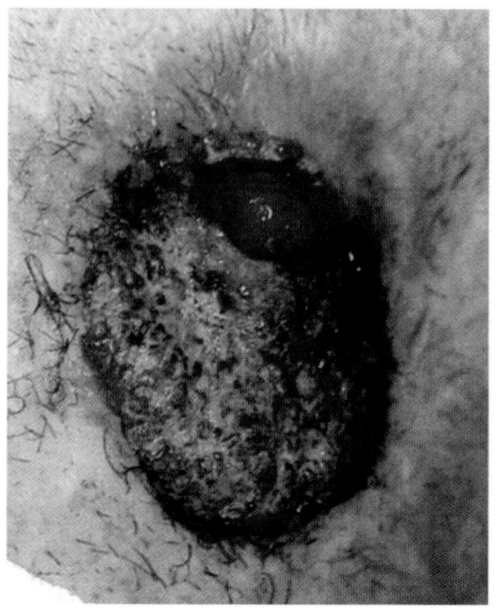

FIGURE 44 ■ (**A**) Recurrent adenocarcinoma around sigmoid colostomy. (**B**) Exophytic polypoid friable mass adjacent to and partially surrounding the ileostomy. *Source*: (**B**) from Ref. 193.

further biopsy. Treatment consists of wide excision of the abdominal wall circumferential to the ileostomy, adjacent ileal resection, and creation of a new ileostomy. Of the 16 patients with adenocarcinoma in an ileostomy found in the literature by Carey et al. (197), only two patients were found to have lymph node metastases. Two patients developed local recurrence, and four patients died, one of an unresectable local recurrence and three others of widespread metastases.

■ QUALITY OF LIFE

Over time, people change, as do their needs. When faced with the diagnosis of carcinoma or debilitating chronic disease and the hope of cure, a stoma may seem a small price to pay. However, in the longer term, some patients do well and some find life more difficult. Quality is measured by considering physical health, functional status, and the psychological well-being of an individual. Psychological adaptation is reflected in a return to previous activities and social relationships, which is generally quite possible. In patients who have been ill for extended periods prior to operation, the level of social activities and sports participation increases following recovery. However, there are reports of significant morbidity in ostomy patient adaptation. Therefore psychological adaptation cannot be left to happenstance. Recognizing the pitfalls and supportive interventions assists adaptation in the long term.

Sexuality is a frequently reported concern. In men, the concern about impotence and infertility requires attention. Damage to nerves during operation for carcinoma of the rectum may impair erection and ejaculation. However, in benign disease, the incidence of sexual dysfunction following proctectomy is significantly less. Based on the disease and risk of sexual dysfunction, patients may wish to "bank" sperm or avoid proctectomy with Hartmann's pouch. In women, dyspareunia may result because of the decreased lubrication or decrease in vaginal size that may occur following proctectomy for malignancy. However, preoperative libido and an interested partner are probably the two most important factors in reestablishing sexual intimacy following operation. Individuals, both heterosexual and homosexual, who have undergone a proctectomy and who had once engaged in anal intercourse must be informed that the stoma cannot be used as a substitute for the anus (198).

An alteration in body image has a huge impact on the ostomate's ability to progress through the rehabilitation process. Helman (199) refers to body image as an individual's perception of a combination of concepts or "maps" that help us to understand the structure and function of our bodies. When a patient undergoes surgery resulting in the creation of a stoma, the map of his body is changed. Furthermore, the creation of stoma can make a private issue public in the event of leakage, and an internal function external with the constant need for an external collecting device. Ostomy patients are subject to the stigma attached to any deviation from norm that dictates youth and physical beauty. They experience the dichotomy of looking normal on the outside while not feeling normal because of the hidden changes of their body (199). This shift in body image can have an impact on interpersonal relationships due to fear and embarrassment. Carlsson (200) studied a group of 21 patients with ileostomies between the ages of 36 and 65 and found that their most intense concerns were intimacy, access to quality medical care, energy level, loss of sexual drive, producing odor, being a burden to others, ability to perform sexually, attractiveness and feelings about their body.

Psychosocial support continues on the long term. Providing the opportunity for patients and family to express concerns and problem solving is essential. Frequently, concerns about technical issues that may impair social contacts can be resolved. Ostomy support group members may demonstrate a positive attitude to encourage the patient. Occasionally it is appropriate to refer a patient for therapeutic counseling. Whatever the circumstances, quality referrals and ongoing monitoring can assist the patient in psychological adaptation.

Karadag et al. (201) examined the problems faced by patients with irrigating colostomies ($n = 16$), nonirrigating colostomies ($n = 15$), and ileostomies ($n = 15$). The digestive disease quality of life questionnaire 15 (DDQ-15) was used to analyze quality of life before and three months after stomatherapy. A second questionnaire consisting of 11 questions with yes/no answers was also used before and three months after stoma therapy to define more specifically the stoma-related problems of each patient as well as the frequency of each issue in a patient group at a given time. Cumulatively the mean quality of life score was significantly higher after stomatherapy than before. Before stomatherapy, the irrigating colostomy patients had the highest quality of life score and the ileostomy group the lowest. Quality of life scores three months after stomatherapy, were significantly higher in all patients than before. Again, the irrigating colostomy patients had a significantly higher score than the nonirrigating colostomy and ileostomy patients. Cumulatively all of the items improved significantly after stomatherapy, such as getting dressed, bathing, and participating in sports. These findings confirm that colostomy or ileostomy has a profoundly negative impact on quality of life but specialized counseling of these patients by a dedicated team improves quality of life significantly.

More recently, Karadag et al. (202) documented their results with colostomy irrigation on the quality of life. When successful irrigation offers a regular, predictable elimination pattern and only a small covering is needed for security between irrigations. The DDQ-15 and short-form-36 were used to analyze quality of life before and 12 months after stomatherapy in a series of 25 irrigating patients with permanent end colostomies. During the same time period, 10 similar patients with left-sided colostomies who also received counseling but did not consent to colostomy irrigation were also analyzed for comparison. Colostomy irrigation was found to be effective for achieving fecal continence in selected patients with end colostomies with no complications or significant side effects. The DDQ-15 score improved significantly in the both groups after stomatherapy. The poststomatherapy DDQ-15 score of the irrigating group was also significantly higher than that of the nonirrigating group. Although none of the poststomatherapy item scales of short-form-36 differ significantly between the two groups, stomatherapy with colostomy irrigation resulted in significant improvements in role limitation due to physical problems, social functioning, role limitation due to emotional problems, general mental health, vitality, and bodily pain. On the contrary, the nonirrigation patient group showed significant improvements only in social functioning and general mental health.

■ SPECIAL PROCEDURES

Changing a Pouching System

The pouch is changed once every four to seven days or whenever it is leaking. It is best to change the pouch when there is the least amount of output from the stoma. This is usually early in the morning or before meals. The best place to perform a pouch change is in the bathroom, where there is good visibility and counterspace. Patients in wheelchairs should perform the procedure in the chair. (When the patient is in a health care facility and a nurse is providing care, the best position for the patient is supine. Universal precautions are then used.)

Set Up Equipment

- Pouching system
- Stoma measuring guide
- Closure clip
- Soft tissues
- Scissors, if needed
- Pouch pattern (optional)
- Paste (optional)
- Powder (optional)
- Preps (optional)
- Plastic disposal bag

Assemble Equipment

1. Close the spout on the pouching system by securing the closure clip.
2. If the opening on the pouching system requires cutting, use the pouch pattern to trace the size onto the pouch skin barrier. Cut out the opening.
3. Remove the paper covering the adhesive.
4. If a skin barrier paste is to be used, apply a small ring of paste around the opening on the pouch.

Remove the Soiled Pouch

1. Moisten the adhesive and gently begin removing the pouch. Support the skin while pulling the adhesive away.
2. Discard the soiled pouch in the plastic bag. Save the closure clip and any other reusable parts.

Apply the Clean Pouching System

1. Use a dry tissue to remove any mucus, stool, or paste from the stoma and skin.
2. Cleanse the peristomal skin by rinsing with water and a soft tissue. Avoid scrubbing and the use of greasy soaps.
3. Keep soft tissues handy to contain stool if the stoma begins to function.
4. Ensure the peristomal skin is completely dry
5. Apply powder on any reddened or irritated skin—remove excess with a tissue
6. Apply the pouch. Smooth the edges to avoid wrinkles in the adhesive.
7. Apply gentle pressure over the system with your hand to be sure that the seal is in contact with the skin.
8. During changing of the appliance, oftentimes the ileostomy functions thus soiling the field. One trick that can be used to control ileostomy effluent is the insertion of a tampon while the skin is being cleaned and the faceplate is being reapplied. Then just prior to application of the appliance, the tampon is removed thereby allowing a clean field of work. The use of a water-soluble lubricant will aid in the insertion of the tampon.

Colostomy Irrigation Procedure

Routine colostomy irrigation is performed to regulate bowel function. It is performed at approximately the same time each day and requires approximately one hour. A patient teaching sheet for colostomy irrigation follows:

1. Prepare equipment by setting up an irrigation set with a cone tip.
2. Fill the water bag with approximately 1000 mL tepid tap water. Hang the bag on a hook in the bathroom so it is visible.
3. Sit on a chair in front of the toilet.
4. Remove the colostomy pouch.
5. Put on the irrigation sleeve, centering the stoma in the middle of the ring.
6. Place the end of the sleeve in the toilet. Sleeves may be attached by belts or adhesive or attached to a flange.
7. Remove air in the tubing by running water through and into the sleeve.
8. Lubricate the cone tip with a water-soluble lubricant.
9. Insert the cone tip gently into the stoma.
10. Hold the tip firmly in the stoma so that no water is running back during the procedure.
11. Run the water into the colon slowly. It usually requires five minutes. If cramping is a problem, stop the water flow until comfortable. If you begin to feel lightheaded, stop the water, sit quietly, or have a glass of water. Light-headedness is usually a sign of water running in too quickly or using cold water.
12. Once the water is into the colon, remove the cone tip and clip the top of the sleeve closed.
13. It is important to sit on the toilet for approximately 15 minutes while the initial return passes into the sleeve and then into the toilet. The toilet may be flushed during the procedure.
14. When there is no further discharge of stool from the colon, rinse out the sleeve and clip the bottom closed. It is now permissible to leave the bathroom with the sleeve in place.
15. Usually, the sleeve is worn for approximately 45 minutes to collect stool that may be discharged. At the end of this period, a clean pouching system can be applied. The sleeve is rinsed and cleaned with a mild soap.

Ileostomy Lavage Procedure

An ileostomy lavage may be performed in an attempt to dislodge a food bolus obstruction. It is most frequently performed in the emergency room.

1. Set up equipment: 500 mL of saline, disposable irrigation sleeve, 60 mL syringe, cone tip or catheter, basin, and water-soluble lubricant.
2. Remove the ileostomy pouching system.
3. Rinse and dry the peristomal skin.
4. Attach the disposable irrigation sleeve.
5. Lubricate the cone tip or catheter.
6. Fill the syringe with saline and attach to the catheter.
7. Insert the cone tip or catheter into the stoma and slowly instill the fluid.
8. Repeat instillations of saline and allow the fluid to drain.

This is not a retention enema. The patient may become very uncomfortable if fluid is retained. Allow the saline to discharge between installations.

■ STOMA MANAGEMENT PRODUCTS

Adhesives

Adhesives are used to attach the pouching system to peristomal skin and include paper tape used to support the pouching system. Most pouches have adhesive backings. Adhesive is also a component of a solid-form skin barrier. Yet adhesive may be required when solid skin barriers are not in use or when additional tack is needed. Faceplates require application of adhesive. Adhesives are available in disk, tape, spray, and cement forms.

Deodorizers

Internal and external forms of deodorant are available. Internal forms are over-the-counter preparations (e.g., bismuth subgallate and chlorophyllin) taken orally multiple times a day. External deodorizers are available in liquid, powder, tablet, and spray forms. Liquid, powder, and tablet forms are indicated for use within the pouch. Sprays are used as room deodorizers.

Irrigation Equipment

Colostomy irrigation or bowel preparation equipment is packaged in a set, and replacement parts are available.

Pouching Systems

Also known as appliances, pouching systems are external collection devices that contain effluent. They may be disposable or reusable, adhesive or nonadhesive, drainable or closed at the bottom, or clear or opaque. Closed pouches are indicated for patients who have a colostomy, irrigate, or have a mucous fistula. Most closed and drainable pouches are offered with or without a charcoal filter to release gas without odor. There are also "clipless" drainable pouches whose spouts are secured without the use of a rigid plastic clip. Pouching systems can be one piece or twopiece (Fig. 45). The majority of ostomy patients prefer a two piece system.

Skin Barriers

Skin barriers protect the peristomal skin from effluent and adhesives. Skin barriers are available as pastes, powders, sealants, and rings and wafers.

Pastes

Paste skin barriers are used to caulk or fill in uneven surfaces in the peristomal field, usually at the base of the stoma. Examples include Stomahesive Paste and Hollister Premium Barrier Paste.

Powders

Commonly made of pectin or karaya, powder barriers are absorptive substances used to treat peristomal skin. They are composed of materials similar to skin-barrier wafers.

Sealants

These products consist of a copolymer liquid film used on the peristomal skin or any skin surface that is to be taped. Sealants reduce mechanical injury, protect the skin from moisture, and fix powders and medications on the skin. Skin-barrier sealants are available in 2 × 2-in. wipes, dabber bottles, and sprays. Most contain alcohol and therefore they should not be used on reddened or irritated skin.

Rings and Wafers

Also referred to as solid-form skin barriers, these products are available in disks, wafers, and strips for protection of peristomal skin from effluent and perspiration. They are

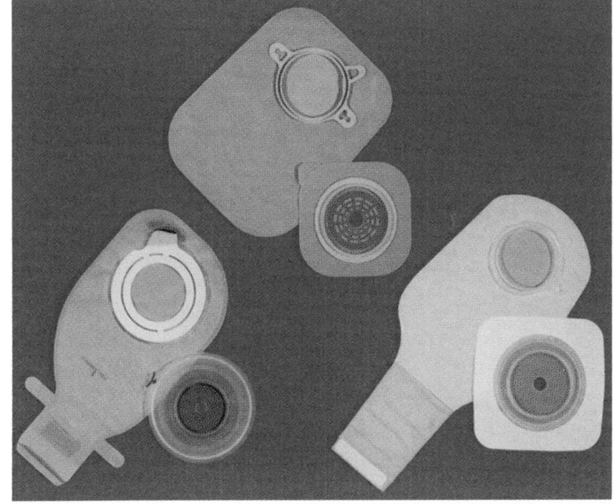

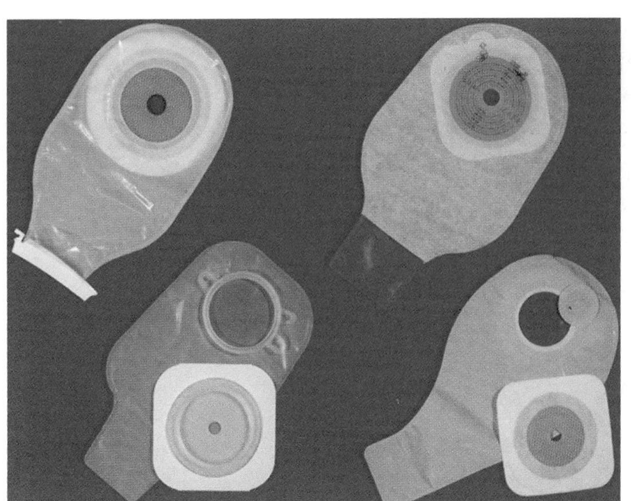

FIGURE 45 ■ Pouching systems. (**A**) Clipless drainable and closed pouch. (**B**) Drainable systems one and two piece.

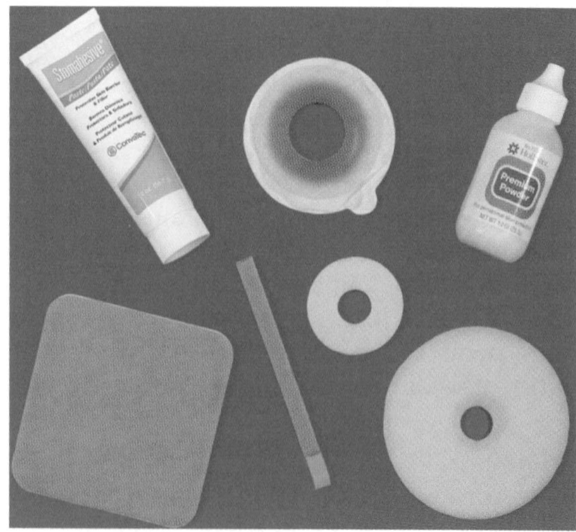

FIGURE 46 ■ Wafer skin barriers.

available as single pieces or attached to the adhesive backing of a pouch. They may be composed of pectin and gelatin or karaya. Solid skin barriers come with a plastic flange for attaching the pouch (Figs. 46 and 47).

Accessories

Belts

Two types of belts are available: ostomy and abdominal support belts. Ostomy belts attach to or around the pouching system, creating pressure at the stoma base. Abdominal support belts are 3- to 9-in. wide and have an opening that surrounds the pouching system in the peristomal field (see Fig. 27).

Closure Clips

Plastic, rubber, and metal clips are used to close the bottom of a spout on the drainable pouch.

Colostomy Plugs

Occlusive colostomy plugs are inserted into the stoma and snapped onto an intact skin barrier flange. They are indicated only after careful assessment of the patient and require close follow-up.

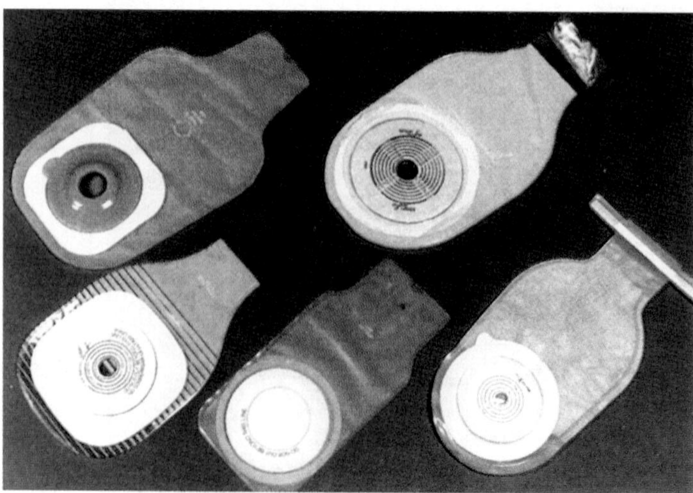

FIGURE 47 ■ Pouch skin barrier combinations.

Pouch Covers

These are fabric garments designed to fit around the base of the pouching system and cover the plastic of the pouch so that the patient's skin is not in contact with plastic.

Skin Care Products

Adhesive solvents, skin cleansers, moisturizers, and antifungal preparations are available. Indiscriminate use is to be avoided. They are not considered essential in routine patient management.

■ OSTOMY PRODUCT MANUFACTURERS

3M, 3M Center, Building 275-4W-02, St. Paul, MN 55133-3275, 1-800-228-3957

Compagnie 3M Canada, 680, Avenue Lepine, Dorval, Quebec, Canada H9P 2S5, 1-800-650-4035, www.mmm.com

Bard Medical Division, 8195 Industrial Boulevvard, Covington, GA 3001, 1-800-367-2273

Coloplast Canada, #12-3330 Ridgeway Drive, Mississauga, ON L5L 5Z9, 1-877-820-7008, www.coloplast.ca

Coloplast Corp., 1955 West Oak Circle, Marietta, GA 30062, 1-800-533-0464

Convatec, A Bristol-Myers Squibb Company, P.O. Box 5254, Princeton, NJ 08543-5254, 1-800-422-8811

Convatec, Division de la Societe Bristol-Myers Squibb, 110-555 Dr Frederik Phillips, Montreal, Quebec, Canada H4M 2X4, 1-866-331-3134, www.convatec.com

Cymed Inc., Micro Skin Ostomy Pouching Systems, 1336-A Channing Way, Berkeley, CA 947402

Dansac Ostomy Products Co., Inc., 307-A South Westgate Drive, Greensboro, NC 27407, 1-800-538-0890

Hollister, Inc., 2000 Hollister Drive, Libertyville, IL 60048, 1-800-323-4060

Hollister Limited, 95 Mary Street, Aurora, Ontario, Canada L4G 1G3, 1-800-263-7400, www.hollister.com

Marlen Manufacturing & Development Co., 5150 Richmond Road, Bedford, OH 44146, 1-216-292-7060

Mentor Corporation, 5425 Hollister Avenue, Santa Barbara, CA 93111, 1-800-328-3863

Mentor Canada, 1129 Wentworth St. W., Unit B2, Oshawa, Ont, Canada L1J 8P7

Nu-Hope Laboratories, Inc., P.O. Box 331150, Paicoima, CA 913333-1150, 1-800-899-5017

Parthenon Company, Inc., 3311 West 2400 South, Salt Lake City, UT 84119, 1-800-453-8898

Perma-Type Company, Inc, 83 Northwest Drive, Plainville, CT 06602, 1-800-242-4234

Rystan Company Inc., 47 Center Avenue, Little Falls, NJ 07424, 1-201-256-3737

Smith & Nephew United, Inc., P.O.Box 1970, Largo, FL 33779-1970, 1-800-876-1261

Smith & Nephew Inc., 4707 Rue Levy, St Laurent, Quebec, Canada H4R 2P9

VPI, A Cook Group Company, 127 South Main Street, P.O. Box 266, Spencer, IN 47460, 1-800-843-4851

■ OTHER RESOURCES

American Cancer Society, 1599 Clifton Road, NE, Atlanta, GA 30329, 1-800-ACS-2345

Canadian Cancer Society, Ontario Division, 1639 Yonge Street, Toronto, Ontario, Canda M4T 2W6, 1-888-939-3333

Crohn's and Colitis Foundation of America, 386 Park Avenue South, 17th Floor, New York, NY 10016, www.ccfa.org

Crohn's and Colitis Foundation of Canada, 60 St. Clair Avenue E., Suite 600,, Toronto, Ontario, Canada M4T 1N5, 1-800-387-1479, ccfc@ccfc.ca

United Ostomy Association, 19772 McArthur Blvd., Suite 200, Irvine, CA 92612-2405, 1-800-826-0826, www.uoa.org

United Ostomy Association of Canada Inc., P.O. Box 825-50 Charles St. E., Toronto, Ontario, Canada M4Y 2N7, 1-888-969-9698, uoacan@astral.magic.ca

World Council of Enterostomal Therapists, 6 Ferrands Close, Harding Bingley, W. Yorkshire BD16 1JA, UK

Wound, Ostomy, Continence Nurses Society, Bristol Street, Suite 110, Costa Mesa, CA 92626, 1-714-476-0268, www.wocn.org

National Digestive Diseases Information, Clearinghouse, 2 Information Way, Bethesda, MD 20892-3570, 1-301-654-3810

National Institute of Diabetes, Digestive and Kidney Diseases, 2 Information Way, Bethesda, MD 20892

REFERENCES

1. Hurny C, Holland J. Psychosocial sequelae of ostomies in cancer patients. CA Cancer J Cin 1985; 35:170–183.
2. Klopp AL. Body image and self-concept among individuals with stomas. J Enterostom Ther 1990; 17:98–105.
3. Rolstad B, Wilson G, Rothenberger DA. Sexual concerns in the patient with an ileostomy. Dis Colon Rectum 1983; 26:170–171.
4. Keltikangas-Järvinen L, Loven E, Möller C. Psychic factors determining the long-term adaptation of colostomy and ileostomy patients. Psychother Psychosom 1984; 41:153–159.
5. Franks K. Colectomy or resection of the large intestine for malignant disease. Med Chir Trans 1889; 72:211–232.
6. Brown JY. The value of complete physiological rest of the large bowel in the treatment of certain ulcerative and obstructive lesions of this organ. Surg Gynecol Obstet 1913; 16:610–613.
7. Warren R, McKittrick LS. Ileostomy for ulcerative colitis. Technique, complications and management. Surg Gynecol Obstet 1951; 93:555–567.
8. Crile G Jr, Turnbull RB. The mechanism and prevention of ileostomy dysfunction. Ann Surg 1954; 140:459–466.
9. Brooke BN. The management of an ileostomy including its complications. Lancet 1952; 2:102–104.
10. Goligher JC. Extraperitoneal colostomy or ileostomy. Br J Surg 1958; 46:97–103.
11. Kock NG, Brevinge H, Philipson BM, et al. Continent ileostomy: the present technique and long-term results. Ann Chir Gynaecol 1986; 75:63–70.
12. Tang CL, Yunos A, Leong APK, Seow-Choen F, Goh HS. Ileostomy output in the early post-operative period. Br J Surg 1998; 82:607–608.
13. Soybel DI. Adaptation to ileal diversion. Surgery 2001; 129:123–127.
14. Tang CL, Yunos A, Leong APK, et al. Ileostomy output in the early postoperative period. Br J Surg 1995; 82:607.
15. Ladas SD, Isaacs PE, Murphy GM, Sladen GE. Fasting and post-prandial ileal function in adapted ileostomates and normal subjects. Gut 1986; 27: 906–912.
16. Hallgren T, Oresland T Andersson H, Hulten L. Ileostomy output and bile acid excretion after intraduodenal administration of oleic acid. Scand J Gastroenterol 1994; 29:1017–1023.
17. Steinhart AH, Jenkins DJA, Mitchell S, Cuff D, Prokipchuk EJ. Effect of dietary fiber on total carbohydrate losses in ileostomy effluent. Am J Gastroenterol 1992; 87:48–54.
18. MacGregor IL, Wiley ZD, Sleisenger MH. The role of bile acids in determining ileal flow rates in normal subjects and following ileostomy. Digestion 1978; 18:192–200.
19. Gorbach SL, Nahas L, Weinstein L. Studies of intestinal microfloral. IV. The microfloral of ileostomy effluent: a unique microbial ecology. Gastroenterology 1967; 53:874–880.
20. Soper NJ, Orkin BA, Kelly KA, Phillips SF, Brown ML. Gastrointestinal transit after proctocolectomy with ileal pouch-anal anastomosis or ileostomy. J Surg Res 1989; 46:300–305.
21. Pemberton JH, van Heerden JA, Beart RW Jr, Kelly KA, Phillips SF, Taylor BM. A continent ileostomy device. Ann Surg 1983; 197:618–626.
22. Bruewer M, Stern J, Herrmann S, Senninger N, Herfarth C. Changes in intestinal transit time after proctocolectomy assessed by the lactulose breath test. World J Surg 2000; 24:119–124.
23. Mibu R, Itoh H, Nakayama F. Effect of total colectomy and mucosal proctectomy on intestinal absorptive capacity in dogs. Dis Colon Rectum 1987; 30: 47–51.
24. Wright HK, Cleveland JC, Tilson MD, Herskovic T. Morphology and absorptive capacity of the ileum after ileostomy in man. Am J Surg 1969; 117: 242–245.
25. Scott R, Freeland R, Mowat W, et al. The prevalence of calcified upper urinary tract stone disease in a random population—Cumbernauld Health Survey. Br J Urol 1977; 49:589–595.
26. Smith LH. Application of physical, chemical and metablolic factors to the management of urolithiasis. In: Fleisch H, Robertson WG, Smith LH, Vahlensleck W, eds. Urolithiasis Research. New York: Premium Press, 1976:199–211.
27. Christie PM, Knight GS, Hill GL. Comparison of relative risks of urinary stone formation after surgery for ulcerative colitis: conventional ileostomy vs. J-pouch. A comparison study. Dis Colon Rectum 1996; 39:50–54.
28. Miettinen TA, Peltokallio P. Bile salt, fat, water, and vitamin B_{12} excretion after ileostomy. Scan J Gastroenterol 1971; 6:543–552.
29. Huibregtse K, Hoek F, Sanders GT, Tytgat GN. Bile acid metabolism in ileostomy patients. Eur J Clin 1977; 7:137–140.
30. Ritchie JK. Ileostomy and excisional surgery for chronic inflammatory disease of the colon: a survey of one hospital region. I. Results of complications of surgery. Gut 1971; 12:528–540.
31. Kurchin A, Ray JE, Bluth EI, et al. Cholelithiasis in ileostomy patients. Dis Colon Rectum 1984; 27:585–588.
32. Kusuhara K, Kusunoki M, Okamoto T, et al. Reduction of the effluent volume in high output ileostomy patients by a somatostatic analogue, SMS 201–995. Int J Colorectal Dis 1992; 7:202–205.
33. Gracey M, Burke V, Oshin A. Reversible inhibition of intestinal sugar transport by deconjugated bile salt in vitro. Biochim Biophys Acta 1971; 225:308–314.
34. Keating J, Kelly EW, Hunt I. Save the skin and improve the scar: a simple technique to minimize the scar from a temporary stoma. Dis Colon Rectum 2003; 46:1428–1429.
35. Kittur DS, Talamini M, Smith GW. Eversion of difficult ileostomies by Guy Rope suture technique. Am J Surg 1989; 157:593–594.
36. Carlsen E, Bergan A. Technical aspects and complications of end-ileostomies. World J Surg 1995; 19:632–636.
37. Williams NS, Nasmyth DG, Jones D, et al. De-functioning stomas: a prospective controlled trial comparing loop ileostomy with loop transverse colostomy. Br J Surg 1986; 73:566–570.
38. Altomare DF, Pannarale OC, Lupo L, et al. Protective colostomy closure: the hazards of a "minor" operation. Int J Colorectal Dis 1990; 5:73–78.
39. Winslet MC, Drolc Z, Allan A, et al. Assessment of the defunctioning efficiency of the loop ileostomy. Dis Colon Rectum 1991; 34:699–703.
40. Chen F, Stuart M. The morbidity of defunctioning stomata. Aust N Z J Surg 1996; 66:218–221.
41. Alexander-Williams J. Loop ileostomy and colostomy for faecal diversion. Ann R Coll Surg Engl 1974; 54:141–148.
42. Fasth S, Hulten L. Loop ileostomy: a superior diverting stoma in colorectal surgery. World J Surg 1984; 8:401–407.
43. Marcello PW, Roberts PL, Schoetz DJ Jr, et al. Obstruction after ileal pouch-anal anastomosis: a preventable complication?. Dis Colon Rectum 1993; 36:1105–1111.
44. Prasad ML, Pearl RK, Orsay CP, et al. Rodless loop ileostomy. A modified loop ileostomy. Dis Colon Rectum 1984; 27:270.
45. Sitzmann JV. A new alternative to diverting double barreled ileostomy. Surg Gynecol Obstet 1987; 165:461–464.
46. Kestenberg A, Becker JM. A new technique of loop ileostomy closure after endorectal ileoanal anastomosis. Surgery 1985; 98:109–111.
47. van de Pavoordt HDWM, Fazio VW, Jagelman DG, et al. The outcome of loop ileostomy closure in 293 cases. Int J Colorec Dis 1987; 2:214–217.
48. Abrams JS. Abdominal stomas. Indications, operative techniques and patient care. In: Wright J, ed. Spontaneous Fistula to Continent Ileostomy. Littleton, MA: PSG, 1984:19–24.
49. Miles WE. A method of performing abdominoperineal excision for carcinoma of the rectum and of the terminal portion of the pelvic colon. Lancet 1908; 2:1812–1813.
50. Heald RJ. Towards fewer colostomies—the impact of circular stapling devices on the surgery of rectal cancer in a district hospital. Br J Surg 1980; 67: 198–200.
51. Khubchandani IT, Trimpi HD, Sheets JA. The magnetic stoma device: a continent colostomy. Dis Colon Rectum 1981; 24:344–350.
52. Clague MB, Heald RJ. Achievement of stomal continence in one-third of colostomies by use of a new disposable plug. Surg Gynecol Obstet 1990; 170: 390–394.
53. Prager E. The continent colostomy. Dis Colon Rectum 1984; 27:235–237.
54. Fielding LP, Stewart-Brown S, Hittinger R, et al. Covering stoma for elective anterior resection of the rectum: an outmoded operation?. Am J Surg 1984; 147:524–530.
55. Stone HH, Fabian TC. Management of perforating colon trauma. Randomization between primary closure and exteriorization. Ann Surg 1979; 190: 430–436.
56. Gordon PH. The chemically defined diet and anorectal procedures. Can J Surg 1976; 19:511–513.
57. Robertson HD. Use of an elemental diet as a nutritionally complete "medical colostomy.". South Med J 1983; 76:1005–1007.
58. Corman ML. Colon and Rectal Surgery. 2nd ed. Philadelphia: JB Lippincott, 1989.
59. Goldstein SD, Salvati EP, Rubin RJ, et al. Tube cecostomy with cecal extraperitonealization in the management of obstructing left sided carcinoma of the large intestine. Surg Gynecol Obstet 1986; 162:379–380.
60. Benacci JC, Wolff BG. Cecostomy: therapeutic indications and results. Dis Colon Rectum 1995; 38:530–534.
61. Haaga JR, Bick RJ, Zollinger RM Jr. CT guided percutaneous catheter cecostomy. Gastrointest Radiol 1987; 12:166–168.

62. Ponsky JL, Aszoki A, Perse D. Percutaneous endoscopic cecostomy: a new approach to nonobstructive colonic dilation. Gastrointest Endosc 1986; 32:108–111.
63. Winkler MJ, Volpe PA. Loop transverse colostomy—the case against. Dis Colon Rectum 1982; 25:321–326.
64. Hopkins JE. Transverse colostomy in the management of cancer of the colon. Dis Colon Rectum 1971; 14:232–236.
65. Abrams BL, Alsikafi FH, Waterman NG. Colostomy: a new look at morbidity and mortality. Am Surg 1979; 45:462–464.
66. Rosenberg L, Gordon PH. Tube cecostomy revisited. Can J Surg 1986; 29:38–40.
67. Fontes B, Fontes W, Utiyama EM, et al. The efficacy of loop colostomy for complete fecal diversion. Dis Colon Rectum 1988; 31:298–302.
68. Schofield PF, Cade D, Lambert M. Dependent proximal loop colostomy: does it defunction the distal colon? Br J Surg 1986; 67:201–202.
69. Morris DM, Rayburn D. Loop colostomies are totally diverting in adults. Am J Surg 1991; 161:668–671.
70. Turnbull RB, Weakley FL, Hawk WA, et al. Choice of operation for toxic megacolon phase of nonspecific ulcerative colitis. Surg Clin North Am 1970; 50:1151–1169.
71. Prasad ML, Pearl RK, Abcarian H. End-loop colostomy. Surg Gynecol Obstet 1984; 158:381–382.
72. Unti JA, Abcarian H, Pearl RK, et al. Rodless end-loop stomas: seven-year experience. Dis Colon Rectum 1991; 34:999–1004.
73. Parks SE, Hastings PR. Complications of colostomy closure. Am J Surg 1985; 149:672–675.
74. Williams RA, Csepani E, Hiatt J, et al. Analysis of the morbidity, mortality, and cost of colostomy closure in traumatic compared to nontraumatic colorectal diseases. Dis Colon Rectum 1987; 30:164–167.
75. Thal ER, Yeary EC. Morbidity of colostomy closure following colon trauma. J Trauma 1980; 20:287–291.
76. Velmahos GC, Degiannis E, Wells M, et al. Early closure of colostomies in trauma patients—a prospective randomized trial. Surgery 1995; 118: 815–820.
77. Whittaker M, Goligher JC. A comparison of the results of extraperitoneal and intraperitoneal techniques for construction of terminal iliac colostomies. Dis Colon Rectum 1976; 19:342–344.
78. Sjödahl R, Anderberg B, Bolin T. Parastomal hernia in relation to site of the abdominal stoma. Br J Surg 1988; 75:339–341.
79. Ortiz H, Sara MJ, Armendariz P, et al. Does the frequency of paracolostomy hernias depend on the position of the colostomy in the abdominal wall?. Int J Colorectal Dis 1994; 9:65–67.
80. Antrum RM, Price JJ. Use of skin staples for fashioning colostomies. Br J Surg 1988; 75:736.
81. Burke TW, Weiser EB, Hoskins WJ, et al. End colostomy using the end-to-end anastomosis instrument. Obstet Gynecol 1987; 69:156–159.
82. Porter JA, Salvati EP, Rubin RJ, et al. Complications of colostomies. Dis Colon Rectum 1989; 32:299–303.
83. Feustel H, Hennig G. Kontinent Kolostomie durch Magnetverschluss. Dtsch Med Wochenschr 1975; 100:1063–1064.
84. Husemann B, Hager TH. Experience with the Erlangen magnetic ring colostomy-closure system. Int Surg 1984; 69:297–300.
85. Cazador AC, Pinol M, Marti Rogue J, et al. Multicentre study of a continent colostomy plug. Br J Surg 1993; 80:930–932.
86. Schmidt E. The continent colostomy. World J Surg 1982; 6:805–809.
87. Mileski WJ, Rege RV, Joehl RJ, et al. Rates of morbidity and mortality after closure of loop and end colostomy. Surg Gynecol Obstet 1990; 171:17–21.
88. Mosdell DM, Doberneck RC. Morbidity and mortality of ostomy closure. Am J Surg 1991; 162:633–637.
89. Pearce NW, Scott SD, Karran SJ. Timing and method of reversal of Hartmann's procedure. Br J Surg 1992; 79:839–841.
90. Keck JO, Collopy BT, Ryan PJ, et al. Reversal of Hartmann's procedure: effect of timing and technique on ease and safety. Dis Colon Rectum 1994; 37: 243–248.
91. Livingston DH, Miller FB, Richardson JD. Are the risks after colostomy closure exaggerated?. Am J Surg 1989; 158:17–20.
92. Khoury DA, Beck DE, Opelka FG, et al. Colostomy closure: Ochsner Clinic experience. Dis Colon Rectum 1996; 39:605–609.
93. Allen-Mersh TG, Thomson JPS. Surgical treatment of colostomy complications. Br J Surg 1988; 75:416–418.
94. Leenen LP, Kuijpers JH. Some factors influencing the outcome of stoma surgery. Dis Colon Rectum 1989; 32:500–504.
95. Carlstedt A, Fasth S, Hulton L, et al. Long-term ileostomy complications in patients with ulcerative colitis and Crohn's disease. Int J Colorectal Dis 1987; 2:22–25.
96. Khoo REH, Cohen MM, Chapman GM, et al. Loop ileostomy for temporary fecal diversion. Am J Surg 1994; 167:519–522.
97. Stothert JC Jr, Brubacher L, Simonowitz DA. Complications of emergency stoma formation. Arch Surg 1982; 117:307–309.
98. Feinberg SM, McLeod RS, Cohen Z. Complications of loop ileostomy. Am J Surg 1987; 153:102–107.
99. Grobler SP, Hosie KB, Keighley MRB. Randomized trial of loop ileostomy in restorative proctocolectomy. Br J Surg 1992; 79:903–906.
100. Wexner SD, Taranow DA, Johansen OB, et al. Loop ileostomy is a safe option for fecal diversion. Dis Colon Rectum 1993; 36:349–354.
101. Leong APK, Londono-Schimmer EE, Phillips RKS. Life-table analysis of stomal complications following ileostomy. Br J Surg 1994; 81:727–729.
102. Senapati A, Nicholls RJ, Ritchie JK, et al. Temporary loop ileostomy for restorative proctocolectomy. Br J Surg 1993; 80:628–630.
103. Kaidar-Person O, Person B, Wexner SD. Complications of construction and closure of temporary loop ileostomy. J Am Coll Surg 2005; 201:759–73.
104. Hughes ESR, McDermott FT, Masterton JP. Intestinal obstruction following operation for inflammatory disease of the bowel. Dis Colon Rectum 1979; 22:469–471.
105. Bubrick MP, Jacobs DM, Levy M. Experience with the endorectal pull-through and S-pouch for ulcerative colitis and familial polyposis in adults. Surgery 1985; 98:689–699.
106. Francois Y, Dozois RR, Kelly KA, et al. Small intestinal obstruction complicating ileal pouch-anal anastomosis. Ann Surg 1989; 209:46–50.
107. Anderson DN, Driver CP, Park KGM, et al. Loop ileostomy fixation: a simple technique to minimize the risk of stomal volvulus. Int J Colorectal Dis 1994; 9:138–140.
108. Snyder CL, Kaufman DB. A simple technique for assessing the viability of stomas of the intestines. Surg Gynecol Obstet 1991; 172:399–400.
109. Fleischer I, Bryant D. Melanosis coli or mucosal ischemia? A case report. Ostomy/Wound Management 1995; 41:44, 46–47.
110. Malt RA, Bartlett MK, Wheelock FC. Subcutaneous fasciotomy for relief of stricture of the ileostomy. Surg Gynecol Obstet 1984; 159:175–176.
111. Todd IP. Mechanical complications of ileostomy (Part 4). Clin Gastroenterol 1982; 11:268–273.
112. Fleshman JW, Lewis MG. Complications and quality of life after stoma surgery: a review of 16,470 patients in the UOA Data Registry. Semin Colon Rectal Surg 1991; 2:66–72.
113. Park JJ, Pino AD, Orsay CP, et al. Stoma complications: the Cook County Hospital Experience. Dis Colon Rectum 1999; 42:1575–1580.
114. Cheung MT. Complications of an abdominal stoma: an analysis of 322 stomas. Aust N Z J Surg 1995; 65:808–811.
115. Zinkin LD, Rosin JD. Button colopexy for colostomy prolapse. Surg Gynecol Obstet 1981; 152:89–90.
116. Rubin MS. Parastomal Hernias. In: Cataldo PA, MacKeigan JM, eds. Intestinal Stomas: Principles, Techniques, and Management. 2nd ed. : Marcel Dekker, 2004:277–305.
117. Botet X, Boldo E, Llaurado JM. Colonic parastomal hernia repair by translocation without formal laparotomy. Br J Surg 1996; 83:981.
118. Carne PW, Robertson GM, Frizelle FA. Parastomal hernia. Br J Surg 2003; 90:784–93.
119. Birnbaum W, Ferrier P. Complication of abdominal colostomy. Am J Surg 1952; 83:64–67.
120. Grier WRN, Postel AH, Syarse A, Localio SA. An evaluation of colonic stoma management without irrigations. Surg Gynecol Obstet 1964; 119: 1234–1242.
121. Marks CG, Ritchie JK. The complications of synchronous combined excision for adenocarcinoma of the rectum at St. Mark's Hospital. Br J Surg 1975; 62:901–905.
122. Von Smitten K, Husa A, Kyllonen L. Long-term results of sigmoidostomy in patients with anorectal malignancy. Acta Chir Scand 1986; 152:211–213.
123. Williams JG, Etherington R, Hayward MWJ, Hughes LE. Paraileostomy hernia: a clinical review and radiological study. Br J Surg 1990; 77: 1355–1357.
124. Oritz H, Sara MJ Armendariz P, deMiguel M, Marti J, Chocarro C. Does the frequency of paracolostomy hernias depend on the position of the colostomy in the abdominal wall?. Int J Colorect Dis 1994; 9:65–67.
125. Londono-Schimmer EE, Leong APK, Phillips RKS. Life table analysis of stomal complications following colostomy. Dis Colon Rectum 1994; 9: 916–920.
126. Cataldo P, Mackeigan JM. Intestinal stomas. Dekker, 2004.
127. Balslev AI. Parakolostomihernier. Ugeskr Laeger 1973; 135:2799–2804.
128. Cheung MT, Chai NH, Chiu WY. Surgical treatment of parastomal hernia complicating sigmoid colostomies. Dis Colon Rectum 2001; 2:266–270.
129. Bayer I, Kyzer S, Chaimoff CH. A new approach to primary strengthening of colostomy with Marlex mesh to prevent paracolostomy hernia. Surg Gynecol Obstet 1986; 163:579–580.
130. Sugarbaker PH. Prosthetic mesh repair of large hernias at the site of colonic stomas. Surg Gynecol Obstet 1980; 150:577–578.
131. Stephenson BM, Phillips RKS. Parastomal hernia: local resiting and mesh repair. Br J Surg 1995; 82:1395–1396.
132. Geisler DJ, Reilly JC, Vaughan SG, Glennon EJ, Kondylis PD. Safety and outcome of use of nonabsorbable mesh for repair of fascial defects in the presence of open bowel. Dis Colon Rectum 2003; 46:1118–23.
133. Steele SR, Lee P, Martin MJ, Mullenix PS, Sullivan ES. Is parastomal hernia repair with polypropylene mesh safe? Am J Surg 2003; 185:436–440.
134. Janes A, Cengiz Y, Israelsson LA. Randomized clinical trial of the use of a prosthetic mesh to prevent parastomal hernia. Br J Surg 2004; 91:280–282.
135. Stelzner S, Hellmich G, Ludwig K. New method for paracolostomy hernia repair. Dis Colon Rectum 1999; 42:823.

136. Amin SN, Armitage NC, Abercrombie JF, Scholefield JH. Lateral repair of parastomal hernia. Ann R Coll Surg Engl 2001; 83:206–208.
137. Rubin MS, Schoetz DJ Jr, Mathews JB. Parastomal hernia. Is stoma relocation superior to fascial repair? Arch Surg 1994; 129:413–419.
138. Greatorex RA. Simple method of closing a paraileostomy fistula. Br J Surg 1988; 75:543.
139. Wiesner RH, LaRusso NT, Dozois RR, et al. Peristomal varices after proctocolectomy in patients with primary sclerosing cholangitis. Gastroenterology 1986; 90:316–322.
140. Strong SA. Colonic anorectal and peristomal varices. Semin Colorectal Surg 1994; 5:50–58.
141. Roberts PL, Martin FM, Schoetz DJ Jr, et al. Bleeding stomal varices: the role of local treatment. Dis Colon Rectum 1990; 33:547–549.
142. Peck JJ, Boydena AM. Exigent ileostomy hemorrhage. A complication of proctocolectomy in patients with chronic ulcerative colitis and primary sclerosing cholangitis. Am J Surg 1985; 150:153–158.
143. Grundfest-Broniatowski S, Fazio V. Conservative treatment of bleeding stomal varices. Arch Surg 1983; 118:981–985.
144. Morgan TR, Feldshon SD, Tripp MR. Recurrent stomal variceal bleeding. Successful treatment using injection sclerotherapy. Dis Colon Rectum 1986; 29:269–270.
145. Hesterberg R, Stahlknecht CD, Roher HD. Sclerotherapy for massive enterostomy bleeding resulting from portal hypertension. Dis Colon Rectum 1986; 29:275–277.
146. Samaraweera RN, Feldman L, Widrich WC, et al. Stomal varices: percutaneous transhepatic embolization. Radiology 1989; 170: 779–782.
147. Fitzgerald JB, Chalmers N, Abbott G, et al. The uses of TIPS to control bleeding caput medusae. Br J Radiol 1998; 71:558–560.
148. Shibata D, Brophy DP, Gordon FD, Asnastopoulos HT, Sentovich SM, Bleday R. Transjugalar intrahepatic portosystemic shunt for treatment of bleeding ectopic varices with portal hypertension. Dis Colon Rectum 1999; 42:1581–1585.
149. Korelitz BI, Cheskin LJ, Sohn N, et al. The fate of the rectal segment after diversion of the fecal stream in Crohn's disease: its implications for surgical management. J Clin Gastroenterol 1985; 7: 37–43.
150. Harig JM, Soergel KH, Komorowski RA, et al. Treatment of diversion colitis with short chain-fatty acid irrigation. N Engl J Med 1989; 320:23–28.
151. Pokorny H, Herkner H, Jakesz R, Herbst F. Mortality and complications after stoma closure. Arch Surg 2005; 140:956–960.
152. Moug SJ, Robertson E, Angerson WJ, Horgan PG. Socioeconomic deprivation has an adverse effect on outcome after ileostomy closure. Br J Surg 2005; 92:376–377.
153. Bosshardt TL. Outcomes of ostomy procedures in patients aged 70 years and older. Arch Surg 2003; 138:1077–1082.
154. Edwards DP, Leppington-Clarke A, Sexton R, Heald RJ, Moran BJ. Stoma-related complications are more frequent after transverse colostomy than loop ileostomy: a prospective randomized clinical trial. Br J Surg 2001; 88:360–363.
155. Kairaluoma M, Rissanen H, Kultti V, Mecklin JP, Kellokumpu I. Outcome of temporary stomas. A prospective study of temporary intestinal stomas constructed between 1989 and 1996. Dig Surg 2002; 19:45–51.
156. Duchesne JC, Wang YZ, Weintraub SL, Boyle M, Hunt JP. Stoma complications: a multivariate analysis. Am Surg 2002; 68:961–966.
157. Cataldo PA. History of enterostomal therapy. Perspect Colon Rectal Surg 1996; 9:117–123.
158. Walsh BA, Grunert BK, Telford GL, et al. Multidisciplinary management of altered body image in the patient with an ostomy. J WOCN 1996; 22: 227–236.
159. Rolstad BS. Facilitating psychosocial adaptation. J Enterostom Ther 1987; 14:28–34.
160. Piwonka A, Merino J. A multidimensional modelling of predictors influencing the adjustment to a colostomy. J WOCN 1999; 26:298–305.
161. Standards of Care: Patient with Ileostomy. Costa Mesa, CA: Wound Ostomy and Continence Nurses Society (WOCN), 1990.
162. Standards of Care: Patient with Colostomy. Costa Mesa, CA: Wound Ostomy and Continence Nurses Society (WOCN), 1989.
163. Persson E, Severinsson E, Hellstrom AL. Spouses perception of and reaction to living with partner who undergone surgery for rectal cancer resulting in a stoma. Cancer Nurs 2004; 27:85–90.
164. O'Shea H. Teaching the adult ostomy patient. J WOCN 2001; 28:47–54.
165. Jeter KF. Perioperative teaching and counseling. Cancer 1992; 70:1346–1349.
166. Pieper B, Mikols C. Predischarge and postdischarge concerns of persons with an ostomy. J WOCN 1996; 23:106–109.
167. Klopp AL. Gastrointestinal and digestive care plans: fecal ostomy. In: Gulanick M, Klopp A, Galanes S, et al., eds. Nursing Care Plans: Nursing Diagnosis and Intervention. 3rd ed. St. Louis: Mosby, 1994:308–310.
168. Corman ML. Preoperative considerations. In: MacKeigan JM, Cataldo PA, eds. Intestinal Stomas: Principles Techniques, and Management. St Louis: Quality Medical Publishing, 1993:52–59.
169. Lavery IC, Erwin-Toth P. Stoma therapy. In: MacKeigan JM, Cataldo PA, eds. Intestinal Stomas: Principles Techniques and Management. St Louis: Quality Medical Publishing, 1993:60–84.
170. Banks N, Razor B. Preoperative stoma site assessment and marking: trained RNs can improve ostomy outcome. AJN 2003; 103:64A–64B.
171. Turnbull R, Weakley F. . Atlas of Intestinal Stomas. St. Louis: CV Mosby, 1967:7–9.
172. Weakley FL. A historical perspective of stomal construction. J WOCN 1994; 21:59–75.
173. Boarini J. Gastrointestinal cancer: colon, rectum, and anus. In: Groenwald SL, Frogge MH, Goodman M, et al., eds. Cancer Nursing: Principles an2d Practice. 2nd ed. Boston: Jones and Bartlett, 1990:792–807.
174. Rolstad BS, Boarini J. Principles and techniques in the use of convexity. Ostomy/Wound Management 1996; 42:24–26.
175. Crina F. Dietary choices of people with ostomies. J WOCN 2001; 28: 28–31.
176. Rolstad BS, Hoyman K. Continent diversions and reservoirs. In: Hampton B, Bryant R, eds. Ostomies and Continent Diversions: Nursing Management. St. Louis: Mosby-Year Book, 1992:129–162.
177. Erwin-Toth P, Doughty DB. Principles and procedures of stomal management. In: Hampton B, Bryant R, eds. Ostomies and Continent Diversions: Nursing Management. St. Louis: Mosby-Year Book, 1992:103.
178. Association Francaise d'Enterostoma- Therapeutes. Guide des Bonnes Pratiques en Stomatherapie Chez L'adulte- Enterostomies. Citron Marine, France 2003:135.
179. Turnbull G. Managing Oversight of Colostomy Irrigation in Long Term Care Facilities. OWM 2002; 49:13–14.
180. Jao S-W, Beart RW Jr, Wendorf LJ, et al. Irrigation management of sigmoid colostomy. Arch Surg 1985; 120:916–917.
181. Dini D, Venturini M, Forno G, et al. Irrigation for colostomized cancer patients: a rational approach. Int J Colorectal Dis 1991; 6:9–11.
182. Sanada H, Kawashima K, Tsuda M, et al. Natural evacuation versus irrigation. Ostomy/Wound Management 1992; 38:24, 26–30.
183. Follick MJ, Smith TW, Turk DC. Psychosocial adjustment following ostomy. Health Psychol 1984; 3:505–517.
184. McLeod RS, Lavery IC, Leatherman JR, et al. Patient evaluation of the conventional ileostomy. Dis Colon Rectum 1985; 28:152.
185. Turnbull G. The Evolution, Current Status and Regulation of Ostomy Products in the United States. J WOCN 2001; 28:18–24.
186. Milne CT, Corbett LQ, Dubuc DL. Wound, Ostomy, and Incontinence Nursing Secrets. Philadelphia: Hanley Belfus Inc., 2003:305.
187. Thompson G. Financial resources for persons with an ostomy. CAET J 1999; 18:7–16.
188. Tucker SB, Smith DB. Dermatologic conditions complicating ostomy care. In: Smith DB, Johnson DE, eds. Ostomy Care and the Cancer Patient. Orlando, FL: Grune & Stratton, 1986:139–153.
189. Canadian Ostomy Assessment Guide. Peristomal Skin Guide. Ville St-Laurent: Canvatec 2000:4.
190. Brady E. Severe peristomal pyoderma gangrenosum: a case study. J WOCN 1999; 26:306–311.
191. Sibbald G, Orstead H, Schultz G, et al. Preparing the wound bed 2003: focus on infection and inflammation. OWM 49:24–51.
192. Kiran RP, O'Brien-Ermlich B, Achkar JP, Fazio VW, Delaney CP. Management of peristomal pyoderma gangrenosum. Dis Colon Rectum 2003: 1397–1403.
193. Vasilevsky CA, Gordon PH. Adenocarcinoma arising at the ileocutaneous junction occurring after proctocolectomy for ulcerative colitis. Br J Surg 1986; 73:378.
194. Starke J, Rodriguez-Bigas M, Marshall W, et al. Primary adenocarcinoma arising in an ileostomy. Surgery 1993; 114:125–128.
195. Iizuka T, Sawada T, Hayakawa K, Hashimoto M, Udagawa H, Watanabe G. Successful local excision of ileostomy adenocarcinoma after colectomy for familial adenomatous polyposis: report of a case. Surg Today 2002; 32: 638–41.
196. Shibuya T, Uchiyama K, Kokuma M. Metachronous adenocarcinoma at a colostomy site after abdominalperineal resection for rectal carcinoma. J Gastroenterology 2002; 37:387–390.
197. Carey PD, Suvarna SK, Baloch KG, et al. Primary adenocarcinoma in an ileostomy: a late complication of surgery for ulcerative colitis. Surgery 1993; 113:712–715.
198. Zmijewski HC. Sexual counselling by the ET nurse: if not you, then who?. J WOCN 2002; 29:184–185.
199. Helman CG. The body image in health and disease: exploring patient's maps of body and self. Patient Educ Counsel 1995; 26:169–175.
200. Carlsson E. Body Composition and Quality of Life in Patients with IBD, Ileostomy and Short Bowel Syndrome. Department of Surgery Goteborg University. Goteborg: Tryckt av Intellect Docusys, 2003:36.
201. Karadag A, Mentes BB, Uner A, Irkorucu O, Ayaz S, Ozkan S. Impact of stomatherapy on quality of life in patients with permanent colostomies or ileostomies. Int J Colorectal Dis 2003; 18:234–8.
202. Karadag A, Mentes BB, Ayaz S. Colostomy irrigation: results of 25 cases with particular reference to quality of life. J Clin Nurs 2005; 14:479–85.

33 Constipation

W. Rudolf Schouten and Philip H. Gordon

INTRODUCTION

Devoting an entire chapter to a single symptom might at first appear unwarranted. Nevertheless, the magnitude of the problem in patients who have sustained a long-standing history of constipation of "idiopathic" origin is great. Enthusiastic physicians report studies designed to shed light on the problem, but much of the information is incomplete or contradictory. The pharmacology of the various medications used in the treatment of constipation frequently is poorly understood.

From a review of four different surveys, Sonnenberg and Koch (1) assessed the epidemiology of constipation in the United States. They estimated that four million people in the United States have frequent constipation, a prevalence rate of approximately 2%. Cathartics and laxatives were prescribed for two to three million patients yearly. Approximately 900 persons died annually from diseases associated with or related to constipation. Constipation was three times more common in women than men and increased markedly after the age of 65 years. Nonwhites were affected 1.3 times more frequently than whites. Constipation more frequently affected people in the southern United States, people from lower income families, and those with a lower educational level. The authors suggested that factors in addition to dietary fiber content and psychogenic influences might be involved in the causation of constipation.

A survey among a representative community from Olmsted County, Minnesota, revealed that constipation is indeed a common complaint, especially in elderly subjects (2). Nearly one in two women and one in three men, aged 65 years and older, had symptoms of constipation or took laxatives and enemas. The results of this survey further suggest that the type of constipation alters with age and differs from that observed in a younger population. Elderly subjects reported more frequent symptoms of obstructed defecation, such as prolonged straining, self-digitation, and feelings of incomplete evacuation.

Robson et al. (3) described the prevalence of constipation and determined risk factors for the development of constipation in a large population of nursing home residents who were at least 65 years of age and who had assessments at baseline and three months ($n = 21{,}012$). The variables examined included medications, mobility, comorbid illness, and nutrition. The mean age of nursing home residents was 83 ± 8 years [standard deviation (SD)] and the population was 70% female and 83% white. At baseline, the prevalence of constipation was 12.5% ($n = 2627$). By the three-month assessment, 7% ($n = 1291$) of nursing home residents had developed constipation. The factors associated independently with the development of constipation were, in order of magnitude, race, decreased fluid intake, pneumonia, Parkinson's disease, and the presence of allergies. Congestive heart failure and the use of feeding tube were two factors identified as having a protective effect.

Constipation is an age-old and worldwide problem for which a variety of treatments have been tried. For example, in ancient times, the Chinese technique for handling constipation consisted of massaging the abdomen with wooden rollers (Fig. 1). Today patients, often young women, may be in distress for days and even weeks before having a bowel movement. The use of a great variety of different laxatives and/or suppositories, with or without the regular use of enemas, becomes the rule in many of these troubled patients.

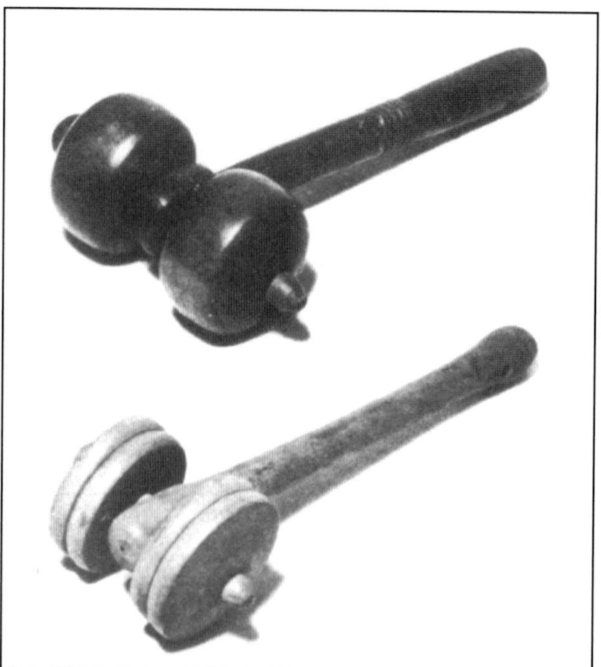

FIGURE 1 ■ Wooden rollers. *Source*: Courtesy of Wellcome Trustees, London.

During the past two decades, new modalities of investigation have added to the knowledge of colonic and anorectal dysfunction, which has resulted in a better understanding of the basic pathophysiology of constipation and disturbed defecation. Despite this fact, a uniform attitude regarding the value of the different diagnostic tools and the benefits of biofeedback is still lacking. It has been suggested that for some patients with constipation, there may be a sound indication for a surgical approach to their problem. However, even the hint of operative treatment of constipation is still controversial. Consequently, it is worthwhile to review the etiology of constipation and to discuss the controversies, especially those involving diagnosis, biofeedback, and surgical treatment.

DEFINITION

Constipation is a symptom, with a different meaning for different patients. Thus, what is meant by this complaint must be determined. To one individual the term may imply that the stools are too small, too hard, or too difficult to expel and to others that defecation is difficult, with characteristic symptoms such as prolonged and repeated straining at stool more than 25% of the time, rectal fullness, the sense of incomplete evacuation, or the necessity for manual assistance (4). Individuals' perceptions of constipation were studied by Moore-Gillon (5), who found that almost 50% considered constipation purely in terms of frequency of bowel actions, almost 25% in terms of straining, pain, and hard stool, and 30% in terms of both. Although symptoms such as fruitless straining and incomplete evacuation are rather subjective and unreliable, an international team of experts included these symptoms in its definition of constipation. This "Rome" definition requires two or more of the following criteria to be reported: (i) straining on more than 25% of bowel movements; (ii) feeling of incomplete evacuation after more than 25% of bowel movements; (iii) hard stool on more than 25% of bowel movements; and (iv) infrequent defecation with three or fewer bowel actions weekly (6).

Probert et al. (7) compared a validated estimate of the whole gut transit time with self-perceived constipation and the "Rome" definition and found little agreement between the definitions. Of 101 women classified as constipated by one or both of the subjective definitions, 64 had normal transit times. Based on these and other data the authors questioned the validity of the "Rome" definition and any other definition based on individual's perceptions, except for infrequency of defecation. Many subjects perceive themselves as constipated, only because they have straining and incomplete evacuation. These symptoms also occur in irritable bowel syndrome (8). Therefore, it seems reasonable to use stool frequency as a clinical guide. Drossman et al. (9) surveyed 789 students and hospital employees and found that 4.2% passed two or fewer stools per week. At present, some use the term constipation exclusively for the description of slow colonic transit, resulting in a stool frequency of fewer than two times per week and reserve the term disturbed or obstructed defecation for all the symptoms associated with impaired evacuation. Devroede (10) believes that a patient should be considered constipated under any of the following circumstances: (i) if the stool weight is less than 35 g per day; (ii) if fewer than three stools for women and five for men are passed per week while following a high residue diet (30 g of dietary fiber); or (iii) if more than three days pass without a bowel movement. Recently, Agachan et al. (11) developed a constipation scoring system based on the following aspects: stool frequency, evacuation difficulties, abdominal pain, time spent in the lavatory per attempt, assistance required for evacuation, number of unsuccessful attempts per 24 hours, and duration of constipation. Although the authors reported that their scoring system was found to be accurate, it is questionable whether such a complex and time-consuming scoring system has any impact on therapeutic decision making. Because these parameters are unreliable or difficult to evaluate, stool frequency remains as a clinical guide.

ETIOLOGY

The causes of constipation are numerous and diverse. Various classifications have been described, and most are either oversimplified or excessively detailed (10,12,13). The classification presented in the box although not exhaustive, is fairly comprehensive.

■ FAULTY DIET AND HABITS

Of outstanding importance are the epidemiologic studies of Burkitt, Painter, Walker, and others (14–17), which have shown that the fiber content of our foodstuffs is the prime factor that determines the fecal weight or bulk and the rate of transit through the colon. Inadequate dietary fiber, common in the Western diet, produces sparse, inspissated stools, whereas populations with a high fiber diet may have a normal bowel habit of two or three large, soft motions per day (17). Because peristaltic movements are stimulated by distention of the intestine, they tend to be sluggish when the food bulk is insufficient to cause a normal amount of distention. Excessive ingestion of foods that harden stools, such as processed cheese, and inadequate fluid intake may be contributing factors. Lack of exercise also decreases colonic activity.

Repeatedly ignoring the call to stool results in insensitivity of the reflex initiated by a fecal mass in the rectum. This in turn results in adaptation of the sensory mechanism so that arrival of further propulsive waves fails to produce an adequate call to stool. Ultimately, all natural periodic urges disappear (Box 1).

One of the imagined causes of constipation is the belief that a daily stool is necessary for good health. This belief may lead to the chronic abuse of harsh laxatives. After the bowel has been completely emptied by a purgative, it generally takes two days for fecal material to accumulate in sufficient quantity to stimulate the desire for a bowel action. Although this may seem self-evident, the absence of a bowel movement often increases the distress of a patient whose attention is focused on his or her bowel function. Further purgation (because of the failure to have a bowel movement the very next day) will unnecessarily abuse the intestine and ultimately lead to a complete loss of natural bowel habits (cathartic colon).

Environmental circumstances such as unfavorable working conditions, travel, and admission to the hospital may cause the patient to ignore the call to stool. Some are obviously only temporary problems.

■ STRUCTURAL OR FUNCTIONAL DISORDERS

Constipation may be only one of several symptoms with which a patient with disorders of bowel structure will present. Constipation in association with other symptoms will lead the examining physician to the appropriate diagnosis, often with the aid of certain investigative modalities. Clearly, obstructive lesions explain constipation, but patients with these lesions may have alternating constipation and diarrhea. Similarly, individuals with, painful anal lesions suppress the call to stool because of the fear of the pain of defecation. This suppression only aggravates the problem because the stool becomes harder and more difficult to pass (a detailed discussion of each cause in this section is provided under the specific heading either later in this chapter or in relevant chapters).

Through the use of radiopaque markers, a slow transit rate—particularly along the transverse, descending, and sigmoid colon—can be demonstrated. Its exact cause is unclear. Patients with idiopathic megabowel have a dilated rectum or distal colon, but ganglion cells are present. Transit studies also can show abnormalities. Patients with irritable bowel syndrome have the dominant complaint of abdominal pain, with constipation only an associated finding. Constipation is not an uncommon symptom associated with diverticular disease and may result from the tendency of the colon to form closed high-pressure segments.

BOX 1 ■ Classification of Causes of Constipation

Faulty Diet and Habits
Inadequate bulk (fiber)
Excessive ingestion of foods that harden stools (e.g., cheese)
Lack of exercise
Ignoring call to stool
Laxative abuse
Environmental changes (e.g., hospitalization, vacation)

Structural or Functional Disorders
- Colonic obstruction
  - Neoplasm, volvulus, inflammation (diverticulitis), ameboma, tuberculosis, syphilis, lymphogranuloma venereum, ischemic colitis, anastomotic stricture, endometriosis
- Diverticular disease
- Anorectal outlet obstruction
  - Anal obstruction (stenosis, fissure)
  - Rectocele
  - Spastic pelvic floor syndrome (anismus)
- Visceral neuropathy or myopathy
  - Congenital aganglionosis (Hirschsprung's disease)
  - Acquired aganglionosis (Chagas' disease)
  - Slow-transit constipation (colonic inertia)
  - Megarectum (sometimes with megacolon)
  - Chronic intestinal pseudo-obstruction
  - Acute Intestinal pseudo-obstruction (Ogilvie's Syndrome)
- Irritable bowel syndrome (visceral hypersensitivity)

Neurologic Abnormalities (Outside Colon)
Central nervous system (cerebral neoplasm, Parkinson's disease)
Trauma
Spinal cord (neoplasm, multiple sclerosis)
Defective innervation (resection of nervi erigentes)

Psychiatric Disorders
Depression
Psychoses
Anorexia nervosa

Iatrogenic Causes
Medication (codeine, antidepressants, iron, anticholinergics)
Immobilization

Endocrine and Metabolic Causes
Hypothyroidism
Hypercalcemia
Pregnancy
Diabetes mellitus
Dehydration
Hypokalemia
Uremia
Pheochromocytoma
Hypopituitarism
Lead poisoning
Porphyria
Mucoviscidosis

Aganglionosis, whether it occurs congenitally in patients with Hirschsprung's disease or is acquired because of the neurotoxin of *Trypanosoma cruzi*, will cause constipation.

■ NEUROLOGIC ABNORMALITIES

Defects of innervation such as those that follow pelvic surgery and occur with diseases of the spinal cord and brain are factors contributing to constipation. Severe constipation occurs in all patients who sustain a spinal cord injury. Menardo et al. (18) demonstrated that patients with injuries between C4 and T12 have a marked prolongation of transit at the level of the left colon and rectum, with minor degrees of transit delay at the level of the right colon. Several surveys have revealed that constipation in patients with spinal cord injury has a significant impact on their quality of life (19,20).

■ PSYCHIATRIC DISORDERS

Psychiatric disturbances often are associated with constipation. However, the medications used in the treatment of psychiatric illnesses very frequently contribute to or cause constipation in their own right. Some patients may become obsessed with their bowel function or lack thereof and resort to excessive laxative abuse. In addition, certain psychiatric patients will deny bowel actions while, in fact, their bowels are moving. Such patients can be detected with the use of radiopaque markers.

■ IATROGENIC CAUSES

A host of medications can contribute to constipation (frequent offenders are listed in box 1). Bedpans are uncomfortable and should be replaced by bedside commodes whenever feasible.

■ ENDOCRINE AND METABOLIC CAUSES

Patients with various endocrine abnormalities with their characteristic clinical patterns may cause constipation. Also included in this group are those patients who are pregnant.

INVESTIGATION

■ HISTORY

The diagnosis of constipation must be confirmed first because the patient's presenting symptoms may be more imagined than real. A simple history will determine the patient's stool frequency. When a patient has two or fewer bowel actions a week, the diagnosis of constipation is considered. The question is whether the reported stool frequency is reliable enough to diagnose constipation. Ashraf et al. (21) investigated 45 subjects complaining of infrequent defecation with fewer than two bowel actions weekly. The authors found a striking discrepancy between the reported stool frequencies on the one hand and objective measures on the other hand. More than half the patients who professed constipation were found to have underestimated stool frequency by three or more bowel actions weekly. In this group, a past history of psychiatric problems was common, and bowel symptoms correlated poorly with colonic transit time. Next, the onset of symptoms is determined because onset in childhood may point to a congenital cause such as Hirschsprung's disease, whereas a more recent onset might point to one of the specific disorders of bowel structure. A recent onset in an adult, especially with blood loss and mucus, is more commonly associated with significant colorectal pathology. Specific questions about dietary and bowel habits, laxative ingestion, other associated symptoms, and prior abdominal or pelvic surgery may lead to the correct diagnosis. Characteristic symptoms such as prolonged and repeated straining at stool, rectal fullness, sense of incomplete evacuation, and necessity for manual assistance may suggest a defecation disorder.

■ PHYSICAL EXAMINATION

In most patients with constipation, abdominal findings will be unremarkable. A stool-filled colon may be palpated. Rarely, a mass suggestive of a carcinoma or hepatomegaly suggestive of metastases may be found.

The anal region should be inspected carefully for findings such as fissures, hemorrhoids, fistulas, and abscesses. Digital examination might reveal a mass suggestive of a rectal neoplasm or a rock-hard fecaloma. In female patients with a rectocele, the pocket-like defect of the anterior rectal wall can be demonstrated just above the anal sphincter. Almy (22) has pointed out that the absence of stool in the rectum suggests that the difficulty lies above the rectum and makes a disorder of defecation unlikely. This observation is not valid if the patient is using laxatives, enemas, or suppositories.

Anal sensitivity and reflexes should be checked. Deficient sensation may represent a neurogenic disorder and cutaneosphincteric reflexes may be absent. In patients with Hirschsprung's disease, profuse fecal discharge occurs characteristically after rectal examination.

■ STOOL EXAMINATION

Gross examination of the stool might reveal a large, hard mass or possibly the pellet-like stools characteristically seen in patients with diverticular disease or irritable bowel syndrome. Stool also should be examined for occult blood, and any positive findings should be investigated further. It has been suggested that determination of stool weight and examination of stool form are mandatory in the evaluation of constipation, because both aspects are closely correlated with colonic transit time (21,23).

■ BIOCHEMICAL EXAMINATION

Routine biochemical examination, including values for electrolytes, calcium, phosphate, urea, creatinine, triiodothyronine, and thyroxine, is necessary to exclude those endocrine and metabolic disorders that can cause constipation.

Special biochemical investigations such as of gastrointestinal neuropeptides would be of interest, but they are not readily available. Interest has grown in the effect of these neuropeptides on gastrointestinal motility. Using sensitive and specific radioimmunoassays, the concentration of gastrointestinal neuropeptides can be determined quantitatively (24). The effect of these neuropeptides on the motor activity of the upper gastrointestinal tract (stomach, duodenum, and small intestine) has been established (24), but the exact role of some of these peptides in the regulation of colonic motor activity has not been determined (Table 1).

It has been suggested that gastrin and motilin have a stimulating effect on the peristaltic activity of the colon (24). Patients with constipation have a smaller rise in circulating blood levels of gastrin and motilin after a meal (25), whereas reduced motilin levels have been reported in pregnancy, when there is a tendency toward constipation (26). However, it is still unknown whether or not these phenomena are primary or secondary. The pharmacokinetics, catabolism, and release of these hormones are very complex. For example, the release of vasoactive intestinal peptide (VIP) from intramural neurons, especially those neurons in the lamina propria and circular muscle of the gut, is induced by stimulation of preganglionic parasympathetic fibers (24). This finding demonstrates the complex interaction between hormonal and neurogenic factors. Further investigation is necessary to determine the exact role of gastrointestinal hormones, especially in patients with slow-transit constipation.

TABLE 1 ■ Effect of Gastrointestinal Neuropeptides on Colonic Motility

In Vivo Effect	Gastrointestinal Neuropeptides
Stimulation	Gastrin Motilin Cholecystokinin (CCK) Oxytocin Corticotropin releasing factor (CRF) Neuropeptide Y Serotonin
Inhibition	Glucagon Somatostatin Secretin Calcitonin gene-related peptide (CGRP) Enkephalins Peptide YY
Unknown	Galanin Gastrin-releasing peptide (GRP) Vasoactive intestinal polypeptide (VIP) Neurotensin Substance P Bombesin
None	Gastric inhibitory polypeptide (GIP) Pancreatic polypeptide

■ PROCTOSIGMOIDOSCOPY

Endoscopic examination is mandatory to rule out the presence of a neoplasm. Nevertheless, in the vast majority of patients complaining of constipation, proctosigmoidoscopic examination will not reveal any abnormality. Frequently, patients with long-standing laxative abuse, mainly involving laxative ingredients of the anthracene family, will demonstrate melanosis coli, a discoloration of the mucosa that may range from light brown to black. In other patients, a solitary rectal ulcer, sometimes associated with anterior mucosal prolapse, will be found.

■ BARIUM ENEMA EXAMINATION

Although plain films of the abdomen occasionally show the extent of fecal accumulation, the main diagnostic tool to demonstrate structural abnormalities in the colon is the barium enema or colonoscopy. In constipation of recent origin, a barium enema study or colonoscopy is mandatory. Sometimes an unusually redundant colon is noted; other times an unusually dilated rectum and/or colon is found. The normal range for the width of the rectum and the colon has been established, with the upper limit of the rectosigmoid in a lateral view at the pelvic brim being 6.5 cm (27).

■ DEFECOGRAPHY

In the 1960s, cineradiography was developed for the dynamic investigation of the defecation mechanism. Some of the techniques used in that period were relatively complex, requiring time and sophisticated radiologic equipment. Currently, simplified techniques such as defecography and balloon proctography are available. Studies have shown that these techniques are reliable and simple to perform (28,29).

Defecography or evacuation proctography is an established radiologic technique to image the dynamic changes in rectal anatomy during attempted expulsion of barium paste (Fig. 2). This method offers the possibility of visualizing abnormalities such as anterior rectal wall prolapse, rectal intussusception, rectocele, and enterocele (30,31). Another application of this technique is the measurement of the anorectal angle. It is generally accepted that this angle, which depends on the tone of the puborectalis muscle, becomes more obtuse during attempted evacuation due to relaxation of the pelvic floor. Failure to increase the anorectal angle on straining, sometimes associated with accentuation of the puborectalis impression, is considered a radiologic sign of anismus. In patients with fecal incontinence the anorectal angle is widened even at rest (Fig. 3). It has been argued, however, that visual assessment of the anorectal angle is rather subjective and, therefore, unreliable. Several authors found wide interobserver and intraobserver variations in the measurement of this angle and concluded that its quantification has only limited clinical value (32,33). Defecography also enables the determination of the position of the pelvic floor by calculating the distance between the anorectal junction and the pubococcygeal line. Demonstrating a drop in the anorectal junction of several centimeters or more below the pubococcygeal line signifies the pathologic descent of the pelvic floor. Evacuation proctography also provides a valid estimate of the rate and degree of rectal emptying (34). These parameters can also be assessed utilizing scintigraphic methods (35) (Fig. 4). The investigation of rectal emptying is considered a major step in the evaluation of constipation, because many patients with infrequent bowel movements also present varying degrees of defecatory impairment. It has been argued, however, that the estimation of time and degree of rectal emptying is rather inaccurate (36). Furthermore, it is questionable whether a delayed and incomplete evacuation on proctography really represents impaired rectal emptying. Karlbom et al. (37) analyzed the relations between proctography findings, rectal emptying, and colonic transit time in 80 constipated patients. The correlation between a sense of obstruction and rectal evacuation as evaluated by defecography was found to be very poor. Patients who claimed emptying difficulties actually had the most efficient evacuation. It has also been suggested that incomplete and prolonged evacuation on proctography may be caused by inability to raise intra-abdominal pressure, thereby simply reflecting inadequate straining (38). Despite these and other objections, evacuation proctography is still considered as one of the most useful tools in the investigation of patients with constipation and disturbed defecation.

■ COLONIC TRANSIT TIME

A major step in the evaluation of constipation is the measurement of colonic transit time. The technique can establish an abnormality but also can demonstrate a normal transit time in a patient with a bowel neurosis or in the occasional patient who denies having bowel actions. With the original method described by Hinton, Lennard-Jones, and Young (39), 20 radiopaque markers of similar specific gravity to feces were ingested on one occasion on the first day before breakfast. Stools were collected and studied with radiography for 7 days or longer until all the pellets had been observed on a radiograph. A variation of this method has been described by Cummings and Wiggins (40). Markers of different shapes were ingested on three consecutive days. Subsequently, all markers present in a single stool collected on the fourth day were counted. This technique reduces the effect of day-to-day variation in transit time by providing three-day transit studies from one

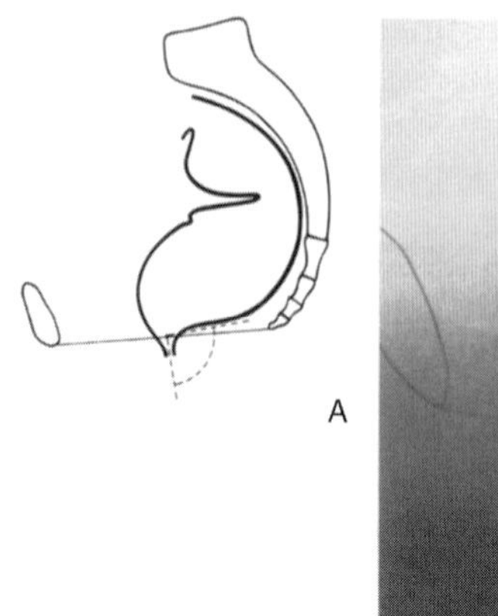

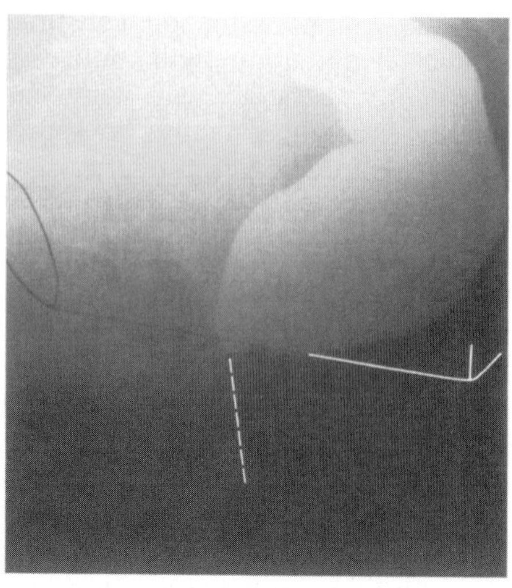

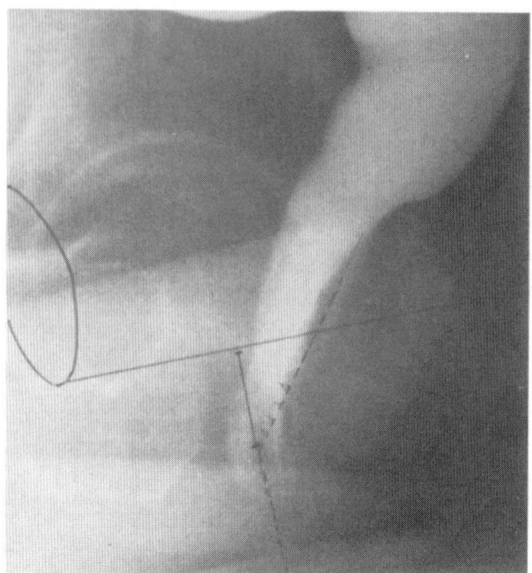

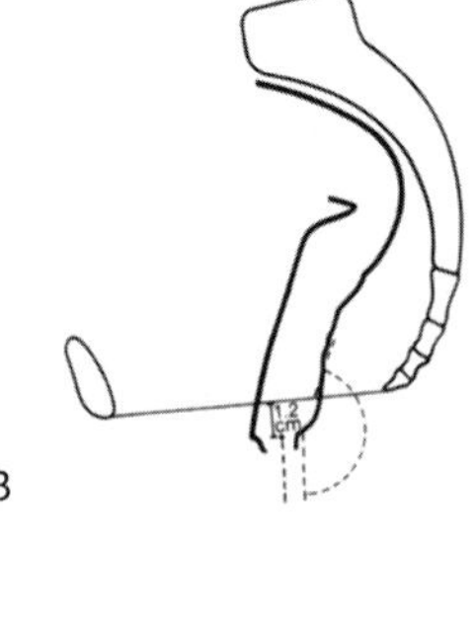

FIGURE 2 ■ Defecography in a normal patient. (**A**) At rest, x-ray film and diagram showing a normal anorectal angle of 92°. (**B**) During straining, x-ray film and diagram showing anorectal angle widens to 137°.

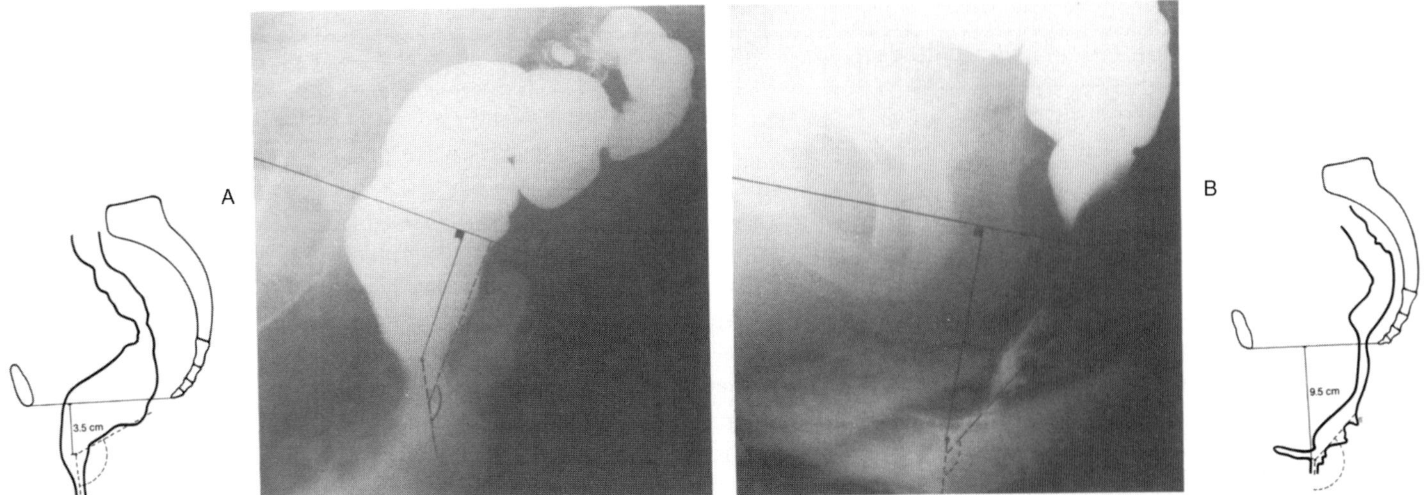

FIGURE 3 ■ Defecography in an incontinent patient. (**A**) At rest, loss of anorectal angle and widening of anal canal, pool of barium escaping beyond anal sphincter, and pathologic descent of perineum (anus well below pubococcygeal line) are noted. (**B**) During straining.

radiograph. Although these marker-appearance methods do not provide accurate data on transit through the different colonic regions, they can be used as a simple test to assess whole-gut transit time. With the Hinton technique, Evans et al. (41) found that 95% of normal male and female subjects pass less than 20% of markers within 12 hours and more than 80% of markers within 120 hours. This finding was similar to the original observation of Hinton et al. (39) in male subjects. It has been argued that it is more convenient to measure the disappearance of a marker from the colon rather than its appearance in the stool. Therefore, Martelli et al. (42) described a technique whereby the patient ingests a single dose of 20 markers. The progression of the markers is followed by daily films of the abdomen until complete expulsion is noted or for a maximum of seven days after ingestion of the markers. Normally all the markers have passed within 7 days. The arrival and disappearance of markers in three regions of the colon (right, left, and rectosigmoid) are assessed. For this purpose the spinal processes and two lines from the fifth lumbar vertebra to the pelvic inlet serve as landmarks (Fig. 5). Transit time is considered prolonged when more than 20% of the markers are still present within the colon, 5 days after ingestion. A drawback of interpretation of such studies is that evaluation of transit of contents in any segment is dependent on the amount of markers received from the proximal bowel.

To reduce the radiation exposure, Metcalf et al. (43) developed a somewhat different technique by giving differently shaped markers on three successive days and taking

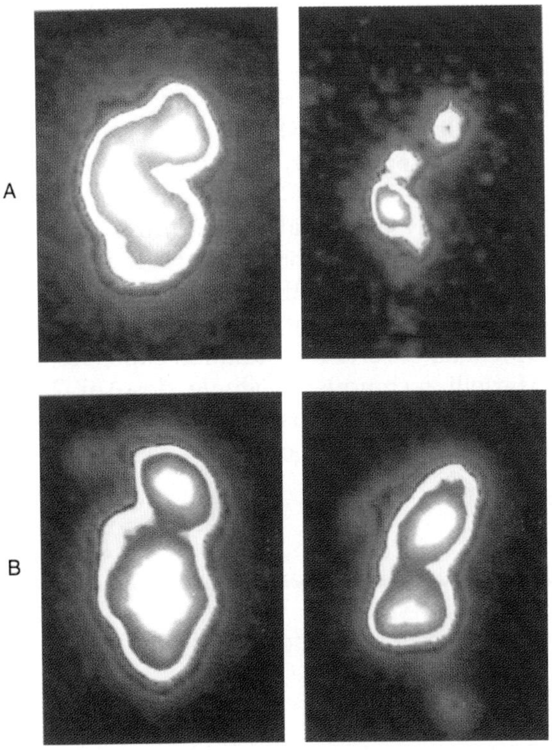

A

B

FIGURE 4 ■ Scintigraphic defecography. A semisolid mixture of beaten cooked eggs, the albumin of which is tagged with Tc sulfur colloid (1 mCi per 350 cc volume) and placed into the rectum by catheter. (**A**) Normal evacuation; (*Left*) Preevacuation; (*Right*) postevacuation (95% evacuation). (Normal values, 85–95% evacuation). (**B**) Incomplete evacuation; (*Left*) Preevacuation; (*Right*) postevacuation (58% evacuation, 42% retention). *Source*: Paul Belliveau, M.D., Montreal, Quebec).

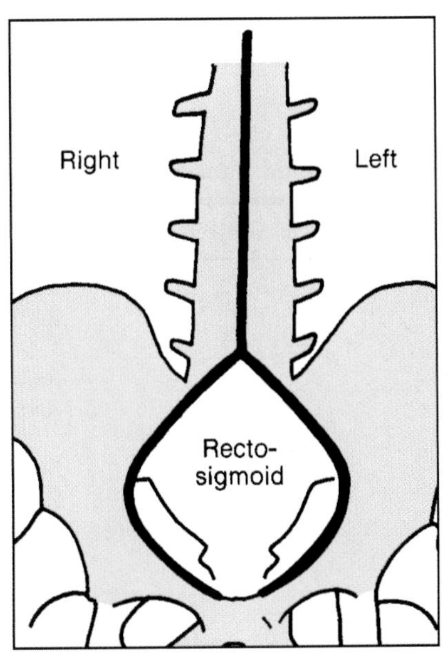

FIGURE 5 ■ Landmarks for markers used to determine transit time.

TABLE 2 ■ **Normal Values for Whole-Gut Transit Time, Expressed in Hours**

Author(s)	No. of Subjects	Method	Mean ± SD	Upper Limit
Cummings and Wiggins (40) (1976)	12	Radiopaque markers	54±9	72
Metcalf et al. (43) (1987)	21	Radiopaque markers	53±8	70
Evans et al. (41) (1992)	43	Radiopaque markers	120±ns	168
Basile et al. (49) (1992)	12	Magnetic markers	56±5	ns
van der Sijp et al. (45) (1993)	12	Radioisotopes	ns	103

Abbreviations: SD, standard deviation; ns, not stated.

an abdominal radiograph on the fourth day after ingestion and if necessary on days 7 and 10. Chaussade et al. (44) modified this technique by giving identical markers on three consecutive days. The quantification of regional colonic transit with these methods has been validated in healthy subjects. It is questionable, however, whether infrequent radiographs allow correct assessment of the site of delay in constipated patients with irregular mass movements, because the results will be very different if a radiograph is taken just before or just after such an event. It has been suggested that the use of radioisotopes provides more accurate information about regional colonic transit, because multiple images can be obtained with a low radiation dose. An additional advantage of scintigraphy is the clear delineation of the different colonic regions, even in subjects with a significant overlap of bowel segments. The use of a radiolabeled meal also yields information about gastric emptying and small bowel transit (45). The radioisotope can also be administered in a coated capsule, which is designed to dissolve at the pH found in the distal part of the small bowel (46), or as a liquid through a tube placed to instill it in the cecum or the ascending colon (47).

Another technique to measure intestinal transit was developed by Ewe et al. (48). They followed a metal particle on its way through the gastrointestinal tract by means of a portable detector. Basile et al. (49) used a magnetized steel sphere and localized this particle with biomagnetic instruments. With this technique they were able to demonstrate that the total colonic transit time in healthy volunteers was 44 ± 5 hours (mean ± SD). Similar figures have been reported by others. The normal values for whole-gut transit time, total colonic transit time, and segmental colonic transit time are listed in Tables 2, 3 and 4.

For the investigation of our own patients, one author has adopted the technique of Martelli et al. (42) and uses commonly available markers (Sitz-marks). The patient is instructed to consume 30 g of dietary fiber daily, and to refrain from the use of laxatives, enemas, and all other nonessential medications for at least 48 hours before and during the investigation. The progression of the markers is followed by daily films of the abdomen until complete expulsion of the markers occurs for a maximum of 7 days after ingestion. The markers are counted in three segments of the large bowel: right, left, and rectosigmoid (see Fig. 5). The transit times of the whole gut and of each segment of the colon are compared with normal values. In this way, patients with colonic inertia, in whom a prolonged whole-gut transit time is found, with markers distributed throughout the large bowel from the cecum to the rectum, can be distinguished from those suffering from anorectal outlet obstruction, in which the markers proceed quickly along the colon but accumulate in the rectum. Another group of patients may exhibit a pattern in which the markers proceed to and then accumulate along the left colon.

The other author has recently adopted the technique described by Dorval et al. (54). All subjects ingest 10 similar radiopaque markers every morning for six consecutive days. On the seventh day an abdominal radiograph is taken. Total and segmental transit times are calculated according to Arhan's method (transit time, $2.4 \times n$). n is the number of markers in the considered zone. This technique is more convenient for the patient. Only one radiograph is taken, and the radiation exposure is minimal. If the Martelli technique (a single dose of 20 markers, followed by daily films) is used in a patient with slow-transit constipation, you might observe a rather normal transit

TABLE 3 ■ **Normal Values for Total Colonic Transit Time, Expressed in Hours**

Author(s)	No. of Subjects	Method	Sex	Mean ± SD	Upper Limit
Arhan et al. (50) (1981)	38	Radiopaque markers		39±5	93
Metcalf et al. (43) (1987)	73	Radiopaque markers	M	31±18	66
			F	39±18	75
Chaussade et al. (51) (1989)	22	Radiopaque markers		34±16	67
Meir et al. (52) (1992)	128	Radiopaque markers	M	30±2	44
			F	41+3	77
Basile et al. (49) (1992)	12	Magnetic markers		44±5	ns
Escalante et al. (53) (1993)	18	Radiopaque markers		28±ns	ns
Dorval et al. (54) (1994)	82	Radiopaque markers	M	25±ns	77
			F	47±ns	91
Bouchoucha et al. (55) (1995)	11	Radiopaque markers		36±3	ns

Abbreviations: F, female; M, male; ns, not significant; SD, standard deviation.

TABLE 4 ■ Normal Values of Segmental Colonic Transit Time, Expressed in Hours

Author(s)	No. of Subjects	Sex	Right Colon	Left Colon	Recto-sigmoid
Arhan et al. (50) (1981)	38		14	14	11
Metcalf et al. (43) (1987)	73	M	9	9	13
		F	13	14	12
Chaussade et al. (51) (1989)	22		7	9	18
Basile et al. (49) (1992)	12		27	15	12
Escalante et al. (53) (1993)	18		7	10	11
Dorval et al. (54) (1994)	82		8	13	12
		M	7	8	8
		F	10	21	17
Bouchoucha et al. (55) (1995)	11		7	16	14

Abbreviations: F, female; M, male.

time when, after a long period, the patient has his or her first bowel movement, just a few days after the ingestion of the markers. The Dorval technique eliminates the influence of such an "accidental" bowel movement.

■ ANORECTAL MANOMETRY

A number of authors advocate the use of anorectal manometry during the initial evaluation of constipation and disturbed defecation to develop individualized and more effective modes of treatment (56,57).

In patients with Hirschsprung's disease, rectal distention does not induce internal sphincter relaxation; hence manometry can be used as a reliable test in the diagnosis of Hirschsprung's disease (58,59). Although manometry is clearly useful in discriminating Hirschsprung's disease from other forms of constipation, its role in the evaluation and management of non-Hirschsprung's constipation remains unclear. There are few data correlating manometric findings with clinical symptoms and outcome of treatment. Studying encopretic children, Loening-Baucke (56) was able to demonstrate that the response to different treatment modalities could be predicted by manometric findings. Borowitz et al. (60) studied 44 children with chronic constipation and encopresis. Spasm of the external anal sphincter during attempted defecation was correlated with the patient's age at onset, duration of symptoms, and the frequency of fecal soiling. All other manometric parameters did not correlate; either with the frequency of bowel movements, or with the other reported symptoms. These observations suggest that manometric findings are not representative of the natural defecation act. They also question the conceptual understanding of childhood constipation, based on the assumption that a diminished sense of rectal distention and paradoxical contraction of the external anal sphincter are the principal causes of constipation and obstructed defecation. In adults, similar conflicting findings have been observed. Pluta et al. (61) studied 24 female patients with severe and disabling slow-transit constipation who underwent a subtotal colectomy followed by ileorectal anastomosis. No correlation was noted between the results of the operation and the manometric parameters, except in one case. Patients requiring abnormally high pressures inside a distending rectal balloon for sensory perception and internal anal sphincter relaxation did poorer than the others. Another striking predictive factor, noted by these authors, was a history of psychiatric illness.

TABLE 5 ■ Resting Anal Pressure in Patients with Non-Hirschsprung's Constipation

Author(s)	Method	Resting Anal Pressure
Arhan et al. (63) (1972)	Balloon system	Normal
Meunier et al. (64) (1979)	Open-tipped catheter	Elevated
Iwai et al. (65) (1979)	Open-tipped catheter	Elevated
Taylor et al. (66) (1980)	Open-tipped catheter	Elevated
Suzuki et al. (67) (1980)	Open-tipped catheter	Normal
Loening-Baucke and Younoszai (68) (1982)	Microtransducer	Normal
Molnar et al. (69) (1983)	Balloon system	Elevated
Read et al. (70) (1986)	Open-tipped catheter	Reduced
Roe et al. (71) (1986)	Microballoon	Normal
Shouler and Keighley (72) (1986)	Balloon system	Normal

TABLE 6 ■ Amplitude of Internal Sphincter Reflex in Patients with Non-Hirschsprung's Constipation

Author(s)	Method	Amplitude
Clayden and Lawson (73) (1976)	Open-tipped catheter	Less
Taylor et al. (66) (1980)	Open-tipped catheter	Normal
Suzuki et al. (67) (1980)	Open-tipped catheter	Normal
Loening-Baucke and Younoszai (68) (1982)	Microtransducer	Less
Read et al. (70) (1986)	Open-tipped catheter	Normal

Many demonstrable pressure abnormalities can be detected by anorectal manometry in patients with idiopathic constipation. The reflex may be normal, the amplitude of relaxation may be less than in normal controls, or the reflex may be totally absent. The resting pressure of the anal canal may be greater than expected and occasionally is accompanied by a rectoanal inhibitory reflex with an amplitude greater than normal (62).

In several studies, elevated anal resting pressures have been found in patients with idiopathic constipation, but in other studies no pressure abnormalities could be detected (Table 5). Although some authors suggested a normal amplitude of the internal sphincter reflex, these findings are not supported by the results of two other studies that showed the amplitude of relaxation is less in patients with idiopathic constipation than in normal controls (Table 6). In patients with severe chronic constipation without megarectum, the threshold for the internal sphincter reflex apparently was normal, whereas in patients with a megarectum the threshold was elevated (Table 7).

Despite the conflicting published data, manometry should continue as part of the evaluation of the severely constipated patient. Only by the continued study of these patients will there be a resolution of the discrepancies that have been reported to date.

During the last decade, attention has been focused on rectal wall properties. Grotz et al. investigated rectal wall contractility in controls and in patients with chronic severe constipation. They found that in patients with constipation the increase in rectal tone following a meal and after the

TABLE 7 ■ Threshold for Internal Sphincter Reflex in Patients with Non-Hirschsprung's Constipation

Author(s)	Method	Threshold	
		With Megarectum	Without Megarectum
Arhan et al. (63) (1972)	Balloon	Elevated	
Meunier et al. (64) (1979)	Open-tipped catheter	Normal	Normal
Taylor et al. (66) (1980)	Open-tipped catheter	Elevated	
Suzuki et al. (67) (1980)	Open-tipped catheter	Elevated	Normal
Loening-Baucke and Younoszai (68) (1982)	Microtransducer		Normal
Molnar et al. (69) (1983)	Balloon		Normal
Shouler and Keighley (72) (1986)	Balloon		Elevated

administration of a cholinergic agonist was significantly blunted. According to these authors, the reduced rectal tone contributes to the inability of these patients to expel stool (74). Other workers from the Netherlands used an electronic barostat assembly to examine rectal tone in response to an evoked urge to defecate. Under radiological control an infinitely compliant polyethylene bag was inserted over a guide wire into the proximal part of the rectum. Additionally, a latex balloon was introduced into the distal part of the rectum. This latex balloon was inflated until an urge to defecate was experienced. Simultaneously, rectal wall tone was assessed by measuring the variations in bag volume. These variations were expressed as percentage changes from the baseline volume. Comparing female controls and women with obstructed defecation, a significant difference was found regarding mean distending volume required to elicit an urge to defecate (median values: 125 vs. 320 cc of air). Twenty-four patients (24%) did not feel an urge to defecate at all. In all controls, the evocation of an urge to defecate induced a pronounced increase in rectal tone, proximal to the distending balloon. In the patients, this increase in rectal tone was significantly lower. Thirty-one patients (31%) showed no increase in rectal tone at all (75). It has been shown that rectal tone increases after a meal. This phenomenon is absent or blunted in women with obstructed defecation (76). These data indicate that the sensorimotor function of the rectum is impaired in patients with obstructed defecation. Afferent parasympathetic nerves are thought to mediate rectal filling sensations. These nerves run from the rectum through branches, which are situated on each side of the rectum around the cervix uteri and both lateral vaginal surfaces. This extensive network of nerve fibres can be damaged during hysterectomy and also during rectopexy with division of the lateral ligaments. It is well known that in some women, obstructed defecation starts following pelvic surgery. Varma et al. studied rectal function in 14 women with intractable constipation following hysterectomy. These patients had significantly decreased rectal sensory perception (77). It has been shown that constipation occurs more frequently, the more radical a hysterectomy is performed (78). Based on an experimental study in dogs, Shafik et al. addressed the important role of the parasympathetic nervous system in the defecation mechanism (79). These and other data do suggest that a deficit of the afferent parasympathetic nerves contribute to the impaired sensorimotor function of the rectum in women with obstructed defecation.

■ ELECTROMYOGRAPHY

Electromyography (EMG) can be used as a functional test for the investigation of muscle activity and is a proven reliable method for the evaluation of electrical activity in the external anal sphincter and puborectalis muscles (80) (Chapter 2).

Through electrophysiologic techniques it has been shown that damage can occur to the nerve supply of the external sphincter and the puborectalis muscle in patients with chronic constipation; this damage is probably due to perineal descent during defecation straining (81). Paradoxical contraction of the pelvic floor during attempted evacuation is considered as the principal cause of obstructed defecation. The terms most frequently used to describe this condition are anismus, spastic pelvic floor syndrome, and nonrelaxing puborectalis syndrome. Despite many limitations EMG is probably the most specific test providing the best assessment of pelvic floor activity during straining (see Fig. 18, Chapter 2).

■ BALLOON EXPULSION TEST

The balloon expulsion test is another method commonly used to reach the diagnosis of anismus. This simple test was introduced by Preston and Lennard-Jones in 1985 (82). It has been reported that almost all controls are able to expel a water-filled rectal balloon; whereas many constipated patients fail to do so. Although this observation underscores the difference between controls and patients, it does not signify that the inability to expel a balloon represents anismus. Normal rectal evacuation requires adequate intrarectal pressure, which can be raised by increasing intrapelvic pressure, achieved by voluntary contraction of the diaphragm and abdominal wall muscles. Propulsive contractile activity of the rectal wall is another contributing factor. It has been reported that constipated patients with both prolonged evacuation and reduced pelvic floor descent on proctography are not able to void a small nondeformable rectal balloon because they fail to raise intrarectal pressure (38). This finding suggests that failure to raise intrapelvic pressure is a major cause of inadequate evacuation.

The aforementioned diagnostic tests are generally recommended, because it is difficult to differentiate subgroups of constipation based on symptoms alone. Despite this recommendation, the clinical utility of these tests is still not known. Recently, Rao and coworkers conducted a systematic review of studies assessing the clinical value of these tests in patients with constipation. Their search revealed no methodologically sound studies. Their review identified several pitfalls. Firstly, no single test appears to provide a pathophysiological basis for constipation. Often, several tests are required to identify the underlying mechanism. Secondly, the inclusion criteria for patients with constipation were either not defined or when available there were significant inter-study differences. Thirdly, a reference or gold standard test is still missing. Despite these pitfalls, the authors concluded that, "there is good evidence to support the use of these tests in order to define subtypes of constipation and aid treatment" (83).

■ SPECIAL EXAMINATIONS

Routine Histologic Examination

In patients with solitary rectal ulcer syndrome, performing a biopsy is mandatory to confirm the diagnosis. Histologic examination will reveal fibromuscular obliteration of the lamina propria, hypertrophy of the muscularis mucosa, and displacement of glands into the submucosa (84,85) (Fig. 6).

When Hirschsprung's disease is suspected, a biopsy is indicated because, classically, aganglionosis is diagnostic of Hirschsprung's disease (Fig. 7). There is no consensus as to whether the best biopsy technique is the superficial punch biopsy, deep full-thickness biopsy, or mucosal suction biopsy. Usually biopsy specimens are taken 2 to 3 cm above the dentate line, as recommended by Aldridge and Campbell (86), who demonstrated a normal hypoganglionic zone in the region of the internal sphincter. This hypoganglionic zone extends proximally from the dentate line an average of 4 mm in the myenteric plexus, 7 mm in the deep submucous plexus, and 10 mm in the superficial submucous plexus. In two studies, it was suggested that the optimal level at which the biopsy should be taken is 1.0 to 1.5 cm above the dentate line (87,88). The authors chose this lower range because taking rectal biopsy specimens at a higher level may result in a missed diagnosis of ultrashort-segment aganglionosis (87). It is not certain how the measurements in these reports from pediatric patients might apply to the adult.

Several difficulties arise in the histopathologic interpretation of biopsy specimens. First, the distal segment of bowel does not contain neurons for up to 25 mm from the distal edge of the internal sphincter, and the normal value for adults is unknown. Second, the severity of the clinical course correlates poorly with the length of the aganglionic segment. A third problem of the histopathologic interpretation lies in the potential existence of "skip" lesions. A fourth problem concerns the qualitative appearance of the nervous plexus (62). Fifth, quantitatively hypoganglionosis causes constipation, but the range of the normal number of ganglion cells is not known (89). Finally, the diagnostic accuracy with routine hematoxylin and eosin staining on superficial biopsies is low, as was demonstrated in a study showing an accuracy rate of only 61% (87).

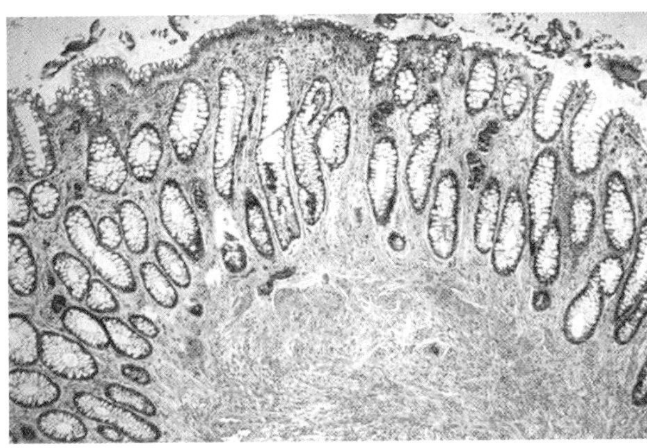

FIGURE 6 ■ Solitary ulcer syndrome demonstrated by microscopic biopsy of edge of ulcer with thickened lamina propria.

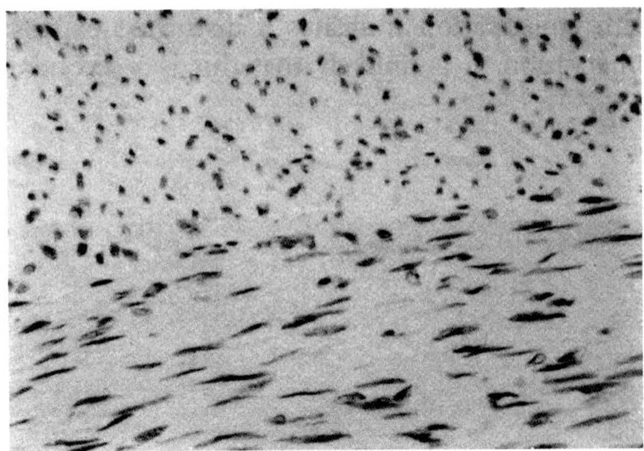

FIGURE 7 ■ Hirschsprung's disease.

Ultrastructural studies of colonic biopsies from patients with a history of long-term laxative abuse, primarily involving anthraquinone derivatives or bisacodyl, indicated that submucosal nerve fibers might be severely damaged. These alterations may correlate morphologically to the clinically evident disturbance of gut motility (90).

Acetylcholinesterase Staining

Increased acetylcholinesterase activity has been demonstrated in patients with Hirschsprung's disease (91–94). With acetylcholinesterase staining, an increased number of enlarged, brown-stained nerve fibers can be found in either the submucosa or the lamina propria (Fig. 8). According to Ikawa et al. (87), this technique has many advantages over routine hematoxylin and eosin staining. The authors demonstrated 99% accuracy in the differentiation of patients with Hirschsprung's disease from patients with idiopathic constipation. Park et al. (95) demonstrated a 97% diagnostic accuracy compared with a 74% accuracy of hematoxylin and eosin staining. Routine hematoxylin and eosin staining of superficial biopsy specimens failed to reveal ganglion cells in 39% of their patients

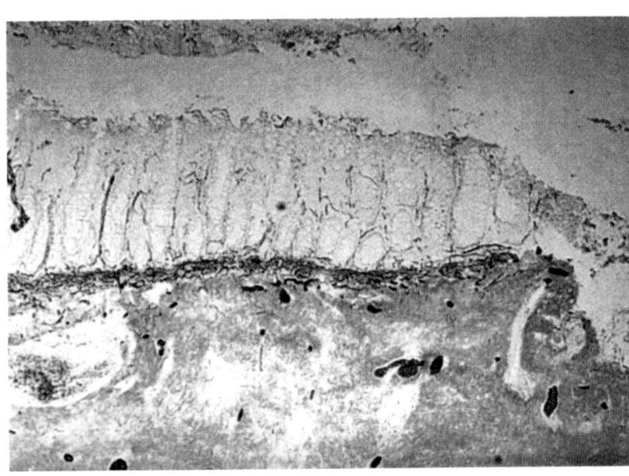

FIGURE 8 ■ Acetylcholinesterase staining used to demonstrate parasympathetic nerve. Note axon bundles with dark staining in center of microphotograph, with staining of small filaments in periphery.

without Hirschsprung's disease, all of whom required repeat superficial biopsy studies or even deep full thickness biopsies while under general anesthesia. Using acetylcholinesterase staining, this problem can be eliminated. Even if the submucosa is not included in the superficial biopsy, the diagnosis still can be made by studying the lamina propria. The histochemical demonstration of acetylcholinesterase activity in suction rectal biopsy specimens is considered an accurate technique and has been recommended in screening for Hirschsprung's disease (96).

Monoclonal Antineurofilament Antibodies

It has been proposed that a distinct visceral neuropathy may be present in patients with idiopathic slow-transit constipation and in patients with idiopathic megacolon. However, with the use of conventional light microscopy (hematoxylin and eosin staining), no abnormalities have been found. Examining resected colon specimens with silver staining (Smith's method), Preston et al. (97) demonstrated complete loss of the argyrophil plexus with a marked increase in Schwann cells, indicating that extrinsic damage to the plexus had occurred. Based on these findings, the authors theorized that the myenteric plexus abnormality is not the primary cause but may be the result of long-standing laxative use. Using conventional light microscopy, Krishnamurthy et al. (98) found no apparent abnormalities of the myenteric plexus in 12 patients who underwent subtotal colectomy for constipation. In contrast, silver stains of the myenteric plexus showed quantitatively reduced numbers of argyrophilic neurons in 10 patients, morphologically abnormal argyrophilic neurons in 11, decreased numbers of axons in 11, and increased numbers of variable-sized nuclei within ganglia in all 12. Thus, severe idiopathic constipation is associated with a pathologically identifiable abnormality of the myenteric plexus (98).

Koch et al. (99) found decreased colonic VIP in patients with idiopathic chronic constipation. This finding could not be confirmed by Tzavella et al. (100), who found normal levels of VIP and decreased levels of the excitatory neurotransmitter substance P in rectal biopsies from patients with slow-transit constipation.

An immunostaining technique using monoclonal antibodies raised against neurofilament (NF_2F_{11}; Sanbio) has been described for the investigation of bowel innervation anomalies (101). In the normally functioning bowel, some axons of the submucous plexus and the myenteric plexus do stain with these monoclonal antibodies (Table 8) (Fig. 9A). In contrast to this subtotal (partial) staining in normal bowel, heavy total axon-bundle staining has been found in the aganglionic segment of patients with Hirschsprung's disease (Table 8) (Fig. 9B).

Schouten et al. (102) were able to demonstrate that in 29 out of 39 patients with slow-transit constipation, the apparently normal axon bundles in the myenteric plexus stained markedly less than normal or failed to stain at all with the monoclonal antibody. In 17 patients this reduced or absent neurofilament expression was found along the entire length of the colon, whereas in 12 patients only a portion of the colon was affected. The same picture was found in the proximal ganglionic segment in 18 of 22 patients with persistent constipation after colectomy for aganglionosis

TABLE 8 ■ Immunostaining with Antineurofilament Monoclonal Antibody NF_2F_{11}

	Hematoxylin–Eosin–Staining Antibody	NF_2F_{11}
Normal colon		
Ganglion cells	+	–
Meissner axons	+	+
Auerbach axons	+	++
Hirschsprung's disease		
Ganglion cells	–	–
Meissner axons	–	+++
Auerbach axons	–	+++
Slow-transit constipation		
Ganglion cells	+	–
Meissner axons	+	–
Auerbach axons	+	–

+ = Positive result; – = negative result.

(103) (Fig. 9C). Because intrinsic innervation is lacking in patients with Hirschsprung's disease, the stained axon bundles in the aganglionic segment can only be of extrinsic origin. Therefore, the lack of axonal staining in patients with constipation indicates a disturbed extrinsic innervation. It is unlikely that this is a secondary phenomenon caused by laxatives because the same condition was found in neonates with severe constipation who were never treated with laxatives.

Two studies have revealed increased serotonin levels in the colonic mucosa and normal serotonin levels in the colonic muscularis propria of patients with slow-transit constipation (104,105). The question is why colonic motility is reduced and transit is prolonged despite local high and normal serotonin levels. It has been suggested that abnormal expression of the serotonin receptors in the colonic wall contributes to colonic inertia. Recently, Zhao et al. were able to demonstrate a reduced expression of serotonin receptors in the left colon of patients with this type of constipation (106). Wedel and coworkers compared the colonic enteric nervous system of patients with slow-transit constipation with the enteric nervous system of controls. They performed a morphometric analysis of the submucous plexus and the myenteric plexus. This analysis was based on Protein Gene Product 9.5 immunohistochemistry. In patients with slow-transit constipation, the total ganglionic area and neuronal number per intestinal length as well as the mean neuron count per ganglion were significantly decreased within the myenteric plexus and the external part of the submucous plexus. The ratio of glia cells to neurons was increased in myenteric ganglia but not in submucous ganglia. The observed quantitative alterations of the colonic enteric nervous system resemble the histologic features by oligoneuronal hypoganglionosis (107). Two recent studies provide further evidence for these findings. Bassotti et al. examined the surgical specimens from 26 patients with slow-transit constipation. They used conventional and immunohistochemical methods. Comparing patients and controls they found a significant decrease in enteric neurons, glial cells, and interstitial cells of Cajal in the constipated subjects (108). Similar findings have been reported by Lee et al. (109). Although all these data provide evidence

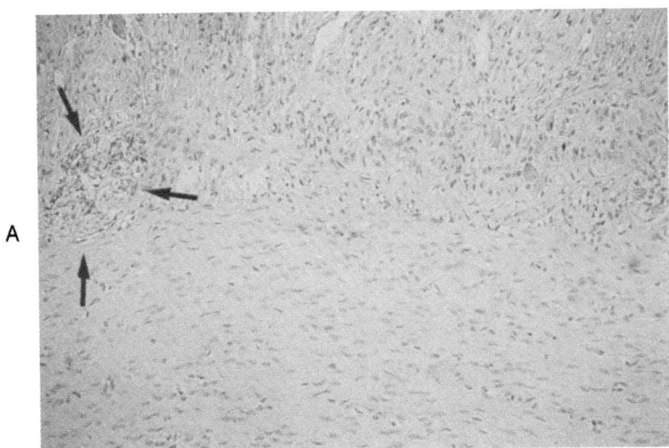

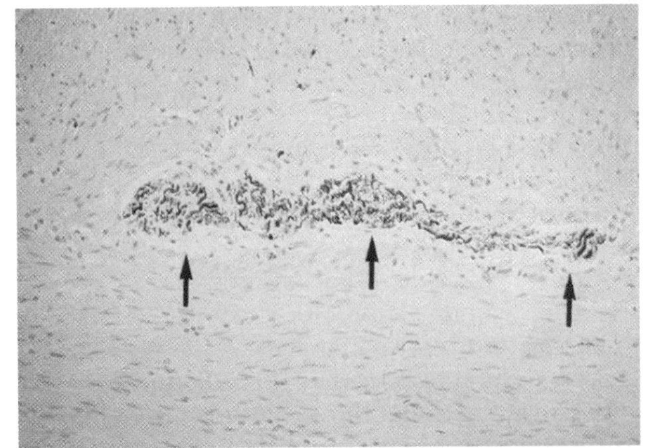

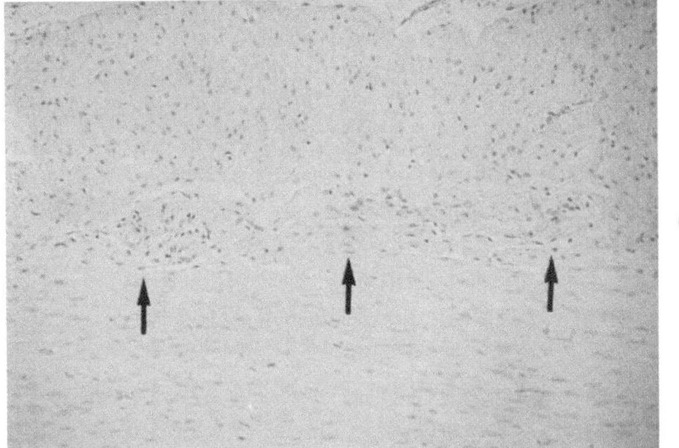

FIGURE 9 ■ Monoclonal antineurofilament antibody. (**A**) Normal: subtotal staining of axonal fibers in myenteric plexus (*arrows*). (**B**) Hirschsprung's disease: deep stain (increased) in myenteric plexus (*arrows*). (**C**) Idiopathic slow-transit constipation: absence of staining in myenteric plexus (*arrows*).

for the neuropathologic deficit in patients with slow-transit constipation, it is still not known whether these alterations of the colonic enteric nervous system are secondary to long-standing constipation or represent a primary defect.

■ PSYCHOLOGICAL EVALUATION

The exact role of psychological factors as related to bowel function has not been defined clearly, but suggestions of such influence have been made. Tucker et al. (110) suggested that stool weight and bowel frequency correlated with personality as much as with variations in fiber intake. Heavier stools tended to be produced by individuals who were more socially outgoing, more energetic and optimistic, and less anxious and who described themselves in more favorable terms than others. A common cause of withholding stool during childhood has been attributed to conflict between parent and child over bowel function.

It is well known that constipation and disturbed defecation occur primarily in women. It is still not clear why these conditions are characterized with such preponderance. One explanation might be the relationship between hysterectomy and changes in bowel habits. Another explanation for the female preponderance might be the fact that women are prone to develop a symptomatic rectocele. It is unlikely, however, that the adverse side effects of hysterectomy and the defecation difficulties due to rectoceles account for all the cases of constipation and disturbed defecation. It is well known that many patients use somatization as a defensive strategy for dealing with psychological distress. This unconscious defense mechanism can be uncovered by several psychological tests such as the Minnesota Multiphasic Personality Inventory (MMPI). In 1989 Devroede et al. (111) used the MMPI to compare women with idiopathic (functional) constipation and women with arthritis. The authors reported that many constipated women demonstrated a "conversion V" profile pattern, which indicates the presence of a somatization defense structure. This finding has been confirmed by others (112). In 1990, Drossman et al. (113) demonstrated that a history of sexual and physical abuse is a frequent experience in women seen in a referral-based gastrointestinal practice and is particularly common in those with functional gastrointestinal disorders. Of 209 consecutive female patients, 89 (44%) reported a history of abuse, but only 17% had informed their physicians. This extremely high prevalence of a past history of sexual abuse is similar to that found by Leroi et al. (114), who reported that 40% of patients suffering from functional disorders of the lower gastrointestinal tract gave a history of having been victims of sexual abuse in contrast to only 10% of patients with organic disease. The prevalence was similar in private practice and university hospital settings. The most frequent symptom of abused patients was constipation. The prevalence of abuse was four times greater in patients with lower rather than upper functional motor disorders. The risk of having a history of sexual abuse was nine times greater among patients with manometric evidence of anismus. The clinical implications of these findings are noteworthy. Because the vast majority of abused patients do not report their hidden history, this type of information must be actively sought.

Dykes and coworkers performed a psychological enquiry among patients with chronic constipation. These patients were assessed for evidence of previous and current affective disorders. A previous episode of psychiatric illness was noted in 64% of the patients, whereas a current affective disorder was observed in 61% of the subjects. Based on these findings the authors suggest that patients who present to surgical departments with chronic intractable constipation should routinely have a psychological assessment (115). It is well known that the vast majority of patients with constipation, especially those with a slow colonic transit, are women (116). It has been suggested that aspects of female identity provide clues to the underlying nature of this condition. Mason et al. conducted a study to examine possible emotional difficulties related to female identity in women with idiopathic constipation and compared the findings with an age-matched group of healthy women and with an age-matched group of women with Crohn's disease. Women with idiopathic constipation were found to have increased psychological and social morbidity, characterized by anxiety, depression, and social dysfunction. They also had increased somatization, less satisfaction in their sexual life, and an altered perception about female self (117). It has been shown that this type of morbidity is associated with altered rectal mucosa blood flow, indicating autonomic dysfunction (118). Chan et al. observed defective use of coping strategies in patients with functional constipation. These differing coping mechanisms were reflected in an absent or blunted rectal sensory perception (119).

It has been shown that biofeedback alone is not successful in the treatment of abused patients with anismus (120). The clinical outcome could be improved by adding psychotherapy to biofeedback conditioning.

Patients with mental defects are liable to the development of megacolon, and constipation may be a presenting symptom of a depressive illness. Patients with anorexia often develop intractable constipation, presumably caused in part by inadequate food intake. A patient may deny the passage of stool, although a transit study may demonstrate clearly that defecation actually has occurred. The denial of passage of stool emphasizes the need to obtain objective evidence of a prolonged transit time before any operative treatment is contemplated.

WHY TREAT CONSTIPATION?

DISPELLING MYTHS

Patients first must be reassured that there is a wide variation of normality with regard to the frequency of bowel movements. The folklore and mythology associated with the need for daily evacuation must be dispelled. Advertising encourages self-purgation by making people feel guilty about constipation and by portraying daily bowel movements as the secret to a healthy and happy life. Erroneous concepts such as the belief that toxic substances may be absorbed into the body without a daily bowel movement must be cast aside.

ASSOCIATED SYMPTOMS AND DAILY ACTIVITY

Martelli et al. (42) noted that constipation is not without associated symptoms and complications. The authors noted the disappearance of a multitude of symptoms after successful surgical treatment of constipation. Symptoms described included hard stools, stools difficult to evacuate, abdominal distention and bloating, and anorexia. Signs included fecalomas, abdominal masses, and abdominal tenderness. To this list, Thompson (121) added foul breath, furred tongue, flatulence, headache, and irritability. Regardless of the cause of constipation, absence of the numerous associated symptoms should allow the patient to function better in his usual daily activity.

POTENTIAL DISEASE

Although the immediate adverse effect of low-fiber diets may be constipation, the long-term adverse effects may include diverticular disease and malignancy, as noted in studies that link the low-fiber content of the usual Western diet with an increased risk of colon carcinoma and diverticulosis (122). Three studies suggest the link between carcinoma and constipation (123–125). More women with carcinoma of the colon had antecedent constipation than a comparable group of controls without constipation. More men with carcinoma of the rectum had a history of constipation. In a study by Wynder and Shigematsu (125), having three stools per week for a long period of time was considered a risk factor. However, in a penetrating review Cranston et al. (126) examined the evidence linking dietary fiber to gastrointestinal disease. They noted that fiber increases stool weight, decreases whole-gut transit time, and lowers colonic intraluminal pressure. Although fiber may be of benefit in the treatment of constipation, irritable bowel syndrome, and diverticular disease, its role in the prevention or treatment of other gastrointestinal disease has not been established.

The most recent effort to evaluate the association between dietary fibre intake and risk of colorectal carcinoma was reported by Park et al. (127). From 13 prospective cohort studies included in the Pooling Project of Prospective Studies of Diet and Carcinoma, 725,628 men and women were followed for up to 6 to 20 years across studies. In this large pooled analysis, dietary fiber intake was inversely associated with risk of colorectal carcinoma in age-adjusted analyses. However, after accounting for other dietary risk factors, high dietary fiber intake was not associated with reduced risk of colorectal carcinoma.

No available data substantiate the claim that volvulus of the large bowel is frequently preceded by long-standing constipation. In many cases, hard stools with straining are the initiating factors in the development of fissures and hemorrhoids.

ECONOMIC CONSIDERATIONS

Constipation creates an economic problem of staggering proportions. In 2005, purchases of laxatives in ethical and proprietary markets (drugstores and hospitals), excluding other points of sale, totaled an astounding sum of $79,504,000 in Canada and $650,624,300 in the United States (IMS Canada Drug Store and Hospital purchases, 2005. IMS America, Drug Store audit and provider perspective. Rhodes D. Personal communication, 2006). Because these values do not include the consumption of all laxatives, the true figures are undoubtedly much higher.

A common misconception is that nonprescription medication is totally safe and without adverse effects. However, if a bowel movement is induced by a laxative, it may be several days before enough stool is present for another bowel movement. Therefore, when an individual attempts to maintain a daily bowel movement with the prolonged use of laxatives, a vicious cycle may develop in which either more of the same laxative or a more potent one must be used. A "cathartic colon" then may develop. Such long-standing use of laxatives creates a varying degree of financial burden on a given patient.

TREATMENT

Almy (22) described the goals in the treatment of a patient with chronic constipation as follows: restoration of normal frequency and consistency of stools, freedom from the discomforts ordinarily associated with constipation, maintenance of reasonably regular elimination without artificial aids, and relief of any generalized illness of which constipation may be a symptom. Although these goals are the ideal, they should be achieved if at all possible.

Traditionally, the mainstay of treatment has included laxatives, suppositories, and enemas. It is now being recognized that surgery has an increasing role to play in the management of these patients. Therefore, medical treatment is discussed first, followed by consideration of the role of surgery.

MEDICAL TREATMENT

General Recommendations

Specific metabolic and endocrinologic problems such as hypothyroidism must be treated on their own merits. A favorite recommendation is for the patient to sit on the toilet at regular intervals and for prolonged periods, regardless of whether there is an urge to defecate or not. However, the value of such a ritual is open to debate. Antispasmodics may relieve cramping in individuals with irritable bowel syndrome.

Correction of Faulty Diet and Habits

Because the most common causes of constipation are faulty diet and habits, management often requires no more than careful examination and reassurance, together with simple guidance. Patients should be advised not to ignore the call to stool because neglect only disrupts the normal adaptive relaxation mechanism of the rectum, yielding fecal stasis. Regular exercise should be encouraged; some patients claim an easier and more satisfactory bowel action with nothing more than a regular walk in the morning or evening. Environmental factors such as working conditions are often difficult to change. Other factors, such as meal patterns (e.g., omission of breakfast), shift work, and dependence on fast foods, may contribute to abnormal bowel function. If the patient's history reveals excessive ingestion of foods that cause hardened stools, such as processed cheese, such foods might be eliminated or at least reduced in quantity. An adequate daily intake of fluids is encouraged up to 2 to 3 liters if need be. Finally, cultural habits and norms may influence an individual's perception of what is abnormal as opposed to normal function.

Fiber-containing foodstuffs have hydrophilic properties that soften the stool. The increased volume of feces favors the stimulation of a natural peristaltic reflex. Cereals, especially bran, are good agents in this regard. The most inexpensive cereal with the highest concentration of crude fiber is unprocessed bran, or Miller's bran (128). This easily obtainable material is effective in lowering intraluminal pressure and decreasing transit time in patients with constipation and diverticular disease. Coarser bran is more beneficial because of its greater water-holding capacity (129). Of the various fiber components, pectin has the greatest water-holding capacity but produces the smallest change in fecal weight, whereas bran has the lowest water-holding capacity and the largest fecal weight changes (130). An inverse relationship between water-holding and fecal bulking suggests that dietary fiber does not exert its effect on fecal weight simply by retaining water in the gut. There are four ways in which dietary fiber might cause stool bulking (131). First, the amount of fiber determines the number of bacteria, which are estimated to form 30% to 50% of feces, and there is a direct relationship between stool weight and pentose-containing polysaccharides. Second, water may be absorbed by undigested hydrophilic components of fiber, but the importance of this is questionable. Third, short-chain fatty acids produced by fermentation of dietary fiber accelerate transit and leave less time for the colonic mucosa to reabsorb water. Fourth, stool weight may increase merely because of the increase in undigested residue. In any event, the diet should contain generous portions of vegetables and fruits. Foods with fat (not excessive) are of value. Patients who are unable to achieve adequate intake of fiber-containing foods should supplement their diets with hydrophilic preparations such as psyllium seed extracts, which act in a similar fashion.

In his diet trial, Devroede recommended that patients ingest an average of 14.4 g of crude fiber per day (42). Today the concept of ingesting dietary fiber is generally accepted. Dietary fiber is the residue derived from plant foods that is resistant to human digestive enzymes (132). The main components of dietary fiber include the structural materials of the plant cell wall (i.e., cellulose, hemicellulose, pectin substances, and lignin) and nonstructural polysaccharides (i.e., gums, mucilages, algal polysaccharides, and modified celluloses). Furthermore, fiber can be considered insoluble or water-soluble. The physical and chemical properties of each component of fiber are important in determining the physiologic response to it. For example, the water-insoluble fibers, which include lignin, cellulose, and hemicelluloses, accelerate intestinal transit, augment fecal weight, slow starch hydrolysis, and delay glucose absorption. Water-soluble fibers, which include pectin and gums, delay intestinal transit, gastric emptying, and glucose absorption and decrease serum cholesterol concentration.

Foods rich in dietary fiber contain a mixture of these fiber components, which are present in the form of a matrix. Food sources of fiber are complex, and the amount of fiber detected varies depending on the plant species and the method used to analyze the fiber content. Crude fiber analysis does not accurately reflect the total amount of dietary fiber in food materials and, in general, underestimates

TABLE 9 ■ Fiber Content of Various Foods

1 cup (250 ml) cornflakes = .7 g fiber (total) vs. 1 cup (250 ml) raisin bran = 6.7 g fiber (total)
1 slice white bread = .6 g fiber (total) vs. 1 slice whole wheat bread = 2.0 g fiber (total)
1 cup (250 ml) shredded lettuce = .9 g fiber (total) vs. 1 cup coleslaw = 1.9 g fiber (total)
1 chocolate chip cookie = .4 g fiber (total) vs. 1 date square 2.1 g fiber (total)

	Dietary Fiber (g)	
High Fiber Breakfast Cereals and Bread	**Total**	**Insoluble**
Fiber 1½ cup (125 ml-refer to label)	14.0	
All Bran ½ cup (125 ml)	11.8	10.2
Grape Nuts ½ cup (125 ml)	6.0	4.8
Harvest Crunch (raisin-almond) ½ cup (125 ml)	3.1	2.1
Muffets (2)	4.9	4.2
Fruit N Fiber (date-raisin-nut) ½ cup (125 ml)	4.2	
Shredded Wheat (Spoon-size) ½ cup (125 ml)	3.2	2.6
Shredded Wheat (1 biscuit)	3.0	2.5
Multigrain bagel (large-refer to label)	7.0	
Whole wheat bread (1 slice)	2.0	
Bran muffin (commercial mix)	1.5	
High Fiber Fruit		
Pear 1 fresh (170 g)	5.1	3.4
Prunes, cooked ½ cup (125 ml)	4.8	
Orange 1 (150 g)	4.4	
Mango 1 fresh	4.1	2.2
Raspberries (raw) ½ cup (125 ml)	3.2	1.0
Raisins ½ cup (125 ml)	3.1	2.0
Apple 1 with skin (138 g)	2.6	1.7
Fig 1 dried	2.3	
Blueberries (raw) ½ cup (125 ml)	2.0	1.5
Banana 1 medium	2.0	1.1
Strawberries (raw) ½ cup (125 ml)	1.7	1.0
Peaches canned slices ½ cup (125 ml)	1.7	.6
Applesauce ½ cup (125 ml)	1.5	1.0
High Fiber Snacks		
Peanuts ½ cup (125 ml)	5.6	2.8
Nuts, mixed, no peanuts ½ cup (125 ml)	4.2	
Popcorn 1 cup	1.4	
High Fiber Vegetables		
Beans, red kidney ½ cup (125 ml)	6.1	3.3
Peas, green, fresh, cooked ½ cup (125 ml)	5.6	4.2
Corn, fresh, 1 cob (120 g)	4.5	
Lentils, cooked ½ cup (125 ml)	4.4	4.2
Chick peas cooked ½ cup (125 ml)	4.0	3.0
Lima beans, cooked ½ cup (125 ml)	4.0	
Cabbage, red, shredded, raw 1 cup (250 ml)	3.8	
Potato, baked with skin	3.4	1.1
Corn, fresh, niblets, cooked ½ cup (125 ml)	3.2	
Sweet potato, mashed, cooked ½ cup (125 ml)	3.1	1.9
Brussels sprouts, fresh, cooked ½ cup (125 ml)	3.0	1.6
Carrots, fresh, cooked ½ cup (125 ml)	2.2	1.0
Turnip, cooked ½ cup (125 ml)	2.4	
Broccoli, fresh, ½ cup (125 ml) cooked	2.4	1.5
Squash, winter, cooked ½ cup (125 ml)	1.9	1.3
Tomato, 1 medium	1.5	1.0
Celery, raw, chopped ½ cup (125 ml)	1.0	0.6
Lettuce, chopped 1 cup (250 ml)	0.9	0.5

Source: Data from Brault Dubuc M, and Caron Lahaie L, Nutritive Value of Foods, third edition, National Library, Ottawa 2004. ISBN 2-9801138-6-7.

TABLE 10 ■ Sample Menu Additions for High Fiber Diets[a]

	Dietary Fiber (g)	
25 g Dietary Fiber	**Total**	**Insoluble**
Breakast		
½ cup spoon-size Shredded Wheat	3.2	2.6
2 slices whole wheat toast	4.0	
1 orange	4.4	
Lunch		
Tossed green salad including:		
1 cup chopped lettuce	0.9	0.5
1 tomato, sliced	1.5	1.0
1 pear	5.1	3.4
Supper		
½ cup mashed sweet potato	3.1	1.9
1 cup fresh strawberries	3.4	2.0
Total	**25.6**	11.4
30 g Dietary Fiber		
Breakfast		
1 sliced banana	2.0	1.1
½ cup Fruit N Fiber cereal	4.2	
Lunch		
1 multigrain bagel	7.0	
Fruit salad including:		
1 mango	4.1	2.2
½ cup raspberries	3.2	1.0
Supper		
1 baked potato	3.4	1.1
½ cup cooked carrots	2.2	1.0
Snack		
½ cup mixed nuts	4.2	
Total	**30.3**	6.4
35 g Dietary Fiber		
Breakfast		
½ cup All Bran cereal	11.8	10.2
½ cup raisins	3.1	2.0
Lunch		
Lentil soup (with ½ cup lentils)	4.4	4.2
2 slices whole wheat bread	4.0	
1 apple	2.6	1.7
Supper		
½ cup green peas	5.6	4.2
½ cup blueberries	2.0	1.5
1 date square	2.1	1.2
Total	**35.6**	25.0

[a]The above listings are *additions* to daily menus to show how high-fiber foods can be incorporated easily into regular meals. They do not represent a complete well-balanced meal but demonstrate how high-fiber intake can be achieved. Insoluble fiber has been specified when values were available.

Note: **The authors wish to thank Ms. Peggy Williams, B.A.Sc., P.Dt., who researched the fiber values of the foodstuffs and prepared these sample diets.**

the total amount of fiber in a range from unity to a ratio of 7:1, depending on the specific components of a given food (133).

"How much dietary fiber the average person should consume daily?" is a difficult question to answer. It has been estimated that the average dietary fiber consumed is approximately 19 g/day. For a beneficial effect on stool weight, consumption of 30 to 60 g/day has been suggested, but this estimate would vary from individual to individual. Soluble fiber, which can be readily degraded by bacteria, contributes only a modest increase in fecal bulk. However, insoluble fiber, which is resistant to bacterial degradation, is responsible for the major contribution to fecal bulk. During a diet trial, patients are instructed to record each bowel movement. They also are instructed to stop taking drugs, if not essential, particularly laxatives, and not to resort to enemas. A diet containing 30 g of dietary fiber from a wide variety of sources is continued for one month. Dietary recommendations emphasize the ingestion of sources of insoluble fiber (134). Sources of fiber and sample diets are shown in Tables 9 and 10. Patients who fail to respond to a change in diet (e.g., three or more stools per week) may require further studies such as colonic transit time evaluation and manometry. Patients who do respond are encouraged to adopt a high fiber diet with a generous fluid intake as a daily habit, to prevent constipation.

Laxatives

Laxatives are compounds that facilitate the passage and elimination of feces from the colon and rectum. In addition to the treatment of constipation, valid indications for the use of laxatives include preparation for gastrointestinal investigations and surgery.

With the almost countless number of laxatives available on the market today, classification of such drugs becomes extremely important but correspondingly difficult. More than 700 proprietary laxative preparations are available in almost every dosage form. The most meaningful method is based on the mechanism of action of the drug. The classification shown in Box 2 is a modification of the ones presented by Brunton (135) and Curry (136).

The use of all cathartics is contraindicated in a patient with abdominal cramps, colic, nausea, vomiting, or any undiagnosed abdominal pain.

Because the drugs in each group act similarly, they are described in groups.

Stimulants

Drugs in this group chemically stimulate the intestinal wall to increased peristaltic activity and hence cause gripping, intestinal cramps, increased mucous secretion, and excessively rapid evacuation in some patients. The mechanism of action is by irritation of the intestinal mucosa or by selective action on the enteric nervous system or intestinal smooth muscle. Increased water and electrolyte excretion is attributed to more rapid transit of feces through the intestine. The initiation of the irritant activity may occur in either the small intestine or the large bowel. Although it might be expected that the colon always must be the site of laxative irritant activity, this is not the case. Any agent that increases the propulsive activity of the small intestine necessarily accelerates large bowel peristalsis.

These agents are useful in the treatment of acute constipation as well as constipation caused by prolonged bed rest or hospitalization and preparation for radiologic examinations. Abuse, however, may lead to cathartic colon, that is, a poorly functioning large intestine; hence prolonged use should be discouraged. It may be that it was induced by laxatives that are no longer in use (137). Anthranoid-containing laxatives—aloe, cascara, frangula, and rheum—may play a role in colorectal carcinoma. Clinical epidemiologic studies have evaluated the carcinoma risk in patients who have abused anthranoid laxatives over a long period. Pseudomelanosis coli is a reliable parameter of chronic laxative abuse (more than 9–12 months) and is specific for anthranoid drugs. In a retrospective study of 3049 patients who underwent diagnostic colorectal endoscopy, the incidence of pseudomelanosis coli was 3.13% in patients without pathologic changes (138). In those with colorectal adenomas, the incidence increased to 8.64%, and in those with colorectal carcinoma it was 3.29%. In a prospective study of 1095 patients, the incidence of pseudomelanosis coli was 6.9% for patients with no abnormality seen on endoscopy, 9.8% for patients with adenomas, and 18.6% for patients with colorectal carcinomas. From these data a relative risk of 3.04 can be calculated for colorectal carcinoma, as a result of anthranoid laxative abuse.

Mechanical Cleansers

Laxatives in this group increase propulsive activity by either increasing the bulk of the stool or changing the

BOX 2 ■ Classification of Laxatives

Stimulants
Anthracene (emodin, anthraquinone)
- Cascara sagrada
- Senna (Senokot)
- Danthron
- Rhubarb

Castor oil
Diphenylmethane cathartics
- Bisacodyl (Dulcolax)
- Phenolphthalein
- Oxyphenisatin acetate

Mechanical Cleansers
Saline laxatives
- Magnesium sulfate (Epsom salt), milk of magnesia, magnesium citrate, magnesium carbonate, sodium sulfate (Glauber's salt), sodium phosphate, and potassium sodium tartrate (Rochelle salt)

Bulk-forming agents
- Psyllium seed preparations (plantago), Metamucil, Konsyl, LA formula, Hydrocil, Mucilose, Sibliny
- Synthetic mucilloids (methylcellulose, and sodium carboxymethyl cellulose)
- Agar
- Tragacanth

Mineral oil
Surface-active agents
- Dioctyl sodium sulfosuccinate (Colace, Doxinate, Bulax, and DOSS)
- Poloxalkol
- Dioctyl calcium sulfosuccinate (Surfak)

Miscellaneous
Lactulose

Obsolete cathartics
Calomel, aloe, podophyllum, jalap, colocynth, elaterin, ipomea, gambage, croton oil, and sulfur

consistency of the stool. Traditional teaching dictates that hypertonic salts attract and retain a large volume of isotonic fluid in the gastrointestinal tract, thus stimulating peristalsis in the small intestine, reducing transit time, and causing the passage of a watery stool. Saline cathartics stimulate the release of cholecystokinin, stimulating small bowel motility, and inhibiting absorption of fluid and electrolytes from the jejunum and ileum (139). These laxatives should be given with adequate amounts of water for two reasons: (i) the holdover in the stomach is shortened; and (ii) the patient suffers less dehydration. With oral administration, laxation occurs in three to six hours.

The laxative effect of bulk-forming agents is due to the absorption and retention of large amounts of water. Mechanical distention caused by this increased residue of unabsorbed material promotes peristalsis and facilitates the passage of stool. The laxative effect usually occurs within 24 hours of ingestion but may take up to three days. Side effects are relatively rare. Minor adverse effects include frequent flatulence and borborygmi. Esophageal, gastric, small intestinal, and colonic obstructions and fecal impactions have been reported with their use. Therefore, this group of agents should be taken with generous amounts of fluids to avoid such problems.

Liquid petrolatum retards the absorption of water from the stool and thus softens fecal material. The onset of action is approximately six to eight hours. This substance can be administered orally or as an enema. The usual dose is 15 to 45 mL. Mineral oil should not be taken at bedtime because of the dangers of aspiration and is best taken between meals to obviate any tendency for interference with absorption of fat-soluble vitamins. A patient with dysphagia should not take it because of the threat of lipoid pneumonia. Pruritus ani and anal leakage are minor annoying side effects.

With its sodium or calcium salt, dioctyl sulfosuccinate lowers surface tension at the oil-water interface of the stool, thereby softening the stool by permitting a greater penetration of feces by water and fat. It has been suggested that dioctyl sulfosuccinate stimulates fluid and electrolyte secretion as well (140). The calcium salt has been reported as more effective than the sodium salt (141). The usual daily dose is 100 to 200 mg. They act within 24 to 48 hours.

Lactulose is a synthetic disaccharide not digested by small intestinal or pancreatic enzymes. In the colon, it is metabolized by microflora with resultant acidification of the stool and release of gas. It is effective in treating constipation and changes the nature of the colonic flora. The resultant anions may cause osmotic catharsis; for this reason the agent might be classified with the saline laxatives. However, it is too costly for routine administration, and with long-term use, superinfection is a risk (121).

Several potential adverse effects may result from overconsumption of laxatives. In fact, the ill effects of laxative abuse may be greater than those of constipation. Such effects include (i) dehydration and electrolyte disturbance, (ii) hypokalemia, (iii) hypermagnesemia, (iv) nausea, vomiting, and abdominal distress, (v) malabsorption, (vi) paraffinomas, (vii) lipoid pneumonia, (viii) intestinal obstruction, (ix) specific toxic effect, (x) anal stenosis, (xi) dependence, and (xii) colonic structural injury. Colonic nerve plexus damage attributed to the long-term use of sennosides has been questioned, and experimental evidence does not support this hypothesis (137). The morphologic changes noted may very well be on an entirely different basis.

Suppositories

Suppositories are useful for evacuating the lower bowel, and their use instead of an enema has been advocated. Although they are probably not as effective as enemas, they are more acceptable to both patient and nurse. The insertion of an inert cylinder such as a glycerin suppository often initiates a defecation response, usually within 30 minutes, which apparently is a reflex act. Other suppositories contain bisacodyl, dioctyl sodium sulfosuccinate, senna, or carbon dioxide.

Other Pharmacologic Agents

The use of agents that enhance the normal propulsive action of the bowel is more appealing than the use of agents whose mechanism of action is by irritation. A number of agents that fall into this category are summarized in Table 11.

Cholinomimetics have not yet gained general usage. The newest groups of agents that enhance the intrinsic motor function of the gut have been classified as the prokinetic agents. Although metoclopramide induces colonic contractions, it is rarely useful in the treatment of constipated patients except when upper intestinal symptoms predominate. Cisapride has been found effective in treating some patients (142). In a randomized double-blind study, the Bavarian Constipation Study Group concluded that cisapride improves bowel habits in patients with idiopathic constipation and reduces laxative consumption (143). This innovative concept requires confirmation through other studies.

Johanson et al. (144) evaluated the efficacy, safety, and tolerability of tegaserod (Zelnorm^{TM}, Novartis) a serotonin subtype 4-receptor, partial agonist in patients with chronic constipation in a randomized double blind, placebo-controlled study. Responder rates for complete spontaneous

TABLE 11 ■ Agents Affecting Neurotransmission

General Class	Mechanisms of Action	Subclass	Example
Cholinomimetics	Stimulate cholinergic receptors, predominantly muscarinics	Cholinergic agents	Bethanechol
		Cholinesterase inhibitors	Neostigmine
Prokinetic agents	Facilitate release of acetylcholine and antagonize dopamine receptors		Metoclopramide
	Facilitate only neurotransmitter		Cisapride
Opioid antagonists	Selectively inhibit peripheral opioid receptors		Naloxone

Source: From Ref. 142.

bowel movements during weeks one to four were significantly greater in the tegaserod 2 mg twice daily (41.4%) and 6 mg twice daily groups (43.2%) versus placebo (25.1%). This effect was maintained over 12 weeks. No rebound effect was observed after treatment withdrawal. Tegaserod was well tolerated; headache and nasopharyngitis, the most frequent adverse events, were more common in the placebo group than in either tegaserod group. Kamm et al. (145) also investigated the efficacy, safety, and tolerability of tegaserod in the treatment of chronic constipation. They randomized 1264 patients to tegaserod or placebo. Responder rates for the primary efficacy variable were 35.6% for tegaserod 2 mg b.i.d., 40.2% for 6 mg b.i.d., and 26.7% for placebo. Tegaserod 6 mg b.i.d. reduced straining, abdominal bloating/distension, and abdominal pain/discomfort during the 12-week treatment period compared with placebo. Significant improvements were also seen in stool form and in global assessment of bowel habits and constipation. The most common adverse events, headache and abdominal pain, were more frequent with placebo than with tegaserod.

Enemas

Clinical indications for enemas include preparation for endoscopic examination, surgery, or childbirth, removal of fecal impaction and barium, and certain cases of acute constipation. Warm tap water or warm saline enemas are preferred. Soapsuds and hydrogen peroxide enemas are quite irritating to the colonic mucosa and should be avoided. Hypertonic phosphate salts also are irritating to the colonic mucosa and tend to stimulate the rectum to produce a large amount of mucus, which may interfere with evaluation of the state of the mucosa. Enemas work within approximately five minutes and act by causing distention and by osmotic activity. Hypertonic enemas may give rise to sodium retention. However, the practical advantage of the packaged enemas makes their use ideal in a busy office practice. Enemas should be administered with the patient lying on his or her left side or prone and with the enema bag two feet above the level of the rectum. Material should be introduced slowly with as many temporary interruptions as necessary to prevent cramps. Repositioning the patient on his or her right side might help ensure adequate distribution of the enema fluid.

Certain dangers are involved with enemas, including electrolyte depletion, water intoxication, colonic perforation, and even psychological dependence.

■ SURGICAL TREATMENT

The indications for operation in patients with constipation of recent origin are relatively clear, and they are related to the underlying cause of the constipation such as carcinoma or diverticular disease. On the other hand, the indications for operation in patients with chronic constipation are poorly defined and controversial at best. During the last two decades, there has been an increasing recognition of serious psychological and psychiatric disorders, particularly in female patients with functional disorders of the lower digestive tract. According to some authors, it is naive to believe that operation could cure these conditions. Despite an increasing skepticism regarding the potential role of surgery, some surgeons still believe that there is a sound indication for operative treatment in selected cases. The high cost of treating constipation and the uncontrolled use of laxatives seems to support the contention that no patient should need to resort to a lifelong consumption of laxatives and administration of enemas if another solution is available. Martelli et al. (42) have classified patients with constipation of unknown origin in terms of the segment of bowel with the disordered function. The authors described three groups: (i) outlet obstruction—impaired rectal evacuation; (ii) hindgut dysfunction—the right colon empties very well, but markers accumulate in the left colon, sigmoid colon, and rectum; and (iii) colonic inertia—the entire large bowel fails to propel contents. Prior to operation, delineation of patients with colonic inertia from those with obstructed defecation is advocated. At first sight, distinction between the first two types of constipation seems logical because it has an obvious impact on the treatment. However, many patients present with symptoms suggestive of both abnormalities. Although it has been suggested that good results can be achieved by adequate selection of patients, it is still not known how to treat subjects with both colonic inertia and obstructed defecation.

Slow-Transit Constipation (Colonic Inertia)

At the beginning of the twentieth century, Sir William Arbuthnot Lane (146) was probably the first to perform colectomy with ileorectal anastomosis in patients with colonic inertia. Initially, colectomy was performed only in patients with idiopathic megacolon because many surgeons were reluctant to remove a normal-sized colon. It has been shown that colectomy also might be beneficial in patients with severe constipation without megacolon. The effort to compare results is probably not entirely justified because series are not comparable. In particular, some series are of patients with megacolon, others are of patients without megacolon, and most are of both. In addition, the extent of resection varies from series to series and within a given series. Despite the fact that the reported results are apparently good, the exact role of colectomy has yet to be defined (147–154).

Slow-Transit Constipation with Megacolon and/or Megarectum

Some patients with severe, intractable constipation have a markedly dilated rectum and/or colon. This condition, also called idiopathic megarectum and/or megacolon, affects males and females in equal proportion. Most patients have the onset of symptoms in childhood or early adult life. Various segments of the large bowel may become dilated, but the process usually begins in the rectum. The etiology of this condition is still unknown. It has been suggested that rectal dilation may result from a behavioral defecatory problem in childhood. Although the muscle layers of the dilated segment and their intrinsic and extrinsic innervation appear grossly normal, subtle neural and muscular abnormalities have been reported (155). Koch et al. (156) reported that VIP levels are decreased in the external muscle layer from idiopathic megacolon. Similar findings have been reported by Gattuso et al. (157). Koch et al. (158) were able to demonstrate that diminished VIP levels are associated with a depletion of the tissue antioxidant, glutathione. This depletion probably permits the free radical-induced alteration of VIP-containing neurons. In another study, the same authors observed a diminished release of nitric oxide in circular smooth muscle from patients with idiopathic megacolon (159). Meier-Ruge examined surgical specimens obtained from patients with idiopathic megacolon. In all specimens, she observed a lack of connective tissue in the muscularis propria. Normally, this connective tissue, consisting of collagen Type III, enables contraction and relaxation of the circular and longitudinal muscle layers. According to Meier-Ruge, the absence of this tissue affects normal peristalsis, resulting in stasis of fecal material and dilatation of the large bowel, despite a normal enteric nervous system (160). Recently, Lee et al. reported a decreased density of interstitial cells of Cajal in resected sigmoid specimens of patients with acquired megacolon (109). Based on a retrospective study among 63 operated patients with megarectum and/or megacolon, Gattuso and Kamm concluded that patients with megarectum differ clinically, diagnostically, and in their outcome from those with megacolon. Patients with megarectum are younger and develop symptoms in childhood. Half of the patients with megacolon become symptomatic as adults. All patients with megarectum present with fecal impaction associated with soiling and fecal incontinence. Manual disimpaction is frequently reported by these patients. The symptoms of those with a megacolon are variable. The authors were able to confirm these findings in a prospective study among 29 patients with idiopathic megarectum and/or idiopathic megacolon (161).

The diagnosis of idiopathic megabowel can only be made after exclusion of recognized neurologic, toxic, and degenerative pathology such as Hirschsprung's disease, myotonic dystrophy, Chagas' disease, and systemic sclerosis. Digital examination almost invariably shows that the rectum is full of feces (162). Radiographic findings are also characteristic, because almost all patients have rectal dilation down to the pelvic floor, with no distal narrow segment. Patients with idiopathic megarectum have normal small bowel transit and abnormal colonic transit, with delay occurring predominantly in the dilated segment (163). The initial management of patients with idiopathic megarectum and/or megacolon should be medical. The aim of treatment is to prevent fecal impaction, either by inducing a semiliquid stool using osmotic laxatives or by regular use of enemas or suppositories. The use of senna laxatives may prove helpful to these patients. In some patients, however, manual disimpaction is inevitable. This is not without risk, because it has been shown that manual disimpaction, performed under general anesthesia, may damage the anal sphincters. This damage further affects continence and compromises the outcome of operative treatment (164). If laxatives and enemas are poorly tolerated or ineffective, operative treatment should be considered.

Colectomy with cecorectal or ileorectal anastomosis is the most commonly performed operation in patients with idiopathic megarectum and/or megacolon. Stabile et al. (165) reported a series of 40 patients in whom the rectum was moderately dilated, measuring 7 to 10 cm in diameter on a lateral radiograph. Twenty-two patients had a cecorectal anastomosis, 11 had an ileorectal anastomosis and seven had a sigmoid resection. When considering all patients, 80% developed a normal stool frequency, and most patients no longer needed to use laxatives. These results are similar to those previously reported by Lane and Todd (166). In patients with a grossly dilated rectum, a colectomy with ileorectal anastomosis seems less appropriate. In these patients, the Duhamel procedure is the most commonly performed operation. The outcome of this operation appears to be less favorable than previously reported. In a series of 20 patients, Stabile et al. (167) documented persistent constipation in seven patients and, of these, five required further operation. Based on the assumption that the physiological abnormalities are confined to the dilated part of the bowel, it seems reasonable to perform a coloanal anastomosis after complete resection of the distal dilated segment down to the level of the pelvic floor. Stabile et al. (168) reported that five of seven patients experienced a return to normal bowel frequency after coloanal anastomosis. Stewart et al. (169) observed a favorable outcome in 8 of 10 patients who underwent coloanal anastomosis. The overall results, as reported in the literature, are listed in Table 12. In their review of the literature, Pfeifer et al. (171) found 84 patients with megabowel in whom the success rate for subtotal colectomy and ileorectal anastomosis was 88%.

Suilleabhain et al. (172) reported on several operative procedures used to treat idiopathic megabowel in 28 patients. All patients had conservative treatment for six months. Those failing to improve underwent full thickness biopsy of the anorectal junction, anorectal physiology studies, colonic transit studies, and evacuation proctography. Surgery involved excision of the abnormal large bowel and formation of an anastomosis (coloanal or ileoanal) using "normal" bowel, identified either by a defunctioning stoma or colonic motility studies. Eight patients responded to conservative management. Two of the 17 patients who underwent full thickness biopsy were cured by the procedure. Anorectal physiology, and colonic transit and evacuation studies did not aid selection of the operative procedure performed in 15 patients: proctectomy and coloanal anastomosis (six), restorative proctocolectomy (three), pan-

TABLE 12 ■ Results of Colonic Resection for Slow-Transit Constipation with Megacolon

Author(s)	Treatment	No. of Cases	Success Rate (%)[a]
Lane and Todd (166) (1977)	Subtotal colectomy	9	88
	Hemicolectomy	2	50
	Sigmoid resection	3	33
Hughes et al. (147) (1981)	Subtotal colectomy	7	100
Belliveau et al. (148) (1982)	Subtotal colectomy	29	76
Hughes et al. (149) (1982)	Segmental resection	5	100
Klatt (150) (1983)	Subtotal colectomy	3	100
Barnes et al. (162) (1986)	Subtotal colectomy	16	69
	Segmental colectomy	4	50
Vasilevsky et al. (154) (1988)	Subtotal colectomy	14	93
Stabile et al. (165) (1991)	Subtotal and segmental resections	40	80
Stabile et al. (167) (1991)	Duhamel procedure	20	35
Stabile et al. (168) (1992)	Coloanal anastomosis	7	71
Keighley (170) (1993)	Ileoanal anastomosis	6	83
	Coloanal anastomosis	10	70
Stewart et al. (169) (1994)	Coloanal anastomosis	10	80

[a]Regular defecation without the use of laxatives.

proctocolectomy (one), and defunctioning stoma (five). At a median follow-up of 3.6 years, 13 of 15 evaluable patients had a satisfactory outcome. They concluded, approximately 40% of patients with megabowel referred for surgery responded to conservative treatment. The remaining patients may be treated successfully by operation.

Based on a recent systemic review, Gladman et al. concluded that the outcome data of surgery for idiopathic megarectum and/or megacolon should be interpreted with caution due to limitations of the reviewed studies. None of these studies were comparative. Most series involved only a small number of patients without long-term follow-up (173). Although recommendations based on clear evidence cannot be given, Gladman et al. advocate subtotal colectomy with ileorectal anastomosis as the optimum procedure in patients with a nondilated rectum. For patients presenting with a dilatation of their colon and rectum, restorative proctocolectomy seems to be the most suitable procedure. For patients with dilatation confined to the rectum, Gladman et al. advocate a vertical reduction rectoplasty. This novel procedure involves transsection of the rectum in a vertical direction along its antimesenterial border and excision of the anterior portion, thereby reducing rectal capacity. In a small series, significant improvements in bowel frequency was obtained in eight out of ten patients (174).

An alternative to these major resections involves the formation of a stoma either as a primary procedure or after a previous operation has failed. One should realize that only the creation of a stoma proximal to the dilated segment would relieve the constipation.

Slow-Transit Constipation without Megacolon

Slow-transit constipation without megacolon is a condition that is almost entirely confined to women (116,151). Other terms used to describe this syndrome are colonic inertia or Arbuthnot Lane's disease. In tertiary referral centres about 20% to 40% of the patients with constipation will be found to have slow-transit constipation (51,175). In the majority of patients, symptoms arise de novo in childhood. A proportion of patients present later in life. Some of these subjects have no obvious trigger for their complaints, whereas others report symptoms following events such as hysterectomy and childbirth (176). Patients with this syndrome have infrequent defecation with two or fewer bowel actions each week. Although these patients have a normal-sized colon, their colonic transit time is markedly prolonged. In most patients, the constipation is associated with a general sense of malaise, bloating, abdominal pain, nausea, and vomiting, which interferes with the ability to work and enjoy social activities. Many of these women have associated gynecologic problems such as irregular menstrual periods, ovarian cysts, and galactorrhea (151). In addition, a delay in gastric emptying and small bowel transit has been found, indicating that inertia of the large bowel might be the colonic manifestation of a pangastrointestinal motility disorder (177,178). Hemingway et al. (179) used cholecystokinin-augmented hepatic 2,6-dimethyliminodiacetic acid (HIDA) scans to measure gall bladder ejection fraction in patients with constipation. The authors found a significant difference between patients with idiopathic slow-transit constipation and those with other causes of constipation, indicating that colonic inertia is associated with biliary dyskinesia. Penning et al. evaluated gall bladder motility in 16 patients with slow-transit constipation and in 20 healthy controls. They observed that patients with slow-transit constipation have smaller fasting gall bladder volumes, impaired gall bladder responses to vagal cholinergic stimulation, but normal gall bladder responses to hormonal stimulation with cholecystokinin. These findings indicate that gall bladder motility is disturbed in patients with slow-transit constipation, probably due to impaired neural responsiveness (180). Mollen et al. reported abnormalities of antroduodenal motility, characterized by absence or prolonged duration of the migrating motor complex, an increased number of clustered contractions and a decreased motility during late Phase 2 of the migrating motor complex (181). Similar findings have been reported by others (182). In contrast with these observations, Penning et al. reported that patients with slow-transit constipation have generally well-preserved antroduodenal motility with only minor alterations (183). It is still unclear whether these anomalies of the proximal digestive tract are primary or not. These abnormalities may very well be primary, because it has been shown that delayed gastric emptying persists in the majority of the patients after subtotal colectomy with ileorectal anastomosis (184). Alternatively they may be secondary to the colonic inertia itself, because it has been shown that inflation of a balloon in the rectum inhibits the motor activity of the entire gastrointestinal tract (185). The observation that women with slow-transit constipation may also have functional urologic problems has prompted the investigation of sacral spinal cord function. In 15 women with colonic inertia, Varma and Smith (77) observed blunted rectal defecatory sensation and increased rectal compliance. In addition, the latency of the pudendoanal reflex was significantly prolonged. Based on these findings, a central neurogenic deficit was postulated. Kerrigan et al. (186) assessed the integrity of evoked spinal reflexes relaying in the conus medullaris (S2–S4). One or more of these reflexes were absent in 75% of the authors' patients. The results of this study indicate that the integration of sensory information within the sacral cord may be impaired in slow-transit constipation. Extramural damage to the pelvic parasympathetic nerves has also been considered a major contributing factor. Colonic branches, arising from the inferior hypogastric plexus, enter the wall of the large bowel at the rectosigmoid junction and extend in the intramuscular plane both caudad and cephalad. In humans it has been demonstrated that these intramural nerves extend cephalad up to 80% of the large intestine (176). Canine studies sectioning pelvic nerves have demonstrated abolition of high amplitude propagating contractions (HAPC's), a decrease in proximal colonic motility, and abnormal bowel movements, characterized by the passage of smaller harder stools with associated straining (187). In patients with slow-transit constipation the number, amplitude, and duration of HAPC's are reduced (188,189). In many patients with slow-transit constipation, rectal sensory perception is reduced. In some patients, this rectal hyposensitivity may be partly explained by abnormal rectal compliance. In other patients, however, rectal wall properties are normal. This latter finding is suggestive of impairment of afferent nerves (190). A significant group of patients with slow-transit constipation have symptoms that started after pelvic surgery, especially hysterectomy, or after childbirth. It has been assumed that extramural damage to the parasympathetic nerves occur during hysterectomy and childbirth (191). Women with slow-transit constipation show impaired sweating after acetylcholine application. It has been suggested that this abnormality is the manifestation of a systemic autonomic dysfunction (192).

On the other hand, alterations in the enteric nervous system have also been cited as a possible explanation for the disturbed motility in colonic inertia. Silver-staining methods and modern techniques with monoclonal antibodies raised against neurofilament have revealed distinctive abnormalities in the enteric nervous system.

According to Wedel et al. the underlying defect is morphologically characterized by oligoneuronal hypoganglionosis of the myenteric plexus and the external submucous plexus, associated with an increased number of thickened submucous nerve fibers (107). Bassotti et al. also observed abnormalities of the enteric nervous system. These abnormalities were not confined to the neurons of the myenteric and submucous plexus. They also found a decreased number of interstitial cells of Cajal as well as a decreased number of enteric glial cells (108). A decreased density of interstitial cells of Cajal has also been reported by others (109,193). Toman et al. could not confirm these reports. They used quantitative immunohistochemistry and did not find a decreased number of interstitial cells of Cajal in patients as compared to controls (194). The neuroendocrine system of the digestive tract has also been subject of several studies. Most of these studies have concentrated on the colonic neuroendocrine system and their results are rather contradictory. Both peptide YY cell-density and serotonin cell-density in the large bowel have been reported to increase or decrease in patients with slow-transit constipation (195). Another study has shown that the large bowel of patients with slow-transit constipation is more densely innervated by nitric oxide nerves (196). Although some of the reported data are conflicting, most studies indicate that there is a subgroup of patients in whom constipation is associated with a dysfunctioning enteric nervous system. Slater et al. (197), in an effort to better understand the pathophysiology of idiopathic slow-transit constipation, studied abnormalities in the contractile properties of colonic smooth muscle. The authors found a hypersensitivity to cholinergic stimulation and suggested the existence of a smooth muscle myopathy in this condition. Rao et al. performed ambulatory 24-hour colonic manometry in 21 patients with slow-transit constipation and 20 healthy controls. Constipated patients showed fewer pressure waves than controls during daytime. Motility induced by waking or meal was decreased in patients. HAPCs were detected in 43% of the patients compared to 100% of the controls and with a much lower incidence (198). Similar findings have been reported by others (199). To date, these techniques have been applied only to resected colon specimens. These methods are, therefore, not suitable to determine preoperatively whether the neuropathologic abnormalities affect only a portion of the colon or its entire length. It has been shown that substance P levels are decreased in both rectal mucosa and submucosa of patients with slow-transit constipation (200). It seems likely that this finding will become more diagnostically relevant, because biopsies can easily be obtained in contrast to transmural sampling. It remains unclear whether the alterations in the enteric nervous system are congenital or acquired due to a possible neurotoxic effect of certain laxatives. These and other controversies indicate that the precise pathogenesis of slow-transit constipation is still an enigma.

Dietary measures and medical treatment including laxatives and enemas usually fail to relieve the distressing symptoms of this syndrome. Battaglia et al. (201) assessed the medium- and long-term effects of biofeedback and muscle straining in patients with slow-transit constipation in 10 patients who were unresponsive to conventional treatments. At 1 year follow-up, beneficial effect was seen in only 20% of these patients and there was no improvement in colonic transit time.

For these reasons, operative intervention is frequently considered. The most common technique is subtotal colectomy with ileorectal anastomosis. According to enthusiastic reports, this procedure seems to be highly effective with success rates of greater than 90%, as shown in Table 13. In their review of the literature, Pfeifer, Agachan, and Wexner (171) found 444 patients without megabowel, and

TABLE 13 ■ Results of Subtotal Colectomy with Ileorectal Anastomosis for Colonic Inertia (Without Megacolon)

Author(s)	No. of Cases	Mean Follow-Up (Yr)	Success Rate
Hughes et al. (147) (1981)	10	ns	80
Klatt (150) (1983)	6	2.1	100
Krishnamurthy et al. (98) (1985)	12	ns	100
Todd (202) (1985)	16	ns	88
Preston and Lennard-Jones (203) (1986)	16	3.5	81
Roe, Bartolo, and McC Mortenson (71) (1986)	7	0.7	71
Beck et al. (153) (1987)	14	1.2	100
Leon, Krrishnamurthy, and Shuffler (204) (1987)	13	2.6	77
Walsh et al. (205) (1987)	19	3.2	65
Åkervall et al. (206) (1988)	12	3.4	66
Kamm et al. (207) (1988)	33	2.0	50
Vasilevsky et al. (154) (1988)	24	4.0	71
Zenilman et al. (208) (1989)	12	2.0	100
Yoshioka and Keighley (209) (1989)	32	3.0	58
Coremans (210) (1990)	10	3.8	60
Kuijpers (211) (1990)	12	ns	50
Pemberton et al. (212) (1991)	38	ns	100
Takahashi et al (213) (1994)	37	3.0	97
Redmond et al. (214) (1995)	34	7.5	90
Piccirillo et al. (215) (1995)	54	2.2	94
Pluta et al. (61) (1996)	24	5.5	92
de Graaf, et al. (216) (1996)	24	4.0	33
Nyam et al. (217) (1997)	74	5.5	90
Fan (218) (2000)	24	1	88
Mollen (219) (2001)	21	5	76
Nyland (220) (2001)	40	11	73
Pikarsky (221) (2001)	30	9	100
Webster (222) (2001)	55	1	89
Glia (223) (2004)	17	5	86

Note: Regular defecation without the use of laxatives.
Abbreviation: ns, not significant.

the success rate for subtotal colectomy and ileorectal anastomosis was 83%. Because the selection of patients with constipation for colectomy may prove difficult, Sunderland et al. (224) evaluated the role of video proctography. The authors suggested that when true idiopathic slow-transit constipation is identified on the basis of delayed markers and the ability to expel liquid on proctography, an excellent result could be anticipated from colectomy and ileorectal anastomosis.

Mollen et al. (219) assessed the results of preoperative functional evaluation of patients with severe slow-transit constipation in relation to functional outcome in 21 patients who underwent colectomy and ileorectal anastomosis. Mean colorectal transit time was 156 hours (normal < 45 hours). Small bowel transit time was normal in 10 patients and delayed in five patients. Morbidity was 33%. Small bowel obstruction occurred in six patients; relaparotomy was done in four patients. Follow-up varied from 14 to 153 (mean 62) months. After 3 months, defecation frequency was increased from one bowel movement per 5.9 days to 2.8 times per day. Seventeen patients continued to experience abdominal pain, and 13 still used laxatives and enemas. Satisfaction rate was 76%. After 1 year defecation, frequency was back at the preoperative level in five patients. An ileostomy was created in two more patients because of incontinence and persistent diarrhea but 52% still felt improved. They concluded the patients should be informed that despite an increase in defecation frequency, abdominal symptoms might persist.

Despite the fact that the reported results of subtotal colectomy are apparently good, some authors have questioned the exact role of this procedure in patients with colonic inertia. In 1988, Kamm et al. (207) reviewed the results obtained in 44 female patients. Subtotal colectomy produced improvement in 22 patients (50%) as defined by more frequent stools. However, 17 patients experienced diarrhea, three-fourths of the patients had persistent abdominal pain, six patients had some degree of incontinence, five patients had persistent constipation, eight patients required an operation for obstruction caused by adhesions, and six patients required an ileostomy, three for persistent constipation and three for intractable diarrhea. Ten patients needed psychiatric treatment. The authors also found that impaired balloon expulsion and signs of anismus did not correlate with the clinical outcome (207).

Similar findings have been documented by Ghosh et al. They also reported a high complication rate during long-term follow-up. For example, 71% of their patients experienced at least one episode of small intestinal obstruction and 42% of these episodes resulted in laparotomy. The incidence of this complication is significantly higher among patients with slow-transit constipation as compared to patients who underwent colectomy for another reason (225). Recently, FitzHarris et al. reviewed the charts and operative reports of all their patients who underwent subtotal colectomy for slow-transit constipation during one decade. Seventy-five subjects returned their questionnaire. Although 81% of these patients were at least somewhat pleased with the final outcome, 41% cited persistent abdominal pain, 21% fecal incontinence, and 46% diarrhea. These problems adversely affected their quality of life (226).

These data suggest that subtotal colectomy in patients with colonic inertia produces new problems of its own. Persistent constipation and abdominal discomfort after this procedure might be derived from small bowel involvement, which is masked by the predominant symptom of constipation, becoming apparent only after the colon has been resected (227). Glia et al. found a trend toward better long-term results after subtotal colectomy with ileorectal anastomosis in constipated patients with normal antroduodenal motility as compared to those with abnormal manometric findings (223). In a study, de Graaf et al. (216) evaluated the clinical outcome of subtotal colectomy in a consecutive series of 24 patients with colonic inertia. Seventeen patients regained normal stool frequency. However, persistent abdominal discomfort and disabling diarrhea with incontinence were noted in 63% and 25%, respectively. Similar results have been reported by others (204). It has been suggested that these rather disappointing results are due to poor selection of patients. In a prospective study, Wexner et al. (228) evaluated 163 patients with chronic constipation. All patients underwent colonic transit time studies, anorectal manometry, evacuation proctography, and EMG of the pelvic floor. Colonic inertia was defined as a diffuse marker delay on transit study without evidence of paradoxic puborectalis contraction on proctography. Only 16 patients fulfilled these criteria and underwent a subtotal colectomy. At a mean follow-up of 15 months, patient satisfaction was good or excellent in 94% of the cases. Pluta et al. (61) noted that patients with a psychiatric history or physiologic evidence of a defect in afferent innervation of the rectum had poorer results. Åkervall et al. (206) found that patients with normal rectal sensory function had a satisfactory functional result after subtotal colectomy, whereas patients with blunted sensation did not improve. The authors suggested that determination of the distention pressures required to elicit rectal sensation is an important step in selecting patients, suitable for subtotal colectomy and ileorectal anastomosis. Similar findings have been reported by others (229).

Many experts consider anismus an absolute contraindication to colectomy and expect it to fail. However, objective evidence for this conclusion can only be provided by a prospective study aimed at evaluating the effect of colectomy both in patients with and without evidence of anismus. Duthie and Bartolo (230) performed a subtotal colectomy in 32 patients with slow-transit constipation. One-half of their patients demonstrated proctographic evidence of anismus. No specific attempt had been made to improve pelvic floor function prior to operation. The clinical outcome was reassessed after five years. Overall, 67% of the patients thought that their life had been significantly improved. Comparing patients with and without radiologic signs of anismus, no differences were noted with regard to the final results. Similar findings have been reported by others (207,217). Based on these observations, it might be concluded that anismus in the setting of slow-transit constipation may in essence be ignored when considering operative intervention.

Most surgeons perform subtotal colectomy, mainly based on the recommendations of Preston et al. (151), who concluded that subtotal colectomy was successful in 11 of 16 patients. However, eight of these 16 patients continued having abdominal pain, 10 had bloating, and six experienced episodes of fecal incontinence. These symptoms were not included in the evaluation of the clinical outcome. Five further patients underwent partial colectomy. In two of these patients, a partial left-sided colectomy was performed and in three a sigmoid resection. None of these five patients were selected on the basis of segmental colonic transit time studies.

In contrast to the detailed discussion regarding the clinical outcome after subtotal colectomy, the authors stated only that patients who had partial colectomy did not improve. Despite a hesitation to perform a segmental resection, most surgeons point to the significance of segmental colonic transit time studies. In our opinion, it does not make sense to quantify regional transit if subtotal colectomy is the only preferable option for patients with slow-transit constipation. de Graaf et al. (216) conducted a prospective study to investigate the value of segmental colonic transit times in the decision-making process prior to operative intervention. Based on the results of the transit time studies, 18 patients underwent partial left-sided colectomy and 24 subtotal colectomy. Comparing both groups, no significant differences were found with regard to recurrent constipation and persistent abdominal pain (216). Kamm et al. (231) and Lundin et al. (232) noted the same favorable experience with left hemicolectomy in selected patients. It would seem germane to consider regional transit in the decision-making process. If markers pass through the right colon but are only held up in the descending and sigmoid colon, a left hemicolectomy would be deemed appropriate because it would accomplish the task of removing the poorly functioning portion of the colon while obviating the potential complications of subtotal colectomy.

It has been demonstrated that proximal gastrointestinal function is normal in the majority of patients with onset of their symptoms after pelvic surgery or childbirth (233). Based on this finding it has been argued that these patients are more suitable for surgical treatment.

Because the functional results of total colectomy and ileorectal anastomosis with the treatment of chronic constipation caused by colonic inertia are often considered unsatisfactory due to the frequency of postoperative diarrhea and the high rate of postoperative small bowel obstruction, Sarli et al. (234) assessed the functional results of eight females who underwent subtotal colectomy with antiperistaltic cecorectal anastomosis. Before antiperistaltic cecorectal anastomosis all ten patients were laxative-dependant, with a mean bowel frequency of 10 days; eight of them had distention, seven bloating, and three abdominal pain. One month after antiperistaltic cecorectal anastomosis, bowel frequency was a mean of 2.2 per day with a semiliquid stool consistency. After one year, bowel frequency was a mean of 1.3 per day with a solid stool consistency; laxatives continued to be used by two patients with paradoxical puborectalis contraction. All 10 patients reported a good or improved quality of life.

After subtotal colectomy with ileorectal anastomosis, approximately 10% of the patients require a stoma because of intractable diarrhea or persistent constipation associated with abdominal discomfort. The creation of a stoma can also be considered as a primary procedure. Until now, little information has been available regarding the results of stoma formation in patients with slow-transit constipation, van der Sijp et al. (235) studied 39 patients who were treated at some stage with either a colostomy or an ileostomy. The authors noted that many symptoms persisted after the creation of a stoma. However, those with the best results were patients who had a primary stoma as the first treatment for their colonic inertia.

Restorative Proctocolectomy

In the desperate situation in which a patient has severe idiopathic constipation for which all medical treatment has failed and total colectomy and ileorectal anastomosis have not resolved the problem, Nicholls and Kamm (236) have described the use of the proctocolectomy with a restorative ileoanal reservoir. The authors suggest that in the very small group of patients who do not show improvement after colectomy and ileorectal anastomosis and who are not prepared to accept an ileostomy; consideration should be given to a pouch procedure that the authors have performed with satisfactory results. Hosie et al. (237) performed a restorative proctocolectomy in 13 patients. Eight of those patients had recurrent constipation after colectomy and five had constipation and overflow incontinence associated with megarectum and megacolon. Despite a high complication rate, 85% of the patients experienced improved symptoms and quality of life. In their review of the literature, Pfeifer et al. (171) found 10 patients who underwent a pouch procedure with an 82% success rate. Thakur et al. (238) reviewed the hospital records of five patients with persistent symptomatic idiopathic colonic inertia. Each of the patients had undergone extensive medical management, and eventually four underwent one or more colonic resections to relieve the recurrent abdominal distention and pain. Three of the patients eventually received a distal ileostomy, which functioned well. Anorectal manometric studies were within normal range for each of the five patients. Restorative proctocolectomy (J-pouch) was performed for each. With a mean follow-up of 42 months after restorative proctocolectomy, each of the five patients was relieved of constipation and small bowel distension. The average number of bowel movements per 24 hours at 6 months was 4.8. All patients were able to discriminate flatus from stool, could hold back for up to 1.5 hours after the initial urge to defecate, and had total daytime continence. Each returned to work or school within three months and each reported greater satisfaction of bowel function than with the ileostomy.

Recently, Kalbassi et al. assessed the outcome of proctocolectomy among 15 patients. Two patients required pouch excision because of intractable pelvic pain. The authors noted improvement in lifestyle scores in the categories of physical function, social function, and pain (239). It is not clear whether this procedure is an appropriate option, because the reported results are rather conflicting.

Sacral Neuromodulation

Sacral neuromodulation has been used successfully in the treatment of patients with urologic disorders and of those with fecal incontinence. Some of these patients noted increased stool frequency and improved rectal evacuation. Based on this observation, Malouf and coworkers implanted a temporary percutaneous electrode in the third sacral foramen of eight women with slow-transit constipation. The electrode was attached to an external stimulator for 3 weeks. A bowel symptom diary card, anorectal physiology studies, and a radiopaque marker transit study were completed before and during the test stimulation. Only two patients clinically responded, both reporting a marked improvement in stool frequency and symptoms. These two patients had an immediate return to prestimulation symptoms after removal of the stimulating leads. Colonic transit did not return to normal in any patient, including the two responders. The test stimulation resulted in a significant improvement of rectal sensory perception, which was the only parameter to change (240). Kenefick et al. described four women with a permanent implant for intractable slow-transit constipation. A good clinical response was obtained in three of them at a median follow-up of 4.5 months. The number of evacuations per week increased from a mean of 1.1 to 5.8. The Cleveland Clinic constipation score improved from 21.5 to 9.2 (241). Kenefick et al. also carried out a double-blind crossover study in two women, who were implanted with a permanent stimulator twelve months previously. The study consisted of two weeks interval with subsensory stimulation either "on" or "off." The patients and the investigator were blinded. The number of evacuations per week changed from one to five and from two to five, respectively, when the stimulator was turned on. Abdominal pain and bloating improved with increased frequency of defecation. This finding suggests that there was no placebo effect (242).

Antegrade Continent Enema Procedure

The antegrade continent enema procedure involves the formation of a continent conduit suitable for intermittent catheterisation, allowing antegrade irrigation of the colon. The procedure was first described by Malone in 1990 for the treatment of neuropathic constipation in pediatric practice. There are some data regarding the short-term outcome of this procedure in the treatment of constipation in adults. Hill et al. described early results in six patients, all of who were successfully relieved of constipation (243). Krogh and Laurberg reported a successful outcome in four of six patients after a follow-up of up to 39 months (244). Rongen et al. reported a successful outcome in eight of twelve patients after a median follow-up of 532 days (245). Recently, Lees et al. described the long-term results of this procedure, obtained in 32 patients. They observed a high rate of conduit reversal or major revision. Satisfactory function was ultimately achieved in 47% of the patients (246). This long-term result indicates that this procedure is less beneficial for patients with slow-transit constipation than previously thought.

Anorectal Outlet Obstruction

Anismus

In 1964, Wasserman (247) described four patients with obstructed defecation due to a "type of stenosis of the anorectum caused by a spasm of a component of the external anal sphincter muscle" and named it "puborectalis syndrome." Since then, a wide variety of appellations have been devised to describe this condition. The most frequently used terms are anismus, spastic pelvic floor syndrome, and nonrelaxing puborectalis syndrome. Most experts believe that symptoms such as prolonged and repeated straining at stool, the necessity of manual assistance, the sensation of incomplete evacuation, and the need for suppositories and enemas are suggestive of this condition. It has to be emphasized, however, that an almost identical pattern of symptoms might be observed in women with a large rectocele. Therefore, the history of the patient is inconclusive in establishing nonrelaxation of the pelvic floor during attempted evacuation. Although paradoxic contraction of the puborectalis muscle has been reported to be easily assessed by physical examination during straining, most investigators do not rely on palpation and advocate the use of specific tests to document anismus. EMG, evacuation proctography, and balloon expulsion test are the most commonly used methods. Much controversy, however, exists relative to the optimal diagnostic test. No single method has been proven to be pathognomonic for anismus or superior to the others. Despite several limitations, EMG is considered the most specific test, providing the best assessment of puborectalis activity during straining. In most studies, EMG is performed with the patient in the left lateral position. However, straining in this position after the painful insertion of a needle and without a natural desire to defecate is rather unphysiologic. Duthie and Bartolo (248) found evidence of anismus on EMG recordings in 11 patients with constipation during attempted defecation on a commode in the laboratory. However, during home recordings the pelvic floor relaxed during straining in all but three patients. These findings support the view that the inability to relax the pelvic floor might represent the inability to comply with the request in the unfamiliar and unphysiologic circumstances of the laboratory.

If anismus represents the principal cause of obstructed defecation, then increased EMG activity of the puborectalis muscle should be observed exclusively in patients with evacuation difficulties. Moreover, recruitment of EMG activity should be associated with a more acute anorectal angle on evacuation proctography and subsequent failure to expel a rectal balloon. Between 1985 and 1993, 10 studies were published regarding EMG evidence of anismus in controls. In only three studies did none of the controls show evidence of paradoxic contraction of the pelvic floor. In the other seven studies, the incidence of anismus varied between 12% and 61% (249). Pezim et al. (250), for example, reported that nearly 50% of their controls exhibited either a paradoxic increase in EMG activity or no suppression during straining. Jones et al. (251) found EMG evidence of anismus in 76% of patients with constipation, 50% of patients with solitary rectal ulcer syndrome, and 48% of subjects with anorectal pain. All patients with anorectal pain had a normal defecation pattern. In 74 patients with functional constipation, Kuijpers (211) found evidence of anismus on EMG and evacuation proctography in 74% and 74% of patients, respectively. Such an excellent agreement between EMG and the other diagnostic tests could not be demonstrated by others (252,253). In a prospective evaluation of a consecutive series of 112 patients with constipation associated with obstructed defecation, Jorge et al. (254) observed evidence of anismus based on EMG and evacuation proctography in 38% and 36% of patients, respectively.

Based on these data, one might suppose that the correlation between the two tests is almost optimal. However, 33% of the patients with evidence of anismus on evacuation proctography showed a normal EMG, whereas 30% of the patients with an EMG diagnosis had a normal evacuation proctography. These observations support the view that the signs of anismus are not specific for constipation and/or obstructed defecation and that EMG results are poorly correlated with evacuation proctography and balloon expulsion test. A study conducted by Schouten et al. also revealed that EMG has a very poor agreement with the other diagnostic modalities (255).

The efficacy of biofeedback has been used as an argument to support the clinical significance of anismus. Loening-Baucke (256) investigated the results of biofeedback in 38 children presenting with chronic constipation and encopresis. All these children showed contraction of the pelvic floor during straining. Twenty-eight children learned to relax their pelvic floor. Despite this beneficial effect of biofeedback, 14 of these children did not recover from constipation. The author also reported that the nonrecovered patients who learned to relax their pelvic floor had significantly decreased rectal and anal responsiveness to rectal distention when compared with the recovered patients. Keck et al. (257) reported the results of biofeedback in 12 constipated patients. Although all subjects could be taught to relax their sphincter in response to bearing down, only one patient reported resolution of symptoms. Turnbull and Ritvo (258) reported a successful outcome after biofeedback in 8 of 10 female patients with constipation. However, five of these patients showed persisting and continuing anismus on objective testing. These findings are not in accordance with the assumption that anismus is the principal cause of obstructed defecation and that biofeedback is successful solely because it corrects the "paradoxic" contraction of the pelvic floor.

Lubowski et al. (259) developed a new scintigraphic method to assess both colonic and rectal function during normal defecation. The authors found that colonic emptying is an integral part of normal defecation and that defecation is not a process of rectal emptying alone. They suggested that, "obstructed defecation may occur in some patients as a result of a disorder of colonic function rather than a disorder of the rectum or the pelvic floor muscles." It seems obvious that the popular concept that obstructed defecation is mainly due to pelvic floor muscle incoordination has little scientific basis. In an earlier EMG study of the pubococcygeus muscles in patients with obstructed defecation, Lubowski et al. (260) concluded that the puborectalis muscle did not cause obstructed defecation and that the concept of "paradoxic" contraction of this muscle is questionable.

In recent years, attention has been focused on the rectal wall properties in women with obstructed defecation. As discussed earlier in this chapter, there is growing evidence that rectal sensory perceptions as well as rectal motility are impaired in these patients, probably due to extramural damage to the efferent and afferent nerves. It seems likely that this damage to the rectal innervation results in "rectal akinesia," as described by Faucheron and Dubreuil (261).

BIOFEEDBACK TRAINING ■ During the last two decades, biofeedback therapy has gained in popularity as the foremost treatment for obstructed defecation. Bleijenberg and Kuijpers (262) achieved good results in 7 of 10 women with spastic pelvic floor syndrome. It has been argued, however, that the length of the hospital admission (2 weeks) and the rather extensive psychotherapy may have been more beneficial than the biofeedback itself. In the same period, Weber et al. (263) reported a successful outcome in 12 of 25 constipated patients (48%) after biofeedback on an outpatient basis. Since then, spectacular results have been reported with success rates of up to 100% (Table 14). There are some data indicating that biofeedback is more effective in patients with obstructed defecation than in patients with colonic inertia. At one-year control Battaglia et al. found that 50% of their patients with obstructed defecation still maintained a beneficial effect from biofeedback, whereas only 20% of those with slow-transit constipation did so (201). Chiarioni et al. reported similar findings. Six months after biofeedback the outcome was successful in 71% of the patients with obstructed defecation. Only 8% of the patients with slow-transit constipation were satisfied with the effect of biofeedback (280). Palsson et al. reviewed the literature in order to assess the efficacy of biofeedback for functional anorectal disorders. They qualified 38 studies on obstructed defecation and/or functional constipation for review. The overall average probability of successful treatment was 62.4% (281). In contrast to the high percentage of controlled studies found in the pediatric literature, only four adult studies randomly assigned patients to different treatment protocols. Koutsomanis et al. randomly assigned 60 patients with obstructed defecation either to EMG biofeedback with balloon defecation training or to balloon

TABLE 14 ■ **Outcome of Biofeedback Training in Patients with Obstructed Defecation**

Author(s)	No. of Cases	Follow-up (mo)	Success Rate (%)
Bleijenberg and Kuijpers (262) (1987)	10	>6	70
Weber et al. (263) (1987)	25	6	48
Dahl et al. (253) (1991)	14	6	93
Kavimbe et al. (264) (1991)	15	6	100
Loening-Baucke (256) (1991)	38	1	37
Lestar et al. (265) (1991)	16	15	69
Turnbull and Ritvo (258) (1992)	10	3	71
West et al. (266) (1992)	18	12	100
Wexner et al. (267) (1992)	18	9	89
Fleshman et al. (268) (1992)	9	6	89
Keck et al. (257) (1994)	12	8	8
Papachrysostomou and Smithes (269) (1994)	22	ns	86
Koutsomanis et al. (270) (1995)	60	3	40
Ho et al. (271) (1996)	62	15	90
Park et al. (272) (1996)	57	24	55
Glia et al. (273) (1997)	20	6	75
Rao et al. (274) (1997)	25	ns	76
Karlbom et al. (275) (1997)	28	14	43
McKee et al. (276) (1999)	28	ns	21
Lau et al. (277) (2000)	108	ns	55
Dailianas et al. (278) (2000)	11	6	64
Rhee et al. (279) (2000)	45	ns	69
Battaglia et al. (201) (2004)	14	12	50
Chiarioni et al. (280) (2005)	34	6	71

Abbreviation: ns, not stated.

defecation training alone and found no significant differences (270). In a randomized study of 20 patients with obstructed defecation, Bleijenberg and Kuijpers found EMG biofeedback to be superior to balloon defecation training (282). Heymen at al. compared four different biofeedback protocols and found no differences among the treatment strategies (283). Glia et al. found EMG biofeedback to be superior to pressure biofeedback with balloon training (273). Of these four studies, Koutsomanis' study is the only one with a sufficient sample size to provide meaningful conclusions.

There is, much controversy regarding the objective effects of biofeedback on anorectal function. Kavimbe et al. (264) observed a significant reduction in the anismus index after biofeedback training, which was intended as a relearning process in which the inappropriate contraction of the pelvic floor was gradually suppressed. There was an associated reduction in the time spent straining at stool and in the difficulty of defecation as well as an increased stool frequency. Papachrysostomou and Smith (269) demonstrated that various parameters related to the obstructive defecation syndrome showed significant change at the end of the biofeedback training period. However, these changes were also observed in those patients (14%) who did not admit to any clinical improvement. Ho et al. (271) studied 62 patients with obstructed defecation. In 40 patients, signs of anismus were observed, whereas 20 subjects had no evidence of anismus. The outcome of biofeedback was similar in both groups. Dahl et al. (253) reported that paradoxic anal contraction disappeared in all their patients after biofeedback. All but one patient improved considerably and learned to defecate spontaneously (Table 15). In other studies, symptom relief has been noted without evidence of correction of anismus (256–258). Rao et al. reported that biofeedback improves objective parameters such as balloon expulsion time and rectal sensory perception (274). It has been demonstrated that coexistent abnormalities such as rectocele and rectal intussusception do not adversely affect the outcome of biofeedback in patients with obstructed defecation (277). Leroi et al. (120) reported that biofeedback alone was not successful in the majority of sexually abused women with anismus. The authors noted that the outcome was markedly better if biofeedback was combined with psychotherapy. This finding suggests that the resolution of symptoms may be attributed to other factors, such as the psychological effects of encouragement and positive verbal feedback.

TABLE 15 ■ Effect of Biofeedback Training on Paradoxic Puborectalis Contraction and Symptoms of Obstructed Defecation

Author(s)	No. of Cases	Evidence of Anismus (%) Before	After	Successful Outcome
Loening-Baucke (256) (1991)	38	100	24	37
Dahl et al. (253) (1991)	14	100	0	93
Tumbull and Ritvo (258) (1992)	10	100	70	80
Papachrysostomou and Smith (269) (1994)	22	100	0	86
Keck et al. (257) (1994)	12	100	0	8
Glia et al. (273) (1997)	20	100	10	75

It has been noted that many patients use the biofeedback sessions to talk about psychosocial distress. So, it might be possible that the behavioral and psychological aspects of therapy are just as important for a successful outcome.

BOTULINUM TOXIN ■ In 1988, Hallan et al. (284) reported seven patients with anismus, diagnosed by EMG, and evacuation proctography. The symptoms of anismus resolved in six patients after the injection of botulinum toxin into the left and right sides of both the puborectalis muscle and the external sphincter. The most important side effect was fecal incontinence, occurring in two patients. Joo et al. (285) reported their experience with four patients who failed to respond to biofeedback. All four patients improved between one and three months after botulinum injections. This improvement was sustained for a longer period of time in only two subjects. Maria et al. treated three patients with animus by injecting 30 units of Type A botulinum toxin in both limbs of the puborectalis muscle. These three patients experienced symptomatic relief. In one patient the treatment had to be repeated twice because of recurrent symptoms (286). Ron et al. treated 25 patients with obstructed defecation by local injection of 10 units of botulinum toxin to each side of the puborectalis muscle. Only 37% of the patients were satisfied with the overall results. Straining, which was the main complaint, decreased in only 29% of the cases. Defecation frequency did not increase after the injection. Based on these disappointing results, the authors concluded that, "injection of botulinum toxin into the puborectalis muscle has limited therapeutic effect on patients suffering from anismus" (287).

DIVISION OF THE PUBORECTALIS MUSCLE ■ In the 1960s, Wasserman (247) and Wallace and Madden (288) advocated partial resection of the puborectalis muscle at the posterior midline in patients with anismus. Although their early results were promising, two other studies revealed very disappointing results after partial division of the puborectalis muscle (152,289). Dissatisfied with the poor outcome after partial division at the posterior midline, Kamm et al. (290) reported on 15 patients with severe constipation and three patients with megarectum who underwent an almost complete uni- or bilateral division of the puborectalis muscle. Only four patients had symptomatic improvement. It was remarkable that this information did not correlate with the ability to expel a balloon. In contrast to the current opinion that division of the puborectalis muscle is not appropriate, Yu and Cui (291) from China believe that there is still a sound indication for this procedure. The authors reported on 18 patients with anismus associated with puborectalis hypertrophy in which a partial resection at the posterior midline was performed. According to Yu and Cui (291), this procedure was successful in 83% of the patients studied (Table 16).

SACRAL NEUROMODULATION ■ Ganio et al. reported their experience with sacral neuromodulation in 16 patients with chronic outlet constipation. Following successful test stimulation all these patients were implanted with a permanent stimulator. Prior to the procedure the overall Wexner score was 14.6 (range 8–20). This score dropped to 2.7 (range 3–16) at 12 months follow-up (293). Until now these promising results have not been confirmed by others.

TABLE 16 ■ Results of Division of the Puborectalis Muscle for Anismus

Author(s)	No. of Cases	Procedure	Success Rate (%)
Keighley and Shouler (152) (1984)	7	PPD	14
Barnes et al. (289) (1985)	9	PPD	24
Kawano et al. (292) (1987)	7	PPR	43
Kamm et al. (290) (1988)	18	CLD	24
Yu and Cui (291) (1990)	18	PPR	83

Abbreviations: CLD, Complete lateral division; PPD, posterior partial division; PPR, posterior partial resection.

Rectal Intussusception

Intussusception of the rectum, or internal procidentia, is considered to be a preliminary stage in the development of complete rectal prolapse. Although complete rectal prolapse is readily apparent, the diagnosis of intussusception may be difficult to demonstrate by physical examination, endoscopy, or barium contrast examination. Evacuation proctography is the most useful diagnostic procedure for identifying intussusception. The radiologic features are characteristic. The rectum begins to intussuscept a few centimeters above the pelvic floor. A typical funnel-like configuration is seen in Figure 10.

In the past, rectal intussusception was considered one of the principal causes of obstructed defecation. In 1984, Hoffman et al. (294) suggested that a modified Ripstein procedure was adequate to relieve symptoms of obstructed defecation. However, the authors' follow-up was short and concerned only a small group of patients. Johansson et al. (295) reported a series of 23 patients who presented for operation because of obstructed defecation. Thirty-five percent of those patients had worsening of their symptoms after rectopexy (295). Similar results have been described by others (296). There is growing evidence that a posterior rectopexy induces rectal evacuation disturbances, especially when the lateral ligaments of the rectum are divided (297,298). Moreover, it has been shown that rectal intussusception is a common finding on evacuation proctography in normal volunteers (299). Based on these and other observations, it has been suggested that intussusception is the result, rather than the cause of obstructed defecation. Operative correction of intussusception in patients with obstructed defecation has not been met with good results. A discussion of the problem was presented in Chapter 21.

Rectocele

A rectocele is a herniation of the anterior rectal wall into the lumen of the vagina. The significance of rectoceles in the pathogenesis of obstructed defecation remains debatable. Some experts believe that rectoceles are merely a secondary manifestation of chronic straining on a rectovaginal septum weakened both by obstetric trauma and progressive pelvic floor deficiency, as part of the aging process. Others believe that rectoceles are indeed an important cause of obstructed defecation. They assume that trapping of feces in the rectocele results in obstructed evacuation and that further straining aggravates the problem by pushing the stool further from the anal opening. Usually the rectocele does not become symptomatic until the fourth or fifth decade of life. During straining, the apex of the rectocele moves inferiorly and anteriorly. Stool is trapped in this sacculation, and straining aggravates the problem by pushing the stool further from the anal opening. Most patients with a symptomatic rectocele have a normal daily urge to defecate, but they "can't get it out." To empty the bowel, some patients use manual pressure on the side or front of the anal outlet or they insert a finger against the posterior vaginal wall to assist defecation. A rectocele may be associated with other symptoms such as rectal fullness, incomplete evacuation, pain, bleeding, protrusion, and soiling. The diagnosis is made by obtaining an adequate history and by bimanual or rectovaginal palpation. A hooked finger pressed on the anterior rectal wall can detect the pocket-like defect located just above the anal sphincter. This mechanism can be demonstrated on evacuation proctography (Fig. 11).

A wide variety of anatomic and functional changes on defecography have been observed in patients with a so-called symptomatic rectocele (300). It has to be emphasized that it is very difficult to determine whether a defecographic finding is the cause or the result of excessive straining. This makes the ultimate therapeutic decision a difficult task. It is generally accepted that rectoceles less

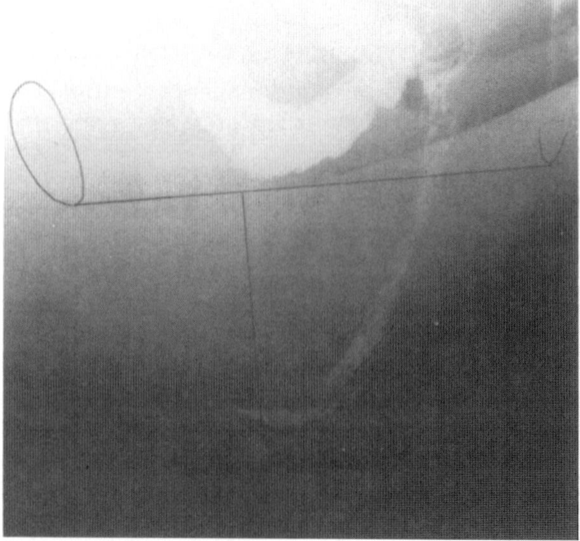

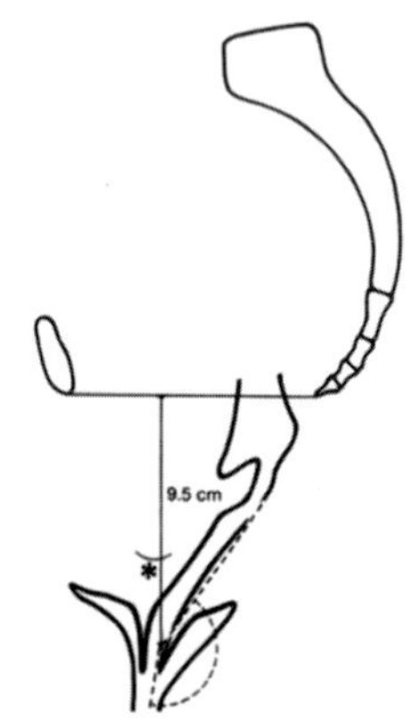

FIGURE 10 ■ Defecography in a patient with, rectal intussusception.

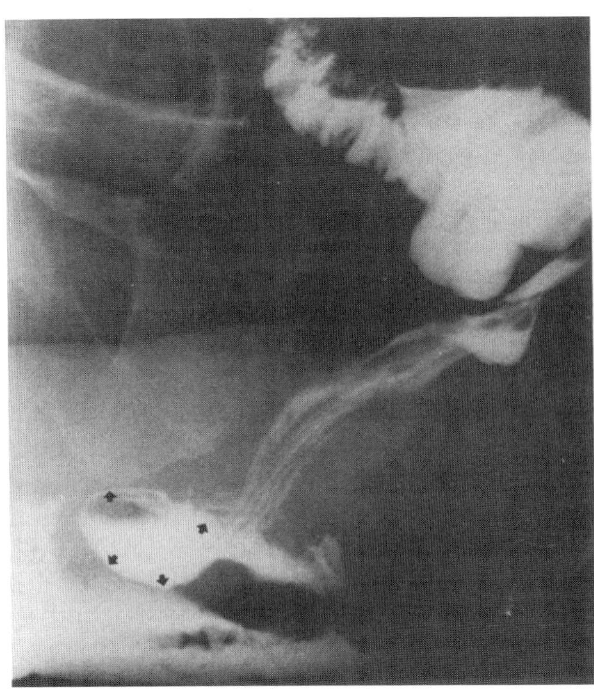

FIGURE 11 ■ Defecography in a patient with rectocele (*arrows*).

than 2 cm in size are not clinically significant (299,301). Only rectoceles more than 3 cm in depth are considered abnormal. It has been shown that larger rectoceles are more likely to retain contrast than smaller ones (300). However, the size of the rectocele and the extent of barium trapping have not been shown to correlate with the degree of symptoms or with the outcome of rectocele repair (300–303). Johansson et al. (304) have suggested that anismus is a causative factor in the formation of a rectocele. The authors stated that rectocele repair in patients with concomitant anismus cannot be successful, because the underlying cause for obstructed defecation persists. van Dam et al. (305) conducted a prospective study to evaluate the prevalence of anismus in patients with a symptomatic rectocele and to investigate the impact of this phenomenon on the outcome of operative repair. The results of rectocele repair in patients with anismus were similar to those obtained in patients without evidence of anismus. This finding was irrespective of the method of diagnosing anismus.

Several authors have tried to assess specific features encountered in women with a symptomatic rectocele. Siproudhis et al. (306) found that patients with a rectocele differed significantly from those without a rectocele in having frequent vaginal digitation, more frequent symptoms of urinary incontinence, and a history of hysterectomy. Delayed rectal emptying, incomplete rectal emptying, and manometric signs of anismus were more frequently encountered in the rectocele group. Murthy et al. (307) adopted a selective approach, based on several criteria, including the sensation of a vaginal mass or bulge that required digital support, barium trapping in the rectocele, and the presence of a very large rectocele associated with anterior rectal wall prolapse. The authors claim that the selection of patients based on these criteria results in a very good clinical outcome. Karlbom et al. (308) observed that the need for vaginal or perineal digitation preoperatively was related to a good result, whereas a previous hysterectomy, a large rectal area on defecography, and the preoperative use of enemas and laxatives related to a poor outcome. In contrast, Mellgren et al. (309) found that preoperative vaginal digitation was not mandatory for a good postoperative result. The authors also demonstrated that delayed colonic transit was related to a less favorable outcome. This finding has been confirmed by others (300,308). Stojkovic et al. compared women with a successful rectocele repair to those with persistent symptoms. There was no difference in age between the two groups. There was also no difference in size of rectocele, degree of emptying, the presence of another defecographic abnormality, and the need to self-digitate between the two groups (310).

Some authors are reluctant to repair a completely emptying rectocele, whereas others report that some patients still derive benefit from operative treatment. These reflections illustrate that many questions regarding the specific features of rectoceles and the selection criteria for repair are still unanswered.

Rectoceles can be repaired by several approaches: transvaginal, transanal (or a combination of both), transperineal, and abdominal. Recently the use of a mesh has been introduced for rectocele repair. Until now it is unknown which treatment modality is the most optimal one.

TRANSVAGINAL REPAIR ■ For more than one century the history of rectocele repair was written by gynecologists. They performed a posterior colporrhaphy combined with levator plication and some form of perineorrhaphy. Nonrandomized studies suggest that this approach is associated with a 25% incidence of dyspareunia after the procedure and that one-third of the patients suffer from persistent evacuation difficulties after the operation (311). Arnold et al. performed a retrospective review of 64 rectocele repairs. Both the transvaginal and the transanal approach were used in 26 and 35 patients, respectively. They found no difference in complications between the techniques. Forty-seven patients could be contacted for follow-up. Although improvement was reported by 80% of the patients, persistent obstructed defecation was noted by 54% of the women. New onset dyspareunia was noted by 22% of the patients. There was no difference in results and complications between the two approaches (312). Nieminen et al. compared the transvaginal approach to the transanal approach. Thirty female patients with a symptomatic rectocele were enrolled in a randomized controlled trial. The need to digitally assist rectal emptying decreased in the transvaginal group from 73% to 7% and in the transanal group from 66% to 27%. The respective recurrence rates were 7% and 40%. In contrast with other studies, none of the patients reported new onset dyspareunia (313). Recently, the use of a mesh has been introduced for transvaginal rectocele repair. Tayrac et al. used a polypropylene mesh. Mesh infection and rectovaginal fistulas were not encountered. The procedure was successful in 92% of the patients (314). Altman et al. designed a study to evaluate transvaginal rectocele repair using porcine collagen mesh (Pelvicol™, CR Bard, Murray Hill, New Jersey, U.S.A.). The outcome was assessed in 29 women. At 12-month follow-up, defecography revealed a persistent or recurrent rectocele in 15 patients. At 6-month follow-up, many patients experienced a significant decrease in rectal evacuation difficulties. This beneficial effect was less pronounced at 12-month follow-up. New onset dyspareunia was not observed. Based on these findings the authors concluded that, although transvaginal rectocele repair with a collagen mesh improves anatomic support, there is a substantial risk for recurrence. It is obvious that further evaluation is warranted before the use of biomaterial mesh can be adopted into clinical practice (315).

TRANSANAL REPAIR ■ Marks was one of the first to note persistent evacuation difficulties following traditional transvaginal rectocele repair (316). He also noted that many women with a symptomatic rectocele had a "thinning" of the anterior rectal wall, including the muscle layers, and an enlarged rectal ampulla. Based on these observations he advocated repair of the rectal side of the rectocele. Although there are several variations and modifications, the principal goal of the procedure is to remove or plicate redundant rectal mucosa and to plicate the anterior rectal wall.

Advantages attributed to the transanal approach are that it is a procedure of lesser magnitude than the gynecologic approach, it affords the opportunity to correct associated anorectal pathology, and there is a more direct access to the suprasphincteric area. The disadvantage of this approach is the inability to correct a cystocele simultaneously.

For transanal repair, the patient is placed in the prone jackknife position. The submucosal plane of the anterior wall is infiltrated with an epinephrine-containing solution such as 0.5% lidocaine (Xylocaine) in 1:200,000 epinephrines. A midline incision is made at a point starting just above the dentate line and is carried upward in the rectum approximately 7 to 8 cm, depending on the size of the rectocele (Fig. 12A). Alternatively, a rectangular flap of mucosa and submucosa is elevated. Mucosal flaps are developed on each side. A further option is a simple transverse mucosal incision 1 cm above the dentate line (317). Meticulous hemostasis is obtained with cautery. The musculofascial defect in the anterior wall is plicated in a transverse manner with interrupted absorbable sutures such as 2–0 Vicryl (318,319) (Figs. 12B and C). If weakness of the anterior wall persists, another row of similar sutures can be placed (Fig. 12D). This row may be supplemented with three or four vertical sutures of the same material (320,321) (Fig. 12E). The technique adopted by Sullivan et al. (320) consists of longitudinal plication of the circular muscle of the anterior rectal wall with five or more slowly absorbed sutures such as 2–0 Dexon or Vicryl (Figs. 12F and G). For large rectoceles, the authors recommend the initial use of three or four transverse sutures to pull the levator ani muscles medially. The transverse apposition is then reinforced by a longitudinal plication (Fig. 12E). The authors have entirely abandoned the use of transverse sutures in favor of longitudinal plication (Sullivan ES. Personal communication, 1997). This decision was based on a subsequent prospective study of 100 patients, in which the authors noted sepsis and separation of the wound when the combined technique was used, especially in patients who were having large rectoceles repaired. Sarles et al. (317) use interrupted polyglycolic acid sutures (2–0), with "bites" of rectal muscle wall taken every 5 mm. Their rationale is that the anatomic lesion is due to weakness of the circular muscle, the horizontal fibers of which are spread apart and attenuated by progressive distention of the anterior rectal wall. Thus, vertical plication sutures are more likely to reconstitute the rectovaginal septum. The excess mucosa is excised, and the mucosal flaps are closed with a continuous absorbable suture (Fig. 12H).

Block described a modification, characterized by simple plication of the redundant mucosa without excision (322). This technique is less popular because some patients complain of persistent tenesmus, and urge to defecate if the excess mucosa is not removed. In addition, necrosis of the plicated rectal mucosa may result in postoperative infection (323). Transanal repair can also be performed using a linear stapler. The results of this modified technique have been reported recently (324). A major concern after transanal repair is the impairment of fecal continence. Arnold et al. reported that 38% of their patients developed incontinence (312). This serious side effect may occur because of an occult sphincter defect that becomes symptomatic or may develop as a result of the anal dilatation and stretching during the procedure. It has been shown that transanal rectocele repair results in a decline of anal resting pressure as well as anal squeeze pressure (325). van Dam et al. evaluated the impact of a combined transvaginal/transanal rectocele repair on fecal continence in a consecutive series of 89 women. They observed deterioration of continence in 7% of the patients (326). Another concern after transanal repair is the development of dyspareunia. Schapayak et al. observed this complication in 20% of their patients (319). van Dam et al. found new onset dyspareunia following a combined transvaginal/transanal repair in 17 out of 41 sexually active patients (41%) (326). Similar figures have been reported by others (327).

Most series, except those reported by Arnold et al. (312), have revealed promising short-term results after transanal rectocele repair. Recent studies, however, do suggest that the medium- and long-term outcome is less favorable (see Table 17).

TRANSPERINEAL REPAIR ■ Rectoceles can also be repaired by a transperineal approach. This type of repair is usually performed through a transverse perineal incision. The anorectal-vaginal plane is dissected and the rectocele is plicated with a running suture. After this plication a levatorplasty is performed. With respect to symptoms of obstructed defecation such a transperineal repair, seems to be as effective as the transanal and the transvaginal repair. Hirst et al. reported a successful outcome in 64% of their patients (333). In another study, the short-term outcome was good in 91% of the cases. However, five years after the procedure the success rate had dropped to 70%. The same study revealed new onset dyspareunia in 17% of the cases (335). Similar figures have been reported by others (336). The transperineal route avoids anal instrumentation and allows the surgeon to perform a sphincter repair in patients who have associated fecal incontinence (311). Ayabaca et al. reported that fecal continence improved in 74% of their patients after a transperineal rectocele repair with concomitant sphincteroplasty (337). In 1996, Watson et al. were the first to describe a transperineal mesh repair, which was successful in eight out of nine women (338). More recently, similar results have been reported by others. One year after mesh

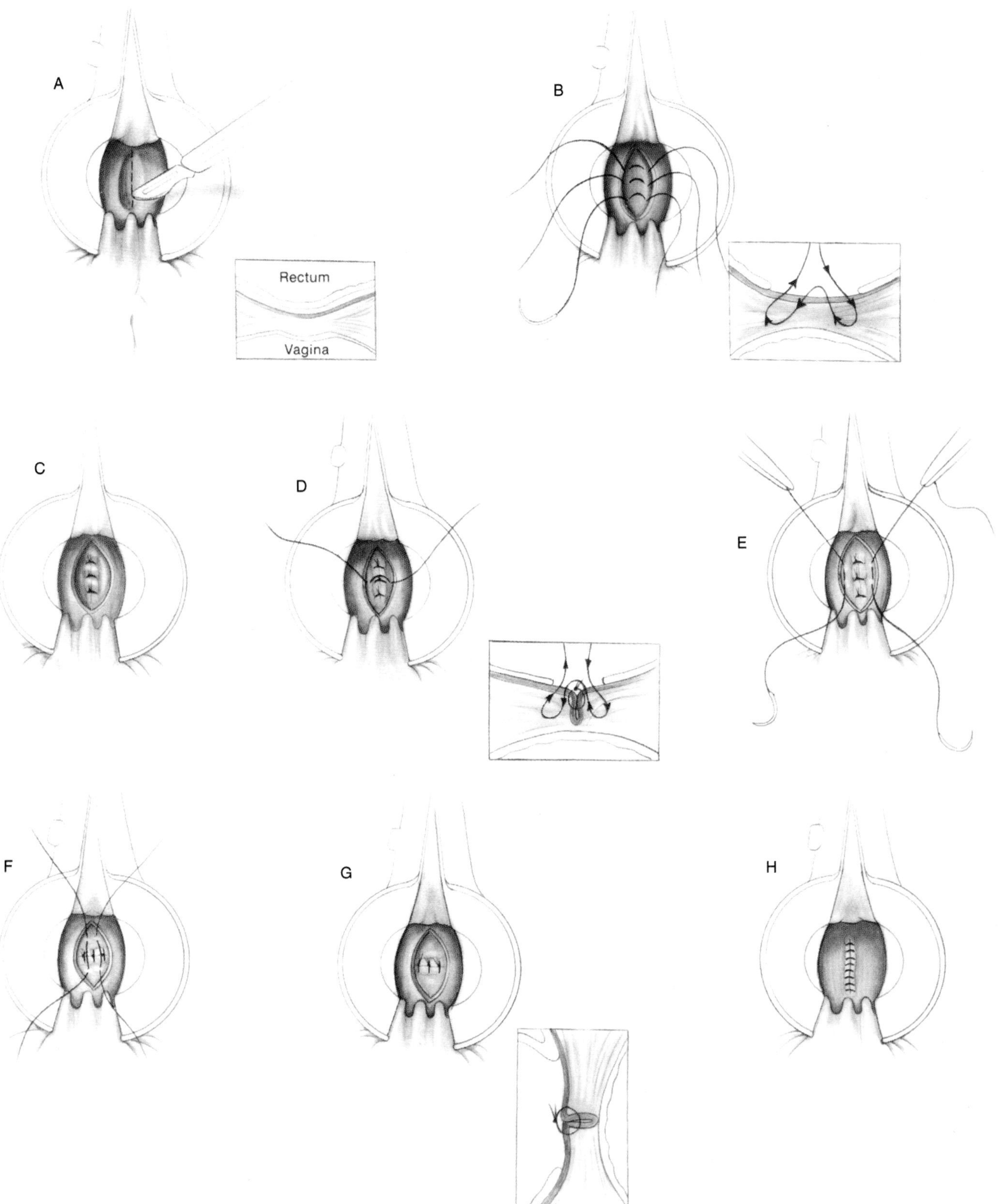

FIGURE 12 ■ Rectocele repair. (**A**) Mucosal incision over rectocele. (**B**) and (**C**) Transverse plication of defect. (**D**) Second row of sutures for persistent anterior defect. (**E**) Supplemental repair by vertical sutures. (**F**) and (**G**) Sullivan's technique for repair of rectocele. (**H**) Mucosal reapproximation.

repair, Mercer-Jones et al. noted a successful outcome in 77% of their patients. They encountered two superficial wound infections and one deep infection, all responding to antibiotic therapy. In their series no mesh had to be removed (339). Lechaux et al. reported a successful outcome in 80% of the cases (340).

ABDOMINAL REPAIR ■ Correction of a rectocele by an abdominal approach is most often employed by gynecologists, when repair of an accompanying enterocele or vault prolapse is indicated. Usually the dissection is performed in the rectovaginal space to expose the posterior vaginal wall down to the perineal body. The fascial defect resulting

TABLE 17 ■ Results of Rectocele Repair

Author(s)	No. of Cases	Procedure	Follow-Up (Yr)	Success Rate (%)[a]
Sullivan et al. (320) (1968)	151	TAR	1.5	80
Capps (318) (1975)	51	TAR	ns	94
Khubchandani et al. (321) (1983)	59	TAR	1.5	80
Sehapayak (319) (1985)	355	TAR	ns	85
Sarles et al. (317) (1989)	16	TAR	1.6	94
Arnold et al. (312) (1990)	35	TAR	ns	46
	29	TVR	ns	46
Janssen and van Dijke (328) (1994)	76	TAR	1.0	87
Mellgren et al. (309) (1995)	25	TVR	1.0	88
Karlbom et al. (308) (1996)	344	TAR	0.9	79
van Dam et al. (305) (1996)	75	TAR + TVR	4.0	71
Murthy et al. (307) (1996)	31	TAR	2.5	92
Khubchandani et al. (329) (1997)	123	TAR	n.s.	82
Tjandra et al. (330) (1999)	59	TAR	1.5	78
Ayav et al. (324) (2004)	21	TAR[b]	5	71
Heriot et al. (331) (2004)	45	TAR	2	55
Thornton et al. (327) (2005)	40	TAR	3.5	63
Abbas et al. (332) (2005)	107	TAR	4	72
Hirst et al. (333) (2005)	42	TAR	2	48
Roman and Michot (334) (2005)	71	TAR	6	50

[a]Excellent (asymptomatic) or good (considerable improvement).
[b]Using a linear stapler.
Abbreviations: ns, not significant; TAR, transanal repair; TVR, transvaginal repair; n.s., not stated.

in the rectocele is repaired by reattaching the posterior vagina bilaterally to the superior fascia of the levator ani, from the perineal body to the uterosacral ligament. In a retrospective matched cohort study, Thornton et al. compared transanal repair to abdominal correction. They found a statistically greater alleviation of obstructed defecation after transanal repair (68% vs. 28%, respectively). New onset dyspareunia was encountered by 36% of the patients following transanal repair and by 22% of the patients after abdominal correction (327). In another recent study, Vermeulen et al. evaluated the results of anterolateral rectopexies for rectocele repair. Twenty patients were included. Defecography, performed postoperatively, revealed that all rectoceles were restored or at least diminished to normal size. Despite this observation, only 40% of the patients experienced resolution of symptoms. New onset dyspareunia was encountered by 50% (341).

Although the role of rectocele as a cause of difficult defecation has been long misunderstood or unrecognized, it should not be dismissed. By the same token, the presence of a rectocele in a patient with constipation does not necessarily indicate that the anatomic abnormality is causative. The simple detection of a rectocele is not in its own right an indication for operation. Sarles et al. (317) list three points of importance in correctly defining the role of rectocele in constipation: (i) the necessity for digital vaginal maneuver for evacuation, (ii) defecography demonstrating not only the rectocele but also presenting evidence of retention of stool, and (iii) defecography permitting the recognition of associated lesions, especially internal rectal procidentia.

Short-Segment Hirschsprung's disease

When classic Hirschsprung's disease is treated by restorative anterior resection of the rectum (Rehbein's procedure), a short aganglionic segment remains, and symptoms of constipation persist. These residual symptoms can be treated by anorectal dilatation. Based on these findings, Bentley recommended using anorectal myectomy for the treatment of short-segment Hirschsprung's disease, which is one of the causes of anorectal outlet obstruction (342). He assumed that the therapeutic effect of the anorectal myectomy could be compared to that of gastroesophageal myotomy (Heller's procedure) in patients with esophageal achalasia. Because his preliminary results were promising, other authors started to treat patients with short-segment Hirschsprung's disease as well as patients with non-Hirschsprung's constipation by anorectal myectomy (Table 18). Anorectal myectomy can be expected to be effective only if patients with high anal basal tone in association with normal transit and impaired rectal emptying are selected. Anorectal myectomy alone or in combination with anterior resection was curative in a small number of patients reported by Fishbein et al. (351).

Idiopathic Megarectum

The entity of idiopathic megarectum was described in the section of slow-transit constipation. The question of which patients might be candidates for operative therapy is difficult to answer. Indications for operation are based on colonic function, taking into account an abnormally low frequency of defecation, delayed transit time of radiopaque markers, and/or abnormalities detected with anorectal manometry. These abnormalities include an absent rectoanal inhibitory reflex, anal contraction instead of relaxation when the rectum is distended, spontaneous variations of pressure in the rectum and anal canal, a hypertonic anal canal, abnormalities of the rectoanal inhibitory reflex with sometimes lesser and other times greater amplitudes of relaxation, and pressure exceeding predistention values before returning to the resting level (overshoot).

TABLE 18 ■ Clinical Results of Anorectal Myectomy

	Short-Segment Hirschsprung's Disease		Non-Hirschsprung's Constipation	
Author(s)	No. of Patients	Success Rate (%)	No. of Patients	Success Rate (%)
Thomas et al. (343) (1970)	11	45		
Lynn and van Heerden (344) (1975)	28	93		
Clayden and Lawson (73) (1976)	10	100	11	82
Shermeta and Nilprabhassorn (345) (1977)	9	78		
Martelli et al. (62) (1978)			62	77
McCready and Beart (346) (1980)	13	62		
Freeman (347) (1984)			61	86
Hamdy and Scobie (348) (1984)	6	66		
Mishalany and Wooley (349) (1984)			25	76
Pinho et al. (350) (1990)	12	17	39	17

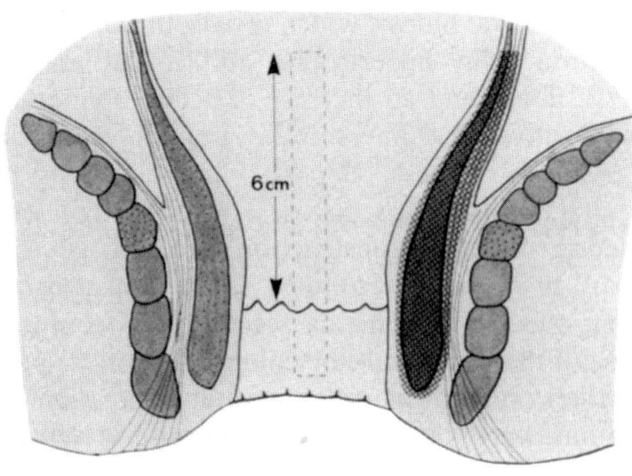

FIGURE 13 ■ Anorectal myectomy.

Anorectal myectomy appears to have a limited role in the treatment of megarectum. The technique consists of submucosal resection of a 1 cm wide strip of internal sphincteric muscle up to at least 6 cm above the dentate line (Fig. 13).

In the series by Martelli et al. (62), anorectal myectomy was performed in 62 patients; 62% of the 50 patients who had fewer than three stools per week had more than three per week one year after myectomy. The six patients operated on because of the abnormal transit of radiopaque markers and the six operated on because of abnormal manometric findings were asymptomatic. Of the 26% of patients who were incontinent preoperatively, two-thirds became continent postoperatively. However, 16% of the patients who were continent preoperatively became incontinent postoperatively. In a more recent report, Poisson and Devroede (352) stated that the results of anorectal myectomy have been disappointing. In their experience, this condition responds well to a Boley pull-through procedure. Yoshioka and Keighley (353) reported the results of anorectal myectomy in 29 patients with chronic constipation. The improvement in 62% of patients correlated with a decrease in the maximal resting anal pressure associated with outlet obstruction. The results of other reports are summarized in Table 18. Martelli et al. (62) recommend performing a Soave procedure in patients who have undergone an anorectal myectomy with no success and in whom markers have demonstrated delayed transit time in the descending and sigmoid colon. Kimura et al. (354) performed posterior myectomy of the remaining aganglionic rectal muscular cuff in patients with persistent rectal achalasia after Soave endorectal pull-through procedure. Following this procedure, five patients had remarkable relief of constipation, distention, and enterocolitis.

Theory based on rather extensive experience with lateral internal sphincterotomy in the treatment of fissure-in-ano suggests that a lateral internal sphincterotomy results in fewer problems than a posterior sphincterotomy. In addition, a sphincterotomy probably also would suffice rather than performing a myectomy. But these opinions are only conjecture at this time.

Adult Hirschsprung's Disease

A certain number of patients with Hirschsprung's disease do not present themselves for medical care until adulthood. Recognition of this childhood disease in an adult is difficult. The patients are usually men in their twenties with a lifelong history of constipation necessitating frequent use of laxatives and enemas. Plain films of the abdomen show distention of the distal colon. A barium enema study reveals a narrowed rectum with proximal colonic distention. The diagnosis depends on the patient's history, barium enema results, anorectal manometry, and rectal biopsy, which reveals the absence of ganglion cells, hypertrophy and hyperplasia of nerve fibers, and an increase of acetylcholinesterase-positive nerve fibers in the lamina propria and muscularis mucosa. Reported complications of adult Hirschsprung's disease are severe fecal impactions leading to obstruction, hemorrhage, volvulus of the colon secondary to an elongated colonic mesentery, ischemia secondary to compromise of the vasculature by colonic distention, perforation, superficial inflammation, ulceration of the mucosa by fecalomas, compromise of venous return, and decreased diaphragmatic excursion leading to pulmonary atelectasis (355).

Several procedures have been used to treat adult Hirschsprung's disease. Although conclusions are difficult to reach regarding the appropriate operative therapy, at the present time the operation of choice is the Duhamel procedure (162,346,356–359). In a comprehensive review of the literature, Wheatley et al. (360) found that for the Duhamel operation, the complication rate was 10% for major complications and 2% for minor complications, and the results were good in 91%, fair in 7%, and poor in 2%. A more recent report by Kim et al. (359) on 11 patients undergoing a Duhamel procedure revealed three major postoperative complications—two fistula-in-ano and one ileus, each resolving without operation. The long-term results were excellent except in one patient who developed impotence. Luukkonen et al. (361) reported eight patients with adult Hirschsprung's disease, seven of whom underwent a Duhamel procedure and one who underwent an anterior resection later converted to a Soave procedure. None of the patients experienced constipation, but five had occasional soiling. These results can be compared to Swenson's operation, in which major complications occurred in 33%, minor complications in 7%, and impotence in 7%, with results good in 80% and poor in 20%. Endorectal pull-through operations result in major complications in 25% and minor complications in 13%, with results good in 85%, fair in 6%, and poor in 9%. The Duhamel operation obviates any extensive pelvic dissection and avoids the damage to the sensory fibers of the rectum that may be encountered during the Swenson procedure. It also avoids the mucosal dissection of the rectum required by the Soave procedure. Wu et al. (362) reported on three patients who underwent resection of the diseased bowel, rectal mucosectomy, and coloanal anastomosis with good results.

Introduction of stapling devices has facilitated performance of the Duhamel procedure. An improved technique involving use of the curved EEA, GIA, and TA 55 staplers has simplified the operation (363). The operation is performed with the patient in the modified lithotomy position. The colon is mobilized, freeing a portion of the aganglionic segment of bowel and any markedly dilated bowel that appears decompensated proximal to the aganglionic segment. The presacral space is entered and a tunnel is created down to the levator ani muscle. Extensive dissection in the pelvis should be avoided, with only enough room made for delivery of the proximal bowel into this space. Mobilization of the proximal colon should be carried out only if there is inadequate length to reach the lower rectum. A 2–0 Prolene pursestring suture is inserted at the proximal line of resection.

Attention is then directed to the perineum, where a suitable retractor (Parks or Pratt) is inserted into the anal canal. A curved circular stapler with the trocar in place is inserted through the anus. The trocar can be extruded through the posterior rectal wall just above the levator ani muscle (Fig. 14A). The trocar is removed (depending on the instrument used), the anvil is reengaged in the central shaft, and the anastomosis is created (Fig. 14B). Inspection reveals that proximal tissue removed is the familiar "ring" but that distal tissue comes out in the form of a disk, because no suture was applied (Fig. 14C).

With the 90 or 100 mm anastomosing stapler, a single application through the anus should suffice to create the side-to-side anastomosis (Fig. 14D and E) between the rectum and the proximal ganglionic bowel. A second application, if necessary, is made by making an opening in the proximal colon and the adjacent rectum. It is probably better not to have divided the rectum before this point because it is a convenient "handle" during this step of the procedure. The rectal stump is then transected with a linear stapling instrument. If an abdominal application of the anastomosing instrument was necessary, the residual opening is closed with sutures or another application of the linear stapling instrument. At the end of the procedure the pelvis is filled with saline, and sigmoidoscopy is performed. The bowel is insufflated with air to ensure that no leak is present. No "covering" colostomy is necessary.

Megacolon Secondary to Chagas' Disease

Chagas' disease is an endemic clinical entity caused by *Trypanosoma cruzi*, a parasite that is transmitted to humans by the hematophagic *Triatominae* insects. It affects several million people in Latin America, mostly in Brazil, Argentina, Chile, Paraguay, and Bolivia. Megacolon, the most common complication of intestinal trypanosomiasis, results in severe constipation, for which operation is indicated. The two main complications are fecaloma and volvulus of the sigmoid colon. A variety of procedures have been proposed for the correction of this disabling condition, including sigmoidectomy, abdominal rectosigmoidectomy, left colectomy, and subtotal colectomy. On long-term follow-up, however, these operations have proved to be inadequate in a significant number of cases, apparently due to preservation of the dyskinetic rectum that continues to act as a functional obstacle to the progression of the fecal bolus. Pull-through operations, which include the removal of all or almost all of the dyskinetic rectum, or the exclusion of the rectum, as in the Duhamel-Haddad operation, have been demonstrated to be superior (364). Functional results are satisfactory. Anal continence is normal in the vast majority of cases, and sexual disturbances are rare.

Neuronal Intestinal Dysplasia

Neuronal intestinal dysplasia is a specific congenital innervation defect of the intestinal wall belonging to the group of dysganglionosis (365). Type A is characterized by aplasia or hypoplasia of the sympathetic innervation leading to constipation and spasticity of the intestinal wall. This form is observed only in children and not in adults. Type B is characterized by dysplasia of the submucous plexus because of impaired development. The clinical manifestation is a weak propulsive motility and consequently constipation. This form is observed in adults as well as children. Classic histologic features show hyperplasia and giant ganglia with 7 to 10 nerve cells that show a variable enzyme activity. Enzymehistochemical examination reveals a dense network of parasympathetic nerve fibers with increased acetylcholinesterase activity. Conservative treatment is usually unavailing and operative intervention is needed—most often subtotal colectomy.

SPECIAL CONSIDERATIONS

■ PREVENTION

In certain clinical circumstances, straining at stool presents an added hazard to the patient. Patients who have had a myocardial infarction and patients with cerebral and cardiovascular disease and thromboembolic disease are at special risk. These patients should be given bulk forming agents, either those found in natural foodstuffs or in a psyllium seed preparation.

■ FECAL IMPACTION

Fecal impaction is a serious crisis that may constitute an intestinal obstruction. Ninety-eight percent of fecal impactions occurs in the rectum. The most common complications associated with fecal impaction include fecal incontinence, urinary tract infections, intestinal obstruction, and ischemic necrosis and stercoral ulcerations that may lead to bleeding or perforation (366). Fecal impaction in an undistressed individual can be evacuated with oral laxatives such as senna (six tablets twice daily). More likely, administration of enemas will be required, and tap water or sodium phosphate enemas are effective. The use of mineral oil and dioctyl sodium sulfosuccinate has been advocated, although the effectiveness of these agents is probably due to the fluid volume. In an acutely distressed individual, digital evacuation can be achieved with the use of moderate sedation. For more proximal impactions, water-soluble contrast material in 20% to 50% solutions will stimulate hyperperistalsis and draw water into the bowel and lubricate the fecal mass (366). Whole-gut irrigation with 2 L of isosmotic solution of polyethylene glycol has been used in nonemergency cases without complete obstruction.

Recurrent fecal impaction should be prevented by reviewing the background factors that have led to the impaction and eliminating or avoiding them in the future. Dietary management and prescription of suppositories and senna preparations may be necessary. Lactulose, 10 mL twice a day, is useful, especially in the unusual case in which fecalomas pack the large bowel all the way to the cecum.

Endoscopic or radiologic examination of the colon is indicated to rule out the presence of a neoplasm. An endocrine or metabolic screen also may be appropriate.

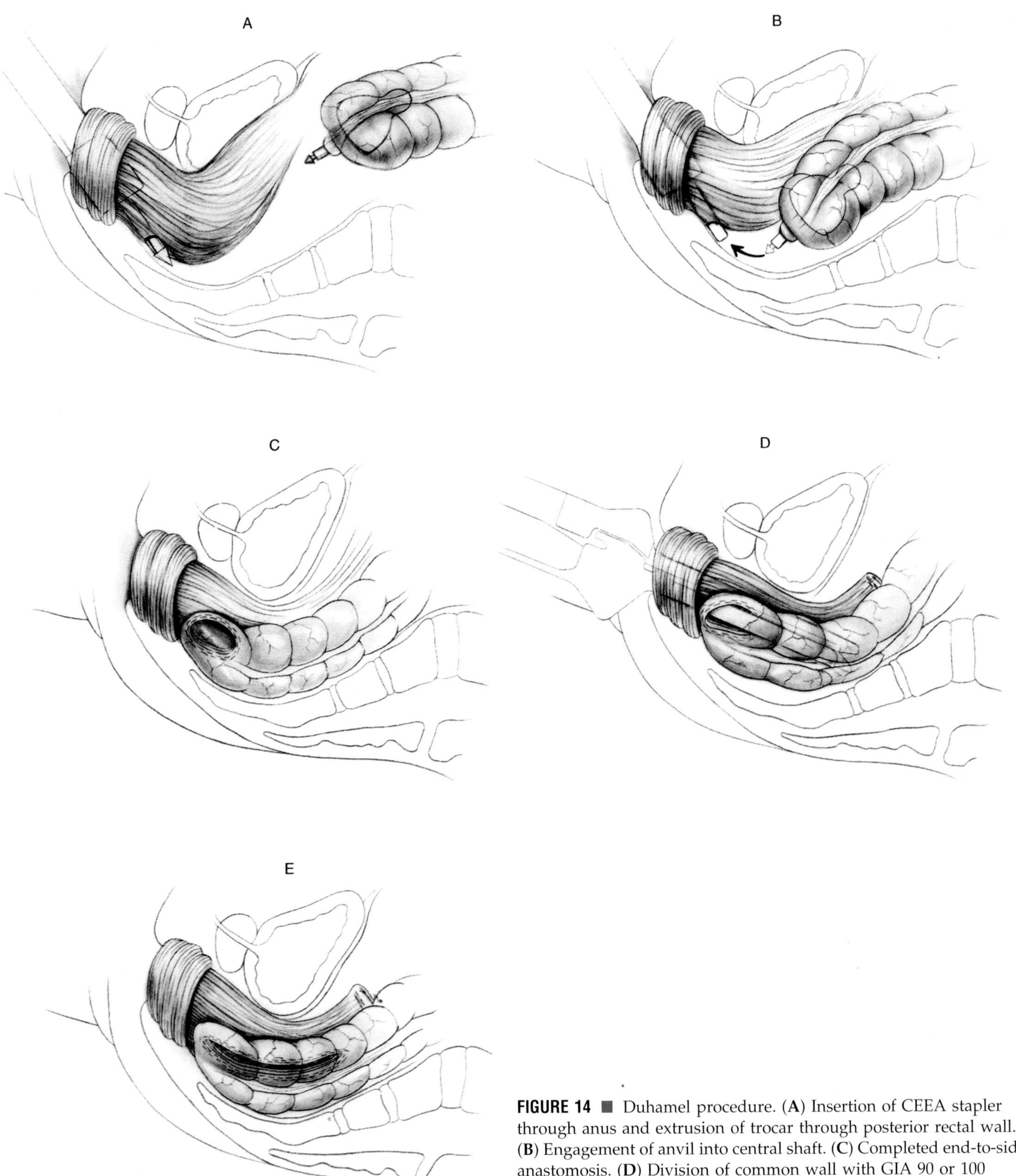

FIGURE 14 ■ Duhamel procedure. (**A**) Insertion of CEEA stapler through anus and extrusion of trocar through posterior rectal wall. (**B**) Engagement of anvil into central shaft. (**C**) Completed end-to-side anastomosis. (**D**) Division of common wall with GIA 90 or 100 instrument. (**E**) Completed procedure.

■ PSYCHIATRIC STATES

As noted previously, various psychiatric states are associated with constipation. The clinician also should remember that various antidepressant drugs are constipating. Constipation resulting from the latter cause is amenable to stimulant laxatives. An organic cause of constipation must not be overlooked in psychiatric patients.

■ SPINAL CORD INJURIES

Severe constipation often follows spinal cord injury. Several mechanisms may be involved in the pathogenesis, including the lack of conscious urge to defecate, forced body immobilization, associated motor paralysis of the abdominal and perineal muscles, and possible motor alterations at the level of the colon, rectum, and anus. Although a minor degree of transit delay may be present in the right colon in virtually all patients, there is either no or abnormally slow transit in the left colon and rectum (18). Constipation in patients with paraplegia and transection of the spine between C4 and T12 vertebral levels is due to alteration in bowel segments innervated by the parasympathetic sacral outflow.

Longo et al. (367), in a review of the functional alterations of the denervated hindgut, summarized their findings as follows. The foregut and midgut are innervated by parasympathetic fibers in the vagus and sympathetic fibers from the lower six thoracic vertebrae. In contrast, the hindgut is innervated by parasympathetic fibers arising from the sacral plexus and by sympathetic fibers from the lumbar spinal column. Consequently, in most spinal cord injuries the foregut and midgut remain normally innervated, whereas the hindgut loses input from cerebral and spinal cord sources. In high-cord lesions this results in decreased colonic motility. In low-cord injuries there is loss of inhibitory influences that normally regulate left colonic and rectosigmoid sphincter activity downward. This increased motility causes a loss of left colonic compliance and increases left colonic transit, thus leading to chronic constipation. In both high- and low-cord injuries, reflex activity of the anorectum is left unregulated by cerebral input. Once stimulated by distention, the rectum spontaneously evacuates its contents. Thus, fecal impaction and incontinence in these patients principally results from loss of inhibitory influences on rectosigmoid sphincter activity and rectal reflex activity.

Constipation is a major problem in the management of patients with spinal cord transection. To avoid overflow, fecal incontinence, and the necessity for frequent disimpaction, these patients may benefit from a bowel training regimen in which the defecation reflex is initiated at fixed time intervals.

Approximately the third or fourth night after the injury, a laxative is given and followed, if necessary, by a suppository the next morning. Administration of the laxative and/or the suppository is continued until a regular bowel habit is achieved. Digital removal and one or two enemas may be required in the first or second week. The goal is bowel evacuation every other day. Diet should contain plentiful amounts of fiber-containing foods. A chemical stimulant such as senna or bisacodyl should be administered on alternate nights. Stimulation to initiate defecation might include body movement, eating, drinking, massage of the abdomen, anal digital stimulation, or insertion of a suppository.

In their review, Safadi et al. (368) found that 27% to 62% of patients with spinal cord injury have complaints related to the gastrointestinal tract that require treatment or alter lifestyle. One of the common problems cited was colonic dysmotility. For patients who fail lesser measures, the formation of an intestinal stoma is effective in the treatment of colonic dysmotility associated with spinal cord injuries. Safadi et al. (368) reviewed the records 45 spinal cord injury patients with intestinal stomas. A left-sided colostomy was performed in 21 patients, right-sided colostomy in 20, and ileostomy in 7. Three of the patients in the right colostomy group ultimately underwent total abdominal colectomy and ileostomy. The indications for stoma formation and colonic transit times were different in the three groups. Bloating, constipation, chronic abdominal pain, and difficulty in evacuation with prolonged colonic transit time were the main indications in 95% of patients in the right colostomy group, 43% of patients in the left colostomy group, and 29% in the ileostomy group. Management of complicated decubitus ulcers, perineal, and pelvic wounds was the primary indication in 43% of patients in the left colostomy group, 5% in the right colostomy group, and none in the ileostomy group. Preoperative total and right colonic transit times were longer in the right colostomy group compared with the left colostomy group: 128 versus 83 hours and 54 versus 29 hours, respectively. At a mean follow-up of 5.5 years after stoma formation, most patients were satisfied with their stoma (right colostomy 88%; left colostomy 100%; ileostomy 83%) and the majority would have preferred to have the stoma earlier (right colostomy, 63%; left colostomy, 77%; ileostomy, 63%). The quality of life index significantly improved in all groups (right colostomy 49 to 79; left colostomy 50 to 86, and ileostomy 60 to 82), as well as the health status index (right colostomy 58 to 83; left colostomy 63 to 92; ileostomy 61 to 88). The average daily time for bowel care was significantly shortened in all groups (right colostomy 102 to 11 minutes; left colostomy 123 to 18 minutes; and ileostomy 73 to 13 minutes). They concluded, regardless of the type of stoma, most patients had functional improvement postoperatively. The successful outcome noted in all groups suggest that preoperative symptoms and colonic transit time studies may have been helpful in optimal choice of stoma site selection.

■ GERIATRIC POPULATION

Read et al. (369) conducted a survey of 453 people living in Sheffield, U.K., and found that the prevalence of constipation was 12% but increased to 41% of patients in acute geriatric wards and to more than 80% of patients in long-term geriatric wards. The authors attributed the abnormally increased incidence in hospitalized patients to immobility, chronic illness, neurologic or psychiatric disease, colonic disease, and drug ingestion rather than solely a consequence of aging. In his doctoral thesis on constipation in the elderly, Kinnunen (370) recorded the complaint of constipation and the use of laxatives separately. He found incidences of 79% and 76%, respectively, in a geriatric hospital, 59% and 60% in an "old people's home," 29% and 31% in a day hospital, 38% and 20% in elderly people living at home, and 12% and 5% in middle-aged people living at home. An increased risk of constipation was found in persons with poor mobility and advancing age and in those living in institutions.

Delay in transit time, incomplete emptying, diminished awareness, and neglect of the call to stool are the four most commonly occurring causes of constipation in the elderly (371). Because this group comprises elderly, physically inactive individuals, often immobile in bed, a loss of muscle tone makes it difficult to empty the bowel completely without straining at stool. A possible cause or explanation of the association of constipation and old age may be autonomic nerve fiber degeneration, especially in diabetics (372) or those who suffer strokes (369).

Jones and Godding (13) pointed out that there are several complications of constipation more likely to occur in the elderly. They include cardiovascular changes, gastrointestinal effects (including pain that simulates angina pectoris), and fecal impaction. As a consequence of fecal impaction, fecal incontinence may occur; if its cause is unrecognized, it may result in unnecessary institutionalization of a patient. Kinnunen (370) conducted a retrospective screening of one-year duration on 245 hospitalized geriatric patients and identified 65 periods of diarrhea that continued for at least three days, 32% of which recurred. Fecal impaction was associated with diarrhea in 55% of the patients, and laxative-induced diarrhea was found in 20%. Other consequences of impaction included intestinal obstruction, restlessness, confusional states, rectal hemorrhage resulting from stercoral ulceration, and urinary retention.

In a review of colonic disease in the elderly, Brocklehurst (373) stressed three important complications of constipation: (i) fecal impaction and intestinal obstruction; (ii) idiopathic megacolon and sigmoid volvulus; and (iii) fecal incontinence.

Therapeutic measures have emphasized reassurance with bowel retraining, encouragement of physical activity, intake of adequate fluids, and dietary alterations, and avoidance of constipation and treatment of known underlying diseases, especially hypothyroidism. Such recommendations infer a readily curable problem, but when the patient is elderly, such hope is unrealistic (374). Elderly patients usually require laxatives; the agents of choice are stimulant laxatives such as senna or bisacodyl. Saline purgatives may disturb water and electrolyte balance, and the hazards of liquid paraffin are well recognized. Bulk-forming agents must be accompanied by adequate amounts of fluids but are contraindicated when fecal accumulations are already present. The use of stool softeners may be inappropriate if the stool is already soft; instead, the neuromuscular responses in the colon need stimulation. Successful therapy is an individual trial-and-error proposition. Encouragement comes from a study at one geriatric center, where supplementation of the total dietary fiber proved effective in preventing constipation in 60% of the residents, with the institution's pharmacy reporting a saving of $44,000 in expenditures for laxatives (375). Similar results were experienced by Hope and Down (376), who found that in elderly institutionalized patients, a daily fiber intake of 25 g per person and controlled fluid intake improved bowel function and almost eliminated aperient use with no adverse effects on body weight or nutritional or mineral status. Kinnunen (370) found magnesium hydroxide to be more efficient than bulk-forming laxatives in treating constipation in elderly long-term patients.

For the nursing home patient who is debilitated and unable to heed the call to stool promptly, an acceptable routine for management includes the regular use of enemas. Tap water enemas administered every 3 to 5 days will keep the colon empty and the patient comfortable.

OBSTETRIC PATIENTS

Multiple etiologic factors are implicated in the occurrence of constipation during pregnancy. Decreased physical activity, changes in hormonal concentration (possibly contributing to atony of the gut muscle), decreased bulk in the diet, and the use of drugs such as iron, all may contribute. During pregnancy the aim should be prevention of constipation, and this is best accomplished with dietary fiber. Anderson and Whichelow (377) have shown that therapeutic supplementation bringing dietary fiber intake to 27 g per day is effective in treating constipation in pregnancy. Increased fluid intake is widely recommended. Laxatives are best avoided, but if necessary, the choice is between bisacodyl and senna. Senna is safe for both mother and baby with no known adverse effects on nutrition or lactation (378). Soft stools passed without straining may help prevent the problems of hemorrhoids and anal fissures so frequently associated with pregnancy. In the puerperium a simple, safe, and inexpensive method of preventing constipation is the use of senna.

TERMINALLY ILL PATIENTS

Lamberton (379) has reported that patients, who are dying, especially from carcinomatosis, present an often neglected problem. Their constipation, frequently aggravated by the universal administration of an opiate analgesic, leads to the distressing symptoms of abdominal distention and excessive gas, with added pain and even vomiting. These patients will benefit from a suppository (glycerin or bisacodyl) or from an enema. Greater attention should be paid to making their dying days more comfortable and peaceful. They should receive a laxative prophylactically with the opiate analgesic.

Patients with carcinoma often suffer from constipation, a symptom that can be considered in one of three categories (380): (i) the direct result of the malignancy itself, with intraluminal or extraluminal encroachment on the bowel or interference with its innervation; (ii) the result of the effects of therapy (e.g., chemotherapy); or (iii) the result of factors indirectly related to the carcinoma. An example of the last category is the general debility accompanying advanced disease, marked by diminished oral intake, immobility, and depression, which predisposes to constipation. An intestinal visceral neuropathy may be a paraneoplastic effect of some carcinomas (381). The results of organ failure such as uremia can have a compounding effect. Therapy with opiates or drugs with anticholinergic effects (e.g., antidepressants and neuroleptics) further complicates the problem.

REFERENCES

1. Sonnenberg A, Koch TR. Epidemiology in the United States. Dis Colon Rectum 1989; 32:1–8.
2. Talley NJ, Fleming KC, Evans JM, et al. Constipation in an elderly community: A study of prevalence and potential risk factors. Am J Gastroenterol 1996; 91:19–25.
3. Robson KM, Kiely DK, Lembo T. Development of constipation in nursing home residents. Dis Colon Rectum 2000; 43:940–943.
4. Lennard-Jones JE. Pathophysiology of constipation. Br J Surg 1985; 72(suppl):S7–S8.
5. Moore-Gillon V. Constipation: What does it mean? J R Soc Med 1984; 77: 108–110.
6. Drossman DA, Thompson WG, Talley NJ, Funch-Jensen P, Janssens J, Whitehead WE. Identification of sub-groups of functional gastrointestinal disorders. Gastroenterol Int 1990; 3:159–172.

7. Probert CSJ, Emmett PM, Cripps HA, Haton KW. Evidence for the ambiguity of the term constipation: the role of irritable bowel syndrome. Gut 1994; 35:1455–1458.
8. Heaton KW, Ghosh S, Braddon FEM. How bad are the symptoms and bowel dysfunction of patients with the irritable bowel syndrome? A prospective, controlled study with emphasis on stool form. Gut 1991; 32:73–79.
9. Drossman DA, Sandler RS, McKee DC, Lovitz AJ. Bowel patterns among subjects not seeking health care. Gastroenterology 1982; 83:529–534.
10. Devroede G. Constipation: Mechanisms and management. In: Sleisenger MH, Fordtran JS, eds. Gastrointestinal Disease, 3rd ed. Philadelphia: WB Saunders, 1983.
11. Agachan F, Chen T, Pfeifer J, Reissman P, Wexner SD. A constipation scoring system to simplify evaluation and management of constipated patients. Dis Colon Rectum 1996; 39:681–685.
12. Hinton JM, Lennard-Jones JE. Constipation: definition and classification. Post Grad Med J 1968; 44:720.
13. Jones FA, Godding EW. Management of Constipation. London: Blackwell Scientific Publications, 1972.
14. Burkitt DP. Epidemiology of the cancer of the colon and the rectum. Cancer 1971; 28:3–13.
15. Painter NS, Burkitt DP. Diverticular disease of the colon: A deficiency disease of western civilization. Br Med J 1971; 2:450.
16. Schneeman BO. Soluble Vs. insoluble fiber—Different physiological responses. Food Technol 1987; 41:81–82.
17. Walker ARP, Walker BF, Richardson BD. Bowel transit times in Bantu populations. Br Med J 1970; 3:48.
18. Menardo G, Bausano G, Corazziari E, et al. Large-bowel transit in paraplegic patients. Dis Colon Rectum 1987; 30:924–928.
19. Levi R, Hultling C, Nash MS, Seiger A. The Stockholm spinal cord injury study: Medical problems in a regional SCI population. Paraplegia 1995; 33:308–315.
20. Glickman S, Kamm MA. Bowel dysfunction in spinal-cord-injury patients. Lancet 1996; 347:1651–1653.
21. Ashraf W, Park F, Lof J, Quigley EMM. Examination of the reliability of reported stool frequency in the diagnosis of idiopathic constipation. Am J Gastroenterol 1996; 91:26–32.
22. Almy TP. Constipation. In Slesenger MH, Fordtran JS, eds. Gastrointestinal Disease. Philadelphia: WB Saunders, 1973.
23. Heaton KW, O'Donnell KJD. An office guide to whole gut transit time. Patient's reflection of their stool form. J Clin Gastroenterol 1994; 19:28–30.
24. Thompson JC, Marx M. Gastrointestinal hormones. Curr Probl Surg 1984; 21:6.
25. Preston DM, Adrian TE, Christofides ND, Lennard-Jones JE, Bloom SR. Positive correlation between symptoms and circulating motilin, pancreatic polypeptides and gastrin levels in functional bowel disorders. Gut 1985; 26:1059–1064.
26. Christofides ND, Ghatei MA, Bloom SR, Borberg C, Gillmer MDG. Decreased plasma motilin concentrations in pregnancy. Br Med J 1982; 285:1453–1454.
27. Preston DM, Lennard-Jones JE, Thomas BM. Towards a radiological definition of idiopathic megacolon. Gastrointest Radiol 1985; 10:167–169.
28. Mahieu P, Pringot J, Bodart P. Defecography. I. Description of a new procedure and results in normal patients. Gastrointest Radiol 1984; 9:247–251.
29. Mahieu P, Pringot J, Bodart P. Defecography. II. Contribution to the diagnosis of defecation disorders. Gastrointest Radiol 1984; 9:253–261.
30. Agachan F, Pfeifer J, Wexner SD. Defecography and proctography. Results of 744 patients. Dis Colon Rectum 1966; 39:899–905.
31. Mellgren A, Bremmer S, Johansson C, et al. Defecography. Results of investigations in 2816 patients. Dis Colon Rectum 1994; 37:1133–1141.
32. Ferrante SL, Perry RE, Schreiman JS, Cheng SC, Frick MP. The reproducibility of measuring anorectal angle in defecography. Dis Colon Rectum 1991; 34: 51–55.
33. Penninckx F, Debryune C, Lestar B, Kerremans R. Intra-observer variation in the radiological measurement of the anorectal angle. Gastrointest Radiol 1991; 16:73–76.
34. Halligan S, McGee S, Bartram CI. Quantification of evacuation proctography. Dis Colon Rectum 1994; 37:1151–1154.
35. Barkel DC, Pemberton JH, Pezim ME, Phillips SF, Kelly KA, Brown ML. Scintigraphic assessment of the anorectal angle in health and after ileal pouch-anal anastomosis. Ann Surg 1988; 208:42–49.
36. Freimanis M, Wald A, Caruana B, Bauman D. Evacuation proctography in normal volunteers. Invest Radiol 1991; 26:581–585.
37. Karlbom U, Pahlman L, Nilsson S, Graf W. Relationships between defecographic findings, rectal emptying, and colonic transit time in constipated patients. Dis Colon Rectum 1995; 36:907–912.
38. Halligan S, Thomas J, Bartram C. Intrarectal pressures and balloon expulsion related to evacuation proctography. Gut 1995; 37:100–104.
39. Hinton JM, Lennard-Jones JE, Young AC. A new method for studying gut transit time using radio-opaque markers. Gut 1969; 10:842–847.
40. Cummings JH, Wiggins HS. Transit through the gut measured by analysis of a single stool. Gut 1976; 17:219–223.
41. Evans RC, Kamm MA, Hinton JM, Lennard-Jones JE. The normal range and a simple diagram for recording whole gut transit time. Int J Colorectal Dis 1992; 7:15–17.
42. Martelli H, Devroede G, Arhan P, Duguay C, Dormic C, Faverdin C. Some parameters of large bowel motility in normal man. Gastroenterology 1978; 75:612–618.
43. Metcalf AM, Phillips SM, Zinsmeister AR, MacCarty RL, Beart RW, Wolff BG. Simplified assessment of segmental colonic transit. Gastroenterology 1987; 92:40–47.
44. Chaussade S, Guerre J, Couturier D. Measurement of colonic transit. Gastroenterology 1987; 92:2053.
45. van der Sijp JRM, Kamm MA, Nightingale JMD, et al. Radioisotope determination of regional colonic transit in severe constipation: Comparison with radio-opaque markers. Gut 1993; 34:402–408.
46. Stivland T, Camilleri M, Vassallo M, Proano M, Rath D, Brown M, Thomforde G, Pemberton J, Phillips SM. Scintigraphic measurement of regional gut transit in idiopathic constipation. Gastroenterology 1991; 101:107–115.
47. Krevsky B, Maurer AH, Fisher RS. Patterns of colonic transit in chronic idiopathic constipation. Am J Gastroenterol 1989; 84:127–132.
48. Ewe K, Press G, Dederer W. Gastrointestinal transit of undigestible solids measured by metal detector EAS II. Eur J Clin Invest 1989; 19:291–297.
49. Basile M, Neri M, Carriero A, et al. Measurement of segmental transit through the gut in man. Dig Dis Sci 1992; 37:1537–1543.
50. Arhan P, Devroede G, Jehannin B, et al. Segmental colonic transit time. Dis Colon Rectum 1981; 24:625–629.
51. Chaussade S, Khyari A, Roche H, et al. Determination of total and segmental colonic transit time in constipated patients. Dig Dis Sci 1989; 34:1168–1172.
52. Meir R, Beglinger C, Dederding JP, et al. Age and sex-specific standard values of colonic transit time in healthy subjects. Schwiz Med Wochenschr 1992; 122:940–943.
53. Escalante R, Sorgi M, Salas Z. Total and segmental colonic transit time. Clinical and prospective study using radiopaque markers in normal subjects. GEN 1993; 47:88–92.
54. Dorval D, Barbieux JP, Picon L, Alison D, Codjovi P, Rouleau P. Mesure simplifiée du temps de transit colique par une seule radiographie de l'abdomen et un seul type de marqueur. Gastroenterol Clin Biol 1994; 18:141–144.
55. Bouchoucha M, Devroede G, Renard P, Arhan P, Barbier JP, Cugnenc PH. Compartmental analysis of colonic transit reveals abnormalities in constipated patients with normal transit. Clin Sci 1995; 89:129–135.
56. Loening-Baucke V. Factors determining outcome in children with chronic constipation and faecal soiling. Gut 1989; 30:999–1066.
57. Benninga MA, Buller HA, Taminiau JA. Biofeedback training in chronic constipation. Arch Dis Child 1993; 68:126–129.
58. Loening-Baucke V, Pringle KC, Ekwo EE. Anorectal manometry for the exclusion of Hirschsprung's disease in neonates. J Pediatr Gastroenterol Nutr 1985; 4:596–603.
59. Low PS, Quak SH, Prabhakaran K, Joseph VT, Chiang GS, Aiyathurai EJ. Accuracy of anorectal manometry in the diagnosis of Hirschsprung's disease. J Pediatr Gastroenterol Nutr 1989; 9:432–436.
60. Borowitz SM, Sutphen J, Ling W, Cox DJ. Lack of correlation of anorectal manometry with symptoms of chronic childhood constipation and encopresis. Dis Colon Rectum 1996; 39:400–405.
61. Pluta H, Bowes KL, Jewell LD. Long-term results of total abdominal colectomy for chronic idiopathic constipation. Value of preoperative assessment. Dis Colon Rectum 1996; 39:160–166.
62. Martelli H, Devroede G, Arhan P, Duguay C. Mechanisms of idiopathic constipation: Outlet obstruction. Gastroenterology 1978; 75: 623–631.
63. Arhan P, Faverdin C, Thouvenot J. Anorectal motility in sick children. Scand J Gastroenterol 1972; 7:309–314.
64. Meunier P, Marechal JM, Jeabert de Beaujeau M. Recto-anal pressures and rectal sensitivity studies in chronic childhood constipation. Gastroenterology 1979; 77:330–336.
65. Iwai N, Ogita S, Kida M. A manometric assessment of anorectal pressures and its significance in the diagnosis of Hirschsprung's disease and idiopathic megacolon. Jpn J Surg 1979; 9:234–240.
66. Taylor I, Hammond P, Darby C. An assessment of anorectal motility in the management of adult megacolon. Br J Surg 1980; 67:754–756.
67. Suzuki H, Amano S, Honzumi M, Saijo H, Sakakura K. Recto-anal pressures and rectal compliance in constipated infants and children. Z Kinderchir 1980; 4:330–336.
68. Loening-Baucke VA, Younoszai MK. Abnormal anal sphincter response in chronically constipated children. J Pediatr 1982; 100:213–218.
69. Molnar D, Taitz LS, Urwin OM, Wales JKH. Anorectal manometry results in defecation disorders. Arch Dis Child 1983; 58:257–261.
70. Read NW, Timms JM, Barfield LJ, Donnelly TC, Bannister JJ. Impairment of defecation in young women with severe constipation. Gastroenterology 1986; 90:53–60.
71. Roe AM, Bartolo DC, Mortenson NJ. Diagnosis and surgical management of intractable constipation. Br J Surg 1986; 73:854–861.
72. Shouler P, Keighley MRB. Changes in colorectal function in severe idiopathic chronic constipation. Gastroenterology 1986; 90:414–420.
73. Clayden GS, Lawson JON. Investigation and management of long-standing chronic constipation in childhood. Arch Dis Child 1976; 57: 918–923.

74. Grotz RL, Pemberton JH, Levin KE, Bell AM, Hanson RW. Rectal wall contractility in healthy subjects and in patients with chronic severe constipation. Ann Surg 1993; 218:761–768.
75. Schouten WR, Gosselink MJ, Boerma MO, Ginai AZ. Rectal tone in response to an evoked urge to defecate. Dis Colon Rectum 1998; 41:473–479.
76. Gosselink MJ, Schouten WR. The gastrorectal reflex in women with obstructed defecation. Int J Colorectal Dis 2001; 16:112–118.
77. Varma JS, Smith AN. Neurophysiological dysfunction in young women with intractable constipation. Gut 1988; 29:963–968.
78. Gurnari M, Mazziotti F, Corazziari E et al. Chronic constipation after gynaecological surgery: a retrospective study. Br J Gastroenterol 1988; 20:183–186.
79. Shafik A, El-Sibai O, Ahmed I. Parasympathetic extrinsic reflex: role in defecation mechanism. World J Surg 2002; 26:737–741.
80. Swash M, Snooks SJ. Electromyography in pelvic floor disorders. In: Henry MM, Swash M, eds. Coloproctology and the Pelvic Floor. London: Butterworth, 1985.
81. Snooks SJ, Barnes PRH, Swash M, Henry MM. Damage to the innervation of the pelvic floor musculature in chronic constipation. Gastroenterology 1985; 89:977–981.
82. Preston DM, Lennard-Jones JE. Anismus in chronic constipation. Dig Dis Sci 1985; 30:413–418.
83. Rao SSC, Ozturk R, Laine L. Clinical utility of diagnostic tests for constipation in adults: a systemic review. Am J Gastroenterol 2005; 100:1605–1615.
84. Madigan MR, Morson BC. Solitary ulcer of the rectum. Gut 1969; 10:871–887.
85. Martin CJ, Parks TG, Biggart JD. Solitary rectal ulcer syndrome in Northern Ireland 1971–80. Br J Surg 1981; 68:744–747.
86. Aldridge RT, Campbell PE. Ganglion cell distribution in the normal rectum and anal canal. A basis for the diagnosis of Hirschsprung's disease by anorectal biopsy. J Pediatr Surg 1968; 3:475–490.
87. Ikawa H, Kim SH, Hendren H, Donahoe PK. Acetylcholinesterase and manometry in the diagnosis of the constipated child. Arch Surg 1986; 121:435–438.
88. Venupogal S, Mancer K, Shandling B. The validity of rectal biopsy in relation to morphology and distribution of ganglion cells. J Pediatr Surg 1981; 16: 433–437.
89. Weinberg AG. The anorectal myenteric plexus: Its relation to hypoganglionosis of the colon. Am J Clin Pathol 1970; 54:637–642.
90. Riemann JF, Schmidt H, Zimmermann W. The fine structure of colonic submucosal nerves in patients with chronic laxative abuse. Scand J Gastroenterol 1980; 15:761–768.
91. Causse E, Vaysse P, Fabre J, Valdiquie P, Thouvenot JP. The diagnostic value of acetylcholinesterase/butylcholinesterase ratio in Hirschsprung's disease. Am J Clin Path 1987; 88:477–480.
92. Goto S, Ikeda K, Nagasaki A, Tomokiyo A, Kusaba M. Hirschsprung's disease in an adult. Special reference to histochemical determination of the acetylcholinesterase activity. Dis Colon Rectum 1985; 27:319–320.
93. Meier-Ruge W, Latterbeck P, Herzog B. Acetylcholinesterase activity in suction biopsies of the rectum in the diagnosis of Hirschsprung's disease. J Pediatr Surg 1972; 7:11–17.
94. Robey SS, Kuhajda FP, Yardley JH. Immunoperoxidase stains of ganglion cells and abnormal mucosal nerve proliferations in Hirschsprung's disease. Hum Pathol 1988; 19:432–437.
95. Park WH, Choi SO, Kwon KY, Chang ES. Acetylcholinesterase histochemistry of rectal suction biopsies in the diagnosis of Hirschsprung's Disease. J Korean Med Sci 1992; 7:353–359.
96. Barr LC, Booth J, Filipe MI, Lawson JON. Clinical evaluation of the histochemical diagnosis of Hirschsprung's disease. Gut 1985; 26:393–399.
97. Preston DM, Butler MG, Smith B, Lennard-Jones JE. Neuropathology of slow transit constipation. Gut 1983; 24:A997.
98. Krishnamurthy S, Schuffler MD, Rohrmann CA, Pope CE. Severe idiopathic constipation is associated with distinctive abnormality of the colonic myenteric plexus. Gastroenterology 1985; 88:26–34.
99. Koch TR, Carney JA, Go L, Go VLW. Idiopathic chronic constipation is associated with decreased colonic vasoactive intestinal peptide. Gastroenterology 1988; 94:300–310.
100. Tzavella K, Riepl RL, Klauser AG, et al. Decreased substance P levels in rectal biopsies from patients with slow transit constipation. Eur J Gastroenterol Hepatol 1996; 8:1207–1211.
101. Kluck P, van Muyen GNP, van der Kamp AWM, et al. Diagnosis of Hirschsprung's disease with monoclonal antineurofilament antibodies on tissue sections. Lancet 1984; 24:652–653.
102. Schouten WR, ten Kate FJW, de Graaf EJR, Gilberts ECAM, Simons JL, Kluck P. Visceral neuropathy in slow transit constipation: An immunohistochemical investigation with monoclonal antibodies against neurofilament. Dis Colon Rectum 1993; 36:1112–1127.
103. Kluck P, Tibboel D, Leendertse-Verloop K, et al. Disturbed defecation after colectomy for aganglionosis investigated with monoclonal antineurofilament antibody. J Pediatr Surg 1986; 21:845–847.
104. Lincoln J, Crowe R, Kamm MA, Burnstock G, Lennard-Jones JE. Serotonin and 5-hydroxyindolacetic acid are increased in the sigmoid colon in severe idiopathic constipation. Gatroenterology 1990; 98:1219–1225.
105. Zhao RH, Baig MK, Wexner SD, et al. Enterochromaffin and serotonin cells are abnormal for patients with colonic inertia. Dis Colon Rectum 2000; 43:858–863.
106. Zhao RH, Baig MK, Thaler KJ, et al. Reduced expression of serotonin receptors in the left colon of patients with colonic inertia. Dis Colon Rectum 2003; 46: 81–86.
107. Wedel T, Roblick UJ, Ott V, et al. Oligoneuronal hypoganglionosis in patients with slow transit constipation. Dis Colon Rectum 2002; 45:54–62.
108. Bassotti G, Villanacci V, Maure CA, Fisogni S, Di Fabio F, et al. The role of glial cells and apoptosis of enteric neurons in the neuropathology of intractable slow transit constipation. Gut Online, published on July 24 as 10.1136/gut.2005.073197.
109. Lee JI, Park H, Kamm MA, Talbot IC. Decreased density of interstitial cells of Cajal and neuronal cells in patients with slow transit constipation and acquired megacolon. J Gastroenterol Hepatol 2005; 20:1292–1298.
110. Tucker DM, Sanstead HH, Logan GM Jr. Dietary fiber and personality factors as determinants of stool output. Gastroenterology 1981; 81:879–883.
111. Devroede G, Gilles G, Bouchoucha M. Idiopathic constipation by colonic dysfunction: Relationship with personality and anxiety. Dig Dis Sci 1989; 34: 1428–1433.
112. Heyman S, Wexner SD, Gulledge AD. MMPI assessment of patients with functional bowel disorders. Dis Colon Rectum 1993; 36:593–596.
113. Drossman DA, Leserman J, Nachman G, et al. Sexual and physical abuse in women with functional or organic disorders of the lower gastrointestinal tract. Ann Intern Med 1990; 113:828–833.
114. Leroi AM, Bernier C, Watier A, et al. Prevalence of sexual abuse among patients with functional disorders of the lower gastrointestinal tract Int J Colorectal Dis 1995; 10:200–206.
115. Dykes S, Smilgin-Humphreys S, Bass C. Chronic idiopathic constipation: a psychological inquiry. Eur J Gastroenterol Hepatol 2001; 13:39–44.
116. Knowles CH, Scott SM, Rayner C, et al. Idiopathic slow transit constipation: an almost exclusively female disorder. Dis Colon Rectum 2003; 46:1716–1717.
117. Mason HJ, Serrano-Ikkos E, Kamm MA. Psychological morbidity in women with idiopathic constipation. Am J Gastroenterol 2000; 95:2852–2857.
118. Emmanuel AV, Mason HJ, Kamm MA. Relationship between psychological state and level of activity of extrinsic gut innervation in patients with a functional gut disorder. Gut 2001; 49:209–213.
119. Chan AOO, Cheng C, Hui WM, Hu WHC, Wong NYH et al. Differing coping mechanisms, stress level and anorectal physiology in patients with functional constipation. World J Gastroenterol 2005; 11:5362–5366.
120. Leroi AM, Duval V, Roussignol C, Berkelmans I, Peninque P, Denis P. Biofeedback for anismus in 15 sexually abused women. Int J Colorectal Dis 1996; 11:187–190.
121. Thompson WG. Constipation and catharsis. Can Med Assoc J 1976; 114: 927–931.
122. Painter NS, Burkitt DP. Diverticular disease of the colon: A deficiency disease of Western civilization. Br Med J 1971; 2:450.
123. Bjelke E. Epidemiologic studies of cancer of the stomach, colon and rectum. Scand J Gastroenterol 1974; 9(suppl):31.
124. Higginson J. Etiological factors in gastrointestinal cancer in man. J Natl Cancer Inst 1966; 37:527–545.
125. Wynder EL, Shigematsu T. Environmental factors of cancer of the colon and rectum. Cancer 1967; 20:1520–1561.
126. Cranston D, McWhinnie D, Collin J. Dietary fiber and gastrointestinal disease. Br J Surg 1988; 75:508–512.
127. Park Y, Hunter DJ, Spiegelman D, et al. Dietary fiber intake and risk of colorectal cancer. JAMA 2005; 294:2849–2857.
128. Med Lett 1973; 15:98.
129. Kirway KO, Smith AN, McConnell AA, Mitchell MO, Eastwood MA. Action of different bran preparations on colonic function. Br Med J 1974; 4: 187–189.
130. Stephen AM, Cummings JH. Water-holding by dietary fiber in vitro and its relationship to fecal output in man. Gut 1979; 10:722–729.
131. Ornstein MH, Baird IM. Dietary fibre and the colon. Mol Aspects Med 1987; 9:41–67.
132. Trowell HC. The development of the concept of dietary fibre in human nutrition. Am J Clin Nutr 1978; 3I:S3–S11.
133. McNutt K. Prospective-fiber. J Nutr Ed 1976; 8:150.
134. Dubuc MB, Lahaie LC. Nutritive Value of Foods. Ottawa: National Library, 1987:16–158.
135. Brunton LL. Laxatives. In: Gilman AG, Goodman LS, Bal TN, Murd F, eds. Goodman and Gilman's the pharmacological basis of therapeuties, 7th ed. New York: Macmillan, 1985, 994–1003.
136. Curry CE. Handbook of Non-Prescription Drugs, 8th ed. Washington, D.C.: American Pharmaceutical Association, 1986:75–97.
137. Müller-Lissner SA. Adverse effects of laxatives: Fact and fiction. Pharmacology 1993; 47(suppl 1):138–145.
138. Siegers C, von Hertzberg-Lottin E, Otte M, Schneider B. Anthroid laxative abuse—A risk of colorectal cancer?. Gut 1993; 34:1099–1101.
139. Harvey RF, Read AF. Mode of action of the saline purgatives. Am Heart J 1975; 89:810–813.
140. Donowitz M, Binder HJ. Effect of dioctyl sodium sulfosuccinate on colonic fluid and electrolyte movement. Gastroenterology 1975; 69:941–950.
141. Fain AM, Susat R, Herring M, Dorton K. Treatment of constipation in geriatric and chronically ill patients: A comparison. South Med J 1978; 71:677–680.

142. Ogorek CP, Reynolds JC. Chronic constipation. Diagnosis and treatment. Endosc Rev 1987; 4(6):47.
143. Müller-Lissner SA, Bavarian Constipation Study Group. Treatment of constipation with cisapride and placebo. Gut 1987; 28:1033–1038.
144. Johanson JF, Wald A, Tougas G, et al. Effect of tegaserod in chronic constipation: a randomized, double-blind, controlled trial. Clin Gastroenterol Hepatol 2004; 2:769–805.
145. Kamm MA, Muller-Lissner S, Talley NJ, et al. Tegaserod for the treatment of chronic constipation: a randomized, double-blind, placebo-controlled multinational study. Am J Gastroenterol 2005; 100:362–72.
146. Lane WA. Chronic intestinal stasis. Br Med J 1912; 2:1125–1130.
147. Hughes ESR, McDermott FT, Johnson WR, Polglase AL. Surgery for constipation. Aust N Z. J Surg 1981; 51:144–148.
148. Belliveau P, Goldberg SM, Rothenberger DA, Nivatvongs S. Idiopathic acquired megacolon: the value of subtotal colectomy. Dis Colon Rectum 1982; 25:118–127.
149. Hughes ESR, McDermott FT, Johnson WR, Polglase A. Surgery for constipation. In: Heberer G, Denecke H, eds. Colorectal Surgery. Berlin: Springer-Verlag, 1982:11–17.
150. Klatt GR, Role of subtotal colectomy in the treatment of incapacitating constipation. Am J Surg 1983; 145:623–625.
151. Preston DM, Hawley PR, Lennard-Jones JE, Todd IP. Results of colectomy for severe idiopathic constipation in women (Arbuthnot Lane's disease). Br J Surg 1984; 71:547–552.
152. Keighley MRB, Shouler P. Anorectal outlet syndrome: Is there a surgical option?. J R Soc Med 1984; 77:559–563.
153. Beck DE, Jagelman DG, Fazio VW. The surgery of idiopathic constipation [review]. Gastroenterol Clin North Am 1987; 16:143–156.
154. Vasilevsky CA, Nemer FD, Balcos EG, Christenson CE, Goldberg SM. Is subtotal colectomy a viable option in the management of chronic constipation. Dis Colon Rectum 1988; 31:679–681.
155. Gattuso JM, Kamm MA, Abassi M, Talbot IC. First description of the pathology of idiopathic megarectum and megacolon. Gut 1993; 34:S49.
156. Koch TR, Schulte-Bockholt A, Telford GL, Otterson MF, Murad TM, Stryker SJ. Acquired megacolon is associated with alteration of vasoactive intestinal peptide levels and acetylcholinesterase activity. Regul Pept 1993; 48:309–319.
157. Gattuso JM, Hoyle CHV, Milner P, Kamm MA, Burnstock G. Enteric innervation in idiopathic megarectum and megacolon. Int J Colorectal Dis 1996; 11:264–271.
158. Koch TR, Schulte-Bockholt A, Otterson MF, et al. Decreased vasoactive intestinal peptide levels and glutathione depletion in acquired megacolon. Dig Dis Sci 1996; 41:1409–1416.
159. Koch TR, Otterson MF, Telford GL. Nitric oxide production is diminished in colonic circular muscle from acquired megacolon. Dis Colon rectum 2000; 43:821–828.
160. Meier-Ruge WA. Idiopathic megacolon. Histopathologic and musculomechanical causes. Der Chirurg 2000; 71:927–931.
161. Gattuso JM, Kamm MA. Clinical features of idiopathic megarectum and idiopathic megacolon. Gut 1997; 41:93–99.
162. Barnes PRH, Lennard-Jones JE, Hawley PR, Todd IP. Hirschsprung's disease and idiopathic megacolon in adults and adolescents. Gut 1986; 27:534–541.
163. Gattuso JM, Phil M, Kamm MA, Morris G, Britton KE. Gastrointestinal transit in patients with idiopathic megarectum. Dis Colon Rectum 1996; 39:1044–1050.
164. Gattuso JM, Phil M, Kamm MA, Halligan SM, Bartram CI. The anal sphincter in idiopathic megarectum. Dis Colon Rectum 1996; 39:435–439.
165. Stabile G, Kamm MA, Hawley PR, Lennard-Jones JE. Colectomy for idiopathic megarectum and megacolon. Gut 1991; 32:1538–1540.
166. Lane RHS, Todd IP. Idiopathic megacolon: A review of 42 cases. Br J Surg 1977; 64:305–310.
167. Stabile G, Kamm MA, Hawley PR, Lennard-Jones JE. Results of the Duhamel operation in the treatment of idiopathic megarectum and megacolon. Br J Surg 1991; 78:661–663.
168. Stabile G, Kamm MA, Phillips RKS, Hawley PR, Lennard-Jones JE. Partial colectomy and coloanal anastomosis for idiopathic megarectum and megacolon. Dis Colon Rectum 1992; 35:158–162.
169. Stewart J, Kumar D, Keighley MRB. Results of anal or low rectal anastomosis and pouch construction for megarectum and megacolon. Br J Surg 1994; 81:1051–1053.
170. Keighley MR, Megacolon and megarectum. In: Keighley MR, Williams NS, eds. Surgery of the Anus, Rectum and Colon, vol 1. London: WB Saunders, 1993:658–673.
171. Pfeifer J, Agachan F, Wexner SD. Surgery for constipation. A review. Dis Colon Rectum 1996; 39:444–460.
172. Suilleabhain CB, Anderson JH, McKee RF, Finlay IG. Strategy for the surgical management of patients with idiopathic megarectum and megacolon. Br J Surg 2001; 88:1392–1396.
173. Gladman MA, Scott SM, Lunniss PJ, Williams NS. Systemic review of surgical options for idiopathic megarectum and megacolon. Ann Surg 2005; 241: 562–574.
174. Gladman MA, Williams NS, Scott SM, Ogunbiyi OA, Lunniss PJ. Medium-term results of vertical reduction rectoplasty and sigmoid colectomy for idiopathic megarectum. Br J Surg 2005; 92:624–630.
175. Surrenti E, Rath DM, Pemberton JH, Camilleri M. Audit of constipation in a tertiary referral gastroenterology practice. Am J Gastroenterol 1995; 90: 1471–1475.
176. Knowles CH, Martin JE. Slow transit constipation: a model of human gut dysmotility. Review of possible aetiologies. Neurogastroenterol Mot 2000; 12: 181–196.
177. Watier A, Devroede G, Duvanceau A, et al. Constipation with colonic inertia. A manifestation of systemic disease?. Dig Dis Sci 1983; 28:1025–1033.
178. Panagamuwa B, Kumar D, Ortiz J, Keighley MR. Motor abnormalities in the terminal ileum of patients with chronic constipation. Br J Surg 1994; 81:1685–1688.
179. Hemingway D, Neilly JB, Finlay IG. Biliary dyskinesia in idiopathic slow transit constipation. Dis Colon Rectum 1996; 39:1303–1307.
180. Penning C, Gielkens HA, Delemarre JB, Lamers CB, Masclee AA. Gall bladder emptying in severe idiopathic constipation. Gut 1999; 45:264–268.
181. Mollen RM, Hopman WP, Kuijpers HH, Jansen JB. Abnormalities of upper gut motility in patients with slow transit constipation. Eur J Gastroenterol Hepatol 1999; 11:701–708.
182. Glia A, Lindberg G. Antroduodenal manometry findings in patients with slow transit constipation. Scand J Gastroenterol 1998; 33:55–62.
183. Penning C, Gielkens HA, Hemelaar M, et al. Prolonged ambulatory recording of antroduodenal motility in slow transit constipation. Br J Surg 2000; 87: 211–217.
184. Mollen RM, Hopman WP, Oyen WJ, Kuijpers HH, Edelbroek MA, Jansen JB. Effect of subtotal colectomy on gastric emptying of a solid meal in slow transit constipation. Dis Colon Rectum 2001; 44:1189–1195.
185. Warren SJ, Lord MG, Rogers J, Williams NS. Neural medication of the human rectocolon inhibitory reflex. Gut 1994; 35:S31.
186. Kerrigan DD, Lucas MG, Sun WM, Donnelly TC, Read NW. Idiopathic constipation associated with impaired urethrovesical and sacral reflex function. Br J Surg 1989; 76:748–751.
187. Ishikawa M, Mibu R, Iwamoto T, Knomi H, Oohata Y, Tanaka M. Change in colonic motility after extrinsic autonomic denervation in dogs. Dig Dis Sci 1997; 42:1950–1956.
188. Waldron DJ, Kumar D, Hallan RI, Wingate DL, Williams NS. Evidence for motor neuropathy and reduced filling of the rectum in chronic intractable constipation. Gut 1990; 31:1284–1288.
189. Bassotti G, Roberto G, Castellani D, Sediari L, Morelli A. Normal aspects of colorectal motility and abnormalities in slow transit constipation. World J Gastroenterol 2005; 11:2691–2696.
190. Gladman MA, Dvorkin LS, Lunniss PJ, Williams NS, Scott SM. Rectal hyposensitivity: a disorder of the rectal wall or afferent pathway? An assessment using the barostat. Am J Gastroenterol 2005; 100:106–114.
191. Knowles CH, Scott M, Lunniss PJ. Slow transit constipation. A disorder of pelvic autonomic nerves? Dig Dis Sci 2001; 46:389–401.
192. Altomare D, Pilot MA, Scott M, Williams N, Rubino M, Ilincic L. Detection of subclinical autonomic neuropathy in constipated patients using a sweat test. Gut 1992; 33:1539–1543.
193. Lyford GL, He CL, Soffer E, Hull TL, Strong SA et al. Pan-colonic decrease in interstitial cells of Cajal in patients with slow transit constipation. Gut 2002; 51:496–501.
194. Toman J, Turina M, Ray M, Petras RE, Stromberg AJ, Galandiuk S. Slow transit colon constipation is not related to the number of interstitial cells of Cajal. Int J Colorectal Dis 2005; October 18: Epub ahead of print.
195. El-Salhy M. Chronic idiopathic slow transit constipation: pathophysiology and management. Colorectal Disease 2003; 5:288–296.
196. Tomita R, Fujisaki S, Ikeda T, Fukuzawa M. Role of nitric oxide in the colon of patients with slow transit constipation. Dis Colon Rectum 2002; 45:593–600.
197. Slater BJ, Varma JS, Gillespie JJ. Abnormalities in the contractile properties of colonic smooth muscle in idiopathic slow transit constipation. Br J Surg 1997; 84:181–184.
198. Rao SSC, Sadeghi P, Beaty J, Kavlock R. Ambulatory 24-hour colonic manometry in slow transit constipation. Am J Gastroenterol 2004; 99:2405–2416.
199. Hagger R, Kumar D, Benson M, Grundy A. Colonic motor activity in slow transit constipation as identified by 24-hour pancolonic ambulatory manometry. Neurogastroenterol Motil 2003; 15:515–522.
200. Goldin E, Karmelli F, Selinger ZVI, Rachmilewitz D. Colonic substance P levels are increased in ulcerative colitis and decreased in chronic severe constipation. Dig Dis Sci 1989; 34:754–757.
201. Battaglia E, Serra AM, Buonrfede G, et al. Long-term study on the effects of visual biofeedback and muscle training as a therapeutic modality in pelvic floor dyssynergia and slow-transit constipation. Dis Colon Rectum 2004; 47:90–95.
202. Todd IP. Constipation: Results of surgical treatment. Br J Surg 1985; 72: S12–S13.
203. Preston DM, Lennard-Jones JE. Severe chronic constipation of young women: Idiopathic slow transit constipation. Gut 1986; 27:41–48.
204. Leon SH, Krishnamurthy S, Shuffler MD. Subtotal colectomy for severe idiopathic constipation. Dig Dis Sci 1987; 32:1249–1254.
205. Walsh PV, Pebbles-Brown DA, Watkinson G. Colectomy for slow transit constipation. Ann R Coll Surg Engl 1987; 69:71–75.
206. Åkervall S, Fasth S, Nordgren S, Oresland T, Hulten L. The functional results after colectomy and ileorectal anastomosis for severe constipation (Arbuthnot

Lane's disease) as related to rectal sensory function. Int J Colorectal Dis 1988; 3:96–101.
207. Kamm MA, Hawley PR, Lennard-Jones JE. Outcome of colectomy for severe idiopathic constipation. Gut 1988; 29:969–973.
208. Zenilman ME, Dunnegan DL, Super NJ, Becker JM. Successful surgical treatment of idiopathic colonic dysmotility. Arch Surg 1989; 124:947–951.
209. Yoshioka K, Keighley MR. Clinical results of colectomy for severe constipation. Br J Surg 1989; 76:600–604.
210. Coremans GE. Surgical aspects of severe chronic non-hirschsprung constipation. Hepatogastroenterology 1990; 37:588–595.
211. Kuijpers HC. Application of the colorectal laboratory in diagnosis and treatment of functional constipation. Dis Colon Rectum 1990; 33:35–39.
212. Pemberton JH, Rath DM, Ilstrup DM. Evaluation and surgical treatment of severe chronic constipation. Ann Surg 1991; 214:403–413.
213. Takahashi T, Fitzgerald SD, Pemberton JH. Evaluation and treatment of constipation. Rev Gastroenterol Mex 1994; 59:133–138.
214. Redmond JM, Smith GW, Barofsky I, Ratych RE, Goldsborough DC, Schuster M. Physiological tests to predict long-term outcome of total abdominal colectomy for intractable constipation. Am J Gastroenterol 1995; 90:748–753.
215. Piccirillo MF, Reissman P, Carnavos R, Wexner SD. Colectomy as treatment for constipation in selected patients. Br J Surg 1995; 82:898–901.
216. de Graaf EJR, Gilberts ECAM, Schouten WR. Role of segmental colonic transit time studies to select patients with slow transit constipation for partial left-sided colectomy or subtotal colectomy. Br J Surg 1996; 83:648–651.
217. Nyam DCNK, Pemberton JH, Illstrup DM, Rath DM. Long-term results of surgery for chronic constipation. Dis Colon Rectum 1997; 40:273–279.
218. Fan CW, Wang JY. Subtotal colectomy for colonic inertia. Int Surg 2000; 85:309–312.
219. Mollen RM, Kuijpers HC, Claassen AT. Colectomy for slow-transit constipation: preoperative functional evaluation is important but not a guarantee for a successful outcome. Dis Colon Rectum 2001; 44:577–580.
220. Nyland G, Oresland T, Fasth S, Nordgren S. Long-term outcome after colectomy in severe idiopathic constipation. Colorectal Dis 2001; 3:253–258.
221. Pikarsky AJ, Singh JJ, Weiss EG, Nogueras JJ, Wexner SD. Long-term follow-up of patients undergoing colectomy for colonic inertia. Dis Colon Rectum 2001; 4:179–183.
222. Webster C, Dayton M. Results after colectomy for colonic inertia: a sixteen-year experience. Am J Surg 2001; 182:639–644.
223. Glia A, Åkerlund JE, Lindberg G. Outcome of colectomy for slow transit constipation in relation to the presence of small bowel motility. Dis Colon rectum 2004; 47:96–102.
224. Sunderland GT, Poon FW, Lander J, Finlay JG. Videoproctography in selecting patients with constipation for colectomy. Dis Colon Rectum 1992; 35:235–237.
225. Ghosh S, Papachrysostomou M, Batool M, Eastwood MA, Long-term results of subtotal colectomy and evidence of noncolonic involvement in patients with slow transit constipation. Scand J Gastroenterol 1996; 31:1083–1091.
226. FitzHarris G, Garcia-Aguilar J, Parker S, et al. Quality of life after subtotal colectomy for slow transit constipation: both quality and quantity count. Dis Colon Rectum 2003; 46:433–440.
227. Schuffler MD, Krishnamurthy S. Constipation and colectomy. Dig Dis Sci 1988; 33:1197–1198.
228. Wexner SD, Daniel N, Jagelman DG. Colectomy for constipation: Physiologic investigation is the key to success. Dis Colon Rectum 1991; 34:851–856.
229. Aldulaymi BH, Rasmussen OO, Christiansen J. Long-term results of subtotal colectomy for severe slow transit constipation in patients with normal rectal function, Colorectal Dis 2001; 3:392–395.
230. Duthie GS, Bartolo DCC. Slow transit constipation and anismus. In: Wexner SD, Bartolo DCC, eds. Constipation: Etiology, Evaluation and Management. Oxford: Butterworth-Heinemann, 1995.
231. Kamm MP, van de Sijp JRM, Hawley PR, Phillips RK, Lennard-Jones JE. Left hemicolectomy with rectal excision for severe idiopathic constipation. Int J Colorectal Dis 1991; 6:49–51.
232. Lundin E, Karlbom U, Pahlman L, Graf W. Outcome of segmental colonic resection for slow transit constipation. Br J Surg 2002; 89:1270–1274.
233. MacDonald A, Baxter JN, Bessent RG, Gray HW, Finlay IG. Gastric emptying in patients with constipation following childbirth and due to idiopathic slow transit. Br J Surg 1997; 84:1141–1143.
234. Sarli L, Costi R, Sarli D, Roncoroni L. Pilot study of subtotal colectomy with antiperistaltic cecoproctostomy for the treatment of chronic slow-transit constipation. Dis Colon Rectum 2001; 44:1514–1520.
235. van der Sijp JRM, Kamm MA, Evans RC, Lennard-Jones JE. The results of stoma formation in severe idiopathic constipation. Eur J Gastroenterol Hepatol 1992; 4:137–140.
236. Nicholls RJ, Kamm MA. Proctocolectomy with restorative ileoanal reservoir for severe idiopathic constipation: A report of two cases. Dis Colon Rectum 1988; 31:968–969.
237. Hosie KB, Kmiot WA, Keighley MRB. Constipation: Another indication for restorative proctocolectomy. Br J Surg 1990; 77:801–802.
238. Thakur A, Fonkalsurd EW, Buchmiller T, French S. Surgical treatment of severe colonic inertia with restorative protocolectomy. Am Surg 2001; 67:36–40.
239. Kalbassi MR, Winter DC, Deasy JM. Quality of life assessment of patients after ileal pouch-anal–anastomosis for slow transit constipation. Dis Colon Rectum 2003; 46:1508–1512.
240. Malouf AJ, Wiesel PH, Nicholls T, NichollsRJ, Kamm MA. Short-term effects of sacral nerve stimulation for idiopathic slow transit constipation. World J Surg 2002; 26:166–170.
241. Kenefick NJ, Nicholls RJ, Cohen RG, Kamm MA. Permanent sacral nerve stimulation for treatment of idiopathic constipation. Br J Surg 2002; 89: 882–888.
242. Kenefick NJ, Vaizey CJ, Cohen CRG, Nicholls RJ, Kamm MA. Double-blind placebo-controlled crossover study of sacral nerve stimulation for idiopathic constipation. Br J Surg 2002; 89:1570–1571.
243. Hill J, Stott S, MacLennan I. Antegrade enemas for the treatment of severe idiopathic constipation. Br J Surg 1994; 81:1490–1491.
244. Krogh K, Laurberg S. Malone antegrade continence enema for fecal incontinence and constipation in adults. Br J Surg 1998; 85:974–977.
245. Rongen MJ, van der Hoop AG, Baeten CG. Cecal access for antegrade colon enemas in medically refractory slow transit constipation: a prospective study. Dis Colon Rectum 2001; 44:1644–1649.
246. Lees NP, Hodson P, Hill J, Pearson RC, MacLennan I. Long-term results of the antegrade continent enema procedure for constipation in adults. Colorectal Dis 2004; 6:362–368.
247. Wasserman JF. Puborectalis syndrome: Rectal stenosis due to anorectal spasm. Dis Colon Rectum 1964; 7:87–98.
248. Duthie GS, Bartolo DCC. Anismus: The cause of constipation?. Results of investigation and treatment. World J Surg 1992; 16:831–835.
249. Schouten WR. Diagnosis and treatment of constipation and disturbed defecation. Perspect Colon Rectal Surg 1996; 9:71–85.
250. Pezim ME, Pemberton JH, Levin KE, Litchy WJ, Phillips SF. Parameters of anorectal and colonic motility in health and in severe constipation. Dis Colon Rectum 1993; 35:484–491.
251. Jones PN, Lubowski DZ, Henry MM, Swash M. Is paradoxical contraction of puborectalis muscle of functional importance?. Dis Colon Rectum 1987; 30: 667–670.
252. Miller R, Duthie GS, Bartolo DCC, Roe AM, Locke-Edmunds J, McC Mortensen NJ. Anismus in patients with normal and slow transit constipation. Br J Surg 1991; 78:690–692.
253. Dahl J, Linguist BL, Tysk C, Leissner P, Philipson L, Järnerot G. Behavioral medicine treatment in chronic constipation with paradoxical anal sphincter contraction. Dis Colon Rectum 1991; 34:769–776.
254. Jorge JMN, Wexner SD, Ger GC, Salanga VD, Nogueras JJ, Jagelman DG. Cinedefecography and electromyography in the diagnosis of nonrelaxing puborectalis syndrome. Dis Colon Rectum 1993; 36:668–676.
255. Schouten WR, Briel JW, Auwerda JJA, et al. Anismus: Fact or fiction? Dis Colon Rectum 1997; 40:1033–1041.
256. Loening-Baucke V. Persistence of chronic constipation in children after biofeedback treatment. Dig Dis Sci 1991; 36:153–160.
257. Keck JO, Staniunas RJ, Coller JA, et al. Biofeedback training is useful in fecal incontinence but disappointing in constipation. Dis Colon Rectum 1994; 37:1271–1276.
258. Turnbull GK, Ritvo PG. Anal sphincter biofeedback relaxation treatment for women with intractable constipation symptoms. Dis Colon Rectum 1992; 37:1271–1276.
259. Lubowski DZ, Meagher AP, Smart RC, Butler SP. Scintigraphic assessment of colonic function during defecation. Int J Colorectal Dis 1995; 10:91–93.
260. Lubowski DZ, King DW, Finlay IG. Electromyography of the pubococcygeus muscles in patients with obstructed defecation. Int J Colorectal Dis 1992; 7:184–187.
261. Faucheron JL, Dubreuil A. Rectal akinesia as a new cause of impaired defecation. Dis Colon Rectum 2000; 43:1545–1549.
262. Bleijenberg G, Kuijpers JHC. Treatment of the spastic pelvic floor syndrome with biofeedback. Dis Colon Rectum 1987; 30:108–111.
263. Weber J, Ducrotte PH, Touchais JY, Roussignol C, Denis PH. Biofeedback training for constipation in adults and children. Dis Colon Rectum 1987; 30:844–846.
264. Kavimbe BM, Papachrysostomou M, Binnie NR, Clare N, Smith AN. Outlet obstruction constipation managed by biofeedback. Gut 1991; 32: 1175–1179.
265. Lestar B, Penninckx F, Kerremans R. Biofeedback defecation training for anismus. Int J Colorectal Dis 1991; 6:202–207.
266. West L, Abell TL, Cutts T. Long-term results of pelvic floor muscle rehabilitation in the treatment of constipation. Gastroenterology 1992; 102:A533.
267. Wexner SD, Cheape JD, Jorge JMN, Heymen S, Jagclman DG. Prospective assessment of biofeedback for the treatment of paradoxical puborectalis contraction. Dis Colon Rectum 1992; 35:145–150.
268. Fleshman JW, Dreznik Z, Meyer K, Fry R, Carney R, Kodner I. Outpatient protocol for biofeedback therapy of pelvic floor outlet obstruction. Dis Colon Rectum 1992; 35:1–7.
269. Papachrysostomou M, Smith AN. Effects of biofeedback on obstructive defecation: Reconditioning of the defecation reflex?. Gut 1994; 35:252–256.
270. Koutsomanis D, Lennard-Jones JE, Roy AAJ, Kamm MA. Controlled randomized trial of visual biofeedback versus muscle training without a visual display for intractable constipation. Gut 1995; 37:95–99.
271. Ho YH, Tan M, Goh HS. Clinical and physiologic effects of biofeedback in outlet obstruction constipation. Dis Colon Rectum 1996; 39:520–524.

272. Park UC, Choi SK, Piccirillo MF, Verzaro R, Wexner SD. Patterns of anismus and the relation to biofeedback therapy. Dis Colon Rectum 1996; 39: 768–773.
273. Glia A, Glyin M, Gullberg K, Lindberg G. Biofeedback retraining in patients with functional constipation and paradoxical puborectalis contraction: comparison of anal manometry and sphincter electromyography for feedback. Dis Colon Rectum 1997; 40:889–895.
274. Rao SSC, Welcher KD, Pelsang RE. Effects of biofeedback therapy on anorectal function in obstructive defecation. Dig Dis Sci 1997; 42:2197–2205.
275. Karlbom U, Hallden M, Eeg-Olofsson KE, Pahlman L, Graf W. Results of biofeedback in constipated patients: a prospective study. Dis Colon Rectum 1997; 40:1149–1155.
276. McKee RF, McEnroe L, Anderson JH, Finlay IG. Identification of patients likely to benefit from biofeedback for outlet obstruction defecation. Br J Surg 1999; 86:355–359.
277. Lau CW, Heymen S, Alabaz O, Iroatulum AJ, Wexner SD. Prognostic significance of rectocele, intussusception and abnormal perineal descent in biofeedback treatment for constipated patients with paradoxical puborectalis contraction. Dis Colon Rectum 2000; 43:478–482.
278. Dailianas A, Skandalis N, Rimikis MN, Koutsomanis D, Kardasi M, Archimandritis A. Pelvic floor study in patients with obstructed defecation: influence of biofeedback. J Clin Gastroenterol 2000; 30:176–180.
279. Rhee PI, Choi MS, Kim YH, Son HJ, Kim JJ et al. An increased rectal maximum tolerable volume and long anal canal are associated with poor short-term response to biofeedback therapy for patients with anismus with decreased bowel frequency and normal colonic transit time. Dis Colon Rectum 2000; 43:1405–1411.
280. Chiarioni G, Salandini L, Whitehead WE. Biofeedback benefits only patients with outlet dysfunction, not patients with isolated slow transit constipation. Gastroenterology 2005; 129:86–97.
281. Palsson OS, Heymen S, Whitehead WE. Biofeedback treatment for functional anorectal disorders: A comprehensive efficacy review. Applied Psychophysiology and Biofeedback 2004; 29:153–174.
282. Bleijenberg G, Kuijpers HC. Biofeedback treatment of constipation: a comparison of two methods. Am J Gastroenterol 1994; 89:1021–1026.
283. Heymen S, Wexner S, Vickers D, Nogueras J, Weiss E, Pikarsky A. Prospective randomized trial comparing four biofeedback techniques for patients with constipation. Dis Colon Rectum 1999; 42:1388–1393.
284. Hallan RI, Williams NS, Melling J, Waldron DJ, Womack NR, Morrison JFB. Treatment of anismus in intractable constipation with botulinum. Lancet 1988; 2:714–717.
285. Joo JS, Agachan F, Wolff B, Nogueras JJ, Wexner SD. Initial North American experience with botulinum toxin type A for treatment of anismus. Dis Colon Rectum 1996; 39:1107–1111.
286. Maria G, Brisinda G, Bentivoglio AR, Cassetta E, Albanese A. Botulinum toxin in the treatment of outlet obstruction constipation caused by puborectalis syndrome. Dis Colon Rectum 2000; 43:376–380.
287. Ron Y, Avni Y, Lukovetski A, et al. Botulinum toxin type-A in therapy of patients with anismus. Dis Colon Rectum 2001; 44:1821–1826.
288. Wallace WC, Madden WM. Experience with partial resection of the puborectalis muscle. Dis Colon Rectum 1969; 12:196–200.
289. Barnes PRH, Hawley PR, Preston DM, Lennard-Jones JE. Experience of posterior division of the puborectalis muscle in the management of chronic constipation. Br J Surg 1985; 72:475–477.
290. Kamm MA, Hawley PR, Lennard-Jones JE. Lateral division of the puborectalis muscle in the management of severe constipation. Br J Surg 1988; 75:661–663.
291. Yu DH, Cui FD. Surgical treatment of puborectalis syndrome. J Pract Surg 1990; 10:1599–1600.
292. Kawano M, Fujioshi T, Takagi K. Puborectalis syndrome. J Jpn Soc Coloproctol 1987; 40:612.
293. Ganio E, Masin A, Ratto C, Basile M, Realis LA, Lise G et al. Sacral nerve modulation for chronic outlet constipation. http:/www.colorep.it (May 2003).
294. Hoffman MJ, Kodner IJ, Fry RD. Internal intussusception of the rectum. Diagnosis and surgical management. Dis Colon Rectum 1984; 27:435–441.
295. Johansson C, Ihre T, Ahlback SO. Disturbances in the defecation mechanism with special reference to intussusception of the rectum (internal procidentia). Dis Colon Rectum 1985; 28:920–924.
296. Fleshman JW, Kodner IJ, Fry RD. Internal intussusception of the rectum: A changing perspective. Neth J Surg 1989; 41:145–148.
297. Speakman CT, Madden MV, Nicholls RJ, Kamm MA. Lateral ligament division during rectopexy causes constipation but prevents recurrence: Results of a prospective randomized study. Br J Surg 1991; 78:1431–1433.
298. Broden G, Dolk A, Holmström B. Evacuation difficulties and other characteristics of rectal function associated with the procidentia and the Ripstein operation. Dis Colon Rectum 1988; 31:283–286.
299. Shorvon PJ, McHugh S, Diamant NE, Somers S, Stevenson G. Defecography in normal volunteers: Results and implications. Gut 1989; 30:1737–1749.
300. van Dam JH, Ginai AZ, Gosselink MJ, Huisman WM, Bonjer HJ, Hop WCJ, Schouten WR. Role of defecography in predicting clinical outcome of rectocele repair. Dis Colon Rectum 1997; 40:201–207.
301. Halligan S, Bartram CI. Is barium trapping in rectoceles significant? Dis Colon Rectum 1995; 38:764–768.
302. Kelvin FM, Maglinte DD, Hornback JA. Pelvic floor prolapse: Assessment with evacuation proctography. Radiology 1992; 184:547–551.
303. Siproudhis L, Robert A, Lucas J. Defecatory disorders, anorectal and pelvic floor dysfunction: A polygamy? Radiologic and manometric studies in 41 patients. Int J Colorectal Dis 1992; 7:102–107.
304. Johansson C, Nilsson BY, Holmström B, Dolk A, Mellgren A. Association between rectocele and paradoxical sphincter response. Dis Colon Rectum 1992; 35:503–509.
305. van Dam JH, Schouten WR, Ginai AZ, Huisman WM, Hop WCJ. The impact of anismus on the clinical outcome of rectocele repair. Int J Colorectal Dis 1996; 11:238–242.
306. Siproudhis L, Dautrème S, Ropert A, et al. Dyschezia and rectocele. A marriage of convenience? Physiologic evaluation of the rectocele in a group of 52 women complaining of difficulty in evacuation. Dis Colon Rectum 1993; 36:1030–1036.
307. Murthy VK, Orkin BA, Smith LE, Glassman LM. Excellent outcome using selective criteria for rectocele repair. Dis Colon Rectum 1996; 39:374–378.
308. Karlbom U, Graf W, Nilsson S, Pählman L. Does surgical repair of a rectocele improve rectal emptying? Dis Colon Rectum 1996; 39:1296–1302.
309. Mellgren A, Anzén B, Nilsson BY, et al. Results of rectocele repair. A prospective study. Dis Colon Rectum 1995; 38:7–13.
310. Stojkovic SG, Balfour L, Burke D, Finan PJ, Sagar PM. Does the need to self-digitate or the presence of a large or nonemptying rectocele on proctography influence the outcome of transanal rectocele repair? Colorectal Disease 2003; 5:169–172.
311. Zbar AP, Lienemann A, Fritsch H, Beer-Gabel M, Pescatori M. Rectocele: pathogenesis and surgical management. Int J Colorectal Dis 2003; 18:369–384.
312. Arnold MW, Stewart WRC, Aguilar PS. Rectocele repair: Four years' experience. Dis Colon Rectum 1990; 33:684–687.
313. Nieminen K, Hiltunen KM, Laitinen J, Oksala J, Heinonen PK. Transanal or transvaginal approach to rectocele repair: a prospective randomized pilot study. Dis Colon Rectum 2004; 47:1636–1642.
314. De Tayrac R, Picone O, Chauveaud-Lambling A, Fernandez H. A 2-year anatomical and functional assessment of transvaginal rectocele repair using a polypropylene mesh. Int Urogynecol J 2005 May 21, Epub ahead of print.
315. Altman D, Zetterström J, López A, et al. Functional and anatomic outcome after transvaginal rectocele repair using collagen mesh: A prospective study. Dis Colon rectum 2005; 48:1233–1242.
316. Marks MM. The rectal side of the rectocele. Dis Colon Rectu 1967; 10:387–388.
317. Sarles JC, Arnaud A, Selezneff I, Olivier S. Endorectal repair of rectocele. Int J Colorectal Dis 1989; 4:167–171.
318. Capps WF. Rectoplasty and perineoplasty for the symptomatic rectocele. A report of fifty cases. Dis Colon Rectum 1975; 18:237–243.
319. Sehapayak S. Transrectal repair of rectocele: An extended armamentarium of colorectal surgeons. A report of 355 cases. Dis Colon Rectum 1985; 28:422–433.
320. Sullivan ES, Leaverton GH, Hardwick CE. Transrectal perineal repair: An adjunct to improved function after anorectal surgery. Dis Colon Rectum 1968; 11:106–114.
321. Khubchandani IT, Hakki AR, Sheets JR, Stasik JJ. Endorectal repair of rectocele. Dis Colon Rectum 1983; 26:792–796.
322. Block IR. Transrectal repair of rectoceles using obliterative sutures. Dis Colon Rectum 1986; 29:707–711.
323. Cundiff GW, Fenner D. Evaluation and treatment of women with rectocele: focus on associated defecatory and sexual dysfunction. Obstetrics and gynecology 2004; 104:1403–1421.
324. Ayav A, Bresler L, Brunaud L, Boissel P. Long-term results of transanal repair of rectocele using linear stapler. Dis Colon Rectum 2004; 47:889–894.
325. Ho YH, Ang M, Nyam D, Tan M, Seow-Choen F. Transanal approach to rectocele repair may compromise anal sphincter pressure. Dis Colon Rectum 1998; 41:354–358.
326. van Dam JH, Huisman WM, Hop WCJ, Schouten WR. Fecal continence after rectocele repair: a prospective study. Int J Colorectal Dis 2000; 15:54–57.
327. Thornton MJ, Lam A, King DW. Laparoscopic or transanal repair of rectocele? A retrospective matched cohort study. Dis Colon Rectum 2005; 48:792–798.
328. Janssen LWM, van Dijke CF. Selection criteria for anterior rectal wall repair in symptomatic rectoceles and anterior rectal wall prolapse. Dis Colon Rectum 1994; 37:1100–1107.
329. Khubchandani IT, Clancey JP, Rosen L, Riether RD, Stasik JJ. Enorectal repair of rectocele revisited. Br J Surg 1997; 84:89–91.
330. Tjandra JJ, Ooi BS, Tang CL, Dwyer P, Carey M. Transanal repair of rectocele corrects obstructed defecation if it is not associated with animus. Dis Colon Rectum 1999; 42:1544–1550.
331. Heriot AG, Skull A, Kumar D. Functional and physiological outcome following transanal repair of rectocele. Br J Surg 2004; 91:1340–1344.
332. Abbas SM, Bissett IP, Neill ME, Macmillan AK, Milne D, Parry BR. Long-term results of the anterior Delorme's operation in the management of symptomatic rectocele. Dis Colon Rectum 2005; 48:317–322.
333. Hirst GR, Hughes RJ, Morgan AR, Carr ND, Patel B, Beynon J. The role of rectocele repair in targeted patients with obstructed defecation. Colorectal Dis 2005; 7:159–163.
334. Roman H, Michot F. Long-term outcomes of transanal rectocele repair. Dis Colon Rectum 2005; 48:510–517.

335. López A, Anzén B, Bremmer S, Mellgren A, Nilsson BY et al. Durability of success after rectocele repair. Int Urogynecol J 2001; 12:97–103.
336. Lamah M, Ho J, Leicester RJ. Results of anterior levatorplasty for rectocele. Colorectal Dis 2001; 3:412–416.
337. Ayabaca SM, Zbar AP, Pescatori M. Anal continence after rectocele repair. Dis Colon Rectum 2002; 45:63–69.
338. Watson SJ, Loder PB, Halligan S, Bartram CI, Kamm MA, Phillips RK. Transperineal repair of symptomatic rectocele with Marlex mesh: a clinical, physiological and radiologic assessment of treatment. J Am Coll Surg 1996; 183:257–261.
339. Mercer-Jones MA, Sprowson A, Varma JS. Outcome after transperineal mesh repair of rectocele: A case series. Dis Colon Rectum 2004; 47:468–468.
340. Lechaux JP, Lechaux D, Bataille P, Bars I. Ann Chir 2004; 129:211–217.
341. Vermeulen J, Lange JF, Sikkenk AC, van der Harst E. Anterolateral rectopexy for correction of rectoceles leads to good anatomical but poor functional results. Tech Coloproctol 2005; 9:35–41.
342. Bentley JFR. Posterior excisional anorectal myotomy in management of chronic fecal accumulation. Arch Dis Childhood 1966; 41:144.
343. Thomas CG, Bream CA, de Connick P. Posterior sphincterotomy and rectal myotomy in the management of Hirschsprung's disease. Ann Surg 1970; 171:796–810.
344. Lynn HB, van Heerden JA. Rectal myectomy in Hirschsprung's disease. A decade of experience. Arch Surg 1975; 110:991–994.
345. Shermeta D, Nilprabhassorn P. Posterior myectomy for primary and secondary short segment aganglionosis. Am J Surg 1977; 133:39–41.
346. McCready RA, Beart RW Jr. Adult Hirschsprung's disease: Results of surgical treatment at Mayo Clinic. Dis Colon Rectum 1980; 23:401–407.
347. Freeman NV. Intractable constipation in children treated by forceful anal stretch or anorectal myectomy: Preliminary communication. J R Soc Med 1984; 77(suppl 3):6–8.
348. Hamdy MH, Scobie WG. Anorectal myectomy in adult Hirschsprung's disease: A report of six cases. Br J Surg 1984; 71:611–613.
349. Mishalany HG, Wooley MG. Chronic constipation. Manometric patterns and surgical considerations. Arch Surg 1984; 119:1257–1259.
350. Pinho M, Yoshioka K, Keighley MGB. Long-term results of anorectal myectomy for chronic constipation. Dis Colon Rectum 1990; 33:795–797.
351. Fishbein RH, Handelsman JC, Schuster MM. Surgical treatment of Hirschsprung's disease in adults. Surg Gynecol Obstet 1986; 163:458–464.
352. Poisson J, Devroede G. Severe chronic constipation as a surgical problem. Surg Clin North Am 1983; 63:193–217.
353. Yoshioka K, Keighley MRB. Anorectal myectomy for outlet obstruction. Br J Surg 1987; 74:373–376.
354. Kimura K, Inomata Y, Soper RT. Posterior sagittal rectal myectomy for persistent rectal achalasia after the Soave procedure for Hirschsprung's disease. J Pediatr Surg 1993; 28:1200–1201.
355. McGarity WC, Cody JE. Complications of Hirschsprung's disease in the adult. Am J Gastroenterol 1974; 61:390–393.
356. Elliot MS, Todd IP. Adult Hirschsprung's disease: Results of the Duhamel procedure. Br J Surg 1985; 72:884–885.
357. Hung WT, Chiang TP, Tsai YW, et al. Adult Hirschsprung's disease. J Pediatr Surg 1989; 24:363–366.
358. Steichen FM, Talbert JL, Ravitch MM. Primary side-to-side colorectal anastomosis in the Duhamel operation for Hirschsprung's disease. Surgery 1968; 64:475–483.
359. Kim CY, Park JG, Park KW, Park KJ, Cho MH, Kim WK. Adult Hirschsprung's disease. Results of the Duhamel procedure. Int J Colorectal Dis 1995; 10: 156–160.
360. Wheatley MJ, Wesley JR, Coran AG, Polley TZ Jr. Hirschsprung's disease in adolescents and adults. Dis Colon Rectum 1990; 3:662–669.
361. Luukkonen P, Heikkinen M, Huikuri K, Jarvinen H. Adult Hirschsprung's disease. Clinical features and functional outcome after surgery. Dis Colon Rectum 1990; 33:65–69.
362. Wu JS, Schoetz DJ Jr, Collcr JH, Veidenheimer MC. Treatment of Hirschsprung's disease in the adult. Report of five cases. Dis Colon Rectum 1995; 38:655–659.
363. Gordon PH. An improved technique for the Duhamel operation using the EEA stapler. Dis Colon Rectum 1983; 26:690–692.
364. Cutait DE, Cutait R. Surgery of Chagasic megacolon. World J Surg 1991; 15:188–197.
365. Stoss F, Meier-Ruge W. Experience with neuronal intestinal dysplasia (NID) in adultsEur J Pediatr Surg 1994; 4:298–302.
366. Wrenn K. Fecal impaction. N Engl J Med 1989; 321:658–662.
367. Longo WE, Ballantyne GH, Modlin IM. The colon, anorectum, and spinal cord patient. A review of the functional alterations of the denervated hindgut. Dis Colon Rectum 1989; 32:261–267.
368. Safadi BY, Rosito O, Nino-Murcia M, Wolfe VA, Perkash I. Which stoma works better for colonic dysmotility in the spinal cord injured patient? Am J Surg 2003; 186:437–442.
369. Read NW, Celik AF, Katsinelos P. Constipation and incontinence in the elderly. J Clin Gastroenterol 1995; 20:61–70.
370. Kinnunen O. Constipation in the elderly, with special reference to treatment with magnesium hydroxide and a bulk laxative. Acta Univ Guluensis. Series D. Medica 1990; 211.
371. Hinton JM. Studies with drugs and hormones on the human colon. Proc R Soc Med 1967; 60:215.
372. Katz LA, Spiro H. Gastrointestinal manifestations of diabetes. N Engl J Med 1966; 275:1350–1361.
373. Brocklehurst JC. Colonic disease in the elderly. Clin Gastroenterol 1985; 14:725–747.
374. Palmer ED. "Presbycolon" problems in the nursing home. JAMA 1976; 235:1150.
375. Hull C, Greco RS, Brooks DL. Alleviation of constipation in the elderly by dietary fiber supplementation. J Am Geriatr Soc 1980; 28:410–414.
376. Hope AK, Down EC. Dietary fiber and fluid in control of constipation in a nursing home population. Med J Aust 1986; 144:306–307.
377. Anderson AS, Whichelow M. Constipation during pregnancy: Dietary fiber intakes and the effect of fibre supplementation. Hum Nutr Appl Nutr 1985; 39A:202–207.
378. Shelton MG. Cited by Jones FA, Godding EW. Management of Constipation. London: Blackwell Scientific Publications, 1972.
379. Lamberton R. Resurrected by an enema. Nurs Times 1976; 72:1653.
380. Portenoy RK. Constipation in the cancer patient: Causes and management. Med Clin North Am 1987; 71:303–311.
381. Schuffler MD, Baird HW, Flemming CR. Intestinal pseudoobstruction as the presenting manifestation of small cell carcinoma of the lung: A paraneoplastic neuropathy of the gastrointestinal tract. Ann Intern Med 1983; 98: 129–134.

34 Traumatic Injuries

Lee E. Smith

Trauma is the fourth leading cause of death in North America and accounts for more lost years of useful life than any other cause (1). It is the number one killer in people up to age 44. With penetrating abdominal trauma, the colon and rectum are often injured because of the large area they occupy. Diagnostic and therapeutic endoscopic procedures may cause perforation from within the lumen, and external penetrating or blunt injury may cause perforation from without.

The desire to improve the results of treatment for penetrating traumatic injuries received in battle has been the driving force of surgical progress throughout history. The treatment of colonic trauma is an example of this advancement, for the mortality rate from colonic injuries has decreased with each war from the Civil War to Vietnam (Table 1).

ETIOLOGY

PENETRATING TRAUMA

External penetrating trauma may result from a bullet, shotgun pellets, a knife, a piercing instrument, or impalement. A bullet wound is the most frequent wound type, outnumbering knife wounds by a ratio of 10 to 1 (7). Inexpensive low-velocity weapons known as "Saturday night specials" have been the usual weapons used in criminal assault in the past. In recent years, high-velocity weapons (with bullets traveling at more than 2000 ft/sec) have become increasingly available and are now common throughout society. Velocity is the dominant factor in determining the amount of tissue damage within the body (8,9). The other factor that determines wound ballistics (motion of the bullet within the tissues) is the mass of the bullet. Velocity (V) and mass (M) can be expressed in the formula for kinetic energy (KE):

$$\text{KE} = \frac{1}{2} M \times V^2$$

The prime factor in kinetic energy is velocity, since it is expressed as the square. As the bullet travels through tissue, it creates a temporary high-pressure cavity around itself, resulting in secondary tissue damage away from the direct path of the bullet. The bullet may tumble (yaw) in its trajectory, also expanding the injury diameter (Fig. 1).

Shotguns are smooth-bore weapons that discharge a number of small projectiles. The velocity of the pellets diminishes rapidly so that deep penetration in most instances does not occur if the weapon is fired more than 7 yards away from the person, but if a shotgun wound is

TABLE 1 ■ Mortality from Colonic Trauma in War

War	Mortality Rate (%)
U.S. Civil War	90
Spanish-American War	90
World War I	58
World War II	37
Korean War	15
Vietnam War	9

Source: From Refs. 2–6.

inflicted at close range, extensive tissue loss occurs. Close-range shotgun wounds require extensive local debridement.

Large, bowel impalement injuries are caused by falling onto or running into an object that penetrates the abdomen or rectum. The rectal injury usually occurs after the individual falls with the legs astride the penetrating object such as a picket fence or a stake.

■ BLUNT TRAUMA

Blunt trauma accounts for approximately 4% of colorectal injuries. Most injuries in this category result from motor vehicle accidents, with the steering wheel being the primary source of injury. Seat belts do save lives, but colonic or rectal injury can occur secondary to the use of seat belts, which cause pelvic fracture with a rectal tear or a compression of the colon between the anterior abdominal wall and the vertebral column, resulting in a "blow out" injury (10). Direct force across the abdomen occurs when the belt either rides up from below the iliac crest or the person has slid down on the seat beneath the belt, creating free abdominal exposure. Shearing from rapid deceleration may cause an injury in which the fixed mesenterica peritoneum suspends the free-floating colon. In addition, hematoma and vascular injury may cause delayed perforation; thus, perforation after blunt trauma must be considered to avoid delay in treatment (11,12). Automobiles striking pedestrians, motorcycle accidents, falls, being crushed under a heavy object, and athletic injuries result in similar damage. Also, blunt trauma to the perineum can disrupt the rectosigmoid and anal canal from the levator muscular sling (11,12).

■ IATROGENIC INJURY

Few organ systems are as accessible for diagnosis and treatment as is the large bowel. This accessibility places it at risk for unintended injury. Diagnostic and therapeutic procedures performed for colon and rectal disease can result in injury if they are performed improperly or if the tissues investigated are weakened by disease.

Injury from Operative Procedures

Intraoperative injury to the colon and rectum can occur during any procedure in the pelvis or abdomen because the colorectum extends into every quadrant.

By proximity, gynecologic procedures can lead to colorectal injury. Perforation may occur during routine dilatation and curettage of the uterus, and the adjacent colorectum is vulnerable to puncture. More complicated procedures that are performed frequently, such as total abdominal hysterectomy and vaginal hysterectomy, also may result in colorectal injury or fistulization. During laparoscopic sterilization electrocoagulation may be used, possibly leading to bowel injury; deaths associated with this procedure have been reported (13). Intrauterine devices have been known to erode into the peritoneal cavity and subsequently into the colon, creating a localized septic inflammatory process (14).

Anorectal injuries can result from simple anorectal surgery, including operations for hemorrhoids, fistulas, and fissure. Resulting complications may include anal stenosis, ectropion, or incontinence. Already there are several reports of leaks and sepsis following the new stapling procedures for hemorrhoids (15–18). The surgical correction of these complications is specifically addressed in Chapters 15 and 36.

Urologic surgery can cause colorectal trauma. Percutaneous nephrostomy is ordinarily a safe and reliable procedure for decompressing the urinary collecting system; however, LeRoy et al. (19) reported on two perforations of the colon that occurred during nephrostomy surgery. Perineal prostatectomy, suprapubic prostatectomy, or transurethral resection of the prostate can be associated with injury of the adjacent rectum (20,21).

During surgery in which electrocautery is used, explosions have occurred in the presence of combustible colonic

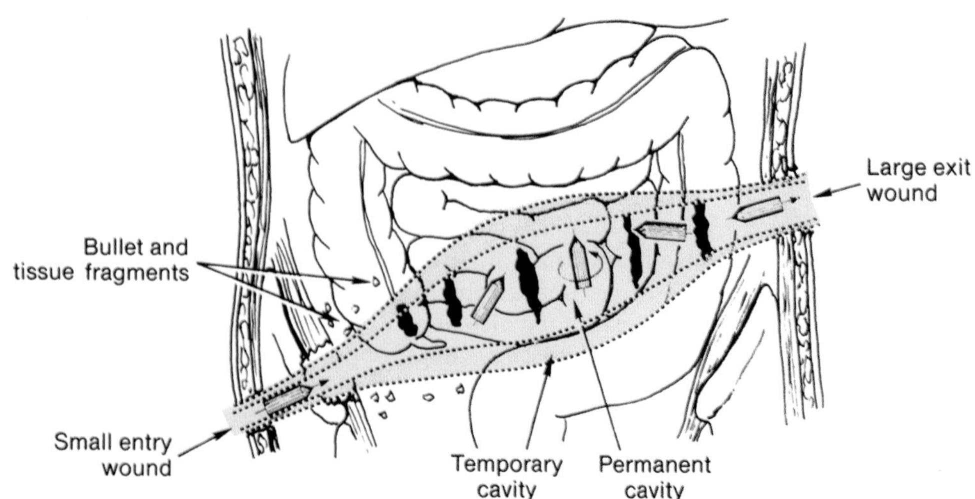

FIGURE 1 ■ Bullet traversing the abdomen. Note tumbling and yawing of the bullet. Area of destruction also results from a combination of cavitation and trajectory of secondary particles.

gases, resulting in large perforations and deaths (22,23). Both the hydrogen from the mannitol bowel preparation and the methane sometimes naturally present within the colon are combustible.

Colorectal injury can occur with neurosurgical and orthopedic operations. Inserting ventriculoperitoneal shunts in infants with hydrocephalus is a standard treatment to reduce intracerebral pressure, but on rare occasions the bowel has been perforated during placement of the peritoneal limb (7,24,25). During internal fixation of a hip fracture, there have been instances of nails being too deep, causing injury to the rectum (26).

Colorectal stents have been employed in obstruction secondary to carcinoma for either palliation or as a bridge to surgery. Khot et al. reviewed the literature and found 29 case series covering 598 stent insertion attempts. Perforation occurred in 22 (4%) (27).

Endoscopically Induced Trauma

Rigid Proctosigmoidoscopy

Proctosigmoidoscopic perforation of the bowel was reviewed in 1967 by Befeler (28). He found reports on 125 cases of iatrogenic perforation of the colon and rectum. Most were near the peritoneal reflection of the rectosigmoid, and in most instances the tear was in a diseased bowel, with a mortality rate >25%. Andresen (29) reported on a series of 94 proctosigmoidoscopic injuries and concluded that mortality was related directly to the time between injury and operative intervention. The mortality rate was only 8% if operation for the perforation was performed within six hours, but if the delay between perforation and operation was greater than 12 hours, death ensued in 20% of cases. In a more recent review by Nelson et al. (30), only three perforations occurred during 16,325 examinations, but one of the three patients died.

In 1953, Klein and Scarborough (31) reported on 50 perforations of the rectum and distal colon by proctosigmoidoscopy. A number of these perforations occurred during purely diagnostic procedures. Factors associated with perforation included blind introduction beyond the anal margin, reinsertion of the obturator to overcome spasm, injudicious use of long cotton-tipped applicators, and the attempted forceful dilatation of rectal strictures with the proctosigmoidoscope. These authors also noted that the mortality rate was dependent on the tune lapse between perforation and definitive operative treatment. Although it is generally believed that injuries to the rectum often are caused by an inexperienced physician, perforation can occur at the hands of experts. Common sense dictates that all endoscopists perform these examinations gently, obtain biopsies judiciously, and insufflate minimally. Examiners frequently err when attempting to overcome an area of spasm by forceful compression of the insufflation bulb. Not only does this method fail to dilate the spastic bowel, but it results in dilatation of the proximal bowel and pain. Few perforations accompany a screening examination but do happen more often during biopsy or therapeutic intervention in elderly patients with acute disease.

Thorbjarnarson (32) reported on 10 iatrogenic perforations of the large bowel, five of which resulted from the use of biopsy forceps or a snare. Two perforations resulted from taking a full-thickness biopsy of a sessile colonic lesion; another resulted from obtaining a biopsy specimen from a thin-walled ulcer, and two resulted from performing snare polypectomy.

Traumatic consequences from biopsy and polypectomy occur far more frequently above the peritoneal reflection. When complete penetration is made, peritonitis may ensue, necessitating emergency surgery. Perforation occurring below the 10-cm level from the anal verge infrequently causes serious complications.

Fiberoptic Sigmoidoscopy and Colonoscopy

The major complications of colonoscopy are hemorrhage and perforation (33–35). Fortunately, the clotting mechanism and healing properties of the body minimize the need for operation in the bleeding patient.

Bleeding can accompany abrasion or laceration of the colonic wall during diagnostic colonoscopy, but this is unusual, and it is rare that it requires operation. Even biopsy with the standard 2-mm biopsy tip rarely leads to bleeding significant enough to require operation. Snare polypectomy is the most frequent source of bleeding in therapeutic colonoscopy and can result in a brisk primary or secondary bleed. Primary hemorrhage occurs as the snare cuts through the polyp when electrocoagulation is inadequate or cuts through it too rapidly while a cutting type of electrical current is being used. Sometimes the patient has been receiving anticoagulant therapy, which contributes to the bleeding. Secondary hemorrhage may occur within a few hours or several days. An adequate clotting mechanism usually stops the hemorrhage; however, blood transfusions, arteriograms for Pitressin drip or embolization, and operation may be considered if bleeding does not prove to be self-limited.

The risk of perforation during colonoscopy and sigmoidoscopy was determined by study of a random sample of 5% of Medicare beneficiaries covered by the Surveillance, Epidemiology, and End Results (SEER) Program registries. After 39,286 colonoscopies, there were 77 perforations, and after 35,298 sigmoidoscopies there were 31 perforations (36). In another study of 26,162 consecutive colonoscopies, 65% diagnostic and 35% therapeutic procedures, there were perforations in 11 (0.06%) diagnostic and 10 (0.11%) therapeutic colonoscopies (37). Another consecutive series of 34,620 colonoscopies resulted in 31 (0.09%) perforations (38).

Perforation during diagnostic colonoscopy can occur when the "slide-by" technique is used, when the tip is forcefully introduced into a large diverticulum, or with insufflation of air into a diverticulum while the scope tip is placed tightly over the diverticular os. Other situations in which perforation can occur include maneuvers such as dilatation of a stenosis or overstretching and splitting a fixed colonic segment with a looping scope (34,39,40).

The slide-by technique works well until the tip becomes entrapped. At that point, the visualized mucosa stops rippling by the scope tip and blanches. Applying continued pressure will rupture the wall. The most likely sites of scope-tip entrapment are the rectosigmoid, midsigmoid, and the angle created by the junction of the descending colon and the sigmoid colon.

False diverticula by definition do not contain all the layers of the bowel wall. Pressure over these diverticula will cause perforation more easily than at a healthy site in the colon. When the scope tip is deflected (i.e., doubled back 180° on the shaft), constant force exerted against the bowel wall may result in a tearing injury over the arc of flexure. If the scope will not advance, the colon must stretch or burst at that point. The shaft of the scope also may form a broad loop in which the pressure of introduction of the scope is transmitted to the wall if the tip is not moving at the rate the shaft is introduced. In addition, improper use of an external splinting device may cause injury. Force should not be used to advance the splint, and the colonoscope should be withdrawn a short length to straighten the scope so that it will accept the splint more safely. Fluoroscopic aid is invaluable for this maneuver.

More frequently, colonoscopic injuries occur with biopsy or therapeutic procedures (41). Seldom does use of the tiny biopsy forceps result in perforation; however, if electrocoagulation to stop bleeding or a hot biopsy forceps is used, a full-thickness burn and necrosis with perforation may ensue. Likewise, the snare may cut a pedunculated polyp, especially a thick stalk, too flush with the colonic wall, causing a full-thickness burn (42). Treating a sessile polyp is a greater risk for the same reasons. Taking <2.0-cm pieces of a sessile polyp and coagulating them in short two-second bursts, allowing cooling periods in between, minimizes the perforation risk. A burn may be created if a pedunculated polyp touches a small site on a wall opposite the stalk. That small site may ground the current, necrose the wall, and result in an acute or delayed perforation.

Snare application is potentially dangerous during performance of polypectomy. A snare may pick up an adjacent fold, cutting or burning a hole in the wall near the polyp. Resistance on closing the snare may be a clue that extra tissue is caught within the snare.

Explosions can result from the use of cautery during endoscopy (43,44). The injuries may vary from none to severe lacerations and perforation. A bowel explosion with colonic perforation was reported when an argon plasma coagulation was employed for hemorrhagic radiation proctitis (45). The gases found frequently in the distal bowel include hydrogen, methane, and hydrogen sulfide. These gases should be evacuated from the colon and rectum by suctioning the lumen before any kind of electrical or laser coagulation treatment is begun. Suctioning gas and insufflation of room air should be repeated frequently during a long coagulation process. Some endoscopists also add an inert nonflammable gas such as nitrogen or carbon dioxide during the coagulation treatment. If an explosion does occur, the patient should be monitored for signs and symptoms of abdominal or shoulder pain and tenderness. Serial abdominal X-ray studies are indicated to look for free abdominal air that would require emergency laparotomy.

A "silent" perforation is manifested by air in the retroperitoneum or free air in the peritoneal cavity (46–51). Although patients with condition often have no symptoms, ileus is the most common symptom that occurs. This condition may be present more frequently than reported since it is usually found on "routine" X-ray studies of the chest or abdomen that were scheduled and unrelated to the endoscopy. If a silent injury is found, antibiotics should be prescribed and the patient observed for evidence of infection or peritonitis. The treatment of 43 perforations in 57,028 colonoscopies was analyzed (52). Prompt surgery in 40 resulted in no deaths. They were treated with primary repair or primary anastomosis generally. Three were asymptomatic and were treated nonoperatively.

Injury from Rectal Thermometer

Obtaining rectal temperature is a routine procedure. Rectal thermometers are well-known causes of perforation during the first few days of a newborn's life. In 1965, Fonkalsrud and Clatworthy (53) reported on 10 accidental perforations of the intestine in infants. The authors pointed out that the distance between the anus and the peritoneal cul-de-sac over the rectosigmoid in newborns is <3 cm and that half the perforations occur at this low level. Horwitz and Bennett (54) reported on an outbreak of peritonitis in a neonatal nursery that was caused by a nurse's perforating the rectum with a thermometer while taking rectal temperatures (Fig. 2).

Perforation by Therapeutic Enema

Even procedures such as giving a simple enema are subject to human error. Usually, perforation results from insertion of the enema tip by an unskilled or careless attendant or during self-insertion. A spectrum of anorectal injuries can occur during insertion of an enema tip (55,56). Perforation from enemas can be classified into five types: (i) anal perforation, (ii) submucosal perforation, (iii) extraperitoneal perforation, (iv) intraperitoneal perforation, and (v) perforation into adjacent organs. The majority of rectal perforations from enema tips are on the anterior wall. Extraperitoneal perforation can cause abscess, fistula, or severe hemorrhage.

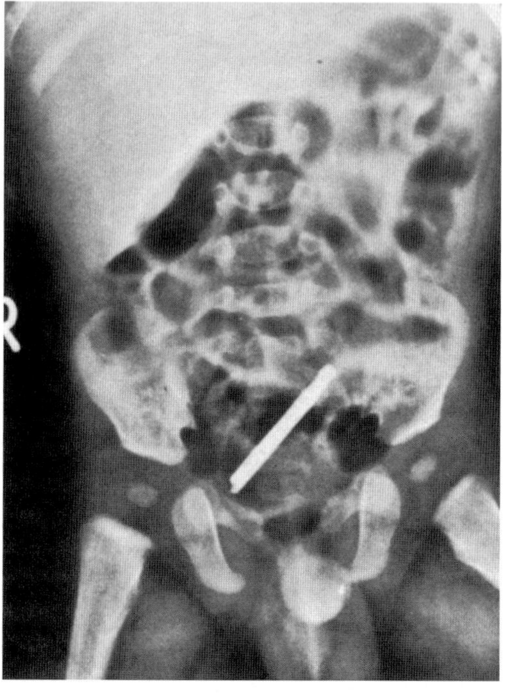

FIGURE 2 ■ Broken rectal thermometer in the rectosigmoid.

Gayer et al. (57) reported 14 rectal perforations secondary to cleansing enemas. Abdominal pain and fever were the common symptoms. All had computerized tomography (CT) with the findings of extraluminal air in the perianal and perirectal fat. No leak was seen on any CT. The CT was of help, because the physician did not suspect the etiology. Ten were subjected to surgery, but five died. The four treated conservatively all died.

Installation of the wrong liquid, such as scalding water, can cause severe burns; the wrong solution, such as formaldehyde instead of paraldehyde, can cause sloughing and rectal bleeding.

Injury from Barium Enema

A variety of complications have been associated with barium enema studies (58). Two of the most serious of these complications are mechanical perforation of the bowel, either intraperitoneally or extraperitoneally by direct penetration of the enema tip, and overinflation of the rectal balloon, causing pneumatic rupture of the rectum (59). Other complications include the formation of barium granulomas within the rectal wall, necrotizing proctitis, and barium embolism.

Kiser et al. (60) reported that one perforation of the colon occurred in 1250 barium enemas administered at the Ellis Fischell State Cancer Hospital in Columbia, Missouri. Most perforations are ruptures through ulcers, neoplasms, diverticula, hernias, inflammatory bowel disease, or other areas of disease. Rosenklint et al. (61) reported on six extraperitoneal perforations that occurred from barium extravasation during 20,000 barium enema examinations. Four of the six patients died, and the other two have permanent colostomies. None of the patients had disease in the colon or rectum. Obtaining tissue for a simple rectal biopsy weakens the bowel enough that a barium enema may complete a perforation. A seven-day wait allows sealing and helps protect against perforation. Biopsy specimens obtained through the rigid sigmoidoscope easily can be 5 mm in size; those taken through the colonoscope can be only 2 to 3 mm (62). Thus, deeper biopsies afford greater risk to proceed to full-thickness perforation.

When small amounts of barium are injected submucosally, a simple barium granuloma results, which may be asymptomatic or cause pain. Sterile barium causes little inflammatory reaction when injected into the subcutaneous and retroperitoneal tissues, the wall of the rectum, or the peritoneal cavity. Several years later, it may present as isolated rectal nodules in a patient who has been asymptomatic (63,64). Larger amounts of barium injected in the same manner can result in severe inflammatory reaction, abscess formation, or even necrotizing proctitis. Ultimately, retroperitoneal barium causes dense retroperitoneal fibrosis. Perforation above the peritoneal reflection results in intraperitoneal contamination by both barium and residual stool from the bowel. Even when perforation reaches into the free peritoneal cavity, the injury may not be suspected immediately because of the lack of symptoms suggesting that a free perforation has occurred. However, symptoms of peritoneal irritation occurring minutes or hours after the enema should be considered as possibly resulting from the barium enema study. During repeat abdominal radiograph, most of these cases show the presence of free air and/or evidence of barium outside the lumen of the bowel. Perforation also may be retroperitoneal.

Unlike the sometimes benign course of endoscopic biopsy perforation, the combination of barium and feces is a dreaded complication (64–68). When barium is combined with significant bacterial contamination from the bowel, a massive, and often overwhelming, inflammatory response occurs. Sisel et al. (69) experimented on rabbits, producing colonic rupture after a barium enema or an enema performed with a water-soluble contrast material. Without treatment, both types were uniformly fatal. Surgical repair of the rupture with concomitant peritoneal lavage resulted in only a 10% survival rate in animals with feces and barium contamination. Fifty percent of the animals with Gastrografin and feces contamination survived if surgery was performed promptly. Zheutlin et al. (70) reported on a collected series of 53 patients in whom barium mixed with feces spilled into the peritoneal cavity. The mortality rate in this group was 51%. Nelson et al. (30) reported a 100% mortality rate with this type of perforation. Based on these data, water-soluble contrast material is the preferred type for use in patients with suspected perforations, or suspected leaks in recent anastomoses.

Barium embolism is rare, but when it happens, a fatal outcome is likely. The pathophysiology begins with intravasation of barium into the veins of the rectum, resulting in pulmonary embolism and sudden death (71). Not performing a barium enema on patients with acute inflammatory bowel disease or on patients who have had recent endoscopic procedures with biopsy or polypectomy will decrease the incidence of this rare occurrence.

A barium enema sometimes is used therapeutically to reduce intussusceptions in infants. Unfortunately, the hydrostatic force introduced into the colon perforated six of 1000 colons in one series (72).

Obstetric Trauma

Cephalopelvic disproportion and the stretching of local anatomy that takes place during childbirth result in trauma to some degree in almost every vaginal delivery (73,74). A deep laceration may occur in the perineum after parturition that involves not only the vagina but also the perineal body, the rectum, and the anal canal, including the anal sphincter mechanism. An episiotomy during delivery will decrease the tendency for third-degree lacerations involving the anal sphincter. If the episiotomy is performed in the posterior midline of the vagina, harm to the sphincteric mechanism is more likely than if it is directed laterally. The size of the infant, the flexibility of the pelvic tissues, the parity of the patient, the weight of the patient, the skill of the obstetrician, and the decision whether or not to use instrumentation are factors that influence incidence of anorectal trauma during childbirth (74).

Precise repair of a third-degree tear is a necessary skill for those who practice obstetrics; a colorectal surgeon seldom is needed to repair such an injury on an emergency basis. Most repairs will heal uneventfully; however, if incontinence is a postdelivery problem, a secondary repair by sphincteroplasty is indicated. See Chapter 15 for details of repair.

Rectovaginal fistulas also may result from difficult parturition, and laceration. Pressure necrosis of the rectovaginal wall, forceps delivery, and midline episiotomies are often associated factors. See Chapter 16 for repair details.

Irradiation-Induced Proctitis

Irradiation of neoplasms of the pelvis may cause both immediate and delayed complications. Irradiation proctitis is an anticipated sequela after radiation of common neoplasms that originate from the uterus, ovary, bladder, prostate, anus, or rectum. Quan (75) reviewed 65 patients who underwent irradiation therapy for pelvic malignancy, 52 of whom had carcinoma of the cervix. Often, radiation damages both the bladder and the intestine simultaneously. The acute findings are edema, inflammation, erythema, and friability of the rectal mucosa, which may progress to ulceration or necrosis (76). As the rectum heals, granulation tissue, fibrosis, and telangiectasia may result. Full rectal wall necrosis may develop, and in women a rectovaginal fistula may occur if necrosis is severe anteriorly. The radiation injury site may form a stricture as part of the healing phase. Microscopic examination of these tissues reveals underlying irradiation-induced endarteritis leading to tissue hypoxia, resulting in the above sequence of macroscopic events. Likewise, lymphatic channels are destroyed.

The onset of symptoms after radiotherapy varies from immediately to years after treatment, with rectal bleeding as the most common symptom. In a review of 80 patients by Quan (75), implantation of iodine-125 radioactive seeds was compared to external beam therapy; none of the patients treated by implantation developed rectal symptoms. Twenty-one of the patients treated by external beam underwent colostomy; 11 were permanent and 10 were temporary. Indications for colostomy were excessive bleeding; radiation necrosis of the rectum; fistulization to the vagina, bladder, or bowel; and obstruction caused by stenosis from radiation. The anterior rectal wall was the site of the most severe radiation-induced changes. The extent of damage depended on the size of the area treated, the total dose delivered, overall treatment time, and fractionation of the dosage. Individual techniques affect the outcome as well.

Mild proctitis usually requires no treatment. Sherman et al. (77) reported good results from using corticosteroid enemas in the management of patients with acute and chronic irradiation proctitis. Henriksson et al. (78) performed a double-blind, placebo-controlled trial using oral sucralfate, an aluminum hydroxide complex of sulfonated sucrose, for two weeks after onset of radiation and continued for six weeks. Bowel movements were significantly improved with treatment and fewer patients required antidiarrheal medications. Colonic obstruction caused by irradiation colitis or proctitis is rare, but if such complications do occur, colostomy is indicated (79). When bleeding becomes incessant oozing from the injured surface, the laser, the argon plasma coagulator, or topical formalin have been effectively used over the entire face to stop the hemorrhage (80–82).

Van Nagell et al. (83) reported on rectal injury in a series of patients with uterine carcinoma requiring irradiation. An increasing incidence of proctitis was noted in patients who had pre-existing hypertensive vascular disease or diabetes mellitus. No rectal injuries occurred when the total dose to the rectum was < 4000 rads. The authors also stressed that severe proctitis often preceded bladder or other bowel complications. Fractionation of the remaining irradiation dosage over longer periods of time prevented much of the later irradiation changes. A two-week rest period in the middle of the treatment course using topical steroids and cleansing enemas lessened acute injury symptoms.

■ INGESTED FOREIGN BODIES

Perforation of the gastrointestinal tract from ingestion of foreign bodies is rare. Natural foods, such as pits, thorns, seeds, or soft bones, undergo significant digestion by the time they reach the colon. However, hard particulate matter, such as chicken and other animal bones, toothpicks, portions of glass, shells, or other sharp objects, may pass through the intestinal tract into the colon and cause injury to the rectum and anus. Infants, children, and mentally deranged adults are at higher risk because of objects they may put in their mouths and subsequently swallow. Of course, anyone could inadvertently swallow an object that enters the mouth; parts of dentures sometimes break off and are swallowed. To prevent such injuries, potentially dangerous objects should be kept out of the reach of infants, children, and mentally incompetent adults.

The complications secondary to ingested foreign bodies include perforation, hemorrhage, abscess formation, bowel obstruction, and death (84,85). Less than 1% of foreign bodies that become entrapped cause perforation. Observation and expeditious gastrointestinal endoscopy are the two best forms of therapy. The physician must decide if it is preferable to watch the foreign body pass spontaneously or to perform endoscopic removal within one or two hours of ingestion. Surgical intervention is required for the 1% of patients who experience perforation or obstruction because of these objects. Seventy-five percent of gastrointestinal perforations occur at the ileocecal valve and the appendix. Sequential abdominal roentgenograms show that most objects exit the gastrointestinal tract within one week. Failure of the foreign body to exit is another indication for surgery. Close observation for the development of the rare complication is a safe approach. Early endoscopic removal of selected easily reached objects may be an acceptable approach.

The illegal drug traffic in North America has led to multiple ways drug dealers have developed to import their product secretly. A health hazard is created if a packet of a pure narcotic is placed into a body orifice (Fig. 3). If swallowed, large packets of the drug may obstruct the gastrointestinal tract. During the attempt to remove them endoscopically or surgically, special care should be exercised to avoid rupturing the packets because if they open in the gut, the patient may suffer overdose.

■ FOREIGN BODIES AND SEXUAL TRAUMA

An amazing variety of objects have been inserted into the rectum and have become entrapped above the anal sphincter musculature. Practically any object that can be contemplated as fitting into the rectum has at one time been used for sexual stimulation. Some of the more "fashionable" foreign bodies that have been placed in the rectum include vibrators, plastic phalluses, cucumbers, baby powder cans,

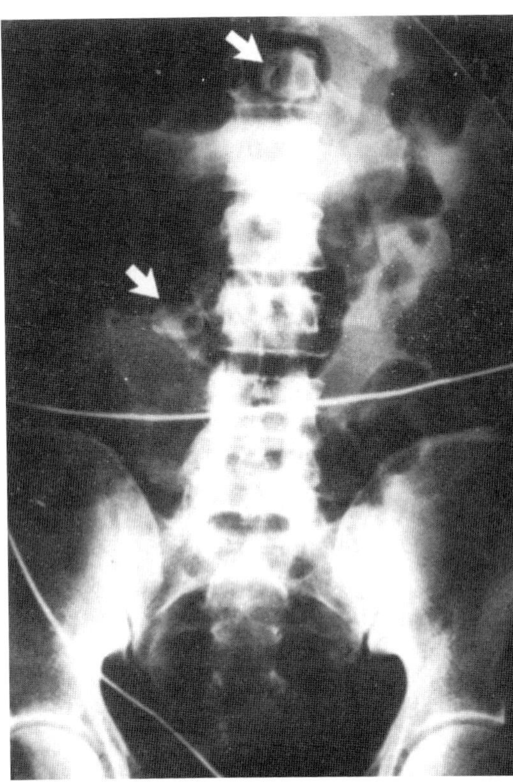

FIGURE 3 ■ Ingested packets of narcotic (*arrows*). These are associated with local bowel obstruction, often at the ileocecal value. Rupture of a packet results in a drug overdose.

balls, bottles of all shapes and sizes, glasses, flashlight batteries, flashlights, test tubes, screwdrivers, ballpoint pens, paperweights, and thermometers (Fig. 4). The entrapment of the object causes the patient not only social embarrassment but also significant physical pain. Serious

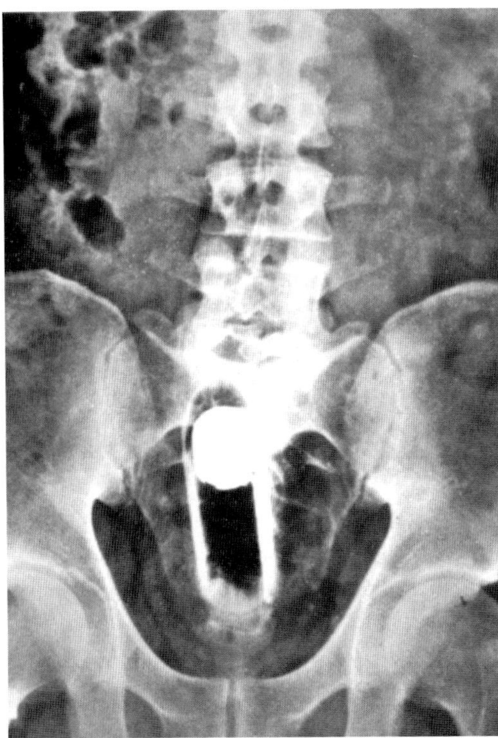

FIGURE 4 ■ Vibrator lodged in the rectosigmoid. Objects such as this are pushed into the anus and cannot be retrieved.

injuries to the rectum, rectosigmoid, and other intraperitoneal structures can occur. Death resulting from placement of foreign bodies in the rectum has been reported by numerous authors (86–90). Eftaiha et al. (89) found it useful to classify the level of entrapment of the foreign body. Most objects lying in the rectum at the low or middle level (up to 10 cm) can be removed transanally, but celiotomy may be needed to remove objects that become lodged in the upper rectum or lower sigmoid.

Beall and DeBakey (91), Barone et al. (87), and Sohn et al. (90) have reported independently on rectosigmoid perforation caused by insertion of foreign bodies. Such injury may be incurred by the patient in an attempt at autoeroticism or may be delivered by a sexual partner or during a criminal assault. Splitting of the rectosigmoid results in peritoneal contamination and peritonitis. Presenting with an acute abdomen, the patient may hide the history of sexual or assaultive action.

Plain radiographs should be part of the emergency evaluation when such injuries are reported or suspected. Anteroposterior and lateral abdominal and pelvic views should be used to determine the type, number, and location of the foreign bodies; however, radiolucent objects may not be visualized.

■ SEXUAL ASSAULT

Sexual assault is one of the fastest growing violent crimes in the United States. Over 500,000 women and 49,000 men report being assaulted each year (92). The assault may be criminal and may be intended to harm, or it may be the result of a vigorous sexual act that was intended to be enjoyed by both partners. Whatever the motive, sexual assault can cause significant injury to the extraperitoneal or intraperitoneal rectum or rectosigmoid.

Sohn et al. (90) reported a previously undescribed act termed "fist fornication" or "fisting" in 11 patients over a four-year interval. Fist fornicators force a closed clenched fist through the intact anus into the rectum for sexual gratification. The rectum or sigmoid colon was the site of injury. Six patients had mucosal lacerations in the rectum that bled, but no sphincteric laceration was noted. Only simple suturing of the mucosal laceration was necessary for these patients. Four patients developed an acute abdomen requiring celiotomy, resection, and a Hartmann pouch. One patient had complete anal sphincteric incontinence from severe sphincteric laceration.

■ CHILD ABUSE

Anorectal trauma in children is rare, but when found, it is usually due to abuse (93). Sexually abused boys experience anorectal trauma in 7% to 16% of cases of this type of abuse, and they are abused at a younger age than girls. Anal sexual acts account for injury in 54.5% of abused boys. Only 3.7% of abused girls suffer anal injury (94).

Black et al. (94) reported on 617 rape victims. Twenty-four percent were younger than 16 years old, and 33% had anal trauma. The medical community must be alert to recognize these criminal acts and report them to prevent more physical and emotional morbidity to the child and his or her siblings (95).

The examiner should keep accurate records as legal evidence, and a one-on-one interview should take place.

Signs of trauma around the anus or elsewhere on the body should be noted. Anal trauma may be the only visible trauma site because no resistance is offered if the assailant is known to the victim. Sperm and acid phosphatase should be sought in any material retrieved (96). Venereal disease testing should be performed if the circumstances make the physician suspicious.

Sedation may be necessary to perform an anal or rectal examination if there is pain or great distress. Obtaining abdominal films to look for free air is warranted if the abdomen is tender.

UNUSUAL PERFORATIONS

Hard impacted stool sometimes perforates the rectum, or the rectosigmoid colon by ischemic necrosis, a condition termed "stercoral perforation." The blood supply to a site in the colorectum is impaired by pressure of the hard bolus of stool pressed against an unyielding organ (97,98).

Rarely, spontaneous perforation will occur in the rectosigmoid or cecum from either distention or spasm. The possibility of perforation is well recognized in pre-existing disease such as inflammatory bowel disease, diverticulitis, or carcinoma, but sometimes spontaneous perforation occurs in the absence of pathologic disease (99).

Cain et al. (100) reported on five bizarre cases of trauma resulting from children sitting on a swimming pool drain. Suction caused perforation of the rectosigmoid, followed by small bowel evisceration and loss of much small bowel.

Electrocution may immediately or subsequently perforate the bowel but most often the colon. If celiotomy is performed as part of therapy, careful exploration for burned bowel is mandatory (101). During sexual antics, people have directed compressed air toward and into the anus so that a hole is blown in the proximal colon (102). Thermal injury of the gastrointestinal tract is rare, but there has been a report of instillation of hot water into a stoma, causing a mucosal burn that subsequently formed a stenosis (103). Improper insertion of a stomal irrigation tube or forceful insertion of a catheter to empty a continent reservoir pouch (Kock's pouch) may cause perforation, which may be unrecognized initially since little or no pain may occur. The design of cone tips for ostomy irrigation prevents deep insertion and bowel injury.

MANAGEMENT

In the last two decades, much thought has been given to the management of the traumatized patient. Through the Advanced Trauma Life Support courses a systematic approach has been promoted, which is divided into four phases: primary survey, resuscitation, secondary survey, and definitive care (Table 2) (104). These principles can be applied to both the military combat situation and civilian trauma.

The primary survey comprises rapid clinical diagnosis of life-threatening conditions such as an occluded airway, inadequate respirations, cardiac failure, arrhythmias, and hemorrhage. The resuscitation phase involves using procedures immediately to save lives. Chest tube placement, pericardiocentesis, intubation of the airway, control of obvious severe hemorrhage, and placement of lines must be performed without delay before time-consuming laboratory examinations are begun.

TABLE 2 ■ Phases of Management in Trauma

Phase	Action	Pertinence of Colorectal Injury
1	Primary survey—diagnosis of life-threatening conditions	
2	Resuscitation	
3	Secondary survey—diagnosis of trauma	Diagnosis of colorectal injury
4	Definitive care	Surgery to repair colorectal injury

During the secondary survey the colorectal injuries are identified, leading to the final phase, definitive care. These two phases are dealt with in depth in the following sections. Without the secondary survey, more subtle perineal and rectal wounds may be overlooked, and delay in diagnosis and late treatment lead to increased morbidity and mortality (105).

DIAGNOSIS OF TRAUMA (SECONDARY SURVEY PHASE)

History

An alert and cooperative patient may be questioned about the circumstances of the trauma. However, the patient with a head injury or multiple trauma may be unable to communicate. At times the trauma is obvious, but a history from someone at the scene (if available) may prove helpful. The observer—a paramedic, ambulance driver, litter bearer, helicopter pilot, corpsman, or a relative—may be able to relate important details of the trauma, specifically the type of trauma, the wounding agent, and the interval of time that has elapsed. For example, knowing whether the injury was caused by an ice pick or a bayonet, a low-velocity 22-caliber pistol or a high-velocity M16 rifle, a fall from 5 feet or 50 feet, or a fall from a golf cart or a motorcycle traveling at high speed, or whether it occurred 20 minutes or 20 hours previously would aid in making the decisions about appropriate diagnostic tests and the extent of treatment.

Patients with isolated anorectal trauma may complain of perineal, anorectal, or abdominal pain. Usually pain begins precisely at the time of injury. Less often, the pain may be delayed in a patient with small extraperitoneal perforations of the rectum or after a foreign body cannot be removed from the rectum. Dull lower abdominal pain may be the only manifestation of an upper rectal or rectosigmoid tear with perforation. Rectal bleeding denotes rectal trauma, and its presence warrants a thorough examination (87,89,106). Wounds of the colon and rectum may be lethal if not recognized promptly. The patient who is hemodynamically stable may deteriorate one or two days later if sepsis results from an overlooked rectal or colonic injury, which may be recognized only when such a patient becomes septic and hypotensive. Crepitus and soft tissue manifestations may denote gas gangrene. When sepsis is not recognized until it is in its late stages, patient survival is less likely.

Physical Examination

During resuscitation, a nasogastric tube and transurethral catheter are inserted as part of the "place a tube in every orifice" dictum. Blood in the nasogastric aspirate directs the examiner to look for intra-abdominal injury. Blood in the urine calls attention to the retroperitoneum and the pelvis. The bladder may be penetrated via the rectum in patients with impalement or other penetrating injuries, so examination of the urine is imperative (107). In the patient with multiple trauma, anorectal and other pelvic organ injuries may be overlooked because of preoccupation of the resuscitation team with cranial and thoracic injury or massive hemorrhage. Thus, looking at the back and perineum should be part of the routine assessment. Furthermore, a wound below the nipple line on the chest or just below the scapular tips represents abdominal entry in 15% of stab wounds and 50% of gunshot wounds (108). Abdominal injury is considered with any thoracoabdominal penetration. This area extends from the nipples to the inguinal ligaments and from the scapular tips to the buttocks.

Multiple trauma from high-speed vehicle injuries or major blunt injuries on the battleground is a prime example of a situation in which less obvious wounds may be overlooked. A conscious patient can indicate whether or not abdominal pain is present. Thorough examination includes inspection of the abdominal wall and palpation for crepitus and hematoma formation. In a patient with penetrating trauma, both the entry and exit wounds should be sought. The surmised track of the penetration provides clues as to organs that may be injured and directs the exploration at laparotomy.

Anal examination can be performed with the patient in the supine or lateral position. It should be noted whether the anus is in its normal position, for blunt trauma sometimes detaches it from muscular sling (109). Even with no observable evidence of perineal trauma, a digital examination should be performed in the usual fashion. In a series by Mangiante et al. (110), blood was evident on rectal examination in 80% of patients with rectal gunshot wounds. A loose sphincteric tone might suggest a central nervous system injury. Specifically, in patients with blunt trauma the levator attachments should be palpated to verify that they are intact. Hematoma may create bogginess around the prostate, or the prostate may be dislocated by severe blunt trauma. In female patients, a vaginal examination should be performed to be certain that the injury does not involve the genital tract. If rectal injury is suspected because bright red blood is present, anoscopy and sigmoidoscopy should be performed to attempt visualization of the lower part of the rectum and anal canal. Positioning of the multiply traumatized patient is difficult, but before operation it is necessary to know whether and where the rectum is injured. Irrigation and suction may allow clearance of stool and blood to at least the peritoneal reflection level (15 cm). The injured site can be specifically identified in 91% of rectal injuries (104). The insufflation of large volumes of air should be avoided when the rectum is filled with blood, because stool and contaminated blood can be forced into the peritoneal cavity or extraperitoneal soft tissues if a perforation is present.

Pelvic and rectal trauma also should direct the examiner to evaluate for neurologic integrity. The sciatic nerve is at risk, and appropriate neurologic assessment should be performed. Impotence may be a neurologic sequela of pelvic trauma that is not noted until later (4).

Radiologic Study

Flat and upright abdominal films and lateral films of the pelvis usually are helpful. They aid in defining the location and trajectory of a bullet. Visualization of free intraperitoneal air, extraperitoneal or extrarectal soft tissue densities, or extraluminal gas shadows may point to colonic or rectal injury. Diastasis of the symphysis pubis or pelvic fracture often is associated with injury to the rectum or other pelvic organs (105).

If the patient's condition permits and the clinical suspicion so indicates, diagnostic contrast studies can be performed; however, they are not performed if the patient has an acute abdomen and operative intervention is planned. Use of water-soluble substances such as diatrizoate sodium (e.g., Gastrografin or Hypaque) is preferred over the use of barium. The radiologist, aware of the possibilities of colorectal injury, should instill the contrast material carefully during the fluoroscopic examination and should stop immediately at the first sign of bowel perforation.

Peritoneal Lavage

Peritoneal lavage may be used for evaluation of patients with blunt abdominal trauma. Peritoneal lavage is most often used for the unstable patient who needs assessment for intra-abdominal bleeding. Currently, computed tomography or ultrasound has replaced peritoneal lavage as the diagnostic tool of choice. However, in a patient with an indication for surgery, such as free air, obvious deep intra-abdominal penetration, increasing abdominal distention, or the physical findings of an acute abdomen, peritoneal lavage creates unnecessary delay (111,112). In patients with penetrating trauma, Obeid et al. (113) showed that lavage was positive only 70% of the time in colonic injuries that were proven by operative intervention. On the other hand, there are times when clinical examination is not possible. Even the clinical assessment has been maligned as being wrong 45% of the time in patients with blunt trauma (114). Peritoneal lavage gives a reasonably accurate reading of intraperitoneal trauma but not of retroperitoneal injury. Lavage, computed tomography, or ultrasound may be useful in a patient with a head injury, a patient with spinal cord damage, an intoxicated patient, or a patient suffering from drug overdose who has an equivocal abdominal examination. They are also indicated in patients with wounds of the low chest in which the diaphragm may be penetrated or when concomitant injuries requiring general anesthesia make serial abdominal examinations impossible. Insertion of the lavage tube may be performed by the closed, open, or semi-open technique (115–117).

Finding gross blood during the initial aspiration is an indication for celiotomy. If lavage fluid is withdrawn, it can be classified as strongly positive, weakly positive, or negative (114). Twenty milliliters of fluid with 100,000 red blood cells/mm^3 is considered strongly positive. Most of these patients have significant injury. A weakly positive study is a red blood cell count that is positive but $< 100{,}000/\text{mm}^3$, and the patient deserves closer observation. Twenty-five percent of these patients will require a celiotomy subsequently. A negative lavage is a great aid in deciding that there is minimal damage; then the patient can be either discharged or observed for a longer interval. Elevated levels of white blood cells to $> 500/\text{mm}^3$ in the lavage return may take several hours to appear. Krausz et al. (118) observed that finding > 500 white blood cells/mm^3 of lavage fluid in four patients in a series of 100 patients suffering blunt abdominal trauma identified intestinal perforation in the four. A suspected obscure bowel injury, especially in the noncommunicative patient, warrants performing lavage later in the observation period.

Computed Tomography and Sonography

Ultrasound, like peritoneal lavage, depends on detection of intraperitoneal fluid; so its specificity is low. It is noninvasive but it is operator dependent.

CT scans are highly sensitive in the nonoperative diagnosis of solid organ injury. Very small volumes of free air are detectable suggesting a hollow viscous injury. Fluid collections in the absence of solid organ injury may mean hollow organ injury. Given time, a triple contrast CT, using oral, intravenous, and rectal contrast may be performed. This gives some evaluation of retroperitoneal portions of the colon. Accuracy of CT in the detection of blunt bowel and mesenteric injuries have been reported as 80% for sensitivity and 78% for specificity (119).

These special studies are of particular value in the evaluation of patients who are delayed in presentation (120). Septic sites in both the pelvis and abdomen, such as pelvic or ischioanal abscesses, may be identified by either CT or ultrasonography. Furthermore, percutaneous drainage of fluid collections can be guided by CT or ultrasound.

■ LAPAROSCOPY

Minimally invasive techniques should be more specific as compared to peritoneal lavage. Presuming a trajectory directs where to look for wounds, laparoscopy often gives a definitive diagnosis. Injury to the flank is problematic and may give a tangential trajectory, not entering the peritoneal cavity. Diagnostic laparoscopy may spare the victim a laparotomy. The same dilemma is created by a back wound. Thus laparoscopy may permit a look at the retroperitoneum as well as the intraperitoneum.

Laparoscopy is a valuable diagnostic technique when assessing stab wounds. Because two-thirds of stab wounds do not result in intra-abdominal injury a stepwise approach is taken. A means of determining entry into the abdomen is exploration of the wound tract under local anesthesia. If penetration of the fascia is recognized, further examination by laparoscopy is useful. If the peritoneum is entered, laparotomy is then needed.

■ SURGICAL TREATMENT (DEFINITIVE CARE PHASE)

A spectrum of treatments exists for traumatic wounds that involve the colon, rectum, and anus. The most important factors in determining treatment for penetrating injuries are these: (i) the general physical condition of the patient, (ii) the mechanism by which the injury was incurred, (iii) the interval between the injury and operative intervention, (iv) the presence of shock or hemodynamic instability, (v) the presence of peritoneal contamination, (vi) any injury or avulsion of the mesentery of the colon or rectum, and (vii) the presence of multiple organ injury.

The difference in the mortality rates of war and civilian trauma series is based on the velocity of the missiles, the extent of contamination after injury to the colon, the interval between the injury and definitive care, and the early use of antibiotics. In a series of war injuries, Dent and Jena (121) reported that two factors resulted in increased mortality: high-velocity bullets and colonic injury. The mortality rate with high-velocity wounds of the colon was 52%, yet the mortality rate from all other penetrating wounds was only 6%.

An isolated colonic injury occurs in approximately 25% of penetrating wounds. Both the morbidity and mortality rates of colonic injuries are directly related to the number of other organs traumatized. Two-thirds of the deaths in patients who have colorectal trauma are due to injury to other organs in the body. The other organs most frequently injured are the small intestine, liver, stomach, lung, and bladder (122).

Intraperitoneal Rectal and Colonic Injury

Penetrating trauma usually demands exploration (123). Gunshot wounds of the anterior abdomen enter the peritoneal cavity 85% of the time and after entry strike an important structure 95% of the time. On the other hand, stab wounds enter the peritoneal cavity only 66% of the time, and of this number serious injury occurs in $< 50\%$ (124). Thus, only a quarter of the time may a celiotomy be required for a stab wound of the abdomen. Yet once the peritoneal cavity has been soiled, an acute abdomen will ensue. Exploratory laparotomy for repair of the injury to the intraperitoneal rectum or colon is necessary.

Preoperative broad-spectrum antibiotics for both anaerobic and aerobic flora should be given early after the injury (125). Thadepalli et al. (126) concluded that anaerobic bacteria are a significant cause of infection in the abdominal cavity after abdominal trauma. Fullen et al. (127) reviewed infection rates in 295 patients with penetrating abdominal wounds. The authors found a 7% infection rate in 116 patients who were given prophylactic antibiotics before operation and a 33% infection rate in 98 patients who were given intraoperative antibiotics. This study reinforces the concept of early administration of prophylactic antibiotics bactericidal for both anaerobic and aerobic organisms (128–130). Antibiotic administration should be continued for at least four days if the bowel is injured. Triple antibiotic therapy would include intravenous ampicillin, an aminoglycoside, and metronidazole. Broad-spectrum single-drug agents that are effective include cefotetan, cefoxitin, and ampicillin/sulbactam.

The conduct of the operation is the same whether the patient is in a war zone or in a civilian institution. The patient should be positioned in stirrups especially if there is a question about rectal or other pelvic injury. The ability to perform endoscopy on the operating table with the abdomen open should always be available. The operation is performed through a midline incision that may be extended to the xiphoid or the symphysis pubis to gain better access to the injured organs. First stopping hemorrhage to aid in resuscitation is accomplished and hemodynamic stability is established. Then contamination from an open intestine must be controlled. Noncrushing bowel clamps isolate the open wound. Holes are closed quickly with running sutures or staples to stop contamination. Thereafter, complete exploration identifies all injuries before repair of any one is undertaken. The "rule of two" applies when following a bullet track. Both an entry wound and an exit wound should be found in each organ. If an odd number of holes are found, either a tangential wound occurred or the bullet is still located in the organ. The surgeon must be convinced that no hole has been missed. Hematoma around the colon and retroperitoneal air require exposure of the retroperitoneal colon. The missile may be left in place unless the colon is traversed. A feces-contaminated bullet may act as a nidus for subsequent infections (131). The wound and the abdominal cavity should be irrigated liberally to remove spillage from the colon. The entry and exit wounds should be debrided.

Mature judgment and a disciplined approach allow the patient to be placed in the proper treatment group. Better categorization of colonic injury has been attempted by Flint et al. (132), who recommend a three-level grading system. Grade 1 is an isolated colonic injury with minimal contamination, no shock, and minimal delay. Grade 2 includes through-and-through perforations and lacerations with moderate contamination. Grade 3 comprises severe tissue loss, devascularization, and heavy contamination.

Another method to quantitate severity of injury, a scale called the Penetrating Abdominal Trauma Index (PATI), has been created by Moore et al. (133). The organ injury is estimated on a scale from 1 to 5: 1, minimal; 2, minor; 3, moderate; 4, major; and 5, maximal. In addition to this general PATI scale, a colon injury scale (CIS) was devised; grade 1, serosal injury; grade 2, single wall injury; grade 3, $<25\%$ wall involvement; grade 4, $>25\%$ wall involvement; and grade 5, whole colonic wall involvement and blood supply injury. The authors plan their surgical management based on the score of injury. Grades 1 to 3 may be eligible for primary repair. New statistical models to accurately predict mortality from trauma have been devised. The newest is a physiologic trauma score, which is easily calculable at bedside, used along with other commonly used indices (134).

In the civilian population, penetrating trauma of the colorectum occurs frequently from a low-velocity weapon, the interval from injury to treatment is short, and only the colon or rectum is perforated by a small single bullet. Such an injury is often ideal for primary closure (Fig. 5) (103,135). The wound can be debrided and blood supply assured. Primary repair can be running or interrupted sutures, single or double layer, but the standard requirements are that the closure is water tight, there is no tension on the anastomosis, and the blood supply is intact.

Although the literature supports primary repair in most colon injuries, unfavorable cases must be recognized and primary repair avoided. Relative contraindications to the use of primary closure without colostomy are the following: (i) delay in operation associated with spreading peritonitis, (ii) high-velocity bullet wounds, (iii) explosive or shotgun injuries with shattering wounds of the colon and rectum, (iv) tissue destruction with extensive intramural hematomas or mesenteric vascular damage, and (v) multiple organ injury (136). Stone and Fabian (137) defined the criteria for obligatory colostomy formation. The patients who did not meet the criteria for exclusion were randomized to primary closure alone (Fig. 5) or primary closure plus colostomy or ileostomy (Fig. 6). In the final analysis, the complication and mortality rates were comparable. Table 3 presents a composite list of criteria for ostomy formation (136–138).

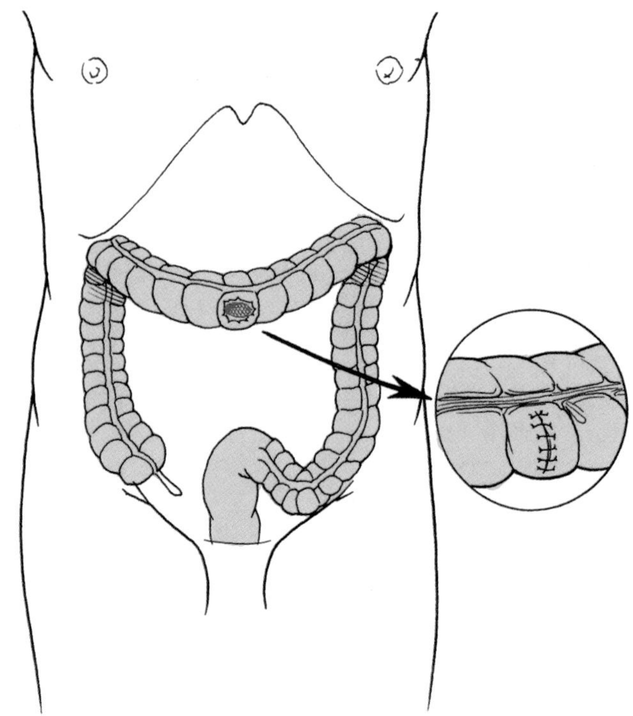

FIGURE 5 ■ Primary repair.

Some differences between war injuries and civilian injuries must be emphasized. In battle, special conditions are to be expected. Multiple casualties may be admitted almost simultaneously; delays in operation occur because of triage priorities; follow-up is seldom performed by the same physician; transportation from the war zone as soon as the patient is stabilized is imperative; and stops while in transit, especially if an ocean must be crossed, are almost a certainty. After World War II, some authors advocated primary closure of colonic wounds without fecal diversion, but the mortality rates with this method exceeded 20% (91,139–142). Thus, results dictated that primary closure of colorectal injuries alone is not safe. In general, wounds must be resected with ostomy creation, exteriorized, or, if that is not possible, protected by diversion (Figs. 6–8). The evidence to support this policy is based on reports from war zones in the past (6,143–146). The dictum of colostomy applied to war wounds has carried over to civilian wounds, even though there has been a safe record for primary repair in properly selected colon injuries.

Controversy still exists as to whether colon injuries require a colostomy or whether primary repair is preferable. Many retrospective and some prospective studies have shown a trend toward favoring primary repair. These studies have been faulted by inherent biases in the trial designs. Five prospective randomized trials have been conducted to answer this question. These are listed in Table 4.

Stone and Fabian (147), in the first of the prospective randomized trials, decided on six conditions that were necessary to be included: (i) shock never < 80 mmHg, (ii) blood loss < 1000 cm^3, (iii) no more than two intra-abdominal organs injured, (iv) no significant fecal soilage, (v) < 8-hour delay to operation, and (vi) an extent of injury to the colon or abdominal wall that did not require a resection of the structure. Forty-eight percent of patients were thus excluded.

No selective criteria were part of the experimental design by Chappuis et al. (148). Their incidence of complications was not increased by primary repair. Unfortunately, the study size (56 patients) was small.

The prospective randomized study by Falcone et al. (149) had exclusion criteria of no delay > 8 hours and patients not deemed admissible by the surgeons. Again the number of patients enrolled in the study, only 22 patients, was a very small sample.

In a trial reported in 1995 by Sasaki et al. (150), 71 patients were randomized, with 60% receiving primary repair. The authors' analysis of multiple factors showed only one factor, the PATI score, which correlated with complications. A PATI score of > 25 meant morbidity. Those patients with PATI scores > 25 had a 33% complication rate after primary repair and 93% after diversion. There were only seven stab wounds and two shotgun injuries as opposed to 62 gunshot wounds. Thus, the mechanism of injury was not delineated with regard to stab and shotgun wounds. The authors' study group was young, so advanced age must be investigated. Because the authors' patients were all operated on within 90 minutes, the

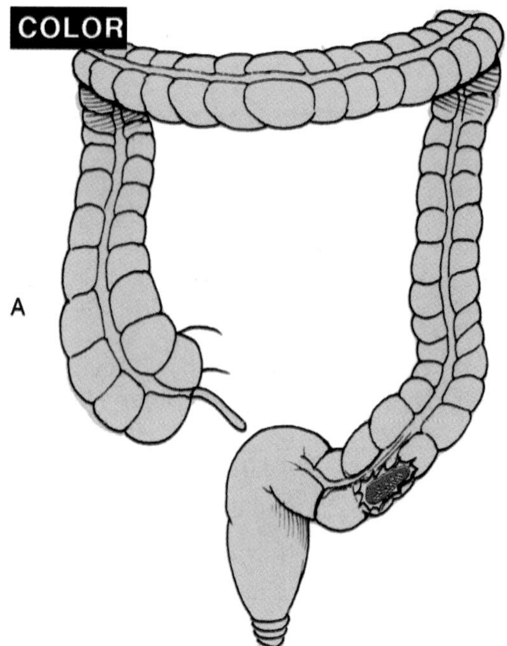

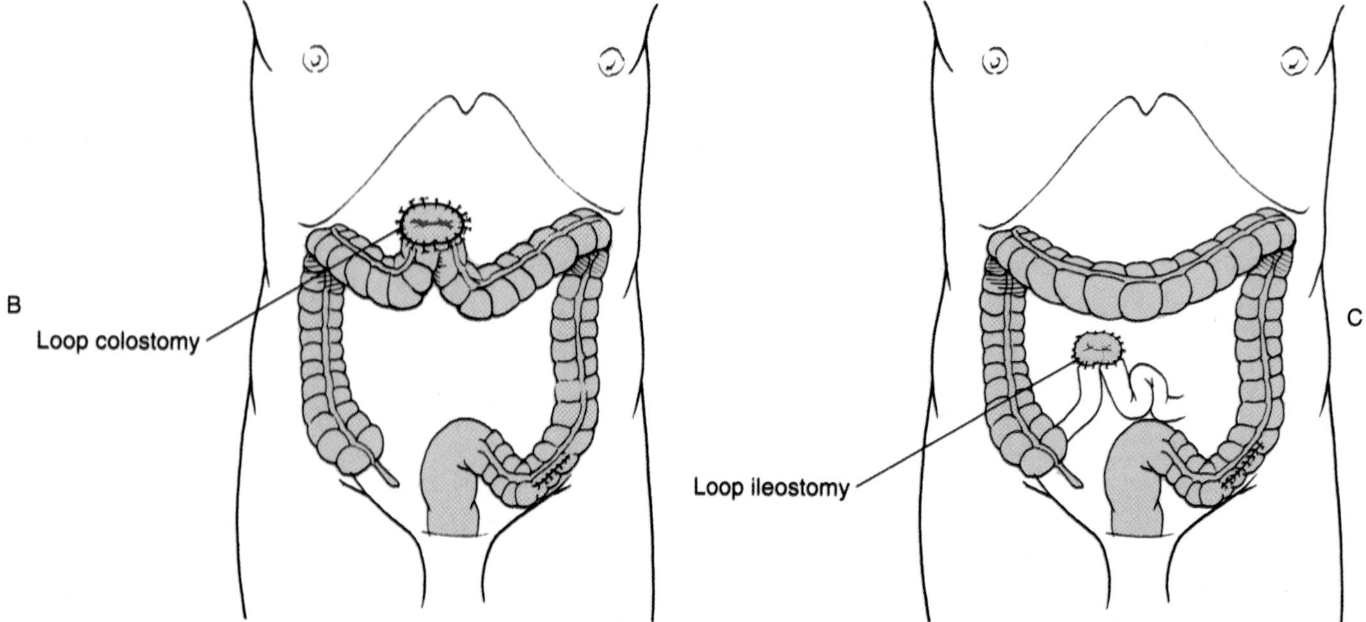

FIGURE 6 ■ Primary repair with proximal diversions. (**A**) Sigmoid colon wound. (**B**) Primary repair with loop colostomy. (**C**) Primary repair with loop ileostomy.

TABLE 3 ■ **Criteria for Use of an Ostomy**

Injuring agent factors
- High-velocity bullet wounds
- Shotgun wounds
- Explosive blast wounds
- Crush injury

Patient factors
- Presence of tumor
- Radiated tissue
- Medical condition
- Advanced age

Injury factors
- Inflamed tissue
- Advanced infection
- Distal obstruction
- Local foreign body
- Impaired blood supply
- Mesenteric vascular damage
- Shock with blood pressure <80/60 mmHg
- Hemorrhage >1000 mL
- More than two organs injured (especially kidney pancreas, spleen, and liver)
- Interval to operation >12 hours
- Extensive injury requiring resection
- Major abdominal wall loss
- Thoracoabdominal penetration

problem of delay in surgery was not a factor in this study. Of special note in this study is that the extent of colon injury did not predict outcome.

The most recent trial by Gonzalez et al. (151) in 2000 with 181 patients is the largest series to date. Their randomization was independent of severity of colon injury, presence of hypotension, blood loss, extent of fecal contamination, and the time from injury to operation. An area of controversy in this study is the removal of five patients initially entered, but died in less than 24 hours of other causes. The PATI for the diversion group was 22.7 and for the primary group 23.7. Septic complications were 18 (21%) in the diversion group and 16 (18%) in the primary repair group. Their conclusion was that all penetrating colon injuries should be managed by primary repair.

Singer and Nelson (152) performed meta-analysis of the five randomized trials found in Table 4. The total patients were 467 with 241 randomized to the primary closure group and 226 randomized to the fecal diversion group. They included the five early deaths that Gonzalez et al. (151) excluded. The outcomes evaluated were mortality, total complications, infectious complications, intra-abdominal infections, wound complications, penetrating abdominal trauma index, and length of stay. The mortality in both the primary anastomosis group and the diverted group were the same. However, all other complication groups showed primary anastomosis to be superior, including the septic complications of intra-abdominal wound infection, dehiscence, generalized sepsis, and peristomal abscess. Thus, they conclude that primary anastomosis is arguably the choice in all penetrating abdominal trauma. More recently, Fealk et al. (153) came to the same conclusion. They believe that the emerging dictum for traumatic colon injuries is primary repair. Questions remain as to whether primary repair is the safest option for all colon injuries. The PATI score, CIS grade, and multiple other factors should be included in the decision-making algorithm with an emphasis on primary repair.

Primary resection has the most value when there is a large hole or an area in which several holes in the colon are adjacent and lend themselves to excision in a short segment (Fig. 9). The open ends are anastomosed only if the patient otherwise meets the criteria for a primary repair. Drains are not used because they do not prevent infections and if placed near an anastomosis, promote leaks. Stewart et al. (154) reported a 14% leak rate after primary resection and anastomosis in 60 patients with destructive colon wounds. The key factors in their review were the presence of underlying medical illness or massive blood transfusion. The leak rate in patients who had one or more of these factors was 42%. The results of ileocolostomy were just as bad as those of colocolostomy. The policy I favor for primary repair or primary anastomosis is not based on the site of injury in the colon but rather on the criteria set forth in Table 3.

The exteriorized repair is out of favor with most trauma surgeons. However, the results of exteriorized repair (repaired loop colostomy as in Fig. 10) were compared with loop colostomy by Nallathambi et al. (155). Potential leak sites were excluded from the abdomen in both types of procedures, but the mortality rate was greater and the hospitalization was longer in the colostomy group. The advantage of a repaired exteriorization is that a leak can be converted to a colostomy by opening the repaired wound. Success can be expected in patients at least 50% of the time if care is taken to keep the colon clean and moist with saline-soaked gauze. The colon can be replaced in the abdomen in 7 to 10 days; thus, the patient can leave the hospital earlier, and only a single hospitalization is necessary (156). The colon often can be replaced in the abdomen with the patient under a local anesthetic. The literature generally supports the view that intraperitoneal soilage with a wound that cannot be exteriorized is safely managed with a repair and proximal diverting colostomy. The sites selected for the colostomy should be located away from the incision, other wounds, bony prominences, and other skin creases.

Iatrogenic injuries, such as those associated with colonoscopy, often can be closed primarily (157,158). However, the criteria in Table 3 apply to the management decisions.

The fascia of the incision should be closed with a monofilament suture or wire. The skin and subcutaneous tissue are left open if fecal contamination is present, and secondary closure may be effected in 5 to 6 days if the patient is doing well.

The primary complication of colonic surgery for trauma is sepsis. Leak of any repair or anastomosis, intra-abdominal abscess, fistula formation, and wound infection must be managed by proper drainage. Diversion of the fecal stream is warranted in patients with anastomotic leaks.

Extraperitoneal Rectal Injury

If the injury to the rectum is partial thickness or a hematoma is found without mucosal injury, no treatment is required. With a small full-thickness perforation in a relatively clean bowel, such as in one prepared for

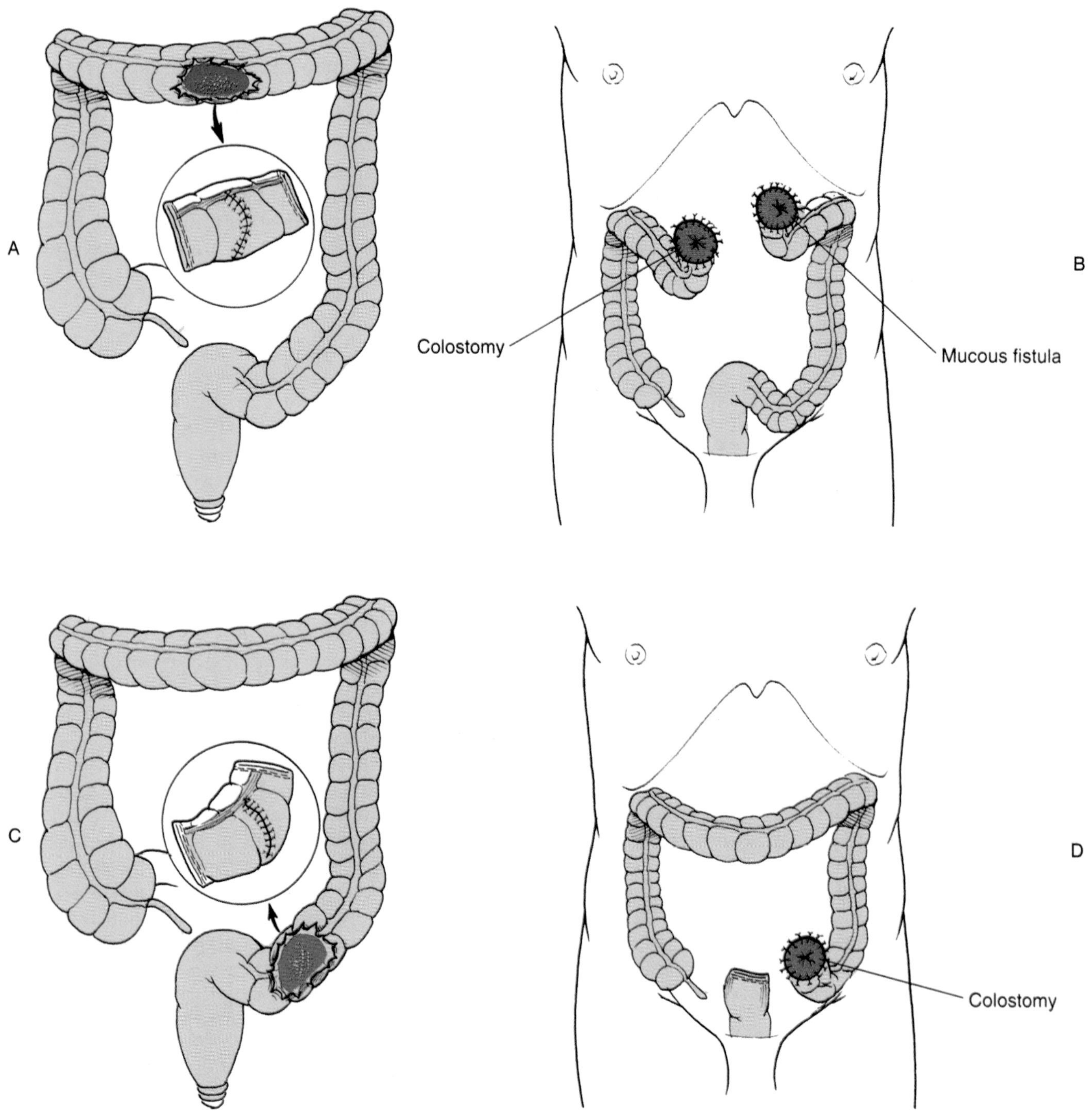

FIGURE 7 ■ Transverse colon wound with excision (**A**), followed by colostomy and mucous fistula (**B**). Sigmoid colon wound with excision (**C**), followed by sigmoid colostomy and Hartmann closure (**D**).

polypectomy, the defect can be closed primarily and the patient placed on antibiotics. Even with penetrating injuries with minimal contamination, Levine et al. (159) primarily repaired five rectal injuries by transanal approach. Two were the result of gunshot, two from prostate biopsy, and one from a foreign object. These five were carefully selected from a total of 30 such injuries. In cases of significant soft tissue injury or pelvic fracture, thorough debridement of devitalized tissue and foreign bodies, adequate retrorectal drainage, closure of the rectal wound (if possible), irrigation of the distal colon and rectum, and construction of a proximal diverting colostomy have evolved as the therapeutic principles of choice (Fig. 11) (160). Copious irrigation with saline or antibiotic solutions into the contaminated tissues should be performed (161–163). To gain access to the anus, the patient must be positioned in stirrups.

Studies from wartime experience have shown that the treatment just described is associated with the lowest mortality and morbidity rates. Armstrong et al. (2) showed from the Vietnam War experience that of 32 patients with missile injuries to the extraperitoneal rectum four died, indicating a mortality rate of 12.5%. An associated intraperitoneal injury occurred in 18 of these patients. If colostomy alone was performed, the incidence of pelvic abscess was 36%, but when colostomy, closure of the primary wound, and transperineal drainage were added to the regimen, the incidence of pelvic abscess was 0%. Armstrong et al. (2) used the washout technique to clear stool from the distal

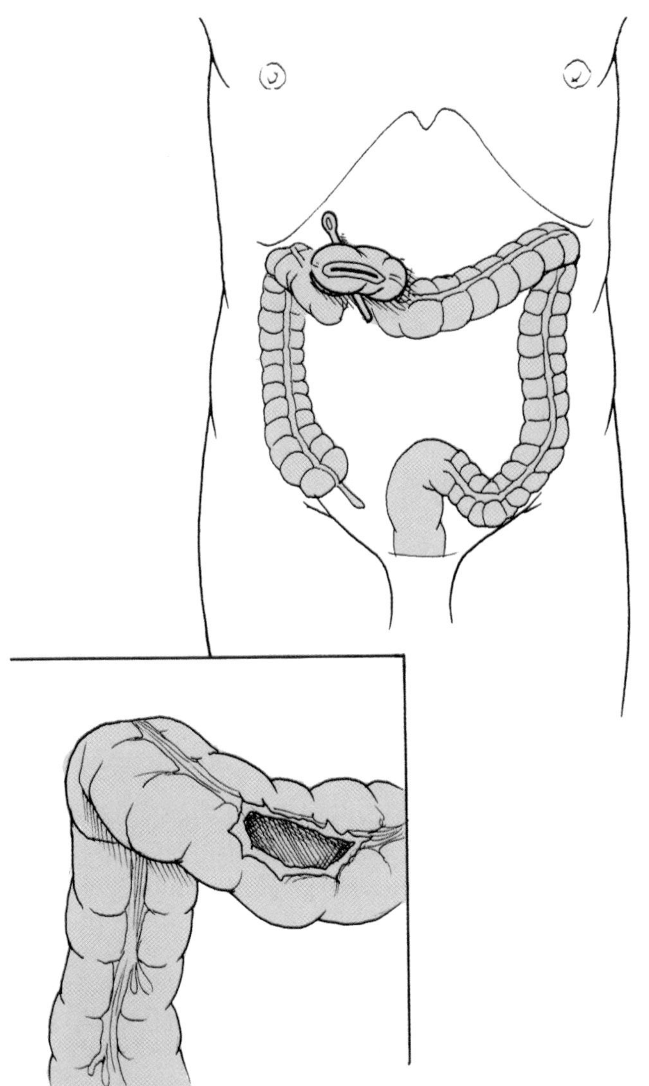

FIGURE 8 ■ Transverse colon wound and enteriorization.

segment of the injured rectum, thus preventing persistent contamination of the perirectal tissues. Washout is aided by dilatation of the anus to allow egress of the feces and solution introduced via the distal limb of the ostomy. For low rectal wounds, the closure of the injured site may be accomplished by per anal suturing technique. The authors recommended using a pericoccygeal drain but did not advocate the performance of coccygectomy, since excision of the coccyx opens new tissue planes and creates the possibility of osteomyelitis. Allen (139) reported on 65 cases of high-velocity extrarectal injuries from combat in Vietnam. He stressed the importance of adequate debridement, posterior-dependent drainage, and evacuation of all retained fecal material from the distal segment. Foreign bodies such as bone, clothing, missiles, and stool must be removed from the pelvis.

Several other authors writing from both civilian and military experience reported a death rate of >20% in patients with extraperitoneal rectal injuries and showed the importance of performing distal washout to decrease the incidence of further sepsis (139,164–166). Other authors fear that washout will push feces out the perforation hole into adjacent tissues. However, if the hole is closed well, the washout should be of benefit. A diverting descending colostomy also is recommended. When a loop colostomy was created, complications occurred in 47% of the patients, with a 5.5% mortality rate, compared with patients with a completely diverting colostomy in whom complications from sepsis occurred in 29%, with a 0% mortality rate. Although creation of a mucous fistula is preferred, constructing a Hartmann pouch is also acceptable. Other organs frequently injured in rectal trauma include the bladder, urethra, vagina, small bowel, and colon (146,161,162). Death rates reflect the association with injuries to other organs and with sepsis, that is, with wound infection, urinary tract infection, respiratory distress syndrome, pancreatitis, osteomyelitis, fistulas, strictures, dehiscence, and pelvic abscess (162,163). If damage to the sacrum opens the dura and the central nervous system is exposed to contamination, ligation of the dura may become necessary (65). The late complications include fecal incontinence, impotence, urinary incontinence, perianal pain, and perineal deformity.

Extensive damage to the rectum and perineum such as with crush compression requires debridement of necrotic tissue and foreign bodies. The sphincter may be sewn together with absorbable sutures. Uncontrollable bleeding may require that packs be left in place. Return to the operating room is necessary to complete debridement and remove packs applied earlier for bleeding. Sometimes abdominoperineal resection may be the best first procedure to perform if the sphincter is not repairable and sepsis and bleeding are out of control.

Attention to a few details prevents local sepsis. Suture materials, when their use is necessary, should be absorbable rather than permanent, since permanent ones may induce chronic sinus tract formation. At the end of the repairs, our policy is to irrigate the peritoneal cavity with up to 10 L of saline solution. The fascia and peritoneum of the incision are closed in one layer, but the skin and subcutaneous tissue are left open if there is intra-abdominal

TABLE 4 ■ **Prospective Randomized Trials of Primary Repair versus Colostomy**

Authors	No. of Patients	Primary Repair No. (%)	Diverting Ostomy No. (%)	Morbidity Primary Repair (%)	Morbidity Ostomy (%)	Mortality Primary Repair (%)	Mortality Ostomy (%)
Stone and Fabian (147)	139	67 (48)	72 (52)	43 (64)	71 (99)	1 (2)	1(1)
Chappuis et al. (148)	56	28 (50)	28 (50)	10 (20)	18 (64)	0	0
Falcone et al. (149)	22	11 (50)	11 (50)	8 (73)	10 (91)	1 (9)	0
Sasaki et al. (150)	71	43 (60)	28 (40)	9 (21)	24 (86)	0	0
Gonzalez et al. (151)	181	92 (51)	89 (49)	21 (23)	21 (24)	5 (5)	3(3)

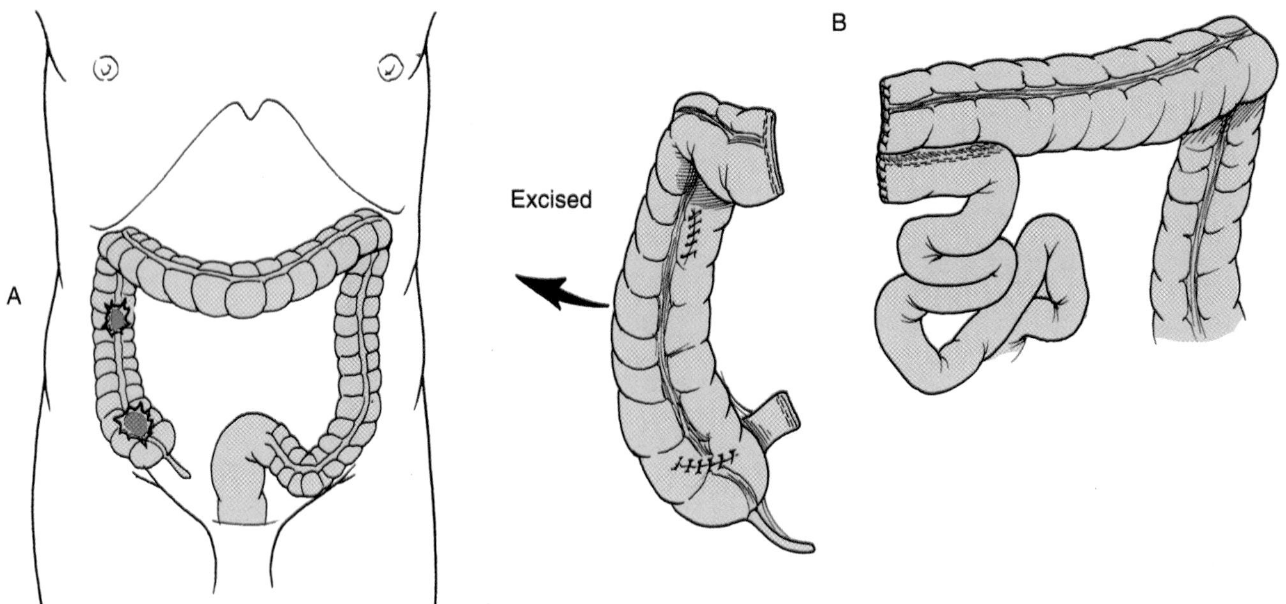

FIGURE 9 ■ (**A**) Two wounds in the right colon. (**B**) Resection of right colon with functional end-to-end anastomosis.

contamination. Entry and exit wounds should be debrided, the peritoneum and fascia should be closed in the base of these wounds, and the skin and subcutaneous tissues should be left open. The incision nearest to the colostomy must be closed for a short length to allow the ostomy appliance to fit better.

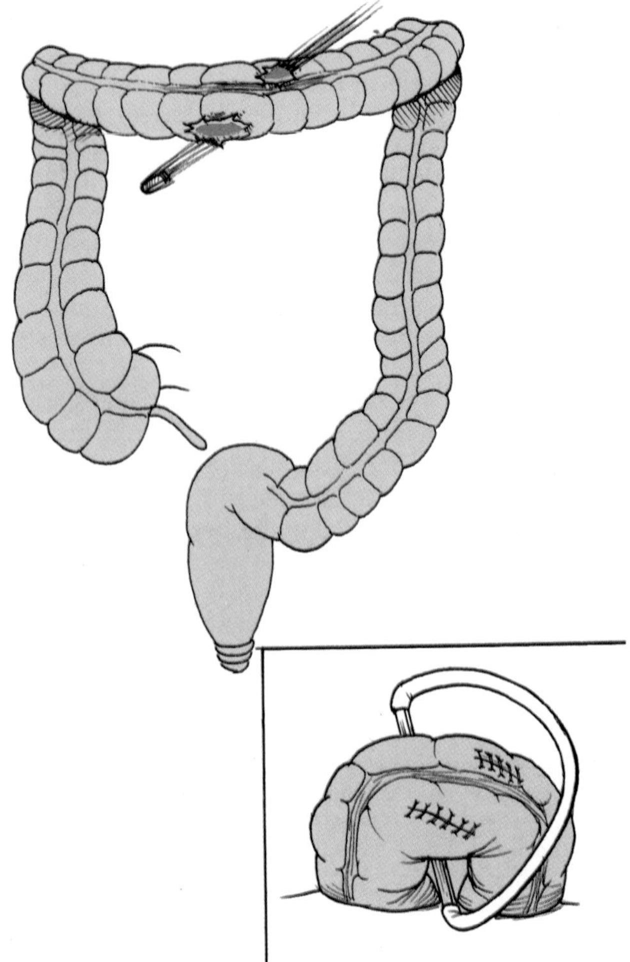

FIGURE 10 ■ Gunshot wound of transverse colon. Exteriorization of the two closed wounds.

Schrock and Christensen (6) and Gustavson (167) have pointed out the septic complications and the mortality rate in patients with extraperitoneal rectal injuries. In a series from Vietnam by Lavenson and Cohen (164), the complication rate caused by sepsis was 60%. Schrock and Christensen (6) noted that half of their patients with rectal injuries were hospitalized for more than 50 days and four patients were hospitalized for more than 100 days. Use of systemic antibiotics is absolutely necessary, and those effective against both anaerobic and aerobic floras should be used (87,127,128).

Massive rectal bleeding that is not responsive to transfusion can be localized by arteriography via the inferior mesenteric artery and iliac vessels. Once the bleeding point has been localized, embolization of autologous clots or Gelfoam may be used to reduce or stop the bleeding. If therapeutic arteriography fails to work, suture ligation or temporary packing of the rectum with gauze usually suffices to control diffuse bleeding. Splitting the symphysis pubis to gain direct visualization of the pelvis allows direct hemostasis. Ligation of the internal iliac arteries has had mixed results in affecting uncontrollable hemorrhage (4). Rarely, massive rectal bleeding secondary to trauma is unresponsive to supportive or arteriographic measures; abdominoperineal resection as an emergency procedure then may be required to stop the bleeding (140). Extensive wounds secondary to a shattered rectum with marked contamination are another indication for performing abdominoperineal resection (164).

The management of rectal impalement is similar to that for other perforations. Initially leaving the impaling object in place is the key to treatment of such injuries (168). The intra-abdominal organs can be examined and explored, and the impaling object can be removed under direct visualization, reducing contamination and damage to the colon and adjacent organs. The specific repair

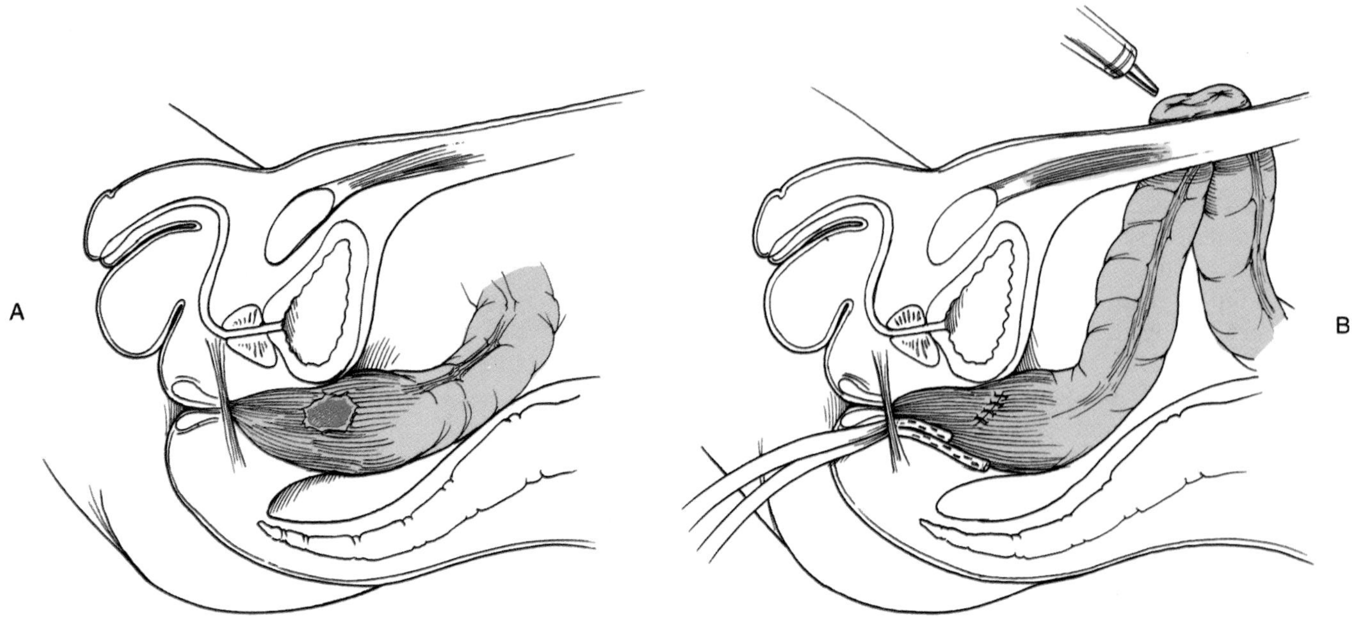

FIGURE 11 ■ (**A**) Wound in the extraperitoneal rectum. (**B**) Colostomy, washout, closed wound and drains.

depends on the contamination and the amount of injury to the rectum, colon, and other organs.

Management of Barium Enema Perforation

If the extraperitoneal rectum has been perforated during the performance of a barium enema examination, a regimen of intravenous fluids, broad-spectrum antibiotics, and observation should be started. Fortunately, in this situation the bowel has been cleared of stool in preparation for the study. If peritoneal findings or signs of sepsis appear, a diverting colostomy with distal irrigation and drainage should be performed (67). Removal of the barium is necessary. However, the barium sometimes is tightly adherent to the wall of loops of bowel. To remove this contamination, excising the bowel and diversion may be necessary. Prevention of this complication depends on several factors: (i) keeping the "head of pressure" of the barium <1 m, (ii) not overinflating the balloon, (iii) keeping the balloon tip minimally inserted, and (iv) deferring the barium enema in patients who have recently undergone a biopsy or polypectomy of the colon or rectum.

Management of Blunt Trauma

In deciding whether a patient had an intraperitoneal or an extraperitoneal rectal injury from blunt abdominal trauma, Perry et al. (169) and Gumbert et al. (170) used diagnostic peritoneal lavage to detect colorectal injuries intraperitoneally. If such lavage is properly performed, the incidence of false positive and false negative lavages is approximately 4%. In recent years, ultrasonography has become a primary diagnostic tool in the assessment of blunt abdominal trauma (171). However, this study is operator dependent. Some investigators have used CT to diagnose perforation (172); however, ultrasonography is often available to the surgeon and thus is faster to obtain and inexpensive. The ability to better assess the patient has led to decreasing the number of laparotomies.

Injuries to the colon and rectum constitute only approximately 10% of all blunt injuries to the abdomen, and only 3% are full-thickness perforations (11). Carillo et al. (12) believe that primary repair without ostomy can be performed if criteria similar to those for penetrating trauma are observed (i.e., no gross fecal contamination, few associated extra-abdominal injuries, a stable vital condition, and no delay in operation) (11).

The literature generally supports the view that intraperitoneal soilage or a large wound is more safely managed with a diverting colostomy, which is believed to be superior to a loop colostomy in preventing sepsis and further complications. When a blunt force is great enough to fracture the pelvic bones and cause major perineal wounds, the resultant trauma should be treated as a major extraperitoneal rectal injury, with the use of colostomy (123). Mesenteric injury and contamination mandate resection of open colonic wounds with colostomy formation. If a nonexpanding intraperitoneal hematoma is found during laparotomy, it should not be opened. The rectum should be evaluated for injury by sigmoidoscopy. Major bleeding from the pelvis or presacral plexus often accompanies penetrating injuries into the pelvis. Control of bleeding can be accomplished by packing, angiographic embolization, balloon tamponade and thumbtack occlusion. Sometimes, a balloon catheter can be introduced to the site of bleeding, the balloon can be inflated, and if in good position, it can be sewn in place. If stable after five days, the balloon can be deflated. It is left in place in case rebleeding ensues. The mortality rate in patients with a blunt colon injury, as in patients with penetrating trauma, is proportional to the number and severity of injury to other organs (173).

Strate and Grieco (173) reported on 109 patients with colonic or rectal injuries. Of the four colon-related deaths, two patients died from anastomotic leaks after resection and primary anastomosis. The other two deaths resulted from a delay in readmission and misdiagnosis. Patients with blunt trauma may present with a delayed colocutaneous fistula and post-traumatic stenosis (174).

Anal Sphincter Injury

The anal sphincter can be injured by a blunt or penetrating force. If there is an isolated sphincteric injury, performing primary repair without colostomy is acceptable, but if the perineal injury is extensive, an associated colostomy becomes necessary. Polyglycolic acid or polyglactin sutures should be used instead of permanent sutures to prevent chronic suture sinuses. Other surgeons prefer to use a delayed repair, especially if the patient has other life-threatening injuries and the abdomen is already open, because sphincteric injuries alone are rarely life-threatening (175,176). If the patient's condition is critical, a delayed repair is preferable. A diverting colostomy can be constructed quickly and protects the anorectal area.

After healing, a post-traumatic assessment by anorectal physiologic testing (manometry and electromyography), anal endosonography, and sometimes examination under general anesthesia are complementary in determining the structural and functional integrity of the anal sphincters. In the study by Engel et al. (177), overlapping repair for traumatic external sphincter damage led to a good clinical outcome in 69% of patients; however, perfect continence was achieved in only 33%.

Sphincteric injury from a blast in war is particularly troubling. In 1970, Lung et al. (4) studied wounds of the rectum sustained by 24 patients during the Vietnam War and stressed using a primary repair of the anal sphincteric musculature. However, the authors noted that hospitalizations were complicated and prolonged, with a mean time of 207 days and an average of 3.2 operations per patient. For details of sphincteric repair, refer to Chapter 15.

Removal of Foreign Bodies

After, the diagnosis of a foreign body in the rectum has been made, the task of removing the object must be undertaken (178). Although certain tried methods are discussed in this section, new ideas may be formulated for ways to remove foreign bodies and minimize the trauma.

Appropriate relaxation and sedation of the patient are necessary for removal of the object. If these measures fail, anesthesia to relax the patient and to relax the anal sphincter muscles totally is required. The anesthetic can be administered in the physician's office, the outpatient area of the emergency room, or the operating room. Use of local anesthetic serves a twofold purpose: analgesia and sphincteric relaxation. After local anesthesia has been achieved, the examiner can insert instruments more easily to examine the patient and to remove the object. Often intravenous sedation can be administered adjunctively. Use of a tranquilizer for sedation is helpful, and narcotics may be necessary if the patient complains of pain. Since the patient is awake he or she can voluntarily perform a Valsalva maneuver, assisting the extraction. Objects that lodge in the low or middle rectum usually can be removed via the anus with the patient under local anesthesia.

A major effort should be made to remove the object per anum, with the anal sphincter kept intact. However, performing an internal anal sphincterotomy or opening the external sphincter muscles to allow extraction of large foreign bodies may be necessary. Thereafter the muscles must be repaired. Having the patient in the lithotomy position is beneficial because performance of the Valsalva maneuver and abdominal manipulation may prove useful. Regardless of the method used for extraction, complete lubrication of the anal area is a great aid.

A variety of unique ways to remove foreign bodies through the anus have been suggested. Peet (179) recommended using obstetric forceps to remove impacted foreign bodies from the rectum. Vadlamundi et al. (180) recommended using a Foley catheter inserted above the object, then inflating the balloon and using it to pull the object down for retrieval. This method breaks the suction formed by the foreign body against the rectosigmoid wall. Hughes et al. (181) recommended the use of a special well-padded pliers for removal of hollow objects, and Sachdev (182) has used plaster of paris inserted into hollow objects, with a string or a clamp inserted into the plaster for use as a handle after it hardens. Occasionally, the proctoscope (and less often the colonoscope) may be used to retrieve foreign bodies. The Sengstaken–Blakemore tube passed through the proctoscope and wedged into a glass provides a handle for removal. After removal of the object via the anus, proctosigmoidoscopy should be performed to check for perforations and bleeding. The patient should be admitted for inpatient observation if there has been difficulty with extraction, because delayed symptoms of perforation may not be evident for several hours.

If a physician fails to remove the object with the patient under local anesthesia, the next step is to attempt removal after administering a caudal or regional anesthetic, which should be performed in the operating room. The approach is the same as that used with a patient under local anesthesia.

Celiotomy is used only as a last resort, after the failure of all anal manipulations, and is performed with the patient under general anesthesia. Objects that lodge in the upper rectum or the lower rectosigmoid may require abdominal celiotomy. The patient is prepared for celiotomy in the usual fashion, which includes the use of antibiotics. The patient's legs are placed in stirrups because the procedure requires both an abdominal and transanal approach. Often no mobilization of the rectum or the sigmoid is necessary. The foreign body can be "milked down" into the middle or lower rectum through the intact rectosigmoid so that the surgeon can remove the object by hand or with instruments. If this procedure fails, a colotomy on the anterior wall of the rectum or the rectosigmoid may be needed for manual extraction of the object. In patients with rectosigmoid perforation caused by a foreign body, the injury is managed as with other intraperitoneal injuries of the colon and rectum. Primary closure alone is rarely recommended because delay is involved and a large contusion with contamination of the peritoneal cavity is usually associated. Most often the laceration or split is repaired, but possibly excised. The wound is usually deep in the pelvis and cannot be exteriorized; therefore, constructing a proximal diverting colostomy and mucous fistula is recommended. The distal washout technique discussed earlier may be used. Sphincteric avulsion caused by a large object or a fist forced through the anus may be repaired primarily (58).

Lake et al. reviewed ninety-three cases of transanally introduced, retained foreign bodies (183). They identified 87 patients. Bedside, extraction was successful in 74%.

Ultimately, 23 patients were taken to the operating room for removal of their foreign body. In total, 17 examinations under anesthesia and eight laparotomies were performed (two patients initially underwent examination under anesthesia before laparotomy). In the eight patients who underwent exploratory laparotomy, only one had successful delivery of the foreign object into the rectum for transanal extraction. The remainder required repair of perforated bowel or retrieval of the foreign body via a colotomy. In that review, a majority of cases had objects retained within the rectum; the rest were located in the sigmoid colon. Fifty-five percent of patients (6/11) presenting with a foreign body in the sigmoid colon required operative intervention versus 24% of patients (17/70) with objects in their rectum ($p = 0.04$). This is the largest single institution series of retained colorectal foreign bodies.

REFERENCES

1. Committee on Trauma Research. Injury in America. Washington, D.C.: National Academy Press, 1985:1.
2. Armstrong RG, Schmitt HJ Jr., Patterson LT. Combat wounds of the extraperitoneal rectum. Surgery 1973; 74:570.
3. Ganchrow MI, Lavenson GS, McNamara JJ. Surgical management of traumatic injuries of the colon and rectum. Arch Surg 1970; 100:515.
4. Lung JA, Turk RP, Miller RE, et al. Wounds of the rectum. Ann Surg 1970; 172:985.
5. Morton JH. Perineal and rectal damage following nonpenetrating abdominal trauma. J Trauma 1972; 12:347.
6. Schrock TR, Christensen N. Management of perforating injuries of the colon. Surg Gynecol Obstet 1972; 135:65.
7. Abu-Dalu K, Pode D, Hadani M, et al. Colonic complications of ventriculoperitoneal shunts. Neurosurgery 1983; 13:167.
8. Amato JJ, Billy LJ, Lawson NS, et al. High velocity missile injury. Am J Surg 1974; 127:454.
9. Sykes LN, Champion HR, Fouty W. Wound ballistics. Contemp Surg 1986; 29:23.
10. Appleby JP, Nagy AG. Abdominal injuries associated with the use of seat belts. Am J Surg 1989; 157:457.
11. Ross SE, Cobean RA, Hoyt DB, et al. Blunt colonic injury: a multicenter review. J Trauma 1992; 33:379.
12. Carillo EH, Somberg LB, Ceballos CE, et al. Blunt traumatic injuries to the colon and rectum. J Am Coll Surg 1996; 183:548.
13. Peterson HB, Ory HW, Greenspan JR, et al. Deaths associated with laparoscopic sterilization by unipolar electrocoagulating devices. Am J Obstet Gynecol 1981; 139:141.
14. Cohen PL, Sutcliffe TJ. Letter-bowel perforation by an intrauterine contraceptive device. S Afr Med J 1982; 62:973.
15. Mohoy RG, Kingsmore D. Life threatening pelvic sepsis after stapled hemorrhoidectomy. Lancet 2000; 355:810.
16. Roos P. Hemorrhoid surgery revised [letter]. Lancet 2000; 355:1648.
17. Ripetti V, Caricato M, Arulani A. Rectal perforation, retropneumoperitoneum, and pnenumomediastinum after stapling procedure for prolapsed hemorrhoids: report of a case and subsequent considerations. Dis Colon Rectum 2002; 45:268–270.
18. Wong L, Jiang J, Chang S, Lin J. Rectal perforation: a life threatening complication of stapled hemorrhoidectomy. Dis Colon Rectum 2003; 46:116–117.
19. LeRoy AJ, Williams HJ, Bender CE, et al. Colon perforation following percutaneous nephrostomy and renal calculus removal. Radiology 1985; 155:83.
20. Borland RN, Walsh PC. Management of rectal injury during radical retropubic prostatectomy. J Urol 1992; 147:905.
21. Lassen PM, Kearse WS. Rectal injuries during radical perineal prostatectomy. Urology 1995; 45:266.
22. Bonnet YY, Haberer JP, Schutz R, et al. Intestinal gas explosion during operation. Ann Fr Anesth Reanim 1983; 2:431.
23. Zanoni CE, Bergamini C, Bertoncini M, et al. Whole-gut lavage for surgery: a case of intraoperative colonic explosion after administration of mannitol. Dis Colon Rectum 1982; 25:580.
24. Fischer G, Goebel H, Latta E. Penetration of the colon by a ventriculoperitoneal drain resulting in intra-cerebral abscess. Zentralbl Neurochir 1983; 44:155.
25. Sathyanarayana S, Wylen EL, Baskaya MK, Nanda A. Spontaneous bowel perforation after ventriculo-peritoneal shunt surgery: case report and review of 45 cases. Surgical Neurol 2000; 54(5):388–396.
26. Seitz WHJ, Berardis JM, Giannaris T, et al. Perforation of the rectum by a Smith–Petersen nail. J Trauma 1982; 22:339.
27. Khot UP, Lang AW, Murali K, Parker MC. Systematic review of the efficacy and safety of colorectal stents. Br. J Surg 2002; 89(9):1096–1102.
28. Befeler D. Proctoscopic perforation of the large bowel. Dis Colon Rectum 1967; 10:376.
29. Andresen AFR. Perforations from proctoscopy. Gastroenterology 1947; 9:32.
30. Nelson RL, Abcarian H, Prasad ML. Iatrogenic perforation of the colon and rectum. Dis Colon Rectum 1982; 25:305.
31. Klein RR, Scarborough RA. Traumatic perforations of rectum and distal colon. Am J Surg 1953; 86:515.
32. Thorbjarnarson B. Iatrogenic and related perforations of the large bowel. Arch Surg 1962; 84:608.
33. Jacobsohn WZ, Levy A. Colonoscopic perforation: its emergency treatment. Endoscopy 1976; 8:15.
34. Smith LE, Nivatvongs S. Complications in colonoscopy. Dis Colon Rectum 1975; 18:214.
35. Smith LE. Fiberoptic colonoscopy: complications of colonoscopy and polypectomy. Dis Colon Rectum 1976; 19:407.
36. Gatto NM, Frucht H, Sundararajan V, Jacobson JS, Grann VR, Neuget A. Risk of perforation after colonoscopy and sigmoidoscopy: a population-based study. J Natl Cancer Inst 2003; 95:230–236.
37. Gatto NM, Frucht H, Sundararajan V, Jacobsen JS, Grann VR, Nergut AI. Risk of perforation after colonoscopy and sigmoidoscopy: a population-based study. J Natl Cancer Inst 2003; 95:230–236.
38. Tran DQ, Rosen L, Kim R, Richter RD, Stasik JJ, Khubchandani IT. Actual colonoscopy: what are the risks of perforation? Am Surg 2001; 67(9):845–847.
39. Araghizadeh FY, Timmcke AE, Opelka FG, Hicks TC, Beck DE. Colonoscopic perforations. Dis Colon Rectum 2001; 44(5):713–716.
40. Thomson SR, Fraser M, Stupp C, et al. Iatrogenic and accidental colon injuries—what to do? Dis Colon Rectum 1994; 37:496–502.
41. Rogers BHG, Silvis SE, Nebel OT, et al. Complications of flexible colonoscopy and polypectomy. Gastrointest Endosc 1975; 22:73.
42. Nivatvongs S. Complications in colonoscopic polypectomy: experience with 1555 polypectomies. Dis Colon Rectum 1986; 29:825–830.
43. Bigard MA, Garcher P, Lasalle C. Fatal colonic explosion during colonic polypectomy. Gastroenterology 1979; 77:1307.
44. Ghazi A, Grossman M. Complications of colonoscopy and polypectomy. Surg Clin North Am 1982; 62:889.
45. Soussan EB, Mathieu N, Roque I, Antonietti M. Bowel explosion with colonic perforation during argon plasma coagulation for hemorrhagic radiation induced proctitis. Gastrointest Endosc 2003; 57(3):412–413.
46. Amshel AL, Shonberg IL, Gopal IA. Retroperitoneal and mediastinal emphysema as a complication of colonoscopy. Dis Colon Rectum 1982; 25:167.
47. Ecker MD, Goldstein M, Hoexter B, et al. Benign pneumoperitoneum after fiberoptic colonoscopy. Gastroenterology 1977; 73:226.
48. Humphreys F, Hewetson KA, Dellipiani AW. Massive subcutaneous emphysema following colonoscopy. Endoscopy 1982; 16:160.
49. Lezak MB, Goldhammer M. Retroperitoneal emphysema after colonoscopy. Gastroenterology 1974; 66:118.
50. Overholt BF, Hargrove RL, Farris RK, et al. Colonoscopic polypectomy: silent perforation. Gastroenterology 1976; 70:112.
51. Taylor R, Weakley FL, Sullivan BH. Non-operative management of colonoscopic perforation with pneumoperitoneum. Gastrointest Endosc 1978; 24:124.
52. Farley DR, Bannon MP, Zietlow SP, Pemberton JH, Ilstrup DM, Larson DR. Management of colonoscopic perforations. Mayo Clin Proc 1997; 72(8):729–733.
53. Fonkalsrud EW, Clatworthy HW Jr. Accidental perforation of the colon and rectum in newborn infants. N Engl J Med 1965; 272:1097.
54. Horwitz MA, Bennett JV. Nursery outbreak of peritonitis with pneumoperitoneum probably caused by thermometer-induced rectal perforation. Am J Epidemiol 1976; 104:632.
55. Hool GJ, Bokey FI, Pheils MT. Enema-nozzle injury of the rectum. Med J Aust 1980; 364:381.
56. Weiss Y, Grunberger P, Aronowitz S. Asymptomatic rectal perforation with retroperitoneal emphysema. Dis Colon Rectum 1981; 24:545.
57. Gayer G, Zissin R, apter S, Oscadchy A, Hertz M. Perforations of the recto sigmoid colon induced by cleansing enema: CT findings in 14 patients. Abdomin Imaging 2002; 27(4):453–457.
58. Critchlow JF, Houlihan MJ, Landoit CC, et al. Primary sphincter repair in anorectal trauma. Dis Colon Rectum 1985; 28:945.
59. Nelson JA, Daniels AV, Dodds WJ. Rectal balloons: complications, causes, and recommendations. Invest Radiol 1979; 14:48.
60. Kiser JL, Spratt JS Jr., Johnson CA. Colon perforations occurring during sigmoidoscopic examinations and barium enemas. Mo Med 1968; 65:969.
61. Rosenklint A, Buemann B, Hansen P, et al. Extraperitoneal perforations of the rectum during barium enema. Scand J Gastroenterol 1975; 10:87.

62. Harned RK, Corsigny PM, Cooper NB, et al. Barium enema examination following biopsy of the rectum or colon. Radiology 1982; 145:11.
63. Kay S, Choy SH. Results of intraperitoneal injection of barium sulfate contrast medium: an experimental study. Arch Pathol 1955; 59:388.
64. Sanders AW, Kobernick SD. Fate of barium sulfate in the retroperitoneum. Am J Surg 1957; 93:907.
65. Beerman PJ, Gelfend DW, Ott DJ. Pneumomediastinum after double-contrast barium enema examination: a sign of colonic perforation. AJR 1981; 36:197.
66. Brunton FJ. Retroperitoneal emphysema as a complication of barium enema. Clin Radiol 1960; 11:197.
67. Levy MD, Hanna EA. Extraperitoneal perirectal extravasation of barium during a barium enema examination. Am Surg 1980; 46(7):382.
68. Peterson N, Rohrmann CA, Leonard ES. Diagnosis and treatment of retroperitoneal perforation complicating the double contrast barium enema examination. Radiology 1982; 144:249.
69. Sisel RJ, Donovan AJ, Yellin AE. Experimental fecal peritonitis: influence of barium sulfate or water-soluble radiographic contrast material on survival. Arch Surg 1972; 104:765.
70. Zheutlin N, Lasser EC, Rigler LG. Clinical studies on effect of barium in the peritoneal cavity following rupture of the colon. Surgery 1952; 32:967.
71. Rosenberg LS, Fine A. Fatal venous intravasation of barium during a barium enema. Radiology 1959; 73:771.
72. Ein SH, Mercer S, Humphrey A, et al. Colon perforation during attempted barium enema reduction of intussusception. J Pediatr Surg 1981; 16:313.
73. Sultan AH, Kamm MA, Bartram CL, et al. Anal sphincter trauma during instrumental delivery. Int J Gynaecol Obstet 1993; 43:263.
74. Richter HE, Brumfield CG, Cliver SP, Burgio KL, Neely CL, Varner RE. Risk factors associated with anal sphincter fear: a comparison of primiparous patients, vaginal births after caesarian deliveries and patients with previous vaginal delivery. Am J Obstet of Gynecol 2002; 187(5):1194–1198.
75. Quan SH. Factitial proctitis due to irradiation for cancer of the cervix uteri. Surg Gynecol Obstet 1968; 126:70.
76. Sedgwick DM, Howard GC, Ferguson A. Pathogenesis of acute radiation injury to the rectum. A prospective study in patients. Int J Colorectal Dis 1994; 9:23–30.
77. Sherman LF, Prem KA, Mensheha NM. Factitial proctitis: a restudy at the University of Minnesota. Dis Colon Rectum 1971; 14:281.
78. Henriksson R, Franzen L, Littbrand B. Effects of sucralfate on acute and late bowel discomfort following radiotherapy of pelvic cancer. J Clin Oncol 1992; 10:969–975.
79. Otchy DP, Nelson H. Radiation injuries of the colon and rectum. Surg Clin North Am 1993; 73:1017.
80. Ahlquist DA, Gostout CJ, Viggiano TR, et al. Laser therapy for severe radiation-induced rectal bleeding. Mayo Clin Proc 1986; 61:927.
81. Alexander TJ, Dwyer TM. Endoscopic Nd:YAG laser treatment of severe radiation injury of the gastrointestinal tract. Gastrointest Endosc 1985; 31:152.
82. Buchi KN, Dixon JA. Argon laser treatment of hemorrhagic radiation proctitis. Gastrointest Endosc 1987; 33:27.
83. VanNagell JR Jr., Parker JC Jr., Maruyama Y, et al. Bladder or rectal injury following radiation therapy for cervical cancer. Am J Obstet Gynecol 1974; 119:727.
84. Fry RD. Anorectal trauma and foreign bodies. Surg Clin North Am 1994; 74:1491.
85. Schwartz GF, Polsky HS. Ingested foreign bodies of the gastrointestinal tract. Am Surg 1976; 42:236.
86. Abcarian H, Lowe R. Colon and rectal trauma. Surg Clin North Am 1978; 58:519.
87. Barone JE, Sohn N, Nealon TF. Perforations and foreign bodies of the rectum. Report of 28 cases. Ann Surg 1976; 184:601.
88. Benjamin HB, Klamecki B, Haft JS. Removal of exotic foreign objects from the abdominal orifices. Am J Proctol 1969; 20:413.
89. Eftaiha M, Hambrick E, Abcarian H. Principles of management of colorectal foreign bodies. Arch Surg 1977; 112:691.
90. Sohn N, Weinstein MA, Gonchar J. Social injuries of the rectum. Am J Surg 1977; 134:611.
91. Beall AC, DeBakey ME. Injuries and foreign bodies of the colon and rectum. Turell RDiseases of the colon and anorectum. 2nd ed Philadelphia: WB Saunders, 1969.
92. American Academy of Pediatrics, Committee on Adolescence. Sexual assault and the adolescent. Pediatrics 1994; 94:761.
93. McCann J, Voris J. Perianal injuries resulting from sexual abuse: a longitudinal study. Pediatrics 1993; 91:390–393.
94. Black CT, Pokorny CW, McGill CW, et al. Anorectal trauma in children. J Pediatr Surg 1982; 17:501.
95. Schiff AF. Attending the child "rape" victim. S Med J 1979; 72:906.
96. Dziegelewski M, Simich JP, Ritten house-Olsen. Use of a Y chromosome probe as an aid in forensic proof of sexual assault. J Forensic Sci 2002; 47(3):601–604.
97. Bauer JJ, Weiss M, Dreiling DA. Stercoraceous perforation of the colon. Surg Clin North Am 1972; 52:1047.
98. Wang SY, Sutherland JC. Colonic perforation secondary to fecal impaction: report of a case. Dis Colon Rectum 1977; 20:355.
99. Lyon DC, Sheiner HJ. Idiopathic rectosigmoid perforation. Surg Gynecol Obstet 1969; 128:991.
100. Cain WS, Howell CG, Ziegler MM, et al. Rectosigmoid perforation and intestinal evisceration from transanal suction. J Pediatr Surg 1983; 18:10.
101. Williams DB, Karl RC. Intestinal injury associated with low-voltage electrocution. J Trauma 1981; 21:246.
102. Raina S, Machiedo GW. Multiple perforations of colon after compressed air injury. Arch Surg 1980; 115:660.
103. Jackson FR, Ott DJ, Gelfand DW. Thermal injury of the colon due to colostomy irrigation. Gastrointest Radiol 1981; 6:231.
104. Committee on Trauma, American College of Surgeons. Advanced trauma life support. Chicago: The College, 1981.
105. Berman AT, Tom L. Traumatic separation of the pubic symphysis with associated fatal rectal tear: a case report and analysis of mechanism of injury. J Trauma 1974; 14:1060.
106. Wolfe WG, Silver D. Rectal perforation with profuse bleeding following an enema. Arch Surg 1966; 92:715.
107. Johnson PA. Rectal impalement with perforation of the bladder. Br Med J 1971; 2:748.
108. Moore JB, Moore EE, Thompson JS. Abdominal injuries associated with penetrating lower chest injuries. Am J Surg 1980; 140:724.
109. Kusminsky RE, Shbeeb I, Makos G, et al. Blunt pelviperineal injuries. Dis Colon Rectum 1982; 25:787.
110. Mangiante EC, Graham AD, Fabian TC. Rectal gunshot wounds. Am Surg 1986; 52:37.
111. Bagwell CE, Ferguson WW. Blunt abdominal trauma: exploratory laparotomy or peritoneal lavage? Am J Surg 1980; 140:368.
112. Thompson JS, Moore EE. Peritoneal lavage in the evaluation of penetrating trauma. Surg Gynecol Obstet 1981; 153:861.
113. Obeid FN, Sorensen V, Vincent G, et al. Inaccuracy of diagnostic peritoneal lavage in penetrating colonic trauma. Arch Surg 1984; 119:906.
114. Olsen WR, Hildreth DH. Abdominal paracentesis and peritoneal lavage in blunt abdominal trauma. J Trauma 1971; 11:824.
115. Lazarus HM, Nelson JA. A technique, for peritoneal lavage without risk or complication. Surg Gynecol Obstet 1979; 149:889.
116. Manganaro AJ, Pachter HL, Spencer FC. Experience with routine open abdominal paracentesis. Surg Gynecol Obstet 1978; 146:795.
117. Soderstrom CA, DuPriest RW, Cowley RA. Pitfalls of peritoneal lavage in blunt abdominal trauma. Surg Gynecol Obstet 1980; 151:513.
118. Krausz MM, Manny J, Vtsunomiya T, et al. Peritoneal lavage in blunt abdominal trauma. Surg Gynecol Obstet 1981; 152:327.
119. Elton C, Riaz AA, Young N, Schamschula R, Papadopoulos B, Malka V. Accuracy of computed tomography in the detection of blunt bowel and mesenteric injuries. Br J Surg 2005; 92(8):1024–1028.
120. Nguyen BD, Beckman L. Silent rectal perforation after endoscopic polypectomy: CT features. Gastrointest Radiol 1992; 17:271–273.
121. Dent RI, Jena GP. Missile injuries of the abdomen in Zimbabwe-Rhodesia. Br J Surg 1980; 67:305.
122. Grablowsky OM, Gage JO, Ray JE, et al. Traumatic colonic and rectal injuries. Dis Colon Rectum 1973; 16:296.
123. Moore EE, Moore JB, Van Duzer-Moore S, et al. Mandatory laparotomy for gunshot wounds penetrating the abdomen. Am J Surg 1980; 140:847.
124. Thompson JS, Moore EE, Van Duzer-Moore S, et al. The evolution of abdominal stab wound management. J Trauma 1980; 20:478.
125. Wittmann DH, Schein M, Condon RE. Management of secondary peritonitis. Am Surg 1992; 224:10–18.
126. Thadepalli H, Gorbach SL, Broido PW, et al. Abdominal trauma, anaerobes, and antibiotics. Surg Gynecol Obstet 1973; 137:270.
127. Fullen WD, Hunt J, Altemeier WA. Prophylactic antibiotics in penetrating wounds of the abdomen. J Trauma 1972; 12:282.
128. Altemeier WA. Bacteriology of traumatic wounds. JAMA 1944; 124:413.
129. Mandal AK, Thadepalli HT, Matory E, et al. Evaluation of dentibiotic therapy and surgical techniques in cases of homicidal wounds of the colon. Am Surg 1984; 50:254.
130. Polk HC Jr., Miles AA. The decisive period in the primary infection of muscle by *Escherichia coli*. Br J Exp Pathol 1973; 54:99.
131. Poret HA, Fabian TC, Croce MA, et al. Analysis of septic morbidity following gunshot wounds to the colon: the missile is an adjuvant for abscess. J Trauma 1991; 31:1088–1095.
132. Flint LM, Vitale GC, Richardson JD, et al. The injured colon: relationships of management to complications. Ann Surg 1981; 193:619.
133. Moore EE, Dunn EL, Moore JB, et al. Penetrating abdominal trauma index. J Trauma 1981; 21:439.
134. Kuhls DA, Malone DL, McCarter RJ, Napolitano LM. Predictors of mortality in adult trauma patients: the physiologic trauma score is equivalent to the trauma and injury severity score. J Am Coll Surg 2002; 194:695–704.
135. Shannon FL, Moore EE. Primary repair of the colon: when is it a safe alternative? Surgery 1985; 98:851.
136. Thompson JS, Moore EE, Moore JB. Comparison of penetrating injuries of the right and left colon. Ann Surg 1981; 193:414.
137. Stone HH, Fabian TC. Management of perforating colon trauma. Randomization between primary closure and exteriorization. Ann Surg 1980; 190:430.

138. Adkins RB, Zirkle PK, Waterhouse G. Penetrating colon trauma. J Trauma 1984; 24:491.
139. Allen BD. Penetrating wounds of the rectum. Tex Med 1973; 69:77.
140. Getzen LC, Pollak EW, Wblfman EF. Abdominoperineal resection in the treatment of devascularizing rectal injuries. Surgery 1977; 82:310.
141. Imes PR. War surgery of abdomen. Surg Gynecol Obstet 1945; 81:608.
142. Woodhall JP, Ochsner A. The management of perforating injuries of the colon and rectum in civilian practice. Surgery 1951; 29:305.
143. Whelan TJ, ed. Emergency war surgery. Washington, D.C.: U.S. Government Printing Office, 1975.
144. Josen AS, Ferrer JM Jr., Forde KA, et al. Primary closure of civilian colorectal wounds. Ann Surg 1972; 176:782.
145. LoCicero J III, Tajima T, Drapanas T. A half-century of experience in the management of colonic injuries: changing concepts. J Trauma 1975; 15:575.
146. Trunkey D, Hays RJ, Shires GT. Management of rectal trauma. J Trauma 1973; 13:411.
147. Stone HH, Fabian TC. Colon trauma: further support for primary repair. Am J Surg 1979; 190:430–433.
148. Chappuis CS, Frey DJ, Dietzen CD, et al. Management of penetrating colon injuries: a prospective randomized trial. Ann Surg 1991; 213:492–494.
149. Falcone RE, Wanamaker SR, Santanello SA, et al. Colorectal trauma: primary repair or anastomosis with intracolonic by pass vs. ostomy. Dis Colon Rectum 1992; 35:957–963.
150. Sasaki LS, Allaban RD, Golwala R, et al. Primary repair of colon injuries: a prospective randomized study. J Trauma 1995; 39:895–901.
151. Gonzalez RP, Falimirski ME, Holevat MR. Further evaluation of colostomy in penetrating colon injury. Am Surg 2000; 66:342–347.
152. Singer MA, Nelson RL. Primary repair of colon injuries: a systematic review. Dis Colon Rectum 2002; 45:1579–1587.
153. Fealk M, Osipov R, Foster K, Caruso D, Kassir A. The conundrum of traumatic colon injury. Am J Surg 2004; 188:663–670.
154. Stewart RM, Fabian TC, Croce MA, et al. Is resection with primary anastomosis following destructive colon wounds always safe? Am J Surg 1994; 168:316–319.
155. Nallathambi MN, Ivatury RR, Shah PM, et al. Aggressive definitive management of penetrating colon injuries: 136 cases with 3.7 per cent mortality. J Trauma 1984; 24:500.
156. Nallathambi MN, Ivatury RR, Rohman M, et al. Penetrating colon injuries: exteriorized repair vs. loop colostomy. J Trauma 1987; 27:876.
157. Vincent M, Smith LE. Management of perforation due to colonoscopy. Dis Colon Rectum 1983; 26:61.
158. Gedebou TM, Wong RA, Rappaport WD, et al. Clinical presentation and management of iatrogenic colon perforations. Am J Surg 1996; 172:454.
159. Levine JH, Longo WE, Pruitt C, et al. Management of selected rectal injuries by primary repair. Am J Surg 1996; 172:575.
160. Levy RD, Strauss P, Aladgem D, et al. Extraperitoneal rectal gunshot injuries. J Trauma 1995; 38:273.
161. Grasberger RC, Hirsch EF. Rectal trauma: a retrospective analysis and guidelines for therapy. Am J Surg 1983; 145:795.
162. Tuggle D, Huber PJ. Management of rectal trauma. Am J Surg 1984; 148:806.
163. Weil PH. Injuries of the retroperitoneal portions of the colon and rectum. Dis Colon Rectum 1983; 26:19.
164. Lavenson GS, Cohen A. Management of rectal injuries. Am J Surg 1971; 122:226.
165. Vannix RS, Carter R, Hinshaw DB, et al. Surgical management of colon trauma in civilian practice. Am J Surg 1963; 106:364.
166. Wanebo HJ, Hunt TK, Matthewson C Jr. Rectal injuries. J Trauma 1969; 9:712.
167. Gustavson RG. Rectal injuries. Am Surg 1973; 39:456.
168. Kaufer N, Shein S, Levowitz BS. Impalement injury of the rectum: an unusual case. Dis Colon Rectum 1967; 10:394.
169. Perry JF Jr., DeMeules JE, Root HD. Diagnostic peritoneal lavage in blunt abdominal trauma. Surg Gynecol Obstet 1970; 131:742.
170. Gumbert JL, Froderman SE, Mercho JP. Diagnostic peritoneal lavage in blunt abdominal trauma. Ann Surg 1967; 165:70.
171. McKenney M, Lentz M, Nunez D, et al. Can ultrasound replace diagnostic peritoneal lavage in the assessment of blunt trauma? J Trauma 1994; 37:439.
172. Sherck J, Shatney C, Sensaki K, et al. The accuracy of computed tomography in the diagnosis of blunt small bowel perforation. Am J Surg 1994; 168:670.
173. Strate RG, Grieco JG. Blunt injury to the colon and rectum. J Trauma 1983; 23:384.
174. McKenzie AD, Bell GA. Nonpenetrating injuries of the colon and rectum. Surg Clin North Am 1972; 52:735.
175. Goligher JC. Injuries of the rectum and colon. Goligher JCSurgery of the anus, rectum and colon. 3rd ed Springfield, Ill.: Charles C Thomas, 1975.
176. Large PG, Murkheiber WJ. Injury to rectum and anal canal by enema syringes. Lancet 1956; 2:596.
177. Engel AF, Kamm MA, Hawley PR. Civilian and war injuries of the perineum and anal sphincters. Br J Surg 1994; 81:1069.
178. Shillingstad RB, Marks JM, Ponsky JL. Endoscopic management of gastrointestinal foreign bodies. Contemp Surg 1997; 50:87–92.
179. Peet TND. Removal of impacted foreign body with obstetric forceps. Br Med J 1976; 1:500.
180. Vadlamundi K, VanBockstaele P, McManus J. Foley catheter in removal of a foreign body from the rectum. JAMA 1972; 221:1412.
181. Hughes JP, Marice HP, Gathright JB. Method of removing a hollow object from the rectum. Dis Colon Rectum 1976; 19:44.
182. Sachdev YV. An unusual foreign body in the rectum. Dis Colon Rectum 1967; 10:220.
183. Lake JP, Essoni R, Petrone P, Kaiser AM, Asensio J, Beart RW Jr. Management of retained colorectal foreign bodies: predictors of operative intervention. Dis Colon Rectum. 2004; 47:1694–1698.

35 Complications of Colonic Disease and Their Management

Santhat Nivatvongs

ACUTE COLONIC OBSTRUCTION

GENERAL CONSIDERATIONS

Large bowel obstruction can result from the progression of a number of colonic diseases. The most common cause of large bowel obstruction in adults (78%) is adenocarcinoma of the colon and rectum. It is followed by noncolonic carcinoma, diverticulitis, volvulus, and inflammatory bowel disease (1).

Carcinoma

Colorectal obstruction from carcinoma is not common. In a series of 908 cases, Serpell et al. (2) reported that 16% of the patients had complete obstruction and 31% had partial obstruction. Of 4583 patients in the Large Bowel Cancer Project of the United Kingdom, obstruction was noted in 16% (3). In this series, the splenic flexure was the site of 49% of the cases, followed by the left colon (23%), the right colon (23%), and the rectum and rectosigmoid colon (6%). In the series by Buechter et al. (1), the sigmoid colon was the most common site of obstruction, accounting for 38%, followed by the descending colon, splenic flexure, transverse colon, rectum, cecum, ascending colon, and hepatic flexure. The sigmoid colon was also noted by Kyllonen (4) as the predominant site of obstruction.

Diverticular Disease

Some degree of colonic obstruction occurs in approximately two-third of the patients with acute diverticulitis. This is usually partial obstruction caused by inflammation with spasm and edema plus an element of adynamic ileus. Complete obstruction occurs in approximately 10% of the cases and is the second most frequent cause of acute colonic obstruction. Complete obstruction usually implies abscess formation with encroachment of the lumen or repeated episodes of diverticulitis with fibrosis and stenosis or both.

Crohn's Disease

Colonic obstruction in patients with Crohn's disease is caused by strictures that result from the transmural nature of Crohn's disease inflammation and the attendant fibrosis and scarring. Thus strictures, which may be primarily inflammatory or fibrotic, are part of the natural progression of the disease. As the bowel lumen narrows, symptoms of stricture eventually occur.

Volvulus

Volvulus of the sigmoid, cecum, and transverse colon causes at least partial obstruction of the colon or the small bowel. In an extensive review, Ballantyne (5) found that 9.6% of 1206 cases of colonic obstruction were caused by sigmoid volvulus in the United States. Cecal volvulus accounts for 1% of all cases of intestinal obstruction (6). If the volvulus does not relieve spontaneously, strangulation results, and an acute colonic or ileal obstruction occurs.

Acute Pseudo Obstruction of the Colon

Acute pseudo obstruction of the colon is a condition in which the colon becomes massively dilated without apparent mechanical obstruction. The mechanism of its occurrence is not clear but is believed to relate to sacral parasympathetic nerve dysfunction (7–9). In fact, an acute pseudo obstruction of the colon is a form of an ileus that typically starts in the left transverse colon. The dysfunction part of the colon is collapsed and has minimal or no air. The proximal part is functionally normal. This is different from an extensive generalized ileus in which the small intestine, the colon, and the rectum are dilated with air.

Acute pseudo obstruction of the colon is secondary to a myriad of diseases and conditions. Limited examples are intra-abdominal sepsis, abdominal and pelvic surgery, normal pregnancy or delivery, cesarean section, retroperitoneal disease, pneumonia, hip fractures, organ transplantation, thoracic and cardiovascular surgery, posttraumatic syndrome, neurologic disease, and chemotherapy (7,10).

Intussusception

Intussusception is the invagination (telescope or accordion) of the segment of the bowel (intussusception) into an adjacent segment distal to it (intussuscipiens) (11). As the intussusception enters into the intussuscipiens, the mesentery is carried with it and is trapped between the overlapping layers of the bowel. This often produces vascular compression with an eventual ischemic necrosis unless a timely intervention is undertaken.

Adult intussusception is rare. In 30 years at Massachusetts General Hospital in Boston, there were 58 cases of surgically proven adult intussusception (12). Adult intussusception accounts for 1% to 5% of all intestinal obstruction and 5% of all intussusception (95% occur in children) (12,13). Approximately 90% of the cases are secondary to a definable lesion, while the opposite is true in children (12,13). Adult intussusception occurs at any age, with a mean age of 47 to 54 years (12,13). Of the 58 cases reported by Azar and Berger (12), 44 were small bowel and 14 colonic; 48% of the small bowel lesions were malignant, compared with 43% of the colonic lesions (Table 1). Intussusception may present as acute or chronic.

Sarcoidosis

Hilzenrat et al. (14) reported a case of colonic obstruction secondary to sarcoidosis. Two areas of narrowing are in

TABLE 1 ■ Etiology of Intussusception

Enteric (n = 43)	No. of Patients	Colonic (n = 12)	No. of Patients
Benign (n = 22)		Benign (n = 6)	
Postoperative	11	Lipoma	3
Meckel's diverticulum	3	Adenoma	2
Lipoma	3	Lymphoid hyperplasia	1
Peutz-Jeghers syndrome	2		
Neurofibroma	1		
Scleroderma	1		
Idiopathic	1		
Malignant (n = 21)		Malignant (n = 6)	
Metastatic melanoma	13	Adenocarcinoma	
Metastatic lymphoma	3	Stage B1	5
Metastatic sarcoma	2	Stage C1	1
Metastatic squamous cell carcinoma	1		
Undifferentiated carcinoma	1		
Jejunal adenocarcinoma	1		

Source: From Ref. 12.

the rectum and another at the splenic flexure, through which a colonoscope could not pass but biopsies demonstrated sarcoidosis. Despite the abdominal and proximal bowel distension, treatment with oral prednisone resulted in symptomatic improvement in three days. Follow-up colonoscopy one month later was essentially normal and the patient avoided operation.

■ CLINICAL MANIFESTATIONS

Vomiting in a patient with large bowel obstruction is a late manifestation unless there is an associated small bowel obstruction. Abdominal tenderness associated with peritoneal irritation is caused by distension of the colon and the small bowel and perhaps by edema of the mesentery. Marked abdominal pain, peritoneal irritation out of proportion, and a white blood cell count greater than 20,000 per milliliter may be signs of ischemia or gangrene of the bowel.

To understand the origin of abdominal pain, it is important to distinguish between visceral and somatic pain. Visceral pain originates in the organs such as the colon and is vaguely localized to the regions of the body. Colonic distension produces pain, usually colicky, in the lower abdomen. The pain may be associated with reflexive nausea. Somatic pain occurs when an inflammatory process such as sigmoid diverticulitis reaches the peritoneum and is sensed by afferent fibers there (15).

■ DIAGNOSIS AND CLINICAL EVALUATION

Obtaining a plain film of the abdomen is the simplest procedure for diagnosing obstruction of the large bowel and gives the most information. although it does not provide reliable information about the site of the obstruction (16). Initially, the large bowel is distended. If there is a cutoff between the distended colon and the collapsed colon, the diagnosis of large bowel obstruction can be entertained, although the specific cause cannot be established. As the obstruction progresses, air will fill the small bowel also, and a picture of small bowel obstruction may supervene. Distention of the right and transverse colon associated with minimal gas in the left colon suggests acute pseudo-obstruction of the colon. However, if the distension is severe, differentiating it from a cecal or sigmoid volvulus may be difficult, and a water-soluble enema should be ordered.

A water-soluble contrast enema (with Gastrografin or Hypaque) examination is the method of choice to delineate the location of the obstruction and to evaluate the degree of obstruction. Another benefit of Gastrografin is its cleansing effect in the colon. Use of a barium enema is not recommended for an acute large bowel obstruction because it makes cleansing of the colon and rectum difficult and may lead to barium impaction; in addition, the complication rate with its use is high if the bowel is perforated. The aim of performing a water-soluble enema is to confirm the diagnosis of acute large bowel obstruction and its location (Fig. 1). Accurate mucosal detail and the nature of the obstruction are of secondary importance. In an acute pseudo obstruction of the colon, the left colon has a normal caliber, air-fluid level is absent, and there is a free flow of the Gastrografin solution to the cecum (Fig. 2). In the case of a volvulus, the "bird's beak" sign is diagnostic.

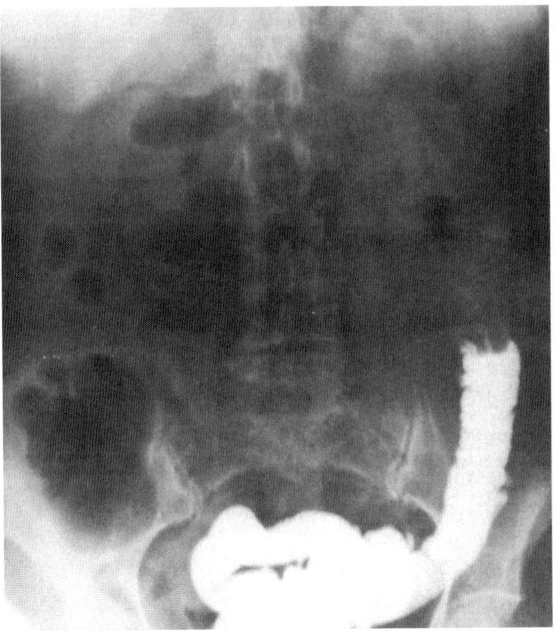

FIGURE 1 ■ Gastrografin enema demonstrating an obstruction of the descending colon caused by a carcinoma.

In a series of 117 patients with the clinical diagnosis of acute large bowel obstruction, Stewart et al. (16) showed that a water-soluble contrast enema was helpful in confirming the diagnosis and in accurately locating the site of obstruction with no false positive results. In 80% of the cases, the water-soluble contrast enema confirmed the presence of a mechanical obstruction and was more accurate than plain films in localizing the site.

A computed tomography (CT) scan of the abdomen is the most accurate test for intussusception and is often preferred to barium enema. In an early stage, it is seen as a "target" mass. The intussusception is the center and the edematous intussuscipiens forms the external ring. In a later stage, the bowel wall becomes thickened. In the

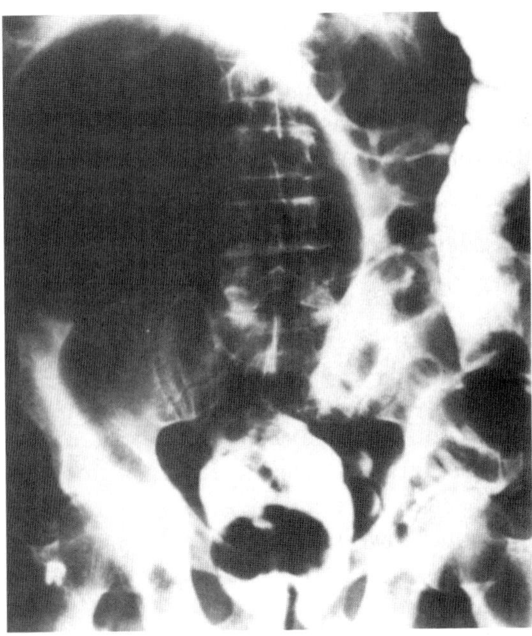

FIGURE 2 ■ Acute pseudoobstruction of the colon. Note the marked dilation of the right colon.

gangrenous stage, the intussusception consists of an amorphous mass with varied density and is surrounded by extensive intraperitoneal fluid (11,12,15,17).

If diverticular disease is suspected, it is worthwhile to perform a CT scan of the abdomen. CT provides an entirely new approach to diverticular diseases. This noninvasive technique permits the radiologist to tell the surgeon the exact extent of the extramural disease. CT-guided percutaneous abscess drainage can be used to convert a two- or three-stage surgical sequence into a one-stage sigmoid colon resection. Occasionally, patients who refuse an operation or those with prohibitive risks may be spared an operation altogether (18).

The distinction between benign strictures and carcinomas producing narrowing of the colon cannot always be made. Colonoscopic examination is helpful if it is possible to pass the scope to or through the stricture. It is also highly successful to reduce sigmoid volvulus. An intussusception can be recognized as a reddish polypoid mass with a coil-spring appearance (19). Other benign and malignant lesions can also be identified.

■ MANAGEMENT

It is essential that the diagnosis be established and confirmed. Sigmoid volvulus is treated best by detorsion of the volvulus, using a proctoscope, flexible sigmoidoscope, or colonoscope as the first step. If this fails, an exploratory celiotomy is indicated. Performing detorsion of the cecum by colonoscopy is unpredictable and has a significant risk of complications. Once the diagnosis has been made, an exploratory celiotomy should be considered (Chapter 29).

Acute pseudo obstruction of the colon is a self-limited condition if the underlying cause is eliminated. However, waiting for the condition to cease on its own is not recommended because the colonic dilatation may persist. Air in the distended colon is swallowed air; therefore, the first step in the management is placement of a nasogastric tube. All potentially implicated medication should be discontinued and fluid and electrolyte disorders corrected. The main goal of treatment is to prevent cecal perforation. It is generally accepted that the critical size of the cecum is 12 cm (7). Treatment with colonoscopic decompression is effective in 85% to 88% of the cases with a low morbidity rate (7,8,20). Repeating the procedure many times may be necessary because of recurrence (7,20).

Neostigmine has been used with impressive results and may become the first-line treatment of choice. Neostigmine is a parasympathomimetic drug. The dosage is 2.0 to 2.5 mg given intravenously over 3 minutes (9,21). The response is usually within minutes. Severe abdominal cramps may precede passing a large amount of gas. The procedure should be performed with close monitoring of cardiac rhythm and blood pressure. Atropine should be readily available in the event of severe bradycardia. Neostigmine should not be given to patients who have been on beta-blockers and those who are acidotic or have had a recent myocardial infarction, because they are prone to cardiac dysrhythmias. Prolonged recurrent acute pseudo obstruction in the colon may signify intra-abdominal complications such as abscess or peritonitis, in which case further investigations are indicated.

Ponec et al. (21) conducted a prospective, randomized trial to evaluate the success rate of neostigmine in patients with acute pseudo-obstruction of the colon. The study involved 21 patients; all had abdominal distension and radiographic evidence of colonic dilatation, with cecal diameter of at least 10 cm, and had no response to at least 24 hours of conservative treatment. The authors randomly assigned 11 to receive 2.0 mg of neostigmine intravenously and 10 to receive intravenous saline. The results showed that 10 of 11 patients who received neostigmine had prompt colonic decompression, as compared with none of the 10 patients who received placebo ($p < 0.001$). The median time to response was four minutes (range, 3 to 30). Side effects of neostigmine included abdominal pain, excess salivation, and vomiting. Symptomatic bradycardia developed in two patients and was treated with atropine.

Before deciding to treat the patient with neostigmine, it is vital to rule out a mechanical obstruction. If there is any doubt, a diatrizoate meglumine (Hypaque, Cystografin) enema should be done. Diatrizoate meglumine may result in therapeutic success (22). If the cecum is 12 cm or larger and nonoperative treatment is not successful, a tube cecostomy is the procedure of choice. The traditional use of a Foley catheter is not effective because of its very small lumen. Using an endotracheal tube is a better technique (22). A transverse colostomy is seldom necessary. A colectomy is indicated only when there is colonic ischemia or perforation. A laparoscopic tube cecostomy can be performed (23).

The diagnosis of intussusception in the adult is difficult because of the various presentations. In 50% of the patients, the diagnosis is bowel obstruction (12). The treatment for an adult is surgical resection. Because almost 50% of the intussusceptions are caused by malignant lesions, on exploration, the intussusception should not be reduced, but one should proceed with bowel resection.

Complete or near-complete obstruction of the colon from carcinoma, diverticular disease, or Crohn's disease requires an urgent exploratory celiotomy.

FREE PERFORATION

■ GENERAL CONSIDERATIONS

Free perforation of the large bowel from colonic diseases is uncommon but it is a very serious and life-threatening condition that requires an emergency operation. Untreated, the patient will die from generalized peritonitis or sepsis. This section discusses patients with free intraperitoneal perforation causing generalized purulent or fecal peritonitis. Patients with a confined or extraperitoneal perforation are not considered.

Diverticular Disease

Most diverticula are situated in the sigmoid colon. Perforation of mesenteric diverticula is confined to the extraperitoneum or between the leaves of the sigmoid colon mesentery, causing an abscess or a phlegmon. Intraperitoneal perforation causing purulent or fecal peritonitis is uncommon. Krukowski and Matheson (24) found that this type of problem was seen, on an average, less than once per year at the Lahey Clinic in Boston, twice per year at the

Mayo Clinic, and seven times per year at Birmingham, United Kingdom. In a prospective study of acute diverticulitis treated throughout Australia and New Zealand, 248 patients were accepted for the survey (25). Of them, 214 had peritonitis: serous in 82 (38%), purulent in 104 (49%), and fecal in 28 (13%).

Carcinoma

Perforation from carcinoma of the colon and rectum is also uncommon. It occurs in 3.3% to 9.5% (26,27) of the cases. There are two types of perforation that may develop: perforation of the carcinoma itself, and less often, perforation of the colon proximal to the carcinoma, especially the cecum, which may occur from overdistention by air.

In the series of Mandava et al. (27), of 1551 patients, 51 (3.3%) presented with perforation, 61% had localized perforation with abscess, and 39% had free perforation. The site of perforation was most often at the carcinoma site (82%). In the remaining patients (18%), the perforation occurred proximal to the obstructed primary lesion.

Ulcerative Colitis

Free perforation resulting from ulcerative colitis without toxic megacolon is unusual and usually occurs in the course of a severe attack of colitis, often during the initial attack itself (28). Among the 1928 patients with ulcerative colitis in one study, perforation of the colon was noted in only five (0.3%), mostly in the sigmoid colon (28).

Crohn's Colitis

Free perforation resulting from small bowel Crohn's disease is rare. In one series it occurred in 1% to 2% of the cases (29). Free perforation in a patient with Crohn's colitis is even more unusual. A 10-year review at the Royal Infirmary of Edinburgh identified 198 patients diagnosed as having Crohn's disease of the colon (30). Six patients (3%) developed free perforation. Out of 679 patients with large bowel Crohn's disease in the series from Oslo, Norway, seven (1%) had free perforations (28).

Toxic Megacolon

Toxic megacolon is a serious condition in which the inflamed colon becomes dilated, causing abdominal distention and serious illness. Although it is typically associated with ulcerative colitis Crohn's colitis, other bacterial colitides, including *C. difficile* colitis, are emerging as important causes of toxic megacolon. Untreated delayed operative intervention may lead to perforation. In a series of 70 patients with toxic megacolon reported by Heppell et al. (31), 15 (21%) had sealed or free perforation.

■ CLINICAL MANIFESTATIONS

Free perforation of the colon and rectum into the peritoneal cavity has a sudden onset, with classic signs and symptoms of acute abdominal pain, distention, peritoneal irritation, fever, and chills. In spite of its severity, the typical presenting signs and symptoms of perforation may be absent and nonspecific. In elderly debilitated patients or patients receiving steroids, the traditional signs and symptoms of an inflammatory process or peritonitis are often muted, and the perforation may go unrecognized until the condition has progressed to unexplained sepsis and multiple organ failure. A sudden or gradual deterioration in a patient should alert physicians and surgeons to the clinical diagnosis of an "acute abdomen."

■ DIAGNOSIS AND CLINICAL EVALUATION

Upright and flat plate films of the abdomen and lateral decubitus x-ray films should be taken. However, pneumoperitoneum, the pathognomonic sign of a perforated viscus, is found in only 20% to 50% of the cases (26,30). Bleeding, presumably from the site of perforation, may be present but usually is minimum or moderate in amount. Proctoscopy, flexible sigmoidoscopy, and colonoscopy are contraindicated because of the risk of enlarging the size of the perforation and further contamination of the peritoneal cavity. CT scan of the abdomen is unnecessary. A water-soluble enema such as Hypaque or Gastrografin is helpful in locating the site of perforation and is particularly useful in establishing the diagnosis in patients with peritonitis confined to the left lower quadrant (32).

■ MANAGEMENT

Free perforation of the colon and rectum into the peritoneal cavity is a true emergency condition. The operative mortality rate is high, ranging from 6% to 29% for diverticular disease (24), 14% to 71% for carcinoma (26,27,33), and 27% for toxic megacolon (31). Once free perforation is diagnosed or suspected, exploratory surgery should be performed as soon as possible. The aim of the operation is to remove the perforated colon or rectum to stop further contamination and to wash the entire abdominal cavity, including performing debridement of fibrin and necrotic tissues. A primary anastomosis should not be performed. The significant prognostic factors are age above >65 years, organ failure, and septic state (34).

NEUTROPENIC ENTEROCOLITIS

Although rare in adults, neutropenic enterocolitis is a potentially fatal condition that deserves to be included as a separate entity. Neutropenic enterocolitis is now a commonly recognized complication of potent combinations of chemotherapy. Surgeons will be increasingly called upon to evaluate neutropenic patients with abdominal pain. Although most cases are associated with chemotherapy, the disease has been described with immunosuppression therapy in transplant recipients, benign cyclic neutropenia, and aplastic anemia (35,36).

Neutropenia is defined as <1000 neutrophils/mm^3 and severe neutropenia as <100 neutrophils/mm (3,37). The condition was first described by Cooke in 1933 (38) and the term neutropenic enterocolitis was first used by Moir and Bale in 1976 (39). This entity has also been called typhlitis (typhlon in Greek is cecum), necrotizing enterocolitis, agranulocyte colitis, and neutropenic enteropathy (36). The process has a predilection for the terminal ileum and cecum, but any segment of the bowel can be involved (36).

The exact pathogenesis of neutropenic enterocolitis is unknown. The neutropenia may allow bacterial invasion of the bowel wall leading to necrosis of various layers of the bowel (35,36). The common signs and symptoms are abdominal pain, fever, diarrhea, abdominal distention, blood in stool nausea, and vomiting (40). Although these symptoms are nonspecific, their presence in patients with neutropenia should alert physicians and surgeons to suspect neutropenic enterocolitis.

The accurate diagnosis is often difficult since other acute abdominal diseases can also occur, such as pancreatitis, appendicitis, and hepatic abscess (36). Besides, the lack of significant intrapertoneal inflammatory response due to neutropenia makes it difficult to diagnose the extent of the acute abdomen. The severity of the enterocolitis ranges from mucosal ulceration to transmural necrosis and perforation. CT scan showed abnormality of the ileocecal area in only 46% of the patients in the series of Wade et al. (36). However, CT scan is the most accurate method of diagnosis. In a typical case, the CT scan shows a dilated cecum with thickened wall and spiculation of pericolonic fat (40). The finding of pneumatosis intestinalis supports the diagnosis but is not specific (41).

The management of neutropenic enterocolitis is most challenging. Needless surgery must be avoided in these very sick patients. On the other hand, delayed operation only increases the risk of mortality. Not all neutropenic patients with abdominal pain require operation. Medical treatment includes nasogastric suction to rest the bowel, broad-spectrum antibiotics, fluid, electrolytes, intravenous nutrition, and consideration of granulocyte transfusion (35). In the meta-analysis of randomized controlled trials (42) ciprofloxacin combined with a β-lactam antimicrobial agent is superior to the more commonly used aminoglycoside/β-lactam in the management of hospitalized febrile neutropenic patients. In addition, this combination is less nephrotoxic and is less expensive.

There are evidences suggesting that the disease may resolve when the number of white blood cells rises (36). If the condition does not improve within a few days, operation is indicated. Patients with signs of localized or generalized peritonitis should be operated on. The bowel should be resected without anastomosis. All dead bowel, regardless of how extensive, has to be resected. A questionable viable small bowel may require a second-look operation within 24 hours (43).

Wade et al. (36) reported 50 patients with neutropenic enterocolitis. The overall mortality rate was 60%. The mortality rate of 37 patients treated medically was 70% and of 17 patients treated surgically, 41%. Abdominal distention was a significant risk to the outcome; 60% of the patients who died had abdominal distention compared with 20% of the patients who did not have abdominal distention and survived. Localization of pain or tenderness and diarrhea had no predictive value to the outcome. Overwhelming sepsis was the major cause of death.

MASSIVE BLEEDING

GENERAL CONSIDERATIONS

Massive colonic bleeding is defined as bleeding that has become life threatening, usually requiring approximately five units of transfused blood. The site of the bleeding is difficult to pinpoint, because bleeding from the gastroduodenum and small bowel can present as bright red rectal bleeding. During the past 20 years, the diagnosis of massive colonic bleeding has changed remarkably. The use of arteriography and nuclear medicine tracers not only identifies the source and site of bleeding in many cases, but may prove therapeutic as well. The recent introduction of emergency colonoscopy has changed the method of diagnosis and treatment further.

Angiectasia

Prompted by the reports of small cecal vascular abnormalities by other authors (44,45), Boley et al. (46) set out to study the blood vessels of the right colon in 1977. They found that in patients with a clinical and angiographic diagnosis of bleeding from colonic vascular lesions, the most consistent and apparently the earliest abnormality noted in all lesions was the presence of dilated, often huge, submucosal veins. The colonic mucosa overlying the lesion was very thin, often separated from the dilated vessels by a single layer of endothelium. Boley et al. (46) believed that the lesions were acquired vascular ectasias, resulting from degenerative changes that accompany aging. This theory accounts both for the higher incidence in older persons and for the multiplicity of lesions.

According to the authors' concept, the direct cause of the ectasias is chronic, partial, and intermittent low-grade obstruction of the submucosal veins, especially where these veins pierce the circular and longitudinal muscular layers of the colon. This obstruction occurs repeatedly over many years during muscular contraction and distention of the cecum and the right colon. Because of the lower pressure within the veins, they can become occluded while higher arterial pressure maintains arterial inflow. Ultimately, repeated episodes of transiently elevated pressure within a submucosal vein result in dilatation and tortuosity of these vessels and later of the venules and capillaries of the mucosal units draining into it. Finally, as the responsible rings dilate, competency of the precapillary sphincters is lost, producing a small arteriovenous communication (Fig. 3). The latter is for the "early" filling veins. Examination of colon resected from those patients older than 60 years without a history of gastrointestinal bleeding or obstruction found submucosal vascular ectasia in 53% and mucosal ectasia in 27% of specim. These findings support the concept that these are degenerative lesions of aging in an older population.

Although aortic stenosis and gastrointestinal bleeding have been noted and blamed as the cause of angiectasia, Boley et al. (46) believed that the low-perfusion pressure from aortic stenosis might cause ischemic necrosis of the single layer of endothelium that often separates ectatic vessels from the colonic lumen. Angiectasia tends to cause slow repeated bleeding from the large bowel. Patients present with anemia or weakness. This is in sharp contrast to diverticular bleeding that is abrupt, more impressive, and less chronic (47).

With increased awareness of angiectasia, more and more lesions have been recognized. Colonoscopy is a safe and effective test for making the diagnosis (47,48).

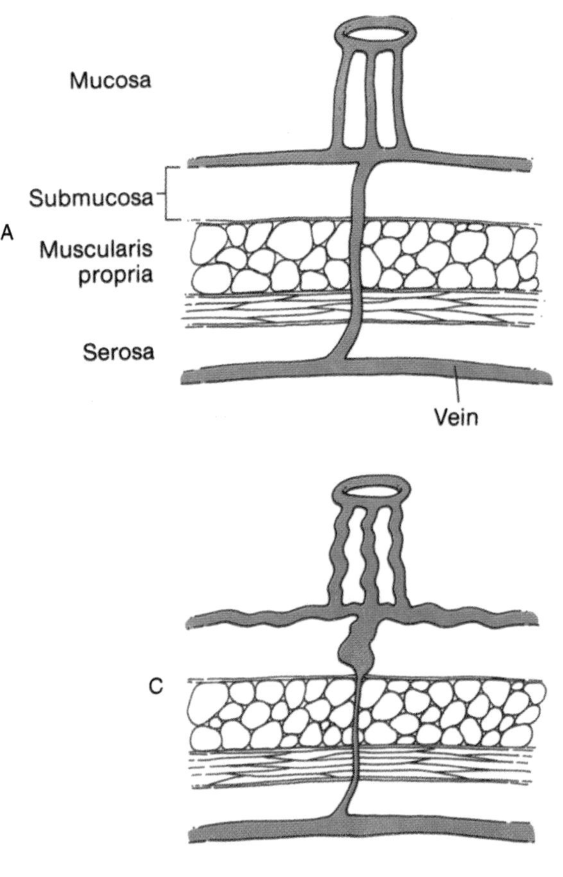

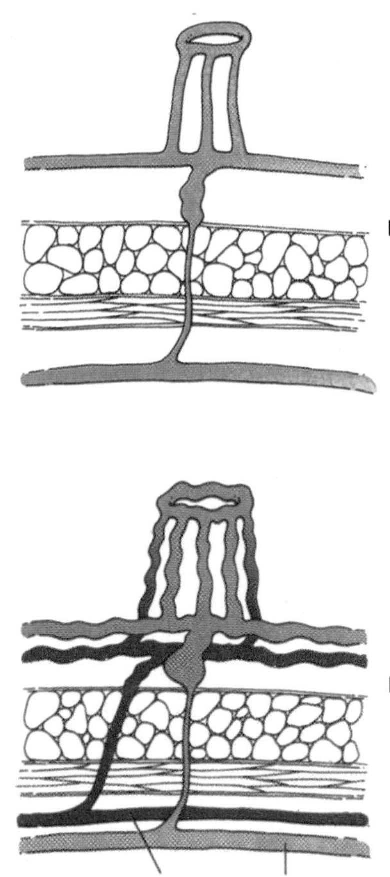

FIGURE 3 ■ Diagrammatic illustration of proposed concept of development of angiectasia. (**A**) Normal state of vein perforating muscular layer of the colonic wall. (**B**) Vein is obstructed partially as a result of muscular contraction or increased intraluminal pressure. (**C**) After repeated episodes over many years, the submucosal and mucosal venules become dilated and tortuous. (**D**) Ultimately, the capillary ring becomes dilated, the precapillary sphincter becomes incompetent, and a small arteriovenous communication is present through the ectasia. *Source*: From Ref. 46.

Angiectasia can be recognized easily via colonoscopy as a distinct red mucosal patch consisting of capillaries (Fig. 4). The size may vary from 2 mm to 1.5 cm. The histology of angiectasia shows tortuous and dilated capillaries in the lamina propria (Fig. 5). Angiectasia discovered incidentally does not need to be treated. When angiectasias with active bleeding are found during colonoscopy in patients with massive lower gastrointestinal bleeding, colon resection should be considered. Electrocoagulation can be performed but the current bleeding is in the range of 40% to 50% with a significant risk of perforation (47). More than 70% of angiectasia was found in the right colon on colonoscopy, 22% in the descending and sigmoid colon, and 6% in the transverse colon in the series of 437 lesions studied by Jensen and Machicado (49).

Diverticular Disease

Approximately 50% of the people over the age of 60 years have radiologic evidence of diverticula. Up to 20% bleed during their lifetime, and 5% have massive bleeding, which recurs in 25%, if the colon is not resected (50). Although most diverticula are in the sigmoid colon, 50% to 95% of bleeding diverticula are to the right of the splenic flexure (51,52). Before the 1960s it was thought that inflammation of the diverticula caused bleeding. Noer et al. (53) were the first to note that most bleeding comes from noninflamed diverticula.

McGuire (52) studied 79 patients with severe bleeding diverticulosis and found that bleeding stopped spontaneously in 76%. Emergency operation was required in 24%. In patients who required no more than three units of blood

FIGURE 4 ■ Angiectasia of the cecum as seen through the colonoscope.

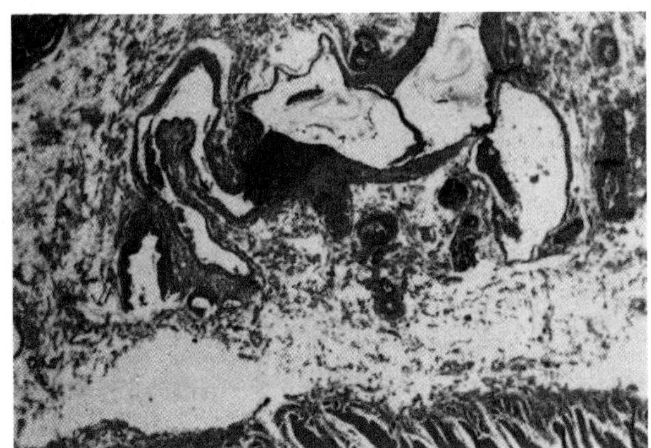

FIGURE 5 ■ Histology of angiectasia shows tortuous and dilated capillaries in the lamina propria.

transfusion on any day, 98.5% stopped spontaneously. In patients who required four or more transfusions on any day, 60% required emergency operation. In those patients who did not require operation, the recurrence rate was 38%, and in 79% of these patients, again, bleeding stopped spontaneously. Bokhari et al. (54) reported that of 115 elderly patients with a mean age of 79 years admitted to the hospital with bleeding diverticulosis and who required blood transfusion, 18% required colon resection. The postoperative mortality rate was 9%.

In the study of acute bleeding diverticulosis by Meyer et al. (55), who used arteriographic and microangiographic techniques, the serial histologic sections revealed that the bleeding was the result of rupture of the vasa recta, which passed around the dome of the diverticulum. The vasa recta at the site of rupture had eccentric intimal thickening associated with thinning of the media and duplication of the internal elastic lamina. These arterial changes probably represent a nonspecific response to repeated arterial injury. The increased frequency of bleeding from the right-sided colonic diverticula remains a puzzling fact. Although the anatomic relationships of the vasa recta to diverticula are similar throughout the colon, one feature distinguishes right-sided from left-sided diverticula. Those on the right have wider necks and domes. Their vasa recta are, therefore, exposed over a greater length to any injurious factors arising from the colon. The nature of the injurious factors has not been determined yet. In addition, the true cause of the bleeding may be an unrecognized vascular ectasia.

Carcinoma

Colonic bleeding is common with carcinoma of the colon and rectum, and ranges from a small amount of intermittent bright red rectal blood to chronic occult or gross bleeding causing anemia. The incidence of massive bleeding from a patient with colorectal carcinoma varies from series to series. In the series reported by Rossini et al. (57), 311 patients with massive colonic bleeding underwent emergency colonoscopy; carcinoma caused the bleeding in 21%. Jensen and Machicado (49), using urgent colonoscopy, found that severe bleeding was caused by colorectal carcinomas and polyps in 11% of the patients. Leitman et al. (56), using emergency arteriography, found carcinoma as the cause of massive bleeding in 10% of 55 patients.

Polyps

Although polyps of the colon and rectum are common, their causing massive bleeding is uncommon, with the incidence ranging from 2% to 10% (49,56,57).

Ischemic Colitis

Ischemic colitis may be acute, transient, or gressive (58). The patient usually presents with bleeding per rectum, diarrhea, and abdominal pain; acute abdomen usually designates gangrene or perforation. In a series of 54 patients with massive lower gastrointestinal hemorrhage who were undergoing emergency arteriography, Leitman et al. (56) found three patients with intestinal ischemia. Using urgent colonoscopy in 74 patients with severe hematochezia, Jensen and Machicado (49) found no case of ischemic colitis. On the other hand, Rossini et al. (57) reported that 21 out of 311 patients with massive, active lower gastrointestinal hemorrhage had ischemic colitis.

Inflammatory Bowel Disease

Ulcerative colitis is characterized by bloody diarrhea in more than 95% of the cases, but severe or massive hemorrhage is quite rare, occurring less commonly than other complications such as toxic megacolon, colonic perforation, or neoplastic degeneration (59). Nevertheless, massive hemorrhage occasionally represents the principal indication for emergency operation. The frequency of severe hemorrhage reported in the literature ranges from 0% to 4.5%. However, this relatively rare complication accounts for approximately 10% of all urgent colectomies for ulcerative colitis (57). In the series by Rossini et al. (57), 45 of 311 patients (14%) with massive lower gastrointestinal bleeding diagnosed by emergency colonoscopy had ulcerative colitis.

The incidence of massive bleeding in patients with Crohn's disease has been reported as 1% to 13% (60). Active bleeding caused by Crohn's colitis is uncommon. In the series reported by Robert et al. (61), 21 of 1526 patients (1.3%) with Crohn's disease developed severe gastrointestinal hemorrhage. The frequency of bleeding was significantly higher among patients with colonic involvement (17 of 929, 1.9%) than among those with small bowel disease alone (4 of 597, 0.7%). Primary bleeding episodes subsided without operation in 10 of 21 patients, but three of the 10 patients (30%) rebled massively. By contrast, primary excisional surgery was followed by recurrent hemorrhage in only one of the 11 cases (9%). Although the differences in mortality and in recurrent bleeding rates were not statistically significant, they favor surgical removal of the diseased bowel at the time of the first episode of massive hemorrhage (61). A review of literature by Cirocco et al. (62) showed that operation was necessary to prevent life-threatening hemorrhage in 30 of 33 patients (91%).

■ CLINICAL MANIFESTATIONS

Massive lower gastrointestinal bleeding is generally defined as bleeding per rectum that requires three to six units of transfused blood within 24 hours (56) or bleeding that results in a hemoglobin level of below 10 g% (57). A large amount of blood acts as a cathartic and will be evacuated accordingly. The color of the stool ranges from bright red to dark red, depending on the speed of bleeding. Symptoms of these patients reflect the underlying disease. Bleeding caused by diverticular disease, ulcerative colitis, polyps, or carcinomas is usually asymptomatic except for some abdominal cramps from the cathartic effect of the blood. Bleeding caused by ischemic colitis is usually associated with severe abdominal cramps. Other signs of severe blood loss such as tachycardia, pallor, and weakness are apparent.

■ DIAGNOSIS AND MANAGEMENT

Massive bleeding per rectum is a life-threatening condition. The most important parts of management are the initial resuscitation with blood and volume replacement and the monitoring of vital systems. These steps must be performed immediately. Any blood dyscrasia should be ruled out and treated accordingly. The next critical item is marking an accurate and early diagnosis. The diagnosis of massive colonic bleeding is usually difficult because the diagnostic techniques are not completely efficient or reliable. Knowing the exact site of bleeding is more important than knowing what causes the bleeding.

In approximately 85% of all patients who have acute gastrointestinal bleeding, the bleeding stops spontaneously. This fact should be known by all involved in the care of these patients (63). Shock from massive gastrointestinal bleeding is usually from gastroduodenal rather than small intestinal or colonic sources.

Nasogastric Suction

The most common cause of massive gastrointestinal bleeding remains peptic ulcer disease. All patients with gastrointestinal hemorrhage should have a nasogastric tube placed in the stomach to rule out an upper gastrointestinal source. If blood returns, a gastroduodenal source is confirmed. The nasogastric return must contain bile to rule out a bleeding duodenal ulcer. A bloody nasogastric aspirate has the highest specificity for high-risk lesions. A clear nasogastic aspirate reduces the possibility significantly (64). If any doubt remains, gastroduodenoscopy should be performed.

Proctoscopy

The rectum and anal canal can be examined quickly with a proctoscope to rule out a local source of the bleeding and to confirm the presence of blood proximal to the rectum. Most of the blood can be washed out, and an adequate examination can be usually done without much difficulty. Any active bleeding from a specific source in the anorectum can be treated with electrocautery or suture ligation.

Technetium-99m Scintigraphy

The detection of colonic bleeding with nuclear medicine tracers depends on the intravenous infusion of technetium, which will stay within the blood pool for a reasonable period of time so that the source of the bleeding, which often is intermittent, can be detected. This procedure was first performed using sulfur colloid. However, because sulfur colloid collects in the liver and spleen, bleeding that occurs in the upper or middle abdomen such as in the stomach, duodenum, and transverse colon was often obscured. For this reason, red blood cells (RBCs) labeled with technetium-99m (^{99m}Tc) are now used. A small sample of the patient's own RBCs is withdrawn, labeled with ^{99m}Tc sodium pertechnetate, and reinjected. Scintigraphic images are then obtained in the hope of identifying the source of bleeding. Even if the patient is not bleeding at the moment of injection, bleeding over the next 12 or more hours can be detected by repeat scanning. With ^{99m}Tc-labeled RBCs, bleeding at a rate of 0.1 mL/min can be detected (57) (Fig. 6). Nuclear medicine tracers are efficient for detecting bleeding that has slowed down and bleeding that is intermittent, but it requires several hours to follow the patient. RBC-tagged scanning is 30% to 90% accurate in localizing the bleeding point (65,66). One of the major problems is that the tagged RBC study depends heavily on the technique and the radiologist. The poor results may be the result of an incorrect scanning interval because of the intermittent nature of bleeding or because the blood moves distally by peristalsis.

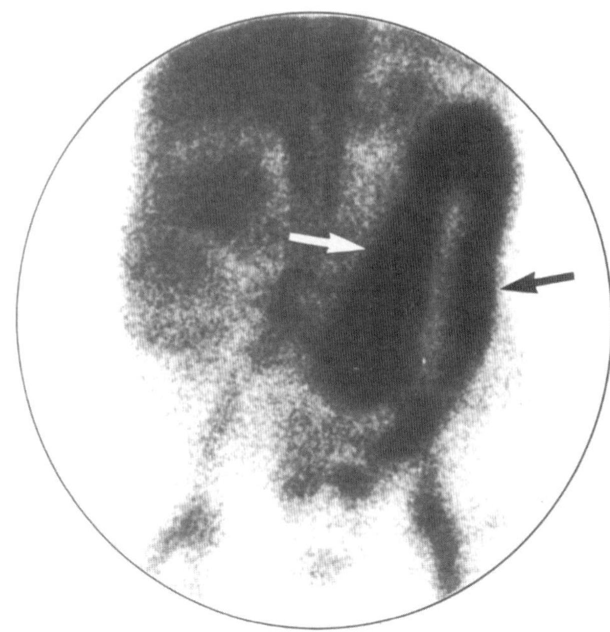

FIGURE 6 ■ A technetium-99m-labeled red blood cell-tagged scan shows hyperactivity of the blood in the left transverse colon, splenic flexure, and descending colon (*arrows*). *Source*: Courtesy of Michael McKusick, M.D., Rochester, Minnesota, U.S.A.

In the series by Nicholson et al. (67), the test sensitivity was as high as 97%, and the specificity was 85%. The predictive values were 94% and 92% when the scans were positive and negative, respectively. These impressive results are also shared by other authors (68,69). Suzman et al. (69) emphasize using a delayed periodic scintigraphic imaging technique. In this technique the images are acquired at five-minute intervals for the first hour and at 15-minute intervals for up to four hours and stored in a dynamic mode. If needed, the patient is imaged every 90 minutes thereafter for up to 24 hours. Scan results demonstrating extravasation to tagged erythrocytes into the bowel lumen are read as positive. Fifty patients who required surgical intervention to control hemorrhage had a bleeding site confirmed by both clinical and pathologic examinations. Forty-eight of these patients (96%) had a bleeding site determined preoperatively. Of 37 patients with bleeding sites localized preoperatively by scintigraphy, 36 (97.3%) had correct localization based on surgical pathology. Only one patient required a subtotal colectomy solely because of nonlocalized bleeding. There was no recurrent postoperative bleeding, and there was no mortality in either operated or nonoperated patients.

A newer technique of CT angiography demonstrated the ability to detect angioectasia, with a sensitivity, specificity, and positive predictive value of 70%, 100%, and 100%, respectively (70,71). However, it remains to be seen whether this newer technique can pinpoint the site of an active colonic bleeding.

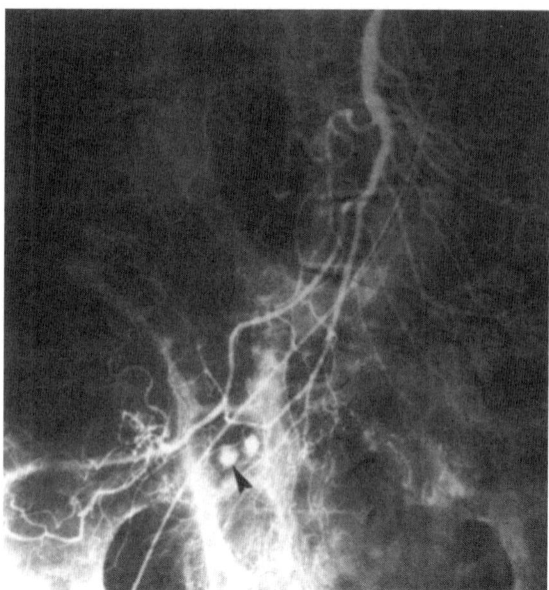

FIGURE 7 ■ Mesenteric arteriography shows extravasation of contrast material into bowel lumen from diverticular bleeding in transverse colon (*arrow*). *Source*: Courtesy of Michael McKusick, M.D., Rochester, Minnesota, U.S.A.

Selective Mesenteric Arteriography

Selective mesenteric arteriography is an invasive method that can detect lower gastrointestinal bleeding provided that the bleeding is active and brisk (0.5–1 mL/min) at the time of the test. Intermittent bleeding or minimal rates of bleeding may be missed by this method. In a patient with active bleeding, the contrast medium can be seen extravasated into the bowel lumen (Fig. 7). Arteriography, when positive, can localize the site the bleeding. The angiographic pattern of the vasculature may also suggest a malignancy, a diverticulum, a vascular malformation, or angiectasia.

In a patient with massive and continuing bleeding, mesenteric arteriography should be used as the primary test, provided that the facilities for the technique are available and can be mobilized quickly. Another important advantage of mesenteric arteriography is its potential therapeutic applications. It is important to adequately resusitate the patient with adequate intravenous fluid and blood transfusion maintain good blood pressure. Once the bleeding site is detected, the transcatheter treatment using a vasopressin drip or emboli can be accomplished (72). If successful, it may convert an emergency exploratory celiotomy into an elective one, or it may avert an operation altogether (Fig. 8). The action of vasopressin is two-fold. It produces both arteriolar contraction and bowel wall contraction, which help to stop the bleeding (73).

However, the use of selective vasoconstrictive agent infusion is associated with high recurrence rates and complication of ischemia of the gastrointestinal tract. Recently, improved microcatheters that allow selective cannulation of secondary vessels and embolization agents such as poly vinyl alcohol (PVA) and metal coils have been used with much greater success.

The incidence of ischemia has markedly decreased due to the use of larger PVA or metal coils and increased experience. Most series since 1997 reported ischemia that required resection of less than 5% (72).

Khanna et al. (72) conducted a meta-analysis of 25 identified publications reporting the use of embolization and an unpublished series of 12 consecutive patients with lower gastrointestinal bleeding from their own institution. Six published series and the authors' series met selection criteria for the analysis. The results showed that embolization for diverticular bleeding was successful in 85% of patients (no recurrence after 30 days). In contrast, rebleeding after embolization for angioextasia and other nondiverticular bleeding occurred in 45%.

Angiographic evidence of angiectasia included clusters of small arteries frequently located along the entire mesenteric border of the cecum and ascending colon, a vascular tuft (representing the degeneration of mucosal venules), and an early filling vein (Fig. 9). Because the natural history of ectasias is one of recurrent bleeding, Boley et al. (74) recommended that all patients who have bleeding and have an ectasia demonstrated by angiography should undergo colonic resection. It is difficult to determine the frequency of bleeding in patients with

A

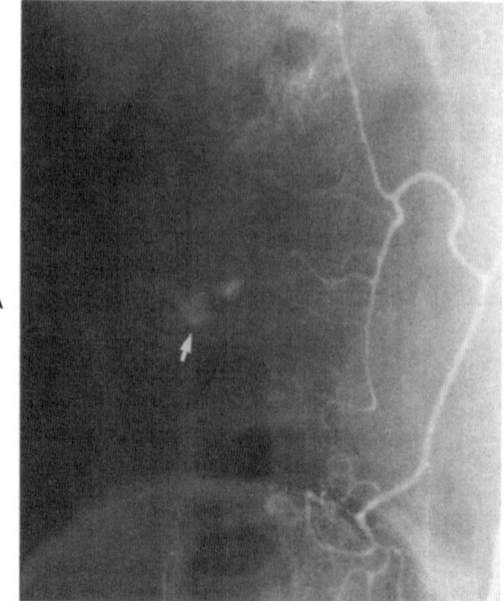

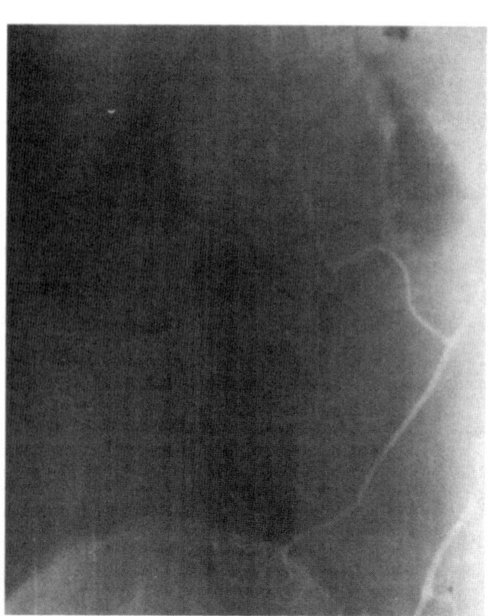

B

FIGURE 8 ■ (**A**) Mesenteric arteriography shows bleeding in the ascending colon from colonoscopic polypectomy (*arrow*). (**B**) Bleeding stopped by vasospasm after vasopressin (Pitressin) drip.

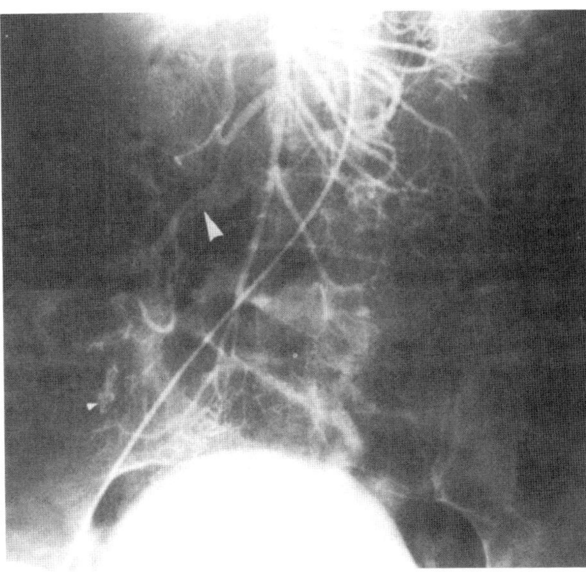

FIGURE 9 ■ Mesenteric arteriography shows vascular tuft in the right colon from angiectasia (*small arrow*) and early filling vein (*large arrow*). *Source*: Courtesy of Michael McKusick, M.D., Rochester, Minnesota, U.S.A.

TABLE 2 ■ Clinical Diagnosis at Emergency Colonoscopy for Massive Colonic Bleeding

Condition	No. of Cases
Diverticular disease	56
Solitary diverticulum of the right colon	4
Ulcerative colitis	45
Ulcerative colitis plus carcinoma or polyp	2
Radiation colitis	15
Ischemic colitis	21
Ulcerated carcinoma	66
Polyp	34
Angioma	2
Solitary ulcer	5
Angiectasia	16
Anastomotic recurrence of carcinoma	22
Recurrence of Crohn's disease (ileotransversostomy)	4
Endometriosis	3
Postpolypectomy hemorrhage (4–5 days after operation)	14
Lymphoma	1
Ureterosigmoidostomy plus ulcerated carcinoma	1
Total	311

Source: From Ref. 57.

diverticular disease and angiectasia, because both occur in the elderly and often the bleeding stops during angiography or colonoscopy.

One advantage of angiography as opposed to scintigraphy or colonoscopy for this particular patient population is that no special preparation is necessary such as labeling of erythrocytes and bowel cleansing. Even hemodynamically unstable patients can be studied while resuscitation efforts are under way, including the administration of intravenous fluids and/or blood products. It is critical that no oral contrast agents be administered fore angiography because it may obscure a subtle bleeding (75).

Urgent Colonoscopy

The use of a colonic lavage (GoLytely or CoLyte) as a gut cleanser has opened a new approach to colonic bleeding. In the hands of a growing number of physicians, urgent colonoscopy has become the first choice of investigative modality in the diagnosis and therapy of massive colonic bleeding. As soon as the patient has been resuscitated and upper gastrointestinal bleeding has been ruled out, GoLytely or CoLyte is rapidly instituted via the nasogastric tube or orally. The entire colon can be cleansed within two hours. Alternatively, oral Phospho-soda can be administered to accomplish the same goal. Colonoscopy can be performed immediately. In a series reported by Jensen and Machicado (76), in 80 consecutive patients with severe, ongoing rectal bleeding (mean, $6\frac{1}{2}$ units of transfused blood) from an unknown source, urgent colonoscopy was performed after oral purge. In all cases the cecum was reached. Seventy-four percent of the patients had bled from the colon (angiomas, 30%; diverticulosis, 17%; polyps or carcinomas, 11%; focal ulcers, 9%; others, 7%), 11% had upper gastrointestinal lesions, and 9% had presumed small bowel lesions. In only 6% was the cause of bleeding not identified. No complications resulted from colonoscopic or colonoscopic hemostatic procedures, although four patients had clinically significant fluid overload and early heart failure during the cleansing procedure. Rossini et al. (57) performed 409 emergency colonoscopies for massive colonic bleeding. The sites and causes of bleeding were found in 311 cases (76%). There was a wide range of causes of the bleeding (Table 2). In 85% of the cases, the bleeding was in the left colon, 4% in the transverse colon, and 11% in the right colon. Only two patients had complications, one developed increasing hemorrhage from ulcerative colitis and one developed diverticulitis. There was no perforation.

One of the greatest advantages of successful colonoscopy is its providing an access to therapy. Colonoscopic hemostatic techniques can be divided into two categories: nonthermal and thermal modalities. The nonthermal techniques involve injection of vasoconstricting agents such as a dilute epinephrine solution and vaso destructive agents alone or in combination with such agents as absolute alcohol, morrhuate sodium, and sodium tetradecyl sulfate. A wide variety of thermal modalities, including electrocoagulation, laser photocoagulation, and heater probe coagulation, are available.

Urgent colonoscopy for massive colonic bleeding has emerged as a practical and efficient method to diagnose and control some causes of colonic bleeding. The gastrointestinal bleeding team established at the Mayo Clinic on October 1, 1988 provides a very useful team approach to the treatment of gastrointestinal bleeding. The bleeding-team contact begins within an hour of the patient's clinical presentation. The triage team determines whether the patient should be admitted to the intensive care unit or whether the team should proceed with evaluation, deciding on the timing of colonoscopy. Emergency colonoscopy is performed after a rapid (1–2-hr) lavage with GoLytely or CoLyte (77). Several lessons can be learned from this study. A total of 417 patients were evaluated. Fifty-six percent of the patients were seen from 8 AM to 5:00 PM, 34% from 5:00 PM to 12 AM, and 10% from

12 AM to 8 AM. Of the 417 patients, 56% developed bleeding while hospitalized. Upper gastrointestinal bleeding accounted for 82%. The five most common etiologies included gastric ulcers (83 patients), duodenal ulcers (67 patients), gastric erosions (41 patients), esophageal varices (35 patients), and diverticulosis (29 patients). Nonsteroidal anti-inflammatory drugs (NSAIDs) were implicated in 53% of gastroduodenal ulcers.

Twenty-nine patients with bleeding diverticulosis involved the oldest patient group, with an average age of 77 years. Diverticula were limited to the left colon in 52% (15 patients). Eventual cessation of bleeding was commonplace and occurred in 27 patients (93%). Four patients (14%) experienced rebleeding during the hospitalization. Only one patient required operation for rebleeding.

From the Mayo Clinic study, it is unclear whether urgent colonoscopy for acute colonic bleeding will alter outcome, especially if majority of the bleeding is from diverticulosis. The very high rates of spontaneous cessation, the low relative transfusion requirements, and absent mortality, argue for initial observation as an appropriate and cost-effective approach. Colonoscopy might more appropriately be performed on an elective basis.

With the better technique of RBC-tagged scan, using dynamic scanning technique, the very high accuracy of both the detection of gastrointestinal bleeding and the localization of the site of bleeding has made it the choice as the primary test (69,78). Another advantage of RBC-tagged scanning is that when the scan is negative, those patients (7.3%) rarely require operative intervention (66). At the present time, it appears that the trend has shifted from urgent or emergent colonoscopy to an emergency RBC-tagged scan or selective mesenteric arteriography as the primary test for acute lower gastrointestinal bleeding (69,72).

Exploratory Celiotomy

Determining when to operate on patients with massive and continuous colonic bleeding requires astute clinical judgment. Generally, an exploratory celiotomy is considered seriously when a patient requires five units of blood transfused within 24 hours or less, if the patient's condition deteriorates. Ironically, greater aggressiveness in deciding to operate earlier is appropriate in treating older and unfit patients. Patients who have recurrent active bleeding that has stopped spontaneously or after nonoperative treatment also should undergo an operation.

Known Bleeding Site

A segmental resection is indicated when the site of bleeding is known, whether the knowledge comes from scintigraphic, arteriographic, or colonoscopic information. The rate of recurrent bleeding after definitive resection has ranged from 0% to 11% (average, 4%), and the reported operative mortality rate has ranged from 0% to 22% (average, 10%) (56,79–83).

Unknown Bleeding Site

It is not uncommon that despite all the efforts and the availability of modern technology, the site of the bleeding still is not ascertained and the bleeding continues. Under these circumstances, exploratory celiotomy should be performed. The entire gastrointestinal tract must be examined carefully for abnormalities. Small bowel lesions such as leiomyoma, lymphoma, and those of Crohn's disease are occasional sources. If they are not present, an intraoperative endoscopy should follow. A sterilized colonoscope is introduced via an enterotomy in the proximal jejunum. An alternative is to pass a clean but nonsterilized colonoscope through the mouth into the stomach and duodenum. The surgeon then guides the scope throughout the entire small bowel into the cecum. The entire small bowel mucosa is examined. At the same time, the surgeon can examine the bowel by transillumination (84,85). Angiectasia can be recognized by its abnormal vasculature. If these are found, they can be ligated with interrupted structures. Other abnormalities can also be effectively visualized (86). If colonoscopy has not been accomplished preoperatively, an intraoperative colonoscopy also should be performed.

When intraoperative endoscopy or thorough examination of the entire gastrointestinal tract is negative and evidence points to colonic bleeding at an unknown site, a subtotal colectomy is performed. Some investigators have argued that blind segmental resection of the right colon may be a better surgical option than blind total colectomy, especially if there are suggestions of right-sided bleeding such as blood primarily in the right colon. This argument is strengthened by a negative preoperative examination of the left colon. Blind right hemicolectomy has had the lowest mortality (less than 5%), and the lowest frequency of rebleeding among segmental resections, and it does not incur the risk of incontinence or diarrhea, especially in elderly patients (83). However, the risk of rebleeding is still significant, and I feel more confident with a total abdominal colectomy. Farner et al. (87) conducted a retrospective study comparing 50 limited colon resections to 27 total/subtotal colon resections for acute lower gastrointestinal bleeding (receiving two or more units of packed red blood cells). They found that recurrent bleeding after the operation was more common in the limited colon resection group (18% vs. 4%; $p < 0.05$).

Torrential lower gastrointestinal bleeding from an unknown site should be explored as soon as possible. If there is no obvious source of bleeding in the small intestine, a total abdominal colectomy should be performed. The recurrent bleeding has ranged from 0% to 6%, and the mortality rate from 0% to 50% (average, 22%) (56,79,80,83,88–91). Because most of the high morbidity and mortality are from anastomotic leaks (90–92) an anastomosis should not be performed in this circumstance. Another risk factor is the delay of surgery. The operation should be performed before 10 units of blood are needed (91).

A schematic approach to massive colonic bleeding is shown in Fig. 10.

FISTULA

GENERAL CONSIDERATIONS

A fistula is an abnormal communication between two epithelialized surfaces. Thus it can be described accurately according to the structures it connects, for example, colovesical, colocutaneous, coloduodenal, and rectovaginal.

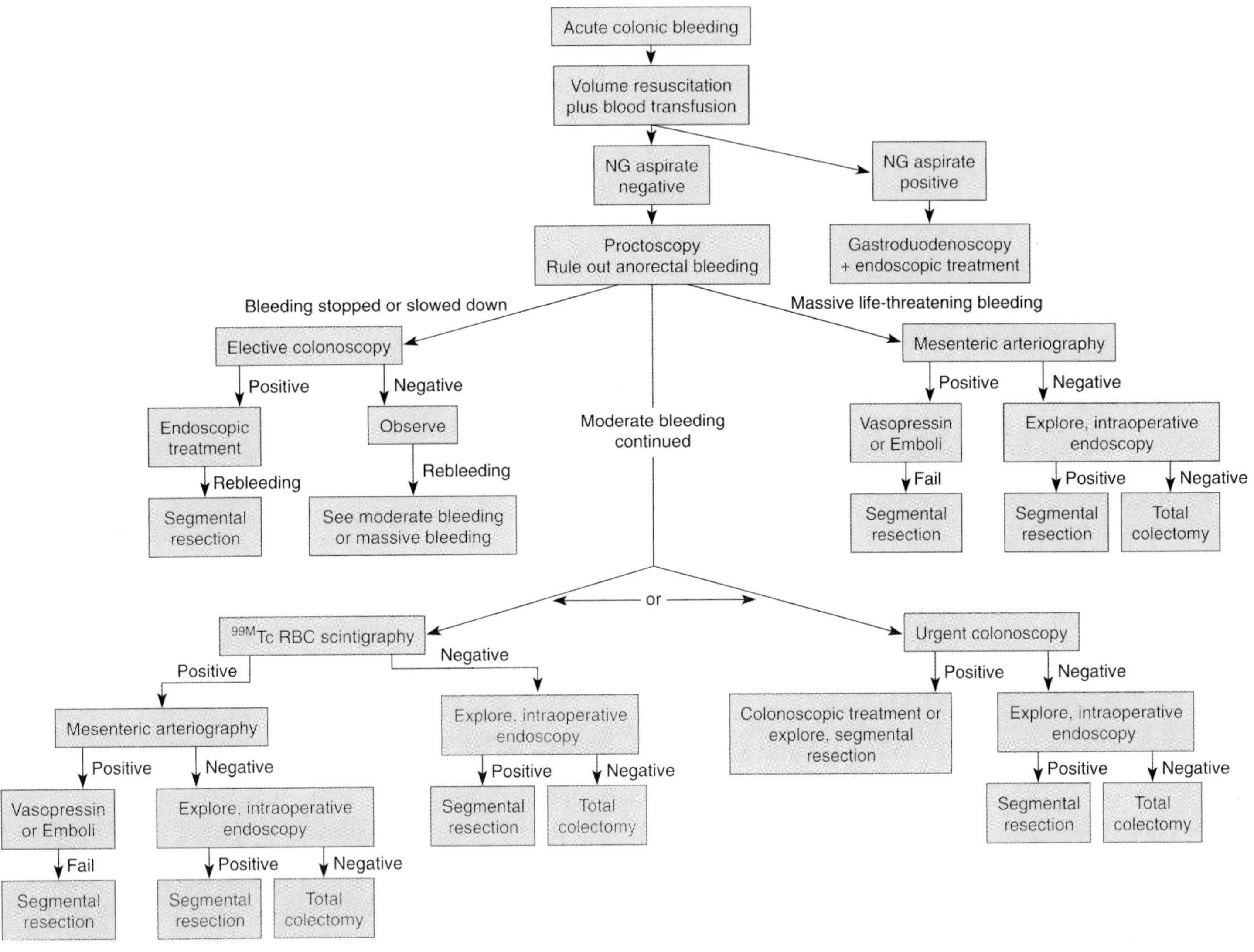

FIGURE 10 ■ Schematic approach to treatment of massive colonic bleeding.

Diverticulitis is by far the most common cause of internal fistulas followed by carcinoma, Crohn's disease, irradiation colitis, and a foreign body (93). In general, colonic fistulas are low-output fistulas. Occasionally, this may not be true when the fistula communicates with the small bowel. Colonic fistulas typically have fewer complications than fistulas located at any other segment of the gastrointestinal tract. Sepsis is often localized and amenable to surgical intervention. Obstruction is uncommon in colonic fistulas as well (94).

Diverticulitis

Diverticulitis complicated by a phlegmon or an abscess may adhere to an adjacent organ and eventually produce perforation into it, causing a fistula. Internal fistulas in patients with diverticulitis are fairly common. Of 412 patients with diverticular disease treated at the Cleveland Clinic, 84 (25%) had internal fistulas (95). The most common type of internal fistula encountered was the colovesical fistula, which accounted for 65%, followed by colovaginal fistulas (25%), colocutaneous fistulas (7%), and colouterine fistulas (3%). Of females with colovesical and colovaginal fistulas, 50% and 83%, respectively, had undergone a hysterectomy previously.

A colocutaneous fistula from diverticular disease is not uncommon. Most of these colocutaneous fistulas result from complications of an operation for diverticulitis, especially anastomotic leaks. Of 93 patients with colocutaneous fistulas associated with diverticulitis reported by Fazio et al. (96), 88 patients developed fistulas after operation for diverticulitis, and in only five patients did the fistulas develop spontaneously. In the series reported by McIntyre et al. (97), of 12 patients with colocutaneous fistulas from diverticular disease, only one fistula was spontaneous, and the rest were from postoperative complications.

Carcinoma

Transmural carcinomas of the colon and rectum may adhere to adjacent organs and eventually invade directly to develop a fistula. Such an event is uncommon today, because most carcinomas are diagnosed and treated before this advanced stage develops.

Carcinoma of the colon is the second most common cause of colovesical fistulas. In the series reported by Pollard et al. (93), this was the cause in 8 of 66 patients with fistulas. Coloenteric fistulas, especially coloduodenal and colojejunal fistulas are rare (98,99). There were only five cases of coloduodenal fistulas from carcinoma of the transverse colon seen in a 28-year period at Massachusetts General Hospital (98), and only two cases of colojejunal fistulas were reported in the literature up to 1982 (99).

Spontaneous colocutaneous fistulas from carcinoma of the colon are rare. In the series reported by Zera et al. (100), of 68 enterocutaneous fistulas, none was from carcinoma of the colon.

Radiation-Associated Fistulas

Radiation-induced fistulas usually develop years after radiation therapy for a gynecologic or urologic malignancy. They develop spontaneously after perforation of the irradiated intestine, with development of an abscess in the pelvis that subsequently drains into an adjacent viscus or to the exterior via the vagina or abdominal wall. Radiation-associated fistulas are usually complex and often involve more than one organ, for example, colon or rectum to bladder, vagina, small bowel, or skin in any combination (101).

Crohn's Disease

The transmural nature of the inflammation characteristic of Crohn's colitis often results in adherence to other organs such as the small intestine and vagina. Subsequent erosion into adjacent organs then can give rise to a fistula. A pericolic abscess eventually may rupture into an adjacent organ and, similarly, give rise to an internal fistula. Fistulous formation in patients with Crohn's disease is common, accounting for 32% to 35% of these patients (102,103). However, most fistulas come from Crohn's disease of the small intestine.

Solem et al. (104) reported 78 patients (56% men) with Crohn's disease complicated with fistulas to the urinary system: fistulas originated from the ileum, 64%; colon, 21%; rectum, 8%; and multiple sites, 7%. Urinary tract sites included the bladder, 88%; urethra, 6%; urachus, 3%; ureter, 1%; and otehr, 1%. A total of 90% required surgery.

Approximately 20% to 30% of all enterocutaneous fistulas are due to Crohn's disease (105). The process is similar to that of an internal fistula in which the diseased bowel adheres to the abdominal wall and invades through the skin or an abscess breaks through the skin. In a series of 39 patients with enterocutaneous fistulas from Crohn's disease reported by Hawker et al. (106), eight were colocutaneous fistulas. In the series reported by Zera et al. (100) of 68 patients with colocutaneous fistulas, only one case was due to Crohn's disease. Of 46 enterocutaneous fistulas from Crohn's disease reported by Michelassi et al. (103), none of them was from the colon.

The locations of intra-abdominal fistulas in patients operated on for complications of Crohn's disease are listed in Table 3.

TABLE 3 ■ Location of 290 Intra-abdominal Fistulas in 22 Patients Operated on for Complications of Crohn's Disease

Location	No. of Fistulas (%)
Internal	
Enteroduodenal	14 (5)
Enteroenteric	51 (18)
Enterocolonic	83 (29)
Enterosigmoid	49 (17)
Enterovesical	36 (12)
Colosigmoid	5 (2)
Enterosalpingeal	2 (2)[a]
Total internal	240 (83)
External	
Enterocutaneous	46 (16)
Enterovaginal	4 (2)[a]
Total external	50 (17)
Total fistulas	290

[a]The percentage is based on the number of fistulas in women.
Source: From Ref. 103.

■ CLINICAL MANIFESTATIONS

Unlike fistulas from the small bowel, colorectal fistulas have low output, and patients seldom develop nutritional problems. Once the fistulas have developed, most patients with an associated abscess are relieved of their sepsis since the abscess spontaneously drains through the fistula. This may not be true if there is significant residual infection. Patients with coloenteric fistulas may present with intra-abdominal infection, diarrhea, abdominal pain, or an abdominal mass. A colocutaneous fistula is easy to recognize by its fecal drainage, which is usually minimal.

■ DIAGNOSIS AND CLINICAL EVALUATION

Every attempt should be made to determine the nature of the underlying disease that caused the fistula, the extent of the disease, and the location or type of the fistula and to rule out associated diseases. The diagnosis of internal fistula can be difficult or impossible. In the series of 290 intra-abdominal fistulas (including 46 enterocutaneous fistulas) reported by Michelassi et al. (103), fistulas were diagnosed preoperatively in 69% of the patients by a combination of history, physical examination, radiographic investigation, and endoscopic procedures. In the remaining patients, a fistula was discovered intraoperatively in 27% or only after careful examination of the specimen in 4%. Ileovesical fistulas are most likely to occur with Crohn's disease, whereas colovesical fistulas are more commonly associated with diverticulitis and rectovesical fistulas are most frequently associated with malignancy (107).

Computed Tomography

CT provides an excellent approach to the diagnosis of complicated diverticular disease. Diverticulitis and its complications are essentially extraluminal events. CT is unique in that it images the transmural extent of the disease process and provides objective information about the surrounding organs and tissue planes. Moreover, in conjunction with the use of oral and rectal contrast material, the intraluminal contour of the gastrointestinal tract and the relationship of its extraluminal pathologic processes can be defined best by CT (108,109). CT has become an initial choice for examining patients with complicated diverticulitis. In a series reported by Labs et al. (108). CT correctly identified 100% of intra-abdominal abscesses and 92% of colovesical fistulas. Air or contrast material in the bladder is diagnostic of a colovesical fistula and can be recognized easily by CT (Fig. 11). Another benefit of CT is its application for CT-guided percutaneous drainage of an intra-abdominal abscess (110,111). For evaluating patients with Crohn's colitis and colorectal carcinoma, however, CT is unnecessary and has no advantage over a barium enema examination or colonoscopy.

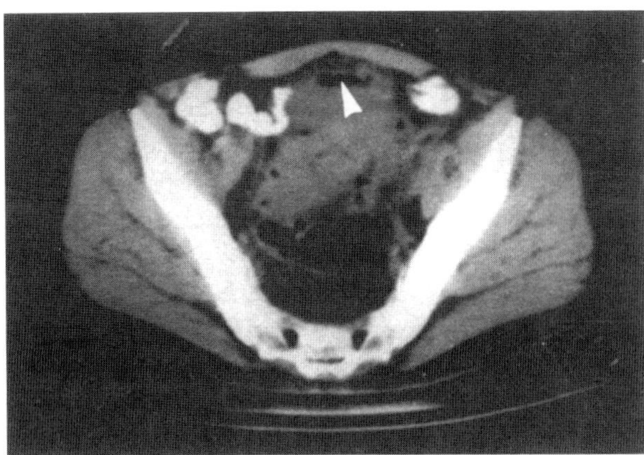

FIGURE 11 ■ A colovesical fistula. A computed tomography of the pelvis shows air in the bladder (*arrow*).

Barium Enema

A barium enema examination is essential in evaluating most internal fistulas. Although it is not always helpful to demonstrate the fistula, the nature and extent of the disease can be usually determined. A series by Woods et al. (95) showed that a barium enema examination demonstrated the fistulas in 42%, 48%, 40%, and 0% for colovesical, colovaginal, coloenteric, and colouterine fistulas, respectively. With Crohn's disease, use of a barium meal to examine the stomach, duodenum, and the entire small intestine is also indicated.

Colonoscopy

Colonoscopy can complement the barium enema examination. When indicated, a biopsy can also be performed to confirm the nature of the disease. Colonoscopy is seldom helpful in diagnosing a fistula.

Cystoscopy

Cystoscopy is essential for diagnosing a colovesical fistula, mainly to rule out malignancy, because cystoscopy gives the best yield for diagnosing or suggesting the presence of a colovesical fistula. In a study reported by Pollard et al. (93) the fistular orifice was seen in 48%, and the bladder appeared abnormal with inflammation and edema in 92% of the patients. Cystoscopy confirmed enterovesical fistulas in 75% of the patients in the series reported by Pontari et al (107). Daniels et al. (112) also recommended cystoscopy and urine cytology for fecal material as the first-line investigations in all patients with a suspected enterovesical fistula.

Fistulography

A fistulogram in conjunction with other examinations, particularly a barium enema examination, is useful to delineate the presence of a colocutaneous fistula. The fistulogram in itself confirms the clinical diagnosis but cannot determine the nature and the extent of disease.

■ MANAGEMENT

Colonic fistulas of the internal organs or of the skin seldom require an emergency or urgent operation unless there is sepsis, severe fluid loss from diarrhea, or bowel obstruction. In the series of 50 patients with colovesical fistula reported by Solka et al. (113), not a single documented case of septicemia occurred despite untreated for a period of 6 months, although 88% of patients had a urinary tract infection. Resection of the diseased bowel is necessary. For colovesical fistulas caused by diverticulitis or Crohn's disease, wide excision of the bladder is not necessary unless it is performed for a technical purpose. Enterocutaneous fistula is a feared complication of abdominal surgery. Such fistulas usually occur soon after surgery, although inflammatory bowel disease, diverticulitis, radiotherapy, trauma, ischemic bowel, and malignancy commonly contribute (114). Favorable outcome relies on early control of sepsis, adequate nutritional support, and skin protection. Enterocutaneous fistulas have traditionally been associated with a high risk of morbidity and death, related to sepsis, malnutrition, fluid, electrolyte, or metabolic disturbance (114).

High fistula output is defined by fluid loss of more than 500 mL/day and low output by fluid loss of less than 500 mL/day (115). Of 277 patients with enterocutaneous fistulas reported by Hollington et al. (114), 103 were high output fistulas, 164 were low-output fistulas, and 10 were not recorded. The small intestine was the most common source of fistulization; the ileum was involved in 128 patients, the duodenum or jejunum in 53, unclassified small bowel in 33, stomach in 1, and colon in 47, site not recorded in 15 patients.

Early and aggressive treatment of sepsis is very important (114,116,117), as the sepsis caused the majority of deaths in 23 of 30 patients in the series of Hollington et al (114). Similarly, adequate nutritional support is recognized as a key factor in reducing mortality rate associated with both conservative and operative management. Fistula output, mortality, and spontaneous closure rates are all improved with nutritional support (114,116,117).

Definitive surgical management is performed only after restitution of normal physiology and nutritional improvement, usually after at least six months, but often for longer periods. Signs that enough time has lapsed (mature of the fistula) are the return of a "soft" abdomen, as well as prolapse of the fistulating bowel, indicating the formation of neopertioneum, and with any residual induration being limited to the perifistula region. All diseased bowel is resected and renanstomosis only performed between healthy ends, irrespective of the amount of bowel lost (114). In malignant fistulas, an en bloc radical excision of both the primary and secondary organs is indicated (118).

Patients with coloduodenal or colojejunal fistulas caused by carcinoma of the colon should have colonic resection with en bloc resection of the fistula and the other organs involved. This even may mean performing a Whipple procedure (118).

Surgery for radiation-induced colorectal fistulas can be difficult. In severe cases, the colorectal and adjacent organs are matted together with no natural planes, making mobilization and resection hazardous. In this situation, a diverting proximal colostomy or ileostomy is advisable. In milder cases where resection can be safely performed, a descending anal anastomosis with or without a colonic J pouch can be performed. Detailed management of radiation injury to the intestine is described in Chapter 31.

REFERENCES

1. Buechter KJ, Boustany C, Caillouette R, Cohn I Jr. Surgical management of the acutely obstructed colon. A review of 127 cases. Am J Surg 1988; 156:163–168.
2. Serpell JW, McDermott FT, Katrivessis H, Hughes ESR. Obstructing carcinomas of the colon. Br J Surg 1989; 76:965–969.
3. Phillips RKS, Hittinger R, Fry JS, Fielding LP. Malignant large bowel obstruction. Br J Surg 1985; 72:296–302.
4. Kyllonen LEJ. Obstruction and perforation complicating colorectal carcinoma. Acta Chir Scand 1987; 153:607–614.
5. Ballantyne GH. Review of sigmoid volvulus. Clinical patterns and pathogenesis. Dis Colon Rectum 1982; 25:823–830.
6. Anderson MJ Sr., Okike N, Spencer RJ. The colonoscope in cecal volvulus: report of three cases. Dis Colon Rectum 1978; 21:71–74.
7. Nivatvongs S, Vermeulen FD, Fang DT. Colonoscopic decompression of acute pseudo-obstruction of the colon. Ann Surg 1982; 196:598–600.
8. Vanek VW, Al-Saeti M. Acute pseudo-obstruction of the colon (Ogilvie's syndrome). An analysis of 400 cases. Dis Colon Rectum 1986; 29:203–210.
9. Trevisani GT, Hyman NH, Church JM. Neostigmine safe and effective treatment for acute colonic pseudo-obstruction. Dis Colon Rectum 2000; 43: 599–603.
10. Kahi CJ, Rex DK. Bowel obstruction and pseudo-obstruction. Gastroenterol Clin N Am 2003; 32:1229–1247.
11. Bar-Ziv J, Solomon A. Computed tomography in adult intussusception. Gastrointest Radiol 1991; 16:264–266.
12. Azar T, Berger DL. Adult intussusception. Ann Surg 1997; 226:134–138.
13. Begos DG, Sander A, Modlin IM. The diagnosis and management of adult intussusception. Am J Surg 1997; 173:88–94.
14. Hilzenrat Z, Spanier A, Lamourex F, Bloom C, Sherker A. Colonic obstruction secondary to sarcoidosis: nonsurgical diagnosis and management. Gatroenterology 1995; 108:1556–1559.
15. Harris NL, McNeely WF, Shepard JO, Ebeling SH, Ellender SM, Peters CC. Case records of the Massachusetts General Hospital case 26–2002. N Engl J Med 2002; 347:601–606.
16. Stewart J, Finan PJ, Courtney DF, Brennan TG. Does a water-soluble contrast enema assist in the management of acute large bowel obstruction: a prospective study of 117 cases. Br J Surg 1984; 71:799–801.
17. Iko BO, Teal JS, Siram SM, Chinwuba CE, Roux VJ, Scott VF. Computed tomography of adult colonic intussusception: clinical and experimental studies. Am J Roentgenol 1984; 143:769–772.
18. Neff CC, van Sonnenberg E. CT of diverticulitis. Diagnosis and treatment. Radiol Clin North Am 1989; 27:743–752.
19. Chang FY, Cheng JT, Lai KH. Colonoscopic diagnosis of ileocolic intussusception in an adult. S Afr Med J 1990; 77:313–314.
20. Geller A, Petersen BT, Gostout CJ. Endoscopic decompression for acute colonic pseudo-obstruction. Gastrointest Endosc 1996; 44:144–150.
21. Ponec RJ, Saunder MD, Kimmey MB. Neostigmine for the treatment of acute colonic pseudo-obstruction. N Engl J Med 1991; 341:137–141.
22. Schermer CR, Hanush JJ, Davis M, Pitcher DE. Ogilvie's syndrome in the surgical patient: A new therapeutic modality. J Gastrointest Surg 1999; 3:173–177.
23. Duh QY, Way LW. Diagnostic laparoscopy and laparoscopic cecostomy for colonic pseudo-obstruction. Dis Colon Rectum 1993; 36:65–70.
24. Krukowski ZH, Matheson NA. Emergency surgery-for diverticular disease complicated by generalized and fecal peritonitis: a review. Br J Surg 1984; 71:921–927.
25. Killingback M. Management of perforative diverticulitis. Surg Clin North Am 1983; 63:97–115.
26. Badia JM, Sitges-Serra A, Pla J, Rague JM, Rogueta F, Sitges-Creus A. Perforation of colonic neoplasms. A review of 36 cases. Int J Colorectal Dis 1987; 2:187–189.
27. Mandava N, Kumar S, Pizzi WF, Aprile IJ. Perforated colorectal carcinomas. Am J Surg 1996; 172:236–238.
28. Softley A, Clamp SE, Bouchier IAD, Myren J, Watkinson G, De-Dombal FT. Perforation of the intestine in inflammatory bowel disease. An OMGE survey. Scand J Gastroenterol 1988; 23(suppl 144):24–26.
29. Abascal J, Diaz-Rojas F, Jorge J. Free perforation of the small bowel in Crohn's disease. World J Surg 1982; 6:200–216.
30. Bundred NJ, Dixon JM, Lumsden AB, Gilmour HM, Davies GC. Free perforation in Crohn's colitis. A ten-year review. Dis Colon Rectum 1985; 28:35–37.
31. Heppell J, Farkouh E, Dube S, Peloquin A, Morgan S, Bernard D. Toxic megacolon. An analysis of 70 cases. Dis Colon Rectum 1986; 29:789–792.
32. Wexner SD, Dailey TH. The initial management of left lower quadrant peritonitis. Dis Colon Rectum 1986; 29:635–638.
33. Kriwanek S, Armbruster C, Dittrich K, Beckerhinn P. Perforated colorectal cancer. Dis Colon Rectum 1996; 39:1409–1414.
34. Kriwanek S, Armbruster C, Beckerhinn P, Dittrich K. Prognostic factors for survival in colonic perforation. Int J Colorectal Dis 1994; 9:158–162.
35. Mulholland MW, Delaney JP. Neutropenic colitis and aplastic anemia: a new association. Ann Surg 1983; 197:84–90.
36. Wade DS, Douglass H Jr., Nava HR, Piedmonte M. Abdominal pain in neutropenic patients. Arch Surg 1990; 125:1119–1127.
37. Bodey GP, Buckley M, Sathe YS, Freireich EJ. Quantitative relationships between circulating leukocytes and infection in patients with acute leukemia. Ann Intern Med 1996; 64:328–340.
38. Cooke JV. Acute leukemia in children. JAMA 1993; 101:432–435.
39. Moir DM, Bale PM. Necropsy findings in childhood leukemia emphasizing neutropenic enterocolitis and cerebral calcification. Pathology 1976; 8:247–258.
40. Keidan RD, Fanning J, Gatenby RA Weese JL. Recurrent typhlitis. A disease resulting from aggressive chemotherapy. Dis Colon Rectum 1989; 32:206–209.
41. Kernagis LY, Levine MS, Jacobs JE. Pneumatosis intestinals: correlation of CT findings with viability of the bowel. Am J Roent 2003; 180:733–736.
42. Bliziotis IA, Michalopoulos A, Kasiakou SK, et al. Ciprofloxacin vs. an aminoglycoside in combination with a β-lactam for the treatment of febrile neutropenia: A meta-analysis of randomized controlled trials. Mayo Clin Proc 2005; 80:1146–1156.
43. Cunnigham SC, Fakhry K, Bass BL, Napolitano LM. Neutropeniz enterocolitis in adults: Case series and review of the literates. Dif Dis Sci 2005; 50:215–220.
44. Margulis AR, Heinbecker P, Bernard HR. Operative mesenteric arteriography in the search for the site of bleeding in unexplained gastrointestinal hemorrhage. Surgery 1960; 48:534–539.
45. Baum S, Nusbaum MH, Blakemore WS. The preoperative radiographic demonstration of intra-abdominal bleeding from undetermined sites by percutaneous selective celiac and superior mesenteric arteriography. Surgery 1965; 58:797–805.
46. Boley SJ, Sammartano R, Adams A, DiBiase A, Kleinhaus S, Sprayregen S. On the nature and etiology of vascular ectasias of the colon. Degenerative lesions of aging. Gastroenterology 1977; 72:650–660.
47. Church JM. Angiodysplasia. Semin Colon Rectal Surg 1994; 5:43–49.
48. Roberts PL, Schoetz DJ Jr, Coller JA. Vascular ectasia. Diagnosis and treatment by colonoscopy. Am Surg 1988; 54:56–59.
49. Jensen DM, Machicado GA. Endoscopic diagnosis and treatment of bleeding colonic angiomas and radiation telangiectasia. Perspect Colon Rect Surg 1989; 2:99–113.
50. McGuire HH Jr, Haynes BW Jr. Massive hemorrhage from diverticulosis of the colon: Guidelines for therapy based on bleeding patterns observed in fifty cases. Ann Surg 1972; 175:847–855.
51. Casarella WJ, Galloway SJ, Taxin RN. "Lower" gastrointestinal tract hemorrhage: New concepts based on arteriography. Am J Roentgenol 1974; 121:357–368.
52. McGuire HH Jr. Bleeding colonic diverticula. A reappraisal of natural history and management. Ann Surg 1994; 220:653–656.
53. Noer RJ, Hamilton JE, Williams DJ. Rectal hemorrhage: Moderate and severe. Ann Surg 1962; 155:794–805.
54. Bokhari M, Vernava AM, Ure T, Longo WE. Diverticular hemorrhage in the elderly—Is it well tolerated? Dis Colon Rectum 1996; 39:191–195.
55. Meyer MA, Alonso DR, Gray GF, Baer JW. Pathogenesis of bleeding colonic diverticulosis. Gastroenterology 1976; 71:577–583.
56. Leitman IM, Paull DE, Shires GT III. Evaluation and manage ment of massive lower gastrointestinal hemorrhage. Ann Surg 1989; 209:175–580.
57. Rossini FP, Ferrari A, Spandre M, et al. Emergency colonoscopy. World J Surg 1989; 13:190–192.
58. Chou YH, Hsu SE, Wang CY, Chen CL, How SW. Ischemic colitis as a cause of massive lower gastrointestinal bleeding and peritonitis. Report of five cases. Dis Colon Rectum 1989; 32:1065–1070.
59. Robert JH, Sachar DB, Aufses AH, Greenstein AJ. Management of severe hemorrhage in ulcerative colitis. Am J Surg 1990; 159:550–555.
60. Renison DM, Forouhar FA, Levine JB, Breiter JR. Filiform polyposis of the colon presenting as massive hemorrhage: An uncommon complication of Crohn's disease. Am J Gastroenterol 1983; 78:413–416.
61. Robert JR, Sachar DB, Greenstein AJ. Severe gastrointestinal hemorrhage in Crohn's disease. Ann Surg 1991; 213:207–211.
62. Cirocco WC, Reilly JC, Rusin LC. Life-threatening hemorrhage and exsanguination from Crohn's disease. Report of four cases. Dis Colon Rectum 1995; 38:85–95.
63. Gostout CJ. Acute gastrointestinal bleeding—A common problem revisited. Mayo Clin Proc 1988; 63:596–604.
64. Aijebreen AM, Fallone CA, Barkun AN. Nasogastric aspirate predicts high-risk endoscopic lesions in patients with acute upper- GI bleeding. Gastrointest Endosc 2004; 59:172–178.
65. Forde KA, Webb WA. Acute lower gastrointestinal bleeding. Perspect Colon Rectal Surg 1988; 1(1):105–112.
66. Bentley DE, Richardson JD. The role of tagged red blood cell imaging in the localization of gastrointestinal bleeding. Arch Surg 1991; 126:821–824.
67. Nicholson ML, Neoptolemos JP, Sharp JF, Wafkin EM, Fossard DP. Localization of lower gastrointestinal bleeding using in vivo technetium-99m-labelled red blood cell scintigraphy. Br J Surg 1989; 76:358–361.
68. Ryan P, Styles CB, Chmiel R. Identification of the site of severe colon bleeding by technetium-labeled red-cell scan. Dis Colon Rectum 1992; 35:219–222.
69. Suzman MS, Talmor M, Jennis R, Binkert B, Barie P. Accurate localization and surgical management of active lower gastrointestinal hemorrhage with technetium-labeled erythrocyte scintigraphy. Ann Surg 1996; 224:29–36.
70. Junguera R, Quiroga S, Saperas E, et al. Accuracy of helical computed tomographic angiography for the diagnosis of colonic angiodysplasia. Gastroenterology 2000; 119:293–299.

71. Horton KM, Fishman EK. CT angiography of the G1 tract. Gastrointest Endosc 2002; 55:537–541.
72. Khanna A, Ognibene SJ, Koniaris LG. Embolization as first-line therapy for diverticulosis-related massive lower gastrointestinal bleeding: Evidence from a meta-analysis. J Gastrointest Surg 2005; 9:343–352.
73. Athanasoulis CA. Angiography in the management of patients with gastrointestinal bleeding. Adv Surg 1983; 16:1–20.
74. Boley SJ, DiBiase A, Brandt LJ, Sammartano RJ. Lower intestinal bleeding in the elderly. Am J Surg 1979; 137:57–64.
75. Zuckerman DA, Bocchini TP. The role of angiography in the diagnosis and treatment of vascular disorders of the lower gastrointestinal tract. Semin Colon Rectal Surg 1994; 5:15–26.
76. Jensen DM, Machicado GA. Diagnosis and treatment of severe hematochezia. The role of urgent colonoscopy after purge. Gastroenterology 1988; 95:1569–1574.
77. Gostout CJ, Wang KK, Ahlquist DA, et al. Acute gastrointestinal bleeding. Experience of a specialized management team. J Clin Gastroenterol 1992; 14: 260–267.
78. Margolin DA, Opelka FG. The role of radionuclide scintigraphy in the management of lower gastrointestinal bleeding. Semin Colon Rectal Surg 1997; 8: 156–160.
79. Colacchio TA, Forde KA, Patsos TJ, Nunez D. Impact of modern diagnostic methods in the management of active rectal bleeding—Ten year experience. Am J Surg 1982; 143:607–610.
80. Britt LG, Warren L, Moore OF III. Selective management of lower gastrointestinal bleeding. Am Surg 1983; 49:121–125.
81. Browder W, Cerise EJ, Litwin MS. Impact of emergency angiography in massive lower gastrointestinal bleeding. Ann Surg 1986; 204:530–536.
82. Parkes BM, Obeid FN, Sorensen VJ, Horst HM, Fath JJ. The management of massive lower gastrointestinal bleeding. Am Surg 1993; 59:676–678.
83. Klas JV, Madoff RD. Surgical options in lower gastrointestinal bleeding. Semin Colon Rectal Surg 1997; 8:172–177.
84. Bowden TA Jr., Hooks VH III, Mansberger AR Jr. Intraoperative gastrointestinal endoscopy. Ann Surg 1980; 191:680–687.
85. Lau WY, Wong SY, Yuen WK, Wong KK. Intraoperative enteroscopy for bleeding angiodysplasias of small intestine. Surg Gynecol Obstet 1989; 168: 341–347.
86. Szold A, Katz LB, Lewis BS. Surgical approach to occult gastrointestinal bleeding. Am J Surg 1992; 163:90–93.
87. Farner R, Lichliter N, Kuhn J, Fisher T. Total colectomy versus limited colonic resection for acute lower gastrointestinal bleeding. Am J Surg 1999; 178:587–591.
88. Giafrancisco JA, Abcarian H. Pitfalls in the treatment of massive lower gastrointestinal bleeding with "blind" subtotal colectomy. Dis Colon Rectum 1982; 25:441–445.
89. Farrands PA, Taylor I. Management of acute lower gastrointestinal hemorrhage in a surgical unit over a 4-year period. J R Soc Med 1987; 80:79–82.
90. Setya V, Singer JA, Minken SL. Subtotal colectomy as a last resort for unrelenting, unlocalized, lower gastrointestinal hemorrhage experience with 12 cases. Am Surg 1992; 58:295–299.
91. Bender JS, Wiencek RG, Bouwman DL. Morbidity and mortality following total abdominal colectomy for massive lower gastrointestinal bleeding. Am Surg 1991; 57:536–541.
92. Terry BG, Beart RW Jr. Emergency colectomy with primary anastomosis. Dis Colon Rectum 1981; 24:1–4.
93. Pollard SG, Macfarlane R, Greatorex R, Everett WG, Hartfoll WG. Colovesical fistula. Ann R Coll Surg Engl 1987; 69:163–165.
94. Foster CE III, Lefor AT. General management of gastrointestinal fistulas. Recognition, stabilization, and correction of fluid and electrolyte imbalances. Surg Clin North Am 1996; 76:1019–1033.
95. Woods RJ, Lavery IC, Fazio VW, Jagelman DG, Weakley FL. Internal fistulas in diverticular disease. Dis Colon Rectum 1988; 31:591–596.
96. Fazio VW, Church JM, Jagelman DG, et al. Colocutaneous fistulas complicating diverticulitis. Dis Colon Rectum 1987; 30:89–94.
97. McIntyre PB, Ritchie JK, Hawley PR, Bartram CI, Lennard-Jones JE. Management of enterocutaneous fistulas: a review of 132 cases. Br J Surg 1984; 71:293–296.
98. Welch JP, Warshaw AL. Malignant duodenocolic fistulas. Am J Surg 1977; 133:658–661.
99. Torosian MH, Zins JE, Rombeau JL. Malignant colojejunal fistula: Case report and review of malignant coloenteric fistula. Dis Colon Rectum 1982; 25: 222–224.
100. Zera RT, Bubrick MP, Sternquist JC, Hitchcock CR. Enterocutaneous fistulas. Effects of total parenteral nutrition and surgery. Dis Colon Rectum 1983; 26:109–112.
101. Lavery IC. Colonic fistulas. Surg Clin North Am 1996; 76:1183–1190.
102. McNamara MJ, Fazio VW, Lavery IC, Weakley FL, Farmer RG. Surgical treatment of enterovesical fistulas in Crohn's disease. Dis Colon Rectum 1990; 33:271–276.
103. Michelassi F, Stella M, Balestracci T, Giuliante F, Marogna P, Block GE. Incidence, diagnosis, and treatment of enteric and colorectal fistula in patients with Crohn's disease. Ann Surg 1993; 318:660–666.
104. Solem CA, Loftus EV, Tremaine WJ, Peruberton JH, Wolff BG, Saudborn WJ. Fistulas to the urinary system in Crohn's disease: clinical features and outcomes. Am J Gastroenterol 2002; 97:2300–2305.
105. Keighley MRB, Heyen F, Winslet MC. Enterocutaneous fistulas and Crohn's disease. Acta Gastroenterol Belg 1987; 50:580–600.
106. Hawker PL, Givel JC, Keighley MRB, Alexander-Williams J, Allan RN. Management of enterocutaneous fistulae in Crohn's disease. Gut 1983; 24:284–287.
107. Pontari MA, McMillen MA, Garvey RH, Ballantyne GH. Diagnosis and treatment of enterovesical fistulae. Am Surg 1992; 58:258–265.
108. Labs JD, Sarr mg, Fishman EK, Siegelman SS, Cameron JL. Complications of acute diverticulitis of the colon: Improved early diagnosis with computerized tomography. Am J Surg 1988; 155:331–336.
109. Thomas HA. Radiologic investigation and treatment of gastrointestinal fistulas. Surg Clin North Am 1996; 76:1081–1094.
110. Schreyer AG, Seitz J, Feuerbach S, Rogler G, Herfarth H. Modern imaging using computer tomography and magnetic resonance imaging for inflammatory bowel disease CIBD. Inflamm Bowel Dis 2004; 10:45–54.
111. Bernini A, Spencer MP, Wong WD, Rothenberger DA, Madoff RD. Computed tomography-guided percutaneous abscess drainage in intestinal disease: factors associated with outcome. Dis Colon Rectum 1997 40(9):1009–1013.
112. Daniels IR, Bekdash B, Scott HJ, Marks CG, Donaldson DR. Diagnostic lessons learnt from a series of enterovesical fistulae. Colorectal Dis 2002; 4:459–462.
113. Solkar MH, Forshaw MJ, Sankararajah D, Stewart M, Parker MC. Colovesical fistula—Is a surgical approach always justified? Colorectal Dis 2005; 7: 467–471.
114. Hollington P, Mawlsley J, Lime W, Gabe SM, Forbes GA, Urindsor AJ. An 11-year experience of enterocutaneous fistula. Br J Surg 2004; 91:1646–1651.
115. Sitges-Serra A, Jaurrieta E, Sitges-ceus A. Management of postoperative enterocutaneous fistulas. The role of parenteral nutrition and surgery. Br J Surg 1989; 69:147–150.
116. Simmang C. Intestinal fistulas. Clin Colon Rectal Surg 2003; 16:213–220.
117. Lynch AC, Delaney CP, Senagove AJ, Connor JT, Remgi FH, Fazio VW. Clinical outcome and factors predictive of recurrence after enterocutaneous fistula surgery. Ann Surg 2004; 240:825–831.
118. Munoz M, Nelson H, Harrington J, Tsiotos G, Devine R, Engen D. Management of acquired rectourinary fistulas. Outcome according to cause. Dis Colon Rectum 1998; 41:1230–1238.

36 Complications of Anorectal and Colorectal Operations

Santhat Nivatvongs

INTRODUCTION

Surgery of the anorectum and the colorectum is prone to the development of complications. Not only is the colon a source of infection, but also improper operative technique can easily cause ischemia, which may result in a leak or a stricture. Operation changes both the anatomy and the physiology of the large bowel. Knowledge of the complications of each procedure is essential, particularly the causes, methods of management, and means of prevention. This chapter is not intended to cover all the complications of anorectal and colorectal operations but to highlight the complications commonly seen or the complications that are uncommon but important ones.

EARLY COMPLICATIONS OF ANORECTAL OPERATIONS

■ BLEEDING

Early postoperative bleeding, which is usually the result of a technical error, is not common. The most common early bleeding is from the external hemorrhoidal area and, therefore, can be detected easily and controlled by placement of a suture; the suturing can be performed at bedside or in a treatment room with local anesthetic used. In other cases, the patient should be returned to the operating room, where the anorectum is examined with the patient under local, regional, or general anesthesia as appropriate. Acute bleeding from the anal canal usually is from insecure stick tying of the hemorrhoidal or fistulotomy pedicles.

■ SEVERE ANAL PAIN

For most patients, the pain following anorectal operations is moderate and requires analgesics during the first 1 to 2 postoperative days. Intolerable pain despite adequate analgesics is uncommon. However, because such pain may be a sign of a perianal hematoma, inspection of the anal wound is required. Even a light dressing around the anus may aggravate the pain, and so it should be removed a few hours after the operation. Anorectal packing has no place in modern anorectal surgery. Warm heat directed toward the perineum will help to relieve the pain during the first 24 hours after operation. The next day warm sitz baths can be used as treatment. Most pain following hemorrhoidectomy comes from anal sphincter spasm. Another source of pain is the closure of the anoderm and anal verge with tension. It is better to leave the wound open than to close it with tension. It has been suggested, but not proven, that anal stretching and sphincterotomy may decrease postoperative pain. However, the risk of anal incontinence makes this practice undesirable. Furthermore, dilatation when added to hemorrhoidectomy does not improve the cure rate of hemorrhoids when compared to hemorrhoidectomy alone (1).

■ URINARY RETENTION

To minimize urinary retention, a preoperative assessment with good history taking will identify patient with voiding problems such as prostatic, pertrophy, an000d urethral stricture. These should corrected prior to embarking on an elective rectal procedure.

Urinary retention after hemorrhoidectomy is common, but it is unusual following fistulotomy and lateral internal sphincterotomy. Following hemorrhoidectomy, urinary retention has been reported to be as low as 3.5% to 10% if the patient is given a limited amount of intravenous fluid during the operation (2,3). A retrospective review of 1026 patients who underwent anal operative care over a 5-year period at the Mayo Clinic, revealed a urinary retention of 34% for hemorrhoidectomy, 4% for internal sphincterotomy, 5% for incision and drainage of perianal abscesses, and 2% for fistulotomy. Anorectal surgery may dull the sacral parasympathetic nerve fibers controlling contraction of the detrusor muscle of the bladder. Pain from surgery may stimulate the sympathetic nerve, to the urethral sphincter causing spasms (5).

The rationale of fluid restriction is to avoid distention of the bladder for as long as possible because many patients are unable to void for several hours after anorectal operations. Friend and Medwell (6) have shown that for hemorrhoidectomy in an outpatient setting, urinary retention is uncommon (1%) and that it is not related to the amount of the fluid given during the procedure. The type of anesthesia does not seem to affect urinary retention. The reason for the low incidence of urinary retention in the outpatient setting is unclear, but could involve the psychological effect of the home or hotel environment. The author believe that if the excises are not beyond the anorectal ring, urinary retention is uncommon. Witness the rare urinary retention in a transsphincteric fistulotomy in which the pain is significant. Witness the frequent urinary relation in a transanal excision of low rectum in which there is almost no pain.

Using no catheterization, unless the bladder is markedly distended, may endanger the bladder single episode of overdistention of the bladder produce chronic changes of irreversible damage to the detrusor muscle (7). Avoidance of acute bladder overdistention by the judicious use of sterile intermittent catheterization in the postoperative period would appear to involve a low risk of inducing bacteremia and may prevent bladder decompensation (8). Using bethanechol chloride (Urecholine) to stimulate the detrusor muscle does not help to prevent or correct urinary retention after hemorrhoidectomy (9,10). Similarly, using prazosin, an α-adrenergic blocker, to release the bladder neck spasm is also not effective (11).

For practicality, all patients should void just before undergoing operation. The intravenous fluid during surgery as well as the first few hours after the operation should be limited to 300 mL. Patients should not be pushed or rushed to void, which may cause anxiety. Anal dressing should be removed and a pad used instead.

■ FEVER, BACTEREMIA, AND LIVER ABSCESS

It is common for a patient to have a transient low-grade fever after anorectal operations, particularly hemorrhoidectomy, usually during the first one to two days. This could be in response to the anal wound. Despite an unprepared bowel and the fecal load, abscess formation following anorectal operations is rare. In a series of 500 closed hemorrhoidectomies reported on by Buls and Goldberg (3), there were no abscesses recorded. In a study by Bonardi et al.

(12), 36 patients had serial blood drawn every six hours for 24 hours after hemorrhoidectomy; 39% of the patients developed a fever above 99°F (37.2°C) in the first six hours, 67% between 99°F (37.2° C) and 101°F (38.3°C), and one patient had a temperature higher than 101°F (38.3°C). Three patients (8%) had positive blood cultures in the immediate postoperative samples but none in the subsequent samples. The significance of fever and bacteremia after hemorrhoidectomy is probably trivial because none of the patients developed further septic complications.

Inpatients with high fever, other signs of sepsis such as chills, leukocytosis, malaise, and jaundice may be signs of serious complications. Parikh et al. (13) reported that two cases of liver abscesses occurred within one week after an uncomplicated hemorrhoidectomy. In both cases, the diagnosis was confirmed by computed tomography (CT) scan of the abdomen and both were successfully treated with CT-guided percutaneous drainage and antibiotics. The bacteria found were *Streptococcus viridans*, *Peptostreptococcus*, and *Klebsietlla pneumoniae*. Pyogenic liver abscess after hemorrhoidectomy is extremely rare. Only four cases have been reported. It is important to be aware of the possibility, because the mortality rate of undrained liver abscesses is between 94% and 100%. Even with treatment, the mortality rate reached 20%.

DELAYED COMPLICATIONS OF ANORECTAL OPERATIONS

Delayed complications are defined as those that occur more than 1 week after the operation. Most patients would have been discharged from the hospital by that time.

BLEEDING

Delayed massive bleeding occurs in 0.8% to 4% of patients after hemorrhoidectomy, usually between 4 and 14 days (3,14,15). The rate of occurrence is much lower for other anorectal procedures. It has been speculated that the bleeding is caused by the breakdown of the granulating wound during defecation or by infection disrupting the blood vessels and the pedicle of the wound in the anal canal. The patient should be admitted to the hospital and given appropriate intravenous fluids. Patients may be in shock, and some patients may require blood transfusions (15). Of note is that one third of patients with posthemorrhoidectomy bleeding were being anticoagulated with medication such as acetylsalicylic acid (ASA), nonsteroidal anti-inflammatory drugs (NSAIDs), or warfarin (Coumadin) in the series reported by Rosen et al. (15).

Most, bleeding stops after bed rest. If bleeding continues, some surgeons use a 30 mL balloon Foley catheter to create a tamponade of the anal canal (16). However, this method is crude and may cause severe anorectal pain. Rosen et al. (15) successfully treated delayed posthemorrhoidectomy bleeding with packing in 20 of 20 patients. They used a rolled, slightly moistened absorbable gelatin sponge (Gelfoam) packing in the anal canal. However, late complications requiring reoperation developed in 15%.

I prefer taking the patient to the operating room, where the anal canal can be explored with the patient under local, regional, or general anesthesia. Hemostasis is controlled with 3–0 Vicryl or Dexon sutures. Frequently, after all blood clots have been removed, the bleeding point cannot be identified except for a friable anal wound. In these situations, a deep stick-tie should be placed at the pedicle of the anal wound; if oozing blood is noted, the suture line should be redone. Besides providing an immediate control of bleeding, cleaning the anorectum stops the patients from passing old blood, which often makes it difficult to tell whether the bleeding has stopped.

In a high-risk group of patients for postoperative bleeding, such as patients who are on chronic hemodialysis, a well-planned anorectal procedure, including hemorrhoidectomy, fistulotomy drainage of perianal abscess, and lateral internal sphincterotomy, can be safely performed. Sheikh et al. (17) performed these anorectal procedures in 18 patients with chronic renal failure; who were undergoing hemodialysis.

Two patients developed postoperative hemorrhage. Only one of them required surgical hemostasis in the operating room on the third postoperative day. None of the patients had delayed wound healing. The authors recommend certain measures to minimize the problems. The final preoperative dialysis should be performed within 24 hours. The bleeding diathesis in patients with chronic renal failure is due to a platelet defect that is corrected by dialysis. They recommend a template bleeding time assessment in addition to standard prothrombin time and partial thromboplastin time testing. Profound anemia (average, 6.1 g% in this series) is generally well tolerated by these patients. Preoperative transfusions to raise the hemoglobin level are usually unnecessary and even inadvisable, because transfusion subjects the patient to risk of potassium administration, congestive heart failure, and hepatitis. Intraoperative fluid administration should be severely restricted, and solutions containing potassium avoided. Arteriovenous fistula thrombosis is a frequent and troublesome complication requiring careful positioning of the involved area during surgery. Infusion or measuring blood pressure in that arm should be avoided. It is desirable to delay hemodialysis in the immediate postoperative period because heparin is required for the extracorporeal circuit (17).

FECAL IMPACTION

Many patients develop constipation after anorectal procedures, particularly hemorrhoidectomy, partly because of the fear of pain and the lack of the image to defecate. Patients who require a large amount of analgesics, particularly morphine, are also prone to constipation. Codeine is contraindicated in anorectal surgery because it severely disturbs the motility of the gastrointestinal tract. Prevention of constipation is the best treatment. Eating plenty fruits and vegetables along with other high-roof age foods is ideal advice. Psyllium seed preparations may not prove beneficial for all patients, especially if such preparations have not been prescribed preoperatively. Laxatives should be given early usually on the first postoperative day, and the dosage should be increased gradually to the maximum until the patient has a good bowel movement. Corman (18) found senna (Senokot) to be and efficient for this purpose. If chemical laxatives are unsuccessful, tap water enemas should be given. A reliable patient can follow instruction home, but it may be best to keep an unreliable patient in the hospital until a normal stool has been passed.

Fecal impaction may be difficult to diagnosis in the postoperative period. Usual symptoms are in creasing pain or pressure in the perineum and sometimes diarrhea from overflow of stool around the impaction. Pain out of proportion is a good indication of fecal impaction. Digital rectal examination will reveal a fecal bolus in the anorectum. If the pain is severe, the surgeon may use a small cotton swab lubricated with KY jelly instead of the finger. If the patient has fecal impaction, and laxatives and enemas have failed to work, it may be necessary to evacuate the impaction in the operating room with the patient under anesthesia. Tap water or other kinds of enemas often do not work in that situation because water cannot be passed into the rectum.

Fecal impaction is a serious complication following anorectal operations. Fortunately, it is uncommon. Impaction occurs in only 0.4% of patients, usually after hemorrhoidectomy (3). The low incidence should be credited to careful attention to bowel movements after anorectal operations, a common practice among colorectal surgeons.

■ ANAL WOUND ABSCESS

Despite continuing fecal contamination after operation, abscess in the anal wound is rare. In a report on 500 patients who underwent closed hemorrhoidectomy, Buls and Goldberg (3) recorded no abscesses. Walker et al. (19) reported a perianal abscess in 2% of 306 patients, following internal sphincterotomy for anal fissure and anal stenosis.

■ FECAL INCONTINENCE

Most patients experience some degree of incontinence, particularly of gas and liquid stool, after anorectal procedures for anal fissure, fistula-in-ano, and hemorrhoids. Anal sensation is partially impaired, leading to some degree of incontinence in up to 50% of patients after hemorrhoidectomy, but it usually resolves within 6 weeks (20). Persistent incontinence after operation for a transsphincteric or extrasphincteric fistulotomy may be improved by a sphincteroplasty (see Chapter 15).

■ ANAL STRICTURE

Stricture or narrowing of the anal canal after hemorrhoidectomy is the direct result of excising too much anoderm and mucosa. Even in circumferential prolapsed hemorrhoids, a standard three-quadrant hemorrhoidectomy is all that is necessary. The redundant mucosa can be trimmed, but there is no need to denude the anal canal.

Mild anal stricture can be treated by the surgeon with a Hegar dilator, or a rectal dilator can be inserted by the patient at home. Severe stricture will require a lateral internal sphincterotomy or a lateral sphincterotomy with an island flap anoplasty.

■ ANAL SKIN TAGS

Some excess skin around the anus does not cause any problem. After hemorrhoidectomy, the anal verge frequently becomes swollen and engorged with edema. On occasion, a thrombosed external hemorrhoid develops. With time, this swollen skin will partially resolve, and the patient is left with a residual skin tag. The skin tag may lead to irritation, discomfort, and difficulty in personal hygiene. Unless symptomatic, skin tags can be left alone; otherwise, a simple excision can be performed in the office with the patient under local anesthesia.

■ ECTROPION

Ectropion is a deformity of the anal canal characterized by protrusion of rectal mucosa through the anus at rest (Fig. 1). It is a complication resulting from an improperly performed Whitehead hemorrhoidectomy, in which the mucosa is pulled down to the anoderm for suturing instead of mobilizing the anoderm upward for suturing to the rectal mucosa (21). The mucosa secretes mucusa, which causes irritation and a "wet" anus. Excision with resuture of the mobilized skin into the upper anal canal may solve the problem. In most sever cases, an island flap anoplasty is the procedure of choice (Fig. 2).

■ MUCOSAL PROLAPSE

This is a late complication of hemorrhoidectomy resulting from inadequate excision of the redundant rectal mucosa or from the rectal mucosa being pulled down too far during suturing. In mild cases, rubber band ligation is effective. In severe cases, excision or anoplasty is necessary.

■ UNHEALED WOUND

Healing following a closed hemorrhoidectomy occurs rapidly. If the wound is closed without tension, it should heal completely within 2 weeks. If the wound is partially separated, it will take longer to heal. For open hemorrhoidectomy, the wound should heal within 4 to 6 weeks. Occasionally the wounds following both open and closed hemorrhoidectomy do not heal, leaving an unhealed ulcer. The same is true for fistulotomy wounds, which in most cases are open ones. Most of the unhealed wounds are found in the posterior midline of the anal canal. Initially

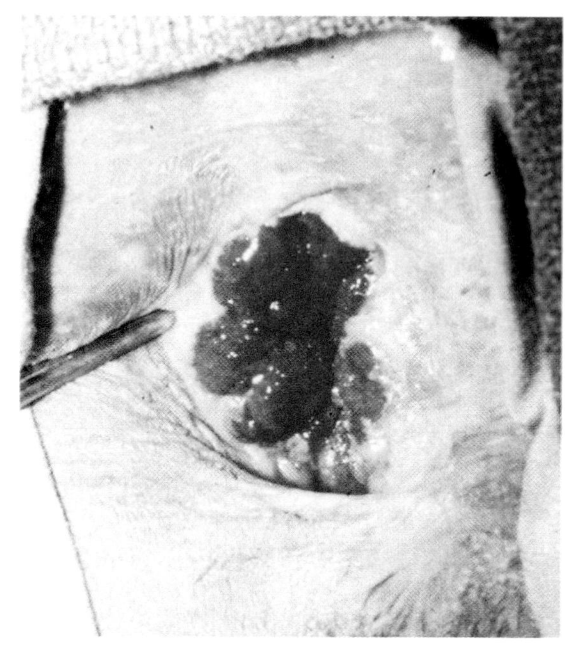

FIGURE 1 ■ Ectropion following a hemorrhoidectomy.

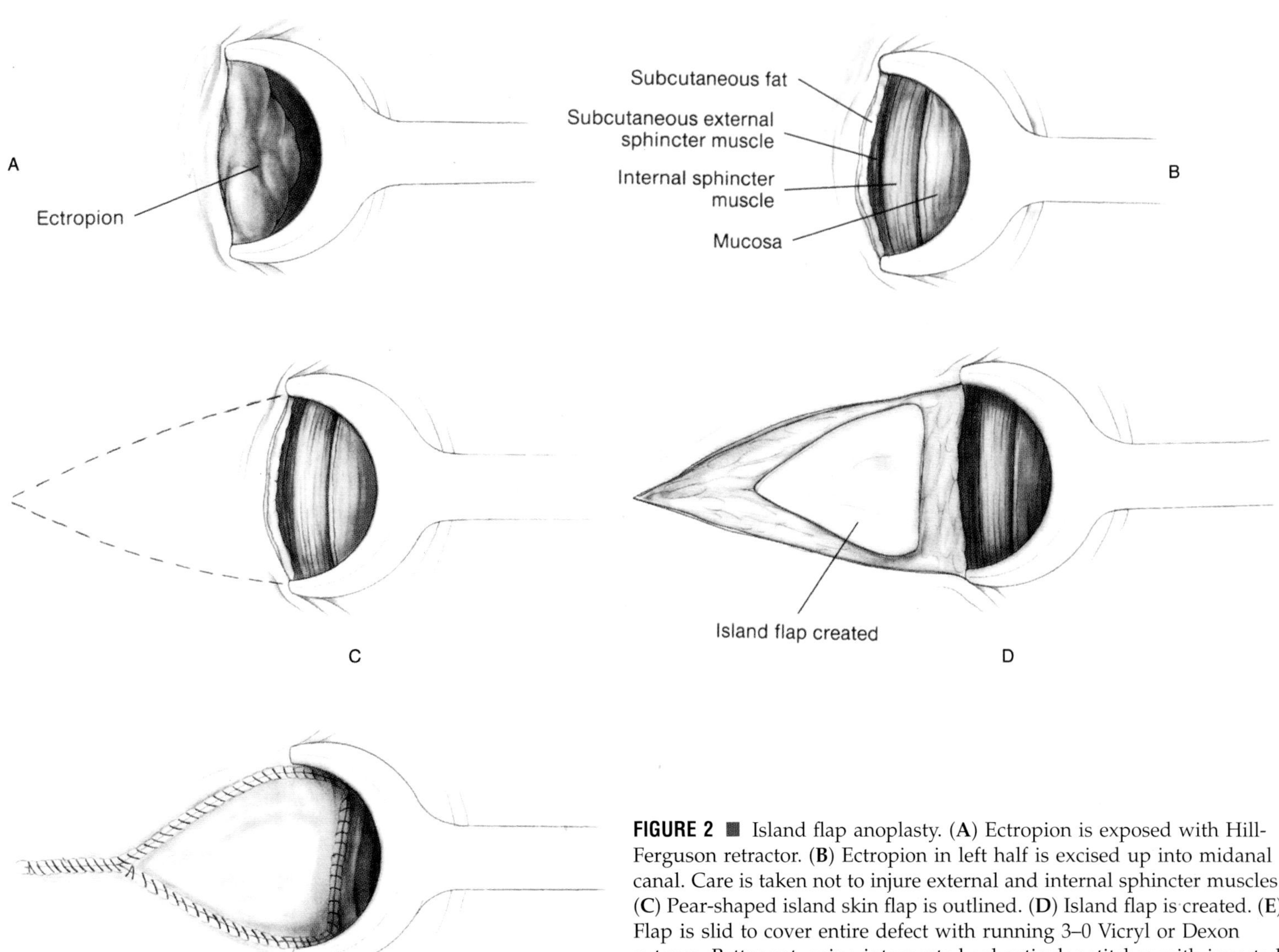

FIGURE 2 ■ Island flap anoplasty. (**A**) Ectropion is exposed with Hill-Ferguson retractor. (**B**) Ectropion in left half is excised up into midanal canal. Care is taken not to injure external and internal sphincter muscles. (**C**) Pear-shaped island skin flap is outlined. (**D**) Island flap is created. (**E**) Flap is slid to cover entire defect with running 3–0 Vicryl or Dexon sutures. Better yet, using interrupted subcuticular stitches with inverted knots, 3–0 PDS or Maxon, makes the wound heal neater. For circumferential ectropion, the other half is performed in same manner.

anal hygiene and curettage of granulation tissue should be tried. If this fails after several months of adequate local care, excision with a sliding skin flap to cover the wound should be performed. Because an unhealed wound that progresses may be an indication of Crohn's disease, a complete gastrointestinal investigation may be necessary.

COMPLICATIONS OF COLORECTAL OPERATIONS

■ THROMBOEMBOLISM IN INFLAMMATORY BOWEL DISEASE

Thromboembolism is a general complication that may follow any operation and as such will not be discussed here. However, because thromboembolism that occurs in inflammatory bowel disease (IBD) is unique, it is essential for surgeons to have some knowledge of this phenomenon and to recognize the problem.

The incidence of thromboembolism associated with IBD is 1% to 7% in various series (22). In autopsy studies, it has been reported as 7% to 39% (22). In a series from the Mayo Clinic, an incidence of 1.3% among 7199 patients with IBD was reported (23). Thromboembolism proved to be a grave complication in IBD patients because 25% of them died. In one autopsy series pulmonary embolism and venous thrombosis ranked third in frequency (9%) as a cause of death in patients with ulcerative colitis, behind peritonitis (38%), and malignant neoplasm (12%) (24).

Thromboses can be venous or arterial. These have been reported to be found in the brain, retinal arteries, mesenteric veins (25), portal veins (26), skin, and peipheral deep veins. Of 92 thromboembolic episodes in the Mayo Clinic series, 66% were peripheral or deep venous thromboses, pulmonary emboli, or both (23). Risk of thromboembolic complications seems to increase with increased disease activities, and thrombosis may recur with another episode. Of 113 patients with thromboembolic complications and other vasculitis, 72 (64%) had active disease at the time and 7 (6%) had a history of recurrent thromboembolic episodes with exacerbated IBD.

The mechanism of thrombosis in IBD is not clear. Most authors point to a hypercoagulable state associated with exacerbations of IBD, including thrombocytosis; elevations in factor V, fact VIII, and fibrinogen; and a decrease in antithrombin. In contrast, patients with inactive chronic IBD showed no evidence of coagulopathy that might predispose to clotting (22). A study by Hudson et al. (27) showed that the most consistent abnormality is an increase in plasma VII:C concentrations, particularly in patients with Crohn's disease. Increased concentrations of plasma VII:C might lead to complications such as microvascular damage and inflammation in the intestinal wall by augmenting focal fibrin deposition on the luminal surface of inflamed vessels. There is no evidence that the plasma VII:C concentration is an acute phase reactant.

No controlled trials of anticoagulation have been performed in patients with thrombosis associated with IBD. No data exist on the acute effects of colectomy on the course of thrombosis, and there are no comparisons of lasting medical treatment vs. immediate colectomy for thrombosis. In an autopsy series reported by Graef et al. (24), medically treated patients had a significantly higher incidence of venous thrombosis (45%) than those who underwent operation (29%). In the series reported by Talbot et al. (23) 15 stable patients underwent resection of diseased bowel after an episode of deep venous thrombosis or pulmonary embolism. None died postoperatively and, of the 13 patients who were followed up, 12 remain free of recurrent thrombosis 2 to 9 years later. Operation in the acute setting, however, actually may increase the risk of thrombosis and is no guarantee that further trouble will not develop.

The use of subcutaneous heparin for prophylaxis in hospitalized patients with acute IBD should be evaluated, with the judgment made against the risk of severe colonic bleeding. Using heparin may help to prevent thrombosis in the postoperative period. For patients with severe deep venous thrombosis of the lower extremities and the pelvis, a caval filter should be considered before colonic resection is performed.

■ SPLENIC INJURY

Operative injury to the spleen accounts for 20% to 40% of all splenectomies performed in hospitals, in the United States. Neither the incidence of this mishap nor its complications have lessened appreciably in the last three decades (28).

Splenic injury can occur during both colorectal operations (0.8%) and operations in which mobilization of the spleen is performed (3%) (29). The injury is invariably an avulsion of the splenic capsule caused by tearing the normal splenic attachments (i.e., gastrosplenic, splenocolic, phrenicosplenic, and phrenicocolic ligaments), or it may be caused by traction on the greater omentum. In one series, half of the splenic injuries were due to traction on an omental band leading to the spleen (29). Injury can occur even before mobilization of the splenic flexure. A common site of capsular tear is a small area (approximately 1 cm) on the anterior or medial aspect of the lower pole of the spleen. Often, there is a definite peritoneal band running medially from the lower pole of the spleen to the greater omentum and adjacent to the greater curvature of the stomach. The band does not become prominent until the stomach is drawn across to the right. Very little traction is needed to pull the band from the spleen and cause bleeding. This band, for which there seems to be no detailed description in most textbooks, usually will be noted if the surgeon looks for it. Lord and Gourevitch (30) have given it the name "lieno-omental band of peritoneum."

Another area where a splenic tear commonly occurs is the hilum. The greater omentum, as it passes to the left, becomes continuous with the gastrosplenic ligament. In most individuals the greater omentum divides, giving rise to an anterior sheet of omentum that hangs down as an apron of variable length from the greater curvature, partially marking the gastrosplenic ligament (30). This anterior or presplenic omental fold can be torn if the stomach or the greater omentum is pulled to the right.

To avoid capsular tear, these omental fold should be incised before any traction is placed on the greater omentum and stomach and before mobilization of the splenic flexure is begun. For save exploration of the left upper quadrant and mobilization of the splenic flexure, it is important cing to have adequate exposure and assistant help. Plato the patient in stirrups, with the operator standing between the patient's legs, will facilitate the procedure, especially in obese patients.

Every attempt should be made to save the spleen. Most capsular tears can be managed by compressing the bleeding points with microfibrillar collagen pledgets (e.g., Avitine). It may be necessary to completely mobilize the spleen in order to adequately compress it. A splenectomy is reserved as a last resort only. Most extensive iatrogenie splenic injuries can be controlled by a partial splenectomy. Morgenstern and Shapiro (31) have recommended the following very useful techniques: control of splenic vasculature and control of renchymatous bleeding.

Control of Splenic Vasculature

The entire spleen should be mobilized medially toward the anterior abdominal wall. The splenic artery is identified as it courses above the pancreas. This artery should be isolated and encircled with a vessel loop for occlusion if necessary. No attempt is made to isolate the fragile splenic veins. The use of vascular clamps for temporary control of the splenic pedicle is not advised because they produce trauma and may result in venous injury. The splenic arterial branches are carefully dissected at or near the splenic hilum. The most constant branch is the superior polar artery, which arises one to several centimeters from the hilum as the first branch of the splenic artery before it enters the spleen. For injury of the superior pole, the superior polar vessel is doubly tied with 2–0 silk. Tying the segmental artery results in almost immediate blanching of the dearterialized segment. Arteries to the lower pole of the spleen may be identified and ligated if branching takes place outside the spleen. For a lower pole injury, if segmental arteries cannot be identified, it may be necessary to tie the main splenic artery distal to the superior pole. Once the segmental branch or branches have been ligated, a scalpel incision is made into the splenic parenchyma at the line of demarcation.

Control of Parenchymatous Bleeding

If excessive bleeding occurs as the initial incision is made, partial control may be achieved by temporarily occluding the splenic artery with the thumb on the vessel loop. The dissection is performed with the back of the scalpel handle, a suction tip, or a peanut sponge. As the vessels are encountered, they are clipped and divided. Large segmental veins should be spared. Following the transection of the splenic parenchyma, a number of bleeding sites will remain. Arterial bleeders are grasped with forceps and clipped. If this is not successful, a figure-of-eight suture should be used. Open linear venous channels are controlled with running sutures. The residual sinusoidal bleeding can be controlled by the use of topical microfibrillar collagen pledgets. Electrocautery is unsatisfactory for maintaining splenic parenchymal hemostasis. However, occasionally it may be useful for minor capsular bleeding points. Heat-induced coagulum poses the threat of delayed bleeding when it sloughs. If such control cannot be achieved, through and through parenchymal sutures are necessary, with 2–0 chromic catgut used on a straight or curved gastrointestinal needle.

PREVENTION AND TREATMENT OF POSTSPLENECTOMY INFECTION

Fulminant, potentially life-threatening infection is a major long-term risk after splenectomy. Splenic macrophages have an important filtering and phagocytic role in removing bacteria and parasitized red blood cells from the circulation. Although the liver can perform this function in the absence of a spleen, higher levels of specific antibody and an intact complement system are probably required. The ability of a splenic patient to mount an adequate protective antibody response may relate more to the indication for or age at splenectomy and to the presence of underlying immune suppression than to the absence of the spleen.

Most instances of serious infection are due to encapsulated bacteria such as *Streptococcus pneumoniae* (pneumococcus), *Haemophilus influenzae* type B, and *Neisseria meningitidis* (meningoccocus). Pneumococcal infection is most common and carries a mortality rate of up to 60%. Infection with *H. influenzae* type B is much less common but nonetheless significant, particularly in children. Meningococcus may also be associated with serious infection. Other infections include *Escherichia coli,* malaria, babesiosis (a rare tick-borne infection), and *Capnoytophaga* canimorsus (DF-2 bacillus), which is associated with dog bites (32).

Pneumococcal Immunization

The current available polyvalent pneumococcal vaccine contains purified capsular polysaccharide from the 23 most prevalent serotypes. The vaccine is >90% effective in healthy adults under the age of 55 years. The patient should be immunized as soon as possible after recovery from the operation and before discharge from hospital. Immunization, however, should be delayed at least six months after immune-suppressive chemotherapy, during which time prophylactic antibiotics should be given. Reimmunization of asplenic patients is currently recommended every 5 to 10 years (32).

H. influenzae Type B Immunization

Most children in the United Kingdom, the United States, and Canada have received *H. influenzae* type B vaccine. Most patients older than 18 years of age will have acquired some immunity through natural exposure, but this may not provide adequate protection in the absence of a spleen. The need for reimmunization is unclear (32).

Meningococcal Immunization

Meningococcal immunization is not routinely recommended for asplenic patients except when traveling to areas where there is an increased risk of group A infection.

Influenza Immunization

Influenza vaccine is recommended yearly.

Antibiotic Prophylaxis

Amoxicillin has been recommended more recently. Phenoxymethyl penicillin is better tolerated in young children. Patients who are allergic to penicillin should be offered erythromycin (Table 1).

Lifelong prophylactic antibiotics should be offered in all cases, especially in the first two years after splenectomy, for all children 16 years of age or younger and when there is underlying impaired immune function. For patients not allergic to penicillin, a supply of amoxicillin should be kept at home and used immediately if infective symptoms of raised temperature, malaise, or shivering develop. Local resistance pattern may dictate the need to use other antibiotics, including for *H. influenzae*, which is not sensitive to phenoxymethyl penicillin or amoxicillin (32).

Treatment of Acute Infection

In suspected pneumococcal, meningococcal, or other serious infections, immediate medical attention is required. An immediate dose of intramuscular or intravenous benzylpenicillin is given before transfer to hospital, and then intravenous administration should be continued. Patients, who have been receiving antibiotic prophylaxis, those allergic to penicillin, those with possible resistant organisms, and children less than 5 years of age, should be given cefotaxime or ceftriaxone instead. Patients allergic to penicillin and who are also allergic to cephalosporins may be given chloramphenicol (32).

Key Guidelines (32)[a]:

1. All splenectomy patients and those with functional hyposplenism should receive pneumococcal immunization[b,c]
2. Documentation, communication, and reimmunization require attention[b,c]
3. Patients not previously immunized should receive *H. influenzae* type B vaccine[b,c]
4. Meningococcal immunization is not routinely recommended[c]
5. Influenza immunization may be beneficial
6. Lifelong prophylactic antibiotics are recommended (oral phenoxymethyl penicillin or an alternative)[b,c]
7. Asplenic patients are at risk for severe malaria[b]
8. Animal and tick bites may be dangerous[b]
9. Patients should be given a leaflet and a car alert health professionals to their risk for over whelming infection[b,c]
10. Patients developing infection despite measures must be given a systemic antibiotic and should be urgently admitted to hospital[b,c]

[a] There are no randomized controlled trials or case-control studies on this issue.

[b] Based on published evidence.

[c] Expert opinion.

TABLE 1 ■ Dosing Regimens for Antibiotic Prophylaxis and Treatment

Antibiotic	Oral Prophylaxis	Treatment for Suspected Infection[a]
Penicillin		
Adult	250–500 mg every 12 hr[b]	1.2 g every 4–6 hr
Child 5–14 yrs	250 mg every 12 hr[c]	200–300 mg/kg/day in six divided doses (maximum, 6 g)
Child < 5 yrs[d]	125 mg every 12 hr[c]	
Erythromycin (base)		
Adult or child > 8 yrs	250–500 mg/day	0.5–1.0 g every 6 hr by mouth or intravenously or 250 mg every 6 hr by mouth
Child 2–8 yrs	250 mg/day	12.5 mg/kg/day by mouth or intravenously by infusion in four divided doses
Child < 2 yrs	125 mg/day	12.5 mg/kg/day intravenously by infusion in four divided doses
Amoxicillin/co-Amoxiclav (doses according to amoxicillin content)		
Adult	250–500 mg/day	0.5–1.0 g every 8 hr by mouth or intravenously
Child 5–14 yrs	125 mg/day	250 mg every 8 hr by mouth or 90 mg/kg/day intravenously in three divided doses
Child 1–5 yrs	10 mg/kg/day	125 mg every 8 hr by mouth or 90 mg/kg/day intravenously in three divided doses
Child < 1 yrs	10 mg/kg/day	62.5 mg every 8 hr by mouth or 90 mg/kg/day intravenously in three divided doses
Cefotaxime		
Adult	Not suitable	2 g every 8 hr intravenously
Child < 14 yrs	Not suitable	100 mg/kg/day intravenously in three divided doses (maximum, 12 g)
Ceftriaxone		
Adult	Not suitable	1–2 g once daily intravenously
Child < 14 yrs	Not suitable	80 mg/kg/day intravenously in a single dose (maximum, 4 g)
Chloramphenicol (only patients allergic to penicillins and cephalosporins)		
All patients	Not suitable	Expert advice

[a]Established infection may require much higher doses given in the hospital.
[b]If compliance is a problem, 500 mg once daily is acceptable.
[c]Phenoxymethyl penicillin (oral).
[d]Benzylpenicillin (intravenous).
[e]Seek expert advice for neonatal doses.
Source: From Ref. 32.

■ PROGNOSIS OF COLORECTAL CARCINOMA IN ASPLENIC PATIENTS

It has been shown that splenectomy is associated with a significant decrease in survival of 5 years patients with Dukes' stage C colorectal adenocarcinoma. The mechanism responsible for this adverse impact of splenectomy is undefined (33).

■ PRESACRAL HEMORRHAGE

During mobilization of the rectum, presacral bleeding can occur if the presacral fascia is stripped and the presacral vein is torn. Although the bleeding is brisk, it usually can be controlled with packing, a stick-tie, or electrocautery, ballon tamponade, breast implant tamponade, and muscle fragment welding (34–38). Bleeding from the spongy bone of the sacrurm is usually mild and only a nuisance. On rare occasions, it can be massive and life threatening.

A study by Wang et al. (39) revealed that in 15% of Chinese patients the basivertebral vein connects the presacral vein and the internal vertebral vein and is usually located at the level of S3 to S5 (Fig. 3). Bleeding from this vein is not only massive but also cannot be controlled by packing, electrocautery, stick-tie, or occlusion with bone wax because of the high pressure. The only effective method of temporarily stopping this type of bleeding is occluding the bleeding point with the index finger. For the permanent arrest of this type of hemorrhage, a thumbtack can be used (40).

To be successful, the pin has to be driven into the hole in the sacrum to plug it. A thumbtack made of material compatible with the body, such as titanium, is preferred (40) (Figs. 4 and 5) (37). Other successful methods are also available. Xu and Lin (37) originally used a piece of rectus muscle fragment holding against the bleeding point of the perineal vein with a long forceps. The muscle was then indirectly electrocoagulated using high current until it melted and sealed the bleeding point. Harrison et al. (41)

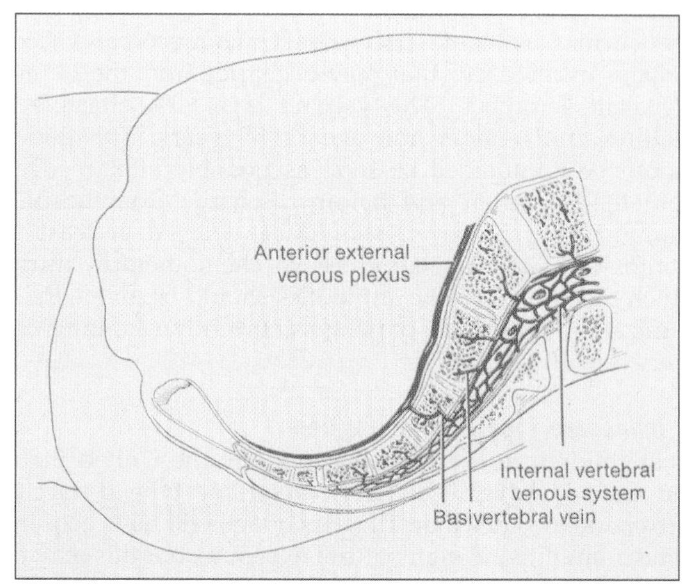

FIGURE 3 ■ Venous system of sacrum. *Source*: From Ref. 40.

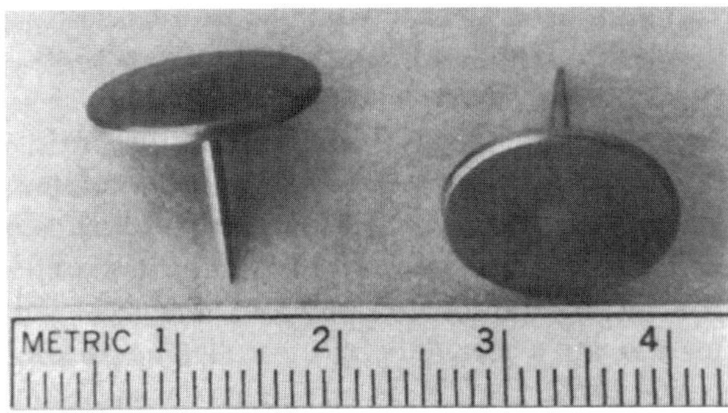

FIGURE 4 ■ Homemade titanium thumbtacks, not commercially available. Hemorrhage occluder pin, commercially available from Surgin Surgical Instrument, Inc. (Tustin, CA, U.S.A.), comes with set of two pins. *Source*: From Ref. 40.

successfully used this technique in 8 patients with basivertebral bleeding. Remzi et al. (42) harvested a 4 × 2 × 1 cm piece of rectus abdominus and sutured the presacral fascia onto the bleeding point to tamponade it. They reported success in two patients.

The diagnosis of bleeding from the basivertebral vein is not difficult. The blood rapidly fills the pelvis. The location is almost always between S3 and S5. The bleeding point can be felt with the index finger as a crater or an opening about 5 mm in size. This potentially fatal complication can be avoided by preserving the presacral fascia during mobilization of the rectum. Sharp dissection of the posterior rectum with scissors or electrocautery is recommended rather than conventional blunt dissection by hand.

■ ANASTOMOTIC BLEEDING

Early postoperative bleeding from a colorectal or an ileocolic anastomosis is uncommon regardless of whether the technique is a one layer anastomosis, a two layer anastomosis, or a stapled anastomosis, provided there is no bleeding diathesis. All techniques of anastomosis involve some degree of hemostasis. The oozing of blood at the cut ends of the bowel should not be disturbed unless there is an active arterial pumper, in which case the pumper is individually ligated or cauterized. Suture line bleeding following the application of the anastomotic stapler is not uncommon and can be controlled easily with suture ligatures or reinforcement of the anastomosis with an absorbable suture.

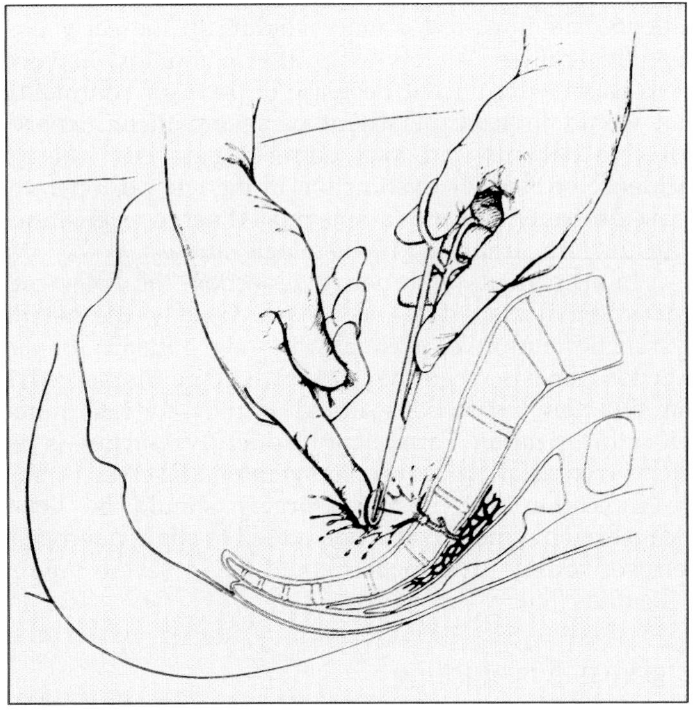

FIGURE 5 ■ Technique of occluding basivertebral vein of sacrum with thumbtack. *Source*: From Ref. 40.

The diagnosis of anastomotic bleeding in the early postoperative period is difficult and usually is determined by deduction. Always, upper gastrointestinal bleeding must be excluded. Proctoscopy or flexible sigmoidoscopy should be performed to rule out the presence of any lesion in the anorectum. Even if the anastomosis is in the lower left colon, it can be examined. Colonoscopy should not be performed for a high anastomosis in the early postoperative period because of the danger of disruption of the anastomosis. Selective arteriography is one option, with the possibility of stopping the bleeding with vasopressin. However, vasopressin may involve the risk of ischemia and eventual anastomotic leak.

Initially, the management of anastomotic hemorrhage is conservative. The patient must be closely monitored and resuscitated. Bleeding diathesis must be corrected. Bleeding from a low anastomosis in the anorectum can be controlled by a peranal approach with suture of the bleeding point. Most high colonic anastomoses require an exploratory celiotomy. Reinforcement sutures art applied, but a resection and reanastomosis may be necessary.

■ INJURY TO URETER

Because of the proximity of the ureters to the colon, intraoperative injury to the ureters can occur particularly when there are severe adhesions in that region from multiple previous operations, a malignancy, an inflammatory process, or previous radiation. However, intraoperative ureteral injuries are not common during colorectal operations. It is important to note that only 20% to 30% of iatrogenic ureteral injuries are recognized or detected at the time of operation (43). This is crucial because immediate repair of the injury results in good healing. When recognition of the problem is delayed, the outcome becomes unpredictable and the incidence of nephrectomy increases sevenfold. It is helpful to remember that "the venial sin is injury to the ureter, but the mortal sin is failure of recognition" (44).

Mechanisms of Injury

For practical purposes, the ureter can be considered as two segments of approximately equal length: the abdominal ureter and the pelvic ureter. The abdominal ureter originates from the renal pelvis and courses downward on the anterior surface of the psoas muscle. As the ureter enters the pelvis, it crosses the iliac artery at the junction of the internal and external iliac arteries. The ureter then tracks posteriorly and inferiorly along the curvature of the pelvis down to the levator ani muscle, where it crosses under the superior vesical artery before entering the posterior aspect of the bladder. In the female, the pelvic ureter lies in the ureterosacral ligament as it courses behind the ovary and then continues inferiorly in the portion of the broad ligament.

Most intraoperative ureteral injuries result from gynecologic procedures and occur at the pelvic brim, but they also may result from colorectal operations. In a series reported by Higgins (44), 61 of 87 iatrogenic ureteral injuries resulted from gynecologic procedures, 12 from colorectal procedures (11 abdominoperineal resections and 1 sigmoid colostomy), 8 from vascular procedures, 5 from urologic procedures, and 1 from an orthopedic procedure. In colonic operations, the left ureter is more commonly injured than the right (45). Types of injuries include ligation, crush injury, transection (partial or complete), and ischemic injury (46).

There are four specific situations that involve the risk of injury to the ureter during colorectal procedures: (i) ligation of the inferior mesenteric artery, (ii) procedures performed near the cul-de-sac, where the ureter crosses the vas deferens ai of the sacral promontory, (iii) division of the lateral stalks of the rectum, and (iv) reperitonealization when the ureter may be included in ligatures (44).

Recognition of Intraoperative Injury

Visual inspection is the most reliable means of assessing ureteral integrity. If there is doubt, methylene blue can be injected intravenously. Extravasation of blue-tinged urine or dye will confirm diagnosis. For delayed diagnosis, retrograde pyelography is the most sensitive radiographic tool for identifying ureteral extravasation or obstruction from ligation (46).

Ureteral Repair

Repair of ureteral injuries is a delicate matter that requires good judgment, experience, and skill. It should be performed by a surgeon who is thoroughly familiar with this type of repair.

In general, injuries detected intraoperatively or within the first few days postoperatively in a stable patient should be repaired immediately. When patient is unstable or the detection is delayed for several days or weeks, the patient should undergo immediate proximal urinary diversion followed by delayed repair. In most cases, proximal urinary diversion can be achieved by placement of a percutaneous nephrostomy catheter (46).

When the ureter has been inadvertently ligated intraoperatively, often all that is necessary is removal of the suture. If the ureter has been crushed by a clamp, the likelihood of injury is higher. The adventitia must be inspected carefully for discoloration because ischemic injury may take several days to manifest itself fully. If the adventitia is non viable, a repair should be performed.

The general principles of ureteral repair include debridement of nonviable tissues, tension anastomosis, and mucosa-to-mucosa reapproximation. Partial transection often can be managed by primary closure with interrupted 4–0 or 5–0 absorbable sutures. Usually complete transection and ischemic injuries can be repaired by resection of the injured segment followed by ureteroureterostomy. All ureteral repairs (primary closures or ureteroureterostomies) should be drained extiaperioneally. All complete transections and most partial transections should be stented, such as with a double J stent. Complete transection of the pelvic ureter or extensive ischemic injury will often be best handled by ureteral reimplantation (46). Various methods of repairs for ureteral injuries have been described by Hamawy et al. (47).

When a difficult operation is anticipated, as may occur with a large malignant mass, an inflammatory mass in the pelvis, or in those who have undergone severe radiation, the risk of ureteral injury can be minimized by preoperative placement of ureteral catheters. This measure will make identification of the ureters easier, although there is no guarantee that injury can be eliminated completely. The complications of preoperative ureteral placement are trivial (48). In the series reported by Bothwell et al. (48), ureteral catheterization was attempted in 92 patients who underwent a left colectomy. It was successful bilaterally in 87% and unilaterally in 98%. A transmural ureteral injury occurred in 0.43%. Surgical injury to the ureter occurred in one patient (1.1%) despite ureteral placement.

■ BLADDER DYSFUNCTION

Problems with bladder function are encountered in 20% to 30% of patients undergoing colon and rectal procedures (49). Several causes of urinary retention include anesthesia and sedation, stimulation of the anovesical reflex by operation, local pain, and anal packing.

Micturition is a reflex process. Parasympathetic nerves innervate the detrusor muscle. Sympathetic nerves innervate the bladder neck, trigone, and urethral area (49). Injury to the autonomic nerves in the pelvis causes bladder dysfunction. Moreover, loss of the posterior support of the bladder after low anterior resection or abdominoperineal resection may add to the problem (50,51). Kinn and Ohman (50) studied 26 patients who underwent resection for rectal carcinoma. All patients had undergone urodynamic studies preoperatively and 6 months postoperatively; interviews concerning bladder and sexual function also were obtained. Seven of 26 patients had impaired urinary voiding in the early postoperative course. At follow-up after 6 months, however, there was no significant decrease of detrusor contractility that would indicate persistent parasympathetic denervation. No patients had total detrusor paralysis. The low incidence of bladder dysfunction in the late postoperative phase probably indicates a time related nerve regeneration, which is also supported by histologic studies.

In all patients with pelvic dissection, the Foley catheter is left in place for 4 to 5 days. Usually, the bladder dysfunction improves gradually. In some patients, the dysfunction persists when they are ready to be discharged. In this situation, instructions should be given for intermittent self catheterization. Permanent bladder dysfunction is rare after a colorectal procedure. In symptomatic cases in men, the indication for prostatic surgery should be liberal because even minor obstruction added to slight neurogenic detrusor muscle dysfunction could cause severe voiding difficulties (50).

■ SEXUAL DYSFUNCTION

As in bladder dysfunction, injuries to pelvic parasympathetic and sympathetic nerves give rise to impotence. The degree and pattern of impotence depends on the nerve involved and can be partial or complete. Potency is defined as the ability to achieve an erection sufficient for vaginal penetration and orgasm. Usually for most patients, sexual dysfunction following operation resolves gradually during the first year. Thus the minimum follow-up interval for determining whether a patient is potent is 1 year (52).

Penile erection is mediated by a coordinated vascular and neurologic event that results in increased inflow of blood to the corpora cavernosa, dilatation of venous sinusoids within the pelvis, and decreased outflow from the corpora cavernosa (52). In addition to the important role of the parasympathetic nerves in initiating the vascular events required to achieve full erection, the somatic nervous system (pudendal nerve) also plays an important role in penile rigidity. Stimulation of the dorsal nerve of the penis will trigger the bulbo-cavernosus reflex. Contraction of the ischiocavernosus muscle compresses the proximal corpora cavernosa and further increases the intracavernous pressure to a level well above the systolic pressure, resulting in the penile rigidity commonly occurring during the heights of masturbation or sexual intercourse (53). The pudendal nerves, which are well protected by the endopelvic fascia, are not usually damaged during a colorectal procedure. The neurologic input for erection is primarily from the parasympathetic nerves (nervi erigentes). Emission and ejaculation are mediated predominantly by sympathetic nerves that travel from the thoracolumbar region of the spinal cord along the sympathetic ganglia and down the hypogastric nerves to the pelvic plexus (52).

Injury to the hypogastric nerves in the retroperitoneal space just above the promontory of the sacrum may result in ejaculatory dysfunction. Excessive traction on the rectum with anterior displacement of the rectum secondary to mobilization posterior to the rectum may result in neurapraxia or avulsion of sacral roots two, three, and four (nervi erigentes). Depending on the severity of injury, this could result in temporary or permanent bladder and/or erectile dysfunction. Such injuries may be prevented by recognizing these possibilities and avoiding excessive traction (52).

Direct injuries to the pelvic plexus may occur during division of the rectal ligaments. The location of the pelvic plexus may be identified intraoperatively by its relationship to the tip of the seminal vesicles. Experience with radical prostatectomy has shown that it is possible to preserve erectile function (and therefore, possible bladder function) despite wide unilateral resection of these nerves. Injuries to the cavernous nerves during perineal dissection of the rectum may result in erectile dysfunction as well. After division of the rectourethralis muscle in the midline anterior to the rectum, the neurovascular bundles may be seen in association with the lateral prostatic fascia coursing from the urethra along the posterolateral surface of the prostate. These neurovascular bundles are anterolateral to the rectum. Excessive use of cautery or posterolateral in this region may result in injury to these nerves (52).

It is important to remember that during any pelvic operation, ligation of the anterior division or distal branch of the internal iliac artery may result in vasculogenic impotence, especially if bilateral ligation of the internal pudendal vessels occurs (52).

The incidence of sexual dysfunction following operation of the rectum depends on many factors. These include the age of the patient, the nature of the disease, and the extent of the procedure. A review of the literature by Walsh and Schlegel (52) showed that erectile dysfunction occurred in 46% of 641 men undergoing abdominoperineal resection for carcinoma and in 15% of those who underwent low anterior resection. Ejaculatory dysfunction occurred in 35% and 44% in to groups, respectively. Havenga et al. (54) of Memorial Sloan-Kettering Cancer Center in New York reported the results of radical total mesorectal excision with an abdominoperineal resection and low anterior resection, with autonomic nerve preservation for carcinoma of the rectum. The autoholds retrospectively studied postoperative sexual and urinary function in 136 patients (82 men and 54 women). Patients who had preoperative dysfunction were excluded. The ability to engage in intercourse was maintained by 86% of the patients younger than 60 years of age and by 67% of patients 60 years of age or older. Eighty-seven percent of male patients maintained their ability to achieve orgasm. An abdominoperineal resection had a higher incidence of erectile dysfunction than an anterior resection. Of the female patients, 85% were able to experience arousal with vaginal lubrication, and 91% could achieve orgasm. Serious urinary dysfunction such as a nevrogenic bladder was not encountered. Excellent results were also obtained by Masui et al. (55) when the autonomic nerve preserving technique was used.

Sexual dysfunction following proctectomy for benign diseases such as ulcerative colitis has a much lower incidence. The incidence of impotence in men who had undergone an ileoanal pouch procedure was 1.6% to 2.0% and retrograde ejaculation was 2.0% to 2.3% (56). The incidence of dyspareunia in women was 7.0% to 8.3% (56–58). These lower incidences reflect the less extensive dissection and the younger age group of patients, usually in their early thirties. Lindsey et al. (59) found no difference in damage to pelvic sexual nerves between close rectal dissection (dissection within mesorectum, close to rectal wall) and anatomical mesorectal plane, in rectal excision for inflammatory bowel disease. In their series of 156 patients, total impotence occurred in 3.8%; they were all in the 50-year-old to 70-year-old age group, and there were no ejaculatory difficulties. Minor diminution of erectile function occured in 13.5%, where sexual activity was still possible. The median follow-up was 74.5 months. Age was the most important risk factor for postoperative impotence.

■ PERONEAL NERVE INJURY

The so-called synchronous position is now standard for an abdominoperineal resection, total proctocolectomy, low anterior resection with stapled anastomosis, low anterior resection with coloanal anastomosis, and ileoanal pouch procedures. The patient is placed on his or her back with both legs on stirrups. Lloyd Davies stirrups commonly have been used for positioning the patient. The problem with this equipment is its lack of support of the feet, which makes it necessary to put the patient's calves on the resting pads. If the positioning is not carefully adjusted or if the procedure lasts longer than 6.5 hours (60), the risk of excessive compression to the calf muscle or peroneal nerve is increased. This varies according to how the patient is positioned and how heavy the patient is. Lloyd Davies stirrups have now been replaced by Allen stirrups or Yellofin stirrups in the United States.

The common peroneal nerve leaves the posterior aspect of the knee and extends laterally around the head of the fibula, where it is extremely superficial and prone to injury. The surgeon must be thoroughly familiar with the patient's history, physical and laboratory findings, and even occupation. Before operation the patient with a peripheral nerve lesion may have had any of the several conditions (e.g., diabetes, arteriosclerosis, herniated disk, aneurysm, neuritis, or neuroma) that could be responsible for the nerve dysfunction now manifested. Diseased nerves will not withstand even short periods of compression, ischemia, or slight degrees of trauma that would be withstood readily by normal nerves (61). The common sign of peroneal nerve injury is footdrop, often associated with an area of sensory loss in the lateral surface of the leg and dorsum of the foot. A rapid test can be performed to rule out a peroneal nerve injury: If dorsiflexion of the big toe is present, the peroneal nerve is intact (61). In the series reported by Herrera-Ornelas et al. (62), of 10 injuries in eight patients, seven resolved without deficit on conservative management alone.

■ COMPARTMENT SYNDROME

Another important complication is prolonged compression of the calf muscle that results in development of a compartment syndrome.

Acute compartment syndrome is a condition in which raised pressure within closed and unyielding facial space reduces capillary perfusion below a level necessitates tissue viability leading to muscle and nerve ischemia within a few hours.

Etiology

Pressure has been seen to rise in the compartments of the leg after some ileoanal pouch procedures lasting 6 to 9 hours (63). The compartment pressure is increase there is head down, tilt into the Trendelenburg position. Pressures have been shown to rapidly return to normal on taking the legs down from the stirrups and placing the legs into the supine position. This manoeuvre has been recommended during operations lasting for more than five hours (63). Trendelenburg with a 15° head down tilt results an immediate fall in leg profusion. Perfusion returns to normal on positioning the legs flat. Acidosis, intraoperative hypotension and vasoconstricting agents may increase intracompartmental ischemia.

The height of elevation of the legs above the level of the heart is crucial. For every centimeter, the calves are raised above the right atrium mean arteriolar pressure is reduced by 0.78 mmHg. A 15° head down tilt has been shown to cause an additional significant decline in blood flow to the limb. If the extreme knee-chest position is used, it can lead to direct compression of blood supply to the lower limb. The calf compartmental pressure can rise from a normal value of 20 up to 240 mmHg in the lithotomy position. Compartmental pressure may increase even further when adequate tissue profusion is restored by returning the patient to the supine position, because a reperfusion injury develops. This postoperative hyperemia reaches its peak 2 hours after completing operation.

Risk Factors

Cited risk factors for the compartment syndrome include: lithotomy position, compromise of blood supply to the periphery, compression of pelvic blood vessels, hypotension, hypovolemia, vasoconstriction, hypothermia, obesity, and ischemic time greater than 6 hours (64).

Diagnosis

The diagnosis of an impending compartment syndrome may be considered with any of the "6Ps." (i) Progressive pain out of proportion to the clinical situation, (ii) paraesthesia in peripheral nerve distribution, (iii) paresis and pain on passive stretch of muscles, (iv) pink skin, (v) presence of pulse until the compartment pressure exceeds arterial inflow pressure, and (vi) compartment pressure of >30 mmHg in any osteofascial compartment. The presence of myoglobin in the urine, suggests an impending compartment syndrome. Serum creatine kinase may be elevated. A definitive diagnosis is made by directly measuring the compartment pressure. The critical compartment pressure value is controversial. A pressure of less than 45 mmHg can be tolerated and a fasciotomy spared, while others recommend a fasciotomy at 30 mmHg. A pressure of 50 to 55 mmHg for 4 to 8 hours will certainly cause irreversible muscle damage (64).

A compartment syndrome may be difficult to differentiate from a nerve injury or an arterial occlusion. Primary nerve injury is expected to produce a deficit in neuromuscular function, but it should not be progressive after the initial injury. Furthermore, signs and symptoms of ischemia and increased tissue pressure should be absent in primary nerve injury.

Acute arterial occlusion may mimic a compartment syndrome by producing signs of compartment ischemia and loss of neuromuscular function. Peripheral pulses are frequently normal in a compartment syndrome because intracompartmental pressure is usually insufficient to affect arterial flow. The presence of Doppler signal distal to the compartment provides no information about the adequacy of compartment perfusion but may indicate an arterial occlusion. When in doubt about the diagnosis of a compartment syndrome, it may be necessary to perform tissue pressure measurements of the calf and direct nerve stimulation (65).

Once the diagnosis of a compartment syndrome has been established, operative decompression is indicated. It is preferable to open all compartments—anterior, lateral, superficial, and deep posterior—through a single lateral incision without removing the fibula (66). Any devitalized tissue should be debrided. The wound should be left open. The patient should be taken to the operating room three to five days later for reexamination and possible closure if this can be performed without tension.

Prevention

These measures include the careful positioning of the lower extremities to avoid excessive angulation of the hips, the use of stirrups that support the leg at the ankle rather than

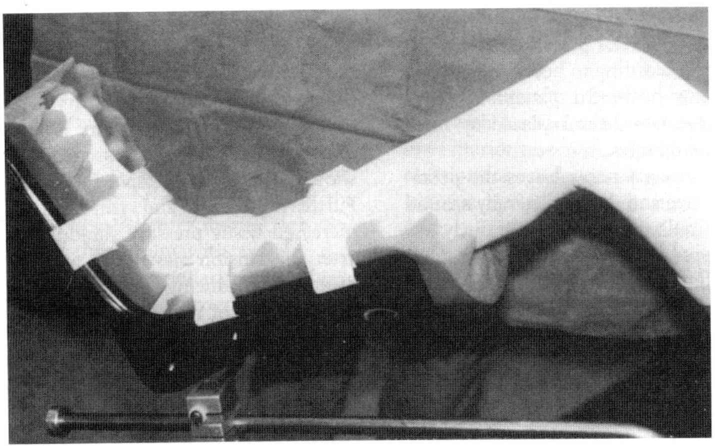

FIGURE 6 ■ Allen stirrups, showing leg resting on foot without compression of calf.

at the calf, and maintaining the Trendelenburg position for only that portion of the operation, during which pelvic dissection is actually occurring a avoidance of intraoperative hypotension.

The Allen or Yellofin Universal stirrups are designed so that compression of the legs does not occur because the legs rest on the feet (Fig. 6) and have gel pads (viscoelastic polymer) as protector. The knees should be slightly flexed and in a neutral position, without internal or external rotation of the hip. The legs must be comfortably rested on the there should be no pressure of the calves resting on the stirrups. Because, the leg support the stirrups are short, compression of the peroneal nerve is eliminated. When the legs are properly placed, the risk of leg injury in the lithotomy position should be very low.

■ FEMORAL NEUROPATHY

Femoral nerve injury is uncommon, but it may be underestimated because the majority of cases are not severe and are self-limited. The injury is caused by the commonly used Balfour and Buck-water self-retaining abdominal retractors. In the first period of a prospective study conducted by Goldman et al. (56) during two 5-year periods, there were 282 cases of postoperative femoral neuropathy following 3736 abdominal hysterectomies. The neuropathy was attributed to the use of the self-retaining retractor. In the second 5-year period, no self-retaining retractors were used. The authors reported a 0.7% incidence of femoral neuropathy. Recently, Brasch et al. (67) reported three cases of femoral neuropathy following colon resections.

Anatomically, the femoral nerve is the largest branch of the lumbar plexus. Branches of the lumbar plexus innervate the psoas major muscle before formation of the femoral nerve. The nerve passes obliquely downward through the psoas major muscle to emerge laterally between the psoas major and iliacus, deep to the iliacus fascia. The femoral nerve enters the thigh lateral to the femoral artery and sheath, where it divides into terminal motor and sensory branches.

The signs and symptoms of femoral neuropathy consist of paresis, quadriceps femoris atrophy, hypoesthesia of the anteromedial thigh, and absent or decreased patellar tendon reflex. In a series of 17 patients with femoral neuropathy reported by Kvist-Poulsen and Borel (68), 94% of patients exited sensory deficits, and 41% had a decrease absent patellar reflex or an inability to perm: straight leg raising. The prognosis is good. In a series of 282 patients, 265 spontaneously recovered, whereas 17 exhibited mild symptoms for as long as 116 days (56). A review of 40 patients with postoperative femoral neuropathy in the literature by Celebrezze et al. (69) revealed that 24 patients fully recovered spontaneously; 2 patients had permanent deficits; 8 patients had permanent sensory deficits; 5 patients had partial motor deficits; and one patients was lost to follow-up.

Retractor injury results from direct compression of the psoas major muscle or impingement of femoral nerve and psoas major against the lateral pelvic wall. Patients who are thin, short statured, or poorly developed rectus muscles are prone to this injury. Retractor injury is preventable, given a thorough understanding of femoral nerve anatomy and repeated evaluation of the placement blades during the operative procedure. Retractor pressure should be minimized and the shortest blade used to permit adequate exposure (67).

■ ANASTOMOTIC LEAK

A bowel anastomosis should heal per primum: the capacity of anastomotic healing is dependent on the patient's general and local condition. Conditions such as malnutrition, particularly hypoalbuminemia, diabetes, irradiation, shock, severe blood loss, and immune deficiency. Technical factors at the time of anastomosis are of equal importance, and these vary depending on how the anastomosis is performed.

Important technical factors that must be considered during bowel anastomosis include blood supply, tension, condition of bowel lumen, condition of bowel ends, and technique of anastomosis.

Blood Supply

The mesentery at or near the transected bowel must be properly dissected, with the surgeon making certain that there is at least an arcade of vessels supplying the area. The fatty tissue should be cleared no more than 5 to 6 mm from the edge. Adequate blood supply is one of the most important factors for proper anastomotic healing.

Tension

Too much tension at the anastomosis not only causes dehiscence of the anastomosis but also compromises its blood supply.

Condition of Bowel Ends

Both bowel ends must be in healthy condition. Bowel that is inflamed and thickened from diverticulitis or radiation enteritis and IBD must be adequately resected until each end has become soft and thin. A generalized edema and thickened bowel from chronic obstruction or malnutrition is a sign of a potential problem.

Technique of Anastomosis

When performed properly, the bowel anastomosis should heal well. There is no longer an issue of whether the anastomosis is performed with one layer or two layers, with interrupted or continuous sutures, and with a stapling device. These methods are all acceptable. Most anastomotic leaks are from resection of rectosigmoid colon with low anastomosis. The incidence varies from 3% to 15% and the mortality is 2% to 7% (69,70). This wide variation reflects the site of anastomosis, definition of leak, the diligence in its detection, and whether the procedure is performed as an elective or emergency situation. The highest risk of anastomotic leak is at the level below 7 cm (70–72). In a prospective study by Law et al. (73), 196 pateints with carcinoma of rectum at 3–12 cm from the anal verge were treated by low anterior resection with total mesorectum excision. The only significant factors affecting anastomotic leak were male gender and a diverting stoma. Although surgical technique is important, there are other adverse factors as well, such as chronic obstructive pulmonary disease, peritonitis, bowel obstruction, malnutrition, the use of corticosteroids, and perioperative blood transfusions, smoking, and excessive alcohol abuse (74).

Management

An anastomotic leak usually becomes apparent between five and seven days postoperatively. Early dehiscence (within 48 hours) is usually serious because adhesions have not developed. Fecal spillage gives rise to generalized peritonitis. The early signs of an anastomotic leak are those of sepsis, including fever, leukocytosis, localized or generalized tenderness, generalized ileus with abdominal distention, and tachycardia or even shock. The evaluation for an anastomotic leak depends on the patient's condition. In generalized peritonitis is obvious, along with other signs of sepsis, an indication of an urgent or emergent exploratory celiotomy. Any investigation to confirm the diagnosis is unnecessary and only delays treatment. Antibiotic coverage for both aerobes and anaerobes should be started immediately.

For an anastomotic leak that develops after 48 hours, pus or fecal material may be apparent if drain is still in place. Plain abdominal films are useful in stapled anastomoses. If anastomotic dehiscence has occurred, the line or the ring of staples is broken. If the anastomotic leak is not apparent but is suspected, a gentle Gastrografin enema is the most accurate method of identifying the leak. Proctoscopy or flexible sigmoidoscopy may or may not be useful in identifying the dehiscence. A CT scan cannot be used to determine the location of an anastomotic leak, but the presence of accumulated fluid may suggest that a leak has occurred.

For practical purposes, the discussion will be limited to leaks that cause generalized peritonitis in the anterior or low anterior resection.

The goal of management is to limit morbidity and mortality and to effectively treat the leak and the resulting sepsis (75,76). The level of treatment depends on the intraoperative findings.

A leak that is caused by necrosis or ischemia at the anatamosis requires its disconnection and a Hartmann procedure. A dehiscence of more than one-third of the circumference should also be disconnected, and a Hartmann procedure performed. Smaller leaks (< 1 cm) can be locally repaired with sutures if the edges of the bowel are healthy, and covered with a piece of omentum if it is available.The area is drained, and a loop ileostomy performed. If the surrounding area of the anastomosis is cemented from dense inflammation, a suction drain should be placed nearby and a loop ileostomy performed.

The fibrins coated on the peritoneum and on the bowel wall should be scraped off with wet sponges as much as possible. The debris in the abscess cavity is curretted and a suction drain placed. The abdominal cavitiy is irrigated with copious amounts of normal saline solution.

■ ANASTOMOTIC STRICTURE

Several factors that contribute to the formation of anastomotic strictures include ischemia, radiation, anastomotic leakage, and recurrent disease (e.g., carcinoma or Crohn's disease). The complication rate has been especially prevalent following low anterior resection of the rectum. From a survey of the members of the American Society of Colon and Rectal Surgeons, Smith (77) found a stenosis incidence of 9% of 3594 patients who underwent an anastomosis with the end-to-end anastomosis (EEA) stapler. Graffner et al. (78) reported that the risk of stricture formation is increased by the establishment of a proximal diverting colostomy. In a series of 73 patients, Gordon and Vasilevsky (79) reported a 20% incidence of stenosis using the circular stapler. Stenosis was defined as failure of the 19 mm sigmoidoscope to pass freely through the anastomosis. Review of the literature reveals that the incidence of rectal anastomotic narrowing varies from 0% to 30% (80). Few authors have given their definition of stenosis. Kyzer and Gordon (80) considered as stenotic any anastomosis that does not accept the 19 mm sigmoidoscope. Leff et al. (81) and Fazio (82) have defined a stricture, as a narrowing that does not allow passage of the 15 mm sigmoidoscope. It was postulated that the narrowing was based on ischemia caused by excessive cleaning of the mesentery adjacent to the anastomosis (80). By limiting the clearing of the bowel edges, Kyzer and Gordon (80) noted that the incidence of narrowing was reduced to 12.5%, and in the last 72 cases, this incidence was further reduced to 4.2%.

Fortunately, most anastomotic strictures are asymptomatic and dilate spontaneously during the first postoperative year. When strictures are symptomatic, several procedures have been tried, namely Hegar dilators, operative intervention, and more recently, balloon dilatation. Some strictures are thin or membranous and can easily be corrected by a single digital dilatation or sigmoidoscopy following which, bulk forming agent's help to maintain patency. Kyzer and Gordon (80) reported a series of 215 anastomoses created, following which 27 patients developed stenosis, but only eight patients were stenosis permanent and only three among them were symptomatic. Each of those patients was treated with balloon dilatation. Johansson (83) performed endoscopic balloon dilatation of postoperative or radiation-induced rectal strictures on 49 occasions in 18 patients. Of the 114 evaluable patients, 12 were relieved of symptoms. The method is simple and can be accomplished with a number of commercially available balloons. It can be performed as an outpatient procedure. The complication rate is acceptable, and one perforation was reported in the Johansson series.

In the colon, anastomotic strictures are uncommon. In a series of 223 anastomoses reported. Kyzer and Gordon (84) there were no strictures noted. The authors' review of the literature revealed reports of stenosis ranging from 0% to 1.1%.

■ FECAL INCONTINENCE

The technical ability to construct anastomoses at lower and lower levels in the pelvis has resulted in the potential imposition of yet another complication, namely fecal incontinence. It has been suggested that as many as 5% of patients may have total incontinence and 25% may have changed their bowel habits, such as soiling or an increase stool frequency that may affect their daily lifestyle (85). Another review suggested 10% to 50% patients who have undergone sphincter-saving operations complain of "incomplete function" (86), continence rates as high as 60% to 80% following low anterior resection have also been suggested. Restoration of abnormal anoneorectal function parameters over a period of one year following operation is believed to occur, but approximately to 47% continue to suffer incontinence (87).

Many factors may contribute to postoperative dysfunction. Stapling devices may harm the sphincter muscles, and rectal mobilization may damage innervation of the sphincter. The high frequency of bowel movements after operation is related to loss of reservoir capacity. Decreased compliance of the neorectum is a consistent finding in all studies (88).

Otto et al. (85) studied 17 patients with rectal neoplasms and found that immediately after operation, 14 of 17 patients showed a certain degree of incontinence but recovered during follow-up with only two patients reporting minor soiling. Anorectal manometric evaluation revealed that resting and squeeze pressures were moderately reduced after operation and increased during the following 6 months without regaining preoperative levels. This suggests damage to sphincter muscle fibers or innervation. The rectoanal inhibitory reflex was present in 94.4% of patients before operation and in about 25% after operation, but was not associated with incontinence. Rectal sensation was significantly reduced as a result of what was believed to be a loss in reservoir capacity, and its recovery was well correlated with a decrease in the frequency of bowel movements.

In a clinicophysiologic study, Ikeuchi et al. (86) found that stapled coloanal anastomoses resulted in a poorer outcome than anterior resection or low anterior resection in terms of soiling and urgency at 12 months. The authors noted that incomplete evacuation was frequently observed in the stapled coloanal anastomoses and low anterior resection groups. Anal manometric parameters recovered in the anterior resection group but not in the other two groups. The authors concluded that the clinical outcome was related to the anastomotic level. This is not universally agreed upon (87).

Ikeuchi et al. (86) related the length of the rectal remnant to the pelvic nervous system. Following anterior resection, the external and internal sphincters, the superior inferior rectal branch, and approximately 10 cm of the rectum remained; following low anterior resection, the external and internal sphincters, the inferior rectal nerve branch, and 4 cm of the rectum remained; and following stapled coloanal anastomoses, the external and internal sphincters, part of the inferior rectal branches, and 2 cm of the rectum remained. Clinically, the daily frequencies of bowel movement and incomplete evacuation were disturbed in the patients who underwent the low anterior resection or stapled coloanal anastomosis procedures. With anterior resection, the remnant rectum and superior rectal branch were longer than with low anterior resection and stapled coloanal anastomosis. The soiling frequency also increased as a result of dissection of the inferior rectal branch. The ability to differentiate between flatus and feces recovered with time. In the early postoperative period, significant differences were observed according to the anastomotic level. No physiologic parameter was shown to be closely related to the change in the frequency of urgency in these patients. However preservation of the inferior rectal branch may have been involved in the recovery from urgency in the low anterior group by 12 months. Both the maximum resting pressure and maximum squeeze pressure showed identical patterns of recovery, indicating that anal sphincter was preserved in all three procedures. Threshold volume was reported to be correlated with difficult evacuation in patients with a coloanal anastomosis. Threshold volume in the stapled coloanal anastomotic group was significantly lower than in either of the other groups. The only parameter that was significantly higher in the stapled coloanal anastomotic group than in the other groups was the soiling frequency. The authors' study demonstrated that the preserved anal sphincter alone was not sufficient to control either bowel movement frequency or urgency. The reservoir function of the neorectum, which is composed of the colorectal muscle layer and nervous components, plays a role in the maintenance of fecal function.

In another physiologic study, Rao et al. (87) concluded that major incontinence is secondary to neurotensin of the inferior mesenteric ganglia and the hypogastric plexus, whereas minor incontinence represents a localized neurotensin/neurapraxia of the inferior mesenteric plexus. Surely other factors play a role in postoperative incontinence, and only time and further studies will clarify the pathogenesis of the problem.

■ EARLY POSTOPERATIVE ILEUS AND SMALL BOWEL OBSTRUCTION

Ileus

Postoperative ileus is a form of temporary bowel motor dysfunction that regularly follows operative procedures in the abdomen. It also occurs after operations remote from the abdomen such as lower extremity arthroplasty (88) and particularly surgery of the brain (89). Prolonged postoperative ileus is one of the most common causes of prolonged hospital stay after a colorectal resection. Not all segments in the gastrointestinal tract are equally affected by postoperative ileus. The average paralytic state lasts between 0 and 24 hours in the small intestine, 24 and 48 hours in the stomach, and between 48 and 72 hours in the colon after major abdominal surgery. The effective duration of ileus is, therefore, mainly dependent on the return of colonic motility and, in particular, motility of the left colon. The difference between right-sided and left-sided colonic procedures on the duration of ileus remains uncertain (90).

Ileus has been demonstrated to be related to the degree of surgical manipulation and the magnitude of the inflammatory response (91). The inhibitory sympathetic reflexes are of major importance in the pathogenesis of ileus. This has substantial clinical implications as these reflexes are subject to modification by epidural blockade.

Various neurotransmitters such as vasoactive intestinal peptide (VIP) and substance P, and inflammatory factors such as leucocyte-derived nitric oxide have been established as inhibitory neurotransmitters in the gut nervous system. However, their relative roles in the initiation and resolution of ileus remain obscure (90).

The definition of ileus and methods of assessment are not well defined. A correlation between some of the widely used clinical end points, such as bowel sounds, passage of flatus and stool, is also controversial. Bowel sounds are nonspecific because they may originate in the small bowel as well as in the large bowel, and also require frequent auscultation for assessment. Passage of flatus is highly dependent on reporting by patients, and the correlation between passage of flatus and the propulsive bowel movement is unclear. Passage of stool, although manifest as a clinical sign, is not specific, as it may indicate only distal bowel emptying and not necessarily the function of the entire gastrointestinal tract. The most adequate definition of resolution probably depends on a combined functional outcome of normalization of food intake and bowel function (90,92).

Can the duration of postoperative ileus be shortened? No proven pharmacological means of accelerating recovery of intestinal motor activity exists. When examined critically, agents used to antagonize sympathetic hyperactivity or to promote parasympathetic activity have not reliably shortened the duration of postoperative ileus. Although a recent report suggests that the acetylcholinesterase inhibitor neostigmine may facilitate resolution of colonic pseudoobstruction, it is unclear whether these findings can extend it to physiological ileus. Drugs commonly used to enhance motility, such as metoclopramide, cisapride (has been withdrawn from U.S. market due to arrhythmic side effects), and erythromycin, do not consistently hasten resolution of ileus and are, therefore, not routinely used in the postoperative setting (93).

The insertion of nasogastric tube does not shorten time of ileus and is not recommended for routine use (94,95); however, if the prolonged physiologic ileus is complicated with abdominal distention or nausea, nasogastric tube is the most effective treatment.

Contrary to popular belief, physical exercise does not improve colonic motility in healthy volunteers. Neither does mobilization itself shorten the duration of postoperative ileus. The commonly practiced prolonged immobilization after surgery has never been proven to be beneficial. In fact, prolonged bed rest may enhance the risk of postoperative complications and prolonged recovery, and so should be avoided for reasons other than recovery of gastrointestinal function (90).

Food intake elicits a reflex response that is propulsive in action. In addition, the presence of food stimulates the secretion of various intestinal hormones, with an overall stimulating effect of gastrointestinal motility. Traditionally, oral feeding has been delayed after an abdominal operation until any ileus has resolved clinically. At that point, a liquid diet is administered, gradually progressive to solid food. However, trials to investigate the effect of early oral feeding have showed conflicting results (90).

Theoretically, epidural blockade with local anesthetic may improve postoperative ileus by several mechanisms: blockade of afferent and efferent inhibitory reflexes, efferent sympathetic blockade with concomitant increase in splanchnic blood flow, and anti-inflammatory effects via systemic absorption of local anesthetics. Several randomized studies in patients undergoing abdominal procedures have evaluated the effect of epidural thoracic local anesthetics compared with systemic opioids. In most studies, the epidural bupivacaine led to reduction of the duration of ileus (90).

It is well known that opioids have a profound inhibitory affect on resting and post-traumatic gastrointestinal motility, primarily mediated through μ opioid receptors within the enteric nervous system. Alvimopan is a novel opioid receptor antagonist (not yet commercially available). It has limited ability to cross the blood-brain barrier. Wolff et al. (96) conducted a randomized, double blind, placebo controlled parallel group study involving 34 centers in North America to evaluate the efficacy and safety of Alvimopan (6 or 12 mg) in recovering of gastrointestinal function after bowel resection or radical hysterectomy. A total of 510 patients scheduled for bowel resection or radical hysterectomy were randomized to receive Alvimopan 6 mg, Alvimopan 12 mg, or placebo orally ≥ 2 hours before surgery, then twice a day until hospital discharge or for up to seven days. The primary efficacy end point was a composite of time to recovery of upper and lower gastrointestinal (GI) function. An associated secondary end point was time to hospital discharge. The results showed that time to recovery of GI function were accelerated for the Alvimopan 6 mg and 12 mg compared to placebo. The time to hospital discharge was also accelerated in the Alvimopan 12 mg group. The incidence of adverse events was similar among treatment groups. Delaney et al. (97) have confirmed these positive results, with an addition that Alvimopan 12 mg reduced the incidence of postoperative nausea by 53%. Alvimopan may have a good potential for clinical use in the future if it is approved by the Federal Drug Administration.

A randomized observer-blinded multicenter trial of the effects of intravenous fluid restriction on postoperative complications conducted by Brandstrup et al. (98) revealed that restricted intravenous fluid regimen significantly reduced overall postoperative complications. Lobo et al. (99) studied the effect of salt and water balance on recovery of gastrointestinal function after elective colonic resection in a randomized controlled trial. This is a small study of 10 patients who were randomly allocated to receive postoperative intravenous fluids in accordance with present hospital practice (≥3 L water and 154 mmol sodium per day) and 10 to receive a restricted intake (≤2 L water and 77 mmol sodium per day). The primary end point was solid and liquid-phase gastric emptying time, measured by dual isotope radionuclide scintigraphy on the fourth postoperative day. Secondary end points included time to first bowel movement and length of postoperative hospital stay. The results showed that median solid and liquid phase gastric emptying time on the fourth postoperative day was significantly longer in the standard group than in the restricted group. Median passage of flatus was 1 day later; median passage of stool 2.5 days later; and median postoperative hospital stay three days longer in the standard group than in the restricted group. One patient in the restricted group developed hypokalemia, whereas seven patients in standard group had side effects or complications. The results showed that by the end of day 4, after correction for insensible losses, fluid balance was positive by 3 L in the standard group compared with zero in the restricted group. Serial weighting is the best measure of fluid balance. The authors were unable to determine whether these effects were a result of fluid gain, hypoalbuminemia, or both, because the two are inseparable even in healthy people who have striking falls in the concentration of albumin in the serum with crystalloid infusions. Although patients in the restricted group received less salt and water than those in the standard group, the urine output did not differ in the first few days, and none of the patients in the restricted group became oliguric or had a higher urea in the blood than normal.

The concentrations of the gastrointestinal hormones cholecystokinin, peptide YY, and motilin did not differ between groups, suggesting that the longer gastric emptying and delayed passage of flatus and feces in the standard group is a mechanical effect of gastrointestinal edema produced by the salt and the water excess. This is useful information to avoid the worldwide common practice of giving excessive fluid during or after the operation.

In summary, postoperative ileus after colorectal resection is a physiologic event that lasts for a few days. In a symptomatic ileus, the primary treatment is a nasogastric tube. It usually resolves with time. Prolonged postoperative ileus (more than 1 week) may be a sign of an abnormal condition such as overuse of narcotic drugs, fluid and electrolyte imbalances, intraoperative abscess or peritonitis, excessive aerophagia, and a mechanical small bowel obstruction.

There has been no reliable medications to treat prolonged postoperative ileus. Preventive measures should be instituted particularly refraining from excessive use of opioids, and avoid excessive intravenous fluid during and after the operation. Oral intake should not be started until the patient has begun to diurese and the excessive body weight has returned to normal. Edema of bowel or mesentery from excessive intravenous fluid during or after surgery is one of the common causes of prolonged physiologic ileus (99).

Although epidural analgesia has been shown to shorten duration of postoperative ileus, it failed to demonstrate a shorter hospital stay or reduction in hospital cost in gastrointestinal surgery. It has its own problems such as epidural catheter migration, pruritus, nausea, and respiratory depression. It also requires expert anesthesiologists particularly for thoracic epidural analgesia. Thoracic epidural analgesia has reduced hospital cost and stay in patients at high risk of cardiac and pulmonary complications (100).

Early Mechanical Small Bowel Obstruction

Mechanical small bowel obstruction can occur after any exploratory celiotomy, particularly procedures performed below the transverse mesocolon. Early postoperative small bowel obstruction from operations on organs above the mesocolon, such as biliary tract procedures, is uncommon (101). In the series reported by Stewart et al. (101), the incidence of early postoperative small bowel obstruction (within 30 days after operation) that required re-operation after a right colectomy was 1.5% and for a left colectomy and resection of rectum was 3%. A series from Menzies and Ellis (102) showed that the incidence of small bowel obstruction in all cases of exploratory celiotomy was 3.2%. However, operations accounting for the majority of early postoperative adhesive obstructions are large bowel, rectal, and appendiceal procedures as well as gynecologic surgery. In the series by Menzies and Ellis (102), 39% of small bowel obstructions occurred within one year of the abdominal surgery, 21% within 1 month, and 21% more than 10 years after operation.

Diagnosis

The diagnosis or early postoperative small bowel obstruction is difficult and is usually impossible to differentiate from postoperative ileus. For this reason, Pickleman and Lee (103) defined an early postoperative small bowel obstruction as one occurring between 7 and 30 days after the operation. A typical patient with early postoperative small bowel obstruction cannot tolerate removal of the nasogastric tube after seven days following the operation or would have already started a liquid or soft diet and has developed abdominal distention associated with nausea and vomiting. Ninety percent of postoperative small bowel obstructions occurred during the first two weeks after the operation (103).

Because the clinical signs of small bowel obstruction (abdominal distention, colicky pain, nausea, and vomiting) are nonspecific, the plain film radiographic demonstration of dilated, lated loops of small intestine with air-fluid levels, and no or minimal colonic gas has been considered essential. Unfortunately, plain film examination is diagnostic in only 46% to 80% of cases. The lower percentage probably reflects radiographic findings at the patients' initial presentation, and the high percentage includes patients who underwent follow-up plain film studies (104).

Management

The management of an early postoperative small bowel obstruction is nasogastric suction and administration of fluid and electrolytes. Nasogastric suction can be continued as long as there is no increased distention of the abdomen, abdominal cramps are not worse, and the body temperature and white blood count are not elevated. With careful monitoring the obstruction can be treated with nasogastric decompression safely for 10 to 14 days (103). A total parenteral nutrition should be considered after one week of unresolved small bowel obstruction.

In a series of 101 patients with early postoperative small bowel obstruction reported by Pickleman and Lee (103), obstruction was successfully resolved in 78 patients by nasogastric decompression: 70% resolved within one week, 26% within two weeks, and 4% within three weeks. Five percent of patients died during treatment, but none of the deaths resulted from strangulation or gangrene of the bowel. Among 23 patients with obstruction who underwent exploratory celiotomy, 14 patients (61%) had obstructive bands, seven patients (31%) had a phlegmon, one patient (4%) had an abscess, and one patient (4%) had intussusception. Three patients (13%) died after the operation, but none of the deaths was from strangulation or ischemia.

When to Operate?

There are three situations in early postoperative small bowel obstruction that require surgical intervention: unresolved obstruction after a prolonged nasogastric tube, a high-grade or complete small bowel obstruction, and ischemic or strangulated small bowel. All these conditions require an expert judgment based on clinical evaluation and interpretation of essential work-up. As shown by Pickleman and Lee (103), 2 weeks' time should be a cutting point to consider an exploratory celiotomy, but sooner if the condition deteriorates.

A high-grade or total small bowel obstruction seldom responds to prolonged conservative treatment and has a danger to become ischemia or perforation. A plain and upright abdomen and erect chest x-ray as an initial evaluation with subsequent serial films give useful and important information. A gasless colon and a stepladder pattern to air-fluid levels on the dilated small intestine signifies complete small bowel obstruction; the "ground glass" appearance and the gasless small bowel and large bowel is the picture of a closed-loop obstruction (105). Nauta (105) used clinical examination, leukocyte count, and the plain film radiography to determine when to operate and when to treat conservatively. In a retrospective review of 413 patients with small bowel obstruction (not an early postoperative small bowel obstruction), 72 patients underwent immediate operation because of the diagnosis of a complete small bowel obstruction, 47 patients required an operation after a period of observation ranging from 3 to 15 days, and 294 patients resolved without an operation. Of the 72 patients who underwent immediate operation, 22 bowel resections were required: 6 for obstructive carcinoma, 12 for ischemic bowel, and 4 for extensive adhesions. Two postoperative deaths occurred within 30 days, both in the bowel resection group; one of these was from an aspiration pneumonia established preoperatively and the other was from acute renal failure established preoperatively. In the 294 patients who were successfully treated conservatively, the readmission and reoperation rates were comparable with those reported in series in which earlier operation was undertaken (56 patients were readmitted with seven requiring operation in 6-year period). The author concluded that plain abdominal films of the abdomen can accurately differentiate between complete and partial small bowel obstruction and that partial small bowel obstruction can be safely treated conservatively with close observation. Although this series does not fit the topic of early postoperative small bowel obstruction, it gives a good lesson on how to simply use abdominal films to diagnose a complete small bowel obstruction that requires an immediate operation.

Ischemic bowel is an urgent indication for surgery. The diagnosis, however, is difficult.

A prospective study was conducted by Sarr et al. (106) to evaluate numerous parameters that might be useful in predicting strangulation versus a simple small bowel obstruction before exploratory celiotomy. No parameter has proved to be more sensitive than 52%, either when used alone or in combination. Parameters studied included continuous abdominal pain (as opposed to colicky pain), bloody bowel movements, duration of symptoms, location of abdominal pain, time interval since last bowel movement, surgical history, fever (greater than 100°F), white blood count greater than 10,000, and tachycardia. Some laboratory studies, such as those used to determine the presence of metabolic acidosis and elevation of serum creatine phosphokinase, have a predictive value of 75%. Hyperamylasemia and hyperphosphatemia were of no diagnostic value. Even the preoperative diagnosis of senior experienced surgeons proved disappointing: sensitivity for recognition of strangulation was only 48% ± 22%.

Review of literature by Sajja et al. (107) showed that in multiple series of early postoperative small bowel obstruction that required an operation, the incidence of intestinal strangulation ranges from 0% to 12% and the mortality ranges from 2% to 18%. The incidence of strangulation is relatively low in early postoperative small bowel obstruction compared to small bowel obstruction from incarcerated hernias because more of these are from adhesions (107).

CT has played an important role in the diagnosis of complicated small bowel obstruction. Mallo et al. (108) conducted a systematic and comprehensive review of the scientific literature using MEDLINE and Cochrane databases for a period from 1966 to 2004. For a report on CT diagnosis of ischemia in small bowel obstruction included 743 patients. The sensitivity was 83% (range 63–100%) and the specificity was 92% (range 61–100%). The positive predictive value (PPV) was 79% (range 69–100%) and the negative predictive value (NPV) was 93% (range 33–100%).

For complete or high-grade obstruction including 408 patients, the sensitivity was 92% (range 81–100%) and the specificity of 94% (range 68–100%). The PPV was 92% (range 84–100%) and the NPV was 93% (range 76–100%).

The CT abdomen has largely replaced the small bowel follow-through or enteroclysis study. The emerging CT enterography (106,109) may improve the accuracy of the conventional CT abdomen for the diagnosis of complicated small bowel obstruction.

Preventing Adhesions

Because of the frequency of postoperative adhesions and the substantial suffering and morbidity endured by patients in addition to the enormous cost in terms of medical care and lost income, the prevention of adhesion formation has been the subject of countless studies. None has offered much hope until the publication by Becker et al. (110) who studied the use of a sodium hyaluronate and carboxymethylcellulose, bioresorbable membrane (Seprafilm Genzyme Corp., Cambridge, MA, U.S.A.). The authors randomly assigned 183 patients with ulcerative colitis or familial adenomatous polyposis (FAP), who were scheduled colectomy and ileal pouch-anal anastomosis diverting loop ileostomy to receive or not receive the membrane placed under the midline incision At the ileostomy closure 8 to 12 weeks later, one aparoscopy was used to evaluate the incidence, extent and severity of adhesion formation. Data analyzed from 175 assessable patients revealed that only 6% of control patients had no adhesions, whereas 51% of patients receiving the membrane were free of adhesions. Dense adhesions were observed in 58% of control patients but in only 15% of those receiving the membrane. This study represents the first controlled prospective evaluation of postoperative abdominal adhesion formation and prevention after general abdominal surgery using standardized direct peritoneal visualization. The membrane was safe with no reported adverse effects.

The results that it is safe and has fewer adhesions have been confirmed by the prospective, randomized, multicenter, controlled studies conducted by Beck et al. (111) and Cohen et al. (112). However, wrapping the anastomosis with Seprafilm should be avoided as it has a higher risk of anastomosis leak rate (111). In the most recent report on the subject, Fazio et al. (113) published their prospective, randomized, multicenter, multinational, single blind, controlled study on 1701 patients who underwent intestinal resection to determine whether Seprafilm usage would translate into a reduction in adhesive small bowel obstruction. Before closure of the abdomen, patients were randomized to receive Seprafilm or no treatment. Seprafilm was applied to adhesiogenic tissues throughout the abdomen. The mean follow-up time for the occurrence of adhesive small bowel obstruction was 3.5 years. There was no difference between the treatment and control groups in overall rate of bowel obstruction. However, the incidence of adhesive small bowel obstruction requiring reoperation was significantly lower for Seprafilm patients compared with no treatment patients; 1.8% vs. 3.4%.

■ ABDOMINAL WOUND INFECTION

Many studies have shown no benefit of mechanical bowel preparation for colorectal resection in terms of wound infection or anastomotic leak; some studies even showed its adverse effects (114–116).

The appropriate use of prophylactic antibiotics for wound injection that cover aerobic and anaerobic bacteria has markedly reduced the incidence of wound infection and abdominal abscess after colorectal operation. These measures, however, must be combined with good operative technique. The risk of the patient developing a wound infection is determined by the interaction of the following factors: (i) amount and nature of bacterial contamination the wound; (ii) the condition of the wound at determination of the operation, which depends on both the pathologic process and the adequacy technique; (iii) the innate ability of the host to deal with infection; (iv) the specific antimicrobial agents present in the wound tissues (117).

Surgical operations call upon the phagocytes involved in host defense responses to respond to traumatized tissue and contaminating bacteria, either element is present in excess; host defer may be strained. If both are present in excess, defense mechanism may be overwhelmed, resulting in a wound abscess. Antibiotics help in defense against bacteria but can do nothing to minimize the effects of excessive trauma to the wound tissues. The amount of tissue damage correlates negatively with the number of bacteria required to in duce infection. Following closure of the wound, its environment is sealed off from the body as a result of local intravascular coagulation and the mechanisms of early inflammation. Any blood remaining within the wound may harbor and nourish bacteria. Pathogens within the wound are protected from host defense and antimicrobial agents by the inflammatory diffusion barrier, explaining why postoperative administration of antibiotics is ineffective in preventing wound infection. Administered preoperatively at the right time, antibiotics diffuse into the peripheral compartment, or in this case, the wound fluid during the operation. The antibiotics must be present in a wound early enough to reduce the ability of contaminating bacteria to cause postoperative infection. If the antibiotic is given too early, it may diffuse into and then be eliminated from the tissues before the incision is made and may not be available in the wound during the vulnerable period. Prophylactic antibiotics are effective only when given immediately (i.e.) preoperatively but not when given after the termination of the operation (118).

Operative wounds have been classified into four different types (119). In a clean wound (type I), the bowel content is not exposed (e.g., an exploratory celiotomy or a simple lysis of adhesions). With a clean contaminated wound (type II), the bowel is open but there is no gross spilling of the gastrointestinal content (e.g., colon resection and anastomosis). In a contaminated wound (type III), there is a gross spilling of gastrointestinal content during the procedure. With a dirty wound (type IV), there is existing infection (e.g., perforated diverticulitis).

The incidence of wound infection in a clean wound is very low (1–3%) and usually results from exogenous contamination with gram-positive organisms such as staphylococci (120). In type II, III, and IV wounds, the risk of wound infection is between 3% and 16% (117,119,121). The common pathogens found in the colon and rectum are *E. coli*, *Klebsiella*, *Enterobacter*, *Bacteroides fragilis*, *peptostreptococci*, and *Clostridia* (118).

The reliable management of dirty wounds is to delay the wound closure or to leave it open altogether, which may take a few months to heal. However, if the healing wound is clean, a secondary skin closure can be done. An alternative is to use vacuum-assisted wound closure. This technique has been successfully used in trauma patients that require to leave the abdomen open (122).

Nosocomial infection is still a major cause of surgical wound infection (117). However, this fact is frequently overlooked. Every effort must be made to minimize this type of infection, and adherence to a few basic principles will help.

From the working group that developed guidelines for prevention of surgical infection at the Centers for Disease Control and Prevention, Polk et al. (117) outlined the preparation of patients for operation as follows: (i) For elective operation, all bacterial infections that are identified should be treated and controlled before the operation, excluding ones for which the operation is performed. (ii) The preoperative hospital stay should be as short as possible. Many tests and therapies can be performed on an outpatient basis. (iii) For elective operation, a grossly malnourished patient should receive preoperative oral or parenteral hyperalimentation. (iv) For elective operation, the patient should bathe or be bathed the night before the operation with an antiseptic soap. Unless hair near the operative site is thick enough to interfere with the surgical procedure, it should not be removed. If hair removal is necessary, it should be performed as close to the time of operation as possible, preferably immediately before. The entire operative field and the adjacent area should be scrubbed with a detergent solution and then covered with an antiseptic solution. Tincture of chlorhexidine iodophors and tincture of iodine are recommended. Plain soap, alcohol, or hexachlorophene is not recommended as a single agent for operative site preparation unless the patient's skin is sensitive to the recommended antiseptic products. Other control measures that must be observed are the preparation of the surgical team and the checking of ventilation and air quality in the operating room, which should be established and standardized in all hospitals.

Factors that have proven or probable influence on the frequency of wound infections are the use of antibiotic prophylaxis, the duration of surgery, the defense mechanisms of the host, the use of ultraclean air in the operating room, the presence of hyporolemia, diabetes mellitus, or adiposity in the patient, the patient's nutritional status, the use of blood transfusion, and pain control. The importance of each factor, however, is difficult to detemine (123).

The maintenance of a normal temperature in the patient during surgery has been reported to decrease the infection rate by two-thirds (124) and the use of supplemental oxygen decreased the rate by half using 30% oxygen during and 2 hours after surgery (125).

The decisive period for the development of surgical wound infection is during surgery and for the first few hours thereafter (123).

■ ABDOMINAL WOUND DEHISCENCE

Abdominal wound dehiscence formerly was a fairly common complication of intra-abdominal operations and was associated with a high morbidity and mortality. At present it is an uncommon problem, partly because of better suture materials, improved techniques, and better antibiotics to control wound infection. In most series the incidence of abdominal dehiscence varies from 0% to 4% (126–129). However, the incidence of incisional hernia is much higher and is directly related to the duration of follow-up. The incidence ranged from 3% in the series reported by Schoetz et al. (126) to 21% in the series reported by Wissing et al. (130) This wide range of complications probably reflects the different techniques of closure and the varying suture size and material used. The most common cause of abdominal wound dehiscence is related to improper closure technique (127). Three major causes of wound dehiscence are tissue tear, suture break, and knot slippage. Other factors include the following: male older than 60 years, severe obstructive pulmonary disease, malnutrition, emergency abdominal procedures, complicated neoplastic and inflammatory bowel disease, and acute abdominal distention (128,129). Patients with jaundice also were found to have healing of abdominal incision as well as visceral wounds, seriously impaired (131). In some patients, dehiscence occurred as a result of deep abdominal wound infection, with necrosis of the fascia.

Unless there is evisceration, the dehiscence may not be apparent. Initially the patient develops ileus, which causes abdominal distention. Nausea and vomiting may mimic small bowel obstruction. Later, serosanguineous fluid leaks through the abdominal wound. Examination of the abdominal wound reveals separation of the fascia. Skin sutures should not be removed because this maneuver will only convert a fascial dehiscence to a complete evisceration. There is no urgency to repair a fascial dehiscence, especially in a relatively sick patient. One can accept an incisional hernia that can be repaired at a later date. In the face of a complete evisceration, it is best to take the patient to the erating room for exploration under general anesthesia. Clinical observation showed that in 88 patients, the sutures were in a disrupted wound intact, having pulled through the fascia (132), the wound should be properly resutured. Although tension sutures probably do not prevent the dehiscence from recurring, they should be considered in some conditions, such as severe obstructive pulmonary disease or lack of good ant fascia.

Many studies have been conducted in a randomized prospective manner and are helpful when applied to the techniques of abdominal wound sure, as described below.

Midline vs. Transverse Incision

In a randomized controlled clinical trial by Greenall et al. (133), on 579 patients under major celiotomy there was no difference incidence of abdominal wound dehiscence between midline vertical incision and transverse incision These authors also showed that postoperative pulmonary complications were not influenced by the direction of the incision (134).

Layered Closure vs. Mass Closure

It is now generally accepted that closure of the peritoneal layer is unnecessary (135). Ellis and Heddle (131) used a mass closure technique that included all layers of the abdominal wall apart from and incorporates wide bites of tissue on either of the line of incision, placed close together under no tension. Only one burst abdomen (0.4%) was noted. This rate compared favorably with 2.5% incidence of burst abdomen in two-layer closure. Mass closure, however, is not perfect, 3% of these patients developed an incisional hernia within six months of follow-up.

How Tight to Pull Sutures

In a prospective randomized trial on retentio tures, the flush-tied sutures (tight) were associated with a higher incidence of wound dehiscence than were loosely tied sutures (over three fingers) (136). Experimental studies in male rats showed that tight closure of sutures on fascia caused overlap of tissue, whereas loosely closed sutures afforded proper alignment of the wound edges and had greater proliferative activity in the cleft of the wounds. The tensile strength and energy-to-failure studies showed, loosely approximated wounds to be far stronger. However, no statistically significant difference was found in hydroxyproline assays of the two groups (137). In practice, it is important to approximate the abdominal fascia, not to strangulate it.

Continuous vs. Interrupted Sutures

A randomized prospective multicentric study was organized to compare results between techniques using continuous sutures and interrupted sutures in closing abdominal midline incisions (138). The suture material employed was polyglycolic acid. This study included 3135 patients who were randomized between the two methods of closure and stratified according to the type of wound (i.e., clean, clean contaminated, and contaminated). The overall dehiscence rate was 1.6% in the continuous suture group versus 2% in the interrupted suture group. In six trials comparing continuous versus interrupted technique (irrespective of suture type), there was no statistical difference in the rate of wound infection or wound dehiscence (139). Meta-analyses of various randomized trials showed that continuous slowly absorbable sutures (such as PDS) gave the best results in terms of less pain, fewer sinuses, with a follow-up of 1 year (140).

At the present time, many surgeons favor running sutures for closing abdominal wounds, not only because they are cheaper to do but also faster. The use of running sutures consumes only half the time needed for interrupted sutures. Continuous sutures, however, are more prone to be pulled too tight either by the surgeon or the assistant. It is important that any type of abdominal closure have the tissue bites 1.5 cm from the fascial edges (127).

Suture Materials

An extensive review of the literature by Poole (141), which included 111 references, made him conclude that chromic catgut should be abandoned for abdominal wound closure because of its unreliable strength by early suture dissolution or breakage Braided organic nonabsorbable materials, such as silk and cotton, have fallen into disfavor because of the intense inflammatory response they elicit and because of the propensity for bacteria to grow in the interstices of the suture, resulting in an increased incidence of wound infection and delayed check in the formation of suture sinuses (126). Most studies indicate that synthetic absorbable sutures have demonstrated strength equal to that of permanent sutures (139). Monofilament sutures are preferred for their lack of reactivity, prolonged tensile strength, and resistance to infection. There is a higher incidence of incisional hernia formation when braided absorbable suture material is used (142).

Laboratory evaluation of a monofilament PDS has shown that its strength prior to implantation exceeds that of nonabsorbable monofilament sutures. Furthermore, its strength is maintained in vivo much longer than that of braided synthetic absorbable sutures. Size 00 PDS suture retained 70% of its breaking strength following in vivo residence of 28 days and still retained 13% of its original strength at 56 days. In contrast, braided synthetic absorbable sutures retained only 1% to 5% of strength at 28 days. Cellular responses are found only in the vicinity of the implant site and are predominately mononuclear in character (143). A No. 1 monofilament synthetic absorbable suture is available and is suitable for a secured abdominal wound closure. A prospective study conducted by Israelsson and Jonsson (144) comparing continuous sutures in midline abdominal incisions using PDS-2 vs. No. 1 nylon showed that PDS suture was as good as nylon.

Retention Sutures

Retention sutures are heavy, non-absorbable sutures that are placed with wide tissue bites through all layers of the abdominal wall including the skin and are tied over a buttress device for skin protection to reduce tension on the wound edges. They are often used to repair postoperative fascial dehiscence. They have also been recommended to reduce the rate of wound dehiscence after major abdominal operations, particularly in those patients who are at increased risk (145).

Rink et al. (145) conducted a controlled randomized study in 95 patients with infective or malignant intra-abdominal diseases that required major abdominal operations. Abdominal midline incisions ($n = 92$) were closed by a mass technique using interrupted multifilament polyglactin. Transverse incisions were closed by a two-layer technique with a running suture of the peritoneum and the deep sheath of the fascia, and an interrupted suture of the superficial fascial sheath using the same suture material.

The retention sutures were placed through all layers of the abdominal wall. Plastic coated wire sutures and buttresses were used.

Forty-four patients were randomized to have the retention sutures, and 51 to act as controls. The results showed that postoperative pain was more severe with retention sutures ($p = 0.003$). Twelve of 44 patients with retention sutures developed local complications of the sutures, and 21 of the 44 had to have them removed prematurely, in most cases because of intolerable pain.

This study showed that retention sutures cause inconvenience and pain. However, whether retention sutures are beneficial in preventing evisceration in a subgroup of patients with high risk of wound complications, such as patients who have been on long-term steroids, is not known.

■ UNHEALED PERINEAL WOUND

After a controlled trial designed to compare the results of healing following packing the perineal wound open and after closure with drainage of the pelvis following an abdominoperineal resection or a total proctocolectomy, Irvin and Goligher (146) concluded that primary closure was the procedure of choice. At the present time, most surgeons completely close the perineal wound in abdominoperineal resection for carcinoma of the rectum and in total proctocolectomy for ulcerative colitis and Crohn's disease. A closed suction drain is placed in the presacral space and preferably brought out through a separate stab wound in the lower abdomen. Campos et al. (147) found that closure of the pelvic peritoneum and perineal wound with a drain results in a higher rate of perineal wound infection and in a longer hospital stay than closure of the perineum without closure of the pelvic peritoneum. Other complications, including bowel obstruction, are not significantly different.

Bullard et al. (148) reviewed 160 patients who underwent abdominoperineal resection with primary closure of perineal wound, for carcinoma of rectum. Seventy-three percent of patients received preoperative radiation. Major wound complication rate was 35%. Delayed healing was the most common complication (24%), followed by infection (10%). Radiation therapy increased the risk of major wound complication (41% vs. 19%), and risk of infection (14% vs. 0%). Christian et al. (149) reviewed their experience in patients who underwent abdominoperineal resection. In the subgroup of 120 patients with carcinoma of rectum, the predictors for major wound complications were increasing BMI and diabetes. Chemoradiation did not appear to increase the complications.

In patients with preoperative sepsis of the perineum, such as those with multiple perineal fistulas or perianal abscesses, the perineal subcutaneous tissue and the skin should be packed open. When there is significant fecal spillage of the pelvis and perineum during the procedure, or in patients who continue to ooze blood in the pelvis or perineum at the end of the procedure, the surgeon must judge whether the wound should be packed open or closed with suction drainage. Delalande et al. (150) showed that although the incidence of wound infection was higher after primary closure, the long-term benefit was better, particularly if the patient required postoperative adjuvant therapy because the delayed wound healing in the group whose wounds were packed was long. The authors argued that it is worthwhile to take a chance and reopen the wound if it becomes infected.

Primary healing of the closed perineal wound is achieved in 45% to 95% of patients (151–154). Patients with IBD have a greater tendency toward perineal wound breakdown than patients with carcinoma of the rectum unless a high dose of preoperative radiation has been given. Most postoperative perineal wounds that are infected should be opened, and those wounds that were left open initially should eventually heal, although this may take a few months. From 4% to 20% of perineal wounds remain open 1 year after the operation (155).

Patients with unhealed perineal wounds require evaluation of the gastrointestinal tract to rule out recurrence or flare-up of Crohn's disease; such patients with carcinoma should be evaluated for a recurrent carcinoma of the pelvis or the perineum The wound should be curetted and examined for any foreign bodies such as stitches. The wound should be carefully packed and the hair in that region shaved. If these basic measures fail, a further procedure should be considered. If small and shallow wounds are present, it may be wise to have the patient live with them.

Recent advances in reconstructive surgery have allowed various muscle flap procedures to be performed with reliable success. Baird et al. (156) used the inferior gluteal myocutaneous flap with eventual healing in 15 out of 16 patients who have had recalcitrant perineal wounds. Anthony and Mathes (155) used the gracilis, gluteus maximus (inferior and superior half), gluteal thigh, and rectus abdominis muscle flaps with long-term (3.5 year follow-up) success of 92%. Others also found them useful as a primary closure or treatment on non-healing perineal wound (157,158). The flap of choice depends on three factors: muscle flaps available, the size of the wound, and amount of skin required for closure (155).

A persistent perineal size is a common problem after an abdominoperineal resection. It is usually small and deep, with the track running into the presacral space. In this situation the sinus track can be unrooted by excising the coccyx and caudal part of the sacrum. A vacuum-assisted closure is then employed. The VAC removes exudate serum, bacteria and thus accelerates wound healing and eventually closes the wound in 95% of cases (159).

For large sacral and perineal defects following an abdominoperineal resection with or without radiation, the trend is to use the rectus abdominis myocutaneous flap. This type of flap has been used extensively in the head and neck, chest wall, breast, extremity, and groin. It provides a wide arc of rotation based on the deep inferior epigastric vessels. It provides a large bulk of tissue to fill the pelvis and perineum and results in minimal donor site morbidity (160,161). See the discussion of Operative Technique in chapter 24.

POSTOPERATIVE PERINEAL HERNIA

Perineal hernia, a protrusion of intra-abdominal viscera through a defect in the pelvic floor, is a rare complication following abdominoperineal resection or pelvic exenteration. In an excellent review So et al. (162) discussed the subject of postoperative perineal hernia and elaborated or their experience with this problem. The following account draws heavily from their review. The exact incidence is unknown but symptomatic herniation is estimated to occur in $<1\%$ of patients with abdominoperineal resection and in approximately 3% after pelvic exenteration. Barium x-ray studies reveal perineal hernias in 7% but most are as symptomatic and do not require repair. So et al. (158) summarized the factors that have been postulated to predispose a patient to perineal hernia formation. These include coccygectomy, previous hysterectomy, pelvic irradiation, excessive length of small bowel mesentery, the larger size of the female pelvis, failure to close the peritoneal defect, and excision of the levators. Symptoms associated with a perineal hernia include a dragging feeling, a sensation of bulging, and discomfort in the perineum. More serious problems such as skin breakdown, urinary symptoms, and bowel obstruction may occur.

Management of the condition is difficult. Symptoms may be controlled with a T bandage or a firm pair of underpants. Repair of this hernia poses a challenging surgical problem. The surgical principles are the same as those for other hernias (i.e., mobilize the sac, reduce its contents, excise the sac, and repair the defect). A perineal approach is attractive because it is simple and the abdominal cavity is not entered. Nevertheless, exposure is limited, so it may be difficult to exclude recurrent carcinoma, to mobilize adherent small bowel, or to repair injured viscera. With an abdominal approach, mesh can be sutured to the bony pelvis under direct vision. It is best reserved for patient with recurrent hernia or for those in whom laparotomy is necessary for other reasons. A combined abdominoperineal approach may provide the best exposure, although it is probably unnecessary except in unusual circumstances.

Operative techniques via the perineum may include simple layered closure, insertion of a synthetic mesh, creation of a gluteus maximus flap, and retroflexion of uterus. Via the abdominal approach, a layered closure may be performed, a mesh inserted, or the bladder or uterus retroflexed. It is not likely that the levators can be approximated because, following excision for malignancy, the defect is likely too large. The bladder or uterus may be sutured to the posterior pelvic wall, thus obliterating the defect. A prosthetic mesh may be sutured to the musculofascial tissue around the pelvic outlet

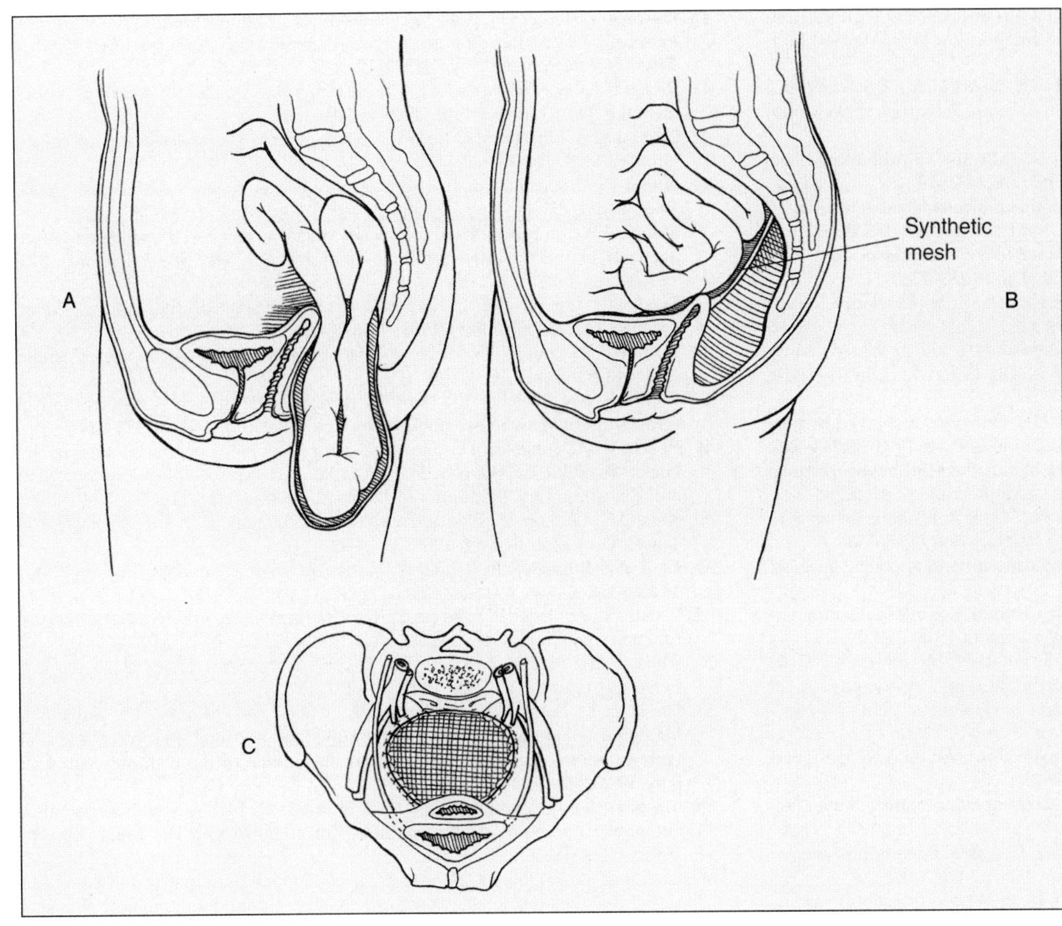

FIGURE 7 ■ Synthetic mesh repair of perineal hernia. (**A**) Sagittal view of pelvis demonstrating perineal hernia with incarcerated small bowel. (**B**) Sagittal view of pelvis with synthetic mesh in place. (**C**) View of the pelvis from above with synthetic mesh in place. *Source*: From Ref. 163.

via a perineal or transabdominal approach. Flaps of fascia lata, gracilis, rectus abdominis, or gluteus maximus can be used to close the pelvic defect.

Beck et al. (163) recommended that the mesh be sutured from the vagina or the prostatic capsule to the presacral fascia and periosteum at or below the level of S3 (Fig. 7). Care should be taken to avoid large vessels. The attachment should be below the level of the ureters. An obturator may be placed into the vagina to aid in the operative identification of the vaginal cuff, and ureteral stents may be inserted preoperatively to identify the ureters. Suction drainage can be used to obliterate dead space below the mesh. Beck et al. (163) used Marlex mesh to repair perineal hernias in eight patients—two perineal and six abdominal. Both perineal hernias and one abdominal hernia recurred (37.5%) and were re-repaired through the abdominal approach. The authors believe that the best method of repair involves the placement of a mesh across the pelvic inlet through an abdominal approach. Brotschi et al. (164) used a gracilis muscle graft tunneled subcutaneously from the thigh and attached to the sacrum.

So et al. (162) reported on 21 patients with perineal hernia. The authors' estimated incidence of symptomatic perineal recurrence following abdominoperineal resection was 0.62%. The original perineal wound was left partially open in 69% and completely open in 10% of patients. The peritoneal defect was closed in 53%, and the levators closed in 21% of patients. A perineal repair was accomplished in 13 patients, an abdominal approach was used in three patients, and a combined approach was used in three patients. Methods of repair included simple closure of pelvic defect in 10 patients; mesh insertion in five, gluteus flap in one, retroflexion of the uterus in one, and retroflexion of the bladder in one. The recurrence rate was 16% after a median 12-month follow-up. All patients had undergone a perineal repair.

Sarr et al. (165) used a combined abdominal and perineal approach allowing mobilization and reduction of herniated viscera. The mesh was sutured transabdominally to the sacrum posteriorly and to the lateral pelvic wall, to the pelvic rami anteriorly from above and from below.

It appears that the perineal approach (with or without mesh) is successful in the majority of cases and that the abdominal approach is best reserved for recurrent hernias or when access to the abdomen or pelvic contents is required.

REFERENCES

1. Mortensen PE, Olsen J, Pedersen IK, Christiansen J. A randomized study on hemorrhoidectomy combined with anal dilatation. Dis Colon Rectum 1987; 30:755–757.
2. Bailey HR, Ferguson JA. Prevention of urinary retention fluid restriction following anorectal operations. Dis Colon Rec turn 1976; 19:250–252.
3. Buls JG, Goldberg SM. Modern management of hemorrloids Surg Clin North Am 1978; 58:469–478.
4. Zaheer S, Reilly WT, Pemberton JH, Ilstrup D. Urinary retention after operation for benign anorectal diseases. Dis Colon Rectum 1998; 41:696–704.
5. Petrol JG, Malleen JK, Howe K, Rimm EB, Robillard R. Patient-controlled analgesia and postoperative urinary retention after open appendectomy. Surg Gynecol Obstet 1993; 177:172–175.
6. Friend WG, Medwell SJ. Outpatient anorectal surgery. Perspect Colon Rectal Surg 1989; 2(1):167–173.
7. Hinman F. Postoperative overdistension of the bladder. Gynecol Obstet 1976; 142:901–902.

8. Blute ML. Urinary retention in men after total hip arthroplasty [editorial]. In Coventry MB, ed. Year Book of Orthopedics Chicago: Year Book Medical Publishers, 1987:121–122.
9. Bowers FJ, Hartmann R, Khanduja KS, Hardy TG Jr., Arguilar PS, Stewart WC. Urecholine prophylaxis for urinary retention in anorectal surgery. Dis Colon Rectum 1987; 30:41–42.
10. Finkbeiner AE. Is bethanechol chloride clinically effective in promoting bladder emptying? A literature review. J Urol 1985; 134:443–449.
11. Cataldo PA, Senagore AJ. Does alpha-sympathetic blockade prevent urinary retention following anorectal surgery. Disco lon Rectum 1991; 34:1113–1116.
12. Bonardi RA, Rosin JD, Stonesifer GL Jr., Bauer FW. Bacterc associated with routine hemorrhoidectomies. Dis Colon turn 1976; 19:233–236.
13. Parikh SR, Molinelli B, Dailey TH. Liver abscess after he rhoidectomy. Report of two cases. Dis Colon Rectum 1994; 37:189.
14. Ganchrow MI, Mazier WP, Friend WG, Ferguson JA. He morrhoidectomy revisited—a computer analysis of 2038 cases. Dis Colon Rectum 1971; 14: 128–133.
15. Rosen L, Sipe P, Stasik JJ, Riether RD, Trimpi HD. Outcome of delayed hemorrhage following surgical hemorrhoidectomy. Colon Rectum 1993; 36:743–746.
16. Basso L, Pescatori M. Outcome of delayed hemorrhage following surgical hemorrhoidectomy [letter to the editor]. Dis Colon Rectum 1994; 37:288–289.
17. Sheikh F, Khubchandani IT, Rosen L, Sheets JA, Stasik JJ. Is anorectal surgery on chronic dialysis patients risky? Dis Colon Rectum 1992; 35:56–58.
18. Corman ML. Management of postoperative constipation in anorectal surgery. Dis Colon Rectum 1979; 22:149–151.
19. Walker WA, Rothenberger DA, Goldberg SM. Morbidity of internal sphincterotomy for anal fissure and stenosis. Dis Colon Rectum 1985; 28:832–835.
20. Roe AM, Bartolo DCC, Vellacott KD, Lock-Edmunds J, Mortensen NJ McC. Submucosal versus ligation excision hemorrhoidectomy: A comparison of anal sensation, anal sphincter manometry, and postoperative pain and function. Br J Surg 1987; 74:948–951.
21. Wolff BG, Culp CE. The Whitehead hemorrhoidectomy. An unjustly maligned procedure. Dis Colon Rectum 1988; 31:587–590.
22. Koenigs KP, McPhedran P, Spiro HM. Thrombosis in inflammatory bowel disease. J Clin Gastroenterol 1987; 9:627–631.
23. Talbot RW, Heppell J, Dozois RR, Beart RW Jr. Vascular complications in inflammatory bowel disease. Mayo Clin Proc 1986; 61:140–145.
24. Graef V, Baggenstoss AH, Sauer WG, Spittell JA Jr. Venous thrombosis occurring in nonspecific ulcerative colitis. A necropsy study. Arch Intern Med 1966; 117:377–382.
25. Fichera A, Cicchiello LA, Mendelrson DS, Greenstein AJ, Heimann TM. Superior mesenteric vein thrombosis after colectomy for inflammatory bowel disease. A not uncommon cause of postoperative acute abdominal pain. Dis Colon Rectum 2003; 46:643–648.
26. Remzi FH, Fazio VW, Oncel M, et al. Portal vein thrombi after restorative proctocolectomy. Surgery 2002; 132: 655–662.
27. Hudson M, Chitolie A, Hutton RA, Smith MSH, Pounder RE, Wakefield AJ. Thrombotic vascular risk factors in inflammatory bowel disease. Gut 1996; 38:733–737.
28. Morgenstern L. The avoidable complications of splenectomy. Surg Gynecol Obstet 1977; 145:525–528.
29. Langevin JM, Rothenberger DA, Goldberg SM. Accidental splenic injury during surgical treatment of the colon and rectum. Surg Gynecol Obstet 1984; 159:139–144.
30. Lord MD, Gourevitch A. The peritoneal anatomy of the spleen, with special reference to the operation of partial gastrectomy. Br J Surg 1965; 52: 202–204.
31. Morgenstern L, Shapiro S. Techniques of splenic conservation. Arch Surg 1979; 114:449–454.
32. Working Party of the British Committee for Standards in Hematology Clinical Hematology Task Force. Guidelines for the prevention and treatment of infection in patients with an absent or dysfunctioned spleen. Br Med J 1996; 312:430–433.
33. Davis EJ, Ilstrup DM, Pemberton JH. Influence of splenectomy on survival rate of patients with colorectal cancer. Am J Surg 1988; 155:173–179.
34. Zama N, Fazio VW, Jagelman DG, et al. Efficacy of pelvic packing in maintaining hemostasis after rectal excision for cancer. Dis Colon Rectum 1988; 31: 923–928.
35. Metzger PP. Modified packing technique for control of presacral pelvic bleeding. Dis Colon Rectum 1988; 31:981–982.
36. McCourtney JS, Hussain N, Mackenzie I. Balloon tamponade for control of massive presacral hemorrhage. Br J Surg 1996; 83:222.
37. Xu J, Lin J. Control of presacral hemorrhage with electrocautery through a muscle fragment pressed on the bleeding vein. J Am Coll Surg 1994; 179:351–352.
38. Braley SC, Schneider PD, Bold RJ, Goodnight JE Jr., Khatri P. Controlled tamponade of severe presacral venous hemorrhage: use of a breast implant sizer. Dis Colon Rectum 2002; 45:140–142.
39. Wang O, Shi W, Zhaw Y, Zhou W, He Z. New concepts in severe presacral hemorrhage during proctectomy. Arch Surg 1985; 120:1013–1020.
40. Nivatvongs S, Fang DT. The use of thumbtacks to stop massive presacral hemorrhage. Dis Colon Rectum 1986; 29:589–590.
41. Harrison J, Hooks VH, Pearl RK, et al. Muscle fragment welding for control of massive presacral bleeding during rectal mobilization. A review of eight cases. Dis Colon Rectum 2002; 46:1115–1117.
42. Remzi FH, Oncel M, Fazio VW. Muscle tamponade to control presacral venous bleeding. Dis Colon Rectum 2002; 45:1109–1111.
43. Zinman LM, Libertino JA, Roth RA. Management of operative ureteral injury. Urology 1978; 12:290–303.
44. Higgins CC. Ureteral injuries during surgery. A review of 87 cases. JAMA 1967; 199:82–88.
45. Melick WF. Complications of colonic and rectal surgery—The causes and management of postoperative urologic complications. Dis Colon Rectum 1973; 16:7–11.
46. Presti JC, Carroll PR. Intraoperative management of the injured ureter. Perspect Colon Rectal Surg 1988; 1(2):98–106.
47. Hamawy K, Smith JJ III, Libertino JA. Injurioes of the distal ureter. Semin Colon Rectal Sug 2000; 11:163–179.
48. Bothwell WN, Bleicher RJ, Dent TL. Prophylactic uretera catheterization in colon surgery. A five-year review. Dis Colon Rectum 1994; 37:330–334.
49. Roach MB, Donaldson DS. Urologic complications of colorectal surgery. In: Hicks TC, Beck DE, Opelka PG, Timmke AE, eds. Complications of Colon and Rectal Surgery. Baltimore: Williams & Wilkins, 1996:99–117.
50. Kinn AC, Ohman U. Bladder and sexual function after surgery for rectal cancer. Dis Colon Rectum 1986; 29:43–48.
51. Cass AS, Bubrick MP. Ureteral injuries in colonic surgery. Urology 1981; 18:359–364.
52. Walsh PC, Schlegel PN. Radical pelvic surgery with preservation of sexual function. Ann Surg 1988; 208:391–400.
53. Aboseif SR, Matzel KE, Lue TF. Sexual dysfunction after rectal surgery. Perspect Colon Rectal Surg 1990; 3(1):157–172.
54. Havenga K, Enker WE, McDermott K, Cohen AM, Minsky BD, Guillem J. Male and female sexual and urinary function after total mesorectal excision with autonomic nerve preservation for carcinoma of the rectum. J Am Coll Surg 1996; 182:495–502.
55. Masui H, Ike H, Yamaguchi S, Oki S, Shimada H. Male sexual function after autonomic nerve-preserving operation for rectal cancer. Dis Colon Rectum 1996; 39:1140–1145.
56. Goldman JA, Feldberg D, Dicker D, et al. Femoral neuropathy subsequent to abdominal hysterectomy: a comprehensive study. Eur J Obstet Gynecol Reprod Biol 1985; 20:385–392.
57. Platell FE, Thompson PJ, Makin GB. Sexual health in women following pelvic surgery for rectal cancer. Br J Surg 2004; 91:465–468.
58. Young-Fadok TM, Wolff BG. Long-term functional outcome with ileal pouch-anal anastomosis. Semin Colorectal Surg 1996; 7:114–120.
59. Lindsey I, George BD, Kettlewell MGW, Mortensen NJMEC. Importance after mesorectal and close rectal dissection for inflammatory bowel disease. Dis Colon Rectum 2001; 44:831–835.
60. Lydon JC, Spielman FJ. Bilateral compartment syndrome following prolonged surgery in the lithotomy position. Anesthesiology 1984; 60:236–238.
61. Nicholson MJ, McAlpine FS. Neural injuries associated with surgical positions and operations. In: Martin JT, ed. Positioning in Anesthesia and Surgery. Philadelphia: WB Saunders, 1978:193–224.
62. Herrera-Ornelas L, Tolls RM, Petrelli NJ, Piver S, Miffelman A. Common peroneal nerve palsy associated with pelvic surgery for cancer: an analysis of 11 cases. Dis Colon Rectum 1986; 29:392–397.
63. Schofield PF, Grace RH. Acute compartment syndrome of the legs after colorectal surgery. Colorectal Dis 2004; 6:285–287.
64. Mumtaz FH, Chew H, Gelister JS. Lower limb compartment syndrome associated with the lithotomy position: concepts and perspectives for the urologist. BJU Int 2002; 90:792–799.
65. Masten FA III. Compartmental Syndromes. New York: Grune & Stratton, 1980:1–162.
66. Masten FA, Winquist RA, Krugmire RB. Diagnosis and management of compartmental syndromes. J Bone Joint Surg [Am] 1980; 62:286–291.
67. Brasch RC, Bufo AJ, Kreienberg PF, Johnson GP. Femoral neuropathy secondary to the use of self-retaining retractor. Report of three cases and review of the literature. Dis Colon Rectum 1995; 38:1115–1118.
68. Kvist-Poulsen H, Borel J. Iatrogenic femoral neuropathy subsequent to abdominal hysterectomy: incidence and prevention. Obstet Gynecol 1982; 60:516–520.
69. Celebrezze JP Jr., Pidala MJ, Porter JA, Slezak FA. Femoral neuropathy: an infrequently reported postoperative complication. Dis Colon Rectum 2000; 43:419–422.
70. Pollard CW, Nivatvongs S, Rojanasakul A, Ilstrup DM. Carcinoma of the rectum. Profiles of intraoperative and early postoperative complications. Dis Colon Rectum 1994; 37:866–874.
71. Eriksen MT, Wibe A, Norstern J, Haffuer J, Wiigs JN, on behalf of the Norwegian rectal cancer group. Colorect Dis 2005; 7:51–57.
72. Matthiessen P, Hallbook O, Andersson M, Rutegard J, Sjodahl R. Risk factors for anatomotic leak after anterior resection of the rectum. Colorect Dis 2004; 6:462–469.
73. Law W, Chu K, Ho J, Chan C. Risk factors for anastomotic leakage after low anterior resection with total mesorectal excision. Am J Surg 2000; 179:92–95.

74. Sorensen LT, Jorgensen T, Kirkety LT. Smoking and alcohol abuse are major risk factors for anastomotic leakage in colorectal surgery. Br J Surg 1999; 86:927–931.
75. Soeters PB, DeZoete JPJGM, Dejong CHC, Williams NS, Baeten CGMI. Colorectal surgery and anastomotic leakage. Dig Surg 2002; 19:150–155.
76. Parc Y, Frileux P, Schmitt G, Dehni N, Olliver JM, Parc R. Management of Postoperative peritonitis after anterior resection. Experience from a referral intensive care unit. Dis Colon Rectum 2000; 43:579–589.
77. Smith LE. Anastomoses with EEA stapler after anterior colonic resections. Dis Colon Rectum 1981; 24:236–242.
78. Graffner H, Fredlund P, Olsson SA, et al. Protective colostomy in low anterior resection of the rectum using the EEA stapling instrument: a randomized study. Dis Colon Rectum 1983; 26:87–90.
79. Gordon PH, Vasilevsky CA. Experience with stapling in rectal surgery. Surg Clin North Am 1984; 64:555–566.
80. Kyzer S, Gordon PH. Experience with the use of the circular stapler in-rectal surgery. Dis Colon Rectum 1992; 35:696–706.
81. Leff EL, Hoexter B, Labow B, et al. The EEA stapler in low colorectal anastomoses: initial experience. Dis Colon Rectum 1982; 25:704–707.
82. Fazio VW. Advances in the surgery of rectal carcinoma utilizing the circular stapler. In: Spratt JS, ed. Neoplasms of the Colon, Rectum, and Anus. Philadelphia: WB Saunders, 1984:268–288.
83. Johansson C. Endoscopic dilation of rectal strictures. A prospective study of 18 cases. Dis Colon Rectum 1996; 39:423–428.
84. Kyzer S, Gordon PH. The stapler functional end-to-end anastomosis following colonic resection. Int J Colorectal Dis 1992; 7:125–131.
85. Otto IC, Ito K, Ye C, et al. Causes of rectal incontinence after sphincter–preserving operations for rectal cancer. Dis Colon Rectum 1996; 39:1423–1427.
86. Ikeuchi H, Kasunoki M, Shoji Y, et al. Clinicophysiological results after sphincter–saving resection for rectal carcinoma. Int J Colorectal Dis 1996; 11: 172–176.
87. Rao GN, Drew PJ, Lee PWR, et al. Anterior resection syndrome is secondary to sympathetic denervation. Int J Colorectal Dis 1996; 11:250–258.
88. Bederman SS, Betsy M, Winiarsky R, Seldes RM, Sharrock NE, Seulco TP. Postoperative ileus in the lower extremity athroplasty patient. J Arthroplasty 2001; 16:1066–1070.
89. Condon RE, Cowles VE, Schulte WJ, Frantzides CT, Mahoney J, Sarna SK. Resolution of postoperative ileus in humans. Ann Surg 1986; 203:574–581.
90. Holte K, Kehlet H. Postoperative ileus: a preventable event. Br J Surg 2000; 87:1480–1493.
91. Kalff JC, Turler A, Schwartz NT, et al. Intra–abdominal activations of a local inflammatory response within the human muscularis externa during laparotomy. Ann Surg 2003; 237:301–315.
92. Waldhawen JH, Shaffrey ME, Skenderis BS II, Jones RS, Schirmer BD. Gastrointestinal myoelectric. Ann Surg 1990; 211:777–784.
93. Prasad M, Matthews JB. Deflating postoperative ileus [editorial]. Gastroenterology 1999; 117:489–492.
94. Cheatham ML, Chapman WC, Key SP, Sawyers JL. A meta analysis of selective versus routine mesogastric decompression after elective laparotomy. Ann Surg 1995; 221:469–476.
95. Wolff BG, Pemberton JH, van Heerden JA, et al. Elective colon and rectal surgery without nasogastric decompression: a prospective, randomized trial. Ann Surg 1989; 209:670–675.
96. Wolff BG, Michelassi F, Gerkin TM, et al. Alvimopan, a novel, peripherally acting in opioid antagonist. Results of a multicutes, randomized, double–blind, placeto–controlled, phase III trial of major abdominal surgery and postoperative ileus. Ann Surg 2004; 240:728–735.
97. Delaney CP, Weese JL, Hyman NH, et al. Dis Colon Rectum 2005; 48:1114–1129.
98. Brandstrup B, Tonnesen H, Beier–Holgersen R, et al. The Danish Study Group on perioperative fluid therapy Ann Surg 2003; 238:641–648.
99. Lobo DN, Bostock KA, Neal KR, Perkins AC, Rowlands BJ, Allison SP. Effects of salt and water balance on recovery of gastrointestinal function after elective colonic resection: a randomized controlled trial. Lancet 2002; 359:1812–1818.
100. Fotiadis RJ, Badvie S, Weston MD, Allen–Mersh TG. Epidural analgesia in gastrointestinal surgery. Br J Surg 2004; 91:828–841.
101. Stewart RM, Page CP, Brender J, Schwesinger W, Eisenhut D. The incidence and risk of early postoperative small bowel obstruction. A cohort study. Am J Surg 1987; 154:643–647.
102. Menzies D, Ellis H. Intestinal obstruction from adhesions—How big is the problem? Ann R Coll Surg Engl 1990; 72:60–63.
103. Pickleman J, Lee RM. The management of patients with suspected early postoperative small bowel obstruction. Ann Surg 1989; 210:216–219.
104. Frager DH, Baer JW. Role of CT in evaluating patients with small-bowel obsruction. Semin Ultrasound CT MR 1995; 16:127–140.
105. Nauta RJ. Advanced abdominal image is not required to exclude strangulation of complete small bowel obstruction undergo prompt laparotomy. J Am Coll Surg 2005; 200:904–911.
106. Sarr MG, Buckley GB, Zuidema GD. Preoperative recog of intestinal strangulation obstruction: Prospective evaluation of diagnostic capability. Am J Surg 1983; 145:176–182.
107. Sajja SBS, Sehein M. Early postoperative small-bowel obstruction. Br J Surg 2004; 91:683–691.
108. Mallo RD, Salen L, Lalani T, Flum DR. Computed tomography diagnosis of ischemia and complete obstruction in small bowel obstruction: a systematic review. J Gastrointest Surg 2005; 9:690–694.
109. Boudiaf M, Jaff A, Soyer P, Bouhrik Y, Hamzi L, Rymer R. Small–bowel disease: protective evaluation of multi–detector row helical CT enteroclysis in 107 consecutive patients. Radiology 2004; 233:338–344.
110. Becker JM, Daton MT, Fazio VM, et al. Prevention of postoperative abdominal adhesions by sodium hyaluronate–based bio resorbable membrane: a prospective, randomized, double–blind multi–center study. J Am Coll Surg 1996; 183:297–306.
111. Beck DE, Cohen Z, Fleshman JW, Kaufman HS, van Goor H, Wolff BG, for the Adhesion Study Group Steering Committee. Dis Colon Rectum 2003; 46:1310–1319.
112. Cohen Z, Senagore AJ, Dayton MT, et al. Prevention of postoperative abdominal adhesives by a novel, glycerol/sodium hyaluronate/carboxymethylcellulose–based bioabsorable membrane: A prospective, randomized, evaluator–fluided multicenter study. Dis Colon Rectum 2005; 48:1130–1139.
113. Fazio VW, Cohen Z, Fleshman JW, et al. Reduction in adhesive small–bowel obstruction by Seprafilm adhesive barrier after intestinal resection. Dis Colon Rectum 2006; 49:1–11.
114. Fa-Si-Oen P, Roumen R, Buitenweg J, et al. Mechanical bowel preparation or not? Outcome of a multicenter, randomized trial in elective open colon surgery. Dis Colon Rectum 2005; 48:1509–1516.
115. Bucher P, Gervaz P, Soravia C, Mermillod B, Erne M, More P. Randomized clinical trial of mechanical bowel preparation versus no preparation before elective left-sided colorectal surgery. Br J Surg 2005; 92:409–414.
116. Wille-Jorgensen P, Guenaga KF, Matos D, Castro AA. Pre-operative mechanical bowel cleansing or not? an updated meta-analysis. Colorectal Dis 2005; 7: 304–310.
117. Polk HC Jr., Simpson CJ, Simmons BP, Alexander JW. Guide lines for prevention of surgical wound infection. Arch Surg 1983; 118:1213–1217.
118. Ulnalp K, Condon RE. Antibiotics prophylaxis for scheduled operative procedures. Surg Clin North Am 1992; 6:613–625.
119. Farnell MB, Worthington–Self S, Mucha P Jr., Ilstrup DM Mc Ilrath DC. Closure of abdominal incisions with subcutaneous catheters. Arch Surg 1986; 121:641–648.
120. Nichols RL, Holmes JWC. Prophylactic and therapeutic antibiotics in colon and rectal surgery. Perspect Colon Recta 1990; 3(1):183–195.
121. Olson M, O'Connor M, Schwartz ML. Surgical wound infections. A 5–year prospective study of 20,193 wounds at the Minneapolis VA Medical Center. Ann Surg 1984; 199:253–259.
122. Miller PR, Meredith JW, Johnson JC, Chang MC. Prospective evaluation of vaccum–assisted fascial closure after open abdomen. Planned ventral hermia rate is substantially reduced. Ann Surg 2004; 239:608–616.
123. Gottrup F. Prevention of surgical wound infections. Editorial. N Engl J Med 2000; 342:202–204.
124. Kurz A, Sessler DI, Lenhardt R. Perioperative normothermia to reduce the incidence of surgical wound infection and shorten hospitalization. N Eng J Med 1996; 334:1209–1215.
125. Greif R, Akea O, Horn EP, Kurz A, Sessler DI. For outcome Research Group. Supplemental perioperative oxygen to reduce the incidence of surgical wound infection. N Engl J Med 2000; 342:161–167.
126. Schoetz DJ Jr., Coller JA, Veidenheimer MC. Closure of abdominal wounds with polydioxanone. A prospective study. Arch Surg 1988; 123:72–74.
127. Richards PC, Balch CM, Aldrete JS. Abdominal wound closure. A randomized prospective study of 571 patients comparing continuous vs. interrupted suture techniques. Ann Surg 1983; 238–243.
128. Penninckx FM, Poelmans SV, Kerremans RP, Beckers JP. Abdominal wound dehiscence in gastroenterological surgery. Ann Surg 1979; 189:345–352.
129. Greenburg AG, Saik RP, Peskin GW. Wound dehiscence. Patho physiology and prevention. Arch Surg 1979; 114:143–146.
130. Wissing J, van Vroonhoven TJ, Schattenkerk ME, Veen F Ponsen RJ, Jeekel J. Fascia closure after midline laparotomy results of a randomized trial. Br J Surg 1987; 74:738–741.
131. Ellis H, Heddle R. Closure of the abdominal wound. R Soc Med 1979; 77:17–18.
132. Alexander HC, Prudden JF. The causes of abdominal wound disruption. Surg Gynecol Obstet 1966; 122:1223–1229.
133. Greenall MJ, Evans M, Pollock AV. Midline or transverse laparotomy? A random controlled clinical trial. Part I: Influence on healing. Br J Surg 1980; 67:188–190.
134. Greenall MJ, Evans M, Pollock AV. Midline or transverse laparotomy? A random controlled clinical trial. Part II: Influence on postoperative pulmonary complications. Br J Surg 1980; 67:191–194.
135. Hugh TB, Nankivell C, Meagher AP, Li B. Is closure of the peritoneal layer necessary–in the repair of midline surgical abdominal wounds? World J Surg 1990; 14:231–234.
136. Rosenberg IL, Brennan TG, Giles GR. How tight should tension sutures be tied? A controlled clinical trial. Br J Surg 1975; 62:950–951.
137. Stone IK, von Fraunhofer JA, Masterson BJ. The biomechanical effects of tight suture closure upon fascia. Surg Gynecol Obstet 1986; 163:448–452.
138. Fagniez PL, Hay JM, Lacaine F, Thomsen C. Abdominal midline incision closure. A multicentric randomized prospective trial of 3135 patients, comparing continuous vs. interrupted polyglycolic acid sutures. Arch Surg 1985; 120:1351–1353.

139. Hodgson NC, Malthaner RA, Ostbye T. The search for an ideal method of abdominal fascial closure. A meta-analysis. Ann Surg 2000; 231:436–442.
140. van't Riet M, Steyerberg EW, Nellensteyn J, Bonjer HJ, Jeekel J. Meta-analysis of techniques for closure of midline abdominal incisions. Br J Surg 2002; 89:1350–1356.
141. Poole GV Jr. Mechanical factors in abdominal wound closure: their prevention of fascial dehiscence. Surgery 1985; 97:631–639.
142. Rucinski J, Margolis M, Panagopoulos G, Wise L. Closure of the abdominal midline fascia: meta-analysis delineates the optimal technique. Am Surg 2001; 67:421–426.
143. Ray JA, Doddi N, Regula D, Williams JA, Melveger A. Polydioxanone (PDS), a novel monofilament synthetic absorbable suture. Surg Gynecol Obstet 1981; 153:497–507.
144. Israelsson LA, Jonsson T. Closure of midline laparotomy incisions with polydioxanine and nylon: the importance of suture technique. Br J Surg 1994; 81:1606–1608.
145. Rink AD, Goldschmidt D, Dietrich J, Nagelschmidt M, Vestweber KH. Negative side-effects of retention sutures for abdominal wound closure. A prospective randomised study. EWC J Surg 2000; 166:932–937.
146. Irvin TT, Goligher JC. A controlled clinical trial of three different methods of perineal wound management following excision of the rectum. Br J Surg 1975; 62:287–291.
147. Campos RR, Ayllon JC, Paricio PP, et al. Management of perineal wound following abdominoperineal resection: prospective study of three methods. Br J Surg 1992; 79:29–31.
148. Bullard RM, Trudel JL, Baxter NN, Rothenberger DA. Primary perineal normal closure after preoperative radiotherapy and abdominoperineal resection has a high incidence of wound failure. Dis Colon Rectum 2005; 48: 438–443.
149. Christian CK, Kwaan MR, Betensky RA, Breen EM, Zinner MJ, Bleday R. Risk factors for perineal wound complications following abdominoperineal resection. Dis Colon Rectum 2005; 48:438–443.
150. Delalande JP, Hay JM, Fingerhut A, Kohlmann GC, Paquet JC. French Association for Surgical Research. Perineal wound management after abdominoperineal rectal excision for carcinoma with unsatisfactory hemostasis or gross septic contamination; Primary closure vs. packing. A multicenter, control trial. Dis Colon Rectum 1994; 37:890–896.
151. Baudot P, Keighley MRB, Alexander-Williams J. Perineal wound healing after proctectomy for carcinoma and inflammatory disease. Br J Surg 1980; 67: 275–276.
152. Elliott M, Todd IP. Primary suture of the perineal wound using constant suction and irrigation, following rectal excision for inflammatory bowel disease. Ann R Coll Surg Engl 1985; 67:6–7.
153. Oakley JR, Fazio VW, Jagelman DG, Lavery IC, Weakley FL, Easley K. Management of the perineal wound after rectal excision for ulcerative colitis. Dis Colon Rectum 1985; 28:885–888.
154. Tompkins RG, Warshaw AL. Improved management of the perineal wound after proctectomy. Ann Surg 1985; 202:760–776.
155. Anthony JP, Mathes SJ. The recalcitrant perineal wound after rectal extirpation. Arch Surg 1990; 125:1371–1377.
156. Baird WL, Hester TR, Nahai F, Bostwick J III. Management of perineal wounds following abdominoperineal resection with inferior gluteal flaps. Arch Surg 1990; 125:1486–1489.
157. Galandink S, Jordon J, Mahid S, McCafferty MH, Tobin G. The use of tissue flaps as an adjunct to pelvic surgery. Am J Surg 2005; 190:186–190.
158. Menon A, Clark MA, Shatari T, Keh C, Keighley MRB. Pedicled flaps in the treatment of nonhealing perineal wounds. Colorect Dis 2005; 7:441–444.
159. Pemberton JH. How to treat the persistent perineal sinus after rectal excision. Colorect Dis 2003; 5:486–489.
160. Loessin SJ, Meland NB, Devine RM, Wolff BG, Nelson H, Zimcke H. Management of sacral and perineal defects following abdominoperineal resection and radiation with transpelvic muscle flaps. Dis Colon Rectum 1995; 38: 940–945.
161. Temple L, Lindsay RL, Temple WJ, Magi E, Ketcham AS. Rectus myocutaneous flaps for primary repair of composite defects of the pelvis. Perspect Colon Rectal Surg 1993; 6:171–174.
162. So JB, Palmer MT, Shellito PC. Postoperative perineal hernia. Dis Colon Rectum 1997; 40:954–957.
163. Beck DE, Fazio VW, Jagelman DG, Lavery JC, McGonagle BA. Postoperative perineal hernia. Dis Colon Rectum 1987; 30:21–24.
164. Brotschi E, Noe JM, Silen W. Perineal hernias after proctectomy. A new approach to repair. Am J Surg 1985; 149:301–305.
165. Sarr MG, Stewart JR, Cameron JC. Combined abdominoperineal approach to repair of postoperative perineal hernia. Dis Colon Rectum 1982; 25:597–599.

37 Unexpected Intraoperative Findings

Philip H. Gordon, Santhat Nivatvongs, and Lee E. Smith

INTRODUCTION

The ever-expanding technology available to the practicing physician has made possible the luxury of defining intra-abdominal pathology well in advance of a laparotomy. Nevertheless, from time to time surprises do arise with additional disease states or anatomic variations and the surgeon must make important decisions rapidly. This chapter highlights some unusual or unexpected findings and offers suggestions for managing them. We fully recognize that the management of many of these problems is controversial; in fact, that is precisely why these subjects have been selected. Although we are well aware that the list of surprises could extend almost without limit, we have chosen to focus on subjects that are not particularly uncommon yet present a dilemma to the surgeon. Suggested therapy may represent only a consensus of the authors.

The gynecologist often discovers large bowel pathology under one of the following circumstances: (1) during the operative treatment of established gynecologic pathology, (2) when acute or chronic pelvic sepsis is demonstrated as due to complications of large bowel disease, (3) when the true nature of an abdominal pelvic neoplasm is determined at laparotomy. Since appropriate bowel preparation most likely will not have been performed in such situations, definitive treatment may result in higher postoperative morbidity than would result under ideal conditions. The dilemma involved is that the surgeon is faced with one of several challenging situations: (1) unprepared bowel, which involves the inherent risk of increased sepsis in colorectal operations, (2) established sepsis with the obvious concern of creating an anastomosis, or (3) possible catastrophic outcome if sepsis should ensue following an associated operation (e.g., as for an abdominal aortic aneurysm).

Some of the following case examples will be all too familiar to many readers.

CASE 1: CARCINOMA OF RECTUM AND UNEXPECTED SYNCHRONOUS CARCINOMA OF HEPATIC FLEXURE

At laparotomy, a 72-year-old patient being operated on for carcinoma of the rectosigmoid is found to have a previously unsuspected mass in the hepatic flexure deemed to represent a synchronous carcinoma. There is no evidence of metastatic disease. What is the most appropriate operation?

With a patient having synchronous carcinomas, a number of options are open. The surgeon could proceed with the planned low anterior resection and assess the right colonic mass postoperatively through a barium enema or colonoscopic evaluation. Alternatively, the surgeon could allow a recovery period of several weeks before a right hemicolectomy is performed. Both options are inappropriate.

The only two viable options are (1) to proceed immediately with a total abdominal colectomy and ileorectal anastomosis or (2) to perform two resections, the planned low anterior resection and a right hemicolectomy. There is no question that the first option is appealing because it rids the patient of both carcinomas through only one anastomosis. Furthermore, it might be best for a patient who already harbors two malignancies of the colon to be liberated from an organ with demonstrated propensity to neoplasia. The short rectal stump would make follow-up of the remaining bowel simple for both the patient and the surgeon. The risk of one anastomosis may be less than the risk of two anastomoses. For patients with carcinomas that are both located more proximally in the bowel (i.e., anywhere from the cecum to the proximal to middle sigmoid colon), this option would seem to be the treatment of choice. If synchronous carcinomas are located in an area of similar lymph node drainage, the respective hemicolectomy is indicated. For patients with malignancies involving different drainage areas in the lymphatic system of the colon, subtotal colectomy or total proctocolectomy and ileostomy (if the distal rectum is involved) should be performed.

There are several proponents of subtotal colectomy (1–3). However, an overriding consideration, especially in the older patient, is what the functional results would be (4). Exactly how much distal bowel is necessary for an adequate reservoir is not certain, and it is unquestionable that the amount will vary from patient to patient. Experience with patients with familial adenomatous polyposis suggests that an anastomosis performed at the level of the sacral promontory has resulted in an acceptable frequency of defecation. It must be noted that for the most part this experience has been accumulated in young individuals.

The patient in question is older, and the proposed anastomosis would need to be performed at a considerably lower level. Under these circumstances, it would be anticipated that functional results would not be good, and therefore we would strongly favor a double resection (i.e., the planned low anterior resection and a concomitant right hemicolectomy at the same operation). With the use of repeated colonoscopy, little trouble would be encountered in following the residual colon for metachronous neoplasia.

CASE 2: CARCINOMA OF RIGHT COLON AND UNEXPECTED MAJOR SINGLE HEPATIC METASTASIS

An unexpected 5 cm mass is found deep in the right lobe of the liver during laparotomy for resection of a right colonic carcinoma. Preoperative liver function tests were normal. What is the recommended management?

The philosophy of the management of patients with metastatic disease to the liver has changed dramatically in the past 20 years. The goal of therapy in any operation for malignancy is the removal of all detectable disease. In this situation, the operation would encompass both a right hemicolectomy and a right hepatic lobectomy, a procedure that is of greater magnitude than is indicated under the circumstances. Prior to hepatic resection, it would be necessary to determine the extent of other metastatic disease, if present. It also would be appropriate to discuss with the patient the potential risks of a partial hepatic resection of this magnitude. If the lesion were one that was suitable for simple wedge excision or left lateral segmentectomy, it would be fitting to do either procedure in association with the right hemicolectomy.

Even in the presence of metastatic disease in the liver, the primary colonic carcinoma should be removed because of the risk of later complications such as bleeding and obstruction. The addition of postoperative systemic chemotherapy is of dubious benefit with respect to prolongation of useful life. The insertion of a catheter via the gastroduodenal artery for hepatic infusion of a chemotherapeutic agent is another option that is of questionable value with respect to the overall potential long-term benefit. For the patient with extensive hepatic involvement, the latter mode of therapy may be considered, but it is not the best form of treatment in patients with isolated liver metastasis. The most appropriate approach to the situation is resection of the primary lesion and biopsy of the hepatic lesion to confirm that it represents metastatic disease. If available, intraoperative ultrasonography may prove to be the most valuable investigative modality to determine the extent of intrahepatic metastatic disease.

Postoperative investigations should include a computed tomography (CT) scan of the abdomen and the chest to rule out the presence of other metastatic disease. If there is no other evidence of metastasis and after the matter has been discussed with the patient, a right hepatic lobectomy should be performed 4 to 6 weeks later. An argument has been offered for waiting as long as six months to permit identification of biologically favorable lesions and resecting only those lesions. However, there seems to be no advantage to this course of action. Indeed, there may be some disadvantage, because metastases can occur from liver metastases. Therefore it would be inappropriate to delay treatment unduly since a 5-year survival rate of 25% to 40% can be achieved following resection of solitary liver metastases (5–7).

CASE 3: SIGMOID MASS THAT PROVES TO BE ENDOMETRIOMA INSTEAD OF CARCINOMA

A 42-year-old woman presented with a six-month history of abdominal cramps. Barium enema study revealed narrowing in the sigmoid colon, and colonoscopy was unsuccessful because the scope could not be negotiated through the narrow portion. A laparotomy was performed for the presumed diagnosis of carcinoma of the sigmoid, but extrinsic pressure from a partially encompassing blue-brown mass was seen. Further inspection revealed purple specks on the pelvic structures. A presumptive diagnosis of endometriosis was made. What would be the appropriate management?

Endometriotic implants on pelvic structures are a common finding during pelvic laparotomy for gynecologic disease. Once the intestinal involvement has become symptomatic, the only successful treatment that prevents subsequent recurrence of symptoms is resection of the affected segment combined with total abdominal hysterectomy and bilateral salpingo-oophorectomy (8–10). If the diagnosis of endometriosis had been suspected preoperatively and the patient was informed of the possibility, resection is the treatment of choice. However, under the current circumstances, we would suggest limitation of treatment to sigmoid resection. We would be reluctant to perform a total abdominal hysterectomy and bilateral salpingo-oophorectomy without the patient's knowledge.

Simple retreat with hope of relief of symptoms by hormonal administration is inappropriate because once intestinal symptoms have developed, scarring has advanced to the point where endocrine treatment will be ineffective (11,12). Similar operative treatment would be endorsed for the patient who still desires a family. If the implant is well circumscribed, local excision of the colonic endometrioma may be effective (9,13). Gonadotropin-releasing hormone antagonists such as leuprolide (Lupron) and nafarelin (Synarel) have demonstrated efficacy in the treatment of small endometrial implants but do not have a major impact on large deposits (10).

CASE 4: EXPLORATION FOR APPENDICITIS THAT PROVES TO BE CARCINOMA OF CECUM

The patient is a 51-year-old man presenting with right lower quadrant pain and scheduled to undergo a laparotomy via McBurney's incision for the diagnosis of acute appendicitis. The patient is found to have a mass interpreted as a walled-off perforated carcinoma of the cecum. How should the patient's management be handled?

The discovery of unexpected disease at laparotomy often taxes the judgment and ingenuity of the surgeon. This is especially true for emergency operations, which are often performed at night. It is estimated that 10% to 15% of right colonic carcinomas will first appear as acute abdomen. It is not too uncommon for a patient to undergo exploration and have a preoperative diagnosis of appendicitis only for the surgeon to find a carcinoma of the cecum causing obstruction and resulting appendicitis, a perforated carcinoma of the cecum or ascending colon with a normal appendix, an acute appendicitis with a more distal obstructing carcinoma of the hepatic flexure or the sigmoid colon, or an adenocarcinoma of the appendix itself. The surgeon is faced with the unprepared bowel and the prospect of contamination from perforation of the bowel if a resection is performed immediately. One choice would be to close the abdomen and return after the patient has undergone adequate bowel preparation, which offers a theoretic advantage for operation. However, there is the risk of progression of the inflammatory process with potential aggravation during bowel preparation. A free perforation may even result. Therefore, whenever the surgeon is faced with the situation that carcinoma is suspected, a right hemicolectomy should be performed.

Next, the surgeon must decide whether McBurney's incision is adequate for the revised operation. Some surgeons would close the incision and make a formal midline incision to gain greater exposure. However, extension of McBurney's incision across the rectus muscle to the midline creates more than ample exposure for performing a right hemicolectomy. In an elderly patient with a less certain diagnosis, a lower midline incision might be considered. After that procedure has been performed, the surgeon is faced with the question of whether to perform a primary anastomosis or to bring out the two ends of bowel. Considerable evidence suggests that it is safe to proceed with a primary anastomosis following emergency right hemicolectomy (14). Appropriate operative treatment should not be postponed because of lack of bowel preparation. Even the presence of walled-off pus rarely contraindicates resection and anastomosis. In the face of generalized peritonitis following excision of the diseased segment of bowel, consideration should be given to performing an end-loop stoma. Of course, appropriate antibiotic coverage is indicated.

Usually, the major problem under these circumstances is making the diagnosis. The ileocecal region is notorious for inflammatory masses that are difficult to distinguish from carcinoma. When appendicitis is present, it is understandable that the surrounding induration may be attributed to the associated inflammatory process without suspicion of an underlying malignancy. The degree of difficulty in making a diagnosis at the time of appendectomy is underscored by the fact that less than one-half of the cases reported in the literature were diagnosed at initial laparotomy. The average delay in diagnosis is 4 to 6 months (15–17). Postoperative clues to the true nature of the underlying disease include cecal fistulas, recurrent abscesses, and discharging sinus following appendectomy. These circumstances dictate further investigation of the colon.

CASE 5: PELVIC LAPAROTOMY FOR GYNECOLOGIC MASS THAT PROVES TO BE CARCINOMA OF SIGMOID

A 43-year-old woman is undergoing laparotomy for a pelvic mass presumed to be of ovarian origin. The gynecologist finds the ovaries to be normal, and the mass proves to be a hard 7 cm lesion in the middle sigmoid colon that is compatible with either carcinoma or diverticular disease. You are called to the operating room and asked to consider removing the lesion. The bowel has not been prepared and hard stool can be palpated throughout the colon. What is your decision?

The options in this case include (1) performing a resection and a colostomy, (2) performing a resection and an anastomosis, (3) doing nothing and having the patient return for an elective resection at a later date, after the bowel has been prepared and the patient has been evaluated fully, or (4) performing a resection, on-table lavage, and anastomosis. If the lesion were in the right colon, a right hemicolectomy with anastomosis would seem appropriate since this procedure can be accomplished without preparation and with minimum morbidity (18,19).

Emergency or unplanned resection of the left colon is much more controversial, particularly in the presence of fecal loading. If the patient has an impending obstruction, resection must be performed immediately. In this circumstance, waiting for time to perform a mechanical bowel preparation and elective resection may not be feasible, and the bowel preparation actually may provoke complete obstruction.

Whether obstruction is imminent or not, once a decision has been made to proceed with resection, a second choice must be made between performing an anastomosis or creating a colostomy. Although primary anastomosis in select patients has been advocated by some authors (20), others have emphasized the prevalence of septic complications and anastomotic leaks when anastomosis is performed in unprepared bowel (21,22). If a colostomy is to be performed, creating an end colostomy and Hartmann's pouch is preferable. The alternative of creating a proximal colostomy with distal anastomosis leaves a column of stool and bacteria between the colostomy and the anastomosis and does not completely protect against septic anastomotic complications. In addition to resection and anastomosis or resection and colostomy, a third option is resection with anastomosis and intraoperative fecal washout (23). One variation is to perform a subtotal excision of the colon to a point in the distal sigmoid colon and to achieve washout of the rectosigmoid per anum to permit a safe anastomosis of the ileum to the distal sigmoid.

Since favorable results have been reported with each of these options, any one of them can be considered acceptable. A growing number of surgeons will favor resection, on-table lavage, and primary anastomosis. This has become our preference. Some surgeons prefer resection and anastomosis and this course of action is supported by publications stating that bowel preparation is not mandatory. If concern of integrity of anastomosis arises, a diverting ileostomy might be in order. This topic has been described in detail in Chapter 4 on bowel preparation.

CASE 6: EXPLORATION FOR ACUTE APPENDICITIS THAT PROVES TO BE SIGMOID PHLEGMON

A 40-year-old man is undergoing exploration for appendicitis through a McBurney's incision. The appendix, cecum, and terminal ileum are found to be perfectly normal. A small amount of serous fluid is found in the peritoneal cavity but the sigmoid colon is noted to be acutely inflamed. What should the management be?

There is controversy regarding the most effective method of managing the perforated diverticular segment. When there is a major unsealed perforation with fecal contamination, immediate resection for the involved segment is appropriate. But in the vast majority of cases with generalized peritonitis from perforated diverticular disease, there is no evidence of fecal contamination, and the perforation is already sealed or cannot be found at laparotomy. Possibly only a phlegmon is present. In this circumstance, it is unclear whether immediate definitive resection is required. Many surgeons favor this policy because the patient is already committed to undergoing laparotomy. On the other hand, some would argue that if the diagnosis had been known preoperatively and if the patient was responding to medical treatment, an urgent operation would not have been offered to the patient and therefore no resection should be performed. It is perhaps important to know whether the patient had experienced previous symptoms of diverticular disease because this would tip the scale in favor of resection. In the minds of some surgeons, a patient younger than the age of 40 and even younger than the age of 50 years should undergo resection. Stefansson et al. (24) found that in patients with a phlegmonous diverticulitis or abscess, the postoperative complications were threefold greater (13% vs. 4%) in those who did not undergo resection. If resection is considered, then a decision must be made as to which of the several options would be the most appropriate—Hartmann's procedure, a primary resection with anastomosis with or without on-table lavage, or a primary resection and anastomosis with proximal diversion. If the patient was previously symptomatic, resection with on-table lavage would probably best serve the patient. Even if the patient had not had symptoms attributable to diverticular disease, the complication rate for phlegmonous diverticulitis reported by Stefansson et al. (24) would persuade us to choose the resection option.

CASE 7: CARCINOMA OF RECTUM WITH INCIDENTAL CHOLELITHIASIS

A 79-year-old man is undergoing anterior resection with a low pelvic anastomosis for adenocarcinoma of the rectum located 9 cm from the dentate line. The liver is normal but the gallbladder contains multiple stones. There is no clear-cut history of symptomatic gallbladder disease, and cholelithiasis was not suspected preoperatively. Should the gallbladder be removed?

The decision of whether to proceed with cholecystectomy must take into account the added morbidity and mortality of this procedure, the risks of symptomatic gallbladder disease developing in the immediate or late postoperative period, and the medicolegal liability of performing such an added procedure. In point of fact, it is not likely that the surgeon is unaware of the presence of gallstones because the preoperative investigation of the patient with carcinoma most likely included ultrasonography or a CT scan of the liver, in which case the gallstones will have been identified. The question that arises as to the propriety of the cholecystectomy and these considerations are discussed.

Most studies have emphasized that although complication rates range from 20% to 41% when cholecystectomy is added to another intra-abdominal procedure, complications specifically related to the cholecystectomy occur in $\leq 3\%$ of these cases, and the mortality rate is not increased (25–27). All of this assumes, however, that the cholecystectomy is performed during a procedure that has gone well, that the patient is stable, and that the incision does not need to be significantly extended. The assumption is that the scope and magnitude of the operation are not significantly increased or that the operation was inordinately prolonged. Shennib et al. (28), in a study of 25 patients who underwent simultaneous cholecystectomy and colectomy, concluded that the addition of cholecystectomy was safe when performed during the course of an elective colonic resection if the patient was stable. The authors do not recommend performing cholecystectomy during the course of emergency colectomy in an ill patient with an unprepared bowel.

It is possible that patients with cholelithiasis discovered incidentally at the time of another abdominal operation may be at greater risk for developing symptomatic gallbladder disease than similar individuals not undergoing operation. In one study the risk of cholecystitis or symptomatic gallbladder disease developing within six months of operation was found to be as high as 70% among 23 patients with cholelithiasis who did not have incidental cholecystectomy during an abdominal operation (25). Acute cholecystitis developing in the immediate postoperative period in similar patients also has been noted (25). Whether this relationship is fortuitous in the above studies or whether it is related to postoperative mechanical or metabolic factors is unclear.

Overall, it does appear reasonable and appropriate to proceed with cholecystectomy in the patient described here if favorable conditions exist This would mean that the anterior resection and anastomosis proceeded without complication, that the patient's condition remained stable throughout the procedure, and that the gallbladder can be reached easily through the original incision. Usually, cholecystectomy is technically feasible from both vertical or transverse incisions as long as the initial incision is generous and the patient is not obese. If the incision needs to be significantly extended to achieve adequate exposure for cholecystectomy, the overall scope of the operation is being expanded and the possibility of having a significant increase in postoperative complications becomes a factor. In these circumstances, it is best to leave the gallbladder intact.

From a medicolegal point of view it appears safe to proceed with a previously unplanned cholecystectomy when unsuspected cholelithiasis is identified, since a surgeon is ordinarily protected by the legal doctrine of "extension of informed consent" (29). The low morbidity and negligible mortality when cholecystectomy is performed, along with the alternative risks of postoperative symptomatic gallbladder disease when cholecystectomy is not performed, reinforce the validity of an intraoperative decision to proceed with cholecystectomy. Nevertheless, since this does constitute removal of an organ without the patient's prior consent, it is especially important that the cholecystectomy be performed only under favorable conditions without increasing the magnitude of the operation. Legally, the safest course is to discuss the possibility of cholecystectomy or removal of other tissues with the patient at the time that consent for colectomy is obtained.

CASE 8: CARCINOMA OF RECTUM WITH INVASION OF URINARY BLADDER

An otherwise healthy 56-year-old man is scheduled to undergo a low anterior resection of the rectum, but at laparotomy the carcinoma is found to have invaded the base of the bladder and the prostate. There is no evidence of distal spread. The patient has not been informed about the possibility of a pelvic exenteration. Should a pelvic exenteration be performed?

The recommendations made here are what we believe to be in the best interest of the patient. However, following them may result in procedures being performed without the patient's fully informed consent. This discussion is not intended to cover that legal aspect of the problem.

Pelvic exenteration for colorectal carcinoma involves en bloc removal of the colon and/or anorectum, the bladder and distal ureters with creation of an ileal conduit, a pelvic lymph node dissection, and removal of internal reproductive organs as indicated. It is a formidable procedure with high morbidity and mortality rates. A review of the literature by Eckhauser et al. (30) showed a mortality rate of 12%. In a large series of pelvic exenterations for colorectal, gynecologic, and urologic diseases reported by Jakowatz et al. (31), there was a major complication rate of 49%, including gastrointestinal fistulas or obstruction, urinary tract fistulas, infection or obstruction, wound dehiscence, and/or hemorrhages. The complications rate was highest (67%) when patients received preoperative radiation and lowest (26%) when radiation was not given. However, the operative mortality rate was only 2.9%. Other reports support the justification of pelvic exenteration or en bloc excision of a T4 lesion, if the procedure can be performed with an intention of cure (32–35).

There are two major justifications for aggressive surgical treatment of patients with locally advanced primary and recurrent rectal carcinoma in the absence of gross distant metastases. First, many of these patients will die with catastrophic symptomatic consequences of uncontrolled pelvic carcinoma, primarily pain and tenesmus. Symptoms are only temporarily abated with radiation therapy alone. Second, autopsy studies suggest that 25% to 50% of such patients have carcinoma limited to the pelvis at the time of death. Hence, aggressive efforts at local control may not only avoid painful recurrence in such patients, but disease-free and overall survival may be improved (36).

Colorectal carcinoma with direct invasion into the bladder but without distant metastases is uncommon, accounting for only 5% of cases (37). This type of lesion cannot be cured by nonoperative management such as chemotherapy or radiation therapy. Preoperative radiation for a clinically resectable lesion will not change the extent of the resection (38), and it may only increase the complication rate (31). When patients are properly selected, the five-year survival rate can be expected to be 45% to 50% (37,39). Ideally, the lesion should be limited locally without lymph node metastases. En bloc resection of the rectum and the adjacent involved organs was performed in 65 patients in a series reported by Orkin et al. (39). Of those patients, 26% underwent a cystectomy. There were no perioperative deaths. Postoperative complications developed in 20% of patients, and the overall five-year survival rate was 52%. Talamonti et al. (40) reviewed the records of 70 patients who underwent resection of a carcinoma of the colon and rectum with en bloc total cystectomy (36 patients) or partial cystectomy (34 patients) because of malignancy directly extending into the urinary bladder. Sixty-four patients with negative resection margins had a median survival of 34 months and a five-year actuarial survival rate of 51.8%. In contrast, the median survival period for six patients who had positive margins was 11 months, with no survivors at five years.

The only hope for cure in colorectal carcinoma with invasion into the bladder is to perform pelvic exenteration. This is an extensive operation with potentially high morbidity, mortality, and prolonged postoperative recovery.

In properly selected patients, the operation is worthwhile in terms of long-term survival and symptomatic relief. Patients with distant metastases should not be considered for pelvic exenteration.

At the time of exploration, the surgeon must accurately establish the extent of pelvic disease and the surgeon's ability to remove it. Actual histologic invasion of adjacent structures can be very difficult to differentiate from inflammatory reaction without pathologic confirmation. Complete excision of the neoplasm with a portion or all of any apparently involved organs appears to result in the best possibility of complete excision and thus cure. A team approach consisting of a colorectal surgeon, a gynecologic surgeon, and a urologic surgeon helps achieve optimal results (39).

The bulkiness of the lesion should not deter surgeons. Size and local extension do not correlate with long-term survival. The most important predictors of survival are lymph node status and involvement of the resection margins. In fact, the overall survival in patients with T4 carcinomas who underwent radical resection is not significantly different from that in those with T3 carcinomas, even in N1 stages (34).

Armed with this information, what should the surgeon do for the patient? Ideally, a discussion is held with the patient preoperatively, but since the intraoperative findings were a surprise, this cannot be done. The options are to proceed with an exenteration or close the abdomen and discuss the recommendation with the patient. It is technically easier to proceed at the original operation because repeat operations are more difficult. Most often, a portion of the mobilization has already been accomplished, and it is quite possible that the best technical operation can be accomplished at this time. However, because of the magnitude of the procedure, the potential high complication rate, and the life-altering style for the patient we would favor aborting the procedure and discuss the advantages of a pelvic exenteration with the patient.

CASE 9: CONCOMITANT CARCINOMA OF RECTUM AND ABDOMINAL AORTIC ANEURYSM

A 75-year-old man is scheduled to undergo low anterior resection of the rectum for a carcinoma. At laparotomy, an unexpected abdominal aortic aneurysm, approximately 6 cm in size, is felt. What is the appropriate management? Should the two conditions be treated simultaneously? Should the surgeon proceed with the resection originally planned and let the aneurysm be resected at a later date, or should the aneurysm be resected immediately and the carcinoma resected later?

The occurrence of synchronous colorectal carcinoma and abdominal aortic aneurysm (AAA) is uncommon. At the Mayo Clinic from 1975 to 1986, approximately 3500 patients with AAA underwent repair, but only 17 patients were found to have a simultaneous colorectal carcinoma (41). Most lesions were discovered before the operation and thus the management could be planned. More recently, Baxter et al. (42) reviewed 435 Mayo Clinic patients with a history of colorectal carcinoma and abdominal aortic aneurysm of which 83 patients had concomitant abdominal aortic aneurysm and colorectal carcinoma. In 64 patients, the colorectal carcinoma was treated first, and 44 of these patients had an abdominal aortic aneurysm <5 cm in diameter (average $=$ 3.8 cm). No abdominal aortic aneurysm ruptured in the postoperative period. Median delay in colorectal carcinoma surgery from diagnosis was four days. There were 20 patients with abdominal aortic aneurysm of 5 cm or greater (average $=$ 5.4 cm) who were treated for colorectal carcinoma first. In two of these patients (with abdominal aortic aneurysms sized 5 and 6.4 cm), the abdominal aortic aneurysm ruptured in the early postoperative period. Median delay in colorectal carcinoma resection was eight days. There were 12 patients who had both an abdominal aortic aneurysm and colorectal carcinoma treated at the same time. The average size of the abdominal aortic aneurysm was 6.4 cm. Median delay from colorectal carcinoma diagnosis to resection was 15 days. No documented cases of graft infection occurred in this group; median follow-up was 3.2 years. There were seven patients who underwent abdominal aortic aneurysm repair before resection of their colorectal carcinoma; in two patients, colorectal carcinoma was found at the time of resection. The average size of the abdominal aortic aneurysm was 6 cm and median delay to treatment of colorectal carcinoma was 122 days, a statistically significant longer delay than in the other two groups. They concluded that in patients with colorectal carcinoma and abdominal aortic aneurysms of 5 cm or more, treatment of colorectal carcinoma first may result in life-threatening rupture, whereas treatment of the abdominal aortic aneurysm first may significantly delay treatment of the colorectal carcinoma. Concomitant treatment seems to be a safe alternative. If anatomically suitable, the abdominal aortic aneurysm may be considered for endovascular repair followed by a staged colon resection. The presence of an abdominal aortic aneurysm less than 5 cm does not affect colorectal carcinoma treatment. Herald et al. (43) also described the use of endovascular placement of a graft for the treatment of abdominal aortic aneurysms in association with rectal carcinoma.

In general, it has been recommended to resect the lesion that causes symptoms first, with an option to resect the second lesion at the same time or at a later date (44). Frequently, however, the patients are generally free of symptoms, and one lesion is discovered incidentally at the elective resection of the other. What should be done? If neither symptoms nor aneurysm size establish priority, the relative indolent course of colon carcinoma favors aneurysmectomy with colectomy in 2 to 4 weeks (41).

The advantages of concomitant resections of colorectal carcinoma and AAA is the avoidance of a second operation and the elimination of the possibility of a ruptured AAA postoperatively if left untreated. The major risk of this approach is a possible aortic graft infection, which can be life threatening. The risk of ruptured AAA after laparotomy is real (41,45). Some attribute this to the increased activity of the proteolytic enzymes collagenase and elastase (45–47), although this is only speculation. In a series by Nora et al. (41), eight patients had colorectal resection without resection of the AAA. Three patients died from complications of the aneurysm, including two ruptured aneurysms and one thrombotic aneurysm. The remaining five patients also died, four from disseminated carcinoma, with death occurring 6, 12, 18, and 48 months later; the other patient died from sepsis 36 hours postoperatively. It appears that for long-term survival both lesions must be resected aggressively (41).

The size of the aneurysm plays an important role in the decision-making process. It is generally agreed that an AAA >7 cm poses a risk of rupture in the near future and tends to rupture soon after colonic resection (48). Therefore, such an aneurysm should be resected first, unless the colorectal carcinoma is obstructing. Velanovich and Andersen (44) recommend that when both lesions are asymptomatic and the aneurysm is 4 to 5 cm in diameter, it should be resected first, if the colorectal carcinoma has a less than 5% chance of obstruction or perforation, as is found in non-circumferential lesions. When the aneurysm is >5 cm, it should be resected first if the carcinoma has a less than 22% chance of obstructing or perforating, as with circumferential lesions. Simultaneous resection should be considered for patients with aneurysms >5 cm and carcinomas with a greater than 75% to 80% chance with obstruction or perforation, provided the dual procedures can be performed with a less than 10% operative mortality and less than 50% complication rate. If it is deemed that there is an impending obstruction by the carcinoma, both the aneurysm and the carcinoma should be resected simultaneously (49). The AAA should be resected first and the retroperitoneum closed, with interposition of omentum between the graft and the peritoneum before resection of the colon and rectum to minimize the risk of graft infection. An elective simultaneous resection of AAA and a right colectomy can be safely performed. The risk of anastomotic leak is higher for a left colectomy. For a low anterior resection, unless the procedure is easy, a complementary loop ileostomy should be considered, or a colostomy and Hartmann's pouch procedure should be performed.

A 5 cm diameter abdominal aortic aneurysm has a 4.1% annual risk of rupture if left untreated, and this risk increases exponentially with increasing aneurysm diameter so that a 7 cm abdominal aortic aneurysm has a 19% yearly risk of rupture (50). In situations where the carcinoma shows no symptoms of obstruction and the aneurysm is also asymptomatic and <6 cm in diameter, it has traditionally been taught that the aneurysm should be resected first because of the risk of post-laparotomy rupture of the aneurysm, which has been reported to be as high as 33.8% (44).

The surgeon must be certain that the two ends of bowel have good blood supply. After sacrificing the inferior mesenteric artery, there is usually enough blood supply from the marginal artery Drummond as well as branches from the iliac arteries. It has been shown that colonic ischemia is usually the result of perioperative low cardiac output and the use of α-adrenergic vasopressive agents (51,52). In this situation, an anastomosis should not be performed.

In the patient with a small AAA, the carcinoma should be resected first and the AAA should be resected at a later date.

CASE 10: PROPRIETY OF INCIDENTAL APPENDECTOMY

The patient is a 72-year-old man who is undergoing sigmoid resection for an annular carcinoma. Should an incidental appendectomy be performed?

When not inflamed, the appendix is easy to remove. Therefore, it is one of the most common organs removed incidentally after completion of the primary abdominal operation mission. The rationale for removing a normal appendix is to avoid the development of appendicitis in the future. The diagnosis of acute appendicitis has remained a problem for the past 100 years, with a false positive rate of 20% to 25% and a delay in diagnosis leading to perforation in as many as 25% to 30% of patients (53). Approximately 7% of the population will have acute appendicitis sometime during their lifetime (54). The morbidity rate of appendicitis is significant. In nonperforated appendicitis the infection rate is 8% (55). For perforated appendicitis the septic rate is 32%, with a wound infection rate of 25% and an intra-abdominal abscess rate of 7% (56). Incidental appendectomy thus eliminates future problems that may occur.

Whether an incidental appendectomy should be performed has been a subject of debate for many years. There are both pros and cons (57,58), largely based on philosophical reasons rather than facts, that are impossible to obtain. Several prospective-controlled studies have shown that incidental appendectomy does not increase morbidity and mortality rates compared with the primary abdominal operation alone (59–61). It must be emphasized that in these studies when incidental appendectomy was performed, the appendix was readily exposed and removed without much time and effort. One should also note that some series show a higher rate of infection when the incidental appendectomy is performed in patients older than 50 years (62,63).

Approximately 250,000 cases of appendicitis occurred annually in the United States between 1979 and 1984. The highest incidence of appendectomy for appendicitis is found in persons who range in age from 10 to 19 years (23.3 per 100,000 population per year). Men have a higher rate of appendicitis than women in all age groups. Appendicitis rates are 1.5 times higher in whites than in non-whites. The highest rate (15.4 per 10,000 population per year) is in the West North Central region of the United States and is 11.3% higher in the summer than in the winter months (64).

The highest rate of incidental appendectomy is found in women from 35 to 44 years of age (43.8 per 10,000 population per year) or 12.1 times higher than the rate in men of the same age. Presumably, this rate is influenced by the same rate of gynecologic procedures in this specific population. Between 1970 and 1984, the incidence of appendicitis decreased by 14.6%; the reasons for this decline are unknown. A life-table model suggests that the lifetime risk of appendicitis is 8.6% for men and 6.7% for women; the lifetime risk of appendectomy is 12% for men and 23.1% for women. Overall, an estimated 36 incidental procedures are performed to prevent one case of appendicitis (64).

The preventive value of each incidental appendectomy performed in different age groups can be estimated using the life-table analysis. For example, 1000 incidental appendectomies can be expected to prevent 52 cases of appendicitis when performed in women from 15 to 19 years of age, 24 cases when performed in women from 35 to 39 years of age, and eight cases when performed in women from 60 to 64 years of age (64).

Although the highest rate of appendicitis is observed in persons from 10 to 19 years of age, most incidental appendectomies are performed in persons older than 35 years of age, which is well past the age of greatest risk for appendicitis, and in women, who are at lower risk than men. To prevent a single lifetime case of acute appendicitis in persons 35 years of age, 59 incidental appendectomies are required. For those 59 years of age, 166 procedures are required. Although the overall rate of incidental appendectomy declined sharply between 1979 and 1984, little change is noted among the elderly, for whom the procedure has the lowest preventive value (64).

In the less recent literature several papers showed that patients with previous appendectomy had a higher incidence of carcinoma of the colon than a comparable control group (65–67). It was believed that lymphoid tissues of the appendix produced immunity against development of malignant disease of the colon and other sites in the body. This issue was put to rest by the prospective study by Moertel et al. (68), who found no evidence to suggest that appendectomy posed a higher risk for development of large bowel carcinoma.

A study by Rutgeerts et al. (69) of Belgium revealed that appendectomy is a protective factor against ulcerative colitis. The authors found that in a group of 174 patients with ulcerative colitis, only one patient had undergone appendectomy, compared with 25% of the case-control group. The authors postulated that normal adult appendiceal lymphocyte reactivity is predominated by helper T cells. The appendix is mainly a helper organ. Resection of the appendix could tip the balance in favor of preventing or suppressing an inappropriate response (69,70).

It is reasonable to remove a normal appendix up to the age of 35 to 40 years, provided it can be performed without difficulty and without the necessity to extend the abdominal incision. However, with a patient of any age, if the appendix contains a mass, an appendicolith, or a calculus, an appendectomy should be performed since carcinoid, adenocarcinoma, lymphoma, mucinous cystadenomas, parasites, metastatic carcinoma, and many other abnormalities may be found (71,72). Appendicoliths and calculi of the appendix often are associated with complicated appendicitis, being present in 18% of patients with perforated appendicitis and in 42% of patients with appendiceal abscesses (73). Some authors have reported on patients with appendiceal calculi who developed abdominal pain mimicking appendicitis but who did not require an operation, only to return some time later with acute appendicitis (73,74). Since appendiceal fecoliths and calculi play a role in the pathogenesis of acute appendicitis and are associated with complicated appendicitis, particularly perforation and abscess, an incidental appendectomy should be considered seriously.

CASE 11: PROPRIETY OF INCIDENTAL MECKEL'S DIVERTICULECTOMY

A 52-year-old woman is undergoing resection for recurrent bouts of diverticulitis. At laparotomy, a Meckel's diverticulum is noted in the ileum 2 feet from the ileocecal junction. Should the diverticulum be resected?

Meckel's diverticulum is the persistence of a portion of the embryonic omphalomesenteric duct. The incidence of this disease is 0.3% to 4% at autopsy and 0.14% to 4.5% at laparotomy. Most Meckel's diverticula are located in the terminal ileum within 90 cm of the ileocecal junction, although there have been reports of their occurrence in the appendix and the jejunum (75).

Complications from Meckel's diverticula occur most often in children. The most common complication is small bowel obstruction followed by bleeding. In the adult, inflammation is the most common problem, followed by small bowel obstruction and bleeding. Inflammation of a Meckel's diverticulum most often is caused by ectopic tissues, namely, gastric and pancreatic cells, which occur in 23% of cases (76). The gastric cells are much more common and may lead to bleeding, ulceration, and perforation. Most obstruction is caused by a fibrous band from the Meckel's diverticulum, intussusception, and volvulus (75,77).

Recognizing a 2% incidence of Meckel's diverticula in the general population, the surgeon can use life-table analysis to calculate the risk of the development of future complications from Meckel's diverticulum. At age 10 years, the risk is 3%. This gradually drops to 0% at 75 years. At age 50 years, the risk is 1% (Fig. 1) (78). In a collective series, the average risk of morbidity from incidental Meckel's diverticulectomy was 4% (range, 2–30%) and the mortality rate was 0.2% (range, 0–0.8%) (79). It appears that incidental Meckel's diverticulectomy for a normal Meckel's diverticulum in patients older than 50 years of age is not indicated. However, if there is evidence of ectopic tissue, which usually can be palpated as thickened tissue, or if there is a fibrous band or a very long Meckel's diverticulum that may cause bowel obstruction or volvulus, excision should be considered strongly (80).

Park et al. (81) reviewed the Mayo Clinic experience with patients who had Meckel's diverticulum to determine which diverticula should be removed when discovered incidentally during abdominal surgery. They found 1476 patients to have a Meckel's diverticulum during operation from 1950 to 2002. Among the 1476 patients, 16% of the Meckel's diverticula were symptomatic. The most common clinical presentation in adults was bleeding; in children, obstruction. Among patients with a symptomatic Meckel's diverticulum, the male–female ratio was approximately 3:1. Clinical or histologic features most commonly associated with symptomatic Meckel's diverticula were patients aged

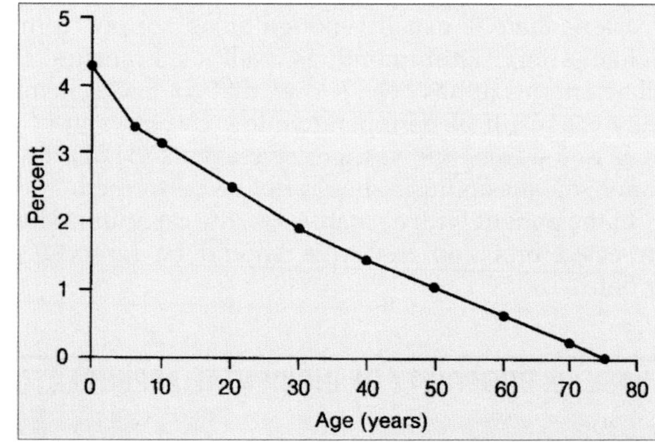

FIGURE 1 ■ Risk of developing a complication from a Meckel's diverticulum from age 0 to 75 years. *Source*: From Ref. 78.

younger than 50 years (odds ratio = 3.5), male sex (odds ratio = 1.8), diverticulum length > 2 cm (odds ratio = 2.2), and the presence of histologically abnormal tissue (odds ratio = 13.9). After analyzing their data, they neither support nor reject the recommendation that all Meckel's diverticula found incidentally should be removed, although the procedure today has little risk. If a selective approach is taken, they recommend removing all incidental Meckel's diverticula that have any of the four features most commonly associated with symptomatic Meckel's diverticula.

CASE 12: RECTAL PROLAPSE AND UNEXPECTED OVARIAN MASS

During the procedure to repair a rectal prolapse in a 67-year-old woman, a mass is found in the right ovary. With the patient under general anesthesia, the bowel is prepared and the patient's condition is stable. There is no obvious evidence of other intra-abdominal disease. How should the surgeon proceed?

An initial impression may be supported by deciding whether the mass is neoplastic, inflammatory, functional, or congenital. It is likely that an inflammatory mass would be associated with fever, pain, and an elevated white blood cell count. A congenital or functional mass might be cystic and regular in shape. Patients younger than age 40 would be more likely to have a benign mass. Benign masses may be removed locally, with care taken to preserve the ovary in young patients. This elderly patient would be more likely to have an ovarian carcinoma or metastatic carcinoma. An elderly patient would have atrophic, tiny ovaries, and a hard, enlarged ovary points to a neoplasm. The large variety of ovarian neoplasms have been classified, and the reader is referred to the World Health Organization's classification and the International Federation of Gynecologists and Obstetrics classification (82,83).

All adnexal masses must be considered to be neoplasms until proven otherwise because approximately 30% to 40% of them are malignant. The greatest frequency of ovarian carcinoma is in the sixth and seventh decades, as in the case of this patient.

Careful exploration of the abdomen should be performed to locate unrecognized primary malignancies or metastases. Any suspicious site should be excised or biopsied. Consultation with a surgeon experienced with gynecologic oncology is ideal but not always possible.

If the mass appears to be benign, unilateral salpingo-oophorectomy is appropriate therapy. The principal operation for ovarian carcinoma is total hysterectomy with bilateral salpingo-oophorectomy (84). The procedure may be quite complicated if the carcinoma is adherent to other organs or to the retroperitoneum. The formal operation may be performed for aggressive removal of the mass(es) (debulking) and omentectomy.

To obtain the most information from the operation, staging procedures should be performed (84,85). Since ovarian metastases float freely in the abdomen, biopsies of the diaphragm, omentum, and retroperitoneal nodes are recommended. Washings of the peritoneal cavity may provide cytologic evidence.

The remaining question is: What is to be done for the prolapse? If the mass was deemed benign, the surgeon should proceed with the operation planned for the prolapse. If the mass proved malignant and it was clear that the patient's condition was incurable, consideration can still be given to repair of the prolapse, since the symptoms of rectal procidentia may make the patient's quality of life miserable, and some patients will live for several years. If the patient showed marked symptoms from prolapse, a proctopexy without bowel resection might be performed. If the surgeon believes that a curative total abdominal hysterectomy and a bilateral salpingo-oophorectomy have been performed, it is reasonable to proceed with repair of the prolapse, but a procedure might be selected for a repair that does not involve the use of a foreign body. If the malignant disease is widely disseminated, consideration can be given to terminate the operation and not treating the prolapse.

CASE 13: VAGINAL HYSTERECTOMY AND INTRAOPERATIVE PERFORATION OF RECTUM

While a 55-year-old woman is undergoing a vaginal hysterectomy, the gynecologist notices an inadvertent perforation of the rectum. You are asked to step in and help solve the problem. Inspection confirms the finding of fecal material in the vagina but the source is not evident. What course of action would you take?

First, the patient should be administered intravenous antibiotics appropriate for a colorectal operation. Second, sigmoidoscopy should be performed. The specific site of perforation may be localized; if found, its size can be appreciated. If the patient is immunocompromised or has diseased bowel at the site of the injury, the surgeon diverts the fecal stream. However, the other questions ordinarily associated with trauma, including time from injury to operation and the velocity of the injury agent, are as favorable as can be expected.

Contamination is the major factor that will influence modifying the operative approach. Ideally, the gynecologist will have performed a preoperative bowel preparation. In general, gynecologists who expect a difficult dissection will plan ahead for inadvertent enterotomy by bowel preparation.

A low-lying, distal rectal, and distal vaginal perforation may be repaired in layers via the anus and/or the vagina (86–88). The contamination will predicate the need for colostomy. If an upper rectal wound has occurred, laparotomy is necessary to repair it and a colostomy often is warranted. The vaginal and rectal repairs may be separated by omentum or a peritoneal flap.

If trauma to the bowel at any point in the free peritoneal cavity occurs, primary closure is the treatment of choice. On the other hand, if perforation is found below the peritoneal reflection in conjunction with gross contamination of the freshly opened planes for the pelvic surgery and the dissection to find and repair the hole, morbidity from infection is likely. This is the ideal model for subsequent cellulitis, abscess, and suture leak. Since a leak will quickly convert the situation to a rectovaginal fistula, diversion of the fecal stream is the safest approach (88).

In addition, the contaminated planes should be drained. Our choice is a soft, closed sump-type drain that can be brought out through separate stab wounds on the abdominal wall.

An important issue for patients with major contamination is distal rectal washout. If a local repair is selected, an effort should be made to evacuate the rectal ampulla in order to remove retained stool. If a primary repair was instituted at laparotomy, the colon proximal to the injury can be emptied by an on-table preparation if there is a fecal load (86). A tube for infusion can be placed into the terminal ileum and advanced into the cecum; thus, liters of saline can be flooded through the bowel. The saline may be allowed to egress from the colorectum by insertion of an anal retractor so that the sphincter mechanism is gently opened. If the situation merits the construction of a colostomy, the distal bowel can be irrigated to empty it of any stool.

CASE 14: EXPLORATION FOR APPENDICITIS WITH UNEXPECTED PSEUDOMYXOMA PERITONEI

A 39-year-old man is undergoing an emergency laparotomy for suspected appendicitis. A cecal mass is identified. During mobilization of the mass, it ruptures, and pools of mucin are discovered. How should this patient be managed?

The true source of this mucin is unknown. It may be mucin accumulated within the dilated lumen of an obstructed appendix, a mucocele, or produced by proliferative epithelial cells, a cystadenoma, or mucinous cystadenocarcinoma. Since this is an unexpected finding, these sources may be indistinguishable. Appendicitis is the presenting clinical diagnosis in 25% (89). Gelatinous deposits or mucinous ascites is termed pseudomyxoma peritonei. If the mucin is secondary to rupture of a simple mucocele, the removal of the appendix is curative. On the other hand, mucin on the basis of cystadenocarcinoma often persists or recurs. The primary treatment of these mucin-producing lesions is resection, and the prognosis is based on the completeness of removal (90,91). On occasion, a thin-walled, distended appendix is recognized; removal of the obstructed appendix is curative. However, sometimes the appendix is surrounded by neoplastic deposits. Then a right colectomy, applying the principles of en bloc resection, is the treatment of choice.

If a diffuse process is discovered on further exploration, and all disease cannot be removed, the patient may be closed and sent to a surgeon who is familiar with debulking and chemotherapy for these neoplasms. Generally, all gross gelatinous implants should be removed. The omentum is part of the diffuse process and should be removed (92,93). Some authors suggest using an irrigation of 5% dextrose solution, a mucolytic agent (94). If the patient is female, the ovaries should be removed in cases of pseudomyxoma peritonei because they may be a hidden source of the process or harbor metastases (95).

Adjuvant therapy is unproven because of the small number of these cases. Because adjuvant treatments may include intraperitoneal chemotherapy, appropriate catheters for introduction and removal of the agents should be placed in the peritoneal cavity and brought out through separate stab wounds. Other adjuvant therapy includes radiogold colloid or systemic chemotherapy, but rarely radiation therapy. Recurrence leads to repeated debulking, cytoreductive operations, and chemotherapy, either systemic or intraperitoneal (93,94,96,97).

CONCLUSION

It is hoped that discussions of these challenge case examples will serve as a useful backdrop enabling surgeons faced with similar difficult operative decisions to reach practical and appropriate conclusions.

REFERENCES

1. Enker WE, Dragacevic S. Multiple carcinomas of the large bowel: A natural experiment in etiology and pathogenesis. Ann Surg 1978; 187:8–11.
2. Fogler R, Weiner E. Multiple foci of colorectal carcinoma. Argument for subtotal colectomy. NY State J Med 1980; 80:47–51.
3. Welch IP. Multiple colorectal tumors. An appraisal of natural history and therapeutic options. Am J Surg 1981; 142:274–280.
4. Ottinger LW. Frequency of bowel movements after colectomy with ileorectal anastomosis. Arch Surg 1978; 113:1048–1049.
5. Adson MA, van Heerden JA, Adson MH, Wagner IS, Ilstrup DM. Resection of hepatic metastases from colorectal cancer. Arch Surg 1984; 119:647–651.
6. Foster JH, Berman MM. Solid liver tumours. Major problems in clinical surgery. Philadelphia: WB Saunders, 1977.
7. Taylor B, Langer B, Falk RE, Ambus U. Role of resection in the management of metastases to the liver. Can J Surg 1983; 26:215–217.
8. Dmowski WP. Current concepts in the management of endometriosis. Obstet Gynecol Annu 1981; 10:279–311.
9. Groom RD, Donovan M, Schwesinger WH. Intestinal endometriosis. Am J Surg 1984; 148:660–667.
10. Bailey HR. Colorectal endometriosis. Perspect Colon Rectal Surg 1992; 5: 251–259.
11. Meyers WC, Kelvin FM, Jones SR. Diagnosis and surgical treatment of colonic endometriosis. Arch Surg 1979; 114:169–175.
12. Perry EP, Peel ALG. The treatment of obstructing intestinal endometriosis. J R Soc Med 1988; 81:172–173.
13. Forsgren H, Lindhagen I, Melander S, Wagermark J. Colorectal endometriosis. Acta Chir Scand 1983; 149:431–435.
14. Peck JJ. Management of carcinoma discovered unexpectedly at operation for acute appendicitis. Am J Surg 1988; 155:683–685.
15. Hill J, Leppard DJ. Acute appendicitis and carcinoma of the colon. J R Soc Med 1986; 79:678–680.
16. Sumpio BE, Ballantyne GH, Zdon MJ, Modlin IM. Perforated appendicitis and obstructing colonic carcinoma in the elderly. Dis Colon Rectum 1986; 29: 668–670.
17. Arabjornsonn E. Acute appendicitis as a sign of a colorectal carcinoma. J Surg Oncol 1982; 30:17–20.
18. Kovalcik RJ, Simstein NL, Cross GH. Ileocecal masses discovered unexpectedly at surgery for appendicitis. Am Surg 1978; 44:279–281.
19. Peck JJ. Management of carcinoma discovered unexpectedly at operation for acute appendicitis. Am J Surg 1988; 155:683–685.
20. Goodall RG, Park M. Primary resection and anastomosis of lesions obstructing the left colon. Can J Surg 1988; 31:167–168.
21. Irvin GL, Horsley JS, Caruana JA Jr. The morbidity and mortality of emergency operation for colorectal disease. Ann Surg 1984; 199:598–601.
22. Terry BG, Beart RW Jr. Emergency abdominal colectomy with primary anastomosis. Dis Colon Rectum 1981; 24:1–4.
23. Thow GB. Emergency left colon resection with primary anastomosis. Dis Colon Rectum 1980; 23:17–24.
24. Stefansson T, Pahlman L, Ekbom A, Yuen J. Surgery in acute diverticulitis, a retrospective population based study. 130 patients operated in the University Hospital in Uppsala, Sweden, 1969–1989. Acta Universitatis Upsaliensis Uppsala, 1994.
25. Thompson JS, Philben VJ, Hodgson PE. Operative management of incidental cholelithiasis. Am J Surg 1984; 148:821–823.
26. Kovalcik PJ, Burrell MJ, Old WL Jr. Cholecystectomy concomitant with either intraabdominal operations. Assessment of risk. Arch Surg 1983; 118:1059–1062.
27. Juhasz ES, Wolff BG, Meagher AP, et al. Incidental cholecystectomy during colorectal surgery. Ann Surg 1994; 219:467–474.

28. Shennib H, Fried GM, Hampson LG. Does simultaneous cholecystectomy increase the risk of colonic surgery? Am J Surg 1986; 151:266–268.
29. Rosoff AJ. Informed consent: A guide for health care providers. Rockville, Md.: Aspen Systems Corp., 1981.
30. Eckhauser FE, Lindehauer MS, Morley GW. Pelvic exenteration for advanced rectal carcinoma. Am J Surg 1979; 138:411–414.
31. Jakowatz JG, Porudominsky D, Riihimaki DU, et al. Complications of pelvic exenteration. Arch Surg 1985; 120:1261–1265.
32. Rodriguez-Bigas MA, Petrelli NJ. Pelvic exenteration and its modification. Am J Surg 1996; 171:293–301.
33. Izbicki JR, Hosch SB, Knoefel WT, Passlick B, Bloechle C, Bloelsch CE. Extended resections are beneficial for patients with locally advanced colorectal cancer. Dis Colon Rectum 1995; 38:1251–1256.
34. Poeze M, Houbiers JGA, Van De Velde CJH, Wobbes TH, von Meyenfeldt ME. Radical resection of locally advanced colorectal cancer. Br J Surg 1995; 82: 1386–1390.
35. Plukker TTH, Aalders JG, Mensink HJA, Oldhoff J. Total pelvic exenteration: A justified procedure. Br J Surg 1993; 80:1615–1617.
36. Cohen AM, Minsky BD. Aggressive surgical management of locally advanced primary and recurrent rectal cancer. Dis Colon Rectum 1990; 33:432–438.
37. Boey J, Wong J, Ong GB. Pelvic exenteration for locally advanced colorectal carcinoma. Ann Surg 1982; 195:513–518.
38. Lopez MJ, Kraybill WG, Downey RS, Johnston WD, Bricker EM. Exenterative surgery for locally advanced rectosigmoid cancers. Is it worthwhile? Surgery 1987; 102:644–651.
39. Orkin BA, Dozois RR, Beart RW Jr, et al. Extended resection for locally advanced primary adenocarcinoma of the rectum. Dis Colon Rectum 1989; 32:286–292.
40. Talamonti MS, Shumate CR, Carlson GW, Curley SA. Locally advanced carcinoma of the colon and rectum involving the urinary bladder. Surg Gynecol Obstet 1993; 177:481–487.
41. Nora JD, Pairolero PC, Nivatvongs S, et al. Concomitant abdominal aortic aneurysm and colorectal carcinoma: priority of resection. J Vase Surg 1989; 9:630–636.
42. Baxter NN, Noel AA, Cherry K, Wolf BG. Management of patitents with colorectal cancer and concomitant abdominal aortic aneurysm. Dis Colon Rectum 2002; 45:165–170.
43. Herald JA, Young CJ, White GH, Solomon MJ. Endosurgical treatment of synchronous rectal cancer and abdominal aortic aneurysm, without laparatomy. Surgery 1998; 124:932–933.
44. Velanovich V, Andersen CA. Concomitant abdominal aortic aneurysm and colorectal cancer: a decision analysis approach to a therapeutic dilemma. Ann Vasc Surg 1991; 5:449–455.
45. Swanson RJ, Littooy FN, Hunt TK, et al. Laparotomy as a precipitating factor in the rupture of intra-abdominal aneurysms. Arch Surg 1980; 115:299–304.
46. Busuttil RW, Abou-Zamzam AM, Machleder HI. Collagenase activity of the human aorta: a comparison of patients with or without abdominal aortic aneurysms. Arch Surg 1980; 115:1373–1378.
47. Cohen JR, Mandell C, Nargolis I, Chang J, et al. Altered aortic protease and antiprotease activity in patients with ruptured abdominal aortic aneurysm. Surg Gynecol Obstet 1987; 164:355–358.
48. Lobbato VJ, Rothenberg RE, LaRaja RD, et al. Coexistence of abdominal aortic aneurysm and carcinoma of the colon: a dilemma. J Vasc Surg 1985; 2:724–726.
49. Morris HL, da Silva AF. Co-existing abdominal aortic aneurysm and intra-abdominal carcinoma. Br J Surg 1998; 85:1185–1190.
50. Taylor LM Jr., Porter JM. Basic data related to clinical decision-making in abdominal aortic aneurysms. Ann Vasc Surg 1987; 1:502–504.
51. Meissner MH, Johansen KH. Colon infarction after ruptured abdominal aortic aneurysm. Arch Surg 1992; 127:979–985.
52. Barnett MG, Longo WE. Intestinal ischemia after aortic surgery. Semin Colon Rectal Surg 1993; 4:229–234.
53. Nivatvongs S. Diseases of the appendix. Curr Opin Gastroenterol 1989; 5:76–79.
54. Fisher KS, Ross DS. Guidelines for therapeutic decision in incidental appendectomy. Surg Gynecol Obstet 1990; 171:95–98.
55. Coleman RJ, Blackwood JM, Swan KG. Role of antibiotic prophylaxis in surgery for nonperforated appendicitis. Am Surg 1987; 53:584–586.
56. Pieper R, Forsell P, Kager L. Perforation of appendicitis. A nine-year survey of treatment and results. Acta Chir Scand Suppl 1986; 530:51–57.
57. Nockerts SR, Detmer DE, Fryback DG. Incidental appendectomy in the elderly? No. Surgery 1980; 88:301–306.
58. Tranmer BI, Graham AM, Sterns EE. Incidental appendectomy?—Yes. Can J Surg 1981; 24:191–192.
59. Parsons AK, Sauer MV, Parsons MT, et al. Appendectomy at cesarean section. A prospective study. Obstet Gynecol 1986; 68:479–482.
60. Strom PR, Turkleson ML, Stone HM. Safety of incidental appendectomy. Am J Surg 1983; 145:819–822.
61. Ikard RW. Prospective analysis of the effect of incidental appendectomy on infection rate after cholecystectomy. South Med J 1987; 80:292–295.
62. Warren JL, Penberthy LT, Addiss AG, McBeam AM. Appendectomy incidental to cholecystectomy among elderly Medicare beneficiaries. Surg Gynecol Obstet 1993; 177:288–294.
63. Andrew MH, Roty AR Jr. Incidental appendectomy with cholecystectomy: is the increased risk justified? Am Surg 1987; 53:553–557.
64. Addis DG, Shaffer N, Fowler BS, Tauxe RV. The epidemiology of appendicitis and appendectomy in the United States. Am J Epidemiology 1990; 132: 910–925.
65. Gross L. Incidence of appendectomies and tonsillectomies in cancer patients. Cancer 1966; 19:849–852.
66. McVay JR Jr. The appendix in relation to neoplastic disease. Cancer 1964; 17:929–937.
67. Bierman HR. Human appendix and neoplasia. Cancer 1968; 21:109–118.
68. Moertel CG, Nobrega FT, Elveback LR, Wentz JR. A prospective study of appendectomy and predisposition to cancer. Surg Gynecol Obstet 1974; 138: 549–553.
69. Rutgeerts P, D'Haens G, Hiele M, Geboes K, Vantrappen G. Appendectomy protects against ulcerative colitis. Gastroenterology 1994; 106:1251–1253.
70. Logan R. Appendectomy and ulcerative colitis: what correlation? Gastroenterology 1994; 106:1382–1384.
71. Khfu W. Value of routine histopathological examination of appendices in Hong Kong. J Clin Pathol 1987; 40:429–433.
72. Westermann C, Mann WJ, Chumas J, et al. Routine appendectomy in extensive gynecologic operations. Surg Gynecol Obstet 1986; 162:307–312.
73. Nitecki S, Karmeli R, Sarr MG. Appendiceal calculi and fecoliths: are they an indication for appendectomy? Surg Gynecol Obstet 1990; 171:185–188.
74. Brady BM, Carroll DS. Significance of calcified appendiceal fecoliths. Radiology 1957; 68:648–653.
75. DeBartolo HM Jr., van Heerden JA. Meckel's diverticulum. Ann Surg 1976; 183:30–33.
76. Ludtke FE, Mende V, Kohler H, Lepsien G. Incidence and frequency of complications and management of Meckel's diverticulum. Surg Gynecol Obstet 1989; 169:537–542.
77. Bemelman WA, Hugenholtz E, Heij HA, Wiersma PH, Obertop H. Meckel's diverticulum in Amsterdam: experience in 136 patients. World J Surg 1995; 19:734–737.
78. Soltero MJ, Bill AH. The natural history of Meckel's diverticulum and its relation to incidental removal. Am J Surg 1976; 132:168–173.
79. Peoples JB, Lichtenberger EJ, Dunn MM. Incidental Meckel's diverticulectomy in adults. Surgery 1995; 118:649–652.
80. Longo WE, Vernava AM III. Clinical implications of jejunoileal diverticular disease. Dis Colon Rectum 1992; 35:381–388.
81. Park JJ, Wolff BG, Tollefson MK, Walsh EE, Larson DR. Meckel diverticulum: the Mayo Clinic experience with 1476 patients (1950–2002). Ann Surg 2005; 241:529–533.
82. Jones HW III. Ovarian cysts and tumors. In: Jones HW III, Wentz AC, Burnett LS, eds. Novak's textbook of gynecology. 11th ed. Baltimore: Williams & Wilkins, 1988:783.
83. Pernoll ML, Benson RC, eds. Current obstetric and gynecologic diagnosis and treatment. Los Altos, CA: Appleton & Lange, 1987:670–714.
84. Lewis JL Jr. Unexpected adenocarcinoma of ovary and uterus. In: Nichols DH, Anderson GW, eds. Clinical problems, injuries, and complications of gynecologic surgery. Baltimore: Williams & Wilkins, 1988:265–267.
85. Ozols RF, Rubin SC, Gillian T. Epithelial ovarian cancer. In: Hoskins WJ, Perez CA, Young RD, eds. Principles and practices of gynecologic oncology, 2nd ed. Philadelphia: Lippincott-Raven, 1997:939–941.
86. Nelson RL, Abcarian H, Prasad ML. Iatrogenic perforation of the colon and rectum. Dis Colon Rectum 1982; 25:305–309.
87. Grasberger RC, Hirsch ER. Rectal trauma. Am J Surg 1983; 145:795–798.
88. Haas PA, Fox TA. Civilian injuries of the rectum and anus. Dis Colon Rectum 1979; 22:17–23.
89. Yeh H, Shafir MK, Slater G, et al. Ultrasonography and computed tomography of pseudomyxoma peritonei. Radiology 1984; 153:507–510.
90. Novell R, Lewis A. Role of surgery in the treatment of pseudomyxoma peritonei. J R Coll Surg Edinb 1990; 35:21–24.
91. Smith JW, Kemeny N, Caldwell C, et al. Pseudomyxoma-peritonei of appendiceal origin: the Sloan-Kettering Cancer Center experience. Cancer 1992; 70: 396–401.
92. Gough DB, Donohue JH. Pseudomyxoma peritonei: long-term patient survival with an aggressive regional approach. Ann Surg 1994; 219:112–119.
93. Sugarbaker PH, Landy D, Jaffe G, et al. Histologic changes induced by intraperitoneal chemotherapy with 5-FU and mitomycin C in patients with peritoneal carcinomatosis from cyst adenocarcinomas of the colon or appendix. Cancer 1990; 1:1495–1501.
94. Mann WJ, Wagner J. The management of pseudomyxoma peritonei. Cancer 1990; 66:1636–1640.
95. Young RH, Gilks CB, Scully RE. Mucinous tumors of the appendix associated with mucinous tumors of the ovary and pseudomyxoma peritonei. Am J Surg Pathol 1991; 15:415–429.
96. Sindelar WF, DeLaney TF, Tochner Z, et al. Technique of ph dynamic therapy for disseminated intraperitoneal malignant neoplasms. Phase I study. Arch Surg 1991; 126:318–324.
97. Nast MF, Kemp GM, Given FT. Pseudomyxoma peritonei: treatment with intraperitoneal 5-fluorouracil. Eur J Gynaecol Obstet 1993; 14:213–217.

38 Laparoscopic Colon and Rectal Surgery

Lee E. Smith and Philip H. Gordon

BACKGROUND AND RATIONALE

HISTORICAL REVIEW

Laparoscopic approaches to operation vaulted into our surgical armamentarium much faster than other technologic innovations and without the clinical scrutiny of other therapeutic modalities. For example, laparoscopic cholecystectomy catapulted from almost an experimental procedure to the gold standard in a few short years, without rigid studies of its advantages and disadvantages. From that procedure stemmed a whole catalog of operations and now virtually every abdominal organ is deemed fair game for a laparoscopic approach. One of the most exciting technologies to be introduced into the armamentarium of colon and rectal surgeons is that of minimal access surgery. Although introduced over a decade ago in 1991, the acceptance of laparoscopic surgery in the field of colon and rectal surgery has been slower when compared with other areas of surgery. Several technical factors have played a role in this development (1). Some of the issues have been the uniquely complex technical nature of the colon resection, the necessity of doing a bowel anastomosis in most circumstances, the necessity to divide large blood vessels, and the need for extraction of a bulky specimen. Many of the early learning curve-related issues have been overcome and with the availability of new instrumentation, the safety and technical feasibility of this approach has now been confirmed. No doubt, with increasing expertise and better instrumentation, the laparoscopic approach will become more attractive for an even broader range of conditions.

The first series of 20 patients who underwent laparoscopic-assisted colectomy was published in 1991 by Jacobs et al. (2). The authors provided a detailed description of their technique. Other investigators were then stimulated to follow their lead. In the same year, others reported on laparoscopic colon operations (3–8). Subsequently, the literature has been replete with reports of series of varying sizes, innovative techniques for virtually every colorectal operation, and the results, complications, and consequences associated with the new technology.

Colectomy is termed an advanced laparoscopic technique because the colon is a large, mobile organ, spanning each abdominal quadrant, a specimen must be removed intact, and an anastomosis is often required; therefore, the visualization and dissection of the colon must move from abdominal quadrant to quadrant. The ability to see the magnified, slightly distorted anatomy is the initial major hurdle to overcome.

ADVANTAGES

Advocates of laparoscopic colectomy cite numerous potential advantages. Among those are less pain postoperatively, faster patient recovery with less postoperative disability, shorter hospitalization, less intraoperative trauma, the technical capability to perform an operation comparable to an open technique, earlier return to work, better cosmetic results, a reduction in postoperative adhesions, and a better quality of life for the patient. Proponents believe that these considerations are sufficient reason to support adoption of the new technology. However, attempts to quantify these parameters have not been unequivocally demonstrated.

One of the benefits attributed to laparoscopic procedures is early postoperative feeding, with some patients permitted fluids as early as the evening of the day of operation, with diet advanced as tolerated. However, a number of investigators have suggested that early feeding might not be a unique benefit of laparoscopic procedures. In a randomized prospective trial, Ortiz et al. (9) found that patients who underwent a standard midline incision tolerated feedings equally well. A frequently cited advantage of laparoscopic colectomy is a shorter postoperative ileus. Hotokezaka et al. (10) studied this issue by placing recording electrodes in the distal antrum, the proximal side of the colonic anastomosis, and the rectosigmoid for postoperative myoelectric recordings. In this study, the potential benefit of using a laparoscopic approach to colon resection was not clearly confirmed because it only offered modest increases in the rapidity of recovery of gastrointestinal function. Early feeding and early discharge from the hospital may be encouraged to satisfy the surgeon, but it may be that this philosophy is equally applicable to open procedures. The same arguments apply to the length of time until the patient returns to work. In this regard, motivation may be the critical factor since self-employed individuals tend to return to work much more quickly than individuals, compensated by "sick leave."

Using serum levels of interleukin (IL)-6, IL-10, C-reactive protein, and granulocyte elastase as indicators of surgical stress, Hildebrandt et al. (11) showed significantly lower levels of these markers after laparoscopic colon resection which was most evident for IL-6 and granulocyte elastase. By using these parameters they found a significant reduction in surgical trauma after laparoscopic surgery compared with the open procedure.

Duepree et al. (12) defined the incidence of access-related complications in a cohort of 716 consecutive patients undergoing either laparoscopic-assisted bowel resection ($n = 211$) or open bowel operation ($n = 505$). The mean follow-up in the laparoscopic-assisted and open groups were 2.7 years and 2.4 years, respectively. The incidence of wound hernia was significantly higher in open cases (12.9%) compared with laparoscopic-assisted ones (2.4%). The incidence of surgical repair of ventral hernia was also significantly higher in the open group (5.5%) compared with the laparoscopic-assisted group (1.9%). Postoperative small bowel obstruction requiring hospitalization with conservative management occurred significantly less frequently in laparoscopic-assisted patients (1.9%) compared with the open resection (6.1%). The need for surgical release of small bowel obstruction was similar between the open and laparoscopic-assisted groups (1.6% vs. 1.4%). The overall reoperation rate for these two complications was two times higher in the open group than in the laparoscopic-assisted group (7.7% vs. 3.8%). The data demonstrate that laparoscopic access for bowel operation significantly reduces the incidence of ventral hernia and small bowel obstruction rates compared with laparotomy.

It is uncertain whether cost should be considered under the heading of advantage or disadvantage. Advocates of laparoscopic colectomy believe that the shorter hospital stay and better quality of life clearly qualify as advantages, but equipment is clearly more expensive, and an exact evaluation is often difficult because of the sometimes-perverted calculations that may involve actual cost or charges to patients. Nevertheless, the decreased length of hospital stay is usually stated to more-than-compensate for the expensive technology and results in overall decreased health care costs. On the other hand, if the case has to be converted to an open procedure, the costs of both laparoscopic and open operation are incurred.

Recently the hand-assisted technique has been employed with some added advantages beyond those of standard laparoscopy. The tactile sense permits locating pathology easier, evaluation of the abdomen for metastases, better retraction, the ability for isolation and control of the vessels, and ease of blunt dissection.

DISADVANTAGES

Laparoscopic colectomy is technically demanding and may be more difficult. The learning curve may be steep and prolonged. An analysis of total operative time as an indication of learning shows that approximately 11 to 15 completed laparoscopic-assisted colectomies are needed to comfortably learn the procedure (13). Another report suggested that the learning curve is longer than appreciated by many surgeons, requiring as many as 35 to 50 procedures to decrease operative time to baseline (14). However, complications can be kept at an acceptably low level while on the curve if a cautious approach is taken. In a series of 60 laparoscopic colectomies, Fowler and White (3) reported a morbidity rate of 11.6% (small bowel obstruction, anastomotic staple line bleeds) and a mortality rate of 1.6% (pulmonary embolus). Length of stay, complications, and operative time all decreased with experience, suggesting a steep learning curve. For example, because of small bowel obstruction, these investigators recommended closure of mesenteric defects. Agachan et al. (15) also studied the impact of surgical experience on complications. Over successive time periods, the total complication rate decreased from 29% during the first period to 11% by the second period and to 7% during the third period. Thus, the learning curve appeared to have required more than 50 cases for the surgeon to become proficient.

A major disadvantage of the laparoscopic approach is the loss of tactile sensation. Operative times are often very prolonged. As opposed to most other laparoscopic procedures, laparoscopic colorectal surgery requires dissection in more than one quadrant and there is need for intraoperative repositioning of instruments, ports, and personnel. The colonic mesentery includes numerous large vessels and vascular control requires considerable time and quite often much more cost than do other procedures. An anastomosis is required for any colorectal operation and retrieval of the resected segment of colon with its attached mesentery requires an incision with the exception of an abdominoperineal resection. Furthermore, it involves specialized equipment. The hand-assisted technique has become popular with some surgeons by restoring some tactile ability and facilitating the operation (16–20). However, a 6- to 7-cm incision is necessary to admit the hand.

PATIENT INFORMATION

The surgeon should discuss with the patient the reasonable expectations for the pathologic condition for which the patient is undergoing the operation. The patient should be informed that intraoperative circumstances may mandate conversion of the technique to an open operation. Because of the new nature of this technology, some patients will decline the option of a laparoscopic approach. Age is not a contraindication as older patients fare as well as younger ones (21).

INDICATIONS

The reputed advantages of laparoscopic operations have been discussed but despite the cited advantages, clear-cut indications for such an approach are far from accepted. Some protagonists forge ahead with evangelical fervor, whereas some ultra-conservative surgeons only grudgingly concede its existence. The following discussion attempts to present a balanced portrayal of current evidence. What is certain is that the indications for operation in any given condition should not be modified simply because of the availability of a minimally invasive technique.

Virtually the entire spectrum of colorectal disorders has been approached laparoscopically. But does the capability to perform a procedure laparoscopically mean that all procedures should be conducted in this fashion? Almost certainly not. Cogent concerns from an oncologic view have been raised against adopting this technique for malignancy. Is the lengthy time required for a restorative proctocolectomy justified? These, among other questions, have made the subject controversial, and only time and critical evaluation of currently performed procedures will permit the establishment of reasonable indications for the use of the laparoscopic approach.

Procedures such as sigmoid resection, rectopexy, abdominoperineal resection, Hartmann's reversal, or laparoscopic-assisted right hemicolectomy have been reported to show potential advantages. Complex procedures such as restorative proctocolectomy and completely intracorporeal right hemicolectomy require advanced technical expertise, and an advantage over open procedures has been questioned (22). For all procedures, the sometimes rather steep "learning curve" must be passed before the benefits of comparable operative times, morbidity, and shorter hospital stay can be achieved. Certainly, initially it would seem prudent to limit laparoscopic colectomy to elective situations.

Disease processes for which the laparoscopic approach has been applied include colonic polyps not amenable to colonoscopic excision, carcinoma, diverticulitis, Crohn's disease, rectal procidentia, volvulus, and diversion ileostomy or colostomy. Absolute contraindications include carcinoma infiltrating into adjacent structures, a large phlegmenous mass and perforation. Factors that could contraindicate laparoscopic approach include urgent intervention, mid-rectal carcinomas, locally advanced carcinomas, previous intestinal surgery, and carcinomas greater than 10 cm in size. Severe uncorrectable coagulopathy is also a contraindication.

Contraindications may be relative or absolute and depend on the experience of the surgeon. Relative contraindications include obstruction, marked obesity, multiple previous laparotomies, extensive intra-abdominal adhesions, and carcinomatosis.

CARCINOMA

In recent years, studies have suggested that laparoscopic resection is equivalent to open resection when the extent of colon margins and the number of lymph nodes retrieved from the specimen are compared. Of more importance is the finding of no clinically significant difference in recurrence rates or survival.

Furthermore, it is unclear whether the difference in lymph node count is clinically significant because the number of lymph nodes harvested has not been shown to affect survival. A number of studies have reported that the lymphovascular clearance in laparoscopic-assisted colectomy is similar to an open operation. In a detailed histopathologic study of laparoscopic-assisted right hemicolectomy specimens, Moore et al. (23) found no clinically significant difference between the groups in terms of margins of clearance or the number of lymph nodes harvested.

The hand-assisted technique reestablishes tactile sense in operations for malignancies. The exploration to find the carcinoma and search for metastases is markedly improved. The surgeon's actions parallel open technique, but the patient's outcome is comparable to a laparoscopic procedure.

Peritoneal dissemination of malignant cells must be considered to have an eventual fatal outcome. The early studies called attention to port-site recurrences. This has not been evident in recent studies (24). Twenty-one patients with emergent complications for advanced colorectal carcinoma were reviewed by Gonzalez et al. (25). Ten patients with perforation, 7 with bleeding, and 4 with obstruction were given a proximal ostomy, and 18 had concomitant colectomy. The complication rate was 30% and mortality was zero.

BENIGN NEOPLASMS

A number of benign neoplasms such as adenomas or lipomas have been removed either through a colotomy or resection.

DIVERTICULAR DISEASE

The feasibility of laparoscopic colectomy for diverticulitis has been reported by several authors (26). Not all patients with diverticulitis are suitable candidates for laparoscopic colectomy. It would seem that patients with a large mass or very dense adhesions would be more safely treated with resection by an open operation. A colovesical or colovaginal fistula is not an absolute contraindication but may require intracorporeal suturing.

With the growth and development of laparoscopic surgery, the ability to perform even more complex intestinal operations via minimal access techniques has become more common. Nowhere is this more evident than in the operative treatment of diverticular disease. Technological advances both in the development of new instruments as well as techniques have made the minimal access treatment of all aspects of diverticular disease feasible. The latest generation of harmonic scalpels, the ligasure device, and the improvement in endoscopic staplers has allowed for safe and relatively rapid division of the bowel intracorporally with minimal conversion. The advent of hand-assisted techniques in the performance of laparoscopic intestinal surgery has dramatically enhanced our ability to perform the most difficult diverticular operations. By restoring tactile sense and proprioception, as well as assisting with retraction of adjacent organs and dissecting inflamed tissue, hand-assisted laparoscopic surgery (HALS) has facilitated the treatment of complicated diverticular disease. Furthermore, the surgery is accomplished with a reduced operating time. Perhaps, most importantly the hand-assisted technique significantly flattens out an otherwise steep learning curve for these otherwise difficult operations.

Hartmann's reversal is a good operation for the surgeon acquiring laparoscopic experience. The advantages are that there is no resection and little mesenteric dissection. A potential disadvantage is that the initial inflammatory reaction may have resulted in dense adhesions that necessitate conversion to an open operation.

INFLAMMATORY BOWEL DISEASE

Patients with Crohn's disease affecting the ileocecal region have frequently been amenable to a laparoscopic approach. Other segments of the colon have also been approached from a laparoscopic point of view. In patients with ulcerative colitis, laparoscopic-assisted total abdominal colectomy with ileorectal anastomosis or even a total proctocolectomy with pouch-anal anastomosis has been performed.

RECTAL PROCIDENTIA

Among the numerous procedures available for the repair of rectal procidentia, the ones that have been applied laparoscopically have included anterior resection, rectopexy, and sacral fixation with a mesh.

COLONIC INERTIA

For patients with colonic inertia, total abdominal colectomy and ileorectal anastomosis or a formal left hemicolectomy can be conducted laparoscopically.

VOLVULUS

For patients with either a cecal or sigmoid volvulus, an appropriate laparoscopic resection can be performed. Fixation procedures through the laparoscope have also been performed.

INTESTINAL STOMAS FOR DIVERSION

Among the less often challenged indications for a laparoscopic approach are procedures for benign disorders. The morbidity associated with nonresectional operations is less than that encountered with resectional cases requiring an anastomosis; hence, stoma creation seems ideally suited. Indications for laparoscopic-assisted diverting ileostomy cited by Luchtefeld (27) include protection of a tenuous colorectal anastomosis, protection of a complex fistula or sphincter repair, severe constipation, and distal obstruction. For a diverting colostomy, indications include anal incontinence, distal obstruction, complex pelvic and perianal sepsis, and protection of a tenuous colorectal anastomosis.

REPAIR OF COLONOSCOPIC PERFORATION

For a patient who sustains a colonic perforation during diagnostic or therapeutic colonoscopy, laparoscopic repair has been reported (28). The laceration can be sutured and the peritoneal cavity lavaged with saline solution. Reinforcement of the suture line with omentum has been suggested (29).

MISCELLANEOUS

Miscellaneous indications for laparoscopic colon operations have included cecostomy or cecopexy for cecal volvulus. Laparoscopic-guided decompression of the cecum in Ogilvie's syndrome has been described. In desperately ill patients with intestinal obstruction, cecostomy for obstruction has been considered (30). Resection for patients with massive lower gastrointestinal bleeding has also been proposed.

EQUIPMENT AND INSTRUMENTATION

During the past five years, the engineering and design of the equipment used for laparoscopy have been changing rapidly. Purchase of equipment is based on acceptable quality versus budget. If the purchaser waits for the final best system, he or she will wait forever. The best way to select equipment is to use it in the operating room and to give all potential users the opportunity to evaluate it. One should avoid buying equipment based on the salesperson's recommendations. Generally, the various pieces of equipment are stacked on a cart with wheels (Fig. 1A) for ease of use and movement between operating rooms (31). Soon many hospitals will invest in dedicated laparoscopy rooms (Fig. 1B), which will contain overhead booms to hold all the equipment and permit easier placement of equipment for different procedures. The following section describes these pieces of equipment.

LAPAROSCOPE

Laparoscopes must deliver a high-quality image to be safe and effective (i.e., perfect vision is necessary for dissection and for identifying bleeding points). Not much has changed from the Hopkins rod-lens introduced in the early 1950s. Laparoscopes in diameters of 5, 7, and 10 mm are available. Viewing angles may be 0°, 12°, 30°, 45°, 70°, 90°, and 120°. Most surgeons use the 0° and 30° views. A flexible-tipped laparoscope is available. For diagnosis, a new class of minilaparoscopes that measure as small as 1.9 mm in diameter and pass through a 2 mm trocar are now available. Laparoscopes with larger rods deliver more light. Brighter light is a trade-off for depth of field and visual acuity. If the laparoscope is inserted cold, the tip fogs up, so it should be warmed before operation. If it becomes fogged, the lens can be cleaned with a sponge saturated with an alcohol-based antifog solution.

Currently, the most used light source is an automatic xenon high-intensity machine; 200, 300, or 400 W lamps may be used. The life of these lamps is 400 to 500 hours. Spare lamps must be available for an unexpected light failure. The machine dispenses automatic light control, but it may be regulated manually. Smaller, less expensive xenon lamps have been designed for purposes requiring less light, as in the case of a choledochoscope, or to provide light behind the mesentery to help define the blood vessels.

Light is transmitted via either fiber or fluid cables. The fiber cable is a bundle of glass fibers bound in a metal jacket that makes them rigid. These may be steam sterilized. The bundles are 1.6, 2.5, 3.5, or 4.5 mm. The cable bundle should be slightly larger than the lens system. However, if the fiber bundle is too large, light intensity is reduced. Fiberoptic cables suppress blue, and the illumination provides a yellow tinge. If 15% of fibers are fractured, a new cable should be obtained.

Fluid cables transmit more light, but are rigid and difficult to use. The fluid tends to turn yellow if gassed, so fluid cables must be soaked to sterilize them. If the fluid is yellowed or the quartz is cracked, it must be replaced.

VIDEO CAMERA

In advanced procedures, such as colon resection, the assistant and primary surgeon work from the same monitor image. The perfect camera is still being sought, but many of the goals are being approached. An ideal camera will be sturdy, small, lightweight, simply controlled, sterilizable by soaking if necessary, well insulated and will bring forth a sharp, high-resolution, true-colored picture. The life of a good camera is approximately two years or 400 cases. Multiple types of cameras have been designed that use single-chip, single-chip digitized, three-chip, three-chip digitized with interchangeable sized focus lenses, zoom lenses, beam splitters, and viewers.

Expensive three-dimensional systems are exciting to view, but the first generation requires use of special image glasses, which are uncomfortable, or nauseating for the surgeon. The second-generation three-dimensional cameras with special viewing monitors are under development, thus avoiding the need for special glasses. In the final analysis, the users of this equipment must conduct trials in the operating room to see which characteristics best suit them with regard to providing good vision and thus better and safer operations.

VIDEO MONITORS

The monitor must generate high-resolution images with connectors to S-VHS systems. The monitor's horizontal resolution should exceed that of the camera. Most single-chip cameras produce 400 to 600 lines, which is twice that of standard consumer monitors. The size of the monitor screen is based on how close the surgeon works from it. Screen sizes vary from 8 to 20 in., but for colon surgery, the surgeon works 6 to 7 ft. away using a 19 in. screen. Generally, a second monitor is placed to face assistants on the opposite side of the operating table.

RECORDING MEDIA

Recording is a part of most laparoscopic systems, but it can exhaust the budget. The best recordings today are obtained by expensive digitized images stored on magnetic or optical disks. However, inexpensive videotapes or films in analog form are most often used. The original VHS, U-Matic, Beta-cam recorders are being replaced by S-VHS, which gives good quality with 400 horizontal lines at a reasonable price.

The best quality video photography for making 35 mm slides for publications or lecturing is taken from 35 mm single-reflex cameras attached to the telescopic eyepiece. This method is superior, but is inconvenient. To match most

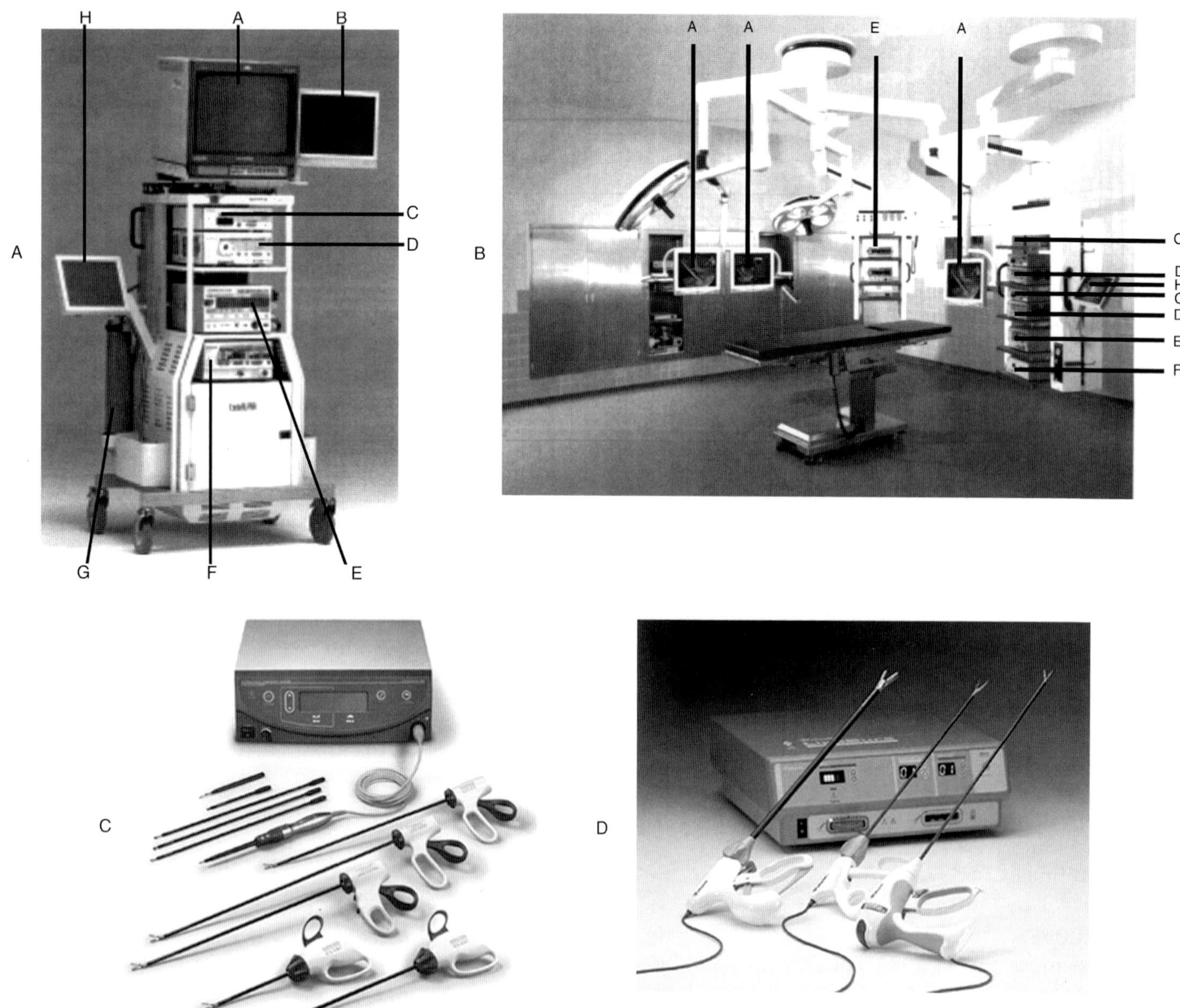

FIGURE 1 ■ (**A**) The laparoscopy cart may contain a monitor (*A*), a component monitor or picture in picture (*B*), camera box (*C*), light source (*D*), electrosurgical unit (*E*), carbon dioxide insufflator (*F*), carbon dioxide tank (*G*), and control panel (*H*) (Courtesy of Olympus Corp.). (**B**) New laparoscopy room with equipment mounted on a five-arm beam. Same labels as in (**A**) (Courtesy of Olympus Corp.). (**C**) Vessel sealing/cutting unit, harmonic scalpel (Courtesy of Ethicon Endosurgery). (**D**) Vessel sealing/cutting unit with graspers. (Courtesy of Ligasure, Valley Laboratory, Boulder, Colorado, U.S.A.)

surgeon's preferences (i.e., fast and easy techniques) electronic photography using the video signal from a still video recorder with a 35 mm camera may be used to capture the field of a moving video image. There are video printers to match the budget. These vary from inexpensive low-resolution printers to high-resolution digital printers.

■ INSUFFLATORS

Insufflation machines should be able to generate a flow of at least 10 L/min. Carbon dioxide is the gas usually used because it is not combustible and is readily absorbed. The machine should have automatic pressure and volume regulators to maintain a constant intraperitoneal pressure.

An acoustic and visual alarm system should be a standard part of the machine, which is activated if the preselected settings are exceeded. Gauges keep the surgeon apprised of insufflation pressure, gas flow per minute, intra-abdominal pressure, and gas volume used.

■ POWER INSTRUMENTS

Cutting and dissecting may be achieved using water jet, electricity, laser, or harmonic vibration instruments (see Chapter 7 for the principles of electrosurgery and laser). Currently, the most commonly used method is monopolar electrocoagulation. No particular advantage has been shown for using lasers in laparoscopic surgery.

Harmonic scalpels (Fig. 1C) and shears use high-energy ultrasonic vibrations to mechanically denature proteins in tissues, thus sealing vessels and causing cavitation. Cutting–coagulation requires vibration frequencies of 55,500/sec. Ultrasonic shears with a blunt vibrating blade and a narrow closure blade have been developed. These shears can coagulate most vessels encountered. As cells are selectively fragmented, leaving nerves, ducts, and larger blood vessels, the cell debris and liquid are suctioned away. The new generation of more efficient harmonic scalpels fit 5 mm ports, have hand control buttons, and seal up to 5 mm vessels. Further advantages include minimal vapor production and increased safety. Avoidance of electric monopolar currents through the body reduces the possibility of burns, but the harmonic scalpel becomes hot enough to burn adjacent bowel if touched.

A vessel-sealing device (Ligasure; Valley Laboratory, Boulder, Colorado, U.S.A.) delivers an electrical energy through special graspers (Fig. 1D). A high coaptive pressure with a temperature $<100°C$ denatures collagen and elastin forming a permanent seal of the vessel walls. This seal has a high tensile strength. The device has a trigger-operated blade to cut and separate the sealed vessel ends.

Waterjet (hydrodynamic) dissection separates and fragments parenchymatous tissues with low collagenous fiber content. Its best use is in solid organs. It is less useful for endoscopic surgery because of mist obscuring the visual field, a limited cutting depth, potential contamination of the accumulated fluid, adjacent tissue bloating, and because hemostasis is not achieved.

■ INSUFFLATION NEEDLES

The Veress needle, invented in 1938, is the most popular needle for establishing pneumoperitoneum (32). These needles are available in 10, 12, and 15 cm lengths with a diameter of 1.8 mm. The outer needle is sharp for cutting through the abdominal wall, and there is a blunt-tipped, spring-loaded inner stylet, which pops out beyond the tip when the sharp needle enters the free peritoneal cavity, preventing puncture of internal organs. The needle usually has an indicator that can be seen when the bare needle point is exposed without protrusion of the blunt internal stylet. The needle has a stopcock for connection to a carbon dioxide source. In turn, the carbon dioxide is insufflated into the needle, which egresses from a hole in the tip of the blunt stylet.

■ CANNULAS AND TROCARS

Access to the abdominal cavity is provided by a large variety of trocars and cannulas. The sizes vary, but colon surgery is performed with a variety of 5, 10, 12, and 15 mm cannulas. The design of these important instruments hinges on changes in the valves and "safety shields." The cost of these instruments depends on whether they are reusable or disposable. Reusable trocars are more expensive, but require much labor to clean and maintain them. Because they are reusable the long-term cost is less. Disposable instruments generally have new, uninjured valves and sharp tips. Trumpet, trap-door, flap, chip, ball, slit, and leaflet valves have been devised. The sharp trocars present a risk for injury to abdominal viscera; so "safety shields" were developed to minimize that risk. There are variations on the principal theme of immediate shielding of the sharp trocar tip when it penetrates to the free peritoneal cavity. The new trocar points are not sharp.

Modular port systems have been designed so that parts of a port that wear can be interchanged. This concept saves money and is particularly beneficial for cleaning and sterilization.

Cannulas are held in place by several "anchor concepts." Knitted sleeves, threaded sleeves, balloons, and mechanical expanders maintain the cannula in place and prevent gas leaks during a procedure.

Flexible cannulas permit the insertion of curved instruments. The flexibility is afforded by creating a trocar from a tightly coiled spring. These instruments usually, require an outer distender sheath to fix them in place and prevent gas leak.

■ HAND-ASSISTED PORTS

Hand-assisted laparoscopic surgery (HALS) is a technique that involves the intra-abdominal placement of a hand or a forearm through a mini-laparotomy incision while pneumoperitoneum is maintained. In this way, the hand can be used in a manner similar to an open procedure to palpate organs, retract viscera, identify vessels, provide traction to permit dissection in the appropriate plane, and apply finger pressure to control bleeding points. This approach may be more economical than a totally laparoscopic approach, reducing both the number of laparoscopic ports and number of instruments required. Some advocates of the technique claim that it is easier to learn and perform than totally laparoscopic approaches and that it may increase patient safety (33).

Using a new generation of hand-access devices that extend the options for hand-assisted techniques, these devices facilitate hand insertion, protect the wound, act as the retrieval site for the specimen and serve as the portal for construction of extracorporeal anastomoses. In addition, these new devices can serve as laparoscopic trocar sites. This permits selective use of hand-assisted and laparoscopic-assisted techniques at various times in the same operation (34). Hand-assisted laparoscopic (HAL) colectomy has evolved into a clinically useful surgical technique. It enables the easy insertion and handling of a large surgical towel inside the peritoneal cavity (35). The towel successfully retracts the small intestine and enables the surgeon to concentrate the use of his or her hand on the targeted structures.

With the introduction of HALS, a series of hand ports have been devised. Six have been Food and Drug Administration approved and are sold for use in HALS. These include Lapdisc (Ethicon Endosurgery Inc., Cincinnati, Ohio, U.S.A.), Handport (Smith & Nephew Endoscopy, Andover, Massachusetts, U.S.A.), Gelport (Applied Medical, Rancho Santa Margarita, California, U.S.A.), Omniport (Advanced Surgical Concepts, Dublin, Ireland), Pneumosleeve (Dexterity Inc., Roswell, Georgia, U.S.A.), and Intromit (Applied Medical). These products need be compared in regard to size, ease of hand insertion, comfortability to introduce instruments, and rapidity of specimen extraction. These devices each have their own advantages and disadvantages. Ideally, the hand port provides easy passage of the hand into the abdominal cavity, protects the wound, maintains a pneumoperitoneum with or without a hand in, and allows easy extraction of the specimen.

Nakajima et al. (36) reviewed 33 HALS colorectal procedures including total colectomy ($n = 16$) and low anterior resection ($n = 10$). In their study, 9.1% of 33 HALS procedures were converted to open surgery and 13.3% of 30 HALS procedures required minimal enlargement of incisions to facilitate extracorporeal procedures. The average operative time was 263 minutes. There were 9.1% major complications and 21% minor wound infections noted postoperatively. The mean hospital stay was 7.9 days. They concluded Gelport HALS is safely and reliably applicable for various colorectal procedures.

Chang et al. (37) compared the outcome of 66 patients undergoing HAL sigmoid resection with that of 85 undergoing laparoscopic sigmoid resection. There were slight differences in operative time favoring hand-assisted (189 minutes vs. 205 minutes) and the extraction incision was larger in the hand-assisted group (8.1 cm vs. 6.2 cm). There was no difference in time for return of bowel function (hand-assisted 2.5 days vs. laparoscopic 2.8 days) or length of hospital (hand-assisted 5.2 days vs. laparoscopic 5.0 days). Complications were similar in the two groups (hand-assisted 21% vs. laparoscopic 23%), but there were fewer conversions in the hand-assisted group (0% vs. 13%). They concluded HAL sigmoid resection yields the same outcomes as standard laparoscopic techniques but with fewer conversions. Hand-assistance is a helpful innovation that may expand the application of laparoscopic colectomy.

OPERATING INSTRUMENTS

Retractors

Colon surgery requires movement from one abdominal site to another. To achieve this mobility with vision, it is necessary to retract adjacent organs, especially the small bowel. The positioning of the table makes gravity direct organs dependently, while a pneumoperitoneum helps "push" and hold organs away. Yet, some retraction locally often becomes necessary. Retractors should be blunt and should have atraumatic tips and blunt edges (Fig. 2A). Unfortunately, for an instrument to fit through a cannula, it must be blade-like. The blades may be made to curve, curl, or fan out, but the edges are still potentially sharp and must be checked for position frequently during an operation. Inflatable retractors may help solve the problem of sharp edges.

Graspers

For the purposes of colon surgery, grasping forceps to push, pull, and dissect are necessary. Although forceps are available with traumatic or atraumatic tip designs, the atraumatic jaws required to avoid colon injury are most often needed. In general, the shafts can be rotated 360° to direct the tip appropriately. The tips can be electrified for electrocoagulating bleeding points. The diameter of the graspers is 5 or 10 mm, and they fit through cannulas of like diameter.

Clip Appliers

Clips are used to occlude larger vessels. The clip appliers may be single load or multifire. Generally, the single load is reusable and the multifire are disposable. In a colon resection, multiple clips are needed, so a multifire clip applier is appropriate. The clips may be metal, such as titanium, or be absorbable.

Staplers

Laparoscopic linear staplers (Fig. 2B) apply rows of staples, and cut between them. The staple lines may be 3 to 6 cm long. The 6-cm stapler only fits through a 12-mm cannula, and the 3-cm stapler fits through a 10-mm cannula. These are used for transecting bowel or performing functional end-to-end anastomoses. Flexible distal stapler shafts allow deeper insertion into the pelvis for rectal stapling with transection. Power driven staplers have been created that perform actions comparable to hand-powered staplers (Fig. 2C).

End-to-end circular staplers may be used in laparoscopic-assisted anastomoses. The anvil is pursestring sutured into the proximal bowel, which is drawn through a small incision, and the stapler is inserted via the anus. Some of these staplers are extra long and reach well up into the abdomen. Special staplers with tighter and closer rows and shorter staple lines have been designed for use on

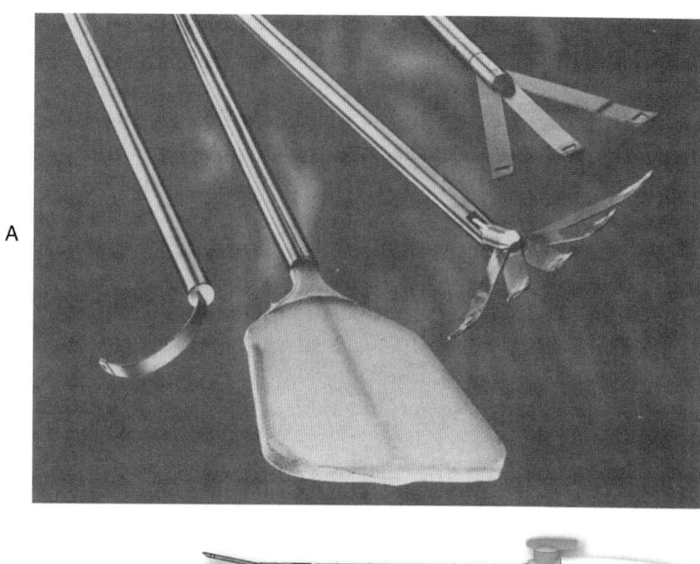

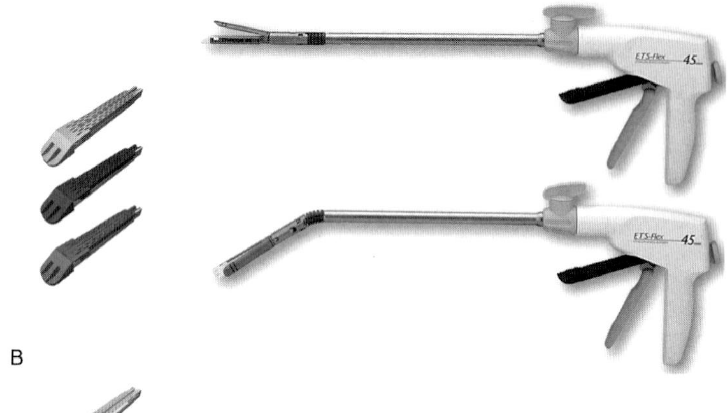

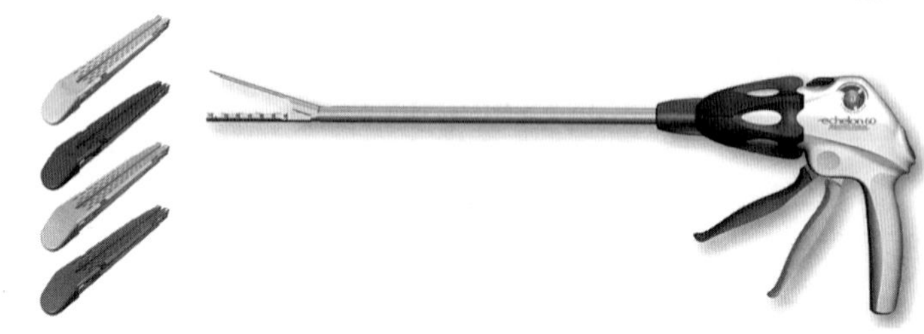

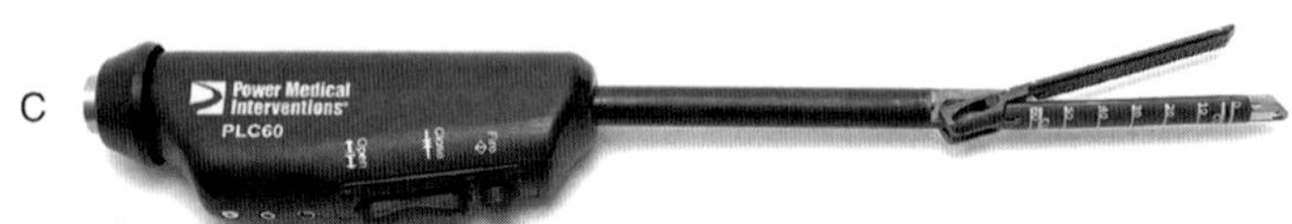

FIGURE 2 ■ (**A**) Laparoscopic retractors. (**B**) Laparoscopic staplers. (Courtesy of Ethicon Endosurgery, Cincinnati, Ohio, U.S.A.) (**C**) Reusable 60 mm linear cutter. (Courtesy of Power Medical Interventions, Langhorne, PA.)

larger vessels; however, these are expensive and add significant costs if many are used.

Needles and Sutures

Standard gastrointestinal needles and sutures generally can be used. Ski-shaped needles have been developed for ease of use with certain needle holders. For running suture and extracorporeal knot tying, polydiaxanone or polypropylene is best.

Automatic sewing devices are being introduced. Needle shuttling devices are available, but they present enough problems and the applications are not well defined; so their use has been minimal. Fortunately, suturing is seldom needed for colectomy.

OPERATIVE PROCEDURE

■ PREOPERATIVE PREPARATION

The mechanical and antibiotic preparation of the colon is the same as that for laparotomy as discussed in Chapter 4. Generally, this entails the use of laxatives, most commonly sodium phosphate, and enemas. Oral polyethylene glycol solutions are used less frequently. In some patients the laparoscopy procedure is converted to an open procedure, and the informed consent should reflect that.

■ PREOPERATIVE EVALUATION

Because the internal organs cannot be palpated during standard laparoscopy, the viscera must be inspected by other means. Colonoscopy is used to determine the pathology that is evident from the mucosal surface. Tattoos around the pathology are very helpful. Computed tomography (CT) scans are used to evaluate the liver and may reveal other pathology or enlarged lymph nodes. A CT scan is more meaningful if oral and intravenous contrast dyes are used, in concert. If the rectum contains pathology, endoluminal ultrasonography is used to help define the relationships of that pathology to the layers of the rectal wall and other pelvic organs.

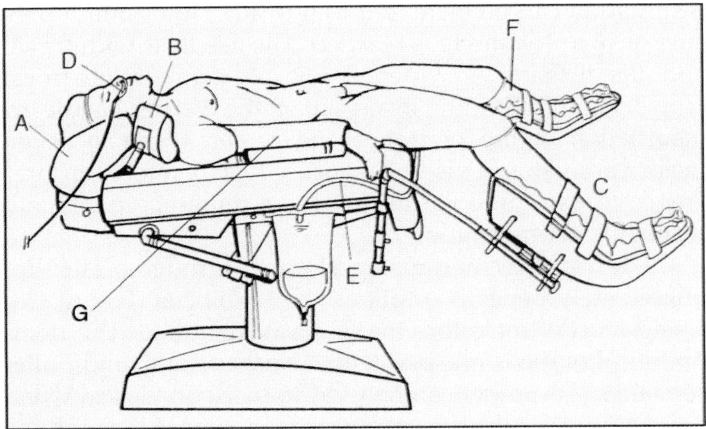

FIGURE 3 ■ Ready position may include "bean bag" torson holder (*A*), shoulder braces (*B*), stirrups with thighs level and legs angled down (*C*), nasogastric or orgastric tube (*D*), urinary catheter (*E*), compression stockings (*F*), and the arms are padded and tucked at the patient's side (*G*).

■ POSITIONING AND READYING THE PATIENT

The table is equipped with devices to hold the patient in place, even when marked tilting of the table is necessary (Fig. 3). A "bean bag" torso holder and shoulder braces work well. The patient is placed in a modified supine position with the legs in stirrups. The perineum is placed just off the inferior end of the table to allow access if intraoperative colonoscopy is deemed necessary and to facilitate a stapled anastomosis. The patient's legs are positioned so that the surgeon or the assistant can stand between the legs. The hips and knees are flexed less than usual to avoid impediment to the surgeon's arm movement and to keep the patient's thigh from obstructing the movement of instruments. The legs are wrapped in compression, stockings (pneumatic if available) to enhance blood flow. The stirrups may be of further help if there is a need to cleanse the colorectum or mark a neoplasm. Both arms are tucked and padded to the sides, permitting more mobility by the surgeons. A gastric tube is inserted and removed at the end of the case, and a urinary catheter is inserted. The rectum may be washed out if rectal pathology is the reason for the operation. The abdomen is washed, prepared, and draped just as for celiotomy. Larger drapes have been designed which cover the legs and body, have straps to tether all the lines and tubes, have a perineal pouch, and a large opening to accommodate well-separated cannulas.

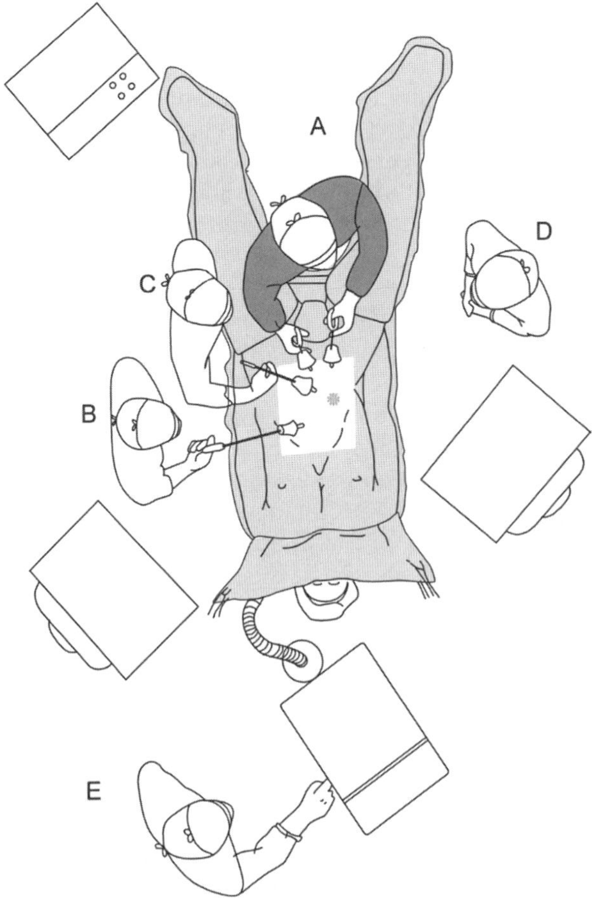

FIGURE 4 ■ Orientation of the operating team. The surgeon's sight, instruments, body, and monitor are aligned across the point of operation. This changes if the point of operation moves to a different abdominal quadrant The team is the surgeon (*A*), assistant surgeon (*B*), cameraman (*C*), scrub nurse (*D*), and anesthesiologist (*E*). Note that the surgeon uses a two-hand technique.

■ OPERATING ROOM SETUP AND CONDUCT OF OPERATION

The placement of the operating team around the table varies with the site of the pathology (Fig. 4). The specifics of personnel placement and port placement are described later for individual colorectal procedures. However, generally the surgeon stands diagonally opposite the pathology. The first assistant stands opposite the surgeon. The cameraman is next to the surgeon, but positions change, depending on where the surgeon moves (i.e., to the right side, left side, or between the patient's legs). The cameraman has responsibility for several functions. Because the view is critical, the laparoscope must be white-balanced, focused, and defogged. If the tip is fogged, the tip can be warmed, the cold CO_2 lines can be moved to another cannula, and additional anti-fog solution can be applied to the tip. The view is frequently changed by moving the laparoscope close to the field for magnification or drawn back to give a wide-angle view. At the beginning of the procedure, the entry sites for trocars must be observed during insertion, and at the end to see whether there is bleeding from the port sites internally as cannulas are withdrawn. The sterile operating room technician must have access to both the instrument table and the operating field. This technician must assemble the selected laparoscopic instruments, plus have instruments available if the laparoscopic procedure is converted to an open procedure. The significant amount of equipment results in clutter on the operating field; thus creating a standard positioning and arrangement of the various tubes and lines aids in smoother start of the operation. The larger pieces of equipment such as the camera, insufflation machine, and photography equipment are stacked on a mobile cart (Fig. 1A). The monitors are placed on the side opposite from the surgeon and assistant so that a direct view is possible without the need to turn his or her head. The camera should face the monitor that the surgeon uses.

■ PNEUMOPERITONEUM

Pneumoperitoneum is achieved with either the Veress needle or the open technique. The Veress needle is easy to introduce, but it is a "blind" technique. For safety, the open technique is used. It is certainly preferred in cases of reoperative surgery, bowel obstruction with distended loops, known adhesions, and pregnancy.

The easiest site for placement of the Veress needle is at the inferior midline margin of the umbilicus, where the fascia is most accessible (Fig. 5). A small incision is made with a No. 11 blade. Sharp, pointed towel clips are used to grasp the skin and umbilical fascia so that both can be lifted and essentially fixed. Without fixation, the peritoneum is more likely to "tent up" off the needle tip and fail to penetrate. The stopcock is opened, and the Veress needle is grasped like a pen, using the other fingers as supports to prevent a rapid thrust into the abdomen. By gentle advancement at 90° to the abdominal wall, the needle traverses the fascia and peritoneum. As the needle penetrates free into the peritoneal cavity, the "pop" of the blunt stylet springing forward to protect the sharp, tip is felt, and heard. When the stopcock is opened, a hiss may be heard.

Simple tests should be performed to verify correct placement of the Veress needle in the free peritoneal cavity. The aspiration test, using a syringe half filled with water,

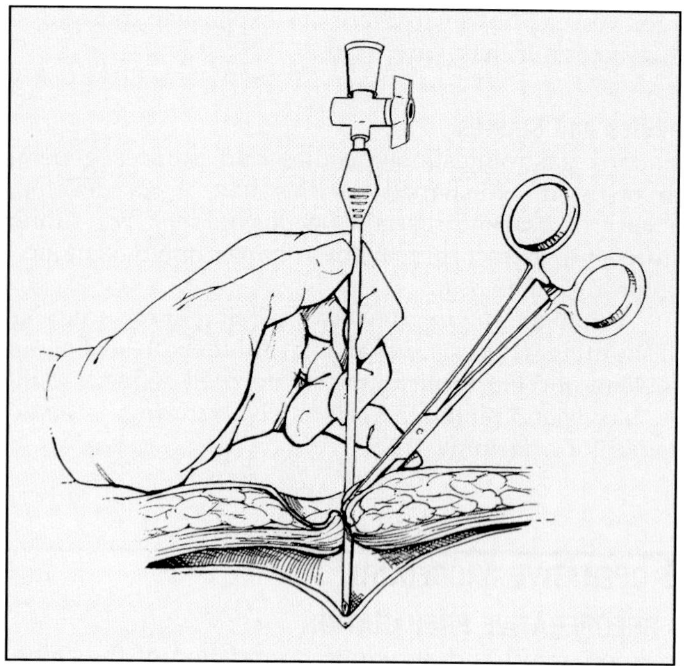

FIGURE 5 ■ Veress needle insertion. The needle is held like a pen with the hand braced on the abdominal wall. The towel clip is used to provide counter traction.

determines whether blood or gas enters the syringe, suggesting that either a blood vessel or the bowel has been penetrated. If neither blood nor gas returns, the fluid is easily injected into the peritoneal cavity. The drop test is performed by placing a drop of saline on the top of the needle with the stopcock closed. When the stopcock is opened, the negative pressure in the abdomen draws the fluid down. If this is not observed, the towel clips may be lifted, creating a negative pressure, and the drop of fluid should be drawn in. If these tests confirm correct placement in the free peritoneal cavity, the insufflation tube is attached to the stopcock. However, initially, the settings should be at a low pressure of 5 mmHg and a low volume of 1 L/min of carbon dioxide. The pressure should read 0 mmHg. If the pressure is >5 mmHg or rises rapidly, the needle tip is likely in the preperitoneal space. When the site of the tip is properly shown to be in place, the rate of carbon dioxide insufflation can be increased to 6 to 10 L/min until a pressure of 10 to 15 mmHg is reached. The needle is withdrawn, and the incision is widened for insertion of the trocar. However, the "blind" insertion of the Veress needle for insufflation of the peritoneal cavity can result in severe major vascular and visceral injuries. It is therefore our preference to use the open technique to minimize potentially avoidable complications.

The open technique is performed through an incision immediately beneath or above the umbilicus (Fig. 6) (38). Using narrow retractors the fascia is identified. The dense umbilical raphe is grasped with a Kocher clamp and pulled cephalad. A scissors can be used to incise the fascia where the umbilical raphe joins it. Sutures are placed through the fascia on each side, which are tied onto the cannula to prevent accidental extraction. Penetration into the free peritoneum can be seen; thus the blunt Hasson trocar–cannula can be inserted under direct vision. The cannulas are generally sewn into place with a heavy fascial suture. This

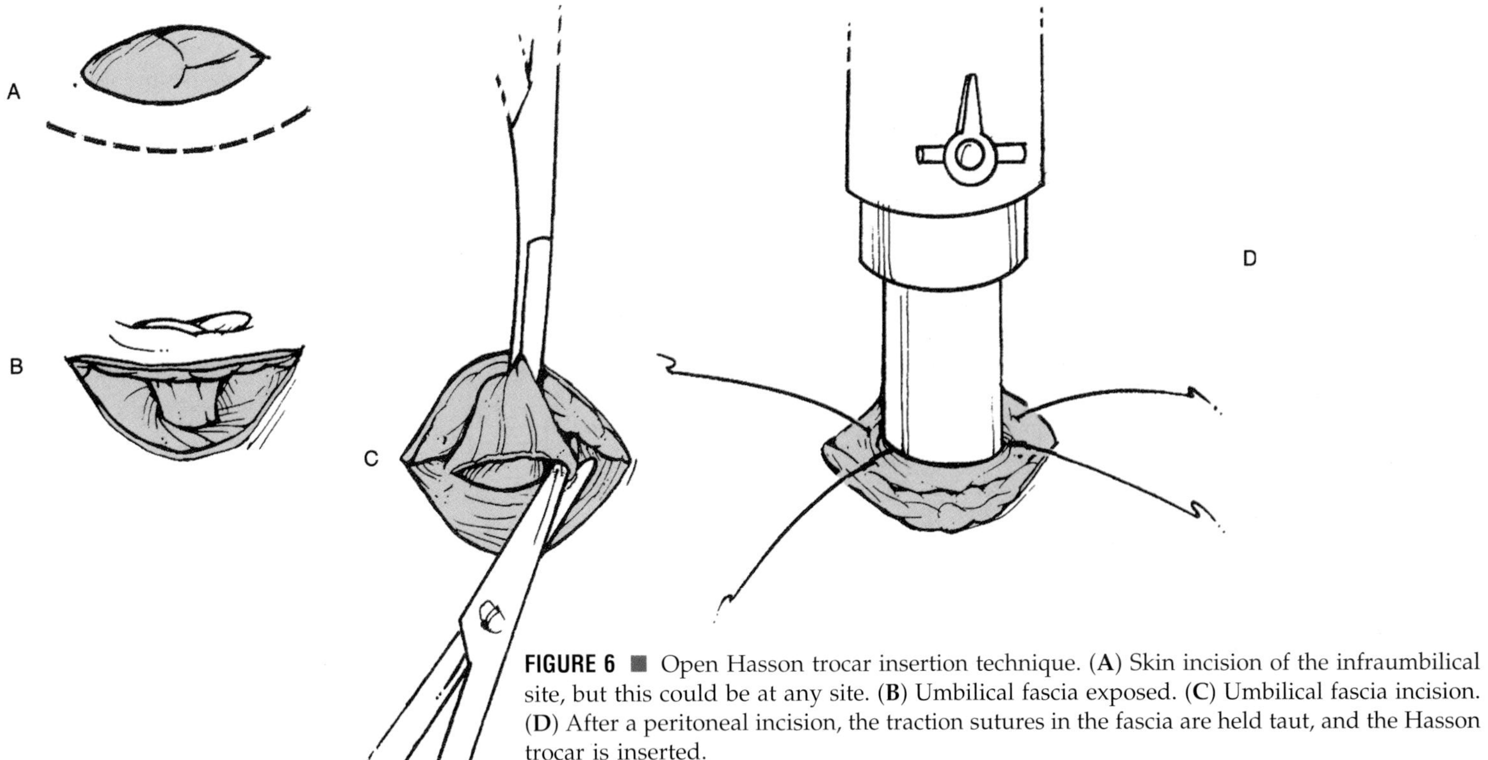

FIGURE 6 ■ Open Hasson trocar insertion technique. (**A**) Skin incision of the infraumbilical site, but this could be at any site. (**B**) Umbilical fascia exposed. (**C**) Umbilical fascia incision. (**D**) After a peritoneal incision, the traction sutures in the fascia are held taut, and the Hasson trocar is inserted.

suture through the fascia may be used for closure later. Thereafter, the abdomen can be insufflated rapidly up to a pressure of 15 mmHg.

■ GASLESS LAPAROSCOPY

Some surgeons have devised methods to perform laparoscopy without the pneumoperitoneum (39). These methods depend on a mechanical means of pulling or lifting the abdominal wall. Various rods, pins, and bars may be configured through the abdominal wall or through the peritoneal cavity and attached to wires connected to a pulley system, which draws up the abdominal wall. Then small incisions can be made or cannulas can be inserted through which the surgeon can work.

Hydraulic lifters were invented to simplify gas-less pneumoperitoneum. In this technique, a small incision is made and blades are inserted, fanned out, and attached to the power lifter so that an anterior space is created.

■ TROCAR–CANNULA INSERTION

The patient is placed in Trendelenburg position with complete pneumoperitoneum. For insertion of the trocar, the intraperitoneal pressure may be increased to 20 mmHg, but after insertion, the pressure is decreased to the 12 to 15 mmHg level. The infraumbilical site of the Veress needle is usually selected for the camera when this technique is used. The incision is widened to a size slightly greater than the cannula. The cannula with the stopcock closed is grasped between the index and middle fingers like a syringe, with the heel of the hand positioned over the trocar base (Fig. 7A). The shield mechanism is checked to ensure that it is "armed." The other hand is used at the entry point into the skin as a brace to prevent sudden thrusts. The clamps holding the fascia are lifted by the assistant to fix the entry point. The sharp point of the trocar is impaled into the fascia at a 90° angle, but is redirected to an angle 30° inferior toward the pelvis. A rotating and twisting motion is used to advance easily. As the trocar enters the free cavity, the safety shield springs over the tip, causing a pop that can be felt and heard. A prewarmed laparoscopic camera is introduced, and the organs are checked for injury. The newer trocars do not have blades; thus tissue is separated rather than cut (Fig. 7B).

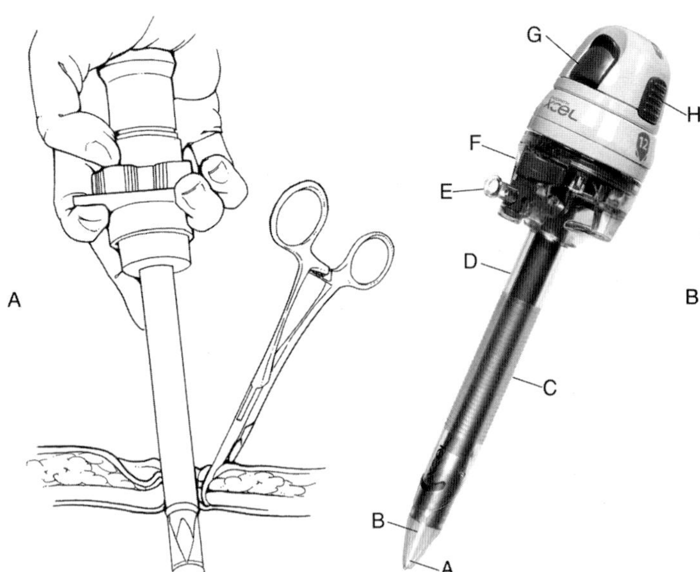

FIGURE 7 ■ (**A**) The penetrating trocar insertion. The thenar eminence is placed over the base of the trocar using the index finger as a guide. The other hand is used as a brace. The camera must focus on the entry site to be indicated when the trocar point is safely within. (**B**) Penetrating trocar. The components are optically guided tip (*A*), bilateral tissue separators (*B*), stability threads (*C*), clear cannula (*D*), insufflation valve (*E*), stopcock (*F*), friction lock for the laparoscope (*G*), and obturator release button (*H*).

■ ADDITIONAL PORTS

For colon surgery, usually three additional 10 to 12 mm ports are needed but 5 mm ports are often adequate except when stapling instruments are required: two for the surgeon's instruments and one for the assistant's instruments. The use of large ports permits the interchange and reposition of the camera and instruments. Port placement must be planned so that the ports are directed at the pathology in a semicircle. Placing the ports at least 7 to 8 cm apart, a hand's width, is preferred to prevent instruments from crossing ("sword fighting") (Fig. 8B). Before insertion, the camera should be used to transilluminate the site to identify large underlying abdominal wall vessels. With the camera in place, the other trocars can be observed as they penetrate the abdominal wall. The strategic placement of ports permits their incorporation into a later incision for specimen retrieval or stoma creation, if needed.

Hand-Assisted Port

When the hand-assisted technique is chosen (Fig. 8A), the number of ports can be decreased to a laparoscope port and two instrument ports for the surgeon. This requires the surgeon with a hand in the abdomen to be thoroughly familiar with the anatomy. The hand port is usually placed through the midline or through the rectus toward the pathology. The surgeon chooses the site based upon the need to mobilize and retract the specimen with the hand, but also draw the end of the bowel into the wound to permit preparation for anastomosis. The incision length is just short of the surgeon's glove size. In the midline, the skin, subcutaneous tissue, and fascia are incised. The hand-assisted device generally can be directly introduced. If the chosen site is off midline, the skin, subcutaneous fat, and anterior and posterior rectus fascias are incised. To approach the posterior fascia the rectus muscle must either be retracted or split. The peritoneum and fascia are bound by sutures at each end and the midpoints of the incision to permit introduction of the hand-port without inadvertent splitting of any tissue plane with the deep edge of the device. Careful hemostasis is needed to avert hidden hematomas or hidden hemorrhage into the peritoneal cavity. The gloves used for the internal hand should be of dark color to prevent glare.

■ SPECIMEN LOCALIZATION

Visual cues such as erythema, puckering of the serosa, or adhesions may identify the point of pathology. Because palpation is not possible, localization may depend on the use of the colonoscope. Preoperatively, dye, preferably India ink, may be injected on a margin of the pathology; the mark may be seen on the serosal surface. If the site is uncertain, the colonoscope can be passed during the operation, and the site can be marked where the colonoscope light is placed adjacent to the pathology. Monson et al. (40) recommend a preoperative barium enema to confirm the location of the colonoscopically diagnosed lesions because of the inability to palpate the colon directly during laparoscopic-assisted colectomy.

The identification of small neoplasms or areas presenting lesions associated with previous endoscopic polypectomy is one of the major problems in laparoscopic colon resection. Munegato et al. (41) evaluated the effectiveness of tattooing with India ink, to identify the area of the colon that is the site of the lesion in order to be able to perform colonic resections with oncologically correct margins. Marking was performed during preoperative colonoscopy in 84 patients by injecting 1 mL of the India ink solution with a sclerotherapy needle into each of the four quadrants of the colon wall. This method invariably allowed easy identification of the site of the neoplasm at laparoscopic colon resection. Only one complication due to paucisymptomatic microperforation was discovered during the operation.

Feingold et al. (42) reviewed 50 consecutive patients with colorectal neoplasms who underwent endoscopic tattooing prior to laparoscopic resection. No complications related to endoscopy or tattooing were incurred. Tattoos were visualized intraoperatively and accurately localized the neoplasm in 88% of patients. In the context of laparoscopic colorectal resection, preoperative endoscopic tattooing is a safe and reliable method of localizing colon lesions and may be preferable to other localizing techniques including intraoperative endoscopy.

Zmora et al. (43) evaluated the use of intraoperative lower endoscopy in 233 patients who underwent laparoscopic segmental colectomy. Lower endoscopy was employed in 24% of them compared with 17% in the laparotomy-matched group. The diseased segment was successfully identified in all of the patients in whom the main indication for endoscopy was localization (65% of cases). Endoscopy was judged to have changed the operative management in 66% of the 57 cases in whom it was employed and especially in 88% of the 37 patients for whom the main indication had been localization.

■ COMPLETION OF LAPAROSCOPY

The camera is used to look in all quadrants for injury or hemorrhage. As cannulas are moved, the site is observed for bleeding, and the skin site is plugged to maintain pneumoperitoneum. All port sites $\geq$10 mm usually have the fascia closed to prevent hernias. The skin is closed with subcuticular sutures and adhesive strips or skin staples.

SPECIFIC COLORECTAL PROCEDURES

■ DIAGNOSTIC LAPAROSCOPY

Diagnostic laparoscopy is valuable when the etiology is unknown or suspected in a patient who is ill from a possible intra-abdominal disease (44). A simple peek may resolve the issue. Such an examination may be combined with colonoscopy, upper endoscopy, ultrasonography, washings, and/or biopsy (45). The patient is positioned supine in stirrups as previously described.

To perform diagnostic laparoscopy, pneumoperitoneum is obtained by the previously described techniques. The size of the cannula to be inserted is predicated on the size of the camera to be used. If looking around the abdomen is the only activity, a very small camera inserted through a 2.5 to 3.0 mm needle may be used. Larger cannulas or secondary cannulas are needed if instruments are to be inserted. To insert a laparoscopic ultrasonographic probe, a 10 to 12 mm cannula is needed at the infraumbilical site.

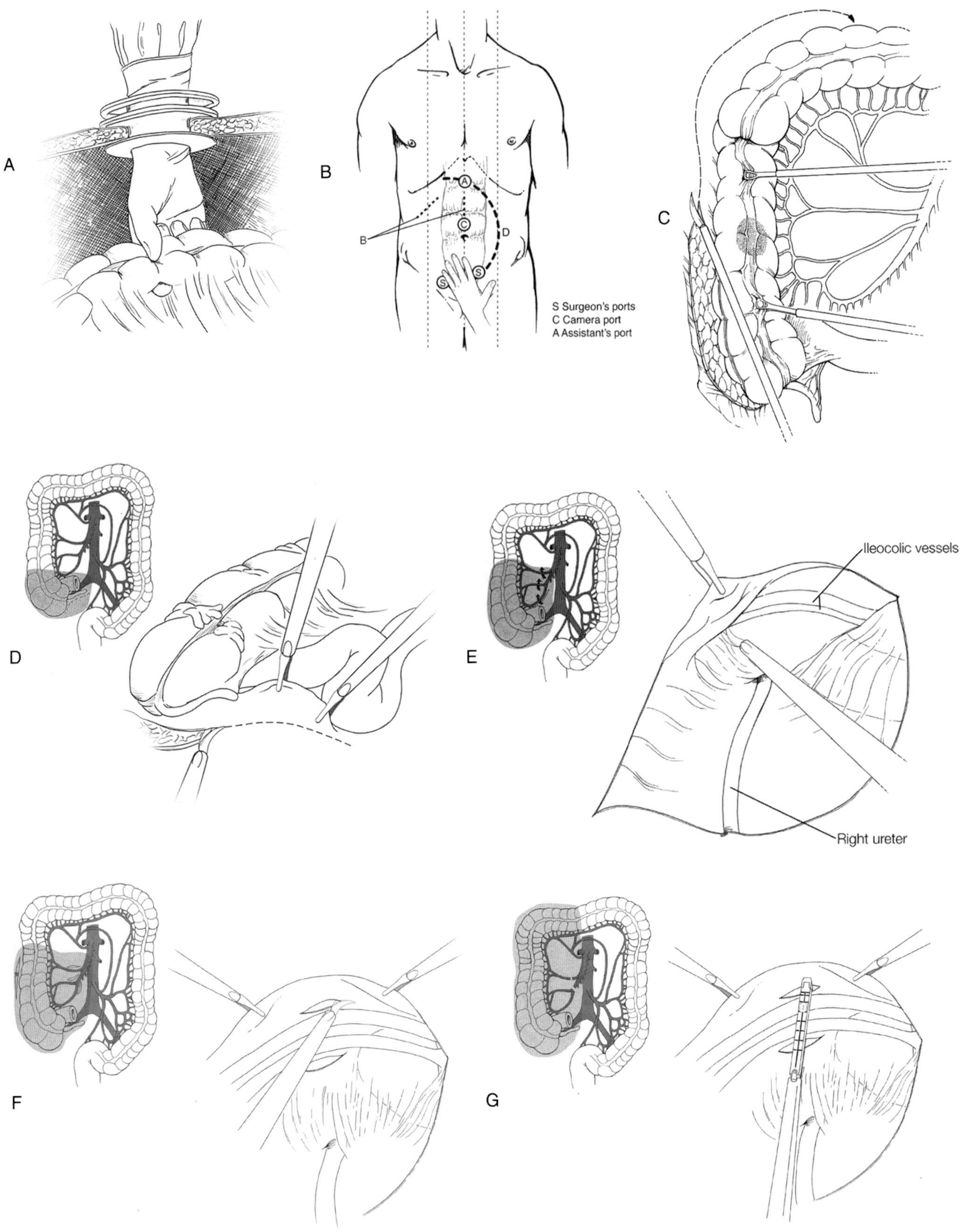

FIGURE 8 ■ (**A**) The hand port is inserted into a short incision, measured in centimeters to match the glove size, with the intent for hand mobilization, specimen and tissue retraction, and anastomosis construction. The touch sensation is reestablished. (**B**) Port placements for a right colectomy: ports are separated by the width of the fingers of a hand. Ports are placed along an imaginary semicircular line (*D*) facing the pathology. The initial port for the camera is usually placed above or below the umbilicus hatched lines (*B*) represent incision sites for either hand port or specimen retrieval. (**C**) Mobilization of the right colon, lateral to medial approach. (**D**) Alternative mobilization of the right colon, medial to lateral approach. First, the peritoneum is incised at the base of the ileal mesentery. (**E**) Alternative mobilization of the right colon, medial to lateral. Dissection separating the retroperitoneum from the right colon mesentery, pushing the ileocolic and right colic vessels anterior, the ureter posterior, and the duodenum medially. (**F**) Alternative mobilization of the right colon, medial to lateral. The ileocolic and right colic vessels are isolated and divided prior to incising the right lateral line of Toldt. (**G**) Alternative mobilization of the right colon, medial to lateral. The vessels are divided.

After the camera has been inserted, all four quadrants are carefully inspected. Exploration is the first step after the ports are placed. The finding of marked adhesions, abnormal anatomy, or carcinoma characteristics may prompt early conversion to hand-assisted or open laparotomy. If colonoscopy has not been completed, the colonoscope tip can be followed in its movements, and sometimes a grasping instrument may help negotiate loops and turns in the colon. The small bowel should be clamped to prevent reflux filling in the event that the ileocecal valve is incompetent. In cases in which a malignancy is suspected, effort must be made to see the entire liver surface. To see over the dome of the liver, a 30° laparoscope or flexible-tipped scope may be used. Intraoperative ultrasound probes have been designed to fit through 10 to 12 mm cannulas, which permits sharper images for the detection of hepatic metastases (46). If the liver has a suspicious site visible on direct inspection, previous or intraoperative ultrasonography, or CT scan, a biopsy may be needed. If the lesion is visible, a biopsy needle can be inserted percutaneously or through a small port aimed directly over the site to be biopsied. If the lesion is not visible, an ultrasonography-guided biopsy can be performed. If a specimen is to be obtained, suction, irrigation, and electrocautery equipment as well as clips and staplers should be immediately available in the operating room if hemorrhage control is necessary.

To look directly into the pelvis and see the depths of the cul-de-sac, a rigid sigmoidoscope can be used to point out the rectum and its junction into the peritoneal cavity. The uterus can be pushed up and out of the posterior pelvis by a special uterine manipulator introduced transvaginally.

The small bowel may be inspected directly by "running the bowel" techniques. Either the terminal ileum at the cecum or the jejunum at the ligament of Treitz is chosen as a beginning point. Two grasping instruments at well-separated cannula sites are used in hand-over-hand fashion along the small bowel. Pneumoperitoneum must be well maintained, and the table may need to be rotated and/or tilted to use gravity to keep the bowel separated and fixed in a quadrant.

■ RIGHT-SIDED COLECTOMY

The principles of right colectomy should be the same as in the open procedure; the difference is access (47). As in all laparoscopic colectomy procedures, the patient is placed in supine position with the legs in stirrups. A gastric tube and a urinary catheter are placed. The abdomen is prepared and draped in sterile fashion, just as if open colectomy were to be performed.

The surgeon stands on the left side facing the right upper quadrant. The surgeon may move to a position between the patient's legs. Likewise, the camera operator and assistant surgeon take other positions as needed. The scrub technician is positioned over the patient's right leg. A monitor is placed facing the right shoulder position for the surgeon. Most of the team uses this monitor. The second monitor can be placed over the left shoulder. If one member of the team is positioned in the right upper quadrant site for retraction, that person uses the second monitor.

As with all laparoscopic colon operations, a variety of trocar positionings have been recommended. These choices are often selected because of individual preference, the specific site of the pathology in the colon, previous operations, incisions that may steer the surgeon away from a particular area, or the body habitus of the patient (Fig. 8B). The first trocar site is placed at an infraumbilical or supraumbilical site with the patient in a head-down position. A 10 to 12 mm trocar is used to accommodate the laparoscope. Other trocars are placed in a semicircle to create a triangle with the pathology as the apex of the triangle. Ports may be placed in the right lower quadrant, midline at a suprapubic site, a left upper abdominal site in the midclavicular line, and high in the midline. These ports are placed so that the surgeon and first assistant can both use a two-handed technique. The 10 to 12 mm trocars may be used for all ports, but 5 mm ports are usually adequate for grasping and dissecting functions. At least one should be a 10 to 12 mm port for possible rapid clip application in the event of acute hemorrhage, or possibly the application of a vascular stapler. The hand-assisted technique may be chosen, which permits tactile sensation, provides the best of retractors, the human hand, and permits guiding and checking of instrument tip position. The site for the hand port is usually the upper midline or through the right, upper rectus. The hand-assisted device is inserted, and it also serves as a wound protector during specimen extraction.

The patient is placed in steep head-down position and rolled to the left. This causes the small bowel to fall away from the cecum and terminal ileum. The patient is repositioned to the head-up position as the operative field moves up the right colon to the hepatic flexure and the transverse colon. Even in this instance the Trendelenburg position may be preferred to prevent the omentum from falling into the field of vision.

The dissection begins in the right lower quadrant with dissection to free up the terminal ileum and appendix (Fig. 8C). As this mobilization progresses superiorly along the white line of Toldt, the right colon mobilizes medially. As the cecum is lifted, the ureter and gonadal vessels should be avoided. The right ureter is often not visualized during mobilization. As the hepatic flexure is approached, the table is tilted to a head-up position, which helps keep the small bowel dependent toward the pelvis by gravity. The duodenum is evident posteriorly as the transverse colon is mobilized by taking down the gastrocolic ligament. Electrosurgical scissors are most often used for the dissection; graspers are used to reflect and hold the bowel. Some surgeons prefer to use the harmonic scalpel for dissection. When mobilization is complete, the colon is suspended by the mesentery where the three named vessels (i.e., the ileocolic, right colic, and right branch of the middle colic vessels) reside; these must be cut. These vessels are individually freed up and clipped, ligated, or stapled (Fig. 9). The ileocolic vessels are always present, but the right colic is often absent and the middle colic is quite variable. When the vessels are divided, windows are evident in the mesentery. The mesentery is divided from the selected point for transection on the ileum to the point on the transverse colon (Fig. 10).

An alternative is the medial to lateral approach. In the beginning, the terminal ileal mesentry is lifted anteriorly so that an incision can be made from the caudal and dorsal

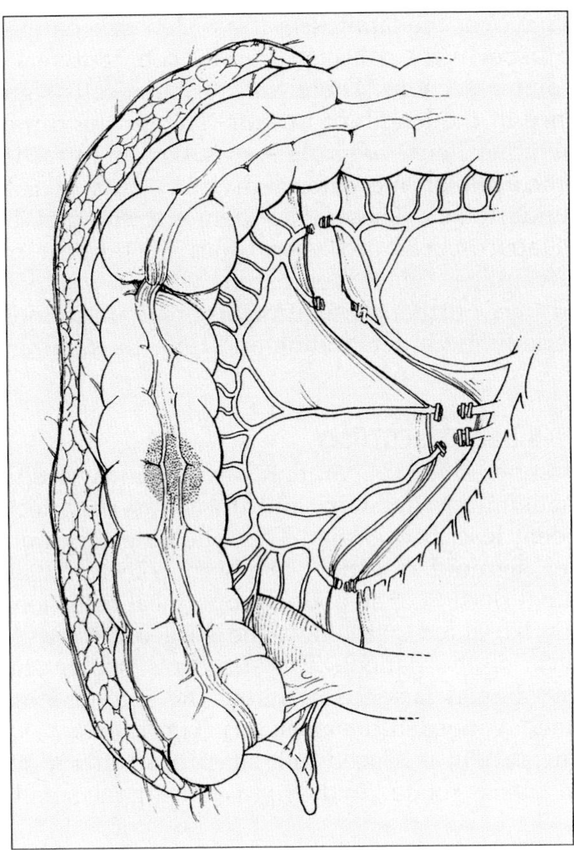

FIGURE 9 ■ Division of the vessels in the lateral to medial approach.

attachments of the cecum up medially toward the duodenum (Fig. 8D). An avascular plane behind the ileocolic vessels can be bluntly separated revealing the ureter and gonadal vessels that are swept posteriorly (Fig. 8E). This dissection proceeds anterior to Gerota's fascia, and extends cephalad to the liver and medially to the second portion of the duodenum, which is pushed medially. By pulling the cecum laterally the ileocolic vessels are drawn taut and stand out so that they can be traced from their origins at the superior mesenteric vessels to the cecum (Fig. 8F). Thus, they can be divided 1.0 to 1.5 cm from their origins. If the right colic vessels exist, they can be isolated and divided near their origins (Fig. 8G). Care is always necessary to spare the superior mesenteric vessels. The hepatic branches of the middle colic artery are encountered and divided as dissection proceeds to the transverse colon. Likewise, the marginal vessels adjacent to the colon are divided. The omentum is hanging from the transverse colon and may be incised, separating it off close to the colon in an avascular plane. Now only the lateral attachments of the white line need be taken down. Bowel transections and the remainder of the operation proceeds as in the lateral to medial approach, either as pure laparoscopic or laparoscopic-assisted technique.

Colectomy can be performed with a laparoscopic-assisted technique (4,48–52). In fact, our preference is laparoscopic-assisted surgery, which means that when adequate mobilization has been accomplished to allow delivery of the bowel to the surface, a 6-cm incision is made in the mid abdominal wall for specimen removal. If the procedure is performed for carcinoma, the incision should be shielded by a wound protector to avoid contamination by malignant cells. Mesenteric vessel ligation can be achieved through this incision. Via this incision, the bowel can be transected, usually with staplers, and anastomosis

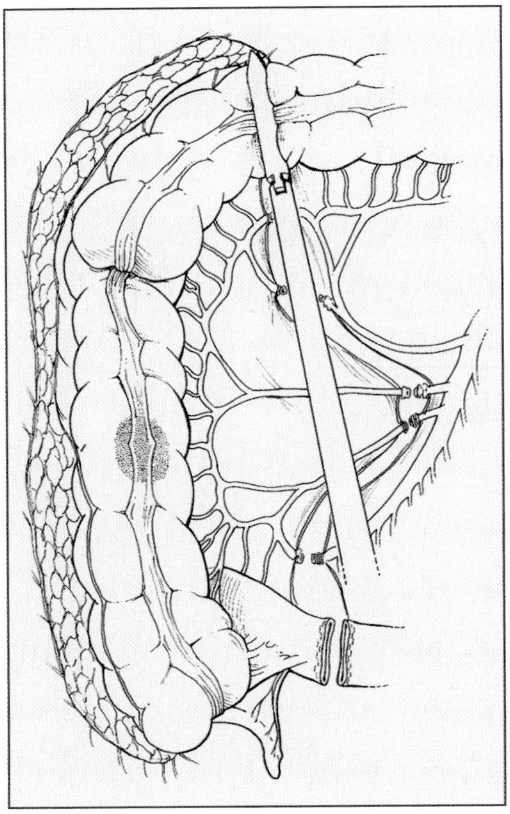

FIGURE 10 ■ Intracorporeal division of the ileum and transverse colon.

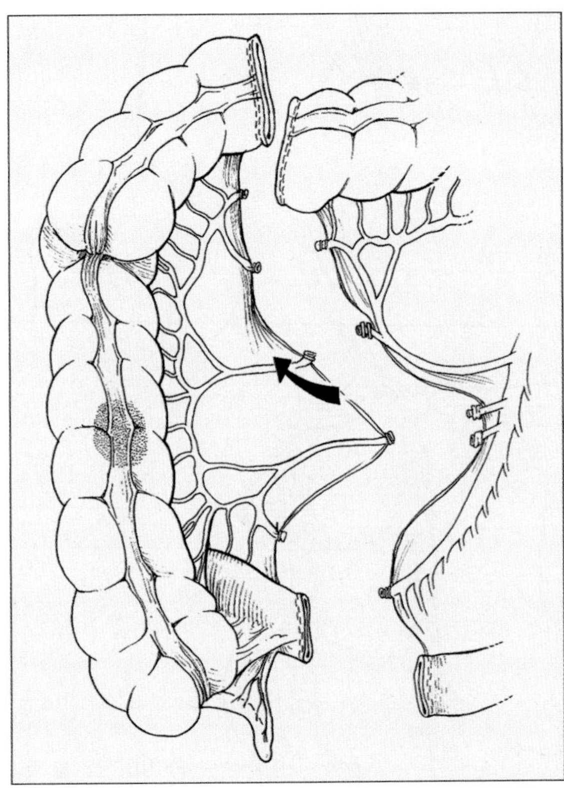

FIGURE 11 ■ Specimen freed for removal.

accomplished, usually with a functional end-to-end anastomosis using staplers (53). This type of stapled anastomosis should be performed as shown in Chapter 23. Subsequently, the mesenteric defect may be closed, but many surgeons do not make an effort to close this defect. Extracorporeal anastomosis and vascular ligation have the advantage of laparoscopic mobilization and avoid the difficulties associated with time-consuming intracorporeal mesenteric dissection, ligation, and anastomosis.

The right hemicolectomy may be performed entirely intraperitoneally, except for specimen removal. The resected tissue specimen may be placed in a special specimen bag and removed later through an incision. Linear cutting endoscopic staplers can be used to divide the bowel (Fig. 10) and the disease-bearing portion of colon removed (Fig. 11). Then the two limbs of bowel can be positioned end to end for an anastomosis with endoscopic stapling (i.e., functional end-to-end stapling). The antimesenteric corner of each transected and stapled bowel end is excised (Fig. 12A) to permit insertion of each limb of the linear laparoscopic stapler (Fig. 12B). When the side-to-side anastomosis has been created (Fig. 12C), the remaining opening at the tip can be closed with the linear stapler (Fig. 12D).

Bernstein et al. (54) reported that intracorporeal division of the mesentery and anastomosis confer no advantage over the laparoscopic-assisted procedures. Data were prospectively collected on 102 consecutive laparoscopic colon resections. There was no statistically significant difference in the length of hospital stay or the duration of postoperative ileus, regardless of whether intracorporeal or extracorporeal mesenteric division and anastomosis were undertaken. These data demonstrate that a completely laparoscopic procedure does not appear to offer any advantage when compared with a laparoscopic-assisted one. Furthermore, intracorporeal anastomoses are considerably more demanding and time-consuming.

■ LEFT-SIDED COLECTOMY

The preoperative preparation, evaluation, positioning, setup, pneumoperitoneum, and trocar insertion technique have been described earlier. The following techniques are used for sigmoid resection, left hermicolectomy, and the abdominal portion of an abdominoperineal resection (2,55).

For left-sided pathology, the surgeon stands on the right side of the patient. The surgeon's hands and eyes must be aligned facing a monitor. The second monitor is positioned as needed for assistants (Fig. 13A).

The patient is placed in a steep head-down position, and the table is rotated to the right, causing the small bowel

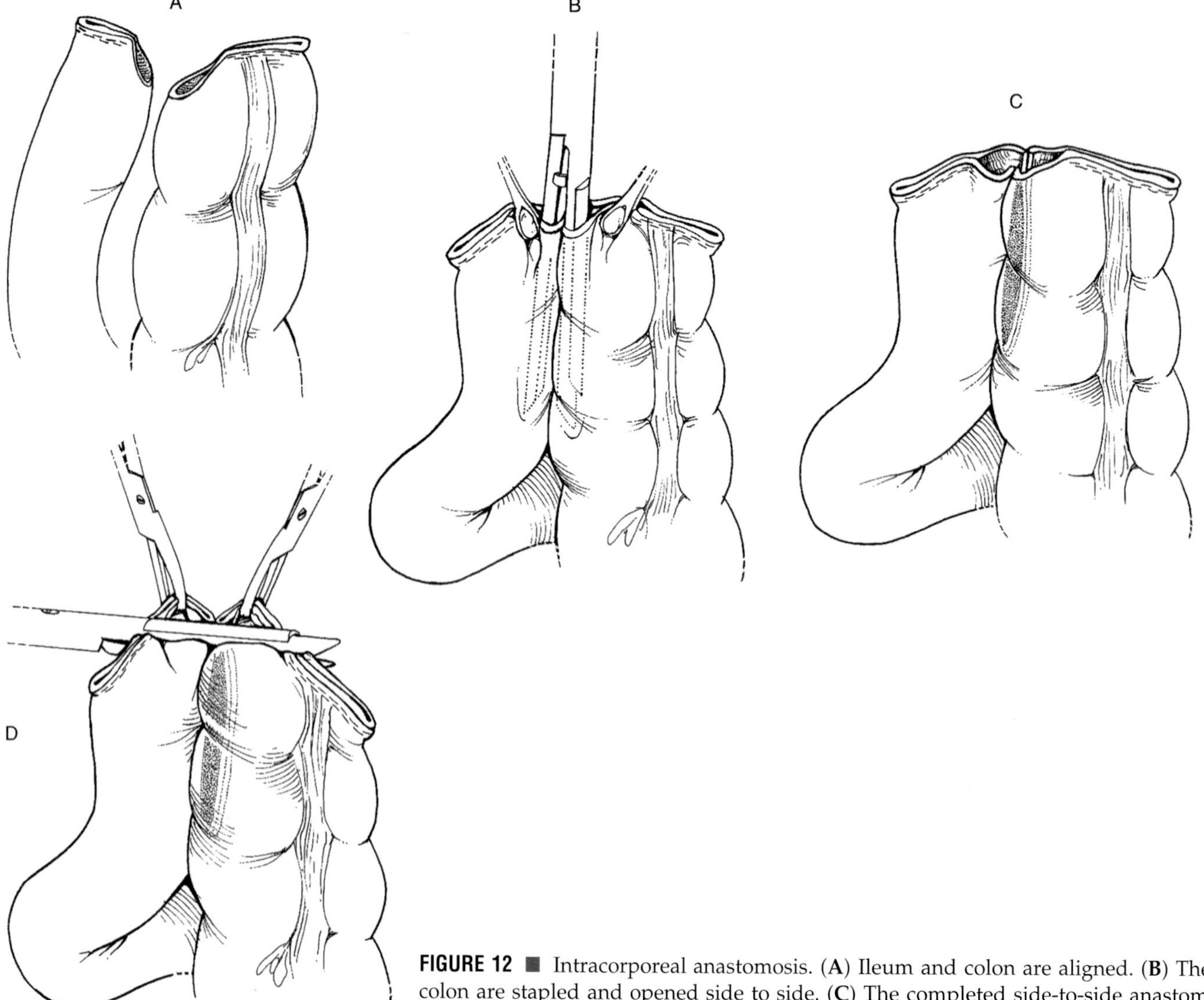

FIGURE 12 ■ Intracorporeal anastomosis. (**A**) Ileum and colon are aligned. (**B**) The ileum and colon are stapled and opened side to side. (**C**) The completed side-to-side anastomosis. (**D**) The open ends are stapled.

to fall away from the left lower quadrant. If great difficulty is encountered in retracting the small bowel out of the pelvis during a left-sided resection, the cecum may be mobilized to facilitate the exclusion of the small bowel from the operative field (Dr. Jaap Bonjer, personal communication). Ports are placed in a semicircle around the umbilical port, which usually holds the camera (Fig. 13B). A site for an incision to remove the specimen or for assisted resection is planned; the incision generally incorporates one or two of the port sites.

Depending on whether the sigmoid colon alone or the descending colon or rectum is also to be resected, the length of mobilization varies and port placement is modified. To resect the sigmoid colon, ports are placed below the umbilicus and in the right lower quadrant, right upper quadrant adjacent to the umbilicus, and left upper

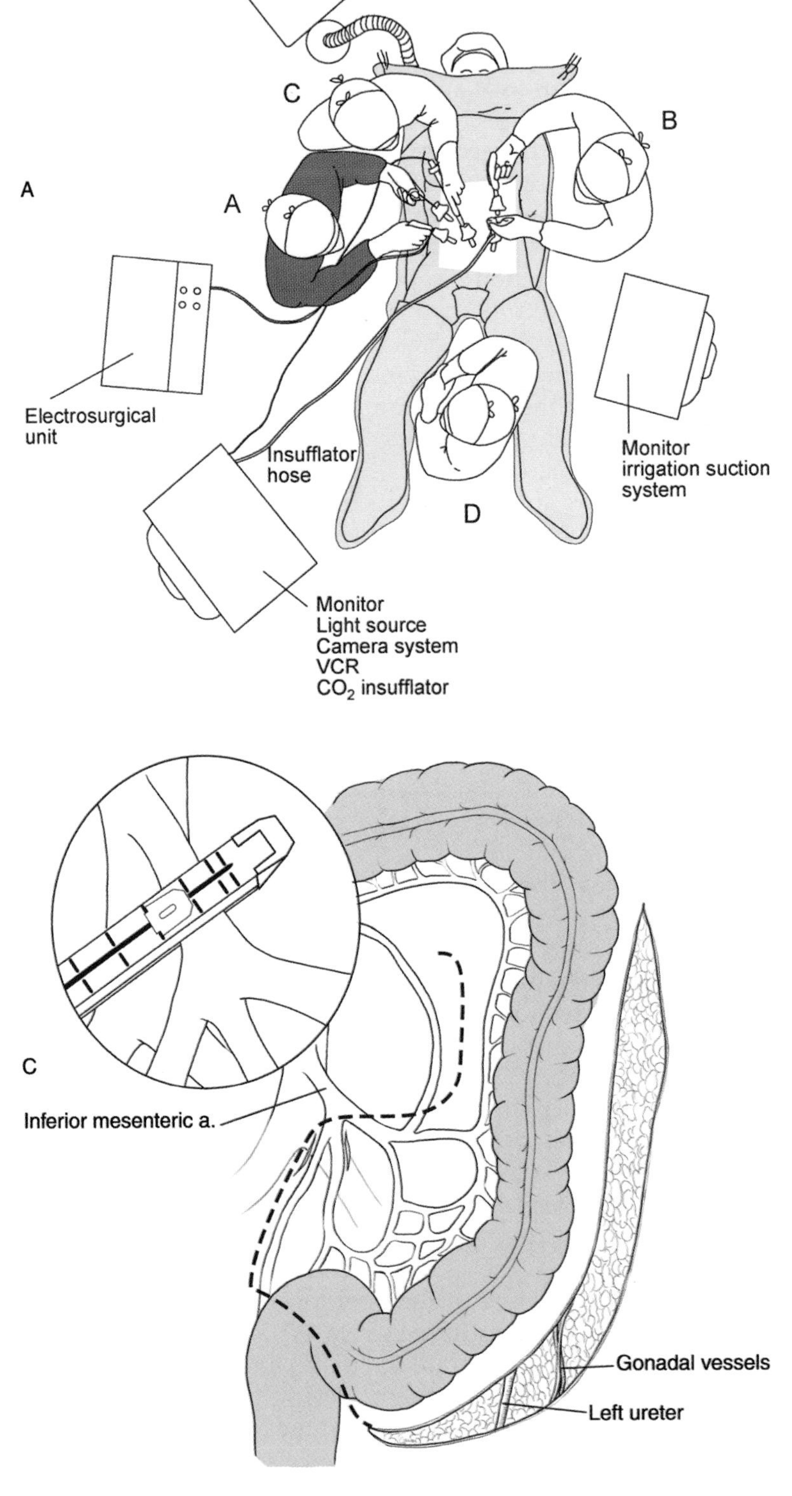

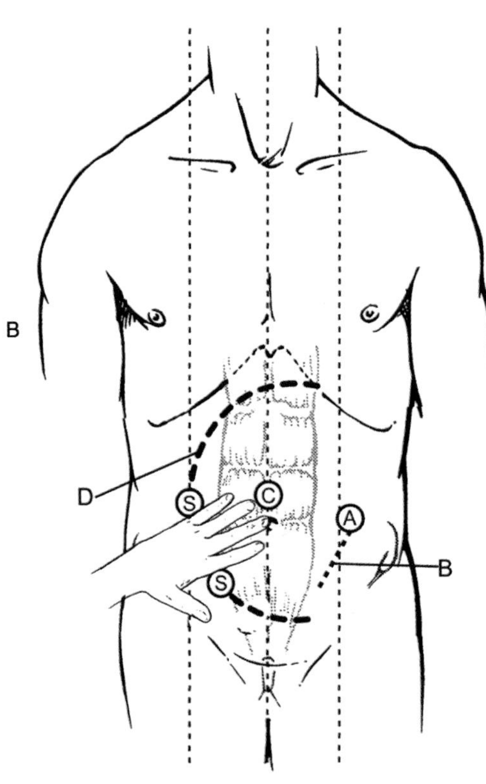

FIGURE 13 ■ (**A**) Positioning for left colectomy or sigmoid colectomy. (*A*) Surgeon; (*B*) first assistant; (*C*) cameraman; (*D*) nurse; (*E*) anesthetist. (**B**) Port placement and specimen removal incision or hand port (*B*). The incision is made early in the procedure if it is to serve as a hand port or late in the procedure if it is for specimen removal. (*D*) is the imaginary semicircular line facing the pathology; (*S*) is the surgeon's port; (*C*) is the camera port; (*A*) the assistant's port. (**C**) Mobilization of the left colon and sigmoid, lateral to medial approach. *Insert*: Division of the inferior mesenteric vessels, lateral to medial approach.

quadrant adjacent to the umbilicus. Frequently, a left lower quadrant trocar is added so that the assistant can aid in retraction and traction on the colon. For the hand-assisted technique, the hand port is made in the left lower quadrant or midline and is used in place of the left-sided ports.

If the patient is thin, the ureters may be visible, especially on the right; thus an incision medial to the ureter can be made as a marker to exclude the ureter during further dissection. The left ureter is more difficult to find, but as mobilization proceeds, the gonadal structures and ureter on the left must be identified and separated from the specimen. If a dense, adherent phlegmon is expected, ureteral stents may be inserted prior to beginning. This aids the surgeon if hand-assisted techniques are employed or the procedure is converted to an open approach.

The sigmoid is retracted medially, exposing the left lateral attachments of the descending colon and sigmoid colon. An electrified scissors or harmonic scalpel is used to incise the white line of Toldt (Fig. 13C). After the left lateral attachments are freed down to the rectum, the sigmoid is retracted laterally, exposing the vessels, taut under the traction. The mesentery is scored across their base near the aorta, and the incision is carried down along the rectum on the right. The vessels are skeletonized and ligated, clipped, or stapled with a vascular stapler (Fig. 13C insert). Either ligatures or clips or both may be used.

An alternative approach is the medial to lateral mobilization. The sigmoid mesentery is pulled anteriorly and inferiorly to make the inferior mesenteric vessels and sigmoid vessels taut and thus stand out. On the right side of the mesorectum an incision is made beneath these vessels near the sacral promentory. By bluntly dissecting across the retroperitoneum the nerve plexuses can be swept posteriorly and the vessels can be pushed anteriorly. As the dissection progresses toward the left side, the ureter and gonadal vessels are identified so that they can be swept lateral and posterior to the specimen (Fig. 14A). The vessels under stretch stand out so that the lateral mesenteric attachments can be taken down permitting the inferior mesenteric vessels to be encircled. The vessels can be divided using previously mentioned methods while carefully observing that the ureter is not picked up (Fig. 14B). Thereafter, the lateral white line can be incised as high as necessary to permit an anastomosis without tension. The operation then proceeds in the same fashion as lateral to medial resections. Patients requiring the takedown of the colonic splenic flexure to facilitate a left hemicolectomy have an initial incision in the mesentery medial to the inferior mesenteric vein, ligation of vessels in no-touch isolation fashion, subsequent medial-to-lateral extension of retroperitoneal dissection along Gerota's fascia, opening of the lesser sac by transection of the gastrocolic ligament, dissection of the mesenteric root of the distal transverse colon, and the final separation of splenocolic ligament and the lateral attachments of the descending colon (56).

If an anterior resection or a left colon resection is necessary, the splenic flexure is mobilized. The team must change position, and the monitors must be realigned. The surgeon usually stands between the patient's legs and uses the left-sided ports for the instruments. The assistant moves to the right upper quadrant to grasp the bowel. The camera person is in the right lower quadrant. The table is shifted to a head-up position to cause the small bowel to slide low and to the right. Traction on the splenic flexure exposes the attachments to the side wall, spleen, omentum, and stomach. Layer after layer is incised until the splenic flexure descends easily. Dissection close to the transverse colon along the omentum is relatively bloodless. Care must be taken to avoid pulling on the spleen and causing a capsular tear and hemorrhage. Reissman et al. (45) described the use of a colonoscope to retract the splenic or hepatic flexures to facilitate exposure, dissection, and mobilization of these flexures.

Dissection into the pelvis is performed under direct vision, using electrocautery or harmonic scalpel. Some surgeons use vessel sealing devices serially down the lateral stalks for cutting and coagulation (Fig. 15). The nerves at the pelvis can be seen and spared. If the rectum must be mobilized, the lateral attachments of the rectum are incised to the pelvic floor. The rectum is pulled anterior so that the presacral space can be entered over the sacral prominence. The rectum is separated from the presacral fascia down to the coccyx (Fig. 15A). The lateral stalks are cut, with special attention to coagulating the middle hemorrhoidal vessels. Anteriorly, the dissection is carried down the rectovaginal septum or below the seminal vesicles. The dissection is the same as that in the open procedure. When the two sites for transection are decided upon (i.e., the colon and rectum), the mesenteric fat is dissected off in preparation for an anastomosis. The transection of the mesorectum is performed with harmonic scalpel, vascular stapler, or a vessel sealing device. In the case of malignancy, the total mesorectal excision (TME) is performed as an en bloc resection. This is extremely difficult in the narrow male pelvis and the fat laden pelvis. The bowel can be transected with a 30 to 60 mm linear or laparoscopic stapler.

An alternative approach is to use laparoscopic-assisted colectomy techniques. In those cases, the planned incision for specimen removal is made, and the mobilized colon is drawn into the wound. Then the vessels can be transected, transection sites dissected clean of fat, and standard stapler transection accomplished (Fig. 15D).

The hand-assisted technique is valuable for pathology that is adherent to the peritoneal side walls. Detecting points where the colon is adherent and where retraction is necessary are more readily and speedily decided (58).

Anastomosis can be performed using a double-stapling technique. The anastomosis may be made at low levels if dissection can be carried out and a staple line applied. Laparoscopic staplers today can be directed squarely across the bowel with the aid of flexible stapler shafts. Often more than one application is necessary to staple completely across rectum or enlarged colon. The laparoscopic-assisted colectomy permits the proximal colon to be drawn out of the incision where a pursestring suture is applied and tightened around the shaft of a standard end-to-end stapler anvil (Fig. 15D). The colon is returned to the abdominal cavity and the pneumoperitoneum is reestablished. The stapler can be introduced via the anus and the stapler trocar opened to penetrate the distal linear staple line. The anvil and stapler trocar are connected (Fig. 15E). The stapler is closed, fired, opened, and withdrawn. The rings of excised tissue ("doughnuts") are inspected for completeness, and

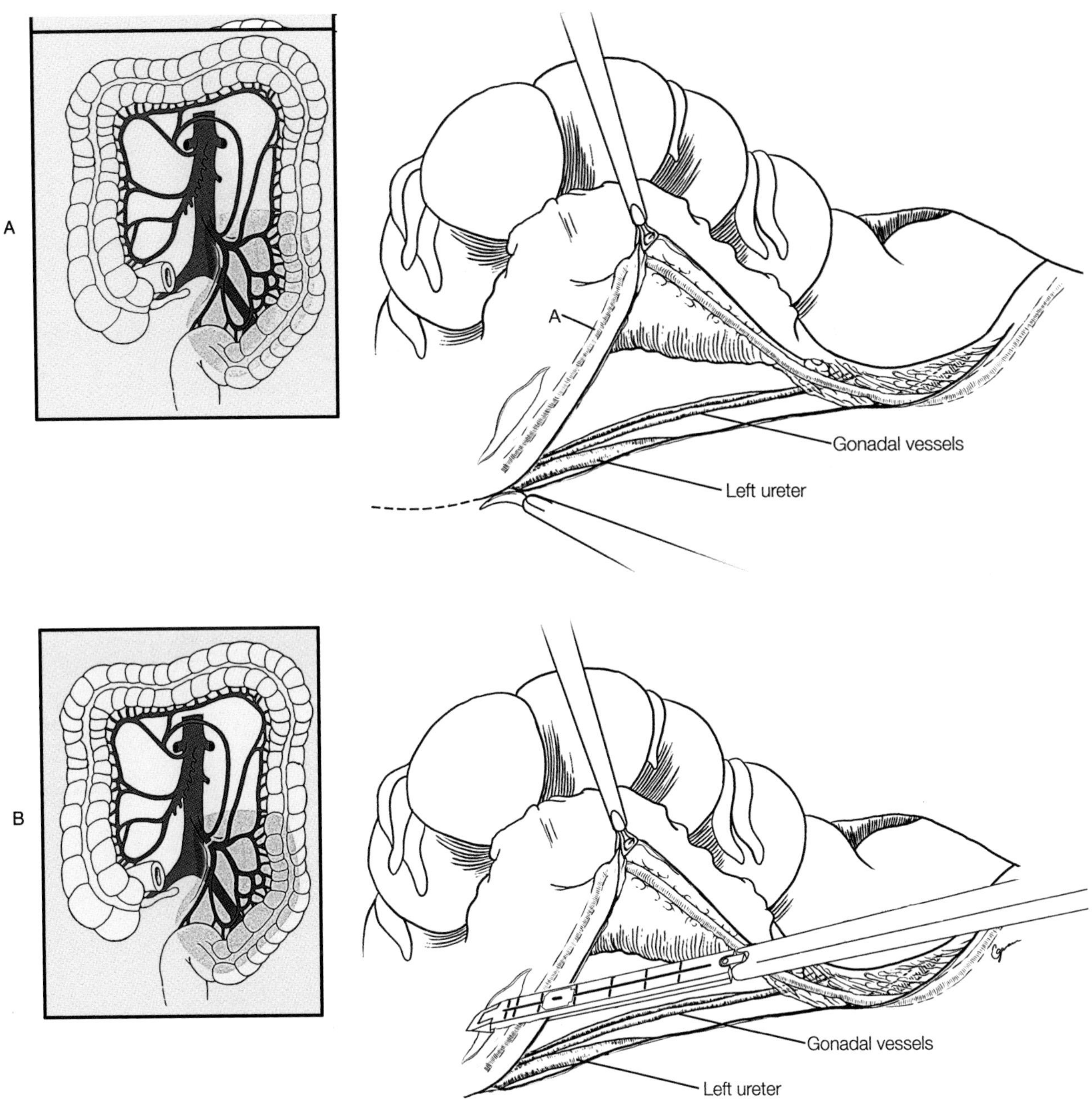

FIGURE 14 ■ (**A**) Alternative mobilization of the left colon, medial to lateral. Early exposure of the left ureter beneath the inferior mesenteric and sigmoid vessels. (**B**) Alternative mobilization of the left colon, medial to lateral. Early division of the inferior mesenteric vessels, prior to lateral mobilization along the left line of Toldt.

the anastomosis is tested by cross-clamping above the anastomosis and introducing air under pressure via the sigmoidoscope (Fig. 15F). Bubbles will be seen if water is placed over the anastomosis and a leak is present. With respect to another approach, there is a report of performing a low extracorporeal anastomosis with the rectal stump everted (57). Generally, laparoscopic surgeons believe that a left-sided colectomy is more technically demanding than a right hemicolectomy because with the latter procedure the bowel can be more easily delivered to the abdominal incision. For low anterior resections and for patients who had neoadjuvant chemoradiation a proximal, diverting ostomy, usually a loop ileostomy, is created.

■ ABDOMINOPERINEAL RESECTION

Equipment and personnel positioning is shown in Figure 16. In laparoscopic abdominoperineal resection of the rectum, an abdominal incision is completely avoided because the carcinoma is delivered through the perineal incision. However, hand-assisted laparoscopy through a low abdominal incision can be useful for retraction, control of hemorrhage and decrease the operation time. Darzi et al. (59) believe that the view provided in the pelvis by laparoscopy is significantly better than at laparotomy and allows excellent anatomic definition and meticulous dissection. In an abdominoperineal resection, a colostomy is created at a properly selected site (i.e., away from bones, scars, creases, and umbilicus) (60–62). A small 3-cm-diameter disk of skin is removed, and the opening is carried down through the subcutaneous fat, fascia, muscle, and peritoneum. A Babcock clamp is inserted through the hole, and the tip of the colon is grasped and drawn through the wall. After wound closures, the colostomy is matured. Ideally, one of the trocar sites should be planned as the colostomy site. Then

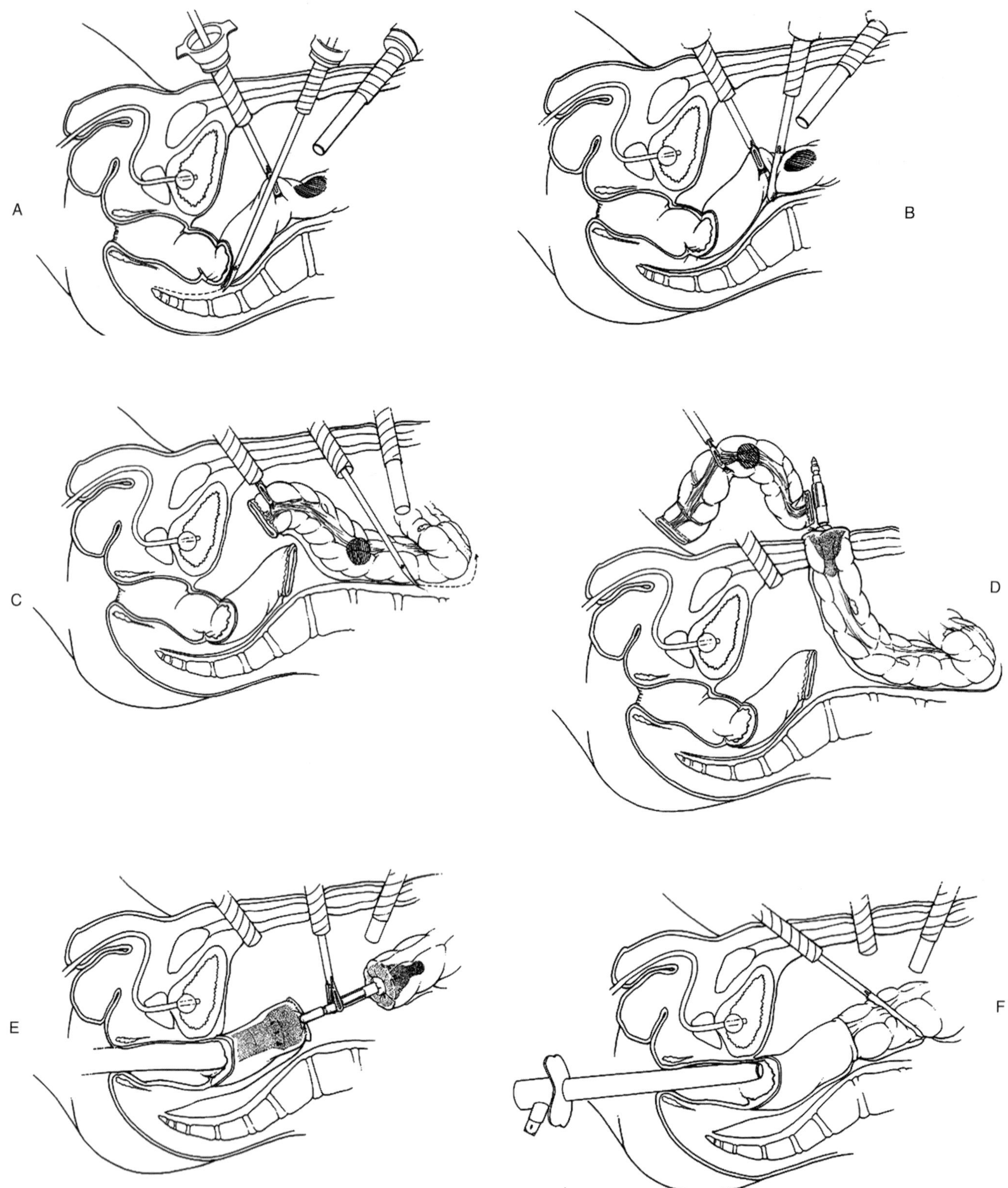

FIGURE 15 ■ Anterior resection. (**A**) The rectum is mobilized. (**B**) The bowel is divided below the pathology with a margin. (**C**) The colon and splenic flexure are mobilized. (**D**) The specimen is pulled through a small incision, and the anvil of the circular stapler is inserted into the proximal colon. (**E**) The stapler is introduced through the anus and aligned with the anvil. (**F**) The double-stapled anastomosis is completed and tested.

the trocar site can be widened to accept the colon with its partial mesentery. The perineal resection is conducted as in the open abdominoperineal resection. Often the perineal dissection is more difficult, because dissection from the abdominal side may not have been carried as far distally as it might have been with the open technique.

■ LAPAROSCOPIC RECTOPEXY

In a benign disease such as rectal prolapse, laparoscopic surgery can be especially effective. The conduct of the operation and port placement are like those of an anterior resection (63,64). In general, the rectum is mobilized, identifying the ureters and preserving the lateral stalks. The

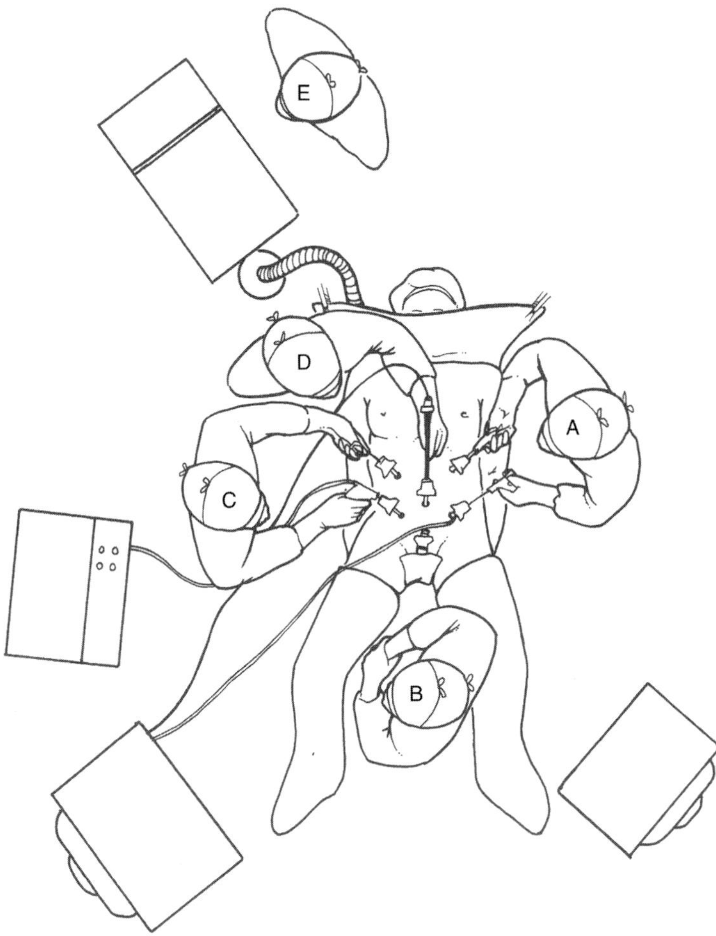

FIGURE 16 ■ Positioning for abdominoperineal resection: (*A*) surgical assistant, (*B*) scrub nurse, (*C*) surgeon, (*D*) cameraman, (*E*) anesthesiologist.

sacrum is cleared of overlying tissues on the sacral promontory (Fig. 17A). The lateral stalks are sewn to the cleaned site on the sacrum, which pulls and holds the rectum up in the pelvis. Usually two sutures are applied through each lateral stalk. In time, the rectum will adhere, and further prolapse is prevented (65). If the patient has had significant constipation, a laparoscopic-assisted anterior resection may be included (66). The technique is like that described for a left colon resection.

Some authors use a mesh to fix the rectum to the sacrum (Fig. 17B) (67,68). First, the mesh is attached to the sacrum; a device for applying tacks to hold the mesh to the sacrum has been devised. Then the mesh is wrapped around the posterior half of the rectum and sewn to it, leaving the anterior half of the rectum unwrapped. Scarring of the rectum to the sacrum will fix it and prevent future prolapse.

The operative technique for the mesh proctopexy as described by Darzi et al. (69) is as follows. A nasogastric tube and urinary catheter are inserted when the patient is anesthetized. Three 12-mm ports are introduced into the abdomen, one umbilical and one in each of the lower quadrants. An additional 10-mm port is inserted suprapubically. The camera is inserted into the right iliac fossa port and the rectosigmoid is grasped by a Babcock clamp passed through the left iliac suprapubic port. The peritoneal reflection is divided with scissors, and the avascular plane between the rectum and presacral fascia is developed. The lateral ligaments are divided. The pelvic nerves are identified posteriorly and preserved. In a woman, anterior dissection is facilitated by holding the cervix upward through the vagina. After complete mobilization, mesh is introduced into the presacral space and stapled to the sacrum with an endoscopic hernia stapler introduced into the right iliac fossa port. After three or four staples have been inserted, the rectum is held on light tension with a Babcock forceps, and each limb of the mesh is sutured to the serosa of the rectum using two or three sutures on each side (Fig. 17B).

■ STOMA CREATION

The site for an ostomy is planned using the basic principles of bringing the stoma through the rectus muscle, but avoiding bones, scars, the umbilicus, and folds. An ileostomy is created through the right lower quadrant, a

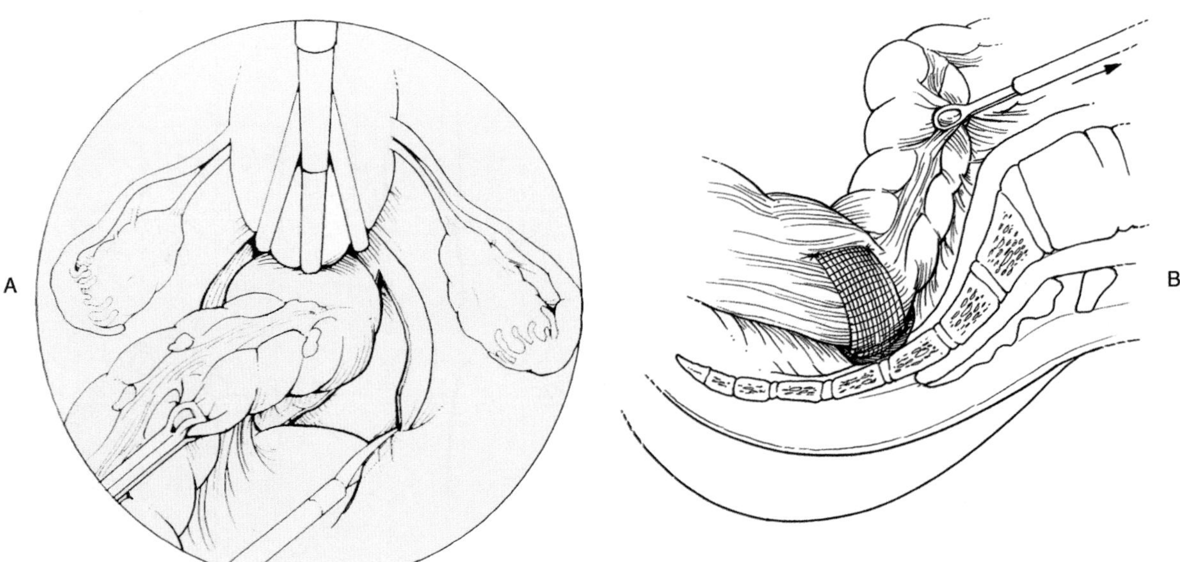

FIGURE 17 ■ Laparoscopic rectopexy. (**A**) The rectum is mobilized and the sacral promontory is exposed. (**B**) Mesh is sewn or stapled into place.

sigmoid colostomy through the left lower quadrant, and a transverse colostomy through the upper quadrants (70–73). The ports are placed at different sites for the various ostomies (Fig. 18).

A 10-mm trocar is inserted through an umbilical site. After diagnostic laparoscopy has been completed, a 10-mm trocar is inserted through the previously selected stoma site. An additional one or two 5-mm trocars are introduced. The segment of bowel is selected, and an umbilical tape is passed through the mesentery, at the point at which the ostomy is to be opened (Fig. 19A). The tape around the loop of bowel is passed through the cannula at the preselected ostomy site. Some surgeons simply grasp the bowel with a Babcock clamp and hold it in position while the opening around the cannula is enlarged (Fig. 19B). The segment of bowel is drawn up to determine whether the loop will reach through the abdominal wall. If it does not reach, mesenteric attachments, adhesions, or vessels may need to be divided.

To open the abdominal wall, the pneumoperitoneum is released. A 3-cm-diameter disk of skin around the cannula site is excised and the subcutaneous fat is retracted. A 2×2 cm gridiron incision is made through the fascia. With the camera observing from the abdominal side, the bowel is pulled through the wound. The bowel may be fixed to the fascia with interrupted sutures. The cannula sites are closed. The ostomy is then matured as for a loop ostomy.

Mattingly et al. (74) evaluated the possibility of performing fecal diversion with the assistance of a colonoscope and without the additional morbidity of abdominal exploration or general anesthesia. There were 15 patients diverted using a colonoscope to identify a site of the sigmoid colon that could be approximated to the anterior abdominal wall as confirmed by transillumination of the abdominal wall. A small skin disk was then removed at this location and a loop colostomy was made. The colonoscope was also used as a guide to identify the proximal and distal limbs of the loop colostomy.

■ STOMA CLOSURE

When a stoma is necessary, the stoma and mucous fistula or the oversewn distal bowel may be placed at sites apart from each other after the diseased segment is resected. The divided, separated bowel may be brought back together at a later date if the patient's health status permits. For the properly selected patient, laparoscopy may be the operation of choice (75–79). The extent of adhesions secondary to extensive surgery, inflammation, or contamination may make laparoscopy a poor choice for closure. When the camera is inserted, the anticipated level of difficulty may be assessed, and the decision to open or not can be made.

For reestablishing intestinal continuity the patient is placed on the table in stirrups as described earlier. The surgeon often has better control positioned between the patient's legs. The assistants are placed on the patient's left with monitors at the patient's upper right and left shoulders. The surgeon lines up the laparoscope, ileostomy, previously transected colon, and the monitor.

The ileostomy is taken down via a circumferential incision, which is gradually carried down into the peritoneal cavity. Adhesions around the stoma are lysed. A 10-mm cannula is inserted through the opening, and a pursestring suture is applied and tied tightly to hold a pneumoperitoneum. When pneumoperitoneum has formed, the camera is inserted. The table is placed head down with rotation to the left. The table is rolled to the right or left, depending on which way the small bowel is

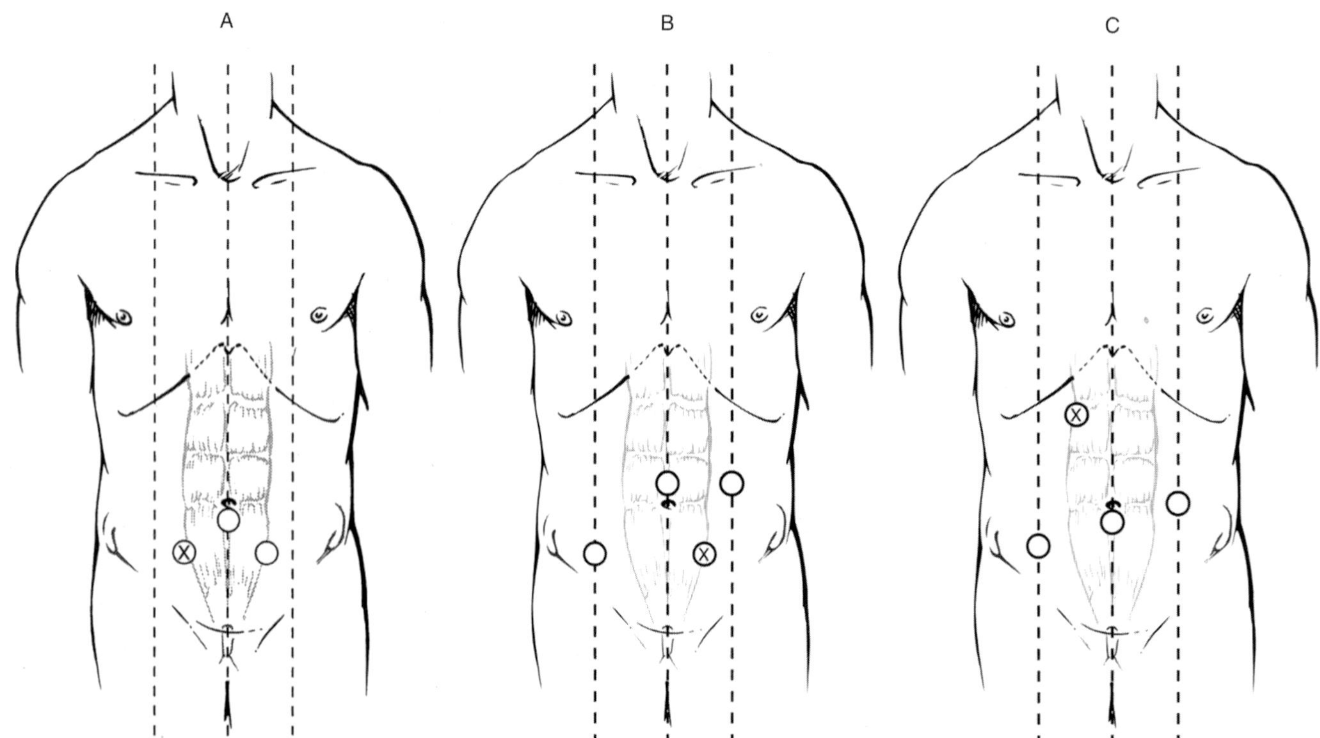

FIGURE 18 ■ Trocar placements for ostomies. (**A**) Loop ileostomy or end ileostomy. (**B**) End-sigmoid colostomy or loop-sigmoid colostomy. (**C**) Loop transverse colostomy.

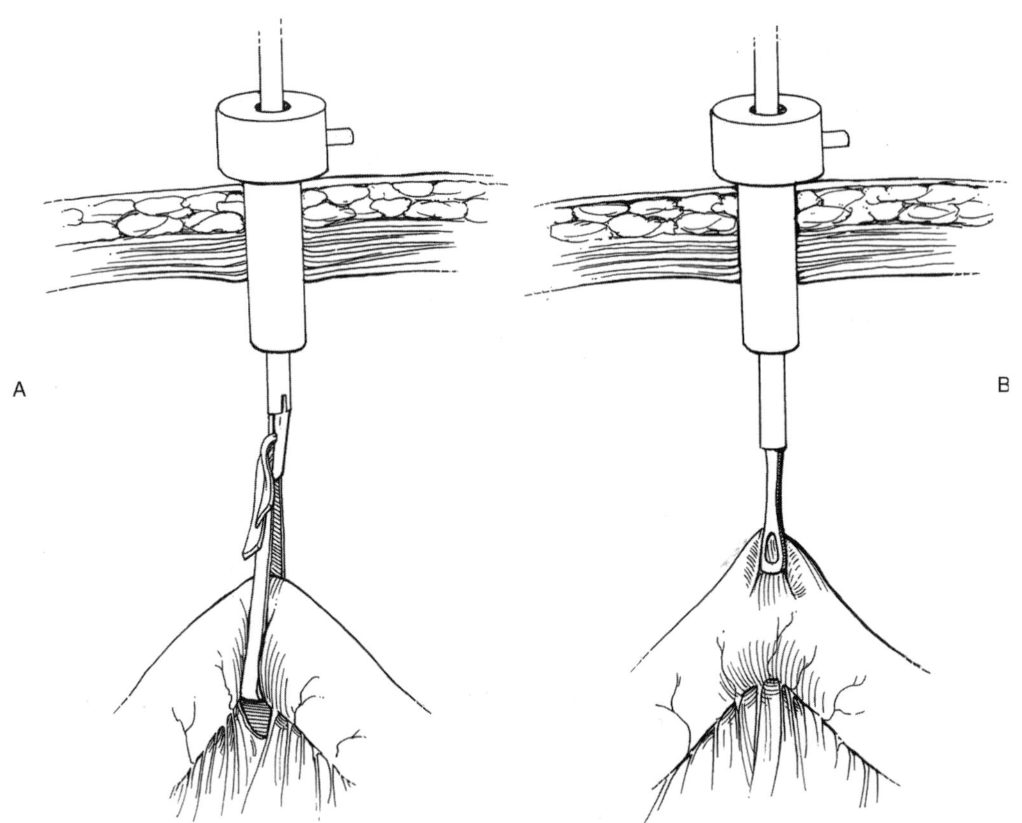

FIGURE 19 ■ Laparoscopic ileostomy. (**A**) Tape holds the ileum beneath the cannula at the proposed site of the ileostomy. (**B**) Babcock clamp pulls the ileum into position beneath the cannula.

most easily shifted. After visual exploration, the decision to proceed with a laparoscopic or an open procedure is made. If laparoscopy is possible, ports are placed in the suprapubic midline, the left lower quadrant, and the left upper quadrant. The ileum is dissected free so that it easily reaches to the colon for anastomosis. A small incision is made around the mucous fistula and carried down into the peritoneal cavity or opened over the closed proximal end of the colon. The two ends are pulled into the same wound, where a functional end-to-end anastomosis can be performed extracorporeally.

For a sigmoid colostomy, closure is performed with the patient in the supine position in stirrups as described previously. The surgeon stands on the patient's right side with an assistant on the left. The table is tilted head down and to the right. The surgeon, stoma, and monitor are lined up. The procedure starts with mobilization of the colostomy. Through this opening, a cannula can be introduced. Ports are placed in the right lower quadrant, right upper quadrant, left upper quadrant, and possibly suprapubic sites. Adhesions are freed up. Often the vagina, uterus, or bladder have become adherent across the pelvis. A sigmoidoscope can be used to identify the rectal or bowel stump (Fig. 20A). Inserting a sizer or other suitable instrument into the vagina may help identify the vaginal vault. A place on the distal bowel must be cleaned of adhesions and fat for an end-to-end stapled anastomosis. The largest possible anvil is pursestringed into the proximal colon (the old colostomy segment). The stapler is introduced through the anus and brought into the previously selected point for anastomosis. The trocar is opened through the wall of the cleaned distal segment, the anvil is snapped onto the stapler, and a standard stapling anastomosis is completed (Fig. 20B). The anastomosis is checked for leaks by insufflating air through a sigmoidoscope. The fascia of the colostomy site is closed, but the skin is left open. The port sites are closed both at the fascia and at the skin.

■ TOTAL ABDOMINAL COLECTOMY AND ILEORECTAL ANASTOMOSIS

Laparoscopic total abdominal colectomy with ileorectal anastomosis requires that many of the previously described resections be performed at one operation (80). Thus the steps to achieve this are reviewed.

The patient is positioned in stirrups with the perineum accessible off the end of the operating table. The position of the patient's knees is low in the stirrups so that they will not interfere with arm motion of the surgeon standing between the patient's legs. The team will frequently need to shift positions, and thus move the monitors and tilt and rotate the table, depending on the segment of bowel being mobilized or resected.

After pneumoperitoneum, the patient is placed in a head-down position while the infraumbilical trocar is inserted. With the laparoscope in place, cannulas are placed in the right upper quadrant, left upper quadrant, left lower quadrant, right lower quadrant, and suprapubic sites according to the surgeon's preference. With the hand-assisted approach, the two most caudad port sites are replaced with an incision of about the length of the surgeon's glove size in the low midline or Pfannenstiel site (81). The ureters must be seen at some point, and it is preferable to locate them early and score the peritoneum along each side of the rectum so that the ureters are known to be out of the operative field.

The rectum is mobilized by incising the peritoneum on each side of the rectum medial to the ureters and

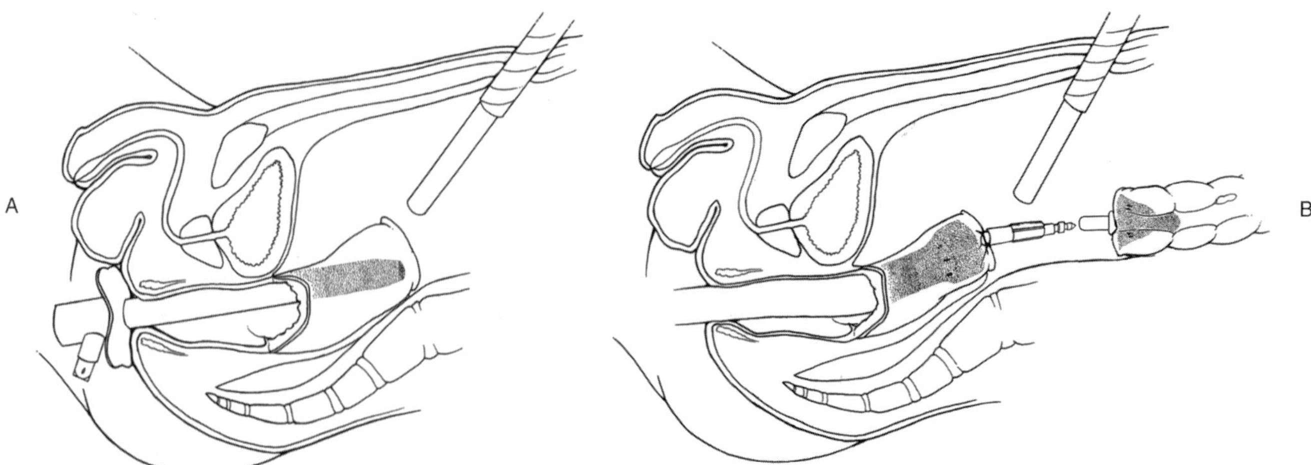

FIGURE 20 ■ Colostomy closure. (**A**) A rigid sigmoidoscope introduces light to aid in identification of the rectal stump, and it may lever the rectum up to aid in lysis of adhesions. (**B**) The stapler is inserted via the anus and the anastomosis is completed.

extending the incision downward on each side to connect anteriorly in the cul-de-sac. When the rectum has been retracted, the attachments are divided and the rectum is freed up off the sacral promontory. The incision is carried to the base of the inferior mesenteric vessels. The vessels are seen as they become taut when the rectum is pulled inferiorly. The peritoneum can be scored across the base of these vessels to a point on their right where the mesentery is very thin. This thin spot in the mesentery is opened and, through this window, the posterior aspect of the inferior mesenteric vessels is exposed.

When the rectum has been freed up, it can be stapled. A rigid sigmoidoscope can be introduced to mark the 15-cm level where it is cleared of fat. The laparoscopic stapler can be fired once or more to transect it. Some surgeons select a site for specimen removal and open it early to use standard staplers for the rectal and ileal transection. The wound is closed to make the abdomen gas-tight again.

Attention is turned to taking down the left-sided attachments of the rectum and sigmoid colon. The rectum and sigmoid colon are tethered by the inferior mesenteric vessels. These vessels are divided together or separately by a vascular stapler, ligations, or clips.

The left colon is mobilized medially and laterally as high as possible around the splenic flexure. The surgeon may move to a position between the patient's legs and the assistants to a right-sided position. The table may need to be tilted head up and to the right to approach the splenic flexure.

When the left colon has been mobilized, the table is rolled to the left to expose the cecum and right colon. The head of the table may need to be shifted head down to move the small bowel out of the way. Often the inferior margins of the ileum, appendix, and cecum are exposed earlier and freed up during exposure of the inferior mesenteric vessels. The surgeon stands between the patient's legs, and the assistants move to the left side.

The ileum is grasped and lifted to expose the ileocolic, attachments, which are taken down. The terminal ileum is cleaned of fat and transected with the laparoscopic linear stapler. With the right colon pulled medially, the white line of Toldt is incised to a point around the hepatic flexure. The table is shifted from a head-down to a head-up position as the dissection progresses. The ileocolic vessels are transected and the right mesentery is taken down. The right colic vessels, if present, are transected. As the colon is mobilized medially, the duodenum is seen and avoided. The ligaments attaching the liver to the colon are divided. The omentum can be removed from the transverse colon in a relatively bloodless plane immediately adjacent to the colon. As the transverse colon mesentery is mobilized, the lesser sac is entered. The middle colic vessels, which can be stapled, ligated, or clipped, will be evident. The remainder of the dissection entails removal of the attachments along the greater curvature of the stomach and the spleen.

When the colon has been totally freed up, an incision is made in the lower abdomen through which the colon is removed. If a previous incision was made for stapling, it is reopened for colon removal. The terminal ileum is drawn out of the wound, opened, and a pursestring suture applied. The largest possible stapler anvil is inserted, and the pursestring suture is tied tight around the anvil shaft. The stapler is introduced through the anus, and the anastomosis is completed using the standard double-stapling technique.

■ RESTORATIVE PROTOCOLECTOMY

This procedure entails combining procedures, the total colectomy described in the previous section and the rectal resection described in the section on "Left-sided Colectomy." The major vessels are serially ligated and transected, the mesentery is serially incised, and the omentum is separated off the transverse colon. The proctectomy dissection is carried down to the levator muscles. An incision must be made in the low abdomen for removal of the specimen and creation of the J-pouch.

Some surgeons believe that the operation should be purely laparoscopic. We believe that since an incision is to be made, any uses of the incision are acceptable to aid in the safe and expeditious completion of the procedure. For example, a hand can be inserted to aid in dissection or a stapler could be inserted to transect the anorectal junction where laparoscopic staplers do not angle into the pelvis well and require more than one application.

The J-pouch is constructed and anastomosed as described for the conventional open approach in Chapter 26.

■ CLOSURE OF COLONOSCOPIC PERFORATION

Goh et al. (82) described the closure of a colonoscopic perforation of the sigmoid colon with the use of the endoscopic stapler to obtain closure in a transverse manner. A colonoscope is passed into the sigmoid colon and air is insufflated to test the integrity of the closure. The peritoneal cavity is then copiously irrigated until the return is clear. Repair can also be secured using a suture technique (83).

Yamamoto et al. (84) described their laparoscopic repair of colonoscopic perforation of the sigmoid or cecum using sutures threaded transversely through all layers of the margin of the defect and pulled up with forceps to align the margins following which the defect was stapled with an endoscopic linear stapler.

■ MISCELLANEOUS PROCEDURES

In a series of 76 laparoscopic-assisted cases, Pera et al. (85) noted a clinical anastomotic dehiscence rate of 10.6%. Among the seven patients who required reoperation, the anastomosis was taken down in only one case. In four of these cases, the reoperation was performed laparoscopically including peritoneal lavage and the creation of a diverting stoma. There were no complications resulting from the use of laparoscopy in the early postoperative period.

Duepree et al. (86) described their experience with planned complete laparoscopic management of deep pelvic endometriosis with bowel involvement. The series consisted of 51 patients with a history of early abdominal operation in 66.7%. Preoperative symptoms were present as dysmenorrhea (85.3%), dyspareunia (55.9%), rectal pain (41.2%), constipation (44.1%), rectal bleeding (14.7%), bloating (29.4%), and tenesmus (8.8%). Management of the bowel disease included superficial excision of the serosal endometriosis implants ($n=26$), bowel resection ($n=18$), and disk excision ($n=5$). Median operating room time was 187 minutes and the median length of stay was two days. One-third of excisions were outpatient procedures. Postoperative complications occurred in 10.3%; 7.8% were converted to formal laparotomy and 7.7% were readmitted within 30 days. Only seven of 47 patients with a uterus (14.9%) required abdominal hysterectomy or bilateral salpingo-oophorectomy. Postoperatively, 87% of patients reported clinically significant improvement of their symptoms.

Prohm et al. (87) described an endoscopic polypectomy using the assistance of a laparoscope on six patients whose colorectal polyps were in an anatomically unfavorable location and at high risk for perforation. The affected area of the colon, the sigmoid, and the left flexure were mobilized and stretched as much as possible to enable a simultaneous and low-risk endoscopic polypectomy. They concluded that laparoscopic-assisted polypectomy is a safe method to remove even complicated polyps in anatomically unfavorable locations.

Rispoli et al. (88) described extraction of a foreign body (a cigar container 22 cm in length and 3.5 cm in diameter), which was introduced into the rectum and migrated upwards to the distal colon, by combining laparoscopic and anal approaches. The foreign body was mobilized laparoscopically, pushed down the rectum, and then extracted transanally with the aid of a dilator anoscope.

ROBOTICS

Robotics has been applied to clinical surgery in the past few years, including colectomy. Weber et al. (89) presented the first two reported cases of telerobotic-assisted laparoscopic colectomies performed on March 6 and 8, 2001—a sigmoid colectomy for diverticulitis and a right colectomy for cecal diverticulitis. The Da Vinci telerobotic surgical system was used in both cases to mobilize the bowel. The mesenteric division, bowel transection, and anastomoses were accomplished with standard laparoscopic-assisted techniques. Both operations were completed with a three trocar technique. They found that the Da Vinci system adequately replaced the camera holder. The combination of the three-dimensional imaging and the hand-like motions of the telerobotic surgical instruments facilitated dissection. Operative time for the sigmoid colectomy was 340 minutes and for the right hemicolectomy 228 minutes. Merola et al. (90) compared the use of voice-controlled robotic camera holder (AESOP 3000; Computer Motion, Inc., Santa Barbara, California, U.S.A.) to a human camera holder in a series of laparoscopic colectomies. The use of the voice-controlled robotic camera did not alter the length of the operative procedure, the patient's length of stay, or postoperative morbidity. However, surgeons often have a subjective sense that there is less smudging, fogging, and inadvertent movements of the laparoscope when it is controlled by a robotic system.

Advocates suggest that advantages include a three-dimensional view and easy instrument manipulation. The disadvantages are the current need for large diameter instruments and the availability of only three robotic arms. Major problems to be solved are the tactile feedback to the operator and the need for more arms. Ultimately, the value of robotics will need to be expressed in terms of safety, operating time, cost, and outcomes. The capital cost is significant with a purchase cost of over US $1,300,000 and maintenance costs of over US $100,000 annually (91,92).

Munz et al. (93) operated on six patients with full-thickness rectal prolapse using the robotic-assisted suture rectopexy. All operations were completed successfully using the robotic system. There were no major complications and no deaths. Mean set-up time was 28 minutes, mean operation time was 127 minutes, and mean hospital stay was 6 days. At 3 to 6 months of follow-up there were no signs of recurrence.

Delaney et al. (92) reported six robot-assisted laparoscopic operations (two right hemicolectomies, three sigmoid colectomies, and one Wells rectopexy) using standard laparoscopic procedures with robot-assisted laparoscopic colon mobilization and vascular ligation. There was no associated morbidity. Operative time was increased from a median of 108 minutes for standard laparoscopic colorectal surgery to 165 minutes for robot-assisted laparoscopic procedures. Blood loss, length of stay, and hospital costs were not significantly different between groups. Additional direct equipment costs for robot-assisted colectomy cases included robotic laparoscopic instruments and sterile drapes (approximately US $350.00 per case) without including acquisition and maintenance cost for the robot. They concluded robot-assisted laparoscopic colectomy is a feasible and safe procedure. Although three-dimensional vision and dexterity are facilitated, operative time is increased, and the overall additional expense of robotics is of concern.

D'Annibale et al. (94) compared the traditional laparoscopic approach and robotic techniques with the Da Vinci robotic system (Intuitive Surgical) in the treatment of colorectal diseases in 106 patients (53 in each group). No differences were observed in the total time of operation (laparoscopic group 222 minutes vs. robotic group 240 minutes), the specimen length (laparoscopic group 29 cm vs. robotic group 27 cm), or the number of lymph nodes retrieved (laparoscopic 16 vs. robotic 17). It took significantly longer to prepare the operating room and patient in the robotic group (24 minutes in the robotic group vs. 18 minutes in the laparoscopic group). There were three conversions to laparotomy in the laparoscopic group and in the robotic group two cases were converted to laparoscopy and three to hand-assisted laparoscopy. No significant differences were observed between the two groups in terms of recovery of bowel function and postoperative hospital stay. They found that because of its dexterity and three-dimensional view, the Da Vinci system was particularly useful in specific stages of the procedure, e.g. takedown of the splenic flexure, dissection of a narrow pelvis, identification of nervous plexus, and hand-sewn anastomosis.

Hanly et al. (95) used the robot to assist in 35 colon resections in cases that did not require multiquadrant dissection. They believe the robot may play a role in shortening the learning curve. Gutt et al. (96) reviewed all papers about telemanipulators used in visceral surgery. Most papers presented case series demonstrating the feasibility of robotic technology in performing a specific procedure. Comparative studies of robot-assisted surgery versus standard laparoscopic or open surgery were usually matched cohort studies. They generally showed an increased operating time for robot-assisted procedures but with similar rates of conversion, intraoperative and postoperative complications, and mortality in comparison with those of laparoscopic surgery. Consistent long-term follow-up data were missing and only one randomized clinical trial was conducted. Robot-assisted surgery appears safe and feasible for certain standard surgical procedures. However, they concluded that at its current level of development, it offers no clear, significant advantage over standard laparoscopic techniques.

POSTOPERATIVE CARE

The nasogastric tube is removed following completion of the procedure. Postoperative feeding has been initiated as early as the night of the operation, but the rush for this seems unfounded. Oral intake can often begin on the first or second postoperative day if there is no evidence of nausea or abdominal distention. Progression of diet is introduced as tolerated. Pain control is the same as that used after the open technique with a patient-controlled analgesia pump or systemic medication, but less medication is usually required.

RESULTS

Assessing and comparing the results of laparoscopic colorectal resections are Herculean tasks. Authors tend to lump procedures together, disparate disease processes together, and simple and complicated cases together. Therefore, a clear picture for a given procedure in a given disease process is almost never presented. Notwithstanding these limitations, a number of selected reports have been reviewed.

CONVERSION RATES

Information about conversion rates and the reasons for conversion is possibly not representative of the overall experience of surgeons performing laparoscopic procedures. Publications at this stage of evolution of the art are presented by those most highly skilled in laparoscopic procedures. Although this criticism may be true of many publications, it is probably more applicable to laparoscopic operations. Notwithstanding this limitation, information is available. Reasons cited for conversion from a laparoscopic to an open procedure include poor exposure for whatever reason (often adhesions or obesity), uncontrollable bleeding, injury to other structures (viscera or vessels), absence of a lesion in the resected specimen, instrumentation difficulties, or lack of progress. The presence of an extensive carcinoma has also been cited, but the wisdom of using an initial laparoscopic approach under these circumstances might best be questioned. Conversion to an open technique should not be viewed as a failure but more appropriately as exercising good surgical judgment. Conversion rates between 0% and 42% (average 14%) have been reported in a review of 26 studies on laparoscope resection colon carcinoma (97). Conversion rates clearly decrease with experience. Patient selection and operative expertise profoundly influence conversion rates. Slim et al. (98) reviewed 16 of 65 laparoscopic-assisted colorectal operations that were converted to open procedures. When compared with 252 planned open operations, a higher postoperative morbidity rate (50% vs. 21%) and more anastomotic leaks (25% vs. 8%) were apparent in the group who underwent conversion to an open procedure. Operating time, postoperative ileus, and hospital stay were longer in those requiring a converted operation. The authors' poor results suggest the need for careful preoperative patient selection and for rapid decision to convert difficult cases to open procedures.

Pandya et al. (99) reviewed their indications for conversion to laparotomy during laparoscopic colectomy. From a registry of 200 patients who underwent laparoscopic colon surgery, 23.5% were converted. The 200 patients were divided into four cohorts of 50 consecutive patients to analyze changes with time. The conversion rate was statistically greater in the first quarter (36.0%) than in the subsequent quarters (16%). The rate of conversion to laparotomy for segmental resection of the ascending and descending colon (20.3%) has been equivalent and less than the conversion rate for other procedures (48.5%). The distribution of patients by operative indication has been fairly constant. The indication for operation has not influenced the need for conversion. The indications for conversion were technical problems in 15 patients (hypercarbia, unclear anatomy, and stapler misfire), laparoscopic complications in 9 patients (bleeding, cystotomy, and enterotomy), and problems that exceeded the limits of laparoscopic dissection in 23 patients (phlegmon, adhesions, obesity, and adjacent organ involvement by carcinoma). Although obesity accentuates the technical limitations of a laparoscopic dissection, it is an infrequent cause for conversion to laparotomy.

Marusch et al. (100) reported on the significance of conversion for the results obtained with laparoscopic colorectal surgery and identified the risk factors that established the need for conversion. Within the framework of the Laparoscopic Colorectal Surgery Study Group, a total of 1658 patients were recruited to a multicenter study. The observed conversion rate was 5.2%. The patients requiring conversion were significantly heavier [body mass index (BMI) 26.5 vs. 24.9] than those undergoing pure laparoscopy. Resections of the rectum were associated with a higher risk for conversion (20.9% vs. 13%). Intraoperative complications occurred significantly more frequently in the conversion group (27.9% vs. 3.8%). The duration of the operation was significantly increased after conversion in a considerable portion of the procedures performed. Postoperative morbidity (47.7% vs. 26.1%), mortality (3.5% vs. 1.5%), recovery time, and postoperative hospital stay were all negatively influenced by conversion. Institutions with experience of more than 100 laparoscopic colorectal procedures proved to have a significantly lower conversion rate than those with experience of fewer than 100 such interventions (4.3% vs. 6.9%). Although of itself, conversion is not considered to be a complication of laparoscopic surgery, it is true that the postoperative course after conversion is associated with appreciably poorer results in terms of morbidity, mortality, convalescence, blood transfusion requirement, and postoperative hospital stay.

Conversion rates following laparoscopic colorectal surgery vary widely between studies, and the outcome of converted patients remains controversial.

Gervaz et al. (101) conducted a comprehensive search of the English-language literature in which 28 studies of 3232 patients were considered for analysis. The overall conversion rate was 15.38%. Seventy-nine percent of the studies did not include a definition for conversion; in these studies the conversion rate was significantly lower than in the studies where a specific definition was considered (13.7% vs. 18.9%). Converted patients had a prolonged hospital stay (11.4 vs. 7.4 days) and operative time (209 minutes vs. 189 minutes) in comparison with laparoscopically completed patients. The factors associated with an increased rate for conversion were left colectomy (odds ratio = 1.06), anterior resection of the rectum (odds ratio = 1.09), diverticulitis (odds ratio = 1.30), and carcinoma (odds ratio = 2.94). They concluded the rate of laparoscopically completed colorectal resections is close to 85% in nonrandomized studies. Because converted patients have a distinct outcome, a clear definition of conversion is required to compare the results of randomized trials.

Schlachta et al. (102) developed a simple model for clinical use in predicting the individual risk of conversion to open surgery in patients undergoing laparoscopic colorectal resections. From their experience of 367 laparoscopic colon resections, a scoring system was developed on the basis of the three factors found to be predictive of the risk of conversion to open surgery: diagnosis of malignancy (odds ratio 3.23; one point), surgeon experience with 50 cases or fewer (odds ratio 2.26; one point), and weight level (odds ratio 3.42; 60 to 90 kg, one point, 90 kg or more, two points). The predicted conversion rates for the cumulative scores of 0 to 4 points were 1.1%, 3.3%, 9.8%, 25.4%, and 49.7%, respectively.

More recently, Tekkis et al. (103) developed a mathematical model for predicting the conversion rate for patients undergoing laparoscopic colorectal surgery using clinical data collected from 1253 patients undergoing laparoscopic surgery. Exclusion criteria for laparoscopic colectomy included a BMI > 50, lesion diameter exceeding 15 cm, and multiple prior major laparotomies (exclusive of appendectomy, hysterectomy, and cholecystectomy). The average conversion rate for the study population was 10%. The independent predictors of conversion of a laparoscopic to open surgery were the BMI (odds ratio 2.1 per 10 American Society of Anesthesiology (ASA) units increase), ASA grade 3 or 4, 1 or 2 (odds ratio 3.2, 5.8), type of resection (low rectal, left colorectal, right colonic vs. small/other bowel procedures; odds ratio 8.82, 4.76, 2.98), presence of intraoperative abscess (odds ratio 3.6), or fistula (odds ratio 4.73), and surgeon seniority (junior vs. senior staff, odds ratio 1.56).

Casillas et al. (104) conducted a study to determine whether conversion is associated with increased morbidity and higher hospital costs. In a series of 430 laparoscopic colectomies (12%) of cases were converted to open operation. There were no significant differences between the groups for age, male to female ratio, or American Society of Anesthesiology score. Conversions occurred before defining the major vascular pedicle/ureter (50%), in relation to intracorporeal vascular ligation (15%), or during bowel transection or presacral dissection (35%). Specific indications for conversion were technical (41%), followed by adhesions (33%), phlegmon or abscess (23%), bleeding (6%), and failure to identify the ureter (6%). Median hospital stay was 5 days for both groups. In-hospital complications (converted 11.6%; open 8%), 30-day readmission rate (converted 13% vs. 8%), and direct costs were similar between groups. There were no mortalities. They concluded, conversion of a laparoscopic colectomy does not result in inappropriately prolonged operative times, increased morbidity or length of stay, increased direct costs or unexpected readmissions compared with similarly complex laparotomies.

■ POSTOPERATIVE ILEUS

Basse et al. (105) assessed gastrointestinal transit in 32 patients randomized to laparoscopic or open colonic resection. They received 4 MGq of 111 indium diethylenetriamine pentaacetic acid, a tracer, at the end of operation. Images of the abdomen were obtained 24 and 48 hours postoperatively. Defecation occurred on median day 2 postoperatively in both groups. At 48 hours postoperatively, 53% of the tracer was excreted by patients in the laparoscopic group when compared with 26% in the open group. Postoperative ileus and gastrointestinal transit normalized within 48 hours after colonic resection in the patients who received multimodal rehabilitation (epidural analgesia, early oral nutrition and mobilization, and laxative use). No significant difference was observed between the patients who underwent the laparoscopic procedure than those who underwent the open procedure.

Kasparek et al. (106) investigated whether colonic motility increases more rapidly following laparoscopic-assisted sigmoid resection in 11 patients compared with open sigmoid colectomy in nine patients. During operation, a manometry catheter was inserted into the colon via the anus, and the tip was placed in the splenic flexure. Continuous manometric recordings were performed from the day of operation until postoperative day 3 with a four-channel microtransducer manometry system combined with a portable data logger. The postoperative colonic motility was 101, 199, and 163 mmHg/min on days 1, 2, and 3 after laparoscopic-assisted sigmoid resection, respectively, which was increased compared with indexes of 53, 71, and 76 following open sigmoid colectomy. The amplitude but not the frequency of contractions was higher following laparoscopic-assisted sigmoid resection compared with open sigmoid colectomy. Following laparoscopic-assisted sigmoid colectomy, patients requested a similar amount of pain medication but resumed oral food more rapidly on postoperative days 2 and 3 and they were discharged from the hospital earlier. Colonic motility in particular and the patient's condition in general seem to improve more rapidly following laparoscopic-assisted sigmoid colectomy compared with the open procedure.

In a novel study Asao et al. (107) evaluated the effect of gum chewing as a convenient method to enhance postoperative recovery from ileus after laparoscopic colectomy. A total of 19 patients were randomly assigned to one of two groups: a gum-chewing group ($n=10$) or control group ($n=9$). The patients in the gum-chewing group chewed gum three times a day from the first postoperative morning until oral intake. The first passage of flatus was seen, on average, on postoperative day 2.1 in the gum-chewing group and day 3.2 in the control group. The first defecation was 2.7 days sooner in the gum-chewing group (postoperative day 3.1) than in the control group (5.8 days). All patients tolerated gum-chewing on the first operative morning. They concluded gum-chewing aids early recovery from postoperative ileus and is an inexpensive and physiologic method for stimulating bowel motility.

Raue et al. (108) reported their experience with a multimodal rehabilitation program ("fast-track") with epidural analgesia, early oral feeding, and enforced early mobilization following laparoscopic colorectal resection. Twenty-nine standard-care patients and 23 fast-track patients were evaluated. On the first postoperative day, pulmonary function was improved in fast-track patients. Oral feeding was achieved early and defecation occurred earlier in the fast-track group. Visual analogue scale scores for pain were similar for the two groups, but fatigue was increased in the standard-care group on the first and second postoperative days. Morbidity was not different for the two groups. Fast-track patients were discharged on day 4 and standard-care patients on day 7. They concluded, multimodal rehabilitation can improve further on the excellent results of laparoscopic sigmoidectomy and decrease the postoperative hospital stay.

■ LAPAROSCOPIC PROCEDURES IN THE ELDERLY

Reissman et al. (109) assessed the outcomes of laparoscopic colorectal operations in patients younger than 60 years with those older than 60 years. There were no statistically significant differences relative to the incidence of complications (11% vs. 14%), conversion (8% vs. 11%), length of ileus (2.8 days vs. 4.2 days), or length of hospitalization (5.2 days vs. 6.5 days).

Peters and Fleshman (110) evaluated 103 patients aged 65 years of age or older who underwent attempted minimally invasive colectomy (right colectomy, 53; left colectomy, sigmoid colectomy, or anterior resection, 36; abdominoperineal resection, 12; and total proctocolectomy with ileostomy, 2). Eighty-one procedures were successfully completed. Complications occurred in 23% of patients converted to laparotomy (including one death) and in 25% undergoing successful minimally invasive colectomy (two deaths). The average length of postoperative stay was 5.3 days in the minimally invasive colectomy group and 8.1 days in patients converted to laparotomy. These results compare favorably with published results of traditional colectomy for elderly patients.

Delgado et al. (111) found that morbidity rates were similar in patients less than 70 years of age but found a significantly lower incidence of complications after laparoscopic colectomy compared with open colectomy in patients over 70 years of age. There may be a selected benefit of laparoscopic left colectomy in the elderly and laparoscopic right hemicolectomy in the young (112). Law et al. (113) also found laparoscopic colorectal resections a safe operation for elderly patients and is especially associated with more favorable short-term outcomes in terms of early return of bowel function, earlier resumption of diet and shorter hospital stay as well as associated with less cardiopulmonary morbidity.

Seshadri et al. (114) identified 62 octogenarians from a large prospective database comprising 507 consecutive laparoscopic colorectal resections. The mean age and weight were 85 years and 63 kg, respectively. Seven patients (11%) were converted to an open procedure. Four (6%) intraoperative complications occurred in four patients (one colon perforation, one small bowel perforation, one burned gallbladder serosa, and one missed lesion), necessitating two conversions. Twenty-four postoperative complications occurred in 19 patients (31%) [six ileus (10%), five wound infections (8%), five cardiac problems (8%), two urinary retentions (3%), two hemorrhages (3%), one abscess (2%), one pneumonia (2%), and two other (3%)]. Intraoperative complications did not increase postoperative morbidity. Three patients (5%) died within 30 days of operation. When the procedure was completed laparoscopically, the overall median postoperative hospital stay was 10 days; occurrence of a postoperative complication increased the median length of stay to 15 days. They concluded these results are superior to the published historical controls involving open colorectal resections in octogenarians. Overall mortality, lung, and urinary tract complications were decreased and there were no reoperations for small bowel obstruction.

Vignali et al. (115) defined the benefits in terms of early outcome for laparoscopic colectomy in patients over 80 years old compared with open colectomy. They matched 61 patients undergoing laparoscopic colectomy for colorectal carcinoma with 61 open colectomy patients. The mean age was 82 years in the laparoscopy group and 83 years in the open group. The conversion rate was 6.1%. Operative time was 49 minutes longer in the laparoscopy group. The overall mortality rate was 2.4%. The morbidity rate was 21.5% in the laparoscopy group and 31.1% in the open group. Patients in the laparoscopy group had a faster recovery of bowel function and a significant reduction of the mean length of hospital stay (9.8 days vs. 12.9 days for the open group). Laparoscopy allowed a better preservation of postoperative independence status compared with that of the open group. They concluded laparoscopic colectomy for carcinoma in octogenarians is safe and beneficial.

■ LEARNING CURVE

The learning curve may be defined in different ways but is essentially that point when the operating time, conversion rates, and complications have stabilized. The consensus number appears to be about 30 laparoscopic colon resections (97).

Schlachta et al. (116) reviewed their data to define the learning curve for laparoscopic colorectal resections. A total of 461 consecutive resections were evenly distributed among three surgeons. Cases 1 to 30 were considered "early experience" whereas cases 31 and higher were combined as "late experience." There were greater proportions of rectal resections performed (14% vs. 32%) in the late experience. Trends toward declining rates of intraoperative complications (9% vs. 7%) and conversion to open surgery (13.5% vs. 9.7%) were observed with experience. Median operative time (180 vs. 160 minutes), and overall length of postoperative hospital stay (6.5 vs. 5 days) declined significantly with experience. There was no difference in the rate of postoperative complications between the early and late experience (30% vs. 32%). They concluded the learning curve for performing colorectal resections was approximately 30 procedures in their study.

Bennett et al. (117) reported that there is a learning curve for laparoscopic-assisted colectomy with respect of intraoperative and postoperative outcomes. As might be expected surgeons who performed higher volumes of laparoscopic-assisted colectomy have lower rates of intraoperative and postoperative complications. They analyzed data of 1194 patients operated on by 114 surgeons from a prospective registry sponsored by the American Society of Colon and Rectal Surgeons. In 75% of cases, operation was completed laparoscopically with no difference between high-volume surgeons (≥40 cases) and low-volume surgeons. Length of stay (average 6 days) did not vary according to surgeon volume. Postoperative complications occurred in 15% of cases with a significantly lower rate for high-volume surgeons (10% vs. 19%). Intraoperative complications occurred in 5% of cases, with a nonsignificant trend toward a lower rate of high-volume surgeons (3.7% vs. 6.3%). A multivariate regression analysis, adjusting for type of disease (carcinoma vs. inflammatory vs. polyps) and for level of difficulty of the procedure (high vs. low) showed that for high-volume surgeons, there is a lower probability of both intraoperative complications (adjusted odds ratio 0.56) and postoperative complications (adjusted odds ratio 0.48).

Dincler et al. (118) defined a multidimensional learning curve for sigmoid resection performed by two surgeons with experience in laparoscopic surgery. Surgeon A performed 199 and surgeon B 139 sigmoid resections. The operation time decreased from 225 minutes to 169 minutes after approximately 90 operations for surgeon A and from 270 minutes to 223 minutes after 110 operations for surgeon B. Based on a decline in intraoperative complications and conversion rate, the steady state was reached after approximately 70 to 80 interventions for both surgeons. They concluded the assessment of a learning curve should not be limited to measurement of a decrease in operation time but also should include the conversion and complication rates.

Concern for prevention of untoward sequelae associated with the "learning curve" prompted establishment of the Laparoscopic Bowel Surgery Registry by the American Society of Colon and Rectal Surgeons, The Society of American Gastrointestinal Endoscopic Surgeons, and The American College of Surgeons Commission on Cancer to identify as early as possible the pattern of practice and acute complications of laparoscopic colectomy (119). Cases were voluntarily registered by community and academic surgeons. Of 1056 cases contributed by 118 surgeons, 763 patients were completed laparoscopically. Indications for operation were carcinoma (43%), inflammatory diseases (23%), polyps (19%), other diagnoses (13%), and unknown indication (2%). The site of pathology was the right colon in 36%, sigmoid colon in 28%, rectum in 15%, left colon in 8%, transverse colon in 2%, and small bowel in 3%. Resection was performed in 91%, bypass in 4%, and polypectomy in 1%. The operative procedure was not reported in 4%. Completion of the intended procedure was possible in 73%. Extracorporeal anastomoses (61%) and intracorporeal anastomoses (18%) were performed. Laparoscopic-initiated procedures were converted to open laparotomies in 24%. Reasons stated for conversion to open operation were unclear anatomy in 23%, bleeding in 4%, perforation in 2%, and other reasons in 42%. No precise reason for conversion was stated in 2%. Intraoperative laparoscopic complications developed in 5%. Intraoperative bleeding, perforation, or contamination occurred with overall rates of 1.2%, 1.1%, and 0.1%, respectively. The overall incidence of postoperative complications was 15% and conforms to other experiences in open operation. The incidence of postoperative complications directly related to the laparoscopic approach was 2.7%. Patients whose bowel operation was performed and completed laparoscopically averaged 5.6 days of hospitalization postoperatively, whereas those converted to open laparotomy went home an average of 8.4 days postoperatively.

In an invited editorial regarding the registry, Abcarian noted that laparoscopic colectomy has been associated with an array of complications heretofore rare in "open" colectomy. These include division of the ureters, perforation of the aorta, vena cava, and iliac artery and vein, perforation of the small bowel and colon, gross contamination of the peritoneal cavity with feces and carcinoma, uncontrolled bleeding, and recurrence at the trocar or port sites. The rate of these complications in the literature is significant and cannot be reconciled with data presented at the registry. Abcarian continues to note that anecdotal reports of complications heard in the hallways of hospitals and meeting rooms during any surgical society meeting far exceed those reported in the registry, even if one takes into consideration the infamous "learning curve." When cases are contributed to a registry on a voluntary basis, the registry is subject to a worst case bias because surgeons are inherently reluctant to report worst case scenarios. Another gross misrepresentation in the registry is the personal subjective opinion of surgeons performing laparoscopic colectomy and declaring that they did not violate the principles of oncologic surgery in 88% of cases. Abcarian stated that in the absence of objective data, such as proximal and distal margins, extent and number of lymph nodes removed, local, regional, anastomotic, or port-site recurrences, and most important, without prospective data comparing the 5-year survival rates of colon carcinoma patients operated on in conventional open technique vs. laparoscopic procedure, the data presented in the registry are unacceptable because of the lack of scientific merit. It must be remembered that data from a registry are probably not representative of results in the general population of surgeons. Participants are surgeons experienced in laparoscopic procedures.

Kuhry et al. (120) assessed the impact of hospital case volume on short-term outcome after laparoscopic operation for 536 colon carcinoma patients within the Colon Cancer Laparoscopic or Open Resection (COLOR) trial. Median operating time was 240, 210, and 188 minutes in centers with low, medium, and high case volumes, respectively. A significant difference in conversion rate was observed among low, medium, and high case volume hospitals (24% vs. 24% vs. 9%). A higher number of lymph nodes were harvested at high case volume hospitals. After operation, fewer complications and a shorter hospital stay were observed in patients treated at hospitals with high caseloads. They concluded laparoscopic operation for colon carcinoma at hospitals with high caseloads appears to be associated with improved short-term results.

■ MORBIDITY AND MORTALITY

Most publications consist of patients with grouped pathologic processes and procedures. However, several authors have addressed individual disease processes or procedures and hence will be presented accordingly. Attempts were made to quote the most recent work from an institution with multiple publications and when possible to use reports with substantial numbers of patients.

Combined Reports

Jacobs et al. (2) reported the first series of laparoscopic-assisted colectomies. Of the 20 patients, 9 patients underwent a right hemicolectomy; 8 a sigmoid colectomy, and 1 each underwent a low anterior resection, Hartmann's procedure, and abdominoperineal resection. Indications for operation were large villous adenomas or adenocarcinoma in 12 patients, diverticular disease in 5, sigmoid endometrioma in one, cecal volvulus in one, and inflammatory bowel disease (IBD) in one. Eighty percent of patients were able to tolerate a liquid diet on the first postoperative day, and 70% were discharged within 96 hours after operation eating a regular diet and having normal bowel movements. There were three operative complications. A patient with a 3-unit postoperative bleed was managed without operation, one patient developed marked edema of the rectosigmoid anastomosis requiring decompression with a rectal tube, and one individual with metastatic colon carcinoma was operated on for a mechanical small bowel obstruction 7 days after the initial laparoscopic operation.

Wexner et al. (121) reported the results of their first 140 consecutive patients who underwent laparoscopic or laparoscopic-assisted colorectal operations. Indications for operation included IBD in 47 patients, colorectal carcinoma in 19, diverticular disease in 17, polyps in 16, familial polyposis in 7, colonic inertia in 7, feed incontinence in 11, sigmoidocele in 3, irradiation proctitis in 3, rectal prolapse in 2, intestinal lymphoma in 2, and miscellaneous conditions in 6. The procedures included 38 total abdominal colectomies (ileoanal reservoir in 28, ileorectal anastomosis in 8, and end ileostomy in 2); 70 segmental resections of the colon, small bowel, and rectum; 18 diverting stoma creations; 10 reversals of Hartmann's procedure; and four other procedures. In 15 cases, the laparoscopic procedure was converted to a laparotomy (11%). Thirty-one patients (22%) sustained 37 complications, which included enterotomies (seven), hemorrhage (10), intra-abdominal abscess (four), prolonged ileus (six), wound infection (four), intestinal obstruction (two), anastomotic leak (one), aspiration (one), cardiac arrhythmia (one), and upper intestinal bleeding (one). There was no morality. The overall complication rate in total abdominal colectomy cases was significantly higher (42%) when compared with all other procedures (segmental resection, 17%; others, 9%). The mean length of operating time was 4.0 hours (range, 2.5 to 6.5 hours) for total abdominal colectomy, 2.6 hours (range, 1.5 to 5.5 hours) for segmental colonic resections, and 1.7 hours (range, 0.7 to 4 hours) for all other procedures. The length of ileus was 3.5 days (range, 2 to 7 days) after total abdominal colectomy, 3 days (range, 2 to 7 days) after the segmental resections, and 2 days (range, 1 to 4 days) after the other procedures. The mean length of hospital stay was 6.8 days (range, 2 to 40 days)(8.4, 6.5, and 6.3 days for total abdominal colectomies, segmental resections, and other procedures, respectively).

Ramos et al. (122) studied the role of laparoscopy in colorectal surgery and found that of 200 patients assessed, 94% were considered appropriate for laparoscopic surgery, 65% of which were successfully completed (right hemicolectomy, 24 of 30; sigmoid resection, 22 of 36; appendectomy, 9 of 10; anterior resection, 3 of 8; abdominoperineal resection, 3 of 5; and left hemicolectomy, 1 of 2). Complications attributed to laparoscopy were 6.3%. Overall morbidity was 28% in the open procedure group, 18% in the converted group, and 15% in the laparoscopic group.

Huscher et al. (123) reported on 200 patients who received laparoscopic colorectal resections for benign (54) or malignant (146) lesions. Twenty-one of 200 patients were converted to open surgery (10.5%), 37 patients had a complete laparoscopic procedure (17.1%), 137 had an assisted resection (68.5%), and the remaining five patients had a facilitated resection. The mean operative time was 208 minutes (range, 90 to 480 minutes) for assisted resection and 275 minutes (range, 54 to 550 minutes) for complete laparoscopic resection. The mortality rate was 1.7% and the overall morbidity rate was 19.6% (the rate of major complications was 11.2%). All patients quickly became ambulatory and demonstrated a prompt resumption of gastrointestinal functions and less postoperative pain compared with converted cases. The average number of lymph nodes was 12.1 (range, 1 to 32 nodes). The mean hospital stay was 8.6 days (range, 5.0 to 14.5 days). The mean follow-up was 16 months (range, 6 to 24 months). The recurrence rate was 11.7%.

Begos et al. (124) reported on their first 50 patients undergoing laparoscopic techniques. These patients were compared with 34 consecutive patients undergoing open resections during the same time period. Overall, 33 patients (66%) were completed laparoscopically. This rate increased to 87% after the first 20 patients. Patients undergoing laparoscopic procedures showed significant improvement compared with patients undergoing open and converted procedures in several areas. Operative blood loss was decreased. Patients ate sooner (3.7 days) and required less postoperative pain medication. Major complications were less common after laparoscopic operations. The average length of stay was 8.3 days compared with 13.9 days and 14.5 days in the converted and open groups, respectively. There was no difference in the operative time between laparoscopic and open cases; the time for converted cases was significantly longer. There was no difference in lymph node counts in patients who underwent resection for carcinoma.

Zucker et al. (51) reported on 65 patients who underwent attempted laparoscopic colon resection. Indications for surgical intervention included carcinoma in 39 patients, adenomatous polyps in 14, diverticulosis in 10, stricture in one, and foreign-body perforation in one. A laparoscopic-assisted technique in which the specimen was removed and the anastomosis was completed outside the abdomen was used in all patients. A dilated umbilical opening was used for right-sided lesions and a left lower quadrant muscle-splitting incision was used for descending and sigmoid colon resections. Two patients required conversion to open laparotomy. There were no deaths and only four complications (one case each of pneumonia, urinary tract infection, prolonged ileus, and subfascial abscess). The mean postoperative stay was 4.4 days (range, 3.0 to 8.0 days), and the average interval for return to normal activity was 8 days.

Tucker et al. (125) retrospectively analyzed the results of their first 114 laparoscopic-assisted bowel procedures. The procedures performed consisted of partial colectomy in 85 patients, total or subtotal abdominal colectomy in eight, total proctocolectomy with J-pouch ileal reservoir in 11, and diverting procedures in 10. Forty-nine procedures were performed for malignancy. The rate of conversion to laparotomy was 13.2%. Oral feedings were resumed in 2.4 days (range, 1.0 to 5.0 days), and bowel function returned in 3.8 days (range, 2.0 to 8.0 days). The average length of stay was 4.2 days for partial colectomy and 6 days for total, subtotal, and proctocolectomy. The mean return to normal activity for all groups was 16.7 days (10.8 days for partial colectomy). There were no deaths. Major morbidity (6%) consisted of abscess (three), anastomotic leak (two), and hemorrhage (one). Mean operative costs analyzed for the initial 37 patients were higher for laparoscopic colectomy when compared with traditional colectomy; however, the mean total hospital costs were less for laparoscopic procedures.

Lumley et al. (126) summarized the outcome for the first 240 patients who underwent a laparoscopic colorectal procedure. All laparoscopic data were collected prospectively, and in selected studies data were compared with open surgical controls. Nineteen patients required open conversion (7.9%). There was a significant decrease in wound infection rates in patients who underwent laparoscopic-assisted colectomy (3.6%) compared with historical controls (7.9%). There were five anastomotic leaks, five laparotomies performed for postoperative adhesive obstruction, and four perioperative deaths. A total of 103 patients had a procedure for colorectal carcinoma. Of the 79 potentially curative procedures, there have been five (6.3%) recurrences to date.

Slim et al. (127) reported their initial 40 cases of laparoscopic-assisted colorectal resection that were prospectively evaluated. The operations were performed for colonic neoplasms of the right segment (four), sigmoid (11), or rectum (seven), diverticular disease (17), and chronic constipation (one). Of 22 neoplasms, 11 were malignant. The operative procedures were four right hemicolectomies, 28 segmental left colectomies, five anterior resections, two abdominoperineal resections, and one total colectomy. Thirty-one patients (77.5%) underwent a successfully completed laparoscopic-assisted resection. The reasons for conversion in the majority of the cases (66.6%) were difficulties in dissection. In the entirely laparoscopic-assisted procedures, the mean time until passage of flatus was postoperative day 3, the mean postoperative hospitalization was 10.7 days, and there were eight complications in seven patients (25%). Two patients were reoperated 2 and 3 months later for adhesion and ischemic stenosis of the colon above the anastomosis. There was one death in the laparoscopic-assisted group (3.2%). The length of operative specimen was 19.6 cm, and the mean number of resected lymph nodes was six. The authors concluded that in contrast to laparoscopic biliary surgery, the benefits of laparoscopic-assisted colorectal surgery are not obvious.

Fleshman et al. (128) compared laparoscopy with minilaparotomy approaches to colorectal diseases. Minilaparotomy was performed in 35 patients to achieve right colectomy (14), left colectomy (eight), total colectomy (two), low anterior resection (six), abdominoperineal resection (two), colostomy (one), and ileal resection (one). Laparoscopic techniques were used in 52 patients to perform right colectomy (20), left colectomy (11), low anterior resection (five), abdominoperineal resection (seven), total colectomy (three), ileal resection (one), colostomy (three), transverse colectomy (one), and colostomy closure (one). Mean operative times were 69 minutes for minilaparotomy (range, 33 to 180 minutes) and 173 minutes for laparoscopy (range, 60 to 300 minutes). Mean incision lengths were 12 cm (range, 8 to 18 cm) and 8 cm (range, 0 to 25 cm); mean time to bowel movement was 4 days (range, 1 to 7 days) and 3.9 days (range, 0 to 8 days); mean day of discharge was 6.9 days (range, 3 to 15 days), and 6 days (range, 1 to 15 days) postoperatively, respectively. Laparoscopy procedures were completed in 39 of 52 patients (75%); the mean time to bowel movement was 3.5 days (range, 0 to 6 days), and the mean day of discharge was 5.3 days (range, 1 to 14 days). The authors concluded that the use of a small incision, whether by minilaparotomy or by laparoscopy, results in similar early return of function and discharge.

An effort to summarize data from such diverse reports in which authors evaluate different aspects and place emphasis on different elements of this new technology is easier said than done. Notwithstanding this difficulty, values for certain relevant concerns have been published. Of paramount importance is the complication rate, which ranges from 6.9% to 25% (2,51,121–123,127), with an average of approximately 15% (119). Reported conversion rates for laparoscopic colectomy to open colectomy range from 3% to 13.2% (51,121,123,125,126), with most reports in the upper range. The operative time varies with the type of procedure performed and is recorded to be from 60 to 390 minutes, with most in the 175- to 200-minute range (121,123,127). Return of bowel function ranges from 1 to 8 days, with an average of approximately 4 days (121,125,127). Postoperative feeding has been offered as early as the first postoperative day and is believed to be possible sooner than with open colectomy, an average 2.4 to 3.7 days (range, 1 to 5 days) (2,124). The hospital length of stay ranges from 2 to 40 days (2,121,123,125,127,129) but averages 5.6 days (119). The operative mortality rate is noted to be 0% to 3.2% (51,123,126,127). Less postoperative medication is required (124). Patients return to normal activity in approximately 17 days (125). Understandably, laparoscopic colectomy costs are higher than for open colectomy (125).

Deguili et al. (130) reviewed 108 patients undergoing laparoscopic colorectal surgery for large bowel disease. Conversion to open was necessary in 4.6% of patients whereas a mandatory conversion was needed in 9.2% of patients because of advanced carcinoma. The overall morbidity rate was 11.9%. There were no anastomotic leaks. In two patients (1.85%) a complication developed that required reoperation. Postoperative mortality was nil. Mean postoperative stay was 7.2 days. No trocar site recurrences were observed in the carcinoma patients.

Senagore et al. (131) reviewed the outcome of the standardization of all the intraoperative and postoperative processes used in their department for the performance of laparoscopic sigmoid colectomy for all colonic pathologies. Criteria for exclusion for an attempted laparoscopic sigmoid colectomy were BMI > 35 and prior major abdominal operations (exclusive of hysterectomy, cholecystectomy, appendectomy). Conversion was performed when a sequential step could not be completed in a reasonable time frame. A standard perioperative care plan was used. A total of 207 colectomies were performed with a 12.1% conversion rate. Indications for the laparoscopic sigmoid colectomies were diverticular disease (115), colonic neoplasia (32), prolapse (14), endometriosis (10), and other (10). Mean operative time was 119 minutes. Mean length of stay was 2.9 days for completed cases and 6.4 days for converted cases. Anastomotic leaks occurred in two patients (1.1%), one of whom died of multisystem organ failure yielding an operative mortality of 0.6%. The overall complication rate was 6.6% and the 30-day readmission rate was 8%.

Lezoche et al. (132) reported a prospective nonrandomized study based on a series of 469 consecutive patients (73.6% with malignant lesions) for laparoscopic and open approach. There were 166 patients who underwent right hemicolectomy (RHC) and 303 left hemicolectomy (LHC). In the RHC group, 108 patients underwent laparoscopic approach and 58 underwent an open operation (26 vs. 13 for benign lesions and 82 vs. 45 for adenocarcinomas, respectively). Left hemicolectomy was performed by laparoscopy in 202 patients and by laparotomy in 101 (55 vs. 30 for benign lesions and 147 vs. 71 for adenocarcinomas, respectively). There were no conversions to open operation in laparoscopic right hemicolectomy while 10 patients (4.9%) in the laparoscopic LHC group required conversion: three of 34 performed for diverticular disease and seven of 147 performed for malignancy. Mean operative time for laparoscopic surgery was longer than for open surgery (182 vs. 140 minutes for RHC and 222 vs. 190 minutes for LHC, respectively), but with increasing expertise this decreased significantly. Mean hospital stay in patients who underwent laparoscopic procedures was significantly shorter both in right hemicolectomy and left hemicolectomy groups (9.2 vs. 13.2 days and 9.9 vs. 13.2 days, respectively). Similar major complication rates were observed between the two laparoscopic and open groups (1.8% vs. 1.7% for RHC and 4.1% vs. 4.9% for LHC, respectively). Mean follow-up time was 57.3 months in the RHC group and 57.5 months in the LHC group. The local recurrence rate was lower after laparoscopic surgery in both arms (7% vs. 8.8% for RHC and 3.3% vs. 7% for LHC, respectively), but the differences were not statistically significant. Two port-site recurrences were observed in the laparoscopic group, one after a palliative right hemicolectomy, one after a Dukes C left hemicolectomy converted to open operation (1.7% vs. 0.9%, respectively). Metachronous metastases rates were similar between the laparoscopic and open groups (20.9% vs. 17.6% for RHC and 4.4% vs. 5.3% for LHC, respectively). Cumulative survival probability at 72 months after laparoscopic right hemicolectomy was 0.79 when compared with 0.77 after open operation and 0.96 after laparoscopic left hemicolectomy compared with 0.88 after open operation. Cumulative survival probability for Dukes A, B and C in the laparoscopic right hemicolectomy group was 0.88, 0.85, and 0.73 when compared with 0.9, 0.89, and 0.6 after open surgery, respectively. Cumulative survival probability for Dukes A, B and C in the laparoscopic left hemicolectomy was 0.1, 0.97, and 0.89 when compared with 0.1, 0.94 and 0.7 after open operation, respectively. Their results suggest that laparoscopic hemicolectomy for both benign and malignant lesions can be performed safely. Oncologic outcomes were comparable with those of open operation.

Schlachta et al. (133) reviewed the 10-year experience of a surgical group from university teaching hospitals in three centers. There were 750 laparoscopic colon and rectal procedures attempted of which 669 were completed laparoscopically. Malignant disease was the indication for operation in 49.6% of cases. Right hemicolectomy and sigmoid colectomy accounted for 54.5% of procedures performed. Intraoperative complications occurred in 8.3% with 29% of these resulting in conversion to open operation. The overall rate of conversion to open operation was 10.8%, most commonly for oncologic concerns. Median operative time was 175 minutes for all procedures. Postoperative complications occurred in 27.5% of procedures completed laparoscopically but were mostly minor wound complications. Pulmonary complications occurred in only 1%. The anastomotic leak rate was 2.5%. The early reoperation rate was 2.4%. Postoperative mortality was 2.2%. No port-site metastases have yet been detected. The median postoperative length of stay was 5 days.

Lauter and Froines (134) reported their experience with 155 procedures. Mean operative time for completed laparoscopic-assisted colectomy, converted procedures, right and sigmoid resections were 164, 203, 121, and 177 minutes, respectively. Twenty-two patients had additional concurrent laparoscopic procedures. Thirty-nine had undergone previous abdominal operation. The conversion rate was 12%. Mean length of stay for all patients was 4.5 days. There were eight major and 16 minor complications. There were no port-site metastases. Major complications and conversion rate decreased from the first 50 cases to the last 50 cases.

Seshadri et al. (135) compared the outcomes of laparoscopic total abdominal colectomy and laparoscopic total proctocolectomy with institutional open procedures used as controls. A total of 73 total abdominal colectomies for various disease processes including IBD and neoplasia were evenly distributed between laparoscopic ($n=37$) and open ($n=36$) approaches. The median operative time was longer with the laparoscopic method (270 vs. 178 minutes) but the median length of hospital stay was significantly shorter (6 vs. 9 days). The short-term postoperative complication rate up to 30 days from operation was not statistically different (25% vs. 44%), although there was a clear trend toward a reduced number of overall complications in the laparoscopic group (9 vs. 24). Wound complications were significantly fewer (0% vs. 19%) and postoperative pneumonia was nonexistent in laparoscopic patients. Long-term complications also were less common in the laparoscopic group (20% vs. 64%) largely because of reduced incidence of impotence, incisional hernia, and ileostomy complications. Total proctocolectomy was performed laparoscopically in 15 patients and with an open procedure in 13 patients over the same period. Median operating time was longer for the laparoscopic patients (400 minutes vs. 235 minutes) whereas the length of hospital stay and morbidity and mortality were not significantly different. The results indicate that laparoscopic total abdominal colectomy can be performed safely with a statistically significant reduction in wound and long-term postoperative complications when compared with its open counterpart.

Kockerling et al. (136) investigated the results of laparoscopic colorectal surgery in 500 consecutive patients operated on by unselected surgeons in 18 centers; 269 operations were performed for benign indications and 231 for carcinoma (palliative and curative). An anastomosis was performed in 84% with an overall leakage rate of 5.3% (colon 3.6% and rectum 11.8%), which required operative reintervention in 1.7%. The mean operating time was 176 minutes and showed a decrease in tendency over the period under study. The conversion rate was 7.0% and the overall complication rate 21.4%. The reoperation rate was 6.6; the most common cause was bleeding. There was one ureteral lesion (0.2%), but urinary tract infections were fairly common (4.8%). A postoperative pneumonia was diagnosed in 1.6% of cases. No thromboembolic complications were reported. The 30-day mortality rate was 1.4% and overall hospital mortality 1.8%.

Kockerling et al. (137) investigated the safety of laparoscopic colorectal surgery as reflected by the anastomotic insufficiency rates in the various sections of the bowel and compared these rates with those of open colorectal surgery. From this prospective multicenter study, the 24 participating centers treated 1143 patients. In all, 626 operations were performed for benign indications and 517 for carcinoma. Most procedures involved the sigmoid colon and rectum (80.9%). An anastomosis was performed in 83% of the operations. Most of the anastomoses were laparoscopic-assisted using the stapling technique. They observed an overall leakage rate of 4.3% (colon 2.9%; rectum 12.7%) and surgical reintervention was required in 1% of the cases. The rate of conversion to open surgery was 5.6%. Intraoperative complications occurred in 5.9% and reoperation was necessary in 4.1% of cases. The overall morbidity rate was 22.3% and the 30-day mortality rate was 1.6%. Morbidity and mortality rates with this method approximate those seen with conventional colorectal surgery.

Schwenk et al. (138) conducted a Cochrane review to compare laparoscopic and conventional colorectal resection with regards to possible benefits of the laparoscopic method in the short-term postoperative period (up to 3 months post-surgery). All randomized controlled trials were included regardless of the language of publication. Operative time was longer in laparoscopic surgery, but intraoperative blood loss was less than in conventional surgery. Intensity of postoperative pain and duration of postoperative ileus were shorter after laparoscopic colorectal resection and pulmonary function was improved after a laparoscopic approach. Total morbidity and local (surgical) morbidity were decreased in the laparoscopic groups. General morbidity and mortality were not different between groups. Until the 30th postoperative day, quality of life was better in the laparoscopic patients. Postoperative hospital stay was less in the laparoscopic patients. These authors concluded that under traditional perioperative treatment, laparoscopic colonic resections show clinically relevant advantages in selected patients. Furthermore, if the long-term oncologic results of laparoscopic and conventional resection of colonic carcinoma show equivalent results, the laparoscopic approach should be preferred in patients suitable for this approach to colectomy.

Carcinoma

Since the introduction of laparoscopic colon surgery, the propriety of adopting this technology to carcinoma has been questioned. Are sound oncologic principles of colorectal resection violated by this approach? Is there a different pattern of recurrence? Is disease-free survival compromised? Many publications have advocated the procedure but were often retrospective small series with relatively short follow-up.

Patankar and Lee (1) recently conducted a comprehensive review of published data. In their assessment of oncologic equivalency of laparoscopic resection they reviewed 10 publications with respect to the resection margins and lymph node yield and on both accounts found that laparoscopic resection achieves the same oncologic resection as open operation. Several prospective and retrospective reviews have reported survival to be comparable with those of open resections.

Retrospective and Prospective Reviews

Long-term survival data has been reported by three large studies, two of these are retrospective case reviews and one is a prospective randomized controlled trial (139–141). Lujan et al. (140) reported the oncologic results of 122 consecutive patients undergoing laparoscopic colon resection for carcinoma at one institution that had complete 5-year survival data. The National Cancer Database (NCDB) of the American College of Surgeons was chosen for comparison because the American College of Surgeons uses date of treatment initiation as the starting point, and their 5-year relative survival rates were analyzed separately for each stage of disease. The 5-year survival rates in the laparoscopic resection group compared favorably with the open resections performed in the same institute as well as to the NCDB reported stage-specific rates. Interestingly, there was a 9% to 11% survival benefit between stage III laparoscopic patients and the open and the NCDB groups. The authors stated that the lumping of colon and rectum together may have affected the survival rates and they also raised the concern regarding the confounding effects of adjuvant therapy.

Pantankar et al. (141) reported their experience with 172 curative intent, laparoscopic colorectal resections. The open resection group was a computerized case-matched control group at the same institution. The survival data was also compared with the two most authoritative sources of information on carcinoma incidence and survival in the United States, the NCDB of the American College of Surgeons Commission on Cancer and the American Cancer Society, and the Surveillance Epidemiology and End Results (SEER) Program of the National Cancer Institute. The data from SEER reports 5-year overall relative survival rates as ranging from 60% to 62%. The data available from the NCDB reports the overall 5-year relative survival for years 1993–1998 to be 62%. The overall 5-year survival rate in this study was 69% for the laparoscopic group and 64% for the open group and compares favorably with the SEER and NCDB statistics. The 5-year survival rates were also analyzed separately for the colon versus rectum sites, and for each stage. Separate analysis was undertaken to avoid the confounding effect of adjuvant therapy with possible interruptions and/or partial treatments. The results show that, in strictly comparable patients as possible through the limitations of nonrandomized study design, the survival with laparoscopic approach was no different from the open resections.

Clinical Trials

There are currently several multi-institutional, large-scale prospective, randomized trials comparing laparoscopic-assisted to open colon resection in patients with colon carcinoma. The National Institutes of Health trial [Clinical Outcomes of Surgical Therapy (COST) Study Group] begun in 1995, proposed to study 1200 patients randomly assigned to laparoscopic or open colectomy for curable colon carcinoma has recently been published and detailed below (142).

The Colon Carcinoma Laparoscopic or Open Resection (COLOR) trial is a European multicenter randomized trial which began in September 1997. The COLOR trial prospectively randomized 1248 patients with colon carcinoma to laparoscopic or open colon resection in 29 participating centers. All patients will be followed for a minimum of 5 years. The primary outcome measure is carcinoma-free survival at 3 years with secondary outcome measures being morbidity, port-site recurrences, quality of life, cost, resection margins, and harvesting of lymph nodes. The short-term outcomes have recently been published (143) (Tables 1 and 5). They concluded that laparoscopic surgery can be used for safe and radical resection for carcinoma in the right, left, and sigmoid colon.

The Medical Research Council Conventional versus Laparoscopic-Assisted Surgery in Colon Carcinoma (MRC CLASICC) trial opened recruitment in 1995. It involved 27 hospitals in the United Kingdom. The aim was to recruit 1000 patients, but ultimately 794 patients were recruited. The primary endpoints are pathological resection margins, mortality, local recurrence rates, disease-free survival and overall survival at 3 years. The secondary outcome measures include quality of life and cost-effectiveness. This trial included patients with carcinoma of both the colon and rectum. The short-term endpoints of this trial have also recently been reported (151).

Abraham et al. (173) conducted a meta-analysis of randomized clinical trials comparing the short-term outcomes of laparoscopic with those of open resection for colorectal carcinoma. The outcomes of 2512 procedures from 12 trials were analyzed. Laparoscopic resection took on average 32.9% longer to perform than open resection but was associated with lower morbidity rates. Specifically, wound infection rates were significantly lower (odds ratio 0.47). In patients undergoing laparoscopic resection, the average time to passage of first flatus was reduced by 33.5%, that to tolerance of a solid diet by 23.9% and that to 80% recovery of peak expiratory flow by 44.3%. Early narcotic analgesia requirements were also reduced by 36.9%, pain at rest by 34.8% and during coughing by 33.9%, and hospital stay by 20.6%. There were no significant differences in perioperative mortality or oncological clearance. They concluded laparoscopic resection for colorectal carcinoma is associated with lower morbidity, less pain, a faster recovery and a shorter hospital stay than open resection without compromising oncologic clearance.

Prospective Randomized Studies

Stage et al. (174) prospectively randomized 34 patients with potentially curable colon carcinoma to laparoscopic ($n=18$) or open surgery ($n=16$). Conversion rate was 16.7%. Patients in the laparoscopic surgery group experienced significantly longer operative times (150 vs. 95 minutes), less pain, shorter hospital stay (5 vs. 8 days), and more rapid return to self care. There were no differences between the two groups and size of specimen removed, number of lymph node glands removed, the Dukes' classification, complications, postoperative reduction in pulmonary function or level of fatigue. Immunodepression as measured by

TABLE 1 ■ Bowel Activity Following Laparoscopic Resection for Colon and Rectal Carcinoma

Author (Ref.)	Year	Type of Study	Procedure	Oral Intake	Bowel Activity
Ramos et al. (144)	1997	RC	Laparoscopic	–	2.5
			Open	–	3.9
Khalili et al. (145)	1998	RC	Laparoscopic	3.9	–
			Open	4.9	–
Hong et al. (146)	2001	RC	Laparoscopic	2.1	1.8
			Open	4	3
Baker et al. (147)	2002	RC	Laparoscopic	–	1.4
			Open	–	1.2
Champault et al. (148)	2002	PNR	Laparoscopic	1.8	1.4
			Open	4.2	3.2
Curet et al. (149)	2000	PR	Laparoscopic	2.7–4.1[a]	–
			Open	4.4–5.8	–
Lacy et al. (139)	2002	PR	Laparoscopic	2.3	–
			Open	3.5	–
Leung et al. (150)	2004	PR	Laparoscopic	4.2	2.4–4.0[b]
			Open	4.9	3.1–4.6
COLOR (143)	2005	PR	Laparoscopic	2.9	3.6
			Open	3.8	4.6
CLASICC, Guillou et al. (151)	2005	PR	Laparoscopic	6	5
			Open	6	6

[a]Fluids–regular diet.
[b]Gas–bowel movement.
Abbreviations: RC, retrospective comparative; PNR, prospective nonrandomized; PR, prospective randomized.

IL-6 and serum C-reactive protein levels, was more pronounced in the laparoscopic group.

Milsom et al. (175) prospectively randomized 109 patients with adenocarcinoma or large polyps to laparoscopic surgery ($n=55$) or open surgery ($n=54$). Conversion was required in 6.8% of patients. There were no differences in the two groups in surgical margins, stage of disease, and length of stay. On average, 19 lymph nodes were resected in the laparoscopic group compared with 25 in the open surgery group. Fifteen percent of patients in each group experienced complications and mortality was similar in both groups. The laparoscopic group experienced less blood loss (252 vs. 344 mL), longer operative time (200 vs. 125 minutes), quicker return of pulmonary function (3 vs. 6 days), less need for analgesia in the first two days postoperatively (0.78 vs. 0.92 mg/kg of morphine) and faster return of flatus (3 vs. 4 days). There were no local or port-site recurrences in the laparoscopic group compared with the two wound recurrences in the open group. Carcinoma-related deaths occurred in three laparoscopic surgery patients and four open surgery patients.

Lacy et al. (139) randomized 219 patients with colon carcinoma (111 laparoscopic group, 108 open group) over 5 years. Median length of follow-up was 43 months. Conversion rate was 11%. Number of lymph nodes resected was similar in the two groups (11.1). Operative time was longer (142 vs. 118 minutes) and intraoperative blood loss lower (105 vs. 193 mL) in the laparoscopic group. The patients in the laparoscopic group had quicker return of gastrointestinal function (54 vs. 85 hours), shorter hospital stay (5.2 vs. 7.9 days), and less morbidity (10.8% vs. 28.7%). One patient developed a port-site metastasis. Overall, mortality was similar between the two groups but carcinoma-related mortality was significantly lower in the laparoscopic group (9% vs. 21%). The probability of overall survival and the probability of carcinoma-related survival were significantly higher in the laparoscopic group. The Cox model showed that laparoscopic-assisted colectomy was independently associated with reduced risk of carcinoma relapse (hazard ratio 0.39), death from any cause (0.48), and death from carcinoma-related causes (0.38) compared with open colectomy. This superiority of laparoscopic-assisted colectomy was due to differences in patients with stage III carcinoma. The differences were so pronounced that data on the stage III patients approached outcomes for stage II patients in the laparoscopic group. The authors postulate that decreased stress and improved immune function associated with a minimally invasive approach may account for these differences.

Delgado et al. (111) prospectively randomized patients with colorectal carcinoma to receive either laparoscopic-assisted colectomy ($n=129$) or open colectomy ($n=126$). They analyzed data by whether patients were younger than 70 years of age or 70 years and older thus ending up with four groups of comparison. There was a higher incidence of co-morbid factors, right colon lesions, and right colectomies in the older group but the distribution was similar in the laparoscopic-assisted and the open group. The conversion rate in the laparoscopic-assisted group was 11.4% in the younger groups and 17% in the older groups. Mean operating time was significantly longer and blood loss significantly lower in the laparoscopic-assisted colectomy than the open colectomy group with no difference in the two age groups. Return of gastrointestinal function was earlier and length of stay was shorter in the laparoscopic-assisted group compared with the open colectomy group with these differences seen in both age groups. Complication rates in the younger group were similar for the laparoscopic-assisted and open colectomy patients. However, in the older age group, complication rates for laparoscopic-assisted patients were significantly less than for the open patients (10.1% vs. 31.3%) because of differences in wound infections (5% vs. 12%).

Hasegawa et al. (176) randomized 59 patients with T2 or T3 colorectal carcinomas who underwent curative resection to laparoscopic-assisted colectomy ($n=29$) or open colectomy ($n=30$). The patients in the laparoscopic group experienced longer operative times (275 vs. 188 minutes), less blood loss (58 vs. 137 mL), smaller incisions (5.9 vs. 17.8 cm), faster progression to oral intake (1.6 vs. 3.2 days), less analgesic requirement (1.7 vs. 3.4 days), and shorter hospital stay (7.1 vs. 12.7 days). No differences in morbidity rates were found between the two groups. C-reactive protein levels were lower in the laparoscopic-assisted group on postoperative days 1 and 4 while there were no differences between the two groups with respect to IL-6 and leukocyte count and natural killer cell activity.

Weeks et al. (177) reported the results of short-term quality of life based on data obtained from the National Institute of Health Trial based on 449 patients from 37 centers with clinically resectable colon carcinoma. In an intention-to-treat analysis, the global rating scale score at 2 weeks postoperative was higher for the laparoscopic group than the open group (76.9 vs. 74.4). These differences disappeared by the two month time analysis period. The laparoscopic surgery patients required fewer days of parenteral analgesics (3.2 vs. 4.0 days) and oral analgesics (1.9 vs. 2.2 days) and were hospitalized for a shorter period of time (5.6 vs. 6.4 days). The conversion rate was 25.7% and these patients reported slightly poorer quality of life results than patients who were not converted. These surprising results could be due to the fact that the instruments used to measure quality of life were not sensitive enough to identity true differences. Also, sample size could have been a factor. The analysis on intention-to-treat resulted in patients who were converted being analyzed in the laparoscopic group, which could also have resulted in skewing of the results. Finally, it is possible that the overriding factor in quality of life in patients who have malignancy is the malignancy and their worries about survival, thus obscuring differences seen with operative approach.

Schwenk et al. (178) prospectively randomized 60 patients with primary colorectal carcinomas to laparoscopic ($n = 30$) or open ($n = 30$) surgery. Length of stay was similar because no patient was discharged before postoperative day 7 to collect complete data. The laparoscopic group required less postoperative analgesics (0.78 vs. 1.38 mg/kg), had lower pain score (507 vs. 755), and lower postoperative fatigue scores (322 vs. 531).

Inflammatory Response

The inflammatory and immune responses to laparoscopic colectomy have been studied in both animal and human trials (179). Carcinoma patients may already have a suppressed immune system and therefore any further attenuation may be potentially harmful. Immunosuppression is mediated by a number of factors, and multiple serological factors have been measured, including C-reactive protein, IL-6, IL-8, and tumor necrosis factor. IL-6 is a major indicator of tissue damage and a major mediator of acute phase protein response. Several authors have found that serum levels of IL-6 reveal the greatest differences between laparoscopic-assisted and open colectomy groups concluding that the acute phase response is attenuated in the laparoscopic-assisted colectomy patients. Similarly, several authors have found a significant decrease in the systemic inflammatory response, specifically IL-6, C-reactive protein, and granulocyte elastase, leading them to conclude that laparoscopic colectomy is less traumatic than open colectomy. Although the blood levels of the cytokines are lower in the laparoscopic group, peritoneal fluid levels are the same, suggesting that the peritoneal trauma is the same despite the lower systemic response. The short-term benefits of laparoscopy may be due at least in part to a lower systemic inflammatory response.

In parallel with the MRC CLASICC trial, Tang et al. (180) evaluated systemic immune response in patients having laparoscopic-assisted colectomy ($n = 118$) compared with those undergoing conventional open operation ($n = 118$) for colorectal carcinoma. Operative time was 18 minutes longer for the laparoscopic-assisted patients (88 vs. 70 minutes) and the incision length was shorter (9 cm vs. 15 cm). There were no significant differences in morbidity rates between the two groups. There were no differences in T-cell, B-cell CD4:CD8 ratios, immunoglobulin (Ig)G, IgM, IgA, natural killer cell, or nitroblue tetrazolium test between the two groups. There were marginal differences in C3 and C4 complement levels, which did not reach statistical significance. Duke's classification, size of carcinoma, wound length, and operating time had little influence on the postoperative immune parameters.

Low Anterior Resection

Delgado et al. (181) reported their results of laparoscopic techniques in 220 patients with rectal carcinoma. Neoadjuvant chemoradiotherapy was used in 59% of their patients. In more than 75% of the patients, a surgical procedure with sphincter preservation was performed. The rate of conversion to the open approach was 20%. Ten patients had intraoperative complications. Postoperative complications developed in 26.3% of patients. The length of hospital stay was 6.8 days. The distribution of stages was as follows: stage I, 16.8%; stage II, 33.6%; stage III, 26.4%; stage IV, 19.1%. The mean number of lymph nodes was 13.8. The incidence of local relapse was 5.3% with a follow-up of 18 months. They concluded, laparoscopic surgery can be safely performed in patients with adenocarcinoma of the rectum with good short-term results.

Yamamoto et al. (160) examined the short-term results of laparoscopy in the treatment of 70 curative cases of rectosigmoid and rectal carcinoma. Mesorectal transection was performed at least 5 cm below the lesion for rectosigmoid and upper rectal carcinomas and a TME was performed for lower carcinomas. Primary anastomosis was performed by a double-stapling technique, or a handsewn coloanal anastomosis was performed. The median follow-up was 23 months. An anastomosis was performed in 93% of the operations. Oral intake was started on median postoperative day 1, and the median length of hospitalization was 8 days. Two patients needed conversion to conventional open operation. A total of 15 postoperative complications occurred in 13 patients (18.6%), including anastomotic leakage in six (8.6%) and bowel obstruction in three (4.3%). Reoperation was required in six patients. Two patients developed recurrence of their carcinoma at the anastomotic site. The expected 5-year survival and disease-free survival rates were 100% and 92%, respectively.

Morino et al. (161) conducted a prospective consecutive series of 100 laparoscopic TMEs for low mid-rectal carcinomas. All patients had a sphincter-saving procedure. The distal limit of the rectal neoplasm was on average 6.1 cm from the anal verge. The mean operative time was 250 minutes. The conversion rate was 12%. The mean postoperative stay was 12 days. The 30-day mortality was 2% and the overall postoperative morbidity was 36% including 17 anastomotic leaks. With a median follow-up of 45.7 months, 18.5% died of carcinoma and 8.5% are alive with metastatic disease. The port-site metastases rate was 1.4%. The local regional pelvic recurrence was 4.2%. This series confirms the safety of the procedure while oncologic results are comparable with the open published series.

Law et al. (182) reported on the early outcomes of 100 patients with laparoscopic resection for rectal carcinoma with TME. Operations included 91 anterior resections, eight abdomino-perineal resections, and one Hartmann's procedure. Conversion was required in 15 patients but none with APR. Postoperative complications occurred in 31%—anastomotic leak in three patients and one patient required reoperation for small bowel obstruction.

Zhou et al. (183) conducted a prospective randomized controlled trial to assess the feasibility and efficacy of the laparoscopic approach of TME with anal sphincter preservation in 82 patients by the laparoscopic procedure and 89 patients by the open technique. In the laparoscopic group, 30 patients in whom the low anterior resection was performed had the anastomosis below the peritoneal reflection and more than 2 cm above the dentate line, 27 patients in whom ultra-low anterior resection was performed had anastomotic height within 2 cm of the dentate line, and 25 patients in whom coloanal anastomosis was performed had the anastomosis at or below the dentate line. In the open group, the numbers were 35, 27, and 27, respectively. There was no statistical difference in operation time, administration or parenteral analgesics, start of food intake, and mortality rate between the two groups. However, blood loss was less, bowel function recovered earlier and hospitalization time was shorter in the laparoscopic group.

Leroy et al. (184) assessed the feasibility, safety and long-term outcome of laparoscopic rectal carcinoma resections following the principles of TME in 102 consecutive unselected patients. Conversion to an open approach was required in 3%. The overall morbidity and mortality rates were 27% and 2%, respectively, with an overall anastomotic leak of 17%. In 91.8% the resection was considered curative. Mean follow-up was 36 months. There were no trocar-site recurrences. The local recurrence rate was 6%, and the carcinoma-specific survival of all curatively resected patients was 75% at 5 years. The overall survival rate of all curatively resected patients was 65% at 5 years.

Rullier et al. (185) reported on the feasibility of laparoscopic rectal resection in patients with mid- or low-rectal carcinoma with regard to quality of mesorectal excision, autonomic pelvic nerve preservation, and anal sphincter preservation. Laparoscopic rectal excision was performed in 32 patients (21 men) with rectal carcinoma located 5 cm from the anal verge. The operative procedure was performed 6 weeks after radiotherapy and included TME, intersphincteric resection, transanal coloanal anastomosis with coloplasty and loop ileostomy. Three patients needed conversion to a laparotomy. Postoperative morbidity occurred in 10 patients, related mainly to coloplasty. Macroscopic evaluation showed an intact mesorectal excision in 29 of 32 excised specimens; microscopically, 30 of the 32 resections were R0. Sphincter preservation was achieved in 31 patients. The hypogastric nerves and pelvic plexuses were identified and preserved in 24 of the 32 patients. Sexual function was preserved in 10 of 18 evaluable men. They concluded a laparoscopic approach can be considered in most patients with mid- or low-rectal carcinoma.

Tsang et al. (162) examined outcomes after patients with mid- or low-rectal carcinomas underwent laparoscopic TME with construction of a colonic J-pouch in 44 patients. There was no conversion to an open procedure. The median distance of the anastomosis from the anal verge was 4 cm. No procedure-related death occurred. Four patients developed significant complications that required reoperation. With a median follow-up period of 15 months, no port-site recurrence was noted. Five patients developed distant metastases and two had local recurrence in the pelvis. Bowel function was satisfactory at 6, 12, and 18 months after ileostomy closure.

Jayne et al. (186) assessed bladder and sexual function in patients who had undergone laparoscopic rectal, open rectal or laparoscopic colonic resection as part of the UK MRC CLASICC trial, using the International Prostatic Symptom Score, the International Index of Erectile Function and the Female Sexual Function Index. Sexual and bladder function data from the European Organization for Research and Treatment of Cancer QLQ-CR38 collected in the CLASICC trial were used for comparison. Questionnaires were completed by 71.2% of the 347 patients. Bladder function was similar after laparoscopic and open rectal operations for rectal carcinoma. Overall, sexual function and erectile function tended to be worse in men after laparoscopic rectal surgery than after open rectal surgery (overall function: difference –11.18; erectile function: difference –5.84). Total mesorectal excision was more commonly performed in the laparoscopic rectal group than in the open rectal group. TME (odds ratio 6.38) and conversion to open operation (odds ratio 2.86) were independent predictors of postoperative male sexual dysfunction. No differences were detected in female sexual function. Laparoscopic rectal resection did not adversely affect bladder function, but there was a trend toward worse male sexual function. This may be explained by the higher rate of TME in the laparoscopic rectal resection group.

Advanced Colorectal Carcinoma

Milsom et al. (187) reported a prospective analysis of 30 patients with incurable colorectal carcinoma who underwent laparoscopic surgery for palliative purposes. Resection of a single segment of the bowel was performed in 15 patients. One patient underwent both right colectomy and sigmoidectomy because of double lesions. Stoma creation only was performed in 11 patients. Three patients were converted to an open procedure. For resection, median operative time was 170 minutes. For stoma creation median operative time was 60 minutes. There were two postoperative deaths. Median time to passage of flatus was 2 days and of stool 5 days after resection and 2 days for both flatus and stool after stoma creation. Median time to discharge was 8 days after resection and 7 days after stoma creation. They concluded the laparoscopic approach for patients with incurable colorectal carcinoma can provide effective palliation with avoidance of a major laparotomy in the majority of cases.

Gonzalez et al. (25) also evaluated the feasibility and outcomes of the laparoscopic approach for the palliation of advanced complicated colorectal carcinoma. They reviewed 21 laparoscopic palliative procedures for emergent complications of advanced colorectal carcinoma. Indications for operation included perforation ($n = 10$), bleeding ($n = 7$), and obstruction ($n = 4$). A proximal diverting procedure was performed in all patients, and a concomitant colon resection was performed in 18 patients (86%). The mean operative time was 181 minutes. The average length of hospital stay was 8.6 days and time to first bowel movement was 61 hours. The complication rate and the 30-day mortality rates were 33% and 0%, respectively.

Leung et al. (150) reported on their detailed comprehensive study in which 403 patients with rectosigmoid carcinoma were randomized to receive either laparoscopic-assisted ($n = 203$) or conventional open ($n = 200$) resection.

Survival and disease-free interval were the main endpoints. The demographic data of the two groups were similar after curative resection, the probabilities of survival at 5 years of the laparoscopic and open resection groups were 76.1% and 72.9%, respectively. The probabilities of being disease-free at 5 years were 75.3% and 78.3%, respectively. The operative time for the laparoscopic group was significantly longer whereas postoperative recovery was significantly better than for the open resection, but these benefits were at the expense of higher direct costs. The distal margin, the number of lymph nodes found in the resected specimen, overall morbidity and overall mortality did not differ between groups. They concluded, laparoscopic resection of rectosigmoid carcinoma does not jeopardize survival and disease control of patients.

In Summary

In their comprehensive review of the literature, Kieran and Curet (179) found in most reports length of stay has been 5 to 6 days for laparoscopic cases compared to 7 to 8 days for open cases. Operative times ranged from 88 to 275 minutes (with most in the 170 to 190 range) compared with 95 to 201 minutes (with most in the 120 to 150 range) for open cases. In general, morbidity rates have been similar between the two groups ranging from 2% to 46% (average 17.6%) for laparoscopic cases and 2% to 60% (average 22.9%) for open cases. Of note is that small bowel perforation, ureteral injury, trocar site injury, and mesenteric and epigastric vessel injury have been reported with laparoscopic-associated complications. Lacy (139) found a higher complication rate in open vs. the laparoscopic group (30% vs. 10.5%) primarily because of a higher incidence of wound complications (16.7% vs. 7.2%). Delgado found similar results in patients <70 or >70 years of age (188). Anastomotic leaks were also similar in the two groups (188). Conversion varied widely from 0% to 40% with most reports in the 15% to 20% range. Cited reasons for conversion include bulky disease, invasion of carcinoma, obesity, adhesions, inability to mobilize the splenic flexure, bleeding, ureteral injury, unclear anatomy, prolonged operative time, stapler malfunction, and anastomotic defects (179). Conversion rates decrease with increasing experience. The cost issue is unclear. Intraoperative costs are certainly higher for the laparoscopic approach but some argue that the total cost is less because of the shorter hospital stay. However, hospital stay may not be substantially shorter or enough to compensate for the increased instrument costs. Lymph node harvests are similar with average range 6–23 laparoscopically and 6–26 open. Resection margins are also similar with the two techniques.

Lacy et al. (139) reported a randomized study with an unforeseen better long-term survival for node positive patients treated by laparoscopic colectomy. Similarly, Capussotti et al. (189) conducted a prospective nonrandomized trial in which they compared short- and long-term results of laparoscopic and open curative resection for adenocarcinoma of the left colon or rectum in 255 consecutive patients. A total of 74 patients underwent a laparoscopic resection and 181 an open resection. The carcinoma was in the descending colon in 32 cases, the sigmoid colon in 98 cases, and the rectum in 125 cases including 87 mid–low-rectal carcinomas. Ten laparoscopic resection-procedures (13.5%) were converted to open surgery. The hospital mortality was 0.08%, and in hospital morbidity was 16.2% for laparoscopic resection and 13.3% for open resection. The median postoperative stay was 1 day shorter for laparoscopic resection (9 days) than for open resection (10 days). The mean number of lymph nodes retrieved were 13.8 for open resection and 12.7 for laparoscopy resection. Age exceeding 70 years, T stage, N stage, grading, mid–low-rectal site, and laparoscopy were found by multivariate analysis to be significant prognostic factors for disease-free and carcinoma-related survival. When patients were stratified by stage, a trend toward a better disease-free and carcinoma-related survival was identified in stage III patients undergoing laparoscopic resection. Overall, disease-free and carcinoma-related 5-year actuarial survivals were 48.5%, 50.5%, and 56.5%, respectively, for the open and 68.2%, 65.2%, and 76.4% for the laparoscopic group. Node positive patients who completed the laparoscopic resection had a longer 5-year disease-free survival (73% vs. 47.8%), carcinoma-related (82.1% vs. 54.5%) survival. There was a trend toward a reduction in the laparoscopic group, a finding similar to that of Lacy et al. (139). Capussotti also noted a trend toward a decreased incidence of distant metastases (189).

COST Trial and Expert Consensus

The long awaited results of the landmark COST trial have recently been published and at the time of writing considered the definitive study (142). Minimally invasive laparoscopic-assisted surgery was first considered in 1990 for patients undergoing colectomy for carcinoma. Concern that this approach would compromise survival by failing to achieve proper oncologic resection or adequate staging or by altering patterns of recurrence (based on frequent reports of recurrences within surgical wounds) prompted a controlled trial evaluation. Members of the COST study group conducted a trial with 48 institutions and randomly assigned 872 patients with carcinoma of the colon to undergo open or laparoscopic-assisted colectomy performed by credentialed surgeons. The median follow-up was 4.4 years. The primary endpoint was the time to recurrence of the carcinoma. Operating times were significantly longer in the laparoscopic surgery group than in the open colectomy group (150 vs. 95 minutes). Bowel margins were less than 5 cm in 6% of patients in the open colectomy group and 5% in the laparoscopic surgery group. In each group, the median number of lymph nodes examined was 12. Perioperative recovery was faster in the laparoscopic surgery group than in the open colectomy group as reflected by a shorter median hospital stay (5 vs. 6 days) and briefer use of parenteral narcotics (3 vs. 4 days) and oral analgesics (1 vs. 2 days). The rates of intraoperative complications (2% in open colectomy group and 4% laparoscopic group), 30-day postoperative mortality (1% open vs. 0.5% laparoscopic), complications at discharge and 60 days (open 20% vs. laparoscopic 21%), hospital readmission (open 10% vs. laparoscopic 12%), and reoperation (both $<2\%$) were very similar between groups. The percentage of patients receiving chemotherapy did not differ significantly between groups and paralleled the rate of stage III disease. At 3 years, the rates of recurrence were similar in the two groups—16% among patients in the group that underwent laparoscopic-assisted surgery and 18% among patients in the open colectomy group (hazard ratio for recurrence 0.86). Recurrence rates in surgical wounds were less than 1% in both groups. The overall survival rate at 3 years was also very similar in the two groups (86% in the laparoscopic group and 85% in the open colectomy group), hazard ratio for death in the laparoscopic group, 0.91; with no significant difference between the groups in the time to recurrence or overall survival for patients with any stage of carcinoma. They concluded in this multi-institutional study, the rates of recurrent carcinoma were similar after laparoscopic-assisted colectomy and open colectomy suggesting that the laparoscopic approach is an acceptable alternative to open surgery for colon carcinoma.

Based on this study, The American Society of Colon & Rectal Surgeons Executive Council held a special meeting May 12, 2004 to develop a position statement on "Laparoscopic Colectomy for Curable Cancer." The following statement was unanimously approved by the ASCRS Executive Council and endorsed by The Society of American Gastrointestinal Endoscopic Surgeons (SAGES).

Laparoscopic colectomy for curable cancer results in equivalent cancer-related survival to open colectomy when performed by experienced surgeons. Adherence to standard cancer resection techniques including but not limited to complete exploration of the abdomen, adequate proximal and distal margins, ligation of the major vessels at their respective origins, containment and careful tissue handling, and en bloc resection with negative tumor margins using the laparoscopic approach will result in acceptable outcomes. Based upon the COST trial, prerequisite experience should include at least 20 laparoscopic colorectal resections with anastomosis for benign disease or metastatic colon cancer before using the technique to treat curable cancer. Hospitals may base credentialing for laparoscopic colectomy for cancer on experience gained by formal graduate medical education training or advanced laparoscopic experience, participation in hands on training courses and outcomes.

The European Association of Endoscopic Surgery (EAES) initiated a consensus development conference on the laparoscopic resection of colon carcinoma (97). A systematic review of the current literature was combined with the opinions of experts in the field of colon carcinoma surgery to formulate evidence-based statements and recommendations on the laparoscopic resection of colon carcinoma. Advanced age, obesity, previous abdominal operations, were not considered absolute contraindications for laparoscopic colon surgery. The most common cause for conversion is the presence of a bulky or invasive carcinoma. Laparoscopic operation takes longer to perform than the open counterpart but the outcome is similar in terms of specimen size and pathological examination. Immediate postoperative morbidity and mortality are comparable for laparoscopic and open colonic surgery for carcinoma. The laparoscopic-operated patients had less postoperative pain, better preserved pulmonary function, earlier restoration of gastrointestinal function, and earlier discharge from the hospital. The postoperative stress response is lower after laparoscopic colectomy. The incidence of port-site metastases is $<1\%$. Survival after laparoscopic resection of colon carcinoma appears to be at least equal to survival after open resection. The costs of laparoscopic surgery for colon carcinoma are higher than those for open surgery. They concluded, laparoscopic resection of colon carcinoma is a safe and feasible procedure that improved short-term outcome. Results regarding the long-term survival of patients enrolled in large multicenter trials will determine its ultimate role.

A panel of worldwide recognized experts in laparoscopic colectomy was assembled and a consensus document was published (97). In brief, their findings are documented as follows. Reported morbidity with laparoscopic colon resection for carcinoma has varied widely but has not differed from that after open colectomy (97). Rates range from 1.5% to 28% with most in the 10% to 15% range (97). In a review of 11 studies, rates of wound infection were 5.7%, respiratory problems 3.1%, cardiac problems 2.9%, hemorrhage 1.9%, anastomotic leak 1.5%, urinary tract injury and small bowel perforations 0.6%, port-site herniation and hematoma 0.4%, and septicemia, peritonitis, anastomotic stricture, anastomotic edema, hypoxia, acute renal failure, renal insufficiency, urinary retention, deep venous thrombosis, small bowel obstruction, phlebitis, intra-abdominal abscess, each 0.2%. Mortality rates after laparoscopic colectomy were also similar to that of open colectomy (97). In most but not all reports, length of stay after laparoscopic colectomy is shorter than after open colectomy (97). Duration ranged from 5.7 to 18.7 days with differences in hospital stay between laparoscopic and open colectomy groups varying from 1 to 7 days. Analgesia needs have been measured by the number of doses per day required or the number of days analgesics are needed. Less analgesia is needed for laparoscopic colectomy. Gastrointestinal function has been measured in several ways, mainly, time to first bowel movement, time to passage of flatus, or time to resume oral intake. By all parameters, recovery is quicker with laparoscopic colorectal operations. Time to flatus ranged 1.5 to 4.5 days; time to bowel movement ranged 1.5 to 4.7 days, and time to oral intake 2.1 to 6.9 days (Table 1). Postoperative pulmonary function is less impaired after laparoscopic resection for colon carcinoma. Overall and disease-free survival following laparoscopic resections are equivalent to open resection (Tables 2–5). Attempts were made to quote the most recent work from an institution with multiple publications and reports with substantial numbers of patients.

With respect to quality of life, effects are most pronounced in the early days after operation. The operative costs for laparoscopic resection of colon carcinoma are higher because of longer operating times and the use of more expensive disposable devices. Furthermore, the stress response after laparoscopic colectomy is lower.

Abdominoperineal Resection

Darzi et al. (59) compared the adequacy of excision of the first 12 patients undergoing laparoscopic abdominoperineal resection of the rectum to the previous 16 patients undergoing open abdominoperineal resection. In all patients, the procedure was carried out with curative intent. The data demonstrate similar nodal harvest in both groups as well as extent of radial excision.

Chindasub et al. (62) reported on 10 patients who underwent laparoscopic abdominoperineal resection with

TABLE 2 ■ Long-term Results of Retrospective Noncomparative Studies of Laparoscopic Resection for Colon and Rectal Carcinoma

Author (Ref.)	Year	n	Conversion Rate (%)	Operating Time (min)	Morbidity (%)	Mortality (%)	LOS (days)	F/U (MOS)	Recurrence (%) Overall	Recurrence (%) Port-site	Recurrence (%) Local	Recurrence (%) Distant	Survival (%) Overall	Survival (%) DFS
Melotti et al. (152)	1999	163	20.4		15.1	0	–	36[a]		1.2			79	69
Franklin et al. (153)	2000	50[b]	6		14	2	–	24	40	0	6	34	39	49
Schiedeck et al. (154)	2000	399	6.3		37	1.8	14	30	8	0.3	1.5	6.3	–	98–86–89[c]
Anderson et al. (155)	2002	93	–	166–228[d]	22	2	8	40.3	15	1	–	–	100–77–52[c]	–
Lechaux et al. (156)	2002	166	11	150	12	2	–	65	11	0.6	–	–	79	61
Lujan et al. (140)	2002	102	7.8		23	1	–	64	14.7	2	2.9	10.7	64	–
Lumley et al. (157)	2002	154				1.1		71	13.6	0.6	2.6	10.3	91–83–74[c]	
Poulin et al. (158)	2002	80[e]				2.5		31	–	0	4.3		72.1	
		AR 52	27	205			6.5						93–87–53[c]	
		APR 28	35	210			8.0							
Scheidbach et al. (159)	2002	292	5.5	172	22.3	2.7		25.2	11.6	0	3.4	8.2	81	–
Yamamoto et al. (160)	2002	70[f]	2.9	–	18.6	–	8	23	2.9	0	–	2.9	100	92
Morino et al. (161)	2003	100[e]	12	250	36	2	12	46	–	1.4	4.2	–	73	81
Tsang et al. (162)	2003	44[e]	0	180	–	0	–	15	–	0	4.5	11.4	80	–
Watanabe et al. (163)	2003	130	2.3		14.6	0	8	61	–	0	2.3	1.5	97.9	–

[a]Stage III only.
[b]Includes all resections (RHC-APR—all procedures).
[c]Stage I, II, III.
[d]Varied with type of resection.
[e]Rectal carcinoma.
[f]T_{is}, T_1, T_2 only rectal.
Abbreviations: LOS, length of stay; F/u, follow-up; MOS, months of survival; DFS, disease-free survival; AR, anterior resection; APR, abdominoperineal resection.

TABLE 3 ■ Long-term Results of Retrospective Comparative Studies of Laparoscopic Resection for Colon and Rectal Carcinoma

Author (Ref.)	Year	Method	n	Conversion Rate (%)	Operation Time (min)	Morbidity (%)	Mortality (%)	LOS (days)	F/U (MOS)	Recurrence (%) Overall	Recurrence (%) Port-site	Recurrence (%) Local	Recurrence (%) Distant	Survival (%) Overall	Survival (%) DFS
Ramos et al. (144)	1997	L	18[a]	10	229	22.2	0	7.4			0	5.5	–	–	–
		O	18		208	16.6	5.5	12.9			0	16.5			
Bouvet et al. (164)	1998	L	91[b]	42	240	24	2.2	6	26		0	–	–	–	93
		O	57		150	21		7							98
Khalili et al. (145)	1998	L	80	7.5	161				21	13	0	3	10	88	–
		O	90	–	163				18	18	0	6	11	85	
Schwandner et al. (165)	1999	L	32[a]			31.3	–	–	33.1	12.5	0	0	12.5	–	–
		O	32			31.3			32.1	15.6	0	0	15.6		
Hong et al. (146)	2001	L	98	12.2	140	27	3.1	6.9	30.6	20.6	0	12.2	9.1	78.5	43.5
		O	219		129	39	1.8	10.9	21.6	17.8	1.4	8.7	9.2	78.5	43.5
Baker et al. (147)	2002	L	28[a]	25			3.6	13	35.6	32.1	0	14.3	7.1	42% at 41 mos	
		O	61				3.3	18	30.8	37.7	0	13.1	4.9	32% at 31 mos	
Anthuber et al. (166)	2003	L	101	11	218	31	0	14.4		7	0	2	5		
		O	334		219	65	5	19.9			0				

[a]Carcinoma rectum – APR
[b]All procedures.
[c]Right hemicolectomy.
Abbreviations: LOS, length of stay; L, laparoscopic; O, open; MOS, months of survival; DFS, disease-free survival.

TABLE 4 ■ Long-term Results of Prospective Nonrandomized Comparative Studies of Laparoscopic Resection for Colon and Rectal Carcinoma

										Recurrence (%)				Survival (%)	
Author (Ref.)	Year	Method	*n*	Conversion Rate (%)	Operation Time (min)	Morbidity (%)	Mortality (%)	LOS (days)	F/U (MOS)	Overall	Port-site	Local	Distant	Overall	DFS
Franklin et al. (167)	1996	L	191[a]			23.8		5.7			0			87	90
		O	224			17		9.7			–			81	92
Santoro et al. (168)	1999	L	50			14	0			20	2.5	–	–	–	73.2
		O	50			14	0			23	2.3	–	–	–	70.1
Hartley et al. (169)	2001	L	42[b]	33	180	28.6	0	13.5	38	–	0	5	–	71	–
		O	22		125	18	0	15			0	4.5	–	77	–
Champault et al. (148)	2002	L	74	8.1	145	13.5	0	8.2	52	24.3	2.7	–	–	63.1	
		O	83		125	33.7	0	12.3	56	25	–	–	–	59.1	
Feliciotti et al. (170)	2002	L	104	4.8			1.9		49	13.1	1	1.3	10.8	89	87
		O	93				1.1			0	0	2.7	10.7	87	87
Lezoche et al. (171)	2002	RHC L	55	0	190	1.9		9.2	42		2.7	5.4	–	86.5	
		RHC O	44	–	140	2.3		13.2		–		9	–	81.8	
		LHC L	86	7	240	7.5		10		1.5	1.5	1.5	–	97.1	
		LHC O	63	–	190	6.3		13.2		–	–	7.5	–	85.7	
Feliciotti et al. (172)	2003	L	81[b]	12.3			0		43.8	–	0	20.8	18.2	70.9	62.5
		O	43				0				0	16.6	21.2	60.6	60.6
Patankar et al. (141)	2003	L	172				1.2		52	16.3	0.6	3.5	12.2	69	–
		O	172				2.4		59	13.4	0	2.9	10.5	64	–

[a]All procedures.
[b]Rectal carcinoma.
Abbreviations: LOS, length of stay; L, laparoscopic; O, open; MOS, months of survival; DFS, disease-free survival; RHC, right hemicolectomy; LHC, left hemicolectomy.

only two complications: postoperative bleeding that required open operation and one case of colostomy ischemia from a tight aperture.

Kockerling et al. (190) analyzed the results of 116 patients who underwent laparoscopic abdominoperineal resections, 84.5% of which were performed with curative intent. The mean operating time was 226 minutes. Intraoperative complications occurred in 6% which in more than half of the cases was a vascular injury involving the presacral venous plexus; the conversion rate was 3.4%. Postoperatively, the overall morbidity rate was 34.4%. Reoperation was necessary in 5.2% of patients performed for bleeding in one half of the cases and ileus in the other half. Postoperative mortality was 1.7%. In most of the curative resections an oncologically radical operation with high transection of the inferior mesenteric artery and a complete dissection of the pelvis down to the floor was performed. The median number of lymph nodes investigated was 11.5. At least one follow-up examination was performed in 81% of patients with a mean follow-up period being

TABLE 5 ■ Long-term Results of Prospective Randomized Comparative Studies of Laparoscopic Resection for Colon and Rectal Carcinoma

										Recurrence (%)				Survival (%)	
Author (Ref.)	Year	Method	*n*	Conversion Rate (%)	Operation Time (min)	Morbidity (%)	Mortality (%)	LOS (days)	F/U (MOS)	Overall	Port-site	Local	Distant (%)	Overall	DFS
Curet et al. (149)	2000	L	25[a]	28	210	4	4	5.2	59	5.8	0	–	–	68	
		O	18		138	27.8	0	7.3		–	0	–	–	39	
Lacy et al. (139)	2002	L	111	11	142	10.8	0.9	5.2	44	17	0.9	6.6	8.8	82	91
		O	108	–	118	28.7	2.8	7.9	43	27	0	6.6	13.7	74	79
COST (142)	2004	L	435	21	150	21.1	0.5	5	53	17.5	0.5			86 } 3 yr	
		O	428		95	19.9	0.9	6		19.6	0.2			85	
Leung et al. (150)	2004	L	203[b]	23	190	17.2	2	8.2	39	22	0	6.6	18	76	75
		O	200		144	20.5	1	8.7	35	18	0	4.1	15	73	78
COLOR, Veldkamp et al. (143)	2005	L	627	17	202 (50–540)	21	1	8.2							
		O	621		170 (45–580)	20	2	9.3							
CLASICC, Guillou et al. (151)	2005	L	526	29	180 (140–220)	13 C-8, R-18	5	C-9 R-11							
		O	268		135 (100–175)	11 C-8, R-14	4	C-9 R-13							

[a]All procedures.
[b]Rectosigmoid carcinoma.
[c]Gas, bowel movement.
Abbreviations: C, colon; R, rectum; LOS, length of stay; L, laparoscopic; O, open; MOS, months of survival; DFS, disease-free survival.

491 days. Local recurrence developed in 7% of patients and distant metastases developed in 6% of patients. The recurrence-free survival rate was 71%.

Crohn's Disease

Laparoscopic techniques are increasingly being used in the operative management of patients with Crohn's disease. The inflammatory process associated with Crohn's disease often makes dissection difficult, even in open procedures. For uncomplicated Crohn's disease, conversion rates have been low (in the range of 4%) but rise dramatically with complicated Crohn's disease being about 25% with abscess or fistula and over 50% if a palpable phlegmon has been identified (191).

Reissman et al. (192) reported on 51 patients who underwent a laparoscopic or a laparoscopic-assisted procedure for Crohn's disease. The indications included terminal ileitis in 31 patients, colitis in 11, perianal disease in four, duodenal disease in three, and rectovaginal fistula and rectourethral fistula in one patient each. Thirty-two patients underwent an ileocolic resection. Total abdominal colectomy with ileorectal anastomosis was performed in six patients with end ileostomy in one, takedown of end ileostomy and ileorectal anastomosis in three, duodenal bypass gastrojejunostomy in three, and loop ileostomy in six patients. The mean operating time was 2.4 hours (range, 0.6 to 4.5 hours) and the mean length of hospital stay was 5.1 days (range, 3 to 18 days). Eight complications were noted in seven patients (14%), which included enterotomy in two patients, bleeding in two, stoma obstruction in two, pelvic sepsis in one, and efferent limb obstruction in one. The procedure was converted to laparotomy in seven patients (14%) due to a large inflammatory mass in five and bleeding in two patients. There were no mortalities. The authors concluded that laparoscopic surgery is a feasible, versatile, safe modality in the surgical management of Crohn's disease.

Bergamaschi et al. (193) reported on the long-term outcomes of 39 patients who underwent laparoscopic ileocolic resection for Crohn's disease compared with 53 patients who had previously undergone open ileocolic resection by the same surgeons at the same institution. At 5-year follow-up, 90.5% of open ileocolic resection patients and 92.3% of laparoscopic ileocolic resection patients were available. Five-year small bowel obstruction rates were 35.4% and 11.1%, respectively, in open ileocolic and laparoscopic ileocolic patients. Five-year recurrence rates were 29.1% and 27.7%. Median time to recurrence was 48 and 56 months, respectively, following open ileocolic resection and laparoscopic ileocolic resection.

Hasegawa et al. (194) assessed the feasibility of laparoscopic surgery for recurrent Crohn's disease and the role of laparoscopy in reoperation. Laparoscopic operations were attempted in 52 patients with ileal or ileocolic Crohn's disease. Of these 16 procedures were performed for recurrence at the anastomotic site. The remaining 45 operations were performed as primary procedures. The median follow-up was 48 months. The median time to reoperation was 46 months. The incidence of enteric fistula and the conversion rate did not differ significantly between the two groups. Although the operating time was significantly longer in the recurrent group, there were no differences in the rate of postoperative complications and hospital stay. They concluded that laparoscopic surgery for recurrent Crohn's disease is feasible in selected patients without an increase in conversion rate or postoperative complications.

Wu et al. (195) conducted a study to determine whether the presence of an abscess, phlegmon, or recurrent disease at a previous ileocolic anastomosis for Crohn's disease was a contraindication to a successful laparoscopic-assisted ileocolic resection. They attempted 46 laparoscopic-assisted ileocolic resections. Fourteen patients had an abscess or phlegmon treated with bowel rest before operation (group 1), 10 patients had recurrent Crohn's disease at the previous ileocolic anastomosis (group 2), and 22 patients had no previous operation and no phlegmon or abscess associated with their disease (group 3). These groups were compared with each other and with 70 consecutive open ileocolic resections for Crohn's disease during the same time period (group 4). Operative blood loss and time were greater in group 4 than in groups 1, 2, and 3 (245 vs. 151, 131, and 195 mL, respectively, and 202 vs. 152, 144, and 139 minutes, respectively). Conversion to open procedure occurred in five patients (group 1, 7%; group 2, 20%; group 3, 9%). Morbidity was highest in group 4 (21% vs. 0%, 10%, and 10%, respectively). Only one patient died (group 4, 1%). Length of hospital stay was longest in group 4 (7.9 days vs. 4.8, 3.9, and 4.5 days, respectively). They concluded co-morbid preoperative findings such as abscess, phlegmon, or recurrent disease at the previous ileocolic anastomosis are not contraindications to a successful laparoscopic-assisted ileocolic resection in selected patients.

Moorthy et al. (196) conducted a study to identify factors that would predict conversion to patients undergoing laparoscopic surgery for Crohn's disease. Data were collected from 48 patients who underwent 57 laparoscopic procedures—26 for recurrent disease. The conversion rate was 42.3% for recurrent disease and 13% for primary disease. Surgery for recurrence, time from diagnosis and the presence of a clinical mass were factors that predicted conversion.

Benoist et al. (197) reported that laparoscopic ileocecal resection in Crohn's disease is safe and effective even in fistulizing disease. There are no significant differences between laparoscopic and open ileocecal resection especially in terms of morbidity and mortality rates. Consequently, because laparoscopic surgery seems to offer cosmetic advantages, it should be considered the procedure of choice for patients with ileocecal Crohn's disease.

A summary of results of laparoscopic resection for Crohn's disease are summarized in Tables 6 and 7.

Ulcerative Colitis

As experience is gained in performing laparoscopic colon resection, procedures of increasing complexity such as total abdominal colectomy and laparoscopic-assisted restorative proctocolectomy are being performed by individuals with great skill and experience (207,208). Laparoscopic total abdominal colectomy for acute colitis has also been reported (209). The benefits of a hand-assist in restorative proctocolectomy have been published (210).

TABLE 6 ■ **Results of Laparoscopic Resection for Crohn's Disease**

Author (Ref.)	Year	Procedure	n	Conversion Rate (%)	Operating Time (min)	Resumption PO Intake (days)	Bowel Activity (days)	Morbidity: Intraop (%)	Morbidity: Postop (%)	Mortality (%)	LOS (days)
Canin-Endres et al. (198)	1999	Ileocolic	70	1	183	1	–	–	74	–	4.2
		Small bowel resection	13								
		Right hemicolectomy	3								
		Subtotal colectomy	3								
		Sigmoid resection	5								
Hamel et al. (199)	2001	Ileocolic	109	17	167		3.2	7	25	–	8.8
Evans et al. (200)	2002	Ileocolic	84	18	145	–	–	–	10.7	–	5.6
		Subtotal colectomy	21	24	231		3.3	29	33	–	8.8

Abbreviations: PO, per os; LOS, length of stay.

Apart from an obviously better cosmetic situation there is controversy in the actual benefit of a laparoscopic and laparoscopic-assisted techniques in restorative proctocolectomy. Kienle et al. (211) reported 59 consecutive patients with ulcerative colitis and familial polyposis who were treated by laparoscopic-assisted restorative proctocolectomy. The colon was mobilized laparoscopically with a four-trocar technique facilitating vascular dissection, rectal resection, an ileo-anal pouch construction to be done through a Pfannenstiel incision. A protective ileostomy was constructed only in patients where the operation was difficult or where the anastomosis was under tension. Laparoscopic mobilization was successful in 91.2% of patients. Two patients had to be primarily converted because of exceeding the set time limits; three other patients had to have an additional median laparotomy. These five patients all had an increased body mass index (BMI) which was a statistically significant risk factor for failure of the laparoscopic technique. Major complications developed in 18.6% of patients. Nine patients required secondary ileostomies, all of them either were under high dose immunosuppression or had an increased BMI. They subsequently reported 50 consecutive patients with familial adenomatous polyposis (FAP) or ulcerative colitis who underwent laparoscopic restorative protocolectomy using only a small perumbilical incision of 4 cm or less for vascular dissection and pouch formation; all other steps were performed entirely laparoscopically (212). In four patients (8%), the operation was converted to an open procedure. The diagnosis of ulcerative colitis was associated with a higher overall rate of complications, and an increased body mass index with a higher rate of major complications. The occurrence of wound infection was related to the diagnosis of ulcerative colitis. Conversion resulted in greater blood loss, but not in a higher complication rate. Patients with an increased BMI and those taking immunosuppressive therapy had a longer hospital stay.

Ky et al. (207) examined the results of one-stage laparoscopic-assisted restorative proctocolectomy in 32 patients—29 with mucosal ulcerative colitis, and three with

TABLE 7 ■ **Results of Retrospective Comparative Studies of Laparoscopic Ileocolic Resection for Crohn's Disease**

Author (Ref.)	Year	Method	n	Conversion Rate (%)	Operating Time (min)	Resumption PO Intake (days)	Bowel Activity (days)	Morbidity (%)	Mortality (%)	LOS (days)
Alabaz et al. (201)	2000	L	26	11.5	150	–	–	15.3		7
		O	48		91	–	–	16.6		9.6
Bemelman et al. (202)	2000	L	30	6.6	138	2.8	3.4	10	–	5.7
		O	48		104	3.3	3.5	14.6	–	10.2
Milsom et al. (203)	2001	L	31	6.5	140	–	3	16.1	0	5
		O	29		85	–	3.3	31	9	6
Tabet et al. (204)	2001	L	32	12.5	124	–	–	9.4	–	–
		O	29		122			24.1	–	–
Young-Fadok et al. (205)	2001	L	33	5.9	147	0–2[a]	–	–	–	4
		O	33		124	3–5[b]			–	7
Duepree et al. (206)	2002	L	24	4.8	–	0[a]	2	14.3	–	3
		O	21		–	2	4	16.7	–	5
Benoist et al. (197)	2003	L	24	17	179	2.8	2.5	20	0	7.7
		O	32	–	198	3.5	3.3	10	0	8
Bergamaschi et al. (193)	2003	L	39	0	105	–	–	10.2	–	5.6
		O	53	–	85	–	–	9.4	–	11.2

[a] Day of operation.
[b] Clear liquids–solids.
Abbreviations: PO, per oral; LOS, length of stay; L, laparoscopic; O, open.

FAP. There were no conversions to open operation. There were two intraoperative complications and inconsequential rectal perforation during mobilization and one staple line misfire. There were 11 postoperative complications: three obstruction/ileus, two pouchitis, two wound infections, two strictures, one pelvic abscess, and one pouch leak (at the top of the J). Three patients required reoperation (one temporary ileostomy, one lysis of adhesions, and one trans-pouch drainage). The median number of bowel movements was 7 per day. They concluded a one-stage laparoscopic-assisted restorative proctocolectomy can be performed effectively and safely.

Bell and Seymour (213) reviewed the records of 18 patients with poorly controlled fulminant colitis on aggressive immunosuppressive therapy who underwent laparoscopic subtotal colectomy. Postoperative complications occurred in six patients (33%). Postoperative length of stay was 5 days versus 8.8 days for a group of six patients who had undergone open subtotal colectomy for the same indications. The relatively high morbidity rate in these patients is likely related to their compromised status at the time of operation. Laparoscopic subtotal colectomy in patients with fulminant colitis allows for earlier hospital discharge, facilitates subsequent pelvic pouch construction, and provides an excellent alternative to conventional two- or three-stage surgical treatment.

Hasegawa et al. (214) reviewed 18 patients with ulcerative colitis who underwent laparoscopic restorative proctocolectomy. Five trocars were placed. After the entire colon and rectum were mobilized and the vessels, divided intracorporally, the rectum was divided with the use of a laparoscopic linear stapler. A pouch-anal anastomosis was fashioned with the use of a double-stapling technique. A diverting loop ileostomy was fashioned. There were no conversions to the open procedure. Median operative time was 360 minutes. Six postoperative complications occurred (two wound sepsis; one bowel obstruction; two anastomotic strictures; one pouchitis). In one patient bowel obstruction developed 3 months after operation which was managed conservatively. Median length of hospital stay was 9 days.

Dunker et al. (215) assessed the feasibility and the safety of emergency laparoscopic colectomy in IBD patients with severe acute colitis. A total of 42 consecutive patients underwent an emergency colectomy with end ileostomy. Ten patients had laparoscopic-assisted colectomy and 32 had open colectomy. There were no conversions in the laparoscopic group. The operation time was longer in the laparoscopic group than in the open group (271 minutes vs. 151 minutes) but the hospital stay was shorter (14.6 days vs. 18.0 days). Complications were similar in the two groups. They concluded laparoscopic-assisted colectomy in IBD patients with severe acute colitis is feasible and as safe as open colectomy.

Rivadeneira et al. (210) evaluated the effectiveness of a hand-assisted laparoscopic approach compared with a conventional laparoscopic method in patients undergoing restorative proctocolectomy. They compared 23 patients comprising 10 hand-assisted and 13 conventional laparoscopic patients. There were no differences in incision size between the hand-assisted and conventional laparoscopic cases (8 cm). The median operative time was significantly shorter in the hand-assisted group (247 minutes) compared with the conventional laparoscopic group (300 minutes). The length of stay was similar between the two groups (hand-assisted 4 days vs. conventional 6 days). Complications occurred in four hand-assisted patients (40%; two ileus, mechanical obstruction, and dehydration) and in four patients undergoing conventional laparoscopic method (31%; two anastomotic leaks, ileus, and mechanical obstruction). They concluded the hand-assisted method resulted in a significant reduction in operative time without detriment to bowel function, length of stay, or patient outcome and is likely to replace conventional laparoscopic methods as a preferred laparoscopic approach for this technically challenging procedure.

A summary of the results of laparoscopic total colectomy for acute nonfulminant colitis is summarized in Table 8 and the results of laparoscopic total proctocolectomy and ileal pouch-anal anastomosis are summarized in Table 9.

Stomas

Fuhrman and Ota (72) reported their early experience with 17 patients who had successfully undergone laparoscopic intestinal diversion. The mean follow-up of this group was 24.3 weeks. Seven patients had their stomas created as part of a laparoscopic abdominoperineal resection, six patients underwent palliative laparoscopic colostomy for an obstructing carcinoma of the rectum or a colorectal-genitourinary fistula, and four patients treated by local excision of a carcinoma were believed to require a proximal protecting fecal diversion. All six patients treated with palliative intent experienced successful relief from their obstruction or fistula and were able to resume enteral nutrition. Complications included prolapse in one patient and paracolostomy hernia in another. Neither the complication required further operative correction.

TABLE 8 ■ **Results of Laparoscopic Total Colectomy for Acute Nonfulminant Colitis**

Author (Ref.)	Year	Method	*n*	Conversion Rate (%)	Operating Time (min)	Bowel Activity (days)	Morbidity (%)	LOS (days)
Marcello et al. (209)	2001[a]	L	19	0	210	1	16	4
		O	29		120	2	24	6
Bell et al. (213)	2002[b]	L	18	0	220–360 (range)	–	33	5
		O	6					8.8

[a]Crohn's disease and chronic ulcerative colitis.
[b]Chronic ulcerative colitis.
Abbreviations: LOS, length of stay; L, laparoscopic; O, open.

TABLE 9 ■ Results of Laparoscopic Total Proctocolectomy and Ileal Pouch-Anal Anastomosis

Author (Ref.)	Year	Method	n	Conversion Rate (%)	Operating Time (min)	Resumption PO Intake (days)	Bowel Activity (days)	Morbidity (%)	Mortality (%)	LOS (days)
Schmitt et al. (216)	1994	L	22[a]	–	240	3.6	4.2	55	0	8.7
		O	20	–	120	4.3	3.3	30	0	8.9
Marcello et al. (208)	2000	L	20	0	330	–	2	20	–	7
		O	20		230	–	4	25	–	8
Araki et al. (217)	2001	L	21	–	215	–	1.7	33.3	–	3.6
		O	11		198	–	5.4	45.5	–	3.9
Hasegawa et al. (214)	2002	L	18	0	360	–	–	33.3	–	9
Ky et al. (207)	2002	L	32	0	315	–	4.4	34.4	–	6
Pace et al. (218)	2002	L	13	8	255	–	–	46	0	7

[a]13 MUC + 7 FAP.
Abbreviations: PO, per oral; LOS, length of stay; L, laparoscopic; O, open.

Oliveira et al. (219) reviewed 32 patients who underwent laparoscopic intestinal diversion (25 loop ileostomies, four loop colostomies, and three end colostomies). Indications for fecal diversion were fecal incontinence (11), Crohn's disease (six) unresectable rectal carcinoma (four), pouch-vaginal fistula (three), rectovaginal fistula (two), colonic inertia (two), radiation proctitis (one), anal stenosis (one), Kaposi's sarcoma of the rectum (one), and tuberculous fistula (one). Conversion was required in five patients (15.6%) because of the presence of adhesions (three), enterotomy (one), or colotomy (one). Major postoperative complications occurred in two patients (6%) and both cases consisted of stoma outlet obstruction after construction of a loop ileostomy. One patient underwent reoperation, at which time a rotation of the terminal ileum at the stoma site was found. The other patient had narrow fascial opening that was successfully managed with 2 weeks of self-intubation of the stoma. The mean operative time was 76 minutes (range, 30 to 210 minutes), the mean length of hospitalization was 6.2 days (range, 2 to 13 days), and stoma function started after a mean 3.1 days (range, 1 to 6 days). The authors concluded that the laparoscopic creation of intestinal stomas is safe, feasible, and effective. Care must be taken to ensure adequate fascial opening and correct limb orientation.

Ludwig et al. (191) reported their initial experience in assessing the safety and efficacy of laparoscopic stoma procedures. A simple two-cannula technique was used in 24 such procedures (16 loop ileostomies, six end-sigmoid colostomies, one transverse colostomy, and one loop-sigmoid colostomy). Indications for diversion were rectovaginal fistula (seven), perianal sepsis (seven), incontinence (four), advanced rectal or colon carcinoma (four), and complicated pelvic infection (two). There were 15 women and nine men with a median age of 44 years (range, 25 to 88 years). The median operative time was 60 minutes (range, 20 to 120 minutes) and the median blood loss was 50 mL (range, 0 to 150 mL). There were no intraoperative complications. One case was converted to a laparotomy because of dense adhesions. The median time to passage of both flatus and stool was 1 day (range, 1 to 3 days) for ileostomy patients, 2 days (range, 2 to 4 days) for flatus, and 3 days (range, 2 to 6 days) for stool after colostomy. The median time to discharge was 6 days (range, 2 to 28 days) and was often delayed by the primary disease process or ostomy teaching. One major postoperative complication, a pulmonary embolism, occurred 8 days after operation in a patient with near obstructing, widely metastatic colon carcinoma. This patient later died of pulmonary failure. All stomas functioned well, with no revisions required. The authors concluded that laparoscopic fecal diversion procedures can be performed safely, simply, and effectively.

Swain and Ellis (220) conducted a retrospective review of the medical records of 53 consecutive patients who underwent laparoscopic-assisted creation of a loop ileostomy as an adjunct to anorectal or perineal surgery. The average duration of operation for laparoscopy-assisted creation of a loop ileostomy was 47 minutes with no conversion to laparotomy. All patients were able to tolerate a regular diet on the first postoperative day. Closure was accomplished 69 days later with an average operative time of 52 minutes. One patient developed an ileus after takedown of his stoma. The other 52 patients were able to tolerate a regular diet by the second postoperative day. They concluded laparoscopy-assisted creation of loop ileostomy is an effective method for temporary fecal diversion in patients undergoing anorectal surgery.

Liu et al. (221) assessed the results of laparoscopic stoma creation for fecal diversion in 80 patients. The most common indications were unresectable advanced colorectal carcinoma ($n=20$), pelvic malignancy (e.g., ovarian, cervix and prostate, $n=16$), and perianal Crohn's disease with complex fistulas ($n=16$). Only in one female patient with pelvic malignant disease the procedure was converted to laparotomy due to obesity (conversion rate 1.3%). Laparoscopic stoma creation included loop ileostomy ($n=30$), loop sigmoid colostomy ($n=40$), and sigmoid colostomy ($n=9$). Postoperative complications were documented in nine patients (overall morbidity rate, 11.4%), including four minor complications treated conservatively (two cases of prolonged atonia and one case each of pneumonia and urinary tract infection) and five major complications requiring reoperation (reoperation rate, 6.3%): one parastomal abscess (drainage), one stoma retraction following rod dislocation (laparoscopic stoma recreation), small bowel obstruction in two patients (small bowel resection), one port-site hernia (fascial closure), and hemorrhage (managed by relaparoscopy). Mean operative time was 74 minutes. Patients were discharged from hospital after a mean of 10.3 days. They believe laparoscopic stoma creation is the method of choice for fecal diversion.

Hartmann's Closure

Sosa et al. (75) reported their experience with laparoscopic-assisted Hartmann's reversal attempted in 18 patients and completed in 14 patients. The average hospital stay in the laparoscopic-completed group was 6.3 days (range, 4 to 10 days). This group had a 0% mortality rate and a 14.3% morbidity rate. Sixty-five patients undergoing reversal of Hartmann's procedure by laparotomy had an average hospital stay of 9.5 days (range, 6 to 34 days). The authors concluded that laparoscopic-assisted Hartmann's reversal results in comparable morbidity, but may be associated with a shorter hospital stay when compared with laparotomy.

Regadas et al. (222) reported on 20 cases of laparoscopic-assisted colorectal anastomoses. The mean length of procedure was 130 minutes. There were two intraoperative complications, a rectal perforation with the stapler and an incomplete anastomosis. Six patients (30%) said that they had no postoperative pain. Bowel sounds occurred in a mean time of 18.2 hours, flatus in 26.4 hours, and bowel movement in an average of 2.5 postoperative days. Liquid diet was started after an average of 1.5 days, and the mean hospital stay was 4 days. There were three conversions (15%) because of excessive pelvic adherence, pelvic neoplastic invasion, and rectal perforation with a stapler. Postoperative complications occurred in seven cases (35%), an incisional hernia, two wound infections, one wound bleeding, an acute renal failure, an undetermined peritonitis, and a small pelvic abscess. No mortality occurred in these cases.

In a review of six series of colostomy closure, Luchtefeld (27) found that overall complication rates ranged from 4.3% to 34% with wound infection in 4.9% to 24% of patients, anastomotic leak and/or fistula in 0% to 10%, and small bowel obstruction in 1.3% to 4.3% of patients. When compared with open colectomy, laparoscopic-assist colectomy was found to have comparable morbidity and mortality rates.

Delgado et al. (223) reported laparoscopy reversal of Hartmann's procedure in 11 patients who had been treated for inflammatory disease or carcinoma of the colon. Restoration of intestinal continuity was achieved in 10 of them. There were no postoperative complications. The mean operative time was 144 minutes and the mean duration of postoperative ileus was 48 hours. The mean hospital stay was 7 days.

Diverticular Disease

Advantages of the adoption of the laparoscopic technique for the treatment of diverticular disease have been reported by many authors. The first surgeons to do so were Bruce et al. (224) who conducted a retrospective comparison of laparoscopic and conventional operation in patients with chronic diverticulitis to assess morbidity, recovery from operation, and cost. Laparoscopic resection involved complete intracorporeal dissection, bowel division, and anastomosis with extracorporeal placement of an anvil. Resections were performed laparoscopically in 25 patients and by open technique in 17 patients by two independent operating teams. In the laparoscopic group, three operations were converted to open laparotomy (12%) because of unclear anatomy. Major complications occurred in two patients who underwent laparoscopic resection, both requiring laparotomy, and in one patient in the conventional surgery group who underwent CT-guided drainage of an abscess. Patients who underwent laparoscopic resection tolerated a regular diet sooner than patients who underwent conventional operation (3.2 vs. 5.7 days) and were discharged from the hospital earlier (4.2 vs. 6.8 days). Overall costs were higher in the laparoscopic group than the open group (US $10,230 vs. $7068) because of a significantly longer total operating room time (397 vs. 115 minutes). Follow-up studies with a mean of 1 year revealed two port-site infections in the laparoscopic group and one wound infection in the open group. Of patients undergoing conventional resection, one patient experienced a postoperative bowel obstruction that was managed nonoperatively and one patient developed an incarcerated. incisional hernia that required urgent laparotomy. The authors concluded that the higher cost of operating room usage time makes the laparoscopic technique difficult to justify economically.

Since then many surgeons have reported the results of their experience (Tables 10 and 11), while others have reported comparative results of laparoscopic and open techniques (Table 12). Several publications have addressed issues specifically to the laparoscopic approach to diverticular disease. Not unexpectedly, patients who suffer from complicated diverticular disease would be expected to encounter a higher complication and conversion rate.

Vargas et al. (233) reported uncomplicated disease was associated with a 14% conversion rate whereas patients with complicated diverticular disease defined as fistula, perforation, stricture and previous percutaneous drainage of diverticular abscess, sustained a 61% conversion rate. Similarly, Kockerling et al. (227) reported a 4.8% conversion rate for patients with less severe diverticulitis defined as those with less severe peridiverculitis, stenosis, or recurrent attacks of inflammation compared with an 18.2% conversion rate for patients with complicated diverticulitis defined as those with perforated diverticulitis and those with fistula and bleeding.

Schwandner et al. (241) reported on laparoscopic surgery for acute complicated diverticulitis, chronically recurrent diverticulitis, sigmoid stenosis or outlet obstruction caused by chronic diverticulitis. In a series of 396 patients who underwent laparoscopic colectomy, the most common reasons for conversion were directly related to the inflammatory process, abscess or fistulas. The total complication rate was 18.4%, with the major complication rate being 7.6%. The most common complication requiring operation was hemorrhage in 3.3%. Anastomotic leakage occurred in 1.6%. Minor complications were noted in 10.7%, late-onset complications occurred in 2.7%. Despite the complicated nature of their patients, they believe laparoscopic colectomy is safe, feasible and effective.

Scheidbach et al. (237) reported the results of laparoscopic treatment of 1545 patients with sigmoid diverticulitis from the data collected in an ongoing prospective multicenter study carried out by the Laparoscopic Colorectal Surgery Study Group. The institutions participating in the study were divided into groups by experience (group I, >100 procedures; group II, 30–100 procedures; group III <30 procedures). Uncomplicated diverticulitis was present in 87.6% of patients, whereas 12.4% had a complicated form of diverticular disease (Hinchey I–IV, diverticular bleeding, fistula formation). Cases of complicated diverticulitis were

TABLE 10 ■ **Results of Laparoscopic Sigmoid Resection for Uncomplicated Diverticulitis**

Author (Ref.)	Year	*n*	Conversion Rate (%)	Operating Time (min)	PO Intake (days)	Bowel Activity (days)	Morbidity (%)	Mortality (%)	LOS (days)
Stevenson et al. (225)	1998	100	8	180	2	2	21	0	4
Berthou et al. (226)	1999	110	8.2	167	–	2.3	7.3	0	8.2
Kockerling et al. (227)	1999	304[a]	7.2	–	–	–	14.8	1.1	–
Schlachta et al. (228)	1999	70	4	150	3	–	27.1	–	5
Smadja et al. (229)	1999	54	9.2	298	–	2.3	14.3	0	6.4
Siriser et al. (230)	1999	65	4.6	179	2.6	2.2	17	0	7.6
Burgel et al. (231)	2000	56	14	300	–	2.4	16	0	9.4
Carbajo et al. (232)	2000	52	3.8	130	2.5	–	15	–	5.5
Vargas et al. (233)	2000	69[a]	26	158	3.5	2.9	10.1	0	4.2
Bouillot et al. (234)	2002	179[a]	13.9	223	3.3	2.5	14.9	0	9.3
Trebuchet et al. (235)	2002	170	4.1	141	3.4	2.5	12.4	0	8.5
Pugliese et al. (236)	2004	49	2.0	175	4.5	3.5	12.2	0	9.2
Scheidbach et al. (237)	2004	Group I, 153[b]	4.4	153	–	–	15.9	0.2	–
		Group II, 169	6.7	169	–	–	16.6	0.5	–
		Group III, 184	7.7	184	–	–	18.6	0.4	–
Bartus et al. (238)	2005	149	5	176	–	–	–	–	4.4

[a]Some were complicated (48).
[b]Group I >100 procedures; group II 30–100 procedures; Group III <30 procedures.
Abbreviations: PO, per os; LOS, length of stay.

significantly more frequently operated on at institutions with greater experience (group I, 20.8%; group II, 8.7%; group III, 7.9%). Despite this fact, these institutions still had better intraoperative complication rates (Table 10). As expected, conversion rates were higher for complicated (10.9%) versus uncomplicated (5.5%) cases. They concluded an increase in experience is associated with an expansion of laparoscopic indications to include complicated forms of diverticulitis with comparable intraoperative and postoperative complication rates, operating time, and mortality rates. Furthermore, the morbidity and mortality rates for patients with uncomplicated disease was 14.8% and 1.1%, respectively; the corresponding rates for complicated diverticular disease being 28.9% and 2.2%.

O'Sullivan et al. (251) reported the use of laparoscopic peritoneal lavage in conjunction with parenteral fluids and antibiotic therapy in the management of eight patients with generalized peritonitis secondary to perforated diverticular disease of the colon. All patients made a complete recovery with resumption of normal diet within 5 to 8 days. No patient has required operative intervention during the 12- to 48-month follow-up.

Franklin et al. (239) reported their experience treating 43 patients with acute complicated diverticulitis, including emergency cases. These patients included: eight with colonic diverticular perforation (Hartmann's procedure in six, omental patch closure in two), 18 patients who underwent diagnostic laparoscopy with drainage and lavage only without resection, four patients with laparoscopic colonic resection for recurrent bleeding, six patients who underwent laparoscopic resection and reanastomosis for colonic fistula and finally, seven patients who underwent laparoscopic resection and colostomy for colonic obstruction. The morbidity rate was 37% but there was no mortality. They felt that the laparoscopic approach led to improvement in postoperative patient status, decreasing the risk of wound infection, atelectasis, and the overall length of hospital stay in these patients.

Obesity is recognized as being associated with increased operative difficulty. Tuech et al. (252) assessed the outcome of laparoscopic colectomy for sigmoid diverticulitis in normal weight, overweight, and obese patients. The patients were divided into three groups: group 1 ($n=29$) consisted of healthy normal weight patients

TABLE 11 ■ **Results of Laparoscopic Sigmoid Resection for Complicated Diverticulitis**

Author (Ref.)	Year	*n*	Conversion Rate (%)	Operating Time (min)	PO Intake (days)	Bowel Activity (days)	Morbidity (%)	Mortality (%)	LOS (days)
Franklin et al. (239)	1997	58	25.8	–	–	–	37.2	0	10.7
Schlachta et al. (228)	1999	22	14	165	3	–	22.7	–	5
Menenakos et al. (240)	2003	18	5.5	237	–	2.9	27.7	0	10
Pugliese et al. (236)	2004	54	3.7	195	5.3	3.5	7.4	0	10.2
Scheidbach et al. (237)	2004	192	10.9	–	–	–	17.4	0.4	–
Schwandner et al. (241)	2004	396	6.8	193	–	6.8	18.4	0.5	11.8
Bartus et al. (238)	2005	36	25	220	–	–	–	–	6.2
Laurent et al. (242)	2005	16	18.8	172	–	–	12.5	0	5.7

Abbreviations: PO, per os; LOS, length of stay.

TABLE 12 ■ Results of Comparative Studies of Laparoscopic Sigmoid Resection for Diverticulitis

Author	Year	Method	*n*	Conversion Rate (%)	Operating Time (min)	PO Intake (days)	Bowel Activity (days)	Morbidity (%)	Mortality (%)	LOS (days)
Bruce et al. (224)	1996	L	25	12	397	3.2	4.2	16	–	4.2
		O	17		115	5.7	6.8	23	–	6.8
Liberman et al. (26)	1996	L	14	–	192	2.9	2.9	14	0	6.3
		O	14		183	6.1	6	14	0	9.2
Sher et al. (243)	1997	L	6 Hinchey-I	0	215	–	–	0	–	5
		O	12 Hinchey-II–III	50	213	–	–	33.3	–	6
			18	–	137	–	–	–	–	7–10
Kohler et al. (244)	1998	L	27	7.5	165	4.5	3.7	16	0	7.9
		O	34		121	5.8	5.3	61.8	0	14.3
Faynsod et al. (245)	2000	L	20	30	251	1	–	10	–	4.8
		O	20		243	5	–	10	–	7.8
Tuech et al. (246)	2000	L	22	9	234	–	–	18	–	13.1
		O	24		136	–	–	50	–	20.2
Senagore et al. (247)	2002	L	61	6.6	109	–	–	–	1.6	3.1
		O	71		101	–	–	–	0	6.8
Dwivedi et al. (248)	2002	L	66	19.7	212	2.9	–	18	0	4.8
		O	88		143	4.9	–	24	0	8.8
Lawrence et al. (249)	2003	L	56	7.1	170	–	–	9	0	4.1
		O	215		140	–	–	27	1.4	9
Gonzalez et al. (250)	2004	L	95	–	170	–	2.8	19	1	7
		O	80		156	–	3.7	32	4	12

Abbreviations: PO, per os; LOS, length of stay; L, laparoscopic; O, open.

(BMI 18–24.9); group 2 ($n=27$) consisted of overweight patients (BMI 25–29.9), group 3 ($n=21$) consisted of obese patients (BMI 30–39.9). There was no difference among the three groups in ASA classification, postoperative length of hospital stay or in-patient rehabilitation. The operating time did not differ for groups 1 and 2 (187 minutes vs. 210 minutes) but it was shorter in group 1 than group 3 (187 vs. 247 minutes). The conversion rate was similar for all three groups, 17.2% in group 1, 14.8% in group 2, and 19% in group 3. The postoperative period during which parenteral analgesics were required, did not differ between groups 1 and 2 (5.7 vs. 7.7 days), but it was longer for group 3 (8.5 days). The morbidity rate was similar for all three groups, 17.2% in group 1, 14.8% in group 2, and 19% in group 3. There were no perioperative deaths. They concluded that laparoscopic colectomy for sigmoid diverticulitis can be applied safely in overweight and obese patients.

Thaler et al. (253) compared the impact of surgical access to sigmoid resection on recurrence rates in patients with uncomplicated diverticulitis of the sigmoid at a minimum follow-up of 5 years. Recurrence after surgery was defined as left lower quadrant pain, fever, and leukocytosis with consistent CT and enema findings on admission and at 6 weeks, respectively. Seventy-nine patients undergoing laparoscopic sigmoid resection were compared with 79 matched controls with open sigmoid resection. There were no significant differences in rates of flexure mobilization, specimen length, and rates of inflammation present at proximal resection margin in 10 recurring and 145 nonrecurring patients. The rate of teniae coli present at distal resection margin was significantly increased in recurring patients (7% vs. 43%). Median time of recurrence after operation was 29 months. Two of the 11 recurrences occurred after 5 years. Surgical access to sigmoid resection for uncomplicated diverticulitis of the sigmoid is unlikely to have an impact on recurrence rates provided that the oral bowel end is anastomosed to the proximal rectum rather than to the distal sigmoid.

The laparoscopic treatment of generalized peritonitis due to perforated sigmoid diverticula is an interesting alternative to the traditional treatment. It is less aggressive and allows a second-stage elective laparoscopic resection. Feranda et al. (254) reported 18 patients who underwent emergency laparoscopic treatment for generalized peritonitis due to perforated diverticula. Eight of these patients had previously had diverticulitis attacks. By peritoneal cavity exploration and following full peritoneal lavage (average 15 L), the infected sigmoid lesion was stuck with biologic glue. A drain was inserted at the site of the lesion and in some cases also in other abdominal zones. No colostomy was necessary. Antibiotic treatment was started at diagnosis and continued for a minimum of 7 days. There was no mortality. Morbidity was limited to three patients (two cases of lymphagitis and one of pulmonary disease). No patient had a wound abscess or residual deep collections. The mean hospitalization was 8 days. Fourteen patients underwent elective laparoscopic sigmoid resection with a delay of 3.5 months.

Natarajan et al. (255) evaluated the relationship between the time interval from an acute attack of diverticulitis to laparoscopic colectomy and surgical outcomes. From a total of 120 patients the mean interval from acute diverticulitis to operation was 64 days. Median number of episodes of diverticulitis before colectomy was 3. Conversion from laparoscopic to open colectomy was required in 11% of patients. Neither interval from acute attack to operation nor number of prior episodes of diverticulitis was associated with any significantly increased rate of conversion to open colectomy, complication rate, operative time, or recovery period.

LeMoine et al. (256) analyzed the causes and consequences of conversion in 168 consecutive patients who underwent laparoscopic-assisted colectomy for diverticular disease. Postoperative mortality, morbidity, conversion, and reoperation rates were 0%, 21.4%, 14.3%, and 3%, respectively. The reasons for conversion were presence of intraperitoneal adhesions and/or inflammatory pseudotumor ($n=21$), an intraoperative diagnosis of sigmoid carcinoma ($n=1$), hypercapnia ($n=1$), and abdominal bleeding ($n=1$). Three preoperative factors were associated with a significant higher risk of conversion: surgical expertise, the presence of sigmoid stenosis or fistula, and the severity of diverticulitis on pathological examination. Morbidity was no different between laparoscopic sigmoidectomy (20.8%) and converted procedures (25%). Open conversion was associated with a longer operative time and significantly delayed patient recovery and hospital discharge.

Rectal Procidentia

Rose et al. (257) reported the findings of a prospective multicenter observational study carried out by the study group for Laparoscopic Colorectal Surgery on 150 patients undergoing laparoscopic or laparoscopic-assisted surgery for rectal prolapse (124 received rectopexy combined with resection and 26 rectopexy alone). In 85 patients, a mesh was employed during rectopexy. The conversion rate was 5.3%. Perioperative complications (21 surgical and 35 general perioperative) were recorded in 24.7% of patients. The reoperation rate was 5.3% (bleeding, two; anastomotic leak, two; ileus, four). No procedure-specific perioperative complications were observed. Postoperative cardiopulmonary problems arose in 3.3%.

Madbouly et al. (258) conducted a study to make a direct comparison of outcomes from laparoscopic resection with rectopexy and laparoscopic Wells' repair using a selected symptom-based choice of operative procedure. Patients with a history of constipation or normal bowel habits with normal continence underwent laparoscopic resection with rectopexy whereas those with diarrhea and anal incontinence underwent laparoscopic Wells' procedure. Continence was scored using the Cleveland Clinic scoring system. Of the 24 patients, 11 underwent laparoscopic resection rectopexy and 13 had laparoscopic Wells' procedure. The laparoscopic resection rectopexy patients were significantly younger (48.6 vs. 63.9 years). Both operative time and length of stay were significantly longer in the resection rectopexy group (operative time 128.5 vs. 69.9 minutes; length of stay 3.6 vs. 2.2 days). All patients in the laparoscopic resection rectopexy group had constipation, preoperative and no patients were incontinent clinically. Preoperatively, seven of the 13 patients in the laparoscopic Wells' group had preoperative diarrhea and one patient had clinical constipation. Five patients experienced clinical symptoms of fecal incontinence, manifested in different degrees. Postoperative complications occurred only in the laparoscopic resection rectopexy group (one case of abdominal wall hematoma and two cases of prolonged ileus). During a mean follow-up period of 18.1 months, there were no recurrences; 10 of the 11 laparoscopic resection rectopexy patients had correction of constipation and four of five of the incontinent laparoscopic Wells' procedure patients had improvement in their symptoms. Constipation developed in one laparoscopic Wells' patient. They concluded clinical assessment of preoperative bowel function and continence allows accurate selection of appropriate laparoscopic technique for rectal prolapse without the added expense of anal physiologic testing.

Solomon et al. (259) compared both subjective and clinical outcomes and the objective stress response of laparoscopic and open abdominal rectopexy in 30 patients with full-thickness rectal prolapse. Patients agreed to conform to a clinical pathway of liquid diet and full mobility on day 1, solid diet on day 2, and discharge before day 5. Some 75% of all clinical pathway objectives of early recovery were achieved in the laparoscopic group compared with 37% in the open group. Significant differences in favor of laparoscopy were noted with regard to narcotic requirements, pain and mobility scores. Differences in objective measures of stress response favoring laparoscopy were found for urinary catecholamines, IL-6, serum cortisol, and C-reactive protein. No differences were noted in respiratory function but significant respiratory morbidity was greater in the open group. None of the measured outcomes, subjective or objective, favored the open group apart from operating time which was significantly shorter (153 vs. 102 minutes).

Heah et al. (260) analyzed 25 patients who underwent laparoscopic rectopexy with full-thickness rectal prolapse (Table 13). With respect to function, 60% of patients either improved or remained unchanged with respect to continence. There was an improvement in 50% of patients among those with continence grade 2 or more. Twenty-eight percent remained incontinent. No patient became more incontinent after operation. Constipation which was present in 36% of patients preoperatively, affected 44% of patients after rectopexy. Postoperative morbidity included a port-site hernia and deep venous thrombosis in one patient and repaired rectal perforation, a retroperitoneal hematoma with prolonged ileus and a superficial wound infection. One patient with solitary rectal ulcer in the laparoscopic surgery group remained unhealed despite resolution of the rectal prolapse after rectopexy and required abdominoperineal resection. Two patients, one laparoscopic and one open, had severe constipation after operation and both required loop colostomies. There were no cases of operative mortality or recurrent prolapse.

Boccasanta et al. (269) compared the functional and clinical results of open Wells' rectopexy (13) and laparoscopic Wells' rectopexy (22). Mean follow-up was 37.1 months in the open and 25.7 months in the laparoscopic group. In both groups, dyschezia and fecal incontinence improved significantly after the operation. The basal pressure of the anal sphincter squeeze and rectoanal reflex improved without significance, and anal-perineal pain was not significantly reduced. In the laparoscopic group, the postoperative hospital stay was lower than in the open group with a reduction in costs. They concluded laparoscopic Wells' rectopexy has the same clinical and functional results as laparotomy and rectopexy but with a shorter hospital stay and lower costs.

Himpens et al. (270) reported 37 patients undergoing laparoscopic Wells' rectopexy for rectal prolapse.

TABLE 13 ■ Results of Laparoscopic Operations for Complete Rectal Procidentia

Author (Ref.)	Year	Procedure	*n*	Conversion Rate (%)	Operation Time (min)	PO Intake (days)	Bowel Activity (days)	Complications (%)	Mortality (%)	LOS (days)	F/U (MOS)	Recurrence (%)
Stevenson et al. (261)	1998	Resection rectopexy	30	0	185	2	2	13	3	5	18	7 (mucosal)
Kessler et al. (262)	1999	Suture rectopexy	32[a]	–	150	–	–	9	0	5	33	6.3
Heah et al. (260)	2000	Suture rectopexy	25	16	96	–	4	16	0	7	26	0
Kellokumpu et al. (263)	2000	Resection rectopexy	17	0	255	–	–	14	0	5	24	0
		Suture rectopexy	17	0	150	–	–	41	0	5		7
Benoist et al. (264)	2001	Mesh rectopexy	14	0	114	2.7	2.3	14	0	5.6	47	2% (mucosal)
		Resection rectopexy	18	0	133	3.6	2.5	11	0	6.7	20	5% (mucosal)
		Suture rectopexy	16	0	107	2.6	2	19	0	5.7	24	4% (mucosal)
Bergamaschi et al. (265)	2003	Resection	30	–	180	3	–	20	–	4.5	34	3.3
Kairaluoma et al. (266)	2003	Resection rectopexy	27[a]	0	270	–	3	23	0	5	12	0
		Suture rectopexy	26	0	128	–	3		0	4.5		6
Madbouly et al. (258)	2003	Resection rectopexy	11	0	129	–	–	27	0	3.6	18	0
		Wells' rectopexy	13	0	70	–	–	0	0	2.8	18	0
D'Hoore et al. (267)	2004	Ventral rectopexy	42	5	60–240	–	–	5	0	5.8	61	5
Ashari et al. (268)	2005	Resection rectopexy	117	1	110–180	–	2	9	1	4–5	62	3

[a]Four patients had an additional resection.
Abbreviations: PO, per os; LOS, length of stay; F/U, follow-up.

Incontinence was seen in 33% of patients. Laparoscopy was successful in all but one case. Follow-up was available in 32 of 37 patients. Prolapse was cured in all patients and the incontinence resolved in 11 of 12. In addition, 38% of patients experienced significant constipation preoperatively versus 5% postoperatively.

Xynos et al. (271) compared laparoscopic resection rectopexy in 10 women to eight women with open resection rectopexy. The duration of operation was longer in the laparoscopic than in the open group. Morbidity was lower and hospital stay was shorter after the laparoscopic than in the open group. Prolapse was cured in all cases. Postoperatively, anal resting and squeeze pressures and rectal compliance increased significantly in both groups of patients. In all patients, the operation resulted in acceleration of large bowel transit and in more obtuse anorectal angles at rest. Preoperatively incontinence was present in 13 patients (seven laparoscopic and six open) and persisted in four of them after rectopexy (two laparoscopic and two open). They concluded resection rectopexy for rectal prolapse can be performed safely via the laparoscopic route with similar functional results.

Bruch et al. (272) assessed the outcome of both laparoscopic suture rectopexy and resection rectopexy in the treatment of complete and incomplete rectal prolapse, outlet obstruction or both. There were 72 patients with indications for operation being rectal prolapse in 21 patients, rectal prolapse combined with outlet obstruction in 36 patients and outlet obstruction alone in 15 patients. A sigmoid resection was added in 40 patients. Mean duration of operation was 227 minutes for rectopexy and 258 minutes for resection rectopexy. Conversion was necessary in 1.4%. Overall complication rate was 9.7% and the mortality rate was 0. Mean postoperative hospitalization was 15 days with a mean follow-up of 30 months. No recurrence of rectal prolapse was recognized. Sixty-four percent of patients with incontinence before operation were continent or had improved continence. In patients experiencing constipation preoperatively, constipation was improved or completely eliminated in 76%. No additional symptoms of constipation occurred after operation.

With respect to functional results Stevenson et al. (261) reported that with a median follow-up of 18 months, 92% of patients felt that the operation had improved their symptoms, that incontinence was improved in 14 of 20 patients with impaired continence (70%) and that constipation was improved in 64%. Symptoms of incomplete emptying and the need to strain at stool were both improved in 62% and 59% of patients, respectively. No full-thickness recurrences have occurred, but two patients have had mucosal prolapse detected (7%) and treated.

In a comparison of laparoscopic-assisted resection rectopexy and sutured rectopexy, Kellokumpu et al. (263) reported that incontinence improves significantly regardless of which method was used. The main determinant of constipation was excessive straining at defecation. Constipation was cured in 70% of patients in the rectopexy group and 64% in the resection rectopexy group. Symptoms of difficult evacuation improved but the changes were significant only after resection rectopexy. Two patients (7%) developed recurrent total prolapse during a median follow-up of 2 years.

Postoperative constipation is a common problem with most mesh suspension techniques used to correct rectal prolapse. Autonomic denervation of the rectum subsequent to its complete mobilization has been suggested as a contributory factor.

D'Hoore et al. (267) assessed the long-term outcome of patients who underwent a novel, autonomic nerve-sparing, laparoscopic technique for rectal prolapse in 42 patients. A peritoneal incision is made over the right side of the sacral promontory and extended in an inverted J-form along the rectum and over the deepest part of the pouch of Douglas. Denonvilliers' fascia is incised and the rectovaginal septum is broadly opened. A strip of Marlex (Bard®, Crawley, U.K.) is sutured to the ventral aspect of the distal rectum and further fixed to the sacral promontory. There is no posterior mobilization. There were no major postoperative complications. After a median follow-up of 61 months late recurrence developed in two patients. In 28 of 31 patients with incontinence, there was a significant improvement in continence. Symptoms of obstructed defecation resolved in 16 of 19 patients. During follow-up, new onset of mild obstructed defecation was noted in only two patients. Symptoms suggestive of slow-transit colonic constipation were not induced. They concluded laparoscopic ventral rectopexy is an effective technique for the correction of rectal prolapse and appears to avoid severe postoperative constipation.

Using meta-analytical techniques, Purkayastha et al. (273) compared open rectopexy and laparoscopic abdominal rectopexy used to treat full-thickness rectal prolapse in adults. Six studies consisting of a total of 195 patients (98 open and 97 laparoscopic) were included. Analysis of the data suggested that there is no significant difference in recurrence and morbidity between laparoscopic abdominal rectopexy and open abdominal rectopexy. Length of stay was significantly reduced in the laparoscopic group by 3.5 days whereas the operative time was significantly longer in this group by approximately 60 minutes.

The results of laparoscopic-selected operations for complete rectal procidentia are summarized in Table 13.

Enteric Fistulas

Regan and Salky (274) conducted a retrospective chart review of 72 patients with complicated diverticular and Crohn's disease who underwent 73 laparoscopic-assisted bowel resections for enteric fistulas. Ninety percent of patients had Crohn's disease, the average age was 39, and the male/female ratio was 38/34. Patients had a history of prior abdominal surgery in 39.7% of cases. Multiple fistulas were present in 30% of patients and 12.3% underwent multiple resections at the time of operation. Mean operating time was 199 minutes, and the conversion rate was 4.1%. Average length of stay was 5.2 days. There were no mortalities in this series, but overall morbidity was 11%. They concluded laparoscopic management of enteric fistula disease is safe and effective.

Poulin et al. (275) compared the outcomes of 13 patients with Crohn's disease or sigmoid diverticulitis with enteric fistulas treated laparoscopically (group I) with 13 patients treated by conventional operation (group II). Mean operative time was 183 minutes in group I vs. 154 minutes in group II. No significant difference was found between groups I and II in the number of patients with major postoperative complications (3 vs. 5) or postoperative stay (7.6 vs. 9.2 days). Conversion to open laparotomy occurred in one (7.7%) patient from group I. No patient required readmission for secondary operation in group I and two patients were admitted and underwent reoperation for complications in group II. They also concluded that laparoscopic treatment of selected cases of enteric fistulas is safe.

Watanabe et al. (276) examined the technical feasibility in 20 patients with Crohn's disease with a total of 31 intestinal fistula (14 ileoileal, six ileocolonic, five ileorectal, two ileovesical, two ileocutaneous, one gastrocolic, and one ileoduodenal) who underwent 25 operations. Fistulas were divided intracorporeally, except for ileoileal fistulas. Fifteen patients underwent ileocecal resection; six underwent strictureplasty; six underwent partial resection of the small intestine; three underwent segmental colonic resection; and one underwent a resection of an anastomotic recurrence. Four complications were observed in 25 patients (16%) including one intestinal obstruction/ileus, two wound infections, and one intra-abdominal abscess. There were no intraoperative or postoperative deaths. Four of the five operations were converted to open surgery (16%).

Bartus et al. (238) reported on 40 patients who were operated upon for colovesical or colovaginal fistulas secondary to diverticular disease. These results were then compared to results from a group of patients who had undergone elective laparoscopic colectomy for recurrent diverticulitis during the same period by the same group of surgeons. Patient demographics were similar among the group with recurrent diverticulitis ($n = 149$). The average hospital stay was 6.2 days for the fistula group and 4.4 days for the recurrent diverticulitis group. The average operating time was 220 minutes for the fistula group versus 176 minutes for the uncomplicated group. The conversion rate was significantly higher in the fistula group (25% vs. 5%). There were no postoperative anastomotic leaks or bleeding episodes requiring reoperation in the fistula group. They concluded diverticular fistula should no longer be considered a contraindication for laparoscopic colectomy.

Constipation

Sample et al. (277) reviewed 14 patients who underwent laparoscopic subtotal colectomy for colonic inertia with a mean age of 38.5 years; 93% of the patients were women. The common presenting symptoms included abdominal pain (93%), bloating (100%), constipation (100%), and nausea (57%). Mean duration of symptoms before operation was 4.5 years (range 1 to 30 years). Subtotal colectomy was completed laparoscopically in 13 patients. There was one conversion (7%) because of adhesions.

Eleven patients (78.6%) had undergone previous abdominal surgery. The mean operating room time was 153 minutes (range 113 to 210 minutes). The median time to full bowel action was 2 days. One patient developed postoperative small bowel obstruction that required open exploration. Complete follow-up was available for 11 patients at a median follow-up of 18 months (range 2 to 98 months). Ninety-one percent of the patients reported excellent satisfaction with operation and their bowel movement frequency ranged from 1.2 per week preoperatively to 17.2 per week postoperatively. Three patients (27%) continued to report abdominal pain and three patients (27%) continued to require laxatives postoperatively. Laparoscopic subtotal colectomy provides excellent symptom relief in patients with colonic inertia who do not respond to medical measures.

Endometriosis

Jerby et al. (278) reported their laparoscopic management of colorectal endometriosis in 30 patients. Twelve required superficial excision of colon and rectal endometriomas. Proctectomy/proctosigmoidectomy was done in seven cases, and rectal disc excision was performed in five patients. Four cases required conversion due to the overall severity of the pelvic disease. For those who did ($n = 12$) and did not ($n = 18$) require full-thickness excision/resections, the median operative time was 180 minutes and 110 minutes, respectively; the median length of hospitalization was 4 days and 1 day, respectively. A major complication occurred in one patient (colovaginal fistula). At the median follow-up of 10 months, 28 patients were improved and 24 of these had near or total resolution of preoperative symptoms.

Familial Adenomatous Polyposis

Milsom et al. (279) described their results in a series of 16 patients undergoing laparoscopic total abdominal colectomy with ileorectal anastomosis for FAP. Procedures were entirely intracorporeal, with a 3- to 6-cm specimen extraction incision. Median operative time was 232 minutes. The only intraoperative complication, a twisted ileorectal anastomosis was noted intraoperatively and revised. There were no conversions to conventional laparotomy. The median postoperative interval to passage of flatus was 3 days and for bowel movements it was also 3 days. Median hospital stay was 5 days. One case of early postoperative small bowel obstruction was treated nonoperatively and one case of brachial plexus neuropraxia resolved spontaneously.

Miscellaneous

Safadi (280) reviewed his institution's experience with the laparoscopic repair of nine parastomal hernias (five ileal conduits, two ileostomies, and two sigmoid colostomies). Their average age was 66 years. A single piece of Gore-Tex Dual Mesh with a slit to accommodate the stoma was used in seven of nine patients; in the other two patients, two pieces of mesh were used. Concurrent incisional hernias were repaired in three of nine patients. The average operating time was 243 minutes. The average postoperative length of stay was 4.7 days. Immediate postoperative complications occurred in three patients (one ileus, one urinary retention, and one ulnar neuropathy). Recurrences developed in four patients (44.4%), and in one patient (11.1%) the stoma was prolapsed. In this series, laparoscopic repair of parastomal hernias failed in 56% of patients, all within 6 months of the operation. Although the laparoscopic approach has potential advantages compared with the conventional open methods, the initial results are disappointing.

Navsaria et al. (281) reviewed the management of isolated civilian extraperitoneal rectal gunshot injuries using a protocol of diagnostic laparoscopy and abdominal wall trephine diverting loop colostomy. A rectal injury was confirmed by digital examination and proctosigmoidoscopy. Missile peritoneal violation was excluded by diagnostic laparoscopy. Normal laparoscopy was followed by creation of a diverting loop-sigmoid colostomy through an abdominal wall trephine, without laparotomy. No distal rectal washout or presacral drainage was performed. Of the 104 patients admitted with 106 rectal injuries, 20 qualified for inclusion in the study. All had sustained low-velocity gunshot injuries of which 18 exhibited a transpelvic trajectory. Diagnostic laparoscopy was normal and a trephine diverting loop-sigmoid colostomy was performed in all 20 patients. No pelvic sepsis occurred. Two patients developed rectocutaneous fistulas, both of which resolved without surgical treatment. Nineteen stomas have since been closed.

■ HAND-ASSISTED TECHNIQUES

Kang (20) compared the perioperative parameters and outcomes achieved with hand-assisted laproscopic (HAL) colectomy (30) versus open colectomy (30) for the management of benign and malignant colorectal disease, including carcinoma patients treated with curative intent. The HAL colectomy patients had significantly shorter hospital stays and incision lengths, faster recovery of gastrointestinal function, less analgesic use and blood loss, and lower pain scores on postoperative days 1, 3, and 14. There were no significant differences in operative time, complications, or time to return to normal activity.

Cobb et al. (282) examined the results of HAL colon surgery for benign disease in 37 patients. Indications for operation were: polyp (thirteen), uncomplicated diverticular disease (eight), complicated diverticular disease (i.e. colovesical fistula, phlegmon, etc.) (seven), chronic constipation (four), rectal prolapse (two), ulcerative colitis (one), endometriosis (one), and fecal incontinence (one). Procedures performed were sigmoidectomy (fourteen), right colectomy (nine), lower anterior resection (seven), subtotal colectomy (five), cecectomy (one), and transverse colectomy (one). There were no deaths. One case was converted to celiotomy (unable to rule out malignancy). The median operative time was 122 minutes. Return of flatus was noted (median) at postoperative day 3 and the median length of stay after operation was 4 days. One patient developed a superficial wound infection and there was one pelvic abscess (drained percutaneously) and one patient developed urinary retention. There were no reoperations.

Nakajima et al. (283) compared the outcomes in 23 patients who underwent total proctocolectomy or total abdominal colectomy using either a HAL technique or laparoscopic-assisted operation. There were 12 hand-assisted (five total proctocolectomy and seven total abdominal colectomy) and 11 laparoscopic-assisted (seven total proctocolectomy and four total abdominal colectomy) for ulcerative colitis ($n=17$), familial polyposis ($n=5$), and colonic inertia ($n=1$). One laparoscopic case was converted (9.1%). The operative time was shorter for the hand-assisted cases (210 vs. 273 minutes). Blood loss and incision length were similar. Postoperative recovery and morbidity rates were comparable. They concluded HAL surgery reduces the operative time but patient morbidity rates and recovery are similar to laparoscopic cases. The hand-assisted technique may be preferable for extensive colorectal procedures such as total proctocolectomy and total abdominal colectomy.

Targarona et al. (284) performed a prospective randomized trial comparing laparoscopic-assisted colectomy and hand-assisted colectomy. A total of 54 patients were enrolled in this study, 27 laparoscopic and 27 hand-assisted. The operative times were similar but hand-assisted was associated with a far lower conversion rate, 7% vs. 23%. Immediate clinical outcomes, oncologic features, and costs were similar for the two procedures but hand-assisted was associated with a significantly greater increase in IL-6 and C-reactive protein than the conventional laparoscopic procedure. This comparative study shows that hand-assisted simplifies difficult intraoperative situations reducing the need for conversion.

■ OBESITY

Senagore et al. (285) compared the outcome of laparoscopic bowel resection in obese and nonobese patients for all patients who underwent a segmental colectomy for any pathologic condition. Patients with a body mass index (BMI) above 30 were defined as obese and patients with a body mass index below 30 were defined as nonobese. A total of 260 patients were evaluated, 77.3% in the nonobese group and 22.7% in the obese group. The obese group had significantly more conversions to an open procedure (23.7% vs. 10.9%), a longer operative duration (109 vs. 94 minutes), a higher morbidity rate (22% vs. 13%), and a higher anastomotic leakage rate (5.1% vs. 1.2%). Despite higher conversion rates and increased risk of pulmonary complications and anastomotic leakages in obese patients, they parallel those of open operation and laparoscopic colectomy can be performed safely in both obese and non-obese patients with the similar benefit of a shorter hospital stay in both groups.

Using the same definition of obesity, Schwandner et al. (286) compared the outcome of laparoscopic colorectal surgery in obese and non-obese patients. All patients who underwent laparoscopic operation for both benign and malignant disease and were laparoscopically completed were analyzed. A total of 589 patients were evaluated, including 95 patients in the obese group and 494 in the non-obese group. There was no significant difference in conversion rate (7.3% in the obese group vs. 9.5% in the non-obese group). No significant differences were observed with respect to age, diagnosis, procedure, duration of operation, and transfusion requirements. In terms of morbidity there were no significant differences related to overall complication rates with respect to BMI (23.3% in the obese group vs. 24.5% in the non-obese group). Major complications were more common in the obese group without showing statistical significance (12.8% in the obese group vs. 6.6% in the non-obese group). Conversely, minor complications were more frequently documented in the non-obese group (8.1% in the obese group vs. 15.5% in the non-obese group). In the postoperative course, no differences were documented in terms of return of bowel function, duration of analgesics required, oral feeding and length of hospitalization. They concluded these data indicate that laparoscopic colorectal surgery is feasible and effective in both obese and non-obese patients.

Delaney et al. (287) conducted a case-matched study comparing outcomes after open and laparoscopic colectomy in 94 patients with a BMI >30. By using intention-to-treat-type analysis, there was no difference in median operating time (100 vs. 110 minutes), complication (21% vs. 24%), readmission (17% vs. 10.6%), reoperation rates (6.4% vs. 4.3%), or direct costs (median US $3368 vs. US $3552; mean US $4003 vs. US $4037) between laparoscopic colectomy or open colectomy; however, a median length of stay (3 vs. 5.5 days) was significantly shorter after laparoscopic colectomy. Twenty-eight patients required conversion for adhesions ($n=11$), bleeding ($n=3$), obesity hindering vision or dissection ($n=9$), large phlegmon or neoplasm ($n=4$), and ureteric injury ($n=1$). The mean operating time for conversions was 142 minutes and length of stay was 6.4 days. Compared with laparoscopically completed cases, the median length of stay (5 vs. 2 days) and median operating times (150 vs. 95 minutes) were significantly higher in the converted group, but there was no difference in the complication, readmission, or reoperation rates. Compared with open colectomy, the operating time was significantly higher in the converted group but there was no significant difference in the length of stay, complication, readmission, or reoperation rates. They concluded, laparoscopic colectomy can be performed safely in obese patients although obesity is associated with a high conversion rate.

■ QUALITY OF LIFE

Adachi et al. (288) evaluated the quality of life of patients who had undergone laparoscopic or open colonic resection for carcinoma. The study included 26 patients with laparoscopic colectomy and 87 with conventional open colectomy for cure. Quality of life was estimated by the 9-item questionnaire with scoring system of 1 (high), 2 (fair), and 3 (low). Laparoscopic colectomy was significantly different from open colectomy with regard to C-reactive protein level (6.34 vs. 11.15 mg/dL) on postoperative day 1, albumin level (3.54 vs. 3.36 g/dL) and lymphocyte count (1354/mm^3 vs. 995/mm^3) on postoperative day 7 and weight loss on postoperative day 14 (3.95% vs. 5.45%). Total score of the quality-of-life questionnaire was not significantly different between the two groups (10.95 vs. 11.81). Both laparoscopic and open colonic resections were similarly accepted by the patients as a good operation that they would recommend to others (1.105 vs. 1.206). These results indicate that although laparoscopic colonic resection for carcinoma was less invasive than conventional open colectomy, both laparoscopic and open colonic resections were favorably accepted by the patients and quality of life after operation was not significantly different between the two procedures.

Thaler et al. (289) compared laparoscopic colectomy and open colectomy in terms of outcome and health-related quality of life. Forty-nine patients who underwent laparoscopic right hemicolectomy or sigmoid resection for benign polyps or uncomplicated diverticular disease were evaluated. Health-related quality of life was assessed by the SF-36 Physical and Mental Component Summary Score (PCS, MCS) and by the SF-36 Health Survey, which measures eight different health-quality domains, including physical and social function (PF, SF), general health perception (GH), physical and emotional limitations (RP, RE), body pain (BP), vitality (VT), and mental health (MH). There were significant differences between the two groups in resection type (26 right hemicolectomy:23 sigmoid resection in laparoscopic colectomy vs. 16 right hemicolectomy: 34 sigmoid resection in open colectomy) and length of follow-up (median 39, and 53.5 months, respectively) but neither parameters were predictive of the main SF-36 scores (PCS and MCS). There were no differences between the groups in recurrence rates (8% in laparoscopic colectomy vs. 11% open colectomy) or surgery-related complications including incisional hernias (16.3% in laparoscopic colectomy vs. 17% in open colectomy) and small bowel obstructions (2% in laparoscopic colectomy vs. 10.5% in open colectomy). None of the eight SF-36 Health Survey domains or the PCS or MCS scores showed significant differences between laparoscopic colectomy and open colectomy patients in health-related quality of life. However, occurrence of hernia after operation was predictive of lower SF-36 scores, specifically in physical functioning, general health perception, social functioning, mental health, and mental component summary score. In addition, small bowel obstruction was significantly associated with lower scores in body pain, general health perception, social functioning, emotional role limitations, mental health, and mental component summary score. Laparoscopic colectomy was not different from open colectomy for selected indications that measure long-term outcome and health-related quality of life. SF-36 appears to be an appropriate instrument to measure postoperative health-related quality of life, showing responsiveness to changes in objective outcome measures.

Weeks et al. (177) compared short-term quality of life outcomes after laparoscopic-assisted colectomy vs. open colectomy for colon carcinoma in a multicenter randomized controlled trial (COST). Of 449 patients, 428 provided quality of life data. In an intention-to-treat analysis comparing Symptoms Distress Scale (SDS) pain intensity, SDS summary, Qualify of Life Index summary, and global rating scale scores, the only statistically significant difference observed between groups was the global rating scale score for 2 weeks postoperatively. The mean (median) global rating scale scores for 2 weeks postoperatively were 76.9 for laparoscopic-assisted colectomy vs. 74.4% for open colectomy. While in the hospital patients assigned to laparoscopic-assisted colectomy required fewer days of both parenteral analgesics compared with patients assigned to open colectomy (mean 3.2 vs. 4.0 days) and oral analgesics (mean 1.9 vs. 2.2 days). Only minimal short-term quality of life benefits were found with laparoscopic-assisted colectomy for colon carcinoma compared with standard open colectomy.

Dunker et al. (290) assessed the functional outcome of quality of life of laparoscopic-assisted ileal pouch-anal anastomosis compared with conventional ileal pouch-anal anastomosis. Sixteen patients who underwent laparoscopic-assisted ileal pouch-anal anastomosis were matched with 19 patients who had a conventional ileal pouch-anal anastomosis. Patients were matched for time period after operation, distribution of FAP/ulcerative colitis and one-/two-stage procedure. Quality of life was measured with the SF-36 Health Survey questionnaire and the Gastrointestinal Quality of Life Index. The Body Image questionnaire was used to measure patients' perceptions of and satisfaction with their own body and their attitude toward their bodily appearance (body image) and the degree of satisfaction of patients with respect to physical appearance of the scar (cosmesis). Patients in the conventional group were older than the patients in the laparoscopic-assisted group (mean 39.2 vs. 30.6 years). No differences were found in functional outcome and quality of life. Satisfaction with the cosmetic result of the scar was significantly higher in the laparoscopic-assisted group compared with the conventional group. Body image score was higher in the laparoscopic-assisted group compared with the conventional group although not significant. In the long term, better cosmesis is the most important advantage after laparoscopic surgery.

■ COST ISSUES

Cost issues have been a growing reality in the practice of medicine but there has been no randomized clinical trial of the costs of laparoscopic colon resection compared with those of open colon resection in the treatment of colonic carcinoma. A subset of Swedish patients included in the COLOR trial was included in a prospective analysis; costs were calculated up to 12 weeks after operation (291). All relevant costs to society were included. Two hundred and ten patients were included in the primary analysis, 98 of whom had laparoscopic colon resection and 112 open resection. Total cost to society did not differ significantly between the two groups (difference in means for laparoscopic colon resection vs. open colon resection, €1846). The cost of operation was significantly higher for laparoscopic colon resection than for open colon resection (difference in means €1171), as was the cost of the first admission (difference in means €1556) and the total cost to the healthcare system (difference in means €2244). Within 12 weeks of surgery for colonic carcinoma there was no difference in total cost to society incurred by laparoscopic colon resection and open colon resection. The laparoscopic colon resection procedure, however, was more costly to the healthcare system.

Delaney et al. (292) performed a comparison of outcome and costs after laparoscopic and open colectomy with 150 patients in each group. American Society of Anesthesiologists classification, body mass index, diagnosis, complications, and rate of readmission within 30 days were similar for both groups. Operating room costs were significantly higher after laparoscopic colectomy but length of hospital stay was significantly lower. This resulted in significantly lower total costs owing to lower pharmacy, laboratory, and ward nursing costs. They concluded laparoscopic colectomy results in significantly lower direct costs compared with open colectomy for carefully matched patients.

Senagore et al. (247) compared the direct cost structure of elective open ($n=71$) and laparoscopic resection ($n=61$) for sigmoid diverticulitis. Indirect costs and total costs were not addressed. Operating time was similar (109 minutes for the laparoscopic procedure vs. 101 minutes for open procedures). The laparoscopic group had a significantly shorter length of stay (3.1 vs. 6.8 days), fewer pulmonary complications (1.6% vs. 5.6%) and fewer wound infections (0% vs. 7%). Conversion to open colectomy was required in 6.6% of patients. Readmission occurred in 4.9% of laparoscopic colectomy patients and 5.6% of open colectomy patients. Operative death occurred in 1.6% of the laparoscopic patients and there were no deaths in the open group. Total direct cost per case was significantly less for laparoscopic procedures (US $3458) than for open colectomies (US $4321). Their data demonstrates that laparoscopic colectomy is a cost-effective means of electively managing sigmoid diverticular disease.

In a similar study, Dwivedi (248) found that although the mean operating room charges were greater in the laparoscopic sigmoid colectomy patients (US $9566), the mean hospital charges were less (US $13,958). In the laparoscopic-assisted approach to ileocecal Crohn's disease, Duepree (206) found that the direct cost per case was significantly lower for the laparoscopic resection group (US $2547 vs. $2985) than for open operation and thus proved to be economically advantageous. Young-Fadok et al. (205) also compared the costs of laparoscopic ileocolic resection for Crohn's disease to open operation. The laparoscopic group had significantly lower direct costs (US $8684 vs. $11,373) and indirect costs (US $1358 vs. $2349) than the open group. This resulted in total costs of US $9895 for laparoscopic versus US $13,268 for open procedures. There were significant postoperative benefits in terms of resolution of ileus, narcotic use, and hospital stay. In their study the laparoscopic approach translated into cost savings of more than US $3300 for laparoscopic patients. In a study comparing laparoscopic versus open sigmoid colectomy for diverticulitis, Lawrence et al. (249) found that the average total hospital charges were US $25,700 for open sigmoid colectomy and US $17,414 for laparoscopic colectomy.

LAPAROSCOPIC COMPLICATIONS AND THEIR PREVENTION

As minimally invasive procedures become more popular, it is inevitable that complications will arise. This is certainly true of operations on the colon. This section alerts the reader to the types of complications that might be encountered and provides suggestions about how the frequency of these complications might be minimized.

Larach et al. (293) reviewed whether the techniques learned during their early learning experience proved to be effective in reducing the complications related to laparoscopic colorectal surgery. They divided 195 laparoscopic operations into "early" and "latter" groups. The incidence of conversions required because of iatrogenic injuries showed a decline from 7.3% in the early group to 1.4% in the latter group. Postoperative complications were observed in 30.3% of patients. Complications specifically related to the technique of laparoscopic surgery occurred in nine (4.6%) of patients. These were postoperative bleeding in three patients, port-site hernias in five patients and left ureteric stricture in one patient. Eight (6.5%) of these complications occurred in the early group whereas only 1.1 (1.4%) occurred in the latter group. Analyzing the conversions caused by intraoperative iatrogenic injuries and the specific postoperative complications together, revealed that the incidence of 13.8% in the early group was reduced to 2.8% in the latter group.

TROCAR COMPLICATIONS

Many complications of laparoscopic procedures occur during trocar insertion. Instrumentation has been designed in an effort to eliminate this complication but no device nor entry technique is entirely safe. Shielded blades, radial-expandable and optical trocars have been recommended. Even the open technique with the Hassan-type cannula may be associated with small bowel or vascular injury.

Procedure-based surveys of laparoscopic entry access injury show a reassuringly low incidence varying from 5 per 10,000 to 3 per 1000 (294). Chandler et al. (294) used existing injury-based reporting systems to access a uniquely large number of entry injuries to define the nature and outcomes of such events. Between 1980 and 1999, 594 structural organs were injured in 506 patients, resulting in 65 deaths (13%). Bowel and retroperitoneal vascular injuries comprised 76% of all injuries incurred in the process of establishing a primary port. Nearly 50% of both small and large bowel injuries were unrecognized for 24 hours or longer. Delayed recognition along with age >59 years and major visceral vascular injuries were each independent significant predictors of death.

In a recent review of the literature, Van der Voort (295) calculated the incidence of laparoscopy-induced gastrointestinal injury to be 0.13% (430 of 329,935) and of bowel perforation 0.22% (66 of 29,532). The small intestine was most frequently injured (55.8%), followed by the large intestine (38.6%). In at least 66.8% of bowel injuries, the diagnosis was made during the laparoscopy or within 24 hours thereafter. A trocar or Veress needle caused the most bowel injuries (41.8%), followed by a coagulator or laser (25.6%). In 68.9% of instances of bowel injury, adhesions or a previous laparotomy were noted. Management was mainly by laparotomy (78.6%). The mortality rate associated with laparoscopy-induced bowel injury was 3.6%.

Trocar injuries to abdominal viscera occur if the viscera are unusually close to the point of trocar insertion. Distances between parietal peritoneum and underlying viscera can be increased by lifting the abdominal wall at the umbilicus with towel clips. Levrant et al. (296) reported that 59% of patients with previous midline incisions and 28% of patients with previous suprapubic and transverse incisions have anterior wall adhesions. Omentum was involved in 96% of adhesions while bowel was included in 29%. In addition, a full bladder or stomach can be injured if not emptied prior to Veress needle or trocar insertion.

The Swiss Association for Laparoscopic and Thoracoscopic Surgery (SALTS) prospectively collected the data on 14,243 patients undergoing various standard laparoscopic procedures between 1995 and 1997 (297). They found 22 trocar and four needle injuries (incidence, 0.18%). Nineteen lesions involved visceral organs; the remaining seven were vessel injuries. The small bowel was the single-most affected organ (six cases), followed by the large bowel and the liver (three cases each). All vascular lesions except for one laceration of the right iliac artery, occurred as venous bleeding of either the greater omentum or the mesentery. Nineteen trocar injuries were recognized intraoperatively; diagnosis of two small bowel and one bladder injuries were made postoperatively. Only five injuries could be repaired laparoscopically; there was one death among the 26 injuries (4.0%). In the Swiss review, 331 patients (2.3%) had intraoperative bleeding complications (298). Whereas 44 patients suffered from an external bleed of the abdominal wall, the bleeding was internal in the remaining 287. Thirty-three patients with internal bleeding required blood transfusion with a mean blood loss of 1630 mL. Surgical hemostasis was necessary in 68% of external and 91% of internal bleeds. There were 250 patients (1.8%) with postoperative bleeding complications. External bleeding occurred in 143 patients and 107 patients developed internal bleeding. External bleeding was mainly treated conservatively (92%), whereas 50% of internal bleeds required further surgical intervention. Major vascular injuries occurred in 12 patients (incidence 0.08%) with open treatment being necessary in all cases.

The key to minimizing morbidity in cases of access injury is immediate recognition. Upon recognition, a standard repair of visceral injuries should be carried out, and in some cases this can be accomplished laparoscopically but there should be no hesitation to convert to open. In cases of vascular injury, conversion to open is usually necessary. The epigastric vessels are the most commonly injured, followed by injuries to the greater omentum and mesenteric vessels, and least common are injuries to the retroperitoneal vessels (297). Injury to a major visceral vessel (i.e. portal vein, hepatic artery, gastroduodenal artery) can carry a mortality rate of up to 44% (294).

Bhoyrul et al. (299) analyzed risk factors associated with injuries resulting from use of disposable trocars with safety shields as reported to the Food and Drug Administration. They analyzed the 629 trocar injuries reported from 1993 through 1996. There were three types of injury: 408 injuries of major blood vessels, 182 other visceral injuries (mainly bowel injuries), and 30 abdominal wall hematomas. Of the 32 deaths, 81% resulted from vascular injuries and 19% resulted from bowel injuries. Eighty-seven percent of deaths from vascular injuries involved the use of disposable trocars with safety shields and 9% involved disposable trocars with a direct viewing feature. The aorta (23%) and inferior vena cava (15%) were the vessels most commonly traumatized in the fatal vascular injuries. Ninety-one percent of bowel injuries involve trocars with safety shields and 7% involve direct view trocars. The diagnosis of an enterotomy was delayed in 10% of cases and the mortality rate in this group was 21%. In 10% of cases, the surgeon initially thought the trocar had malfunctioned but in only one instance was malfunction subsequently found when the device was examined. These data show that safety shields and direct view trocars cannot prevent serious injuries. Bowel injuries often went unrecognized in which case they were highly lethal. Device malfunction was rarely a cause of trocar injuries.

■ VISCERAL INJURY

Small bowel injury, including the duodenum, may occur because of a grasping or cauterizing instrument. Of course, any viscera or vessel may be injured during trocar insertion. Such injuries might be minimized by cannula insertion using the open technique and subsequent cannula insertions under vision of the laparoscope.

Splenic injury may be minimized by exercising caution during traction in the left upper quadrant to obtain exposure of the splenic flexure of the colon.

■ VASCULAR INJURY

Injury to the mesenteric, iliac, or epigastric vessels may be encountered during trocar insertion. Again, insertion under direct vision of the laparoscope will hopefully minimize these injuries. Also, insertion of cannulas lateral to the rectus muscle will avoid epigastric vessels. Visualization of the undersurface of the anterior abdominal wall with the laparoscope will help avoid unnamed vessels.

A case of superior mesenteric artery and portal vein thrombosis following laparoscopic-assisted right hemicolectomy has been reported (300). The patient presented with severe abdominal pain 10 days after a seemingly uneventful operation. After 10 days of abdominal pain, a CT scan revealed the diagnosis, and the patient underwent thrombolytic therapy and treatment with heparin with ultimate resolution of the thrombosis. Factors possibly contributing to this unique complication included decreased splanchnic flow with carbon dioxide pneumoperitoneum or mechanical compression of the colon and mesentery with vascular compression when the area was exteriorized for anastomosis.

■ URINARY TRACT INJURY

Ureteral injury (either from direct transection or diathermy) has been observed with laparoscopic colectomy. In the presence of a phlegmonous mass, ureters may be drawn up into the mass and injured during dissection. Sackier (301) suggested the insertion of an illuminated ureteral catheter preoperatively to permit visualization of the illuminated ureter in its entirety.

Bladder injury has also been reported during abdominoperineal resection (302). This may be encountered because the perineal portion of dissection is usually greater in extent in procedures performed laparoscopically.

■ ABDOMINAL WALL (PORT-SITE) RECURRENCE

One of the concerns of adopting the laparoscopic approach to colorectal malignancy is the reported development of recurrence noted at a port site and not necessarily the one through which the specimen was retrieved or even one created during the operation in question (303–305). An initial review reported the incidence to vary from 1.5% to 21.0% (304), although most authors report laparoscopic colectomies for carcinoma without any evidence of port-site implantations. At least 30 port-site recurrences have been described, but the number of procedures performed is unknown, and hence the exact incidence of this complication is unknown but was initially estimated to be 4% (304). Another concern is that this development has occurred in patients with Dukes' A, B, and C lesions, not necessarily those undergoing palliative resection. Furthermore, most of these recurrences present within the first year after operation.

The exact reason for these abdominal wall metastases has not definitely been elucidated and is probably multifactorial. Some offered explanations include seeding of malignant cells from intraoperative manipulation and instrumental contamination. Gas flow generated during pneumoperitoneum may spread malignant cells. Gas leaking around a port may lead to malignant cells lodging in wounds. The chimney effect, operative technique, and excessive manipulation may be contributing factors. Experimentally, pneumoperitoneum with carbon dioxide stimulates the growth of malignant colonic cells (306). In the hamster model, pneumoperitoneum increased implantation in mesenteric and midline incisions (307).

Over the past decade the incidence of port-site recurrence has diminished suggesting that the incidence may be related in part to operative technique. The use of bags to remove the specimen and irrigation of the ports with different solutions has been advocated. Irrigation of the peritoneal cavity with various solutions has been suggested. Amongst those listed are povidone-iodine, heparin, methotrexate, cyclophosphamide, taurolidine, distilled water, saline, heparin + 5-FU. Much of this information is only animal tested (97). The use of wound protectors is currently recommended.

Balli et al. (308) suggested a number of techniques to prevent port-site metastases. In addition to the general oncologic principles after resection, consider irrigation of trocar sites with 5% Betadine before removal, bag the specimen, protect extraction site and irrigation of trocar sites with Betadine and water.

In a Medline search, Curet (309) identified over 100 articles published during the last 15 years regarding the history incidence, etiology, and prevention of port-site metastases. The incidence of port-site metastases, initially thought to be as high as 21% is now thought to be closer to the incidence of wound metastases after open operation.

There are four reported prospective randomized trials examining the incidence of wound recurrence following laparoscopic versus open resections for carcinoma. Stage et al. (174) have followed up for a median of 14 months, 18 patients who underwent laparoscopic-assisted colectomy versus 16 who were treated with standard open colectomy and found no incisional wound or port-site recurrences. Lacy et al. (310) reported no incisional wound or port-site recurrences after a median follow-up period of 21 months in a randomized study of 91 segmental resections, 44 of which were performed laparoscopically. Milsom et al. reported two cases of abdominal wall wound recurrences associated with widespread disease of 42 patients followed up for a median of 1.7 years after undergoing open colectomy. Conversely, no wound ecurrences were found in any of 38 patients treated with laparoscopic-assisted colectomy after a median follow-up period of 1.5 years (175). These studies have not been seen as providing definitive answer to the issue because of the small sample size. However, Lacy (139) reported the results of a large randomized controlled trial that had 106 patients in the laparoscopy arm versus 102 in the open colectomy group. The strengths of the study include power analysis to identify sample size necessary to show statistical significance, clearly defined inclusion and exclusion criteria, and endpoints of the study. The median length of follow-up was 43 months. No statistically significant difference in the occurrence of port-site recurrences was identified in this study.

Silecchia et al. (311) reported the results of the Italian Prospective Registry of Laparoscopic Colorectal Surgery confirm that the incidence of abdominal wall recurrences is similar to that reported in open studies, i.e. <1% in 1753 cases of carcinoma. Ziprin reviewed 27 studies, each with a minimum of 50 cases from 1993 to 2001 and found an overall incidence of only 0.715 with an incidence as the only evidence of metastatic disease of 0.33% (312). Ziprin's study suggests that the incidence of port-site metastases after laparoscopic surgery is similar to that seen after open surgery. Two of the prospective randomized trials found no port-site metastases at follow-up ranging from 1.5 to 2 years (175,310).

In a recent review of 29 publications involving 5305 patients, the incidence of port-site metastases was 0.72% (97). In another recent review by Patankar and Lee (1) collated information from 23 reports showed wound recurrence rates following laparoscopic colectomy to be low—between 0% and 2.4% and compared favorably to their review of eight reports following open resection with rates ranging from 0.9% to 3.3%.

Specific reference to the incidence of wound implantation following open colectomy is seldom made. Hughes et al. (313) described a 1% incidence of metastases to the surgical access wound. Most of these patients had advanced disease at the time of the initial operation. Reilly et al. (314) reviewed 1711 patients with primary carcinoma treated for cure and found that 0.6% of patients had documented incisional recurrences. Nine of 11 patients were found to have multiple sites of recurrence, suggesting that it is usually a harbinger of diffuse abdominal disease. From the registry initiated under the auspices of The American Society of Colon and Rectal Surgeons, the American College of Surgeons Commission on Cancer, and the Society of American Gastrointestinal Endoscopic Surgeons, recurrences were evaluated by the primary surgeon and reported to the registry (315). A minimum follow-up of 1 year was obtained for 480 of 493 evaluable patients (97.4%). Wound recurrence was identified in five patients (1.1%).

■ BLEEDING

Bleeding, either intraoperatively or postoperatively, is not a complication unique to laparoscopic procedures. Bleeding may be mesenteric in origin or may originate in other locations. Anastomotic bleeding may arise whether the anastomosis is created with sutures or staples or whether it is performed extracorporeally or intracorporeally.

■ ANASTOMOTIC DEHISCENCE

Anastomotic complications following bowel operations are a dreaded but well-recognized occurrence. Fistula formation may also arise. There is no documented evidence to suggest that the incidence of these complications has increased with the use of laparoscopic procedures.

Rotation of a loop involved in an anastomosis is a rare but known complication after open resection. Rotation of the terminal ileum after a laparoscopic-assisted right hemicolectomy has been described (316). To prevent this complication, inspection of the terminal ileum before exteriorization and again after completion of the anastomosis is recommended (316). If the anastomosis is performed extracorporeally closure of the mesentery prior to the anastomosis will also obviate this complication.

■ MISSED LESIONS

A frustrating situation for the surgeon is the inability to identify the pathology at the time of laparoscopic colectomy. Where serosal involvement is absent, definitive recognition of the pathology is difficult or may be impossible. This limitation has resulted in the resection of a wrong segment of colon. If in doubt, intraoperative colonoscopy with transillumination should identify the location of the pathology. The preoperative injection of carbon particles into the normal colonic wall around the lesion may permit accurate delineation of the lesion and avoid time-consuming colonoscopy (307). Unrecognized synchronous carcinomas have also been reported (318).

Reported success rates for the detection of neoplasms after tattooing vary between 78.6% and 98% (97). Nizam et al. (319) reviewed the world literature. A total of 734 citations on India ink alone were present. Nine major studies were identified and reviewed. Various India ink preparations were used. Ink was unsterilized in 57%, autoclaved 42%, and gas sterilized in 1% of cases. Prophylactic antibiotics were used in 1% of cases. Dilution of India ink varied from undiluted to 1:100 (with 0.9% saline). The volume injected range from 0.1 to 2 mL per site injected, commonly with tangential needle insertion and delivery of ink into the submucosa in the majority of cases. Intraoperative localization was easier with multiple tattoo injections. Five reports of complications have been made. In only one instance did overt clinical complications develop. Risk of a clinical complication with colonic tattooing with India ink is 0.22%. Injection into the peritoneal space has been reported in 0.5% to 8% (320,321).

■ ELECTROSURGICAL INJURY

Electrosurgical injuries occur during laparoscopic operations and are potentially serious. The overall incidence of recognized injuries is between one and two patients per 1000 operations. The majority of such injuries go unrecognized at the time of the electrical insult and commonly present 3 to 7 days afterward with fever and pain in the abdomen. Because of the delayed presentation they often carry a high mortality. Since these injuries appear late, the pathophysiology remains speculative. Nduka et al. (322) conducted a comprehensive review of the physics of electrosurgery and provided the surgeon with an insight to the mechanisms responsible in each type of injury. The authors summarized the main causes of electrosurgical injuries as inadvertent touching or grasping of tissue during current application, direct coupling between a portion of intestine and a metal probe that is touching the activated probe, insulation breaks in the electrodes, direct sparking to the intestine from the diathermy probe, and current passage to the intestine from recently coagulated electrically isolated tissue. The majority of injuries, not surprisingly, are caused by monopolar diathermy. Bipolar diathermy is safer and should be used in preference to monopolar diathermy, especially in anatomically crowded areas. An awareness of the hazards of diathermy together, with an understanding of the mechanisms of injury should enable the surgeon to dissect tissue and achieve hemostasis, and at the same time, decrease the risk of serious complications for the patient.

■ ULTRASONIC ENERGY INJURY

Ultrasonic energy can be used instead of electrosurgery and its utilization can replace mechanical surgical clips and scissors. Ultrasonically activated devices can cut and coagulate tissues (Harmonic Scalpel®, Ethicon Endosurgery Inc.; Autosonix®, US Surgical Corporation, Norwalk, Connecticut, U.S.; Sonosurg®, Olympus Corp.). These devices can coagulate vessels up to 5 mm in diameter (323).

■ WOUND

As with any incision, wound infection is always a possibility. This may occur in a port site or through the incision created for specimen retrieval. The antibiotic prophylaxis used for a colon operation should minimize this complication.

Richter's hernia developing at a port site is possible when using cannulas 10 mm or larger in size. It is therefore important to make every effort to close the fascia through which a 10-mm or larger cannula has been inserted. This does not appear necessary for 5-mm cannulas. Patients may, indeed, require laparotomy for correction of such a hernia.

Winslow et al. (324) randomized 37 patients to laparoscopic colectomy and 46 to open colonic resection. Seven patients in the laparoscopic group were converted to open. Laparoscopic colectomy was performed using a limited midline incision for anastomosis and specimen extraction. Incision length was significantly greater in the open group (19.4 cm) compared with the laparoscopic extraction site (6.3 cm). Wound infections occurred in 13.5% of patients after laparoscopic (2.7% trocar, 10.8% extraction sites) and in 10.9% of patients after open colectomy. Over a mean follow-up period of 30.1 months, incisional hernias developed in 24.3% of patients after laparoscopic colectomy and 17.4% after open colectomy. In the laparoscopic group, extraction sites accounted for 85.7% of all wound complications. They concluded the extraction site for laparoscopic colectomy is associated with a high incidence of complications comparable to open colectomy.

In their review Hackert et al. (325) noted there is no standardized retrieval technique for the different procedures. Specimen retrieval after colonic resection is difficult due to the large size of the specimen usually resected. Three major complications are described in the literature: wound infection (0.9%), hernias (0–2%), and incision site recurrence (0–1.3%). In laparoscopic surgery for malignant disease retrieval is usually performed using a plastic bag, whereas retrieval can be performed hand-assisted without a bag during operations for benign diseases. Wound-edge protectors are recommended by several authors yet there is no standard system which is accepted broadly. The morbidity rate for specimen retrieval complications ranges between 0% and 9%.

Kercher et al. (326) reviewed the outcomes for patients with and without the use of a wound protector in 141 patients who underwent laparoscopic-assisted colectomy (98 for benign/malignant neoplasms, 35 for diverticular disease, and 8 for Crohn's disease). There were no differences between the wound protector group ($n=84$) and the no-wound protector group ($n=57$) with respect to mean age, average body mass index, gender, indication for operation, co-morbidities, antibiotics used, or mean operative time. Nine patients in the wound protector group and eight in the no-wound protector group developed a wound infection at the colon extraction site. Patients undergoing resection for Crohn's disease or diverticulitis had a higher infection rate (18.6%) than patients undergoing resection for polyps or carcinoma (9.2%). No-wound recurrence of carcinoma was observed in either group at a mean follow-up of 23 months. They concluded that the wound protector, although useful for mechanical retraction of small wounds, does not significantly diminish the rate of wound infection.

■ MISCELLANEOUS

Brachial plexus injury attributed to the Trendelenburg position during prolonged laparoscopic procedures has been reported (128). Care should be exercised to avoid excessive hyperextension of the patient's shoulder.

■ NONSPECIFIC COMPLICATIONS

A host of nonspecific complications have been reported to be associated with laparoscopic colectomy. These may include cardiac arrhythmias such as atrial fibrillation, urinary tract infection, urinary retention, pulmonary embolus, pneumonia, atelectasis, cerebral vascular accident, and stress gastritis. Pneumoperitoneum may cause mechanical pressure on the inferior vena cava which reduces cardiac filling and potentially reduces blood pressure. Pulmonary effects may be mechanical with direct pressure on the diaphragm or metabolic due to increased CO_2 that needs to be disposed via ventilation. Patients should be monitored for hypercarbia and the risk of CO_2 embolus exists. Physiologic changes associated with pneumoperitoneum are often controlled by the anesthesiologist. Frequently, cervical emphysema, pneumothorax, and pneumomediastinum are attributed to the passage of insufflating gas through defects in the diaphragm. The anesthesiologist must maintain a high index of suspicion for these potential complications and must undertake appropriate monitoring. If there is clinical evidence of a tension pneumothorax, immediate chest tube decompression is indicated.

Cottin et al. (327) reported seven cases of carbon dioxide embolism during laparoscopic surgery. None of the cases involved colorectal operations, but this complication is not procedure specific. In the seven cases cited, gas embolism occurred during insufflation or a few minutes later. All the patients had a previous abdominal or pelvic surgical history. Five patients presented with cardiac bradycardia or arrhythmia. Cardiovascular collapse or cyanosis was the first manifestation in three cases. Sudden bilateral mydriasis was the earliest neurologic sign and was present in five cases. The gas embolism complication was lethal in two cases.

Baixauli et al. (328) reported a case of portal vein thrombosis in a patient with no other demonstrable hypercoagulable states or risk factors who underwent an uneventful laparoscopic sigmoid colectomy. They suggest that heparin prophylaxis may be advisable to avoid these kinds of complications, especially if a past history of coagulable disorders is present.

REFERENCES

1. Patankar SK, Lee W. Current status of laparoscopic resection for colorectal cancer. J Clin Gastroenterol 2004; 38:621–627.
2. Jacobs M, Verdeja JC, Goldstein HS. Minimally invasive colon resection (laparoscopic colectomy). Surg Laparosc Endosc 1991; 1:144–150.
3. Fowler DL, White SA. Laparoscopic-assisted sigmoid resection. Surg Laparosc Endosc 1991; 1:183–188.
4. Schlinkert RT. Laparoscopic-assisted right hemicolectomy. Dis Colon Rectum 1991; 34:1030–1031.
5. Saclarides TJ, Ko ST, Airan M, et al. Laparoscopic removal of a large colonic lipoma. Report of a case. Dis Colon Rectum 1991; 34:1027–1029.
6. Cooperman AM, Katz V, Zimmon D, et al. Laparoscopic colon resection: a case report. J Laparoendosc Surg 1991; 1:221–224.
7. Nezhat C, Pennington E, Nezhat F, et al. Laparoscopically assisted anterior rectal wall resection and reanastomosis for deeply infiltrating endometriosis. Surg Laparosc Endosc 1991; 1:106–108.
8. Lange V, Meyer G, Schardey HM, et al. Laparoscopic creation of a loop colostomy. J Laparoendosc Surg 1991; 1:307–312.
9. Ortiz H, Armendariz P, Yarnoz C. Early postoperative feeding after elective colorectal surgery is not a benefit unique to laparoscopic-assisted procedures. Int J Colorectal Dis 1996; 11:246–249.
10. Hotokezaka M, Dix J, Mentis EP, et al. Gastrointestinal recovery following laparoscopic vs. open colon surgery. Surg Endosc 1996; 10:485–489.
11. Hildebrandt U, Kessler K, Plusczyk T, Pistorius G, Vollmar B, Menger MD. Comparison of surgical stress between laparoscopic and open colonic resections. Surg Endosc 2003; 17:242–246.
12. Duepree HJ, Senagore AJ, Delaney CP, Fazio VW. Does means of access affect the incidence of small bowel obstruction and ventral hernia after bowel resection? Laparoscopy versus laparotomy. J Am Coll Surg 2003; 197: 177–181.
13. Simons AJ, Anthone GH, Ortega AK. Laparoscopic-assisted colectomy learning curve. Dis Colon Rectum 1995; 38:600–603.
14. Wishner JD, Baker JW Jr., Hoffman GC, et al. Laparoscopic assisted colectomy. The learning curve. Surg Endosc 1995; 9:1179–1183.
15. Agachan F, Joo JS, Weiss EG, et al. Intraoperative laparoscopic complications: Are we getting better? Dis Colon Rectum 1996; 39:S14–S19.
16. Romanelli JR, Litwin DEM. Hand-assisted laparoscopic surgery. Prob Gen Surg 2001; 18:45–51.
17. Southern Surgeons Club Study Group. Handoscopic surgery. A prospective, multicenter trial of minimally invasive techniques for complex abdominal surgery. Arch Surg 1999; 34:477–486.
18. HALS Study Group. Hand-assisted laparoscopic surgery vs standard laparoscopic surgery for colorectal disease. Surg Endosc 2000; 14:896–901.
19. Taragona EM, Gracia E, Garriga J, et al. Prospective randomized trial comparing conventional laparoscopic colectomy with hand-assisted laparoscopic colectomy. Surg Endosc 2002; 16:234–239.
20. Kang JC, Chung MH, Chao PC, et al. Hand-assisted laparoscopic colectomy vs open colectomy: a prospective randomized study. Surg Endosc 2004; 18: 577–581.
21. Senagore AJ, Madbouly KM, Fazio VW, Duepree HJ, Brady KM, Delaney CP. Advantages of laparoscopic colectomy in older patients. Arch Surg 2003; 138:252–256.
22. Schmitt SL, Cohen SM, Wexner SD, et al. Does laparoscopic-assisted ileal pouch anal anastomosis reduce the length of hospitalization? Int I Colorectal Dis 1994; 9:134–137.
23. Moore JWE, Bokey EL, Newland RC, et al. Lymphovascular clearance in laparoscopically assisted right hemicolectomy is similar to open surgery. Aust N Z J Surg 1996; 66:605–607.
24. Jacquet P, Sugarbaker PH. Wound recurrence after laparoscopic colectomy for cancer. New rationale for intraoperative intraperitoneal chemotherapy. Surg Endosc 1996; 16:295–296.

25. Gonzalez R, Smith CD, Ritter EM, et al. Laparoscopic palliative surgery for complicated colorectal cancer. Surg Endosc 2005; 19:43–46.
26. Liberman MA, Phillips EH, Carroll BJ, et al. Laparoscopic colectomy vs. traditional colectomy for diverticulitis. Outcome and costs. Surg Endosc 1996; 10:15–18.
27. Luchtefeld MA. Laparoscopic-assisted stoma formation and takedown. Perspect Colon Rectal Surg 1996; 9:43–60.
28. Miyahara M, Kitano S, Shimoda K, et al. Laparoscopic repair of a colonic perforation sustained during colonoscopy. Surg Endosc 1996; 16:352–353.
29. Mehdi A, Closset J, Gay F, et al. Laparoscopic treatment of a surgical perforation after colonoscopy. Case report and review of literature. Surg Endosc 1996; 10:616–617.
30. Sackier JM. Laparoscopy: applications to colorectal surgery. Semin Colon Rectal Surg 1992; 3:2–8.
31. Sackier JM. Laparoscopic equipment and basic techniques. Perspect Colon Rectal Surg 1993; 6:175–189.
32. Veress J. Neues instrument zur ausfahrung von brust- oder bauchpunktionen und pneumothoraxbehandlung. Dtsch Med Wochenschr 1938; 41:1480–1481.
33. Darzi A. Hand-assisted laparoscopic colorectal surgery. Surg Endosc 2000; 14:999–1004.
34. Ballantyne GH, Leahy PR. Hand-assisted laparoscopic colectomy: evolution to a clinically useful technique. Dis Colon Rectum 2004; 47:753–765.
35. Nakajima K, Milsom JW, Margolin DA, Szilagy EJ. Use of the surgical towel in colorectal hand-assisted laparoscopic surgery (HALS). Surg Endosc 2004; 18:552–553.
36. Nakajima K, Lee SW, Cocilovo C, et al. Hand-assisted laparoscopic colorectal surgery using GelPort. Surg Endosc 2004; 18:102–105.
37. Chang YJ, Marcelle PW, Rusin LC, Roberts PL, Sohoetz DJ. Hand-assisted laparoscopic sigmoid colectomy: helping hand or hindrance? Surg Endosc 2005; 19:655–661.
38. Hasson HM. Modified instrument and method for laparoscopy. Am J Obstet Gynecol 1971; 110:886–887.
39. Nisii H, Hirai T, Ohara H, et al. Laparoscopic-assisted colon surgery by abdominal wall lifting with newly developed lifting bars. Surg Endosc 1997; 11:754–757.
40. Monson JRT, Hill ADK, Darzi A. Laparoscopic colonic surgery. Br J Surg 1995; 82:150–157.
41. Munegato G, De Min V, Schiano di Visconte M, Salemi S, Barbaresco S, Mazzarolo G. The diagnosis of non-palpable lesions in laparoscopic surgery of the colon. Chir Ital 2003; 55:657–661.
42. Feingold DL, Addona T, Forde KA, et al. Safety and reliability of tattooing colorectal neoplasms prior to laparoscopic resection. J Gastrointest Surg 2004; 8:543–546.
43. Zmora O, Dinnewitzer AJ, Pikarsky AJ, et al. Intraoperative endoscopy in laparoscopic colectomy. Surg Endosc 2002; 16:808–811.
44. Sackier JM, Berci G, Paz-Partlow M. Elective diagnostic laparoscope Am J Surg 1992; 161:326–331.
45. Reissman P, Teoh TA, Piccirillo M, et al. Colonoscopic-assisted laparoscopic colectomy. Surg Endosc 1994; 8:1352–1353.
46. John TG, Greig RD, Crosbie JL, et al. Superior staging of liver tumors with laparoscopy and laparoscopic ultrasound. Ann Surg 1994; 220:711–719.
47. Franklin ME, Ramos R, Rosenthal D, et al. Laparoscopic colonic procedures. World J Surg 1993; 17:51–53.
48. Van Ye TM, Cattery RP, Henry LG. Laparoscopically assisted colon resections compare favorably with open technique. Surg Laparosc Endosc 1994; 4:25–31.
49. Scoggin SD, Frazee RC, Snyder SK, et al. Laparoscopic-assisted bowel surgery. Dis Colon Rectum 1993; 36:747–750.
50. Quattlebaum JK, Flanders HD, Usher CH, et al. Laparoscopically assisted colectomy. Surg Laparosc Endosc 1993; 3:81–87.
51. Zucker KA, Pitcher DE, Martin DT, et al. Laparoscopic-assisted colon resection. Surg Endosc 1994; 8:12–18.
52. Puente I, Sosa JL, Sleeman D, et al. Laparoscopic assisted colorectal surgery. J Laparoendosc Surg 1944; 4:1–7.
53. Steichen FM. The use of staplers in anatomical side-to-side and functional end-to-end enteroanastomoses. Surgery 1968; 64:948–952.
54. Bernstein MA, Dawson JW, Reissman P, et al. Is complete laparoscopic colectomy superior to laparoscopic assisted colectomy? Am Surg 1996; 62: 507–511.
55. Larson DW, Nelson H. Laparoscopic colectomy for cancer. J Gastrointest Surg 2004; 8:636–642.
56. Liang JT, Lai HS, Lee PH. Laparoscopic medial-to-lateral approach for the curative left hemicolectomy. Dis Colon Rectum 2005 Sept 16 [Epub ahead of print].
57. Tanaka J, Ito M, Shindo Y, et al. Laparoscopically assisted resection of the lower rectum. Surg Endosc 1996; 10:338–340.
58. Loungnorath R, Fleshman J. Hand-assisted laparoscopic colectomy techniques. Semin Laparosc Surg 2003; 10:219–230.
59. Darzi A, Lewis C, Mengies-Gow N, et al. Laparoscopic abdominoperineal excision of the rectum. Surg Endosc 1995; 9:414–417.
60. Decanini C, Milsom JW, Bohm B, et al. Laparoscopic oncologic abdominoperineal resection. Dis colon Rectum 1994; 37:552–558.
61. Larach SW, Salomon MC, Williamson PR, et al. Laparoscopic-assisted abdominoperineal resection. Surg Laparosc Endosc 1993; 3:115–118.
62. Chindasub S, Charntaracharmnong C, Nimitvanit C, et al. Laparoscopic abdominoperineal resection. J Laparoendosc Surg 1994; 4:17–21.
63. Munro W, Avramovic J, Roney W. Laparoscopic rectopexy. J Laparoendosc Surg 1993; 3:55–58.
64. Berman IR. Sutureless laparoscopic rectopexy for procidentia. Dis colon Rectum 1992; 35:689–693.
65. Graf W, Stefansson T, Arvidsson D, et al. Laparoscopic suture rectopexy. Dis Colon Rectum 1995; 38:211–212.
66. Baker R, Senagore AJ, Luchtefeld MA. Laparoscopic-assisted vs. open resection rectopexy offers excellent results. Dis Colon Rectum 1995; 38:199–201.
67. Cuschieri A, Shimi SM, Vander-Velpen G, et al. Laparoscopic prosthesis fixation rectopexy for complete rectal prolapse. Br J Surg 1994; 81:138–139.
68. Poen AC, de Brauw M, Felt-Bersma RJF, et al. Laparoscopic rectopexy for complete rectal prolapse. Clinical outcome and anorectal function tests. Surg Endosc 1996; 10:904–908.
69. Darzi A, Henry MM, Guillou PJ, et al. Stapled laparoscopic rectopexy for rectal prolapse. Surg Endosc 1995; 9:301–303.
70. Lange V, Meyer G, Schardey HM, et al. Laparoscopic creation of a loop colostomy. J Laparoendosc Surg 1991; 1:217–220.
71. Khoo RE, Montrey J, Cohen MM. Laparoscopic loop ileostomy for temporary fecal diversion. Dis Colon Rectum 1993; 36:966–968.
72. Fuhrman GM, Ota DM. Laparoscopic intestinal stomas. Dis Colon Rectum 1994; 37:444–449.
73. Lyerly HK, Mault JR. Laparoscopic ileostomy and colostomy. Ann Surg 1994; 219:317–322.
74. Mattingly M, Wasvary H, Sacksner J, Deshmukh G, Kadro O. Minimally invasive, endoscopically assisted colostomy can be performed without general anesthesia or laparotomy. Dis Colon Rectum 2003; 46:271–273.
75. Sosa JL, Sleeman D, Puente I, et al. Laparoscopic-assisted colostomy closure after Hartmann's procedure. Dis Colon Rectum 1994; 37:149–152.
76. Constantino GN, Mukalian GG. Laparoscopic reversal of Hartmann procedure. J Laparoendosc Surg 1994; 4:429–433.
77. Vernava AM, Liebscher G, Longo WE, et al. Laparoscopic restoration of intestinal continuity after Hartmann procedure. Surg Laparosc Endosc 1995; 5:129–132.
78. Anderson CA, Fowler DL, White S, et al. Laparoscopic colostomy closure. Surg Laparosc Endosc 1993; 3:69–72.
79. Khan AL, Ah-See AK, Crofts TJ, et al. Reversal of Hartmann's colostomy. J R Coll Surg Edinb 1994; 39:239–242.
80. Wexner SD, Johansen OB, Nogueras JJ, et al. Laparoscopic total abdominal colectomy. A prospective trial. Dis Colon Rectum 1992; 35:651–655.
81. Nakajima K, Lee SW, Cocilovo C, et al. Laparoscopic total colectomy. Hand-assisted vs standard technique, Surg Endosc 2004; 18:582–586.
82. Goh PMY, Kum CK, Chia YW, et al. Laparoscopic repair of perforation of the colon during colonoscopy. Gastrointest Endosc 1994; 37:496–497.
83. Schlinkert RT, Rasmussen TE. Laparoscopic repair of colonoscopic perforation of the colon. J Laparoendosc Surg 1994; 4:51–54.
84. Yamamoto A, Ibusuki K, Koga K, Taniguchi S, Kawano M, Tanaka H. Laparoscopic repair of colonic perforation associated with colonoscopy: use of passing sutures and endoscopic linear stapler. Surg Laparosc Endosc Percutan Tech 2001; 11:19–21.
85. Pera M, Delgado S, Garcia-Valdecasas JC, et al. The management of leaking rectal anastomoses by minimally invasive techniques. Surg Endosc 2002; 16:603–606.
86. Duepree HJ, Senagore AJ, Delaney CP, Marcello PW, Brady KM, Falcone T. Laparoscopic resection of deep pelvic endometriosis with rectosigmoid involvement. J Am Coll Surg 2002; 195:754–758.
87. Prohm P, Weber J, Bonner C. Laparoscopic-assisted colonoscopic polypectomy. Dis Colon Rectum 2001; 44:746–748.
88. Rispoli G, Esposito C, Monachese TD, Armellino M. Removal of a foreign body from the distal colon using a combined laparoscopic and endoanal approach: report of a case. Dis Colon Rectum 2000; 43:1632–1634.
89. Weber PA, Merola S, Wasielewski A, Ballantyne GH. Telerobotic-assisted laparoscopic right and sigmoid colectomies for benign disease. Dis Colon Rectum 2002; 45:1689–1694.
90. Merola S, Weber P, Wasielewski A, Ballantyne GH. Comparison of laparoscopic colectomy with and without the aid of a robotic camera holder. Surg Laparosc Endosc Percutan Tech 2002; 12:46–51.
91. Corcione F, Esposito C, Cuccurulo D, et al. Advantages and limits of robot-assisted laparoscopic surgery. Surg Endosc 2005; 19:117–119.
92. Delaney C, Lynch A, Senagore A, et al. Comparison of robotically performed and traditional laparoscopic colorectal surgery. Dis Colon Rectum 2003; 46:1633–1639.
93. Munz Y, Moorthy K, Kudchadkar R, et al. Robotic assisted rectopexy. Am J Surg 2004; 187:88–92.
94. D'Annibale A, Morpurgo E, Fiscon V, et al. Robotic and laparoscopic surgery for treatment of colorectal disease. Dis Colon Rectum 2004; 47:2162–2168.
95. Hanly EJ, Talamini MA. Robotic abdominal surgery. Am J Surg 2004; 188(4A suppl):19S–26S.
96. Gutt CN, Oniu T, Mehrabi A, Kashfi A, Schemmer P, Buchler MW. Robot-assisted abdominal surgery. Br J Surg 2004; 91:1390–1397.
97. Veldkamp R, Gholghesaei M, Bonjer HJ, et al. European Association of Endoscopic Surgery (EAES). Laparoscopic resection of colon cancer: consensus of

the European Association of Endoscopic Surgery (EAES). Surg Endosc 2004; 18:1163–1185.
98. Slim K, Pezet D, Riff D, et al. High morbidity rate after converted laparoscopic colorectal surgery. Br J Surg 1995; 82:1406–1408.
99. Pandya S, Murray JJ, Coller JA, Rusin LC. Laparoscopic colectomy: indications for conversion to laparotomy. Arch Surg 1999; 134:471–475.
100. Marusch F, Gastinger I, Schneider C, et al. Laparoscopic Colorectal Surgery Study Group (LCSSG). Importance of conversion for results obtained with laparoscopic colorectal surgery. Dis Colon Rectum 2001; 44:207–214.
101. Gervaz P, Pikarsky A, Utech M, et al. Converted laparoscopic colorectal surgery. Surg Endosc 2001; 15:827–832.
102. Schlachta CM, Mamazza J, Seshadri PA, Cadeddu MO, Poulin EC. Predicting conversion to open surgery in laparoscopic colorectal resections. A simple clinical model. Surg Endosc 2000; 14:1114–1117.
103. Tekkis PP, Senagore AJ, Delaney CP. Conversion rates in laparoscopic colorectal surgery: a predictive model with 1253 patients. Surg Endosc 2005; 19: 47–54.
104. Casillas S, Delaney CP, Senagore AJ, Brady K, Fazio VW. Does conversion of a laparoscopic colectomy adversely affect patient outcome? Dis Colon Rectum 2004; 47:1680–1685.
105. Basse L, Madsen JL, Billesbolle P, Bardram L, Kehlet H. Gastrointestinal transit after laparoscopic versus open colonic resection. Surg Endosc 2003; 17: 1919–1922.
106. Kasparek MS. Muller MH, Glatzle J, et al. Postoperative colonic motility in patients following laparoscopic-assisted and open sigmoid colectomy. J Gastrointest Surg 2003; 7:1073–1081.
107. Asao T, Kuwano H, Nakamura J, Morinaga N, Hirayama I, Ide M. Gum chewing enhances early recovery from postoperative ileus after laparoscopic colectomy. J Am Coll Surg 2002; 195:30–32.
108. Raue W, Haase O, Junghans T, Scharfanberg M, Muller JM, Schwenk W. 'Fast-track' multimodal rehabilitation program improves outcome after laparoscopic sigmoidectomy: a controlled prospective evaluation. Surg Endosc 2004; 18:1463–1468.
109. Reissman P, Agachan F, Wexner SD. Outcome of laparoscopic colorectal surgery in older patients. Am Surg 1996; 62:1060–1063.
110. Peters WR, Fleshman JW. Minimally invasive colectomy in elderly patients. Surg Laparosc Endosc 1995; 5:477–479.
111. Delgado S, Lacy AM, Garcia-Valdecasas JC, et al. Could age be an indication for laparoscopic colectomy in colorectal cancer? Surg Endosc 2000; 14:22.
112. Sklow B, Read T, Birnbaum E, Fry R, Fleshman J. Age and type of procedure influence the choice of patients for laparoscopic colectomy. Surg Endosc 2003; 17:923–929.
113. Law WL, Chu KW, Tung PHM. Laparoscopic colorectal resection: A safe option for elderly patients. J Am Coll Surg 2002; 195:768–773.
114. Seshadri PA, Mamazza J, Schlachta CM, Cadeddu MO, Poulin EC. Laparoscopic colorectal resection in octogenarians. Surg Endosc 2001; 15: 802–805.
115. Vignali A, Di Palo S, Tamburini A, Radaelli G, Orsenigo E, Staudacher C. Laparoscopic vs. open colectomies in octogenarians: a case-matched control study. Dis Colon Rectum 2005 Aug 3; [Epub ahead of print].
116. Schlachta CM, Mamazza J, Seshadri PA, Cadeddu M, Gregoire R, Poulin EC. Defining a learning curve for laparoscopic colorectal resections. Dis Colon Rectum 2001; 44:217–222.
117. Bennett CL, Stryker SJ, Ferreira MR, Adams J, Beart RW Jr. The learning curve for laparoscopic colorectal surgery. Preliminary results from a prospective analysis of 1194 laparoscopic-assisted colectomies. Arch Surg 1997; 132: 41–44.
118. Dincler S, Koller MT, Steurer J, Bachmann LM, Christen D, Buchmann P. Multidimensional analysis of learning curves in laparoscopic sigmoid resection: eighth-year results. Dis Colon Rectum 2003; 46:1371–1378.
119. Ortega AK, Beart RW Jr, Steel GD Jr, et al. Laparoscopic bowel surgery registry: preliminary results. Dis Colon Rectum 1995; 38:681–686.
120. Kuhry E, Bonjer HJ, Haglind E, et al. COLOR Study Group. Impact of hospital case volume on short-term outcome alter laparoscopic operation for colonic cancer. Surg Endosc 2005; 19:687–692.
121. Wexner SD, Reissman P, Pfeifer J, et al. Laparoscopic colorectal surgery: an analysis of 140 cases. Surg Endosc 1996; 10:133–136.
122. Ramos JM, Beart RW Jr, Goes R, et al. Role of laparoscopy in colorectal surgery. A prospective evaluation of 200 cases. Dis Colon Rectum 1995; 38:494–501.
123. Huscher C, Silecchia G, Croce E, et al. Laparoscopic colorectal resection. A multicentre Italian study. Surg Endosc 1996; 10:875–879.
124. Begos DG, Arsenault J, Ballantyne GH. Laparoscopic colon and rectal surgery at a VA hospital. Analysis of the first 50 cases. Surg Endosc 1996; 10:1050–1056.
125. Tucker JG, Ambroze WL, Orangio GR, et al. Laparoscopically assisted bowel surgery. Analysis of 114 cases. Surg Endosc 1995; 9:297–300.
126. Lumley JW, Fielding GA, Rhodes M, et al. Laparoscopic-assisted colorectal surgery: lessons learned from 240 consecutive patients. Dis Colon Rectum 1996; 39:155–159.
127. Slim K, Pezet D, Stenci J, et al. Prospective analysis of 40 initial laparoscopic colorectal resections: a plea for a randomized trial. J Laparoendosc Surg 1994; 4:241–245.
128. Fleshman JW, Fry RD, Birnbaum EH, et al. Laparoscopic-assisted and minilaparotomy approaches to colorectal diseases are similar in early outcome. Dis Colon Rectum 1996; 39:15–22.
129. Gagnon J, Poulin EC. Beware of the Trendelenburg position during prolonged laparoscopic procedure. Can J Surg 1993; 36:505–506.
130. Degiuli M, Mineccia M, Bortone A, Arrigoni A, Pennazio M, Spandre M, Cavallero M, Calvo F. Outcome of laparoscopic colorectal resection. Surg Endosc 2004; 18:427–432.
131. Senagore AJ, Duepree HJ, Delaney CP, Brady KM, Fazio VW. Results of a standardized technique and postoperative care plan for laparoscopic sigmoid colectomy: a 30-month experience. Dis Colon Rectum 2003; 46:503–509.
132. Lezoche E, Feliciotti F, Guerrieri M, et al. Laparoscopic versus open hemicolectomy. Minerva Chir 2003; 58:491–502, 502–507.
133. Schlachta CM, Mamazza J, Gregoire R, Burpee SE, Poulin EC. Could laparoscopic colon and rectal surgery become the standard of care? A review and experience with 750 procedures. Can J Surg 2003; 46:432–440.
134. Lauter DM, Froines EJ. Initial experience with 150 cases of laparoscopic-assisted colectomy. Am J Surg 2001; 181:398–403.
135. Seshadri PA, Poulin EC, Schlachta CM, Cadeddu MO, Mamazza J. Does a laparoscopic approach to total abdominal colectomy and proctocolectomy offer advantages? Surg Endosc 2001; 15:837–842.
136. Kockerling F, Schneider C, Reymond MA, et al. Early results of a prospective multicenter study on 500 consecutive cases of laparoscopic colorectal surgery. Laparoscopic Colorectal Surgery Study Group (LCSSG). Surg Endosc 1998; 12:37–41.
137. Kockerling F, Rose J, Schneider C, et al. Laparoscopic colorectal anastomosis: risk of postoperative leakage. Results of a multicenter study. Laparoscopic Colorectal Surgery Study Group (LCSSG). Surg Endosc 1999; 13:639–644.
138. Schwenk W, Haase O, Neudecker J, Muller JM. Short term benefits for laparoscopic colorectal resection. Cochrane Database Syst Rev 2005; July 20(3): CD003145.
139. Lacy AM, Garcia-Valdecasas JC, Delgado S, et al. Laparoscopic-assisted colectomy vs. open colectomy for treatment of non-metastatic colon cancer: a randomized trial. Lancet 2002; 359:2224–2229.
140. Lujan HJ, Plasencia G, Jacobs M, et al. Long-term survival after laparoscopic colon resection for cancer. Dis Colon Rectum 2002; 45:491–501.
141. Patankar S, Larach S, Ferrara A, et al. Prospective comparison of laparoscopic vs. open resections for colorectal adenocarcinoma over a ten-year period. Dis Colon Rectum 2003; 46:601–611.
142. The Clinical Outcomes of Surgical Therapy Study Group. A comparison of laparoscopically assisted and open colectomy for colon cancer. NEJM 350:2050–2059.
143. Veldkamp R, Kuhry E, Hop WC, et al., Colon Cancer Laparoscopic or Open Resection Study Group (COLOR). Laparoscopic surgery versus open surgery for colon cancer: short-term outcomes of a randomized trial. Lancet Oncol 2005; 6:477–484.
144. Ramos JR, Petrosemolo RH, Valory EA, Polania FC, Pecanha R. Abdominoperineal resection: laparoscopic versus conventional. Surg Laparosc Endosc 1977; 7:148–152.
145. Khalili TM, Fleshner PR, Hiatt JR, et al. Colorectal cancer: comparison of laparoscopic with open approaches. Dis Colon Rectum 1998; 41:832–838.
146. Hong D, Tabet J, Anvari M. Laparoscopic vs. open resection for colorectal adenocarcinoma. Dis Colon Rectum 2001; 44:10–18.
147. Baker RP, White EE, Titu L, Duthie GS, Lee PW, Monson JR. Does laparoscopic abdominoperineal resection of the rectum compromise long-term survival? Dis Colon Rectum 2002; 45:1481–1485.
148. Champault GG, Barrat C, Raselli R, Elizalde A, Catheline JM. Laparoscopic versus open surgery for colorectal carcinoma: a prospective clinical trial involving 157 cases with a mean follow-up of 5 years. Surg Laparosc Endosc Percutan Tech 2002; 12:88–95.
149. Curet MJ, Putrakul K, Pitcher DE, Josloff RK, Zucker KA. Laparoscopically assisted colon resection for colon carcinoma: perioperative results and long-term outcome. Surg Endosc 2000; 14:1062–1066.
150. Leung KL, Kwok SP, Lam SC, et al. Laparoscopic resection of rectosigmoid carcinoma: prospective randomised trial. Lancet 2004; 10;363(9416): 1187–1192.
151. Guillou PJ, Quirke P, Thorpe H, et al., MRC CLASICC trial group. Short-term endpoints of conventional versus laparoscopic-assisted surgery in patients with colorectal cancer (MRC CLASSIC trial): multicentre, randomized controlled trial. Lancet 2005; 365:1718–1726.
152. Melotti G, Tamborrino E, Lazzaretti MG, Bonilauri S, Mecheri F, Piccoli M. Laparoscopic surgery for colorectal cancer. Semin surg Oncol 1999; 16:332–336.
153. Franklin ME, Kazantsev GB, Abrego D, Diaz-E JA, Balli J, Glass JL. Laparoscopic surgery for stage III colon cancer: long-term follow-up. Surg Endosc 2000; 14:612–616.
154. Schiedeck TH, Schwandner O, Baca I, et al. Laparoscopic surgery for the cure of colorectal cancer: results of a German five-center study. Dis Colon Rectum 2000; 43:1–8.
155. Anderson CA, Kennedy FR, Potter M, et al. Results of laparoscopically assisted colon resection for carcinoma. Surg Endosc 2002; 16:607–610.
156. Lechaux D, Trebuchet G, Le Calve JL. Five-year results of 206 laparoscopic left colectomies for cancer. Surg Endosc 2002; 16:1409–1412.

157. Lumley J, Stitz R, Stevenson A, Fielding G, Luck A. Laparoscopic colorectal surgery for cancer: intermediate to long-term outcomes. Dis Colon Rectum 2002; 45:867–872.
158. Poulin EC, Schlachta CM, Gregoire R, Seshadri P, Cadeddu MO, Mamazzsa J. Local recurrence and survival after laparoscopic mesorectal resection for rectal adenocarcinoma. Surg Endosc 2002; 16:989–995.
159. Scheidbach H, Schneider C, Huegel O, et al. Laparoscopic sigmoid resection for cancer: curative resection and preliminary medium-term results. Dis Colon Rectum 2002; 45:1641–1647.
160. Yamamoto S, Watanabe M, Hasegawa H, Kitajima M. Prospective evaluation of laparoscopic surgery for rectosigmoidal and rectal carcinoma. Dis Colon Rectum 2002; 45:1648–1654.
161. Morino M, Parini U, Giraudo G, Salval M, Contul BR, Garrone C. Laparoscopic total mesorectal excision: a consecutive series of 100 patients. Ann Surg 2003; 237:335–342.
162. Tsang WW, Chung CC, Li MK. Prospective evaluation of laparoscopic total mesorectal excision with colonic J-pouch reconstruction for mid and low rectal cancers. Br J Surg 2003; 90:867–871.
163. Watanabe M, Hasegawa H, Yamamoto S, Baba H, Kitajima M. Laparoscopic surgery for stage I colorectal cancer. Surg Endosc 2003; 17:1274–1277.
164. Bouvet M, Mansfield PF, Skibber JM, et al. Clinical, pathologic, and economic parameters of laparoscopic colon resection for cancer. Am J Surg 1998; 176(6):554–558.
165. Schwandner O, Schiedeck TH, Killaitis C, Bruch HP. A case-control-study comparing laparoscopic versus open surgery for rectosigmoidal and rectal cancer. Int J Colorectal Dis 1999; 14:158–163.
166. Anthuber M, Fuerst A, Elser F, Berger R, Jauch KW. Outcome of laparoscopic surgery for rectal cancer in 101 patients. Dis Colon Rectum 2003; 46:1047–1053.
167. Franklin ME Jr, Rosenthal D, Abrego-Medina D, et al. A prospective comparison of open vs laparoscopic colon surgery for carcinoma: five-year results. Dis Colon Rectum 1996; 39:S35–S46.
168. Santoro E, Carlini M, Carboni F, Feroce A. Colorectal carcinoma: laparoscopic versus traditional open surgery. A clinical trial. Hepatogastroenterology 1999; 46:900–904.
169. Hartley JE, Mehigan BJ, Qureshi AE, Duthie GS, Lee PW, Monson JR. Total mesorectal excision: assessment of the laparoscopic approach. Dis Colon Rectum 2001; 44:315–321.
170. Feliciotti F, Guerrieri M, Paganini AM, Sanctis A, Campagnacci R, Lezoche E. Results of laparoscopic vs open resections for colon cancer in patients with a minimum follow-up of 3 years. Surg Endosc 2002; 16:1158–1161.
171. Lezoche E, Feliciotti F, Paganini AM, et al. Laparoscopic vs open hemicolectomy for colon cancer. Surg Endosc 2002; 16:596–602.
172. Felicitti F, Guerrieri m, Paganini AM, et al. Long-term results of laparoscopic versus open resections for rectal cancer for 124 unselected patients. Surg Endosc 2003; 17:1530–1535.
173. Abraham NS, Young JM, Solomon MJ. Meta-analysis of short-term outcomes after laparoscopic resection for colorectal cancer. Br J Surg 2004; 91:1111–1124.
174. Stage JG, Schulze S, Moller P, et al. Prospective randomized study of laparoscopic versus open colonic resection for adenocarcinoma. Br J Surg 1997; 84:391.
175. Milsom JW, Böhm B, Hammerhofer KA, Fazio V, Steiger E, Elson PA. Prospective, randomized trial comparing laparoscopic versus conventional techniques in colorectal cancer surgery: a preliminary report. J Am Coll Surg 1998; 187:46.
176. Hasegawa H, Kabeshima Y, Watanabe M, Yamamoto S, Kitajima M. Randomized controlled trial of laparoscopic versus open colectomy for advanced colorectal cancer. Surg Endosc 2003; 17:636.
177. Weeks JC, Nelson H, Gelber S, Sargentfor AD, The Clinical Outcomes of Surgical Therapy (COST) Study Group, Schroeder G. Short-term quality-of-life outcomes following laparoscopic-assisted colectomy vs open colectomy for colon cancer: a randomized trial. JAMA 2002; 287:321.
178. Schwenk W, Böhm B, Müller JM. Postoperative pain and fatigue after laparoscopic or conventional colorectal resections. Surg Endosc 1998; 12:1131.
179. Kieran JA, Curet MJ. Laparoscopic colon resection for colon cancer. J Surg Res 2004; 117:79–91.
180. Tang CL, Eu KW, Tai BC, Soh JG, MacHin D, Seow-Choen F. Randomized clinical trial of the effect of open versus laparoscopically assisted colectomy on systemic immunity in patients with colorectal cancer. Br J Surg 2001; 88:801.
181. Delgado S, Momblan D, Salvador L, et al. Laparoscopic-assisted approach in rectal cancer patients: lessons learned from >200 patients. Surg Endosc 2004; 18:1457–1462.
182. Law WL, Chu KW, Tung HM. Early outcome of 100 patients with laparoscopic resection for rectal neoplasm. Surg Endosc 2004; 18:1592–1596.
183. Zhou ZG, Hu M, Li Y, et al. Laparoscopic versus open total mesorectal excision with anal sphincter preservation for low rectal cancer. Surg Endosc 2004; 18:1211–1215.
184. Leroy J, Jamali F, Forbes L, Smith M, Rubino F, Mutter D, Marescaux J. Laparoscopic total mesorectal excision (TME) for rectal cancer surgery: long-term outcomes. Surg Endosc 2004; 18:281–289.
185. Rullier E, Sa Cunha A, Couderc P, Rullier A, Gontier R, Saric J. Laparoscopic intersphincteric resection with coloplasty and coloanal anastomosis for mid and low rectal cancer. Br J Surg 2003; 90:445–451.
186. Jayne DG, Brown JM, Thorpe H, Walker J, Quirke P, Guillou PJ. Bladder and sexual function following resection for rectal cancer in a randomized clinical trial of laparoscopic versus open technique. Br J Surg 2005; 92:1124–1132.
187. Milsom JW, Kim SH, Hammerhofer KA, Fazio VW. Laparoscopic colorectal cancer surgery for palliation. Dis Colon Rectum 2000; 43:1512–1516.
188. Delgado S, Lacy AM, Garcia Valdecasas JC, Balague C, Pera M, Salvador L, et al. Could age be an indication for laparoscopic colectomy in colorectal cancer? Surg Endosc 2000; 14:22–26.
189. Capussotti L, Massucco P, Murator A, Amisano M,. Bima C, Zorzi D. Laparoscopic as a prognostic factor in curative resection for node positive colorectal cancer: results for a single-institution nonrandomized prospective trial. Surg Endosc 2004; 18:1130–1135.
190. Kockerling F, Scheidbach H, Schneider C, et al. Laparoscopic abdominoperineal resection: early postoperative results of a prospective study involving 116 patients. The Laparoscopic Colorectal Surgery Study Group. Dis Colon Rectum 2000; 43:1503–1511.
191. Ludwig KA, Milsom JW, Garcia-Ruiz A, et al. Laparoscopic techniques for fecal diversion. Dis Colon Rectum 1996; 39:285–288.
192. Reissman P, Salky BD, Edye M, et al. Laparoscopic surgery in Crohn's disease. Surg Endosc 1996; 10:1201–1204.
193. Bergamaschi R, Pessaux P, Arnaud JP. Comparison of conventional and laparoscopic ileocolic resection for Crohn's disease. Dis Colon Rectum 2003; 46:1129–1133.
194. Hasegawa H, Watanabe M, Nishibori H, Okabayashi K, Hibi T, Kitajima M. Laparoscopic surgery for recurrent Crohn's disease. Br J Surg 2003; 90: 970–973.
195. Wu JS, Brinbaum EH, Kodner IJ, Fry RD, Read TE, Fleshman JW. Laparoscopic-assisted ileocolic resections in patients with Crohn's disease: are abscesses, phlegmons, or recurrent disease contraindications? Surgery 1997; 122:682–688.
196. Moorthy K, Shaul T, Foley RJ. Factors that predict conversion in patients undergoing laparoscopic surgery for Crohn's disease. Am J Surg 2004; 187:47–51.
197. Benoist S, Panis Y, Beaufour A, Bouhnik Y, Matuchansky C, Valleur P. Laparoscopic ileocecal resection in Crohn's disease: a case-matched comparison with open resection. Surg Endosc 2003; 17:814–818.
198. Canin-Endres J, Salky B, Gattorno F, Edye M. Laparoscopically assisted intestinal resection in 88 patients with Crohn's disease. Surg. Endosc 1999; 13: 595–599.
199. Hamel CT, Hildebrandt U, Weiss EG, Feifelz G, Wexner SD. Laparoscopic surgery for inflammatory bowel disease. Surg Endosc 2001; 15:642–645.
200. Evans J, Poritz L, MacRae H. Influence of experience on laparoscopic ileocolic resection for Crohn's disease. Dis Colon Rectum 2002; 45:1595–1600.
201. Alabaz O, Iroatulam AJ, Nessim A, Weiss EG, Norgueras JJ, Wexner SD. Comparison of laparoscopically assisted and conventional ileocolic resection for Crohn's disease. Eur J Surg 2000; 166:213–217.
202. Bemelman WA, Slors JF, Dunker MS, et al. Laparoscopic-assisted vs. open ileocolic resection for Crohn's disease. A comparative study. Surg Endosc 2000; 14:721–725.
203. Milsom JW, Hammerhofer KA, Bohm B, Marcello P, Elson P, Fazio VW. Prospective, randomized trial comparing laparoscopic vs. conventional surgery for refractory ileocolic Crohn's disease. Dis Colon Rectum 2001; 44:1–8.
204. Tabet J, Hong D, Kim CW, Wong J, Goodacre R, Anvari M. Laparoscopic versus open bowel resection for Crohn's disease. Can J Gastroenterol 2001; 15:237–242.
205. Young-Fadok TM, HallLong K, McConnell EJ, Gomez Rey G, Cabanela RL. Advantages of laparoscopic resection for ileocolic Crohn's disease. Improved outcomes and reduced costs. Surg Endosc 2001; 15:450–454.
206. Duepree HJ, Senagore AJ, Delaney CP, Brady KM, Fazio VW. Advantages of laparoscopic resection for ileocecal Crohn's disease. Dis Colon Rectum 2002; 45:605–610.
207. Ky AJ, Sonoda T, Milsom JW. One-stage laparoscopic restorative proctocolectomy: an alternative to the conventional approach? Dis Colon Rectum 2002; 45:207–210.
208. Marcello PW, Milsom JW, Wong SK, et al. Laparoscopic restorative proctocolectomy: case-matched comparative study with open restorative proctocolectomy. Dis Colon Rectum 2000; 43:604–608.
209. Marcello PW, Milsom JW, Wong SK, Brady K, Goormastic M, Fazio VW. Laparoscopic total colectomy for acute colitis: a case-control study. Dis Colon Rectum 2001; 44:1441–1445.
210. Rivadeneira DE, Marcello PW, Roberts PL, et al. Benefits of hand-assisted laparoscopic restorative proctocolectomy: a comparative study. Dis Colon Rectum 2004; 47:1371–1376.
211. Kienle P, Weitz J, Benner A, Herfarth C, Schmidt J. Laparoscopically assisted colectomy and ileoanal pouch procedure with and without protective ileostomy. Surg Endosc 2003; 17:716–720.
212. Kienle P, N'graggen K, Schmidt J, Benner A, Weitz J, Buchler MW. Laparoscopic restorative proctocolectomy. Br J Surg 2005; 92:88–93.
213. Bell RL, Seymour NE. Laparoscopic treatment of fulminant ulcerative colitis. Surg Endosc 2002; 16:1778–1782.
214. Hasegawa H, Watanabe M, Baba H, Nishibori H, Kitajima M. Laparoscopic restorative proctocolectomy for patients with ulcerative colitis. J Laparoendosc Adv Surg Tech A 2002; 12:403–406.

215. Dunker MS, Bemelman WA, Slors JF, van Hogezand RA, Ringers J, Gouma DJ. Laparoscopic-assisted vs open colectomy for severe acute colitis in patients with inflammatory bowel disease (IBD): a retrospective study in 42 patients. Surg Endosc 2000; 14:911–914.
216. Schmitt SL, Cohen SM, Wexner SD, Nogueras JJ, Janelman DG. Does laparoscopic-assisted ileal pouch anal anastomosis reduce the length of hospitalization? Int J Colorectal Dis 1994; 9:134–137.
217. Araki Y, ishibashi N, Ogata Y, Shirouzu k, Isomoto H. The usefulness of restorative laparoscopic-assisted total colectomy of ulcerative colitis. Kurume Med J 2001; 48:99–103.
218. Pace DE, Seshadri PA, Chiasson PM, Poulin EC, Schlachta CM, Mamazza J. Early experience with laparoscopic ileal pouch-anal anastomosis for ulcerative colitis. Surg Laparosc Endosc Percutan Tech 2002; 12:337–341.
219. Oliveira L, Reissman P, Nogueras J, et al. Laparoscopic creation of stomas. Surg Endost 1997; 11:19–23.
220. Swain BT, Ellis CN Jr. Laparoscopy-assisted loop ileostomy: an acceptable option for temporary fecal diversion after anorectal surgery. Dis Colon Rectum 2002; 45:705–707.
221. Liu J, Bruch HP, Farke S, Nolde J, Schwnadner O. Stoma formation for fecal diversion: a plea for the laparoscopic approach. Tech Coloproctol 2005; 9: 9–14.
222. Regadas FSP, Siebra JA, Rodrigues LV, et al. Laparoscopically assisted colorectal anastomoses post-Hartmann's procedure. Surg Lap'arosc Endosc 1996; 1:1–4.
223. Delgado Gomis F, Garcia Lozano A, Domingo del Pozo C, Grau Cardona E, Martin Delgado J. Laparoscopic reconstruction of intestinal continuity following Hartmann's procedure. Rev Esp Enferm Dig 1998; 90:499–502.
224. Bruce CJ, Coller JA, Murray JJ, et al. Laparoscopic resection for diverticulitis disease. Dis Colon Rectum 1996; 39:51–56.
225. Stevenson AR, Stitz RW, Lomley JW, Fielding GA. Laparoscopically assisted anterior resection for diverticular diseases: follow-up of 100 consecutive patients. Ann Surg 1998:335–342.
226. Berthou JC, Charbonneau P. Elective laparoscopic management of sigmoid diverticulitis. Results in a series of 110 patients. Surg Endosc 1999; 13: 457–460.
227. Kockerling F, Schneider C, Reymond MA, et al. Laparoscopic resection of sigmoid diverticulitis. Results of a multicenter study. Laparoscopic Colorectal Surgery Study Group. Surg Endosc 1999; 13:567–571.
228. Schlachta CM, Mamazza J, Poulin EC. Laparoscopic sigmoid resection for acute and chronic diverticultis. An outcomes comparison with laparoscopic resection for nondiverticular disease. Surg Endosc 1999; 13:649–653.
229. Smadja C, Sbai Idrissi M, Tahrat M, et al. Elective laparoscopic sigmoid colectomy for diverticulitis. Results of a prospective study. Surg Endosc 1999; 13: 645–648.
230. Siriser F. Laparoscopic-assisted colectomy for diverticular sigmoiditis. A single-surgeon prospective study of 65 patients. Surg Endosc 1999; 13: 811–813.
231. Burgel JS, Navarro F, Lemoine MC, et al. Elective laparoscopic colectomy for sigmoid diverticultis. Prospective study of 56 cases. Ann Chir 2000; 125: 231–237.
232. Carbajo Caballero MA, Martin del Olmo JC, Blanco Alvarez JI, et al. Acute diverticulitis and diverticular disease of the colon: a safe indication for laparoscopic surgery. Rev Esp Enferm Dig 2000; 92:718–725.
233. Vargas HD, Ramirez RT, Hoffman GC, et al. Defining the role of laparoscopic-assisted sigmoid colectomy for diverticulitis. Dis Colon Rectum 2000; 43: 1726–1731.
234. Bouillot JL, Berthou JC, Champault G, et al. Elective laparoscopic colonic resection for diverticular disease: results of a multicenter study in 179 patients. Surg Endosc 2002; 16:1320–1323.
235. Trebuchet G, Lechaux D, Lacalve JL. Laparoscopic left colon resection for diverticular disease. Surg Endosc 2002; 16:18–21.
236. Pugliese R, Di Lernia S, Sansonna F, et al. Laparoscopic treatment of sigmoid diverticultis. A retrospective review of 103 cases. Surg Endosc 2004; 18: 1344–1348.
237. Scheidbach H, Schneider C, Rose J, et al. Laparoscopic approach to treatment of sigmoid diverticulitis: changes in the spectrum of indications and results of a prospective, multicenter study on 1,545 patients. Dis Colon Rectum 2004; 47:1883–1888.
238. Bartus CM, Lipof T, Sarwar CM, Vignati PV, Johnson KH, Sardella WV, Cohen JL. Colovesical fistula: not a contraindication to elective laparoscopic colectomy. Dis Colon Rectum 2005; 48:233–236.
239. Franklin ME Jr, Dorman JP, Jacobs M, Plasencia G. Is laparoscopic surgery applicable to complicated colonic diverticular disease? Surg Endosc 1997; 11:1021–1025.
240. Menenakos E, Hahnloser D, Nassioloulos K, Chanson C, Sinclair V, Petropoulos P. Laparoscopic surgery for fistulas that complicate diverticular disease. Langenbeck Arch Surg 2003; 388:189–193.
241. Schwandner O, Farke S, Fischer F, Eckmann C, Schiedeck TH, Bruch HP. Laparoscopic colectomy for recurrent and complicated diverticulitis: a prospective study of 396 patients. Langenbecks Arch Surg 2004; 389:97–103.
242. Laurent SR, Detroz B, Detry O, Degauque C, Honore P, Meurisse M. Laparoscopic sigmoidectomy for fistulized diverticulitis. Dis Colon Rectum 2005; 48:148–152.
243. Sher ME, Agachan F, Bortul M, Nogueras JJ, Weiss EG, Wexner SD. Laparoscopic surgery for diverticulitis. Surg Endosc 1997; 11:264–267.
244. Kohler L, Rixen D, Troidl H. Laparoscopic colorectal resection for diverticulitis. Int J Colorectal Dis 1998; 13:43–47.
245. Faynsod M, Stamos MJ, Arnell T, Borden C, Udani S, Vargas H. A case-control study of laparoscopic versus open sigmoid colectomy for diverticulitis. Am Surg 2000; 66:841–843.
246. Tuech JJ, Pessaux P, Rouge C, Regenet N, Bergamaschi R, Arnaud JP. Laparoscopic vs open colectomy for sigmoid diverticulitis: a prospective comparative study in the elderly. Surg Endosc 2000; 14:1031–1033.
247. Senagore AJ, Duepree HJ, Delaney CP, Dissanaike S, Brady KM, Fazio VW. Cost structure of laparoscopic and open sigmoid colectomy for diverticular disease: similarities and difference. Dis Colon Rectum 2002; 45:485–490.
248. Dwivedi A, Chahin F, Agrawal S, et al. Laparoscopic colectomy vs. open colectomy for sigmoid diverticular disease. Dis Colon Rectum 2002; 45:1309–1314.
249. Lawrence DM, Pasquakle MD, Wasser TE. Laparoscopic versus open sigmoid colectomy for diverticulitis. Am Surg 2003; 69:499–503.
250. Gonzalez R, Smith CD; Matter SG, et al. Laparoscopic vs open resection for the treatment of diverticular disease. Surg Endosc 2004; 18:276–280.
251. O'Sullivan GC, Murphy D, O'Brien MG, Ireland A. Laparoscopic management of generalized peritonitis due to perforated colonic diverticula. Am J Surg 1996; 171:432–434.
252. Tuech JJ, Regenet N, Hennekinne S, Pessaux P, Bergamaschi R, Arnaud JP. Laparoscopic colectomy for sigmoid diverticulitis in obese and nonobese patients: a prospective comparative study. Surg Endosc 2001; 15: 1427–1430.
253. Thaler K, Weiss EG, Nogueras JJ, Arnaud JP, Wexner SD, Bergamaschi R. Recurrence rates at minimum 5-year follow-up: laparoscopic versus open sigmoid resection for uncomplicated diverticulitis. Surg Laparosc Endosc Percutan Tech 2003; 13:325–327.
254. Faranda C, Barrat C, Catheline JM, Champault GG. Two-stage laparoscopic management of generalized peritonitis due to perforated sigmoid diverticula: eighteen cases. Surg Laparosc Endosc Percutan Tech 2000;. 10:135–138.
255. Natarajan S, Ewings EL, Vega RJ. Laparoscopic sigmoid colectomy after acute diverticulitis: when to operate? Surgery 2004;. 136:725–730.
256. Le Moine MC, Fabre JM, Vacher C, Navarro F, Picot MC, Domergue J. Factors and consequences of conversion in laparoscopic sigmoidectomy for diverticular diseases. Br J Surg 2003; 90:232–236.
257. Rose J, Schneider C, Scheidbach, et al. Laparoscopic treatment of rectal prolapse: experience gained in a prospective multicenter study. Langenbecks Arch Surg 2002; 387:130–137.
258. Madbouly KM, Senagore AJ, Delaney CP, Duepree HJ, Brady KM, Fazio VW. Clinically based management of rectal prolapse. Surg Endosc 2003; 17:99–103.
259. Solomon MJ, Young CJ, Eyers AA, Roberts RA. Randomized clinical trial of laparoscopic versus open abdominal rectopexy for rectal prolapse. Br J Surg 2002; 89:35–39.
260. Heah SM, Hartley JE, Hurley J, Duthie GS, Monson JR. Laparoscopic suture rectopexy without resection is effective treatment for full-thickness rectal prolapse. Dis Colon Rectum 2000; 43:638–643.
261. Stevenson AR, Stitz RW, Lumley JW. Laparoscopic-assisted resection-rectopexy for rectal prolapse: early and medium follow-up. Dis Colon Rectum 1998; 41:46–54.
262. Kessler H, Jerby BL, Milsom JW. Successful treatment of rectal prolapse by laparoscope suture rectopexy. Surg Endosc 1999; 13:858–861.
263. Kellokumpu IH, Vironen J, Scheinin T. Laparoscopic repair of rectal prolapse: a prospective study evaluating surgical outcome and changes in symptoms and bowel function. Surg Endosc 2000; 14:634–640.
264. Benoist S, Taffinder N, Gould S, Chang A, Darzi A. Functional results two years after laparoscopic rectopexy. Am J Surg 2001; 182:168–173.
265. Bergamaschi R, Lovvik K, Marvik R. Preserving the superior rectal artery in laparoscopic sigmoid resection for complete rectal prolapse. Surg Laparosc Endosc Percutan Tech 2003; 13:374–376.
266. Kairaluoma MV, Viljakka MT, Kellokumpu IH. Open vs. Laparoscopic surgery for rectal prolapse: a case-controlled study assessing short-term outcome. Dis Colon Rectum 2003; 46:353–360.
267. D'Hoore A, Cadoni R, Penninckx F. Long-term outcome of laparoscopic ventral rectopexy for total rectal prolapse. Br J Surg 2004; 91:1500–1505.
268. Ashari LH, Lumley JW, Stevenson AR, Stitz RW. Laparoscopically-assisted resection rectopexy for rectal prolapse: ten years' experience. Dis Colon Rectum 2005; 48:982–987.
269. Boccasanta P, Venturi M, Reitano MC, et al. Laparotomic vs. laparoscopic rectopexy in complete rectal prolapse. Dig Surg 1999; 16:415–419.
270. Himpens J, Cadiere GB, Bruyns J, Vertruyen M. Laparoscopic rectopexy according to Wells. Surg Endosc 1999; 13:139–141.
271. Xynos E, Chrysos E, Tsiaoussis J, Epanomeritakis E, Vassilakis JS. Resection rectopexy for rectal prolapse. The laparoscopic approach. Surg Endosc 1999; 13:862–864.
272. Bruch HP, Herold A, Schiedeck T, Schwandner O. Laparoscopic surgery for rectal prolapse and outlet obstruction. Dis Colon Rectum 1999; 42: 1189–1194.

273. Purkayastha S, Tekkis P, Athanasiou T, et al. A comparison of open vs. laparoscopic abdominal rectopexy for full-thickness rectal prolapse: a meta-analysis. Dis Colon Rectum 2005; 48:1930–1940.
274. Regan JP, Salky BA. Laparoscopic treatment of enteric fistulas. Surg Endosc 2004; 18:252–254.
275. Poulin EC, Schlachta CM, Mamazza J, Seshadri PA. Should enteric fistulas from Crohn's disease or diverticulitis be treated by laparoscopic or by open surgery? A matched cohort study. Dis Colon Rectum 2000; 43:621–626.
276. Watanabe M, Hasegawa H, Yamamoto S, Hibi T, Kitajima M. Successful application of laparoscopic surgery to the treatment of Crohn's disease with fistulas. Dis Colon Rectum 2002; 45:1057–1061.
277. Sample C, Gupta R, Bamehriz F, Anvari M. Laparoscopic subtotal colectomy for colonic inertia. J Gastrointest Surg 2005; 9:803–808.
278. Jerby BL, Kessler H, Falcone T, Milsom JW. Laparoscopic management of colorectal endometriosis. Surg Endosc 1999; 13:1125–1128.
279. Milsom JW, Ludwig KA, Church JM, Garcia-Ruiz A. Laparoscopic total abdominal colectomy with ileorectal anastomosis for familial adenomatous polyposis. Dis Colon Rectum 1997; 40:675–678.
280. Safadi B. Laparoscopic repair of parastomal hernias: early results. Surg Endosc 2004; 18:676–680.
281. Navsaria PH, Shaw JM, Zellweger R, Nicol AJ, Kahn D. Diagnostic laparoscopy and diverting sigmoid loop colostomy in the management of civilian extraperitoneal rectal gunshot injuries. Br J Surg 2004; 91:460–464.
282. Cobb WS, Lokey JS, Schwab DP, Crockett JA, Rex JC, Robbins JA. Hand-assisted laparoscopic colectomy: a single-institution experience. Am Surg 2003; 69:578–580.
283. Nakajima K, Lee SW, Cocilovo C, Foglia C, Kim K, Sonoda T, Milsom JW. Laparoscopic total colectomy: hand-assisted vs standard technique. Surg Endosc 2004; 18:582–586.
284. Targarona EM, Gracia E, Garriga J, et al. Prospective randomized trial comparing conventional laparoscopic colectomy with hand-assisted laparoscopic colectomy: applicability, immediate clinical outcome, inflammatory response, and cost. Surg Endosc 2002; 16:234–239.
285. Senagore AJ, Delaney CP, Madboulay K, Brady KM, Fazio VW. Laparoscopic colectomy in obese and nonobese patients. J Gastrointest Surg 2003; 7: 558–561.
286. Schwandner O, Farke S, Schiedeck TH, Bruch HP. Laparoscopic colorectal surgery in obese and nonobese patients: do difference in body mass indices lead to different outcomes? Surg Endosc 2004; 18:1452–1456.
287. Delaney CP, Pokala N, Senagore AJ, et al. Is laparoscopic colectomy applicable to patients with body mass index >30? A case-matched comparative study with open colectomy. Dis Colon Rectum 2005; 48:975–981.
288. Adachi Y, Sato K, Kakisako K, et al. Quality of life after laparoscopic or open colonic resection for cancer. Hepatogastroenterology 2003;. 50: 1348–1351.
289. Thaler K, Dinnewitzer A, Mascha E, et al. Long-term outcome and health-related quality of life after laparoscopic and open colectomy for benign disease. Surg Endosc 2003; 17:1404–1408.
290. Dunker MS, Bemelman WA, Slors JF, van Duijvendijk P, Gouma DJ. Functional outcome, quality of life, body image, and cosmesis in patients after laparoscopic-assisted and conventional restorative proctocolectomy: a comparative study. Dis Colon Rectum 2001; 44:1800–1807.
291. Janson M, Bjorholt I, Carlsson P, et al. Randomized clinical trial of the costs of open and laparoscopic surgery for colonic cancer. Br J Surg 2004; 91: 409–417.
292. Delaney CP, Kiran RP, Senagore AJ, Brady K, Fazio VW. Case-matched comparison of clinical and financial outcome after laparoscopic or open colorectal surgery. Ann Surg 2003; 238:67–72.
293. Larach SW, Patankar SK, Ferrara A, Williamson PR, Perozo SE, Lord AS. Complications of laparoscopic colorectal surgery. Analysis and comparison of early vs. later experience. Dis Colon Rectum 1997; 40:592–596.
294. Chandler JG, Corson SL, Way LW. Three spectra of laparoscopic entry access injuries. J Am Coll Surg 2001;. 192:478–490.
295. Van der Voort M, Heijnsdijk EA, Gouma DJ. Bowel injury as a complication of laparoscopy. Br J Surg 2004; 91:1253–1258.
296. Levrant SG, Bieber EJ, Barnes RB. Anterior abdominal wall adhesions after laparotomy or laparoscopy. J Am Assoc Gynecol Laparosc 1997; 4:353–356.
297. Schafer M, Lauper M, Krahenbuhl L. Trocar and Veress needle injuries during laparoscopy. Surg Endosc 2001; 15:275–280.
298. Schafer M, Lauper M, Krahenbuhl L. A nation's experience of bleeding complications during laparoscopy. Am J Surg 2000; 180:73–77.
299. Bhoyrul S, Vierra MA, Nezhat CR, Krummel TM, Way LW. Trocar injuries in laparoscopic surgery. J Am Coll Surg 2001; 192:677–683.
300. Millikan KW, Szczerba SM, Dominguez JM, et al. Superior mesenteric portal vein thrombosis following laparoscopic-assisted right hemicolectomy. Dis Colon Rectum 1996; 39:1171–1175.
301. Sackier JM. Visualization of the ureter during laparoscopic colonic resection. Br J Surg 1993; 80:1332.
302. Williams IM, Haray PN, Lloyd-Davies E, et al. Bladder injury during laparoscopic abdominoperineal resection. Br J Surg 1995; 82:1207.
303. Fusco MA, Paluzi MW. Abdominal wall recurrence after laparoscopic-assisted colectomy for adenocarcinoma of the colon. Dis Colon Rectum 1993; 36:858–861.
304. Wexner SD, Cohen SM. Port site metastases after laparoscopic colorectal surgery for cure of malignancy. Br J Surg 1995; 82:295–298.
305. Ugarte F. Laparoscopic cholecystectomy port seeding from a colon carcinoma. Am Surg 1995; 61:820–821.
306. Jacobi CA, Sabat R, Böhm B, et al. Pneumoperitoneum with carbon dioxide stimulates growth of malignant colonic cells. Surgery 1997; 121:72–78.
307. Jones DB, Guo LW, Reinhard MK, et al. Impact of pneumoperitoneum on trocar site implantation of colon cancer in hamster model. Dis Colon Rectum 1995; 38:1182–1188.
308. Balli JE, Franklin ME, Alameida A, et al. How to prevent port-site metastases in laparoscopic colorectal surgery. Surg Endosc 2000; 14:1034.
309. Curet MJ. Port site metastases. Am J Surg 2004; 187:705–712.
310. Lacy AM, Delgado S, García-Valdecasas JC, et al. Port site metastases and recurrence after laparoscopic colectomy. A randomized trial. Surg Endosc 1998; 12:1039.
311. Silecchia G, Perrotta N, Giraudo G, et al., For the Italian Registry of Laparoscopic Colorectal Surgery. Abdominal wall recurrence after colorectal resection for cancer: results of the Italian registry of laparoscopic colorectal surgery. Dis Colon Rectum 2002; 45:1172–1177.
312. Ziprin P, Ridgway PF, Peck DH, Darzi AW. The theories and realities of port-site metastases: a critical appraisal. J Am Coll Surg 2002; 195:395.
313. Hughes ESR, McDermott FT, Polglase AL, et al. Tumor recurrence in the abdominal wall scar tissue after large bowel cancer surgery. Dis Colon Rectum 1983; 26:571–572.
314. Reilly WT, Nelson H, Schroeder G, et al. Wound recurrence following conventional treatment of colorectal cancer. A rare but perhaps underestimated problem. Dis Colon Rectum 1996; 39:200–207.
315. Vukasin P, Ortega AK, Greene FL, et al. Wound recurrence following laparoscopic colon cancer resection: results of The American Society of Colon and Rectal Surgeons Laparoscopic Registry. Dis Colon Rectum 1996; 39:S20–S23.
316. Bonjer HJ, Lange JF. Rotation of the terminal ileum in laparoscopic right hemicolectomy. Surg Endosc 1993; 7:534.
317. Kitamura K, Yamane T, Oyama T, et al. Rapid and accurate method for delineating cancer lesions in laparoscopic colectomy using activated carbon injection. J Surg Oncol 1995; 58:31–34.
318. McDermott JP, Devereaux DA, Caushaj PF. Pitfall of laparoscopic colectomy: an unrecognized synchronous cancer. Dis Colon Rectum 1994; 37:602–603.
319. Nizam R, Siddiqi N, Landas SK, Kaplan DS, Holtzapple PG. Colonic tattooing with India ink: benefits, risks, and alternatives. Am J Gastroenterol 1996; 91:1804–1808.
320. Coman E, Brandt LS, Brenner S, et al. Fat necrosis and inflammatory pseudotumor due to endoscopic tattooing of the colon with India ink. Gastrointest Endosc 1991; 37:65–68.
321. Park SI, Genta RS, Romeo DP, Weesner RE. Colonic abscess and focal peritonitis secondary to India ink tattooing of the colon. Gastrointest Endosc 1991; 37:68–71.
322. Nduka CC, Sager PA, Monson JRT, et al. Cause and prevention of electrosurgical injuries in laparoscopy. J Am Coll Surg 1994; 179:161–170.
323. Hoenig DM, Chrostek CA, Amaral JF. Laparosonic coagulating shears: alternative method of hemostatic control of unsupported tissue. J Endourol 1996; 10:431–433.
324. Winslow ER, Fleshman JW, Birnbaum EH, Brunt LM. Wound complications of laparoscopic vs open colectomy. Surg Endosc 2002; 16:1420–1425.
325. Hackert T, Uhl W, Buchler MW. Specimen retrieval in laparoscopic colon surgery. Dig Surg 2002; 19:502–506.
326. Kercher KW, Nguyen TH, Harold KL, et al. Plastic wound protectors do not affect wound infection rates following laparoscopic-assisted colectomy. Surg Endosc 2004; 18:148–151.
327. Cottin V, Delafosse B, Viale JP. Gas embolism during laparoscopy. A report of seven cases in patients with previous abdominal surgical history. Surg Endosc 1996; 10:166–169.
328. Baixauli J, Delaney CP, Senagore AJ, Remzi FH, Fazio VW. Portal vein thrombosis after laparoscopic sigmoid colectomy for diverticulitis: report of a case. Dis Colon Rectum 2003; 46:550–553.

39 Miscellaneous Entities

Philip H. Gordon

COCCYGODYNIA

Coccygodynia (coccydynia, coccyalgia) denotes pain in the coccyx, which may be functional in origin or organic. Patients complain of aching, cramping, or sharp pain that is localized in the region of the coccyx or sometimes radiates to the buttocks or down the backs of the thighs. At times, the attacks of pain can become sharp, shooting, or breathtaking. Patients with symptoms of coccygodynia usually make the rounds of orthopedic surgeons, gynecologists, neurologists, and colon and rectal surgeons to seek help.

De Andres and Chaves (1) recently reviewed this subject and much of the following information was obtained from that detailed review. Coccydynia mainly affects women. Some authors attribute this to the more posterior location of the sacrum and coccyx and the characteristics of the ischial tuberosities that leave a woman's coccyx more exposed and susceptible to trauma both in common situations (sitting position) and during childbirth. The coccyx is larger in women than in men and is therefore more susceptible to injuries. A high incidence of the disorder has also been reported in debilitated elderly patients.

ANATOMIC REVIEW

The coccyx is composed of one to four bony segments joined to the distal portion of the sacrum by means of the sacrococcygeal joint, the latter constituting a synarthrosis or fibrous joint. The sacrococcygeal joint is bound by sacrococcygeal ligaments and this fibrous tissue encloses the sacral cornua that form the last intervertebral foramen, through which the fifth sacral roots exit. The first and second coccygeal segments are potentially mobile, a fact that predisposes to possible pathologic hypermobility. Posterior luxation is a common feature if there is obesity or a history of trauma. The S5 roots exit above the first coccygeal vertebra to contribute to the coccygeal plexus, which is formed from the anterior division of L5 and a small filament from L4 that joins with the coccygeal nerve. These lay anterior to the sacrum and coccyx but posterior to the pelvic organs, an area rich in somatic and autonomic nerve endings. These autonomic structures consist of the so-called ganglion impar (ganglion of Walther) and the superior and inferior hypogastric plexus. Pain around the coccyx is felt with stimulation of S4, S5 and coccygeal roots. In some patients the coccyalgia is related to the S3 distribution, because the stimulation of this root is felt in the perianal region, rectum, and genitalia.

ETIOLOGY AND PATHOGENESIS OF COCCYGODYNIA

The classification of coccygodynia is based on the time course of the disorder. The most common sources of acute pain are the coccygeal disks or joints in 70% of the cases with four different causes: coccygeal spicules, anterior luxation, coccygeal hypermobility, and subluxation or luxation. Acute local trauma related to a fall in the sitting position or childbirth is a common etiology. This presentation usually responds well to conservative management with anti-inflammatory drugs and rest. The duration of pain is limited. The condition is considered chronic when it has persisted for more than two months and the underlying cause is often uncertain. Treatment response is variable.

Coccygodynia has been classified according to the characteristics of pain. Conditions associated with somatic pain have included idiopathic hypermobility of the coccyx, luxation of the coccyx, myofascial syndromes, depression and somatization, septic conditions, arthritis, osteitis, and sacral hemangioma. Those associated with neuropathic pain included idiopathic lumbar disk herniation, intradural schwannoma, neurinoma, arachnoid cysts, and glomus neoplasms. Mixed presentations may be associated with chordoma, bone metastases, and neoplastic visceral processes.

DIAGNOSIS

Diagnosis is based on the clinical manifestations. Patients should be questioned about the characteristics of pain, because the information obtained might help to determine the underlying pathogenic mechanism. All patients should be asked for a history of precipitating trauma and the time at which it occurred, presence of sudden and acute pain when passing from sitting to standing, and type of seat that makes the pain worse. Comprehensive personality/behavioral assessment may be recommended to show possible abnormal personality traits or psychologic impairment as indicative of anxiety or depression.

In cases of coccygodynia involving somatic pain, the coccyx is found to be painful and tender to palpation. The pain is intensified on sitting on a hard surface and the diagnosis of cyccygodynia should be questioned when the pain fails to disappear on lying down. Somatic pain at coccygeal level is related to body posture and is accentuated with coccygeal movements during rectal digital examination.

Neuropathic pain in turn manifests as poorly localized coccygeal pain accompanied by a burning or lancing sensation and is occasionally associated with loss of sensitivity or paresthesias. In such cases, the pain increases in response to palpation, but no pain is recorded on mobilizing the coccyx. The pain tends to exhibit a segmental distribution when originating from the sacral root or peripheral nerve. In cases of spinal involvement, the pain characteristically intensifies with coughing, sneezing, or defecation. In cases of spinal (lumbar) involvement, the pain can also be triggered by lumbar movements.

Radiographic studies usually include a lateral X-ray view of the coccyx. X-rays can identify fractures, luxations, osteoarthritis, and osteolytic lesions caused by neoplasms. In dynamic radiographic imaging, hypermobolity of the coccyx is defined as more than 25° of flexion on the lateral view. Luxation is defined as more than 25% movement (backward displacement) of the coccyx from the standing to the sitting view. Measurement of the intercoccygeal angle, the angle formed between the first coccygeal segment and the last coccygeal segment can provide an objective measurement of forward inclination of the coccyx. Magnetic resonance imaging might be used for better visualization of the shape of the coccyx, especially the tip, for visualization of a dorsal bursitis and also to discard cysts, neoplasms, or neural lesions. Isotope bone scans of the sacrococcygeal area might be useful.

Kim and Suk (2) compared the clinical and radiological differences between 19 patients with traumatic coccygodynia and 13 patients with idiopathic coccygodynia. The outcome of treatment was assessed by a visual analog scale based on the pain score. There were no statistically significant differences between the traumatic and idiopathic coccygodynia groups in terms of age, sex ratio, and the number of coccyx segments. There were significant differences between the traumatic and idiopathic coccygodynia groups in terms of the pain score (pain on sitting: 82 vs. 47), pain on defecation (39 vs. 87), the intercoccygeal angle (47.9° vs. 72.2°), and the satisfactory outcome of conservative treatment (47.4% vs. 92.3%).

■ FUNCTIONAL COCCYGODYNIA

For functional coccygodynia, more frequently seen in highly nervous people, no organic pathology has been described. Spasm of the coccygeus and piriformis muscles has been mentioned as an accompaniment. The condition has been tagged as "TV watcher's disease," with the implication that sitting for long periods of time on sofas or soft chairs may be a causative factor. Sitting on hard chairs, frequent changes of position, supportive measures for reassurance, and occasionally, tranquilizers are recommended measures. Performing surgery (coccygectomy) is never indicated because the pain often decreases without treatment or is increased by any treatment.

Maroy (3) described a novel and imaginative systematic study of the association of coccygodynia with depression. For six months he followed 313 patients who had signs of depression or spontaneous or evoked pain in the coccygeal area. A highly significant correlation was found between the following evoked parameters: pain and depressive status in noncoccygodynic patients, coccygodynia and evoked pain, and coccygeal and paracoccygeal muscular spasm. Seventy-nine percent of patients with spontaneous pain and 66% without pain had coccygeal pain evoked by rectal digital examination, and 71% of patients with spontaneous pain and 56% without spontaneous pain had paracoccygeal pain evoked by rectal digital examination. Among severely depressed patients, 76% had evoked pain and 80% coccygeal pain (either spontaneous or evoked). By comparison, in 120 consecutive patients who had colonic radiographic examination and no depressive signs, only two had coccygeal pain during rectal touch. In 57% all signs disappeared within six months when the patients were treated with various antidepressants. Two percent were failures, 14% were lost to follow-up, and 27% did not return after the first consultation. In a few patients, signs recurred after treatment was stopped but disappeared when treatment was administered again. Of the 59% of patients followed to the end of the study, 96% recovered completely. Accordingly, Maroy has proposed rectal pain evoked by digital examination as an "objective" diagnostic sign for masked depression.

■ ORGANIC COCCYGODYNIA

Organic coccygodynia may arise either from rigidity of the sacrococcygeal joint or from traumatic arthritis. Fracture and dislocation of the coccyx with displacement are usually a result of direct violence but may occur during difficult childbirth. Coccygodynia has also been attributed to so-called pericoccygeal glomus tumors (4). However, an autopsy study of 20 coccyges from fetuses, infants, and adults revealed intracoccygeal glomera in six of nine pediatric specimens and all 11 adult specimens. All were microscopic structures, and none appeared to cause bony destruction or erosion. Their role in the pathogenesis of coccygodynia is therefore questionable.

The symptoms of local pain during sitting and during defecation are attributed to spasm of the surrounding muscles. Pain is exquisite, and tenderness is sharply localized over the coccyx. In a patient with a recent injury, swelling and ecchymosis may be found over the lower sacral region. The diagnosis is made if abnormal mobility at the coccygeal articulation and accompanying sensitivity, and tenderness are present (5). Other symptoms include pelvic floor muscle spasms, referred pain from lumbar pathology, arachnoiditis of the lower sacral nerve roots, local post-traumatic lesions, and somatization (1). Marx (6) suggested that if the injection of a mixture of local anesthetic (4 mL 1% lidocaine and 4 mL 0.5% bupivacaine) with a depository steroid (100 mg prednisone) into the pericoccygeal soft tissue resulted in relief of pain within a few minutes, the diagnosis of coccygodynia is confirmed. Coccygeal pain resulting from acute trauma responds well to conservative management with nonsteroidal anti-inflammatory drugs and sitting aids (donut pillow).

Treatment generally consists of reduction by digital manipulation through the rectum, but that may fail because of the muscle forces continually in play (5). Bed rest for approximately one week is usually sufficient to alleviate majority of the symptoms. Tight cross-strapping of the buttocks lessens pain in some patients, but in others it exacerbates pain.

The patient should sit on an inflated rubber ring. Sitting on one buttock at an angle may be sufficient to eliminate the discomfort of sitting squarely on both ischial tuberosities. Some patients prefer a hard surface that allows the ischia alone to bear the body weight (5). Sitz baths help relieve muscle spasm, and stool softeners should be provided so that constipation does not aggravate symptoms.

Other therapeutic possibilities include blockade of the ganglion of Walther (or ganglion impar), electrical spinal cord stimulation, and selective nerve root stimulation (1). Coccygectomy should be considered for those patients who have severe disability following a coccygeal fracture (5). To determine whether surgery probably will be beneficial, Steindler advised infiltrating the region of the coccyx with a local anesthetic; if temporary relief is obtained, then coccygectomy probably will relieve the pain (5). Wray et al. (7) conducted a five-year prospective trial involving 120 patients to investigate the etiology and treatment of coccydynia. The cause lies in some localized musculoskeletal abnormality in the coccygeal region. The condition is genuine and distressing and they found no evidence of neurosis in their patients. Physiotherapy was of little help in treatment, but 60% of the patients responded to local injections of corticosteroid and local anesthesia. Manipulation and injection was even more successful and cured about 85%. Coccygectomy was required in almost 20% and had a success rate of over 90%.

TABLE 1 ■ Success of Treatment of Coccygodynia

	Local Injection[a]		Coccygectomy	
	No. of Injections (n)	Percent Success (%)	No. of Injections (n)	Percent Success (%)
Wray et al. (7)	120	60	24	90
Grosso et al. (9)	–	–	9	89
Ramsey et al. (12)	24	78	15	87
Hodges et al. (11)	17	–	11	82
Doursounian et al. (10)	–	–	61	87

[a]Injection of steroids ± local anesthetic.

Operation is contraindicated for acute sacrococcygeal injuries even when the coccyx is severely angulated anteriorly. Operation is also contraindicated when the low back is painful because occasionally coccygodynia or rectal pain is an early symptom of pathologic change in the lumbosacral disc (8).

Operative removal of the coccyx is accomplished through a paramedian incision that extends from the sacrococcygeal junction distally (5). The sacrococcygeal joint is disarticulated and dissection is continued distally along each side of the bone. The sharp distal margin of the sacrum should be beveled so that no prominence remains. The pelvic diaphragm is repaired by reanchoring the structures stripped from the coccyx, and the gluteus maximus muscle is reattached to the posterior sacral aponeurosis.

Grosso and van Dam (9) reported on nine patients who underwent total coccygectomy. There was one postoperative wound infection. With an average follow-up of 56 months, three patients reported complete relief of pain, five reported marked improvement, and one reported slight improvement.

Doursounian et al. (10) operated on 61 patients with instability-related coccygodynia. There were 49 women and 12 men, with a mean age of 45.3 years. Twenty-seven patients had hypermobility of the coccyx and 33, subluxation. In all cases, the unstable portion was removed through a limited incision directly over the coccyx. Follow-up was between 12 months and more than 30 months. The outcome was rated excellent or good in 53 patients, fair in one, and poor in seven. There were nine patients with infection requiring reoperation. Hodges et al. (11) assessed the outcomes after conservative and surgical therapy in 32 patients presenting with symptoms of coccydynia. Patients completed visual analog pain scales and the Oswestry functional capacity index. Of the 32 patients, 13% were treated with nonsteroidal anti-inflammatory drugs alone, 53% were treated with NSAIDs followed by local injections, and 34% underwent coccygectomy after failure of NSAIDs or local injection. Patients undergoing operation had significantly greater pretreatment VAS scores (8.3 vs. 5.4). Surgical patients also had greater OSW scores, but not significantly (36.6 vs. 24.2). Marked improvement was reported by 82% of the surgical patients. Wound infections developed in 27% of the surgical patients and 9% developed wound dehiscence. All infections resolved following irrigation and debridement and a short course of oral antibiotics. Ramsey et al. (12) reviewed the clinical results of the treatment of coccygodynia. Twenty-four patients were treated with local injections and 15 patients treated with coccygectomy. Local injections were successful in 78% and coccygectomy was successful in 87% of the patients. Perkins et al. (13) reviewed 13 patients who had coccygectomy. Pain was assessed by the numerical rating scale and function by Oswestry Low Back Disability Score at a mean of 43 months. The mean age was 45 years. There were two complications. The numerical rating scale improved from 7.3 to 3.6 and the Oswestry Low Lack Disability Score improved from 55 to 36. The results of treatment for coccygodynia are summarized in Table 1. De Andres and Chaves (1) offered the algorithm presented in Figure 1 for the diagnosis and therapeutic approach to coccygodynia.

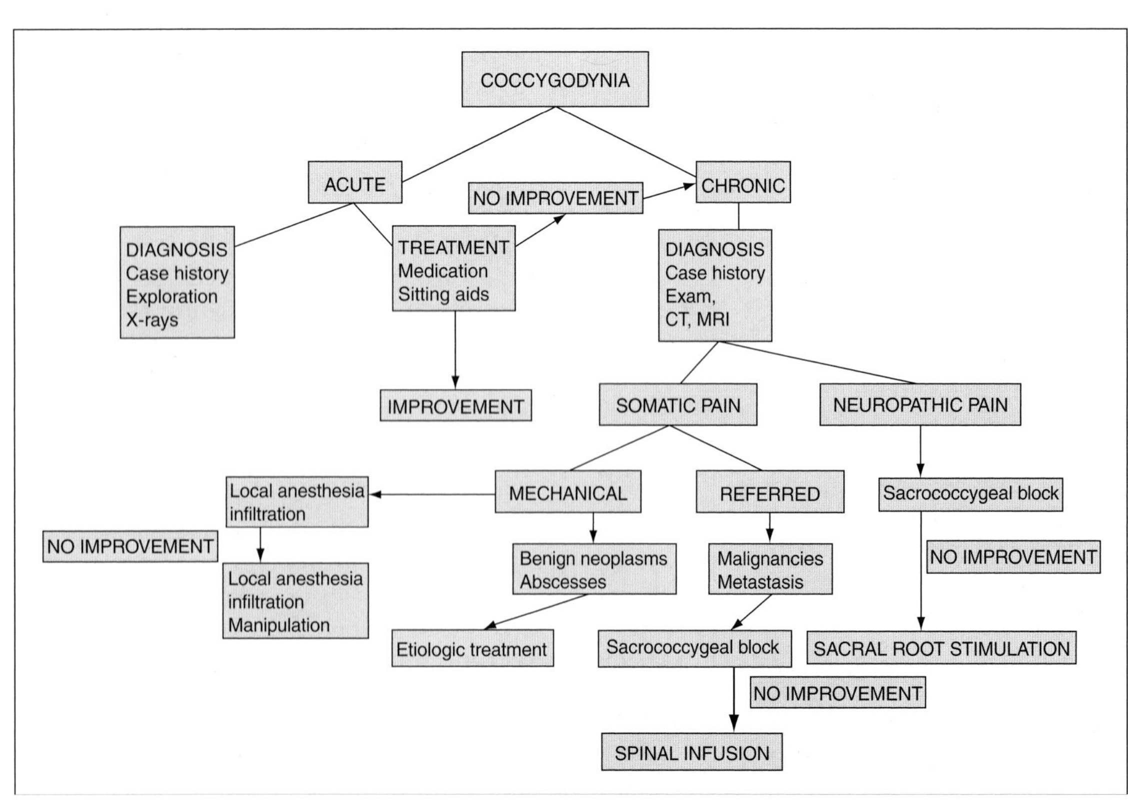

FIGURE 1 ■ Algorithm for diagnosis and therapeutic approach to coccygodynia.

ENDOMETRIOSIS

Although major advances have been made in the medical and surgical treatment of endometriosis, the pathophysiology of this disorder remains an enigma (14). The availability of the laparoscope for evaluating various gynecologic disorders has provided a new perspective on the incidence of endometriosis and on the anatomic distribution of endometriotic implants (15). An estimate of the incidence of endometriosis is approximately 4% to 17% of women in the reproductive age group (16). Endometriosis is found in decreasing order of frequency on the ovaries, the posterior broad ligament, the anterior cul-de-sac, the posterior cul-de-sac, the uterosacral ligaments, and the anterior wall of the rectosigmoid colon (15). Although the incidence of colorectal involvement in women with endometriosis has been reported as high as 50%, involvement severe enough to necessitate bowel resection is <10% (16).

COLORECTAL INVOLVEMENT

Histogenesis

The pathogenesis of endometriosis has been and continues to be controversial. Prevailing theories include transtubal regurgitation of menstrual blood; the coelomic metaplasia doctrine; lymphatic dissemination; and hematogenous spread.

Pathology

The lesions of endometriosis are typically multiple and vary in size from minute hard nodules to extensive areas of cystic hemorrhagic necrosis and fibrosis. They are generally serosal, sometimes intramural, and only rarely mucosal. At operation intestinal endometriosis appears either as a puckered scarred area, often on the antimesenteric surface of the bowel, or as a nodular constricting lesion extending into the wall or encircling it (16). Further inspection may reveal rusty brown or purplish specks. Frequently, implants are seen on other pelvic structures. Palpation discloses thickening of the colonic wall. The focus of endometriosis may enlarge to present as a mass; hence the designation as an endometrioma. The mucosal surface is usually intact, but on occasion ulceration may be evident.

Microscopically, multiple foci of endometrial glands and stroma are present in the muscularis propria and in the subtending mesentery in which there is reactive fibrosis and scarring. Smooth muscle hyperplasia is produced by the endometrioma (17). The overlying mucosa is usually normal. However, the mucosa overlying endometrial deposits may be abnormal with crypt irregularity with branching and sometimes shortening of the tubules, crypt abscesses and an increase in lamina propria mononuclear cells, or mucosal atrophy (18). Endometriosis of the large bowel can masquerade as inflammatory bowel disease or ischemic changes, but the possibility should be borne in mind, particularly with very focal histologic changes (19).

Clinical Features

Endometriosis is characteristically a disease of the reproductive years of life and occurs most frequently in women 30 to 40 years of age. Prystowsky et al. (20), in a review of 1573 consecutive patients with endometriosis diagnosed at laparoscopy or celiotomy, found that only 85 patients (5.4%) had gastrointestinal involvement and only 11 patients (0.7%) required bowel resection as a result of recurrent gastrointestinal symptoms (usually obstructive in nature) and/or suspicion of malignancy. In a review of 1616 operations for endometriosis, Bailey (16) reported only 16 involved bowel resections (1%). Endometriosis may mimic malignancy in that it is characterized by local disease and distant "spread." Gastrointestinal involvement commonly affects those segments of bowel in proximity to the genital organs, with the rectosigmoid region more frequently involved than the ileum (17). Bailey (16) reported the most common areas of intestinal involvement to be rectum and rectosigmoid (88%), sigmoid colon (7%), cecum (3%), and terminal ileum (2%), followed by proximal colon. He noted that other authors have reported small bowel involvement as high as 27%. In most instances there is only serosal involvement, and the diagnosis is made incidentally at the time of laparotomy for other reasons. Under these circumstances the patient's state of well-being is not affected, and no treatment is necessary. If intestinal symptoms are present, endometriosis is probably extensive, and resection is almost always required. The diagnosis of small intestinal endometriosis is rarely made prior to operation (18). A history of colicky abdominal pain might be suggestive (21).

Patients may be asymptomatic, but a wide variety of intestinal symptoms may occur. These include intermittent abdominal crampy pain, rectal or pelvic pain, cyclical rectal bleeding, tenesmus, constipation (especially with menses), decreased stool caliber, bloating, nausea, vomiting, diarrhea, and even bleeding from an umbilical nodule during menses (17). Extensive intestinal wall involvement can result in occasional bleeding or obstructive symptoms, in which case a diagnosis of neoplasm or inflammatory bowel disease requires exclusion.

The cyclic nature of the symptoms with exacerbations just before or during menstruation yields a clue to the diagnosis. Associated gynecologic symptoms of dysmenorrhea, cyclic lower abdominal and pelvic pain, dyspareunia, menometrorrhagia, infertility, and findings of characteristic tender pelvic nodularity and cul-de-sac induration and thickening during physical examination further point to the diagnosis (17). Rigid sigmoidoscopy may reveal a flattened or puckered mucosa or rarely a mass secondary to infiltration of the submucosa, along with extrinsic fixation and angulation of the rectosigmoid (16). In their review of the literature, Groom et al. (17) found that endometrial implants in the proximal intestine or appendix may serve as the lead point for intussusception or that associated inflammatory adhesions may produce obstruction by stenosis, kinking, or volvulus. Varras et al. (22) reported a case of endometriosis causing extensive intestinal obstruction simulating carcinoma of the sigmoid colon. A point not commonly appreciated is that intestinal endometriosis may produce symptoms long after menopause with an incidence as high as 7% (16).

Investigation

Unfortunately, no radiologic tests are diagnostic of endometriosis. Barium enema studies may reveal a narrowed luminal caliber in the affected portion of the bowel, mainly in the sigmoid or rectosigmoid area, with extrinsic pressure or an irregular asymmetric appearance but no mucosal destruction. An intramural, intraluminal polypoid filling defect may be demonstrated (17). In the advanced stage, even complete obstruction with proximal distention may occur. Endoscopy, either sigmoidoscopy or colonoscopy, may similarly reveal a stenotic lumen with normal mucosa. A mass or polypoid lesion may be visualized (23). Occasionally, bluish submucosal discoloration may be apparent. Obtaining an intravenous pyelogram also should be considered because ureteral involvement can occur in the presence of a pelvic mass, estimated at 15% (16). A small intestinal series may be helpful when symptoms are more suggestive of small bowel involvement; ideally, it is obtained just before or during the menstrual period. Computed tomography (CT) and ultrasonography may help delineate the extent and location of the disease. Intrarectal ultrasonography has been of limited help because of tenderness of rectal nodules and angulation or narrowing of bowel, which makes insertion of probe difficult (16). Laparoscopy may permit direct visualization of the pelvic organs for determination of the extent of the disease and allow performance of a biopsy of the lesions for histologic diagnosis (14).

Differential Diagnosis

The differential diagnosis includes primary bowel carcinoma, diverticulosis, other chronic inflammatory bowel diseases, carcinoids, benign intramural neoplasms, metastases from occult intra-abdominal malignancies, pelvic abscess, ischemic stricture, radiation colitis, pelvic (ovarian) and mesenteric neoplasms, and cysts (17,21).

Treatment

Endocrine treatment has proved ineffective in patients with intestinal endometriosis that produces symptoms (16,21,24). The growth and development of endometriosis is dependent on cyclic stimulation by the ovarian hormones estrogen and progesterone. Hormonal therapy is designed to induce a state of pseudopregnancy or pseudomenopause. Danazol is an effective antiestrogen agent but its androgenic side effects have distressed many patients. More recently, gonadotropin-releasing hormone antagonists such as leuprolide (Lupron) and nafarelin (Synarel) have demonstrated equal antiestrogen activity with fewer side effects (16). Unfortunately, the cost of these drugs is not inconsequential. These agents are quite effective in the treatment of small endometrial implants of the peritoneal surfaces but do not have a major impact on large deposits. They are of value in the preoperative preparation of patients for infertility operations because they decrease the vascularity of implants (16). In patients with endometriosis, fibrosis is considerable, and this extensive scarring usually produces the symptoms in patients with intestinal endometriosis. For patients with obstructive symptoms, most authors advocate resection. This recommendation is based on the need to rule out malignancy as well as the observation that fibrotic lesions are unlikely to respond to endocrine manipulation. Resection may also prevent later development of endometrial carcinoma (16).

In an effort to define the indications for resection, Prystowsky et al. (20) found that of 63 patients with gastrointestinal involvement at sites other than the appendix who did not undergo bowel resection, only two patients had gastrointestinal symptoms at the time of diagnosis (neither patient had obstructive symptoms). Follow-up revealed that only one patient developed significant gastrointestinal symptoms. The authors concluded that indications for resection included the presence of clear-cut obstructive symptoms or the inability to exclude malignancy. Indeed, the absence of symptoms appeared predictive of the absence of clinically significant intestinal endometriosis. They also found that appendiceal endometriosis apparently is an incidental finding and one that is not clinically important. Others have reported the value of sigmoid colon affected by symptomatic endometriosis (25).

The only successful mode of treatment for gastrointestinal endometriosis that prevents subsequent recurrence is resection of the affected segment and a total abdominal hysterectomy and bilateral salpingo-oophorectomy (14,17). An exception to this recommendation is the clinical situation in which the patient still desires to have a family, in which case resection of the involved intestinal segment along with excision of the area of pelvic endometriosis may be appropriate (17). Occasionally, local excision of a colonic endometrioma may be an effective treatment (17,26). A biopsy of asymptomatic serosal lesions found incidentally should be performed and the diagnosis confirmed by frozen section. Coronado et al. (27) presented 77 consecutive patients with deep colorectal endometriosis treated with a full thickness resection. Gynecologic procedures included conservative laparotomies for preserving fertility (39 patients); hysterectomy with bilateral salpingo-oophorectomy (29 patients); bilateral salpingo-oophorectomy (2 patients); left salpingo-oophorectomy (1 patient); and resection of pelvic endometriosis in patients with previous ablative surgery (6 patients). A low anterior resection was performed in 68 patients (88.3%); a disc excision of the anterior rectal wall in five (6.5%); sigmoid resection in three (3.9%), and partial cecal resection in one (1.3%). The postoperative febrile morbidity was 10.4%, with no apparent anastomotic leaks. Of 33 patients who attempted to conceive postoperatively, 13 achieved a term pregnancy (39.4%). Complete relief of pelvic symptoms was obtained in 49%; improvement in 39%; no improvement in 10%; and worsening of symptoms in 1%. There has been no recurrence of symptomatic bowel endometriosis during one to nine years of follow-up.

Urbach et al. (28) reported 29 patients undergoing bowel resection for severe (American Fertility Society Stage IV) endometriosis. The most frequent symptoms were pelvic pain, abdominal pain, rectal pain, and dysmenorrhea. Nearly all patients (93%) underwent low anterior resection of the rectum and distal sigmoid. Other intestinal procedures were appendectomy, terminal ileal resection, cecectomy, and sigmoid resection. Simultaneous total abdominal hysterectomy and bilateral salpingo-oophorectomy were performed in 34% of the patients. All patients reported subjective improvement. Forty-six percent of the patients were cured according to the prospectively applied definition (resolution of symptoms without need for further medical or surgical therapy). The only variable analyzed that was associated with cure was concomitant total abdominal hysterectomy and bilateral salpingo-oophorectomy (odds ratio 12).

Nezhat et al. (29) reported on laparoscopic disk excision and primary repair of the anterior rectal wall to treat eight patients with infiltrative symptomatic endometriosis. Complete relief was obtained in six patients.

Woods et al. (30) described the use of the circular stapler to accomplish a disk excision of the anterior rectal wall for small endometrial implants—a procedure that can be accomplished either by laparotomy or laparoscopy.

Koh and Janik (31) reviewed the controversy regarding the extent of rectal wall resection necessary to affect a cure in women with rectovaginal endometriosis. They consider deep rectovaginal endometriosis to be present when a bulky lesion is present in the cul-de-sac or has invaded the muscularis of the vagina or rectum or both. The understanding of the frequent location and extension of the lesions in deep endometriosis allows for a logical and consistent approach to its resection with a high degree of success. The most common area of involvement of deep endometriosis is the uterosacral ligament. With increasing infiltration laterally, the cardinal ligament and the proximate peri-ureteral tissue become involved, leading to constriction of the ureter. It is very rare for the ureteral muscularis to be part of this process. Medial extension begins to incorporate the serosa and later the outer muscularis of the adjacent rectum but infrequently to the rectal mucosa. Anterior extension involves posterior cervix and vagina ipsilaterally.

Redwine and Wright (32) found 73% of the patients with obliteration of the cul-de-sac had histologically proved rectal endometriosis. To ensure complete removal of all tissue, intestinal surgery is required in most patients with complete obliteration of the cul-de-sac.

The preoperative diagnosis of severe ureteral and rectal wall involvement would aid in surgical preparation. Coronado et al. (27) evaluated patients who underwent colectomy by laparotomy for bowel endometriosis and found only two biopsy-positive lesions at proctosigmoidoscopy in 74 exams and extrinsic compression or nonspecific abnormality in 18 of 73 barium studies. Transrectal ultrasonography has been used in the assessment of rectovaginal endometriosis with a sensitivity and specificity of 97% and 96% respectively, in the identification of rectal and vaginal wall infiltration (33).

Knowledge of the extent of the disease may help guide the surgeon to the appropriate operative approach. A determination is made of the depth of infiltration of the rectum. Partial thickness resection should only be performed when the outer longitudinal muscularis is involved and can be peeled mechanically from the inner circular muscularis. The inner muscularis cannot be peeled from the mucosa and any resection will be incomplete. A full thickness disk resection is performed when the inner muscularis or mucosa is involved and the lesion is less than 3 to 4 cm. With larger lesions or multifocal lesions, a colectomy with end-to-end stapled anastomosis is performed. Koh and Janik (31) evaluated over 400 cases of deep infiltrating endometriosis of the cul-de-sac. Of these, 105 had rectal disease; 22 required laparoscopic colectomy; 17 had full thickness anterior rectosigmoid resection, and 56 had partial thickness resection. All cases were laparoscopic except for one colectomy early in the series. Following operation, only one serious complication occurred and that was a rectal perforation, which was treated with a diverting colostomy. A 48% fertility rate was achieved. Their management of deep infiltrating endometriosis has evolved from what they term indiscriminate and often ineffective hysterectomy and oophorectomy to radical excision of all fibrotic endometriosis with disease-free margins.

Kavallaris et al. (34) evaluated the microscopic extent of endometriosis in surgical en bloc specimens of 50 patients with intestinal pain, and palpable disease in the rectovaginal septum who underwent combined laparoscopic vaginal en bloc resection of the cul-de-sac with partial resection of the posterior vaginal wall and rectum with re-anastomosis by mini-laparotomy. The mean length of the bowel specimen was 7.5 cm. Endometriosis involved the serosa and muscularis propria in all patients, the submucosa in 34% of the patients and the mucosa in 10% of the patients. After a mean follow-up of 32 months, 90% of the patients reported a considerable improvement or were completely free of symptoms and the rate of recurrence was 4%.

Malignant Transformation

Only 21.3% of the cases of malignant transformation of endometriosis occur at extragonadal pelvic sites (35). Yantiss et al. (36) characterized the clinicopathologic features of neoplasms arising in gastrointestinal endometriosis. They reported 17 cases of gastrointestinal endometriosis complicated by neoplasms (14 cases) or precancerous changes (three cases). Nine patients had a long history of endometriosis, 11 patients had hysterectomies, and eight of these had also received unopposed estrogen therapy. The lesions involved the rectum (six), sigmoid (six), colon, unspecified (two) and small intestine (three), and comprised eight endometrioid adenocarcinomas, four mullerian adenosarcomas, one endometrioid stromal sarcoma, one endometrioid adenofibroma of borderline malignancy with carcinoma in situ, two atypical hyperplasias and one endometrioid adenocarcinoma in situ. Up to 2002, 40 cases of endometriosis-associated intestinal carcinoma had been reported in the literature. Of these, 17 cases were primary adenocarciomas arising in the rectosigmoid colon. In eight of the 17 case reports, the patients were using unopposed estrogen replacement therapy. Jones et al. (35) reported the ninth case of a patient with malignant transformation of endometriosis in the literature.

Cho et al. (37) reported the case of endometrial stromal sarcoma of the sigmoid colon arising in endometriosis with a review of six additional cases of endometrial stromal sarcoma arising in intestinal endometriosis found in the English literature. The patients ranged in age from 36 to 64 years. Presenting symptoms were pain, bloody diarrhea, and tenesmus. Most of the sarcomas arose in the rectosigmoid colon.

■ PERIANAL ENDOMETRIOMA

Despite the fact that the presence of endometriosis is common, the finding of a perianal endometrioma is no more than a surgical curiosity even in the practice of a busy colorectal surgeon. Shickele (38), in 1923, apparently was the first to report a case of perineal endometriosis. Pollack et al. (39) in 1988, reviewed the literature and found only 58 cases of endometriosis involving the perineum.

Histogenesis

Although the histogenesis of perianal endometrioma is not clear, it is best explained by the implantation theory, a variation of the "retrograde menstruation" theme (40). Confounding the issue is a unique case of perineal endometriosis reported in a patient with primary infertility (39).

Pathology

Perianal endometriomas vary in size from microscopic lesions to lesions 1 to 2 cm in diameter and in color from reddish blue to yellowish brown. They may enlarge and coalesce. Because of the irritative effect of the blood, the nodules may provoke a marked fibroblastic proliferation, resulting in dense, fibrous nodules. Because of periodic bleeding into the "cystic structures," the cysts have become known as "chocolate cysts." Paradoxically, making the diagnosis can be most difficult in the advanced, florid, long-standing cases because, as the disease advances, the fibroproliferative response progressively obliterates recognizable features. A definitive histologic diagnosis usually requires two of the following three features: stroma, glands, and hemosiderin pigment, with the stroma being the most important element. Microscopically, edematous endometrial stroma with an inflammatory infiltrate is often characteristic. Glands with their endometrial epithelial lining can be demonstrated together with hemosiderin-laden macrophages, which may be seen frequently. Collections of blood also are often present.

Clinical Features

Gordon et al. (41) described the varied manifestations of perianal endometrioma. The clinical manifestations of endometriosis depend on the functional activity of the involved tissue. The lesion may present as an asymptomatic mass or, in the classic fashion, as a painful mass, especially during menstruation. The mass, in fact, may become noticeable only at the time of menstruation, when it becomes larger and more painful. It subsides several days after the termination of menses. During physical examination the lesions are usually found in old episiotomy scars. Endoanal sonography can be used to assess the relationship to the sphincter mechanism and determine whether any sphincter injury has already been incurred (42). The onset of symptoms has become apparent as early as 45 days and as late as 14 years from the time of delivery and perineal trauma (38). The diagnosis is based on the results of a microscopic section.

Included in the differential diagnosis are anal fistula with abscess formation, thrombosed hemorrhoids, perianal melanoma, and other neoplastic and inflammatory conditions (41).

Treatment

Because this lesion is so readily accessible and because its exact nature is frequently not known pre-operatively, the treatment of choice undoubtedly is local excision. Great care must be taken during local excision not to injure the anal sphincteric mechanism, because these lesions frequently are associated intimately with the muscle. Plastic repairs and reinforcements of the sphincter may be necessary in the area where the lesion is excised, because the sphinteric muscle may be considerably thinned there. Control of symptoms, especially for patients with incompletely excised lesions, has been obtained through hormonal manipulations (43). Hormonal therapy uses progestational compounds to attain necrosis and atrophy of the deposited endometrial tissue, thus achieving the beneficial effect. Danazol or, more recently, luteinizing hormone-releasing hormone analogs have been used for this purpose (14). The use of ovarian ablative therapy also may be considered.

Dougherty and Hull (44) agree that primary sphincteroplasty for patients with perineal endometriosis with anal sphincter involvement seems to be the best chance of cure with good functional results. It should be considered particularly in younger patients to obviate the need of the long-term subsequent hormonal therapy or re-excision for symptomatic recurrences. In contracts, they believe patients closer to menopause (when endometriosis tends to regress) may be treated optimally by narrow excision to avoid the risks of significant anal sphincter resection.

PROCTALGIA FUGAX AND LEVATOR SYNDROME

Proctalgia fugax may be defined as pain, seemingly arising in the rectum, that recurs at irregular intervals and is unrelated to organic disease (45). The term "proctalgia fugax" was first introduced by Thaysen (46) in 1935, and Schuster (47) has provided an excellent description of the clinical presentation. The onset of pain during the day or night is abrupt, and patients may be awakened with pain several hours after falling asleep. The pain appears suddenly mostly at night without any particular warning and disappears completely without any objective traces. The pain varies in severity but often is excruciating. Symptoms last from only a few minutes to less than half an hour, and their duration, although variable from patient to patient, is constant in a given patient. Pain is described variously as gnawing, grinding, cramplike, sharp, or tight. It is localized in the rectal region above the anus, varying in location from person to person but remaining constant in a given person. Symptoms disappear spontaneously without residue except for a weak, washed-out feeling after particularly severe attacks. There are no associated intestinal disturbances such as alteration in bowel habits, tenesmus, or paresthesia.

The etiology of proctalgia fuga is unknown, although it has been suggested that it is due to spasms of the levator ani muscles (45). A unique study was reported by Harvey (48), who obtained intraluminal pressure recordings from the rectum and sigmoid colon in two patients experiencing attacks of proctalgia fugax. In each case the pain appeared to result from contractions of the sigmoid colon and not from spasm of the levator ani muscles.

Kamm et al. (49) reported a newly identified myopathy of the internal anal sphincter in a family in which at least one member from each of five generations had severe proctalgia fugax. Anal endosonography revealed a grossly thickened internal anal sphincter. Manometric assessment demonstrated an increased maximal anal canal pressure with marked ultraslow wave activity. Two patients were treated by internal anal sphincter strip myectomy; one showed marked improvement and one was relieved of the constipation but had only slight improvement of pain. The authors believe that this entity is an autosomal-dominant inherited myopathy of the internal anal sphincter responsible for the symptoms of proctalgia fugax and constipation.

Celik et al. (50) described a second family with hereditary proctalgia fugax and internal anal sphincter hypertrophy associated with constipation. Physiologic studies showed deep, ultraslow waves and an absence of internal anal sphincter relaxation on rectal distention in the two most severely affected family members, suggesting the possibility of a neuropathic origin. Both these patients had an abnormally high blood pressure. After treatment with a sustained release formulation of the calcium antagonist, nifedipine, their blood pressure returned to normal, anal tone was reduced, and the frequency and intensity of anal pain was suppressed. The presence of a megarectum (and nonrelaxing internal sphincter) in these patients may bring up a question whether these patients might have some other condition such as short-segment Hirschsprung's disease.

A third report of hereditary internal anal sphincter myopathy was described by Konig and co-workers (51). Guy et al. (52) reported a case of a distinctive familial internal anal sphincter myopathy with unique histologic and radiologic features. A 67-year-old woman presented with a 20-year history of proctalgia fugax and outlet obstruction; other family members were similarly affected. Computed tomography and magnetic resonance imaging demonstrated a grossly hypertrophied internal anal sphincter. Strip myectomy of the sphincter was carried out with improvement in evacuation but little relief in proctalgia. Further relief of symptoms was obtained using oral and transdermal nitrates and a calcium antagonist. Histological examination of the excised muscle revealed hypertrophy and an abnormal arrangement of fibres in whorls; many fibres contained vacuoles with inclusion bodies positive for periodic acid-Schiff.

Takano (53) reported his experience with 68 patients with proctalgia fugax, among who, 55 patients had tenderness along the pudendal nerve. The location, character, and degree of pain caused by digital examination were confirmed by all of them to be similar to that which they experienced at times of paroxysm. After administration of a nerve block, symptoms disappeared completely in 65% of the patients and decreased in 25%. His data suggest that the pathogenesis of proctalgia fugax is neuralgia of the pudendal nerves.

The condition occurs in approximately 14% of healthy people and is more common in women (17.3%) than in men (8.8%) (54). Between attacks no consistent physical abnormality is evident. The absence of any objective abnormality suggests that at least a portion, if not all, of these cases are of psychogenic origin. A study of 48 patients with proctalgia fugax by Pilling et al. (55) revealed that the majority of the patients had professional or managerial occupations. They were found to be perfectionistic, anxious, and tense; had a relatively high incidence of neurotic symptoms in childhood; and were of above-average intelligence. The authors believed that the tendency of this anxious, perfectionistic group to somatize emotional conflicts by pain in the gastrointestinal tract is strong evidence that proctalgia fugax is of psychogenic origin.

Treatment of this condition is unsatisfactory. Firm upward pressure on the anus can provide relief. Other measures that have been used include taking hot sitz baths, having a bowel movement, inserting a finger into the anus, massaging the muscles, or administering an enema. Such maneuvers probably only pass the time for patients who have a condition in which the duration of pain is self-limited. Inhalation of amyl nitrite or sublingual nitroglycerin has also been used. Eckardt et al. (56) conducted a randomized, double-blind, placebo-controlled, crossover trial of inhaled salbutamol in 18 patients with proctalgia fugax and found that salbutamol inhalation shortened the duration of severe pain. Interestingly, in the asymptomatic state there were no changes in anal resting pressure, anal relaxation during distention, or rectal compliance. For patients who have frequent repeated nocturnal attacks, nightly doses of quinine have been recommended (46). Anesthetics, sedatives, and spasmolytic agents have been employed (56). Peleg and Shvartzman (57) described a case where a single dose of an intravenous lidocaine infusion completely stopped pain attacks. Katsinelos et al. (58) described a case of proctalgia fugax responding to anal sphincter injection of Clostridium botulinum type A toxin. Lowenstein and Cataldo (59) reported a case of proctalgia fugax that responded to 0.3% nitroglycerin ointment Sinaki et al. (60) reported that diazepam was helpful in 40% of their patients.

Making the correct diagnosis is important to avoid a mistaken diagnosis and subsequent misguided treatment and to assure the perplexed and anxious victim that his or her condition is recognized and is neither a symptom nor a precursor of malignancy. Unfortunately, Douthwaite's skeptical but realistic appraisal (45) holds true: proctalgia fugax "is harmless, unpleasant, and incurable."

A closely allied condition, if not a variation of the same theme, is the so-called levator syndrome. Individuals with this syndrome experience a dull ache or pressure in the rectum, sometimes describing the sensation as "sitting on a ball" or "having a ball in my rectum." The pain is worse during sitting and disappears when the patient stands or lies down. Precipitating factors have included the trauma of a long-distance ride in a car, childbirth, lumbar disc surgery, low anterior resection or abdominoperineal resection of the rectum, gynecologic operations, and occasionally sexual intercourse (61). Often no etiologic factor can be elicited, and a large component of the condition has been attributed to a psychologic overlay. The prevalence of this condition has been reported in 6.6% of the general population in the United States (62).

The syndrome occurs more commonly in women, usually in the fourth to sixth decades of life. The diagnosis is made by the demonstration of tenderness and spasm of the affected muscle, which are usually unilateral and on the left side.

Treatment consists of puborectalis muscle massage up to 50 times, performed in a firm manner based on the patient's tolerance and carried out at three to four week intervals. Warm baths and short-term judicious use of diazepam also can be of value. For patients who do not respond to these measures, Sohn et al. (63) first described the use of electrogalvanic stimulation as a treatment. The rationale for this therapy is based on the fact that a low-frequency oscillating current applied to a muscle induces fasciculation and fatigue, which breaks the spastic cycle. The treatment is painless, and no adverse side effects are known. Success rates of 60% to 94% have been reported (61,63–65). Recurrence rates are significant. In the series by Billingham et al. (65) only 25% of the patients remained symptom-free. Further improvement can be obtained through retreatment (64). Less-favorable results were reported by Hull et al. (66) In a series of 52 patients, 50% received fewer than four one-hour treatments, 33% received four to six treatments, and 17% received more than six treatments. The treatment was painless in 77%. With an 88% follow-up with a mean of 28 months, there was symptom relief in 19% of the patients, partial relief in 24%, and no relief in 57%. Total treatment failures may be due to a large psychologic component and should be treated accordingly (61). Hull et al. (66) found that misdiagnoses included recurrent pelvic carcinoma and fissure-in-ano. Recognition of this disorder is important to avoid unnecessary and expensive diagnostic investigations, or worse, totally needless operations.

Heah et al. (67) assessed the effects of biofeedback on pain relief in 16 consecutive patients (nine men, seven woman, mean age 50 years) with levator ani syndrome. Mean duration of pain was 32.5 months. All underwent a full course of biofeedback using a manometric balloon technique. Mean follow-up was 12.8 months. Pain score was administered prospectively by an independent observer. After biofeedback the pain score was significantly improved (median 8 vs. 2). Analgesic requirements were also significantly reduced (all 16 patients needed nonsteroidal anti-inflammatory drugs before biofeedback; only two patients needed NSAIDs after biofeedback).

OLEOGRANULOMA

Oleogranuloma (lipoid granuloma, paraffinoma) is a foreign body reaction that usually results from the inflammatory reaction induced by unabsorbed, oil-based sclerosing agents used in the injection treatment of hemorrhoids (68). Mineral oil enemas also may cause a rectal oleogranuloma (69). Retention of injected oil and consequent fibrosis have been held responsible for stricture formation in persons who have previously received such an injection.

Lipoid granulomas are seen rarely today because the trend has been away from injection treatment of internal hemorrhoids. Their symptoms are rectal pressure, a sensation of incomplete evacuation, and occasionally a sensation of partial obstruction of the bowel. Oleogranuloma generally occurs as a round submucous mass in the anal canal just above the dentate line (Fig. 2), but annular and even ulcerating lesions have been described (70,71).

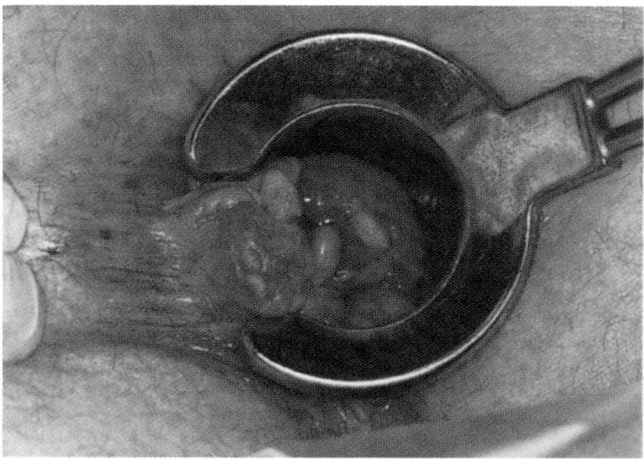

FIGURE 2 ■ Macroscopic features of an oleogranuloma.

The lesions may extend as high as the rectosigmoid junction because the injected oil can track upward in the submucosal layer.

The histology of oleogranuloma is characteristic (72), with conspicuous fibrosis and a variable degree of inflammatory cell infiltration dependent on the age of the lesion. In the early stages, the acute inflammatory response includes many eosinophils. Rounded spaces lined by large mononuclear or multinucleate histiocytes are scattered throughout the oleogranuloma (Fig. 3). These spaces contain oil that is removed from the tissues during the course of histologic preparation but can be demonstrated in frozen sections of formalin-fixed material. An unsuspected oleogranuloma may be found in a hemorrhoidectomy specimen. Its histologic appearance may be confused with that of lymphangioma and with that of cystic pneumatosis, although the latter shows no fibrous or inflammatory reaction.

The principal interest in this entity is from the standpoint of differential diagnosis. Clinically, the polypoid appearance can simulate adenomas or even carcinomas. The most common distinguishing feature is that the overlying mucosa is usually intact when an oleoma is present in contradistinction to the usual ulceration of the mucosa when a carcinoma is present. Knowing the patient's history of previous injections is of some help.

Simple excision is the recommended treatment, but because of the fixation and scarring, operative removal may be rather difficult (73).

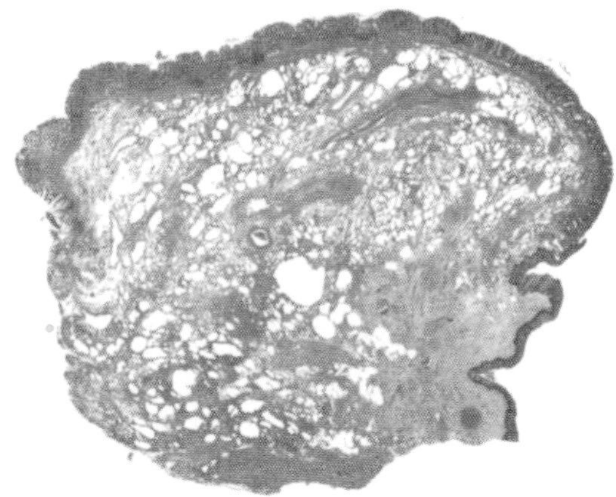

FIGURE 3 ■ Microscopic appearance of an oleogranuloma.

MELANOSIS COLI

Melanosis coli is characterized by a deep pigmentation of the mucosa of the colon and rectum caused by the presence of a melanin-like pigment. It may involve the large bowel from the rectum to the ileocecal valve, with a sharp demarcation at this point. This dramatic demarcation is seen at an ileocolic anastomosis (Fig. 4). The color of the mucosa varies from shades of yellowish brown to black (Fig. 5). It is seen in the appendix but not the terminal ileum. Examination reveals adenomatous polyps and adenocarcinomas rendered strikingly apparent by their lack of pigmentation against the blackish background of the surrounding mucosa (Fig. 6) (74). Moreover, nonpigmented areas of mucosa that are not grossly abnormal ultimately prove to be adenomatous hyperplasia.

Melanosis may be obvious to the naked eye, but the vast majority of cases are apparent only on microscopic examination. Histologically, the melanin-like pigment is found in histocytes within the lamina propria. A few may be seen in the sub-mucosa and even in the regional lymph nodes (75). There is a lack of inflammatory change in the colon. Walker et al. (76) reported an electron microscopic study that showed apoptosis of colonic surface epithelial cells and phagocytosis of resulting apoptotic bodies by intraepithelial macrophages. The latter migrated to the lamina propria where intracellular degradation of the apoptotic bodies resulted in formation of lipofuscin, characteristic of this condition.

Ewing et al. (77) reported the case of a patient who underwent a left hemicolectomy for colonic adenocarcinoma and was found incidentally to have melanosis coli associated with long-term use of the herbal laxative Swiss Kriss, not only in his colonic mucosa, but also in the colonic submucosa and in his pericolic lymph nodes. To their knowledge, the presence of identical pigment in macrophages of pericolonic lymph nodes has been reported in only four other patients in the English literature.

Use of a member of the laxative family, which consists of derivatives of anthraquinone (cascara, aloes, rhubarb, senna, and frangula), contributes to this pigmentation (74).

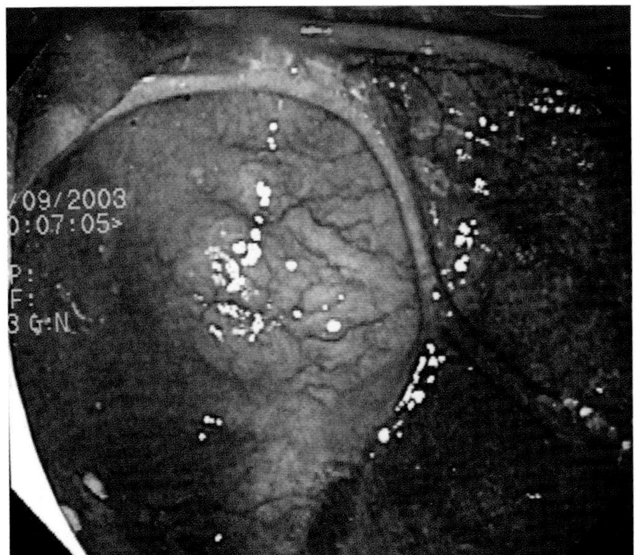

FIGURE 4 ■ Dramatic demarcation of melanosis coli at an ileocolic anastomosis.

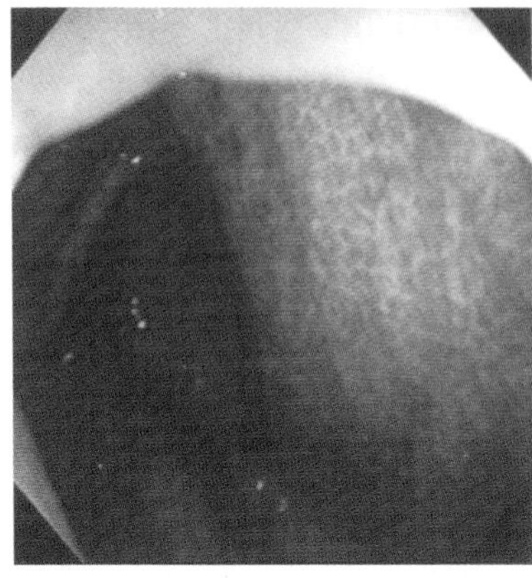

FIGURE 5 ■ Characteristic appearance of moderately severe melanosis coli.

In most instances the laxative had been taken almost daily for one year or more. This distinct group of cathartics owes its activity to the presence of an irritating anthracene or emodin. The exact mechanism of pigment formation is uncertain. Perhaps the active ingredient of these laxatives contains a pigment or elaborates a pigment within the colon that is phagocytized by the deep mucosal cells.

Pardi et al. (78) reported 25 patients with inflammatory bowel disease and melanosis coli, 20% of whom had documented laxative use. Most patients had ulcerative colitis (72%) or Crohn's colitis (24%), and the mean duration of inflammatory bowel disease was more than seven years. These data raise the possibility that chronic colitis could cause melanosis coli even in the absence of laxative use.

Reports of the incidence of melanosis coli vary from 1 % to 5% (74), and in unselected constipated patients it has been observed in 12% to 31% (79). Melanosis coli occurs in all races. In a histologic study of 200 autopsy cases, Koskela et al. (80) found a prevalence of 60% for melanosis coli, a prevalence that increased with age: 20 to 54 years, 30% and >75 years, 71%. Melanosis was more common in the proximal part of the colon: ascending colon, 49%; sigmoid, 18%; and rectum, 6%. Earlier writers suggested that melanosis coli is found in the older age group; however, this, probably, is related to the duration of the ingestion of these laxatives. There is a female preponderance of from 3:1 to 8:1, which probably reflects the greater incidence of constipation and habitual use of laxative agents among women patients.

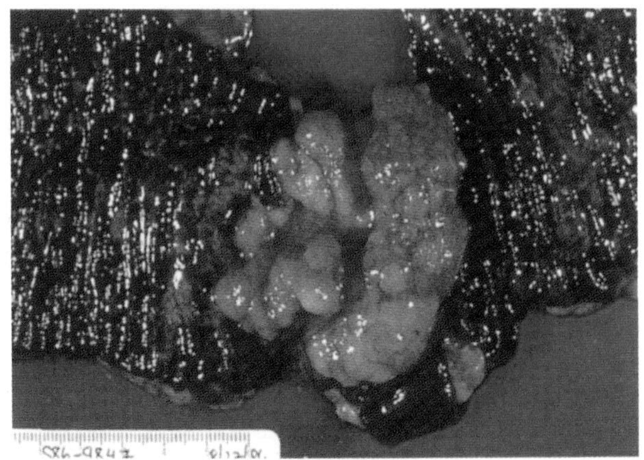

FIGURE 6 ■ Carcinoma of the colon in a patient with melanosis coli. Note the lack of pigmentation of the neoplastic lesion on a pigmented background. *Source*: Courtesy Steven J. Stryker, M.D., Chicago, Illinois, U.S.A.

Morganstern et al. (74) found that pigment-bearing macrophages are absent from benign and malignant neoplasms and from surrounding normal mucosa. They postulated that the neoplastic epithelium elaborates some substance that inhibits the aggregation or function of macrophages. How this might be related to neoplasia, if at all, is unknown.

Melanosis coli cannot be held responsible for any known symptom complex. A history of constipation is present almost universally, for it is in constipated patients that the laxatives are initially ingested. As a rule, the pigmentation disappears within a period of 4 to 12 months after discontinuation of all anthracene laxatives.

In a colonoscopic study of 2277 patients, Nusko et al. (81) found no significant increase in colorectal carcinoma rate either in laxative users or in patients with melanosis coli.

Subsequently Nusko et al. (82) performed a prospective case control study to investigate the risk of anthranoid laxative use for the development of colorectal adenomas or carcinomas. A total of 202 patients with newly diagnosed colorectal carcinomas, 114 patients with adenomatous polyps, and 238 patients (controls) who had been referred for total colonoscopy were studied. The use of anthranoid preparations was assessed by standardized interviews, and endoscopically visible or microscopic melanosis coli was studied by histopatological examination. Neither anthranoid laxative use, even in the long-term, nor macroscopic or microscopic melanosis coli was associated with any significant risk for the development of colorectal adenoma or carcinoma.

The associations between colorectal carcinoma and constipation, anthranoid laxative use, and melanosis coli are controversial. Nascimbeni et al. (83) investigated the relationship between sigmoid carcinoma and constipation, anthranoid laxative use, and melanosis coli using aberrant crypt foci analysis as an additional tool of investigation. Fifty-five surgical patients with sigmoid carcinoma, 41 surgical patients with diverticular disease, 96 age and sex matched patients without intestinal disease (controls) were interviewed on their history of constipation and anthranoid laxative use. Constipation and anthranoid laxative use were similar between patients with sigmoid carcinoma (30.9% and 32.7% respectively) and those with diverticular disease (39% and 28.6%) but higher than among controls (18.8% and 8.3%). Melanosis coli was found in 38.2% of the patients with sigmoid carcinoma and 39% of those with diverticular disease. Mean aberrant crypt foci frequency was higher in patients with sigmoid carcinoma (0.24/cm^2) than in those with diverticular disease (0.10 cm^2); and it did not vary according to constipation, laxative use, or melanosis coli in either group. This study confirms the association of aberrant crypt foci frequency with colon carcinoma and does not support the hypothesis of a causal effect relationship of colorectal carcinoma with constipation, anthranoid laxative use, or melanosis coli.

COLITIS CYSTICA PROFUNDA

Colitis cystica profunda (CCP) is a benign disease characterized by varying sizes of mucin-filled cysts located deep at the muscularis mucosae. The chief importance of this entity is its differentiation from colonic mucinous adenocarcinoma. Failure to recognize this benign condition may lead to unnecessary radical operation.

AGE AND SEX

The incidence and prevalence of CCP are unknown, but the disease is uncommon. Patients with this condition, once believed to be preponderantly female, usually present in the third and fourth decades (84,85). However, a review of the world literature disclosed that CCP occurs equally often in men and women (86).

ETIOLOGY

The etiology of CCP remains unclear. A plausible explanation is that the condition is the result of invagination of the mucosa during the healing phase of an ulcer. Rutter and Riddell (87) believe that the term "colitis cystica profunda" should be used as a purely descriptive term and should be recognized for what it is: an unusual complication of several different lesions. The causes of the ulcer might include ulcerative colitis, bacterial colitides, resolution of lymphoid abscesses in the submucosa, radiation, instrumentation, biopsy of the colonic mucosa, and polypectomy (88) and Crohn's disease (89).

Others consider the lesions to be inverted polyps, either acquired or congenital. If the condition were congenital, one would expect to find it in pediatric patients, but this has not been the case. Despite the suggestions of those who believe that CCP is of congenital origin, representing hamartomal formation, chronic inflammation has been accepted by most investigators as the primary etiologic factor in its pathogenesis (90).

CLINICAL FEATURES

Hematochezia, mucous discharge, diarrhea, tenesmus, and pain (either vague abdominal or perineal) may occur alone or in combination for many months or years before CCP is diagnosed (85,86,88). Other indications include rectal pain, weight loss, and previous rectal surgery (90). Involvement may vary from the dentate line to 15 cm from the anal verge, most frequently on the anterior rectal wall from 6 to 7 cm (85). Rectal examination may reveal single or multiple nodules that frequently have a rubbery consistency. Polypoid masses may be sessile, slightly raised, or pedunculated and may be single or multiple (86). When multiple, they may be confluent, with a diameter of several centimeters. Sigmoidoscopy may reveal that the mucosa overlying the cysts has irregularly distributed areas of edema, hyperemia, hypertrophy, and atrophy, with occasional superficial ulceration or central umbilication or a white "cap" (85,86). The mucosa is generally intact, but it may be ulcerated, in which case it may resemble a carcinoma. Stenosis and rectal prolapse have been found, and ulcerative colitis also may be present. An unusual presentation with a complete colonic obstruction due to an intussusception with a rectosigmoid inflammatory mass associated with distal ulcerative colitis has been reported (91).

PATHOLOGY

The mucin-containing cysts in the submucosa of the colon and rectum in a patient with CCP may present as a localized process, a segmental process, or may be diffusely distributed (92). Of 144 cases reviewed, 123 were localized, and 21 were diffusely distributed (86). Grossly, there are nodular polypoid or plaque-like areas measuring 1 to 3 cm in diameter that are covered by intact mucosa. In the classic lesion, mucus-filled cystic spaces are present, but in the early stages, thickening of the submucosa is present.

Microscopically, the cysts, which are deep at the muscularis mucosae, are lined with normal-appearing columnar epithelium and may be filled with mucus that stains faintly basophilic. The overlying mucosa may be histologically unremarkable or may show focal ulceration. The surrounding submucosa is invariably fibrotic and contains a mixed inflammatory infiltrate of mild to moderate intensity (88). Differentiating CCP from a well-differentiated mucinous adenocarcinoma may be difficult. Silver and Stolar (93) stressed that multilayering of cystic mucosa with cellular atypia and prominent intraglandular papillation and budding are seen in patients with carcinoma, whereas the mucosal lining of the cysts in patients with CCP is usually unicellular or absent.

Its distribution distinguishes CCP from colitis cystica superficialis, in which multiple tiny mucous cysts are scattered throughout the colon but are confined to the mucosa. The latter condition usually is associated with pellagra (88).

■ DIAGNOSIS

The results of barium enema studies may appear normal, or there may be single or multiple radiolucent filling defects of various sizes or longitudinal thickened mucosal folds (94). Rarely, partial intestinal obstruction may supervene. Endorectal ultrasonography identifies multiple cysts in the rectal submucosa with areas of echorefringent fibrosis between cysts, and confirms the absence of lymph node involvement or invasion of the muscular layer (95). With CT, the lesion appears as a noninfiltrating entity in the submucosa. With magnetic resonance imaging (MRI), nodulations produce intense signals that illustrate the mucoprotein content of the cysts. Included in the differential diagnosis are a variety of rectal neoplasms: adenomatous polyps, endometriosis, multiple polyposis, lipoma, leiomyoma, sarcoma, polypoid inflammatory granulomas such as those that occur with schistosomiasis, ulcerative colitis, and Crohn's disease, ischemic proctitis or colitis with submucosal hemorrhage and edema, infectious disorders, drug-induced colitides, and, most important, a mucus-producing adenocarcinoma (86,90). Differentiation among these entities is possible with an adequate biopsy.

Patients may undergo numerous barium enema examinations, sigmoidoscopies, and removal of rectal polyps before CCP is diagnosed. Colonoscopy may aid in the diagnosis of CCP involving the colon. A definitive diagnosis is made based on the typical histologic findings of this disorder and the absence of histologic features of malignancy (86).

■ TREATMENT

Valenzuela et al. (95) reported that re-education of bowel habits aimed at avoiding straining and a high fiber diet with bulk laxatives can lead to remission of lesions in 6 to 18 months. Steroid enemas have been used to treat the condition, but operation is generally the treatment of choice (86). For patients with associated rectal procidentia, an operation designed to correct the procidentia should be performed. The localized form, for which the treatment of choice is local excision (85,92,96), is usually found in the rectum. Excision through the anus or the Kraske approach can be used. The use of a mucosal sleeve resection and coloanal pull-through has been reported for circumferential involvement of the rectum (84). The higher segmental form of the disease can be treated by segmental resection (85,90,92). For diffuse involvement, an exceedingly rare situation usually associated with ulcerative colitis, a more extended resection is necessary, with the extent of resection depending on the extent of involvement. Management by diverting colostomy has also been reported, but this would seem to be a rather desperate maneuver (92).

DESCENDING PERINEUM SYNDROME

As a result of study of the disordered physiology of patients with rectal prolapse, a distinct condition was recognized in which perineal descent is caused by excessive straining. The pelvic floor muscles become weakened by repeated straining and stretching, and perineal descent occurs; this condition is referred to as the descending perineum syndrome (97).

■ PATHOGENESIS

The possibility of perineal descent as an etiologic factor in fecal incontinence has arisen from the observation that denervation changes occur in the pelvic floor and external sphincteric muscles of patients with idiopathic fecal incontinence (98). Some patients with perineal descent have the same histologic and electrophysiologic abnormalities as recorded in patients with fecal incontinence (99). In patients with perineal descent 20% to 30% stretching of the pudendal nerve occurs. Since irreversible nerve damage develops when nerves are stretched, it is possible that stretching of the nerves leads to secondary neuropathic damage to these muscles.

■ CLINICAL FEATURES

Symptomatology

Abdominal straining is such a potent inhibitor of pelvic muscle tone that if the individual persists in straining at stool over many years, the effectiveness of the postdefecation reflex will be reduced considerably. As a result, during the straining effort of defecation, stool is passed, followed by the anterior rectal wall mucosa. Further straining then follows in an effort to pass it. In advanced cases prolapsing anterior rectal mucosa becomes so large that it occludes the upper end of the anal canal, giving a feeling of anal blockage and preventing further defecation through straining. The patient typically relates that after partial emptying of the rectum a sense of obstruction develops that cannot be overcome except by ceasing all straining. Indeed, some of these patients develop frank anal obstruction and may pass a finger into the anal canal to temporarily reduce this obstruction and allow defecation. If straining is repeated and prolonged, the anterior rectal wall mucosa will ultimately protrude.

A vague, dull, aching pain in the perineum and sacral region may follow defecation because of the anterior rectal wall mucosa's presence in the upper anal canal, and the patient may continue straining fruitlessly in an endeavor to relieve it. The sensation of incomplete evacuation ensues. Mucosa that prolapses becomes irritated and secretes mucus, causing perineal moisture, soreness, and irritation. The prolapsing mucosa may bleed, and anal leakage with soiling of the clothes and secondary pruritus may occur. Partial incontinence also may be present.

In the clinical review by Harewood et al. (100), 39 patients (38 women, one man), mean age 53 years, presented with constipation (97%), incomplete rectal evacuation (92%), excessive straining (97%), digital evacuation (38%), and fecal incontinence (15%). Associated features included female gender (96%) multiparity with vaginal delivery (55%), hysterectomy or cystocele/rectocele repair (74%).

Pucciani et al. (101) evaluated the effect of abdominal hysterectomy on patients affected by the descending perineum syndrome. They studied 89 female patients affected by the descending perineum syndrome and 10 healthy women with normal bowel habits. All subjects underwent clinical evaluation, computerized anorectal manometry, and defecography. Dyschezia was found predominantly in subjects who had not undergone a hysterectomy. Fecal incontinence was significantly higher in patients who had undergone a hysterectomy. The worst anal resting pressure was found in incontinent patients. Rectoanal intussusception was a significant defecographic sign in subjects who had undergone abdominal hysterectomy. They suggested a possible link between fecal incontinence and abdominal hysterectomy in patients affected by the descending perineum syndrome.

Physical Signs

In the normal individual, the anal margin lies just below a line drawn between the coccyx and the symphysis pubis. In patients with this syndrome, the anal canal is either situated several centimeters below this line or it rapidly descends 3 or 4 cm when a straining effort is made. Digital examination reveals a lack of muscle tone, but the most characteristic change occurs when the patient is asked to strain. The puborectalis muscle descends sharply and can no longer be felt as a separate bar constituting the anorectal ring. Henry (98) stated that the descending perineum syndrome could be defined simply as being present when the plane of the perineum extends beyond that of the ischial tuberosities during a straining effort. On sigmoidoscopy during straining, the anterior wall bulges down into the instrument and follows it as it is withdrawn. Solitary ulceration may be seen on the anterior rectal mucosa in these patients (87).

■ INVESTIGATIONS

Anorectal Manometry

Continent patients with the descending perineum syndrome have normal sphincteric pressures, whereas incontinent patients with perineal descent and similar obstructive symptoms exhibit abnormally low pressures (102). Thus the obstructive symptoms apparently are not related to the anal tone. The rectal inhibitory reflex is abnormally sensitive in both continent and incontinent patients (102). Laboratory tests conducted by Harewood et al. (100) showed anal sphincter resting pressure was 54 ± 26 mmHg, and squeeze pressure was 96 ± 35 mmHg; expulsion from the rectum of a 50 mL balloon required >200 g added weight in 27%.

Radiologic Studies

Perineal descent may occur in both continent and incontinent patients. Patients with obstructed defecation may have a normal or an obtuse anorectal angle (102). In patients with the descending perineum syndrome, defecography usually demonstrates a descent of the anal canal >3.5 cm from its resting position at the inferior plane of the ischial tuberosities (103). Harewood et al. found perineal descent was 4.4 ± 1 cm (normal <4 cm) by scintigraphy. Scintigraphic evacuation, rectoanal angle change during defecation, and perineal descent were abnormal in 23%, 57%, and 78% of the patients, respectively. The most prevalent abnormality on testing is perineal descent of >4 cm; rectal balloon expulsion is an insensitive screening test for the descending perineum syndrome.

Electromyographic Studies

In the normal person there is, at first, increased electrical activity in the sphincteric muscles during straining, followed after several seconds by inhibition, which may be partial or complete. As soon as the straining ceases, there is a sharp return of exaggerated activity, which is called the closing reflex. In patients with a descending perineum, the postural reflex (i.e., the continuous activity of the pelvic floor at rest) is usually normal, but during straining, inhibition occurs once the pelvic muscles are relaxed and allows rapid pelvic floor descent (97). Reflex recovery after straining may be delayed or grossly diminished.

■ TREATMENT

The chief aim is to prevent further damage by eliminating all straining during defecation. Laxative use is of limited value because many of these patients have persistently liquid stool; a combination of liquid stool with lax sphincters causes soiling and sometimes partial incontinence. Patients in whom the stool is hard are instructed to use liquid paraffin or a hydrophilic laxative, either of which is sufficient to soften the stool. Usually the most successful method of facilitating rectal emptying is use of a glycerin or bisacodyl irritant suppository. Suppositories are inserted daily, and the patient is instructed to stop straining. The origin of these repeated urges to defecate is explained to the patient, who is told that once the bowel has emptied, all further urges should be ignored. Muscle weakness may be corrected partially by sphincteric exercises, but many weeks may pass before any effect is noted. Submucosal injection of sclerosants, such as phenol in oil, or the application of rubber band ligatures may relieve symptoms and hopefully will stop the bleeding and mucous discharge and relieve the sensation of tenesmus. Harewood et al. (100) reported 17 patients who underwent pelvic floor retraining. At two-year median follow-up (range, one to six years), 12 still experienced constipation or excessive straining; their perineal descent was greater than in patients who responded to retraining. Pelvic floor retraining is a suboptimal treatment for this chronic disorder of rectal evacuation; the extent of perineal descent appears to be a useful predictor of response to retraining. The potential role for biofeedback has not been clarified.

In patients with large hemorrhoids, an extended hemorrhoidectomy performed to remove the redundant lower rectal mucosa may be of benefit, but the results are rarely sustained (102).

When severe weakness of the perineal muscles results in anal incontinence, the postanal repair described by Parks is recommended (98). The effect of this operation is to raise the level of the pelvic floor and reduce the anorectal angle. The operation is not the end of the treatment because it is essential that the patient avoid straining during defecation so as not to stretch the repair.

PNEUMATOSIS COLI

The term "pneumatosis coli" is applied to the condition pneumatosis cystoides intestinalis (PCI) when it is limited to the large intestine. This rare condition is characterized by cystic accumulations of gas in the submucosa or subserosa of the bowel. The peak incidence is between 40 and 50 years of age (104). The male-female ratio has been reported from 3.5:1 to 1:1 (104–106). The condition may be seen in all sections of the gut but is most common in the small intestine. In a collected series, colonic involvement was reported in 36% of the cases (104). The entire colon and rectum or only a part of the large intestine, more commonly the left side than the right, can be affected.

ETIOLOGY

The etiology of this condition is unknown, but the three most frequent hypotheses are the mechanical, pulmonary, and bacterial theories (107). Other proposed hypotheses have included biochemical, neoplastic, and nutritional theories, but they have had little support.

Mechanical Hypothesis

It has been suggested that gastrointestinal gas, under abnormal pressure because of obstruction, is forced through mucosal defects, enters the submucosal lymphatics, and is distributed distally in the submucosa by peristalsis (105). Marshak et al. (108) reported pneumatosis of the descending colon after sigmoidoscopy without biopsy, and they suggested that the use of instruments in the bowel may produce mucosal defects that lead to localized pneumatosis. Other authors also have reported the development of pneumatosis coli after ulcerations such as a perforated duodenal ulcer, perforated jejunal diverticula, trauma such as colonoscopy, intestinal anastomoses, and jejunoileal bypass (109–111). Smith and Welter (112) reported mucosal ulcerations or necrosis in 45% of their patients, although Koss (105) and others reported that they found no demonstrable mucosal lesions.

Pulmonary Hypothesis

Keyting et al. (111) noted an association of pneumatosis intestinalis with chronic pulmonary disease. They postulated that severe coughing produces alveolar rupture and pneumomediastinum. Gas then dissects downward to the retroperitoneum and along perivascular spaces to the bowel wall and accumulates in a subserosal location. Artificial inflation of the lungs is capable of initiating dissection of the air. Asthma and pulmonary fibrosis also have been associated with PCI. The hydrogen content of cystic gas does not support the pulmonary theory since this gas is not present in large quantities in alveoli.

Bacterial Hypothesis

This theory implicates gastrointestinal bacteria as the origin of gas found in the bowel wall. The typical location of gas in patients with pulmonary disease is subserosal, whereas pneumatosis secondary to gastrointestinal disease is linear in distribution and is located in the submucosa. PCI has been produced experimentally in the guinea pig by injecting a mixture of *Escherichia coli, Aerobacter aerogenes,* and *Clostridium welchii* into the bowel wall (113). Yale and Balish (114) readily produced PCI in the germ-free rat by inoculating its peritoneal cavity with a pure culture of either *C. perfringens* or *C. tertium.* Similar inoculation of the germ-free animal with any one of eight other clostridial species does not result in the formation of PCI. The authors believed, therefore, that the bacterial theory for the formation of at least some cases of PCI has been established and that treatment should be directed at controlling a possible clostridial infection. High hydrogen levels in cysts suggest a bacterial cause since hydrogen is a product of bacterial metabolism (115).

ASSOCIATED CONDITIONS

In approximately 15% of the cases there are no associated medical conditions, and PCI is considered primary. It is estimated that associated abnormalities occur in the remaining 85% of cases and these are considered secondary. Yale (116) listed a large number of conditions that have been found in association with PCI. Included among the pulmonary conditions were chronic lung disease, emphysema, and pneumomediastinum. PCI is more frequently seen in association with gastrointestinal conditions, most commonly with peptic ulceration, carcinoma of the gastrointestinal tract, and pyloric stenosis. Galandiuk and Fazio (117), in their review of the literature, added the following associated conditions: necrotizing enterocolitis, pseudomembranous enterocolitis, diverticulitis, intestinal strangulation, appendicitis, gallstones, volvulus, Crohn's disease, ulcerative colitis, esophageal stricture, tuberculous enteritis, scleroderma, blunt abdominal trauma, diaphragmatic hernia, and jejunoileal bypass. PCI has been reported as occurring with renal and hepatic transplantation and with the use of lactulose, steroids, and chemotherapeutic regimens (118). Samson and Brown (119) reported PCI associated with AIDS-associated cryptosporidiosis and suggested that the infection may be pathogenetically involved in the pneumatosis and not merely incidental as the pneumatosis resolved upon treatment of the cryptosporidiosis. (Characteristically the right side of the colon is affected.) Colonoscopic polypectomy has been associated with PCI (120). PCI has been described with needle catheter jejunostomy (121,122). PCI has also been associated with dermatomyosites (123), lactulose administration (124), celiac disease (125), polymyositis (126), *C. difficile* pseudomembranous colitis (127), previous intestinal anastomosis (128).

CLINICAL FEATURES

Symptoms and Signs

The symptomatology and prognosis of PCI are generally those of the associated condition. The presence of PCI is not associated with any characteristic clinical picture, and when symptoms do occur, they are nonspecific. Manifestations range from the case found incidentally in an asymptomatic individual to the more severe form that may cause partial intestinal obstruction. Bouts of diarrhea, diarrhea alternating with constipation, constipation alone, melena, and flatulence are common. Patients may complain of mucus, colicky lower abdominal pain, incontinence, occasional flecks of bright red blood on the stools, urgency, malabsorption, or weight loss (117).

Complications of PCI occur in approximately 3% of the cases and include volvulus, pneumoperitoneum, intestinal obstruction, intussusception, tension pneumoperitoneum, hemorrhage, and intestinal perforation (117).

Physical findings occasionally include an abdominal mass. Rectal examination may reveal cysts in the rectum.

The length of the history of a patient with PCI may vary from a few months to a few years (105).

In adults the clinical features are usually quite benign, but in children they often are associated with necrotizing enterocolitis, in which case there is usually a fulminant presentation with a high mortality rate (117).

Radiology

Radiographically, the cysts may be suspected when a plain film of the abdomen reveals radiolucent clusters along the contours of the bowel and in the region of the mesentery. These clusters are more common in the sigmoid mesentery, and they shift in position in different projections. The presence of a pneumoperitoneum in an asymptomatic patient without a clinical perforation syndrome should suggest the disease; indeed, it is almost pathognomonic of the disease. Making a correct diagnosis will prevent an unnecessary operation. The diagnosis can be made from a chest film in which air cysts can be seen in the splenic or hepatic flexure of the colon. Multiple transparent bubbles between the liver and right diaphragmatic dome are called the Moreau-Chilaiditi sign and are present in 15% of the patients with small bowel pneumatosis (104). Retroperitoneal air may be present beneath the diaphragm bilaterally, showing no shift regardless of the position in which the films are taken, and producing no specific symptoms. Portal vein gas is generally an ominous sign and is often indicative of ischemic bowel, but it can also be a benign condition in adults (129) in association with PCI. Barium enema studies demonstrate large polypoid defects on the wall of the intestine or smooth filling defects that change in shape with distention or compression of the bowel (108). Sometimes the barium practically obliterates the cysts, and they are not visualized well except on the postevacuation film on which the mucosa appears swollen, suggesting ulcerative colitis. The gas may also be evident as a linear radiolucent strip along the intestinal margin (Fig. 7). Streaks of air may separate loops of bowel, and gas may be seen in the portal and mesenteric veins (117). Sonography shows multiple immobile linear or spotty high echoes in the thickened colonic wall (130).

CT scanning has been reported as useful in evaluating patients with PCI and distinguishing it from other conditions such as abdominal abscess, mesenteric or biliary air, and bowel infarction (131). Endoscopic ultrasonography has been used to diagnose colonic pneumatosis (132). MRI is less sensitive and specific than CT in this setting (129).

Pathology

The cysts vary in size from a few millimeters to a few centimeters in diameter. They may occur either singly or in clusters. Apparently they do not communicate with the intestinal lumen or with each other.

Day et al. (133) described the macroscopic appearance of a surgical specimen of cystic pneumatosis as characteristic. The mucosal surface has a coarse cobblestone appearance resulting from a large number of submucosal cysts, the apices of which may show intramucosal hemorrhage. Cysts also project from the serosal surface. The gas appears to be under pressure because rupture of cysts viewed through the sigmoidoscope or in fresh surgical specimens causes a popping sound. Although submucosal cysts predominate in the colon, sub-serous cysts are frequently found in the small bowel.

Rectal biopsy appearances are distinctive (133). Cystic spaces lying in the submucosa immediately beneath the muscularis mucosae are lined by large macrophages, some of which may be multinucleate with much eosinophilic cytoplasm (Fig. 8). The connective tissue between the cysts, which are often multilobular, shows little or no evidence of inflammation. The covering mucosa is attenuated and sometimes contains small hemorrhages. The

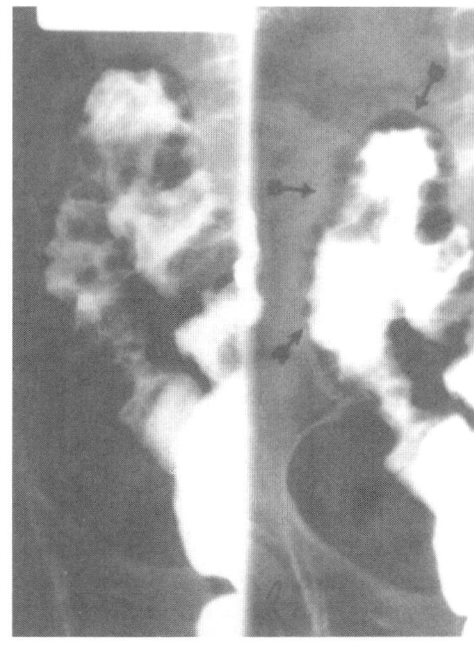

FIGURE 7 ■ Pneumatosis coli. Barium enema shows a linear radiolucent strip of gas along the sigmoid colon (*arrows*).

appearance is most likely to be confused with that of lymphangioma and oleogranuloma. In a patient with a lymphangioma there are no macrophages, and the lymphatic spaces are lined by a flattened endothelium without any interstitial inflammation. In a patient with an oleogranuloma, there is a macrophage response, but also present is much inflammation and fibrosis around fat-filled spaces.

Diagnosis

Very rarely, during examination, a palpable colon may be found. Rectal examination may reveal gaseous cysts. Sigmoidoscopic examination may disclose the clusters of cysts protruding into the bowel's lumen. A simple radiograph of the abdomen may show the very striking appearance of pneumatosis coli. For more proximal involvement, colonoscopic examination will reveal the cysts that project into lumen-like sessile polyps (Fig. 9).

This examination might be useful when the diagnosis is in doubt, such as when considering the differential diagnosis of familial adenomatous polyposis (134). A barium enema study will confirm the diagnosis.

The differential diagnosis with a barium enema study may include familial adenomatous polyposis. Other causes of intestinal perforation in patients presenting with a pneumoperitoneum should be considered. The presence of rectal bleeding may suggest carcinoma. In symptomatic patients with abdominal pain the condition may be mistaken for appendicitis. Diffuse emphysema is usually distributed in all tissue spaces. Other conditions include enterogenous intestinal cysts, emphysematous gastritis, lymphangioma, and sclerosing lipogranulomatosis (117).

Careful sigmoidoscopic and radiologic examinations and a biopsy should be performed to avoid errors in diagnosis and thus avoid unnecessary operations.

■ TREATMENT

Asymptomatic PCI does not call for any treatment. Indeed, spontaneous remission can occur (135). Historically, symptomatic patients were treated by operation. The problem of differentiating pneumatosis coli from polyposis and other neoplastic conditions led Calne to favor operation (134).

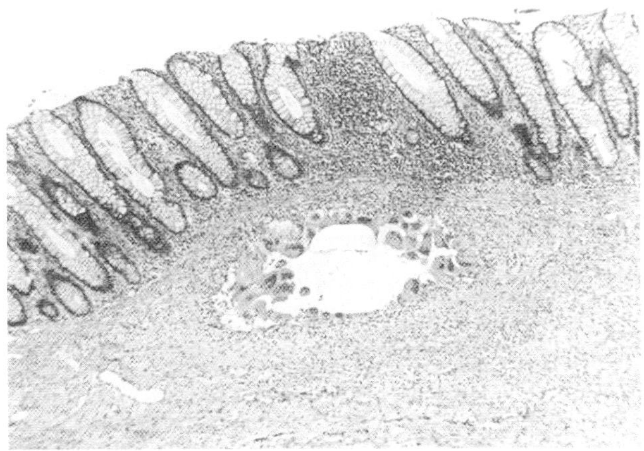

FIGURE 8 ■ Microscopic appearance of pneumatosis cystoides intestinalis; the cystic space in the submucosa is lined by large macrophages.

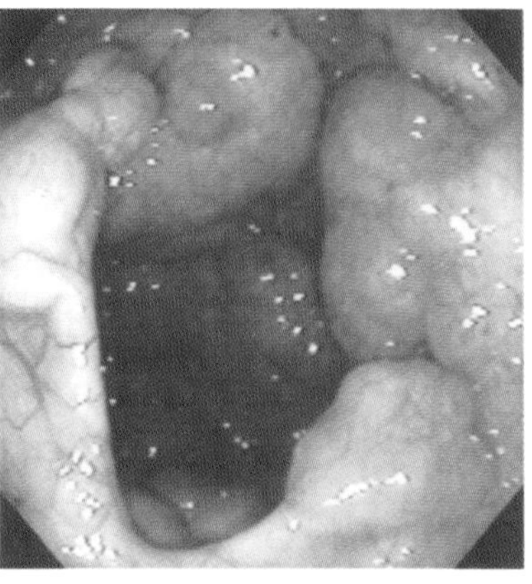

FIGURE 9 ■ Colonoscopic appearance of pneumatosis coli with multiple protruding cystic lesions of varying size. *Source*: Courtesy of Carol-Ann Vasilevsky, M.D., Montreal, Quebec.

He believed that the distinction was academic since the treatment of resection was common to both gaseous cysts and familial adenomatous polyposis.

For the asymptomatic patient with established PCI, e.g., a CT scan, revealing characteristic air-filled cysts in the intestinal wall and free intraperitoneal air, a nonoperative management is appropriate (136). If the patient does not have an acute abdomen or findings requiring emergency laparotomy, supportive care is adequate. The sole finding of free air with PCI does not mandate exploratory laparotomy.

Therapy for secondary pneumatosis should be directed at the underlying disease process. For example, patients with SLE have had resolution of their PCI with high-dose steroids, pulse intravenous cyclophosphamide, and octreotide therapy (129).

For patients with PCI secondary to cytotoxic or immunosuppressive treatment for hematologic or oncologic disorders, treatment with broad-spectrum antibiotics and possible parenteral nutrition has been suggested until recovery from the myelo-suppression (137). For patients with pneumatosis intestinalis and AIDS-associated infections—cryptosporidiosis, CMV, and toxoplasmosis, Gelman and Brandt advocated conservative management (138).

In 1973 Forgacs et al. (106) described a method of treatment that was both simple and effective. It consisted of administering oxygen by face mask for a few days. The treatment is based on the theoretic consideration of gas exchange between the cysts and the surrounding tissues. The authors predicted that the cysts could be deflated if the total pressure of gases in venous blood is lowered by the patient's prolonged breathing of a gas mixture containing a high concentration of oxygen. Successful therapy has subsequently been reported by others (117,139–144).

The paradoxic persistence of gas-filled cysts in the bowel wall implies that they are replenished at a rate that equals or exceeds the rate of absorption. Since a direct communication with the lumen of the bowel has never been demonstrated, gas presumably enters the cysts by diffusion. The rate of diffusion from bowel gas to cyst and from cyst to capillaries is determined by the partial pressure of gases in each of these compartments, their solubility in tissue fluid, and the dimensions of the diffusing surface represented by the tissues separating them.

The object of treatment is to alter the balance between the diffusion of gases into and out of the cysts in favor of absorption. This can be accomplished by lowering the total pressure of gases in venous blood by breathing oxygen, thereby increasing the pressure gradient between the cysts and the surrounding tissues. Investigators have described using different quantities of intracystic gaseous constituents. Oxygen content varied from 2.5% to 16%, nitrogen content from 80% to 90%, and carbon dioxide content from 0.3% to 7.5% (145,146). Hydrogen content from 2% to 50% has been reported,[a] whereas normal intestinal gas contains 14% hydrogen (148). Breathing 100% oxygen washes nitrogen out of the lungs and the tissues, leaving only oxygen and carbon dioxide in arterial blood. Most of the oxygen is metabolized by the tissues so that the total pressure of gases at the venous end of the capillary is less than 100 mm Hg and the gas mixture in the cysts remains at or above atmospheric pressure. The pressure gradient, which determines the rate of removal of gases from the cyst, is thus increased several fold. This approach has been used to hasten reabsorption of gases from a pneumothorax, to relieve postoperative abdominal distention, and to prevent abdominal pain in airmen flying over high altitudes.

Down and Castleden (149) suggested that the reason such therapy works is that the cysts are created and maintained by a fastidious anerobic gas-forming organism that provides gas at a rate that exceeds the rate of absorption until an equilibrium is reached. The high tissue oxygen tension achieved with oxygen therapy kills the organisms, and the gas is then reabsorbed in the same way as gas contained within any natural or artificially created space in the body.

Pure oxygen cannot be administered safely over long periods because it damages the lungs. The concentration of oxygen in the gas mixture is therefore kept below 75%, with nitrogen comprising the rest. To prevent the entry of atmospheric nitrogen into the lung, the administration of oxygen must be continuous. Humidified oxygen at 8 L/min is delivered via a suitable mask resulting in an inspired oxygen rate of 70% to 75% and the arterial oxygen tension (Pa_{O_2}) levels in excess of 300 mmHg (150). Breaks in oxygen breathing of half an hour are allowed four times each day to permit the patient to eat meals and to attend to other necessities; however, the patient must receive at least 4 hours of unbroken oxygen administration, and the mask must be worn all night.

Daily abdominal and chest X-ray studies are performed. The plain radiograph will show gradual diminution in size of the cysts, and a chest X-ray film will exclude the presence of atelectasis related to oxygen therapy.

The method of administration of oxygen, the amount given, and the length of time for which it is given, are important practical issues that have not been defined fully. Masks and nasal cannulas are more acceptable to patients than oxygen tents. Aggressive oxygen therapy for six days was initially recommended, but it should be continued for at least 48 hours after complete radiologic disappearance of all cysts has been obtained (106). Disappearance of gas-filled cysts has been accomplished after three to five days of oxygen therapy (139,140).

A two-week treatment with an elemental diet also results in cystic resolution and disappearance of symptoms (151). The rationale of this treatment is that it reduces bacterial hydrogen production. Recurrences are common after a regular diet is resumed. The use of an eight-week course of metronidazole has been reported as an easy ambulatory alternative to high-pressure oxygen therapy. The appropriate dose has not been determined, but doses of 250 to 500 mg three times daily for several months have been used (129). Successful resolution of the symptomatic and radiologic features of PCI has been documented with the added bonus of avoiding hospitalization and the potential for oxygen toxicity (142,152,153).

Operation is indicated when PCI is associated with necrosis of the bowel or sepsis or when complications of volvulus, intestinal obstruction, or severe rectal bleeding supervene. A unique case of pneumatosis coli with extensive colon and rectal involvement that did not respond to inhalation oxygen therapy and metronidazole was successfully managed by restorative proctocolectomy (154). Treatment of obstructive pneumatosis coli has been treated by endoscopic rupture and sclerotherapy with 1 to 2 mL of aethoxy sclerol (1%) applied within cysts and cyst walls (155). Colonoscopic needle deflation alone has been used (133).

Gagliardi et al. (156) reviewed the management of 25 cases treated over a 30-year period. Treatment with antidiarrheals and anti-inflammatory drugs in 14 patients resulted in improvement in nine cases (64%). Oxygen therapy in nine patients always alleviated symptoms but there was a high rate of recurrence (78%). With further courses of therapy, lasting remission was achieved in five patients. Two patients underwent colectomy.

HIDRADENITIS SUPPURATIVA

Hidradenitis suppurativa, also known as Verneuil's disease, is an acute or chronic infection of the apocrine glands of the skin. In its chronic form it is an indolent inflammatory disease of the skin and subcutaneous tissue characterized by abscesses and sinus formation. It may be located wherever apocrine sweat glands are found such as at the nape of the neck and in the axilla, mammary, inguinal, genital, perianal, scalp, and periumbilical regions (157).

CLINICAL FINDINGS

Hidradenitis suppurativa is essentially a disease of adult life because apocrine glands are activated at the time of puberty (158). It most often occurs in the third and fourth decades of life and affects both sexes (157,159) but most authors report that perianal disease is more common in men (157,160–164). The disease is more prevalent in the black race than in other races (157,159). Affected individuals frequently have a seborrheic type of skin, are usually overweight, and perspire profusely.

A number of associated abnormalities, including acne vulgaris, diabetes mellitus, hypercholesterolemia, a low basal metabolic rate, interstitial keratitis, anemia, and atopic reactions, have been reported in patients with hidradenitis suppurativa (165). To these have been added poor personal hygiene, irritation from tight clothing, close shaving, fat skin, excessive sweating, and Cushing's syndrome (159). In one series, 70% of the patients were smokers (164). In addition, patients with this infection can be simultaneously affected in other parts of their body.

[a] Refs. 106, 115, 116, 141, 142, 147.

■ ETIOLOGY

The etiology of hidradenitis suppurativa remains unclear. Certain predisposing factors have been mentioned and include mechanical irritation, trauma, and contact dermatitis (166). Attanoos et al. (167) undertook a pathologic study of 118 skin resection specimens from 101 patients with hidradenitis suppurativa. Follicular occlusion was identified in all the specimens regardless of disease duration (one month to 18 years) but was not identified in axillary and inguinal skin of controls. The authors therefore regard follicular occlusion by keratinous material, with subsequent active folliculitis and secondary destruction of skin adnexae and subcutis, as an integral step in the pathogenesis of hidradenitis suppurativa. The stimulus for initial follicular occlusion remains undetermined. Obesity is common in patients with hidradenitis and may be a contributing factor. Occlusion of the apocrine ducts by keratin with subsequent sepsis may be hormonally induced. A functional disorder of the hypothalmopituitary axis was described (168). In a response to a combined thyrotrophin-releasing hormone and gonadotrophin-releasing hormone test, the prolactin and thyroid-stimulating hormone responses were significantly greater in patients with hidradenitis suppurativa than in controls. The results may reflect a disturbance of feedback signals from peripheral hormones.

A strong temporal relationship between the initiation of treatment with certain oral contraceptives and the onset of hidradenitis suppurativa has been reported (169). Resolution of symptoms occurred in some patients when the contraceptive pill was discontinued. Other patients benefited when the pill was changed to one that contained a higher estrogen-to-progesterone ratio. The presence of androgens is apparently a prerequisite for the development of hidradenitis suppurativa, and raised testosterone concentrations have been found in these women (170). The androgenic properties of the oral contraceptives also can be overcome by the administration of preparations that contain a higher estrogen-to-progesterone ratio. Barth et al. (171) studied endocrine factors in pre- and postmenopausal women and found no supporting evidence for biochemical hyperandrogenism in women with hidradenitis suppurativa. But there is clearly a relationship between sex hormones and hidradenitis suppurativa. The failure of hidradenitis suppurativa to develop before puberty, the general decline in disease activity during the climacteric, and the improvement during pregnancy and the menstrual cycle, all suggest a condition dependent on hormones (170). Clinical assessment of 134 patients with hidradenitis suppurativa revealed clinical evidence to support an androgen-based endocrine disorder underlying the condition (172). Such features included post-pubertal onset that is maximal during the third decade; female preponderance (13:5), premenstrual flare in 57% of the women, absence of this flare associated with irregular or anovulatory menstrual cycles, and an increased incidence of obesity and acne.

Konig et al. (173) performed a matched-pair case-control study to evaluate the influence of smoking habits on the manifestation of hidradenitis suppurativa. Of 63 subjects (27 men, 36 women), the rate of active cigarette smokers was 88.9% whereas 6.4% of the subjects had never smoked and 4.8% of the patients stated to be ex-smokers. The rate of smokers in the matched-pair control group was 46%. The significantly higher proportion of active smokers among patients with hidradenitis suppurativa can be expressed by an odds ratio of 9.4. The expected smoking prevalence in Germany was 26.7%. Seventy-three percent of their patients had no family history of hidradenitis suppurativa whereas 27% reported at least one affected first-degree relative. From the exceedingly high rate of smokers among patients with this condition, they concluded that cigarette smoking is a major triggering factor of hidradenitis suppurativa.

■ BACTERIOLOGY

Adams and Haisten (166) reported the organisms usually found include *Staphylococcus aureus*, *Streptococcus viridans*, and coliforms. The results of cultures from the series of 104 patients with hidradenitis suppurativa reported by Thornton and Abcarian (157) revealed no growth in 48%, *Staphylococcus epidermidis* in 44%, *E. coli* in 19%, a-streptococcus in 15%, and other flora in 22%. *Proteus* species and diphtheroids also have been found (160). It is uncertain whether the link between *Chlamydia trachomatis* is a direct cause or a predisposing factor (174).

■ DIAGNOSIS

Clinically the diagnosis of hidradenitis suppurativa is made by the above clinical features. One of the key features of hidradenitis suppurativa is multiple-sinuses (Figs. 10 and 11). Making the pathologic diagnosis may be difficult because the apocrine glands have been destroyed by abscess formation. The condition may be confused with anal fistulas, Crohn's disease of the perianal skin, furunculosis, and pilonidal disease (161). An important point of differentiation between a fistulous track of hidradenitis suppurativa and a fistula-in-ano is that the former does not communicate with the intersphincteric plane. Tracking of hidradenitis suppurativa lies superficial to the internal sphincter and bears no relationship to the dentate line. The lack of gastrointestinal symptoms, a normal sigmoidoscopic examination, and negative contrast studies should help in ruling out Crohn's disease. The abscess of hidradenitis suppurativa lacks the necrotic plug or "core" of a furuncle. A lack of midline pits in the coccygeal area should rule out pilonidal disease.

■ CLINICAL COURSE

Hidradenitis suppurativa may start insidiously with burning, itching, local heat, and hyperhidrosis, and may eventually progress to produce pain. As the inflammatory process develops, subcutaneous nodules may be palpable, and reddening or cyanotic discoloration of the skin may be present. The inflammatory process may resolve slowly with or without operative or spontaneous drainage, over a period of several weeks, or, more commonly, adjacent nodules may appear and coalesce to form a network of sinus tracts. Suppuration is usually slight, and only a few drops of pus may be evacuated from a nodule. Resolution and scarring may occur, or a series of recurrences and remissions may ensue, with the formation of considerable induration, abscesses, and deep sinus tracts. Discharge

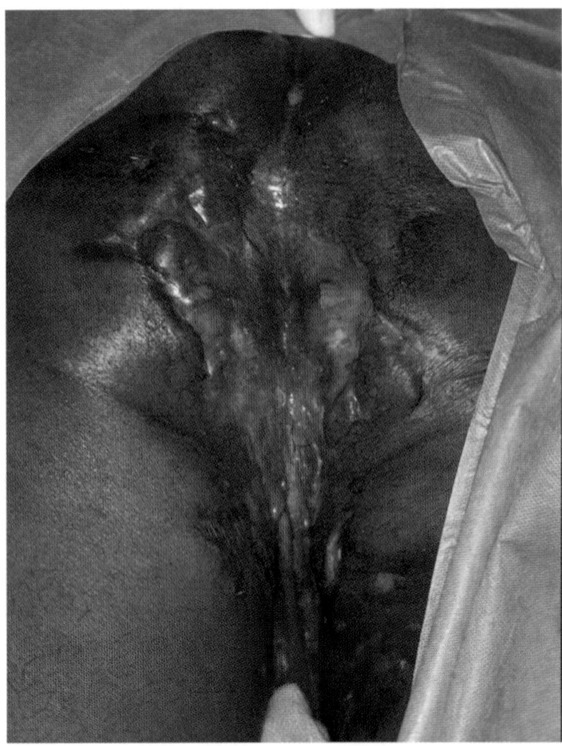

FIGURE 10 ■ Severe perianal and perineal hidradenitis suppurativa. *Source*: Courtesy of Dr. Nancy Morin, Montreal, Quebec.

may persist, and in later stages, ulceration may occur. Pitted scars are characteristic in patients with hidradenitis suppurativa and are due to the retraction of skin as a result of fibrotic contraction (161). The average duration of the disease is many years. The foul odor and discharge from the lesions may interfere with the patient's employment and normal social activities.

■ ASSOCIATED CONDITIONS

The arthritis associated with hidradenitis suppurativa is rare and most commonly affects the peripheral joints (175,176). The axial skeleton is less frequently involved

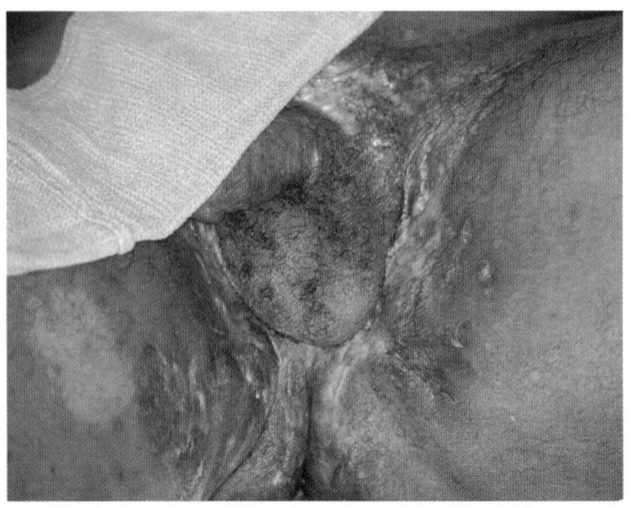

FIGURE 11 ■ Severe perianal, perineal, and inguinal hidradenitis suppurativa. *Source*: Courtesy of Dr. Nancy Morin, Montreal, Quebec.

and is often asymptomatic. Hidradenitis suppurativa has been reported in association with Crohn's disease (177,178). The coexistence of hidradenitis suppurativa and Crohn's disease may affect patient care in three ways (178). Patients with hidradenitis suppurativa may be mistakenly diagnosed as having Crohn's disease and appropriate operative treatment may be withheld, or inappropriate treatment may be given. Conversely, patients with Crohn's disease may be diagnosed as having hidradenitis suppurativa although this is unlikely because perianal or perineal Crohn's disease is usually associated with colorectal involvement. Such a misdiagnosis may lead to a more aggressive operation than would be wise. Finally, hidradenitis suppurativa may affect the clinical course of patients with Crohn's disease leading, for example, to persistent perineal skin sepsis after proctectomy. Most surgeons treat perineal Crohn's disease conservatively. Sepsis stemming from hidradenitis suppurativa justifies a more aggressive approach.

■ PATHOLOGY

This chronic inflammatory condition affects the skin and subcutaneous tissues. The affected area of skin has a red and white blotchy appearance and is thick and edematous, with watery pus draining from multiple openings of sinus tracts. The persistent chronic nature of the disease leads to ulceration and scarring. Lesions may be localized, or they may involve large areas of perianal skin extending onto the buttocks. Microscopic examination of excised specimens shows an inflammatory exudate consisting of plasma cells, lymphocytes, and occasionally, giant cells of the foreign body type, with the formation of sinus tracts (Fig. 12). The tracts become lined by squamous epithelium by downgrowth from the surface skin (163). In long-standing cases squamous cell carcinoma has been found (157,166,179–182).

In their review of the literature, Perez-Diaz et al. (159) found 26 patients with squamous cell carcinoma associated with hidradenitis suppurativa. The average age at diagnosis was 47 years with a predominance of males (77%). The average duration of the disease before carcinoma was 20 years. Wide local excision was the most frequent treatment but abdominoperineal resections were performed in some patients and some were given radiotherapy. Disease-free survival at one year was 31%. Cosman et al. (183) described the second case of verrucous carcinoma arising in hidradenitis suppurative of the anal margin in a nonimmunosuppressed man. The ability of anal and genital hidradenitis suppurativa to form squamous and verucous carcinomas reinforces the argument for early and complete resection (183,184).

■ TREATMENT

Initially warm baths and cleansing agents are used to maintain hygiene. Both systemic and topical antibiotics have been used based on culture results (185,186). Jemec and Wendelboe (187) compared topical clindamycin with systemic tetracycline in the treatment of 46 patients with stage 1 or 2 hidradenitis suppurativa in a double-blind, double-dummy controlled trial. No significant difference was found between the two types of treatment. If the patient presents while she is taking an oral contraceptive,

A 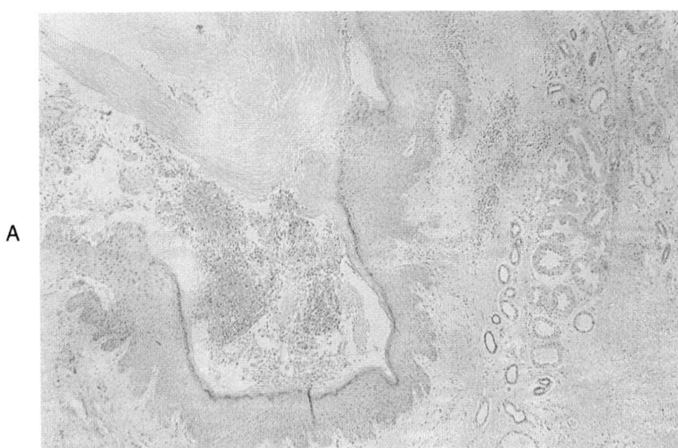 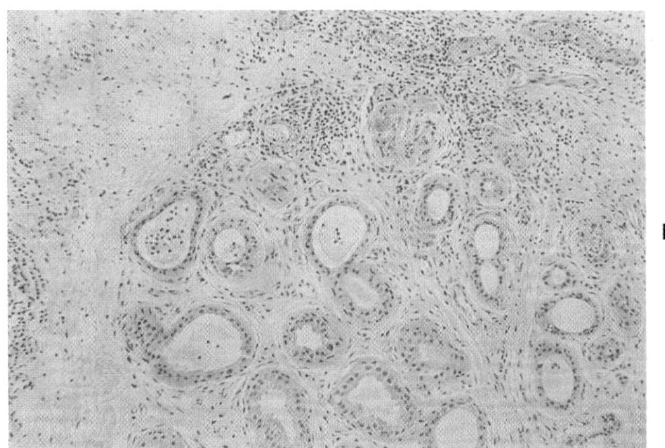 B

FIGURE 12 ■ (**A**) Dilated hair follicle pore with a mixed keratin and inflammatory exudate plug. Dilated apocrine glands (oxyphilic staining) and the darker stained cuboidal cells lining the eccrine glands are noted. (**B**) High power demonstrating a dilated ductal lumen indicating obstruction of the hair follicle and dilated ductules—some filled with inflammatory exudate. There is some distortion of the cellular wall and peristromal inflammation. *Source*: Courtesy H. Srolovitz, M.D., Montreal, Quebec.

cessation of the medication or a change to an alternative form with greater estrogenic properties may be indicated (159). Based on their belief that hidradenitis suppurativa is a cutaneous manifestation of a variably expressed androgen excess, Mortimer et al. (188) have provided a rationale for the treatment of early disease with cyproterone acetate. The use of steroids to decrease inflammation and androgen production and leuprolide acetate to reduce androgen production have been reported (185).

Sullivan et al. (189) noted patients' self-reported disease activity scores for hidradenitis suppurativa were significantly decreased following infliximab infusion treatment for rheumatoid arthritis and psoriasis. This correlated with physician observed clinical improvement. They believe infliximab is a promising agent for the treatment of hidradenitis suppurativa.

The surgical treatment of hidradenitis suppurativa in its acute phase is incision and drainage of a localized abscess. In neither the acute nor the chronic phase are antibiotics considered of value as definitive therapy (157,160).

Surgical treatment in the chronic stage may consist of (i) wide excision with the defect left open to granulate and epithelialize (157,164,186), (ii) excision and primary closure (165), (iii) excision and split-thickness skin grafting (158,164,190,191), and (iv) excision and closure with a pedicle flap (192,186). Each of these procedures has its advocates, and each may have its use, depending on the location and extent of the pathology. In mild chronic cases, unroofing of the area may be considered (161,179), but in most cases a better and wiser plan would be excision of the diseased skin and subcutaneous tissues. Excision and primary closure are usually suitable for a small wound located in a relatively clean area (i.e., the axilla). Because of the contaminated environment, many surgeons are reluctant to close perineal wounds primarily and they can simply be left open. A combination of both procedures is demonstrated in Figure 13.

If there is extensive infection with abscess formation, incision and drainage may be necessary as a preliminary procedure. Following this, wide excision should include all sinus and epithelial skin bridges, along with all of the fibrous and inflamed portions of the subcutaneous fat. In the past, split-thickness skin grafts have been applied (158), but they seldom have been necessary; Bocchini et al. (193) presented the results of management of extensive hidradenitis suppurativa in gluteal, perineal and inguinal areas in 56 patients (93% male) with a mean age of 40 years. Gluteal and perineal diseases were present in 37.6% and 30.6% respectively. Squamous cell carcinoma and Crohn's disease were observed in one patient each. Wide surgical excision was performed in all. Healing by secondary intention was the choice in 57%, whereas 43% of the patients underwent delayed skin grafting. Diverting colostomy was used in 41% of the patients. Mean time for complete healing in the nongrafted group was 10 weeks and in the skin-grafted group was six weeks. New resection was performed in 9% of the patients. Partial graft loss was 38% and recurrence was observed in only one patient.

The establishment of a colostomy, as recommended by some authors, is generally unnecessary (174). A similar result can be obtained through adequate bowel preparation and placement of the patient on an elemental diet and obstipating medications as described by Gordon (194).

In fact, Thornton and Abcarian (157) found that even this measure is unnecessary. In an effort to clarify conflicting information and to establish principles of operative treatment, they reviewed the records of 104 patients with perianal and perineal hidradenitis suppurativa who were treated at Cook County Hospital in Chicago. With the patient in the prone jackknife position, their operative procedure consisted of wide excision of the involved area down to normal fat or fascia, with electrocautery used. Wounds were packed with iodoform gauze, and an occlusive dressing was applied. Diverting colostomy or skin grafts were not used routinely, nor were antibiotics administered. In only one of their 104 patients was a diverting colostomy deemed necessary. Sitz baths were instituted four times a day, and patients were discharged when comfortable—an average hospital stay of 7.2 days. Average healing times ranged from 3.5 to 7 weeks. Only four patients were operated on for recurrence in the five-year period of the authors' study. The extensive experience of

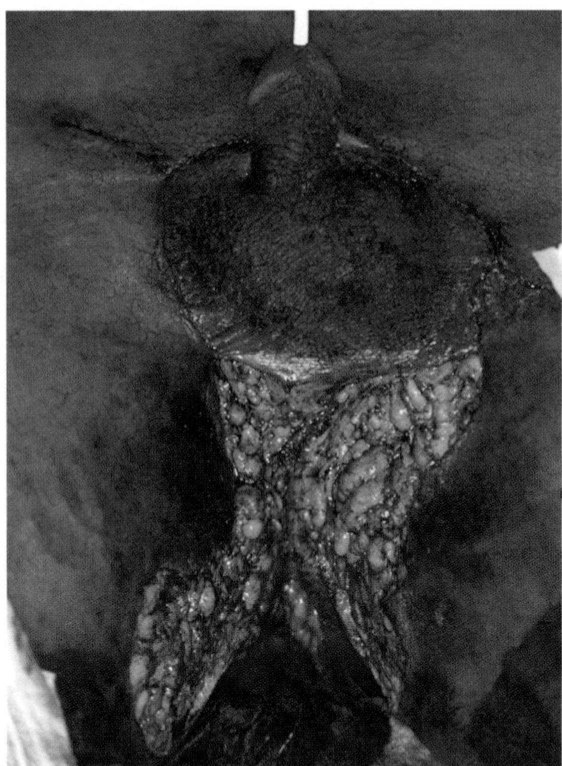

FIGURE 13 ■ Wide local excision of perianal and perineal hidradenitis suppurativa with partial suture of inguinoscrotal skin. *Source*: Courtesy of Dr. Nancy Morin, Montreal, Quebec.

Thornton and Abcarian and their excellent results indicate that the wide excision along with packing is followed by rapid healing without ancillary measures and is the treatment of choice. Other authors concur (164,186). Harrison et al. (162) recommended the use of a Silastic foam dressing to avoid the pain of dressing changes with gauze. Reported recurrence rates after excision of perianal hidradenitis suppurativa have varied from almost nil (186) to 67% (164).

Lapins et al. (195) used a carbon dioxide laser technique for stepwise horizontal vaporization in the management of hidradenitis suppurativa in various anatomic locations. In 24 patients followed for an average of 27 months, healing occurred in four weeks and only two patients developed recurrences. Despite these results, the authors state that in most cases wide local excision is the method of choice. Others have also used this method with success (182).

ANAL LEUKOPLAKIA

Anal leukoplakia is a rare and ill-understood condition. Donaldson et al. (196) reviewed the clinical findings and pathology of 27 patients who ranged in age from 31 to 79 years and presented with pruritus or an anal lump. The male-to-female ratio was 20:7. Macroscopically, the lesions were circumscribed or circumferential white plaques surrounded by moist, thickened perianal skin. Histologic findings were characterized by hyperkeratosis, acanthosis, "spiky" downgrowth of rete ridges, and bandlike chronic inflammatory cell infiltrate at the dermoepidermal junction. A synchronous keratinizing squamous cell carcinoma was found in nine patients, and a metachronous lesion occurred 11 years later in one patient. Operative treatment consists of excision with or without skin grafts or flaps, but leukoplakia recurs in majority of the cases. Anal leukoplakia has been reported to cause anal stenosis (197). Careful follow-up is necessary.

DIVERSION COLITIS

"Diversion colitis" is a term used to describe the clinical entity of nonspecific inflammation of excluded colonic and rectal mucosa. The condition was first described by Glotzer et al. (198) in 1981. Its importance lies in the inability to differentiate it from other types of proctitis and may result in inappropriate therapy and reluctance to recommend stoma closure. Of clinical consequence is the fact that there is complete resolution of the inflammatory process when intestinal continuity is restored.

In a study of 53 patients, Whelan et al. (199) reported a 91% incidence. Ferguson and Siegal (200) noted that 70% of 20 patients demonstrated diversion colitis. Whelan et al. (199) reported that age, type of stoma, or indication for operation play no role in the incidence of the disease. However, Haas et al. (201) found diversion colitis in 25% after operations for carcinoma and 86% after diverticulitis.

The etiology of this condition has not been definitely established, but it is thought to be a deficiency of short-chain fatty acids, which are preferred nutrients of the colonic mucosal cell. Butyrate, a SCFA generated by microbial fermentation of dietary substrates, is produced in the colon of humans (202). Butyrate is absorbed by colonocytes in the proximal colon via passive diffusion and by active transport mechanisms, which are linked to various ion exchange transporters. In the distal colon, the main mechanism of absorption is passive diffusion of the lipid-soluble form. Butyrate and other SCFA are important for the absorption of electrolytes by the large intestine and may play a role in preventing certain types of diarrhea. The mechanism by which butyrate and other SCFA exerts control over fluid and electrolyte fluxes in the colon is not well delineated though it may occur through an energy generated fuel effect, the up-regulation of various electrolyte transport systems, as well as possible effects on neuroendocrine factors. Butyrate regulates colonic motility, increases colonic blood flow and may enhance colonic anastomosis healing. Butyrate may reduce the symptoms from diversion colitis and it may prevent the progression of colitis in general. Harig et al. (203) demonstrated low levels of short-chain fatty acids in the diverted colon and noted that daily irrigation of the diverted segment with a solution of short-chain fatty acid results in improvement in the endoscopic appearance of the excluded bowel. Bacterial overgrowth by normal colonic flora or invasion by a specific pathogenic organism has been postulated as a cause of diversion colitis. Winslet et al. (204) reported that the onset or resolution of diversion proctitis was not associated with any significant changes in colonic cellular proliferation, glycoprotein synthesis, or mucosa-associated or luminal flora.

Rarely has diversion colitis caused clinical problems and for the most part is seldom clinically significant. The reported frequency of symptoms related to diverted bowel have varied greatly from asymptomatic to 50% (199–201). Whelan et al. (199) noted symptoms in only 6% of 53 patients studied. Orsay et al. (205) noted that 76% of patients demonstrated mild to severe colitis on an average of 30 weeks following diversion. From the largest series of reported patients with diversion colitis, Haas, Fox, and Szilagy (201) found that almost half of the 85 patients were symptomatic. The most prominent symptom is rectal bleeding, which is usually modest in amount but may be significant enough to require transfusion. Other symptoms include tenesmus, mucous discharge, and abdominal pain. The onset of symptoms may occur any time from one month to 22 years after fecal diversion (206).

Diversion colitis is a frequent, persistent, and sometimes problematic complication in patients with myelopathy who have also had colostomies (207).

Endoscopic examination may reveal abnormal findings in up to 80% of the patients (208). It may be impossible to distinguish defunctioned proctitis from inflammatory bowel disease. The simplest procedure to detect underlying disease is flexible fiberoptic sigmoidoscopy. Endoscopic examination reveals a colitic picture ranging from mild to severe. Haas, Fox, and Szilagy (201) found abnormal endoscopic findings in 80% of the patients with diversion colitis but these included mucous plugs and scybala. In the study by Whelan et al. (199) endoscopic mucosal findings included contact irritation or bleeding (98%), focal erythema (77%), sessile pale polypoid lesions (60%), petechiae (52%), ulcerations (29%), edema (23%), and blood in the lumen (13%). In majority of the patients, the colitis does not uniformly involve the mucosal surface. Instead, patches of inflammation are found interspersed between areas of normal mucosa (199). In one-fourth of the cases, inflammatory changes are limited to the rectum, whereas in three-fourths, the inflammatory process involves the rectum and the more proximal diverted colon (199).

Histologic findings noted in descending order of frequency include mild chronic inflammation, focal inflammation, lymphoid nodule, crypt changes, lymphoid follicle, and glandular atrophy. Other features may include crypt abscesses, epithelial degeneration, crypt regeneration, and aphthoid ulcers (204). Mucin granulomas are also a histologic feature (209). It has been suggested that lymphoid hyperplasia is a striking distinctive feature of diversion colitis (210). Asplund et al. (211) reviewed the histologic findings in the defunctioned rectums of 84 consecutive patients. All excised rectal specimens had ulcers and erosions, usually with prominent mucosal lymphoid aggregates, often with mucosal atrophy, diffuse mucin depletion, and marked mucosal architectural distortion. The transmural lymphoid aggregates were identified in 67% and were graded as moderate or marked in 42%. Ten rectal specimens contained non-necrotizing granulomas. No feature in the defunctioned rectum was associated with the original diagnosis or duration of defunctionalization. Granulomas in a defunctioned rectum were associated with an original diagnosis of Crohn's disease. Transmural lymphoid aggregates were common in defuctioned rectums in patients with inflammatory bowel disease and did not indicate Crohn's disease. Nonetheless, biopsies appear to have little or no role in establishing the diagnosis.

The investigation of such patients might include bacterial cultures, search for ova and parasites, and *Clostridium difficile* toxin, but these yield negative results in diversion colitis.

Asymptomatic endoscopic disease requires no pharmacologic treatment. For permanently diverted symptomatic patients, irrigation with a solution of short-chain fatty acids is recommended twice daily for two to four weeks (203). Other less successful treatments have included oral steroids and steroid enemas. Treatment with 5-ASA enemas has reportedly resulted in both endoscopic and histologic resolution (208). Definitive treatment consists of stoma closure following which full resolution can be expected. This has been observed in all 21 patients in whom the stoma was closed by Whelan et al. (199) and in 34 patients closed by Orsay et al. (205). An increased vascular pattern may persist but is asymptomatic (199). Winslet et al. (204) found macroscopic improvement in all patients after restoration of intestinal continuity but histologic evidence of disease remained in 50% of the patients. Colostomy closure need not be delayed in these patients.

Patients in whom the diversion is permanent should undergo periodic endoscopic examinations since polyps and malignancy can arise in out-of circuit large bowel. This is especially true if the original operation was performed for neoplastic disease. In this case both proximal "incontinuity" bowel and distal "diverted" bowel need inspection. Haas et al. (201) underscore the importance of follow-up surveillance. In their series of 85 patients, follow-up detected four patients with polyps and seven cases of carcinoma. Lim et al. (212) have suggested that diversion colitis may be a risk factor for the development of ulcerative colitis.

SEGMENTAL OR DIVERTICULA-ASSOCIATED COLITIS

A clinical syndrome of chronic colitis unique to the sigmoid colon harboring diverticula has been reported. Peppercorn (213) reported the clinical presentation, endoscopic, radiologic, and pathologic features, and response to therapy in eight patients more than 60 years old who presented with segmental chronic active colitis associated with sigmoid diverticula. Each patient presented with rectal bleeding and mucus and complaints of constipation alternating with loose stools, often with a sense of incomplete evacuation. Crampy lower abdominal pain and excessive flatulence were frequently described, but nausea, vomiting, fever, and weight loss were absent. None of the patients had prior similar complaints, or any symptoms of perirectal disease. Stools for bacterial pathogens, ova and parasites, and *C. difficile* toxin were negative in all eight patients.

Endoscopic appearance consisted of patchy, nonconfluent areas of hemorrhage and exudate limited to the sigmoid colon in an area of multiple diverticula 20 to 50 cm from the anus. The areas of visible inflammation were not contiguous with the diverticular orifices. No gross ulcerations or polypoid lesions were noted. Upper gastrointestinal series and small bowel X-ray studies were normal in all eight patients. From each patient, biopsies of endoscopically involved areas showed focal chronic active colitis without granulomas. Each patient had biopsies from grossly normal-appearing mucosa in the rectum and proximal to the sigmoid colon. The patients were treated with sulfasalazine in doses ranging from 2 to 4 g/day. In each case, there was full resolution of symptoms within six weeks of initiating therapy.

Makapugay and Dean (214) analyzed the clinical and pathologic features of 23 patients (age range, 38–87 years; median age, 72 years) with diverticular disease-associated chronic colitis. Nineteen presented with hematochezia; four had abdominal pain. Colonoscopic visualization of the mucosa showed patchy or confluent granularity and friability affecting the sigmoid colon encompassing diverticular ostia. Colonic mucosae proximal and distal to the sigmoid were endoscopically normal. Mucosal biopsy specimens showed features of idiopathic inflammatory bowel disease that included plasma cellular and eosinophilic expansion of the lamina propria (100%), neutrophilic cryptitis (100%) with crypt abscesses (61%), basal lymphoid aggregates (100%), distorted crypt architecture (87%), basal plasmacytosis (61%), surface epithelial sloughing (61%), focal Paneth cell metaplasia (48%), and granulomatous cryptitis (26%). Concomitant rectal biopsies obtained in five patients demonstrated histologically normal mucosa. Fourteen patients treated with high-fiber diet or antibiotics or both improved clinically, as did nine patients who received sulfasalazine or 5-ASA. Five patients underwent sigmoid colonic resection, three for stricture with obstruction and two for chronic blood loss anemia. Among a control population of 23 age- and gender-matched patients with diverticular disease without luminal surface mucosal abnormality, none required resection during the same follow-up period. In addition, three patients developed ulcerative proctosigmoiditis, 6, 9, and 17 months after the onset of diverticular disease-associated colitis. The data indicate that diverticular disease-associated chronic sigmoid colitis expresses morphologic features traditionally reserved for idiopathic inflammatory bowel disease. Its clinical and endoscopic profiles permit distinction from Crohn's disease and ulcerative colitis. Patients with chronic colitis in conjunction with diverticula are at increased risk for sigmoid colonic resection. Diverticular disease-associated chronic colitis may also precede the onset of conventional ulcerative proctosigmoiditis in some cases.

Gore et al. (215) described an endoscopic appearance of the sigmoid colon characterized by mucosal swelling, erythema, and hemorrhage strictly localized to the crescentic mucosal folds. In a five-year period these changes were seen in 34 of 2380 colonoscopies and fiberoptic sigmoidoscopies (1.42%). Majority of the patients were middle-aged or elderly. Diverticular disease was present in most (82%), but the abnormalities were confined to the crescentic mucosal folds with sparing of the diverticular orifices. The majority of patients presented with a history of bleeding per anus. Histologically there was a spectrum of changes varying from minor vascular congestion to florid active inflammatory disease with crypt architectural abnormalities mimicking ulcerative colitis, but rectal biopsies were invariably normal. Three patients later progressed to typical distal ulcerative colitis and two other patients presenting with endoscopic crescentic fold disease had a previous histologically documented history of distal ulcerative colitis. In three patients the histologic features were of mucosal prolapse. Approximately half the patients required some form of therapy to control their symptoms. Steroids and/or sulfasalazine were of value, although two patients subsequently underwent sigmoid resection, one to control bleeding and the second for a diverticulosis-associated stricture. Although endoscopic crescentic fold disease represents a specific endoscopic appearance, the clinical and histologic features indicate a wide spectrum of disease.

Imperiali et al. (216) evaluated the incidence of segmental colitis associated with diverticular in patients undergoing colonoscopy in a multi-center prospective study. Patients with inflammatory bowel disease-like lesions limited to colonic segments with diverticula were enrolled. Patients were treated with oral and topical 5-ASA until remission was achieved. A total of 5457 consecutive colonoscopies were recorded at five participating institutions; 20 patients (0.36%) met the endoscopic criteria for segmental colitis associated with diverticula. All had lesions in the left colon and one also had lesions in the right colon. Hematochezia was the main clinical feature and no relation with gender, age, or smoking habit was found. Blood chemistries were generally normal and the rectum was spared. The histological features were nondiagnostic and most patients did not complain of any abdominal symptoms 12 months after enrollment.

Guslandi (217) noted the term "segmental colitis" often mimicks inflammatory bowel disease at histological examination. The observed rectal sparing suggests a possible form of Crohn's disease, but no other similarities between segmental colitis and Crohn's colitis are detectable. Medical treatment for segmental colitis, empirically carried out with drugs such as sulfasalazine and mesalazine, is mostly successful and, when surgery is required, postoperative recurrences are infrequent. Although the existence of segmental colitis as a true clinical entity remains questionable, it appears unlikely that this condition represents an atypical form of inflammatory bowel disease.

In summary the unusual coexistence of an inflammatory bowel disease and diverticular disease, sometimes with stricturing, suggests a distinct entity. The possible coexistence of Crohn's disease and diverticular disease has been elaborated upon on p. 962.

AORTOENTERIC FISTULA

A primary aortoenteric fistula is a rare clinical entity that results in fatal exsanguination if undiagnosed. Saers and Scheltinga (218) reviewed the literature to determine whether management and survival have altered over time. The classic triad (gastrointestinal bleeding, pain, and a pulsating mass) was present in only 11% of 81 patients. Most primary aortoenteric fistulas were caused by an aneurysmal aorta and were almost always (94%) heralded by repetitive gastrointestinal bleeds. Computed tomography provides images superior to those of other diagnostic modalities, such as gastroduodenoscopy or conventional angiography. Operative mortality rates were lower in later years possibly owing to improvements in perioperative care and the advent of endovascular techniques. The concluded gastrointestinal bleeding combined with a negative endoscopy in the presence of an aneurysmal aorta suggests primary aortoenteric fistula and requires urgent evaluation by CT. Endovascular operation is an attractive treatment option.

COLON INTERPOSITION

From time to time the colorectal surgeon will be called upon to partake in an operation that requires esophageal replacement or bypass by the colon. The following is a brief resume of the important considerations needed to participate in that procedure. Much of the information has been obtained from the excellent description by Rice (219).

INDICATIONS FOR COLON INTERPOSITION

The indications for esophageal replacement by the colon are varied. For the most part, colon interposition after resection for primary esophageal carcinoma is indicated only if the stomach is unacceptable for this substitution. Although gastric replacement for benign esophageal disease is equivalent or superior to colon replacement, other indications have included congenital atresia, corrosive strictures, recurrent hiatal herniation, short esophagus with gastroesophageal reflux, and columnar lined esophagus with marked dysplasia (220).

ADVANTAGE AND DISADVANTAGES

Advantages of colon replacement include the fact that an adequate length of colon is usually available and the blood supply is easily assessed and generally adequate. Disadvantages of colon replacement are multiple. The preoperative evaluation and preparation of the colon are more demanding than the evaluation or preparation of either the stomach or jejunum because of the frequent occurrence of intrinsic colonic disease and the abundant bacterial colonization of the colon. Colon replacement is a more complex operation than either gastric or simple jejunum replacement. Three anastomoses are mandatory to re-establish gastrointestinal continuity in colon replacement; only one anastmosis is required in gastric substitution. The early complication of colonic graft necrosis is uniformly lethal if it is not recognized early and treated by excision of the necrotic colon. There is a propensity to late complications as a result of the limited acid resistance of the colonic mucosa and the tendency of the colon replacement to dilate and form redundant loops.

PREOPERATIVE PREPARATIONS

A history of significant colonic symptoms, treatment of primary colonic disorders, or previous abdominal operations, suggest that the colon may be unsatisfactory for esophageal replacement. Severe constipation, especially in elderly patients, should signal that the colon might not be an appropriate esophageal substitute. It is essential that the colonic mucosa be inspected before it is used. Colonoscopy provides examination of the mucosa and it allows a biopsy of the mucosal abnormalities to be performed and any colonic polyps to be removed.

Because the arterial blood supply and venous drainage of the colon play such a vital role in a successful operation, many surgeons consider preoperative angiography to be a prerequisite examination. Although three colonic branches of the superior mesenteric artery are seen in 68% of the patients, anomalies in this arterial blood supply are common (219). In order of frequency, these anomalies are: (i) absence of the right colic artery (12.4%), (ii) multiple right colic arteries (8.9%), (iii) multiple middle colic arteries (6.2%), (iv) absence of the middle colic artery (3.6%), and (v) multiple middle and right colic arteries (0.5%). A discontinuous marginal artery of the right colon has been reported in 5% to 70% of the patients. Absence of the marginal artery, which connects the superior and inferior mesenteric arteries at the splenic flexure, is infrequent. In one report, this anomaly was seen in 2% of the patients. Even though this portion of the marginal artery is constant, the inferior mesenteric artery and its branches are susceptible to atherosclerosis. In patients with significant peripheral vascular disease, the inferior mesenteric artery and its branches may be occluded. In this situation, although the left colon usually is adequately supplied through the marginal artery, it is unacceptable for esophageal replacement.

The venous drainage follows the arterial supply in the colonic mesentery. The superior mesenteric vein drains directly into the portal vein. A lack of sufficient marginal venous drainage in the right colon has been implicated in the complications of colon infarction and anastomotic leakage in as many as 25% of the patients who undergo right colonic esophageal replacement. The left colic vein drains into the splenic vein. Excellent marginal venous drainage of the left colon is reported in 100%.

The more constant reliable arterial supply and venous drainage of the left colon led to its preferential use for esophageal replacement (Fig. 14). The smaller diameter of the left colon more closely approximates the esophageal diameter and this may be a beneficial attribute in colon replacement. When a colon replacement is indicated, the right or transverse colon should be reserved and used when the left colon is not available or is inadequate for esophageal substitution.

The length of colon required for esophageal substitution is determined by the extent of the esophageal resection and the route of reconstruction. Meticulous colon preparation is required and should consist of both mechanical and an antibiotic component.

OPERATIVE TECHNIQUE

The segment of colon used (e.g., right, transverse, or left) and the direction of replacement (e.g., isoperistaltic or antiperistaltic) are determined by the state of the colon and the surgeon's preference and experience. The mesentery should be inspected to ensure that there is adequate length with no mesenteric shortening or fibrosis. The arterial supply of the segment of colon to be used is inspected and transilluminated to guarantee an adequate and complete marginal artery. When it is confirmed that the colon is

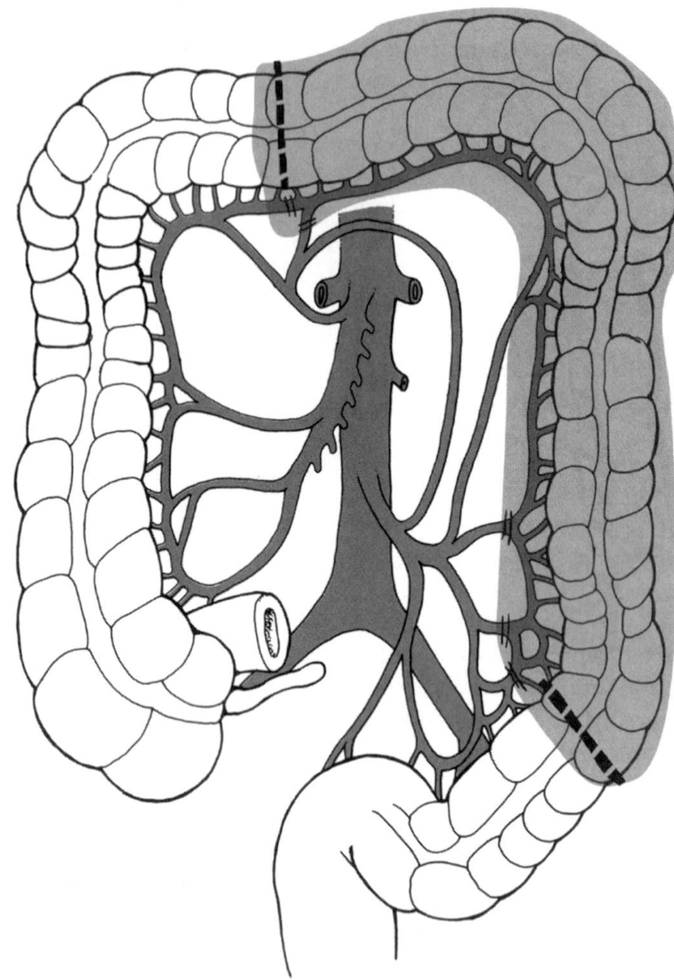

FIGURE 14 ■ The anatomy of the colon in relation to its blood supply that demonstrate the appropriate vascular pedicles required for various lengths of colon used in interposition surgery.

acceptable for esophageal substitution, the esophageal resection is completed.

Left Colon

The greater omentum is removed from the splenic flexure and the distal two-thirds of the transverse colon (219). The arterial supply of the omentum from the stomach and hepatic flexure is maintained so that the omentum is available for later use if required.

The length of colon necessary for esophageal replacement is estimated by the placement of an umbilical tape along the prepared surface of the skin over the proposed route of reconstruction from the mid portion of the gastric remnant (or the jejunal loop if the stomach has been removed) to the distal end of the esophagus or pharynx. This marked length of umbilical tape is then placed along the antimesenteric border of the colon to provide an approximate estimate of the length of colon needed. The marginal artery proximal and distal to these marked areas is exposed. If the proximal line of transection is to the right of the middle colonic artery, the base of this artery must be exposed proximal to the marginal artery. Atraumatic vascular clamps are then placed on the proximal and distal segments of the marginal artery and, if necessary, the middle colic artery.

Once adequate vascularity of the left colon segment has been determined, the middle colic artery is ligated and divided (if required) proximal to its branching into the marginal artery, and the proximal and distal portions of marginal artery are ligated and divided (Fig. 15). The peritoneum and mesentery are divided from the colonic wall to the base of the mesentery at the proposed proximal and distal areas of transaction. The colon segment is then isolated by transaction of the colon at the proximal and distal margins with a linear cutting stapler. If the segment of colon does not have an adequate supply, an alternate segment of colon or a different organ of substitution must be sought.

Furst et al. (220) described an alternative colon interposition procedure in which the ascending and transverse colon is used as graft but still relies on the left colonic artery for blood supply. They state that the standard procedure to obtain a left colon interposition graft requires ligation of the middle colic artery and mobilization of the left and right flexure. This approach carries a risk because preparation of the left flexure may damage arterial or venous collaterals located at this site that are crucial for graft perfusion. The authors modified the standard technique so that mobilization of the left flexure is no longer necessary. To obtain a colon interposition graft that is long enough, the ascending colon was included into the graft by ligating the middle and right colic arteries. The left colic artery remained the blood-supplying vessel. An intact left colic artery including its collaterals at the splenic flexure, supplies significant blood supply to the proximal ascending colon after central ligation to the middle and right colic arteries. Even without mobilization of the left flexure, a sufficient graft length can be obtained. Preliminary complication rates with the use of this technique for colon interposition are in the range of those found for the standard colon interposition. These modifications may represent an alternative to established procedures for creating a colon interposition graft.

Right Colon

The greater omentum is removed from the hepatic flexure and the proximal two-thirds of the transverse colon (219). The arterial supply of the omentum from the stomach and splenic flexure is maintained so that the omentum is available for later use if required. The length of colon necessary for esophageal replacement is estimated as previously described. The marginal artery proximal and distal to these marked areas is exposed. The base of the ileocolic, right colic, and ileal (if required) arteries are exposed proximal to the marginal artery. Atraumatic vascular clamps are then placed on these arteries and the viability of this segment of colon, now supplied solely by the middle colic artery, is assessed.

Once adequate vascularity of the right colon segment has been ensured, the ileocolic and right colic arteries are ligated and divided proximal to their branching to form the marginal artery, and the proximal and distal portions of the marginal artery are ligated and divided (Fig. 16). The peritoneum and mesentery are divided from the colonic wall to the base of the mesentery at the proposed proximal and distal areas of transection. The colon segment

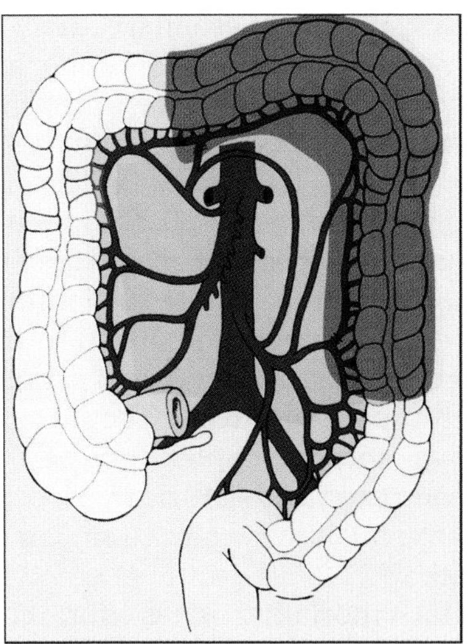

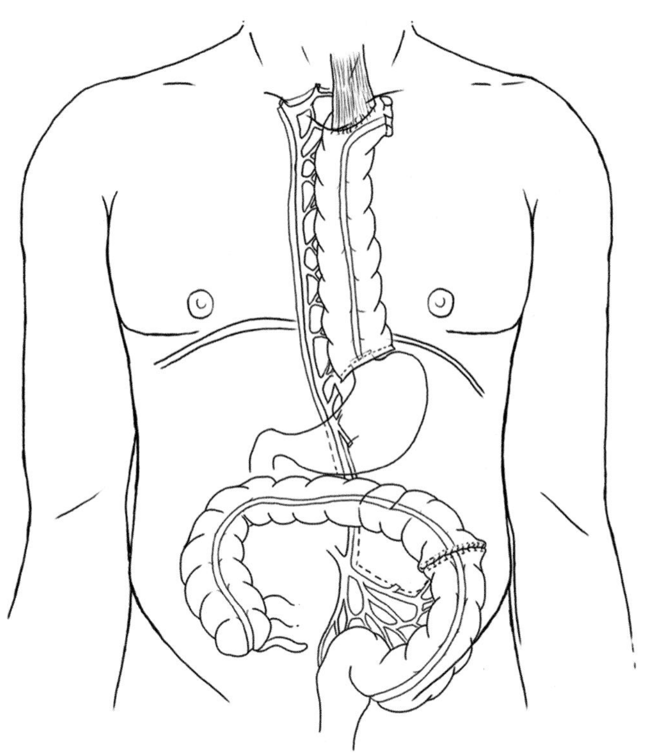

FIGURE 15 ■ An isoperistaltic subcutaneous left colon replacement of the esophagus. The preparation of the arterial supply based on the left colic artery (*left insert*). Anteroposterior view of this isoperistaltic left colon replacement.

is then isolated by transection of the colon at the proximal distal margins with a linear cutting stapler.

Transverse Colon

The transverse colon is used much less frequently than the left or right colon segments for esophageal substitution. The greater omentum is removed from the transverse colon and the hepatic and splenic flexures (219). The arterial supply of the omentum from the stomach is maintained so that the omentum is available for later use if required. The length of colon necessary for esophageal replacement is estimated as previously described. If the segment is based on the left colic artery, mobilization is similar to that described for a left colon replacement. If it is based on the middle colic artery, mobilization is similar to that described for a right colon replacement.

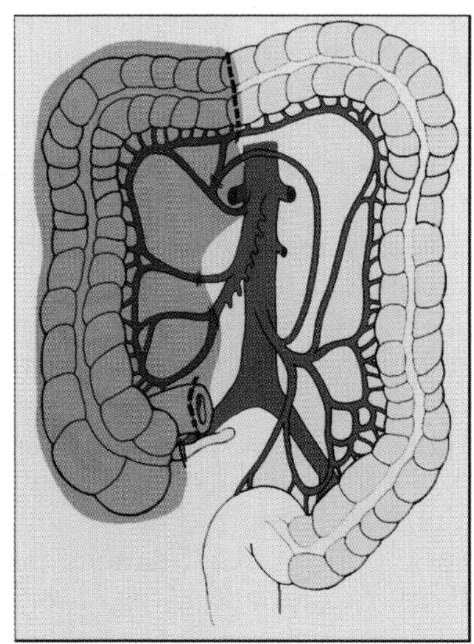

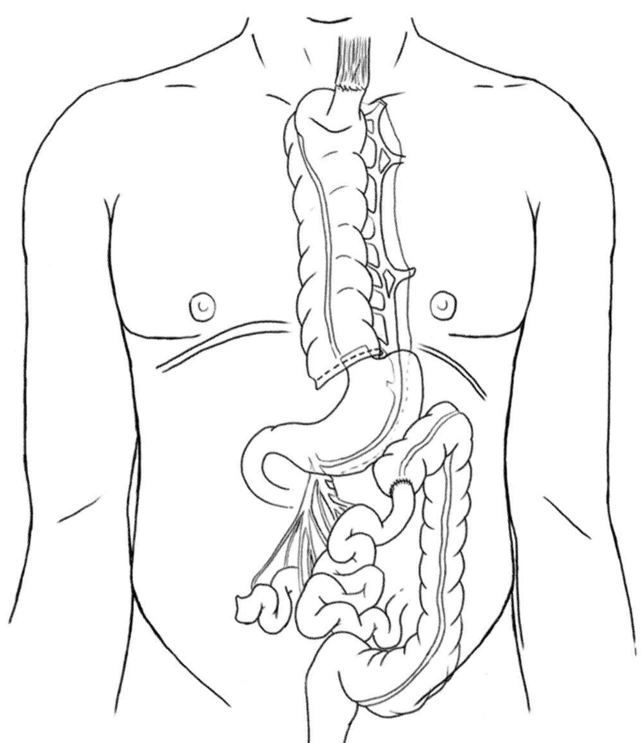

FIGURE 16 ■ Isoperistaltic retrosternal right colon replacement of the esophagus. Preparation of the arterial blood supply is based on the middle colic artery (*left insert*). Anteroposterior view of this istoperistaltic right colon replacement.

Completion of Procedure

The thoracic surgeon prepares the route for the interposed colon. It may be subcutaneous, transpleural, or retrosternal. The colon segment is inspected and prepared for passage through the tunnel. This is facilitated by the placement of the colon segment into a large sterile plastic bag, and the bag is drawn through the prepared replacement route. The proximal esophagocolic anastomosis is contructed usually in an end-to-side fashion along the antimesenteric tenia of the colon with an interrupted sutured anastomosis of single-layer monofilament absorbable suture. The colon is tacked to the edges of the tunnel (diaphragm) with three stitches, each applied to one of the tenia. Any excess colon is excised. The cologastric or colojejunal anastomosis is then constructed. To minimize reflux into the colon replacement, the anastomosis can be constructed on the posterior gastric wall at the junction of the upper and middle thirds of the gastric remnant. The anterior wall of the stomach is an alternative site for the cologastric anastomosis. The cologastric anastomosis is amenable to stapling. The last of the three anastamoses re-establishes gastrointestinal continuity and is either ileocolic or colocolic. The colonic mesenteric defect is then closed with absorbable sutures. A feeding jejunostomy should be constructed at this time.

Results

A review of the results was described by Rice (219). As many as 65% of patients experience postoperative complications after colon interposition. In addition to the complications that may occur after any thoracic operation, the specific early complications of colon replacement of the esophagus are anastomotic leak and necrosis of the colon graft. Anastomotic leakage is variable and complicates 2% to 40% of the operations. As with other gastrointestinal anastomoses, the reasons for the failure of an anastomosis in a colon replacement are multi-factorial. Commonly implicated factors include ischemia, technical error, anastomotic tension, infection, and distraction of the anastomosis as a result of swallowing and excessive head and neck motion. Anastomotic leakage usually occurs at the esophagocolic anastomosis. It is uncommon to have failure of the cologastric, colojejunal, ileocolic, or colocolic anastomoses. Therapy requires the placement of the anastomosis at rest, adequate drainage, administration of antibiotics, and nutritional support. In the absence of complete disruption of the anastomosis, proximal colonic necrosis, or mediastinitis, surgical intervention is seldom required. Most fistulas heal spontaneously, but as many as 50% are complicated by anastomotic strictures that require dilatation. Repeated surgery with anastomotic revision is uncommon.

Vascular compromise is usually precipitated by venous insufficiency and thrombosis, and less commonly by arterial insufficiency. This problem is magnified by the bacterial contamination of the colon and results in necrosis of the colon graft in up to 16% of the patients, a significantly greater incidence than that seen with gastric replacement (1%). This complication is uniformly fatal if not recognized and treated with immediate graft excision. Colon necrosis is a major cause of death after this procedure.

Davis et al. (221) compared 42 patients who underwent colonic interposition with 959 patients who underwent gastric transposition after esophagectomy. Greater blood loss and longer operation duration were encountered in the colon group. They found no difference in cardio-pulmonary complications but they found significantly greater incidences of anastomotic leakage (14.3% vs. 3.9%) and intra-abdominal septic complications (9.5% vs. 0.2%) in the colon group. Conduit ischemia developed in 0.5% in the stomach group and 2.4% in the colon group. Hospital mortality rates included 16.7% in the colon group and 10.6% in the stomach group. Median survival was 12.8 and 10.4 months in the stomach and colon groups respectively. They concluded colon interposition is a more complex procedure with increased morbidity compared with gastric transposition. Overall, mortality and survival, however, were similar to those for gastric transposition.

Hospital mortality rates for colon replacement vary from 0% to 23% (219). The incidence of operative death has decreased with time, in part because of the improved preoperative preparation, operative technique, and postoperative care but also as a result of better patient selection.

The major late complications of colon replacement of the esophagus are stricture, graft redundancy, and poor function of the colon replacement. In addition, reflux of gastric contents may cause ulceration and stricture of the lower portion of the replacement. Peptic ulcer of the esophagus occurs in 0.5% to 8% of the patients.

Briel et al. (223) determined the risk factors for graft ischemia and anastomotic leakage in 363 patients undergoing esophageal anastomosis with gastric or colonic reconstructions. After esophagectomy, 10% of the patients will develop conduit ischemia or anastomotic leak and 22% will develop anastomotic stricture. Anastomotic leak and strictures are more common and the strictures are more severe after gastric pull-up compared with colon interposition. Dilatation is a safe and effective treatment.

Renzulli et al. (224) reported the results of 19 patients undergoing colon interposition for esophageal replacement. Surgical morbidity was 36.8%. Anastomotic insufficiency and fatal mediastinal bleeding occurred in one patient each (5.3%). No cases of graft necrosis were observed, and no re-operations were necessary. In-hospital mortality was 15.8%, twice due to surgical complications (abdominal sepsis, mediastinal bleeding) and once due to pulmonary and cardiac failure. As a late complication, four patients (21.1%) developed anastomotic strictures that necessitated repeated endoscopic dilatation.

Yildirim et al. (225) compared gastric pull-up with colon interposition in terms of graft function and patient satisfaction. Of 62 patients undergoing esophagectomy, reconstruction was performed by colonic interposition in 11, and gastric pull-up in 51. Among patients undergoing gastric pull-up, regurgitation was observed in 22% to 27% during follow-up. None of the patients with colonic interposition had reflux or regurgitation. No esophagitis was observed in patients with colonic interposition during the same period. Overall, satisfaction was superior in patients undergoing colonic interposition.

Late re-operation rates as high as 37% have been reported in the management of persistent symptoms and anastomotic complications (219). Domreis et al. (226) reviewed the charts of six patients who underwent one or more revisions of a colon interposition at a mean follow-up of 16 years. Symptoms of problems with the colon interposition were dysphagia (67%), regurgitation (67%), pneumonia (40%), and chest pain (33%). Findings that accounted for failure were colonic redundancy (67%), and gastrocolonic reflux (50%). The approach was resection of redundant colon or management of reflux. Four patients underwent segmental resection of the colon preserving blood supply. Three patients had gastric resection or diversion of bile and acid for management of reflux.

Adenocarcinoma in colonic replacements is uncommon; it has been reported in 1% of the patients (227,228).

Dysfunction of a colon replacement results in persistent dysphagia or development of upper GI and respiratory symptoms. Cense et al. (229) assessed the quality of life in patients at least six months after esophageal carcinoma resection and colon interposition without signs of recurrent disease. Based on the SF-36 questionnaire, patients after colon interposition by necessity have a poor general quality of life. Even long after the operation, they have a broad spectrum of persisting symptoms. Prior to operation patients should be informed about the disabling long-term functional outcome of a colon interposition. On the other hand, good to excellent results with colon replacement are achieved in 75% to 85% of the patients with benign esophageal disease (219). Perhaps the best determination of a successful colon replacement is the ability of a patient to gain and maintain weight.

REFERENCES

1. De Andres J, Chaves S. Coccygodynia: a proposal for an algorithm for treatment. J Pain 2003; 4:257–266.
2. Kim NH, Suk KS. Clinical and radiological differences between traumatic and idiopathic coccygodynia. Yonsoi Med J 1999; 40(3):215–220.
3. Maroy R. Spontaneous and evoked coccygeal pain in depression. Dis Colon Rectum 1988; 31:210–215.
4. Albrecht S, Hicks HI, Antalffy B. Intracoccygeal and pericoccygeal glomus bodies and their relationship to coccygodynia. Surgery 1994; 115:1–6.
5. Kane WJ. Fractures of the pelvis. In: Rockwood CA, Green DP, eds. Fractures. 2nd ed. Philadelphia: JB Lippincott, 1984:1124–1125.
6. Marx FA. Coccydynia/levator syndrome. A therapeutic test. Tech Coloproctol 1996; 4:91.
7. Wray CC, Easom S, Hoskinson J. Cocydynia. Aetiology and treatment. J Bone Joint Surg Br 1991; 73:335–338.
8. Wood GW. Lower back pain and disorders of intervertebral disc. In: Crenshaw AH, ed. Campbell's Operative Orthopedics. 7th ed. St. Louis: CV Mosby, 1987:3289–3299.
9. Grosso NP, van Dam BE. Total coccygectomy for the relief of coccygodynia: a retrospective review. J Spinal Disord 1995; 8:328–330.
10. Doursounian L, Maigne JY, Faure F, Chatellier G. Coccygectomy for instability of the coccyx. Int Orthop 2004; 28:176–179.
11. Hodges SD, Eck JC, Humphreys SC. A treatment and outcomes analysis of patients with coccydynia. Spine J 2004; 4:138–140.
12. Ramsey ML, Toohey JS, Neidre A, Stromberg LJ, Roberts DA. Coccygodynia: treatment. Orthopedics 2003; 26:403–405.
13. Perkins R, Schofferman J, Reynolds J. Coccygectomy for severe refractory sacrococcygeal joint pain. J Spinal Disord Tech 2003; 16(1):100–103.
14. Dmowski WP. Current concepts in the management of endometriosis. Obstet Gynecol Annual 1981; 10:279–311.
15. Jenkins S, Olive DL, Hany AF. Endometriosis: pathogenetic implications of the anatomic distribution. Obstet Gynecol 1986; 67:335–338.
16. Bailey HR. Colorectal endometriosis. Perspect Colon Rectal Surg 1992; 5:251–259.
17. Groom RD, Donovan M, Schwesinger WH. Intestinal endometriosis. Amar J Surg 1984; 148:660–667.
18. Rowland R, Langman JM. Endometriosis of the large bowel: a report of 11 cases. Pathology 1989; 21:259–265.
19. Larglois NE, Park KG, Keenan RA. Mucosal changes in the large bowel with endometriosis: a possible cause of misdiagnosis of colitis? Hum Pathol 1994; 25:1030–1034.
20. Prystowsky JB, Stryker SJ, Ujiki GT, Poticha SM. Gastrointestinal endometriosis. Incidence and indications for resection. Arch Surg 1988; 123:855–858.
21. Singh KK, Lessells AM, Adam DJ, et al. Presentation of endometriosis to general surgeons: a 10-year experience. Br J Surg 1995; 82:1349–1351.
22. Varras M, Kostopanagiotou E, Katis K, Farantos CH, Angelidou-Manika Z, Antoniou S. Endometriosis causing extensive intestinal obstraction simulating carcinoma of the sigmoid colon: a case report and review of the literature. Eur J Gynaecol Oncol 2002; 23(4):353–357.
23. Bozdech JM. Endoscopic diagnosis of colonic endometriosis. Gastrointest Endosc 1992; 38:568–570.
24. Perry EP, Peel AL. The treatment of obstructing intestinal endometriosis. J R Soc Med 1988; 81:172–173.
25. Verspyck E, Lefranc JP, Guyard B, Blondon J. Treatment of bowel endometriosis: a report of six cases of colorectal endometriosis and a survey of the literature. Eur J Obstet Gynecol Reprod Biol 1997; 71(1):81–84.
26. Forsgren H, Lindhagen J, Melander S, Wagermark J. Colorectal endometriosis. Acta Chir Scand 1983; 149:431–435.
27. Coronado C, Franklin RR, Lotze EC, Balley HR, Valdes CT. Surgical treatment of symptomatic colorectal endometriosis. Fertil Steril 1990; 53(3):411–416.
28. Urbach DR, Reedijk M, Richard CS, Lie KI, Ross TM. Bowel resection for intestinal endometriosis. Dis Colon Rectum 1998; 41(9):1158–1164.
29. Nezhat C, Nezhat F, Pennington E, et al. Laparoscopic disk excision and primary repair of the anterior rectal wall for the treatment of full-thickness bowel endometriosis. Surg Endosc 1994; 8:682–685.
30. Woods RJ, Heriot AG, Chen FC. Anterior rectal wall excision for endometriosis using the circular stapler. ANZ J Surg 2003; 73(8):647–678.
31. Koh CH, Janik GM. The surgical management of deep rectovaginal endometriosis. Curr Opin Obstet Gynecol 2002; 14(4):357–364.
32. Redwine DB, Wright JT. Laparoscopic treatment of complete obliteration of the cul-de-sac associated with endometriosis: long-terms follow-up of en bloc resection. Fertil Steril 2001; 76(2):358–365.
33. Fedele L, Bianchi S, Portuese A, Borruto F, Dorta M. Transrectal ultrasonography in the assessment of rectovaginal endometriosis. Obstet Gynecol 1998; 91(3):444–448.
34. Kavallaris A, Kohler C, Kuhne-Heid R, Schneider A. Histopathological extent of rectal invasion by rectovaginal endometriosis. Hum Reprod 2003; 18(6):1323–1327.
35. Jones KD, Owen E, Berresford A, Sutton C. Endometrial adenocarcinoma arising from endometriosis of the rectosigmoid colon. Gynecol Oncol 2002; 86(2):220–222.
36. Yantiss RK, Clement PB, Young RH. Neoplastic and pre-neoplastic changes in gastrointestinal endometriosis: a study of 17 cases. Am J Surg Pathol 2000; 24:513–524.
37. Cho HY, Kim MK, Cho SJ, Bae JW, Kim I. Endometrial stromal sarcoma of the sigmoid colon arising in endometriosis: a case report with a review of literatures. J Korean Med Sci 2002; 17(3):412–414.
38. Shickele M. Endometriosis of the perineum: review of the literature and case report. Am J Obstet Gynecol 1957; 73:890–893 (quoted by Prince LN, Abrams J).
39. Pollack R, Gordon PH, Ferenczy A, Tulandi T. Perineal endometriosis: a case report and review of the literature. J Reprod Med 1990; 2:109–112.
40. Sampson JA. Perforating hemorrhagic (chocolate) cysts of the ovary: their importance and especially their relation to pelvic adenomas of endometrial type ("adenomyoma") of the uterus, rectovaginal septum, sigmoid, etc.). Arch Surg 1921; 3:245–323.
41. Gordon PH, Schottler JL, Balcos EG, Goldberg SM. Perianal endometrioma: report of 5 cases. Dis Colon Rectum 1976; 19:260–265.
42. Hernandez-Margo PM, Villanueva Saenz E, Alvarez-Tostado Fernandez F, Luis Rocha Ramirez J, Valdes Ovalle M. Endoanal sonography in the assessment of perianal endometriosis with external anal sphincter involvement. J Clin Ultrasound 2002; 30(4):245–248.
43. Hambrick E, Abcarian H, Smith D. Perineal endometrioma in episiotomy incisions: clinical features and management. Dis Colon Rectum 1979; 22:550–552.
44. Dougherty LS, Hull T. Perineal endometriosis with anal. sphincter involvement: report of a case. Dis Colon Rectum 2000; 43:1157–1160.
45. Douthwaite AH. Proctalgia fugax. Br Med J 1962; 2:164–165.
46. Thaysen TEH. Proctalgin fugax. Lancet 1935; 2:243–246.
47. Schuster MM. Constipation and anorectal disorders. Clin Gastroenterol 1977; 6(0):643–658.
48. Harvey RF. Colonic motility in proctalgia fugax. Lancet 1979; 2:713–714.
49. Kamm MA, Hoyle CH, Burleigh DE, et al. Hereditary internal anal sphincter myopathy causing proctalgia fugax and constipation. Gastroenterology 1991; 100:805–810.
50. Celik AF, Katsinelos P, Read NW, Khan MI, Donnelly TC. Hereditary proctalgia fugax and constipation: report of a second family. Gut 1995; 36:581–584.
51. Konig P, Ambrose NS, Scott N. Hereditary internal anal sphincter myopathy causing proctalgia fugax and constipation: further clinical and histological characterization in a patient. Eur J Gastroenterol Hepatol 2000; 12(1):127–128.
52. Guy RJ, Kamm MA, Martin JE. Internal anal sphincter myopathy causing proctalgia fugax and constipation: further clinical and radiological characterization in a patient. Eur J Gastroenterol Hepatol 1997; 9(2):221–224.

53. Takano M. Proctalgia fugax: caused by pudendal neuropathy? Dis Colon Rectum 2005; 48:114–120.
54. Thompson WG, Heaton K. Proctalgia fugax. J R Coll Physicians Lond 1980; 14:147–148.
55. Pilling LF, Swenson WM, Hill JR. The psychologic aspects of proctalgia fugax. Dis Colon Rectum 1965; 8:372–376.
56. Eckardt VF, Dodt O, Kanzler G, Bernhard G. Treatment of proctalgia fugax with sulbutamol inhalation. Am J Gastroenterol 1996; 91:686–689.
57. Peleg R, Shvartzman P. Low-dose intravenous lidocaine as treatment for proctalgia fugax. Reg Anesth Pain Med 2002; 27(1):97–99.
58. Katsinelos P, Kalomenopoulou M, Christodoulou K, et al. Treatment of proctalgia fugax with botulinum A toxin.Eur J Gastroenterol Hepatol 2001; 13(11):1371–1373.
59. Lowenstein B, Cataldo PA. Treatment of proctalgia fugax with topical nitroglycerin: report of a case. Dis Colon Rectum 1998; 41(5):667–668.
60. Sinaki M, Merritt J, Stillwell GK. Tension myalgia of the pelvic floor. Mayo Clin Proc 1977; 52:717–722.
61. Salvati EP. The levator syndrome and its variant. Gastroenterol Clin North Am 1987; 16:71–78.
62. Drossman DA, Li Z, Andruzzi E, et al. US householder survey of functional gastrointestinal disorders. Prevalence, sociodemography, and health impact. Dig Dis Sci 1993; 38:1569–1580.
63. Sohn N, Weinstein MA, Robbins RD. The levator syndrome and its treatment with high-voltage electrogalvanic stimulation. Am J Surg 1982; 144:580–582.
64. Nicosia JF, Abcarian H. Levator syndrome—a treatment that works. Dis Colon Rectum 1985; 28:406–408.
65. Billingham RP, Isler JT, Friend WG, Hostetler J. Treatment of levator syndrome using high-voltage electrogalvanic stimulation. Dis Colon Rectum 1987; 30:584–587.
66. Hull TL, Milsom JW, Church J, Oakley J, Lavery I, Fazio V. Electrogalvanic stimulation for levator syndrome: how effective is it in the long-term? Dis Colon Rectum 1993; 36:731–733.
67. Heah SM, Ho YH, Tan M, Leong AF. Biofeedback is effective treatment for levator ani syndrome. Dis Colon Rectum 1997; 40(2):187–189.
68. Graham-Stewart CW. Injection treatment of hemorrhoids. Br Med J 1962; 1:213–216.
69. Neshat AA, Stone DH, Price HP. Self-induced lipoid granuloma of the rectum: report of a case. Dis Colon Rectum 1974; 17:696–699.
70. Hernandez V, Hernandez IA, Berthrong M. Oleogranuloma simulating carcinoma of the rectum. Dis Colon Rectum 1967; 10:205–209.
71. Webb AJ. Oleocysts presenting as rectal tumors. Br J Surg 1966; 53:410–413.
72. Day DW, Jass JR, Price AB, et al. eds. In: Morson BC and Dawson MP. Gastrointestinal Pathology. 4th ed. Oxford: Blackwell Scientific Publications, 2003: 669–670.
73. Mazier WP, Sun KM, Robertson WG. Oil-induced granuloma (eleoma) of the rectum: report of four cases. Dis Colon Rectum 1978; 21:292–294.
74. Morganstern L, Shemen L, Allen N, Amodeo P, Michel SL. Melanosis coli. Changes in appearance when associated with colonic neoplasia. Arch Surg 1983; 118:62–67.
75. Day DW, Jass JR, Price AB, et al. eds. In: Morson BC and Dawson MP. Gastrointestinal Pathology. 4th ed. Oxford: Blackwell Scientific Publications 2003: 635–636.
76. Walker NI, Smith MM, Smithers BM. Ultrastructure of human melanosis coli with reference to its pathogenesis. Pathology 1993; 25:120–123.
77. Ewing CA, Kalan M, Chucker F, Ozdemirli M. Melanosis coli involving pericolonic lymph nodes associated with the herbal laxative Swiss Kriss: a rare and incidental finding in a patient with colonic adenocarcinoma. Arch Pathol Lab Med 2004; 128(5):565–567.
78. Pardi DS, Tremaine WJ, Rothenberg HJ, Batts KP. Melanosis coli in inflammatory bowel disease. J Clin Gastoenterol 1998; 26(5):167–170.
79. Müller-Lissner SA. Adverse effects of laxatives: fact and fiction. Pharmacology 1993; 47(suppl 1):138–145.
80. Koskela E. Kulju T, Collan Y. Melanosis coli. Prevalence, distribution, and histologic features in 200 consecutive autopsies at Kuopio University Central Hospital. Dis Colon Rectum 1989; 32:235–239.
81. Nusko G, Schneider B, Muller G, et al. Retrospective study on laxative use and melanosis coli as risk factors for colorectal neoplasms. Pharmacology 1993; 47(suppl 1):234–241.
82. Nusko G, Schneider B, Schneider I, Wittekind C, Hahn EG. Anthranoid laxative use is not a risk factor for colorectal neoplasia: results of a prospective case control study. Gut 2000; 46:651–655.
83. Nascimbeni R, Donato F, Ghirardi M, Mariani P, Villanacci V, Salerni B. Constipation, anthranoid laxatives, melanosis coli, and colon cancer: a risk assessment using aberrant crypt foci. Cancer Epidemiol Biomarkers Prev 2002; 11(8):753–737.
84. Guy PJ, Hall M. Colitis cystica profunda of the rectum treated by mucosal sleeve resection and coloanal pullthrough. Br J Surg 1988; 75:289.
85. Martin JK, Culp CE, Weiland LH. Colitis cystica profunda. Dis Colon Rectum 1980; 23:488–491.
86. Guest CB, Reznick RK. Colitis cystica profunda. Review of the literature. Dis Colon Rectum 1989; 32:983–988.
87. Rutter KRP, Riddell RH. The solitary ulcer syndrome of the rectum. Clin Gastroenterol 1975; 4:505–530.
88. Tedesco FJ, Sumner HW, Kassens WD. Colitis cystica profunda. Am J Gastroenterol 1976; 65:339–343.
89. Madan A, Minocha A. First reported case of colitis cystica profunda in association with Crohn's disease. Am J Gastroenterol 2002; 97:2472–2473.
90. Green GI, Ramos R, Bannayan GA, McFee AS. Colitis cystica profunda. Am J Surg 1974; 127:749–752.
91. Freeman HJ. Colitis cystica profunda complicated by complete colorectal obstruction. Can J Gastroenterol 1994; 8:326–330.
92. Herman AH, Nabseth DC. Colitis cystica profunda, localized, segmental and diffuse. Arch Surg 1973; 106:337–341.
93. Silver H, Stolar J. Distinguishing features of well-differentiated mucinous adenocarcinoma of the rectum and colitis cystica profunda. Am J Clin Pathol 1969; 59:493–500.
94. Rosengren JE, Hildell J, Lindstrom CO, Leandoer L. Localized colitis cystica profunda. Gastrointest Radiol 1982; 7:79–83.
95. Valenzuela M, Martin-Ruiz JL, Alvarez-Cienfuegos E, et al. Colitis cystica profunda: imaging diagnosis and conservative treatment. Report of two cases. Dis Colon Rectum 1996; 39:587–590.
96. Wayte DM, Helwig EB. Colitis cystica profunda. Am J Clin Pathol 1967; 48:159–169.
97. Parks AG, Porter NH, Hardcastle JD. The syndrome of the descending perineum. Proc R Soc Med 1966; 59:477–482.
98. Henry MM. Descending perineum syndrome. Henry MM, Swash M, eds. Coloproctology and the Pelvic Floor. Pathophysiology and Management. London: Butterworth, 1985:299–302.
99. Henry MM, Parks AG, Swash M. The pelvic floor musculature in the descending perineum syndrome. Br J Surg 1982; 69:470–472.
100. Harewood GC, Coulie B, Camilleri M, Rath-Harvey D, Pemberton JH. Descending perineum syndrome: audit of clinical and laboratory features and outcome of pelvic floor retraining. Am J Gastroenteral 1999; 94:126–130.
101. Pucciani F, Boni D, Perna F, Bassotti G, Bellini M. Descending perineum syndrome: are abdominal hysterectomy and bowel habits linked? Dis Colon Rectum 2005; 22; [Epub ahead of print].
102. Bartolo D, Roe A. Disorders of the bowel: obstructed defecation. Br J Hosp Med 1986; 35:225–236.
103. Karasick G, Karasick D, Karasick SR. Functional disorders of the anus and rectum: findings on defecography. Am J Roentgenol 1993; 160:777–782.
104. Jamart J. Pneumatosis cystoides intestinalis: a statistical study of 919 cases. Acta Hepato-Gastroenterol 1979; 26:419–422.
105. Koss LG. Abdominal gas cysts (pneumatosis cystoides intestinalorum hominis). Arch Pathol 1952; 53:523–549.
106. Forgacs P, Wright PH, Wyatt AP. Treatment of intestinal gas cysts by oxygen breathing. Lancet 1973; 1:579–582.
107. Rayna R, Soper RT, Condon RE. Pneumatosis intestinalis: report of twelve cases. Am J Surg 1973; 125:667–671.
108. Marshak RH, Linder AE, McKlansky D. Pneumatosis cystoides coli. Gastrointest Radiol 1977; 2:85–89.
109. Bryk D. Unusual causes of small bowel pneumatosis: perforated duodenal ulcer and perforated jejunal diverticula. Radiology 1973; 106:299–302.
110. Ghahremani GG, Port RB, Beachley ML. Pneumatosis coli in Crohn's disease. Dig Dis Sci 1974; 19:315–323.
111. Keyting WS, McCarver RR, Kovarik JL, et al. Pneumatosis intestinalis: a new concept. Radiology 1961; 76:733–741.
112. Smith BH, Welter LH. Pneumatosis intestinalis. Am J Clin Pathol 1967; 48:455–465.
113. Stone HH, Allen WB, Smith RB III, et al. Infantile pneumatosis intestinalis. J Surg Res 1968; 8:301–307.
114. Yale CE, Balish E. Pneumatosis cystoides intestinalis. Dis Colon Rectum 1976; 19:107–111.
115. Read NW, Al-Janabi NM, Cann PA. Is raised breath hydrogen related to the pathogenesis of pneumatosis coli. Gut 1984; 25:839–845.
116. Yale CE. Etiology of pneumatosis cystoides intestinalis. Surg Clin North Am 1975; 55:1297–1302.
117. Galandiuk S, Fazio VW. Pneumatosis cystoides intestinalis: review of the literature. Dis Colon Rectum 1986; 29:358–363.
118. Janssen DA, Kalayoglu M, Sollinger HW. Pneumatosis cystoides intestinalis following lactulose and steroid treatment in a liver transplant patient with an intermittently enlarged scrotum. Transplant Proc 1987; 19:2949–2952.
119. Samson VE, Brown WR. Pneumatosis cystoides intestinalis in AIDS–associated cryptosporidiosis. More than an incidental finding? J Clin Gastroenterol 1996; 22:311–312.
120. McCollister DL, Hammerman HJ. Air, air everywhere: pneumatosis cystoides coli after colonoscopy. Gastrointest Endosc 1990; 36:75–76.
121. North JH, Nava HR. Pneumatosis intestinalis and portal venous air associated with needle catheter jejunostomy. Am Surg 1995; 61:1045–1048.
122. Wolthuis AM, Vanrijkel JP, Aelvoet C, De Weer F. Needle catheter jejunostomy complicated by pneumatosis intestinalis: a case report. Acta Chir Belg 2003; 103:631–632.

123. Selva-O'Callaghan A, Martinez-Costa X, Solans-Laque R, Mauri M, Capdevila JA, Vilardell-Tarres M. Refractory adult dermatomyositis with penumatosis cystoids intestinalis treated with infliximab. Rheumatology (Oxford) 2004; 43:1196–1197.
124. Goodman RA, Riley TR III. Lactulose-induced pneumatosis intestinalis and pneumoperitoneum. Dig Dis Sci 2001; 46:2549–2553.
125. Terzic A, Holzinger F, Klaiber C. Pneumatosis cystoides intestinalis as a complication of celiac disease. Surg Endosc 2001; 15:1360–1361.
126. Kuroda T, Ohfuchi Y, Hirose S, Nakano M, Gejyo F, Arakawa M. Pneumatosis cystoides intestinalis in a patient with polymyositis. Clin Rheumatol 2001; 20:49–52.
127. Kreiss C, Forohar F, Smithline AE, Brandt LJ. Pneumatosis intestinalis complicating C. difficile pseudomembranous colitis. Am J Gastroenterol 1999; 94:2560–2561.
128. Horiuchi A, Akamatsu T, Mukawa K, Ochi Y, Arakura N, Kiyosawa K. Case report: pneumatosis cystoides intestinalis associated with post-surgical bowel anastomosis: a report of three cases and review of the Japanese literature. J Gastroenterol Hepatol 1998; 13:534–537.
129. Boerner RM, Fried DB, Warshauer DM, et al. Pneumatosis intestinalis: two case reports and a retrospective review of the literature from 1985 to 1995. Dig Dis Sci 1996; 41:2272–2285.
130. Sato M, Ishida H, Konno K, et al. Sonography of pneumatosis cystoides intestinalis. Abdom Imaging 1999; 24(6):559–561.
131. Quiroz ES, Flannery MT, Martinez EJ, et al. Pneumatosis cystoides intestinalis in progressive systemic scleroses: a case report and literature review. Am J Med Sci 1995; 310:252–255.
132. Bansal R, Bude R, Nostrant TT, et al. Diagnosis of colonic pneumatosis cystoides intestinalis by endosonography. Gastrointest Endosc 1995; 42:90–93.
133. Day DW, Jass JR, Price AB, Shepherd NA, Sloan JM, Talbot IC, Warren BF, Williams GT, eds. In: Morson BC and Dawson MP. Gastrointestinal Pathology. 4th ed. Oxford: Blackwell Scientific Publications, 2003: 636–637.
134. Spigelman AD, Williams CB, Ansell JK, et al. Pneumatosis coli: a source of diagnostic confusion. Br J Surg 1990; 77:155.
135. Bloch C. The natural history of pneumatosis coli. Radiology 1977; 123:311–314.
136. Hwang J, Reddy VS, Sharp KW. Pneumatosis cystoides intestinalis with free intraperitoneal air: a case report. Am Surg 2003; 69(4):346–349.
137. Galm O, Fabry U, Adam G, Osieka R. Pneumatosis intestinalis following cytotoxic or immunosuppressive treatment. Digestion 2001; 64:128–132.
138. Gelman SF, Brandt LJ. Pneumatosis intestinalis and AIDS: a case report and review of the literature. Am J Gastroenterol 1998; 93:646–650.
139. Born A, Inouye T, Diamant N. Pneumatosis coli: case report documenting time from x-ray appearance to onset of symptoms. Dig Dis Sci 1981; 26:855–859.
140. Elberg JJ. Oxygen therapy for pneumatosis coli, symptomatic and radiologic remission of colonic gas cysts after breathing high concentration oxygen. Acta Chir Scand 1985; 151:399–400.
141. Gillon J, Tadesse K, Logan RF, et al. Breath hydrogen in pneumatosis cystoides intestinalis. Gut 1979; 20:1008–1011.
142. Gruenberg JC, Batra SK, Priest RJ. Treatment of pneumatosis cystoides intestinalis with oxygen. Arch Surg 1977; 112:112–116.
143. Masterson JS, Fratkin JB, Osler TR, et al. Treatment of pneumatosis cystoides intestinalis with hyperbaric oxygen. Ann Surg 1978; 187:245–247.
144. van Leeuwen JCJ, Nossent JC. Pneumatosis intestinalis in mixed connective tissue disease. Neth J Med 1992; 40:299–304.
145. Lee SP, Coverdale HA, Niccholson GI. Oxygen therapy for pneumatosis coli: a report of 2 cases and a review. Aust N Z J Med 1977; 7:44–46.
146. Mujahed Z, Evans JA. Gas cysts of the intestine (pneumatosis intestinalis). Surg Gynecol Obstet 1958; 107:151–160.
147. Hughes DT, Gordon MC, Swann JC, et al. Pneumatosis cystoides intestinalis. Gut 1966; 7(5):553–557.
148. Ecker JA, Williams RG, Clay KL. Pneumatosis cystoides intestinalis: bullous emphysema of the intestine. Am J Gastroenterol 1971; 56:125–136.
149. Down RHL, Castleden WM. Oxygen therapy for pneumatosis coli. Br Med J 1975; 1:493–494.
150. Wyatt AP. Prolonged symptomatic and radiological remission of colonic gas cysts after oxygen therapy. Br J Surg 1975; 62:837–839.
151. Van der Linden W, Marsell R. Pneumatosis cystoides coli associated with high H_2 excretion: treatment with an elemental diet. Scand J Gastroenterol 1979; 14:173–174.
152. Jauhonen P, Lehtola J, Karttunen T. Treatment of pneumatosis coli with metronidazole. Dis Colon Rectum 1987; 30:800–801.
153. Miralbes M, Hinojosa J, Alonso J, et al. Oxygen therapy in pneumatosis coli: What is minimum oxygen requirement. Dis Colon Rectum 1983; 26:458–460.
154. Woodward A, Lai L, Burgess B, et al. A case of pneumatosis coli managed by restorative proctectomy and ileal pouch–anal anastomosis. Int J Colorectal Dis 1995; 10:181–182.
155. Johannson K, Lindstrom E. Treatment of obstructive pneumatosis coli with endoscopic sclerotherapy: report of a case. Dis Colon Rectum 1991; 34:94–96.
156. Gagliardi G, Thompson JW, Hershman MJ, et al. Pneumatosis coli: a proposed pathogenesis based on a study of 25 cases and review of the literature. Int J Colorectal Dis 1996; 11:111–118.
157. Thornton JP, Abcarian H. Surgical treatment of perianal and perineal hidradenitis suppurativa. Dis Colon Rectum 1978; 21:573–577.
158. Chalfant WP III, Nance FC. Hidradenitis suppurativa of the perineum: treatment by radical excision. Am Surg 1970; 36:331–334.
159. Perez-Diaz D, Calvo-Serrano M, Martinez-Hijosa E, et al. Squamous cell carcinoma complicating perianal hidradenitis suppurativa. Int J Colorectal Dis 1995; 10:225–228.
160. Broadwater JR, Bryant RL, Petrino RA, et al. Advanced hidradenitis suppurativa. Review of surgical treatment in 23 patients. Am J Surg 1982; 144:668–670.
161. Culp CE. Chronic hidradenitis suppurativa of the anal canal. A surgical skin disease. Dis Colon Rectum 1983; 26:669–676.
162. Harrison BJ, Harding KD, Hughes LE. Surgical management of perianal hidradenitis suppurativa. Br J Surg 1985; 72(suppl):S143.
163. Day DW, Jass JR, Price AB, Shepherd NA, Sloan JM, Talbal IC, Warren BF, Williams CT, eds. In: Morson BC and Dawson MP. Gastrointestinal Pathology. 4th ed. Oxford: Blackwell Scientific Publications, 2003; 651.
164. Wiltz O, Schoetz DJ, Murray JJ, et al. Perianal hidradenitis suppurativa. The Lahey Clinic Experience. Dis Colon Rectum 1990; 33: 731–734.
165. Bell BA, Ellis H. Hidradenitis suppurativa. J R Soc Med 1978; 71:511–515.
166. Adams JD, Haisten AS. Perianal hidradenitis suppurativa. Surg Clin North Am 1972; 52:467–472.
167. Attanoos RL, Appleton MA, Douglas-Jones AG. The pathogenesis of hidradenitis suppurativa: a closer look at apocrine and apoeccrine glands. Br J Dermatol 1995; 133:254–258.
168. Harrison BJ, Kumar S, Reed GF, et al. Hidradenitis suppurativa: evidence for an endocrine abnormality. Br J Surg 1985; 72:1002–1004.
169. Stellon AJ, Wakeling M. Hidradenitis suppurativa associated with the use of oral contraceptives. Br Med J 1989; 298:28–29.
170. Mortimer PS, Dawber RP, Gales MA, et al. Mediation of hidradenitis suppurativa by androgens. Br Med J 1986; 292:245–248.
171. Barth JH, Layton AM, Cunliffe WJ. Endocrine factors in pre-and postmenopausal women with hidradenitis suppurativa. Br J Dermatol 1996; 134:1057–1059.
172. Harrison BJ, Reed GF, Hughes LE. Endocrine basis for the clinical presentation of hidradenitis suppurativa. Br J Surg 1988; 75:972–975.
173. Konig A, Lehmann C, Rompel R, Happle R. Cigarette smoking as a triggering factor of hidradenitis suppurativa. Dermatology 1999; 198:261–264.
174. Bendahan J, Paran H, Kolman S, et al. The possible role of *Chlamydia trachomatis* in perineal suppurativa hidradenitis. Eur J Surg 1992; 158: 213–215.
175. Bhalla R, Sequeira W. Arthritis associated with hidradenitis suppurativa. Ann Rheum Dis 1994; 53:64–66.
176. Rosner JA, Burg CG, Wisnieski JJ, et al. The clinical spectrum of the arthropathy associated with hidradenitis suppurativa and acne carglobate. J Rheumatol 1993; 20:684–687.
177. Tsianos EV, Dalekos GN, Tzermias C, et al. Hidradenitis suppurativa in Crohn's disease. A further support of this association. J Clin Gastroenterol 1995; 20:151–153.
178. Church JM, Fazio VW, Lavery FC, et al. The differential diagnosis and comorbidity of hidradenitis suppurativa and perianal Crohn's disease. Int J Colorectal Dis 1993; 8:117–119.
179. Brown SC, Kazzazi N, Lord PH. Surgical treatment of perianal hidradenitis suppurativa with special reference to recognition of the perianal form. Br J Surg 1986; 73:978–980.
180. Malaquarnera M, Pontillo T, Pistone G, et al. Squamous-cell cancer in Verneciolí's disease. (Hidradenitis suppurativa). Lancet 1994; 348:1449.
181. Dufresne RC Jr, Ratz JL, Bergfeld WF, et al. Squamous cell carcinoma arising from the follicular occlusion triad. J Am Acad Dermatol 1996; 35:475–477.
182. Finlay EM, Ratz JL. Treatment of hidradenitis with carbon dioxide laser excision and second-intention healing. J Am Acad Dermatol 1996; 34:465–469.
183. Cosman BC, O'Grady TC, Pekarske S. Verrucous carcinoma arising in hidradentis suppurativa. In J Colorectal Dis 2000; 15:342–346.
184. Altunay IK, Gokdemir G, Kurt A, Kayaoglu S. Hidradenitis suppurativa and squamous cell carcinoma. Dermatol Surg 2002; 28:88–90.
185. Rubin RJ, Chinn BT. Perianal hidradenitis suppurativa. Surg Clin North Am 1994; 74:1317–1325.
186. Banerjee AK. Surgical treatment of hidradenitis suppurativa. Br J Surg 1992; 79:863–866.
187. Jemec GB, Wendelboe P. Topical clindamycin versus systemic tetracycline in the treatment of hidradenitis suppurativa. J Am Acad Dermatol 1998; 39:971–974.
188. Mortimer PS, Dawber RP, Gales MA, et al. A double blind controlled crossover trial of cyproterone acetate in females with hidradenitis suppurativa. Br J Dermatol 1986; 115:263–268.
189. Sullivan TP, Welsh E, Kerdel FA, Burdick AE, Kirsner RS. Inflximab for hidradenitis suppurativa. Br J Dermatol 2003; 149:1046–1049.
190. Rosenfeld N, Babar A. Hidradenitis suppurativa of the perineal and gluteal regions, treated by excision and skin grafting. Plast Reconstr Surg 1976; 58:98–99.
191. Shaughnessy DM, Greminger RR, Margolis JB. Hidradenitis suppurativa: a plea for early operative treatment. JAMA 1972; 222:320–321.

192. Liron-Ruiz R, Torralba-Martinez JA, Pellicer-Franco E, et al. Treatment of long-standing entersive perianal hidradentis suppurativa using double rotation plasty, V-Y Plasty, and free grafts. Int J Colorectal Dis 2004; 19:73–78.
193. Bocchini SF, Habr-Gama A, Kiss DR, Imperiale AR, Araujo SE. Gluteal and perianal hidradenitis suppurativa: surgical treatment by wide excision. Dis Colon Rectum 2003; 46:944–949.
194. Gordon PH. The chemically defined diet and anorectal procedures. Can J Surg 1976; 19:511–513.
195. Lapins J, Marcussor JA, Emtestam L. Surgical treatment of chronic hidradenitis suppurativa: CO_2 laser stripping—secondary intention technique. Br J Dermatol 1994; 131:551–556.
196. Donaldson DR, Jass JR, Mann CV. Anal leukoplakia. Gut 1987; 28:A1368.
197. Katsinelos P, Christodoulou K, Pilpilidis I, et al. Anal leukoplakia: an unusual case of anal stenosis. Endoscopy 2001; 33:469.
198. Glotzer DJ, Glick ME, Goldman H. Proctitis and colitis following diversion of the fecal stream. Gastroenterology 1981; 80:438–441.
199. Whelan RL, Abramson D, Kim DS, Hashmi HF. Diversion colitis. A prospective study. Surg Endosc 1994; 8:19–24.
200. Ferguson CM, Siegal RJ. A prospective evaluation of diversion colitis. Am Surg 1991; 57:46–49.
201. Haas PA, Fox TA, Szilagy EJ. Endoscopic examination of the colon and rectum distal to a colostomy. Am J Gastroenterol 1990; 85:850–854.
202. Velazquez OC, Lederer HM, Rombeau JL. Butyrate and the colonocyte. Production, absorption, metabolism, and therapeutic implications. Adv Exp Med Biol 1997; 427:123–134.
203. Harig JM, Soergel KH, Komorowski RA, Wood CM. Treatment of diversion colitis with short-chain fatty acid irrigation. N Engl J Med 1989; 320:23–28.
204. Winslet MC, Poxon V, Young S, et al. A pathophysiologic study of diversion colitis. Surg Gynecol Obstet 1993; 177:57–60.
205. Orsay CP, Kim DO, Pearl RK, Abcarian H. Diversion colitis in patients scheduled for colostomy closure. Dis Colon Rectum 1993; 36:366–367.
206. Ona FU, Boger J. Rectal bleeding due to diversion colitis. Am J Gastroenterol 1985; 80:40–41.
207. Frisbie JH, Ahmed N, Hirano I, Klein MA, Soybel DI. Diversion colitis in patients with myelopathy: clinical, endoscopic, and histopathological findings. J Spinal Cord Med 2000; 23:142–149.
208. Tripodi J, Gorcey S, Burakoff R. A case of diversion colitis treated with 5-aminosalicylic acid enemas. Am J Gastroenterol 1992; 87:645–647.
209. Murray FE, O'Brien MJ, Birkett DH, et al. Diversion colitis. Pathologic findings in a resected sigmoid colon and rectum. Gastroenterology 1987; 93:1404–1408.
210. Yeong ML, Bethwaite PB, Prasad J, Isbister WH. Lymphoid follicular hyperplasia—a distinctive feature of diversion colitis. Histopathology 1991; 19:55–61.
211. Asplund S, Gramlich T, Fazio V, Petras R. Histologic changes in defunctioned rectums in patients with inflammatory bowel disease: a clinicopathologic study of 82 patients with long-term follow-up. Dis Colon Rectum 2002; 45:1206–1213.
212. Lim AG, Langmead FL, Feakins RM, Rampton DS. Diversion colitis: a trigger for ulcerative colitis in the in-stream colon? Gut 1999; 44:279–282.
213. Peppercorn MA. Drug-responsive chronic segmental colitis associated with diverticula: a clinical syndrome in the elderly. Am J Gastroenterol 1992; 87:609–612.
214. Makapugay LM, Dean PJ. Diverticular disease-associated chronic colitis. Am J Surg Pathol 1996; 20:94–102.
215. Gore S, Shepherd NA, Wilkinson SP. Endoscopic crescentic fold disease of the sigmoid colon: the clinical and histopathological spectrum of a distinctive endoscopic appearance. Int J Colorectal Dis 1992; 7:76–81.
216. Imperiali G, Meucci G, Alvisi C, et al. Segmental colitis associated with diverticula: a prospective study. Gruppo di Studio per le Malattie Infiammatorie Intestinali (GSMII). Am J Gastroenterol 2000; 95:1014–1016.
217. Guslandi M. Segmental colitis: so what? Eur J Gastroenterol Hepatol 2003; 15:1–2.
218. Saers SJ, Scheltinga MR. Primary aortoenteric fistula. Br J Surg 2005; 92(2): 143–152.
219. Rice TW. Colon replacement. In: Esophageal Surgery. Pearson FG, Cooper JD, Deslaurier J, Ginsberg RJ, Hiebert CA, Patterson GA, Urschel HC Jr, eds. 2nd ed. Philadelphia: Churchill Livingstone, 2002:917–930.
220. Furst H, Hartl WH, Lohe F, Schildberg FW. Colon interposition for esophageal replacement: an alternative technique based on the use of the right colon. Ann Surg 2000; 231:173–178.
221. Davis PA, Law S, Wong J. Colonic interposition after esophagectomy for cancer. Arch Surg 2003; 138:303–308.
222. Jeyasengher K. Long term results of colon replacement. In: Esophageal Surgery. Pearson FG, Cooper JD, Deslaurier J, et al. (eds) 2nd ed. Philadelphia: Churchill Livingstone, 2002; 931–937.
223. Briel JW, Tamhankar AP, Hagen JA, et al. Prevalance and risk factors for ischemia, leak, and structure of esophageal anastomosis: gastric pull-up versus colon interposition. J Am Call Surg 2004; 198:536–541.
224. Renzulli P, Joeris A, Strobel O, et al. Colon interposition for esophageal replacement: a single-center experience. Langenbecks Arch Surg 2004; 389:128–133.
225. Yildirim S, Koksal H, Celayir F, Erdem L, Oner M, Baykan A. Colonic interposition vs. gastric pull-up after total esophagectomy. J Gastrointest Surg 2004; 8:675–678.
226. Domreis JS, Jobe BA. Aye RW, Deveney KE, Sheppard BC, Deveney CW. Management of long-term failure after colon interposition for benign disease. Am J Surg 2002; 183:544–546.
227. Liau CT, Hsueh S, Yeow KM. Primary carcinoma arising in esophageal colon interposition: report of a case. Hepatogastroenterology 2004; 51:748–749.
228. Goyal M, Bang DH, Cohen LE. Adenocarcinoma arising in interposed colon: report of a case. Dis Colon Rectum 2000; 43:555–558.
229. Cense HA, Visser MR, van Sandick JW, de Boer AG, Lainme B, Obertop H, van Lanschot JJ. Quality of life after colon interposition by necessity for esophageal cancer replacement. J Surg Oncol 2004; 88:32–38.

Index